ACS SURGERY 7

ACS SURGERY 7

2014

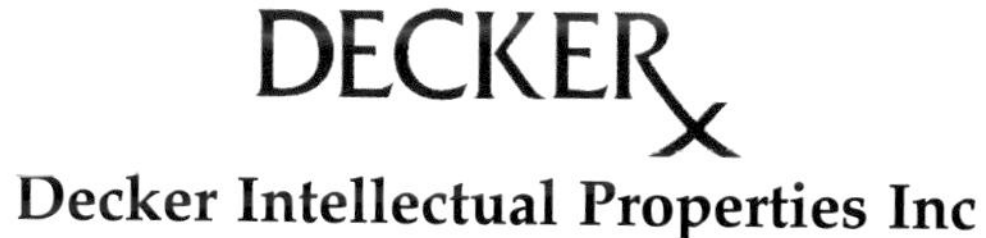

Decker Intellectual Properties Inc

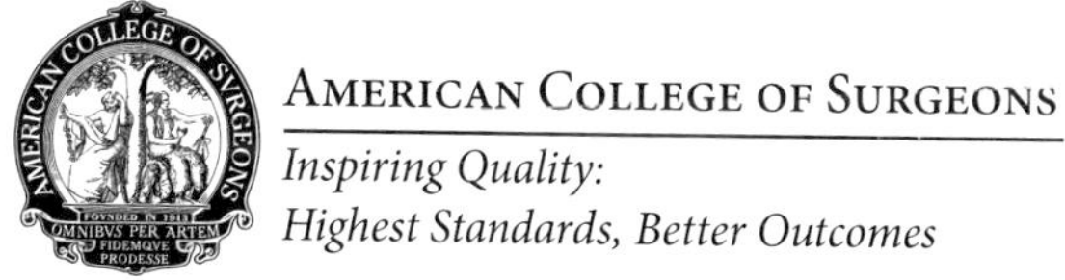

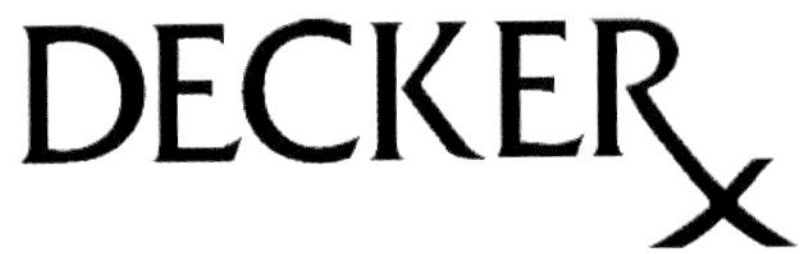

Decker Intellectual Properties Inc
69 John Street South, Suite 310
Hamilton, Ontario L8N 2B9 CANADA
1-855-647-6511
E-mail: customercare@deckerip.com
www.deckerip.com

14 15 16 17/SN/9 8 7 6 5 4 3 2 1

ISBN 978-0-615-85974-3
Printed in India by S. Narayan & Sons
Managing Editor: Ben Shragge; Publisher: Brian C. Decker

Sales and Distribution

Western Hemisphere
Decker Intellectual Properties Inc.
69 John Street South, Suite 310
Hamilton, Ontario L8N 2B9

Europe, Middle East, Africa, Asia
Eurospan Group
3 Henrietta Street
London, United Kingdom WC2E 8LU
44 (0) 1767 604972
E-mail: info@eurospangroup.com
www.eurospan.co.uk

ACS Surgery: Principles and Practice is sponsored by the American College of Surgeons and written by individuals who are recognized experts.The text represents the authors' approaches to clinical problems and to other important issues in surgical practice. It should be used as a general reference with other sources in the formation of an integrated care plan.

Notice: The authors, editors, and publisher have conscientiously and carefully tried to ensure that recommended measures and drug dosages in these pages are accurate and conform to the standards that prevailed at the time of publication. The reader is advised, however, to check the product information sheet accompanying each drug to be familiar with any changes in the dosage schedule or in the contraindications. This advice should be taken with particular seriousness if the agent to be administered is a new one or one that is infrequently used. *ACS Surgery: Principles and Practice* describes basic principles of diagnosis and therapy. Because of the uniqueness of each patient and the need to take into account a number of concurrent considerations, however, this information should be used by physicians only as a general guide to clinical decision making.

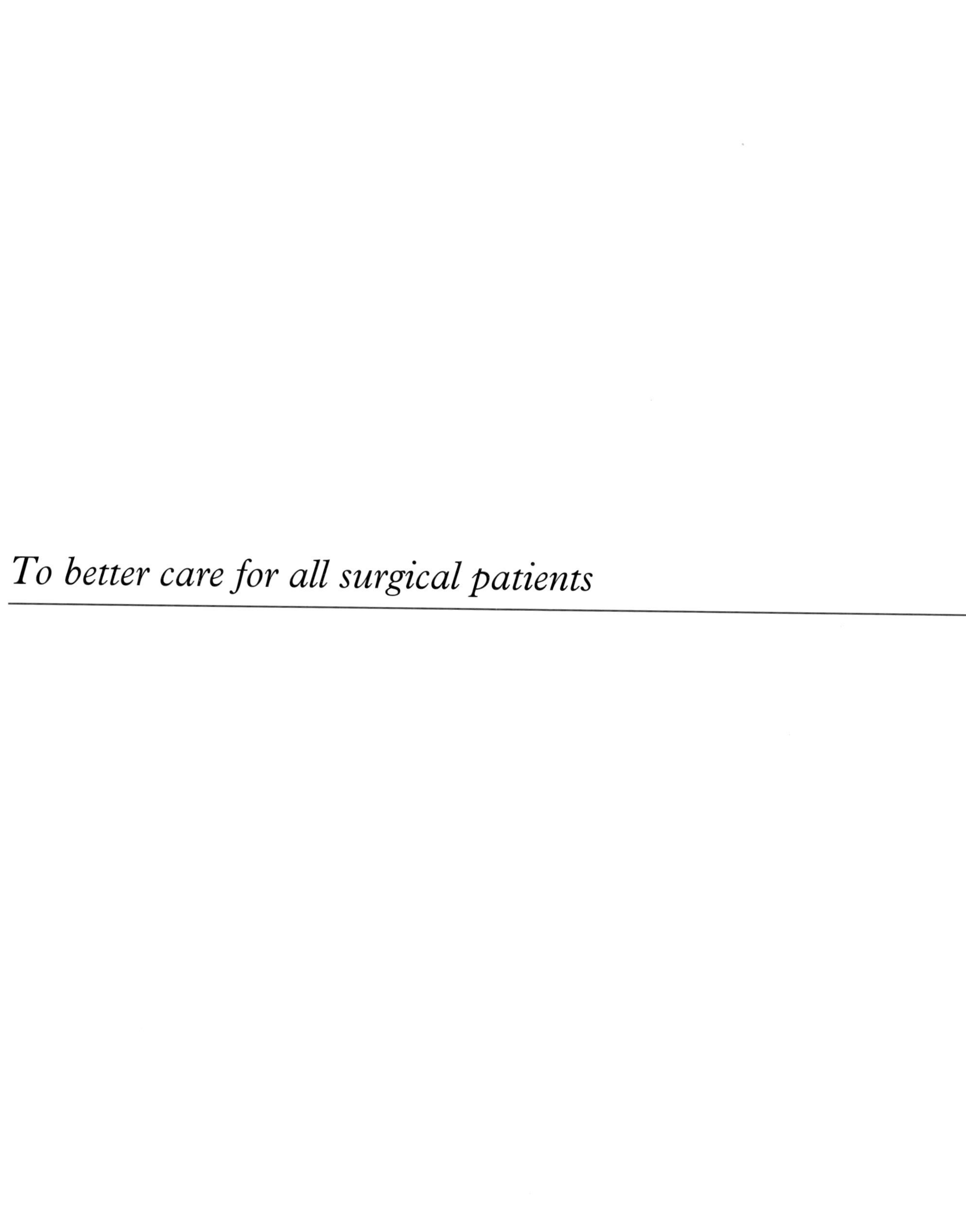

To better care for all surgical patients

CONTENTS

VOLUME 1

1. COMPETENCY-BASED SURGICAL CARE

2. BASIC SURGICAL AND PERIOPERATIVE CONSIDERATIONS

3. HEAD AND NECK

4. BREAST, SKIN, AND SOFT TISSUE

5. THE THORAX

6. GASTROINTESTINAL TRACT AND ABDOMEN

7. VASCULAR SYSTEM

VOLUME 2

8. TRAUMA AND THERMAL INJURY

9. CRITICAL CARE

CONTRIBUTORS

Ahmed M. Abou-Zamzam Jr, MD
Loma Linda University Medical Center, Loma Linda, CA

Ali F. AbuRahma, MD
Robert C. Byrd Health Sciences Center, West Virginia University, Charleston, WV

Bekele Afessa, MD
Mayo Clinic, Rochester, MN

Suresh K. Agarwal, MD, FACS, FCCM
University of Wisconsin School of Medicine and Public Health, Madison, WI

Sonya P. Agnew, MD
Northwestern University Feinberg School of Medicine, Chicago, IL

Shannon H. Allen, MD
Temple University School of Medicine, Philadelphia, PA

Paul Alvord, MD
Naval Medical Center, San Diego, CA

John B. Ammori, MD
Case Western Reserve University, Cleveland, OH

Shahriyour Andaz, MD, FACS, FRCS
New York College of Medicine, Westbury, NY

John T. Anderson, MD, FACS
University of California Davis School of Medicine, Sacramento, CA

Rafael S. Andrade, MD, FACS
University of Minnesota, Minneapolis, MN

Donald J. Annino Jr, MD, DMD
Brigham and Women's Hospital, Boston, MA

Stanley W. Ashley, MD, FACS
Harvard Medical School, Boston, MA

Shazad Ashraf, MD
University of Oxford, Oxford

Sean M. Bagshaw, MD, MSc, FRCPC
Austin Hospital, Heidelberg, Victoria

Talia B. Baker, MD, FACS
Northwestern University Feinberg School of Medicine, Chicago, IL

Chad G. Ball, MD, FRCSC
University of Calgary, Calgary, AB

Farzaneh Banki, MD
The University of Texas Medical School at Houston, Houston, TX

Rafal Barczak, MD
University of Connecticut School of Medicine, Farmington, CT

Alan Barkun, MD, MSc, FRCPC
McGill University, Montreal, QC

Jeffrey Barkun, MD, MSc, FRCSC
McGill University, Montreal, QC

Katherine A. Barsness, MD
Northwestern University Feinberg School of Medicine, Chicago, IL

Robert H. Bartlett, MD, FACS, FCCM, FCCP
University of Michigan, Ann Arbor, MI

Davis E. Beck, MD, FACS, FASCRS
Ochsner Clinic Foundation, New Orleans, LA

Rinaldo Bellomo, MD, FRACP, FJFICM
University of Melbourne, Melbourne

John J. Bergan, MD, FACS
University of California, San Diego School of Medicine, San Diego, CA

Simon Bergman, MD, MSc, FACS, FRCSC
McGill University, Montreal, QC

William R. Berry, MD, MPH, FACS
Harvard School of Public Health, Boston, MA

Noelle L. Bertelson, MD
Mayo Clinic, Phoenix, AZ

Palmer Q. Bessey, MD
Weill Cornell Medical College, New York, NY

Neil Bhattacharyya, MD, FACS
Harvard Medical School, Boston, MA

Phillip A. Bilderback, MD
Virginia Mason Medical Center, Seattle, WA

Karl Y. Bilimoria, MD, MS
The University of Texas MD Anderson Cancer Center, Houston, TX

John D. Birkmeyer, MD
University of Michigan Medical School, Ann Arbor, MI

Nancy J.O. Birkmeyer, PhD
University of Michigan Medical School, Ann Arbor, MI

Ermelinda Bonaccio, MD
State University of New York at Buffalo, Buffalo, NY

Karen R. Borman, MD, FACS
Temple University School of Medicine, Philadelphia, PA

Bryon J. Boulton, MD
Emory University, Atlanta, GA

Wilbur B. Bowne, MD
State University of New York Downstate College of Medicine, New York, NY

Carol R. Bradford, MD, FACS
University of Michigan, Ann Arbor, MI

Karen J. Brasel, MD, FACS
Medical College of Wisconsin, Milwaukee, WI

Bruce M. Brenner, MD, FACS
University of Connecticut Health Center, Farmington, CT

David C. Brooks, MD, FACS
Harvard Medical School, Boston, MA

L. Michael Brunt, MD, FACS
Washington University School of Medicine, St Louis, MO

Ayesha S. Bryant, MSPH, MD
University of Alabama at Birmingham, Birmingham, AL

Sara Buckman, MD, PharmD
University of Wisconsin School of Medicine and Public Health, Madison, WI

Clay Cothren Burlew, MD, FACS
University of Colorado, Denver, CO

Sigrid Burruss, MD
David Geffen School of Medicine, University of California, Los Angeles, CA

John Byrne, MCh, FRCSI (Gen)
Albany Medical College, Albany, NY

Richard P. Cambria, MD
Harvard Medical School, Boston, MA

Guilherme M. Campos, MD, FACS
University of Wisconsin School of Medicine and Public Health, Madison, WI

Helen Cappuccino, MD, FACS
University of Buffalo School of Medicine, Buffalo, NY

Eden Cardozo, MD
Northwestern University Feinberg School of Medicine, Chicago, IL

Franco Carli, MD, PhD, FRCA, FRCPC
McGill University, Montreal, QC

Kathleen Casey, MD
University of Medicine and Dentistry of New Jersey, Newark, NJ

Jason A. Castellanos, MD
Vanderbilt University Medical Center, Nashville, TN

Susan M. Cera, MD, FACS
Cleveland Clinic Florida, Weston, FL

Robert James Cerfolio, MD, FACS, FCCP
University of Alabama at Birmingham, Birmingham, AL

Ara A. Chalian, MD, FACS
University of Pennsylvania Health System, Philadelphia, PA

Prosanto Chaudhury, MD, CM, MSc (Oxon), FRCSC, FACS
McGill University, Montreal, QC

Herbert Chen, MD, FACS
University of Wisconsin, Madison, WI

Kathryn T. Chen, MD
Temple University School of Medicine, Philadelphia, PA

Clifford S. Cho, MD, FACS
University of Wisconsin School of Medicine and Public Health, Madison, WI

Nicolas V. Christou, MD
McGill University, Montreal, QC

Robert R. C[illegible], MD, MA
Mayo Clinic College of Medicine, Rochester, MN

G. Patrick Clagett, MD, FACS
University of Texas Southwestern Medical Center, Dallas, TX

Thomas E. Clancy, MD, FACS
Harvard Medical School, Boston, MA

Panna A. Codner, MD, FACS
Medical College of Wisconsin, Milwaukee, WI

Jeffrey L. Cohen, MD, FACS, FASCRS
University of Connecticut Health Center, Farmington, CT

Mark F. Conrad, MD, MMSc
Harvard Medical School, Boston, MA

Craig M. Coopersmith, MD, FACS
Emory University School of Medicine, Atlanta, GA

Aimee M. Crago, MD
Memorial Sloan-Kettering Cancer Center, New York, NY

David Crippen, MD, FCCM
University of Pittsburgh School of Medicine, Pittsburgh, PA

Thomas A. D'Amico, MD
Duke University Medical Center, Durham, NC

T. Forcht Dagi, MD, MPH, FACS, FCCM
Uniformed Services University of the Health Sciences, Bethesda, MD

Svetlana Danovich, DO, PhD
Stony Brook University Medical Center, Stony Brook, NY

Alan Dardik, MD, PhD, FACS
Veterans Affairs Connecticut Healthcare Systems, New Haven, CT

R. Clement Darling III, MD
Albany Medical College, Albany, NY

Marcelo C. DaSilva, MD
Harvard Medical School, Boston, MA

Ingemar J.A. Davidson, MD, PhD, FACS
University of Texas Southwestern Medical Center, Dallas, TX

Mark G. Davies, MD, PhD, MBA, FACS
Methodist DeBakey Heart & Vascular Center, The Methodist Hospital, Houston, TX

John Mihran Davis, MD
University of Medicine and Dentistry of New Jersey, Newark, NJ

E. Patchen Dellinger, MD, FACS
University of Washington, Seattle, WA

Achilles A. Demetriou, MD, PhD, FACS
Case Western Reserve University School of Medicine, Cleveland, OH

Sara M. Demola, MD
University of Texas Medical Branch, Galveston, TX

Tina R. Desai, MD, FACS
University of Chicago, Chicago, IL

Ravi Dhanisetty, MD
Oregon Health & Science University, Portland, OR

Justin B. Dimick, MD, MPH
University of Michigan Medical School, Ann Arbor, MI

Joseph J. Disa, MD, FACS
Memorial Sloan-Kettering Cancer Center, New York, NY

Gerard M. Doherty, MD
Boston University, Boston, MA

Robert B. Dorman, MD, PhD
University of Minnesota, Minneapolis, MN

Gregory A. Dumanian, MD, FACS
Northwestern University Feinberg School of Medicine, Chicago, IL

Brian J. Dunkin, MD, FACS
Weill Cornell Medical College, New York, NY

Geoffrey Dunn, MD, FACS
Hamot Medical Center, Erie, PA

Kelli Bullard Dunn, MD, FACS, FACRS
University at Buffalo, The State University of New York, Buffalo, NY

Joseph R. Durham, MD, FACS
John H. Stroger, Jr. Hospital of Cook County, Chicago, IL

Samuel H. Eaton, MD
Northwestern University Feinberg School of Medicine, Chicago, IL

Stephen B. Edge, MD, FACS
University at Buffalo, The State University of New York, Buffalo, NY

Matthew S. Edwards, MD, FACS
Wake Forest Baptist Health Medical Center, Winston-Salem, NC

Dina Elaraj, MD
Northwestern University Feinberg School of Medicine, Chicago, IL

Dawn Emick, MD
Duke University Medical Center, Durham, NC

Mark E. Engelstad, DDS, MD
University of Washington, Seattle, WA

Guillermo A. Escobar, MD
University of Michigan, Ann Arbor, MI

Mark K. Eskandari, MD, FACS
Northwestern University Feinberg School of Medicine, Chicago, IL

David A. Etzioni, MD, MSHS, FACS
Mayo Clinic, Phoenix, AZ

Heather L. Evans, MD, MS, FACS
University of Washington, Seattle, WA

Amy R. Evenson, MD
Beth Israel Deaconess Medical Center, Boston, MA

Timothy C. Fabian, MD, FACS
University of Tennessee Health Science Center, Memphis, TN

Lee D. Faucher, MD, FACS
University of Wisconsin School of Medicine and Public Health, Madison, WI

Liane S. Feldman, MD, FRCS(C), FACS
McGill University, Montreal, QC

David V. Feliciano, MD, FACS
Emory University School of Medicine, Atlanta, GA

Luis A. Fernandez, MD, FACS
University of Wisconsin School of Medicine and Public Health, Madison, WI

James R. Fink, MD
University of Washington, Seattle, WA

William R. Finkelmeier, MD, FACS
Veinsolutions, Corvasc, Carmel, IN

Samuel R.G. Finlayson, MD, MPH
Dartmouth Medical School, Hanover, NH

David P. Foley, MD
University of Wisconsin School of Medicine and Public Health, Madison, WI

Yuman Fong, MD, FACS
Memorial Sloan-Kettering Cancer Center, New York, NY

Seth D. Force, MD
Emory University, Atlanta, GA

Elizabeth Franco, MD, MPH&TM
Uniformed Services University of the Health Sciences, Bethesda, MD

Heidi L. Frankel, MD, FACS, FCCM
University of Texas Southwestern Medical Center, Dallas, TX

Julie A. Freischlag, MD
The Johns Hopkins Hospital, Baltimore, MD

Gerald M. Fried, MD, FRCS(C), FACS
McGill University, Montreal, QC

Jonathan S. Friedstat, MD
University of North Carolina, Chapel Hill, NC

Michael E. Friscia, MD
Hospital of the University of Pennsylvania, Philadelphia, PA

Jonathan P. Fryer, MD
Northwestern Memorial Hospital, Chicago, IL

Mark W. Fugate, MD
University of Tennessee College of Medicine, Chattanooga, TN

Luke M. Funk, MD, MPH
Brigham and Women's Hospital, Boston, MA

Susan Galandiuk, MD, FACS, FASCRS
University of Louisville School of Medicine, Louisville, KY

Joseph M. Galante, MD
University of California Davis School of Medicine, Sacramento, CA

Robert D. Galiano, MD
Northwestern University Feinberg School of Medicine, Chicago, IL

Atul Gawande, MD, MPH
Brigham and Women's Hospital, Boston, MA

Racheed J. Ghanami, MD
Wake Forest Baptist Health Medical Center, Winston-Salem, NC

Nicole S. Gibran, MD, FACS
University of Washington School of Medicine, Seattle, WA

Angela L. Gibson, MD, PhD
University of Wisconsin Hospitals and Clinics, Madison, WI

Donald M. Glenn, PA-C
North Shore Vascular Associates, Northfield, IL

Christopher J. Godshall, MD, FACS
Wake Forest Baptist Health Medical Center, Winston-Salem, NC

Laura A. Goguen, MD, FACS
Brigham and Women's Hospital, Boston, MA

John F. Golan, MD, FACS
Northwestern University Feinberg School of Medicine, Chicago, IL

Vita Golubovskaya, PhD
Roswell Park Cancer Institute, Buffalo, NY

J.C. Goslings, MD, PhD
University of Amsterdam, Amsterdam

Robert C. Gosselin, MT
University of California Davis Medical Center, Sacramento, CA

Vivienne M. Gough, MB, CHB
Wythenshawe Hospital, Manchester

Jon C. Gould, MD, FACS
University of Wisconsin School of Medicine and Public Health, Madison, WI

Caprice C. Greenberg, MD, MPH, FACS
Harvard Medical School, Boston, MA

Jacob A. Greenberg, MD, EdM
University of Wisconsin Hospital and Clinics, Madison, WI

Joel A. Gross, MD
University of Washington School of Medicine, Seattle, WA

Angela Gucwa, MD
Medical College of Georgia, Augusta, GA

Jose G. Guillem, MD, MPH, FACS
Weill Cornell Medical College, New York, NY

Eric G. Halvorson, MD
Brigham and Women's Hospital, Boston, MA

Fadi T. Hamadani, MD
McGill University, Montreal, QC

Allen D. Hamdan, MD, FACS
Harvard Medical School, Boston, MA

Maxim D. Hammer, MD
University of Pittsburgh School of Medicine, Pittsburgh, PA

Kimberley J. Hansen, MD, FACS
Wake Forest Baptist Health Medical Center, Winston-Salem, NC

Alden H. Harken, MD
University of California, San Francisco, CA

J. Garrett Harper, MD
Emory University, Atlanta, GA

Karem Harth, MD, MHS
University Hospitals Case Medical Center, Cleveland, OH

Heitham T. Hassoun, MD
The Methodist Hospital Research Institute, Houston, TX

Herbert B. Hechtman, MD
Harvard Medical School, Boston, MA

Melissa Heffler, MD
University at Buffalo, The State University of New York, Buffalo, NY

David M. Heimbach, MD, FACS
University of Washington School of Medicine, Seattle, WA

W. Scott Helton, MD, FACS
Virginia Mason Medical Center, Seattle, WA

Peter K. Henke, MD, FACS
University of Michigan, Ann Arbor, MI

Hung S. Ho, MD, FACS
University of California Davis Medical Center, Sacramento, CA

Andrew W. Hoel, MD
Northwestern University Feinberg School of Medicine, Chicago, IL

James W. Holcroft, MD, FACS
University of California Davis School of Medicine, Sacramento, CA

Joe C. Hong, MD
David Geffen School of Medicine, University of California, Los Angeles, CA

Richard A. Hopper, MD, MS
University of Washington, Seattle, WA

J. Jason Hoth, MD, FACS
Wake Forest University School of Medicine, Winston-Salem, NC

Steven K. Howard, MD
Stanford University School of Medicine, Stanford, CA

Thomas J. Howard, MD, FACS
Indiana University School of Medicine, Indianapolis, IN

Tjasa Hranjec, MD, MS
University of Virginia, Charlottesville, VA

Richard C. Hsu, MD, PhD
Danbury Hospital Department of Surgery, Danbury, CT

Matthew O. Hubbard, MD
Case Western Reserve School of Medicine, Cleveland, OH

Eric S. Hungness, MD, FACS
Northwestern University Feinberg School of Medicine, Chicago, IL

Roger Hurst, MD
University of Chicago Pritzker School of Medicine, Chicago, IL

Sayeed Ikramuddin, MD, FACS
University of Minnesota, Minneapolis, MN

Ramin Jamshidi, MD
University of California, San Francisco, CA

William D. Jordan Jr, MD
University of Alabama Medical Center, Birmingham, AL

Rohan A. Joseph, MD
Methodist Institute for Technology, Houston, TX

Gregory J. Jurkovich, MD, FACS
University of Washington School of Medicine, Seattle, WA

Larry R. Kaiser, MD, FACS
The University of Texas Medical School at Houston, Houston, TX

Kiran Kakarala, MD
Harvard Medical School, Boston, MA

Patrick S. Kamath, MD
Mayo Clinic College of Medicine, Rochester, MN

Lewis J. Kaplan, MD, FACS, FCCM, FCCP
Yale University School of Medicine, New Haven, CT

Sahil K. Kapur, MD
University of Wisconsin School of Medicine and Public Health, Madison, WI

Mark T. Keegan, MD
Mayo Clinic, Rochester, MN

Aoife N. Keeling, FFRRCSI
Northwestern University Feinberg School of Medicine, Chicago, IL

Henrik Kehlet, MD, PhD, FACS (Hon)
Copenhagen University, Copenhagen

Rachel R. Kelz, MD, MSCE, FACS
University of Pennsylvania Perelman School of Medicine, Philadelphia, PA

Gregory D. Kennedy, MD, PhD
University of Wisconsin School of Medicine and Public Health, Madison, WI

Jason D. Keune, MD, MBA
Washington University School of Medicine, St. Louis, MO

Melina R. Kibbe, MD
Northwestern University Feinberg School of Medicine, Chicago, IL

Billy J. Kim, MD
New York University School of Medicine, New York, NY

Kee D. Kim, MD
University of California Davis School of Medicine, Sacramento, CA

Min P. Kim, MD
The University of Texas MD Anderson Cancer Center, Houston, TX

Sylvia S. Kim, MD, FACS
State University of New York Downstate College of Medicine, New York, NY

Edward H. Kincaid, MD, FACS
Wake Forest University School of Medicine, Winston-Salem, NC

Timothy W. King, MD, PhD
University of Wisconsin School of Medicine and Public Health, Madison, WI

Dennis R. Klassen, MD, FRCS(C), FACS
Dalhousie University Faculty of Medicine, Halifax, NS

Nancy Klauber-DeMore, MD, FACS
University of North Carolina, Chapel Hill, NC

Matthew B. Klein, MD, MS, FACS
University of Washington, Seattle, WA

Mary E. Klingensmith, MD, FACS
Washington University School of Medicine, St. Louis, MO

Charles H. Knowles, MBBChir, PhD, FRCS
Queen Mary University, London

M. Margaret Knudson, MD, FACS
University of California, San Francisco, CA

Ira J. Kodner, MD, FACS, FACSRS
Washington University School of Medicine, St. Louis, MO

Marin H. Kollef, MD
Washington University School of Medicine, St. Louis, MO

Matthew C. Koopmann, MD
University of Wisconsin School of Medicine and Public Health, Madison, WI

John C. Kucharczuk, MD
Hospital of the University of Pennsylvania, Philadelphia, PA

Swati Kulkarni, MD, FACS
State University of New York at Buffalo, Buffalo, NY

Constantinos B. Kyriakides, MD
St. Mary's Hospital, London

Eric S. Lambright, MD
Vanderbilt University Medical Center, Nashville, TN

Miriam N. Lango, MD, FACS
Temple University Health System, Philadelphia, PA

Andy Lee, MD
Harvard Medical School, Boston, MA

Linda G. Lesky, MD, MA
George Washington University, Washington, DC

Keith D. Lillemoe, MD, FACS
Indiana University School of Medicine, Indianapolis, IN

Harrison W. Lin, MD
Harvard Medical School, Boston, MA

D. Scott Lind, MD
Medical College of Georgia, Augusta, GA

Philip A. Linden, MD, FACS
Case Western Reserve School of Medicine, Cleveland, OH

David C. Linehan, MD, FACS
Washington University Medical School, St. Louis, MO

Spencer S. Liu, MD
Copenhagen University, Copenhagen

Susan Logan, MD, MPP
Washington University Medical School, St. Louis, MO

Dana C. Lynge, MD, FACS
University of Washington School of Medicine, Seattle, WA

Robyn A. Macsata, MD, FACS
Georgetown University Hospital, Washington, DC

Michael A. Maddaus, MD, FACS
University of Minnesota, Minneapolis, MN

Robert D. Madoff, MD, FACS, FACSRS
University of Minnesota, Minneapolis, MN

Mark A. Malangoni, MD, FACS
University of Pennsylvania School of Medicine, Philadelphia, PA

Thomas S. Maldonado, MD
New York University School of Medicine, New York, NY

James D. Maloney, MD, FACCP
University of Wisconsin School of Medicine and Public Health, Madison, WI

Joseph Mamazza, MDCM, FRSC
University of Ottawa, Ottawa, ON

Paul E. Marik, MD, FCCP, FCCM
Eastern Virginia Medical School, Norfolk, VA

Jovan N. Markovic, MD
Duke University School of Medicine, Durham, NC

Jeffrey Marks, MD, FACS
University Hospitals Case Medical Center, Cleveland, OH

Deborah L. Marquardt, MD, FACS
General Surgery, Bremerton, WA

John C. Marshall, MD, FACS, FRCSC
University of Toronto, Toronto, ON

Jon S. Matsumura, MD, FACS
University of Wisconsin School of Medicine and Public Health, Madison, WI

Kazuhide Matsushima, MD
University of Texas Southwestern Medical School, Dallas, TX

Adrian A. Maung, MD, FACS
Yale University School of Medicine, New Haven, CT

Haggi Mazeh, MD
University of Wisconsin School of Medicine and Public Health, Madison, WI

Christopher R. McHenry, MD, FACS
Case Western Reserve University School of Medicine, Cleveland, OH

Jonathan L. Meakins, MD, DSc, FACP
University of Oxford, Oxford

Nipun B. Merchant, MD, FACS
Vanderbilt University Medical Center, Nashville, TN

J. Wayne Meredith, MD, FACS
Wake Forest University School of Medicine, Winston-Salem, NC

Joshua D. Mezrich, MD
University of Wisconsin School of Medicine and Public Health, Madison, WI

Fabrizio Michelassi, MD
Weill Cornell Medical College, New York, NY

Magdy P. Milad, MD, MS, FACOG
Northwestern University Feinberg School of Medicine, Chicago, IL

Lillian Min, MD, MSHS
University of Michigan, Ann Arbor, MI

Christian Minshall, MD, PhD, FACS
University of Texas, Southwestern Medical School, Dallas, TX

J. Gregory Modrall, MD
Harvard Medical School, Boston, MA

Gregory L. Moneta, MD
Oregon Health & Science University, Portland, OR

Ernest E. Moore, MD, FACS
University of Colorado, Denver, CO

Francis D. Moore Jr, MD
Brigham and Women's Hospital, Boston, MA

Frederick A. Moore, MD, FACS
Weill Cornell Medical College at Methodist Hospital, Houston, TX

Laura J. Moore, MD, FACS
Weill Cornell Medical College at Methodist Hospital, Houston, TX

Molly E. Moore, PharmD
University of Cincinnati, Cincinnati, OH

Wesley S. Moore, MD, FACS
David Geffen School of Medicine, University of California, Los Angeles, CA

Neil J. Mortensen, MD
John Radcliffe Hospital, Oxford

Anne C. Mosenthal, MD, FACS
New Jersey Medical School, Newark, NJ

Michael J. Mosier, MD
University of Washington Burn Center, Seattle, WA

Eric W. Mueller, PharmD
University of Cincinnati, Cincinnati, OH

J. Paul Muizelaar, MD, PhD
University of California Davis School of Medicine, Sacramento, CA

Scott Musicant, MD
Private Practice Vascular Surgery, La Mesa, CA

Robert B. Nadler, MD, FACS
Northwestern University Feinberg School of Medicine, Chicago, IL

Alex Nagle, MD, FACS
Northwestern University Feinberg School of Medicine, Chicago, IL

David M. Nagorney, MD
Mayo Clinic College of Medicine, Rochester, MN

Attila Nakeeb, MD, FACS
Indiana University School of Medicine, Indianapolis, IN

Brian Nam, MD
University of Wisconsin Hospital and Clinics, Madison, WI

Peter A. Naughton, MD
Northwestern University Feinberg School of Medicine, Chicago, IL

Heather B. Neuman, MD, MS
University of Wisconsin School of Medicine and Public Health, Madison, WI

William B. Newton III, MD
Wake Forest Baptist Health Medical Center, Winston-Salem, NC

Valerie Ng, MD, PhD
University of California San Francisco-East Bay, Oakland, CA

Paul L. O'Donnell, DO
Physicians of Southern New Jersey, Vineland, NJ

Patrick J. O'Hara, MD, FACS
Cleveland Clinic Lerner College of Medicine, Cleveland, OH

Bert W. O'Malley Jr, MD, FACS
University of Pennsylvania Health System, Philadelphia, PA

Patrick B. O'Neal, MD
Brigham and Women's Hospital, Boston, MA

Ann P. O'Rourke, MD, MPH
University of Wisconsin School of Medicine and Public Health, Madison, WI

David W. Ollila, MD, FACS
University of North Carolina, Chapel Hill, NC

Raymond P. Onders, MD, FACS
Case Western Reserve School of Medicine, Cleveland, OH

James A.W. Orr, MD, FACS
University of Wisconsin School of Medicine and Public Health, Madison, WI

Satoru Osaki, MD, PhD
University of Wisconsin School of Medicine and Public Health, Madison, WI

David M. Ota, MD, FACS
Duke University, Durham, NC

John T. Owings, MD, FACS
University of California Davis Medical Center, Sacramento, CA

Pauline K. Park, MD, FACS, FCCM
University of Michigan, Ann Arbor, MI

Luigi Pascarella, MD
Vein Institute of La Jolla, La Jolla, CA

Vivek Patel, MBBS
University of Pittsburgh Medical Center, Pittsburgh, PA

Taine T.V. Pechet, MD, FACS
University of Pennsylvania, Philadelphia, PA

Erik Peltz, DO
University of Colorado School of Medicine, Denver, CO

John H. Pemberton, MD, FACS
Mayo Clinic, Rochester, MN

Brian G. Peterson, MD, FACS
Saint Louis University Health Sciences Center, St. Louis, MO

William C. Pevec, MD, FACS
University of California Davis School of Medicine, Sacramento, CA

Ancil Philip, MD
University of Wisconsin School of Medicine and Public Health, Madison, WI

K.J. Ponsen, MD
University of Amsterdam, Amsterdam

Jeffrey L. Ponsky, MD, FACS
Case Western Reserve University, Cleveland, OH

Eric C. Poulin, MD, MSc, FACS, FRCSC
University of Ottawa, Ottawa, ON

Mark E.P. Prince, MD, FRCSC
University of Michigan, Ann Arbor, MI

Clinton D. Protack, MD
Veterans Affairs Connecticut Healthcare Systems, New Haven, CT

Roni B. Prucz, MD
University of Washington, Seattle, WA

Jennifer L. Rabaglia, MD
University of Texas Southwestern Medical School, Dallas, TX

Charlotte Rabl, MD
Paracelsus Private Medical University, Salzburg

Krishnan Raghavendran, MD, FACS
University of Michigan, Ann Arbor, MI

Alexandra Reiher, MD
University of Wisconsin, Madison, WI

H. David Reines, MD, FACS
Virginia Commonwealth University, Falls Church, VA

Louis Reines, MD, MBA
University of Connecticut General Surgery Residency, Farmington, CT

Caroline E. Reinke, MD, MSHP
University of Pennsylvania Perelman School of Medicine, Philadelphia, PA

Robert Y. Rhee, MD
Maimonides Medical Center, Brooklyn, NY

Robert S. Rhodes, MD, FACS
University of Pennsylvania School of Medicine, Philadelphia, PA

Taylor S. Riall, MD, PhD, FACS
University of Texas Medical Branch, Galveston, TX

Charles L. Rice, MD, FACS
Uniformed Services University of the Health Sciences, Bethesda, MD

Rocco Ricciardi, MD, FACS
Tufts University Medical School, Boston, MA

John A. Ridge, MD, PhD, FACS
Temple University School of Medicine, Philadelphia, PA

Jennifer Roberts, MD
Medical College of Wisconsin, Milwaukee, WI

Bryce R.H. Robinson, MD, FACS
University of Cincinnati, Cincinnati, OH

Sean Ronnekleiv-Kelly, MD
University of Wisconsin School of Medicine and Public Health, Madison, WI

Michael J. Rosen, MD, FACS
University Hospitals Case Medical Center, Cleveland, OH

Matthew R. Rosengart, MD, MPH
University of Pittsburgh, Pittsburgh, PA

David A. Rothenberger, MD, FACS
University of Minnesota, Minneapolis, MN

Madhuchhanda Roy, MD, PhD
University of Wisconsin School of Medicine and Public Health, Madison, WI

Daniel T. Ruan, MD
Brigham and Women's Hospital, Boston, MA

James Sampson, MD
University of Alabama at Birmingham, AL

Russell H. Samson, MD, FACS, RVT
Florida State University Medical School, Sarasota, FL

Juan R. Sanabria, MD, MSc, FACS
Case Western Reserve University School of Medicine, Cleveland, OH

Naveed U. Saqib, MD
University of Texas Medical School at Houston, Houston, TX

Robert G. Sawyer, MD, FACS, FIDSA, FCCM
University of Virginia, Charlottesville, VA

Ramesh Saxena, MD, PhD
University of Texas Southwestern Medical Center, Dallas, TX

Keith G. Saxon, MD, FACS
Harvard Medical School, Boston, MA

Christopher Scally, MD
University of Michigan, Ann Arbor, MI

William Schecter, MD, FACS, FCCM
University of California, San Francisco, CA

Christopher M. Schlachta, MDCM, FACS, FRSCS
University of Western Ontario, London, ON

David F. Schneider, MD, MS
Loyola University Medical Center, Maywood, IL

Michael J. Schurr, MD, FACS
University of Colorado, Denver, CO

Margaret L. Schwarze, MD, MPP, FACS
University of Wisconsin School of Medicine and Public Health, Madison, WI

Jessica Secor, MD
University of Wisconsin Hospitals and Clinics, Madison, WI

Matthew J. Sena, MD, FACS
University of California Davis School of Medicine, Sacramento, CA

Neha D. Shah, MD
Rush University Medical Center, Chicago, IL

Kiarash Shahlaie, MD, PhD
University of California Davis School of Medicine, Sacramento, CA

Jo Shapiro, MD, FACS
Harvard Medical School, Boston, MA

Cynthia K. Shortell, MD, FACS
Duke University School of Medicine, Durham, NC

Margo Shoup, MD, FACS
Loyola University Medical Center, Maywood, IL

Joseph B. Shrager, MD, FACS
Stanford University School of Medicine, Stanford, CA

Anton N. Sidawy, MD, MPH, FACS
George Washington University Hospital, Washington, DC

Samuel Singer, MD, FACS
Memorial Sloan-Kettering Cancer Center, New York, NY

Rebecca S. Sippel, MD, FACS
University of Wisconsin School of Medicine and Public Health, Madison, WI

Anton I. Skaro, MD, PhD, FRCSC
Northwestern University Feinberg School of Medicine, Chicago, IL

Randi Smith, MD
University of California San Francisco-East Bay, Oakland, CA

Ryan K. Smith, BA
Virginia Mason Medical Center, Seattle, WA

Sumona V. Smith, MD
University of Texas Southwestern Medical Center, Dallas, TX

Linda Sohn, MD, MPH
UCLA School of Medicine/Geriatrics, Los Angeles, CA

Julie Ann Sosa, MA, MD, FACS
Yale University School of Medicine, New Haven, CT

Wiley W. Souba, MD, ScD, MBA, FACS
The Ohio State University College of Medicine, Columbus, OH

Sharon L. Stein, MD
University Hospitals Case Medical Center, Cleveland, OH

Steven M. Steinberg, MD, FACS
The Ohio State University College of Medicine, Columbus, OH

Jose P. Sterling, MD
Parkland Medical Center, Dallas, TX

Richard H. Sterns, MD
University of Rochester School of Medicine and Dentistry, Rochester, NY

Karyn B. Stitzenberg, MD, MPH
University of North Carolina, Chapel Hill, NC

Patrick A. Stone, MD
Robert C. Byrd Sciences Center, West Virginia University, Charleston, WV

Robert T. Stovall, MD
University of Colorado School of Medicine, Denver, CO

Steven M. Strasberg, MD, FACS, FRCS(C), FRCS(Ed)
Washington University School of Medicine, St. Louis, MO

Cord Sturgeon, MD
Northwestern University Feinberg School of Medicine, Chicago, IL

William D. Suggs, MD, FACS
Albert Einstein College of Medicine, Yeshiva University, New York, NY

Stephen R. Sullivan, MD, MPH
Brown University Warren Alpert Medical School, Providence, RI

R. Sudhir Sundaresan, MD, FRCSC, FACS
University of Ottawa, Ottawa, ON

Pasithorn A. Suwanabol, MD
University of Wisconsin School of Medicine and Public Health, Madison, WI

Scott J. Swanson, MD
Harvard Medical School, Boston, MA

Mark S. Talamonti, MD, FACS
NorthShore University Health System, Evanston, IL

Kenneth Tanabe, MD
Harvard Medical School, Boston, MA

Roger P. Tatum, MD, FACS
University of Washington School of Medicine, Seattle, WA

Ali Tavakkolizadeh, MD, FRCS, FACS
Harvard Medical School, Boston, MA

Lloyd M. Taylor Jr, MD, FACS
Oregon Health & Science University, Portland, OR

Ezra N. Teitelbaum, MD
Northwestern University Feinberg School of Medicine, Chicago, IL

Theodore H. Teruya, MD
Loma Linda University Medical Center, Loma Linda, CA

[illegible], MD, FACS, FRACS (Hon)
University of Texas Southwestern Medical School, Dallas, TX

Areti Tillou, MD
David Geffen School of Medicine, University of California, Los Angeles, CA

Patrick Twomey, MD
University of California San Francisco-East Bay, Oakland, CA

Gilbert R. Upchurch Jr, MD
University of Michigan, Ann Arbor, MI

Caesar Ursic, MD
University of California, San Francisco, CA

Garth H. Utter, MD, MSc, FACS
University of California Davis Medical Center, Sacramento, CA

O.M. van Delden, MD, PhD
University of Amsterdam, Amsterdam

Erik G. Van Eaton, MD, FACS
University of Washington, Seattle, WA

Alex J. Vanni, MD
University of Washington, Seattle, WA

Ara Vaporciyan, MD, FACS
The University of Texas MD Anderson Cancer Center, Houston, TX

Frank J. Veith, MD, FACS
Cleveland Clinic Lerner College of Medicine of Case Western Reserve University, Cleveland, OH

P. James Villeneuve, MDCM, PhD, FRCSC
University of Ottawa, Ottawa, ON

Todd R. Vogel, MD, MPH, FACS
University of Missouri Hospital and Clinics, Columbia, MO

Philip Wai, MD
Loyola University Medical Center, Maywood, IL

Thomas W. Wakefield, MD, FACS
University of Michigan, Ann Arbor, MI

J. Patrick Walker, MD, FACS
Houston County Surgical Associates, Crockett, TX

Tracy S. Wang, MD, MPH, FACS
Medical College of Wisconsin, Milwaukee, WI

Jennifer A. Wargo, MD
Harvard Medical School, Boston, MA

Jeffrey D. Wayne, MD, FACS
Northwestern University Feinberg School of Medicine, Chicago, IL

Sharon Weber, MD, FACS
University of Wisconsin School of Medicine and Public Health, Madison, WI

Jon O. Wee, MD, FACS
Harvard Medical School, Boston, MA

Tracey L. Weigel, MD, FACS, FACCP
University of Wisconsin School of Medicine and Public Health, Madison, WI

Jordan A. Weinberg, MD, FACS
University of Tennessee Health Science Center, Memphis, TN

John P. Welch, MD, FACS
University of Connecticut, Farmington, CT

Hunter Wessells, MD, FACS
University of Washington, Seattle, WA

Steven D. Wexner, MD, FACS, FRCS, FRCS (Ed)
University of South Florida, Tampa, FL

Daniel C. Wiener, MD
Tufts Medical Center, Boston, MA

J. Graham Williams, MCh, FRCS
New Cross Hospital, Wolverhampton

Emily R. Winslow, MD
University of Wisconsin School of Medicine and Public Health, Madison, WI

David H. Wisner, MD, FACS
University of California Davis School of Medicine, Sacramento, CA

Sook-Bin Woo, DMD, MMSc
Harvard School of Dental Medicine, Boston, MA

Cameron D. Wright, MD, FACS
Massachusetts General Hospital, Boston, MA

Timothy Wu, MD
University of Chicago, Chicago, IL

Dai Yamanouchi, MD, PhD
University of Wisconsin School of Medicine and Public Health, Madison, WI

George P. Yang, MD, PhD, FACS
Stanford University School of Medicine, Stanford, CA

Michael W. Yeh, MD, FACS
David Geffen School of Medicine, University of California, Los Angeles, CA

Min C. Yoo, MD
University of Tennessee/Methodist Transplant Institute, Memphis, TN

Tonia Young-Fadok, MD, MS
Mayo Clinic College of Medicine, Scottsdale, AZ

Barbara Zarebczan, MD
University of Wisconsin School of Medicine and Public Health, Madison, WI

Michael E. Zenilman, MD, FACS
State University of New York Downstate College of Medicine, New York, NY

Linda P. Zhang, MD
Washington University School of Medicine, St. Louis, MO

Marike Zwienenberg-Lee, MD
University of California Davis School of Medicine, Sacramento, CA

FOREWORD

ACS Surgery is being offered in a new seventh edition, available in classical hard cover as well as Web-based online versions. It provides a comprehensive reference work across all stages of surgical training and practice, from the surgical resident to the experienced practitioner. There are several features to this excellent new edition that bear comment.

The new edition not only covers all traditional areas of surgical practice but also has a number of novel and innovative sections. At the outset, Competency-Based Surgical Care (Section 1) deals with professionalism, performance-based measurement, surgical safety, cost-effective care, and health care economics. The Trauma and Critical Care chapters (Sections 8, 9) have been expanded with several new chapters and are supplemented by Section 10, which details the specific care needed by several less common and high-risk population groups. This includes a new chapter on the relevant aspects of transplantation needed by the general surgeon.

Scientific Foundations (Section 11) has virtually all new material. Two chapters deal with clinical trial design/statistics and evidence-based medicine. Several chapters deal with the unique needs and care of the aging patient and related subjects involving questions of advance directives, do not resuscitate orders, and so forth. Additional chapters deal with the technical details and physiology of laparoscopic and robotic surgery.

Overall, there are more than 50 new chapters added to the book, ensuring that the material is relevant to current needs and cutting edge in its relevance to today's practice. As with previous editions of the book, the illustrations, diagrams, tables, and algorithms are extremely well done and serve to enhance and clarify concepts outlined in the text. In addition, the practice in the online version of updating chapter content on a continuing basis, so that the full textbook is continually renewed with updated and new material on a 4-year cycle, provides assurance of continuing currency of the material.

A unique feature of this text is that it has established links with the curriculum established by the Surgical Council on Resident Education (SCORE) and has provided linkage between the written text and the SCORE curriculum, which is in use by more than 90% of surgical residency programs.

Dr. Ashley and the Editorial Board are to be commended for the excellent content and organization of this edition and for the selection of several younger but experienced and authoritative authors for the new sections of the text. It can be highly recommended to surgical practitioners of all ages.

Frank R Lewis, MD, FACS
Executive Director
American Board of Surgery
Philadelphia, PA
October 2013

PREFACE

With this new edition, *ACS Surgery* continues the traditions of excellence that the work has embodied since its inception. The only surgical textbook bearing the imprimatur of the American College of Surgeons, it has continued to evolve to meet the needs of both the practicing surgeon and the trainee.

Our emphasis remains the same—to provide a comprehensive and accessible reference covering the entire field of general surgery. With this goal in mind, we have made several changes since our previous edition. In addition to new editorial board members and new authors who have brought fresh perspectives, we have expanded not only the chapters focusing on medical knowledge and patient care, but also those devoted to the other competencies—professionalism, interpersonal communication, systems-based practice, and practice-based learning and improvement.

We have also capitalized on a unique effort by the Surgical Council for Resident Education (SCORE), a collaborative of US surgical education stakeholders, to develop a comprehensive curriculum for general surgery, outlining diseases and conditions, as well as the operations that the general surgeon should be competent to perform. With each chapter update, we have asked authors to incorporate this curriculum, a process that has often added new information or changed the emphasis. Moving away from the text's historic organization by clinical presentations and operations, new chapters provide an integrated approach to disease processes and their treatment.

The text continues to be offered in two formats—this classic hardbound volume and a Web version (www.acssurgery.com) available to purchasers of the text on a 3-month trial basis. Whereas the hardbound version is as current as the date of printing, the online version is continuously updated, with new revisions and state-of-the art information added on a monthly basis. Special features of the online version include a monthly column entitled *What's New in ACS Surgery* and an interactive CME program focusing on the updated chapters. Surgeons who rely on *ACS Surgery* for CME will find that they also satisfy the American Board of Surgery's requirement for Maintenance of Certification.

ACS Surgery occupies a unique niche among surgical textbooks, and it is our intention to continue to adapt to the changing needs of general surgeons in training and in practice.

Stanley W Ashley
Boston, MA
October 2013

1 PROFESSIONALISM IN SURGERY

Jo Shapiro, MD, FACS, Steven M. Steinberg, MD, FACS, and Wiley W. Souba, MD, ScD, MBA, FACS

Over the past decade, the American health care system has had to cope with and manage an unprecedented amount of change. As a consequence, the medical profession has been challenged along the entire range of its cultural values and its traditional roles and responsibilities. It would be difficult, if not impossible, to find another social issue directly affecting all Americans that has undergone as rapid and remarkable a transformation—and oddly, a transformation in which the most important protagonists (i.e., the patients and the doctors) remain dissatisfied.[1]

Nowhere is this metamorphosis more evident than in the field of surgery. Marked reductions in reimbursement, explosions in surgical device biotechnology, a national medical malpractice crisis, and the disturbing emphasis on commercialized medicine have forever changed the surgical landscape, or so it seems. The very foundation of patient care—the doctor-patient relationship—is in jeopardy. Surgeons find it increasingly difficult to meet their responsibilities to patients and to society as a whole. In these circumstances, it is critical for us to reaffirm our commitment to the fundamental and universal principles and values of medical professionalism.

The concept of medicine as a profession grounded in compassion and sympathy for the sick has come under serious challenge.[2] One eroding force has been the growth and sovereignty of biomedical research. Given the high position of science and technology in our societal hierarchy, we may be headed for a form of medicine that includes little caring but becomes exclusively focused on the mechanics of treatment, so that we deal with sick patients much as we would a flat tire or a leaky faucet. In such a form of medicine, healing becomes little more than a technical exercise, and any talk of morality that is unsubstantiated by hard facts is considered mere opinion and therefore carries little weight.

The rise of entrepreneurialism and the growing corporatization of medicine also challenge the traditions of virtue-based medical care. When these processes are allowed to dominate medicine, health care becomes a commodity. As Pellegrino and Thomasma remark, "When economics and entrepreneurism drive the professions, they admit only self-interest and the working of the marketplace as the motives for professional activity. In a free-market economy, effacement of self-interest, or any conduct shaped primarily by the idea of altruism or virtue, is simply inconsistent with survival."[2]

Another profound change in the practice of medicine is the shift from a largely autonomous focus, with the surgeon both shouldering tremendous personal responsibility and wielding considerable control and independence, to a complex, team-based focus. Within this new paradigm, leadership of a surgical team requires vastly different competencies than were previously required or even valued. Many surgeons have flourished in this new environment: leading a cohesive team dedicated to excellent outcomes is highly rewarding. Unfortunately, however, as a profession, we have not explicitly taught these teamwork and leadership skills, nor have we always helped our colleagues remediate deficiencies in such skills.

The Meaning of Professionalism

Professionalism is the basis of our contract with society. A profession is a collegial discipline that regulates itself by means of mandatory, systematic training. It has a base in a body of technical and specialized knowledge that it both teaches and advances; it sets and enforces its own standards; and it has a service orientation, rather than a profit orientation, enshrined in a code of ethics.[3–5] To put it more succinctly, a profession has cognitive, collegial, and moral attributes. These qualities are well expressed in the familiar sentence from the Hippocratic oath: "I will practice my art with purity and holiness and for the benefit of the sick."

Historically, the legitimacy of medical authority is based on three distinct claims[2,6]: first, that the knowledge and competence of the professional have been validated by a community of peers; second, that this knowledge has a scientific basis; and third, that the professional's judgment and advice are oriented toward a set of values. These aspects of legitimacy correspond to the collegial, cognitive, and moral attributes that define a profession.

The American College of Surgeons (ACS) Task Force on Professionalism has developed a Code of Professional Conduct,[7] which emphasizes the following four aspects of professionalism:

1. A competent surgeon is more than a competent technician.
2. Whereas ethical practice and professionalism are closely related, professionalism also incorporates surgeons' relationships with patients and society.
3. Unprofessional behavior must have consequences.
4. Professional organizations are responsible for fostering professionalism in their membership.

Specifically, the ACS Code of Professional Conduct includes tenets of professionalism that relate to both our care of individual patients and our role in society [*see Table 1*].

The Accreditation Council on Graduate Medical Education (ACGME) has identified six competencies that must be demonstrated by the surgeon: (1) patient care; (2) medical knowledge; (3) practice-based learning and improvement; (4) interpersonal and communication skills; (5) professionalism; and (6) systems-based practice. These competencies are now being integrated into the training programs of all accredited surgical residencies.

Being a professional demands unwavering personal integrity and a commitment to lifelong learning and improvement. It

Table 1 American College of Surgeons' Code of Professional Conduct[27]

During the continuum of pre-, intra-, and postoperative care, we accept responsibilities to
- Serve as effective advocates for our patients' needs;
- Disclose therapeutic options, including their risks and benefits;
- Disclose and resolve any conflict of interest that might influence the decisions of care;
- Be sensitive and respectful of patients, understanding their vulnerability during the perioperative period;
- Fully disclose adverse events and medical errors;
- Acknowledge patients' psychological, social, cultural, and spiritual needs;
- Encompass within our surgical care the special needs of terminally ill patients;
- Acknowledge and support the needs of patients' families; and
- Respect the knowledge, dignity, and perspective of other healthcare professionals.

Our profession is also accountable to our communities and to society. In return for their trust, as Fellows of the American College of Surgeons, we accept responsibilities to
- Provide the highest quality of surgical care;
- Abide by the values of honesty, confidentiality, and altruism;
- Participate in lifelong learning;
- Maintain competence throughout our surgical careers;
- Participate in self-regulation by setting, maintaining, and enforcing practice standards;
- Improve care by evaluating its processes and outcomes;
- Inform the public on subjects within our expertise;
- Advocate strategies to improve individual and public health by communicating with government, healthcare organizations, and industry;
- Work with society to establish a just, effective, and efficient distribution of healthcare resources;
- Provide necessary surgical care without regard to gender, race, disability, religion, social status, or ability to pay; and
- Participate in educational programs addressing professionalism.

places the responsibility to serve (care for) others above self-interest and reward [*see Sidebar* Elizabeth Blackwell: A Model of Professionalism[8]].

Regrettably, examples of unprofessional behavior exist. An excerpt from a note from a third-year medical student to the core clerkship director reads as follows: "I have seen attendings make sexist, racist jokes or remarks during surgery. I have met residents who joke about deaf patients and female patients with facial hair. [I have encountered] teams joking and counting down the days until patients die" (personal communication, 2004). This kind of exposure to unprofessional conduct and language can influence young people negatively, and it must change.

Most of us went to medical school because we wanted to help and care for people who are ill. This genuine desire to care is unambiguously apparent in the vast majority of personal statements that medical students prepare as part of their application process. To quote William Osler, "You are in this profession as a calling, not as a business; as a calling which extracts from you at every turn self-sacrifice, devotion, love and tenderness to your fellow man. We must work in the missionary spirit with a breath of charity that raises you far above the petty jealousies of life."[9] To keep medicine a calling, we must explicitly incorporate into the meaning of professionalism those nontechnical practices, habits, and attributes that the compassionate, caring, and competent physician exemplifies. We must remind ourselves that a true professional places service to the patient above self-interest and above reward.

One of the core tenets of professionalism is being consistently respectful not only toward our patients and their families but also toward our colleagues and other health care team members. Although no one would argue with this in principle, there are many factors that challenge our ability to hold true to this precept, including poor interpersonal communication skills, lack of training in conflict resolution, resource constraints, and cultural tradition.

Given that professionalism is so multifaceted, it is not surprising that various important professional values may conflict with one another, creating tension sometimes internally and at other times between various groups. For example, the patient may want a specific treatment that is not yet supported by evidence but may be of benefit. Meeting the patient's expectations and needs may directly conflict with the expectation that we are advocates for "efficient distribution of health care resources." Another direct challenge to several professionalism obligations is trying to balance the important adherence to the duty hours mandate with the equally important value of continuity of care.[10]

The underpinning of medicine as a compassionate, caring profession is the doctor-patient relationship, a relationship that has become jeopardized and sometimes fractured over the past decade. Our individual perceptions of what this relationship is and how it should work will inevitably have a great impact on how we approach the care of our patients.[2]

The view of the physician-patient relationship as a covenant does not demand devotion to medicine to the exclusion of other responsibilities and is not inconsistent with the fact that medicine is also a science, an art, and a business.[2] Nevertheless, in our struggle to remain viable in a health care environment that has become a commercial enterprise, efforts to preserve market share cannot take precedence over the provision of care that is grounded in charity and compassion. It is exactly for this reason that medicine always will be, and should be, a relationship between people. To fracture that relationship by exchanging a covenant based on charity and compassion for a contract based solely on the delivery of goods and services is something none of us would want for ourselves. The nature of the healing relationship is itself the foundation of the special obligations of physicians as physicians.[2]

Translation of Theory into Practice

It is encouraging to note that many instances of unprofessional conduct that once were routinely overlooked—such

Elizabeth Blackwell: A Model of Professionalism[8]

Elizabeth Blackwell was born in England in 1821, the daughter of a sugar refiner. When she was 10 years old, her family emigrated to New York City. Discovering in herself a strong desire to practice medicine and care for the underserved, she took up residence in a physician's household, using her time there to study using books in the family's medical library.

As a young woman, Blackwell applied to several prominent medical schools but was snubbed by all of them. After 29 rejections, she sent her second round of applications to smaller colleges, including Geneva College in New York. She was accepted at Geneva—according to an anecdote, because the faculty put the matter to a student vote, and the students thought her application a hoax. She braved the prejudice of some of the professors and students to complete her training, eventually ranking first in her class. On January 23, 1849, at the age of 27, Elizabeth Blackwell became the first woman to earn a medical degree in the United States. Her goal was to become a surgeon.

After several months in Pennsylvania, during which time she became a naturalized citizen of the United States, Blackwell traveled to Paris, where she hoped to study with one of the leading French surgeons. Denied access to Parisian hospitals because of her gender, she enrolled instead at La Maternité, a highly regarded midwifery school, in the summer of 1849. While attending to a child some 4 months after enrolling, Blackwell inadvertently spattered some pus from the child's eyes into her own left eye. The child was infected with gonorrhea, and Blackwell contracted a severe case of ophthalmia neonatorum, which later necessitated the removal of the infected eye. Although the loss of an eye made it impossible for her to become a surgeon, it did not dampen her passion for becoming a practicing physician.

By mid-1851, when Blackwell returned to the United States, she was well prepared for private practice. However, no male doctor would even consider the idea of a female associate, no matter how well trained. Barred from practice in most hospitals, Blackwell founded her own infirmary, the New York Infirmary for Indigent Women and Children, in 1857. When the American Civil War began, Blackwell trained nurses, and in 1868 she founded a women's medical college at the Infirmary so that women could be formally trained as physicians. In 1869, she returned to England and, with Florence Nightingale, opened the Women's Medical College. Blackwell taught at the newly created London School of Medicine for Women and became the first female physician in the United Kingdom Medical Register. She set up a private practice in her own home, where she saw women and children, many of whom were of lesser means and were unable to pay. In addition, Blackwell mentored other women who subsequently pursued careers in medicine. She retired at the age of 86.

In short, Elizabeth Blackwell embodied professionalism in her work. In 1889 she wrote, "There is no career nobler than that of the physician. The progress and welfare of society is more intimately bound up with the prevailing tone and influence of the medical profession than with the status of any other class."

as mistreating medical students, speaking disrespectfully to coworkers, and fraudulent behavior—are now being dealt with. Still, from time to time, an incident is made public that makes us all feel shame. In March 2003, the *Seattle Times* carried a story about the chief of neurosurgery at the University of Washington, who pleaded guilty to a felony charge of obstructing the government's investigation and admitted that he asked others to lie for him and created an atmosphere of fear in the neurosurgery department.[11] According to the US Attorney in Seattle, University of Washington employees destroyed reports revealing that university doctors submitted inflated billings to Medicare and Medicaid. The department chair lost his job, was barred from participation in Medicare, and, as part of his plea bargain, had to pay a $500,000 fine, perform 1,000 hours of community service, and write an article in a medical journal about billing errors. The university spent many millions in legal fees and eventually settled the billing issues with the federal government for one of the highest Physicians at Teaching Hospitals (PATH) settlements ever.

Fortunately, such extreme cases of unprofessionalism are quite uncommon. Nevertheless, there are numerous reports in the literature of other types of unprofessional behavior, such as disruptive behavior,[7] that can lead to patient safety risks.[12–14] To this end, The Joint Commission has mandated that all of our hospitals have zero tolerance for disruptive behavior. Regardless of the practice setting, it remains our responsibility as professionals to prevent such behaviors from developing and from being reinforced. A study published in 2004 demonstrated an association between displays of unprofessional behavior in medical school and subsequent disciplinary action by a state medical board.[15] The authors concluded that professionalism is an essential competency that students must demonstrate to graduate from medical school. Who could disagree? Yet we know that throughout our careers, there will be challenges, both personal and external, to our consistently behaving professionally.

In addition to the reports recounting acts of unprofessional behavior, various publications describing methods of teaching and assessing professionalism have begun to appear in the past few years.[16,17] As an example, Kumar and colleagues found that using ACS case-based multimedia materials enhanced the ability of residents to recognize and discuss matters related to professional behavior.[18] Surgical residents who viewed these materials scored higher on an assessment tool than did residents with the same level of experience who did not use the materials. An additional encouraging finding was that residents of all years were able to define the components of professionalism. In another publication, Gauger and colleagues described an evaluation instrument used to evaluate residents with respect to the aspects of professionalism.[19] They divided the concept of professionalism into 15 domains and modified a standard resident evaluation form to assess the faculty's perception of resident performance in each domain. This evaluation tool proved to be internally consistent, but in the absence of any other gold standard tools with which to compare it, its validity could not be determined.

Hickson developed a system to monitor patient complaint data and use this to improve the behavior of individual physicians.[20] Others have developed 360 assessment tools to give feedback to physicians regarding how their professionalism skills are perceived by their team members.[21]

Assessment tools and formal courses alone are not enough to support the significant adaptive challenge[22] that is involved in maintaining a culture of professionalism.[10] Several authors have argued for a nuanced approach to supporting professional behaviors—one that acknowledges that professionalism is not a fixed trait but rather a set of developmental skills that need to be continuously taught, role-modeled, and reflected on throughout one's career.[23] Understanding that professional behavior is contextual and situation dependent is crucial to developing programs to support professionalism.

The Future of Surgical Professionalism

It is often subtly implied—or even candidly stated—that no matter how well we adjust to the changing health care environment, the practice of surgery will never again be quite as rewarding as it once was. This need not be the case. The ongoing advances in surgical technology, the increasing opportunities for community-based surgeons to enrol their patients into clinical trials, the growing emphasis on lifelong learning, and the increased focus on teamwork and shared responsibility are factors that not only help satisfy social and organizational demands for quality care but also are in the best interest of our patients.

In the near future, maintenance of certification for surgeons will involve much more than taking an examination every decade. The ACS is taking the lead in helping to develop new measures of competence. Whatever specific form such measures may take, displaying professionalism and living up to a set of uncompromisable core values[24] will always be central indicators of the performance of the individual surgeon and the integrity of the discipline of surgery as a whole.

Although surgeons vary enormously with respect to personality, practice preferences, areas of specialization, and style of relating to others, they all have one role in common: that of healer. Indeed, it is the highest of privileges to be able to care for the sick. As the playwright Howard Sackler once wrote, "To intervene, even briefly, between our fellow creatures and their suffering or death, is our most authentic answer to the question of our humanity."[25] Inseparable from this privilege is a set of responsibilities that are not to be taken lightly: a pledge to offer our patients the best care possible and a commitment to teach and advance the science and practice of medicine. Commitment to the practice of patient-centered, high-quality, cost-effective care is what gives our work meaning and provides us with a sense of purpose.[26] As surgeons, we must participate actively in the current evolution of integrated health care. By doing so, we help build our own future.

Jo Shapiro, MD, FACS, has disclosed a potential conflict of interest as follows: grants and/or salary by Health Dialog

References

1. Fein R. The HMO revolution. Dissent 1998;Spring:29.
2. Pellegrino ED, Thomasma DC. Helping and healing. Washington (DC): Georgetown University Press; 1997.
3. Brandeis LD. Familiar medical quotations. In: Strauss M, editor. Business—a profession. Boston: Little Brown & Co; 1986. p. 17.
4. Cogan ML. Toward a definition of profession. Harv Educ Rev 1953;23:33.
5. Greenwood E. Attributes of a profession. Social Work 1957;22:44.
6. Starr PD. The social transformation of American medicine. New York: Basic Books; 1982.
7. Gruen RI, Arya J, Cosgrove EM, et al. Professionalism in surgery. J Am Coll Surg 2003;197:605.
8. Speigel R. Elizabeth Blackwell: the first woman doctor. Snapshots in science and medicine. Available at: http://science-education.nih.gov/snapshots.nsf/story?openform&pds~Elizabeth_Blackwell_Doctor (accessed March 21, 2012).
9. Hinohara S, Niki H, editors. Osler's "Way of Life" and other addresses, with commentary and annotations. Durham (NC): Duke University Press; 2001.
10. Lucey C, Souba W. The problem with the problem of professionalism. Acad Med 2010;85:1018–24.
11. Ostrom CM. A neaurosurgeon 'crisis': Insurer drops doctors' group. The Seattle Times 2003 June 7.
12. Rosenstein AH, O' Daniel M. A survey of the impact of disruptive behaviors and communication defects on patient safety. Jt Comm J Qual Patient Saf 2008;34:464–71.
13. Rosenstein AH, O'Daniel M. Disruptive behavior and clinical outcomes. Am J Nurs 2005;105:54–64.
14. The Joint Commission. Behaviors that undermine a culture of safety. Sentinel Event Alert 2008;40:1–3.
15. Papadakis M, Hodgson C, Teherani A, Kohatsu ND. Unprofessional behavior in medical school is associated with subsequent disciplinary action by a state medical board. Acad Med 2004;79:244.
16. Papadakis MA, Osborn EH, Cooke M, Healy K. A strategy for the detection and evaluation of unprofessional behavior in medical students. University of California, San Francisco School of Medicine Clinical Clerkships Operation Committee. Acad Med 1999;74:980–90.
17. Yao D, Wright S. National survey of internal medicine residency program directors regarding problem residents. JAMA 2000;284:1099–104.
18. Kumar A, Shibru D, Bullard K, et al. Case-based multimedia program enhances the maturation of surgical residents regarding the concepts of professionalism. J Surg Educ 2007;64:194.
19. Gauger P, Gruppen L, Minter R, et al. Initial use of a novel instrument to measure professionalism in surgical residents. Am J Surg 2005;189:479.
20. Hickson G, Pichert JW, Webb LE, Gabbe SG. A complementary approach to promoting professionalism: identifying, measuring and addressing unprofessionalism behaviors. Acad Med 2007;82:1040–8.
21. Harmon L, Gregory P, Hiller N, Batista L. PULSE (Physicians Universal Leadership Skills Education Survey) technical report executive summary. Physicians Development Program, Miami, FL; 2010 (Unpublished proprietary manuscript).
22. Heifetz R, Linsky M. Leadership on the line. Boston: Harvard Business Press; 2002.
23. Lesser C, Lucey C, Egener B, et al. A behavioral and systems view of professionalism. JAMA 2010;304:2732–7.
24. Souba W. Academic medicine's core values: what do they mean? J Surg Res 2003;115:171.
25. Rosenow EC. The art of living...the art of medicine: the wit and wisdom of life and medicine: a physician's perspective. Victoria BC: Trafford; 2003. p. 128.
26. Souba W. Academic medicine and our search for meaning and purpose. Acad Med 2002;77:139.
27. American College of Surgeons. Code of professional conduct. Available at: www.facs.org/memberservices/codeofconduct.html (accessed March 21, 2012).

2 PERFORMANCE MEASUREMENT IN SURGERY

Justin B. Dimick MD, MPH, and John D. Birkmeyer MD

With growing recognition that the quality of surgical care varies widely, good measures of performance are in high demand. Patients and their families are looking to make informed decisions about where and from whom to get their surgical care.[1] Employers and payers need measures on which to base their contracting decisions and pay-for-performance initiatives.[2] Finally, clinical leaders need measures that can help them identify "best practices" and guide their quality improvement efforts. An ever-broadening array of performance measures is being developed to meet these different needs.

However, considerable uncertainty remains about which measures are most useful for measuring surgical quality. Current measures are remarkably heterogeneous, encompassing different elements of health care structure, process of care, and patient outcomes. Although each of these three types of performance measures has unique strengths, each is also associated with conceptual, methodological, and/or practical problems. The baseline risk and frequency of the procedure are obviously important considerations in weighing the strengths and weaknesses of different measures.[3] So too is the underlying purpose of performance measurement. Measures that work well when the primary intent is to steer patients to the best hospitals or surgeons (selective referral) may not be optimal for quality improvement purposes and vice versa.

Expanding on other recent reviews of performance measurement,[3–5] this chapter provides an overview of measures commonly used to assess surgical quality, considers their main strengths and limitations, and closes with recommendations for selecting the optimal quality measure [*see Table 1*].

Overview of Current Measures

The number of performance measures that have been developed for the assessment of surgical quality is already large and continues to grow. Many surgical quality indicators are already used in hospital accreditation, pay-for-performance, or public reporting efforts. Over the past few years, the National Quality Forum (NQF) has emerged as the leading organization endorsing quality measures. Many influential organizations, including the Joint Commission on Accreditation of Healthcare Organizations (JCAHO) and the Centers for Medicare and Medicaid Services (CMS), rely on the endorsement of the NQF before applying a measure to practice. The number of measures relevant to surgery that have been endorsed by the NQF has grown rapidly.

Although the NQF is the central organization for evaluating quality measures, many organizations develop candidate measures and submit them for endorsement. The Agency for Healthcare Research and Quality (AHRQ) has focused primarily on quality measures that take advantage of readily available administrative data, such as the hospital discharge data sets comprising the Healthcare Cost and Utilization Project (HCUP) [*see Table 2*]. Because little information on process of care is available in these data sets, these measures are mainly structural (e.g., hospital procedure volume) or outcome based (e.g., risk-adjusted mortality).

The Leapfrog Group (http://www.leapfroggroup.org), a coalition of large employers and purchasers, has developed perhaps the most visible set of surgical quality indicators for its value-based purchasing initiative. The organization's original standards focused exclusively on procedure volume but later expanded its standards to include selected process variables (e.g., the use of beta blockers in patients undergoing abdominal aortic aneurysm repair) and outcome measures, such as mortality. Most recently (2010), the Leapfrog Group began using a composite of operative mortality and hospital volume, the so-called "Survival Predictor," as the primary measure for its evidence-based hospital referral initiative. Such composite measures are discussed further below.

Several surgical professional organizations have played a large part in developing many of the quality measures endorsed by the NQF. The Society of Thoracic Surgeons (STS) has been a leader in the development of quality measures for cardiac and thoracic procedures [*see Table 3 and Table 4*]. These measures include the structure, process, and outcomes of cardiac surgical care. In addition, the STS recently developed a composite measure that combines all of these domains of quality into a single hospital rating. The National Surgical Quality Improvement Program (NSQIP) has also developed measures for colectomy, lower extremity bypass, and elderly surgical patients [*see Table 3 and Table 4*]. Finally, the Society for Vascular Surgery (SVS) has acted as the steward for measures of process of care for carotid endarterectomy [*see Table 4*].

Structural Measures of Quality

Health care structure reflects the setting or system in which care is delivered. Many structural measures describe hospital-level attributes, such as the physical plant and resources or staff coordination and organization (e.g., nurse-to-bed ratios, designation as a Level I trauma center). Other structural measures reflect attributes associated with the relative expertise of individual physicians (e.g., board certification, subspecialty training, or procedure volume).

STRENGTHS

From a measurement perspective, structural measures of quality have several attractive features. First, many of these

Table 1 Primary Strengths and Limitations of Structure, Process, and Outcome Measures

	Structure	*Process*	*Outcomes*
Examples	Procedure volume, intensivist-managed ICUs	Appropriate use of prophylactic antibiotics	Risk-adjusted mortality rates for CABG from state or national registries
Strengths	Expedient, inexpensive Efficient—one measure may relate to several outcomes For some procedures, better predictor of subsequent performance than other measures	Reflect care that patients actually receive—buy-in from providers Directly actionable for quality improvement activities Do not need risk adjustment for many measures	Face validity Measurement alone may improve outcomes (i.e., Hawthorne effect)
Limitations	Limited number of measures Generally not actionable Do not reflect individual performance, considered unfair by providers	Many measures hard to ascertain with existing databases Variable extent to which process measures link to important patient outcomes Lack of high leverage, procedure-specific processes	Sample size constraints Expense of clinical data collection Concerns about risk adjustment with administrative data

CABG = coronary artery bypass grafting; ICU = intensive care unit.

Table 2 Surgical Performance Measures that Apply to Multiple Surgical Procedures Endorsed by the National Quality Forum

Diagnosis or Procedure	*Performance Measure*	*Steward*
All surgical procedures	Appropriate antibiotic prophylaxis (selection, timing, and duration)	AMA
	Hair clipping prior to surgery	CMS
	Appropriate venous thromboembolism prophylaxis	AMA/CMS
	Perioperative temperature management	CMS
	Preoperative beta blockers continued after surgery	CMS
	Urinary catheter removed postoperative day 2	CMS
	Risk-adjusted surgical mortality or major complications in elderly patients	ACS/NSQIP
	Accidental puncture or laceration	AHRQ
	Iatrogenic pneumothorax	AHRQ
	Wound dehiscence	AHRQ
	Postoperative respiratory failure	AHRQ
	Failure to rescue	AHRQ
	Postoperative venous thromboembolism	AHRQ
	Foreign body left after procedure	AHRQ
	Superficial surgical site infection	CDC
Cardiac and thoracic surgery	Participation in a systematic quality improvement database	STS
Pediatric surgery	Risk-adjusted mortality in neonates undergoing noncardiac surgery	CHOP

ACS = American College of Surgeons; AHRQ = Agency for Healthcare Research and Quality; AMA = American Medical Association; CDC = Centers for Disease Control and Prevention; CHOP = Children's Hospital of Pennsylvania; CMS = Centers for Medicare and Medicaid Services; JCAHO = Joint Commission on Accreditation of Healthcare Organizations; NSQIP = National Surgical Quality Improvement Program; STS = Society of Thoracic Surgeons.

measures are strongly related to patient outcomes. For example, with esophagectomy and pancreatic resection, operative mortality rates at very high-volume hospitals are as much as 10% lower, in absolute terms, than at lower-volume centers.[6,7] In some instances, structural measures such as procedure volume are more predictive of subsequent hospital performance than any known processes of care or direct mortality measures[8] [*see Figure 1*].

A second advantage is efficiency. A single structural measure may be associated with numerous outcomes. For example, with some types of cancer surgery, hospital or surgeon procedure volume is associated not only with lower operative mortality but also with lower perioperative morbidity and higher late survival rates.[9–11] Intensivist model intensive care units are linked to shorter length of stay and reduced resource use, as well as lower mortality.[12,13]

The third and perhaps most important advantage of structural variables is expediency. Many can be assessed easily with readily available administrative data. Although some structural measures require surveying hospitals or providers, such data are much less expensive to collect than measures requiring patient-level information.

Table 3 Surgical Performance Measures Endorsed by the National Quality Forum that Apply to Specific Cardiac and Vascular Procedures

Diagnosis or Procedure	*Performance Measure*	*Steward*
Coronary artery bypass grafting	Hospital volume	STS
	Risk-adjusted mortality rate	STS
	Postoperative renal failure	STS
	Internal mammary artery use	STS
	Preoperative beta blockade	STS
	Postoperative glucose controlled by 6 am the day after surgery	JCAHO
	STS composite measure	STS
	Reoperation for tamponade, bleeding, or other cardiac reason	STS
	Antiplatelet therapy at discharge	STS
	Beta-blocker therapy at discharge	STS
	Antilipid therapy at discharge	STS
	Deep sternal wound infection rate	STS
	Prolonged intubation	STS
	Stroke	STS
Aortic valve replacement	Risk-adjusted mortality rate	STS
	Hospital volume	STS
Mitral valve replacement/repair	Risk-adjusted mortality rate	STS
	Hospital volume	STS
Pediatric heart surgery	Hospital volume	AHRQ
	Risk-adjusted mortality rates	AHRQ
Abdominal aneurysm repair	Hospital volume	AHRQ
	Risk-adjusted mortality rates	AHRQ
Lower extremity bypass	Risk-adjusted mortality or major complications	CMS
Carotid endarterectomy	Perioperative antiplatelet therapy	SVS
	Patch closure of arteriotomy	SVS

AHRQ = Agency for Healthcare Research and Quality; CMS = Center for Medicare and Medicaid Services; JCAHO = Joint Commission on Accreditation of Healthcare Organizations; STS = Society of Thoracic Surgeons.

DISADVANTAGES OF STRUCTURAL VARIABLES

Among the downsides, there are relatively few structural measures that may be potentially useful as quality indicators. Second, in contrast to process measures, most structural measures are not readily actionable. For example, a small hospital can increase the number of surgical patients receiving antibiotic prophylaxis but cannot readily make itself a high-volume center. Thus, although selected structural measures may be useful for selective referral initiatives, they have limited value for quality improvement purposes.

Finally, structural measures generally describe groups of hospitals or providers with better performance but do not adequately discriminate performance among individuals. For example, in aggregate, high-volume hospitals have much lower mortality rates than lower-volume centers for pancreatic resection. However, some individual high-volume hospitals may have high mortality rates. Although difficult to confirm empirically (for sample size reasons), some low-volume centers may have excellent performance.[14] For this reason, structural measures are viewed as "unfair" by many providers.

Process of Care Measures

Processes of care are the clinical interventions and services provided to patients. Process measures have long been the predominant quality indicators for both inpatient and outpatient medical care, and their popularity as quality measures for surgical care is growing rapidly. Perhaps the best example of the trend toward using process measures is the CMS Surgical Care Improvement Program (SCIP). The SCIP mandates all hospitals to collect and publicly report process measures related to prevention of surgical site infections (SSIs), postoperative cardiac events, venous thromboembolism (VTE), and respiratory complications.

STRENGTHS

Given that processes of care reflect the care that physicians deliver, they have face validity and enjoy greater buy-in from providers. They are usually directly actionable and thus good substrate for quality improvement activities.

Although risk adjustment may be important for outcomes, it is not required for many process measures. For example, when measuring appropriate prophylaxis

Table 4 Surgical Performance Measures Endorsed by the National Quality Forum that Apply to Specific General Surgical Procedures

Diagnosis or Procedure	*Performance Measure*	*Steward*
Esophageal resection	Hospital volume	AHRQ
	Risk-adjusted mortality	STS/AHRQ
	Preoperative assessment of performance status	STS
Pancreatic resection	Hospital volume	AHRQ
	Risk-adjusted mortality rates	AHRQ
Colon resection	Risk-adjusted mortality or major complications	ACS/NSQIP
	For cancer, adjuvant chemotherapy within 4 months for lymph node–positive disease	ACS
	For cancer, at least 12 lymph nodes are harvested	ACS
	For cancer, complete pathology reporting	ACS
Melanoma	Coordination of care	AMA
Breast cancer	Post–breast conservation radiation	ACS
	Appropriate axillary staging	Intermountain Healthcare
	Adjuvant hormonal therapy in receptor-positive patients	ACS
	Adjuvant chemotherapy in appropriate patients	ACS
	Needle biopsy to establish diagnosis of cancer precedes surgical excision/resection	ACS
Appendicitis	Proportion with perforation	AHRQ
	Incidental appendectomy in the elderly	AHRQ

ACS = American College of Surgeons; AHRQ = Agency for Healthcare Research and Quality; AMA = American Medical Association; NSQIP = National Surgical Quality Improvement Program; STS = Society of Thoracic Surgeons.

against postoperative VTE, one of the SCIP measures, it is not necessary to account for patient differences in risk. Given that virtually all patients undergoing open abdominal surgery should be offered some form of prophylaxis, there is little need to collect detailed clinical data about illness severity for the purpose of risk adjustment.

Finally, process measures are generally less constrained by sample size problems than direct outcome measures. Whereas important outcomes (e.g., perioperative death) are relatively rare, most targeted process measures are relevant to a larger proportion of patients. Moreover, because they generally target aspects of general perioperative care, process measures can often be assessed on patients undergoing numerous different procedures, increasing sample sizes and measurement precision.

LIMITATIONS

At the current time, a major limitation of process measures is the lack of a reliable data infrastructure for ascertaining them. Administrative data sets lack the requisite clinical detail and specificity for this purpose. Measurement systems based on clinical data, including that of the NSQIP,[15] focus on patient characteristics and outcomes and do not collect information on process of care. Presently, pay-for-performance programs rely on self-reported information from hospitals, but the reliability of such data is uncertain (particularly when reimbursement is at stake).

Even if this limitation were overcome, a second limitation remains to be considered—namely, that process variables are limited in their ability to explain observed variations in mortality. A growing body of empirical data supports this statement. Most of the data come from the literature on medical diagnoses (e.g., acute myocardial infarction), where the link between process and outcome is much stronger than it is in surgery.[16–18] For example, the JCAHO/CMS process measures for acute myocardial infarction explained only 6% of the observed variation in risk-adjusted mortality for this condition.[17]

There is reason to believe that existing process measures explain very little of the variation in important outcomes in surgery. First, most process measures currently used in surgery relate to secondary rather than primary outcomes. For example, although the value of antibiotic prophylaxis in reducing the risk of superficial SSI should not be underestimated, this process is not among the most important adverse events of major surgery (including death). Second, process measures in surgery often relate to complications that are very rare. For example, there is a consensus that prophylaxis for VTE is necessary and important. Accordingly, the SCIP measures, endorsed by the NQF, include the use of appropriate prophylaxis. However, pulmonary embolism is very uncommon; therefore, improving adherence to these measures will not avert many deaths.

Several recent empirical studies on the relation between SCIP processes and patient outcomes support this assertion. For example, Nicholas and colleagues examined the relation between hospital SCIP process compliance and risk-adjusted rates of mortality, thromboembolism, and surgical infection.[19] Despite wide variation in process compliance, there was no association between adherence to SCIP measures

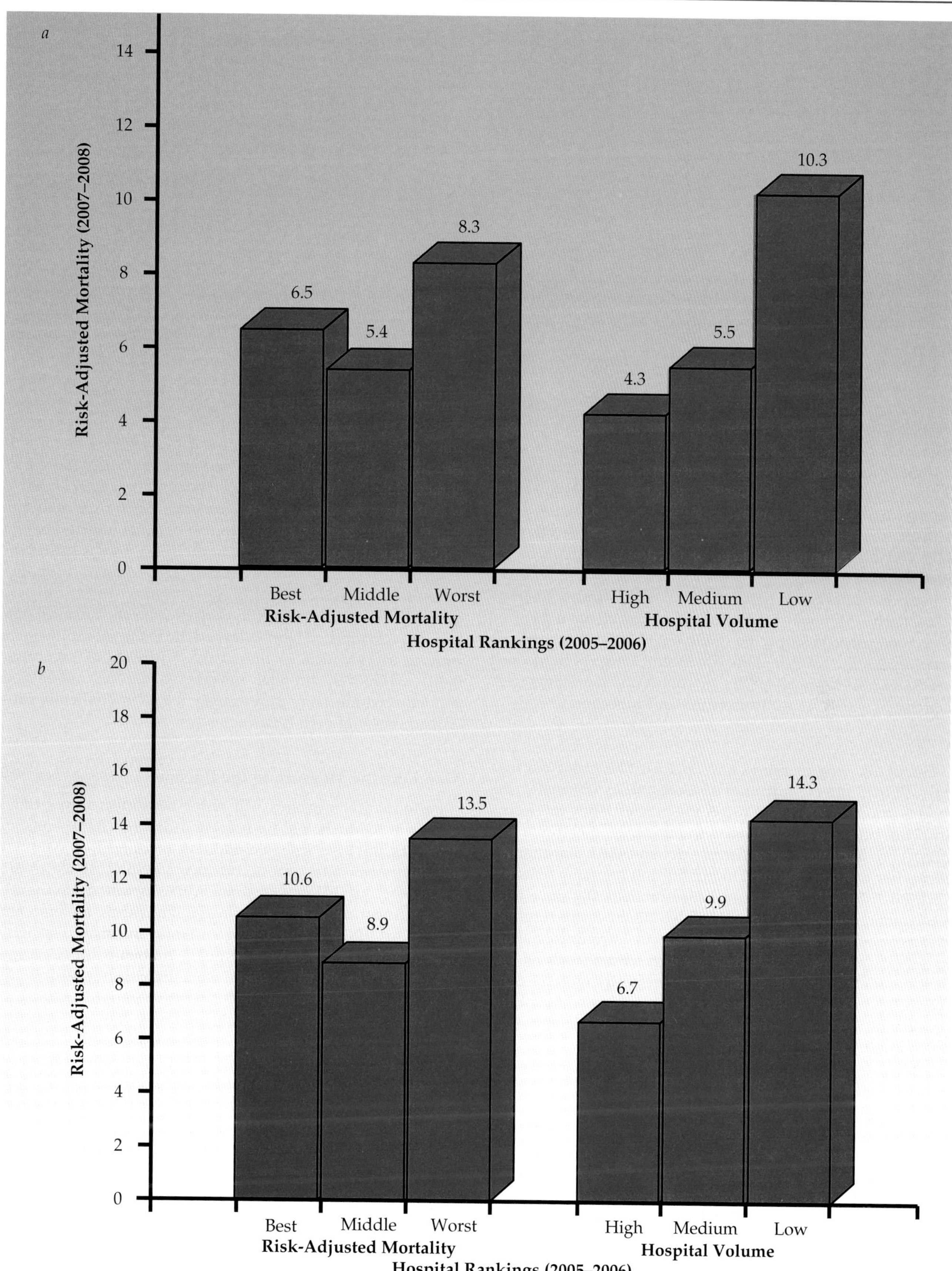

Figure 1 **Relative ability of historical (2005–2006) measures of hospital volume and risk-adjusted mortality to predict subsequent (2007–2008) risk-adjusted mortality in US Medicare patients. (*a*) Pancreatic resection. (*b*) Esophageal resection.**

and any of these risk-adjusted outcomes. Until a better understanding is achieved regarding which details account for variations in the most important complications, especially those adverse events leading to death, process measures will continue to be of limited usefulness in surgical quality improvement.

Direct Outcome Measures

Direct outcome measures reflect the end result of care, from a clinical perspective or as judged by the patient. Although mortality is by far the most commonly used measure in surgery, other outcomes that could be used as quality indicators include complications, hospital readmission, and a variety of patient-centered measures of satisfaction or health status.

There are several ongoing, large-scale initiatives involving direct outcomes assessment in surgery. Proprietary health care rating firms (e.g., Healthgrades) and state agencies are assessing risk-adjusted mortality rates using Medicare or state-level administrative data sets. However, most of the current interest in outcomes measurement involves large clinical registries. Cardiac surgery registries in New York, Pennsylvania, and a growing number of other states are perhaps the visible examples. At the national level, the STS and the American College of Cardiology (ACC) have implemented systems for tracking morbidity and mortality with cardiac surgery and percutaneous coronary interventions, respectively. Although most outcomes measurement efforts have been procedure specific (and largely limited to cardiac procedures), the NSQIP of the American College of Surgeons (ACS) assesses hospital-specific morbidity and mortality rates aggregated across surgical specialties and procedures.[16]

STRENGTHS

Direct outcome measures have at least two major advantages. First, direct outcome measures have obvious face validity and thus are likely to get the greatest "buy-in" from hospitals and surgeons. Second, outcomes measurement alone may improve performance—the so-called Hawthorne effect. For example, surgical morbidity and mortality rates in Veterans Affairs' hospitals have fallen dramatically since implementation of NSQIP in 1991.[15] No doubt many surgical leaders at individual hospitals made specific organizational or process improvements after they began receiving feedback on their hospitals' performance. However, it is very unlikely that even a full inventory of these specific changes would explain such broad-based and substantial improvements in morbidity and mortality rates.

DISADVANTAGES OF DIRECT OUTCOME MEASURES

Hospital- or surgeon-specific outcome measures are severely constrained by small sample sizes. For the large majority of surgical procedures, very few hospitals (or surgeons) have sufficient adverse events (numerators) and cases (denominators) for meaningful, procedure-specific measures of morbidity or mortality. For example, Dimick and colleagues used data from the Nationwide Inpatient Sample to study seven procedures for which mortality rates have been advocated as quality indicators by the AHRQ.[20] For six of these procedures, a very small proportion of US hospitals had adequate caseloads to rule out a mortality rate twice the national average. Although identifying poor quality outliers is an important function of outcomes measurement, focusing on this goal alone significantly underestimates problems with small sample sizes. Discriminating among individual hospitals with intermediate levels of performance is even more difficult.

Other limitations of direct outcomes assessment depend on whether outcomes are being assessed from administrative data or clinical information abstracted from medical records. For outcomes measurement based on clinical data, the major problem is expense. For example, it costs over $100,000 annually for a private sector hospital to participate in the NSQIP.

With administrative data, the adequacy of risk adjustment remains a major concern. High-quality risk adjustment may be essential for outcome measures to have face validity with providers. It may also be useful for discouraging gaming, for example, hospitals or providers avoiding high-risk patients to optimize their performance measures. However, it is not clear how much the scientific validity of outcome measures is threatened by imperfect risk adjustment with administrative data. Although administrative data lack clinical detail on many variables related to baseline risk,[21–24] it is not clear to what extent case mix varies systematically across hospitals or surgeons. Among patients undergoing the same surgical procedure, there is often surprisingly little variation. For example, we examined risk-adjusted mortality rates for hospitals performing coronary artery bypass grafting in New York State, as derived from their clinical registries.[25] Unadjusted and adjusted hospital mortality rates were nearly identical in most years (correlations exceeding 0.90). Moreover, hospital rankings based on unadjusted and adjusted mortality were equally useful in predicting subsequent hospital performance.

Matching the Measure to the Purpose

Performance measures will never be perfect. Over time, analytical methods will be refined. Access to higher-quality data may improve with the addition of clinical elements to administrative data sets or broader adoption of electronic medical records. However, some problems with performance measurement, including sample size limitations, are inherent and not fully correctable. Thus, clinical leaders, patient advocates, payers, and policy makers will not escape having to make decisions about when imperfect measures are good enough to act upon.

A measure should be implemented only with the expectation that acting will result in a net improvement in health quality. Thus, the direct benefits of implementing a particular measure cannot be outweighed by the indirect harms. Unfortunately, these benefits and harm are often difficult to measure and heavily influenced by the specific context and who—patients, payers, or providers—is doing the accounting. For this reason, there is no simple answer for where to "set the bar."

It is important to ensure a good match between the performance measure and the primary goal of measurement. The right measure depends on whether the underlying goal is (1) quality improvement or (2) selective referral—directing patients to higher-quality hospitals and/or providers. Although many pay-for-performance initiatives have both goals, one often predominates For example, the ultimate objective of CMS's pay-for-performance initiative with prophylactic antibiotics is improving quality at all hospitals—not directing patients to those centers with high compliance rates. Conversely, although it may indirectly incentivize quality improvement, the Leapfrog Group's efforts in surgery are primarily aimed at getting patients to hospitals likely to have the best outcomes (selective referral).

For quality improvement purposes, a good performance measure—most often a process of care variable—must be actionable. Measurable improvements in the given process should translate to clinically meaningful improvements in patient outcomes. Although quality improvement activities are rarely "harmful," their major downsides relate to their opportunity cost. Initiatives hinged on bad measures siphon away resources (e.g., time and focus of physicians and other staff) from more productive activities.

With selective referral, a good measure will steer patients to better hospitals or physicians (or away from worse ones). As one basic litmus test, a measure based on prior performance should reliably identify providers likely to have superior performance now and in the future. At the same time, an ideal measure would not incentivize perverse behaviors (e.g., surgeons doing unnecessary procedures to meet a specific volume standard) or negatively affect other domains of quality (e.g., patient autonomy, access, and satisfaction).

Measures that work well for quality improvement may not be particularly useful for selective referral, and vice versa. For example, appropriate use of perioperative antibiotics in surgical patients is a good measure for quality improvement. This process of care is clinically meaningful, linked to lower risks of SSIs, and directly actionable. Conversely, antibiotic use would not be particularly useful for selective referral purposes. It is unlikely that patients would use this information to decide where to have surgery. More importantly, surgeons with high rates of appropriate antibiotic use may not necessarily do better with more important outcomes (e.g., mortality). Physician performance with one quality indicator is often poorly correlated with other indicators for the same or other clinical conditions.[26]

As a counter example, the two main quality indicators for pancreatic cancer—hospital volume and operative mortality—are very informative in the context of selective referral. Patients would markedly improve their odds of surviving surgery by selecting hospitals highly ranked by either measure [*see Figure 1*]. However, neither measure would be particularly useful for quality improvement purposes. Volume is not readily actionable; mortality rates are too unstable at the level of individual hospitals (because of small sample size problems) to identify top performers, identify best practices, or evaluate the effects of improvement activities.

Many believe that a good performance measure must discriminate performance at the individual level. From the provider perspective in particular, a "fair" measure must reliably reflect the performance of individual hospitals or physicians. Unfortunately, as described earlier, small caseloads (and sometimes case-mix variation) conspire against this objective for most procedures. Patients, however, should value information that improves their odds of good outcomes on average. Many measures meet this latter interest while failing on the former.

For example, Krumholz and colleagues used clinical data from the Cooperative Cardiovascular Project to assess the usefulness of Healthgrades' hospital ratings for acute myocardial infarction (based primarily on risk-adjusted mortality rates from Medicare data).[27] Relative to one-star (worst) hospitals, five-star (best) hospitals had significantly lower mortality (16% versus 22%, $p < .001$) after risk adjustment with clinical data. They also discharged significantly more (appropriate) patients on aspirin, beta blockers, and angiotensin-converting enzyme (ACE) inhibitors, all recognized quality indicators. However, the Healthgrades' ratings poorly discriminated among any two individual hospitals. In only 3% of head-to-head comparisons did five-star hospitals have statistically lower mortality rates than one-star hospitals.

Thus, some performances measures that clearly identify groups of hospitals or providers with superior performance may be limited in their ability to discriminate individual hospitals from one another. There may be no simple solution to resolving the basic tension implied by performance measures that are unfair to providers yet informative for patients. However, it underscores the importance of being clear about both the primary purpose (quality improvement or selective referral) and whose interests are receiving top priority (provider or patient).

Future of Performance Measurement

Although great progress has been made, the science of surgical quality measurement is still in its infancy. Several barriers must be overcome before performance measures can be optimally used to improve patient care. Perhaps the biggest barrier is the lack of an accurate and affordable measurement infrastructure. One practical solution that may reduce the expense of detailed data collection with clinical registries is to create hybrid systems that join data elements from administrative and clinical data sets. Although administrative data are criticized for their lack of accuracy in identifying coexisting diseases, they can reliably identify the type of procedure performed, certain demographic variables (e.g., age, gender, and race), and some outcome variables (e.g., vital status, discharge to a skilled nursing facility, and length of stay). This set of variables could then be linked to a limited set of clinical risk factors that would allow robust risk adjustment. This solution will be even more attractive as administrative data come to contain more accurate information (e.g., present-on-admission codes to distinguish complications from coexisting problems).[28]

In addition to improving the efficiency of data collection, it would be worthwhile to rethink how existing registries are designed so as to make them less expensive and more useful. For example, although the ACS-NSQIP is in a key position to become the leading measurement platform for surgical quality improvement, several changes could be made to ensure its success.[29] First, the burden of data collection could be reduced; this would substantially decrease the costs of participating. The number of data elements could be reduced by creating more parsimonious risk adjustment models.[30] Second, the sampling strategy could be changed to sample 100% of the most important operations; this change would allow assessment of procedure-specific outcomes. Ultimately, participating hospitals would need procedure-specific outcome data to target specific operations for improvement. Third, clinical processes of care could be added to the data collection process; this would allow hospitals to respond to national pay-for-performance mandates and to provide more actionable quality measures. This last change would require the ACS-NSQIP to manifest a level of flexibility that it has not exhibited to date. With the flexibility to change data measurement periodically, the ACS-NSQIP would not only be able to add other measures that are used in national mandates (e.g., SCIP) but also to evaluate their importance.

One of the biggest limitations of surgical quality measurement is the statistical noise from the small sample sizes at most hospitals. An emerging technique, reliability adjustment, directly addresses the problem of statistical noise. This technique, based on hierarchical modeling, quantifies and subtracts statistical noise from the measurement process.[31] Essentially, it "shrinks" a provider's performance back toward average, unless they deviate to such an extreme that it is safe to assume that they are truly different. In this way, it gives providers the benefit of the doubt. For example, Figure 2 shows the risk-adjusted mortality and morbidity rates for colon resection in 20 ACS-NSQIP hospitals before and after reliability adjustment. Prior to reliability adjustment, rates of mortality and morbidity vary greatly across these hospitals. After reliability adjustment, however, the "noise" has been removed and rates of morbidity and mortality vary much less, yielding a range of performance that is clinically more realistic. These reliability-adjusted mortality rates are much more accurate at capturing true performance, as assessed by their ability to predict future performance.

Despite increasing use in other fields, such as ambulatory care, reliability adjustment is only beginning to find applications in surgery. Perhaps the most prominent example is the Massachusetts cardiac surgery report card, which publishes reliability-adjusted mortality rates for each hospital. This approach will also likely be applied to general and vascular surgery, as described with other changes in a recent "blueprint" for a new NSQIP, discussed above. As the advantages of this technique become more widely known, there is no doubt that it will become the standard technique for reporting risk-adjusted outcomes.

Another barrier to improving surgical performance is the lack of good global measures of performance. With the proliferation of pay-for-performance pilot programs, various stakeholders have been confronted with the problem of how to make sense of multiple competing measures of quality. Most have responded by combining multiple domains to create a composite measure of performance. The Premier/CMS Hospital Quality Incentive Demonstration uses a composite of process and outcome as a quality measure for coronary artery bypass surgery. The STS's Task Force on Quality Measurement advocates a composite score based on a set of outcome and process measures endorsed by the NQF.[32] In these composite approaches, the different measures are essentially weighted equally, with no empirical determination of which ones are the most important. There are, however, emerging techniques that use empirically derived weighting to create a composite score that optimally predicts future mortality for high-risk surgery.[33] As such methods become more fully developed, composite measures will no doubt continue to gain popularity.

Given that most existing quality improvement efforts focus on optimizing measurement of technical quality, it is important not to lose sight of the fact that many quality concerns arise upstream from the operation itself—that is, with the decision to operate in the first place. While variations in the use of surgery have long been recognized. Some of these variations are attributable to differences in disease prevalence and physician practice style. Some, however, arise from overuse, underuse, or misuse of surgical management. For a full accounting of surgical quality, it will be necessary to develop reliable means of measuring the appropriateness of surgical treatment and the extent to which patient preferences are incorporated into clinical decisions, in addition to measures assessing how well patients do after surgery.

Dr. Dimick and Dr. Birkmeyer are both equity owners and paid consultants for ArborMetrix, Inc.

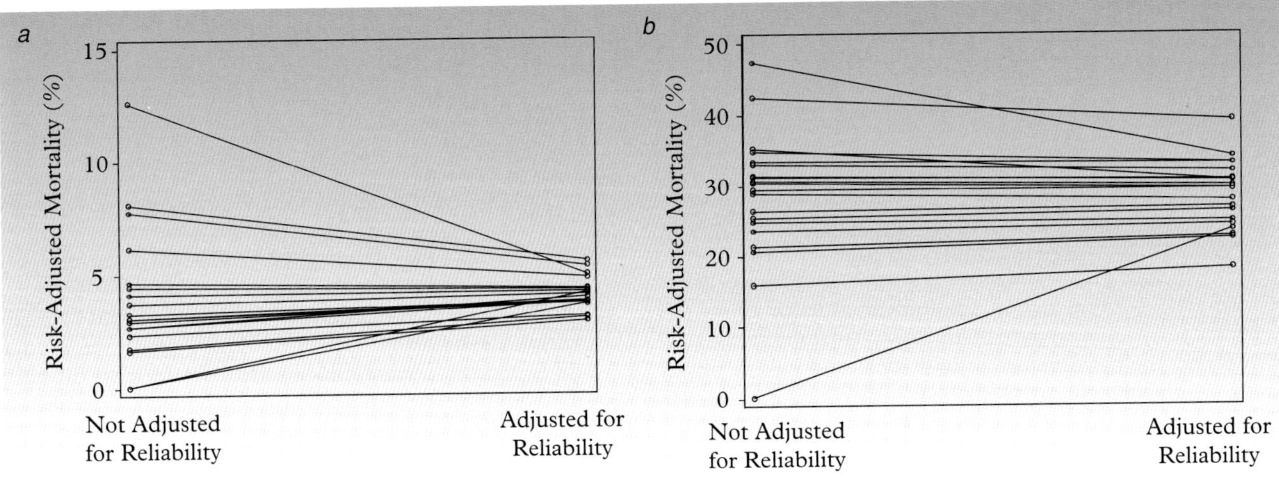

Figure 2 **Risk-adjusted (*a*) mortality and (*b*) morbidity rates for colon resection at individual hospitals before and after adjustment for reliability. Data are from the 2007 American College of Surgeons National Surgical Quality Improvement Program (ACS-NSQIP).**

References

1. Lee TH, Meyer GS, Brennan TA. A middle ground on public accountability. N Engl J Med 2004;350:2409–12.
2. Galvin R, Milstein A. Large employers' new strategies in health care. N Engl J Med 2002;347:939–42.
3. Birkmeyer JD, Birkmeyer NJ, Dimick JB. Measuring the quality of surgical care: structure, process, or outcomes? J Am Coll Surg 2004;198:626–32.
4. Landon BE, Normand SL, Blumenthal D, Daley J. Physician clinical performance assessment: prospects and barriers. JAMA 2003;290:1183–9.
5. Bird SM, Cox D, Farewell VT, et al. Performance indicators: good, bad, and ugly. J R Statist Soc 2005;168:1–27.
6. Halm EA, Lee C, Chassin MR. Is volume related to outcome in health care? A systematic review and methodologic critique of the literature. Ann Intern Med 2002;137:511–20.
7. Dudley RA, Johansen KL, Brand R, et al. Selective referral to high volume hospitals: estimating potentially avoidable deaths. JAMA 2000;283:1159–66.
8. Birkmeyer JD, Dimick JB, Staiger DO. Operative mortality and procedure volume as predictors of subsequent hospital performance. Ann Surg 2006;243:411–7.
9. Bach PB, Cramer LD, Schrag D, et al. The influence of hospital volume on survival after resection for lung cancer. N Engl J Med 2001;345:181–8.
10. Begg CB, Reidel ER, Bach PB, et al. Variations in morbidity after radical prostatectomy. N Engl J Med 2002;346:1138–44.
11. Finlayson EVA, Birkmeyer JD. Effects of hospital volume on life expectancy after selected cancer operations in older adults: a decision analysis. J Am Coll Surg 2002;196:410–7.
12. Pronovost PJ, Angus DC, Dorman T, et al. Physician staffing patterns and clinical outcomes in critically ill patients: a systematic review. JAMA 2002;288:2151–62.
13. Pronovost PJ, Needham DM, Waters H, et al. Intensive care unit physician staffing: financial modeling of the Leapfrog standard. Crit Care Med 2004;32:1247–53.
14. Shahian DM, Normand SL. The volume-outcome relationship: from Luft to Leapfrog. Ann Thorac Surg 2003;75:1048–58.
15. Khuri SF, Daley J, Henderson WG. The comparative assessment and improvement of quality of surgical care in the Department of Veterans Affairs. Arch Surg 2002;137:20–7.
16. Fink A, Campbell DJ, Mentzer RJ, et al. The National Surgical Quality Improvement Program in non-Veterans Administration hospitals: initial demonstration of feasibility. Ann Surg 2002;236:344–53.
17. Fonarow GC, Abraham WT, Albert NM, et al. Association between performance measures and clinical outcomes for patients hospitalized with heart failure. JAMA 2007;297:61.
18. Bradley EH, Herrin J, Elbel B, et al. Hospital quality for acute myocardial infarction: correlation among process measures and relationship with short-term mortality. JAMA 2006;296:72.
19. Nicholas LH, Osborne NH, Birkmeyer JD, Dimick JB. Hospital process compliance and surgical outcomes in Medicare beneficiaries. Arch Surg 2010;145:999–1004.
20. Dimick JB, Welch HG, Birkmeyer JD. Surgical mortality as an indicator of hospital quality: the problem with small sample size. JAMA 2004; 292:847–51.
21. Finlayson EV, Birkmeyer JD, Stukel TA, et al. Adjusting surgical mortality rates for patient comorbidities: more harm than good? Surgery 2002;132:787–94.
22. Fisher ES, Whaley FS, Krushat WM, et al. The accuracy of Medicare's hospital claims data: progress, but problems remain. Am J Public Health 1992;82:243–8.
23. Iezzoni LI, Foley SM, Daley J, et al. Comorbidities, complications, and coding bias. Does the number of diagnosis codes matter in predicting in-hospital mortality? JAMA 1992; 267:2197–203.
24. Iezzoni LI. The risks of risk adjustment. JAMA 1997;278:1600–7.
25. Dimick JB, Birkmeyer JD. Ranking hospitals on surgical quality: does risk-adjustment always matter? J Am Coll Surg 2008;207:347–51.
26. Palmer RH, Wright EA, Orav EJ, et al. Consistency in performance among primary care practitioners. Med Care 1996;34(9 Suppl):SS52–66.
27. Krumholz HM, Rathore SS, Chen J, et al. Evaluation of a consumer-oriented Internet health care report card: the risk of quality ratings based on mortality data. JAMA 2002;287:1277–87.
28. Fry DE, Pine M, Jordan HS, et al: Combining administrative and clinical data to stratify surgical risk. Ann Surg 2007;246:875.
29. Birkmeyer JD, Shahian DM, Dimick JB, et al. Blueprint for a new American College of Surgeons: National Surgical Quality Improvement Program. J Am Coll Surg 2008;207:777–82.
30. Dimick JB, Osborne NH, Hall BL, et al. Risk adjustment for comparing hospital quality with surgery: how many variables are needed? J Am Coll Surg 2010;210:503–8.
31. Dimick JB, Staiger DO, Birkmeyer JD. Ranking hospitals on surgical mortality: the importance of reliability adjustment. Health Serv Res 2010;45:1614–29.
32. O'Brien SM, Shahian DM, DeLong ER, et al. Quality measurement in adult cardiac surgery: part 2—statistical considerations in composite measure scoring and provider rating. Ann Thorac Surg 2007;83(4 Suppl): S13–26.
33. Dimick JB, Staiger DO, Baser O, Birkmeyer JD. Composite measures for predicting surgical mortality in the hospital. Health Aff (Millwood) 2009;28:1189–98.

3 STRATEGIES FOR IMPROVING SURGICAL QUALITY

Nancy J.O. Birkmeyer, PhD

Surgical morbidity and mortality are major public health concerns. At least 1 million surgical patients die, and many times more experience a serious complication each year worldwide.[1] The outcomes of surgery have been shown to differ among providers[2–7] and according to provider attributes such as procedure volume[8–10] and subspecialty training.[11–13] This variability in the outcomes of surgical procedures has long suggested opportunities to improve the quality of surgical care. For this reason, many large-scale quality improvement efforts target patients undergoing surgery.

Payers, health care policy makers, and surgeons' professional organizations have implemented a range of strategies to improve surgical quality. With selective referral, payers use various methods to try to steer patients to providers that they have deemed to be of higher quality. Pay-for-performance programs, such as the Surgical Care Improvement Project (SCIP), provide incentives for providers' compliance with specific evidence-based processes of perioperative care. Many professional organizations, including the American College of Surgeons National Surgical Quality Improvement Program (NSQIP), have instituted outcomes measurement and feedback programs to stimulate quality improvement at the local level. Regional collaborative quality improvement programs go beyond outcomes measurement and feedback to broad-scale implementation of quality improvement interventions.

These strategies, which we refer to as selective referral, process compliance, outcomes measurement and feedback, and regional collaborative quality improvement, are the current, dominant approaches to surgical quality improvement in the United States. This chapter reviews these strategies and some of the major ongoing initiatives in each [*see Table 1*]. In addition, the evidence to date for the effectiveness of each of these strategies in improving surgical quality is summarized.

Selective Referral

Selective referral includes strategies that aim to identify and steer patients toward providers with the best results for certain procedures. Payers' selective referral programs may involve the use of tiered health plans and benefits packages that give patients' financial incentives (e.g., lower copayments or monthly premiums) for selecting providers that they have deemed to be of higher quality. Some payers restrict their enrollees' choice of providers to selected Centers of Excellence (COE) for certain high-risk procedures, whereas others simply provide information about approved COE to their enrollees without restricting choice. Examples of selective referral programs include the Leapfrog Group's Evidence-Based Hospital Referral program, Blue Cross and Blue Shield Association Blue Distinction Centers for Specialty Care, and bariatric surgery COE programs of the American College of Surgeons and the American Society for Metabolic and Bariatric Surgery.

The extent to which selective referral programs result in improvements in surgical quality has been assessed in a number of recent studies. One group of studies has examined whether COE programs successfully identify hospitals with better outcomes. For example, one study investigated whether Medicare patients undergoing major cancer resections (1994 to 1999) at National Cancer Institute (NCI) cancer centers have lower mortality rates than patients at control hospitals matched for procedure volume.[14] NCI cancer centers had significantly lower adjusted surgical mortality rates than control hospitals for four of the six procedures assessed, including colectomy, pulmonary resection, gastrectomy, and esophagectomy. Trends toward lower adjusted operative mortality rates at NCI cancer centers were also observed for cystectomy and pancreatic resection. However, there were no important differences in subsequent 5-year mortality rates between NCI cancer centers and control hospitals for any of the procedures. A subsequent study including Survival, Epidemiology, and End Results (SEER)-Medicare patients from 1999 to 2003 did find improved survival rates for patients undergoing surgery for colorectal cancer at NCI cancer centers compared with other hospitals, reflecting perhaps the difference in time periods between the two studies and/or the ability to control for tumor stage with the data source used in the later study.[15] In bariatric surgery, two studies found that bariatric COE hospitals do not have lower rates of surgical complications than other hospitals.[16,17]

Two recent studies considered whether selective referral programs have altered referral patterns for high-risk surgery and whether these trends have resulted in improvements in operative mortality with those procedures. One study found that increased market concentration was strongly associated with declining mortality with some high-risk cancer operations [*see Figure 1*], including pancreatectomy, esophagectomy, and cystectomy.[18] A smaller proportion of mortality improvements could be attributed to market concentration for lung resection, abdominal aortic aneurysm repair, and aortic valve replacement, but trends in market concentration had no role in declining mortality with coronary artery bypass grafting (CABG) and carotid endarterectomy. A study based on data from Washington State found that the proportion of patients undergoing surgery in hospitals meeting the Leapfrog Groups' volume standard had significantly increased for pancreatectomy and esophagectomy, but not aortic aneurysm repair, since

Table 1 Characteristics of Different Strategies for Improving Surgical Quality

	Selective Referral	*Process Compliance*	*Outcomes Measurement and Feedback*	*Regional Collaborative Quality Improvement*
Mechanism	Steer patients to best hospitals or surgeons	Increase compliance with evidence-based processes of care	Spur internal quality improvement with feedback on benchmarked outcomes	Identify and broadly implement best practices
Examples	Leapfrog Group's Evidence-Based Hospital Referral Program Payers' Center of Excellence (COE) programs	Surgical Care Improvement Project (SCIP) Surgical Checklist projects	National Surgical Quality Improvement Program (NSQIP) Society of Thoracic Surgeons (STS) National Cardiac Surgery Database	Northern New England Cardiovascular Disease Study Group Blue Cross and Blue Shield of Michigan/Blue Care Network Value Partnership program
Evidence: pro	Effective for relatively rare procedures with strong evidence linking provider characteristics (e.g., procedure volume) and outcomes	Programs that involve active participation of surgeons and other clinicians (e.g., check-lists) may be effective regardless of actual content of intervention	Effective for motivating internal quality improvement efforts among low-performing providers	Improved outcomes in the areas where it has been tried: cardiovascular procedures, other general and vascular surgery, and bariatric surgery
Evidence: con	COE programs based on self-reported, unreliable data not effective in identifying higher-quality providers	Disappointing results for other process compliance interventions	Do not provide guidance for how to improve either to low-performing providers or others	Strategy has not been widely adopted perhaps because expense and complexity and lack of a natural sponsor

implementation of the Leapfrog Groups' Evidence-Based Hospital Referral Program.[19] Although mortality rates tended to be lower for hospitals meeting the volume thresholds, statewide mortality rates did not improve over the time period.[19]

Selective referral is arguably the most controversial of the quality improvement strategies discussed in this chapter. Although selective referral strategies are effective in improving outcomes in a number of procedures, they are less useful for many others. This strategy is also highly divisive, with many arguing that providers should be judged by their own clinical outcomes rather than having their outcomes judged by imperfect proxy measures, such as volume.[20] Selective referral is probably best reserved for high-risk procedures where a strong relation between provider structural characteristics (such as procedure volume or subspecialty training) and outcomes has been demonstrated. Selective referral programs should not rely on self-reported and/or unverifiable information to determine which providers have the highest quality.[16,17,21]

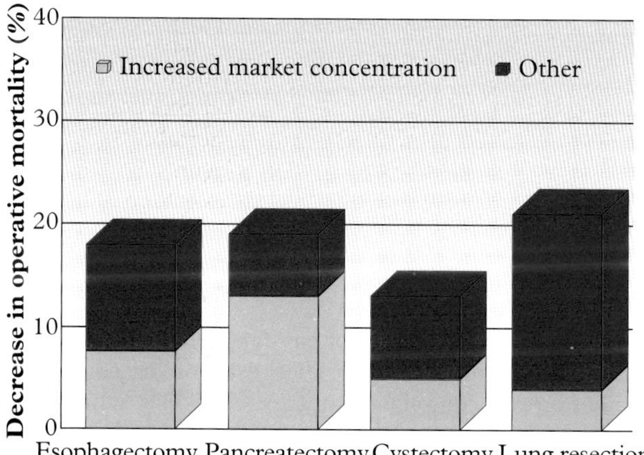

Figure 1 **Percent of mortality decline for esophagectomy, pancreatectomy, cystectomy, and lung resection attributable to increases in market concentration, based on 2001 to 2008 national Medicare data.[18]**

Process Compliance

Another strategy for improving surgical quality is for hospitals to increase their use of evidence-based processes of care. Public and private payers' ongoing pay-for-performance programs, which provide financial incentives for high rates of compliance, best exemplify this strategy. The largest pay-for-performance program targeting surgery is the SCIP, which links Medicare hospital reimbursement to satisfactory adherence to processes for reducing rates of surgical site infection, postoperative cardiac events, venous thromboembolism, and ventilator-associated pneumonia.

SURGICAL CARE IMPROVEMENT PROJECT (SCIP)

The relation between SCIP measure compliance and outcomes has been assessed in a number of studies [*see Table 2*]. Nicholas and colleagues used national Medicare data to examine whether rates of compliance with the SCIP measures were associated with rates of surgical site infection, venous thromboembolism, or surgical mortality for patients undergoing high-risk cancer or cardiovascular procedures.[22] Although process compliance ranged from 53.7% for hospitals in the bottom tercile to 91.4% for hospitals in the top tertile, there was no relation between rates of process compliance and rates of surgical site infection, venous thromboembolism, or surgical mortality overall or for any of

Table 2 Evidence Regarding the Relation between Compliance with Surgical Care Improvement Project (SCIP) Measures and Clinical Outcomes

Study, Year	*Data Sources (Year)*	*Patient Population (n)*	*SCIP Measure**	*Infection*	*VTE*	*Mortality*
Nicholas et al, 2010[22]	2000 US hospitals/ Medicare/Hospital Compare (2005–2006)	6 high-risk procedures (325,052)	SCIP INF/VTE-Composite	No	No	No
Ingraham et al, 2010[23]	200 ACS-NSQIP hospitals/ Hospital Compare (2008)	General and vascular surgery (81,524)	SCIP INF-1 SCIP INF-2 SCIP INF-3 SCIP INF-6	No Yes No No		No No No No
Stulberg et al, 2010[25]	398 Premier Inc. hospitals/ Hospital Compare (2006–2008)	Inpatient surgery (405,720)	SCIP INF-1 SCIP INF-2 SCIP INF-3 SCIP INF-4 SCIP INF-6 SCIP INF-7 SCIP INF-Composite	No No No No No No Yes		
Lehtinen, 2010[41]	1 ACS-NSQIP hospital (2006–2009)	Gastrointestinal surgery (469)	SCIP INF-10	No		
Pastor, 2010[42]	1 US hospital (2006–2008)	Colorectal surgery (491)	SCIP INF-Composite	No		
Hawn et al, 2008[26]	95 Veterans Affairs hospitals (2005–2006)	Elective orthopedic, colon, and vascular surgery (9,195)	SCIP INF-1	No		
[illegible] et al, [illegible][27]	1 Canadian hospital (2004–2007)	Major hepatobiliary or colorectal surgery ([illegible])	SCIP INF-Composite	Yes—NS		
Berenguer, 2010[29]	1 ACS-NSQIP hospital (2006–2008)	Colorectal surgery (197)	SCIP INF-Composite			
Hedrick et al, 2007[28]	1 hospital (2000–2005)	Colorectal surgery (307)	SCIP INF-Composite	Yes		

ACS-NSQIP = American College of Surgeons-National Surgical Quality Improvement Program; NS = not statistically significant; VTE = venous thromboembolism.
*SCIP measures: SCIP INF-1: prophylactic antibiotic received within 1 hour prior to surgical incision; SCIP INF-2: prophylactic antibiotic selection for surgical patients; SCIP INF-3: prophylactic antibiotics discontinued within 24 hours after surgery end; SCIP INF-4: cardiac surgery patients with controlled 6 am postoperative blood glucose; SCIP INF-6: surgery patients with appropriate hair removal; SCIP INF-7: colorectal surgery patients with immediate postoperative normothermia; SCIP INF-10: surgery patients with perioperative temperature management; SCIP VTE-1: surgery patients with recommended venous thromboembolism prophylaxis ordered; SCIP VTE-2: surgery patients who received appropriate venous thromboembolism prophylaxis within 24 hours prior to surgery to 24 hours after surgery.

the six procedures individually. Numerous studies have examined the relation between the subset of SCIP measures related to the prevention of surgical site infection (SCIP INF) and clinical outcomes. Of these, one found that just one of the measures (SCIP 2: appropriate antibiotic given) was associated with rates of surgical site infection.[23] Another study found that only SCIP 1 (antibiotic given within 1 hour of surgery) was associated with rates of surgical site infection among colorectal surgery patients.[24] Another study found that none of the individual SCIP INF measures were associated with rates of surgical site infection but that a global composite measure was.[25] The other studies found no relation between SCIP INF measures and clinical outcomes.[26]

Taken as a whole, these studies provide scant evidence for the effectiveness of process compliance in improving outcomes in surgery. Given that the SCIP measures were chosen on the basis of randomized trials supporting their effectiveness, these findings are somewhat counterintuitive. One explanation may be that in the randomized trials, these interventions were assessed under tightly controlled conditions (e.g., patient populations, hospital environments) that simply are not representative of their use in general practice. This is sometimes referred to as the difference between the effectiveness and the efficacy of an intervention. Another plausible explanation is that high rates of compliance or improvements in rates of compliance are really indicative of better documentation rather than actual compliance or clinical care processes. The three single-site studies[27–29] showing the effectiveness of these process changes in the prevention of surgical site infections for colorectal surgery patients at their sites following changes in clinical care would support this explanation.

Checklists

Although not yet a target of pay-for-performance or other incentive programs, surgical checklists can be considered another process compliance strategy. Checklists, which have long been used in aviation, came to be used in health care following the publication of a study documenting their effectiveness for the prevention of catheter-related bloodstream infections in intensive care units.[30] Surgical checklists range from simple preoperative "timeouts" to prevent rare but dreadful errors, such as operating on the wrong site or patient, to broad lists of practices known to reduce complications and/or improve teamwork.

Checklists have been the subject of two recent process compliance studies in surgery. A study supported by the World Health Organization (WHO) tested the effects of a 19-item intraoperative checklist among nearly 4,000 patients undergoing noncardiac surgery at eight large hospitals around the world using a pre/post study design.[31] The second study evaluated the effects of a comprehensive checklist (11-part instrument with more than 100 items, encompassing all phases of care) in six regional and tertiary care centers and five control hospitals in the Netherlands.[32] Despite differences in the extensiveness of checklists and in the scientific rigor of the study designs, both studies found that the use of a surgical checklist resulted in dramatic reductions in surgical morbidity and mortality. In the WHO study, mortality was reduced by almost 50% and complications dropped from 11% to 7%. In the de Vries and colleagues study, mortality was also cut in half and rates of complications were reduced from 15% to 11%.[32]

In each of the two surgical checklist studies, all types of complications were reduced rather than just those that would be expected based on the content of the checklists. This suggests that checklists may have indirect effects that may be as, if not more important, than their specific content. For example, checklists could reduce the rates of surgical complications by improving hospitals' safety culture, lead to more effective communication and/or handoffs between different types of providers, or reduce distractions in the operating room. The durability of improvements in outcomes attained with checklists is yet to be determined as neither of the two studies had a very long duration of postintervention study time (3 to 6 months). It is also to be determined what specific items are essential for an effective surgical checklist. Nonetheless, checklists should be considered among the more promising interventions for improving rates of morbidity and mortality with surgery.

Outcomes Measurement and Feedback

Many of the professional organizations in surgery have focused their quality improvement efforts on the development and dissemination of clinical registries for tracking surgical outcomes. The goal of these efforts is to provide benchmarking data with which hospitals and surgeons can compare their outcomes with those of their peers. The rationale for benchmarking performance is to allow hospitals to identify opportunities for quality improvement and therefore to be motivated to engage in internal quality improvement activities. The Society of Thoracic Surgeons (STS) is considered a pioneer in this area, and virtually all US hospitals involved in cardiac surgery now participate in its registry. The NSQIP is the largest outcomes measurement platform in noncardiac surgery. The NSQIP was developed for use in Veterans Affairs (VA) hospitals, but since being adapted for use in the private sector by the American College of Surgeons, several hundred private sector hospitals now participate. Finally, a number of states have been measuring and publicly reporting risk-adjusted outcomes for certain high-risk procedures, most frequently coronary bypass surgery.

There is strong evidence that outcomes measurement and feedback are an effective strategy for reducing rates of surgical morbidity and mortality. For example, surgical complication rates decreased by more than 40% in VA hospitals following the implementation of the NSQIP.[33] Surgical complication rates also dropped among private sector hospitals after the implementation of NSQIP, although much less dramatically than in the VA hospitals.[34] Mortality among Medicare patients undergoing coronary bypass surgery in the state of New York declined by 41% between 1989 and 1992 with the implementation of the New York State Department of Health Cardiac Reporting Systems.[35] During this same time period, mortality among Medicare patients undergoing coronary bypass nationally declined by only 13%.[36] Another study assessed rates of mortality with coronary artery bypass with (Ohio, New Jersey, New York, and Pennsylvania) and without public outcomes reporting systems between 1994 and 1999.[37] Coronary bypass mortality rates in states with public reporting systems decreased between 20 and 33% more than those in states without these systems.

Outcomes measurement and feedback can be an effective way to improve surgical care. However, certain conditions are necessary for the success of this approach, including mandatory reporting of all hospitals, audits of data quality, a neutral third party to analyze and report data, and some kind of pressure (e.g., public reporting) for poor performers to improve.[38] It also probably works best for procedures where the primary outcomes occur within the perioperative period and can be measured and verified at a relatively low cost. Finally, the way that this approach works is by stimulating improvements among low-performing providers. However, it does not provide those institutions in need of improvement with information they will need to accomplish that goal. Outcomes measurement and feedback programs also do not provide the motivation or the information required to improve care overall.

Regional Collaborative Quality Improvement

Regional collaborative quality improvement goes beyond the measurement and feedback of outcomes data with region-wide implementation of explicit quality improvement interventions. Similar to outcomes measurement and feedback programs, regional collaborative quality improvement programs are based on clinical registry data, which are used to provide regular feedback on performance. Where regional collaborative quality improvement programs differ from straight outcomes measurement and feedback programs is that they convene regularly to review and interpret registry data with a specific focus on areas of variation in practice or outcomes. Once the processes that are associated with the best outcomes (best practices) are identified, they are broadly implemented throughout the region. The Northern New England Cardiovascular Disease Study Group, which started in 1987, is the original regional collaborative quality improvement collaborative. In Michigan, Blue Cross and Blue Shield of Michigan/Blue Care Network (BCBSM/BCN) has funded similar programs in many clinical areas, including surgery (cardiac, bariatric, and other types of general and vascular surgery).

For many years, the only evidence for the effectiveness of regional collaborative quality improvement has been from the Northern New England Cardiovascular Disease Study Group. During the first 5 years of the collaborative (1987 to 1992), the group received regular feedback on outcomes and training in continuous quality improvement techniques, and teams from each of the hospitals engaged in round robin site visits to observe perioperative care for CABG patients at other sites.[39] The CABG mortality rate decreased by 24% over the study time period. A subsequent study based on Medicare data showed that northern New England and New York State had a combination of the lowest CABG mortality rates in 1992 and the greatest improvement in mortality rates over this time period in the country.[36]

With the funding of numerous regional collaborative quality improvement programs in the state of Michigan, there are now many more data on which to gauge the effects of this approach.[40] For example, risk-adjusted morbidity rates among patients undergoing general or vascular surgery in hospitals participating in ACS-NSQIP in Michigan fell from 13.1% in 2005 to 10.5% in 2009 ($p < .001$). In contrast, morbidity rates in non-Michigan hospitals participating in ACS-NSQIP remained essentially flat between 2005 and [illegible] at approximately 12.5%, before dipping slightly to 11.5% in 2009. Risk-adjusted 30-day mortality with bariatric surgery in Michigan fell from 0.21% in 2007 to 0.02% in 2009 ($p = .004$) [*see Figure 2*]. During this time period, bariatric surgery mortality at non-Michigan hospitals participating in ACS-NSQIP did not improve significantly (0.18% to 0.11%). In cardiac surgery, during its initial reporting periods (2006 to 2007 and 2007 to 2008), composite quality scores for Michigan hospitals as a whole were statistically indistinguishable from national benchmarks. Michigan hospitals have now achieved a three-star rating from the STS (on an 11-item composite quality measure, which includes risk-adjusted mortality, complications, internal mammary graft use, and several other important processes of care, as defined by the Adult Cardiac Surgery Registry of the STS), indicating that its aggregate performance exceeded national norms and falls within the top 10th of hospitals nationwide.

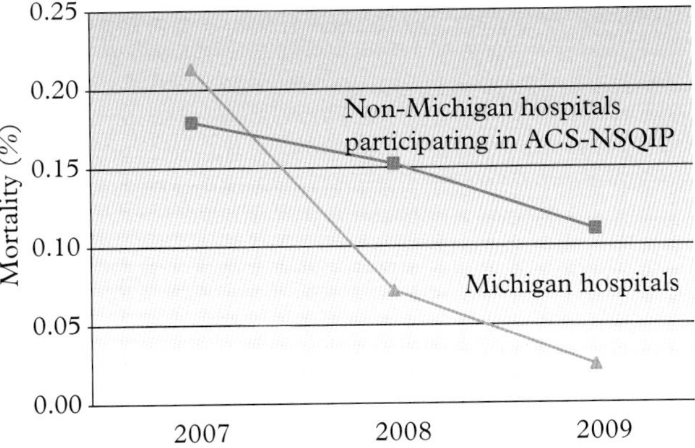

Figure 2 **Mortality after (30-day) bariatric surgery: Michigan hospitals versus non-Michigan hospitals participating in the American College of Surgeons-National Surgical Quality Improvement Program (ACS-NSQIP), based on data from the 2007 to 2009 Michigan Bariatric Surgery Collaborative and national ACS-NSQIP registries.[40]**

Despite growing evidence of the effectiveness of regional, collaborative quality improvement, this approach has not been widely adopted because it is expensive, is complicated to coordinate, and lacks a natural sponsor. The programs in Michigan exist because the state's largest private insurer has not only funded the costs of running them but has also offered additional financial incentives for hospitals to participate. Convincing others, including other private payers, public payers, purchasers, and provider systems, to invest in regional, collaborative quality improvement will require a convincing demonstration of return on investment. Although there are substantial obstacles to more widespread adoption, this is the only approach that works by reducing variation in practice and improving quality overall. In contrast, the other strategies aim to improve performance among poor performers or, in the case of selective referral, to steer patients away from them.

Summary

Each of the approaches to surgical quality improvement addressed in this chapter has advantages and disadvantages. Selective referral strategies are probably best reserved for relatively rare procedures for which outcomes [illegible] shown to vary dramatically according to provider factors such as procedure volume. COE programs that rely on self-reported and unaudited information have not been effective in identifying high-quality providers. As they are currently configured, process compliance programs have mainly focused on improving adherence to a small number of evidence-based practices in perioperative care. That many of the results for process compliance programs have been disappointing may reflect that what these programs have improved is the documentation of clinical care practices rather than the actual clinical care processes. Process compliance efforts involving surgical checklists and the active participation of surgeons and other members of operative teams are having more promising results. Outcomes measurement and feedback programs, especially where they are publicly reported, can motivate local quality improvement efforts among hospitals with poor performance. Finally, regional collaborative quality improvement programs may accelerate improvement by having the ability to rapidly identify and broadly implement best practices. However, this strategy has not been widely adopted, perhaps because of the expense and complexity of these programs as well as their lack of a natural sponsor.

Financial Disclosures: None Reported

References

1. Weiser T, Makary M, Haynes A, et al. Standardized metrics for global surgical surveillance. Lancet 2009;374:1113–7.
2. Birkmeyer JD, Dimick JB. Understanding and reducing variation in surgical mortality. Annu Rev Med 2009;60: 405–15.

3. Dimick JB, Cowan JA Jr, Ailawadi G, et al. National variation in operative mortality rates for esophageal resection and the need for quality improvement. Arch Surg 1305; 138:1305–9.
4. Dimick JB, Pronovost PJ, Cowan JA Jr, et al. Variation in postoperative complication rates after high-risk surgery in the United States. Surgery 2003;134:534–40.
5. Dimick JB, Stanley JC, Axelrod DA, et al. Variation in death rate after abdominal aortic aneurysmectomy in the United States: impact of hospital volume, gender, and age. Ann Surg 2002;235:579–85.
6. Ghaferi AA, Birkmeyer JD, Dimick JB. Variation in hospital mortality associated with inpatient surgery. N Engl J Med 1368;361:1368–75.
7. Mukherjee D, Wainess RM, Dimick JB, et al. Variation in outcomes after percutaneous coronary intervention in the United States and predictors of periprocedural mortality. Cardiology 2005;103:143–7.
8. Luft H, Bunker J, Enthoven A. Should operations be regionalized? The empirical relation between surgical volume and mortality. N Engl J Med 1979;301:1364–9.
9. Birkmeyer J, Siewers A, Finlayson E, et al. Hospital volume and surgical volume in the United States. N Engl J Med 2002;346:1128–37.
10. Birkmeyer J, Stukel T, Siewers A, et al. Surgeon volume and operative mortality in the United States. N Engl J Med 2003;349:2117–27.
11. Goodney P, Lucas F, Stukel T, Birkmeyer J. Surgeon specialty and operative mortality with lung resection. Ann Surg 2005;241:179–84.
12. Callahan M, Christos P, Gold H, et al. Influence of surgical subspecialty training on in-hospital mortality for gastrectomy and colectomy patients. Ann Surg 2003;238:629–36.
13. Hannan E, Popp A, Feustel P. Association of surgical specialty and processes of care with patient outcomes for carotid endarterectomy. Stroke 2001;32:2890–7.
14. Birkmeyer N, Goodney P, Stukel T, et al. Do cancer centers designated by the National Cancer Institute have better surgical outcomes? Cancer 2005;103:435–41.
15. Paulson E, Mitra N, Sonnad S, et al. National Cancer Institute designation predicts improved outcomes in colorectal cancer surgery. Ann Surg 2008;248:675–86.
16. Birkmeyer N, Dimick J, Share D, et al. Hospital complication rates with bariatric surgery in Michigan. JAMA 2010; 304:435–42.
17. Livingston E. Bariatric surgery outcomes at designated centers of excellence vs nondesignated programs. Arch Surg 2009;144:319–25.
18. Finks JF, Osborne NH, Birkmeyer JD. Trends in hospital volume and operative mortality for high-risk surgery. N Eng J Med 2011;364:2128–37.
19. Massarweh N, Flum D, Symons R, et al. A critical evaluation of the impact of Leapfrog's evidence-based hospital referral. J Am Coll Surg 2011;212:150–9.
20. Finlayson S. The volume-outcome debate revisited. Am Surg 2006;72:1038–42.
21. Kernisan L, Lee S, Boscardin W, et al. Association between hospital-reported Leapfrog safe practices scores and inpatient mortality. JAMA 2009;301:1341–8.
22. Nicholas L, Osborne N, Birkmeyer J, Dimick J. Hospital process compliance and surgical outcomes in Medicare beneficiaries. Arch Surg 2010;145:999–1004.
23. Ingraham A, Cohen M, Bilimoria K, et al. Association of surgical care improvement project infection-related process measure compliance with risk-adjusted outcomes: implications for quality measurement. J Am Coll Surg 2010;211: 705–14.
24. Nguyen N, Yegiyants S, Kaloostian C, et al. The Surgical Care Improvement Project (SCIP) initiative to reduce infection in elective colorectal surgery: which performance measures affect outcome. Am Surg 2008;74:1012–6.
25. Stulberg J, Delaney C, Veuhauser D, et al. Adherence to Surgical Care Improvement Project measures and the association with postoperative infections. JAMA 2010;303: 2479–85.
26. Hawn M, Itani K, Gray S, et al. Association of timely administration of prophylactic antibiotics for major surgical procedures and surgical site infection. J Am Coll Surg 2008; 206:814–21.
27. Forbes S, Stephen W, Harper W, et al. Implementation of evidence-based practices for surgical site infection prophylaxis: results of a pre- and postintervention study. J Am Coll Surg 2008;207:336–41.
28. Hedrick T, Heckman J, Smith R, et al. Efficacy of protocol implementation on incidence of wound infection in colorectal operations. J Am Coll Surg 2007;205:432–8.
29. Berenguer C, Ochsner M, Lord S, Senkowski C. Improving surgical site infections: using National Surgical Quality Improvement Program data to institute surgical care improvement project protocols in improving sugical outcomes. J Am Coll Surg 2010;210:737–43.
30. Pronovost P, Needham D, Berenholtz S, et al. An intervention to decrease catheter-related bloodstream infections in the ICU. N Engl J Med 2006;355:2725–32.
31. Haynes A, Weiser T, Berry W, et al. A surgical safety checklist to reduce morbidity and mortality in a global population. N Engl J Med 2009;360:491–9.
32. de Vries E, Prins H, Crolla R, et al. Effect of a comprehensive surgical safety system on patient outcomes. N Engl J Med 2010;363:1928–37.
33. Khuri S, Daley J, Henderson W. The comparative assessment and improvement of quality of surgical care in the Department of Veterans Affairs. Arch Surg 2002;137:20–7.
34. Hall B, Hamilton B, Richards K, et al. Does surgical quality improve in the American College of Surgeons National Surgical Quality Improvement Program: an evaluation of all participating hospitals. Ann Surg 2009;250:363–76.
35. Hannan E, Kilburn HJ, Racz M, et al. Improving the outcomes of coronary artery bypass surgery in New York State. JAMA 1994;271:761–6.
36. Peterson E, DeLong E, Jollis J, et al. The effects of New York's bypass surgery provider profiling on access to care and patient outcomes in the elderly. J Am Coll Cardiol 1998;32:993–9.
37. Hannan E, Vaughn Sarrazin M, Doran D, Rosenthal G. Provider profiling and quality improvement efforts in coronary artery bypass graft surgery: the effect on short-term mortality among Medicare beneficiaries. Med Care 2003; 41:1164–72.

38. Chassin M. Achieving and sustaining improved quality: lessons for New York State and cardiac surgery. Health Aff 2002;21:40–51.
39. O'Connor G, Plume S, Olmstead E, et al. A regional prospective study of in-hospital mortality associated with coronary artery bypass grafting: the Northern New England Cardiovascular Disease Study Group. JAMA 1991;266:803–9.
40. Share DA, Campbell DA, Birkmeyer N. et al. How a regional collaborative of hospitals and physicians in Michigan cut costs and improved the quality of care. Health Aff (Millwood) 2011;30:636–45.
41. Lehtinen SJ, Onicescu G, Kuhn KM, et al. Normothermia to prevent surgical site infections after gastrointestinal surgery: Holy grail or false idol? Ann Surg 2010;252:696–704.
42. Pastor C, Artinyan A, Varma MG, Kim E, et al. An increase in compliance with the Surgical Care Improvement Project measures does not prevent surgical site infection in colorectal surgery. Dis Colon Rectum 2010;53:24–30.

4 EVIDENCE-BASED SURGERY

Samuel R.G. Finlayson, MD, MPH

Evidence-based surgery describes the consistent and judicious use of the best available scientific evidence in making decisions about the care of surgical patients. Evidence-based surgery is part of a broader movement—evidence-based medicine—to apply the scientific method to medical practice. This movement has its historical roots in the pioneering work of the Scottish epidemiologist Archibald Cochrane (1909–1988), for whom the preeminent international organization for research in evidence-based medicine, the Cochrane Collaboration, is named. The term "evidence-based medicine" itself was popularized through a landmark article advocating a new approach to medical education that appeared in the *Journal of the American Medical Association* in 1992.[1] This article urged the de-emphasis of "intuition, unsystematic clinical experience, and pathophysiologic rationale as sufficient grounds for clinical decision making." In essence, advocates of evidence-based medicine seek to demote "expert opinion" to the least valid basis for clinical decision making. The practice of surgery, once driven more by the eminence of tradition than the evidence of science, now increasingly requires its students to adopt evidence-based scientific standards of practice.

The imperative that surgical care be delivered in accordance with the best available scientific evidence is only one facet of evidence-based surgery. In addition, evidence-based surgery refers to systematic efforts to establish standards of care supported by science, as well as the movement to popularize evidence-based practice. Systematic reviews of the literature are often generated by independent researchers or collaborative study groups (e.g., Cochrane collaborations) and published as review articles in journals or disseminated as practice guidelines. The movement to propagate evidence-based surgical practice is a relatively recent phenomenon exemplified by the collaborative efforts to develop the Surgical Care Improvement Project Core Measure Set[2] and by the US federal government's efforts to reward best practices with "pay for performance" policies.[3] Although researchers are charged with generating and disseminating scientific evidence, the greatest responsibility for the success of evidence-based surgery is ultimately with individual surgeons, who must not only practice evidence-based surgery but also understand and appropriately interpret an immense surgical literature.

This chapter provides a framework for evaluating the strength of evidence for surgical practices, the validity of scientific studies in surgery, and the role of evidence-based surgery in assessing and improving the quality of surgical care. The intent is to provide the reader with conceptual and analytic tools that a modern, evidence-based surgeon needs to navigate the surgical literature and implement practices that are based on sound science.

Guidelines and Secondary Sources of Scientific Evidence

To meet the growing demand for evidence-based practice information, a market has developed around the work of pooling and interpreting "best scientific evidence." Scientific reviews serve as secondary sources for evidence-based practice and are increasingly found in journals, in books, and on the Internet. Prominent examples include *Clinical Evidence* (published semiannually by the *British Journal of Medicine* and continually updated online[4]), the *Cochrane Database of Systematic Reviews*,[5] and the Institute for Healthcare Improvement.[6] For surgical practices specifically, the Surgical Care Improvement Project serves as a clearinghouse for evidence-based guidelines.

Efforts to summarize and disseminate information about evidence-based surgery provide a convenient "user interface" for the surgical literature that can be very helpful to practicing surgeons. However, because such aids are far from complete and new evidence emerges continually, surgeons cannot rely on these sources entirely. The modern "evidence-based surgeon" must learn to assess the quality of individual scientific studies and interpret their implications for his or her practice.

Levels of Evidence

Evidence for surgical practice comes in many forms with variable reliability. At one end of the spectrum is an empirical impression that a practice makes physiologic sense and seems to work well. Much of what surgeons do in practice falls into this category and has not been formally tested. At the other end of the spectrum is evidence accumulated from multiple carefully conducted scientific experiments with consistent and reproducible results. The task of the evidence-based surgeon is to judge the reliability of scientific evidence and select practices that conform to the best evidence available.

To help clinicians judge the strength of scientific evidence, researchers have attempted to create hierarchies of evidence, which range from those sources that are most reliable to those that are least sure. With the understanding that not all practices have been subjected to the highest levels of scientific scrutiny, clinicians are advised to base practices on evidence gleaned from studies as high on the evidence hierarchy as possible.

A commonly cited example of such a hierarchy is the "levels of evidence" system popularized by the U.S. Preventive Medicine Task Force (USPMTF) [*see Table 1*].[7] Since its inception, the hierarchy of scientific evidence created by the USPMTF has become common parlance among clinicians. Hence, frequently heard references to "level 1 evidence" refer to well-conducted randomized controlled trials. However, almost as soon as the USPMTF released its evidence grading system, debate about its adequacy began.[8] The predominant criticism has been that the system is too simple and inflexible to accurately describe the strength of evidence for clinical practices. Although the system identifies the design of the study from which the evidence is drawn, it does not describe important factors that influence the quality of the study. For example, in the USPMTF system, the same grade is awarded to a randomized, double-blind, placebo-controlled trial with 50,000 subjects as to an unblinded randomized trial with 30 subjects. The latter trial would, in turn, be graded higher than a well-designed and conducted, multi-institution, prospective cohort study with 10,000 subjects.

In response to these deficiencies, numerous alternative grading systems have been developed that take into account factors other than study design, such as quality, consistency, and completeness. However, it is widely recognized that no single grading system is perfect,[9] and surgeons are often required to judge the quality and applicability of scientific evidence for themselves.

Appraising Scientific Evidence

Specific study designs are associated with different levels of confidence about cause and effect. The clinical study design that is considered to have the greatest potential for determining causation is the randomized, controlled clinical trial.

Table 1 Levels of Evidence, as Stratified by the U.S. Preventive Services Task Force

Level of Evidence	Source of Evidence
I	At least one properly randomized controlled trial
II – 1	Well-designed controlled trials without randomization
II – 2	Well-designed cohort or case-control analytic study, preferably from more than one center or research group
II – 3	Multiple time-series with or without intervention or possibly dramatic results from uncontrolled trials (e.g., penicillin treatment in the 1940s)
III	Opinions from respected authorities based on clinical experience, descriptive studies and case reports, or committees of experts
Category of Recommendation	**Basis of Recommendation**
Level A	Good and consistent scientific evidence
Level B	Limited or inconsistent scientific evidence
Level C	Consensus and/or expert opinion

This simple categorization scheme is generally considered inadequate but is still frequently referenced.

However, even studies with this design can lead to erroneous conclusions if they are not performed properly. Evaluating the quality of clinical evidence requires a close look at how the study that produced it was conceived, implemented, analyzed, and interpreted.

Scientific evidence from studies of clinical practice relies on two important inferences. The first inference is that the observed outcome is the result of the practice and cannot be attributed to some alternative explanation. When this inference is deemed true, the study is considered to have *internal validity*. The second inference is that what was observed in the clinical study is relevant to scenarios outside the study where the surgeon seeks to implement the practice. The extent to which this is true is called *external validity* or *generalizability*. Whereas internal validity relies on how well the study is conducted and the results analyzed, external validity relies on how well the study plan reflects the real-world clinical question that inspired it and how well the study's conclusions apply to real-world scenarios outside the study [*see Figure 1*]. Poor external validity can also refer to the difference between an intervention's efficacy (how well it works when applied perfectly) and its effectiveness (whether it has the same effect when applied generally in an uncontrolled environment).

Evaluating the Quality of a Study: Internal Validity

Assessment of the internal validity of a study requires an understanding of the potential influences of *chance*, *bias*, and *confounding* [*see Table 2*]. Chance refers to unpredictable randomness of events that might mislead researchers. Bias refers to systematic errors in how study subjects were selected or assessed. Confounding refers to differences in the comparison groups (other than the intended exposure) that lead to differences in outcomes.

CHANCE

In clinical studies that compare outcomes between two or more groups, the assumption that there is no difference in outcomes is called the *null hypothesis*. Erroneous conclusions with regard to the null hypothesis can sometimes occur by chance alone. There are two types of chance-related errors: type I and type II. Type I error (also called α error) occurs when researchers erroneously reject the null hypothesis, that is, infer that there is a difference in outcomes when there is really no difference. Type II error (also called β error) occurs when researchers erroneously confirm the null hypothesis, that is, infer that there is no difference in outcomes when, in reality, a difference exists.

Type I Errors

Statistical testing is used to quantify the likelihood of a type I error. A "p value" indicates the probability that observed differences between groups might be due to chance alone. The threshold for "statistical significance" is conventionally set at a p value of .05, signifying that the likelihood of the observed differences being due to chance alone is 5 out of 100. Although a likelihood of 5% falls short of absolute certainty, this level of confidence is generally accepted as scientific proof.

An alternative expression of statistical likelihood is confidence intervals. Confidence intervals show the range of

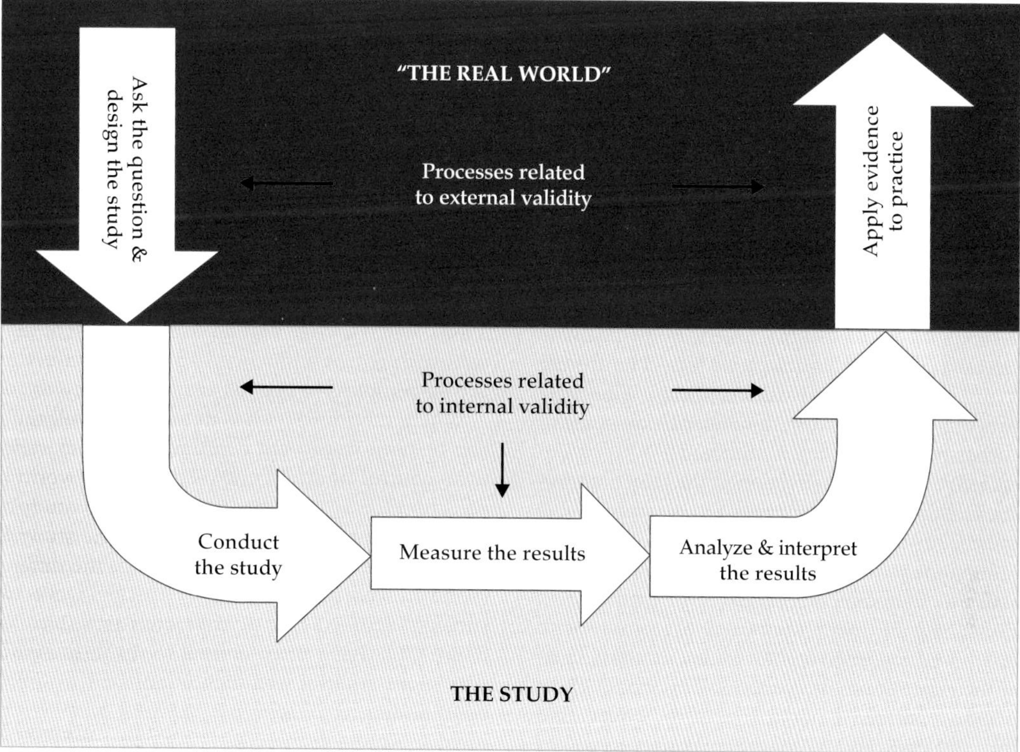

Figure 1 **Processes that affect the internal and external validity of a clinical study.**

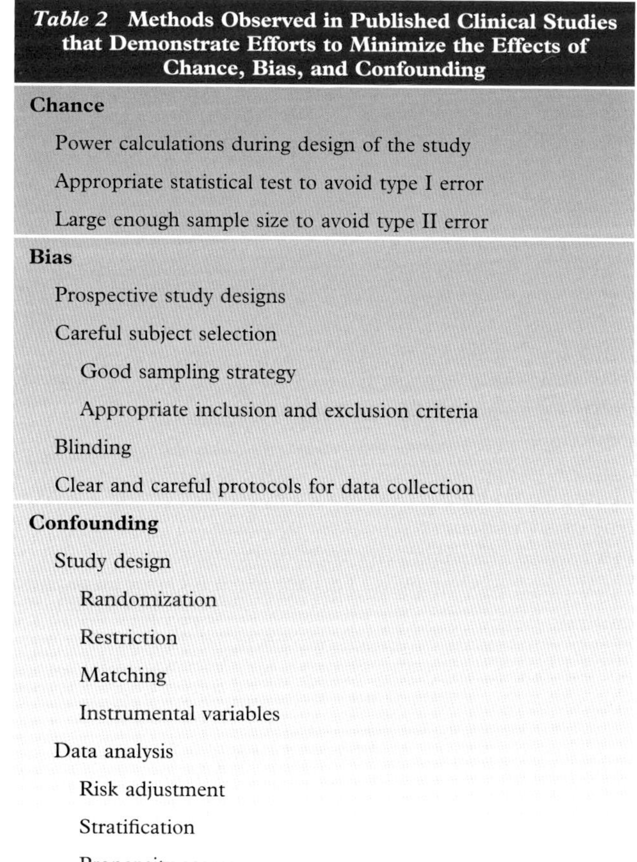

Table 2 Methods Observed in Published Clinical Studies that Demonstrate Efforts to Minimize the Effects of Chance, Bias, and Confounding

Chance
Power calculations during design of the study
Appropriate statistical test to avoid type I error
Large enough sample size to avoid type II error
Bias
Prospective study designs
Careful subject selection
Good sampling strategy
Appropriate inclusion and exclusion criteria
Blinding
Clear and careful protocols for data collection
Confounding
Study design
Randomization
Restriction
Matching
Instrumental variables
Data analysis
Risk adjustment
Stratification
Propensity scores

the observed difference that would be expected if the same study were repeated an infinite number of times. For example, a 95% confidence interval would include the observed difference 95% of the times that the study was repeated.

Many statistical tests can be used to calculate p values and confidence intervals. The appropriate statistical test must be selected according to several factors, including the number of observations in the comparison groups, the number of groups being compared, whether two or more groups are being compared with each other or one group is being compared with itself after some interval of time, what kind of numerical data are being analyzed (e.g. continuous, categorical), or whether risk adjustment is required. Although most surgeons are unlikely to fully comprehend all of the nuances of more complex statistical analyses, most clinical surgical studies are designed simply enough to employ statistical tests that are within reach of the nonstatistician. Fortunately, several useful and concise texts are available that can help surgeons become conversant in basic statistical methods.[10–12]

Type II Errors

Type II errors (erroneously accepting the null hypothesis) often occur when sample size is simply insufficient to detect small but clinically important differences in outcomes. When a study's sample size is too small to detect differences in outcomes between comparison groups, it is said to lack sufficient statistical power. Once a study is complete, no amount of analysis can correct for insufficient statistical power. Before starting a study, researchers should perform a "power calculation," which involves determining the minimum size of a meaningful difference in outcomes and then calculating the number of observations required to show that difference statistically. Surgeons should be particularly cautious when evaluating studies with null findings, particularly when no power calculation is explicitly reported. An evidence-based surgeon is wise to remember the adage, "No evidence for effect is not necessarily evidence of no effect."

BIAS

Bias refers to a systematic problem with a clinical study that results in an inaccurate estimate of the differences in outcomes between comparison groups. There are two general types of bias: *selection bias* and *measurement bias*. The former results from errors in the choice of study subjects. The latter results from errors in the way information about exposures or outcomes (or other pertinent data) is obtained.

Selection bias refers to any imperfection in the selection process that results in either the wrong types of subjects (people who are not typical of the target population) or a sample of subjects that is for some reason (unrelated to the intervention) more likely to have the outcome of interest. For example, paid volunteer subjects may be more motivated to comply with treatment regimens and report favorable results, resulting in an overestimate of the effect of an intervention. This would affect both internal validity (inference about size of the effect) and external validity (generalizability to other populations). As another example, selecting subjects from among diners at a Szechuan Chinese restaurant for a trial of medical versus surgical treatment of gastroesophageal reflux might lead to results favoring medical treatment (people with reflux who consume Szechuan Chinese food are more likely to have symptoms that are already well-controlled medically). When assessing the validity of scientific evidence, surgeons must carefully consider the characteristics of the subjects selected for study.

Measurement bias refers to problems caused by the way information about outcomes or other pertinent data is obtained. For example, in a study of sexual function after surgery for rectal cancer, subjects may report symptoms differently in an in-person interview than they would in an anonymous mailed survey. As another example, using surgeons to assess hernia repair outcomes in their own patients might result in erroneous reported rates of chronic pain. Retrospective studies are particularly prone to a variety of types of measurement bias. For example "recall bias" may occur because of subjects' selective memory of past events, and "ascertainment bias" may occur if the outcome is likely to influence how hard observers look for information about exposures. Sources of measurement bias may be more subtle than selection bias and require careful attention to reported study methods. Efforts to control measurement bias include blinding (not telling the subject or assessor what intervention was performed) and prospective study design.

Confounding

Confounding refers to differences in outcomes that occur because of differences in the baseline risks of the comparison groups. Confounding is often the result of selection bias. For example, a comparison of mortality after open versus laparoscopic colectomy might be skewed because of the greater likelihood of open colectomy being performed as an emergency in a critically ill patient. In this example, the severity of the illness confounds the observed association between mortality and surgical approach.

In evaluating the strength of evidence in a published study, readers must assess how well the researchers accounted for the potential effect of confounding. Confounding can be minimized in several ways, both in the design of the study and in the analysis of the study's results. In the design of a study, confounding is most effectively addressed with *randomization*. When subjects are randomized, potentially confounding variables (both recognized and unrecognized) are likely to be evenly distributed across comparison groups. Thus, whereas the baseline rate of outcomes in the entire cohort might be influenced by these factors, the differences across comparison groups are less likely to be affected.

Where randomization is not practical, *restriction* or *matching* can be used to prevent confounding. Restriction refers to the tight control of study entry criteria (e.g., enter only elective colectomy cases in the study described above). However, restrictive entry criteria can sometimes limit generalizability. Matching refers to using a comparison group of unexposed (control) subjects who are identical to the exposed (case) subjects across a set of characteristics (e.g., age, sex, residence) that have the potential to result in confounding.

A more complicated technique used to limit the effect of confounding is *instrumental variable analysis*. This approach involves studying the effect of a given exposure on outcomes by comparing groups with different levels of a third factor (the instrumental variable) that is highly correlated with the exposure but does not independently affect the outcome.[13] For example, an observational study of the effect of catheterization and revascularization on mortality following acute myocardial infarction is prone to confounding related to differences in baseline health characteristics of the populations receiving or not receiving these treatments. To limit this potential source of confounding, a group of researchers studied the effect of these treatments (the exposure) on mortality after myocardial infarction (the outcome) by comparing groups of patients living at different distances from hospitals providing these services (the instrumental variable).[14] The researchers assumed that potentially confounding health characteristics would be distributed randomly geographically and that geographic distance would affect mortality only indirectly through its correlation with access to treatment. In a way, they used distance to "randomize" their study population to different levels of treatment for acute myocardial infarction.

In addition to minimizing confounding through good study design, confounding can also be addressed during the analytic phase of a study. The most common approach is the use of *statistical risk adjustment* techniques, typically with multivariate regression analysis. This approach involves taking into account differences in the prevalence of recognized confounders across comparison groups. However, statistical risk adjustment has two important limitations. First, only recognized confounders can be addressed. Second, every potential confounding variable added to a statistical model decreases the model's statistical power and thereby increases the chance of resulting in a type II error.

Other analytic techniques used to address confounding include *stratification* (subanalyses in which subjects with similar risk profiles are compared) and *propensity score risk adjustment.*[15] The latter technique addresses the problem created by unequal chances of receiving treatment caused by differences in health characteristics. In an observational study of the outcomes of a given treatment, a propensity score is a scalar summary of all observed confounders that predict the probability of receiving the treatment. Propensity scores are typically calculated using multivariate regression models and are used as the basis for stratified analysis or for matching cases and controls in observational studies.

Interpreting and Applying Evidence to Practice: External Validity

Once one is convinced that a clinical study is internally valid (i.e., that the observed outcome is the result of the exposure or intervention and cannot be attributed to some alternative explanation), then the challenge to the surgeon is judging the study's external validity (i.e., determining whether the findings are applicable to the clinical scenario he or she faces). An assessment of external validity requires attention to several components of a clinical study, including the patient population, the intervention, and the outcome measure. In the discussion that follows, a large prospective randomized clinical trial of laparoscopic versus open inguinal hernia repair performed in the Veterans Administration (VA) will be used as an illustrative example.[16] This trial concluded that outcomes of open repair are superior to those of laparoscopic repair. The trial was well designed and well conducted but generated substantial discussion about the generalizability of the results.

As noted above, subject selection bias can adversely affect the external validity (or generalizability) of a study's results. If the population studied is in some important measure different from the population for which a surgeon is making clinical decisions, he or she may not achieve similar results. In the VA hernia trial, subjects were military veterans, who tend to be, on average, older than the nonveteran general population. If older subjects are more prone to the risks of laparoscopic hernia repair (e.g., general anesthesia), one might expect that the difference in morbidity outcomes would be exaggerated in the VA trial. In this respect, a surgeon might consider the evidence provided by the trial applicable to his or her older patients but reserve judgment on the use of laparoscopy to repair hernias in younger, healthier patients.

A striking example of the potential effect of selection bias on generalizability comes from the Asymptomatic Carotid Artery Stenosis (ACAS) trial.[17] In this large prospective randomized study, volunteers for the trial were substantially younger and healthier than the average patient who undergoes carotid endarterectomy. As a result, the observed perioperative mortality rate in the trial was considerably lower than that observed in the general population or even in the very hospitals where the trial was conducted.[18] Although the results of the ACAS trial significantly changed practice, one could argue that the evidence provided by the ACAS trial may have been generalizable only to younger populations.

The external validity of a clinical study can also be affected by who provides the intervention and by what type of intervention is provided. In the VA hernia trial, surgeons had variable experience with the laparoscopic approach, and the trial reported twofold differences in hernia recurrences between surgeons who had done more than 250 cases and surgeons who had less experience. Surgeons deciding whether evidence supports the use of laparoscopic repair would need to examine their own experience before determining the generalizability of this study to their practices. Furthermore, some have argued that one of the laparoscopic techniques commonly used in the VA trial (transabdominal preperitoneal repair) is outmoded and more hazardous.[19] Surgeons who avoid using this approach might reasonably question the generalizability of this study to their practices.

The type of outcome measured can also affect the generalizability of clinical studies. Outcomes chosen for clinical studies may be those that are most convenient or most easily quantified and may not be the outcomes of greatest interest to patients. In the VA hernia trial, several outcomes were studied, including operative complications, hernia recurrence, pain, and length of convalescence. Some of the outcome differences favored open repair, whereas some favored laparoscopic repair. The interpretation of the trial evidence for one type of repair versus the other involves implicit value judgments regarding which outcomes are most important to patients. Surgeons applying the VA hernia trial evidence to decisions about hernia repair must examine the specific outcomes measured before knowing whether a study is generalizable to an individual patient with specific values and interests.

Evidence-Based Surgery and Quality of Care

In clinical studies, the efficacy of a surgical practice is measured in terms of the resulting patient outcomes. Similarly, efforts to assess the quality of surgical care have until recently focused almost exclusively on clinical outcomes. In recent years, however, the movement to promote evidence-based surgery has offered an alternative measure of surgical quality: adherence to processes of care (e.g., routine use of perioperative antibiotics) supported by the best available scientific evidence.

The question of whether efforts to assess quality should focus on evidence-based processes of care or clinical outcomes is as much practical as philosophical. The practical argument against outcomes is largely driven by a growing recognition that individual hospitals and surgeons generally have too few adverse outcomes to provide enough statistical power to show meaningful differences between providers.[20] The practical argument against evidence-based processes of care is driven by the paucity of high-leverage, procedure-specific processes for which sound evidence is available, as well as the logistical challenge of measuring such processes. A more complete discussion of this topic is provided elsewhere [*see 1:2 Performance Measurement in Surgery*].

Given its current momentum, the evidence-based surgery movement will likely play a progressively larger role in efforts to assess and improve quality of surgical care. Furthermore, as payers increasingly turn to "pay for performance" strategies to improve quality and control costs, the demand for evidence-based practice guidelines will continue to grow. More importantly, efforts to identify and implement evidence-based surgical practices will ultimately provide patients with safer, better care.

Financial Disclosures: None Reported

References

1. Evidence-Based Medicine Working Group. Evidence-based medicine: a new approach to teaching the practice of medicine. JAMA 1992;268:2420–5.
2. Surgical Care Improvement Project Core Measures. Available at http://www.jointcommission.org/PerformanceMeasurement/PerformanceMeasurement/SCIP+Core+Measure+Set.htm (accessed January 29, 2009).
3. Payment and Performance Improvement Programs Committee on Redesigning Health Insurance Performance Measures. Rewarding provider performance: aligning incentives in medicare. Washington (DC): National Academies Press; 2007.
4. Clinical Evidence. Available at http://www.clinicalevidence.bmj.com (accessed January 29, 2009).
5. The Cochrane Collaboration. Available at http://www.cochrane.org/ (accessed January 29, 2009).
6. Institute for Healthcare Improvement. Available at http://www.ihi.org (accessed January 29, 2009).
7. Harris RP, Helfand M, Woolf SH, et al. Current methods of the US Preventive Services Task Force: a review of the process. Am J Prev Med 2001;20 Suppl 3:21–35.
8. Woloshin S. Arguing about grades. Eff Clin Pract 2000;3:94–5.
9. Atkins D, Eccles M, Flottorp S, et al. Systems for grading the quality of evidence and the strength of recommendations I: Critical appraisal of existing approaches—the GRADE Working Group. BMC Health Serv Res 2004;4:38.
10. Glanz S. Primer of biostatistics. 6th ed. New York: McGraw-Hill Medical; 2005.
11. Motulsky H. Intuitive biostatistics. New York: Oxford University Press; 1995.
12. Dawson B, Trapp R. Basic & clinical biostatistics. 4th ed. New York: McGraw-Hill Medical; 2004.
13. Stukel TA, Fisher ES, Wennberg DE, et al. Analysis of observational studies in the presence of treatment selection bias: effects of invasive cardiac management on AMI survival using propensity score and instrumental variable methods. JAMA 2007;297: 278–85.
14. McClellan M, McNeil B, Newhouse J. Does more intensive treatment of acute myocardial infarction in the elderly reduce mortality? Analysis using instrumental variables. JAMA 1994;272:859–66.
15. Braitman LE, Rosenbaum PR. Rare outcomes, common treatments: analytic strategies using propensity scores. Ann Intern Med 2002;137:693–5.
16. Neumayer L, Giobbe-Hurder O, Johansson O, et al. Open mesh versus laparoscopic mesh repair of inguinal hernia. N Engl J Med 2004;350:1819–27.
17. Executive Committee for the Asymptomatic Carotid Atherosclerosis Study. Endarterectomy for asymptomatic carotid artery stenosis. JAMA 1995;273:1421–8.
18. Wennberg DE, Lucas FL, Birkmeyer JD, et al. Variation in carotid endartectomy mortality in the Medicare population: trial hospitals, volume, and patient characteristics. JAMA 1998;279:1278–81.
19. Grunwaldt LJ, Schwaitzberg SD, Rattner DW, Jones DB. Is laparoscopic inguinal hernia repair an operation of the past? J Am Coll Surg 2005;200:616–20.
20. Dimick JB, Welch HG, Birkmeyer JD. Surgical mortality as an indicator of hospital quality: the problem with small sample size. JAMA 2004;292:847–51.

5 PATIENT SAFETY IN SURGICAL CARE: A SYSTEMS APPROACH

Robert S. Rhodes, MD, FACS, and Caprice C. Greenberg, MD, MPH, FACS

High-profile catastrophes such as the explosion of the nuclear power plant at Chernobyl, the near meltdown of the nuclear power plant at Three Mile Island, the explosion of a chemical plant in Bhopal, numerous aviation disasters, and the loss of the space shuttles *Challenger* and *Columbia* share important characteristics. First, the casualties are notable for their number, their celebrity, or both. Second (and more germane to this chapter), each occurred as a result of multiple failures within complex systems. Human errors played a role in all of these failures, but the errors were not single acts of negligence as much as they were magnifications of multiple seemingly small interactions, the significance of which was initially unrecognized or underestimated.

Until about a decade ago, medical errors, unlike the above events, rarely received much publicity. This was in part because they affected only one patient at a time, and, as a result, their aggregate number was neither recognized nor well publicized. Another factor has been the tendency to regard error in medicine as a special case of medicine rather than as a special case of error.[1] The unfortunate result of this view has been the isolation of medical errors from much of the body of theory, analysis, and application that has been developed to deal with error in other high-risk work domains such as aviation and nuclear power.

Yet at least two factors now appear to be changing this view. One, the 1999 report of the Institute of Medicine (IOM), *To Err Is Human: Building a Safer Health System*, made national headlines with its estimates of the frequency and severity of adverse events in health care, including that as many as 98,000 medical error–related deaths occur each year in the United States.[2] This estimate far exceeds the number of casualties from more publicized nonmedical disasters, and if it is accurate, then medical errors would be one of the leading causes of death in the United States. Moreover, surgical adverse events represent over half of all adverse events experienced by hospitalized patients, and 75% of those have their origin in the operating room.[3] This highlights the critical importance of patient safety in surgical care, particularly in the operating room.

A second factor affecting this view was advances in cognitive psychology that greatly increased the understanding of the influences that lead to error and affect human performance. The observation that the basic principles of human error are highly applicable to clinical practice has markedly advanced our understanding and willingness to address error in this setting. Medical errors are not a special case of medicine, and their underlying causes are not unique to medical practice.

These factors also challenged the notion that medical injury is primarily the result of "bad apples" and that safety can be improved largely by ridding the system of these persons. Undoubtedly, bad apples exist, but it is increasingly clear that health care–related injuries represent system failures and are rarely solely the result of negligence on the part of a single provider. Furthermore, there is a growing recognition that modern health care systems are as complex as—if not more complex than—the systems associated with nuclear power, aviation, and space flight.[1] The cognitive and technical complexity of the tasks performed in the operating room, the intensive care unit, and the emergency department certainly rivals that of these other endeavors. Furthermore, optimal patient care increasingly requires coordination among an expanding number of participants. For instance, in the early 20th century, it is estimated that health care involved the interaction of three persons, on average; a century later that number had risen to 16.

This chapter seeks to address the characteristics of systems in general and the system of surgical care in particular. It describes the growing knowledge of factors that affect human performance and how these factors contribute to adverse surgical outcomes. The chapter also outlines current obstacles to improving safety, identifies systems approaches to making improvements, and discusses ways in which surgeons can take the lead in overcoming these obstacles. An overall goal is that acceptance of error and a willingness to investigate its underlying causes will allow health care professionals to make use of the lessons learned from study of nonmedical systems. Although issues of patient safety are often intertwined with those of the overall cost-effectiveness and quality of surgical care,[4] the latter are discussed in greater detail elsewhere.

Nature and Magnitude of Adverse Events in Surgical Care

For most of the important concepts bearing on patient safety in the surgical setting, generally accepted definitions exist [*see Sidebar* Definitions of Terms Related to Patient Safety]; the ensuing discussion is based on these definitions.[5] A solid understanding of the key concepts—such as the distinctions between an adverse event (or adverse outcome), an error, and negligence—is critical for managing errors as system failures rather than as isolated incidents.[6] In particular, such an understanding can help in navigating the often turbulent emotional milieu that can surround adverse patient events. Given their motivation to help patients, physicians tend to be highly sensitive to issues of causation, and this

Definitions of Terms Related to Patient Safety[5]

- An *adverse event* is an injury that was caused by medical management and that results in measurable disability.
- An *error* is the failure of a planned action to be completed as intended or the use of a wrong plan to achieve an aim. Errors can include problems in practice, products, procedures, and systems.
- A *preventable adverse event* is an adverse event that is attributable to error.
- An *unpreventable adverse event* is an adverse event resulting from a complication that cannot be prevented given the current state of knowledge.
- A *near miss* is an event or situation that could have resulted in accident, injury, or illness but did not, either by chance or through timely intervention.
- A *medical error* is an adverse event or near miss that is preventable with the current state of medical knowledge.
- A *latent error* is a condition of the system that is removed from the adverse event, such as poorly designed equipment, management decisions, or physical plan of the operating room. Latent errors set up the conditions in which an adverse event can occur, but their impact is not directly recognized.
- An *active error* is an action that directly leads to the adverse event.
- A *system* is a regularly interacting or interdependent group of items forming a unified whole.
- A *systems error* is an error that is not the result of an individual's actions but the predictable outcome of a series of actions and factors that make up a diagnostic or treatment process.

sensitivity can then interfere with the recognition and management of safety issues.

The two most widely cited estimates of adverse medical events derive from the Harvard Medical Practice Study (HMPS)[7] and from a study in Colorado and Utah.[3] The HMPS, a population-based study of patients hospitalized in New York State during 1984, found that nearly 4% of patients experienced an adverse event and that about half of such events occurred in surgical patients. The Colorado/Utah study, which randomly sampled 15,000 nonpsychiatric discharges during 1992, found that the annual incidence of adverse surgical events was 3.0% and that 54% of these events were preventable. Nearly half of all adverse surgical events were accounted for by technique-related complications, wound infections, and postoperative bleeding. This study also identified common operations that were associated with a significantly higher risk of an adverse event and a significantly higher risk of a preventable event.

Other studies yielded comparable or higher estimates,[8] and still others evaluated the rates at which specific events occurred, as follows:

- Retained sponges or surgical instruments were estimated to occur at a rate between one in 8,801 and one in 18,760 inpatient procedures at nonspecialty acute care hospitals.[9]
- Wrong-site surgery is more than just an isolated event,[10] and the apparent increased frequency at which such events are currently being reported probably reflects previous underreporting.
- Medication errors (e.g., wrong drug, wrong dose, wrong patient, wrong time, or wrong administration route) are alarmingly frequent.[11,12] The US Pharmacopeia monitors these events through its reporting programs (www.usp.org/patientsafety). In 2001, these programs received reports of 105,603 errors, 2,539 (2.4%) of which resulted in patient injury. Of these, 353 necessitated hospitalization or prolonged its duration, 70 necessitated interventions to sustain life, and 14 resulted in a patient's death. The main contributing factors were distractions (47%), workload increases (24%), and staffing issues (36%). Miscalculating patient weight conversions (e.g., from pounds to kilograms) and subsequent improper dosing are all too common among pediatric patients. Errors in the administration of radiopharmaceuticals are also frequent and may involve the wrong isotope (68.9%), the wrong patient (24%), the wrong dose (6.5%), or the wrong route (0.6%).[12] One study estimated that the US rates would have to be reduced by one third to match the benchmark rates in Germany and the United Kingdom with regard to medical mistakes, medication errors, or laboratory test errors.[13]
- Blood transfusions continue to be plagued by patient misidentification.
- Device-related deaths and serious injuries also occur at an alarming rate, even after premarket safety testing.[14] The Food and Drug Administration (FDA) maintains a registry of the thousands of such injuries that occur each year. A survey noted that 35% of physicians and 42% of the public said that they had experienced a medical mistake in their own care or in the care of a family member.[15]

As might be expected, the IOM report prompted a great deal of debate. Some medical professionals questioned the accuracy of the estimates, whereas others disagreed with the definitions of medical error and adverse event, with the extent to which either or both were considered preventable. Still others argued that adverse events that are caused by conceptual errors (e.g., a contraindicated, unsound, or inappropriate approach) should be differentiated from the side effects of an intended action that is correct in the circumstances (e.g., an indicated diagnostic or therapeutic procedure).[16] The aim of this argument was to sharpen the distinction between accidents (i.e., unplanned, unexpected, and undesired events) and true side effects (which result from correct management and which are often accepted as reasonable therapeutic tradeoffs).

The HMPS attempted to address these issues by characterizing adverse events as either preventable or unpreventable in the light of the prevailing state of knowledge. Preventable errors were further subclassified as either diagnostic errors or treatment errors; treatment errors included preventive errors such as failure of prophylaxis and failure to monitor and follow treatment.[7,17] The HMPS found that preventability varied according to the type of event: 74% of early surgical adverse events were judged preventable, compared with 65% of nonsurgical adverse events, and more than 90% of late surgical failures, diagnostic mishaps, and nonprocedural therapeutic mishaps were judged preventable.

The above estimates of patient injury rates have also raised speculations about trends in the frequency of these events. To some, the observation that the rate of such events was lower in the Colorado/Utah study than in the HMPS suggests that patient safety was improving even before the IOM report. Although there may be some improvements in care, wide gaps in quality persist (www.healthgrades.com/business/study/quality.aspx).

Regardless of any actual trend, there is agreement that progress since the IOM report has been slow, that the results have been modest at best, and that the gap between the best possible care and the care actually being delivered remains large.[18–20] Although the lack of more evident improvement has been somewhat disappointing, clear progress has nevertheless been made with respect to (1) understanding the complexities of medical care systems, (2) identifying the challenges to improving these systems, and (3) developing new perspectives on the assessment of errors. Thus, an increase in estimates of the incidence of adverse events may simply reflect improved reporting rather than actual increases in their occurrence.

Nature and Characteristics of Systems

A system may be broadly defined as a regularly interacting or interdependent group of items that form a unified whole. System functions or tasks usually involve sequential steps that have human, technological, and logistical components. The overall probability of a system failure (i.e., an adverse outcome), then, is a function of the probability of error within each step, the total number of steps, and the degree to which the steps are coupled. The degree of coupling is the extent to which an error at one step can propagate through subsequent steps and adversely affect the final outcome. Loosely coupled systems tend to have built-in redundancy that acts as a safety barrier to prevent errors from propagating to subsequent steps. As a result, satisfactory outcomes in such systems are far less dependent on successful completion of each step. Errors in loosely coupled systems are more readily "trapped" by these safety barriers.

In contrast to loosely coupled systems, tightly coupled systems have relatively little redundancy and relatively few fail-safe mechanisms. Consequently, successful outcomes in tightly coupled systems are highly dependent on the success of each step in essentially a factorial fashion. Thus, the probability of success in a tightly coupled linear 20-step process with a 1% likelihood of error at each step is equivalent to 0.99 factored 20 times, or 0.818. Thus, even though the probability of error for each step is .01, the overall likelihood of an unintended outcome is 0.182.

Given that safety barriers are generally more numerous in loosely coupled than in tightly coupled systems, it is relatively unusual for an isolated error to produce an injury or system failure in the former. Thus, failures in loosely coupled systems typically involve malfunctions at multiple steps. A tradeoff with the level of redundancy in loosely coupled systems is that it makes the system more complex, and the added complexity can introduce its own errors.

James Reason was the first to distinguish between active and latent system errors and their individual importance in understanding the overall role in system failures.[21] Active errors are what might be traditionally associated with the term "error": a discrete action that produces an immediate effect. Latent errors, on the other hand, are structural characteristics of the system, features of the environment, or decisions or plans that are removed from the point of care. They do not produce an immediate result but rather set up the conditions in which a given result can arise. The importance of a system's latent failures as contributing factors in adverse outcomes may be illustrated by considering a general schema of an injury [*see Figure 1*].[21] Whereas overt system problems are relatively easy to identify and correct, latent failures are insidious and often do not become evident until a seemingly improbable series of events produces errors in otherwise routine processes. Latent failures tend to be introduced by persons who work at the "blunt end" of the system (e.g., management or housekeeping) but do not actively participate in the main processes of care. A typical injury pathway is one in which organizational processes introduce latent failures, which in turn produce system defects, which in turn interact with external events so that persons who work at the "sharp end" of the system (e.g., anesthesiologists, nurses, or surgeons) commit unsafe acts. These unsafe acts precipitate an active failure that then penetrates the final safety barrier or barriers.[22] Indeed, the greatest risk of an adverse event in a complex system may come not from a breakdown of one or more major subsystems or from isolated operator errors but from the presence or accumulation of latent failures.[21,23,24]

Surgical Care as a System

The characteristics of systems already discussed (see above) have many attributes directly applicable to medicine in general and to surgery and anesthesiology in particular. In addition to the parallels between the habitats associated with surgery (e.g., the operating room, the intensive care unit, and the emergency department) and those associated with many high-tech, high-risk nonmedical endeavors, strong parallels exist between observed behavior in the operating room and behavioral issues in an airplane cockpit.[25,26]

The nature of the operating room as a system and the complexity of the interactions that occur there have been studied extensively. The performance of the operating room system depends on the individual performance of practitioners, the interactions of those individuals or teamwork, and the environment in which the practitioners work. It is important to note the interdependence of each of these components of the system. To understand the role that each plays, we examine each and their impact on surgical safety in turn: individual performance, teamwork, and environmental or structural factors.

Factors that Affect Performance

COGNITIVE PSYCHOLOGY OF INDIVIDUAL PERFORMANCE

Because human factors play a major role in system failure, any attempt to improve patient safety must be based on an understanding of the factors that affect human performance and their relation to human error.[27] Major advances in the field of cognitive psychology over the past several decades have greatly enhanced the understanding of human performance. A widely accepted schema classifies such performance into the following three types,[28] in descending order of familiarity with the specific task:

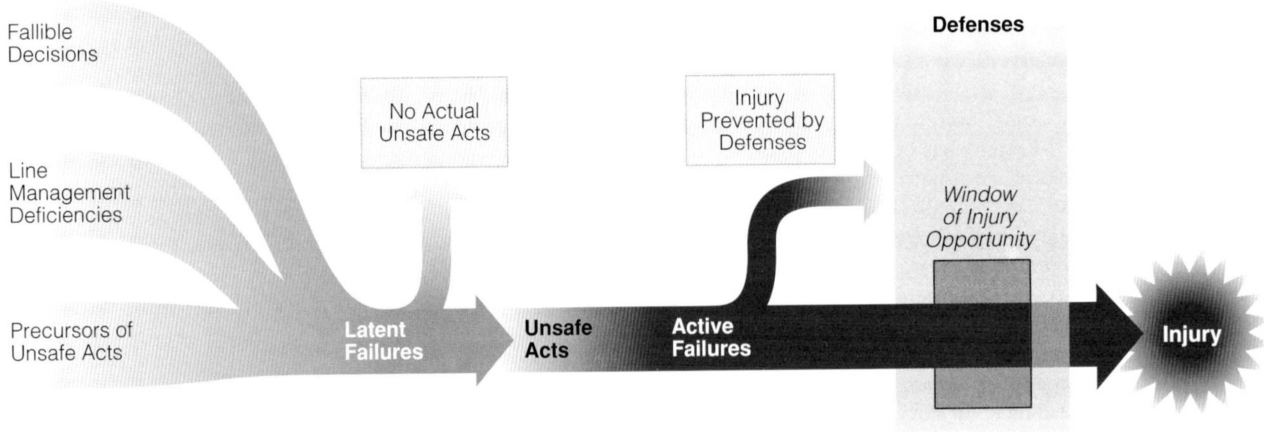

Figure 1 **Schematic depiction of the process by which system failures (latent and active) may lead to injury. Defenses may be inadequate if they allow the formation of a window of injury opportunity.**

1. *Skill-based performance.* This type of performance is governed by stored patterns of preprogrammed instructions. It occurs without conscious control and uses long-term memory.
2. *Rule-based performance.* This type involves solving problems by means of stored rules of the if-then variety. Like skill-based performance, it uses long-term memory; however, unlike skill-based performance, it is associated with a consciousness that a problem exists.[23] The rules are usually based on experience garnered from previous similar situations and are structured hierarchically, with the main rules on top; their strength appears to be a function of how recently and how frequently they are used.[27] Rule-based performance varies according to expertise: novices tend to rely on a few main rules, whereas experts have many side rules and exceptions.
3. *Knowledge-based performance.* This type involves conscious analytic processes and stored knowledge. It relies on working memory, which is comparatively slow and of relatively limited capacity. Typically, people resort to knowledge-based performance when their existing skills are not applicable or their repertoire of rules has been exhausted.

Successful performance or problem solving has three main phases: planning, storage, and execution. Errors resulting from failures in performance may be classified as slips, lapses, or mistakes,[21] depending on which phase of the problem-solving sequence is involved. Slips are failures of the execution phase, the storage phase, or both, and they may occur regardless of whether the plan from which they arose was adequate. Lapses are failures of the storage phase. Generally, slips are overt, whereas lapses are covert. Mistakes are failures of planning, reflecting basic deficiencies or failures in selecting an objective or specifying the means to achieve it, regardless of how well the plan was executed.

A key concept is that specific types of error tend to be associated with specific modes of failure [*see Table 1*].[21] Slips and lapses are failures of skill-based performance and generally precede recognition of a problem. Mistakes may be either failures of knowledge-based performance (i.e., attributable to lack of expertise) or failures of rule-based performance (i.e., attributable to failure of expertise). They typically arise during attempts to solve a problem. Mistakes tend to be more subtle,

Table 1 Common Modes of Failure Associated with Specific Types of Performance[21]

Failures of Skill-Based Performance
Inattention
Double-capture slips
Omissions following interruptions
Reduced intentionality
Perceptual confusions
Interference errors
Overattention
Omissions
Repetitions
Reversals
Failures of Rule-Based Performance
Misapplication of good rules
First exceptions
Countersigns and nonsigns
Informational overload
Rule strength
General rules
Redundancy
Rigidity
Application of bad rules
Encoding deficiencies
Action deficiencies
Wrong rules
Inelegant rules
Inadvisable rules
Failures of Knowledge-Based Performance
Selectivity
Workspace limitations
Out of sight, out of mind
Confirmation bias
Overconfidence
Biased reviewing
Illusory correlation
Halo effects
Problems with causality
Problems with complexity

more complex, and less well understood than slips or lapses and thus more dangerous. It has been suggested that experienced surgeons are more prone to slips and lapses and that junior surgeons and trainees are more prone to mistakes.[29]

Underspecification of the problem is common in clinical practice and clearly affects performance. A problem may seem underspecified when limited attention is paid, when the wrong cues are picked up, when the problem is truly ill-defined, or when the problem falls outside the known rules. Underspecification is more likely to occur in situations where cues change dynamically or are ambiguous and is associated with two types of error forms: similarity matching and frequency bias (or frequency gambling). In similarity matching, a present situation is thought to resemble a previous one and consequently is addressed in the same way (which is not necessarily appropriate). In frequency gambling, a course of action is chosen that has worked before, and the more often that course of action has been successfully used, the more likely it is to be chosen. These behavior patterns have been confirmed among anesthesiologists, who, like many dynamic decision makers, use approximation strategies (or heuristics) to handle ambiguous situations.[1]

Confirmation bias is another characteristic problem of performance. It may be defined as the propensity to stick with a chosen diagnosis or course of action and either to interpret new information so as to favor the original choice or to disregard such information entirely. It is also referred to as cognitive fixation, cognitive lockup, or fixation error and is often associated with knowledge-based performance.[30] Confirmation bias is particularly likely when the situation is unusual or evolving and when there is concomitant pressure to maintain coherence[31]—again, situations frequently encountered in surgical practice. A well-known adage is relevant here: good surgeons believe what they see; bad ones see what they believe.[32] The issue of how cognitive psychology affects diagnostic and clinical reasoning has been addressed in detail elsewhere.[33–35]

Confirmation bias may be considered an error of perception; other errors may be classified as errors of cognition or execution. Thus, classification schemes may be modified to meet specific needs.[36] For instance, some experts categorize errors according to whether they can be addressed by engineering, design, societal, or procedural changes; others prefer to emphasize psychological intervention and modification; and still others classify errors by their mode of appearance—for example, as errors of omission, errors of insertion, errors of repetition, or errors of substitution (e.g., misadministration of lidocaine, heparin, or potassium chloride as a result of poor package labeling).

RELATION OF INDIVIDUAL PERFORMANCE TO SURGICAL ERROR

To many, the concepts of performance and error, as they relate to patient care, seem straightforward—obvious, even. To others, however, it is crucial to make a distinction between human error and human performance, both because the assignment of error is often retrospective and thus subject to hindsight bias and because the term "error" is inherently prejudicial.

Important advances in our understanding of the role of surgeon performance in error come from an analysis of surgeon-reported errors[37] and a review of closed malpractice claims.[38] In the former, cognitive factors (primarily involving errors in judgment or vigilance) were involved in 86% of the incidents, whereas inexperience or lack of competence contributed to 53% of errors. The latter study reported similar findings: errors in judgment, failure of vigilance or memory, and lack of technical competence or knowledge were factors in 66%, 63%, and 41% of the cases, respectively.

Further analysis revealed that 65% of the technical errors were linked to manual error, 9% to errors in judgment or knowledge, and 26% to both manual and judgment or knowledge error.[39] Seventy-three percent of technical errors occurred with experienced surgeons operating within their field of expertise, and over 80% were performing routine operations but often under extenuating circumstances, such as complicated patient factors (61%) or systems failures (21%). Current approaches to decreasing technical performance include such interventions as volume-based referral or regionalization, increased specialization, and more stringent credentialing for high-risk procedures. The results of this study, however, suggest that these approaches are unlikely to lead to significant improvement. Rather, attention should be paid to improving technical performance (including both manual and judgment) in general but particularly when operating under complicated conditions.

In one sense, a surgeon's performance is a system factor, but in another sense, their cognitive and technical abilities make up a large part of the system's safety barriers. There is much that can be learned about human performance by studying how providers compensate when things start to go wrong and return the system to a safe state. Legal concerns aside, it is vital that surgeons not overemphasize the first sense and interpret it as an excuse for avoiding responsibility for complications.[40] Nevertheless, placing too much emphasis on surgeons' individual role retards rather than advances understanding of system failure and tends to evoke defensiveness rather than constructive action.[22,23,41] Regardless of whether these adverse events are performance failures or errors, eliminating them entirely is an impossible goal; a more realistic goal is to gain a better understanding of the contributing and compensatory factors and then to minimize—or possibly even eliminate—their consequences. The overall implication here is that to achieve meaningful improvements in safety, it is necessary to shift the focus from fallible individuals to the situational and organizational circumstances through which human performance leads to medical errors.[26]

Another important consideration in performance is an individual's physical and psychological well-being. The effects of sleep deprivation and fatigue on performance and learning have been particularly studied.[42–46] Fatigue, by impairing vigilance, can accentuate confirmation bias. In addition, errors increase as time on task increases; no other hazardous industry permits—let alone requires—employees to work the regular long hours common in hospitals.[30] Stress may increase the likelihood of error, but it is clearly neither necessary nor sufficient for cognitive failure.[21] Unfortunately, physicians tend to have unrealistic beliefs about their ability to deal with stress and fatigue and so may not seek help even when they clearly need it.[47] Recent studies have highlighted the striking prevalence of burnout among surgeons and the high degree of correlation between burnout and medical errors.[48] Surgeons also appear to have only a limited ability to assess their own learning needs, with those who are least skilled and those who are most confident being the worst at this task.[49] As a corollary, surgical skill is positively related to the ability to detect errors.[29]

The mental overload that can occur in situations involving a plethora of tasks may compromise the ability to respond to secondary tasks. Errors related to loss of vigilance include not observing a data stream at all, not observing a data stream sufficiently frequently, and not observing the particular data stream that is optimal for the existing situation. In watching for rare occurrences (a not uncommon situation in medicine), it is difficult to remain fully alert for longer than 10 to 20 minutes. Knowing when and how to verify data is an important metacognitive skill. An analysis of intraoperative safety identified high workloads, poor workload leveling, and multiple competing tasks as a major threat to performance and safety.[50]

In addressing these types of errors, a great deal of emphasis has been placed on reducing work hours, but there seems to have been relatively little consideration of the impact of workload and workflow on medical errors.[37] Yet data on resident work activities indicate that residents experience extremely fragmented workflows that result in frequent interruptions and changes in focus.[51] Moreover, the current limit on resident work hours does not appear to have improved patient safety[52] or reduced the incidence of technical complications.[53] Thus, demands for greater productivity within a health care system that is increasingly constrained by cost considerations may also contribute to an increase in medical errors.

Psychological framing effects also play a role in judgment. Examples of such effects are the irrational preference for established treatments when outcomes are framed in terms of gain (e.g., survival) and the similarly irrational preference for risky treatments when outcomes are framed in terms of loss (e.g., mortality). The impetus to "do the right thing" can adversely affect medical judgment.[54]

RELATION OF SYSTEM FACTORS TO SURGICAL ERROR

Teamwork and Communication

Teamwork and communication among team members also play essential roles in determining performance, particularly when there is a lack of cohesion and mutual support among team members.[1,30] On the one hand, a team structure that is too informal tends to undermine patterns of authority and responsibility and to hinder effective decision making. On the other hand, a hierarchy that is too strong may make it excessively difficult for juniors to question decisions made by those at higher levels of authority. Rigid behavior may impair the ability to cope with unforeseen events and discourage initiative.

Teamwork can be an especially complex matter in the operating room. The crews from nursing, surgery, and anesthesia often have fundamentally different perceptions of their respective roles, and these perceptual differences can adversely affect situational awareness. For example, anesthesiologists and nurse anesthetists are much more likely to feel that a preoperative briefing is important for team effectiveness than are surgeons and surgical nurses. In aviation, concern that junior team members would not question the decisions of more senior staff led to significant policy changes and safety enhancements.[55] Given the traditional surgical hierarchy, similar attitudes may exist in the operating room. Such varying perceptions can not only compromise patient safety but also hinder teaching and learning. Unfortunately, there is no broad consensus on how to achieve optimal team coordination in this setting.

The critical role of communication in surgical errors has been described in a number of studies. Two or more clinicians substantially contributed to error in 70% of surgeon-reported errors, and three or more were involved in 18% of the incidents.[37] Communication breakdowns contributed to approximately one quarter of surgical errors that led to patient injury as detected on malpractice claims analysis.[56] These tended to be verbal communications between two or more people and were equally as likely to be cross-disciplinary as intradisciplinary. They occurred with equal frequency in the pre-, intra-, and postoperative period, and the surgical attending physician was most often involved either as the transmitter or the receiver. Intraoperative field observations suggest that communication breakdowns and failures are pervasive in the operating room, occurring in up to one third of communication events.[50,57]

Environmental and Organizational Factors

The importance of the structural characteristics of the system in which care is provided is underscored by the relation between variations in the frequency of risk-adjusted outcomes among institutions and differences in the systems of care in place within those institutions.[58] The substantial similarities between medical and nonmedical systems notwithstanding, the complex content and organizational structure of health care make it distinctive. Many system concepts that derive primarily from analyses of human-engineered, highly technical, nonbiologic systems may not be fully applicable to the more complex issues of patient safety.[59] Linearly engineered systems are likely to be far more predictable than biologic systems, in which appropriate processes do not always result in good outcomes. Patients frequently differ greatly from each other in terms of their ability to communicate relevant issues, their severity of illness, their comorbidities, and their responses to diagnosis and treatment. When a system is not expected to work perfectly at all times—as health care is not—it becomes more difficult to distinguish problems related to individual error from problems related to flaws in the system. This distinction between nonmedical mechanical systems and medical systems may be akin to the distinction between complicated and complex endeavors.[60]

Differences in organizational structure between medical and nonmedical systems may be particularly relevant. A nonmedical system is typically a single structure that is managed vertically through hierarchical control. Patient care, in contrast, tends to consist of numerous diverse subsystems that may be only loosely aggregated.[61] These subsystems tend to function in isolation, and intrasystem changes tend to be managed laterally across individual subsystems. The resulting loose structure often leads to the creation of ineffective or even contradictory policies, all of which increase the chances of error.

The potential role of a systems approach in improving safety is further suggested by data that correlate improved outcomes with higher hospital or surgeon volume.[62,63] Whether these findings are explained by "practice makes perfect" or by "perfect makes practice" is yet to be resolved, but in either case, it seems likely that the improved outcomes reflect better care systems. That some high-volume hospitals and surgeons have below-average outcomes and many low-volume hospitals and surgeons have excellent ones is consistent with the role of systems.[64]

The physical characteristics of the system in which care is provided can influence the safety of the system. Issues such as ergonomics, lighting, equipment malfunctions, noise levels, and interruptions can increase the vulnerability to error and adverse outcomes.

A system's results may be summed up as follows: "Whether your output is good or bad, it is, nonetheless, the only output of which your systems, processes, and methods are currently capable."[59] Otherwise stated, every system is perfectly designed for the results it gets.

Lessons from Other High-Risk Domains

A systems approach to safety improvement has led to major advances in a number of other high-risk work environments, such as aviation and other transportation domains. As we start to understand health care as a system and the role of human factors in system performance, we can learn from the advances made in these other fields. Patterson and colleagues identified handoff strategies that were identified in other settings with high consequences for failure (space shuttle mission control, nuclear power, railroad and ambulance dispatchings) that could be applied to improve the safety of handoffs in health care [*see Table 2*].[65]

Significant advances have been made in adopting the technique of crew resource management (CRM) from aviation to health care and surgery. CRM was first used by the aviation industry to improve airline crew coordination, and the IOM report *To Err Is Human: Building a Safer Health System* identified it as a strategy to reduce medical errors and improve patient safety.[2] Since this call for its implementation, the use of CRM has been evaluated in various health care fields, including operating room teams. In one study, teams underwent an 8-hour training course that covered six key areas of CRM: managing fatigue; creating and managing a team; recognizing adverse situations; cross-checking and communication techniques; developing and applying shared mental models for decision making; and giving and receiving performance feedback.[66] Although 95% of respondents agreed that the training would reduce errors in their workplace, cultural barriers still exist within surgery. Whereas only 26% of pilots denied that fatigue has a detrimental effect on performance, 70% of surgeons and 47% of anesthesiologists felt that they can perform effectively even when fatigued.[67] In the same study, only about half of attending surgeons favored a flat hierarchy in which junior members of a team could question decisions made by senior team members, whereas 94% of pilots advocated for this approach. Perhaps more broad adoption of CRM will help bridge this cultural divide.

Table 2 Handoff Coordination and Communication Objectives and Relevant Strategies[65]

Improve handoff update effectiveness
1. Face-to-face verbal update with interactive questioning
2. Additional update from practitioners other than one being replaced
3. Limit interruptions during update
4. Topics initiated by incoming and outgoing team members
5. Limit initiation of operator actions during update
6. Include outgoing team's stance toward changes to plans and contingency plans
7. Readback to ensure that information was correctly received
Improve handoff update efficiency and effectiveness
8. Outgoing writes summary before handoff
9. Incoming assesses current status
10. Update information in the same order every time
11. Incoming scans historical data before update
12. Incoming reviews automatically captured changes to sensor-derived data before update
13. Intermittent monitoring of system status while "on call"
14. Outgoing has knowledge of previous shift activities
Increase access to data
15. Incoming receives primary access to the most up-to-date information
16. Incoming receives paperwork that includes handwritten annotations
Improve coordination with others
17. Unambiguous transfer of responsibility
18. Make it clear to others at a glance which personnel are responsible for which duties at a particular time
Enable error detection and recovery
19. Overhear others' updates
20. Outgoing oversees incoming's work following update
Delay transfer of responsibility during critical activities
21. Delay the transfer of responsibility when concerned about status/stability

Approaches to Improving Patient Safety

Given the similarities between medical and nonmedical systems, it should not be surprising that many safety improvement techniques derived from nonmedical settings have been successfully applied in medical contexts [*see Table 3*].[68,69] Other useful strategies include prioritization of tasks, distribution of the workload over time or resources, changing the nature of the task, monitoring and checking all available data, effective leadership, open communication, mobilization and use of all available resources, and team building.[1] The

Table 3 Nonmedical System Techniques Also Applicable to Medical Systems

Simplify or reduce handoffs
Reduce reliance on memory
Standardize procedures
Improve information access
Use constraining or forcing functions
Design for errors
Adjust work schedules
Adjust the environment
Improve communication and teamwork
Decrease reliance on vigilance
Provide adequate safety training
Choose the right staff for the job

general idea behind many of these approaches is to redesign the problem space to reduce the cognitive workload.[28,70]

A vital early step in improving patient safety is to establish a safety culture throughout the workplace. An important development in this area is the ability to make valid measurements of an organization's safety climate.[71] An appropriate organizational culture views errors as signals for needed changes and focuses on learning rather than on accountability. If the team or organization is designed to learn from and benefit from experience, its collective wisdom should be greater than the sum of the wisdom of its individual members. Needed changes often involve difficult choices among strategic factors and sometimes introduce new latent flaws.[37,72] Accordingly, once a change in procedure or policy has been implemented, its impact must be monitored closely.[73] New latent failures may result from either oversimplification[31] or redundancy. As noted (see above), the latter enhances reliability, but its benefits are often offset by greater complexity and a consequent increase in the risk of human failure.[30] In addition, the more complex the system, the greater the chance that a change will have more than local effects. How to control some errors without relaxing control over others is a general problem in error management.[30,74]

Good teamwork requires that team members share a clear understanding of what is happening and what should happen (i.e., situational awareness).[30] Unfortunately, there is a common tendency to believe that the prevailing level of situational awareness is greater than it actually is. For example, the aviation industry further improved its safety record when it identified and removed barriers that impeded junior officers from communicating with the captain. This achievement is noteworthy because these improvements took place after good communication was already thought to exist.[75]

Even though physicians have increasing access to information technology in practice (www.hschange.org/CONTENT/891), physician acceptance of computerization has been neither easy nor universal, and medicine is far behind other industries in terms of the extent to which it has adopted such technology. Studies from the past few years suggest that only about one third of physicians receive any data (process data, outcome data, or patient surveys) about the quality of care they provide.[76] This finding may be partly explained by the cost of introducing information technology (which can become outmoded relatively quickly).

Another possible factor here is concern that caregivers might become too dependent on computerized advice-giving systems and thus might start making a habit of perfunctorily acceding to the computer's advice rather than trusting their own judgment. Issues of legal liability then arise: how much computer advice is too much, and is relying on such advice tantamount to abandoning responsibility for critical independent thought? A related concern is that many patient care tasks may be too complex for computerization and thus may be better suited to human performance. The tradeoff for retaining the human ability to deal with such complexity is the human susceptibility to error: systems that rely on error-free human performance are destined to experience failures. Because the kinds of transitory mental states that cause errors are both unintended and largely unpredictable, they are the last and least manageable links in the error chain.

A further approach to improving patient safety has been the development of specific tools and indicators for identifying common safety problems. Examples of these are the Patient Safety Indicators from the Agency for Healthcare Research and Quality (AHRQ) (www.ncbi.nlm.nih..gov/bookshelf/br.fcgi?book=techrev5) [*see Table 4*] and the serious reportable event list from the National Quality Forum (NQF) (www.qualityforum.org/Projects/s-z/SRE_Maintenance_2006/Fact_Sheet_-_Serious_Reportable_Events_in_Healthcare_2005-2006_Update.aspx) [*see Table 5*]. The lists are similar in some respects but not identical: the NQF further subcategorizes events into surgical events, product or device events, patient protection events, care management events, environmental events, and criminal events. Both lists specify clearly identifiable and readily measurable events, both include a variety of causes in addition to medical errors that lead to such adverse events, and both were developed by panels of experts. Yet a recent study indicated that, relative to risk managers, physicians were less aware of error-reporting systems in their hospitals or the adequacy of such mechanisms.[77]

Techniques for Identifying System Flaws

Intensive examination of system flaws is most often triggered by a catastrophic failure or, less often, by a near miss. The appropriate investigation of such events is known as root cause analysis (RCA). The Joint Commission (formerly the JCAHO) (www.jointcommissioninternational.org/Books-and-E-books/Root-Cause-Analysis-in-Health-Care-Tools-and-Techniques-Fourth-Edition/1502) has a matrix for RCA, and experience with RCA in health care institutions has been reported.[78,79]

In the case of an actual failure, the next steps are to identify all the relevant subsystems and to assemble a team whose members represent all of the components. Determining all of the components within a complex system can be challenging, and it may prove necessary to add members to the team as more subsystems are identified. In this regard, it is better to err on the side of inclusiveness rather than exclusivity to minimize the chances of missing latent flaws and maximize the number of possible solutions. Studies that relate nurse staffing to quality of care illustrate the important roles that

Table 4 **Agency for Healthcare Quality and Research Patient Safety Indicators**
Complications of anesthesia
Death in low-mortality diagnosis-related group
Decubitus ulcer
Failure to rescue
Foreign body left during procedure
Iatrogenic pneumothorax
Selected infections
Postoperative hip fracture
Postoperative hemorrhage or hematoma
Postoperative pulmonary embolism or deep vein thrombosis
Postoperative sepsis
Postoperative wound dehiscence
Accidental puncture or laceration
Transfusion reaction
Obstetric trauma

Table 5 National Quality Forum List of Health Care Facility–Related Serious Reportable Events

Category	Event
Surgical	A. Surgery performed on the wrong body part B. Surgery performed on the wrong patient C. Wrong surgical procedure on a patient D. Unintended retention of a foreign object in a patient after surgery or other procedure E. Intraoperative or postoperative death in an ASA class I patient
Product or device	A. Patient death or serious disability associated with use of contaminated drugs, devices, or biologics B. Patient death or serious disability associated with use or function of a device in patient care, in which the device is used or functions otherwise than intended C. Patient death or serious disability associated with intravascular air embolism
Patient protection	A. Infant discharged to the wrong person B. Patient death or serious disability associated with patient elopement (disappearance) C. Patient suicide or attempted suicide resulting in serious disability
Care management	A. Patient death or serious disability associated with a medication error B. Patient death or serious disability associated with a transfusion reaction C. Maternal death or serious disability associated with labor and delivery in a low-risk pregnancy D. Patient death or serious disability associated with hypoglycemia E. Death or serious disability associated with failure to identify or treat neonatal hyperbilirubinemia F. Stage 3 or 4 pressure ulcer acquired after admission G. Patient death or serious disability associated with spinal manipulative therapy H. Artificial insemination with wrong donor sperm or wrong egg
Environmental	A. Patient death or serious disability associated with electrical shock B. Any incident in which a line designated for oxygen or other gas to be delivered to a patient contains the wrong gas or is contaminated by toxic substances C. Patient death or serious disability associated with a burn incurred from any source D. Patient death or serious disability associated with a fall E. Patient death or serious disability associated with the use of restraints or bedrails
Criminal	A. Any care ordered by someone impersonating a physician or other licensed health care provider B. Abduction of a patient of any age C. Sexual assault of a patient D. Death or significant injury of a patient or staff member from a physical assault

ASA = American Society of Anesthesiologists.

other members of the health care team play in ensuring patient safety.[80–82] In some situations, it may be difficult to generate interest in RCA because the circumstances are so unusual that they are unlikely ever to combine in the same way again.

Systems analyses in the presence of a near miss, or in the absence of any specific event, require a more global approach to help avoid future errors. Areas where such analyses might be fruitful include those identified by AHRQ [*see Table 4*], the NQF [*see Table 5*], and the Joint Commission. Another source for specific topics is AHRQ WebM&M (www.webmm.ahrq.gov), an AHRQ-developed Web site that provides expert analysis of medical errors in five specialty areas (including surgery), as well as interactive learning modules. AHRQ has also created extensive lists of other quality measures (www.qualitymeasures.ahrq.gov) and tools for improving patient safety. The next steps in this situation are to decide on measures for analysis and to identify appropriate data sources. Medical record audits yield far greater detail than claims data but are expensive, labor intensive, and time-consuming. Moreover, information on the environment or behavior in medical records may be irrelevant or even contradictory. This problem can sometimes be mitigated by employing appropriate screening criteria.[83] Some of the shortcomings of medical record audits can be avoided by using administrative data, but such data often lack sufficient accuracy or depth. Electronic health records can potentially simplify this process and possess a number of other advantages.[84,85] RCA can be automated,[86] but the potential advantages of doing so may be offset by a dependence on the developer's interpretation of the risk reduction process or by the factors identified as the principal event.

Regardless of the data source, the process is likely to be evolutionary: rarely is a perfect set of measures available from the start. Although the findings from such an analysis might seem to offer little benefit to the institution in which they occurred, such incidents may occur frequently enough at a regional or national level to make the analysis worthwhile.

Other analyses associated with successful quality improvement efforts include patient notification systems,[87] patient safety systems,[88] analyses of system failures in laparoscopic surgery,[89] and analyses of medical microsystems.[72] Critical analyses of evidence-based practices also identified 11 surgically relevant quality improvement practices for which the data were strong enough to support more widespread implementation [*see Table 6*].[90,91] A note of caution that should be sounded here is that exclusive emphasis on evidence-based data could skew safety priorities and might actually prevent relatively few adverse events.[92] Another potential area for review involves changes in policy or equipment that might introduce unanticipated problems or unexplained variations in a relevant outcome measure. Every change in a system necessitates a new learning cycle, and the new environment may be conducive to failures from new latent errors.[93]

Table 6 **Surgically Relevant Quality Improvement Practices Appropriate for Widespread Implementation**[90]
Appropriate use of prophylaxis to prevent venous thromboembolism in patients at risk
Use of perioperative beta blockers in appropriate patients to prevent perioperative morbidity and mortality
Use of maximum sterile barriers while placing central venous catheters to prevent infection
Appropriate use of antibiotic prophylaxis to prevent postoperative infections
Requesting that patients recall and state what they have been told during the informed consent process
Continuous aspiration of subglottic secretions to prevent ventilator-associated pneumonia
Use of pressure-relieving bedding materials to prevent pressure ulcers
Use of real-time ultrasound guidance during central line placement to prevent complications
Patient self-management for warfarin to achieve appropriate outpatient anticoagulation and prevent complications
Appropriate provision of nutrition, with particular emphasis on early enteral nutrition in critically ill and surgical patients
Use of antibiotic-impregnated central venous catheters to prevent catheter-related infections

Successes and Obstacles to Success

In view of the complexities of health care, taking a systems approach to safety improvement may seem a daunting endeavor. Nevertheless, there are a number of cases in which this task has been successfully accomplished. For the purposes of illustration, it is worthwhile to review these examples briefly.

Anesthesiologists were among the first physicians to take a systems approach to patient safety, and their success is irrefutable: anesthesia-related mortality fell from approximately two in 10,000 to the current one in 200,000 to one in 300,000[94–96]—a degree of safety approaching that advocated for nonmedical industries (i.e., < 3.4 defects or errors/10^6 products or events).[97] This improvement primarily resulted from a broad effort involving teamwork, practice guidelines, automation, simplification of procedures, and standardization of equipment and many functions. For instance, before the anesthesiologists' safety initiatives, design standards for anesthesia machines did not exist. As a result, it was not unusual to have one machine in which turning a valve in a given direction would increase gas flow and other machines in which turning it in the same direction would decrease flow; in fact, both types might be present in the same hospital. Equipment manufacturers subsequently worked together to standardize anesthesia equipment, and these kinds of arbitrary design variations are no longer seen.

The experience with safety efforts in anesthesiology underscores the importance of understanding the human-technology interface and the ergonomics of equipment design.[98] To improve patient safety, it is necessary to understand the devices and techniques employed, the ways in which individual persons use the technology, and the means by which these users interact with other aspects of the system.[98,99] Similar considerations should be applied to innovative practices.[100]

Another example is the recent high-profile application of procedural checklists. These checklists serve as the cornerstone of system-based interventions aimed at improving safety. A Michigan-wide collaborative targeting best practices around central line placement markedly reduced the morbidity and mortality associated with central lines in an intensive care setting.[101] A surgical safety checklist implemented in eight international hospitals similarly was associated with a decrease in death and complications from nonpediatric surgical procedures.[102] A number of different mechanisms may underlie the association between the checklists and improved outcomes, including better communication, less reliance on individual knowledge and memory, and increases in situational awareness and a shared mental model; however, whatever the mechanism, the use of checklists, adopted from aviation, changes the system in which care is delivered and the behavior and interactions of the team and individual practitioners.

Another emerging success is the use of technological adjuncts in the tracking of surgical sponges. The traditional approach to preventing retained objects following surgery depends on several members of the surgical team manually counting every item that is introduced onto the sterile field and again at the end of the operation. These protocols have been shown to be labor intensive as well as unreliable.[103] Seventy to 88% of cases of retained surgical equipment are associated with a correct count.[9] The recognition that manual counts will not be sufficient to completely ameliorate retained objects after surgery, making it a true "never event," has led to the development of several technological solutions. Radiofrequency identification tags and bar codes are two examples of such solutions. A randomized, controlled trial suggests that bar-coding sponges can improve the ability to track sponges during an operation.[104]

These examples of success are encouraging, but considerable obstacles to improving patient safety still exist. Specific obstacles include (1) a residual lack of awareness that a problem exists; (2) a traditional medical culture based on individual responsibility and blame (and shame); (3) a perceived vulnerability to legal discovery and liability; (4) primitive medical information systems; (5) the time and expense involved in defining and implementing evidence-based practice; (6) inadequate resources for quality improvement and error prevention; (7) the local nature of health care; and (8) the perception of a poor return on investment (i.e., the lack of a business case).[105] Although the need to redefine health care on the basis of value seems obvious, the current environment still appears to focus primarily on cost; value (i.e., quality per unit cost) is not part of the equation.[106]

One hindrance to improving patient safety is the idea that traditional improvement methods are adequate to address the problem. The persistence of patient safety problems in the face of the ongoing use of these methods should be a sufficient argument for the inadequacy of existing approaches. For instance, morbidity and mortality (M & M) conferences are perhaps the most traditional venue for discussion of adverse events, but they often do not consider all complications, are not consistently well attended, do not categorize complications systematically, and often do not involve extensive debriefing.[37,107–109] One study that compared NSQIP with traditional M & M conferences noted that the latter failed to consider about 50% of the deaths and about 75% of the complications.[110] Furthermore, M & M conferences tend to be intradepartmental and thus provide little opportunity for discussion of system problems that involve other departments (e.g., anesthesiology or nursing). M & M conferences also typically do not consider near misses (i.e., close calls), even though such events can identify important actual and potential system flaws. Finally, M & M conferences have a tradition of focusing on the actions of individuals rather than on the circumstances within which the individuals acted. This tradition serves to perpetuate a defensive attitude among trainees that is counterproductive. It is possible, however, that a more systematized review process could improve the value of the M & M conference.[111,112]

Joint Commission accreditation of hospitals is based on analyses of safety and quality information (www.jointcommissionreport.org). However, it has been observed that the Joint Commission's accreditation program lacks the ability to identify many patient safety problems.[113]

Peer review organizations were originally intended as a mechanism for professional self-evaluation but subsequently became subject to anticompetitive abuse and other undesired consequences.[114] The potential for inequity was a particular concern in that physicians who relinquished privileges on their own initiative might be treated more leniently than those against whom action was initiated by a peer review committee. Moreover, the data reviewed by peer review organizations were often legally discoverable, and this lack of anonymity and confidentiality tended to deter voluntary participation. Even when peer review organizations identified problems, they were often unable to implement solutions. Peer review organizations have now been largely supplanted by quality improvement organizations, although it is not yet clear whether the latter are substantially more effective.[115,116]

Hospital incident reports have much the same shortcomings as the peer review process. They place limited emphasis on close calls and tend to lack systematic follow-up. Individuals also may be reluctant to file reports out of fear that their employment might be jeopardized or that the reported party might seek retribution.

The present professional liability system is particularly controversial with respect to whether it facilitates or hinders improvements in patient safety. This system has its basis in the traditional paradigm of surgical care (see below), which holds the individual surgeon accountable as the "captain of the ship." This paradigm has enabled many great achievements in surgical care, but it has also probably fostered a dangerous sense of infallibility. As a consequence, errors tend to be equated with negligence, and questions of professional liability tend to involve blaming individuals. Indeed, the very willingness of professionals to accept responsibility for their actions makes it convenient to focus more on individual errors than on collective ones[22]; an individual surgeon is a more satisfactory target for the anger and grief of a patient or family than a faceless organization would be. This is certainly not to say that surgeons should avoid responsibility; rather, the point is that focusing on the errors of individual surgeons without addressing flaws in the underlying system does little to improve health care.

Another notable flaw in the liability process is that judgments of causality or fault are vulnerable to hindsight bias, which can skew experts' assessments of quality of care. This tendency was illustrated by a study of anesthetic care in which differences in outcome significantly influenced the perception of negligence, even when the care provided was equivalent.[117] Hindsight bias focuses too narrowly on adverse outcomes and pays insufficient attention to the processes of care. Yet another defect of the liability process is that it can be emotionally devastating for physicians (and their families),[118-120] often adversely affecting their problem-solving abilities. To the extent that experience with or fear of a liability action deters efforts at quality improvement, it is counterproductive. Defensive medicine, with its attendant costs, adds very little value to health care.[121]

Many believe that major reform of the professional liability system is a prerequisite for achieving any significant improvements in quality. Undoubtedly, tort reform is highly desirable; however, the real prerequisite for improving identification and correction of system failures is the provision of increased protection for privileged discussion of such failures. The federal Patient Safety and Quality Improvement Act of 2005 (Public Law 109-41) was enacted for the purpose of improving patient safety by encouraging voluntary and confidential reporting of events that adversely affect patients. This act creates patient safety organizations whose goal is to collect, aggregate, and analyze confidential information reported by health care providers. It also calls for establishing a network of patient safety databases as an interactive, evidence-based management resource. The act limits the use of this information in criminal, civil, and administrative proceedings and includes provisions imposing monetary penalties for violations of confidentiality or privilege protections. The notion that a reduction in liability concerns may facilitate disclosure and discussion of mistakes is suggested by international comparisons of health care systems. In one study, patients in New Zealand, which has no-fault medical malpractice, were the most likely to report error discussions with their physicians.[13]

It is to be hoped that the tort reform movement and the patient safety movement can seek and find common ground.[122] The improvements in patient safety achieved by anesthesiologists speak for the benefits of such an approach. Instead of pushing for laws to protect them against patients' lawsuits, anesthesiologists focused on improving patient safety. As a result, they pay less for malpractice insurance today, in constant dollars, than they did more than 20 years ago.[123]

Even before the enactment of the Patient Safety Act, the view that open discussion of medical errors was appropriate appeared to be gaining adherents.[21] Today, there is even more evidence that such open communication may reduce the likelihood of legal action and enhance public confidence in health care providers.[124,125] Unfortunately, some hospitals persist in separating risk management from quality assurance issues, to the detriment of both.[126]

The obvious need for liability reform notwithstanding, there are issues involved in enhancing safety and quality that are too complex to be addressed solely by changes in the liability system. Major safety and quality problems exist in nations where professional liability is not an issue; however, the higher rates of adverse events in these countries should not be taken as evidence of the benefits of the current US liability system. Physicians tend to act defensively even in a no-fault liability system. To minimize such defensiveness, greater emphasis must be placed on measurement for improvement than on measurement for judgment.[127]

Changing the Traditional Surgical Paradigm

Contemporary surgical practice requires that surgeons rethink the traditional paradigm of surgical practice (see above). The burgeoning growth of knowledge, the accompanying increase in specialization, the expanding role of technology, and the rising complexity of practice are making surgeons more and more dependent on persons or factors beyond their immediate control. As a result, surgeons are finding it more and more difficult even to appreciate, let alone manage, the larger context within which they provide care. The traditional surgical paradigm, despite its past successes, is no longer entirely adequate to the task now at hand [*see Table 7*].[128] Paradoxically, surgeons seeking to improve patient safety must acquire a deeper understanding of patient care systems at the very time when those systems are becoming increasingly difficult to understand.

To achieve the requisite understanding, it is necessary to have a reporting system that collects, tabulates, and analyzes data on the frequency and nature of both adverse events and near misses.[129] The primary function of a patient safety reporting system should be to identify both real and potential adverse consequences of latent flaws and make them visible to others. Once these real and potential adverse events are identified and made visible, the system can be redesigned so as to eliminate or minimize them.

A successful reporting system such as the highly successful Aviation Safety Reporting System (ASRS) is typically nonpunitive, confidential (and preferably anonymous), independent, timely, systems oriented, and responsive.[22,88,130] In addition, it includes expert analysis, meaning that reports are evaluated by persons who understand the relevant circumstances and are trained to recognize underlying system-based causes. A successful reporting system usually also tabulates seemingly rare incidents (including near misses) even if there seems to be little direct or immediate benefit to doing so; in addition to their potential value in larger contexts, such analyses may help institutions predict and thereby avoid errors and system failures. The absence of a punitive focus reduces health care workers' concerns that reports might be used against them and thus minimizes underreporting.[36,131,132] The concerns about the possible adverse consequences of a reporting system are quite strong—so much so that many believe that a health care reporting system can succeed only if legal immunity is available.[133] The fear of being sued is widespread among physicians; however, the perceived risk of being sued is three times greater than the actual risk, and there is no good correlation between hospitals' claims ratings and their injury rates.[72]

A mandatory, anonymous, confidential, and nondiscoverable reporting system has been instituted in the state of Pennsylvania. Founded in 2003, the Pennsylvania Patient Safety Reporting System, a statewide database maintained by the Pennsylvania Patient Safety Authority, collects over 200,000 annual reports of near miss and adverse events. (http://patientsafetyauthority.org). The events are evaluated, summarized, and analyzed to identify patterns that can be used to develop patient safety solutions and interventions.

Whether such reporting should be voluntary or mandatory is still a matter of debate. On the one hand, voluntary reporting has a high inaccuracy rate even when mandated by state or federal regulations. On the other hand, many surgeons believe that mandatory reporting may increase the pressure to conceal errors rather than analyze them; that it is unworkable in the current legal system; and that it may result not in constructive error-reducing solutions but merely in more punishment or censure.[134]

Some argue that patient safety efforts should focus (at least initially) on medical injury rather than on medical errors.[135,136] A focus on medical injury recognizes the difficulties of identifying medical errors and is based on a public health improvement model that has been useful in addressing other types of injuries; it also recognizes that most medical injuries are not caused by negligence. Such an approach may be more compatible with the current liability system and may help restore physicians' stature as patient advocates. Moreover, placing the initial focus on medical errors rather than injuries might divert attention from other system flaws, with the result that such flaws go uncorrected. Although, ultimately, a successful reporting system must focus both on errors and on injuries, an initial focus on injury may achieve greater initial buy-in from surgeons and may therefore be a more pragmatic first step. The issues associated with reporting errors or injuries must also be distinguished from those associated with reporting outcomes to the public. The latter type of report is currently being seen with increasing frequency, but it may have unintended consequences.[137]

The complexities involved in understanding and improving health care systems make it likely that patients' expectations of improved safety may grow faster than they can be met.[138,139] This potential disparity between expectations and performance may be further exacerbated by the likelihood that errors have been substantially underreported.[140] A reporting system that is punitive or not anonymous may discourage appropriate reporting of medical errors. Underreporting of adverse events is also more likely if side effects are delayed or unpredictable, if there is a longer survival or latency interval, or if a patient has been transferred from one facility to another. In addition, inadequate doses of drugs or anesthetics may not be reported if they cause no immediately evident injury.

Another challenge facing surgeons is how to incorporate current concepts of performance and error into undergraduate and residency education.[141] The optimal basis for such education might be an objective-based curriculum that

Table 7 Contrasting Characteristics of Medical Practice in the 20th and 21st Centuries[129]

20th century characteristics
Autonomy
Solo practice
Continuous learning
Infallibility
Knowledge
21st century characteristics
Teamwork/systems
Group practice
Continuous improvement
Multidisciplinary problem solving
Change

provides defined skills, rules, and knowledge.[142,143] The blame-and-shame approach must be eliminated from both the educational setting and the practice atmosphere. If, instead, educators focus on making residents aware of their tendencies in the presence of uncertainty, residents (like pilots) may be able to develop better responses to underspecified situations. In addition, it is vital to monitor the residents to ensure that they learn to assess and address knowledge deficits, as well as acquire healthy and effective techniques for dealing with errors. Such monitoring will make the learning curve less painful for all concerned.[144]

There is some question as to whether safety improvements are more likely to result from compliance with standards (i.e., individual performance) or from improvements in the system. Better training of individual physicians will certainly improve performance, but only so far. For substantial improvements in safety, it is probably necessary to make use of both approaches.[145] If every system is perfectly designed to achieve the results it gets, the obvious conclusion is that to obtain the desired results, it is necessary to change the system. Determining what form the new system should take is a critical step.[106,146]

Conclusions

Reducing adverse events during the course of medical care is a dauntingly complex topic, and the progress made in reducing such errors has, in many cases, been disappointingly slow. Roughly a century ago, surgeons were called on to report their results, but over the intervening years, this call largely went unheeded.[147] It must be said, however, that at the beginning of the 20th century, the basic principles of human performance and error were not as well understood as they currently are, and the tools necessary for systems analysis did not exist. A further difference between then and now is the increase in public awareness of safety issues, as well as the potential consequences of this awareness.[13,148] For instance, the growing concern about safety is changing the way in which patients select providers: there has been a substantial increase in the percentage of patients who would choose a highly rated surgeon whom they had not seen before over a less highly rated surgeon whom they had seen before (www.ahrq.gov/qual/kffhigh00.htm). Improving patient safety thus becomes a matter of self-interest for the provider. It also may have a direct bearing on the maintenance of physicians' social contract with their patients.

The systems approach to improving patient safety is based on three principles: (1) human error, as an inherent aspect of human work, is unavoidable; (2) faulty systems allow human error to injure patients; and (3) systems can be designed that prevent or detect human error before such injuries occur.[149,150] Support for a systems approach to patient safety will come from patients, purchasers from both the public and the private sector, professional societies, and specialty boards.[151] It is crucial for all of these parties to acknowledge that most medical errors are attributable to system flaws rather than incompetence or neglect. It is also essential to recognize that the current systems of surgical care are shaped by the larger system within which all of these parties interact. This means that any worthwhile effort to improve such systems is likely to require substantial collaboration among the parties involved,[152] as well as significant change in the larger system.

Medical errors have a substantial impact on 90-day costs and outcomes of surgical patients.[153] Moreover, there appears to be a business case for investing in patient safety.[154] Physicians, with their history of patient advocacy and scientific innovation, are in the best position to provide the leadership necessary for such changes.[87,155] To restore the public's trust in the health care system, safety and quality must be made high priorities,[156] and transparency must be ensured.[157] If physicians do not take the opportunity to lead the movement to improve the safety and quality of care, they may anticipate further erosion of public trust and further loss of professional autonomy.

Financial Disclosures: None Reported

References

1. Gaba DM. Human error in dynamic medical domains. In: Bogner MS, editor. Human error in medicine. Hillsdale (NJ): Lawrence Erlbaum Associates; 1994. p. 197–224.
2. Kohn LT, Corrigan JM, Donaldson MS, editors. To err is human: building a safer health system. Washington (DC): Institute of Medicine, National Academy Press; 2000.
3. Gawande AA, Thomas EJ, Zinner MJ, et al. The incidence and nature of surgical adverse events in Colorado and Utah in 1992. Surgery 1999;126:66–75.
4. Khuri S. Safety, quality, and the National Surgical Quality Improvement Program. Am Surg 2006;72:994–8.
5. Doing what counts for patient safety: federal actions to reduce medical errors and their impact. Report of the Quality Interagency Task Force (QuIC) to the President, February 2000. Available at: http://www.quic.gov/report/errors6.pdf. (accessed Oct 26, 2010).
6. Espin S, Levinson W, Regehr G, et al. Error or "act of God"? A study of patients and operating room team members' perceptions of error definition, reporting, and disclosure. Surgery 2006;139:6–14.
7. Brennan TA, Leape LL, Laird NM, et al. Incidence of adverse events and negligence in hospitalized patients, results of the Harvard Medical Practice Study I. N Engl J Med 1991;324:370–6.
8. Mills DH, editor. Report of the California Medical Insurance Feasibility Study. San Francisco: California Medical Association; 1977.
9. Gawande A, Studdert DM, Orav EJ, et al. Risk factors for retained instruments and sponges after surgery. N Engl J Med 2003; 348:229–35.
10. Seiden SC, Barach P. Wrong-side/wrong-site, wrong procedure and wrong-patient adverse events: are they preventable? Arch Surg 2006;141:931–9.
11. Bates DW, Cullen DJ, Laird N, et al. Incidence of adverse drug events and potential adverse drug events. Implications for prevention. ADE Prevention Study Group. JAMA 1995;274:29–34.
12. Serig DI. Radiopharmaceutical misadministrations: what's wrong? In: Bogner MS, editor. Human error in medicine. Hillsdale (NJ): Lawrence Erlbaum Associates; 1994. p. 179–96.
13. Schoen C, Davis K, How SKH, Schoenbaum SC. US health system performance: a national scorecard. Health Aff (Millwood) 2006;25 Suppl:w457–75.
14. Feigal DW, Gardner SN, McLellan M. Ensuring safe and effective medical devices. N Engl J Med 2003;348:191–2.
15. Blendon RJ, DesRoches CM, Brodie M, et al. Views of practicing physicians and the public on medical errors. N Engl J Med 2002;347:1933–40.
16. Perper JA. Life-threatening and fatal therapeutic misadventures. In: Bogner MS, editor. Human error in medicine. Hillsdale (NJ): Lawrence Erlbaum Associates; 1994. p. 27–52.
17. Leape L. The preventability of medical injury. In: Bogner MS, editor. Human error in medicine. Hillsdale (NJ): Lawrence Erlbaum Associates; 1994. p. 13–26.
18. Longo DR, Hewett JE, Ge B, et al. The long road to patient safety—a status report. JAMA 2005;294:2858–65.

19. Leape LL, Berwick DM. Five years after To Err Is Human—what have we learned? JAMA 2005;293:2384–90.
20. Wachter RM. Patient safety at ten: unmistakable progress, troubling gaps. Health Aff (Millwood) 2010;29:1–9.
21. Reason JT. Human error. Cambridge (UK): Cambridge University Press; 1990.
22. Reason JT. Foreword. In: Bogner MS, editor. Human error in medicine. Hillsdale (NJ): Lawrence Erlbaum Associates; 1994. p. vii–xv.
23. Cook RI, Woods DD. Operating at the sharp end. In: Bogner MS, editor. Human error in medicine. Hillsdale (NJ): Lawrence Erlbaum Associates; 1994. p. 255–310.
24. Rasmussen J. Afterword. In: Bogner MS, editor. Human error in medicine. Hillsdale (NJ): Lawrence Erlbaum Associates; 1994. p. 385–94.
25. Ewell MG, Adams RJ. Aviation psychology, group dynamics, and human performance issues in anesthesiology. In: Proceedings of the Seventh International Symposium on Aviation Psychology, Columbus, Ohio, 1993. Ohio State University Department of Aviation. p. 499–504.
26. Howard SK, Gaba DN, Fish KJ, et al. Anesthesia crisis resource management: teaching anesthesiologists to handle critical incidents. Aviat Space Environ Med 1992; 63:763–70.
27. Ternov S. The human side of medical mistakes. In: Spath PL, editor. Error reduction in health care: a systems approach to improving patient safety. San Francisco: Jossey-Bass; [illegible]
28. Rasmussen J. Skills, rules, knowledge: signals, signs and symbols and other distinctions in human performance models. IEEE Trans Syst Man Cybern 1983;257.
29. Bann S, Mansoor K, Datta V, Darzi A. Surgical skill is predicted by the ability to detect errors. Am J Surg 2005;19:412–5.
30. Moray N. Error reduction as a systems problem. In: Bogner MS, editor. Human error in medicine. Hillsdale (NJ): Lawrence Erlbaum Associates; 1994. p. 67–92.
31. Leape LL. Error in medicine. JAMA 1994; 272:1851–7.
32. Cook RI. Seeing is believing. Ann Surg 2003;237:472–3.
33. LeBlanc VR, Brooks LR, Norman GR. Believing is seeing: the influence of a diagnostic hypothesis on the interpretation of clinical features. Acad Med 2002;10 Suppl: S67–9.
34. Croskerry P. The importance of cognitive errors in diagnosis and strategies to minimize them. Acad Med 2003;78:775–80.
35. Redelmeir DA. The cognitive psychology of missed diagnoses. Ann Intern Med 2005; 142:115–20.
36. Senders JW. Medical devices, medical errors, and medical accidents. In: Bogner MS, editor. Human error in medicine. Hillsdale (NJ): Lawrence Erlbaum Associates; 1994. p. 159–78.
37. Gawande A, Zinner MJ, Studdert DM, et al. Analysis of errors reported by surgeons at three teaching hospitals. Surgery 2003;133: 614–21.
38. Rogers SO, Gawande AA, Kwaan M, et al. Analysis of surgical errors in closed malpractice claims at 4 liability insurers. Surgery 2006;140:25–33.
39. Regenbogen, SE, Greenberg CC, Studdert DM, et al. Patterns of technical error among surgical malpractice claims: an analysis of strategies to prevent injury to surgical patients. Ann Surg 2007;246:705–11.
40. Lillemoe KD. To err is human, but should we expect more from a surgeon? Ann Surg 2003;237:470–1.
41. Gaba DM. Human error in dynamic medical domains. In: Bogner MS, editor. Human error in medicine. Hillsdale (NJ): Lawrence Erlbaum Associates; 1994. p. 197–224.
42. Barger LK, Ayas NT, Cade BE, et al. Impact of extended-duration shifts on medical errors, adverse events, and attentional failures. PLoS Med 2006;3:2440–8.
43. Landrigan CP, Rothschild JM, Cronin JW, et al. Effect of reducing interns' work hours on serious medical errors in intensive care units. N Engl J Med 2004;351:1838–48.
44. Lockley SW, Cronin JW, Evans EE, et al. Effect of reducing interns' weekly work hours on sleep and attentional failures. N Engl J Med 2004;351:1829–37.
45. Gaba DM, Howard SK. Fatigue among clinicians and the safety of patients. N Engl J Med 2002;347:1249–55.
46. Cao CG, Weinger B, Slagle J, et al. Differences in night and day shift clinical performance in anesthesiology. Hum Factors 2008;50:276–90.
47. Helmreich RL, Schaefer H-G. Team performance in the operating room. In: Bogner MS, editor. Human error in medicine. Hillsdale (NJ): Lawrence Erlbaum Associates; 1994. p. 225–54.
48. Shanafelt TD, Balch CM, Bechamps G, et al. Burnout and medical errors among American surgeons. Ann Surg 2010;251: 995–1000.
49. Davis DA, Mazmanian PE, Fordis M, et al. Accuracy of physician self-assessment compared with observed measures of competence: a systematic review. JAMA [illegible]
50. Christian CK, Gustafson ML, Roth EM, et al. A prospective study of patient safety in the operating room. Surgery 2006;139:159–73.
51. Gabow PA, Karkhanis A, Knight A, et al. Observations of residents' work activities for 24 consecutive hours: implications for workflow resign. Acad Med 2006;81: 766–75.
52. Poulose BK, Ray WA, Arbogast PG, et al. Resident work hour limits and patient safety. Ann Surg 2005;241:847–60.
53. Naylor RA, Rege RV, Valentine RJ. Do resident duty hour restrictions reduce technical complications of emergency laparoscopic cholecystectomy? J Am Coll Surg 2005;201:724–31.
54. Vaughan D. The Challenger launch decision: risky technology, culture, and deviance at NASA. Chicago: University of Chicago Press; 1996.
55. Heimreich RL. Cockpit management attitudes. Hum Factors 1984;26:583–9.
56. Greenberg CC, Regenbogen SE, Studdert DM, et al. Patterns of communication breakdowns resulting in injury to surgical patients. J Am Coll Surg 2007;204:533–40.
57. Lingard L, Espin S, Whyte S, et al. Communication failures in the operating room: an observational classification of recurrent types and effects. Qual Saf Health Care 2004;13:330–4.
58. Daley J, Forbes MG, Young GJ, et al. Validating risk-adjusted surgical outcomes: site visit assessment of process and structure. National VA Surgical Risk Study. J Am Coll Surg 1997;185:341–51.
59. Scholtes PR. The leader's handbook: making things happen, getting things done. New York: McGraw-Hill; 1998.
60. Westley F, Zimmerman B, Patton QP. Getting to maybe: how the world is changed. Toronto: Random House; 2006.
61. Van Cott H. Human errors: their causes and reductions. In: MS, editor. Human error in medicine. Hillsdale (NJ): Lawrence Erlbaum Associates; 1994. p. 53–66.
62. Interpreting the volume-outcome relationship in the context of health care quality. Institute of Medicine workshop summary. Washington (DC): National Academy of Sciences; 2000.
63. Interpreting the volume-outcome relationship in the context of cancer care. Institute of Medicine workshop summary. Washington (DC): National Academy of Sciences; 2001.
64. Dudley RA, Johansen KL. Physician responses to purchaser quality initiatives for surgical procedures (invited commentary). Surgery 2001;130:425–8.
65. Patterson ES, Roth EM, Woods DD, et al. Handoff strategies in settings with high consequences for failure: lessons for health car operations. Int J Qual Health Care 2004; 16:125–32.
66. Grogan EL, Stiles RA, France DJ, et al. The impact of aviation-based teamwork training on the attitudes of health-care professionals. J Am Coll Surg 2004;199:843–8.
67. Sexton BJ, Thomas EJ, Helmreich RL. Error, stress, and teamwork in medicine and aviation: cross sectional surveys. BMJ 2000; 320:745–9.
68. Spath PL. Reducing errors through work system improvements. In: Spath PL, editor. Error reduction in health care: a systems approach to improving patient safety. San Francisco: Jossey-Bass; 2000. p. 199–234.
69. Risser DT, Simon R, Rice MM, et al. A structured teamwork to reduce clinical [illegible] Error reduction in health care: a systems approach to improving patient safety. San Francisco: Jossey-Bass; 2000. p. 235–78.
70. DaRosa D, Bell RH Jr, Dunnington GL. Residency program models, implications, and evaluation: results of a think tank consortium on resident work hours. Surgery 2003;133:13–33.
71. Makary M, Sexton JB, Freischlag JA, et al. Patient safety in surgery. Ann Surg 2006; 243:628–35.
72. Donaldson MS, Mohr JJ. Exploring innovation and quality improvement in health care micro-systems: a cross-case analysis. Washington (DC): National Academy of Sciences; 2001.
73. Larson EB. Measuring, monitoring, and reducing medical harm from a systems perspective: a medical director's personal reflections. Acad Med 2002;77:993–1000.
74. Dörner D. The logic of failure: recognizing and avoiding error in complex situations. Cambridge (MA): Perseus Books; 1996.
75. Nance J. Establishing a safety culture. Presented at the Conference on the Role and Responsibility of Physicians to Improve Patient Safety; 2001 Sep; Arlington (VA).
76. Audet AJ, Doty M, Shamasdin J, et al. Measure, learn, and improve: physicians' involvement in quality improvement. Health Aff (Millwood) 2005;24:843–53.
77. Loren DJ, Garbutt J, Claiborne W, et al. Risk managers, physicians, and disclosure of harmful medical errors. J Qual Patient Safety 2010;36:101–8.
78. Spencer FC. Human error in hospitals and industrial accidents: current concepts. J Am Coll Surg 2000;191:410–8.
79. Bagian JP, Gosbee J, Lee CZ, et al. The Veterans Affairs root cause analysis system in action. Jt Comm J Qual Improv 2002; 28:531–45.
80. Needleman J, Buerhaus P, Mattke S, et al. Nurse staffing levels and the quality of

care in hospitals. N Engl J Med 2002;346: 1715–22.
81. Aiken LH, Clarke SP, Sloane DM, et al. Hospital nurse staffing and patient mortality, nurse burnout, and job dissatisfaction. JAMA 2002;288:1987–93.
82. Vincent C. Understanding and responding to adverse events. N Engl J Med 2003;348: 1051–6.
83. Karson AS, Bates DW. Screening for adverse events. J Eval Clin Pract 1999;5: 23–32.
84. Liang L. The gap between evidence and practice. Health Aff (Millwood) 2007;26: w119–21.
85. Platt R. Speed bumps, potholes, and tollbooths on the road to panacea: making best use of data. Health Aff (Millwood) 2007;26: w153–5.
86. Latino RJ. Automating root cause analysis. In: Spath PL, editor. Error reduction in health care: a systems approach to improving patient safety. San Francisco: Jossey-Bass; 2000. p. 155–64.
87. Becher EC, Chassin MR. Taking back health care: the physician's role in quality improvement. Acad Med 2002;77:953.
88. Manuel BM, editor. Patient safety manual. 3rd ed. Chicago: American College of Surgeons; 2001.
89. Hyman WA. Errors in the use of medical equipment. In: Bogner MS, editor. Human error in medicine. Hillsdale (NJ): Lawrence Erlbaum Associates; 1994. p. 327–48.
90. Making health care safer: a critical analysis of patient safety practices. Evidence Report/ Technology Assessment No. 43. Rockville (MD): Agency for Healthcare Research and Quality; 2001. Publ. No.: 01-E058.
91. Shojania KG, Duncan BW, McDonald KM, et al. Safe but sound: patient safety meets evidence-based medicine. JAMA 2002;288: 508–13.
92. Leape LL, Berwick DM, Bates DW. What practices will most improve safety? Evidence-based medicine meets patient safety. JAMA 2002;288:501–7.
93. Feldman SE, Roblin DW. Accident investigation and anticipatory failure analysis in hospitals. In: Spath PL, editor. Error reduction in health care: a systems approach to improving patient safety. San Francisco: Jossey-Bass; 2000. p. 139–54.
94. Eichhorn JH. Prevention of intra-operative anesthesia accidents and related severe injury through safety monitoring. Anesthesiology 1989;70:572–7.
95. Sentinel events: approaches to error reduction and prevention. Jt Comm J Qual Improv 1998;24:175–86.
96. Orkin FW. Patient monitoring in anesthesia as an exercise in technology assessment. In: Saidman LJ, Smith NT, editors. Monitoring in anesthesia. 3rd ed. London: Butterworth-Heinemann; 1993. p. 439–55.
97. Chassin M. Is health care ready for Six Sigma quality? Milbank Q 1998;76: 565–91.
98. Samore MH, Evans RS, Lassen A, et al. Surveillance of medical device-related hazards and adverse events in hospitalized patients. JAMA 2004;291:325–34.
99. Small SD. Medical device-associated safety and risk. Surveillance and stratagems. JAMA 2004;291:367–70.
100. Strasberg SM, Ludbrook PA. Who sees innovative practice? Is there a structure that meets the monitoring needs of new techniques? J Am Coll Surg 2003;196: 938–48.
101. Pronovost P, Needham D, Berenholtz S, et al. An intervention to decrease catheter-related bloodstream infections in the ICU. N Engl J Med 2007;355:2725–32.
102. Haynes AB, Weiser TG, Berry WR, et al. A surgical safety checklist to reduce morbidity and mortality in a global population. N Engl J Med 2009;360:491–9.
103. Greenberg CC, Regenbogen SE, Lipsitz SR, et al. The frequency and significance of discrepancies in the surgical count. Ann Surg 2008;248:337–41.
104. Greenberg CC, Diaz-Flores, R, Lipsitz SR, et al. Bar-coding surgical sponges to improve safety: a randomized, controlled trial. Ann Surg 2008;247:612–6.
105. Galvin RS. The business case for quality. Health Aff (Millwood) 2001;20:57–8.
106. Porter ME, Teisberg EO. Redefining health care. Creating value-based competition on results. Boston: Harvard Business School Press; 2006.
107. Orlander JD, Barber TW, Fincke BG. The morbidity and mortality conference: the delicate nature of learning from error. Acad Med 2002;77:1001–6.
108. Thompson JS, Prior MA. Quality assurance and morbidity and mortality conference. J Surg Res 1992;52:97–100.
109. McGreevy J, Otten T, Poggi M, et al. The challenge of changing roles and improving surgical care now: crew resource management approach. Am Surg 2006;72:1082–7.
110. Hutter MM, Rowell KS, Devaney LA, et al. Identification of complications and deaths: an assessment of the traditional surgical morbidity and mortality conference compared with the American College of Surgeons-National Surgical Quality Improvement Program. J Am Coll Surg 2006;203:618–24.
111. Goldfarb MA, Baker T. An eight-year analysis of surgical morbidity and mortality: data and solutions. Am Surg 2006;72:1070–81.
112. Pine M, Fry DE. Linking processes and outcomes to improve surgical performance. A new approach to morbidity and mortality peer review. Am Surg 2006;72:1115–9.
113. Miller MR, Pronovost P, Donlithan M, et al. Relationship between performance and accreditation: implications for quality of care and patient safety. Am J Med Qual 2005;20:239–52.
114. Livingston EH, Harwell JD. Peer review. Am J Surg 2001;182:103–9.
115. Rollow W, Lied TR, McGann P, et al. Assessment of the Medicare quality improvement organization program. Ann Intern Med 2006;145:342–53.
116. Snyder C, Anderson G. Do quality improvement organizations improve the quality of care for Medicare beneficiaries? JAMA 2005;293:2900–7.
117. Caplan RA, Posner KL, Cheney FW. Effect of outcome on physician judgments of appropriateness of care. JAMA 1991;65: 1957–60.
118. Andrews LB, Stocking C, Krizek T, et al. An alternative strategy for studying adverse events in medical care. Lancet 1997;349: 309–13.
119. Lang NP. Professional liability, patient safety, and first do no harm. Am J Surg 2002;182:537–41.
120. Manuel BM. Double-digit premium hikes: the latest crisis in professional liability. Bull Am Coll Surg 2001;86:19.
121. Studdert DM, Mello MM, Sage WM, et al. Defensive medicine among high-risk specialist physicians in a volatile malpractice environment. JAMA 2005;293:2609–17.
122. Budetti PP. Tort reform and the patient safety movement: seeking common ground. JAMA 2005;293:2660–2.
123. Once seen as risky, one group of doctors changes its ways. Wall Street J 2005 June 21. p. A1.
124. Stewart RM, Corneille MG, Johnston J, et al. Transparent and open discussion of errors does not increase malpractice risk in trauma patients. Ann Surg 2006;243: 645–51.
125. Kesselheim AS, Ferris TG, Studdert DM. Will physician-level measures of clinical performance be used in medical malpractice litigation? JAMA 2006;295:1831–4.
126. Brennan TA. Physicians' responsibility to improve the quality of care. Acad Med 2002;77:973–80.
127. Donaldson MS, editor. Measuring the quality of health care: a statement by the National Roundtable on Health Care Quality. Washington (DC): National Academy Press; 1999.
128. Shine KI. Health care quality and how to achieve it. Acad Med 2002;77:91–9.
129. Clarke JR. Making surgery safer. J Am Coll Surg 2005;200:229–35.
130. Leape LL. Reporting of adverse events. N Engl J Med 2002;347:1633–8.
131. Leape LL, Bates DW, Cullen DJ, et al. Systems analysis of adverse drug events. ADE Prevention Study Group. JAMA 1995; 274:35–43.
132. Pennachio D. Error reporting does a turn around. Hosp Peer Rev 1998;23:121.
133. Andrus CH, Villasenor EG, Kettelle JB, et al. "To err is human": uniformly reporting medical errors and near misses, a naïve, costly, and misdirected goal. J Am Coll Surg 2003;196:911–8.
134. Roscoe LA, Krizek TJ. Reporting medical errors: variables in the system shape attitudes toward reporting. Bull Am Coll Surg 2002;87:1–17.
135. Layde PM, Cortes LM, Teret SP, et al. Patient safety efforts should focus on medical injuries. JAMA 2002;287:1993–2001.
136. McNutt RA, Abrams R, Aron DC. Patient safety efforts should focus on medical errors. JAMA 2002;287:1997–2001.
137. Werner RM, Asch DA. The unintended consequences of publicly reporting quality information. JAMA 2005;293:1239–44.
138. Galvin R. Pay-for-performance: too much of a good thing? A conversation with Martin Roland. Health Aff (Millwood) 2006;25: w412–9.
139. Grissom TL. Comments during panel discussion at invitational conference on contemporary surgical quality, safety, and transparency. Am Surg 2006;72:1021–30.
140. Heget JR, Bagian JP, Lee CZ, et al. John M. Eisenberg Patient Safety Awards. System innovation: Veterans Health Administration National Center for Patient Safety. Jt Comm J Qual Improv 2002;28:660–5.
141. Volpp KGM, Grande D. Residents' suggestions for reducing errors in teaching hospitals. N Engl J Med 2003;348:851–5.
142. Battles JB, Shea CE. A system of analyzing medical errors to improve GME curricula and programs. Acad Med 2001;76:125–33.
143. Hugh TB. New strategies to prevent laparoscopic bile duct injury—surgeons can learn from pilots. Surgery 2002;132:826–35.
144. Gawande A. The learning curve. New Yorker 2002 Jan 28. p. 52–61.
145. Clarke JR. How a system for reporting medical errors can and cannot improve patient safety. Am Surg 2006;72:1088–91.
146. Enthoven AC, Tollen LA. Competition in health care: it takes systems to pursue quality and efficiency. Health Aff (Millwood) 2005;24 Suppl 3:w5420–33.

147. Codman EA. A study in hospital efficiency. Oakbrook Terrace (IL): Joint Commission on Accreditation of Healthcare Organizations; 1996.
148. Robinson AR, Hohmann KB, Rifkin JI, et al. Physician and public opinions of quality of health care and the problem of medical errors. Arch Intern Med 2002;162:2186–90.
149. Etchells E, O'Neill C, Bernstein M. Patient safety in surgery. World J Surg 2003;27:936–42.
150. Cuschieri A. Nature of human error: implications for surgical practice. Ann Surg 2006;244:642–8.
151. Gallagher TH, Waterman AD, Ebers AG, et al. Patients' and physicians' attitudes regarding the disclosure of medical errors. JAMA 2003;289:1001–7.
152. Birkmeyer NJ, Share D, Campbell DA Jr, et al. Partnering with payers to improve surgical quality: the Michigan plan. Surgery 2005;138:815–20.
153. Encinosa WE, Hellinger FJ. The impact of medical errors on ninety-day costs and outcomes: an examination of surgical patients. Health Serv Res 2008;43:2067–85.
154. Zhan C, Friedman B, Mosso A, et al. Medicare payment for selected adverse events: building the business case for investing in patient safety. Health Affairs 2006;25:1386–93.
155. Berwick DM. Quality of health care. Part 5: payment by capitation and the quality of care. N Engl J Med 1996;335:1227–31.
156. Russell T. Safety and quality in surgical practice. Ann Surg 2006;244:653–5.
157. Polk HC. Presidential address: quality, safety, transparency. Ann Surg 2005;242:293–301.

Acknowledgment

Figure 1 Seward Hung

6 PREOPERATIVE TESTING, PLANNING, AND RISK STRATIFICATION

*Randi Smith, MD, Valerie Ng, MD, PhD, Patrick Twomey, MD, and Alden H. Harken, MD**

In most circumstances in medicine, diagnosis precedes treatment. Consensus statements and regulatory guidelines endorse the long-hallowed practice of identifying patients at increased risk for complications. This is called "prognostic testing." The implication is that the benefit of special risk reduction strategies should be confined to these patients. Most of the cardiovascular (and pulmonary) "screening" tests considered below are of the prognostic type only.

Much more useful than prognostic testing is predictive or directive testing, which means identifying patients who will benefit from a specified, available intervention. By definition, this discriminates a subset of "bad prognosis" patients who can be helped and thus requires the existence of a therapeutic intervention of demonstrated benefit. This often includes identifying those patients who are not too ill but not too well to benefit from the associated therapy.

Proof that a testing strategy is predictive, not merely prognostic, is best demonstrated by randomized trials comparing outcomes in groups receiving best conventional care with or without the proposed test. This is a high standard but has been met in situations such as screening mammography for breast cancer in women ages 50 to 70 and computed tomographic (CT) scans in closed-head injury.

In medicine and surgery, we like to think of ourselves as scientists who make decisions and perform procedures based on the results of studies and clinical trials that support our management strategies. Traditionally, we always obtain a clinical history and perform a physical examination. This interaction with our patients helps us focus and refine our therapies but, equally importantly, promotes the health literacy of our patients.[1] There is good evidence that patients who understand their disease and who participate actively in their therapy will fare better.[1]

However, once we have finished talking with our patients, the data-driven support for the traditional model of preoperative testing begins to break down. We define a "routine test" as a test that we obtain on an asymptomatic, apparently healthy patient in the absence of any specific clinical indication.[2] Then we examine the frequency of abnormal routine test results, but it gets cloudier when we try to determine how often an abnormal test result changes our management. There is almost no information relating a test-driven alteration in management to any benefit in outcome. Intuitively, we do know that the more fragile the patient and the bigger the surgical procedure, the more likely it is that we should anticipate trouble.

In addition to functional capacity and comorbid conditions, age is a robust determinant of operative risk, as is the type of operation. Vascular procedures and prolonged, complicated thoracic, abdominal, or head and neck procedures carry higher levels of risk. None of this is surprising.

The purposes of this chapter are as follows:

1. To explore the tools available to the surgeon for assessing patient vulnerability to operative stress
2. To examine the practical specifics of preoperative functional status testing
3. To analyze methods of quantifying surgical stress
4. To develop patient status and operative insult-specific indications for some "routine" preoperative tests
5. To suggest some strategies to reduce risk in specified groups of patients

Preoperative Laboratory Testing

There are at least 33 reasons why surgeons order preoperative laboratory tests; some are unique to teaching environments, and most are not clinically useful or relevant in the "otherwise healthy patient in the absence of a specific indicator."[3] There is poor correlation between the number of tests ordered and quality of care or physician competence, and the wide variation in test ordering suggests that some, or perhaps many, tests are ordered unnecessarily.[4]

As a corollary, surgeons order preoperative laboratory tests for fear of malpractice, for detection of an unsuspected disease, or because they "have always done it that way." Note that detecting an unsuspected disease in the preoperative period is no different from screening for disease in a population, albeit a selected (preoperative) population.

Comprehensive literature reviews and government publications guiding reimbursement for preoperative testing (or lack thereof)[2,5,6] lament the lack of Level I evidence to guide policy making, but most admit that the preponderance of nonrandomized clinical trial data demonstrates that preoperative testing is not clinically useful. Amazingly, this question has been studied formally for at least 50 years (yes, half a century), with the following strikingly similar conclusions. Preoperative laboratory testing

1. Has no clinical value for asymptomatic healthy individuals, in the absence of a specific clinical indication, such as a diuretic
2. Has only marginal value for those with known disease
3. Will yield abnormal results for 1 to 2% of all test results
4. Yields results that would have been predicted from the underlying patient diseases
5. Does not change treatment when abnormal results are obtained
6. Yields abnormal results that are often ignored by the ordering physician
7. Allows considerable unrealized cost savings derived from not performing these preoperative tests

* The authors and editors gratefully acknowledge the contributions of the previous authors, Cyrus J. Parsa, MD, Andrew E. Luckey, MD, Nicolas V. Christou, MD, to the development and writing of this chapter.

So let us chronologically recapitulate selected studies chosen to demonstrate the evolution of this issue through the lenses of multiple medical specialties. In 1965, pathologists Bold and Corrin published their study titled "Use and Abuse of Clinical Chemistry in Surgery."[7] This study was performed in the early days of clinical pathology, before automated analyzers were commercially available. One hundred fifty of 344 (44%) tests were preoperative tests of "urea and electrolytes and metabolic abnormalities in patients with renal calculi." Almost all of the preoperative test results were within accepted reference ranges and were euphemistically termed "useful negative" results. This study pioneered the acquisition of nonuseful preoperative laboratory data.

Automated clinical laboratory testing became widely available in the late 1960s, exponentially increasing the opportunity for unnecessary laboratory testing. In the early 1980s, several groups assessed preoperative laboratory testing (they termed it "screening") for 2,000 patients. Many tests were ordered "by protocol," including complete blood count (CBC), white blood cell (WBC) differential, prothrombin time (PT), partial thromboplastin time (PTT), platelet count, "six-factor automated multiple analysis" (sodium, potassium, chloride, total carbon dioxide content, serum urea nitrogen, creatinine), and glucose. Of 2,785 routine preoperative admission tests, the authors concluded that approximately [illegible] were "unindicated" (i.e., the patient lacked a recognizable clinical indication for testing). Four results ([illegible]) were substantially significant so as to affect anesthetic or surgical management, yet there was no documentation that care management was altered based on these abnormal laboratory results. Furthermore, there was no documentation by physicians of further exploration of these abnormal results, presumably raising (rather than limiting) issues of legal liability for the ordering physician. The authors concluded that preoperative testing should be performed only for patients with an identified disease or for whom the surgical procedure would be altered based on the result. They extrapolated that approximately 9,000 tests annually could have been avoided, resulting in approximately $147,000 decreased charges and a cost savings of $95,800 (1985 dollar value).

Physicians and surgeons are perhaps guilty of a certain amount of intellectual inertia as similar studies paradoxically concluded that preoperative testing was "useful" even when the authors acknowledged that test abnormalities provoked no clinical consequences. A consistent finding was a 1 to 2% incidence of abnormal results, a lack of clinical consequences, and an absence of physician response to the abnormal laboratory tests.

Anesthesiologists have been the first discipline to substantively engage in the debate. When managed care capitation was introduced and cost containment became critical to the survival and success of health care organizations, anesthesiologists were the first group to responsibly respond. Allison and Bromley assessed the clinical usefulness of preoperative testing in 60 randomly selected veterans prior to ambulatory surgery.[8] They concluded that two thirds of testing was inappropriate and estimated the unnecessary costs at $47 for a veteran and $80 for a community hospital patient (1996 dollar value), with potential savings of $11,757 for their Veterans Affairs Medical Center alone. They concluded that preoperative testing limited exclusively to those patients with clinical indications would have no effect on the quality or safety of care.

In a similar study of 520 patients undergoing elective general, vascular, thoracic, and head and neck surgery, preoperative tests included electrolytes, blood urea nitrogen (BUN), creatinine, glucose, hemoglobin/hematocrit, total protein, albumin, total lymphocyte count, PT, PTT, platelet count, urinalysis, electrocardiography (ECG), and chest radiography.[9] Age, gender, and specific concomitant illnesses were associated with predictably abnormal laboratory tests. Routine preoperative laboratory testing was identified as "neither useful nor cost-effective." Perhaps in response to this wave of data, preoperative testing practice at four institutions over 8 years and for only four surgical procedures was examined. Although wide variations from "operation to operation, test to test and institution to institution," were unexpectedly identified, an approximately 20% decrease in both unnecessary and medically indicated testing was achieved. For the unnecessary tests alone, the authors extrapolated to the entire United States and estimated an approximately $320 million annual savings.

The obvious question is what happens to patients who do not enjoy the safety of preoperative laboratory testing? Narr and colleagues reviewed the outcomes of 1,044 randomly selected patients from [illegible] patients who had no laboratory tests performed within [illegible] days before a surgical procedure. Ninety-seven percent of the patients were "relatively healthy." Zero deaths or major perioperative complications resulted. Furthermore, this group observed that no laboratory test performed intra- or postoperatively changed surgical or medical management "substantially." They concluded that patients who, following a history and physical examination, are "determined to have no preoperative indication for laboratory tests can safely undergo anesthesia and operation with tests obtained only as indicated intra- and postoperatively."

In 1995, laboratory medicine, surgery, and anesthesia practitioners collaborated to develop laboratory testing guidelines before admission for elective surgery.[10] Testing guidelines were developed and categorized into four major groups, as well as by age and gender. The surgeons then agreed to delegate test ordering to nurses and anesthesiologists who evaluated the patients before surgery. Volume and appropriateness of ordered tests were compared before and after guideline adoption. They observed a 67% reduction in the overall number of tests ordered per patient for the first 2 years after guideline implementation, with an improvement in the appropriateness of test ordering (65% were considered "appropriate" prior to guideline implementation and 81 to 86% postimplementation). They noted marked fiscal savings related to this performance improvement initiative, quantified as $66,981 in year 1 and $75,995 in year 2.

In the late 1990s, anesthesiologists Vogt and Henson conducted a prospective, cross-sectional study in a university hospital, studying 312 consecutive patients scheduled for elective surgery and evaluated by an anesthesiologist in a preoperative clinic.[11] The goal of the study was to determine if there was a difference in the ordering of "unindicated preoperative laboratory tests" for healthy (American Society of Anesthesiologists [ASA] physical status I and II) versus sicker (ASA physical status III) patients. The anesthesiologists evaluated the test ordering by surgeons relative to ASA status and concluded that 72.5% of tests ordered by surgeons were considered not indicated by the anesthesiologists. Although there were fewer "unindicated" tests with worsening ASA status, the overall conclusion was that a large proportion of surgeon-ordered preoperative tests were unnecessary. By eliminating unnecessary testing, they estimated an annual cost savings of $80,000 (1997 dollars).

In 2002, the ASA Task Force on Preanesthesia published its review and practice advisory.[5] Regarding laboratory tests, a clear distinction was made between "routine" and "selective" preoperative tests. Routine tests were defined as those intended to discover a disease or disorder in an asymptomatic individual. The task force bluntly stated that routine tests "do not make an important contribution to the process of perioperative assessment and management of the patient by the anesthesiologist." In contrast, the task force recommended performing selective tests, that is, those tests medically indicated because of the history and physical findings, medical record review, and type of invasiveness of the planned procedure and anesthetic, because their results "may assist the anesthesiologist in making decisions about the process of perioperative assessment and management."[5] Clinical studies are very hard to do, and it is easy to criticize them. Perhaps these studies were performed in settings where timely treatment of chronic diseases was available, allowing maximal optimization of patients prior to elective surgery. The recommendations of a conscientious task force are difficult to ignore, however. So what happens to surgical patients in developing countries where no chronic disease management is available?

Pal and colleagues retrospectively studied the benefit of preoperative testing in 216 asymptomatic healthy surgical patients in Pakistan.[12] Their findings were strikingly similar to those of previous studies; the most common preoperative laboratory abnormality was a low hemoglobin in 42 of 216 (19%) patients, almost all females. Chest x-ray abnormalities were the next most common abnormality, present in 11 of 103 (10.6%) patients, followed by mild hypokalemia in 6 of 123 (4.8%) patients and an elevated glucose in 1 of 113 (0.88%) patients. Aside from a single preoperative intervention for a patient with a preoperative hemoglobin of 4.8 g/dL, treatment plans or outcomes were not affected. The authors concluded that the history and physical examination were the most reliable and cost-effective preoperative screening tools available. They endorsed the existing ASA guidelines for class I (asymptomatic healthy) patients, that is, no preoperative testing is recommended.

In 2003, the general medicine and primary care practitioners entered the debate. Smetana and Macpherson reviewed the published literature on preoperative testing and concluded that "almost all "routine" laboratory tests before surgery have limited clinical value."[13] Based on their review, they recommended the following:

- "Clinicians should order tests only if the outcome of an abnormal test will influence management."
- "When an abnormal test results from such testing, it is critical that physicians document their thinking about the result."
- "Physicians should not be criticized for selective test ordering before surgery."
- "Physicians and institutions recommending routine preoperative testing for all patients provide no clinical value to their patients at considerable cost."

A subset of studies have noted specific abnormal laboratory results related to age, gender, and concomitant underlying illnesses. The latter, selective testing for concomitant underlying illnesses, is accepted practice for routine medical care regardless of anticipated surgery. The common theme appears to be that if the physician would request a test in the absence of anticipated surgery, the test is also warranted prior to surgery. Extremes of age and gender do keep reappearing as potential independent predictors of trouble.

AGE

Dzankic and colleagues assessed the importance of preoperative laboratory testing in 544 patients 70 years and older undergoing noncardiac surgery.[14] They observed that 0.5 to 5% had electrolyte and platelet count abnormalities, 12% had elevated serum creatinine (> 1.5 mg/dL), 10% had hemoglobin less than 10 g/dL, and 7% had serum glucose greater than 200 mg/dL. None of these abnormalities were predictive of postoperative adverse outcomes. The ASA classification and surgical risk were stronger univariate predictors for adverse outcome than abnormal serum electrolyte or creatinine values, and only the ASA classification and surgical risk by multivariate logistic regression were predictive of postoperative adverse outcomes. The authors concluded that age alone was not sufficient justification for routine preoperative laboratory testing and recommended using the history and physical examination to guide preoperative testing.

Ophthalmologists Schein and colleagues conducted a landmark study of 9,408 patients aged 80 years and older who underwent 9,626 cataract surgeries without preoperative testing, compared with 9,411 patients undergoing 9,624 operations who had routine preoperative laboratory testing.[15] They found no difference between groups relative to intraoperative or postoperative events. Routine preoperative testing offered no benefit over that attained from ASA classification and medical history. They concluded that routine preoperative testing before cataract surgery did not measurably increase the safety of surgery.

Schein and colleagues noted that cataract surgery was the most commonly performed operation in elderly people in developed countries, with 1.5 million cataract operations in 1996.[15] From their study, it was estimated that the cost of routine preoperative testing prior to cataract surgery exceeded $150 million annually and, given the lack of benefit from testing, suggested that these costs could be saved without a negative effect on patient outcome.

The screening value of preoperative laboratory findings in children is the same as that for adults: not clinically useful for healthy children presenting for minor elective surgery. Burk and colleagues encouraged preoperative coagulation testing to identify rare, undiagnosed congenital or hereditary bleeding disorders in children prior to tonsillectomy.[16] This value, however, was clearly offset by the rarity of the disorders coupled with the high frequency of false positive bleeding histories and laboratory tests.

GENDER

A relatively common finding in many preoperative testing studies was anemia in women of childbearing age. This is the only gender-specific "abnormality" reported and would support preoperative inquiry if the clinical presentation would prompt the clinician to respond to an abnormal result.

Several decades ago, a group at the Mayo Clinic began to realize that subjecting patients to large numbers of preoperative tests did not change surgical results.[17,18] They further observed that when preoperative testing returned an abnormal result, they rarely did anything differently anyway[17] [*see Table 1 and Table 2*].

In summary, the overwhelming majority of studies have concluded that there is little to no value of screening preoperative laboratory tests in asymptomatic patients in the absence of a specific clinical indication [*see Table 3*]. Laboratory tests within 6 months of surgery to gauge surgical and anesthesia risk are acceptable if the patient's condition has not changed clinically in the intervening period. Conversely, if the patient's condition has changed, laboratory testing is medically indicated as specifically dictated by the change in clinical condition.[2,5,6,13]

A color-coded "at a glance" guide modeled on traffic signals (green = consensus to do a test; red = consensus not to do a test; amber = absence of consensus, "consider testing") has been prepared to guide busy practitioners regarding when to order what preoperative test [*see Figure 1*][6]; other similar guides abound [*see Figure 2*[19] *and Table 4*]. Audits[20] of current preoperative laboratory testing practices will remain scrutinized by conscientious investigators, but professional guidelines consistently reveal persistent unnecessary preoperative testing.[21]

Table 1 Effect of Abnormal Screening Results on Physician Behavior[18]

Screening Test	*% Abnormal Test Results*	*% Resulting in Management Change*
Bleeding time	3.8	Abnormal result rarely led to change
Chest x-ray	2.5–3.7	2.1
Coagulation time	4.8	Abnormal result rarely led to change
Electrocardiogram	4.6–31.7	0–2.2
Hemoglobin	5 (for < 10 g/dL; < 9 g/dL was rare)	Abnormal result rarely led to change
Partial thromboplastin time	15.6	Abnormal result rarely led to change
Total leukocyte count	< 1	Abnormal result rarely led to change
Urinalysis	1–34.1	0.1–2.8

Table 2 Minimum Preoperative Test Requirements at the Mayo Clinic (in 1993)[17]

Age (yr)	Tests Required
< 40	None
40–59	Electrocardiography, measurement of creatinine, measurement of glucose
≥ 60	Chest x-ray, complete blood cell count, electrocardiography, measurement of creatinine, measurement of glucose

In addition, the following guidelines apply: (1) a complete blood cell count is indicated in all patients who undergo blood typing and are crossmatched; (2) measurement of potassium is indicated in patients taking diuretics or undergoing bowel preparation; (3) a chest x-ray is indicated in patients with a history of cardiac or pulmonary disease or with recent respiratory symptoms; and (4) spirometry (forced vital capacity) is indicated in patients 40 years of age or older who have a history of cigarette smoking and are scheduled for an upper abdominal or thoracic procedure.

Table 3 American Society of Anesthesiologists' Physical Status Classification[5]

Classification	*Description*	*Examples*
Class I	Healthy patient with no systemic disorder	
Class II	Mild to moderate systemic disorder that need not be associated with the surgical problem	Chronic obstructive pulmonary disease Diet-controlled diabetes Extremes of age Medication-controlled hypertension Moderate obesity
Class III	Severe systemic disease that limits activity but is not incapacitating	Insulin-dependent diabetes Lifestyle-limiting pulmonary insufficiency Morbid obesity Stress-induced angina
Class IV	Incapacitating, life-threatening systemic disease	Active cardiac ischemia Advanced hepatic, pulmonary, or renal disease Refractory arrhythmia Signs of congestive heart failure Unstable angina
Class V	Moribund patient, not expected to survive 24 hours without an operation	Major cerebral trauma with increasing intracranial pressure Major trauma with shock Massive pulmonary embolus Ruptured aortic aneurysm with profound shock

Changing Paradigms of Surgical Success

It is now clear that postoperative survival by itself is no longer an adequate assay of surgical success. Risk must be stratified before operation, and the degree of risk must be evaluated in light of both the quantity and the quality of postoperative life. Cost must then be judiciously assessed relative to a risk-stratified, quality-adjusted postoperative year of life. In 2008, Cohen and colleagues published an assessment of health economics.[22] These authors calculated the cost-effectiveness ratio by dividing the incremental costs of surgical

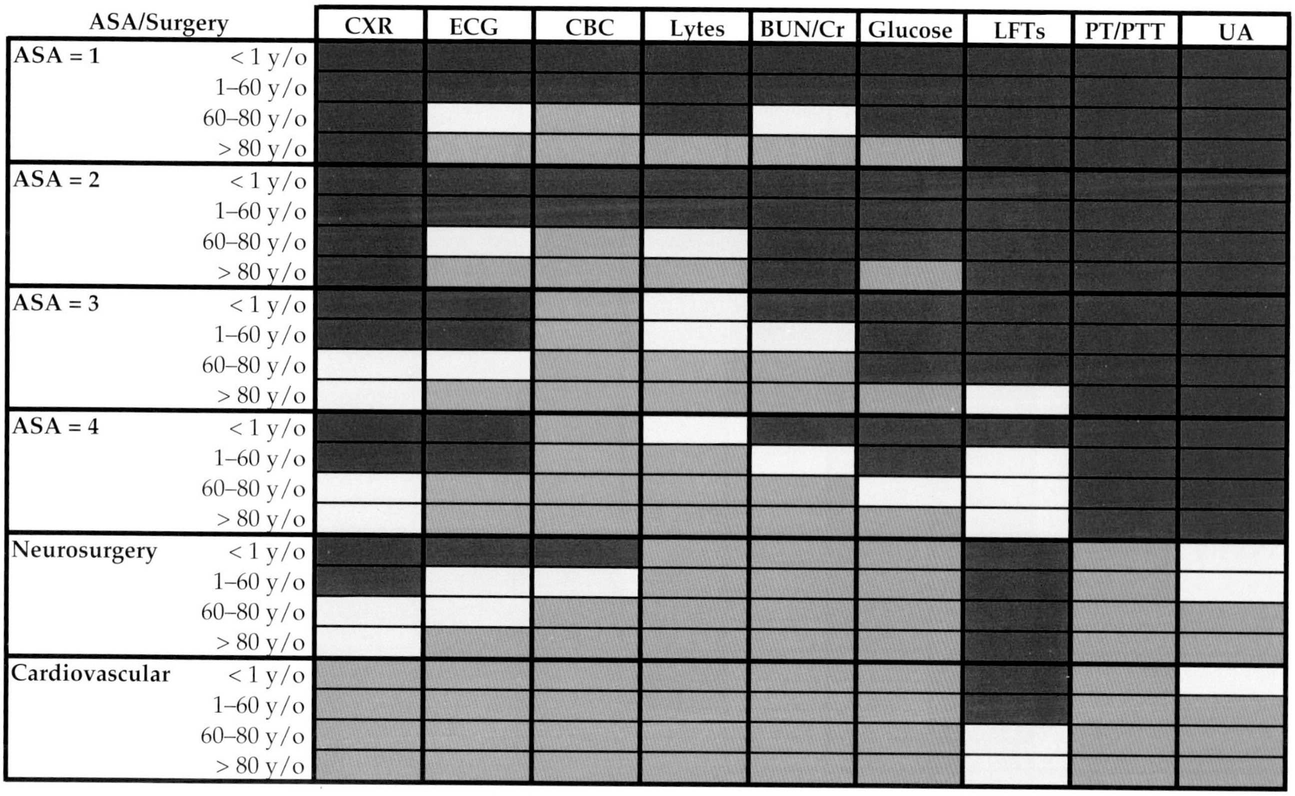

ASA/Surgery		CXR	ECG	CBC	Lytes	BUN/Cr	Glucose	LFTs	PT/PTT	UA
ASA = 1	< 1 y/o									
	1–60 y/o									
	60–80 y/o									
	> 80 y/o									
ASA = 2	< 1 y/o									
	1–60 y/o									
	60–80 y/o									
	> 80 y/o									
ASA = 3	< 1 y/o									
	1–60 y/o									
	60–80 y/o									
	> 80 y/o									
ASA = 4	< 1 y/o									
	1–60 y/o									
	60–80 y/o									
	> 80 y/o									
Neurosurgery	< 1 y/o									
	1–60 y/o									
	60–80 y/o									
	> 80 y/o									
Cardiovascular	< 1 y/o									
	1–60 y/o									
	60–80 y/o									
	> 80 y/o									

Figure 1 Appropriate preoperative tests related to the patient's American Society of Anesthesiology (ASA) classification and age. *Red* indicates that the preponderance of evidence suggests that the test will not be useful (or positively influence patient care); *yellow* indicates that the test is controversial; *green* indicates that the test is useful. BUN = blood urea nitrogen; CBC = complete blood count; Cr = creatinine; CXR = chest x-ray; ECG = electrocardiogram; LFT = liver function test; PT = prothrombin time; PTT = partial thromboplastin time; UA = urinalysis; y/o = years old.

therapy by incremental benefits as quality-adjusted year of life (QALY), compared with standard medical care. They reported that cochlear implants for profoundly deaf children reduced lifetime aggregate costs and improved health; liver transplantation for primary sclerosing cholangitis cost $41,000/QALY; implantation of cardioverter-defibrillators in patients with left ventricular dysfunction cost $52,000/QALY, and surgery in 70-year-old men with a new diagnosis of prostate cancer increased costs and compromised health compared with watchful waiting.[22] Thus, the purposes of this section are to add "dollar cost" and postoperative quality of life to the preoperative risk assessment equations. We also propose to describe the potential preoperative cardiac, pulmonary, and laboratory tests; analyze the significance of abnormal results; and ultimately develop a strategy for relating patient characteristics and the magnitude of the procedure to the menu of preoperative studies.

Although no one ever truly wants to undergo a surgical procedure, the results of surgery can be formidably gratifying to both patient and surgeon when the right operation is performed accurately, expeditiously, and for the right reasons, on the right patient at the right time. In attempting to bring about this state of affairs, surgeons must consciously and honestly balance the physiologic, psychological, social, and financial burdens of surgery against the anticipated benefits.[23] Although surgeons are not the only medical professionals who must perform this kind of balancing act, we are the ones who do it most conspicuously.

Continuing refinement of the methods employed to stratify preoperative risks permits surgeons to "handicap" both patients and surgical procedures with greater precision. Outcome assessment must clearly incorporate the "sickness quotient," which is typically expressed in terms of the ratio of observed to expected outcome (O/E), into the assessment of therapeutic value. If a surgeon were to operate only on Olympic athletes with single-organ diseases (or no disease at all), his or her patients would likely do very well. Those of us who must operate on a more diverse patient population will have less gratifying results.

The most widely used risk classification system was developed by the ASA and is based on the patient's functional status and comorbid conditions (e.g., diabetes mellitus, peripheral vascular disease, renal dysfunction, and/or chronic pulmonary disease) [*see Table 3*].[24] The ASA index generally associates poorer overall health with increased postoperative complications, longer hospital stays, and higher mortality.

In addition to functional capacity and comorbid conditions, age is a robust determinant of operative risk, as is the type of operation. Vascular procedures and prolonged, complicated thoracic, abdominal, or head and neck procedures carry higher levels of risk. None of this is surprising.

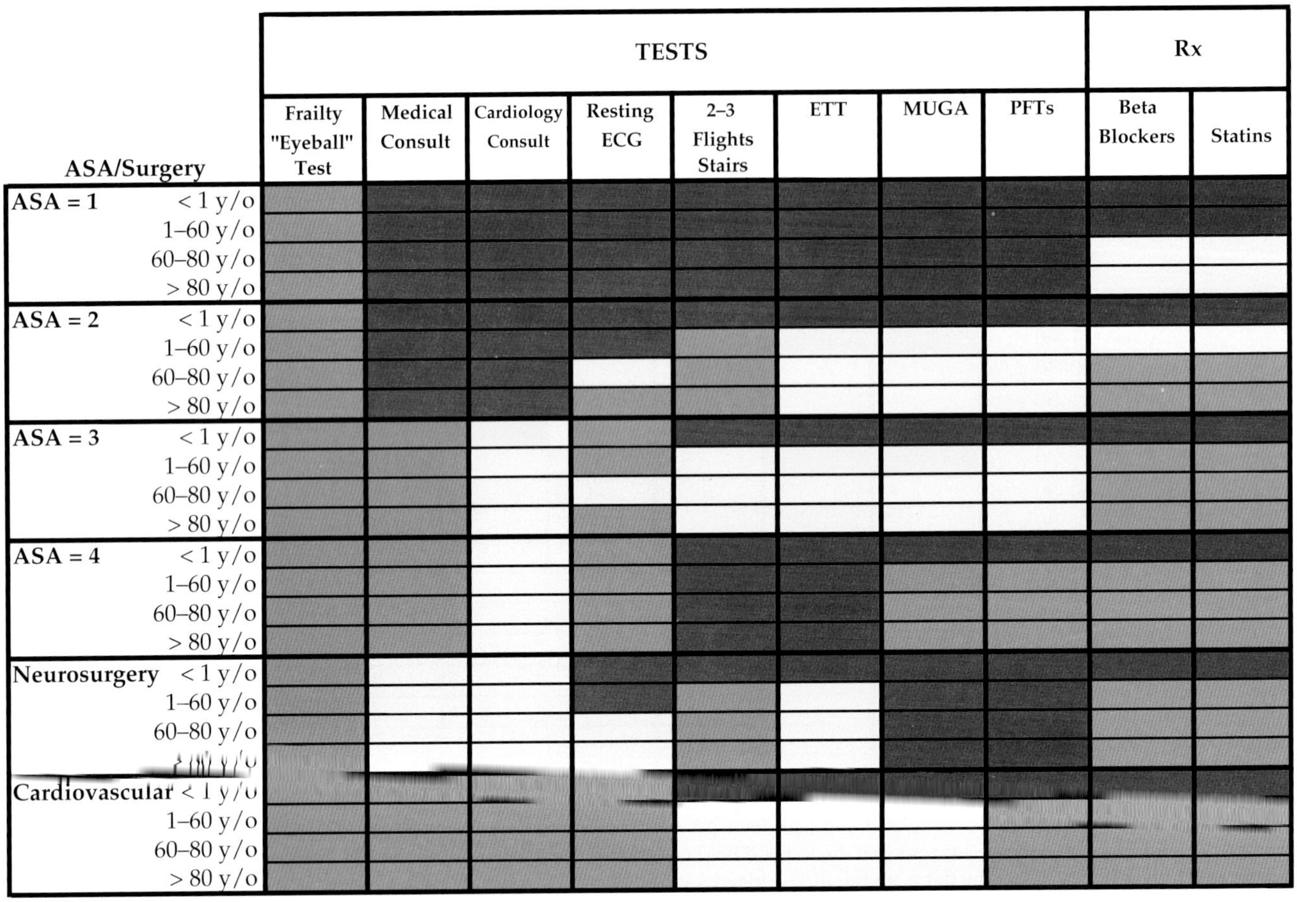

ASA/Surgery		TESTS								Rx	
		Frailty "Eyeball" Test	Medical Consult	Cardiology Consult	Resting ECG	2–3 Flights Stairs	ETT	MUGA	PFTs	Beta Blockers	Statins
ASA = 1	< 1 y/o										
	1–60 y/o										
	60–80 y/o										
	> 80 y/o										
ASA = 2	< 1 y/o										
	1–60 y/o										
	60–80 y/o										
	> 80 y/o										
ASA = 3	< 1 y/o										
	1–60 y/o										
	60–80 y/o										
	> 80 y/o										
ASA = 4	< 1 y/o										
	1–60 y/o										
	60–80 y/o										
	> 80 y/o										
Neurosurgery	< 1 y/o										
	1–60 y/o										
	60–80 y/o										
	> 80 y/o										
Cardiovascular	< 1 y/o										
	1–60 y/o										
	60–80 y/o										
	> 80 y/o										

Figure 2 Preoperative assessment strategies and recommended risk-reducing therapy relative to American Society of Anesthesiologists (ASA) classification performed by the surgeon and age. *Red* indicates that the preponderance of evidence suggests that the strategy or therapy will not be useful (or positively influence patient care); *yellow* indicates that it will be controversial; *green* indicates that it will be useful. Each discipline has its own quasisubjective test for perceived patient fortitude. The anesthesiologists term it the ASA classification; surgeons use the frailty index or the "eyeball" test. Nutritionists refer to the subjective global assessment, whereas oncologists rely on Karnofsky scoring. In each instance, the subjective "eyeball" impression of a seasoned clinician has traditionally proven to be gratifyingly valuable. ECG = electrocardiogram; ETT = exercise tolerance testing; MUGA = multigated acquisition; PFT = pulmonary function test; y/o = years old.

WHAT TO LOOK FOR IN THE PATIENT'S HISTORY

We all deteriorate as we age. In fact, the Mayo Clinic uses age alone as the initial filter in its selection of preoperative tests for "healthy" patients. The anesthesiologists refine this ASA policy by defining the "health" of the patient [*see Table 3*], which requires a search for comorbid disease. The diseases and other indicators that seem to count most are those that reflect cardiovascular compromise: angina, a past myocardial infarction, and surrogates for coronary artery disease, such as diabetes, hypertension, obesity, and advanced age. Nothing else seems to have much effect. Goldman and colleagues first reported this observation in 1977.[25] They followed 1,001 patients through a major surgical procedure and related their preoperative history, physical findings, and routine laboratory work to major complications: perioperative myocardial infarction, cardiogenic pulmonary edema, ventricular tachycardia/fibrillation, and death. They then applied univariate analysis to ascribe varying numbers of points to each preoperative factor that predicted postoperative problems. All of the ominous preoperative signals were those that reflected cardiovascular disease: recent myocardial infarction (10 points), congestive heart failure (11 points), any nonsinus cardiac rhythm (7 points), and advanced age (5 points). These cardiac risk factors were assigned high numbers of points, although, perhaps surprisingly, no other warning signs received more than three—not even carbon dioxide tension (P_{CO_2}) greater than 50 mm Hg, BUN greater than 50 mg/dL, bicarbonate less than 20 mM/L, or potassium less than 3.0 mM/L. Liver function tests were so insensitive that they were deemed insignificant. In 1995, Mangano and Goldman repeated this study and reported the same conclusions.[26]

Many risk stratification systems refer to "otherwise healthy patients." The term "healthy patient" should be translated as "asymptomatic patient." When you are taking the patient's history, you should focus on probing for the indicators of cardiac disease.

INDICATORS OF CARDIAC RISK

In a successful attempt to simplify Goldman and colleagues' equation, Boersma and colleagues refined the Lee and colleagues Revised Cardiac Risk Index (RCRI), which is currently the most widely applied cardiac risk stratification system.[27,28] The RCRI identifies six predictors of major

Table 4 Preoperative Assessment Strategies Related to Purposes and Potential Information Derived

Assessment Strategy	*Information Derived*	*Purpose(s)*	*Indication/Comments*
Medical consultation	Assessment of chronic disease	To stabilize chronic disease	ASA classes III and IV (not typically useful in ASA I, II, or V)
Cardiac clearance	Assessment of chronic cardiac disease	To stabilize chronic cardiopulmonary disease	ASA classes III and IV (not typically useful in ASA I, II, or V)
Frailty ("eyeball") test	Global assessment of surgical risk/benefit	Practical guide to surgical risk/benefit	Useful in assessing necessity/benefits of surgical intervention
Resting ECG	(1) Cardiac rhythm; (2) may reflect prior muscle damage (Q waves)	To determine resting cardiac rhythm	Disappointing indicator of cardiac status
Climbing 2–3 flights of stairs	Practical indicator of strength and cardiopulmonary status	Subjective indicator of cardiopulmonary status	Useful indicator of cardiopulmonary status in sorting out ASA class III patients
Exercise tolerance test	Quantitative indicator of cardiopulmonary status	Objective indicator of cardiopulmonary status	Useful if results might lead to cardiac intervention in the absence of proposed elective general surgery
Multigated acquisition (MUGA) scan	Ejection fraction	To assess ventricular function	Low yield in ASA class I, II, and III patients
Pulmonary function tests (PFTs)	Pulmonary status	To assess medical reversibility of lung dysfunction	Valuable in discriminating patients with equivocal 2–3 flights of stairs climbing test

ASA = American Society of Anesthesiologists; ECG = electrocardiogram.

cardiac complications (high risk surgical procedures, ischemic heart disease, history of congestive heart failure, history of cerebrovascular disease, insulin use and a creatinine greater than 2.0 mg/dL). Scores range from 0 to 5, and the likelihood of major perioperative complications increases with rising scores [*see Table 5*].[25,26] This index has weaknesses. It was derived from calculations that excluded emergency surgical patients and neurosurgical patients, whereas thoracic, vascular, and orthopedic patients were overrepresented. In addition, it classified surgical procedures simplistically into two categories: high risk and non–high risk. Despite these weaknesses, the predictive accuracy of the RCRI has been validated in large cohorts.[27]

Whereas the RCRI documents cardiac risk factors, the American College of Cardiology (ACC)/American Heart Association (AHA) Task Force guidelines (see below) were developed to serve as a national quality initiative for use of the RCRI and optimization of perioperative risk by medical or, rarely, surgical means. The goal of a preoperative cardiac consultation is to determine the most appropriate testing and treatment strategies for optimizing patient care while avoiding unnecessary testing. This represents a definite paradigm shift from the stratification and revascularization strategies commonly employed only a decade ago.

Interestingly, these guidelines are not always followed in clinical practice. One survey found that despite the availability of the guidelines, 40% of cardiology consultations resulted in the simple recommendation to proceed with surgery, without modification of perioperative plans or optimization of risk factors.[29] Patients selected for noninvasive testing do appear to receive more medical therapy (e.g., beta blockers, statins, and platelet inhibitors) than patients who are not referred for further cardiac evaluation.

ACC/AHA TASK FORCE GUIDELINES

Routine preoperative cardiac evaluation and testing suffer significant inherent limitations. The ACC and the AHA have combined task forces to clarify current recommendations for national quality initiatives in perioperative stratification and risk modification.[30] Their strategy bases diagnostic and therapeutic approaches on clinical screening for disease state and functional capacity. Specialized testing is conservatively employed only when additional information provided by the proposed test is likely to impact the outcome. The ACC/AHA consensus guidelines recommend aggressive medical management to provide myocardial protection in the perioperative period to mitigate cardiac risk. This strategy has proven to be both efficient and cost-effective in vascular surgery patients. The most recent update of these guidelines was published in late 2007.[30]

The ACC/AHA guidelines employ a five-step algorithm designed to guide patient risk stratification and subsequently determine appropriate cardiac evaluation. This algorithm is available on the ACC website (http://www.acc.org/clinical/guidelines/perio/update/fig1.htm).

Step 1 involves assessing the urgency of the operation. Step 2 is the process of looking for active cardiac conditions, including unstable coronary syndromes, decompensated heart failure, significant dysrhythmias, and severe valvular disease. If any of these conditions are present and the operation is elective, the patient should be evaluated further and treated according to ACC/AHA guidelines. Step 3 is activated when no active cardiac condition is present and the proposed operation is low risk. In this instance, the surgeon may proceed without further intervention. Step 4 includes operations that are deemed to be of intermediate to high risk. The patient's functional status must be determined [*see Table 6*]. If the patient is asymptomatic and functional status is good, the planned operation may proceed without further intervention. If the patient is symptomatic or functional status is undetermined or poor (defined as the inability to perform activities involving energy expenditure greater than 4 metabolic equivalents [METs]), further investigation is

Table 5 Revised Cardiac Risk Index[26]

No. of Risk Factors	Risk of Major Cardiac Complications (%)
0	0.4
1	0.9
2	7.0
3+	11.0

There are six clinical risk factors: (1) high-risk surgery; (2) ischemic heart disease (myocardial infarction, positive treadmill test, use of nitroglycerin, current chest pain, pathologic Q waves on electrocardiogram); (3) congestive heart failure (documented history, pulmonary edema, paroxysmal nocturnal dyspnea, S_3 or chest x-ray with pulmonary vascular redistribution); (4) cerebrovascular disease (transient ischemic attack or cerebrovascular accident); (5) insulin-dependent diabetes mellitus; and (6) renal failure (progressive serum creatinine > 2.0 mg/dL).

necessary. In step 5, the final step, the surgeon searches for major clinical predictors of specific cardiac risk. As defined by the ACC/AHA Task Force, clinical cardiac risk factors include a history of ischemic heart disease, compensated or previous heart failure, cerebrovascular disease, diabetes mellitus, and/or renal insufficiency.[30] Patients with no history of clinical risk factors may proceed to surgery. Patients with one or two clinical risk factors who are undergoing a vascular procedure or patients with one or more clinical risk factors who are undergoing an intermediate-risk operation have the option of either proceeding with surgery after appropriate beta blockade or receiving additional evaluation, but only if the results might change management. Patients with three or more clinical risk factors who are undergoing a vascular procedure should receive further evaluation, but, again, only if the results might change management.

Identification of Factors Affecting Cardiac Risk

Heart failure is the most common discharge diagnosis in hospitals across the United States. The prevalence of heart failure increases with age, and as our surgical population ages, we treat more and more elderly patients with relevant degrees of heart failure.

Numerous cardiac risk indices have been created over the past three decades. During that period, risk stratification has evolved from the early Goldman and colleagues criteria, the first substantial effort at risk assessment, to the RCRI developed by Lee and colleagues[27] [*see Table 5*]. A review of the initial and updated multivariate analysis of risk predictors prior to noncardiac surgery attributes the lion's share of risk to the cardiovascular system.[25,26] If your patient suffers a major perioperative complication (myocardial infarction, cardiogenic pulmonary edema, sustained ventricular tachycardia/fibrillation, or death), the only organ system that appears to matter much is the heart.

To reiterate, Mangano and Goldman ascribe 11 points to any preoperative evidence of congestive heart failure, 10 points to a myocardial infarction within the last 6 months, 7 points to any ECG rhythm other than sinus rhythm, and

Table 6 Approximate Metabolic Equivalents and Peak Oxygen Intake Related to Common Daily Activities and Stages of the Bruce Protocol (Modified Duke Activity Status Index)

Activities: "Are you able to..."	Metabolic Equivalents (METs)	Peak Oxygen Intake* (mL/kg/min)	Bruce Protocol Correlates		
			Stage	% Grade	mph
Lie in bed with minimal movement (bedridden)?	≈ 1.00	< 10	NA†	NA†	NA†
Sit up in bed independently?	1.25				
Walk around the house?	1.75	10–15	1	10	1.7
Take care of yourself (toilet, feed, bathe, and clothe yourself?)	2.75				
Do light housework, such as washing dishes?	2.75				
Walk two blocks at ground level?	3.00	15–20			
Do moderate housework, such as vacuuming/sweeping floors?	3.50				
Do yard work, such as raking leaves?	4.50	20–25	2	12	2.5
Have sexual relations?	5.25				
Walk up a hill or climb two or three flights of stairs?	6.00				
Participate in moderate recreational activities such as swimming, golf, or slow dancing?	6.00				
Do heavy housework such as lifting or moving heavy furniture?	8.00	> 25	3	14	3.4
Run a short distance?	10.00				
Participate in strenuous sports such as volleyball or basketball, run on a treadmill, or use an elliptical machine?	12.00		4	16	4.2
Run a long distance?	12.00+				

NA = not applicable.
*Estimates of peak oxygen uptake are based on comparison data obtained from various levels of an exercise cardiac stress test (i.e., the Bruce protocol). These numbers vary by age and gender and hence represent estimates for women and men of differing ages.
†Bedridden patients are unable to participate in exercise stress testing. Hence, no data are available for this group in regard to Bruce protocol staging.
A physician may assess functional status as part of a preoperative checklist, but the patient usually provides only a snapshot of his or her most recent activities. Activity levels are not static but, rather, dynamic. Indeed, exercise tolerance can be gained over time with work ("training"). If patients are able to climb the ladder of activity status and tolerate more vigorous exercise, this is the ultimate cardiac stress test. Hence, increasing exercise in patients ("training") is a constructive preoperative formula.

5 points to age greater than 70 years of age (a surrogate for coronary disease).[25,26] No other indices (including a P_{CO_2} greater than 50 mm Hg or a creatinine level greater than 3.0 mg/dL) warrant more than 3 points. So a seemingly innocuous sigmoid resection (abdominal surgery = 3 points) in a 70-year-old gentleman (5 points) in atrial fibrillation (7 points, and 20% of septuagenarians exhibit atrial fibrillation) who suffered just a "little" heart attack 3 months ago (10 points) climbs into the highest risk category with 26 total points. In the Goldman and colleagues and Mangano and Goldman studies, class IV risk (patients scoring more than 25 points) suffered a 26% chance of major complications such as ventricular tachycardia or ventricular fibrillation or death.[25,26]

Now—15 to 30 years later—we may be doing a little better, but the cardiovascular system remains the culprit. The purposes of this section are to review the various tests of cardiovascular function and to develop a practical and safe algorithm for preoperative cardiac evaluation. There are no surprises here. The bigger the operation, the higher the cardiac risk; the older the patient, the riskier the outcome is likely to be. Conversely, even two decades ago, Warner and colleagues reviewed the 30-day mortality of over 45,000 patients undergoing outpatient anesthesia and surgery[31] [*see Figure 3*]. Adjusting for age and gender, these authors concluded that the low-risk surgical procedure provoked no more deaths than would have occurred during a month without surgery. On the other hand, when a surgeon is confronted with a high-risk patient needing a high-risk procedure, a strategic alternative is not a retreat; it is responsible medicine. All too often, however, an elderly patient presents with a clear mesenteric vascular accident, and surgical intervention is the only option. This situation obligates a compassionate explanation to the patient, a sensitive discussion with the family, and a bold acceptance of reality by the surgeon. Most often, however, both the patient and the procedure are solidly positioned in an intermediate gray zone.

Conceptually, cardiac dysfunction may be comfortably discriminated into four broad categories. Each may be defined using standard cardiac function tests. These cardiac dysfunction categories are ventricular systolic compromise, ventricular diastolic compromise, valvular heart disease, and myocardial ischemic disease resulting in electrophysiologic instability.

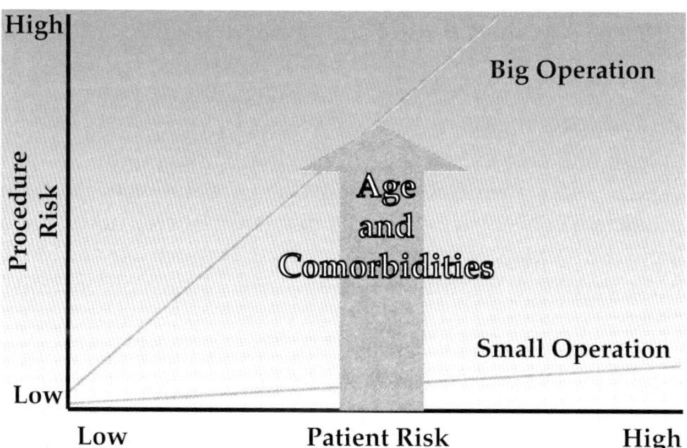

Figure 3 **A low-risk operation (such as a cataract) renders negligible additional morbidity and mortality to a patient (irrespective of American Society of Anesthesiologists [ASA] status) with or without the surgical procedure.**

FUNCTIONAL CAPACITY

Patients who are able to exercise regularly without limitation generally have sufficient cardiovascular reserve to withstand stressful operations. Those with limited exercise capacity are prone to exhibit this poor cardiovascular reserve either during or after noncardiac surgery. Even outside the surgical arena, patients with poor functional status enjoy a shorter life span.[32]

Functional capacity is readily expressed in terms of METs. One MET is equivalent to the energy expended (or the oxygen used) in sitting and reading this chapter (3.5 mL O_2/kg/min). For a 70 kg person, one MET amounts to 70 kg × 3.5 mL O_2/kg/min, or 245 mL O_2/kg/min. Multiples of the baseline MET value can then be used to quantify the aerobic demands posed by specific activities. A modification of the Duke Activity Status Index[33] developed 20 years ago is still a practical guide [*see Table 6*].

Functional status correlates with exercise treadmill testing. Multiple studies have indicated that perioperative cardiac and long-term risks are increased in patients who are unable to meet the 4-MET demand associated with most normal daily activities. This higher-risk status can be signaled by poor performance on a treadmill test protocol [*see Table 7*]. However, just by talking with your patient, you can assess the patient's exercise capacity. This assessment is a practical, inexpensive, and accurate predictor of your patient's ability to tolerate a surgical stress.

RESTING ELECTROCARDIOGRAM

To determine whether a patient or an organ can tolerate a stress, we must stress that organ or patient. Intuitively, it does not make much sense to obtain a resting ECG in an asymptomatic young or middle-aged patient. With older patients, the resting ECG can exhibit abnormal rhythms and an old scar (big Q waves). In a retrospective analysis of 23,036 patients undergoing cardiac surgery, the preoperative ECG improved the predictive value of perioperative cardiac events in comparison with clinical risk stratification alone.[34] This predictive benefit was not apparent in low-risk patients undergoing low-risk procedures.[34] We conclude that a routine resting ECG prior to even major surgery in a young or middle-aged asymptomatic patient (ASA I/II) with no historical red flags is very low yield. Vascular disease, however, is systemic disease. Prior to vascular surgery, patients deserve a resting ECG.

Table 7 **Bruce Protocol Stress Test**

Stage	*% Grade*	*mph*	*METs*
1	10	1.7	4.7
2	12	2.5	7.0
3	14	3.4	10.1
4	16	4.2	12.9
5	18	5.0	15.0

MET = metabolic equivalent.

Current guidelines discourage routine preoperative noninvasive cardiac testing for most intermediate-risk preoperative patients. In a 2006 study, 1,476 patients were stratified according to their RCRI scores.[35] Of these, 770 patients on beta-blocker therapy with tight heart rate control met the criteria for intermediate risk. This intermediate-risk group was split and randomly assigned to receive either cardiac stress testing or continued beta-blocker therapy. Some degree of ischemia was noted in 25.8% of the patients in the testing group, but analysis of the 30-day outcomes after operation found no difference between the two groups with respect to the incidence of major cardiac adverse events. The major difference was that patients in the untested group underwent their procedures 3 weeks sooner than patients in the tested group. Noninvasive cardiac testing even in intermediate-risk patients just takes additional time without discernible benefit.

In general, indications for specialized testing are the same prior to surgery as in the nonoperative setting. If your patient exhibits the kind of cardiac indicators that might warrant coronary revascularization in the absence of an impending surgical procedure, proceed with noninvasive testing; otherwise, do not proceed.

The timing of cardiac testing depends on the urgency of the noncardiac procedure, the risk factors present, and specific considerations associated with the procedure. Coronary revascularization before noncardiac surgery has sometimes been advocated as a way of enabling a patient to tolerate a noncardiac procedure, but it is appropriate only for a very small subset of very high-risk patients.

The ACC/AHA guidelines provide the following summary recommendations. In each instance, evidence is persuasive, or only Level B:

1. Pre- and postoperative resting 12-lead ECG is not indicated in asymptomatic patients undergoing low-risk surgical procedures.
2. Vascular disease is a systemic disease, so resting 12-lead ECG is indicated in patients undergoing vascular surgery.
3. Preoperative resting 12-lead ECG is recommended in patients with the following clinical risk factors: cerebrovascular disease, diabetes mellitus, renal insufficiency, a history of ischemic heart disease, or a history of congestive heart failure.

This leaves a relatively wide gray zone, in which there is only Level C, or "pretty good," evidence:

1. Preoperative resting 12-lead ECG is not helpful in asymptomatic patients undergoing intermediate-risk surgical procedures.
2. Resting 12-lead ECG is recommended in patients with known coronary artery disease prior to intermediate-risk operations.

CARDIAC EXERCISE STRESS TESTING

A monitored exercise stress test would logically appear to be a safe way of reproducing the hemodynamic components of surgical stress. Exercise testing on a treadmill has the advantage that the results can be quantified in METs achieved, and the test (unlike an operation) can be rapidly aborted. The patient walks on a treadmill as the speed and slope are increased [*see Table 7*]. Four outcome variables are continuously monitored: angina, ST-T wave changes, ectopy as a reflection of ischemia, and, most importantly, blood pressure. When a healthy person exercises, the blood pressure should rise. No change, or a decrease in blood pressure, is ominous both for perioperative cardiovascular complications and as a prognostic indicator of nonoperative life expectancy.[32]

In 2009, the ACC collaborated with the AHA Task Force on Practice Guidelines and produced a comprehensive analysis of exercise stress testing for myocardial ischemia and functional capacity.[36] These authors provided a table cataloguing 10 published studies in which high-risk patients prior to peripheral vascular or abdominal aortic aneurysm (high-risk) surgery were subjected to exercise stress testing preoperatively.

When exercise tolerance testing (ETT) is used to identify obstructive coronary disease, the results are disappointing. As many as half of the patients with a single 70% coronary artery stenosis will sail through ETT with a "normal" result. For patients with involvement of all three major coronary arteries or even left main disease, the sensitivity is better at 86%, the specificity remains only 53%.[37]

The mechanics of an ETT are relatively straightforward. A 12-lead ECG is continuously monitored as the patient walks on a treadmill. The Bruce protocol is most commonly used [*see Table 7*]. The patient is required to walk at 1.7 mph (not very fast) on a 10% incline. Every 3 minutes, the incline is increased by 2%, and the treadmill speed is increased, as indicated below.

The patient is questioned continuously concerning chest pain and fatigue, while the blood pressure is determined at the end of each stage. Although the early stages of the Bruce protocol do not seem like a lot of exercise, this may need to be modified to a lower workload for sedentary and elderly patients. Thus, the first two stages of a "modified Bruce protocol" are conducted at 1.7 mph at a zero grade (stage I) and then a 5% grade (stage II).

The inconvenience and expense of formal exercise testing have prompted many investigations to develop more accessible and practical historical questioning and functional testing strategies. Therefore, the ACC and the AHA equate the ability to walk around the block on level ground as stage I (Bruce protocol) or less than 4 METs; walking up two flight of stairs is around 6 METs or stage II (Bruce protocol).[37] Nikolić and colleagues refined stair climbing by monitoring pulse oximetry in 101 patients prior to thoracic surgery as they climbed stairs.[38] Eighty-seven of the 101 patients suffered at least one postoperative complication. Disappointingly, age, gender, and oximetry-monitored stair climbing were not predictive. This is an example of high-risk patients undergoing high-risk surgery, so the experienced surgeon should have been prepared for trouble irrespective of any preoperative tests.

Conversely, multiple groups have linked the graded results of an ETT to a patient's annual mortality.[32] These investigators identified 12% of a medically treated group of patients with coronary artery disease who could manage only stage I of a Bruce protocol. These patients suffered over 5% annual mortality. In this study, 34% of patients carrying the diagnosis of coronary artery disease who could accomplish stage III of a Bruce protocol suffered less than 1% annual mortality. It would appear to be a minor conceptual leap to assume that the risk characteristics predicting a short life are similar to the patient limitations that cause perioperative morbidity and mortality. For example, Myers and colleagues retrospectively studied the ETT results of 6,000 veterans (with and without a diagnosis of coronary artery disease) and compared the maximum METs achieved with annual medically treated mortality data.[32] Again, patients who could achieve 8 METs or more suffered less than half of the mortality of patients who could not complete Bruce protocol stage I. The predictive value of METs in this study also overwhelmed smoking, hypertension, body mass index of 30 or greater, chronic obstructive pulmonary disease (COPD), and diabetes.[32]

So functional capacity, measured in METs, is a comprehensive assessment of cardiopulmonary status and muscle strength and would appear to be superior to tests specific for myocardial ischemia in calibrating a patient's risk for perioperative morbidity and mortality.

VENTRICULAR FUNCTION TESTING

Radionuclide angiography, cardiac ventriculography, gated blood pool imaging, and multigated acquisition (MUGA) scans are different names for the same procedure. An intravenous injection of technetium-99m (pertechnetate) labels the patient's red blood cells (RBCs) in vivo. The patient's heart is then scanned with a gamma camera. Low-level gamma radiation is emitted by RBCs tagged with technetium, and the radiation detected at end-systole is then related to the radiation at end-diastole and thus permits calculation of an ejection fraction. The radiation emitted during a single cardiac cycle is not sufficient signal to reliably calculate the ventricular volumes, so multiple cycles are acquired "gated" to the ECG (thus, "multigated acquisition"). A healthy ventricle ejects about 60% of its end-diastolic volume with each heartbeat.

Exercise MUGA scanning can also be performed, typically with the patient on a stationary bicycle. With exercise, both the patient's blood pressure and ejection fraction should rise.

With advancing age and congestive failure, the increasing stiffness of the ventricles can be measured in terms of the time to peak filling rate. The shorter this interval, the more compliant the ventricle. Diastolic dysfunction is now increasingly recognized as an etiology of heart failure; the ventricle becomes too stiff to fill during diastole. A healthy heart should be capable of filling completely within 130 to 200 milliseconds.

In patients with a normal, healthy exercise capacity, preoperative measurement of ventricular function will be very low yield, and the possibility of modifying any perioperative strategy by virtue of this test is unlikely.

In addition to the obvious patients who present with congestive failure and/or limited functional capacity, the surgeon should be mindful of patients on chemotherapeutic drugs. Two common culprits are doxorubicin (Adriamycin) and immunotherapy (trastuzumab [Herceptin]), which are both frequently cardiotoxic.

STAIR CLIMBING: PUTTING IT ALL TOGETHER

Arguably, climbing stairs incorporates cardiopulmonary status, muscle strength, and "vitality" into a single practical and inexpensive test of performance capacity. Brunelli and colleagues studied 640 patients scheduled for pulmonary resective surgery with a preoperative, symptom-limited stair climbing test.[39] Patients who climbed less than 12 m (less than two flights of stairs) experienced a twofold increase in complications ($p < .0001$) and a 13-fold increase in mortality ($p < .0001$) and incurred costs 2.5 times higher than patients who could manage a climb of 22 m (more than two flights). These investigators then refined the stair climbing test by concurrently measuring finger oximetry. While studying 536 patients breathing room air during stair climbing, they sought to determine whether oxygen saturation less than 90% or desaturation greater than 4% drop from resting level better discriminated the likelihood of postoperative complications. The stair climbing was uniquely suited to elicit oxygen desaturation, and patients exhibiting oxygen desaturation greater than 4% were twice as likely to suffer postoperative problems. Exercise-induced desaturation (> 4%) appeared superior to resting finger oximetry as a predictor of postoperative problems.

Pulmonary Function Tests

Conceptually, pulmonary dysfunction may comfortably be divided into four broad categories: obstructive airway disease, hyperinflation, restriction, and diffusion (compromise). Each of these categories may be defined through the use of standard pulmonary function tests (PFTs).

OBSTRUCTIVE AIRWAY DISEASE

When surgeons receive multiple-page PFT results, we almost always focus first on a single parameter: forced expiratory volume in 1 second (FEV_1). This measurement requires patients to inhale to maximum lung volume (total lung capacity) and then exhale as forcefully and quickly as they are able to [*see Figure 4*]. These tests may require a "race correction" for ethnicity of as much as 6 to 12%. Healthy young adults can exhale almost all of their total lung capacity within a second or two, so a healthy FEV_1 approaches 4 to 5 L! After 2 seconds, healthy lungs have emptied down to residual volume. A patient with asthma or COPD cannot move air through airways that have been constricted by bronchospasm [*see Figure 4*]. So if your patient, following bronchodilators, can only exhale in 1 second (FEV_1) less than 70% of all they can inhale (forced vital capacity [FVC]), they have met the Global Initiative for Obstructive Lung Disease (GOLD) criterion for COPD ($FEV_1/FVC < 70\%$).

In a patient with significantly compromised airway resistance, pulmonary function should also be assessed following inhaled aerosolized bronchodilators. These drugs come in three varieties: short-acting $beta_2$ agonists, such as albuterol; long-acting $beta_2$ agonists, such as salmeterol; and methylxanthines, such as caffeine and theophylline.

Many receptor agonist/antagonist drugs are somewhat, but not absolutely, receptor specific. So in this chapter, when we recommend a $beta_2$ agonist for perioperative bronchodilation and simultaneously encourage a cardiospecific $beta_1$ inhibitor (such as metoprolol or atenolol) for cardioprotection, you may appropriately envision a patient entering the operating room with one foot capably placed on the accelerator while the other foot is simultaneously placed on the brakes.

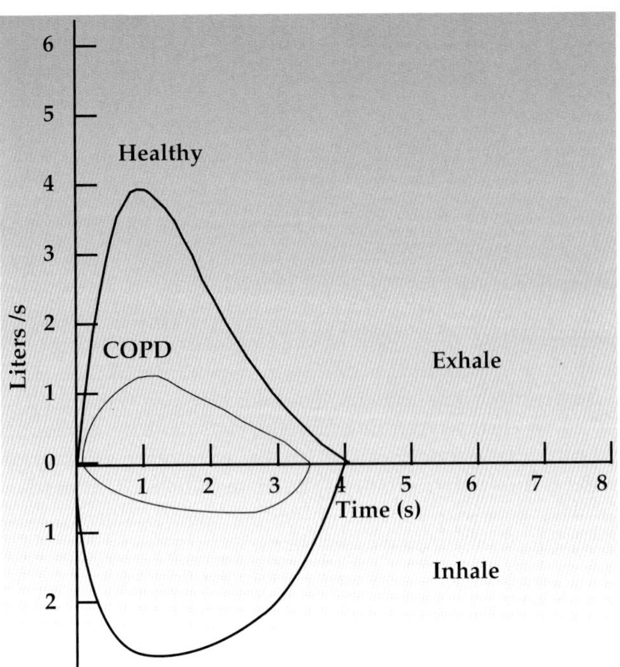

Figure 4 **A flow-volume loop relates volume of exhaled/inhaled gas to time (seconds). Note that the volume of air that a young, healthy person [illegible] forcibly exhale in 1 second (FEV_1) can be as high as 4 to [illegible] L. Chronic obstructive pulmonary disease (COPD) dramatically reduces air flow.**

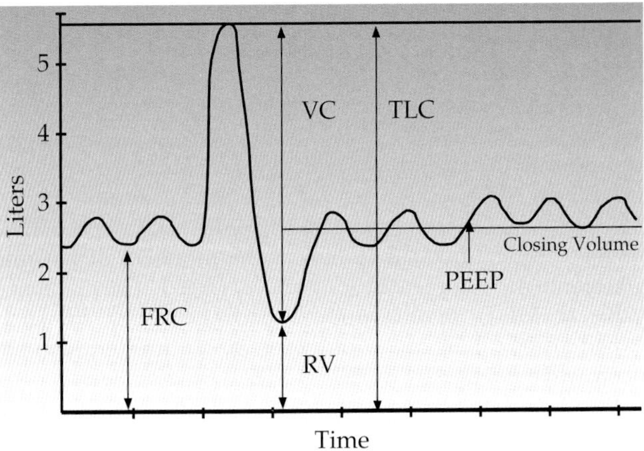

Figure 5 **Spirometric lung volumes. The therapeutic purpose of positive end-expiratory pressure (PEEP) is to raise the functional residual capacity (FRC), or the lung volume following tidal exhalation, above closing volume so that terminal airways never close during tidal exhalation. RV = residual volume; TLC = total lung capacity; VC = vital capacity or the volume of the air exhaled from the TLC to RV.**

HYPERINFLATION

Lung volumes are measured using a relatively simple dilutional principle. For example, 1 L of 100% nondiffusible helium is added to a spirometer and mixed. When the helium concentration gauge reads 10% helium, the volume of the spirometer can be calculated to be 10 L. The respiratory technician then places a tube into the patient's mouth and connects the tube to the spirometer with a handheld valve. The patient is instructed either to achieve total lung capacity (TLC) and exhale down to residual volume (RV) or just to breathe comfortably, initiating each breath from functional residual capacity (FRC) [*see Figure 5*]. When the technician observes the patient to be at the desired lung volume, the technician flips the valve connecting the patient to the spirometer. The increased volume of dilution equals the patient's lung volume at the time the valve was opened. So if the valve is opened at the end of a comfortable tidal breath (FRC) and the helium gauge concentration falls to 8%, then the total volume of dilution must be 12.5 L (spirometer plus FRC volume), or 12.5 L minus 10 L (for the spirometer) equals a 2.5-liter FRC.

If the patient continues to breathe while connected to the spirometer, the helium concentration should stabilize at 8%.

We all sigh frequently. Try not to sigh for several minutes, and you will become surprisingly uncomfortable. When a young patient sighs, the helium concentration will remain at 8% (no increased volume of distribution). But when an elderly patient sighs, the helium concentration, which had previously leveled off at 7.5%, revealing a higher "hyperinflated" FRC of 3.33 L, typically falls a little further, perhaps to 7.35%. The sigh must have uncovered an additional volume of distribution or volume of previously trapped gas. The new total volume of helium distribution is now 13.61 L minus 10 L (spirometer) minus 3.33 L (FRC), and the volume of trapped gas is 280 mL. This volume of trapped gas [illegible] due to [illegible] because collapsed alveoli could not further dilute the helium concentration in the system. Therefore, this additional decrease in helium concentration must be due to previously trapped alveolar gas, producing perfused but not ventilated lung (shunt). Histologically, terminal airways have no cartilaginous rings to hold them open. With age, increasing interstitial lung water (which is characteristic of congestive heart failure), and obesity, these terminal airways collapse at lower lung volumes. The lung volume at which terminal airways collapse is termed "closing volume." Thus, a big barrel chest with a flat diaphragm, an increased anteroposterior diameter, and radiolucent lungs on a chest x-ray is a natural attempt by the patient to set the FRC above the closing volume. When the closing volume is above the FRC, terminal airways close during each tidal breath, creating a transient shunt.

Therapeutically, when we ventilate a patient, we can elevate FRC above closing volume by adding positive end-expiratory pressure (PEEP) [*see Figure 5*]. A decade ago, the Acute Respiratory Distress Syndrome Network (ARDSnet) reported that lower tidal volume ventilation (6 mL/kg) in patients with acute respiratory distress syndrome reduced mortality and increased ventilator-free days compared with traditional tidal volume ventilation (10 to 15 mL/kg).[40] Controversy lingers as to whether these lower tidal volumes promote further airway collapse.

RESTRICTIVE LUNG DISEASE

The ability to expand the lung can be constrained by chest wall scarring (secondary to a large burn), pleural fibrosis (secondary to tuberculosis), or a decrease in lung parenchymal compliance secondary to pulmonary interstitial fibrosis (multiple inflammatory etiologies).

Pulmonary function studies exhibit reduced lung volumes. The patient's vital capacity is reduced, but there is no obstruction to the airway flow, so the exhaled gas (the limited volume that there is) can be exhaled quickly. Therefore, the FEV_1/FVC ratio is normal or may actually be increased.

DIFFUSION COMPROMISE

Once oxygen arrives in an alveolus, it is uncommon for transfer across the alveolar-capillary membrane to be limited. One can imagine, however, circumstances in which this could occur. At extremely high pulmonary blood flow, blood might not linger in the pulmonary capillaries long enough to saturate hemoglobin. Conversely, with anemia, all available hemoglobin might be saturated very early as RBCs traverse the pulmonary capillaries. With hemorrhage into the lung parenchyma, oxygen can be diverted away from pulmonary capillaries. In late-stage emphysema, the alveolar septae are destroyed and the effective alveolar-capillary surface area is reduced, but this is not a diffusion problem. The classic pulmonary diffusion disease is an idiopathic interstitial pneumonitis (Hamman-Rich syndrome). Patients present with nonspecific shortness of breath. A lung biopsy reveals noncellular debris thickening the diffusion distance from alveolus to pulmonary capillary. The measured diffusion of carbon monoxide test (DLCO) should reveal compromised gas diffusion. Fortunately, true limitation of oxygen diffusion across the alveolar-capillary membrane is not common.

For a DLCO test, the patient inhales a tiny concentration of a maximally diffusible gas (carbon monoxide 0.3%) and a small volume of a maximally nondiffusible gas, such as helium, along with a large amount of room air. The patient holds his or her breath for 10 seconds and exhales. Concentrations of carbon monoxide and helium are then measured in the exhaled gas. Both gases will have been diluted by the inhaled breath, so the concentrations of both gases will decrease. Most of the diffusible carbon monoxide should have been transferred to the pulmonary capillary blood. The lower the exhaled carbon monoxide, the better the diffusion capability of the lung. Unfortunately, there are many ways to introduce error into this test. If the patient inhales rapidly, he or she can translocate additional blood into the pulmonary capillaries and falsely enhance the apparent diffusing capacity. Conversely, severe anemia permits rapid saturation of the limited hemoglobin with carbon monoxide, resulting in a false depression in the DLCO. A heavy smoker may live with carboxyhemoglobin as high as 10% and actually excrete carbon monoxide, thus confounding the test. Even most pulmonologists acknowledge that the DLCO is not a very good test.

Testing for Nutritional Abnormalities

For nutritional support, consensus statements and regulatory guidelines endorse the long-hallowed practice of identifying patients at increased risk for complications due to protein or calorie deficits. Again, this is called prognostic testing. The implication is that the benefit of special support will be confined to these patients. Poor functional status ("bedridden, requires assistance to ambulate") is a bad prognostic sign [*see Table 6*]. In cancer patients, functional status is typically more important than nodal status, cytologic differentiation, or surgical margins in predicting morbidity and mortality. But assessing functional status provides no direct information on selection of therapy.

Much more therapeutically useful than prognostic testing is predictive (or directive) testing, which means identifying patients who will benefit from a specified, available intervention. By definition, predictive testing identifies that subset of "bad prognosis" patients who can be helped. This requires the existence of a therapeutic intervention of demonstrated benefit. It also requires the identification of those patients not too ill but not too well to benefit from the associated therapy.

Proof that a testing strategy is predictive or directive, not merely prognostic, is best demonstrated by randomized trials comparing outcome in groups receiving best conventional care with or without the proposed test. This is a high standard but has been met in some situations.

The therapy-prediction conundrum exists in nutritional support where possibly effective therapies have been applied in patients not able to benefit due to absence of an accurate predictive test to select the best target population. For example, identification of the role of vitamin B_{12} in treating anemia awaited the ability to identify macrocytosis and, later, vitamin B_{12} serum levels. Previously, most populations of anemic patients were dominated by those with iron deficiency, and no predictive test was available to find the subset benefiting from vitamin B_{12} supplementation, so the benefit of vitamin B_{12} remained unknown.

A vivid illustration of the difference between prognostic versus predictive/directive testing has recently arisen in breast cancer. The presence in breast tumor cells of human epidermal growth factor receptor type 2 (HER-2) has long been recognized as an indicator of poor prognosis, independent of stage, differentiation, or estrogen receptor status. Initially, nothing could be done in response to this information until the development of a blocker for HER-2, trastuzumab (Herceptin). Suddenly, HER-2 receptor testing permitted identification of a target patient capable of response. Patients with positive receptors given the blocker improved, whereas those with negative receptors did not. Not only was the HER-2 receptor test predictive, its prognostic implication also reversed itself. The receptor-positive patients now do better than average.

In nutrition for surgical patients, a variety of composite scores and indices have been proposed to predict prognosis. One clearly labeled prognostic measure, the Prognostic Nutritional Index (PNI), was proposed in 1980 to quantify surgical risk. This measure was used (in modified form) in the design of a large prospective, randomized trial of preoperative total parenteral nutrition (TPN) in veterans undergoing major general, vascular, or thoracic surgery.[41] Patients judged too well nourished or too malnourished by this screen were omitted from the study, and the remainder, judged "moderately malnourished," were randomized into TPN or no TPN preoperatively. The modified PNI score was composed of albumin and weight loss scores only, which had previously been shown to be prognostic and easy to apply.

Unfortunately, after randomizing and treating 395 patients, the investigators found no outcome difference between the treatment groups, and in this sense, the trial's main result was negative.[42] Retrospective subsetting by degree of severity within "moderate malnutrition" using a Subjective Global Assessment (SGA) tool[43] was then performed. This was interpreted to show that patients not severely enough malnourished to benefit from the extra protein and calories suffered increased septic complications and overall did worse with TPN. In contrast, the more malnourished patients did exhibit a net benefit.

For the studies reviewed in the following section, we use a scoring system that grades the conclusions as follows: Level A, supported by prospective, randomized, controlled trials (PRCTs) or meta-analyses of PRCTs; Level B, supported by nonrandomized, prospective, retrospective, or case-controlled studies; and Level C, supported by uncontrolled published experiences, case reports, or "expert opinion."

PREOPERATIVE TOTAL PARENTERAL NUTRITION

We have defined preoperative TPN to be intravenous provision of calories and nitrogen sufficient to meet metabolic needs for 5 or more days before elective surgery. Fourteen randomized, controlled trials of this approach, involving over 1,100 patients, have been examined,[42,44–49] chiefly involving gastrointestinal cancer patients with at least moderate malnutrition and typically providing at least 7 to 10 days of preoperative TPN. Ten of these 14 studies found a benefit from TPN, which in five reached conventional statistical significance for reduced postoperative morbidity. The pooled results indicate an overall reduction in the risk of postoperative morbidity of about 10% in the TPN groups, that is, a reduction in the rate of complications of approximately 30%. Only one center found a statistically significant reduction in mortality [*see Figure 6*].

Based on these studies, we conclude that for malnourished gastrointestinal cancer patients, 7 to 10 days of preoperative TPN reduces postoperative morbidity (Level A).

POSTOPERATIVE TOTAL PARENTERAL NUTRITION

Routine administration of TPN to general surgical patients in the immediate postoperative period has been studied in nine randomized, controlled trials involving over 700 patients.[46,50–54] No consistent benefit has been demonstrated, and the possibility of harm has been raised. These data are summarized in Figure 7.

Based on these studies, we conclude that, outside of a study situation in defined patient groups, routine use of postoperative TPN is not recommended (Level A).

It is also clear that nutritional support of patients unable to eat for long periods after surgery is needed to prevent starvation. The duration of starvation that can be tolerated without increased morbidity is unknown and depends in part on the previous nutritional status and current metabolic stresses the patient faces. Most feel that, after 5 to 10 days without adequate intake, special support is appropriate (Level C). For stressed or already malnourished patients, this interval will be shorter. Although the enteral route of administration is preferable, if the gut is not working adequately, TPN is needed (Level B).

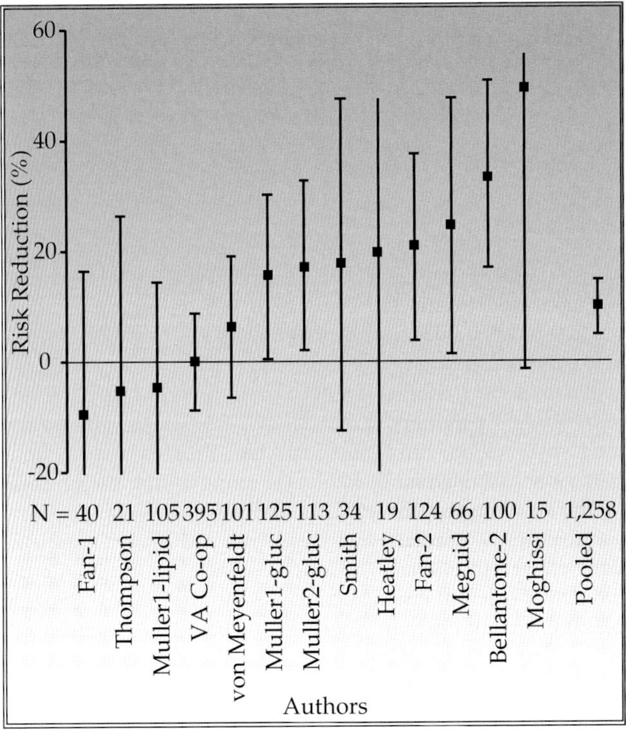

Figure 6 **Effect of preoperative total parenteral nutrition on postoperative complications.[101]**

In the majority of trials summarized here, the quantity and type of substrates given were not what is now thought to be optimal. For example, calories were often given in amounts substantially greater than metabolic needs. It is probable that

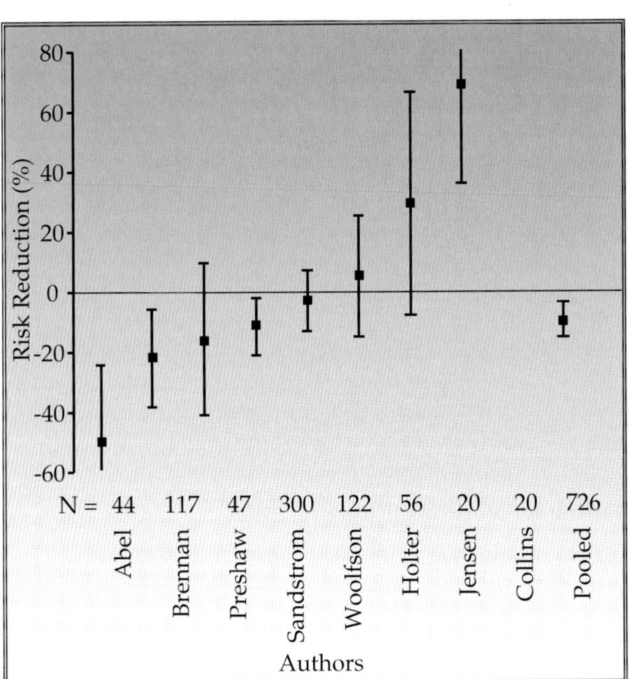

Figure 7 **Effect of early postoperative total parenteral nutrition (TPN) on postoperative complications. These results are disappointing, but the quantity and type of substrates infused in these trials were not what is now thought to be optimal.[101]**

outcomes in many of these trials would improve if the trials were repeated using present-day understanding of caloric needs and other metabolic requirements in specific patient groups (Level C).

SPECIAL ENTERAL FEEDING

Provision of special enteral nutrition via tubes placed in the gastrointestinal tract perioperatively has been studied in 10 randomized trials.[55-57] Five of these compared the enterally supported to patients receiving TPN, and the other five used a comparison group of routine oral feeding. In the enteral nutrition versus TPN trials for postoperative trauma patients, septic morbidity and mortality were minimized with enteral feeding, which is deemed superior to TPN.

One study reported a decrease in mortality in burned children provided with high-protein enteral supplementation compared with standard feeding.[56] A trial of nocturnal tube feeding in malnourished female hip fracture patients demonstrated speedier rehabilitation and shorter hospital stays.[57]

On the basis of the available information, we conclude that special enteral nutrition is helpful in burn and malnourished hip fracture patients (Level A). In trauma patients requiring special support, the enteral route is associated with decreased septic morbidity compared with the parenteral route (Level A).

TIGHT GLUCOSE CONTROL

Extending work from the world of chronic diabetes management, in which ever-tighter glucose regulation is associated with improved outcomes, Van den Berghe and colleagues presented two large randomized trials on intensive care (ICU) patients receiving supplemental calories early in their courses.[58,59] The first of these, on surgical patients (chiefly postoperative cardiac patients), revealed a clear benefit in morbidity—and a raw reduction in mortality of 11%—when glucose levels were maintained below 110 mg/dL. Hypoglycemia in this ICU setting was not a serious problem.[58] A follow-up study from the same authors showed little or no benefit using the same approach in medical ICU patients.[59] Finally, a large (over 6,000 patients) multinational study coordinated from Australia and New Zealand found a worsening of mortality with tight glucose control in similar patients.[60]

The issue of tight control is of obvious importance in TPN patients, and it may be that disappointing results in the perioperative trials summarized above might be improved with better glucose regulation. Tighter glucose control carries risks of hypoglycemia and hypokalemia.[36]

Target glucose levels in recent randomized trials appear to be converging toward about 140 to 150 mg/dL. Until more definitive data are available, this target seems safe for patients treated outside an ICU (Level C).

IMMUNONUTRITION AND "DESIGNER FEEDS"

The provision of special nutrients with the intent of stimulating the immune system, or providing targeted support for a failing liver or kidneys, and thereby reducing septic complications has been studied in a large number of trials that were reviewed by Dhaliwal and Heyland,[61] with variable results. A fundamental problem is the use of ad hoc mixtures of arginine, fish oil, RNA fragments, and sometimes glutamine, in various proportions, for which no rationale is given. The more recent of these trials have been much less encouraging than the earlier reports, with actual harm being reported in several trials of products containing high arginine levels. The recent publication from Holland of a randomized blinded trial of nearly 600 patients testing this strategy is unequivocally negative and may serve to foster a more cautious scientific approach toward evaluating such strategies.[62]

Immunonutrition and "designer" feeds are not supported by a satisfactory evidence base (Level C).

PREOPERATIVE ORAL CARBOHYDRATE LOADING

The traditional dictum of nihil per os (NPO) after midnight for procedures to be performed under general anesthesia has been challenged in some centers in Scandinavia and eastern Europe since the 1990s. In these facilities, anesthesiologists provide several hundred milliliters of carbohydrate-enriched electrolyte solutions swallowed 2 hours prior to surgery. The rationale is that stress-induced insulin resistance is normalized and patient well-being improved by ingestion of these "potions."[63] Interestingly, similar biochemical changes are also produced by glucose-containing intravenous lines in fasting preoperative patients.[64]

Ingestion of 200 mL clear liquids does not increase the risk of aspiration pneumonia as long as there is a delay of 1.5 to 2 hours before anesthesia. A Cochrane Review first published in 2003 concludes that no strong evidence of harm from this practice can be adduced.[65] The generally small sample size in these reports contributes to this conservatism; most reports include fewer than 50 patients per group and are thus not powered to detect rare but catastrophic events. Gastric fluid secretion is traditionally quantified at approximately 100 mL/hr, so the gastric volumes are not likely to be influenced measurably by this preoperative cocktail.

Those concerned about insulin resistance might more easily and conventionally start the usual intravenous line an hour or two earlier and administer glucose by that route. But wetting the patient's thirsty tongue with 200 mL of clear fluid 2 hours prior to surgery is very likely to enhance patient comfort at negligible risk of aspiration (Level B).

How Can We Make Surgery Safer?

The problem with searching the available, conscientiously conducted clinical trials for answers is that the patients recruited for those trials never really fit the patient you are currently considering for surgical therapy. As indicated above [*see Figure 3*], patients undergoing "low-risk" operations will do pretty well even if they present with significant comorbidities—or as well as they would do without surgery.[31] The risk stratification strategies[25,26] [*see Table 3 and Table 5*[27]] each target the patient's cardiovascular system as the overwhelmingly dominant culprit promoting perioperative trouble.

Over the past decades, the scope of perioperative efforts to reduce cardiac risk with cardioprotective therapy has changed. At present, the emphasis is on plaque stabilization, reduction of myocardial oxygen demand (reduction of oxygen delivery to oxygen consumption mismatch), and myocardial protection, with revascularization reserved for a discrete subset of patients who would be candidates for cardiac revascularization regardless of any elective preoperative evaluation. It is hypothesized that the likelihood of coronary artery plaque rupture may be increased by perioperative stressors such as amplified sympathetic activation, vasospasm, disruption of coagulation homeostasis, and oxygen supply-demand mismatch.[66]

Physicians, and perhaps more clearly surgeons, are sufficiently intellectually arrogant that we are more comfortable accepting a conclusion if we can understand the "mechanism" of the recommendation. Thus, if the heart is the organ that most endangers our patients, and we can reduce cardiac work/stress with a beta blocker, why not give this perioperative, antiadrenergic protection to all of our patients—or at least to all surgical patients with cardiovascular disease? Interestingly, and perhaps predictably, perioperative beta blockade produced a significant reduction in mortality in patients undergoing abdominal aortic aneurysmectomy (most likely patients with concurrent coronary artery disease).[67] No such benefit was appreciated in patients who were less likely to suffer comorbid coronary artery disease undergoing esophagectomy, hepatectomy, pancreatectomy, colectomy, gastrectomy, or pulmonary lobectomy.[67] These investigators concluded that evidence-based process measures are "procedure specific" and do not necessarily reflect overall hospital quality.

If some patients do not appear to benefit from perioperative beta blockade, is overuse of this particular therapy likely to hurt them? Some controversy remains regarding appropriate management of patients identified preoperatively as having significant but stable coronary artery disease. Current data support the use of presumptive medical therapy, and this has led to reductions in the extent of preoperative cardiac assessment, thereby decreasing the time from surgical diagnosis to surgical therapy. Perhaps surprisingly, documented coronary stenoses account for only 50% of perioperative myocardial infarctions; the remaining 50% occur in vascular distributions unrelated to documented coronary disease.[68,69] The presence of severe stenosis is more a "marker" of disease, and thus the subset of patients at risk, rather than a finite predictor of endangered myocardial territory. In part, preoperative cardiac testing identifies this "at-risk" subset, even though the stenotic lesion may not be the cause of the postoperative ischemic event. The inability to assess the propensity for coronary plaque rupture proves to be the main challenge in both risk stratification and risk factor modification.

THE BETA-BLOCKER CONTROVERSY

The purported advantages of beta-blocker therapy include prolongation of diastole (and, thus, augmentation of diastolic filling with concurrent accompanying improvement in coronary artery perfusion), reduction of ischemic ventricular dysrhythmias, and reduction of sympathetic tone.[70,71] Despite the plethora of available data, the argument for preoperative use of beta blockers to modify cardiac risk remains controversial. Except in high-risk vascular procedures, perioperative cardiac events are so rare among patients enrolled in randomized, controlled trials of perioperative beta blockade that any absolute reduction in cardiac risk is difficult to detect. However, in high-risk vascular procedures, the data are overwhelmingly persuasive. Poldermans and colleagues screened 1,351 vascular patients (high risk) and identified 846 patients with one or more cardiac risk factors (very high risk).[72] Of this group, 173 patients exhibited positive dobutamine stress echocardiography (very, very high risk). Fifty-nine patients were randomly assigned to perioperative beta blockade and were compared with 53 patients who received "standard" perioperative care. The primary end point of death or nonfatal myocardial infarction occurred in two (3.4%) of the beta-blocker group and in 18 (34%) of the standard care group (3.4% versus 34%; $p < .001$). It is clearly not permissible to extrapolate from this "very, very high risk" procedure-specific group to a "routine" general surgical patient.

Unfortunately, the studies on the opposite end of the risk spectrum are more confusing. Lindenauer and colleagues divided 782,969 patients (a huge number) into high, intermediate, and low risk for major, noncardiac surgery.[73] Again, perioperative beta blockade was associated with reduced risk for in-hospital death in high-risk patients. Perhaps surprisingly, beta blockade appeared to provoke increased trouble in the low-risk group. Subsequent review of this study design suggested that the low-risk patients did not receive beta blockers preoperatively and did not enter the beta-blocker arm of the study until after their operation, at a time when they were treated for a postoperative cardiac event.

The POISE Study Group attempted to resolve any recommendation to liberalize the use of beta blockers in noncardiac surgery by prospectively randomizing 8,351 patients at 190 hospitals in 23 countries.[74] The frighteningly formidable logistics of this study obligated a simplified investigative strategy. A large dose (two to eight times the standard dose) of extended-release metoprolol was given 2 to 4 hours before surgery to 4,174 patients unless their heart rate was below 60 beats/min. Fewer patients in the metoprolol group (5.8%) than in the placebo group (6.9%) reached the primary end point ($p < .0399$), but more patients in the beta-blocker group suffered a stroke (1.0% versus 0.5%) and/or died (3.1% versus 2.3%). In commentary on the POISE study, the 2009 ACC/AHA consensus document endorsed the use of beta blockers in high-risk patients but cautioned that: "routine administration of higher dose long-acting metoprolol in beta-blocker naïve patients on the day of surgery and in the absence of dose titration is associated with an increase in mortality."[75] Clinical investigation is hard to do. To enhance patient recruitment and standardize the POISE experimental protocol, patients with a heart rate over 60 beats/min were given a large dose of an extended-release beta blocker. In high-risk patients, even this regimen provided protection. However, neither we, nor they, should be surprised that a large dose of beta blocker to a patient with a heart rate of 60 beats/min might provoke bradycardia and hypotension with a resultant increase in cerebrovascular accident and even death.

Multiple smaller studies examining noncardiac surgical patients with surrogates for coronary artery disease such as diabetes,[76] mild hypertension,[77] and advanced age[78] have typically reported fewer instances of perioperative myocardial ischemia in the beta-blocker group but were not sufficiently powered to detect more ominous outcomes.

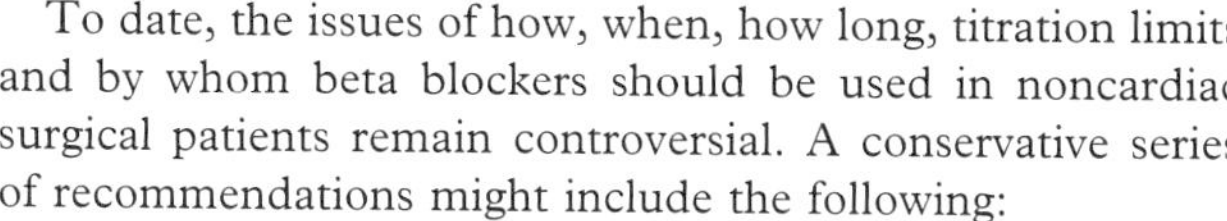

To date, the issues of how, when, how long, titration limits and by whom beta blockers should be used in noncardiac surgical patients remain controversial. A conservative series of recommendations might include the following:

1. When preoperative beta-blocker therapy is used, it is optimally initiated 1 to 2 weeks prior to surgery, targeting a resting heart rate of 60 to 80 beats/min and monitored to avoid hypotension (Level A).
2. Although it is not permissible to extrapolate from patients following a myocardial infarction to patients during noncardiac surgery, Cucherat assembled 17 trials of beta blockers in post–myocardial infarction patients and estimated that each reduction in heart rate of 10 beats/min (in the absence of hypotension) accrued a relative reduction in cardiac death of 30% (Level A).[79]
3. When a patient presents already on beta blockers, do not stop them (Level A).
4. The higher the perceived risk of the (especially vascular surgical) patient, the more likely it is that beta blockers will help (Level A).
5. Untitrated large doses of extended-release beta blockers in drug-naïve, low-risk patients are contraindicated (Level A).
6. This leaves a large middle "gray zone" group of patients in whom surgeons are on their own to use their best judgment.

STATINS

The statin (HMG-CoA [3-hydroxy-3-methylglutaryl coenzyme A] reductase inhibitor) story is complex but becoming clearer. HMG-CoA reductase is the rate-limiting step in cholesterol synthesis. Statins both inhibit cholesterol synthesis and increase expression of low-density lipoprotein (LDL) receptors, which results in an increased clearance of circulating LDL cholesterol. Cholesterol is, however, critically important to cell membrane stabilization. Cholesterol is the glue that holds the functionally important cell membrane phospholipids together. Only 20% of our cholesterol is ingested, whereas over 75% is synthesized by the liver. So, intuitively, it should be dangerous to manipulate this structurally pivotal molecule. Over 40 years ago, the Framingham study first associated hypercholesterolemia with atherosclerotic cardiovascular disease. So it made sense to try judiciously to lower cholesterol a little. A storm of inquiry followed. Law and colleagues recently reviewed several hundred trials and concluded that a reduction of LDL cholesterol by only 1.8 mmol/L conveyed a 60% decrease in ischemic heart disease and a 17% decrease in stroke.[80] Statins not only prevent heart disease; Poynter and colleagues reported a 47% reduction in the relative risk of colorectal cancer after adjusting for other recognized risk factors.[81] If both atherosclerosis and malignant neoplastic degeneration are exacerbated by systemic inflammation, then statins might be effective in pacifying inflamed patients (as evidenced by an elevated C-reactive protein) even independent of absolute LDL levels. And, Albert and colleagues report that they are.[82]

Surgery provokes inflammation. Logically, statins should help. Pan and colleagues and Ouattara and colleagues both reported a significant dose-dependent reduction in adverse cardiovascular outcomes with statins in coronary artery bypass surgery.[83,84] Biccard examined the implications of comorbid disease associated with perioperative cardiovascular risk for patients on statin therapy, the indications for perioperative statin protection, and the efficacy of acute perioperative beta blockade in addition to statin therapy and the effect of perioperative statin withdrawal.[85] Although many of the recent recommendations regarding retrospective reporting of statin trials may minimize some inherent investigator bias, the benefit of perioperative statins appears secure. Statins seem to benefit surgical patients with both cardiovascular and neoplastic disease; age overwhelms both of these indications. Patients who benefit from perioperative beta blockers are the same group that will likely derive advantage from statins. The data here are fuzzier, but in high-risk patients, both beta blockers and statins are useful. The dose and duration of preoperative prophylaxis are not clear, but 2 weeks is better than 2 hours. When a patient is already taking a statin, do not stop it.[85]

Smoking Cessation Programs

It is hard to stop smoking; it is an addiction. Although there is a paucity of data indicating that smoking cessation just prior to surgery changes outcome, there are a lot of data linking smoking to perioperative trouble. So, intuitively, it makes sense to ask your patients to stop. A planned surgical procedure, especially if the purpose is to resect cancer, can provide persuasive incentive. Cooley and colleagues recommended smoking cessation to patients undergoing surgery for lung cancer.[86] Eighty-four patients (89%) were "ever-smokers," and 35 (37%) reported smoking at diagnosis. Forty-six percent of the ever-smokers remained abstinent, 16% continued smoking, and 38% relapsed. In a separate analysis of lung cancer patients, these investigators catalogued the factors associated with failure to stop as young age, depression, and a household member who smokes.[87] A similar study identified the red flags of smoking cessation failure as mentholated cigarettes and a habit of enjoying the first cigarette within 30 minutes of awakening in the morning.[88]

Several groups have tested smoking cessation programs in a prospective, randomized fashion.[89,90] Prior to elective surgery, 210 smokers were randomly allocated to a nicotine replacement group or a "usual care" group. A whopping 73% of dependent smokers (> 10 cigarettes/day) reported (no confirmatory tests) abstinence prior to surgery compared with 56% abstinence in the "usual care" group. The bad news, however, is that 3 months following surgery, 82% and 95% of patients, respectively, were smoking again.[89]

A single puff on a cigarette produces profound vasoconstriction. Some surgical groups believe that it is justified to refuse breast reconstructive surgery to smokers.[91] Although it is clear that smokers suffer more postoperative complications, it is not evident that these problems will vanish if they stop.

The news is not all bad, however. Varenicline is a partial agonist/antagonist selective for alpha$_4$/beta$_2$ nicotinic acetylcholine receptors that is touted as a first-line treatment smoking cessation option. Garrison and Dugan reviewed eight clinical trials and reported continuous abstinence rates ranging from 21.9 to 34.6% at a year.[92] In a very slow race, even the lame can win.

Frailty Index: The "Eyeball" Test

Age is not the distance from the beginning but, more accurately, the proximity to the end. Although "frailty" has not yet achieved a standardized definition, we all recognize the status when we see it. Age and frailty are frequent, but not obligatory, partners. Frailty confers an increased risk of disability, falls, cognitive decline, hospitalization, and perioperative morbidity/mortality. Interestingly, the phenotype of frailty is not concordant with either disability or comorbidity, but the pathogenesis of frailty includes comorbidities, and disability is more the outcome than the cause.

Frailty can now be diagnosed as a medical syndrome.[93] Fried and colleagues identified this entity with three or more of the following: (1) unintentional weight loss of more than 10 pounds over a year; (2) self-reported exhaustion; (3) weak grip strength; and (4) slow walking speed or low physical activity [*see Figure 4*].[94] In this study, frailty was independently (stratifying for comorbidities) predictive (over 3 years) of falls, declining mobility, hospitalization (and intuitively perioperative morbidity/mortality), and death, with hazard ratios ranging from 1.82 to 4.46. Socioeconomic status resurfaces again, with frailty associated with lower education and income. As more statistics are successfully dissociating frailty from age,[95,96] frailty has now been proposed as the missing element in predicting operative mortality.[97]

Makary and colleagues prospectively measured frailty in 594 patients older than 65 years.[98] They used a 5-point scale, including weight loss, weakness, exhaustion, low physical activity, and walking speed. Frailty independently predicted postoperative complications, length of hospital stay, and nursing home discharge. Frailty even enhanced the predictive power of the ASA risk index ($p < .01$).

Although both the ASA and frailty indices aspire to quantitative status, the predictive (albeit subjective) value of the "eyeball" test performed by an experienced surgeon remains invaluable (although not formally tested). We continue to endorse this test.

An exercise prescription as an antidote to frailty[99,100] would make intuitive sense in the preoperative period. Castillo-Garzón and colleagues provided compelling evidence that patient-specific exercise programs can attenuate the negative consequences of frailty.[100]

Financial Disclosures: None Reported

References

1. Rudd RE. Improving Americans' health literacy. N Engl J Med 2010;363:2283–5.
2. Munro J, Booth A, Nicholl J. Routine preoperative testing: a systematic review of the evidence. Health Technol Assess 1997;1(12):i–iv; 1–62.
3. Lundberg GD. Perseverance of laboratory test ordering: a syndrome affecting clinicians. JAMA 1983;249:639.
4. Daniels M, Schroeder SA. Variation among physicians in use of laboratory tests. II. Relation to clinical productivity and outcomes of care. Med Care 1977;15:482–7.
5. American Society of Anesthesiologists Task Force on Preanesthesia Evaluation. Practice advisory for preanesthesia evaluation: a report by the American Society of Anesthesiologists Task Force on Preanesthesia Evaluation. Anesthesiology 2002;96:485–96.
6. National Institute for Clinical Excellence. Preoperative tests. The use of routine preoperative tests for elective surgery. Evidence, methods and guidance. Available at: http://www.nice.org.uk/nicemedia/live/10920/29094/29094.pdf (accessed February 7, 2011).
7. Bold AM, Corrin B. Use and abuse of clinical chemistry in surgery. Br Med J 1965;2:1051–2.
8. Allison JG, Bromley HR. Unnecessary preoperative investigations: evaluation and cost analysis. Am Surg 1996;62:686–9.
9. Narr BJ, Warner ME, Schroeder DR, Warner MA. Outcomes of patients with no laboratory assessment before anesthesia and a surgical procedure. Mayo Clin Proc 1997;72:505–9.
10. Nardella A, Pechet L, Snyder LM. Continuous improvement, quality control, and cost containment in clinical laboratory testing. Effects of establishing and implementing guidelines for preoperative tests. Arch Pathol Lab Med 1995;119:518–22.
11. Vogt AW, Henson LC. Unindicated preoperative testing: ASA physical status and financial implications. J Clin Anesth 1997;9:437–41.
12. Pal KM, Khan IA, Safdar B. Preoperative work up: are the requirements different in a developing country? J Pak Med Assoc 1998;48:339–41.
13. Smetana GW, Macpherson DS. The case against routine preoperative laboratory testing. Med Clin North Am 2003;87:7–40.
14. Dzankic S, Pastor D, Gonzalez C, Leung JM. The prevalence and predictive value of abnormal preoperative laboratory tests in elderly surgical patients. Anesth Analg 2001;93:301–8.
15. Schein OD, Katz J, Bass EB, et al. The value of routine preoperative medical testing before cataract surgery. Study of Medical Testing for Cataract Surgery. N Engl J Med 2000;342:168–75.
16. Burk CD, Miller L, Handler SD, Cohen AR. Preoperative history and coagulation screening in children undergoing tonsillectomy. Pediatrics 1992;89:691–5.
17. Narr BJ, Hansen TR, Warner MA. Preoperative laboratory screening in healthy Mayo patients: cost-effective elimination of tests and unchanged outcomes. Mayo Clin Proc 1991;66:155–9.
18. Macpherson DS. Preoperative laboratory testing: should any tests be "routine" before surgery? Med Clin North Am 1993;77:289–308.
19. Halaszynski TM, Juda R, Silverman DG. Optimizing postoperative outcomes with efficient preoperative assessment and management. Crit Care Med 2004;32(4 Suppl):S76–86.
20. Putnis S, Nanuck J, Heath D. An audit of preoperative blood tests. J Perioper Pract 2008;18:56–9.
21. Mayor S. NICE guidance clarifies when to do preoperative tests in elective surgery. Br Med J 2003;326:1418.
22. Cohen JT, Neumann PJ, Weinstein MC. Does preventive care save money? Health economics and the presidential candidates. N Engl J Med 2008;358:661–3.
23. Harken AH. Enough is enough. Arch Surg 1999;134:1061–3.

24. Dripps RD, Echenhoff JE, Vandam D. Introduction to anesthesia. Philadelphia: WB Saunders; 1988.
25. Goldman L, Caldera DL, Nussbaum SR, et al. Multifactorial index of cardiac risk in noncardiac surgical procedures. N Engl J Med 1977;297:845–50.
26. Mangano DT, Goldman L. Preoperative assessment of patients with known or suspected coronary disease. N Engl J Med 1995;333:1750–6.
27. Boersma E, Kertai MD, Schouten O, et al. Perioperative cardiovascular mortality in noncardiac surgery: validation of the Lee cardiac risk index. Am J Med 2005;118:1134–41.
28. Lee TH, Marcantonia ER, Mangione CM, et al. Derivation and prospective validation of a simple index for prediction of cardiac risk in patients undergoing noncardiac, nonvascular surgery. Circulation 1999;100:1043–9.
29. Katz RI, Cimino L, Vitkun SA, et al. Preoperative medical consultations: impact on perioperative management and surgical outcome. Can J Anaesth 2005;52:697–702.
30. Fleisher LA, Beckman JA, Brown KA, et al. ACC/AHA 2007 guidelines on perioperative cardiovascular evaluation and care for noncardiac surgery. A report of the American College of Cardiology/American Heart Association Task Force on Practice Guidelines (Writing Committee to Revise the 2002 Guidelines on Perioperative Cardiovascular Evaluation for Noncardiac Surgery). Circulation 2007;116:e418–99.
31. Warner MA, Shields SE, Chute MG. Major morbidity and mortality within one month of ambulatory surgery and anesthesia. JAMA 1993;270:1437–41.
32. Myers J, Prakash M, Froelicher V, et al. Exercise capacity and mortality among men referred for exercise testing. N Engl J Med 2002;346:793–801.
33. Hlatky MA, Boineau RE, Higginbotham MB, et al. A brief self-administered questionnaire to determine functional capacity (the Duke Activity Status Index). Am J Cardiol 1989;64:651–4.
34. Noordzij PG, Boersma E, Bax JJ, et al. Prognostic value of preoperative electrocardiography in patients undergoing non-cardiac surgery. Am J Cardiol 2006;97:1103–6.
35. Poldermans D, Bax JJ, Schouten O, et al. Should major vascular surgery be delayed because of preoperative cardiac testing in intermediate-risk patients receiving beta-blocker therapy with tight heart rate control? J Am Coll Cardiol 2006;48:964–9.
36. Van den Berghe G, Schetz M, Vlasselaers D, et al. Clinical review: Intensive insulin therapy in critically ill patients: NICE SUGAR or Leuven blood glucose target? J Clin Endocrinol Metab 2009;94:3163–70.
37. Fleisher LA, Beckman JA, Brown KA, et al. 2009 ACCF/AHA focused update on perioperative beta blockade incorporated into the ACC/AHA 2007 guidelines on perioperative cardiovascular evaluation and care for noncardiac surgery. J Am Coll Cardiol 2009;54:e13–118.
38. Nicolić I, Majerić-Kogler V, Plavec D, et al. Stairs climbing test with pulse oximetry as predictor of early postoperative complications in functionally impaired patients with lung cancer and elective lung surgery: prospective trial of consecutive series of patients. Croat Med J 2008;49:50–7.
39. Brunelli A, Refai M, Xiumé F, et al. Performance at symptom-limited stair-climbing test is associated with increased cardiopulmonary complications, mortality, and costs after major lung resection. Ann Thorac Surg 2008;86:240–7; discussion 247–8.
40. Brower RG, Matthay MA, Morris A, et al; The Acute Respiratory Distress Syndrome Network. Ventilation with lower tidal volumes as compared with traditional tidal volumes for acute lung injury and the acute respiratory distress syndrome. The Acute Respiratory Distress Syndrome Network. N Engl J Med 2000;342:1301–8.
41. Buzby GP, Knox LS, Crosby LO, et al. Study protocol: a randomized clinical trial of total parenteral nutrition in malnourished surgical patients. Am J Clin Nutr 1988;47 (2 Suppl):366–81.
42. Perioperative total parenteral nutrition in surgical patients. The Veterans Affairs Total Parenteral Nutrition Cooperative Study Group. N Engl J Med 1991;325:525–32.
43. Baker JP, Detsky AS, Wesson DE, et al. Nutritional assessment: a comparison of clinical judgment and objective measurements. N Engl J Med 1982;306:969–72.
44. Bellantone R, Doglietto G, Bossola M, et al. Preoperative parenteral nutrition in the high risk surgical patient. JPEN J Parenter Enteral Nutr 1988;12:195–7.
45. Bellantone R, Doglietto G, Bossola M, et al. Preoperative parenteral nutrition of malnourished surgical patients. Acta Chir Scand 1988;22:249–51.
46. Jensen S. Clinical effects of enteral and parenteral nutrition preceding cancer surgery. Med Oncol Tumor Pharmacother 1985;2:225–9.
47. Muller J, Keller H, Brenner U, et al. Indications and effects of preoperative parenteral nutrition. World J Surg 1986;10: 53–63.
48. Smith RC, Hartemink R. Improvement of nutritional measures during preoperative parenteral nutrition in patients selected by the prognostic nutritional index: a randomized controlled trial. JPEN J Parenter Enteral Nutr 1988;12:587–91.
49. von Meyenfeldt M, Meijerink W, Rouflart M, et al. Perioperative nutritional support: a randomised clinical trial. Clin Nutr 1992;11:180–6.
50. Brennan MF, Pisters PW, Posner M, et al. A prospective randomized trial of total parenteral nutrition after major pancreatic resection for malignancy. Ann Surg 1994;220: 436–41.
51. Collins J, Oxby C, Hill G. Intravenous amino acids and intravenous hyperalimentation as protein-sparing therapy after major surgery: a controlled clinical trial. Lancet 1978; 1:778–91.
52. Preshaw R, Attisha R, Hollingworth W. Randomized sequential trial of parenteral nutrition in healing of colonic anastomoses in man. Can J Surg 1979;22:437–9.
53. Sandstrom R, Drott C, Hyltander A, et al. The effect of postoperative intravenous feeding (TPN) on outcome following major surgery evaluated in a randomized study. Ann Surg 1993;217:185–95.
54. Woolfson A, Smith J. Elective nutritional support after major surgery: a prospective randomised trial. Clin Nutr 1989;8:15–21.
55. Ziegler TR. Parenteral nutrition in the critically ill patient. N Engl J Med 2009;361:1088–97.
56. Alexander JW, MacMillan BG, Stinnett JD, et al. Beneficial effects of aggressive protein feeding in severely burned children. Ann Surg 1980;192:505–17.
57. Bastow MD, Rawlings J, Allison S. Benefits of supplementary tube feeding after fractured neck of femur: a randomised controlled trial. Br Med J 1983;187:1589–92.

58. Van den Berghe G, Wouters P, Weekers F, et al. Intensive insulin therapy in critically ill patients. N Engl J Med 2001;345:1359–67.
59. Van den Berghe G, Wilmer A, Hermans G, et al. Intensive insulin therapy in the medical ICU. N Engl J Med 2006;354:449–61.
60. NICE-SUGAR Study Investigators, Finfer S, Chittock DR, Su SY, et al. Intensive versus conventional glucose control in critically ill patients. N Engl J Med 2009;360:1283–97.
61. Dhaliwal R, Heyland DK. Nutrition and infection in the intensive care unit: what does the evidence show? Curr Opin Crit Care 2005;11:461–7.
62. Kieft H, Roos AN, van Drunen JD et al. Clinical outcome of immunonutrition in a heterogeneous intensive care population. Intensive Care Med 2005;31:524–32.
63. Kaska M, Tatana G, Havel E, et al. The impact and safety of preoperative oral or intravenous carbohydrate administration. Wien Klin Wochenschr 2010;122:23–30.
64. Awad S, Constantin-Teodosiu D, Constan D, et al. Cellular mechanisms underlying protective effects of pre-operative feedings. Ann Surg 2010;252:247–53.
65. Brady MC, Kinn S, Stuart P, et al. Preoperative fasting for adults to prevent perioperative complications. Cochrane Database Syst Rev 2003;(5):CD004423.
66. Schouten O, Poldermans D. Cardiac risk in non-cardiac surgery. Br J Surg 2007;94:1185–6.
67. Brooke BS, Meguid RA, Makary MA, et al. Improving surgical outcomes through adoption of evidence-based process measures: intervention specific or associated with overall hospital quality? Surgery 2010;147:481–90.
68. Poldermans D, Boersma E, Bax JJ, et al. Correlation of location of acute myocardial infarct after noncardiac vascular surgery with preoperative dobutamine echocardiographic findings. Am J Cardiol 2001;88:1413–4, A6.
69. Dawood MM, Gutpa DK, Southern J, et al. Pathology of fatal perioperative myocardial infarction: implications regarding pathophysiology and prevention. Int J Cardiol 1996;57:37–44.
70. Cruickshank JM. Beta-blockers continue to surprise us. Eur Heart J 2000;21:354–64.
71. Poldermans D, Boersma E. Beta-blocker therapy in noncardiac surgery. N Engl J Med 2005;353:412–4.
72. Poldermans D, Boersma E, Bax JJ, et al. The effect of bisoprolol on perioperative mortality and myocardial infarction in high-risk patients undergoing vascular surgery. Dutch Echocardiographic Cardiac Risk Evaluation Applying Stress Echocardiography Study Group. N Engl J Med 1999;341:1789–94.
73. Lindenauer PK, Pekow P, Wang K, et al. Pathology of fatal perioperative myocardial infarction: implications regarding pathophysiology and prevention. N Engl J Med 2005;353:349–61.
74. POISE Study Group, Devereaux PJ, Yang H, Yusuf S, et al. Effects of extended-release metoprolol succinate in patients undergoing non-cardiac surgery (POISE trial): a randomised controlled trial. Lancet 2008;371:1839–47.
75. Fleisher LA, Beckman JA, Brown KA, et al. 2009 ACCF/AHA focused update on perioperative beta blockade incorporated into the ACC/AHA 2007 guidelines on perioperative cardiovascular evaluation and care for noncardiac surgery: a report of the American College of Cardiology Foundation/American Heart Association Task Force on Practice Guidelines. Circulation 2009;120:e169–276.
76. Juul AB, Wetterslev J, Gluud C, et al. Effect of perioperative beta blockade in patients with diabetes undergoing major non-cardiac surgery: randomised placebo controlled, blinded multicentre trial. BMJ 2006;332:1482.
77. Stone JG, Foëx P, Sear JW, et al. Risk of myocardial ischaemia during anaesthesia in treated and untreated hypertensive patients. Br J Anaesth 1988;61:675–9.
78. Zaugg M, Tagliente T, Lucchinetti E, et al. Beneficial effects from beta-adrenergic blockade in elderly patients undergoing noncardiac surgery. Anesthesiology 1999;91:1674–86.
79. Cucherat M. Quantitative relationship between resting heart rate reduction and magnitude of clinical benefits in post-myocardial infarction: a meta-regression of randomized clinical trials. Eur Heart J 2007;28:3012–9.
80. Law MR, Wald NJ, Rudnicka AR. Quantifying effect of statins on low density lipoprotein cholesterol, ischaemic heart disease and stroke: systematic review and meta-analysis. BMJ 2003;326:1423.
81. Poynter JN, Gruber SB, Higgins PD, et al. Statins and the risk of colorectal cancer. N Engl J Med 2005;352:2184–92.
82. Albert MA, Danielson E, Rifai N, et al. Effect of statin therapy on C-reactive protein levels: the pravastatin inflammation/CRP evaluation (PRINCE): a randomized trial and cohort study. JAMA 2001;286:64–70.
83. Pan W, Pintar T, Anton J, et al. Statins are associated with a reduced incidence of perioperative mortality after coronary artery bypass surgery. Circulation 2004;110 (11 Suppl 1):II45–9.
84. Ouattara A, Benhaoua H, Le Manach Y, et al. Perioperative statin therapy is associated with a significant and dose-dependent reduction of adverse cardiovascular outcomes after coronary artery bypass surgery. J Cardiothorac Vasc Anesth 2009;23:633–8.
85. Biccard BM. A peri-operative statin update for non-cardiac surgery Part II: Statin therapy for vascular surgery and peri-operative statin trial design. Anaesthesia 2008;63:162–71.
86. Cooley ME, Sarna L, Kotlerman J, et al. Smoking cessation is challenging even for patients recovering from lung cancer surgery with curative intent. Lung Cancer 2009;66:218–25.
87. Cooley ME, Sarna L, Brown JK, et al. Tobacco use in women with lung cancer. Ann Behav Med 2007;33:242–50.
88. Robles GI, Singh-Franco D, Ghin HL. A review of the efficacy of smoking-cessation pharmacotherapies in nonwhite populations. Clin Ther 2008;30:800–12.
89. Wolfenden L, Wiggers J, Knight J, et al. A programme for reducing smoking in pre-operative surgical patients: randomised controlled trial. Anaesthesia 2005;60:172–9.
90. Sadr Azodi O, Lindström D, Adami J, et al. The efficacy of a smoking cessation programme in patients undergoing elective surgery: a randomised clinical trial. Anaesthesia 2009;64:259–65.
91. Bikhchandani J, Varma SK, Henderson NP. Is it justified to refuse breast reduction to smokers? J Plast Reconstr Aesthet Surg 2007;60:1050–4.

92. Garrison GD, Dugan SE. Varenicline: a first-line treatment option for smoking cessation. Clin Ther 2009;31:463–91.
93. Xue QL. The frailty syndrome: definition and natural history. Clin Geriatr Med 2011;27:1–15.
94. Fried LP, Tangen CM, Walston J, et al. Frailty in older adults: evidence for a phenotype. J Gerontol A Biol Sci Med Sci 2001;56:M146–56.
95. Gilleard C, Higgs P. Frailty, disability and old age: a re-appraisal. Health 2010. [Epub ahead of print]
96. Mack MJ. Risk scores for predicting outcomes in valvular heart disease: how useful? Curr Cardiol Rep 2011;13: 107–12.
97. Chikwe J, Adams DH. Frailty: the missing element in predicting operative mortality. Semin Thorac Cardiovasc Surg 2010;22:109–10.
98. Makary MA, Segev DL, Pronovost PJ, et al. Frailty as a predictor of surgical outcomes in older patients. J Am Coll Surg 2010;210:901–8.
99. Liu CK, Fielding RA. Exercise as an intervention for frailty. Clin Geriatr Med 2011;27:101–10.
100. Castillo-Garzón MJ, Ruiz JR, Ortega FB, et al. Anti-aging therapy through fitness enhancement. Clin Interv Aging 2006;1:213–20.
101. Klein S, Kinney J, Jeejeebhoy K. Nutrition support in clinical practice: review of published data and recommendations for future research directions. Summary of a conference sponsored by the National Institutes of Health, American Society for Parenteral and Enteral Nutrition, and American Society for Clinical Nutrition. Am J Clin Nutr 1997;66:683–706.

7 ELEMENTS OF COST-EFFECTIVE NONEMERGENT SURGICAL CARE

Robert S. Rhodes, MD, FACS, Charles L. Rice, MD, FACS, and Julie Ann Sosa, MA, MD, FACS

Citizens of industrialized nations generally enjoy a high level of health, and the positive correlation between life expectancy and per capita income is among the best known relationships in international development.[1] Yet there are differences among the health care systems of these nations with regard to quality, cost, and access to care.[2,3] There also appears to be a dynamic tension among these three characteristics, and the goal of providing broad access to high-quality health care at a reasonable cost is an increasing challenge. One particular challenge is that health care costs tend to rise at a faster pace than the costs of other goods and services. In the United States, for example, health care costs have consistently risen faster than overall inflation for the past 65 years. Interestingly, despite differences in the percentage of gross domestic product (GDP) that nations spend on health care, the slopes of these curves often appear to increase in parallel [*see Figure 1*].

The hyperinflation in health care costs, particularly in the context of the recent economic downturn, often forces choices among social goals (e.g., health care versus education). Such choices may be more readily rationalized when the costs of the chosen goal produce demonstrable value (i.e., if greater health care spending generates measurably better health, it is regarded as worthwhile; if it does not, it is regarded as wasteful). Unfortunately, the latter appears to be the case in the United States. Although the United States spends more on health care as a percentage of its GDP [*see Figure 1*] and per capita [*see Figure 2*] than other industrialized nations, its citizens seem less healthy than those of many nations with respect to indices of population health, such as life expectancy and infant mortality [*see Figure 3 and Figure 4*]. Thus, per capita health care expenditures have only a modest correlation with life expectancy. Although some of this disparity in the apparent value of health care might be explained by specific characteristics of the US population, much of it cannot. Although the United States has slight advantages over some countries in 5-year survival rates for both breast and colorectal cancer, the cost of such benefits seems disproportionately large. Overall, the United States lags behind other nations in measures of illness and some chronic conditions amenable to health care.[4] All of this suggests that the US health care system exhibits a relative lack of cost-effectiveness, the causes of which include higher prices for health care goods and services[5] and waste related to overuse or misuse of resources.

As health care increasingly competes with other social goals for the same funds, individuals, employers, and governments all feel the strain. The impact on US citizens is reflected in the fact that in 2007, over 62% of personal bankruptcies were related to health care issues, up from 46% 6 years earlier.[6] Also, the percentage of nonelderly Americans who lived in

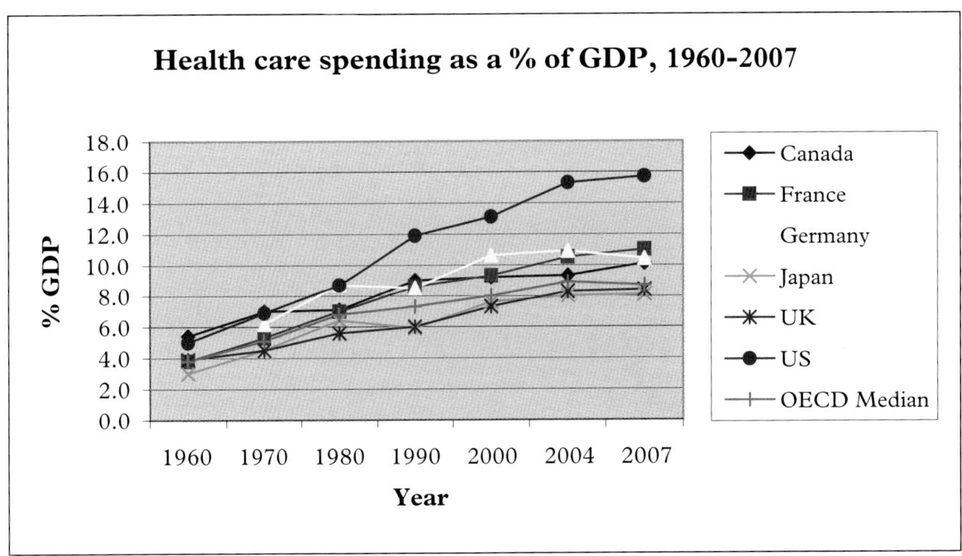

Figure 1 **Health care spending as a percentage of gross domestic product (GDP) among selected countries within the Organisation for Economic Co-operation and Development (OECD). US health care spending has been increasing at a disproportionately faster rate. Note that the *x*-axis scale does not have constant intervals. (www.oecd.org/health/hcqi. accessed July 5, 2010).**

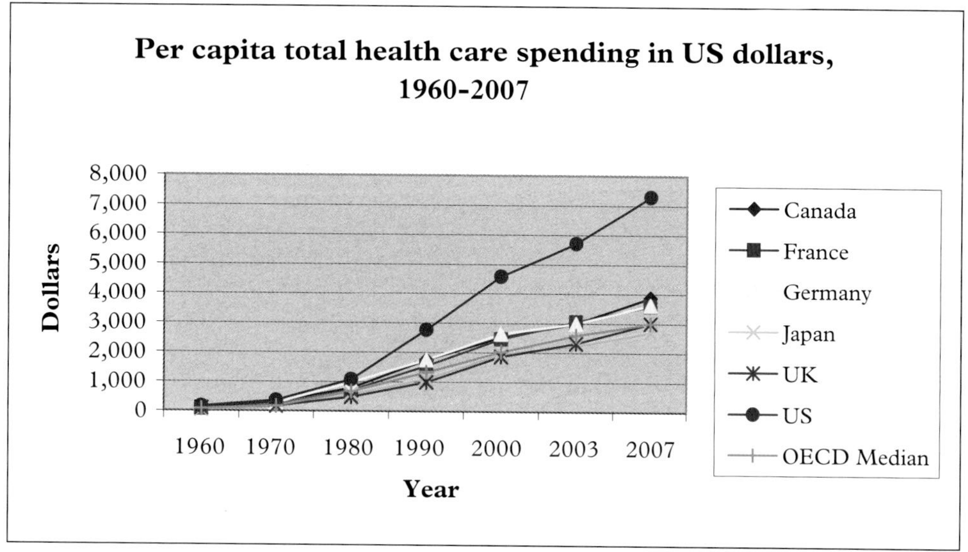

Figure 2 **Health care spending per capita among selected countries within the Organisation for Economic Co-operation and Development (OECD) in US dollars. Again, US health care spending is increasing at a disproportionately faster rate. Note that the *x*-axis scale does not have constant intervals. (www.oecd.org/health/hcqi. accessed July 5, 2010).**

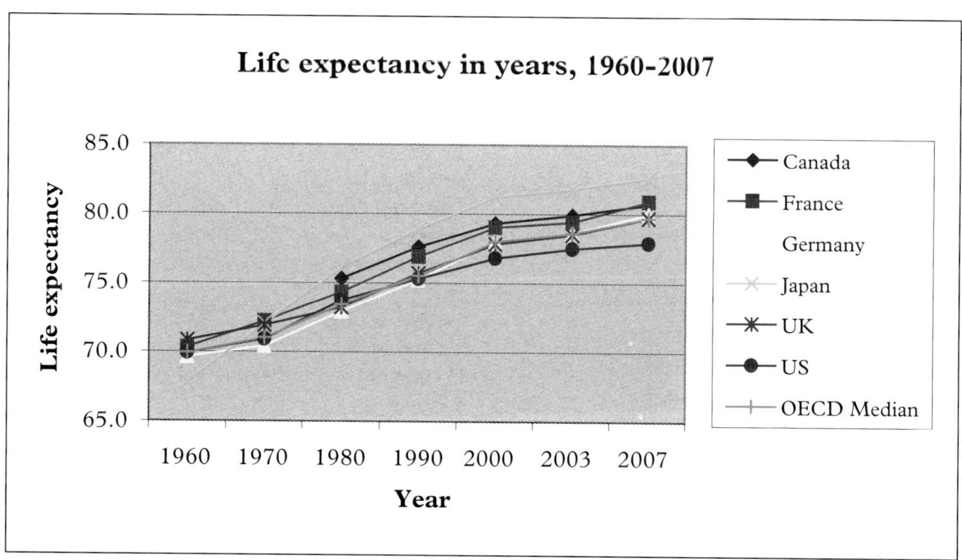

Figure 3 **Life expectancy among selected countries within the Organisation for Economic Co-operation and Development (OECD). The increase in US life expectancy is falling behind the increases seen in other countries. Note that the *x*-axis scale does not have constant intervals. (www.oecd.org/health/hcqi. accessed July 5, 2010).**

families spending more than 10% of their income on health care rose from 14.4% in 2001 to 19.1% in 2006.[7]

The phrase "bending the cost curve" refers to efforts to minimize or eliminate differences in inflation in general and inflation in the cost of health care. Accordingly, there is a long history of attempts to control health care costs that includes price controls (the Nixon era), prospective payment (the Reagan era), and managed care (the Clinton era). Unfortunately, these initiatives had little long-term impact.[8] More recently, concerns about increases in health care costs were sufficient to engender federal legislation aimed at controlling costs; whether this effort will be more successful has yet to be determined.

Many factors contribute to the costs of health care, but physicians' decisions are the largest single factor; they are estimated to account for 75% of these costs. This pronounced impact of physicians on health care costs explains, in turn, why those who pay the bills increasingly seek to identify the most cost-effective physicians. Surgeons in particular are likely to be a target of efforts to contain costs because surgical illnesses often are of relatively short duration, surgical outcomes are readily quantified, and surgeon reimbursement often involves global fees.

Given the impetus to improve the cost-effectiveness of surgical care, the goals of this chapter are to (1) explore the fundamental principles of cost-effectiveness, particularly as

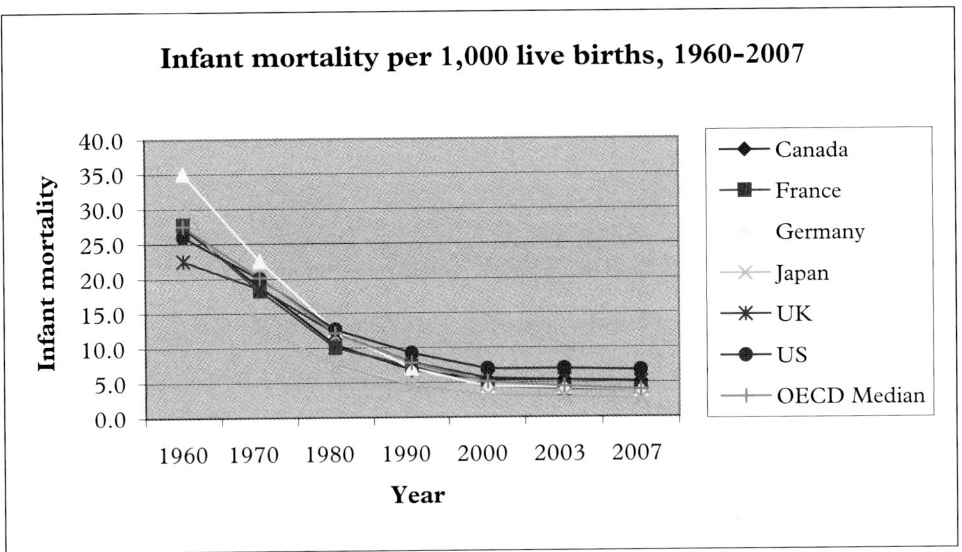

Figure 4 **Infant mortality per 1,000 live births among selected countries in the Organisation for Economic Co-operation and Development (OECD). The decline in US infant mortality is not keeping pace with the declines seen in other countries. Note that the *x*-axis scale does not have constant intervals. (www.oecd.org/health/hcqi. accessed July 5, 2010).**

applied to surgical care; (2) review the attributes and complexities of both cost and quality; (3) review current data on the relationship of cost and quality; and (4) identify specific skills and attributes to help surgeons deliver more cost-effective care.

Fundamental Principles of Cost-effectiveness

Cost-effectiveness expresses the cost of a given strategy (in dollars) relative to a given measure of quality. Developed in the military and in the evaluation of how to spend government monies on different public works projects (e.g., roads, dams, bridges), cost-effectiveness analysis (CEA) was first applied to health care in the mid-1960s. It was introduced with enthusiasm to clinicians in 1977 by Weinstein and Stason[9] but was received with skepticism or reluctance. Cost-effectiveness can be an absolute term, but a more frequent application in health care is to compare the value of two or more clinical strategies. Expressed mathematically, it is the difference in the cost of a new strategy and the cost of current practice divided by the difference in the effectiveness of the new strategy and the effectiveness of current practice. Specific strategies might include assessing one intervention against another, assessing an intervention against no intervention, or assessing early treatment against delayed treatment. An example of the last is a study of appendicitis that concluded that each 10% increase in diagnostic accuracy was associated with a 14% increase in the perforation rate; the greater costs associated with higher morbidity from perforation might offset the cost savings associated with reducing negative appendectomies through greater diagnostic accuracy.[10]

Cost-effectiveness differs from cost-benefit, which measures return on investment (where the numerator and denominator are expressed in dollars), and from efficiency, which is an expression of productivity (with outputs divided by inputs). Comparative effectiveness is another frequently used term that compares the effectiveness of two or more treatments.

Given that cost-effectiveness considers both cost and quality, changes in cost-effectiveness also represent changes in the value of care. The interaction of cost and quality also means that improvements in cost-effectiveness can result from changes in the numerator, the denominator, or both. Moreover, beneficial effects in one component of a strategy can be outweighed by adverse changes in the other, and vice versa. These interactions are represented in Figure 5. Here, strategies that increase quality and lower cost are highly desirable, and maximal cost-effectiveness is the optimal outcome that can be achieved with the least use of resources. Conversely, changes that lower quality and increase cost are clearly undesirable. In contrast, judgments of strategies where costs and quality move in the same direction tend to be controversial.

The controversial nature of such changes was evident during the debate on health care reform. Greater support for cost-effectiveness research was included in the American Reinvestment and Recovery Act (ARRA) of 2009, raising concerns that health care decisions going forward might be made by outside agencies. This fueled at least some of the opposition to health care reform.[11] Moreover, a recent survey indicated that a majority of consumers believed that more care meant higher-quality, better care.[12] Many of these consumer beliefs, values, and knowledge are at odds with what policy makers described as evidence-based health care. These beliefs likely account for the recent pushback on the changes in recommendations proposed by the U.S. Preventive Services Task Force regarding the appropriateness of routine mammography screening for women ages 40 to 49.[13]

Attributes of Health Care Costs

Assessing cost-effectiveness may seem simple, but measures of costs have multiple dimensions that are reflected in the phrase "cost is a noun that never stands alone." Thus,

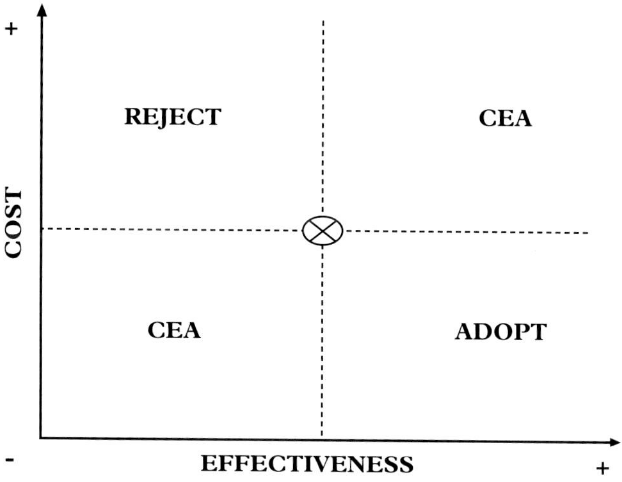

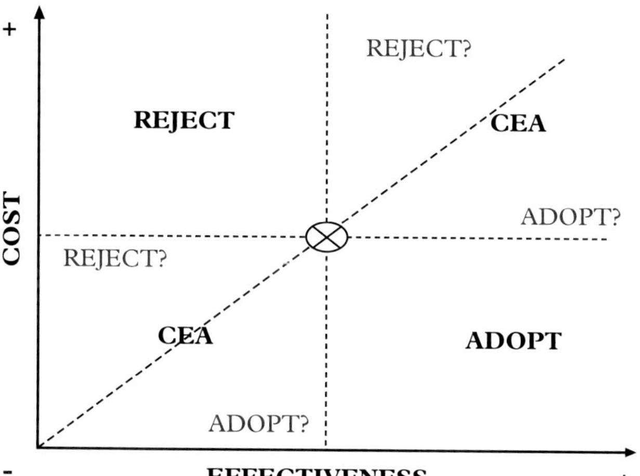

Figure 5 **Cost analysis methods. Adapted from the National Information Center on Health Services Research and Health Care technology of the US National Library of Medicine, National Institutes of Health. Available at: http://www.nlm.nih.gov/nichsr/hta101/ta10106.html. accessed January 10, 2011. CEA = cost-effectiveness analysis.**

assessing the relative cost-effectiveness of a specific strategy requires a precise definition of the costs being considered.[14]

An important first step is to appreciate the distinction between costs and charges. Charges are the price at which a "seller" provides a given product or service, but this price may not reflect the actual cost of that product or service (e.g., a loss leader). Although aggregate hospital costs can be a relatively constant fraction of hospital charges, there are often substantial variations among institutions in the cost-to-charge ratio for specific goods and services. These differences can be attributed to differences in cost attribution among different accounting systems but are also evident within the relatively standardized accounting standards required by the Centers for Medicare and Medicaid Services (CMS). Whether such variations result from differences in efficiency or differences in accounting practices is often not clear.

Third-party reimbursements to hospitals and surgeons reflect contractual agreements and, like charges, also do not reflect costs.

Table 1 lists ways to categorize health care costs. Cost traceability and its behavior in relation to output or activity are particularly important concepts for surgeons and hospitals.[15] Examples of direct costs are salaries, supplies, rents, and utilities, whereas indirect costs might be depreciation and/or administrative costs associated with regulatory compliance. Yet these definitions are not cast in stone, and some indirect costs might be considered direct costs depending on the cost objective.

Cost behavior relative to an output or activity costs can be variable, fixed, semivariable, or semifixed. Variable costs (e.g., supplies) change in a constant, proportional manner with changes in output, whereas fixed costs (e.g., equipment) do not change in response to changes in volume. Semivariable costs (e.g., utilities) include elements of both fixed and variable costs: there is a fixed basic cost per unit of time and a direct, proportional relation between volume and cost. Semifixed costs (also known as step costs) also change with changes in output, but the changes occur in discrete steps rather than linearly. An example of a semifixed cost is the number of full-time equivalents (FTEs) needed to run one operating room; labor costs will be constant whether that room is used all the time or part-time. Conversely, when operating room use is reduced, there may not be any cost savings until a room is completely taken out of service. Unless the step threshold is attained, costs do not change.

Physicians affect hospital costs primarily via their impact on fully variable and semifixed costs. Such costs typically constitute 15 to 35% of total hospital costs, and this range often reflects substantial variations in the use of resources among surgeons for similar types of patients or procedures.

Table 1 **Categories and Types of Hospital Costs**

Category	Type	Example or Definition
Traceability to the object being costed	Direct Indirect	Salaries, supplies, rents, and utilities Depreciation and employee benefits
Behavior of cost in relation to output or activity	Variable Fixed Semivariable Semifixed	Supply Depreciation Utilities Number of full-time equivalents per step in output
Management responsibility for control	—	Often limited to direct, variable costs
Future versus historical	Avoidable costs Sunk costs Incremental costs Opportunity costs	Costs affected by a decision under consideration Costs not affected by a decision under consideration Changes in total costs resulting from alternative courses of action Value forgone by using a resource in a particular way instead of in its next best alternative way

This variability, in turn, can affect the "profitability" of a given disease-related group (DRG). Hospital administrators often are aware of this variability but seem reluctant to bring it to a surgeon's attention. Physicians also affect fixed costs as they influence investments in technology. This is discussed in greater detail in a later section.

Perspectives on costs also vary among payers (e.g., insurers), providers, and patients.[16] Payers' perspectives primarily focus on the impact of price and use, a perspective exemplified by the introduction of laparoscopic cholecystectomy.[17] Lower per procedure hospital costs were offset by an increase in procedure volume and an increase in aggregate costs to payers. This effect often accounts for differing opinions among patients, providers, and insurers regarding the value of new technology. In this context, regional variation in per capita Medicare spending appears to be more related to differences in use than in price.[18]

The interval between an intervention and the point of measurement may also affect estimates of value.[19,20] Patients are likely to view outcomes over the long term, whereas providers and purchasers tend to have a shorter horizon (e.g., the term of a health care contract). To improve the comparability of cost-effectiveness, the Panel on Cost-Effectiveness in Health and Medicine (a nonfederal panel with expertise in CEA, clinical medicine, ethics, and health outcomes measurement convened by the US Public Health Service) recommended that calculations of cost-effectiveness be based on a broad societal perspective rather than on that of patients, providers, or insurers. Such a perspective would more likely include costs incurred by patients or others (e.g., outpatient medication or home care after hospital discharge).

Defining Quality in Health Care

Assessing cost-effectiveness also requires suitable measures of quality. Unfortunately, defining quality can be even more complex than assessing cost.[21,22] Measures such as operative mortality are straightforward but have become increasingly rare; therefore, mortality alone is not useful in the vast majority of cases.

A long-held standard of health care quality was the appropriateness of care, and an individual physician's knowledge was the authority with regard to judging quality. In recent decades, several factors have seriously undermined appropriateness (and perhaps even physician authority) as a primary indicator of quality. These factors included findings that some procedures had a high incidence of inappropriate indications; judgments as to appropriate care relative to groups differed from such judgments relative to individuals[23]; retrospective assessments often judged appropriateness on the basis of outcome without considering processes of care[24]; and a realization that variations in procedure frequency often related to provider capacity (e.g., the number of hospital beds per 1,000 persons). Unexplained variations in the use of health care services across small geographic areas, in particular, have undermined physician authority on quality and are discussed in more detail in a later section.

The overall consequence is that appropriateness is not sufficiently granular to be a useful measure of quality. These shortcomings were addressed by Donabedian, who characterized quality in terms of structure (faculties, equipment, and services), process (content of care), and outcomes.[25] These three components can be measured more objectively than appropriateness and allow application of the quality control techniques pioneered in industry by W. Edwards Deming. These techniques minimize variation in quality by examining production systems. The analogy to health care is that the production systems are the systems of care; the health care systems' structure and processes are independent variables, and patient outcome is a dependent variable.

Although outcomes are unquestionably a more definitive measure of quality than process, the nature of health care is such that measuring processes of care (i.e., what is done to a patient) may be more immediately relevant to improving the quality of care than measuring outcome per se (i.e., what happens to a patient). One reason for placing greater emphasis on process in health care is that all the factors that affect outcomes in biologic systems may not be known or controllable. This differs from mechanical systems such as aircraft, where a given perturbation has a fairly predictable result. Conversely, the adaptability inherent in biologic systems means that a poor outcome may not occur every time there is an incorrect decision or an error in process.[26] Another reason to identify critical processes of care is that it avoids the methodological problems of risk-adjusting outcomes and/or the statistical limitations of comparing outcomes for low-frequency procedures and/or events.

Ultimately, efforts to improve quality will need to account for outcomes, but attempts to improve outcomes without consideration for the relevant processes are likely to prove frustrating. Therefore, it is critically important to identify processes that have the greatest impact on outcomes[27]; the time and effort spent measuring processes not directly linked to outcomes are likely to be wasteful. The ARRA seeks to promote the burgeoning field of cost-effectiveness research, which informs health care decisions by providing evidence on the effectiveness, benefits, and harm of different treatment options, whether they are drugs, medical devices, surgical procedures, or ways to deliver health care. Evidence can come from existing data or by generating new evidence.

Connecting the Dots: Linking Quality to Systems of Care

Given the importance of processes of care, a surgeon's (or hospital's) systems of care reflect the consistency with which the same processes of care are applied to a given situation. Indirect evidence for this link comes from data on the relationship between volume and outcomes for complex procedures; surgeons and/or hospitals that do a given operation more frequently (i.e., high volumes) often have better outcomes.[28–33] Moreover, the relative impact of hospital volume and surgeon volume on outcomes can vary by procedure. Thus, complex, team-dependent procedures such as cardiac surgery, pancreatectomy, and esophagectomy have a stronger relation with hospital volume even if performed by low-volume surgeons; by comparison, carotid endarterectomy and thyroidectomy have a strong relation with surgeon volume. A positive relation with outcomes also has been noted for surgical subspecialty training.[28,32,34]

These volume-outcome relations data are intriguing, although they only represent associations and probabilities, not cause-and-effect relationships.[35] This raises the question of whether practice makes perfect or perfect makes practice. The answer is not known but has produced two schools of thought. The practice makes perfect school of thought advocates that quality improvements on a widespread basis will derive from the adoption of better systems or processes of care. These proponents note that low volume is not always associated with worse outcomes, and high volume is not always associated with improved outcomes. Thus, the findings apply to surgeons in general but not to specific surgeons. This means that good outcomes can be achieved even with low volumes if carried out using good systems. Conversely, high volumes may result in worse outcomes in the presence of poor systems. As a further caveat, the relative applicability of the role of systems to complex care is suggested by findings from the Department of Veterans Affairs' (VA) National Surgical Quality Improvement Project (NSQIP). One study of eight common surgical procedures noted no correlation between hospital operative volume and postoperative mortality.[36]

In comparison, the perfect makes practice school advocates regionalizing care to those centers with better outcomes. Perhaps the best known of these advocates is the Leapfrog Group (www.leapfroggroup.org), a large consortium of major employers. They used empirical observations of cost and outcomes to identify the minimum volumes for procedures such as coronary artery bypass grafting, esophagectomy, carotid endarterectomy, and aortic aneurysm repair that were associated with optimal outcomes. The empirical basis of these determinations is subject to methodological problems.[37] Moreover, changes in technology, such as the advent of endovascular aortic aneurysm repair, have substantially undermined the experience levels that were the basis of the original recommendations.

Other proponents of regionalization are the Institute of Medicine's National Cancer Policy Board and the National Research Council. They concluded that complicated cancer operations had better initial outcomes with high-volume providers.[38] Higher volumes also were associated with improved long-term survival.

Although regionalization has proven effective in trauma care, the basis of the improved quality in this setting may be better systems of care, not higher volume per se.[39] Moreover, the perception of preventability of trauma deaths increased in parallel with the appreciation of the importance of the system. Thus, regionalization of care without a solid understanding of the basis of the volume-outcome relation has the potential to create unintended or adverse consequences for overall care. Consequently, many believe that it is too soon to use volume-outcome data as a surrogate for quality or as criteria for establishing policy.[40] The higher quality of care at level I trauma centers comes with a price; these centers' better outcomes are also more expensive.[41] This reflects both the relative and absolute aspects of cost-effectiveness. Regionalization of trauma care appears to be cost-effective relative to lack of regionalization, with an associated incremental cost of less than $50,000/life-year saved (LYS); LYS is a measure of the number of life-years saved as a result of a health intervention. The $50,000 figure is a threshold conventionally used to ascertain cost-effectiveness. A corollary is that cost-effectiveness does not always equate to cost saving

Linking Processes to Performance

The desire to link processes to performance has become manifest in pay-for-performance (P4P) programs that provide incentives to adopt evidence-based process measures.[42,43] The most conspicuous of these is Medicare's Physician Quality Reporting Initiative (PQRI) (www.cms.hhs.gov/pqri). The list of applicable measures has expanded considerably in the last several years, and some specific measures related to surgical care are listed in Table 2. A recent notable finding is that the infection control measures of the Surgical Care Improvement Project (SCIP), which are closely aligned with similar PQRI measures, appear to be most effective when used in the aggregate rather than as individual measures.[44]

Although the rationale for these programs seems straightforward, there are concerns about their long-term potential effectiveness. One such concern is that only a small number of surgical process measures have been identified so far. In addition, these measures tend to be related to general aspects of care, with many processes of care more specific to the outcome of a given procedure or disease process yet to be identified.

There are also concerns that the magnitude of the cost reductions relative to the incentives is presently not known. This is particularly relevant if health care finance is a zero-sum game. If incentive payments exceed the savings, there will be increased pressure to reduce other payments to maintain budget neutrality. If the savings exceed the incentives, there may be increased pressure to increase the incentives.

A further concern relates to assigning the benefits from P4P. Surgeon-related quality improvements that appear to confer disproportionate financial benefits on the insurer rather than on the surgeon may reduce the incentive for surgeons to implement improvements. This concern also relates to P4P measures where implementation requires coordination of systems among providers rather than an isolated action on the part of an individual or an institution. For example, compliance with the measures for prophylactic antibiotics may reward or penalize a surgeon even though she or he may have little control over whether antibiotics are given in a timely fashion; the hospital systems needed for compliance may be a more important determinant of compliance with this measure. Indeed, one study found that a major barrier to compliance was that no single participant in the perioperative routine had acknowledged responsibility to administer prophylactic antibiotics.[45] The need for coordination among individuals in such situations has been recognized among commercial health maintenance organizations' (HMOs) P4P programs: only 13.3% of the physician-oriented programs focus solely on the individual physician as the unit of payment.[42,43] The need for such coordination has raised concern that the dispersion of patient care among multiple physicians could limit the effectiveness of initiatives that rely on a single retrospective method for assigning responsibility.[46]

Another concern is that P4P may not be so much pay for performance as it is pay for compliance. It is argued that the real goal should be to encourage innovation to optimize cost-effectiveness. Moreover, not all P4P programs focus on evidence-based measures. For example, one study found that 24% of physicians faced incentives derived from patient satisfaction surveys and 14% faced incentives derived from

Table 2 Current Physician Quality Reporting Initiative Measures by Surgical Specialty

General and Perioperative Measures, All Specialties

20. Perioperative Care: Timing of Antibiotic Prophylaxis — Ordering Physician
Percentage of surgical patients aged 18 years and older undergoing procedures with the indications for prophylactic parenteral antibiotics, who have an order for prophylactic parenteral antibiotic to be given within 1 hour (if fluoroquinolone or vancomycin, 2 hours) prior to the surgical incision (or start of procedure when no incision is required)

21. Perioperative Care: Selection of Prophylactic Antibiotic — First- OR Second-Generation Cephalosporin
Percentage of surgical patients aged 18 years and older undergoing procedures with the indications for a first- OR second-generation cephalosporin prophylactic antibiotic, who had an order for cefazolin OR cefuroxime for antimicrobial prophylaxis

22. Perioperative Care: Discontinuation of Prophylactic Antibiotics (Noncardiac Procedures)
Percentage of noncardiac surgical patients aged 18 years and older undergoing procedures with the indications for prophylactic parenteral antibiotics who received a prophylactic parenteral antibiotic and have an order for discontinuation of prophylactic parenteral antibiotics within 24 hours of surgical end time

23. Perioperative Care: Venous Thromboembolism (VTE) Prophylaxis (When Indicated in ALL Patients)
Percentage of patients aged 18 years and older undergoing procedures for which VTE prophylaxis is indicated in all patients, who had an order for low-molecular-weight heparin, low-dose unfractionated heparin, adjusted-dose warfarin, fondaparinux, or mechanical prophylaxis to be given within 24 hours prior to incision time or within 24 hours after surgery end time

30. Perioperative Care: Timely Administration of Prophylactic Parenteral Antibiotics
Percentage of surgical patients aged 18 years and older who receive an anesthetic when undergoing procedures with the indications for prophylactic parenteral antibiotics for whom administration of the prophylactic parenteral antibiotic ordered has been initiated within 1 hour (if fluoroquinolone or vancomycin, 2 hours) prior to the surgical incision (or start of procedure when no incision is required)

46. Medication Reconciliation: Reconciliation after Discharge from an Inpatient Facility
Percentage of patients aged 65 years and older discharged from any inpatient facility (e.g., hospital, skilled nursing facility, or rehabilitation facility) and seen within 60 days following discharge in the office by the physician providing ongoing care who had a reconciliation of the discharge medications with the current medication list in the medical record documented

76. Prevention of Catheter-Related Bloodstream Infections: Central Venous Catheter (CVC) Insertion Protocol
Percentage of patients, regardless of age, who undergo CVC insertion for whom CVC was inserted with all elements of maximal sterile barrier technique (cap AND mask AND sterile gown AND sterile gloves AND a large sterile sheet AND hand hygiene AND 2% chlorhexidine for cutaneous antisepsis [or acceptable alternative antiseptics per current guideline]) followed

114. Preventive Care and Screening: Inquiry Regarding Tobacco Use
Percentage of patients aged 18 years or older who were queried about tobacco use one or more times within 24 months

115. Preventive Care and Screening: Advising Smokers and Tobacco Users to Quit
Percentage of patients aged 18 years and older who are smokers or tobacco users and who received advice to quit smoking

124. Health Information Technology: Adoption/Use of Electronic Health Records (EHRs)
Documents whether provider has adopted and is using health information technology. To qualify, the provider must have adopted and be using a certified/qualified EHR.

193. Perioperative Temperature Management
Percentage of patients, regardless of age, undergoing surgical or therapeutic procedures under general or neuraxial anesthesia of 60 minutes' duration or longer, except patients undergoing cardiopulmonary bypass, for whom either active warming was used intraoperatively for the purpose of maintaining normothermia or at least one body temperature $\geq$36°C (or 96.8°F) was recorded within the 30 minutes immediately before or the 15 minutes immediately after anesthesia end time

Cardiac Surgery

43. Coronary Artery Bypass Graft (CABG): Use of Internal Mammary Artery (IMA) in Patients with Isolated CABG Surgery
Percentage of patients aged 18 years and older undergoing isolated CABG surgery using an IMA graft

44. Coronary Artery Bypass Graft (CABG): Preoperative Beta Blocker in Patients with Isolated CABG Surgery
Percentage of patients aged 18 years and older undergoing isolated CABG surgery who received a beta blocker within 24 hours prior to surgical incision

45. Perioperative Care: Discontinuation of Prophylactic Antibiotics (Cardiac Procedures)
Percentage of cardiac surgical patients aged 18 years and older undergoing procedures with the indications for prophylactic antibiotics who received a prophylactic antibiotic and who have an order for discontinuation of prophylactic antibiotics within 48 hours of surgical end time

164. Coronary Artery Bypass Graft (CABG): Prolonged Intubation (Ventilation)
Percentage of patients aged 18 years and older undergoing isolated CABG surgery who require intubation > 24 hours

165. Coronary Artery Bypass Graft (CABG): Deep Sternal Wound Infection Rate
Percentage of patients aged 18 years and older undergoing isolated CABG surgery who developed deep sternal wound infection (involving muscle, bone, and/or mediastinum requiring operative intervention) within 30 days postoperatively

166. Coronary Artery Bypass Graft (CABG): Stroke/Cerebrovascular Accident (CVA)
Percentage of patients aged 18 years and older undergoing isolated CABG surgery who had a stroke/CVA within 24 hours postoperatively

167. Coronary Artery Bypass Graft (CABG): Postoperative Renal Insufficiency
Percentage of patients aged 18 years and older undergoing isolated CABG surgery who develop postoperative renal insufficiency or require dialysis

168. Coronary Artery Bypass Graft (CABG): Surgical Reexploration
Percentage of patients aged 18 years and older undergoing isolated CABG surgery who require a return to the operating room for mediastinal bleeding/tamponade, graft occlusion (attributable to acute closure, thrombosis, or technical or embolic origin), or other cardiac reason

169. Coronary Artery Bypass Graft (CABG): Antiplatelet Medications at Discharge
Percentage of patients aged 18 years and older undergoing isolated CABG surgery who have antiplatelet medication at discharge

170. Coronary Artery Bypass Graft (CABG): Beta Blockers Administered at Discharge
Percentage of patients aged 18 years and older undergoing isolated CABG surgery who were discharged on beta blockers

171. Coronary Artery Bypass Graft (CABG): Lipid Management and Counseling
Percentage of patients aged 18 years and older undergoing isolated CABG surgery who have antilipid treatment at discharge

***Table 2* Continued**

197. Coronary Artery Disease (CAD): Drug Therapy for Lowering Low-Density Lipoprotein Cholesterol
Percentage of patients aged 18 years and older with a diagnosis of CAD who were prescribed a lipid-lowering therapy (based on current American College of Cardiology/American Heart Association guidelines)

General Surgery/Colorectal Surgery

185. Endoscopy and Polyp Surveillance: Colonoscopy Interval for Patients with a History of Adenomatous Polyps — Avoidance of Inappropriate Use
Percentage of patients aged 18 years and older receiving a surveillance colonoscopy and with a history of colonic polyp(s) in a previous colonoscopy who had a follow-up interval of 3 or more years since their last colonoscopy documented in the colonoscopy report

Ophthalmology

12. Primary Open-Angle Glaucoma (POAG): Optic Nerve Evaluation
Percentage of patients aged 18 years and older with a diagnosis of POAG who have an optic nerve head evaluation during one or more office visits within 12 months

14. Age-Related Macular Degeneration (AMD): Dilated Macular Examination
Percentage of patients aged 50 years and older with a diagnosis of AMD who had a dilated macular examination performed that included documentation of the presence or absence of macular thickening or hemorrhage AND the level of macular degeneration severity during one or more office visits within 12 months

139. Cataracts: Comprehensive Preoperative Assessment for Cataract Surgery with Intraocular Lens (IOL) Placement
Percentage of patients aged 18 years and older with a procedure of cataract surgery with IOL placement who received a comprehensive preoperative assessment of (1) dilated fundus examination; (2) axial length, corneal keratometry measurement, and method of IOL power calculation reviewed; and (3) functional or medical indication(s) for surgery prior to the cataract surgery with IOL placement within 12 months prior to cataract surgery

141. Primary Open-Angle Glaucoma (POAG): Reduction of Intraocular Pressure (IOP) by 15% OR Documentation of a Plan of Care
Percentage of patients aged 18 years and older with a diagnosis of POAG whose glaucoma treatment has not failed (the most recent IOP was reduced by at least 15% from the preintervention level), OR if the most recent IOP was not reduced by at least 15% from the preintervention level, a plan of care was documented within 12 months

191. Cataracts: 20/40 or Better Visual Acuity within 90 Days following Cataract Surgery
Percentage of patients aged 18 years and older with a diagnosis of uncomplicated cataract who had cataract surgery and no significant ocular conditions impacting the visual outcome of surgery and had best-corrected visual acuity of 20/40 or better (distance or near) achieved within 90 days following the cataract surgery

192. Cataracts: Complications within 30 Days following Cataract Surgery Requiring Additional Surgical Procedures
Percentage of patients aged 18 years and older with a diagnosis of uncomplicated cataract who had cataract surgery and any of a specified list of surgical procedures in the 30 days following cataract surgery that would indicate the occurrence of any of the following major complications: retained nuclear fragments, endophthalmitis, dislocated or wrong power IOL, retinal detachment, or wound dehiscence

Orthopedics

24. Osteoporosis: Communication with the Physician Managing Ongoing Care Postfracture of Hip, Spine, or Distal Radius for Men and Women Aged 50 Years and Older
Percentage of patients aged 50 years and older treated for a hip, spine, or distal radial fracture with documentation of communication with the physician managing the patient's ongoing care that a fracture occurred and that the patient was or should be tested or treated for osteoporosis

40. Osteoporosis: Management following Fracture of Hip, Spine, or Distal Radius for Men and Women Aged 50 Years and Older
Percentage of patients aged 50 years and older with fracture of the hip, spine, or distal radius who had a central dual-energy x-ray absorptiometry measurement ordered or performed or pharmacologic therapy prescribed

Otolaryngology

91. Acute Otitis Externa (AOE): Topical Therapy
Percentage of patients aged 2 years and older with a diagnosis of AOE who were prescribed topical preparations

92. Acute Otitis Externa (AOE): Pain Assessment
Percentage of patient visits for those patients aged 2 years and older with a diagnosis of AOE with assessment for auricular or periauricular pain

93. Acute Otitis Externa (AOE): Systemic Antimicrobial Therapy — Avoidance of Inappropriate Use
Percentage of patients aged 2 years and older with a diagnosis of AOE who were not prescribed systemic antimicrobial therapy

94. Otitis Media with Effusion (OME): Diagnostic Evaluation — Assessment of Tympanic Membrane Mobility
Percentage of patient visits for those patients aged 2 months through 12 years with a diagnosis of OME with assessment of tympanic membrane mobility with pneumatic otoscopy or tympanometry

Surgical Oncology

71. Breast Cancer: Hormonal Therapy for Stage IC–IIIC Estrogen Receptor/Progesterone Receptor (ER/PR)-Positive Breast Cancer
Percentage of female patients aged 18 years and older with stage IC through IIIC, ER- or PR-positive breast cancer who were prescribed tamoxifen or aromatase inhibitor during the 12-month reporting period

72. Colon Cancer: Chemotherapy for Stage III Colon Cancer Patients
Percentage of patients aged 18 years and older with stage IIIA through IIIC colon cancer who are referred for adjuvant chemotherapy, are prescribed adjuvant chemotherapy, or have previously received adjuvant chemotherapy within the 12-month reporting period

99. Breast Cancer Resection Pathology Reporting: pT Category (Primary Tumor) and pN Category (Regional Lymph Nodes) with Histologic Grade
Percentage of breast cancer resection pathology reports that include the pT category (primary tumor), the pN category (regional lymph nodes), and the histologic grade

100. Colorectal Cancer Resection Pathology Reporting: pT Category (Primary Tumor) and pN Category (Regional Lymph Nodes) with Histologic Grade
Percentage of colon and rectum cancer resection pathology reports that include the pT category (primary tumor), the pN category (regional lymph nodes), and the histologic grade

Table 2 Continued

112. Preventive Care and Screening: Screening Mammography
Percentage of women aged 40 through 69 years who had a mammogram to screen for breast cancer within 24 months

113. Preventive Care and Screening: Colorectal Cancer Screening
Percentage of patients aged 50 through 75 years who received the appropriate colorectal cancer screening

136. Melanoma: Follow-up Aspects of Care
Percentage of patients, regardless of age, with a new diagnosis of melanoma or a history of melanoma who received all of the following aspects of care within 12 months: (1) patient was asked specifically if he/she had any new or changing moles; AND (2) a complete physical skin examination was performed and the morphology, size, and location of new or changing pigmented lesions were noted; AND (3) patient was counseled to perform a monthly self skin examination

137. Melanoma: Continuity of Care — Recall System
Percentage of patients, regardless of age, with a current diagnosis of melanoma or a history of melanoma whose information was entered, at least once within a 12-month period, into a recall system that includes a target date for the next complete physical skin examination AND a process to follow-up with patients who either did not make an appointment within the specified time frame or who missed a scheduled appointment

138. Melanoma: Coordination of Care
Percentage of patients, regardless of age, with a new occurrence of melanoma who have a treatment plan documented in the chart that was communicated to the physician(s) providing continuing care within 1 month of diagnosis

157. Thoracic Surgery: Recording of Clinical Stage for Lung Cancer and Esophageal Cancer Resection
Percentage of surgical patients aged 18 years and older undergoing resection for lung or esophageal cancer who had clinical TNM staging provided prior to surgery

194. Oncology: Cancer Stage Documented
Percentage of patients, regardless of age, with a diagnosis of breast, colon, or rectal cancer who are seen in the ambulatory setting who have a baseline AJCC cancer stage or documentation that the cancer is metastatic in the medical record at least once within 12 months

Urology

102. Prostate Cancer: Avoidance of Overuse of Bone Scan for Staging Low-Risk Prostate Cancer Patients
Percentage of patients, regardless of age, with a diagnosis of prostate cancer at low risk of recurrence receiving interstitial prostate brachytherapy, OR external-beam radiotherapy to the prostate, OR radical prostatectomy, OR cryotherapy who did not have a bone scan performed at any time since diagnosis of prostate cancer

104. Prostate Cancer: Adjuvant Hormonal Therapy for High-Risk Prostate Cancer Patients
Percentage of patients, regardless of age, with a diagnosis of prostate cancer at high risk for recurrence receiving external-beam radiotherapy to the prostate who were prescribed adjuvant hormonal therapy (GnRH agonist or antagonist)

105. Prostate Cancer: Three-Dimensional Radiotherapy
Percentage of patients, regardless of age, with a diagnosis of clinically localized prostate cancer receiving external-beam radiotherapy as a primary therapy to the prostate with or without nodal irradiation (no metastases; no salvage therapy) who receive three-dimensional conformal radiotherapy (3D-CRT) or intensity-modulated radiation therapy

Vascular Surgery

126. Diabetes Mellitus: Diabetic Foot and Ankle Care, Peripheral Neuropathy — Neurologic Evaluation
Percentage of patients aged 18 years and older with a diagnosis of diabetes mellitus who had a neurologic examination of their lower extremities within 12 months

127. Diabetes Mellitus: Diabetic Foot and Ankle Care, Ulcer Prevention — Evaluation of Footwear
Percentage of patients aged 18 years and older with a diagnosis of diabetes mellitus who were evaluated for proper footwear and sizing

158. Carotid Endarterectomy: Use of Patch During Conventional Carotid Endarterectomy
Percentage of patients aged 18 years and older undergoing conventional (noneversion) carotid endarterectomy who undergo patch closure of the arteriotomy

163. Diabetes Mellitus: Foot Examination
Percentage of patients aged 18 through 75 years with diabetes who had a foot examination

172. Hemodialysis Vascular Access Decision Making by Surgeon to Maximize Placement of Autogenous Arteriovenous (AV) Fistula
Percentage of patients aged 18 years and older with a diagnosis of advanced chronic kidney disease (stage 4 or 5) or end-stage renal disease requiring hemodialysis vascular access documented by surgeon to have received autogenous AV fistula

186. Wound Care: Use of Compression System in Patients with Venous Ulcers
Percentage of patients aged 18 years and older with a diagnosis of venous ulcer who were prescribed compression therapy within the 12-month reporting period

195. Stenosis Measurement in Carotid Imaging Studies
Percentage of final reports for all patients, regardless of age, for carotid imaging studies (neck magnetic resonance angiography, neck computed tomographic angiography, neck duplex ultrasonography, carotid angiography) performed that include direct or indirect reference to measurements of distal internal carotid diameter as the denominator for stenosis measurement

201. Ischemic Vascular Disease (IVD): Blood Pressure Management Control
Percentage of patients aged 18 years and older with IVD who had most recent blood pressure in control (less than 140/90 mm Hg)

202. Ischemic Vascular Disease (IVD): Complete Lipid Profile
Percentage of patients aged 18 years and older with IVD who received at least one lipid profile within 12 months

203. Ischemic Vascular Disease (IVD): Low-Density Lipoprotein (LDL) Cholesterol Control
Percentage of patients aged 18 years and older with IVD who had most recent LDL cholesterol level in control (less than 100 mg/dL)

204. Ischemic Vascular Disease (IVD): Use of Aspirin or Another Antithrombotic
Percentage of patients aged 18 years and older with IVD with documented use of aspirin or other antithrombotic

The number of each measure is that assigned by the Centers for Medicare and Medicaid Services. Available at: https://www.cms.gov/PQRI/Downloads/2010_PQRI_MeasuresList_111309.pdf. accessed January 10, 2011.
AJCC = American Joint Committee on Cancer; GnRH = gonadotropin-releasing hormone.

profiling based on use of medical resources, whereas 19% faced incentives derived from quality of care measures. Patient satisfaction is undoubtedly important, but it is not clear that improved patient satisfaction alone suffices to address problems of cost-effectiveness.

Lastly, there is the issue of how providers might react when there are differences in P4P programs among the various health plans in which they participate. Many providers would prefer health plans to use a single standardized set of measures, but local market environments can make such standardization unlikely.[47] As a result, providers may ignore measures that seem to be contradictory, are perceived as too complex, or derive from health plans from which they get relatively few patients. A related concern is that some P4P programs could have unintended negative consequences if physicians are convinced that the program does not incorporate adequate risk adjustment mechanisms. Providers then might simply opt out of seeing challenging patients.[48,49] To avoid some of these problems, the Agency for Healthcare Research and Quality (AHRQ) has a specific section of their website (www.ahrq.gov/qual/p4pguide.htm) devoted to P4P programs, including a decision guide for purchasers.

P4P and "value-based purchasing" are incentive payment or shared savings programs that are related to "gainsharing." The Office of the Inspector General (OIG) has defined gainsharing as an "arrangement in which a hospital will share with each physician group a percentage of the hospital's cost savings arising from the physician groups' implementation of cost reduction methods."[50] Although intended to encourage physicians to deliver quality care, such gainsharing arrangements can technically look like a model of a kickback; moreover, they are barred by the civil monetary penalty law, which prohibits hospitals from rewarding physicians for reducing services to patients. The Deficit Reduction Act of 2005 directed the CMS to conduct demonstration projects, and these are now under way.

These programs notwithstanding, substantial direct evidence of the link between systems and quality comes from the quality improvement efforts of organizations that analyze and standardize systems of care. Perhaps the most notable of these efforts is the multi-institutional Northern New England Cardiovascular Disease Study Group (NNECVDSG).[51] This group began in 1990 and consisted of cardiac surgical teams (e.g., surgeons, nurses, anesthesiologists, pump technicians) that received feedback on outcomes, were trained in Deming's quality improvement techniques, and site-visited other participating centers. They also periodically met to share data and discuss processes of care. The result has been to substantially reduce morbidity and mortality from cardiac surgery and to minimize the year-to-year mortality variations among the institutions. They also had a low incidence of procedures that did not adhere to recommended indications for surgery.[52]

The group's success can be attributed to several characteristics: there is no ambiguity of purpose, the data are not owned by any member or subgroup of members, members have an established safe place to work, a forum is set up for discussion, and there is regular feedback. This was achieved without personal criticism or an attempt to identify any proverbial "bad apples." Despite concerns that the findings would lead to unfavorable publicity, this did not occur. Three important conclusions to be drawn from these efforts are as follows: physician-initiated interventions can be as effective as external review (and possibly more effective) in improving quality; a systems approach to quality improvement is better than a bad apple approach; and it is possible to conduct quality improvement programs involving practice groups that might otherwise be viewed as competitors.

The VA's NSQIP is another example of a successful quality initiative, achieving a 27% reduction in 30-day mortality after major procedures and a 45% decrease in morbidity.[53] NSQIP found the two most important risk factors for prolonged hospital stay after major elective surgery to be the intraoperative processes of care and postoperative adverse events.[54] Notably, the savings from improved surgical care far exceeded investment in the project.[55] NSQIP has now expanded into the broader community under the auspices of the American College of Surgeons (ACS). NSQIP data also have been used to validate the AHRQ Patient Safety Indicators (www.academyhealth.org/2005/ppt/tsilimingras.ppt).

Other successful surgically related quality improvement efforts include Intermountain Health Systems in Utah; the Maine Medical Assessment Foundation[56]; the Washington State Surgical Clinical Outcomes Assessment Program (SCOAP)[57]; Quality Surgical Solutions in Kentucky[58]; the Michigan Surgical Quality collaborative[59]; the Society for Thoracic Surgery national database, which is now widely accepted as a benchmark for quality in cardiac surgery[60]; the New England Colorectal Cancer Quality Project[61]; the Vascular Study Group of Northern New England[62]; and the National Surgical Infection Collaborative.[45]

The Maine and Michigan efforts are notable in that they have been carried out in conjunction with insurers.[63–65] Moreover, none of these efforts increased liability exposure; indeed, they often reduced it. Because the practice profiles were physician initiated, there was little risk that the findings would be used to make decisions about credentialing, reimbursement, or contracting.[56] It is also noteworthy that the parties that funded these efforts (including insurers) usually agreed to confidentiality in return for the benefit associated with voluntary physician involvement.

Measuring Health Outcomes

As noted above, the primary goal of investigating the structure and process components of care is, ultimately, to improve outcomes. Using outcomes to assess quality can be confounded by a number of factors, however. One such factor is the reduced usefulness of traditional metrics. For instance, mortality is infrequent with most surgical procedures, and morbidity such as wound infection rates can be difficult to assess in an era of early discharges. Other short-term outcome metrics, such as length of stay, readmission, or return to work, are often influenced by deeply rooted social and economic factors. A further issue is that many measures of quality lack standard definitions.[66]

Another factor confounding the measurement of health care outcomes has been the growth of knowledge and technology that has increased surgical care related to chronic and/or degenerative diseases. Recent data show that 133 million people, or almost half of all Americans, live with a chronic condition.[67] That number is projected to increase by more than 1% per year by 2030, resulting in an estimated chronically ill population of 171 million. Moreover, almost half of all people with chronic illnesses have multiple conditions. Integrated health care delivery via the chronic care model is intended to address the many deficiencies in the current management of diseases such as diabetes, heart disease, depression, and asthma. Traditional measures of quality (e.g., 30-day mortality) that are applied to acute conditions such as perforated ulcer are not as applicable here. Given that the number and complexity of treatment options for many surgical conditions have increased, it has become necessary to identify quality metrics for each treatment strategy. There also is increasing emphasis on patient-centered care; given the multicultural nature of US society, the result is substantial heterogeneity in patient perspectives on quality. Overall, there has been little research (i.e., clinical trials) on the quality perspectives of vulnerable populations.

Health care quality in this context is typically assessed in terms of quality-adjusted life years (QALYs),[68,69] a measure that reflects the length of time during which a patient experiences a given health status. The lexicon of research in this area is extensive. Cost-utility analysis is the form of CEA of alternative interventions where costs are measured in monetary units and outcomes in terms of patient utility, usually to the patient, in QALYs. A patient utility is the relative desirability or preference from the patient's perspective for a given health outcome. QALYs are units of health outcomes that adjust gains or losses of years of life subsequent to a health care intervention by the quality of life during those years. Other (although less frequently employed) measures for patient utilities include disability-adjusted life-years (DALYs) and health-year equivalents (HYEs). DALYs are units of health status adjusting age-specific life expectancy by loss of health and years of life attributable to disability from disease or injury, whereas HYEs are the number of years of perfect health considered to be equal to the remaining years of life in their respective health states.

QALYs are applicable to assessing surgical outcomes. They can be calculated by several different methods; some include objective measures (e.g., functional status), whereas others only consider subjective estimates of well-being. Even the objective measures consider patient-desired outcomes to capture the meaningfulness of a given functional status. For instance, a patient may not be able to walk as far as another, but whether the former has a worse quality of life depends on each patient's lifestyle.[70] The result is that QALYs data tend not to follow a normal distribution, and comparative analyses often require use of nonparametric techniques.[71]

Estimates of QALYs can be affected by other factors.[26,72] For instance, estimates of the future value of an outcome measure may vary with the prevailing circumstances at the time of assessment (e.g., acute pain) or with the patient's age (e.g., elderly patients often place great value on the ability to live independently). Calculation of QALYs may also be affected by gender, ethnicity, socioeconomic status, religious beliefs, time away from work, and other factors that affect attitudes about health care. One study noted that surgeons tended to underestimate the importance of patients' social and spiritual themes.[73] Adjusting outcome measures to account for health status and severity of illness before treatment also can be difficult.[74]

As with other aspects of cost-effectiveness, estimates of QALYs are confounded by different perspectives among patients, providers, and payers with regard to the experiential, physiologic, and resource-related dimensions that should apply. Thus, the weight given to clinical probabilities, patient utilities and preferences, and cost will affect the calculations. Assessment of quality is further complicated when there is no consensus across perspectives with regard to the preferred strategy or outcome. Finally, quality of life studies can be compromised by other methodological flaws, such as a relative paucity of validated instruments for measuring health-related quality of life, especially in certain specialty areas.[75] In this context, a 2008 review could not identify a fully validated instrument for assessing postoperative recovery.[76]

INTERPRETING AND/OR INITIATING COST-EFFECTIVENESS ANALYSES

A primer to initiate and/or interpret CEA is available at www.acponline.org/shell-cgi/printhappy.pl/journals/ecp/sepoct00/primer.htm.

Several important principles that must be considered when performing and/or interpreting a CEA are the comparison, perspective, direct and indirect costs, time horizon, discounting, and sensitivity analyses.[77–79] The specific comparison between one health care intervention and another should be precisely defined at the outset of the analysis. Alternative perspectives are of society overall (favored by many), a third party payer, a physician, a hospital, or a patient. CEA should incorporate two types of cost; direct costs represent the value of all goods, services, and other resources consumed in providing health care or dealing with the side effects of the care, whereas indirect costs (or productivity losses) include the costs of lost work attributable to absenteeism or early retirement, impaired productivity at work, or premature mortality. Intangible costs (i.e., pain, suffering, and grief) are often omitted, which is an important limitation of most CEA. The time horizon of a CEA is the time frame of the study and should be long enough to capture streams of health and economic outcomes; depending on the research question, the time horizon might encompass a disease episode, patient life, or even multiple generations. Discounting allows the model to account for the effect of the passage of time on the values of costs and outcomes, such that costs and outcomes are discounted relative to their present value (e.g., at a rate of 3 to 5% per year). Inflation should be a separate consideration. Finally, sensitivity analyses should be performed to determine if plausible variations in the estimates of certain variables thought to be subject to significant uncertainty affect the results of the cost analysis.

Lower values of cost-effectiveness are understood to be "more cost-effective" or have "increased cost-effectiveness." In contrast "less cost-effective" and "decreased cost-effectiveness" refer to higher costs per LYS. Cost-effectiveness that has a negative value implies that money would be saved.

Particular points that warrant consideration are as follows:

- CEA is highly sensitive to the choice of compared strategies: it often involves marginal benefits, and excluding a simple strategy in which the only comparison is between treatment and no treatment can make a particular strategy appear far more cost-effective than it otherwise might seem. CEA does not answer the question of which strategy is economically preferred; rather, it identifies which strategy is more effective in terms of LYS for a given expenditure.[80]

- The quality of supporting evidence is another important consideration. Data garnered in real practice or from a registry are more likely to be generalizable than data that are modeled or collected from a clinical trial.
- Determinations made under optimal circumstances (efficacy) tend to overestimate cost-effectiveness compared with determinations made under real-world conditions (true effectiveness). This distinction between efficacy and effectiveness is reflected in how differences in postoperative stroke rates influence the cost-effectiveness of carotid endarterectomy. Randomized, controlled trials (RCTs) show this procedure to be efficacious when performed by surgeons, with low rates of perioperative stroke and death. As the incidence of stroke and other complications increases with more general use, the procedure becomes less effective or even ineffective.[81–83] If effectiveness can vary over a relatively narrow range of outcomes, there is a strong ethical motivation for surgeons to be familiar with their own clinical outcomes and seek their patients' informed consent based on their personal results.[84] In this context, differences in quality or cost measures may be more a function of patient mix than the abilities of the wider surgeon population.
- There needs to be awareness of recent concerns that there may be a bias related to the funding of the study.

These and other considerations require surgeons to possess fundamental skills related to critical analysis of the medical literature, technology assessment, use of diagnostic testing, and clinical decision analysis. Specifics on these skills are further detailed below.

CRITICAL ANALYSIS OF THE MEDICAL LITERATURE

The medical literature is so expansive that one can keep current only with a small fraction of it. Moreover, the potential value of a given study is assigned a level of evidence based on the study's methodology. Yet even here there are a number of accepted techniques for grading level of evidence that include that from the Centre for Evidence Based Medicine (CEBM; www.cebm.net/index.aspx?o=1025), the U.S. Preventive Health Task Force, or the Grading of Recommendations, Assessment, Development and Evaluation (GRADE) system.[85] The GRADE Working Group is an international collaboration of guideline developers, methodologists, and clinicians whose recommendations on clinical practice guidelines have been increasingly validated in a number of practice settings. Many guideline organizations and medical societies have endorsed the system and adopted it for their guideline processes. Further discussion of guidelines is in the section on Clinical Guidelines below.

RCTs are at the high end of all these scales, and meta-analyses of RCTs have even higher validity. Still, even RCTs have shortcomings: the reporting methods are not fully standardized; their stringent inclusion criteria tend to limit their applicability to highly specific groups of patients (e.g., elderly and/or pregnant patients are often excluded); they can be expensive; and the numbers of patients needed for statistical purposes can be impractical. In addition, study findings that might seem to apply to a particular patient may be difficult to reproduce in settings that differ from the controlled conditions of the original trial. Also, the pressure to enroll patients in such trials has, on occasion, led to questionable ethical behavior by the investigators.

Three particularly valuable sources for identifying studies relevant to cost-effectiveness and judging the quality of those studies are MEDLINE (www.ncbi.nlm.nih.gov/PubMed/medline.html), the Cochrane Collaboration (www.cochrane.org), and the CEBM (www.cebm.net). Each site has relative advantages and disadvantages. The Cochrane Collaboration is an international network of epidemiologists and clinicians who systematically review the best available medical evidence; it includes sources not always accessible through MEDLINE but, in contrast to MEDLINE, requires a subscription. Recent Cochrane Collaboration reviews are abstracted monthly in the *Journal of the American College of Surgeons* (*JACS*).

The ACS also makes several literature resources available. These include *Selected Readings in General Surgery* (*SRGS*), a trusted point of reference that is also available in a Web-based version; and *Evidence Based Reviews in Surgery* (*EBRS*), a Web-based program developed jointly with the Canadian Association of General Surgeons. Each month during the academic year, *EBRS* presents a clinical and methodological article that teaches critical appraisal skills. More information about these programs is available at www.facs.org. A series of publications by the Evidence-Based Medicine Working Group also provides further insight into critical literature analysis (http://jamaevidence.com/resource/520).

The complexities of literature analysis are reflected in a prospective study of the value of computed tomography (CT) in diagnosing appendicitis. This study compared the clinical likelihood of appendicitis (as estimated by the referring surgeon) to the estimated probability of appendicitis (as determined by CT) and the pathologic condition (or absence thereof), which was then confirmed by operation or recovery.[86] The clinical likelihood of appendicitis was assigned to one of four categories: (1) definitely appendicitis (80 to 100% likelihood), (2) probably appendicitis (60 to 79%), (3) equivocally appendicitis (40 to 59%), and (4) possibly appendicitis (20 to 39%). The real-life observed incidence of appendicitis in these four categories was 78%, 56%, 33%, and 44%, respectively. Thus, CT interpretations had a sensitivity of 98%, a specificity of 98%, a positive predictive value of 98%, a negative predictive value of 98%, and an accuracy of 98% for either diagnosing or ruling out appendicitis.

Although these results may seem relatively clear-cut, it is possible that the study could have yielded different results and reached other conclusions if it had been performed at another institution. For example, the clinical diagnosis of appendicitis is more accurate among men than among women, and, as a result, the relative value of CT scanning will vary according to the gender distribution of the study group. Also, variability in the estimates of the clinical likelihood of appendicitis among surgeons in that institution, the availability of less expensive alternatives to in-hospital observation, and use of the emergency department for triage all might lead to substantially different results. The impact of variability in clinical estimates of appendicitis is reflected by the fact that in this report, 53% of the patients had appendicitis; in contrast, other studies have shown that only 30% of patients with an admitting diagnosis of appendicitis eventually underwent appendectomy.[87] The impact of the accuracy of CT or ultrasonography on negative appendectomies also has been reported.[88]

Literature analysis also requires a distinction between relative and absolute risk reduction. The degree of relative improvement is a function of the baseline results such that a treatment that reduces the incidence of an undesired outcome from 5% to 4% and a treatment that reduces it from 50% to 40% both achieve a 20% relative reduction in risk. However, the second treatment achieves a 10-fold greater absolute risk reduction. In addition, the cost-effectiveness of these two treatments is likely to be very different. This distinction between absolute and relative improvement is an important aspect of patient-centeredness in decision making. It is particularly relevant to patients' willingness to participate in trials of adjuvant cancer therapy. Their decisions for or against such therapy may be affected more by the potential for absolute benefit than by relative benefit.

Interpretation of the literature also needs to consider disease staging. Earlier diagnosis may appear to improve long-term survival but actually only identifies the condition for a longer time. This is known as lead-time bias, and it can lead to overestimation of disease prevalence.[89]

Literature assessment skills are also needed to keep pace with patients' growing access to medical information. There are tens of thousands of health-related Web sites, and tens of millions of adults find health information online. Patients also get information from poorly monitored sources, such as disease-specific bulletin boards. At least some of this information will be inaccurate, misleading, out-of-date, incomplete, or unconventional.[90] For example a recent study of thyroid cancer information on the Internet determined that the data pertaining to surgical treatment, in particular, were wanting, and only 38% of Web sites were updated in the previous 2 years. No predictors of quality were identified.[91] Indeed, a study of the methodological quality of economic analyses of surgical procedures concluded that studies of cost-effectiveness in surgery in the medical literature often do not meet established criteria.[92]

TECHNOLOGY ASSESSMENT

The "technological imperative" reflects a prevailing societal attitude that equates the latest with the best and creates considerable pressure to acquire the newest equipment and techniques, even before its value is evident. The explosive growth of technology in recent years has been a particularly important contributor to the rapid growth of health care costs.[93,94] Although many technological advances have undeniably improved surgical care, some new technologies do not prove to be useful. Accordingly, surgeons need to know how to make decisions about technology acquisition[95] and how they may contribute to excess capacity and increase health care costs. The problem begins with providers who succumb to the technological imperative before a technology's value is fully known. Other providers, fearful of being left behind, then follow suit. If the new technology is beneficial, capacity may grow to the point that it exceeds community's needs; if not beneficial, injudicious adoption severely reduces cost-effectiveness. Although some advocate competition among providers as a way of restraining health care costs, competition driven by the technological imperative can contribute to inflationary increases in these same costs. A further consideration is the opportunity costs related to differences in efficiency among competing surgical devices.[96]

Innovations that involve new applications of existing technology are a particular challenge.[97] Laparoscopic cholecystectomy is a striking example of an existing technology that was rapidly and widely adopted into a new surgical procedure before its nuances were fully appreciated or mastered. Although now a relatively safe procedure, the learning curve of laparoscopic cholecystectomy was associated with a number of bile duct injuries; it is conceivable that at least some of these adverse events could have been avoided had the procedure been introduced in a more systematic fashion. Important lessons here come from a study that analyzed the time needed to learn minimally invasive cardiac surgery.[98] Fast-learning teams were characterized by members who worked well together in the past, had gone through the early learning phase together before adding new members, scheduled several of the new procedures close together, discussed each case in detail beforehand and afterward, and carefully tracked results. Notably, surgeons on the fast-learning teams were less experienced than those on the slow-learning teams but were more willing to accept input from others on the team.

Given this background, there are a number of questions that should be asked whenever a new technology or an innovation in surgical care is being considered:

- Has the new technology or innovation been adequately tested for safety and efficacy?
- Is the new technology or innovation at least as safe and effective as existing, proven techniques?
- Is the individual proposing to perform the new procedure fully qualified to do so? This raises issues pertaining to surgeon education, skill acquisition, team identification, credentialing, and systems preparation failure.
- Is the new technology effective for the intended purpose? Does the new technology or innovation improve cost-effectiveness?
- Has allowance been made for appropriate patient selection and informed consent?
- What is the appropriate role of industry in new technology education efforts?
- What role do media and public expectations and desires play in driving the application of new technology?

USE OF DIAGNOSTIC TESTING

Laboratory and imaging studies account for a large share of health care costs, and there are substantial variations in the use of such studies. Improving cost-effectiveness goes beyond just being aware of a test's sensitivity (i.e., the ability to identify patients with a disease) and specificity (i.e., the ability to identify patients without a disease). It also depends on the prevalence of the disease in the population in question.[99] As an example, if a given test has a 98% sensitivity and a 98%

specificity and is applied to a group of patients with a disease prevalence of 10% (i.e., 10% of them has the disease), the results of 49 of 500 patients will be true positives (500 × 0.98 × 0.1) and 9 (500 × 0.02 × 0.9) will be false positives. If this same test is applied to a population with a disease prevalence of 1% (a more likely prevalence in the real world), the results of fewer than five of every 500 patients tested (500 × 0.98 × 0.01) will be true positives and just under 10 (500 × 0.02 × 0.99) will be false positives. Thus, for any given sensitivity, the ratio of false true positives to true positives increases inversely with disease prevalence.

If this example was applied to a screening test, which if positive might then indicate the need for a riskier downstream test, the likelihood is that an increasing number of false positives would be exposed to the cost and safety risks of the follow-up test without potential benefit. This illustrates the shortcomings of appropriateness as a measure of quality where the relation between health care cost and quality was seen exclusively as positive. Given that complications of downstream tests are just as likely to occur among patients with false positives as among patients with true positives, the net effect of such testing is to decrease the slope of the cost-benefit curve and increase the slope of the cost-harm curve. The differential effects of such testing on these curves alter the relation of quality to cost and produce a negative slope [*see Figure 6*].[100] This is more than just a theoretical relation as there are now data to show that hospitals' performance on quality of care is not associated with the intensity of their spending.[101] Another key point is that the slope between two points represents the incremental changes in cost-effectiveness.[80] Thus, changes in cost-effectiveness may vary, depending on which portion of the curve is considered.

This effect of disease prevalence on the incidence of false positives establishes a test's value or utility and explains why a test may have relatively little value as a screening test in general practice (where the disease prevalence is low) but may have high value as a diagnostic tool in a specialty practice (where referrals increase the relative prevalence of the disease). The above calculations illustrate how CEAs can be performed on diagnostic tests and screening techniques as well as more traditional comparisons of treatment.

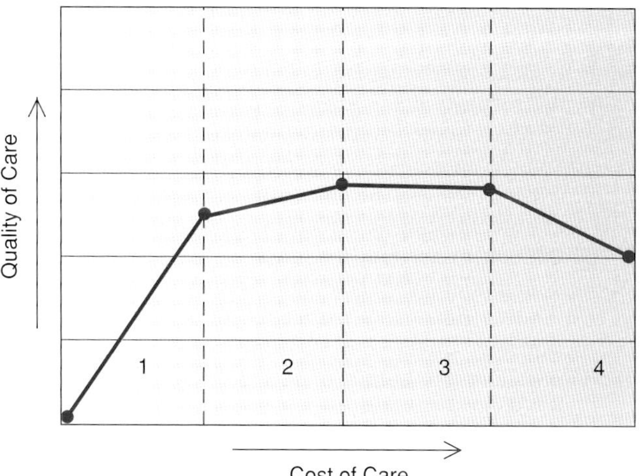

Figure 6 **The new concept of quality and cost.[99] A positive association between quality and cost still exists in zones 1 and 2, but the slope of the curve flattens in zone 3 and actually becomes negative in zone 4. Here, further cost increases are associated with decreasing quality because increased use of sophisticated (albeit riskier) technology in earlier (or even just suspected) stages of disease may result in a flat slope (zone 3) or even a negative one (zone 4).**

A specific example of how test utility might affect clinical decision making is that of the functional assessment of incidental adrenal masses.[102] Biochemical testing of patients with these masses in the absence of concrete signs and symptoms may be of relatively little value. Analyses of many other "routine" preoperative tests also suggest that they may add little value.[103,104] Whether a recent increase in testing noted among cancer patients has added value is unknown.[105]

CLINICAL DECISION ANALYSIS

Clinical decision analysis involves identifying and quantifying the effect or impact of each option involved in a diagnostic or therapeutic decision. On the basis of the best estimates available, the outcome of each decision acquires a probability, and each component of the decision tree carries an explicit assumption that allows an appreciation of how specific factors affect the outcome. Management of penetrating colon trauma[106] and treatment of asymptomatic carotid artery stenosis[107] are two examples subject to such analyses. It is important to emphasize that physicians should not feel unduly constrained by these clinical decision analyses; depending on individual patient circumstances, it may be reasonable to give greater consideration to some options and discount others. Thus, decision trees are not intended as absolute mandates but rather as tools for reducing uncertainty and thereby increasing cost-effectiveness.[108–110]

Some find the mathematics and lexicon of clinical decision analyses intimidating; others may perceive such analyses as exemplifying a "cookbook" approach to health care. Markov modeling involves a set of mutually exclusive states for which there are transition probabilities of moving from one state to another. States have a uniform time period, and transition probabilities remain constant over time, which is often not a realistic circumstance. Nonetheless, it is clear that formal clinical decision analysis yields estimates of the importance of specific facets of health care that might be difficult to obtain otherwise.[111]

PRACTICE GUIDELINES/CRITICAL PATHWAYS

Practice guidelines, also known as critical pathways, intend to indicate the best known processes of care for improving safety and quality. They seek to standardize medical processes, especially in high-volume, high-risk, or complex procedures.[112] Such standardization is intended to minimize the variations in practice that imply consequent variations in the cost and quality of care. These pathways are increasingly developed by specialty societies and consensus conferences; they are also available commercially and through focused publications. Online guidelines are available through the National Guideline Clearinghouse (NGC) of the AHRQ at www.guideline.gov or through evidence-based practice centers. Critical pathways seek to improve cost-effectiveness by displaying optimal goals for both patients and providers. The potential benefit of these pathways can be quantified using deviation-based cost modeling.[113]

These guidelines have been criticized on several accounts: the evidence and knowledge needed for such guidelines are often lacking[114]; there may be a lack of consensus regarding what constitutes "best practice"; guidelines from different sources may be at odds with each other; they may not adhere to established methodological standards[115,116]; they may become quickly outdated[117]; they have been criticized as embodying an overly simplistic approach to health care; the focus on quality and efficiency of care is often adopted after a decision has been made to admit a patient or perform a procedure; and they often do not apply to particular patients and can be difficult to use in patients with other, more urgent medical problems. Finally, there are emerging data calling into question whether published practice guidelines are incorporated adequately into all aspects of day-to-day practice, particularly with regard to vulnerable populations, such as the elderly.[118,119]

In summary, use of these guidelines may not automatically improve quality. Thus, they should best be understood not as rigid rules but rather as ways to codify experiences so that others can avoid mistakes. Accordingly, critical pathways should be considered flexible and should be modified on the basis of experience.

COORDINATION OF CARE

The growing complexity of health care makes teamwork and communication increasingly essential. Lack of coordination can increase costs through the duplication of tests and unnecessary delays; it can also decrease patient satisfaction. One study categorized delays as being attributable to test scheduling (31%), availability of other facilities postdischarge (18%), physician decision making (13%), discharge planning (12%), and surgical scheduling (12%).[120] Moreover, poor coordination of care is a notable factor in professional liability claims against surgeons.[121]

ELECTRONIC MEDICAL RECORDS

Electronic medical records have been advocated as a means of expediting the transfer of important information and improving the coordination of care. Indeed, a key portion of the ARRA was the Health Information Technology for Economic and Clinical Health Act (HITECH), which includes substantial funding for implementation of "meaningful use" of information technology. The goal is to bring US health care fully into the Information Age. To date, the effect of introducing information technology (IT) into hospitals and practices has been a mixed bag. The VA has estimated substantial benefits from its investment,[122] but the benefit of electronic medical records at private sector hospitals and in private practices appears to be marginal. Electronic medical records are not a panacea, and their benefit in reducing failure to inform patients of clinically significant outpatient tests was greatest in practices that already had good processes for recording progress notes and test results.[123]

IT is invaluable in improving safety[124,125] as it facilitates use of strategies to reduce medical errors. Such strategies include tools to improve communication, make information more readily accessible, acquire key pieces of information for subsequent process steps, assist with calculations, perform checks in real time, assist with monitoring information, and provide decision support.[126] Studies of computerized clinical decision support systems indicate that practitioners perform better with systems that provide automatic prompts than systems that first require system activation. Such studies also find that there is a greater likelihood of better performance in systems developed by the authors than in those who were not.[127] Computerized physician order entry has been shown to reduce medication errors[128] and facilitate ventilator weaning[129] but is not foolproof and can introduce other types of errors.[130]

Strategies for Improving Cost-effectiveness

It is human nature that every surgeon believes that she or he is among the best. Yet data often show considerable variations in resource use, cost, and outcomes among surgeons. Moreover, these variations cannot readily be accounted for by differences in disease prevalence or severity. Furthermore, areas with higher frequencies of procedures do not have demonstrably better procedure-related health.[131,132] As a result, these variations are thought to be related more to community signatures or physician uncertainty. Curiously, data on individual surgeon performance are often available to hospital administrators and insurance companies but not the surgeons themselves. The result has been that strategies for cost containment and/or quality improvements often originate at the "blunt" end of a system rather than focusing on direct surgeon involvement. Examples of some of these strategies are outlined in the following sections.

BENCHMARKING CLAIMS DATA

Insurers use claims data to create hospital and physician performance profiles of costs and outcomes. The most favorable data are then used to establish benchmarks. Unfortunately, such benchmarks have limitations. For example, they tend to reflect an ideal or exceptional patient population and may not fully account for severity factors that affect outcome.[133] Adjustments for disease severity are particularly difficult to make on the basis of claims data because in many cases, the requisite data either are not collected or are miscoded.[134] Medical record review is effective at accounting for severity but is more time-consuming and costly. Even with medical record review, the effects of comorbid conditions on cost and outcome can be difficult to sort out. As a result, it is still difficult to account for much of the cost variation.[135] Another limitation of benchmarks is that some differences in cost and length of stay are related to factors that are not under surgeons' direct control, such as patient age, gender, and various cultural, ethnic, or socioeconomic factors extrinsic to the medical care system.[136–138] Selection bias can affect outcome reporting.[139] High rates of functional health illiteracy also can adversely affect compliance and thereby outcomes.[140] In the end, some efforts to meet benchmark performance levels actually have the unintended effect of increasing the risk of adverse outcomes in patients with complicated health problems who need more complex care.

PUBLIC REPORT CARDS

Another approach to improving cost-effectiveness has been to distribute provider outcomes directly to the public in the form of report cards.[141] The rationale is that patients armed with this information will choose providers with better outcomes. Such an effort by the CMS (then the Health Care Financing Administration, or HCFA) in the 1980s calculated mortality data for individual hospitals using a risk adjustment model based on DRGs. Subsequently, however, the CMS acknowledged the flaws in the associated mortality model and stopped releasing these data. Subsequently, the CMS (using Medicare data) and some states publicly disclosed provider-specific data on the outcomes of cardiac surgery. Although these efforts used more criteria than were available through DRGs alone,[142,143] the profiles remained controversial because they still did not adequately account for all the differences in case mix and disease severity. Good surgeons operating on high-risk patients could be adversely affected and less qualified surgeons operating on low-risk patients (or perhaps even without indications for surgery) inappropriately rewarded.

Although release of these data did lower patient mortality, it also might have had the unintended consequence of creating incentives to reduce mortality by avoiding high-risk patients.[144,145] These report cards also appeared to have limited credibility among cardiovascular specialists.[145] Moreover, the data seemed to be of limited value to the target audience (i.e., patients undergoing cardiac surgery) in that there were few changes in market share among the involved institutions.

The success of provider report cards in prompting quality improvement depends on several factors.[146,147] These include the strength of the research design and the ease with which the public can understand the text and/or the data display. Despite their shortcomings, use of report cards has now expanded to other specialties. One Web site (www.healthgrades.com) contains hospital outcomes for cardiac, orthopedic, neurologic, pulmonary, and vascular surgery. Transplantation outcomes are also available from the United Network for Organ Sharing (UNOS) at www.unos.org.

To date, evidence supporting a positive effect from these various strategies remains mixed. A 2002 literature review concluded that, based on limited evidence, explicit incentives placing physicians at financial risk appeared to be effective in reducing resource use.[148] However, the empirical evidence regarding the effectiveness of bonus payments on physician resource use was mixed. A more recent review of the value of publicly reported performance data on effectiveness, safety, and patient-centeredness failed to identify conclusive evidence that such reporting was effective.[149] Moreover, only a minority of providers appear to be participating in the PQRI program. This makes it difficult to assess the effect of the program on overall quality. It is still not clear whether the refusal to pay for some "never events" (i.e., shocking medical errors that should never occur) by Medicare[150] and by some private insurers will beneficially impact quality and safety.

Given the limitations of these externally initiated efforts and the remarkable success of physician-initiated efforts noted above, the most difficult step in enhancing cost-effectiveness may be developing a local willingness to initiate the process. Studies of factors associated with practice change in relation to continuing medical education (CME) consistently emphasize that effective change strategies include reminders, patient-mediated interventions, outreach visits, input from opinion leaders, and multifaceted activities. Specific factors associated with an increased probability of practice change are peer interaction, commitment to change, and assessment of the results of change.[151–153] Successful activities place substantial emphasis on performance change rather than simply on learning.[154,155] Additional evidence suggests that improvement in care is more likely to occur with CME activity that is directly linked to processes of care.[156]

An underlying tenet from the outset should be that improving cost-effectiveness is an ongoing process akin to peeling an onion: initial steps inevitably lead to deeper analyses. A starting place may be as simple as choosing a particularly bad outcome and taking steps to avoid its occurrence or recurrence. Simple data charts may reveal changes or patterns in outcomes or resource consumption that might not otherwise be obvious. On occasion, merely standardizing a process is sufficient to substantially improve outcomes. With time, strategies for optimal practice are likely to emerge. However, the majority of these efforts are unlikely to eliminate all variations in provider outcomes. For instance, when advances in the care of cystic fibrosis were adopted nationwide, outcomes improved for most centers, but some centers still had better risk-adjusted outcomes than others.[157] Identifying the factors responsible for these remaining differences is a difficult but critical undertaking to achieve the next level of improvement.

Improving Cost-effectiveness in the Operating Room

The operating room is a frequent target for efforts to improve efficiency. Delays in room turnover are a common complaint, the responsibility for which is variously ascribed to nurses, anesthesiologists, and surgeons themselves. Maintaining large inventories to satisfy individual surgeon preferences also contributes to higher costs, and the growth of minimally invasive surgery has added new dimensions to this challenge.[158] Key issues in this setting include reusable versus disposable equipment, variations in the costs of different types of equipment used to accomplish the same task, and just-in-time inventory. Major pieces of equipment often are duplicated to allow similar cases to be performed simultaneously in different rooms, but this duplication often means that the equipment may then be idle for relatively long periods. More efficient use of such equipment reduces costs, but this requires levels of cooperation and coordination among surgical staff members that heretofore have been hard to achieve.

To improve efficiency, surgeons, who have heretofore often been steeped in the view that they are the "captain of the ship," must embrace the view that all members of the surgical team have interdependent goals for quality, safety, and efficient use of the operating room. Indeed, the team concept requires abandoning the idea that the operating room is staffed by separate surgical, nursing, and anesthesia crews. Models for achieving greater efficiency have been proposed, largely based on the airline industry and aerospace travel coordination.[159] Successful team efforts have led to cost reductions in trauma care[160,161] and to the development of protocols to guide ventilator weaning.[162,163] More human factors research is needed to identify and overcome insidious barriers to human communication.[164–168]

Ambulatory surgical units often are heralded as cost-effective. However, potential savings are likely to depend on existing operating room capacity and on specific payer issues.[169] By taking less complex cases away from the hospital, there may be fewer cases on which the hospital can amortize fixed costs. Another reason ambulatory surgical units may cost less is that they do not have to maintain standby capability to deal with emergencies. As more surgical procedures are performed on an outpatient basis, there is a growing tension between hospitals and surgeons over the facilities used for such procedures. Independent facilities may be able to eliminate some costs, but they also contribute to excess capacity and probably will not reduce health costs in the long run. This means that sooner or later, surgeons and hospitals will have to address their common interests.[170] Eliminating some of the barriers to gainsharing is likely to facilitate such efforts.

Ethical and Legal Concerns

Efforts to improve cost-effectiveness are often seen as forcing health professionals to face conflicts among the needs of individual patients, the interests of society as a whole, and third parties. Physicians are no strangers to such potential conflicts. Indeed, the vast majority of physicians successfully avoid the temptations inherent in fee-for-service care. The managed care era raised some concerns about conflicts between corporate and patient interests, but these concerns proved to have relatively little foundation and have since abated. Some have suggested that evidence-based data derived from large populations may not readily apply to individual patients, but the rationale for this view is not clear.[23] Thus, physicians should be able to represent both an individual patient's viewpoint and a societal perspective.

The high costs of the terminally ill frequently generate controversy, particularly among patients who require intensive care. To mitigate the dilemmas that may face physicians in making life-ending decisions, increasing emphasis is being placed on patient self-determination. Even the best efforts of physicians and institutions to comply with patient or family choices in the setting of terminal illness may not substantially reduce costs or improve outcomes.[171] Actual savings may be small.[172]

Quality in the Aggregate: Small Geographic Area Variation

Earlier in this chapter, it was noted that physician decisions powerfully impact a large proportion of health care costs. The traditional approach has been to honor physicians' deference in such decisions. An increasing challenge to physicians' authority as an arbiter of quality is the long recognized, poorly explained variation in the frequency of surgical procedures among small geographic areas.[173–175] These variations have been intensively studied and found to remain relatively constant over time. The result is that some communities acquire distinct "surgical signatures"—a finding that supports the idea that many operative decisions are based on opinion rather than on evidence.[176] This idea is further supported by data indicating that variations in procedure frequency are often procedure specific and inversely related to the degree of consensus regarding indications.[177] Procedures with highly specific indications (e.g., repair of a fractured hip or appendectomy) often show minimal frequency variation, whereas procedures with seemingly less definitive indications (e.g., carotid endarterectomy, hysterectomy, and coronary angiography) often show a great deal of variation.[178] Variations in frequency also can have downstream effects[179]; one example of this is the relatively close relation between the intensity of local diagnostic testing and the subsequent performance of invasive cardiac procedures.[180]

One issue of debate in interpreting these geographic frequency variations is whether high rates of use are too high or low rates are too low. The association between variation and the ratio of hospital beds to population has raised concerns that low frequency of use may reflect restricted access to care.[181] In one study where patients in the aggregate received about half the recommended level of care,[182] a lack of access to health services did not appear to be the underlying problem. To date, efforts to find evidence supporting other possible explanations for these variations (e.g., differences in disease incidence and in the appropriateness of use) have not been successful.[183]

Although some might attribute variations in frequency to the potential conflict of interest inherent in a fee-for-service system, similar variations in procedure frequency are known to occur among VA medical care facilities,[184] as well as in countries that do not have fee-for-service reimbursement.

The current belief is that the high use rates are too high and is supported by findings that patients from areas with widely disparate use rates have comparable health status. These findings have led to the conclusion that "marked variability in surgical practices and presumably in surgical judgment and philosophy must be considered to reflect absent or inadequate data by which to evaluate surgical treatment."[185] This was supported by a study in the 1970s that estimated that only about 15% of common medical practices had documented foundations in medical research.[186] Although this does not necessarily mean that only 15% of care is effective, it does raise concerns about the lack of hard evidence for most care. A more recent estimate is that one third of current health care spending may be wasteful.[187]

A related issue is whether these variations should be used to formulate public policy.[188,189] Some discount these variations by arguing that they are not risk adjusted for differences among patients and cannot predict which will be better at saving lives. Others acknowledge that the Dartmouth analyses are not perfect but are better than other existing methods. Both views agree that these variations should not be used as the sole method to set hospital payment rates and that end-of-life data used for these analyses provide only limited insight into the overall quality of care.

The point is that in addition to misuse, overuse and underuse also can reflect quality. Although there has been some improvement in the adoption of processes of proven value (e.g., the optimal timing and duration of perioperative antibiotics), overall progress has been disappointingly slow.[190]

Reassessing the Relationship between Cost and Quality in Health Care

This chapter sought to emphasize that health care costs do not necessarily have to have a direct relation to quality (i.e., better care does not need to be more expensive). Indeed, higher-quality health care can cost less. Unfortunately, US physicians are more likely than physicians in other countries to report that interventions in patient care geared to cost control were threatening the quality of care they could provide their patients.[191] Thus, recognizing that quality does not have to be sacrificed with reductions in cost is essential to overcoming fears that health care reform will adversely affect quality. In this context, it is likely to take time for evidence supporting higher-quality/lower-cost care to evolve. Hopes that such evidence might come quickly have been dashed by reports showing that hospital P4P measures were not strongly associated with better outcomes[192,193] or produced only modest reductions in mortality.[194] On the positive side, there are studies that show an inverse relation between volume and cost.[195,196] Thus, high volume might improve cost-effectiveness by affecting both the numerator and the denominator of the equation.

Although it is clear that more data are needed with regard to the relation between cost and quality in health care, an activity likely to bear fruit is reducing costs by reducing the complications of surgical care. A useful approach here may be to consider the added costs of a complication in a given patient with respect to the frequency of that complication in the entire population undergoing a given treatment.[197] The goal is to establish priorities for quality improvement efforts to prevent complications based on both the incidence of the complication and its contribution to resource use.[198]

Reassessing the relation between cost and quality may also suffer if there is a relative lack of emphasis on the latter by hospital boards.[199] Similarly, a national survey found that 39% of managed care organizations were moderately or largely influenced in their initial physician selection by previous patterns of costs or use, and nearly 70% profiled their member physicians.[200] On the other hand, at least one HMO recognized that practices with high scores on service and quality indicators attracted significantly more new enrollees than practices with lower scores. A challenge in considering both cost and quality is that potential benefits may not occur concurrently. Thus, cost savings may appear before quality improvement, or quality might improve before long-term cost savings are evident.

The Future

All indications are that the efforts to reduce the cost and/or improve the quality of the US health care system will remain strong for the foreseeable future. As an example, large employers increasingly provide incentives to use "high-performance" health provider networks.[201] Physicians may dispute the validity of cost profiling[202] and other challenges to their authority as arbiters of quality; regardless, they will have to bear an increasing burden of proof as to the quality of care. Moreover, health care payers are likely to address substantial variations in frequency and cost of care by using apparent similarities in quality to contract for less expensive care. How this tension will be resolved remains to be determined. One view is that the pressure on physicians will be based on an assumption by payers that physicians will not knowingly or willingly sacrifice quality. Indeed, some believe that value-based competition may spark physicians to provide care that exceeds patients' expectations.[203,204]

In response, physicians need to remain cognizant of a predominant theme of this chapter: physician-led organizations appear to be more successful in improving the cost-effectiveness of care than external policies. Practicing surgeons, who are at the "sharp" end of the system, will need to access data on their performance and participate in the development of better outcome measures. These metrics then can be used to improve performance by redesigning processes of care.[205] Physicians need to acknowledge variations in intervention rates and outcomes and to increasingly make medical decisions that are evidence based. They are the best equipped participants in the health care system to identify cost-effective care because they have the necessary knowledge and skill set. If physicians can respond constructively to these challenges, rather than simply ignore or dismiss them, they stand a good chance of recapturing much of their lost stature and autonomy.

In this context, the fee-for-service payment system may be increasingly criticized because it lacks incentives that reimburse physicians based on quality. It seems likely, therefore, that new payment systems will emerge that are more closely linked to quality than the current P4P programs. In one such approach, the Geisinger Health System established incentives through a warranty program for elective cardiac surgery in which there is no added reimbursement for managing complications occurring within the first 90 days after surgery. Geisinger was able to adopt this approach because many of its patients were also insured through the Geisinger system. This eliminated many of the conflicts that might otherwise be present with third-party payers. In creating this program, Geisinger embedded best practices within their processes of care, and the program's initial success is largely attributed to high compliance rates.[206] Interestingly, Geisinger patients insured by other payers also benefit from this system.[207]

Although such changes may seem daunting, surgeons should recognize that the growing interest in assessing performance is not new. In the early 1900s, Ernest Codman, a Boston surgeon, crusaded for hospitals and surgeons to publicize their results, yet his efforts often met with disinterest, defensiveness, or outright opposition.[208] The current call to assess surgeon performance is clearly here to stay. If physicians respond dismissively or defensively (e.g., explaining variations in outcomes by invoking care for sicker patients), they may miss an important opportunity to reestablish their authority on quality. Surgeons who preemptively familiarize themselves with their own outcomes will be better positioned to participate in efforts to improve the cost-effectiveness of surgical care.

Financial Disclosures: None Reported

References

1. Bloom DE, Channing D. The health and wealth of nations. Science 2000;287:1207–11.
2. Schoen C, Osborn R, Huynh PT, et al. Taking the pulse of health care systems: experiences of patients with health problems in six countries. Health Aff (Millwood) 2005 Jul–Dec;Suppl Web Exclusives:W5-509–25.
3. Reid TR. The healing of America. A global quest for better, cheaper, fairer health care. New York: Penguin Press; 2009.
4. Docteur E, Berenson RA. How does the quality of U.S. health care compare internationally? Robert Wood Johnson Foundation Urban Institute 2009. Available at: http://www.rwjf.org/pr/product.jsp?id=47508 (accessed January 11, 2001).
5. Anderson GF, Reinhardt UE, Hussey PS, et al. It's the price, stupid: why the United States is so different from other countries. Health Aff (Millwood) 2003;22:89–105.
6. Himmelstein DU, Thorne D, Warren E, et al. Medical bankruptcy in the United States, 2007: results of a national study. Am J Med 2009;122:741–6.
7. Cunnigham PJ. The growing financial burden of health care: national and state trends, 2001–2006. Health Aff 2010;29:1037–44.
8. Altman DE, Levitt L. The sad history of health care cost containment as told in one chart. Health Aff (Millwood) [illegible] Dec;Suppl Web Exclusives:W83-4.
9. Weinstein MC, Stason WB. Foundations of cost-effectiveness analysis for health and medical practice. N Engl J Med 1977;296:716–21.
10. Wen SW, Naylor CD. Diagnostic accuracy and short-term surgical outcomes in cases of suspected acute appendicitis. CMAJ 1995;153:888–90.
11. Avorn J. Debate about funding comparative effectiveness research. N Engl J Med 2009;360:1927–9.
12. Carman KL, Maurer M, Yeglan JM, et al. Evidence that consumers are skeptical about evidence-based health care. Health Aff (Millwood) 2010;29:1400–6. Epub 2010 Jun 3.
13. U.S. Preventive Services Task Force recommendation statement on screening for breast cancer. Ann Intern Med 2009;151:716–26.
14. Cleverly WO. Essentials of healthcare finance. 2nd ed. Rockville (MD): Aspen Publishers; 1986.
15. Roberts RR, Frutos PW, Ciavarella GG, et al. Distribution of variable vs fixed costs of hospital care. JAMA 1999;281:644–9.
16. Rhodes RS. How much does it cost? How much can be saved? Surgery 1999;125:102–3.
17. Legorreta AP, Silber JH, Constantino GN, et al. Increased cholecystectomy rate after the introduction of laparoscopic cholecystectomy. JAMA 1993;270:1429–32.
18. Gottlieb DJ, Zhou W, Song Y, et al. Prices don't drive regional Medicare spending variations. Health Aff (Millwood) 2010;29:1–7.
19. Schermerhorn ML, Birkmeyer J, Gould DA, et al. The impact of operative mortality on cost-effectiveness in the UK Small Aneurysm Trial. J Vasc Surg 2000;31:217–26.
20. Heudebert GR, Marks R, Wilcox CM, et al. Choice of long-term strategy for the management of patients with severe esophagitis: a cost-utility analysis. Gastroenterology 1997;112:1078–86.
21. Phelps CE. The methodologic foundations of studies of the appropriateness of medical care. N Engl J Med 1993;329:1241–5.
22. Kassirer JP. The quality of care and the quality of measuring it. N Engl J Med 1993;329:1263–5.
23. Redelmeier DA, Tversky A. Discrepancy between medical decisions for individual patients and for groups. N Engl J Med 1990;322:1162–4.
24. Caplan RA, Posner KL, Cheney FW. Effect of outcome on physician judgments of appropriateness of care. JAMA 1991;265:1957–60.
25. Donabedian A. The definition of quality and approaches to its assessment. explorations in quality assessment and monitoring. Vol 1. Ann Arbor (MI): Health Administration Press; 1980.
26. Brook RH, Kamberg CJ, McGlynn EA. Health system reform and quality. JAMA 1996;276:476–80.
27. Birkmeyer JD, Dimick JB, Birkmeyer NJO. Measuring the quality of surgical care: structure, process, or outcomes? J Am Coll Surg 2004;198:626–32.
28. Sosa JA, Bowman HM, Tielsch JM, et al. The importance of surgeon experience for clinical and economic outcomes from thyroidectomy. Ann Surg 1998;228:320–30.
29. Sosa JA, Bowman HM, Gordon TA, et al. Importance of hospital volume in the overall management of pancreatic cancer. Ann Surg 1998;228:429–38.
30. Birkmeyer JD, Finlayson SRG, Tosteson ANA, et al. Effect of hospital volume on in-hospital mortality with pancreaticoduodenectomy. Surgery 1999;125:250–6.
31. Begg CB, Cramer LD, Hoskins WJ, et al. Impact of hospital volume on operative mortality for major cancer surgery. JAMA 1998;280:1747–51.
32. Pearce WH, Parker MA, Feinglass J, et al. The importance of surgeon volume and training in outcomes for vascular surgical procedures. J Vasc Surg 1999;29:768–78.
33. Harmon JW, Tang DG, Gordon TA, et al. Hospital volume can serve as a surrogate for surgeon volume for achieving excellent outcomes in colorectal resection. Ann Surg 1999;230:404.
34. Porter GA, Soskolne CL, Yakimets WW, et al. Surgeon-related factors and outcome in rectal cancer. Ann Surg 1998;277:157–67.
35. Houghton A. Variance in outcome of surgical procedures. Br J Surg 1994;81:653–60.
36. Khuri SF, Henderson WG, Hur K, et al. Relation of surgical volume to outcome in eight common operations: results from the VA National Quality Improvement Program. Ann Surg 1999;230:414–32.
37. Christian CK, Zinner MJ, Gustafson ML, et al. The Leapfrog volume criteria may fall short in identifying high quality surgical centers. Ann Surg 2003;238:447–57.
38. Institute of Medicine. Interpreting the volume-outcome relationship in the context of cancer care. Available at: www.iom.edu/Reports/2001/Interpreting-the-Volume-Outcome-Relationship-in-the-Context-of-Cancer-Care.aspx (accessed January 10, 2011).
39. Davis JW, Hoyt DB, McArdle MS, et al. An analysis of errors causing morbidity and mortality in a trauma system: a guide for quality improvement. J Trauma 1992;32:660–6.
40. Hannan EL. The relation between volume and outcome in health care. N Engl J Med 1999;340:1677–9.
41. MacKenzie EJ, Weir S, Rivara FP, et al. The value of trauma center care. J. Trauma 2010;69:1–10.
42. Rosenthal MB, Landon BE, Normand S-LT, et al. Pay for performance in commercial HMOs. N Engl J Med 2006;355:1895–902.
43. Rosenthal MB, Dudley RA. Pay-for-performance: will the latest payment trend improve care? JAMA 2007;297:740–4.
44. Stulberg JJ, Delaney CP, Neuhauser DV, et al. Adherence to surgical care improvement project measures and the association with postoperative infections. JAMA 2010;303:2479–85.
45. Dellinger EP, Hausmann SM, Bratzler DW, et al. Hospitals collaborate to decrease surgical site infection. Am J Surg 2005;190:9–15.
46. Pham HH, Schrag D, O'Malley AS. Care patterns in Medicare and their implications for pay for performance. N Engl J Med 2007;356:1130–9.
47. Trude S, Au M, Christianson JB. Health plan pay-for-performance strategies. Am J Manag Care 2006;12:537–42.
48. Fisher ES. Paying for performance—risks and recommendations. N Engl J Med 2006;355:1845–7.
49. Casalino LP, Elster A. Will pay-for-performance and quality reporting affect health care disparities? Health Aff (Millwood) 2007;26:W405–14.
50. Gainsharing arrangements and CMPs for hospital payments to physicians to reduce or limit services to beneficiaries. Available at: http://oig.hhs.gov/fraud/docs/alertsandbulletins/gainsh.htm (accessed Jan 9, 2011).
51. O'Connor GT, Plume SK, Olmstead EM, et al. A regional intervention to improve the hospital mortality associated with coronary artery bypass graft surgery. JAMA 1996;275:841–6.
52. O'Connor GT, Olmstead EM, Nugent WC, et al. Appropriateness of coronary artery bypass graft surgery performed in northern New England. J Am Coll Cardiol 2008;51:2323–8.
53. Khuri S. Safety, quality, and the National Surgical Quality Improvement Program. Am Surg 2006;72:994–8.
54. Collins TC, Daley J, Henderson WH, et al. Risk factors for prolonged length of stay after major elective surgery. Ann Surg 1999;230:251–9.
55. Khuri SF, Daley J, Henderson W, et al. Relation of surgical volume to outcome in eight common operations: results from the VA National Surgical Quality Improvement Program. Ann Surg 1999;230:414–29.
56. Keller RB, Griffin E, Schneiter EJ, et al. Searching for quality in medical care: the Maine Medical Assessment Foundation model. Rockville (MD): Agency for Healthcare Research and Quality; 2000. Publ. No.: 00-N002.
57. Flum DR, Fisher N, Thompson J, et al. Washington State's approach to variability in surgical processes/outcomes: Surgical Clinical Outcomes Assessment Program (SCOAP). Surgery 2005;138:821–8.
58. Shively EH, Heine MJ, Schell RH, et al. Practicing surgeons lead in quality care, safety, and cost control. Ann Surg 2004;239:752–60.
59. Campbell DA. Quality improvement is local. J Am Coll Surg 2009;209:141–3.

60. Ferguson TB, Peterson ED, Coombs LP, et al. Use of continuous quality improvement to increase use of process measures in patients undergoing coronary artery bypass graft surgery. JAMA 2003;290:49–56.
61. Hyman NH, Ko CY, Cataldo PA, et al. The New England Colorectal Cancer Quality Project: a prospective multi-institutional feasibility study. J Am Coll Surg 2006; 202:36–44.
62. Cronenwett JL, Likosky DS, Russell MT, et al. A regional registry for quality assurance and improvement: the Vascular Study Group of Northern New England (VSGNNE). J Vasc Surg 2007;46:1093–101; discussion 1101–2. Epub 2007 Oct 24.
63. Birkmeyer NJ, Share D, Campbell DA, et al. Partnering with payers to improve surgical quality: the Michigan plan. Surgery 2005; 138:815–20.
64. Englsebe MJ, Dimick JB, Sonneday CJ, et al. The Michigan Surgical Quality Collaborative: will a statewide quality improvement initiative pay for itself? Ann Surg 2007; 246:1100–3.
65. Campbell DA, Dellinger EP. Multihospital collaborations for surgical quality improvement. JAMA 2009;302:1584–5.
66. Bruce J, Russell EM, Mollison J, et al. The measurement and monitoring of surgical adverse events. Health Technol Assess 2001;5:1–194.
67. Partnership for Solutions: Johns Hopkins University, Baltimore, MD for the Robert Wood Johnson Foundation (September 2004 update). Chronic conditions: making the case for ongoing care. Available at: http://www.rwjf.org/files/research/chronicbook.pdf (accessed on January 13, 2011).
68. Russell LB, Gold MR, Siegel JE, et al. The role of cost-effectiveness analysis in medicine. JAMA 1996;276:1172–7.
69. Testa MA, Simonson DC. Assessment of quality of life outcomes. N Engl J Med 1996; 334:835–40.
70. Velanovich V. Behavior and analysis of 36-item short-form health survey data for surgical quality-of-life research. Arch Surg 2007;142:473–8.
71. Leplege A, Hunt S. The problem of quality of life in medicine. JAMA 1997;278:47–50.
72. Garvin DA. Afterword: Reflections on the future. In: Berwick DM, Godfrey AB, Roessner J, editors. Curing health care: new strategies for quality improvement: a report on the National Demonstration Project on Quality Improvement in Health Care. San Francisco (CA): Jossey-Bass; 1990. p. 159–219.
73. Ammerman DJ, Watters J, Clinch JJ, et al. Exploring quality of life for patients undergoing major surgery: the perspectives of surgeons, other healthcare professionals, and patients. Surgery 2007;141:100–9.
74. Kreder HJ, Wright JG, McLeod R. Outcomes studies in surgical research. Surgery 1996;121:223–6.
75. Velanovich V. The quality of quality of life studies in general surgical journals. J Am Coll Surg 2001;193:288–96.
76. Kluivers KB, Riphagen I, Vierhout ME, et al. Systematic review on recovery specific quality of life instruments. Surgery 2008; 143:206–15.
77. Byford S, Palmer S. Common errors and controversies in pharmacoeconomic analyses. Pharmacoeconomics 1998;13:659–66.
78. Drummond MF, Jefferson TO. Guidelines for authors and peer reviewers of economic submissions to the BMJ. The BMJ Economic Evaluation Working Party. BMJ 1996; 313:275–83.
79. Gold MR, Siegel JE, Russell LB, Weinstein MC. Cost-effectiveness in health and medicine. New York: Oxford University Press; 1996.
80. Mark DH. Visualizing cost-effectiveness analysis. JAMA 2002;287:2428–9.
81. Tu JV, Hannan EL, Anderson GM, et al. The fall and rise of carotid endarterectomy in the United States and Canada. N Engl J Med 1998;339:1441–7.
82. Wennberg DE, Lucas FL, Birkmeyer JD, et al. Variation in carotid endarterectomy in the Medicare population: trial hospitals, volumes, and patient characteristics. JAMA 1998;279:1278–81.
83. Chassin MR. Appropriate use of carotid endarterectomy. N Engl J Med 1998;339: 1468–71.
84. Burger I, Schill K, Goodman S. Disclosure of individual surgeon's performance rates during informed consent: ethical and epistemological considerations. Ann Surg 2007; 245:507.
85. Atkins D, Best D, Eccles M; GRADE. Working Group. Grading quality of evidence and strength of recommendations. BMJ 2004;328:1490–4.
86. Rao PM, Rhea JT, Novelline RA, et al. Effect of computed tomography of the appendix on treatment of patients and use of hospital resources. N Engl J Med 1998; 338:141–6.
87. Gill BD, Jenkins JR. Cost-effective evaluation and management of the acute abdomen. Surg Clin North Am 1996;76:71–82.
88. The SCOAP Collaborative. Negative appendectomy and imaging accuracy in the Washington State Surgical Care and Outcomes Assessment Program. Ann Surg 2008;248:557–63.
89. Black WC, Welch HG. Advances in diagnostic imaging and overestimations of disease prevalence and the benefits of therapy. N Engl J Med 1993;328:1237–43.
90. Soot LC, Moneta GL, Edwards JM. Vascular surgery and the Internet: a poor source of information. J Vasc Surg 1999;30:84–91.
91. Yeo H, Roman S, Air M, et al. Filling a void: thyroid cancer information on the Internet. World J Surg 2007;31:1165–91.
92. Kruper L, Kurichi JE, Sonnad SS. Methodologic quality of cost-effectiveness of surgical procedures. Ann Surg 2007;245: 147–51.
93. Aaron HJ, Ginsburg PB. Is health spending excessive? If so, what can be done about it? Health Aff (Millwood) 2009;28:1260–1275. DOI: 10.1377/hlthaff.28.5.1260.
94. Baker L, Birnbaum H, Geppert J, et al. The relationship between technology availability and health care spending. Health Aff (Millwood) 2003 Jul–Dec;Suppl Web Exclusives:W3-537–51.
95. Laupacis A, Feeny D, Detsky AS, et al. How attractive does a new technology have to be to warrant adoption utilization? Tentative guidelines for using clinical and economic evaluations. CMAJ 1992;146:473–81.
96. Chatterjee A, Payette MJ, Demas, CP, et al. Opportunity cost: a systematic application to surgery. Surgery 2009;146:818–22.
97. Strasberg SM, Ludbrook PA. Who oversees innovative practice? Is there a structure that meets the monitoring needs of new techniques? J Am Coll Surg 2003;196:938–48.
98. Pisano GP, Bohmer RMJ, Edmondson AC. Organizational differences in rates of learning: evidence from the adoption of minimally invasive cardiac surgery. Manage Sci 2001;47:752.
99. Rigelman RK. Studying a study and testing a test: how to read the medical literature Boston: Little, Brown & Co; 1981.
100. Stoline AM, Weiner JP. The new medical market-place: a physician's guide to the health care system in the 1990s. Baltimore (MD): Johns Hopkins University Press; 1993. p. 138.
101. Yasaitis L, Fisher ES, Skinner JS, et al. Hospital quality and intensity of spending: is there an association? Health Aff 2009; 28:W566–72. DOI: 10.1377/hlthaff.28.4.W566–72.
102. Ross NS, Aron DC. Hormonal evaluation of the patient with the incidentally discovered adrenal mass. N Engl J Med 1990;323: 1401–3.
103. Velanovich V. Preoperative laboratory test evaluation. J Am Coll Surg 1996;183: 79–87.
104. Marcello PW, Roberts PL. "Routine" preoperative studies: which studies in which patients? Surg Clin North Am 1996;76: 11–23.
105. Dinan MA, Curtis LH, Hammill BG, et al. Changes in the use and costs of diagnostic imaging among Medicare beneficiaries with cancer, 1999–2006. JAMA 2010;303: 1625–31.
106. Brasel KJ, Borgstrom DC, Weigelt JA. Management of penetrating colon trauma: a cost-utility analysis. Surgery 1999;125: 471–9.
107. Cronenwett JL, Birkmeyer JD, Nackman GB, et al. Cost-effectiveness of carotid endarterectomy in asymptomatic patients. J Vasc Surg 1997;25:298–311.
108. Sox HC, Blatt MA, Higgins MC, et al. Medical decision making. Boston: Butterworth-Heinemann; 1988.
109. Birkmeyer JD, Welch HG. A reader's guide to surgical decision analysis. J Am Coll Surg 1997;184:589–95.
110. Millilli JJ, Philiponis VS, Nusbaum M. Predicting surgical outcome using Bayesian analysis. J Surg Res 1998;77:45–9.
111. Birkmeyer JD, Birkmeyer NO. Decision analysis in surgery. Surgery 1996;120:7–15.
112. Ferraco K, Spath PL. Measuring performance of high risk processes. In: Spath PL, editor. Error reduction in health care: a systems approach to improving patient safety. San Francisco (CA): Jossey-Bass; 2000. p. 17.
113. Vanounou T, Pratt W, Fischer JE, et al. Deviation-based cost modeling: a novel model to evaluate the clinical and economic impact of clinical pathways. J Am Coll Surg 2007;204:570–9.
114. Tricoci P, Allen JM, Kramer JM, et al. Scientific evidence underlying the ACC/AHA clinical practice guidelines. JAMA 2009;301:839–41.
115. Shaneyfelt TM, Mayo-Smith MF, Rothwangl J. Are guidelines following guidelines? The methodological quality of clinical practice guidelines in the peer-reviewed medical literature. JAMA 1999;281:1900–5.
116. Cook D, Giacomini M. The trials and tribulations of clinical practice guidelines. JAMA 1999;281:1950–1.
117. Shekelle PG, Ortiz E, Rhodes S, et al. Validity of the Agency for Healthcare Research and Quality clinical practice guidelines: how quickly do guidelines become outdated? JAMA 2001;286:1461–7.
118. Famakinwa O, Wang TS, Roman SA, et al. ATA practice guidelines for the management of differentiated thyroid cancer: were they being followed in the United States? Am J Surg 2010;199:189–98.
119. Park HS, Roman SA, Sosa JA. Treatment patterns of aging Americans with differentiated thyroid cancer. Cancer 2010;116: 20–30.
120. Selker HP, Beshansky JR, Paulker SG, et al. The epidemiology of delays in teaching hospitals. Med Care 1989;27:112–29.

121. Griffen FD, Stephens LS, Alexander JB, et al. The American College of Surgeons' closed claims study: new insights for improving care. J Am Coll Surg 2007;204:561–9.
122. Byrne CM, Mercincavage LM, Pan EC, et al. The value from investments in health information technology at the U.S. Department of Veterans Affairs. Health Aff (Millwood) 2010;29:629–38.
123. Casalino LP, Dunham D, Chin MH, et al. Frequency of failure to inform patients of clinically significant outpatient test results. Arch Intern Med 2009;169:1123–9.
124. Moray N. Error reduction as a systems problem. In: Bogner MS, editor. Human error in medicine. Hillsdale (NJ): Lawrence Erlbaum Associates; 1994. p. 67.
125. Sheridan TB, Thompson JM. People versus computers in medicine. In: Bogner MS, editor. Human error in medicine. Hillsdale (NJ): Lawrence Erlbaum Associates; 1994. p. 141.
126. Bates DW, Gawande AA. Improving safety with information technology. N Engl J Med 2003;348:2526–34.
127. Garg AX, Adhikari NKJ, McDonald H, et al. Effects of computerized clinical decision support systems on practitioner performance and patient outcomes: a systematic review. JAMA 2005;293:1223–8.
128. Kuperman GJ, Teich JM, Gandhi TK, et al. Patient safety and computerized medication ordering at Brigham and Women's Hospital. Jt Comm J Qual Improv 2001;27:509–21.
129. Horst HM, Mouro D, Hall-Jenssens RA, et al. Decrease in ventilation time with a standardized weaning process. Arch Surg 1998;133:483–8; discussion 488–9.
130. Koppel R, Metlay JP, Cohen A, et al. Role of computerized order entry systems in facilitating medication errors. JAMA 2005;293:1197–203.
131. Fisher ES, Wennberg DE, Stukel TA, et al. The implications of regional variations in Medicare spending. Part 1: the content, quality, and accessibility of care. Ann Intern Med 2003;138:273–87.
132. Fisher ES, Wennberg DE, Stukel TA, et al. The implications of regional variations in Medicare spending. Part 2: health outcomes and satisfaction with care. Ann Intern Med 2003;138:288–98.
133. Rutledge R. An analysis of 25 Milliman & Robertson guidelines for surgery: data-driven versus consensus-driven clinical practice guidelines. Ann Surg 1998;228:579–87.
134. Iezzoni LI, editor. Risk adjustment for measuring health care outcomes. Ann Arbor (MI): Health Administration Press; 1994.
135. Horn SD, Sharkey PD, Buckle JM, et al. The relationship between severity of illness and hospital length of stay and mortality. Med Care 1991;29:305–17.
136. Rhodes RS, Sharkey PD, Horn SD. Effect of patient factors on hospital costs for major bowel surgery: implications for managed health care. Surgery 1995;117:443–50.
137. Kalman PG, Johnston KW. Sociological factors are major determinants of prolonged hospital stay following abdominal aneurysm repair. Surgery 1996;119:690–3.
138. Salem-Schatz S, Moore G, Rucker M, et al. The case for case-mix adjustment in practice profiling: when good apples look bad. JAMA 1994;272:871–4.
139. Melton JL. Selection bias in the referral of patients and the natural history of surgical conditions. Mayo Clin Proc 1985;60:880–5.
140. Williams MV, Parker RM, Baker DW, et al. Inadequate functional health literacy among patients at two public hospitals. JAMA 1995;274:1677–82.
141. Steinbrook R. Public report cards—cardiac surgery and beyond. N Engl J Med 2006;355:1847–9.
142. Hannan EL, Kilburn H, Racz M, et al. Improving the outcomes of coronary artery bypass surgery in New York State. JAMA 1994;271:761–6.
143. Green J, Wintfeld N. Report cards on cardiac surgeons: assessing New York State's approach. N Engl J Med 1995;332:1229–32.
144. Chaissin MR, Hannan EL, DeBuono BA. Benefits and hazards of reporting medical outcomes publicly. N Engl J Med 1996;334:394–8.
145. Schneider EC, Epstein AM. Influence of cardiac surgery performance report cards on referral practices and access to care. N Engl J Med 1996;335:251–6.
146. Mehrotra A, Bodenheimer T, Dudley RA. Employers' efforts to measure and improve hospital quality: determinants of success. Health Aff (Millwood) 2003;22:60–71.
147. Hibbard JH, Stockard J, Tusler M. Does publicizing hospital performance stimulate quality improvement efforts? Health Aff (Millwood) 2003;22:84–94.
148. Armour BS, Pitts MM, Maclean R, et al. The effect of explicit financial incentives on physician behavior. Arch Intern Med 2002;162:612–3.
149. Fung CH, Lim Y-W, Mattke S, et al. Systematic review: the evidence that publishing patient care performance data improves the quality of care. Ann Intern Med 2008;148:111–23.
150. Milstein A. Ending extra payments for 'never events'—stronger incentives for patient safety. N Engl J Med 2009;360:2388–90.
151. Bradley EH, Holmboe ES, Mattera JA, et al. A qualitative study of increasing beta-blocker use after myocardial infarction: why do some hospitals succeed? JAMA 2001;285:2604–11.
152. Mazmanian PE, Daffron SR, Johnson RE, et al. Information about barriers to planned change: a randomized, controlled trial involving continuing medical education lectures and commitment to change. Acad Med 1998;73:882–6.
153. Mazmanian PE, Johnson RE, Zhang A, et al. Effects of signature on rates of change: a randomized, controlled trial involving continuing medical education and the commitment-to-change model. Acad Med 2001;76:642–6.
154. Davis, DA, O'Brien MJT, Freemantle N, et al. Impact of formal continuing medical education: do conferences, workshops, rounds, and other traditional activities change physician behavior or health care outcomes? JAMA 1999;282:867–74.
155. Mazmanian PE, Davis DA. Continuing medical education and the physician as learner: guide to the evidence. JAMA 2002;288:1057–60.
156. Verstappen WHJM, van der Weijden T, Sijbrandij J, et al. Effect of a practice-based strategy on test ordering performance of primary care physicians: a randomized trial. JAMA 2003;289:2407–12.
157. Gawande A. The bell curve. The New Yorker 2004 Dec 6; 82.
158. Newman RM, Traverso LW. Cost-effective minimally invasive surgery: what procedures make sense? World J Surg 1999;23:415–21.
159. Sokal SM, Chang Y, Craft DL, et al. Surgeon profiling: a key to optimum operating room use. Arch Surg 2007;142:365–70.
160. Taheri PA, Wahl WL, Butz DA, et al. Trauma service cost: the real story. Ann Surg 1998;227:720–5.
161. Taheri PA, Butz DA, Watts CM, et al. Trauma services: a profit center? J Am Coll Surg 1999;188:349–54.
162. Horst HM, Mouro D, Hall-Jenssens RA, et al. Decrease in ventilation time with a standardized weaning process. Arch Surg 1998;13:483–9.
163. Thomsen GE, Pope D, East TD, et al. Clinical performance of a rule-based decision support system for mechanical ventilation of ARDS patients. Proc Annu Symp Comput Appl Med Care 1993;339–43.
164. Coats RD, Burd RS: Intra-operative communication of residents with faculty: perception versus reality. J Surg Res 2002;104:40–5.
165. Lingard L, Espin S, Whyte S, et al. Communication failures in the operating room: an observational classification of recurrent types and effects. Qual Saf Health Care 2004;13:330–4.
166. Patterson ES. Communication strategies from high-reliability organizations. Translation is hard work. Ann Surg 2007;245:170–2.
167. Lingard L, Regehr G, Orser B, et al. Evaluation of a preoperative checklist and team briefing among surgeons, nurses, and anesthesiologists to reduce failures in communication. Arch Surg 2008;143:12–7.
168. Varpio L, Hall P, Lingard L, et al. Interprofessional communication and medical error: a reframing of research questions and approaches. Acad Med 2008;83(10 Suppl):S76–81.
169. Rhodes RS. Ambulatory surgery and the societal cost of surgery. Surgery 1994;116:938–40.
170. Berenson RA, Ginsburg PB, May JH. Hospital-physician relations: cooperation, competition, or separation. Health Aff 2007;26:W31–43. DOI: 10.1377/hlthaff.26.1.w310.
171. A controlled trial to improve care for seriously ill hospitalized patients. The study to understand prognoses and preferences for outcomes and risks of treatment. The SUPPORT Principal Investigators [published erratum appears in JAMA 1996;275:1232]. JAMA 1995;274:1591–8.
172. Emanuel EJ, Emanuel LL. The economics of dying—the illusion of cost saving at the end of life. N Engl J Med 1994;330:540–4.
173. Wennberg J, Gittelsohn A. Variations in medical care among small areas. Sci Am 1982;246:120–34.
174. Chaissin MR, Brook RH, Park RE, et al. Variations in the use of medical and surgical services by the Medicare population. N Engl J Med 1986;314:285–90.
175. The Dartmouth atlas of health care. Chicago: American Hospital Publishing; 1998.
176. Muir Gray JA. Evidence-based health care: how to make health policy and management decisions. New York: Churchill Livingstone; 1997.
177. Eddy DM. Variations in physician practice: the role of uncertainty. Health Aff (Millwood) 1984;3:74–89.
178. Birkmeyer JD, Sharp SM, Finlayson SR, et al. Variation profiles of common surgical procedures. Surgery 1998;124:917–23.
179. Verrilli D, Welch GH. The impact of diagnostic testing on therapeutic interventions. JAMA 1996;275:1189–91.
180. Wennberg DE, Kellett MA, Dickens JD, et al. The association between local diagnostic intensity and invasive cardiac procedures. JAMA 1996;275:1161–4.
181. Health Services Research Group. Small area variations: what are they and what do they mean? CMAJ 1992;146:467–70.

182. McGlynn EA, Asch SM, Adams J, et al. The quality of health care delivered to adults in the United States. N Engl J Med 2003; 348:2635–45.
183. Leape LL, Park RE, Solomon DH, et al. Does inappropriate use explain small-area variations in the use of health care services? JAMA 1990;263:669–72.
184. Ashton CM, Petersen NJ, Souchek J, et al. Geographic variations in utilization rates in Veterans Affairs hospitals and clinics. N Engl J Med 1999;340:32–9.
185. Bunker JP. Surgical manpower: a comparison of operations and surgeons in the United States and in England and Wales. N Engl J Med 1970;282:135–44.
186. Williamson JW, Goldschmidt PG, Jillson IA. Medical Practice Information Demonstration Project: final report. Office of the Asst Secretary of Health, US Department of Health, Education, and Welfare, contract #282-77-0068GS. Baltimore (MD): Policy Research Inc; 1979.
187. Orszag PR, Ellis P. Addressing rising health care costs—a view from the Congressional Budget Office. N Engl J Med 2007;357: 1885–7.
188. Bach P. A map to bad policy—hospital efficiency measures in the Dartmouth Atlas. N Engl J Med 2010;362:569–73.
189. Skinner J, Staiger D, Fisher ES. Looking back, moving forward. N Engl J Med 2010; 362:569–73.
190. Wachter RM. Patient safety at ten: unmistakable progress, troubling gaps. Health Aff (Millwood) 2010;29:165–173. Epub 2009 December 1.
191. Blendon R, Schoen C, Donelan C, et al. Physicians views on quality of care: a five country comparison. Health Aff (Millwood) 2001;20:233–43.
192. Werner RM, Bradlow ET. Relationship between Medicare's Hospital Compare performance measures and mortality rates. JAMA 2006;296:2694–702.
193. Horn SD. Performance measures and clinical outcomes. JAMA 2006;296:2731–2.
194. Lindenauer PK, Remus D, Roman S, et al. Public reporting and pay for performance in hospital quality improvement. N Engl J Med 2007;356:486–96.
195. Trends in the concentration of six surgical procedures under PPS and their implications for patient mortality and Medicare cost. Technical report #E-87-08. Chevy Chase (MD): Project Hope; 1988.
196. Gordon TA, Burleyson GP, Tielsch JM, et al. The effect of regionalization on cost and outcome for one general high-risk surgical procedure. Ann Surg 1995;221: 43–9.
197. Dimick JB, Pronovost PJ, Cowan JA, et al. Complications and costs after high-risk surgery: where should we focus quality improvement initiatives? J Am Coll Surg 2003;196:671–8.
198. Schilling PI, Dimick JB, Birkmeyer JD. Prioritizing quality improvement in general surgery. J Am Coll Surg 2008;207:698–704.
199. Jha AK, Epstein AM. Hospital governance and the quality of care. Health Aff (Millwood) 2010;29(1):182–7. Epub 2009 Nov 6. DOI: 10.1377/hlthaff.2009.0297.
200. Gold MR, Hurley R, Lake T, et al. A national survey of the arrangements managed-care plans make with physicians. N Engl J Med 1995;333:1678–83.
201. Matthews AW. Doctors slam insurers over their rankings. Wall Street Journal 2010; July 20. Available at: http://online.wsj.com/article/SB10001424052748704720004575377523886401684.html (accessed on January 13, 2011).
202. Adams JL, Mehrotra A, Thomas WJ, et al. Physician cost profiling—reliability and risk of misclassification. N Engl J Med 2010; 362:1014–21.
203. Porter ME. A strategy for health care reform—toward a value-based system. N Engl J Med 2009;361:109–12.
204. Porter ME, Teisberg EO. How physicians can change the future of health care. JAMA 2007;297:1103–11.
205. Audet A-MJ, Doty MM, Shamasdin J, et al. Measure, learn, and improve: physicians' involvement in quality improvement. Health Aff (Millwood) 2005;24:843–53.
206. Abelson R. In a bid for better care, surgery with a warranty. New York Times 2007; May 17. Available at: http://www.nytimes.com/2007/05/17/business/17quality.html (accessed January 11, 2011).
207. Abelson R. A health insurer pays more to save. New York Times 2010 Jun 21. Available at: http://www.nytimes.com/2010/06/22/business/22geisinger.html (accessed January 11, 2011).
208. Passaro E, Organ CH. Ernest A. Codman: the improper Bostonian. Bull Am Coll Surg 1999;84:16–22.

8 HEALTH CARE ECONOMICS: THE BROADER CONTEXT

*Linda G. Lesky, MD, MA, Robert S. Rhodes, MD, FACS, and Charles L. Rice, MD, FACS**

In a companion chapter [*search ACS Surgery for information on cost-effective nonemergency surgical care*], we review the principles of cost-effective surgical care and discuss the implications of such principles for health care spending. Our primary focus there is on the interaction between an individual surgeon and an individual patient. In this chapter, we explore some of the issues surrounding health care spending on a larger (i.e., national) scale. It is important for surgeons to have a broad understanding of these issues, in particular because such concerns are increasingly becoming the subject of political debate.

US Health Care Expenditures and Health Outcomes

In 2009, US national health expenditures amounted to $2.5 trillion (approximately 17.6% of the gross domestic product [GDP]).[1] According to data from the World Health Organization, if the current level of US health care spending were treated as a separate economy, it would be the seventh largest economy in the world, nearly equal to the GDPs of France and the United Kingdom.[2] This level of spending translates into a per capita expenditure of $8,086, which is more than double the average of other Organisation for Economic Co-operation and Development (OECD) countries and which surpasses the per capita expenditure of the next highest-spending country, Switzerland, by more than 30%. Between 1950 and 2001, US per capita spending on health care in constant dollars increased more than 11-fold.

Since the end of World War II, the growth rate of health care spending has exceeded the overall growth of the economy. Although the rate of growth of per capita health care spending has slowed over the past 4 years, there is reason to believe that this slowing trend will be short-lived.[3] Over the past 30 years, total national spending on health care has more than doubled as a share of GDP. According to Congressional Budget Office (CBO) projections, total health care spending will reach $4 trillion by 2015, and in the absence of a significant change in the long-term trends, the share of GDP will double again by 2035, to 31% of GDP. Only a small percentage of this spending growth can be attributed to general inflation, growth in the size of the population, and changes in the age distribution of the population.[4] The majority is projected to be attributable to rising costs of care and increasing amounts of care.

Economists differ on the extent to which such spending represents a risk to the overall economic well-being of the United States. Those who are concerned about both the amount that is spent on health care and the rate at which this amount is growing cite a number of concerns:

1. In spending more on health care, society spends less on other goods and services—a process referred to as displacement. Thus, health care consumes resources that might otherwise have been allocated to services such as education or public safety.
2. The health care sector of the economy is so large—not only in terms of the amounts of money involved but also in terms of the number of people employed—that short-term changes in its growth rate (in either direction) necessarily exert substantial and painful economic effects. Moreover, the potential magnitude of these effects thwarts political consideration of potential changes to the system.
3. As costs increase, voluntary participation by employers in the provision of health insurance to employees and retirees comes under increasing pressure, with the result that employers either shift more and more of the costs of insurance to employees or decide to stop providing health insurance altogether. Between 2001 and 2006, the contribution of households to health care expenditures increased by more than 35%.[3]
4. A specific concern also relates to the extent to which spending on Medicare threatens the long-term solvency of the US government. In 2009, Medicare spending grew 7.9% to $502.3 billion. Absent policy change, the CBO estimates that Medicare spending will grow at an average of 7% each year from 2010 to 2018, rising to $879 billion annually and 4% of GDP. The rate of growth of Medicare spending over the long term is predicted to exceed the rate of growth of federal revenues and the overall economy,[5] which most believe is unsustainable. As a result, discussions of health care reform have focused not only on reducing the number of uninsured but also on "bending the health care cost curve" to reduce the rate of growth of health care spending (see below).

Others dismiss these concerns and argue that the health care share of GDP has no natural limit as long as health care is more highly valued than the goods and services that it displaces.[6] Proponents of this viewpoint distinguish between spending that is affordable (i.e., sustainable) and spending that the country is unwilling to sustain.

The proponents of these two perspectives agree that increases in spending should reflect the increased value placed on health care services relative to non–health care goods and services that are forgone. There is substantial evidence, however, that increased health care expenditures are not invariably associated with demonstrable improvements in health outcomes. Although the United States

* The views expressed are those of the authors and do not reflect the official policy or position of the Uniformed Services University of the Health Sciences, the Department of Defense, the United States Government, or the American Board of Surgery.

spends more on health care than any other OECD country, its health status rankings do not compare well with those of other industrialized countries. OECD data indicate that of the 30 OECD countries, the United States has the highest rate of obesity and ranks 15th in infant mortality, 13th in cancer mortality, 21st in mortality from ischemic heart disease, and 15th in life expectancy at 65 years.[7] An analysis of mortality from causes that were potentially avoidable with timely and effective health care in 19 industrialized countries found that the United States ranked last in the level of decline in these deaths between 1997 and 2002.[8]

Within the United States, several major studies have shown that patients treated in higher-spending regions do not have either better health outcomes or greater satisfaction with their care than patients treated in lower-spending regions.[9] One such study reported that the differences in spending were largely attributable to the higher frequency of physician visits, the tendency to consult specialists more readily, the ordering of more tests, the performance of more minor procedures, and the more extensive use of hospital and intensive care services in the higher-spending regions. The authors could find no evidence that these types of increased use resulted in improved survival, better functional status, or enhanced satisfaction with care. These findings have profound implications for efforts aimed at containing the further growth of health care spending.

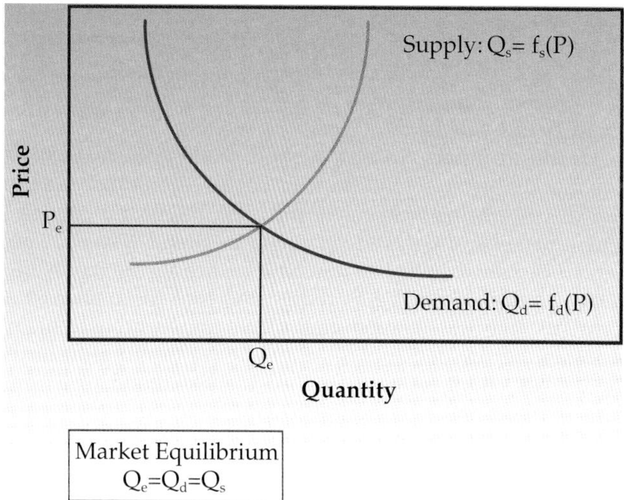

Figure 1 **The model of supply and demand determines the quantity produced at a given price. Illustrated here is the application of this model to health care. Persons who fall below the equilibrium point on the demand curve cannot afford health care at the market price and must either do without care or seek it in the safety-net health care system. P = price; Q = quantity; Q_d (quantity demanded) = $f_d(P)$ (the demand equation, which includes price); Q_s (quantity supplied) = $f_s(P)$ (the supply equation, which includes price).**

Discrepancy between Costs and Outcomes

Many factors influence the cost of health care and the health outcomes of a population. The increase in the size of the uninsured population is often cited as contributing to poorer health outcomes of US residents and the slow decline in the US amenable mortality.[8] Wider availability of advanced technology, an increasingly older population, newer and more expensive prescription drugs, inefficiencies in health care delivery, and the rising costs of medical malpractice insurance are all contributors to rising health care costs. However, the single factor that distinguishes health care in the United States from that in other developed countries is the market-based delivery system that characterizes US health care. With the exception of the aging of the population, the health care market influences all of the factors that contribute to the cost of health care and health care outcomes in the United States. A simple review of how the health care market functions reveals why a market-based health care delivery system contributes to rising costs and poor health outcomes.

MODEL OF SUPPLY AND DEMAND

The model of supply and demand is a useful tool for understanding the behavior of buyers and sellers in a market [*see Figure 1*]. With price on the vertical axis and quantity of a particular good or service on the horizontal axis, the demand curve represents the total demand by all consumers for that good or service. The downward slope of this curve reveals that as price decreases, consumers are willing to purchase more. The demand curve also shows the amount of a good or service that the market is willing and able to purchase at a given price. Similarly, the supply curve represents the total quantity of a good or service that suppliers are willing to produce at a given price. The point where the two curves intersect represents the equilibrium price and quantity of the good or service.

This equilibrium between supply and demand gives markets their most valued attributes. A competitive market price forces producers to satisfy consumers' demands for a quality product with the least-cost methods of production. Markets also ensure the most efficient and least wasteful allocation of resources in that only the quantity demanded at a specific price is produced. Markets assume, however, that consumers who cannot afford to pay the market price either will find a less expensive substitute product or will do without. They also assume that consumers can be knowledgeable enough about a product to assess its quality and appropriateness for their needs. Finally, markets exist to maximize both the utility of consumers through the purchase of goods and services and the profits of suppliers. Research and the development of innovative products are driven by the opportunity to be the first to enter a market with a new or improved product and thus reap maximum profits.

A key question is whether the features that are normally associated with well-functioning markets in other areas are also applicable to health care. Further analysis of the supply-and-demand model as it relates to the health care market may shed some light on this question.

AFFORDABILITY OF HEALTH CARE

Despite the massive growth of employer-sponsored health insurance, the universal coverage of the Medicare population over the age of 65, the addition of more than 1 million disabled persons under Medicare, and widespread coverage of the poor under Medicaid, more than 45 million US citizens (almost one of every six) have no health insurance coverage.

Health insurance, in and of itself, leads to distortions in the market because consumers of health care do not see the actual price being paid for health care goods and services. This creates a situation referred to as moral hazard. This term originated with the purchase of fire insurance in the 19th century, when it was recognized that the owner of a property that was insured might have an incentive to incur a loss either by deliberately setting a fire (a moral hazard) or by not taking steps to reduce the likelihood of a fire. The implication of the moral hazard effect for health care spending is that those who are insured (or more generously insured) will tend to use more health services without regard to cost. Insurers seek to reduce the extent of the moral hazard problem by increasing the coinsurance and making the consumer pay a larger share of the full cost.

A more significant economic and ethical concern centers on those persons with no health insurance coverage, who fall below the equilibrium point on the demand curve [*see Figure 1*]. In a well-functioning market, it is expected that those who cannot afford to pay the market price for a good or service will do without, but our society seems unwilling to allow this when it comes to health care. The result is a patchwork of substitute care that serves the uninsured and underinsured. The so-called safety-net health care system comprises hospitals, community health centers, "free" clinics, and emergency departments. The Institute of Medicine estimated that in 2001, the safety-net health care system cost $99 billion in direct services and $65 to $130 billion in lost productivity.[10] Under current arrangements, the costs of this care are built into the prices charged to those who do have the ability to pay. A 1992 analysis of the distribution of the health care financing burden associated with the US health care system showed that the greatest financial burden fell on those in the middle class: the fourth to seventh income deciles devoted approximately 12% of their cash income to finance health care, whereas the highest income decile devoted about 8%.[11]

Despite this degree of public spending, the safety-net health care system does not ensure continuity of care or access to all needed care, and as a consequence, the uninsured have poorer health outcomes than those with continuous health insurance coverage.[12] Not only does this safety-net system cost a great deal and result in suboptimal health outcomes for the population it serves, but there is also increasing evidence that in the United States, all patients seeking emergency care for critical conditions wait longer for needed attention as a consequence of overcrowding and the use of emergency departments by uninsured patients who lack a regular source of health care.[13] The structure of any market assumes that there are those who cannot or will not pay for the good or service at the market price. As long as a market structure for health care delivery is maintained, there will be those who will not have access to appropriate health care.

ASYMMETRICAL KNOWLEDGE

Consumers rely heavily on the advice of their physicians for guidance regarding diagnosis and treatment. In this setting, not only do physicians function as suppliers of health care services, but they also play a major role in determining the level of demand for these services. For example, physicians advise patients about the frequency of office visits, the types of diagnostic tests to undergo, and the treatment or treatments that may be needed. Asymmetry of knowledge between patients and their physicians forces patients to rely on this advice for health care decisions.

Substantial evidence exists to support the notion that physicians do increase the demand for health care. Supply-and-demand theory dictates that the entry of more sellers into a market should result in increased competition, lower prices, and lower total costs for goods and services. Yet in health care, it has been demonstrated repeatedly that an increased supply of health care services results in an increased demand for services and an increase in costs. Initial concerns about this unusual market behavior stemmed from the observation that in geographic areas that were similar with respect to demographics, socioeconomic characteristics, and burden of disease, hospital use rates were higher in areas with a greater supply of hospital beds.[14] In a study of the supply of surgeons and the demand for surgery, it was estimated that a 10% increase in the supply of surgeons, as measured by the surgeon-to-population ratio, led to a 3% increase in the per capita surgery rate.[15] A number of other studies have addressed the effect of physician ownership on health care use rates. In a study examining the issue of physician ownership of ancillary services, 50% more visits were ordered at physician-owned physical therapy clinics in Florida than were ordered at clinics that received no referrals from owners.[16] The authors of the study could find no discernible difference in the quality of care across ownership structures. An analysis of more than 65,000 insurance claims found that doctors who owned imaging machines ordered more than four times more imaging studies than those who referred to independent radiologists.[17] Finally, in a study addressing the impact of the 1990 Medicare physician reimbursement changes on thoracic surgeons who were predicted to lose substantial income if surgical volumes remained unchanged, the Medicare fee cuts led to volume increases in both Medicare and private-pay patients, to the point where 70% of the fee loss from Medicare was recaptured through higher patient volume.[18]

These findings make supplier-induced demand (SID) one of the most controversial issues in health economics. If SID exists to a substantial extent, economic analysis would then suggest that competitive markets are useless as a means of managing health care delivery and reducing costs [*see Figure 2*]. Although numerous other hypotheses have been offered to explain the empirical findings of the increases in demand associated with increased supply, none disprove SID.

Physicians find the SID hypothesis disturbing because it suggests that they manipulate the demand for health care to advance their own economic interests. Most physicians are aware of the relation between service volume and income, but various other factors (e.g., rapidly evolving technologies, medical uncertainties at all levels of care, and defensive practices to avoid the risk of litigation) make it impossible to determine the exact impact of SID. The concept of target

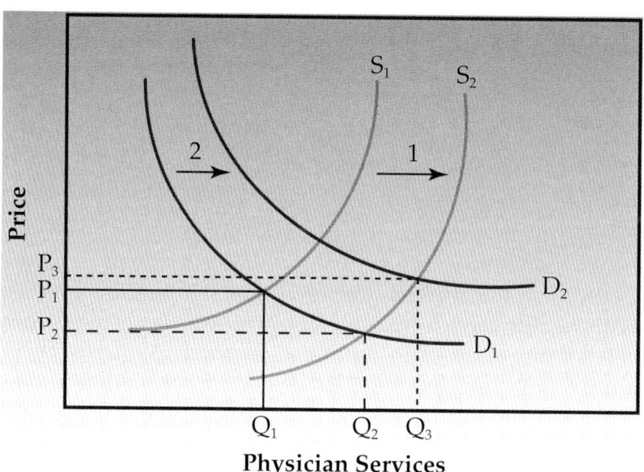

Figure 2 Given an initial supply and demand for physician services at S_1 and D_1, assume that the number of physicians increases (*arrow 1*), thereby shifting the supply curve to the right. In normal economic conditions, the quantity of physician services would increase (to Q_2), and the price would fall (to P_2). Empirical evidence, however, suggests that the demand for services also increases, shifting the demand curve to D_2 (*arrow 2*) and resulting in an increase in both price (P_3) and quantity (Q_3). D = demand; P = price; Q = quantity; S = supply; subscripts 1, 2, and 3 reflect the order in which quantity and price change in response to a change in supply (*arrow 1*) followed by a change in demand (*arrow 2*).

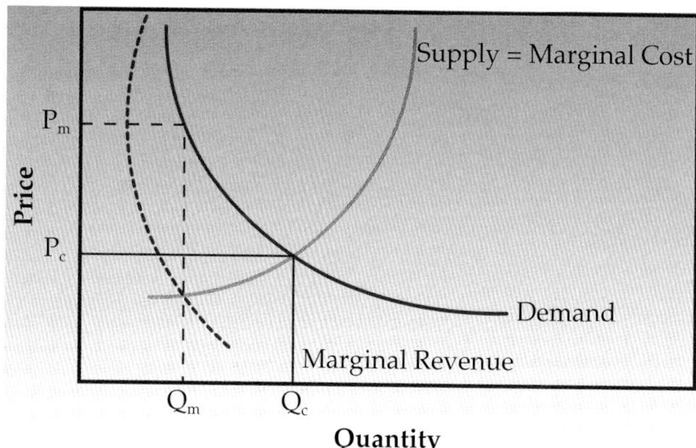

Figure 3 Monopolies set prices to maximize profits by equating the marginal cost of production and the marginal revenue. This process results in higher prices and lower levels of production than would be found in a competitive market. P_c = competitive price; P_m = monopoly price; Q_c = competitive quantity; Q_m = monopoly quantity.

incomes is certainly known to be a factor in other arenas of the economy. Regardless of the true extent of SID's impact on the cost of health care, it is the market-based structure of health care that creates incentives for physicians to influence the demand for health care.

MARKETS, MONOPOLIES, NEW DRUGS, AND TECHNOLOGY

The market is uniquely effective in fostering innovation and technological advances. Firms compete to introduce new products, and in doing so, they gain monopoly power and enhance profits through increased market share and monopoly pricing. Unlike competitive markets, where supply and demand determine the price of a good or service, monopolies set their own price. The profit-maximizing price is achieved by equating the marginal cost of producing one additional unit to the marginal revenue from selling one additional unit [*see Figure 3*]. This results in a higher price and a lower level of production than would be achieved in a competitive market. Monopoly profits are typically short-lived because as more suppliers enter the market, the marginal revenue curve shifts so that it eventually equals the demand curve, thereby reducing the price and increasing the quantity supplied.

In virtually every other sector of the economy, the introduction of new technology tends to reduce the cost of a particular good or service. Health care is one of the few exceptions to this general rule. A 2003 analysis of the relation between the availability of advanced technologies and health care spending found that for certain technologies (e.g., diagnostic imaging, cardiac catheterization facilities, and intensive care facilities), increased availability was often accompanied by increased use (and hence increased spending).[19] Similarly, expenditures on prescription drugs doubled between 1990 and 2000 and are expected to account for one seventh of total health care costs by 2012 [*see Table 1*].[20] Moreover, whereas consumers pay less than 3% of hospital service costs out of their own pockets, they pay about 32% of pharmaceutical costs.

One of the factors contributing to these increased costs is the presence of legal restrictions, in the form of patents afforded to pharmaceuticals and medical devices that prevent other firms from entering the market with a similar product. Patents give pharmaceutical companies and device manufacturers legal monopolies for a period of 20 years. The purpose of this law, as expressed in Article 1, Section 8 of the US Constitution, is "to promote the progress of science and the useful arts by securing for limited times to inventors the exclusive right to their respective discoveries." In addition, at the end of the patent period, pharmaceutical companies can switch their products from prescription to over-the-counter status and gain 3 additional years of market exclusivity if they can demonstrate that any misuse of a drug will not endanger a consumer's health. During these protected periods, companies work to establish brand loyalty among physicians and consumers.

Pharmaceutical companies and device manufacturers argue that the costs of research, development, and testing would be impossible to recoup without these legal

Table 1 Major Components of Health Spending, 1999–2009

	1990	*1993*	*1997*	*2000*	*2003*	*2006*	*2009*
Hospital care	9.6	8.0	3.6	5.6	7.5	7.0	5.1
Physician and clinical services	12.8	8.5	4.6	7.0	8.5	5.9	4.0
Prescription drugs	12.8	8.2	11.1	15.3	10.5	8.5	5.3

Adapted from Martin A et al.[38]

protections. Others, however, are concerned that companies are using their monopoly power to raise prices, restrict output, and earn excessive profits. Since 1980, the rate of growth in drug prices has exceeded consumer price inflation rates. In addition, the profitability of drug firms has been consistently higher than that of the manufacturing industry average.[21]

Again, pharmaceutical companies argue that the high rate of profit observed in the industry is justified by the significant risk and cost of innovations. However, not all innovations are costly to the company, risky to investors, or beneficial to society. One of the most notable examples of profiteering by a pharmaceutical company was the introduction of the "new little purple pill." The original purple pill, Prilosec (a trade name for omeprazole), was introduced in 1989 by AstraZeneca. In 2000, it was the best-selling drug in the world, with over $6 billion in sales per year. When the patent was due to expire in 2001, the company applied for a patent for the "new little purple pill," Nexium (esomeprazole magnesium), which was simply a chemical isomer of Prilosec. Despite the Food and Drug Administration's determination that Nexium offered no significant clinical advance over Prilosec, a patent was awarded. The company launched a very successful marketing campaign, and in 2006, sales of Nexium exceeded $5 billion. The price of Prilosec for [illegible] is $30 per month, whereas that of Nexium is $200 per month. The current market-based model of new product development accompanied by long periods of monopoly protection can be predicted to increase the costs of health care substantially.

PRICE TRANSPARENCY

For most goods and services, price transparency leads to lower and more uniform prices, a view consistent with standard economic theory. Currently, there is considerable variation in prices for similar procedures. For example, a comprehensive metabolic panel costs $97 at San Francisco General Hospital and $1,733 at Doctors Hospital in Modesto, California. A single Percocet tablet costs $6.68 at San Francisco General, $15.00 at UC Davis in Sacramento, and $35.50 at Doctors Hospital in Modesto.[22] If evidence from other markets could be applied to health care, then reforms that increase transparency should result in lower and more uniform prices.[23,24] However, there are reasons to be concerned that greater price transparency would not have the desired effect. Health care differs from other consumer goods in ways that make it difficult to apply empirical evidence from other markets. For one, patients with insurance pay little of the cost of their medical care and are therefore less price sensitive. In addition, there is evidence to suggest that price acts as a proxy for quality in health care, with many believing that higher-cost care is better care.[25] Second, physicians typically make choices for patients, such as what tests to order, whether and where to hospitalize, and which specialists to recommend. Patients are unlikely to challenge this advice to save a few dollars. Finally, transparency could create an incentive to raise prices. Hospitals that charge different payer types different prices would be inclined to publish the higher price. For these reasons, pricing may have a more muted effect on the health care market than it has on other markets, and improvements in price transparency may be less effective. So far, preliminary data from New Hampshire[26] and California[22] suggest that this is the case. Neither state demonstrated any effect of hospital price transparency 2 years after initiation.

ADMINSTRATIVE COSTS

In general economic terms, markets function best and society benefits most when multiple suppliers compete to produce the highest-quality product at the lowest cost. With health care, however, this process has resulted in a bewildering array of insurers and contracts. Virtually every physician in the United States has had to expend considerable time and effort dealing with complicated, arcane, and apparently deliberately confusing rules and requirements.

The repeal in 1986 of laws that sought to regulate the growth of the health care industry resulted in an abandonment of all efforts to constrain market-based entrepreneurship in health care. Not-for-profit hospitals and health maintenance organizations converted to for-profit status. Consolidation of the insurance industry reduced the number of plans available in a market area, thus affording insurers monopoly power and leading to higher prices. The cost of administering private health insurance in the United States reached $143 billion in 2005.[27] For-profit insurance companies have reaped impressive profits and gains in stock value, as well as significant political power.

As a reaction to this state of affairs, [illegible] critics of the US system have asserted that the adoption of a simplified, Canadian-style, single-payer health insurance system would yield large savings in administrative costs, which could then be used to expand coverage to those who are currently uninsured. A 2003 study compared administrative health care costs in the United States with those in Canada.[28] In 1999, per capita health administration costs amounted to $1,059 in the United States (for a total cost of $294 billion), in contrast to $307 in Canada [*see Table 2*]. The authors arrived at these figures by analyzing data from governments, hospitals, insurance companies, and physicians. They argued that much of the difference between the two countries was accounted for by the multiple sources of health coverage in the United States, as opposed to the single source in the Canadian system. This analysis has not been replicated by others, and an accompanying editorial questioned the methodology used.[29] Nevertheless, the author of the editorial did agree that the current system is "an administrative monstrosity, a truly bizarre mélange of thousands of payers with payment systems that differ for no socially beneficial reason."

THE PATIENT PROTECTION AND AFFORDABLE CARE ACT AND OTHER LEGISLATIVE INITIATIVES

The most significant impact of the Patient Protection and Affordable Care Act (ACA) is that an estimated 32 million Americans will gain insurance coverage by 2019. The health reform law mandates that currently uninsured Americans obtain health insurance. Medicaid eligibility is expanded and substantial subsidies are provided to make insurance more affordable for those ineligible for public insurance programs. Currently, the uninsured rely heavily on the safety-net health care system, which is associated with

Table 2 Administrative Costs of Health Care: United States versus Canada

Administrative Cost Category	*United States*		*Canada*	
	Total Cost ($ billion)	*Per Capita Cost ($)*	*Total Cost ($ billion)*	*Per Capita Cost ($)*
Insurance overhead	72	259	1.43	47
Employer costs	15.9	57	0.257	8
Hospital administration	87.6	315	3.1	103
Practitioners	89.9	324	3.3	107
Total	294.3	1,059	9	307

higher costs and poorer health outcomes. If previous trends hold, the newly insured will enjoy better health outcomes, but the cost implications of health care reform are less clear.

Both the Centers for Medicaid & Medicare Services (CMS) and the CBO have projected that health care reform will result in an expansion of national health care expenditures.[30,31] The ACA includes a number of mechanisms to offset the new spending, including a reduction in the update factor for Medicare hospital reimbursement, a reduction in the overpayment to Medicare Advantage insurers, an assessment on employers whose employees use subsidies rather than employer-sponsored insurance, and an increase in the Medicare tax for high-income families. The CBO estimates that the revenue increases will exceed the increased costs and ultimately reduce the federal deficit by more than $100 billion in the first decade and more than $1 trillion in the second decade.[22] However, critics argue that although these measures may pay for health care reform, they do nothing to rein in the growth of health care costs. Health care spending in the United States already accounts for 17% of GDP. At the current rate of growth, it will reach 38% of GDP by 2075. The ACA includes a variety of provisions intended to lower the rate of cost growth (bend the health care cost curve), including physician payment reform, incentives to coordinate care for patients with chronic conditions, increased access to electronic health records, and funding for comparative effectiveness research, but there is currently little evidence that any of these measures actually work.

A second implication of increased access to health insurance is the need for a larger primary care workforce. Numerous studies have demonstrated that access to primary care is associated with improved outcomes at reduced cost. Although primary care physicians provide 57% of all patient visits, they represent only 35% of the US physician workforce.[32] Even without the new demands created by health care reform, the aging of the population and the increasing proportion of the population with a chronic medical condition have strained the capacity of the primary care workforce. The 2008 Medicare Payment Advisory Commission (MedPAC) beneficiary survey found that 28% of beneficiaries without a primary care physician reported a problem finding one.[33] This represented a 17% increase from 2006. The number of beneficiaries reporting a problem finding a new specialist declined. The Massachusetts experience with expanded health insurance coverage illustrates the disconnection between access to health insurance and access to care. The average wait time for a new patient to obtain an appointment to see an internist in Massachusetts was 31 days in 2008, up from 17 days in 2005.[34] Patients without access to primary care will be forced to continue to seek care at high-cost, poor-continuity sites, such as emergency departments. General surgery also faces shortages that are likely to be exacerbated by health care reform. The overall number of general surgeons has declined by 26% over the past 25 years.[35] Rural areas are most acutely affected. The income gap between generalist and subspecialist careers and rising medical student debt account for most of the decline in medical student interest in both of these generalist careers.

The ACA and the American Recovery and Reinvestment Act of 2009 include several provisions aimed at highlighting the importance of primary care and general surgery. The economic stimulus package provided about $500 million for training programs in health professions, including $300 million for expanding the National Health Service Corps, a program that offers scholarships and loan repayment for health professionals who agree to serve in shortage areas for 2 to 5 years. The ACA includes additional funding to support training of primary care providers, redistributes approximately 900 unfilled residency positions into primary care and general surgery, provides a 10% bonus under the Medicare fee schedule for primary care providers, and requires that states increase Medicaid payment to Medicare rates for primary care services. Notably missing in the provisions is a lifting of the cap on the total number of residency positions, which were frozen by the Balanced Budget Amendment of 1997. In the absence of an expansion of total residency training positions, it is not clear that the provisions will make a significant dent in the projected primary care and general surgery shortages.

Implications for Surgeons

Market-based health care has not only increased the costs of care but has also changed the professional behavior of physicians. Organized medicine's priorities place the financial interests of physicians above access to and quality of care. Hospitals invest in programs that promise a high return on investment with less regard for evidence of benefit or greater societal need. The fragmentation of the profession into over 130 specialties and subspecialties has resulted in competition among disciplines, further promoting self-interest over best practices. In this environment and despite advances in evidence-based medicine, individual physicians are equally tempted to place their own interests above those of patients by recommending interventions of limited value. A 2007 study highlighted these disturbing trends by revealing that median wait times for both routine and urgent dermatology appointments were nearly four times longer than wait times for an appointment to receive cosmetic botulinum toxin injections.[36] Patients with a potentially cancerous skin lesion wait a median of 26 days to be seen by a dermatologist.

Adam Smith's 1776 book *An Inquiry into the Nature and Causes of the Wealth of Nations* is considered the first full-scale treatise in classical economics. In it, Smith espoused the virtues of the market as a means toward national wealth. He made the case that self-interest leads naturally to greater public good: "It is not from the benevolence of the butcher, the brewer, or the baker, that we expect our dinner, but from their regard for their own interest. We address ourselves, not to their humanity, but to their self-love and never talk to them of our own necessities but to their advantages."[37] However, Smith was also quick to draw a distinction between self-interest and greed. He criticized those who desired excessive wealth, for whom "the chief enjoyment of riches consists in the parade of riches, which in their eyes is never so complete as when they appear to possess those decisive marks of opulence which nobody can possess but themselves." In his view, the market's ability to foster the growth of a nation depended on social cooperation, discipline, and respect for others. Greed denied others and thereby weakened the whole.

Finally, Smith understood the intrinsic failure of the market to ensure equity and the vital role of government in this regard:

> Is this improvement in the circumstances of the lower ranks of the people to be regarded as an advantage or as an inconveniency to the society? The answer seems at first sight abundantly plain. Servants, labourers, and workmen of different kinds, make up the far greater part of every great political society. But what improves the circumstances of the greater part can never be regarded as an inconveniency to the whole. No society can surely be flourishing and happy, of which the far greater part of the members are poor and miserable. It is but equity, besides, that they who feed, clothe, and lodge the whole body of the people, should have such a share of the produce of their own labour as to be themselves tolerably well fed, clothed, and lodged.[37]

Arguably, health care is as necessary to the prosperity of a society as food and lodging are.

Although individual physicians can do little to fix the society-wide problems created by market-based health care, surgeons can help restore confidence in the profession by helping to develop and then adhering to evidence-based approaches to surgical intervention. Communication skills and attention to the needs of patients should be stressed as vital to the best patient care. Equally important is remembering that the profession of medicine is not merely another way of making a living. The importance of education in evidence-based and compassionate care, preferably one on one, for the training of surgical residents and students must also be emphasized. Mastery of these skills, which place patient interests ahead of surgeon interests, truly defines professionalism.

Financial Disclosures: None Reported

References

1. Centers for Medicaid & Medical Services. World Health Statistics 2009. Available at: http://www.cms.hhs.gov/NationalHealthExpendData/02_NationalHealthAccountsHistorical.asp (accessed March 18, 2011).
2. World Health Organization. World health statistics 2009. Available at: http://www.who.int/whosis/whostat/2009/en/index.html (accessed November 15, 2011).
3. Ginsberg PB. Don't break out the champagne: continued slowing of health care spending growth unlikely to last. Health Aff (Millwood) 2008;27:30–2.
4. Congressional Budget Office. The long-term outlook for health care spending. Congress of the United States, November 2007. Washington (DC): Government Printing Office; 2007.
5. Congressional Budget Office. The budget and economic outlook: fiscal years 2008 to 2018. Available at: http://www.cbo.gov/ftpdocs/89xx/doc8917/01-23-2008_BudgetOutlook.pdf (accessed March 18, 2011).
6. Chernow ME, Hirth RA, Cutler DM. Increased spending on health care: how much can the United States afford? Health Aff (Millwood) 2003;22:15–25.
7. Organisation for Economic Co-operation and Development. OECD health data 2007. Statistics and indicators for 30 countries. Available at: http://www.oecd.org/health/healthdata (accessed March 18, 2011).
8. Nolte E, McKee CM. Measuring the health of nations: updating an earlier analysis. Health Aff (Millwood) 2008;27:58–71.
9. Fisher ES, Wennberg DE, Stukel TA, et al. The implications of regional variations in Medicare spending. Part 2: Health outcomes and satisfaction with care. Ann Intern Med 2003;138:288–98.
10. Committee on the Consequences of Uninsurance. Hidden costs, value lost. Washington, DC: Institute of Medicine of the National Academy of Sciences; June 2003.
11. Holohan J, Zedlewski S. Who pays for health care in the United States? Implications for health system reform. Inquiry 1992;29:231–48.
12. Committee on the Consequences of Uninsurance. Care without coverage. Washington, DC: Institute of Medicine of the National Academy of Sciences; May 2002.
13. Wilper AP, Woolhandler S, Lasser KE, et al. Waits to see an emergency department physician: U.S. trends and predictors, 1997–2004. Health Aff (Millwood) 2008;27: w84–95.
14. Roemer MI. Bed supply and hospital utilization. Hospitals 1961;35:36–42.
15. Fuchs VR. The supply of surgeons and the demand for operations. J Hum Resour 1978;13 Suppl:35–56.
16. Mitchell JM, Sass TR. Physician ownership of ancillary services: independent demand inducement or quality assurance. J Health Econ 1995;14:263–89.
17. Hillman BJ, Joseph CA, Mabry MR, et al. Frequency and costs of diagnostic imaging in office practice: a comparison of self-referring and radiologist referring physicians. N Engl J Med 1990;323:1604–8.
18. Yip W. Physicians responses to medical fee reductions: changes in the volume and intensity of supply of coronary artery bypass graft surgeries in Medicare and the private sector. J Health Econ 1998;17:675–700.

19. Baker L, Birnbaum H, Geppert J, et al. The relationship between technology availability and health care spending. Health Aff (Millwood) 2003;(Suppl Web Exclusives):W3-537–51. Available at: http://content.healthaffairs.org/content/early/2003/11/05/hlthaff.w3.537.citation (accessed March 18, 2011).
20. Heffler S, Smith S, Keehan S, et al. Health spending projections for 2002–2012. Health Aff (Millwood) 2003; (Suppl Web Exclusives): W3-54–65. Available at: http://content.healthaffairs.org/content/early/2003/02/07/hlthaff.w3.54.citation (accessed March 19, 2011).
21. Comanor WS, Schweitzer SO. Pharmaceuticals. In: Adams W, Brock J, editors. The structure of American industry. Englewood Cliffs (NJ): Prentice Hall; 1995.
22. Austin DA, Gravelle JG. CRS Report for Congress. Does price transparency improve market efficiency? Implications of empirical evidence in other markets for the health sector. April 29, 2008. Available at: http://www.fas.org/sgp/crs/misc/RL34101.pdf (accessed March 18, 2011).
23. Sinaiko AD, Rosenthal MB. Increased price transparency in health care—challenges and potential effects. N Engl J Med 2011;364:891–4.
24. Cutler DM, Dafny L. Designing transparency systems for medical care prices. N Engl J Med 2011;364: 894–5.
25. Waber RL, Shiv B, Carmon Z, et al. Commercial features of placebo and therapeutic efficacy. JAMA 2008;299:1016–7.
26. Tu HT, Lauer J. Impact of health care price transparency on price variation: the New Hampshire Experience. Issue brief no. 128. Washington (DC): Center for Studying Helath System Change; 2009. Available at: http://hschange.org/CONTENT/1095/1095.pdf (accessed March 18, 2011).
27. Centers for Medicare & Medicaid Services. National health expenditures by type of service and source of funds, CY 1960–2005. Available at: http://www.cms.hhs.gov/NationalHealthExpendData/02_NationalHealthAccountsHistorical.asp#TopOfPage (accessed March 18, 2011).
28. Woolhandler S, Campbell T, Himmelstein DU. Costs of health care administration in the United States and Canada. N Engl J Med 2003;349:768–75.
29. Aaron HJ. The costs of health care administration in the United States and Canada—questionable answers to a questionable question. N Engl J Med 2003;349:801–3.
30. Center for Medicare & Medicaid Services. Projected national health expenditure data. Available at: https://www.cms.gov/NationalHealthExpendData/03_NationalHealthAccountsProjected.asp (accessed March 18, 2011).
31. Letter from Douglas W. Wilmendorf to House Speaker Nancy Pelosi, March 20, 2010. Available at: http://www.cbo.gov/ftp docs/113xx/doc11355/hr4872.pdf (accessed March 18, 2011).
32. Cherry DK, Hing E, Woodwell DA, Rechtsteiner EA. National Ambulatory Medical Care Survey: 2006 summary. Hyattsville (MD): National Center for Health Statistics; 2008. National Health Statistics Report no. 3.
33. Medicare Payment Advisory Commission. Report to the Congress: Medicare payment policy. Washington (DC): MedPAC; March 2009.
34. Massachusetts Medical Society. 2008 Physician Workforce Study. Waltham (MA): Massachusetts Medical Society; October 2008.
35. Lynge DC, Larson EH, Thompson MJ, et al. A longitudinal analysis of the general surgery workforce in the United States, 1981-2005. Arch Surg 2008;143:345–50.
36. Resneck JS Jr, Lipton S, Pletcher MJ. Short wait times for patients seeking cosmetic botulinum toxin appointments with dermatologists. J Am Acad Dermatol 2007;57:985–9.
37. Smith A. An inquiry into the nature and causes of the wealth of nations. Vol I, book 1. New York: Random House; 1994.
38. Martin A, Lassman D, Whittle L, Catlin A, and the National Health Expenditure Accounts Team. Recession contributes to slowest annual rate of increase in five decades. Health Aff 2011;30:11–22.

9 MINIMIZING VULNERABILITY TO MALPRACTICE CLAIMS

*William R. Berry, MD, MPH, FACS**

No surgeon wants to be sued. The threat of a medical malpractice suit is, however, a reality for everyone who practices surgery. Lawsuits can extract a tremendous price from those who are sued. The surgeon who has been sued bears the burden of the lawsuit for a period of years while it slowly works its way through a system that is not designed for speed or efficiency. Life decisions are often postponed. Sometimes careers are forever changed. Confidence is shaken, and sleep is lost. For some, there is no relief until it is over; for others, it repeatedly intrudes on life. It is better to never be sued. The situation, however, is not totally out of the surgeon's control—nor is it hopeless. Armed with knowledge of the legal system and an understanding of why patients seek the courts, the surgeon can decrease the likelihood of ever being named. This chapter provides strategies for avoiding lawsuits and advice for dealing with a suit if one is ever filed against you.

What Is Medical Malpractice?

Medical malpractice law is a subset of the law of torts or law that concerns itself with civil injuries as a result of negligent behavior or a failure to practice due diligence. For a medical malpractice suit to be successful, a number of elements must be satisfied. A plaintiff (the patient or the patient's estate) must prove, by a preponderance of the evidence, that the defendant (the surgeon) was negligent or failed to exercise due care in the circumstances. A plaintiff must also show that the defendant's negligence caused his injuries and that he has suffered injuries or quantifiable damages as a result.

Four conditions must be met:

1. There must be a "relationship" of some kind between the patient and the surgeon. The relationship can be a direct one, in which the surgeon operated on the patient, or a more indirect one, in which the surgeon only consulted.
2. The surgeon must be "negligent," which means that he or she did not perform to the "standard of care." The definition of the standard of care varies from state to state but usually means that the surgeon failed to perform in a manner consistent with the care that would be given by the average physician practicing in the same specialty. To help the judge and the jury understand the evidence in relation to the standard of care, both sides use "expert" witnesses to provide opinions about the care.
3. The surgeon's negligence must have been the cause of the injuries that the patient sustained.
4. The injuries that the patient has suffered must have caused measurable damage. This reflects the civil nature of malpractice, whereby injuries are compensated with a payment.

The judge and/or the jury are responsible for determining whether each of these conditions has been met and uses a standard of "more likely than not." Unlike criminal law, the evidence does not have to reach the level of "beyond a reasonable doubt"—only that there is a greater than 50% chance that the conditions were met. In our judicial system, the judge and the jury interpret and decide whether the "standard of care" was met.

Malpractice lawsuits often begin with the filing of suit papers that are delivered or "served" to those being sued. A written demand for compensation for an injury from the patient or an attorney is usually called a claim and can precede the filing of a suit. Suits and claims can end in different ways, and not all involve a jury trial. They can be dropped by the patient at any time; denied by the insurance carrier and not pursued by the patient; settled with a payment before, during, or after a trial; dismissed by the court; or ended with a jury verdict.

Personal Issues for the Defendant Physician

How physicians cope personally with being a defendant in a medical malpractice suit varies, but a number of factors come to bear on the amount of stress that litigation inflicts. These factors include the physician's previous exposure to litigation claims, degree of familiarity with the legal system and the litigation process, and previous experience testifying in the courtroom or in depositions; the size of the claim as measured by the seriousness of the alleged injury; and the presence or absence of a claim for punitive damages—which, of course, are not insured by professional liability policies. Some physicians experience a sense of profound isolation when they are first named in a suit, particularly when service of suit papers is accompanied by the standard instruction from their risk management office or legal counsel not to discuss the case with anyone.

Allegations of negligence or substandard care, in and of themselves, are bitter pills to swallow, but they are all the more painful when they are accompanied with a claim for punitive damages. Such claims, announced in the formal complaint, are then typically followed promptly with a grim

* The author and editors gratefully acknowledge the contributions of the previous authors, Grant H. Fleming Esq and Wiley W. Souba, MD, ScD, FACS, to the development and writing of this chapter.

letter to the defendant physician from the insurers involved, reminding the physician that there is no coverage for punitive damages awarded. The allegations in the plaintiff's complaint necessary to support a claim for punitive damages are hurtful and sometimes outrageous; the physician is accused of willful, reckless, and wanton behavior bordering on intent to injure the plaintiff. The awards sought in such cases reach far beyond fair compensation for the injured plaintiff. Rather, punitive damages are calculated to punish the defendant physician—the perceived wrongdoer—and to serve as public sanctions. The physician against whom punitive damages are sought then undergoes pretrial discovery, sometimes shortly after suit is filed. This process involves requests (interrogatories) for detailed accounting of personal assets that might be available to be attached in the event of a judgment in the plaintiff's favor.

Whether or not punitive damages are sought, it is difficult for most physicians to regard being harpooned by a medical malpractice claim as merely a cost of doing business, and for many, the arduous and seemingly never-ending nature of the claim is distracting and potentially debilitating.

Who Brings Medical Malpractice Claims?

Brennan and colleagues have shown that there is no relation between the occurrence of adverse events and the assertion of claims, nor is there any association between adverse events and negligent or substandard care.[1] These authors did, however, find a relation between the degree of disability and the payment of claims. They found that patients who were injured through negligent care usually did not file suit and that the patients who did file suit often did not suffer from negligent care. Further, they also found that patients do turn to the courts when they are disabled in the course of medical care. The need to pay for long term care for themselves or a dependent often contributes to the filing of the suit.

Only a small fraction of patients who are injured through substandard care or treatment actually bring claims or suits.[2] Localio and colleagues concluded that although 1% of hospitalized patients sustain a significant injury as a result of negligent care, fewer than 2% of these patients initiate a malpractice claim.[3] Other authors have found that only 2 to 4% of patients injured through negligence file claims, yet five to six times as many patients who sustained injuries that do not meet the threshold for malpractice also file malpractice claims.[4]

Strategies for Preventing Malpractice Suits

Clearly, not every malpractice suit can be prevented. When catastrophic injuries follow surgery or treatment, the emotional impact of the tragedy, coupled with overwhelming economic pressures, can create an environment in which a claim is likely. On the other hand, not all adverse outcomes from treatment result in claims. Why is it that some patients and families sue for adverse outcomes and some do not? Why do some patients sue for adverse outcomes that are expected and that occur in the context of high-quality care? The answers to those questions typically have to do with physician-patient relationships rather than professional skill.

It has become increasingly clear that surgeons can reduce the likelihood of litigation by adopting a few key habits and practices with their patients and their patients' families. These include building trust through open communication, making effective use of the informed consent process, keeping accurate and complete medical records, and educating office staff.

COMMUNICATION AND INTERPERSONAL SKILLS IN THE PHYSICIAN-PATIENT RELATIONSHIP

Although advancing medical technology has elevated patients' level of expectation regarding treatment outcome, easy public access to medical information on the Internet has encouraged patients to become partners with their physicians in their own care. Experience with juries over the past few decades continues to support the belief that, in general, laypersons have a high regard for physicians and a deep respect for their superior level of knowledge and training. At the same time, patients expect and deserve to receive thorough understandable explanations from their physicians regarding their diagnosis, their treatment plan, and the risks and benefits of their treatment. Even when the disease process is beyond the physician's control, the physician can create an environment for effective communication with the patient. Years of listening to patients and their family members relate their experiences at depositions and trials have confirmed that the quality of communication and the presence of trust between physician and patient are the most important factors in the patient's decision to file a medical malpractice suit.

Several researchers have analyzed physician-patient communication and its relation to claims for damages for alleged professional negligence. Beckman and colleagues studied 45 deposition transcripts of plaintiffs in settled malpractice suits, focusing on the question of why these plaintiffs decided to bring malpractice actions.[5] They concluded that the process of care, rather than the adverse outcome, determined the decision to bring the claim. They found that 71% of the depositions revealed problems with physician-patient communication in four major categories: (1) perceived unavailability ("You never knew where the doctor was," "You asked for a doctor and no one came," "No one returned our calls"); (2) devaluing of the patient's or the family's views (e.g., perceived insensitivity to cultural or socioeconomic differences); (3) poor delivery of medical information (e.g., lack of informed consent, failure to keep patients informed during care, or failure to explain why a complication occurred); and (4) failure to understand the patient's perspective.

Vincent and colleagues examined the reasons patients and their relatives take legal action in a survey of 227 patients and relatives.[6] Over 70% of respondents were seriously affected by incidents that gave rise to litigation. However, the decision to take legal action was determined not only by the original injury but also by insensitive handling and poor communication after the original incident. Patients taking legal action wanted greater honesty, an appreciation of the severity of the trauma they had suffered, and assurances that lessons had been learned from their experiences.

Levinson and colleagues studied specific communication behaviors associated with malpractice history.[7] Although they did not discover a relation between those two factors in the surgeons they studied, they found that primary care physicians who had no claims filed against them used more statements of orientation (i.e., they educated patients about what to expect), used humor more with their patients, and employed communication techniques designed to solicit their patients' level of understanding and opinions (i.e., they encouraged patients to provide verbal feedback).

Hickson and colleagues studied specific factors that led patients to file malpractice claims after perinatal injuries by surveying patients whose claims had been closed after litigation.[8] Dissatisfaction with physician-patient communication was a significant factor: 13% of the sample believed that their physicians would not listen, 32% felt that their physicians did not talk openly, 48% believed that their physicians had deliberately misled them, and 70% indicated that their physicians had not warned them about long-term developmental problems.

The American College of Surgeons' Patient Safety and Professional Liability Committee performed a closed claims study of 460 liability claims between April 2004 and February 2006.[9] Ninety of the claims (19.8%) were filed because of failures in communication that predominantly involved patients or their families. Among some of the claims, the standard of care was clearly met. However, defendants suffered litigation solely because they failed to spend the time required to provide the insight and satisfaction necessary to defuse anger and mistrust.

Many defense attorneys recount stories of surgeons who had developed a positive rapport with their patients and were not named in a suit, whereas other physicians involved in the patient's care were named. Patients apparently made these decisions without regard to the extent of each defendant's factual involvement in the case but instead sued physicians with whom they had poor or weak relationships. A component of the motivation to sue may be simply an unsatisfactory or incomplete explanation of how and why an adverse outcome occurred. Patients who remain uninformed often assume the worst: that their physician is uncomfortable talking about the complication because he or she made a mistake, was careless, or is hiding something. Malpractice plaintiffs have sometimes claimed that when they sat through the process of jury education during the trial, it was the first time they received any explanation of the complication for which they had brought suit. Physicians should make a point of explaining to patients and their families how and why adverse conditions arose, independent of any possible deficiencies in the quality of care received at home or in patient compliance. Patients and their families are keenly sensitive to unintended inferences that blame for the bad outcome rests with them.

The principles of good communication are the same, whether or not an adverse event has occurred. They include the following:

1. *Educating and informing the patient.* Convey medical information in descriptive terms that patients can understand, using illustrations, sketches, and diagrams. Ask about the response to the therapeutic regimen. Provide counseling and instruction if no improvement is observed. Inform the patient about specific steps in the examination or treatment plan.
2. *Ensuring patient understanding.* Ask patients whether they understand what they have been told; check the understanding by listening to the patient after providing an explanation. Demonstrate respect for any cultural or socioeconomic differences that may be impeding the patient's understanding.
3. *Emotionally engaging the patient.* Demonstrate concern and understanding of the patient's complaints. Express empathy; use humor where appropriate. Demonstrate awareness of the patient's occupation, social circumstances, hobbies, or interests.
4. *Following up with the patient.* Return telephone calls. Explain the protocol for substitute or resident coverage and introduce patients to other personnel who may be following their care. During longer hospitalizations, keep the patient and the family informed of the patient's progress or treatment plan. Keep the referring physician promptly informed by providing treatment or discharge summaries. In the event of a patient's death, meet with the family several weeks later to review and explain autopsy findings and answer questions that they might have about what happened to their loved one.

Further guidelines apply when an adverse outcome occurs. In the hospital setting, prompt disclosure of an untoward or unexpected event that causes injury or harm is mandated by the Joint Commission on the Accreditation of Healthcare Organizations (JCAHO). JCAHO standards require disclosure of unanticipated outcomes "whenever those outcomes differ significantly from the anticipated outcome."[10] The responsibility to communicate lies with both the attending physician and, in the case of a complication incident to surgery, the person accountable for securing consent for the procedure.

When possible, it may be advisable to invite other responsible caregivers to take part in the discussion of the adverse event with the patient and the family. Consideration should also be given to inviting other persons who may be sources of support for the patient and could benefit from the disclosure. During the discussion, express regret for the occurrence, without ascribing blame, fault, or neglect to oneself or any other caregiver. Describe the decisions that led to the adverse event, including those in which the patient participated. Explain and outline the course of events, using factual, nontechnical language, without admitting fault or liability or ascribing blame to anyone else. Do not speculate or hypothesize. State the nature of the mistake or error, if one was made, and highlight the expected consequences and prognosis, if known. Outline the plan of corrective action with respect to the patient. In the event that certain information is unknown at the time of the discussion (e.g., the etiology of the condition, suspected equipment malfunction in the absence of controlled testing, or pending laboratory test results), tell the patient and family that such information is currently unknown and offer to share the information with them when it becomes available.

A special case exists when children suffer injuries. Parents may seek subconsciously to avoid blaming themselves and so may attempt to transfer the responsibility to the health care providers. After a complication or adverse event arises in a pediatric case, the physician should speak openly with the parents. The discussion should cover possible or known causes or mechanisms of the injury or death that are independent of any care rendered by the parents, including prenatal care or home care of a chronically ill child.

THE INFORMED CONSENT PROCESS

Effective informed consent can reduce the risk of litigation. The informed consent process is an extension of good communication practices, albeit one that is mandated by law. The tort of informed consent is derived from the concept of battery—for example, unauthorized touching. Patients are deemed not to have consented to a procedure unless they have been advised of all the risks involved in it and all the alternatives to it. Although differing somewhat from state to state, in most jurisdictions, the standard is objective rather than subjective. In other words, the risks and alternatives that must be disclosed are those that a "reasonable patient, in similar circumstances"—not necessarily the plaintiff—would regard as material to the decision whether to undergo the surgery in question. With procedures for which the statistical incidence of risks has been published or is known, the physician has a duty to quantify for the patient the likelihood of the risk being realized. If the patient's particular condition or situation is such that the likelihood of the risk occurring is higher than average, the physician has the duty to so inform the patient.

Many physicians ignore another critical element in the required informed consent discussions: describing the range of reasonable alternative procedures or modalities other than the procedure in question that are available to the patient. The hazard that such omissions entail is illustrated by a case in which the physician performed a transesophageal balloon dilatation of the esophagus to address achalasia that had not responded to conservative medical therapy. The risk of esophageal perforation was disclosed as part of informed consent, and the procedure was performed totally within the standard of care, but the patient suffered perforation of the esophagus with serious permanent and long-term disability. Although an alternative approach, via thoracotomy, was a known option, it was not used at the defendant hospital, and the informed consent discussion therefore did not include the surgical alternative. The defendants were forced to settle the case for a significant amount of money, even though there had been no negligence and the patient acknowledged that the risk of esophageal perforation had been thoroughly disclosed. A breach of informed consent was easily established because one of the reasonable alternatives was not disclosed to the patient. The argument that a reasonable person would probably have rejected the surgical alternative had it been disclosed was not a valid defense; nondisclosure of a reasonable alternative, in and of itself, created strict liability.

Some surgeons regard the informed consent discussion as an inconvenient imposition on their time. However, the few minutes needed for this discussion pale in comparison with the time needed to defend a lawsuit involving a breach of informed consent, either as the central claim or as an ancillary one. In addition, given that the surgeon's personal interaction with a patient may be significantly limited in comparison with that of the primary care physician, obstetrician, gynecologist, or medical specialist, the informed consent discussion presents an important opportunity for the surgeon to develop a rapport and a positive relationship with the patient. Such a rapport can be invaluable in the event of a later complication or adverse outcome. An effective informed consent discussion may reduce the likelihood of a claim for a particular adverse outcome if the patient remembers that the risk of its occurrence was disclosed and discussed.

Informed consent is not the consent form; it is the process of informing the patient. The form is merely a piece of evidence documenting that informed consent occurred; the critical factor is the content of the discussion. For the form to be effective, it must cogently summarize the discussion in a manner that makes it difficult for the patient later to refute, in a "he said, she said" controversy, the version of the discussion that the physician may be rendering in the courtroom under oath.

An effective discussion of informed consent based on custom and habit is essential because of the slow pace of the legal system. In most jurisdictions, the statute of limitations for bringing claims involving adult patients is 2 years. By the time the defendant physician's pretrial deposition is taken, another 1 to 3 years may have elapsed, and after that, even more time passes before the conversation will have to be relayed under oath if the claim goes to trial. It is exceedingly rare that physicians can actually recall the informed consent discussion in question at the time of the suit. However, the content of the communication can be proved more reliably through custom and habit than through direct recollection, particularly when the elements of the discussion are corroborated with a comprehensive and clear form signed by the patient.

In some cases, physicians encourage the showing of a patient education video that explains the intended procedure; such a video should also communicate the risks of the procedure. The use of educational videos can provide additional evidence to support the defense that the patient gave informed consent. Each version of the video should be labeled with the dates when it was routinely used and should not be discarded when it is replaced with updated versions. The patient's chart should reflect that the patient watched the video and had no questions after a review of its contents.

The physician who will perform the procedure, not the nurse or resident who will assist at it, has the duty to secure the patient's consent. However, information provided by other health care providers can be used by the defense as evidence.

DOCUMENTATION

Along with effective communication techniques and informed consent protocols, good documentation practices can minimize a surgeon's risk of becoming a defendant in a medical malpractice suit, or at least provide a more effective defense if litigation is commenced. Although the purpose of keeping medical records is to provide subsequent caregivers with important information relevant to the patient's condition and treatment, in the context of litigation, medical records are used to demonstrate what care was or was not rendered. A standard question that plaintiffs' attorneys ask defendants at pretrial depositions is whether the defendant agrees with the adage, "If it is not documented, it wasn't done." Time and time again, otherwise defensible cases are compromised meritless claims, regardless of cost, on the assumption that strong and successful defenses against such claims will discourage future meritless claims against the physicians they insure.

From the standpoint of an insured physician who is a named defendant, the risk of an adverse verdict is, or should be, an important consideration, as should the emotional wear and tear incurred in preparing for and enduring the stresses of a trial; the time spent away from work and family; the degree to which a settlement, as opposed to a successful verdict, may affect future insurance premiums; and the extent to which a favorable jury verdict will result in clearing of the physician's good name and restoration of his or her professional reputation. How these considerations affect the decision between settlement and trial is strongly influenced by the psychological makeup of the defendant physician: a physician with a strong emotional support structure who also has a personality capable of standing up to the emotional stress and rigors of the courtroom is more suited to participation in a trial than a physician with a more fragile personality who is intolerant of criticism and distrustful of the jury and the legal system. A physician who favors going to trial over settling the claim should be willing to become fully invested in preparing the case for trial, should have a high degree of confidence in the preparation and skills of the defense attorney trying the case, and should be willing to spend the time required to read the voluminous pretrial discovery depositions, medical literature, and medical records associated with the case.

Many physicians would rather have professional negligence claims judged by other physicians than by laypersons from all walks of life and of different education levels. These attitudes have their roots in the 19th century, when the judicial system was struggling to resolve the claims of injured patients against a backdrop of inconsistent medical standards, relatively unsophisticated scientific knowledge and information technology, and antiquated means of communicating medical concepts to laypersons, many of whom were illiterate and lacked what would currently be considered a minimal education. Today, the situation is different: jurors with college degrees are the norm, rather than the exception, in many venues, and the expanded use of technology in the courtroom enables illustrations, concepts, and documentation to be displayed clearly and effectively while witnesses discuss and interpret them for the jury. Accordingly, it is likely that at least some of the traditional suspicion of lay juries may be misplaced. As Struve has noted, "Juries' liability determinations in malpractice cases are not random; rather, studies find some degree of correlation between jury outcomes and medical reviewers' findings of negligence and causation."[11] The statistics released for the year 2005 demonstrate that in Pennsylvania, more than 80% of the verdicts in malpractice trials courts continue to be rendered in favor of the defendant.[12]

It is noteworthy that medical malpractice cases seem to account for a far higher share of tort trials than other types of tort actions do. For example, in Philadelphia County in 1996, malpractice accounted for only 3% of tort case filings but 18.7% of tort trials. To make the comparison in another way, about one of every eight malpractice filings went to trial, compared with about one of every 100 automobile accident filings.[13]

Preparing for a Deposition

Depositions are part of the process of gathering evidence and information in preparation for a malpractice trial. They are often held in an attorney's office. State law controls depositions, so there is some variation, but, in general, they follow similar guidelines. During a deposition, you will usually be questioned by the plaintiff's attorney first, with follow-up questions asked by your own counsel during cross-examination. Additional questions by both attorneys are possible to further clarify points. The entire proceeding will be transcribed by a court reporter, and objections are allowed in most states. It is important to prepare for your deposition by reviewing the available records so that you are familiar with them. It is also important to take the time to understand the questions that you are being asked and to answer them carefully. Depositions may be used at trial to demonstrate inconsistencies in your answers to questions, so it is important to carefully consider answers before you give them. Your attorney can help you in your preparation for the deposition and is usually present while it is being taken.

How Should Surgeons Act When They Are Defendants or Witnesses in a Courtroom Trial?

Although the experience of a medical malpractice trial is not inevitable for all practicing physicians, it is a significant possibility for many. If the suit is held to have merit, no settlement has been arrived at and the case goes to trial, an understanding of what to expect at trial is helpful. In addition, strategies for more effectively, credibly, and persuasively presenting the defense of a medical case to a jury of laypersons charged with the duty to arrive at a verdict can be useful.

Many witnesses who have to testify in court feel frightened or intimidated as they approach the witness stand to be sworn in. Sometimes the truth that the witness is attempting to tell is distorted because of this fear and because of the tactics of the opposing lawyer. The perception and judgment of the jurors who listen to the witness are affected not only by what the witness says but also by the manner in which the testimony is given, the degree to which the witness is acclimated to the facts of the case, and the demeanor of the witness on and off the witness stand. Rightly or wrongly, how the witness testifies is often more critical than what he or she actually says. The jury members' responsibility is to weigh the facts that they are presented with and to come to a judgment. The trust that they have in the witnesses is a crucial element of this process.

Preparation for an appearance in the courtroom is critical for any physician testifying in a trial to best use the opportunity to present the facts in a fair and convincing light. Not surprisingly, under the stress of the moment, intelligent, experienced, and articulate witnesses often abandon their habits of good judgment and solid common sense the moment they walk into a courtroom. The guidelines presented are applicable to both physicians who are actual defendants in a medical malpractice trial and those who are merely witnesses.

GENERAL PREPARATION

Most persons who have rarely or never been a witness in a trial are nervous and anxious at the thought of testifying in front of a jury. A major reason for this reaction is the fear that one's words will be twisted by the opposing lawyer or that the intended testimony will be unfairly distorted or misrepresented as a result of deceptively phrased trick questions. You can overcome, or at least alleviate, this nervousness and anxiety by preparing painstakingly and familiarizing yourself with the case well before the trial, as well as by concentrating on and paying close attention to the content of any questions posed by opposing counsel during your testimony.

Defense counsel should discuss the key case issues with you in detail before your appearance, but, obviously, not all questions and answers can be (or should be) rehearsed. For your part, you should make sure that you are thoroughly familiar with the portions of the medical records for which you are responsible (either directly or in a supervisory capacity). You should also read and study your pretrial deposition transcript to prevent inconsistencies in your trial testimony. If possible, you should review the pretrial depositions of other witnesses in the case. Stenographers are now able to generate word index transcripts that allow you to search the index of another witness's deposition, quickly find all locations in that deposition where the witness or the examiner mentions your name, and then focus on any portion of the testimony that has a bearing on you or your involvement in the case. Currently available trial presentation software also allows such searches to be linked to corresponding segments of the video portion of a videotaped deposition, with the written transcript appearing below the video as the witness testifies. This approach can be an extremely effective tool for a trial lawyer during cross-examination, in that it facilitates demonstration of inconsistencies in a witness's statements through verbal and visual comparison of trial testimony with a pretrial deposition.

Unless a sequestering order has been issued, you should try, if possible, to come to court to watch other witnesses testify before you. This will not only familiarize you with the process of cross-examination but will also help you feel more comfortable with the courtroom environment as a whole by the time you testify. Of course, if you are a named defendant in the case, you will have been there almost all the time during all phases of the trial anyway.

BEHAVIOR AT TRIAL

During Jury Selection

If you are a named defendant, it is very important that you be present during jury selection, a process known as voir dire, which is used in most states. At this time, you will first be introduced to the jurors who will be hearing the case. Some information is elicited from the potential jurors before the selection process actually takes place. You will have an opportunity to communicate with your counsel if you have any preferences or concerns about any individual potential juror. Each party to the case generally has a limited number of so-called peremptory challenges. This means that your counsel can eliminate a preset number of potential jurors for virtually any reason. In addition, each party has an unlimited number of so-called challenges for cause, which involve making the argument that a particular potential juror cannot sit on the case fairly and impartially. If the reasons underlying this argument are demonstrated to the satisfaction of the judge during the questioning of the juror, the challenge is upheld; if not, it is denied.

Ideally, before the selection process begins, you and your counsel should spend some time discussing the qualities your team would like your jurors to have and developing a consensus on what responses to questions should be considered favorable and what responses should not. You should feel free to offer suggestions to your counsel regarding questions to ask the jurors, even if the questions you think of may seem obvious. In some instances, your counsel may retain jury consultants to assist in developing voir dire questions aimed at identifying positive or adverse jurors. In the last analysis, jurors are generally selected on the basis of nothing more than a hunch. Most of the time, decisions made during the selection process are based mainly on a "gut feeling" derived from observing the jurors as they react to the lawyer's questions during voir dire.

During Lawyers' Opening Statements

After the jury is empaneled, each side has the opportunity to make an opening statement to the jury before the evidence is actually presented. An effective opening statement can go a long way toward persuading the jury to accept one side's view of the case, even though the jury is cautioned by the judge to withhold judgment until all the evidence is heard. If you are not a named party to the case but merely a witness, you should still try to be present during the opening statements; doing so will help you quickly develop a feel for the case and will alert you to the issues you may face when you testify on the witness stand a few days later. In some instances, however, you may not have this option. Certain trial judges may allow opposing counsel to obtain a sequestering order preventing witnesses (but not parties) from being present during the opening statements or during the testimony of other witnesses.

During Presentation of Evidence

Because the burden of proof is on the plaintiff, the plaintiff's case commences first, after the opening statements. Sometimes the first witness called is not the plaintiff but the defendant (or one of the defendants if the suit was brought against multiple physicians). Plaintiffs' lawyers like to use this tactic early in the case, when the witnesses are likely to be more nervous and have not yet had time to observe and warm up to the pace and facts of the case. By applying this tactic, they hope to take advantage of the initial unfamiliarity with the testifying process, sometimes attempting to strong-arm a nervous or inexperienced witness or manipulate his or her testimony. Sometimes all the plaintiff's attorney is trying to accomplish is simply to make the witness appear unsettled, evasive, or defensive so as to prejudice the jury against that witness.

The upside of being called in the plaintiff's case as one of the first witnesses is that it gives you an excellent opportunity to present the defense's side before the plaintiff's points are firmly established in the jurors' minds. Although the questions asked in this situation are, of course, under the control of the plaintiff's lawyer, they may—depending on how narrowly they are phrased—yield you an opening through which you can make the central points of the defense at the outset of the case.

respect. This nonverbal communication with the jury is important because it is representative of your caring and respectful attitude toward the entire case. If you are asked to identify an exhibit, you should take the time to examine it carefully before verbally identifying it.

When you are asked to show the exhibit to the jury or to explain something while using the exhibit, you should first ask for permission to step down from the witness box and then place the exhibit on an easel or otherwise position it and yourself in such a way that you do not obstruct any juror's view of the exhibit as you are testifying. During your testimony, you have an excellent opportunity to make eye contact with each juror and build a rapport. Sometimes, in dealing with an exhibit, you will have to face away from the court reporter. Therefore, you should make sure that you always speak loudly enough to be heard easily by the court reporter so that the key portions of your testimony will not be interrupted by the court reporter's requests for you to repeat a statement or to speak louder.

Conduct While Not Testifying

When your testimony is concluded, or when the judge orders a pause, you should not attempt to communicate nonverbally with any of the attorneys, parties, or other witnesses. You should walk away from the witness chair with an erect and confident posture and resume the seat you occupied before you testified (unless you have been dismissed from the courtroom by the judge).

While other witnesses are testifying in the courtroom, you must avoid any emotional facial expressions signaling either approval or disapproval of the witnesses or the attorneys. Facial expressions showing exasperation, disbelief, approval, or other emotions will be seen by the jury as contrived and self-serving and may cause you to be perceived as less objective, factual, and trustworthy. You should also endeavor to distance yourself physically from other defense witnesses who are in the room to avoid the appearance of collusion. If you are a defendant or the physician whose care is being called into question, you should not wave to or acknowledge any other witnesses (including the defense expert) who may come into the courtroom during the proceedings when the jury is in the room.

You should not stare or smile at the jurors: they will resent any attempt, subtle or overt, to influence or curry favor with them. Especially if you are sitting at the counsel table, it is a good idea to take notes occasionally during the proceedings or to have something in front of you at the table to read. If you have a suggestion to make to your attorney during another witness's testimony, you should write it down and hand the note to the attorney or else discuss the matter during the next recess.

During recesses, at lunch, in the elevator, or en route to or from the courtroom, you must be extremely careful not to discuss the case with anyone if there is a risk that you may be overheard by a juror or a friend of the plaintiff. During recess, when the jury is not in the courtroom, you may want to converse with courtroom personnel, witnesses, attorneys, or other persons in the courtroom. Once the bailiff has called for the jurors, however, you should return to your seat promptly, before the jurors return to the courtroom. Again, you should be careful not to stare at the jurors as they leave and enter.

Financial Disclosures: None Reported

References

1. Brennan TA, Sox CM, Burstin HR. Relation between negligent adverse events and the outcomes of medical malpractice litigation. N Engl J Med 1996;335:1963–7.
2. Brennan TA, Leape LL, Laird NM, et al. Incidence of adverse events and negligence in hospitalized patients. N Engl J Med 1991;324: 370–6.
3. Localio AR, Lawthers AG, Brennan TA, et al. Relations between malpractice claims and adverse events due to negligence: results of the Harvard Medical Practice Study III. N Engl J Med 1991;325:245–51.
4. Hickson GB, Pichert JW, Federspiel CF, et al. Development of an early identification and response model of malpractice prevention. Law Contemp Probl 1997;60:7.
5. Beckman HB, Markakis KM, Suchman AL, et al. The doctor-patient relationship and malpractice: lessons from plaintiff depositions. Arch Intern Med 1994;154:1365–70.
6. Vincent C, Young M, Phillips A. Why do people sue doctors? A study of patients and relatives taking legal action. Lancet 1994; 343:1609–13.
7. Levinson W, Roter DL, Mullooly JP, et al. Physician-patient communication: the relationship with malpractice claims among primary care physicians and surgeons. JAMA 1997;277:553–9.
8. Hickson GB, Clayton EW, Githens PB, et al. Factors that prompted families to file medical malpractice claims following perinatal injuries. JAMA 1992;267:1359–63.
9. Griffen FD. ACS closed claims study reveals critical failures to communicate. Bull Am Coll Surg 2007;92:11–6.
10. Joint Commission for the Accreditation of Health Care Organizations. Comprehensive accreditation manual for hospitals: the official handbook. Chicago: Joint Commission Resources; 2002. p. R1–10.
11. Struve CT. Expertise in medical malpractice litigation: special courts, screening panels, and other options. Project on Medical Liability in Pennsylvania. 2003. Available at: http://www.pewtrusts.org/uploadedFiles/wwwpewtrustsorg/Reports/Medical_liability/medical_malpractice_101603.pdf (accessed on April 5, 2011).
12. Medical malpractice jury verdicts: January 2005 to December 2005. News release of the Administrative Office of Pennsylvania Courts. April 25, 2006.
13. Bovbjerg RR, Bartow A. Understanding Pennsylvania's medical malpractice crisis: facts about liability insurance, the legal system, and health care in Pennsylvania. The Project on Medical Liability in Pennsylvania (funded by The Pew Charitable Trusts). June, 2003. p. 44.

10 SURGICAL PALLIATIVE CARE: CLINICAL AND ETHICAL CONSIDERATIONS

Anne C. Mosenthal, MD, FACS, and Geoffrey Dunn, MD, FACS

The last 15 years have seen a renewed interest in and concern about the end of life and the care of the dying, both in American society and in the practice of medicine and surgery. This can be traced to the growth of the hospice movement, patient-centered care, and the change in demographics permitting many more adults to live longer with chronic, life-limiting illness. Simultaneously, it can also be seen as a reaction to the increasing emphasis of American medicine on technology, cure and prolongation of life at the expense of the relief of suffering, humanism, and the "art" of medicine. The last decades of the 20th century saw an unprecedented growth in life-prolonging technology but also an increasing awareness of the erosion of the doctor-patient relationship, the dehumanizing effect of much of medical care, and the shift from physician as healer to physician as technician and gatekeeper. The Study to Understand Prognoses and Preferences for Outcomes and Risks of Treatments (SUPPORT) in the 1990s observed that most Americans died in institutions, usually on life support, with untreated pain and suffering,[1,2] yet most Americans wish to die at home and fear untreated pain and artificial extension of life.[3] At the same time, ethical and judicial decisions that emphasize patient autonomy provided the legal foundation for the care of the dying today, ensuring that physicians can both relieve suffering and avoid burdensome or futile treatments for their patients at the end of life. The convergence of these developments has perhaps fostered the renewal of the twin goals of medicine and surgery: the relief of suffering alongside life-prolonging, curative therapy.

Surgical palliative care has evolved in this context over the last 10 years, drawing not only from the fields of hospice and palliative medicine but also surgery itself. The emergence of this field of surgery has in one sense reclaimed the long surgical traditions of palliation and compassion from a time when to bear witness and relieve suffering were all the surgeon could offer, attributable in part to the limitations of medical knowledge or surgical technique. Historically, much of surgery and surgical care has focused not on cure but on palliation of symptoms and restoration of quality of life, with burn care, vascular surgery, and surgical oncology being prime examples. The contemporary practice of surgery now includes the integration of technical competence with knowledge and skill in relief of suffering, restoration of quality-of-life, communication, and, when the end of life is near, appropriate decision making and withholding or withdrawing of life support. The following chapter describes the evolution of surgical palliative care, its ethical basis, and its approach and clinical applications in surgical practice.

Evolution of Surgical Palliative Care

The roots of surgical palliative care can be traced first to the hospice movement founded by Dr. Cicely Saunders in the 1960s. She focused on the needs of the terminally ill, particularly their intense suffering from untreated pain at the end of life. She defined the model of "Total Pain" and distinguished "pain" from "suffering." She described the four dimensions of pain as physical, psychological, social/economic, and spiritual, which lead to suffering. Hospice care developed to treat all four aspects of pain, for both patient and family, at the end of life. This model focused initially on those dying of cancer, where the trajectory of illness encouraged the aggressive treatment of suffering only when death was imminent or life-prolonging care had been exhausted.

During the 1980s and 1990s, palliative care extended this model of care to patients dying of other illnesses, such as dementia, cardiovascular disease, and organ failure, where the trajectory of decline is long and unpredictable and the dichotomy of cure versus comfort is blurred. Concomitantly, other concepts of suffering, such as that proposed by Eric Cassell, brought the realization that medical care itself might be the cause of suffering rather than the relief. He described suffering as arising from a threat to the integrity or wholeness of a person. Cassell noted that "the relief of suffering and the cure of disease must be seen as twin obligations of a medical profession that is truly dedicated to the care of the sick. Physicians' failure to understand the nature of suffering can result in medical intervention that (though technically adequate) not only fails to relieve suffering but becomes a source of suffering itself."[4] Now palliative care has evolved to a model of interdisciplinary care that aims to relieve suffering and improve quality of life for patients with advanced illness and their families. It is offered simultaneously with all other appropriate medical treatment.

In 2010, surgical palliative care has evolved from these trends in palliative care and long traditions in surgical care. Although the goal of cure is paramount in much of surgical care, the relief of suffering and palliation of symptoms are equally important. The core values of surgical culture include ethical decision making, preservation of hope, nonabandonment, relief of suffering, and improvement in quality of life. Certainly, surgeons have always prided themselves as being the doctors of last resort, taking on the most difficult cases and thereby maintaining hope and presence when others have "given up." Coronary artery bypass graft for the treatment of angina, organ transplantation, and vascular surgery were developed as palliative procedures, with their primary goal to improve quality of life as well as prolong it. Fields such as burn care, trauma, and critical care are examples of surgical specialties that emphasize not only aggressive, technology-based, lifesaving care but also aggressive attention to pain relief, rehabilitation, and quality of life. Both are considered equally important, neither is mutually exclusive, and usually both are delivered simultaneously to patients.[5,6] It is no surprise, therefore, that surgical palliative care would be embraced as a specialty inasmuch as it is a renewal of core surgical values and the adoption of other disciplines.

Contemporary practice of end-of-life care was officially recognized in the surgical profession when the American College of Surgeons endorsed its *Statement of Principles Guiding Care at the End of Life* in 1998 [*see Table 1*].[7] Over the next decade, the principles of end-of-life care were integrated into the surgical canon, and the palliative approach to care was moved upstream to include those patients with chronic, serious illness and the critically ill, not just those who are imminently dying. In 2005, the American College of Surgeons endorsed the *Statement of Principles of Palliative Care* [*see Table 2*],[8] thereby codifying a new discipline of surgery. Over the last 10 years, the field of surgical palliative care has grown, culminating in recognition by the American Board of Surgery and the American Board of Medical Specialties as a distinct discipline with board certification.

Table 1 American College of Surgeons Statement of Principles Guiding Care at the End of Life

Respect the dignity of both patient and caregivers.
Be sensitive to and respectful of the patient's and family's wishes.
Use the most appropriate measures that are consistent with the choices of the patient or the patient's legal surrogate.
Ensure alleviation of pain and management of other physical symptoms.
Recognize, assess, and address psychological, social, and spiritual problems.
Ensure appropriate continuity of care by the patient's primary and/or specialist physician.
Provide access to therapies that may realistically be expected to improve the patient's quality of life.
Provide access to appropriate palliative care and hospice care.
Respect the patient's right to refuse treatment.
Recognize the physician's responsibility to forego treatments that are futile.

Adapted from the American College of Surgeons.[7]

Table 2 Statement of Principles of Palliative Care

1.	Respect the dignity and autonomy of patients, patients' surrogates, and caregivers.
2.	Honor the right of the competent patient or surrogate to choose among treatments, including those that may or may not prolong life.
3.	Communicate effectively and empathically with patients, their families, and caregivers.
4.	Identify the primary goals of care from the patient's perspective and address how the surgeon's care can achieve the patient's objectives.
5.	Strive to alleviate pain and other burdensome physical and nonphysical symptoms.
6.	Recognize, assess, discuss, and offer access to services for psychological, social, and spiritual issues.
7.	Provide access to therapeutic support, encompassing the spectrum from life-prolonging treatments through hospice care, when they can realistically be expected to improve the quality of life as perceived by the patient.
8.	Recognize the physician's responsibility to discourage treatments that are unlikely to achieve the patient's goals and encourage patients and families to consider hospice care when the prognosis for survival is likely to be less than a half-year.
9.	Arrange for continuity of care by the patient's primary and/or specialist physician, alleviating the sense of abandonment patients may feel when "curative" therapies are no longer useful.
10.	Maintain a collegial and supportive attitude toward others entrusted with care of the patient.

Adapted from American College of Surgeons.[8]

Ethical and Legal Foundations of Palliative Care

The current practice of palliative and end-of-life care is guided by bioethical principles and established judicial decisions. The vast majority of deaths in America now occur in hospitals and institutions, where active decisions must be made to withhold or withdraw interventions to allow a "natural" death. Over 70% of patients dying in an intensive care unit have at least one intervention withheld or withdrawn prior to death.[9] Surgeons must be familiar with the ethical principles and judicial decisions that form the basis of this practice.

Clinical decisions in palliative care are grounded in the four ethical principles that guide all of modern medicine: autonomy, beneficence, nonmaleficence, and justice [*see Table 3*].[10] Each clinical situation requires consideration of all four principles for each patient; however, frequently, fulfillment of one principle conflicts with fulfillment of others. For example, a surgeon may perform a surgical procedure that can successfully remove a cancer (beneficence) but may cause pain or even death from complications (nonmaleficence). Treatment of pain may be beneficial but can theoretically hasten death in some cases. Patients may refuse lifesaving surgery (autonomy) even if it means imminent death or disability. The ethical principle of double effect allows the surgeon to perform surgery and aggressively treat pain and suffering at the end of life if the *intent* is to do good, even though the side effect of the treatment may harm the patient. The bad effect may be a foreseen, but not intended, consequence or purpose of the treatment.

In Western culture in general, and the United States in particular, the principle of autonomy has been codified and supported by the judicial and legal system as the prevailing ethical principle to guide medical decision making. Patient autonomy is considered a fundamental right of Americans; this includes the right to be informed about medical illness, prognosis, and treatment options and the right to choose or refuse these options even if they are lifesaving. The Patient Self-Determination Act of 1990, passed by the US Congress, legally ensures that patients have the right to facilitate their own health care decisions, accept or refuse medical treatment, and create an advance directive. This allows patients to determine their future health care decisions by completing a living will. Surgeons are ethically and legally bound to observe the wishes set forth in a living will in the event the patient becomes incapable of making such decisions. In practice, however, this is complicated by the reality that specific clinical scenarios are rarely laid out in a living will, situations

Table 3 Common Ethical Issues in the Practice of Surgical Palliative Care

Issue	Commentary
Disclosure of bad news	Broad legal and ethical consensus supports disclosure of bad news when permitted by patient or surrogate. Disclosure of bad news does not "take away hope" if conveyed with empathy in the spirit of nonabandonment. Empathic truth telling fosters trust, which is the basis of hope.
Perioperative do-not-resuscitate (DNR) orders	The American College of Surgeons, the Association of Operating Room Nurses, and the American Society of Anesthesiologists support a policy of "required reconsideration" of DNR orders in the perioperative period. This is a preoperative discussion between patient/surrogate and anesthesiologist and surgeon to clarify goals and limits of care, with either revision or continuation of the DNR order in the operating and recovery room. Automatic rescinding of DNR orders during surgery is not recommended.
Withholding/withdrawal of life support	The withholding of medical treatments is considered legally and ethically equivalent to withdrawal. This is based on the principle of autonomy. In practice, for both physicians and surrogates, it is more difficult to withdraw a life-supporting treatment once it has been started than to withhold it. A surrogate's persistent reluctance to consider termination of life support is usually related to the fear that he or she will be "killing the patient" or the fear that withdrawing life support will cause suffering. Legally and ethically, termination of undesired medical treatment of the properly informed patient/surrogate is not considered homicide, suicide, or euthanasia.
Aggressive symptom management	Aggressive management of unbearable symptoms at the end of life is a moral imperative, even at the risk of hastening or causing death, as long as causing death is not the intention of treatment. The risk of hastening death is present with any surgical treatment for serious illness, including attempts to cure. The rule of double effect, broadly accepted by ethicists, is invoked: • The act must be good or morally neutral. • Bad effects are foreseen but not intended. • A good end cannot justify a bad means. • The risk/benefit ratio must be reasonable.
Donation after cardiac death (DCD)	Ethical and legal principles support DCD, invoking principles of autonomy and double effect. DCD should be considered for patients where withdrawal of life support is contemplated. The Organ Procurement Organization personnel should be consulted prior to decision making to evaluate feasibility and medical suitability before approaching this option.

arise that are unforeseen, and written documents cannot substitute for informed discussions between physician and patient. This reality has led to reliance on surrogate decision makers and health care proxies to interpret a patient's living will or advance directive in consultation with the physician. Although the Patient Self-Determination Act did not specifically address the issue of surrogate decision maker or the ethical basis of substituted judgment in medical decision making, the legal and ethical basis has been clearly established by the Supreme Court decisions of the Karen Anne Quinlan and Nancy Cruzan cases.[11–13] These two cases established that it is consistent with autonomy, beneficence, nonmaleficence, and justice if a surrogate decision maker acts based on the patient's best interest and/or in accordance with the patient's previously expressed wishes. This provides the legal basis for decisions to withhold or withdraw life support in patients who are incapacitated, as long as these principles are maintained.

The Practice of Surgical Palliative Care

Surgical palliative care is the treatment of suffering and the restoration of quality of life for seriously ill or terminally ill patients with surgical disease, regardless of the prognosis. The surgeon brings all the tools in his or her armamentarium to treat distress, not just disease. The measure of surgical palliative skill in this context is not disease specific, such as complications, morbidity, or mortality, but rather patient centered. Quality of life, relief of symptoms, and the opportunity for spiritual comfort or closure at the end of life are more important measures of success in this discipline. This constitutes a cultural shift in surgery, where the morbidity and mortality conference reinforces the notion that death is a "failure" of the surgeon and brings "shame" on him or her.[14] It is not a large leap to see how this stigma would cause some surgeons to view end-of-life care as the sine qua non of "giving up" and therefore distinct from their aggressive, life-prolonging care. Surgical palliative care is currently moving away from this false dichotomy to an affirmative concept upstream in the patient's care, when symptom control and restoration of quality of life can be delivered alongside life-prolonging surgery.

PALLIATIVE CARE ASSESSMENT

The first goal of the assessment for palliative care is to gauge the level of overall distress. The assessment is, in a sense, a "staging procedure" to determine the scope and severity of palliative care needs. Palliative care assessment includes the identification of the current illness, treatments, and likely prognosis; sources of pain in all dimensions; personal, social, and spiritual resources; and individual values and hopes. The patient's decision-making capacity, advance directives, and health care proxy should be identified as well. Table 4, adapted from the American Medical Association Education for Physicians on End-of-Life Care Curriculum (EPEC), describes the domains of palliative care assessment

Table 4 Ethical Principles in Palliative Care

Principle	Ethical Imperative
Autonomy	Respect the capacity of individuals to make their own choices and act accordingly
Beneficence	Relieve pain and suffering, foster the interests and well-being of other persons and society
Nonmaleficence	Do no harm; do not inflict pain or suffering
Justice	Act fairly; distribute benefits and harms equitably

Adapted from Beauchamp TL and Childress JF.[10]

with sample questions for each. Immediate relief of pressing symptoms should be a priority and initiated concurrently with the assessment if necessary. Further discussions around goals of care cannot ensue if untreated symptoms are allowed to persist. Who should be included in the discussions should also be established at this time as the patient may or may not want family present.

The assessment of physical symptoms is usually the first priority in palliative care. This is focused on pain and nonpain symptoms, that is, the patient's subjective report, not on disease processes or disease-based review of systems (Table 5). The patient's self-report is the gold standard. Validated pain assessment tools using numeric scoring from 0 to 10 are the most common. Assessment tools are also available for nonpain symptoms but are generally validated for specific disease or patient populations. The Edmonton Symptom Assessment Scale (ESAS) is a validated tool for palliative care patients and includes assessment for nonpain symptoms such as fatigue, thirst, dyspnea, and nausea.[15,16] Assessment should include not only the severity of the symptom but also questions as to the level of distress the symptom causes.

GOALS OF CARE

The patient's goals of care that emerge from this initial assessment and discussion should guide the scope of all further surgery and treatments. The goals of care are generated by the patient's preferences and wishes in the context of the medical realities and the prognosis. Goals may be fluid and evolve over time. Singer and colleagues identified five domains of quality of life that patients with life-limiting illness hope for: adequate pain and symptom management, avoidance of inappropriate prolongation of dying, sense of control, relief of burdens, and strengthening of relationships with loved ones.[3] More recent studies suggested that seriously ill patients weigh treatment options based on the treatment burden, treatment outcome, and likelihood of the outcome, with cognitive or severe functional impairment often considered more unacceptable outcomes than death.[17] Although the surgeon must elicit preferences from the patient, he or she must provide the medical information and prognosis to the patient, especially likely and unlikely outcomes from contemplated therapy. Physicians are notoriously poor at prognostication, but ranges of life expectancy can be provided, keeping in mind that in some disease trajectories, death may be years away, but chronic, debilitating decline may be the life-limiting feature. Some trajectories are more predictable, such as cancer, and assessment of function, or progression of symptoms, is an indication of life expectancy. The Karnofsky Performance Scale score is a widely used scale for the assessment of function and prognosis in cancer patients.[18] Patients with congestive heart failure or chronic respiratory failure who may be contemplating surgery have a more unpredictable trajectory to death but will need prognostic information about the likely decline in quality of life over time, with or without surgery.

All therapy should be evaluated by both patient and surgeon based on the goals of care established. Surgery or procedures are weighed, not by their defined complications or indications but by their benefits or burdens for the patient, in the context of his or her goals. Palliative surgery to relieve malignant bowel obstruction should be considered based on the likelihood of eating again and the relief of nausea, vomiting, and pain (benefit) versus the likelihood of pain, open wounds, infection, or death in the operating room or the hospital (burdens). The patient's decision will depend on his or her goals ("I want to die at home," "I want to see my daughter's wedding"), as well as the information the surgeon provides about the surgery and alternatives. Each treatment or therapy should be considered independent of other therapies and based solely on its benefits or burdens. Patients who want do-not-resuscitate (DNR) orders in the event of cardiopulmonary arrest will still need symptom relief or simple, life-extending treatments. Surgery to relieve malignant obstruction or antibiotics to treat pneumonia would still meet their goals, even if they do not want cardiopulmonary resuscitation (CPR).

Establishing goals of care can be a difficult transition for both patient and surgeon. The surgeon is often consulted as the last hope and held up as the "rescuer," bringing lifesaving surgery or other "miracles." It is not difficult to see that changing the goals of care is, in a sense, breaking this "covenant for cure"; the surgeon may feel that he or she is "taking away hope" or abandoning the patient by not performing futile surgery that would only add burden, not benefit.[14,19] Conversely, the surgeon may have a long relationship with a patient, always focusing on aggressive, life-prolonging care, but now the prognosis has shifted, and a transition to comfort and relief of suffering changes this role. This is further complicated if the patient's condition has changed after surgery because of complications or iatrogenic events; this is frequently the case in the intensive care unit when unforeseen postoperative events have changed the course or patients linger with multiple organ failure and uncertain prognosis. The ability of the surgeon to reflect on his or her own sense of failure or loss is the first step in making a transition in goals of care. The surgeon has the unique role of helping the patient and family find new hope, whether it is hope for symptom relief or time with family. If likely outcomes are uncertain, the surgeon can convey this range of possibilities, and goals of care can include a focus on relief of suffering alongside other life-prolonging therapies, not in an either/or fashion.

INTERDISCIPLINARY TEAM

The relief of "total pain" or suffering requires an interdisciplinary approach, particularly if suffering is extreme. The collaboration of pain medicine specialists, clinical pharmacists, palliative medicine and nursing colleagues, and spiritual and psychosocial care providers is essential. Surgeons may not be familiar with nonsurgical alternatives for treatment of nonpain symptoms. Similarly, the best approach to breaking

Table 5 Palliative Care Assessment

Domain	Sample Questions to Ask the Patient
Illness/treatment summary	Tell me what you know about your illness. Could you give me an account about your illness and treatment you have had until now? Tell me what stands out in your memory (about your illness, about treatment to date). I will review (have reviewed) your medical history in your chart, but I am really interested in hearing about it from your point of view.
Physical symptoms	How long have you had (symptom)? Are you having this (symptom) all the time or on and off? How would you describe what you are feeling? Is the (symptom) staying the same, getting better, or getting worse? Using a scale (provide a scale), what is the lowest you have been in the past day? The highest? Where are you now? Does anything make the (symptom) better? Worse? To what extent does the (symptom) interfere with what you want to do? Is the (symptom) causing problems in your relations to others? Have any treatments helped your (symptom)? How much? What do you think is causing it (symptom)? Does it (symptom) frighten you? Why?
Psychological symptoms	Does everything happening make any sense to you? What do you think will happen next? How has your illness affected your life? What do you see as the biggest problem facing you now? What frightens you most about your illness? How would you describe your mood? How well do you think you are coping now? Do you feel depressed? Have you ever thought of taking your life? Do you have a plan? Have you been sad? Frightened? Anxious? Are you afraid of being a burden to others? How have you handled tough times in your life previously? Whom do you turn to for support in tough times? Have you ever had problems with depression, alcohol, or other psychological difficulties before your illness? Did you ever have treatment for these? Are you afraid we won't be there when you need us?
Spiritual issues	Do you consider yourself a religious or spiritual person? How important is your faith or belief in your life? Do you belong to a community of faith? What sustains your hope? Do you have religious or spiritual beliefs that help you through difficulty? What gives your life meaning? Does your faith influence your feelings about your illness? Your surgery? Do you see any possible conflicts between your health care and your beliefs? Do you have any specific observances or rituals we should be mindful of during your care?
Social/cultural context	Can you tell me about other people in your everyday life, at work, at home, etc.? What language is spoken in your home or community? Do you have a community or spiritual leader whom you would like to involve in your medical decisions?
Communication preferences	Is it your preference to be alone or have someone close to you present when we discuss important matters? Is there anyone with whom you would like me to discuss your care? If I am approached by family members with questions about your situation, do I have your permission to discuss it? To what extent?
Decision making	Who will make decisions about your medical care if (when) you are not able to? What would you like them to know?
Practical concerns	Where do you hope to go after this hospitalization? When you are ready for home, will your home be ready for you? Are you concerned about being a financial burden on your family?
Anticipatory planning	Have you given any thought of what comes after your hospitalization ? What plans have you made for your future? Are there things you need to know right now for planning for the future? Would it be helpful for us to schedule a meeting with us and your family to plan your future treatment and care?

Adapted from palliative care assessment in EPEC, American Medical Association's Education for Physicians on End-of-life Care. 1999.

bad news, communication under conflict, or relief of existential pain may be beyond the scope of the usual surgical practice. In palliative care, the patient and family are considered part of the unit of care. Attention to bereavement, grief, and the needs of family at the end of life is especially important. Studies show that the nature of communication, access to the dying patient, and the patient's relief of distressing symptoms all affect the bereavement outcome of family members.[20,21] Furthermore, the majority of hospitalized patients, particularly in the intensive care unit, are incapacitated and cannot make any medical or end-of-life decisions for themselves. Decision making generally falls on their surrogates, who are likely in crisis themselves because of the illness of a loved one. Emotional and educational support for their decision-making role is critical in avoiding conflict or prolonging the dying process, whether in the form of bereavement counselors, pastoral care, or other members of the palliative care team. Studies clearly show that interdisciplinary communication, whether in the form of family meetings, ethics, or palliative care consultation, has a salutary effect on both patient and family psychosocial outcomes.[22–24] Surgeons may also benefit from this team approach as they seek balance in the dual imperatives to rescue and to relieve suffering. The death of a patient is also a loss for the surgeon; reflection and the ability to seek support are important steps for adapting to the multiple roles of the surgeon in palliative care.

COMMUNICATION

Shared decision making between the physician and the patient/family is the foundation of end-of-life care. Communication of bad news, along with treatment of distressing symptoms, is perhaps the fundamental "procedure" of palliative care. The emphasis on patient autonomy, the patient-doctor relationship, and professionalism and the realization that clinical and litigation outcomes are improved now require competency in communication skills in all aspects of surgical practice. Although as late as the 1960s, most physicians did not reveal a distressing diagnosis to their patients, it is now the expectation and legal obligation that all medical information be disclosed, no matter how upsetting. Communication around death and dying can be one of the most stressful aspects of practice. Surgical myths and fears abound: surgeons are poor communicators or lack empathy, truth telling will take away hope, talking is too time consuming—all further compound these stressful encounters. In fact, good communication is a skill. Increasing studies demonstrate that patients and families' satisfaction and understanding of the illness are improved when physicians do less talking and more listening, impart information clearly and simply, allow time and space for emotion, connect the emotional distress with its source (the medical information), and provide support.[25–27] Several communication protocols for delivering bad news or conducting a family meeting have been proposed and studied.[28,29] The SPIKES protocol developed by Baile and colleagues is one example, as shown in Table 6.[29] All of these emphasize preparation for the meeting, the appropriate setting, providing a "warning shot" for bad news, clear delivery of information, empathic reflection of emotion, and concluding with recommendations for treatment. Following these steps will provide support to the patient and family and allow for further communication. This is particularly important when end-of-life decisions will be discussed. If initial communications are not clear and compassionate, conflicts around withdrawal and withholding of life support can ensue. The timing of communication is important, particularly with families of critically ill or injured patients. Family meetings to discuss prognosis and end-of-life decisions in the intensive care unit are more effective if held within 72 hours of admission.[22,30]

***Table 6* SPIKES: A Six-Step Protocol for Delivering Bad News**

Step 1: S – Setting Up the Interview Arrange for some privacy Involve significant others Sit down Make connection with the patient Manage time constraints and interruptions
Step 2: P – Assessing the Patient's Perception
Step 3: I – Obtaining the Patient's Invitation
Step 4: K – Giving Knowledge and Information to the Patient Avoid medical jargon Give information in small amounts at a time
Step 5: E – Addressing the Patient's Emotions with Empathetic Responses Allow time for expression of emotion Identify patient's emotion Identify cause of emotion Connect emotion with cause of emotion
Step 6: S – Strategy and Summary Discuss goals of care Treatment plans Future meetings

Adapted from Baile WF et al.[29]

WITHDRAWING AND WITHHOLDING OF LIFE SUPPORT

The vast majority of deaths in the United States, whether in the hospital or at home, now occur in the setting of withdrawing or withholding of life support. Although use of hospice during the last months of life has increased in the last decade, multiple studies suggest that the largest percentage of Centers for Medicare and Medicaid Services expenditures result from high-technology care in hospitals and intensive care units in the last 6 months of life.[31] Death after end-of-life decision making and withholding or withdrawing of life support have become the norm, and expertise in this area is now part of standard surgical practice.

The process of withholding or withdrawing life support is based on shared decision making around end-of-life issues between patient, family, physician, and other health care providers. The decision should be based on patient preferences and goals, knowledge of the likely outcome of continuing life support versus withdrawing it, and the benefits and burdens of each option. Conducting these discussions requires skill in communication and knowledge of the ethical issues, symptoms, and therapies available to treat them. There continues to be misunderstanding around the difference between withdrawal of life support, euthanasia, and physician-assisted suicide. Families may worry that if they decide to withdraw the ventilator they "are killing the patient"; similarly, they fear that their loved one may "suffocate." Part of the discussion should include assurances that dyspnea, pain, and other symptoms can be treated successfully and that physicians will not abandon the patient once a decision is made. The "DNR discussion" can be particularly difficult; following available guidelines is helpful.[32] These include the basic steps of good communication: preparation, appropriate setting, and reflecting troubling emotions around difficult issues. It is helpful to describe CPR as a procedure with certain indications, benefits, and burdens and to make a recommendation about whether or not to withhold it based on the medical prognosis and condition.

Confusion on the part of physicians still exists about their role in withholding and withdrawing life support. Many are more comfortable withholding therapy rather than withdrawing it because of unfounded fears that they may be causing death, abandoning the patient, or vulnerable to litigation. Historically, several studies have noted high variability in physician practice around DNR orders, withdrawal, and withholding, with some preferring to withhold rather than withdraw, whereas others withdraw therapy in a particular sequence or avoid withdrawal of the ventilator altogether.[33–36] Ethical and legal precedents are clear that withdrawing is equivalent to withholding and the decision for each therapy should be based on patient's preference (autonomy) and burdens and benefits.[37]

Withdrawal of the ventilator deserves special consideration as it is a procedure that continues to cause anxiety among physicians. Several protocols have been developed for this procedure, which include family and patient preparation, use of terminal wean versus direct extubation, and guidelines for the use of opioids and benzodiazepines for the treatment of refractory dyspnea.[38] It is ethically and legally sound to aggressively treat dyspnea with opioids based on the principle of double effect. The fears of hastening death by administration of opioids or benzodiazepines have not been borne out in several studies, where the time to death was equivalent for patients who did and did not receive these medications after withdrawal of the ventilator.[39,40]

The practice of withdrawing life support can be perceived as a conflict between the patient-centered goals of palliative care and societal goals of organ donation. In fact, the two are not mutually exclusive. If the patient is likely to proceed to brain death and organ donation is possible, efforts to stabilize and support a patient can coincide with attention to patient's pain relief and comfort and family support until brain death protocols are completed. In other clinical situations near the end of life, once the surgeon contemplates withdrawing or withholding life support for a patient, the issue of organ donation must also be considered. With the advent of donation after cardiac death (DCD), it is theoretically possible for patients to donate organs if cardiac death ensues after withdrawal of the ventilator or pressors. For some families, the prospect of organ donation is comforting in the face of otherwise bad news. Organ Procurement Organization personnel should be contacted prior to any communication with the family about this option to evaluate if medically appropriate. Any request for organ donation should be made by the organ procurement organization, not the physician caring for the patient. The decision to withdraw life support should be made before and separately from any consideration of organ donation. With DCD, organ donation may increasingly become part of the end-of-life decisions around withdrawal of life support.

Financial Disclosures: None Reported

References

1. The SUPPORT Principal Investigators. A controlled trial to improve care for seriously ill hospitalized patients: the Study to Understand Prognoses and Preferences for Outcomes and Risks of Treatments. JAMA 1995; 274:1591–8.
2. Desbiens NA, Wu AW, Brost SK, et al. Pain and satisfaction with pain control in seriously ill hospitalized adults: findings from the SUPPORT research investigations. Crit Care Med 1996;24:1953–61.
3. Singer PA, Martin DK, Kelner M. Quality end-of-life care: patients perspectives. JAMA 1999;281:163–8.
4. Cassell EJ. The nature of suffering and the goals of medicine. N Engl J Med 1982; 306:639–45.
5. Dunn G. Introduction: is surgical palliative care a paradox? In: Dunn G, Johnson A, editors. Surgical palliative care. New York: Oxford University Press; 2004. p. 3–15.
6. Mosenthal AC, Murphy PA. Trauma care and palliative care: time to integrate the two? J Am Coll Surg 2003;197:509–16.
7. American College of Surgeons. Statement of principles guiding care at the end of life. Bull Am Coll Surg 1998;83.
8. American College of Surgeons. Statement of principles of palliative care. Bull Am Coll Surg 2005;90.
9. Prendergast TJ, Luce JM. Increasing incidence of withholding and withdrawal of life support from the critically ill. Am J Respir Crit Care Med 1997;155:15–20.
10. Beauchamp TL, Childress JF. Principles of biomedical ethics. 3rd ed. New York: Oxford University Press; 1989.
11. In re Quinlan, 355 A2d 647 (JN), 429 US 922 (1976).
12. Cruzan v Director, Missouri Department of Health 497 US 261 (1990).
13. Annas GJ. Nancy Cruzan and the right to die. N Engl J Med 1990;323:670–3.
14. Buchman TG, Cassell J, Ray SE, Wax M. Who should manage the dying patient? Rescue, shame and the surgical ICU dilemma. J Am Coll Surg 2002;194:665–3.
15. Bruera E, Kuehn N, Miller MJ, et al. The Edmonton Symptom Assessment System (ESAS): a simple method for the assessment of palliatve care patients. J Palliat Care 1991; 7:6–9.
16. Bruera E, Macdonald S. Audit methods: the Edmonton Symptom Assessment System. In: Higginson I, Hanks GW, editors. Clinical audit in palliative care. New York: Radcliffe Medical Press; 1993. p. 61–77.
17. Fried TR, Bradley EH, Towle VR, Allore H. Understanding the treatment preferences of seriously ill patients. N Engl J Med 2002; 346:1061–6.
18. Yates JW, Chalmer B, McKegney FP. Evaluation of patients with advanced cancer using the Karnofsky performance status. Cancer 1980;45:2220–4.
19. Nuland SB. How we die: reflections on life's final chapter. New York: Alfred A Knopf; 1994.
20. Azoulay E, Pochard F, Kentish-Barnes N, et al. Risk of post-traumatic stress symptoms in family members of intensive care unit patients. Am J Respir Crit Care Med 2005; 171:987–94.
21. Gelfman LP, Meier DE, Morrison RS. Does palliative care improve quality? A survey of bereaved family members. J Pain Symptom Manage 2008;36:22–8.
22. Mosenthal AC, Murphy PA, Barker LK, et al. Changing the culture around end-of-life care in the trauma intensive care unit. J Trauma 2008;64:1587–93.
23. Lautrette A, Darmon M, Megarbane B, et al. A communication strategy and brochure for relatives of patient dying in the ICU. N Engl J Med 2007;356:469–78.
24. Schneiderman LJ, Gilmer T, Teetzel HD, et al. Effect of ethics consultation on nonbeneficial life-sustaining treatments in the intensive care setting: a randomized controlled trial. JAMA 2003;290:1166–72
25. Schaefer KG, Block SD. Physician communication with families in the ICU: evidence-based strategies for improvement. Curr Opin Crit Care 2009;6:569–77.
26. Barclay JS, Blackhall LJ, Tulsky JA. Communication strategies and cultural issues in the delivery of bad news. J Palliat Med 2007; 10:958–77.
27. Tulsky JA. Interventions to enhance communication among patients, providers, and families. J Palliat Med 2005;8 Suppl 1:S95–102.

toward the patient's head), the left side of the screen is oriented toward the head, with the right side toward the feet. When the marker is turned toward the patient's right for transverse imaging, the patient's right side is on the left side of the screen, and the head would now be toward the top of the screen. Holding transducers incorrectly results in serious errors in interpretation of the images. Other tricks for obtaining the best possible images (in addition to those listed above) include darkening the room as much as possible; sliding, tilting, and rocking the transducer on the skin rather than picking it up and moving it abruptly; using gentle but firm pressure; applying graded compression when air is present; or repositioning the patient if needed. Most importantly, the surgeon sonographer should take his or her time to obtain the best possible images under the circumstances. Rushing through an examination is the most common source of error.

Although ultrasound technology has an excellent safety profile, with the added benefit of high image quality and portability without radiation, there is still the possibility to inflict harm on a patient. Each unit must be well maintained and checked routinely to be sure that the ALARA principle (As Low As Reasonably Achievable) is adhered to, in reference to power and exposure time while obtaining the necessary clinical information. Tissues will heat up during lengthy examinations, and cavitation is also possible if the power is too high. Each transducer should be inspected regularly for breaks in the housing or cable that could potentially produce an electrical shock. After each examination, the transducers should be thoroughly cleaned using a solution recommended by the manufacturer so that blood or fluids are not transmitted from one patient to the next. Surgeons must also be involved in performance improvement programs where diagnostic decisions and procedures performed using ultrasound are reviewed for accuracy and patient safety.

USE OF ULTRASONOGRAPHY IN TRAUMA

The FAST Scan

The use of ultrasonography to query the pericardium and peritoneal cavity for blood has become standard in trauma centers. Referred to as the FAST examination (Focused Assessment for the Sonographic examination of the Trauma patient), it has rapidly replaced diagnostic peritoneal lavage as the preferred method for detecting hemoperitoneum in the unstable patient following blunt trauma.[1] It is also appropriate for pregnant and pediatric patients, for whom radiation exposure is more dangerous. In penetrating trauma, the abdominal portion of the FAST examination is not always helpful, because the amount of intra-abdominal fluid associated with hollow viscous injuries (most likely to be injured in penetrating trauma) is often too small to detect with ultrasonography. On the other hand, a limited echocardiographic examination is extremely sensitive in detecting penetrating injuries to the heart associated with pericardial fluid and has replaced all other noninvasive (e.g., central venous pressure [CVP], serial electrocardiograms) and invasive (i.e., pericardial window) methods of initial evaluation.[2]

Technique Sonographic detection of pericardial effusion is straightforward, requiring no specialized knowledge of echocardiographic cardiac anatomy. This echocardiographic portion of the FAST examination is performed using a curved array transducer (2.0–5.0 MHz) with a small footprint held in the subxiphoid position at 30° to the skin and aimed toward the left shoulder [*see Figure 1*]. Note that for all views, the marker groove points toward the left side of the screen. From this same position, the transducer is rotated transversely, and a four-chamber view can be seen in most patients depending on body habitus. The third view is obtained from the left parasternal area (long axis of the heart) with the transducer oriented along a line between the right shoulder and the left hip. Pleural effusions may be confused with pericardial effusions, but this is minimized in the subcostal view because there is no pleural reflection between the liver and the heart. Additionally, intrapericardial fluid will conform to the contour of the heart. Viewing the heart in more than one plane will also help reduce interpretation errors. Echocardiography can also be used to detect the presence of cardiac motion when no blood pressure is obtainable after trauma (pulseless electrical activity [PEA]). Following penetrating trauma, the detection of PEA may be an indication for emergency department thoracotomy, particularly in the presence of pericardial tamponade.

The abdominal portion of the FAST examination begins in the right upper quadrant with the transducer placed in sagittal orientation along the right anterior midaxillary line between the 11th and 12th ribs. The liver, diaphragm, and right kidney are imaged and, in particular, the Morison pouch (between the kidney and liver) is examined for fluid. In the supine position, this is the most likely spot for fluid or blood to accumulate [*see Figure 2*]. On the left side, the spleen and left kidney are found in the posterior midaxillary line slightly higher (between the ninth and 10th ribs). Once again, the transducer is oriented in a sagittal plane. It is extremely important to examine not only the space between the spleen and the kidney but also the space between the left hemidiaphragm and the spleen, where many splenic injuries will manifest. Because rib shadows may prevent full visualization of the spleen, having a cooperative patient take a deep breath can be helpful. The final abdominal image is of the pelvis. Here the bladder serves as an acoustic window and must contain fluid to be seen. The transducer is oriented for transverse sections over the pubis, aimed at the feet. If a Foley catheter is in place, fluid should be instilled into the bladder to facilitate detection of pelvic fluid [*see Figure 2*].

Detection of Hemothorax

Other uses for ultrasonography following injury include scanning for the presence of hemothorax, or pneumothorax, and in serial follow-up of intra-abdominal solid organ injuries being managed conservatively. Surgeons from Emory University were among the first to describe the evaluation of the pleural space using a standard 3.5 MHz transducer in the trauma room as part of the FAST examination.[3] Briefly, the transducer is held in the sagittal position and advanced in the midaxillary line from the 10th and 11th intercostal spaces (where the liver, diaphragm, and kidney are seen) cephalad until the supradiaphragmatic space is visualized. Fluid in the pleural space will appear as a black triangle above the hyperechoic (white) diaphragm [*see Figure 3*]. On the left side, the spleen and kidney are first viewed at approximately the ninth or 10th intercostal space in the posterior axillary line, and the transducer is simply advanced cephalad until the left hemidiaphragm and the supradiaphragmatic space are identified. The 97.5%

a

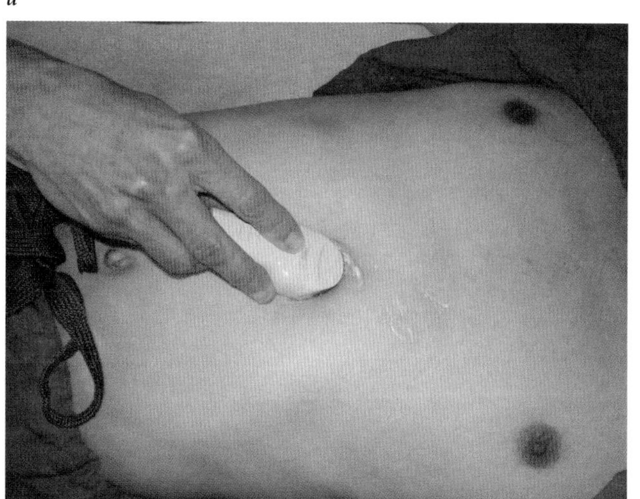

b

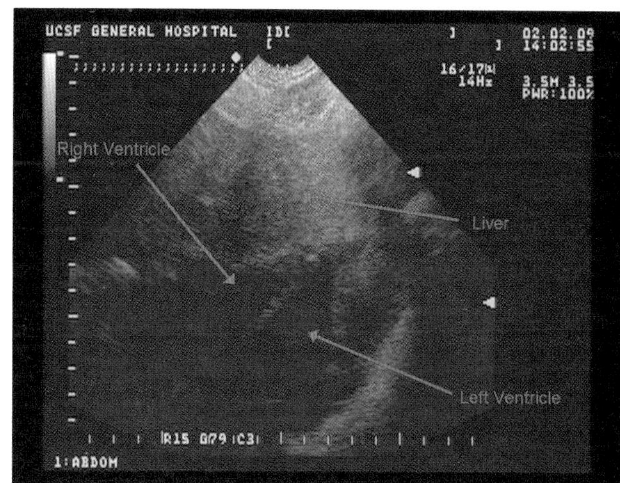

c

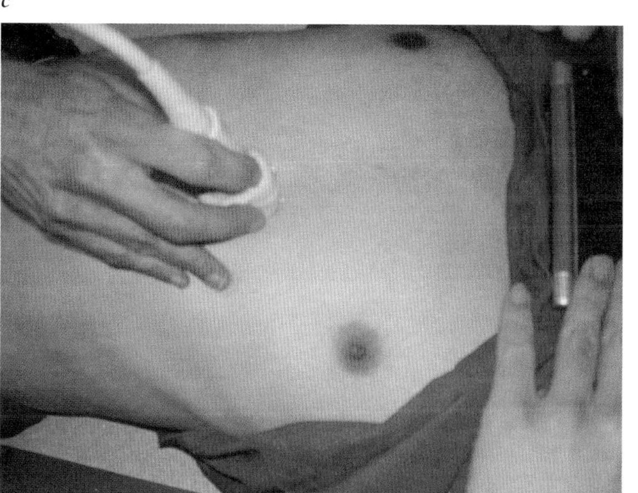

d

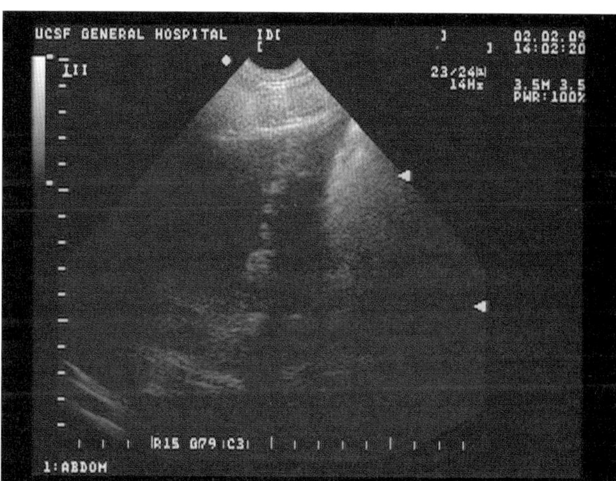

e

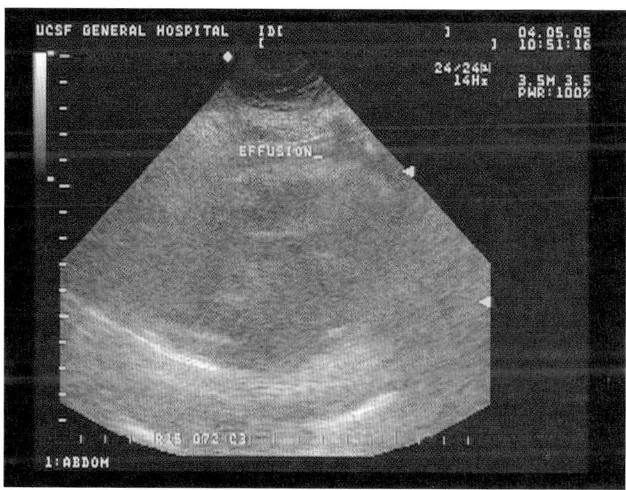

Figure 1 **(*a*) Transducer position for a subxiphoid view of the heart. (*b*) Normal four-chamber view of the heart from the subxiphoid position. (*c*) Transducer position for a parasternal long view of the heart. Note orientation along a line between the right shoulder and the left hip. (*d*) Normal parasternal long view. (*e*) Positive echocardiogram showing pericardial fluid.**

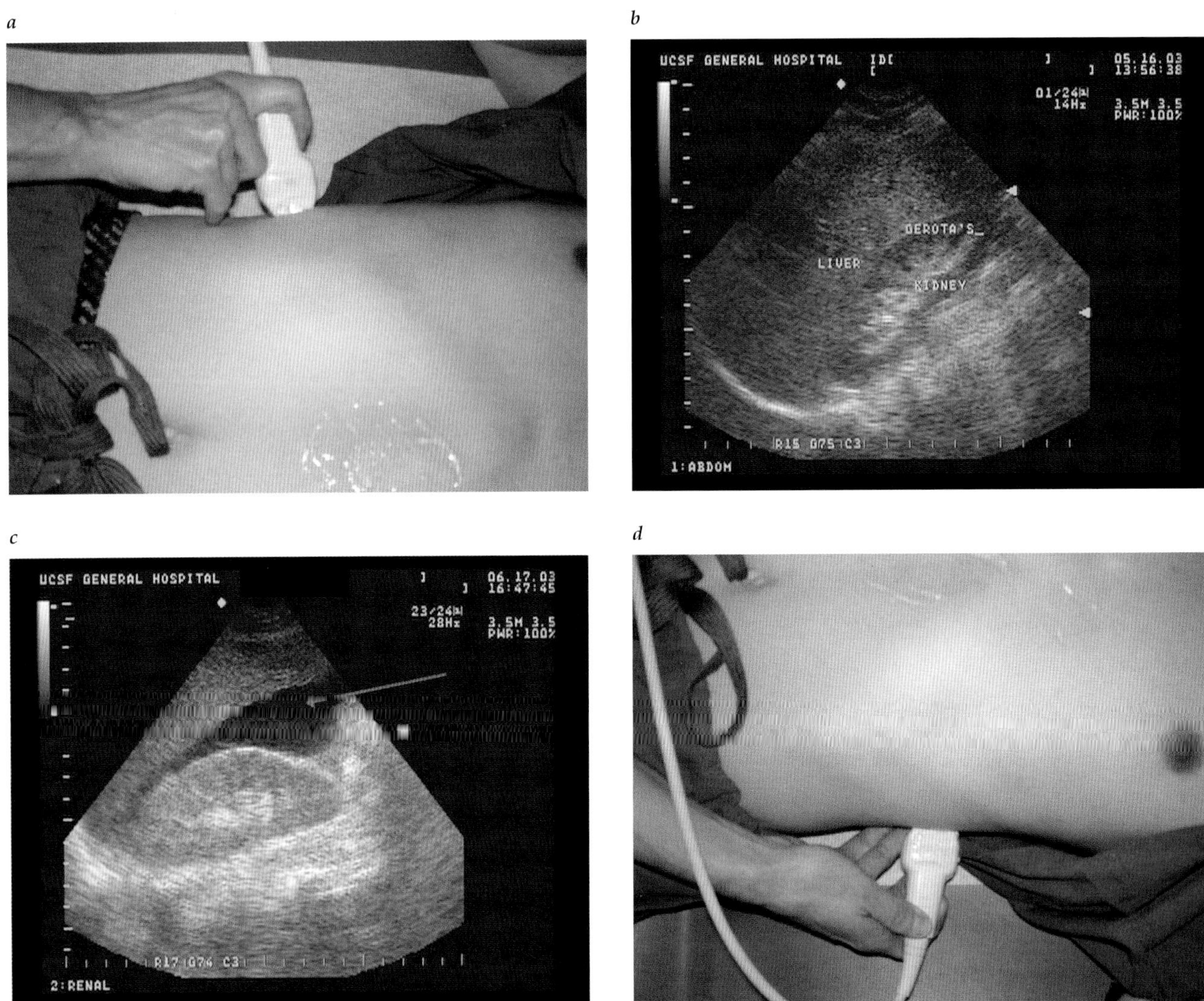

Figure 2 **(*a*) Transducer position for the right upper quadrant (RUQ) portion of the FAST examination for trauma. (*b*) Normal RUQ scan showing the liver and kidney. (*c*) Fluid seen in the Morison pouch in an RUQ scan (*arrow*). (*d*) Transducer position for the left upper quadrant (LUQ) portion of the FAST examination for trauma. Note the slightly higher position and more posterior than that for the RUQ.**

sensitivity and 99.7% specificity observed for thoracic ultrasonography were similar to those for portable chest x-rays in the trauma bay. The accuracy of this technique was only slightly less when used in the critical care setting to detect pleural effusion (94% accuracy).[4]

Detection of Pnemothorax

Using ultrasonography to detect pneumothorax is slightly more challenging as it requires recognition of the "absence" of the normal findings seen with an expanded lung. To perform this examination, a 3.5 MHz phased array transducer is held in a sagittal orientation in the second intercostal space in the midclavicular line. The examination is performed over several respiratory cycles. A normal lung will demonstrate a "lung-sliding" sign, seen as a to-and-fro motion at the interface between the visceral and parietal pleura with respirations [*see Figure 4*]. A comet tail artifact, manifested by hyperechoic streaks extending down from the visceral and the parietal pleural interface, is also commonly seen when imaging a normal lung. In the absence of these two findings, a pneumothorax will be present 99% of the time.[5,6] Visualizing of the lung slide can be enhanced by using a linear array transducer (7.5 MHz) oriented for sagittal sections and applying power color Doppler mode ("power slide").[7] Although neither of these methods eliminates completely the need for a chest x-ray, they may be very useful in situations such as the operating room, the intensive care unit (ICU), or an austere environment when an x-ray is delayed or unavailable.

Evaluation of Patients with Solid Organ Injuries

The treatment of a stable patient with a solid organ injury (liver, spleen, kidney) identified on a computed tomographic

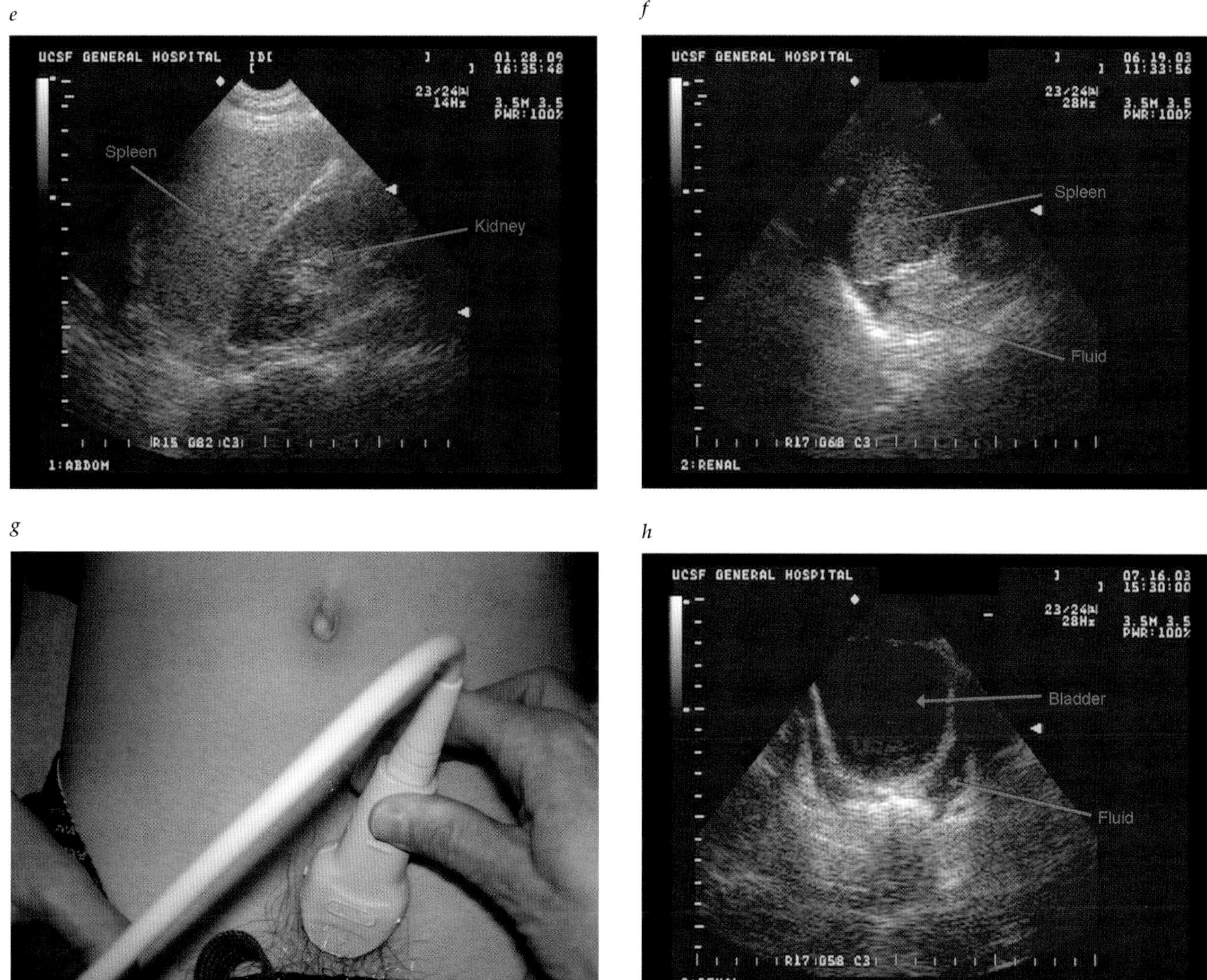

Figure 2 **(*e*) Normal LUQ view showing the spleen and kidney. (*f*) Positive LUQ scan showing fluid around the spleen (*arrow*). (*g*) Transducer position for a pelvic image of the FAST examination (sitting on the pubic bone and aimed toward the feet). (*h*) Fluid in the pelvis using a full bladder as the acoustic window.**

(CT) scan is most often observational. However, the need for follow-up imaging to identify patients whose injuries have progressed and/or those who have developed complications is controversial. Abdominal CT scanning, although extremely accurate, is expensive and delivers additional radiation (of particular concern in the management of pediatric trauma). We hypothesized that surgeon sonographers could successfully follow these injuries using ultrasonography. The surgeons involved in our study had considerable training and experience in performing ultrasound examinations, but we were only able to visualize the actual organ injury approximately one third of the time.[8] However, we successfully detected 13 of the 15 complications, including intra-abdominal abscesses, arterial pseudoaneurysms, and bilomas. More importantly, we were able to assess the amount of hemoperitoneum present during serial examinations and thus determine more accurately than by following hematocrits that patients were still bleeding.

USE OF ULTRASONOGRAPHY IN THE SURGICAL ICU

Central Line Placement Using Ultrasound Guidance

In the United States, an estimated 5 million central venous catheters are inserted annually for the purposes of monitoring hemodynamic variables, administering fluids and medications, or providing parenteral nutrition.[9] Unfortunately, the use of central venous catheters is associated with a number of complications, which are both hazardous for the patient and expensive to treat. Mechanical complications occur in 5 to 19% of patients, infectious complications in 5 to 26%, and thrombotic events in 2 to 26%. Using ultrasound guidance during insertion of an internal jugular (IJ) catheter has been demonstrated to reduce the time required for insertion, the rates of unsuccessful attempts, and the number of carotid artery punctures. A recent meta-analysis of 18 trials concluded that the use of ultrasonography to place central lines resulted in a significant reduction

a

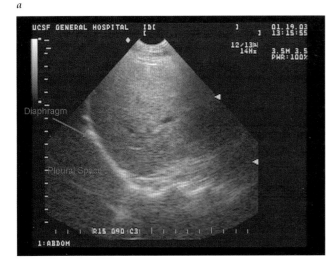

b

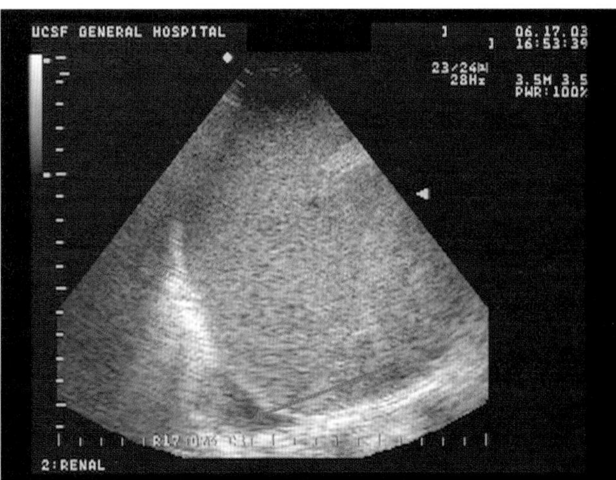

Figure 3 **(*a*) Normal ultrasound view of the pleural space (*arrow at diaphragm*). (*b*) Ultrasound view of a hemothorax (*arrow*).**

a

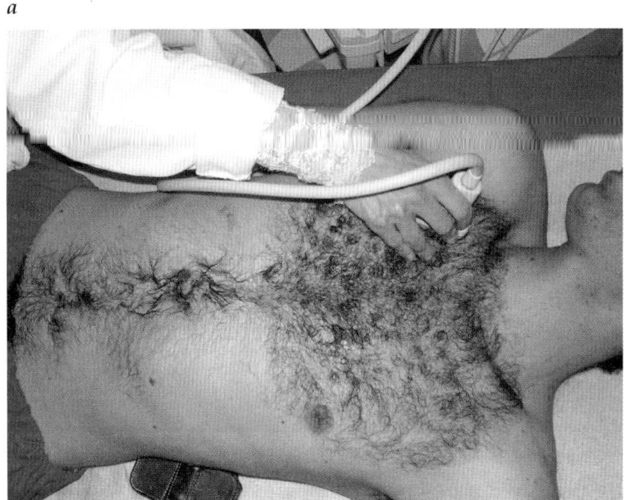

b

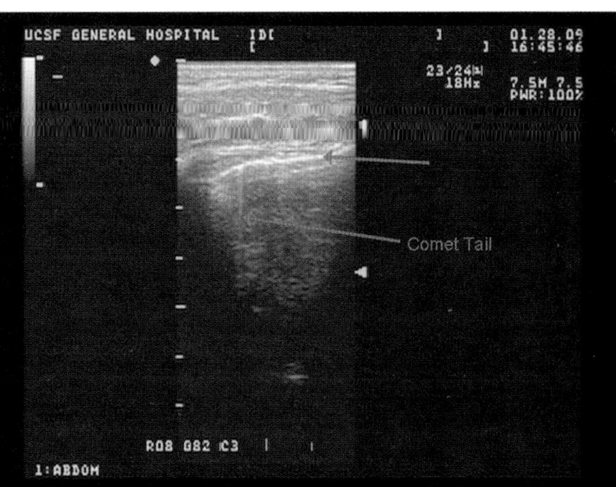

Figure 4 **(*a*) A 7.5 MHz transducer in the second intercostal space for evaluation of a potential pneumothorax. (*b*) Normal lung markings. Note the "comet tail" effect from a normal air artifact. The interface between the parietal and visceral pleura is marked with the upper *arrow* (point of observation for the "lung slide").**

in failure rates (risk difference –12, 95% confidence interval [CI] –0.18 to –0.06), the number of attempts (risk reduction 1.41, 95% CI 1.15 to 1.67), and arterial puncture rates (risk difference –0.07, 95% CI –0.10 to –0.03).[10] Ultrasonongraphy improved outcomes most convincingly for IJ vein cannulation (as opposed to the subclavian vein) and when used by clinicians less experienced at line placement. Karakitsos and colleagues performed a prospective comparison of the landmark technique versus real-time ultrasound-guided catheterization of the IJ veins in critically ill patients.[11] This randomized study included 450 patients in each of the two study arms. There were no significant differences between the two groups in gender, body mass index, previous catheterization, skeletal deformities, or other factors that could make line placement difficult. The clinicians involved in the study had considerable experience in inserting central lines (10 years on average). Cannulation of the IJ vein was accomplished in all 450 patients using ultrasound guidance versus 425 patients using surface landmark techniques ($p < .001$). The time for line placement and the number of attempts were also significantly reduced in the ultrasound group. In the landmark group, hematoma formation occurred in 8.4%, hemothorax in 1.7%, pneumothorax in 2.4%, and central venous catheter–associated bloodstream infection in 18%, which were all significantly more common than in the ultrasound group ($p < .001$).

Technique of Placing an IJ Catheter Under Ultrasound Guidance

Step 1: Assemble the equipment listed in Table 2.

Step 2: Don personal protective gear and a sterile gown and gloves.

Step 3: Place the patient in the head-down position if possible.

Table 2 Equipment Needed for Central Line Placement

Standard commercial central catheter insertion kit
Large barrier drape
Sterile gown/gloves
Mask, eyewear, hat (personal protective gear)
7.5 linear array transducer connected to standard ultrasound unit
Sterile conduction gel
Sterile plastic sheath/probe cover

Step 4: Standing at the head of the bed, identify the relevant surface anatomy: the mastoid process, clavicle, and clavicular and sternal heads of the sternocleidomastoid muscle.

Step 5: Prepare the area widely with chlorhexidine and drape widely.

Step 6: Insert the ultrasound transducer into the sterile sheath after placing conduction gel into the bottom of the probe cover.

Step 7: Place a small amount of sterile conduction gel on the skin surface at the junction of the two heads of the sternocleidomastoid muscle.

Step 8: Holding the transducer parallel to and just above the clavicle, locate the IJ vein. It will be larger and flatter than the adjacent carotid artery, which is located medial to the vein [*see Figure 5a*]. A patent IJ vein should be compressible if it does not contain thrombus. Rarely, color flow or Doppler applications may be needed. Once the vein is located, orient the probe so that the vein appears on the right side of the screen (for right IJ vein cannulation) or on the left side of the screen if the left IJ vein is used. This will minimize confusion during the procedure.

Step 9: Continue to visualize the vein holding the transducer with one hand while introducing the needle with the other hand. The direction of the needle must be at right angles to the middle of the transducer and at an angle of 45° to the skin [*see Figure 5b*].

Step 10: Once the needle is seen to enter the vein, aspirate back with a syringe to confirm free venous flow [*see Figures 5c to 5e*].

Step 11: Pass the guide wire through the needle, monitoring for any cardiac arrhythmias (should they occur, pull the guide wire back). The needle can now be withdrawn from the vein, leaving the wire intact.

Step 12: Using a blade, make a small skin incision at the entrance of the wire and pass the catheter-dilator assembly over the wire into the vein. The catheter can also be visualized by ultrasonography.

Step 13: Remove the dilator and wire together, then use a syringe to aspirate air from the catheter, confirm venous return, and demonstrate that fluid can be infused without excessive pressure.

Step 14: Suture the catheter securely in place.

Step 15: Confirm the position with x-ray.

Complications associated with placement of an IJ catheter The most common immediate complications of central venous catheter placement are arterial puncture, hematoma formation, and pneumothorax. A chest radiograph should be obtained immediately after any central venous catheterization attempt to evaluate for pneumothorax and to confirm proper catheter position prior to its use. Arterial puncture, which occurs in 6 to 9% of attempts, is more common with IJ line placement than with subclavian catheterization. If arterial puncture is recognized at the time of needle placement, it is managed by withdrawing the needle and maintaining gentle pressure over the artery for several minutes while observing for hematoma formation. If the injury is recognized after the dilator is in place, it should be left in place and a vascular surgeon consulted; removal of the catheter may require endovascular stenting or suture closure of the carotid artery. Pneumothorax (incidence of 0.2 to 1% with IJ catheters) is slightly less likely than with subclavian lines and is generally caused by advancing the needle too far in search of the vein instead of withdrawing to reassess the position and course of the needle. Small pneumothoraces (< 10%) may be observed and reevaluated with chest imaging 6 hours later; larger or symptomatic pneumothoraces require tube thoracostomy.

Assessment of Volume Status in the ICU with Ultrasound Techniques

Surgeons are beginning to use bedside ultrasonography to assess cardiac function and to estimate volume status in the ICU. One simple measure is to note the relative collapse of the right ventricle in a patient who is volume depleted. Another method is to measure the diameter of the inferior vena cava (IVC) during resuscitation. Using a standard abdominal transducer held for sagittal scanning, the anteroposterior diameter of the IVC can be measured just below the diaphragm in the hepatic segment.[12] Given that the diameter will change with respiration, it should be measured in both phases. A second measurement is taken in a transverse orientation [*see Figure 6*]. Yanagawa noted that the IVC diameter was significantly smaller (average 6.5 mm) in patients who became hypotensive again after an initial response to fluid resuscitation (so-called transient responders) as opposed to stabilized patients, in whom the IVC diameter averaged 10.7 mm.[12] In a more advanced study, Gunst and colleagues measured both stroke volume and IVC diameter using ultrasonography and compared their estimates of cardiac index based on ultrasound data compared with the results found with more directly measured indices using pulmonary artery catheterization.[13] These surgeons were very accurate in estimating cardiac index and CVP; however, each of these investigators had completed 2 days of focused cardiac ultrasound training and had 5 to 15 years of ultrasound training prior to participating in this study. Nonetheless, it is clear that the utility of bedside ultrasonography in estimating volume status will continue to expand in the near future.

Ultrasound-guided Thoracentesis

Pleural effusions can be easily diagnosed and aspirated under ultrasound guidance in the ICU.[14] In one recent study of ultrasound-guided thoracentesis in patients receiving mechanical ventilation, pneumothorax occurred in only 1.3% of the 232 patients who underwent this procedure.[15] Pigtail catheters can

a

b

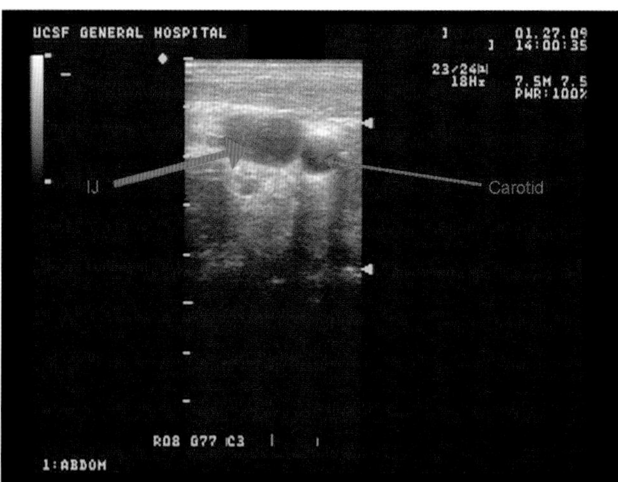

c

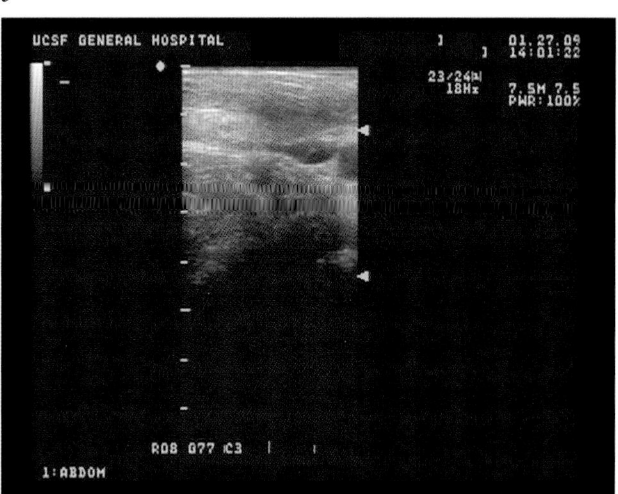

d

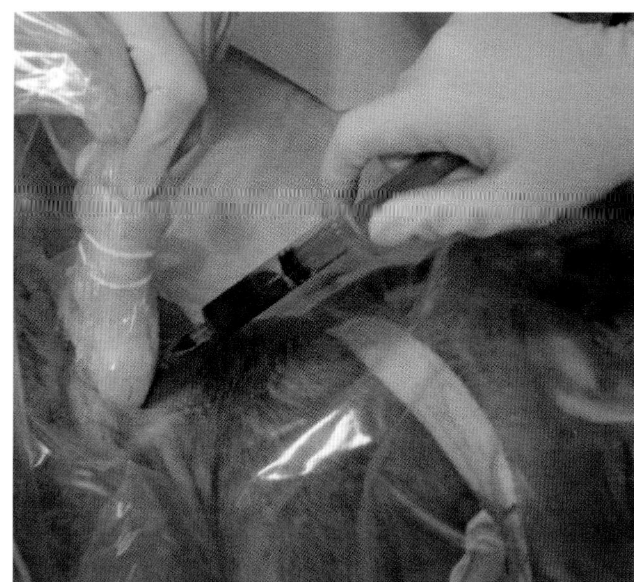

e

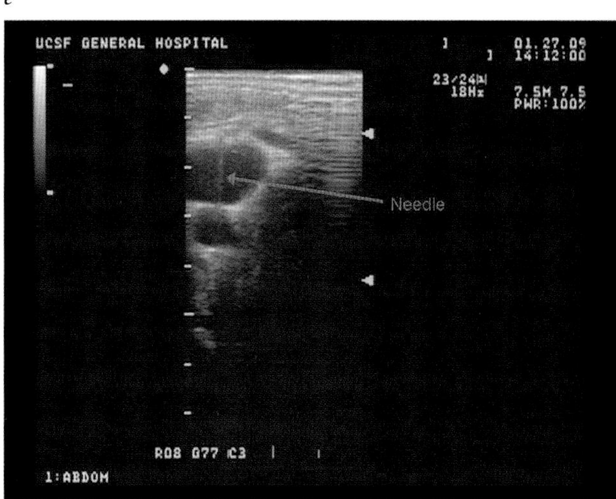

Figure 5 **(*a*) A 7.5 MHz transducer in a sterile bag for real-time imaging during placement of a central line. Note the acoustic gel inside the bag and the rubber band occlusion technique to avoid an air artifact. (*b*) Ultrasound image of the right carotid artery and internal jugular (IJ) vein. (*c*) Internal jugular vein collapsed with gentle pressure (normal). (*d*) Angle of the needle relative to the transducer. Note that the needle aims for the middle of the transducer and must enter at 90° to the transducer to be imaged on a sonogram. (*e*) Needle seen on a sonogram in the internal jugular vein (*arrow*).**

a

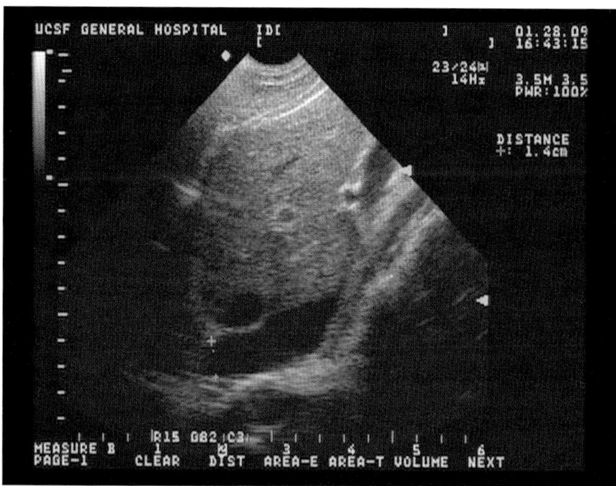

b

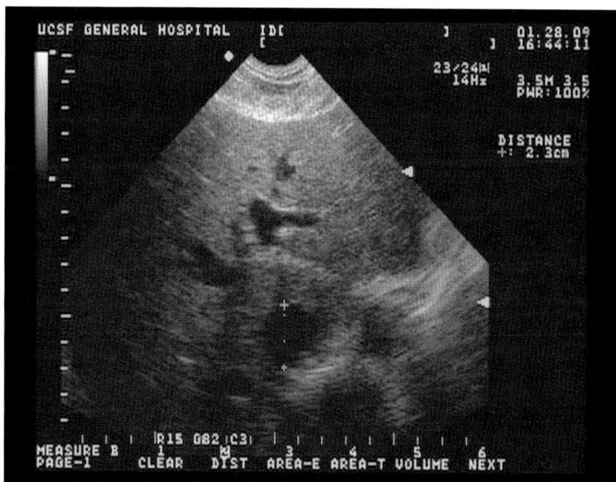

Figure 6 **(*a*) Measurement of the inferior vena cava diameter (sagittal) at the level of the diaphragm (+ markings are calibers). (*b*) Transverse measurement of the inferior vena cava at the same level.**

Table 3 Equipment Needed for Thoracentesis/Paracentesis
Standard central line insertion kit
Large barrier drape
Sterile gown/gloves
Mask, eyewear, hat (personal protective gear)
Caldwell needle (15 gauge)
Sterile extension tubing
Syringe
Scalpel
Local anesthetic

also be inserted using ultrasonography.[16] The equipment needed for these procedures is outlined in Table 3.

Technique for Performing Ultrasound-Guided Thoracentesis

Step 1: Position the patient either in the lateral decubitus (the affected side up) or the supine position. Elevation of the head of the bed may also be useful.

Step 2: Perform the ultrasound examination (using a 3.5 MHz convex transducer) to locate the diaphragm, liver (or spleen), and targeted pleural fluid.

Step 3: If possible, switch to a 7.5 MHz linear probe to visualize the ribs and vascular structures within the chest.

Step 4: Choose a puncture site allowing at least one rib space of fluid above and below.

Step 5: Mark the site, prepare the chest, and then inject the area generously with local anesthesia, including the pleural surface.

Step 6: Insert a 18- to 20-gauge sheath needle into the targeted area, confirming the location of the needle with ultrasonography, and perform the aspiration.

Step 7: Once the fluid has been completely removed, withdraw the needle while applying constant negative pressure to minimize the chance of pneumothorax.

Step 8: If prolonged drainage is necessary, a larger catheter can be advanced into this area using the Seldinger technique, attaching the catheter to a water-sealed drainage system.[17]

Ultrasound and Paracentesis

Paracentesis is another useful technique that is also made safer under ultrasound guidance. In the ICU, paracentesis can be used to sample abdominal fluid for diagnosis (blood, intestinal contents, infection) or as a method of relieving pressure (ascites or secondary intra-abdominal hypertension following burns or overzealous resuscitation). The right and left lower quadrants are the most dependent locations and the easiest to access (generally above and medial to the superior iliac spine). Safe entry points for paracentesis that avoid the inferior epigastric vessels were mapped out recently by Saber and colleagues.[18]

Technique for Performing Ultrasound-Guided Paracentesis

Step 1: Assemble the equipment listed in Table 3.

Step 2: The abdomen is scanned using a 3.5 MHz curved array transducer to locate the fluid collection(s).

Step 3: Place the patient in a supine position of comfort.

Step 4: Don personal protective gear, including a gown and gloves.

Step 5: Scrub the anterior abdominal wall with chlorhexidine solution and drape the region.

Step 6: Infiltrate the skin of the intended puncture site with local anesthetic.

Step 7: Use the scalpel to make a nick in the skin to allow passage of the needle.

Step 8: Advance the Caldwell needle through the abdominal wall while aspirating with a syringe (note: ultrasonongraphy can be used to guide the needle into the fluid collection).

Step 9: Once fluid is seen to enter the syringe, stop advancing the needle. The drainage catheter should be advanced over the needle into the fluid and the needle removed.

Step 10: If prolonged drainage is required (as with tense ascites), the catheter can be attached to a collection canister.

Step 11: Observe the wound for ascetic leak and/or the development of a hematoma, and then dress it with a transparent dressing.

Complications of thoracentesis and paracentesis

The principal complications of thoracentesis are pneumothorax and hemothorax. Drainage of very large effusions may also lead to reexpansion pulmonary edema, although this is a rare entity. In one recent study of ultrasound-guided thoracentesis in patients receiving mechanical ventilation, pneumothorax occurred in only 1.3% of the 232 patients who underwent this procedure.[15] As noted above with IJ cannulation, small pneumothoraces may be observed, but larger (> 10%) or symptomatic cases require tube thoracostomy. Hemothorax complicating thoracentesis is particularly troubling because it suggests injury to an intercostal vessel, which may bleed significantly and potentially require operative ligation. A routine chest radiograph should be obtained following the procedure, and attention should be paid to significant hematoma or oozing from the puncture site.

Paracentesis may be complicated by abdominal wall hemorrhage and by hemodynamic instability resulting from fluid shifts. Large volume paracentesis leads to fluid and protein losses with accompanying hypovolemia, hypotension, and even acute renal insufficiency. Empiric replacement of proteinaceous solute by infusion of salt-poor albumin is generally practiced (50 mL of 25% albumin for each liter of ascites drained). If the puncture site is not carefully selected, inferior epigastric vessel injury may occur, leading to expanding abdominal wall hematoma and/or hemoperitoneum. If this occurs and the hematoma does not tamponade the bleeding, exposure and ligation of the vessels will be necessary.

Detection of Venous Thrombosis with Duplex Ultrasonography

Critically ill and injured patients are at high risk for potentially lethal venous thromboembolism. Unfortunately, the current methods of venous thromboembolism prophylaxis are often contraindicated in the patients who are at greatest risk, and surveillance for deep vein thrombosis (DVT) is frequently used even in the absence of symptoms. Additionally, an immediate DVT scan can be helpful when pulmonary embolism is suspected in ICU patients. The sensitivity and specificity for duplex ultrasonography in symptomatic patients are very high, and this study has now replaced venography as the primary imaging procedure for the detection of DVT. Compressibility under probe pressure is the most accurate test, reaching 97 to 100% sensitivity and 99% specificity for the diagnosis of femoral and popliteal DVT.[19] In contrast, the visibility of the thrombus as a fixed, echoic image within the lumen has a sensitivity of only 50%. DVT should also be suspected when there is a lack of augmentation of flow above the area being compressed. As with any ultrasound examination, the accuracy is highly dependent on the expertise of the examiner, and we do not mean to imply that surgeons will have the same excellent results as registered vascular technicians. However, focused venous ultrasound examinations should be within the skill set of a general surgeon.

Technique for Performing a Venous Ultrasound Examination

Step 1: Position the patient in a supine and reversed Trendelenburg position (if possible), with the leg abducted and externally rotated and the knee flexed.

Step 2: Using a 7.5 MHz linear transducer held in a transverse position, identify the common femoral vein and artery at the level of the inguinal ligament.

Step 3: The initial imaging should be done using the B-mode (grayscale).

Step 4: Focusing on the vein, apply pressure until the vein collapses. Follow the vein down in a transverse plane, using serial compression applied at 1 to 2 cm intervals.

Step 5: The vein will dive deep above the knee but can be visualized again posterior to the knee.

Step 6: Although the hallmark of DVT is a lack of compressibility, occasionally, a thrombus will be visible within the lumen [*see Figure 7*].

Step 7: Flow can be visualized within the vein by applying color and Doppler imaging. With the transducer still in a transverse orientation, find the common femoral vein or artery and apply color flow. Keeping the vein in view, orient the transducer for longitudinal imaging. Once flow is visualized in the thigh, squeezing the calf muscles should increase the flow signal. Clinically significant DVT below the level of the thigh is unlikely if augmentation is present.

Step 8: Repeat these same steps on the opposite side and compare images and results.

Other Bedside Procedures

PERCUTANEOUS TRACHEOSTOMY

Operative tracheostomy has been performed for several centuries, and the typical modern technique was standardized by Jackson in 1909. A percutaneous Seldinger technique was developed in the 1980s by Ciaglia and colleagues and has gained popularity in recent years because of its suitability for performance at the bedside.[20] Use of videobronchoscopic guidance has reduced immediate complications, but it should be recognized that operative ("open") tracheostomy remains the gold standard as it allows for more control and has lower rates of long-term complications, such as subglottic stenosis.[21,22]

Indications for tracheostomy include orofacial trauma, resection of head or neck malignancy, and the need for prolonged mechanical ventilation. The timing of tracheostomy in critically ill patients has long been debated, and ongoing clinical trials strive to determine the optimal timing. The basic principle is to perform the procedure early enough to facilitate subacute care and reduce oropharyngeal, sinus, and pulmonary complications; however, performing tracheostomy too early in a course of mechanical ventilation will lead to unnecessary procedures on those patients who were nearing extubation at the time of operation. The TracMan clinical trial conducted at Oxford University randomized over 900 critically ill patients to early (days 1 to 4) versus late (day 10 or later) tracheostomy. This represents the largest coordinated effort yet to determine the optimal timing of tracheostomy; recruitment completed in December 2008, and the results are expected to be reported in 2009.[23]

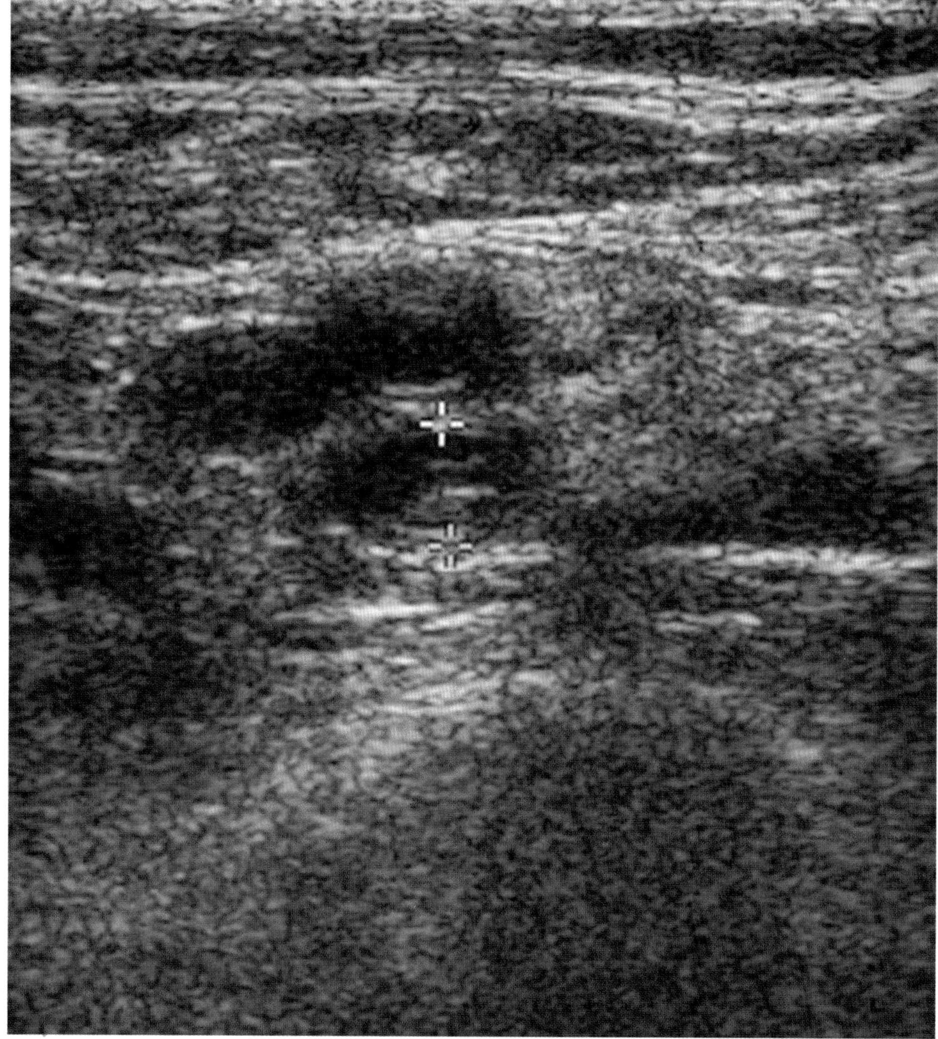

Figure 7 **Ultrasound image of a femoral vein deep vein thrombosis (*markers*).**

Tracheostomy is a clean-contaminated operation because the respiratory tract is entered. These wounds are far from sterile as there is considerable contamination by respiratory secretions and saliva. However, infections are infrequent, and there is no role for prolonged courses of antibiotic therapy beyond a single preincision dose, as is the general recommendation for clean-contaminated operations.

Technique for Percutaneous Tracheostomy

Step 1: Assemble the equipment listed in Table 4.
Step 2: Position the patient so as to slightly raise the shoulder off the bed and extend the neck.
Step 3: Don personal protective gear, including a sterile gown and gloves.
Step 4: Scrub the anterior neck from the chin to the sternal notch with chlorhexidine solution and place sterile drapes.
Step 5: Ask the bronchoscopist to advance the scope down the endotracheal tube and visualize the carina and then withdraw the scope to a position a centimeter below the vocal folds. Maintain this endoluminal view of the trachea.

Table 4 **Equipment Needed for Percutaneous Tracheostomy**
Large barrier drape
Sterile gown/gloves
Mask, eyewear, hat (personal protective gear)
Bronchoscope
Laryngoscope and endotracheal tube
Tracheostomy tube (at least two sizes)
Seldinger tracheostomy kit with dilator
Skin suture and needle holder
Ventilator tubing adapter for bronchoscope and accordion extension for tracheostomy
Scalpel
Syringe

Step 6: Withdraw the endotracheal tube so that the tip is repositioned just distal to the bronchoscope tip.

Step 7: Identify a point in the midline of the anterior neck, midway between the cricothyroid membrane and sternal notch. Apply local anesthetic to this site and then use an 18-gauge needle attached to a 10 mL syringe to puncture the trachea. It is critical that the puncture be visualized by the bronchoscope and be in the midline of the anterior trachea and not too close to the cricothyroid cartilage [*see Figure 8*].

Step 8: Pass the guide wire through the needle into the trachea and remove the needle.

Step 9: Make a 2 cm transverse skin incision centered on the wire. Do not cut deep to the skin as bleeding from the thyroid or thyroid vessels can be problematic and require operative repair.

Step 10: Apply generous sterile lubricant to the assembled tracheostomy tube–dilator device, then pass it over the wire and twist it while pushing posteriorly to dilate the tracheal puncture site and pass the tracheostomy tube. Once in the trachea (visualized by the bronchoscope), immediately remove the dilator while holding the tracheostomy tube in place.

Step 11: Confirm proper ventilation through the tracheostomy tube and then remove the endotracheal tube.

Step 12: Suture the flange of the tracheostomy tube to the adjacent skin and further secure it with a necklace-type tie around the neck.

Step 13: Remove instruments for reprocessing and dispose of sharp waste.

Complications of percutaneous tracheostomy Following tracheostomy, patients should initially be cared for in an ICU owing to the potential severity of complications. The site should be observed for bleeding, cellulitis, or development of subcutaneous emphysema. Dislodgment or misplacement of the tracheostomy tube must be immediately corrected as this will lead to death in short order. If possible, the tube should be reinserted, but often the safest approach is to resecure the airway by orotracheal intubation and then convert to a formal ("open") tracheostomy in the operating room. Significant bleeding around the tracheostomy tube usually signifies injury to the thyroid parenchyma or one of its vessels; if this does not abate with hematoma tamponade in a matter of minutes, this, too, requires operative intervention.

A first tracheostomy tube change should be avoided at all costs during the first 10 days as there is the potential for fatal airway loss. Even after 10 days, any tracheostomy tube change should be performed with airway rescue equipment and supplemental oxygen available, an informed nurse at the bedside to assist as needed, knowledge of the patient's native anatomy by the surgeon (i.e., is the larynx patent, thus permitting orotracheal intubation), and a spare tracheostomy tube one size smaller than the one in the patient's airway. The presence of a respiratory therapist is encouraged, especially for the first change.

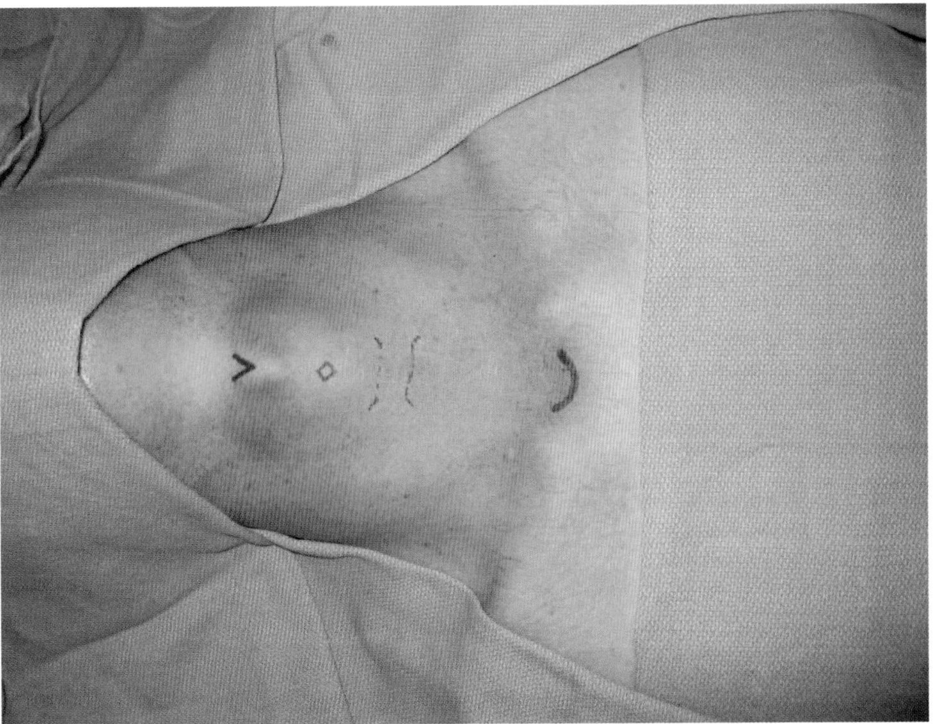

Figure 8 **Anatomic land markings of the neck. V = thyroid notch; box at the cricothyroid membrane; broken line at the thyroid isthmus; solid line at the first tracheal ring; curved line at the sternal notch.**

TUBE THORACOSTOMY

Thoracostomy tubes ("chest drains" or "chest tubes") are placed to evacuate air or fluid in the pleural space and have become a primary treatment modality for pleural disease since first described by Hewett in 1876. Pneumothorax may occur spontaneously, following injury, or as the - result of instrumentation, such as with percutaneous biopsy or thoracentesis. Pneumothoraces can be treated with standard chest tubes (of any size) or with pigtail catheters inserted using a Seldinger technique. Fluid can accumulate in the pleural space as a result of many different processes, including trauma, pneumonia, malignancy, and congestive cardiac disease. Drains placed for simple fluid may be of smaller caliber, but those placed for hemothorax should be larger to prevent blockage by coagula (typically 36 French for adults).

All hemothoraces should be promptly drained to prevent fibrothorax and possible trapped lung. Failure to promptly drain blood in the pleural space will render this technique ineffective, and formal decortications (i.e., via video-assisted thoracic surgery) will be required. Other fluid collections should be drained and the underlying pathology addressed to prevent recurrent accumulation. Special caution should be taken when addressing malignant effusions because these have a tendency to reaccumulate after drain removal. If the underlying disease is not going to be treated, the patient should generally either be treated with pleurodesis (to obliterate the pleural space and prevent recurrence) or placement of a chronic, tunneled pleural drain.[24]

These chest procedures must always be performed in as sterile a fashion as possible, although the immediacy of tension physiology may sometimes require the surgeon to forgo fastidious draping. It remains unclear whether presumptive or prophylactic antibiotics prevent empyema related to chest drain placement. Although the answer remains unclear, a recent multicenter trial in trauma patients failed to demonstrate a benefit of antibiotic administration.[25] If antibiotics are administered, they should be given prior to beginning the procedure and be limited to one dose of a first-generation cephalosporin.

Technique for Tube Tracheostomy

Step 1: Assemble the equipment listed in Table 5. If the patient is stable, consider administering an intravenous narcotic.

Step 2: Position the patient with the affected side tilted up and the ipsilateral arm raised above the head [*see Figure 9*].

Table 5 **Equipment Needed for Tube Thoracostomy**
Large barrier drape
Sterile gown/gloves
Mask, eyewear, hat (personal protective gear)
Standard commercial central catheter insertion kit
Suitably sized chest tube
Scalpel, large hemostat, needle driver
Heavy silk or nylon suture
Local anesthetic
Drain trap/suction regulator
Occlusive dressing

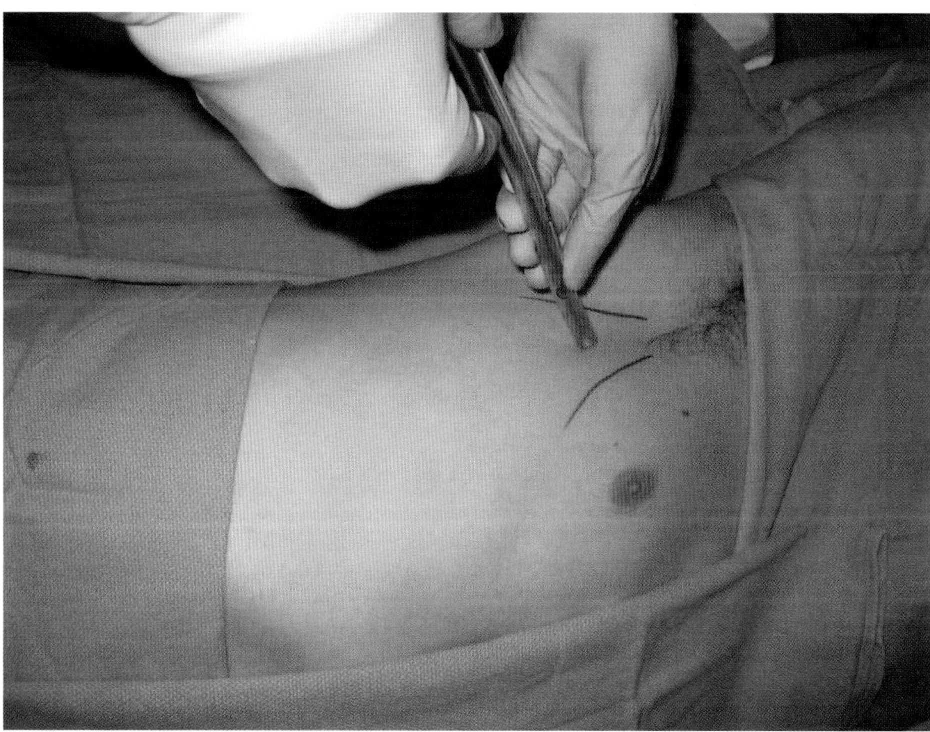

Figure 9 **Correct position for placement of a chest tube. Note that the tube is directed posterior and cephalad and the right arm is raised above the head.**

Step 3: Don personal protective gear, including a sterile gown and gloves.

Step 4: Scrub the anterolateral chest wall with chlorhexidine solution and drape the region.

Step 5: Palpate the chest wall to identify an intercostal space around the fifth rib. In men, the nipple is a useful surface landmark to indicate the height of the dome of the diaphragm, below which one should generally not stray.

Step 6: Infiltrate the skin with local anesthetic and make a skin incision at the interspace below the intended thoracostomy site. Bluntly separate the subcutaneous tissue and overlying muscle to arrive at the rib and intercostal musculature. Infiltration of local anesthetic in the periosteum and pleura is a useful but often ignored step.

Step 7: Blunt spreading over the top of a rib allows puncture through the pleura into the intercostal space, after which the tube can be slid in while pointing it superiorly and posteriorly. Creation of a proper subcutaneous tract and direction of the tube toward the thoracic apex decrease the likelihood of the tube entering a pulmonary fissure.

Step 8: Secure the tube to the adjacent skin with a heavy suture of silk or nylon.

Step 9: Connect the tube to the drain trap–suction device and apply an occlusive dressing.

Step 10: Remove instruments for reprocessing and dispose of sharp waste.

For a visual reference, readers are referred to the video featured in the *New England Journal of Medicine*.[26]

Traditionally, all chest drains were initially placed to suction (20 cm water) and subsequently transitioned to water seal (a one-way safety valve with no applied suction) as the volume of output decreased. For many chest tube indications, a growing body of evidence supports placement of chest drains to water seal from the outset. This has been demonstrated to accelerate the resolution of air leaks and duration of chest tubes.[27]

Complications of tube thoracostomy The most common immediate complication of this procedure is a malpositioned tube, whether in an interlobar fissure, occluded by a kink, or even placed completely within the chest wall rather than the pleural space. A chest radiograph should be obtained after the placement of any chest drain to verify tube position and to determine if the pleural air or fluid is beginning to drain properly. Inadequate tube position may sometimes be addressed by sterile withdrawal and resuturing, but once a tube has been placed, it should never be advanced. Much more rarely, tube placement may cause injury to the pulmonary parenchyma or bleeding from an intercostal or pulmonary vessel. The latter should be suspected with persistent voluminous bloody output and/or any hemodynamic instability after tube placement. Such vascular injuries require operative intervention for definitive control.

Removal of chest tubes should be done with care not to allow air to entrain into the pleural space. This is primarily accomplished by maintaining an occlusive dressing over the tube site and asking the patient to cooperate with tube removal. Some prefer tube removal during forced expiration to increase intrapleural pressure and thus decrease the risk of recurrent pneumothorax. With this approach, however, some patients suddenly gasp with surprise or pain, suddenly dropping the intrapleural pressure and potentially drawing air in through the tube tract. Another school of thought is to remove the tube while the patient maintains maximal inspiration.

Principles and Process of Documenting Competency in Surgical Skills

Although documenting knowledge in surgery has been standardized by the American Board of Surgery, demonstration of skills has not as yet become part of the certification process. How one acquires, practices, and perfects a surgical skill is an area of great interest to educators and the public alike. Although, certainly, the time spent learning and practicing will vary with the task, with each new skill, the essentials include the following:

1. A period of didactic, hands-on instruction by an expert
2. A period of practice, often while being mentored
3. Demonstration of acquisition of the skill
4. Continued practice-based learning including participation in performance improvement programs and continued education

The Surgical Institutes, currently being developed through the Education Division of the American College of Surgeons (ACS), will form the basis for development of a standard curriculum (including skills training) for each level of residency. Another group that has been very proactive in this arena is the Society of Gastrointestinal Surgeons (SAGES), which has developed and propagated the "Fundamentals of Laparoscopic Surgery" course. In ultrasonography, the ACS Ultrasound Education Committee has developed a series of courses including Level I certification (attendance at the course), Level II certification (passing a skill set), and Level III certification (acquisition of skills under proctorship until reaching the expert or instructor level). In particular, the skills-oriented postgraduate course "Ultrasound in the Surgical ICU" is an excellent model for introducing bedside ultrasound techniques. Once learned, how many examinations are necessary before proficiency is attained is unclear but certainly varies with the nature of the examination. In trauma, 25 FAST examinations performed under supervision is generally considered adequate, although it is important that some of those examinations include patients with positive findings. The American Society of Breast Surgeons requires at least 100 breast ultrasound examinations prior to applying for credentialing. There has been limited success in using simulators to introduce ultrasound skills.[28] Recently, Hutton and Wong documented improvement in placement of chest tubes by junior house staff after practicing on a patient simulator.[29] A recent systematic review concluded that simulation-based training seems to be transferable to the operating room.[30] In this era of decreased time spent in training, surgical educators are challenged to develop more efficient methods of ensuring that general surgeons have acquired competency in both operative and bedside skills, with patient safety and satisfaction as the ultimate measures of success.

Financial Disclosures: None Reported

References

1. Rozycki GS, Ballard RB, Feliciano DV, et al. Surgeon-performed ultrasound for assessment of truncal injuries: lessons learned from 1540 patients. Ann Surg 1998;228:557–67.
2. Rozycki GS, Feliciano DV, Ochsner G, et al. The roles of ultrasound in patients with possible penetrating cardiac wounds: a prospective multicenter study. J Trauma 1999;46:543–51.
3. Sisley AC, Rozycki GS, Ballard RB, et al. Rapid detection of traumatic effusion using surgeon-performed ultrasonography. J Trauma 1998;44:291–7.
4. Rozycki GS, Pennington SD, Feliciano DV. Surgeon-performed ultrasound in the critical care setting: its use as an extension of the physical examination to detect pleural effusion. J Trauma 2001;50:636–42.
5. Dulchavsky SA, Schwarz KL, Kirkpatrick AW, et al. Prospective evaluation of thoracic ultrasound in the detection of pneumothorax. J Trauma 2001;50:201–5.
6. Knudtson JL, Dort JM, Helmer SD, Smith RS. Surgeon-performed ultrasound for pneumothorax in the trauma suite. J Trauma 2004;56:527–30.
7. Cunningham J, Kirkpatrick AW, Nicolaou S, et al. Enhanced recognition of "lung sliding" with power color Doppler imaging in the diagnosis of pneumothorax. J Trauma 2002;52:769–71.
8. Rozycki GS, Knudson MM, Shackford SR, Dicker R. Surgeon-performed bedside organ assessment with sonography after trauma (BOAST): a pilot study from the WTA multicenter group. J Trauma 2005;59:1356–64.
9. McGee DC, Gould MK. Preventing complications of central venous catheterization. N Engl J Med 2003;348:1123–33.
10. Keenan SP. Use of ultrasound to place central lines. J Crit Care 2002;17:126–37.
11. Karakitsos D, Labropoulos N, De Groot E, et al. Real-time ultrasound-guided catheterization of the internal jugular vein: a prospective comparison with the landmark technique in critical care patients. Crit Care 2008;10:R162.
12. Yanagawa Y, Sakamoto T, Okada Y. Hypovolemic shock evaluated by sonographic measurement of the inferior vena cava during resuscitation in trauma patients. J Trauma 2007;63:1245–8.
13. Gunst M, Ghaemmaghami V, Sperry J, et al. Accuracy of cardiac function and volume status estimates using the bedside echocardiographic assessment in trauma/critical care. J Trauma 2008;65:509–16.
14. Bouhemad B, Zang M, Lu Q, Rouby JJ. Clinical review: bedside lung ultrasound in critical care practice. Crit Care 2007;11:205.
15. Mayo PH, Goltz HR, Tafreshi M, Doelken P. Safety of ultrasound-guided thoracentesis in patents receiving mechanical ventilation. Chest 2004;125:1059–62.
16. Liang SJ, Tu CY, Chen HJ, et al. Application of ultrasound-guided pigtail catheter for drainage of pleural effusions in the ICU. Intensive Care Med 2009;35:350–4.
17. Nicolaou S, Talsky A, Khastoggi JD, et al. Ultrasound-guided interventional radiology in critical care. Crit Care Med 2007;35:5186–97.
18. Saber AA, Meslemani AM, Davis R, Pimentel R. Safety zones for anterior abdominal wall entry during laparoscopy: a CT scan mapping of epigastric vessels. Ann Surg 2004;239:182–5.
19. Gaitini D. Current approaches and controversial issues in the diagnosis of deep vein thrombosis via duplex Doppler ultrasound. J Clin Ultrasound 1996;34:289–97.
20. Ciaglia P, Firsching R, Syniec C. Elective percutaneous dilational tracheostomy: a new simple bedside procedure; preliminary report. Chest 2005;128:816–20.
21. Norwood S, Vallina VL, Short K, et al. Incidence of tracheal stenosis and other late complications after percutaneous tracheostomy. Ann Surg 2000;232:233–41.
22. Raghuraman G, Rajan S, Marzouk JK, et al. Is tracheal stenosis caused by percutaneous tracheostomy different from that by surgical tracheostomy? Chest 2005;127:879–85.
23. TracMan. Tracheostomy management in critical care. Available at: http://www.tracman.org.uk (accessed December 2008).
24. Trembly A, Michaud G. Single-center experience with 250 tunnelled pleural catheter insertions for malignant pleural effusion. Chest 2006;129:363–8.
25. Maxwell RA, Campbell DJ, Fabian TC, et al. Use of presumptive antibiotics following tube thoracostomy for traumatic hemopneumothorax in the prevention of empyema and pneumonia-a multi-center trial. J Trauma 2004;57:742–9.
26. Nascimiento B, Simone C, Chien V. Videos in clinical medicine: chest-tube insertion. N Engl J Med 2007;357:e15.
27. Cerfolio RJ, Bryant AS, Singh S, et al. The management of chest tubes in patients with a pneumothorax and an air leak after pulmonary resection. Chest 2005;128:816–20.
28. Knudson MM, Sisley AC. Training residents using simulation technology: experience with ultrasound for trauma. J Trauma 2000;48:659–65.
29. Hutton IA, Wong C. Using simulation to teach junior doctors how to insert chest tubes: a brief and effective teaching module. Intern Med J 2008;38:887–91.
30. Sturm LP, Wiindsor JA, Cosman PH, et al. A systematic review of skills transfer after surgical simulation training. Ann Surg 2008;248:166–79.

12 ETHICAL ISSUES IN SURGERY

Jason D. Keune, MD, MBA, Ira J. Kodner, MD, FACS, and Mary E. Klingensmith, MD, FACS

As sociologist Charles Bosk put it in the introduction to his seminal study on the culture of surgical training, "If they taught me nothing else, the surgeons taught me that delivering high-quality humane care is hard work."[1] The care that Bosk describes is hard, not only because of the technical difficulty of the surgical cases or the long hours required to care for surgical patients. It is hard because the work is conducted in an ethical framework that is both unique to and important to surgeons. To be a good surgeon, one must be technically good and scientifically sound, but also ethical to the degree that has traditionally been demanded by our profession.

In this chapter, we discuss what ethical problems in surgery are and how they might be approached. We then scrutinize several contemporary problems in surgical ethics. This chapter is not meant to be an exhaustive treatment of surgical ethics but a survey highlighting the most common ethical problems.

What Is an Ethical Problem?

Discussion about clinical ethics in surgery and the discovery of ethical problems proceeds in the same way that it does for most other physicians. Clinical care is conducted on a daily basis against a background of historical ethical problems for which stable solutions have been found. The moral intuition of most surgeons today, for example, includes the importance of obtaining informed consent prior to performing a surgical operation. Although historically, appropriate informed consent was not always obtained, today, almost no one would find it efficient or necessary to dispute the need to obtain informed consent. The entirety of the clinical care of patients tends to proceed in this manner: we strive for an ethical practice of surgery that meets the demands of contemporary morality.

Occasionally, however, the moral intuitions of clinicians will disagree: what one surgeon views as right, another will view as wrong. In this disagreement lies an ethical problem that is worthy of scrutiny. In this scrutiny, we shift our modes of thinking from everyday moral intuition, which is part of every professional's mode of thought, to moral reasoning, which requires a special process of explicit thinking. In moral reasoning, the thinker attempts to reach a well-supported answer to a distinct moral question. Skill at moral reasoning is something that can be learned and practiced. A surgical education should equip future surgeons with both a sound moral intuition and an introduction to moral reasoning so that resolution of ethical problems can be obtained in a professional and fruitful manner.

In what follows, we review clinical ethics as it pertains to surgeons. We focus on the normative questions of practical ethics; that is, we try to use ethical norms and methods of reasoning to answer the question of how to act when an ethical problem arises. This is important because, as surgeons, often situations arise that require action, but which action is the right one is not clear or not agreed on by all involved. The situations can intensify when there is time pressure (as when a patient is bleeding) and because the stakes can be very high (life and death), making a right decision of great importance.

Ethical Theories and Principles

The history of ethical thought is expansive. Ancient Greece is where the first instances of highly developed ethical thought that have survived to compete with contemporary ethical theories appear. Several of these theories are reviewed below.

PRINCIPLISM

Principlism is the name given to the set of four principles that have emerged from the common morality of health care workers. Although not the only approach to health care ethics, the four principle approach, defended by Tom Beauchamp and James Childress, forms the backbone of most discourse in clinical medical ethics.[2] The four principles that Beauchamp and Childress espouse as being starting points for clinical medical ethics are respect for autonomy, nonmaleficence, beneficence, and justice.

Respect for Autonomy

The principle of respect for autonomy requires clinicians to allow individuals to make decisions regarding their medical care that are at once fully informed and free from outside coercion. The principle of respect for autonomy is best exemplified in the practice of obtaining informed consent from patients prior to performing an operation on them. One quality that is respected in obtaining informed consent is that of *liberty*: the patient is left to decide whether the operation should be performed. We value offering patients such choices that are free of coercion. Another quality that is fundamental to respect for autonomy that is exemplified in the obtaining of informed consent is that of *agency*: the operation and its risks are carefully explained to the patient in such a way that he or she has the details needed to make a decision that is fully informed.

Nonmaleficence

The principle of nonmaleficence requires physicians to refrain from causing harm. The obligation not to harm becomes important in drawing distinctions between killing and letting die and when weighing the risks and benefits of a specific procedure. The notion that one ought not harm others in the course of care is often cited as one of the most fundamental to an ethical practice of medicine and is often associated with the aphorism *Primum non nocere*, "First do no harm." Harming should be thought of not only in the active sense but also in the passive, as when a physician is negligent.

Beneficence

The principle of beneficence implores physicians to contribute to the welfare of others. It is distinct from nonmaleficence but exists on the same spectrum. It is well established that not harming is not enough, but physicians should also do positive acts that benefit others. In the practice of medicine, beneficence can conflict with the respect for autonomy. A physician, intent on doing good for a patient, might override a patient's wishes for his or her own care. When a physician's actions derive from the principle of beneficence but violate the principle of respect for autonomy, the actions can be called *paternalistic*. Also, just what degree of beneficence is required of physicians is measured. Supererogatory acts, or acts that go "beyond the call of duty," are rarely morally required of physicians.

Justice

Justice is concerned with inequality. The notion of justice in health care requires physicians to be cognizant of the fact that there are great disparities in the baseline health of patients, the abilities that patients have to seek care, and the outcomes of the treatments that physicians provide. The argument about what justice should look like in health care today ranges from whether citizens have a right to a minimum, basic amount of health care to the allocation of scarce resources, such as kidneys for transplantation.

The history of ethical thought is marked by the emergence of several distinct theories, which are frameworks through which different ethical problems can be understood. The most popular and long-standing theories are presented briefly here; all of them have proponents in contemporary dialogue on ethics.

CONSEQUENTIALISM/UTILITARIANISM

The theory of consequentialism is based on the idea that what one ought to do is based entirely on the consequences of one's actions. The foundations of consequentialism were developed by Jeremy Bentham (1748–1832) and John Stewart Mill (1806–1873). Both thinkers supported the idea that the morally right act was the one that would produce the most happiness. Later consequentialist thinkers proposed a broader goal: that acts should result in maximization of the good or of utility in general, not just happiness. Debates exist too about whether acts should be evaluated on their intended consequences or their actual consequences.

DEONTOLOGY

The ethical thought of Immanuel Kant (1724–1804) was focused on moral reasoning that did not have to do with the consequences of one's actions. The rightness of actions under deontology stem from a consideration of whether the reasons for the action would apply to anyone else in a similar situation. In the simplest form of his "categorical imperative," Kant recommends that one "act only according to that maxim whereby you can, at the same time, will that it should become a universal law."[3] The substantial contribution that Kant made to ethical thought with the introduction of deontology is that morality is strictly grounded in reason, not in tradition, intuition, or desire. The result of Kant's work contrasts to consequentialism in that instead of outcomes being important, what is important are the rules that one generates based on the categorical imperative. Any ethical theory that takes rules to be the most important factor in ethical decision making can be called deontologic.

VIRTUE ETHICS

The roots of virtue ethics lie in the writings of Plato and Aristotle. Although virtue ethics formed the backbone of Western ethical thought until the Enlightenment, it disappeared from ethical dialogue until interest in it was reignited in the mid-20th century. In contrast to deontology, which emphasizes rules and duties, and consequentialism, which emphasizes outcomes of actions, virtue ethics emphasizes character. In most versions of virtue ethics, the concept of "the good life" or "human flourishing" is emphasized as the primary goal. The way to obtain this good life is through living a life in full accordance with virtue. Most virtue ethics emphasize that virtues that are necessary to obtain a good life, such as courage or generosity, are not just simple character traits but richly complex ones that affect one's emotions, actions, desires, and interests.

"ETHICS OF CARE" OR FEMINIST ETHICS

Feminist ethics starts by recognizing that there are several groups whose moral experience is not recognized in traditional moral thought, the first among these being women. The feminist ethical thought that has been most often applied to medicine is the "ethics of care." In contrast to traditional ethics, which involves itself with justice, rights, and rules, the feminist ethics of care asserts that an ethics rooted in relationships and responsibilities would be more appropriate for the medical setting.

CASUISTRY

Finally, casuistry is a mode of ethical reasoning that begins not with principles or theories but with cases. Although casuistry has been used in a pejorative fashion to criticize modes of thought as being "shallow," recent thinkers have embraced casuistry as appropriate for bioethical thought. The argument for casuistry is that although people will often disagree at the level of theory, when it comes to cases, moral intuitions often converge. Such convergence for paradigm cases causes us to recognize a level of confidence and stability in our shared moral beliefs and thus can prove useful in a pluralistic society in which people of vastly different worldviews are brought together to address ethical issues. As Stephen Toulmin, who was involved as philosophy consultant to the first presidential commission on research ethics noted, agreement was obtained on several contentious issues with a casuist approach, which otherwise would have been impossible if consensus had depended on agreement at the theoretical or religious level.[4]

Ethical Issues Associated with the End of Life

Surgeons frequently find themselves at the bedside of patients who are near death. The trauma surgeon takes care of patients who have life-threatening injuries, many of whom do not survive. Oncologists, even after a flawless operation, often find that patients succumb to the disease with which they presented. The acute care surgeon faces patients who have a life-threatening condition that may be more advanced than surgical therapy can ameliorate. Skill with decision making at the end of life should therefore be part of every surgeon's armamentarium.

SURROGATE DECISION MAKING

An ethical problem arises when a patient, once competent to make decisions about his or her own care, becomes incompetent. The response to such a situation is rooted in the respect for the patient's autonomy. Someone else must be entrusted to make decisions on the patient's behalf. Several questions beset the surgeon faced with this problem:

1. Who should make the decisions for the patient?
2. How should the surrogate decision maker best decide?

Advanced directives are instructions that are provided by patients that provide direction to caretakers about how decisions should be made should the patient become impaired.[5] Frequently, a surgeon finds himself or herself at the bedside of a patient who has lost decisional capacity and is also dying. Competence regarding advanced directives and surrogate decision making is therefore important.

There are a variety of standard ways that patients may express their end-of-life preferences. The first is through a living will. A living will is a document prepared by a still-competent patient that details what the patient's preferences would be should he or she lose decisional capacity. Living wills can span a spectrum from a simple statement indicating that a patient would like to die a natural death and not be kept alive by heroic measures to one in which the patient indicates that he or she would like life to be prolonged, whatever the method or cost. Living wills can also give specific directions as to which medical therapies should and should not be used. In many states, the activation of a living will requires death to be imminent before the terms are activated.

In 1991, the Physician Order for Life-Sustaining Treatment (POLST) Paradigm Initiative was brought into existence as an alternative to the advanced directive.[6] It was recognized that the diversity and lack of uniformity among advanced directives led to uneven realization of patients' end-of-life preferences.[7] The POLST Paradigm Initiative was a taskforce centered at Oregon Health and Sciences University composed of stakeholders from across the spectrum of health care. The result was the development of a standardized form, released in 1995, known as "the POLST form," which could serve as a set of portable physician orders and would be placed in the front of a patient's chart. A sample POLST form is shown in Figure 1.

Another method by which a patient's preferences can be expressed is by the appointment of a durable power of attorney for health care. A durable power of attorney is a person who is appointed in advance by the patient to act as a surrogate decision maker if a patient should lose decisional capacity. The "durable" aspect refers to the fact that the power of attorney will be able to continue to make decisions for the patient should he or she become incapacitated.

A problem exists, however, if a durable power of attorney has not been designated and the patient has not prepared a living will. In this instance, a surrogate decision maker must be identified. Laws regarding how such surrogate decision makers are identified differ from state to state. A hierarchy is often specified in such laws (e.g., spouse, adult children, siblings). Once identified, it should be verified that the surrogate decision maker is interested in acting in the best interest of and according to the wishes and values of the patient. It is commonly accepted that a durable power of attorney who is selected by the patient or a family member who knows the patient well is superior to a living will document because a person who is familiar with the patient's preferences can respond to the complexities of treatment in a way that a static document cannot. If no relative or other suitable surrogate decision maker can be located, most states allow physicians to seek a court-appointed conservator, who may make decisions for the patient. In most states, a conservator is not required, however, and health care facilities are usually allowed to make decisions for such patients as long as the decisions made are within the ethical guidelines of the institution.

Once a surrogate decision maker is identified, how should he or she decide what should be done? Two standards apply in this situation: the standard of substituted judgment and the best interest standard. In applying the standard of substituted judgment, the decision maker bases the decision on his knowledge of the patient and of other, perhaps similar decisions that the patient has made in the past. The decision, then, is based on what the surrogate decision maker imagines that the patient would want were the patient competent. In applying the best interest standard, decision makers decide based on what, in the decision maker's opinion, would be best for the patient without trying to determine what the patient would want. This mode is most useful when decision makers lack comfort in making a determination about what the patient would want in the given circumstances, possibly because their knowledge about the patient is not that intimate.

FUTILITY

The concept of futility arises commonly in a surgical practice that revolves around surgical intervention. When does a proposed treatment have such a small chance of being efficacious that the surgeon should refrain from performing it? There is a range of definitions of what is considered "futile" care, usually focusing on lack of efficaciousness, lack of therapeutic "success," or care that is so burdensome that it vastly outweighs any therapeutic benefit. The lack of strict definition is difficult in part because there is disagreement about what death is. Given that surgeons and families may view death differently, the meaning of what life-sustaining treatment is may also be different.

Early attempts to deal with the problem of futility were made by defining it in terms of specific clinical criteria, qualitative judgments comparing patients with other similar patients in whom similar treatments have been useless, or the use of physiologic goals. There was a failure of such approaches because specific clinical criteria are hard to link to specific outcomes, what "useless" means is disputable, and physiologic goals can be quite arbitrary.[8] A second phase

HIPAA PERMITS DISCLOSURE TO HEALTH CARE PROFESSIONALS & ELECTRONIC REGISTRY AS NECESSARY FOR TREATMENT

Physician Orders for Life-Sustaining Treatment (POLST)

Follow these orders until orders change. These medical orders are based on the patient's **current** medical condition and preferences. Any section not completed does not invalidate the form and implies full treatment for that section. With significant change of condition new orders may need to be written. *Guidance for Health Care Professionals.* http://www.ohsu.edu/polst/programs/documents/Guidebook.pdf.

Patient Last Name:		Patient First Name	Middle Int.
Date of Birth: (mm/dd/yyyy) ____ ____ ____	Gender: ☐ M ☐ F	Last 4 SSN: ☐☐☐☐	
Address: (street / city / state / zip)			

A *Check One* — **CARDIOPULMONARY RESUSCITATION (CPR):** ***Patient has no pulse and is not breathing.***

- ☐ **Attempt Resuscitation/CPR**
- ☐ **Do Not Attempt Resuscitation/DNR**

When not in cardiopulmonary arrest, follow orders in **B** and **C**.

B *Check One* — **MEDICAL INTERVENTIONS:** ***If patient has pulse and/or is breathing.***

- ☐ **Comfort Measures Only** (Allow Natural Death). Relieve pain and suffering through the use of any medication by any route, positioning, wound care and other measures. Use oxygen, suction and manual treatment of airway obstruction as needed for comfort. ***Patient prefers no transfer to hospital*** *for life-sustaining treatments.* ***Transfer*** *if comfort needs cannot be met in current location.* **Treatment Plan: Maximize comfort through symptom management.**
- ☐ **Limited Additional Interventions** In addition to care described in Comfort Measures Only, use medical treatment, antibiotics, IV fluids and cardiac monitor as indicated. No intubation, advanced airway interventions, or mechanical ventilation. May consider less invasive airway support (e.g. CPAP, BiPAP). ***Transfer*** *to hospital if indicated. Generally avoid the intensive care unit.* **Treatment Plan: Provide basic medical treatments.**
- ☐ **Full Treatment** In addition to care described in Comfort Measures Only and Limited Additional Interventions, use intubation, advanced airway interventions, and mechanical ventilation as indicated. ***Transfer to hospital*** *and/or intensive care unit if indicated.* **Treatment Plan: Full treatment including life support measures in the intensive care unit.**

Additional Orders: ____________

C *Check One* — **ARTIFICIALLY ADMINISTERED NUTRITION:** ***Offer food by mouth if feasible.***

- ☐ No artificial nutrition by tube.
- ☐ Defined trial period of artificial nutrition by tube.
- ☐ Long-term artificial nutrition by tube.

Additional Orders: ____________

D — **DOCUMENTATION OF DISCUSSION:**

- ☐ Patient (Patient has capacity)
- ☐ Parent of minor
- ☐ Court-Appointed Guardian
- ☐ Health Care Representative or legally recognized surrogate
- ☐ Surrogate for patient with developmental disabilities or significant mental health condition (Note: Special requirements for completion. See reverse side.)
- ☐ Other____________

Signature of Patient or Surrogate

Signature: ***recommended***	Name (print):	Relationship (write "self" if patient):

This form will be sent to the POLST Registry unless the patient wishes to opt out, if so check opt out box ☐

E — **SIGNATURE OF PHYSICIAN / NP/ PA**

My signature below indicates to the best of my knowledge that these orders are consistent with the patient's **current** medical condition and preferences.

Print Signing Physician / NP / PA Name: ***required***	Signer Phone Number:	Signer License Number: *(optional)*
Physician / NP / PA Signature: ***required***	Date: ***required***	Office Use Only

SEND FORM WITH PATIENT WHENEVER TRANSFERRED OR DISCHARGED, SUBMIT COPY TO REGISTRY

HIPAA PERMITS DISCLOSURE TO HEALTH CARE PROFESSIONALS & ELECTRONIC REGISTRY AS NECESSARY FOR TREATMENT

Information for patient named on this form PATIENT'S NAME: ____________

The POLST form is **always voluntary** and is usually for persons with advanced illness or frailty. POLST records your wishes for medical treatment in your current state of health. Once initial medical treatment is begun and the risks and benefits of further therapy are clear, your treatment wishes may change. Your medical care and this form can be changed to reflect your new wishes at any time. However, no form can address all the medical treatment decisions that may need to be made. The Oregon Advance Directive is recommended for all capable adults, regardless of their health status. An Advance Directive allows you to document in detail your future health care instructions and/or name a Health Care Representative to speak for you if you are unable to speak for yourself.

Contact Information

Surrogate (optional):	Relationship:	Phone Number:	Address:

Health Care Professional Information

Preparer Name:	Preparer Title:	Phone Number:	Date Prepared:
PA's Supervising Physician:		Phone Number:	
Primary Care Professional:			

Directions for Health Care Professionals

Completing POLST

- Completing a POLST is always voluntary and cannot be mandated for a patient.
- Should reflect current preferences of persons with advanced illness or frailty. Also, encourage completion of an Advance Directive.
- Verbal / phone orders are acceptable with follow-up signature by physician/NP/PA in accordance with facility/community policy.
- Use of original form is encouraged. Photocopies, faxes, and electronic registry forms are also legal and valid.
- A person with developmental disabilities or significant mental health condition requires additional consideration before completing the POLST form; refer to *Guidance for Health Care Professionals* at http://www.ohsu.edu/polst/programs/documents/Guidebook.pdf.

Sending to Oregon POLST Registry (Required unless "Opt Out" box is checked)

For the Oregon POLST Registry the following must be completed:

- Patient's full name
- Date of birth
- Section A
- MD / DO / NP / PA signature
- Date signed

Send a copy of both sides of this POLST form to the Oregon POLST Registry.

FAX or eFAX: 503-418-2161
or
Mail: Oregon POLST Registry
CDW-EM
3181 SW Sam Jackson Park Rd.
Portland, OR 97239

Date Submitted ____ /____ /____

MAY PUT REGISTRY ID STICKER HERE:

Registry Phone: 503-418-4083
*Please allow up to 10 days from receipt for processing into the Registry. Mailed confirmation packets may take four weeks for delivery.

Reviewing POLST

This POLST should be reviewed periodically and if:

- The patient is transferred from one care setting or care level to another, or
- There is a substantial change in the patient's health status, or
- The patient's treatment preferences change, or
- The patient's primary care professional changes.

Voiding POLST

- A person with capacity, or the valid surrogate of a person without capacity, can void the form and request alternative treatment.
- Draw line through sections A through E and write "VOID" in large letters if POLST is replaced or becomes invalid.
- Send a copy of the voided form to the POLST Registry as above (required).
- If included in an electronic medical record, follow voiding procedures of facility/community.

For permission to use the copyrighted form contact the OHSU Center for Ethics in Health Care. Information on the POLST program is available online at www.polst.org or at polst@ohsu.edu.

SEND FORM WITH PATIENT WHENEVER TRANSFERRED OR DISCHARGED, SUBMIT COPY TO REGISTRY

Figure 1 **Sample Physician Order for Life Sustaining Treatment (POLST) form.**

in the history of dealing with the problem of futility is best represented by the American Medical Association Council on Ethical and Judicial Affairs recommendation that a process-based approach to futility determinations is taken.[9]

This approach, which is summarized below, does not require a definition of what is considered futile but rather describes a process in which such definitions might be recognized and agreed on locally. The procedural approach has been incorporated into legislation in several states. The approach begins with a serious attempt, on the part of the patient, the physician group, and the patient's proxies, to determine what constitutes futility. If there is serious disagreement that cannot be resolved, it is recommended that transfer to another institution be arranged. If agreement on this topic is achieved, then decision making must proceed with the use of outcomes data and must take into account the physician's and the patient's, or patient's proxy's, goals for treatment. If substantial disagreement results from this deliberation, the Council recommends that assistance of an individual ethics consultant be obtained, who might facilitate a discussion in the hope of a resolution. If resolution is not achieved with one consultant, the next step as proposed by the Council is to involve the institutional ethics committee. The committee should include significant involvement of the patient or the patient's proxy. If care cannot be agreed on after such an ethics committee hearing, it is reasonable to transfer the patient to the care of a different physician group within the same hospital. If one cannot be found, however, a transfer to another institution can be arranged if an institution can be found that will honor the patient's wishes. If no physician and no institution can be found that will honor the patient's wishes, then it can be considered that the patient's request is likely not consistent with a majority view regarding medical ethics and professional standards. In such a setting, the proposed intervention need not be provided. The Council points out, however, that the legal ramifications of such a decision are not clear. The problem of futility therefore has not been fully resolved in the contemporary era.

"DO NOT RESUSCITATE" ORDERS IN THE OPERATING ROOM

Consider an elderly patient with clear "do not resuscitate/do not intubate" (DNR/DNI) orders who presents to you with a bowel obstruction. The cause of the obstruction is found to be a sigmoid volvulus. He wants a sigmoidectomy to ameliorate the problem. Should you rescind the DNR/DNI order?

Although DNR orders are very valuable in the end-of-life setting, they are difficult to interpret when a surgical operation is being considered. The performance of surgery relies heavily on a wide variety of life support techniques, without which most surgery would not be possible. For this reason, many advocate rescinding the DNR order during an operation. One problem with rescinding DNR orders in this fashion, however, is that it is unclear when they should be restarted. The decision to restart DNR orders as soon as the patient is extubated or arrives in the postanesthesia care unit or after 48 hours has passed is one that should be made through discussion with the patient and the patient's family.

Conflicts of Interest, Industry Payments, and Surgical Innovation

A conflict of interest is a state in which a dynamic interaction exists between two differing interests in the same person, such that his or her interest in one impacts the ability to realize, and possibly execute, a pure motive in the other. Conflicts of interest come to light as an ethical problem for physicians when one of the interests is financial and the other is patient care. The idea of obtaining extramural support from industry becomes increasingly attractive as federal research funding available to surgeons diminishes. Surgeons are at once common targets of marketing efforts by such companies and valuable consultants without whom new device development would be impossible.

Many institutions in the field of medicine and biomedical research, such as the American Medical Association,[10] Pharmaceutical Research and Manufacturers of America (PhRMA),[11] and the National Institutes of Health,[12] as well as most universities, have published guidelines that serve to give their members guidance with regard to financial conflict of interest and relationships with industry. The American College of Surgeons (ACS) has a conflict of interest policy that went into effect in 2002.[13] Guidelines for the management of conflicts of interest have also been put forth by the Institute of Medicine[14] and the Association of American Medical Colleges.[15]

Where financial conflicts of interest in medicine are concerned, the worry is that physicians who receive payments from industry cannot properly manage this financial interest when it conflicts with patient care. Is it possible to have a conflict of interest and yet be resistant to the type of bias that would negatively impact patient care? There is no term to describe conflicts of interest properly managed, but the proper management of all conflicts of interest seems to be common to the successful practice of surgery. The fact that financial conflicts of interest are of heightened concern compared with other interests, such as academic promotion, advancement of original ideas in diagnosis or therapy, and balance between family and work life, is interesting. One potential reason for the focus on financial conflicts of interest is that money is quantifiable and therefore easier to regulate. A question that remains is whether something more than just the quantifiability of money warrants a nearly exclusive focus on this conflict of interest.

One solution to the problem of financial conflicts of interest in medicine that has been put forth is that of disclosure. Two of us (M.E.K. and J.D.K.) recently published a summary and categorization of 4 years of disclosures (2006–2009) given by presenters at the annual Clinical Congress of the ACS. We found that in the 3,122 disclosures made by 490 individuals, colorectal surgeon was the most common profession of disclosers and the most common type of disclosure was consulting. The company most commonly disclosed was Covidien. Disclosers used 195 different terms to describe their relationships, making the need for a standardized nomenclature necessary.[16] In another study, only 71% of disclosers at a national meeting of orthopedic surgeons believed that their relationships with industry involved any conflict.[17]

The concept of disclosure as a solution to conflict of interest problems in many complex professional environments is rooted in the words of Justice Louis Brandeis, who said, "Sunlight is said to be the best of disinfectants."[18] For several years prior to the passage of the Patient Protection and Affordable Care Act (PPACA), attempts at legislation of the physician financial conflicts of interest problem were made by members of the US Congress, led by US Senator Charles Grassley, who has made openness and disclosure across industries a focus of his legislative effort. The PPACA, which became law on March 23, 2010, includes a section known as the "Physician Payment Sunshine Provision."[19] The provision requires drug, biologic, and medical device companies to report all payments and other transfers of value to physicians and teaching hospitals. The minimum value required for reporting is $10 per instance or $100 per year. The first reports will be due on March 31, 2013. Figure 2 is extracted from the PPACA and shows what types of financial relationships will be counted.

Financial conflicts of interest among surgeons represent a special case that stands out against the financial conflicts of interest of other physicians. The innovation and mass production of safe and effective surgical devices, which have marked the progress of surgery of the last several decades, require the involvement of surgeons who are in active practice. There is a necessity for a relationship between such surgeons and industry given that the means of production in the United States is in the private sector. Innovation and device development are difficult to conceive of without such a relationship, and it is difficult to imagine how surgeons should engage with industry without an exchange of remuneration for expertise and ideas.

Informed Consent

Informed consent is a process that allows respect for a patient's autonomy to be preserved. American courts have long held that a patient's informed consent to a medical or surgical procedure or diagnostic test is essential. Informed consent should be obtained from a patient every time a procedure is performed, except in some emergency settings. Informed consent should be composed of a detailed description of the procedure and accompanied by the procedure's inherent risks, benefits, and alternatives, including the alternative of not being treated. Additionally, true informed consent should not be done in one sitting but should be part of an ongoing conversation between patient and physician. Beauchamp and Childress have broken the informed consent process down into seven elements [*see Table 1*].[2]

The "threshold elements" (competence and voluntariness) are the preconditions necessary for appropriate informed consent. In its most basic sense, competence means the "ability to perform a task."[20] To exercise autonomy, a person

H. R. 3590

One Hundred Eleventh Congress of the United States of America

AT THE SECOND SESSION

Begun and held at the City of Washington on Tuesday, the fifth day of January, two thousand and ten

An Act

Entitled The Patient Protection and Affordable Care Act.

Be it enacted by the Senate and House of Representatives of the United States of America in Congress assembled,

"SEC. 1128G. TRANSPARENCY REPORTS AND REPORTING OF PHYSICIAN OWNERSHIP OR INVESTMENT INTERESTS.

"(a) TRANSPARENCY REPORTS.—

"(1) PAYMENTS OR OTHER TRANSFERS OF VALUE.—

"(A) IN GENERAL.—On March 31, 2013, and on the 90th day of each calendar year beginning thereafter, any applicable manufacturer that provides a payment or other transfer of value to a covered recipient (or to an entity or individual at the request of or designated on behalf of a covered recipient), shall submit to the Secretary, in such electronic form as the Secretary shall require, the following information with respect to the preceding calendar year:

"(i) The name of the covered recipient.

"(ii) The business address of the covered recipient and, in the case of a covered recipient who is a physician, the specialty and National Provider Identifier of the covered recipient.

"(iii) The amount of the payment or other transfer of value.

"(iv) The dates on which the payment or other transfer of value was provided to the covered recipient.

"(v) A description of the form of the payment or other transfer of value, indicated (as appropriate for all that apply) as—

"(I) cash or a cash equivalent;

"(II) in-kind items or services;

"(III) stock, a stock option, or any other ownership interest, dividend, profit, or other return on investment; or

"(IV) any other form of payment or other transfer of value (as defined by the Secretary).

H. R. 3590—572

"(vi) A description of the nature of the payment or other transfer of value, indicated (as appropriate for all that apply) as—

"(I) consulting fees;

"(II) compensation for services other than consulting;

"(III) honoraria;

"(IV) gift;

"(V) entertainment;

"(VI) food;

"(VII) travel (including the specified destinations);

"(VIII) education;

"(IX) research;

"(X) charitable contribution;

"(XI) royalty or license;

"(XII) current or prospective ownership or investment interest;

"(XIII) direct compensation for serving as faculty or as a speaker for a medical education program;

"(XIV) grant; or

"(XV) any other nature of the payment or other transfer of value (as defined by the Secretary).

"(vii) If the payment or other transfer of value is related to marketing, education, or research specific to a covered drug, device, biological, or medical supply, the name of that covered drug, device, biological, or medical supply.

"(viii) Any other categories of information regarding the payment or other transfer of value the Secretary determines appropriate.

Figure 2 Excerpt from the Patient Protection and Affordable Care Act.

Table 1 Seven Elements of Informed Consent[2]

I. Threshold elements (preconditions)
   1. Competence (to understand and decide)
   2. Voluntariness (in deciding)

II. Transformation elements
   3. Disclosure (of material information)
   4. Recommendation (of a plan)
   5. Understanding (of 3 and 4)

III. Consent elements
   6. Decision (in favor of a plan)
   7. Authorization (of the chosen plan)

must be competent. Whether a patient is competent to make decisions regarding medical care depends on his or her ability to comprehend information, his or her overall cognitive ability, and the ability to consider the consequences of the proposed treatment. The judging of competence in marginal cases is a complex task that should be approached with seriousness because a patient deemed not competent to make his or her own medical decisions will not be offered the opportunity to make decisions about his or her medical care. The other threshold element is voluntariness, that is, the condition in which decision making can be considered free from outside coercive influence.

The "transformation elements" are a second preliminary requirement for informed consent. Disclosure of material information is a fundamental part of the informed consent process and is often regarded as the main requirement of informed consent. Beauchamps and Childress sketched the basic information that should be disclosed in an informed consent; this includes the fourth element, recommendation [*see Table 2*].[2]

The final transformation element preliminary to informed consent is establishing that the patient understands the disclosure and the recommendation.

The "consent elements" comprise the action portion of the informed consent process that occurs after all of the preliminary conditions are met. A decision that is free from coercion must now be made by the patient. Finally, for the informed consent process to be complete, the patient must signify, usually in the form of a signed document, his or her authorization that the procedure may be carried out.

There is a legal perspective on informed consent that differs slightly from the ethical view just presented. Although the ethical basis of informed consent is a respect for autonomy, the courts have long focused on the disclosure element. Many civil litigation suits have been brought because of a lack of appropriate disclosure that was later shown to cause injury. There are three main norms that govern the disclosure of information to patients, and much of the legal environment surrounding informed consent has focused on these. The first is the "reasonable person standard," which

Table 2 The Transformation Elements[2]

1. Those facts or descriptions that patients or subjects usually consider material in deciding whether to refute or consent to the proposed intervention or research
2. Information the professional believes to be material
3. The professional's recommendation
4. The purpose of seeking consent
5. The nature and limits of consent as an act of authorization

suggests that what should be disclosed is that which an imaginary "reasonable person" would expect to be disclosed. Although this standard has gained traction in the courts, it has been criticized for its abstract nature: how should a reasonable person be imagined, and by whom? The second is the "subjective standard," which suggests that what should be disclosed is that which is required by the individual being consented. The third, the "professional practice standard" or the "reasonable doctor standard," suggests that what should be disclosed is simply that which is customary for the profession. The testimony that would count the most as evidence in a case in which the professional practice standard is emphasized is that of the other members of the profession. This version is problematic as well as it leaves out the patient entirely.

Refusal of Care

The care that surgeons provide is often invasive, visible, and temporarily, or even permanently, disabling. The principles surrounding the refusal of care by patients are therefore important for surgeons to know and to understand. There are several situations in which patients may refuse surgery or even certain elements of care. In this section, we review this central topic in surgical ethics.

Sometimes treatments that are considered to be the "standard of care" by contemporary surgeons are refused by patients based on their values and beliefs. Often such refusal can cause dissonance between surgeon and patient and can alter the outcome of surgery. One common such refusal is that of blood products by Jehovah's Witnesses. The guiding organization of the church of Jehovah's Witnesses, the Watchtower Society, introduced the policy regarding refusal of blood transfusions in 1945. The prohibition was initially enforced by "disfellowshipping" or expelling members who willingly accepted prohibited blood products, which included red and white blood cells, platelets, and plasma. In 2000, however, a directive was issued by the Watchtower Society stating that members would no longer be disfellowshipped if they did not comply with the refusal of blood.[21] Despite this policy change, the Jehovah's Witness who willingly accepts blood products can still be shunned by other members of this group.

A landmark case that established the right of any patient with sound decisional capacity to refuse treatment was *Schloendorff v. Society of New York Hospital*.[22] In 1914, Mary Schloendorff sued New York Hospital when a surgeon, who had consented her for an "exam under ether," surgically removed a fibroid tumor. Schloendorff suffered an infection and gangrene of several fingers, which ultimately led to their amputation in the postoperative period. Schloendorff alleged that the surgeon acted against her express wishes. Justice Cardozo of the New York Court of Appeals, who ruled in favor of Ms. Schloendorff, included the following statement in his decision:

> In the case at hand, the wrong complained of is not merely negligence. It is trespass. Every human being of adult years and sound mind has a right to determine what shall be done with his own body; and a surgeon who performs an operation without his patient's consent commits an assault, for which he is liable in damage.[22]

The strict observation of patient autonomy can break down when patients do not refuse entire recommended procedures (such as coronary artery bypass grafting) but rather pick and choose elements of the care necessary to perform such procedures (such as the administration of blood products). Most practicing surgeons are careful to standardize their practice in such a way that consistent outcomes are produced and outcomes from one patient to the next can be compared. The patient who refuses one element of that standard of care causes the surgeon to enter into clinical territory with which he or she is not familiar. Calculating the risk of doing cardiac surgery without blood transfusion, for example, is difficult as blood transfusion is common to the standard practice of that procedure. It is therefore difficult to appropriately consent a patient who refuses specific elements of care.

In the setting of major surgery, the refusal of blood products can be associated with a major risk of death, making the decision to operate on such patients a difficult one. In all cases, however, the patient's autonomy must prevail over almost every other consideration when the patient is competent and not a minor. In cases where the physician considers the patient not to be competent to make such a major decision, he or she may seek a court order permitting the blood transfusion. If a reasonable argument is presented that the negative effects of transfusion are outweighed by the positive, the court may permit the transfusion of blood.

The ethics also change when the patient is a minor and the patient's parents attempt to block the transfusion of blood products or other elements of care. This is probably the most common situation in which a court order is sought and the one for which court orders to transfuse are most commonly granted. Traditionally, the power to consent to or withhold medical treatment from a child lies with the child's parents or guardians. Unless the decision is made in the emergency setting, parental consent is necessary to perform any procedure on a child. Although courts have primarily granted these rights to parents, based on the right to raise children as a parent sees fit and the right to religious freedom, there are limits to these rights that rest on a parents' duty to promote the health of their children. In a 1944 US Supreme Court case, the groundwork for government oversight of child well-being was laid.[23] The following excerpt from the court's ruling summarizes it well: "Parents may be free to become martyrs themselves. But it does not follow they are free, in identical circumstances, to make martyrs of their children before they have reached the age of full and legal discretion when they can make that choice for themselves."[23]

Surgical Disparities

Justice is a fundamental principle in biomedical ethics that has specific applications in surgery; its fundamental meaning is "to be fair." Given that surgery is as much a social institution as it is a system of scientific thought, John Rawls's claim that justice "is the first virtue of social institutions, as truth is of systems of thought"[24] is apropos. When surgical outcomes are studied with regard to racial and socioeconomic lines, disparities seem to emerge that defy biology. Such studies suggest that members of racial minority groups and those of lower socioeconomic standing have worse outcomes than whites of higher socioeconomic standing.

The problem of disparities in surgical outcomes has been studied. In patients with nonmetastatic breast cancer,[25] rectal cancer,[26] and non–small cell lung cancer[27] in South Carolina, it was found that African-American race is an independent predictor of underuse of surgery.[25] Furthermore, blacks with colon cancer, breast cancer, and lung cancer are more likely than whites to present with advanced disease.[28] Selwyn Rogers and colleagues showed that although African-American race is associated with greater comorbidities and cardiac or renal complications, race itself is not an independent predictor of mortality after the most common general surgery procedures, implying that surgeons should focus on more effective treatment of comorbidities in these populations.[29]

The advent of large, collaborative, national databases has allowed researchers to gain insight into national trends. A recent National Surgical Quality Improvement Project (NSQIP) study showed that black, Hispanic, and American Indian/Alaskan Native surgical patients were more likely to have comorbidities, more likely to undergo more complex resections, and more likely to have longer postoperative hospital stays.[30] In another National Trauma Data Bank study, it was found that in 311,568 traumatically injured patients, those who presented to hospitals that treated a high percentage of minority patients had higher mortality rates.[31] In a different study, researchers studying kidney transplantation found that African-American patients with end-stage renal disease were 35 to 76% less likely to undergo kidney transplantation than their white counterparts.[32] All of these studies controlled for confounding variables that might cause minority patients to have such different outcomes.

Surgical outcomes have also been shown to differ in patients of differing socioeconomic status. A study performed at the Harvard School of Public Health in 2011 noted that uninsured patients in a National Trauma Data Bank sample had markedly lower odds of being transferred to a skilled nursing facility, home with home health, or a rehabilitation facility.[33] Low socioeconomic status and lack of insurance have also been linked to disparities in outcome for thyroid,[34] colon,[35] and lung cancer.[36]

Just what a surgeon's response to these injustices should be has not been fully elucidated. The important concepts that are being weighed against each other when answering this question are those of liberalism and justice. The idea of liberalism saturates American culture. It is the idea that individuals should be completely free from interference with respect to their activity, autonomous, and self-directed. Contrast this to notions of justice, which may require individuals to give up certain freedoms to ensure an egalitarian society. Attempts to increase levels of justice within a society can sometimes be seen as diminishing other individuals' liberty.

The view that most strongly supports an egalitarian view is known as "the justice perspective" on public health.[37] It aims to ameliorate wrongs within our health care infrastructure that arose outside of it. The justice perspective hopes to provide a counterweight to a prevailing opinion that health is simply a matter of personal, individual responsibility.

Here, reaching outside of what is usually considered the health care system seems necessary. The root causes of ill health are many and are often rooted in deeper socioeconomic circumstances, many of which test the limits of the expertise of the medical community. For example, it is known that people in severe urban poverty in the United States have little or no access to fresh fruits and vegetables.[38] Other so-called social determinants of health include access to fresh water, levels of health literacy, birth weight, and chronic stress, among others. Several studies have shown that the effect of race on cancer stage at presentation might be confounded by socioeconomic factors, including education, income, and insurance status.[39,40]

Another view of justice in health care is that disparities that exist due to social determinants of health should not be allowed to propagate within the health care system but may not be amenable to intervention given the limits of medicine. Patients may present with different starting conditions, but the treatment they receive will be equivalent, and when controlling for the severity of disease, outcomes will be equal for all comers.

A third view is to see health solely as a matter of personal responsibility. Here, although disparities in outcomes might be acknowledged, they should not be the concern of the health care community. Rather, such disparities arise from inequities that will persist despite the efforts of the medical establishment. In this view, it is not incumbent on the health care industry to equalize outcomes for those who present for care. Instead, money should buy better care, and those who can afford it will buy better care that will lead to better outcomes for them.

Unconscious bias may play a role in disparities in outcomes. One survey studying the unconscious biases of medical students entering the Johns Hopkins School of Medicine revealed that 69% had implicit preferences toward white persons and 89% toward persons of the upper class.[41] It is possible that freshman medical students arrive at medical school with such views already solidified. If this is a way that disparities might arise, it is incumbent upon surgeons to work with student populations in such a way so as to determine the influence of these unconscious biases in patient care.

In its *Statement on Healthcare Disparities*, the ACS states that "ethnic and racial health care disparities have no role in a humane and just society, and are ethically and morally antithetical to the practice of medicine and surgery."[42] The recent strong scholarship being done in the field of racial and socioeconomic disparities in surgical outcome and this 2010 statement by the ACS suggest that such problems are becoming more prominent in the contemporary era and are being taken seriously.

Racial Diversity in the Surgical Workforce

Diversity is a descriptive characteristic of a group of people who exhibit differences in their demographic makeup, cultural identities or ethnicity, and training and expertise.[43] Scholars have suggested that diverse groups are better at solving problems and making predictions if the diversity of the group is appropriately leveraged.[44,45] It is not presently known what the degree of racial or socioeconomic diversity is in the contemporary American surgical workforce.

The problem of disparities seems related to the problem of diversity in the surgical workforce. Understanding how they are related is a major challenge in contemporary surgical ethics. A common misconception is an oversimplification, in which it is suggested that underserved racial minorities, if recruited into medical specialties, will, out of obligation, return to practice in the communities from which they came. Proponents of such thinking suggest that if we could only recruit minorities, this will likely lead to a decrease in health care disparities through this duty of obligation. The lack of diversity in the workforce, however, is probably related to the problem of disparities in health in a more complex way. Although it may be true that a more diverse surgical workforce will lead to improvements in the disparities in health outcomes discussed above, it should not be out of a moral obligation imposed on physicians from minority backgrounds.

The causative factors that might lead to the lack of racial diversity in the medical workforce have been studied. Andriole and Jeffe recently published the results of a retrospective study in which 97,445 US medical school matriculants were examined for causative factors that might lead to suboptimal performance outcomes.[46] It was found that nonwhite race/ethnicity and premedical debt greater than $50,000 were independently associated with a greater likelihood of academic withdrawal or dismissal and graduation without first-attempt passing scores on the US Medical Licensing Examination Step 1 and/or Step 2 Clinical Knowledge. This study suggests that the details of potential surgeons' lives, even before they are in a position to apply for residency training, might play as large a role as anything in what lack of diversity in the surgical workforce there may be.

In contrast to the relative interest in racial and socioeconomic disparities in surgical outcomes, the data regarding diversity in the workforce are scant. As Cohen and colleagues pointed out, the US research agenda is predominantly set by investigators who become curious about scientific problems in a way that is very dependent on "personal culture and ethnic filters."[47] This statement is certainly applicable to the scientific progress of surgery. Lee Bollinger, president of Columbia University, has argued that nurturing an educational setting that is rich in ethnic and cultural diversity is the most important way to prepare students to work in a diverse society and that simply learning about cultural and ethnic diversity is not enough: students must be immersed in a learning environment that is rich with such diversity.[48] US medical schools should strive to enrich the ethnic and sociocultural diversity of their student bodies, thereby developing environments in which not only will the future physicians they produce be best able to function in the diverse society in which we live, but also physician-investigators will find their interests being sparked by a broader and richer set of problems.

Surgeons have addressed the problem of diversity in the workforce. The ACS currently supports a committee on diversity issues, which exists to "study the educational and professional needs of underrepresented surgeons and surgical trainees and the impact that its work may have on the elimination of health disparities among diverse population groups."[49] The ACS, which is the largest organization of surgeons in the United States, however, does not currently collect data on the racial identification of its members. This, in combination with the American Board of Surgery's similar stance on collecting demographic data, makes it difficult to know just how diverse the surgical workforce is. The diversity of the surgery workforce may parallel that of the overall physician workforce in terms of racial distribution, however, which is known. In 2008, although blacks, Hispanics, and Native American populations comprised 12.8%, 15.4%, and 1%, respectively, of the US population in total,[50] these groups comprised only a mere 3.5%, 4.8%, and 0.1%, respectively, of the total number of physicians in the United States.[51]

The recent academic interest in racial disparities in surgical outcome may reflect an increased level of sensitivity regarding these issues in the surgical workforce. The challenge is to increase the level of diversity in the surgical workforce while also recognizing at what level this increased diversity can be leveraged to decrease disparities in surgical outcomes. Once this is realized, it is likely that many other benefits of a diverse workforce will be realized.

Equipoise and Research Ethics

The surgical profession in the United States has a strong tradition of research. The simple notion that surgery is "scientific" has its roots in the fact that much of what surgeons do is based on a foundation generated from research. Research ethics is therefore a fundamental part of surgical ethics.

Human subjects research is a socially valuable component of surgical practice that can be morally troublesome because some of this research exposes subjects to risk. The question of what makes research ethically justifiable has been subject to scrutiny over the last several decades. The evolution of the concept of what makes research ethical has primarily been a response to events that occurred in the historical conduct of research. The Nuremberg Code, for example, was written as part of a judicial ruling in response to atrocious Nazi human experiments conducted during the 20th century.[52] Other such documents include the Belmont Report,[53] the Declaration of Helsinki,[54] and the International Ethical Guidelines for Biomedical Research Involving Human Subjects.[55]

In many clinical research settings, there is an emphasis on informed consent. Often this emphasis can eclipse other ethical issues that might be salient. Emanuel and colleagues offered an exhaustive list of conditions that make clinical research ethically justifiable [*see Table 3*].[56] First, the research must have, as its goal, an end point that will improve health or increase knowledge. Second, ethical research must be designed in a scientifically valid way so that the results of the research will be reliable enough that it will satisfy the first requirement. Part of ensuring that research is scientifically valid is to verify that true clinical equipoise exists (discussed below). Third, justice must be observed in that vulnerable populations are not made the only subjects of risky research and that participation in potentially beneficial research be made possible for all members of society. Fourth, a favorable risk-to-benefit ratio should be achieved in that risks should be minimized and proportional to the benefits gained for the individual, as well as the benefits for society. Fifth, the research should be subject to independent review and be made publicly accountable, such as by review by an Institutional Review Board (IRB). Sixth, informed consent should be obtained out of respect for the study subjects' autonomy. Finally, the welfare and privacy of study subjects should be monitored and protected. It is generally accepted that clinical research should not go ahead unless these criteria are met.

Given that clinic research is a complex and continuously changing endeavor, it is necessary for public policy and review committees to ensure that ongoing research meets ethical standards. The most common way for this to be achieved is through IRBs. IRBs are entities empowered by the Department of Health and Human Services to approve or disapprove proposed research studies in their institutions. IRBs are governed by Title 45 Code of Federal Regulations Part 46, "Protection of Human Subjects."[57] IRBs are positioned in universities and other research institutions, including those in the private sector. They consist of individuals who are able to understand research protocols and others, including members who are part of the community but not part of the institution. They serve to rule on whether a research protocol proposed to it satisfies the ethical requirements laid out in the aforementioned Title 45 Code.[58]

Special mention should also be made of the notion of clinical equipoise. Clinical equipoise is the situation in which there is consensus among experts that clinical evidence does not weigh in favor of either of the treatments being compared. The reason that this is ethically important is that if one of the two treatments is found to be more efficacious, then it would be wrong not to offer it to patients. The notion itself has undergone some evolution. The original concept of equipoise was put forth by Charles Fried.[59] Fried's characterization of equipoise required individual researchers to have genuine uncertainty about the relative merits of each arm of a trial. The notion of clinical equipoise was introduced by Benjamin Freedman in 1987 in a *New England Journal of Medicine* article in which he argued that the standard put forth by Fried is simply too difficult to adhere to as most researchers have some rudimentary data that might push them in favor of one treatment or another.[60] In clinical equipoise, the "moral locus" is shifted from the individual researcher to the community of responsible researchers, who must honestly disagree about which treatment arm is preferred.

The notion of equipoise becomes most important when physician-researchers begin to enrol their own patients into clinical trials that they are conducting. In this setting, the clinician must question whether the proposed treatment (whether or not it is an experimental one) is the best one for the patient. When research comes into play, the clinician must maintain a standard of beneficence and must believe that no matter which treatment arm the patient is enrolled into, the same potential for benefit exists. In 1987, Appelbaum and colleagues introduced the concept of the therapeutic misconception.[61] The term refers to the false belief, on

Table 3 Seven Requirements for Determining Whether a Research Trial Is Ethical[56]

1	Value	The research must have an end point that will improve health or increase knowledge
2	Validity	Results of the research must be reliable enough to satisfy the first requirement
3	Fair selection	Justice must be observed in the selection of study subjects
4	Risk-to-benefit ratio	A favorable risk-to-benefit ratio should be achieved
5	Independent review	The research should be made publically accountable through independent review
6	Informed consent	Appropriate informed consent should be obtained
7	Respect for subjects	Welfare and privacy of study subjects should be monitored and protected

the part of research subjects who are also patients, that a research protocol in which they are enrolled is designed to benefit them directly, not only to test competing therapies or produce scientific knowledge. Even subjects who understand randomization, blinding, and placebo controls often falsely believe that they will be placed into the more therapeutic arm of a trial. It is incumbent upon the physician-researcher to minimize the degree of therapeutic misconception in patients when enrolling them in a clinical trial.

Summary

A tradition of ethics is embedded in the practice of surgery. The principles outlined in this chapter are substantial and can be taught. In the plural societies in which most surgeons practice, there will be times at which moral intuitions disagree. Therefore, not only moral knowledge but also moral reasoning is of utmost importance. Moral reasoning can be learned, practiced, and honed in much the same way that surgical skills can. It is important that ethics be a part of surgical training and be incorporated into every surgical practice.

Financial Disclosures: None Reported

References

1. Bosk CL. Forgive and remember: managing medical failure. 2nd ed. Chicago: University of Chicago Press; 2003.
2. Beauchamp TL, Childress JF. Principles of biomedical ethics. 6th ed. New York: Oxford University Press; 2008.
3. Gregor M, Timmermann J, Kosgaard C, editors. Kant: Groundwork of the metaphysics of morals (Cambridge texts in the history of philosophy). 2nd ed. New York: Cambridge University Press; 2012.
4. Toulmin S. How medicine saved the life of ethics. Perspect Biol Med 1982;25:736–50.
5. Jaworska A. Advance directives and substitute decision-making. In: Zalta EN, editor. The Stanford encyclopedia of philosophy. 2009. Available at: http://plato.stanford.edu/archives/sum2009/entries/advance-directives/ (accessed September 13, 2012).
6. Center for Ethics in Health Care, Oregon Health and Sciences University. History of the POLST Paradigm Initiative. 2008. Available at: http://www.ohsu.edu/polst/developing/history.htm (accessed September 13, 2012).
7. Perkins HS. Controlling death: the false promise of advance directives. Ann Intern Med 2007;147:51–7.
8. Burns JP, Truog RD. Futility: a concept in evolution. Chest 2007;132:1987–93.
9. Plows CW, Tenery RM Jr, Hartford A, et al. Medical futility in end-of-life care - report of the Council on Ethical and Judicial Affairs. JAMA 1999;281:937–41.
10. American Medical Association. Conflict of interest policy and statement on disclosure of affiliations. 1999. Available at: http://www.ama-assn.org/ama1/pub/upload/mm/37/coi-policy.doc (accessed December 21, 2009).
11. Pharmaceutical Research and Manufacturers of America (PhRMA). Code on interactions with healthcare professionals. 200[illegible]. Available at: http://www.phrma.org/files/attachments/PhRMA%20Marketing%20Code%202008.pdf (accessed December 21, 2009).
12. National Institutes of Health Ethics Program. Conflict of interest. 2008. Available at: http://ethics.od.nih.gov/topics/coi.htm (accessed December 21, 2009).
13. American College of Surgeons. Conflict of interest policy. Officers, officers-elect, board of regents, board of governors executive committee, editor-in-chief of the American College of Surgeons and its affiliated organizations. June 2002. Available at: http://www.facs.org/about/policy.pdf (accessed October 3, 2012).
14. Institute of Medicine. Conflict of interest in medical research, education, and practice. Washington (DC): National Academies Press; 2009. Available at: http://www.iom.edu/en/Reports/2009/Conflict-of-Interest-in-Medical-Research-Education-and-Practice.aspx (accessed October 30, 2009).
15. Association of American Medical Colleges. Industry funding of medical education report of an AAMC task force. Available at: http://services.aamc.org/publications/showfile.cfm?file=version114.pdf&prd_id=232 (accessed October 30, 2009).
16. Keune JD, Vig S, Hall BL, et al. Taking disclosure seriously: disclosing financial conflicts of interest at the American College of Surgeons. J Am Coll Surg 2011;212:215–24.
17. Okike K, Kocher MS, Wei EX, et al. Accuracy of conflict-of-interest disclosures reported by physicians. N Engl J Med 2009;361:1466–74.
18. Brandeis L. What publicity can do. Harper's Weekly 1913; Dec 20: 1.
19. Patient Protection and Affordable Care Act (PPACA), Pub. L. 111-148, 124 Stat. 119 through 124 Stat. 1025 (March 23, 2010).
20. Culver CM, Gert B. Philosophy in medicine. New York: Oxford University Press; 1982.

21. Muramoto O. Bioethical aspects of the recent changes in the policy of refusal of blood by Jehovah's Witnesses. BMJ 2001;322:37–9.
22. Mary E. Schloendorff, Appellant, v. The Society of the New York Hospital, Respondent Court of Appeals of New York, 211 N.Y. 125; 105 N.E. 92 (1914).
23. Prince v. Massachusetts, Supreme Court of the United States, 321 U.S. 158 (1944).
24. Rawls J. A theory of justice. Oxford (UK): Oxford University Press; 1999.
25. Esnaola NF, Knott K, Finney C, et al. Urban/rural residence moderates effect of race on receipt of surgery in patients with nonmetastatic breast cancer: a report from the South Carolina central cancer registry. Ann Surg Oncol 2008;15: 1828–36.
26. Esnaola NF, Gebregziabher M, Finney C, Ford ME. Underuse of surgical resection in black patients with nonmetastatic colorectal cancer: location, location, location. Ann Surg 2009;250:549–57.
27. Esnaola NF, Gebregziabher M, Knott K, et al. Underuse of surgical resection for localized, non-small cell lung cancer among whites and African Americans in South Carolina. Ann Thorac Surg 2008;86:220–6; discussion 227.
28. Siegel R, Ward E, Brawley O, Jemal A. Cancer statistics, 2011: the impact of eliminating socioeconomic and racial disparities on premature cancer deaths. CA Cancer J Clin 2011;61:212–36.
29. Esnaola NF, Hall BL, Hosokawa PW, et al. Race and surgical outcomes: it is not all black and white. Ann Surg 2008; 248:647–55.
30. Parsons HM, Habermann EB, Stain SC, et al. What What happens to racial and ethnic minorities after cancer surgery at American College of Surgeons National Surgical Quality Improvement Program hospitals? J Am Coll Surg 2012;214: 539–-47; discussion 547-9.
31. Haider AH, Ong'uti S, Efron DT, et al. Association between hospitals caring for a disproportionately high percentage of minority trauma patients and increased mortality: a nationwide analysis of 434 hospitals. Arch Surg 2012;147:63–70.
32. Hall EC, James NT, Garonzik Wang JM, et al. Center-level factors and racial disparities in living donor kidney transplantation. Am J Kidney Dis 2012;59:849–57.
33. Sacks GD, Hill C, Rogers SO Jr. Insurance status and hospital discharge disposition after trauma: inequities in access to postacute care. J Trauma 2011;71:1011–5.
34. Lim II, Hochman T, Blumberg SN, et al. Disparities in the initial presentation of differentiated thyroid cancer in a large public hospital and adjoining university teaching hospital. Thyroid 2012;22:269–74.
35. Halpern MT, Ward EM, Pavluck AL, et al. Association of insurance status and ethnicity with cancer stage at diagnosis for 12 cancer sites: a retrospective analysis. Lancet Oncol 2008;9:222–31.
36. Yorio JT, Xie Y, Yan J, Gerber DE. Lung cancer diagnostic and treatment intervals in the United States: a health care disparity? J Thorac Oncol 2009;4:1322–30.
37. Gostin LO, Powers M. What does social justice require for the public's health? Public health ethics and policy imperatives. Health Aff (Millwood) 2006;25:1053–60.
38. Algert SJ, Agrawal A, Lewis DS. Disparities in access to fresh produce in low-income neighborhoods in Los Angeles. Am J Prev Med 2006;30:365–70.
39. Hegarty V, Burchett BM, Gold DT, et al. Racial differences in use of cancer prevention services among older Americans. J Am Geriatr Soc 2000;48:735–40.
40. Bradley CJ, Given CW, Roberts C. Disparities in cancer diagnosis and survival. Cancer 2001;91:178–88.
41. Haider AH, Sexton J, Sriram N, et al. Association of unconscious race and social class bias with vignette-based clinical assessments by medical students. JAMA 2011;306:942–51.
42. American College of Surgeons. Statement on healthcare disparities. November 16, 2010. Available at: http://www.facs.org/fellows_info/statements/st-67.html (accessed February 16, 2012).
43. Hong L, Page SE. Groups of diverse problem solvers can outperform groups of high-ability problem solvers. Proc Natl Acad Sci U S A 2004;101:16385–9.
44. Thomas DA, Ely RJ. Making differences matter: a new paradigm for managing diversity. Harvard Business Rev 1996;74:79–90.
45. Page SE. The difference: how the power of diversity creates better groups, firms, schools, and societies. Princeton (NJ): Princeton University Press; 2008.
46. Andriole DA, Jeffe DB. Prematriculation variables associated with suboptimal outcomes for the 1994-1999 cohort of US medical school matriculants. JAMA 2010;304:1212–9.
47. Cohen JJ, Gabriel BA, Terrell C. The case for diversity in the health care workforce. Health Aff (Millwood) 2002;21:90–102.
48. Bollinger LC. The need for diversity in higher education. Acad Med 2003;78:431–6.
49. American College of Surgeons. Committee on Diversity Issues. Committees of the American College of Surgeons. Available at: http://www.facs.org/about/committees/index.html#diversity (accessed April 1, 2012).
50. US Census Bureau. Population, race – Hispanic origin. The 2012 statistical abstract: USA statistics in brief. Available at: http:/www.census.gov/compendia/statab/brief.html (accessed April 1, 2012).
51. Smart DR. Physician characteristics and distribution in the US, 2010. Chicago: American Medical Association; 2010.
52. The Nuremberg Code. JAMA 1996;276:1691.
53. National Commission for the Protection of Human Subjects of Biomedical and Behavioral Research. The Belmont report. Washington (DC): US Government Printing Office; 1979.
54. World Medical Association. Declaration of Helsinki. JAMA 1997;277:925–6.
55. Council for International Organizations of Medical Sciences. International ethical guidelines for biomedical research involving human subjects. Geneva: Council for International Organizations of Medical Sciences; 1993.
56. Emanuel EJ, Wendler D, Grady C. What makes clinical research ethical? JAMA 2000;283:2701–11.
57. Department of Health and Human Services. Code of Federal Regulations. Title 45 public welfare. Part 46. Protection of Human Subjects. Available at: http://www.hhs.gov/ohrp/humansubjects/guidance/45cfr46.html (accessed October 17, 2012).

58. Jonsen AR, Siegler M, Winslade WJ. Clinical ethics: a practical approach to ethical decisions in clinical medicine. 7th ed. New York (NY): McGraw-Hill; 2010.
59. Fried C. Medical experimentation: personal integrity and social policy. Amsterdam: North Holland; 1974.
60. Freedman B. Equipoise and the ethics of clinical research. N Engl J Med 1987;317:141–5.
61. Appelbaum PS, Roth LH, Lidz CW, et al. False hopes and best data: consent to research and the therapeutic misconception. Hastings Cent Rep 1987;17(2):20–4.

1 PREVENTION OF POSTOPERATIVE INFECTION

Jonathan L. Meakins, MD, DSc, FACS

Epidemiology of Surgical Site Infection

Historically, the control of wound infection depended on antiseptic and aseptic techniques directed at coping with the infecting organism. In the 19th century and the early part of the 20th century, wound infections had devastating consequences and a measurable mortality. Even in the 1960s, before the correct use of antibiotics and the advent of modern preoperative and postoperative care, as much as one quarter of a surgical ward might have been occupied by patients with wound complications. As a result, wound management, in itself, became an important component of ward care and of medical education. It is fortunate that many factors have intervened so that the so-called wound rounds have become a practice of the past. The epidemiology of wound infection has changed as surgeons have learned to control bacteria and the inoculum and to focus increasingly on the patient (the host) for measures that will continue to provide improved results.

The following three factors are the determinants of any infectious process[1]:

1. The infecting organism (in surgical patients, usually bacteria)
2. The environment in which the infection takes place (the local response)
3. The host defense mechanisms, which deal systemically with the infectious process

Wounds are particularly appropriate for analysis of infection with respect to these three determinants. Because many components of the bacterial contribution to wound infection now are clearly understood and measures to control bacteria have been implemented, the host factors become more apparent. In addition, interactions between the three determinants play a critical role, and with limited exceptions (e.g., massive contamination), few infections will be the result of only one factor [*see Figure 1*].

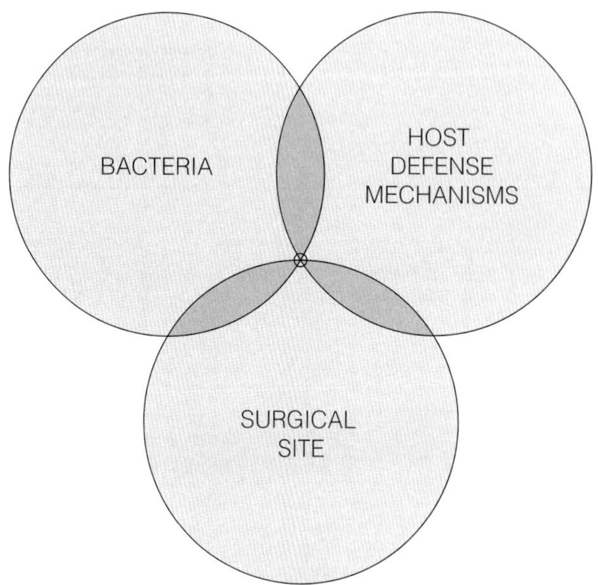

Figure 1 **In a homeostatic, normal state, the determinants of any infectious process—bacteria, the surgical site, and host defense mechanisms (represented by three circles)—intersect at a point indicating zero probability of sepsis.**

Definition of Surgical Site Infection

Wound infections have traditionally been thought of as infections in a surgical wound occurring between the skin and the deep soft tissues—a view that fails to consider the operative site as a whole. As prevention of these wound infections has become more effective, it has become apparent that definitions of operation-related infection must take the entire operative field into account; obvious examples include sternal and mediastinal infections, vascular graft infections, and infections associated with implants (if occurring within 1 year of the procedure and apparently related to it). Accordingly, the Centers for Disease Control and Prevention currently prefers to use the term *surgical site infection* (SSI). SSIs can be classified into three categories: superficial incisional SSIs (involving only skin and subcutaneous tissue), deep incisional SSIs (involving deep soft tissue), and organ or space SSIs (involving anatomic areas other than the incision itself that are opened or manipulated in the course of the procedure) [*see Figure 2*].[2,3]

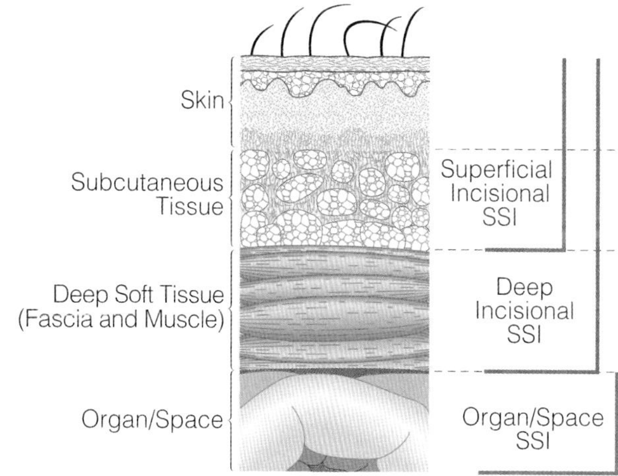

Figure 2 **Surgical site infections (SSI) are classified into three categories, depending on which anatomic areas are affected.**[3]

Epidemiology of Surgical Site Infection

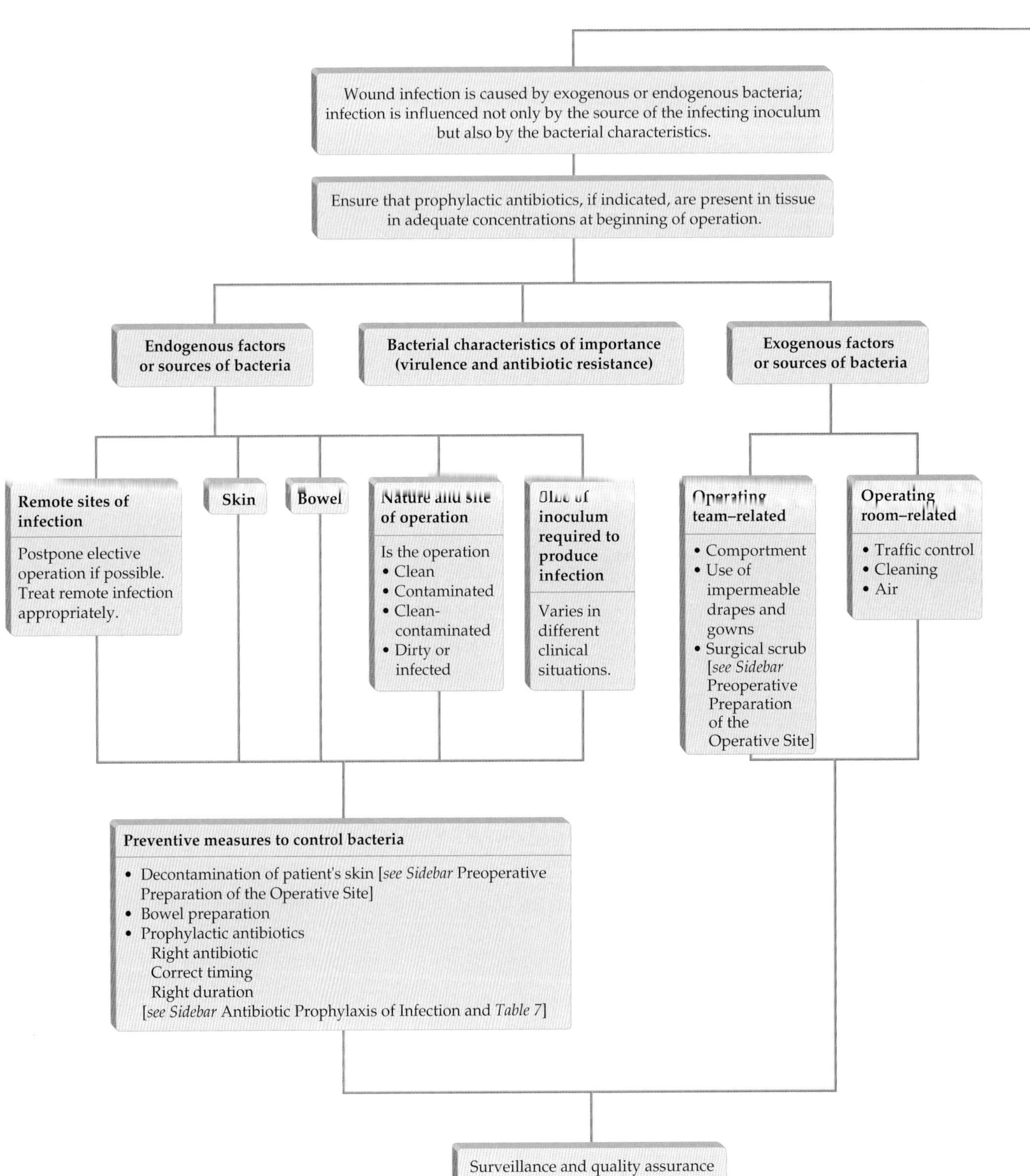

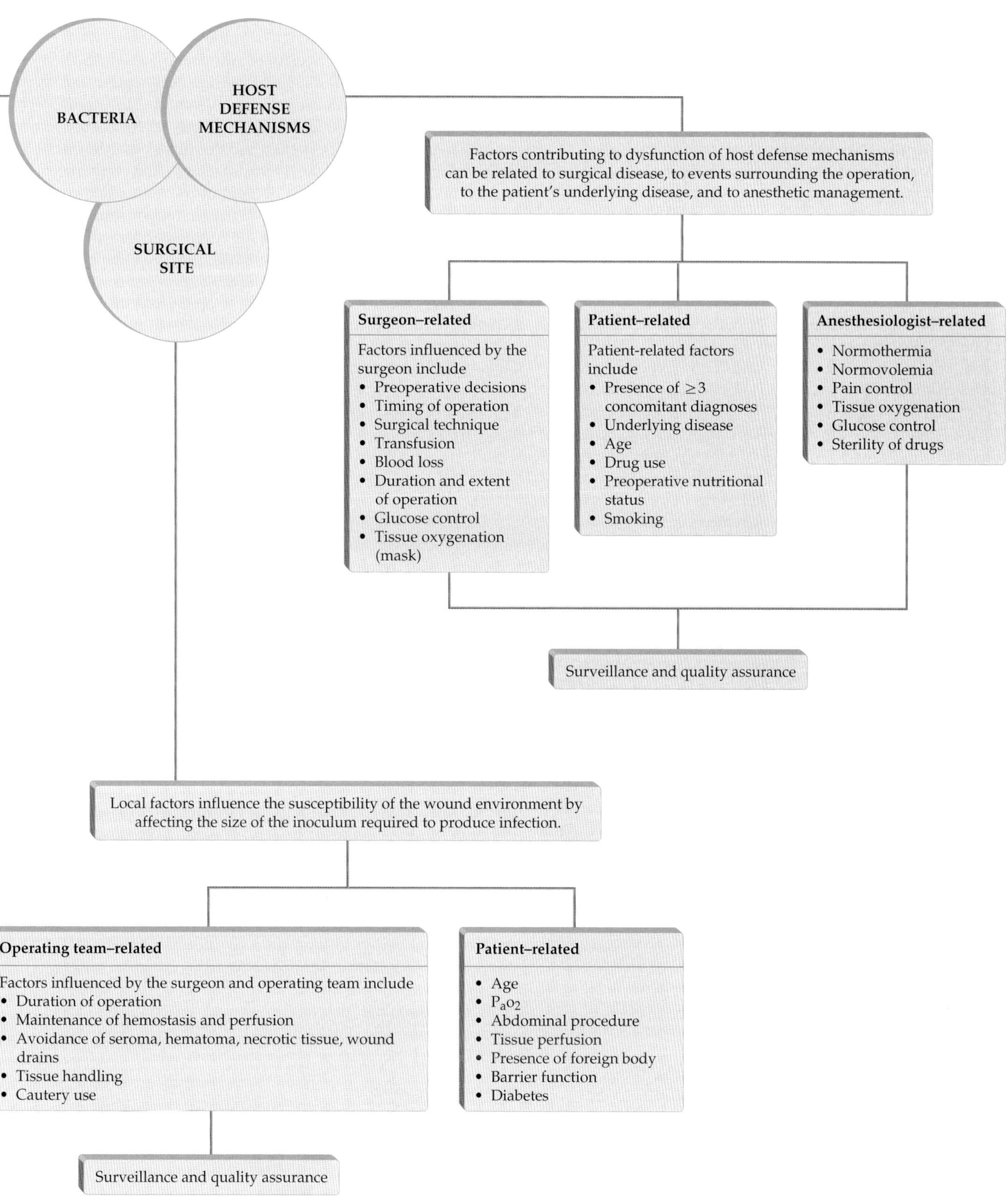
BACTERIA
HOST DEFENSE MECHANISMS
SURGICAL SITE
Factors contributing to dysfunction of host defense mechanisms can be related to surgical disease, to events surrounding the operation, to the patient's underlying disease, and to anesthetic management.
Surgeon–related
Factors influenced by the surgeon include
• Preoperative decisions
• Timing of operation
• Surgical technique
• Transfusion
• Blood loss
• Duration and extent of operation
• Glucose control
• Tissue oxygenation (mask)
Patient–related
Patient-related factors include
• Presence of ≥3 concomitant diagnoses
• Underlying disease
• Age
• Drug use
• Preoperative nutritional status
• Smoking
Anesthesiologist–related
• Normothermia
• Normovolemia
• Pain control
• Tissue oxygenation
• Glucose control
• Sterility of drugs
Surveillance and quality assurance
Local factors influence the susceptibility of the wound environment by affecting the size of the inoculum required to produce infection.
Operating team–related
Factors influenced by the surgeon and operating team include
• Duration of operation
• Maintenance of hemostasis and perfusion
• Avoidance of seroma, hematoma, necrotic tissue, wound drains
• Tissue handling
• Cautery use
Patient–related
• Age
• P_aO_2
• Abdominal procedure
• Tissue perfusion
• Presence of foreign body
• Barrier function
• Diabetes
Surveillance and quality assurance

Standardization in reporting will permit more effective surveillance and improve results, as well as offer a painless way of achieving quality assurance. The natural tendency to deny that a surgical site has become infected contributes to the difficulty of defining SSI in a way that is both accurate and acceptable to surgeons. The surgical view of SSI recalls one judge's (probably apocryphal) remark about pornography: "It is hard to define, but I know it when I see it." SSIs are usually easy to identify. Nevertheless, there is a critical need for definitions of SSI that can be applied in different institutions for use as performance indicators.[4] The criteria on which such definitions must be based are more detailed than the simple apocryphal remark just cited; they are outlined more fully elsewhere [*see 2:6 Preparation of the Operating Room*].

STRATIFICATION OF RISK FOR SSI

The National Academy of Sciences–National Research Council classification of wounds [*see Table 1*], published in 1964, was a landmark in the field.[5] This report provided incontrovertible data to show that wounds could be classified as a function of probability of bacterial contamination (usually endogenous) in a consistent manner. Thus, wound infection rates could be validly compared from month to month, between services, and between hospitals. As surgery became more complex in the following decades, however, antibiotic use became more standardized and other risk variables began to assume greater prominence. In the early 1980s, the Study on the Efficacy of Nosocomial Infection Control (SENIC) identified three risk factors in addition to wound class: location of the operation (abdomen or chest), duration of the operation, and patient clinical status (three or more diagnoses on discharge).[6] The National Nosocomial Infection Surveillance (NNIS) study reduced these four risk factors to three: wound classification, duration of the operation, and American Society of Anesthesiologists (ASA) class III, IV, or V.[7,8] Both risk assessments integrate the three determinants of infection: bacteria (wound class), local environment (duration), and systemic host defenses (one definition of patient health status), and they have been shown to be applicable outside the United States.[9] However, the SENIC and NNIS assessments do not integrate other known risk variables, such as smoking, tissue oxygen tension, glucose control, shock, and maintenance of normothermia, all of which are relevant for clinicians (although they are often hard to monitor and to fit into a manageable risk assessment). In addition, they do not incorporate a variety of other host variables or operation characteristics derived from the Patient Safety in Surgery Study/National Surgical Quality Improvement Program (NSQIP). These give high, medium, and low probabilities of SSI, which appear to be more accurate but more complex to ascertain than NNIS prediction [*see* Integration of Determinants *below*].[10]

Table 1 National Research Council Classification of Operative Wounds[5]

Clean (class I)	Nontraumatic No inflammation encountered No break in technique Respiratory, alimentary, or genitourinary tract not entered
Clean-contaminated (class II)	Gastrointestinal or respiratory tract entered without significant spillage Appendectomy Oropharynx entered Vagina entered Genitourinary tract entered in absence of infected urine Biliary tract entered in absence of infected bile Minor break in technique
Contaminated (class III)	Major break in technique Gross spillage from gastrointestinal tract Traumatic wound, fresh Entrance of genitourinary or biliary tracts in presence of infected urine or bile
Dirty and infected (class IV)	Acute bacterial inflammation encountered, without pus Transection of "clean" tissue for the purpose of surgical access to a collection of pus Traumatic wound with retained devitalized tissue, foreign bodies, fecal contamination, delayed treatment, or all of these or from dirty source

Bacteria

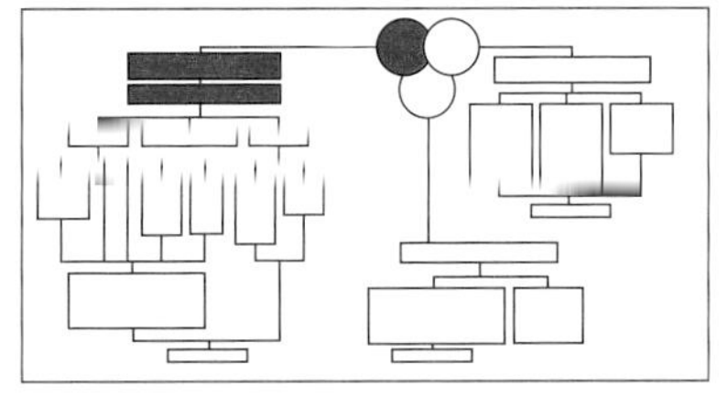

Clearly, without an infecting agent, no infection will result. Accordingly, most of what is known about bacteria is put to use in major efforts directed at reducing their numbers by means of asepsis and antisepsis. The principal concept is based on the size of the bacterial inoculum.

Wounds are traditionally classified according to whether the wound inoculum of bacteria is likely to be large enough to overwhelm local and systemic host defense mechanisms and produce an infection [*see Table 1*]. One study showed that the most important factor in the development of a wound infection was the number of bacteria present in the wound at the end of an operative procedure.[11] Another quantitated this relation and provided insight into how local environmental factors might be integrated into an understanding of the problem [*see Figure 3*].[12] In the years before prophylactic antibiotics, as well as during the early phases of their use, there was a very clear relation between the classification of the operation (which is related to the probability of a significant inoculum) and the rate of wound infection.[5,13] This relation is now less dominant than it once was; therefore, other factors have come to play a significant role.[6,14]

CONTROL OF SOURCES OF BACTERIA

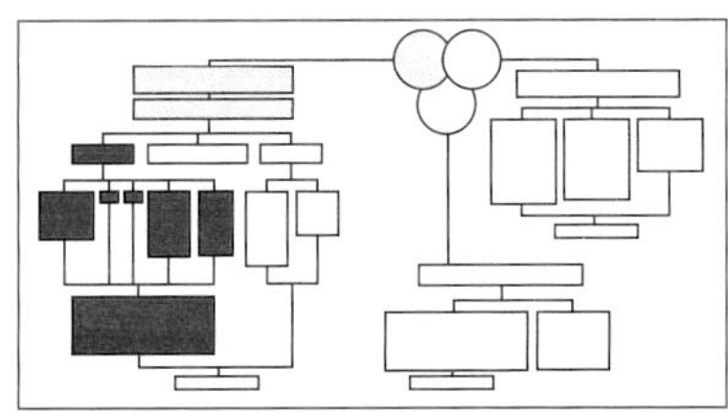

Endogenous bacteria are a more important cause of SSI than exogenous bacteria. In clean-contaminated, contaminated, and dirty-infected operations, the source and

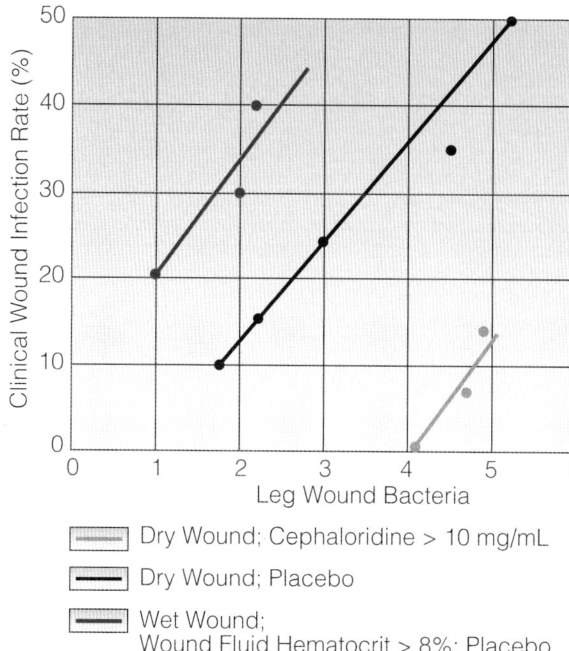

Figure 3 **The wound infection rate is shown here as a function of bacterial inoculum in three different situations: a dry wound with an adequate concentration of antibiotic (cephaloridine > 10 µg/mL), a dry wound with no antibiotic (placebo), and a wet wound with no antibiotic (placebo, wound fluid hematocrit > 8%).**[12]

the amount of bacteria are functions of the patient's disease and the specific organs being operated on.

Operations classified as infected are those in which infected tissue and pus are removed or drained, providing a guaranteed inoculum to the surgical site. The inoculum may be as high as 10^{10} bacteria/mL, some of which may already be producing an infection. In addition, some bacteria could be in the growth phase rather than the dormant or lag phase and thus could be more pathogenic. The heavily contaminated wound is best managed by delayed primary closure. This type of management ensures that the wound is not closed over a bacterial inoculum that is almost certain to cause a wound infection, with attendant early and late consequences.

Patients should not have elective surgery in the presence of remote infection, which is associated with an increased incidence of wound infection.[5] In patients with urinary tract infections, wounds frequently become infected with the same organism. Remote infections should be treated appropriately, and the operation should proceed only under the best conditions possible. If the operation cannot be appropriately delayed, the use of prophylactic and therapeutic antibiotics should be considered [*see Sidebar* Antibiotic Prophylaxis of Infection *and Tables 2 through 4*].

Preoperative techniques of reducing patient flora, especially endogenous bacteria, are of great concern. Bowel preparation, antimicrobial showers or baths, and preoperative skin decontamination have been proposed frequently. These techniques, particularly preoperative skin decontamination [*see Sidebar* Preoperative Preparation of the Operative Site], may have specific roles in selected patients during epidemics or in units with high infection rates. As a routine for all patients, however, these techniques are unnecessary, time-consuming, and costly in institutions or units where infection rates are low.

The preoperative shave is a technique in need of reassessment. It is now clear that shaving the evening before an operation is associated with an increased wound infection rate. This increase is secondary to the trauma of the shave and the inevitable small areas of inflammation and infection. If hair removal is required,[15] clipping is preferable and should be done in the OR or the preparation room just before the operative procedure. Shaving, if ever performed, should not be done the night before the operation.

In the past few years, the role of the classic bowel preparation [*see Table 5*] has been questioned [*see* Discussion, Infection Prevention in Bowel Surgery, *below*].[16–21] The suggestion has been made that selective gut decontamination (SGD) may be useful in major elective procedures involving the upper gastrointestinal (GI) tract and perhaps in other settings. At present, SGD for prevention of infection cannot be recommended in either the preoperative or the postoperative period.

When infection develops after clean operations, particularly those in which foreign bodies were implanted, endogenous infecting organisms are involved, but the skin is the primary source of the infecting bacteria. The air in the operating room (OR) and other OR sources occasionally become significant in clean cases; the degree of endogenous contamination can be surpassed by that of exogenous contamination. Thus, both the operating team—surgeon, assistants, nurses, and anesthetists—and OR air have been reported as significant sources of bacteria [*see 2:6 Preparation of the Operating Room*]. In fact, personnel are the most important source of exogenous bacteria.[22–24] In the classic 1964 study by the National Academy of Sciences–National Research Council, ultraviolet light (UVL) was efficacious only in the limited situations of clean and ultraclean cases.[5] There were minimal numbers of endogenous bacteria, and UVL controlled one of the exogenous sources.

Clean air systems have very strong advocates, but they also have equally vociferous critics. It is possible to obtain excellent results in clean cases with implants without using these systems. However, clean air systems are here to stay. Nevertheless, the presence of a clean air system does not mean that basic principles of asepsis and antisepsis should be abandoned, because endogenous bacteria must still be controlled.

The use of impermeable drapes and gowns has received considerable attention. If bacteria can penetrate gown and drapes, they can gain access to the wound. The use of impermeable drapes may therefore be of clinical importance.[25,26] When wet, drapes of 140-thread-count cotton are permeable to bacteria. It is clear that some operations are wetter than others, but, generally, much can be done to make drapes and gowns impermeable to bacteria. For example, drapes of 270-thread-count cotton that have been waterproofed are impermeable, but they can be washed only 75 times.

Antibiotic Prophylaxis of Infection

Selection

Spectrum. The antibiotic chosen should be active against the most likely pathogens. Single-agent therapy is almost always effective except in colorectal operations, small bowel procedures with stasis,emergency abdominal operations in the presence of polymicrobial flora, and penetrating trauma; in such cases, a combination of antibiotics is usually used because anaerobic coverage is required.

Pharmacokinetics. The half-life of the antibiotic selected must be long enough to maintain adequate tissue levels throughout the operation.

Administration

Dosage, route, and timing. A single preoperative dose that is of the same strength as a full therapeutic dose is adequate in most instances. The single dose should be given IV immediately before skin incision. Administration by the anesthetist is most effective and efficient.

Duration. A second dose is warranted if the duration of the operation exceeds either 3 hours or twice the half-life of the antibiotic. No additional benefit has been demonstrated in continuing prophylaxis beyond the day of the operation, and mounting data suggest that the preoperative dose is sufficient. When massive hemorrhage has occurred (i.e., blood loss equal to or greater than blood volume), a second dose is warranted. Even in emergency or trauma cases, prolonged courses of antibiotics are not justified unless they are therapeutic.[79,114]

Indications

CLEAN CASES

Prophylactic antibiotics are not indicated in clean operations if the patient has no host risk factors or if the operation does not involve placement of prosthetic materials. Open heart operation and operations involving the aorta of the vessels in the groin require prophylaxis.

Patients in whom host factors suggest the need for prophylaxis include those who have more than three concomitant diagnoses, those whose operations are expected to last longer than 2 hours, and those whose operations are abdominal.[6] A patient who meets any two of these criteria is highly likely to benefit from prophylaxis. When host factors suggest that the probability of a surgical site infection is significant, administration of cefazolin at induction of anesthesia is appropriate prophylaxis. Vancomycin should be substituted in patients who are allergic to cephalosporins or who are susceptible to major immediate hypersensitivity reactions to penicillin.

When certain prostheses (e.g., heart valves, vascular grafts, and orthopedic hardware) are used, prophylaxis is justified when viewed in the light of the cost of a surgical site infection to the patient's health. Prophylaxis with either cefazolin or vancomycin is appropriate for cardiac, vascular, or orthopedic patients who receive prostheses.

Catheters for dialysis or nutrition, pacemakers, and shunts of various sorts are prone to infection mostly for technical reasons, and prophylaxis is not usually required. Meta-analysis indicates, however, that antimicrobial prophylaxis reduces the infection rate in CSF shunts by 50%.[115] Beneficial results may also be achievable for other permanently implanted shunts (e.g., peritoneovenous) and devices (e.g.,long-term venous access catheters and pacemakers); however, the studies needed to confirm this possibility will never be done, because the infection rates are low and the sample sizes would have to be prohibitively large. The placement of such foreign bodies is a clean operation, and the use of antibiotics should be based on local experience. A recent meta-analysis indicates that antibiotic prophylaxis (cefazolin) prevents SSI in breast surgery.[116]

CLEAN-CONTAMINATED CASES

Abdominal procedures. In biliary tract procedures (open or laparoscopic), prophylaxis is required only for patients at high risk: those whose common bile duct is likely to be explored (because of jaundice,bile duct obstruction, stones in the common bile duct, or a reoperative biliary procedure); those with acute cholecystitis; and those older than 70 years. A single dose of cefazolin is adequate. In hepatobiliary and pancreatic procedures, antibiotic prophylaxis is always warranted because these operations are clean-contaminated, because they are long, and because they are abdominal, Prophylaxis is also warranted for therapeutic endoscopic retrograde cholangiopancreatography. In gastroduodenal procedures, patients whose gastric acidity is normal or high and in whom bleeding, cancer, gastric ulcer, and obstruction are absent are at low risk for infection and require no prophylaxis; all other patients are at high risk and require prophylaxis. Patients undergoing operation for morbid obesity should receive double the usual prophylactic dose[117]; cefazolin is an effective agent.

Operations on the head and neck (including the esophagus). Patients whose operation is of significance (i.e., involves entry into the oral cavity, the pharynx, or the esophagus) require prophylaxis.

Gynecologic procedures. Patients whose operation is either high-risk cesarean section, abortion, or vaginal or abdominal hysterectomy will benefit from cefazolin. Aqueous penicillin G or doxycycline may be preferable for first-trimester abortions in patients with a history of pelvic inflammatory disease. In patients with cephalosporin allergy, doxycycline is effective for those having hysterectomies and metronidazole for those having cesarean sections. Women delivering by cesarean section should be given the antibiotic immediately after cord clamping.

Urologic procedures. In principle, antibiotics are not required in patients with sterile urine. Patients with positive cultures should be treated. If an operative procedure is performed, a single dose of the appropriate antibiotic will suffice.

(continued)

Economics plays a role in the choice of drape fabric because entirely disposable drapes are expensive. Local institutional factors may be significant in the role of a specific type of drape in the prevention of SSI.

PROBABILITY OF CONTAMINATION

The probability of contamination is largely defined by the nature of the operation [*see Table 1*]. However, other factors contribute to the probability of contamination; the most obvious is the expected duration of the operative procedure, which, whenever examined, has been significantly correlated with the wound infection rate.[6,11,13] The longer the procedure lasts, the more bacteria accumulate in a wound; the sources of bacteria include the patient, the operating team (gowns, gloves with holes, wet drapes), the OR, and the equipment. In addition, the patient undergoing a longer operation is likely to be older, to have other diseases, and to have cancer of—or to be undergoing an operation on—a structure with possible contamination. A longer duration, even of a clean operation, represents increased time at risk for contamination. These points, in addition to pharmacologic considerations, suggest that the surgeon should be alert to the need for a second dose of prophylactic antibiotics [*see Sidebar* Antibiotic Prophylaxis of Infection].

Abdominal operation is another risk factor not found in the NNIS risk assessment.[6,8] Significant disease and age are

Antibiotic Prophylaxis of Infection (*continued*)

CONTAMINATED CASES

Abdominal procedures. In colorectal procedures, antibiotics active against both aerobes and anaerobes are recommended. In appendectomy, SSI prophylaxis requires an agent or combination of agents against both aerobes and anaerobes; a single dose of cefoxitin, 2 g IV, or, in patients who are allergic to β-lactam antibiotics, metronidazole, 500 mg IV, is effective. A combination of an aminoglycoside and clindamycin is effective if the appendix is perforated; a therapeutic course of 3 to 5 days is appropriate but does not seem warranted unless the patient is particularly ill. A laparotomy without a precise diagnosis is usually an emergency procedure and demands preoperative prophylaxis. If the preoperative diagnosis is a ruptured viscus (e.g., the colon or the small bowel), both an agent active against aerobes and an agent active against anaerobes are required.

Trauma. The proper duration of antibiotic prophylaxis for trauma patients is a confusing issue—24 hours or less of prophylaxis is probably adequate, and more than 48 hours is certainly unwarranted. When laparotomy is performed for nonpenetrating injuries, prophylaxis should be administered. Coverage of both aerobes and anaerobes is mandatory. The duration of prophylaxis should be less than 24 hours. In cases of penetrating abdominal injury, prophylaxis with either cefoxitin or a combination of agents active against anaerobic and aerobic organisms is required. The duration of prophylaxis should be less than 24 hours, and in many cases, perioperative doses will be adequate. For open fractures, management should proceed as if a therapeutic course were required. For grade I or II injuries, a first-generation cephalosporin will suffice, whereas for grade III injuries, combination therapy is warranted; the duration may vary. For operative repair of fractures, a single dose of cefazolin may be given preoperatively, with a second dose added if the procedure is long. Patients with major soft tissue injury with a danger of spreading infection will benefit from cefazolin, 1 g IV every 8 hours for 1 to 3 days.

DIRTY OR INFECTED CASES

Infected cases require therapeutic courses of antibiotics; prophylaxis is not appropriate in this context. In dirty cases, particularly those resulting from trauma, contamination and tissue destruction are usually so extensive that the wounds must be left open for delayed primary or secondary closure. Appropriate timing of wound closure is judged at the time of débridement. Antibiotics should be administered as part of resuscitation. Administration of antibiotics for 24 hours is probably adequate if infection is absent at the outset. However, a therapeutic course of antibiotics is warranted if infection is present from the outset or if more than 6 hours elapsed before treatment of the wounds was initiated.

Prophylaxis of Endocarditis

Studies of the incidence of endocarditis associated with dental procedures, endoscopy, or operations that may result in transient bacteremia are lacking. Nevertheless, the consensus is that patients with specific cardiac and vascular conditions are at risk for endocarditis or vascular prosthetic infection when undergoing certain procedures; these patients should receive prophylactic antibiotics.[118,119] A variety of organisms are dangerous, but viridans streptococci are most common after dental or oral procedures, and enterococci are most common if the portal of entry is the GU or GI tract. Oral amoxicillin now replaces penicillin V or ampicillin because of superior absorption and better serum levels. In penicillin-allergic patients, clindamycin is recommended; alternatives include cephalexin, ceftriaxone, azithromycin, and clarithromycin. When there is a risk of exposure to bowel flora or enterococci, oral amoxicillin may be given. If an IV regimen is indicated, ampicillin may be given, with gentamicin added if the patient is at high risk for endocarditis. In patients allergic to penicillin, vancomycin is appropriate, with gentamicin added in high-risk patients. These parenteral regimens should be reserved for high-risk patients undergoing procedures with a significant probability of bacteremia. [*see Tables 3 and 4*]

The new recommendations of the American Heart Association have reduced the cardiac conditions needing prophylaxis and the procedures that warrant antibiotics.[118,119] There should be a reduction in antibiotic use as a result.

additional factors that play a role in outcome; however, because the major concentrations of endogenous bacteria are located in the abdomen, abdominal operations are more likely to involve bacterial contamination.

For some years, postoperative contamination of the wound has been considered unlikely. However, one report of SSI in sternal incisions cleaned and redressed 4 hours postoperatively clearly shows that wounds can be contami-

Table 2 Parenteral Antibiotics Recommended for Prophylaxis of Surgical Site Infection

	Antibiotic	Dose	Route of Administration
For coverage against aerobic gram-positive and gram-negative organisms	Cefazolin	1 g	IV or IM (IV preferred)
If patient is allergic to cephalosporins or if methicillin-resistant organisms are present	Vancomycin	1 g	IV
Combination regimens for coverage against gram-negative aerobes and anaerobes	Cefoxitin *or* Cefazolin *plus* Metronidazole *or* Ampicillin/sulbactam	1–2 g 1–2 g 0.5 g 3 g	IV IV IV IV
Allergic to penicillin or cephalosporins	Clindamycin *plus* Gentamicin, ciprofloxacin, aztreonam	600 mg	IV
For single-agent coverage against gram-negative aerobes and anaerobes	Cefoxitin	1–2 g	IV

Table 3 Conditions and Procedures that Require Antibiotic Prophylaxis against Endocarditis[118,119]

Conditions that Warrant Prophylaxis
Prosthetic cardiac valve or prosthetic material used for cardiac valve repair
Previous infective endocarditis
Congenital heart disease (CHD)
- Unrepaired cyanotic CHD, including palliative shunts and conduits
- Complete repaired congenital heart defect with prosthetic material or device, whether placed by surgery or by catheter intervention, during the first 6 months after the procedure
- Repaired CHD with residual defects at the site or adjacent to the site of a prosthetic patch or prosthetic device (which inhibit endothelialization)

Cardiac transplantation recipients who develop cardiac valvulopathy

Procedures that Warrant Prophylaxis
Dental or oropharyngeal procedures that
1. manipulate gingival tissue or the periapical region of the teeth
2. perforate the oral mucosa

Incision and drainage, manipulation, or débridement of infected sites regardless of location
Gastrointestinal (GI) or genitourinary (GU) procedures for which antibiotics to prevent surgical site infection would be administered
Endoscopy of GI tract or uninfected GU tract prophylaxis is NO longer recommended

nated and become infected in the postoperative period.[27] Accordingly, use of a dry dressing for 24 hours seems prudent.

BACTERIAL PROPERTIES

Not only is the size of the bacterial inoculum important; the bacterial properties of virulence and pathogenicity are also significant. The most obvious pathogenic bacteria in surgical patients are gram-positive cocci (e.g., *Staphylococcus aureus* and streptococci). With modern hygienic practice, it would be expected that *S. aureus* would be found mostly in clean cases, with a wound infection incidence of 1 to 2%; however, it is, in fact, an increasingly common pathogen in SSIs. Surveillance can be very useful in identifying either wards or surgeons with increased rates. Operative procedures in infected areas have an increased infection rate because of the high inoculum with actively pathogenic bacteria.

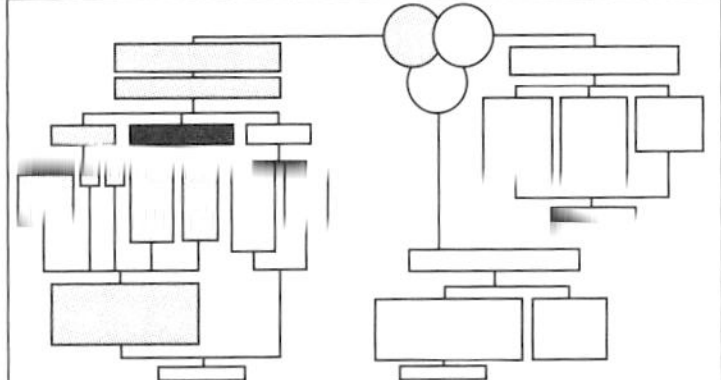

Table 4 Antibiotics for Prevention of Endocarditis[118,119]

	Prophylactic Regimen*	
Manipulative Procedure	**Usual**	**In Patients with Penicillin Allergy**
Dental procedures likely to cause gingival bleeding; operations or instrumentation of the upper respiratory tract	Oral Amoxicillin 2 g 1 hr before procedure	Oral Clindamycin,† 600 mg 1 hr before procedure *or* Cephaloxin,† 1 g 1 hr before procedure *or* Azithromycin or clarithromycin, 500 mg1 hr before procedure
	Parenteral Ampicillin, 2 g IM or IV 30 min before procedure *or* Cefazolin or ceftriaxone 1 g IM or IV	Parenteral Clindamycin, 600 mg IV within 30 min before procedure *or* Cefazolin or ceftriaxone, 1 g IM or IV within 30 min before procedure
Infected gastrointestinal or genitourinary operation; abscess drainage	Oral Amoxicillin, 2 g 1 hr before procedure	
	Parenteral Ampicillin, 2 g IM or IV within 30 min before procedure; if risk of endocarditis is considered high, add gentamicin, 1.5 mg/kg (to maximum of 120 mg) IM or IV 30 min before procedure	Parenteral Vancomycin, 1 g IV infused slowly over 1 hr, beginning 1 hr before procedure; if risk of endocarditis is considered high, add gentamicin, 1.5 mg/kg (to maximum of 120 mg) IM or IV 30 min before procedure‡

*Pediatric dosages are as follows: oral amoxicillin, 50 mg/kg; oral or parenteral clindamycin, 20 mg/kg; oral cephalexin or cefadroxil, 50 mg/kg; oral azithromycin or clarithromycin, 15 mg/kg; parenteral ampicillin, 50 mg/kg; parenteral cefazolin, 25 mg/kg; parenteral gentamicin, 2 mg/kg. *The total pediatric dose should not exceed the total adult dose.*
†Patients with a history of immediate-type sensitivity to penicillin should not receive these agents.
‡High-risk patients should also receive ampicillin, 1 g IM or IV, or amoxicillin, 1 g PO, 6 hours after the procedure.

Preoperative Preparation of the Operative Site

The sole reason for preparing the patient's skin before an operation is to reduce the risk of wound infection. A preoperative antiseptic bath is not necessary for most surgical patients, but their personal hygiene must be assessed and preoperative cleanliness established. Multiple preoperative baths may prevent postoperative infection in selected patient groups, such as those who carry *Staphylococcus aureus* on their skin or who have infectious lesions. Chlorhexidine gluconate is the recommended agent for such baths.[120]

Hair should not be removed from the operative site unless it physically interferes with accurate anatomic approximation of the wound edges.[15] If hair must be removed, it should be clipped in the OR.[15] Shaving hair from the operative site, particularly on the evening before operation or immediately before wound incision in the OR, increases the risk of wound infection. Depilatories are not recommended, because they cause serious irritation and rashes in a significant number of patients, especially when used near the eyes and the genitalia.[121]

In emergency procedures, obvious dirt, grime, and dried blood should be mechanically cleansed from the operative site by using sufficient friction. In one study, cleansing of contaminated wounds by means of ultrasound débridement was compared with highpressure irrigation and soaking. Both ultrasound débridement and high-pressure irrigation were also effective in reducing the wound infection rate in experimental wounds contaminated with a subinfective dose of *S. aureus* and colloidal clay.[122]

For nonemergency procedures, the necessary reduction in microorganisms can be achieved by using povidoneiodine (10% available povidoneiodine and 1% available iodine) or chlorhexidine gluconate both for mechanical cleansing of the intertriginous folds and the umbilicus and for painting the operative site. Which skin antiseptic is optimal is unclear. The best option appears to be chlorhexidine gluconate or an iodophor.[123] The patient should be assessed for evidence of sensitivity to the antiseptic (particularly if the agent contains iodine) to minimize the risk of an allergic reaction. What some patients report as iodine allergies are actually burns. Iodine in alcohol or in water is associated with an increased risk of skin irritation,[96] particularly at the edges of the operative field, where the iodine concentrates as the alcohol evaporates. Iodine should therefore be removed after sufficient contact time with the skin, especially at the edges. Iodophors do not irritate the skin and thus need not be removed.

The preoperative hospital stay has frequently been found to make an important contribution to wound infection rates.[13] The usual explanation is that during this stay, either more endogenous bacteria are present or commensal flora is replaced by hospital flora. More likely, the patient's clinical picture is a complex one, often entailing exhaustive workup of more than one organ system, various complications, and a degree of illness that radically changes the host's ability to deal with an inoculum, however small. Therefore, multiple factors combine to transform the hospitalized preoperative patient into a susceptible host. Same-day admission should eliminate any bacterial impact associated with the preoperative hospital stay.

Table 5 Effect of Surveillance and Feedback on Wound Infection Rates in Two Hospitals[29]

		Period 1	Period 2*
Hospital A	Number of wounds	1,500	1,447
	Wound infection rate	8.4%	3.7%
Hospital B	Number of wounds	1,746	1,939
	Wound infection rate	5.7%	3.7%

*Periods 1 and 2 were separated by an interval during which feedback on wound infection rates was analyzed.

Bacteria with multiple antibiotic resistance (e.g., methicillin-resistant *S. aureus* [MRSA], *Staphylococcus epidermidis*, and vancomycin-resistant enterococci [VRE]) can be associated with significant SSI problems. In particular, staphylococci, with their natural virulence, present an important hazard if inappropriate prophylaxis is used.

Many surgeons consider it inappropriate or unnecessary to obtain good culture and sensitivity data on SSIs; instead of conducting sensitivity testing, they simply drain infected wounds, believing that the wounds will heal. However, there have been a number of reports of SSIs caused by unusual organisms[24,27,28]; these findings underscore the usefulness of culturing pus or fluid when an infection is being drained. SSIs caused by antibiotic-resistant organisms or unusual pathogens call for specific prophylaxis, perhaps other infection control efforts, and, if the problem persists, a search for a possible carrier or a common source.[22–24,27,28]

SURGEONS AND BACTERIA

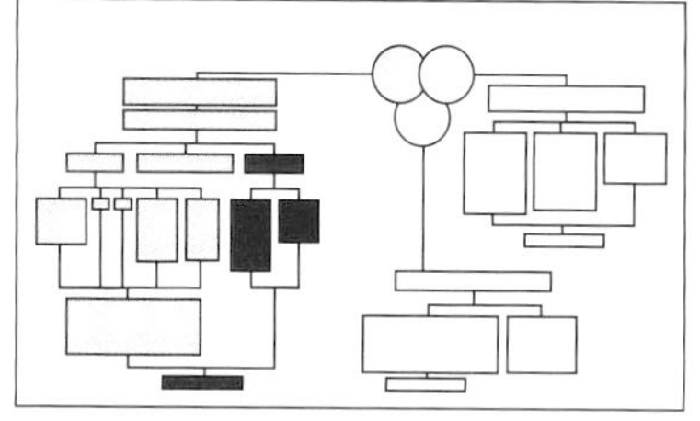

The surgeon's perioperative rituals are designed to reduce or eliminate bacteria from the operative field. Many old habits are obsolete [*see 2:6 Preparation of the Operating Room* and Discussion, Hand Washing, *below*]. Nonetheless, it is clear that surgeons can influence SSI rates.[14] The refusal to use delayed primary closure or secondary closure is an example. Careful attention to the concepts of asepsis and antisepsis in the preparation and conduct of the operation is important. Although no single step in the ritual of preparing a patient for the operative procedure is indispensable, it is likely that certain critical standards of behavior must be maintained to achieve good results.

The measurement and publication of data about individuals or hospitals with high SSI rates have been associated with a diminution of those rates [*see Table 6*].[13,14,29] It is uncertain by what process the diffusion of these data relates to the observed improvements. Although surveillance has unpleasant connotations, it provides objective data that individual surgeons are often too busy to acquire but that can contribute to improved patient care. For example, such data can be useful in identifying problems (e.g., the presence of MRSA, a high SSI incidence, or clusters), maintaining quality assurance, and allowing comparison with accepted standards.

Environment: Local Factors

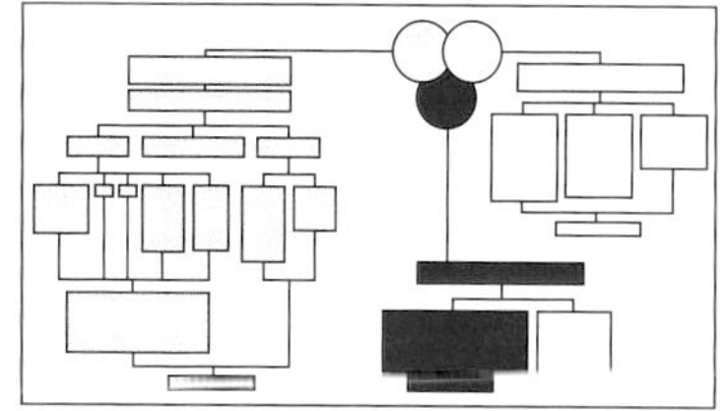

Local factors influence SSI development because they affect the size of the bacterial inoculum that is

Table 6 Determinants of Infection and Factors that Influence Wound Infection Rates[29]

Variable	Determinant of Infection		
	Bacteria	Wound Environment (Local Factors)	Host Defense Mechanisms (Systemic Factors)
Bacterial numbers in wound	a		
Potential contamination	a		
Preoperative shave	a		
Presence of three or more diagnoses			c
Age		b	c
Duration of operation	a	b	c
Abdominal operation Relative value unit > 10 Emergency surgery	a	b	c
ASA class III, IV, or V			c
O_2 tension		b	
Glucose control			c
Normothermia		b	c
Shock		b	c
Smoking		b	c
Diabetes[10]		b	c
Dyspnea[10]			c
Steroid use[10]		b	c
Serum albumin ≤ 3.5 g/L[10]			c
Age ≥ 40[10]			c
Radiotherapy[10]			c
> 2 alcoholic drinks[10]			c

ASA = American Society of Anesthesiologists.

required to produce an infection: in a susceptible wound, a smaller inoculum produces infection [*see Figure 2*].

THE SURGEON'S INFLUENCE

Most of the local factors that make a surgical site favorable to bacteria are under the control of the surgeon. Although Halsted usually receives, deservedly so, the credit for having established the importance of technical excellence in the OR in preventing infection, individual surgeons in the distant past achieved remarkable results by careful attention to cleanliness and technique.[30] The halstedian principles dealt with hemostasis, sharp dissection, fine sutures, anatomic dissection, and the gentle handling of tissues. Mass ligatures, large or braided nonabsorbable sutures, necrotic tissue, and the creation of hematomas or seromas must be avoided, and foreign materials must be judiciously used because these techniques and materials change the size of the inoculum required to initiate an infectious process. Logarithmically fewer bacteria are required to produce infection in the presence of a foreign body (e.g., suture, graft, metal, or pacemaker) or necrotic tissue (e.g., that caused by gross hemostasis or injudicious use of electrocautery devices).

The differences in inoculum required to produce wound infections can be seen in a model in which the two variables are the wound hematocrit and the presence of an antibiotic [*see Figure 3*]. In the absence of an antibiotic and in the presence of wound fluid with a hematocrit of more than 8%, 10 bacteria yield a wound infection rate of 20%. In a technically good wound with no antibiotic, however, 1,000 bacteria produce a wound infection rate of 20%.[12] In the presence of an antibiotic, 10^5 to 10^6 bacteria are required.

Drains

The use of drains varies widely and is very subjective. All surgeons are certain that they understand when to use a drain. However, certain points are worth noting. It is now recognized that a simple Penrose drain may function as a drainage route but is also an access route by which pathogens can reach the patient.[31] It is important that the operative site not be drained through the wound. The use of a closed suction drain reduces the potential for contamination and infection.

Many operations on the gastrointestinal (GI) tract can be performed safely without employing prophylactic drainage.[32] A review and meta-analysis from 2004 concluded that (1) after hepatic, colonic, or rectal resection with primary anastomosis and after appendectomy for any stage of appendicitis, drains should be omitted (recommendation grade A), and (2) after esophageal resection and total gastrectomy, drains should be used (recommendation grade D). Additional randomized, controlled trials will be required to determine the value of prophylactic drainage for other GI procedures, especially those involving the upper GI tract.

Duration of Operation

In most studies, contamination certainly increases with time (see above).[6,11,13] Wound edges can dry out, become macerated, or in other ways be made more susceptible to infection (i.e., requiring fewer bacteria for development of infection). Speed and poor technique are not suitable approaches; expeditious operation is appropriate.

Electrocautery

The use of electrocautery devices (but not the harmonic scalpel) has been clearly associated with an increase in the incidence of superficial SSIs. However, when such devices are properly used to provide pinpoint coagulation (for which the bleeding vessels are best held by fine forceps) or to divide tissues under tension, there is minimal tissue destruction, no charring, and no change in the wound infection rate.[31]

PATIENT FACTORS

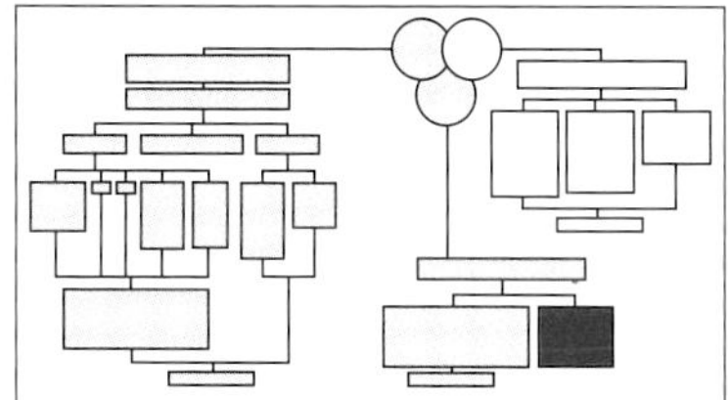

Local Blood Flow

Local perfusion can greatly influence the development of infection, as is seen most easily in the tendency of the patient with peripheral vascular disease to acquire infection of an extremity. As a local problem, inadequate perfusion reduces the number of bacteria required for infection, in part because inadequate perfusion leads to decreased tissue levels of oxygen. Shock, by reducing local perfusion, also greatly enhances susceptibility to infection. Fewer organisms are required to produce infection during or immediately after shock [*see Figure 4*].

To counter these effects, the arterial oxygen tension (P_aO_2) must be translated into an adequate subcutaneous oxygen level (determined by measuring transcutaneous oxygen tension)[33]; this, together with adequate perfusion, will provide local protection by increasing the number of bacteria required to produce infection. Provision of supplemental oxygen in the perioperative period may lead to a reduced SSI rate, probably as a consequence of increased tissue oxygen tension,[34] although the value of this practice has been questioned.[35] If the patient is not intubated, a mask, not nasal prongs, is required.[36]

Barrier Function

Inadequate perfusion may also affect the function of other organs, and the resulting dysfunction will, in turn, influence the patient's susceptibility to infection. For example, ischemia-reperfusion injury to the intestinal tract is a frequent consequence of hypovolemic shock and bloodstream infection. Inadequate perfusion of the GI tract may also occur during states of fluid and electrolyte imbalance or when cardiac output is marginal. In experimental studies, altered blood flow has been found to be associated with the breakdown of bowel barrier function—that is, the inability of the intestinal tract to prevent bacteria, their toxins, or both from moving from the gut lumen into tissue at a rate too fast to permit clearance by the usual protective mechanisms. A variety of experimental approaches aimed at enhancing bowel barrier function have been studied; at present, however, the most clinically applicable method of bowel protection is initiation of enteral feeding (even if the quantity of nutrients provided does not satisfy all the nutrient requirements) and administration of the amino acid glutamine [*see 11:19 Nutritional Support*]. Glutamine is a specific fuel for enterocytes and colonocytes and has been found to aid recovery of damaged intestinal mucosa and enhance barrier function when administered either enterally or parenterally.

Advanced Age

Aging is associated with structural and functional changes that render the skin and subcutaneous tissues more susceptible to infection. These changes are immutable; however, they must be evaluated in advance and addressed by excellent surgical technique and, on occasion, prophylactic antibiotics [*see Sidebar* Antibiotic Prophylaxis of Infection]. SSI rates increase with aging until the age of 65 years, after which point, the incidence appears to decline.[37]

Host Defense Mechanisms

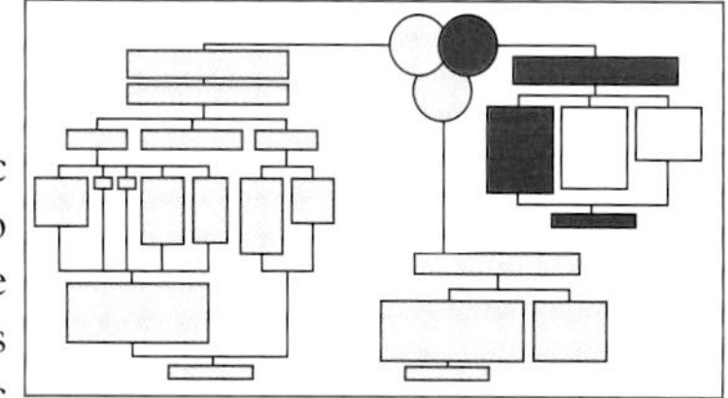

The systemic response is designed to control and eradicate infection. Many factors can inhibit systemic host defense mechanisms; some are related to the surgical disease and others to the patient's underlying disease or diseases and the events surrounding the operation.

SURGEON-RELATED FACTORS

There are a limited number of ways in which the surgeon can improve a patient's systemic responses to surgery. Nevertheless, when appropriate, attempts should be made to modify the host. The surgeon and the operation are both capable of reducing immunologic efficacy; hence, the operative procedure should be carried out in as judicious a manner as possible. Minimal blood loss, avoidance of shock, and maintenance of blood volume, tissue perfusion, and tissue oxygenation will minimize trauma and will reduce the secondary, unintended immunologic effects of major procedures.

Diabetes has long been recognized as a risk factor for infection and for SSI in particular. Three studies from the past decade demonstrated the importance of glucose control for reducing SSI rates in both diabetic and nondiabetic patients who underwent operation,[38,39] as well as in critically ill intensive care unit patients.[40] Glucose control is required throughout the entire perioperative period. The beneficial effect appears to lie in the enhancement of host defenses. The surgical team must also ensure maintenance of adequate tissue oxygen tension[33,34] and maintenance of normothermia.[41]

When abnormalities in host defenses are secondary to surgical disease, the timing of the operation is crucial to outcome. With acute and subacute inflammatory processes, early

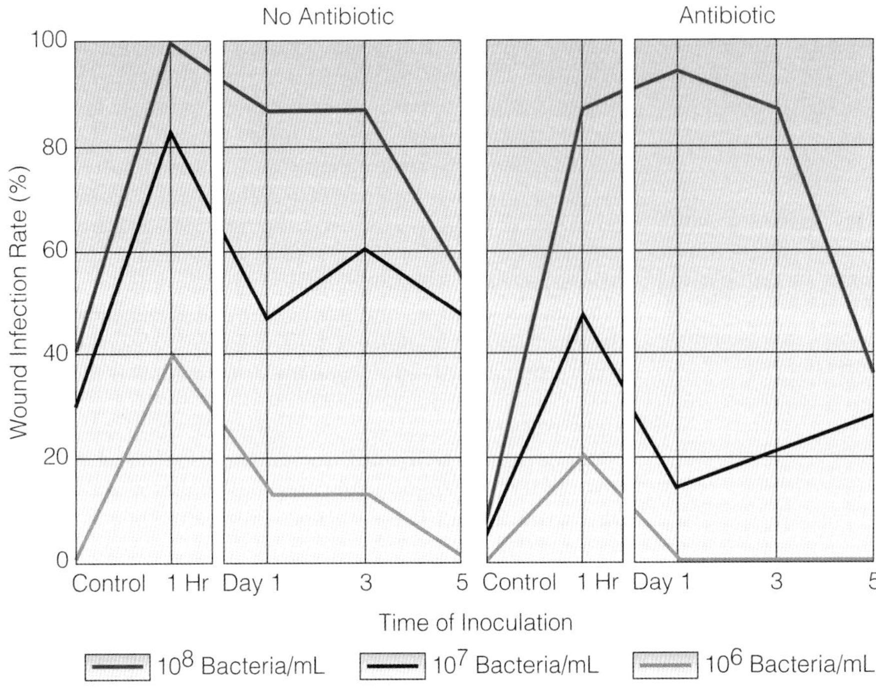

Figure 4 **Animals exposed to hemorrhagic shock followed by resuscitation show an early decreased resistance to wound infection. There is also a persistent influence of shock on the development of wound infection at different times of inoculation after shock. The importance of inoculum size (10^6/mL to 10^8/mL) and the effect of antibiotic on infection rates are evident at all times of inoculation.[109]**

operation helps restore normal immune function. Deferral of definitive therapy frequently compounds problems.

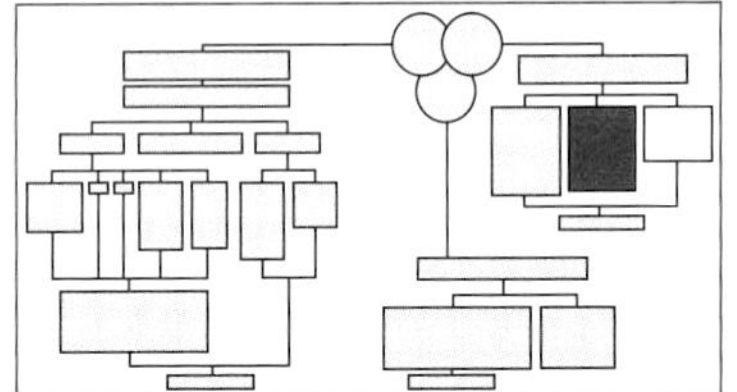

PATIENT FACTORS

Surgeons have always known that the patient is a significant variable in the outcome of operation. Various clinical states are associated with altered resistance to infection. In all patients, but particularly those at high risk, SSI creates not only wound complications but also significant morbidity (e.g., reoperation, incisional hernia, secondary infection, impaired mobility, increased hospitalization, delayed rehabilitation, or permanent disability) and occasional mortality.[23] SENIC has proposed that the risk of wound infection be assessed not only in terms of probability of contamination but also in relation to host factors.[6,7,9] According to this study, patients most clearly at risk for wound infection are those with three or more concomitant diagnoses; other patients who are clearly at risk are those undergoing a clean-contaminated or contaminated abdominal procedure and those undergoing any procedure expected to last longer than 2 hours. These last two risk groups are affected by a bacterial component, but all those patients who are undergoing major abdominal procedures or lengthy operations generally have a significant primary pathologic condition and are usually older, with an increased frequency of concomitant conditions. The NNIS system uses most of the same concepts but expresses them differently. In the NNIS study, host factors in the large study are evaluated in terms of the ASA score. The duration of the operation is measured differently as well, with a lengthy operation being defined by the NNIS as one that is at or above the 75th percentile for operating time. Bacterial contamination remains a risk factor, but the operative site is eliminated.[8]

Shock has an influence on the incidence of wound infection [*see Figure 4*]. This influence is most obvious in cases of trauma, but there are significant implications for all patients in regard to maintenance of blood volume, hemostasis, and oxygen-carrying capacity. The effect of shock on the risk of infection appears to be not only immediate (i.e., its effect on local perfusion) but also late because systemic responses are blunted as local factors return to normal.

Advanced age, transfusion, and the use of steroids and other immunosuppressive drugs, including chemotherapeutic agents, are associated with an increased risk of SSI.[42,43] Often, these factors cannot be altered; however, the proper choice of operation, the appropriate use of prophylaxis, and meticulous surgical technique can reduce the risk of such infection by maintaining patient homeostasis, reducing the size of any infecting microbial inoculum, and creating a wound that is likely to heal primarily.

Smoking is associated with a striking increase in SSI incidence. As little as 1 week of abstinence from smoking will make a positive difference.[44]

Pharmacologic therapy can affect host response as well. Nonsteroidal anti-inflammatory drugs that attenuate the production of certain eicosanoids can greatly alter the adverse effects of infection by modifying fever and cardiovascular effects. Operative procedures involving inhalational anesthetics result in an immediate rise in plasma cortisol concentrations. The steroid response and the associated immunomodulation can be modified by using high epidural anesthesia as the method of choice; pituitary adrenal activation will be greatly attenuated. Some drugs that inhibit steroid elaboration (e.g., etomidate) have also been shown to be capable of modifying perioperative immune responses. Using this vast database of NSQIP, Neumayer and colleagues integrated most of these variables into an expanded risk assessment [*see Table 6*].[10]

ANESTHESIOLOGIST-RELATED FACTORS

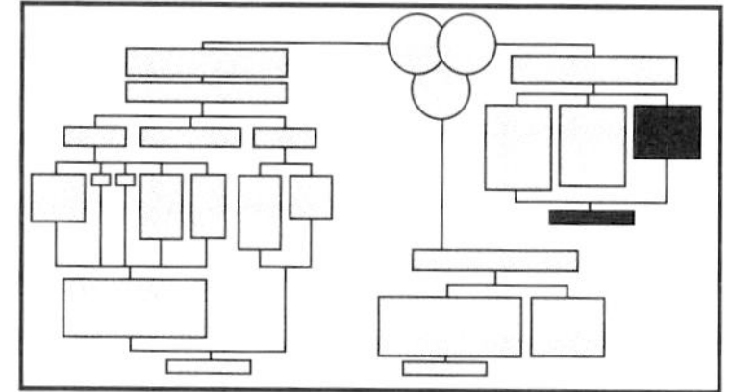

A 2000 commentary in *The Lancet* by Donal Buggy considered the question of whether anesthetic management could influence surgical wound healing.[45] In addition to the surgeon- and patient-related factors already discussed (see above), Buggy cogently identified a number of anesthesiologist-related factors that could contribute to better wound healing and reduced wound infection. Some of these factors (e.g., pain control, epidural anesthesia, and autologous transfusion) are unproven but nonetheless make sense and should certainly be tested. Others (e.g., tissue perfusion, intravascular volume, and—significantly—maintenance of normal perioperative body temperature) have undergone formal evaluation. Very good studies have shown that dramatic reductions in SSI rates can be achieved through careful avoidance of hypothermia.[41,46] Patient-controlled analgesia pumps are known to be associated with increased SSI rates, through a mechanism that is currently unknown.[47] Infection control practices are required of all practitioners; contamination of anesthetic drugs by bacteria has resulted in numerous small outbreaks of SSI.[48,49]

As modern surgical practice has evolved and the variable of bacterial contamination has come to be generally well managed, the importance of all members of the surgical team in the prevention of SSI has become increasingly apparent. The crux of Buggy's commentary may be expressed as follows: details make a difference, and all of the participants in a patient's surgical journey can contribute to a continuing decrease in SSI. It is a systems issue.

INTEGRATION OF DETERMINANTS

As operative infection rates slowly fall, despite the performance of increasingly complex operations in patients at greater risk, surgeons are approaching the control of infection with a broader view than simply that of asepsis and antisepsis. This new, broader view must take into account many variables, of which some have no relation to bacteria, but all play a role in SSI [*see Table 6 and Figure 1*].

To estimate risk, one must integrate the various determinants of infection in such a way that they can be applied to patient care. Much of this exercise is vague. In reality, the day-to-day practice of surgery includes a risk assessment that is essentially a form of logistic regression, although not recognized as such. Each surgeon's assessment of the probability of whether an SSI will occur takes into account the determining variables:

$$\text{Probability of SSI} = x + a\ (\text{bacteria}) + b\ (\text{environment: local factors}) + c\ (\text{host defense mechanisms: systemic factors})$$

Discussion

ANTIBIOTIC PROPHYLAXIS OF SSI

It is difficult to understand why antibiotics have not always prevented SSI successfully. Certainly, surgeons were quick to appreciate the possibilities of antibiotics; nevertheless, the efficacy of antibiotic prophylaxis was not proved until the late 1960s.[12] Studies before then had major design flaws—principally, the administration of the antibiotic some time after the start of the operation, often in the recovery room. The failure of studies to demonstrate efficacy and the occasional finding that prophylactic antibiotics worsened rather than improved outcome led in the late 1950s to profound skepticism about prophylactic antibiotic use in any operation.

The principal reason for the apparent inefficacy was inadequate understanding of the biology of SSIs. Fruitful study of antibiotics and how they should be used began after physiologic groundwork established the importance of local blood flow, maintenance of local immune defenses, adjuvants, and local and systemic perfusion.[50]

The key antibiotic study, which was conducted in guinea pigs, unequivocally proved the following about antibiotics[51]:

1. They are most effective when given before inoculation of bacteria.
2. They are ineffective if given 3 hours after inoculation.
3. They are of intermediate effectiveness when given between these times [*see Figure 5*].

Although efficacy with a complicated regimen was demonstrated in 1964,[52] the correct approach was not defined until 1969.[12] Established by these studies are the philosophical and practical bases of the principles of antibiotic prophylaxis of

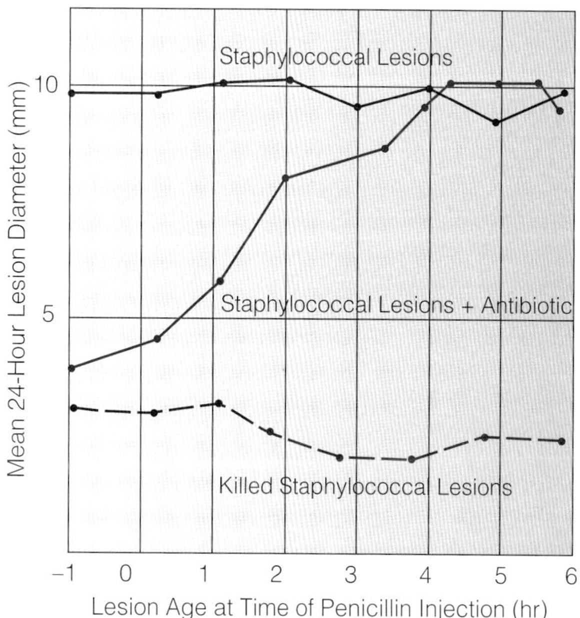

Figure 5 **In a pioneer study of antibiotic prophylaxis,[51] the diameter of lesions induced by staphylococcal inoculation 24 hours earlier was observed to be critically affected by the timing of penicillin administration with respect to bacterial inoculation.**

SSI in all surgical arenas[12,51]: that prophylactic antibiotics must be given preoperatively within 2 hours of the incision, in full dosage, parenterally, and for a very limited period. These principles remain essentially unchanged despite minor modifications from innumerable subsequent studies.[53–57] Prophylaxis for colorectal operations is discussed elsewhere [*see* Infection Prevention in Bowel Surgery, *below*].

Principles of Patient Selection

Patients must be selected for prophylaxis on the basis of either their risk for SSI or the cost to their health if an SSI develops (e.g., after implantation of a cardiac valve or another prosthesis). The most important criterion is the degree of bacterial contamination expected to occur during the operation. The traditional classification of such contamination was defined in 1964 by the historic National Academy of Sciences–National Research Council study.[5] The important features of the classification are its simplicity, ease of understanding, ease of coding, and reliability. Classification is dependent on only one variable—the bacterial inoculum—and the effects of this variable are now controllable by antimicrobial prophylaxis. Advances in operative technique, general care, antibiotic use, anesthesia, and surveillance have reduced SSI rates in all categories that were established by this classification.[6,13,14,51]

In 1960, after years of negative studies, it was said, "Nearly all surgeons now agree that the routine use of prophylaxis in clean operations is unnecessary and undesirable."[58] Since then, much has changed: there are now many clean operations for which no competent surgeon would omit the use of prophylactic antibiotics, particularly as procedures become increasingly complex and prosthetic materials are used in patients who are older, sicker, or immunocompromised.

A separate risk assessment that integrates host and bacterial variables (i.e., whether the operation is dirty or contaminated, is longer than 2 hours, or is an abdominal procedure and whether the patient has three or more concomitant diagnoses) segregates more effectively those patients who are prone to an increased incidence of SSI [*see* Integration of Determinants of Infection, *below*]. This approach enables the surgeon to identify those patients who are likely to require preventive measures, particularly in clean cases, in which antibiotics would normally not be used.[6]

The prototypical clean operation is an inguinal hernia repair. Technical approaches have changed dramatically over the past 10 years, and most primary and recurrent hernias are now treated with a tension-free mesh-based repair. The use of antibiotics has become controversial. In the era of repairs under tension, there was some evidence to suggest that a perioperative antibiotic (in a single preoperative dose) was beneficial.[59] Current studies, however, do not support antibiotic use in tension-free mesh-based inguinal hernia repairs.[60,61] On the other hand, if surveillance indicates that there is a local or regional problem[62] with SSI after hernia surgery, antibiotic prophylaxis (again in the form of a single preoperative dose) is appropriate. Without significantly more supportive data, prophylaxis for clean cases cannot be recommended unless specific risk factors are present.

Data suggest that prophylactic use of antibiotics may contribute to secondary *Clostridium difficile* disease; accordingly, caution should be exercised when widening the indications for prophylaxis is under consideration.[63] If local results are poor, surgical practice should be reassessed before antibiotics are prescribed.

Antibiotic Selection and Administration

When antibiotics are given more than 2 hours before operation, the risk of infection is increased.[53,55] IV administration in the OR or the preanesthetic room guarantees appropriate levels at the time of incision. The organisms likely to be present dictate the choice of antibiotic for prophylaxis. The cephalosporins are ideally suited to prophylaxis: their features include a broad spectrum of activity, an excellent ratio of therapeutic to toxic dosages, a low rate of allergic responses, ease of administration, and attractive cost advantages. Mild allergic reactions to penicillin are not contraindications for the use of a cephalosporin.

Physicians like new drugs and often tend to prescribe newer, more expensive antibiotics for simple tasks. First-generation cephalosporins (e.g., cefazolin) are ideal agents for prophylaxis. Third-generation cephalosporins are not: they cost more, are not more effective, and promote emergence of resistant strains.[64,65]

The most important first-generation cephalosporin for surgical patients continues to be cefazolin. Administered IV in the OR at the time of skin incision, it provides adequate tissue levels throughout most of the operation. A second dose administered in the OR after 3 hours will be beneficial if the procedure lasts longer than that. Data on all operative site infections are imprecise, but SSIs can clearly be reduced by this regimen. No data suggest that further doses are required for prophylaxis.

Fortunately, cefazolin is effective against both gram-positive and gram-negative bacteria of importance, unless significant anaerobic organisms are encountered. The significance of anaerobic flora has been disputed, but for elective colorectal surgery,[66] abdominal trauma,[67,68] appendicitis,[69] or other circumstances in which penicillin-resistant anaerobic bacteria are likely to be encountered, coverage against both aerobic and anaerobic gram-negative organisms is strongly recommended and supported by the data.

Despite several decades of studies, prophylaxis is not always properly implemented.[53,55,69,70] Unfortunately, didactic education is not always the best way to change behavior. Preprinted order forms[71] and a reminder sticker from the pharmacy[72] have proved to be effective methods of ensuring correct use.

The commonly heard decision "This case was tough; let's give an antibiotic for 3 to 5 days" has no data to support it and should be abandoned. The extended duration is associated with an increase in MRSA SSIs.[73] Differentiation between prophylaxis and therapeusis is important. A therapeutic course for perforated diverticulitis or other types of peritoneal infection is appropriate. Data on casual contamination associated with trauma or with operative procedures suggest that 24 hours of prophylaxis or less is quite adequate.[74–76] Mounting evidence suggests that a single preoperative dose is good care and that additional doses are not required.

Trauma Patients

The efficacy of antibiotic administration on arrival in the emergency department as an integral part of resuscitation has been clearly demonstrated.[77] The most common regimens have been (1) a combination of an aminoglycoside and clindamycin and (2) cefoxitin alone. These two regimens or variations thereof have been compared in a number of studies.[41,68,76,77] They appear to be equally effective, and either regimen can be recommended with confidence. For prophylaxis, there appears to be a trend toward using a single drug: cefoxitin or cefotetan.[56] If therapy is required because of either a delay in surgery, terrible injury, or prolonged shock, the combination of an agent that is effective against anaerobes with an aminoglycoside seems to be favored. Because aminoglycosides are nephrotoxic, they must be used with care in the presence of shock.

In many of the trauma studies just cited, antibiotic prophylaxis lasted for 48 hours or longer. Subsequent studies, however, indicated that prophylaxis lasting less than 24 hours is appropriate.[75,76,78] Single-dose prophylaxis is appropriate for patients with closed fractures.[79]

Complications

Complications of antibiotic prophylaxis are few. Although data linking prophylaxis to the development of resistant organisms are meager, resistant microbes have developed in every other situation in which antibiotics have been used, and it is reasonable to expect that prophylaxis in any ecosystem will have the same result, particularly if selection of patients is poor, if prophylaxis lasts too long, or if too many late-generation agents are used.

A rare but important complication of antibiotic use is pseudomembranous enterocolitis, which is induced most commonly by clindamycin, the cephalosporins, and ampicillin [*see 9:13 Hospital Infections*].[63] The common denominator among different cases of pseudomembranous enterocolitis is hard to identify. Diarrhea and fever can develop after administration of single doses of prophylactic antibiotics. The condition is rare, but difficulties occur because of failure to make a rapid diagnosis.

Current Issues

The most significant questions concerning prophylaxis of SSIs already have been answered.

The problem has been the implementation of the strategies known to work. Table 7 outlines seven measures known with hard data to be important in the reduction of SSI. These management approaches are integrated into the Surgical Care Improvement Project[80] and the Surgical Infection Prevention Project.[81] Single hospitals have used these criteria in ongoing quality improvement programs.[82] More impressive is the collaborative reported by Dellinger and colleagues in which 56 hospitals tracked, monitored, and internally fed back the seven variables in Table 7 and demonstrated that as compliance increased, SSI rates came down.[83] An important remaining issue is the proper duration of prophylaxis in complicated cases, in the setting of trauma, and in the presence of foreign bodies. No change in the criteria for antibiotic prophylaxis is required in laparoscopic procedures; the risk of infection is lower in such cases.[84,85] Cost factors are important and may justify the endless succession of studies that compare new drugs in competition for appropriate clinical niches.

Further advances in patient selection may take place but will require analysis of data from large numbers of patients and a distinction between approaches to infection of the wound, which is only part of the operative field, and approaches to infections directly related to the operative site. These developments will define more clearly the prophylaxis requirements of patients whose operations are clean but whose risk of wound or operative site infection is increased.

Table 7 Quality Improvement Objectives to Reduce Surgical Site Infections[80,83]

Timeliness of antibiotics
Appropriate selection of antibiotics
Correct duration of antibiotics
Preventing hyperglycemia
Maintaining normothermia
Optimizing oxygen tension
Avoidance of shaving surgical site

A current issue of some concern is loss of infection surveillance capability. Infection control units have been shown to offer a number of benefits in the institutional setting, such as the following:

1. Identifying epidemics caused by common or uncommon organisms[24,27,57]
2. Establishing correct use of prophylaxis (timing, dose, duration, and choice)[53,56,74]
3. Documenting costs, risk factors, and readmission rates[86,87]
4. Monitoring postdischarge infections and secondary consequences of infections[88–90]
5. Ensuring patient safety[91]
6. Managing MRSA and VRE[92]

S. aureus—in particular, MRSA—is a major cause of SSI.[92] Cross-infection problems are a concern, in a manner reminiscent of the preantibiotic era. Hand washing (see below) is coming back into fashion, consistent with the professional behavior toward cross-infection characteristic of the preantibiotic era. At present, hard evidence is lacking, but clinical observation suggests that *S. aureus* SSIs are especially troublesome and destructive of local tissue and require a longer time to heal than other SSIs do. When *S. aureus* SSIs occur after cardiac surgery, thoracotomy, or joint replacement, their consequences are significant. Prevention in these settings is important. When nasal carriage of *S. aureus* has been identified, mupirocin may be administered intranasally to reduce the incidence of *S. aureus* SSIs.[93]

The benefits of infection surveillance notwithstanding, as the business of hospital care has become more expensive and financial control more rigid, the infection control unit is a hospital component that many administrators have come to consider a luxury and therefore expendable. Consequently, surveillance as a quality control and patient safety mechanism has been diminished.

It is apparent that SSIs have huge clinical and financial implications [*see Sidebar* Patient Safety and Antibiotic Use]. Patients with infections tend to be sicker and to undergo more complex operations. Therefore, higher infection rates translate into higher morbidity and mortality as well as higher cost to the hospital, the patient, and society as a whole. With increasingly early discharge becoming the norm, delayed diagnosis of postdischarge SSI and the complications thereof

Patient Safety and Antibiotic Use

Prophylactic antibiotics have been considered to be a harmless manner in which to prevent surgical site infections. The evidence is that a single dose of prophylactic antibiotics can precipitate *Clostridium difficile* pseudomembraneous enterocolitis.[63] These can be as malignant as the same entity caused by therapeutic antibiotic regimens.

Although the principles of delivery of added prophylactic antibiotics and their duration have been established for a long time, the evidence is clear that adherence to these principles is frequently poor. Two areas that are primarily at fault are the timing of administration of the first dose and whether it gets given and the duration of use of prophylactic antibiotics.[43,70–72] The principles are (1) that the drug must be at the site of the wound at the time of incision and (2) a duration longer than 24 hours has no positive impact on SSI and may have a negative one. The inability of hospitals around the world to ensure the short postoperative duration of prophylaxis is a puzzle but is clear in all studies thus far performed.

Although prophylactic antibiotics are not the only stimulus to produce resistant microflora, their control and correct management will contribute to decreasing the incidence of methicillin-resistant *Staphylococcus aureus* (MRSA) and vancomycin-resistant enterococcus (VRE). MRSA, in particular, is now found in community practice clearly as a result of excessive antibiotic use. The key to effective prophylactic antibiotics use and decreased pressure for antibiotic resistance can be simplified to the right drug, the right timing, and the right duration. The increased use of third- and fourth-generation antibiotics is to be strongly discouraged.

The new recommendations for the use of antibiotics in the prevention of infective endocarditis in association with either dental or other operative procedures are clear. The number of conditions has been reduced and clarified, and the recommendations regarding procedures have been greatly simplified.[118,119]

All recommendations for prophylactic antibiotics, whatever the indication, suggest the use of first- or second-generation cephalosporins, ampicillin or its derivatives, metronidazole, and first-generation erythromycins and aminoglycosides.[56,118]

is a growing problem.[88–90] Effective use of institutional databases may contribute greatly to identification of this problem.[89]

Clearly, the development of effective mechanisms for identifying and controlling SSIs is in the interests of all associated with the delivery of health care.[91] The identification of problems by means of surveillance and feedback can make a substantial contribution to reducing SSI rates [*see Table 6*].[13,91]

HAND WASHING

The purpose of cleansing the surgeon's hands is to reduce the numbers of resident flora and transient contaminants, thereby decreasing the risk of transmitting infection. Although the proper duration of the hand scrub is still subject to debate, evidence suggests that a 120-second scrub is sufficient, provided that a brush is used to remove the bacteria residing in the skin folds around the nails.[94] The nail folds, the nails, and the fingertips should receive the most attention because most bacteria are located around the nail folds and most glove punctures occur at the fingertips. Friction is required to remove resident microorganisms that are attached by adhesion or adsorption, whereas transient bacteria are easily removed by simple hand washing.

Solutions containing either chlorhexidine gluconate or one of the iodophors are the most effective surgical scrub preparations and have the fewest problems with stability, contamination, and toxicity.[95] Alcohols applied to the skin are among the safest known antiseptics, and they produce the greatest and most rapid reduction in bacterial counts on clean skin.[96] All variables considered, chlorhexidine gluconate followed by an iodophor appears to be the best option [*see Table 8*].

The purpose of washing the hands after surgery is to remove microorganisms that are resident, that flourished in the warm, wet environment created by wearing gloves, or that reached the hands by entering through puncture holes in the gloves. On the ward, even minimal contact with colonized patients has been demonstrated to transfer microorganisms.[97] As many as 1,000 organisms were transferred by simply touching the patient's hand, taking a pulse, or lifting the patient. The organisms survived for 20 to 150 minutes, making their transfer to the next patient clearly possible.

A return to the ancient practice of washing hands between each patient contact is warranted. Nosocomial spread of numerous organisms—including *C. difficile*; MRSA, VRE, and other antibiotic-resistant bacteria; and viruses—is a constant threat.

Hand washing on the ward is complicated by the fact that overwashing may actually increase bacterial counts. Dry, damaged skin harbors many more bacteria than healthy skin and is almost impossible to render even close to bacteria free. Although little is known about the physiologic changes in skin that result from frequent washings, the bacterial flora is certainly modified by alterations in the lipid or water content of the skin. The so-called dry hand syndrome was the impetus behind the development of the alcohol-based gels now available. These preparations make it easy for surgeons to

Table 8 Characteristics of Three Topical Antimicrobial Agents Effective against Both Gram-Positive and Gram-Negative Bacteria[96]

Agent	Mode of Action	Antifungal Activity	Comments
Chlorhexidine	Cell wall disruption	Fair	Poor activity against tuberculosis-causing organisms; can cause ototoxicity and eye irritation
Iodine/iodophors	Oxidation and substitution by free iodine	Good	Broad antibacterial spectrum; minimal skin residual activity; possible absorption toxicity and skin irritation
Alcohols	Denaturation of protein	Good	Rapid action but little residual activity; flammable

clean their hands after every patient encounter with minimal damage to their skin.

INFECTION PREVENTION IN BOWEL SURGERY

At present, the best method of preventing SSIs after bowel surgery is, once again, a subject of debate. There have been three principal approaches to this issue, involving mechanical bowel preparation in conjunction with one of the following three antibiotic regimens[56,98–103]:

1. Oral antibiotics (usually neomycin and erythromycin),[16–21,102]
2. Intravenous antibiotics covering aerobic and anaerobic bowel flora,[16–21,56,100,101] or
3. A combination of regimens 1 and 2 (meta-analysis suggests that the combination of oral and parenteral antibiotics is best).[103]

With respect to mechanical bowel preparation, there are now many trials that in modern times have failed to be supportive.[16–19] Meta-analysis suggests no value in the prevention of infection and the possibility of increasing complications.[16,21] The increased SSI and leak rates noted have been attributed to the complications associated with vigorous bowel preparation, leading to dehydration, overhydration, or electrolyte abnormalities.

An observational study reported a 26% SSI rate in colorectal surgery patients.[104] Intraoperative hypotension and body mass index were the only independent predictive variables. All patients underwent mechanical bowel preparation the day before operation and received oral antibiotics and perioperative IV antibiotics. Half of the SSIs were discovered after discharge. Most would agree that the protocol was standard. These and other results suggest that a fresh look at the infectious complications of surgery—and of bowel surgery in particular—is required.

INTEGRATION OF DETERMINANTS OF INFECTION

The significant advances in the control of wound infection during the past several decades are linked to a better understanding of the biology of wound infection, and this link has permitted the advance to the concept of SSI.[2] In all tissues at any time, there will be a critical inoculum of bacteria that would cause an infectious process [*see Figure 3*]. The standard definition of infection in urine and sputum has been 10^5 organisms/mL. In a clean dry wound, 10^5 bacteria produce a wound infection rate of 50% [*see Figure 3*].[12] Effective use of antibiotics reduces the infection rate to 10% with the same number of bacteria and thereby permits the wound to tolerate a much larger number of bacteria.

All of the clinical activities described are intended either to reduce the inoculum or to permit the host to manage the number of bacteria that would otherwise be pathologic. One study in guinea pigs showed how manipulation of local blood flow, shock, the local immune response, and foreign material can enhance the development of infection.[105] This study and two others defined an early decisive period of host antimicrobial activity that lasts for 3 to 6 hours after contamination.[51,105,106] Bacteria that remain after this period are the infecting inoculum. Processes that interfere with this early response (e.g., shock, altered perfusion, adjuvants, or foreign material) or support it (e.g., antibiotics or total care) have a major influence on outcome.

One investigation demonstrated that silk sutures decrease the number of bacteria required for infection.[107] Other investigators used a suture as the key adjuvant in studies of host manipulation,[108] whereas a separate study demonstrated persistent susceptibility to wound infection days after shock.[109] The common variable is the number of bacteria. This relation may be termed the inoculum effect, and it has great relevance in all aspects of infection control. Applying knowledge of this effect in practical terms involves the following three steps:

1. Keeping the bacterial contamination as low as possible via asepsis and antisepsis, preoperative preparation of patient and surgeon, and antibiotic prophylaxis
2. Maintaining local factors in such a way that they can prevent the lodgment of bacteria and thereby provide a locally unreceptive environment
3. Maintaining systemic responses at such a level that they can control the bacteria that become established

These three steps are related to the determinants of infection and their applicability to daily practice. Year-by-year reductions in wound infection rates, when closely followed, indicate that it is possible for surgeons to continue improving results by attention to quality of clinical care and surgical technique, despite increasingly complex operations.[5,14,29–31] In particular, the measures involved in the first step (control of bacteria) have been progressively refined and are now well established.

The integration of determinants has significant effects [*see Figures 3 and 4*]. When wound closure was effected with a wound hematocrit of 8% or more, the inoculum required to produce a wound infection rate of 40% was 100 bacteria [*see Figure 3*]. Ten bacteria produced a wound infection rate of 20%. The shift in the number of organisms required to produce clinical infection is significant. It is obvious that this inoculum effect can be changed dramatically by good surgical technique and further altered by use of prophylactic antibiotics. If the inoculum is always slightly smaller than the number of organisms required to produce infection in any given setting, the results are excellent. There is clearly a relation between the number of bacteria and the local environment. The local effect can also be seen secondary to systemic physiologic change, specifically shock. One study showed the low local perfusion in shock to be important in the development of an infection.[105,106]

One investigation has shown that shock can alter infection rates immediately after its occurrence [*see Figure 4*].[109] Furthermore, if the inoculum is large enough, antibiotics will not control bacteria. In addition, there is a late augmentation of infection lasting up to 3 days after restoration of blood volume. These early and late effects indicate that systemic determinants come into play after local effects are resolved. These observations call for further study, but, obviously, the combined abnormalities alter the outcome.

Systemic host responses are important for the control of infection. The patient has been clearly implicated as one of the four critical variables in the development of wound infection.[6] In addition, the bacterial inoculum, the location of the procedure and its duration, and the coexistence of three or more diagnoses were found to give a more accurate prediction of the risk of wound infection. The spread of risk is defined better with the SENIC index (1 to 27%) than it is with the traditional classification (2.9 to 12.6%). The importance of the number of bacteria is lessened if the other factors are considered in addition to inoculum. The inoculum effect has to be considered with respect to both the number of organisms and the local and systemic host factors that are in play. Certain variables were found to be significantly related to the risk of wound infection in three important prospective studies.[6,11,13] It is apparent that the problem of SSI cannot be examined only with respect to the management of bacteria. Host factors have become much more significant now that the bacterial inoculum can be maintained at low levels by means of asepsis, antisepsis, technique, and prophylactic antibiotics.[110]

Important host variables include the maintenance of normal homeostasis (physiology) and immune response. Maintenance of normal homeostasis in patients at risk is one of the great advances of surgical critical care.[110] The clearest improvements in this regard have come in maintenance of blood volume, oxygenation, and oxygen delivery.

One group demonstrated the importance of oxygen delivery, tissue perfusion, and P_aO_2 in the development of wound infection.[111] Oxygen can have as powerful a negative influence on the development of SSI as antibiotics can.[112] The influence is very similar to that seen in other investigations. Whereas a P_aO_2 equivalent to a true fractional concentration of oxygen in inspired gas (F_IO_2) of 45% is not feasible, maintenance, when appropriate, of an increased F_IO_2 in the postoperative period may prove an elementary and effective tool in managing the inoculum effect.

Modern surgical practice has reduced the rate of wound infection significantly. Consequently, it is more useful to think in terms of SSI, which is not limited to the incision but may occur anywhere in the operative field; this concept provides a global objective for control of infections associated with a surgical procedure. Surveillance is of great importance for quality assurance. Reports of recognized pathogens (e.g., *S. epidermidis* and group A streptococci) and unusual organisms (e.g., *Rhodococcus* [Gordona] *bronchialis*, *Mycoplasma hominis*, and *Legionella dumoffii*) in SSIs highlight the importance of infection control and epidemiology for quality assurance in surgical departments.[22–24,27,28] (Although these reports use the term *wound infection*, they are addressing what we now call SSI.) The importance of surgeon-specific and service-specific SSI reports should be clear [*see Table 6*][13,14,113] and their value in quality assurance evident.

Financial Disclosures: None Reported

References

1. Meakins JL. Host defence mechanisms: evaluation and roles of acquired defects and immunotherapy. Can J Surg 1975;18:259.
2. Consensus paper on the surveillance of surgical wound infections. The Society for Hospital Epidemiology of America; the Association for Practitioners in Infection Control; the Centers for Disease Control; the Surgical Infection Society. Infect Control Hosp Epidemiol 1992;13:599.
3. Horan TC, Gaynes RP, Martone WJ, et al. CDC definitions of nosocomial surgical site infections, 1992: a modification of CDC definitions of surgical wound infections. Infect Control Hosp Epidemiol 1992;13:606.
4. Wilson APR, Gibbons C, Reeves BC, et al. Surgical wound infection as a performance indicator: agreement of common definitions of wound infection in 4773 patients. BMJ 2004;329:720.
5. Report of an Ad Hoc Committee of the Committee on Trauma, Division of Medical Sciences, National Academy of Sciences-National Research Council. Postoperative wound infections: the influence of ultraviolet irradiation of the operating room and of various other factors. Ann Surg 1964; Suppl 1:160.
6. Haley RW, Culver DH, Morgan WM, et al. Identifying patients at high risk of surgical wound infection: a simple multivariate index of patient susceptibility and wound contamination. Am J Epidemiol 1985;121:206.
7. Mangram AJ, Horan TC, Pearson ML, et al. The Hospital Infection Control Practices Advisory Committee: guideline for prevention of surgical site infection, 1999. Infect Control Hosp Epidemiol 1999;20:247.
8. Culver DH, Horan TC, Gaynes RP, et al. Surgical wound infection rates by wound class, operative procedure and patient risk index. Am J Med 1991;91(Suppl 3B):153S.
9. Farias-Alvarez C, Farias C, Prieto D, et al. Applicability of two surgical-site infection risk indices to risk of sepsis in surgical patients. Infect Control Hosp Epidemiol 2000;21:633.
10. Neumayer L, Hosokawa P, Itani K, et al. Multivariable predictors of postoperative surgical site infection after general and vascular surgery: results from the Patient Safety in Surgery Study. J Am Coll Surg 2007;204:1178.
11. Davidson AIG, Clark C, Smith G. Postoperative wound infection: a computer analysis. Br J Surg 1971;58:333.
12. Polk HC Jr, Lopez-Mayor JF. Postoperative wound infection: a prospective study of determinant factors and prevention. Surgery 1969;66:97.
13. Cruse PJE, Foord R. The epidemiology of wound infection: a 10-year prospective study of 62,939 wounds. Surg Clin North Am 1980;60:27.
14. Olson M, O'Connor M, Schwartz ML. Surgical wound infections: a 5-year prospective study of 20,193 wounds at the Minneapolis VA Medical Center. Ann Surg 1984;199:253.
15. Tanner J, Woodings D, Moncaster K. Preoperative hair removal to reduce surgical site infection. Cochrane Database Syst Rev (3): CD004122, 2006.
16. Ram E, Sherman Y, Weil R, et al. Is mechanical bowel preparation mandatory for elective colon surgery? A prospective randomized study. Arch Surg 2005;140:285.
17. Bretagnol F, Alves A, Ricci A, et al. Rectal cancer surgery without mechanical bowel preparation. Br J Surg 2007;94:1266.
18. Jung B, Pahlman L, Nystrom PO, et al. Multicentre randomized clinical trial of mechanical bowel prepartion in elective colonic resection. Br J Surg 2007;94:689.
19. Contant CME, Hop WCJ, van't Sant HP, et al. Mechanical bowel preparation for elective colorectal surgery. Cochrane Database Syst Rev (1):CD001544, 2005.
20. Guenaga KF, Matos D, Castro AA, et al. Mechanical bowel preparation for elective colorectal surgery. Cochrane Database Syst Rev 2005 Jan 25;(1):CD001544.
21. Slim K, Vicaut E, Pais Y, et al. Meta-analysis of randomized clinical trials of colorectal surgery with or without mechanical bowel preparations. Br J Surg 2004;91:1125.
22. Boyce JM, Potter-Bynoe G, Opal SM, et al. A common-source outbreak of Staphylococcus epidermidis infections among patients undergoing cardiac surgery. J Infect Dis 1990;161:493.
23. Mastro TD, Farley TA, Elliott JA, et al. An outbreak of surgical-wound infections due to group A streptococcus carried on the scalp. N Engl J Med 1990;323:968.
24. Richet HM, Craven PC, Brown JM, et al. A cluster of Rhodococcus (Gordona) bronchialis sternal-wound infections after coronary-artery bypass surgery. N Engl J Med 1991;324:104.
25. Moylan JA, Kennedy BV. The importance of gown and drape barriers in the prevention of wound infection. Surg Gynecol Obstet 1980;151:465.
26. Garibaldi RA, Maglio S, Lerer T, et al. Comparison of nonwoven and woven gown and drape fabric to prevent intraoperative wound contamination and postoperative infection. Am J Surg 1986;152:505.
27. Lowry PW, Blankenship RJ, Gridley W, et al. A cluster of Legionella sternal-wound infections due to postoperative topical exposure to contaminated tap water. N Engl J Med 1991;324:109.
28. Wilson ME, Dietze C. Mycoplasma hominis surgical wound infection: a case report and discussion. Surgery 1988;103:257.

29. Cruse PJE. Surgical wound sepsis. Can Med Assoc J 1970;102:251.

30. Wangensteen OH, Wangensteen SD. The rise of surgery: emergence from empiric craft to scientific discipline. Minneapolis: University of Minnesota Press; 1978.

31. Cruse PJE. Wound infections: epidemiology and clinical characteristics. In: Howard RJ, Simmons RL, editors. Surgical infectious disease. 2nd ed. Norwalk, CT: Appleton and Lange; 1988. p. 319–330.

32. Petrowsky H, Demartines N, Rousson V, et al. Evidence-based value of prophylactic drainage in gastrointestinal surgery: a systematic review and meta-analyses. Ann Surg 2004;240:1074.

33. Hopf HW, Hunt TK, West JM, et al. Wound tissue oxygen tension predicts the risk of wound infection in surgical patients. Arch Surg 1997;132:997.

34. Greif R, Akca O, Horn EP, et al. Supplemental perioperative oxygen to reduce the incidence of surgical-wound infection. Outcomes Research Group. N Engl J Med 2000;342:161.

35. Pryor KO, Fahey TJ, Lien CY, et al. Surgical site infection and the routine use of perioperative hyperoxia in a general surgical population: a randomized controlled trial. JAMA 2004;291:79.

36. Gottrup F. Prevention of surgical-wound infections. N Engl J Med 2000;342:202.

37. Kaye KS, Schmit K, Pieper C, et al. The effect of increasing age on the risk of surgical site infection. J Infect Dis 2005;191:1056.

38. Latham R, Lancaster AD, Covington JF, et al. The association of diabetes and glucose control with surgical-site infections among cardiothoracic surgery patients. Infect Control Hosp Epidemiol 2001;22:607.

39. Furnary AP, Zerr KJ, Grunkemeier GI, et al. Continuous intravenous insulin infusion reduces the incidence of deep sternal wound infection in diabetic patients after cardiac surgical procedures. Ann Thorac Surg 1999;67:352.

40. Van Den Berghe G, Wouters P, Weekers F, et al. Intensive insulin therapy in critically ill patients. N Engl J Med 2001;345:1359.

41. Kurz H, Sessler DI, Lenhardt R. Perioperative normothermia to reduce the incidence of surgical wound infection and shorten hospitalization. N Engl J Med 1996;334:1209.

42. Nichols RL, Smith JW, Klein DB, et al. Risk of infection after penetrating abdominal trauma. N Engl J Med 1984;311:1065.

43. Jensen LS, Andersen A, Fristup SC, et al. Comparison of one dose versus three doses of prophylactic antibiotics, and the influence of blood transfusion, on infectious complications in acute and elective colorectal surgery. Br J Surg 1990;77:513.

44. Møller AM, Villebro N, Pedersen T, et al. Effect of preoperative smoking intervention on postoperative complications: a randomised clinical trial. Lancet 2002;359:114.

45. Buggy D. Can anaesthetic management influence surgical wound healing? Lancet 2000;356:355.

46. Melling AC, Ali B, Scott EM, et al. Effects of preoperative warming on the incidence of wound infection after clean surgery: a randomised controlled trial. Lancet 2001; 358:876.

47. Horn SD, Wright HL, Couperus JJ, et al. Association between patient-controlled analgesia pump use and postoperative surgical site infection in intestinal surgery patients. Surg Infect 2002;3:109.

48. Bennett SN, McNeil MM, Bland LA, et al. Post-operative infections traced to contamination of an intravenous anesthetic: propofol. N Engl J Med 1995;333:147.

49. Nichols RL, Smith JW. Bacterial contamination of an anesthetic agent. N Engl J Med 1995;333:184.

50. Miles AA, Miles EM, Burke J. The value and duration of defense reactions of the skin to the primary lodgment of bacteria. Br J Exp Pathol 1957;38:79.

51. Burke JF. The effective period of preventive antibiotic action in experimental incisions and dermal lesions. Surgery 1961;50:161.

52. Bernard HR, Cole WR. The prophylaxis of surgical infection: the effect of prophylactic antimicrobial drugs on incidence of infection following potentially contaminated wounds. Surgery 1964;56:151.

53. Classen DC, Evans RS, Pestotnik SC, et al. The timing of prophylactic administration of antibiotics and the risk of surgical-wound infection. N Engl J Med 1992;326:282.

54. Scottish Intercollegiate Guidelines Network. Antibiotic prophylaxis in surgery. Available at: http://www.show.scot.nhs.uk/sign/guidelines/fulltext/45/section1.html (accessed December 11, 2004).

55. Burke JP. Maximizing appropriate antibiotic prophylaxis for surgical patients: an update from LDS Hospital, Salt Lake City. Clin Infect Dis 2001;33(Suppl):78.

56. Antimicrobial prophylaxis for surgery: treatment guidelines. Med Lett 2006;4:83.

57. Kaiser AB. Surgical wound infection. N Engl J Med 1991;324:123.

58. Finland M. Antibacterial agents: uses and abuses in treatment and prophylaxis. RI Med J 1960;43:499.

59. Platt R, Zaleznik DF, Hopkins CC, et al. Perioperative antibiotic prophylaxis for herniorrhaphy and breast surgery. N Engl J Med 1990;322:153.

60. Taylor EW, Duffy K, Lee K, et al. Surgical site infection after groin hernia repair. Br J Surg 2004;91:105.

61. Aufenacker TJ, van Geldere D, Bossers AN, et al. The role of antibiotic prophylaxis in prevention of wound infection after Lichtenstein open mesh repair of primary inguinal hernia: a multicenter double-blind randomized controlled trial. Ann Surg 2005;240:955.

62. Perez AR, Roxas MF, Hilvano SS. A randomized, double-blind placebo-controlled trial to deter effectiveness of antibiotic prophylaxis for tension-free mesh herniorrhaphy. J Am Coll Surg 2005; 200:393.

63. Yee J, Dixon CM, McLean APH, et al. Clostridium difficile disease in a department of surgery: the significance of prophylactic antibiotics. Arch Surg 1991;126:241.

64. Meijer WS, Schmitz PI, Jeekel J. Meta-analysis of randomized, controlled clinical trials of antibiotic prophylaxis in biliary tract surgery. Br J Surg 1990;77:283.

65. Rotman N, Hay J-M, Lacaine F, et al. Prophylactic antibiotherapy in abdominal surgery: first- vs third-generation cephalosporins. Arch Surg 1989;124:323.

66. Washington JA III, Dearing WH, Judd ES, et al. Effect of preoperative antibiotic regimen on development of infection after intestinal surgery. Ann Surg 1974;180:567.

67. Fullen WD, Hunt J, Altemeier WA. Prophylactic antibiotics in penetrating wounds of the abdomen. J Trauma 1972; 12:282.

68. Gentry LO, Feliciano DV, Lea AS, et al. Perioperative antibiotic therapy for penetrating injuries of the abdomen. Ann Surg 1984;200:561.

69. Heseltine PNR, Yellin AE, Appleman MD, et al. Perforated and gangrenous appendicitis: an analysis of antibiotic failures. J Infect Dis 1983;148:322.

70. Bratzler DW, Houck PM, Richards C, et al. Use of antimicrobial prophylaxis for major surgery. Arch Surg 2005;140:174.

71. Girotti MJ, Fodoruk S, Irvine-Meek J, et al. Antibiotic handbook and pre-printed perioperative order forms for surgical prophylaxis: do they work? Can J Surg 1990;33:385.

72. Larsen RA, Evans RS, Burke JP, et al. Improved perioperative antibiotic use and reduced surgical wound infections through use of computer decision analysis. Infect Control Hosp Epidemiol 1989;10:316.

73. Manian FA, Meyer PL, Setzer J, et al. Surgical site infections associated with methicillin-resistant *Staphylococcus aureus*: do postoperative factors play a role? Clin Infect Dis 2003;36:863.

74. Stone HN, Haney BB, Kolb LD, et al. Prophylactic and preventive antibiotic therapy: timing duration and economics. Ann Surg 1978;189:691.

75. Fabian TC, Croce MA, Payne LW, et al. Duration of antibiotic therapy for penetrating abdominal trauma: a prospective trial. Surgery 1992;112:788.

76. Sarmiento JM, Aristizabal G, Rubiano J, et al. Prophylactic antibiotics in abdominal trauma. J Trauma 1994;37:803.

77. Hofstetter SR, Pachter HL, Bailey AA, et al. A prospective comparison of two regimens of prophylactic antibiotics in abdominal trauma: cefoxitin versus triple drug. J Trauma 1984;24:307.

78. Dellinger EP. Antibiotic prophylaxis in trauma: penetrating abdominal injuries and open fractures. Rev Infect Dis 1991;13: 5847.

79. Boxma H, Broekhuisen T, Patka P, et al. Randomized controlled trial of single-dose antibiotic prophylaxis in surgical treatment of closed fractures: the Dutch Trauma Trial. Lancet 1996;347:1133.

80. Surgical Care Improvement Project (SCIP) Module 1: infection prevention update. Available at: http://medqic.org/dcs/ContentServer?cid=1101332573904&pagename=Medqic%2FMQLiterature%2FLiteratureTemplate&c=MQLiterature. (accessed January 22, 2008).

81. Fry DE. The Surgical Infection Prevention (SIP) project: processes, outcomes, and future impact. Surg Infect 2006;7:S-17.

82. Hedrick TL, Turrentine, FE, Smith RL, et al. Single-institutional experience with the Surgical Infection Prevention (SIP) project in intra-abdominal surgery. Surg Infect 2007;8:425.

83. Dellinger EP, Hausmann SM, Bratzler DW, et al. Hospitals collaborate to decrease surgical site infections. Am J Surg 2005; 190:9.

84. Illig KA, Schmidt E, Cavanaugh J, et al. Are prophylactic antibiotics required for elective

laparoscopic cholecystectomy? J Am Coll Surg 1997;184:353.

85. Richards C, Edwards J, Culver D, et al. Does using a laparoscopic approach to cholecystectomy decrease the risk of surgical site infection? Ann Surg 2003;237:358.

86. Kirkland KB, Briggs JP, Trivette SL, et al. The impact of surgical-site infection in 1990's: attributable mortality, excess length of hospitalisation, and extra costs. Infect Control Hosp Epidemiol 1999;20:725.

87. Gaynes RP. Surveillance of surgical-site infections: the world coming together? Infect Control Hosp Epidemiol 2000;21: 309.

88. Weiss CA, Statz CL, Dahms RA, et al. Six years of surgical wound infection surveillance at a tertiary care center. Arch Surg 1999;134:1041.

89. Sands K, Vineyard G, Livingston J, et al. Efficient identification of postdischarge surgical site infections: use of automated pharmacy dispensing information, administrative data, and medical record information. J Infect Dis 1 1999;79:434.

90. Platt R. Progress in surgical-site infection surveillance. Infect Control Hosp Epidemiol 2002;23:361.

91. Burke JP. Infection control—a problem for patient safety. N Engl J Med 2003;348:651.

92. Simor AE, Ofner-Agostini M, Bryce E, et al. The evolution of methicillin-resistant Staphylococcus aureus in Canadian hospitals: 5 years of national surveillance. CMAJ 2001;165:21.

93. Perl TM, Cullen JJ, Wenzel RP, et al. Intranasal mupirocin to prevent post-operative Staphylococcus aureus infections. N Engl J Med 2002;346:1871.

94. Lowbury EJL, Lilly HA, Bull JP. Methods for disinfection of hands and operation sites. Br Med J 1964;2:531.

95. Aly R, Maibach HI. Comparative antibacterial efficacy of a 2-minute surgical scrub with chlorhexidine gluconate, povidone-iodine, and chloroxylenol sponge-brushes. Am J Infect Control 1988;16:173.

96. Larson E. Guideline for use of topical antimicrobial agents. Am J Infect Control 1988;16:253.

97. Casewell M, Phillips I. Hands as route of transmission for Klebsiella species. Br Med J 1977;2:1315.

98. Jagelman DG, Fabian TC, Nichols RL, et al. Single dose cefotetan versus multiple dose cefoxitin as prophylaxis in colorectal surgery. Am J Surg 1988;155(Suppl 5A): 71.

99. Periti P, Mazzei T, Tonelli F, et al. Single dose cefotetan versus multiple dose cefoxitin—antimicrobial prophylaxis in colorectal surgery. Dis Colon Rectum 1989;32:121.

100. Norwegian Study Group for Colorectal Surgery Should antimicrobial prophylaxis in colorectal surgery include agents effective against both anaerobic and aerobic micro-organisms? A double-blind, multicenter study. Surgery 1985;97:402.

101. Song J, Glenny AM. Antimicrobial prophylaxis in colorectal surgery: a systematic review of randomized controlled trials. Br J Surg 1998;85:1232.

102. Condon RE, Bartlett JG, Greenlee H, et al. Efficacy of oral and systemic antibiotic prophylaxis in colo-rectal operations. Arch Surg 1983;118:496.

103. Lewis RT. Oral versus systemic antibiotic prophylaxis in elective colon surgery: a randomized study and meta-analysis send a message from the 1990's. Can J Surg 2002;45:173.

104. Smith RL, Bohl JK, McElearney ST, et al. Wound infection after elective colorectal resection. Ann Surg 2004;239:599.

105. Miles AA, Miles EM, Burke J. The value and duration of defence reactions of the skin to the primary lodgement of bacteria. Br J Exp Pathol 1957;38:79.

106. Miles AA. The inflammatory response in relation to local infections. Surg Clin North Am 1980;60:93.

107. Alexander JW, Alexander WA. Penicillin prophylaxis of experimental staphylococcal wound infections. Surg Gynecol Obstet 1965;120:243.

108. Polk HC Jr. The enhancement of host defenses against infection: search for the holy grail. Surgery 1986;99:1.

109. Livingston DH, Malangoni MA. An experimental study of susceptibility to infection after hemorrhagic shock. Surg Gynecol Obstet 1989;168:138.

110. Meakins JL. Surgeons, surgery and immunomodulation. Arch Surg 1991; 126:494.

111. Knighton D, Halliday B, Hunt TK. Oxygen as an antibiotic: a comparison of the effects of inspired oxygen concentration and antibiotic administration on in vivo bacterial clearance. Arch Surg 1986;121:191.

112. Rabkin J, Hunt TK. Infection and oxygen. In: Davis JC, Hunt TK, editors. Problem wounds: the role of oxygen. New York: Elsevier; 1987. p. 1.

113. Olson MM, Lee JT Jr. Continuous, 10-year wound infection surveillance: results, advantages, and unanswered questions. Arch Surg 1990;125:794.

114. Oreskovich MR, Dellinger EP, Lennard ES, et al. Duration of preventive antibiotic administration for penetrating abdominal trauma. Arch Surg 1982;117:200.

115. Langely JM, Le Blanc JC, Drake J, et al. Efficacy of antimicrobial prophylaxis in placement of cerebrospinal fluid shunts: meta-analysis. Clin Infect Dis 1993;17:98.

116. Tejirian T, DiFronzo LA, Haigh PI. Antibiotic prophylaxis for preventing wound infection after breast surgery: a systematic review and metaanalysis. J Am Coll Surg 2006;203:729.

117. Forse RA, Karam B, MacLean LD, et al. Antibiotic prophylaxis for surgery in morbidly obese patients. Surgery 1989;106: 750.

118. Wilson W. Taubert KA, Gewitz M, et al. Prevention of infective endocarditis: guidelines from the American Heart Association. Circulation 2007;116:1736.

119. Major changes in endocarditis prophylaxis for dental, GI and GU procedures. Med Lett Drug Ther 2007;49:99.

120. Hayek LJ, Emerson JM, Gardner AMN. A placebo-controlled trial of the effect of two preoperative baths or showers with chlorhexidine detergent on postoperative wound infection rates. J Hosp Infect 1987;10:165.

121. Hamilton HW, Hamilton KR, Lone FJ. Preoperative hair removal. Can J Surg 1977; 20:269.

122. McDonald WS, Nichter LS. Debridement of bacterial and particulate-contaminated wounds. Ann Plast Surg 1994;33:142.

123. Edwards PS, Lipp A, Holmes A. Preoperative skin antiseptics for preventing surgical wound infections after clean surgery. Cochrane Database Syst Rev (3):CD003949, 2004.

Acknowledgment

Figures 3 and 4 Albert Miller.
The author would like to thank Byron J. Masterson, MD, FACS for his contribution to a previous iteration of this chapter, on which the current version is partially based.

2 BLEEDING AND TRANSFUSION

Garth H. Utter, MD, MSc, FACS, Robert C. Gosselin, MT, and John T. Owings, MD, FACS

Approach to the Patient with Massive Hemorrhage

A surgeon is frequently one of the first people to be called when a patient experiences massive hemorrhage. "Massive hemorrhage" is usually not hard to recognize in practice, but it can be defined as hemorrhage requiring at least 10 units of cellular blood products within 24 hours. To treat such a patient appropriately, the surgeon must rapidly and simultaneously accomplish three tasks: identify the source or cause of the bleeding, stop or limit the bleeding, and restore the patient's circulation.

Causes fall into two main categories: (1) conditions involving loss of vascular integrity, such as a patient with bleeding from a peptic ulcer or a trauma patient with a severe liver laceration, and (2) conditions involving a derangement of the hemostatic process. Typically, massive hemorrhage begins with a loss of vascular integrity, but derangements of hemostasis frequently develop as a secondary problem and play a major role in the exacerbation of such hemorrhage. In this section, we focus on the immediate concerns to keep the patient alive with particular attention to how to address the associated coagulopathy. We consider derangements of hemostasis that are not associated with massive hemorrhage in the next section, "Approach to the Patient with a Derangement of Hemostasis."

Control of the Source of Bleeding

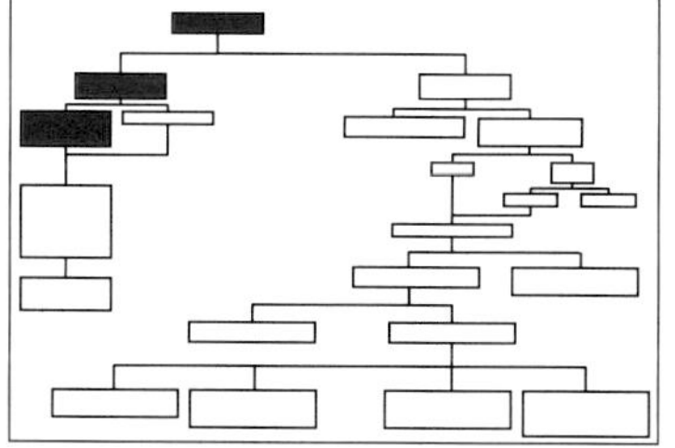

If a coagulopathy develops as a result of uncontrolled hemorrhage from loss of vascular integrity, attempting to treat the coagulopathy without controlling the source is an exercise in futility. Other sections of this text address the anatomic and technical considerations involved in controlling different sites of bleeding [see subcategories under "Bleeding" in the Index]. However, in contrast to the routine conduct of operations, control of the source of massive bleeding requires a fundamentally different mindset.

The goals of operative conduct change from definitive management of all issues to "damage control," in which the salient objective is to address immediately life-threatening problems: restoration of vascular integrity and, to the extent necessary and prudent, restoration of the circulation of the viscera and limbs. Other goals, such as reestablishment of intestinal continuity or closure of the wound, become secondary and can be addressed later if the patient survives. Even selected, more drastic maneuvers for exposure of the site of bleeding should be considered when the patient is at appreciable risk of death; these apply even if the hemorrhage developed during an elective procedure. For example, right nephrectomy may be warranted to afford exposure of the infrahepatic inferior vena cava, or deliberate division of a common iliac artery may be necessary to expose bleeding from the corresponding common iliac vein. Temporary vascular shunts may be helpful to rapidly restore blood flow to ischemic limbs if it is still possible to salvage the limb. However, reperfusion of a large volume of ischemic tissue in the setting of shock can cause severe systemic problems, so expert judgment is necessary to decide whether to try to preserve or amputate the limb in such situations.

Sometimes, the best option to control massive hemorrhage is not necessarily an open operation. Increasingly, interventional radiologic and endovascular techniques are serving important roles: although long used for control of bleeding from sites not easily managed with open procedures, such as pelvic fractures, they have recently become an accepted approach for some problems traditionally managed with open procedures, such as ruptured abdominal aortic aneurysms,[1] because of the speed of access by an experienced interventionalist. However, the surgeon should be actively involved in decisions to use minimally invasive techniques and should never hesitate to operate if that is the best option in a given situation. Surgeons must individualize their approach to each patient based on their expertise, available resources, and the most current standards of care but be willing to use all tools in their armamentarium.

Restoration of the Blood Volume

Just as massive hemorrhage should lead the surgeon to reprioritize the goals of an operation, it should also prompt a major shift in the fluid resuscitation strategy. Initially, when there is massive hemorrhage that can be addressed with an operation, resuscitation with blood products and other intravenous (IV) fluids should be implemented only as an adjunct while attempts are made to stop the loss of blood. Although surgeons continue to debate the merits of "permissive hypotension" (the concept that fluid resuscitation before control of hemorrhage should be minimized because it will lead to increased bleeding[2]), attempts at fluid resuscitation should not delay procedures to control massive hemorrhage, even temporarily.

When massive bleeding exists and direct control of the site of bleeding is under way, the decision to transfuse should be based primarily on hemodynamic status rather than on the hemoglobin or hematocrit level. These laboratory values do

Approach to the Patient with Hemorrhage

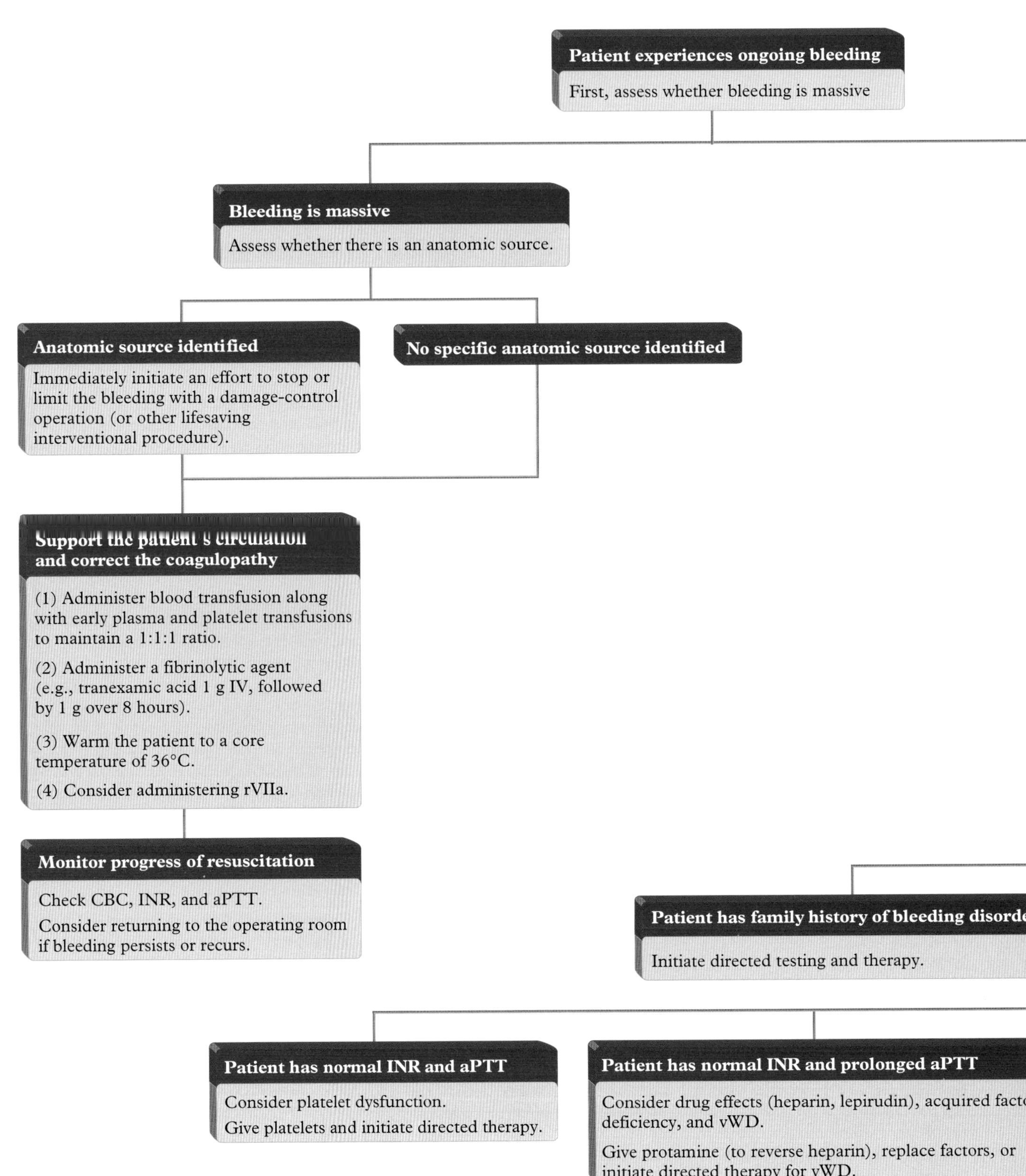
Patient experiences ongoing bleeding
First, assess whether bleeding is massive
Bleeding is massive
Assess whether there is an anatomic source.
Anatomic source identified
Immediately initiate an effort to stop or limit the bleeding with a damage-control operation (or other lifesaving interventional procedure).
No specific anatomic source identified
Support the patient's circulation and correct the coagulopathy
(1) Administer blood transfusion along with early plasma and platelet transfusions to maintain a 1:1:1 ratio.
(2) Administer a fibrinolytic agent (e.g., tranexamic acid 1 g IV, followed by 1 g over 8 hours).
(3) Warm the patient to a core temperature of 36°C.
(4) Consider administering rVIIa.
Monitor progress of resuscitation
Check CBC, INR, and aPTT.
Consider returning to the operating room if bleeding persists or recurs.
Patient has family history of bleeding disorde
Initiate directed testing and therapy.
Patient has normal INR and aPTT
Consider platelet dysfunction.
Give platelets and initiate directed therapy.
Patient has normal INR and prolonged aPTT
Consider drug effects (heparin, lepirudin), acquired facto
deficiency, and vWD.
Give protamine (to reverse heparin), replace factors, or initiate directed therapy for vWD.

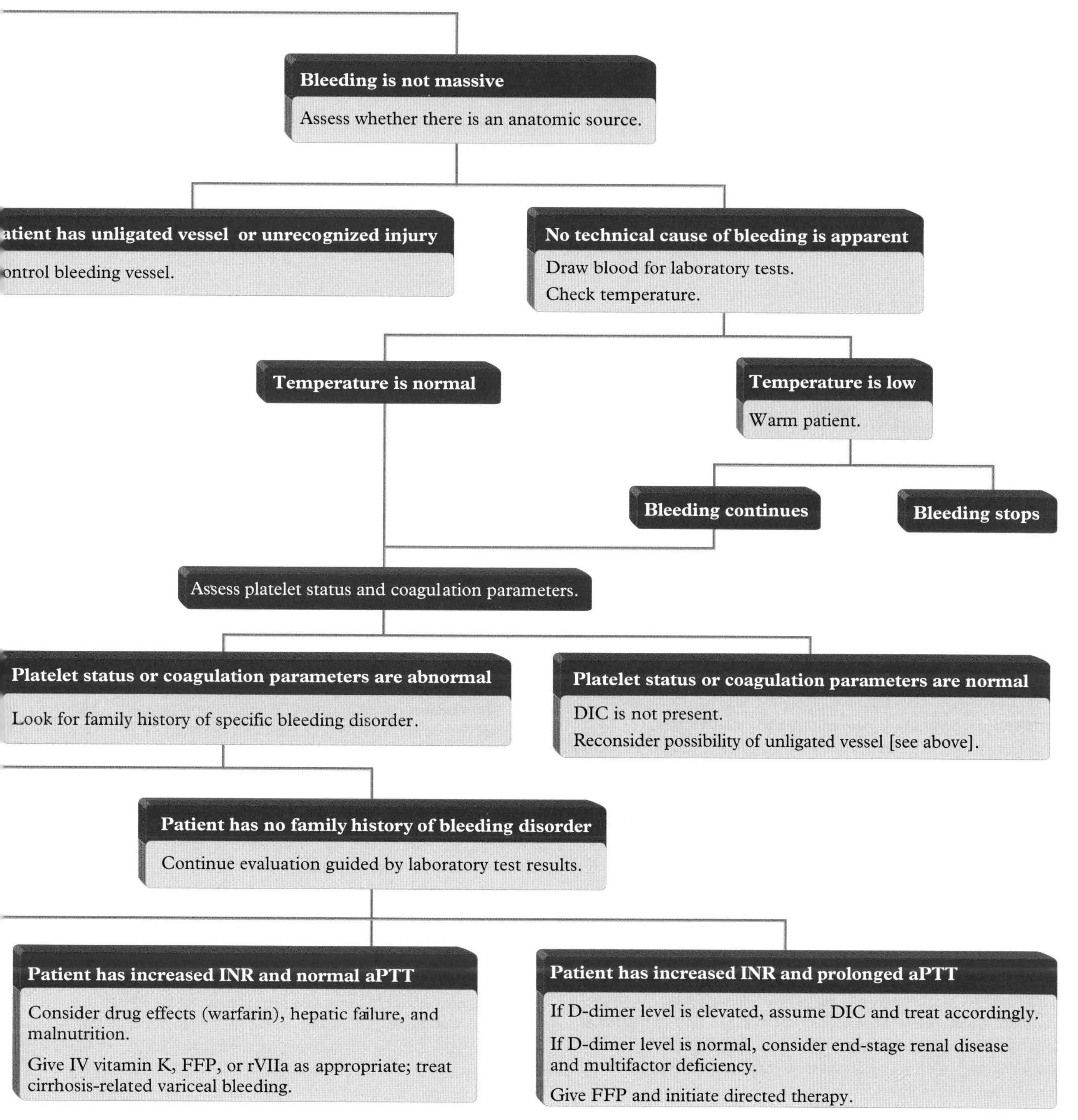
Bleeding is not massive
Assess whether there is an anatomic source.
atient has unligated vessel or unrecognized injury
ontrol bleeding vessel.
No technical cause of bleeding is apparent
Draw blood for laboratory tests.
Check temperature.
Temperature is normal
Temperature is low
Warm patient.
Bleeding continues
Bleeding stops
Assess platelet status and coagulation parameters.
Platelet status or coagulation parameters are abnormal
Look for family history of specific bleeding disorder.
Platelet status or coagulation parameters are normal
DIC is not present.
Reconsider possibility of unligated vessel [see above].
Patient has no family history of bleeding disorder
Continue evaluation guided by laboratory test results.
Patient has increased INR and normal aPTT
Consider drug effects (warfarin), hepatic failure, and malnutrition.
Give IV vitamin K, FFP, or rVIIa as appropriate; treat cirrhosis-related variceal bleeding.
Patient has increased INR and prolonged aPTT
If D-dimer level is elevated, assume DIC and treat accordingly.
If D-dimer level is normal, consider end-stage renal disease and multifactor deficiency.
Give FFP and initiate directed therapy.

not reflect acute hemorrhage because there is a time lag before these levels equilibrate from fluid shift between the extravascular and vascular compartments and from administration of IV fluids. The goals of transfusion are therefore as much to increase the intravascular volume as to prevent the development of profound deficits in oxygen-carrying capacity. Stabilized patients who are at high risk for recurrent bleeding (e.g., those with a massive liver injury or gastrointestinal (GI) hemorrhage from an unknown source) should receive transfusions up to a level at which, should bleeding recur, enough reserve oxygen-carrying capacity would be available to allow diagnosis and correction of the hemorrhage without significant compromise of oxygen delivery (we advocate a target hematocrit of roughly 30% during this phase). The standard restrictive transfusion strategy used in stable intensive care unit (ICU) patients [*see* Approach to the Patient with Anemia, *below*] warrants modification in these circumstances because of the higher likelihood of occult active hemorrhage.

Management of the Coagulopathy

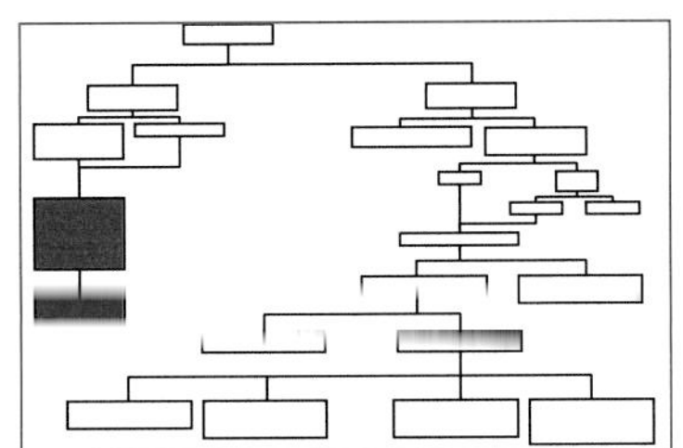

It is true that coagulopathy may promote massive hemorrhage and that massive hemorrhage causes a coagulopathy. As a rule, the massively hemorrhaging patient has a coagulopathy out of proportion to the abnormalities reflected with in vitro laboratory tests such as the prothrombin time (PT, commonly expressed as an international normalized ratio [INR]) or activated partial thromboplastin time (aPTT). Coagulopathy most typically occurs when there is massive hemorrhage in concert with injury to a large volume of tissue. Although the nature of this coagulopathy is not precisely defined, it probably involves a number of factors: (1) platelet dysfunction and diminished availability of platelets at the interface between the vascular endothelium and luminal flow; (2) dysfunctional formation of thrombi in the setting of acidosis and hypothermia; (3) accelerated thrombolysis (attributable to dysfunctional thrombosis); and, eventually, (4) consumption of clotting factors.

Increased recognition of this coagulopathy has prompted enthusiasm for administration of plasma and platelets early in the treatment of the patient with massive hemorrhage. This practice, frequently incorporated into a massive transfusion protocol, is described as "1:1:1 transfusion" because the goal is to transfuse one unit of plasma and one of platelets along with each unit of red blood cells (RBCs) such that the ratio stays balanced throughout the resuscitation phase. (Adjustment of these ratios is necessary for centers that use pooled quantities of plasma and/or platelets.) The rationale is that patients are already extensively coagulopathic by the time they manifest thrombocytopenia or prolongation of the INR or aPTT. Thus, during the first several hours during and after massive hemorrhage, plasma and platelets are necessary independent of the laboratory tests and help address a significant contributing factor for persistent hemorrhage.

The concept of liberal, early use of plasma and platelets developed in large part from the recent US-led military campaigns in Iraq and Afghanistan. Initially in those conflicts, the lack of a reliable supply of blood products near the scene of injury—and platelets especially—led to the use of fresh whole blood transfusion. Although fresh whole blood would be impractical in the civilian setting because of logistical issues and the risk of transmitting transfusion-related infections, the perception of improved outcomes associated with its use prompted military surgeons to advocate 1:1:1 transfusion.

Proponents of this approach argue that it restores hemostatic capacity and helps limit hemorrhage, leading to improved survival. Indeed, observational studies suggest that mortality is reduced.[3] However, the ratios examined in these studies typically have been calculated retrospectively over relatively long (e.g., 12- or 24-hour) time periods after hemorrhage. Critics emphasize that patients who do not survive long enough to receive early plasma and platelets bias such observational comparisons (i.e., they are classified as receiving a large ratio of RBCs to plasma or platelets because they died early) and that plasma and platelets carry theoretical harms of transfusion-related acute lung injury and bacterial infection, respectively. Despite some uncertainty about the actual merits of the 1:1:1 approach, given that military conflicts have frequently spurred advances in transfusion medicine, it appears likely that the approach will be adopted more widely if the availability of blood products does not limit its application. In the absence of sufficient availability of blood products to allow a 1:1:1 approach, aggressive correction of abnormalities of the INR, aPTT, and platelet count are warranted for patients with massive hemorrhage.

More convincing information supports the use of antifibrinolytic agents in the setting of massive hemorrhage. Aprotinin, tranexamic acid, and ε-aminocaproic acid (Amicar) are known to reduce transfusion requirements in the setting of elective operations (primarily cardiac procedures). Furthermore, a recent large randomized trial, the CRASH-2 trial, showed that patients with or at risk for significant bleeding (i.e., hypotension or tachycardia) from traumatic injury had decreased all-cause and bleeding-related mortality when they received tranexamic acid within 8 hours of injury.[4] In this study, tranexamic acid was administered intravenously as a 1 g loading dose, followed by an infusion of an additional 1 g over 8 hours. Tranexamic acid did not increase the likelihood of major vascular occlusion events (myocardial infarction, stroke, and pulmonary embolism).

Recombinant activated factor VII (rVIIa) is approved for the treatment of hemophilia in the United States. It has also been advocated for off-label use early in the course of uncontrolled hemorrhage[5] and intracranial hemorrhage. Although rVIIa can be a rapid and highly specific form of treatment in certain instances of bleeding (e.g., traumatic brain injury in a patient on warfarin), the rationale for its use is not as highly targeted in the setting of massive hemorrhage, during which factor deficiencies are not typically an early abnormality. Two sponsor-initiated international randomized trials of rVIIa in severely injured trauma patients have been performed, and their results—although neither had overwhelming power to detect improved survival—suggest that rVIIa decreases blood transfusions but does not reduce mortality.[6,7] One recent report suggested that off-label use of rVIIa in certain populations significantly increased the risk of arterial thromboembolic complications.[8] In the absence of better designed and conducted studies of patients with massive bleeding, surgeons will need to decide whether use of rVIIa is warranted despite its costs and incompletely understood efficacy and safety profile in this setting. Consensus recommendations have attempted to define appropriate use in light of insufficient evidence.[9]

There is relatively little controversy over the management of hypothermia. As a series of chemical reactions, the coagulation cascade slows with decreasing temperature.[10] Thus, a patient with a temperature lower than 35°C (95°F) clots more slowly and less efficiently than one with a temperature of 37°C (98.6°F). The resulting coagulopathy cannot be detected by laboratory tests because the laboratory warms the sample to 37°C to run the coagulation assays (INR and aPTT). Thus, bleeding hypothermic patients should be rewarmed, and active measures are warranted if the core temperature is 34.5°C (94.1°F) or lower.[11]

Relatively new agents have been promulgated to facilitate hemostasis at sites of focal bleeding. QuikClot (Z-Medica, Newington, CT), a granular substance containing the mineral zeolite, and HemCon (HemCon, Inc., Portland, OR), a chitosan-based dressing, have been used in the setting of military trauma. Preliminary information suggests that whereas QuikClot appears to cause superficial burns, HemCon may carry few disadvantages.[12]

Approach to the Patient with a Derangement of Hemostasis

Not infrequently, surgeons encounter patients with actual or suspected derangements of hemostasis short of massive hemorrhage. These situations range from the preoperative assessment of asymptomatic patients potentially at risk for coagulopathic bleeding to the postoperative management of patients with an observed bleeding diathesis. Although it is still important to rule out the possibility of technical causes of bleeding, surgeons should also be able to recognize coagulopathic bleeding and know how to prevent it when possible or evaluate and manage its most common etiologies when it occurs.

Coagulopathies are varied in their causes, treatments, and prognoses. Although specialized hematologic tests exist to identify rare congenital or acquired clotting abnormalities, our goal in this section is to outline a practical, effective approach to the coagulopathies surgeons see most frequently. The vast majority of these coagulopathies can be diagnosed by means of a brief patient and family history, a review of medications, physical examination, and commonly used laboratory studies—in particular, PT (commonly expressed as an INR), aPTT, complete blood count (CBC), and D-dimer assay.

In the Discussion section later in this chapter, we present an overview of the physiology of hemostasis and consider some of the rarer conditions and theoretical considerations in greater detail.

Exclusion of Technical Causes of Bleeding

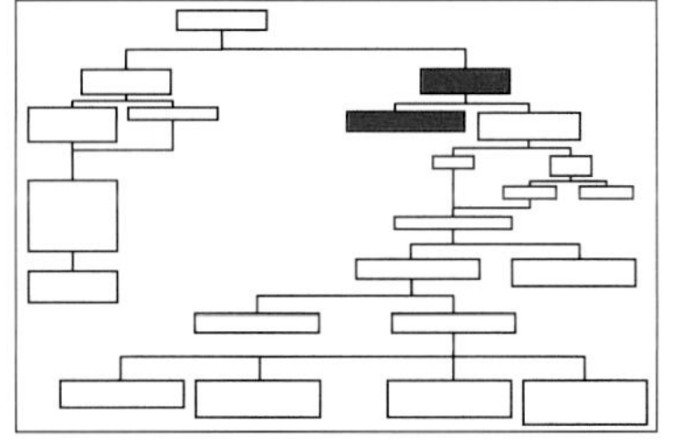

It is critical to emphasize that the most common causes of postoperative bleeding, even when it is not massive, are technical: an unligated vessel or an unrecognized injury is much more likely to be the cause of a falling hematocrit than either a drug effect or an endogenous hemostatic defect. Furthermore, if an unligated vessel is treated as though it were an endogenous hemostatic defect (i.e., with transfusions), the outcome is frequently disastrous. For these reasons, in all cases of ongoing bleeding, the first consideration must always be to exclude a surgically correctable cause.

Ongoing bleeding may be surprisingly difficult to diagnose. Healthy young patients can usually maintain a normal blood pressure until their blood loss exceeds 40% of their blood volume (roughly 2 L). If the bleeding is from a laceration to an extremity, it will be obvious; however, if the bleeding is occurring internally, there may be few physiologic signs until the patient is at high risk for death.

Even when a technical cause of bleeding has seemingly been excluded, the possibility should be reconsidered periodically throughout assessment. Patients who are either unresuscitated or underresuscitated undergo vasospasm that results in decreased bleeding. As resuscitation proceeds, the catecholamine-induced vasospasm subsides and bleeding may recur. Only when the surgeon is confident that a missed injury or unligated vessel is not the cause of the bleeding should other potential causes be investigated.

Initial Assessment of Potential Coagulopathy

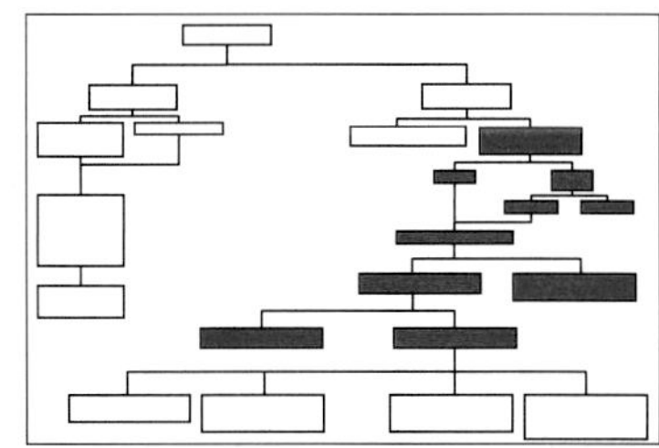

The first step in the assessment of a stable patient with a potential coagulopathy is to draw a blood sample. The blood should be drawn into a tube containing ethylenediaminetetraacetic acid (EDTA) for a CBC and into a citrated tube for coagulation analysis (these tubes commonly have purple and blue tops, respectively).

Concomitant with these laboratory tests, it is essential to obtain a personal and family history of bleeding tendencies. A patient who has had dental extractions without major problems or who had a normal adolescence without any history of bleeding dyscrasias is very unlikely to have a congenital or hereditary bleeding disorder.[13] Alternatively, previous bleeding events and a familial history of bleeding are both suggestive of a congenital coagulopathy and warrant further testing to diagnose and treat the disorder [*see* Discussion, Bleeding Disorders, *below*]. Mucosal and superficial bleeding is suggestive of platelet abnormalities, and deep bleeding is suggestive of a factor deficiency. A thorough medication inventory is necessary to assess the possible impact of drugs on laboratory and clinical presentations. In the patient history query, it is advisable to ask explicitly about nonprescription drugs—using expressions such as "over-the-counter drugs," "cold medicines," and "Pepto-Bismol"—because unless specifically reminded, patients tend to equate the term "medications" with prescription drugs. If this is not done, many drugs that are capable of influencing hemostasis in vivo and in vitro (e.g., salicylates, cold and allergy medicines, and herbal supplements) may be missed.

Interpretation of Coagulation Parameters

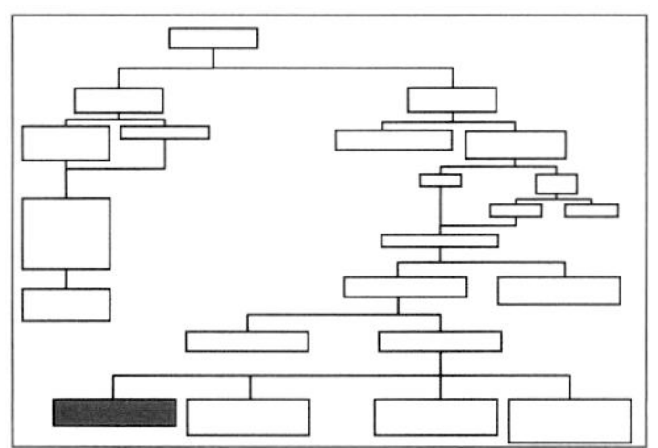

NORMAL INR, NORMAL APTT

Patients with a normal INR and a normal aPTT who exhibit unexpected bleeding may have an impaired platelet activity. Inadequate platelet activity is frequently manifested as persistent oozing from wound edges or as low-volume bleeding. Such bleeding is rarely the cause of exsanguinating hemorrhage, although it may be life-threatening when it occurs in certain locations (e.g., inside the cranium or the pericardium). Inadequate platelet activity may be attributable to an insufficient number of platelets, platelet dysfunction, or a platelet inhibitor. In the absence of a major surgical insult or concomitant coagulopathy, a platelet count of 20,000/μL or higher is usually adequate for normal coagulation.[14,15] There is some disagreement regarding the threshold for platelet transfusion in the absence of active bleeding. Patients undergoing procedures in which even small-vessel oozing is potentially life-threatening (e.g., craniotomy) should be maintained at a higher platelet count (i.e., > 20,000/μL). Patients without ongoing bleeding who are not specifically at increased risk for major complications from low-volume bleeding may be safely watched with platelet counts as low as 10,000/μL.[16]

Oozing in a patient who has an adequate platelet count and normal coagulation parameters may be a signal of platelet dysfunction. The now-routine administration of acetylsalicylic acid (aspirin) and clopidogrel (Plavix) to reduce the risk of myocardial infarction and stroke has led to a rise in the incidence of drug-induced platelet dysfunction. Aspirin causes irreversible platelet dysfunction through the cyclooxygenase pathway. It takes approximately 10 days for sufficient numbers of new platelets to be formed such that the effect of aspirin lapses; however, because the half-life of aspirin is on the order of 2 to 5 hours, new platelet transfusions should be unaffected if at least a day has passed since the last use of aspirin. The platelet dysfunction caused by other nonsteroidal antiinflammatory drugs (e.g., ibuprofen) is reversible and consequently does not generally last as long as that caused by aspirin.

Newer platelet-blocking agents have been found to be effective in improving outcome after coronary angioplasty.[17] These drugs function through different mechanisms. Some, such as abciximab (ReoPro), eptifibatide (Integrilin), and tirofiban (Aggrastat), block the platelet surface receptor glycoprotein (GP) IIb-IIIa, which binds platelets to fibrinogen. Others, such as clopidogrel, ticlopidine (Ticlid), and prasugrel (Effient), target the $P2Y_{12}$ receptor (also known as the adenosine diphosphate [ADP] receptor). Clopidogrel, the most commonly used among this group, permanently prevents the association of $P2Y_{12}$ receptors into functional oligomeric complexes. As a result, there is no way to inactivate this medication if the patient experiences bleeding during its therapeutic window, which typically lasts about 5 days from the last dose. In the face of life-threatening bleeding during this interval, it is reasonable to administer platelets based on the rationale that, in large-enough quantities, they may eventually bind all of the active metabolite. Some of the newest drugs in the $P2Y_{12}$ inhibitor class (which have not yet been evaluated for use in the United States), for example, ticagrelor, are reversible, which may help avoid such difficulties in the future.

von Willebrand disease (vWD), although sometimes associated with a slight prolongation of the aPTT (as a result of decreased factor VIII activity), most commonly shows no abnormalities with both the INR and the aPTT. The clinical expression is variable, but von Willebrand factor (vWF) levels of less than 30% are more likely associated with clinically important bleeding. Confirmation of the diagnosis can be obtained by specialized tests [*see* Discussion, Bleeding Disorders, *below*]. Correction is accomplished by administering desmopressin, directed therapy (vWF/factor VIII), or cryoprecipitate.

In patients with platelet dysfunction caused by an inhibitor of platelet function, such as an elevated blood urea nitrogen (BUN) level or aspirin, 1-desamino-8-D-arginine vasopressin (desmopressin) is capable of significantly improving the platelet dysfunction.[18] The mechanism of this effect is not entirely understood but appears to involve more complex changes than simply increased release of factor VIII and vWF.

Supratherapeutic effects of the low-molecular-weight heparins (LMWHs) may also manifest with a normal INR and aPTT [*see* Normal INR, Prolonged aPTT, *below* for a discussion of both unfractionated heparin and the LMWHs].

Less common causes of bleeding in patients with a normal INR and a normal aPTT include factor XIII deficiency, hypofibrinogenemia or dysfibrinogenemia, and derangements in the fibrinolytic pathway [*see* Discussion, Mechanics of Hemostasis, *below*].

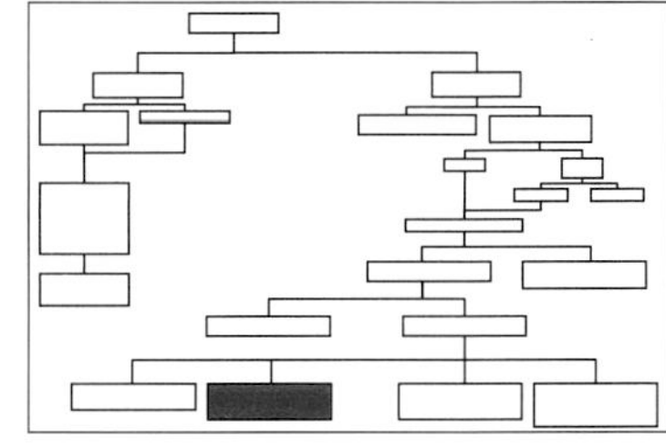

NORMAL INR, PROLONGED APTT

In the absence of a history of significant bleeding, patients with a normal INR and an abnormal aPTT are likely to have a drug-induced coagulation defect. The agent most commonly responsible is unfractionated heparin. Reversal of the heparin effect, if desired, can be accomplished by administering protamine sulfate. Protamine should be given with caution, however, because it may induce both hyper- and hypocoagulable states.[19] Protamine should also be used with caution because of the potential for allergic reactions, including anaphylaxis. Patients can become sensitized to impurities in protamine if they have previously received it. Also, diabetic patients have been described to become sensitized through their exposure to similar impurities in protamine-containing insulin formulations (e.g., neutral protamine Hagedorn, or "NPH," insulin).[20]

Importantly, the aPTT does not detect the anticoagulant activity of LMWHs. Because such heparins exert much of their anticoagulant effect by potentiating antithrombin to inactivate factor Xa rather than factor IIa, an assay that measures anti-Xa activity is needed to measure the anticoagulant effect. However, the anti-Xa effect of the LMWHs may not be as effectively reversed by protamine as the anti-IIa effect of unfractionated heparin. It is currently unclear which agent is best for reversal of LMWHs, but both protamine and rVIIa have been advocated. Whether or not bleeding has occurred, because the standard coagulation tests do not detect the effect of the LMWHs, suspicion for a supratherapeutic effect should be aroused if there is a concern that excessive doses have been administered or clearance has decreased (e.g., renal insufficiency).

One nuance of the anti-Xa laboratory assay is that it may not truly measure the degree of anticoagulation in vivo; rather, anti-Xa results for some of the available assays should be interpreted merely as the concentration of LMWH in plasma. Because heparins (including LMWHs) function to a large extent by catalyzing the activity of antithrombin, the therapeutic effect of heparin is critically dependent on adequate antithrombin levels. In fact, acquired antithrombin deficiency (as occurs with trauma and other critical illnesses) is the most common reason for LMWH to have an inadequate effect. The anti-Xa laboratory assay may not account for in vivo antithrombin levels, because some methods involve the addition of antithrombin to the test sample as a reagent. Consequently, the results of this assay may not be a reliable guide to the patient's coagulation status.

An additional crucial point is that the administration of plasma (e.g., fresh frozen plasma [FFP]) will not correct the anticoagulant effect of either unfractionated heparin or LMWHs. In fact, given that plasma contains antithrombin and that both unfractionated heparin and LMWHs act by potentiating antithrombin, administration of FFP could actually enhance the heparins' anticoagulant effect.

A variety of direct thrombin inhibitors (e.g., bivalirudin [Hirulog], lepirudin, argatroban, and dabigatran) are currently available in Europe, Asia, and North America.[21] Many of them cause prolongation of the aPTT. Dabigatran is a new oral direct thrombin inhibitor that has been recently approved for use in the United States for atrial fibrillation. As an oral alternative to warfarin that does not require frequent laboratory tests to monitor its anticoagulant effect, dabigatran may become widely used. It has a variable impact on coagulation assays: the aPTT is typically elevated but may be only moderately prolonged with supratherapeutic levels of dabigatran.[22] One disadvantage shared by most of the direct thrombin inhibitors is that the effects are not reversible; if thrombin inhibition is no longer desired, FFP should be given to attempt to correct the aPTT. Because the inhibitor that is circulating but not bound at the time of FFP administration will bind the prothrombin in the FFP, the amount of FFP required to correct the aPTT may be greater than would be needed with a simple factor deficiency.

Hemophilia is also associated with prolongation of the aPTT. It can cause spontaneous bleeding or prolonged bleeding after a surgical or traumatic insult. As noted, hemophilia is rare in the absence of a personal or family history of the disorder. Although hemophilia can occur as an acquired autoimmune condition with production of antibodies against clotting factors, the most common forms of hemophilia are inherited and involve deficiencies of factors VIII, IX, and XI (hemophilia A, hemophilia B [Christmas disease], and hemophilia C, respectively). As X-linked recessive disorders, hemophilias A and B occur almost exclusively in males. The clinical presentations of hemophilia A and hemophilia B are similar: hemarthroses are the most common clinical manifestations, ultimately leading to degenerative joint deformities. Spontaneous bleeding may also occur, resulting in intracranial hemorrhage, large hematomas in the muscles of extremities, hematuria, and GI bleeding. Certain types of vWD can result in a deficiency of factor VIII and thus present like hemophilia A. Factor XI deficiency is relatively common in Jewish persons but rarely results in spontaneous bleeding. Such deficiency may result in bleeding after oral operations and trauma; however, a number of major procedures (e.g., cardiac bypass surgery) do not result in postoperative bleeding in this population.[23]

In contrast to depletion of natural anticoagulants such as antithrombin and protein C, depletion of procoagulant factors rarely gives rise to significant manifestations until it is relatively severe. Typically, no laboratory abnormalities result from depletion of procoagulant factors until factor activity levels fall below 40% of normal, and clinical abnormalities are frequently absent even when factor activity levels fall to only 10% of normal. This tolerance for subcritical degrees of depletion is a reflection of the built-in redundancies in the procoagulant pathways.

If hemophilia is suspected, specific factor analysis is indicated. Appropriate therapy involves administering the deficient factor or factors. Hemophiliac patients who have undergone extensive transfusion therapy may pose a particular challenge: massive transfusions frequently lead to the development of antibodies that make subsequent transfusion or even directed therapy impossible. Accordingly, several alternatives to transfusion or directed factor therapy (e.g., rVIIa) have been developed for use in this population.

Other conditions may also have an isolated effect on the aPTT. Drotrecogin alfa (i.e., activated protein C), a medication approved for treatment of certain subgroups of patients with sepsis, may prolong the aPTT. Its use is contraindicated in the presence of active hemorrhage, but if bleeding should arise during its use, cessation of the infusion should suffice as a result of its short half-life. Lupus anticoagulant and contact factor deficiency can also cause prolongation of the aPTT; however, these phenomena do not clinically result in a hypocoagulable state.

INCREASED INR, NORMAL APTT

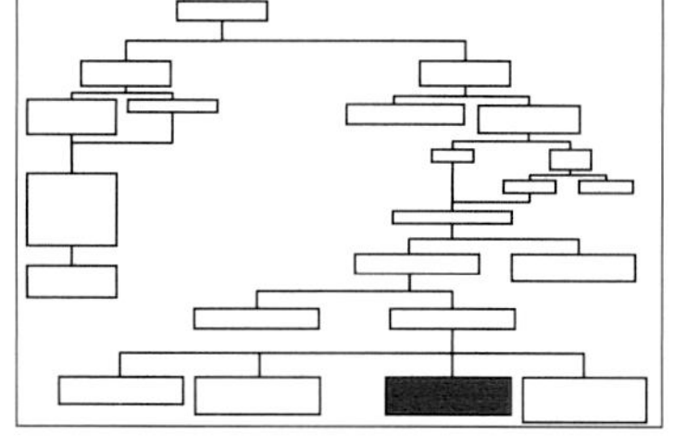

An increased INR in association with a normal aPTT is potentially a more ominous finding in a patient with a coagulopathy. Any of a number of causes, all centering on factor deficiency, may be responsible.

An elevated INR occurs with the administration of vitamin K antagonists (e.g., warfarin), with variable effects on the aPTT. If the aPTT is normal, this usually demonstrates that warfarin was only recently started (usually < 3 days of treatment) or has been underdosed. Such a coagulopathy is the result of a pure factor deficiency, and its degree is proportional to the prolongation of the INR. Because warfarin acts by disrupting vitamin K metabolism, the coagulopathy may be corrected by giving vitamin K [*see Table 1*], but this process takes several hours for additional proteins to be synthesized.[24] If the patient is actively bleeding, vitamin K should still be given, but the primary corrective measures should be to administer FFP and/or rVIIa. FFP should be administered in an amount proportional to the patient's size and the relative increase in the INR, whereas rVIIa should be administered at a dose of 15 to 90 µg/kg. The INR should subsequently be rechecked to ensure that correction has been achieved. Because rVIIa has a relatively short half-life, in general, it should be used as an adjunct to FFP rather than a replacement for it. Aside from the time delay involved, the main potential disadvantage of vitamin K replacement therapy is that if the patient is to be reanticoagulated with warfarin in the near future, dosing will be difficult because the patient will exhibit resistance to warfarin for a variable period.

Cirrhosis is arguably the most serious of the causes of an elevated INR. It is a major problem not so much because of the coagulopathy itself but because of the associated deficits in wound healing and immune function that result from dysfunction of reticuloendothelial cells and hepatocytes. Generally, factor replacement should be instituted with FFP, but use of rVIIa is reasonable in the setting of active hemorrhage or any intracranial hemorrhage. Although to date there is little information on its efficacy in this particular setting, the administration of rVIIa, 20 to 40 µg/kg, would be a reasonable approach. If the bleeding is a manifestation of portal hypertension (as in variceal bleeding), emergency portal decompression—typically via transjugular intrahepatic portosystemic shunting—should be considered. Modest elevations of the INR in patients with cirrhosis who are not actively bleeding, have not recently undergone operation, and are not specifically at increased risk for life-threatening hemorrhage may be observed without correction.

INCREASED INR, PROLONGED APTT

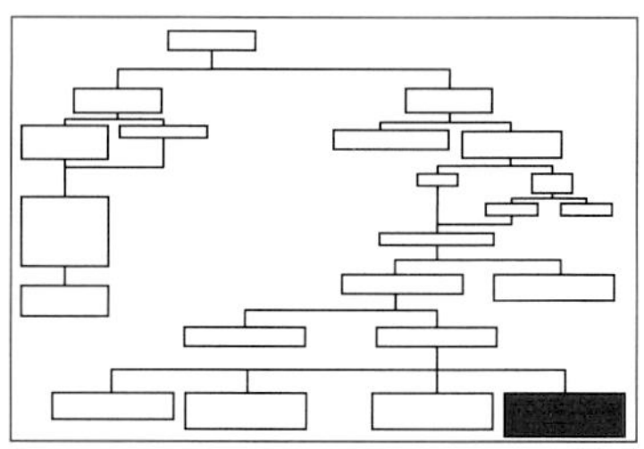

Increases in both the INR and the aPTT may be the most problematic finding of all. When both assays show increases, the patient is likely to have multiple factor deficiencies; possible causes include disseminated intravascular coagulation (DIC), severe hemodilution, and renal failure with severe nephrotic syndrome. However, when dramatic elevations of the aPTT and the INR occur that are out of proportion to the patient's clinical status, the problem may simply be that the specimen tube was not adequately filled. If a life-threatening coagulopathy seems unlikely, the blood sample should be redrawn and the tests repeated.

Hemodilution and nephrotic syndrome result in a coagulopathy that is attributable to decreased concentration of coagulation proteins. Dilutional coagulopathy may occur when a patient who is given a large volume of packed RBC units is not also given coagulation factors.[25] Because of the tremendous redundancy of the hemostatic process, pure dilutional coagulopathy is rare. It is considered an unlikely diagnosis until after one full blood volume has been replaced (as when a patient requires 10 units of packed RBCs to

Table 1 **Management of the Patient with an Increased International Normalized Ratio**

Indication		Recommended Treatment
No significant bleeding	INR above therapeutic range but < 5.0	Lower or hold the next dose
	INR > 5.0 but < 9.0	
	Rapid reduction of INR is not required	In the absence of additional risk factors for bleeding, withhold next 1–2 doses; alternatively, withhold next dose and give vitamin K, 1.0–2.5 mg orally
	Rapid reduction of INR is required	Give vitamin K, 1.0–2.0 mg p.o.; expected reduction of INR should occur within 24 hr
	INR > 9.0	Give vitamin K, 3.0–5.0 mg p.o.; expected reduction of INR should occur within 24 hr
Serious bleeding	Any elevation of INR	Give vitamin K, 10 mg IV, supplemented with FFP, prothrombin complex concentrate, or rVIIa; further vitamin K supplementation may be required every 12 hr
Life-threatening bleeding	Any elevation of INR	Give FFP, prothrombin complex concentrate, or rVIIa supplemented with vitamin K 10 mg IV, repeated as necessary

FFP = fresh frozen plasma; INR = international normalized ratio; rVIIa = recombinant activated factor VII.

maintain a stable hematocrit). Nephrotic syndrome is associated with loss of plasma proteins (including coagulation factors) from the kidneys.

Both hemodilution and nephrotic syndrome should be distinguished from DIC (which is a consumptive rather than a dilutional process[26]), although, on occasion, this distinction is a difficult one to make. A blood sample should be sent for D-dimer assay. If the D-dimer level is low (< 1,000 ng/mL), DIC is unlikely; if it is very high (> 2,000 ng/mL) and there is no other clear explanation (e.g., a complex pelvic fracture), DIC is more likely than dilutional coagulapathy. Treatment of dilutional coagulopathy should be directed at replacement of lost factors. FFP should be given first, followed by cryoprecipitate, calcium, and platelets. Transfusion should be continued until the coagulation parameters are corrected and the bleeding stops.

The term "DIC" refers to the phenomenon of diffuse, disorganized activation of the clotting cascade within the vascular space. It does not occur as an isolated process; rather, it is always secondary to an underlying problem. It typically results either from an overwhelming clotting stimulus (e.g., massive crush injury, overwhelming infection, or transfusion reaction) or from a more moderate clotting stimulus in the context of shock. The underlying problem that manifests as DIC has a range of severity, with mild and moderate cases represented by anything from a subclinical process to the development of organ dysfunction. One school of thought is that the systemic inflammatory response syndrome and DIC are simply different manifestations of the same process. However, severe cases are what surgeons traditionally think of as DIC: bleeding in the context of fibrinolysis and consumption of coagulation factors. Severe DIC arises when congestion of the microvasculature with thrombi occurs, resulting in large-scale activation of the fibrinolytic system. This fibrinolytic activity results in breakdown of clot at previously hemostatic sites of microscopic injury (e.g., endothelial damage) and macroscopic injury (e.g., IV catheter sites, fractures, or surgical wounds), as well as degradation of fibrinogen systemically. Bleeding and reexposure to tissue factor stimulate activation of factor VII with increased coagulation activity; thus, microthrombi are formed, and the vicious circle continues.

Beyond recognition and correction of the underlying problem causing DIC and the associated coagulopathy, the diagnosis of DIC represents something of an academic exercise because there is no specific treatment for the condition. Scoring systems that assess the severity of DIC are most useful for distinguishing DIC from other causes of coagulopathy (e.g., hypothermia, dilution, and drug effects) [*see Table 2*]. Heparin, antifibrinolytic agents, and antithrombotics

Table 2 **Coagulopathy (DIC) Score**

Score	INR (s)	aPTT (s)	Platelets (1,000/µL)	Fibrinogen (mg/dL)	D-Dimer (ng/mL)
0	< 1.2	< 34	> 150	> 200	< 1,000
1	> 1.2	> 34	< 150	< 200	< 2,000
2	> 1.4	> 39	< 100	< 150	< 4,000
3	> 1.6	> 54	< 60	< 100	> 4,000

aPTT = activated partial thromboplastin time; DIC = disseminated intravascular coagulopathy; INR = international normalized ratio.

(e.g., antithrombin and protein C) have been used. Despite improvements in laboratory measures with some of these agents, they do not appear to improve survival. One interpretation of the PROWESS trial[27] that evaluated drotrecogin alfa (recombinant activated protein C) as treatment for sepsis is that the observed improvement in survival resulted from containment of intravascular coagulation. However, the mortality benefit in that study has not been replicated in other trials and may not apply to patients undergoing operations. Currently, the most appropriate treatment of severe DIC is removal of the clotting stimulus and aggressive transfusion to restore blood loss and clotting factor deficits. The high mortality associated with severe DIC probably relates more to the underlying pathology than to the hematologic derangement per se.

An increased INR with a prolonged aPTT may also be caused by various isolated factor deficiencies of the common pathway. Congenital deficiencies of factors X and V and prothrombin are very rare. Acquired factor V deficiencies have been observed in patients with autoimmune disorders. Acquired hypoprothrombinemia has been documented in a small percentage of patients with lupus anticoagulants who exhibit abnormal bleeding. Factor X deficiencies have been noted in patients with amyloidosis.

Several anticoagulant medications can affect both the INR and the aPTT. Patients receiving large doses of unfractioned heparin may have a prolonged INR, depending on the specific reagents used in the test, and the related oral anti-Xa inhibitors (e.g., rivaroxaban) may also prolong both the INR and the aPTT.[28] The oral direct thrombin inhibitors typically prolong the aPTT but can also affect the INR. Stabilized warfarin therapy will increase both the INR and the aPTT. Several rodenticides in the vitamin K antagonist class with warfarin (e.g., brodifacoum) exert the same effect; however, because they have a considerably longer half-life than warfarin, the reversal of the anticoagulation effect with vitamin K or FFP may be correspondingly longer.[29] Animal venoms may also increase the INR and the aPTT.

Approach to the Patient with Anemia

Anemia is common among hospitalized surgical patients. In large prospective cohort studies, the average hemoglobin level in surgical ICU patients was 11.0 g/dL,[30] and 55% of surgical ICU patients received transfusions.[31] Anemia results from at least three factors: (1) blood loss related to the primary condition or to the operation, (2) serial blood draws (totaling, on average, approximately 40 mL/day in the ICU),[30] and (3) diminished erythropoiesis related to the primary illness.

Treatment of anemia has evolved over the past few decades. Cellular transfusions have long been a common, available means to treat anemia in the perioperative and critical care setting, but recognition in the 1980s that blood products were transmitting fatal viral infections changed the risk-benefit analysis. The blood-banking community in the United States and most developed countries adapted and systematically reduced the risk of transmission of the most likely infectious agents by restricting the eligible donor pool and routinely testing blood products for serologic and nucleic acid evidence of pathogens.[32] Currently, the possibility that an unpredictable new pathogen might emerge, such as a novel or mutated virus, is thought to pose a greater risk to the safety of the blood supply than such recognized pathogens as HIV, hepatitis B virus (HBV), and hepatitis C virus (HCV). These latter viruses are now so rarely transmitted in developed countries that the incidence of transfusion-related infection is difficult to quantify.

Transfusion of allogeneic blood products has also been associated with significant dysfunction of the immune system and inflammatory processes. These immunomodulatory effects are presumably much more frequent than rare cases of viral transmission, but it is not clear whether they are causally related to poorer outcomes [*see* Discussion, Mechanism and Significance of Transfusion-Related Immunomodulation, *below*]. Furthermore, transfusion also may not augment oxygen delivery as assumed as a result of a variety of changes that occur with red cell storage.

Moreover, randomized trials comparing a restrictive RBC transfusion protocol (hemoglobin concentration maintained at 7.0 to 9.0 g/dL) with a more liberal protocol (hemoglobin maintained at 10.0 to 12.0 g/dL) for critically ill patients have not demonstrated harm with the restrictive approach.[33] In fact, as suggested by the Transfusion Requirements in Critical Care (TRICC) study, the restrictive approach may even improve survival for younger or less severely ill patients.[34]

Thus, for a variety of reasons, the conventional wisdom is to try to limit blood transfusions when possible. The decision whether to transfuse should be based on the patient's current and predicted need for additional oxygen-carrying capacity [*see Figure 1*]. First, it is important to determine whether significant hypovolemia or active bleeding is present. In such patients, liberal transfusion is indicated as a means of increasing intravascular volume and preventing the development of profound deficits in oxygen-carrying capacity [*see* Approach to the Patient with Massive Hemorrhage, *above*].

In a hemodynamically stable but critically ill patient without evidence of active hemorrhage, it is appropriate to take a more restrictive approach and administer transfusion only when the hemoglobin concentration is less than 7.0 g/dL (hematocrit 21%). Less acutely ill patients can even be followed for hemoglobin concentrations below 7.0 g/dL, especially if they are asymptomatic and at minimal risk for hemorrhage. In the absence of transfusion, iron supplementation should be considered, particularly for menstruating women. There is no specific hemoglobin concentration or hematocrit (i.e., transfusion trigger) at which all patients should receive transfusions.

The above approach should apply to most patients, but there are two groups for whom a more aggressive RBC transfusion policy should be considered. Although opinion is divided, patients who have acute coronary artery ischemic syndromes and those with acute neurologic conditions may benefit from a more liberal transfusion strategy. To date, relatively few such patients have been included in the randomized trials on this topic.

Acute Coronary Artery Ischemic Syndromes

Currently, there is no consensus regarding the most appropriate transfusion strategy for patients with acute coronary artery ischemic syndromes, such as active myocardial infarction and unstable angina. The results of observational studies have been mixed,[35,36] and no clinical trial has yet addressed this specific subgroup of patients. Some distinction should be drawn between patients who have acute coronary artery ischemic syndromes and those who merely have a history of coronary artery or other atherosclerotic disease. Although the TRICC trial did not enrol patients admitted after a routine cardiac surgical procedure,[34] it included enough patients with cardiovascular disease to allow a sizable subgroup analysis.[37] This post hoc analysis suggested that in patients with cardiovascular disease as a primary diagnosis or an important comorbid condition, survival was essentially the same regardless of whether a liberal transfusion protocol or a restrictive one was followed. In patients with confirmed ischemic heart disease, however, a nonsignificant decrease in survival was noted, generating some concern that adverse cardiovascular events (e.g., myocardial infarction and stroke) might increase in frequency at lower hemoglobin levels. Consequently, a target hemoglobin of 10 g/dL is generally considered acceptable for patients with acute coronary artery ischemic syndromes or significant coronary artery disease.

Neurologic Conditions

Some have argued that just as the heart may be sensitive to decreases in oxygen-carrying capacity, the injured central nervous system may be vulnerable to further damage from anemia because anemia may limit the delivery of oxygen to damaged tissue. According to this view, patients with traumatic brain injury, stroke, or spinal cord injury may be vulnerable to anemia-related damage; however, as yet, the clinical evidence—mostly from observational studies with significant methodological weaknesses—is insufficient either to support or to refute liberal transfusion of such patients.[38]

Symptomatic Anemia

An additional consideration in the decision to transfuse blood is the oxygen-carrying capacity that is necessary to prevent patient fatigue or discomfort. Typical symptoms of anemia include lightheadedness, tachycardia, and tachypnea either during activity or at rest. Clearly, some degree of tachycardia is to be expected in any patient who has undergone a major operation or sustained a serious injury. The key judgment to make in deciding whether to treat symptomatic anemia with transfusion is whether the anemia is truly compromising the patient's health or recovery. It is not always easy, however, to determine whether symptoms or signs attributed to anemia will actually improve as a result of transfusion. For example, a liberal transfusion approach does not appear to lead to earlier discontinuation of mechanical ventilation.[39] A major randomized trial that is near completion, the Functional Outcomes in Cardiovascular Patients Undergoing

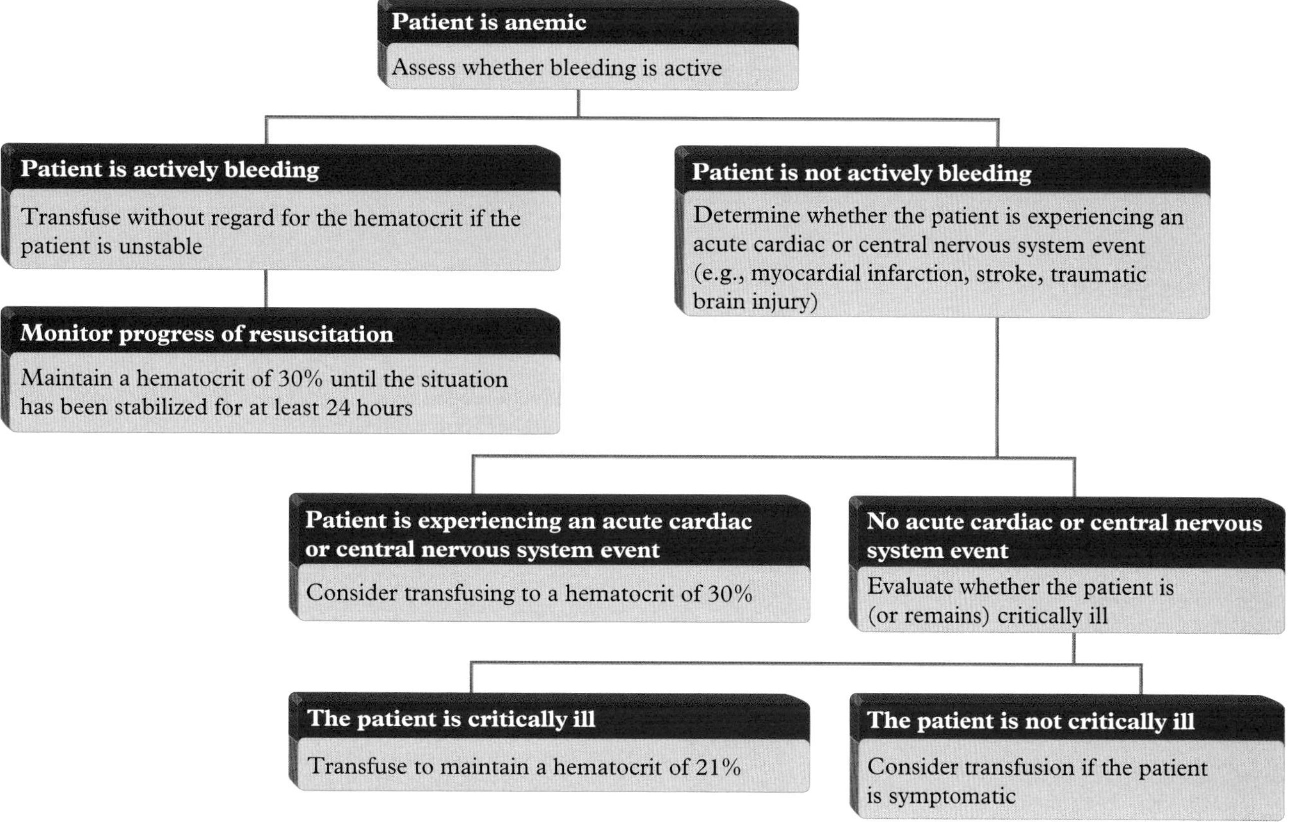

Figure 1 **Algorithm depicting the decision-making process for transfusion in anemic patients.**

Surgical hip fracture repair (FOCUS) study, is addressing the issue of functional recovery. Its primary aim is to determine whether liberal transfusion improves walking ability among anemic patients with a history of cardiovascular disease who undergo operative repair of a hip fracture.[40]

Observation of Anemia

Although it is now standard practice to observe patients with hemoglobin concentrations of 6 to 7 g/dL, data suggest that the benefits of transfusion probably outweigh the risks below this level.

For all patients, if the hemoglobin level drops low enough, cellular metabolism cannot be sustained and death becomes a certainty. Followers of certain religious faiths who decline blood transfusion even when death is the probable or certain consequence have provided valuable observational data on the effects of severe anemia that would otherwise be unethical to obtain. Such cases have challenged surgeons and intensive care physicians to find techniques for supporting life at extremely low hemoglobin concentrations and have helped define the limits beyond which anemia may be fatal. Reviews of patients who have refused transfusion suggest that a hemoglobin below 5 g/dL results in substantial increases in mortality, especially in elderly persons and patients with cardiovascular disease.[41]

When RBC transfusion is not possible (whether because the patient declines transfusion or because compatible blood is unavailable), a number of temporizing measures can be used. First, steps should be taken to minimize additional iatrogenic blood loss. Laboratory tests should be restricted to those that are most likely to benefit the patient and should be conducted with the smallest amount of blood possible (e.g., pediatric specimen tubes). Nonemergency operations that are likely to involve appreciable blood loss should be postponed if possible. Second, any impediments to native erythropoiesis should be removed: iron should be supplemented (orally if possible), and the administration of recombinant erythropoietin should be considered. Third, 100% oxygen should be administered because oxygen dissolved in plasma contributes a significant proportion of oxygen delivery at very low hemoglobin levels. Fourth, in extreme cases, consideration should be given to decreasing oxygen demand. Because the mechanical work of respiration itself becomes a significant contributor to oxygen demand in severely anemic patients, mechanical ventilation and even neuromuscular blocking agents should be considered to reduce oxygen demand from skeletal muscle. The metabolic rate can be further reduced by inducing hypothermia.

For decades, efforts have been in progress to augment oxygen-carrying capacity using RBC substitutes. Various different substitutes have been evaluated, some of which remain under investigation. None have been approved for routine use by the US Food and Drug Administration (FDA), largely because of significant adverse effects. The main categories of substitutes are those based on hemoglobin and those based on perfluorocarbons. Unmodified, acellular hemoglobin is nephrotoxic, so hemoglobin-based blood substitutes involve either attempts to modify the hemoglobin molecule or encapsulate hemoglobin within synthetic membranes. Even with such modifications, however, these substitutes appear to increase the risk of death and myocardial infarction.[42,43] Perfluorocarbon-based substitutes have attempted to take advantage of the high solubility of oxygen in these liquids, but their development has been impeded by practical hurdles in their production and storage as well as adverse effects with their use.[44] Thus, although blood substitutes promise a number of advantages (increased shelf life, availability that is not limited by donor supply, and reduced or eliminated risk of incompatibility reactions and pathogen transmission), the extent to which they will ever be a suitable treatment for anemia in surgical patients is unclear.

Discussion

Mechanics of Hemostasis

Hemostasis is the term for the process by which cellular and plasma components interact in response to vessel injury to maintain vascular integrity and promote wound healing. The initial response to vascular injury (primary hemostasis) involves the recruitment and activation of platelets, which then adhere to the site of injury. Subsequently, plasma proteins, in concert with cellular components, begin to generate thrombin, which causes further activation of platelets and converts fibrinogen to fibrin monomers that polymerize into a fibrin clot (secondary hemostasis). The final step is the release of plasminogen activators that induce clot lysis and tissue repair.

The cellular components of hemostasis include endothelium, subendothelial cells and substrate, white blood cells (WBCs), RBCs, and platelets. The plasma components include a number of pro- and anticoagulant proteins that, once activated, can accelerate or downregulate thrombin formation or clot lysis to facilitate wound healing. In normal individuals, these hemostatic components are in a regulatory balance; thus, any abnormality involving one or more of these components can result in a pathologic state, whether of uncontrolled clot formation (thrombosis) or of excessive bleeding (hemorrhage). These pathologies can result from either hereditary or acquired causes.

CELLULAR COMPONENTS

Endothelium and Subendothelial Tissue

The endothelium has both procoagulant and anticoagulant properties. At baseline, in its normal, undamaged state, the endothelial surface is covered with endogenous antithrombins (antithrombin III, heparan sulfate, dermatan sulfate, and others) that protect against pathologic coagulation, thus providing a barrier between prothrombotic factors in the plasma and thrombogenic subendothelial factors. However, when vascular injury occurs, the endothelium and subendothelial tissues serve as a nidus for recruitment, adhesion, and aggregation of platelets. Disruption of the endothelium exposes collagen fibrils, to which platelets adhere, and tissue factor (TF), which serves as an integral, potent clotting stimulus [*see* Procoagulants, *below*]. TF is pervasive on the cell surfaces of subendothelial tissue and especially concentrated on such tissue as vascular adventitia, cerebral cortex, lung parenchyma, visceral organ capsules, and epidermis.[45] Damaged or activated endothelial cells express adhesion molecule receptors (E-selectin and P-selectin), and release of vWF from the Weibel-Palade bodies of endothelial cells causes platelets to adhere to their surface. The presence of interleukin-1β (IL-1β), tissue necrosis factor (TNF), interferon gamma, and thrombin also promotes expression of TF on the endothelium.[46,47] TF activates factors X and VII, and these activated factors generate additional thrombin, which increases both fibrin formation and platelet aggregation.

The endothelium also acts in numerous ways to downregulate coagulation.[48] Heparan sulfate and thrombomodulin are both downregulators of thrombin formation. In the presence of thrombin, the endothelium responds by expressing or releasing (1) membrane-bound thrombomodulin, which forms a complex with thrombin to activate protein C; (2) endothelium-derived relaxing factor (i.e., nitric oxide[49]) and prostacyclin, which have vasodilating and platelet aggregation-inhibiting effects, respectively; and (3) tissue plasminogen activator (t-PA) or urokinase-type plasminogen activator (u-PA), either of which converts the zymogen plasminogen to its active form, plasmin, that degrades fibrin and fibrinogen.[47,50] Heparan sulfate, on the endothelium wall, forms a complex with plasma antithrombin to neutralize thrombin. The endothelium is also the source of tissue factor pathway inhibitor (TFPI), which downregulates TF-VIIa-Xa complexes.

Erythrocytes and Leukocytes

The nonplatelet cellular components of blood play indirect roles in hemostasis. RBCs contain thromboplastins that are potent stimulators of various procoagulant proteins. In addition, in the setting of laminar flow, a sufficient concentration of RBCs within the bloodstream (i.e., the hematocrit) assists in primary hemostasis by physically forcing the platelets toward the endothelial surfaces. When the RBC count is low enough, there is a reduction in this force, which results in inadequate endothelium-platelet interaction and subsequently a bleeding diathesis.

Leukocytes have several functions in the hemostatic process. The interaction between the adhesion molecules expressed on both leukocytes and endothelium results in cytokine production, initiation of inflammatory responses, and degradation of extracellular matrix to facilitate tissue healing. In the presence of thrombin and other stimuli, monocytes express TF, potentiating coagulation. Neutrophils and activated monocytes bind to stimulated platelets and endothelial cells that express P-selectin. Adhesion and rolling of neutrophils, mediated by fibrinogen and selectins on the endothelium, appear to help restore vessel integrity but may also lead to inflammatory responses.[51,52] Lymphocytes also adhere to endothelium via adhesion molecule receptors and appear to be responsible for cytokine production and inflammatory responses.

Platelets

Platelets facilitate hemostasis and subsequent fibrin formation both by generating the initial platelet plug and by providing a phospholipid surface on which the activation of coagulation factors is localized. Activation of platelets by agonists such as adenosine triphosphate (ATP), ADP, epinephrine, thromboxane A_2, collagen, and thrombin causes platelets to undergo morphologic changes and degranulation. Degranulation releases procoagulants (e.g., thrombospondin, vWF, fibrinogen, ADP, ATP, and serotonin) that promote further platelet adhesion and aggregation and surface expression of P-selectin, which induces cellular adhesion. Platelet degranulation also results in the release of β-thromboglobulin, platelet factor 4 (which has antiheparin properties), various growth factors, and calcium, as well as the formation of platelet microparticles. Plasminogen activator inhibitor–1 (PAI-1) released from degranulated platelets neutralizes the fibrinolytic pathway by forming a complex with t-PA.

On exposure to vascular injury, platelets adhere to the exposed endothelium via binding of vWF to the GPIb-IX-V complex.[53] Conformational changes in the GPIIb-IIIa complex on the activated platelet surface enhance fibrinogen binding, which results in platelet-to-platelet aggregation and complex morphologic changes. The end result of these changes is a platelet plug with such dense adherence of platelets and such dramatic changes in platelet shape that, on electron microscopy, each platelet resembles a piece within a three-dimensional jigsaw puzzle. The phospholipid surface of the membranes of activated platelets then anchors activated IXa-VIIIa and Xa-Va complexes, thereby localizing thrombin generation.[54]

PLASMA COMPONENTS

Procoagulants

In primary hemostasis, circulating plasma vWF—in addition to the vWF secreted by endothelial cells in response to injury—facilitates adhesion of platelets to the endothelium. Plasma vWF also serves as the carrier protein for factor VIII, preventing its neutralization by the protein C regulatory pathway.

Secondary hemostasis involves numerous plasma components. Traditional diagrams of the coagulation cascade depict two distinct pathways, the intrinsic and extrinsic pathways, that join in a final common pathway. The historical reason for depicting the coagulation cascade this way is to emphasize differences between the aPTT test (which is prolonged in the absence of sufficient quantities of components in the intrinsic pathway: factor XII, prekallikrein, and high-molecular-weight kininogen) and the INR (which measures clotting time in response to the extrinsic stimulus, TF). In vivo, however, the primary stimulus for secondary hemostasis is the exposure of TF (i.e., the extrinsic pathway), and the thrombin generated from this process activates factor VIII, effectively bypassing the initial steps in the intrinsic pathway. Accordingly, our focus is not on the standard view of intrinsic and extrinsic pathways but rather on the different roles contact factors (part of the intrinsic cascade) and TF play in coagulation.

The main role of the contact factors (factor XII, prekallikrein, and high-molecular-weight kininogen) appears to be in downregulation of coagulation rather than the generation of thrombin. Even in patients completely lacking these factors, who have a markedly prolonged aPTT, abnormal bleeding does not occur. However, the contact factors activate the bradykinin (BK) pathway, which exerts profibrinolytic effects by stimulating endothelial release of plasminogen activators. It also stimulates endothelial production of nitric oxide and prostacyclin, which play vital regulatory roles in vasodilation and regulation of platelet activation.[55]

The key initiator of plasma procoagulant formation is the expression of TF on cell surfaces.[46,56] TF activates factor VII and binds with it to form the TF-VIIa complex, which activates factors X and IX. Factor Xa enhances its own production by activating factor IX, which in turn converts more factor X to Xa. Factor Xa also produces minimal amounts of thrombin by cleaving the prothrombin molecule. The thrombin generated from this process cleaves the coagulation cofactors V and VIII to enhance production of the factor complexes IX-VIIIa (intrinsic tenase) and Xa-Va (prothrombinase), which dramatically catalyzes conversion of prothrombin to thrombin [*see Figure 2*].[57]

Thrombin has numerous effects, including pro- and antithrombotic functions. Its procoagulant properties include cleaving fibrinogen, activating the coagulation cofactors V and VIII, inducing platelet aggregation, inducing expression of TF on cell surfaces, and activating factor XIII. In cleaving fibrinogen, thrombin causes the release of fibrinopeptides A and B (fibrin monomer). The fibrin monomer undergoes conformational changes that expose the α and β chains of the molecule, which then polymerize with other fibrin monomers to form a fibrin mesh. Activated factor XIII cross-links the polymerized fibrin (between the α chains and the χ chains) to stabilize the fibrin clot and delay fibrinolysis.

Fibrin(ogen)olysis

Plasminogen is the primary fibrinolytic zymogen that circulates in plasma. In the presence of t-PA or u-PA (released from the endothelium), plasminogen is converted to the active form, plasmin. Plasmin cleaves fibrin (or fibrinogen) between the molecule's D and E domains, causing the formation of X, Y, D, and E fragments from fibrinogen degradation, and D-dimers from polymerized fibrin degradation. The secondary function of the fibrinolytic pathway is the activation by u-PA of matrix metalloproteinases that degrade the extracellular matrix.[58]

Endogenous Antithrombotic Factors

In persons with normal coagulation status, downregulation of hemostasis occurs simultaneously with the production of procoagulants (e.g., activated plasma factors, stimulated endothelium, and stimulated platelets). In addition to their procoagulant activity, both thrombin and contact factors stimulate downregulation of the coagulation process. Thrombin forms a complex with endothelium-bound thrombomodulin to activate protein C, which inhibits factors Va and VIIIa. The thrombin-thrombomodulin complex also regulates the fibrinolytic pathway by activating a circulating plasma protein

Acquired platelet abnormalities, both qualitative (i.e., dysfunction) and quantitative (i.e., decreases in absolute numbers), are common occurrences. Many acquired thrombocytopathies are attributable to medications (e.g., aspirin, ibuprofen, other nonsteroidal antiinflammatory drugs, various antibiotics, certain antihistamines, and phenytoin). Newer classes of antiplatelet drugs function by inhibiting platelet receptors [*see* Interpretation of Coagulation Parameters, Normal INR, Normal aPTT, *above*].[70] Thrombocytopenia can be primary or secondary to a number of clinical conditions. Primary bone disorders (e.g., myelodysplastic or myelophthisic syndromes) and spontaneous bleeding may arise when platelet counts fall below 10,000/μL.

Thrombocytopenia can be associated with immune causes (e.g., immune thrombocytopenic purpura and heparin-induced thrombocytopenia) or such conditions as a deficiency in the plasma metalloproteinase ADAMTS13 (a disintegrin and metalloproteinase with a thrombospondin type 1 motif, member 13) (thrombotic thrombocytopenic purpura). Acquired platelet dysfunction (e.g., acquired vWD) that is not related to dietary or pharmacologic causes has been observed in patients with immune disorders or cancer.

Multifactorial coagulopathies are common as well. Patients with severe renal disease typically exhibit platelet dysfunction (from excessive amounts of uremic metabolites), factor deficiencies associated with impaired protein synthesis and protein loss (as with increased urinary excretion), or thrombocytopenia (from diminished thrombopoietin production).[71,72] Patients with severe hepatic disease commonly have impairment of coagulation factor synthesis, increases in circulating levels of paraproteins, and splenic sequestration of platelets.

Massive cellular transfusion can dilute the levels of clotting factors if more than 10 packed RBC units are given within a short period without plasma supplementation. In addition, because RBC units contain citrate as an anticoagulant, massive transfusion can induce a coagulopathy from hypocalcemia. Immunologic reactions to ABO/Rh mismatches can induce immune-mediated hypercoagulation. Acquired multifactorial deficiencies associated with extracorporeal circuits (e.g., cardiopulmonary bypass, hemodialysis, and continuous venovenous dialysis) can arise as a consequence of hemodilution from circuit priming fluid or activation of procoagulants after exposure to thrombogenic surfaces. Thrombocytopenia can result from platelet destruction and activation caused by circuit membrane exposure or can be secondary to the presence of heparin antibody.

Animal venoms can be either pro- or antithrombotic. The majority of the poisonous snakes in the United States (rattlesnakes in particular) have venom that works by activating prothrombin, but cross-breeding has produced a number of new venoms with different hemostatic consequences. The clinical presentation of coagulopathies associated with snakebites generally mimics that of consumptive coagulopathies.[73]

Drug-induced factor deficiencies are common, particularly as a result of anticoagulant therapy. The most commonly used anticoagulants are heparin and warfarin. Heparin does not cause a factor deficiency; rather, it accelerates production of antithrombin, which inhibits factor IXa, factor Xa, and thrombin, thereby prolonging clot formation. Warfarin reduces procoagulant potential by inhibiting vitamin K synthesis, thereby reducing carboxylation of factor VII, factor IX, factor X, prothrombin, and proteins C and S. Newer drugs that may also cause factor deficiencies include direct thrombin inhibitors (e.g., lepirudin and bivalirudin[74]) and fibrinogen-degrading drugs (e.g., ancrod[75]).

Isolated acquired factor deficiencies are relatively rare. Clinically, they present in exactly the same way as inherited factor deficiencies, except that there is no history of earlier bleeding. In some cases, there is a secondary disease (e.g., lymphoma or an autoimmune disorder) that results in the development of antibody to a procoagulant (e.g., factor V, factor VIII, factor IX, vWF, prothrombin, or fibrinogen).

Disseminated Intravascular Coagulation

DIC is a complex coagulation process that involves massive activation of the coagulation system with deposition of fibrin in the microvasculature that causes the subsequent activation of the fibrinolytic pathway. The overwhelming microvascular fibrin deposition is the cause of both the activation of the fibrinolytic system (which promotoes more bleeding) and eventually multiple organ dysfunction syndrome (MODS). The activation occurs at all levels, including platelets, endothelium, and pro- and anticoagulants. It is crucial to emphasize that DIC is an acquired disorder that occurs secondary to an underlying clinical event (e.g., child birth complicated by amniotic fluid embolism, severe gram-negative infection, shock, severe traumatic brain injury, polytrauma, severe burns, or cancer). As noted [*see* Interpretation of Coagulation Parameters, Increased INR, Prolonged aPTT, *above*], there is some controversy regarding the best approach to therapy, but there is no doubt that treating the underlying cause of DIC is paramount to patient recovery.

DIC is not always clinically evident: low-grade DIC may lack clinical symptoms altogether and manifest itself only through laboratory abnormalities, even when thrombin generation and fibrin deposition are occurring. In an attempt to facilitate recognition of DIC, the disorder has been divided into three phases, distinguished on the basis of clinical and laboratory evidence. In phase I DIC, there are no clinical symptoms, and the routine screening tests (i.e., INR, aPTT, fibrinogen level, and platelet count) are within normal limits.[76] Secondary testing (i.e., measurement of antithrombin, prothrombin fragment, thrombin-antithrombin complex, and soluble fibrin levels) may reveal subtle changes indicative of thrombin generation. In phase II DIC, there are usually clinical signs of bleeding around wounds, suture sites, IV sites, or venous puncture sites, and decreased function is noted in specific organs (e.g., lung, liver, and kidneys). The INR is increased, the aPTT is prolonged, and the fibrinogen level and platelet count are decreased. Other markers of thrombin generation and fibrinolysis (e.g., D-dimer level) show sizable elevations. In phase III DIC, MODS is observed, the INR and the aPTT are markedly increased, the fibrinogen level is markedly depressed, and the D-dimer level is dramatically increased. A peripheral blood smear shows large numbers of schistocytes, indicating RBC shearing from fibrin deposition.

The activation of the coagulation system seen in DIC appears to be primarily caused by TF. The brain, the placenta, and solid tumors are all rich sources of TF. Gram-negative endotoxins also induce TF expression. The exposure of TF on cellular surfaces causes activation of factors VII and

IX, which ultimately leads to thrombin generation. Circulating thrombin is rapidly cleared by antithrombin. Moreover, the coagulation pathway is downregulated by activated protein C and protein S. However, constant exposure of TF (as a result of underlying disorders) results in constant generation of thrombin, and these regulator proteins are rapidly consumed. TAFI and PAI also contribute to fibrin deposition by restricting fibrinolysis and subsequent fibrin degradation and clearance. Finally, it is likely that release of cytokines (e.g., IL-6, IL-10, and TNF) may play some role in causing the sequelae of DIC by modulating or activating the coagulation pathway.

Laboratory Assessment of Bleeding

Patients with massive or life-threatening hemorrhage should be treated presumptively and without a delay to obtain the results of laboratory tests [*see* Approach to the Patient with Massive Hemorrhage, *above*]. However, these tests serve an integral role in the diagnostic algorithm for patients with more modest bleeding. If the patient is not experiencing massive or life-threatening hemorrhage, blood samples for coagulation testing should be drawn before administering blood products or medication intended to promote coagulation. The CBC (including platelet count and differential count), the INR, and the aPTT tests should be the primary laboratory tests for differentiating coagulopathies [*see Figure 3*]. Technological advances have made it possible to perform these and other diagnostic laboratory tests outside the confines of the clinical laboratory ("near-care" or "point-of-care" testing). Whatever tests of coagulation are employed, it is important to recognize their limitations.

Several technical factors can influence the results of the INR and aPTT. These tests involve adding activators, phospholipids, and calcium to plasma in a test tube (or the equivalent) and determining the time to clot formation. Time to clot formation is a relative value in that it is compared with the time in a normal population, and each laboratory must periodically adjust the reference range accordingly. Poor sampling techniques (e.g., hemolysis, inadequately filled coagulation tubes, excessive tourniquet time, and clotted or activated samples) can influence the results. Hemolysis from poor phlebotomy technique can release thromboplastins from RBC membranes that initiate the coagulation process. An elevated hematocrit or inadequately filled specimen tube can prolong test results because the excess citrate chelates the calcium added in the assay. Hemolysis, jaundice, and lipemia can all interfere with the optical systems that modern instruments use to detect clot. In addition, factor VIII in particular is relatively labile, so failure to process and run coagulation samples expeditiously can prolong the aPTT.

Not all coagulation tests are functionally equivalent: different laboratory methods may yield differing results.[77] For most laboratories, coagulation reagents have been selected in such a way as to ensure that the tests are sensitive to factor VIII and IX deficiencies (i.e., diagnosis and monitoring of hemophilia) and the effects of warfarin and heparin. As a consequence, a normal aPTT in a patient with an abnormal INR may not exclude the possibility of common pathway deficiencies (e.g., deficiencies of factors X, V, and II), and most current methods of determining the INR and the aPTT

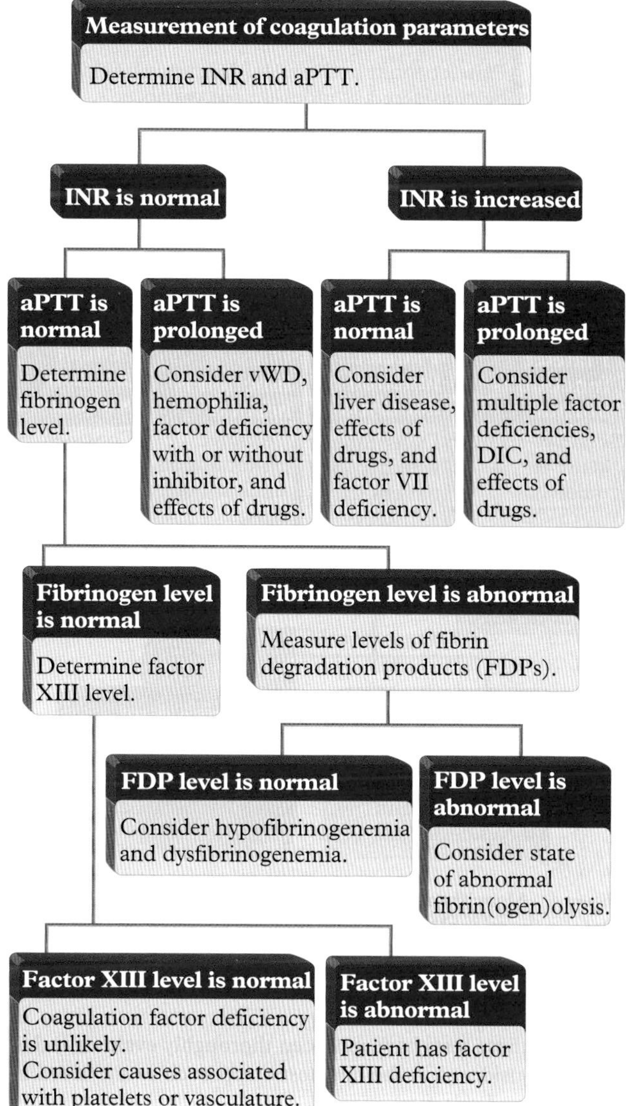

Figure 3 **Algorithm depicting the use of coagulation parameters in assessment of coagulopathies. aPTT = activated partial thromboplastin time; DIC = disseminated intravascular coagulation; INR = international normalized ratio; vWD = von Willebrand disease.**

do not detect low fibrinogen levels. In this chapter, we have assumed that the methods used with the INR and aPTT tests result in abnormalities when factor activity levels fall below 0.4 IU/mL.

Assessment of platelets also involves certain pitfalls. Platelet count and platelet function should be considered as completely independent metrics [*see Figure 4*]. Patients with congenital thrombocytopathies often have normal platelet counts; therefore, assessment of platelet function is required as well. Historically, the bleeding time has been used to assess platelet function. However, this test is grossly insensitive, yielding normal results in as many as 50% of patients with congenital thrombocytopathies.[78,79] Numerous rapid tests of platelet function are currently available that can be used to screen for platelet defects; although the accuracy and clinical

However, this study has been criticized for several methodologic issues, and many consider the issue unsettled. Transfusion-related acute lung injury (which some define very broadly to include underrecognized cases of immunomodulation) appears to be caused in some cases by donor antibodies to recipient leukocyte antigens. This has led some blood centers to exclude individuals likely to have such antibodies (e.g., previously pregnant women) from plasma donation.[82]

A plethora of observational studies and some randomized trials have attempted to evaluate the role of blood transfusion in the recurrence of resected malignancies and postoperative infection. Most of the observational studies have compared the outcomes of transfused cohorts with those of nontransfused cohorts. The randomized trials, however, have mostly evaluated different kinds of blood transfusions against one another (e.g., autologous versus allogeneic and leukoreduced versus nonleukoreduced). The literature is extensive, but many methodologic issues have been identified that limit the validity of the studies.[83] Accordingly, the evidence appears to be insufficient to establish a causal connection between allogeneic blood transfusion and either increased cancer recurrence or postoperative infection. Nonetheless, the heterogeneity of the study results and the finding of a major randomized trial, the TRICC trial, that a restrictive transfusion policy may improve survival in some patients continue to fuel debate over whether the avoidance or modification of allogeneic blood transfusion may improve patient outcomes.

Financial Disclosures: None Reported

References

1. Rayt HS, Sutton AJ, London NJ, et al. A systematic review and meta-analysis of endovascular repair (EVAR) for ruptured abdominal aortic aneurysm. Eur J Vasc Endovasc Surg 2008;36:536–44.
2. Bickell WH, Wall MJ Jr, Pepe PE, et al. Immediate versus delayed fluid resuscitation for hypotensive patients with penetrating torso injuries. N Engl J Med 1994;331:1105–9.
3. Stansbury LG, Dutton RP, Stein DM, et al. Controversy in trauma resuscitation: do ratios of plasma to red blood cells matter? Transfus Med Rev 2009;23:255–65.
4. Shakur H, Roberts I, Bautista R, et al. Effects of tranexamic acid on death, vascular occlusive events, and blood transfusion in trauma patients with significant haemorrhage (CRASH-2): a randomised, placebo-controlled trial. Lancet 2010;376:23–32.
5. Martinowitz U, Kenet G, Segal E, et al. Recombinant activated factor VII for adjunctive hemorrhage control in trauma. J Trauma 2001;51:431–8; discussion 8–9.
6. Boffard KD, Riou B, Warren B, et al. Recombinant factor VIIa as adjunctive therapy for bleeding control in severely injured trauma patients: two parallel randomized, placebo-controlled, double-blind clinical trials. J Trauma 2005;59:8–15; discussion 15–8.
7. Hauser CJ, Boffard K, Dutton R, et al. Results of the CONTROL trial: efficacy and safety of recombinant activated factor VII in the management of refractory traumatic hemorrhage. J Trauma 2010;69:489–500.
8. Goodnough LT, Shander AS. Recombinant factor VIIa: safety and efficacy. Curr Opin Hematol 2007;14:504–9.
9. Shander AS, Goodnough LT, Ratko T, et al. Consensus recommendations for the off-label use of recombinant human factor VIIa (NovoSeven) therapy. Pharmacol Ther 2005;30:644–58. Available at: http://ptcommunity.com/ptjournal/fulltext/30/11/PTJ3011644.pdf (accessed January 2011).
10. Gubler KD, Gentilello LM, Hassantash SA, Maier RV. The impact of hypothermia on dilutional coagulopathy. J Trauma 1994;36:847–51.
11. Gentilello LM, Jurkovich GJ, Stark MS, et al. Is hypothermia in the victim of major trauma protective or harmful? A randomized, prospective study. Ann Surg 1997;226:439–47; discussion 47–9.
12. Cox ED, Schreiber MA, McManus J, et al. New hemostatic agents in the combat setting. Transfusion 2009;49 Suppl 5:248S–55S.
13. Rapaport SI. Blood coagulation and its alterations in hemorrhagic and thrombotic disorders. West J Med 1993;158:153–61.
14. Practice guidelines for blood component therapy: a report by the American Society of Anesthesiologists Task Force on Blood Component Therapy. Anesthesiology 1996;84:732–47.
15. Heckman KD, Weiner GJ, Davis CS, et al. Randomized study of prophylactic platelet transfusion threshold during induction therapy for adult acute leukemia: 10,000/microL versus 20,000/microL. J Clin Oncol 1997;15:1143–9.
16. Slichter SJ. Relationship between platelet count and bleeding risk in thrombocytopenic patients. Transfus Med Rev 2004;18:153–67.
17. Spinler SA. Oral antiplatelet therapy after acute coronary syndrome and percutaneous coronary intervention: balancing efficacy and bleeding risk. Am J Health Syst Pharm 2010;67(15 Suppl 7):S7–17.
18. Despotis GJ, Levine V, Saleem R, et al. Use of point-of-care test in identification of patients who can benefit from desmopressin during cardiac surgery: a randomised controlled trial. Lancet 1999;354:106–10.
19. Levy JH, Schwieger IM, Zaidan JR, et al. Evaluation of patients at risk for protamine reactions. J Thorac Cardiovasc Surg 1989;98:200–4.
20. Stewart WJ, McSweeney SM, Kellett MA, et al. Increased risk of severe protamine reactions in NPH insulin-dependent diabetics undergoing cardiac catheterization. Circulation 1984;70:788–92.
21. Fenton JW 2nd, Ofosu FA, Brezniak DV, Hassouna HI. Thrombin and antithrombotics. Semin Thromb Hemost 1998;24:87–91.
22. van Ryn J, Stangier J, Haertter S, et al. Dabigatran etexilate—a novel, reversible, oral direct thrombin inhibitor: interpretation of coagulation assays and reversal of anticoagulant activity. Thromb Haemost 2010;103:1116–27.
23. Bolton-Maggs PH. The management of factor XI deficiency. Haemophilia 1998;4:683–8.
24. Ansell J, Hirsh J, Hylek E, et al. Pharmacology and management of the vitamin K antagonists: American College of Chest Physicians Evidence-Based Clinical Practice Guidelines (8th Edition). Chest 2008;133(6 Suppl):160S–98S.
25. Murray DJ, Pennell BJ, Weinstein SL, Olson JD. Packed red cells in acute blood loss: dilutional coagulopathy as a cause of surgical bleeding. Anesth Analg 1995;80:336–42.
26. Holcroft JW, Blaisdell FW, Trunkey DD, Lim RC. Intravascular coagulation and pulmonary edema in the septic baboon. J Surg Res 1977;22:209–20.
27. Bernard GR, Vincent JL, Laterre PF, et al. Efficacy and safety of recombinant human activated protein C for severe sepsis. N Engl J Med 2001;344:699–709.
28. Hillarp A, Baghaei F, Blixter IF, et al. Effects of the oral, direct factor Xa inhibitor rivaroxaban on commonly used coagulation assays. J Thromb [illegible]
29. Weitzel JN, Sadowski JA, Furie BC, et al. Surreptitious ingestion of a long-acting vitamin K antagonist/rodenticide, brodifacoum: clinical and metabolic studies of three cases. Blood 1990;76:2555–9.
30. Vincent JL, Baron JF, Reinhart K, et al. Anemia and blood transfusion in critically ill patients. JAMA 2002;288:1499–507.
31. Corwin HL, Gettinger A, Pearl RG, et al. The CRIT Study: Anemia and blood transfusion in the critically ill—current clinical practice in the United States. Crit Care Med 2004;32:39–52.
32. Busch MP, Kleinman SH, Nemo GJ. Current and emerging infectious risks of blood transfusions. JAMA 2003;289:959–62.
33. Carless PA, Henry DA, Carson JL, et al. Transfusion thresholds and other strategies for guiding allogeneic red blood cell transfusion. Cochrane Database Syst Rev (Online) 2010;(10):CD002042.
34. Hebert PC, Wells G, Blajchman MA, et al. A multicenter, randomized, controlled clinical trial of transfusion requirements in critical care. Transfusion Requirements in Critical Care Investigators, Canadian Critical Care Trials Group. N Engl J Med 1999;340:409–17.
35. Rao SV, Jollis JG, Harrington RA, et al. Relationship of blood transfusion and clinical outcomes in patients with acute coronary syndromes. JAMA 2004;292:1555–62.
36. Wu WC, Rathore SS, Wang Y, et al. Blood transfusion in elderly patients with acute myocardial infarction. N Engl J Med 2001;345:1230–6.
37. Hebert PC, Yetisir E, Martin C, et al. Is a low transfusion threshold safe in critically ill patients with cardiovascular diseases? Crit Care Med 2001;29:227–34.
38. Utter GH, Shahlaie K, Zwienenberg-Lee M, Muizelaar JP. Anemia in the setting of traumatic brain injury: The arguments for and against liberal transfusion. J Neurotrauma 2011;28:155–65.

39. Hebert PC, Blajchman MA, Cook DJ, et al. Do blood transfusions improve outcomes related to mechanical ventilation? Chest 2001;119:1850–7.
40. ClinicalTrials.gov. US National Library of Medicine ClinicalTrials.gov Web site. Available at: http://clinicaltrials.gov/ct2/show/NCT00071032?term=NCT00071032&rank=1 (accessed January 2011).
41. Carson JL, Noveck H, Berlin JA, Gould SA. Mortality and morbidity in patients with very low postoperative Hb levels who decline blood transfusion. Transfusion 2002;42: 812–8.
42. Natanson C, Kern SJ, Lurie P, et al. Cell-free hemoglobin-based blood substitutes and risk of myocardial infarction and death: a meta-analysis. JAMA 2008;299:2304–12.
43. Moore EE, Moore FA, Fabian TC, et al. Human polymerized hemoglobin for the treatment of hemorrhagic shock when blood is unavailable: the USA multicenter trial. J Am Coll Surg 2009;208:1–13.
44. Castro CI, Briceno JC. Perfluorocarbon-based oxygen carriers: review of products and trials. Artif Organs 2010;34:622–34.
45. Drake TA, Morrissey JH, Edgington TS. Selective cellular expression of tissue factor in human tissues. Implications for disorders of hemostasis and thrombosis. Am J Pathol 1989;134:1087–97.
46. Edgington TS, Mackman N, Brand K, Ruf W. The structural biology of expression and function of tissue factor. Thromb Haemost 1991;66:67–79.
47. Mantovani A, Sozzani S, Vecchi A, et al. Cytokine activation of endothelial cells: new molecules for an old paradigm. Thromb Haemost 1997;78:406–14.
48. Vane JR, Anggard EE, Botting RM. Regulatory functions of the vascular endothelium. N Engl J Med 1990;323:27–36.
49. Ignarro LJ, Buga GM, Wood KS, et al. Endothelium-derived relaxing factor produced and released from artery and vein is nitric oxide. Proc Natl Acad Sci U S A 1987;84:9265–9.
50. ten Cate JW, van der Poll T, Levi M, et al. Cytokines: triggers of clinical thrombotic disease. Thromb Haemost 1997;78:415–9.
51. Brunetti M, Martelli N, Manarini S, et al. Polymorphonuclear leukocyte apoptosis is inhibited by platelet-released mediators, role of TGFbeta-1. Thromb Haemost 2000;84: 478–83.
52. Cerletti C, Evangelista V, de Gaetano G. P-selectin-beta 2-integrin cross-talk: a molecular mechanism for polymorphonuclear leukocyte recruitment at the site of vascular damage. Thromb Haemost 1999;82:787–93.
53. Stel HV, Sakariassen KS, de Groot PG, et al. Von Willebrand factor in the vessel wall mediates platelet adherence. Blood 1985;65: 85–90.
54. Michelson AD, Barnard MR. Thrombin-induced changes in platelet membrane glycoproteins Ib, IX, and IIb-IIIa complex. Blood 1987;70:1673–8.
55. Motta G, Rojkjaer R, Hasan AA, et al. High molecular weight kininogen regulates prekallikrein assembly and activation on endothelial cells: a novel mechanism for contact activation. Blood 1998;91:516–28.
56. Osterud B, Rapaport SI. Activation of factor IX by the reaction product of tissue factor and factor VII: additional pathway for initiating blood coagulation. Proc Natl Acad Sci U S A 1977;74:5260–4.
57. Mann KG. Biochemistry and physiology of blood coagulation. Thromb Haemost 1999; 82:165–74.
58. Collen D, Lijnen HR. Basic and clinical aspects of fibrinolysis and thrombolysis. Blood 1991;78:3114–24.
59. Chetaille P, Alessi MC, Kouassi D, et al. Plasma TAFI antigen variations in healthy subjects. Thromb Haemost 2000;83:902–5.
60. Esmon CT, Owen WG. Identification of an endothelial cell cofactor for thrombin-catalyzed activation of protein C. Proc Natl Acad Sci U S A 1981;78:2249–52.
61. Broze GJ Jr, Warren LA, Novotny WF, et al. The lipoprotein-associated coagulation inhibitor that inhibits the factor VII-tissue factor complex also inhibits factor Xa: insight into its possible mechanism of action. Blood 1988;71:335–43.
62. Schmidt B, Mitchell L, Ofosu FA, Andrew M. Alpha-2-macroglobulin is an important progressive inhibitor of thrombin in neonatal and infant plasma. Thromb Haemost 1989; 62:1074–7.
63. Juhan-Vague I, Valadier J, Alessi MC, et al. Deficient t-PA release and elevated PA inhibitor levels in patients with spontaneous or recurrent deep venous thrombosis. Thromb Haemost 1987;57:67–72.
64. Korninger C, Lechner K, Niessner H, et al. Impaired fibrinolytic capacity predisposes for recurrence of venous thrombosis. Thromb Haemost 1984;52:127–30.
65. Shovlin CL. Molecular defects in rare bleeding disorders: hereditary haemorrhagic telangiectasia. Thromb Haemost 1997;78: 145–50.
66. Nichols WL, Hultin MB, James AH, et al. von Willebrand disease (VWD): evidence-based diagnosis and management guidelines, the National Heart, Lung, and Blood Institute (NHLBI) Expert Panel report (USA). Haemophilia 2008;14:171–232.
67. Nurden P, Nurden AT. Congenital disorders associated with platelet dysfunctions. Thromb Haemost 2008;99:253–63.
68. Lind B, Thorsen S. A novel missense mutation in the human plasmin inhibitor (alpha2-antiplasmin) gene associated with a bleeding tendency. Br J Haematol 1999;107:317–22.
69. Minowa H, Takahashi Y, Tanaka T, et al. Four cases of bleeding diathesis in children due to congenital plasminogen activator inhibitor-1 deficiency. Haemostasis 1999;29: 286–91.
70. Bhatt DL, Topol EJ. Current role of platelet glycoprotein IIb/IIIa inhibitors in acute coronary syndromes. JAMA 2000;284: 1549–58.
71. Humphries JE. Transfusion therapy in acquired coagulopathies. Hematol Oncol Clin North Am 1994;8:1181–201.
72. Zachee P, Vermylen J, Boogaerts MA. Hematologic aspects of end-stage renal failure. Ann Hematol 1994;69:33–40.
73. Boyer LV, Seifert SA, Clark RF, et al. Recurrent and persistent coagulopathy following pit viper envenomation. Arch Intern Med 1999; 159:706–10.
74. Eriksson BI, Kalebo P, Ekman S, et al. Direct thrombin inhibition with Rec-hirudin CGP 39393 as prophylaxis of thromboembolic complications after total hip replacement. Thromb Haemost 1994;72:227–31.
75. Sherman DG, Atkinson RP, Chippendale T, et al. Intravenous ancrod for treatment of acute ischemic stroke: the STAT study: a randomized controlled trial. Stroke Treatment with Ancrod Trial. JAMA 2000;283:2395–403.
76. Muller-Berghaus G, ten Cate H, Levi M. Disseminated intravascular coagulation: clinical spectrum and established as well as new diagnostic approaches. Thromb Haemost 1999;82:706–12.
77. Lawrie AS, Kitchen S, Purdy G, et al. Assessment of Actin FS and Actin FSL sensitivity to specific clotting factor deficiencies. Clin Lab Haematol 1998;20:179–86.
78. Lind SE. The bleeding time does not predict surgical bleeding. Blood 1991;77:2547–52.
79. Mammen EF, Comp PC, Gosselin R, et al. PFA-100 system: a new method for assessment of platelet dysfunction. Semin Thromb Hemost 1998;24:195–202.
80. Opelz G, Sengar DP, Mickey MR, Terasaki PI. Effect of blood transfusions on subsequent kidney transplants. Transplant Proc 1973;5:253–9.
81. Koch CG, Li L, Sessler DI, et al. Duration of red-cell storage and complications after cardiac surgery. N Engl J Med 2008;358: 1229–39.
82. Triulzi DJ, Kleinman S, Kakaiya RM, et al. The effect of previous pregnancy and transfusion on HLA alloimmunization in blood donors: implications for a transfusion-related acute lung injury risk reduction strategy. Transfusion 2009;49:1825–35.
83. Vamvakas EC, Blajchman MA. Deleterious clinical effects of transfusion-associated immunomodulation: fact or fiction? Blood 2001;97:1180–95.

Acknowledgments

Figures 1, 3, and 4 Marcia Kammerer
Figure 2 Seward Hung

3 POSTOPERATIVE MANAGEMENT OF THE HOSPITALIZED PATIENT

Deborah L. Marquardt, MD, FACS, Roger P. Tatum, MD, FACS, and Dana C. Lynge, MD, FACS

At the beginning of the modern era of surgery, operative procedures commonly took place in an operating theater, performed by plainclothes surgeons in aprons for audiences of students and other onlookers. Afterward, patients were typically cared for at home or in a hospital ward, with scarcely any monitoring and little to help them toward recovery besides their own strength and physiologic reserve. In the current era, surgery is a high-tech, rapid-paced field, with new knowledge and technological advances seemingly appearing around every corner. Many of these new discoveries have allowed surgeons to work more efficiently and safely, and as a result, a number of operations have now become same-day procedures. In addition, some very complex operations that were once thought to be impossible or to be associated with unacceptably high morbidity and mortality have now become feasible thanks to advances in surgical technique, anesthesia, postoperative management, and critical care. The focus of our discussion is on the postoperative considerations that have become essential for successful recovery from surgery.

Each patient is unique, and each patient's case deserves thoughtful attention; no two patients can be managed in exactly the same way. Nevertheless, certain basic categories of postoperative care apply to essentially all patients who undergo surgical procedures. Many of these categories are discussed in greater detail elsewhere in *ACS Surgery*. Our objective in this chapter is to provide a complete yet concise overview of each pertinent topic.

Disposition

The term disposition refers to the location and level of care and monitoring to which the patient is directed after the completion of the operative procedure. Although disposition is not often discussed as a topic in its own right, it is an essential consideration that takes into account many important factors. It may be classified into four general categories as follows:

1. Home or same-day surgery via the recovery room
2. The intensive care unit (ICU), with or without a stay in the recovery room
3. The surgical floor via the recovery room
4. The telemetry ward via the recovery room

The disposition category that is appropriate for a given patient is determined by considering the following four factors:

1. The patient's preoperative clinical status (including both the condition being treated and any comorbid conditions), as indicated by the history, the physical examination, and the input of other medical practitioners
2. The operative procedure to be performed
3. The course and duration of the operative procedure
4. The patient's clinical status at the completion of the procedure, as managed with the help of anesthesia colleagues

The initial phase of disposition planning begins preoperatively. After a full history has been obtained and a complete physical examination carried out, the procedure to be performed is decided on. This decision then initiates a discussion of the complexity and potential complications associated with the procedure, as well as of the concerns and special needs related to any comorbid conditions that may be present. If, as is often the case, the surgeon requires some assistance with planning the operation around the patient's other health problems, input from appropriate medical and surgical colleagues can be extremely helpful. Key factors to take into consideration include the potential complications related to the procedure and the urgency of their treatment; the level of monitoring the patient will require with respect to vital signs, neurologic examination, and telemetry; and the degree of care that will be necessary with respect to treatments, use of drains, and wound care. Relatively few published references describe specific criteria for the various disposition categories; however, most hospitals and surgery centers will have developed their own policies specifying a standard of care to be provided for each category.

SAME-DAY SURGERY

Same-day surgery is appropriate for patients who (1) have few or no comorbid medical conditions and (2) are undergoing a procedure that involves short-duration anesthesia or local anesthesia plus sedation and that carries a low likelihood of urgent complications. Operations commonly performed on a same-day basis include inguinal or umbilical hernia repair, simple laparoscopic cholecystectomy, breast biopsy, and small subcutaneous procedures.

The growth in the performance of minor and same-day procedures has led to the development of various types of short-stay units or wards. The level of care provided by a short-stay ward is generally equivalent to that provided by a regular nursing ward; however, the anticipated duration of care is substantially shorter, typically ranging from several hours to a maximum of 48 hours. Short-stay wards also undergo some modifications to facilitate the use of streamlined teaching protocols designed to prepare patients for home care. Many hospitals now have short-stay units, as do some independent surgery centers.

SURGICAL FLOOR

The vast majority of patients receive the postoperative care they require on the surgical floor (or regular nursing ward). Assessment of vital signs, control of pain, care of wounds, management of tubes and drains, and monitoring of intake and output are addressed every 2 to 8 hours (depending on the variable). Assignment of the patient to the regular nursing ward presupposes that he or she is hemodynamically stable and does not need continuous monitoring.

The telemetry ward is a variant of the regular nursing ward. The care provided in the telemetry ward is generally equivalent to that provided on other floor wards except that patients undergo continuous cardiac monitoring. Patients commonly assigned to the telemetry ward after operation include (1) those with a known medical history of arrhythmias that may necessitate intervention, (2) those with intraoperative arrhythmias or other electrocardiographic (ECG) changes who are not believed to require ICU monitoring but who do need this form of cardiac follow-up, and (3) those making the transition from the ICU to a regular ward who are hemodynamically stable but who require ongoing follow-up of a cardiac issue.

INTENSIVE CARE UNIT

When early postoperative complications may necessitate urgent intervention and close observation is therefore essential, patients should be admitted to the ICU for postoperative care. Postoperative ICU admission may also be appropriate for patients who are clinically unstable after the procedure; these patients often require ongoing resuscitation, intravenous (IV) administration of vasoactive agents, ventilatory support, or continuous telemetry monitoring for dysrhythmias. In addition, admission to the ICU should be considered for patients in whom the complexity of drain management, wound care, or even pain control may necessitate frequent postoperative monitoring that is not available on a regular nursing ward. At present, there is no single set of accepted guidelines directing ICU admission. There are, however, published sources that can provide some guidance. For example, a 2003 article supplied recommendations for the various services to be provided by differing levels of ICUs.[1] Published recommendations of this sort may be adopted or modified by individual hospitals and surgery centers as necessary.

Care Orders

Nurses and other ancillary personnel provide the bulk of the care received by patients after a surgical procedure; accordingly, it is essential that they receive clear and ample instructions to guide their work. Such instructions generally take the form of specific postoperative orders directed to each ancillary service. Services for which such orders may be appropriate include nursing, respiratory therapy, physical therapy (PT), occupational therapy (OT), and diet and nutrition. In what follows, we briefly outline some of the common tasks that require orders to be directed toward these services.

NASOGASTRIC TUBES

Nasogastric (NG) tubes are commonly placed after gastrointestinal (GI) operations, most frequently for drainage of gastric secretions when an ileus is anticipated or offloading of the upper GI tract when a fresh anastomosis is located close by. Although NG tubes have often been placed routinely after abdominal surgery, the current literature cites a number of reasons why routine use is inadvisable and selective use is preferable. For example, significantly earlier return of bowel function, a trend toward fewer pulmonary complications, and enhanced patient comfort and decreased nausea are reported when NG tubes are not routinely placed or when they are removed within 24 hours after operation.[2]

When postoperative placement of an NG tube is considered appropriate, an order from a physician is required, along with direction regarding the method of drainage. Sometimes NG tubes are placed to low continuous suction; more often, however, they are placed to low intermittent suction to eliminate the chance of continuous suction against a visceral wall and to promote generalized drainage. If large volumes of secretions are not expected, continuous gravity may be used instead of suction. A key concern with NG tubes is maintenance of the patency of both the main port and the sump port. Should either port become blocked, the tube will be rendered ineffective. This concern should be discussed with the nursing staff. At times, it may be necessary to issue specific orders to ensure that this concern is appropriately addressed. As a rule, surgical nurses are well acquainted with tube maintenance; however, if thick secretions are expected, orders for routine flushing may be indicated. When the tube is no longer indicated, its removal may be ordered.

URINARY CATHETERS

Urinary catheters can serve a large variety of purposes. In the setting of bladder or genitourinary surgery, they are often employed to decompress the system so that it will heal more readily. After general surgical procedures—and many other surgical procedures as well—they are used to provide accurate measurements of volume output and thus, indirectly, to give some indication of the patient's overall volume and resuscitation status. Furthermore, after many procedures, patients initially find it extremely difficult or impossible to mobilize for urination, and a urinary catheter may be quite helpful during this time.

Their utility and importance notwithstanding, urinary catheters are associated with the development of nosocomial urinary tract infections (UTIs). As many as 40% of all hospital infections are UTIs, and 80 to 90% of these UTIs are associated with urinary catheters [*see* Postoperative Complications, *below*]. Accordingly, when catheterization is no longer deemed necessary, prompt removal is indicated. As a rule, orders specifically pertaining to urinary catheter care are few, typically including gravity drainage, flushing to maintain patency (if warranted), and removal when appropriate. At times, irrigation is employed after urologic procedures or for the management of certain infectious agents.

OXYGEN THERAPY

Supplemental administration of oxygen is often necessary after a surgical procedure. Common indicators of a need for postoperative oxygen supplementation include shallow breathing and pain, atelectasis, operative manipulation in the chest cavity, and postoperative impairment of breathing mechanics. Because supplemental oxygen is considered a medication, a physician's order is required before it can be administered. In many cases, oxygen supplementation is ordered on an as-needed basis with the aim of enabling the patient to meet specific peripheral oxygen saturation criteria. In other cases, it is ordered routinely in the setting of known preoperative patient oxygen use.

An important factor to keep in mind is that oxygen supplementation protocols may vary from one nursing unit to another. Different units may place different limitations on the amount of supplemental oxygen permitted, depending on their specific monitoring and safety guidelines. Another important factor is that patients with known obstructive pulmonary disease and carbon dioxide retention are at increased risk for respiratory depression with hyperoxygenation; accordingly, particular care should be exercised in ordering supplemental oxygen for these patients.

DRAINS

Drains and tubes are placed in a wide variety of locations for a number of different purposes—in particular, drainage of purulent materials, serum, or blood from body cavities. Several types are commonly used, including soft gravity drains (e.g., Penrose), closed-suction drains (e.g., Hemovac, Jackson-Pratt, and Blake), and sump drains, which draw air into one lumen and extract fluid via a companion lumen. Traditionally, surgeons have often made the decision to place a drain on the basis of their surgical training and practice habits rather than of any firm evidence that drainage is warranted. Multiple randomized clinical trials have now demonstrated that routine use of drains after elective operations—including appendectomies and colorectal, hepatic, thyroid, and parathyroid procedures—does not prevent anastomotic and other complications (although it does reduce seroma formation). Consequently, it is recommended that drains, like NG tubes, be employed selectively.[3–5] Once a drain is in place, specific orders must be issued for its maintenance. These include use of gravity or suction (and the means by which suction is to be provided if ordered), management and measurement of output, stripping, and care around the drain exit site.

Biliary tract drains include T tubes, cholecystostomy tubes, percutaneous drains of the biliary tree, and nasobiliary drains. Daily site maintenance, flushing, and output recording are performed by the nursing staff. Most biliary tract drains are removed by the practitioner or other trained midlevel staff members.

T tubes are generally placed after operative exploration or repair of the common bile duct (CBD). The long phalanges are left within the CBD, and the long portion of the tube is brought out to the skin for drainage. The tube is left in place until the CBD is properly healing and there is evidence of adequate distal drainage (signaled by a decrease in external drainage of bile). Before the T tube is removed, a cholangiogram is recommended to document distal patency and rule out retained gallstones or leakage.[6]

Cholecystostomy tubes are placed percutaneously—typically under ultrasonographic guidance and with local anesthesia—to decompress the gallbladder. Generally, they are used either (1) when cholecystectomy cannot be performed, because concomitant medical problems make anesthesia or the stress of operation intolerable, or (2) when the presence of severe inflammation leads the surgeon to conclude that dissection poses too high an operative risk. Particularly in the latter setting, delayed elective cholecystectomy may be appropriate; if so, the cholecystostomy tube may be removed at the time of the operation.

Nasobiliary tubes are placed endoscopically in the course of biliary endoscopy. They are used to decompress the CBD in some settings. They are usually placed to gravity and otherwise are managed in much the same way as NG tubes.[7]

WOUND CARE

The topic of wound care is a broad one. Here we focus on initial postoperative dressing care, traditional wet-to-dry dressings, and use of a vacuum-assisted closure device (e.g., VAC Abdominal Dressing System, Kinetic Concepts, Inc., San Antonio, TX). These and other components of wound care are discussed in more detail elsewhere.

Initial wound management after an operative procedure generally entails placement of a sterile dressing to cover the incision. The traditional recommendation has been to keep this dressing in place and dry for the first 48 hours after operation; because epithelialization is known to take place within approximately this period, the assumption is that this measure will reduce the risk of wound infection. Although most surgeons still follow this practice, especially in general surgical cases, supporting data from randomized clinical studies are lacking. In addition, several small studies that evaluated early showering with closed surgical incisions found no increases in the rate of infection or dehiscence.[8,9] It should be kept in mind, however, that these small studies looked primarily at soft tissue and other minor skin incisions that did not involve fascia. Thus, even though the traditional approach to initial dressing management is not strongly supported, the data currently available are insufficient to indicate that it should be changed.

Wet-to-dry dressings are used in a variety of settings. In a surgical context, they are most often applied to a wound that cannot be closed primarily as a consequence of contamination or inability to approximate the skin edges. Wet-to-dry dressings provide a moist environment that promotes granulation and wound closure by secondary intention. Moreover, their removal and replacement cause débridement of excess exudate or unhealthy superficial tissue. Postoperative orders should specify the frequency of dressing changes and the solution used to provide dampness. For most clean open incisions, twice-daily dressing changes using normal saline solution represent the most common approach. If there is excess wound exudate to be débrided, dressing changes may be performed more frequently. If there is particular concern about wound contamination or superficial colonization of organisms, substitution of dilute Dakin solution for normal saline may be considered.

A new era of wound management arrived in the late 1990s with the introduction of negative-pressure wound therapy (NPWT). In NPWT, a vacuum-assisted wound closure device places the wound under subatmospheric pressure conditions, thereby encouraging blood flow, decreasing local wound edema and excess fluid (and consequently lowering bacterial counts and encouraging wound granulation), and increasing wound contraction.[10,11] Since the first published animal studies, NPWT has been successfully employed for a multitude of wound types, including complex traumatic and surgical wounds, skin graft sites, and decubitus wounds. Before vacuum-assisted closure is used, however, it is necessary to consider whether and to what extent the wound is contaminated, the proximity of the wound to viscera or vascular structures, and the potential ability of the patient to tolerate dressing changes. Wounds that are grossly contaminated or contain significant amounts of nonviable tissue probably are not well suited to an occlusive dressing system of this type given that frequent evaluation and possibly débridement may be needed to prevent ongoing tissue infection and death. Furthermore, the suction effect of the standard vacuum sponge may cause serious erosion of internal viscera or exposed major blood vessels. Some silicone-impregnated nonadherent sponges are available that may be suitable in this setting, but caution should be exercised in using them. Finally, because of the adherence of the sponge and the occlusive adhesive dressing, some patients may be unable to tolerate dressing changes without sedation or anesthesia.

Nutrition

The patient's nutritional status has a significant effect on postoperative morbidity and even mortality. After most operative procedures that do not involve the alimentary tract or the abdomen and do not affect swallowing and airway protection, the usual practice is to initiate the return to full patient-controlled oral nutrition as soon as the patient is fully awake. In these surgical settings, therefore, it is rarely necessary to discuss postoperative nutrition approaches to any great extent.

After procedures that do involve the alimentary tract or the abdomen, however, the situation is different. The traditional practice has been to institute a nihil per os (NPO) policy, with or without NG drainage, after all abdominal or alimentary tract procedures until the return of bowel function, as evidenced by flatus or bowel movement, is confirmed. The routine application of this practice has been challenged, however, especially over the past 15 years. Data from prospective studies of high statistical power are lacking, but many smaller studies evaluating early return to enteral nutrition after alimentary tract procedures have yielded evidence tending to favor more routine use of enteral intake within 48 hours after such procedures.

Issues related to postoperative nutritional support are discussed further and in greater detail elsewhere.

NPO STATUS

In the setting of elective colorectal surgery, it is well-accepted practice to initiate a return to patient-controlled enteral-oral feeding within 24 to 48 hours after operation; this practice yields no increase in the incidence of postoperative complications (e.g., anastomotic leakage, wound and intra-abdominal infection, and pneumonia) or the length of hospital stay and, according to some reports, may even decrease them.[12] In the setting of upper GI surgery (specifically, gastric resection, total gastrectomy, and esophagectomy), the situation is less clear-cut. Traditional concerns—in particular, the need to avoid distention stress on gastric or gastrojejunal anastomoses after gastric resection, the more tenuous nature of a esophagojejunostomy after total gastrectomy, and the delayed gastric conduit emptying, aspiration risk, and anastomotic stress seen after esophagectomy or resection—have led to the current practice of instituting NG drainage and placing the patient on NPO status postoperatively until evidence of the return of bowel function is apparent, as well as, in some cases, investigating the anastomosis for possible leakage by means of contrast fluoroscopy. There are no clinical trial data to support this approach. In fact, many surgeons routinely remove the NG tube within 24 hours after gastric resection and early feeding without incurring increased complications. However, there are also no clinical trial data indicating that the current approach is potentially ineffective or harmful. Consequently, traditional management methods after upper GI procedures still are often endorsed in the literature.[13,14]

ENTERAL NUTRITION

Enteral nutrition may be delivered via several routes. Most patients who have undergone an operation are able to take in an adequate amount of calories orally. When they are unable to do so, whether because of altered mental status, impaired pulmonary function, or some other condition, the use of enteral feeding tubes may be indicated. In the acute setting, NG and nasojejunal feeding tubes are the types most commonly employed to deliver enteral solutions into the GI tract. Either type is appropriate for this purpose; the two types are equivalent overall as regards their ability to provide adequate nutrition, and there are no significant differences in outcome or complications. In cases where prolonged inability to take in adequate calories orally is expected, the use of an indwelling feeding tube, such as a gastrostomy or jejunostomy tube, may be indicated. These tubes must be placed either at the time of operation or subsequently via surgical or percutaneous means, and there is some potential for complications. The specific indications for the use of such tubes are patient derived; they are not routinely associated with the performance of specific procedures.

TOTAL PARENTERAL NUTRITION

Total parenteral nutrition (TPN) is a surrogate form of nutrition in which dextrose, amino acids, and lipids are delivered via a central venous catheter. It is a reliable method in that it delivers nutrients and calories regardless of whether the patient's gut is functioning. Nevertheless, multiple studies over the past 20 years have shown that when the patient has a functioning intestinal tract, enteral feeding is clearly preferable to TPN. Although the specific mechanisms are not fully understood, enteral nutrition is known to foster gut mucosal integrity, to support overall immune function, and to be associated with lower complication rates and shorter hospital stays. In contrast, TPN is known to be associated with altered immune function, an increased rate of infectious complications, and, in some studies, a higher incidence of anastomotic complications after GI surgery. Moreover, there are as yet no data to indicate that acute use of TPN during short periods of starvation benefits patients who are adequately nourished preoperatively. TPN may, however, be lifesaving in patients who are malnourished and who do not have functioning GI tracts (e.g., those with short gut syndrome, severe gut dysmotility or malabsorption, mesenteric vascular insufficiency, bowel obstruction, high-output enteric fistulas, or bowel ischemia).[15]

CALORIC GOALS

Once a route of nutritional support has been decided on, overall goals for caloric and protein intake may be established on the basis of the patient's ideal body weight (IBW) and expected postoperative metabolic state. One approach is to rely on a general estimate; a commonly used formula is 25 kcal/kg IBW. Another approach is to calculate a basal energy requirement by using the Harris-Benedict equation. This calculation is separate from the calculation of protein needs. A daily protein intake goal may be calculated on the basis of the patient's estimated level of physical stress. A well-nourished unstressed person requires a protein intake of approximately 1.0 g/kg IBW/day. A seriously ill patient under ongoing severe physical stress, however, may require 2.0 g/kg IBW/day; in some settings (e.g., extensive burns), a protein intake as high as 3.0 g/kg IBW/day may be recommended. Once the patient's specific needs have been calculated, the amount and type of nutrient solution to be provided enterally or via TPN are determined. If the patient is on a full oral diet, a calorie count or recording of the percentage of items eaten at each meal or snack may be made by the nursing staff and used to estimate the patient's intake, with nutritional supplementation provided as needed.[16]

Patients who require assistance with nutritional intake should be monitored to determine whether the interventions being carried out are having the desired effect. The most common method of monitoring patients' nutritional status with nutritional supplementation is to measure the serum albumin and prealbumin (transthyretin) concentrations. Albumin has a half-life of approximately 14 to 20 days and thus serves as a marker of longer-term nutritional status. A value lower than 2.2 g/dL is generally considered to represent severe malnutrition, but even somewhat higher values (< 3.0 g/dL) have been associated with poorer outcomes after elective surgery. Although the serum albumin concentration is a commonly used marker, it is not always a reliable one. Because of albumin's relatively long half-life, the serum concentration does not reflect the patient's more recent nutritional status. In addition, the measured concentration can change quickly in response to the infusion of exogenous albumin or to the development of dehydration, sepsis, and liver disease despite adequate nutrition. Prealbumin is a separate serum protein that has a half-life of approximately 24 to 48 hours and thus can serve as a marker of current and more recent nutritional status. Like the albumin concentration, the prealbumin concentration can be affected by liver and renal disease. Overall, however, it is more immediately reliable in following the effects of nutritional intervention.

Fluid Management

IV fluids may be classified into two main categories: resuscitation and maintenance. Supplemental fluids constitute a third category.

RESUSCITATION FLUIDS

Resuscitation fluids maintain tissue perfusion in the setting of hypovolemia by restoring lost volume to the intravascular space. They may be further classified into two subcategories: crystalloids and colloids.

Crystalloids

Crystalloid solutions are water-based solutions to which electrolytes (and, sometimes, organic molecules such as dextrose) have been added. The crystalloid solutions used for resuscitation are generally isotonic to blood plasma and include such common examples as 0.9% sodium chloride, lactated Ringer solution, and Plasma-Lyte (Baxter Healthcare, Round Lake, IL). The choice to use one solution over another is usually inconsequential, but there are a few notable exceptions. For example, in the setting of renal dysfunction, there is a risk of hyperkalemia when potassium-containing solutions such as lactated Ringer solution and Plasma-Lyte are used. As another example, the administration of large volumes of 0.9% sodium chloride, which has a pH of 5.0 and a chloride content of 154 mmol/L, can lead to hyperchloremic metabolic acidosis. Regardless of which crystalloid solution is used, large volumes may have to be infused to achieve a significant increase in the circulating intravascular volume. Only one third to one quarter (250 to 330 mL/L) of the fluid administered stays in the intravascular space; the rest migrates by osmosis into the interstitial tissues, producing edema and potential impairment of tissue perfusion (the latter is a theoretical consequence whose existence has not yet been directly demonstrated).[17]

Colloids

Colloid solutions are composed of microscopic particles dispersed in a second substance in such a way that they are suspended and do not separate by normal filtration. Colloids are derived from three main forms of semisynthetic molecules: gelatins, dextrans, and hydroxyethyl starches. All of the commonly used synthetic colloids are dissolved in crystalloid solution. Nonsynthetic colloids also exist, including human albumin solutions, fresh frozen plasma, plasma-protein fraction, and immunoglobulin solutions. Compared with crystalloid solutions, colloid solutions increase the circulating intravascular volume to a much greater degree per unit of volume infused. In this respect, the various colloids may be thought of as a single group; however, in practice, they are most often given selectively on the basis of secondary characteristics other than their volume-increasing action, such as effect on hemostasis, risk of allergic reaction, and cost.

Crystalloids versus Colloids

The debate over whether crystalloids or colloids are superior for resuscitation has been going on for at least 30 years. Although multiple randomized, controlled trials have compared the two types of solutions in a variety of settings, including sepsis, trauma, burns, and surgery, the evidence accumulated to date has not established that one is clearly better than the other in terms of overall outcome. Supporters of crystalloid resuscitation cite the risk of altered hemostasis, the increased likelihood of drug interactions and allergic reactions, the potential for volume overload, and the relatively high cost as factors arguing against the use of colloids. Supporters of colloid resuscitation cite the large volume of crystalloid needed to produce significant volume effects, the subsequent tissue edema, and the potential for impaired tissue perfusion and oxygenation as factors arguing against the use of crystalloids. Current recommendations favor crystalloid for resuscitation, with colloid an acceptable substitute when its secondary effects are desired in specific situations.[17,18]

MAINTENANCE FLUIDS

Maintenance fluids provide required daily amounts of free water and electrolytes (e.g., sodium, potassium, and chloride) to balance expected daily losses and maintain homeostasis. A basic rule of thumb used by many practitioners to calculate the infusion rate for maintenance IV fluids is the so-called 4, 2, 1 rule:

- 4 mL/kg/hr for the first 10 kg of body weight
- 2 mL/kg/hr for the next 10 kg of body weight and
- 1 mL/kg/hr for every 1 kg of body weight above 20 kg

Generally accepted maintenance requirements include 30 to 35 mL/kg/day for free water, 1.5 mEq/kg/day for chloride, 1 mEq/kg/day for sodium, and 1 mEq/kg/day for potassium. In the setting of starvation or poor oral intake, dextrose 5% is often added to maintenance fluids to inhibit muscle breakdown. In regular practice, however, these specific values are not commonly used; more often, a rough estimate is made of expected daily fluid requirements, and solutions are ordered in accordance with this estimate. Although this practice is unlikely to cause noticeable harm in the majority of postoperative patients, there are situations where inaccurate calculations can lead to dehydration and volume overload. Three studies from the early 2000s evaluated patients undergoing elective colorectal surgery with the aim of determining whether providing higher volumes of fluid perioperatively had an impact on outcome.[19–21] In all three, the data supported the use of smaller fluid volumes perioperatively, which was shown to result in earlier return of gut function after operation, shorter hospital stays, and overall decreases in cardiopulmonary and tissue-healing complications.

SUPPLEMENTAL FLUIDS

Supplemental fluids are given to replace any ongoing fluid loss beyond what is expected to occur via insensible loss and excretion in urine and stool. They are most commonly required by patients with prolonged NG tube output, enterocutaneous fistulas, diarrhea, high-output ileostomies, or large open wounds associated with excessive insensible fluid loss. In each case, the amount of fluid lost daily should be calculated, and replacement fluid should be given in a quantity determined by this measurement (either as a whole or in part) and by the patient's overall intravascular volume status. The particular solution to be used depends on the characteristics of the fluid loss. The components and volume of the fluids produced in the GI tract are different at different sites [*see Table 1*].

Pain Control

The topic of postoperative pain control covers a broad spectrum of possible interventions that serve a wide range of purposes. The most obvious purpose is simply to relieve the suffering and stress associated with postoperative pain. Another is to improve the patient's overall postoperative status. Bringing the patient closer to the baseline sensory state by reducing pain allows him or her to engage in activities that promote healing and prevent complications, including mobilization to help prevent deep vein thrombosis (DVT) and deep breathing and coughing to help prevent pneumonia. Common methods of pain relief include IV infusion of narcotics, epidural analgesia using local anesthetics with or without narcotics, oral administration of narcotics, and the use of nonnarcotic oral medications such as nonsteroidal antiinflammatory drugs (NSAIDs) and acetaminophen (see below). These and other issues related to postoperative pain control are discussed in greater detail elsewhere.

IV NARCOTIC ANALGESIA

IV narcotics may be administered either by the medical staff or, if patient-controlled analgesia (PCA) is feasible, by the patient. In most cases, with the exception of brief hospital stays (< 48 hours) and ICU settings where the patient may not be alert enough to manage a patient-controlled system, PCA is now generally considered preferable to as-needed nurse-administered IV narcotic analgesia. Numerous studies and reviews have shown that PCA is safe and is no more likely to cause side effects (e.g., oversedation, overdose, itching, and nausea) than nurse-administered IV narcotic analgesia is. In addition, the use of PCA improves patients' subjective perceptions of the efficacy of pain relief and the timeliness of drug administration.[22]

EPIDURAL ANALGESIA

Epidural analgesia usually makes use of a local anesthetic (e.g., bupivicaine) with or without the addition of a narcotic (e.g., fentanyl). The anesthetic solution is instilled into the epidural space, bathing the nerve roots in a given region and thereby providing pain relief. Until the past decade or so, epidural analgesia was considered a more dangerous method of pain relief and was not routinely employed outside the ICU. With time and further observation has come the recognition that epidural analgesia is safe and effective for postoperative pain control in a routine floor setting if managed by the proper supporting team of physicians.

There has been some debate regarding whether epidural analgesia leads to earlier return of bowel function after GI surgery or reduces the incidence of pulmonary complications; at present, this debate remains unresolved. There is clear evidence, however, that patients subjectively experience less pain with epidural analgesia, both at rest and in the course of activities such as mobilization and coughing. Moreover, in patients who have sustained traumatic rib fractures, early use of epidural analgesia in place of IV narcotic analgesia has been shown to reduce the incidence of associated pneumonia and shorten the time for which mechanical ventilation is required.[23] Epidural analgesia does have certain drawbacks, including an increased incidence of orthostatic episodes and a need for more frequent adjustments of the medication dosage. Nevertheless, it can be highly effective and can be a reasonable option when judged appropriate by the anesthesiologist and agreed to by the patient.[24,25]

ORAL ADMINISTRATION OF NARCOTICS

Oral administration of narcotics is one of the oldest methods of providing postoperative pain relief. Numerous

Table 1 **Electrolyte Content and Rate of Production of Fluids Secreted in the Gastrointestinal Tract**

Source of Secretion	Electrolyte Concentration (mEq/L)					Rate of Production (mL/day)
	Na^+	K^+	Cl^-	HCO_3^-	H^+	
Salivary glands	50	20	40	30		100–1,000
Stomach						
Basal	100	10	140		30	1,000
Stimulated	30	10	140		100	4,000
Bile	140	5	100	60		500–1,000
Pancreas	140	5	75	100		1,000
Duodenum	140	5	80			100–2,000
Ileum	140	5	70	50		100–2,000
Colon	60	70	15	30		

different narcotic agents are now available for use in this setting. When deciding which narcotic to prescribe, however, physicians typically do not select freely from the entire available range; rather, they tend to choose from a small subset of agents that they know well and are comfortable with. A key point to keep in mind is that in some formulations, narcotics are combined with other compounds (e.g., acetaminophen or aspirin), and these added medications can have side effects of their own if taken in excessively high doses. Such formulations may require more careful titration than narcotics alone would. Another key point is that many narcotics are available in both short-acting and long-acting versions. In patients who are experiencing substantial postoperative pain, a combination of long-acting agents and short-acting agents may yield more sustained and predictable pain relief than either type alone would.

Finally, for patients who have a history of chronic pain conditions and who regularly used pain medications preoperatively, the assistance of an acute pain service management team may be invaluable in treating pain postoperatively.

NSAIDS AND ACETAMINOPHEN

NSAIDs are available both by prescription and over the counter. They not only provide effective analgesia for pain from minor procedures but also may be a powerful adjunct to narcotics in more acute hospital settings. Their major disadvantages, which in some contexts are substantial enough to limit their use, include their propensity to cause gastric irritation and ulceration; their antiplatelet effects, which increase the tendency toward bleeding; and their potential nephrotoxic effects in some formulations. When employed in settings where these disadvantages are not considered to pose a high risk, NSAIDs can be a useful addition to narcotics, both by providing further pain relief and by reducing the required narcotic doses (and thus the incidence of narcotic-related side effects).

Like the NSAIDs, acetaminophen provides minor pain relief and is an antipyretic, but unlike the NSAIDs, it has no antiinflammatory effect. Acetaminophen also is often added to narcotic regimens or formulations to reduce the need for narcotics. Its greatest potential side effect is hepatic toxicity with excessive use. Accordingly, the dosage should be less than 2 g/day in patients with normal hepatic function and even lower in those with impaired hepatic function. It is particularly important to keep these dose limits in mind when narcotic-acetaminophen combinations are prescribed on an as-needed basis; in this situation, safe dosage limits may well be exceeded if sufficient care is not taken.

Glycemic Control

Over the last decade, blood glucose control in the postoperative period has become a topic of great interest. Many studies, beginning with that of Van den Berghe and colleagues in 2001,[26] have found that strict glucose control reduces morbidity and mortality in critically ill surgical ICU patients. Although most of the data currently available are derived from ICU patients rather than from the surgical population as a whole, the principle of tight glycemic control has been generalized to apply to most postoperative patients.

The target glucose range has been the subject of debate, with most institutions using a range of 80 to 140 mg/dL. The ability to achieve this target range and the means of achieving it vary according to the level of nursing care that is provided. Options include continuous IV insulin infusion and combinations of subcutaneous injections that use various long- and short-acting insulin formulations. Episodes of hypoglycemia are an ever-present risk with tight glucose control; accordingly, the use of standard dosage regimens and careful monitoring are recommended to reduce the risk of such episodes.

The debate over the specifics of glycemic control notwithstanding, it is generally well accepted that this issue should be addressed in all patients who have undergone major operative procedures, regardless of whether they carry a preoperative diagnosis of diabetes mellitus.[26,27]

Postoperative Complications

Numerous complications may arise in the postoperative period. Many of these are specific to particular operative procedures and hence are best discussed in connection with those procedures. Many others, however, may develop after virtually any operation and thus warrant a general discussion in this chapter (see below). Prompt discovery and treatment of these latter complications rely heavily on a sufficiently high index of suspicion.

POSTOPERATIVE FEVER

Postoperative temperature elevations are quite common, occurring in nearly one third of patients after surgery. Only a relatively small number of these are actually caused by infection. Fevers that are caused by infections (e.g., pneumonias, wound infections, or UTIs) tend to reach higher temperatures (> 38.5°C [101.3°F]), usually are associated with moderate elevation of the white blood cell (WBC) count 3 or more days after operation, and typically extend over consecutive days. Noninfectious causes of postoperative fevers include components of the inflammatory response to surgical intervention, reabsorption of hematomas, and (possibly) atelectasis.[28]

Beyond checking the WBC count, a shotgun approach to the workup of postoperative fever probably is not warranted. A focused approach based on well-directed questioning and a careful physical examination is more likely to obtain the highest diagnostic yield. Coughing, sputum production, and respiratory effort should be noted, and the lungs should be auscultated for rales. All incisions should be inspected for erythema and drainage, and current and recent IV sites should be checked for evidence of cellulitis. If a central line has been placed, particularly if it has been in place for several days, the possibility of a line infection should be considered. Patients who have undergone prolonged NG intubation may have sinusitis, which is most readily diagnosed through computed tomography (CT) of the sinuses. Further workup for fever may include, as indicated, chest x-ray, sputum cultures, urinalysis, blood cultures, or CT of the abdomen (after procedures involving laparotomy—especially bowel resections—where intra-abdominal abscess is a possible complication).

PNEUMONIA

Respiratory infections in the postoperative period are generally considered nosocomial pneumonias and, as such, are potentially serious complications. The estimated incidence of postoperative pneumonia varies significantly, with many estimates tending to run high. A 2001 study of more than 160,000 patients undergoing major noncardiac surgery provided what may be a reasonable overall figure, finding the incidence of postoperative pneumonia to be approximately 1.5%.[29] In the 2,466 patients with pneumonia, the 30-day mortality was 21%. Thoracic procedures, upper abdominal procedures, abdominal aortic aneurysm repair, peripheral vascular procedures, and neurosurgical procedures were all identified as placing patients at significantly increased risk for pneumonia. Patient-specific risk factors included age greater than 60 years, recent alcohol use, dependent functional status, long-term steroid use, and a 10% weight loss in the 6 months preceding the operation.[29]

The diagnosis of postoperative pneumonia is based on the usual combination of index of suspicion, findings from the history and physical examination (e.g., fever, shortness of breath, hypoxia, productive cough, and rales on lung auscultation), imaging, and laboratory evaluation. Appropriate workup, directed by the clinical findings, typically starts with chest x-rays (preferably in both posteroanterior and lateral views, if possible) and sputum cultures, sometimes accompanied by CT scanning of the chest and, possibly, bronchoscopy with bronchoalveolar lavage (which may be useful in directing antibiotic therapy when sputum cultures are nondiagnostic). Empirical broad-spectrum antibiotic therapy is typically initiated before the causative organism is identified; this practice has been shown to reduce mortality. Piperacillin-tazobactam, which is effective against *Pseudomonas aeruginosa*, is commonly used for this purpose; however, when Gram staining of the sputum identifies gram-positive cocci, vancomycin or linezolid may be used initially instead.[30] Once the causative organism is identified, specific antibiotic therapy directed at that organism is indicated, as in treatment of other infectious processes. Drainage of parapneumonic effusions may also be necessary, and this measure may be helpful in diagnosing or preventing the development of empyema.

SURGICAL SITE INFECTION

Surgical site infection (SSI) is one of the most common postoperative complications and may occur after virtually any type of procedure. Rates of infection vary widely (from less than 1% to approximately 20%) depending on the procedure performed, the classification of the operative wound (clean, clean-contaminated, contaminated, or dirty), and a host of patient-related and situation-specific factors. The majority of SSIs, regardless of site, are caused by skin-based flora, most commonly gram-positive cocci (e.g., staphylococci). Gram-negative infections are also commonly seen after GI procedures, and anaerobes may be present after pharyngo-esophageal procedures.[31] With SSI, as with other postoperative infectious complications, prompt recognition of the signs and symptoms is the key to successful management. Hence, regular examination of the wound, particularly in the setting of postoperative fever, is critical. Erythema and induration (indicative of cellulitis) are obvious signs of SSI, as is active drainage of pus from the wound. A more subtle sign is pain that is greater than expected, especially when the pain seems to be increasing several days after operation.

In most cases, it is necessary to open and drain the wound (which is easily done at the bedside or in the clinic in most cases) and allow it to heal via secondary intention. Generally, wet-to-dry dressing changes with saline are employed; however, larger wounds may benefit from NPWT [*see* Care Orders, Wound Care, *above*]. Success with NPWT has been widely reported, and this technique has been used to treat difficult wounds such as exposed vascular grafts and sternotomy infections.[32,33] The use of antibiotics depends on the presence and degree of cellulitis. The initial choice of an agent should be guided by the likelihood that particular organisms will be present, which is estimated on the basis of the site of the operation and the type of procedure being performed. Whenever possible, any purulent material in the SSI should be cultured; this step may permit more targeted antimicrobial therapy.

DEEP VEIN THROMBOSIS AND PULMONARY EMBOLISM

In the absence of appropriate prophylaxis, the incidence of DVT may be as high as 30% in abdominal and thoracic surgery patients and that of fatal pulmonary embolism (PE) may be as high as 0.9%. Thus, prophylaxis against thromboembolism is clearly of high importance in the postoperative care of many patients. Major risk factors for DVT and PE in this setting include the operation itself, physical immobility, advanced age, the presence of a malignancy, obesity, and a history of smoking.[34]

DVT should be suspected postoperatively whenever a patient complains of lower-extremity pain or one leg is noticeably more swollen than the other. The gold standard for diagnosis remains a venous duplex examination, which has a sensitivity of 97% for detecting DVT of the femoral and popliteal veins.[35] In most cases, treatment involves starting a heparin infusion (typically without a loading bolus in the postoperative setting), targeting a partial thromboplastin time (PTT) that is double to triple the normal PTT (i.e., approximately 60 to 80 seconds), and then switching to warfarin therapy when the patient is stable and able to tolerate oral medications.

PE should be suspected whenever a postoperative patient experiences a decrease in oxygen saturation or shortness of breath; this decrease may be accompanied by chest pain, tachycardia, and diaphoresis, all of which may also be seen in the setting of myocardial infarction (MI). When PE is suspected, it may be appropriate to start heparin therapy even before the diagnosis has been confirmed, depending on the degree of suspicion and the relative risk anticoagulation may pose to the patient. Currently, the principal means of diagnosing acute PE is spiral CT. This modality has relatively wide availability, can be performed fairly rapidly, and has a sensitivity of 53 to 100% and a specificity of 81 to 100%. In addition, it is readily usable in most critically ill patients, including those undergoing mechanical ventilation (although the amount of IV contrast material it requires may limit its use in patients with renal insufficiency). Greater diagnostic yield may be obtained by combining spiral CT with a lower-extremity venous duplex examination.[36] For most patients with postoperative PE, anticoagulation is administered in the form of heparin. Low-molecular-weight heparins (LMWHs) are also generally safe and effective; however, because their effect cannot be turned off in the same way as that of IV unfractionated heparin, they may be less useful in the period after operation.[37] In patients with massive PE, surgical embolectomy or suction-catheter embolectomy may be considered as conditions warrant. Thrombolytic therapy is generally contraindicated in the postoperative setting.

CARDIAC COMPLICATIONS

Cardiac dysrhythmias may occur after a wide variety of surgical procedures; as one might imagine, they are most common after cardiac operations. Predisposing factors and possible causes are numerous and various, including underlying cardiac disease, perioperative systemic stress, electrolyte and acid-base imbalances, hypoxemia, and hypercarbia. Thus, controlling such conditions to the extent possible both preoperatively and postoperatively is an important part of preventing and managing postoperative cardiac dysrhythmias. Treatment generally involves first achieving hemodynamic stability and then converting the rhythm back to sinus if possible.

Supraventricular tachycardias (SVTs) are the dysrhythmias most commonly seen in the postoperative period, occurring after approximately 4% of noncardiac major operations. Atrial fibrillation and atrial flutter account for the majority of SVTs.[38] Ventricular rate control may be achieved pharmacologically by infusing diltiazem. Digoxin has long been used for this purpose but is less effective in acute settings than diltiazem is. Amiodarone, which is used to treat ventricular dysrhythmias, may also be used to restore sinus rhythm postoperatively in some cases, especially after cardiac procedures.[39] When pharmacologic rate control is not possible, particularly in hypotensive patients, cardioversion is indicated.

Approximately one third of patients who undergo noncardiac surgery in the United States have some degree of coronary artery disease and thus are at increased risk for perioperative MI. The incidence of coronary artery disease is even higher in certain subpopulations, such as patients who undergo major vascular procedures.[40,41] In the perioperative setting, however, the pathophysiology of coronary ischemia is different from that in nonsurgical settings, where plaque rupture is the most common cause of MI. Approximately 50% of all MIs occurring in surgical patients are caused by increased myocardial oxygen demand in the face of inadequate supply resulting from factors such as fluid shifts, physiologic stress, hypotension, and the effects of anesthesia. The majority of cardiac ischemic events occur in the first 4 days of the postoperative period.[41]

Perioperative beta blockade for patients at risk for MI is now routine. Multiple trials and meta-analyses have demonstrated that this practice yields significant risk reductions in terms of both cardiac morbidity and mortality[42,43] and that these risk reductions are achieved regardless of the type of surgery being performed. Although there has been some variation in the protocols used by these trials and the results reported, there is general agreement that beta blockade should be initiated preoperatively, delivered at the time of surgery, and continued postoperatively for up to 1 week.[42]

Diagnosis of postoperative MI is complicated by the fact that as many as 95% of patients who experience this complication may not present with classic symptoms (e.g., chest pain). Identification of MI may be further hindered by the ECG changes brought on by the stress of the perioperative period (including dysrhythmias). Ultimately, the most useful signal of an ischemic cardiac event in the postoperative period is a rise in the levels of cardiac enzymes, particularly troponin I. Accordingly, cardiac enzyme activity should be assessed whenever there is a high index of suspicion for MI or a patient is considered to be at significant perioperative risk for MI.[40]

Treatment of postoperative MI focuses on correcting any factors contributing to or exacerbating the situation that led to the event (e.g., hypovolemia or hypotension). Typically, although antiplatelet agents (e.g., aspirin) are sometimes given, thrombolytic therapy is avoided because of concerns about postoperative bleeding. Acute percutaneous coronary intervention is also associated with an increased risk of bleeding but has nonetheless been used successfully in the perioperative setting and is recommended by some physicians.[44] Beta blockade is often advocated as a means of treating postoperative MI, although it is probably more effective when used both preoperatively and perioperatively as a means of preventing MI.[40]

Discharge

Planning for discharge from the hospital is clearly an essential part of perioperative care. In the best of circumstances, discharge planning starts before admission for elective surgery and is discussed with the patient and family as part of preoperative patient education. Starting the process early enables the provider to estimate the patient's probable needs at the end of acute hospitalization and thus to make preliminary arrangements as needed. For example, if it appears likely that the patient will have to stay in a skilled nursing or extended care facility or will require prolonged physical therapy and rehabilitation, these matters can be addressed to the mutual satisfaction of both patient and physician in advance of hospital discharge. In this way, delays in discharge and unnecessary days of acute hospitalization can be avoided, at least in some instances.

Criteria for discharge or transfer from acute hospital care vary widely depending on the procedure, the provider, and the patient; rarely are they codified. For example, in a 2005 survey of 16 surgeons performing open colorectal resections within one hospital, only two factors—absence of complications and reported postoperative bowel movement—were considered criteria for early discharge by most (but not all) of the surgeons.[45] There was wide disagreement on all other criteria, including postoperative mobility and the ability to tolerate a general diet. Given such variation in discharge criteria for even one category of procedure, it is clear that a discussion of specific criteria for each type of surgery is well beyond the scope of this chapter. It is worth pointing out, however, that the various discharge criteria now in use, despite their differences, have a common basis—namely, the idea that at discharge, the patient should ideally be able to manage basic self-care activities (e.g., feeding, wound care, and mobility) without advanced assistance and that the likelihood of readmission should be minimized to the extent possible. Identification, investigation, and control of factors such as nausea, pain, fever, deconditioning, and fatigue are important in determining whether a patient is at risk for a return to the hospital in the postoperative period.[46]

Over the past two decades, critical pathways, which are organized plans that outline the sequence of patient care and discharge, have been increasingly used in managing postoperative care after a variety of procedures from all disciplines. They have been shown to reduce hospital stays and maintain safety in patients undergoing common procedures (e.g., colectomy), patients undergoing complex procedures (e.g., esophagectomy),[47] and patients with high comorbidity.[48] Individual pathways are typically specific to a hospital or health care system; thus, the discharge criteria are those agreed on by the providers involved in the care of eligible patients at that particular institution. Critical pathways can be helpful not only by standardizing care and improving the relative appropriateness of postoperative discharge but also, in many cases, by decreasing the overall length of postoperative hospitalization.[46] In a 2003 study of 27 postoperative critical pathways used at the Johns Hopkins Hospital, the authors found that seven (27%) of the pathways were associated with significant (5 to 45%) decreases in length of stay.[49]

Regardless of whether critical pathways are implemented, if discharge planning is not addressed preoperatively, addressing it as early as possible in the postoperative period is extremely valuable not only for ensuring an appropriate length of stay but also for maintaining the satisfaction and comfort of both patient and family. Specific issues should be addressed at this point as needed, including the home resources and support available to the patient, wound care, ostomy care, management of feeding tubes and drains, IV antibiotic therapy, and physical rehabilitation. Thus, as soon as it appears that a patient is on track either for discharge home or for transfer to a rehabilitation or skilled nursing facility, a discussion with the appropriate social work or discharge planning personnel should be scheduled. PT/OT evaluations early in the postoperative course can also be of great assistance in determining a patient's needs on discharge, and such evaluations are essential for any patient who may need a stay in an inpatient rehabilitation facility. Typically, it requires at least 1 day to set up services such as home health care and outpatient PT, and it may take this long or longer to obtain a bed at an appropriate rehabilitation or skilled nursing facility. Consequently, the earlier these plans are made, the better. For many surgical patients, formal discharge planning and PT/OT evaluations are not actually necessary. Brief discussions with the patient, the family, or the nursing staff caring for the patient will assist in determining which surgical patients are most likely to benefit from this approach.

Current Controversies in Postoperative Management

OBSTRUCTIVE SLEEP APNEA

Obstructive sleep apnea (OSA) has rapidly become the most prevalent sleep disorder over the last 20+ years. At present, estimates suggest that it affects 9% of women and 24% of men in the United States. Additionally, estimates also suggest that as many as 82% of men and 92% of women affected do not carry the formal diagnosis of OSA.[50,51] Despite the large percentage of the population affected, no well-vetted specific guidelines are present in the current literature. That being said, there is a wealth of discussion of the issue from which several more general guidelines may be drawn.

Preoperative screening for OSA is the first and most critical step in management. As a majority of affected patients have not been formally diagnosed, this allows the operative team the opportunity to detect the greatest number of patients at risk and to adjust their operative plan of care accordingly.[52] Most commonly, screening is done by anesthesiology in the preanesthesia setting using one of a number of available screening tools. In addition to this, it is important for the surgeon to also consider the potential presence of OSA as this may significantly affect the choice of surgical setting and postoperative setting planned.[53] Although, again, there are no set guidelines provided in the literature dictating criteria for outpatient versus inpatient surgical settings, for patients with known or suspected OSA requiring significant sedation or general anesthesia, using a setting with access to difficult airway carts, advanced respiratory care, and the option of a prolonged postanesthesia recovery unit (PACU) observation is recommended.[54]

The two greatest issues in postoperative management are the level of monitoring provided and the use of sedatives and narcotic analgesics. The choice of surgical/postoperative setting is best made after consideration of known or potential OSA, any associated comorbidities, and the type of surgery to be performed. Patients with severe OSA generally require inpatient monitoring postoperatively. Outside of known severe OSA, the time observed in the PACU may also provide further information on which to base ongoing care or discharge.[51] Any patient who currently uses a home continuous positive airway pressure (CPAP) or bilevel positive airway pressure (BiPAP) device should use this in the immediate postoperative period.[55] In the inpatient setting, the use of continuous pulse oximetry and telemetry should be considered, and supplemental oxygen should be used with caution.[53,55]

Anesthetics and sedatives depress the central nervous system, inhibit respiration, depress skeletal muscle tone, and relax the upper airway.[55] Opiate drugs can depress respiratory drive and rate, decrease tidal volume, and lead to decreased sensitivity to arousal. Thus, the use of sedatives postoperatively should be avoided or used with great caution. Narcotic agents need to be titrated to adequate pain relief but should be used only when nonnarcotic agents are ineffective. Additionally, the need for opiates may be significantly decreased with the use of nonnarcotic agents such as acetaminophen, centrally acting agents such as tramadol hydrochloride, NSAIDs, or topical anesthetics when appropriate.[53]

The prevalence of OSA is only likely to increase given current trends in associated comorbidities such as obesity. Further prospective data are needed for more definitive future recommendations, particularly regarding postoperative monitoring and admission status.

POSTOPERATIVE ILEUS

Ileus, or the cessation of bowel function and transit in the absence of mechanical obstruction, is a common postoperative phenomenon particularly after abdominal surgery and occurs in virtually all patients undergoing bowel resection. Its causes are multifactorial, including an overall increase in sympathetic tone, the inflammatory response to bowel as a result of direct manipulation, and the well-known effects of narcotic analgesics on GI motility.[56] Although the typical duration of postoperative ileus averages around 3 days, in up to 32% of patients, return of bowel function may be particularly delayed.[57]

Multiple strategies have been employed in attempts to decrease the length of postoperative ileus, such as early feeding, the use of chewing gum, and pharmacologic agents particularly directed at blocking the GI effects of narcotics. Feeding patients early (i.e., before evidence of return of bowel function) after abdominal surgery has been demonstrated to be generally safe and forms an element of many postoperative pathways. However, various studies comparing early feeding with awaiting return of bowel function have yielded mixed results, and no clear recommendation for early feeding can be made across all procedures.[56,58] Chewing gum is thought to represent a sham-feeding condition that may have benefit in stimulating GI motility after abdominal surgery. It is safe; has few, if any, significant risks; and is well tolerated by patients. A recent meta-analysis of seven randomized, controlled trials comparing chewing gum with no gum after abdominal surgery concluded that gum leads to a clinically significant improvement in return of bowel function as represented by a sooner return of flatus.[59] However, not all individual trials have demonstrated a benefit.[56] Of the pharmacologic agents that have been investigated in the treatment of postoperative ileus, alvimopan, which is a selective antagonist of the peripheral opioid mu receptor, appears to confer the most significant benefit and was recently approved by the Food and Drug Administration for this indication. The recommended dose is 12 mg orally given twice daily for up to 7 days.[57,60,61] Alvimopan was shown to reduce the time to [illegible] function after bowel resection by 12 hours compared with placebo in a meta-analysis of five randomized, controlled trials involving a total of 1,877 patients.[62] Further, it does not appear to have serious side effects.

Postoperative ileus remains a major factor in determining the length of hospital stay after abdominal surgery, particularly after bowel resection. Both chewing gum and alvimopan appear to provide some benefit in reducing the time to bowel recovery after surgery, with the former being the most simple and cost-effective to implement. None of these measures eliminate the effects of surgical intervention on GI motility entirely, however, and this will continue to be an area of active investigation in improving the care of the postoperative patient.[56–62]

Financial Disclosures: None Reported

References

1. Haupt M, Bekes C, Brilli R, et al. Guidelines on critical care services and personnel: recommendations based on a system of categorization of three levels of care. Crit Care Med 2003;31:2677.
2. Nelson R, Edwards S, Tse B. Prophylactic nasogastric decompression after abdominal surgery (review). Cochrane Database Syst Rev 2006;(3):1.
3. Pothier DD. The use of drains following thyroid and parathyroid surgery: a meta-analysis. J Laryngol Otol 2005;119:669.
4. Petrowksy H, Demartines N, Rousson V, et al. Evidence-based value of prophylactic drainage in gastrointesinal surgery. Ann Surg 2004;240:1074.
5. Jesus EC, Karliczek A, Matos D, et al. Prophylactic anastamotic drainage for colorectal surgery. Cochrane Database Syst Rev 2006;(18):1.
6. Halpin V, Soper N. The management of common bile duct stones. In: Cameron J, editor. Current surgical therapy. 7th ed. St. Louis: CV Mosby, Inc; 2001. p. 435–40.
7. Fakhry SM, Rutherford EJ, Sheldon GF. Routine postoperative management of the hospitalized patient. In: Souba WW, Jurkovich GJ, Fink MP, et al, editors. ACS surgery. New York: WebMD Inc; 2006. p. 90.
8. Heal C, Buettner P, Raasch B, et al. Can sutures get wet? Prospective randomized controlled trial of wound management in general practice. BMJ 2006;332:1053.
9. Noe JM, Keller M. Can stitches get wet? Plast Reconstr Surg 1988;81:82.
10. Morykwas MF, Argenta LC, Shelton-Brown ET, et al. Vacuum-assisted closure: a new method for wound treatment: animal studies and basic foundation. Ann Plast Surg 1997; 38:553.
11. Venturi ML, Attinger CE, Mesbahi AN, et al. Mechanisms and clinical application of the vacuum assisted closure (VAC) device. Am J Clin Dermatol 2005;6:185.
12. Lewis SJ, Egger M, Sylvester PA, et al. Early enteral feeding vs "nil by mouth" after gastrointestinal surgery: systematic review and meta-analysis of controlled trials: BMJ 2001; 323:1.
13. Lassen K, Revhaug A. Early oral nutrition after major upper gastrointestinal surgery: why not? Curr Opin Clin Nutr Metab Care 2006;9:613.
14. Ward N. Nutrition support to patients undergoing gastrointestinal surgery. Nutr J 2003;2: 18.
15. Zaloga G. Parenteral nutrition in adult inpatients with functioning gastrointestinal tracts: assessment of outcomes. Lancet 2006; 367:1101.

16. Heyland DK, Dhaliwal R, Drover JW, et al. Canadian clinical practice guidelines for nutritional support in mechanically ventilated patients. JPEN J Parenter Enteral Nutr 2003; 27:355.
17. Grocott MPW, Hamilton MA. Resuscitation fluids. Vox Sanguinis 2002;82:1.
18. Roberts I, Alderson P, Bunn F, et al. Colloids versus crystalloids for fluid resuscitation in critically ill patients (review). Cochrane Database Syst Rev 2006;(3):1.
19. Tambyraja AL, Sengupta F, MacGregor AB, et al. Patterns and clinical outcomes associated with routine intravenous fluid administration after colorectal resection. World J Surg 2004;28:1046.
20. Brandstrup B, Tennesen H, Beier-Holgersen R. Effects of intravenous fluid restriction on postoperative complications: comparison of two perioperative fluid regimens. Ann Surg 2003;238:641.
21. Lobo DN, Bostock KA, Neal KR, et al. Effect of salt and water balance on recovery of gastrointestinal function after elective colonic resection: a randomized controlled trial. Lancet 2002;359:1812.
22. Macintyre PE. Safety and efficacy of patient-controlled analgesia. Br J Anaesth 2001;87: 36.
23. Bulger EM, Edwards T, Klotz P, et al. Epidural analgesia improves outcome after multiple rib fractures. Surgery 2004;136:426.
24. Mann C, Pouzeratte Y, Boccara B, et al. Comparison of intravenous or epidural patient-controlled analgesia in the elderly after major abdominal surgery. Anesthesiology 2000;92:433.
25. Flisburg P, Rudin A, Linner R, et al. Pain relief and safety after major surgery: a prospective study of epidural and intravenous analgesia in 2696 patients. Acta Anaesthesiol Scand 2003;47:457.
26. Van den Berghe G, Wouters P, Weekers F, et al. Intensive insulin therapy in critically ill patients. N Engl J Med 2001;345:1345.
27. Hammer L, Dessertaine G, Timsit JF, et al. Intensive insulin therapy in the medical ICU [letter]. N Engl J Med 2006;354:2069.
28. De la Torre S, Mandel L, Goff BA. Evaluation of postoperative fever: usefulness and cost effectiveness of routine workup. Am J Obstet Gynecol 2003;188:1642.
29. Arozullah AM, Khuri SF, Henderson WG, et al. Development and validation of a multifactorial risk index for predicting postoperative pneumonia after major noncardiac surgery. Ann Intern Med 2001;135:847.
30. Mehta RM, Niederman MS. Nosocomial pneumonia. Curr Opin Infect Dis 2002;15: 387.
31. Barie PS, Eachempati SR. Surgical site infections. Surg Clin North Am 2005;85:1115.
32. Dosluoglu HH, Schimpf DK, Schultz R, et al. Preservation of infected and exposed vascular grafts using vacuum assisted closure without muscle flap coverage. J Vasc Surg 2005;42:989.
33. Cowan KN, Teague L, Sue SC, et al. Vacuum-assisted wound closure of deep sternal infections in high-risk patients after cardiac surgery. Ann Thorac Surg 2005;80:2205.
34. Anaya DA, Nathens AB. Thrombosis and coagulation: deep vein thrombosis and pulmonary embolism prophylaxis. Surg Clin North Am 2005;85:1163.
35. Michiels JJ, Gadisseur A, van der Planken M, et al. Screening for deep vein thrombosis and pulmonary embolism in outpatients with suspected DVT or PE by the sequential use of clinical score: a sensitive quantitative D-dimer test and noninvasive diagnostic tools. Semin Vasc Med 2005;5:351.
36. Cook D, Douketis J, Crowther MA, et al. The diagnosis of deep vein thrombosis and pulmonary embolism in medical-surgical intensive care unit patients. J Crit Care 2005;20:314.
37. Piazza G, Goldhaber SZ. Acute pulmonary embolism: part II: treatment and prophylaxis. Circulation 2006;114:42.
38. Heintz KM, Hollenberg SM. Perioperative cardiac issues: postoperative arrhythmias. Surg Clin North Am 2005;85:1103.
39. Samuels LE, Holmes EC, Samuels FL. Selective use of amiodarone and early cardioversion for postoperative atrial fibrillation. Ann Thorac Surg 2005;79:113.
40. Akhtar S, Silverman DG. Assessment and management of patients with ischemic heart disease. Crit Care Med 2004;32(4 Suppl): S126.
41. Grayburn PA, Hillis DL. Cardiac events in patients undergoing noncardiac surgery: shifting the paradigm from noninvasive risk stratification to therapy. Ann Intern Med 2003;138:506.
42. Schouten O, Shaw LJ, Boersma E, et al. A meta-analysis of safety and effectiveness of perioperative beta-blocker use for the prevention of cardiac events in different types of noncardiac surgery. Coron Artery Dis 2006;17:173.
43. McGory ML, Maggard MA, Ko CY. A meta-analysis of perioperative beta blockade: what is the actual risk reduction? Surgery 2005; 138:171.
44. Obal D, Kindgen-Milles D, Schoebel F, et al. Coronary artery angioplasty for treatment of peri-operative myocardial ischaemia. Anaesthesia 2005;60:194.
45. Nascimbeni R, Cadoni R, Di Fabio F, et al. Hospitalization after open colectomy: expectations and practice in general surgery. Surg Today 2005;35:371.
46. Kiran RP, Delaney CP, Senagore AJ, et al. Outcomes and prediction of hospital readmission after intestinal surgery. J Am Coll Surg 2004;198:877.
47. Cerfolio RJ, Bryant AS, Bass C, et al. Fast tracking after Ivor-Lewis esophagogastrectomy. Chest 2004;126:1187.
48. Delaney CP, Fazio VW, Senagore AJ, et al. 'Fast track' postoperative management protocol for patients with high co-morbidity undergoing complex abdominal and pelvic colorectal surgery. Br J Surg 2001;88:1533.
49. Dy SM, Garg PP, Nyberg D, et al. Are critical pathways effective for reducing postoperative length of stay? Med Care 200;41:637.
50. Chung F, Elsaid H. Screening for obstructive sleep apena before surgery: why is it important? Curr Opin Anesthesiol 2009;22: 405–11.
51. Gali B, Whalen FX, Schroeder DR, et al. Identification of patients at risk for postoperative respiratory complications using a preoperative obstructive sleep apnea screening tool and postanesthesia care assessment. Anesthesiology 2009;110:869–77.
52. Hwang D, Shakir N, Limann B, et al. Association of sleep-disordered breathing with postoperative complications. Chest 2008,133: 1128–34.
53. Mickelson S. Anesthetic and postoperative management of the obstructive sleep apnea patient. Oral Maxillofac Surg Clin North Am 2009;21:425–34.
54. Stephan P, Mercier D, Coleman J, et al. Obstructive sleep apnea: implications for the plastic surgeon and ambulatory surgery centers. Plast Reconstr Surg 2009;124:652–5.
55. Jain S, Dhand R. Perioperative treatment of patients with obstructive sleep apnea. Curr Opin Pulm Med 2004;10:482–8.
56. Stewart D, Waxman K. Management of postoperative ileus. Am J Ther 2007;14:561–6.
57. Yeh YC, Klinger EV, Reddy P. Pharmacologic options to prevent postoperative ileus. Ann Pharmacother 2009;43:1474–85. Epub 2009 Jul 14.
58. Augestad KM, Delaney CP. Postoperative ileus: impact of pharmacological treatment, laparoscopic surgery and enhanced recovery pathways. World J Gastroenterol 2010;16: 2067–74.
59. Fitzgerald JE, Ahmed I. Systematic review and meta-analysis of chewing-gumtherapy in the reduction of postoperative paralytic ileus following gastrointestinal surgery. World J Surg 2009;33:2557–66.
60. Tan EK, Cornish J, Darzi AW, Tekkis PP. Meta-analysis: alvimopan vs. placebo in the treatment of post-operative ileus. Aliment Pharmacol Ther 2007;25:47–57.
61. Becker G, Blum HE. Novel opioid antagonists for opioid-induced bowel dysfunction and postoperative ileus. Lancet 2009;373: 1198–206.
62. Senagore AJ, Bauer JJ, Du W, Techner L. Alvimopan accelerates gastrointestinal recovery after bowel resection regardless of age, gender, race, or concomitant medication use. Surgery 2007;142:478–86.

4 POSTOPERATIVE PAIN

Spencer S. Liu, MD, and Henrik Kehlet, MD, PhD, FACS (Hon)

Clinical Approach to the Patient with Postoperative Pain

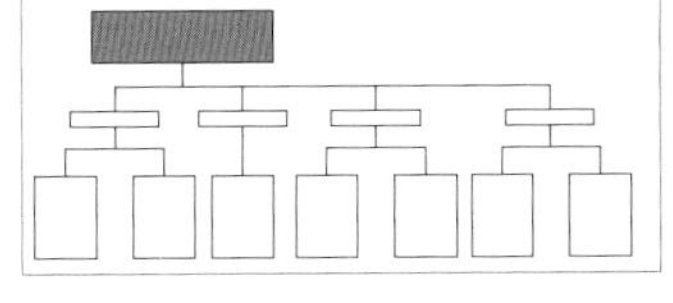

Postoperative pain consists of a constellation of unpleasant sensory, emotional, and mental experiences associated with autonomic, psychological, and behavioral responses precipitated by the surgical injury. Pain management has received increasing attention, and multiple government agencies and medical specialty organizations have now created guidelines for treatment of postoperative pain.[1] In 2001, the Joint Commission on Accreditation of Healthcare Organizations (JCAHO) introduced standards for pain management,[2] stating that patients have the right to appropriate evaluation and management and that pain must be assessed.

Postoperative pain relief has two practical aims. The first is provision of subjective comfort, which is desirable for humanitarian reasons. The second is inhibition of trauma-induced nociceptive impulses to blunt autonomic and somatic reflex responses to pain and to enhance subsequent restoration of function by allowing the patient to breathe, cough, and move more easily. Because these effects reduce pulmonary, cardiovascular, thromboembolic, and other complications, they may lead secondarily to improved postoperative outcome.

Inadequate Treatment of Pain

A common misconception is that pain, no matter how severe, can always be effectively relieved by opioid analgesics. It has repeatedly been demonstrated, however, that in a high proportion of postoperative patients, pain is inadequately treated.[3,4] This discrepancy between what is possible and what is practiced can be attributed to a variety of causes [*see Table 1*], which to some extent can be ameliorated by increased teaching efforts. Recent evidence also indicates that overreliance on opioid therapy may be inherently limiting because of development of both acute tolerance and opioid-induced hyperalgesia.[5] The ability of opioids in high doses or with chronic administration to potentially induce pain illustrates the importance of using multimodal analgesic regimens that target multiple analgesic pathways.

Guidelines for Postoperative Pain Treatment

In the past few years, efforts have been made to develop procedure-specific perioperative pain management guidelines. The impetus for these efforts has been the realization that the analgesic efficacy may be procedure dependent and that the choice of analgesia in a given case must also depend on the benefit-to-risk ratio, which varies among procedures. In addition, it is clear that some analgesic techniques will be considered only for certain specific operations (e.g., peripheral nerve blocks and intraperitoneal local anesthesia).[6–8] At present, these procedure-specific guidelines are still largely in a developmental state and are available for laparoscopic cholecystectomy, open colon surgery, hysterectomy, inguinal hernia repair, thoracotomy, mastectomy, hemorrhoidectomy, and knee and hip replacement.[9,10]

THORACIC PROCEDURES

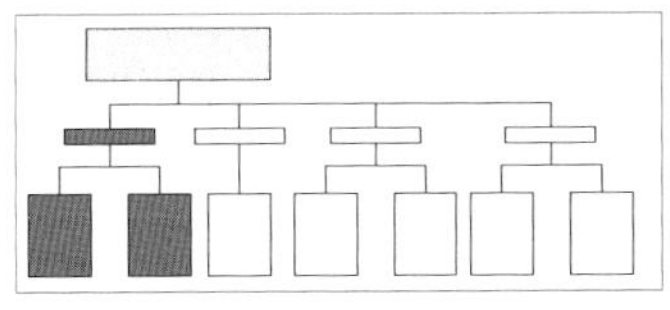

Pain after thoracotomy is severe, and pain therapy should therefore include a combination regimen, preferably comprising epidural local anesthetics and opioids[11] combined with systemic nonsteroidal antiinflammatory drugs (NSAIDs) or cyclooxygenase-2 (COX-2) inhibitors (depending on risk factors) [*see algorithm*]. If the epidural regimen is not available, then comparable analgesia may be achieved with continuous thoracic paravertebral block, with

Table 1 Contributing Causes of Inadequate Pain Treatment
Insufficient knowledge of drug pharmacology among surgeons and nurses
Uniform (p.r.n.) prescriptions
Lack of concern for optimal pain relief
Failure to give prescribed analgesics
Fear of side effects
Fear of addiction

the potential for lesser incidence of urinary retention and postoperative nausea and vomiting.[12] Although comparable, the continuous paravertebral technique may be more technically difficult. If neither regional analgesic technique is available, then the inferior regimen of NSAIDs and systemic opioids may be used. Cryoanalgesia is not recommended as it is less effective.[10] Acetaminophen is recommended as a basic analgesic for multimodal analgesia. Pain after cardiac operation with sternotomy is less severe, and systemic opioids plus NSAIDs are recommended. The combined regimen of epidural local anesthetics and opioids or parasternal wound catheters with continuous administration of local anesthetics[13] is recommended when more effective pain relief is necessary, and it may reduce cardiopulmonary morbidity and perhaps length of stay.[14]

ABDOMINAL PROCEDURES

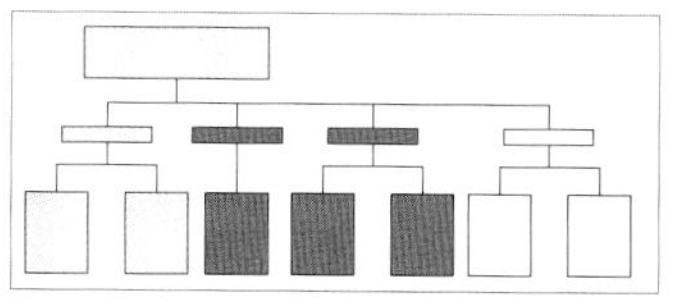

Pain after major and upper open abdominal operations is severe, and a combined regimen of epidural local anesthetics and opioids is recommended because it has proved to be superior to systemic opioids and to have few and acceptable side effects.[10,11,15] Furthermore, the epidural regimen will reduce postoperative pulmonary complications and ileus compared with treatment with systemic opioids.[16] Systemic NSAIDs or COX-2 inhibitors are added when needed. Acetaminophen is recommended as a basic analgesic for multimodal analgesia.

After gynecologic lower abdominal or pelvic operations,[10] systemic opioids plus NSAIDs or COX-2 inhibitors are recommended except in patients in whom more effective pain relief is desirable. In such patients, the combined regimen of epidural local anesthetics and opioids is preferable. Acetaminophen is recommended as a basic analgesic for multimodal analgesia.

Pain following prostatectomy is usually not severe and may be treated with systemic opioids combined with NSAIDs or COX-2 inhibitors and acetaminophen. However, blood loss and thromboembolic complications are reduced when epidural local anesthetics are administered. This method is therefore recommended intraoperatively and continued in selected high-risk patients for pain relief after open prostatectomy and transurethral resection. In low-risk patients, systemic opioids with NSAIDs or COX-2 inhibitors and acetaminophen alleviate postoperative pain.

PERIPHERAL PROCEDURES

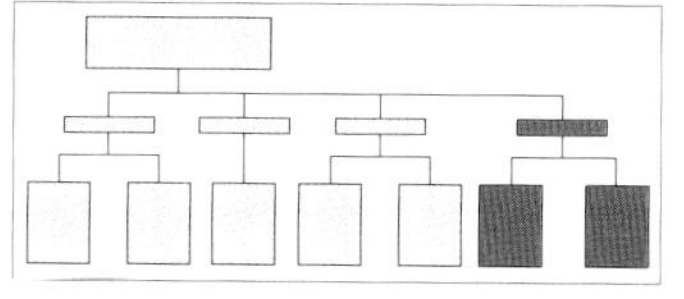

After vascular procedures, postoperative pain control is probably best achieved with epidural local anesthetic–opioid mixtures, combined with systemic NSAIDs or COX-2 inhibitors.[11] Acetaminophen is recommended as a basic analgesic for multimodal analgesia. This regimen will be effective, and the increase in peripheral blood flow that is documented to occur with epidural local anesthetics may lower the risk of graft thrombosis.

Pain relief after major joint procedures (e.g., hip and knee operations)[10] may involve an epidural regimen in certain high-risk patients because such regimens have been shown to reduce thromboembolic complications and intraoperative blood loss and to improve physical rehabilitation when compared with systemic opioid regimens.[17,18] However, the severe pain noted after knee replacement is probably best treated with peripheral nerve blocks.[10,19] Most of the benefit of continuous femoral nerve analgesia may also be achieved with a single-injection femoral nerve block.[20] Total hip replacement is a less painful procedure, but when pain is severe, a continuous lumbar plexus or femoral nerve block can be used.[10,21] Alternatively and with less technical expertise, a single intrathecal dose of local anesthetic and low-dose morphine will provide effective analgesia for the first 8 to 16 hours,[10] after which NSAIDs or COX-2 inhibitors may be added. Acetaminophen is provided as a basic analgesic for multimodal analgesia.

Treatment Modalities

COMPLEMENTARY AND ALTERNATIVE MEDICINE INTERVENTIONS

Cognitive, behavioral, alternative, or social interventions should be used in combination with pharmacologic therapies to prevent or control acute pain, with the goal of such interventions being to guide the patient toward partial or complete self-control of pain.[22,23] A recent survey by the American Hospital Association indicated that 27% of member hospitals offered complementary and alternative medications (CAMs).[24] Use of nonpharmacologic adjunctive analgesics has been endorsed by advisory bodies such as the Anesthesia Patient Safety Foundation and Institute of Healthcare Improvement.[25,26]

Psychological preparation in patients with postoperative pain has been demonstrated to shorten hospital stay and reduce postoperative narcotic use [*see Table 2*].[27] Guided imagery, relaxation, and music techniques have been demonstrated to reduce postoperative opioid use and affective pain.[22] Acupuncture and acupressure has been successfully used as an adjunct for postoperative analgesia and reduces pain scores, anxiety levels, and postoperative nausea.[28] Alternative techniques

Table 2 Psychological Preparation of Surgical Patients

Procedural information
Give a careful and relevant description of what will take place.
Sensory information
Describe the sensations that will be experienced either during or after the operation.
Pain treatment information
Outline the plan for administering sedative and analgesic medication and encourage patients to communicate concerns and discomforts.
Instructional information
Teach patients postoperative exercises, such as leg exercises, and show them how to turn in bed or move so that pain is minimal.
Reassurance
Reassure those who are mentally, emotionally, or physically unable to cooperate that they are not expected to take an active role in coping with pain and will still receive sufficient analgesic treatment.

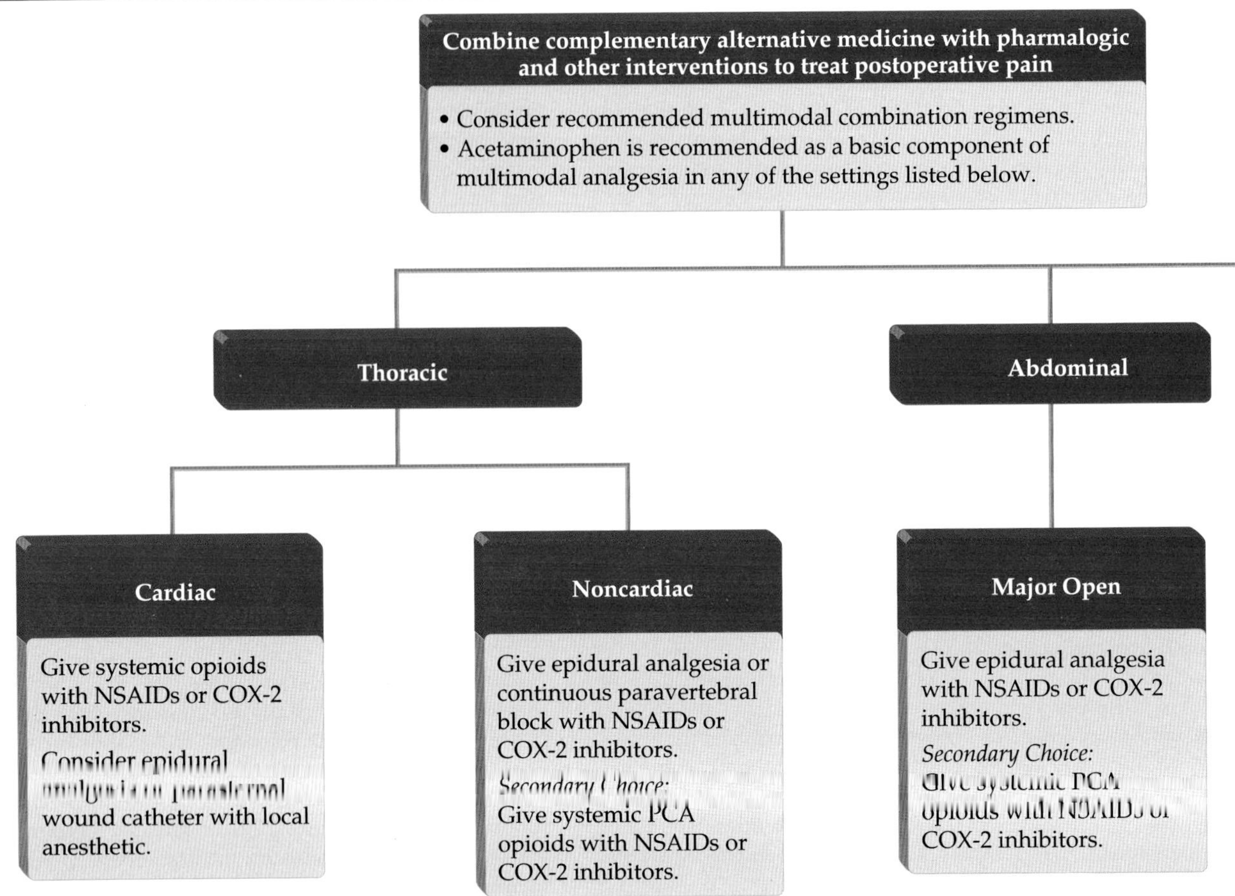

Combine complementary alternative medicine with pharmalogic and other interventions to treat postoperative pain
• Consider recommended multimodal combination regimens.
• Acetaminophen is recommended as a basic component of multimodal analgesia in any of the settings listed below.
Thoracic
Abdominal
Cardiac
Give systemic opioids with NSAIDs or COX-2 inhibitors.
Consider epidural
wound catheter with local anesthetic.
Noncardiac
Give epidural analgesia or continuous paravertebral block with NSAIDs or COX-2 inhibitors.
Give systemic PCA opioids with NSAIDs or COX-2 inhibitors.
Major Open
Give epidural analgesia with NSAIDs or COX-2 inhibitors.
Secondary Choice:
COX-2 inhibitors.

COX-2 = cyclooxygenase-2, NSAIDs = nonsteroidal antiinflammatory drugs; PCA = patient-controlled analgesia.

Clinical Approach to the Patient with Postoperative Pain

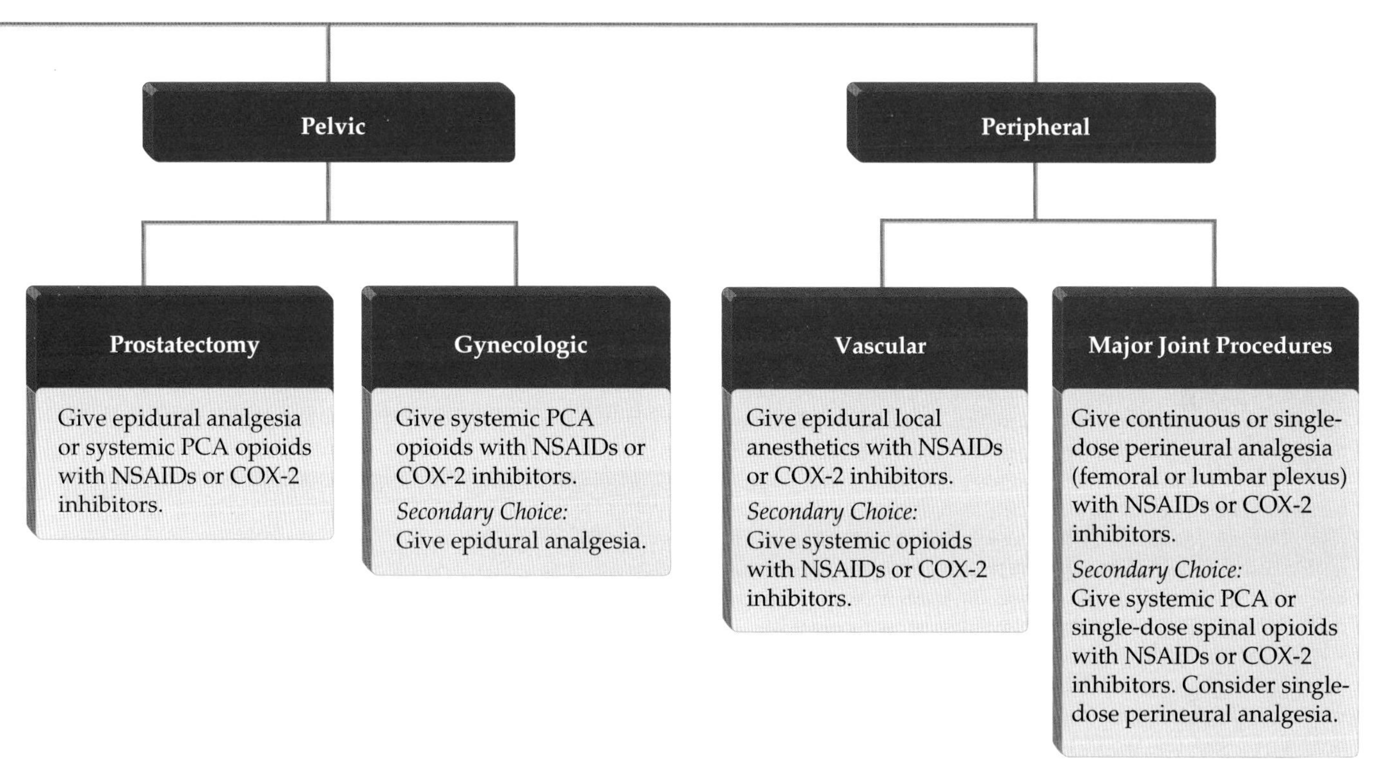

Pelvic
Peripheral
Prostatectomy
Give epidural analgesia or systemic PCA opioids with NSAIDs or COX-2 inhibitors.
Gynecologic
Give systemic PCA opioids with NSAIDs or COX-2 inhibitors.
Secondary Choice:
Give epidural analgesia.
Vascular
Give epidural local anesthetics with NSAIDs or COX-2 inhibitors.
Secondary Choice:
Give systemic opioids with NSAIDs or COX-2 inhibitors.
Major Joint Procedures
Give continuous or single-dose perineural analgesia (femoral or lumbar plexus) with NSAIDs or COX-2 inhibitors.
Secondary Choice:
Give systemic PCA or single-dose spinal opioids with NSAIDs or COX-2 inhibitors. Consider single-dose perineural analgesia.

Table 3 Opioid Receptor Types and Physiologic Actions

Receptor Type	Prototypical Ligand		Physiologic Actions
	Endogenous	Exogenous	
Mu^1	ß-Endorphin	Morphine	Supraspinal analgesia
Mu^2	ß-Endorphin	Morphine	Respiratory depression
Delta	Enkephalin	—	Spinal analgesia
Kappa	Dynorphin	Ketocyclazocine	Spinal analgesia, sedation, visceral analgesia

should be combined with pharmacologic or other interventions, but care must be taken to ensure that the pharmacologic treatment does not compromise the mental function necessary for the success of the planned psychological intervention.

SYSTEMIC OPIOIDS

Mechanisms of Action

Opioids produce analgesia and other physiologic effects by binding to specific receptors in the peripheral and central nervous system (CNS) [*see Table 3*]. These receptors normally bind a number of endogenous substances called opioid peptides. These receptor-binding interactions mediate a wide array of physiologic effects.[29] Three types of opioid receptors and their subtypes have been discovered: mu, delta, and kappa receptors. The most commonly used opioids bind to mu receptors. The mu receptor is responsible for the production of opioid-induced analgesia, whereas the mu_2 receptor appears to be related to the respiratory depression, cardiovascular effects, and inhibition of GI motility commonly seen with opioids.

The discovery of peripheral opioid receptors has led to investigation into potential clinical applications. Phase III studies with alvimopan (a peripheral opioid antagonist that does not cross the blood-brain barrier) have demonstrated reduced ileus and hospitalization after abdominal surgery.[30]

Other studies have also investigated the analgesic effects of applying opioids to wound sites in an attempt to provide peripheral analgesia without central side effects. Unfortunately, neither incisional[31] nor intra-articular[32] opioid administration has demonstrated significant beneficial effect.[30] This finding may be attributable to the need for chronic inflammatory mediators to facilitate expression of peripheral opioid receptors.[33]

The relation between receptor binding and the intensity of the resultant physiologic effect is known as the intrinsic activity of an opioid. Most of the commonly used opioid analgesics are agonists. An agonist produces a maximal biologic response by binding to its receptor. Other opioids, such as naloxone, are termed antagonists because they compete with agonists for opioid receptor-binding sites. Still other opioids are partial agonists because they produce a submaximal response after binding to the receptor. (An excellent example of a submaximal response produced by partial agonists is buprenorphine's action at the mu receptor.)

Drugs such as nalbuphine, butorphanol, and pentazocine are known as agonist-antagonists or mixed agonist-antagonists.[29] These opioids simultaneously act at different receptor sites: their action is agonistic at one receptor and antagonistic at another [*see Table 4*]. The agonist-antagonists have certain pharmacologic properties that are distinct from those of the more common mu agonists: (1) they exhibit a ceiling effect and cause only submaximal analgesia compared with mu agonists and (2) administration of an agonist-antagonist with a complete agonist may cause a reduction in the effect of the complete agonist.[29]

Agents

Morphine Morphine is the opioid with which the most clinical experience has been gained. Sufficient pharmacokinetic and pharmacodynamic data are available. Use of this agent is recommended; it may be given orally, intravenously (IV), or intramuscularly (IM).

Meperidine Detailed and sufficient pharmacokinetic and pharmacodynamic data on meperidine are available. It is less suitable than morphine as an analgesic because its active

Table 4 Intrinsic Activity of Opioids

Opioid	Mu	Kappa	Delta
Agonists			
Morphine	Agonist	—	
Meperidine (Demerol)	Agonist	—	
Hydromorphone (Dilaudid)	Agonist		
Oxymorphone (Numorphan)	Agonist		
Levorphanol (Levo-Dromoran)	Agonist		
Fentanyl (Duragesic)	Agonist		
Sufentanil (Sufenta)	Agonist		
Alfentanil (Alfenta)	Agonist		
Methadone (Dolophine)	Agonist		
Agonist-Antagonists			
Buprenorphine (Buprenex)	Partial agonist		
Burtorphanol (Stadol)	Antagonist	Agonist	Agonist
Nalbuphine (Nubain)	Antagonist	Partial agonist	Agonist
Pentazocine (Talwin)	Antagonist	Agonist	Agonist
Dezocine (Dalgan)	Partial agonist		
Antagonists			
Naloxone (Narcan)	Antagonist	Antagonist	Antagonist

metabolite, normeperidine, can accumulate, even in patients with normal renal clearance, and this accumulation can result in CNS excitation and seizures.[29] Other agents should be used before meperidine is considered. Like morphine, meperidine can be given orally, IV, or IM.

Side Effects

By depressing or stimulating the CNS, opioids cause a number of physiologic effects in addition to analgesia. The depressant effects of opioids include analgesia, sedation, and altered respiration and mood; the excitatory effects include nausea, vomiting, and miosis.

All mu agonists produce a dose-dependent decrease in the responsiveness of brainstem respiratory centers to increased carbon dioxide tension (Pco_2). This change is clinically manifested as an increase in resting Pco_2 and a shift in the CO_2 response curve. Agonist-antagonist opioids have a limited effect on the brainstem and appear to elicit a ceiling effect on increases in Pco_2.

Opioids also have effects on the gastrointestinal (GI) tract. Nausea and vomiting are caused by stimulation of the chemoreceptor trigger zone of the medulla. Opioids enhance sphincteric tone and reduce peristaltic contraction. Delayed gastric emptying is caused by decreased motility, increased antral tone, and increased tone in the first part of the duodenum. Delay in passage of intestinal contents because of decreased peristalsis and increased sphincteric tone leads to greater absorption of water, increased viscosity, and desiccation of bowel contents, which cause constipation and contribute to postoperative ileus. Opioids also increase biliary tract pressure. Finally, opioids may inhibit urinary bladder function, thereby increasing the risk of urinary retention.

Several long-acting, slow-release oral opioids are currently available, but their role (in particular, their safety) in the setting of moderate to severe postoperative pain remains to be established. In addition, modern principles of treatment increasingly emphasize the use of opioid-sparing analgesic approaches to enhance recovery (see below).

CLINICAL APPLICATION OF SYSTEMIC OPIOIDS

Traditional IM dosing of opioids is a suboptimal means of analgesia.[34] IM dosing does not result in consistent blood levels, because opioids are absorbed at a variable rate from the vascular bed of muscle. Moreover, administration of traditional IM regimens results in opioid concentrations that exceed the concentrations required to produce analgesia only about 30% of the time during any 4-hour dosing interval. The optimal means to treat moderate to severe postoperative pain with systemic opioids is via IV patient-controlled analgesia (PCA). This delivery system compensates for the wide inter- and intraindividual variability in analgesic needs and blood levels after opioid administration. Self-delivery helps produce timely titration of analgesia and reduces administrative delay from conventional delivery (e.g., p.r.n.). Systematic reviews have noted that IV PCA delivery of opioids reduces pain scores and improves patient satisfaction over conventional delivery.[34] Typical regimens are provided in Table 5. Recent advances in iontophoretic technology have led to commercial release of a transdermal fentanyl iontophoretic PCA system. This system delivers 40 μg fentanyl over 10 minutes after patient demand. Onset is rapid because of the active electrical current driving the fentanyl transdermally. The system deactivates after 24 hours or 80 administrations. Several clinical trials have reported equivalence between the fentanyl system and IV PCA opioid.[35] One pooled analysis suggested less analgesic gaps with the fentanyl system because of fewer technical failures and administrative delays than the IV PCA device[36]; however, the role of this fentanyl system remains to be fully defined.

EPIDURAL AND SUBARACHNOID OPIOIDS

Opioids were first used in the epidural and subarachnoid spaces in 1979. Since that time, they have become the mainstay of postoperative management for severe pain. Epidural opioids may be administered in a single bolus or via continuous infusions. They are usually combined with local anesthetics in a continuous epidural infusion to enhance analgesia.[37]

Mechanisms of Action

Opioids injected into the epidural or subarachnoid space cause segmental (i.e., selective, spinally mediated) analgesia by binding to opioid receptors in the dorsal horn of the spinal cord.[38] The lipid solubility of an opioid, described by its partition coefficient, predicts its behavior when introduced into the epidural or subarachnoid space. Opioids with low lipid solubility (i.e., hydrophilic opioids) have a slow onset of action and a long duration of action. Opioids with high lipid solubility (i.e., lipophilic opioids) have a quick onset of action but a short duration of action. This is attributable to more rapid diffusion across the dura into the spinal cord but also more rapid systemic uptake and clearance via uptake into

Table 5 Typical Intravenous Patient-Controlled Analgesia Regimens

Drug Concentration	Size of Bolus	Lockout Interval (min)
Agonists		
Morphine (1 mg/mL)		
Adult	0.5–2.5 mg	5–10
Pediatric	0.01–0.03 mg/kg (max. = 0.15 mg/kg/hr)	5–10
Fentanyl (0.01 mg/mL)		
Adult	10-20 ug	4–10
Pediatric	0.5–1 μg/kg (max. = 4 μg/kg/hr)	5–10
Hydromorphone (0.2 mg/mL)		
Adult	0.05–0.25 mg	5–10
Pediatric	0.003–0.005 mg/kg (max. = 0.02 mg/kg/hr)	5–10

epidural and spinal cord blood vessels. In fact, current evidence suggests that a major site of action of spinal lipophilic opioids is not the spinal cord but the brain via systemic uptake.[39] Thus, lipophilic opioids as sole epidural analgesic agents are becoming less frequently recommended.

Subarachnoid opioids should be used when the required duration of analgesia after surgery is relatively short (< 24 hours) because of typical single-injection delivery. When protracted analgesia is required, epidural administration is preferred; repeated injections may be given through epidural catheters, or continuous infusions may be used. Smaller doses of subarachnoid opioids are generally required to produce analgesia. Ordinarily, no more than 0.1 to 0.25 mg of morphine should be used to provide 12 to 24 hours of analgesia. These doses, which are about 10 to 20% of the size of comparably effective epidural doses, provide reliable pain relief with few side effects.[40] Fentanyl has also been extensively used in the subarachnoid space in a dose range of 6.25 to 25 µg to provide 3 to 6 hours of analgesia. Recently, an extended duration formulation of epidural morphine has been commercially released.[41–43]

This formulation consists of morphine encased in multivesicular lipid with predictable sustained release. Clinical studies have overall supported the efficacy and general safety of this formulation (10–15 mg doses) without demonstrating marked superiority over conventional central neuraxial opioid therapy. Thus, the role of this preparation remains to be determined.

Side Effects

The chief side effects associated with epidural and subarachnoid opioids are respiratory depression, nausea and vomiting, pruritus, and urinary retention.[38,40,44] The poor lipid solubility of morphine is responsible for its protracted duration of action but also allows morphine to undergo cephalad migration in the cerebrospinal fluid (CSF). This migration can cause delayed respiratory depression, with a peak incidence 3 to 10 hours after an injection. The high lipid solubility of lipophilic opioids such as fentanyl allows them to be absorbed into lipids close to the site of administration. Consequently, the lipophilic opioids do not migrate rostrally in the CSF and cannot cause delayed respiratory depression. Of course, the high lipid solubility of lipophilic opioids allows them to be absorbed into blood vessels, which may cause early respiratory depression, as is commonly seen with systemic administration of opioids. Overall, the typical incidence of respiratory depression is similar to that seen with systemic opioids at approximately 0.2%.[44]

Naloxone reverses the depressive respiratory effects of spinal opioids. In an apneic patient, 0.4 mg IV will usually restore ventilation. If a patient has a depressed respiratory rate but is still breathing, small aliquots of naloxone (0.2 to 0.4 mg) can be given until the respiratory rate returns to normal.

Nausea and vomiting are caused by transport of opioids to the vomiting center and the chemoreceptor trigger zone in the medulla via CSF flow or the systemic circulation. Nausea can usually be treated with antiemetics or, if severe, with naloxone (in 0.2 mg increments, repeated if necessary).

Pruritus is probably the most common side effect of the spinal opioids. Although not fully defined, the mechanism likely involves activation of "itch-specific" opioid receptors on spinal sensory neurons.[45] Although pruritus is commonly treated with antihistamines, there is minimal evidence for mechanism-specific effectiveness. An alternative and probably superior treatment is use of a mixed opioid agonist antagonist to directly block the opioid receptor–induced itching while maintaing opioid analgesias. Doses of 5 mg of nalbuphine IV or 2 to 4 mg of butorphanol intranasally or IV every 6 hours is commonly used.[45]

The mechanism of spinal opioid–induced urinary retention involves inhibition of volume-induced bladder contractions and blockade of the vesical reflex. Naloxone administration is the treatment of choice, although bladder catheterization is sometimes required.

CLINICAL APPLICATION OF EPIDURAL AND SUBARACHNOID OPIOIDS

As stated earlier, subarachnoid opioids are limited in the duration of analgesia because of typical single-injection delivery. Epidural administration allows prolonged delivery of opioids, and typical regimens are listed in Table 6. However, side effects from opioids are common, and it is better to combine epidural opioids with local anesthetics to obtain multimodal and synergistic analgesia. This allows smaller doses of both agents to be used with better analgesia and fewer side effects. Typical regimens are listed in Table 7.

EPIDURAL LOCAL ANESTHETICS AND OTHER REGIONAL BLOCKS

Local anesthetic neural blockade is unique among available analgesic techniques in that it may offer sufficient afferent neural blockade, resulting in relief of pain; avoidance of sedation, respiratory depression, and nausea; and, finally, efferent sympathetic blockade, resulting in increased blood flow to the region of neural blockade.[46]

Table 6 Typical Dosing of Neuraxial Opoids

Drug	Intrathecal or Subarachnoid Single Dose	Epidural Single Dose	Epidural Continuous Infusion
Fentanyl	5–25 µg	50–100 µg	25–100 µg/hr
Sufentanil	2–10 µg	10–50 µg	10–20 µg/hr
Morphine	0.1–0.3 mg	1–5 mg	0.1–1 mg/hr
Hydromorphone	—	0.5–1 mg	0.1–0.2 mg/hr
Meperidine	10–30 mg	20–60 mg	10–60 mg/hr

Lower doses may be effective when administered to the elderly or when injected in the cervical or thoracic region. Units vary across agents for single dose (mg versus µg) and continuous infusion (mg/hr versus µg/hr).

Table 7 Typical Patient-Controlled Epidural Analgesia Regimens

Analgesic Solution	Continuous Rate (mL/hr)	Demand Dose (mL)	Lockout Interval (min)
0.0625–0.125% bupivacaine + 2–5 µg/mL fentanyl	4–6	3–4	10–15
0.125–0.125% bupivacaine + 2–5 µg//mL sufentanil	3–5	2–3	12
0.1–0.2% ropivacaine + 2–4 µg//mL fentanyl	3–5	2–5	10–20

Mechanism of Action

Local anesthetic neural blockade is a nondepolarizing block that reduces the permeability of cell membranes to sodium ions.[47] Whether different local anesthetics have different effects on different nerve fibers is debatable.

Choice of Drug

For optimal management of postoperative pain, the anesthetic agent should provide excellent analgesia of rapid onset and long duration without inducing motor blockade. The various local anesthetic agents all meet one or more of these criteria; however, the ones that come closest to meeting all of the criteria are bupivacaine, ropivacaine, and levobupivacaine. This should not preclude the use of other agents, because their efficacy has also been demonstrated. Ropivacaine and levobupivacaine may have a better safety profile, but the improvement may be relevant only when high intraoperative doses are given.[47]

Side Effects

The main side effects of epidural local anesthesia are hypotension caused by sympathetic blockade, vagal overactivity, and decreased cardiac function (during a high thoracic block). Under no circumstances should epidural local anesthetics be used before a preexisting hypovolemic condition is treated. Hypotension may be treated with ephedrine, 10 to 15 mg IV, and fluids, with the patient tilted in a head-down position. Atropine, 0.5 to 1.0 mg IV, may be effective during vagal overactivity.

Urinary retention occurs in 20 to 100% of patients, and urinary catheterization is typically used during epidural analgesia. Motor blockade may delay mobilization; however, its incidence can be reduced by using the weakest concentration of local anesthetic that is compatible with adequate sensory blockade.

The routine complications associated with the epidural catheter are minimal when proper nursing protocols are followed [*see Table 8*]. The decision to employ epidural local anesthetics in such patients should be made only after the risks[44,48] are carefully compared with the documented advantages of such anesthetics.[49,50]

Spinal hematoma attributable to the combination of epidural analgesia and anticoagulants is rare, but the risk may be increased by specific agents. Guidelines on the use of epidural analgesia and anticoagulation are currently listed on the American Society of Regional Anesthesia and Pain Medicine Web site.[48] Most anticoagulants can be safely managed with epidural analgesia; however, special care must be taken with thrombolytics, low-molecular-weight heparins, and newer antiplatelet, antithrombin, and anti–factor Xa agents.

CLINICAL APPLICATION OF CONTINUOUS EPIDURAL ANALGESIA

Typical regimens are listed in Table 7. As is similar with IV PCA, patient-controlled epidural analgesia (PCEA) has been demonstrated to provide superior analgesia, decreased analgesic consumption, and decreased side effects.[51] The safety of PCEA regimens for hospital wards has been well documented.[52] As all epidural analgesic agents are deliberately segmental (limited in anatomic spread) in nature, it is important for the vertebral site of epidural placement to match the site of surgery. For example, lumbar epidurals offer inferior analgesia to thoracic epidurals for thoracic surgery. Suggested epidural sites are also listed in Table 9.

OTHER REGIONAL ANALGESIA TECHNIQUES

Intraperitoneal administration of local anesthetics cannot be recommended for typical postoperative analgesia, because they are not efficacious,[53] except in laparoscopic cholecystectomy.[8,10] Intraincisional administration of bupivacaine or other long-acting local anesthetics, which has negligible side effects and demands little or no surveillance, is recommended for patients undergoing relatively minor procedures.

Continuous administration of local anesthetics into the wound via a catheter directly placed at the end of surgery is a simple and efficacious means to provide postoperative analgesia. A recent systematic review noted that wound catheters improved postoperative analgesia, reduced opioid

Table 8 Procedures for Maintenance of Epidural Anesthesia for Longer than 24 Hours

1. Administer appropriate drug in appropriate dosage at selected infusion rate as determined by physician
2. Nurse evaluates vital signs and intake and output as required for a postoperative patient
3. Nurse checks infusion pump hourly to ensure that it is functioning properly, that infusion rate is proper, and that alarm is on
4. Nurse also assesses
    - Bladder—for distention, if patient is not catherized
    - Lower extremities—for status of motor function
    - Central nervous system—for signs of toxicity or respiratory depression
    - Skin integrity on back (breakdown may occur if motor function is not present)
    - Tubing and dressing (disconnection of tubing or dislodgment of catheter may occur)
5. Every 48 hr, the catheter dressing should be removed, the catheter entrance site cleaned, and topical antibiotic applied (much as in care of a central venous catheter)

Table 9 Recommended Location of Catheter Insertion for Surgical Procedures

Location of Incision	Examples of Surgical Procedures	Congruent Epidural Catheter Placement
Thoracic	Lung reduction, radical mastectomy, thoracotomy, thymectomy	T4–8
Upper abdominal	Cholecystectomy, esophagectomy, gastrectomy, hepatic section, Whipple procedure	T6–8
Middle abdominal	Cystoprostatectomy, nephrectomy	T7–10
Lower abdominal	Abdominal aortic aneurysm repair, colectomy, radical prostatectomy, total abdominal hysterectomy	T8–11
Lower extremity	Femoropopliteal bypass, total hip or total knee replacement	L1–4

L = lumbar; T = thoracic.

use, and decreased opioid-related side effects in a variety of procedures.[13] However, there is still a need for more procedure-specific data before general recommendations can be made as a wide variety of surgical procedures, catheter locations, and analgesic regimens were included in the systematic review.

Continuous peripheral nerve blocks are growing in popularity, and the analgesic treatment may be continued after discharge.[54,55] A systematic review has documented multiple benefits from the use of continuous perineural analgesia versus systemic opioids, such as reduced pain scores at rest and with activity, reduced opioid use, reduced opioid-related side effects, and increased patient satisfaction.[illegible] Use of outpatient perineural analgesia is also growing in popularity, and studies have observed that this form of analgesia reduces unplanned hospital admission after ambulatory procedures, improves patients quality of life at home, and may facilitate conversion of hospital procedures to short-stay procedures (e.g., total knee replacement).[56] A growing body of literature surveying the use of thousands of perineural catheters for postoperative analgesia documents a low incidence of complications and overall safety of this technique.[57] More recently, a high-volume infiltration technique with dilute concentrations of local anesthetics with or without adjuvants seems promising because of its apparent efficacy, simplicity, and safety.[58,59]

NSAIDS, COX-2 INHIBITORS, AND ACETAMINOPHEN

NSAIDs and COX-2 inhibitors are modest analgesics that have both peripheral and central analgesic mechanisms and antiinflammatory effects [*see Table 10*]. Although these agents are typically less effective as sole analgesic agents than opioids,[60] they have an excellent efficacy to safety profile and are generally recommended after all kinds of operations for low-risk patients.[61,62] Several reviews and systematic reviews report that NSAIDs and COX-2 inhibitors decrease systemic morphine use by approximately 13 to 18 mg over a 24-hour period.[61,62] More importantly, these reviews indicate that NSAIDs decrease pain scores by approximately 1 cm on a 10 cm visual analogue scale pain score and reduce opioid-related side effects of sedation and nausea by approximately 30%. Conventional NSAIDs inhibit both COX-1 and COX-2. Selective COX-2 inhibitors, which do not inhibit COX-1, have the potential to achieve analgesic efficacy comparable to that of conventional NSAIDs but with fewer minor side effects.[63–65]

Only a few of the NSAIDs may be given parenterally. The data now available on the use of NSAIDs for postoperative pain are insufficient to allow definitive recommendation of any agent or agents over the others, and selection therefore may depend on the convenience of delivery, duration, and cost.[66] All of the NSAIDs have potentially serious side effects: GI and surgical site hemorrhage, renal failure, impaired bone healing, and asthma. The endoscopically verified superficial ulcer formation seen within 7 to 10 days after the initiation of NSAID therapy is not seen with selective COX-2 inhibitor treatment in volunteers. The clinical relevance of these findings for perioperative treatment remains to be established, however, given that acute severe GI side effects (bleeding, perforation) are extremely rare in elective cases.

Because prostaglandins are important for regulation of water and mineral homeostasis by the kidneys in the dehydrated patient, perioperative treatment with NSAIDs, which inhibit prostaglandin synthesis, may lead to postoperative renal failure. So far, specific COX-2 inhibitors have not been demonstrated to be less nephrotoxic than conventional NSAIDs.[62,67] Although little systematic evaluation has been done, extensive clinical experience with NSAIDs suggests that the renal risk is not substantial.[68] Nonetheless, conventional NSAIDs and COX-2 inhibitors should be used with caution in patients who have preexisting renal dysfunction.[62]

Although conventional NSAIDs prolong bleeding time and inhibit platelet aggregation, there generally does not seem to

Table 10 Typical Dosing for Common NSAIDs, COX-2 Inhibitors, and Acetaminophen

Drug	Typical Dose for Postoperative Analgesia	Maximum Recommended Dose (mg/day)
Acetaminophen	650–1,000 mg q 6 hr	4,000
Celecoxib	100–200 mg q 12 hr	400
Diclofenac	50 mg q 8 hr	150
Ibuprofen	400 mg q 6 hr	3,200
Indomethacin	25–50 mg q 8 hr	200
Ketorolac	10 mg q 4–6 hr	40
Ketorolac (intravenous)	15–30 mg q 6 hr	120
Meloxicam	7.5–15 mg q day	15
Naproxen	250 mg q 6–8 hr	1,375
Paracetamol (intravenous)	1,000 mg q 6 hr	4,000

COX-2 = cyclooxygenase; NSAIDs = nonsteroidal antiinflammatory drugs.

be a clinically significant risk of increased bleeding. However, in some procedures for which strict hemostasis is critical (e.g., tonsillectomy, cosmetic surgery, and eye surgery), these drugs have been shown to increase the risk of bleeding complications and should therefore be replaced with COX-2 inhibitors, which do not inhibit platelet aggregation.[69] The observation that prostaglandins are involved in bone and wound healing has given rise to concern about potential side effects in surgical patients. Although there is experimental evidence that both conventional NSAIDs and COX-2 inhibitors can impair bone healing,[70] the clinical data available at present are insufficient to document increased wound or bone healing failure with these drugs.[71] This is a particularly important issue for future study in that many orthopedic surgeons remain reluctant to use NSAIDs.

Currently, there is widespread concern about the increased risk of cardiovascular complications associated with long-term treatment with selective COX-2 inhibitors. Generally, such side effects have appeared only after 1 to 2 years of treatment and led to the withdrawal of rofecoxib in 2004 and valdecoxib in 2005 from the US market.[72] In the past few years, however, two studies of patients undergoing coronary artery bypass grafting (CABG) found that the risk of cardiovascular complications was increased significantly (two- to threefold) in this setting and led to the label change for COX-2 inhibitors and NSAIDs indicating that these agents are contraindicated in CABG patients.[72] The larger question is whether these drugs should also be contraindicated for perioperative use, or at least used with caution, in high-risk cardiovascular patients who are undergoing procedures other than CABG. At present, the data are insufficient to allow final conclusions; nonetheless, reviews suggest that the benefits of short-term use of these agents in patients without cardiovascular risk factors probably outweigh the potential (low) risk of complications. Until further studies are performed, use in patients with cardiovascular risk factors should be cautious.[72]

Acetaminophen also possesses analgesic capability, both peripherally and centrally. Its analgesic effect is somewhat (about 20 to 30%) weaker than those of conventional NSAIDs and COX-2 inhibitors. For example, use of acetaminophen typically reduces morphine consumption by approximately 9 mg over a 24-hour period,[61] which may be insufficient to significantly reduce opioid-related side effects or dramatically improve analgesia. However, acetaminophen lacks the side effects typical of NSAIDs.[62] Combining acetaminophen with NSAIDs may improve analgesia, especially in smaller and moderate-sized operations[73,74]; accordingly, this agent is recommended as a basic component of multimodal analgesia in all operations.

OTHER ANALGESICS

Glucocorticoids are powerful antiinflammatory agents and have proven analgesic value in less extensive procedures,[75,76] especially dental, laparoscopic, and arthroscopic operations. In addition, they have profound antiemetic effects.[77] Concerns about possible side effects in the setting of perioperative administration have not been borne out by the results of randomized studies.[75,76]

Tramadol is a weak analgesic that has several relatively minor side effects (e.g., dizziness, nausea, and vomiting) and possesses weak opioid agonist activity and inhibits reuptake of serotonin and norepinephrine.[78] It can be used as an intravenous analgesic but is less potent than opioids (morphine, meperidine)[79] and is a poor sole agent for control of postoperative pain.[80]

Several systematic reviews have suggested that some analgesic and perioperative opioid-sparing effects can be achieved by adding an *N*-methyl-d-aspartate (NMDA) receptor antagonist (e.g., ketamine), gabapentin, or pregabalin [*see* Combination Regimens, *below*].[34,81]

TRANSCUTANEOUS ELECTRICAL NERVE STIMULATION

Transcutaneous electrical nerve stimulation (TENS) is the application of a mild electrical current through the skin surface to a specific area, such as a surgical wound, to achieve pain relief; the exact mechanism whereby it achieves this effect is yet to be explained but may involve spinal gating and activation of opioid receptors. Although several randomized controlled trials have reported efficacy after inguinal herniotomy,[82] thoracotomy,[83] and other procedures,[84] the specific values and the proper uses of the various stimulation frequencies, waveforms, and current intensities have not been determined. In addition, blinding of subjects is difficult with TENS studies, and this effect of bias is difficult to assess. Overall, the effect of TENS on acute pain is too imprecise to warrant a recommendation for routine use.[85]

COMBINATION REGIMENS

Because no single pain treatment modality is optimal, combination regimens (e.g., balanced analgesia or multimodal treatment) offer major advantages over single-modality regimens, whether by maintaining or improving analgesia, by reducing side effects, or by doing both.[86] Combinations of epidural local anesthetics and morphine,[15,44] of NSAIDs and opioids,[66,87,88] of NSAIDs and acetaminophen,[73,74] of acetaminophen and opioids,[89] of acetaminophen and tramadol,[90] and of a selective COX-2 inhibitor and gabapentin[91] or pregabalin[81] have been reported to have additive effects. At present, information on other combinations (involving ketamine, clonidine, glucocorticoids, and other agents) is too sparse to allow firm recommendations; however, multimodal analgesia is undoubtedly promising, and multidrug combinations should certainly be explored further.

The potential of combination regimens is especially intriguing with respect to the concept of perioperative opioid-sparing analgesia. The use of one or several nonopioid analgesics in such regimens may enhance recovery in that the concomitant reduction in the opioid dosage will lead to decreased nausea, vomiting, and sedation.[92–95] Both the adverse events associated with postoperative opioid analgesia and the relatively high costs of such analgesia argue for an opioid-sparing approach.[96,97] The ability to reduce opioid-related and non–opioid-related side effects by use of multimodal analgesia may become especially attractive for several reasons. First, there is growing evidence that the use of opioids as sole analgesics can lead to opioid-induced hyperalgesia, whereby overstimulation of opioid receptors creates a nociceptive state (i.e., opioids increase sensitivity to painful stimuli).[98] Also, in light of the JCAHO pain initiative and overall increased focus on reducing pain,[1] a concern exists that these initiatives may precipitate increased use of opioids and thereby an increased risk of side effects.[99,100]

Discussion

Physiologic Mechanisms of Acute Pain

The noxious stimuli from iatrogenic surgical injury or accidental trauma set a cascade of events in motion cumulating in the perception of "pain." Many interrelated components contribute to the processing of nociceptive stimuli. Clinicians should recognize that the neurobiology of nociception is extremely complex, with multiple levels of redundancy, such that there is no "hardwired" or "final common" pathway for the process of nociception of acute pain. The basic mechanisms are (1) afferent transmission of nociceptive stimuli through the peripheral nervous system after tissue damage, (2) modulation of these injury signals by control systems in the dorsal horn, and (3) modulation of the ascending transmission of pain stimuli by a descending control system originating in the brain [*see Figure 1*].[101–103]

PERIPHERAL PAIN RECEPTORS AND NEURAL TRANSMISSION TO THE SPINAL CORD

Peripheral pain receptors (nociceptors) can be identified by function but cannot be distinguished anatomically. The responsiveness of peripheral pain receptors may be enhanced by endogenous algesic substances (e.g., prostaglandins, serotonin, bradykinin, nerve growth factor, and histamine), as well as by increased efferent sympathetic activity.[101] Antidromic release of substance P may amplify the inflammatory response and thereby increase pain transmission. The peripheral mechanisms of visceral pain are different from somatic or neuropathic nociception and likely involve transient receptor potential vanilloid 1 receptors, acid-sensing ion channels, and tachykinins.[104] Peripheral opioid receptors have been demonstrated to appear in inflammation on the peripheral nerve terminals but probably have little clinical relevance.[31–33] Somatic nociceptive input is transmitted to the CNS through A-delta and C fibers, which are small in diameter and either unmyelinated or thinly myelinated. Visceral pain is transmitted through afferent sympathetic pathways; the evidence that afferent parasympathetic pathways play a role in visceral nociception is inconclusive.[104,105]

DORSAL HORN CONTROL SYSTEMS AND MODULATION OF INCOMING SIGNALS

All incoming nociceptive traffic synapses in the gray matter of the dorsal horn (Rexed laminae I to IV). Several substances may be involved in primary afferent transmission of nociceptive stimuli in the dorsal horn: substance P, enkephalins, somatostatin, neurotensin, γ-aminobutyric acid (GABA), glutamic acid, angiotensin II, vasoactive intestinal polypeptide (VIP), and cholecystokinin octapeptide (CCK-8).[102,106] From the dorsal horn, nociceptive information is transmitted through the spinothalamic tracts to the hypothalamus, through spinoreticular systems to the brainstem and reticular formation, and finally to the cerebral cortex.

DESCENDING PAIN CONTROL SYSTEM

A descending control system for sensory input originates in the brainstem and reticular formation and in certain higher brain areas. The main neurotransmitters in this system are norepinephrine, serotonin, acetylcholine, and enkephalins. Stimulation or augmentation of this descending system enhances analgesia. Epidural-intrathecal administration of alpha-adrenergic agonists (e.g., clonidine) or of anticholinesterases (e.g., neostigmine) works in this manner to provide pain relief.[94]

SPINAL REFLEXES

Nociception may be enhanced by spinal reflexes that affect the environment of the nociceptive nerve endings. Thus, tissue damage may provoke an afferent reflex that causes muscle spasm in the vicinity of the injury, thereby increasing nociception. Similarly, sympathetic reflexes may cause decreased microcirculation in injury tissue, thereby generating smooth muscle spasm, which amplifies the sensation.

POSTINJURY CHANGES IN PERIPHERAL AND CENTRAL NERVOUS SYSTEMS

After an injury, the afferent nociceptive pathways undergo physiologic, anatomic, and chemical changes.[102,103] These changes include increased sensitivity on the part of peripheral nociceptors, as well as the growth of sprouts from damaged nerve fibers that become sensitive to mechanical and alpha-adrenergic stimuli and eventually begin to fire spontaneously. Moreover, excitability may be increased in the spinal cord, which leads to expansion of receptive fields in dorsal horn cells. Such changes may lower pain thresholds, may increase afferent barrage in the late postinjury state, and, if normal regression does not occur during convalescence, may contribute to a chronic pain state.[102]

Neural stimuli have generally been considered to be the main factor responsible for initiation of spinal neuroplasticity; however, it now appears that such neuroplasticity may also be mediated by cytokines released as a consequence of COX-2 induction.[103] Improved understanding of the mechanisms of pain may serve as a rational basis for future drug development and may help direct therapy away from symptom control and toward mechanism-specific treatment.[107]

In experimental studies, acute pain behavior or hyperexcitability of dorsal horn neurons may be eliminated or reduced if the afferent barrage is prevented from reaching the CNS. Preinjury neural blockade with local anesthetics or opioids can suppress excitability of the CNS; this is called preemptive analgesia. Although this has been a consistent finding in laboratory studies, clinical studies have been less dramatic. A critical analysis of controlled clinical studies that compared the efficacy of analgesic regimens administered preoperatively with the efficacy of the same regimens administered postoperatively concluded that preemptive analgesia does not always provide a clinically significant increase in pain relief.[108,109] Nonetheless, it is important that pain treatment be initiated early to ensure that patients do not wake up with high-intensity pain.

Effects of Pain Relief

SELECTED PHYSIOLOGIC RESPONSES TO OPERATION

Cardiovascular

It has traditionally been thought that an imbalance of myocardial oxygen supply and demand, such as an increase in

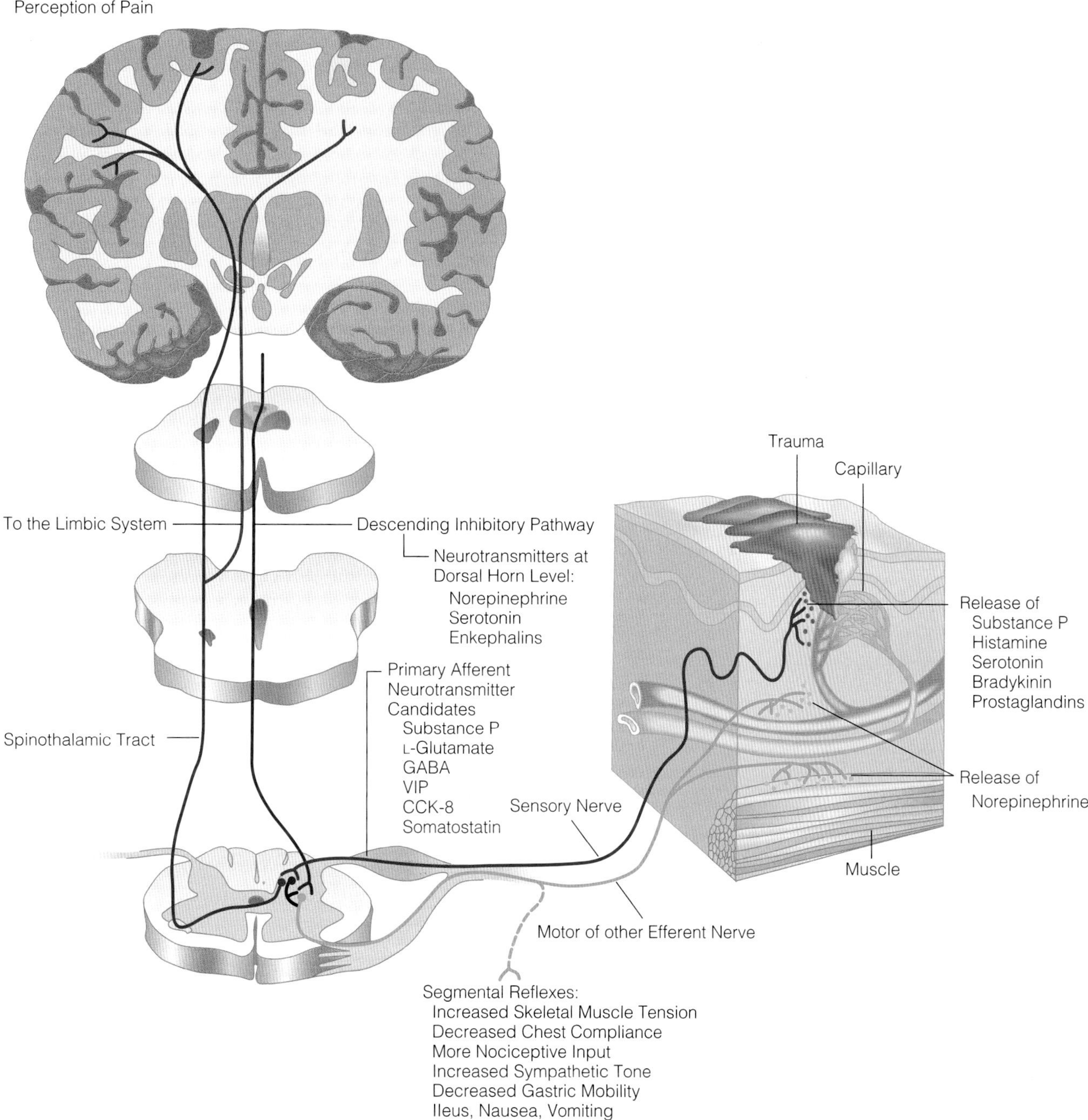

Figure 1 **Shown are the major neural pathways involved in nociception. Nociceptive input is transmitted from the periphery to the dorsal horn via A-delta and C fibers (for somatic pain) or via afferent sympathetic pathways (for visceral pain). It is then modulated by control systems in the dorsal horn and sent via the spinothalamic tracts and spinoreticular systems to the hypothalamus, to the brainstem and reticular formation, and eventually to the cerebral cortex. Ascending transmission of nociceptive input is also modulated by descending inhibitory pathways originating in the brain and terminating in the dorsal horn. Nociception may be enhanced by reflex responses that affect the environment of the nociceptors, such as smooth muscle spasm. CCK = cholecystokinin-octapeptide; GABA = γ -aminobutyric acid; VIP = vasoactive intestinal peptide.**

demand (e.g., increase in heart rate or blood pressure) or a decrease in supply (e.g., decreased coronary blood flow to the vulnerable subendocardial areas), may contribute to perioperative cardiac events, particularly in patients with decreased cardiac reserve.[110] Although many factors may contribute to an imbalance of myocardial oxygen supply and demand, uncontrolled postoperative pain may be especially detrimental and contribute to cardiac morbidity through activation of the sympathetic nervous system, other surgical stress responses, and the coagulation cascade. Increased sympathetic nervous system activity can increase myocardial oxygen demand by increasing heart rate, blood pressure, and contractility or even decrease myocardial oxygen supply, which, in turn, may lead to angina, dysrhythmias, and areas of myocardial infarction.[110] In addition, sympathetic activation may enhance perioperative hypercoagulability, which may contribute to perioperative coronary thrombosis or vasospasm, thus reducing myocardial oxygen supply.[111]

Pulmonary

The pathophysiology of pulmonary dysfunction after surgery is multifactorial. Relevant factors include disruption of normal respiratory muscle activity, which may result from either surgery or anesthesia, reflex inhibition of phrenic nerve activity with subsequent decrease in diaphragmatic function, and uncontrolled postoperative pain, which may contribute to voluntary inhibition of respiratory activity, or splinting.[112] Although the pathophysiology of breathing and respiratory muscle function following surgery is complex, it is clear that anesthetic or analgesic agents administered in the perioperative period affect the central regulation of breathing and activities of respiratory muscles. This incoordination of respiratory muscle function (which may last well into the postoperative period) will impair lung mechanics, increasing the risk of hypoventilation, atelectasis, and pneumonia. Visceral stimulation may decrease phrenic motoneuron output, which results in a decrease in diaphragmatic descent and lung volumes.[112]

Gastrointestinal

Although decreased GI motility is expected after abdominal surgery, return of GI function usually occurs within several days postoperatively. Some patients will develop paralytic ileus, a protracted and more severe state of GI immotility. Although the pathophysiology of postoperative ileus and decreased GI motility is multifactorial, the primary mechanisms include neurogenic (spinal, supraspinal adrenergic pathways), inflammatory (i.e., local inflammatory responses initiate neurogenic inhibitory pathways), and iatrogenic pharmacologic (e.g., opioids) mechanisms.[113] In the acute postoperative phase, neurogenic (spinal and supraspinal) mechanisms are primary mediators of decreased GI motility.[113] Activation of splanchnic afferents and increased sympathetic outflow, along with the possible use of opioids, are the predominant mechanisms for decreased GI motility immediately following surgery. However, over the subsequent postoperative days, a prolonged phase of postoperative ileus occurs. The presumed etiology of the latter is distinct and involves an enteric molecular inflammatory response that impairs local neuromuscular function and activates neurogenic inhibitory pathways.[113] Our understanding of the mechanisms of postoperative ileus is not complete, and it is likely that these three mechanisms are not discrete phenomena but interrelated.

Coagulation

It is recognized that hypercoagulability occurs in association with surgical procedures. Although the pathophysiology of coagulation-related events (e.g., formation of deep vein thrombosis has essentially been unchanged since Virchow's initial description of the triad of stasis, blood vessel injury, and hypercoagulability, our current understanding of the coagulation system is that it is a complex system with many other functions, including tissue repair, autoimmune regulation, arteriosclerosis, and tumor growth and metastasis.[114] Nevertheless, the primary components of the coagulation systems comprise cellular (e.g., platelets, endothelial cells, monocytes, and erythrocytes) and molecular (e.g., coagulation factors and inhibitors, fibrinolysis factors and inhibitors, adhesive and intercellular proteins, acute-phase proteins, immunoglobulins, phospholipids, prostaglandins, and cytokines) components.[114] The normal process of coagulation involves several steps, including initiation (damaged vascular endothelium expresses tissue factor, which ultimately leads to generation of thrombin), amplification (augmentation of the effects of thrombin), propagation (formation of clot), and stabilization (formation of a stable fibrin meshwork that protects clot from fibrinolytic attack).[114] However, following surgery, the normal process of coagulation may become unbalanced, which may result in a tendency toward thrombosis. Immediately after surgical incision, there are increases in the levels of tissue factor, tissue plasminogen activator, plasminogen activator inhibitor–1, and von Willebrand factor, which contribute to a hypercoagulable and hypofibrinolytic state postoperatively.[114] Many of these detrimental responses may be reduced by excellent postoperative analgesia and in particular by the sympathetic and afferent block provided by thoracic epidural analgesia with local anesthetics.

POSTOPERATIVE MORBIDITY

Despite excellent theoretical reasons why high-quality analgesia should improve postoperative physiology and outcomes, the effects of nociceptive blockade and pain relief on postoperative morbidity remain controversial.[16] There are several likely reasons why these effects are difficult to assess. Primarily, surgical techniques and perioperative care are constantly evolving and improving, with subsequent reduction in baseline morbidity and mortality. Thus, the positive effects of analgesia on outcomes may be apparent only on selected high-risk patients or procedures. Several systematic reviews have examined this question and have reached the following conclusions. For open major vascular and thoracic procedures, there is good evidence from systematic reviews and large randomized controlled trials that thoracic epidural analgesia may reduce cardiovascular and pulmonary morbidity when compared with systemic opioids.[16] There is good evidence from meta-analyses that intraoperative spinal or epidural local anesthetics in lower-body procedures reduce estimated blood loss by about 30%.[17,115] Finally, the duration of postoperative ileus is reduced by approximately 24 to 36 hours with the use of epidural analgesia with local anesthetic–containing solutions after major open abdominal procedures.[16] This effect may be of major significance in that reduction of ileus allows earlier oral nutrition,[50] which has been demonstrated to improve outcome.

Another key feature in the difficulties assessing the impact of postoperative analgesia is that most studies to date have focused on the effects of a single factor (i.e., epidural analgesia) on overall postoperative morbidity. In current medical practice, this is probably too simplistic an approach as overall postoperative outcome is known to be determined by multiple factors.[116–118] Besides postoperative pain relief, reinforced psychological preparation of the patient, reduction of stress by performing neural blockade or opting for minimal invasive procedures, and enforcement of early oral postoperative feeding and mobilization may all play a significant role in determining outcome.[118] Prevention of intraoperative hypothermia, avoidance of fluid overloading, and avoidance of hypoxemia may be important as well.[118,119] Therefore, although adequate pain relief is obviously a prerequisite for good outcome, the best results are likely to be achieved by combining analgesia with all of the aforementioned factors in a multimodal rehabilitation effort.

DEVELOPMENT AND PREVENTION OF CHRONIC POSTOPERATIVE PAIN

Although not all nociceptive input results in a pathologic process, a substantial percentage of patients who undergo certain surgical procedures will exhibit prolonged central sensitization and chronic pain [*see Table 11*]. Pathologic nociceptive input may cause central sensitization, which is marked by hyperexcitable spinal neurons that exhibit a decreased threshold for activation, increased and prolonged response to noxious input, expansion of receptive fields, possible spontaneous activity, and activation by normally non-noxious stimuli.[120]

Induction and maintenance of central sensitization emphasize different receptor-neurotransmitter combinations, including NMDA receptors, prostaglandins, and neuropeptides (substance P, calcitonin gene–related peptide, neurokinin A).[121] Ultimately, transcriptional changes (including induction of genes), structural changes in synaptic connections (e.g., contact between low-threshold afferent and nociceptive neurons), and loss of inhibitory interneurons may result in a persistent state of central sensitization.[122]

Multiple studies and reviews have noted that more severe acute postoperative pain is a risk factor for development of chronic postoperative pain.[61,123] Although optimal strategies for prevention of chronic pain have not been identified, promising modalities include preemptive regional analgesia such as thoracic epidural local anesthetics, NMDA antagonists, and anticonvulsant analgesia adjuncts such as gabapentin.[61,124,125] Future studies will need to define optimal strategies for high-risk procedures and patients.

BARRIERS TO EFFECTIVE POSTOPERATIVE ANALGESIA

In general, multiple advisory and supervisory organizations (e.g., JCAHO, World Health Organization) recognize the importance of adequate pain control.[1] Partially in response to these initiatives, there has been a marked increase in the creation and requirement of acute pain treatment services within hospitals across the world.[126] Work continues on attempting to create efficient and simple delivery techniques and technologies for postoperative analgesia. In addition to economic constraints, significant concerns regarding potential for opioid tolerance and addiction remain as a barrier.[1] Continued exposure of an opioid receptor to high concentrations of opioid will cause tolerance. Tolerance is the progressive decline in an opioid's potency with continuous use, so higher and higher concentrations of the drug are required to cause the same analgesic effect. Physical dependence refers to the production of an abstinence syndrome when an opioid is withdrawn. It is defined by the World Health Organization as follows:

> A state, psychic or sometimes also physical, resulting from interactions between a living organism and a drug, characterized by behavioural and other responses that always include a compulsion to take the drug on a continuous or periodic basis in order to experience its psychic effects, and sometimes to avoid discomfort from its absence.[127]

This definition is very close to the popular concept of addiction. It is important, however, to distinguish addiction (implying compulsive behavior and psychological dependence) from tolerance (a pharmacologic property) and from physical dependence (a characteristic physiologic effect of a group of drugs). Physical dependence does not imply addiction. Moreover, tolerance can occur without physical dependence; the converse does not appear to be true. The possibility that the medical administration of opioids could result in a patient becoming addicted has generated much debate about the use

Table 11 Approximate Incidences and Risk Factors for Development of Postoperative Chronic Pain

Surgical Procedure	Incidence of Chronic Pain (%)	Risk Factors
Thoracotomy	30–70	Increased acute pain
		Open vs thoracoscopic
		Not using thoracic epidural analgesia with local anesthetics
		Intercostal nerve injury
Mastectomy	11–60	Increased acute pain
		Increased acute opioid consumption
		Immediate adjuvant radiation therapy
		Axillary dissection vs sentinel node biopsy
Inguinal hernia repair	0–37	Increased acute pain
		Preoperative pain
		Female gender
		Surgery for recurrent hernia
		Open vs laparoscopic

95. Romsing J, Moiniche S, Mathiesen O, Dahl JB. Reduction of opioid-related adverse events using opioid-sparing analgesia with COX-2 inhibitors lacks documentation: a systematic review. Acta Anaesthesiol Scand 2005;49:133–42.
96. Wheeler M, Oderda GM, Ashburn MA, Lipman AG. Adverse events associated with postoperative opioid analgesia: a systematic review. J Pain 2002;3:159–80.
97. Philip BK, Reese PR, Burch SP. The economic impact of opioids on postoperative pain management. J Clin Anesth 2002;14:354–64.
98. Chu LF, Angst MS, Clark D. Opioid-induced hyperalgesia in humans: molecular mechanisms and clinical considerations. Clin J Pain 2008;24:479–96.
99. Frasco PE, Sprung J, Trentman TL. The impact of the joint commission for accreditation of healthcare organizations pain initiative on perioperative opiate consumption and recovery room length of stay. Anesth Analg 2005;100:162–8.
100. Taylor S, Voytovich AE, Kozol RA. Has the pendulum swung too far in postoperative pain control? Am J Surg 2003;186:472–5.
101. Kidd BL, Urban LA. Mechanisms of inflammatory pain. Br J Anaesth 2001;87:3–11.
102. Carr DB, Goudas LC. Acute pain. Lancet 1999;353:2051–8.
103. Woolf CJ, Salter MW. Neuronal plasticity: increasing the gain in pain. Science 2000;288:1765–9.
104. Cervero F, Laird JM. Understanding the signaling and transmission of visceral nociceptive events. J [illegible] 2004;61:45–54.
105. Chen SL, Wu XY, [illegible] ZJ, et al. Subdiaphragmatic vagal afferent nerves modulate visceral pain. Am J Physiol Gastrointest Liver Physiol 2008;294:G1441–9.
106. Julius D, Basbaum AI. Molecular mechanisms of nociception. Nature 2001;413:203–10.
107. Woolf CJ. Pain: moving from symptom control toward mechanism-specific pharmacologic management. Ann Intern Med 2004;140:441–51.
108. Moiniche S, Kehlet H, Dahl JB. A qualitative and quantitative systematic review of preemptive analgesia for postoperative pain relief: the role of timing of analgesia. Anesthesiology 2002;96:725–41.
109. Ong CK, Lirk P, Seymour RA, Jenkins BJ. The efficacy of preemptive analgesia for acute postoperative pain management: a meta-analysis. Anesth Analg 2005;100:757–73.
110. Warltier DC, Pagel PS, Kersten JR. Approaches to the prevention of perioperative myocardial ischemia. Anesthesiology 2000; 92:253–9.
111. Parker SD, Breslow MJ, Frank SM, et al. Catecholamine and cortisol responses to lower extremity revascularization: correlation with outcome variables. Perioperative Ischemia Randomized Anesthesia Trial Study Group. Crit Care Med 1995;23: 1954–61.
112. Warner DO. Preventing postoperative pulmonary complications: the role of the anesthesiologist. Anesthesiology 2000;92:1467–72.
113. Bauer AJ, Boeckxstaens GE. Mechanisms of postoperative ileus. Neurogastroenterol Motil 2004;16 Suppl 2:54–60.
114. Bombeli T, Spahn DR. Updates in perioperative coagulation: physiology and management of thromboembolism and haemorrhage. Br J Anaesth 2004;93:275–87.
115. Rodgers A, Walker N, Schug S, et al. Reduction of postoperative mortality and morbidity with epidural or spinal anaesthesia: results from overview of randomised trials. BMJ 2000;321:1493.
116. Kehlet H, Wilmore DW. Multimodal strategies to improve surgical outcome. Am J Surg 2002;183:630–41.
117. Kehlet H, Dahl JB. Anaesthesia, surgery, and challenges in postoperative recovery. Lancet 2003;362:1921–8.
118. Kehlet H, Wilmore DW. Evidence-based surgical care and the evolution of fast-track surgery. Ann Surg 2008;248:189–98.
119. White PF, Kehlet H, Neal JM, et al. The role of the anesthesiologist in fast-track surgery: from multimodal analgesia to perioperative medical care. Anesth Analg 2007;104:1380–96.
120. Scholz J, Woolf CJ. Can we conquer pain? Nat Neurosci 2002;5 Suppl:1062–7.
121. Schaible HG, Richter F. Pathophysiology of pain. Langenbecks Arch Surg 2004; 389:237–43.
122. Wu CL, Garry MG, Zollo RA, Yang J. Gene therapy for the management of pain: Part I: methods and strategies. Anesthesiology 2001;94:1119–32.
123. Kehlet H, Jensen TS, Woolf CJ. Persistent postsurgical pain: risk factors and prevention. Lancet 2006;367:1618–25.
124. Fassoulaki A, Melemeni A, Stamatakis E, et al. A combination of gabapentin and local anaesthetics attenuates acute and late pain after abdominal hysterectomy. Eur J Anaesthesiol 2007;24:521–8.
125. Fassoulaki A, Triga A, Melemeni A, Sarantopoulos C. Multimodal analgesia with gabapentin and local anesthetics prevents acute and chronic pain after breast surgery for cancer. Anesth Analg 2005;101:1427–32.
126. Werner MU, Soholm L, Rotboll-Nielsen P, Kehlet H. Does an acute pain service improve postoperative outcome? Anesth Analg 2002;95:1361–72.
127. World Health Organization. WHO expert committee on drug dependence. Sixteeth Report. World Health Organ Tech Rep Ser 1969;407:1–28.
128. Porter J, Jick H. Addiction rare in patients treated with narcotics. N Engl J Med 1980;302:123.

Acknowledgments

Figure 1 Carol Donner.

5 ACUTE WOUND CARE

*Roni B. Prucz, MD, Stephen R. Sullivan, MD, MPH, and Matthew B. Klein, MD, MS, FACS**

Acute wounds are the result of local trauma and may be associated with severe life-threatening injuries. The approach to a patient with an acute wound begins with assessment of the ABCs (airway, breathing, and circulation). Life-threatening injuries are addressed first. Only after more urgent problems have been corrected is the wound itself addressed. A complete history is obtained and a thorough physical examination is performed, with special attention paid to both local and systemic wound environment factors that may affect healing. Information about the cause of injury is sought. In the case of a hand injury, the patient's hand dominance and occupation are determined. All patients with acute wounds should be assessed for malnutrition, diabetes, peripheral vascular disease, neuropathy, obesity, immune deficiency, autoimmune disorders, connective tissue diseases, coagulopathy, hepatic dysfunction, malignancy, smoking practices, medication use that could interfere with healing, and allergies. The local wound environment should be evaluated to determine the extent and complexity of injury, the tissues involved, the degree of contamination by microorganisms or foreign bodies, and the extent of damage related to previous irradiation or injury to surrounding tissues.

The wound is carefully examined, with particular attention paid to size, location, bleeding, arterial or venous insufficiency, tissue temperature, tissue viability, and foreign bodies. Latex- and powder-free gloves are worn to prevent allergic reactions, and a shielded mask should also be used to protect the practitioner from body fluids.[1] The possibility of damage to vessels, nerves, ducts, cartilage, muscles, or bones in proximity to the injury is assessed. X-rays and a careful motor and sensory examination may be required to rule out such injuries. While these tests are being performed, moist gauze should be applied to wounds to prevent desiccation.

The goal of acute wound management is to create a healing wound that will result in the best functional and aesthetic outcome. In what follows, we address the key considerations in management of the acute wound, including anesthesia, choice of repair site (e.g., operating room or emergency department), hemostasis, irrigation, débridement, closure materials, timing and methods of closure, adjunctive treatment (e.g., tetanus and rabies prophylaxis, antibiotics, and nutritional supplementation), appropriate closure methods for specific wound types, dressings, postoperative wound care, and potential disturbances of wound healing. We conclude by briefly reviewing the physiology of wound healing.

* The authors and editors gratefully acknowledge the contributions of the previous author, Loren H. Engrav, MD, FACS, to the development and writing of this chapter.

Wound Preparation

ANESTHESIA

After conducting a careful motor, sensory, and vascular examination, adequate general or local anesthesia must be instituted before definitive exploration and treatment can begin. General anesthesia in the operating room should be employed in any of the following circumstances: if the patient is unable to tolerate local anesthesia; adequate pain control cannot be achieved with a local block; the wound requires significant débridement, exploration, or repair; bleeding cannot be controlled; or the required local anesthetic dose for adequate pain control exceeds the maximum safe dose. Local anesthesia is usually sufficient for débridement and closure of most small traumatic wounds. Often the local anesthetic may be injected directly into wounded tissue. However, direct wound injection may be less reliable in inflamed or infected tissue or may distort important anatomic landmarks used to align wound edges. In these situations, regional nerve blocks directed at specific sensory nerves outside the injured field may be employed instead.

Injectable anesthetics can be broadly divided into amides and esters [*see Table 1*]. An easy way to remember which category an agent belongs to is to recall that the amides all have two i's in their generic name, whereas the esters have only one. Lidocaine, an amide, is the most commonly used local anesthetic. Its advantages include a rapid onset of action (< 2 minutes), extended duration of effect (60 to 120 minutes), relative safety in comparison with more potent anesthetics (e.g., bupivacaine), and availability in multiple forms (e.g., liquid, jelly, and ointment) and concentrations (e.g., 0.5, 1.0, and 2.0%). In addition, lidocaine rarely causes allergic reactions, whereas ester anesthetics (e.g., tetracaine) are metabolized to para-aminobenzoic acid, which may cause allergic reactions in some patients. Bupivacaine (Marcaine) should be considered when longer periods of anesthesia are desired (e.g., length of action, dosing).

Vasoconstriction can be produced by adding epinephrine to a local anesthetic, usually in a dilution of 1:100,000 or 1:200,000 (5 to 10 μg/mL). Through vasoconstriction, epinephrine prolongs the anesthetic agent's duration of action, allows a larger dose to be safely administered, and aids in hemostasis.[2] Traditionally, local anesthetics with epinephrine have not been used in finger and toe wounds because of the theoretical risk of ischemia and tissue loss. Nevertheless, these adverse effects have not yet been clinically reported or documented by any prospective studies.[3]

Local anesthetics can cause systemic toxicity when injected intravascularly or given in excessive doses. Manifestations of systemic toxicity begin with central nervous system effects (e.g., vertigo, tinnitus, sedation, and seizures) and may progress to cardiovascular effects (e.g., hypotension, cardiac conduction abnormalities, and cardiovascular collapse). Treatment for systemic toxicity is supportive with oxygen, airway support,

Patient presents with acute wound

Obtain complete history and perform thorough physical examination. Life-threatening conditions take priority over wound care.
Examine local wound environment, look for local and systemic factors that may impair wound healing, and identify wounded structures.
Consider antibiotics prophylaxis for clean or clean-contaminated wounds if factors likely to impair wound healing are present [see Tables 4, 8, and 9].
Initiate antibiotic prophylaxis for contaminated and dirty wound and for wounds with extensive devitalized tissue.

Initial measures are complete and wound care is initiated

Prepare wound:
Anesthesia: use local anesthesia in most cases. Use general anesthesia if pain cannot be controlled with local anesthesia or if local anesthetic dose needed would be unsafe, if wound requires extensive exploration, débridement, or significant repair, or if bleeding cannot be controlled.
Hemostasis: use pressure, cauterization, or ligation (but do not ligate lacerated arteries proximal to amputated part). Place drain if there is risk of hematoma or fluid collection.
Irrigation: use only nontoxic solutions, avoiding antibiotic and strong antiseptic solutions. Low pressure is generally preferable to high pressure (but bulb syringe is inadequate).
Débridement: débride necrotic tissue and remove foreign bodies. If there is questionably viable tissue, defer débridement and initiate dressing changes.

Abrasion

Remove foreign bodies to prevent traumatic tattooing.
Allow healing by secondary intention.
Antibiotics rarely indicated.

Laceration

Close immediately if patient presents with clean wound within 8 hours of injury or up to 24 hours for simple facial injury (see Table 3). Otherwise, allow the wound to heal by secondary intention.
Cover with sterile dressing for 48 hours.
Antibiotics may be indicated.

Puncture/Penetrating

Remove all foreign bodies and consider operative exploration.
Allow to heal by secondary intention.
Antibiotics often indicated.

Crush injury

Severity of injury is not always apparent.
Monitor for compartment syndrome and treat urgently.
Antibiotics often indicated.

Complex wounds

Includes stellate, degloving, avulsion, open fractures, and mutilation injuries.
Consider operative exploration with débridement and delayed primary closure if significant nonviable or questionably viable tissue is present.
Closure or dressing should be applied by 6–8 hours but may be delayed up to 24 hours for transfer to skilled trauma facility.
Antibiotics often indicated (required for all open fractures).

Extravasation injury

Conservative management (i.e., elevation, ice, and monitoring) suffices in most cases.
Injury involving high volume, high osmolarity, or chemotherapeutic agent may necessitate additional measures (e.g., hydrocortisone, incision and drainage, hyaluronidase or saline injection, or aspiration). Antibiotics rarely indicated.

Consider tetanus treatment, antibiotic prophylaxis, or both.
Apply dressings as appropriate for individual wound type.

Abrasion

Use occlusive dressings to provide warm moist environment.
Avoid dry dressings and scab formation

Laceration, complex wound closed primarily, injection injury, projectile wound, bite wound, or sting

Consider three-layer dressings for open draining wounds with inner nonadherent layer, middle absorbent layer, and outer binding layer.
Consider antibacterial ointment if there is minimal drainage or in areas not amenable to a dressing (e.g., scalp).
Dressings are only required for 48 hours after wound closure if minimal drainage.
Consider temporary immobilization for wounds that cross joints.

Approach to Acute Wound Management

Wound is ready for closure

Select closure materials: sutures (see Table 2), staples, tapes, or adhesives.
Determine timing and method of closure (see Table 3):

- Primary intention: clean wound without contraindications to closure
- Secondary intention: wound with contamination or contraindications to closure, wounds with significant amounts of devitalized tissue, wounds older than 8–24 hours, patient who cannot tolerate closure, or wounds for which closure is not needed.
- Tertiary closure: contaminated wound, wound with questionably viable tissue, or patient who cannot tolerate immediate closure
- Skin grafting: large superficial wound
- Tissue transfer: large wound with exposed vital structure

Formulate specific closure approach suitable for individual wound type.

Injection injury

Wound appearance is often deceptively benign.
Examine wound area carefully and obtain appropriate radiographs.
Treat aggressively with incision, wide exposure, débridement, and removal of foreign bodies.
Allow healing by secondary intention.
Antibiotics may be indicated.

Bite wound

Take into account risk of rabies, bacterial and viral infections, and envenomation.
Obtain x-rays to evaluate for fractures and joint involvement.
Treat with exploration, irrigation, débridement, and close observation.
Wounds should be allowed to heal by secondary intention or delayed primary closure except in certain circumstances (e.g., facial wounds).
Consider rabies treatment, rabies prophylaxis, or both (see Tables 6 and 7). Consider antivenom when indicated.
Antibiotics often indicated (see Table 8).

Projectile wounds

Wound appearance is often deceptively benign (high-velocity injuries cause extensive tissue damage).
Foreign bodies are frequently present, and operative exploration is typically required.
Obtain appropriate radiographs.
Wound should be allowed to close by secondary intention or delayed primary closure.
Antibiotics indicated except in soft tissue only injuries.

Stings

Take into account risk of envenomation.
Symptoms may be local or systemic.
Treatment is usually directed toward local symptoms (i.e., analgesia) and wound care.
For systemic reactions, epinephrine, antihistamines, corticosteroids, and supportive care may be required.
The wounded area should be elevated and iced
Antibiotics rarely indicated.

Complex wound left open or closed after delay

Wet-to-dry dressings, wet-to-wet, or negative pressure wound therapy is indicated for contaminated wounds or wounds with questionably viable tissue (negative pressure therapy should not be used over exposed blood vessels or bowel).
Topical antimicrobials may be used in significantly contaminated wounds.
Avoid compression dressings in wounds with questionably viable tissue.

Extravasation injury or crush injury

Avoid compression dressings.

Table 1 Common Injectable Anesthetics[3]

Common Injectable Anesthetics
Amides
Lidocaine (Xylocaine)
Bupivacaine (Marcaine)
Mepivacaine (Carbocaine)
Prilocaine (Citanest)
Etidocaine (Duranest)
Phenocaine
Dibucaine (Nupercainal)
Ropivacaine (Naropin)
Levobupivacaine (Chirocaine)
Esters
Procaine (Novocain)
Chloroprocaine (Nesacaine)
Tetracaine (Pontocaine)
Benzocaine (multiple brands)
Propoxycaine (Ravocaine)
Cocaine

and cardiovascular bypass (if necessary) until the anesthetic has been metabolized. The maximum safe dose of lidocaine is 3 to 5 mg/kg without epinephrine and 7 mg/kg with epinephrine. Doses as high as 55 mg/kg have been used without toxicity for tumescent anesthesia in patients undergoing liposuction[4]; however, in this scenario, some of the anesthetic is aspirated by the liposuction lowering the effective dose. The lidocaine doses used for local wound injection should be substantially smaller than those used in liposuction. To prevent local anesthesia from causing systemic toxicity, the recommended safe doses of the anesthetics should not be exceeded and aspiration should be performed before injection to ensure that the agent is not injected intravascularly.

The pain associated with injection of the local anesthetic can be minimized by using a small-caliber needle (27 to 30 gauge), warming the anesthetic, injecting the agent slowly, using a subcutaneous rather than an intradermal injection technique,[5] providing counterirritation, buffering the anesthetic with sodium bicarbonate to reduce acidity (in a 1:10 ratio of sodium bicarbonate to local anesthetic),[6] and applying a topical local anesthetic before injection. Topical local anesthetics (e.g., TAC [tetracaine, adrenaline (epinephrine), and cocaine] and EMLA [a eutectic mixture of lidocaine and prilocaine]) are as effective as injectable anesthetics when applied to an open wound.[7] EMLA requires approximately 60 minutes to induce sufficient anesthesia for open wounds; TAC requires approximately 30 minutes.[8] EMLA is more effective than TAC for open wounds of the extremity. Benzocaine 20% (in gel, liquid, or spray form) can also be used for topical anesthesia and is frequently employed before endoscopic procedures. It is poorly absorbed through intact skin but well absorbed through mucous membranes and open wounds. A 0.5- to 1-second spray is usually recommended, although even with a standardized spray duration, the delivered dose can vary considerably.[9] A 2-second spray results in a statistically, although not clinically, significant increase in methemoglobin levels.[10] Methemoglobinemia is a rare but life-threatening complication of benzocaine spray use. If symptoms of methemoglobinemia develop (e.g., cyanosis or elevated methemoglobin levels on cooximetry), prompt treatment with intravenous (IV) methylene blue, 1 to 2 mg/kg, is indicated.[9]

EXPLORATION

After anesthesia is achieved, the wound should be thoroughly explored. Injuries to the hand should raise a high suspicion for nerve, muscle, tendon, and vascular injuries. In general, complex hand wounds should be explored under tourniquet control in the operating room. Injuries to the abdomen or chest, especially penetrating wounds, should be explored for violation of the abdominal fascia, pleura, or mediastinal spaces. Potential for damage to organs should be assessed, and a low threshold for operative exploration should be maintained. Finally, injuries to the face should elicit high suspicion for nerve (both sensory and motor) or duct injuries (e.g., the parotid duct or the lacrimal duct) that may require probing. Any potential vascular injuries to the extremities should be assessed by measuring an ankle-brachial index (considered abnormal if < 0.9). Radiographs should be obtained to rule out fracture, joint involvement, and embedded foreign material.

HEMOSTASIS

In most wounds, hemorrhage can be readily controlled with pressure, cauterization, or ligation of vessels. Direct pressure with one to two fingers is often all that is needed to stop active bleeding. Avoid placing large amounts of gauze or other absorptive materials on an actively bleeding wound as they may make applying direct pressure difficult and aid little in hemostasis. When direct pressure fails, wound exploration with cauterization or ligation of transected vessels may be appropriate. Lacerated arteries proximal to amputated parts such as fingers or ears, however, should not be ligated because an intact vessel is necessary for microsurgical replantation. In general, vessels greater than 1.5 mm in diameter should be preserved when possible.[11] If ligation is to be performed, the divided end of the vessel should be isolated, clamped with a small hemostat, and ligated with a synthetic absorbable braided suture. Packing, wrapping, and elevating can help control hemorrhage temporarily. If necessary (although the need should be rare, and only in cases of life-threatening hemorrhage), a tourniquet may be applied to an injured extremity. It should be applied before the development of shock. Data from combat situations suggest that survival may be increased and that tourniquet use time of less than 1 hour does not have any significant adverse effects except for transient nerve palsy (rate $< 2\%$).[12]

Hemostasis prevents hematoma formation, thereby decreasing the risk of infection and wound inflammation. If there appears to be a potential risk of hematoma or fluid collection, drains should be placed. Although drains may help prevent accumulation of blood or serum in the wound, they are not a replacement for meticulous hemostasis. Drains facilitate approximation of tissues, particularly under flaps; however, they also tend to potentiate bacterial colonization because they serve as retrograde conduits for bacteria.[13] As a rule, drains can be safely removed when drainage reaches levels of 25 to 30 mL/day. If a hematoma or seroma forms, the subsequent course of action depends on the size of the fluid collection. Small hematomas and seromas usually are reabsorbed and can be treated conservatively. Larger fluid collections provide a significant barrier to healing, and treatment may include reopening the wound and placing drains. Intermittent sterile aspirations, followed by application of a compressive dressing, may also be indicated.

IRRIGATION

After débridement of necrotic tissue and foreign bodies, the next step is irrigation of the wound. This may be accomplished by several different methods, including bulb syringe irrigation, gravity flow irrigation, and pulsatile lavage. These methods can be further divided into high-pressure (15 to 35 psi) and low-pressure (1 to 15 psi) delivery systems. High-pressure pulsatile lavage may reduce bacterial concentrations in the wound more efficiently than low-pressure and bulb syringe systems,[14] but it can also cause disruption to soft tissue structure and deeper penetration with greater retention of bacteria.[15–17] A recent randomized, controlled trial found no benefit with higher pressures in the irrigation of open fractures, but further studies are needed.[18] In general, low-pressure systems should be employed for acute wound irrigation and high-pressure irrigation may be considered for grossly contaminated wounds. Simply running saline over a wound is of little value; thus, to obtain continuous irrigation with pressures as low as 5 to 8 psi, one group recommended using a saline bag in a pressure cuff inflated to 400 mm Hg and connected to IV tubing with a 19-gauge angiocatheter.[19]

Only nontoxic solutions (e.g., 0.9% sterile saline, lactated Ringer solution, sterile water, and tap water) should be used for wound irrigation.[20] Irrigation with an antibiotic solution appears to offer no advantages over a nonsterile soap solution, and the antibiotic solution may increase the risk of wound-healing problems.[21] Strong antiseptics (e.g., povidone-iodine, chlorhexidine, alcohol, sodium hypochlorite, and hydrogen peroxide) should not be placed directly into the wound because they may impede healing. After copious irrigation, the surrounding skin should be prepared with an antibacterial solution to limit further contamination.

DÉBRIDEMENT

Normal healing can proceed only if tissues are viable, the wound contains no foreign bodies, and tissues are free of excessive bacterial contamination. To reduce the risk of infection, necrotic tissue and foreign bodies must be removed.[22] The wound and the surrounding local tissue must be exposed so that necrotic tissue can be identified and débrided. Hair may be trimmed with scissors or an electric clipper or retracted with an ointment or gel to facilitate exposure, débridement, and wound closure. Close shaving with a razor should be avoided because it potentiates wound infections.[23] Clipping of eyebrows should also be avoided, both because the eyebrows may not grow back and because the hair is necessary for proper alignment.

Some wounds contain a significant amount of questionably viable tissue. Models of wound management have defined three zones of injury: zone of necrosis, zone of stasis (vulnerable to necrosis), and zone of hyperemia (viable tissue).[24] If there is enough indeterminately viable tissue to preclude acute débridement, dressing changes may be initiated. When all necrotic tissue has been surgically or mechanically débrided, the wound can be closed. Adjuncts to help delineate viable tissue include the use of methylene blue to stain tissue, photoplethysmography, laser Doppler ultrasonography, and transcutaneous Po_2 monitoring.[11,25] However, skin usually demarcates by 24 hours and muscle by 4 to 5 days.[17]

Most foreign bodies are easily removed either by hand or surgical débridement. Abrasion injuries or gunpowder explosions can cause small foreign body fragments to embed in and beneath the skin. These small foreign bodies are often difficult to extract but should be removed as soon as possible. Irrigation usually suffices for removal of loose foreign bodies, but surgical débridement with a small drill, sharp instrument, or brush may be required for more firmly embedded material. If the interval between injury and treatment exceeds 1 to 2 days, the wounds will begin to epithelialize and the embedded material will be trapped in the skin, resulting in traumatic tattooing. Although débridement within 6 hours remains the standard of care to decrease the risk of infection, some evidence suggests that débridement can be performed anytime within the first 24 hours if the delay is for the purpose of transferring to an experienced trauma center.[26]

Wound Closure Considerations

MATERIALS

Once the appropriate preparatory measures have been taken (as described above), the wound is ready to be closed. The first step is to choose the material to be used for wound closure. The materials currently available include sutures, staples, tapes, and adhesives. Selection of the appropriate material is based on the type and location of the wound, the potential for infection, the patient's ability to tolerate closure, and the degree of mechanical stress imposed by closure. The selected material must provide wound edge approximation until the tensile strength of the wound has increased to the point where it can withstand the stress present.

The majority of wounds are closed with sutures. A suture is a foreign body by definition; thus, it may generate an inflammatory response, interfere with wound healing, and increase the risk of infection. Accordingly, the number and diameter of sutures used to close a wound should be kept to the minimum necessary for coaptation of the wound edges.

Sutures are categorized on the basis of material, tensile strength, number of filaments, absorbability, and time to degradation [*see Table 2*]. Suture material may be either natural or synthetic. Natural fibers (e.g., catgut and silk) cause more intense inflammatory reactions than synthetic materials (e.g., polypropylene).[27] The tensile strength of suture material is defined as the amount of weight required to break a suture divided by the suture's cross-sectional area. It is typically expressed in an integer-hyphen-zero form whereby larger integers correspond to smaller suture diameters (i.e., 3-0 sutures have a greater diameter and more tensile strength than 5-0 sutures).[28] To minimize the amount of foreign body in the wound and to minimize damage to local tissue, suture of the narrowest diameter with sufficient strength should be used and buried sutured knots should be cut short.[29]

Table 2 Types and Characteristics of Suture Material Used for Wound Closure

Suture Type	*Material*	*Comment*	*Configuration*	*Method of Absorption*	*Tensile Strength at 2 wk (%)*	*Time to Degradation*
Absorbable	Plain catgut (bovine intestinal serosa)	Natural; high tissue reactivity	Monofilament	Proteolysis	0	10–14 days
	Chromic catgut (bovine intestinal serosa treated with chromic acid)	Natural; stronger, less reactive, and longer-lasting than plain catgut	Monofilament	Proteolysis	0	21 days
	Fast-absorbing catgut	Natural	Monofilament	Proteolysis	0	7–10 days
	Polyglytone 6211 (Caprosyn)	Synthetic	Monofilament	Hydrolysis	10	56 days
	Glycomer 631 (Biosyn)	Synthetic	Monofilament	Hydrolysis	75	90–110 days
	Polyglycolic acid (Dexon)	Synthetic	Monofilament/ multifilament	Hydrolysis	20	90–120 days
	Polyglactic acid (Vicryl)	Synthetic	Multifilament	Hydrolysis	20	60–90 days
	Polyglyconate (Maxon)	Synthetic	Monofilament	Hydrolysis	81	180–210 days
	Polyglycolide (Polysorb)	Synthetic	Multifilament	Hydrolysis	80	56–70 days
	Polydioxanone (PDS)	Synthetic	Monofilament	Hydrolysis	74	180 days
	Polyglecaprone 25 (Monocryl)	Synthetic	Monofilament	Hydrolysis	25	90–120 days
	Polyglactin 910 (Vicryl RAPIDE)	Synthetic	Multifilament	Hydrolysis	0	7–14 days
Nonabsorbable	Polybutester (Novafil)	Synthetic; low tissue reactivity, elastic; good knot security	Monofilament		High	
	Nylon (Monosof, Dermalon, Ethilon)	Synthetic; low tissue reactivity; memory effect necessitates more knots	Monofilament	—	High	—
	Nylon (Nurolon)	Synthetic; low tissue reactivity	Multifilament	—	High	—
	Nylon (Surgilon)	Synthetic; silicon coated; low tissue reactivity	Multifilament	—	High	—
	Polypropylene (Prolene, Surgilene, Surgipro)	Synthetic; low tissue reactivity; slippery	Monofilament	—	High	—
	Polyethylene (Dermalene)	Synthetic	Monofilament	—	High	—
	Stainless steel	Lowest tissue reactivity of all sutures; poor handling; creates artifact on CT scan; moves with MRI	Monofilament/ multifilament	—	Highest	—
	Cotton	Natural	Multifilament	—	—	—
	Silk (Sofsilk)	Natural; high tissue reactivity; good knot security	Multifilament	—	Poor	—
	Polyester (Dacron, Mersilene, Surgidac)	Synthetic; uncoated; high friction; low tissue reactivity; poor knot security	Multifilament	—	High	—
	Polyester (Ticron)	Synthetic; silicon coated; low tissue reactivity; good knot security	Multifilament	—	High	—
	Polyester (Ethibond)	Synthetic; polybutylate coated; low tissue reactivity; good knot security	Multifilament	—	High	—
	Polyester (Ethiflex, Tevdek)	Synthetic; Teflon coated; low tissue reactivity; good knot security	Multifilament	—	High	—

CT = computed tomographic; MRI = magnetic resonance imaging.

Suture material may be composed of either a single or multiple filaments. Multifilament suture material may either be twisted or braided, which is of clinical importance because the interstices created by braiding may harbor organisms and increase the risk of infection. Monofilament sutures require five knots for security, whereas multifilament sutures are easier to handle and require only three knots. With all sutures, the knots must be square to be secure and must be tight enough only to coapt the wound edges.

Absorbable or nonabsorbable sutures may be appropriate depending on the situation. Absorbable sutures (lose tensile strength within 60 days) are generally used for buried sutures to approximate deep tissues (e.g., dermis, muscle, fascia, tendons, nerves, blood vessels), in areas where removal is difficult (e.g., hair-bearing areas such as the eyebrow), or in patients who will not tolerate removal (e.g., children) or not return for suture removal. Nonabsorbable sutures are typically used in reliable patients and in areas under high tension (e.g., over a joint) or in areas of high cosmetic importance (e.g., face), where inflammation must be minimized to reduce scarring (with the exception of silk). Absorption of synthetic suture material occurs by hydrolysis and causes less tissue reaction than absorption of natural suture material, which occurs by proteolysis. Common rules for closure are that deep tissues should be approximated with 3-0 absorbable sutures and skin should be approximated with 4-0 to 6-0 suture depending on the location [*see Table 3*]. Areas of cosmetic importance (e.g., the face) should be approximated with 5-0 or 6-0 nonabsorbable suture, except in specific patients, as detailed above.

Staple closure is less expensive and significantly faster than suture closure and offers a slightly more acceptable cosmetic outcome when used to close scalp wounds.[30,31] Scalp wounds that are bleeding significantly can be quickly closed with staples to achieve hemostasis while the patient undergoes further evaluation and be revised later if needed. Contaminated wounds closed with staples have a lower incidence of infection than those closed with sutures due to their low level of tissue reactivity, but closure with staples is not a substitute for adequate wound irrigation and débridement.[32] In addition, staple closure eliminates the risk that a health care provider will experience a needle stick, which is a particularly important consideration in caring for a trauma patient with an unknown medical history. Staples are not suitable for wounds with irregular skin edges.

Tapes used for wound closure are either rubber based or employ an acrylate adhesive. Rubber-based tapes (e.g., athletic tape) are a potential irritant to skin; degrade with exposure to heat, light, and air; and are occlusive, thereby preventing transepidermal water loss. Tapes that include acrylate adhesives (e.g., Micropore and Steri-Strip), on the other hand, are hypoallergenic, have a long shelf life, and are porous, thereby allowing water to evaporate.[33] Linear wounds in areas with little tension with even wound edges are easily approximated with tape alone, whereas wounds in areas where the skin is more taut (e.g., the extremities) or uneven generally require that tape skin closure be supplemented by dermal sutures. The use of tape alone is desirable when feasible, especially in children, because it avoids the discomfort associated with suture placement and removal and prevents suture puncture scars.[33] However, tape is not a substitute for multilayered or meticulous wound closure. Tape closure has some other advantages: it may permit earlier suture removal; is easy to perform and comfortable for the patient; leaves no marks on the skin; and yields a lower infection rate in contaminated wounds than suture closure.[34] It also has a few disadvantages: patients may inadvertently remove the tape; wound edge approximation is less precise; tape will not adhere to mobile areas under tension (e.g., the plantar aspects of the feet) or to moist areas (e.g., mucous membranes and groin creases); wound edema can lead to blistering at the tape margins and to inversion of wound edges; and tape may elicit allergic reactions.

The use of tissue adhesives (e.g., octylcyanoacrylate) is a fast, strong, and flexible method of approximating wound

Table 3 Suggested Materials for Wound Approximation Based on Location

Location	*Suggested Closure Material*	*Suggested Time to Removal/Comments*
Deep structures (i.e., fascia, dermis, muscle)	3-0 or 4-0 absorbable suture depending on location	N/A
Oral/buccal mucosa	4-0 chromic gut	N/A
Lip	4-0 plain gut for wet vermillion 6-0 monofilament nonabsorbable for dry vermillion	5 days Ensure proper alignment of "red line" and "white line" of lip
Face	5-0 to 6-0 nonabsorbable monofilament 5-0 to 6-0 fast gut (children)	5 days
Ear	5-0 synthetic absorbable for cartilage 6-0 monofilament nonabsorbable for skin	5–7 days Bolster dressing to prevent hematoma or seroma formation
Scalp	3-0 monofilament nonabsorbable or absorbable suture Staples	10–14 days If injured, the galea must also be approximated with nonabsorbable suture
Other areas	3-0 absorbable or nonabsorbable Staples	7–10 days

N/A = not available.

involving high fluid volumes, high-osmolar contrast agents, or chemotherapeutic drugs can have more serious effects, such as skin ulceration and extensive soft tissue necrosis similar to a chemical burn. Treatment of these injuries is not standardized. It may include conservative management, hydrocortisone cream, incision and drainage, hyaluronidase injection, saline injection, and aspiration by means of liposuction.[71–73]

INJECTION INJURIES

Wounds caused by injection of foreign materials (e.g., paint, oil, grease, or dirty water) can be severe. Injection injuries usually result from the use of high-pressure spray guns (600 to 12,000 psi) and often occur on the nondominant hand.[74,75] On the initial examination, the injury may appear deceptively benign, with only a punctate entry wound visible; however, foreign material is often widely distributed in the deeper soft tissues. Radiographs are obtained to identify any fractures present and, in some cases, to determine the extent to which the injected material is distributed. Injection wounds must be treated aggressively with incision, wide exposure, débridement, and removal of foreign bodies to prevent extensive tissue loss and functional impairment. The functional outcome is determined by the time elapsed between injury and treatment and by the type of material injected. Oil-based paint is more damaging to tissues than water-based paint, oil, grease, water, or air.[10,11]

PROJECTILE WOUNDS

Projectile injuries are divided into low- and high-velocity wounds. Low velocity is defined as speeds up to 350 m/s, whereas high-velocity projectiles travel over 600 m/s. The distinction has clinical importance because with low-velocity projectiles, tissue damage is confined to the bullet tract. On the other hand, high-velocity wounds from explosions or gunshots cause extensive tissue damage due to the release of significant kinetic energy.[17] Small entry wounds are common, but the seemingly benign appearance of such a wound often belies the actual severity. As the bullet travels through the soft tissue, it does not follow a linear path but rather tumbles. Thus, the exit wound and interspace may contain large areas of ischemic and damaged tissue that affect critical structures (e.g., bone and blood vessels). Clothing and dirt may also be transmitted into the deep spaces. Radiographs may identify radiopaque foreign bodies (e.g., metal objects or pieces of leaded glass).[78] Treatment of wounds created by high-velocity missiles involves extensive débridement and identification of injured tissue. Wounds should be left open to heal by secondary or delayed primary closure.[42] Antibiotics are indicated to prevent bacteremia[17] except in soft tissue–only gunshot wounds.[79]

BITE WOUNDS

Treatment of bite wounds involves thorough exploration, irrigation, and débridement. X-rays must be obtained and wounds explored to evaluate the patient for fractures or open joint injuries. If a joint capsule has been violated, the joint must be thoroughly cleaned. Due to the infection risk, wounds may be allowed to heal by secondary intention or delayed primary closure. Primary closure is also possible if thorough débridement is performed,[42] but no prospective data exist, and this area remains highly controversial. Facial wounds may be considered for closure given the area's cosmetic importance and overall lower risk of infection. Delayed primary closure with a 3- to 5-day interval may also be considered as this may give a better cosmetic result than healing by secondary intention. Irrigation is the most important factor in decreasing the bacterial load.[38] Rabies prophylaxis treatment should be considered for patients who have been bitten by wild animals [*see* Adjunctive Wound Treatment, Rabies Prophylaxis, *above*].

Humans and Nonvenomous Animals

Most human bite wounds are clenched-fist wounds sustained by young men.[80] Human bite wounds are considered infected from the moment of infliction and must be treated with antibiotics.[48,49] The antibiotic regimen should be targeted against the bacterial species most likely to be present. Common isolates from bite wounds include *Streptococcus anginosus*, *Staphylococcus aureus*, *Eikenella corrodens*, *Fusobacterium nucleatum*, *Prevotella melaninogenica*, and *Candida* species.[80] To cover these organisms, a broad-spectrum antibiotic or combination of antibiotics (e.g., amoxicillin-clavulanate or moxifloxacin or ciprofloxacin with clindamycin in patients with a penicillin allergy) should be administered.[80] Infections related to human and animal bites develop within 12 to 24 hours of the injury.[38]

Nonhuman primates can cause viral infection, most commonly with cercopithecine herpesvirus type 1. If left untreated, such infection can lead to meningoencephalitis, which carries a 70% mortality. Accordingly, acyclovir prophylaxis is recommended.[81]

Wounds caused by cat bites or scratches are at high (80%) risk for infection that is usually attributable to *Pasteurella multocida*. The aerobic species commonly isolated from such wounds include *Pasteurella*, *Streptococcus*, *Staphylococcus*, *Moraxella*, and *Neisseria*; common anaerobic isolates include *Fusobacterium*, *Bacteroides*, *Porphyromonas*, and *Prevotella*.[50] Patients with severe infection should be treated with parenteral antibiotics (i.e., ampicillin-sulbactam). Acute regional lymphadenitis after a cat scratch is known as cat-scratch disease and is caused by *Bartonella henselae*.[82] It is treated by administering azithromycin.[83] Cat bites should not be closed.

Dog bite wounds are at lower (16%) risk for infection than human bite or cat bite wounds and tend to be less severely contaminated. The aerobic and anaerobic organisms commonly found in cat bite wounds are similar to those found in dog bite wounds, and antibiotic prophylaxis with a combination of a β-lactam antibiotic with a β-lactamase inhibitor (e.g., amoxicillin-clavulanate) is appropriate.[45,50]

Venomous Animals

Snake bites Four types of poisonous snakes are native to the United States. These include the coral snakes (*Micrurus* and *Micruroides* species) from the family Elapidae and three species of pit vipers from the family Viperidae: rattlesnakes (*Crotalus* species), copperheads (*Agkistrodon tortortrix*), and cottonmouths or water moccasins (*Agkistrodon piscivorus*).[84–86] Pit vipers can be identified by the pit between the eye and the nostril on each side of the head, the vertical elliptical pupils, the triangle-shaped head, the single row of subcaudal plates distal to the anal plate, and the two hollow fangs protruding from the maxilla that produce the characteristic fang marks.[87] Coral snakes have rounder heads and eyes and lack fangs. They are identified by their characteristic color pattern consisting of red, yellow, and black vertical bands.

Patients bitten by coral snakes show no obvious local signs when envenomation has occurred. Consequently, the physician must look for systemic signs such as paresthesias, increased salivation, tongue fasciculations, dysphagia, dysarthria, visual disturbances, respiratory distress, convulsions, and shock. These symptoms may not develop until several hours after the bite. On the other hand, patients bitten by pit vipers typically develop local pain and swelling within 30 minutes of the bite. In some cases, these manifestations may take up to 4 hours to appear. Erythema, petechiae, bullae, and vesicles are also sometimes seen. Severe envenomation may induce systemic reactions, including disseminated intravascular coagulation (DIC), bleeding, hypotension, shock, acute respiratory distress syndrome (ARDS), and renal failure.

If signs or symptoms of envenomation are found, appropriate laboratory tests (hematocrit, fibrinogen level, coagulation studies, platelet count, urinalysis, and serum chemistries) should be ordered. Laboratory tests should be repeated every 8 to 24 hours for the first 1 to 3 days to determine whether envenomation is progressing. Severe envenomation can cause decreased fibrinogen levels, coagulopathy, bleeding, and myoglobinuria.

Treatment of venomous snake bites includes immobilization and elevation. If envenomation is suspected or confirmed, antivenin should be administered intravenously as early as possible. Antivenins commonly used in the United States include Antivenin (Crotalidae) Polyvalent (ACP) (Wyeth Pharmaceuticals, Collegeville, PA) and Crotalidae Polyvalent Immune Fab (Ovine) (CroFab, Protherics Inc., Nashville, TN).[88] Fab antivenom (FabAV) is less allergenic and more potent than ACP and thus has largely supplanted it in the United States.[88,89] Patients are treated with a loading dose of four to six vials of FabAV followed by three two-vial maintenance doses at 6, 12, and 18 hours to prevent recurrence of symptoms. If symptoms progress despite antivenin treatment, an additional four to six vials of FabAV are given twice more. If symptoms continue to progress, consideration should be given to using ACP. ACP remains the most effective antivenin for patients with coral snake bites and those who do not respond to FabAV. Before ACP is administered, the patient must be tested for sensitivity. The major complication of antivenin therapy is serum sickness. This complication occurs in approximately 50 to 75% of patients treated with ACP but in only 16% of those treated with FabAV.[88,90,91]

Compartment syndrome is a rare but severe complication of a snake bite. Fasciotomy is sometimes required to relieve extremity compartment syndrome, but it is not necessary for prophylactic purposes. Tourniquets, incision and suction, cryotherapy, and electric shock treatment are of little value for snake bites and may increase complication rates. There is no clear evidence to support antibiotic prophylaxis in this setting.[87]

Spider bites The bites of most spiders found in the United States cause little to no wound or local reaction; however, three types are capable of injecting venom. Brown recluse spiders (*Loxosceles reclusa*) can be identified by a violin-shaped dorsal mark. They are nocturnal, live in dark and dry places, and are found in the central and southern United States. The venom is a phospholipase enzyme that acts as a dermal toxin and almost always causes a local reaction.[92] Local signs and symptoms may be limited to minor irritation, although they may also progress to extreme tenderness, erythema, and edema. The onset of symptoms may be delayed for as long as 8 hours, and tissue necrosis may develop over the following days to weeks. Systemic reactions may include mild hemolysis, mild coagulopathy, and DIC, although severe intravascular hemolytic syndrome and death have also been reported.[92,93] Oral administration of dapsone (50 to 100 mg/day) to minimize tissue necrosis has been advocated by some[94]; however, this treatment is of uncertain efficacy, and no prospective data currently support its use. Moreover, dapsone can cause hemolytic anemia, a potentially life-threatening condition.[93] If systemic symptoms develop, systemic corticosteroid therapy and supportive measures are indicated. Brown recluse antivenin is not available in the United States.

Black widow spiders (*Latrodectus mactans*) can be identified by a red-hourglass ventral mark.[86] They live in dark, dry, and protected areas and are distributed widely throughout the continental United States. The venom is a neurotoxin that produces immediate and severe local pain. Local signs and symptoms include two fang marks, erythema, swelling, and piloerection.[92] Systemic reactions with neurologic signs may develop within 10 minutes and include muscle pain and cramps starting in the vicinity of the bite, abdominal pain, vomiting, tremors, increased salivation, paresthesias, hyperreflexia, and, with severe envenomation, shock. Systemic symptoms may last for days to weeks. High-risk persons (e.g., those who are younger than 16 years, the elderly, pregnant women, hypertensive patients, or persons who continue to show symptoms despite treatment) may experience paralysis, hemolysis, renal failure, or coma. Treatment includes 10% calcium gluconate IV for relief of muscle spasm, methocarbamol or diazepam for muscle relaxation, and a single dose of antivenin. Antivenin causes serum sickness in as many as 9% of patients; consequently, its use is controversial except in high-risk patients.[95]

Hobo spiders (*Tegenaria agrestis*) can be identified by their long hairy legs and a cephalothorax that is marked by two stripes and butterfly markings dorsally and two stripes ventrally. Found throughout the northwestern United States, they live in low places and build funnel-shaped webs in dark spaces. Hobo spiders have been reported to inflict painful bites that lead to wound ulceration, dermonecrosis, and a persistent headache, although the accuracy of such reports has been debated.[93,96,97] A slow-healing ulcer that leaves a central crater has been described. Treatment consists of local wound care.

Scorpions Stings from most scorpion species found in the United States cause only limited local reactions that can be managed conservatively; however, stings from *Centruroides sculpturatus*, which is found in California and many southern states, may be more severe. *Centruroides* has a sting that causes envenomation with a neurotoxin. Erythema, edema, and ecchymosis at the site of the sting are evidence that envenomation did not take place. Instead, envenomation is indicated by an immediate and intense burning pain at the wound site.[98] The initial local pain may then be followed by systemic symptoms such as muscle spasm, excess salivation, fever, tachycardia, slurred speech, blurry vision, convulsions, or death.[92] Treatment consists of icing and elevation of the wounded area followed by administration of barbiturates for control of neuromuscular activity and institution of supportive therapy with antihistamines, corticosteroids, and analgesics.[98]

Centipedes Centipedes are slender, multisegmented, and multilegged arthropods that range in size from 1 to 30 cm and in color from bright yellow to brownish black. The first pair of legs is modified into sharp, stinging structures that are connected to venom glands. Centipedes prefer dark, damp environments and may be found throughout the southern United States. Local symptoms associated with centipede stings include pain, erythema, edema, lymphangitis, lymphadenitis, weakness, and paresthesia. Skin necrosis may occur at the envenomation site. Systemic symptoms may include anxiety, fever, dizziness, palpitations, and nausea.[99] Treatment consists of symptomatic pain control, infiltration of local anesthetics, administration of antihistamines, and local wound care.[99]

Hymenoptera The order Hymenoptera includes wasps, bees, and ants. Wasps, which are found across the United States, live in small colonies and may attack in groups when provoked. Honeybees (*Apis mellifera*) and bumblebees (*Bombus* species), also found across the United States, are generally docile and rarely sting unless provoked. Africanized honeybees (*Apis mellifera scutellata*; also referred to as killer bees) are found primarily in the southwestern states and are far more aggressive than other bees. Fire ants (*Solenopsis invicta* and *Solenopsis richteri*) are wingless, ground-dwelling arthropods that are found in many southern states and attack in an aggressive swarm when provoked.

Although Hymenoptera stingers are small, they can evoke severe local and systemic reactions. The local response to a Hymenoptera sting is a painful, erythematous, and edematous papule that develops within seconds and typically subsides in 4 to 6 hours. Some stingers are barbed and must be removed with a scraping motion, rather than pinching, to prevent the injection of more venom. Systemic reactions occur in about 5% of the population and may lead to anaphylaxis with syncope, bronchospasm, hypotension, and arrhythmias. Wounds and local reactions are treated with ice, elevation, and analgesics. Systemic reactions are treated with subcutaneous epinephrine, diphenhydramine, and supportive airway and blood pressure control.[92] Persons with a history of systemic reactions to insect stings should carry epinephrine kits.

Dressings for Specific Types of Wounds

The functions of a wound dressing include protection, antisepsis, pressure, immobilization, débridement, provision of a physiologic environment, absorption, packing, support, comfort, and aesthetic appearance. More specifically, the functions of a dressing should be tailored to the wound type and the purpose of the dressing must be carefully considered before application. In general, because dry wounds do not epithelialize, a wound with a clean base should be covered with a dressing that retains moisture. If the wound is contaminated or produces a large amount of exudate, an absorptive dressing is needed to remove excess moisture to protect adjacent skin from maceration.

ABRASIONS

Abrasions heal by epithelialization, which is accelerated by the warm, moist environment created by an occlusive dressing.[100,101] Such an environment not only promotes epithelialization but also enhances healing by retaining moisture and a low oxygen tension that promotes the inflammatory phase.[102] A variety of dressings are suitable for treatment of abrasions, including biologic dressings, hydrogels, hydrocolloids, and semipermeable films. These dressings need not be changed as long as they remain adherent. Small, superficial wounds also heal readily when dressed with impregnated gauze dressings (e.g., Xeroform and Scarlet Red, Kendall, Mansfield, MA) that allow exudates to pass through them while maintaining a moist wound bed.[102] These less adherent dressings must be changed more regularly, such as one to two times per day.[103]

Dry dressings (e.g., gauze) should be avoided with abrasions because they facilitate scab formation. Scabs slow epithelialization because advancing cells must enzymatically débride the scab-wound interface to migrate.[104] Wounds covered with a scab also tend to cause more discomfort than wounds covered with occlusive dressings.

LACERATIONS

For sutured wounds, the specific purposes of a dressing are to prevent bacterial contamination, to protect the wound, to manage drainage, and to facilitate epithelialization. Dressings used on such wounds usually consist of three basic layers. The inner (contact) layer is chosen to minimize adherence of the dressing to the wound and to facilitate drainage through itself to the overlying layers. Common choices for this layer include fine-mesh gauze, petrolatum gauze, Xeroform or Xeroflo (Kendall) gauze, and Adaptic (Johnson & Johnson, New Brunswick, NJ). These substances should be applied only as a single layer because when applied in multiple layers, they become occlusive. The middle layer is chosen for absorbency and ability to conform to the shape of the wound. It is usually composed of fluffs, Kerlix (Kendall), or wide-mesh gauze, all of which facilitate capillary action and drainage.[105] Telfa (Kendall) is an example of a simple dressing that combines both a nonadherent layer and an absorbent pad. The middle layer must not become saturated because exudate will collect on the wound surface, causing maceration and possibly bacterial contamination. The outer (binding) layer serves to secure the dressing. Common choices for this layer include Kling (Johnson & Johnson), ACE bandages (BD Medical, Franklin Lakes, NJ), Coban (3M, St. Paul, MN), and Tegaderm (3M).

Dressings are required only until drainage ceases or for 48 hours if draining is minimal. This corresponds with the time that it takes for epithelial cells to seal the superficial layers of the wound. Antibacterial ointments are a viable alternative to dressings in a minimally draining wound [*see* Adjunctive Wound Treatment, Topical Antimicrobials, *above*]. Such ointments are occlusive and maintain a sterile, moist environment for the 48 hours required for epithelialization. In anatomic areas that are difficult to dress (e.g., the scalp), it may be reasonable to forgo a dressing and simply apply ointments or allow a scab to form on the wound surface. Operative wounds are also sometimes covered with an occlusive dressing to optimize epithelialization [*see* Dressings for Specific Types of Wounds, Abrasions, *above*]. Some of these dressings are transparent, allowing observation of the wound. The disadvantage of occlusive dressings is their limited absorptive capacity, which allows drainage from the wound to collect underneath.

COMPLEX WOUNDS

For complex wounds containing necrotic tissue, foreign bodies, or other debris that cannot be removed sharply, wet-to-dry dressings are effective, simple, and inexpensive. A single layer of coarse, wet gauze is applied to a wound, allowed to dry over a period of 6 hours, and removed. Necrotic tissue, granulation tissue, debris, and wound exudate become incorporated within the gauze and are removed with the dressing. The disadvantages of wet-to-dry dressings are pain and possible damage to viable tissue. If the wound bed contains tendons, arteries, nerves, or bone, wet-to-wet dressings should be used to prevent desiccation of these critical structures.

Wet-to-wet dressings, which are not allowed to dry, cause less tissue damage than wet-to-dry dressings. However, they do not produce as much débridement. Most wet-to-wet dressings are kept moist with saline. Wounds with significant bacterial contamination may be treated with dressings that contain antibacterial agents (e.g., Dakin's, mafenide, silver sufadiazine, silver nitrate, or iodine) [*see* Adjunctive Wound Treatment, Topical Antimicrobials, *above*]. Biologic and semipermeable films also maintain a moist wound bed but are difficult to use on deep or irregular wounds and wounds with significant drainage. Enzymatic agents have also been used for wound débridement as an alternative to dressings, but there is a lack of high-quality evidence to guide clinical decisions.[106]

Some wounds are difficult to dress and require special consideration. For wounds with flaps or questionably viable tissue, compression dressings should not be used as they may cause ischemia. Wounds that cross joints are best dressed with plaster splints for temporary immobilization; semipermeable films are flexible and may also be used in this setting. Wounds with high levels of exudates may be dressed with hydrocolloids, hydrogels, or alginates.[102] For large or irregular wounds, NPWT may be beneficial as dressings conform well and remain adherent. Additionally, NPWT uses subatmospheric pressure to remove excess wound fluid, stimulates the formation of granulation tissue, improves peripheral blood flow and tissue oxygenation, reduces the size of the wound, decreases the number of dressing changes, and may even convert a wound not amenable to skin grafting (e.g., exposed bone, tendon, or hardware) to a granulating wound amenable to definitive closure.[37,107,108] Use of NPWT is contraindicated in wounds with exposed blood vessels or bowel due to the risks of vessel desiccation and fistula formation. Although NPWT may be helpful when delayed wound closure is planned,[91] there is no definitive evidence that it leads to better wound healing, and for chronic wounds, there may not be any benefit over simpler dressings.[109]

Postoperative Wound Care

Closed wounds should be kept clean and dry for 24 to 48 hours after repair. Epithelialization begins within hours after wound approximation and forms a barrier to contamination. Tension on the wound should be minimized, and patients should refrain from strenuous activity until the wound has regained sufficient tensile strength. In the first 6 weeks after repair, the wound's tensile strength increases rapidly. After this period, tensile strength increases more slowly, eventually reaching a maximum of 75 to 80% of normal skin strength [*see Figure 2*]. Wounds at risk for infection should be assessed by a medical provider within 48 hours of closure. In addition, the patient should be taught to look for signs of infection (e.g., erythema, edema, pain, purulent drainage, and fever).

The timing of suture or staple removal is determined by balancing the requirements for optimal appearance against the need for wound support. For optimal appearance, sutures should be removed early, before inflammation and epithelialization of suture tracts occur. An epithelialized tract will develop around a suture or staple that remains in the skin for longer than 7 to 10 days. Once the suture or staple is removed, the tract will be replaced by scar.[110] On the other hand, it takes a number of weeks for the wound to gain significant tensile strength, and early removal of wound support can lead to dehiscence of wounds that are under substantial tension. Early suture removal is warranted for some wounds. For example, sutures in aesthetically sensitive areas (e.g., the face) may be removed on day 4 or 5,

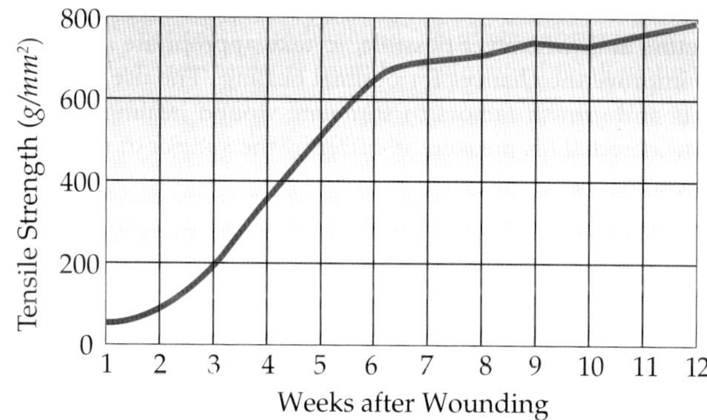

Figure 2 **The tensile strength of skin wounds increases rapidly for approximately 6 weeks after wounding. It then continues to increase slowly for 6 to 12 months, although it never reaches the tensile strength of unwounded tissue. Collagen is remodeled and replaced with highly cross-linked collagen along tissue stress lines. The process of collagen replacement and scar remodeling continues for years.**

1. O_2 delivery = CO × Cao_2
2. $Cao_2 = (1.34 \times Hb \times Sao_2) + (0.003 \times Pao_2)$
3. $P_{A}O_2 = F_{I}O_2(P_B - P_{H2o}) - P_{A}CO_2/R$

where CO = cardiac output, Cao_2 = arterial concentration of oxygen, Hb = hemoglobin, Sao_2 = percent saturation of hemoglobin with O_2, Pao_2 = arterial oxygen tension in mm Hg, $P_{A}O_2$ = alveolar oxygen tension in mm Hg, $F_{I}O_2$ = fraction of inspired oxygen, P_B = barometric pressure in mm Hg, P_{H20} = saturated vapor pressure of water, $P_{A}CO_2$ = alveolar carbon dioxide tension in mm Hg, R = respiratory quotient.

Supplemental administration of oxygen (inspired or hyperbaric) has been shown to have beneficial effects on wound healing in some studies. The incidence of infection in surgical wounds can be reduced by improving the $F_{I}O_2$ with supplemental oxygen.[127] In a study of patients undergoing colon surgery, for example, the wound infection rate was 50% lower when an $F_{I}O_2$ of 0.8 was maintained intraoperatively and for 2 hours postoperatively than when an $F_{I}O_2$ of 0.3 was maintained.[128] Hyperbaric oxygen therapy (i.e., the delivery of oxygen in an environment of increased ambient pressure) has been used for treatment of many types of wounds in which tissue hypoxia may impair healing.[129] It increases tissue oxygen concentrations 10-fold while also causing vasoconstriction, which results in decreased posttraumatic edema and decreased compartment pressures.[130,131] The elevated pressure and hyperoxia induced by hyperbaric oxygen therapy may promote wound healing. For patients with an acute wound, this modality may be a useful adjunct in treating limb-threatening injury, crush injury, and compartment syndrome.[129]

Circulating volume can be improved by administering crystalloids or blood. However, anemia alone is not associated with impaired wound healing unless it is severe enough to limit circulating blood volume.[132] The vasculature may be compromised either systemically (e.g., by diabetes mellitus or peripheral vascular disease) or locally (e.g., by trauma or scar). Vascular bypass may be necessary to improve tissue oxygenation in patients with poor arterial inflow.[113] Transcutaneous Po_2 monitoring may also help determine care as partial pressure of oxygen in tissue should be maintained above 30 mm Hg to promote proper healing.

Tobacco Smoking

Tobacco smoking reduces tissue oxygen concentrations, impairs wound healing, and contributes to wound infection and dehiscence.[133,134] The effects of smoking are attributable to vasoconstriction (caused by nicotine), displacement of oxygen binding (resulting from the high affinity of carbon monoxide for hemoglobin), increased platelet aggregation,[135] impairment of the inflammatory cell oxidative burst,[136] endothelial damage, and the development of atherosclerosis.[133,134,137] All acutely injured patients should stop smoking, and, ideally, all noninjured patients scheduled to undergo surgery should stop smoking at least 3 weeks before an elective surgical wound is made.[136,138] Like smoked tobacco, transcutaneous nicotine patches alter the inflammatory cell oxidative burst and cause vasoconstriction; accordingly, they, too, should not be used when a wound is present.[136]

Malnutrition

On average, hospitalized patients show a 20% increase in energy expenditure.[113] Good nutritional balance and adequate caloric intake (including sufficient amounts of protein, carbohydrates, fatty acids, vitamins, and other nutrients) are thus necessary for normal wound healing.

All patients who have sustained wounds should undergo nutritional assessment,[139] which typically includes measuring serum levels of albumin, protein, prealbumin, transferrin, and insulinlike growth factor–1 (IGF-1).[113] The serum albumin level is one of the best predictors of operative mortality and morbidity.[140] A value lower than 2.5 g/dL is considered severely depressed, and a value lower than 3.4 g/dL is associated with higher perioperative mortality.[141,142] Protein provides an essential supply of the amino acids used in collagen synthesis, and hypoproteinemia results in impaired healing. Consequently, it is not surprising that protein replacement and supplementation can improve wound healing.[143,144] In particular, supplementation specifically with the amino acids arginine, glutamine, and taurine (which are essential for anabolic processes and collagen synthesis) is thought to enhance wound healing.[145–147] Glutamine is the most abundant free amino acid in the body, and under catabolic conditions, it is released from muscle unless provided as a supplement.

Vitamins C, A, K, and D are essential for normal healing. Vitamin C (ascorbic acid) hydroxylates the amino acids lysine and proline during collagen synthesis and cross-linking. A deficiency of this vitamin causes scurvy, marked by failed healing of new wounds and dehiscence of old wounds. Vitamin C supplementation (100 to 1,000 g/day) can improve wound healing.[113,147] Vitamin A (retinoic acid) is essential for normal epithelialization, proteoglycan synthesis, and normal immune function.[148–150] Retinoids and topical tretinoin may help foster acute wound healing by accelerating epithelialization of full- and partial-thickness wounds, activating fibroblasts, increasing type III collagen synthesis, and decreasing metalloprotease activation.[151,152] Oral retinoid treatment significantly increases the decreased hydroxyproline content, tumor growth factor–β (TGF-β) level, and IGF-1 concentration associated with corticosteroids.[151] In addition, all aspects of corticosteroid-impaired healing—other than wound contraction—can be reversed by providing supplemental oral vitamin A at a recommended dosage of 25,000 IU/day.[153] The retinoic acid derivative isotretinoin (13-*cis*-retinoic acid), however, impairs wound epithelialization and delays wound healing.[154] Vitamin K is a cofactor in the synthesis of coagulation factors II, VII, IX, and X, as well as thrombin. Consequently, vitamin K is necessary for clot formation and hemostasis, the first step in acute wound healing. Vitamin D is required for normal calcium metabolism and therefore plays a necessary role in bone healing.

Dietary minerals (e.g., zinc and iron) are also essential for normal healing. Zinc is a necessary cofactor for DNA and RNA synthesis. A deficiency of this mineral can lead to inhibition of cellular proliferation, deficient granulation tissue formation,[155] and delayed wound healing.[156] Zinc replacement and supplementation can improve wound healing.[147] However, daily intake should not exceed 40 mg of elemental zinc, because excess zinc can immobilize macrophages, bind copper, and inhibit healing.[157] Iron is also a cofactor for DNA synthesis, as well as for hydroxylation of proline and lysine in collagen synthesis.[113] However, iron deficiency anemia does not appear to affect wound strength.[158]

Jaundice

The effect of jaundice on wound healing is controversial. Jaundiced patients appear to have a higher rate of postoperative wound-healing complications,[159] as well as a lower level of collagen synthesis. However, obstructive jaundice does not affect healing of blister wounds in humans.[160] Jaundiced animals show a significant delay in collagen accumulation within the wound but no significant reduction in the wound's mechanical strength.[161] Biliary drainage may be considered in jaundiced patients with wounds. This measure will improve collagen synthesis, although it may not have any appreciable effect on the healing rate.[160]

Age

Aging has a deleterious effect on the capacity for wound healing.[162] Increasing age is associated with an altered inflammatory response, impaired macrophage phagocytosis, and delayed healing.[163] Nevertheless, even though the wound healing phase begins later and proceeds more slowly compared to younger individuals, elderly patients are still able to heal most wounds.[164]

Diabetes Mellitus

Diabetes mellitus is associated with poor wound healing and an increased risk of infection. Diabetic neuropathy leads to sensory loss (typically in the extremities) and diminished ability to detect or prevent injury and wounding. Once present, wounds in diabetic patients heal slowly. The etiology of this healing impairment is multifactorial. Diabetes is associated with impaired granulocyte function and chemotaxis, depressed phagocytic function, altered humoral and cellular immunity, peripheral neuropathy, peripheral vascular disease, and various immunologic disturbances.[165–168] In addition, it is associated with a microangiopathy that can limit perfusion and delivery of oxygen, nutrients, and inflammatory cells to the healing wound.[169] Diabetes-induced impairment of healing, as well as the attendant morbidity and mortality, may be reduced by tightly controlling blood sugar levels with insulin.[170] Diabetic patients must also closely monitor themselves for wounds and provide meticulous care for any wounds present.

Obesity

Obesity is a growing epidemic in the United States. Not only is obesity often accompanied by diabetes and peripheral vascular disease, the excess weight itself also can lead to shearing forces across the wound and decrease blood flow, which may increase the risk of ischemia, dehiscence, and infection.[24,171]

Uremia

Uremia and chronic renal failure are associated with weakened host defenses, an increased risk of infection, and impaired wound healing.[172] Studies using uremic animal models show delayed healing of intestinal anastomoses and abdominal wounds.[173] Uremic serum also interferes with the proliferation of fibroblasts in culture.[119,173] Treatment of this wound-healing impairment includes dialysis.

Uremic patients with wounds may experience bleeding complications. In this situation, appropriate evaluation includes determining the prothrombin time (PT), the activated partial thromboplastin time (aPTT), the platelet count, and the hematocrit. Treatment includes dialysis without heparin; administration of desmopressin (0.3 μg/kg), cryoprecipitate, conjugated estrogens (0.6 mg/kg/day IV for 5 days),[174] and erythropoietin; and transfusion of red blood cells to raise the hematocrit above 30%.[175,176]

Uremic patients with hyperparathyroidism may also exhibit the uremic gangrene syndrome (calciphylaxis), which involves the spontaneous and progressive development of skin and soft tissue wounds, usually on the lower extremities. Patients with this syndrome typically are dialysis dependent and have secondary or tertiary hyperparathyroidism. Wound biopsies demonstrate fat necrosis, tissue calcification, and microarterial calcification.[177] Treatment includes local wound care, correction of serum phosphate levels with oral phosphate binders,[178] correction of calcium levels with dialysis, and subtotal parathyroidectomy.[177]

Drugs

Steroids Corticosteroids are antiinflammatory agents that inhibit all aspects of healing, including inflammation, macrophage migration, fibroblast proliferation, protein and collagen synthesis, development of breaking strength, wound contraction, and epithelialization.[119,153,179] In the setting of an acute wound that fails to heal, corticosteroid doses may be reduced, vitamin A administered topically or systemically, and anabolic steroids given to restore steroid-retarded inflammation.[119,153]

Unlike corticosteroids, anabolic steroids accelerate normal collagen deposition and wound healing. Oxandrolone is an oral anabolic steroid and testosterone analogue that is employed clinically to treat muscle wasting and foster wound healing and mitigates the catabolism associated with severe burn injury. Supplementation with this agent leads to significant improvements in the wound-healing rate.[180] In burn patients treated with oral oxandrolone, hospital length of stay is significantly reduced and the number of necessary operative procedures is decreased.[181] In ventilator-dependent surgical patients receiving oxandrolone, however, the course of mechanical ventilation is longer than in those not treated with oxandrolone. It has been suggested that the very ability of oxandrolone to enhance wound healing may increase collagen deposition and fibrosis in the later stages of ARDS and thereby prolong recovery.[182] Acute elevation of liver enzyme levels has been seen in some patients treated with oxandrolone; accordingly, hepatic transaminase concentrations should be intermittently monitored in all patients treated with this medication.[181]

Chemotherapeutic agents Both wound healing and tumor growth depend on metabolically active and rapidly dividing cells. Consequently, chemotherapeutic drugs that hinder tumor growth can also impair wound healing. These agents (which include adrenocorticosteroids, alkylating agents, antiestrogens, antimetabolites, antitumor antibodies, estrogen, progestogens, nitroureas, plant alkaloids, and random synthetics) attenuate the inflammatory phase of wound healing, decrease fibrin deposition, reduce the synthesis of collagen by fibroblasts, and delay wound contraction.[113] Some cytotoxic drugs (e.g., methotrexate and doxorubicin) substantially attenuate the early phases of wound repair and reduce wound strength.[183] The magnitude of these effects is influenced by the timing of the chemotherapeutic agent's delivery in relation to the time when the wound is sustained. Preoperative delivery has a greater adverse effect on healing; for example, doxorubicin impairs wound healing to a greater extent if given before operation than if treatment is delayed until 2 weeks after operation.[184] Chemotherapy also results in myelosuppression and neutropenia that can decrease resistance to infection, allowing small wounds to progress to myonecrosis and necrotizing soft tissue infections.[185] In all acutely wounded patients who have recently been treated with, are currently taking, or will soon begin to take chemotherapeutic agents, the wounds must be closely observed for poor healing and complications.

Other drugs Many other commonly used drugs affect wound healing and thus should be avoided in the setting of an acute wound. Nicotine, cocaine, ergotamine, and epinephrine all cause vasoconstriction and tissue hypoxia. Nonsteroidal antiinflammatory drugs (e.g., ibuprofen and ketorolac) inhibit cyclooxygenase production and reduce wound tensile strength. Colchicine decreases fibroblast proliferation and degrades newly formed extracellular matrix. Antiplatelet agents (e.g., aspirin) inhibit platelet aggregation and arachidonic acid–mediated inflammation. Heparin and warfarin impair hemostasis by virtue of their effects on fibrin formation.[108,186,187] As noted [*see* Factors that May Hinder Wound Healing, Systemic Factors, Malnutrition, *above*], isotretinoin inhibits wound epithelialization and delays wound healing.[154] Vitamin E (α-tocopherol) impairs collagen formation, inflammation, and wound healing,[188] and topical application of this agent can cause contact dermatitis and worsen the cosmetic appearance of scars.[111]

Discussion

PHYSIOLOGY OF WOUND HEALING

Wound healing is not a single event but a continuum of processes that begin at the moment of injury and continue for months. These processes take place in the same way throughout the body and for the purposes of description may be broadly divided into three phases: (1) inflammation, (2) migration and proliferation, and (3) remodeling [*see Figure 3*]. Humans, unlike salamanders, for instance, lack the ability to regenerate specialized structures; instead, they heal by forming a scar that lacks the complex and important skin structures seen in unwounded skin [*see Figure 4*].

Inflammatory Phase

The inflammatory phase of wound healing begins with hemostasis followed by the arrival of neutrophils and then macrophages [*see Figure 5*]. This response is most prominent during the first 24 hours. Signs of inflammation are erythema, edema, heat, and pain. These are generated primarily by changes in the venules on the distal side of the capillary bed. In clean wounds, signs of inflammation dissipate relatively quickly, and few, if any, inflammatory cells are seen after 5 to 7 days. In contaminated wounds, inflammation may persist for a prolonged period.

Because wounds bleed when blood vessels are injured, hemostasis is essential. In the first 5 to 10 minutes after wounding, platelets aggregate and release dense and alpha granules. Dense granules contain vasoactive substances that induce vasoconstriction, contributing to hemostasis, and the skin blanches as a result. Vasoconstriction is mediated by catecholamines (e.g., epinephrine and norepinephrine) and prostaglandins (e.g., prostaglandin $F_{2\alpha}$ [$PGF_{2\alpha}$] and thromboxane A_2 [TXA_2]). As vessels contract, platelets continue to aggregate and adhere to the blood vessel collagen exposed by the injury. Aggregating platelets release alpha-granule proteins that result in further platelet aggregation and trigger further cytokine release. The growth factors and cytokines involved in cutaneous wound healing include epidermal growth factors, fibroblast growth factors, transforming growth factor–β (recruits neutrophils and T cells and stimulates collagen production by fibroblasts), platelet-derived growth factor (exerts chemotactic, activating, and mitogenic effects on neutrophils, fibroblasts, smooth muscle cells, and macrophages), vascular endothelial growth factor (VEGF), tumor necrosis factor–α (TNF-α), interleukin-1 (IL-1), IGF-1, granulocyte colony-stimulating factor, and granulocyte-macrophage colony-stimulating factor.[189] Some of these cytokines have direct effects early in the healing process; others are bound locally and play critical roles in later healing phases. The use of specific cytokines to reverse healing deficits or promote wound healing appears to be a promising clinical tool and is currently the subject of ongoing basic scientific and clinical research.[190] Currently, platelet-derived growth factor is the only topical growth factor approved by the Food and Drug Administration that is used in the treatment of chronic wounds. Cellular therapy research with mesenchymal stromal cells and endothelial progenitor cells is another example of active research.

The coagulation cascade also contributes to hemostasis. The extrinsic pathway is essential to hemostasis and is stimulated by the release of tissue factor from injured tissue. The intrinsic cascade is not essential and is triggered by exposure to factor XII. Both coagulation pathways lead to the generation of fibrin, which interacts with platelets to form a clot in the injured area. Fibrin both contributes to hemostasis and is the primary component of the provisional matrix [*see* Physiology of Wound Healing, Migratory and Proliferative Phase, Provisional Matrix Formation, *below*].

Vasoconstriction and hemostasis are followed by vasodilatation, which is associated with the characteristic signs of inflammation. Vasodilatation is mediated by prostaglandins (e.g., PGE_2 and PGI_2 [prostacyclin]), histamine, serotonin, and kinins.[191–193] As the blood vessels dilate, the endothelial cells separate from one another, thereby increasing vascular permeability. Inflammatory cells initially roll along the endothelial cell lining, subsequently undergo integrin-mediated adhesion, and finally transmigrate into the extravascular space.[192]

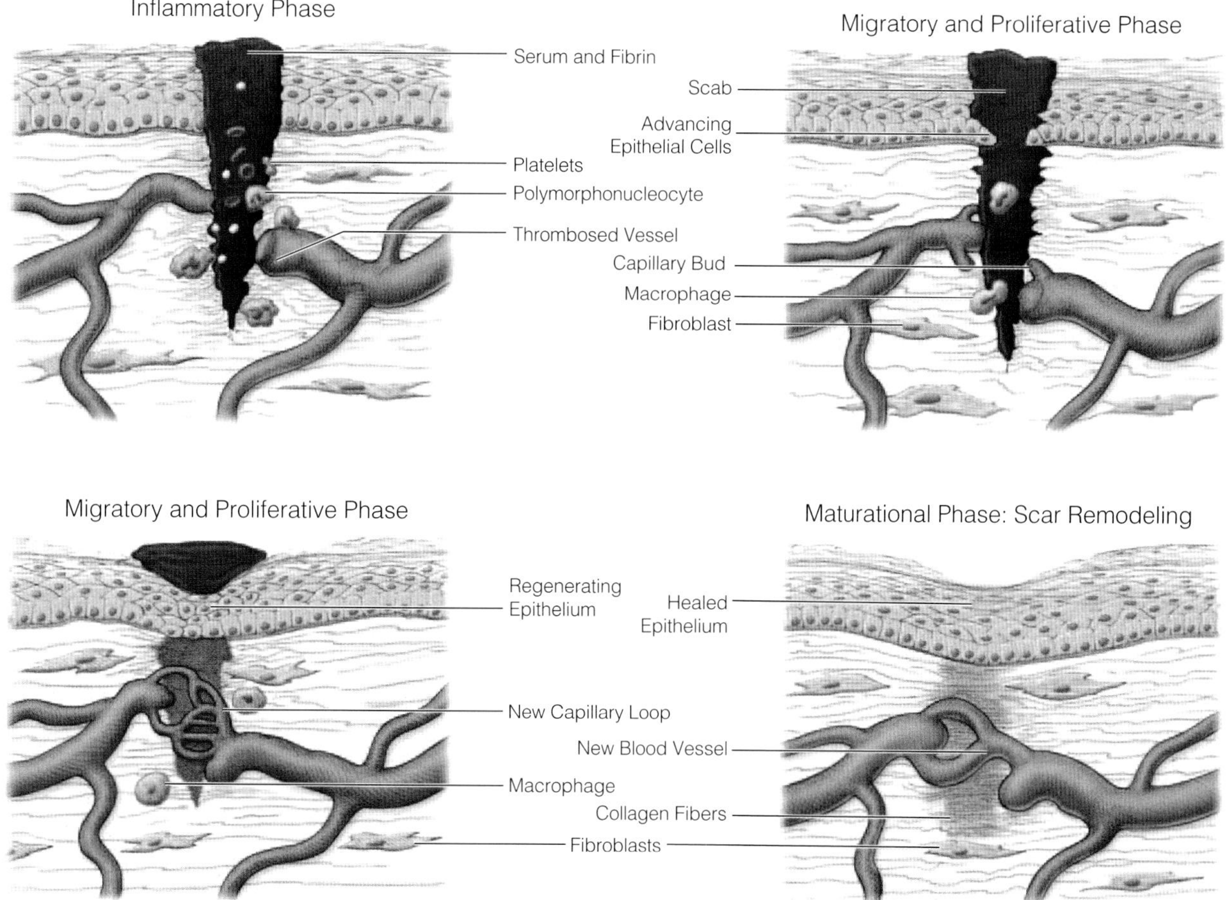

Figure 3 **The phases of wound healing. In the inflammatory phase (*top, left*), platelets adhere to collagen exposed by damage to blood vessels to form a plug. The intrinsic and extrinsic pathways of the coagulation cascade generate fibrin, which combines with platelets to form a clot in the injured area. Initial local vasoconstriction is followed by vasodilatation mediated by histamine, prostaglandins, serotonin, and kinins. Neutrophils are the predominant inflammatory cells (a polymorphonucleocyte is shown here). In the migratory and proliferative phase (*top, right*; *bottom, left*), fibrin and fibronectin are the primary components of the provisional extracellular matrix. Macrophages, fibroblasts, and other mesenchymal cells migrate into the wound area. Gradually, macrophages replace neutrophils as the predominant inflammatory cells. Angiogenic factors induce the development of new blood vessels as capillaries. Epithelial cells advance across the wound bed. Wound tensile strength increases as collagen produced by fibroblasts replaces fibrin. Myofibroblasts induce wound contraction. In the maturational phase (*bottom, right*), scar remodeling occurs. The overall level of collagen in the wound plateaus; old collagen is broken down as new collagen is produced. The number of cross-links between collagen molecules increases, and the new collagen fibers are aligned so as to yield an increase in wound tensile strength.**

For the first 48 to 72 hours after wounding, neutrophils are the predominant inflammatory cells in the wound. About 48 to 96 hours after wounding, monocytes migrate from nearby tissue and blood and transform into macrophages, eventually becoming the predominant inflammatory cells in the wound, typically by 72 hours. Both neutrophils and macrophages engulf damaged tissue and bacteria and digest them. After neutrophils phagocytose damaged material, they cease to function and often release lysosomal contents, which can contribute to tissue damage and a prolonged inflammatory response. Macrophages are essential to wound healing and unlike neutrophils do not cease to function after phagocytosing bacteria or damaged material.[194] In the wound environment, macrophages also secrete collagenase, elastase, and matrix metalloproteinases (MMPs) that break down damaged tissue. Macrophages also produce cytokines that mediate wound-healing processes, as well as IL-1 (which can lead to a systemic response, including fever) and TNF-α.[189]

Migratory and Proliferative Phase

The migratory and proliferative phase is marked by the attraction of epidermal cells, fibroblasts, and endothelial cells to the wound. Cells migrate along the scaffolding of fibrin and fibronectin. This process involves the upregulation of integrin receptor sites on the cell membranes, which allows the cells to bind at different sites in the matrix and pull themselves through the scaffolding. Migration through the provisional matrix is facilitated by proteolytic enzymes. Cytokines and growth factors then stimulate the proliferation of these cells.[189,194]

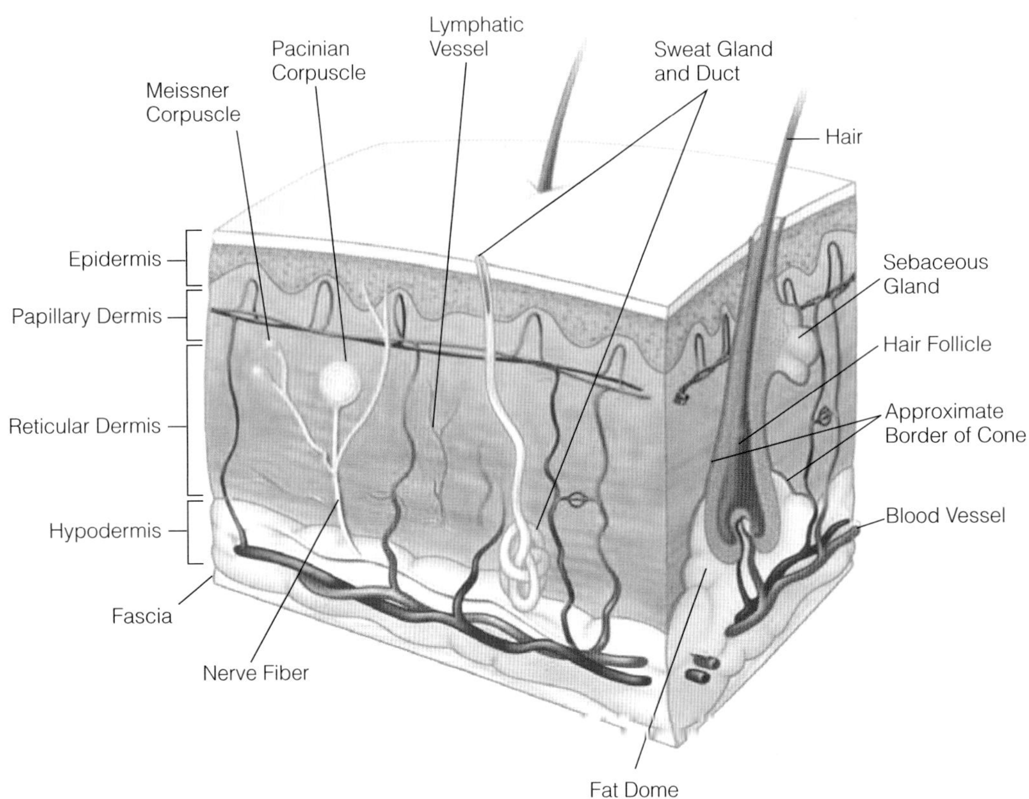

Figure 4 **Key anatomic components of the skin.**

Epithelialization Within approximately 24 hours of injury, epidermal cells from the wound margin and skin appendages begin to migrate into the wound bed. These migrating epidermal cells dissect the wound, separating desiccated eschar from viable tissue.[104] At 24 to 48 hours after wounding, epidermal cells at the wound margin begin to proliferate, producing more migrating cells.[189] As epidermal migration is initiated, the desmosomes that link epidermal cells together and the hemidesmosomes that link the epidermal cells to the basement membrane disappear.[195] Migrating epidermal cells express integrin receptors that allow interaction with extracellular matrix proteins, laminin, collagen, and fibrin clot.[196] When epidermal cells migrating from two areas meet, contact inhibition prevents further migration. The cells making up the epidermal monolayer then differentiate, divide, and form a multilayer epidermis. For incisional wounds closed primarily, reepithelialization is typically complete within 24 to 48 hours.

Angiogenesis and vasculogenesis The growth of new blood vessels begins 2 to 3 days after wounding to support the healing tissue. Angiogenesis is the growth of new blood vessels from existing vessels, whereas vasculogenesis is the de novo formation of blood vessels from endothelial progenitor cells. This process of neovascularization may be stimulated by the hypoxic and acidic wound microenvironment as well as by cytokines (e.g., VEGF) released from epidermal cells and macrophages.[189,197] Endothelial cells from surrounding vessels express fibronectin receptors and grow into the provisional matrix. These migrating endothelial cells create paths in the matrix for developing capillaries by releasing plasminogen activator, procollagenase, heparanase, and MMPs that break down fibrin and basement membranes.[189,198] The budding capillaries join and initiate blood flow. As the wounded area becomes better vascularized, the capillaries consolidate to form larger blood vessels or undergo apoptosis.[199] It is during this phase that the granulation tissue begins to develop, classically described as beefy red tissue. This serves as a sign that the proliferative phase is beginning to predominate.

Provisional matrix formation Formation of the provisional matrix and granulation tissue begins approximately 3 to 4 days after wounding. Lymphocytes begin to predominate around days 4 to 7 and release cytokines, mediating the inflammatory response. T cells are critical to normal wound healing, as demonstrated by the fact that immunosuppressive regimens targeting T cells have detrimental effects on the healing process. Fibroblasts synthesize an extracellular matrix of fibrin, fibronectin, and proteoglycans that supports epidermal and endothelial cell migration and proliferation.[196,200] Proteoglycans (e.g., dermatan sulfate, heparin, heparan sulfate, keratan sulfate, and hyaluronic acid) consist of a protein core that is linked to one or more glycosaminoglycans that anchor proteins and facilitate the alignment of collagen into fibrils.

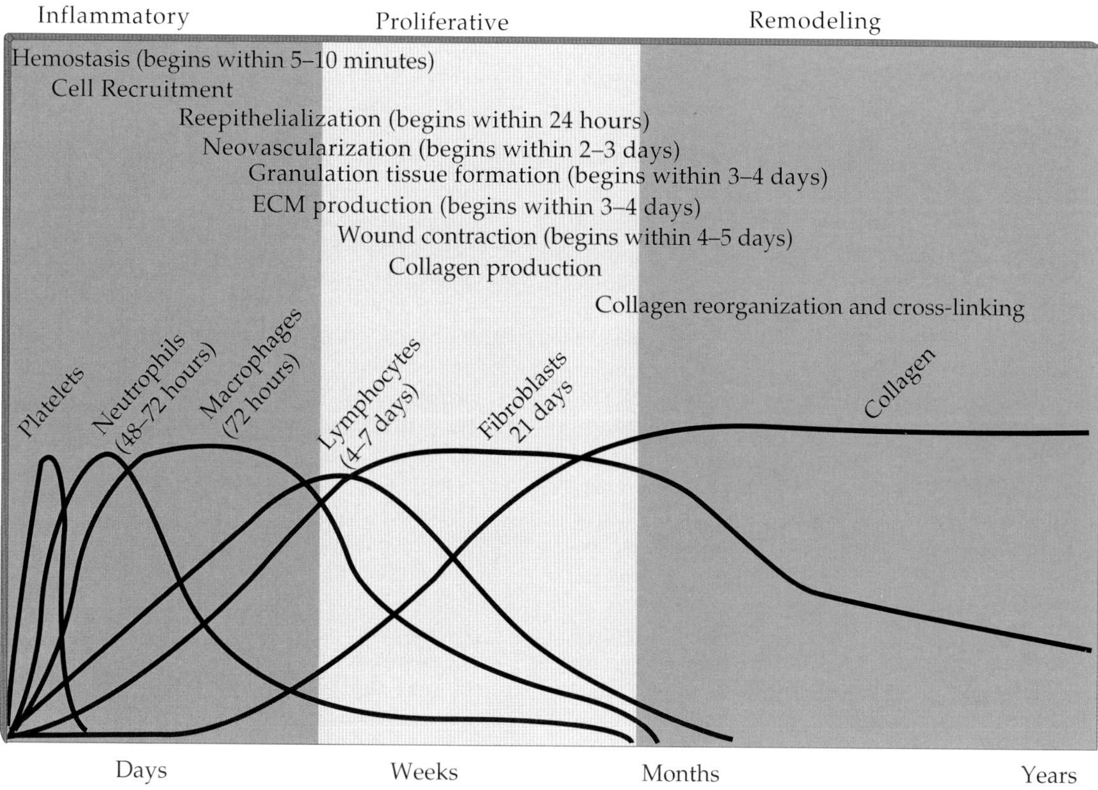

Figure 5 **The phases of wound healing. The inflammatory phase begins within 5 to 10 minutes after wounding with the arrival of platelets. The release of cytokines and chemokines signals other cells to migrate to the injured area. Neutrophils arrive next to engulf damaged material and are soon followed by the arrival of macrophages. Damaged tissue is broken down, and soon epidermal cells, fibroblasts, and endothelial cells migrate to the wound, signaling the beginning of the proliferative phase. Fibroblasts then begin replacing the provisional extracellular matrix (ECM) with a collagen matrix, and the wound gains strength. The rate of collagen synthesis continues at an increased rate for 21 days before gradually declining, marking the beginning of the remodeling phase. Adapted from Figure 1.2 in Herdrich B. Liechty K. Wound healing. In: Porrett P, Frederick J, Roses R, Kaiser L, editors. The surgical review. An integrated basic and clinical science study guide. 3rd ed. Philadelphia: Lippincott Williams & Wilkins; 2010. p. 4.**

Fibrin becomes coated with vitronectin and fibronectin, which are glycoproteins that facilitate the adhesion of migrating fibroblasts and other cells to the provisional extracellular matrix.[201] By influencing cellular attachment, fibronectin helps modulate cell migration into the wound.[202] In addition, the fibrin-fibronectin lattice binds various cytokines that are released at the time of injury and serves as a reservoir for these factors in the later stages of healing.[203]

Fibroblasts then replace the provisional extracellular matrix with a collagen matrix, and the wound gains strength. The rate of collagen synthesis increases greatly after the initial 3 to 5 days and continues at an increased rate for 21 days before gradually declining.[204] Of the many types of collagen, the ones that are of primary importance in the skin are types I and III. Approximately 80 to 90% of the collagen in the skin is type I collagen; the remaining 10 to 20% is type III. The percentage of type III collagen is higher in embryonic skin and in skin that is in the early stages of wound healing. During remodeling, the type III collagen is replaced by type I collagen.

Collagen molecules are synthesized by fibroblasts. Lysine and proline residues within the collagen molecule become hydroxylated after being incorporated into polypeptide chains. This process requires specific enzymes as well as various cofactors (i.e., oxygen, vitamin C, α-ketoglutarate, and ferrous iron). The result is procollagen, which is released into the extracellular space. Individual collagen molecules then align and associate with one another to form fibrils. Covalent cross-links form between various combinations of the hydroxylated residues (lysine and hydroxylysine) in aligned collagen fibrils, with the strongest links occurring between hydroxylysine and hydroxylysine residues. These cross-links are essential to the tensile strength of the wound. Cofactor deficiencies (e.g., vitamin C deficiency in scurvy) and the use of corticosteroids can lead to the synthesis of weak, underhydroxylated collagen that is incapable of generating strong cross-links.

Wound contraction Myofibroblasts are specialized fibroblasts containing alpha–smooth muscle actin microfilaments that contribute to wound contraction.[205,206] The wound edges are pulled together by the contractile forces supplied by the myofibroblast. Wound contraction generally begins in the 4- to 5-day period after wounding and continues for 12 to 15 days or until the wound edges meet. The rate at which contraction occurs varies with the laxity of the tissue and is highest at anatomic sites with redundant tissue. Excessive contraction can lead to contracture, a pathologic scarring that impairs the function and appearance of the scar.

Remodeling Phase

Collagen remodeling begins approximately 3 weeks after wounding. Collagen synthesis is downregulated, and the rates at which collagen is synthesized and broken down reach equilibrium. The wound becomes less cellular as apoptosis occurs. During this process, the extracellular matrix, including collagen, is continually remodeled and synthesized in a more organized fashion along stress lines.[204] Collagen breakdown is mediated by MMPs, and the number of cross-links between collagen fibers increases.[198,207] The realigned and highly cross-linked collagen is much stronger than the collagen produced during the earlier phases of healing. The tensile strength of the wound increases rapidly for 6 weeks after injury, and during this period, heavy lifting and any other activity that applies stress across the wound should be avoided. After the initial 6 weeks, tensile strength increases more slowly for a further 6 to 12 months, although it never reaches the tensile strength of unwounded tissue [*see Figure 2*]. TGF-β's effects on increasing collagen and decreasing extracellular matrix degradation result in increased collagen formation; thus, TGF-β has been linked to the development of pathologic fibrosis and hypertrophic scarring.

Financial Disclosures: None Reported

References

1. Edlich RF, Reddy VR. 5th Annual David R. Boyd, MD Lecture: Revolutionary advances in wound repair in emergency medicine during the last three decades. A view toward the new millennium. J Emerg Med 2001;20: 167–93.
2. Siegel RJ, Vistnes LM, Iverson RE. Effective hemostasis with less epinephrine. An experimental and clinical study. Plast Reconstr Surg 1973;51:129–33.
3. Wilhelmi BJ, Blackwell SJ, Miller JH, et al. Do not use epinephrine in digital blocks: myth or truth? Plast Reconstr Surg 2001;107:393–7.
4. Ostad A, Kageyama N, Moy RL. Tumescent anesthesia with a lidocaine dose of 55 mg/kg is safe for liposuction. Dermatol Surg 1996;22:921–7.
5. Arndt KA, Burton C, Noe JM. Minimizing the pain of local anesthesia. Plast Reconstr Surg 1983;72:676–9.
6. Christoph RA, Buchanan L, Begalla K, Schwartz S. Pain reduction in local anesthetic administration through pH buffering. Ann Emerg Med 1988;17:117–20.
7. Anderson AB, Colecchi C, Baronoski R, DeWitt TG. Local anesthesia in pediatric patients: topical TAC versus lidocaine. Ann Emerg Med 1990;19:519–22.
8. Zempsky WT, Karasic RB. EMLA versus TAC for topical anesthesia of extremity wounds in children. Ann Emerg Med 1997;30:163–6.
9. Moore TJ, Walsh CS, Cohen MR. Reported adverse event cases of methemoglobinemia associated with benzocaine products. Arch Intern Med 2004;164:1192–6.
10. Guertler AT, Pearce WA. A prospective evaluation of benzocaine-associated methemoglobinemia in human beings. Ann Emerg Med 1994;24:626–30.
11. Lee CK, Hansen SL. Management of acute wounds. Surg Clin North Am 2009;89:659–76.
12. Kragh JF Jr, Walters TJ, Baer DG, et al. Survival with emergency tourniquet use to stop bleeding in major limb trauma. Ann Surg 2009;249:1–7.
13. Magee C, Rodeheaver GT, Golden GT, et al. Potentiation of wound infection by surgical drains. Am J Surg 1976;131: 547–9.
14. Brown LL, Shelton HT, Bornside GH, Cohn I Jr. Evaluation of wound irrigation by pulsatile jet and conventional methods. Ann Surg 1978;187:170–3.
15. Boyd JI 3rd, Wongworawat MD. High-pressure pulsatile lavage causes soft tissue damage. Clin Orthop Relat Res 2004:13–7.
16. Hassinger SM, Harding G, Wongworawat MD. High-pressure pulsatile lavage propagates bacteria into soft tissue. Clin Orthop Relat Res 2005;439:27–31.
17. Edlich RF, Rodeheaver GT, Thacker JG, et al. Revolutionary advances in the management of traumatic wounds in the emergency department during the last 40 years: part I. J Emerg Med 2010;38:40–50.
18. Petrisor B, Sun X, Bhandari M, et al. Fluid lavage of open wounds (FLOW): A multicenter, blinded, factorial pilot trial comparing alternative irrigating solutions and pressures in patients with open fractures. J Trauma 2011;71: 596–606.
19. Singer AJ, Hollander JE, Subramanian S, et al. Pressure dynamics of various irrigation techniques commonly used in the emergency department. Ann Emerg Med 1994;24: 36–40.
20. Dulecki M, Pieper B. Irrigating simple acute traumatic wounds: a review of the current literature. J Emerg Nurs 2005;31:156–60.
21. Anglen JO. Comparison of soap and antibiotic solutions for irrigation of lower-limb open fracture wounds. A prospective, randomized study. J Bone Joint Surg Am 2005;87: 1415–22.
22. Haury B, Rodeheaver G, Vensko J, et al. Debridement: an essential component of traumatic wound care. Am J Surg 1978;135:238–42.
23. Mangram AJ, Horan TC, Pearson ML, et al. Guideline for prevention of surgical site infection, 1999. Hospital Infection Control Practices Advisory Committee. Infect Control Hosp Epidemiol 1999;20:250–78; quiz 79–80.
24. Park H, Copeland C, Henry S, Barbul A. Complex wounds and their management. Surg Clin North Am 2010;90: 1181–94.
25. Dorafshar AH, Gitman M, Henry G, et al. Guided surgical debridement: staining tissues with methylene blue. J Burn Care Res 2010;31:791–4.
26. Pollak AN, Jones AL, Castillo RC, et al. The relationship between time to surgical debridement and incidence of infection after open high-energy lower extremity trauma. J Bone Joint Surg Am 2010;92:7–15.
27. Postlethwait RW, Willigan DA, Ulin AW. Human tissue reaction to sutures. Ann Surg 1975;181:144–50.
28. Moy RL, Lee A, Zalka A. Commonly used suture materials in skin surgery. Am Fam Physician 1991;44:2123–8.

29. Edlich RF, Rodeheaver GT, Thacker JG, et al. Revolutionary advances in the management of traumatic wounds in the emergency department during the last 40 years: part II. J Emerg Med 2010;38:201–7.
30. Kanegaye JT, Vance CW, Chan L, Schonfeld N. Comparison of skin stapling devices and standard sutures for pediatric scalp lacerations: a randomized study of cost and time benefits. J Pediatr 1997;130:808–13.
31. Khan AN, Dayan PS, Miller S, et al. Cosmetic outcome of scalp wound closure with staples in the pediatric emergency department: a prospective, randomized trial. Pediatr Emerg Care 2002;18:171–3.
32. Stillman RM, Marino CA, Seligman SJ. Skin staples in potentially contaminated wounds. Arch Surg 1984;119: 821–2.
33. Edlich RF, Becker DG, Thacker JG, Rodeheaver GT. Scientific basis for selecting staple and tape skin closures. Clin Plast Surg 1990;17:571–8.
34. Conolly WB, Hunt TK, Zederfeldt B, et al. Clinical comparison of surgical wounds closed by suture and adhesive tapes. Am J Surg 1969;117:318–22.
35. Singer AJ, Quinn JV, Clark RE, Hollander JE. Closure of lacerations and incisions with octylcyanoacrylate: a multicenter randomized controlled trial. Surgery 2002;131: 270–6.
36. Singer AJ, Thode HC Jr. A review of the literature on octylcyanoacrylate tissue adhesive. Am J Surg 2004;187: 238–48.
37. Janis JE, Kwon RK, Attinger CE. The new reconstructive ladder: modifications to the traditional model. Plast Reconstr Surg 2011;127 Suppl 1:205S–12S.
38. Moran GJ, Talan DA, Abrahamian FM. Antimicrobial prophylaxis for wounds and procedures in the emergency department. Infect Dis Clin North Am 2008;22:117–43, vii.
39. Garrett WE Jr, Seaber AV, Boswick J, et al. Recovery of skeletal muscle after laceration and repair. J Hand Surg [Am] 1984;9:683–92.
40. Trail IA, Powell ES, Noble J. An evaluation of suture materials used in tendon surgery. J Hand Surg [Br] 1989;14: 422–7.
41. Zitelli JA. Wound healing by secondary intention. A cosmetic appraisal. J Am Acad Dermatol 1983;9:407–15.
42. Leaper DJ. Traumatic and surgical wounds. BMJ 2006;332: 532–5.
43. Johnson BW, Scott PG, Brunton JL, et al. Primary and secondary healing in infected wounds. An experimental study. Arch Surg 1982;117:1189–93.
44. Cummings P, Del Beccaro MA. Antibiotics to prevent infection of simple wounds: a meta-analysis of randomized studies. Am J Emerg Med 1995;13:396–400.
45. Cummings P. Antibiotics to prevent infection in patients with dog bite wounds: a meta-analysis of randomized trials. Ann Emerg Med 1994;23:535–40.
46. Cruse PJ, Foord R. The epidemiology of wound infection. A 10-year prospective study of 62,939 wounds. Surg Clin North Am 1980;60:27–40.
47. Gustilo RB, Anderson JT. Prevention of infection in the treatment of one thousand and twenty-five open fractures of long bones: retrospective and prospective analyses. J Bone Joint Surg Am 1976;58:453–8.
48. Peeples E, Boswick JA Jr, Scott FA. Wounds of the hand contaminated by human or animal saliva. J Trauma 1980; 20:383–9.
49. Edlich RF, Rodeheaver GT, Morgan RF, et al. Principles of emergency wound management. Ann Emerg Med 1988;17:1284–302.
50. Talan DA, Citron DM, Abrahamian FM, et al. Bacteriologic analysis of infected dog and cat bites. Emergency Medicine Animal Bite Infection Study Group. N Engl J Med 1999;340:85–92.
51. Fitzgerald RH Jr, Cooney WP 3rd, Washington JA 2nd, et al. Bacterial colonization of mutilating hand injuries and its treatment. J Hand Surg [Am] 1977;2:85–9.
52. Kucan JO, Robson MC, Heggers JP, Ko F. Comparison of silver sulfadiazine, povidone-iodine and physiologic saline in the treatment of chronic pressure ulcers. J Am Geriatr Soc 1981;29:232–5.
53. Dire DJ, Coppola M, Dwyer DA, et al. Prospective evaluation of topical antibiotics for preventing infections in uncomplicated soft-tissue wounds repaired in the ED. Acad Emerg Med 1995;2:4–10.
54. Dixon AJ, Dixon MP, Dixon JB. Randomized clinical trial of the effect of applying ointment to surgical wounds before occlusive dressing. Br J Surg 2006;93:937–43.
55. Davis SC, Cazzaniga AL, Eaglstein WH, Mertz PM. Over-the-counter topical antimicrobials: effective treatments? Arch Dermatol Res 2005;297:190–5.
56. Rhee P, Nunley MK, Demetriades D, et al. Tetanus and trauma: a review and recommendations. J Trauma 2005;58: 1082–8.
57. Updated recommendations for use of tetanus toxoid, reduced diphtheria toxoid and acellular pertussis (Tdap) vaccine from the Advisory Committee on Immunization Practices, 2010. MMWR Morb Mortal Wkly Rep 2011;60: 13–5.
58. Rupprecht CE, Gibbons RV. Clinical practice. Prophylaxis against rabies. N Engl J Med 2004;351:2626–35.
59. Rupprecht CE, Briggs D, Brown CM, et al. Use of a reduced (4-dose) vaccine schedule for postexposure prophylaxis to prevent human rabies: recommendations of the Advisory Committee on Immunization Practices. MMWR Recomm Rep 2010;59:1–9.
60. Warrell MJ, Warrell DA. Rabies and other lyssavirus diseases. Lancet 2004;363:959–69.
61. Iverson PC. Surgical removal of traumatic tattoos of the face. Plast Reconstr Surg 1947;2:427–32.
62. Agris J. Traumatic tattooing. J Trauma 1976;16:798–802.
63. Elek SD. Experimental staphylococcal infections in the skin of man. Ann N Y Acad Sci 1956;65:85–90.
64. Krizek TJ, Davis JH. The role of the red cell in subcutaneous infection. J Trauma 1965;5:85–95.
65. Howe CW. Experimental studies on determinants of wound infection. Surg Gynecol Obstet 1966;123:507–14.
66. Myers MB, Brock D, Cohn I Jr. Prevention of skin slough after radical mastectomy by the use of a vital dye to delineate devascularized skin. Ann Surg 1971;173:920–4.
67. Elliott KG, Johnstone AJ. Diagnosing acute compartment syndrome. J Bone Joint Surg Br 2003;85:625–32.
68. Ulmer T. The clinical diagnosis of compartment syndrome of the lower leg: are clinical findings predictive of the disorder? J Orthop Trauma 2002;16:572–7.

154. Zachariae H. Delayed wound healing and keloid formation following argon laser treatment or dermabrasion during isotretinoin treatment. Br J Dermatol 1988;118: 703–6.
155. Fernandez-Madrid F, Prasad AS, Oberleas D. Effect of zinc deficiency on nucleic acids, collagen, and noncollagenous protein of the connective tissue. J Lab Clin Med 1973;82: 951–61.
156. Andrews M, Gallagher-Allred C. The role of zinc in wound healing. Adv Wound Care 1999;12:137–8.
157. Posthauer ME. Do patients with pressure ulcers benefit from oral zinc supplementation? Adv Skin Wound Care 2005;18:471–2.
158. Macon WL, Pories WJ. The effect of iron deficiency anemia on wound healing. Surgery 1971;69:792–6.
159. Grande L, Garcia-Valdecasas JC, Fuster J, et al. Obstructive jaundice and wound healing. Br J Surg 1990;77:440–2.
160. Koivukangas V, Oikarinen A, Risteli J, Haukipuro K. Effect of jaundice and its resolution on wound re-epithelization, skin collagen synthesis, and serum collagen propeptide levels in patients with neoplastic pancreaticobiliary obstruction. J Surg Res 2005;124:237–43.
161. Greaney MG, Van Noort R, Smythe A, Irvin TT. Does obstructive jaundice adversely affect wound healing? Br J Surg 1979;66:478–81.
162. Lindstedt E, Sandblom P. Wound healing in man: tensile strength of healing wounds in some patient groups. Ann Surg 1975;181:842–6.
163. Swift ME, Burns AL, Gray KL, DiPietro LA. Age-related alterations in the inflammatory response to dermal injury. J Invest Dermatol 2001;117:1027–35.
164. Eaglstein WH. Wound healing and aging. Clin Geriatr Med 1989;5:183–8.
165. Nolan CM, Beaty HN, Bagdade JD. Further characterization of the impaired bactericidal function of granulocytes in patients with poorly controlled diabetes. Diabetes 1978; 27:889–94.
166. Fahey TJ 3rd, Sadaty A, Jones WG 2nd, et al. Diabetes impairs the late inflammatory response to wound healing. J Surg Res 1991;50:308–13.
167. Bagdade JD, Root RK, Bulger RJ. Impaired leukocyte function in patients with poorly controlled diabetes. Diabetes 1974;23:9–15.
168. Greenhalgh DG. Wound healing and diabetes mellitus. Clin Plast Surg 2003;30:37–45.
169. Duncan HJ, Faris IB. Skin vascular resistance and skin perfusion pressure as predictors of healing of ischemic lesion of the lower limb: influences of diabetes mellitus, hypertension, and age. Surgery 1986;99:432–8.
170. van den Berghe G, Wouters P, Weekers F, et al. Intensive insulin therapy in the critically ill patients. N Engl J Med 2001;345:1359–67.
171. Kabon B, Nagele A, Reddy D, et al. Obesity decreases perioperative tissue oxygenation. Anesthesiology 2004;100: 274–80.
172. Cheung AH, Wong LM. Surgical infections in patients with chronic renal failure. Infect Dis Clin North Am 2001; 15:775–96.
173. Colin JF, Elliot P, Ellis H. The effect of uraemia upon wound healing: an experimental study. Br J Surg 1979;66: 793–7.
174. Vigano G, Gaspari F, Locatelli M, et al. Dose-effect and pharmacokinetics of estrogens given to correct bleeding time in uremia. Kidney Int 1988;34:853–8.
175. Mannucci PM. Hemostatic drugs. N Engl J Med 1998;339: 245–53.
176. DeLoughery TG. Management of bleeding with uremia and liver disease. Curr Opin Hematol 1999;6:329–33.
177. Kane WJ, Petty PM, Sterioff S, et al. The uremic gangrene syndrome: improved healing in spontaneously forming wounds following subtotal parathyroidectomy. Plast Reconstr Surg 1996;98:671–8.
178. Gipstein RM, Coburn JW, Adams DA, et al. Calciphylaxis in man. A syndrome of tissue necrosis and vascular calcification in 11 patients with chronic renal failure. Arch Intern Med 1976;136:1273–80.
179. Stephens FO, Dunphy JE, Hunt TK. Effect of delayed administration of corticosteroids on wound contraction. Ann Surg 1971;173:214–8.
180. Demling RH, Orgill DP. The anticatabolic and wound healing effects of the testosterone analog oxandrolone after severe burn injury. J Crit Care 2000;15:12–7.
181. Wolf SE, Edelman LS, Kemalyan N, et al. Effects of oxandrolone on outcome measures in the severely burned: a multicenter prospective randomized double-blind trial. J Burn Care Res 2006;27:131–9; discussion 40–1.
182. Bulger EM, Jurkovich GJ, Farver CL, et al. Oxandrolone does not improve outcome of ventilator dependent surgical patients. Ann Surg 2004;240:472–8; discussion 8–80.
183. Bland KI, Palin WE, von Fraunhofer JA, et al. Experimental and clinical observations of the effects of cytotoxic chemotherapeutic drugs on wound healing. Ann Surg 1984;199:782–90.
184. Lawrence WT, Talbot TL, Norton JA. Preoperative or postoperative doxorubicin hydrochloride (Adriamycin): which is better for wound healing? Surgery 1986;100:9–13.
185. Johnston DL, Waldhausen JH, Park JR. Deep soft tissue infections in the neutropenic pediatric oncology patient. J Pediatr Hematol Oncol 2001;23:443–7.
186. Karukonda SR, Flynn TC, Boh EE, et al. The effects of drugs on wound healing—part II. Specific classes of drugs and their effect on healing wounds. Int J Dermatol 2000;39: 321–33.
187. Karukonda SR, Flynn TC, Boh EE, et al. The effects of drugs on wound healing: part 1. Int J Dermatol 2000;39: 250–7.
188. Ehrlich HP, Tarver H, Hunt TK. Inhibitory effects of vitamin E on collagen synthesis and wound repair. Ann Surg 1972;175:235–40.
189. Singer AJ, Clark RA. Cutaneous wound healing. N Engl J Med 1999;341:738–46.
190. Robson MC. Cytokine manipulation of the wound. Clin Plast Surg 2003;30:57–65.
191. Williams TJ, Peck MJ. Role of prostaglandin-mediated vasodilatation in inflammation. Nature 1977;270:530–2.
192. Ley K. Leukocyte adhesion to vascular endothelium. J Reconstr Microsurg 1992;8:495–503.
193. Ryan GB, Majno G. Acute inflammation. A review. Am J Pathol 1977;86:183–276.
194. Leibovich SJ, Ross R. The role of the macrophage in wound repair. A study with hydrocortisone and antimacrophage serum. Am J Pathol 1975;78:71–100.

195. Gipson IK, Spurr-Michaud SJ, Tisdale AS. Hemidesmosomes and anchoring fibril collagen appear synchronously during development and wound healing. Dev Biol 1988; 126:253–62.
196. Clark RA, Lanigan JM, DellaPelle P, et al. Fibronectin and fibrin provide a provisional matrix for epidermal cell migration during wound reepithelialization. J Invest Dermatol 1982;79:264–9.
197. Detmar M, Brown LF, Berse B, et al. Hypoxia regulates the expression of vascular permeability factor/vascular endothelial growth factor (VPF/VEGF) and its receptors in human skin. J Invest Dermatol 1997;108:263–8.
198. Nadav L, Eldor A, Yacoby-Zeevi O, et al. Activation, processing and trafficking of extracellular heparanase by primary human fibroblasts. J Cell Sci 2002;115:2179–87.
199. Ilan N, Mahooti S, Madri JA. Distinct signal transduction pathways are utilized during the tube formation and survival phases of in vitro angiogenesis. J Cell Sci 1998; 111(Pt 24):3621–31.
200. Greiling D, Clark RA. Fibronectin provides a conduit for fibroblast transmigration from collagenous stroma into fibrin clot provisional matrix. J Cell Sci 1997;110(Pt 7): 861–70.
201. Grinnell F, Billingham RE, Burgess L. Distribution of fibronectin during wound healing in vivo. J Invest Dermatol 1981;76:181–9.
202. Clark RA, Folkvord JM, Wertz RL. Fibronectin, as well as other extracellular matrix proteins, mediate human keratinocyte adherence. J Invest Dermatol 1985;84:378–83.
203. Wysocki AB, Grinnell F. Fibronectin profiles in normal and chronic wound fluid. Lab Invest 1990;63:825–31.
204. Madden JW, Peacock EE Jr. Studies on the biology of collagen during wound healing. 3. Dynamic metabolism of scar collagen and remodeling of dermal wounds. Ann Surg 1971;174:511–20.
205. Gabbiani G, Ryan GB, Majne G. Presence of modified fibroblasts in granulation tissue and their possible role in wound contraction. Experientia 1971;27:549–50.
206. Desmouliere A, Chaponnier C, Gabbiani G. Tissue repair, contraction, and the myofibroblast. Wound Repair Regen 2005;13:7–12.
207. Riley WB Jr, Peacock EE Jr. Identification, distribution, and significance of a collagenolytic enzyme in human tissues. Proc Soc Exp Biol Med 1967;124:207–10.
208. General recommendations on immunization. Recommendation of the Immunization Practices Advisory Committee. Ann Intern Med 1983;98:615–22.
209. Human rabies prevention—United States, 1999. Recommendations of the Advisory Committee on Immunization Practices (ACIP). MMWR Recomm Rep 1999;48:1–21.

Acknowledgments

Figures 1 and 4 Thom Graves
Figure 2 Janet Betries
Figure 3 Carol Donner

6 PREPARATION OF THE OPERATING ROOM

T. Forcht Dagi, MD, MPH, FACS, FCCM, and William Schecter, MD, FACS, FCCM

This chapter concentrates on the general principles of operating room (OR) design and operation. The OR is designed to permit sterile, safe, painless, and effective surgical intervention to improve the lives of patients. Advances in science and technology have significantly increased the complexity of the OR environment. With further advances, the OR will continue to evolve.

The basic aspects of OR design have not changed since the late 19th century, except for changes necessitated by the introduction of complex surgical imaging and monitoring equipment. Effective integration of this equipment into the confined OR space is essential. This chapter focuses on general principles of planning and operation rather than the specific requirements of individual surgical specialties.

Efficient operation of the OR depends on many individuals, some seldom seen, whose skills are essential. They are rarely acknowledged and easily overlooked. Continuous, respectful communication is essential for safe and successful outcomes.

General Principles of OR Design and Construction

PHYSICAL LAYOUT

The basic physical design of the OR is determined first by requirements for patient positioning, illumination, anesthesia, and instrumentation and second by considerations of storage, patient and staff movement, and communication. Basic OR design has not changed substantially over the past century. More recently, however, advances in minimally invasive surgery, intraoperative imaging, patient monitoring, surgical navigation, surgical robotics, and data connectivity have stimulated surgeons and architects to rethink the layout of the OR.

Positioning the Patient

The anesthesia machine is positioned at the head of the table so that the anesthesiologist has an unimpeded view of the machine, monitors, airway, and intravenous (IV) fluids. The suction tubing and electrocautery cords are usually brought off the field toward the feet. However, they may be brought off the side or head of the patient in selected cases depending on equipment location and room orientation.

Laparotomy

The patient is positioned supine on the operating table. The arms may be tucked in at the patient's sides or placed on well-padded arm boards at 90° angles to the table. Care must be taken to avoid hyperextending the arms to avoid injury to the brachial plexus. If the arms are tucked in at the side, the area of the cubital tunnel must be well padded to avoid injury to the ulnar nerve. The surgeon generally stands on the patient's right and the assistant on the left. For pelvic procedures, the right-handed surgeon may elect to stand on the patient's left. The scrub nurse stands next to the instrument tray placed on a Mayo stand over the patient's legs. The back table containing additional instruments is placed at the foot of the bed (Figure 1A).

Two sets of ceiling lights are positioned over the field. In many cases, a head light worn by the surgeon provides additional focused illumination. For pelvic procedures, access to the perineum is either helpful or essential. The patient should be placed in the Lloyd-Davies position. The patient's legs are placed in well-padded leg holders attached to the side of the OR table. The distal portion of the table is lowered to form a right angle with the proximal table. The patient is moved distally so that the sacrum is positioned adjacent to the table brake. Care is taken to protect the airway, arms, and legs during repositioning. A foam pad is placed between the sacrum and the OR table. The leg holders are positioned to avoid abduction of the hips. Care is taken to ensure padding in the area of the peroneal nerves, feet, and calves. Peroneal nerve palsy and compartment syndrome attributable to prolonged pressure are risks. Morbid obesity is a relative contraindication to the Lloyd-Davies position because of the risk of a traction injury to the sciatic nerve.

Thoracotomy

The patient is placed in the full lateral position. A bean bag is a useful device to hold the patient in position. It holds its shape when a suction device is applied. An axillary roll, either a rolled sheet or an IV bag, is placed to protect the brachial plexus. Alternatively, a large pillow may be placed under the axilla and chest. Pillows are useful for supporting the legs. The bottom leg should be slightly flexed and the top leg extended. The position should be secured by the application of 2-inch tape to the area of the iliac crest. Care must be taken to protect the skin from the tape to avoid blister formation. The arms are extended in front of the patient. They may rest on an arm board protected by pillows or sheets. Alternatively, the top arm may be supported by a well-placed "airplane splint." As in laparotomy, the surgeon and assistant stand on either side of the patient and the scrub nurse stands toward the feet. Two lights are positioned over the patient. The use of a head light by the operating surgeon is routine in many situations (Figure 1B).

Thyroidectomy and Parathyroidectomy

Thyroidectomy and parathyroidectomy are the most common neck procedures performed by general surgeons.

a

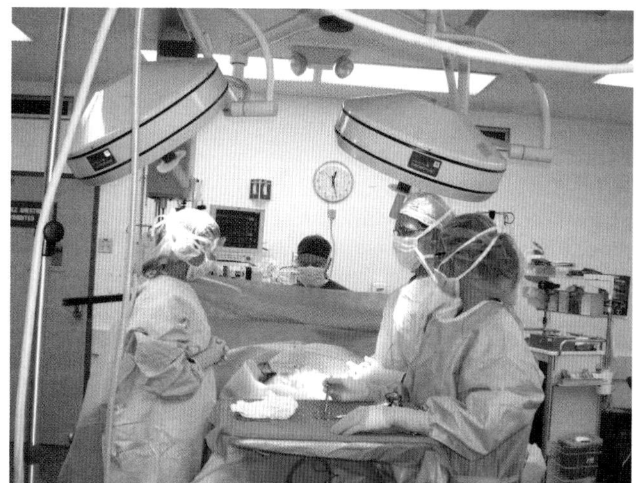

b

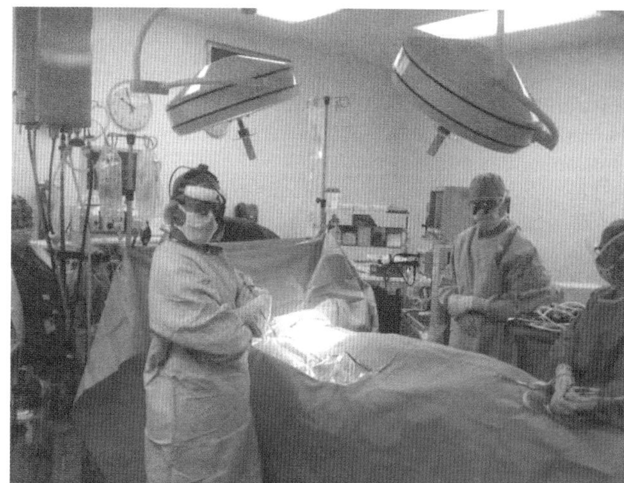

c

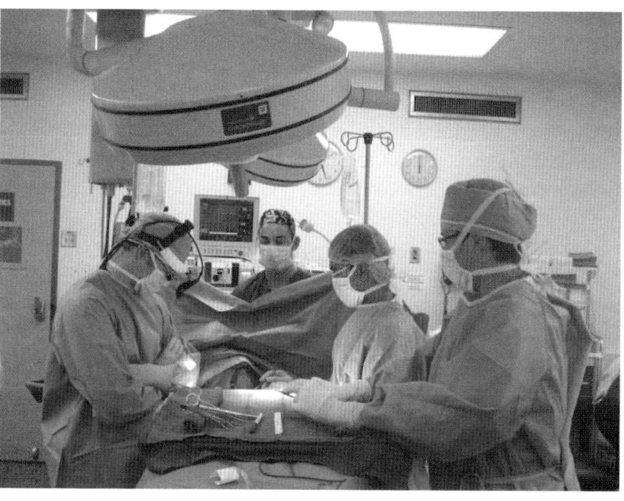

Figure 1 **Patient positioning: (*a*) laparotomy, (*b*) thoracotomy, and (*c*) thyroidectomy.**

Preoperative evaluation should include assessment of cervical spine mobility. The patient is positioned supine on the OR table. After endotracheal intubation, a sheet roll is placed posterior to the scapula. The head is extended and placed on a foam "donut" pad, avoiding excess tension on the cervical spine. Extension of the head should be avoided in the presence of limited cervical spine mobility. The head of the table is elevated to reduce venous pressure. Two ceiling lights are positioned over the neck. Most surgeons use a head light to provide additional focused illumination. The scrub nurse stands next to the Mayo stand holding the instrument tray over the patient's feet (Figure 1C).

A similar position is employed for neck explorations. For unilateral neck exploration, the patient's head is turned away from the side of the planned incision.

DESIGN STANDARDS

Standards for new construction and major remodeling of ORs in the United States generally fall under the jurisdiction of state and local agencies. These agencies, in turn, often incorporate guidelines published by the Department of Health and Human Services,[1] as well as other groups and agencies, such as the Occupational Safety and Health Administration (OSHA) and the Nuclear Regulatory Commission.[2–5]

Numerous articles and books discuss the various aspects of OR design.[6–10] The American Institute of Architects has published a comprehensive set of guidelines for health care facility design that includes a detailed discussion of OR design.[11] Along with such guidelines and recommendations obtained from specialty surgical, anesthesiology, biomedical engineering and nursing associations, the design of new ORs must consider local needs and perspectives. The design of a new OR should be a collaborative effort reflecting the efforts of clinical services, support services, and administration.

DESIGN PROCESS AND CONSIDERATIONS

Designs must accommodate work flow and patient movement. Important considerations include the mix of inpatient and outpatient surgery, the design of the hospital or institution (including proximity to clinical services such as radiology and pathology), the surgical specialties to be served, accessibility to perioperative care units, accessibility of supplies, and removal of waste materials. The need for intraoperative fluoroscopy and sectional imaging, shielding, ceiling mounted microscopes, and surgical robotics and similar advanced technologies will be influential. It is important to allow for flexibility and to anticipate the introduction of new technologies over the life of the design. Time motion studies, simulations, and models may prove helpful and contribute to OR efficiency long term. Balancing flexibility and cost is a continuing challenge.[12]

The geography and physical relationship of clean and less clean areas in the operating suite determine many other aspects of the OR suite. There are two designs in common use. The first involves one or more clean hubs. The ORs are situated centrifugally in spokelike fashion. Clean and sterile equipment and supplies that must be on hand for immediate use are stored in the hub. A peripheral corridor typically affords access to perioperative care units, instrument and anesthesia workrooms, clean storage, staff lounges, and other facilities. Entry and egress from the suite and access to the OR front desk and reception area also involve the peripheral corridor. In the simplest embodiment, four ORs surround a hub. The number can be greater or smaller. Controlled movement through the hub or hubs drives this design.

The second model uses corridors rather than hubs and spokes. Supply rooms are typically situated between adjacent rooms. A less common variation builds a separate supply room next to each individual OR. Older ORs were designed with one door only. Current design favors two, one connecting to the more sterile area and the other to the less sterile area.

The OR must balance the restrictions on access needed for safety and efficiency with freedom of movement for personnel and patients. This balance is equally important in emergency situations and during complex and lengthy operations.

Should ORs be dedicated to specific surgical specialties? There are practical and logistical advantages to dedicated rooms, especially in cardiac surgery, neurosurgery, trauma, and ophthalmology. However, specialty-specific rooms can limit scheduling flexibility. Although it is hard to imagine justifying a room so narrowly designed that it absolutely cannot be used for more than one specialty, dedicated rooms might be emphasized in one institution and versatility in another. Each approach has its advocates. Design and equipment should ultimately reflect expected and projected case mix.

Finally, the design of the OR suite must facilitate cleaning, disinfection and efficient turnover, and the installation and maintenance of installed equipment.

STORAGE

The OR design must provide adequate storage space for urgently required supplies. Storage in hallways and inside the OR can create obstructions and hazards.

CRITICAL DEVICES AND EMERGENCY EQUIPMENT

Critical devices, as well as emergency supplies and instruments, must be prepared and positioned for immediate deployment. Accessories should be stored next to the instruments that need them.

Some hospitals have mass casualty response as part of their mission. These institutions will have special requirements for versatility, equipment, storage, and supplies. The specific design requirements for response to mass casualty events, including nuclear, biological, chemical, and radiation incidents, are not addressed in this chapter.

PHYSICAL REQUIREMENTS

The fundamental model for OR design is a quadrangular room with minimum dimensions of 20 × 20 ft or 7 × 7 m. More often, the dimensions are closer to 30 × 30 ft or 10 × 10 m, so as to accommodate more specialized cardiac, neurosurgical, minimally invasive, orthopedic, and multiteam procedures. Smaller rooms are generally adequate for minor surgery and for procedures such as cystoscopy and eye surgery.

Ceiling height should be at least 10 ft or 3.5 m to allow ceiling mounting of operating lights, microscopes, robots, navigational systems, and other equipment. An additional 1 to 2 ft or 0.5 to 0.75 m of ceiling height may be advisable if x-ray or other boom equipment is to be permanently mounted. In ORs designed to accept intraoperative sectional imaging devices (computed tomography [CT] and magnetic resonance imaging [MRI]), the floors may be elevated to accommodate cabling and wiring for power and data connections. When floors are elevated, the overall height of the OR has to be increased.

Some institutions design or redesign the entire OR suite with the potential to accommodate oversized equipment as well as conduits and cables in both the ceiling and floor. Others prefer to customize individual rooms.

OR and perioperative facilities may be specially constructed to withstand environmental hazards such as earthquakes, tornadoes, and floods or hardened to contend with hostile military or terrorist attack. Standards and specifications for this type of construction fall outside the scope of this chapter.

COMPUTERIZATION, COMMUNICATION, AND DATA EXCHANGE: VOICE, VIDEO, AND DATA

Computers, telephones, imaging, and other systems for data capture, analysis, and exchange should be integrated into the OR design. The ubiquitous deployment of radiology Picture Archiving and Communication Systems (PACS) and the potential of digital pathology to improve surgical pathology services mandate the installation of high-speed broadband connections. Two-way audio with teleconferencing capabilities enables teleconsultation and teaching from and in the OR.

Effective communication systems capable of connecting the OR team, the OR front desk, and the rest of the hospital must be accessible. Emergency communication channels must be tested at regular intervals. Most importantly, systems for communication, data exchange, and data storage retrieval must be available, preferably off-site. Off-site data storage backup is essential for hospitals likely to respond to mass casualty events or subject to environmental hazards.

ASSIMILATING NEW TECHNOLOGIES

Advances in the medical device and information technology (IT) sectors stimulate a constant stream of innovation. Nevertheless, the undisciplined introduction of new technologies can be distracting, contraproductive, and expensive. ORs should be focused on measurable benefit and integration rather than novelty. The introduction of new technologies should reduce complexity and tangibly increase therapeutic benefits and options for patients in ways that have been recognized for more than a decade.[13]

The OR of the future will be characterized by increasing dependence on technology. Although it is essential to track new technologies, they should be assessed and introduced in a disciplined manner. Technology acquisition should be strategic. A full discussion of technology assessment in surgery is outside the purview of this chapter, but the central principles are straightforward. First, the magnitude of unmet needs should be detailed and quantified. Second, the cost-effectiveness of a new technology should be assessed. Next, competitive solutions, including substitutes for the candidate technology acquisition, should be considered. Last, the marginal benefits and burdens of new technology introduction should be quantified.

Patient Safety, OR Efficiency, and Quality Improvement

The OR is a high-stress environment with inherent risk in which members of multiple disciplines temporarily congregate to treat surgical patients. The potential for error and inefficiency is great. Conversion of this group of individuals from disciplines with differing professional cultures and skill sets into a smoothly functioning surgical team is the key to increasing patient safety and efficiency.[14] Surgical team training is an effective method to achieve a "team culture" resulting in improved communication and decreased risk of error.[15] The use of perioperative care protocols reduces failures of communication.[16]

The Joint Commission Universal Protocol became effective on July 1, 2004. The key principles of the Universal Protocol are (1) the preoperative verification process, (2) marking the correct surgical site, (3) taking a "time-out" prior to surgery, and (4) adapting the requirements to non-OR settings. The elements of the time-out concept are evolving and may include introduction of team members; patient identification; review of the patient's history, risk factors, medications, and allergies; availability of appropriate images and equipment; goals of surgery; and potential intra- and postoperative problems. The role of a discussion of planned postoperative care at the completion of the surgical procedure prior to the emergence from anesthesia is not clear at the present time.[17]

The use of a protocol during the hand-over of surgical patients to intensive care results in improved care.[18] Extending the team concept to postanesthesia care has resulted in improved quality of care as measured by intubation times and hospital stay following cardiac surgery.[19] The use of specialty teams during surgery to improve communication and efficiency is logical, but at present, there is a paucity of studies documenting its efficacy. Continuous monitoring is essential to maintain quality.[20]

Patient safety[21] begins with protection of patients from misidentification, physical and chemical hazards, medication error, operative error, and improper positioning.[22] The surgeon is responsible for positioning the patient and preventing positioning injury.[23] The OR team is responsible for procuring and maintaining the equipment for proper positioning and monitoring the patient intraoperatively. The entire team is responsible for preventing falls.[24]

The risks associated with malpositioning deserve further comment. Any bony prominence is subject to injury from excessive pressure. The fragile skin of infants and older patients may be injured by dragging rather than lifting into position. The American Society of Anesthesiologists (ASA) practice advisory on the prevention of perioperative peripheral neuropathies recommends that when practical, patients should be placed in the intended position before induction of anesthesia to test for comfort.[25] Uncomfortable positions should be modified. This is especially important with older patients or patients with degenerative spine and joint disease or skeletal instability.

Two major preventable consequences of malpositioning are neuropathy or plexopathy and skin burns or ulceration. Approximately 80% of surgical procedures are performed with patients in the supine position. Ulnar neuropathy and brachial plexopathy are the two most common complications in this position and constitute 28% and 20% of claims, respectively, in recent closed claims studies.[26–31] Padding of the precondylar groove of the humerus and tucking of the arms or, at the least, restriction of abduction to less than 90° help prevent this problem.[25]

The lithotomy position is used in approximately 9% of cases and is the next most commonly used position.[27,29] Damage to the obturator, sciatic, lateral femoral cutaneous, and peroneal nerves has been observed. These injuries account for 5% of claims for nerve damage in the Closed Claims Data Base. They represent a small but not insignificant risk.[26] Other patient positions have also been associated with malpositioning injuries.

OCCUPATIONAL INJURY TO THE HEALTH CARE TEAM

Professionals engaged in perioperative and surgical care are exposed to biologic, ergonomic, chemical, physical, and psychosocial occupational risks.

Biologic Risks

These risks include (1) parenteral and mucocutaneous exposure to pathogens, (2) respiratory tract exposure to pathogens, (3) exposure to the biologic components of surgical smoke, and (4) exposure to allergens in latex gloves.[32] Strategies to reduce mucocutaneous exposure to pathogens include double-gloving, blunt suture needles, a neutral zone for passage of sharps, and engineered sharps injury prevention devices.[33] The use of N-95 respirator masks reduces the risk of occupational exposure to aerosolized *Mycobacterium tuberculosis* and particulate matter greater than 1 micron in size.[34] Health care workers with allergies to latex should avoid contact with latex gloves and tubing.

Ergonomic Risks

Health problems related to ergonomics, especially back pain, are common. These problems are associated with awkward posture at the operating table, standing for long periods of time, and back injury incurred by lifting patients.

The OR table, monitors, imaging screens, and equipment should be positioned so that the OR team's posture and position are as comfortable as possible within the limits of patient safety. Lifting injury can be minimized by using proper patient transfer techniques and obtaining additional assistance when moving patients in the OR. Repetitive motion injury is a less common but not insignificant risk.[32]

Chemical Risks

Health care workers are exposed to numerous potentially hazardous chemicals in the OR, including anesthetic gases, disinfecting and sterilizing chemicals, specimen preservatives, and chemotherapeutic drugs.[32] Scavenger systems are deployed broadly and have significantly reduced exposure to anesthetic gases.[35] Protective gowns and gloves prevent exposure to other chemicals in the OR.

Physical Risks

Physical risks to patients and the OR team include fire, electrocution, radiation exposure, and laser energy exposure.[32]

Fire The first principle of fire prevention is control of the three elements of the fire triangle: oxygen, fuel, and an ignition source.[36] Air/oxygen mixtures should be adjusted to reduce the fraction of inspired oxygen (FiO_2) to the lowest level consistent with patient safety and satisfactory hemoglobin oxygen saturation.[36] Light, heat, and electrical sources of ignition should be carefully monitored and kept away from paper drapes. The use of alcohol-based skin preparation solutions should be minimized if possible.[37] The use of the electrocautery or laser energy in the airway or in the unprepared intestinal lumen in the presence of high concentrations of oxygen increases the risk of fire.

Radiation exposure Exposure to ionizing radiation is inherently dangerous. For this reason, the extent of exposure must be minimized through the use of all protective means available. Although the hazards of radiation were witnessed early in the 20th century, how exposure was to be calculated and what acute and cumulative doses were dangerous could not be determined until later. In 1928, the International Commission on Radiological Protection (ICRP) was formed to study and set standards for radiation protection. The National Council on Radiation Protection (NCRP) was established in the United States to help set US policy on radiation protection.[37] Until recently, guidelines for radiation exposure have been based on annual exposure limits (maximal permissible yearly dose). The historical means of dosimetry underestimated exposure because of technical limitations and sampling error. For this reason, guidelines now focus on lifetime accumulated exposure as a more useful surrogate for the real risks in those with chronic or prolonged exposure.

Concessions to higher annual dose limits were made for workers allowed higher radiation exposure because of occupational responsibilities. These were called "classified" workers, and they were subjected to strict monitoring and regular examination. Radiologists have been considered classified workers, but not surgeons. Classified workers were permitted more than three times the annual dose than nonclassified.[38]

Empirical data suggest that the typical spinal surgeon performing fluoroscopically guided procedures may receive as much as 1.3-fold the annual whole-body radiation dose allowable for radiologists, although the level of thyroid exposure is less than 10% of the applicable limit specified by the NCRP.[39] A study of endovascular surgeons, in contrast, showed that their radiation exposure fell well within these limits, as well as the limits established by the ICRP.[40]

Another study considered risks to the fetus of the pregnant surgeon. This risk is of particular importance early in gestation, before the pregnancy is recognized. In this study, the calculated accumulative dose received intraoperatively exceeded the threshold dose for the induction of radiation injury by at least two orders of magnitude. Approximately 2100 hours of fluoroscopy are required to reach this threshold.

Childhood cancer is another documented risk of low-dose fetal radiation exposure. The extent of this risk remains controversial. Nevertheless, the ICRP has recommended a maximum dose of 2 mSv and preferably less than 1 mSv during the declared pregnancy. With the protection afforded by a 0.5 mm lead-equivalent apron, however, the calculated expected cumulative fetal dose is less than 0.37 mSv, a figure that extrapolates to a significantly lower dose, and consequently a lower risk, than that derived from natural background radiation.

Surgeons exposed to intraoperative ionizing radiation may avail themselves of several protective strategies. A 1 mm lead-equivalent whole-body shield or apron provides 99% protection. A 0.5 mm lead-equivalent free-standing shield reduces exposure by 90%. A neck (thyroid) shield with 0.25 mm lead equivalence reduces exposure by 60%. Radiation-protective gloves reduce dosage to the hand by up to 40%.[37,41]

Maintaining distance is also protective. Radiation attenuates with the square of the distance. For any given distance from the source of radiation, if the intensity of the radiation at a distance of d = 1, the intensity at any other distance is equal to $1/d^2$. Intensity diminishes as a function of the square of distance.

The effects of distance are manifested quickly. Staff exposure at 1 m distance from a C arm is 1/1000th that of the patient, even without shielding. In a model of femoral fracture, moving from the treated hip side of a patient to the contralateral side reduces exposure by a factor of 57 for the surgeon, 13 for the nurse, and 21 for the anesthetist. If the surgeon remains ipsilateral to the operative site but moves as little as 0.5 m away (cephalad) from the beam, the dose is reduced by a factor of 13, and at 1.5 m away, by a factor of 26. At 2 m from the source of radiation, the scattered radiation received by staff is very small.[42] Nevertheless, because of the problem of accumulated lifetime exposure, no degree of exposure is ever deemed truly innocuous.

Image-guided surgery now plays a major role in many surgical disciplines, including orthopedics, vascular surgery, and urology. The cumulative radiation exposure associated with image guidance may be hazardous. The use of radionuclides for identification of sentinel nodes and intraoperative brachytherapy for the treatment of certain malignancies also creates the potential for radiation exposure.[43]

Exposure to radiation comes from background radioactivity and from radiation sources in the workplace. The ICRP has established recommended yearly limits of radiation exposure for these two categories [*see Table 1*].[44] Recent studies of OR staff indicate that radiation exposure during surgical procedures employing radiation imaging techniques are well within the ICRP limits.[45–47]

All OR personnel should wear radiation safety badges to allow monitoring of radiation exposure on a monthly basis.

Table 1 ICRP-Recommended Radiation Dose Limits[44]

	Dose Limit	
	Occupational	Public
Effective dose	20 mSv/yr averaged over defined periods of 5 yr	1 mSv/yr
Annual equivalent dose in		
Lens of the eye	150 mSv	15 mSv
Skin	500 mSv	50 mSv
Hands and feet	500 mSv	—

ICRP = International Commission on Radiological Protection; mSv = millisievert.

OR personnel should wear protective lead aprons (0.25–0.5 mm in thickness) with thyroid shields during procedures in which fluoroscopy is used. Personnel frequently exposed to radiation should wear lead-containing lenses for eye protection. A mobile shield is useful for additional protection during cine runs.

OR personnel should stand as far away from the x-ray beam as possible to limit exposure. Even a distance of several feet can significantly reduce exposure. Equipment emitting ionizing radiation should be maintained and monitored to ensure proper function.[48] The use of pulsed fluoroscopy and effective collimation of images will help minimize the dose of radiation. Excessive and unnecessary imaging should be eliminated.

Laser exposure Surgical lasers are class 4 lasers that have the potential to irreparably damage the eye and burn the skin. A class 4 laser beam is 1 billion times brighter than a 100 W light bulb.[49] All OR personnel must wear protective glasses with lenses designed specifically for the wavelength of the specific laser being used. Glasses should be inspected prior to use to ensure that there are no scratches on the lens that could render the wearer vulnerable to an eye injury. The windows of the room should be shielded to protect individuals passing by. The number of personnel in a laser therapy room should be kept to a minimum.

Noise and light exposure General environmental hazards include high levels of noise and intense levels of light.[50–52] These hazards are of equal significance to patients and to staff. One early study has indicated that elevated noise levels during orthopedic procedures (above the recommended limits of 110 dBA) were associated with significant hearing loss in orthopedic surgeons.[51] Noise, excessive chatter, and even music can also pose a hazard to the patient by distracting the attention of OR personnel.

Psychosocial risks Perhaps the most underappreciated risks to the perioperative professional are psychosocial. Long hours and nighttime emergencies lead to fatigue. The high level of responsibility, the consequences of error, and the level of oversight have led to high levels of stress and burnout.[53] Unfortunately, violence in the health care workplace, both verbal and physical, is common.[54] Stress reduction can be achieved by team training.[15] Hospitals should have zero tolerance for workplace violence.[55]

OR Design

Advances in videoendoscopic surgery and endoluminal vascular surgery since 1990 have led to the introduction of many complex electronic devices into an OR environment designed at the end of the 19th century. The promise of widespread robotics use in the future may further complicate equipment and use of space within the OR. At the same time, the importance of IT in both the performance of surgery and its documentation will only increase. These changes will inevitably require design adaptations in the OR to ensure adequate power and communication infrastructure support.[56]

The ideal OR of the future will have videoendoscopic monitors, light sources, and CO_2 insufflators mounted on booms that can be introduced or withdrawn from patient care without moving heavy carts or reconnecting cables and power sources. ORs with ceiling- or floor-mounted fluoroscopy permit efficient use of catheter-based endoluminal and intravascular techniques during surgical care. Boom-mounted equipment can be easily moved, permitting more rapid room turnover between cases.

Designing rooms with the flexibility for multidisciplinary use may be more cost effective for many hospitals. In the long run, however, team training for subspecialty fields employing complex imaging equipment and catheter-based therapy may prove to be a more important factor for patient safety and efficiency than any particular OR design.[57] This is a key element in program development. Hospital administration must also commit the capital necessary to complete such a project before proceeding with program development. Balancing OR efficiency, new technology, and cost is a continuous challenge.

Environmental Issues in the OR

TEMPERATURE AND HUMIDITY

In Europe and North America, the OR is typically maintained at 18° to 26°C (64.4° to 78.8°F). A higher temperature is necessary during operations on infants and burn patients to conserve body heat. Fully gowned surgeons prefer the lower temperature of 18°C (64.4°F), but anesthesiologists prefer 21.5°C (70.7°F).[58] The optimum ambient temperature in the OR reflects a compromise between the comfort of gowned and ungowned staff. The ubiquitous deployment of patient warming devices has all but eliminated the problem of hypothermia in the adult during elective surgery.

Recent publications have indicated neurologic benefits from controlled hypothermia in the region of 34°C (93.2°F) in certain cases of asystole, cardiopulmonary arrest, and resuscitation.[59–61] The equipment required for therapeutic hypothermia can be cumbersome.

Humidity in the OR is generally maintained between 50 and 60%. Humidity greater than 60% may cause condensation on cool surfaces. Humidity less than 50% may not suppress static electricity. Static electricity can adversely affect the function of modern computers and smart medical devices.

LIGHTING

ORs are no longer provided with skylights and northern exposure to maximize the benefit of natural illumination.

Nevertheless, effective lighting remains an important factor in reducing stress by providing clear views of the operative field, the anesthesia and monitoring systems, and the nursing area.

The standards for OR illumination were outlined by Dr. William Beck and the Illuminating Engineering Society.[62,63] A general illumination brightness of up to 200 footcandles (ft-c) is desirable in new construction. The lighting sources should be free of glare and nonreflective.[64]

The amount of light required during an operation varies with the surgeon and the operative site. Quantities of light can be measured as a function of the amount beamed on a subject (incident light) or the amount reflected (reflected light). In one study, general surgeons operating on the common bile duct found 300 ft-c sufficient because the reflectance of this tissue area is 15%. The corresponding incident light level would be 2,000 ft-c.[21] Surgeons performing coronary bypass operations require an incident level of 3,500 ft-c.[21] Whether changes in the color of light can improve discrimination of different tissues is unknown.

The powerful lights installed for surgery generate heat through the projection of infrared energy. This is an inefficient but inevitable byproduct of most forms of light appropriate for the OR. Much of the infrared energy can be eliminated by filtration or by heat-diverting dichroic reflectors.

There are several types of overhead lighting designs. For small ORs, a single large overhead light with one or two small satellites may suffice. Larger ORs may benefit more from several large lights with broader orbits. The larger the OR, the more important the installation of multiple light sources that can concentrate light in different areas of the operating field. This consideration is of particular importance where large body areas are exposed or where multiple sites are accessed simultaneously.

The illumination provided by overhead lighting can be usefully amplified and improved with headlights. Headlights have substituted for mobile lights in many OR suites, but both have their place. When headlights are used, spare bulbs must be kept on hand and cabling examined for damage and properly stored after each use.

During microsurgical and laparoscopic procedures, the surgical field is illuminated primarily by dint of the instruments used for visualization. The importance of ambient lighting for the remainder of the OR must not be forgotten.

All ORs should be equipped with battery-powered backup illumination and flashlights for emergency use.

OR EQUIPMENT

The modern OR is replete with medical devices designed to facilitate the work of the surgical team and to support, position, and protect the patient [*see Table 2*]. The equipment in the OR must be chosen and maintained with three concerns in mind: patient safety, surgical efficiency, and reduction of occupational hazards.

ELECTROSURGICAL DEVICES

The common electrosurgical device is a 500 W radiofrequency generator used to cut and coagulate tissue. A current passes from the cutting or coagulating surgical instrument to a dispersion electrode. Heat is generated at the tissue interface as a function of resistance to the flow of current. The vaporization of intracellular water content leads to disintegration of the cell. Heat leads to the coagulation of proteins and hemostasis. Cellular debris is aerosolized. The smoke that is generated is comparable to that accompanying laser use. The smoke and its particulate content may be carcinogenic, allergenic, inflammatory, and infectious. There is little difference between laser plume and electrosurgical smoke.[65]

The electrosurgical instrument requires close supervision.[66] It is very easy to become complacent in its use. The unit generates an electrical arc. In the past, these have been associated with explosions. This risk has been lessened because explosive anesthetic agents are no longer used. Nevertheless, explosion of hydrogen and methane gases in the large bowel remains a threat, especially when surgery must be performed on an unprepared bowel.[67] Because the unit and its arc generate a broad and unfiltered band of radiofrequencies, electrosurgical units may interfere with monitoring devices, most notably the electrocardiographic (ECG) monitor. Interference with cardiac pacemaker activity may occur.[68]

Skin burns are the most frequently reported complication in use. Rarely are they fatal, but they are painful and may require skin grafts, raising the possibility of litigation. The burn site can be at the dispersive electrode, ECG monitoring leads, esophageal or rectal temperature probes, or areas of body contact with grounded objects. The dispersive electrode should be firmly attached to a broad area of dry, hairless skin, preferably over a large muscle mass.[67,68]

Alcohol-based hair care products should be avoided during head and neck surgery because the risk of combustion during the use of electrocautery.

Preparation of the OR should include verification of the proper function and grounding of the unit and proper placement of the dispersive electrode. Smoke evacuators are highly recommended. The National Institute for Occupational Safety and Health (NIOSH) recommends a system that can pull 50 cubic feet per minute with a capture velocity of 100 to 150 feet per minute at the inlet nozzle and positioned within 2 inches of the surgical site.[69] Filters should be installed to capture the contents of the smoke. Used filters are deemed biohazardous. Routine, unfiltered suction is not adequate for this purpose.[69]

LASERS AND LASER SAFETY

Lasers generate focused energy. They have been implicated in skin burns, retinal injuries, endotracheal tube fires, pneumothorax, and damage to viscera and the vasculature.[70] Both patients and staff have suffered injuries.

The laser-safe OR requires specific modifications. The OR should not have windows. Walls, ceilings, and equipment should be nonreflective. Equipment used in the operative field should be nonreflective and nonflammable. A sign warning personnel that a laser is in use should be posted.

Anesthetic technique should also take the use of lasers into consideration. When lasers are used in the vicinity of the face, airway, or chest cavity, the concentration of O_2 and N_2O in the inhaled gases should be reduced to decrease the possibility of fire. Personnel should wear appropriate eye protection. A smoke evacuator will improve visualization, reduce objectionable odor, and decrease the potential for papillomavirus infection or ingestion of toxic fumes from the laser smoke plume.[65,71–74]

Table 2 Devices Used in the Operating Room

Function	Device
Support of patient	Anesthesia delivery devices Ventilator Physiologic monitoring devices Warming devices IV fluid warmers and infusers
Support of surgeon	Sources of mechanical, electrical, and internal power, including power tools and electrocautery, as well as laser and ultrasound instruments Mechanical retractors Lights mounted in various locations Suction devices and smoke evacuators Electromechanical and computerized assistive devices, such as robotic assistants Visualization equipment, including microscopes, endoscopic video cameras, and display devices such as video monitors, projection equipment, and head-mounted displays Data, sound, and video storage and transmission equipment Diagnostic imaging devices (e.g., for fluoroscopy, ultrasonography, MRI, and CT)
Support of OR team	Surgical instruments, usually packaged in case carts before each operation but occasionally stored in nearby fixed or mobile modules Tables for display of primary and secondary surgical instruments Containers for disposal of single-use equipment, gowns, drapes, etc. Workplace for charting and record keeping Communication equipment

CT = computed tomography; IV = intravenous; MRI = magnetic resonance imaging; OR = operating room.

POWERED DEVICES

The surgical table must be properly positioned and adjusted to ensure the safety of the patient and the efficient work of the surgical team. Manually adjustable tables are simple, but those with electrical controls are easier to manage. OR table attachments, such as the arm boards and leg stirrups used to position patients, must be properly maintained and secured to prevent injuries to patients or staff. During transfer to and from the OR table, care must be taken to ensure that the patient is not injured and that life support, monitoring, and intravenous (IV) systems remain connected. Proper transfer technique, adequate staff, and the use of assistive devices such as rollers will help prevent musculoskeletal injuries to the OR staff during this maneuver. Patients with fragile skin, including infants, small children, the ill, and the elderly, should be lifted and not dragged into position.

Other powered surgical instruments common in the OR include those used to obtain skin grafts, open the sternum and the cranium, and perform orthopedic procedures. Powered saws and drills can aerosolize body fluids, thereby creating a potential infection and contamination hazard for OR personnel.[75]

OPERATING MICROSCOPE

Microsurgery is a routine part of many surgical specialties, including neurosurgery, plastic surgery, hand surgery, gynecologic surgery, and ophthalmology. Microscopes may be moved into the OR on wheeled stands or mounted on the ceiling, wall, or floor. Built-in microscopes are best employed in dedicated ORs.[46] All controls and displays must be properly positioned at or below the user's line of sight to allow comfortable and unobstructed viewing.

Modern operating microscopes are servo controlled and counterbalanced. The sequence for properly balancing a microscope should be carefully followed prior to every procedure and each time accessories are added or removed. Improperly balanced instruments have been known to twist or fall, causing injury to patients and staff.

Many commercial microscope drapes are available. Where the laser is mounted to the microscope, it is essential to confirm that the drape is out of the line of fire to avoid contamination, melting, or kindling.

INTRAOPERATIVE IMAGING AND NAVIGATION

The advent of less invasive surgery requires accurate intraoperative confirmation of surgical anatomy through the use of x-ray, CT, MRI, and ultrasonography. These modalities are increasingly accompanied by and aligned with the use of surgical navigation systems. Intraoperative ultrasonography requires a high-quality portable ultrasound unit and specialized probes. Depending on the procedure and the training of the surgeon, the presence of a radiologist and an ultrasound technician may be requested.

The ultrasound unit should be positioned near the patient, and the surgical team must be able to view the image comfortably. In some cases, the image may be displayed on OR monitors by means of a video mixing device. Ultrasound units may also be used to modify the reference image in real time in surgical navigation systems.[76]

Fluoroscopic and x-ray units may be portable or dedicated. Open radiologic units are usually installed either in the OR proper or immediately adjacent to the OR to permit intraoperative imaging of the selected body area. Intraoperative angiography and MRI devices are typically installed in dedicated ORs.[77] Intraoperative CT for neurosurgery, for example, may involve either portable or fixed devices.[78]

The use of sequential compression stockings has become the standard of care for the prevention of venous thromboembolism in the majority of operations for which direct access to the lower extremities is not required [*see 7:6 Venous Thromboembolism*].[79] The air pump often must be placed near the patient on the floor or on a nearby cart. The pressure tubing from the stockings to the pump must be carefully routed so as not to interfere with surgical access.

Suction devices are ubiquitous in the OR. A typical suction apparatus consists of a set of canisters on a wheeled base receiving suction from a wall- or ceiling-mounted source. The surgeon's aspirating cannula is connected sterilely to these canisters. Suction tubing is a common tripping hazard in the OR. In some procedures, the suction canisters may require repeated changing.

EQUIPMENT

Imaging Equipment

Imaging equipment for endovascular surgery can be fixed to the ceiling or portable. The fixed system is also employed in catheterization laboratories and dedicated interventional radiology suites. Portable systems use C-arms with dedicated vascular software packages designed for optimal endovascular imaging. Each of these systems has advantages and disadvantages.

Fixed ceiling-mounted systems have higher power output and smaller focal spot size and provide the highest-quality images. Larger image intensifiers (up to 16 in.) make possible larger visual fields for diagnostic arteriograms. Fewer runs are necessary, with the advantage of reducing the quantity of contrast injected and radiation exposure.

Fixed systems are accompanied by floating angiography tables, which allow the surgeon to move the patient easily beneath the fixed image intensifier. The variable distance between the x-ray tube and the image intensifier allows the intensifier to be placed close to the patient if desired, thereby improving image quality and decreasing radiation scatter. It is generally accepted that such systems afford the surgeon the most control and permit the most effective imaging of patients.

Fixed ceiling-mounted systems are quite expensive (typically $1 to $1.5 million), and major structural renovations are often required for installation in a typical OR. These systems are not particularly flexible. The floating angiography tables and the immobility of the image intensifiers render the rooms unsuitable for most conventional open surgical procedures. As a result, fixed imaging systems are generally restricted to high-volume centers where use rates justify the construction of dedicated endovascular ORs.

The imaging capability and versatility of portable digital C-arms have increased dramatically. State-of-the-art portable C-arms are considerably less expensive than fixed systems ($175,000 to $225,000) while retaining many of their advantages. The variable image intensifier size (from 6 to 12 in.) offers valuable flexibility, with excellent resolution at the smaller end and an adequate field of view at the larger end. With some portable C-arm systems, it is possible to vary the distance between the image intensifier and the x-ray tube, as with a fixed system (see above). Pulsed fluoroscopy, image collimation, and filtration are standard features for improving imaging and decreasing radiation exposure. Sophisticated software packages allow high-resolution digital subtraction angiography, variable magnification, road mapping (i.e., the superimposition of live fluoroscopy over a saved digital arteriogram), image fusion, and a number of other useful features. Improvements in C-arm design allow the surgeon to use a foot pedal to select various imaging and recording modes and to play back selected images and sequences.

Unlike fixed systems, which require patients to be moved on a floating table to change the field of view, C-arm systems require the image intensifier to be moved from station to station over a fixed patient. Although more cumbersome than fixed systems, the newest C-arms have increased mobility and maneuverability. Patients must be placed on a special nonmetallic carbon fiber table. To provide a sufficient field of view and permit panning from head to toe, the tables must be supported at one end and completely clear beneath. Although these tables do not flex, they are sufficient for most operations. Furthermore, they are mobile and may be replaced with conventional operating tables when the endovascular suite is being used for standard open surgical procedures.

Interventional Equipment

The performance of endovascular procedures in the OR requires familiarity with a wide range of devices that may be unfamiliar to OR personnel. These include guidewires, sheaths, specialized catheters, angioplasty balloons, stents, and stent grafts [*see Table 3*]. In a busy endovascular OR, much of this equipment must be stocked for everyday use, with the remainder ordered on a case-by-case basis. The expense of establishing the necessary inventory of equipment can be substantial and can place a considerable burden on smaller hospitals that are already spending sizable amounts on stocking similar devices for their catheterization laboratories and interventional suites. Fortunately, many companies are willing to supply equipment on a consignment and case basis, allowing hospitals to pay for devices as they are used and reducing the volume of devices stocked.

ORs in Other Specialties

Specialty equipment is generally available for permanent installation in ophthalmologic, orthopedic, trauma, neurosurgical, and urologic ORs. The observations offered regarding microscopes, imaging devices and lasers, storage, and physical layout are broadly applicable. The cardiovascular OR and the neurosurgical OR often have complex needs that are more difficult to fill simply by equipping a general-purpose OR. Thus, a neurosurgical OR may need to be equipped for neuronavigation, laser and microsurgery, intraoperative angiography, neurointerventional surgery, and pediatric surgery. In addition, it may need shielding for neurophysiologic recordings necessary for cranial electrostimulation. The presence of fixed or mounted instrumentation per se rarely poses an insurmountable difficulty in adapting a general-purpose OR to specialty use, but the reverse is not the case.

Surgeon's Control of Equipment: Touch Panels, Voice Activation, and Robotics

Inherent shortcomings in the design of OR equipment have been exacerbated by the spread of minimally invasive procedures. Because most of the equipment needed for minimally invasive surgery resides outside the sterile field, the circulating nurse becomes the point person for critical control. Often the circulating nurse is out of the room at the precise moment important equipment adjustments must be made.

Surgeons grow frustrated at the inevitable delays that follow, and nurses often weary of these additional and sometimes distracting responsibilities. As a result, there is great

Table 3 Standard Equipment for Endovascular Operating Rooms

Diagnostic arteriography	Entry needle (16-gauge beveled)
	Entry wire (J wire or floppy-tip wire)
	Arterial sheath (5 Fr)
	Catheters
	  Multipurpose nonselective (pigtail, tennis racquet, straight, etc.)
	  Selective (cobra head, shepherd's crook, etc.)
	Guidewires (floppy, steerable, angled, hydrophilic, etc.)
	Contrast agent (nonionic preferred)
	Power injector

Balloon stent angioplasty	Sheaths (various lengths and diameters)
	Guide catheters
	Balloons (various lengths and diameters)
	Stents
	  Balloon expandable (various lengths and diameters)
	  Self-expanding (various lengths and diameters)
	Inflation device

Endovascular aneurysm repair	Large-caliber sheaths (12–24 Fr)
	Super-stiff guidewires
	Endovascular stent grafts
	  Main body and contralateral iliac limb
	  Aortic and iliac extension grafts
	Endovascular arterial coils

interest in improving the interface of surgical devices with the surgeon. Sterile touchscreens offered the first solution, but many two-handed surgical procedures still make it difficult for a surgeon to control ancillary equipment manually. Voice activation technology offers a potential solution.

Development of voice activation began in the late 1960s. The goal was a simple, safe, and universally acceptable voice recognition system that flawlessly carried out the verbal requests of the user. However, attempts to construct a system capable of accurately recognizing a wide array of speech patterns faced formidable technological hurdles that are only now beginning to be overcome.

In 1998, the first Food and Drug Administration (FDA)-approved voice activation system, Hermes (Computer Motion, Santa Barbara, CA), was introduced into the OR. Designed to provide surgeons with direct access and control of surgical devices, Hermes is operated via either a handheld pendant or voice commands from the surgeon. The challenges of advanced laparoscopic surgery provide a fertile ground for demonstrating the benefits of voice activation [*see Table 4*].

Voice activation offers surgeons immediate access to and direct control of surgical devices. At the same time, it provides the OR team with critical information about the progress of the operation. To operate a device, the surgeon must take approximately 20 minutes to train the recognition system to his or her voice patterns and must wear an audio headset to relay commands. The learning curve for voice control is minimal (two or three cases, on average). Devices that can now be controlled by voice activation software include cameras, light sources, digital image capture and documentation devices, printers, insufflators, OR ambient and surgical lighting systems, operating tables, and electrocauteries.

Infection Control in the OR

Infection control is a major concern in health care in general, but it is a particularly important issue in the sterile environment of the OR, where patients undergo surgical procedures and are at significant risk for perioperative nosocomial infection. Even the best OR design will not compensate for improper surgical technique or failure to pay attention to infection prevention.

Surgical site infection (SSI) is a major cause of patient morbidity, mortality, and health care costs. In the United States, according to the Centers for Disease Control and Prevention (CDC), approximately 2.9% of nearly 30 million

Table 4 Benefits of Voice Activation Technology in the Laparoscopic Operating Room

Benefits to surgical team	Gives surgeons direct and immediate control of devices Frees nursing staff from dull, repetitive tasks Reduces miscommunication and frustration between surgeons and staff Increases OR efficiency Alerts staff when device is malfunctioning or setting off alarm
Benefits to hospital	Saves money, allowing shorter, more efficient operations Contributes to better OR use and, potentially, performance of more surgical procedures Lays foundation for expanded use of voice activation in ORs Allows seamless working environment
Benefit to patient	Reduces operating time, which—coupled with improved optics, ergonomics, and efficiency—leads to better surgical outcome

OR = operating room.

operations are complicated by SSIs each year. This percentage may, in fact, be an underestimate, given the known inherent problems with surgeons' voluntary self-reporting of infections occurring in the ambulatory surgical setting.[80] Each infection is estimated to increase total hospital stay by several days and add materially to costs and charges.

SSIs pose an increasingly difficult problem for institutions with a large Medicare population. Recently, the Centers for Medicare and Medicaid Services (CMS) published the Inpatient Prospective Payment System (IPPS) FY 2009 final rule expanding the list of hospital-acquired conditions (HACs) that will reduce Medicare payments. A number of SSIs figure prominently on this list.[81] State Medicaid directors have also been authorized to deny payment for certain HACs.

The epidemiology and management of SSIs in older adults are receiving increasing attention.[82] SSIs have been divided by the CDC into three broad categories: superficial incisional SSI, deep incisional SSI, and organ or space SSI [*see Table 5 and 2:1 Prevention of Postoperative Infection*].[83]

Factors that contribute to the development of SSI include (1) the patient's health status, (2) the physical environment where surgical care is provided, and (3) clinical interventions that increase the patient's inherent risk. Careful patient selection and preparation, including judicious use of antibiotic prophylaxis, can decrease the overall risk of infection, especially after clean-contaminated and contaminated operations.

HAND HYGIENE

Hand antisepsis plays a significant role in preventing nosocomial infections. When outbreaks of infection occur in the perioperative period, careful assessment of the adequacy of hand hygiene among OR personnel is important. Agents used for surgical hand scrubs should substantially reduce microorganisms on intact skin, contain a nonirritating antimicrobial preparation, possess broad-spectrum activity, and be fast-acting and persistent.[84] The CDC offers the following guidelines[85]:

- Surgical hand antisepsis using either an antimicrobial soap or an alcohol-based hand rub with persistent activity is recommended before donning sterile gloves when performing surgical procedures (evidence level IB).
- When performing surgical hand antisepsis using an antimicrobial soap, scrub hands and forearms for the length of time recommended by the manufacturer, usually 2 to 6 minutes. Long scrub times (e.g., 10 minutes) are not necessary (evidence level IB).
- When using an alcohol-based surgical hand-scrub product with persistent activity, follow the manufacturer's instructions. Before applying the alcohol solution, prewash hands and forearms with a nonantimicrobial soap and dry hands and forearms completely. After application of the alcohol-based product, allow hands and forearms to dry thoroughly before donning sterile gloves.

GLOVES AND PROTECTIVE BARRIERS

There is a high risk of pathogen transfer during surgery. This is a risk from which both the patient and the surgical team must be protected. The risk can be reduced by using protective barriers, such as surgical gloves. Wearing two pairs of surgical gloves rather than a single pair provides an additional barrier and further reduces the risk of contamination. A 2002 Cochrane Review concluded that wearing two pairs of latex gloves significantly reduced the risk of hand exposure. The rate of single-glove perforations is approximately 15%. The rate of inner glove perforation when two pairs of gloves are worn is approximately 5%.[86]

OSHA requires that personal protective equipment be available in the health care setting, and these requirements are specified in the OSHA standard on occupational exposure to bloodborne pathogens, which went into effect in 1992. Among the requirements is the implementation of the CDC's universal precautions, designed to prevent transmission of HIV, hepatitis B virus, and other bloodborne pathogens.[87] These precautions dictate the use of protective barriers (e.g., gloves, gowns, aprons, masks, and protective eyewear) to reduce the risk that the health care worker's skin or mucous membranes will be exposed to potentially infectious materials.

Performance standards for protective barriers are the responsibility of the FDA's Center for Devices and Radiological Health. FDA standards define the performance properties that these products must exhibit, including minimum strength, barrier protection, and fluid resistance. The current CDC recommendation is to use surgical gowns and drapes that resist liquid penetration and remain effective barriers when wet.

These standards are intuitively appealing, but few studies address the comparative benefits of specific types of drapes. A meta-analysis of over 5,000 surgical cases indicated that adhesive drapes increase the risk of SSI (relative risk = 1.23; $p = .03$) and iodine-impregnated drapes had no effect.[88]

Compliance with universal precautions and barrier protection is a challenge. Educational efforts aimed at OR personnel improved compliance significantly, particularly with regard to the use of protective eyewear and double-gloving. These efforts were associated with a reduced incidence of blood and body fluid exposure.[89]

ANTIMICROBIAL PROPHYLAXIS

SSIs are established several hours after contamination.[90] There is a well-recognized "golden period" during which prophylactic antibiotics can be effective. Administration of antibiotics before contamination reduces the risk of infection but is subsequently of little value.[91] Selective use of short-duration, narrow-spectrum antibiotic agents should be considered for appropriate patients to cover the usual pathogens isolated from SSIs [*see Table 6*].[92]

Recommendations for antibiotic prophylaxis are addressed in more detail elsewhere [*see 2:1 Prevention of Postoperative Infection*]. In brief, the principles of optimal surgical antimicrobial prophylaxis include (1) appropriate choice of an antimicrobial agent, (2) proper timing of antibiotic administration before incision, and (3) limited duration of antibiotic administration after operation.

When a preoperative antibiotic is indicated, a single dose of therapeutic strength, administered shortly before incision, usually suffices.[93] The dose may have to be increased if the patient is morbidly obese.[94] A second dose is indicated if the procedure is longer than two half-lives of the drug or if extensive blood loss occurs. Continuation of prophylaxis beyond 24 hours is not recommended.

Table 5 Criteria for Defining a Surgical Site Infection[83]

Superficial incisional SSI

Infection occurs within 30 days after the operation, *and* infection involves only skin or subcutaneous tissue of the incisions, *and* at least *one* of the following:

1. Purulent drainage, with or without laboratory confirmation, from the superficial incision
2. Organisms isolated from an aseptically obtained culture of fluid or tissue from the superficial incision
3. At least one of the following signs or symptoms of infection: pain or tenderness, localized swelling, redness, or heat; *and* superficial incision is deliberately opened by surgeon, *unless* incision is culture negative
4. Diagnosis of superficial incisional SSI by the surgeon or attending physician

Do *not* report the following conditions as SSI:

1. Stitch abscess (minimal inflammation and discharge confined to the points of suture penetration)
2. Infection of an episiotomy or newborn circumcision site
3. Infected burn wound
4. Incisional SSI that extends into the fascial and muscle layers (see deep incisional SSI)

Note: Specific criteria are used for identifying infected episiotomy and circumcision sites and burn wounds.

Deep incisional SSI

Infection occurs within 30 days after the operation if no implant* is left in place or within 1 yr if an implant is in place and the infection appears to be related to the operation, *and* infection involves deep soft tissues (e.g., fascial and muscle layers) on the incision, *and* at least *one* of the following:

1. Purulent drainage from the deep incision but not from the organ/space component of the surgical site
2. A deep incision spontaneously dehisces or is deliberately opened by a surgeon when the patient has at least one of the following signs or symptoms: fever (> 38°C [100.4°F]), localized pain, or tenderness, unless the site is culture negative
3. An abscess or other evidence of infection involving the deep incision is found on direct examination, during reoperation, or by histopathologic or radiologic examination
4. Diagnosis of a deep incisional SSI by a surgeon or attending physician

Notes

1. Report infection that involves both superficial and deep incision sites as deep incisional SSI
2. Report an organ/space SSI that drains through the incision as a deep incisional SSI

Organ/space SSI

Infection occurs within 30 days after the operation if no implant* is left in place or within 1 yr if an implant is in place and the infection appears to be related to the operation, *and* infection involves any part of the anatomy (e.g., organs or spaces), other than the incision, which was opened or manipulated during an operation, *and* at least *one* of the following:

1. Purulent drainage from a drain that is placed through a stab wound† into the organ/space
2. Organisms isolated from an aseptically obtained culture of fluid or tissue in the organ/space
3. An abscess or other evidence of infection involving the organ/space that is found on direct examination, during reoperation, or by histopathologic or radiologic examination
4. Diagnosis of an organ/space SSI by a surgeon or attending physician

SSI = surgical site infection.
*National Nosocomial Infection Surveillance definition; a non–human-derived implantable foreign body (e.g., prosthetic heart valve, nonhuman vascular graft, mechanical heart, or hip prosthesis) that is permanantly placed in a patient during surgery.
†If the area around a stab wound becomes infected, it is not an SSI. It is considered a skin or soft tissue infection, depending on its depth.

The provision of prophylactic antibiotics, where indicated, has been accepted as a measure of surgical quality aimed at a reduction in SSIs.[95,96] A strong economic case has been made for infection control, including prophylactic antibiotics, benefiting the hospital as well as the patient.[97] The perioperative nursing team has a central role, together with the anesthesiologist, in monitoring the administration of preoperative prophylactic antibiotics.[98–100]

NONPHARMACOLOGIC PREVENTIVE MEASURES

Several studies have confirmed that certain nonpharmacologic measures, including maintenance of perioperative normothermia and provision of supplemental perioperative oxygen, are efficacious in preventing SSIs.[101]

Perioperative Normothermia

A 1996 study showed that warming patients during colorectal surgery reduced infection rates.[102] This finding was confirmed in a subsequent observational cohort study that reported a significantly increased incidence of SSI with hypothermia.[103] A randomized, controlled trial of 421 patients, published in 2001, determined that warming patients before short-duration clean procedures (breast, varicose vein, or hernia) reduced infection ($p = .001$) and reduced wound scores ($p = .007$) in this setting as well.[104]

The safest and most effective way of protecting patients from hypothermia is to use forced-air warmers with specialized blankets placed over the upper or lower body. Alternatives include placing a warming water mattress under the patient and draping the patient with an aluminized blanket. Second-line therapy involves warming all IV fluids. Any irrigation fluids used in a surgical procedure should be at or slightly above body temperature before use. Radiant heating devices placed above the operative field may be especially useful during operations on infants. Use of a warmer on the inhalation side of the anesthetic gas circuit can also help maintain the patient's body temperature during an operation.

Supplemental Perioperative Oxygen

Destruction by oxidation, or oxidative killing, is the body's most important defense against surgical pathogens. This

Table 6 Distribution of Pathogens Isolated from Surgical Site Infections: National Nosocomial Infections Surveillance System, 1986–1996[83]

Pathogen	Percentage of Isolates*	
	1986–1989 (N = 16,727)	1990–1996 (N = 17,671)
Staphylococcus aureus	17	20
Coagulase-negative staphylococci	12	14
Enterococcus species	13	12
Escherichia coli	10	8
Pseudomonas aeruginosa	8	8
Enterobacter species	8	7
Proteus mirabilis	4	3
Klebsiella pneumoniae	3	3
Other *Streptococcus* species	3	3
Candida albicans	2	3
Group D streptococci (nonenterococci)	—	2
Other gram-positive aerobes	—	2
Bacteroides fragilis	—	2

*Pathogens representing less than 2% of isolates are excluded.

defensive response depends on oxygen tension in contaminated tissue. An easy method of improving oxygen tension in adequately perfused tissue is to increase the FiO_2. Supplemental perioperative oxygen (i.e., an FiO_2 of 80% instead of 30%) significantly overcomes the decrease in phagocytosis and bacterial killing usually associated with anesthesia and surgery (and significantly reduces postoperative nausea and vomiting). Oxygen tension in wound tissue has been found to be a good predictor of SSI risk.[105]

Avoidance of Blood Transfusion

The association between blood transfusion and increased perioperative infection rates is well documented. In a 1997 study, geriatric hip fracture patients undergoing surgical repair who received blood transfusion had significantly higher rates of perioperative infection than those who did not (27% versus 15%), and this effect was confirmed on multivariate analysis.[106] Another study yielded similar findings in colorectal cancer: the relative risk of infection was 1.6 for transfusion of one to three units of blood and 3.6 for transfusion of more than three units.[107]

A large prospective cohort study published in 2003 evaluated the association between anemia, blood transfusion, and perioperative infection.[108] Regression analysis confirmed that intraoperative transfusion of packed red blood cells was an independent risk factor for perioperative infection (odds ratio 1.06; confidence interval 1.01 to 1.11; $p > .0001$). Furthermore, transfusion of more than four units of packed red blood cells was associated with a ninefold increased risk of infection (confidence interval 5.74 to 15.00; $p < .0001$).

Tight Glycemic Control

Hyperglycemia is common under conditions of physiologic stress, in the intensive care unit (ICU) and in the OR. Tight glycemic control using intensive insulin therapy and continuous glucose monitoring has been shown to reduce infection in the ICU and is emerging as a standard in surgical critical care and intraoperatively.[109,110] It has been associated with a decrease in mortality rate generally in critically ill patients.[111,112] The effects are not restricted to diabetics. In fact, there is evidence to conclude that nondiabetics enjoy more protection than diabetics.[113]

Some questions remain about just how tight control must be to have an effect. There is a small but measurable risk of hypoglycemia with intensive IV insulin therapy, but this risk can be mitigated with continuous or near-continuous glucometry or dynamic scale nomograms.[114]

Housekeeping Procedures

FLOORS AND WALLS

Despite detailed recommendations for cleaning the OR [*see Table 7*], the procedures that are optimal to provide a clean environment while still being cost-effective have not been critically analyzed.[115]

Only a few studies have attempted to correlate surface contamination of the OR with SSI risk. In one randomized, controlled study, for example, the control rooms were cleaned with a germicidal agent and wet-vacuumed before the first case of the day and between cases, whereas in the experimental rooms, cleaning consisted only of wiping up grossly visible contamination after clean and clean-contaminated cases.[116] Both rooms had complete floor cleanup after contaminated or dirty and infected cases. Bacterial colony counts obtained directly from the floors were lower in the control rooms, but counts obtained from other horizontal surfaces did not differ between the two OR groups. Wound infection rates were the same in the control rooms and the experimental rooms and were comparable with rates reported in other series.

Another study found that floor disinfectants decreased bacterial concentration on the floor for 2 hours only. Colony counts return to pretreatment levels as personnel walked about.[117]

Even when an OR floor is contaminated, the rate of redispersal of bacteria into the air is low, and the clearance rate is

Table 7 Operating Room Cleaning Schedules

Areas requiring daily cleaning	Surgical lights and tracks Fixed ceiling-mounted equipment Furniture and mobile equipment, including wheels OR and hall floors Cabinet and push-plate handles Ventilation grills All horizontal surfaces Substerile areas Scrub and utility areas Scrub sinks
Areas requiring routinely scheduled cleaning	Ventilation ducts and filters Recessed tracks Cabinets and shelves Walls and ceilings Sterilizers, warming cabinets, refrigerators, and ice machines

OR = operating room.

high. It seems unlikely, therefore, that bacteria from the floor contribute to SSI. Consequently, routine disinfection of the OR floor between clean or clean-contaminated cases appears to be unnecessary.

According to CDC guidelines for the prevention of SSI, when visible soiling of surfaces or equipment occurs during an operation, an Environmental Protection Agency (EPA)-approved hospital disinfectant should be used to decontaminate the affected areas before the next operation.[83] This statement is in keeping with the OSHA requirement that all equipment and environmental surfaces be cleaned and decontaminated after contact with blood or other potentially infectious materials.

Disinfection after a contaminated or dirty case and after the last case of the day is probably a reasonable practice, although it is not supported by directly pertinent data. Wet-vacuuming of the floor with an EPA-approved hospital disinfectant should be performed routinely after the last operation of the day or night.

DIRTY CASES

Operations are classified or stratified into four groups in relation to the epidemiology of SSIs [*see 2:1 Prevention of Postoperative Infection*][118]:

- Clean operations are those elective cases in which the gastrointestinal (GI) tract or the respiratory tract is not entered and there are no major breaks in technique. The infection rate in this group should be less than 3%.
- Clean-contaminated operations are those elective cases in which the respiratory or the GI tract is entered or during which a break in aseptic technique has occurred. The infection rate in such cases should be less than 10%.
- Contaminated operations are those cases in which a fresh traumatic wound is present or gross spillage of GI contents occurs.
- Dirty or infected operations include those in which bacterial inflammation occurs or in which pus is present. The infection rate may be as high as 40% in a contaminated or dirty operation.

Fear that bacteria from dirty or heavily contaminated cases could be transmitted to subsequent cases has resulted in the development of numerous and costly rituals of OR cleanup. However, there are no prospective studies and no large body of relevant data to support the usefulness of such rituals. In fact, one study found no significant difference in environmental bacterial counts after clean cases than after dirty ones.[119] Numerous authorities have recommended that there be only one standard of cleaning the OR after either clean or dirty cases.[115,119,120] This recommendation is reasonable because of two important considerations:

- Any patient may be a source of contamination caused by unrecognized bacterial or viral infection.
- The second major source of OR contamination is the personnel who work there.

Rituals applied to dirty cases include placing a germicide-soaked mat outside the OR door, allowing the OR to stand idle for an arbitrary period after cleanup of a dirty procedure, and using two circulating nurses, one inside the room and one outside. None of these practices has a sound theoretical or factual basis.

By tradition, dirty cases are scheduled after all of the clean cases of the day have been completed. This restriction, however, reduces the efficiency with which operations can be scheduled and may unnecessarily delay emergency cases. There are no data to support special cleaning procedures or the closing of an OR after a contaminated or dirty operation has been performed.[121] Mats placed outside the entrance to the OR suite show neither a reduction in the number of organisms on shoes and stretcher wheels nor a reduction in SSI risk.[122]

Data Management in the OR

Regular analysis of OR data is essential to monitor efficiency and correct deficiency.[123] OR efficiency is maximized by adherence to several basic principles:

1. The number of ORs available should be matched to the number required to achieve good use.
2. Nurses and anesthesiologists rather than attending surgeons should control access to the surgical schedule.
3. Surgeons should be allowed to follow themselves.

4. Block time should be provided to surgeons.
5. Systems should be established to enable and enforce efficient turnover between cases.[124]

The distinction between efficiency and effectiveness is important. Measures of effectiveness relate achievements to goals. Measures of efficiency relate achievements to cost. The OR must be both efficient and effective.

Data must be both available and rapidly accessible. Automation of OR data is critical and must integrate with the institutional health information system (HIS).[125] Hospital-wide data regarding work flow, staffing, referral patterns, and even parking may yield useful information for improvements in OR efficacy and efficiency.[126]

OR SCHEDULING

OR scheduling systems should be designed to track all of the operational aspects of the OR, including patients, resources, rooms, and staff. They should be fully integrated into the institutional HIS while also interfacing with key elements located in other parts of the hospital (or ambulatory center), including finance, materials management, electronic medical records, radiology, pathology, nursing, the emergency room, labor and delivery, the blood bank, and the pharmacy.

One of the most important purposes of a good OR scheduling system is to allow informed case substitution. Informed case substitution is critical because surgical scheduling must contend with frequent last-minute case cancellations.[127] Different specialties differ widely in their scheduling practices. An understanding of these practices allows the OR to use resources to maximum efficiency.[128]

Information systems that predict and fill unexpected openings already exist in the transportation and manufacturing industries. In the future, such technology may be a useful adjunct to computerized OR scheduling.[127]

QUALITY IMPROVEMENT

The key to increased OR efficiency is increased productivity. Standardization of internal procedures reduces bottlenecks. Computerization speeds the flow of information so that continuous improvement of the system becomes possible. Before a desired improvement can be implemented, the proposed change must be tested quickly so that its effect can be determined, ideally through a small-scale pilot implementation. This requires a collaborative effort, in which the group involved in the change learns how to "plan, do, check, and act." These are the elements of the so-called "PDCA cycle," a classic quality initiative method. During the PDCA cycle, teams are encouraged to strategize and communicate about various solutions and look for changes that can be made. A change is tested, quickly evaluated, and adopted if efficacious. The PDCA cycle depends on integrated surgical teams with open communication and mutual respect. Such teams remain the key to a safe, efficient, and effective OR.[89]

Dr. Dagi is a director for Acela, Inc. and IntelliDx, Inc. His personal investment portfolio includes pharmaceutical and medical device companies, none of whose products have been mentioned in this chapter. He chairs the Scientific Advisory Board for Dupont life sciences. He has received neither financial nor research support from any of these entities.

Dr Schecter has no significant financial or other relationships with pharmaceutical, medical device, or biologics companies relevant to this chapter.

References

1. Guidelines for construction and equipment of hospital and medical facilities. Bethesda (MD): US Department of Health and Human Services; 1984. DHHS Publication No.: (HRS-M-HF) 84-1.
2. Maloney ME. The dermatological surgical suite—design and materials. In: Grekin M, editor. Practical manuals in dermatologic surgery. New York: Churchill Livingstone; 1991.
3. Jolesz FA, Shtern F. The operating room of the future. Report of the National Cancer Institute Workshop "Imaging-Guided Stereotactic Tumor Diagnosis and Treatment." Invest Radiol 1992;27:326.
4. Green FL, Taylor NC. Operating room configuration. In: Ballantyne G, Leahy PF, Modlin IR, editors. Laparoscopic surgery. Philadelphia: WB Saunders; 1994. p. 34.
5. Laufman H. Surgical hazard control: effect of architecture and engineering. Arch Surg 1973;107:552.
6. Johnston D, Hunter A, editors. The design and utilization of operating theatres. London: Edward Arnold; 1984.
7. Klebanoff G. Operating-room design: an introduction. Bull Am Coll Surg 1979; 64(11):6.
8. Smith W. Planning the surgical suite. New York: FW Dodge Corp; 1960.
9. Putsep E. Planning of surgical centres. London: Lloyd-Luke Ltd; 1973.
10. A bibliography of the operating room environment. Chicago: American College of Surgeons; 1995.
11. The American Institute of Architects. Guidelines for construction and equipment of hospital and health care facilities. Washington (DC): The American Institute of Architects Press; 2001.
12. Heslin MJ, Doster BE, Daily SL, et al. Durable improvements in efficiency, safety and satisfaction in the operating room. J Am Coll Surg 2008;206:1083–9, discussion 1089–90.
13. Mathius JM. OR of the future to be less complicated, more efficient. OR Manager 1995;11:7.
14. Davenport DL, Henderson WG, Mosca CL, et al. Risk-adjusted morbidity in teaching hospitals correlates with reported levels of communication and collaboration on surgical teams but not with scale measures of teamwork climate, safety climate, or working conditions. J Am Coll Surg 2007;205: 778.
15. Awad SS, Fagan SP, Bellows C, et al. Bridging the communication gap in the operating room with medical team training. Am J Surg 2005;190:770.
16. Lingard L, Regehr G, Orser B, et al. Evaluation of a pre-operative check list and team briefing among surgeons, nurses and anesthesiologists to reduce failures in communication. Arch Surg 2008;143:12.
17. The Joint Commission. Universal Protocol. Available at: http://www.jointcommission.org/PatientSafety/UniversalProtocol/up_facts.htm (accessed July 29, 2008).
18. Catchpole KR, de Leval MR, McEwan A, et al. Patient handover from surgery to intensive care: using Formula 1 pit-stop and aviation models to improve safety and quality. Paediatr Anaesth 2007;17:470.
19. Ender J, Borger MA, Scholz M, et al. Cardiac surgery fast-track treatment in a postanesthetic care unit: six-month results of the Leipzig fast-track concept. Anesthesiology 2008;109:61.
20. Zohar E, Noga Y, Davidson E, et al. Peri-operative patient safety: correct patient, correct surgery, correct side—a multifaceted, cross-organizational, interventional study. Anesth Analg 2007;105:443.

21. Kern KA. The National Patient Safety Foundation: what it offers surgeons. Bull Am Coll Surg 1998;83:24.
22. Egan MT, Sandberg WS. Auto identification technology and its impact on patient safety in the operating room of the future. Surg Innov 2007;14:41–50, discussion 51.
23. Christian CK, Gustafson ML, Roth EM, et al. A prospective study of patient safety in the operating room. Surgery 2006;139: 159–73.
24. Practice advisory for the prevention of perioperative peripheral neuropathies. Anesthesiology 2000;92:1168.
25. Cheney FW, Domino KB, Caplan RA, et al. Nerve injury associated with anesthesia. Anesthesia 1999;90:1062.
26. Warner ME, LaMaster LM, Thoening AK, et al. Compartment syndrome in surgical patients. Anesthesiology 2001;94:705
27. Barash PG, Cullen BF, Stoelting RK. Clinical anesthesia. 5th edition. Philadelphia: Lippincott, Williams & Wilkins; 2005. p. 639–66.
28. Cucciara RF, Faust RJ. Patient positioning. In: Miller RD, editor. Anesthesia. 5th ed. Philadelphia: Churchill Livingstone; 2000.
29. West JB. Respiratory physiology. 2nd ed. Baltimore: Williams & Wilkins; 1979.
30. Benumof JL. Respiratory physiology and respiratory function during anesthesia. In: Miller RD, editor. Anesthesia. 5th ed. Philadelphia: Churchill Livingstone; 2000.
31. AORN. Position statement on workplace safety. Available at: http://www.aorn.org/PracticeResources/AORNPositionStatements/Position_WorkplaceSafety (accessed July 29, 2008).
32. American College of Surgeons. Statement on sharps safety. Bull Am Coll Surg 2007;92:34–7.
33. Panni MK, Corn SB. Scavenging in the operating room. Curr Opin Anaesthesiol 2003;16:611.
34. Daane SP, Toth BA. Fire in the operating room: principles and prevention. Plast Reconstr Surg 2005;115:73e.
35. Meneghetti SC, Morgan MM, Fritz J, et al. Operating room fires: optimizing safety. Plast Reconstr Surg 2007;120:1701.
36. Batra S, Gupta R. Alcohol based surgical prep solution and the risk of fire in the operating room: a case report. Patient Saf Surg 2008;2:10.
37. Statkiewicz-Sherer MA, Visconti PJ, Ritenour ER, et al. Radiation protection in medical radiography. St. Louis: Mosby; 1998.
38. Hafez MA, Smith RM, Matthews SJ, et al. Radiation exposure to the hands of orthopaedic surgeons: Are we underestimating the risk? Arch Orthop Trauma Surg 2005; 125:330–5.
39. Ul Haque M, Shufflebarger HL, O'Brien M, Macagno A. Radiation exposure during pedicle screw placement in adolescent idiopathic scoliosis: Is fluoroscopy safe? Spine 2006;31:2516–20.
40. Ho P, Cheng SW, Wu PM, et al. Ionizing radiation absorption of vascular surgeons during endovascular procedures. J Vasc Surg 2007;46:455–9.
41. Shapiro J. Radiation protection: A guide for scientists, physicians and regulators. 4th ed. Cambridge (MA): Harvard University Press; 2002.
42. Theocharopoulos N, Damilakis J, Perisinakis K, et al. Image-guided reconstruction of femoral fractures: is the staff progeny safe? Clin Orthop Relat Res 2005;430:182–8.
43. Fuchs M, Schmid A, Eiteljorge T, et al. Exposure of the surgeon to radiation during surgery. Int Orthop 1998;22:153.
44. Radiological protection and safety in medicine: a report of the International Commission of Radiological Protection. Ann ICRP 1996;26:1.
45. Lipsitz EC, Veith FJ, Ohki T, et al. Does endovascular repair of aortoiliac aneurysms pose a radiation safety hazard to vascular surgeons? J Vasc Surg 2000;32:702.
46. Singh PJ, Perera NS, Dega R. Measurement of the dose of radiation to the surgeon during foot and ankle surgery. J Bone Joint Surg Br 2007;89:1060.
47. National Institute for Occupational Safety and Health. Guidelines for protecting the safety and health of healthcare workers. Available at: http://www.cdc.gov/niosh/hcwold5d.html (accessed July 31, 2008).
48. Andersen K. Safe use of lasers in the operating room: what perioperative nurses should know. AORN J 2004;79:171–88.
49. Mehlman CT, DiPasquale TG. Radiaiton exposure to the orthopaedic surgical team during fluoroscopy: how far away is far enough? J Orthop Trauma 11:392–8, 1997.
50. Ray CD, Levinson R. Noise pollution in the operating room: a hazard to surgeons, personnel, and patients. J Spinal Disord 1992; 5:485.
51. Willett KM. Noise-induced hearing loss in orthopaedic staff. J Bone Joint Surg Br 1991;73:113–5.
52. Cowan C Jr. Light hazards in the operating room. J Natl Med Assoc 1992;84:425.
53. Marine A. Rutschlainen J, Serra C, Verbeek J. Preventing occupational stress in healthcare workers. Cochrane Database Syst Rev 2006;(18):CD002892.
54. Lanza ML, Zeiss RA, Rierdan J. Non-physical violence: a risk factor for physical violence in health care settings. AAOHN J 2006;54:397–402.
55. Council on Surgical and Perioperative Safety. Statement on workplace violence. Available at: http://www.cspsteam.org (accessed July 31, 2008).
56. Staylor A. Robotics. Moving surgery into the information age. Windhover Medtech Insight 2007;(October):1–8.
57. Fernsebner B. Building a staffing plan based on OR's needs. OR Manager 1996;12(2):7.
58. Chinyanga HM. Temperature regulation and anesthesia. Pharmacol Ther 1984;26: 147.
59. The Hypothermia after Cardiac Arrest Study Group: Mild therapeutic hypothermia to improve the neurologic outcome after cardiac arrest. N Engl J Med 2001;346: 549–56.
60. Nolan JP, Morley PT, Vanden Hoek TL, Hickey RW. Therapeutic hypothermia after cardiac arrest. An advisory statement by the Advanced Life Support Task Force of the International Liaison Committee on Resuscitation. Circulation 2003;108: 118–21.
61. Polderman, KH. Induced hypothermia and fever control for prevention and treatment of neurological injuries. Lancet 2008;371: 1955–61.
62. Beck WC. Choosing surgical illumination. Am J Surg 1980;140:327.
63. Beck WC. Operating room illumination: the current state of the art. Bull Am Coll Surg 1981;66(5):10.
64. Verrinder J. Use of right lighting levels essential. Health Estate 2007;61(6):31–2.
65. McCormick PW. Bovie smoke. A perilous plume. AANS Neurosurg 2008;17:10–2.
66. AORN Recommended Practices Subcommittee: Recommended practices: electrosurgery. AORN J 1985;41:633.
67. Pearce J. Current electrosurgical practice: hazards. J Med Eng Technol 9:107, 1985
68. Bochenko WJ. A review of electrosurgical units in the operating room. J Clin Eng 1977;2:313.
69. AORN Recommended Practices Committee: Recommended practices for electrosurgery. AORN J 2005;81:616–8, 621–6, 629–32.
70. Lobraico RB. Laser safety in health care facilities: an overview. Bull Am Coll Surg 1991;76(8):16.
71. Gloster HM Jr, Roenigk RK. Risk of acquiring human papillomavirus from the plume produced by the carbon dioxide laser in the treatment of warts. J Am Acad Dermatol 1995;32:436.
72. Wisniewski PM, Warhol MJ, Rando RF, et al. Studies on the transmission of viral disease via the CO2 laser plume and ejecta. J Reprod Med 1990;35:1117.
73. King B, McCullough J. Health hazard evaluation report 2001-0030-3020. NIOSH; 2006.
74. Jewett DL, Heinsohn P, Bennett C, et al. Blood-containing aerosols generated by surgical techniques: a possible infectious hazard. Am Ind Hyg Assoc J 1992;53:228.
75. Patkin M. Ergonomics and the operating microscope. Adv Ophthalmol 1978;37:53.
76. Bates LM, Robb RA. Investigation of ultrasound image based correction of intraoperative brain shift. In: Proceedings of the IEEE 2nd International Symposium on Bioinformatics and Bioengineering Conference. 2001. p. 254–61.
77. Ntoukas V, Krishnan R, Seifert V. The new generation polestar n20 for conventional neurosurgical operating rooms: a preliminary report. Neurosurgery 2008;63(3 Suppl 1):82–9; discussion 89–90.
78. Jacob AL, Regazzoni P, Bilecen D, et al. Medical technology integration: CT, angiography, imaging-capable OR-table, navigation and robotics in a multifunctional sterile suite. Minim Invasive Ther Allied Technol 2007;16:2005–11.
79. Walenga JM, Fareed J. Current status on new anticoagulant and antithrombotic drugs and devices. Curr Opin Pulmon Med 1997; 3:291.
80. Barie PS. Surgical site infections: epidemiology and prevention. Surg Infect 2002;3 (Suppl 1):S9.
81. CMS Office of Public Affairs: CMS improves patient safety for Medicare and Medicaid by addressing never events. Available at: http://www.cms/hhs.gov/apps/media/press/factsheet.asp (accessed August 10, 2008).
82. Young M, Washer L, Malani P. Surgical site infections in older adults: epidemiology and management strategies. Drugs Aging 2008; 25:399–414.
83. Mangram AJ, Horan TC, Pearson ML, et al. The Hospital Infection Control Practices Advisory Committee. Guideline for prevention of surgical site infection, 1999. Am J Infect Control 1999;27:98.
84. AORN. Standards and recommended practices. Denver (CO):AORN; 2008. p. 337–406.
85. Boyce JM, Pittet D, Healthcare Infection Control Practices Advisory Committee, HICPAC/SHEA/APIC/IDSA Hand Hygiene Task Force. Guideline for hand hygiene in health-care settings. Recommendations of the Healthcare Infection Control Practices Advisory Committee and the HICPA/SHEA/APIC/IDSA Hand Hygiene Task Force. MMWR Recomm Rep 2002; 51(RR-16):1.
86. Tanner J, Parkinson H. Double-gloving to reduce surgical cross-infection (Cochrane Review). Cochrane Database Syst Rev 2002,(3).CD003087.

87. Universal precautions for prevention of transmission of human immunodeficiency virus, hepatitis B virus, and other blood-borne pathogens in health-care settings. MMWR Morb Mortal Wkly Rep 1988;37: 377.
88. Webster J, Alghamdi AA. Use of plastic adhesive drapes during surgery for preventing surgical site infection. Cochrane Database Syst Rev 2007;(4):CD006353.
89. Kim LE, Jeffe DB, Evanoff BA, et al. Improved compliance with universal precautions in the operating room following an educational intervention. Infect Control Hosp Epidemiol 2001;22:522.
90. Burke JF. The effective period of preventive antibiotic action in experimental incisions and dermal lesions. Surgery 1961;50:161.
91. Classen DC, Evans RS, Pestotnik SL, et al. The timing of prophylactic administration of antibiotics and the risk of surgical-wound infection. N Engl J Med 1992;326:281.
92. Stewart AH, Eyers PS, Earnshaw JJ. Prevention of infection in peripheral arterial reconstruction: a systematic review and meta-analysis. J Vasc Surg 2007;46: 148–55.
93. Antimicrobial prophylaxis in surgery. Med Lett Drugs Ther 2001;43:92.
94. Forse RA, Karam B, MacLean LD, et al. Antibiotic prophylaxis for surgery in morbidly obese patients. Surgery 1989;106: 750.
95. Bhattacharyya T, Hooper D. Antibiotic dosing before primary hip and knee replace-[illegible] performance measure. J Bone J[illegible] 2007;8[illegible]:287–91.
96. Schoen D. Antibiotic dosing before primary hip and knee replacement as a pay-for-performance measure. Orthopaed Nurs 2007;26:257–8.
97. Perencevich E, Stone P, Wright S, et al. Raising standards while watching the bottom line: making a buisness case for infection control. Infect Control Hosp Epidemiol 2007;28:1121–33.
98. Brendle, T. Surgical care improvement project and the perioperative nurse's role. AORN J 2007;86:94–5, 97–101.
99. The role of anesthesiologist in the selection and administration of perioperative antibiotics: a survey of the American Association of Clinical Directors. Surv Anesthesiol 2007; 51:218.
100. Wiener-Kronish JP. Infection control for the anesthesiologist: is there more than handwashing? ASA Referesher Courses in Anesthesiology. 2007;35:219–25.
101. Sessler DI, Akca O. Nonpharmacological prevention of surgical wound infections. Clin Infect Dis 2002;35:1397.
102. Kurz A, Sessler DI, Lenhardt R. Perioperative normothermia to reduce the incidence of surgical wound infection and shorten hospitalization. Study of Wound Infection and Temperature Group. N Engl J Med 1996;358:876.
103. Flores-Maldonado A, Medine-Escobedo CE, Rios-Rodriguez HM, et al. Mild perioperative hypothermia and the risk of wound infection. Arch Med Res 2001;32:227.
104. Melling AC, Ali B, Scott EM, et al. Effects of preoperative warming on the incidence of wound infection after clean surgery: a randomized controlled trial. Lancet 2001; 358:876.
105. Hopf HW, Hunt TK, West JM. Wound tissue oxygen tension predicts the risk of wound infection in surgical patients. Arch Surg 1997;132:997.
106. Koval KJ, Rosenberg AD, Zuckerman JD, et al. Does blood transfusion increase risk of infection after hip fracture? J Orthop Trauma 1997;11:260.
107. Houbiers JG, van de Velder CJ, van de Watering LM, et al. Transfusion of red cells is associated with increased incidence of bacterial infection after colorectal surgery: a prospective study. Transfusion 1997;37: 126.
108. Dunne J, Malone D, Genuit T, et al. Perioperative anemia: an independent risk factor for infection and resource utilization in surgery. J Surg Res 2002;102:237.
109. Berkers J, Guns J, Vanhorebeek J, Van den Berghe G. Glycaemic control and perioperative organ protection. Best practice and research. Clin Anaesthesiol 2008;22: 135–49.
110. Velmahos GC, Alam HB. Advances in surgical critical care. Curr Probl Surg [illegible] 453–516.
111. Langley J, Adams G. Insulin-based regimens decrease mortality rates in criticall ill patients: a systematic review. Diabetes Metab Res Rev 2007;23:184–92.
112. Vanhorebeek I, Langouche L, Van den Berghe G. Tight blood glucose control: what is the evidence? Crit Care Med 2007; 35(9 Suppl):5496–502.
113. Van den Berghe G, Wilmer A, Hermans G, et al. Intensive insulin therapy in the medical ICU. N Engl J Med 2006;354:449–61.
114. Meijering S, Corstjens AM, Tulleken JE, et al. Towards a feasible algorithm for tight glycaemic control in critically ill patients: a systematic review of the literature. Crit Care 2006;10(1):R19.
115. Peers JG. Cleanup techniques in the operating room. Arch Surg 1973;107:596.
116. Weber DO, Gooch JJ, Wood WR, et al. Influence of operating room surface contamination on surgical wounds: a prospective study. Arch Surg 1976;111:484.
117. Daschner F. Patient-oriented hospital hygiene. Infection 1980;39 Suppl:243.
118. Report of an Ad-Hoc Committee of the Committee of Trauma, Division of Medical Sciences, National Academy of Sciences-National Research Council. Postoperative wound infections: the influence of ultraviolet irradiation of the operating room and of various other factors. Ann Surg 1964;160 Suppl:1.
119. Hambraeus A, Bengtsson S, Laurell G. Bacterial contamination in a modern operating suite: II. Effect of a zoning system on contamination of floors and other surfaces. J Hyg (Lond) 1978;80:57.
120. McWilliams RM. There should be only one way to clean up between all surgical procedures. J Hosp Infect Control 1976;3:64.
121. Nichols RL. The operating room. In: Bennett JV, Brachman PS, editors. Hospital infections. 3rd ed. Boston: Little, Brown & Co; 1992. p. 461.
122. Ayliffe GA. Role of the environment of the operating suite in surgical wound infection. Rev Infect Dis 1991;13(Suppl 10):S800.
123. Overdyck FJ, Harvey SC, Fishman RL, et al. Successful strategies for improving operating room efficiency at academic institutions. Anesth Analg 1998;86:896.
124. Patterson P. Is an 80% to 85% utilization a realistic target for ORs? OR Manager 1997;13(5):1.
125. Mueller J, Marinari B, Kunkel S. Flipping assumptions and revisioning perioperative services. J Nurs Admin 1995;25:22.
126. Epstein RH, Dexter F. Statistical power analysis to estimate how many months of data are required to identify operating room [illegible] solutions to reduce labor costs and [illegible] productivity. Anesth Analg 2002; 94:640.
127. Surgery teams make strides on OR delays. OR Manager 1998;14(1):1.
128. Dexter F, Traub RD. How to schedule elective surgical cases into specific operating rooms to maximize the efficiency of use of operating room time. Anesth Analg 2002; 94:933.

Acknowledgment

The authors wish to acknowledge Rene Lafrenière, MD, CM, FACS, Ramon Berguer, MD, FACS, Patricia C. Seifert, RN, Michael Belkin, MD, FACS, Stuart Roth, MD, PhD, Karen S. Williams, MD, Eric J. De Maria, MD, FACS, and Lena M. Napolitano, MD, FACS, FCCM, who wrote and edited this chapter for the previous version of *ACS Surgery*. This chapter has drawn heavily on their work and generally follows their outline and concept of the subject discussed. Russell Stewart contributed to the research and bibliography.

7 FAST TRACK INPATIENT AND AMBULATORY SURGERY

Liane S. Feldman, MD, FRCS(C), FACS, and Franco Carli, MD, PhD, FRCA, FRCPC

Fast track (also known as accelerated recovery, accelerated rehabilitation, enhanced recovery, or multimodal rehabilitation) surgery involves the use of a coordinated, multidisciplinary perioperative care plan to reduce complications, facilitate earlier discharge from the hospital, and permit faster recovery of the ability to carry out daily activities after elective surgery.[1] This approach is the result of advancements in anesthetic techniques, improved understanding of perioperative organ dysfunction, and the introduction of minimally invasive surgery (MIS). Attenuation of the stress response to surgery (endocrine, metabolic and immunologic) and consequent prevention of some of its negative effects (e.g., increased cardiac demands, decreased gastrointestinal [GI] motility, and pain) underlie many of the benefits of fast track surgery.[2]

A unifying theme in the development and implementation of fast track surgery is the quest to understand and address the factors that keep patients hospitalized after major surgery and impede their return to baseline performance and function.[3] These interrelated factors include the need for parenteral analgesia, the requirement for intravenous (IV) fluids, and lack of mobility.[4] Whereas some of these factors have a physiologic basis (e.g., decreased GI motility from the sympathetic response to surgery), others are related to traditions or cultural aspects of the care of surgical patients (e.g., waiting for GI motility to return before introducing oral intake). The goal is to combine a variety of individual evidence-based elements of perioperative care, each of which may have only modest benefits when used in isolation, into a coordinated effort that can be expected to have a synergistic beneficial effect on surgical outcomes.[5] The term fast track has contributed to the misconception that the primary goal of this approach is cost containment through the reduction of hospital stay; however, the primary goals are in fact to shorten recovery time, decrease morbidity, and improve efficiency.[6,7] The principles of fast track surgery are applicable to both outpatient and inpatient procedures: many procedures that once necessitated hospitalization are now routinely performed in an ambulatory or short-stay setting.

A fast track surgery program encompasses preoperative, intraoperative, and postoperative phases. The principal elements are as follows.

1. Preoperative patient education and preparation for surgery ("prehabilitation").
2. Newer anesthetic, analgesic, and surgical techniques, whose aim is to decrease the surgical stress response, pain and discomfort, and postoperative nausea and vomiting.
3. Aggressive postoperative rehabilitation, including early enteral feeding and ambulation. This also includes changes in the traditional surgical practice concerning the use of drains, tubes and catheters.

Some of these individual elements may be part of evidence-based modern surgical care, but there remains a great deal of variability among surgeons and institutions.[8] Introduction of one or more components in isolation may improve some specific outcomes, but the underlying hypothesis in fast track surgery is that a multimodal approach to care will enhance outcomes further.[4] Although few data are available, the existing evidence is encouraging and suggests that fast track programs are associated with reductions in hospital stay and morbidity.[6] Successful implementation of a formal fast track program at the institutional level, however, requires significant resources and time and involves an organized and coordinated effort on the part of a motivated multidisciplinary team that includes anesthesiologists, surgeons, nurses, physiotherapists, social workers, nutritionists, and patients. This represents a shift from conventional surgical practice, in which perioperative management is primarily dictated by the surgeon's preference.

In this chapter, we describe the constituent elements of a fast track surgery program. We review the organizational steps required to set up such a program and provide specific examples of care plans in digestive surgery.

Preoperative Issues

PHYSICAL OPTIMIZATION

Evaluation and Optimization of Preexisting Organ Function

Postoperative complications are related to preoperative comorbid conditions,[9] including inadequate nutrition.[10] Classification of functional capacity and optimization of organ function are expected to reduce cardiovascular and other complications. The preoperative evaluation is also an opportunity to improve long-term health apart from surgical considerations—for example, by counseling patients who may benefit from long-term beta blockade, smoking cessation, or tightened glycemic control. A substantive discussion of cardiopulmonary risk assessment and reduction is beyond the scope of this chapter; however, various current guidelines and algorithms are available for assessment and reduction of perioperative risk related to cardiac disease,[11] pulmonary complications,[12] obesity,[13] and diabetes.[14]

The perioperative period provides smokers with a good opportunity to quit. Smoking increases the risk of cardiac, respiratory, and wound complications,[15] and abstinence reduces complications.[16,17] Although reduction of pulmonary complications requires an abstinence period of weeks to months, cardiac and wound complications are reduced after shorter periods.[15] Smokers should be advised to quit and referred to resources that will help them do so.

Assessment and Optimization of Nutritional Status

Poor nutritional status is an independent risk factor for complications after surgery. Patients with moderate and severe preoperative undernutrition benefit from preoperative nutritional support, preferably via the enteral route, for at least 7 days preoperatively.[10,18] Patients with less severe malnutrition, including those with diminished oral intake as a consequence of their underlying disease, generally benefit from the addition of oral nutritional supplements to their normal diet.

Improvement of Physical Fitness

The perioperative period may be associated with rapid physical deconditioning, requiring a period of recovery during which patients are fatigued and quality-of-life and activities are curtailed. Given that patients with poor baseline exercise tolerance and physical conditioning are at increased risk for serious perioperative complications[11,19] and prolonged disability,[20,21] it seems reasonable to hypothesize that improving functional capacity by increasing physical activity before surgery may be protective.[22] Physical fitness can potentially be improved significantly while patients are waiting for scheduled procedures; modest improvements in aerobic capacity may be seen in older adults after training only 1 hour a day, four times a week, for 4 weeks.[23] The strategy of augmenting physical capacity in anticipation of an upcoming stressor is termed prehabilitation—as opposed to rehabilitation, which begins only after the injury or operation has taken place.

Preliminary evidence supports the use of exercise prehabilitation before surgery. In one study, adults randomly assigned to exercise for 1 month showed faster healing of a punch-biopsy site than control subjects did.[24] In another, a preoperative exercise program carried out by patients awaiting lung cancer surgery improved exercise capacity to a degree that mitigated the expected postsurgical decline.[25] In yet another study, patients receiving twice-weekly exercise training while waiting for coronary artery bypass graft surgery (CABGS) had shorter hospital stays and better preoperative and postoperative quality of life than control subjects; the quality-of-life differences remained for up to 6 months after surgery.[26] Observational data suggest that simply instructing patients to walk 30 minutes daily in the perioperative period may be beneficial, without the need for a formal individualized exercise program (F. Carli and associates, unpublished data).

Preoperative Fasting

To reduce the risk of tracheal aspiration of gastric contents at the induction of general anesthesia, patients have traditionally had to refrain from oral ingestion of both solids and liquids (nil per os [NPO]) from midnight of the night before the operation. This standard approach is convenient and easy to follow, but it requires patients to spend a long period without hydration or nutrition, especially for operations scheduled in the afternoon. Solids may present a risk, but there is no evidence that oral intake of water and other clear fluids (e.g., tea, coffee, apple juice, and pulp-free orange juice) up to 2 hours preoperatively increases gastric fluid volume or exacerbates the risk of aspiration in otherwise healthy adults.[27,28] Current preoperative fasting guidelines for adult patients undergoing elective surgery recommend a 2-hour fast for liquids and a 6-hour fast for solids.[29] These recommendations do not apply to patients with delayed gastric emptying (e.g., from gastroparesis, GI obstruction, or upper GI tract malignancy).

Preoperative Ingestion of Oral Carbohydrate Drink

That it is safe to administer fluids up to 2 hours before surgery enables the use of high-carbohydrate drinks immediately before operation. Emerging evidence suggests that it may be beneficial to provide a drink containing 100 g of carbohydrate the evening before surgery and a second drink containing a further 50 g 2 to 3 hours before induction of anesthesia. This measure improves preoperative feelings of thirst, hunger, and anxiety[30]; reduces postoperative insulin resistance; and reduces the catabolic stress response to surgery.[31] Compared with control subjects, patients receiving preoperative oral carbohydrate drinks had less muscle loss[32] and better whole-body protein balance[33] after major abdominal surgery and had shorter hospital stays after colorectal surgery.[34] Preoperative carbohydrate drinks reduced nausea and vomiting after laparoscopic cholecystectomy in one trial[35] but not in another.[36]

PATIENT EDUCATION

Preoperative patient education is an essential component of fast track surgery. For many patients, impending major surgery represents a significant psychological stress. Greater preoperative emotional distress, depression, and anxiety are associated with poorer operative outcomes, including increased pain, higher complication rates, poorer wound healing, longer hospital stays, slower return to normal daily activities, and reduced patient satisfaction.[37,38] There is evidence that emotional distress delays wound healing by altering endocrine and inflammatory responses.[39,40] The results from meta-analyses suggest that preoperative patient education and preparation have positive effects on certain outcomes (e.g., pain, psychological distress, and indexes of recovery, including hospital stay), even if the intervention is relatively brief and not individualized.[40] For example, patients who watched a video involving an actor outlining aspects of perioperative care after inguinal hernia surgery experienced improved quality of life and faster resumption of baseline activities in comparison with control subjects.[41]

Patient expectation may also play a role in determining postoperative outcome.[42] Because the fast track recovery program may differ from patients' and caregivers' expectations for and previous experiences with hospitalization and surgery, it is important to specify the active role the patient is expected to play. Such specification includes providing explicit written information about the benefits of the program, the goals for daily nutritional intake and ambulation in the early postoperative period, the discharge criteria, and the expected hospital stay. Information about sensory experiences (e.g., pain, nausea and vomiting, and fatigue) are included in the discussion and the written materials, as well as guidelines regarding what to expect once they leave the hospital.

PREMEDICATION

In the past, preanesthetic medication was administered with the intent of providing sedation and reducing anxiety. Today, with the advent of same-day admission and fast track surgery, premedication may play additional roles, including modulation of intraoperative hemodynamics and attenuation of postoperative side effects.[43]

Benzodiazepines are excellent anxiolytics that possess rapid onset of action and are flexible in use, being available in both IV and oral forms. Doses as small as 2 mg effectively reduce anxiety and anxiety-related complications.[44] They also reduce the amount of anesthetic required and provide comfort. Opioids such as morphine and meperidine are no longer for premedicants in outpatient settings, because of the prolonged duration of action and the high incidence of side effects. Fentanyl has a better profile for fast track surgery and facilitates early hospital discharge. Acetaminophen and cyclooxygenase-2 (COX-2) inhibitors (e.g., celecoxib) can be administered either orally or rectally up to 1 hour before surgery and possess significant perioperative opioid-sparing effects.[45]

Anticholinergics (e.g., atropine and scopolamines) are rarely used today, except for procedures such as laryngoscopy or bronchoscopy, in which reduction of secretions is required. These compounds are not given to elderly patients, because they may trigger delirium; rather, glycopyrrolate (0.3 mg IV), which does not cross the blood-brain barrier, is preferred.

Beta blockers and $alpha_2$ agonists can be used as adjuvants to fast track anesthetic techniques. With their anesthetic and analgesic-sparing effects,[46–49] these medications maintain perioperative hemodynamic stability and reduce postoperative pain, thus facilitating the early recovery process. Beta blockers (e.g., propanolol, atenolol, labetalol, esmolol) attenuate the intraoperative rise in circulating concentrations of catecholamines, promote hemodynamic stability during emergence from anesthesia and in the early postoperative period, and prevent perioperative cardiovascular events in elderly patients undergoing noncardiac surgery[50] and patients with preexisting coronary artery disease.[51,52] In addition, preliminary evidence that beta blockers possess anticatabolic properties and anesthetic and analgesic-sparing effects suggests that they may play a role in accelerating the recovery process.[53] $Alpha_2$ agonists (e.g., clonidine or dexmedetomidine) have also been used as premedicants with the goal of reducing the need for opioid analgesics and attenuating sympathoadrenergic and hypothalamopituitary responses. Clonidine shortens the duration of paralytic ileus after colorectal procedures[54] and decreases the incidence of postoperative nausea and vomiting (PONV). Both clonidine and dexmedetomidine have been shown to reduce the incidence of myocardial ischemia.[55]

Antacids and H_2-receptor antagonists can be administered before surgery in subjects at risk for gastric aspiration (e.g., those who are diabetic, obese, or pregnant; have gastroesophageal reflux disease; or have sustained a stroke). H_2-receptor antagonists are given the evening before surgery and in the morning to decrease the volume and acidity of gastric content. A nonparticulate antacid (e.g., sodium citrate) is given 1 hour before surgery to raise the gastric pH.

Administration of anti-PONV medications such as dexamethasone and odansetron before or during the induction and maintenance of anesthesia is recommended in high-risk subjects and has been shown to facilitate the recovery period and decrease hospital admission after ambulatory surgical procedures.

Intraoperative Issues

ATTENUATION OF SURGICAL STRESS RESPONSE

Surgery initiates a series of metabolic and inflammatory responses that are involved in the pathogenesis of postoperative morbidity and can slow the recovery process. These responses induce a transient but reversible state of insulin resistance, the magnitude of which is linked to the invasiveness of the surgical procedure. This state is characterized by a decrease in peripheral glucose uptake and a concomitant increase in endogenous glucose production. The magnitude of this noxious response can be reduced by perioperative interventions that modify the catabolic response. These interventions can be classified as pharmacologic (high-dose opioids, neural blockade with local anesthetics, beta blockers, glucocorticoids, $alpha_2$ agonists, nonsteroidal anti-inflammatory drugs [NSAIDS]), hormonal (insulin, growth hormone, estrogens), physical (normothermia, MIS), and nutritional. Among these interventions, intraoperative and postoperative blockade of afferent neural nociceptive stimuli by epidural and spinal block using local anesthetics has been shown to be the most powerful modulator of the metabolic and endocrine stress response. To be effective, however, the neural blockade must be established before surgery and continued for a minimum of 48 hours.[56]

For postoperative pain relief, epidural block achieved with a mixture of local anesthetics and opioids provides excellent postoperative analgesia at rest and during movement compared with systemic opioids,[57] thus facilitating resumption of dietary intake and utilization of nutrients,[58] attenuating the loss of body mass, and allowing earlier resumption of exercise.[59] Epidural block also affects insulin resistance, attenuating the hyperglycemic response, facilitating the oxidative utilization of exogenous glucose,[60] and thereby preventing the postoperative loss of aminoacids and saving almost 100 g of lean body mass daily.[61] The extent of protein sparing has been found to be greater than that previously achieved with hormonal and nutritional interventions. Epidural block has anticatabolic effects, and patients can be rendered anabolic with the concomitant administration of glucose and aminoacids[62] or aminoacids alone; the advantage of the latter is that it is not associated with hyperglycemia.[63–65] Preoperative oral or IV carbohydrate administration also reduces postoperative insulin resistance, thus decreasing postoperative catabolism and resulting in less fatigue.[66–68]

A single dose of glucocorticoids given at induction of anesthesia decreases the inflammatory response without causing any significant side effects. Beta blockers also reduce cardiac demands and sympathetic stimulation and have been shown to attenuate catabolism in burn patients.[53] MIS attenuates the inflammatory response but not the endocrine one. Although it is not clear to what extent MIS modulates catabolism, the administration of dextrose after laparoscopic colon surgery results in a significant suppression of endogenous glucose production (an index of gluconeogenesis), with no protein-sparing capacity.[69] This implies enhanced whole body glucose uptake and greater utilization and oxidation of exogenous glucose. Insulin, growth hormones, and anabolic steroids have been shown to improve wound healing, directing aminoacids toward anabolic pathways to enhance lean tissue synthesis.

ANESTHETIC TECHNIQUES

General Anesthesia

After general anesthesia for fast track surgery, the patient should be able to walk out of the hospital with minimal side effects. Therefore, the choice of anesthetic agents should include fast-acting IV drugs and less soluble volatile anesthetics, along with adjuvants to minimize the side effects.

Propofol is the IV agent of choice for induction of fast track anesthesia.[70] For maintenance of anesthesia, highly soluble volatile anesthetic agents, such as desflurane and sevoflurane, offer advantages over propofol and isoflurane, in that they facilitate early recovery.[71–73] Nitrous oxide (50–70%) remains a popular adjuvant during the maintenance period because of its anesthetic- and analgesic-sparing effects, low cost, and favorable pharmacokinetic profile;[74] however, it is not recommended in subjects at risk for PONV, nor is it suitable for laparoscopic surgery when the operating time is longer than 1 hour. Prolonged use of nitrous oxide causes bowel distention (the so-called gas effect) and predisposition to PONV. When general anesthesia is maintained with volatile anesthetic agents, there is an increased risk of PONV in the early postoperative period; accordingly, it is suggested that low-dose droperidol (0.625 mg) and dexamethasone (4–8 mg) should be sued to provide effective antiemetic prophylaxis.[75] Titration of both IV and inhaled anesthetics using cerebral monitoring devices may also facilitate the fast track process,[76–79] except in spontaneously breathing patients.[80]

With regard to opioids, fentanyl remains a good choice, though infusion of the ultra–short-acting opioid remifentanil (0.05–0.15 µg/kg/min) is an increasingly popular alternative for short and painful conditions. Whereas intraoperatively administered fentanyl can maintain some residual effect during the postoperative period, remifentanil is rapidly metabolized; thus, one must remember that as soon as the remifentanil infusion ends, the patient can be in serious pain. Long-acting opioids must therefore be administered in due time. The use of nonopioid analgesics (e.g., NSAIDs, [including COX-2 inhibitors], acetaminophen, $alpha_2$ agonists, glucocorticoids, ketamine, and local anesthetics in the wound) are recommended as part of a multimodal analgesic regimen aimed at reducing opioid-related side effects.[81,82] Adjuvants such as beta blockers and lidocaine have had some success in reducing opioid use during and after laparoscopic surgery. These compounds represent an alternative to short-acting opioids in controlling for any associated acute autonomic responses.[83–85]

Short- or intermediate-acting muscle relaxants are used for fast track surgery because they often do not need to be reversed. A novel agent, sugammadex (a cyclodextrin compound),[86] has been shown to provide faster reversal of nondepolarizing muscle relaxants without anticholinergic side effects,[87] thus facilitating earlier tracheal extubation and reducing postoperative respiratory complications as a result of residual muscle paralysis.

In summary, short-acting anesthetic drugs and adjuvants minimize postoperative side effects and enhance the ability to fast track patients after both ambulatory and major inpatient surgical procedures. Not surprisingly, combining short-acting anesthetic techniques with an educational program has been reported to increase fast tracking significantly in ambulatory centers. Although a majority of adults can be fast-tracked after ambulatory surgery under general anesthesia, minimizing patient discomfort and anxiety is critically important for establishing a successful fast track surgery program for all types of elective surgery.

Regional Anesthesia

Regional anesthetic techniques (spinal, epidural, and peripheral nerve blocks) have several advantages over general anesthesia—including improved pulmonary function, decreased cardiovascular demand, a lower incidence of ileus, and good quality of analgesia at rest and on ambulation—both when used in place of GA and when used as adjuvants. The appropriate combination of a local anesthetic with an adjuvant will facilitate readiness for discharge. Consequently, epinephrine should not be added to spinal local anesthetics, because it might delay time to micturition; however, fentanyl in small doses does not interfere with bladder function.[88,89] Faster recovery of sensory and motor function results when minidose lidocaine (10–30 mg), bupivacaine (3.5–7 mg), or ropivacaine (5–10 mg) spinal anesthetic techniques are combined with a potent opioid analgesic (e.g., fentanyl [10–25 µg] or sufentanil [5–10 µg]).[90,91] However, postoperative side effects (e.g., pruritus, nausea) are increased when intrathecal opioids are used.

Thoracic epidural blockade is the most effective technique for postoperative analgesia. Whether in the form of a continuous infusion or of patient-controlled analgesia (PCA), epidural analgesia results in better static and dynamic pain relief than IV opioid–based PCA delivery systems.[92] Epidural block with local anesthetics reduces the endocrine and metabolic responses to surgery, improves pulmonary outcome after major abdominal and thoracic operations (e.g., aortic surgery[93] and thoracoabdominal esophagectomy),[94] and facilitates the return of bowel function, while resulting in better preservation of perioperative nutritional profiles, higher health-related quality-of-life scores, and improved exercise capacity after colon surgery[59]; however, it has not been found to affect the duration of hospitalization. Over the past 20 years, several randomized controlled studies and meta-analyses have been conducted to study the effect of spinal and epidural block on postoperative outcome. One large meta-analysis reported that morbidity and mortality were significantly lower with spinal and epidural analgesia than with general anesthesia and systemic opioid analgesia,[95] but these benefits could not be demonstrated in several subsequent randomized, controlled trials. However, these studies were not controlled for factors that might influence the stress response, including hypothermia, immunosuppression, hypoxemia, perioperative surgical and nursing care, infection, and the use of drains and tubes. One might therefore assume that the beneficial effects of regional anesthesia on postoperative mortality and morbidity are most apparent when it is used as part of a multimodal therapeutic regimen in which all evidence-based therapeutic strategies have been put in place.

With regard to some biologic outcome measures, thoracic epidural analgesia with a local anesthetic and administration of opioids reduce ileus and lead to faster discharge after colonic surgery in patients enrolled in a fast track program (i.e., in patients being treated with multimodal techniques that include preoperative preparation, attenuation of the intraoperative stress response, multimodal analgesia, early oral feeding and mobilization, and early removal of drains and tubes).[6,96] A role for epidural analgesia as part of a multimodal analgesia technique has also been suggested in the setting of fast track cardiac anesthesia,[97–100] in which epidural local anesthetics have been associated with earlier tracheal extubation, decreased pulmonary complications and cardiac dysrhythmias, reduced postoperative pain and opioid analgesic requirements, shorter stays in the intensive care unit (ICU), and faster recovery of bowel and bladder function.[101–103] However, with advances in MIS, the perioperative use of mu-receptor antagonists and other analgesia adjuvants, and the advent of fast track accelerated recovery programs in which all surgical, anesthetic, and nursing care elements are revised according to scientific evidence, the role of thoracic epidural technique in some types of surgery must be reconsidered.[104]

Incisional Local Anesthesia

Infiltration of local anesthetics into the surgical wound is an effective analgesia technique for minor surgical procedures (e.g., hernia repair, anal surgery, and breast procedures). When possible, local infiltration should be performed before the surgical incision is made and should be a component of all balanced fast track anesthetic techniques.[105,106] Better analgesia results when the infiltration of local anesthetics is supplemented with a peripheral nerve block (e.g., ileoinguinal block for inguinal hernia repair).[106] Compared with neuroaxial or general anesthetic techniques, local anesthetic infiltration techniques reduce the risk of postoperative urinary retention associated with anorectal surgery[107] and inguinal herniorrhaphy.[108,109] The instillation of local anesthetics on the visceral peritoneum during laparoscopy has only weak and short-lasting analgesic effects.[110]

Continuous wound infusion with local anesthetics has been used for abdominal, gynecologic, and thoracic operations, and many studies have shown it to yield improved analgesia, greater patient satisfaction with pain management, reduced PONV, and shorter hospital stay.[111] Continuous infusion of bupivacaine at the median sternotomy incision site after cardiac surgery not only provides good postoperative pain relief but also allows patients to ambulate earlier, leading to a shorter hospital stay.[112,113] A systematic review of randomized trials of the efficacy of continuous wound irrigation with local anesthetics for postoperative analgesia demonstrated good analgesia and opioid-sparing, with reduced side effects.[111] Nevertheless, the quality of analgesia can be highly variable even in a given patient or a given type of surgery, which highlights the difficulty of interpreting the results.

MAINTENANCE OF NORMOTHERMIA

During major surgery, body temperature falls by approximately 1° to 2°C as a result of loss of body heat and inhibition of the thermoregulatory response. Whereas a small drop in core temperature is not a cause for concern in fit and healthy persons, it can be detrimental in elderly, malnourished, or frail persons with cardiorespiratory and metabolic instability. Mild hypothermia elicits a stress response during the recovery period while the patient attempts to regain normothermia by means of shivering and vasoconstriction. It results in increased cardiovascular demands, elevated oxygen consumption, hypoxia, and impaired coagulation and leukocyte formation. Maintenance of intraoperative normothermia with the use of active and passive warming devices in conjunction with aggressive postoperative management of shivering and residual hypothermia decreases the incidence of wound infections, blood loss, myocardial ischemia, and protein breakdown.[114]

FLUID MANAGEMENT

Intraoperative fluid management strategy remains controversial, in that adverse outcomes may be associated with both inadequate and excessive fluid administration.[115–117] Inadequate fluid administration can lead to a reduction in effective circulating volume, with diversion of blood towards the brain and heart and away from the gut, skin, and kidneys. Liberal (as opposed to restrictive) IV fluid administration improves gut perfusion and increases left ventricular stroke volume. In contrast, excessive IV fluid administration may result in adverse effects. Excess fluid in the intravascular compartment leads to increased venous pressure and pulmonary and peripheral edema that may compromise peripheral oxygenation. Two studies have suggested that excessive hydration can increase postoperative morbidity and lengthen the hospital stay after major abdominal surgery.[118,119] In these studies, perioperative water and salt restriction reduced cardiopulmonary and tissue healing complications and prevented hyperchloremic metabolic acidosis after abdominal surgery. On the other hand, after laparoscopic cholecystectomy, large volumes of intraoperative fluid have been associated with reduced side effects (e.g., pulmonary dysfunction, dizziness, drowsiness, thirst, and PONV) and a shorter hospital stay.[120] Although aggressive crystalloid administration during colorectal surgery improves tissue oxygenation,[117] it does not reduce the risk of surgical site infection (SSI).[121]

Perioperative fluid administration should take into account preoperative dehydration resulting from fasting and bowel preparation, replacement of blood loss and secretions, and maintenance hydration. The volume and composition of the fluid, together with the type of surgery performed and the patient's hemodynamic requirements, influence the duration and magnitude of intravascular volume expansion. Intraoperative esophageal Doppler monitoring can facilitate goal-directed fluid administration by targeting specific values for the cardiac index. Several studies have been conducted on different types of surgical procedures, and the outcomes have been positive (shorter length of hospital stay, lower incidence of admission to ICU, and fewer complications) when fluid administration was guided by a predetermined stroke volume and filling pressure.[122,123] Therefore, strategies that avoid both hypovolemia and postoperative fluid overload are important in facilitating the fast track recovery process.

MINIMIZATION OF INCISION SIZE AND USE OF MIS

The size and orientation of the surgical incision are dictated primarily by the location and extent of the pathology, the need for exposure, the requirement for stoma placement (if applicable), the likelihood of further abdominal surgery, and the patient's body habitus. The incision should be as small as possible while allowing adequate exposure. Transverse incisions are used when possible by some fast track colorectal groups (though not by all). A meta-analysis found clinical outcomes after transverse or midline incisions to be similar overall.[124]

Laparoscopic techniques are used when possible. In comparison with conventional open surgery, laparoscopic surgery is associated with better preservation of systemic immune function,[125,126] less pulmonary compromise,[127] a lower incidence of ileus,[128] a shorter hospital stay, and earlier resumption of regular activities.[129–134] In addition, the risk of SSI,[135] incisional hernia,[136,137] and small-bowel obstruction[138] may be reduced with laparoscopic approaches.

In the setting of colorectal surgery, it is unclear at present whether the laparoscopic approach further improves on the short-term recovery benefits already seen with multimodal rehabilitation programs; benefits have been reported in some studies[138,139] but not in others.[140,141]

Postoperative Issues

PAIN MANAGEMENT

Pain remains the most common reason for delaying discharge after ambulatory surgery,[142] while good analgesia accelerates restoration of function and improves recovery [*see 2:4 Postoperative Pain*].[143] Although there is no direct relation between analgesic techniques and postoperative morbidity and mortality,[144] optimal pain control, in combination with other interventions, remains a priority for the physician in the perioperative period. The pathophysiology of postoperative pain is characterized by a combination of nociceptive stimuli from the wound, inflammation and sensitization of peripheral somatic and visceral nerve terminals and central neurons, and inhibition of central descending control. It is therefore necessary to approach pain in a multidisciplinary fashion, whereby different treatment modalities complement each other with the aim of improving analgesia while minimizing the side effects associated with each treatment.

Opioids remain the most successful compounds for postoperative pain control, but they are associated with several important side effects (e.g., acute opioid tolerance, hypoventilation, sedation, ileus, nausea and vomiting, and urinary retention), any of which may delay hospital discharge. Accordingly, it is sensible to consider multimodal analgesia as the next step in providing optimal pain control. In this approach, the synergistic or additive effects of a variety of analgesics are exploited, allowing the individual doses to be reduced and thereby minimizing individual drug-related side effects. Intraoperative use of adjuvants such as ketamine, clonidine, dexmedetomidine, adenosine, gabapentine, dexamethasone, lidocaine, beta blockers, magnesium, and neostigmine has an opioid-sparing effect during the whole perioperative period.

The use of peripheral nerve blocks and conduction blockade for major and minor surgical procedures in combination with adjuvants provides excellent analgesia, though not always consistently. One reason for partial analgesic failures might be that too often, the analgesia regimen has not been optimized for a specific procedure. Accordingly, various procedure-specific analgesic regimens have been developed. On the basis of published evidence, the addition of either NSAIDs or regional analgesia and beta blockers to opioids enhances the quality of analgesia and exerts significant opioid-sparing effects.[145] At present, the evidence does not support adding acetaminophen to an opioid; however, the combination of acetaminophen with an NSAID provides better analgesia than either drug alone. More work is needed to verify whether the combination of several nonopioid analgesics could produce good analgesia with minimal side effects.[81] In the meantime, the current strategy for postoperative analgesia involves a combination of regional and local anesthesia, MIS, and nonopioid pharmacologic interventions.

POSTOPERATIVE NAUSEA AND VOMITING

PONV continues to be a common complication of surgery, with an overall estimated incidence of 20 to 30%. PONV delays discharge from the postanesthesia care unit (PACU) and is the leading cause of unanticipated hospital admission in ambulatory surgical patients. Vomiting increases the risk of aspiration and has been associated with suture dehiscence. Nausea and vomiting remain the most common reasons for poor patient satisfaction during the postoperative period. In one study, a simplified risk factor chart was developed that identified four main risk factors for PONV: female sex, nonsmoking status, a history of PONV, and opioid use.[146] The incidence of PONV in patients with none, one, two, three, or all four of these risk factors was approximately 10%, 20%, 40%, 60%, and 80%, respectively. In a large study of 18,000 ambulatory patients, general anesthesia was associated with an 11-fold higher incidence of PONV than regional or local anesthesia was.[147] The risk of PONV has also been shown to increase with longer operating times.

Consensus guidelines for managing PONV recommend intraoperative pharmacologic strategies designed to compensate for baseline risk factors and modify the incidence of this complication. Currently available antiemetics may act at the cholinergic (muscarinic), dopaminergic (D_2), histaminergic (HI), or serotonergic (5-HT3) receptors. NK-1–receptor antagonists are also being investigated. A 2000 study introduced the concept of a multimodal approach to management of PONV in high-risk patients, utilizing total IV anesthesia (TIVA) with propofol and remifentanil, ketorolac, no nitrous oxide, no neuromuscular blockade, IV hydration, ondansetron, droperidol, and dexamethasone.[148] This approach resulted in a 98% complete response rate (i.e., no PONV and no antiemetic rescue). A subsequent study comprising 5,000 patients employed a multifactorial design to evaluate three antiemetic interventions (ondansetron [4 mg], droperidol [1.25 mg], and dexamethasone [4 mg]) and three anesthetic interventions (TIVA with propofol, omission of nitrous oxide, and substitution of remifentanil for fentanyl) for PONV prophylaxis.[149] Each antiemetic reduced the risk of PONV by approximately 26%. The efficacy of the interventions was dependent on the patient's baseline risk. The greatest absolute risk reduction from the intervention was achieved in the patients at high risk for PONV. Consensus guidelines for management of PONV do not currently recommend prophylaxis for patients at low risk for PONV. For those at moderate risk, combination therapy with two antiemetic agents is recommended. For those at high risk, combination therapy with three antiemetic agents is recommended. In patients who experience PONV despite receiving prophylaxis, an antiemetic regimen acting at a different receptor should be used for rescue within the first 6 hours after surgery.[150] After 6 hours, PONV can be treated with any of the drugs used for prophylaxis except dexamethasone and scopolamine. Other useful adjuvants to standard antiemetic drugs include beta blockers, $alpha_2$ agonists, acupuncture, acupressure, and transcutaneous electrical nerve stimulation (TENS).[151,152]

ILEUS

Postoperative ileus is defined as a temporary paralysis of the gut after major surgical procedures. It occurs as a consequence of sympathetic reflexes resulting from surgery and pain and of production of local and systemic inflammatory mediators. The effect on bowel motility can last up to 72 hours in the colon. Ileus causes discomfort and delays oral food intake, thereby prolonging recovery and the duration of hospitalization. The most effective technique for reducing ileus is continuous thoracic epidural administration of local anesthetics to block sympathetic visceral innervation and reestablish the balance between vagal and sympathetic neural influence on the gut. Other interventions, such as early feeding, prokinetics like metoclopromide and cisapride (currently unavailable because of a high incidence of cardiac dysrhthymias), prophylactic nasogastric intubation, have only minor effects on the occurrence of ileus. In the past few years, there has been some interest in the mu-receptor antagonist alvimopan, which may reduce the effect of opioids on the gut mucosa, favor the restoration of bowel function, and accelerate hospital discharge.[153–155]

Within multimodal programs in GI surgery, the combination of epidural analgesia using diluted concentrations of local anesthetics and minimal amounts of opioids, aggressive PONV prophylaxis, and early oral feeding and mobilization has been found to shorten the duration of ileus.[96] There is also evidence that reduced perioperative sodium administration and avoidance of fluid excess[153] are associated with earlier return of bowel function after abdominal surgery and a shorter hospital stay.[156] IV infusion of lidocaine during surgery and the first 24 postoperative hours has been shown to minimize ileus and facilitate dietary intake.[85,157]

POSTOPERATIVE FEEDING

GI motility is predictably decreased after major abdominal surgery, with colonic motility requiring 3 to 5 days to recover. On the assumption that bowel rest shortens the duration of ileus and protects anastomoses, patients have traditionally been kept fasting until peristalsis has returned throughout the entire GI tract, as evidenced by passage of flatus or stool[158]; a step-wise progression of oral intake is then allowed, resulting in a planned minimum perioperative starvation period of several days. Yet after abdominal surgery, interruption of oral intake is actually neither necessary nor beneficial in most patients.[10] After colorectal surgery, feeding before complete return of peristalsis is tolerated by most patients.[159] Meta-analysis of randomized trials comparing early enteral or oral feeding with fasting after various types of elective GI surgery found no obvious advantages to keeping patients on NPO status, with several studies suggesting that early feeding offered benefits, such as decreased overall infectious complications and reduced length of stay. Although the risk of vomiting is somewhat higher with early feeding, the risk of anastomotic dehiscence is not increased.[160] One caveat is that most studies of early oral feeding involve patients undergoing colorectal resection, which means that the results may not be applicable to patients with upper GI anastomoses.

In fast track surgery, the protocol should be tailored in accordance with the procedure being done and by the patient's tolerance (e.g., as evidenced by PONV and abdominal distention). After most types of abdominal surgery, patients are encouraged to take liquids on the night following the operation, with light solids given on the morning of postoperative day 1 and a normal diet initiated on postoperative day 2. Protein-rich drinks are given between meals. This approach allows patients to resume recommended energy and protein intake in just a few days and preserves lean body mass, particularly when combined with thoracic epidural analgesia and early mobilization.[161] Setting specific daily goals that are understood by the patients and formulating protocol-based orders for the nursing staff are important for achieving adequate oral intake of calories and protein, given that simply starting clear fluids on postoperative day 1 without a structured, written plan does not prevent negative nitrogen balance.[162]

In patients for whom early oral feeding is not possible (e.g., those who have undergone major head and neck surgery, esophageal or gastric anastomoses, or pancreaticoduodenectomy), especially in those who were undernourished preoperatively, enteral tube feeding should be considered. This is done via a tube placed distal to the anastomosis at the time of surgery; either a nasojejunal tube or a feeding jejunostomy may be employed. Enteral feedings are started at a low rate (10–20 mL/hr) within 24 hours after the procedure and are slowly increased over the next few days as the patient's tolerance permits.[10]

In undernourished patients, oral nutritional supplements are continued for 10 weeks after discharge; this approach results in less weight loss, faster weight regain, better preservation of muscle mass and grip strength, and improved quality of life.[163]

MOBILIZATION

Postoperative bed rest should be discouraged. In addition to impairing pulmonary function and predisposing to thrombotic complications,[164] bed rest reduces exercise capacity in a linear fashion[165] and decreases muscle mass[166] and strength[167] (a result that may be related to the development of postoperative fatigue[168]). Although the association of early postoperative mobilization with faster recovery and lower pulmonary and thrombotic complications has been acknowledged since the 1940s,[169] modern surgical patients actually spend very little time out of bed in conventional care plans. For example, patients in the control arm of a trial comparing fast track care with conventional care after

surgery literature, there are no off-the-shelf protocols, and local differences in expertise, experience, and resources will inevitably shape the development of the protocol for each individual center. To further complicate implementation, each surgical procedure or family of procedures requires an individual protocol with specialized input from a team that is experienced in caring for this subset of patients. Even after the protocol is implemented, compliance remains an important issue that necessitates ongoing monitoring and adjustment, particularly to ensure compliance with the post-operative components.[175] Creating the protocol is necessary for success but not sufficient to ensure it; even within a fast track program, patients cared for by surgeons who are new adopters have longer hospital stays than those cared for by surgeons experienced with the protocol.[172]

The implementation process has been well described[1] and includes the following major steps [*see Table 1*]:

1. Assemble the relevant stakeholders (the multidisciplinary team).
2. Examine the evidence for components of perioperative care.
3. Interpret the evidence in the light of local experience, patient population, resources, and so forth.
4. Write, circulate, and revise the protocol.
5. Implement the plan.
6. Measure the outcomes with timely feedback.
7. Revise the protocol in the light of the outcomes.

Once the protocol is introduced, there is an adjustment and learning period for the medical and nursing personnel, which is estimated to last about 1 year.[190]

Examples of multimodal perioperative care plans for inpatient and outpatient surgical procedures are available [*see Table 2, Table 3, Table 4, and Table 5*].

CONTRAINDICATIONS

Whether fast track surgery is applicable to a wide variety of patients and procedures has been questioned. Fast track protocols seem to be feasible for most patients undergoing elective colon surgery, as demonstrated by a report from 24 German centers of various sizes and affiliations that voluntarily adopted the same fast track protocol.[191] Compliance and outcomes were prospectively documented in more than 1,000 patients with a median age of 66 years. More than 30% of the patients had significant comorbid disease (American Society of Anesthesiologists [ASA] class 3 or 4). Compliance with the protocol was high, with more than 85% of the

Table 2 **Sample Multimodal Perioperative Care Plan for Elective Colorectal Resection**

Preoperative assessment and optimization

Evaluation of medication compli[illegible] control of risk factors: hypertension, diabetes, COPD, smoking, alcohol, asthma, CAD, malnutrition, [illegible]

Psychological preparation for surgery and postoperative recovery: explanation of preoperative bowel prep[illegible] clear fluid intake up to 2 hr before surgery, intraoperative and postoperative trajectory and hospital stay (2–4 days for nonrectal surgery, > 4 days for rectal surgery), immediate postoperative mobilization, early oral intake, presence of routine bladder catheter for 24 hr

Physical preparation with exercises at home: anaerobic and resistance 1–2 hr/day, gradual increase from 50% to 80% of maximum capacity, breathing exercises

Surgical considerations: laparoscopic or laparotomy, risk of SSI, drains, bleeding risk, strategies for blood loss reduction.

Familiarization with epidural analgesia: occasional numbness in lower extremities, short spells of hypotension, pain assessment at rest and on coughing and walking, care of the epidural catheter, explanation of possible risks (hematoma and paralysis, pain and abscess)

Nutritional preparation: oral nutritional supplements for patients with diminished oral intake or mild undernutrition

Intraoperative management

Anesthetic management

Allay anxiety with midazolam and good hydration. Insert epidural catheter at appropriate intervertebral level (T7–8 for right, transverse, and left hemicolectomy; T9–10 for sigmoid and rectal resection). Use local anesthetics, and test epidural blockade for bilateral spread. Infuse local anesthetics during surgery. Give minimal amount of IV opioids throughout surgery. Administer prophylactic antiemetics, antibiotics, and DVT prophylaxis. Avoid overhydration. Avoid blood replacement in cancer resection. Maintain normothermia. Use BIS to guide anesthesia titration. Avoid neostigmine to reverse muscle relaxants.

Surgical care

Minimize incision size, and use MIS if possible. Achieve accurate hemostasis and thorough removal of debris. Check integrity of anastomosis. Do not routinely place nasogastric and abdominal drains.

Postoperative strategy

PACU

Discharge criteria: patient alert, cooperative, pain free, warm, normotensive, able to lift legs; urine output > 0.5 mL/kg

Surgical ward

Day of surgery (0–24 hr): Mobilize patient for 2 hr in chair and 2 hr walking, starting 6 hours after operation, and increase by 50% daily. Have patient drink fluids, including nutritional supplements. Hold oral intake if abdomen distended. Place NG tube for persistent PONV (repeated in subsequent days). Confirm working epidural block with VAS for pain at rest, cough, and mobilization. Check skin site (repeated in subsequent days). Give oral acetaminophen, 1 g q. 4 hr, and NSAID (repeated in subsequent days).

Postoperative day 1 (24–48 hr): Remove urinary catheter in the morning. Mobilize patient for at least 6 hr. Institute light oral diet, including nutritional supplement.

Postoperative day 2 and later (> 48 hr): Mobilize patient fully. Institute regular diet. Transition from epidural to oral medication (oxycontin + oxycodone + acetaminophen + NSAIDs) if epidural stop test is successful (repeated in subsequent days if epidural stop test is not successful). Enforce criteria for discharge: passing gas or stool, no fever, minimal pain, walking unattended, eating. If five criteria are fulfilled, patient can go home.

Post discharge

Instructions while recovering at home or on chemotherapy/radiotherapy: normal diet (±supplements), exercise every day for 1–2 hr, no opioids for pain relief, psychological support

Clinic visit on postoperative day 14: check wound and overall recovery; discuss pathology and further treatment; plan further follow-up

BIS = bispectral index monitor; CAD = coronary artery disease; COPD = chronic obstructive pulmonary disease; DVT = deep vein thrombosis; MIS = minimally invasive surgery; NG = nasogastric; NSAID = nonsteroidal antiinflammatory drug; PONV = postoperative nausea and vomiting; SSI = surgical site infection; VAS = visual analog scale.

Table 3 **Sample Multimodal Perioperative Care Plan for Ambulatory Laparoscopic Cholecystectomy**

Preoperative assessment and optimization

Evaluation of medication compliance and control of risk factors: hypertension, diabetes, COPD, smoking, alcohol, asthma, CAD, malnutrition, anemia

Psychological preparation for surgery and postoperative recovery: explanation of perioperative pathway, postoperative out-of-hospital self-care, expectations about duration of recovery period

Day of surgery: drink clear fluids containing carbohydrate up to 2 hr before operation

Preinduction: give acetaminophen 1 gm and NSAID. Provide DVT prophylaxis.

Intraoperative management

Anesthetic management

Induce with propofol, give short-acting opiates for analgesia (e.g., fentanyl), consider adjuvants for analgesia (beta blockers [propanolol, esmolol] or lidocaine), administer rocuronium or desflurane.

Prevent PONV with dexamethasone, ondansetron, or droperidol.

Give normal saline, 2 L IV, over intraoperative and postoperative time.

Keep patient warm.

Surgical care

Provide incisional anesthesia with local anesthetic at beginning and end of case. Keep abdominal insufflation pressure as low as possible (12 mm Hg or less). Maximize use of small (5 mm) trocars.

Postoperative strategy

PACU

Provide analgesia with strong short-acting opioid (e.g., fentanyl). Manage PONV with ondansetron. Encourage postoperative oral fluid intake as soon as possible; do not wait for voiding to discharge from PACU.

> 6 hr after operation[205]

Provide nonopioid analgesia with NSAIDs (e.g., ketorolac, naproxen, COX-2 inhibitor) and acetaminophen. Add oxycodone, 5–10 mg q. 4 hr, if pain persists.

Post discharge

Provide written instructions for postdischarge care; no specific activity limitations need be placed. Schedule follow-up visit at 2 wk after surgery.

CAD = coronary artery disease; COPD = chronic obstructive pulmonary disease; DVT = deep-vein thrombosis; NSAID = nonsteroidal antiinflammatory drug; PACU = postanesthesia care unit; PONV = postoperative nausea and vomiting;

patients undergoing epidural analgesia, oral nutrition, and mobilization on the day of the operation. The median length of stay was 8 days, representing a 40% decrease from conventional German data. Readmissions occurred in 4% of cases. A 2001 study enrolled 60 consecutive patients undergoing elective laparotomy and intestinal surgery over a 6-week period, including many reoperative and complex pelvic cases; only two of the 60 patients had to be excluded from the fast track protocol on the basis of operative findings.[192] Fast track colorectal surgery has been successfully performed in older patients,[193] patients with significant comorbidities (ASA class 3 or 4),[192,194,195] and patients requiring complex operations.[195] Whether these results are applicable to more complex procedures in general is not known. In a study of fast track Ivor-Lewis esophagectomy, 75% of patients older than 70 years failed the protocol.[196]

Readmission is a concern after early discharge from hospital. The rate at which readmission occurs is related to the planned day of hospital discharge, with readmission rates after colon surgery decreasing from 20% to 11% as planned hospital stays increase from 2 days to 3. The difference is mainly attributable to a reduction in readmissions for "social reasons" or observation; no significant differences in complications have ben reported.[197] A systematic review of fast track studies in colon surgery found no overall increase in readmission rates over those seen with conventional care.[6]

RESULTS

There remains significant variability in perioperative care among individual surgeons, institutions, and geographic areas, and overall adherence with evidence-based recommendations and guidelines is still suboptimal.[8] Consequently, it is likely that creation of any standard perioperative care protocol (also referred to as a critical pathway or clinical pathway) that multiple surgeons are willing to buy into may improve efficiency and outcomes simply by removing variability and improving compliance with evidence-based care. This phenomenon has been demonstrated not only for colon surgery[198] but also for more complex procedures such us pancreaticoduodenectomy[199] and aortic surgery.[200] By themselves, however, pathways often are not effective in decreasing the length of stay.[201]

Fast track surgery represents an extension of the critical pathway that integrates new modalities in anesthesia and nutrition, enforces early mobilization and feeding, and emphasizes reduction of the surgical stress response. It is hoped that this approach will not only improve efficiency by shortening the hospital stay and reducing variability, as any standardized protocol might, but also decrease the physiologic impact of major surgery, thereby reducing organ dysfunction and shortening the recovery time. Experience with fast track programs is accumulating in a number of different areas. Most reports are single-center studies focusing on colorectal surgery. A systematic review of three randomized trials and three additional prospective studies of enhanced recovery programs for colon surgery found that fast track protocols were associated with decreased ileus, duration of hospitalization, and morbidity, without any significant increase in the readmission rate.[6] Fewer results are available for other types of abdominal surgery. Preliminary reports, however, suggest that it is possible to implement fast track protocols even for debilitated patients undergoing complex procedures. Some studies have reported dramatically low lengths of stay (e.g., a 3-day median length of stay after open aortic aneurysm repair,[202] a 2-day median length of stay after colon surgery,[96] and an 88% discharge rate on postoperative day 1 after laparoscopic donor nephrectomy[203]). Even if these results are not widely applicable, they might well stimulate us

Table 4 **Sample Multimodal Perioperative Care Plan for Esophageal Resection[206–208]**

Preoperative assessment and optimization

Initial evaluation of medication compliance and control of risk factors: hypertension, diabetes, COPD, smoking, alcohol, asthma, CAD, anemia

Psychological preparation for surgery and postoperative recovery: explanation of pathway, diet and mobilization plan, presence of drains, expectations for length of hospital stay (7–8 days) and postdischarge recovery

Physical preparation with exercises at home: anaerobic and resistance 1–2 hr/day, gradual increase from 50% to 80% of maximum capacity, breathing exercises

Surgical considerations: operative approach individualized on basis of tumor characteristics and location, patient comorbidity, previous surgery

Familiarization with epidural analgesia: occasional numbness in lower extremities, short spells of hypotension, pain assessment at rest and on coughing, walking, care of epidural catheter

Nutritional preparation: oral nutritional supplements for patients with diminished oral intake or mild undernutrition; formal nutritional assessment if malnutrition is more severe

Intraoperative management

Anesthetic management

Insert thoracic epidural catheter. Use local anesthetics, and test epidural blockade for bilateral spread. Infuse local anesthetics during surgery. Provide antibiotics and DVT prophylaxis. Give prophylactic antiemetics. Restrict fluids. Avoid blood transfusion. Maintain normothermia. Perform early extubation (preferably in operating room).

Surgical care

Minimize blood loss. Place feeding jejunostomy. Routinely place NG tube and chest tubes.

Postoperative strategy

Day of surgery (0–24 hr)

Admit to ICU or other unit with continuous monitoring of heart rate and pulse oximetry. Apply strict aspiration precautions; place head of bed at 30°, and place NG tube to suction. Restrict fluids postoperatively as dictated by hemodynamics (~ 1–1.5 mL/kg/hr crystalloid and 20–30 mL/hr urine output if renal function is normal). Place chest tube to suction. Have patient sitting in chair on evening of surgery if possible and ambulating in hall on morning after surgery. Perform incentive spirometry. Monitor chest tube and urinary output q. 4 hr. Obtain hemoglobin level q. 6 hr three times; measure electrolyte concentrations in morning.

Surgical ward

Postoperative day 1: Have patient ambulate 3–4 times daily, obtain physiotherapy consult. Perform incentive spirometry (repeated in subsequent days). Apply strict aspiration precautions; place head of bed at 30°; place NG tube to suction (repeated in subsequent days). Order complete blood count and electrolyte levels in morning (repeated in subsequent days). Obtain chest x-ray (repeated three times in subsequent days). Confirm working epidural block with VAS for pain at rest, cough, and mobilization; check skin site (repeated in subsequent days). Supply jejunal feedings at full concentration, starting at 20 mL/hr.

Postoperative day 2: Increase rate of jejunal feedings by 10 mL/4 hr until achieving target rate is achieved. Request nutritional therapy consult. Remove anterior chest tube. Ambulate a minimum of four times daily until discharge.

Remove bladder catheter unless urinary output is poor.

Postoperative day 3: Remove NG tube if abdomen is not distended and gastric conduit is not dilated on chest x-ray.

Remove last chest tube if drainage < 450 mL/day (reassess in subsequent days if drainage is higher). Transition from epidural to oral/J-tube analgesics (oxycontin + oxycodone + acetaminophen + NSAID) if epidural stop test is successful (repeated in subsequent days if epidural stop test is not successful).

Postoperative day 4 or 5: Transition from epidural to oral/J-tube analgesics (oxycontin + oxycodone + acetaminophen + NSAID) if epidural stop test is successful (repeated in subsequent days if epidural stop test is not successful). Perform sodium amidotrizoate–meglumine amidotrizoate swallow. If there is no leak, advance to full liquid diet with oral supplements. Continue jejunal feedings. Continue aspiration precautions: avoid eating if drowsy, and avoid recumbency within 3 hr of eating.

Postoperative day 5 or 6: Advance to soft diet. If patient is undernourished, start compressing jejunal feedings by increasing rate and turning off for 4 hr/day. Arrange for home nighttime feedings (7 pm to 7 am). Remove central line. Continue physiotherapy and aspiration precautions. Obtain nutritional education from dietitian.

Postoperative day 7: Discharge home on soft diet with aspiration precautions ± nighttime jejunal feedings.

Post discharge

Instructions while recovering at home and/or on chemotherapy/radiotherapy: eating normal diet (± supplements), exercise every day for 1–2 hr, no opioids for pain relief, psychological support

Clinic visit on postoperative day 14 to check wound and overall recovery, discuss pathology and further treatment, and plan further follow-up

CAD = coronary artery disease; COPD = chronic obstructive pulmonary disease; DVT = deep-vein thrombosis; ICU = intensive care unit; NG = nasogastric; NSAID = nonsteroidal antiinflammatory drug.

to question our assumptions about what keeps patients in the hospital after surgery.

More research is required to understand which of the multiple individual components of fast track surgery have the greatest impact.[6] In addition, it remains unclear whether certain patients are more likely than others to benefit from fast track protocols. Several elements of this approach seem relatively consistent among fast track centers, at least with respect to colorectal surgery (e.g., thoracic epidural analgesia and the philosophy of encouraging early oral feeding and ambulation), whereas several others are more variable (e.g., use of probiotics, specific feeding protocols, preoperative carbohydrate administration, bowel preparation, and specific anesthesia protocols). Length of hospital stay is the most common outcome measure used, but this measure can be confounded by nonphysiologic issues: even within fast track programs, only a minority of patients are discharged on the day of functional recovery.[204] Yet little research has been undertaken to achieve a better description of the recovery process, and there is no currently accepted outcome measure to define the length of clinical recovery. More research is also needed in the area of implementation.

Financial Disclosures: None Reported

Table 5 **Sample Multimodal Perioperative Care Plan for Laparoscopic Foregut Surgery**[209]

Preoperative assessment and optimization
Initial evaluation of medication compliance and control of risk factors: hypertension, diabetes, COPD, smoking, alcohol, asthma, CAD, anemia
Psychological preparation for surgery and postoperative recovery: explanation of pathway, diet and mobilization plan, expectations for length of hospital stay (1–2 days) and postdischarge recovery
Nutritional preparation: oral nutritional supplements for patients with diminished oral intake or weight loss
Intraoperative management
Anesthetic management
Address aspiration risk. Give short-acting opioids. Use TIVA with propofol to minimize PONV. Provide good muscle relaxation to facilitate surgical repair. Give prophylactic antiemetics to prevent postoperative retching (dexamethasone, 8 mg; droperidol, 0.625 mg; ondansetron, 4 mg). Provide DVT prophylaxis. Initiate active warming.
Surgical care
Use small trocars. Administer preincisional and postoperative local anesthesia. Avoid lithotomy position (use split table and bean bag). Apply pneumatic compression stockings. Do not routinely place Foley catheter or NG tube.
Give sips of water immediately after operation and fluids the morning after surgery. Request nutritional consult for education on posthiatal surgery diet on postoperative day 1.
Have patient ambulate the night of the operation.
No routine postoperative investigations are required. Take stepwise approach to analgesia: start with NSAIDs and acetaminophen, avoid opiates if possible, and do not use PCA. Assess for discharge criteria after lunch on postoperative day 1 (fluids tolerated, no fever, pain controlled with oral analgesia).

CAD = coronary artery disease; COPD = chronic obstructive pulmonary disease; DVT = deep-vein thrombosis; NG = nasogastric; NSAID = nonsteroidal anti-inflammatory drug; PCA = patient-controlled analgesia; PONV = postoperative nausea and vomiting; TIVA = total intravenous anesthesia.

References

1. Kehlet H, Wilmore DW. Multimodal strategies to improve surgical outcome. Am J Surg 2002;183:630–41.
2. Wilmore DW. From Cuthbertson to fast-track surgery:70 years of progress in reducing stress in surgical patients. Ann Surg 2002;236:643–8.
3. Kehlet H. Labat lecture 2005: surgical stress and postoperative outcome—from here to where? Reg Anesth Pain Med 2006;31: 47–52.
4. Fearon KC, Ljungqvist O, Von Meyenfeldt M, et al. Enhanced recovery after surgery: a consensus review of clinical care for patients undergoing colonic resection. Clin Nutr 2005;24:466–77.
5. Kehlet H. Future perspectives and research initiatives in fast-track surgery. Langenbecks Arch Surg 2006;391:495–8.
6. Wind J, Polle SW, Fung Kon Jin PHP, et al. Systematic review of enhanced recovery programmes in colonic surgery. Br J Surg 2006;93:800–9.
7. Kehlet H, Wilmore DW. Fast track surgery. In: Souba WW, Fink MP, Jurkovich, GJ, et al, editors. ACS surgery CD: principles and practice. Hamilton (ON); BC Decker Inc; July 2008.
8. Kehlet H, Buchler MW, Beart RW Jr, et al. Care after colonic operation: is it evidence based? J Am Coll Surg 2006;202:45–54.
9. Khuri SF, Daley J, Henderson W, et al. The Department of Veterans Affairs' NSQIP: the first national, validated, outcome-based, risk-adjusted, and peer-controlled program for the measurement and enhancement of the quality of surgical care. National VA Surgical Quality Improvement Program. Ann Surg 1998;228:491–507.
10. Weimann A, Braga M, Harsanyi L, et al. ESPEN Guidelines on Enteral Nutrition: Surgery including organ transplantation. Clin Nutr 2006;25:224–44.
11. Fleisher LA, Beckman JA, Brown KA, et al. ACC/AHA 2007 guidelines on perioperative cardiovascular evaluation and care for noncardiac surgery: a report of the American College of Cardiology/American Heart Association Task Force on Practice Guidelines. J Am Coll Cardiol 2007;50: e159–241.
12. Qaseem A, Snow V, Fitterman N, et al. Clinical Efficacy Assessment Subcommittee of the American College of Physicians. Risk assessment for and strategies to reduce perioperative pulmonary complications for patients undergoing noncardiothoracic surgery: a guideline from the American College of Physicians. Ann Intern Med 2006;144:575–80.
13. Ebert TJ. Shankar H. Haake RM. Perioperative considerations for patients with morbid obesity. Anesthesiol Clin 2006;24: 621–36.
14. Robertshaw HJ, Hall GM. Diabetes mellitus: anaesthetic management. Anesthesia 2006;61:1187–90.
15. Warner DO. Tobacco dependence in surgical patients. Curr Opin Anaesthesiol 2007; 20:279–83.
16. Theadom A, Cropley M. Effects of preoperative smoking cessation on the incidence and risk of intraoperative and postoperative complications in adult smokers: a systematic review. Tob Control 2006;15: 352–358.
17. Moller AM, Villebro N, Pedersen T, Tonnesen H. Effect of preoperative smoking intervention on postoperative complications: a randomised clinical trial. Lancet 2002;359:114–7.
18. Wu GH, Liu ZH, Wu ZH, Wu ZG. Perioperative artificial nutrition in malnourished gastrointestinal cancer patients. World J Gastroenterol 2006;12:2441–4.
19. Reilly DF, McNeely MJ, Doerner D, et al. Self-reported exercise tolerance and the risk of serious perioperative complications. Arch Intern Med 1999;159:2185–92.
20. Lawrence VA, Hazuda HP, Cornell JE, et al. Functional independence after major abdominal surgery in the elderly. J Am Coll Surg 2004;199:762–72.
21. Legner VJ, Doerner D, Reilly DF, McCormick WC. Risk factors for nursing home placement following major nonemergent surgery. Am J Med 2004;117:82–6.
22. Carli F, Zavorsky GS. Optimizing functional exercise capacity in the elderly surgical population. Curr Opin Nutr Metab Care 2005;8:23–32.
23. Govindasamy D, Paterson DH, Poulin MJ, Cunningham DA. Cardiorespiratory adaptation with short-term training in older me. Eur J Appl Physiol Occup Physiol 1992; 65:203–208.
24. Emery CF, Kiecolt-Glaser JK, Glaser R, et al. Exercise accelerates wound healing among health older adults: a preliminary investigation. J Gerontol 2005 60A:1432–1436.
25. Jones LW, Peddle CJ, Eves ND, et al. Effects of presurgical exercise training on cardiorespiratory fitness among patients undergoing thoracic surgery for malignant lung lesions. Cancer 2007 Aug 1;110: 590–8.
26. Arthur HM, Dabiels C, McKelvie R, et al. Effect of a preoperative intervention on preoperative and postoperative outcomes in low-risk patients awaiting elective coronary artery bypass graft surgery. A randomized, controlled trial. Ann Intern Med 2000 Aug 15;133:253–62.
27. Brady M, Kinn S, Stuart P. Preoperative fasting for adults to prevent perioperative complications. Cochrane Database Syst Rev 2003;CD004423.
28. Ljungqvist O, Søreide E. Preoperative fasting. Br J Surg 2003;90:400–406.
29. American Society of Anesthesiologist Task Force on Preoperative Fasting. Practice guidelines for preoperative fasting and the use of pharmacologic agents to reduce the risk of pulmonary aspiration: application to healthy patients undergoing elective procedures: a report by the American Society of Anesthesiologist Task Force on Preoperative Fasting. Anesthesiology 1999; 90:896–905.
30. Hausel J, Nygren J, Lagerkranser M, et al. A carbohydrate-rich drink reduces preoperative discomfort in elective surgery patients. Anesth Analg 2001 93:1344–50.
31. Ljungqvist O, Nygren J, Thorell A. Modulation of post-operative insulin resistance by pre-operative carbohydrate loading. Proc Nutr Soc 2002;61:329–36.
32. Yuill KA, Richardson RA, et al. The administration of oral carbohydrate-containing fluid prior to major elective upper gastrointestinal surgery preserves skeletal muscle mass postoperatively. Clin Nutr 2005;24: 32–7.

33. Svanfeldt M, Thorell A, Hausel J, et al. Randomized clinical trial of the effect of preoperative oral carbohydrate treatment on postoperative whole-body protein and glucose kinetics. Br J Surg 2007;94: 1342–50.
34. Noblett SE, Watson DS, Huong W, et al. Pre-operative oral carbohydrate loading in colorectal surgery: a randomized controlled trial. Colorectal Dis 2006;8:563–69.
35. Hausel J, Nygren J, Thorell, et al. Randomized clinical trial of the effects of oral preoperative carbohydrates on postoperative nausea and vomiting after laparoscopic cholecystectomy. Br J Surg 2005;92: 415–21).
36. Bisgaard T, Kristiansen VB, Hjortso NC, et al. Randomized clinical trial comparing an oral carbohydrate beverage with placebo before laparoscopic cholecystectomy. Br J Surg 2004;91:151–8.
37. MacLaren JE, Kain ZN. Perioperative biopsychosocial research: the future is here. J Clin Anesth 2007;19:410–12.
38. Kiecolt-Glaser JK, et al. Psychological influences on surgical recovery. Am Psychol 1998;53;1209–18.
39. Glaser R, Kiecolt-Glaser JK, Marucha PT, et al. Stress-related changes in proinflammatory cytokine production in wounds. Arch Gen Psych 1999;56:450–456.
40. Kiecolt-Glaser JK, Page GG, Marucha PT, et al. Psychological influences on surgical recovery. Am Psychol 1998;53;1209–18.
41. Zieren J, Menenakos, Mueller JM. Does an informative video before inguinal hernia repair influence postoperative quality of life? Results of a prospective randomized study. Qual Life Res 2007;16:725–9,
42. Mondloch MV, Cole DC, Frank JW. Does how you do depend on how you think you'll do? A systematic review of the evidence for a relation between patients' recovery expectations and health outcomes. CMAJ 2001; 165:174–9.
43. White PF. Pharmacologic and clinical aspects of preoperative medication. Anesth Analg 1986;65:693–74.
44. Van Vlymen JM, Sa Rego MM, While PF. Benzodiazepine premedication: can it improve outcome in patients undergoing breast biopsy procedures? Anesthesiology 1999;90:740–7.
45. Elia N, Lysakowski C, Tramer MR. Does multimodal analgesia with acetaminophen, nonsteroidal anti-inflammatory drugs, or selective cyclooxygenase-2 inhibitors and patient-controlled analgesia morphine offer advantages over morphine alone? Meta-analysis of randomized trials. Anesthesiology 2005;103:1296–304.
46. Johansen JW, Flaishon R, Sebel PS. Esmolol reduces anesthetic requirement for skin incision during propofol/nitrous oxide/ morphine anesthesia. Anesthesiology 1997; 86:364–71.
47. Chia YY, Chan MH, Ko NH, Liu K. Role of beta-blockade in anaesthesia and postoperative pain management after hysterectomy. Br J Anaesth 2004;93:799–805.
48. Segal IS, Jarvis DJ, Duncan SR, et al. Clinical efficacy of oral-transdermal clonidine combinations during the perioperative period. Anesthesiology 1991;74:220–5.
49. Arain SR, Ruehlow RM, Uhrich TD, Ebert TJ. The efficacy of dexmedetomidine versus morphine for postoperative analgesia after major inpatient surgery. Anesth Analg 2004; 98:153–8.
50. Zaugg M, Tagliente T, Lucchinetti E, et al. Beneficial effects from beta-adrenergic blockade in elderly patients undergoing noncardiac surgery. Anesthesiology 1999; 91:1674–86.
51. Lindenauer PK, Pekow P, Wang K, et al. Perioperative beta-blocker therapy and mortality after major noncardiac surgery. N Engl J Med 2005;353:349–61.
52. Devereaux P, Beattie W, Choi P, et al. How strong is the evidence for the use of perioperative beta-blockers in patients undergoing noncardiac surgery? A systematic review and metaanalysis. BMJ 2005;331:313–21.
53. Herndon DN, Hart DW, Wolf SE, et al. Reversal of catabolism by beta-blockade after severe burns. N Engl J Med 2001; 345:1223–9.
54. Wu CT, Jao SW, Borel CO, et al. The effect of epidural clonidine on perioperative cytokine response, postoperative pain, and bowel function in patients undergoing colorectal surgery. Anesth Analg 2004; 99:502–9.
55. Wallace AW, Galindez D, Salahieh A, et al. Effect of clonidine on cardiovascular morbidity after noncardiac surgery. Anesthesiology 2004;101:284–293.
56. Carli F, Halliday D. Modulation of protein metabolism in the surgical patient: effect of 48-H continuous epidural blockade with local anaesthetics on leucine kinetics. Reg Anaesthesia 1996;21;430–435.
57. Block MB, Liu SS, Rowlingson AJ, et al. Efficacy of postoperative epidural analgesia: A meta analysis. JAMA 2003;290:2455–63.
58. Holte K, Kehlet H. Epidural anaesthesia and analgesia: effects on surgical stress responses and implications for postoperative nutrition. Clin Nutr 2002;21:199–205.
59. Carli F, Mayo N, Klubien K, et al. Epidural analgesia enhances functional exercise capacity and health-related quality of life. Results of a randomized trial. Anesthesiology 2002;97:540–549.
60. Hjortso R, Lewin MR, Halliday D, Clark C. Effects of extradural administration of local anesthetic agents and morphine on the urinary excretion of cortisol, catecholamines and nitrogen following abdominal surgery. Br J Anaesth 1985;57:400–6.
61. Schricker T, Meterissian S, Lattermann R, Carli F. Postoperative protein sparing with epidural analgesia and hypocaloric glucose. Ann Surg 2004;240:916–21.
62. Schricker T, Wykes L, Eberhart L, et al. The anabolic effect of epidural blockade requires energy and substrate supply. Anesthesiology 2002;97:943–51.
63. Schricker T, Wykes L, Eberhart L, et al. Randomized clinical trial of the anabolic effect of hypocaloric perenteral nutrition after abdominal surgery. Br J Surg 2005;92: 947–53.
64. Donatelli F, Schricker T, Asenjo JF, et al. Intraoperative infusion of amino acids induces anabolism independently of the type of anesthesia. Anesth Analg 2006;103: 1549–56.
65. Donatelli F, Schricker T, Mistraletti G, et al. Postoperative infusion of amino acids induces a positive protein balance independently of the type of analgesia used. Anesthesiology 2006;105:253–9.
66. Nygren J, Thorell A, Soop M, et al. Perioperative insulin and glucose infusion maintains normal insulin sensitivity after surgery. Am J Physiol 1998;275:E140–8.
67. Ljungqvist O, Thorell A, Gutniak M, et al. Glucose infusion instead of preoperative fasting reduces postoperative insulin resistance. J Am Coll Surg 1994;178:329–336.
68. Crowe P, Dennison A, Royle G. The effect of preoperative glucose loading on postoperative nitrogen metabolism. Br J Surg 1984;71:635–637.
69. Carli F, Galeone M, Gzodzic B, et al. Effect of laparoscopic colon resection on postoperative glucose utilization and the protein sparing effect. Arch Surg 2005;140: 593–597).
70. Pavlin DJ, Rapp SE, Polissar NL, et al. Factors affecting discharge time in adult outpatients. Anesth Analg 1998;87:816–26.
71. Tang J, Chen L, White PF, et al. Recovery profile, costs, and patient satisfaction with propofol and sevoflurane for fast-track office-based anesthesia. Anesthesiology 1999;91:253–261.
72. Song D, Joshi GP, White PF. Fast-track eligibility after ambulatory anesthesia: A comparison of desflurane, sevoflurane, and propofol. Anesth Analg 1998;86:267–73.
73. Tang J, White PF, Wender RH, et al. Fast-track office-based anesthesia: A comparison of propofol versus desflurane with antiemetic prophylaxis in spontaneously breathing patients. Anesth Analg 2001;92:95–9.
74. Tang J, Chen L, White PF, et al. A use of propofol for office-based anesthesia: effect of nitrous oxide on recovery profile. J Clin Anesth 1999;11:226–30.
75. White PF. Prevention of postoperative nausea and vomiting – a multimodal solution to a persistent problem. N Engl J Med 2004;350:2441–51.
76. Gan TJ, Glass PS, Windsor A, et al. Bispectral index monitoring allows faster emergence and improved recovery from propofol, alfentanil, and nitrous oxide anesthesia. BIS Utility Group. Anesthesiology 1997;87: 808–17.
77. Song D, Joshi GP, White PF. Titration of volatile anesthetics using bispectral index facilitates recovery after ambulatory anesthesia. Anesthesiology 1997;87:842–8.
78. Song D, van Vlymen J, White PF. Is the bispectral index useful in predicting fast-track eligibility after ambulatory anesthesia with propofol and desflurane? Anesth Analg 1998;87:1245–8.
79. White PF, Ma H, Tang J, et al. Does the use of electroencephalographic bispectral index or auditory evoked potential index monitoring facilitate recovery after desflurane anesthesia in the ambulatory setting? Anesthesiology 2004;100:811–7.
80. Zohar E, Luban I, White PF, et al. Bispectral index monitoring does not improve early recovery of geriatric outpatients undergoing brief surgical procedures. Can J Anaesth 2006;53:20–25.
81. Kehlet H. Postoperative opioid sparing to hasten recovery. What are the issues? Anesthesiology 2005;102:1983–5.
82. White PF. The changing role of non-opioid analgesic techniques in the management of postoperative pain. Anesth Analg 2005;01: S5–22.
83. Coloma M, Chiu JW, White PF, Armbruster SC. The use of esmolol as an alternative to remifentanil during desflurane anesthesia for fast-track outpatient gynecologic laparoscopic surgery. Anesth Analg 2001;92: 352–7.
84. Collard V, Taqi A, Mistraletti G, et al. Intraoperative esmolol infusion in absence of opioids spares postoperative fentanyl in patients undergoing ambulatory laparoscopic cholecystectomy. Anesth Analg 2007; 105:1255–62.
85. Kaba A, Laurent SR, Detroz BJ, et al. Intravenous lidocaine infusion facilitates acute rehabilitation after laparoscopic colectomy. Anesthesiology 2007;106:11–8.
86. Hunter JM, Flockton EA. The doughnut and the hole: a new pharmacological concept for anaesthetists. Br J Anaesth 2006; 97:123–6.
87. Sacan O, White PF, Tufanogullari Sayin B, Klein K. Sugammadex reversal of rocuronium-induced neuromuscular blockade: A

comparison with neostigmine-glycopyrrolate and edrophonium-atrophine. Anesth Analg 2007;104:569–74.
88. Liu S, Chiu AA, Carpenter RL, et al. Fentanyl prolongs lidocaine spinal anesthesia without prolonging recovery. Anesth Analg 1995;80:730–4.
89. Ben-David B, Solomon E, Levin H, et al. Intrathecal fentanyl with small-dose dilute bupivacaine: better anesthesia without prolonging recovery. Anesth Analg 1997; 85:560–5.
90. Ben-David B, Maryanovsky M, Gurevitch A, et al. A comparison of minidose lidocaine-fentanyl and conventional dose lidocaine spinal anesthesia. Anesth Analg 2000;91:865–70.
91. Vaghadia H, McLeod DH, Mitchell GW, et al. Small-dose hypobaric lidocaine-fentanyl spinal anesthesia for short duration outpatient laparoscopy. I. A randomised comparison with conventional dose hyperbaric lidocaine. Anesth Analg 1997;84: 59–64.
92. Wu CL, Cohen SR, Richman JM, et al. Efficacy of postoperative patient-controlled and continuous infusion epidural analgesia versus intravenous patient-controlled analgesia with opioids. Anesthesiology 2005; 103:1079–88.
93. Norris EJ, Beattie C, Perler BA, et al. Double-masked randomized trial comparing alternate combinations of intraoperative anesthesia and postoperative analgesia in abdominal aortic surgery. Anesthesiology 2001;95:1054–67.
94. Brodner G, Pogatzki E, Van Aken H, et al. A multimodal approach to control postoperative pathophysiology and rehabilitation in patients undergoing abdominothoracic esophagectomy. Anesth Analg 1998;86: 228–34.
95. Anthony Rodgers, Natalie Walker, S Schug, et al. Reduction of postoperative mortality and morbidity with epidural or spinal anaesthesia: results from overview of randomised trials. BMJ 2000;321:1493.
96. Basse L, Torbol JE, Lossel K, Kehlet H. Colonic surgery with accelerated rehabilitation or conventional care. Dis Colon Rectum 2004;47:271–8.
97. Zarate E, Latham P, White PF, et al. Fast-track cardiac anesthesia: a comparison of remifentanil plus intrathecal morphine with sufentanil in a desflurane-based anesthetic. Anesth Analg 2000;91:283–7.
98. Bettex DA, Schmidlin D, Chassot PG, Schmid ER. Intrathecal sufentanil-morphine shortens the duration of intubation and improves analgesia in fast-track cardiac surgery. Can J Anaesth 2002;49:711–7.
99. Lena P, Balarac N, Arnulf JJ, et al. Fast-track coronary artery bypass grafting surgery under general anesthesia with remifentanil and spinal analgesia with morphine and clonidine. J Cardiothorac Vasc Anesth 2005; 19:49–53.
100. Liu SS, Block BM, Wu CL. Effects of perioperative central neuroaxial analgesia on outcome after coronary artery bypass surgery: A meta-analysis. Anesthesiology 2004;101:153–61.
101. Djaiani G, Fedorko L, Beattie WS. Regional anesthesia in cardiac surgery: a friend or a foe? Semin Cardiothorac Vasc Anesth 2005; 9:87–104.
102. Ronald A, Abdul Azizb KA, Day TG, Scott M. Best evidence topic — Cardiac general. In patients undergoing cardiac surgery, thoracic epidural analgesia combined with general anaesthesia results in faster recovery and fewer complications but does not affect length of hospital stay. Interact Cardiovasc Thorac Surg 2006;5:207–16.
103. Hansdottir V, Philip J, Olsen MF, et al. Thoracic epidural versus intravenous patient-controlled analgesia after cardiac surgery: a randomized controlled trial on length of hospital stay and patient-perceived quality of recovery. Anesthesiology 2006; 104:142–51.
104. Carli F, Kehlet H. Continuous epidural analgesia for colonic surgery—years from now but what about the future? Reg Anesth Pain Med 2005;30:140–2.
105. Chung F, Ritchie E, Su J. Postoperative pain in ambulatory surgery. Anesth Analg 1997; 85:808–16.
106. Andersen FM, Nielsen K, Kehlet H. Combined ilioinguinal blockade and local infiltration anaesthesia for groin hernia repair-a double-blind randomized study. Br J Anaesth 2005;94:520–3.
107. Li S, Coloma M, White PF, et al. Comparison of the costs and recovery profiles of three anesthetic techniques for ambulatory anorectal surgery. Anesthesiology 2000;93: 1225–30.
108. Song D, Greilich NB, White PF, et al. Recovery profiles and costs of anesthesia for outpatient unilateral inguinal herniorrhaphy. Anesth Analg 2000;91:876–81.
109. Jensen P, Mikkelsen T, Kehlet H. Postherniorraphy urinary retention—effect of local, regional, and general anesthesia: a review. Reg Anesth Pain Med 2002;27:587–89.
110. Moiniche S, Jorgensen H, Wettersley J, Dahl JB. Local anesthetic infiltration for postoperative pain relief after laparoscopy: a qualitative and quantitative systematic review of intraperitoneal, port site infiltration and mesosalpinx block. Anesth Analg 2000;90:899–912.
111. Liu SS, Richman JM, Thirlby R, Wu CL. Efficacy of continuous wound catheters delivering local anesthetic for postoperative analgesia: a quantitative and qualitative systematic review of randomized controlled trials. J Am Coll Surg 2006;203:914–32.
112. Dowling R, Thielmeier K, Ghaly A, et al. Improved pain control after cardiac surgery: results of a randomized, double blind, clinical trial. J Thorac Cardiovasc Surg 2003;126:1271–8.
113. White PF, Rawal S, Latham P, et al. Use of a continuous local anesthetic infusion for pain management after median sternotomy. Anesthesiology 2003;99:918–23.
114. Sessler DI. Mild perioperative hypothermia. N Engl J Med 1997;336:1730–7.
115. Grocott MP, Mythen MG, Gan TJ. Perioperative fluid management and clinical outcomes in adults. Anesth Analg 2005;100: 1093–106.
116. Holte K, Kehlet H. Fluid therapy and surgical outcomes in elective surgery: a need for reassessment in fast-track surgery. J Am Coll Surg 2006;202:971–89.
117. Arkilic CF, Taguchi A, Charma N. Supplemental perioperative fluid administration increases tissue oxygen pressure. Surgery 2003;133:49–55.
118. Brandstrup B, Tonnesen H, Beier-Holgersen R, et al. Effects of intravenous fluid restriction on postoperative complications: comparison of two perioperative fluid regimens. A randomized assessor-blinded multicenter trial. Ann Surg 2003;238: 640–50.
119. Nisanevich V, Felsenstein I, Almogy G, et al. Effect of intraoperative fluid management on outcome after intraabdominal surgery. Anesthesiology 2005;103:25–32.
120. Holte K, Klarskov B, Christensen DS, et al. Liberal versus restrictive fluid administration to improve recovery after laparoscopic cholecystectomy: a randomized, double-blind study. Ann Surg 2004;240:892–9.
121. Kabon B, Akca O, Taguchi A, et al. Supplemental intravenous crystalloid administration does not reduce the risk of surgical wound infection. Anesth Analg 2005;101: 1546–53.
122. Gan TJ, Soppitt A, Maroof M, et al. Goal directed intraoperative fluid administration reduces length of hospital stay after major surgery. Anesthesiology 2002;97:820–6.
123. Venn R, Steele R, Richardson P, et al. Randomized controlled trial to investigate influence of the fluid challenge on duration of hospital stay and perioperative morbidity in patients with hip fractures. Br J Anaesth 2002;88:65–71.
124. Brown SR, Goodfellow PB. Transverse versus midline incisions for abdominal surgery. Cochrane Database Syst Rev 2005; CD005199.
125. Gupta A, Watson DI. Effect of laparoscopy on immune function. Br J Surg 2001; 88:1296–306.
126. Carter JJ, Whelan RL. The immunologic consequences of laparoscopy in oncology. Surg Oncol Clin N Am 2001;10:655–77.
127. Lawrence VA, Cornell JE, Smetana GW; American College of Physicians. Strategies to reduce postoperative pulmonary complications after noncardiothoracic surgery: systematic review for the American College of Physicians. Ann Intern Med 2006;144: 596–608.
128. Holte K. Kehlet H. Postoperative ileus: a preventable event. Br J Surg 87:1480–93, 2000.
129. Memon MA, Cooper NJ, Memon B., et al Meta-analysis of randomized clinical trials comparing open and laparoscopic inguinal hernia repair. Br J Surg 2003; 90:1479–92.
130. Nanidis TG, Antcliffe D, Kokkinos C, et al. Laparoscopic versus open live donor nephrectomy in renal transplantation: a meta-analysis. Ann Surg 2008;247:58–70.
131. Keus F, de Jong JA, Gooszen HG, van Laarhoven CJ. Laparoscopic versus open cholecystectomy for patients with symptomatic cholecystolithiasis. Cochrane Database Syst Rev 2006;(4):CD006231.
132. Nguyen NT, Goldman C, Rosenquist CJ, et al. Laparoscopic versus open gastric bypass: a randomized study of outcomes, quality of life, and costs. Ann Surg 2001;234: 279–89.
133. Schwenk W, Haase O, Neudecker J, Müller JM. Short term benefits for laparoscopic colorectal resection.Cochrane Database Syst Rev 2005;(3):CD003145.
134. Håkanson BS, Thor KB, Thorell A, Ljungqvist O. Open vs laparoscopic partial posterior fundoplication. A prospective randomized trial. Surg Endosc 2007;21:289–98.
135. Boni L, Benevento A, Rovera F, et al. Infective complications in laparoscopic surgery. Surg Infect (Larchmt) 2006;7(Suppl 2): S109–11).
136. Luján JA, Frutos MD, Hernández Q, et al. Laparoscopic versus open gastric bypass in the treatment of morbid obesity: a randomized prospective study. Ann Surg 2004; 239:433–7.
137. Duepree HJ, Senagore AJ, Delaney CP, Fazio VW. Does means of access affect the incidence of small bowel obstruction and ventral hernia after bowel resection? Laparoscopy versus laparotomy. J Am Coll Surg 2003;197:177–81.

138. King PM, Blazeby JM, Ewings P, et al. Randomized clinical trial comparing laparoscopic and open surgery for colorectal cancer within an enhanced recovery programme. Br J Surg 2006;93:300–8.
139. Raue W, Haase O, Junghans T, et al. 'Fast-track' multimodal rehabilitation program improves outcome after laparoscopic sigmoidectomy: a controlled prospective evaluation. Surg Endosc 2004;18:1463–8.
140. Basse L. Jakobsen DH. Bardram L. et al. Functional recovery after open versus laparoscopic colonic resection: a randomized, blinded study. Ann Surg 2005;241:416–23.
141. MacKay G, Ihedioha U, McConnachie A, et al. Laparoscopic colonic resection in fast-track patients does not enhance short-term recovery after elective surgery. Colorectal Dis 2007;9:368–72.
142. Pavlin DJ, Chen C, Penaloza DG, et al. Pain as a factor complicating recovery and discharge after ambulatory surgery Anesth Analg 2002;95:627–34.
143. Wu Cl, Rowlingson AJ, Partin AW, et al. Correlation of postoperative pain to quality of recovery in the immediate postoperative period. Reg Anesth Pain Med 2005;30: 516–22.
144. Liu SS, Wu CL. Effect of postoperative analgesia on postoperative complications. A systematic update of the evidence. Anesth Analg 2007;104:689–702.
145. Curatolo M, Sveticic G. Drug combinations in pain treatment: a review of the Published evidence and a method for finding the optimal combination. Best Pract Res Clin Anaesthesiol 2002;16:507–19.
146. Apfel CC, Laara E, Koivuranta M, et al. A simplified risk score for predicting post-operative nausea and vomiting: conclusions from cross-validations between two centers. Anesthesiology 1999;91:693–700.
147. Sinclair D, Chung F, Mezei G. Can post-operative nausea and vomiting be predicted? Anesthesiology 1999;91:109–18.
148. Scuderi PE, James RL, Harris L, Mims GR 3rd. Multimodal antiemetic management prevents early postoperative vomiting after outpatient laparoscopy. Anesth Analg 2000; 91:1408–14.
149. Apfel CC, Korttila K, Abdalla M, et al. A factorial trial of six interventions for the prevention of postoperative nausea and vomiting. N Engl J Med 2004;350: 2441–51.
150. Gan TJ, Meyer T, Apfel CC, et al. Consensus guidelines for managing postoperative nausea and vomiting. Anesth Analg 2003; 97:62–71.
151. Lee A, Done M. The use of nonpharmacologic techniques to prevent postoperative nausea and vomiting: a meta-analysis. Anesth Analg 1999;88:1362–9.
152. White PF, Issioui T, Hu J, et al. Comparative efficacy of acustimulation (ReliefBand) versus ondansetron (Zofran) in combination with droperidol for preventing nausea and vomiting. Anesthesiology 2002;97:1075–81.
153. Wolff BG, Michelassi F, Gerkin TM, et al. Alvimopan, a novel, peripherally acting mu opioid antagonist: results of a multicenter, randomized, double-blind, placebo-controlled, phase III trial of major abdominal surgery and postoperative ileus. Ann Surg 2004;240:728–34.
154. Delaney CP, Weese JL, Hyman NH, et al. Phase III trial of alvimopan, a novel, peripherally acting, mu opioid antagonist, for postoperative ileus after major abdominal surgery. Dis Colon Rectum 2005;48:1114–25.
155. Viscusi ER, Goldstein S, Witkowski T, et al. Alvimopan, a peripherally acting mu-opiod receptor antagonist, compared with placebo in postoperative ileus after major abdominal surgery. Results of a randomized, double-blind, controlled study. Surg Endosc 2006; 20:64–70.
156. Lobo DN, Bostock KA, Neal KR, et al. Effect of salt and water balance on recovery of gastrointestinal function after elective colonic resection: a randomized controlled trial. Lancet 2002;359:1812–18.
157. Herroeder S, Pecher S, Schonherr ME, et al. Systemic lidocaine shortens length of hospital stay after colorectal surgery. Ann Surg 2007;246:192–200.
158. Mattei P, Rombeau JL. Review of the pathophysiology and management of post-operative ileus. World J Surg 2006;30:1382–91.
159. Han-Geurts IJ, Hop WC, Kok NF, et al. Randomized clinical trial of the impact of early enteral feeding on postoperative ileus and recovery. Br J Surg 2007;94:555–61.
160. Andersen HK, Lewis SJ, Thomas S. Early enteral nutrition within 24h of colorectal surgery versus later commencement of feeding for postoperative complications. Cochrane Database Syst Rev 2006;(4): CD004080.).
161. Henriksen MG, Hansen HV, Hessov I. Early oral nutrition after elective colorectal surgery: influence of balanced analgesia and enforced mobilization. Nutrition 2002;18: 263–7.
162. Brodner G, Van Aken H, Hertle L, et al. Multimodal perioperative management— [illegible] epidural analgesia, [illegible] and oral nutrition reduces hormonal and metabolic stress and improves convalescence after major urologic surgery. Anesth Analg 2001;92:1594–600.
163. Beattie AH, Prach AT, Baxter JP, Pennington CR. A randomised controlled trial evaluating the use of enteral nutritional supplements postoperatively in malnourished surgical patients. Gut 2000;46:813–8.
164. Harper CM, Lyles YM. physiology and complications of bedrest. J Am Geriatr Soc 1988;36:1047–54.
165. Convertino VA. Cardiovascular consequences of bed rest: effect on maximal oxygen uptake. Med Sci Sports Exerc 1997;29:191–196.
166. Adams GR, Caiozzo VJ, Baldwin KM. Skeleteal muscle unweighting:spaceflight and ground-based models. J Appl Physiol 2003;95:197–206.
167. Bloomfield SA. Changes in musculoskeletal structure and function with prolonged bed rest. Med Sci Sports Exerc 1997;29: 197–206.
168. Christensen T, Kehlet H. Postoperative fatigue. World J Surg 1993;17:220–5.
169. Brieger GH. Early ambulation. A study in the history of surgery. Ann Surg 1983;197: 443–449.
170. Gatt M, Anderson AD, Reddy BS, et al. Randomized clinical trial of multimodal optimization of surgical care in patients undergoing major colonic resection. Br J Surg 2005;92:1354–62.
171. Browning L, Denehy L, Scholes RL. The quantity of early upright mobilisation performed following upper abdominal surgery is low: an observational study. Aust J Physiother 2007;53:47–52.
172. Delaney CP, Zutshi M, Senagore AJ, et al. Prospective, randomized, controlled trial between a pathway of controlled rehabilitation with early ambulation and diet and traditional postoperative care after laparotomy and intestinal resection. Dis Colon Rectum 46:851–9, 2003.
173. Basse L, Raskov HH, Hjort Jakobsen D, et al. Accelerated postoperative recovery programme after colonic resection improves physical performance, pulmonary function and body composition. Br J Surg 2002;89: 446–53.
174. Henriksen MG, Jensen MB, Hansen MV, et al. Enforced mobilization, early oral feeding, and balanced analgesia improve convalescence after colorectal surgery. Nutrition 2002;18:147–52.
175. Maessen J, Dejong CH, Hausel J, et al. A protocol is not enough to implement an enhanced recovery programme for colorectal resection. Br J Surg 2007;94:224–31.
176. Nelson R, Edwards S, Tse B. Prophylactic nasogastric decompression after abdominal surgery.Cochrane Database Syst Rev 2007; (3):CD004929.
177. Doglietto GB, Papa V, Tortorelli AP, et al. Nasojejunal tube placement after total gastrectomy: a multicenter prospective randomized trial. Arch Surg 2004;139: 1309–13.
178. Carrère N, Seulin P, Julio CH, et al. Is nasogastric or nasojejunal decompression necessary after gastrectomy? A prospective randomized trial. World J Surg 2007;31: 122–7).
179. Karliczek A, Jesus EC, Matos D, et al. Drainage or nondrainage in elective colorectal anastomosis: a systematic review and meta-analysis. Colorectal Dis 2006;8:259–65.
180. Samraj K, Gurusamy KS. Wound drains following thyroid surgery. Cochrane Database Syst Rev 2007;(4):CD006099.
181. Gurusamy KS, Samraj K, [illegible] Davidson BR. Routine abdominal [illegible] for uncomplicated laparoscopic cholecystectomy. Cochrane Database Syst Rev 2007; (4):CD006004.
182. Gurusamy KS, Samraj K. Routine abdominal drainage for uncomplicated open cholecystectomy. Cochrane Database Syst Rev 2007;(2):CD006003.
183. Gurusamy KS, Samraj K, Davidson BR. Routine abdominal drainage for uncomplicated liver resection. Cochrane Database Syst Rev 2007;(3):CD006232.
184. Conlon KC, Labow D, Leung D, et al. Prospective randomized clinical trial of the value of intraperitoneal drainage after pancreatic resection. Ann Surg 2001;234: 487–93.
185. Benoist S, Panis Y, Denet C, et al. Optimal duration of urinary drainage after rectal resection: a randomized controlled trial. Surgery 1999;125:135–41.
186. Baldini G, Bagry H, Aprikian A, Carli F. Postoperative urinary retention: anesthetic and perioperative considerations. Anesthesiology [In press].
187. Basse L, Werner M, Kehlet H. Is urinary drainage necessary during continuous epidural analgesia after colonic resection? Reg Anesth Pain Med 2000;25:498–501.
188. Bisgaard T, Klarskov B, Kehlet H, Rosenberg J. Recovery after uncomplicated laparoscopic cholecystectomy. Surgery 2002;132:817–25.
189. Guenaga KF, Matos D, Castro AA, et al. Mechanical bowel preparation for elective colorectal surgery [update in Cochrane Database Syst Rev 2005;(1):CD001544]. Cochrane Database Syst Rev 2003; CD001544.
190. King PM, Blazeby JM, Ewings P, et al. The influence of an enhanced recovery programme on clinical outcomes, costs and quality of life after surgery for colorectal cancer. Colorectal Dis 2006;8:506–13.
191. Schwenk W, Günther N, Wendling P, et al. "Fast-track" rehabilitation for elective colonic surgery in Germany—prospective

observational data from a multi-centre quality assurance programme. Int J Colorectal Dis 2008;23:93–9.

192. Delaney CP, Fazio VW, Senagore AJ, et al. 'Fast track' postoperative management protocol for patients with high co-morbidity undergoing complex abdominal and pelvic colorectal surgery. Br J Surg 2001;88: 1533–8.
193. Scharfenberg M, Raue W, Junghans T, Schwenk W. "Fast-track" rehabilitation after colonic surgery in elderly patients—is it feasible? Int J Colorectal Dis 2007;22: 1469–74.
194. Basse L, Hjort Jakobsen D, Billesbolle P, et al. A clinical pathway to accelerate recovery after colonic resection. Ann Surg 2000;232:51–7.
195. Schwenk W, Neudecker J, Raue W, et al. "Fast-track" rehabilitation after rectal cancer resection. Int J Colorectal Dis 2006; 21:547–53.
196. Cerfolio RJ, Bryant AS, Bass CS, et al. Fast tracking after Ivor Lewis esophagogastrectomy. Chest 2004;126:1187–94.
197. Andersen J, Hjort-Jakobsen D, Christiansen PS, Kehlet H. Readmission rates after a planned hospital stay of 2 versus 3 days in fast-track colonic surgery. Br J Surg 2007; 94:890–3.
198. Bradshaw BG, Liu SS, Thirlby RC. Standardized perioperative care protocols and reduced length of stay after colon surgery. J Am Coll Surg 1998;186:501–6.
199. Porter GA, Pisters PW, Mansyur C, et al. Cost and utilization impact of a clinical pathway for patients undergoing pancreaticoduodenectomy. Ann Surg Oncol 2000;7:484–9.
200. Murphy MA, Richards T, Atkinson C, et al. Fast track open aortic surgery: reduced post operative stay with a goal directed pathway. Eur J Vasc Endovasc Surg 2007;34: 274–87.
201. Dy SM, Garg P, Nyberg D, et al. Critical pathway effectiveness: assessing the impact of patient, hospital care, and pathway characteristics using qualitative comparative analysis. Health Serv Res 2005;40:499–516.
202. Abularrage CJ, Sheridan MJ, Mukherjee D. Endovascular versus "fast-track" abdominal aortic aneurysm repair. Vasc Endovasc Surg 2005;39:229–36.
203. Kuo PC, Johnson LB, Sitzmann JV. Laparoscopic donor nephrectomy with a 23-hour stay: a new standard for transplantation surgery. Ann Surg 2000;231:772–9.
204. Maessen JM, Dejong CH, Kessels AG, et al. Length of stay: an inappropriate readout of the success of enhanced recovery programs. World J Surg 2008;[Epub ahead of print].
205. Kehlet H, Gray AW, Bonnet F, et al. A procedure-specific systematic review and consensus recommendations for postoperative analgesia following laparoscopic cholecystectomy. Surg Endosc 2005;19: 1396–415.
206. Low DE, Kunz S, Schembre D, et al. Esophagectomy—it's not just about mortality anymore: standardized perioperative clinical pathways improve outcomes in patients with esophageal cancer. J Gastrointest Surg 2007;11:1395–402.
207. Cerfolio RJ, Bryant AS, Bass CS, et al. Fast tracking after Ivor Lewis esophagogastrectomy. Chest 2004;126:1187–94.
208. Neal JM, Wilcox RT, Allen HW, Low DE. Near-total esophagectomy: the influence of standardized multimodal management and intraoperative fluid restriction. Reg Anesth Pain Med 2003;28:328–34.
209. Ferri LE, Feldman LS, Stanbridge DD, Fried GM. Patient perception of a clinical pathway for laparoscopic foregut surgery. J Gastrointest Surg 2006;10:878–82.

Acknowledgment

Portions of this chapter are based on a previous chapter "Fast Track Surgery" by Henrik Kehlet, MD, PhD, FACS (Hon) and Douglas W. Wilmore, MD, FACS. The authors wish to thank Drs. Kehlet and Wilmore.

1 ORAL CAVITY LESIONS

Kiran Kakarala, MD, Sook-Bin Woo, DMD, MMSc, and Keith G. Saxon, MD, FACS

Approach to Oral Cavity Lesions

The oral cavity is a complex structure that plays a role in many important functions, including mastication, swallowing, speech, and respiration. It extends from the vermilion border of the lips to the oropharynx and is separated from the oropharynx by the anterior tonsillar pillars, the junction of the hard and soft palates, and the junction between the base of the tongue and the oral tongue at the circumvallate papillae. Subsites of the oral cavity include the lips, buccal mucosa, alveolus, retromolar trigone, tongue, floor of the mouth, and hard palate [*see Figure 1*].

In most cases, lesions of the oral cavity reflect locally confined processes, but, on occasion, they are manifestations of systemic disease. The cause of an oral cavity lesion can usually be identified by the history and the physical examination; however, it is most often determined definitively by either a response to a therapeutic trial or a biopsy. A systematic classification of oral cavity lesions facilitates the development of a differential diagnosis. One approach to classification is based on the appearance of the lesion (e.g., white, red, pigmented, ulcerative, vesiculobullous, raised, or cystic). Another approach is first to categorize the lesion as either neoplastic or nonneoplastic and then to further divide the nonneoplastic lesions into various subcategories (e.g., infectious, inflammatory, vascular, traumatic, and tumorlike) [*see Table 1*]. In the following discussion, we adopt the second approach.

Clinical Evaluation

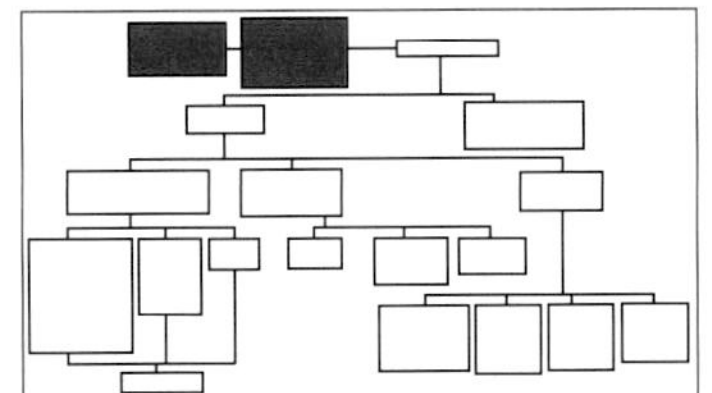

HISTORY

The onset, duration, and growth rate of the oral lesion should be determined. Inflammatory lesions usually have an acute onset and are self-limited, and they may be recurrent. Neoplasms tend to exhibit progressive enlargement; a rapid growth rate is suggestive of malignancy. It is often possible to identify specific events (e.g., upper respiratory tract infection, oral trauma, or medications) that precipitated the lesions. Both malignancies and inflammatory conditions may be associated with various nonspecific symptoms, including pain and dysphagia. Symptoms suggestive of malignancy include trismus, bleeding, a change in denture fit or occlusion, facial sensory changes, and referred otalgia. Fever, night sweats, and weight loss may occur in various settings but are particularly associated with lymphomas and systemic inflammatory conditions. Some oral lesions are identified without presenting signs or symptoms as incidental findings noted during a general dental or medical examination.

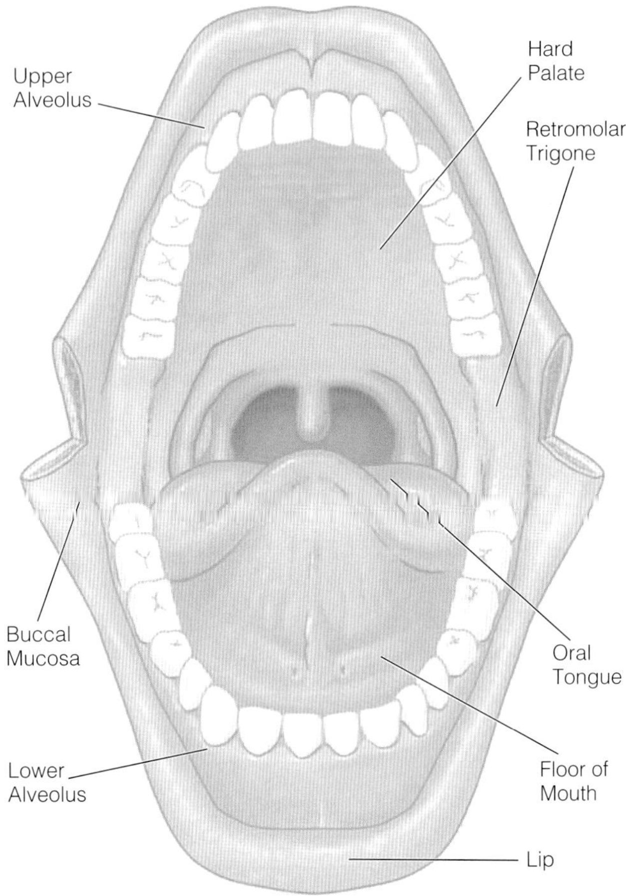

Figure 1 **Depicted are the major anatomic subsites of the oral cavity.**

A review of systems may uncover signs (e.g., rashes or arthritis) that suggest a possible autoimmune disorder. The medical history should always address previous or current connective tissue diseases, malignancies, radiation therapy, chemotherapy, and HIV infection. It is especially important to elicit a medication history because many classes of medications cause drug eruptions that involve the oral mucosa: for instance, well over 100 medications are associated with lichenoid drug reaction, and even more are associated with xerostomia. Use of alcohol or tobacco is a notable risk factor for the development of oral cavity carcinoma, as is a previous head and neck carcinoma. The quantity of alcohol or tobacco consumed should be determined because a dose-response relationship exists between the level of use and the risk of cancer. Other risk factors for oral cavity carcinoma include sun exposure (lip cancer), human papillomavirus infection, and nutritional deficiencies. Radiation exposure is a risk

Table 1 Differential Diagnosis of Oral Cavity Lesions Based on Etiology

- Inflammatory lesions
  - Infectious
    - Viral
      - Herpes simplex
      - Herpes zoster
      - Cytomegalovirus
      - Herpangina
      - Hand, foot, and mouth disease
      - Oral hairy leukoplakia (Epstein-Barr virus)
    - Bacterial
      - Mycobacterial infection
      - Syphilis
      - Gingivostomatitis
    - Fungal
      - Candidiasis
      - Coccidioidomycosis
    - Noninfectious
      - Recurrent aphthous stomatitis
      - Traumatic ulcer
      - Autoimmune disorders
      - Behçet syndrome
      - Systemic lupus erythematosus
      - Wegener granulomatosis
      - Sarcoidosis
      - Amyloidosis
      - Pemphigus and pemphigoid
      - Pyogenic granuloma
      - Necrotizing sialometaplasia
      - Lichen planus
- Tumorlike lesions
  - Mucocele
  - Ranula
  - Tori
  - Fibroma
  - Odontogenic cysts
- Neoplasms
  - Benign
    - Squamous papilloma
    - Minor salivary gland neoplasms
    - Ameloblastoma
    - Hemangioma
    - Granular cell tumor
    - Brown tumor
    - Neuroma, schwannoma, neurofibroma
    - Osteoma, chondroma
  - Malignant
    - Squamous cell carcinoma
    - Verrucous carcinoma
    - Minor salivary gland malignancies
    - Mucoepidermoid carcinoma
    - Adenoid cystic carcinoma
    - Polymorphous low-grade adenocarcinoma
    - Mucosal melanoma
    - Kaposi sarcoma
    - Lymphoma
    - Osteosarcoma

factor for soft tissue sarcoma, lymphoma, and minor salivary gland tumors, and HIV infection is a risk factor for Kaposi sarcoma.

PHYSICAL EXAMINATION

The head and neck should be examined in an organized and systematic manner. Illumination with a headlight or a reflecting mirror facilitates oral examination by freeing the examiner's hands for use in retracting the cheeks and the tongue.

The mucosa of the oral cavity is evaluated at each of the oral subsites. Any trismus should be noted, as should the general health of the teeth and the gingiva. Percussion of carious teeth with pulpitis often elicits pain, although this is not always the case if caries is shallow or pulpal necrosis is present. Palpation of the tongue, the floor of the mouth, and the oral vestibule is an essential component of oral examination. Palpation of the submandibular and submental regions is best performed bimanually.

Oral lesions should be characterized in terms of color, depth, location, texture, fixation, and other applicable attributes. When cancer is present, tenderness, induration, and fixation are common. Invasion of surrounding structures (e.g., the mandible, the parotid duct, or the teeth) by a malignant lesion should be noted. Physical examination is not a definitive means of detecting mandibular invasion, because tumor fixation can be secondary to other factors and cortical invasion can occur with minimal fixation.[1,2] In addition, lesions in some areas of the oral cavity (e.g., the hard palate and the attached gingiva) almost always appear to be fixed.

A history of otalgia warrants otoscopic examination. Otalgia in the absence of any identifiable pathologic condition of the ear often represents referred pain from a malignancy of the upper aerodigestive tract. The presence of otalgia in a middle-aged person should always trigger a search for an underlying cause. The nasal cavity should be examined with a speculum to rule out tumor extension in lesions of the hard palate, and transnasal fiberoptic pharyngoscopy and laryngoscopy should be done if a malignant neoplasm is a possibility or if a systemic condition is suspected that may also affect the nasal or pharyngeal mucosa.

Examination of the neck may reveal enlarged lymph nodes. Lymphadenopathy in an adult should be considered to represent metastatic cancer until proved otherwise. A benign ulcer in the oral cavity may cause a reactive adenopathy as a consequence of the associated inflammation, but in the setting of cervical lymphadenopathy, the initial diagnostic assumptions should emphasize the strong possibility of a primary oral cancer with metastases to the neck. Asymmetrical enlargement of the parotid or submandibular glands may result either from obstruction of the ducts by an oral cavity mass or from enlargement of nodes intimately associated with the glands. Symmetrical enlargement suggests a systemic process (e.g., Sjögren syndrome or HIV infection). The cranial nerves should be examined, with particular attention focused on the trigeminal, facial, and hypoglossal nerves.

Investigative Studies

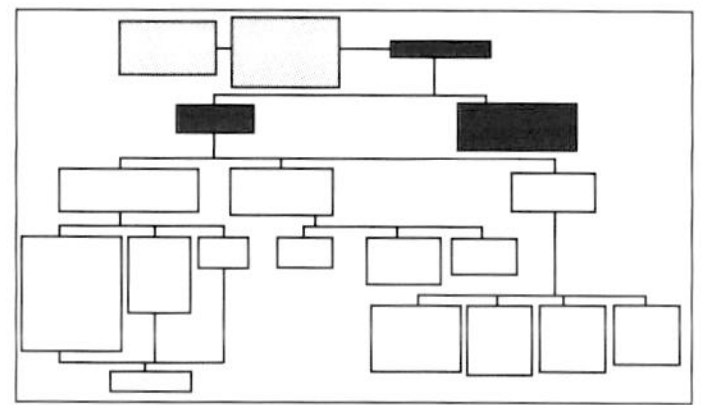

The history and physical examination should narrow down the differential diagnosis and lead to a working diagnosis. If a benign local process (e.g., aphthous stomatitis, traumatic ulcer, or viral infection) is suspected, no further investigation, other than reevaluation, may be needed. If the lesion persists or progresses, further investigation is warranted.

LABORATORY TESTS

Laboratory studies are usually not beneficial in the initial workup of oral cavity lesions. If a connective tissue disease

is suspected, serologic tests [*see Table 2*] and referral to a rheumatologist or another appropriate specialist may be considered.

IMAGING

The value of advanced imaging with computed tomography (CT), magnetic resonance imaging (MRI), or both in the management of oral cavity lesions has not been firmly established. Accordingly, judgment must be exercised. There is evidence to suggest that early oral cavity malignancies can be managed without either CT or MRI. Nevertheless, many clinicians obtain these studies in all cases of malignancy and in most cases of suspected malignancy. CT and MRI can help assess the size and location of the lesion and determine the degree to which surrounding structures are involved. In patients with oral cavity carcinoma, imaging facilitates the staging of tumors and the planning of treatment. In patients with cervical metastases, physical examination augmented by MRI and CT has a better diagnostic yield than physical examination alone. Bone-window CT scans are particularly helpful for assessing invasion of the mandible, the maxilla, the cervical spine, and the base of the skull. CT scans are highly sensitive and specific for detecting mandibular invasion.[1–3] MRI provides better soft tissue delineation than CT, with fewer dental artifacts, and therefore is particularly valuable for assessing malignancies of the tongue, the floor of the mouth, and the salivary glands. Loss of the usual marrow signal on T_1-weighted MRI images suggests bone invasion, although this is not a specific finding. Chest radiography, CT, or both may be employed to search for lung metastases or a second primary tumor.

Positron emission tomography (PET) is playing an increasingly important role in the workup of patients with head and neck carcinoma or mucosal melanoma. PET is useful for confirming the presence of a malignancy, as well as for assessing cervical and distant metastases; it is particularly valuable for detecting recurrent or persistent disease.[4–6] The development of fused PET-CT images has allowed for greater accuracy in anatomically delineating tumors and planning treatment. Drawbacks of PET include frequent false positive results with active inflammation, high cost, and limited availability. In addition, the quality of the images obtained and the level of technical experience available vary considerably among institutions. The role of PET imaging in the initial management and follow-up of head and neck cancer is still being defined.

Table 2 **Serologic Tests for Diagnosing Connective Tissue Disease**

Connective Tissue Disease	Serologic Tests
SLE	CBC, antinuclear antibody, anti–double-stranded DNA antibody, anti-Smith antibody
Sjögren syndrome	Antinuclear antibody, rheumatoid factor, anti-Ro (SS-A) and anti-La (SS-B) antibodies
Wegener granulomatosis	cANCA, serum creatinine level, urine microscopy
Sarcoidosis	Serum calcium and ACE levels

ACE = angiotensin-converting enzyme; cANCA = cytoplasmic antineutrophil cytoplasmic antibodies; CBC = complete blood count; SLE = systemic lupus erythematosus.

BIOPSY

For oral cavity lesions that are suggestive of malignancy or are probably of neoplastic origin, biopsy is usually required. A brief observation period to allow reevaluation, with biopsy withheld, may be warranted if a response to therapy or spontaneous resolution is possible. The potential morbidity associated with a biopsy done in a previously irradiated region should be considered in deciding whether biopsy is advisable. Specimens are usually sent to the pathologist in 10% buffered formalin, but there are notable exceptions. If a lymphoma is suspected, specimens should be sent without formalin for genetic testing and flow cytometry. If an autoimmune disease is suspected, special tests requiring immunofluorescence are indicated, and specimens should be sent either fresh or in Michel solution. In addition, if fungal, mycobacterial, bacterial, or viral infection is suspected, a small portion of a specimen may be sent separately for culture. If there is an associated neck mass, fine-needle aspiration (FNA) may be performed to rule out metastatic disease.[7] In general, FNA is not useful for biopsy of oral lesions: incisional biopsy is often technically easier and provides more tissue.

EXAMINATION UNDER ANESTHESIA AND PANENDOSCOPY

In patients with oral carcinoma, examination under anesthesia (EUA) and panendoscopy should be performed before definitive resection to assess the extent of the primary tumor and identify any synchronous tumors. Both EUA and panendoscopy are commonly performed in the operating room with the patient under general anesthesia. Panendoscopy involves endoscopic examination of the larynx, the oropharynx, the hypopharynx, the esophagus, and, occasionally, the nasopharynx. As a rule, assessment of the tumor and neck is more accurately performed when the patient is relaxed under a general anesthetic.

Diagnosis and Management of Specific Oral Cavity Lesions

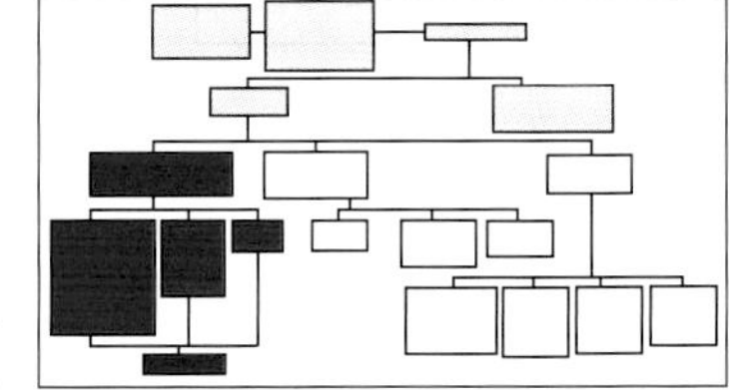

INFLAMMATORY LESIONS

Infectious

Viral stomatitis may be caused by a number of different viruses, including herpes simplex virus (type 1 or type 2), varicella-zoster virus, and coxsackievirus [*see Figure 2, a and b*].[8] It is most common in children and immunocompromised patients. The lesions of viral stomatitis are generally vesicular, occur in the oral cavity and the oropharynx, and erupt over the course of several days to form painful ulcers. Eruption may be preceded by local symptoms (e.g., burning, itching, or tingling) or systemic symptoms (e.g., fever, rash, malaise, or lymphadenopathy). The diagnosis is usually established by the history and the physical examination and may be confirmed by means of biopsy or viral culture.

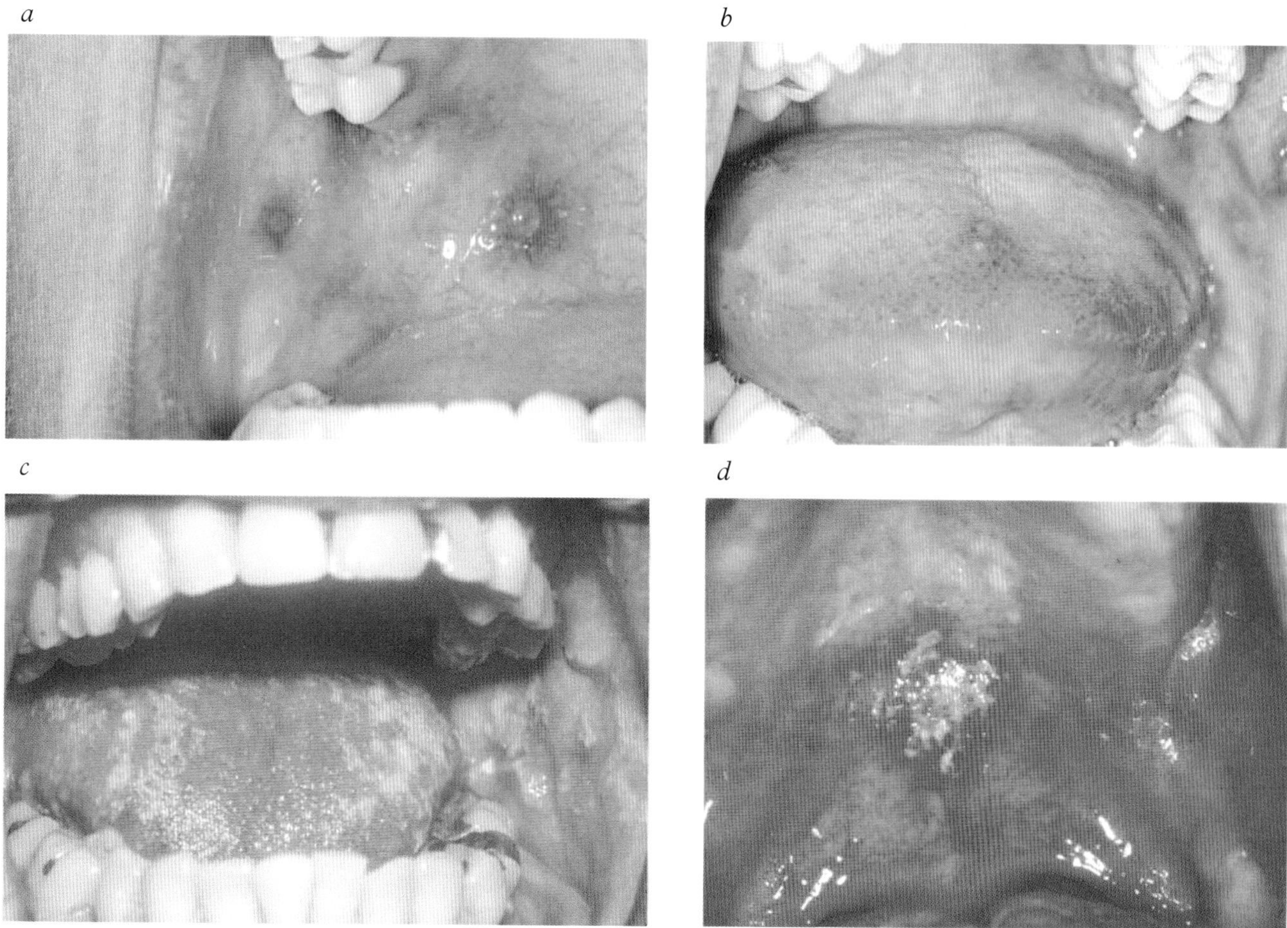

Figure 2 **Shown are infectious lesions of the oral cavity: (*a*) primary herpes stomatitis of the buccal mucosa and soft palate; (*b*) primary herpes stomatitis of the tongue (in the same patient as in frame *a*); (*c*) oral candidiasis (pseudomembranous form); and (*d*) oral candidiasis (erythematous form).**

Treatment of viral stomatitis primarily involves managing symptoms with oral rinses, topical anesthetics, hydration, and antipyretics. Systemic antiviral medications may shorten the course of herpetic stomatitis and are indicated in immunocompromised patients.[9]

Candidiasis is a common fungal infection of the oral cavity [*see Figure 2, c and d*]. *Candida albicans* is the species most commonly responsible; however, other *Candida* species can cause this condition as well, with *Candida glabrata* emerging as a growing problem in immunocompromised hosts. Factors predisposing to oral candidal infection include immunosuppression, use of broad-spectrum antibiotics, diabetes, prolonged use of local or systemic steroids, and xerostomia.[10] Oral candidiasis presents in several different forms [*see Table 3*], of which pseudomembranous candidiasis (thrush) is the most common. This form is characterized by white, curdlike plaques on the oral mucosa that may be wiped off (with difficulty) to leave an erythematous, painful base (the Auspitz sign). Widespread oral and pharyngeal involvement is common. The diagnosis is based on the clinical appearance of the lesion and on evaluation of scrapings with the potassium hydroxide (KOH) test. Culture is generally not useful, because *Candida* is a common commensal oral organism.[11]

Ideally, initial management of oral candidiasis is aimed at reversing the underlying condition, although this is not always possible. Treatment typically involves either topically administered antifungal agents or, if infection is severe or topical therapy fails, systemically administered antifungals. Patients who are immunocompromised or have xerostomia may benefit from long-term prophylaxis.

Table 3 **Clinical Presentation of Oral Candidiasis**

Type of Oral Candidiasis	Presentation
Pseudomembranous	White, curdlike plaques on oral mucosa that when wiped off (with difficulty) leave erythematous, painful base
Hyperplastic	Thick white plaques on oral mucosa that cannot be rubbed off
Erythematous	Red, atrophic areas on palate or dorsum of tongue
Angular cheilitis	Cracking and fissuring at oral commissures

Noninfectious

Recurrent aphthous stomatitis Aphthous stomatitis is a common idiopathic ulcerative condition of the oral cavity [*see Figure 3, a and b*]. The ulcers are typically painful and

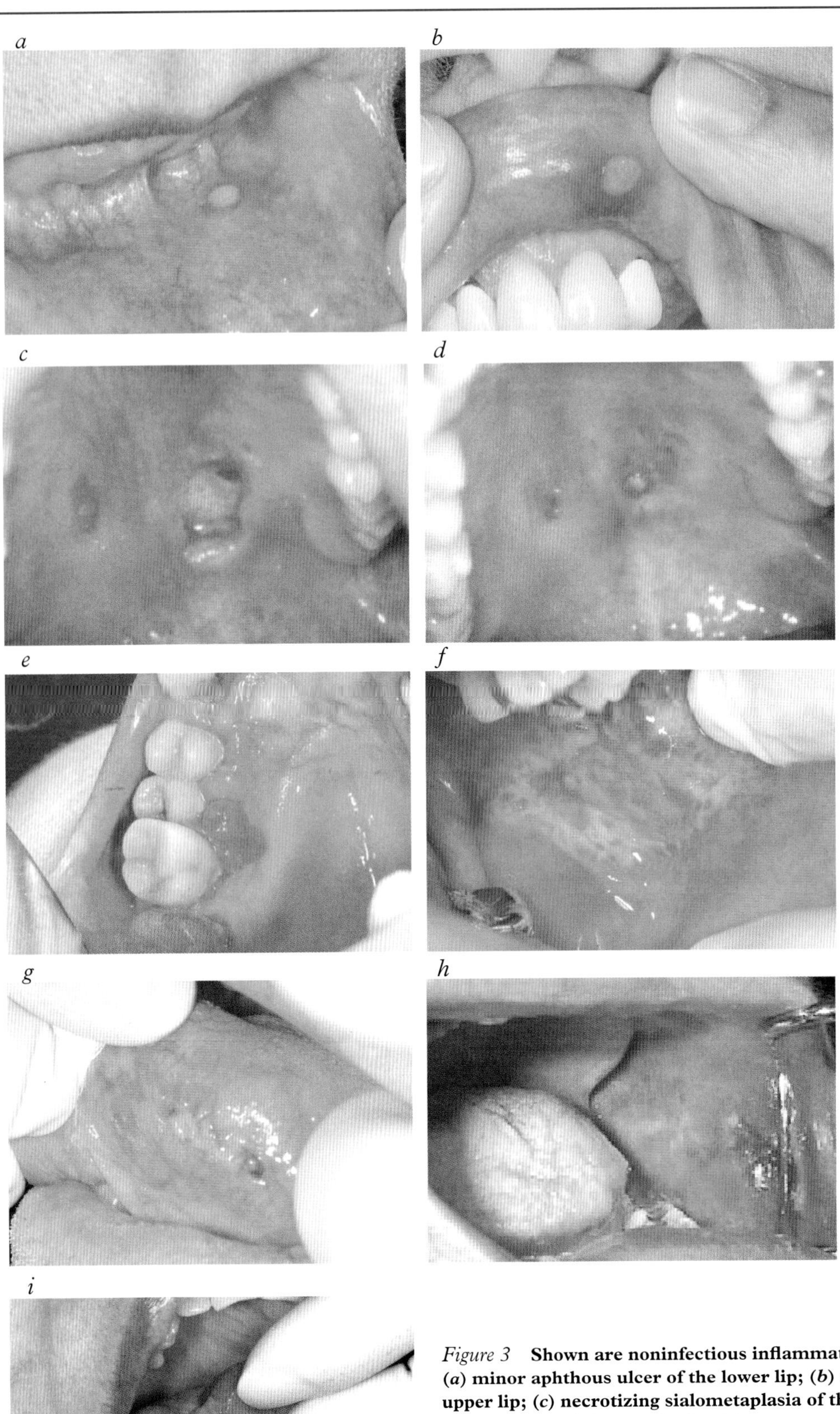

Figure 3 **Shown are noninfectious inflammatory lesions of the oral cavity: (*a*) minor aphthous ulcer of the lower lip; (*b*) minor aphthous ulcer of the upper lip; (*c*) necrotizing sialometaplasia of the hard palate; (*d*) resolution of necrotizing sialometaplasia without treatment (in the same patient as in frame *c*); (*e*) pyogenic granuloma of the upper alveolus; (*f*) reticular lichen planus involving the buccal mucosa; (*g*) lichen planus of the lateral tongue; (*h*) pemphigus vulgaris of the oral cavity, with an erythematous base after rupture of bullae (involving the left lateral tongue, the buccal mucosa, and the lip); and (*i*) traumatic ulcer of the tongue secondary to dental trauma.**

may occur anywhere in the oral cavity and the oropharynx but are rarely found on the hard palate, the dorsal tongue, and the attached gingiva.[9,12] Affected patients often have a history of lesions, beginning before adolescence. There are three different clinical presentations of recurrent aphthous stomatitis, of which minor aphthous ulcers are the most common [*see Table 4*].[9] The diagnosis is made on the basis of the history and the physical examination; biopsy is reserved for lesions that do not heal or that grow in size.

Numerous therapies have been tried for recurrent aphthous stomatitis, most with only minimal success. The majority of aphthous ulcers heal within 10 to 14 days and require no treatment; however, patients with severe symptoms may require medical intervention. Temporary pain relief can be obtained with topical anesthetic agents (e.g., viscous lidocaine). Tetracycline oral suspension and antiseptic mouthwashes have also been used, with varying success.[9,12] Topical steroids are the mainstay of therapy and may shorten the duration of the ulcers if applied during the early phase.[11,12] These agents may be applied either in a solution (e.g., dexamethasone oral suspension, 0.5 mg/5 mL) or in an ointment (e.g., fluocinolone or clobetasol). Ointments work much better in the oral cavity than creams or gels do. Systemic steroids are indicated when the number of ulcers is large or when the outbreak has persisted for a long time.

Necrotizing sialometaplasia Necrotizing sialometaplasia is a rare benign inflammatory lesion of the minor salivary glands that resembles carcinoma clinically and histologically and is readily mistaken for it [*see Figure 3c*].[8] This condition most commonly develops in white males in the form of a deep, sudden ulcer of the hard palate. The presumed cause is ischemia of the minor salivary glands resulting from infection, trauma, surgery, irradiation, or irritation caused by ill-fitting dentures.[9] Biopsy is usually necessary to rule out squamous cell carcinoma or a minor salivary gland malignancy. Review of the tissue by a pathologist well versed in head and neck pathology is essential. Characteristic histologic findings include coagulation necrosis of the salivary gland acini, ductal squamous metaplasia, preservation of the lobular architecture, and a nonmalignant appearance of squamous nests.[13]

Lesions resolve without treatment within 6 to 10 weeks [*see Figure 3d*].

Table 4 **Clinical Presentation of Aphthous Stomatitis**

Type of Aphthous Ulcer	Presentation	Time to Resolution
Minor	Multiple painful, well-demarcated ulcers, < 1.0 cm in diameter, are noted, with yellow fibrinoid base and surrounding erythema; typically involve mobile mucosa, with tongue, palate, and anterior tonsillar pillar the most common sites	7–10 days, without scarring
Major (Sutton disease)	Ulcers, often multiple, may range in size from a few millimeters to 3 cm and may penetrate deeply with elevated margins; typically involve mobile mucosa, with tongue, palate, and anterior tonsillar pillar the most common sites	4–6 wk, with scarring
Herpetiform	Small (1–3 mm) ulcers occur in "crops" but are still limited to movable mucosal surfaces; gingival involvement, if present, is caused by extension from nonkeratinizing crevicular epithelium	1–2 wk

Pyogenic granuloma A pyogenic granuloma is an aggregation of proliferating endothelial tissue [*see Figure 3e*] that occurs in response to chronic persistent irritation (e.g., from a calculus or a foreign body) or trauma.[10] The lesion appears as a raised, soft, sessile or pedunculated mass with a smooth, red surface that bleeds easily and can grow rapidly.[14] Surface ulceration may occur, but the ulcers are not invasive. The gingiva is the most common location, but any of the oral tissues may be involved.

Conservative excision with management of the underlying irritant is the recommended treatment. The classic presentation is in a pregnant woman, and hormonal influences may have an additional influence on recurrence.

Lichen planus Lichen planus is a common immune-mediated inflammatory mucocutaneous disease [*see Figure 3, f and g*].[15] Clinically, idiopathic lichen planus is indistinguishable from lichenoid drug reaction. The reticular form of lichen planus is the most common one and presents as interlacing white keratotic striae on the buccal mucosa, the lateral tongue, and the palate.[15] Lichen planus is usually bilateral, symmetrical, and asymptomatic.[16] The symptomatic phases may wax and wane, with erythematous and ulcerative changes being the primary signs. Cutaneous lesions occur less frequently and appear as small, violaceous, pruritic papules. The diagnosis is generally made on the basis of the history and the physical examination; biopsy is not always necessary.

For asymptomatic lesions, no treatment is required other than observation. For painful lesions, which are more common with the erosive form of the disease, either topical or systemic steroids are appropriate.[16] There is some controversy regarding the risk of malignant transformation; however, long-term follow-up is still recommended.[16] The main risk posed by lichen planus may be the masking effect that the white striae cause, which can prevent the clinician from observing the early leukoplakic and erythroplakic changes associated with epithelial dysplasia.

Ulcer from autoimmune disease Oral ulcers may be the first manifestation of a systemic illness. The most common oral manifestation of systemic lupus erythematosus (SLE) is the appearance of painful oral ulcers in women of childbearing age. Patients with Behçet disease present with the characteristic triad of painful oral ulcers, genital ulcers, and associated iritis or uveitis. Patients with Crohn disease or Wegener granulomatosis frequently manifest oral ulceration during the course of the illness. These disorders should be managed in conjunction with a rheumatologist.

Mucous membrane pemphigoid and pemphigus vulgaris are chronic vesiculobullous autoimmune diseases that frequently affect the oral mucosa [*see Figure 3h*]. In mucous membrane pemphigoid, the antibodies are directed at the mucosal basement membrane, resulting in subepithelial bullae.[16] These bullae rupture after 1 to 2 days to form painful ulcers, which may heal over a period of 1 to 2 weeks but often do not display a predictable periodicity. Oral pain is often the chief complaint, but there may be undetected ocular involvement that can lead to entropion and blindness.

Pemphigus vulgaris is a more severe disease than mucous membrane pemphigoid. In this condition, the antibodies are directed at intraepithelial adhesion molecules, leading to the formation of intraepithelial bullae.[9] The blisters are painful and easily ruptured and tend to occur throughout the oral cavity and the pharynx.[17] The Nikolsky sign (i.e., vesicle formation or sloughing when a lateral shearing force is applied to uninvolved oral mucosa or skin) is present in both pemphigus and pemphigoid. In most cases, biopsy with pathologic evaluation (including immunofluorescence studies) is helpful in establishing the diagnosis. Circulating antibodies may be present in either condition but are more common in pemphigus. Serologic tests may suffice to establish the diagnosis, without any need for biopsy. Management involves administration of immunosuppressive agents, often in conjunction with a dermatologist.

Traumatic ulcer Trauma (e.g., from tooth abrasion, tooth brushing, poor denture fit, or burns) is a common cause of oral mucosal ulceration [*see Figure 3i*]. The ulcers usually are painful but typically are self-limited and resolve without treatment. Topical anesthetic agents may be beneficial if pain is severe enough to limit oral intake.

Tumorlike Lesions

TORUS MANDIBULARIS AND TORUS PALATINUS

Palatal and mandibular tori are benign focal overgrowths of cortical bone [*see Figure 4, a and b*].[10] They appear as slow-growing, asymptomatic, firm, submucosal bony masses developing on the lingual surface of the mandible or the midline of the hard palate.[14] When these lesions occur on the labial or buccal aspect of the mandible and the maxilla, they are termed exostosis.[18] Torus mandibularis tends to occur bilaterally, whereas torus palatinus arises as a singular, often lobulated mass in the midline of the hard palate. Surgical management is required only if the tori are interfering with denture fit.

MUCOCELE AND MUCOUS RETENTION CYST

A mucocele is a pseudocyst that develops when injury to a minor salivary gland duct causes extravasation of mucus, surrounding inflammation, and formation of a pseudocapsule [*see Figure 4, c and d*].[14] Mucoceles are soft, compressible, bluish or translucent masses that may fluctuate in size. They are most commonly seen on the lower lip but also may develop on the buccal mucosa, anterior ventral tongue, and floor of the mouth. Only very rarely do they involve the upper lip; masses in the upper lip, even if they are fluctuant, should be assumed to be neoplastic, developmental, or infectious. Treatment involves excision of the mucocele and its associated minor salivary gland.

A ranula (from a diminutive form of the Latin word for frog) is a mucocele that develops in the floor of the mouth as a consequence of obstruction of the sublingual duct,[19] secondary either to trauma or to sublingual gland sialoliths. If the ranula extends through the mylohyoid muscle into the neck, it is referred to as a plunging ranula. A plunging ranula may present as a submental or submandibular neck mass. Imaging helps delineate the extent of the mass and may confirm the presence of a sialolith. The recommended treatment is excision of the ranula with removal of the sublingual gland and often the adjacent submandibular gland. Marsupialization is an option but is associated with a relatively high recurrence rate.[19,20]

A mucous retention cyst (salivary duct cyst) is usually the result of partial obstruction of a salivary gland duct accompanied by mucous accumulation and ductal dilatation [*see Figure 4e*].[19] It is a soft, compressible mass that may occur at any location in the oral cavity where minor salivary glands are present. Treatment involves surgical excision with removal of the associated minor salivary gland.

FIBROMA

A fibroma is a hyperplastic response to inflammation or trauma [*see Figure 4, f and g*].[8] It is a pedunculated soft or firm mass with a smooth mucosal surface that may be located anywhere in the mouth. Such lesions are managed with either observation or local excision.

ODONTOGENIC CYST

A dentigerous cyst is an epithelium-lined cyst that, by definition, is associated with the crown of an unerupted tooth [*see Figure 4h*]. Such cysts cause painless expansion of the mandible or the maxilla. Treatment involves enucleation of the cyst and its lining and extraction of the associated tooth.[21]

An odontogenic keratocyst is a squamous epithelium–lined cyst that produces keratin. Bone resorption occurs secondary to pressure resorption and to inflammation caused by retained keratin. Management involves either excision or débridement and creation of a well-ventilated and easily maintained cavity.[22]

Neoplastic Lesions

BENIGN

Squamous Papilloma

Squamous papilloma is one of the most common benign neoplasms of the oral cavity [*see Figure 5, a and b*].[13] It usually presents as a solitary, slow-growing, asymptomatic lesion, typically less than 1 cm in diameter. It is well circumscribed and pedunculated and has a warty appearance.[16] The palate and tongue are the sites most frequently affected[13]; occasionally, multiple sites are involved. The presumed cause is a viral infection, most likely human papillomavirus.[23]

Papillomas are managed with complete excision, including the base of the stalk.

Giant Cell Lesions

Central giant cell granulomas, brown tumors of hyperparathyroidism, aneurysmal bone cysts, and lesions associated with genetic diseases (e.g., cherubism) may all be seen in the jaws. Of particular note is the aneurysmal bone cyst that may occur at sites of trauma, which, in theory, is the consequence

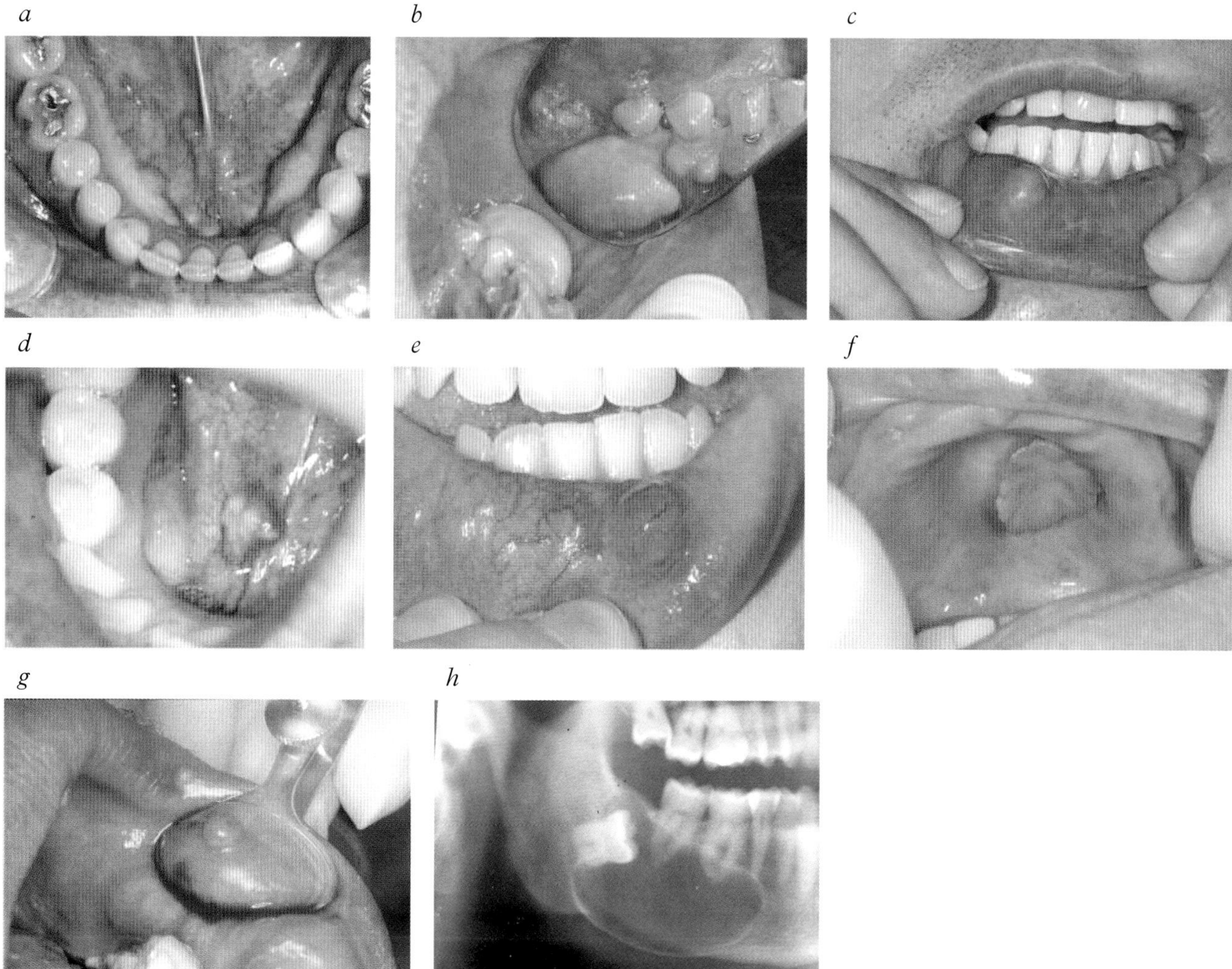

Figure 4 **Shown are tumorlike lesions of the oral cavity: (*a*) torus mandibularis, with bilateral bony protuberances on the lingual surface of the mandible; (*b*) mandibular exostosis, with a unilateral bony protuberance on the labial-buccal surface of the mandible; (*c*) mucocele of the lip (note the bluish hue of the cystic lesion; cf. frame *e*); (*d*) mucocele of the floor of the mouth associated with the sublingual gland (ranula); (*e*) mucous retention cyst of the lower lip (presenting much like mucocele but appearing more transparent); (*f*) fibroma of the hard palate resulting from denture trauma; (*g*) fibroma of the lower lip; and (*h*) dentigerous cyst (a unilocular radiolucency surrounding the crown of an unerupted tooth, with no bone destruction).**

of an organizing hematoma that leads to bony expansion and giant cell proliferation.[24] Eventually, erosion of the buccal cortex may occur with the development of facial swelling.

Management involves enucleation and curettage.[24,25] The surgeon should be prepared for bleeding during treatment. The use of calcitonin or intralesional steroid injections is gaining popularity.[25]

Minor Salivary Gland Neoplasms

The minor salivary glands are small, mucus-secreting glands that are distributed throughout the upper aerodigestive tract, with the largest proportion concentrated in the oral cavity. Minor salivary gland neoplasms are uncommon, but when they do occur, they are most likely to develop in the oral cavity. Within the oral cavity, the hard palate and the soft palate are the most common sites of minor salivary gland neoplasms; however, tumors involving the tongue, the lips, the buccal mucosa, and the gingivae have been described. Approximately 30% of minor salivary gland neoplasms are benign. Of these benign lesions, the most common is pleomorphic adenoma, which presents as a painless, slow-growing submucosal mass [*see Figure 5, c and d*].[13,26]

Pleomorphic adenoma is managed with complete surgical excision to clear margins. This tumor exhibits small, pseudopodlike extensions that may persist and cause recurrence if enucleation around an apparent capsule is attempted.

Granular Cell Tumor

A granular cell tumor is a benign neoplasm that is thought to arise from Schwann cells.[13] It usually presents as a small, asymptomatic, solitary submucosal mass. The lateral border and the dorsal surface of the tongue are the sites where this tumor is most frequently found in the oral cavity.[27] Pathologic examination may reveal pseudoepitheliomatous hyperplasia, which is similar in appearance to well-differentiated squamous cell carcinoma.[28] This similarity has led to reports of

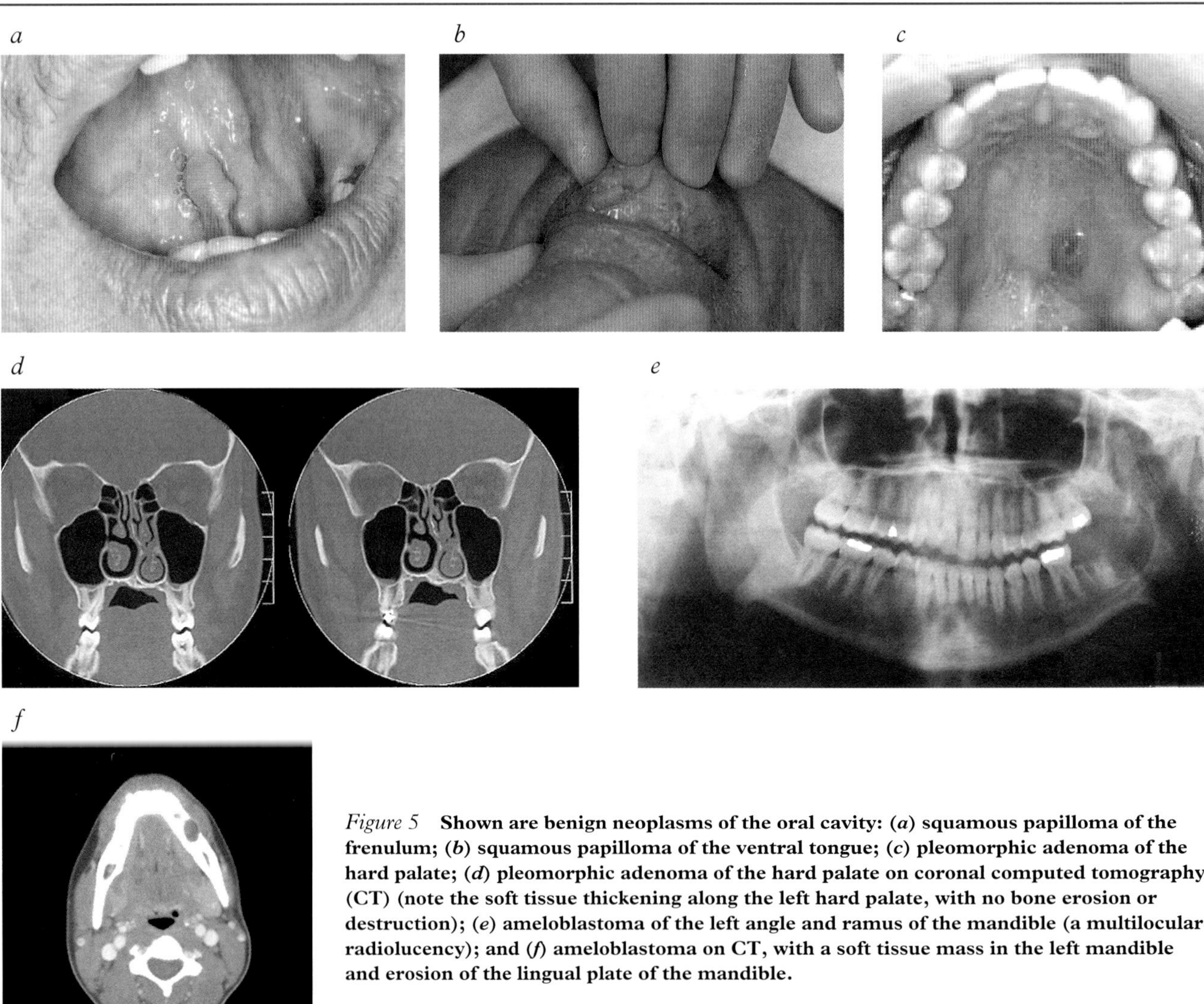

Figure 5 **Shown are benign neoplasms of the oral cavity: (*a*) squamous papilloma of the frenulum; (*b*) squamous papilloma of the ventral tongue; (*c*) pleomorphic adenoma of the hard palate; (*d*) pleomorphic adenoma of the hard palate on coronal computed tomography (CT) (note the soft tissue thickening along the left hard palate, with no bone erosion or destruction); (*e*) ameloblastoma of the left angle and ramus of the mandible (a multilocular radiolucency); and (*f*) ameloblastoma on CT, with a soft tissue mass in the left mandible and erosion of the lingual plate of the mandible.**

misdiagnosis on histopathologic evaluation. Accordingly, given the known rarity of squamous cell carcinoma of the dorsal surface of the anterior two thirds of the tongue, it may be prudent to obtain a second histopathologic opinion whenever a diagnosis of squamous cell carcinoma is rendered in this location. Treatment consists of conservative excision.[27]

Ameloblastoma

Ameloblastoma is a neoplasm that arises from odontogenic (dental) epithelium, most frequently in the third and fourth decades of life [*see Figure 5, e and f*].[8,26] It often presents as a painless swelling with bony enlargement. Approximately 80% of ameloblastomas involve the mandible and 20% the maxilla[29]; the mandibular ramus is the most common site.[29] Ameloblastomas are usually benign but are often locally aggressive and infiltrative. Malignant ameloblastomas are rare but are notable for being associated with pain, rapid growth, and metastases.[11]

On CT and panoramic jaw films, ameloblastomas typically appear as multilocular radiolucent lesions with a honeycomb appearance and scalloped borders.[30] These tumors are often associated with an unerupted third molar tooth and, with the exception of the desmoplastic variant, rarely appear radiopaque. They may also appear unilocular on radiographic imaging.[31] Histologic examination shows proliferating odontogenic epithelium with palisading peripheral cells that display reverse polarization of the nuclei.[13]

Appropriate management of ameloblastomas involves resection to clear margins. For mandibular ameloblastomas, either a marginal or a segmental mandibulectomy is done, depending on the relation of the lesion to the inferior cortical border. Curettage is associated with a high recurrence rate.[29] The prognosis for maxillary multicystic ameloblastoma is relatively poor because of the higher recurrence rate and the greater frequency of invasion of local adjacent structures (e.g., the skull base).[32]

Most types of mesenchymal neoplasms may be found also in the oral region. Benign mesenchymal neoplasms known to occur in the oral cavity include (but are not limited to) hemangiomas, lipomas, schwannomas, neuromas, and neurofibromas. These are relatively rare lesions but should nonetheless be included in the differential diagnosis of intraoral masses. The diagnosis is usually made on the basis of histopathologic examination of biopsy specimens. Benign bone tumors, although uncommon, are not unknown. Chondromas, hemangiomas, ossifying fibromas, and osteomas may all present as intraoral masses with bony expansion and normal overlying mucosa.

PREMALIGNANT

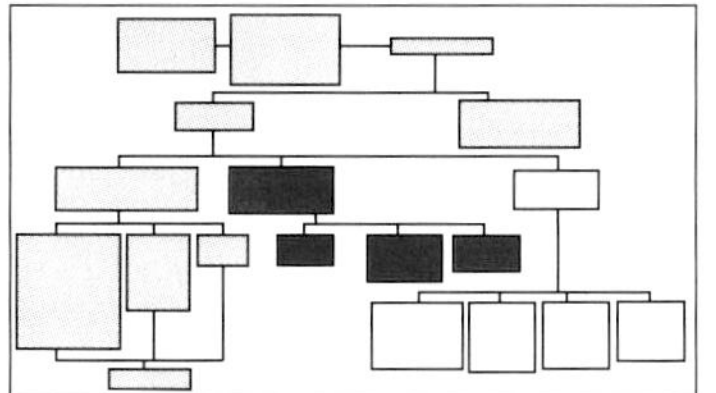

Leukoplakia

Leukoplakia is defined by the World Health Organization as a whitish patch or plaque that cannot be characterized clinically or pathologically as any other disease and that is not associated with any physical or chemical causative agent (except tobacco).[33] It is therefore a clinicopathologic entity of exclusion. It is often considered a potentially premalignant lesion. Leukoplakic lesions vary in size, shape, and consistency; there is usually no relation between morphologic appearance and histologic diagnosis. Histologic examination may reveal hyperkeratosis, dysplasia, carcinoma in situ (CIS), or invasive squamous cell carcinoma, or other pathologic processes.[16] Dysplasia occurs in as many as 30% of leukoplakic lesions.[8] Whereas a small percentage of lesions show invasive squamous cell carcinoma on pathologic examination,[14] 60% of oral mucosa carcinomas present as white, keratotic lesions.[16]

Because leukoplakias are clinicopathologic entities, a biopsy result of "hyperkeratosis, acanthosis with or without inflammation" must be further interpreted by the clinician as to whether the clinical lesion could represent a frictional injury such as morsicatio mucossae oris, benign alveolar ridge keratosis, or some other less well-defined frictional keratosis. This is because it is well known that some so-called "benign leukoplakias" will develop squamous cell carcinoma when followed. Furthermore, the entity "proliferative verrucous leukoplakia" almost always shows benign histology for many years and the majority if not all of such lesions become invasive cancer when followed over time.

All leukoplakic lesions should undergo biopsy. For small areas of leukoplakia, excisional biopsy is usually appropriate. For larger lesions, incisional biopsy is generally preferable: it is important to obtain an adequate-size biopsy specimen in that varying degrees of hyperplasia and dysplasia may occur within the same specimen. There is no consensus regarding the management of "nondysplastic" leukoplakias that in the clinician's opinion are not reactive or inflammatory in nature. Some believe that such hyperkeratotic lesions should be followed on a long-term basis, with rebiopsy performed if there are any changes in size or appearance. Others believe that they should be narrowly excised and, if the lesion recurs, more widely excised. Lesions characterized by dysplasia and CIS should be completely excised to clear margins when possible.

Erythroplakia

Erythroplakia is defined as a red or erythematous patch of the oral mucosa. It is associated with significantly higher rates of dysplasia, CIS, and invasive carcinoma than leukoplakia is.[8] Erythroplakia is managed in much the same fashion as leukoplakia, with biopsy performed to rule out a malignant or premalignant lesion. Complete surgical excision is indicated if either a malignancy or a premalignancy is confirmed, and frequent follow-up is necessary.

MALIGNANT

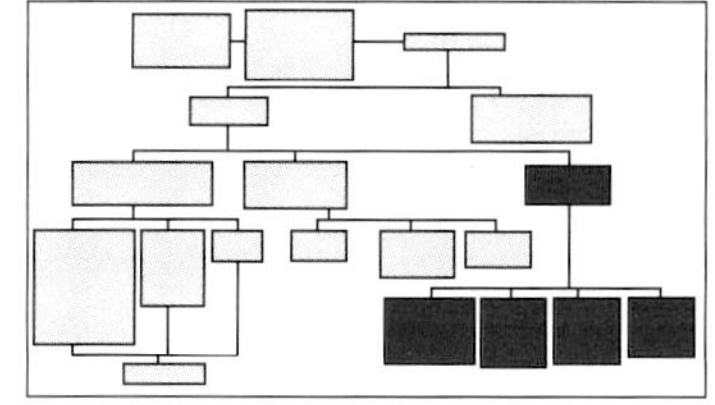

Minor Salivary Gland Malignancies

The majority (60 to 70%) of minor salivary gland neoplasms are malignant, with adenoid cystic carcinoma, mucoepidermoid carcinoma, and adenocarcinoma [*see Figure 6a*] being the most commonly encountered cancers.[26,34] As with benign minor salivary gland neoplasms, the hard and soft palates are the most common sites.[34]

A minor salivary gland malignancy usually appears as a painless, slow-growing, intraoral mass.[35] Nodal involvement at presentation is uncommon.[26] Treatment usually involves surgical excision; adequate margins should be obtained with frozen-section control. Because these malignancies—particularly adenoid cystic carcinoma and polymorphous low-grade adenocarcinoma—have a propensity for perineural spread, frozen-section analysis of the nerves within the field of resection is usually obtained at the time of operation. If perineural spread occurs, postoperative irradiation is usually indicated, and distant metastases are likely to develop despite surgery and locoregional radiotherapy. As a result, it is usually best to limit the extent of the operation if major morbidity is anticipated from a radical resection.

Neck dissection is warranted in the treatment of minor salivary gland malignancies only if there is clinical or radiographic evidence of cervical metastases. Postoperative irradiation is indicated for most patients with high-grade malignancies, positive or close surgical margins, cervical metastases, or pathologic evidence of perineural spread or bone invasion.[35] Studies suggest that postoperative radiotherapy allows improved local control and may lead to longer disease-free survival.[36,37]

Local recurrence and distant metastases are common, often developing many years later; regional recurrence is uncommon.[34] The survival rate for adenoid cystic carcinoma is relatively high (approximately 80%) at 5 years but decreases dramatically over the subsequent 10 to 15 years.[34,38] Various factors predictive of poor survival have been identified [*see Table 5*].[38]

Mucosal Melanoma

After the sinonasal region, the oral cavity is the site at which mucosal melanoma most often occurs in the head and neck.[39] Within the oral cavity, mucosal melanoma is most frequently found involving the upper alveolus and the hard palate.[40] It is most common in men, usually developing in the sixth decade of life.[40] No specific risk factors or premalignant lesions have been identified. There may, however, be an increased risk among certain subsets of East Asian patients.

Oral mucosal melanoma typically appears as a flat or nodular pigmented lesion, frequently associated with ulceration. Amelanotic melanoma is, fortunately, rare.[41] Patients usually seek medical attention at an advanced stage of the

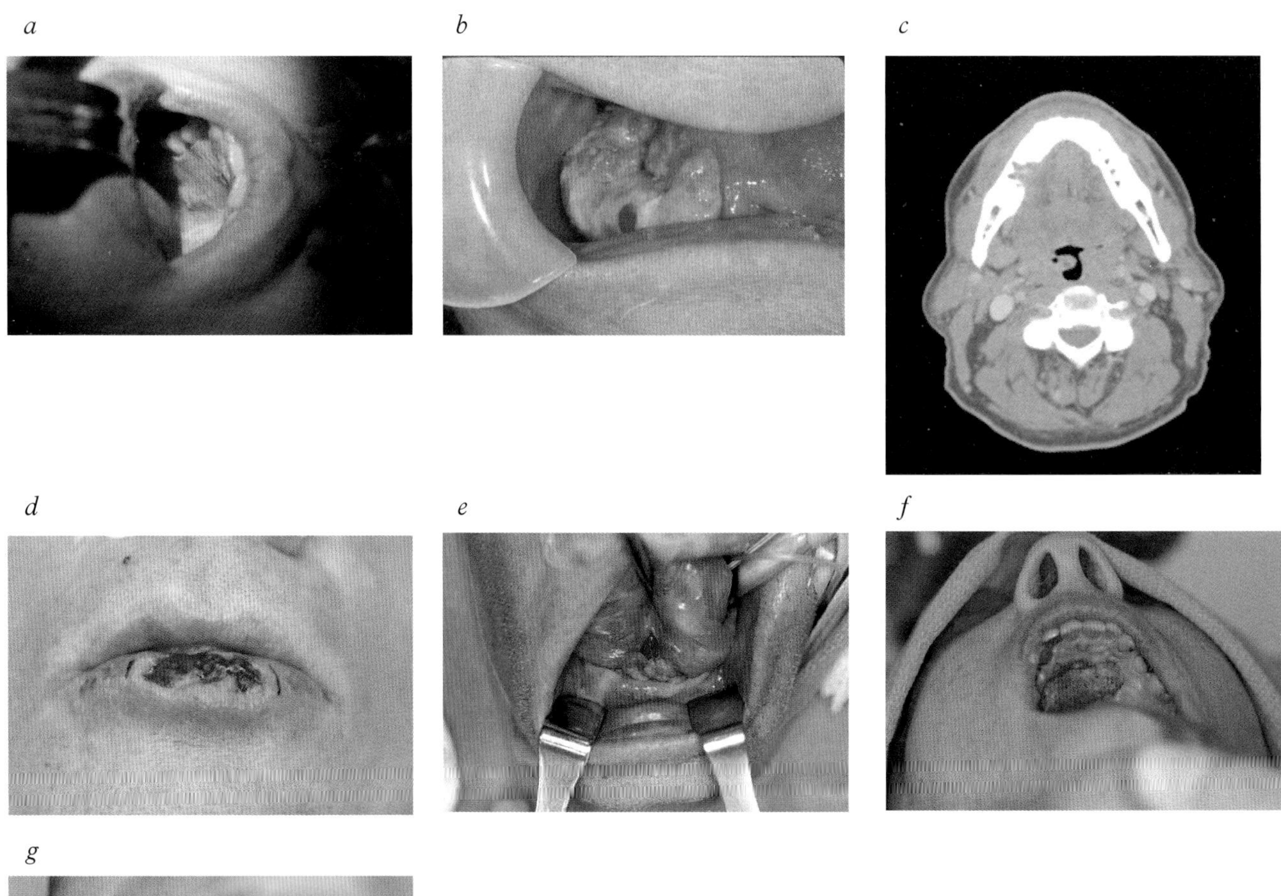

Figure 6 **Shown are malignant lesions of the oral cavity: (*a*) polymorphous low-grade adenocarcinoma of the hard palate (raised, erythematous lesion); (*b*) extensive squamous cell carcinoma of the tongue, the alveolar ridge, and the floor of the mouth; (*c*) squamous cell carcinoma of the right floor of the mouth, with mandibular invasion on computed tomography scan; (*d*) squamous cell carcinoma of the lip (ulcerative lesion); (*e*) squamous cell carcinoma of the floor of the mouth (exophytic lesion); (*f*) squamous cell carcinoma of the hard palate; and (*g*) squamous cell carcinoma of the retromolar trigone.**

disease, when pain develops or when they notice a change in the fit of their dentures. Early asymptomatic lesions are usually identified incidentally by either a physician or a dentist. Approximately 25% of patients have nodal metastases at presentation.[40] Tumors thicker than 5 mm are associated with an increased likelihood of nodal metastases at presentation.[42]

No formal staging system has been developed for mucosal melanoma. The diagnosis is made by means of biopsy and immunohistochemical staining (e.g., for HMB-45 antigen, Melan-A, or S-100 protein). Any suspicious pigmented lesion in the oral cavity should undergo biopsy to rule out melanoma. Amalgam tattoos are common in the oral cavity and can often be diagnosed on the basis of the presence of metallic fragments on dental radiographs.

Table 5 **Poor Prognostic Factors for Minor Salivary Gland Malignancies**

Advanced disease at time of diagnosis
Positive nodes
High-risk histologic type (i.e., high-grade malignancies such as high-grade mucoepidermoid carcinoma, adenocarcinoma, carcinoma ex pleomorphic adenoma, and adenoid cystic carcinoma)
Positive margins
Male sex

Mucosal melanoma is managed primarily with surgical resection. The role of radiation therapy in this setting remains controversial.[39] Some clinicians recommend postoperative radiotherapy for all cases of mucosal melanoma; others recommend it only for patients with close or positive margins. The role of lymph node mapping has not been defined for mucosal melanoma. Because of the high incidence of nodes at presentation and the high regional recurrence rates reported in some studies, consideration should be given to treating the neck prophylactically by extending the postoperative radiation fields to cover this region.[39,40]

The poor prognosis of mucosal melanoma with conventional treatment employing surgery and irradiation is a strong argument for referring patients to a medical oncologist for potential enrolment in postoperative systemic therapy trials. The survival rate for oral mucosal melanomas at 5 years ranges from 15 to 45%,[40,41,43] with most patients dying of distant disease. Nodal involvement further reduces survival.[41] Melanoma of the gingiva has a slightly better prognosis than melanoma of the palate.[41] Several factors predictive of poor survival have been identified [*see Table 6*].[40] The relation between lesion depth and prognosis is not as clearly defined for oral mucosal melanoma as it is for cutaneous melanoma.

Squamous Cell Carcinoma

The incidence of squamous cell carcinoma increases with age, with the median age at diagnosis falling in the seventh decade of life,[44,45] and is higher in men than in women. This cancer may be found at any of a number of oral cavity subsites [*see Figure 6, b through g*]. Lip carcinoma is the most common oral cavity cancer; 80 to 90% of these lesions occur on the lower lip.[13] After the lip, the most common sites for oral cavity carcinoma are the tongue and the floor of the mouth. When the primary lesion is on the tongue, the lateral border is the most common location, followed by the anterior tongue and the dorsum.[8] Approximately 75% of cases of oral cavity squamous cell carcinoma arise from a specific 10% of the mucosal surface of the mouth,[11] an area extending from the anterior floor of the mouth along the gingivobuccal sulcus and the lateral border to the retromolar trigone and the anterior tonsillar pillar.[11] Verrucous carcinoma is a subtype of squamous cell carcinoma and occurs most frequently on the buccal mucosa, appearing as a papillary mass with keratinization.

Between 80 and 90% of patients with oral cavity carcinoma have a history of either tobacco use (cigarette smoking or tobacco chewing) or excessive alcohol intake.[46] A synergistic effect is created when alcohol and tobacco are frequently used together.[46] In Asia, the practice of reverse smoking is associated with a high incidence of palatal carcinoma; betel nut chewing is associated with a high incidence of buccal carcinoma. The incidence of tumors in patients who have never smoked or drunk alcohol is rising, and the role of human papillomavirus in the pathogenesis and prognosis of this disease continues to be defined.[47]

Small lesions tend to be asymptomatic. Larger lesions are often associated with pain, bleeding, poor denture fit, facial weakness or sensory changes, dysphagia, odynophagia, and trismus. Oral intake may worsen the pain, leading to malnutrition and dehydration.

Squamous cell carcinoma of the oral cavity has four different possible growth patterns: ulceroinfiltrative, exophytic, endophytic, and superficial [*see Table 7*].[48] Lip and buccal carcinomas tend to appear as exophytic masses. Ulceration is less common early in the course of cancers arising at these sites, but it may develop as the lesion enlarges. Cancers of the floor of the mouth may be associated with invasion of the tongue and the mandible. Decreased tongue mobility as a result of fixation is an indicator of an advanced tumor.[48,49] Mandibular invasion occurs frequently in carcinomas of the floor of the mouth, the retromolar trigone, and the alveolar ridge as a consequence of the tight adherence of the mucosa to the periosteum in these regions. The risk of mandibular invasion increases with higher tumor stages. The majority (70 to 80%) of alveolar ridge carcinomas occur on the lower alveolus, often in areas of leukoplakia.[50]

Table 6 Poor Prognostic Factors for Mucosal Melanoma

Amelanotic melanoma
Advanced stage at presentation
Tumor thickness > 5 mm
Presence of vascular invasion
Distant metastases

Table 7 Growth Patterns of Squamous Cell Carcinoma of Oral Cavity[48]

Growth Pattern	Characteristics
Ulceroinfiltrative	Most common pattern; appears as ulcerated lesion that penetrates deep into underlying structures with surrounding induration
Exophytic	Common on lip and buccal mucosa; appears as papillary mass that may ulcerate when large
Endophytic	Uncommon; extends deep into soft tissue, with only small surface area involved
Superficial	Flat, superficial appearance; may be either a white patch or a red/velvety patch

Oral cavity carcinoma is generally classified according to the staging system developed by the American Joint Committee on Cancer [*see Table 8 and Table 9*].[51] Staging is based on clinical examination and diagnostic imaging. The diagnosis is made on the basis of biopsy and immunohistochemical staining (e.g., for cytokeratin and epithelial membrane antigen).

Squamous cell carcinoma of the oral cavity is usually managed with surgery, radiation therapy, or a combination of the two. Chemotherapy is increasingly used in combination with radiotherapy for patients at high risk of local or regional recurrence. For localized disease without bone invasion, the cure rate for radiation therapy is comparable to that of surgery.[46] The development of free tissue transfer has allowed for the successful cosmetic and functional reconstruction of large surgical defects of the oral cavity, including the mandible. Advanced tumors of the oral cavity are best managed with both surgery and irradiation. Traditionally, in North America, oral cavity cancer is treated primarily with surgery, and postoperative radiotherapy is added if the disease is advanced or if there are pathologic features indicative of a high risk of recurrence (i.e., positive margins on microscopy, extensive perineural or intravascular invasion, two or more positive nodes or positive nodes at multiple levels, or nodal capsular extension). North American practice is reflected in the guidelines developed by the American Head and Neck Society (www.headandneckcancer.org/clinicalresources/docs/oralcavity.php).

Radiation may be delivered to an oral cavity carcinoma via either external beam radiotherapy or brachytherapy, with the former being more commonly employed. Postoperative radiation, if indicated, should be started 4 to 6 weeks after surgery. The total radiation dose depends on the clinical and pathologic findings; the usual range is between 50 and 70 Gy, administered over 5 to 8 weeks. Primary radiation therapy is indicated for patients with stage I and selected stage II oral

Table 8 **American Joint Committee on Cancer TNM Classification of Head and Neck Cancer**

Primary tumor (T)	TX	Primary tumor cannot be assessed
	T0	No evidence of primary tumor
	Tis	Carcinoma in situ
	T1	Tumor 2 cm or less in greatest dimension
	T2	Tumor more than 2 cm but not more than 4 cm in greatest dimension
	T3	Tumor more than 4 cm in greatest dimension
	T4a	Tumor invades adjacent structures, extending through cortical bone into deep (extrinsic) muscles of tongue, maxillary sinus, or facial skin
	T4b	Tumor invades masticator space, pterygoid plates, or skull base or encases internal carotid artery
Regional lymph nodes (N)	NX	Regional lymph nodes cannot be assessed
	N0	No regional lymph node metastases
	N1	Metastases in a single ipsilateral lymph node ≤ 3 cm in greatest dimension
	N2a	Metastases in a single ipsilateral lymph node > 3 cm but ≤ 6 cm in greatest dimension
	N2b	Metastases in multiple ipsilateral lymph nodes, none > 6 cm in greatest dimension
	N2c	Metastases in bilateral or contralateral lymph nodes, none > 6 cm in greatest dimension
	N3	Metastases in lymph node > 6 cm in greatest dimension
Distant metastases (M)	MX	Distant metastases cannot be assessed
	M0	No distant metastases
	M1	Distant metastases

cavity carcinomas, patients who refuse surgery or in whom surgery is contraindicated, and patients with incurable lesions who require palliative treatment. Radiation therapy is less effective against large or deeply invasive tumors, especially those that are invading bone, and therefore generally is not used alone for curative management of T3 and T4 lesions. For advanced stage tumors of the oral cavity, surgery with postoperative radiotherapy is performed to decrease recurrence rates. Brachytherapy can be used as an adjunct when close or positive margins are noted. Brachytherapy also has a role in the management of recurrence or previously irradiated patients.[52]

The decision regarding which treatment is presented to a patient as the first option is often determined by factors other than the extent of the tumor. Patient factors to be considered include desires and wishes, age, medical comorbidities, and performance status. Disease factors to be considered include tumor grade and stage, extent of invasion, primary site, the presence and degree of nodal or distant metastasis, and previous treatment. It is often helpful to discuss each case at a multidisciplinary treatment planning conference to develop a ranked list of options.

Table 9 **American Joint Committee on Cancer Staging System for Head and Neck Cancer**

Stage	T	N	M
0	Tis	N0	M0
I	T1	N0	M0
II	T2	N0	M0
III	T3 T1, T2, T3	N0 N1	M0 M0
IVA	T4a T1, T2, T3, T4a	N0, N1 N2	M0 M0
IVB	Any T T4b	N3 Any N	M0 M0
IVC	Any T	Any N	M1

Squamous cell carcinoma of the oral cavity tends to spread to regional lymph nodes in a relatively predictable fashion. The primary levels of metastatic spread from oral cavity carcinoma include level I through III nodes and, less frequently, level IV nodes[53–55]; metastases to level V are infrequent.[53,55] The likelihood that cervical node metastases will develop varies depending on the location of the primary tumor in the oral cavity and on the stage of the tumor. Cervical metastases from carcinomas of the lip or the hard palate usually occur only in advanced disease[8]; however, cervical metastases from carcinomas of any of the other oral cavity subsites are common at presentation [*see Table 10*].[8,11,48,50,51,53,56,57] Larger tumors carry a higher risk of cervical metastasis.

The clinically positive neck is usually managed with either a radical or a modified radical neck dissection, depending on the extent of the disease. Some studies have found that for N1 and some N2a patients, a comparable control rate can be achieved with a selective neck dissection encompassing levels I through IV, with postoperative radiation therapy added when indicated.[58,59]

The clinically negative neck can occasionally be managed with observation alone, with treatment initiated only when nodal metastases develop. Alternatively, the nodal basins at risk can be managed prophylactically by means of either surgery or radiation therapy (involving levels I through III and, possibly, IV). The rationale for prophylactic neck management is that treatment initiated while metastases are still

Table 10 **Incidence of Nodal Metastases* at Presentation in Oral Cavity Subsites**

Oral Cavity Subsite	Incidence of Metastases (%)
Lip	10
Tongue	30–40
Floor of the mouth	50
Alveoli	28–32
Buccal mucosa	40–52

*Clinically detectable or occult.

occult is thought to be more effective than treatment initiated after the disease has progressed to the point where it is clinically detectable. For this reason, many clinicians advocate prophylactic neck dissection for patients with oral cavity carcinomas who are at moderate (15–20%) risk for occult metastases at presentation. The selective neck dissection not only addresses any occult metastatic nodes but also functions as a staging procedure that helps in determining the prognosis and assessing the need for postoperative radiotherapy.[60,61] In general, elective neck management is recommended for T2 and higher-stage carcinomas of the tongue, the floor of the mouth, the buccal mucosa, the alveolus, and the retromolar trigone, as well as for advanced (T3 or T4) carcinomas of the lip and the hard palate.[8,11,48,56,57,62,63] Most surgeons now emphasize the depth of invasion of the primary tumor as a critical determinant of the risk of occult nodal metastases. It has been suggested that elective treatment of the neck with surgery or radiation therapy should be considered on the basis of the depth of tumor invasion rather than the surface diameter of the lesion. The tumor depth that is held to warrant investigation varies among published studies, ranging from 2 to 5 mm.[64–66] Bilateral neck dissection may be indicated for midline oral cavity cancers.

The prognosis depends on the location of the tumor in the oral cavity. Overall, if all of the oral cavity subsites are considered together, the presence of cervical metastases decreases survival by approximately 50%. Varying 5-year survival rates have been reported for the different subsites of the oral cavity [*see Table 11*].[8,11,48,50,51,56,67]

Oral Cavity Manifestations of HIV Infection

Infectious and neoplastic oral cavity lesions are often the first manifestation of HIV infection or the first indication of the progression to AIDS.

INFECTIONS

The same organisms that affect the general population cause most of the oral infections seen in the HIV population; however, oral infections in HIV patients tend to be recurrent, comparatively severe, and relatively resistant to treatment.[68] Oral hairy leukoplakia, caused by Epstein-Barr virus, is a common oral infection seen almost exclusively in the HIV population. It presents as an asymptomatic, corrugated, whitish, nonremovable, slightly raised patch on the lateral borders of the tongue. The finding of such a lesion on clinical examination of an HIV patient is suggestive of the diagnosis, but confirmation of the diagnosis requires biopsy. Treatment usually is not necessary. High-dose acyclovir may be given if the patient requests treatment.

Several rare infections of the oral cavity are being seen with increasing frequency in the HIV population, including tuberculosis, syphilis, *Rochalimaea henselae* infection (bacillary angiomatosis), *Borrelia vincentii* infection (acute necrotizing ulcerative gingivitis), cryptococcosis, histoplasmosis, coccidioidomycosis [*see Figure 7*], and human papillomavirus infection.

NEOPLASMS

The two most common intraoral neoplasms in the HIV population are Kaposi sarcoma and non-Hodgkin lymphoma. Kaposi sarcoma occurs most commonly in patients with HIV, although it is not exclusive to this population. It frequently involves the oral cavity, showing a predilection for the attached mucosa of the palate or the gingiva.[68] The characteristic lesions are blue, brown, purple, or red exophytic masses that may be either confined to the oral mucosa or systemic. They are usually asymptomatic but may become painful or obstructive with growth or ulceration. Treatment is aimed at palliation of symptoms and may involve sclerotherapy, intralesional chemotherapy, laser ablation, cryotherapy, surgical excision, or radiation therapy.[69] Systemic chemotherapy may be provided if the disease is systemic.

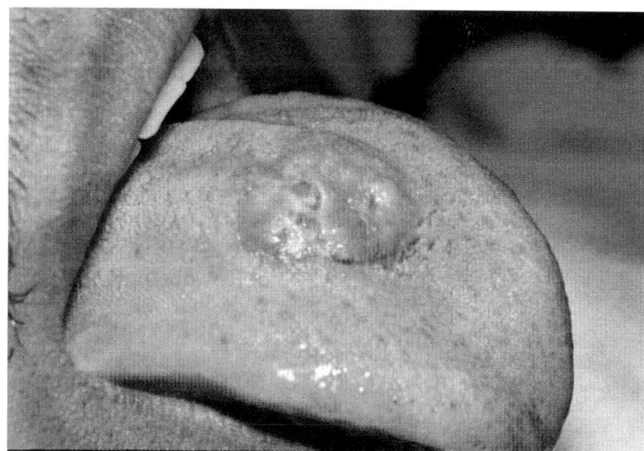

Figure 7 **Shown is coccidioidomycosis of the tongue in an HIV-positive patient.**

The risk of non-Hodgkin lymphoma is much higher in the HIV population than in the general population.[69] It should be suspected in any HIV patient who presents with an intraoral mass or an ulcerated lesion. Non-Hodgkin lymphoma appears as painful lesions that show a predilection for the palate, the retromolar trigone, and the tongue. Associated symptoms include facial paresthesias, loose dentition, fever, night sweats, and weight loss. Local disease is managed with radiation; systemic disease is managed with chemotherapy.

Table 11 **Five-Year Carcinoma Survival Rates for Oral Cavity Subsites**

Oral Cavity Subsite	Survival Rate
Lip	80%; > 90% for early-stage disease
Tongue	30–35% (advanced-stage disease); > 80% (early-stage disease)
Floor of the mouth	85% for stages I and II (T1 lesions > 95%); 20–52% for stages III and IV
Alveoli	50–60%
Retromolar trigone	75% for T1 and T2 lesions; approximately 20–50% for T3 and T4 lesions
Buccal mucosa	49–68%
Palate	85% for T1 lesions; 30% for T4 lesions

Financial Disclosures: None Reported

References

1. Rumboldt Z, Day TA, Michel M. Imaging of oral cavity cancer. Oral Oncol 2006;42: 854–65.
2. Tsue TT, McCulloch TM, Girod DA, et al. Predictors of carcinomatous invasion of the mandible. Head Neck 1994;16:116.
3. Bahadur S. Mandibular involvement in oral cancer. J Laryngol Otol 1990;104:968.
4. Sigg MB, Steinert H, Gratz K, et al. Staging of head and neck tumors: fluorodeoxyglucose positron emission tomography compared with physical examination and conventional imaging modalities. J Oral Maxillofac Surg 2003;61:1022.
5. Zimmer LA, Branstetter BF, Nayak JV, Johnson JT. Current use of 18F-fluorodeoxyglucose positron emission tomography and combined positron emission tomography and computed tomography in squamous cell carcinoma of the head and neck. Laryngoscope 2005;115:2029–34.
6. Lonneux M, Lawson G, Ide C, et al. Positron emission tomography with fluorodeoxyglucose for suspected head and neck tumor recurrence in the symptomatic patient. Laryngoscope 2000;110:1493.
7. Layfield LJ. Fine-needle aspiration in the diagnosis of head and neck lesions: a review and discussion of problems in differential diagnosis. Diagn Cytopathol 2007;35:798–805.
8. Cummings CW, Haughey BH, Thomas JR et al. Otolaryngology head and neck surgery. 4th ed. St. Louis: Mosby; 2004.
9. Murray N, Muller G, [illegible] [illegible] Alexandria, VA: American Academy of Otolaryngology–Head and Neck Surgery Foundation; 2000.
10. Sciubba J, Regezei J, Rogers R III. PDQ oral disease diagnosis and treatment. Hamilton (ON): BC Decker; 2002.
11. Bailey BJ, Calhoun KH, Deskin RW et al. Head and neck surgery–otolaryngology. 4th ed. Philadelphia: Lippincott-Raven; 2006.
12. Scully C, Porter S. Oral mucosal disease: recurrent aphthous stomatitis. Br J Oral Maxillofac Surg 2008;46:198–206.
13. Fu YS, Wenig BM, Abemayor E, et al. Head and neck pathology: with clinical correlations. New York: Churchill Livingstone; 2001.
14. Lumerman H. Essentials of oral pathology. Philadelphia: JB Lippincott; 1975.
15. Scully C, Carrozzo M. Oral mucosal disease: lichen planus. Br J Oral Maxillofac Surg 2008;46:15–21.
16. Giunta JL. Oral pathology. 3rd ed. Toronto: BC Decker; 1989.
17. Casiglia J, Woo S, Ahmed AR. Oral involvement in autoimmune blistering diseases. Clin Dermatol 2001;19:737.
18. Jainkittivong A, Langlais RP. Buccal and palatal exostosis: prevalence and concurrence with tori. Oral Surg Oral Med Oral Pathol Oral Radiol Endod 2000;90:48.
19. Baurmash HD. Mucoceles and ranulas. J Oral Maxillofac Surg 2003;61:369.
20. Patel MR, Deal AM, Shockley WW. Oral and plunging ranulas: what is the most effective treatment? Laryngoscope 2009;119:1501–9.
21. Williams T, Hellstein JW. Odontogenic cysts of the jaws and other selected cysts. In: Fonseca R, editor. Oral and maxillo-facial surgery. Vol 5. Surgical pathology. Philadelphia: WB Saunders; 2000. p. 297.
22. Blanas N, Freund B, Schwartz M, Furst IM. Systematic review of the treatment and prognosis of the odontogenic keratocyst. Oral Surg Oral Med Oral Pathol Oral Radiol Endod 2000;90:553–8.
23. Syrjänen S. Human papillomavirus (HPV) in head and neck cancer. J Clin Virol 2005;32 Suppl 1:S59–66.
24. Slootweg PJ. Lesions of the jaws. Histopathology 2009;54:401–18.
25. de Lange J, van den Akker HP, van den Berg H. Central giant cell granuloma of the jaw: a review of the literature with emphasis on therapy options. Oral Surg Oral Med Oral Pathol Oral Radiol Endod 2007;104:603–15.
26. Yih WY, Kratochvil FJ, Stewart JC. Intraoral minor salivary gland neoplasms: review of 213 cases. J Oral Maxillofac Surg 2005;63: 805–10.
27. Eguia A, Uribarri A, Gay Escoda C, et al. Granular cell tumor: report of 8 intraoral cases. Med Oral Patol Oral Cir Bucal 2006;11: E425–8.
28. Vered M, Carpenter WM, Buchner A. Granular cell tumor of the oral cavity: updated immunohistochemical profile. J Oral Pathol Med 2009;38:150–9.
29. Mendenhall WM, Werning JW, Fernandes R, et al. Ameloblastoma. Am J Clin Oncol 2007; 30:645–8.
30. Katz JO, Underhill TE. Multilocular radiolucencies. Dent Clin North Am 1994;38:63.
31. Wenig B. Atlas of head and neck pathology. Philadelphia: WB Saunders; 1993.
32. Zwahlen RA, Gratz KW. Maxillary ameloblastomas: a review of the literature and of a 15-year database. J Craniomaxillofac Surg 2002;30:273.
33. Fischman SL, Ulmansky M, Sela J, et al. Correlative clinico-pathological evaluation of oral premalignancy. J Oral Pathol 1982;11: [illegible]
34. Jones AS, Beasley NP, Houghton DJ, et al. Tumors of the minor salivary glands. Clin Otolaryngol 1997;22:27.
35. Spiro RH. Salivary neoplasms: overview of a 35 year experience with 2807 patients. Head Neck Surg 1986;8:177.
36. Cianchetti M, Sandow PS, Scarborough LD, et al. Radiation therapy for minor salivary gland carcinoma. Laryngoscope 2009;119: 1334–8.
37. Garden AS, Weber RS, Ang KK, et al. Postoperative radiation therapy for malignant tumors of minor salivary glands: outcome and patterns of failure. Cancer 1994;73:2563.
38. Lopes MA, Santos GC, Kowalski LP. Multivariate survival analysis of 128 cases of oral cavity minor salivary gland carcinomas. Head Neck 1998;20:699.
39. Medina JE, Ferlito A, Pellitteri PK, et al. Current management of mucosal melanoma of the head and neck. J Surg Oncol 2003;83: 116.
40. Mendenhall WM, Amdur RJ, Hinerman RW, et al. Head and neck mucosal melanoma. Am J Clin Oncol 2005;28:626–30.
41. Hicks MJ, Flaitz CM. Oral mucosal melanoma: epidemiology and pathobiology. Oral Oncol 2000;36:152.
42. Umeda M, Shimada K. Primary malignant melanoma of the oral cavity: its histological classification and treatment. Br J Oral Maxillofac Surg 1994;32:39.
43. Wagner M, Morris CG, Werning JW, Mendenhall WM. Mucosal melanoma of the head and neck. Am J Clin Oncol 2008;31:43–8.
44. Funk GF, Hynds Karnell L, Robinson RA, et al. Presentation, treatment, and outcome of oral cavity cancer: a National Cancer Data Base Report. Head Neck 2002;24:165.
45. Teresa Canto M, Devesa SS. Oral cavity and pharynx cancer incidence rates in the United States, 1975-1988. Oral Oncol 2002;38:610.
46. Rhys Evans PH, Montgomery PQ, Gullane PJ. Principles and practice of head and neck oncology. London: Martin Dunitz; 2003.
47. Curado MP, Hashibe M. Recent changes in the epidemiology of head and neck cancer. Curr Opin Oncol 2009;21:194–200.
48. Shah JP, Patel SG. Head and neck surgery and oncology. 3rd ed. London: Mosby; 2003.
49. Hicks WL Jr, Loree TR, Garcia RI, et al. Squamous cell carcinoma of the floor of mouth: a 20 year review. Head Neck 1997; 19:400.
50. Soo KC, Spiro RH, King W, et al. Squamous carcinoma of the gums. Am J Surg 1998;156: 281.
51. Greene FL, Page DL, Fleming ID, et al. AJCC cancer staging manual. 6th ed. New York: Springer; 2002.
52. Narayana A, Cohen GN, Zaider M, et al. High-dose-rate interstitial brachytherapy in recurrent and previously irradiated head and neck cancers—preliminary results. Brachytherapy 2007;6:157–63.
53. Shah JP. Patterns of cervical lymph node metastasis from squamous carcinomas of the upper aerodigestive tract. Am J Surg 1990;1 60:405.
54. Khafif A, Lopez-Garza JR, Medina JE. Is dissection of level IV necessary in patients with T1-T3 N0 tongue cancer? Laryngoscope 2001;111:1088.
55. Shah JP, Candela FC, Poddar AK. The patterns of cervical lymph node metastases from squamous carcinoma of the oral cavity. Cancer 1990;66:109.
56. Ayad T, Guertin L, Soulières D, et al. Con[illegible] trigone carcinoma. Head Neck 2009;31: 398–405.
57. Diaz EM, Holsinger FC, Zuniga ER, et al. Squamous cell carcinoma of the buccal mucosa: one institution's experience with 119 previously untreated patients. Head Neck 2003;25:267.
58. Kolli VR, Datta RV, Orner JB, et al. The role of supraomohyoid neck dissection in patients with positive nodes. Arch Otolaryngol Head Neck Surg 2000;126:413.
59. Majoufre C, Faucher A, Laroche C, et al. Supraomohyoid neck dissection in cancer of the oral cavity. Am J Surg 1999;178:73.
60. Tankere F, Camproux A, Barry B, et al. Prognostic value of lymph node involvement in oral cancers: a study of 137 cases. Laryngoscope 2000;110:2061.
61. Hao S, Tsang N. The role of the supraomohyoid neck dissection in patients of oral cavity carcinoma. Oral Oncol 2002;38:309.
62. Haddadin KJ, Soutar DS, Oliver RJ, et al. Improved survival for patients with clinically T1/T2, N0 tongue tumors undergoing a prophylactic neck dissection. Head Neck 1999;21:517.
63. Zitsch RP, Lee BW, Smith RB. Cervical lymph node metastases and squamous cell carcinoma of the lip. Head Neck 1999; 21:447.
64. Spiro RH, Huvos AG, Wong GY, et al. Predictive value of tumor thickness in squamous carcinoma confined to the tongue and floor of the mouth. Am J Surg 1986;152:345.
65. Kurokawa H, Yamashita Y, Takeda S, et al. Risk factors for late cervical lymph node metastases in patients with stage 1 or 2 carcinoma of the tongue. Head Neck 2002; 24:731.
66. Jones KR, Lodge-Rigal RD, Reddick RL, et al. Prognostic factors in the recurrence of stage I and II squamous cell cancer of the oral cavity. Arch Otolaryngol Head Neck Surg 1992;5:483.
67. Gomez D, Faucher A, Picot V, et al. Outcome of squamous cell carcinoma of the

gingiva: a follow-up study of 83 cases. J Craniomaxillofac Surg 2000;28:331.
68. Laskaris G. Oral manifestations of HIV disease. Clin Dermatol 2000;18:447.
69. Casiglia JW, Woo S. Oral manifestations of HIV infection. Clin Dermatol 2000;18:541.

Acknowledgments

The authors and editors gratefully acknowledge the contributi ons of the previous authors, David P. Goldstein, MD, Henry T. Hoffman, MD, FACS, John W. Hellstein, DDS, and Gerry F. Funk, MD, FACS, to the development and writing of this chapter.

Figure 1 Tom Moore

2 PAROTID MASS

*Harrison W. Lin, MD, and Neil Bhattacharyya, MD, FACS**

Demographics

Major salivary gland tumors constitute 3 to 6% of all tumors of the head and neck in adults,[1] and approximately 85% of these salivary gland tumors are found in the parotid gland. Roughly 16% of these neoplasms are malignant.[2] The spectrum of histopathologic entities encompassed by the term "parotid mass" is exceedingly broad and continues to evolve as our understanding of the origin and clinical behavior of the various tumors arising from the parotid gland expands.

Anatomy

The parotid gland is an irregular, wedge-shaped, unilobular salivary gland residing in the parotid space, a compartment that additionally contains the facial nerve (cranial nerve VII), sensory and autonomic nerves, branches of the external carotid artery and external jugular vein, and lymphovasculature [see Figure 1].[3] The gland itself resides within the split layers of the superficial layer of the deep cervical fascia and overlies the upper one fourth of the sternocleidomastoid muscle, the ramus of the mandible, and the masseter muscle. Approximately 20% of the gland extends medially through the stylomandibular tunnel, which is formed by the posterior edge of the mandibular ramus, the anterior border of the sternocleidomastoid muscle, and the posterior belly of the digastric muscle. At its lower pole, the parotid gland is separated from the submandibular gland by the stylomandibular ligament, which extends from the tip of the styloid process to the angle and the posterior edge of the mandible.

The seventh cranial nerve artificially divides the parotid gland into two surgical zones: tissue lateral to the facial nerve is designated as the superficial lobe, whereas the medial portion is referred to as the deep lobe. Moreover, each lobe has been described to have variable processes, including the condylar, meatal, and posterior processes of the superficial lobe and the glenoid and stylomandibular processes of the deep lobe. Furthermore, a retromandibular portion of the deep lobe resides in the prestyloid compartment of the parapharyngeal space, anterior to the styloid process and associated musculature, the carotid sheath, and cranial nerves IX through XII. Note that the separation of the parotid gland into superficial and deep lobes is not based on a fascial plane. The parotid isthmus, the portion of the gland between the ramus of the mandible and the posterior belly of the digastric muscle, connects the superficial with the deep lobes of the parotid gland.

The parotid (Stensen) duct originates from the superficial lobe of the gland, courses anteriorly on the lateral surface of the masseter muscle, and then turns medially to pierce the buccinator muscle at the level of the second maxillary molar tooth and open into the mouth through the parotid papilla. The expected course of the duct is approximated by a line drawn between the tragus and philtrum of the upper lip, midway between the angle of the mouth and the zygomatic arch.

Etiology

Two predominant theories of the neoplastic pathogenesis of parotid masses have been proposed, including the bicellular and multicellular theories. The former, also referred to as the reserve cell theory, suggests that tumors arise from stem cell populations in both the excretory and intercalated ductal systems. Warthin tumor, mixed tumor, oncocytoma, acinic cell carcinoma, adenoid cystic carcinoma, and oncocytic carcinoma are proposed to arise from stem cells of the intercalated duct, whereas squamous cell carcinoma (SCC) and mucoepidermoid carcinoma are thought to derive from excretory duct stem cells. Alternatively, the multicellular theory suggests that the various parotid tumors arise from the fully differentiated cells within the salivary gland unit. Based on this theory, mucoepidermoid and squamous cell carcinomas derive from excretory duct cells, oncocytic tumors from striated duct cells, acinous tumors from acinar cells, and mixed tumors from intercalated duct cells and myoepithelial cells.[4]

Although the true nature of the neoplastic transformation of parotid gland cells is yet to be fully elucidated, these and other classification systems are founded on the understanding that primary parotid tumors are of epithelial origin. The parotid gland also hosts numerous lymph nodes that serve as a basin for metastatic spread of malignancies of the head. Accordingly, parotid masses will not infrequently represent the presenting sign of a cutaneous SCC or melanoma of the temple or scalp, for example.

Differential Diagnosis

NONNEOPLASTIC CONDITIONS

The causes of nonneoplastic parotid masses include congenital, infectious or inflammatory, and lymphoepithelial conditions. Congenital lesions such as hemangiomas and vascular malformations often present in childhood as a swelling in the preauricular region. First branchial cleft cysts can also present in the pediatric population and can be manifest as a mass inferior to the cartilaginous external auditory canal and with a cyst tract that will have a variable relationship with the branches of the facial nerve.

Inflammatory disorders of the parotid gland can be categorized into acute and chronic processes. Moreover, acute infections of the salivary glands can be further subclassified

* The authors and editors gratefully acknowledge the contributions of the previous author, Ashok R. Shaha, MD, FACS, to the development and writing of this chapter.

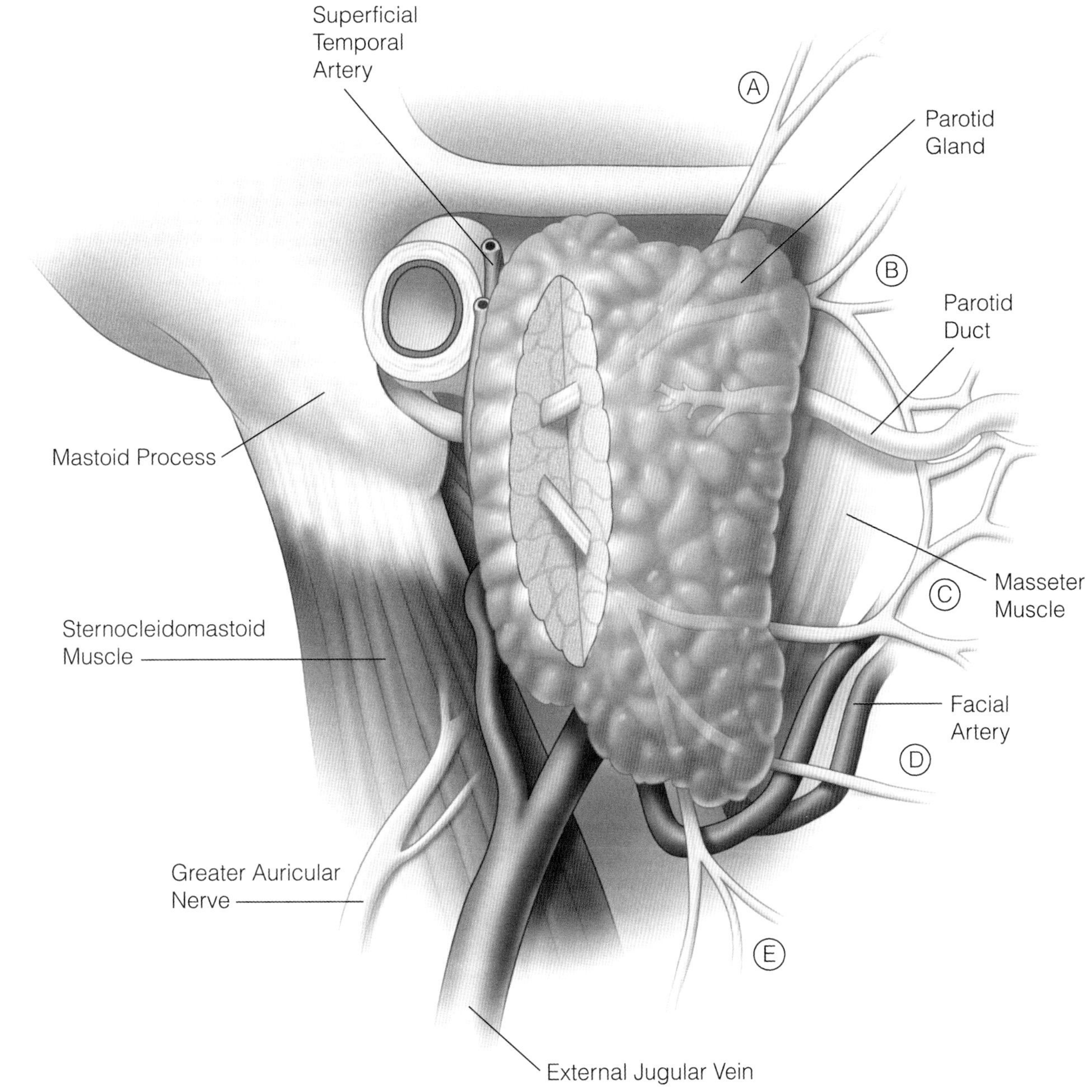

Figure 1 **Anatomy of the parotid region. Branches of the facial nerve: A = temporal; B = zygomatic; C = buccal; D = marginal; E = cervical.**

into viral and bacterial processes. Although viral parotid infections by the RNA virus paramyxovirus resulting in the mumps syndrome are now exceedingly rare following the introduction of the mumps vaccine in 1967, acute viral parotitis from the influenza, parainfluenza, adenovirus, cytomegalovirus, coxsackievirus, and enteric cytopathic human orphan (ECHO) viruses have been reported in the literature.[5] Acute bacterial infections of the parotid gland, however, are by far more common and are believed to be the result of retrograde contamination of the salivary ducts and parenchymal tissues by oral flora combined with stasis of salivary flow, often attributable to dehydration. Additionally, the serous composition of the saliva produced by the parotid gland lacks many of the antibacterial lysosomes, antibodies, and mucins found in the mucinous saliva produced by the other major salivary glands. Accordingly, bacterial sialadenitis most commonly affects the parotid gland. Relatively sudden onset of pain, tenderness, and swelling of the parotid are the most frequent presenting signs and symptoms, and treatment consists of hydration, sialagogues, and systemic antistaphylococcal therapy. If a discrete abscess is suspected and identified on cross-sectional imaging, surgical or radiologically guided needle drainage may be required.

Chronic inflammatory disorders of the parotid gland are frequently manifested by a mildly painful, recurrent, and gradual enlargement of the gland. Of these disorders, chronic sialadenitis is the most frequently encountered and is believed to be the result of reduced rates of salivary production and flow, resulting in frequent subacute suppurative infections, sialectasis, ductal ectasia, and progressive acinar cell loss. Initial treatment is similar to that of acute bacterial sialadenitis, and failure to respond to conservative measures may prompt consideration for surgical interventions, including ductal dilation, ductal ligation, and parotidectomy. In sarcoidosis, salivary gland involvement may cause duct obstruction, pain associated with the duct, xerostomia, or enlargement of the gland. The diagnosis is supported by chest films that show bilateral hilar adenopathy and by elevated levels of angiotensin-converting enzyme. Uveoparotid fever (Heerfordt disease), a subtype of sarcoidosis manifested by the triad of uveitis, parotid enlargement, and facial weakness, can persist for months to years and will often resolve spontaneously and without treatment.[6]

Lymphoepithelial lesions of the parotid gland may be divided into lymphocytic infiltrative diseases and lymphomas. In many cases, patients with lymphocytic infiltrative diseases such as Mikulicz disease, sicca complex, and Sjögren syndrome have had their conditions for long periods and simply believe that their chronic enlargement of bilateral parotid glands was normal facial soft tissue changes associated with age. Eighty percent of patients with primary Sjögren syndrome will experience parotid gland swelling; moreover, malignant transformation to high-grade lymphoma is known to occur. Lymphoepithelial cysts are benign cystic lesions that may arise from lymph nodes or from lymphoid aggregates in the salivary gland. These lesions may be associated with HIV infection.

Primary lymphoma of the salivary gland is uncommon, occurring in fewer than 5% of patients with parotid masses. Suggestive clinical features include (1) the development of a parotid mass in a patient with a known history of malignant lymphoma, (2) the occurrence of a parotid mass in a patient with an immune disorder (e.g., Sjögren syndrome, rheumatoid arthritis, or AIDS), (3) the presence of a parotid mass in a patient with a previous diagnosis of benign lymphoepithelial lesion, (4) the finding of multiple masses in one parotid gland or of masses in both parotid glands, and (5) the association of a parotid mass with multiple enlarged cervical lymph nodes unilaterally or bilaterally.[7]

As discussed, infectious or inflammatory diseases involving the parotid, unlike neoplasms, tend to give rise to pain in their early stages. However, certain parotid malignancies may also present with pain attributable to sensory nerve involvement. Most such inflammatory conditions begin with diffuse enlargement of one or more salivary glands rather than with presentation with a discrete, palpable parotid mass. Although parotitis is generally unilateral, it may be bilateral or affect other salivary glands if a systemic causative condition is involved. The pain reported may be related to the presence of a stone in the salivary duct or to diffuse obstructive parotitis. Chronic parotitis may lead to recurrent infection and inflammation. When recurrent swelling of the salivary gland does occur, it may be directly related to eating and increased salivation.

NEOPLASTIC CONDITIONS

Neoplastic masses may be present for years without causing any symptoms and affect both men and women at similar rates. Benign salivary tumors tend to be more common in younger persons, whereas malignant parotid lesions are more common in the fifth and sixth decades of life.[8] The classic presentation of a benign parotid tumor is that of an asymptomatic parotid mass that has been present for months to years, often exhibiting slow growth.

Benign Neoplasms

Benign neoplasms of the parotid, which include pleomorphic adenoma, basal cell adenoma, myoepithelioma, Warthin tumor, oncocytoma, and cystadenoma, are typically slow-growing and rarely exhibit malignant transformation. However, the observation of rapid growth in a long-standing pleomorphic adenoma (often 10 to 15 years later) is suggestive of malignant transformation. In a 2005 study of 94 patients with pleomorphic adenoma, malignant transformation to carcinoma ex pleomorphic adenoma was documented in 8.5% of cases.[9] Rapid tumor growth, metastasis to lymph nodes, deep fixation, and facial nerve weakness are all strongly suggestive of malignant disease and are indicators of a poor prognosis.[10] Although pain is more often experienced by patients with inflammatory or infectious conditions, it is also reported by some patients with infiltrative malignant tumors. In these patients, pain is another indicator of a poor prognosis.[11,12]

Malignant Neoplasms

Although considerable debate continues to surround the histopathologic classification of malignant parotid tumors, most clinicians currently prefer the classification system of the Armed Forces Institute of Pathology[13] or that of the World Health Organization.[14] Malignant parotid neoplasms include primary SCC, mucoepidermoid carcinoma, acinic cell carcinoma, adenocarcinoma, adenoid cystic carcinoma, carcinoma ex pleomorphic adenoma, and malignant mixed tumor. The presence of facial nerve palsy should raise the index of suspicion for malignancy. Occasionally, patients present with classic Bell palsy. This condition is usually of viral origin, and most patients recover over time. If Bell palsy persists, however, further investigation is required, including imaging or biopsy studies to rule out an associated parotid lesion.[15]

Mucoepidermoid carcinoma is the most common malignant tumor of the parotid gland, comprising roughly one third of all parotid cancers, and is subclassified into low-, intermediate-, and high-grade tumors. For high-grade tumors, selective cervical node dissection may be indicated and postoperative radiation therapy is often required. Combined surgical and radiation therapies for such tumors results in a 5-year survival rate of under 50%. In contrast, low-grade tumors are more circumscribed and contain more mucinous cells. Surgical therapy without radiation yields a 5-year survival rate of 75%.

Adenoid cystic carcinoma is an aggressive salivary gland tumor that exhibits a very high incidence of perineural spread with skip metastasis along the facial nerve and its branches, and the incidence rises with higher tumor stages.[16] The incidence of local recurrence is also very high; therefore, postoperative radiation therapy should be provided to patients who are at high risk for relapse, such as those with close or positive margins and those with perineural invasion. Although

Approach to Evaluation of a Parotid Mass

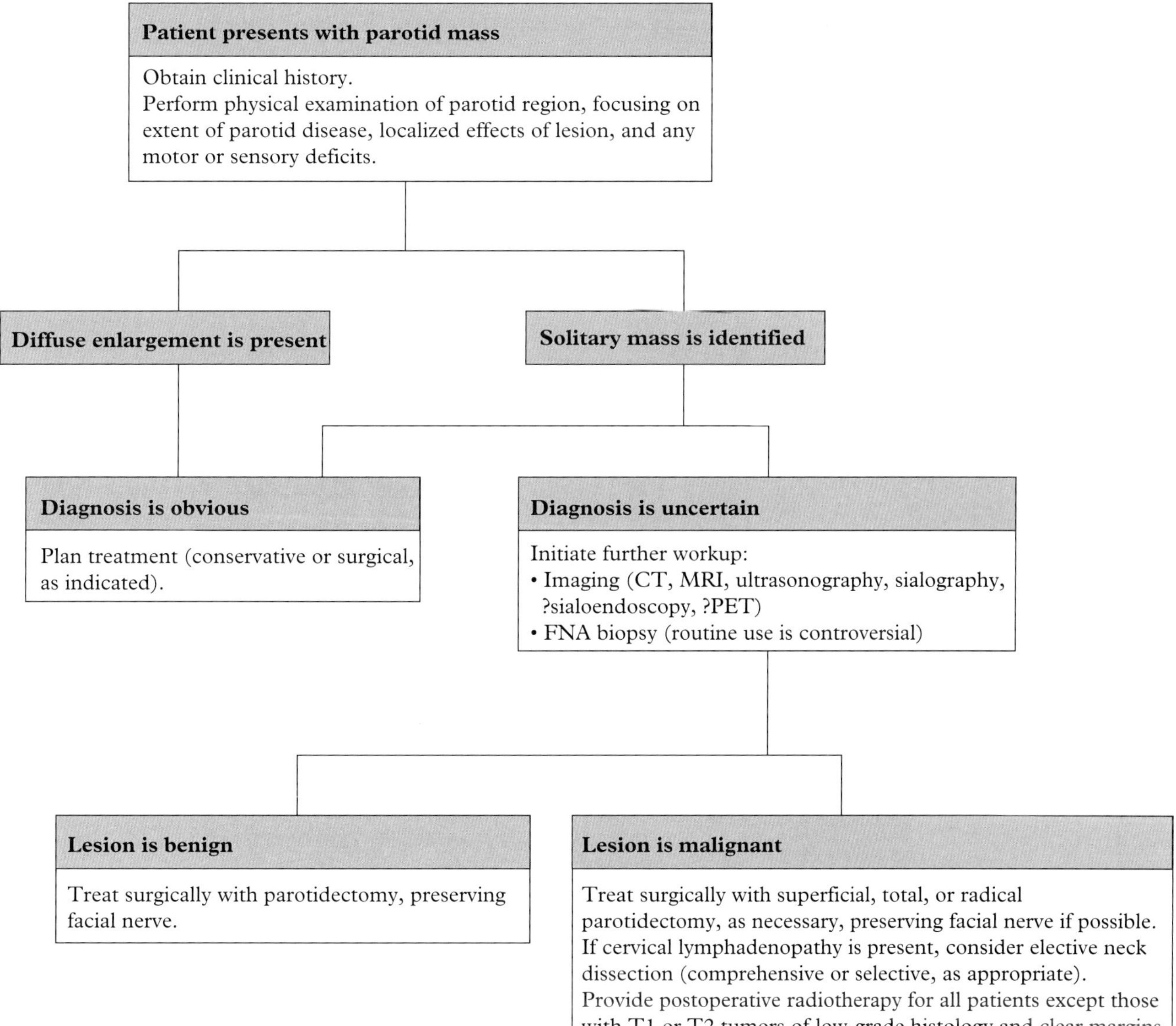
Patient presents with parotid mass
Obtain clinical history.
Perform physical examination of parotid region, focusing on extent of parotid disease, localized effects of lesion, and any motor or sensory deficits.
Diffuse enlargement is present
Solitary mass is identified
Diagnosis is obvious
Plan treatment (conservative or surgical, as indicated).
Diagnosis is uncertain
Initiate further workup:
• Imaging (CT, MRI, ultrasonography, sialography, ?sialoendoscopy, ?PET)
• FNA biopsy (routine use is controversial)
Lesion is benign
Treat surgically with parotidectomy, preserving facial nerve.
Lesion is malignant
Treat surgically with superficial, total, or radical parotidectomy, as necessary, preserving facial nerve if possible.
If cervical lymphadenopathy is present, consider elective neck dissection (comprehensive or selective, as appropriate).
Provide postoperative radiotherapy for all patients except those with T1 or T2 tumors of low-grade histology and clear margins.

the incidence of cervical lymph node metastasis in patients with adenoid cystic carcinoma is relatively low, the incidence of distant metastasis (especially pulmonary metastasis) has been reported to be as high as 38%.[17] Long-term follow-up in these patients is essential.

Adenocarcinoma has been considered a shrinking category as advances in electron microscopy and immunohistochemistry have reclassified many of these tumor variants into other subtypes and histopathologies. Adenocarcinomas are exceedingly aggressive tumors with high rates of facial nerve involvement, regional disease, and distant metastases and, accordingly, should be managed as a high-grade parotid tumor with surgical and radiation therapies.

Acinic cell carcinoma is a low-grade tumor with a female predominance and bilateral presentation approximately 3% of the time. Tumors are frequently well circumscribed, but a small percentage of patients will present with cervical nodal metastases. Patients with acinic cell carcinoma are typically managed with surgical therapy alone, although histopathologic findings to suggest a more aggressive, high-grade tumor have been proposed to serve as indicators for postoperative radiation therapy.[18]

Primary SCC of the parotid gland is quite rare, and most diagnoses of parotid SCC represent skin cancer that has metastasized to the periparotid lymph nodes. Primary SCC has a high malignant potential, and radical surgical extirpation (with preservation of the facial nerve when possible), followed by planned postoperative radiotherapy, is the treatment of choice.[19]

Metastatic Neoplasms to the Parotid

The parotid gland represents the first or second nodal basin for metastatic scalp, temple, and auricular cutaneous malignancies. Although the incidence of metastatic parotid disease is comparatively low in the Northern Hemisphere, it has been reported to be far more common than primary parotid disease in regions of the world with high rates of skin cancers, such as Australia.[20] Cutaneous SCC and melanoma are by far the most frequently encountered metastatic parotid malignancies and, despite treatment, will exhibit local or distant failure in 25 to 50% of cases. Other cancers that have been reported to metastasize to the parotid include basal cell, Merkel cell, and small cell carcinomas.

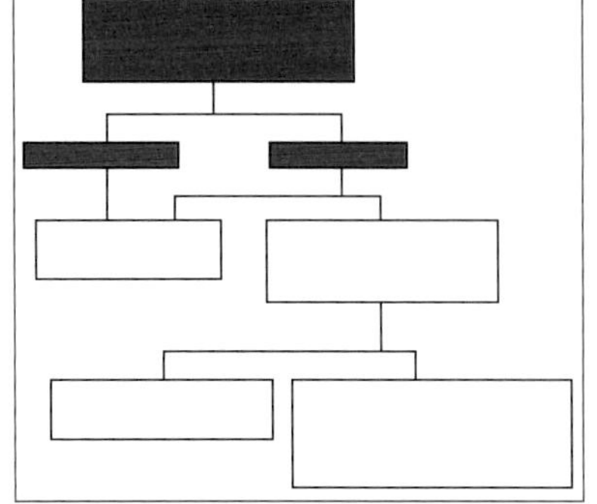

Presentation and Diagnostic Workup

HISTORY

Evaluation of any parotid mass should begin with a detailed clinical history. Comprehensive inquiries regarding the duration of signs and symptoms are paramount as masses resulting in local pain and swelling of recent onset (i.e., within the past few days) are more likely to be infectious or obstructive in nature. If the mass has been present for a longer period (i.e., weeks to months), a neoplasm is more likely. Unfortunately, the presentations of some nonneoplastic conditions resemble those of neoplasms, and distinguishing one type of condition from the other can be challenging. Accordingly, the history should continue with further questions focusing on local or systemic signs and symptoms, the presence of swelling or other masses in the salivary glands, and previous medical conditions, including cancers of the skin.

PHYSICAL EXAMINATION

The physical examination begins with an assessment of the extent of the disease in the parotid region, the neck, and the parapharynx. Extension of a tumor to regional compartments can be manifest as trismus or as motor or sensory deficits resulting from neural invasion. Palpation of the mass will reveal whether it is painless or painful; soft, firm, hard, or cystic; and mobile or fixed to deep tissue or skin. The skin of the scalp, ear, and face should be carefully examined for suspicious lesions, and the neck is palpated for adenopathy. In the oral cavity, the Stensen ducts are examined for discharge or saliva with parotid massage. The oropharynx is examined for asymmetries or lateral wall deviation.

The most common presentation of a parotid mass, whether benign or malignant, is an asymptomatic swelling in the preauricular or retromandibular region. Of note, the location of the parotid mass is a very important diagnostic factor. A benign tumor will classically present as a firm, mobile and marblelike mass in the superficial portion of the gland and not fixed to the deeper structures or to the skin. Parotid tumors that originate in the deep lobe, however, may present as a vague, diffuse swelling behind the angle of the mandible or as a swelling of the parapharyngeal area, resulting in medial displacement of the tonsil, soft palate, or lateral oropharyngeal wall.

Occasionally, patients will present with metastases to one or more of the 17 to 20 intraparotid or periparotid lymph nodes in the substance of the parotid and along its tail. These lymph nodes may be directly affected by metastatic tumors originating from the anterior scalp or the temporal, periocular, or malar regions. It is critical to obtain a detailed history of any previously excised skin lesions, some of which may have been an SCC or a melanoma primary tumor that metastasized to the periparotid nodes. Generally, such metastasis involves multiple superficial lymph nodes and presents as diffuse enlargement of the parotid parenchyma. With massive involvement of the parotid gland, facial nerve palsy is not uncommon in this setting. Although the majority of metastases to the parotid gland derive from cutaneous SCC or melanoma, metastatic spread from the lung, breast, and kidney has also been reported.

As with any patient with an otolaryngologic complaint, a thorough evaluation of the head and neck, including a detailed visualization of the oral cavity and laryngopharynx, is required. Occasionally, a tumor of the oropharynx presents as cervical lymphadenopathy or as metastatic disease in the tail of the parotid. In such cases, it may be difficult to determine whether the patient has a primary salivary gland tumor or a metastatic lesion. The presence of any suspicious pathologic condition in the oropharynx or the base of the tongue is an indication for appropriate endoscopy and biopsy of the suspected primary site.

Physical findings suggestive of malignancy include a large and fixed mass, facial nerve weakness, lymph node metastasis, and skin involvement; patients with advanced parotid malignancies may present with trismus. Although patients with benign parotid tumors rarely exhibit facial nerve weakness, approximately 12 to 15% of patients with parotid malignancies have facial nerve dysfunction at presentation. The most common causes of facial nerve weakness in this setting are adenoid cystic carcinoma, poorly differentiated carcinoma, and SCC.

The presence of cervical lymph node metastasis may direct the clinician's attention to the parotid mass, although less than 20% of persons with parotid malignancies actually have clinically apparent cervical lymph node metastases at the time of the initial presentation.[11,21] The parotid tumors most commonly associated with metastatic disease to the lymph nodes at presentation are undifferentiated carcinoma (89%),[22] high-grade mucoepidermoid carcinoma (42%),[23] and SCC (44%).[24] Lymph node metastases may also derive from high-grade adenocarcinomas (22%) or malignant mixed tumors (16%).[25]

Some patients will present without any symptoms, with the only significant physical examination finding being an oropharyngeal mass, which is suggestive of either a deep-lobe parotid or parapharyngeal tumor. Given that between 80 and 90% of the parotid tissue is superficial to the facial nerve, the majority of parotid tumors, not surprisingly, develop within the superficial lobe of the parotid. However, approximately 10% of parotid masses will be found within the deep lobe. Most deep-lobe parotid tumors are benign, in which case, surgical treatment generally consists of a superficial parotidectomy with dissection and preservation of the facial nerve, followed by removal of the tumor. Occasionally, however, malignant deep-lobe parotid tumors do occur, and such tumors frequently involve the facial nerve. Surgical treatment may require sacrifice of the facial nerve in select circumstances. Most patients who have undergone surgical treatment of a malignant deep-lobe tumor will require postoperative radiation therapy.

Table 1 Salivary and Nonsalivary Pathologic Processes Distinguished by Fine-Needle Aspiration Biopsy

Salivary processes
Benign
Mixed tumor
Warthin tumor
Oncocytoma
Malignant
Primary salivary gland cancer
Adenoid cystic carcinoma
Acinic cell carcinoma
Adenocarcinoma
SCC
Mucoepidermoid carcinoma
Metastatic disease in salivary gland
Melanoma
SCC
Nonsalivary processes
Lipoma
Sebaceous cyst
Lymph node pathology
Metastatic cancer
Lymphoma

SCC = squamous cell carcinoma.

FINE-NEEDLE ASPIRATION CYTOLOGY

Although fine-needle aspiration cytology (FNAC) has been shown to play a vital part in the management of head and neck SCC, the role of FNAC in parotid gland masses has yet to be fully resolved. This is attributable in large part to the perceived minimal impact of FNAC results on therapeutic decision making as most parotid masses, both benign and malignant, will require surgical excision and thereby provide a definitive pathologic diagnosis. Moreover, the variability of histopathologic subtypes, intralesional cellular distribution, and cytopathologist expertise has led some surgeons to question the utility of preoperative FNAC.

However, the ability of FNAC to distinguish masses of benign nature from those of malignant nature, salivary gland origin from those of nonsalivary gland origin (e.g., sarcoid, lymphoma, metastatic melanoma), and, in some cases, low-grade malignancy from high-grade malignancy has been suggested to provide useful guidance for medical and surgical planning [*see Table 1*]. Preoperative discovery of a non-salivary gland neoplasm in a parotid mass may preclude surgical excision in lieu of medical, radiation, or palliative therapies. Additionally, preoperative knowledge of a parotid malignancy has been shown to significantly impact both surgical planning and surgical results. In one study, patients who underwent parotidectomy for an FNAC-diagnosed parotid malignancy had significantly higher rates of both upfront cervical neck dissections and clear pathologic margins.[26] In addition, knowledge of the nature of a parotid mass may greatly influence patient counseling, which may have particular utility in patients who are poor surgical candidates or prefer a watchful-waiting strategy, when appropriate. Accordingly, the use of FNAC in the evaluation of a parotid mass should be strongly considered as it is generally felt to be an excellent investigational tool as long as it is employed in the appropriate clinical context.

IMAGING

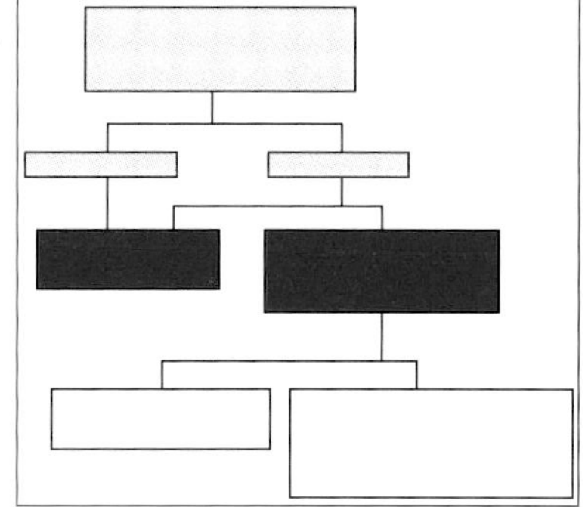

Modern imaging of salivary gland pathology predominantly consists of computed tomography (CT) or magnetic resonance imaging (MRI) or both. As with their characteristics in the imaging of other regions of the body, CT is considered superior to MRI for evaluation of the bony structures, whereas MRI is typically more helpful in soft tissue resolution and in distinguishing between inflammatory conditions and neoplasms. Additionally, MRI may better discern an inferior tail of a parotid mass from an upper cervical mass and detect radiologic signs of malignancy, including irregular, indistinct margins with parotid tissue, low signal intensities on all imaging sequences, and tumor infiltration into muscle, bone, or nerve [*see Figure 2*].

a b

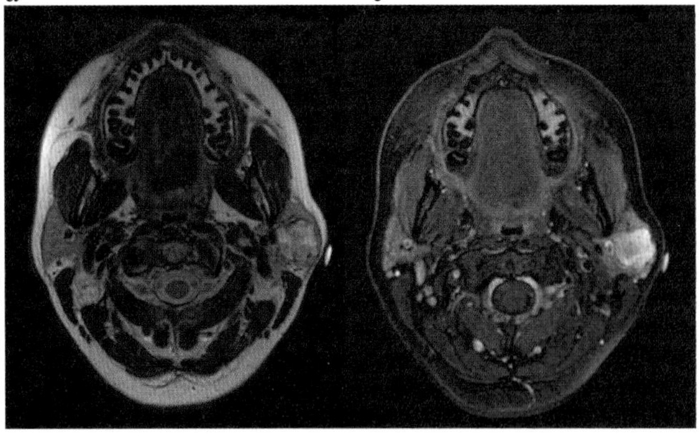

Figure 2 **Axial (*a*) T_1 and (*b*) T_2 magnetic resonance images of a left superficial parotid pleomorphic adenoma demonstrating the classic irregular, bosselated appearance.**

Similar to FNAC, the utility of the various imaging modalities used in the evaluation of a parotid mass continues to be controversial. Many surgeons believe that preoperative ultrasonography, CT, and MRI will provide little to no influence on therapy for a small, mobile, superficial parotid nodule, which would be better assessed with FNAC, surgery, or both. Conversely, management of the more advanced, fixed, aggressive, and deep parotid tumors can be considerably influenced by CT or MRI findings. Patients with diffuse parotid enlargement, tumor extension beyond the superficial lobe, facial nerve weakness, trismus, or deep tumors that are difficult to evaluate clinically should be initially assessed with CT. Fixation to the deeper structures may prompt the need for MRI to evaluate the extent and for parapharyngeal extension or origin. Patients with tumors in close proximity to the facial nerve, external auditory canal, mastoid, mandible, or regional musculature may also benefit from a preoperative MRI, which may influence surgical planning.

Currently, the role of positron emission tomography (PET) in the initial evaluation of a parotid mass remains undefined. This modality may, however, be of some value in the evaluation of suspected recurrent parotid cancers, lymph node metastases, or distant metastases.

Management

BASIC PRINCIPLES

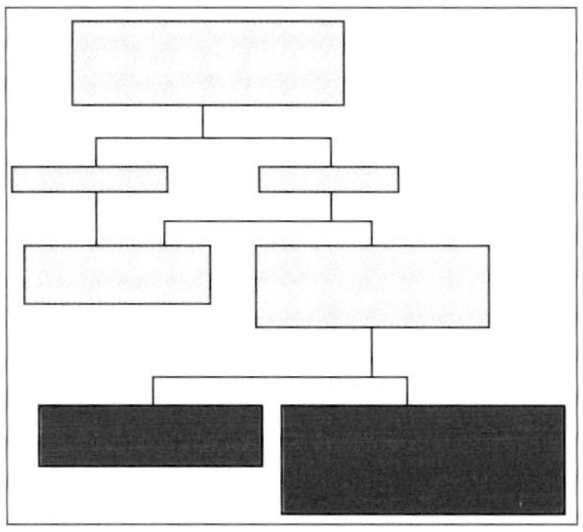

Treatment of a parotid mass depends on the nature and extent of the lesion, which, like most cancers of the body, is categorized and described by a universal staging system. Staging for cancers of the parotid gland is accomplished by means of the familiar tumor-node-metastasis (TNM) system developed by the American Joint Committee on Cancer (AJCC) [*see Table 2 and Table 3*].

Malignant parotid masses are primarily treated surgically according to established oncologic principles [*see Table 4*]. An appropriate parotidectomy with identification and assessment of the facial nerve for tumor involvement is considered the current standard of care. Postoperative radiation therapy is often indicated for more involved and advanced-stage tumors. Moreover, benign parotid masses are frequently managed surgically as well, with exploration of the parotid gland, identification and preservation of the facial nerve, and evaluation of the neoplasm regarded as the customary surgical interventions. Enucleation, once considered an acceptable alternative to superficial parotidectomy for benign pathologies, is now discouraged owing to the possibility of tumor spillage, incomplete removal of the tumor, inadvertent injury to the branches of the facial nerve, and high rates of local recurrence. The need for revision surgery for benign parotid processes is considered unacceptable given the difficulty of surgery on a previously operated tissue bed and consequential increased risk of injury to the facial nerve.

SURGICAL THERAPY

Surgery is the primary treatment modality for nonlymphoid salivary gland neoplasms, both benign and malignant. Optimal surgery for the parotid gland should address both the primary tumor and cervical disease, if present, in a single operation. The minimum surgical intervention for a parotid mass is superficial parotidectomy with identification, dissection, and preservation of the facial nerve, although a subtotal or total parotidectomy and neck dissection may be required for larger tumors that involve the deep lobe of the parotid gland or for patients with clinical or radiologic evidence of regional disease, respectively. If the tumor involves and directly infiltrates the facial nerve, a diagnosis of malignancy, if not previously established preoperatively, should be explored. If a malignant diagnosis is confirmed, a low threshold for nerve sacrifice should be maintained. However, facial nerve preservation despite tumor encroachment on the nerve can be considered as long as all gross disease is removed. With the availability of adjuvant radiation therapy, the surgeon can choose to leave behind microscopic disease, which can be addressed postoperatively. In addition to temporary or permanent facial weakness, patients should be counseled on and consented for other potential complications of parotid surgery, including permanent numbness of the auricle from greater auricular nerve injury and Frey and first-bite syndromes. Frey syndrome, also known as auriculotemporal syndrome or gustatory sweating, is believed to result from misdirected regeneration of cut parasympathetic fibers from the otic ganglion to the parotid gland, leading to the innervation of sweat glands and subcutaneous vasculature. Patients report discomfort, erythema, and perspiration over the parotid bed or neck when eating. First-bite syndrome is a poorly understood complication of surgery in the parapharyngeal space believed to result from injury to the cervical sympathetic chain. A denervation hypersensitivity of parotid myoepithelial cells to parasympathetic neurotransmitters results, leading to supramaximal myoepithelial contraction and consequent pain with the first bite of a meal. Intracutaneous and intraglandular injections of botulinum toxin type A have been shown to provide patients with long-term and effective relief from the symptoms of Frey and first-bite syndromes, respectively.

Table 2 American Joint Committee on Cancer TNM Clinical Classification of Major Salivary Gland Tumors

Primary tumor (T)
- TX: Primary tumor cannot be assessed
- T0: No evidence of primary tumor
- T1: Tumor ≤ 2 cm in greatest dimension without extraparenchymal extension
- T2: Tumor > 2 cm but ≤ 4 cm in greatest dimension without extraparenchymal extension
- T3: Tumor having extraparenchymal extension without seventh nerve involvement and/or > 4 cm but < 6 cm in greatest dimension
- T4a: Tumor invades the skin, mandible, external auditory canal, seventh nerve, and/or > 6 cm in greatest dimension
- T4b: Tumor invades the base of skull, pterygoid plates, carotid artery

Regional lymph nodes (N)
- NX: Regional lymph nodes cannot be assessed
- N0: No regional lymph node metastasis
- N1: Metastasis in a single ipsilateral lymph node, ≤ 3 cm in greatest dimension
- N2: Metastasis in a single ipsilateral lymph node, > 3 cm but ≤ 6 cm in greatest dimension; or in multiple ipsilateral lymph nodes, none > 6 cm in greatest dimension; or in bilateral or contralateral lymph nodes, none > 6 cm in greatest dimension
  - N2a: Metastasis in a single ipsilateral lymph node > 3 cm but ≤ 6 cm in greatest dimension
  - N2b: Metastasis in multiple ipsilateral lymph nodes, none > 6 cm in greatest dimension
  - N2c: Metastasis in bilateral or contralateral lymph nodes, none > 6 cm in greatest dimension
- N3: Metastasis in a lymph node > 6 cm in greatest dimension

Distant metastasis (M)
- MX: Distant metastasis cannot be assessed
- M0: No distant metastasis
- M1: Distant metastasis

An incision in a preauricular skin crease gently curving 2 mm below the auricular lobule and continuing 2 to 3 cm below the mandible is made down to the level of the parotid fascia to prevent lobular distortion and transection of the marginal mandibular branch of the facial nerve, respectively. An anterior flap above the level of the parotid fascia is elevated with a blade or scissors, whereas a posterior flap is raised to expose the tail of the parotid, sternocleidomastoid muscle, and mastoid tip. Dissection then proceeds deeper to identify the posterior belly of the digastric muscle. Identification of the tragal pointer is then accomplished with cautious dissection along the tragal cartilage, and the main trunk of the facial nerve is typically found roughly 1 cm anterior and deep to this important landmark at the level of the digastric muscle. After the nerve is identified, the superficial lobe of the parotid is removed with the mass with careful dissection along the nerve branches.[27] In certain instances, a retrograde approach to facial nerve identification can be used and has been shown to reduce operative time and blood loss and conserve normal parotid tissue without compromising surgical margin status.[28]

Table 3 American Joint Committee on Cancer Staging System for Major Salivary Gland Tumors

Stage	T	N	M
I	T1	N0	M0
II	T2	N0	M0
III	T3 T1, T2, T3	N0 N1	M0 M0
IVA	T4a, T4b T1, T2, T3, T4a	N0, N1 N2	M0 M0
IVB	T4b Any T	Any N N3	M0 M0
IVC	Any T	Any N	M1

Table 4 Principles of Treatment of Parotid Tumors

Adequate local excision of tumor, based on extent of primary lesion
Preservation of facial nerve if possible
Elective neck dissection reserved for selected patients
Postoperative radiotherapy when indicated (in appropriate fields)
Prognosis determined primarily by stage and grade of tumor

High-grade tumors involving the deep lobe or with extension to the parapharyngeal space may require a total parotidectomy. Following removal of the superficial portion of the gland, the facial nerve and its branches are carefully raised off the deep parotid tissue or tumor, and this tissue is subsequently elevated off the masseter muscle and removed. A cervical-parotid approach with exposure of the internal and external carotid arteries, internal jugular vein, and vagus, spinal accessory, and hypoglossal nerves may facilitate identification and excision of parapharyngeal space masses posterior to the stylomandibular ligament. A midline mandibulotomy to provide additional exposure and control of vessels can also be added for tumors extending to the skull base or encasing the carotid artery. If the tumor extends beyond the parotid gland and involves the skin, infratemporal fossa, ascending ramus of the mandible, or mastoid process, more extensive surgical procedures (e.g., composite resection, lateral temporal bone resection, or radical parotidectomy) may become necessary.

Patients with preoperative facial weakness or paralysis will often require sacrifice of the main trunk of the facial nerve. If the tumor involves only an isolated branch of the facial nerve, the surgeon can elect to selectively sacrifice the involved branch alone. Following nerve sacrifice, nerve grafting should be considered in the same procedure. Reconstruction of the facial nerve can be performed with a nerve graft from the greater auricular nerve, medical or lateral antecubial cutaneous nerve, sural nerve, and ansa hypoglossi, among others. The functional results of nerve grafting vary considerably, depending on the age of the patient, the extent of the disease, and the identification of and appropriate anastomosis to the peripheral branches of the facial nerve. If postoperative radiation therapy is envisioned, its potential deleterious effects on nerve regeneration should be considered.

FACIAL NERVE MONITORING

Postoperative facial weakness is a frequent complication of parotid surgery and is the most feared complication for both the patient and the surgeon. Transient facial dysfunction after parotidectomy ranges from 20 to 40%, whereas permanent paralysis has been reported to be as high as 5%. Continuous visual observation of the patient's ipsilateral face by the assistant surgeon or nurse has historically been the traditional method of facial nerve monitoring during a parotidectomy. More recently, however, facial nerve stimulators and continuous electromyographic neuromonitoring of the facial nerve have been employed by surgeons as a means to assist in nerve identification, to provide additional indication for what is "safe" to cut, and to reduce operative time.

Although a few small retrospective case-control comparisons have noted a significant reduction in the rates of temporary and/or permanent facial weakness with the use of these electrophysiologic devices,[29] the vast majority of studies have failed to demonstrate a significant improvement in postoperative facial nerve function outcome.[30,31] Given the exceedingly low incidence of inadvertent permanent facial paralysis in parotid surgery, however, Eisele and colleagues pointed out that a prospective, randomized study would need, at minimum, 1,000 patients to demonstrate a reduction in permanent facial nerve injury from 2% to 1%.[32] Accordingly, the authors suggested that a large, multi-institutional study will be needed to ascertain the benefits and drawbacks of electrophysiologic nerve monitoring technologies and that surgeons who believe that patients will benefit from the information provided should continue to use the devices.

INTRAOPERATIVE FROZEN-SECTION ANALYSIS

The role of intraoperative frozen-section examination in the evaluation of a parotid mass, like that of fine-needle aspiration biopsy, is the subject of considerable debate. Nevertheless, frozen-section examination has been found to be useful for distinguishing salivary processes from nonsalivary processes and benign disease from malignant disease. In 80 to 90% of cases, the findings from intraoperative frozen-section examination correlate with the final pathologic diagnosis.[33] If frozen-section examination shows a benign tumor and confirms the presumed preoperative diagnosis, lateral superficial parotidectomy should be sufficient. If frozen-section examination shows high-grade mucoepidermoid carcinoma in a patient without evidence of cervical disease, selective neck dissection may be considered for staging purposes. Moreover, if frozen-section examination provides a definitive diagnosis of malignancy, further decisions about the extent of parotidectomy and possible selective neck dissection can be made accordingly. If the pathology is unrevealing, the procedure originally planned can be performed, and any further interventions, if required, can be dictated by the final pathologic diagnosis. Notably, significant caution should be exercised when deciding on facial nerve preservation or sacrifice based solely on frozen-section results as frozen-section classification of the wide variety of parotid tumors (both benign and malignant) is often difficult and will often depend on the experience of the frozen-section pathologist.

NECK DISSECTION

Overall, about 10 to 20% of patients with malignant parotid tumors present with clinically detectable cervical lymphadenopathy, most frequently in levels II and III. Nodal metastasis reduces the survival rate by roughly 50%.[11,21,34] Patients with clinically or radiologically positive cervical metastases are treated with either a comprehensive, modified radical, or selective neck dissection, depending on the extent of the disease. However, the surgical management of patients with salivary malignancies who have no detectable cervical lymphadenopathy continues to be a matter of debate. Studies have revealed that only 12 to 16% of patients without clinical evidence of cervical disease demonstrated pathologically positive nodes.[25,35] In view of the low incidence of occult metastases, these investigators do not recommend routine elective treatment of the neck.

Other authors have investigated the patient and tumor factors that may predict the presence of neck disease. Two large population studies identified older age, facial nerve paralysis, extraparotid involvement, higher tumor grade, and perilymphatic invasion as variables predictive of occult cervical disease.[34,36] In addition, Bhattacharyya and Fried determined that tumor size and histopathologic type were also predictors of regional disease and identified adenocarcinoma and SCC as histopathologies with the highest odds ratios for nodal metastases.[34] Similarlly, Regis De Brito Santos and colleagues found that the variables that showed the highest correlation with the incidence of lymph node metastasis were the histopathologic type (i.e., adenocarcinoma, undifferentiated carcinoma, high-grade mucoepidermoid carcinoma, SCC, or salivary duct carcinoma) and tumor stage.[37]

Accordingly, an elective neck dissection may be considered in patients with advanced-stage primary tumors, those whose tumors are of high histologic grades, and those whose tumors are of certain specific histologic types. A selective neck dissection may be performed to remove levels IB, II, III, and the upper part of V for the purposes of staging.[38] However, a more comprehensive neck dissection that encompasses levels I through V may be necessary in patients who present with clinically or radiologically apparent cervical metastases.

RADIATION THERAPY

Candidates for postoperative radiation therapy include patients with advanced-stage disease, a large primary tumor, close or positive margins, nodal disease, perineural spread, soft tissue extension, preoperative facial nerve dysfunction, or

Table 5 Indications for Postoperative Radiation Therapy for Parotid Cancer

Aggressive, highly malignant tumor
Invasion of adjacent tissues outside parotid capsule
Regional lymph node metastases
Deep-lobe cancer
Gross residual tumor after resection
Recurrent tumor after resection
Invasion of facial nerve by tumor

high-grade tumors [*see Table 5*].[39,40] Accordingly, postoperative radiation therapy is suggested for all patients with parotid malignancy other than those with low-grade T1 or T2 tumors and clear surgical margins. Combined surgical and radiation therapy has been shown to result in 5- and 10-year survivals of as high as 95% and 84%, respectively.[41]

A role for radiation therapy for the treatment of an N0 neck in lieu of an elective neck dissection has been proposed, and there is some evidence to suggest that elective irradiation is as effective as elective neck dissection.[25] Some authors have proposed that postoperative patients who will already be requiring radiation therapy for additional primary-site sterilization are excellent candidates for elective radiation of the neck.[42]

Additionally, there is substantial interest in the potential role of neutron radiotherapy as a primary treatment modality for certain parotid malignancies, including advanced inoperable cancers, adenoid cystic carcinomas, and recurrent pleomorphic adenomas, and for poor surgical candidates. Particle radiation may be of particular benefit in adenoid cystic carcinoma to treat perineural extension. Although additional work and further data on survival and related complications await this treatment modality, neutron radiotherapy may be the best option currently available for patients with inoperable parotid cancer.[43]

Table 6 Prognostic Factors for Salivary Gland Tumors

Increasing age at diagnosis
Pain at presentation
Higher T stage
Higher N stage
Skin invasion
Facial nerve dysfunction
Perineural growth
Positive surgical margins
Soft tissue invasion
Treatment type

Survival

Survival of patients with parotid gland malignancies is influenced by multiple factors [*see Table 6*]. The various histopathologies with variable aggressiveness will naturally exert different influences on mean survival durations and rates; histopathologic distributions and survival estimates of parotid gland cancers extracted from a national cancer database are provided in Table 7.[44] In this study, acinar cell carcinomas and mucoepidermoid carcinomas exhibited the best survival, whereas carcinoma ex pleomorphic adenoma, adenocarcinomas, and SCCs displayed substantially poorer survivals. Of note, separate survival analyses of the different grades of mucoepidermoid carcinoma demonstrated statistically significant differences in overall survival according to grade.

In addition to histopathology, increasing age, tumor size, tumor grade, extraglandular extension, and the presence of cervical disease all significantly and negatively impacted survival, whereas the use of external-beam radiation therapy provided a statistically significant survival benefit.[44,45] Moreover, Lima and colleagues concluded in their institutional experience that the presence of facial nerve dysfunction also negatively influenced prognosis.[21]

Financial Disclosures: None Reported

Table 7 Histopathologic Distribution of Major Salivary Gland Malignancies of the Parotid

Histopathology	*n*	%	Mean Survival (mo)	5-Year Actuarial Survival (%)	10-Year Actuarial Survival (%)
Mucoepidermoid carcinoma	367	40.6	105	81.5	63.5
Primary SCC	191	21.2	60	46.1	27.2
Adenocarcinoma	189	20.9	70	65.9	49.7
Acinar cell carcinoma	95	10.5	108	80.0	77.7
Carcinoma ex pleomorphic adenoma	23	2.5	59	40.2	0.0
Malignant mixed tumor	20	2.2	95	73.3	55.0
Adenoid cystic carcinoma	18	2.0	95	70.7	NA
Total	903	100.0	88	66.6	49.7

NA = not available; SCC = squamous cell carcinoma.

References

1. Ward, MJ, Levine, PA. Salivary gland tumors. In: Close LG, Larson DL, Shah JP, editors. Essentials of head and neck oncology. 1st ed. New York: Thieme; 1998. p. 153.
2. Pinkston JA, Cole P. Incidence rates of salivary gland tumors: results from a population-based study. Otolaryngol Head Neck Surg 1999;120:834–40.
3. Janfaza P, Montgomery WW, Fabian RL, et al, editors. Surgical anatomy of the head and neck. Philadelphia: Lippincott Williams and Wilkins, 2001.
4. Califano J, Eisele DW. Benign salivary gland neoplasms. Otolaryngol Clin North Am 1999;32:861–73.
5. McQuone SJ. Acute viral and bacterial infections of the salivary glands. Otolaryngol Clin North Am 1999;32:793–811.

6. Rice DH. Malignant salivary gland neoplasms. Otolaryngol Clin North Am 1999;32:875–86.
7. Barnes L, Myers EN, Prokopakis EP. Primary malignant lymphoma of the parotid gland. Arch Otolaryngol Head Neck Surg 1988;124:573.
8. Kane WJ, McCaffrey TV, Olsen KD, et al. Primary parotid malignancies. A clinical and pathologic review. Arch Otolaryngol Head Neck Surg 1991;117:307.
9. Friedrich RE, Li L, Knop J, et al. Pleomorphic adenoma of the salivary glands: analysis of 94 patients. Anticancer Res 2005;25:1703.
10. Wong DS. Signs and symptoms of malignant parotid tumours: an objective assessment. J R Coll Surg Edinb 2001;46:91.
11. Spiro RH, Huvos AG, Strong EWL. Cancer of the parotid gland: a clinicopathologic study of 288 primary cases. Am J Surg 1975;130:452.
12. Spiro RH. Salivary neoplasms: overview of a 35-year experience with 2,807 patients. Head Neck Surg 1986;8:177–84.
13. Ellis GL, Auclair PL. Tumors of the salivary glands. Atlas of tumor pathology, series 3, fascicle 17. Washington (DC): Armed Forces Institute of Pathology; 1996.
14. Seifert G, Sobin LH. Histological classification of salivary gland tumours. In: World Health Organization. International histological classification of tumours. Berlin: Springer-Verlag; 1991.
15. Quesnel AM, Lindsay RW, Hadlock TA. When the bell tolls on Bell's palsy: finding [illegible] malignancy in acute-onset facial paralysis. Am J Otolaryngol 2010. DOI: 10.1016/j.amjoto.2009.04.003.
16. Vrielinck LJ, Ostyn F, van Damme B, et al. The significance of perineural spread in adenoid cystic carcinoma of the major and minor salivary glands. Int J Oral Maxillofac Surg 1988;17:190.
17. Spiro RH. Distant metastasis in adenoid cystic carcinoma of salivary origin. Am J Surg 1997;174:495.
18. Gomez DR, Katabi N, Zhung J, et al. Clinical and pathologic prognostic features in acinic cell carcinoma of the parotid gland. Cancer 2009;115:2128–37.
19. Lee S, Kim GE, Park CS, et al. Primary squamous cell carcinoma of the parotid gland. Am J Otolaryngol 2001;22:400–6.
20. Bron LP, Traynor SJ, McNeil EB, O'Brien CJ. Primary and metastatic cancer of the parotid: comparison of clinical behavior in 232 cases. Laryngoscope 2003;113:1070–5.
21. Lima RA, Tavares MR, Dias FL, et al. Clinical prognostic factors in malignant parotid gland tumors. Otolaryngol Head Neck Surg 2005;133:702–8.
22. Stennert E, Kisner D, Jungehuelsing M, et al. High incidence of lymph node metastasis in major salivary gland cancer. Arch Otolaryngol Head Neck Surg 2003;129:720–3.
23. Emerick KS, Fabian RL, Deschler DG. Clinical presentation, management, and outcome of high-grade mucoepidermoid carcinoma of the parotid gland. Otolaryngol Head Neck Surg 2007;136:783–7.
24. Ying YL, Johnson JT, Myers EN. Squamous cell carcinoma of the parotid gland. Head Neck 2006;28:626–32.
25. Armstrong JG, Harrison LB, Thaler HT, et al. The indications for elective treatment of the neck in cancer of the major salivary glands. Cancer 1992;69:615.
26. Lin AC, Bhattacharyya N. The utility of fine needle aspiration in parotid malignancy. Otolaryngol Head Neck Surg 2007;136:793–8.
27. Thompson DM, McCafferey TV. Surgical approaches for primary parotid malignancies. Oper Techn Otolaryngol Head Neck Surg 1996;7:358–64.
28. Bhattacharyya N, Richardson ME, Gugino LD. An objective assessment of the advantages of retrograde parotidectomy. Otolaryngol Head Neck Surg 2004;131:392–6.
29. Terrell JE, Kileny PR, Yian C, et al. Clinical outcome of continuous facial nerve monitoring during primary parotidectomy. Arch Otolaryngol Head Neck Surg 1997;123:1081–7.
30. Reilly J, Myssiorek D. Facial nerve stimulation and postparotidectomy facial paresis. Otolaryngol Head Neck Surg 2003;128:530–3.
31. Grosheva M, Klussmann JP, Grimminger C, et al. Electromyographic facial nerve monitoring during parotidectomy for benign lesions does not improve the outcome of postoperative facial nerve function: a prospective two-center trial. Laryngoscope 2009;119:2299–305.
32. Eisele DW, Wang SJ, Orloff LA. Electrophysiologic facial nerve monitoring during parotidectomy. Head Neck 2010;32:399–405.
33. Seethala RR, LiVolsi VA, Baloch ZW. Relative accuracy of fine-needle aspiration and frozen section in the diagnosis of lesions of the parotid gland. Head Neck 2005;27:217–23.
34. Bhattacharyya N, Fried MP. Nodal metastasis in major salivary gland cancer: predictive factors and effects on survival. Arch Otolaryngol Head Neck Surg 2002;128:904–8.
35. Korkmaz H, Yoo GH, Du W, et al. Predictors of nodal metastasis in salivary gland cancer. J Surg Oncol 2002;80:186–9.
36. Frankenthaler RA, Byers RM, Luna MA, et al. Predicting occult lymph node metastasis in parotid cancer. Arch Otolaryngol Head Neck Surg 1993;119:517–20.
37. Regis De Brito Santos I, Kowalski LP, Cavalcante De Araujo V, et al. Multivariate analysis of risk factors for neck metastases in surgically treated parotid carcinomas. Arch Otolaryngol Head Neck Surg 2001;127:56.
38. Ferlito A, Shaha AR, Rinaldo A, et al. Management of clinically negative cervical lymph nodes in patients with malignant neoplasms of the parotid gland. ORL J Otorhinolaryngol Relat Spec 2001;63:123.
39. Harrison LB, Armstrong JG, Spiro RH, et al. Postoperative radiation therapy for major salivary gland malignancies. J Surg Oncol 1990;45:52.
40. Tullio A, Marchetti C, Sesenna E, et al. Treatment of carcinoma of the parotid gland: the results of a multicenter study. J Oral Maxillofac Surg 2001;59:263.
41. Spiro IJ, Wang CC, Montgomery WW. Carcinoma of the parotid gland. Analysis of [illegible] results and patterns of failure after combined surgery and radiation therapy. Cancer 1993;71:2699–705.
42. Gold DR, Annino DJ Jr. Management of the neck in salivary gland carcinoma. Otolaryngol Clin North Am 2005;38:99–105.
43. Laramore GE, Krall JM, Griffin TW, et al. Neutron versus photon irradiation for unresectable salivary gland tumors: final report of an RTOG-MRC randomized clinical trial. Radiation Therapy Oncology Group. Medical Research Council. Int J Radiat Oncol Biol Phys 1993;27:235.
44. Bhattacharyya N, Fried MP. Determinants of survival in parotid gland carcinoma: a population-based study. Am J Otolaryngol 2005;26:39–44.
45. Jeannon JP, Calman F, Gleeson M, et al. Management of advanced parotid cancer. A systematic review. Eur J Surg Oncol 2009;35:908–15.

3 NECK MASS

*Christopher Scally, MD, and Gerard M. Doherty, MD**

Assessment of a Neck Mass

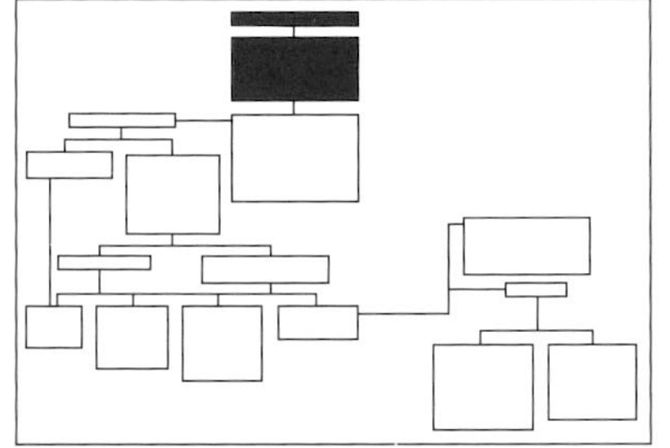

Clinical Evaluation

HISTORY

The evaluation of any neck mass begins with a careful history taken with the differential diagnosis in mind [*see Table 1*] because directed questions can narrow down the diagnostic possibilities and focus subsequent investigations. For example, in younger patients, one might suspect congenital or inflammatory lesions, whereas in older adults, the first concern is often neoplasia.

The duration and growth rate of the mass are important: malignant lesions are more likely to grow rapidly than benign ones, which may grow and shrink. The location of the mass in the neck can also narrow the list of possibilities. This is particularly important for differentiating congenital masses from neoplastic or inflammatory ones because each type usually occurs in particular locations. In addition, the location of a neoplasm has both diagnostic and prognostic significance. The possibility that the mass is an infectious or inflammatory process should also be assessed. One should evaluate for evidence of infection or inflammation (e.g., fever, pain, or tenderness); a recent history of tuberculosis, sarcoidosis, or fungal infection; the presence of dental problems; and a history of trauma to the head and neck. Masses that appear inflamed or infected are far more likely to be benign.

Finally, factors suggestive of cancer include a history of malignancy elsewhere in the head and neck (e.g., a history of skin cancer, melanoma, thyroid cancer, or head and neck cancer); night sweats (suggestive of lymphoma); excessive exposure to the sun (a risk factor for skin cancer); smoking or excessive alcohol consumption (risk factors for squamous cell carcinoma of the head and neck); nasal obstruction or bleeding, otalgia, odynophagia, dysphagia, or hoarseness (suggestive of a malignancy in the upper aerodigestive tract); or exposure to low-dose therapeutic radiation (a risk factor for thyroid cancer).

* The authors and editors gratefully acknowledge the contributions of the previous authors, Barry Roseman, MD, FACS, and Orlo Clark, MD, FACS, to the development and writing of this chapter.

PHYSICAL EXAMINATION

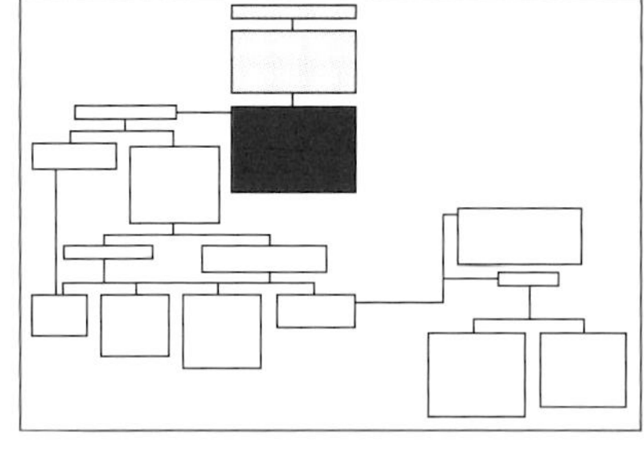

The head and neck examination is challenging because much of the area to be examined is not easily seen. Patience and practice are necessary to master the special instruments and techniques of examination. A head and neck examination is usually performed with the patient sitting in front of the physician. Constant repositioning of the head is necessary to obtain adequate visualization of the various areas. Gloves must be worn during the examination, particularly if the mucous membranes are to be examined. Good illumination is essential. Fiberoptic endoscopy with a flexible laryngoscope and a nasopharyngoscope is a common component of the physical examination for evaluating

Table 1 Etiology of Neck Mass
Inflammatory and infectious disorders
Acute lymphadenitis (bacterial or viral infection)
Subcutaneous abscess (carbuncle)
Infectious mononucleosis
Cat-scratch fever
AIDS
Tuberculous lymphadenitis (scrofula)
Fungal lymphadenitis (actinomycosis)
Sarcoidosis
Congenital cystic lesions
Thyroglossal duct cyst
Branchial cleft cyst
Cystic hygroma (lymphangioma)
Vascular malformation (hemangioma)
Laryngocele
Benign neoplasms
Salivary gland tumor
Thyroid nodules or goiter
Soft tissue tumor (lipoma, sebaceous cyst)
Chemodectoma (carotid body tumor)
Neurogenic tumor (neurofibroma, neurilemmoma)
Laryngeal tumor (chondroma)
Malignant neoplasms
Primary
Salivary gland tumor
Thyroid cancer
Upper aerodigestive tract cancer
Soft tissue sarcoma
Skin cancer (melanoma, squamous cell carcinoma, basal cell carcinoma)
Lymphoma
Metastatic
Upper aerodigestive tract cancer
Skin cancer (melanoma, squamous cell carcinoma)
Salivary gland tumor
Thyroid cancer
Adenocarcinoma (breast, gastrointestinal tract, genitourinary tract, lung)
Unknown primary tumor

Assessment of a Neck Mass

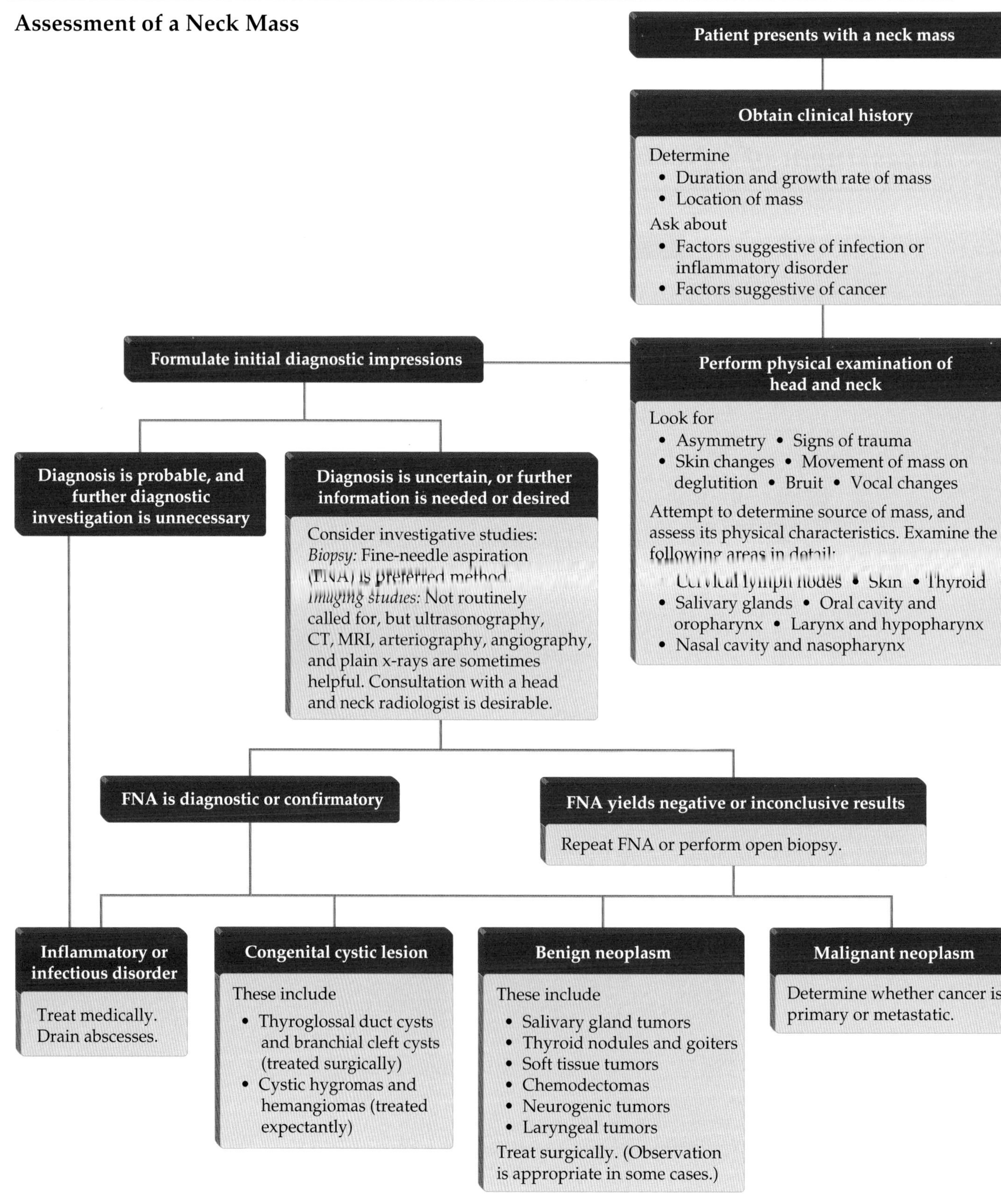

Patient presents with a neck mass
Obtain clinical history
Determine
• Duration and growth rate of mass
• Location of mass
Ask about
• Factors suggestive of infection or inflammatory disorder
• Factors suggestive of cancer
Perform physical examination of head and neck
Look for
• Asymmetry • Signs of trauma
• Skin changes • Movement of mass on deglutition • Bruit • Vocal changes
Attempt to determine source of mass, and assess its physical characteristics. Examine the following areas in detail:
• Cervical lymph nodes • Skin • Thyroid
• Salivary glands • Oral cavity and oropharynx • Larynx and hypopharynx
• Nasal cavity and nasopharynx
Formulate initial diagnostic impressions
Diagnosis is probable, and further diagnostic investigation is unnecessary
Diagnosis is uncertain, or further information is needed or desired
Consider investigative studies:
Biopsy: Fine-needle aspiration (FNA) is preferred method.
Imaging studies: Not routinely called for, but ultrasonography, CT, MRI, arteriography, angiography, and plain x-rays are sometimes helpful. Consultation with a head and neck radiologist is desirable.
FNA is diagnostic or confirmatory
FNA yields negative or inconclusive results
Repeat FNA or perform open biopsy.
Inflammatory or infectious disorder
Treat medically.
Drain abscesses.
Congenital cystic lesion
These include
• Thyroglossal duct cysts and branchial cleft cysts (treated surgically)
• Cystic hygromas and hemangiomas (treated expectantly)
Benign neoplasm
These include
• Salivary gland tumors
• Thyroid nodules and goiters
• Soft tissue tumors
• Chemodectomas
• Neurogenic tumors
• Laryngeal tumors
Treat surgically. (Observation is appropriate in some cases.)
Malignant neoplasm
Determine whether cancer is primary or metastatic.

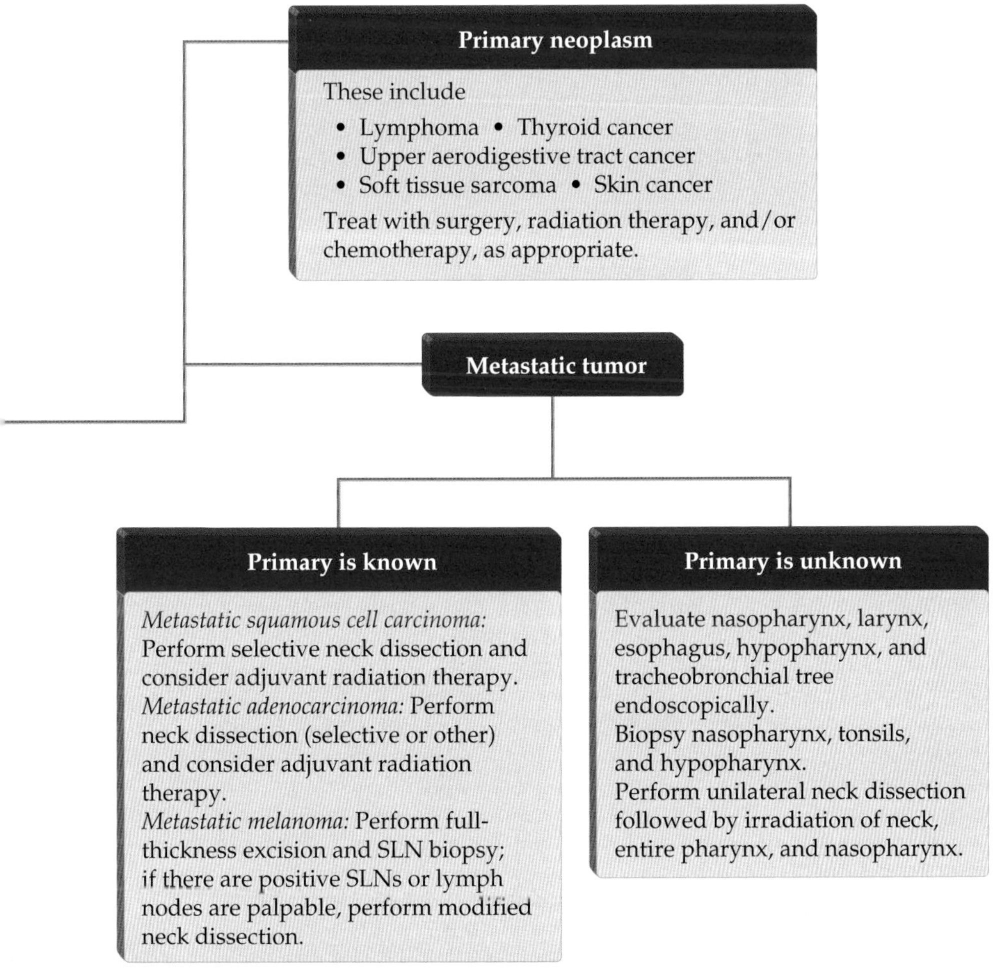

Primary neoplasm

These include

- Lymphoma • Thyroid cancer
- Upper aerodigestive tract cancer
- Soft tissue sarcoma • Skin cancer

Treat with surgery, radiation therapy, and/or chemotherapy, as appropriate.

Metastatic tumor

Primary is known

Metastatic squamous cell carcinoma: Perform selective neck dissection and consider adjuvant radiation therapy.
Metastatic adenocarcinoma: Perform neck dissection (selective or other) and consider adjuvant radiation therapy.
Metastatic melanoma: Perform full-thickness excision and SLN biopsy; if there are positive SLNs or lymph nodes are palpable, perform modified neck dissection.

Primary is unknown

Evaluate nasopharynx, larynx, esophagus, hypopharynx, and tracheobronchial tree endoscopically.
Biopsy nasopharynx, tonsils, and hypopharynx.
Perform unilateral neck dissection followed by irradiation of neck, entire pharynx, and nasopharynx.

the larynx, the nasopharynx, and the paranasal sinuses, especially when these areas cannot be adequately inspected with other techniques.

The examination should begin with inspection for asymmetry, signs of trauma, and skin changes. The examiner should ask the patient to swallow to observe whether the mass moves with deglutition and should palpate the neck from both the front and behind. Auscultation can detect audible bruits. One should also both listen to and ask about the patient's voice, changes in which may suggest either a laryngeal tumor or recurrent nerve dysfunction from locally invasive thyroid cancer.

During the physical examination, one should be thinking about the following questions: What structure is the neck mass arising from? Is it a lymph node? Is the mass arising from a normally occurring structure, such as the thyroid gland, a salivary gland, a nerve, a blood vessel, or a muscle? Or is it arising from an abnormal structure, such as a laryngocele, a branchial cleft cyst, or a cystic hygroma? Is the mass soft, fluctuant, easily mobile, well encapsulated, and smooth? Or is it firm, poorly mobile, and fixed to surrounding structures? Does it pulsate? Is there a bruit? Does it appear to be superficial, or is it deeper in the neck? Is it attached to the skin? Is it tender?

The following areas of the head and neck are examined in some detail.

Cervical Lymph Nodes

The cervical lymphatic system consists of interconnected groups or chains of nodes that parallel the major neurovascular structures in the head and neck. The skin and mucosal surfaces of the head and neck all have specific and predictable nodes associated with them. The classification of cervical lymph nodes has been standardized to comprise six levels [*see Figure 1*]. Accurate determination of lymph node level on physical examination and in surgical specimens not only helps establish a common language among clinicians but also permits comparison of data among different institutions.

The location, size, and consistency of lymph nodes furnish valuable clues to the nature of the primary disease. Other physical characteristics of the adenopathy should be noted as well, including the number of lymph nodes affected, their mobility, their degree of fixation, and their relation to surrounding anatomic structures. One can often establish a tentative diagnosis on the basis of these findings alone. For example, soft or tender nodes are more likely to derive from an inflammatory or infectious condition, whereas hard, fixed, painless nodes are more likely to represent metastatic cancer. Multiple regions of enlarged lymph nodes are usually a sign of systemic disease (e.g., lymphoma, tuberculosis, or infectious mononucleosis), whereas solitary nodes are more often due to malignancy. Firm, rubbery nodes are typical of lymphoma.

The submental and submandibular nodes (level I) are palpated bimanually. The three levels of internal jugular chain nodes (levels II, III, and IV) are best examined by gently rolling the sternocleidomastoid muscle between the thumb and the index finger. The posterior triangle nodes (level V) are palpated posterior to the sternocleidomastoid. The tracheoesophageal groove nodes (level VI) are then palpated.

Skin

Careful examination of the scalp, the ears, the face, the oral cavity, and the neck can identify potentially malignant skin lesions, which may give rise to lymph node metastases.

Thyroid Gland

The thyroid gland is first observed as the patient swallows; it is then palpated and its size and consistency are assessed to determine whether it is smooth, diffusely enlarged, or nodular and whether one nodule or several are present. If it is unclear whether the mass arises from the thyroid, one can clarify the point by asking the patient to swallow and watching to see whether the mass moves upward with the larynx. Signs of superior mediastinal syndrome (e.g., cervical venous engorgement and facial edema) suggest retrosternal extension of a thyroid goiter. Elevation of the arms above the head can elicit this finding in a patient with a substernal goiter (a positive Pemberton sign). The larynx and trachea are examined, with special attention to the cricothyroid membrane, over which Delphian nodes can be palpated. These nodes can be an indication of thyroid or laryngeal cancer.

Major Salivary Glands

Examination of the paired parotid and submandibular glands involves not only palpation of the neck but also an intraoral examination to inspect the duct openings. The submandibular glands are best assessed by bimanual palpation, with one finger in the mouth and one in the neck. They are normally lower and more prominent in older patients. The parotid glands are often palpable in the neck, although the deep lobe cannot always be assessed. A mass in the region of the tail of the parotid must be distinguished from enlarged level II jugular nodes. The oropharynx is inspected for distortion of the lateral walls. The parotid (Stensen) duct may be found opening into the buccal mucosa, opposite the second upper molar.

Oral Cavity and Oropharynx

The lips should be inspected and palpated. Dentures should be removed before the mouth is examined. The buccal mucosa, the teeth, and the gingiva are then inspected. The patient should be asked to elevate the tongue so that the floor of the mouth can be examined and bimanual inspection performed. The tongue should be inspected both in its normal position in the mouth and during protrusion.

Most of the oropharyngeal contents are easily visualized if the tongue is depressed. Only the anterior two thirds of the tongue are clearly visible on examination, however. The base of the tongue is best inspected using a mirror. In most persons, the tongue base can be palpated, although with some discomfort to the patient. The ventral surface of the tongue must also be carefully inspected and palpated.

The hard palate is examined by gently tilting the patient's head backward, and the soft palate is inspected by gently depressing the tongue with a tongue blade. The movement of the palate is assessed by having the patient say "ahh."

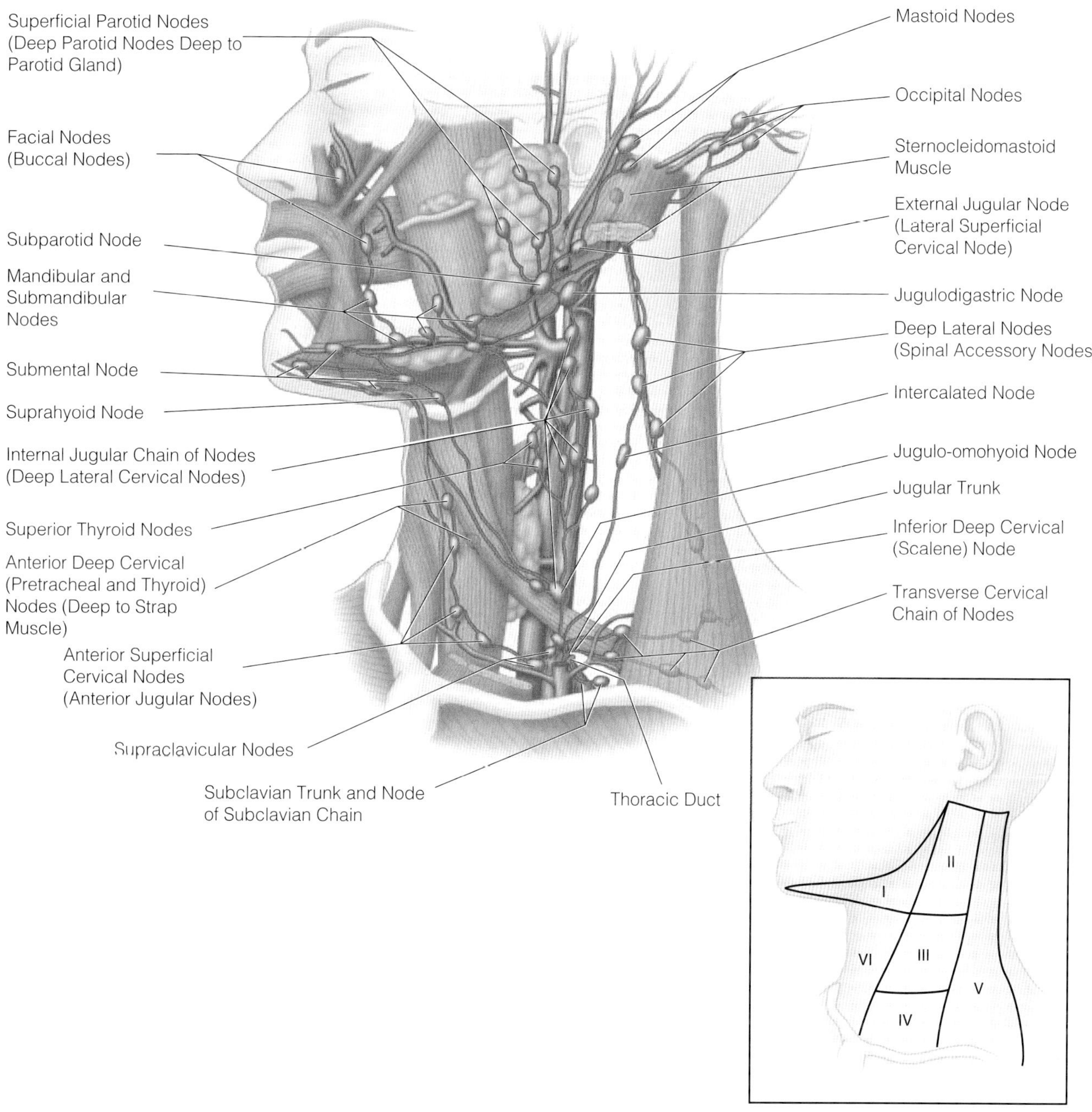

Figure 1 **Cervical lymph nodes. Inset: Classification of cervical lymph nodes by anatomic level.**

The tonsils are then examined. They are usually symmetrical but may vary substantially in size. For example, in young patients, hyperplastic tonsils may almost fill the oropharynx, but in adult patients, this is an uncommon finding. Finally, the posterior pharyngeal wall is inspected.

Larynx and Hypopharynx

The larynx and the hypopharynx are best examined by indirect or direct laryngoscopy. A mirror is warmed, and the patient's tongue is gently held forward to increase the space between the oropharyngeal structures. The mirror is carefully introduced into the oropharynx without touching the base of the tongue. The oropharynx, the larynx, and the hypopharynx can be inspected by changing the angle of the mirror.

The lingual and laryngeal surfaces of the epiglottis are examined. Often the patient must be asked to phonate to bring the endolarynx into view. The aryepiglottic folds and the false and true vocal cords should be identified. The mobility of the true vocal cords is then assessed: their resting position is carefully noted, and their movement during inspiration is recorded. Normally, the vocal cords abduct during breathing and move to the median position during phonation. The larynx is elevated when the patient attempts to say "eeeee"; this allows one to observe vocal cord movement and to better visualize the piriform sinuses, the postcricoid hypopharynx, the laryngeal surface of the epiglottis, and the anterior commissure of the glottic larynx. Passage of a fiberoptic laryngoscope through the nose yields a clear view of the hypopharynx and the larynx. This procedure is well tolerated by almost all patients, particularly if a topical anesthetic is gently sprayed into the nose and swallowed, thereby anesthetizing both the nose and the pharynx.

Nasal Cavity and Nasopharynx

The nasopharynx is examined by depressing the tongue and inserting a small mirror behind the soft palate. The patient is instructed to open the mouth widely and breathe through it to elevate the soft palate. With the patient relaxed, a warmed nasopharyngeal mirror is carefully placed in the oropharynx behind the soft palate without touching the mucosa.

The nasal septum, the choanae, the turbinates, and the eustachian tube orifices are systematically assessed. The dorsum of the soft palate, the posterior nasopharyngeal wall, and the vault of the nasopharynx should also be inspected. The exterior of the nose should be carefully examined, and the septum should be inspected with a nasal speculum. Polyps or other neoplasms can be mistaken for turbinates.

Careful evaluation of the cranial nerves is essential, as is examination of the eyes (including assessment of ocular movement and visual activity), the external ear, and the tympanic membrane.

Additional Areas

The remainder of the physical examination is also important, particularly as regards the identification of a possible source of metastases to the neck. Other sets of lymph nodes—especially axillary and inguinal nodes—are examined for enlargement or tenderness. Women should undergo complete pelvic and rectal examination. Men should undergo rectal, testicular, and prostate examinations; tumors from these organs may metastasize to the neck, albeit rarely.

Developing a Differential Diagnosis

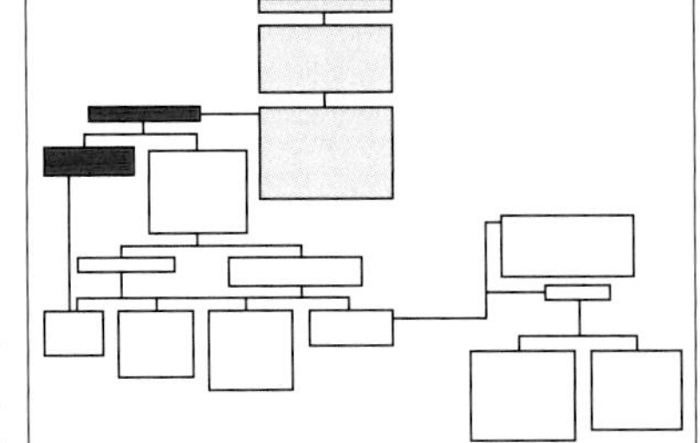

Once a comprehensive history and examination have been performed, one is likely to have a better idea of the etiology of the mass. In some patients, the findings are clear enough to strongly suggest a specific disease entity. For example, a rapidly developing mass that is soft and tender to palpation is most likely a reactive lymph node from an acute bacterial or viral illness. A slow-growing facial mass associated with facial nerve deficits is probably a malignant parotid tumor. A thyroid nodule with an adjacent abnormal lymph node in a young patient probably represents thyroid cancer. In an elderly patient with a substantial history of smoking and alcohol use, a neck mass may be a metastasis from squamous cell carcinoma in the aerodigestive tract.

The initial diagnostic impressions and the degree of certainty attached to them determine the next steps in the workup and management of a neck mass; options include empirical therapy, ultrasonographic scanning, computed tomography (CT), fine-needle aspiration (FNA), and observation alone. For example, in a patient with suspected bacterial lymphadenitis from an oral source, empirical antibiotic therapy with close follow-up is a reasonable approach. In a patient with a suspected parotid tumor, the best first test is a CT scan: the tumor probably must be removed, which means that one will have to ascertain the relation of the mass to adjacent structures. In a patient with suspected metastatic cancer, FNA is a sensible choice: it will confirm the presence of malignancy and may suggest a source of the primary cancer.

Investigative Studies

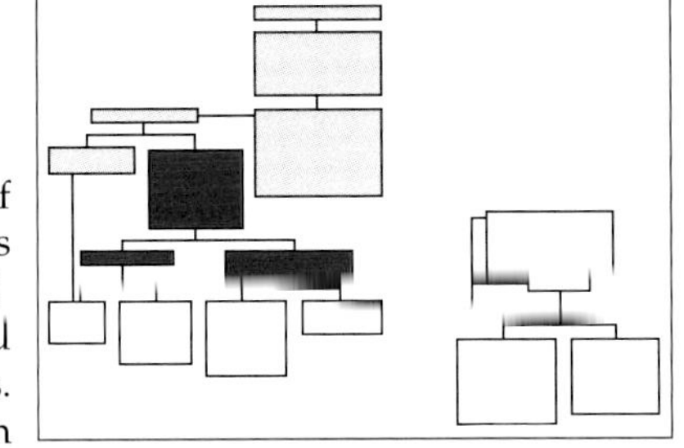

Neck masses of suspected infectious or inflammatory origin may be observed for short periods. Most neck masses in adults, however, are abnormal and are often manifestations of serious underlying conditions. In most cases, therefore, further diagnostic evaluation should be rigorously pursued.

ULTRASONOGRAPHY

Ultrasonography of the neck can be extremely useful in clarifying physical examination findings and supplying additional definitive information. In many clinics, ultrasonography is considered an extension of the physical examination and is applied for nearly all patients with neck masses. Ultrasonography can also be useful to guide tissue sampling and is helpful for mapping of normal or abnormal lymph nodes, for characterizing lesions as cystic or solid, and for defining the risk of some individual lesions (especially thyroid lesions) of being malignant. Ideally, point-of-care ultrasound examination by the treating physician can guide and clarify the subsequent evaluation.

TISSUE SAMPLING

Whether or not the history and the physical examination strongly suggest a specific diagnosis, the information obtained by sampling tissue from the neck mass is often highly useful. In many cases, biopsy establishes the diagnosis or, at least, reduces the diagnostic possibilities. At present, the preferred method of obtaining biopsy material from a neck mass is FNA, which is generally well tolerated and can usually be performed without local anesthesia. Although FNA is, on the whole, both safe and accurate, it is an invasive diagnostic procedure and carries a small but definable risk of potential problems (e.g., bleeding and sampling error). Accordingly, FNA should be done only when the results are likely to influence management.

FNA can be used to sample cystic or solid lesions and can often diagnose malignancy. It has become the standard for making treatment decisions in patients with thyroid nodules and for assessing for suspicious adenopathy for treatment planning. Benign FNA results should not be considered the end point of any search and do not rule out cancer.

Several studies have shown FNA to be approximately 90% accurate in establishing a definitive diagnosis.[1] Lateral cystic neck masses that collapse on aspiration usually represent hygromas, branchial cleft cysts, or cystic degeneration of a metastatic papillary thyroid cancer, although the cystic nature of these lesions is best determined on ultrasonography. Fluid from these masses is sent for cytologic examination. If both cystic and solid components are evident on a sonogram, or if a palpable mass remains after cyst aspiration, then tissue sampling should target the solid component as the morphology of the cells will be better preserved.

If a complete physical examination including ultrasonography has been completed and the FNA is not diagnostic, then an open biopsy may be necessary to obtain a specimen for histologic sections and microbiologic studies. It is estimated that open biopsy eventually proves necessary in about 10% of patients with a malignant mass. For an open biopsy, it is important to orient skin incisions within the boundaries of a neck dissection; the incisions can then, if necessary, be extended for definitive therapy or reexcised if reoperation subsequently proves necessary.

IMAGING

Diagnostic imaging beyond ultrasound studies should be used selectively in the evaluation of a neck mass; imaging studies should be performed only if the results are likely to affect subsequent therapy. Such studies often supply useful information about the location and characteristics of the mass and its relation to adjacent structures. Diagnostic imaging is particularly useful when a biopsy has been performed and a malignant tumor identified. In such cases, these studies can help establish the extent of local disease and the presence or absence of metastases.

CT is useful for differentiating cysts from solid neck lesions and for determining whether a mass is within or outside a gland or nodal chain.[2] In addition, CT can delineate small tongue base or tonsillar tumors that have a minimal mucosal component. Magnetic resonance imaging (MRI) provides much the same information as CT. T_2-weighted gadolinium-enhanced scans are particularly useful for delineating the invasion of soft tissue by tumor: endocrine tumors are often enhanced on such scans. Fluorodeoxyglucose (FDG) positron emission tomography (PET) is increasingly employed in the diagnosis and staging of both primary and metastatic head and neck malignancies, including squamous cell carcinoma, thyroid cancer, lymphoma, and melanoma.[3] FDG-PET is generally reserved for specific situations, however, rather than as a primary imaging modality. FDG-PET-positive, radioiodine-negative, metastatic thyroid cancers are more aggressive than their radioiodine-avid counterparts, for example.

Arteriography is useful mainly for evaluating vascular lesions and tumors fixed to the carotid artery. Angiography is helpful for evaluating the vascularity of a mass, its specific blood supply, or the status of the carotid artery but provides very little information about the physical characteristics of the mass. Plain radiographs of the neck are rarely helpful in differentiating neck masses, but a chest x-ray can often confirm a diagnosis (e.g., in patients with lymphoma, sarcoidosis, or metastatic lung cancer).

It is important to communicate with the radiologist: an experienced head and neck radiologist may be able to offer the surgeon valuable guidance in choosing the best diagnostic test in a specific clinical scenario. Furthermore, providing the radiologist with a detailed clinical history facilitates interpretation of the images.

Management of Specific Disorders

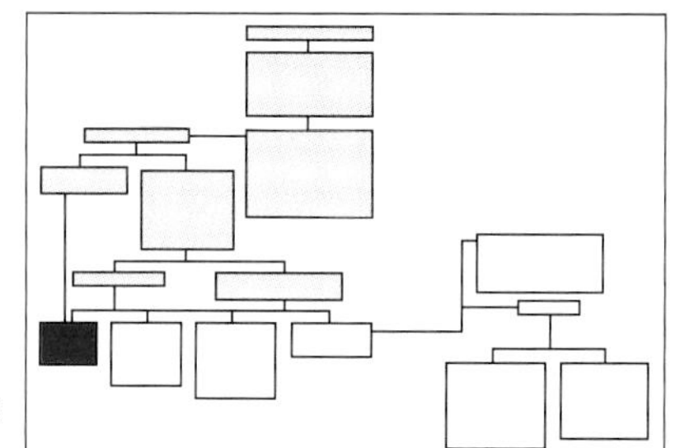

CERVICAL ADENOPATHY

Anatomy

The lymph nodes of the neck are typically divided into six levels [*see Table 2 and Figure 1*], based on common patterns of metastatic spread.[4] These six levels correspond to the submandibular and submental nodes (level I), the jugular nodes (levels II to IV), the posterior triangle nodes (level V), and the anterior triangle nodes (level VI). The boundaries of level I are the mandible superiorly, the anterior belly of the digastric muscle anteriorly, and the stylohyoid muscle posteriorly. Malignant nodes in this level most commonly contain metastases from cancers of the lips, the oral cavity, or the facial skin.

Level II contains nodes located near the upper third of the internal jugular vein. The anterior boundary of level II is the stylohyoid muscle; the posterior boundary is the posterior border of the sternocleidomastoid. Level II extends inferiorly to the level of the hyoid bone. Level III relates to the middle third of the jugular vein. The superior border is the hyoid bone, the inferior border is the level of the cricoid cartilage, and the anterior and posterior borders are the sternohyoid and sternocleidomastoid muscles, respectively. Level II and level III lymph nodes are common sites for lymph node metastases from primary cancers of the oropharynx, the larynx, and the hypopharynx.

Level IV contains nodes relating to the lower third of the internal jugular vein. Its anterior and posterior borders are the same as those for level III; the superior border is the cricoid cartilage, and the inferior border is the superior edge of the clavicle. Metastases in level IV lymph nodes can arise from cancers of the upper aerodigestive tract, cancers of the thyroid gland, or cancers arising below the clavicle.

Level V consists of the posterior triangle of the neck and contains several nodal groups: the spinal accessory, transverse cervical, and supraclavicular nodes. Nodal metastases in the posterior triangle can arise from nasopharyngeal and thyroid cancers and from squamous cell carcinoma or melanoma of the posterior scalp and the pinna of the ear. The eponymous Virchow node in the left supraclavicular region is a common site of distant metastasis. The anterior border of level V is the sternocleidomastoid; the posterior border is the anterior edge of the trapezius muscle. Level V extends

Table 2 Classification of Cervical Lymph Nodes

Level	Nodes	Common Sources of Metastatic Disease
I	Submental nodes Submandibular nodes	Oral cavity and lip, facial skin
II	Upper internal jugular chain nodes	Oropharynx, larynx, hypopharynx
III	Middle internal jugular chain nodes	Oropharynx, larynx, hypopharynx
IV	Lower internal jugular chain nodes	Upper aerodigestive tract, thyroid
V	Spinal accessory nodes Transverse cervical nodes	Remote metastases (Virchow node); posterior scalp
VI	Tracheoesophageal groove nodes	Thyroid, larynx

superiorly from the point at which the sternocleidomastoid and trapezius converge to the clavicle inferiorly.

Level VI contains the lymph nodes of the anterior compartment of the neck. The borders are the hyoid superiorly and the sternal notch inferiorly, and this level extends laterally to the carotid arteries on each side. Nodes in level VI commonly contain metastases from thyroid cancer, as well as from laryngeal cancers.

Investigative and Diagnostic Studies

Lymph node enlargement is a frequent finding with a wide differential diagnosis. Most commonly, lymph node enlargement occurs as a reaction to acute infection; however, given the potential for alternate causes such as malignancy, a benign diagnosis cannot be assumed. A careful history and thorough examination, as well as consideration by the clinician of all potential causes, are essential. Acute infection of the neck (cervical adenitis) is most often the result of dental infection, tonsillitis, pharyngitis, viral upper respiratory tract infection, or skin infection. In this situation, the enlarged lymph nodes are usually just posterior and inferior to the angle of the mandible. Signs of acute infection (e.g., fever, malaise, and a sore mouth or throat) are usually present. A constitutional reaction, tenderness of the cervical mass, and the presence of an obvious infectious source confirm the diagnosis. Treatment should be directed toward the primary disease and should include a monospot test for infectious mononucleosis.

For patients with cervical adenopathy without an obvious acute infection, further investigation is indicated. Various chronic infections (e.g., tuberculosis, fungal lymphadenitis, syphilis, cat-scratch fever, and AIDS) may also involve cervical lymph nodes. Certain chronic inflammatory disorders (e.g., sarcoidosis) may present with cervical lymphadenopathy as well. Because of the chronic lymph node involvement, these conditions are easily confused with neoplasms, especially lymphomas. Biopsy is occasionally necessary; however, skin tests and serologic studies are often more useful for establishing a diagnosis. Treatment of these conditions is primarily medical; surgery is reserved for complications.

In adult patients with cervical adenopathy and no clear infectious etiology, there is a high risk of malignancy, and FNA is recommended. FNA may provide a conclusive diagnosis or further reduce the range of diagnostic possibilities. FNA is also useful in patients with a known distant malignancy in whom confirmation of metastases is needed for staging and for planning therapy, as well as in patients with a primary tumor of the head and neck who are not candidates for operation but in whom a tissue diagnosis is necessary for appropriate nonsurgical therapy to be initiated. A wide variety of primary tumors may metastasize to the cervical lymph nodes, and therapy depends on the primary site and the type and stage of the tumor.

FNA of an enlarged cervical node does have limitations. Sampling error or an inadequate sample may occur; in these cases, a repeat aspiration or an excisional biopsy may be useful.

When lymphoma and metastatic squamous cell carcinoma are diagnostic possibilities, FNA alone is often incapable of determining the precise histologic subtype for lymphoma, but it is usually capable of distinguishing a lymphoproliferative disease from metastatic squamous cell carcinoma. This is a crucial distinction in that the two neoplasms are treated in drastically different ways.

If a lymphoma is suspected, FNA is typically followed by open biopsy, frozen-section confirmation, and submission of fresh tissue for further pathologic characterization. The intact node is placed in normal saline and sent directly to the pathologist for analysis of cellular content and nodal architecture and identification of lymphocyte markers. If, however, metastatic squamous cell carcinoma is suspected, FNA usually suffices for establishing the diagnosis and formulating a treatment plan, which is specific to the site and size of the primary tumor but often includes chemotherapy and radiation initially. In this setting, performing an open biopsy can lead to significant wound healing complications; there is no need to incur this risk when FNA is sufficient to initiate treatment.

THYROID NODULES: BENIGN AND MALIGNANT THYROID DISEASE

Thyroid disease is a relatively common cause of neck mass. Nearly 4% of the population have a palpable thyroid nodule. The majority of thyroid nodules are benign; however, approximately 5% of these lesions are malignant.[5] The evaluation of a thyroid nodule begins with a careful history, focusing on both local symptoms (dysphagia, hoarseness, vocal changes, sleep apnea) and systemic symptoms, as well as a family history of thyroid disease and past exposure to radiation [*see Figure 2*]. A past history of radiation exposure in particular is associated with increased risk of malignancy. After a thorough history and examination, including

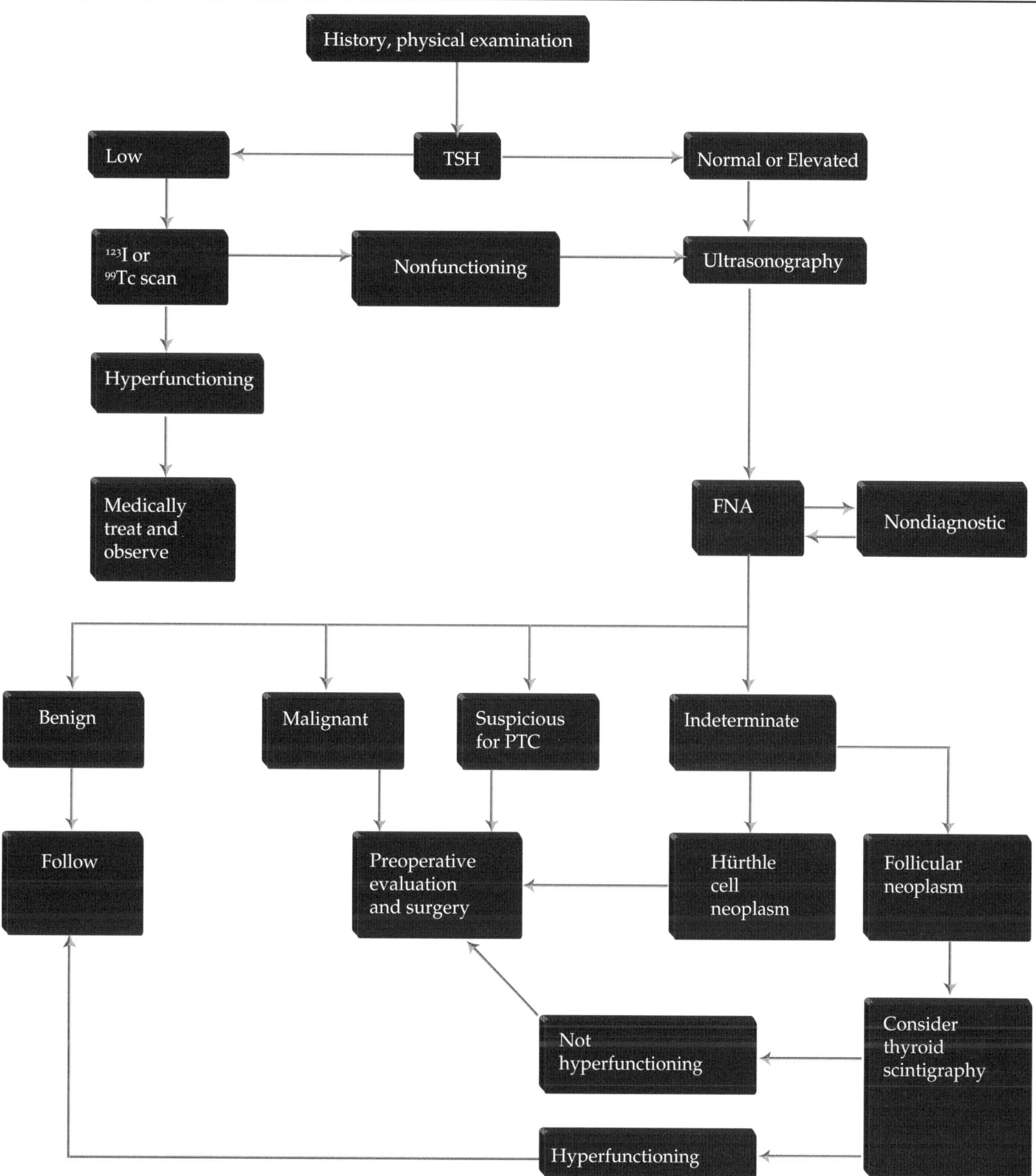

Figure 2 **Management algorithm for thyroid nodules. FNA = fine-needle aspiration; PTC = papillary thyroid cancer; TSH = thyroid-stimulating hormone.**

ultrasonography, further investigation is usually warranted. This can include laboratory studies, further imaging, and cytologic assessment.[6]

A serum thyroid-stimulating hormone (TSH) level should be obtained on any patient with a palpable thyroid nodule or a nodule detected incidentally on imaging. If the serum TSH is low, then radionuclide scanning should be performed. If the nodule is hyperfunctioning, then no further evaluation is needed as the risk of malignancy is low. Patients with a hyperfunctioning nodule, a depressed serum TSH, and clinical symptoms may then be evaluated and medically treated for hyperthyroidism. Additionally, an elevated TSH is associated with a small increased risk of malignancy.

Ultrasonography should be performed for any patient with a palpable thyroid nodule as part of the initial evaluation. Sonography can indicate the size of the nodule and its position within the gland; it can identify features that suggest a benign or malignant nodule. A thorough ultrasound examination may also help the practitioner identify suspicious cervical adenopathy, additional nodules not palpated on examination, or other abnormalities. Findings of microcalcifications, irregular margins, and increased vascularity are suggestive of papillary thyroid cancer. Follicular cancers are often iso- or hyperechoic with a peripheral "halo" of decreased echogenicity.

FNA is recommended for the majority of thyroid nodules detected either by palpation or imaging. Table 3 outlines the current recommendations for FNA based on clinical history, size of the nodule, and imaging characteristics. FNA is not routinely recommended for nodules smaller than 1 cm; however, in patients with a higher risk of malignancy, including those with a family history of thyroid cancer or a history of radiation exposure in childhood or adolescence, FNA of a smaller nodule may be indicated. FNA can be performed either by palpation or ultrasound guidance. The latter is recommended for most nodules as it decreases the occurrence of nondiagnostic results but especially for those that are predominantly cystic, located posteriorly in the thyroid lobe, or nonpalpable. FNA is useful in the evaluation of thyroid nodules in children.[7]

Interpretation of FNA Cytology

FNA results can be classified as nondiagnostic, benign, malignant, suspicious for malignancy, or indeterminate.[8] Nearly 20% of FNAs are nondiagnostic; repeated FNA under ultrasound guidance can lead to a diagnostic cytology specimen in 50 to 75% of these nodules. For nodules that repeatedly yield nondiagnostic samples, surgical excision should be considered, particularly if the nodule is solid rather than cystic. For nodules with FNA findings diagnostic of malignancy, surgical resection is recommended. For benign nodules, no further investigation is required. However, if a benign nodule continues to grow, as demonstrated on follow-up ultrasonography, repeated biopsy should be performed, and a diagnostic thyroid lobectomy may be indicated.

Nodules with indeterminate cytology are typically reported as "cellular atypia," "Hürthle cell neoplasm," or "follicular neoplasm" and are an area of significant debate in terms of management. Many molecular markers and imaging studies have been evaluated for a possible role in improving the diagnostic accuracy in patients with these lesions. Most recently, the role of ^{18}FDG-PET has been explored as a promising method of determining malignant potential; however, the findings of most studies of FDG-PET utility show low specificity. Currently, for indeterminate lesions interpreted as "suspicious for papillary carcinoma" or "Hürthle cell neoplasm," surgical resection is recommended.[6] For the remainder of indeterminate lesions, a radionuclide study can be considered; if the nodule is not hyperfunctioning, then surgical resection may be warranted.

Table 3 Thyroid Nodule Assessment

Nodule Sonographic or Clinical Features	Recommended Size Threshold for FNA
High-risk history	
Nodule with suspicious sonographic features	> 5 mm
Nodule without suspicious sonographic features	> 5 mm
Abnormal cervical lymph nodes	All
Microcalcifications present in nodule	≥ 1 cm
Solid nodule	
And hypoechoic	> 1 cm
And iso- or hyperechoic	≥ 1.5 cm
Mixed cystic-solid nodule	
With any suspicious sonographic features	≥ 1.5–2.0 cm
Without any suspicious sonographic features	≥ 2.0 cm
Purely cystic nodule	FNA not indicated
Spongiform nodule	≥ 2.0 cm

Adapted from Cooper DS et al.[6]
FNA = fine-needle aspiration.

Thyroid Cancer: Overview of Surgical and Medical Management

The procedure of choice for a papillary thyroid cancer that is small (< 1 cm in diameter) and confined to the gland, as well as for minimally invasive follicular thyroid cancer, is a thyroid lobectomy. For the remainder of papillary or follicular cancers, as well as Hürthle cell and medullary thyroid cancer, total or near-total thyroidectomy is preferable. Patients with thyroid nodules and a history of radiation exposure should also undergo a total thyroidectomy as approximately 40% of these patients have at least one additional focus of papillary thyroid cancer. Total thyroidectomy also allows the use of ^{131}I scanning to monitor for recurrence and increases the sensitivity of thyroglobulin and calcitonin assays in posttreatment surveillance. New information regarding the molecular basis for thyroid neoplasia is gradually informing the individualized care for patients with these tumors.[9]

Patients with medullary thyroid cancer should additionally undergo bilateral central neck dissection, screening for *ret* proto-oncogene mutations, and screening for pheochromocytoma.[10] Anaplastic thyroid cancer is best treated with a combination of chemotherapy and radiation therapy, in conjunction with removal of as much of the neoplasm as can be safely excised. Most patients with thyroid lymphomas should receive chemotherapy, radiation therapy, or a combination of the two.

NEOPLASTIC MASSES

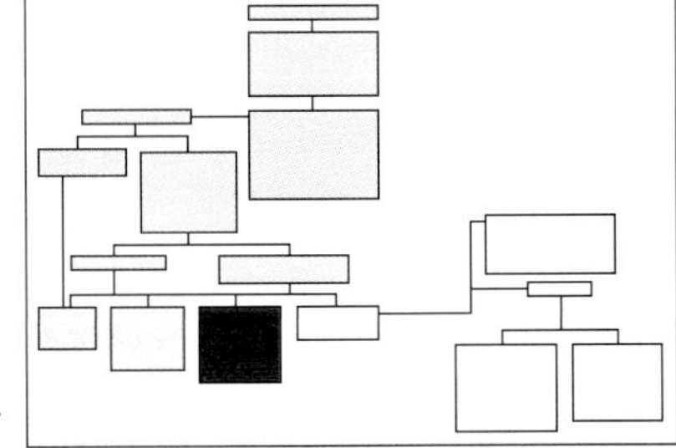

Salivary Gland Tumor

Salivary gland neoplasms usually present as an enlarging solid mass in front of and below the ear, at the angle of the mandible, or in the submandibular triangle. Benign salivary gland lesions are often asymptomatic; malignant ones are often associated with seventh cranial nerve symptoms or skin fixation. Diagnostic imaging studies (CT or MRI) indicate whether the mass is salivary in origin but do not help classify it histologically. The diagnostic test of preference is open biopsy in the form of complete submandibular gland removal or superficial parotidectomy.

With any mass in or around the ear, one should be prepared to remove the superficial lobes of the parotid, the deep lobes, or both and to perform a careful facial nerve dissection. Any less complete approach reduces the chances of a cure: there is a high risk of implantation and seeding of malignant tumors. Benign mixed tumors make up two thirds of all salivary tumors; these must also be completely removed because recurrence is common after incomplete resection. Malignant lesions may require additional therapy with radiation or chemotherapy.[11]

Soft Tissue Tumor (Lipoma, Sebaceous Cyst)

Superficial intracutaneous or subcutaneous masses may be sebaceous (or epidermal inclusion) cysts or lipomas. Final diagnosis and treatment usually involve simple surgical excision, often done as an office procedure with local anesthesia.

Chemodectoma (Carotid Body Tumor)

Carotid body tumors belong to a group of tumors known as chemodectomas (or, alternatively, as glomus tumors or nonchromaffin paragangliomas), which derive from the chemoreceptive tissue of the head and neck. Chemodectomas most often arise from the tympanic bodies in the middle ear, the glomus jugulare at the skull base, the vagal body near the skull base along the inferior ganglion of the vagus, and the carotid body at the carotid bifurcation. They are sometimes familial and can occur bilaterally.[12]

A carotid body tumor presents as a firm, round, slowly growing mass at the carotid bifurcation. Occasionally, a bruit is present. The tumor cannot be separated from the carotid artery by palpation and can usually be moved laterally and medially but not in a cephalocaudal plane. The differential diagnosis includes a carotid aneurysm, a branchial cleft cyst, a neurogenic tumor, and nodal metastases fixed to the carotid sheath. The diagnosis is made by CT or arteriography, which demonstrate a characteristic highly vascular mass at the carotid bifurcation. Neurofibromas tend to displace, encircle, or compress a portion of the carotid artery system, events that are readily demonstrated by carotid angiography.

Biopsy should be avoided. Chemodectomas are sometimes malignant and should therefore be removed in most cases to prevent subsequent growth and pressure symptoms. Fortunately, even malignant chemodectomas are usually low grade; long-term results after removal are generally excellent. Vascular surgical experience is desirable in that the tumors are very vascular and intimately involve the carotid artery, and clamping of the carotid artery may result in a stroke. Expectant treatment may be indicated in older or debilitated individuals. Radiotherapy may be helpful for patients with unresectable tumors.

Neurogenic Tumor (Neurofibroma, Neurilemmoma)

The most common neurogenic tumors in the head and neck, neurilemmomas (schwannomas) and neurofibromas, arise from the neurilemma and usually present as painless, slowly growing masses in the lateral neck. Neurilemmomas can be differentiated from neurofibromas only by means of histologic examination.

Given the potential these tumors possess for malignant degeneration and slow but progressive growth, surgical resection is indicated. This may include resection of the involved nerves, particularly with neurofibromas, which tend to be more invasive and less encapsulated than neurilemmomas.

Laryngeal Tumor

In rare cases, a chondroma may arise from the thyroid cartilage or the cricoid cartilage. It is firmly fixed to the cartilage and may present as a mass in the neck or as the cause of a progressively compromised airway. Surgical excision is indicated.

Lymphoma

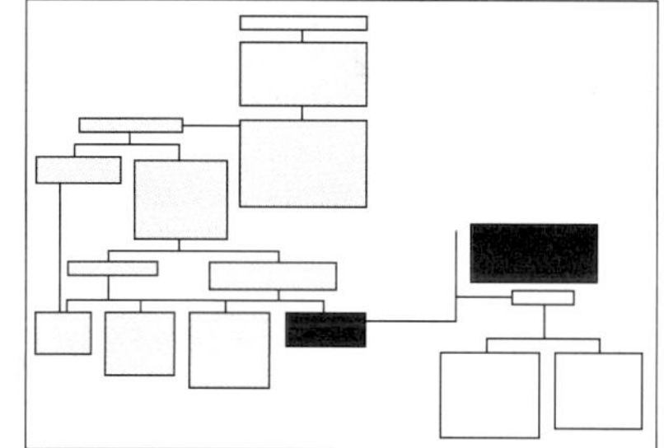

Cervical adenopathy is one of the most common presenting symptoms in patients with Hodgkin and non-Hodgkin lymphoma. The nodes tend to be softer, smoother, more elastic, and more mobile than nodes containing metastatic carcinoma. Rapid growth is common, particularly in non-Hodgkin lymphoma. Involvement of extranodal sites, particularly Waldeyer tonsillar ring, often occurs in patients with non-Hodgkin lymphoma; enlargement of these sites may provide a clue to the diagnosis. The diagnosis is usually suggested by FNA and then confirmed via excisional biopsy of an intact lymph node. Lymphoma is typically treated by radiation therapy, chemotherapy, or both depending on the disease's pathologic type and clinical stage.

Upper Aerodigestive Tract Cancer

Many localized tumors of the aerodigestive tract can be cured with surgery alone. Treatment of locally advanced squamous cell cancers, however, often necessitates a multimodality approach.[13] Such an approach has traditionally consisted of surgery followed by radiation therapy, but recent data indicate that concurrent chemoradiotherapy has an additional beneficial effect as an adjuvant measure.[14,15]

Chemoradiotherapy is also employed for unresectable disease, and induction chemotherapy may be administered preoperatively to reduce operative morbidity. Among the chemotherapeutic agents active against head and neck squamous cell cancers are the taxanes, cisplatin and fluorouracil, and various newer targeted agents (e.g., epidermal growth factor receptor antagonists).

Treatment planning for such patients depends on the tumor's location and stage, the patient's age, and the presence and severity of associated medical conditions, among other factors.[16] Consultation with a specialist in this field is generally required. Therefore, cancers involving the nose, the paranasal sinuses, the nasopharynx, the floor of the mouth, the tongue, the palate, the tonsils, the piriform sinus, the hypopharynx, or the larynx are best managed by an experienced head and neck oncologic surgeon in conjunction with a radiation therapist and a medical oncologist.

Soft Tissue Sarcoma

Malignant sarcomas are not common in the head and neck. The sarcomas most frequently encountered include rhabdomyosarcoma in children, fibrosarcoma, liposarcoma, osteogenic sarcoma (which usually arises in young adults), and chondrosarcoma. The most common head and neck sarcoma, however, is malignant fibrous histiocytoma (MFH). MFH occurs most frequently in the elderly and extremely rarely in children, but it can arise at any age. It is often difficult to differentiate from other entities (e.g., fibrosarcoma). MFH can occur in the soft tissues of the neck or involve the bone of the maxilla or the mandible. The preferred treatment is wide surgical resection; adjuvant radiation therapy and chemotherapy are being studied in clinical trials.

Rhabdomyosarcoma, usually of the embryonic form, is the most common form of sarcoma in children. It generally occurs near the orbit, the nasopharynx, or the paranasal sinuses. The diagnosis is confirmed by biopsy. A thorough search for distal metastases is important before treatment—consisting of a combination of surgical resection, radiation therapy, and chemotherapy—is begun.

Skin Cancer

Basal cell carcinomas are the most common of the skin malignancies. These lesions arise most commonly in areas that have been extensively exposed to sunlight (e.g., the nose, the forehead, the cheeks, and the ears). Treatment consists of local resection with adequate clear margins. Metastases are rare, and the prognosis is excellent. Inadequately excised and neglected basal cell carcinomas may ultimately spread to regional lymph nodes and can cause extensive local destruction of soft tissue and bone. For example, basal cell carcinoma of the medial canthus may invade the orbit, the ethmoid sinus, and even the brain. Periauricular basal cell carcinoma can spread across the cartilage of the ear canal or into the parotid gland. In such cases of locally advanced basal cell cancer or nodal involvement with tumor, patients may require more extensive surgical treatment (i.e., modified neck dissection). Postoperative radiation therapy is often administered to optimize local control and reduce the risk of recurrence.

Squamous cell carcinoma also arises in areas associated with extensive sunlight exposure; the lower lip and the pinna are the most common sites. Unlike basal cell carcinoma, however, squamous cell carcinoma tends to metastasize to both regional and distant sites. This tumor must also be excised with an adequate margin.

Melanoma is primarily classified on the basis of depth of invasion (as quantified by Clark level or Breslow thickness), location, and histologic subtype, although the prognosis is closely related to the thickness of the tumor [*see* Metastatic Disease, Metastatic Melanoma, *below*]. In addition to the typical pigmented, irregularly shaped skin lesions, malignant melanoma can also arise on the mucous membranes of the nose or the throat, on the hard palate, or on the buccal mucosa. The treatment of choice is wide surgical resection. Radiation therapy, chemotherapy, and immunotherapy may be useful in specific situations.

METASTATIC DISEASE

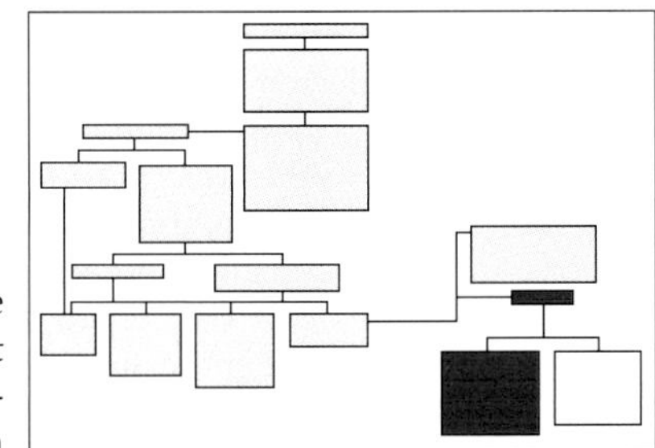

Metastatic Squamous Cell Carcinoma

The basic principle in the management of metastatic squamous cell carcinoma is wide excision of the primary tumor and treatment of all regional lymph node groups at highest risk for metastases by means of surgery or radiation therapy, depending on the clinical circumstances. Selective lymph node dissection can be performed along with wide excision of the primary tumor at the time of the initial operation. Sentinel lymph node (SLN) biopsy may provide a low morbidity staging opportunity for this as in other diseases.[17] For example, carcinomas of the oral cavity are treated with supraomohyoid neck dissection, and carcinomas of the oropharynx, the hypopharynx, and the larynx are treated with lateral neck dissection. If extranodal extension or the presence of multiple levels of positive nodes is confirmed by the pathologic findings, the patient should receive adjuvant bilateral neck radiation therapy for 4 to 6 weeks after operation.

Metastatic Adenocarcinoma

Adenocarcinoma in a cervical node most frequently represents a metastasis from the thyroid gland, the salivary glands, or the gastrointestinal (GI) tract. The primary tumor must therefore be sought through endoscopic and radiologic study of the bronchopulmonary tract, the GI tract, the genitourinary tract, the salivary glands, and the thyroid gland. Other possible primary sites include breast and pelvic tumors in women and prostate cancer in men.

If the primary site is controlled and the tumor is potentially curable, or if the primary site is not found and the neck disease is the only established site of malignancy, neck dissection is the appropriate treatment. Postoperative adjuvant radiation may also be considered. If the patient has thyroid cancer and palpable nodes, lateral neck dissection (levels II to V) and central neck dissection (level VI) are recommended.

Overall survival is low—about 20% at 2 years and 9% at 5 years—except for patients with papillary or follicular thyroid cancer, who have a good prognosis. Two factors associated with a better prognosis are unilateral neck involvement and limitation of disease to lymph nodes above the cricoid cartilage.

Metastatic Melanoma

If the patient has a thin melanoma (Breslow thickness < 1 mm; Clark level I, II, or III), full-thickness excision with 1 cm margins is adequate treatment for the primary site.

Patients with intermediate-thickness melanomas (Breslow thickness 1 to 4 mm; Clark level IV) should have a full-thickness excision with at least a 1.5 cm margin. These patients also have a definable risk of lymph node spread and thus should be concurrently staged with lymphatic mapping and SLN biopsy. All patients with intermediate-thickness melanomas and positive SLNs and all melanoma patients with palpable lymph nodes should undergo complete staging with full-body CT/PET scans. If no other disease is found, modified neck dissection should be performed to obtain optimal local disease control. Because these tumors may metastasize to nodes in the parotid region, superficial parotidectomy is often included in the neck dissection, particularly in the case of melanoma located on the upper face or the anterior scalp. Consultation with a medical oncologist is indicated for all patients with intermediate-thickness or thick (Breslow thickness > 4 mm; Clark level V) melanomas; immunotherapy or chemotherapy may be considered. Radiation therapy is often considered in patients with extensive local or nodal disease following adequate surgical resection.

Metastasis from an Unknown Primary Malignancy

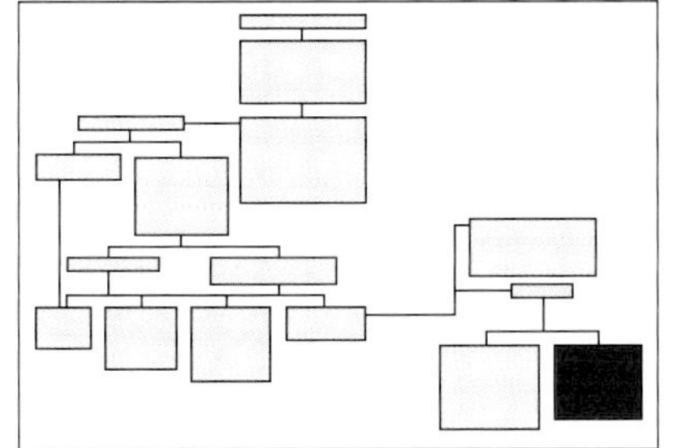

Management of patients with an unknown primary malignancy is challenging for the surgeon. It is helpful to know that when cervical lymph nodes are found to contain metastatic squamous cell carcinoma, the primary tumor is in the head and neck about 90% of the time. Typically, such patients are found to have squamous cell carcinoma on the basis of FNA of an abnormal cervical lymph node; this finding calls for an exhaustive review of systems and a detailed physical examination of the head and neck.

If no primary tumor is identified, the patient should undergo endoscopic evaluation of the nasopharynx, the hypopharynx, the esophagus, the larynx, and the tracheobronchial tree under general anesthesia. Biopsies of the nasopharynx, the tonsils, and the hypopharynx often identify the site of origin (although there is some debate on this point). If the biopsies do not reveal a primary source of cancer, the preferred treatment is unilateral neck dissection, followed by radiation therapy directed toward the neck, the entire pharynx, and the nasopharynx. In 15 to 20% of cases, the primary cancer is ultimately detected. Overall 5-year survival in such cases ranges from 25 to 50%.

If a malignant melanoma is found in a cervical lymph node but no primary tumor is evident, the patient should be asked about previous skin lesions, and a thorough repeat head and neck examination should be done, with particular attention to the scalp, the nose, the oral cavities, and the sinuses. An ophthalmologic examination is also required. If physical examination and radiographic studies find no evidence of metastases, modified neck dissection should be performed on the involved side.

Metastatic adenocarcinoma in a cervical lymph node with no known primary tumor is discussed elsewhere [*see* Metastatic Adenocarcinoma, *above*]. The most common primary sites in the head and neck are the salivary glands and the thyroid gland. The possibility of an isolated metastasis from the breast, the GI tract, or the genitourinary tract must also be rigorously investigated. If no primary site is identified, the patient should be considered for protocol-based chemotherapy and radiation therapy, directed according to what the primary site is most likely to be in that patient.

CONGENITAL NECK MASS

Thyroglossal Duct Cyst

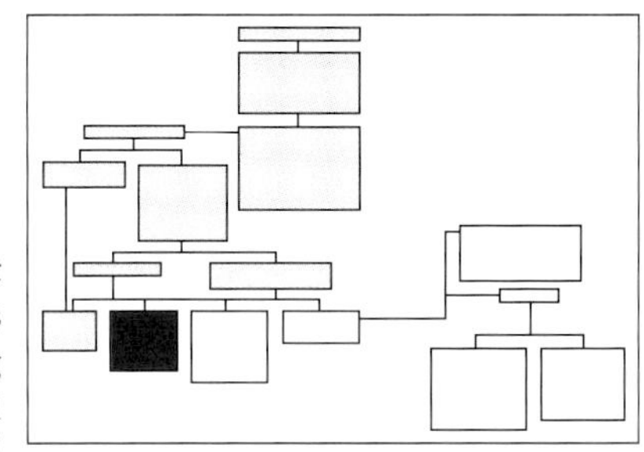

Thyroglossal duct cysts are remnants of the tract along which the thyroid gland descended into the neck from the foramen cecum [*see Figure 3*]. They account for about 70% of all congenital abnormalities of the neck. Thyroglossal duct cysts may be found in patients of any age but are most common in the first decade of life. They may present as a lone cyst, a cyst with a sinus tract, or a solid core of thyroid tissue. They may be so small as to be barely perceptible, as large as a grapefruit, or anything in between. Thyroglossal duct cysts are almost always found in the midline, at or below the level of the hyoid bone; however, they may be situated anywhere from the base of the

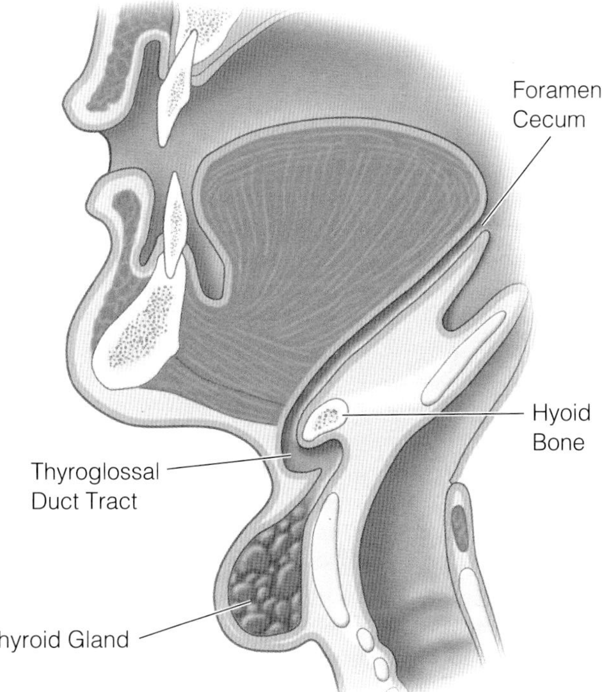

Figure 3 **The course of the thyroglossal duct from the foramen cecum to the pyramidal lobe of the thyroid gland. The operative treatment of thyroglossal duct abnormalities includes removal of the central portion of the hyoid bone to ensure complete tract removal, thus limiting the risk of recurrence.**

tongue to the suprasternal notch. They occasionally present slightly lateral to the midline and are sometimes associated with an external fistula to the skin of the anterior neck. They are often ballotable and can usually be moved slightly from side to side but not up or down; however, they do move up and down when patients swallow or protrude the tongue.

Thyroglossal duct cysts must be differentiated from dermoid cysts, lymphadenopathy in the anterior jugular chain, and cutaneous lesions (e.g., lipomas and sebaceous cysts). Operative treatment is almost always required, not only because of cosmetic considerations but also because of the high incidence of recurrent infection, including abscess formation. About 1% of thyroglossal duct cysts contain cancer; papillary cancer is the neoplasm most commonly encountered, followed by squamous cell carcinoma. About 25% of patients with papillary thyroid cancer in thyroglossal duct cysts have papillary thyroid cancer in other parts of the thyroid gland as well. About 10% have nodal metastases, which in some cases are bilateral.

Branchial Cleft Cyst

Branchial cleft cysts are vestigial remnants of the fetal branchial apparatus from which all neck structures are derived. Early in embryonic development, there are five branchial arches and four grooves (or clefts) between them. The internal tract or opening of a branchial cleft cyst is situated at the embryologic derivative of the corresponding pharyngeal groove, such as the tonsil (second arch) or the piriform sinus (third and fourth arches). The second arch is the most common area of origin for such cysts. The position of the cyst tract is also determined by the embryologic relation of its arch to the derivatives of the arches on either side of it.

The majority of branchial cleft cysts (those that develop from the second, third, and fourth arches) tend to present as a bulge along the anterior border of the sternocleidomastoid muscle, with or without a sinus tract. Branchial cleft cysts may become symptomatic at any age, but most are diagnosed in the first two decades of life. They often present as a smooth, painless, slowly enlarging mass in the lateral neck. Frequently, there is a history of fluctuating size and intermittent tenderness. The diagnosis is more obvious when there is an external fistulous tract and there is a history of intermittent discharge. Infection of the cyst may be the reason for the first symptoms.

Treatment consists of complete surgical removal of the cyst and the sinus tract. Any infection or inflammation should be treated and allowed to resolve before the cyst and the tract are removed.

Cystic Hygroma (Lymphangioma)

A cystic hygroma is a lymphangioma that arises from lymph channels in the neck. Almost always, this condition is first noted by the second year of life; on rare occasions, it is first diagnosed in adulthood. A cystic hygroma may present as a relatively simple thin-walled cyst in the floor of the mouth or may involve all the tissues from the floor of the mouth to the mediastinum. About 80% of the time, there is only a painless cyst in the posterior cervical triangle or in the supraclavicular area. A cystic hygroma can also occur, however, at the root of the neck, in the angle of the jaw (where it may involve the parotid gland), and in the midline (where it may involve the tongue, the floor of the mouth, or the larynx).

The typical clinical picture is of a diffuse, soft, doughy, irregular mass that is readily transilluminated. Cystic hygromas look and feel somewhat like lipomas but have less well-defined margins. Aspiration of a cystic hygroma yields straw-colored fluid. They may be confused with angiomas (which are compressible), pneumatoceles from the apex of the lung, or aneurysms. They can be distinguished from vascular lesions by arteriography. On occasion, a cystic hygroma grows suddenly as a result of an upper respiratory tract infection, infection of the hygroma itself, or hemorrhage into the tissues. If the mass becomes large enough, it can compress the trachea or hinder swallowing.

In the absence of pressure symptoms (i.e., obstruction of the airway or interference with swallowing) or gross deformity, cystic hygromas may be treated expectantly. They tend to regress spontaneously; if they do not, complete surgical excision is indicated. Excision can be difficult because of the numerous satellite extensions that often surround the main mass and because of the association of the tumor with vital structures such as the cranial nerves. Recurrences are common; staged resections for complete excision are often necessary.

Vascular Malformation (Hemangioma)

Hemangiomas are usually considered congenital because they either are present at birth or appear within the first year of life. A number of characteristic findings—bluish-purple coloration, increased warmth, compressibility followed by refilling, bruit, and thrill—distinguish them from other head and neck masses. Angiography is diagnostic but is rarely indicated.

Given that most of these congenital lesions resolve spontaneously, the treatment approach of choice is observation alone unless there is rapid growth, thrombocytopenia, or involvement of vital structures.

Financial Disclosures: None Reported

References

1. Tandon S, Shahab R, Benton JI, et al. Fine-needle aspiration cytology in a regional head and neck cancer center: comparison with a systematic review and meta-analysis. Head Neck 2008;30:1246–52.
2. de Bree R, Castelijns JA, Hoekstra OS, Leemans CR. Advances in imaging in the work-up of head and neck cancer patients. Oral Oncol 2009;45:930–5.
3. Liu T, Xu W, Yan W-L, et al. FDG-PET, CT, MRI for diagnosis of local residual or recurrent nasopharyngeal carcinoma, which one is the best? A systematic review. Radiother Oncol 2007;85:327–35.
4. Robbins KT, Shaha AR, Medina JE, et al. Consensus statement on the classification and terminology of neck dissection. Arch Otolaryngol Head Neck Surg 2008;134:536–8.
5. Hegedus L. Clinical practice. The thyroid nodule. N Engl J Med 2004;351:1764–71.
6. Cooper DS, Doherty GM, Haugen BR, et al. Revised American Thyroid Association management guidelines for

patients with thyroid nodules and differentiated thyroid cancer. Thyroid 2009;19:1167–214.

7. Stevens C, Lee JKP, Sadatsafavi M, Blair GK. Pediatric thyroid fine-needle aspiration cytology: a meta-analysis. J Pediatr Surg 2009;44:2184–91.
8. Baloch ZW, LiVolsi VA, Asa SL, et al. Diagnostic terminology and morphologic criteria for cytologic diagnosis of thyroid lesions: a synopsis of the National Cancer Institute Thyroid Fine-Needle Aspiration State of the Science Conference. Diagn Cytopathol 2008;36:425–37.
9. Melck AL, Yip L, Carty SE. The utility of BRAF testing in the management of papillary thyroid cancer. Oncologist 2010;15:1285–93.
10. Wu LS, Roman SA, Sosa JA. Medullary thyroid cancer: an update of new guidelines and recent developments. Curr Opin Oncol 2011;23:22–7.
11. Rizk S, Robert A, Vandenhooft A, et al. Activity of chemotherapy in the palliative treatment of salivary gland tumors: review of the literature. Eur Arch Otorhinolaryngol 2007; 264:587–94.
12. Dziegielewski PT, Knox A, Liu R, et al. Familial paraganglioma syndrome: applying genetic screening in otolaryngology. J Otolaryngol Head Neck Surg 2010;39:646–53.
13. National Comprehensive Cancer Network, Forastiere AA, Ang KK, et al. Head and neck cancers. J Natl Compr Cancer Netw 2008;6:646–95.
14. Adelstein DJ, Moon J, Hanna E, et al. Docetaxel, cisplatin, and fluorouracil induction chemotherapy followed by accelerated fractionation/concomitant boost radiation and concurrent cisplatin in patients with advanced squamous cell head and neck cancer: a Southwest Oncology Group phase II trial (S0216). Head Neck 2010;32:221–8.
15. Genden EM, Ferlito A, Rinaldo A, et al. Recent changes in the treatment of patients with advanced laryngeal cancer. Head Neck 2008;30:103–10.
16. Wolf GT. Routine computed tomography scanning for tumor staging in advanced laryngeal cancer: implications for treatment selection. J Clin Oncol 2010;28:2315–7.
17. Paleri V, Rees G, Arullendran P, et al. Sentinel node biopsy in squamous cell cancer of the oral cavity and oral pharynx: a diagnostic meta-analysis. Head Neck 2005;27:739–47.

Acknowledgment

Figures 1 and 3 Tom Moore

4 HEAD AND NECK DIAGNOSTIC PROCEDURES

*Donald J. Annino Jr, MD, DMD, and Laura A. Goguen, MD, FACS**

Head and neck diseases can be inflammatory, infectious, congenital, neoplastic, or traumatic. An accurate diagnosis is mandatory and is based on a detailed history and physical examination, as well as ancillary tests. After a detailed history, including the chief complaint, history of present illness, past medical history, current medications, allergies, social history including tobacco and ethanol use, and family history, is obtained, a physical examination should be done.

The physical examination of the head and neck is complicated by the close relationship of structures and the need to examine many of the structures through orifices. The entire mucosal surface of the head and neck needs be examined when evaluating for head and neck cancers. Once a detailed history and physical examination have been done, a differential diagnosis list is created. The correct diagnosis and treatment plan are arrived at with the use of diagnostic procedures including imaging and sampling of the tissue.

Anatomy

The regions of the head and neck are usually divided into the following areas: the ear, the nose and paranasal sinuses, the oral cavity, the pharynx, the larynx, the salivary glands, and the neck, including the thyroid [*see Figure 1*].

EAR

The ear is divided into three parts: the external, middle, and inner ear. The external ear is made of the pinna and external auditory canal. The pinna is the only part of the ear that grows after birth. It is composed of an irregular plate of fibrocartilage tightly covered by skin and a thin layer of subcutaneous tissue. The external auditory canal is a tortuous passage with an average length of 3.7 cm in an adult male. The canal has thicker skin overlying cartilage in the outer half. This skin also has hair and special glands that secrete cerumen. The inner portion of the canal is thin skin over bone. The tympanic membrane is the common wall between the external ear and the middle ear. It is semitranslucent, cone shaped, and concave laterally.

The middle ear is an air-filled chamber that has five bony walls. The sixth wall is the tympanic membrane. Within the middle ear are ossicles. It is connected to the nasopharynx by the eustachian tube. It runs downward and forward and is composed of a cartilaginous segment and a bony segment.

The inner ear is made up of a system of channels and chambers within the otic capsule. It has two parts anatomically and functionally: the vestibular labyrinth and the cochlear. The vestibular system is responsible for balance and the cochlear system for hearing.

Tumors of the ear may present with pain, discharge, decreased hearing, facial nerve involvement, and dizziness.

NOSE AND PARANASAL SINUSES

The external nose is made of two fused nasal bones and four alar cartilages. There are two nasal passages that are separated by a vertical septum composed of cartilage (anteroinferiorly) and bone (the thin perpendicular plate of the ethmoid bone and the vomer). The nose is lined with ciliated respiratory mucoperichondrium, which contains glands and mucus-secreting cells. The cribriform plate forms the roof of the nose, with the hard palate forming its floor. The lateral wall is a partition between the paranasal sinuses and the nasal passages. There are three turbinates on each lateral wall: superior, middle, and inferior. The inferior turbinate is the largest and most vascular. The turbinates divide the nasal passages vertically and create the superior, middle, and inferior meatuses.

There are four paranasal sinuses on each side. The frontal and sphenoid sinuses are midline and frequently are asymmetrical. The ethmoid and maxillary sinuses are placed laterally. The ethmoid sinus is considered the key sinus and can provide access to all the other sinuses [*see Figure 2*]. Its roof is the fovea ethmoidales, which, in conjunction with the cribriform plate, separates the anterior cranial vault from the nose. The sphenoid sinus is the most posterior sinus and has the internal carotid artery, optic nerve, second division of the trigeminal nerve, and vidian nerve all in close proximity.

The symptoms associated with nasal cavity tumors frequently do not occur early in the diseases because much of the nasal cavity and paranasal sinuses is air filled. This can also be a hard area to examine, and the symptoms are usually first attributed to more mundane conditions, such as allergies and sinusitis. The most common symptoms are facial pain, nasal obstruction, epistaxis, nasal discharge, decreased sense of smell, and changes to the orbit.

Oral Cavity

The limits of the oral cavity are the lips anteriorly and the anterior tonsil pillars and circumvallate papillae of the tongue posteriorly. The oral cavity is divided into the vestibules, which is the space between the teeth and cheek; the alveolar ridges, which are the teeth-bearing areas of the maxilla and mandible; the floor of the mouth; the retromolar trigone, which is the triangular area of gum and soft tissue immediately posterior to the lower molars; the buccal mucosa, which

* The authors and editors gratefully acknowledge the contributions of the previous authors, Adam S. Jacobson, MD, Mark L. Urken, MD, FACS, and Marita S. Teng, MD, to the development and writing of this chapter.

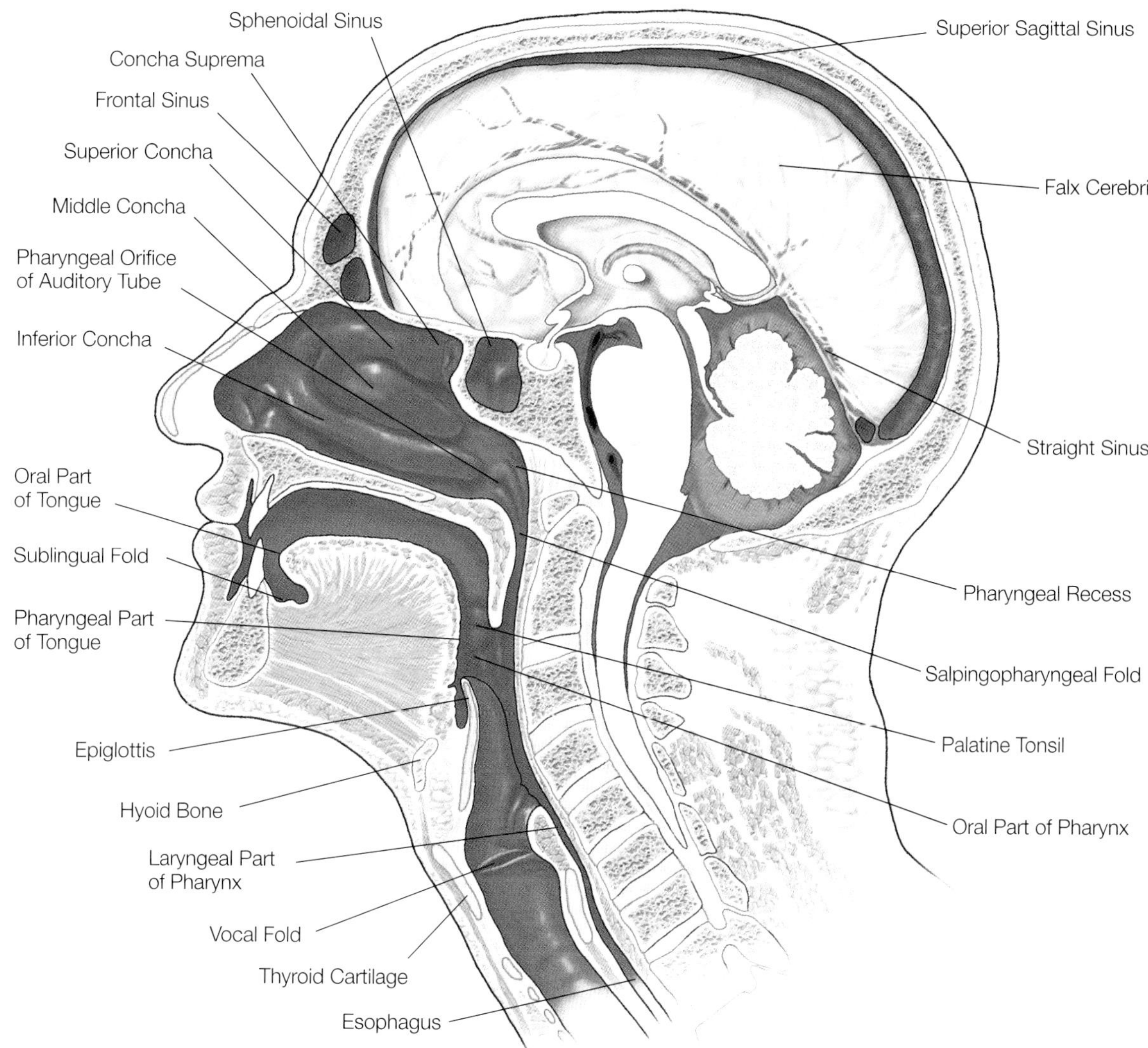

Figure 1 **The anatomic structures of the head and neck are shown.**

is the mucous membrane lining of the cheek; and the oral tongue, which is the anterior two thirds of the tongue. The posterior limit is the circumvallate papillae.

Salivary Glands

Salivary glands are subdivided into major and minor salivary glands. The major salivary glands consist of the parotid glands, submandibular glands, and sublingual glands. The parotid gland is the largest salivary gland. It is incompletely split by the facial nerve into deep and superficial lobes. The main duct runs horizontal to the zygoma on the lateral surface of the masseter and enters the oral cavity opposite the second maxillary molar. It has serous secretions with low mineral content. Approximately 80 to 85% of the neoplasms in the parotid are benign.

The submandibular gland is below the body of the mandible. It lies on the lateral surface of the mylohyoid muscle. The duct passes upward and medially to the anterior floor of the mouth. Its secretions are mixed serous and mucous, and it has a higher mineral content than the parotid gland. Neoplasms in the submandibular glands are more evenly split between malignant and benign.

The sublingual glands are located in the floor of the mouth and frequently have multiple ducts. The secretion is mucous.

Thousands of minor salivary glands are present throughout the oral cavity, pharynx, and epiglottis. Minor salivary gland neoplasms are usually malignant, with quoted rates around 75%.

Pharynx

The pharynx is an incomplete muscular tube from the base of the skull to the inlet of the esophagus. The pharynx is divided into three parts: the nasopharynx, oropharynx, and hypopharynx. The nasopharynx sits behind the nasal cavity, extending from the choanae to the inferior surface of the palate. Adenoid tissue and the eustachian tubes are present in the nasopharynx. Malignancies of the nasopharynx can present as nasal obstruction, epistaxis, tinnitus, headache, diminished hearing, and facial pain.

The oropharynx extends from the junction of the hard and soft palates and the circumvallate papillae to the valleculae. It includes the soft palate and uvula, base of the tongue, pharyngoepiglottic and glossoepiglottic folds, palatine arch

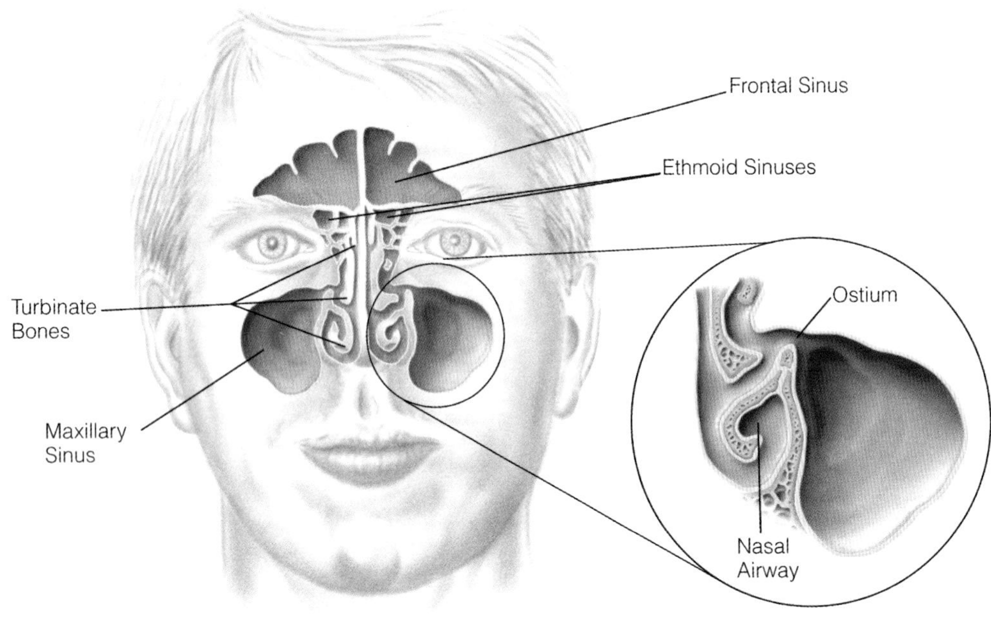

Figure 2 **The paranasal sinuses are shown.**

(which includes the tonsils and the tonsillar fossae and pillars), valleculae, and lateral and posterior oropharyngeal walls. Carcinomas of the oropharynx can present as pain, sore throat, dysphagia, and referred otalgia.

The hypopharynx extends from the superior border of the hyoid bone to the inferior border of the cricoid cartilage. It includes the piriform sinuses, hypopharyngeal walls, and postcricoid region (i.e., the area of the pharyngoesophageal junction). Malignancies of the hypopharynx can present as odynophagia, dysphagia, hoarseness, referred otalgia, and excessive salivation.

LARYNX

The larynx is subdivided into the supraglottis, glottis, and subglottis. It consists of a framework of cartilages that are held together by extrinsic and intrinsic musculature and lined with a mucous membrane that is topographically arranged into two characteristic folds (the false and true vocal cords). The larynx has the following basic functions: (1) to protect the lower airway; (2) to conduct air to the lungs; and (3) to allow vocalization. Neoplasms of the larynx can present as hoarseness, dyspnea, stridor, hemoptysis, odynophagia, dysphagia, and otalgia.

Supraglottis

The supraglottis extends from the tip of the epiglottis to the junction between respiratory and squamous epithelium on the floor of the ventricle (the space between the false and true cords). Carcinomas of the supraglottis can present as sore throat, odynophagia, dysphagia, and otalgia.

Glottis

The space between the free margin of the true vocal cords is the glottis. This structure is bounded by the anterior commissure, true vocal cords, and posterior commissure. The most common symptom of carcinoma of the glottis is hoarseness.

Subglottis

The subglottis extends from the junction of squamous and respiratory epithelium on the undersurface of the true vocal cords (approximately 5 to 10 mm below the true vocal cords) to the inferior edge of the cricoid cartilage. The cricoid is the only complete cartilaginous ring in the airway; therefore, it is the only rigid area in the respiratory tree. The most common symptom of carcinoma of the subglottis is hoarseness.

NECK

The neck is divided into different compartments by fascia. The visceral compartment is in the midline and contains the larynx, pharynx, trachea, thyroid, parathyroid glands, recurrent laryngeal nerves, and cervical esophagus. The neurovascular compartment runs the entire length of the neck from the base of the skull to the esophageal inlet. It contains the carotid artery, internal jugular vein, vagus nerve, and jugular lymph nodes. There are two muscular compartments on each side of the neck. Neoplasms in the neck usually present as masses. Most commonly, they are painless. When malignant, they are usually metastastic from primary malignancies in the aerodigestive tract.

The thyroid gland performs a vital role in regulating metabolic function. It is susceptible to benign conditions (e.g., nodule, goiter, and cyst), inflammatory disease (e.g., thyroiditis), and malignancies. Additionally, congenital anomalies of the thyroid, such as a thyroglossal duct cyst, can present later in life. Thyroid lesions can present as pain, hoarseness, dyspnea, or dysphagia.

On the posterior aspect of the thyroid gland reside the four parathyroid glands. These glands play a vital role in maintaining calcium balance. Parathyroid adenomas and, rarely, carcinomas can develop.

Clinical Evaluation

The diagnostic approach to the upper aerodigestive tract begins with a thorough history, starting with a detailed evaluation of the chief complaint. Once a complete history of the chief complaint has been obtained, the physician should elicit a more comprehensive general medical history from the patient, including pertinent past medical history, past surgical history, medications, allergies, social history (tobacco, ethanol, and intravenous drug use), and family history.

The next step is to perform a comprehensive physical examination. This begins with a thorough inspection of the entire surface of the head and neck. The examination should proceed in an orderly fashion. The exact order is not important, but examiners should determine the order with which they are most comfortable and not deviate from that order. This way, they are unlikely to skip an anatomic area. The mucosal surfaces of the aerodigestive tract are inspected. Endoscopic evaluation of the upper aerodigestive tract is crucial in establishing a definitive diagnosis. The equipment used consists of both rigid and flexible laryngoscopes, bronchoscopes, and esophagoscopes. Many of these techniques can be performed in the office setting, providing the surgeon with an array of methods for gaining the information necessary for a working diagnosis and, in some cases, for performing a therapeutic intervention [*see Figure 3*]. Operative endoscopy is performed to obtain a definitive diagnosis, to stage tumors, and to rule out synchronous lesions. There is no substitute for a thorough examination and biopsy of a lesion with the patient under general anesthesia. Regardless of the endoscopic method used, an adequate biopsy specimen must be obtained for a histologic diagnosis.

An accurate history and a careful physical examination of the head and neck, including the mucosal surfaces, are the most important steps in evaluating a lesion in this part of the body; this clinical evaluation usually provides only a working diagnosis. The head and neck surgeon must then proceed in a stepwise fashion to further clarify the diagnosis and, in the case of a neoplasm, to perform an accurate staging.

Radiographic techniques allow the head and neck surgeon to visualize the mass and determine its characteristics (i.e., to differentiate between solid and cystic lesions), as well as its anatomic associations. Ultrasonography, magnetic resonance imaging (MRI), computed tomography (CT), and dual-modality positron emission tomography (PET)/CT each provide a unique view of the pathology in question and thereby help narrow the differential diagnosis. Acquisition of a tissue specimen for cytologic or histologic analysis, or both, is the next step. Fine-needle aspiration (FNA) is often used at this stage in the workup provided that the location of the mass lends itself to a safe procedure. If the lesion is located deep in the neck near vital structures, image-guided FNA can be attempted before resorting to an open biopsy. If the lesion is on a mucosal surface of the upper aerodigestive tract, an endoscopic biopsy is performed. Often panendoscopy is performed at this point to accurately map the lesion, obtain a tissue specimen, and, in patients with cancer, assess the rest of the upper aerodigestive tract for a synchronous primary tumor.

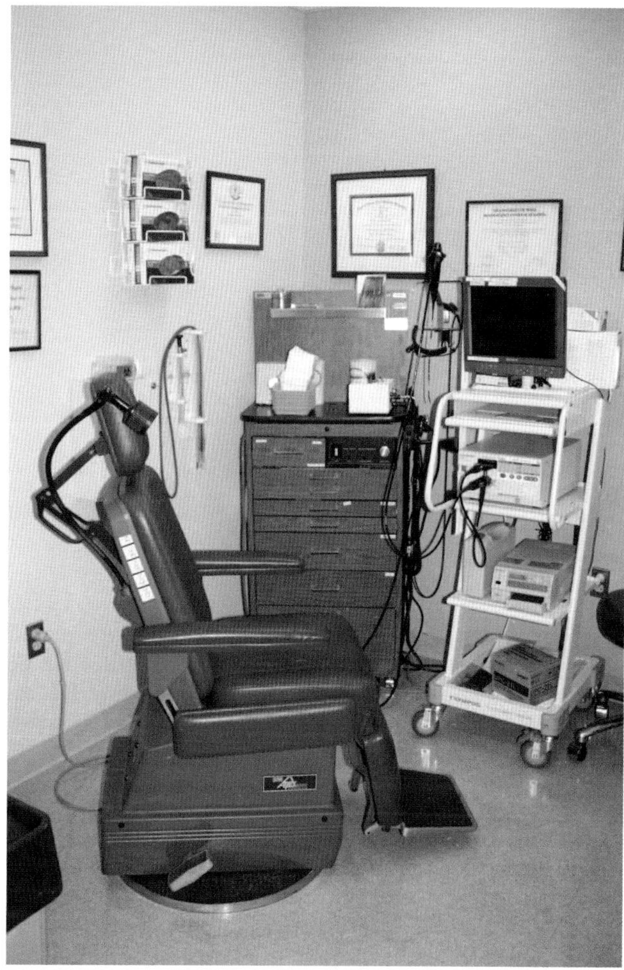

Figure 3 **Otolaryngology clinic office space with needed equipment, including an examination chair, a headlight, and a fiberoptic rhinolaryngoscope.**

After a histologic diagnosis has been made and correlated with imaging, the patient and the physician can have a comprehensive discussion of the pathology, the stage of the disease, and the selection of therapy.

NOSE

Anterior Rhinoscopy

Anterior rhinoscopy is the examination of the nasal cavities with the use of a nasal speculum [*see Figure 4*]. The speculum is used to spread the ala. When done, the speculum should touch only the parts that are covered with skin. Resting the speculum on the nasal mucosa is painful. Anterior rhinoscopy is best done before and after topical vasoconstriction of the nasal mucosa. A good coaxial light source is needed. The more anterior portions of the nasal cavity are most readily examined.

Posterior Rhinoscopy

Posterior rhinoscopy is used to examine the posterior portion of the nasal cavity and, more importantly, the

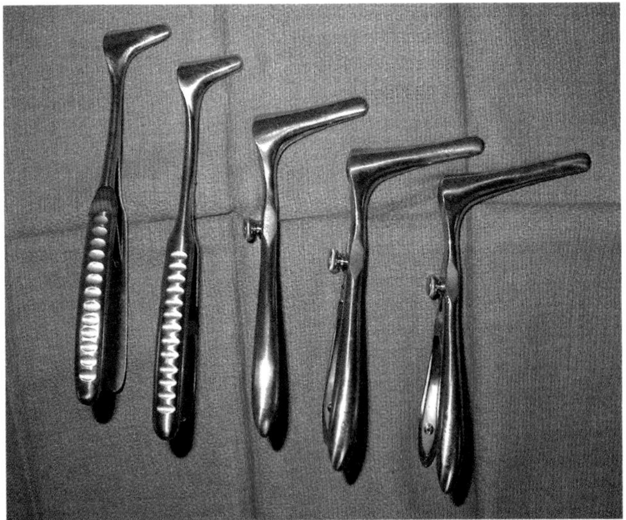

Figure 4 **Shown is an assortment of nasal specula.**

nasopharynx. It is done with a small-angled mirror placed posterior to the palate and uvula. The tongue should be depressed using a tongue blade with the other hand. This examination is limited at times by the patient's gag reflex and the presence of enlarged adenoids.

Rigid Nasal Endoscopy

Rigid nasal endoscopy offers a superior view of the nasal cavity. Topical anesthesia and vasoconstriction are required for a good examination. The image is magnified, and deeper structures are better visualized than with anterior rhinoscopy. The endoscopes come in a variety of lens angles (0, 30, and 90 degrees). This allows inspection of structures that may be blocked from direct line of site. A more complete examination of both the anterior and posterior nasal cavities and nasopharynx is obtained than with anterior and posterior rhinoscopy. Rigid nasal endoscopy has become the examination of choice for a through nasal evaluation.

LARYNX AND PHARYNX

Indirect Laryngoscopy

Indirect laryngoscopy is used to examine the larynx, oropharynx, and hypopharynx. It is done in the clinic under topical or no anesthesia. An angled mirror is used, and the patient needs to be sitting upright with the neck straight and the head thrust slightly forward [*see Figure 5*]. A bright coaxial light source is used. The patient should relax and breathe deeply and rhythmically, as if panting like a dog. The nondominant hand of the examiner grasps the patient's tongue with gauze. The mirror is warmed and placed gently against the soft palate. To optimize the view, the examiner should ask the patient to say "ee." This technique can be performed rapidly and is inexpensive.

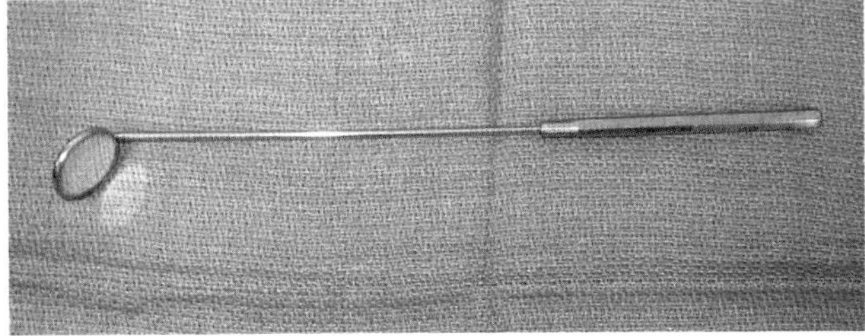

Figure 5 **Shown is a laryngeal mirror, which is used for indirect laryngoscopy.**

Flexible Laryngoscopy

Flexible laryngoscopy is also referred to as flexible rhinolaryngoscopy [*see Figure 6*]. It has become the most common way to examine the nasopharynx, oropharynx, hypopharynx, and larynx and is superior to indirect laryngoscopy. It allows better visualization and assessment of the structures, and since the tongue is not grasped, it allows better assessment of how structures function. The procedure is better tolerated by the patient, with less gagging. It has the disadvantage of requiring more expensive equipment than indirect laryngoscopy. Topical anesthesia is used. Most commonly, an anesthetic and a decongestant are sprayed into the nasal cavity prior to the procedure. The passage of the scope is best tolerated passing just inferior to the middle turbinate. If the patient has a deviated septum, the side with less obstruction is used.

Fiberoptic examinations in the clinic setting are not tolerated by all patients. Even if this examination is tolerated, an exact diagnosis frequently is not reached or a lesion is seen that cannot be biopsied in the clinic. It is recommended that the patients undergo an examination under anesthesia. This is done to look for an occult synchronous tumor and to more accurately examine and map the known tumor. The advantages of doing this under anesthesia are that it is better tolerated by the patient (gagging is eliminated) and allows deeper digital palpation and biopsies as needed. The disadvantage is that it requires general anesthesia and its possible complications as well as the complications of the procedure.

Direct Laryngoscopy

Direct laryngoscopy requires general anesthesia and therefore is done in the operating room. It is done with hollow, metal, rigid tubes [*see Figure 7*]. The laryngoscopes used by otolaryngologists differ from those used by anesthesiologists. They are straight and tubular and have distal lighting. There

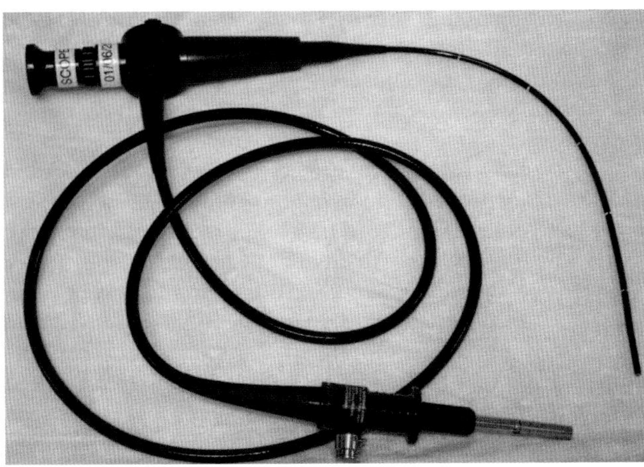

Figure 6 **A small-caliber flexible laryngoscope is used for rhinolaryngoscopy.**

a

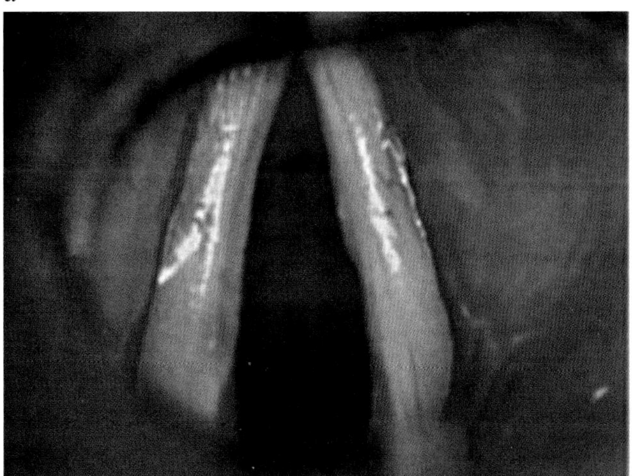

b

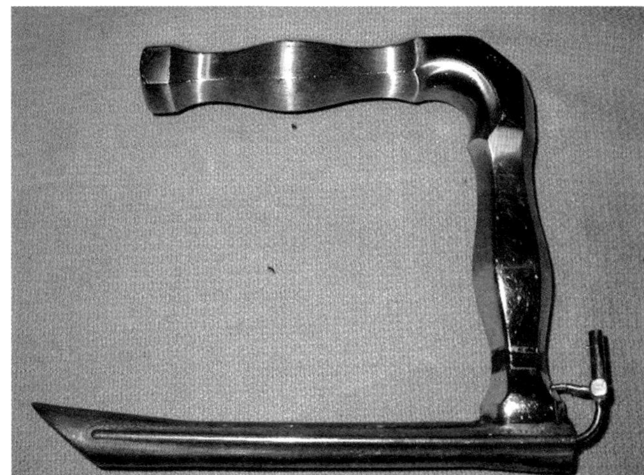

Figure 7 **Shown are (*a*) normal vocal folds directly visualized via (*b*) a rigid laryngoscope.**

are many different laryngoscopes. The sides of the laryngoscope hold surrounding soft tissue out of the way, allowing uninterrupted direct inspection of pharyngeal and laryngeal structures. The teeth are protected with a guard, and the structures in the oral cavity, pharynx, and larynx are all examined. It is best to become accustomed to doing this procedure in a specific order so that it becomes routine and lesions will not be missed. With the use of general anesthesia, palpation of the structures and a lesion can be done. The examination can be improved with suspension of the laryngoscope from a Mayo stand or the use of other suspension devices to allow the surgeon's hands to be free to perform procedures. Increased magnification is possible with the added use of a microscope. This is particularly useful when examining laryngeal lesions and is referred to as suspension microlaryngoscopy. A laser can also be used if needed.

ESOPHAGUS

Esophagoscopy plays an important role in the evaluation of patients with dysphagia, odynophagia, caustic ingestion, trauma, ingested foreign bodies, suspected anomalies, and upper aerodigestive tract malignancies. This procedure may be performed with either a flexible or a rigid scope.

Flexible Esophagoscopy

Flexible esophagoscopy is a diagnostic tool used to examine the esophagus and stomach. It is not well suited to visualizing the pharynx and is usually used in an outpatient setting with sedation and topical anesthesia. It is easier to perform than rigid esophagoscopy in patients who are elderly or have limited neck mobility, short, thick necks, and/or a limited mouth opening. The examination is usually done in the lateral decubitus position with the neck flexed. Air insufflation is important to completely visualize the mucosal surfaces. Tissue sampling is performed with a cup forceps through a working channel or by obtaining a brush biopsy. An endoscopic ultrasound probe can be passed to help define the extent of cancer of the esophagus. It is particularly useful to see the depth to which a tumor has invaded into the wall of the esophagus. If a lesion is found within the esophagus, its location is measured in centimeters from the teeth.

Rigid Esophagoscopy

Rigid esophagoscopy has been used for more than a century [*see Figure 8*]. It is used to diagnose cancer and remove foreign bodies. Unlike flexible esophagoscopy, it needs to be done under general anesthesia. The esophagoscope is a hollow metal tube of varying lengths and widths. The patient is placed supine and the maxillary teeth are protected with a mouth guard. The scope is passed transorally under direct visualization down the right side of the oral cavity and pharynx. If resistance is met, the scope should never be forced. There is a greater chance of perforation than with a flexible scope. As the scope is advanced, the lumen of the esophagus is kept in the center of the field of vision. The lumen has the appearance of a rosette. When advancing the scope, the left thumb is used. The right hand helps direct the scope and is used to pass instruments through its lumen. With rigid esophagoscopy, the removal of the scope is as important, if not more so, than inserting it. Removal allows better visualization of the mucosal surface as it slips over the tip of the instrument as it is removed.

TRACHEA AND LUNGS

Bronchoscopy is the technique of visualizing the trachea and lungs for both diagnostic and therapeutic reasons. Two basic forms of bronchoscopes are available: rigid and flexible. Each has it own advantages and disadvantages.

Rigid Bronchoscopy

The use of rigid bronchoscopy began in the 19th century with Killian. A rigid bronchoscope is a hollow, metal tube that is available in differing widths and lengths [*see Figure 9*].

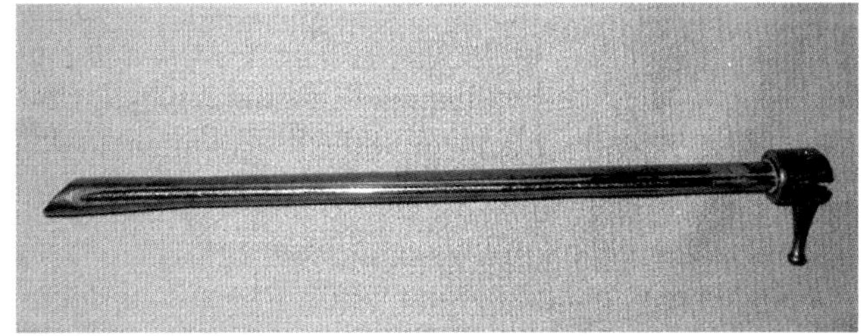

Figure 8 **Shown is a rigid esophagoscope.**

a
b

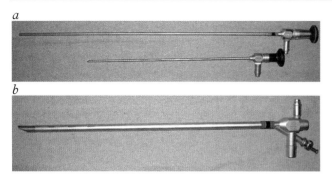

Figure 9 **(*a*) Rigid bronchoscopes incorporate stainless steel tubes of varying lengths and diameters. The beveled distal end of this Hopkins bronchoscope facilitates mobilization of the epiglottis during intubation; the side ports permit ventilation and use of suction catheters. (*b*) Illumination is provided by fiberoptic rods that are inserted into the bronchoscope.**

It is used to examine the trachea and lungs and requires general anesthesia. It is used to remove foreign bodies and to diagnose and biopsy tumors and is better than flexible bronchoscopes for evaluation of large-volume hemoptysis because it allows suctioning and instruments to be used together. The patient is under general anesthesia with the neck hyperextended.

The bronchoscope is passed into the trachea either directly or through a slotted laryngoscope. Once in the airway, ventilation is usually done through a port on the scope. Venturi jet ventilation is also possible through a rigid bronchoscope. The entire trachea and main bronchi of both lungs are easily examined. Bronchial lavage is also possible.

Flexible Bronchoscopy

In the 1970s, Ikeda introduced flexible bronchoscopy. It is usually performed under sedation and is more common than rigid bronchoscopy. The instrument is thinner and longer than a rigid scope. There is a working channel that allows passage of biopsy forceps and brushes and lavage.

Panendoscopy

When visualization of the entire mucosal surface of the aerodigestive tract is needed, then panendoscopy is performed. Panendoscopy is the term used when direct laryngoscopy (with or without microscopic assistance), esophagoscopy, and bronchoscopy are done in the same setting.

Biopsy

After a thorough physical examination and history, tissue sampling should be considered if a lesion has been present for more than 3 to 4 weeks. To make a diagnosis, an open biopsy is not immediately indicated. Other methods are available to help obtain tissue and make a diagnosis. However, a biopsy is not recommended until after the history and physical examination have been done and appropriate imaging has been obtained. Imaging is important prior to a biopsy because the biopsy may cause a distortion of the tissue, such as occurs when a hematoma develops.

When a biopsy is indicated to establish a diagnosis for a neck mass or lesion, the options include FNA, a core biopsy, and an open biopsy. FNA offers the advantages of being simple and quick and can be done in the clinic.

FNA is possible for lesions that can be palpated. A thin-gauge needle is passed into the lesion, allowing a small number of cells to be sampled. It is a safe procedure that can be done under local or no anesthesia. It has not been shown to have an increased risk of seeding of the tumor spread along its tract. However, there is a risk of sampling error. This occurs if the needle does not collect a representative sample from the lesion. In reality, the test has a high sensitivity and specificity. The benefits of FNA include the rapid availability of results.

To optimize sampling, FNA can be done under guidance with CT or ultrasonography. The use of imaging allows direct visualization of the biopsy and therefore increases the likelihood of obtaining an accurate sample.

The procedure is performed with a thin-gauge needle such as a 23-gauge needle. The needle is attached to a 20 mL syringe, which allows negative pressure to be generated [*see Figure 10*]. Multiple passes are made through the lesion prior to removing the needle. Just before the needle is removed from the skin, any negative pressure in the syringe is released and the needle is withdrawn. If a cyst is encountered, it should be completely evacuated and the fluid sent for cytologic analysis. Ideally, for FNA, there should be minimal to no fluid or tissue in the syringe. The cells should be in the needle. The sample is then placed on a glass slide. A smear is made by laying another glass slide on top of the drop of fluid and pulling the slides apart to spread the fluid. Fixative spray is then applied. Alternatively, wet smears are placed in 95% ethyl alcohol and treated with the Papanicolaou technique and stains.

When the lesion is not easily palpated or is close to a delicate structure, FNA may need to be done under imaging. The most common imaging techniques used are ultrasonography and CT. When ultrasonography is used, it allows real-time imaging of the needle's passage. This results in an accurate trajectory and avoidance of vital structures. It also provides an image of the mass, allowing its characterization as solid, cystic, or heterogeneous. With cystic or complex masses, the tip of the needle can be placed into the wall to increase specimen yield.

CT guidance also provides visualization of the needle as it is passed through the tissue and into the underlying mass. It has the disadvantage of requiring ionizing radiation.

Core Biopsy

A core biopsy is a percutaneous biopsy done with a large-bore needle. The needle has a cutting tip and a hollow core. The area is infiltrated with local anesthesia prior to the needle being passed. The procedure can be done with image

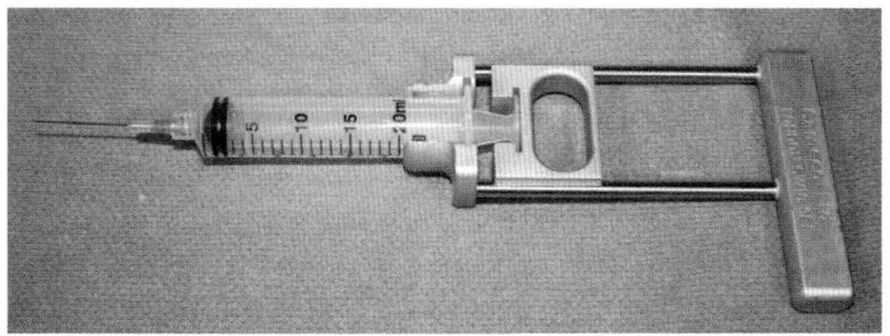

Figure 10 **A 20 mL syringe with a 23-gauge needle attached. The syringe is mounted in a handle to help allow creation of negative pressure.**

guidance if needed. It has the disadvantage of causing more bleeding and has an increased risk of seeding the tumor along the needle tract. For most lesions in the neck, FNA is usually the first choice.

Open Biopsy

An open biopsy is indicated when a needle biopsy or core biopsy is unable to give a diagnosis. This can be done in either the clinic or, more commonly, in the operating room. Whenever possible, open biopsy is usually done after other techniques have not yielded a diagnosis. It has the greatest chance of seeding the tumor along the path of the biopsy.

Imaging

Imaging studies are important in the workup of patients with head and neck complaints. This is true because direct visualization of many structures is difficult because most of the structures are examined through orifices. The most common studies ordered are a barium swallow, CT, MRI, ultrasonography, and dual-modality PET with CT.

ULTRASONOGRAPHY

Ultrasonography offers many advantages. It is inexpensive, offers real-time imaging, and is performed without radiation exposure. Ultrasonography is particularly helpful in differentiating between solid and cystic masses. It allows evaluation of surrounding structures such as blood vessels. It is an excellent tool to follow masses to assess for changes in the size or character of the structure. It can also be used to help guide cytologic evaluation with FNA.

Barium Swallow

A barium swallow is used to examine the esophagus and, to a lesser extent, the stomach. Barium sulfate is swallowed and is used to identify tumors, ulcers, diverticula, and strictures. It is done under fluoroscopy to be able to follow the dynamic passage of the barium through the esophagus and stomach.

Computed Tomography

CT of the neck with contrast is the most common test performed to evaluate a mass in the head and neck. It allows evaluation of the primary tumor and regional metastasis. It is usually used as part of the workup for head and neck malignancies and for surveillance posttreatment.

Magnetic Resonance Imaging

MRI results in superior evaluation of soft tissue compared with CT and does so without ionizing radiation. Instead, its images are attributable to a strong magnetic field that aligns the nuclear magnetization of hydrogen atoms in water. The examination is more difficult for some patients to tolerate compared with CT. The machine can make patients feel more claustrophobic and is noisier during the procedure. It also has the disadvantage that patients with implanted ferromagnetic foreign material are not able to go into the magnetic field. MRI is not as accurate for calcium structures such as bone and teeth.

Positron Emission Tomography/Computed Tomography

PET is a study that measures tissue metabolic activity by using a radioactive tracer. The tracer is fluorodeoxyglucose (FDG), an analogue of glucose. FDG is short acting with a half-life of 110 minutes. The scan works because neoplastic cells have a higher rate of glycolysis; therefore, the tracer is localized in the tissue. Unfortunately, tracer localization is not specific for neoplastic disease and can occur with inflammatory processes as well. Muscle activity will also result in increased uptake of the FDG. The scan is also limited by the inability to identify neoplasms that are smaller than 3 to 4 mm. In this situation, the amount of FDG concentrated is not large enough to stand out from the surrounding structures. The dual-modality scan of PET/CT has, for the most part, replaced the PET scan alone. Performing coregistered scans allows the metabolic activity from the PET scan to be more accurately correlated with the anatomic detail of the CT. PET/CT is most useful in head and neck oncology to look for unknown primary tumors, second primary tumors, and metastatic disease, both regional and distant. In the era of chemoradiotherapy, PET/CT has been used posttreatment to assess for response to treatment. This is most accurately done 2 to 3 months after treatment because the inflammation must resolve first.

Financial Disclosures: None Reported

Recommended Reading

Bailey B. Head and neck surgery—otolaryngology. 3rd ed. Philadelphia: Lippincott Williams & Wilkins; 2001.

Thawley SE, Panje WR, Batsakis JG, Lindberg, RD. Comprehensive management of head and neck tumors. 2nd ed. Philadelphia: W.B. Saunders; 1999.

5 ORAL CAVITY PROCEDURES

Carol R. Bradford, MD, FACS, and Mark E.P. Prince, MD, FRCSC

Preoperative Evaluation

Oral cavity procedures are commonly performed to treat malignancies. Tumors should be assessed preoperatively to allow accurate staging of the disease and to facilitate planning of definitive treatment. In most cases, an examination under anesthesia with endoscopy and biopsy is required to stage the primary tumor and to look for synchronous second primary tumors. Except in the case of very superficial lesions, computed tomography (CT) plays an important role in preoperative planning. In selected cases, plain radiographs (e.g., Panorex views) may be useful in evaluating the mandible. When the lesion is located in the tongue, magnetic resonance imaging (MRI) may provide additional information about the extent of the primary tumor.

Wide surgical margins are necessary for adequate treatment of primary squamous cell carcinoma of the head and neck. A margin of 1 to 2 cm should be achieved whenever possible, ideally with frozen-section control. Current evidence clearly indicates that overall patient outcome improves when clear margins are obtained.

Nodal metastases are common with oral cavity tumors. Accordingly, patients should be assessed for cervical adenopathy both clinically and radiographically. A chest x-ray should be obtained in all cases. CT or MRI can provide valuable information regarding the nodal status of the neck. In patients with advanced disease, a more extensive search for distant metastases should be conducted, including a CT scan of the chest. In some circumstances, combining CT with positron emission tomography (PET) may be useful.

Operative Planning

Surgical management of the neck is an evolving field. In general, if the risk of occult metastasis is greater than 20 to 25%, a selective neck dissection is recommended, particularly if postoperative radiation therapy is not planned. Whenever there is clinical evidence of nodal disease, treatment of the neck must be included in operative planning.

The oral cavity is a major component of a number of important functions, including speech and swallowing. Reconstruction of the anticipated surgical defect must be carefully planned to achieve the best results. Several basic considerations must be kept in mind. Tongue mobility and sensation must be maintained to the extent possible. Maintenance of mandibular continuity (especially in the anterior segment of the mandible) is vital for ensuring postoperative oral competence. Separation of the nasal cavity from the oral cavity is critical for the oral phase of swallowing and speech. Maintenance of the gingivobuccal and gingivolabial sulcus is important for oral function and the fitting of dentures.

As a rule, oral cavity defects should be closed primarily whenever possible. Primary closure has the advantage of using sensate tissue similar in form to the tissue that was excised. With experience and careful judgment, the surgeon can usually determine when a defect is too large for primary closure or when primary closure is likely to cause distortion and tethering of adjacent tissues and result in a significant functional disturbance. In such cases, a flap reconstruction must be considered. In select cases, pedicled flaps may be appropriate. Often, particularly with larger or more complicated defects, free flaps provide the best reconstructive result. Free tissue reconstruction has the advantage of allowing the surgeon to reconstruct the defect with the exact tissue components that were excised, including bone and skin. In addition, free flaps can be reinnervated to achieve a sensate reconstruction.

If the planned surgical procedure involves resection of part of the maxilla or the mandible, appropriate dental consultation should be obtained. If a postoperative splint, obturator, or dental prosthesis is to be placed, it is critical that dental impressions be obtained before operation. Thyroid function should be tested in all patients who have a history of radiation therapy to the neck to confirm that they are euthyroid.

In cooperative patients, small primary lesions of the oral cavity can sometimes be excised with local anesthesia; however, general anesthesia with adequate relaxation is required in the majority of cases. The route of intubation must be carefully considered for each patient. When the planned resection is extensive and when significant postoperative edema is anticipated, a tracheostomy should be performed. Patients with bulky lesions should undergo tracheostomy under local anesthesia before general anesthesia is induced. When a tracheostomy is not planned, nasotracheal intubation is often desirable.

When the excision is limited to the oral cavity, perioperative antibiotics are generally unnecessary. When a graft, a flap, or packing is employed, however, perioperative intravenous administration of antibiotics is advisable. In all cases in which the neck is entered, perioperative antibiotics are recommended. The oral cavity can be prepared preoperatively with chlorhexidine and a toothbrush.

A nasogastric feeding tube should be inserted whenever it is believed that the patient may have a problem maintaining oral nutrition postoperatively. Patients who undergo primary closure or split-thickness skin grafting or whose surgical wound is allowed to heal by secondary intention may be allowed clear liquids in 24 to 48 hours and a pureed diet by postoperative day 3; they can often tolerate a soft diet within 1 week. Patients who undergo flap reconstruction will have to be fed via a nasogastric tube until they have healed to the point where they can resume oral intake.

Patients should be advised to maintain oral hygiene postoperatively by means of frequent irrigation and rinses with either normal saline or half-strength hydrogen peroxide.

Teeth may be gently cleaned with a soft toothbrush until healing has occurred.

Anterior Glossectomy

OPERATIVE PLANNING

Either orotracheal or nasotracheal intubation may be appropriate, depending on the surgical approach and the extent of the planned resection. A tracheostomy should be performed whenever significant postoperative swelling or airway compromise is anticipated.

The depth of the excision and the size of the anticipated defect determine the optimal reconstructive approach. Defects that connect to the neck, unless they are small and can easily be closed primarily, usually necessitate creation of a flap for optimal reconstruction. When the excision extends down to the underlying musculature but there is no connection to the neck, a skin graft may be used. If a postoperative dental splint is planned to hold a skin graft in place, a dental consultation must be obtained before operation.

The patient should be supine in a 20° reverse Trendelenburg position. Turning the table 180° may facilitate access and positioning for the surgeon.

OPERATIVE TECHNIQUE

Step 1: Surgical Approach

Small anterior lesions up to 2 cm in diameter may be approached transorally, as may certain carefully selected larger lesions. Exposure of the tongue is usually achieved with the help of an appropriately sized bite block; alternatively, a specialized retractor (e.g., a Molt retractor) may be used. Retraction of the tongue is facilitated by the use of a piercing towel clip or a heavy silk suture placed through the tip of the tongue.

Access to posterior lesions and most larger lesions is obtained by performing a mandibulotomy through a lip-splitting incision [*see Figure 1*]. A stair-step incision is made in the lip and extended downward straight through the mentum, and a Z-plasty is done at the mental crease. Alternatively, the incision may be carried around the mental subunit.

The mandibular periosteum is elevated and a plate contoured to the mandible before the mandible is divided; this measure ensures exact realignment of the cut ends of the mandible. When possible, the mandibulotomy should be made anterior to the mental foramen to preserve sensation throughout the distribution of the mental nerve. Repair of the mandibulotomy is greatly facilitated by making a stair-step or chevron-type mandibulotomy [*see Figure 2*]. A paralingual mucosal incision is made to allow retraction of the mandible and exposure of the posterior oral cavity.

As an alternative, a visor flap may be created [*see Figure 3*]. Such a flap allows the surgeon to avoid making a lip-splitting incision and provides adequate exposure of small lesions of the anterior oral cavity; however, it is inadequate for exposure of lesions posterior to the middle third of the tongue or in the area of the retromolar trigone. Furthermore, creation of a visor flap results in anesthesia of the lower lip because of the necessity of dividing both mental nerves.

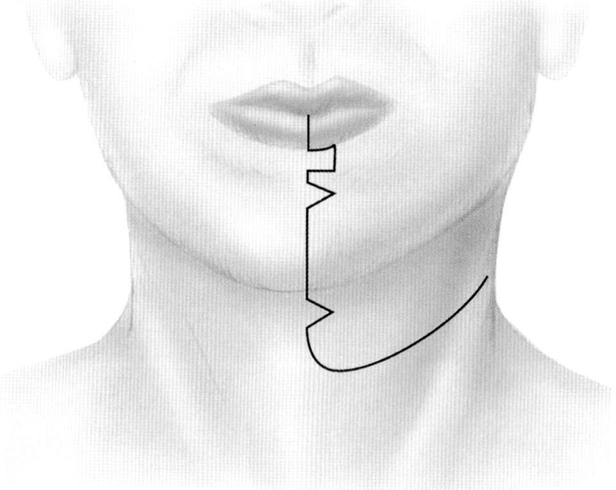

Figure 1 **Anterior glossectomy. A lip-splitting incision is made that extends downward straight through the mentum.**

To create a visor flap, an incision is made from mastoid to mastoid along a skin crease in the neck, with care taken to remain below the marginal mandibular nerves. The skin flap is elevated in the subplatysmal plane to the level of the mandible. The marginal mandibular nerves are preserved. The flap is elevated from the lateral surface of the mandible, and the two mental nerves are divided. An incision is made in the oral cavity mucosa along the gingivolabial sulcus and

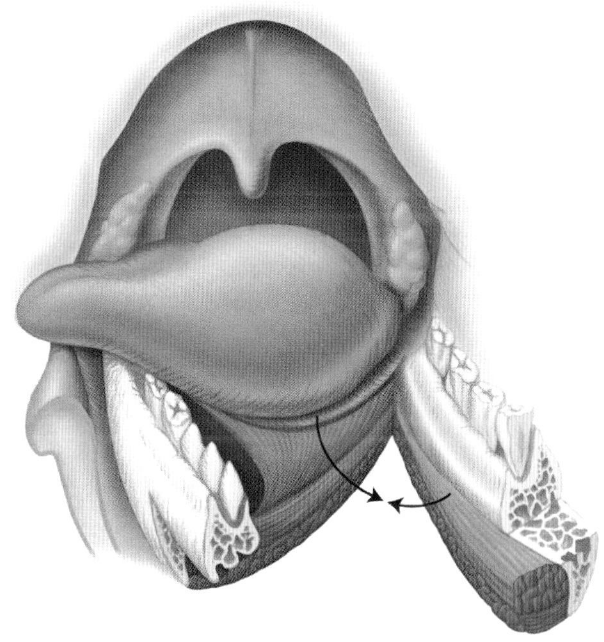

Figure 2 **Anterior glossectomy. A stair-step mandibulotomy is made.**

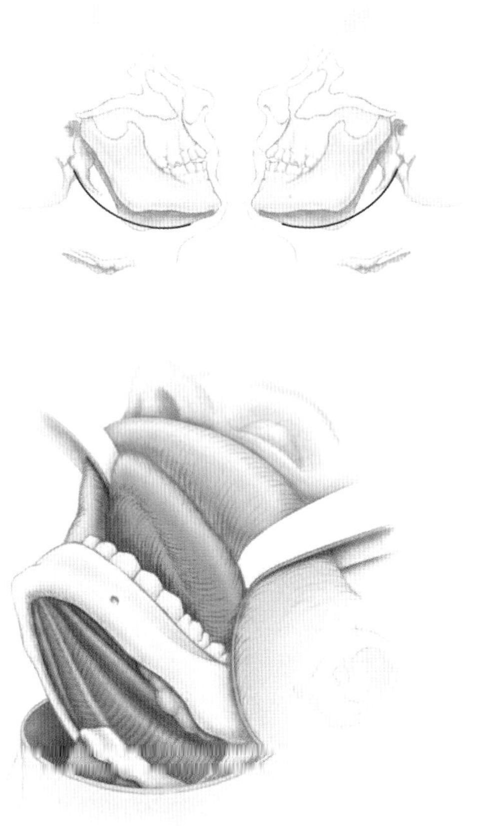

Figure 3 **Anterior glossectomy. As an alternative to a lip-splitting incision with mandibulotomy, a visor flap may be employed for exposure.**

continued so that it connects to the skin incision. The flap is then retracted superiorly to expose the anterior mandible and the oral cavity.

Step 2: Resection

The excision should include a generous mucosal margin around the visible lesion. A significant amount of the tongue musculature surrounding the lesion should be resected as well. Palpation of the lesion is critical for obtaining adequate deep surgical margins.

Resection may be performed with a monopolar electrocautery, with the cutting current used to incise the mucosa and the coagulation current used to cut the muscle. Alternatively, resection may be performed with a scalpel and scissors. Hemostasis is achieved with a monopolar or bipolar electrocautery. Larger vessels are ligated with chromic catgut or Vicryl ties.

Lesions of the lateral tongue should be wedge-excised in a transverse (rather than horizontal) fashion to facilitate closure and enhance postoperative function. With larger lesions, for which either flap reconstruction or healing by secondary intention is typically indicated, the shape of the defect is contoured so as to obtain wide margins around the lesion, and the flap is designed to fill the contoured defect.

Step 3: Reconstruction

After negative margins are confirmed by frozen-section examination, repair of the surgical defect is initiated. Careful preoperative assessment of the anticipated defect lays the groundwork for optimal reconstruction. Many defects can be either repaired primarily or allowed to heal by secondary intention. Free tissue transfer is an excellent reconstructive option in many cases, allowing the maintenance of tongue mobility and the separation of the tongue from the mandible and making sensate reconstruction possible.

In many patients with wedge-excised lateral tongue lesions, primary closure of the defect yields good results. The deep muscle is carefully reapproximated with long-lasting absorbable sutures. The mucosa is also closed with absorbable sutures. Care should be taken not to strangulate tissues by making the sutures too tight. When complete primary closure is not possible or desirable, the tongue may be allowed to granulate and heal by secondary intention. Split-thickness skin grafts, although useful for relining the floor of the mouth, generally do not take well on the tongue.

For large defects of the tongue and those involving the floor of the mouth, flap reconstruction is appropriate. Defects that connect to the neck, unless they are small and can be closed primarily, should also be closed with a flap. Free tissue transfer is frequently the optimal reconstructive approach. Free fasciocutaneous flaps from the radial forearm, the anterior lateral thigh, or the lateral arm are well suited to reconstruction in this area. Pedicled flaps (e.g., myocutaneous flaps from the pectoral muscle) are also used in this setting but are bulkier and harder to contour to the defects.

If a mandibulotomy was made, it is repaired with the previously contoured plate. The lip-splitting incision is closed in three layers (mucosa, muscle, and skin). Great care must be taken to ensure accurate realignment of the vermilion border and the orbicularis oris muscle.

Alternative Procedure: Laser Vaporization

Very superficial and premalignant lesions of the tongue may be vaporized by using a CO_2 laser. The desired depth of tissue destruction for leukoplakia is approximately 1 to 2 mm.

TROUBLESHOOTING

Larger excisions may lead to airway edema. Whenever this possibility is a concern, a tracheostomy should be performed. A single intraoperative dose of steroids may reduce postoperative tongue edema without adversely affecting wound healing. Using a stair-step incision for the lip-splitting incision facilitates accurate reapproximation of the vermilion border. Excessive tongue movement may result in dehiscence of the closure. Voice rest for 3 to 5 days after operation may be beneficial.

POSTOPERATIVE CARE

Patients who undergo primary closure of the tongue may begin a fluid diet on the day after operation; they should remain on a liquid diet for 7 to 10 days. Patients who undergo skin grafting may also begin a liquid diet on postoperative day 1. If a flap was used to close the defect or if there is some question whether the patient will be capable of adequate oral intake, a nasogastric feeding tube should be inserted and maintained until the suture lines heal.

Bolster dressings may be removed and skin grafts inspected after 7 to 10 days. Patients with skin grafts should stay on a soft diet for 2 weeks. If a tracheotomy was performed, the patient may be decannulated when postoperative edema has settled.

Meticulous and frequent oral hygiene is essential. Mouth rinses and irrigation with normal saline or half-strength hydrogen peroxide should be done at least four times a day and after every meal. Teeth may be gently cleaned with a soft toothbrush.

COMPLICATIONS

The main complications of anterior glossectomy are as follows:

1. Injury to the lingual nerve, which causes numbness and loss of the sense of taste in the ipsilateral tongue
2. Injury to the submandibular and sublingual gland ducts, which causes obstruction of the glands, pain and swelling, and possibly ranula formation
3. Injury to the hypoglossal nerve, portions of which are resected with the lesion. Injury to the main trunk of this nerve leads to paralysis and atrophy of the remaining ipsilateral tongue.
4. Tethering and scarring of the tongue, which can lead to difficulties with speech and swallowing. This problem can usually be avoided by careful preoperative planning of reconstruction.

Excision of Floor-of-Mouth Lesions

OPERATIVE PLANNING

Planning for excision of a lesion from the floor of the mouth is essentially the same as that for anterior glossectomy [*see* Anterior Glossectomy, Operative Planning, *above*]. If either or both of Wharton ducts are to be transected without excision of the submandibular glands, consideration must be given to the management of these glands.

OPERATIVE TECHNIQUE

Step 1: Surgical Approach

The surgical approach is the same as that described for glossectomy [*see* Anterior Glossectomy, Operative Technique, Step 1, *above*].

Step 2: Resection

The area to be excised, including adequate margins, is marked. The lesion is then excised with a monopolar electrocautery; as in a glossectomy, the cutting current is used to cut the mucosa and the coagulation current to cut the deeper tissues. Palpation is important for obtaining adequate deep surgical margins.

If the excision cuts across the Wharton duct, the duct should be identified and transected obliquely to create a wider opening. The transected stump is held with a 4-0 chromic catgut suture. Once the resection is complete, the duct is transposed posteriorly to the cut edge of the mucosa of the floor of the mouth and sutured in place with two or three 4-0 chromic sutures. During subsequent reconstruction, care should be taken not to obstruct the orifice of the duct.

Step 3: Reconstruction

After clean surgical margins have been verified by frozen-section examination, repair of the surgical defect is initiated. Small superficial defects of the floor of the mouth may be allowed to heal by secondary intention.

For small defects that do not connect to the neck, reconstruction with a 0.014 to 0.016 inch–thick split-thickness skin graft is appropriate. The graft is cut to size and sutured in place with 4-0 chromic sutures. Several perforations should be made in the graft to allow the egress of blood and serum. A Xeroform gauze bolster is fashioned to fit over the skin graft and sutured in place with 2-0 silk tie-over bolster stitches; alternatively, it may be held in place by a prefabricated dental prosthesis.

For larger defects, particularly those involving the tongue, a flap reconstruction typically yields the best functional results. In select cases, a platysma flap may be used for reconstruction of defects in the floor of the mouth. Other regional flaps tend to be bulky and difficult to shape to the contours of the defect. Free tissue transfer frequently provides the most suitable reconstructive tissue characteristics and the most favorable postoperative results. A free fasciocutaneous radial forearm flap is usually the optimal choice for reconstruction of floor-of-mouth defects when a flap is required.

TROUBLESHOOTING

Special care should be taken to identify the lingual nerve and artery so that these structures are not inadvertently divided. Meticulous hemostasis should be obtained in all cases. Any skin grafts used should be adequately sized and should not "tent up." Generally, skin grafting and bolsters do not work well on mobile structures. Quilting grafts to the underlying tissues with multiple absorbable sutures can eliminate the need for a bolster and result in acceptable graft take.

POSTOPERATIVE CARE

Postoperative care of patients undergoing excision of floor-of-mouth lesions is virtually identical to that of patients undergoing anterior glossectomy [*see* Anterior Glossectomy, Postoperative Care, *above*].

COMPLICATIONS

Excision of floor-of-mouth lesions is associated with the same complications as anterior glossectomy [*see* Anterior Glossectomy, Complications, *above*].

Excision of Superficial or Plunging Ranulas

OPERATIVE PLANNING

Planning for excision of a superficial or plunging ranula resembles that for glossectomy. A Ring-Adair-Elwyn (RAE) tube is inserted orally and taped to the contralateral cheek. Cervical exploration is usually unnecessary because the cervical component of the ranula resolves after removal of the ipsilateral sublingual gland. In select cases, especially those involving disease recurrence after a previous attempt at excision, a transcervical approach should be considered.

OPERATIVE TECHNIQUE

Step 1: Surgical Approach

Ranulas are resected via the transoral approach. A bite block or a Molt retractor is used to gain exposure.

Step 2: Resection

A local anesthetic preparation with epinephrine is infiltrated into the area of the mucosal incisions. A small superficial ranula may be marsupialized and packed with gauze. The ranula is widely unroofed and the contents removed with suction. The margins of the cyst are sutured to the mucosa with 4-0 chromic sutures, and the cavity is packed with iodoform strip gauze. The gauze may be removed in 5 to 7 days.

A plunging ranula is treated with complete surgical excision of the cyst and the sublingual gland [*see Figure 4*]. A mucosal incision is made directly over the cyst. Careful dissection is carried out around the cyst and the associated gland. Hemostasis is achieved with a bipolar electrocautery, with care taken not to injure the adjacent lingual nerve. The submandibular gland duct is cannulated with a lacrimal probe to help guard against inadvertent injury to this structure. The incision is closed with 4-0 chromic suture.

TROUBLESHOOTING

Efforts should be made to identify the lingual nerve and artery to prevent inadvertent division of these structures.

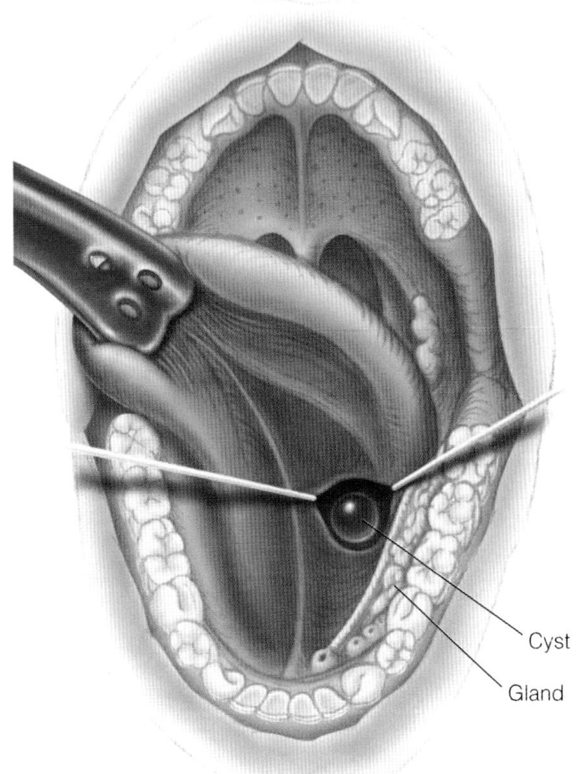

Figure 4 **Excision of plunging ranula. A mucosal incision is made over the cyst, dissection is done around the cyst and the associated sublingual gland, and the cyst and gland are completely excised.**

Meticulous hemostasis should be obtained in all cases. If the submandibular gland duct is injured, it should be transected and the cut end sutured to the adjacent floor-of-mouth mucosa (sialodochoplasty).

COMPLICATIONS

The three main complications of the procedure for excising a ranula are among those that are also associated with anterior glossectomy and excision of floor-of-mouth lesions: injury to the lingual nerve, injury to the submandibular gland duct, and injury to the hypoglossal nerve [*see* Anterior Glossectomy, Complications, *above*].

Removal of Submandibular Gland Duct Stones

OPERATIVE PLANNING

When a submandibular gland duct stone is readily palpable in the floor of the mouth, a transoral approach is appropriate. When the stone is within the hilum of the gland, however, it generally cannot be removed transorally and often must be treated by excising the submandibular gland.

OPERATIVE TECHNIQUE

Step 1: Surgical Approach

The procedure is easily accomplished with local anesthesia in a cooperative patient. The patient is seated upright in the examining chair, and a topical anesthetic is applied to the oral cavity.

Step 2: Resection

A local anesthetic preparation with epinephrine is infiltrated into the floor of the mouth and around the duct in which the stone is palpated. A 2-0 silk suture may be placed around the duct behind the stone to prevent it from migrating back into the hilum of the gland.

A lacrimal probe is inserted into the duct and advanced to the stone in a retrograde manner. A mucosal incision is then made directly over the stone and extended downward to the duct, with the stone and the lacrimal probe serving as guides. The duct is incised and the stone delivered. As a rule, repair of the duct is not required.

TROUBLESHOOTING

Careful dissection directly onto the duct and stone usually serves to prevent inadvertent injury to the lingual nerve.

COMPLICATIONS

The main complications of the procedure are as follows:

1. Injury to the lingual nerve, resulting in numbness and loss of the sense of taste to the ipsilateral tongue
2. Stricture of the submandibular gland duct. This is an unusual complication that can be corrected by transecting the duct posterior to the stricture and suturing it to the mucosa of the floor of the mouth.

Resection of Hard Palate

OPERATIVE PLANNING

Careful evaluation is required to determine whether resection of part of the hard palate will suffice or whether a more extensive dissection (e.g., maxillectomy) will be required. If it is anticipated that a dental prosthesis will be required, a dental consultation should be obtained before operation. When the lesion to be resected is superficial or only a limited amount of the bony hard palate must be resected, the procedure may be performed via the transoral approach.

OPERATIVE TECHNIQUE

Step 1: Surgical Approach

The patient is supine, with the bed turned 180° to facilitate the surgeons' access to the operative site. An oral RAE tube is inserted and taped in the midline. The lesion is approached transorally, and a Dingman or Crowe-Davis retractor is used to obtain exposure.

Step 2: Resection

An incision is made around the periphery of the lesion in such a way to maintain adequate margins; a monopolar electrocautery with a needle tip is ideal for this purpose. The periosteum is elevated away from the underlying bone, and the lesion is removed [*see Figure 5*].

When bone must be resected, the periosteum is elevated away from the incision site. A high-speed oscillating saw or an osteotome is used to make the cuts in the bone, after which the specimen is rocked free and removed.

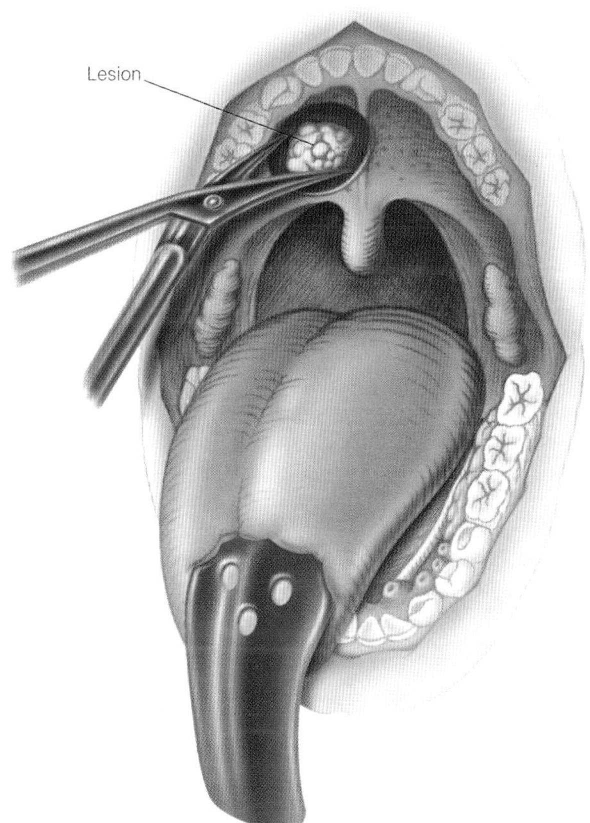

Figure 5 **Resection of hard palate. An incision is made around the lesion, with adequate margins maintained, the periosteum is lifted off the bone, and the lesion is removed.**

Step 3: Reconstruction

After surgical margins have been verified by frozen-section review, repair of the surgical defect is initiated. Small mucosal defects may be allowed to heal by secondary intention. Small through-and-through resections may be closed by placing relaxing incisions laterally and advancing the mucosa to permit primary closure. Larger defects may be closed with palatal mucosal flaps. Many through-and-through defects can be closed quite satisfactorily with a dental obturator.

POSTOPERATIVE CARE

The patient should be maintained on a soft diet postoperatively. Meticulous oral hygiene is important. Oral rinses and flushes with normal saline or half-strength hydrogen peroxide should be performed at least four times daily and after meals.

COMPLICATIONS

The most significant potential complication of hard palate resection is oral antral or oronasal fistula; careful tissue reconstruction and the use of an obturator can prevent this complication.

Maxillectomy

OPERATIVE PLANNING

General anesthesia with muscle relaxation is essential for all types of maxillectomy. Either orotracheal or nasotracheal intubation may be appropriate, depending on the surgical approach. Skin incisions should be marked before the endotracheal tube is taped in place to avoid distortion of facial structures and skin lines. The patient should be supine in a 20° reverse Trendelenburg position. The eyes should be protected carefully (e.g., with a corneal shield or a temporary nylon tarsorrhaphy suture).

Radiographic evaluation plays a vital role in planning the surgical approach and determining the extent of resection required [*see Figure 6*]. Lesions of the infrastructure of the maxilla can be excised by means of partial maxillectomy via the transoral route. More extensive lesions usually must be accessed via facial incisions in conjunction with the transoral approach.

In all cases, a dental consultation should be obtained preoperatively so that a dental impression can be taken and an obturator fashioned for intraoperative use. Antibiotics should be given perioperatively and continued until nasal packing is removed.

OPERATIVE TECHNIQUE

Step 1: Surgical Approach

In addition to the transoral approach, maxillectomy usually requires exposure of the anterior face of the maxilla. There are several options for achieving such exposure, including a Weber-Ferguson incision and midface degloving. Midface degloving has the advantage of eliminating the need for visible facial incisions but yields limited exposure in the ethmoid region. The choice of surgical approach is determined by the extent of the planned resection and by the preferences of the patient and the surgeon.

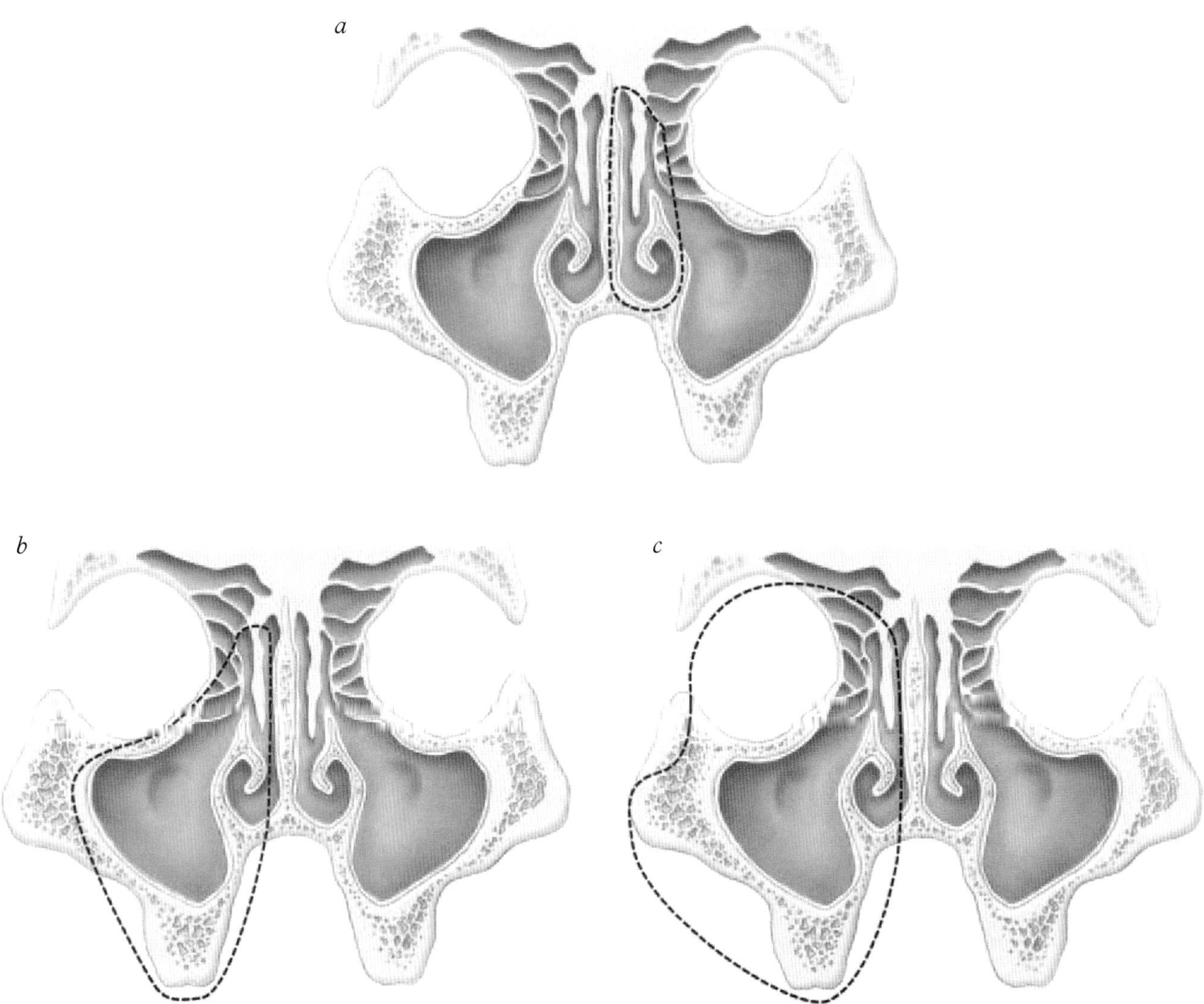

Figure 6 **Maxillectomy. Radiographic assessment helps determine the required extent of resection. Depicted are (*a*) medial maxillectomy, (*b*) subtotal maxillectomy without orbital exenteration, and (*c*) total maxillectomy with orbital exenteration.**

In the Weber-Ferguson approach, the first step is to mark the path of the incision, which begins in the midline of the upper lip; extends through the philtrum; curves around the nasal vestibule and the ala; continues upward along the lateral nasal wall, just medial to the junction of the nasal sidewall and the cheek; and ends near the medial canthus. For added exposure in the ethmoid region, a Lynch extension, in which the incision is continued superiorly up to the medial eyebrow, may be performed. Alternatively, the Weber-Ferguson incision may be continued laterally in the subciliary crease along the inferior eyelid to the lateral canthus of the eye; this extension yields added exposure of the posterolateral aspect of the maxilla.

The skin incisions should initially be made with a scalpel and then continued with an electrocautery. The upper lip is divided through its full thickness, and the incision is continued in the gingivolabial sulcus laterally until the posterolateral aspect of the sinus is exposed. When possible, the infraorbital nerve is identified and preserved. The soft tissues are elevated from the anterior wall of the maxillary sinus; if access to the pterygomaxillary fissure is desired, elevation should be continued up to the zygoma.

In a midface degloving, the skin of the lower face and nose is mobilized and retracted superiorly. A standard transfixion incision is made, transecting the membranous septum. Intercartilaginous incisions are then made bilaterally and connected to the transfixion incision. The incision is then continued laterally along the cephalic border of the lower lateral cartilage and across the floor of the nose. To prevent stenosis, a small Z-plasty or triangle is incised medially just before the transfixion incision is joined. The soft tissues are elevated over the nasal dorsum and the nasal tip with Joseph scissors. An incision is made in the gingivolabial sulcus with the monopolar cautery, and this incision is connected to the floor-of-nose incisions by means of gentle dissection. The soft tissues are then elevated from the anterior maxilla as far as the infraorbital rims and laterally as far as the zygoma.

Step 2: Resection

A Molt retractor is placed on the side opposite the side of the planned excision and opened as wide as possible to expose the hard palate and the alveolus.

The infraorbital rim should be preserved if it is possible to do so safely. Often a thin strip of the rim can be preserved even when the rest of the bone must be resected. If the orbital floor must be resected but the orbital contents can be preserved, the periorbita can be dissected away from the bone of the orbital floor and preserved. If the orbital contents are involved, an orbital exenteration must be performed in conjunction with the maxillectomy.

The cut along the infraorbital rim and superior anterior maxillary wall is made with a high-speed oscillating saw with a fine blade. The level at which this superior cut is made is determined by the extent of the resection. Lesions that are confined to the alveolus or the palate and do not invade the maxilla typically can be removed by excising the infrastructure of the maxilla. The line of transection is continued through the nasal process of the maxilla medially and downward through the piriform aperture. Laterally, the cut extends to the zygomatic process of the maxilla and around the posterolateral aspect of the sinus.

If the pterygoid plates are to be preserved, they are cut free by placing a curved osteotome along the posterior wall of the sinus and sharply dividing the plates from the sinus wall. If the pterygoid plates, part of the pterygoid musculature, or both are to be resected, the soft tissue attachments are cut sharply with curved Mayo scissors once the entire maxillary specimen has been mobilized.

The line of transection in the maxillary alveolus can run between two teeth if a suitable gap is evident. In the majority of cases, however, it is advisable to extract a tooth and make the cut through the extraction site. A power saw is used, and the cut is connected to the transection line through the nasal process of the maxilla and the piriform aperture. The hard palate mucosa is then incised lateral to the proposed cut in the hard palate bone to preserve a flap of mucosa that can be used to cover the raw cut bony edge of the palate. This incision is made with a needle-tip electrocautery and carried down to the bone of the hard palate. It should extend from the maxillary tuberosity posteriorly to the cut bone in the maxillary alveolus anteriorly, with care taken to obtain adequate mucosal margins. The mucosa is elevated for a short distance over the hard palate bone to create a short mucosal flap that is wrapped over the cut bony edge of the palate. The mucosal cut is connected around the maxillary tuberosity to the gingivolabial sulcus incision that was made earlier.

The hard palate is then cut with a power saw. Once all the bone cuts are complete, an osteotome may be used to connect them if necessary. The remaining soft tissue attachments are divided along the posterior hard palate with curved Mayo scissors. The surgical defect is packed to control bleeding. Bleeding from the internal maxillary artery is controlled by ligatures or ligating clips.

Step 3: Reconstruction

All sharp spicules of bone are débrided. The flap of hard palate mucosa is brought up over the cut bony edge of the palate and held in place with several Vicryl sutures. The anterior and posterior cut edges of the soft palate are reapproximated with absorbable sutures.

A split-thickness skin graft, 0.014 to 0.016 inches thick, is harvested and used to line the raw undersurface of the cheek flap. The skin graft is sutured to the mucosal edge of the cheek flap with 3-0 chromic sutures. Superiorly, the graft is not sutured but draped into position and retained by a layer of Xeroform packing and strip gauze coated with antibiotic ointment. Gentle pressure is applied to the packing so that it conforms to the defect. The previously fabricated dental obturator is placed to support the packing and to close the oral cavity from the nasal cavity. In a dentulous patient, the obturator may be wired to the remaining teeth; in an edentulous patient, it may be temporarily fixed in place with two screws placed in the remaining hard palate.

The skin incisions are closed in two layers, with interrupted absorbable sutures used for the deep layers and nonabsorbable monofilament sutures for the skin. If a lip-splitting incision was made, care must be taken to ensure exact reapproximation of the orbicularis oris and the vermilion border.

If the infraorbital rim was resected, it should be reconstructed to yield good aesthetic results. A split calvarial bone graft may be used for this purpose when there is adequate soft tissue coverage for the bone grafts available. When soft tissue coverage is inadequate or the orbital floor must be reconstructed, an osteocutaneous radial forearm or scapular flap may be employed, with excellent results.

Alternative Procedure: Peroral Partial Maxillectomy

The oral cavity is exposed with cheek retractors. An incision is made in the gingivobuccal sulcus and the mucosa of the hard palate, with care taken to maintain adequate margins; a monopolar electrocautery, set to use the cutting current, is suitable for this purpose. Incisions are made circumferentially through all the soft tissues up to the anterior wall of the maxilla and the hard palate. The infraorbital nerve should be preserved if it is not involved with the disease process.

The cut in the hard palate mucosa should be made lateral to the planned cuts in the hard palate bone to create a mucosal flap, which will be used to cover the cut bony edge of the hard palate. If necessary, teeth may be extracted to allow the surgeon to make bone cuts through tooth sockets while preserving adjacent teeth. The bone is cut with a high-speed power saw, and an osteotome is used to divide any remaining bony attachments and deliver the specimen. If the mucosa remaining in the maxillary antrum is not diseased, it need not be removed.

A split-thickness skin graft, 0.014 to 0.016 inches thick, is harvested from the anterolateral thigh and used to reline the raw buccal mucosa area. The graft is sutured to the cut edge of the buccal mucosa with 4-0 chromic catgut. Xeroform and strip gauze coated with antibiotic ointment are gently packed into the defect to secure the skin graft. The previously fabricated dental obturator is wired to the remaining teeth to hold the packing in place.

TROUBLESHOOTING

If a lip-splitting incision is planned, lip contraction can be reduced and vermilion border realignment improved by employing a stair-step lip incision and a Z-plasty. A single intraoperative steroid dose reduces facial edema without compromising wound healing. Retention of the obturator is

Additional Readings

Baurmash H. Submandibular salivary stones: current management modalities. J Oral Maxillofac Surg 2004;62:369.

Brown JD. The midface degloving procedure for nasal, sinus and nasopharyngeal tumors. Otolaryngol Clin North Am 2001;34:1095.

Brown JS, Kalavrezos N, D'Sousa J, et al. Factors that influence the method of mandibular resection in the management of oral squamous cell carcinoma. Br J Oral Maxillofac Surg 2002;40:275.

Campana JP, Meyers AD. The surgical management of oral cancer. Otolaryngol Clin North Am 2006;39:331.

Galloway RH, Gross PD, Thompson SH, et al. Pathogenesis and treatment of ranula: report of three cases. J Oral Maxillofac Surg 1989; 47:299.

Hussain A, Hilmi OJ, Murray DP. Lateral rhinotomy through nasal aesthetic subunits: improved cosmetic outcome. J Laryngol Otol 2002;116:703.

Johnson JT, Leipzig B, Cummings CW. Management of T1 carcinoma of the anterior aspect of the tongue. Arch Otolaryngol 1980; 106:249.

Katz P, Fritsch MH. Salivary stones: innovative techniques in diagnosis and treatment. Curr Opin Otol Head Neck Surg 2003;11:173.

Lanier DM. Carcinoma of the hard palate. In: Bailey BJ, editor. Surgery of the oral cavity. Chicago: Year Book Medical Publishers; 1989. p. 163.

Leipzig B, Cummings CW, Chung CT, et al. Carcinoma of the anterior tongue. Ann Otol Rhinol Laryngol 1982;91:94.

Osguthorpe JD, Weisman RA. "Medial maxillectomy" for lateral nasal neoplasms. Arch Otolaryngol Head Neck Surg 1991;117:751.

Schrag C, Chang YM, Tsai CY, Wei FC. Complete rehabilitation of the mandible following segmental resection. J Surg Oncol 2006;94: 538.

Schramm VL, Myers EN, Sigler BA. Surgical management of early epidermoid carcinoma of the anterior floor of the mouth. Laryngoscope 1980;90:207.

Spiro RH, Gerold FP, Strong EW. Mandibular "swing" approach for oral and oropharyngeal tumors. Head Neck 1981;3:371.

Stern SJ, Geopfert H, Clayman G, et al. Squamous cell carcinoma of the maxillary sinus. Arch Otolaryngol Head Neck Surg 1993; 119:964.

Wald RM, Calcaterra TC. Lower alveolar carcinoma: segmental v. marginal resection. Arch Otolaryngol 1983;109:578.

Acknowledgment

Figures 1 through 8 Alice Y. Chen

6 PAROTIDECTOMY

*Kathryn T. Chen, MD, Shannon H. Allen, MD, and John A. Ridge, MD, PhD, FACS**

Anatomic Considerations

The parotid ("near the ear") gland, the largest of the salivary glands, occupies the space immediately anterior to the ear, overlying the angle of the mandible. It drains into the oral cavity via the Stensen duct, which enters the oral vestibule opposite the upper molars. The gland is invested by a strong fascia, and its "parotid space" is bounded superiorly by the zygomatic arch, anteriorly by the masseter muscle, posteriorly by the external auditory canal and the mastoid process, and inferiorly by the sternocleidomastoid muscle. The masseter muscle, the styloid muscles, the posterior belly of the digastric muscle, and a portion of the sternocleidomastoid muscle lie deep to the parotid [*see Figure 1*]. The parotid gland is separated from the submandibular gland by the stylomandibular ligament, which is a continuation of the investing fascia between the styloid process and the angle of the mandible.

Terminal branches of the external carotid artery, the facial vein, and the facial nerve are found within the gland. Parasympathetic innervation to the parotid is via the otic ganglion, which gives fibers to the auriculotemporal branch of the trigeminal nerve. Sympathetic innervation to the gland originates in the sympathetic ganglia and reaches the auriculotemporal nerve by way of the plexus around the middle meningeal artery.[1]

Lymphatic channels and nodes may be found within the parotid space. The majority of lymph nodes are found in the superficial layer between the gland and fascial layer, but a second lymphatic system exists in the deep space as well. Lymph drainage is to the cervical nodes.

The facial nerve trunk exits the stylomastoid foramen and courses toward the parotid. Once inside the gland, it commonly bifurcates into superior (temporofrontal) and inferior (cervicomarginal) divisions before giving rise to its terminal branches, which innervate the muscles of facial expression. The variations of facial nerve anatomy within the parotid can be complex, but the common patterns are well known and their relative frequencies well established.[2,3] They have little to no impact on the conduct of parotidectomy. The portion of the parotid gland lateral and superficial to the facial nerve (about 80% of the gland) is designated as the superficial lobe; the portion medial and deep to the facial nerve (the remaining 20%) is designated as the deep lobe. Deep lobe tumors often present clinically as retromandibular or parapharyngeal masses, sometimes with displacement of the tonsil or the soft palate appreciated in the pharynx.

* The authors and editors gratefully acknowledge the contributions of the previous author, Leonard R. Henry, MD, to the development and writing of this chapter.

Preoperative Evaluation

When a patient presents with a mass at the angle of the mandible, a neoplasm within the parotid is a strong consideration. The type of resection performed depends on on preoperative clinical suspicion for benign versus malignant disease.

A thorough history should be secured and a complete head and neck examination undertaken. Clinical findings worrisome for malignancy include facial pain, facial nerve palsy, a fixed or nonmobile mass, and cervical lymphadenopathy and should be documented.[4] Ultrasound evaluation cannot adequately demonstrate the deep lobe of the parotid.[5] For parotid masses clinically suspicious for malignancy, computed tomography (CT) with intravenous contrast or magnetic resonance imaging (MRI) with gadolinium encompassing the skull base to clavicle is warranted. Involvement of bone, muscle, or pharyngeal mucosa will require extended resection and may (rarely) necessitate mandibulectomy or maxillectomy. If involvement is suspected, the surgeon should also be prepared to resect the facial nerve, and appropriate counseling regarding anticipated deficits should be provided to the patient. Consultation with a reconstructive surgeon may be prudent if resection will include the mandible or create a substantial cutaneous defect.

Operative Planning

In general, there are three types of operations undertaken for the parotid gland: subtotal, superficial, or total parotidectomy. The term *subtotal parotidectomy* has sometimes been interchangeably used with superficial parotidectomy in the literature but might be considered as any parotid resection less than a total parotidectomy. Obtaining informed consent for parotidectomy entails discussing both the features and the potential complications of the procedure. It is appropriate to address the possibility of facial nerve injury, but in doing so, the surgeon should not neglect other, far more common sequelae, such as cosmetic deformity, earlobe numbness secondary to division of the posterior auricular nerve, and Frey syndrome (gustatory sweating). Even conditions that are expected beforehand may prove distressing or debilitating for the patient. The risk of complications such as nerve injury is greater in cases involving reoperation or resection of malignant or deep lobe tumors. However, the overwhelming majority of parotid tumors are benign and lateral to the facial nerve. Accordingly, in what follows, we focus primarily on superficial parotidectomy, referring to variants of the procedure where relevant.

Excellent lighting, correctly applied traction and countertraction, adequate exposure, and clear definition of the surgical anatomy are essential in parotid surgery. The use of magnifying loupes and headlights is recommended. General anesthesia without muscle relaxation should be employed.

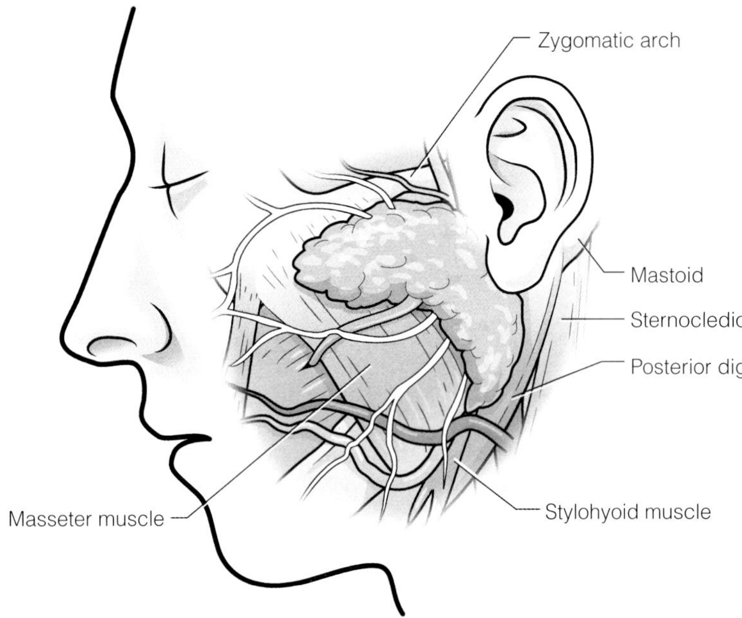

Figure 1 **Anatomic boundaries of parotid space. The parotid space is bounded by the zygomatic arch superiorly, the external auditory canal and mastoid process posteriorly, and the sternocleidomastoid muscle inferiorly. Additionally, the masseter muscle, the styloid muscles, and the posterior belly of the digastric muscle lie deep to the gland.**

The use of electromyography (EMG)-based facial nerve monitoring has not been found to be associated with a lower incidence of long-term permanent facial nerve injury[6,7] and, as such, is not routinely used. However, it may be useful in reoperative cases, where the anatomy of the facial nerve may be distorted and its location obscured by scar.

The patient is placed in the supine position, with the head elevated and turned away from the side undergoing operation and with the neck slightly extended. The table is positioned to allow the first assistant to stand directly above the patient's head while the surgeon faces the operative field. A small cottonoid sponge is placed in the external auditory canal, where it remains for the duration of the procedure to prevent otitis externa from blood clot in the external auditory canal. The skin is painted with an antiseptic agent. A single perioperative dose of an antibiotic is administered.

The patient is draped in a fashion that permits the operating team to see all of the muscle groups innervated by the facial nerve and to move the head if necessary. To this end, we employ a head drape that incorporates the endotracheal tube and anesthesia circuit. This drape secures the airway, keeps the tube from interfering with the surgeon, and permits rotation of the head without tension on the endotracheal tube. The skin of the upper chest and neck is widely painted and draped with a split sheet to allow additional exposure in the unlikely event that a neck dissection or a tracheotomy becomes necessary. The nose, the lips, and the eyes are covered with a sterile transparent drape that allows observation of movement during the procedure and permits access to the oral cavity (if desired) [*see Figure 2*].

Operative Technique

STEP 1: INCISION AND SKIN FLAPS

The incision is planned so as to permit excellent exposure with good cosmetic results. It may usually be placed in a skin crease to help conceal the resulting scar. The incision begins immediately anterior to the ear, continues downward past the tragus, curves back under the ear (staying close to the earlobe), and finally turns downward to descend along the sternocleidomastoid muscle [*see Figure 2*]. All or part of this incision may be used, depending on the circumstances. The incision is marked before draping.

Skin flaps are then created to expose the parotid gland. A tacking suture is placed within the dermis of the earlobe so that it can be retracted posteriorly. Skin hooks are used to apply vertical traction. The anterior flap is created superficial to the parotid fascia to afford access to the appropriate dissection plane. Vertically oriented blunt dissection minimizes the risk of injury to the distal branches of the facial nerve, which become more superficial than the proximal origins [*see Figure 3*]. The face is observed for muscle motion. The flap is raised until the anterior border of the gland is identified. The facial nerve branches are rarely encountered during flap elevation until they emerge from the parenchyma of the parotid. If muscle movement occurs, the flap has been more than adequately developed. The anterior flap is retracted with a suture through the dermis.

The posteroinferior skin flap is then elevated in a similar manner. Careful dissection is performed to define the relationship of the parotid tail to the anterior border of the sternocleidomastoid. During this portion of the procedure, the great auricular nerve is identified coursing cephalad and superficial to the sternocleidomastoid muscle. Uninvolved branches of this nerve should be preserved, if possible, to prevent postoperative numbness of the earlobe.[8,9] The parotid tail is dissected from the sternocleidomastoid muscle and should not be violated. Vertical traction is applied to the gland surface with clamps to facilitate exposure.

A favorable skin crease, if available, may be used for the incision to improve the postoperative cosmetic result; however, it is important to keep the incision a few millimeters from the earlobe itself. A wound at the junction of the

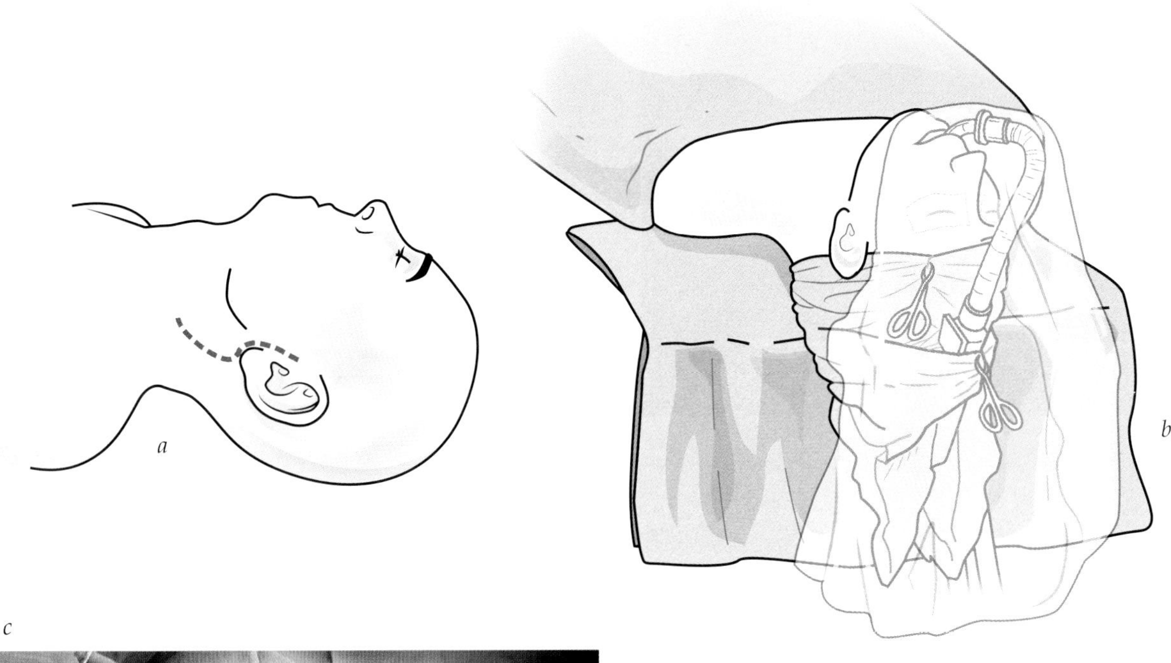

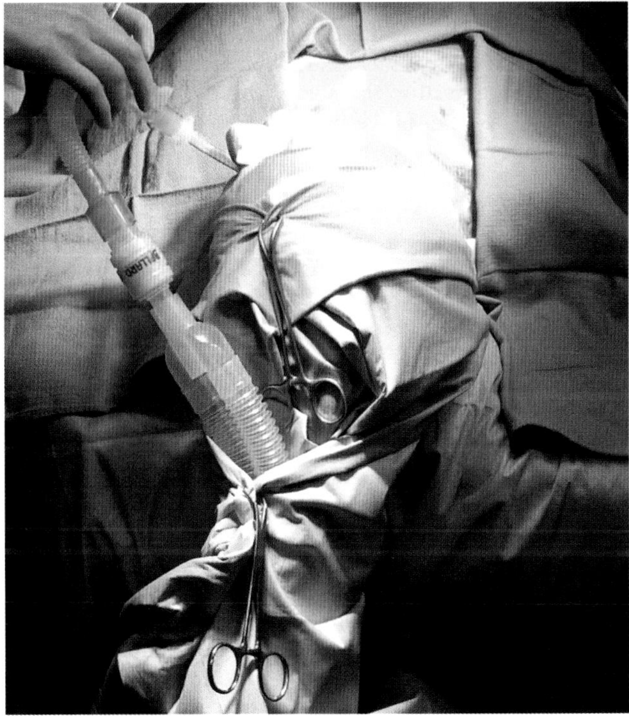

Figure 2 **Parotidectomy. (*a*) The recommended head position and incision. A transparent drape is placed over the eyes, the lip, and the oral cavity. (*b* and *c*) The head drape incorporates the hose from the endotracheal tube.**

earlobe with the facial skin will distort the earlobe and create a visible contour change. An incision behind the tragus may lead to similar problems.

STEP 2: IDENTIFICATION OF FACIAL NERVE

Once the skin flaps have been developed and retracted, the next step is to identify the facial nerve. Usually, the nerve may be identified either at its main trunk (the antegrade approach) or at one of the distal branches, with subsequent dissection back toward the main trunk (the retrograde approach). For a superficial parotidectomy, our preference is to identify the main trunk first (unless it is thoroughly obscured by tumor or scar).

Antegrade Approach

The dissection plane is immediately anterior to the cartilage of the external auditory canal. The gland is mobilized anteriorly by means of blunt dissection. To reduce the

a

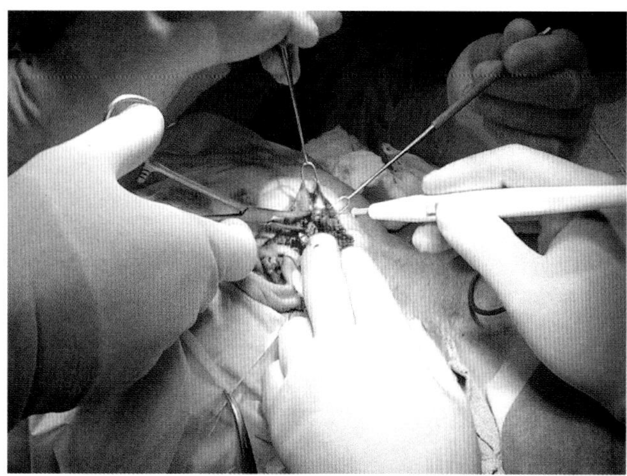

b

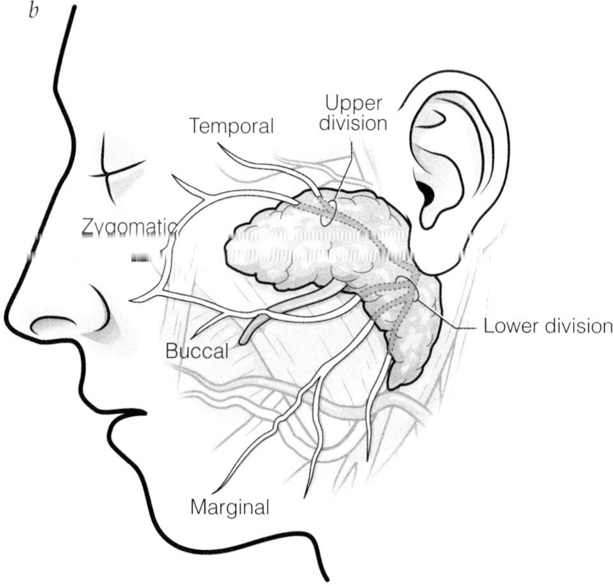

Figure 3 **Parotidectomy. (*a*) The creation of the anterior skin flap superficial to the parotid gland. (*b*) Branches of the facial nerve, including superior and inferior divisions and distal branches.**

risk of a traction injury, tissue is spread in a direction that is perpendicular to the incision and thus parallel to the direction of the main trunk of the nerve [*see Figure 4*]. The nerve trunk can usually be located underlying a point about halfway between the tip of the mastoid process and the ear canal.

Another commonly employed method is to identify the tragal pointer, or the tip of the external canal cartilage. The dictum is that the nerve is typically found slightly anterior and inferior to this landmark and 1.0 to 1.5 cm deep, although distance can vary considerably.[10,11] Other anatomic landmarks that facilitate identification of the nerve include the posterior belly of the digastric muscle and the tympanomastoid suture. Of these, the tympanomastoid suture is closest to the main trunk of the facial nerve.[12] The clinical utility of this landmark is limited, however, because the

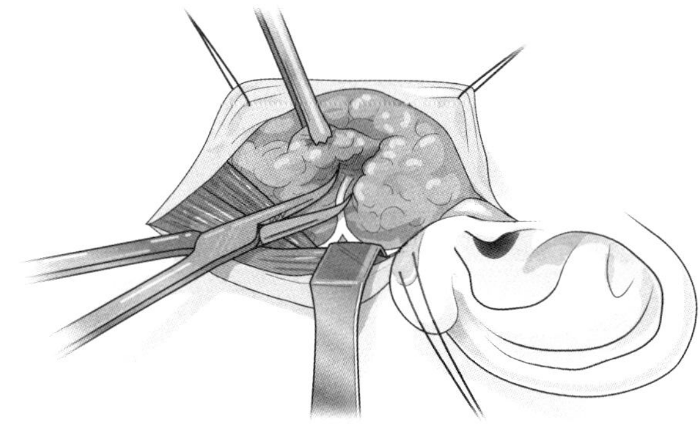

Figure 4 **Parotidectomy. Dissection of the gland parenchyma is carried out over the branches of the facial nerve to minimize the risk of nerve injury. Each division of the substance of the gland should reveal more of the facial nerve.**

tympanomastoid suture is not easily appreciated in every case. In addition, deep lobe tumors may displace the nerve from its normal location. For appropriate and safe exposure of the nerve trunk, it is preferable to mobilize several centimeters of the parotid, thereby creating a trough rather than a deep hole. Small arteries run superficial and parallel to the facial nerve; these must be divided. In particular, the stylomandibular artery enters the stylomastoid foramen alongside and superficial to the nerve. Use of the electrocautery this close to the nerve is potentially hazardous, and bipolar current or suture ligation is preferred. Bleeding is typically minor but nonetheless must be controlled.

Retrograde Approach

As noted, when the main trunk cannot be exposed, the most common alternative method of identifying the facial nerve is to find a peripheral branch and then dissect proximally toward the main trunk. Which branch is sought may depend on factors such as the surgeon's comfort with the anatomy and the known consistency of the nerve branch's location. In this setting, tumor bulk is often the deciding factor.

The anatomic relationships between the nerve branches and various landmarks can be exploited for more efficient identification. For example, the marginal mandibular branch of the facial nerve characteristically lies below the horizontal ramus of the mandible.[13] Often the facial vein can be traced superiorly toward the parotid on the submandibular gland; the nerve branch can then be found coursing perpendicularly across and superficial to the vein [*see Figure 5*]. The buccal branch of the facial nerve has a typical location in the so-called buccal pocket—the area inferior to the zygoma and deep to the superficial musculoaponeurotic layer, which contains the buccal fat pad and Stensen duct in addition to the buccal branch.[13] The zygomatic branch of the facial nerve lies roughly 3 cm anterior to the tragus, and the temporofrontal branch lies at the midpoint between the outer canthus of the eye and the junction of the ear's helix with the preauricular skin.[7] Nerve branches to the eye should be dissected with particular care: even transient weakness of these branches may be associated with substantial morbidity.

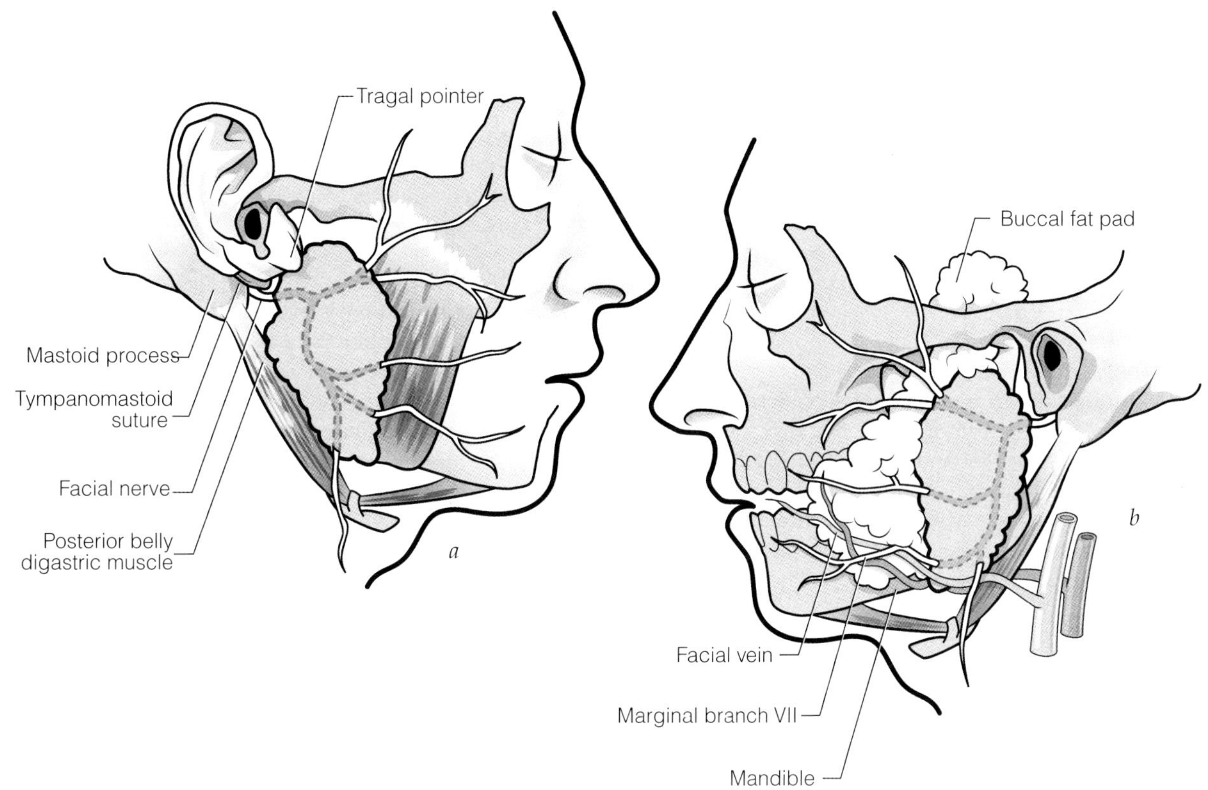

Figure 5 **Dissection of the facial nerve. (*a*) Antegrade approach. Shown are the relationships between the main trunk of the facial nerve, mastoid process, tragal pointer, posterior belly of the digastric muscle, and tympanomastoid suture. (*b*) Retrograde approach. Shown are the relationships between the distal branches of the facial nerve and the horizontal mandibular ramus, facial vein, and buccal fat pad.**

Troubleshooting

Special efforts should be made to ensure that the cartilage of the ear canal is not injured during exposure of the facial nerve trunk. Any injury to this cartilage must be avoided, or else the patient will hear an intense whistling as air enters the closed-suction drain after operation.

The anxiety associated within isolation of the nerve trunk may be alleviated somewhat by keeping in mind that the nerve typically lies deeper than one might expect. In a study of 46 cadaver dissections, the facial nerve was found to lie at a median depth of 22.4 mm from the skin at the stylomastoid foramen (range 16 to 27 mm). The diameter of the nerve trunk was found to range from 1.1 to 3.4 mm.[14] In our experience, the facial nerve trunk is slightly larger than the nearby deep vessels, but their presence limits identification unless they are divided.

Some surgeons advocate the use of a nerve stimulator to aid in identifying the facial nerve trunk or its branches; however, we have substantial reservations about whether this measure should be employed on a regular basis [*see* Complications, Facial Nerve Injury, *below*]. Knowledge of the anatomy and sound surgical technique are the keys to a safe parotidectomy; it is potentially hazardous to rely too much on practices that may diminish them.

STEP 3: PARENCHYMAL DISSECTION

Once identified, the plane of the facial nerve remains uniform throughout the gland (unless the nerve is displaced by a tumor) and serves to guide the parenchymal dissection. Although some surgeons advocate the use of hemostatic devices for parenchymal division,[15,16] our practice is to divide the substance of the parotid gland sharply and use ligatures as appropriate when bleeding is encountered. Usually, there is no significant hemorrhage: loss of more than 30 mL of blood is rare.

The parenchymal dissection proceeds directly over the facial nerve. We favor using fine curved clamps for this portion of the procedure. To prevent trauma to the nerve, care must be taken to resist the tendency to rest the blades of the clamp on the nerve during dissection. Each division of the gland should reveal more of the facial nerve [*see Figure 4*]. When this is the case, the surgeon can continue the parenchymal dissection with confidence that the nerve will not be injured. As a rule, if a parenchymal division does not immediately show more of the facial nerve, it is in an improper (potentially unsafe) plane.

We do not regularly resect the entire lateral lobe of the parotid unless the tumor is large and such resection is required on oncologic grounds. The goal in resecting the substance of the parotid is to obtain sound margins while preserving the remainder of the gland and limiting manipulation of the nerve it harbors. This so-called partial superficial parotidectomy, or subtotal parotidectomy, has been shown to reduce the incidence of Frey syndrome without increasing the rate of recurrence of pleomorphic adenoma.[17] The plane of dissection is developed along facial nerve branches until the lateral margins have been secured. This is the portion of the procedure during which the risk of nerve injury is highest. Once the lateral margins have been secured, the parenchymal dissection can proceed from deep to superficial for the excision of the tumor. The vertical portion of the dissection (perpendicular to the plane of the nerve branches) seldom poses a threat to the integrity of the facial nerve, but care must be taken to maintain appropriate margins. If division of the Stensen duct is required, the distal remnant may be either left open[18] or ligated.

Caution is appropriate in the resection of deep lobe tumors. Tumors medial to the facial nerve may displace it laterally. Thus, after establishing the plane of the facial nerve, the surgeon must remain vigilant when dissecting near the tumor to keep from injuring the nerve. Once the substance of the gland obscuring the tumor has been removed, the nerve branches in the area of the tumor are retracted to allow exposure of the deep portion of the gland and facilitate resection. Traction injury to the nerve may still result in transient facial weakness.

Troubleshooting

Complete superficial parotidectomy with full dissection of all facial nerve branches is seldom necessary, although in some cases, it is mandated by tumor size or histologic findings. Removal of the entire superficial lobe with the intention of obtaining a larger lateral margin is rarely useful because the closest margin is usually where the tumor is nearest the facial nerve. Even temporary paresis of the temporofrontal branch of the facial nerve may have devastating consequences, and dissection near this branch is usually unnecessary in treating a benign tumor in the parotid tail. After complete resection of cancer, any close margins remaining after nerve-preserving resection can be addressed by means of postoperative radiation therapy, usually with excellent results.[19]

The question of whether to sacrifice the facial nerve almost invariably arises in the setting of malignancy. In our view, this measure is seldom necessary. Benign tumors tend to displace the nerve, not invade it. Sacrifice of the nerve probably does not enhance survival.[20,21] Although this issue remains a subject of debate, our practice, like that of others,[22] is to sacrifice only those branches intimately involved with tumor. Repair, if feasible, should be performed [*see* Complications, Facial Nerve Injury, *below*].

STEP 4: DRAINAGE AND CLOSURE

Before closure, absolute hemostasis is confirmed (including hemostasis during the Valsalva maneuver, which is approximated by transiently increasing airway pressure to 30 cm H_2O[1]). We sometimes then confirm the integrity of the facial nerve with a nerve stimulator. A 5 mm closed-suction drain is placed through a stab incision posterior to the inferior aspect of the ear in a hair-bearing area. The tip of the drain is loosely tacked to the sternocleidomastoid muscle, with care taken to avoid direct contact with the facial nerve. The wound is closed with the drain placed on continuous suction. The skin is closed with interrupted 5-0 nylon sutures. Bacitracin is applied to the wound. No additional dressing is necessary or desirable [*see Figure 6*].

The use of interrupted skin sutures instead of a continuous suture allows the surgeon to perform directed suture removal to drain the rare postoperative hematoma or fluid collection instead of reopening the entire wound. We maintain gentle pressure over the surgical bed with an unfolded surgical sponge during extubation to limit bleeding that may be engendered by coughing during extubation.

Postoperative Care

Facial nerve function is evaluated in the recovery room, with particular attention paid to whether the patient is able to close the eyelid. The patient resumes eating when nausea (if any) abates. Pain is generally well controlled by means of oral agents. At discharge, the patient should be warned to protect the numb earlobe against cold injury. The closed-suction drain is kept in place for 5 to 7 days (until the first postoperative visit) to minimize the risk of salivary fistula.

Complications

FACIAL NERVE INJURY

Facial nerve injuries include both intraoperative transection and paralysis. Transection or partial resection of the facial nerve may be intentional, as in the case of a locally advanced cancer with preoperative nerve dysfunction or direct invasion, but can also be inadvertent. If the injury is discovered intraoperatively, it should be repaired if possible. Primary repair—performed with interrupted fine permanent monofilament sutures under magnification[23]—is preferred if sufficient nerve is available for a tension-free anastomosis. If both transected nerve ends are identified but tension-free repair is not feasible, interposition nerve grafts may be used. A sensory nerve harvested from the neck (e.g., the great auricular nerve) is often employed for this purpose. If the nerve is injured (or deliberately sacrificed) in conjunction with treatment of malignancy, use of nerve grafts from distant sites may be indicated[24] but is seldom necessary because uninvolved sensory nerves are almost invariably to be found in the neck Recovery of facial nerve function following grafting occurs at a mean time of 6 to 7 months.[23,25]

Facial nerve function should be assessed immediately in the postanesthesia care unit to establish a baseline as transient paralysis may worsen over time. However, if unexpected facial nerve dysfunction is identified immediately following the operation and if the surgeon is unsure of the anatomic integrity of the nerve (ideally, a rare occurrence), the patient should be returned to the operating room for exploration so that either the continuity of the nerve can be confirmed or the injury to the nerve can be identified and, if possible, repaired. When the surgeon is certain that the nerve is intact, facial nerve dysfunction may be approached expectantly, in anticipation of recovery[24]; however, this may take many months.

Facial nerve paralysis is generally secondary to traction, compression, or ischemic insult. Studies have found that transient paralysis of all or part of the facial nerve occurs in 17 to 100% of patients undergoing parotidectomy[26–29]

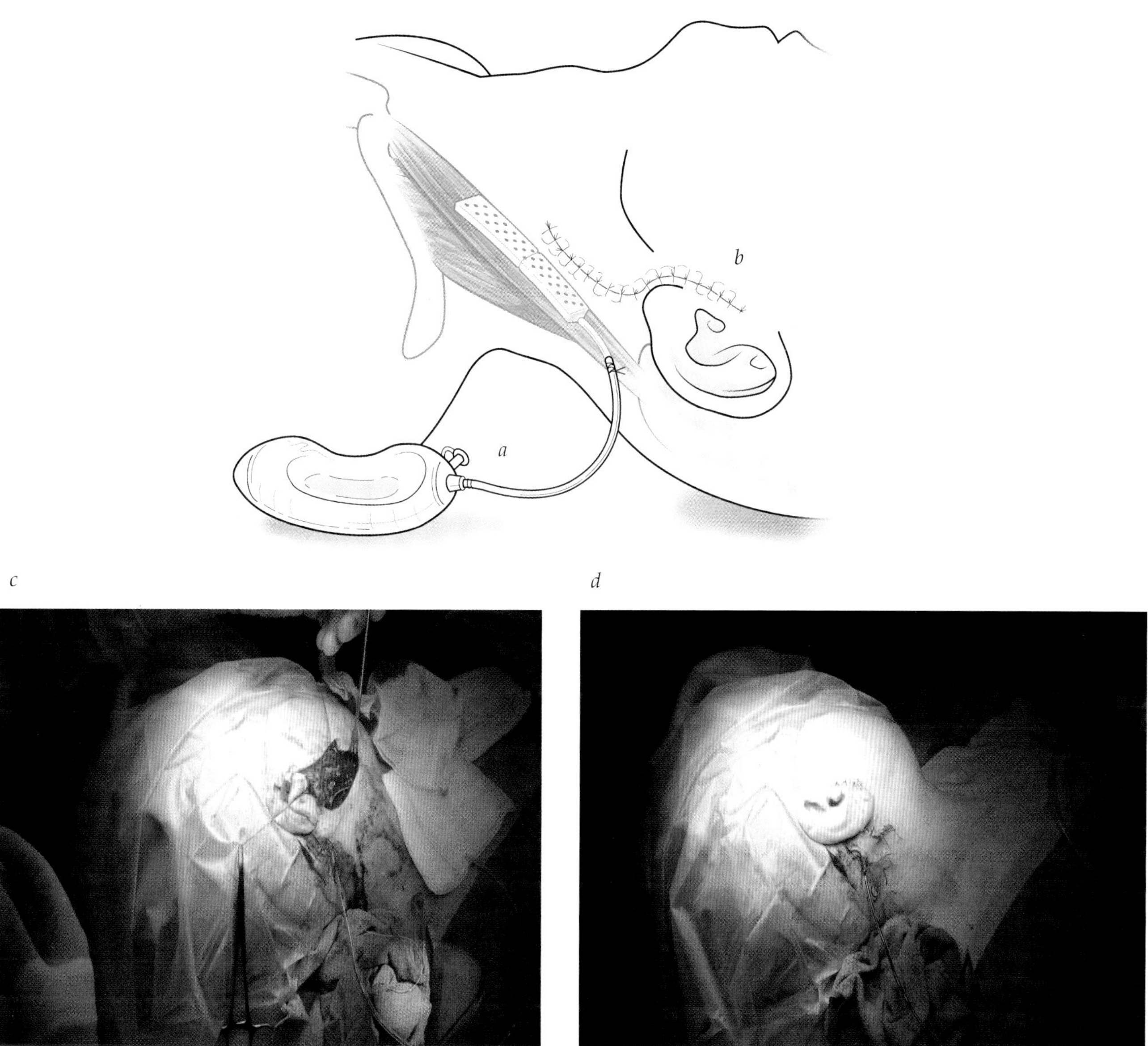

Figure 6 **Parotidectomy. Shown is drainage and closure after parotidectomy. (*a*) A closed-suction drain is placed in the operative bed and loosely tacked to the sternocleidomastoid muscle. (*b*) Interrupted monofilament sutures are used for the skin. Bacitracin is applied. No additional dressings are used. (*c*) Photograph of a patient's wound being drained after parotidectomy. (*d*) Photograph of a patient's wound being closed after parotidectomy.**

depending on the extent of the resection and the location of the tumor. Factors predictive of facial nerve palsy following parotidectomy include prolonged operative time and larger tumor sizes.[28,30] Recovery of nerve function can take between 6 months and 1 year[29–31]; fortunately, permanent paralysis is uncommon, occurring in fewer than 5% of cases.[28,32]

Nerve monitoring has been advocated to reduce the incidence or severity of facial nerve injury, particularly in the setting of resection for a recurrent parotid tumor.[33] To date, however, no randomized trial has demonstrated that intraoperative facial nerve monitoring or nerve stimulators yield any significant reduction in the incidence of facial nerve paralysis after either primary parotidectomy or recurrence surgery. Indeed, indiscriminate use of nerve monitoring and nerve stimulators may imbue the surgeon with a false sense of security and cause him or her to pay insufficient attention to the appearance of nerve tissue. There are grounds to fear that reliance on the nerve monitor may limit the surgeon's ability to identify the appearance of the nerve or its branchses. Transient nerve dysfunction may follow inappropriate (or even appropriate and unavoidable) trauma to or traction and pressure on nerve trunks. Nerve monitoring does not prevent such problems; moreover, it adds to the cost of the procedure and lengthens the operating time.[6,7] Some, in fact, have suggested that nerve stimulators may actually increase transient dysfunction. Accordingly, our use of nerve stimulators is selective and limited to reoperations. Management of enduring facial nerve paralysis (from any cause) is beyond the scope of our discussion and constitutes a surgical subspecialty in itself.

HEMORRHAGE

Hemorrhage is a rare event and is usually secondary to inadequate intraoperative hemostasis. Additional factors that may contribute to bleeding include antiplatelet medications and anticoagulants, which should be discontinued in an appropriate time frame prior to surgery.

Bleeding may manifest postoperatively as a hematoma or persistent oozing at the surgical incision site and almost always presents within the first 24 hours.[34] Although hemostasis may have been established intraoperatively, increased venous return on emergence from anesthesia may disrupt clotted or ligated vessels in the surgical bed (thus, pressure is typically applied at the surgical site during extubation, as noted above). It is important to remember that the parotid space is not easily compressible given the skeletal and muscular boundaries, and pressure is unlikely to resolve an expanding hematoma once it develops. Thus, it is always prudent to return to the operating room for hemostasis when bleeding is suspected postoperatively.

GUSTATORY SWEATING (FREY SYNDROME)

Gustatory sweating, or Frey syndrome, occurs in most patients after parotidectomy; it has been seen after submandibular gland resection as well. The symptom complex includes sweating, skin warmth, and flushing after chewing food and is caused by cross-innervation of the parasympathetic secretomotor fibers supplying the parotid gland and cutaneous sympathetic receptors of the sweat glands and blood vessels in the overlying skin. The reported incidence of Frey syndrome varies greatly, apparently depending on the sensitivity of the test used to elicit it. When Minor's starch iodine test is employed, the incidence of Frey syndrome may reach 95% at 1 year after operation.[35] Fortunately, the majority of patients have only subclinical findings, and only a small fraction complain of debilitating symptoms.[35] Most symptomatic patients are adequately treated with topical antiperspirants; eventually, however, they tend to become noncompliant with such measures, preferring simply to dab the face with a napkin while eating.[35] Despite the relatively low incidence of clinically significant Frey syndrome, there is an extensive literature addressing prevention and additional treatment of this condition.[17,32,36–44]

SIALOCELE (SALIVARY FISTULA)

Sialocele, a collection of salivary fluid underneath the skin flap, and salivary fistulae have been reported to occur after 1 to 15% of parotidectomies.[17,45] Although both conditions are generally minor and self-limited, they may nonetheless be annoying and embarrassing for the patient. The diagnosis is assigned with an increase in clear drainage during eating or mastication or by aspiration of clear fluid with an amylase level sent.[45–47] The incidence of sialocele and fistula can be reduced by maintaining closed-suction drainage for 5 to 7 days (to facilitate adhesion of the skin flaps to the underlying parotid parenchyma). Salivary leaks are usually attributable to gland disruption rather than to duct transection and therefore tend to resolve without difficulty.[48] Once a sialocele has formed, repeated aspiration and compression dressings are generally effective for treatment and typically resolve within 2 weeks.[45] Anticholinergic agents have been used in this setting as well.[46,47,49,50] Low-dose radiation,[51] completion parotidectomy, botulinum toxin injection,[47,52] and tympanic neurectomy[53] have all been employed in refractory cases.

COSMETIC CHANGES

Parotidectomy creates a depression anterior and inferior to the ear, which may extend behind the mandible and may reach a significant size in patients with large or recurrent tumors. This cosmetic change is a necessary feature of the procedure, not a complication; nonetheless, it should be discussed with the patient before operation. Many augmentation methods, using a wide variety of techniques, have been devised for improving postoperative appearance (as well as alleviating Frey syndrome).[37–41,54,55] All of these methods have limitations or drawbacks that have kept them from having wide application and acceptance. None has gained overwhelming favor.

Outcome Evaluation

With proper surgical technique, superficial or partial superficial parotidectomy can be performed safely and within a reasonable operating time. The requirement for blood transfusions should be vanishingly rare. Given adequate exposure, good knowledge of the relevant anatomy, limited trauma to the nerve, and appropriate use of closed-suction drains (see above), complications should be uncommon. Although patients may tolerate parotidectomy on an outpatient basis, we prefer to keep them in the hospital overnight. Patients should be able to leave the hospital with minimal pain, comfortable with their drain care, by the morning of postoperative day 1.

Financial Disclosures: None Reported

References

1. Berkovitz BKG, Moxham BJ. A textbook of head and neck anatomy. Chicago: Year Book Medical Publishers; 1988.
2. Davis BA, Anson BJ, Budinger JM, Kurth LR. Surgical anatomy of the facial nerve and the parotid gland based upon a study of 350 cervicofacial halves. Surg Gynecol Obstet 1956; 102:385–412.
3. Bernstein L, Nelson RH. Surgical anatomy of the extraparotid distribution of the facial nerve. Arch Otolaryngol 1984;110:177–83.
4. Wong DS. Signs and symptoms of malignant parotid tumors: an objective assessment. J R Coll Surg Edinb 2001; 46:91–5.
5. Howlett DC, Kesse KW, Hughes DV, Sallomi DF. The role of imaging in the evaluation of parotid disease. Clin Radiol 2002;57:692–701.

6. Meier JD, Wenig BL, Manders EC, Nenonene EK. Continuous intraoperative facial nerve monitoring in predicting postoperative injury during parotidectomy. Laryngoscope 2006;116:1569–72.
7. Terrell JE, Kileny PR, Yian C, et al. Clinical outcome of continuous facial nerve monitoring during primary parotidectomy. Arch Otolaryngol Head Neck Surg 1997;123:1081–7.
8. Hui Y, Wong DS, Wong LY, et al. A prospective controlled double-blind trial of great auricular nerve preservation at parotidectomy. Am J Surg 2003;185:574–9.
9. Christensen NR, Jacobsen SD. Parotidectomy: preserving the posterior branch of the great auricular nerve. J Laryngol Otol 1997;111:556–9.
10. Cannon CR, Replogle WH, Schenk MP. Facial nerve in parotidectomy: a topographical analysis. Laryngoscope 2004;114:2034–7.
11. Pather N, Osman M. Landmarks of the facial nerve: implications for parotidectomy. Surg Radiol Anat 2006;28:170–5.
12. de Ru JA, van Benthem PP, Bleys RL, et al. Landmarks for parotid gland surgery. J Laryngol Otol 2001;115:122–5.
13. Peterson RA, Johnston DL. Facile identification of the facial nerve branches. Clin Plast Surg 1987;14:785–8.
14. Salame K, Ouaknine GER, Arensburg B, et al. Microsurgical anatomy of the facial nerve trunk. Clin Anat 2002;15:93–9.
15. Colella G, Giudice A, Vicidomini A, Sperlongano P. Usefulness of the LigaSure Vessel Sealing System during superficial lobectomy of the parotid gland. Arch Otolaryngol Head Neck Surg 2005;131:413–6.
16. Jackson LL, Gourin CG, Thomas DS, et al. Use of the harmonic scalpel in superficial and total parotidectomy for benign and malignant disease. Laryngoscope 2005;115: 1070–3.
17. Leverstein H, van der Wal JE, Tiwari RM, et al. Surgical management of 246 previously untreated pleomorphic adenomas of the parotid gland. Br J Surg 1997;84:399–403.
18. Woods JE. Parotidectomy: points of technique for brief and safe operation. Am J Surg 1983;145:678–83.
19. Garden AS, el-Naggar AK, Morrison WH, et al. Postoperative radiotherapy for malignant tumors of the parotid gland. Int J Radiat Oncol Biol Phys 1997;37:79–85.
20. Renehan AG, Gleave EN, Slevin NJ, McGurk M. Clinicopathological and treatment-related factors influencing survival in parotid cancer. Br J Cancer 1999;80:1296–300.
21. Magnano M, Gervasio CF, Cravero L, et al. Treatment of malignant neoplasms of the parotid gland. Otolaryngol Head Neck Surg 1999;121:627–32.
22. Spiro JD, Spiro RH. Cancer of the parotid gland: role of 7th nerve preservation. World J Surg 2003;27:863–7.
23. Eaton DA. Hirsch BE, Mansour OI. Recovery of facial nerve function after repair or grafting: our experience with 24 patients. Am J Otolaryngol 2007;28:37–41.
24. Shindo M. Management of facial nerve paralysis. Otolaryngol Clin North Am 1999;32:945–64.
25. Ozmen OA, Falcioni M, Lauda L, Sanna M. Outcomes of facial nerve grafting in 155 cases: predictive value of history and preoperative function. Otol Neurotol 2011;32:1341–6.
26. Witt RL. Facial nerve monitoring in parotid surgery: the standard of care? Otolaryngol Head Neck Surg 1998;119: 468–70.
27. Reilly J, Myssiorek D. Facial nerve stimulation and postparotidectomy facial paresis. Otolaryngol Head Neck Surg 2003;128:530–3.
28. Dulguerov P, Marchal F, Lehmann W. Postparotidectomy facial nerve paralysis: possible etiologic factors and results with routine facial nerve monitoring. Laryngoscope 1999; 109:754–62.
29. Bron LP, O'Brien CJ. Facial nerve function after parotidectomy. Arch Otolaryngol Head Neck Surg 1997;123:1091–6.
30. Mra Z, Komisar A, Blaugrund SM. Functional facial nerve weakness after surgery for benign parotid tumors: a multivariate statistical analysis. Head Neck 1993;15:147–52.
31. Nouraei SA, Ismail Y, Ferguson MS, et al. Analysis of complications following surgical treatment of benign parotid disease. Aust N Z J Surg 2008;78:134–8.
32. Debets JMH, Munting JDK. Parotidectomy for parotid tumours: 19-year experience from The Netherlands. Br J Surg 1992;79:1159–61.
33. Makeieff M, Venail F, Cartier C, et al. Continuous facial nerve monitoring during pleomorphic adenoma recurrence surgery. Laryngoscope 2005;115:1310–4.
34. Henney SE, Brown R, Phillips D. Parotidectomy: the timing of post-operative complications. Eur Arch Otorhinolaryngol 2010;267:131–5.
35. Linder TE, Huber A, Schmid S. Frey's syndrome after parotidectomy: a retrospective and prospective analysis. Laryngoscope 1997;107:1496–501.
36. Bonanno PC, Palaia D, Rosenberg M, Casson P. Prophylaxis against Frey's syndrome in parotid surgery. Ann Plast Surg 2000;44:498–501.
37. Ahmed OA, Kolhe PS. Prevention of Frey's syndrome and volume deficit after parotidectomy using the superficial temporal artery fascial flap. Br J Plast Surg 1999;52:256–60.
38. Bugis SP, Young JE, Archibald SD. Sternocleidomastoid flap following parotidectomy. Head Neck 1990;12:430–5.
39. Jeng SF, Chien CS. Adipofascial turnover flap for facial contour deformity during parotidectomy. Ann Plast Surg 1994;33:439–41.
40. Govindaraj S, Cohen M, Genden EM, et al. The use of acellular dermis in the prevention of Frey's syndrome. Laryngoscope 2001;111:1993–8.
41. Nosan DK, Ochi JW, Davidson TM. Preservation of facial contour during parotidectomy. Otolaryngol Head Neck Surg 1991;104:293–8.
42. Sinha UK, Saadat D, Doherty CM, Rice DH. Use of AlloDerm implant to prevent Frey syndrome after parotidectomy. Arch Facial Plast Surg 2003;5:109–12.
43. Beerens AJ, Snow GB. Botulinum toxin A in the treatment of patients with Frey syndrome. Br J Surg 2002;89:116–9.
44. Marchese-Ragona R, De Filippis C, Marioni G, Staffieri A. Treatment of complications of parotid gland surgery. Acta Otorhinolaryngol Ital 2005;25:174–8.
45. Wax M, Tarshis L. Post-parotidectomy fistula. J Otolaryngol 1991;20:10–3.
46. Cavanaugh K, Park A. Postparotidectomy fistulas: a different treatment for an old problem. Int J Pediatr Otorhinolaryngol 1999;47:265–8.
47. Vargas H, Galati LT, Parnes SM. A pilot study evaluating the treatment of postparotidectomy sialoceles with

botulinum toxin type A. Arch Otolaryngol Head Neck Surg 2000;126:421–4.
48. Ananthakrishnan N, Parkash S. Parotid fistulas: a review. Br J Surg 1982;69:641–3.
49. Guntinas-Lichius O, Sittel C. Treatment of postparotidectomy salivary fistula with botulinum toxin. Ann Otol Rhinol Laryngol 2001;110:1162–4.
50. Chow TL, Kwok SP. Use of botulinum toxin type A in a case of persistent parotid sialocele. Hong Kong Med J 2003; 9:293–4.
51. Shimms DS, Berk FK, Tilsner TJ, Coulthard SW. Low-dose radiation therapy for benign salivary disorders. Am J Clin Oncol 1992;15:76–8.
52. von Lindern JJ, Niederhagen B, Appel T, et al. New prospects in the treatment of traumatic and postoperative fistulas with type A botulinum toxin. Plast Reconstr Surg 2002;109:2443–5.
53. Davis WE, Holt GR, Templer JW. Parotid fistula and tympanic neurectomy. Am J Surg 1977;133:587–9.
54. Kerawala CJ, McAloney N, Stassen LF. Prospective randomized trial of the benefits of a sternocleidomastoid flap after superficial parotidectomy. Br J Oral Maxillofac Surg 2002;40:468–72.
55. Shridharani SM, Tufaro AP. A systematic review of acellular dermal matrices in head and neck reconstruction. Plast Reconstr Surg 2012;130(5 Suppl 2):35S–43S.

Acknowledgment

Figures 1, 2a, 2b, 3b, 4, 5, 6a, 6b Shannon H. Allen, MD

7 NECK DISSECTION

Miriam N. Lango, MD, FACS, Bert W. O'Malley Jr, MD, FACS, and Ara A. Chalian, MD, FACS

Preoperative Evaluation

In the majority of cases, cancer in the neck is a metastasis from a primary lesion in the upper aerodigestive tract [*see Figure 1*], although metastases from skin, thyroid, and salivary gland neoplasms are also encountered. Lymphomas often present as cervical lymphadenopathy.

When a patient presents with a suspicious lesion in the neck, a careful history and physical examination should be performed, along with a thorough evaluation of the aerodigestive tract aimed at locating the source of possible metastatic disease. Fine-needle aspiration (FNA) of the neck mass should then be done to determine whether the mass is malignant. FNA can often differentiate between epithelial and lymphoid malignancies, and this differentiation will guide subsequent workup. The reported sensitivity of FNA ranges from 92 to 98% and the reported specificity from 94 to 100%.[1,2]

If FNA reveals the presence of atypical lymphoid cells, an excisional lymph node biopsy may be performed if additional tissue is required for adequate tumor typing. However, a lymphoma or leukemia may frequently be typed with FNA biopsy alone.[3] If a Hodgkin lymphoma or low-grade follicular lymphoma is suspected, an open biopsy will be needed to establish the diagnosis. Thus, an excisional biopsy may be performed if the FNA is negative or indeterminate, the surgeon suspects a malignancy, and the rest of the physical examination yields negative results. Routine excisional biopsy of neck masses for diagnostic purposes is not recommended, however, because it may result in tumor spillage into the wound and complicate subsequent definitive resection.

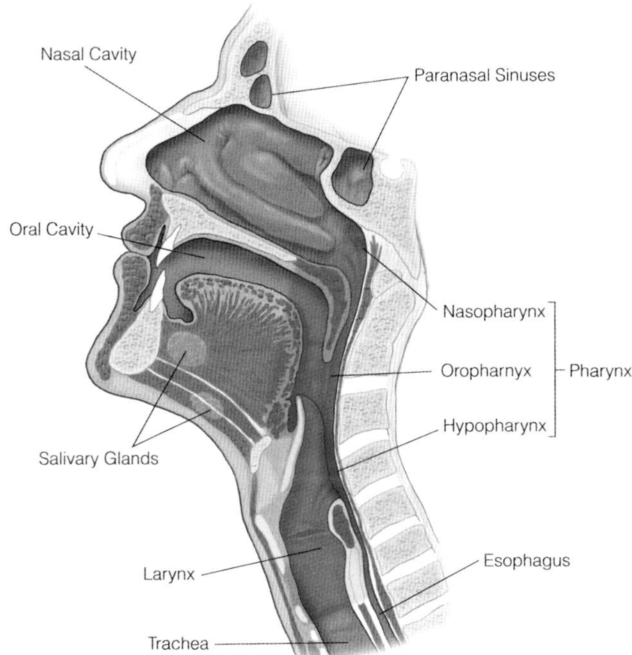

Figure 1 **Sagittal section of the upper aerodigestive tract.**

Once the presence of an epithelial malignancy is established, the primary site of the lesion must be determined. The clinical setting provides clues regarding the source of the cancer. For example, in an elderly patient with a previous history of skin cancer, with abnormal cutaneous lesions over the scalp or face and a nontender, enlarging posterior triangle neck mass, a metastasis from a cutaneous cancer is suspected. Alternatively, in a 50-year-old alcohol abuser with an enlarging level II lymph node also complaining of a several-month history of sore throat and otalgia, a metastasis from a pharyngeal primary cancer should be entertained. In any patient with metastatic cervical adenopathy thought to originate in the upper aerodigestive tract, panendoscopy and biopsy with general anesthesia are mandatory for locating and characterizing the primary source of the tumor and ruling out the presence of synchronous lesions. The most common occult primary sites are the base of the tongue, the tonsils, and the nasopharynx. Imaging studies (e.g., computed tomography [CT] and magnetic resonance imaging) may be helpful in locating the source of a cervical metastasis. Positron emission tomography (PET) detects lesions with increased metabolic activity but has the limitation of being unable to detect lesions smaller than 1 cm in diameter. Primary lesions greater than 1 cm in diameter usually are easily identified on physical examination and other imaging studies; thus, PET scans add little in this setting. In 5 to 10% of patients who present with a metastatic node, the primary lesion is never found despite extensive workup.

INCIDENCE AND IMPACT OF NECK METASTASES

Cutaneous Squamous Cell Carcinoma

The incidence of cervical metastases is governed by many factors. Cervical metastases from cutaneous squamous cell carcinomas are rare, occurring in 2 to 10% of cases. However, certain lesions—those that are greater than 2 cm in diameter; are recurrent; are deeper than 6 mm; involve the ear, the temple, or the classic H zone; occur in an immunocompromised patient; or are poorly differentiated—have a significant occult metastatic rate, ranging from 20 to 60%.[4] The presence of cervical metastases reduces 5-year survival by approximately 50%.[5–7] Nevertheless, postoperative radiation rather than elective lymphadenectomy is usually recommended for high-risk cutaneous squamous cell carcinomas.[8]

Salivary Gland Neoplasms

With salivary gland neoplasms, the incidence of cervical metastases is related to the histopathology and the size of the tumor. The most aggressive salivary gland lesions are squamous cell carcinoma, carcinoma ex pleomorphic adenoma, adenocarcinoma, and salivary ductal carcinoma. Patients with these lesions often have cervical metastases at presentation that warrant a therapeutic neck dissection [*see Table 1*]. How best to manage occult cervical salivary gland metastatic disease is controversial. The occult metastatic rate for aggressive lesions ranges from 25 to 45%. For such lesions, a selective neck dissection is typically incorporated into the surgical approach.[9]

Metastatic Well-Differentiated Thyroid Cancer

The American Thyroid Association Risk of Recurrence Classification recognizes the presence of papillary thyroid cancer metastases to the neck as risk factors increasing the risk of recurrence.[10] The presence of macroscopic metastases detected on imaging studies is more clinically significant than metastatic disease identified incidentally.[11] Less than one half of patients with macroscopic nodal disease in the lateral compartment achieve a complete biochemical response to treatment (defined as a stimulated/unstimulated thyroglobulin level of less than 1 ng/mL and negative imaging, within 24 months of initial treatment).[12] A postoperative stimulated thyroglobulin of 50 ng/mL or more, obtained after surgery but before radioiodine treatment, is a strong predictor of disease persistence in patients with metastatic papillary thyroid carcinoma,[13] but this value is reliable only in patients who have undergone a complete thyroidectomy. Patients with elevated stimulated thyroglobulin levels virtually never achieve a complete biochemical response, more often harbor extranodal extension of cancer, and require additional neck surgery in up to 80% of cases.[12] A careful preoperative ultrasound evaluation of neck compartments is mandatory in patients with metastatic papillary carcinoma. The pattern of metastatic spread has been well described previously.[14,15] The modified radical neck dissection for metastatic thyroid cancer has been shown to be safe with acceptable morbidity[16] and is more effective than so-called cherry-picking operations or limited lymph node excisions, which result in higher rates of recurrence.[5]

Table 1 Incidence of Cervical Metastases in Selected Head and Neck Cancers

Tumor	*Incidence of Cervical Adenopathy (%)*
Cutaneous squamous cell carcinoma	2–10
Salivary gland malignancies Mucoepidermoid carcinoma (high grade)	30–70
Adenoid cystic carcinoma	8
Malignant mixed tumor	25
Squamous cell carcinoma	46
Salivary duct carcinoma	50
Acinic cell carcinoma	40
Metastatic well-differentiated thyroid cancer	10–15
Squamous cell carcinoma of upper aerodigestive tract	
Alveolar ridge	30
Hard palate	10
Oral tongue	30
Anterior pillar/retromolar trigone	45
Floor of mouth	30
Soft palate	44
Tonsillar fossa	76
Tongue base	78
Bilateral	20

Squamous Cell Carcinoma of the Upper Aerodigestive Tract

With upper aerodigestive tract squamous cell carcinomas, the incidence of cervical metastases is related to the site of the primary lesion, the size of the tumor, the degree of differentiation, the depth of invasion,[17,18] and other biologic factors. A significant proportion of head and neck cancer patients who harbor clinically silent primary tumors of the base of the tongue, the tonsils, or the nasopharynx initially present with cervical adenopathy [*see Table 1*]. These sites lack anatomic barriers that limit tumor spread and are supplied by rich lymphatic networks that facilitate metastasis. In contrast, patients with glottic and lip cancers rarely present with clinical adenopathy.

The presence of cervical metastases negatively affects prognosis and has been associated with increased recurrence rates and reduced disease-free and overall survival. The presence of clinical adenopathy decreases survival by 50%. Metastatic tumors that rupture the lymph node capsule—a process known as extracapsular spread (ECS)—are biologically more aggressive. Patients who have palpable cervical lymphadenopathy with ECS manifest a 50% decrease in survival compared with those who have palpable cervical lymphadenopathy without ECS.[19] In addition, about 50% of clinically negative, pathologically positive neck specimens exhibit ECS. Clinically negative, pathologically positive, and ECS-positive specimens are associated with a high risk of regional recurrence and distant metastases.[20–22] The presence of extracapsular extension (ECE) is an indication for adjuvant concurrent chemoradiation, which has been shown to decrease the risk of recurrence and improve survival in randomized clinical trials.[23,24]

Until recently, the presence of ECE in lymph node metastases was considered the single most important prognostic factor in patients with head and neck cancer. Since the identification of human papillomavirus (HPV) in head and neck cancers originating in the oropharynx, ECE has been shown to have a lesser impact on recurrence and disease-free survival than HPV status.[25–27] Indeed, the feasibility of any study attempting to demonstrate a difference in prognosis among patients with HPV-related oropharyngeal cancer will be hampered by the generally favorable outcomes of this subset of patients. Nevertheless, ECE remains an important marker of prognosis among HPV-negative head and neck cancer patients.

STAGING OF NECK CANCER

For most tumor types, the presence of nodal metastases has a significant effect on prognosis and affects subsequent treatment recommendations. The limitations of clinical staging of the neck are well described. In particular, patients with short, thick necks are challenging to stage accurately on physical examination alone. The addition of imaging to clinical examination improves diagnostic sensitivity. The pathologic review of neck dissection specimens, however, remains the gold standard for anatomic staging. Given that elective neck dissection (a compartment-oriented sampling of at-risk neck levels for diagnostic purposes in the absence of clinical or radiographic metastases) carries some morbidity, alternatives to routine elective neck dissection have been investigated. Sentinel lymph node biopsy is now routinely used to stage the regional lymphatics in melanoma and Merkel cell carcinoma. The results from the First International Conference on Sentinel Node Biopsy in Mucosal Head and Neck Cancer revealed that sentinel lymph node biopsy of the clinically negative neck has a sensitivity comparable to that of a staging neck dissection,[28] although this technology is not currently used to stage head and neck cancer in routine clinical practice. Currently, a cooperative group has launched a multi-institutional study to investigate whether the negative PET-CT study can be used to justify withholding an elective neck dissection for patients with head and neck cancers radiographically staged N0. The results should be forthcoming in the next few years.

Staging of the neck for metastatic squamous cell carcinomas of the head and neck is based on the TNM classification formulated by the American Joint Committee on Cancer (AJCC). The N classification applies to cervical metastases from all upper aerodigestive tract mucosal sites except the nasopharynx and mucosal melanoma; in addition, neck staging for cutaneous squamous cell carcinoma, sinonasal, and salivary gland malignancies uses a similar form, characterizing nodal metastases with respect to number (0, 1, or more), size (> 3 or 6 cm), and location (ipsilateral, bilateral, or contralateral neck). For nasopharyngeal carcinoma, nodal disease greater than 6 cm, bilateral and/or involving the supraclavicular fossa, carries a worse prognosis. Thyroid cancer has its own staging system. Given that the AJCC staging is updated every few years, it is important to use the most current system available when assigning tumor stage.

INDICATIONS FOR NECK DISSECTION

The indication for neck dissection may be diagnostic, to identify clinically and radiographically occult nodal metastases in the neck by means of an elective neck dissection, or therapeutic, performed to remove clinically or radiographically identifiable disease. In patients with head and neck cancer, neck dissection may be performed as part of the initial definitive treatment, often combined with resection of the primary cancer. Alternatively, neck dissection may be performed in an adjuvant setting to remove residual cancer in the neck following treatment with radiation or chemoradiation. Regardless, a compartment-oriented approach within anatomically defined cervical levels is recommended in all cases. Six lymph node drainage basins in the neck are formally recognized [*see Figure* 2]. In contrast to comprehensive neck dissections, which involve resection levels I to V, selective neck dissection involves resection of nodal levels removed according to predicted drainage patterns from specific primary sites of the upper aerodigestive tract.[2] Neck

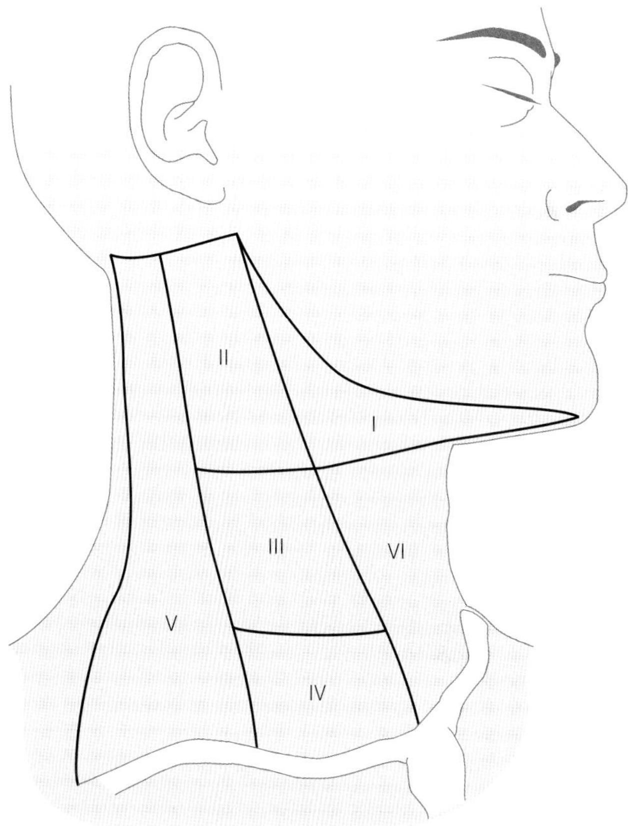

Figure 2 **Cervical lymph nodes are divided into six levels on the basis of their location in the neck.**

dissections may also be extended to remove structures involved by cancer (e.g., hypoglossal nerve, carotid artery). Posterolateral neck dissections that include the resection of postauricular and suboccipial nodes, in addition to the contents of other neck levels, are most often used to manage metastatic cutaneous malignancies arising in the scalp. In managing metastatic cutaneous cancers including melanoma, greater attention to resecting superficial nodes, such as those along the external jugular vein, is necessary. Given that metastatic disease frequently also involves the parotid gland in metastatic cutaneous malignancies, parotidectomy is often indicated as well. Operative reporting should include an account of the nodal levels resected, and anatomic structures that were preserved and sacrificed.

CONTRAINDICATIONS TO NECK DISSECTION

Contraindications to neck dissection can be medical or surgical. A patient can be medically inoperable due to the presence of comorbid medical problems. The only absolute surgical contraindication to neck dissection is surgical unresectability. There is no formal definition of resectability. Nevertheless, the designation suggests that a gross-total resection of the cancer will not be possible on anatomic grounds. The determination of unresectability is made by the operating surgeon either preoperatively, on the basis of imaging studies, or in the operating room. Typically, the presence of Horner syndrome, paralysis of the vagus nerve or the phrenic nerve, or invasion of the brachial plexus or the prevertebral muscles indicates that the tumor is unresectable. The involvement of the carotid artery may be predicted on the basis of imaging studies. Encasement of the carotid artery by tumor suggests direct invasion of the vessel; studies correlating imaging characteristics and pathologic invasion of the carotid have shown that tumors surrounding 180 or more of the carotid's circumference have a higher incidence of carotid invasion than tumors surrounding less than 180 (75% versus 50%). In the absence of direct invasion of the vessel wall, tumor may be peeled off by means of subadventitial surgical dissection. Tumors surrounding 270 of the vessel have an 83% incidence of carotid invasion, necessitating sacrifice of the artery.[29] However, sacrifice of the carotid artery, with or without reconstruction with a vein graft, has been associated with significant morbidity. The survival of patients with such extensive neck disease is uniformly poor.[30]

The presence of skin involvement in nodal disease may be attributed to direct extension or dermal lymphatic infiltration. Although direct extension of cancer, such as ECE, suggests more aggressive disease, skin involvement is not a contraindication to neck dissection per se. However, the presence of dermal metastases, seen more often in the setting of disease recurrence, such as the presence of distant metastases, suggests a very poor prognosis.

Operative Planning

CHOICE OF PROCEDURE

Comprehensive Dissection: Radical and Modified Radical Neck Dissection

The radical neck dissection was first described in 1906 by George Crile, who based his approach on the Halstedian principle of en bloc resection.[31] The procedure was subsequently standardized by Hayes Martin at Memorial Hospital in New York in the 1930s and 1940s. In this latter version of the procedure, lymphatic structures from the strap muscles anteriorly, the trapezius posteriorly, the mandible superiorly, and the clavicle inferiorly are removed. Nonlymphatic structures in this space are also sacrificed, including the spinal accessory nerve, the sternocleidomastoid muscle, the internal and external jugular veins, the submandibular gland, and sensory nerve roots. The routine sacrifice of the spinal accessory nerve, the internal jugular vein, and the sternocleidomastoid muscle contributes to the significant morbidity associated with radical neck dissection.

Since the 1970s, the necessity of en bloc resection for oncologic cure has been reexamined. Structures once routinely sacrificed are now usually preserved unless they are grossly involved with cancer. The various functional, or modified, radical neck dissections are classified according to which structures are preserved. Type I dissections preserve the spinal accessory nerve; type II, the spinal accessory nerve and the internal jugular vein; and type III, both of these structures, along with the sternocleidomastoid muscle. Modified radical neck dissections have proved to be as effective in controlling metastatic disease to the neck as the classic radical neck dissection.[32]

Selective Neck Dissection

In a selective neck dissection, at-risk lymph node drainage basins are selectively removed on the basis of the location of the primary tumor in a patient with no clinical evidence of cervical lymphadenopathy. Cancers in the oral cavity, for example, typically metastasize to levels I through III and, occasionally, IV; laryngeal cancers typically metastasize to levels II through IV. The rationale for selective neck dissection is based on retrospective pathologic reviews of radical neck dissection specimens from patients without palpable lymphadenopathy. These reviews revealed that lymph node micrometastases were confined to specific neck levels for a given aerodigestive tract site.[33]

The advantages of selective neck dissection over radical and modified radical neck dissection are both cosmetic and functional. A selective neck dissection involves less manipulation (and thus less risk of traction-related injury as well as devascularization) of the spinal accessory nerve, thereby decreasing the incidence of postoperative shoulder dysfunction. Preservation of the sternocleidomastoid muscle alleviates the cosmetic deformity seen with a radical neck dissection and provides some protection for the carotid artery. Preservation of the internal jugular vein decreases venous congestion of the head and neck and is necessary if the contralateral internal jugular vein is sacrificed.

The growing focus on preservation of function and limitation of morbidity has led some surgeons to promote the use of selective neck dissection to treat node-positive neck tumors. Although retrospective studies have suggested that a selective neck dissection may be adequate in carefully selected node-positive patients,[34] the effectiveness of this approach is still unproven, and its application remains subject to individual surgical judgment. Of patients with node-positive disease, those with HPV-positive head and neck cancer and low-volume metastases appear to be most appropriate for management with a selective neck dissection.[35] A finding of multiple pathologically positive lymph nodes with or without ECS suggest adjuvant therapy is indicated.[36]

Extended Neck Dissection

Extended neck dissections can be combined with selective or comprehensive neck dissections to remove additional nodal basins, such as the suboccipital and retroauricular nodes. These groups of nodes, which are located in the upper posterior neck, are the first-echelon nodal basins for posterior scalp skin cancers, including melanoma, squamous cell carcinoma, and others. The retroauricular nodes lie just posterior to the mastoid process, and the suboccipital nodes lie near the insertion of the trapezius muscle into the inferior nuchal line. Cancers of the anterior scalp, the temple, and the preauricular skin drain to periparotid lymph nodes; these lymph nodes are removed in conjunction with a parotidectomy. Retropharyngeal nodes may be removed in the treatment of selected cancers originating in the posterior pharynx, the soft palate, or the nasopharynx. A mediastinal lymph node dissection may be combined with a neck dissection in the treatment of metastatic thyroid carcinomas.

Bilateral Neck Dissection

With primary lesions located in the midline in the base of the tongue, the supraglottic larynx, or the medial wall of the piriform sinus, bilateral regional metastases are common, and bilateral neck dissections are therefore indicated. Provided that at least one internal jugular vein is preserved, bilateral neck dissection is well tolerated. In contrast, sacrifice of both internal jugular veins is associated with significant morbidity, including increased intracranial pressure, syndrome of inappropriate antidiuretic hormone secretion, airway edema, and death. Bilateral internal jugular sacrifice is managed by staging the neck dissections or by carrying out vascular repair.

NECK DISSECTION AFTER CHEMORADIATION

The indications for neck dissection have been significantly affected by the increasing use of organ preservation protocols for the treatment of head and neck cancer. Following chemoradiation, neck dissection is reserved for patients with an incomplete clinical response to treatment who are at high risk for cancer recurrence in the neck. Most patients with early nodal disease (N0 or N1) treated according to organ preservation protocols do not require neck dissection. Patients who have advanced neck disease (N2 or N3) are less likely to respond completely to nonsurgical treatment and require a neck dissection. Patients with HPV-related oropharyngeal cancer are more likely to respond completely to treatment with radiation and chemotherapy, both radiographically and clinically.[37] Thus, waiting for the results of a PET-CT scan, obtained 3 months after the completion of radiation, will enable most patients with HPV-positive oropharyngeal cancer to avoid neck dissection.

Early surgery (within 8 to 10 weeks) may be considered for patients unlikely to have a complete response to nonsurgical treatment, such as those with HPV-negative head and neck cancer. Imaging with CT of the neck 4 weeks after radiation can be used to evaluate the clinical response following chemoradiation in high-risk patients. The presence of nodes on a CT scan measuring greater than 1.5 cm or any nodes with focal lucency, enhancement, or calcification has been shown to be a sensitive marker of residual disease in the neck.[38]

Early neck dissection (less than 3 to 4 months after radiation) has several advantages. The absence of soft tissue fibrosis simplifies the surgical dissection and diminishes surgery-related complications. Moreover, surgery also becomes less effective in clearing disease from the neck, and surgical treatment of such so-called neck failures is rarely curative.[39] Observation of necks suspected of harboring residual cancer after chemoradiation is therefore not recommended.

After chemoradiation, neck dissection of levels involved based on imaging studies is the minimum extent of lymphadenectomy. Pathologic reviews of comprehensive neck specimens after chemoradiation reveal that in patients with oropharyngeal cancer, levels I and V are rarely involved in the absence of radiographic abnormalities,[40] which suggests that a selective dissection involving levels II through IV may be sufficient. Patients with residual cancer in the neck following radiation or chemoradiation are at greater risk for recurrence than patients who are found to have negative pathologic specimens after neck dissection.[41] Recurrences less often involve the neck than distant sites.[42] Adjuvant treatment may be beneficial for such high-risk patients and may be treated through a national cooperative study group trial.

RECONSTRUCTION AND RECURRENCE AFTER NECK DISSECTION

The use of microvascular free tissue transfer to reconstruct surgical defects in the head has allowed surgeons to resect large tumors with large margins while simultaneously achieving improved functional results. Preservation of vascular—and, occasionally, neural—structures during neck dissection may facilitate the reconstructive process. Typically, several vessels, including an artery and one or two veins, are required for inflow and outflow into a free flap. The facial artery, the retromandibular vein, and the external jugular vein, which are preserved during level I and level II dissection, are the vessels that are most frequently used for flap revascularization. If these vessels are unavailable as a consequence of high-volume neck disease, the superior thyroid artery and the transverse artery, with companion veins, are suitable substitutes. To date, there is no evidence in the literature that preservation of vascular structures in the neck predisposes patients to regional recurrence. Caution must, however, be exercised in the setting of pathologic lymphadenopathy.

Operative Technique

RADICAL NECK DISSECTION

Step 1: Incision and Flap Elevation

When a radical or modified radical neck dissection is indicated, appropriate neck incisions must be designed so as to facilitate exposure while preserving blood flow to the skin flaps [*see Figure 3*]. The incision provides access to the relevant levels of the neck, affects cosmesis, and determines the extent of lymphedema and postoperative fibrosis ("woody" neck), especially in previously irradiated areas. If a biopsy was previously performed, the tract should be excised and incorporated into the new incision. When a total laryngectomy is done, the stoma may be fashioned separately from the neck incision; in the event of a pharyngocutaneous fistula, the salivary flow will be diverted away from the stoma.

Once the incision is made, subplatysmal flaps are raised. If there is extensive lymphadenopathy or extension of tumor into the soft tissues of the neck, skin flaps may be raised in a supraplatysmal plane to ensure negative surgical margins. Such flaps, however, are not as reliably vascularized as subplatysmal flaps. Clinical judgment must be exercised in these situations. The flaps are raised to the mandible superiorly, the clavicle inferiorly, the omohyoid muscle and the submental region anteriorly, and the trapezius posteriorly. Radical neck dissection for bulky cervical adenopathy typically necessitates wide exposure of levels I through V. If a vertical limb is used [*see Figure 3d*], it must not be centered over the carotid artery, because of the risk of potentially catastrophic dehiscence. Deep utility-type incisions yield more limited exposure of level I but provide reliable vascular inflow to skin flaps.

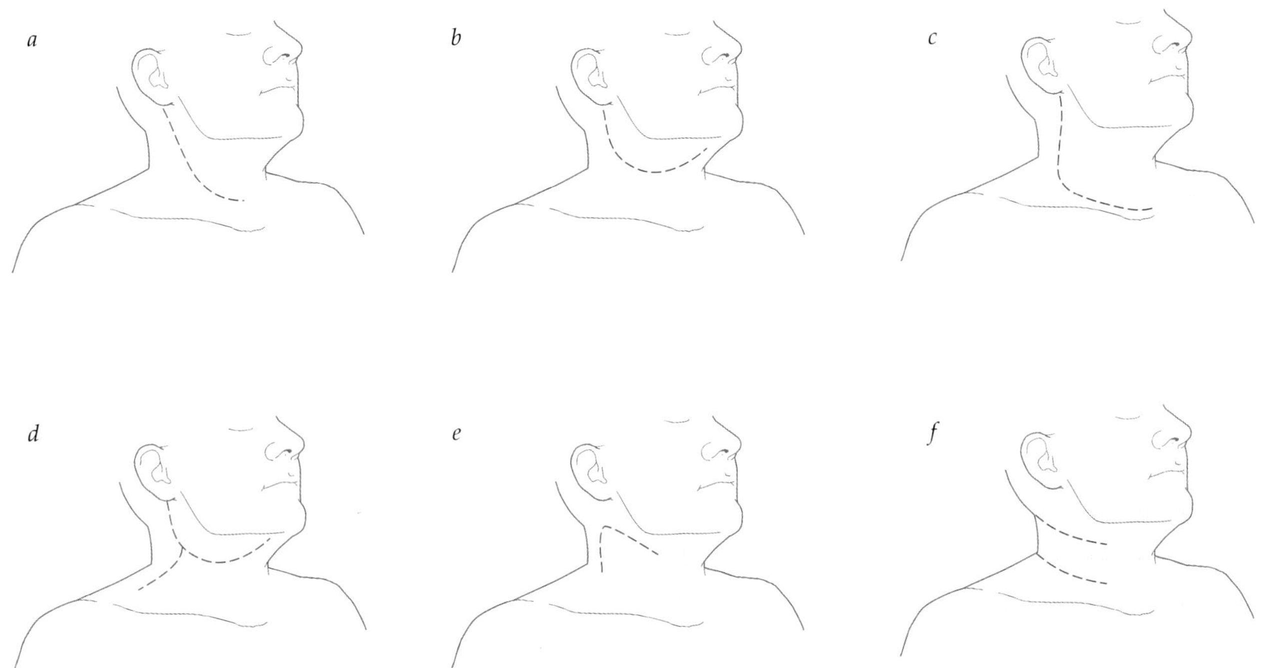

Figure 3 **Incisions used for neck dissections. Incision design is a critical element of operative planning. Incisions are chosen with the aims of optimizing exposure of relevant neck levels and minimizing morbidity. The incisions depicted in (*a*) and (*b*) are useful for selective neck dissections. For the more extensive exposure required in a radical or modified radical neck dissection, a deeper half-apron–style incision (*c*) may be used, or a vertical limb may be dropped from a mastoid-submental incision (*d*), the latter [illegible] vital structures such as the carotid. The incision depicted in (*e*) is also useful for selective neck dissections. The Macfee incision (*f*) provides limited exposure and results in persisent lymphedema in the bipedicled skin flap.**

Step 2: Dissection of Anterior Compartment

Embedded within the fascia overlying the submandibular gland is the marginal mandibular branch of the facial nerve, which must be elevated and retracted to prevent lower lip weakness. The submental fat pad is then grasped, retracted posteriorly and laterally, and mobilized away from the floor of the submental triangle. The omohyoid muscle is identified inferior to the digastric tendon and followed inferiorly to the sternocleidomastoid muscle. The omohyoid muscle forms the anteroinferior limit of the dissection.

Fat and lymphatic structures are dissected away from the digastric muscle and the mylohyoid muscle. The hypoglossal and lingual nerves lie just deep to the mylohyoid muscle and are protected by it [*see Figure 4*]. In this region, the distal end of the facial artery can be identified and preserved as needed for reconstructive purposes. Once the posterior edge of the mylohyoid muscle is visualized, an Army-Navy retractor is inserted beneath the muscle to expose the submandibular duct, the lingual nerve with its attachment to the submandibular gland, and the hypoglossal nerve. The submandibular duct and the submandibular ganglion, with its contributions to the gland, are ligated, and the submandibular gland is retracted out of the submandibular triangle.

The posterior belly of the digastric muscle is then identified inferior to the submandibular gland and skeletonized to the sternocleidomastoid muscle posteriorly, where it inserts on the mastoid tip. The specimen must be mobilized off structures just inferior to the digastric muscle. To prevent inadvertent injury, it is essential to understand the relationships among these structures [*see Figure 4*]. The hypoglossal nerve emerges from beneath the mylohyoid muscle and passes into the neck under the digastric muscle. It then loops around the external carotid artery at the origin of the occipital artery and ascends to the skull base between the external carotid artery and the internal jugular vein. Often the hypoglossal nerve is surrounded by a plexus of small veins, branching off the common facial vein. Bleeding in this region places the hypoglossal nerve at risk. The jugular vein, located just posterior to the external carotid artery and the hypoglossal nerve, may be isolated and doubly suture-ligated at this point. Frequently, the spinal accessory nerve is identified just lateral and posterior to the internal jugular vein, proceeding posteriorly into the sternocleidomastoid muscle.

In a radical neck dissection, the sternocleidomastoid muscle and the spinal accessory nerve are transected at this point and elevated off the splenius capitis and the levator scapulae to the trapezius posteriorly. The anterior edge of the trapezius is skeletonized from the occiput to the clavicle. In a radical neck dissection, the accessory nerve is again transected where it penetrates the trapezius.

Step 3: Control of Internal Jugular Vein Inferiorly; Ligation of Lymphatic Pedicle

The sternal and clavicular heads of the sternocleidomastoid muscle are transected and elevated to expose the anterior belly of the omohyoid muscle. The soft tissue overlying

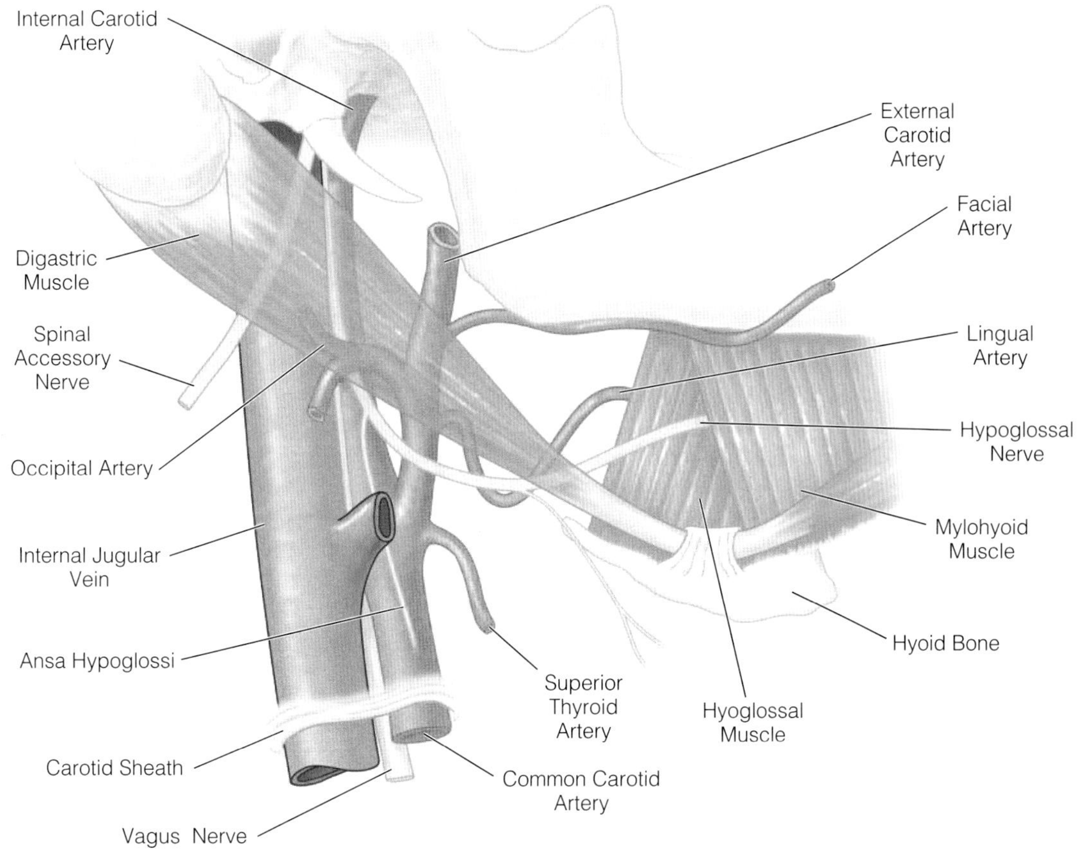

Figure 4 **The key anatomic relationships in levels I and II that must be kept in mind in performing a neck dissection. View is of the right neck.**

the posterior belly of the omohyoid muscle is clamped and ligated as necessary. The omohyoid muscle is then transected, and the jugular vein, the carotid artery, and the vagus nerve are exposed. The jugular vein is isolated and doubly suture-ligated. Care is taken not to transect the adjacent vagus nerve and carotid artery. The lymphatic tissues in the base of the neck adjacent to the internal jugular vein are clamped and suture-ligated 1 cm superior to the clavicle. If a chyle leak is encountered, a figure-eight stitch is placed along the lymphatic pedicle until there is no evidence of clear or turbid fluid on the Valsalva maneuver. Care is taken to avoid inadvertent injury to the vagus nerve or the phrenic nerve, which course through this region.

Step 4: Mobilization of Supraclavicular Fat Pad ("Bloody Gulch")

The fascia overlying the supraclavicular fat pad is incised, and the supraclavicular fat pad is bluntly retracted superiorly so as to free the tissues from the supraclavicular fossa. If transverse cervical vessels are encountered, they are clamped and ligated as necessary. Fascia is left on the deep muscles of the neck, which also envelop the brachial plexus and the phrenic nerve.

Step 5: Dissection and Removal of Specimen

Attention is then turned to the posterior aspect of the neck. Fat and lymphatic tissues are retracted anteriorly with Allis clamps, and the specimen is dissected off the deep muscles of the neck with a blade. Again, a layer of fascia is left on the deep cervical musculature: stripping fascia off the deep cervical musculature results in denervation of these muscles, which adds to the morbidity associated with accessory nerve sacrifice. Once the specimen is mobilized beyond the phrenic nerve, the cervical nerves (C1–C4) may be divided. The specimen is peeled off the carotid artery and removed.

Step 6: Closure

The neck incision is closed in layers over suction drains.

MODIFIED RADICAL NECK DISSECTION

The incision is made and flaps are elevated as in a radical neck dissection. Care must be exercised in elevating the posterior skin flap. Typically, the platysma is deficient in this area, and often no natural plane exists. Dissection deep in the posterior triangle may result in inadvertent injury to the spinal accessory nerve, which travels inferiorly and posteriorly across the posterior triangle in a relatively superficial plane to innervate the trapezius.

A type I modified radical neck dissection begins with dissections of levels I and II, as described for a radical neck dissection (see above). The spinal accessory nerve is identified just superficial or posterior to the internal jugular vein and preserved; the distal spinal accessory nerve is then identified in the posterior triangle. Typically, the spinal accessory nerve can be identified 1 cm superior to the cervical plexus along the posterior border of the sternocleidomastoid muscle. Provided that the patient is not fully paralyzed, the surgeon can distinguish this nerve from adjacent sensory branches by using a nerve stimulator.

Once the spinal accessory nerve is identified, it is dissected and mobilized distally. Proximally, the nerve is dissected through the sternocleidomastoid muscle, which is transected over the nerve. The branch to the sternocleidomastoid muscle is divided with Metz scissors, and the nerve is fully mobilized from the trapezius posteroinferiorly to the posterior belly of the digastric muscle anterosuperiorly and then gently retracted out of the way.

The rest of the neck dissection proceeds as described for a radical neck dissection. If the tumor does not involve the internal jugular vein, it may also be preserved; this constitutes a type II modified radical neck dissection. If the spinal accessory nerve, the internal jugular vein, and the sternocleidomastoid muscle are all preserved, the procedure is a type III modified radical neck dissection. In a type III dissection, the sternocleidomastoid muscle is fully mobilized and retracted with two broad Penrose drains, and the contents of the neck are exposed. The spinal accessory nerve is preserved thoughout its entire course, including the branch to the sternocleidomastoid muscle. The remainder of the neck dissection proceeds as previously described (see above).

SELECTIVE NECK DISSECTION

Levels I to IV

In a selective neck dissection, the posterior triangle is not removed; thus, there is no need to elevate skin flaps posterior to the sternocleidomastoid muscle. Limited elevation of skin flaps is beneficial, particularly for patients who have previously undergone chemoradiation therapy, in whom extensive flap elevation may contribute to significant persistent lymphedema after operation. Subplatysmal skin flaps are raised sufficiently to expose the neck levels to be dissected, with the central compartment left undisturbed. If level I dissection is planned, the fascia overlying the submandibular gland is raised and retracted so as to preserve the marginal nerve. The submental fat pad is grasped and mobilized away from the floor of the submental triangle (composed of the anterior belly of the digastric muscle and the mylohyoid muscle). Inferiorly, the lymphatic tissues are mobilized off the posterior aspect of the omohyoid muscle, which forms the anteroinferior limit of the neck dissection.

Once the digastric tendon and the posterior edge of the mylohyoid muscle are visualized, the mylohyoid is retracted with an Army-Navy retractor so that the submandibular duct, the lingual nerve with its attachment to the submandibular gland, and the hypoglossal nerve are visualized. The submandibular duct and ganglion are ligated, and the submandibular gland is retracted out of the submandibular triangle.

At this point, the facial artery is encountered and suture-ligated. Because the artery curves around the submandibular gland, the facial artery, if not preserved, must be ligated twice (proximally and distally). If the neck dissection is part of a large extirpative procedure involving free flap reconstruction, the facial artery is preserved for use in microvascular anastomosis.

The posterior belly of the digastric muscle is then identified inferior to the submandibular gland. This muscle has been referred to as one of several "resident's friends" in the neck because it serves to protect several critical structures that lie just deep to it, including the hypoglossal nerve, the external carotid artery, the internal jugular vein, and the spinal accessory nerve [*see Figure 5*]. The posterior belly of the digastric muscle is skeletonized to the sternocleidomastoid muscle, where it inserts on the mastoid tip. The specimen is then mobilized away from structures just inferior to the digastric muscle. The hypoglossal nerve emerges from beneath the mylohyoid muscle and passes into the neck just below the digastric muscle, looping around the external carotid artery at the origin of the occipital artery and ascending to the skull base between the external carotid artery and the internal jugular vein. Bleeding from small branches of the common facial vein that envelop the hypoglossal nerve places this structure at risk for injury. The spinal accessory nerve is often visualized just superficial or posterior to the internal jugular vein, extending posteriorly to innervate the sternocleidomastoid muscle.

Next, the fascia overlying the sternocleidomastoid muscle is grasped and unrolled medially throughout its length, starting at the anterior edge of the muscle. The fascia is removed until the spinal accessory nerve is identified at the point where it penetrates the muscle. This nerve is dissected and mobilized superiorly through fat and lymphatic tissues to the digastric muscle. Care must be taken not to inadvertently injure the internal jugular vein, which lies in close proximity to the nerve superiorly. Tissue posterior to the accessory nerve is grasped and freed from the deep muscles of the neck, the digastric muscle superiorly, and the sternocleidomastoid muscle posteriorly. The tissue included in so-called level IIb is passed beneath the spinal accessory nerve and incorporated into the main specimen.

The sternocleidomastoid muscle is retracted, and the fascia posterior to the internal jugular vein is incised. Dissection is carried down to the deep cervical musculature and cervical nerves, which form the floor of the dissection. The specimen is retracted anteriorly. A layer of fascia is left on the deep cervical musculature and the cervical nerves to preserve innervation of the deep muscles of the neck and protect the phrenic nerve as it courses over the anterior scalene muscle.

The specimen is peeled off the internal jugular vein and removed. Dissection too far posteriorly behind the vein may result in injury to the vagus nerve or the sympathetic trunk and predisposes to postoperative thrombosis of the vein. Ligation of internal jugular vein branches should be done without affecting the caliber of the vein or giving the vessel a "sausage link" appearance, which would create turbulent flow patterns predisposing to thrombosis. Overall, gentle dissection around all vessels, with care taken to avoid pulling-related trauma, minimizes the risk of endothelial injury.

A level IV dissection may be facilitated by retracting the omohyoid muscle inferiorly or by dividing it for additional exposure. The tissue inferior to the omohyoid is mobilized and delivered with the main specimen. The lymphatic

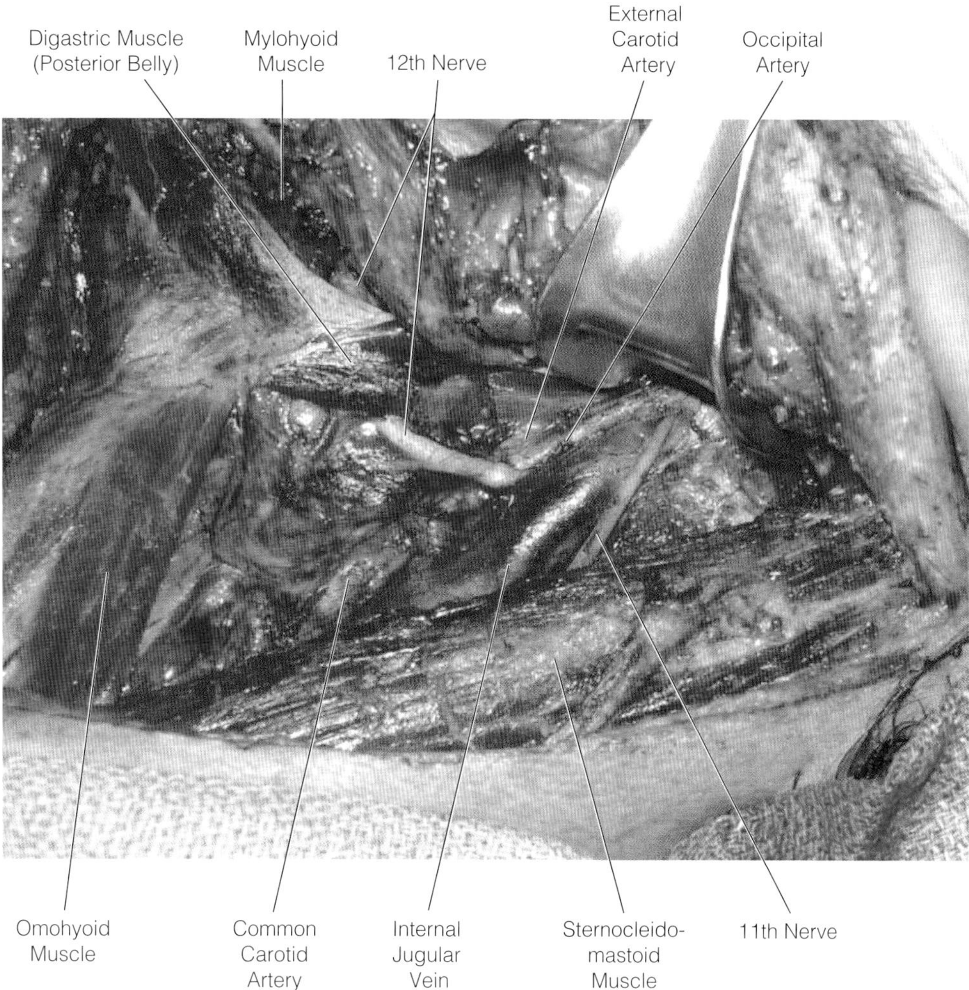

Figure 5 **Selective neck dissection. The posterior belly of the digastric muscle is identified inferior to the submandibular gland. This muscle protects several critical structures just deep to it (the hypoglossal nerve, the carotid artery, the internal jugular vein, and the spinal accessory nerve). View is of a left neck dissection.**

pedicle is clamped and ligated. Care is taken to look for leakage of chyle, particularly when a level IV dissection is performed on the left.

Levels II to IV

When level I is spared, a smaller incision suffices for exposure. Subplatysmal flaps are raised superiorly to the level of the submandibular gland. The inferior flap is raised, exposing the anterior edge of the sternocleidomastoid muscle. Dissection proceeds just inferior to the submandibular gland until the posterior belly of the digastric muscle is identified. The digastric muscle is skeletonized posteriorly to the sternocleidomastoid muscle and anteriorly to the omohyoid muscle, which forms the anterior limit of the dissection. The rest of the neck dissection proceeds as described for a selective neck dissection involving levels I through IV.

Complications

INTRAOPERATIVE

Most intraoperative complications may be prevented by means of careful surgical technique, coupled with a thorough understanding of head and neck anatomy. Injury to the internal jugular vein may occur either proximally or distally. Uncontrolled proximal bleeding endangers adjacent critical structures, such as the carotid artery and the hypoglossal nerve. Occasionally, a laceration extends up to the skull base, and the vessel cannot be controlled with clamping and ligation. In these cases, it is acceptable to pack the jugular foramen for hemostasis.

It is important to gain distal control of the internal jugular vein before repair to prevent air embolism. Harbingers of air embolism include the presence of a sucking sound in the neck, a mill-wheel murmur over the precordium, electrocardiographic changes, and hypotension. Predisposing factors include elevation of the head of the bed and spontaneous breathing, which increase negative intrathoracic pressure and thus promote entry of air into the venous system. Injury to the internal jugular vein is more difficult to control when it occurs distally in the neck or chest at the junction with the subclavian vein. For this reason, ligation of the internal jugular vein in radical and modified radical neck dissection is typically performed 1 cm superior to the clavicle.

Opalescent or clear fluid in the inferior neck suggests the presence of a chyle fistula. Chyle fistulae generally can be prevented by clamping and ligating the lymphatic pedicle at the base of the neck. Those fistulae that occur are repaired at the time of the neck dissection. There is no benefit in isolating individual lymphatic vessels, because these structures are fragile, do not hold stitches, and are prone to tearing. A figure-eight stitch is placed along the lymphatic pedicle until there is no evidence of clear or turbid fluid on the Valsalva maneuver. Care must be taken not to inadvertently injure the vagus nerve or the phrenic nerve during repair of a chyle leak.

POSTOPERATIVE

The best treatment of postoperative complications such as hematoma and chyle leak is prevention. Hematomas, once present, are best managed by promptly returning the patient to the operating room for evacuation. Management of postoperative leakage of chyle depends on the volume of the leak. Low-volume leaks may be managed with packing, wound care, and nutritional supplementation with medium-chain triglycerides.

Wound complications (e.g., infection, flap necrosis, and carotid artery exposure or rupture) share certain interrelated causative factors. Poor nutritional status, advanced tumor stage at presentation, hypothyroidism, and preoperative radiation therapy have all been associated with wound complications. After chemoradiation therapy, the use of smaller incisions and more limited dissection of soft tissues may lower the incidence of postoperative wound problems, including persistent lymphedema and soft tissue fibrosis. Conversely, poor planning of skin incisions may increase the likelihood of wound complications such as wound breakdown, skin flap loss, and exposure of vital structures. Wound complications predispose to carotid artery rupture, the most catastrophic complication of neck dissection.

In some cases, severe edema after planned neck dissections in patients previously treated with chemoradiation may cause respiratory decompensation that necessitates tracheotomy. Postoperative internal jugular vein thrombosis is not uncommon despite preservation at the time of surgery[43] and may exacerbate facial and upper airway edema. Impaired venous outflow predisposes to increased intracranial pressure.[44] This may be a greater concern in patients who require bilateral neck dissections. If a radical neck dissection is performed on one side, the internal jugular vein must be preserved on the other, or the neck dissections must be staged. These problems are further exacerbated when the patient has undergone chemoradiation therapy before operation.

Most neck dissections result in some degree of temporary shoulder dysfunction.[45–48] Patients in whom nerve-sparing procedures are performed can expect function to return within 3 weeks to 1 year, depending on the procedure performed. Shoulder dysfunction and pain are exacerbated when nerves supplying the deep muscles of the neck are also sacrificed. Patients may benefit from physical therapy, which preserves full range of motion in the shoulder while function returns.[49]

Soft tissue fibrosis is a long-term problem for many patients who undergo treatment with radiation or chemoradiation. Patients who additionally undergo neck dissection may have limited neck and shoulder range of motion after multimodality therapy. Physical therapy and lymphedema therapy may be helpful. Soft tissue fibrosis in this patient population also contributes to long-term dysphagia observed in these patients[50,51] and appears to be a cumulative effect of multimodality therapy. Aggressive intervention with speech and swallowing therapy may be helpful.

Financial Disclosures: None Reported

References

1. Wakely PE Jr, Kneisl JS. Soft tissue aspiration cytopathology. Cancer 2000;90:292–8.
2. Carroll CM, Nazeer U, Timon CI. The accuracy of fine-needle aspiration biopsy in the diagnosis of head and neck masses. Ir J Med Sci 1998;167:149–51.
3. Wakely P Jr, Frable WJ, Kneisl JS. Soft tissue aspiration cytopathology of malignant lymphoma and leukemia. Cancer 2001;93:35–9.
4. Veness MJ, Palme CE, Morgan GJ. High-risk cutaneous squamous cell carcinoma of the head and neck: results from 266 treated patients with metastatic lymph node disease. Cancer 2006;106:2389–96.
5. Kraus DH, Carew JF, Harrison LB. Regional lymph node metastasis from cutaneous squamous cell carcinoma. Arch Otolaryngol Head Neck Surg 1998;124:582–7.
6. Ch'ng S, Maitra A, Allison RS, et al. Parotid and cervical nodal status predict prognosis for patients with head and neck metastatic cutaneous squamous cell carcinoma. J Surg Oncol 2008;98:101–5.
7. Hinerman RW, Indelicato DJ, Amdur RJ, et al. Cutaneous squamous cell carcinoma metastatic to parotid-area lymph nodes. Laryngoscope 2008;118:1989–96.
8. Veness MJ, Porceddu S, Palme CE, Morgan GJ. Cutaneous head and neck squamous cell carcinoma metastatic to parotid and cervical lymph nodes. Head Neck 2007;29:621–31.
9. Spiro RH. Management of malignant tumors of the salivary glands. Oncology (Williston Park) 1998;12:671–80; discussion 683.
10. Tuttle RM, Tala H, Shah J, et al. Estimating risk of recurrence in differentiated thyroid cancer after total thyroidectomy and radioactive iodine remnant ablation: using response to therapy variables to modify the initial risk estimates predicted by the new American Thyroid Association staging system. Thyroid 2010;20:1341–9.
11. Moreno MA, Agarwal G, de Luna R, et al. Preoperative lateral neck ultrasonography as a long-term outcome predictor in papillary thyroid cancer. Arch Otolaryngol Head Neck Surg 2011;137:157–62.
12. Lango M, Flieder D, Arrangoiz R, et al. Extranodal extension of metastatic papillary thyroid carcinoma: correlation with biochemical endpoints, nodal persistence and systemic disease progression. Thyroid 2013 Feb 19. [Epub ahead of print]
13. Piccardo A, Arecco F, Puntoni M, et al. Focus on high-risk DTC patients: high postoperative serum thyroglobulin level

is a strong predictor of disease persistence and is associated to progression-free survival and overall survival. Clin Nucl Med 2013;38:18–24.
14. Kupferman ME, Patterson M, Mandel SJ, et al. Patterns of lateral neck metastasis in papillary thyroid carcinoma. Arch Otolaryngol Head Neck Surg 2004;130:857–60.
15. Pingpank JF Jr, Sasson AR, Hanlon AL, et al. Tumor above the spinal accessory nerve in papillary thyroid cancer that involves lateral neck nodes: a common occurrence. Arch Otolaryngol Head Neck Surg 2002;128:1275–8.
16. Kupferman ME, Patterson DM, Mandel SJ, et al. Safety of modified radical neck dissection for differentiated thyroid carcinoma. Laryngoscope 2004;114:403–6.
17. Sparano A, Weinstein G, Chalian A, et al. Multivariate predictors of occult neck metastasis in early oral tongue cancer. Otolaryngol Head Neck Surg 2004;131:472–6.
18. Ganly I, Goldstein D, Carlson DL, et al. Long-term regional control and survival in patients with "low-risk," early stage oral tongue cancer managed by partial glossectomy and neck dissection without postoperative radiation: the importance of tumor thickness. Cancer 2013;119:1168–76. DOI: 10.1002/cncr.27872. Epub 2012 Nov 26.
19. Alvi A, Johnson JT. Extracapsular spread in the clinically negative neck (N0): implications and outcome. Otolaryngol Head Neck Surg 1996;114:65–70.
20. Myers JN, Greenberg JS, Mo V, Roberts D. Extracapsular spread. A significant predictor of treatment failure in patients with squamous cell carcinoma of the tongue. Cancer 2001; 92:3030–6.
21. Johnson JT, Wagner RL, Myers EN. A long-term assessment of adjuvant chemotherapy on outcome of patients with extracapsular spread of cervical metastases from squamous carcinoma of the head and neck. Cancer 1996;77:181–5.
22. Jose J, Coatesworth AP, Johnston C, MacLennan K. Cervical node metastases in squamous cell carcinoma of the upper aerodigestive tract: the significance of extracapsular spread and soft tissue deposits. Head Neck 2003;25:451–6.
23. Cooper JS, Pajak TF, Forastiere AA, et al. Postoperative concurrent radiotherapy and chemotherapy for high-risk squamous-cell carcinoma of the head and neck. N Engl J Med 2004;350:1937–44.
24. Bernier J, Domenge C, Ozsahin M, et al. Postoperative irradiation with or without concomitant chemotherapy for locally advanced head and neck cancer. N Engl J Med 2004; 350:1945–52.
25. Mehra R, Ang KK, Burtness B. Management of human papillomavirus-positive and human papillomavirus-negative head and neck cancer. Semin Radiat Oncol 2012;22: 194–7.
26. Fakhry C, Westra WH, Li S, et al. Improved survival of patients with human papillomavirus-positive head and neck squamous cell carcinoma in a prospective clinical trial. J Natl Cancer Inst 2008;100:261–9.
27. Fakhry C, Gillison ML. Clinical implications of human papillomavirus in head and neck cancers. J Clin Oncol 2006;24: 2606–11.
28. Ross GL, Shoaib T, Soutar DS, et al. The First International Conference on Sentinel Node Biopsy in Mucosal Head and Neck Cancer and adoption of a multicenter trial protocol. Ann Surg Oncol 2002;9:406–10.
29. Jacobs JR, Arden RL, Marks SC, et al. Carotid artery reconstruction using superficial femoral arterial grafts. Laryngoscope 1994;104:689–93.
30. Adams GL, Madison M, Remley K, Gapany M. Preoperative permanent balloon occlusion of internal carotid artery in patients with advanced head and neck squamous cell carcinoma. Laryngoscope 1999;109:460–6.
31. Crile G. Landmark article Dec 1, 1906: Excision of cancer of the head and neck. With special reference to plan of dissection based on one hundred and thirty-two operations. By George Crile. JAMA 1987;258:3286–93.
32. Bocca E, Pignataro O, Oldini C, Cappa C. Functional neck dissection: an evaluation and review of 843 cases. Laryngoscope 1984;94:942–5.
33. Shah JP, Candela FC, Poddar AK. The patterns of cervical lymph node metastases from squamous carcinoma of the oral cavity. Cancer 1990;66:109–13.
34. Andersen PE, Warren F, Spiro J, et al. Results of selective neck dissection in management of the node-positive neck. Arch Otolaryngol Head Neck Surg 2002;128:1180–4.
35. Weinstein GS, Quon H, O'Malley BW Jr, et al. Selective neck dissection and deintensified postoperative radiation and chemotherapy for oropharyngeal cancer: a subset analysis of the University of Pennsylvania transoral robotic surgery trial. Laryngoscope 2010;120:1749–55.
36. Pitman KT, Johnson JT, Myers EN. Effectiveness of selective neck dissection for management of the clinically negative neck. Arch Otolaryngol Head Neck Surg 1997;123:917–22.
37. Chan JY, Sanguineti G, Richmon JD, et al. Retrospective review of positron emission tomography with contrast-enhanced computed tomography in the posttreatment setting in human papillomavirus-associated oropharyngeal carcinoma. Arch Otolaryngol Head Neck Surg 2012;138: 1040–6.
38. Liauw SL, Mancuso AA, Amdur RJ, et al. Postradiotherapy neck dissection for lymph node-positive head and neck cancer: the use of computed tomography to manage the neck. J Clin Oncol 2006;24:1421–7.
39. Narayan K, Crane CH, Kleid S, et al. Planned neck dissection as an adjunct to the management of patients with advanced neck disease treated with definitive radiotherapy: for some or for all? Head Neck 1999;21:606–13.
40. Doweck I, Robbins KT, Mendenhall WM, et al. Neck level-specific nodal metastases in oropharyngeal cancer: is there a role for selective neck dissection after definitive radiation therapy? Head Neck 2003;25:960–7.
41. Lango MN, Andrews GA, Ahmad S, et al. Postradiotherapy neck dissection for head and neck squamous cell carcinoma: pattern of pathologic residual carcinoma and prognosis. Head Neck 2009;31:328–37.
42. Huang SH, O'Sullivan B, Weinreb I, et al. Patterns of failure and histopathologic outcome predictors following definitive radiotherapy and planned neck dissection with residual disease. Head Neck 2012;34:913–22.
43. Leontsinis TG, Currie AR, Mannell A. Internal jugular vein thrombosis following functional neck dissection. Laryngoscope 1995;105:169–74.
44. Lydiatt DD, Ogren FP, Lydiatt WM, Hahn FJ. Increased intracranial pressure as a complication of unilateral radical neck dissection in a patient with congenital absence of the transverse sinus. Head Neck 1991;13:359–62.

45. Witt RL, Rejto L. Spinal accessory nerve monitoring in selective and modified neck dissection. Laryngoscope 2007; 117:776–80.
46. Teymoortash A, Hoch S, Eivazi B, Werner JA. Postoperative morbidity after different types of selective neck dissection. Laryngoscope 2010;120:924–9.
47. Cheng PT, Hao SP, Lin YH, Yeh AR. Objective comparison of shoulder dysfunction after three neck dissection techniques. Ann Otol Rhinol Laryngol 2000;109:761–6.
48. Short SO, Kaplan JN, Laramore GE, Cummings CW. Shoulder pain and function after neck dissection with or without preservation of the spinal accessory nerve. Am J Surg 1984;148:478–82.
49. McGarvey AC, Chiarelli PE, Osmotherly PG, Hoffman GR. Physiotherapy for accessory nerve shoulder dysfunction following neck dissection surgery: a literature review. Head Neck 2011;33:274–80.
50. Lango MN, Egleston B, Ende K, et al. Impact of neck dissection on long-term feeding tube dependence in patients with head and neck cancer treated with primary radiation or chemoradiation. Head Neck 2010;32:341–7.
51. Machtay M, Moughan J, Trotti A, et al. Factors associated with severe late toxicity after concurrent chemoradiation for locally advanced head and neck cancer: an RTOG analysis. J Clin Oncol 2008;26:3582–9.

Acknowledgment

Figures 1, 2, 3, 4 Tom Moore

8 TRACHEOSTOMY

H. David Reines, MD, FACS, and Elizabeth Franco, MD, MPH&TM

History

The word *tracheotomy* first appeared in *Libri Chirgurae 12*, published in 1649, but it was not until Laurence Heruter, a German surgeon, reintroduced it that it became part of modern medicine. It was initially performed as a lifesaving procedure to establish an airway. Alexander the Great is reported to have used his sword to open the trachea of a suffocating soldier. The term *tracheotomy* is defined as a surgical creation of an opening in the anterior trachea that can be reversible and temporary, whereas, technically, *tracheostomy* is the formation of an opening into the trachea by suturing the edges of the opening to the skin of the neck. However, over the years, the two terms have been used interchangeably. For this document, we use the term *tracheostomy* to describe the procedure.

Indications

The indication for a tracheostomy has changed over the years. Originally, it was conceived as a method to obtain an airway for obstruction from infections, neoplasm, or trauma. The most common indications for modern tracheostomy are prolonged ventilation for respiratory failure and airway protection following traumatic brain injury with neurologic dysfunction.

Patients requiring tracheostomy or cricothyroidotomy fall into four categories:

1. Emergency for airway control, that is, airway obstruction from the epiglottis, foreign-body aspiration, laryngeal trauma, or maxillofacial trauma
2. Semielective for patients requiring prolonged intubation or mechanical ventilation for respiratory failure or high spinal cord injury
3. Elective for airway protection, that is, traumatic brain injury, stroke, sleep apnea, or vocal cord problems
4. Elective for long-term airway access. Permanent tracheostomies are used to maintain airway access when patients undergo major head or neck dissection for tumors of the larynx and the base of the tongue.

Patients who arrive with either acute airway compromise from neck trauma or facial burns should first undergo an attempt at oral intubation, and if this fails, an emergent surgical airway is required.

Laryngoscopy should be attempted prior to performing surgical airway. If a patient arrives talking, but there is evidence of hoarseness with increasing airway compromise, the surgeon should be prepared for a surgical airway if oral intubation is unsuccessful. When an attempt at oral intubation fails and ventilation is a problem, immediate cricothyroidotomy should be performed. A semielective surgical airway should be undertaken in a patient whose injuries may result in progressive laryngeal and cervical soft tissue edema prior to decompensation from respiratory distress. Patients with a Glasgow Coma Scale (GCS) less than or equal to 8 cannot protect their airway, and intubation should be performed immediately. If this is not possible, then a surgical airway should be considered prior to transporting the patient.

Early Tracheostomy

If the patient is ventilator dependent or has severe head injury and will need prolonged airway protection, early tracheostomy should be considered when intracranial pressure is not elevated. Early tracheostomy is defined as occurring at or before 7 days, whereas late tracheostomy occurs after 7 days. Early tracheostomy has been associated with decreased incidence of ventilator-associated pneumonia, decreased days of mechanical ventilation, decreased hospital stay, decreased intensive care unit (ICU) length of stay, and increased patient comfort. Although no study has demonstrated a decrease in overall mortality with early tracheostomy, tracheostomy does provide easier access for suctioning and allows patients to be liberated from the ventilator without the loss of an airway.

Pertinent Anatomy

The trachea lies relatively superficially in the anterior neck covered by the strap muscles midline and the platysma. The first tracheal ring is just below the cricothyroid, whereas the next three rings may lie beneath the thyroid isthmus. The sixth through seventh rings lie low in the neck and into the sternal notch [*see Figure 1*]. When performing a tracheostomy, knowledge of the normal and potentially abnormal vasculature is imperative. Care must be taken with a horizontal incision to avoid bleeding from injury to the anterior jugular vein. Other potential causes of hemorrhage may arise from injury to a high-riding innominate artery, a medially placed carotid artery, and the thyroid ima vessels in the midline. Tumors, hematoma, and edema can cause tracheal deviation from midline. Other anatomic variants should also be considered. An obese patient may require deeper dissection, longer instruments, and the use of an extra-long tracheostomy tube. The length of the neck and the distance from the jaw to the thyroid cartilage should also be examined. Patients with a known or potential neck injury or with kyphosis must be positioned without extension. Access to the trachea may be compromised, and plans for dissecting the thyroid isthmus should be considered.

* The authors and editors gratefully acknowledge the contributions of the previous author, Ara A. Chalian, MD, FACS, to the development and writing of this chapter.

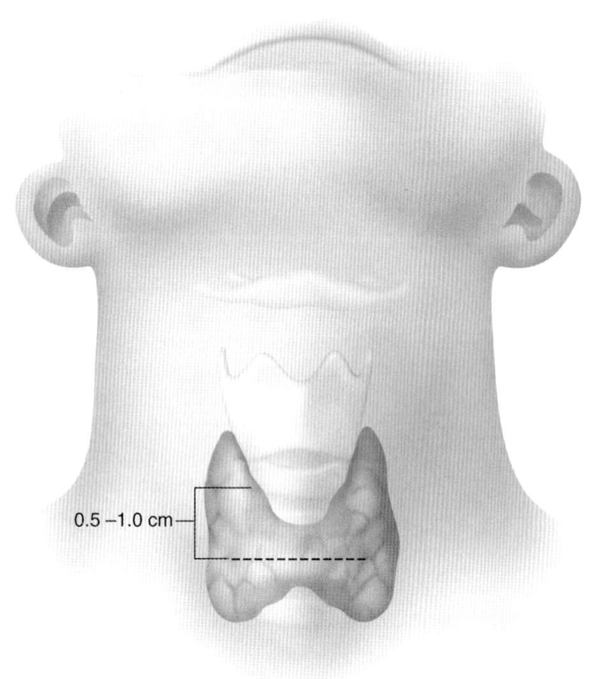

Figure 1 **Surgical tracheostomy. A transverse cutaneous incision is made that is approximately [illegible] to [illegible] cm long (or as long as is necessary for adequate exposure). The extent of flap elevation may be 1 cm or less.**

Physiology

When undergoing a tracheostomy, ideally, the patient should be adequately ventilated and hyperoxygenated in anticipation of a period of apnea during tracheostomy tube placement. An oxygen saturation of 100% and a normal pH and carbon dioxide tension (P_{CO_2}) are desirable at the start of an elective tracheostomy. Use of 100% oxygen during the procedure will help maintain adequate oxygenation throughout the procedure. When an emergency cricothyroidotomy or tracheostomy is necessary, an attempt should be made to preoxygenate and ventilate.

Counseling and Informed Consent

The patient, the family, or both should be advised of the risks and benefits of a tracheostomy. Commonly discussed issues, including pain, mortality, and the range of possibilities of early and late complications (see below), should be on the consent form. A tracheostomy should be proposed as the best option for the patient requiring prolonged mechanical ventilation or airway protection. Tracheostomy contributes to patient comfort, allowing improved oral care, oral alimentation, and speaking as well as the potential for earlier liberation from the ventilator.

Site of the Procedure

Elective open tracheostomy requires good lighting and electrocautery. Some may find open tracheostomy in the ICU more ergonomically difficult than in the operating room (OR) because the patient is on a hospital bed; however, finding OR time and transporting the patient may be inconvenient. Several studies comparing bedside open to percutaneous tracheostomies find the techniques to be essentially equivalent in outcome with the open technique and possibly lower in cost. Percutaneous tracheostomy is most commonly performed at the bedside, in the ICU, and does not require the same lighting or instrumentation and nursing availability that an open tracheostomy does. A cricothyroidotomy is frequently performed in the trauma bay, although it may be executed anywhere and requires the least amount of instrumentation. Emergency tracheostomy and cricothyroidotomy are frequently not performed in the OR.

Anesthesia

Anesthesia can frequently be given as conscious sedation and/or local anesthesia with epinephrine. Paralysis should be avoided when possible in a patient with any spontaneous breathing.

Patient Positioning

Extension of the neck is desirable; however, if the patient has a known or potential cervical spine injury, operation in the neutral position is necessary. When possible, the patient should be placed on an operating table with a shoulder roll and a foam pad (donut) under the head. When the neck can be extended, the head rest of the surgical bed can be lowered and the patient placed in a 30° head elevation position to decrease venous pressure. Extending the head allows better palpation of the landmarks. If cervical spine precautions are necessary, the posterior portion of the cervical collar should remain in place and the head stabilized by a team member. Another alternative is to stabilize the neck with bilateral head rolls with tape over the forehead and chin extending across the bed.

Operative Techniques

EMERGENT SURGICAL AIRWAY

Cricothyroidotomy

Cricothyroidotomy is generally performed for emergent control of the airway. Inability to secure an airway, especially with severe facial trauma, requires immediate access to the trachea. A cricothyroidotomy can be performed rapidly and does not risk the anatomic problems of a tracheostomy because the cricothyroid membrane is thin and closest to the skin directly under the thyroid membrane If a #5 or #6 tracheostomy tube is not available, an endotracheal tube can be introduced for immediate airway access.

Transtracheal Needle Ventilation and Oxygenation

Transtracheal needle access also can be used in emergency situations. A large-bore 12- or 14 gauge angiocatheter or a pulmonary artery catheter introducer sheath is placed through the cricoid membrane and attached to oxygen tubing with the capability of providing oxygen at 50 psi. A hole in the tubing is finger-occluded and intermittently opened to allow for ventilation. Adequate ventilation can be provided for

20 to 30 minutes. This method is best used as a bridge while awaiting the proper equipment and support for an orotracheal or surgical airway.

OPEN TRACHEOSTOMY

Steps

1. *Incision of the skin.* The patient should be assessed for a high-riding innominate artery, abnormally placed vessels, and tracheal deviation. Incision can be made either vertically or horizontally. The horizontal scar heals better than the vertical scar. However, visualization, especially if the neck cannot be extended, is frequently easier in a vertical incision. Damage to the anterior jugular veins likewise is less likely with a vertical incision. In an emergency, a longer vertical incision can facilitate exposure while avoiding the subplatysmal anterior jugular veins [*see Figure 2*]. In general, the incision should be made midway between the cricoid cartilage and the sternal notch. The size of the incision is up to the individual surgeon. However, a minimum of 2 to 2.5 cm is desirable.

   Subsequent dissection must be performed perpendicular to the trachea. A common mistake when dividing the subcutaneous tissue is to deflect in a slightly oblique fashion, arriving lower in the trachea than anticipated.
2. *Retracting the strap muscles.* The midline raphe is divided and an assistant with Senn or Army-Navy retractors or with a self-retraining retractor then retracts the strap muscles laterally. Undermining should be minimized to decrease the potential creation of dead-space areas. In the case of a malignant neoplasm overlying the thyroid compartment, the anatomic landmarks may be less clear. In such a case, palpation of the thyroid cartilage and dissecting caudally are helpful. Care must be taken, especially in women, to palpate the thyroid and not the hyoid cartilage [*see Figure 3*].
3. *Dissection of the thyroid gland.* The thyroid isthmus frequently lies in the field of dissection. Because its size and thickness vary greatly and can vary from 5 to 10 mm in vertical dimension, dissection of this can be undertaken, and, in many cases, immobilizing the trachea and retracting the isthmus either superiorly or inferiorly to place the tracheal incision in the second or third tracheal interspace can be accomplished [*see Figure 4*]. However, if the isthmus is a problem, especially in cases where the neck cannot be extended, it can be divided and the edges ligated either with ties or with a Harmonic scalpel. When there is an isthmus nodule, the isthmus should be removed for diagnostic and therapeutic purposes. Recurrent laryngeal nerves should not be directly in the operative field and are rarely at risk as long as one stays in the midline anterior on the trachea. If significant deviation of the trachea is noted, the nerves may be injured. Because the blood supply to the trachea is laterally based, one should not encounter them. However, a thyroid ima vessel is frequently noted in the lower portion of the isthmus, and this may need to be ligated prior to dissection.
4. *Incision of the trachea.* Tracheostomy should be performed with a sharp blade. The pretracheal tissues may be coagulated with a bipolar electrocautery. The opening of the airway may bring volatile gasses into the operative field; therefore, monopolar electrocautery should be avoided if volatile gasses are in use. Several types of incisions are possible:

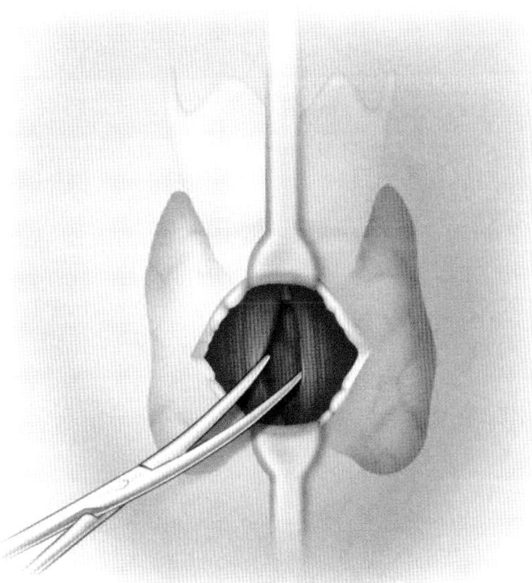

Figure 2 **Surgical tracheostomy. Retractors are placed, the skin is retracted, and the strap muscles are visualized in the midline. The muscles are divided along the raphe and then retracted laterally.**

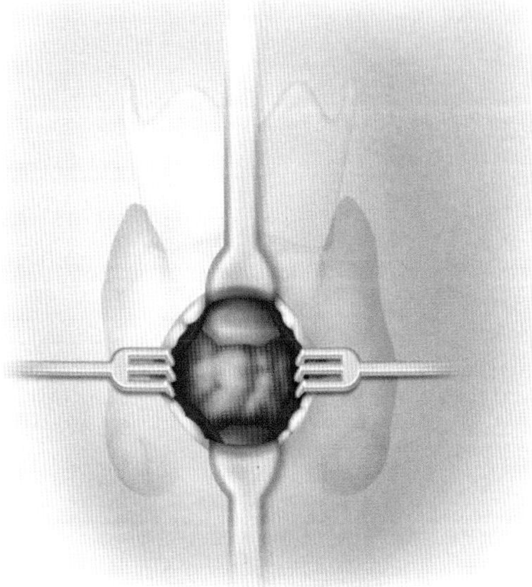

Figure 3 **Surgical tracheostomy. With the strap muscles retracted, the thyroid isthmus is visualized, and the inferior (or superior) edge of the isthmus is dissected down to the trachea. The isthmus is then retracted superiorly (or inferiorly) or divided to permit visualization of the trachea before the tracheal incision is made.**

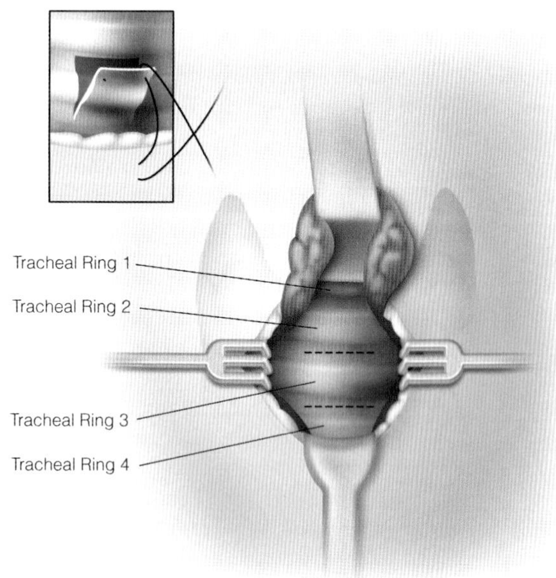

Figure 4 **Surgical tracheostomy. A tracheotomy is made either between the second and third tracheal rings or between the third and fourth rings. A Björk flap (*inset*) may be created by extending the ends of the tracheostomy downward through the next lower tracheal ring in an inverted U shape.**

a. *Linear incision.* This transverse incision is made either between the second and third rings or the third and fourth rings. Stay sutures are then placed superiorly and inferiorly around the tracheal rings [*see Figure 5*].

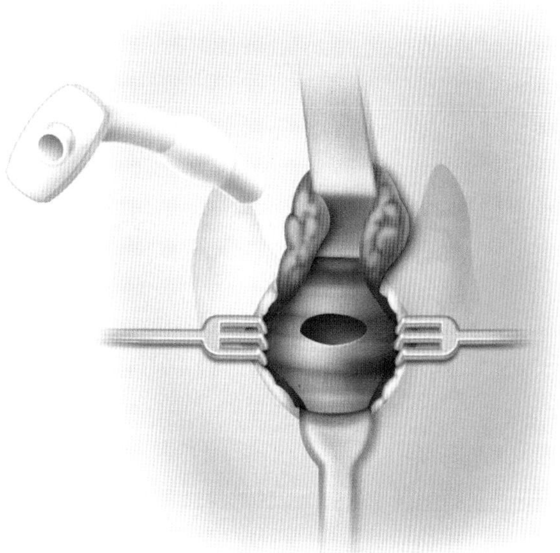

Figure 5 **Surgical tracheostomy. The tracheostomy tube is inserted into the tracheal opening from the side, with the faceplate rotated 90° so that the tube's entry into the airway can be well visualized.**

b. *T-type incision.* This incision is a combination of a vertical incision that crosses the second ring and forms a "T" with a transverse incision below the third tracheal ring. Stay sutures are placed laterally and allow for controlled opening of the trachea with a tracheostomy spreader.
c. *Tracheal window.* Although a tracheal window with removal of a portion of the third tracheal ring has been performed, this is more difficult and may not heal as rapidly as a ring-preserving incision.
d. *Björk flap.* A Björk flap is an inferiorly based U-shaped flap that incorporates the ring below and the tracheal incision [*see Figure 4*]. A U-type incision is made from the third tracheal ring through the second tracheal ring, and the second tracheal ring is then retracted inferiorly and sutured with a dissolvable suture as high in the neck as possible to the skin. The theoretical justification for this is to keep the tracheal incision close to the skin edges in the instance of tracheostomy tube displacement, to ensure ease of airway access. This flap suture can be released 3 to 5 days after creation once the tract has been established or after the first tracheostomy change.

5. *Stay sutures.* Stay sutures using a 2-0 nonabsorbable suture on a UR6 needle can be placed either laterally or inferiorly and superiorly. These help stabilize the tracheostomy during the procedure. The sutures are then taped to the chest and labeled so that they will not be inadvertently removed. Stay sutures may provide access to a fresh tracheostomy if the tracheostomy tube becomes dislodged in the immediate postoperative period. These sutures are left in place until the first tube change.

In adults, a number 8(outside diameter [OD]) or 6(OD) tube is preferable. If there is significant edema or obesity, the use of an extra-long tube is desirable. If a tracheostomy tube is not available, a standard endotracheal tube can be used to intubate the neck. Remember when trimming the tube to spare the pilot balloon.

PERCUTANEOUS TRACHEOSTOMY

Percutaneous tracheostomy was first described over 50 years ago, but the availability of a dilational percutaneous tracheostomy kit prompted widespread use in the 1990s. In many centers, this has become the method of choice for tracheostomy. Although initial contraindications included morbid obesity, inability to extend the neck as in potential cervical spine injuries, short neck, enlarged thyroid isthmus, and previous tracheostomy, these have been disproven with increasing experience. A benefit of the percutaneous approach is the ability to perform the procedure at bedside in the ICU, reducing OR costs and scheduling conflicts. The percutaneous approach has been championed for its ease of performance at the bedside in the ICU; however, several studies comparing cost and personnel use demonstrate open bedside tracheostomy to be more cost-effective with equivalent complications and safety outcomes. The long-term cosmetic effects of percutaneous tracheostomy appear to be better than those of the open technique.

The choice between percutaneous and open tracheostomy remains a decision best left to individual centers.

Operative Technique

Equipment and personnel The personnel necessary for the procedure are a respiratory therapist, a critical care nurse, a surgeon, and a bronchoscopist to safely perform a percutaneous tracheostomy. The equipment required is a bronchoscope and a percutaneous dilation tracheostomy kit. Surgical instruments for an open tracheostomy should be readily available. Maximum sterile barriers are employed, including sterile gown, gloves, and drapes. All participating personnel must wear mask and head covers.

Procedure

1. *Incision.* Once conscious sedation is initiated, the subcutaneous tissue is infiltrated with local anesthetic 1 cm caudal to the cricoid cartilage. A 1 to 1.5 cm incision is made either in a horizontal or a vertical fashion. The subcutaneous tissue is then bluntly dissected using a hemostat to spread the tissue down to the level of the trachea.
2. *Bronchoscopy.* The bronchoscope is advanced to the tip of the endotracheal tube. With the surgeon providing one-finger ballottement at the level of the first or second tracheal ring, the endotracheal tube is slowly withdrawn while maintaining the bronchoscope at the tip of the tube until one-to-one ballottement is appreciated. Every step of the procedure involving instrumentation of the trachea is preferably performed under direct bronchoscopic visualization.
3. *Transcutaneous tracheostomy.* The introducer needle is advanced through the incision at the level where one-to-one ballottement was appreciated. Constant aspiration of the syringe and direct bronchoscopic visualization immediately identify the entrance into the trachea. Once the needle is noted to be in a good position, the guide wire is introduced again under direct bronchoscopic visualization.
4. *Dilation.* Using a modified Seldinger technique, the needle is removed and a stiff conical dilator is introduced and removed. The tract is then dilated with the largest conical dilator to the level marked for the skin. The dilator is removed and fully introduced three times. The tracheostomy tube is then introduced over the snuggest fitting dilator. Once the tracheostomy tube is in place, the guide wire and dilator are removed. Often the endotracheal tube must be withdrawn a short distance to allow for serial dilation and introduction of the tracheostomy tube.
5. *Confirmation of placement.* Once the tracheostomy tube is in place, the bronchoscope is withdrawn from the endotracheal tube and introduced through the tracheostomy tube to confirm placement within the trachea. The endotracheal tube is kept in place until confirmation is complete. The tracheostomy tube is then secured with sutures from the faceplate to the skin and tied in place.

Tracheostomy Management

Tracheal sutures are removed on postoperative day 7. If the patient is on minimal ventilator settings or liberated from the ventilator, the tracheostomy tube is downsized. Once the patient is liberated from the ventilator, the tracheostomy tube cuff is deflated and the patient is placed on humidified air or oxygen. The humidified air can be delivered via a tracheostomy collar or tracheostomy tube. A tracheostomy collar allows more patient freedom and less torque than a T tube when frequent suctioning is not required. Speech pathology consultation should be obtained for swallowing evaluation and speaking valve placement versus capping the tracheostomy tube. The approach depends on the patient's mental status and suctioning requirements. Once the patient is tolerating either tracheostomy tube occlusion or a speaking valve for greater than 24 hours and managing his or her own secretions, the tracheostomy is removed. In preparation for decannulation, the patient should be suctioned and a replacement tracheostomy with a stylet should be available in case of sudden respiratory decompensation. An occlusive dressing is left in place for 24 hours. Generally, no further dressing is required afterward.

Complications

Reported complication rates from tracheostomy range from 5 to 31%, with an average of nearly 12%. Major complications range from 2 to 6%. Mortality is extremely low (0.5%).

EARLY COMPLICATIONS

Displacement

The most dangerous complication is early accidental displacement or decannulation. This can occur when moving the patient to the ICU or recovery room and when patients are turned for care or x-rays in the ICU in the first 5 to 7 days after placement. A loosely tied tracheostomy or one placed in a precarious position can be dislodged, resulting in the inability to ventilate and oxygenate. If this is suspected, the patient should immediately be placed supine and an attempt at ventilation should commence. If the patient cannot be ventilated, an attempt to replace the tube should be tried if stay sutures or a Björk flap is present. Emergency oral intubation should be performed if the attempt fails. Multiple attempts to replace the tube can result in a false passage. The tracheostomy can then later be replaced via the same incision with the proper light and proper retraction. A new tracheostomy tube should be available in the room or above the bed for all patients who have had a fresh tracheostomy.

Pneumomediastinum/Pneumothorax

Pneumomediastinum can occur, especially with a low tracheostomy or if a false passage is created. Pneumothorax is a rare (< 2%) complication that can occur especially in children, in whom the cupola of the lung may ride high. Pneumothorax can also occur in patients who require high ventilatory pressures or who cough vigorously during the procedure. A low tracheostomy and deep dissection potentially increase the risk of pneumothorax.

Bleeding

A small amount of blood via the wound or tracheostomy immediately following the procedure is not alarming. However, the persistence of blood around the trachea implies venous bleeding from either the skin, subcutaneous tissues, or thyroid gland. In general, this can be controlled with gentle packing and the use of a bioabsorbable hemostatic agent. If bleeding continues, the patient should be taken to the OR if possible and reintubated under ideal light and retraction, the tracheostomy should be removed and the bleeding controlled with cautery or sutures if necessary. If hemorrhage is demonstrated via the tracheostomy tube, early careful bronchoscopy should be performed to ascertain the site of bleeding. Significant bleeding from the tracheostomy is usually a late complication and may be related to a tracheoinnominate fistula (see below).

Infection

Tracheostomy infections requiring treatment are much less common than one would imagine, considering the contamination of the bronchial/tracheal tree in many patients who have been intubated for a period of time. The majority of infections can be treated with local wound care, although deep infections from *Staphylococcus aureus* and *Pseudomonas aerigunosa* may require antibiotics and removal of sutures. Placing tracheostomies through burn eschar presents a separate problem.

Acute Obstruction

The most common cause for acute obstruction of a tracheostomy is dislodgment. If that is not the case, the tracheostomy may have accumulated blood or mucus, which can clog the airways. To avoid this, humidified oxygen should always be administered, and gentle careful suctioning should be initiated by experienced personnel. The inner cannula should be removed and examined. Occasionally, bronchoscopy will be necessary to remove and irrigate mucus plugs.

Negative Pressure Pulmonary Edema

A rare complication of upper airway obstruction may occur after a tracheostomy is performed for airway obstruction. Patients generating large negative pressure against resistance, which is suddenly released, can experience a noncardiogenic pulmonary edema. The patient becomes hypoxic, develops rales in the lungs, and can demonstrate pink frothy pulmonary edema via the tube. A chest x-ray may demonstrate bilateral pulmonary edema. This process is usually self-limited and responds to positive end-expiratory pressure (PEEP) and positive pressure ventilation.

LATE COMPLICATIONS

Late complications of tracheostomy are often attributable to the cuff, either from the tracheostomy tube or from the endotracheal tube in place prior to tracheostomy. Complications attributable to cuff injuries are less common now than previously as a result of improvement in technology allowing for lower-pressure cuffs, but they still occur in patients who undergo prolonged endotracheal intubation.

Tracheostomy cuff pressures should be measured daily or more often to prevent tracheal necrosis. X-rays demonstrating a dilated cuff in the trachea require assessment of the tube, cuff, and trachea.

Subglottic Tracheal Stenosis

Tracheal stenosis has a reported incidence of 4 to 18%. Stenosis is associated with a longer hospital stay and prolonged time to tracheostomy. Dyspnea and stridor result when tracheal stenosis is greater than 50% of tracheal diameter. In suspected tracheal stenosis, referral to a specialist for evaluation either by computed tomography (CT) or rigid laryngoscopy is essential for diagnosis. Once the diagnosis is confirmed, treatment may require tracheal reconstruction.

Tracheal Granulation

Tracheal granulation may cause bleeding or occlusion of the tracheostomy tube if a flap of granulation tissue is elevated on exhalation. Granulation tissue may mimic tracheal stenosis. This complication is often easily treatable with removal of the tracheostomy tube. Occasionally, resection of the granulation tissue is necessary.

Vocal Cord Dysfunction

Vocal cord dysfunction occurs in less than 2%, whereas voice changes, including hoarseness and weakness, occur in 10 to 20% of patients. In cases of bilateral vocal cord paralysis, a tracheostomy is necessary until the paralysis resolves. Most complaints of vocal changes are considered minor by patients.

Tracheoesophageal Fistula

Tracheoesophageal fistula occurs in less than 0.3% of patients following tracheostomy. It can occur if a puncture is made into the posterior trachea or a cuff erodes into the esophagus. The combination of a a tracheostomy tube and a stiff nasogastric tube in the esophagus increases the risk of this complication. Symptoms include aspiration and persistent cuff leak around the tracheostomy. Persistent tracheobronchitis or pneumonia may also be present. A swallow study with the cuff deflated or CT and panendoscopy will demonstrate the defect. Definitive therapy is usually necessary.

Tracheoinnominate Fistula

Tracheoinnominate fistula has a reported incidence of 0.4 to 4.5% and presents initially as "sentinel bleeding" that usually develops within the first month following the procedure. Mortality between 50 and 75% has been reported. Risk factors include a low (below the third ring) tracheostomy, caudal migration from leverage on the tube, and the presence of a more cephalad-coursing innominate artery. An attempt to visualize the site of bleeding should be undertaken. If hemorrhage is significant, hyperinflate the cuff and try to compress the vessel against the posterior sternum. If this is unsuccessful, oral intubation should be performed. The tracheostomy tube must be removed and replaced with digital pressure through the tracheostomy to tamponade the bleeding en route to the OR. Often the upper extremity of the person responsible for maintaining digital pressure is prepared into the operative field in preparation for median sternotomy

Tracheocutaneous Fistula

Rarely, the tracheostomy wound does not completely close in 24 to 48 hours. Granulation tissue may be treated topically with silver nitrate with good success. Occasionally, the tracheostomy site must be surgically closed in layers for a nonhealing tracheocutaneous fistula.

Scar

Cosmetic results vary following tracheostomy. Ten to 15% of patients consider scar revision of the tracheostomy site.

Financial Disclosures: None Reported

Additional Reading

American College of Surgeons Committee on Trauma. Airway and ventilatory management. In: Advanced trauma life support for doctors, student edition. Chicago, IL: American College of Surgeons; 2008. p. 25–53.

Clec'h C, Albert C, Vincent F, et al. Tracheostomy does not improve the outcome of patients, requiring prolonged mechanical ventilation: a propensity analysis. Crit Care Med 2007;35: 135–8.

Griffiths J, Barber VS, Morgan L, Young JD. Systematic review and meta-analysis of studies of the timing of tracheostomy in adult patients undergoing artificial ventilation. BMJ 2005;330(7500):1243–50.

Grover A, Robbins J, Bendick P, et al. Open versus percutaneous dilatational tracheostomy: efficacy and cost analysis. Am Surg 2001;67: 297–302.

Marx WH, Ciaglia P, Graniero KD. Some important details in the technique of percutaneous dilatational tracheostomy via the modified Sledinger technique. Chest 1996; 110:762–6.

Pratt LW, Ferlito A, Rinaldo A. Tracheostomy. Historical review. Laryngoscope 2008;1188: 1597–606.

Silva B, Andriolo R, Saconato H, Atalla A. Early versus late tracheostomy for critically ill patients. Cochrane Database and Systematic Reviews 2009;(4).

Silvester W, Goldsmith D, Uchino S, et al. Percutaneous versus surgical tracheostomy: a randomized controlled study with long term follow up. Crit Care Med 2006;34: 2145–52.

Acknowledgments

Figures 1 through 5 Thom Graves

9 THYROID DISEASES

*Karen R. Borman, MD, FACS, and Jennifer L. Rabaglia, MD**

Approach to the Patient with Thyroid Disease

The thyroid plays a central role in normal metabolic and homeostatic processes, including thermomodulation, protein synthesis, carbohydrate and lipid metabolism, and modulation of adrenergic activity. A normal thyroid weighs 15 to 25 g and is firm, mobile, and smooth to palpation. The thyroid contains two distinct, physiologically active cell types. Follicular cells are responsible for thyroid hormone synthesis, whereas parafollicular or C cells produce calcitonin. Patients are most often referred to the surgeon for control of hyperthyroidism or for treatment of euthyroid nodular disease.

APPROACH TO THE PATIENT WITH HYPERTHYROIDISM

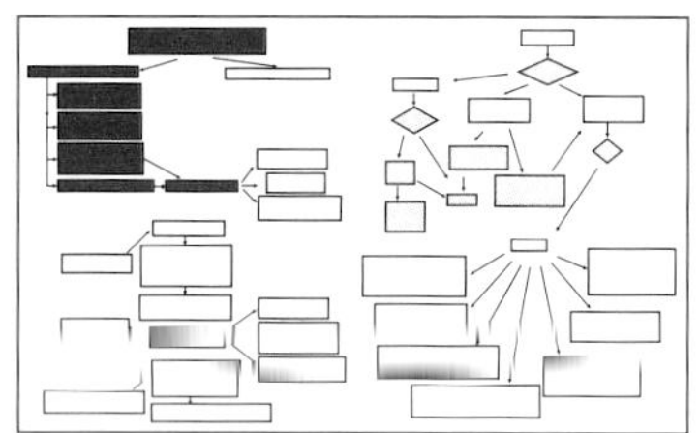

[SCORE] The symptoms of thyroid hormone overproduction are numerous and often nonspecific, including palpitations, heat intolerance, weight changes (gain or loss), increased appetite, poor concentration, decreased libido, and irregular menses. The diagnosis of hyperthyroidism is definitively [SCORE] established by thyroid function testing (TFT); thyroid-stimulating hormone measurement (TSH, thyrotropin) is the single most useful test. TSH normally ranges between 0.3 and 3.0 mU/L; values less than 0.3 indicate hyperthyroidism (excess thyroid hormone causing decreased TSH secretion), and values > 3.0 suggest hypofunction (low levels of circulating thyroid hormone stimulating increased TSH secretion). Free thyroxine (T_4) and triiodothyronine (T_3) levels can provide further confirmation. Total T_4 and T_3 levels are influenced by serum protein derangements and must be interpreted with caution. Thyroglobulin (Tg) and calcitonin determinations are not useful for diagnosing hyperthyroidism.

DIFFERENTIAL DIAGNOSIS

Potential etiologies for hyperthyroidism are numerous, but relatively few lead to surgical referrals. Thyroidectomy as [SCORE] a treatment option is largely confined to three entities: diffuse toxic goiter (Graves disease), toxic nodular goiter (TNG; Plummer disease), and solitary hyperfunctioning nodule. Other forms of hyperthyroidism most often respond to medical management and/or withdrawal of the inciting agent (e.g., amiodarone) while the underlying thyroiditis resolves [*see Table 1*].

* The authors and editors gratefully acknowledge the contributions of the previous authors of "Thyroid and Parathyroid Operations," Wen T. Shen, MD, Gregg H. Jossart, MD, FACS, and Orlo H. Clark, MD, FACS, to the development and writing of this chapter.

Table 1 Etiologies of Hyperthyroidism

Disease	Predominant Treatment
Iodine induced (jodbasedow)	Medical
Subacute thyroiditis (de Quervain)	Medical
Chronic lymphocytic thyroiditis (Hashimoto thyroiditis)	Medical (surgical for compressive symptoms)
Postpartum thyroiditis	Medical
Drug induced (e.g., amiodarone)	Medical (rarely surgical)
Struma ovarii	Surgical (resect ovarian teratoma)
Graves disease	Medical or surgical
Toxic nodular goiter (Plummer disease)	Surgical or medical
Solitary hyperfunctioning nodule	Surgical, rarely medical

CLINICAL EVALUATION

History and Physical Examination

A thorough history may raise considerations of thyroiditis (e.g., amiodarone, pregnancy, iodinated contrast agents) and lead to reconsideration of nonsurgical management. Previous or ongoing treatment with thyroxine or antithyroid medications (ATMs) is noteworthy, along with review of recent TFT results. Factors that could influence treatment choices (e.g., iodine allergy, comorbid diseases) should be identified. Adrenergic symptoms (e.g., palpitations, tremor) are valuable in assessing antithyroid treatment response and readiness for operation. Compression symptoms (dysphagia, nocturnal dyspnea) are more likely with TNG than Graves disease or solitary toxic nodule (STN). Dysphonia is extremely rare with benign disease and should be definitively evaluated before thyroidectomy is recommended.

Examination of the thyroid begins with observation of the neck for goiter, including size and symmetry. Palpation may discriminate the smooth, soft, diffuse Graves gland from the firm, multinodular toxic goiter or the STN. Tenderness to palpation is most consistent with thyroiditis, as is bilateral lymphadenopathy. Unilateral, hard, or fixed cervical or supraclavicular adenopathy should prompt evaluation as outlined below for euthyroid nodular disease. Substernal extension of the goiter and cervical tracheal deviation should be noted when present. A solitary or dominant nodule should be characterized as to its location, size, and mobility. Physical examination should also focus on other signs of hyperthyroidism, including Graves ophthalmopathy (lid lag, lid retraction, proptosis, exophthalmos) and adrenergic excess (tachycardia, bilateral fine tremor of the hands). General medical status should be assessed as for any potential preoperative patient.

[SCORE] Indicates the text is tied to a SCORE learning objective. Please see the HTML version online at www.acssurgery.com.

Imaging

Thyroid scintigraphy reliably characterizes the hyperthyroid processes most often referred to surgeons and should precede any other form of imaging. Technetium pertechnetate (Tc-99m) scanning is rapid and produces sharper images at lower cost than iodine-123 (^{123}I). ^{123}I scintigraphy is superior when precise uptake quantification is required (before radioactive ^{131}I treatment) or when better bone penetration is necessary (substernal goiter).[1] Graves disease appears as homogeneous radionuclide uptake. An enlarged, heterogeneous gland with two or more areas of increased uptake surrounded by areas of normal or decreased uptake is typical of TNG. An STN is confirmed when a single, high-uptake ("hot") focus is seen against a suppressed background. Computed tomography (CT) and magnetic resonance imaging (MRI) have limited utility in hyperthyroidism other than for assessment of substernal goiters, and iodinated contrast administration will interfere with any subsequent ^{131}I treatment. Once the etiology of the hyperthyroidism is established, treatment options may then be considered. TNG and STN are preferentially treated operatively, whereas the algorithm for Graves is a bit more complex; ultrasonography (US) and fine-needle aspiration (FNA) may be indicated to exclude malignancy if nonoperative treatment is chosen.

TREATMENT CONSIDERATIONS

Initial Therapy

Medical management for control of symptoms and signs of hyperthyroidism precedes surgical treatment. ATMs and beta blockers are the most commonly used agents. The thionamides propylthiouracil (PTU) and methimazole limit thyroid hormone synthesis by disrupting organification of iodine. PTU also inhibits peripheral conversion of T_4 to the metabolically more active T_3. Minor side effects (pruritis, fever, gastrointestinal disturbances, and arthralgia) occur in 5 to 25% of patients receiving thionamides, and agranulocytosis affects 0.2 to 0.5% of patients receiving either medication.[2] Rare cases of fulminant hepatic failure and autoimmune vasculitis have been associated with PTU alone.[2-4] Beta blockers (atenolol, propranolol) may be added to ATM for more rapid control of severe adrenergic symptoms when present. Treatment efficacy is monitored by TFTs and clinical evaluation (resolution of tachycardia and tremor). Most patients are rendered euthyroid within 6 weeks of treatment initiation; virtually all are euthyroid at 3 months. PTU is often chosen over methimazole during pregnancy as methimazole is more apt to cross the placenta and has been linked to fetal scalp aplasia cutis.

Preoperative Therapy

Achieving euthyroidism markedly reduces the chance of thyrotoxicosis and thyroid storm intra- or postoperatively. Preoperative treatment goals include normalization of TFTs, a resting heart rate of 60 to 70 beats per minute, and resolution of tremor. In Graves disease patients, inorganic iodine administration in the form of Lugol solution (3 to 5 drops t.i.d.) or saturated solution of potassium iodide (SSKI; 2 to 3 drops t.i.d.) may decrease the size and vascularity of the gland when given for 7 to 10 days immediately preoperatively. Beta blockade alone supplemented by inorganic iodine is somewhat less effective but is rarely used in urgent clinical circumstances or for patients intolerant of thionamides.

Graves Disease

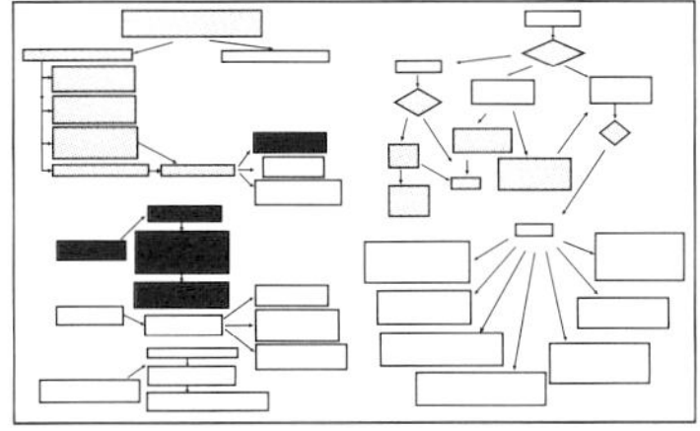

Graves disease is the leading cause of hyperthyroidism in the United States, comprising about 70% of cases. Women between the ages of 20 and 50 years are most commonly affected.[3] There are three effective, long-term treatments for Graves disease: prolonged ATM administration, radioactive iodine (RAI), and thyroidectomy. Factors influencing treatment choice include overall patient status (age, gender, comorbidities, life expectancy); thyroid findings (goiter size, dominant nodule, compression symptoms); health care system characteristics (access to physicians, medications, and laboratory testing); and patient preference.

Prolonged ATM administration Although common in Europe and Asia, this treatment is not often chosen in the United States, perhaps linked to the rare but potentially life-threatening side effect profile of thionamides. This approach also requires a prolonged medication trial (12 to 24 months), and patients often find this less palatable when more rapidly acting treatments with higher success rates are available. Remission (euthyroidism for at least 1 year posttreatment) is achieved initially in approximately 50% of cases, but this success rate declines to 30% at 10 years.[2,3,5] Negative predictors of remission include large goiter, severe biochemical disease, high serum ratio of T_3 to T_4, male gender, multiple relapses, and very high TSH receptor antibody titers.[2,5] Remissions are more common in adults than in children. Prolonged ATM administration should be considered when life expectancy is limited. Here methimazole has the advantage of twice-daily dosing versus PTU, which is given three to four times per day. Patients who fail to achieve remission or who relapse can be salvaged with RAI or surgery.

Radioactive iodine RAI is the definitive management of choice for Graves disease in the United States. Approximately 60% of patients are euthyroid within 6 to 8 weeks after a single oral dose of 5 to 15 mCi, and nearly all the remaining patients become euthyroid within several months.[4] Hyperthyroidism persists or recurs in 5 to 25% of cases and is dose dependent. Posttreatment hypofunction is also dose dependent. The risk of hypothyroidism is 20% within the first year and 3 to 5% per year thereafter. Thus, TFTs must be followed lifelong in all patients treated with RAI. Acute adverse reactions are uncommon after RAI administration. Pain secondary to radiation thyroiditis and nausea are reported most often. Because RAI treatment can trigger thyrotoxicosis, pretreatment with ATM before RAI administration may be appropriate for patients who are elderly or have concurrent heart disease. An exceedingly rare but more serious complication is hypoparathyroidism, which can be detected promptly by monitoring serum calcium.

RAI may not be the preferred treatment for some subgroups of patients with Graves disease. Although little credible evidence supports a generalized oncogenic effect of RAI, parental concerns about future cancers may prompt a choice for prolonged ATM administration or surgery in Graves disease in children and adolescents. RAI may exacerbate eye manifestations in patients with Graves ophthalmopathy,

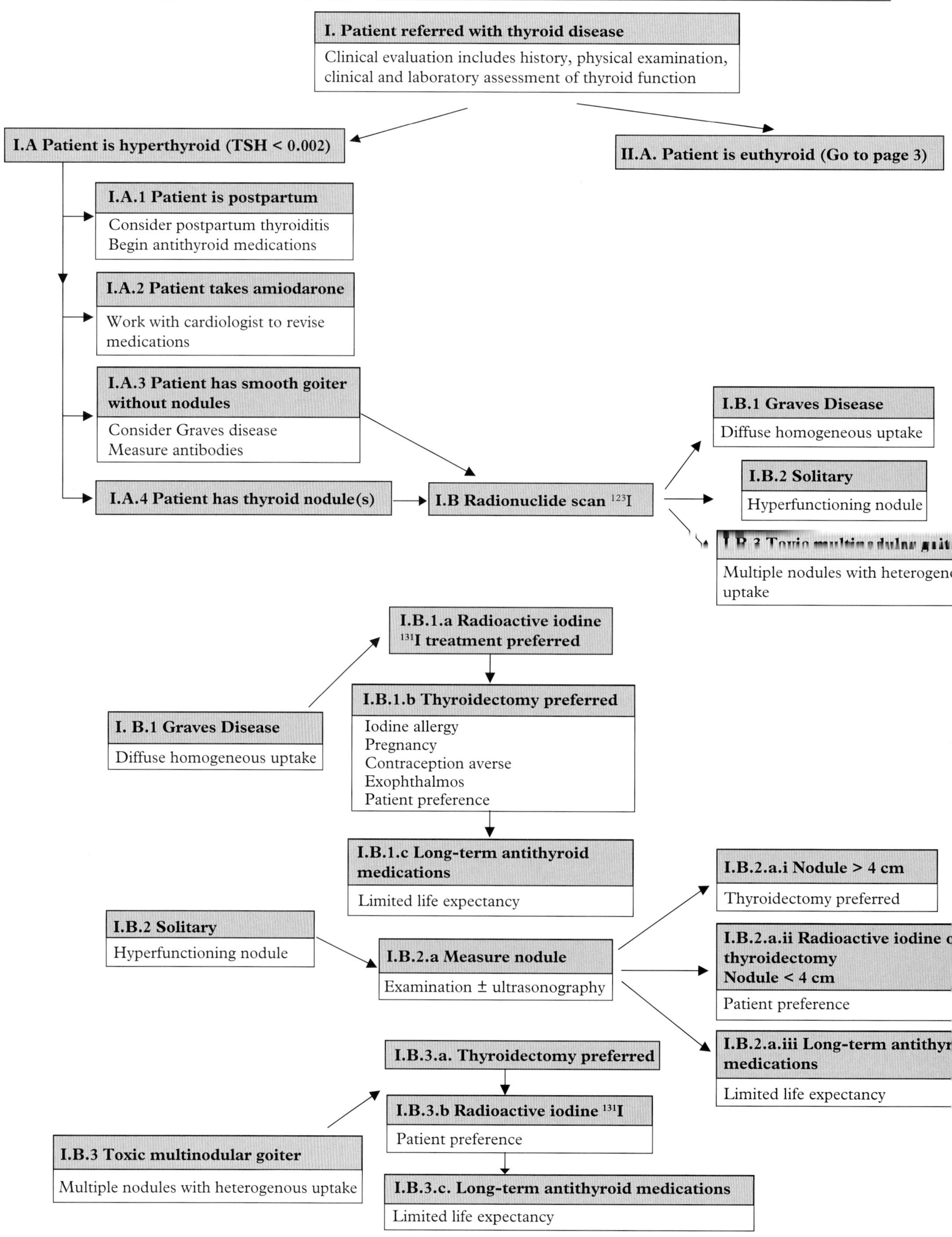
I. Patient referred with thyroid disease
Clinical evaluation includes history, physical examination, clinical and laboratory assessment of thyroid function
I.A Patient is hyperthyroid (TSH < 0.002)
II.A. Patient is euthyroid (Go to page 3)
I.A.1 Patient is postpartum
Consider postpartum thyroiditis
Begin antithyroid medications
I.A.2 Patient takes amiodarone
Work with cardiologist to revise medications
I.A.3 Patient has smooth goiter without nodules
Consider Graves disease
Measure antibodies
I.A.4 Patient has thyroid nodule(s)
I.B Radionuclide scan 123I
I.B.1 Graves Disease
Diffuse homogeneous uptake
I.B.2 Solitary
Hyperfunctioning nodule
Multiple nodules with heterogen
uptake
I.B.1.a Radioactive iodine 131I treatment preferred
I.B.1.b Thyroidectomy preferred
Iodine allergy
Pregnancy
Contraception averse
Exophthalmos
Patient preference
I. B.1 Graves Disease
Diffuse homogeneous uptake
I.B.1.c Long-term antithyroid medications
Limited life expectancy
I.B.2.a.i Nodule > 4 cm
Thyroidectomy preferred
I.B.2 Solitary
Hyperfunctioning nodule
I.B.2.a Measure nodule
Examination ± ultrasonography
I.B.2.a.ii Radioactive iodine
thyroidectomy
Nodule < 4 cm
Patient preference
I.B.2.a.iii Long-term antithy
medications
Limited life expectancy
I.B.3.a. Thyroidectomy preferred
I.B.3.b Radioactive iodine 131I
Patient preference
I.B.3 Toxic multinodular goiter
Multiple nodules with heterogenous uptake
I.B.3.c. Long-term antithyroid medications
Limited life expectancy

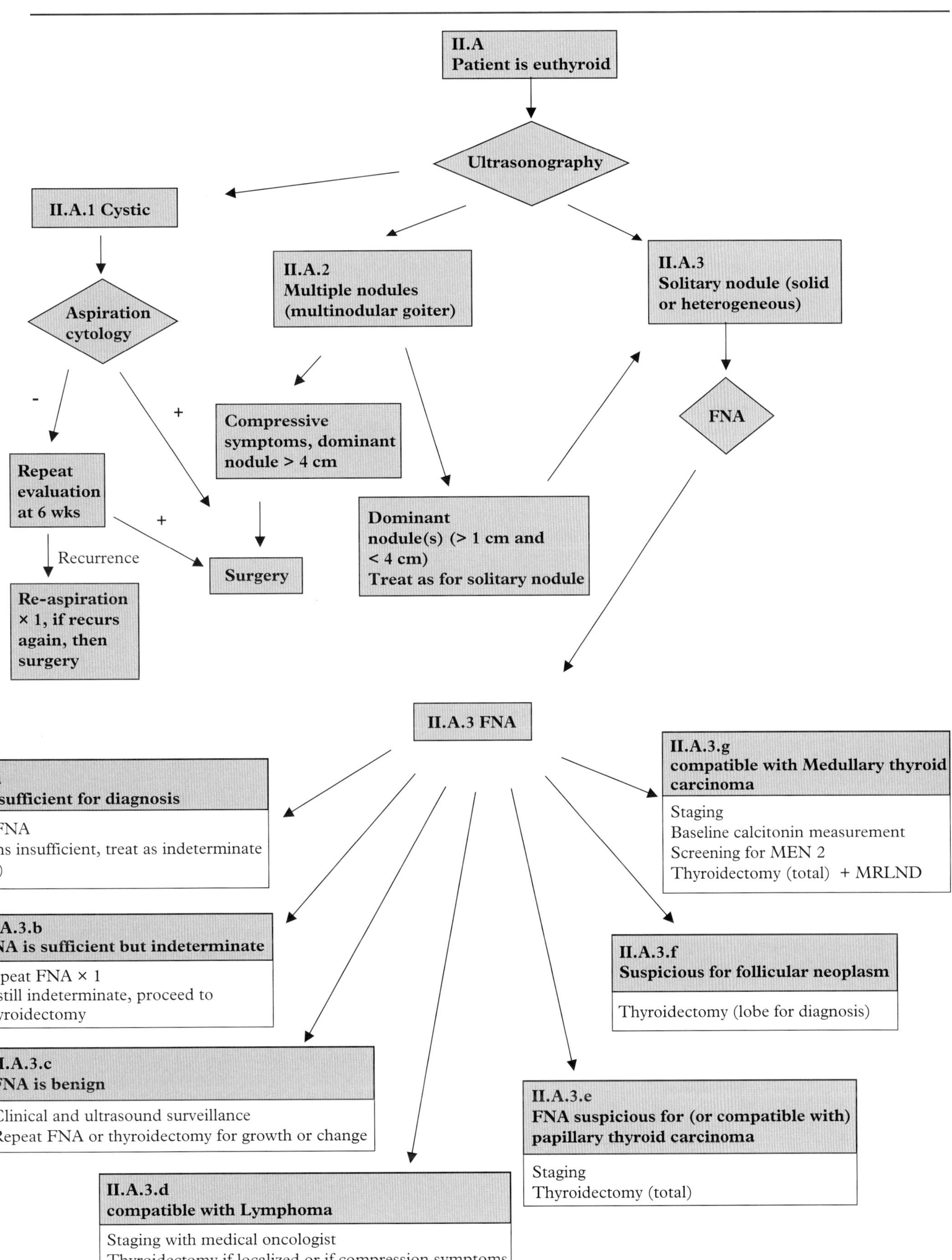
II.A
Patient is euthyroid
Ultrasonography
II.A.1 Cystic
Aspiration cytology
-
+
Repeat evaluation at 6 wks
+
Recurrence
Re-aspiration × 1, if recurs again, then surgery
II.A.2
Multiple nodules (multinodular goiter)
Compressive symptoms, dominant nodule > 4 cm
Surgery
Dominant nodule(s) (> 1 cm and < 4 cm)
Treat as for solitary nodule
II.A.3
Solitary nodule (solid or heterogeneous)
FNA
II.A.3 FNA
.3.a
A insufficient for diagnosis
eat FNA
mains insufficient, treat as indeterminate
gery)
II.A.3.b
FNA is sufficient but indeterminate
Repeat FNA × 1
If still indeterminate, proceed to thyroidectomy
II.A.3.c
FNA is benign
Clinical and ultrasound surveillance
Repeat FNA or thyroidectomy for growth or change
II.A.3.d
compatible with Lymphoma
Staging with medical oncologist
Thyroidectomy if localized or if compression symptoms
II.A.3.e
FNA suspicious for (or compatible with) papillary thyroid carcinoma
Staging
Thyroidectomy (total)
II.A.3.f
Suspicious for follicular neoplasm
Thyroidectomy (lobe for diagnosis)
II.A.3.g
compatible with Medullary thyroid carcinoma
Staging
Baseline calcitonin measurement
Screening for MEN 2
Thyroidectomy (total) + MRLND

particularly in smokers or when hyperthyroidism is severe.[6,7] Concurrent glucocorticoid administration minimizes this risk,[6,7] although moderate to severe ophthalmopathy remains a relative contraindication to RAI therapy, and surgery may be preferred in cases where eye findings of Graves disease are clinically overt. Pregnancy and lactation are absolute contraindications to RAI because ^{131}I crosses the placenta and is secreted into breast milk. Women should defer pregnancy for 6 to 12 months after receiving RAI to allow for stabilization of maternal thyroid function and to prevent transplacental passage of residual radioisotope and subsequent fetal hypothyroidism. RAI therapy is also contraindicated in patients who are allergic to iodine.

Surgery Surgical intervention provides rapid normalization of thyroid function with the lowest rate of recurrent hyperthyroidism while avoiding both the potential risks of prolonged ATM administration and the theoretical risk of ionizing radiation. Surgical treatment is preferred for Graves disease patients with relative or absolute contraindications to RAI, as outlined above, as well as in patients with compressive symptoms and those with concurrent suspicious or indeterminate nodules. Operation also is favored in patients for whom RAI is less likely to be effective, including patients with large goiters, severe biochemical disease, a high serum ratio of T_3 to T_4, male gender, or very high TSH receptor antibody titers. Graves ophthalmopathy frequently stabilizes and sometimes regresses after operation.[8,9] In some cases, patients may choose surgery to avoid ionizing radiation, to simplify family planning, or to minimize the duration of thyrotoxicosis.

Recommendations about the optimal extent of thyroidectomy for Graves disease have evolved over time. Bilateral subtotal resection was historically advocated for its safety profile and control of hyperthyroidism with the potential for euthyroidism without medication. However, estimation of tissue remnant size that will avoid hypothyroidism while minimizing recurrent hyperthyroidism may be difficult. Recent studies suggest similar complication rates following subtotal and total resections, whereas cure rates are substantially higher after total thyroidectomy.[8,10,11] When performed by surgeons with appropriately low morbidity (recurrent laryngeal nerve injury less than 1% and permanent hypoparathyroidism less than 3%[8,10]), total thyroidectomy is now favored over lesser resections.

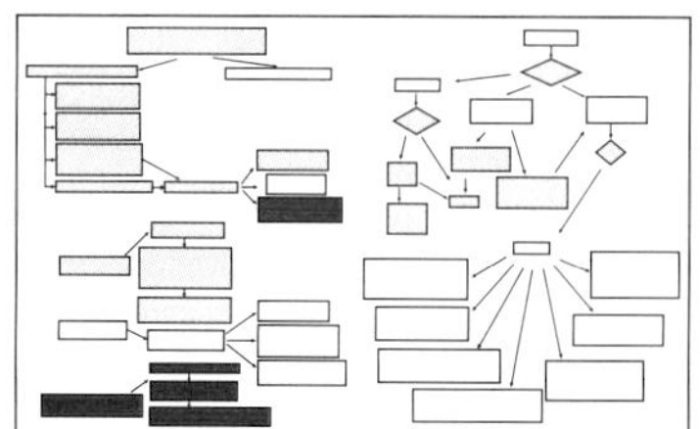

Toxic Nodular Goiter

Much less prevalent than Graves disease, TNG accounts for about 25% of all cases of hyperthyroidism in the United States. TNG is uncommon in patients under 50 years of age but is the most common cause of hyperthyroidism in the elderly.[12] TFT abnormalities are similar to those in Graves disease, although a higher proportion of patients with TNG will have T_3 thyrotoxicosis. Treatment options include ATM, RAI, and surgery.

Prolonged ATM administration TNG results from thyroid hormone production by multiple autonomously functioning nodules without the potential for spontaneous remission. Definitive management of TNG by ATM therefore requires lifelong ATM administration. Because of rare but sometimes life-threatening adverse reactions to the thionamides, only TNG patients with limited life expectancies are suitable for primary ATM treatment.

Radioactive iodine Iodine uptake is lower and less uniform in TNG than in Graves disease, making effective RAI dosing less predictable. Substantially higher initial doses are necessary, and up to 20% of patients require at least one additional RAI treatment.[2] Thus, patients may experience more side effects, including prolonged xerostomia and xerophthalmia, oral ulcers, and sialadenitis.[13] As with Graves disease, the time to euthyroidism is prolonged, and the risk of posttreatment hypothyroidism remains substantial. RAI shrinks the gland in less than half of patients, and radiation thyroiditis may cause serious, symptomatic thyroid edema. As a result, RAI is particularly unsuited for TNG patients with large or substernal goiters or with pretreatment compression symptoms. RAI for treatment of TNG is typically reserved for patients who are poor surgical candidates or those with small, asymptomatic goiters who refuse surgery.

Surgery Thyroidectomy is the treatment of choice for TNG. Surgery allows for rapid control of hyperthyroidism, relief of compressive symptoms, and histologic examination of any dominant or suspicious nodules and avoids any long-term side effects of ionizing radiation. Total thyroidectomy is favored when performed by surgeons with acceptable complication rates and confers the advantages of easy titration of thyroid replacement and a nonexistent recurrence rate. Inorganic iodine (Lugol, SSKI) generally is not given preoperatively in this setting as the variable and unpredictable iodine uptake by TNG raises the risk of triggering acute thyrotoxicosis.

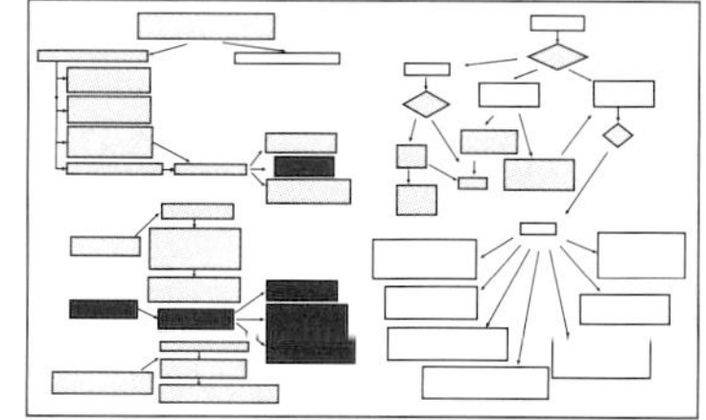

Solitary Toxic Nodule

STN causes less than 5% of all cases of hyperthyroidism in the United States. The frequency of STN is higher in women and increases with age. STNs are usually palpable on physical examination as thyrotoxicosis is rare when nodules are under 3 cm in diameter.[2] Like TNG, STN can be associated with T_3 toxicosis and normal T_4 levels. Treatment choices include ATM, RAI, and surgery.

Prolonged ATM administration Excess thyroid hormone secretion by the autonomously functioning STN will recur after ATM withdrawal. Definitive management of STN by lifelong ATM treatment is an option of last resort because of the rare but sometimes life-threatening adverse reactions to the thionamides, and this is indicated only for patients with limited life expectancy.

Radioactive iodine RAI can be effective definitive treatment for STN but usually is reserved for very-high-risk surgical candidates and for patients who refuse operation. The differential RAI uptake of the surrounding suppressed gland compared with the STN can confound RAI dosing. Intense RAI concentration by the STN itself exposes the adjacent normal thyroid to potentially oncogenic levels of ionizing radiation, with subsequent risk of thyroid neoplasia.

Surgery Thyroidectomy is the treatment of choice for STN. Resection of the affected thyroid lobe promptly controls hyperthyroidism in patients with STN and relieves any symptoms associated with these relatively large nodules. The risks of operation are quite low because lobectomy plus isthmusectomy is sufficient in most cases. When the contralateral remaining lobe is normal, long-term T_4 supplementation is usually unnecessary.

Approach to the Patient with Euthyroid Nodular Disease

Thyroid nodules are very common and represent a wide spectrum of thyroid disease, both benign and malignant [*see Table 2 and Table 3*]. Palpable disease is present in 5 to 7% of women and 1 to 2% of men, whereas cervical US reveals subclinical nodular disease in up to 67% of patients.[14] Most patients with nodules are clinically and biochemically euthyroid. Surgical referral is usually targeted at symptomatic relief in bulky benign disease, definitive diagnosis for indeterminate lesions, and definitive therapy for malignancy. Although the incidence of thyroid cancer has doubled since 1973,[14] 85 to 96% of palpable and subclinical nodules are benign. The rate of malignancy varies with factors including age, gender, family history, and radiation exposure. Screening for thyroid cancer is not cost-effective in the general population but is appropriate for some high-risk groups (e.g., multiple endocrine neoplasia [MEN] kindreds, after substantial radiation exposure). When considering treatment options, near-total (residual tissue < 1 g) and total (removal all visible thyroid) thyroidectomy will be used interchangeably. Subtotal resection refers to residual tissue more than 1 and less than 5 g.

Table 2 Benign Etiologies of Euthyroid Nodular Disease

Disease	Nodularity	Predominant Treatment
Colloid nodule	Solitary or multiple	Observation
Simple cyst	Solitary or multiple	Observation or aspiration if > 4 cm or growing
Follicular adenoma (FA)	Solitary or multiple	Resection (thyroid lobectomy) to exclude malignancy
Multinodular goiter (MNG)	Often with dominant nodule in multinodular gland	Resection for compressive symptoms, dominant nodule > 4 cm, or suspicious dominant nodule
Chronic lymphocytic thyroiditis (Hashimoto disease)	Heterogeneous gland; may have dominant nodule	Resection for compressive symptoms or if suspicious dominant nodule

Table 3 Malignant Etiologies of Euthyroid Nodular Disease

Disease	Percentage
Papillary thyroid cancer (PTC)	80
Follicular thyroid cancer (FTC)	10
Hürthle cell cancer (HCC)	1
Anaplastic thyroid cancer (ATC)	2
Medullary thyroid cancer (MTC)	5
Lymphoma	1
Metastases	< 1

DIFFERENTIAL DIAGNOSIS

The clinical challenge of euthyroid nodular disease is to reliably identify the small subset of patients with substantial likelihood of malignancy while avoiding the risks of surgery for the vast majority of patients with benign disease. Most thyroid nodular disease is more common in women and occurs in middle age, although anaplastic thyroid cancer (ATC), lymphoma, and sporadic medullary thyroid cancer (MTC) peak somewhat later.[15] Papillary (PTC) and follicular (FTC) thyroid cancers are often grouped together as well-differentiated thyroid cancer (WDTC).

CLINICAL EVALUATION

History and Physical Examination

A palpable solitary or dominant nodule should lead to documentation of duration, changes in size, associated symptoms, exposure to ionizing radiation, prior thyroid disease, or prior therapy with T_4. Recent TFT results should be reviewed. Bearing in mind that most WDTCs are slow-growing and asymptomatic, rapid growth with associated symptoms suggests an aggressive process, such as ATC or lymphoma.[16] Dysphagia and dyspnea are more common with multinodular goiter (MNG), whereas pain and hoarseness should heighten concerns for malignancy. Hashimoto disease raises the chance of lymphoma, and exposure to ionizing radiation, especially in childhood or adolescence, increases the likelihood of PTC. Family history should target a history of familial endocrinopathy or other hereditary tumor syndromes linked to thyroid disease, especially in the setting of suspected MTC[17] [*see Table 4*]. A history of prior neck surgery or irradiation should be carefully documented.

On examination, the neck is observed for visible nodule or goiter. Voice quality and volume are noted. Palpation defines thyroid size, symmetry, and consistency, as well as the number, size, location, consistency, tenderness, and mobility of nodules; the number, size, location, and mobility of cervical lymph nodes; and the presence of tracheal deviation or substernal extension. A firm, mobile, solitary nodule is most often a colloid nodule or simple cyst but also may represent follicular adenoma; a hard, fixed mass suggests cancer but may represent Hashimoto disease. Central or unilateral adenopathy favors PTC or MTC. Thyromegaly of variable texture and multiple nodules are most common with MNG; substernal extension may produce cervical tracheal deviation or venous engorgement. General medical status should be assessed as for any potential preoperative patient.

Table 4 Familial Syndromes of Thyroid Disease

Syndrome	Thyroid Disease	Gene/Tumor Marker
MEN type IIA	Medullary thyroid cancer	*ret* proto-oncogene/ calcitonin
MEN type IIB	Medullary thyroid cancer	*ret* proto-oncogene/ calcitonin
FMTC	Medullary thyroid cancer	*ret* proto-oncogene/ calcitonin
Familial adenomatous polyposes	Papillary thyroid cancer	*APC*
Carney complex	Well-differentiated thyroid cancer	*PRKAR1A*
Cowden disease (*PTEN* multiple hamartoma syndrome)	Follicular adenoma/ follicular carcinoma	*PTEN*
Peutz-Jeghers syndrome	Well-differentiated thyroid cancer	*STK 11* or *LKB 1*

FMTC = familial medullary thyroid carcinoma; MEN = multiple endocrine neoplasia.

Ultrasonography

Further assessment is accomplished with US, a safe, noninvasive, cost-effective means of imaging thyroid parenchyma and the cervical nodal basins. Patients are categorized as having solitary or multiple nodules, and lesions are subdivided into cystic, solid, or mixed cystic-solid. In a multinodular thyroid, a particularly large or irregular nodule is termed dominant. Benign nodules typically are round, homogeneous, slightly hypoechoic, and easily separable from surrounding tissue. Malignant nodules are more often irregular in shape, heterogeneous, markedly hypoechoic, and poorly demarcated. Tiny, hyperechoic, "comet tail"–shaped lucencies in a nodule favor benignity, whereas fine internal calcifications or hypervascularity suggests malignancy.[18] Thin-walled cysts without internal echoes are overwhelmingly benign; mixed cystic-solid nodules are indeterminate and grouped with solid lesions for further evaluation.

Fine-Needle Aspiration

FNA provides the most accurate, cost-effective assessment of thyroid nodules. Benign lesions comprise 70% of FNA results, whereas roughly 5% of FNA are read as definitively malignant. Most of the remaining lesions are "follicular aspirates," ranging from hyperplastic nodules to follicular cancer. A benign FNA diagnosis is credible[19,20] and requires no further intervention other than periodic screening. The sensitivity and specificity of FNA for the diagnosis of malignancy approach 94% and 99%, respectively.[21] A standardized thyroid FNA reporting system (Bethesda criteria) has recently been advocated.[22] There are six general diagnostic categories: nondiagnostic or unsatisfactory, benign, atypia of undetermined significance (AUS) or follicular lesion of undetermined significance (FLUS), suspicious for follicular neoplasm, suspicious for malignancy, and malignant. Risk of malignancy varies by category [*see Table 5*]. FNA of solid solitary or dominant nodules greater than 1 cm is appropriate in most cases. Solid lesions 5 to 10 mm may warrant FNA if the nodule is hypoechoic and microcalcifications are present, if the history discloses a high risk for cancer, or if they are found on an

Table 5 Bethesda Classification of FNA Cytology and Associated Malignancy Risk

Bethesda FNA Cytology Class	Risk of Malignancy (%)
Nondiagnostic/unsatisfactory	1–4
Benign	0–3
AUS/FLUS	5–15
Suspicious for follicular neoplasm	15–30
Suspicious for malignancy	60–75
Malignant	97–99

AUS = atypia of undetermined significance; FLUS = follicular lesion of undetermined significance; FNA = fine-needle aspiration.

unrelated fluorodeoxyglucose–positron emission tomographic (FDG-PET) scan.[14,23] When US confirms MNG and compression symptoms are absent, FNA is indicated for the dominant nodule.

Sequencing of Investigations

US typically precedes FNA as US findings may change the FNA target (e.g., an unsuspected suspicious nodule). "Pure" cystic lesions are rare, are overwhelmingly benign, and can be observed without FNA for diagnosis when asymptomatic. When a mixed nodule has a substantial cystic component, US-guided FNA allows fluid aspiration for cytology and FNA of the residual solid component. For solid nodules, US-guided FNA can reduce the rates of nondiagnostic and false negative results when the likelihood of inadequate material or sampling error is high (difficult to palpate, posteriorly located).[14] Operation without FNA is indicated for a solitary or dominant nodule exceeding 4 cm given the substantial chance of malignancy and the possibility of nonrepresentative sampling by FNA (although many clinicians obtain a biopsy for the purpose of operative planning). FNA is also unnecessary when US confirms MNG in a patient with compression symptoms.

MORPHOLOGY-BASED TREATMENT CONSIDERATIONS

Cystic Lesions

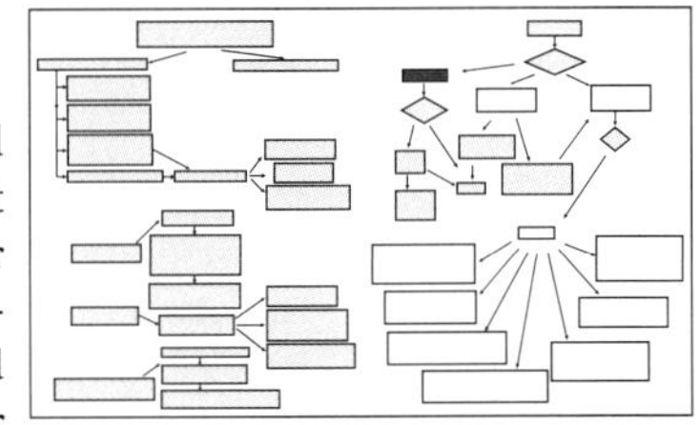

Incidentally discovered simple cysts do not require investigation or treatment. Clinically evident cysts are aspirated dry and the fluid sent for cytology. Benign cysts commonly recur and are reaspirated; thyroid lobectomy is indicated after two failed aspirations or for cysts greater than 4 cm. Percutaneous ethanol injection carries a 20% recurrence rate and is an alternative treatment for smaller cysts.[14] Mixed cystic-solid nodules are managed like solid lesions based on cytology and FNA results.

Multinodular Goiter

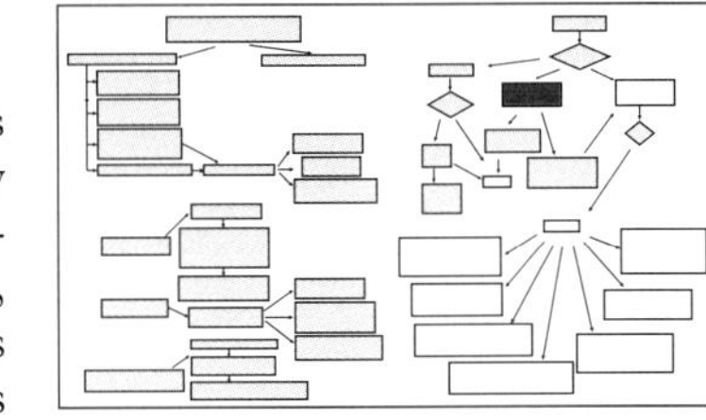

Most MNG patients are managed medically with serial clinical evaluations (examination, TFT, and US) unless compressive symptoms or dominant nodules develop. Thyroidectomy is indicated for patients with US findings of MNG and compressive symptoms. Compressive symptoms are typically associated with markedly asymmetrical goiters or those with substernal extension. When examination or US findings are inconsistent with symptomatology, CT or MRI can help exclude other etiologies. These cross-sectional modalities are also useful to delineate the extent of the mediastinal component if present. Indications for surgery include compressive symptoms, severe or bothersome cosmetic deformity, any dominant nodule greater than 4 cm, or any nodule greater than 1 cm with FNA results that meet the criteria for removal. Total thyroidectomy is preferred over lesser resections to minimize recurrent disease from remnant hypertrophy and is appropriate for these patients when done by surgeons with low complication rates. Nearly all substernal goiters can be safely removed through a generous collar incision, and the remaining few are reached via partial sternotomy. Patients with tracheal deviation or substernal goiters may present endotracheal intubation challenges; airway management is optimized by preoperative dialogue between the surgeon and the anesthesiologist. Frozen section adds little value except when preoperative FNA was nondiagnostic or not performed or when intraoperative findings suggest unexpected malignancy.

Solitary or Dominant Nodule

The management of a solitary nodule is highly dependent on cytologic diagnosis and can be broken down into six categories based on the Bethesda criteria.[22]

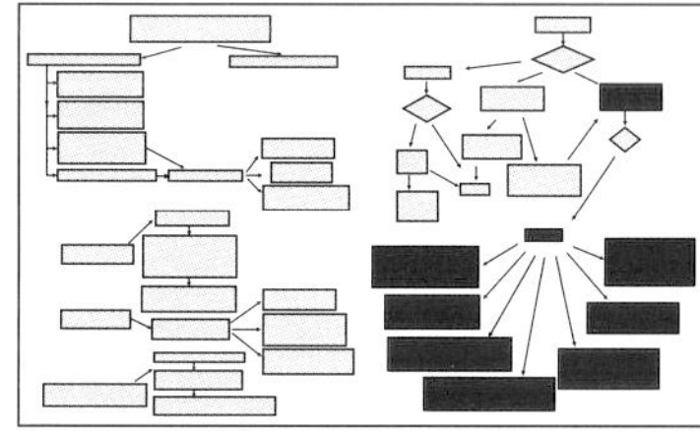

FNA nondiagnostic About 10 to 15% of aspirates are nondiagnostic, most often attributable to technical error, inadequate sampling, or a substantial cystic component. Less than 5% of these are malignant. Repeat FNA often yields adequate and definitive material[24]; US guidance may enhance yields. Persistently insufficient results should prompt lobectomy.

FNA benign A benign diagnosis is rendered in nearly 70% of all specimens, and no intervention is required. The risk of malignancy is 0.5 to 3%.[22] Surveillance by serial clinical evaluations (examination, TFT, and US) is done annually and then less often for stable nodules. Enlarging lesions (50% or more increased volume) warrant repeat FNA.

FNA AUS/FLUS Atypia or follicular lesion of undetermined significance is a heterogeneous subset of cytologically indeterminate nodules; roughly 5 to 15% prove to be malignant.[22] AUS/FLUS is managed like FNA nondiagnostic: repeat FNA and then lobectomy if a definitive diagnosis remains elusive. Molecular markers (e.g., *braf*, *ras*) hold promise for future use in this patient subset; FDG-PET specificity is too low to add clinically relevant value.

FNA suspicious for follicular neoplasm Cancer is present in 15 to 30% of suspicious for follicular neoplasm (SFN),[22] but the distinction between benign follicular adenoma and follicular carcinoma cannot be made by FNA cytology. Assessment for malignancy is based on capsular or vascular invasion, and lobectomy is indicated for tissue diagnosis. Completion thyroidectomy is performed for final diagnoses of follicular cancer or follicular variant of papillary cancer. Some patients opt for total thyroidectomy initially to avoid the need for reoperation; this strategy is reasonable when complication rates are kept low.

FNA suspicious for malignancy A small number of abnormal cells within a sparsely cellular or more benign-looking background characterizes lesions in this category. Malignancy rates are 60 to 75%.[22] Thyroid lobectomy is the minimum adequate treatment, and total thyroidectomy is preferable when complication rates are low.

FNA malignant Roughly 5% of cytologic diagnoses are conclusively malignant, and the positive predictive value of FNA for cancer is 97 to 99%.[22] Comments about the cell type are usually provided. Total thyroidectomy is the preferred treatment for WDTC and MTC, whereas lobectomy suffices for unilateral metastases from other primary sites. Resections for primary thyroid lymphoma and ATC are tailored to the extent of disease, although resection for ATC is usually aimed at palliation only.

High-Risk Patients

Patients exposed to ionizing radiation, especially in childhood or adolescence, have a lifetime increased risk of PTC. Whereas FNA is credible for assessing their nodules, total thyroidectomy should be considered once nodules develop. Patients who retain irradiated thyroids require extremely close surveillance, so noncompliant individuals are better served by operation. A contralateral nodule developing after a lobectomy for cancer most often warrants completion thyroidectomy. Close surveillance is acceptable for compliant patients when FNA is clearly benign. Large (> 4 cm) solitary or dominant nodules should be resected to allow complete histopathologic examination; lobectomy is the minimum acceptable procedure. When intraoperative findings suggest malignancy (e.g., adherence to strap muscles), total thyroidectomy is appropriate for surgeons with low complication rates. For less experienced surgeons or when findings are benign, lobectomy suffices, and further resection decisions are based on the final pathology. Frozen section cannot exclude malignancy in these cases because of the potential sampling error.

Additional Studies

Additional laboratory tests are seldom indicated preoperatively. When the history raises the potential for MTC, the cytopathologist should be alerted and special cytologic stains performed. Any suspicion of MTC on FNA should trigger exclusion of pheochromocytoma and assessment for primary hyperparathyroidism prior to thyroidectomy (plasma or urine metanephrine assays, serum parathyroid hormone and calcium levels). Additional imaging is warranted for palpable cervical adenopathy in the setting of any thyroid malignancy; the modality is selected based on local expertise. US avoids iodinated contrast administration (which confounds postoperative ^{131}I scanning or therapy), but accuracy is more operator dependent than for CT or MRI. FNA is appropriate when other etiologies for adenopathy are present or when documented nodal metastases would change management (e.g., lobectomy only is planned, tertiary care referral). For nodes detected only on preoperative imaging, image-guided FNA is used similarly. Preoperative laryngoscopy to document vocal cord function is indicated for patients with vocal complaints, audible vocal abnormalities, and prior neck operation or radiotherapy, although some surgeons perform laryngoscopy routinely. Vocal cord paralysis or other concerns for tracheal or esophageal invasion should be investigated by endoscopy and imaging. Vocal cord paralysis should also trigger preoperative dialogue about airway management with both the patient and the anesthesiologist. Radionuclide scanning is not useful, and the role of FDG-PET in preoperative staging remains ill-defined.

Intraoperative observations may lead to revision of the operative plan. Strap muscle adherence, adjacent soft tissue invasion, and extracapsular tumor extension are consistent with malignancy and favor total thyroidectomy. Contralateral disease palpable through the strap muscles warrants at least FNA (through the muscles) and consideration of total thyroidectomy. To lessen the morbidity of reoperation, the contralateral strap muscles should not be elevated unless resection is planned at the same operative session. Suspicious nodes may be evaluated by FNA or frozen section. Multiple suspicious central nodes or a positive biopsy result merit central lymphadenectomy [*see Figure 1, Level VI*]. Central neck dissection also should be considered by surgeons with low complication rates for T3 or T4 WDTC tumors even though nodal disease is absent. Proven lateral nodal disease is best treated by level II–IV en bloc functional resection when appropriate surgical expertise is available [*see Figure 1*].

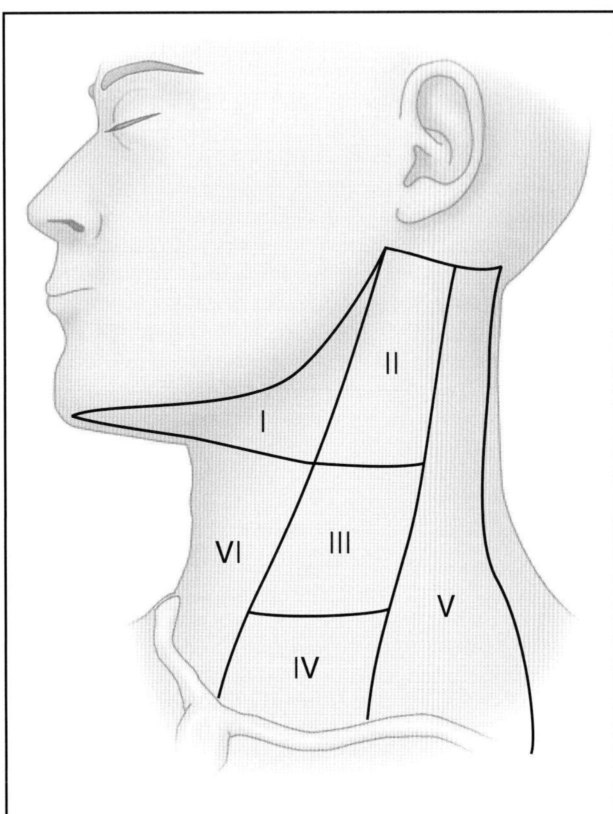

Figure 1 **Cervical lymph nodes can be classified into six levels (*inset*) on the basis of their location in the neck.**

DISEASE-SPECIFIC TREATMENT CONSIDERATIONS

Papillary Thyroid Cancer

PTC is the most common thyroid cancer and carries an excellent prognosis when treated appropriately (> 90% 10-year survival overall). Poor prognostic factors include age less than 20 or more than 60 years, tumor greater than 4 cm, extrathyroidal extension, and the presence of distant metastases.[25,26] Lymphatic spread worsens the prognosis and increases local recurrence risk for patients over 45 years and those with clinically apparent nodal involvement.[14] The tall cell, columnar, diffuse sclerosing, trabecular, and insular variants are more aggressive but uncommon. The follicular variant is more common but behaves more like classical PTC. One quarter of PTCs are multicentric, and lymph nodes are involved at the initial presentation in about one third.[27] Distant metastases, usually pulmonary, are present initially in 5% of cases. PTC rates are sharply increased by ionizing radiation, with a lag time of 15 to 25 years. The high long-term survival rates of PTC patients and paucity of large randomized controlled trials have contributed to inconsistent treatment guidelines and to multiple prognostic scoring systems [*see Table 6*]. Staging should follow the TNM classification [*see Table 7*]. Most scoring systems correlate with recurrent disease, whereas the TNM system links best to mortality. Recent consensus evaluation and treatment recommendations from the American Thyroid Association are achieving widespread recognition.[14]

Total thyroidectomy should be performed for most PTCs exceeding 1 cm[28]; this procedure addresses multicentricity, maximizes the therapeutic impact of postoperative RAI, and facilitates surveillance for recurrences. Lobectomy suffices for small, intrathyroidal PTC discovered incidentally in glands resected for other diagnoses when radiation exposure, nodal disease, and poor prognostic variants are absent. Central neck dissection is added based on FNA or operative findings suggesting lymphatic spread [*see Figure 1, Level VI*]. Judicious addition of prophylactic dissection by surgeons with low complication rates is reasonable, particularly for patients over 45 years, larger tumors (T3–T4), and more aggressive histologies.[14,27] The favorable natural history of PTC and the morbidity of lateral cervical lymphadenectomy suggest that this procedure be added only for pathologically proven lateral nodal disease. An aggressive operative approach should be considered in good operative candidates with PTC invading the trachea or esophagus. A functioning recurrent laryngeal nerve (normal vocal cord function) should seldom, if ever, be sacrificed.

Postoperative administration of RAI for thyroid remnant ablation may also have an adjuvant therapeutic effect on residual microscopic disease in the central neck. RAI ablation is indicated when nodal or distant metastases are known to be present and for T3–T4 tumors.[14] Ablation may also reduce recurrence rates for N1 disease or T2 tumors. Lifelong levothyroxine is given postoperatively at doses sufficient to suppress TSH secretion without causing overt hyperthyroidism. Dose reduction may be required if the osteoporosis risk

Table 6 Elements of Common Prognostic Schemes for Well-Differentiated Thyroid Cancer

Prognostic Scheme	Patient Characteristics		Tumor Characteristics						Operative Factors
	Age	Gender	Size	Histologic Grade	Histologic Subtype	Extrathyroidal Extension	Nodal Metastasis	Distant Metastasis	Completeness of Resection
AGES	+	−	+	+	*	+	−	+	−
AMES	+	+	+	−	+	+	−	+	−
MACIS	+	−	+	−	*	+	−	+	+
MSKCC	+	−	+	+	+	+	+	+	−

+ = variable used in defining risk group; − = variable not used; * = only for papillary thyroid carcinoma; AGES = patient age, tumor grade, extent, and tumor size; AMES = patient age, presence of distant metastases, extent, and tumor size; MACIS = metastatic lesions, patient age, completeness of resection, invasion, and size of tumor; MSKCC = Memorial Sloan-Kettering Cancer Center scheme.

Table 7 Staging of Differentiated Thyroid Cancer

Tumor Type	Stage	Patient Age (yr)	Tumor	Node	Metastasis
PTC/FTC	I	< 45	Any T	Any N	M0
	I	45 or older	T1	N0	M0
	II	< 45	Any T	Any N	M1
	II	45 or older	T2	N0	M0
	III	45 or older	T3	N0	M0
	III	45 or older	T1–3	N1a	M0
	IVA	45 or older	T4a	N0-1a	M0
	IVB	45 or older	T4b	Any N	M0
	IVC	45 or older	Any T	Any N	M1

Adapted from Greene FL, editor. AJCC Cancer Staging Manual, Sixth Edition. New York: Springer-Verlag; 2002.
FTC = follicular thyroid cancer; PTC = papillary thyroid cancer.

is high or atrial fibrillation develops. Postoperative surveillance can include RAI whole body scan, serum Tg levels, and cervical US; test combinations and frequencies are individualized based on tumor staging, estimated recurrence risks, and patient compliance. Anti-Tg antibodies should be measured simultaneously with each Tg assay.

Follicular Thyroid Cancer

FTC comprises 10 to 15% of thyroid malignancies. In contrast to PTC, FTC is typically solitary, and metastasis is more often hematogenous than lymphatic, favoring lung and bone. Poor prognostic factors include age over 50 years and tumors over 3.5 cm. An FTC with a limited area of microscopic capsular invasion and no vascular invasion is termed "minimally invasive" and carries no excess mortality when treated by thyroid lobectomy. Total thyroidectomy is indicated for more extensive capsular invasion or for vascular invasion. Central [*see Figure 1, Level VI*] or lateral lymphadenectomy [*see Figure 1, Level II–IV*] is performed for clinically evident or palpable nodal disease. Staging follows the TNM classification. RAI ablation is indicated for all FTCs except minimally invasive lesions. Levothyroxine suppression is given, and surveillance is performed as for PTC. Stage for stage, FTC and PTC have equivalent prognoses.

Oncocytic (Hürthle Cell) Carcinoma

Hürthle cell carcinomas (HCCs) comprise less than 5% of WDTCs and are a subset of follicular neoplasms. They contain at least 75% oncocytes and demonstrate capsular or vascular invasion. Oncocytic cancers are considered more aggressive than classical FTC because extrathyroidal extension and metastases (nodal and distant) are more common and RAI uptake is often minimal.[15,29] Total thyroidectomy is indicated for nearly all HCCs, although this is often done in a two-stage fashion because FNA cannot provide a definitive diagnosis. Central or lateral lymphadenectomy is performed when nodes are clinically positive. Staging should follow the TNM classification. RAI ablation is indicated for all HCCs, and levothyroxine suppression is given as for FTC. Surveillance includes US and Tg; FDG-PET may be useful when Tg is elevated and a radioiodine whole body scan is negative.

Anaplastic Thyroid Cancer

ATC is rare in the United States, representing less than 2% of thyroid malignancies.[29,30] The median survival for patients with ATC is approximately 6 months.[15,30] ATC is suspected when older patients present with rapidly progressive, bulky, fixed tumors. Diagnosis may require core-needle or incisional biopsy when FNA is inadequate. The vast majority of tumors are unresectable at diagnosis because of locoregional spread. Over 40% of patients have extensive nodal involvement, and nearly 50% present with distant metastases (lung, bone, brain, adrenal).[30] Surgery has little utility other than for establishing an airway for palliation. External beam radiotherapy plus chemotherapy may transiently shrink the tumor;

palliative debulking is occasionally feasible for the few patients with significant and sustained responses.

Medullary Thyroid Carcinoma

Unlike WDTC, MTC is a neuroendocrine tumor that arises from the calcitonin-secreting parafollicular cells. MTC constitutes about 5% of thyroid cancers; most (75%) cases are sporadic, whereas the remainder are hereditary. Sporadic disease presents as a solitary nodule, often with palpable adenopathy. Cytologic features are characteristic and confirmed by immunostaining for calcitonin. Distant metastases to lung, liver, and bone are frequent. Staging follows the TNM classification [*see Table 8*]. Preoperative staging includes neck, chest, and abdominal CT or MRI for all but those with small primary tumors and no adenopathy. Liver and lung lesions are often multiple but sometimes small enough to escape detection via CT. A baseline calcitonin should be measured preoperatively. Testing to exclude pheochromocytoma also is essential because the patient may represent the index case of an unsuspected kindred with MEN. If present, pheochromocytoma must be resected prior to thyroidectomy for MTC. Overall survival in MTC is considerably lower when compared with WDTC. Poor prognostic features include large tumor size, high preoperative calcitonin, advanced age, and mediastinal adenopathy.[28] Surgery is the only effective treatment modality and should consist of total thyroidectomy plus central neck dissection [*see Figure 1, Level 6*] and ipsilateral modified radical neck dissection [*see Figure 1, Levels I–V*]. Contralateral lymphadenectomy is added when bilateral thyroid masses or clinically positive nodes are identified. Extrathyroidal or extranodal tumor extension worsens the prognosis. Calcitonin is followed serially as a tumor marker postoperatively. A subset of patients with persistent or recurrent hypercalcitonemia follow a prolonged course, and reoperation may be indicated when tumor masses are detected by imaging and confirmed by FNA. Aggressive cervical reoperation for persistent hypercalcitonemia alone is controversial. Symptomatic hypercalcitonemia is unusual. RAI has no therapeutic role for MTC.

MTC occurs as a component of three familial syndromes: MEN type IIA, MEN type IIB, and familial medullary thyroid carcinoma (FMTC). MTC associated with MEN type IIB is the most aggressive, followed by MEN type IIA and then FMTC. Hereditary lesions usually are bilateral and are associated with a precursor lesion termed C-cell hyperplasia. MEN type IIA accounts for two thirds of hereditary MTCs. *Ret* proto-oncogene testing is recommended before age 6 within known kindreds. Prophylactic total thyroidectomy and central neck dissection are performed when a *ret* mutation is confirmed, after excluding pheochromocytoma.[31,32] MTC has an earlier age at onset in MEN type IIB, and genetic screening is conducted shortly after birth. Positive *ret* testing is followed by total thyroidectomy and central neck dissection in the first year of life.[31] FMTC is defined by the presence of four or more MTC cases within a family in the absence of associated endocrinopathy. The age at onset of FMTC is delayed compared with that of MEN type II, but FMTC survival is optimized by childhood genetic screening and operation (total thyroidectomy and central neck dissection).

Table 8 Staging of Medullary and Anaplastic Cancer

Tumor Type	Stage	Tumor	Node	Metastasis
MTC	I	T1	N1	M0
	II	T2–3	N0	M0
	III	T1–3	N1a	M0
	IVA	T4a	N0–1a	M0
	IVA	T1–4a	N1b	M0
	IVB	T4b	Any N	M0
	IVC	Any T	Any N	M1
Anaplastic	IVA	T4a	Any N	M0
	IVB	T4b	Any N	M0
	IVC	Any T	Any N	M1

Adapted from Greene FL, editor. AJCC Cancer Staging Manual, Sixth Edition. New York: Springer-Verlag; 2002.
MTC = medullary thyroid cancer.

Primary Thyroid Lymphoma

Primary thyroid lymphoma (PTL) accounts for approximately 1% of thyroid malignancies and 1% of extranodal lymphomas.[27,28] The risk of PTL is increased by Hashimoto thyroiditis. FNA is diagnostic in most cases (80%); core-needle or incisional biopsy may be required for diagnosis or for tumor markers. About 75% of PTL are diffuse large B cell lesions and 25% are mucosa-associated lymphoid tissue (MALT) lymphomas, with MALT lesions carrying a better prognosis.[16] Poor prognostic features include size greater than 10 cm, advanced stage, compressive symptoms, mediastinal involvement, and rapid tumor growth. Constitutional symptoms are rare. PTLs are chemo- and radiosensitive, so multiagent chemotherapy is usually combined with external-beam radiation as definitive treatment. Surgery alone may be appropriate for early-stage MALT tumors.[16,30] If PTL is diagnosed intraoperatively, total thyroidectomy is appropriate.

Metastases

Metastases to the thyroid are rare. Renal cell and breast tumors are common tumors of origin. FNA will suggest metastatic tumor, although perhaps not identify a specific tumor of origin. When the thyroid is the sole site of metastatic disease, thyroidectomy (lobe versus total) may be curative. Palliative resection is seldom, if ever, appropriate. Preoperative evaluation is tailored to the tumor of origin.

Thyroidectomy: Technique, Tips, and Troubleshooting

OPERATIVE TECHNIQUE

Proper Positioning

The first step to a safe thyroidectomy is positioning the patient to optimize operative exposure. A shoulder roll or a sandbag placed between the scapulas allows the neck to be extended and shifted anteriorly. Proper positioning is particularly important in facilitating access to substernal goiters through the cervical approach. Neck extension must be gentle in all patients and should be limited in patients with known cervical disk disease, rheumatoid arthritis, or osteoporosis. The occiput should be stabilized by support with a foam pillow. Neck hyperextension or poor occipital support can result in significant postoperative muscle spasm and associated headache.

General Technical Principles

The thyroidectomy incision is located in a cosmetically sensitive area, but exposure should not be compromised by an inadequate incision. A larger operative field is generally needed for resections for Graves disease and toxic multinodular goiters, for large nontoxic multinodular goiters producing compression symptoms (particularly those with substernal components), when preoperative evaluation suggests extrathyroidal extension of tumor, and when there is a high likelihood of performing a lymphadenectomy.

Operative complications are best avoided by unhurried dissection in a bloodless field.[33,34] If encountered, bleeding can and should be controlled first by pressure so that the relationship of the source vessel to the recurrent laryngeal nerve can be clarified. Early identification of the nerve facilitates safe control of vessels. Suture ligatures should be considered for controlling vessel ends that are likely to retract away from the operative field (e.g., cephalad end of the superior thyroid artery at the superior pole, mediastinal end of a thyroidea ima artery). Operating telescopes (2.5 to 3.5 power magnification) are a useful adjunct during delicate dissection around the recurrent nerve and vascular branches supplying parathyroid glands.

When bilateral resection is planned, dissection should nearly always be done first on the side of the suspected tumor or larger goiter. Should a problem be encountered (e.g., parathyroid involvement by tumor or recurrent nerve operative injury), the operative plan can be revised to a subtotal resection on the contralateral side to enhance protection of the parathyroid glands and recurrent nerve on that side. Rarely, when tumors are known or suspected preoperatively to be very extensive, beginning on the "easy" (less abnormal) side may facilitate identification of and access to the trachea and esophagus.

Step 1: Skin Incision and Subplatysmal Flaps

A collar incision paralleling the normal cervical skin lines offers extensile exposure. Typically, the incision is sited about 1 cm caudad to the cricoid cartilage and extends between the sternocleidomastoid muscles [*see Figure 2*]. Shifting the incision cephalad should be considered when the superior poles are likely to extend significantly upward (e.g., Graves disease) or caudad when a substernal goiter is present. After dividing the platysma, subplatysmal flaps are raised widely in all directions in this bloodless plane, avoiding the anterior jugular veins that may be particularly prominent in patients with Graves disease or substernal goiters.

Tips and troubleshooting Developing the superior flap to 1 to 2 cm above the thyroid cartilage notch will facilitate later access to the superior poles and the pyramidal lobe. Taking the inferior flap until the flat surface of the manubrium is palpable will aid exposure of substernal goiters. A retractor with attachable side-arm blades (e.g., the Mahorner-Hamburger-Brennan) is particularly useful for operations on larger glands but requires a slightly longer skin incision for atraumatic placement into the neck.

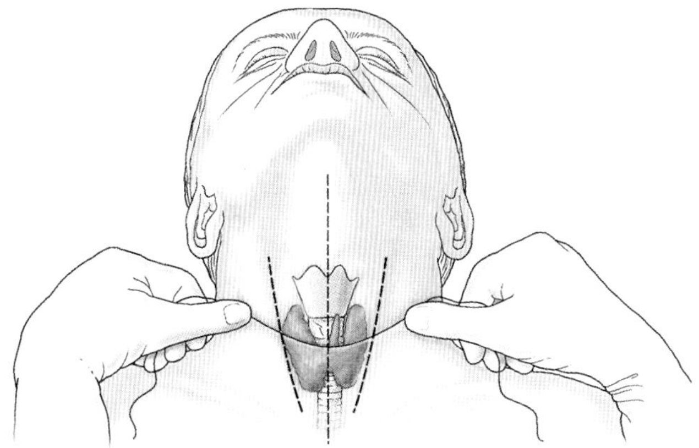

Figure 2 **The initial incision in a thyroidectomy is made 1 cm below the cricoid cartilage and follows normal skin lines. A sterile marking pen is used to mark the midline of the neck, the level of the incision, and the lateral borders of the incision. A 2-0 silk tie is pressed against the neck to mark the incision site itself.**

Step 2: Mobilization of Strap Muscles

The thyroid gland is exposed by dividing the investing and pretracheal layers of the cervical fascia in the midline. The sternohyoid and sternothyroid muscles can then be elevated as a single unit on each side off the thyroid lobe in what is usually a bloodless plane [*see Figure 3*]. The dissection is carried laterally until the lateral border of the sternothyroid muscle is easily seen. Partial or complete division of the sternothyroid muscle at its insertion into the thyroid cartilage can significantly improve exposure of the superior pole while avoiding denervation of the muscle. Routine division of both strap muscles is unnecessary in most cases. Once the strap muscle unit is elevated fully, side-arm blades can be inserted and fixed to the self-retraining retractor for lateral retraction of the strap muscles.

In patients operated on to exclude or to treat malignancy, a deliberate pause prior to further dissection is appropriate after the strap muscle unit is fully elevated from the thyroid lobe. The size, location, color, and consistency of the solitary or dominant nodule should be noted, along with the integrity of the overlying thyroid capsule and the presence of fibrosis in or adherence of adjacent soft tissues to the lobe. The characteristics of visible central neck lymph nodes should be assessed.

Tips and troubleshooting The midline fascia should be opened down to the inferior aspect of the sternal notch, where the interclavicular ligament can be palpated, facilitating later mobilization of substernal goiter, identification of inferior parathyroid glands, and central lymphadenectomy.

Tissue attachments or vessels crossing the plane between the thyroid and the midline strap muscles are concerning for malignancy, and any densely adherent portion of strap muscle should be sacrificed and left attached to the underlying thyroid for en bloc resection. This maneuver will also aid the pathologist later in determining extrathyroidal extension of tumor, a finding that is an important predictor of recurrence. Tissue reaction to a preoperative FNA biopsy can simulate tumor adherence. Benign central lymph nodes should be

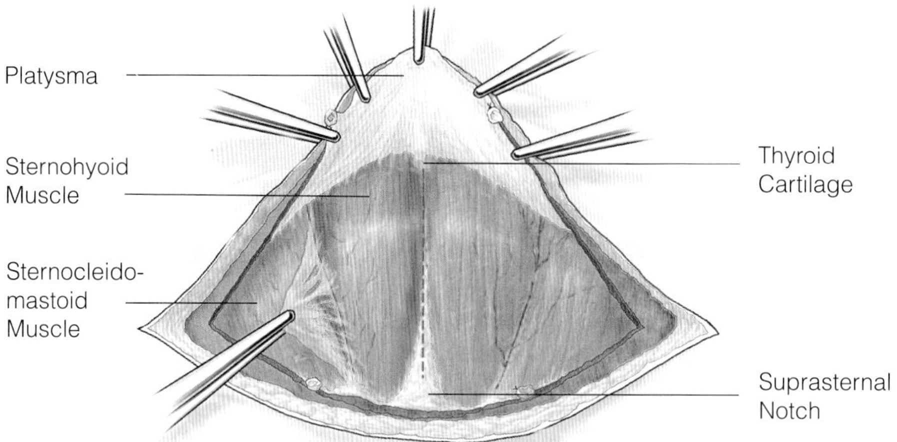

Figure 3 **To expose the thyroid, a midline incision is made through the superficial layer of deep cervical fascia between the strap muscles. The incision is begun at the suprasternal notch and extended to the thyroid cartilage.**

small, firm but not hard, and mobile and have well-defined capsules; nodes appearing otherwise should be regarded as suspicious, and intraoperative FNA should be considered. Benign lymphadenopathy is most often associated with Graves disease and Hashimoto thyroiditis.

Step 3: Initial Mobilization of the Thyroid Lobe and Superior Parathyroid Gland Identification

A 2-0 suture is placed deeply through the thyroid lobe for retraction to facilitate exposure. The stitch should not traverse a thyroid nodule as it is more likely to pull loose and may create artifacts that confound later histopathologic interpretation. The lobe is retracted medially while the filmy soft tissue lateral to the lobe is divided close to the gland. Dissection parallel to the usual course of the recurrent laryngeal nerve is safest. The addition of inferior traction facilitates carrying the dissection up to the superior pole. Vessels are controlled and divided near or on the surface of the lobe whenever feasible, limiting risk to the nerve and minimizing the chance of parathyroid devascularization. The superior thyroid artery is best managed by dividing it at the branch level, controlling the individual branches low on the thyroid gland, which minimizes the risk of injury to the external branch of the superior laryngeal nerve [*see Figure 4*].

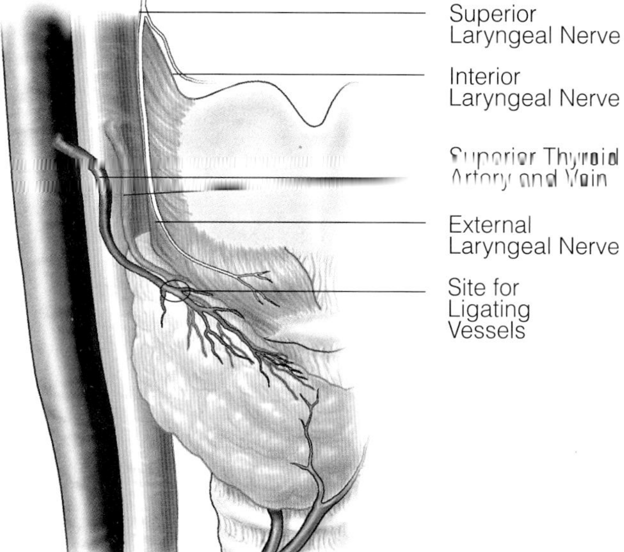

Figure 4 **The superior pole vessels should be individually identified and ligated low on the thyroid gland to minimize the chances of injury to the external branch of the superior laryngeal nerve.**

Tips and troubleshooting A small sponge applied to the gland surface further facilitates lobar retraction and lessens trauma to the thyroid surface, particularly when the gland is hypervascular (e.g., Graves disease). Palpation of the inferior cornu of the hyoid bone is advisable as the lobe is retracted medially and caudally as a guide to the location of the recurrent nerve, which enters the cricothyroid muscle in close proximity to the cornu. As the lobe is rotated medially and the superior pole branches are divided, the superior parathyroid gland usually is easily seen and should be gently freed from the perithyroidal soft tissue [*see Figure 5*]. The parathyroid with its adjacent soft tissue and fat is gently swept away from the thyroid.

Step 4: Recurrent Laryngeal Nerve Identification

It is usually safest to identify the recurrent laryngeal nerve low in the neck and then to follow it to where it enters the cricothyroid muscle through the Berry ligament [*see Figure 6*]. With the thyroid lobe retracted medially and anteriorly, the nerve is put on stretch and can be palpated as a taut, linear structure ("guitar string") slightly inferior to the inferior thyroid artery. The filmy soft tissue overlying the nerve can be lifted anteriorly away from the nerve and divided under direct vision, allowing the nerve to be followed to its cricothyroid entry. Sharp, fine-bladed scissors (e.g., tenotomy, Jameson) and fine-tipped hemostats ("mosquito") are essential instruments for this step. Having looped around the right subclavian artery, the right recurrent nerve follows a more oblique lateral-to-medial course than the left nerve, which follows a straight vertical course somewhat more deeply in the tracheoesophageal groove, having looped around the ductus arteriosus in the mediastinum.

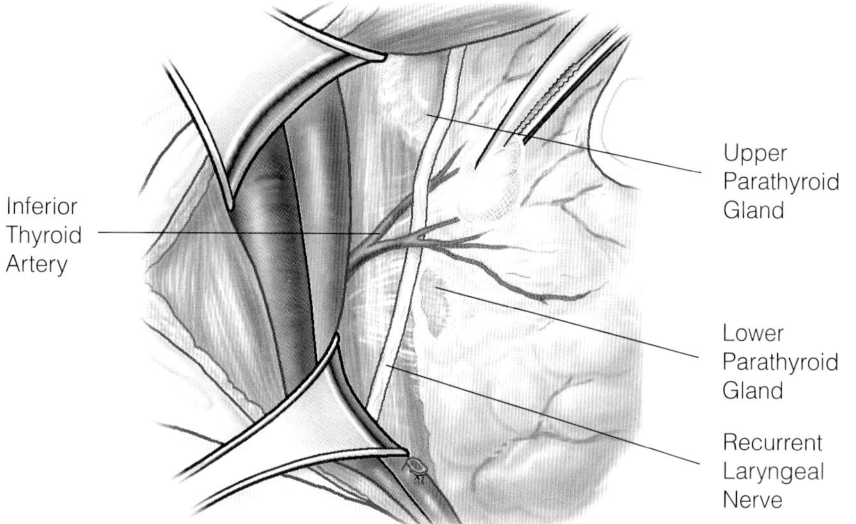

Figure 5 **The upper parathyroid glands are usually situated on either side of the thyroid at the level where the recurrent laryngeal nerve enters the cricothyroid muscle. The lower parathyroid glands are usually anterior to the recurrent laryngeal nerve and inferior to where the inferior thyroid artery crosses this nerve.**

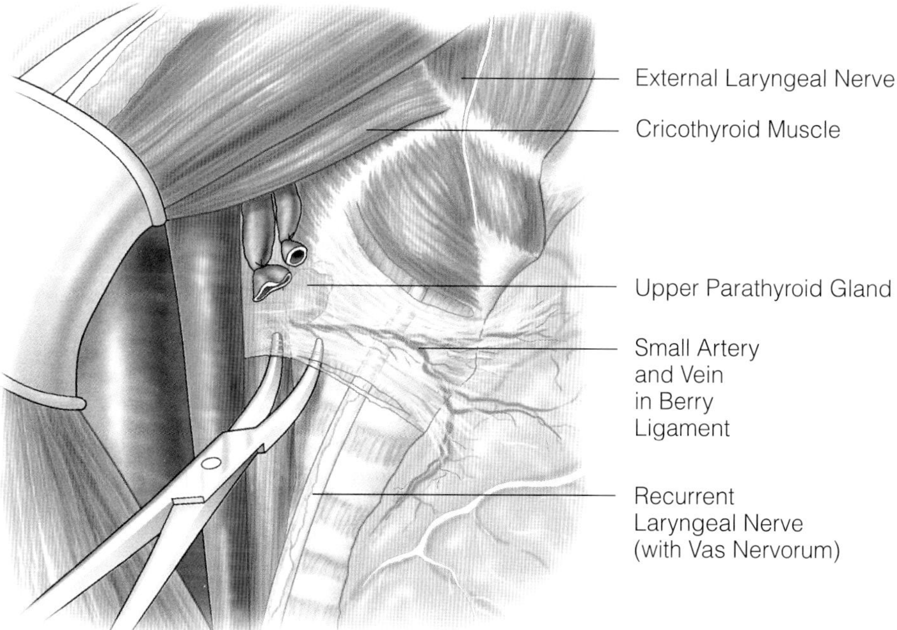

Figure 6 **The recurrent laryngeal nerve enters the cricothyroid muscle at the level of the cricoid cartilage, first passing through the Berry ligament.**

Tips and troubleshooting In about 0.5% of persons, the right recurrent laryngeal nerve is, in fact, "nonrecurrent," arising as a direct branch from the vagus in the midneck and coursing toward the thyroid from either laterally or superiorly.[1] Rarely, both a recurrent and a nonrecurrent nerve are present on the right. Branching of the nerve is common on both sides, and all branches must be preserved because all of the motor fibers of the recurrent laryngeal nerve are usually in the most medial branch. Initial identification of the nerve near the level of the inferior thyroid pole rather than superiorly will usually allow identification of any nerve branches. Some surgeons find intraoperative nerve monitoring to be helpful, but its use is not uniform among endocrine surgeons.[35]

Step 5: Thyroid Mobilization and Identification of Inferior Parathyroid Glands

Once the course of the recurrent laryngeal nerve has been identified, the lobe can be further rotated medially along its length and around the inferior pole, again controlling vessels close to the lobar surface. During this dissection, the inferior parathyroid gland is typically seen. Located in a plane anterior to the recurrent nerve, the parathyroid gland often appears attached to the capsule of the inferolateral thyroid pole. The attachment is filmy and easily separated, but care must be taken to avoid injuring the small vessels to the parathyroid.

Tips and troubleshooting Parathyroid glands should be swept from the thyroid gland on as broad a vascular pedicle as possible to prevent devascularization. If the pedicle is injured or if the parathyroid changes from its normal dark mustard color to a dusky purple, a tiny piece of the gland should be sent for frozen section to confirm its identity as parathyroid. Once confirmed, the gland is resected and put on sterile iced slush for autotransplantation into the sternocleidomastoid muscle just prior to closure.

In patients who have invasive tumors or who require reoperation, extensive scarring is often present. It may be preferable to identify the recurrent laryngeal nerve from a superior and medial approach by dividing the isthmus and the superior thyroid vessels. Careful medial to lateral rotation of the thyroid lobe from the trachea allows visualization of the nerve at its most consistent location (i.e., at its entrance into the larynx immediately posterior to the cricothyroid muscle). Alternatively, the nerve can be approached from laterally by identifying the lateral border of the sternothyroid muscle at the level of the inferior thyroid pole and working medially toward the inferior thyroid artery. The approach is modified to maximize dissection through the least scarred plane.

Step 6: Mobilization of the Pyramidal Lobe

A pyramidal lobe is found in about 80% of patients. This embryologic remnant usually arises from the left thyroid lobe near the midline and extends for a variable distance cranially. Inferior traction on the left lobe will bring most if not all of the pyramidal lobe into the operative field. The pyramidal lobe is dissected free medially and laterally from adjacent soft tissue and is transected at its cephalad termination. It is left attached to the main thyroid mass caudally and resected en bloc. As the pyramidal lobe is mobilized, one or more central neck nodes may be encountered overlying the cricothyroid membrane (so-called Delphian nodes) [*see Figure 7*].

Tips and troubleshooting The pyramidal lobe may extend to the base of the tongue as a thyroglossal duct remnant, but it is often just a fibrotic strand, particularly superior to the hyoid bone. Complete resection of the pyramidal lobe up to the tongue and removal of the middle third of the hyoid bone are important components of the Sistrunk operation for thyroglossal duct cyst. Resection of the pyramidal lobe within the usual thyroidectomy operative field without hyoid excision is sufficient during thyroid resection for other diseases.

Step 7: Completing the Thyroid Resection

Once the lobe has been mobilized superiorly, inferiorly, and laterally, it must be freed from its attachments to the trachea. As the lobe is rolled from lateral to medial, the most challenging part of the dissection involves the thyrotracheal ligament (Berry ligament), connecting the posterior aspect of the lobe to the trachea just caudal to the cricoid cartilage [*see Figure 6*]. A small branch of the inferior thyroid artery traverses the ligament, as do one or more thyroid veins; controlling bleeding from these vessels risks recurrent nerve injury as the nerve passes through or under the ligament. Should bleeding occur, it should be controlled by applying pressure with a gauze pad, avoiding clamps and ligatures until the course of the nerve through the ligament has been clearly delineated. Irrigating the field to limit blood staining of tissues is helpful. In some patients, a lateral projection of the thyroid (the tubercle of Zuckerkandl) overlies the nerve and ligament. Once the thyrotracheal ligament has been divided, the remaining thyroid attachments to the trachea can be divided through what is usually an avascular plane on the tracheal surface.

Division of the isthmus should be done between clamps and the ends suture ligated. When lobectomy is performed, the point of division should be at the junction of the isthmus with the contralateral lobe that will remain in situ. Division of the isthmus may be done earlier in the dissection when doing so will facilitate thyroid retraction or mobilization.

Tips and troubleshooting If bilateral resection will be performed, the isthmus may be left intact until the contralateral lobe is dissected free and the entire gland delivered as a

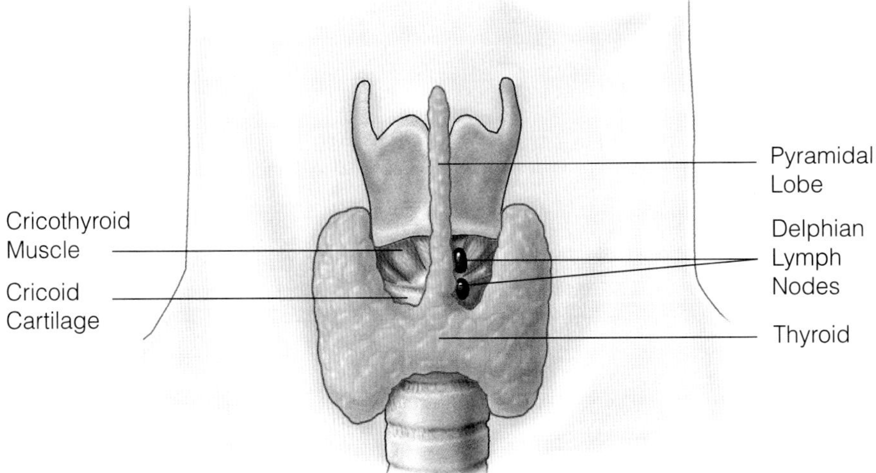

Figure 7 **Delphian lymph nodes may be found just cephalad to the isthmus over the cricothyroid membrane.**

single specimen The thyroid lobe should be carefully examined after removal. If a parathyroid gland is identified with the specimen, a frozen section biopsy is sent for confirmation and the gland is autotransplanted back into the neck unless the parathyroid appears to be involved by thyroid tumor extension (see above). The resected thyroid should be oriented for the pathologist; marking sutures or clips are helpful for this purpose.

Step 8: Closure

The best strategy to avoid a postoperative neck hematoma is taking time to ensure meticulous hemostasis prior to closure. Thorough irrigation of the field followed by precise identification and control of bleeders should be repeated as necessary until the field is hemostatic and dry throughout. The recurrent nerve should always be reidentified prior to placement of clamps or ligatures. The sternothyroid and sternohyoid muscles are reapproximated as separate layers in the midline. The platysma is closed as a separate layer once the subplatysmal flaps have been released from the self-retaining retractor and verified to be hemostatic. The skin can be closed in several ways, including subcuticular suture, butterfly clips, or tissue adhesive; the key factor in cosmesis is gentle tissue handling, not the closure method.

Smooth emergence from anesthesia with avoidance of coughing and retching can reduce the chance of high pressures being transmitted to the neck veins, and administration of an antiemetic during closure can be helpful, along with spraying the oral cavity with a topical local anesthetic. Endotracheal extubation with the patient still in a relatively "deep" plane of anesthesia is also helpful if not otherwise contraindicated. If postoperative laryngoscopy is contemplated, insertion of a nasal pack containing cocaine or another local anesthetic and decongestant during wound closure will facilitate early flexible fiberoptic endoscopy in the operating room or postanesthesia care unit.

Tips and troubleshooting It is not necessary to reattach a divided sternothyroid muscle to its thyroid cartilage insertion. However, the distal sternothyroid segment should be stretched to full length during closure to allow accurate approximation to the contralateral sternothyroid muscle. When both sternothyroid muscles have been divided superiorly, they can be anchored by including bites of both sternohyoid muscles at the cephalad end of the sternothyroid layer closure.

Drainage of the thyroid bed is no substitute for adequate hemostasis. A drain does not prevent wound hematoma, nor does it provide "early warning" of significant wound hemorrhage. A suction drain placed beneath the midline strap muscle closure may be useful when there is a large dead space in the resected thyroid bed (e.g., after excision of very large goiters). The drain is generally removed on postoperative day 1.

When a subcuticular closure is performed, a patient-friendly wound dressing can be created using a clothlike strip (e.g., roller gauze, Cover Strip II) placed directly over the incision and painted with collodion to render it waterproof. The patient is allowed to shower or wash over the wound beginning on the first postoperative day. The dressing separates from the skin at 7 to 10 days and is easily removed by the patient at that time.

EARLY POSTOPERATIVE CARE

Unilateral Resection (Lobectomy)

Thyroid lobectomy is often accomplished successfully on an outpatient or ambulatory basis, particularly when regional anesthesia is used. Patients with multiple comorbidities or those living in remote areas may be candidates for overnight observation, along with those failing to meet ambulatory surgical unit discharge criteria. The patient is maintained in a gentle head-up position (10° to 20°) for the first 24 hours when nonambulatory to enhance venous drainage and minimize edema formation. After regaining consciousness at a level sufficient to protect the airway, the patient is allowed liquid intake and can be advanced to a regular diet by the following morning. Liberal use of antiemetics during the early postoperative period will minimize retching and emesis. Initial patient-controlled analgesia should be transitioned to oral analgesics as soon as smooth swallowing is observed. Unless there has been neck surgery previously, there is no risk of clinically important hypocalcemia after thyroid lobectomy. It is unnecessary to measure serum calcium levels or to prescribe prophylactic calcium supplementation. The quality of the voice and the adequacy of the airway should be assessed in the postanesthesia care unit and prior to discharge to home. If there is any concern about the integrity of recurrent laryngeal nerve function, flexible fiberoptic laryngoscopy should be performed. Finally, if there is any question of a developing neck hematoma, the patient should be kept hospitalized for airway monitoring. A tray with sufficient instruments to reopen the neck incision urgently is kept at the bedside (e.g., tracheostomy tray).

Bilateral Resection

Patients undergoing bilateral thyroid resections are typically observed overnight or admitted for a brief inpatient stay. Patients undergoing removal of extensive tumors, tracheal or esophageal resections, or lymphadenectomies have longer lengths of stay. Positioning, antiemetics, diet, and patient-controlled analgesia are given as for lobectomy. Severe sore throat may be improved by topical anesthetic spray or solution. Voice quality and airway adequacy should be assessed in the postanesthesia care unit and periodically thereafter; any concern about the integrity of recurrent laryngeal nerve function should be evaluated promptly with flexible fiberoptic laryngoscopy. Patients with known coagulation abnormalities or evidence of neck hematoma merit close monitoring in a special care unit for 24 to 48 hours. A tray with sufficient instruments to reopen the neck incision urgently is kept at the bedside (e.g., tracheostomy tray).

Patients undergoing bilateral resections (or completion thyroidectomy after prior lobectomy) are at risk for transient or permanent hypoparathyroidism; the risk is increased with malignancy and by lymphadenectomy. Strategies for detecting and treating hypocalcemia vary among surgeons.[36] Total calcium is more often available and less expensive compared with ionized calcium. In some series, postoperative parathyroid hormone levels are early predictors of hypocalcemia, but parathyroid hormone may not always be available. In the absence of symptoms (perioral tingling, digital paresthesias), there is little reason to measure serum calcium until the morning of postoperative day 1. An exception might be when multiple parathyroid glands have been autotransplanted or when parathyroid tissue is excised deliberately en bloc with tumor. A simultaneous albumin level allows correction of the total calcium level for hemodilution by perioperative fluids; otherwise, ionized calcium alone is the optimal single measurement. An elevated serum phosphate level (> 4.5 mg/dL) denotes an increased risk of parathyroid hypofunction. Magnesium assay is performed when patients are symptomatic because hypomagnesemia can mimic or worsen hypocalcemia. An abnormal calcium value (unexplained by hemodilution) when symptoms are absent merits reassessment in 6 to 8 hours and again on postoperative day 2. Symptomatic patients and those with total calcium values less than 7.5 mg/dL warrant treatment. When symptoms are minimal, oral calcium suffices; calcium citrate is the best absorbed of the calcium salts. Severe symptoms (e.g., dark vision, feelings of doom) or neuromuscular findings (e.g., Trousseau sign or claw hand) merit intravenous calcium; calcium gluconate is the least problematic if extravasated. Calcium is remeasured if treatment is required and reaches a steady state 5 to 6 hours after oral dosing. Vitamin D supplementation is seldom necessary but is useful for patients who have required intravenous calcium or who are marginally controlled by 3 to 4 g calcium citrate total daily doses. 1,25-Dihydroxycholecalciferol is the maximally effective vitamin D agent and is given in one to two doses daily (0.5 to 1.0 μg total daily dose). Some surgeons use a strategy of routine postoperative oral calcium (1.5 to 3 g daily, with or without vitamin D) for all patients after bilateral resections to facilitate early discharge to home. Serum calcium is measured at the first postoperative visit and weaned as tolerated thereafter.

POSTOPERATIVE THYROID HORMONE MANAGEMENT

The half-life of T_4 is long enough that thyroid hormone replacement can be withheld safely until the final surgical pathology results are available. Awaiting the final diagnosis allows efficient, individualized treatment. Previously euthyroid patients seldom become hypothyroid after lobectomy alone. TFT measurement by the patient's primary care physician at 6 months (sooner if hypothyroid symptoms develop) will detect most patients who need T_4 supplementation. Older patients and those with Hashimoto disease are at greatest risk.

Patients will require T_4 therapy after bilateral resections. For patients with benign disease, levothyroxine can be started as soon as the pathology results are known. For patients with cancer, a decision for or against RAI will guide next steps. When RAI will be given, efficient preparation with minimal hypothyroid symptoms is accomplished by giving low-dose T_3 (50 μg b.i.d.) for 3 weeks. One week thereafter, most patients will have a TSH level suitable for RAI administration. Alternatively, patients may be given no thyroid hormone for the 4 weeks prior to RAI administration, but this approach more often results in bothersome symptoms. Patients can also reach appropriately high TSH levels by administration of recombinant human TSH for a brief period prior to giving RAI; this option, however, is very expensive, and the efficacy of RAI using this approach is not conclusively known. A baseline Tg level is most sensitive for the detection of residual thyroid tissue and/or residual WDTC when measured while the patient is thyroprival (TSH is elevated). Anti-Tg antibody assay should be measured along with each Tg level; Tg is unreliable when antibodies are present.

Regardless of the RAI preparation approach chosen, T_4 is started after RAI treatment and/or whole body scan. Replacement, achieving a TSH level within the normal range, is the treatment goal for patients with benign diagnoses. For patients with WDTC, suppression such that TSH is undetectable is the therapeutic target. Lower T_4 doses (less suppression) should be considered for older patients, those with cardiac disease, when osteoporosis risks are increased, or when clinically important hyperthyroid symptoms develop on full suppression. Some clinicians favor full suppression for the first few years postoperatively and then T_4 dose reduction to replacement levels if there is no evidence of recurrent WDTC. A steady-state TSH level is reached at 4 to 6 weeks after starting T_4 or after a dose adjustment.

Patients with MTC, ATC, or lymphoma are started on replacement doses of T_4 postoperatively because there is no proven benefit to TSH suppression in these diseases.

COMPLICATIONS

Thyroidectomy is well tolerated by most patients. General postoperative complications such as atelectasis and deep vein thrombosis or pulmonary embolism are possible but less common than after intracavitary operations. Thyroidectomy is a clean operation, and wound infection should be rare. If wound infection occurs, however, it is potentially quite serious. Infection-related soft tissue edema can lead to airway compromise, and local infection can progress to mediastinitis since the soft tissues of the thoracic inlet are usually opened during thyroidectomy. Thyroidectomy should be postponed if a patient arrives for operation with a recent history or current symptoms of acute pharyngitis.

Complications specific to thyroidectomy include neck hematoma or seroma, recurrent or external laryngeal nerve injury, and transient or permanent hypoparathyroidism. Postoperative bleeding into the neck can produce life-threatening airway compromise, and any postoperative respiratory distress should raise concern for neck hematoma. Urgent bedside decompression by reopening the wound down through the strap muscles is lifesaving when symptoms are sudden and severe. The patient is then returned to the operating room for wound exploration and reclosure under anesthesia. Neck hematoma development with few or no symptoms merits intensive care unit observation for at least 24 hours. Most bleeding occurs within 4 hours of operation, and virtually all occurs within 24 hours. Neck seroma is particularly likely after resection of very large goiters because of the residual dead space, and subplatysmal fluid is ballotable early postoperatively. In the absence of airway symptoms or persistent dysphagia, reassurance of the patient is the only intervention necessary. Percutaneous aspiration is performed for airway or swallowing symptoms or when preferred by the patient for cosmetic or comfort reasons.

Symptoms or signs of airway compromise not attributable to neck hematoma may indicate injury to the recurrent laryngeal nerves. Prompt performance of flexible fiberoptic laryngoscopy allows assessment of vocal cord position and function along with evaluation for other etiologies of respiratory distress (laryngeal edema, laryngospasm). Diagnostic laryngoscopy should not delay securing the airway of a patient with true stridor. Laryngoscopy may, however, be a useful adjunct to rapid, safe reintubation. Paretic or paralyzed vocal cords warrant reintubation. Symptomatic patients who are maintaining their oxygenation without tachypnea may benefit from inhaling a helium-oxygen admixture. The clinical response is rapid, and the admixture should be continued for several hours before attempting weaning to supplemental oxygen alone.

The reintubated patient should be kept in a head-up position for 36 to 48 hours. A parenteral dexamethasone bolus may be useful at the time of reintubation and carries little risk. Once the patient has mobilized his perioperative fluids and has minimal neck edema (usually by 48 hours postoperatively), airway reassessment can be undertaken. The patient who can vocalize and move air through the larynx with the endotracheal tube in place but with the cuff deflated is likely to tolerate extubation. Flexible laryngoscopy should be done immediately postextubation to document vocal cord function and adequate airway lumen. Close observation for an additional 24 to 48 hours is appropriate after successful extubation. For the patient failing extubation, laryngoscopic findings should drive the decision for early tracheostomy or for a second extubation attempt. Vocal cord function sufficient to maintain the airway must be documented before tracheal decannulation.

Some hoarseness or other vocal change is fairly common early postoperatively and can represent intubation trauma rather than recurrent nerve injury. Intubation-related vocal changes improve rapidly postoperatively. Hoarseness that persists at the first outpatient office visit deserves diagnostic laryngoscopy. If vocal cord motion is impaired, consideration should be given to confirmation by a second, independent observer. Voice rest and aspiration precautions should be instituted, and the patient is followed carefully. When symptoms resolve or plateau, laryngoscopy is repeated to document the level of functional return. Interventions such as vocal cord injection are not undertaken until function has clearly stabilized. Nerve dysfunction at 1 year is likely to be permanent.

Superior laryngeal nerve external branch dysfunction typically is more subtle than recurrent nerve injury, and injury rates are not as well established. Referral for comprehensive evaluation of vocal function is appropriate for persistent voice symptoms despite good vocal cord movement or for patients whose livelihoods require normal voices (e.g., a professional singer or storyteller). The impact of routine intraoperative nerve monitoring on recurrent and external branch nerve injury rates is unclear.

Permanent hypoparathyroidism (requirement for calcium supplementation more than 1 year postoperatively) should be uncommon (< 2%) after bilateral thyroid resections. Up to 10% of patients may have transient hypocalcemia that requires treatment, especially with Graves disease or synchronous lymphadenectomy. Resolution is usually fairly rapid (< 6 weeks). Autotransplanted parathyroid tissue is usually functional within 12 weeks postoperatively. Diagnosis and management of hypocalcemia have already been discussed [*see* Early Postoperative Care, Bilateral Resections, *above*].

OUTCOME EVALUATION

Surgeons performing thyroidectomies should track their individual rates of nerve and parathyroid injuries along with wound infections and neck hematomas. Participation in a registry system such as the National Surgical Quality Improvement Program (NSQIP) facilitates recognition of nonspecific complications (e.g., urinary tract infection) and system parameters (e.g., length of stay).

Financial Disclosures: None Reported

References

1. Smith JR, Oates E. Radionuclide imaging of the thyroid gland: patterns, pearls and pitfalls. Clin Nucl Med 2004;29:181–93.
2. Cooper DS. Hyperthyroidism. Lancet 2003; 362:459–68.
3. Schussler-Fiorenza CM, Bruns CM, Chen H. The surgical management of Graves' disease. J Surg Res 2006;133:207–14.
4. Hegedus L. Treatment of Graves' hyperthyroidism: evidence-based and emerging modalities. Endocrinol Metab Clin North Am 2009;38:355–71.
5. Stalberg P, Svensson A, Hessman O, et al. Surgical treatment of Graves' disease: evidence based approach. World J Surg 2008; 32:1269–77.
6. Bartelena L, Marcocci C, Bogazi F, et al. Relation between therapy for hyperthyroidism and the course of Graves' ophthalmopathy. N Engl J Med 1998;338:73–8.
7. Acharya SH, Avenell A, Philip S, et al. Radioiodine therapy (RAI) for Graves' disease and the effect on ophthalmopathy: a systematic review. Clin Endocrinol 2008;69:943–50.
8. Weber KJ, Solorzano CC, Lee JK, et al. Thyroidectomy remains an effective treatment option for Graves' disease. Am J Surg 2006;191:400–5.
9. Jarhult J, Rudberg C, Larsson E, et al. Graves' disease with moderate-severe endocrine ophthalmopathy—long term results of a prospective, randomized study of total or subtotal thyroid resection. Thyroid 2005;15: 1157–64.
10. Palit TK, Miller CC, Miltenburg DM. The efficacy of thyroidectomy for Graves' disease: a meta-analysis. J Surg Res 2000;90:161–5.
11. Boger MS, Perrier ND. Advantages and disadvantages of surgical therapy and optimal extent of thyroidectomy for the treatment of hyperthyroidism. Surg Clin North Am 2004;84:849–74.
12. Porterfield JR Jr, Thompson GB, Farley DR, et al. Evidence-based management of toxic multinodular goiter (Plummer's disease). World J Surg 2008;32:1278–84.
13. Solans R, Bosh JA, Galofre P, et al. Salivary and lacrimal gland dysfunction after radioiodine therapy: clinical thyroidology. J Nucl Med 2001;42:738–43.
14. Cooper DS, Doherty GM, Haugen BR, et al. Revised American Thyroid Association management guidelines for patients with thyroid nodules and differentiated thyroid cancer. Thyroid 2009;19:1167–214.
15. Delellis RA. Pathology and genetics of thyroid carcinoma. J Surg Oncol 2006;94: 662–9.
16. Mack LA, Pasieka JL. An evidence-based approach to the treatment of thyroid lymphoma. World J Surg 2007;31:978–86.
17. Dotto J, Nosé V. Familial thyroid carcinoma. Adv Anat Pathol 2008;15:332–49.
18. Kim TB Orloff LA. Thyroid ultrasonography. In: Orloff LA, editor. Head and neck ultrasonography. 1st ed. San Diego: Plural Publishing; 2008. p. 69–114.
19. Boey J, Hsu C, Collins RJ. False-negative errors in fine-needle aspiration biopsy of dominant thyroid nodules: a prospective follow-up study. World J Surg 1986;10: 623–30.
20. Grant CS, Hay ID, Gough IR, et al. Long-term follow-up of patients with benign thyroid fine-needle aspiration cytologic diagnoses. Surgery 1989;106:980–6.
21. Yang J, Schnadig V, Logrono R, et al. Fine-needle aspiration of thyroid nodules: a study of 4703 patients with histologic and clinical correlations. Cancer 2007;111:306–15.
22. Cibas ES, Ali SZ. The Bethesda system for reporting thyroid cytopathology. Thyroid 2009;11:1159–65.
23. AACE/AME Task Force on Thyroid Nodules. American Association of Clinical Endocrinologists and Associazione Medici Endocinologi medical guidelines for clinical practice for the diagnosis and management of thyroid nodules. Endocr Pract 2006;12: 64–101.
24. Rosen IB, Wallace C, Strawbridge HG, et al. Re-evaluation of needle aspiration cytology in detection of thyroid cancer. Surgery 1981;90: 747–56.
25. Kinder BK. Well differentiated thyroid cancer. Curr Opin Oncol 2003;15:71–7.
26. Ito Y, Miyauchi A. Prognostic factors and therapeutic strategies for differentiated carcinomas of the thyroid. Endocr J 2009;56: 177–92.

27. Mazzaferri EL, Doherty GM, et al. The pros and cons of prophylactic central compartment lymph node dissection for papillary thyroid carcinoma. Thyroid 2009;19:683–9.
28. Bilimoria KY, Bentrem DJ. Extent of surgery affects survival for papillary thyroid cancer. Ann Surg 2007;246:375–84.
29. Thyroid Carcinoma Task Force. AACE/AAES medical/surgical guidelines for clinical practice: management of thyroid carcinoma. Endocr Pract 2001;7:202–20.
30. Green LD, Mack L, Pasieka JL. Anaplastic thyroid cancer and primary thyroid lymphoma: a review of these rare thyroid malignancies. J Surg Oncol 2006;94:725–36.
31. Richards ML. Thyroid cancer genetics: multiple endocrine neoplasia type 2, non-medullary familial thyroid cancer and familial syndromes associated with thyroid cancer. Surg Oncol Clin N Am 2008;18:39–52.
32. Roman S, Mehta P, Sosa JA. Medullary thyroid cancer: early detection and novel treatments. Curr Opin Oncol 2008;21:5–10.
33. Thompson NW, Olsen WR, Hoffman GL. The continuing development of the technique of thyroidectomy. Surgery 1973;73:913–27.
34. Delbridge L. Total thyroidectomy: the evolution of surgical technique. Aust N Z J Surg 2003;73:761–8.
35. Sturgeon C, Sturgeon T, Angelos P. Neuromonitoring in thyroid surgery: attitudes, usage patterns, and predictors of use among endocrine surgeons. World J Surg 2009;33: 417–25.
36. Asari R, Passler C, Kaczirek K, et al. Hypoparathyroidism after total thyroidectomy. a prospective study. Arch Surg 2008;143: 132–7.

Acknowledgment

Figures 2 through 7 Tom Moore

10 PARATHYROID DISEASES AND OPERATIONS

Patrick B. O'Neal, MD, Atul Gawande, MD, MPH, Francis D. Moore Jr, MD, and Daniel T. Ruan, MD

Anatomy/Embryology

SCORE The parathyroid glands arise during the fourth and fifth weeks of gestation from branchial pouches III and IV. The superior glands descend into the neck from branchial pouch IV, whereas the inferior glands descend into the neck from branchial pouch III. In general, the superior glands settle 1 cm superior to the inferior thyroid artery in a posterior position to the thyroid gland, and the inferior glands settle at the lower pole of the thyroid gland in a posterolateral position. The superior and inferior parathyroids are consistently located posterior and anterior to the recurrent laryngeal nerve, respectively.

The parathyroid glands can be found in ectopic locations. Approximately 60% of parathyroids on reoperation are not located in the typical locations. The inferior glands have a higher propensity for this in comparison with the upper glands. Common ectopic locations of the inferior glands at reoperation include the thymus (46%), within the thyroid itself (7%), undescended (4%), and the carotid sheath (1%). Common ectopic locations of the superior glands include the posterior superior mediastinum (40%), the tracheoesophageal groove (17%), within the thyroid (1.5%), and the carotid sheath (1.5%). Of note, the posterior and anterior relation to the recurrent laryngeal nerve is typically preserved in superior and inferior ectopic glands, respectively.

Most commonly, there are four parathyroid glands; however, the incidence of supernumerary glands is around 13%. All four glands derive their blood supply from the inferior thyroid artery. Venous drainage is by the venous network of the thyroid capsule and/or venous pedicles of the thyroid body. The glands are often found embedded in fat. When dissected, normal parathyroid glands have a flat triangular shape with a mustard hue whereas pathologic parathyroids are plump with a reddish-brown hue resembling a grape.

The recurrent laryngeal nerves innervate all intrinsic muscles of the larynx except the cricothyroid muscles. These nerves arise from the vagus nerves in the chest and travel upward on either side of the trachea through the tracheoesophageal groove. They usually cross posterior to the inferior thyroid arteries but can pass anteriorly. They will then cross posterior to or through the Berry ligament to insert into the cricothyroid muscles. Caution should be taken when dissecting this area as the nerve may branch into an anterior motor branch and a posterior sensory branch. One can easily mistake a posterior sensory branch as the only branch and ligate the motor branch causing ipsilateral vocal cord paralysis.

Function

The primary function of the parathyroid glands is to maintain calcium homeostasis within the body. Calcium concentrations in the serum are directly regulated by a sensitive calcium-sensing receptor that is highly expressed on the surface of the parathyroid cells. When ionized calcium is bound within this receptor, release of parathyroid hormone (PTH) is inhibited. In contrast, when ionized calcium levels are low, fewer receptors are bound, and production of PTH is stimulated. PTH is an 84–amino acid protein with multiple effects on calcium homeostasis. PTH increases osteoclast and osteoblast activity, leading to the net release of calcium from bone stores as clastic activity is more affected than blastic activity. Furthermore, PTH increases gastrointestinal absorption and renal calcium retention, primarily in the proximal tubule and the loop of Henle. Lastly, PTH increases renal hydroxylation of 25-hydroxyvitamin D. In addition to increasing serum calcium, PTH also decreases serum phosphate and increases renal bicarbonate excretion.

Dysfunction

Primary hyperparathyroidism (PHPT) results from the inappropriately high secretion of PTH causing hypercalcemia. This is thought to be caused by the spontaneous loss of calcium-sensing receptors in parathyroid tissue. This may be caused by dysfunction in one or multiple parathyroid glands. Approximately 90% of PHPT is caused by adenomas, which can be multiple in approximately 3 to 8% of cases. In contrast, 9% of PHPT is attributable to four-gland hyperplasia and approximately 1% is the result of parathyroid carcinoma. As much as 3% of PHPT is associated with the multiple endocrine neoplasia (MEN) syndromes. PHPT is not caused by renal disease, a history of lithium use, or gastrointestinal malabsorptive syndromes. SCORE

Although PHPT has traditionally been considered to manifest itself by hypercalcemia in the setting of excessive PTH secretion, a less common manifestation of PHPT that has only minimal, intermittent, or even the absence of hypercalcemia is now being recognized. As many at 15% of patients with PHPT will have "normocalcemic hyperparathyroidism." As noted, these patients will have elevated PTH levels but will not have persistently elevated calcium levels. In fact, some may have calcium levels that are consistently within a normal range. They will still exhibit, however, the destructive complications of PHPT. Because one cannot use hypercalcemia as a diagnostic tool for this entity, diagnosis is difficult. Typically, PTH levels are inappropriately elevated in the presence of PHPT complications. Vitamin D deficiency and benign familial hypocalciuric hypercalcemia should be excluded prior to the diagnosis. Additionally, evidence suggests that calcium-loading challenges may assist in identifying these patients. In most normal patients, an oral calcium load has been shown to suppress serum PTH levels by 70% or more, whereas in patients with normocalcemic PHPT, this is usually not the case. Nonetheless, this is not a perfect test and cannot be used alone to identify these patients.

Secondary hyperparathyroidism (SHPT) occurs from the physiologic response to low serum calcium levels of nonparathyroid origin. Although the pathophysiology of SHPT is complex, it is most commonly caused by chronic renal failure, which interferes with vitamin D metabolism, which in turn leads to decreased calcium absorption from nutritional sources. Other causes include "hungry bone syndrome," sprue, chronic vitamin D deficiency, and aluminum toxicity from hemodialysis. Generally, hypercalcemia is not a characteristic of this disease.

Tertiary hyperparathyroidism (THPT) is the long-term consequence of prolonged SHPT after the cause is corrected. It results in autonomously elevated PTH concentrations as a result of the loss of calcium-sensing receptors in parathyroid tissue. The net result of THPT is elevated serum calcium. The typical scenario is the patient with SHPT attributable to end-stage renal disease who undergoes renal transplantation. In this condition, all four glands are treated as hyperplastic glands.

Parathyroid carcinoma is a very rare cause of hyperparathyroidism. It often results in markedly elevated levels of both PTH and calcium. Complications of hyperparathyroidism are more common with parathyroid carcinoma. The incidence of kidney stones is over 50%, whereas severe bone disease is observed in as many as 90% of patients. These lesions are more likely palpable than benign hypersecreting glands, and on gross inspection, they exhibit invasive features. Histologically, parathyroid carcinoma shows features of capsular and vascular invasion, cellular mitoses, thick fibrous bands separating tumor lobules, and a trabecular pattern. Of course, the hallmark of parathyroid carcinoma is its invasive nature. Thirty percent of patients will have nodal metastases on presentation, and the 5-year survival rate approximates 60% with treatment. Posttreatment, recurrent hypercalcemia is a good marker for local recurrence or new metastases.

Complications of Hypercalcemia

The normal serum calcium level is 9 to 10.5 mg/dL. Dysregulation of calcium homeostasis has profound effects on patient well-being. On questioning, patients often complain of a general sense of poor physical performance. This includes symptoms of depression, fatigue, muscle weakness, cognitive deficits, and forgetfulness. In addition, patients may present with gastrointestinal complaints, particularly constipation and gastroesophageal reflux.

More seriously, 30% of patients with PHPT will develop nephrolithiasis and 15% of patients will develop osteoporosis. Occasionally, patients can develop severe osteodystrophy, resulting in bone pain, osteomalacia, pathologic fractures, and osteitis fibrosa cystica (brown tumors of bone).

Interestingly, there is now a growing literature implicating hyperparathyroidism in atherosclerotic disease. Evidence for this includes studies showing increased blood pressure, arterial stiffness, and intima/media thickness in patients with PHPT as well as derangements in a number of metabolic processes leading to the development of cardiovascular disease, including dyslipidemia and impaired glucose metabolism. In fact, cardiovascular complications are the most common cause of death in both treated and untreated patients with PHPT. Estimates of mortality resulting from cardiovascular disease in patients with PHPT range from 53 to 68%. This includes death from myocardial infarction, stroke, and heart failure. Epidemiologic studies suggest that the life expectancy in patients with PHPT is lower than that in matched controls.

Evaluation of Primary Hyperparathyroidism

Although often unrevealing, a thorough history and physical examination should be performed. This may reveal symptoms or complications of hyperparathyroidism that may need to be addressed. Additionally, the information obtained may reveal the need to evaluate patients for familial causes of hyperparathyroidism, particularly the MEN syndromes. Physical examination may reveal a palpable neck mass that may alert the surgeon to the possibility of malignancy. Physical examination findings in chronic PHPT include band keratopathy and intraoral tumors.

Laboratory workup should include serum calcium and PTH levels and 24-hour urinary calcium levels to rule out familial hypocalciuric hypercalcemia. As noted earlier, patients with PHPT typically have elevated serum PTH and serum calcium levels but PTH may fluctuate and near normocalcemic variants have been reported. In these patients, one will see a persistently elevated (as opposed to suppressed) PTH level despite near normal serum calcium or high normal serum calcium levels. Patients with PHPT may have normal but often have high 24-hour urinary calcium levels as the kidneys surpass their threshold for calcium resorption. Patients with benign familial hypocalciuric hypercalcemia will have low 24-hour urinary calcium levels. Additionally, patients with familial hypocalciuric hypercalcemia generally have mildly elevated serum calcium levels. Benign familial hypocalciuric hypercalcemia can be excluded in patients with a history of normal serum calcium levels in the distant past. Hyperparathyroid patients are typically hypophosphatemic, and alkaline phosphatase may predict high-turnover bone disease. 25-Hydroxyvitamin D should be checked to exclude vitamin D deficiency.

Localization studies have improved dramatically over recent years, allowing for progressively fewer invasive surgical options. Because 80% of patients with PHPT have a single adenoma, preoperative localization studies allow far less extensive neck dissection. The mainstays of localization studies are ultrasonography and sestamibi scanning. Ultrasonography has a sensitivity of 79%. Sestamibi scanning has a sensitivity of 88%. When these two modalities are combined, sensitivity increases to greater than 90%. Sestamibi scanning works on the premise that both thyroid and parathyroid absorb tracer but that, as a result of increased blood flow in the thyroid, thyroid tracer washes out more quickly (minutes to 2 hours), allowing for visualization of enlarged parathyroid glands. When comparing early and delayed sestamibi images persistent uptake may be seen in the delayed images at the location of pathologic parathyroid glands. Occasionally, these imaging modalities are insufficient. The advent of four-dimensional computed tomographic (CT) scanning has allowed for the localization of many allusive parathyroid glands. Other options include venous PTH sampling. Although localization studies are useful for surgical planning, they should not be used to establish the biochemical diagnosis.

Treatment

Treatment algorithms depend on the pathology causing hyperparathyroidism. In general, PHPT is treated surgically with removal of all hyperfunctioning parathyroid tissue. There is agreement that all symptomatic disease should be treated surgically. However, the indications for the treatment of asymptomatic disease are less clear-cut. These indications receive a great deal of scrutiny and are periodically revised by National Institutes of Health consensus conferences in response to evolving data. Currently, surgery is recommended for asymptomatic patients with serum calcium levels 1.0 mg/dL above the upper limit of normal, a glomerular filtration rate less than 60 mL/min, T scores less than −2.5 at any site and/or previous fracture fragility, or age less than 50 years. T score refers to the number of standard deviations above or below the normal bone mineral density a person's own bone mineral density is. Normal is defined by a T score above −1. Osteopenia is defined by a T score between −1 and −2.5. Osteoporosis is defined by a T score less than −2.5. It is expected that these criteria for surgery in the asymptomatic patient may be further revised as new data elucidate other complications of hyperparathyroidism, particularly atherosclerotic disease.

For individuals who cannot undergo surgery, patients with persistent hyperparathyroidism in which hyperfunctioning tissue cannot be found, and patients with hypercalcemic crisis, a number of medical therapies may improve hypercalcemia. These include hydration with normal saline, loop diuretics, bisphosphonates, calcitonin, mithramycin, and calcium receptor agonists. SHPT generally is not considered a surgical disease. Instead, these patients are treated with calcimimetics, calcium, and vitamin D replacement. Rarely, with failure of medical management, surgery may be considered. In this case, indications for surgery may include severe pruritis, musculoskeletal pain, renal osteodystrophy, and calciphylaxis.

Tertiary hyperthyroidism is primarily a surgical disease. Because all parathyroid tissue is hyperfunctioning in these patients, the preferred operation is four-gland parathyroidectomy with autotransplantation of half of a single gland or subtotal parathyroidectomy. In the latter case, a parathyroid remnant roughly the size of a normal parathyroid gland is left in situ.

Parathyroid carcinoma absolutely requires surgery if cure is to be achieved. In this case, the operation of choice is en bloc resection of the malignant parathyroid tumor with the overlying musculature and ipsilateral thyroid lobe. Additionally, local recurrences and localized distant metastases should be treated surgically. Systemic chemotherapy and radiation have minimal efficacy and are considered palliative interventions in this context.

Surgical Technique

OPERATIVE PLANNING

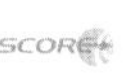

Patients with profound hypercalcemia (serum calcium ≥ 12.5 mg/dL) or mild to moderate renal failure should be hydrated and given furosemide before operation. On rare occasions, such patients require additional treatment—for example, administration of bisphosphonates, mithramycin, or calcitonin. Bisphosphonates should be used with caution as they can exacerbate postoperative hypocalcemia. Electrolyte abnormalities, such as hypokalemia, should also be corrected prior to this elective surgery. Optimally, patients should have any anticoagulation held perioperatively and should be deemed safe from a cardiopulmonary standpoint for anesthesia.

We recommend either bilateral exploration or focused exploration with intraoperative PTH assay for most patients undergoing initial operations for primary sporadic hyperparathyroidism. The latter approach can be taken only when the abnormal gland has been identified by sestamibi scanning and/or ultrasonography. For patients with familial primary or secondary hyperparathyroidism, bilateral exploration is recommended because most of these patients have multiple abnormal parathyroid glands.

Other preoperative localization studies (e.g., magnetic resonance imaging [MRI] and CT scanning) are generally unnecessary: they provide useful information in about 75% of patients but are often not considered cost-effective, because an experienced surgeon can treat hyperparathyroidism successfully without imaging 95 to 98% of the time. Such studies are, however, essential when reoperation for persistent or recurrent hyperparathyroidism is indicated. High-resolution, four-dimensional CT scanning is particularly useful for patients in this setting. Patients requiring reoperation should be considered for direct or indirect laryngoscopy before operation to evaluate vocal cord function.

Optimum exposure of the parathyroid glands is facilitated by placing a soft roll transversely across the scapula and a support under the occiput; in this way, the neck is gently extended and the thyroid or parathyroids can assume a more anterior position. This positioning also facilitates identification of the recurrent laryngeal nerve by placing it under slight tension. The head must be supported to prevent postoperative posterior neck pain. Care also is taken to ensure that no body parts are exposed to undue pressure. The skin is prepared with betadine or chlorhexidine.

OPERATIVE TECHNIQUE

General Troubleshooting

Safe parathyroid operations require good visualization of central neck structures. Therefore, the field should be bloodless and well illuminated, preferably with the use of a headlamp. Operating telescopes (×2.5 or ×3.5 magnification) are also recommended because the recurrent laryngeal nerve can be difficult for some to visualize without magnification. If bleeding occurs, surgeons should avoid grasping or clamping a poorly visualized vessel. A bleeding vessel should be clamped only after it is precisely identified and inclusion of the recurrent laryngeal nerve is excluded. Preoperative localization studies should be available in the operating room to guide the dissection.

Step 1: Incision and Mobilization of Skin Layers

A transverse incision paralleling the normal skin lines of the neck is made approximately 1 cm caudad to the cricoid cartilage [*see Figure 1*]. Preferably, this incision can be placed completely within a skin crease. Such creases can be marked in the preoperative setting with the patient sitting upright with a neutral neck position. As a rule, the incision should be about 4 to 6 cm long and should extend from the anterior border of one sternocleidomastoid muscle to the anterior border of the other. Either sharp dissection or electrocautery can be used to dissect through the subcutaneous layer and platysma muscle. Straight Kelly or small Kocher clamps are placed on the dermis for retraction, which facilitates the creation of flaps in the avascular plane located just deep to the platysmal muscle and anterior to the anterior jugular veins and their branches. These subplatysmal flaps are made in the cephalad direction up to the level of the thyroid cartilage notch and caudally down to the suprasternal notch. Self-retaining retractors are then applied.

Troubleshooting Placing the incision approximately 1 cm below the cricoid locates it precisely over the thyroid isthmus. The course of the incision should conform to or overlay the natural skin creases. The length of the incision should be modified as necessary for good exposure. Patients with short, thick necks or large, low-lying tumors require longer incisions. The lateral margins of the incision should be at equal distances from the midline, and the overall shape of the incision should be symmetrical. Flaps must be created using anterior traction and taking care not to perforate the skin.

Step 2: Midline Dissection and Mobilization of Strap Muscles and Thyroid

The thyroid gland is exposed via a longitudinal midline incision through the deep cervical fascia between the strap muscles. Because the strap muscles are farthest apart low in the neck, the incision is begun at the sternal notch and extended upward to the thyroid cartilage [*see Figure 2*].

On the side where the suspected parathyroid adenoma is located, the more superficial sternohyoid muscle is separated from the underlying sternothyroid muscle by blunt dissection using a Kitner sponge. This typically does not cause bleeding and should extend posterolaterally until the ansa cervicalis becomes visible on the lateral edge of the sternothyroid muscle and on the medial side of the internal jugular vein. The sternothyroid muscle is then dissected free from the thyroid and the prethyroidal fascia with electrocautery until the middle thyroid vein or veins are encountered laterally.

The thyroid is retracted anteriorly and medially and the carotid sheath laterally; this retraction places tension on the middle thyroid veins and helps expose the area posterolateral to the thyroid, where the parathyroid glands and the recurrent laryngeal nerves are situated. The middle thyroid veins are ligated with sutures or with a hemostatic device to mobilize the thyroid and provide exposure behind the superior portion of the thyroid lobe [*see Figure 3*].

Troubleshooting Separation of the sternohyoid muscle from the sternothyroid muscle improves exposure of the operative field and does not worsen postoperative morbidity. The middle thyroid veins should be dissected free to prevent injury to the recurrent laryngeal nerve prior to their ligation. It is always safest to mobilize tissues parallel to the recurrent laryngeal nerve rather than transversely across its anticipated course. If the exposure is so limited that the strap muscles have to be divided, this should be done horizontally and high enough in the neck to preserve innervation to the bulk of the muscles. These muscles can be closed with interrupted figure-of-eight 2-0 absorbable sutures, holding the muscle apposed as the sutures are taken to prevent shredding. The neck can be gently flexed or held in a neutral position at this late stage of the operation to facilitate muscle approximation.

Step 3: Identification of Upper Parathyroid Glands

Dissection is continued superiorly, laterally, and posteriorly with a small Kitner sponge on a clamp. This maneuver can be performed with minimal bleeding when done gently. The superior thyroid artery and veins are identified by retracting the thyroid inferiorly and medially. The tissues posterolateral to the upper lobe of the thyroid and medial to the carotid sheath can be mobilized caudally to the cricothyroid muscle; the recurrent laryngeal nerve enters the larynx just posterior to the Berry ligament at this craniocaudal level [*see Figure 4*]. Berry ligament refers to the lateral ligament suspending the thyroid to the trachea. It is attached to the inferior margin of the cricoid cartilage cornu and extends inferomedially onto the trachea. At the level of the cricoid cartilage, the mean distance between the attachment of the ligament to the cricoid cartilage and the recurrent laryngeal nerve is 1.9 mm. This is the most common location of recurrent laryngeal nerve injury. Caution should be taken when dissecting caudal to the cricoid cartilage in this region, where the recurrent nerve can be encountered.

The tissues posterior and lateral to the superior pole can be easily swept by blunt dissection away from the thyroid gland medially and anteriorly and away from the carotid sheath

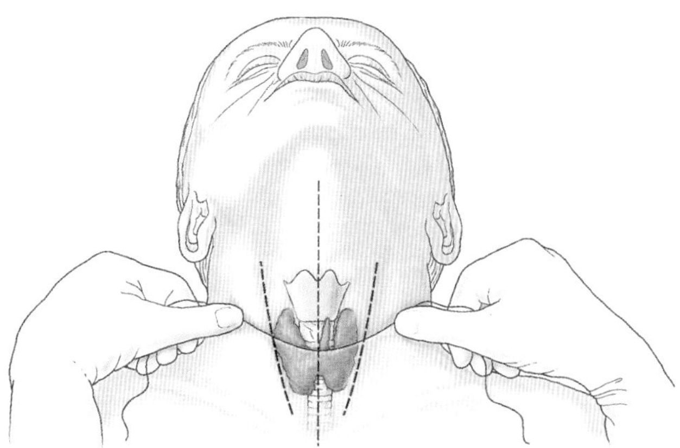

Figure 1 **The initial incision is made 1 cm below the cricoid cartilage and follows normal skin lines. A sterile marking pen is used to mark the midline of the neck, the level of the incision, and the lateral borders of the incision. A 2-0 silk tie is pressed against the neck to mark the incision site itself.**

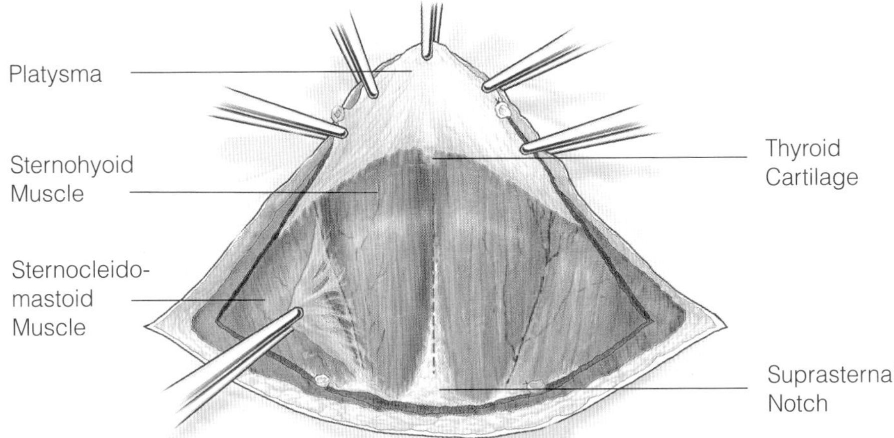

Figure 2 **To expose the thyroid, a midline incision is made through the superficial layer of deep cervical fascia between the strap muscles. The incision is begun at the suprasternal notch and extended to the thyroid cartilage.**

laterally. The upper parathyroid gland is often identified at this time near the level of the cricoid cartilage situated posterior to the recurrent laryngeal nerve.

Step 4: Identification of Recurrent Laryngeal Nerves and Lower Parathyroid Glands

When the thyroid lobe is further mobilized and retracted anteromedially, the lower parathyroid gland is often found anterior to the recurrent laryngeal nerve and inferior to where the inferior thyroid artery crosses the recurrent laryngeal nerve [*see Figure 5*]. The carotid sheath is gently retracted laterally, and the thyroid gland is retracted anteriorly and medially. This retraction puts tension on the inferior thyroid artery and consequently on the recurrent laryngeal nerve, thereby facilitating the identification of the nerve. The recurrent laryngeal nerve is situated more medially on the left in the tracheoesophageal groove and more obliquely on the right. As such, it can be more susceptible to accidental injury on the right side. Dissection should proceed cephalad along the lateral edge of the thyroid. Fatty and lymphatic tissues loosely attached to the thyroid capsule are swept from it with a Kitner sponge on a clamp, and small vessels are ligated. No tissue should be transected until one is sure that it is not the recurrent laryngeal nerve. Some find it helpful to use a nerve monitoring device for this portion of the dissection.

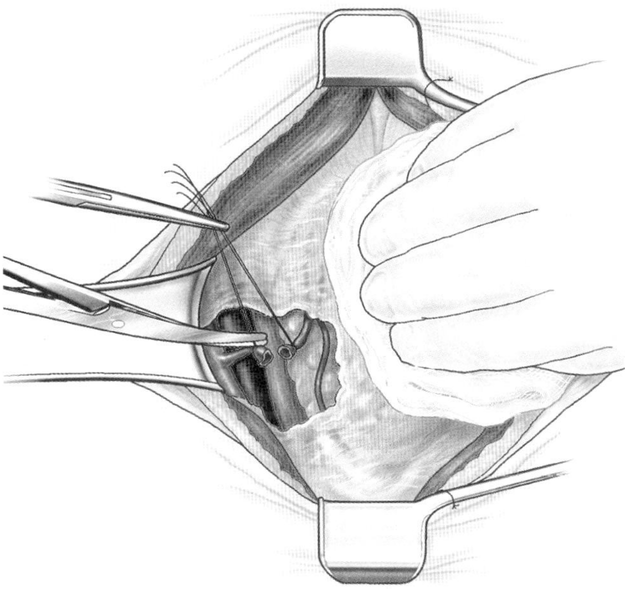

Figure 3 **The middle thyroid veins are divided to give better exposure behind the superior portion of the thyroid lobe.**

Troubleshooting The upper parathyroid glands are usually situated on each side of the thyroid gland just posterolateral to where the recurrent laryngeal nerves enter the cricothyroid muscle [*see Figure 4 and Figure 5*]. Because the recurrent laryngeal nerve enters the larynx posterior to the cricothyroid muscle at the level of the cricoid cartilage, caution should be taken when dissecting caudal to this area.

The right and left recurrent laryngeal nerves should be preserved during every parathyroid operation. Although both nerves enter at the posterior medial position of the larynx in the cricothyroid muscle, their courses vary considerably. The right recurrent laryngeal nerve takes a more oblique course than the left recurrent laryngeal nerve and may pass either anterior or posterior to the inferior thyroid artery. In about 0.5% of persons, the right recurrent laryngeal nerve is nonrecurrent and may enter the thyroid from a superior or lateral direction. On rare occasions, both a recurrent and a nonrecurrent laryngeal nerve may be present on the right. The left recurrent laryngeal nerve almost always runs in the tracheoesophageal groove because of its deeper origin within the thorax as it loops around the ductus arteriosus. Recurrent laryngeal nerves often branch before entering the larynx; the left nerve is more likely to do this. Although all nerve branches should be preserved, the motor fibers of the recurrent laryngeal nerve are usually in the most medial branch.

It is helpful to remember that the recurrent laryngeal nerves are supplied by a small vascular plexus and that a tiny vessel runs parallel to and directly on each nerve, which contrasts with the white color of the nerve [*see Figure 4*]. In young persons, the artery usually is readily distinguished from the recurrent laryngeal nerve. However, in older persons with

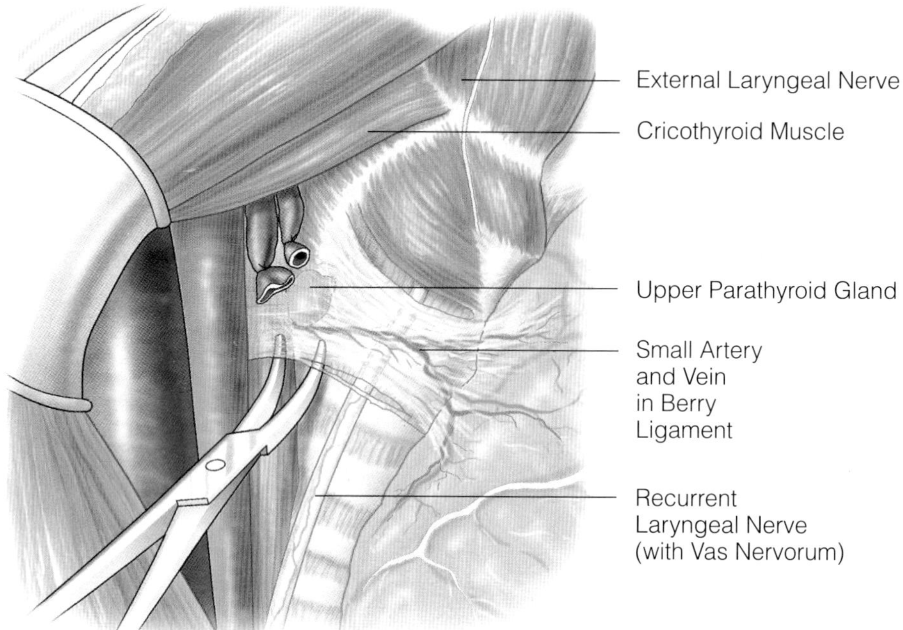

Figure 4 **The recurrent laryngeal nerve enters the cricothyroid muscle at the level of the cricoid cartilage, first passing through the Berry ligament.**

arteriosclerosis, the white-appearing artery may be mistaken for the nerve, and caution should be taken. Lateral traction on the carotid sheath and medial and anterior traction on the thyroid gland place tension on the inferior thyroid artery; this maneuver often helps identify the recurrent laryngeal nerve where it courses lateral to the midportion of the thyroid gland. It is usually safest to identify the recurrent laryngeal nerve low in the neck and then to follow it to where it enters the cricothyroid muscle through the Berry ligament. Sometimes the recurrent laryngeal nerves can be palpated through the surrounding tissue in the neck; they feel like a taut ligature of approximately 2-0 gauge.

About 85% of people have four parathyroid glands, and in about 85% of these persons, the parathyroids are situated on the posterior lateral capsule of the thyroid. Normal parathyroid glands measure about 3 × 3 × 4 mm and are light brown in color. The upper parathyroid glands are more posterior and more constant in position (at the level of the cricoid cartilage) than the lower parathyroid glands, which typically are more anterior (on the posterolateral surface of the thyroid

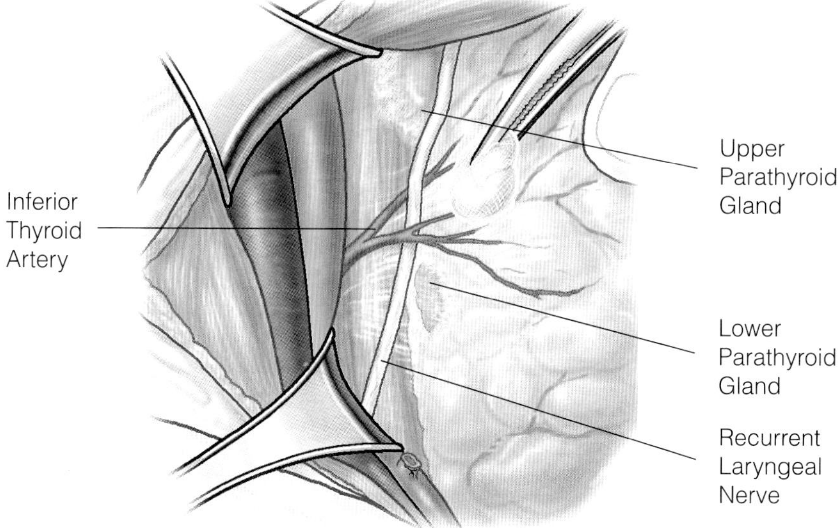

Figure 5 **The upper parathyroid glands are usually situated on either side of the thyroid at the level where the recurrent laryngeal nerve enters the cricothyroid muscle. The lower parathyroid glands are usually anterior to the recurrent laryngeal nerve and inferior to where the inferior thyroid artery crosses this nerve.**

gland). Both the upper and the lower parathyroid glands are supplied by small branches of the inferior and superior thyroid arteries in most patients. About 15% of parathyroid glands are intrathymic, and about 1% are intrathyroidal. Other abnormal sites for the parathyroid glands are (1) the carotid sheath, (2) the anterior and posterior mediastinum, and (3) anterior to the carotid bulb or along the pharynx (undescended parathyroids).

The upper parathyroid glands are usually posterolateral to the recurrent laryngeal nerve at the level of the Berry ligament. When the upper parathyroids are not found at this site, they often can be found in the tracheoesophageal groove or in the posterior mediastinum along the esophagus. The lower parathyroid glands are almost always situated anterior to the recurrent laryngeal nerves and caudal to where the recurrent laryngeal nerve crosses the inferior thyroid artery; they may be surrounded by lymph nodes. When the lower parathyroids are not found at this site, they usually can be found in the anterior mediastinum (typically in the thymus or the perithymic fat).

Step 5: Parathyroid Resection

Abnormal parathyroid glands are then removed. In about 80% of patients with PHPT, one parathyroid gland is abnormal; in about 15%, all glands are abnormal (diffuse hyperplasia); and in about 5%, two or three glands are abnormal and one or two are normal. Parathyroid cancer occurs in about 1% of patients with PHPT.

Troubleshooting In some patients, parathyroid tumors and hyperplastic parathyroid glands are difficult to find. If this is the case, the first step is to explore the sites where the parathyroids are usually located, near the posterolateral surface of the thyroid gland within 1 cm of the point where the inferior thyroid artery crosses the recurrent laryngeal nerve. Typically, the upper and lower parathyroid glands are located posterolateral and anteromedial to the recurrent nerve, respectively. When a lower gland is missing from the usual location, it is often intrathymic in the upper mediastinum or lower neck. Approximately 15% of parathyroids are found within the thymus. If an upper parathyroid gland cannot be located, one should look not only far behind the thyroid gland superiorly but also in a paraesophageal position down into the posterior mediastinum. A thyroid lobectomy should be done on the side where fewer than two parathyroid glands have been located and no abnormal parathyroid tissue has been identified, and the preoperative consent should prepare patients for this possibility. The carotid sheath and the area posterior to the carotid, as well as the retroesophageal area, should also be explored for unidentified upper parathyroids. In rare cases, there may be an undescended parathyroid tumor anterior to the carotid bulb.

Although we do not recommend routine biopsy of more than one normal-appearing parathyroid gland, we do recommend taking a small biopsy of all normal parathyroid glands when no abnormal parathyroid tissue can be found. This can be done by placing a small clip across the apex of the gland followed by sharp dissection; this achieves good hemostasis without devascularizing the gland and permanently marks it for future reference. When four normal parathyroid glands are found in the neck, the fifth (abnormal) parathyroid gland is often in the mediastinum. To minimize the risk of recurrent nerve injury during removal of identified parathyroids, dissection should be directly on the surface of the capsule without disruption. The risk of permanent hypoparathyroidism or injury to the recurrent nerve should be less than 2%.

Step 6: Closure

The strap muscles are approximated with interrupted 3-0 Vicryl sutures, and an opening is left in the midline at the suprasternal notch to make any bleeding that occurs more evident and to allow the blood to exit the central neck. The platysma is reapproximated with interrupted absorbable sutures. The skin is then closed using a deep dermal absorbable stitch, and either a skin adhesive or sterile tape is applied on the epidermis.

SPECIAL CONCERNS

Four-Gland Parathyroidectomy for Hyperplasia

This procedure will render a patient permanently hypocalcemic. We prefer to leave a remnant of the most normal-appearing parathyroid gland in situ. Alternatively, autotransplantation can be done by mincing the most normal parathyroid into 1 mm cubes and placing it in a pocket inside the sternocleidomastoid muscle, subcutaneous tissue, or forearm muscle. Clips can be placed in this location to aid in localization should a second resection become required.

Parathyroid Cancer

Parathyroid lesions that grossly extend into neighboring structures should prompt suspicion of malignancy. Such lesions should be removed en bloc with the ipsilateral thyroid lobe by hemithyroidectomy. On rare occasions, parathyroid cancers may invade the trachea or the esophagus. As much as 5 cm of the trachea can be resected safely, without impairment of the patient's voice. If the invasion is not extensive and is confined to the anterior portion of the trachea, a small section of the trachea that contains the tumor should be excised, and a tracheostomy may be placed at the site of resection. If the invasion is more extensive or occurs in the lateral or posterior portion of the trachea, a segment of the trachea measuring several centimeters long is resected, and the remaining segments are reanastomosed. To prevent tension on the anastomosis, the trachea should be mobilized before resection, the recurrent laryngeal nerves should be preserved and mobilized from the trachea, and the mylohyoid fascia and muscles should be divided above the thyroid cartilage to drop the cartilage. Care must be taken not to injure the internal laryngeal nerves during this dissection, given that these nerves course from lateral to medial just above the lateral aspects of the thyroid cartilage. After resection, the trachea is reapproximated with 3-0 Maxon sutures. One or two Penrose drains should be left near the resection site to allow air to exit. The drains are removed after several days, when there is no more evidence of air leakage.

If the esophagus is invaded by tumor, the muscular wall of the esophagus can be resected along with the tumor, with the inner esophageal layer left in place. If the recurrent nerve is surrounded or invaded by tumor, it is known that it can be dissected free, even with a slight coating of tumor, without adversely affecting the patient's cancer prognosis. However, preoperative direct laryngoscopy or the use of nerve monitoring can allow the surgeon to determine whether the nerve is still functional prior to this dissection by testing proximal to the point of invasion. Knowledge that the nerve is not functioning can then be used to more aggressively resect the tissue in the ipsilateral paratracheal space, including the nerve. In the absence of nerve testing, careful observation can reveal a full, white nerve proximal to the tumor but a collapsed, gray nerve distal to the tumor, in which case, a complete interruption by the tumor can be inferred. In general, a recurrent laryngeal nerve that is functioning normally preoperatively also should be functioning postoperatively.

POSTOPERATIVE CARE

Patients with hyperparathyroidism should have values for serum calcium, phosphorus, and PTH checked in follow-up to evaluate for the possibility of persistent or recurrent hyperparathyroidism. Persistent hyperparathyroidism is considered when hypercalcemia in the setting of elevated PTH levels occurs within 6 months of surgery, whereas recurrent hyperparathyroidism is considered when corrected calcium and PTH levels rise again 6 months or more after surgery. As many as 10% of patients will develop recurrent hyperparathyroidism in their lifetime.

In the immediate postoperative days, patients should receive oral calcium and vitamin D as prophylaxis against hypocalcemia that can occur in the early days after parathyroidectomy. Such temporary calcium supplementation allows the remaining, normal, potentially suppressed parathyroid tissue time to upregulate. Serum calcium level checks during this period of supplementation can be used to guide withdrawal. A typical starting dose for calcium supplementation is 5 days' worth of two calcium citrate tablets four times daily.

COMPLICATIONS

The following are the most significant complications of parathyroidectomy:

1. *Hypocalcemia.* Hypocalcemia after parathyroidectomy has a number of causes, including permanent hypoparathyroidism, transient hypoparathyroidism, and a condition referred to as hungry bone syndrome. Whereas the normal serum calcium is 9.0 to 10.5 mg/dL, anything below that would be considered hypocalcemic. Few people, however, will have symptomatic hypocalcemia with only mildly low serum calcium. Symptoms generally do not occur unless serum calcium is less than 8.0 mg/dL. Additionally, it is important to note that symptomatic hypocalcemia may be related to both the actual serum calcium level as well as its rate of fall. It is important to acknowledge how high a patient's serum calcium level was preoperatively when faced with an individual complaining of hypocalcemic symptoms.

   Hypocalcemia can have a wide range of severity. Mild hypocalcemia may present with perioral numbness and tingling in the fingertips, whereas severe hypocalcemia may present with muscle cramping, spasm, and tetany. Signs of hypocalcemia include Chvostek sign, a twitching of the facial muscles when the cheek is tapped over the facial nerve. Trousseau sign is elicited by inflating a sphygmomanometer above systolic blood pressure, which causes muscular contractions with hyperextension of the fingers in some hypocalcemic patients.

   Hypoparathyroidism may arise as the result of removal, bruising, ischemic injury, or devascularization of the parathyroid glands. These injuries can be avoided by restricting any dissection to the plane nearest the thyroid capsule and then gently teasing tissue away in a posterolateral direction. As noted, hypocalcemia from hypoparathyroidism may be transient or permanent if all four glands are permanently damaged. If one is concerned about the inadvertent devascularization of normal parathyroid tissue intraoperatively, biopsy should be performed on the gland to confirm its identity and then minced pieces should be autotransplanted into a pocket in the sternocleidomastoid muscle. This tissue should not be expected to function immediately; rather, it will begin to function in a matter of weeks. Only about 50% of autotransplanted parathyroid glands survive.

   Laboratory values in postoperative patients with hypoparathyroidism are likely to show low serum calcium, high phosphorus, and low or even undetectable PTH levels. It is also important to note magnesium levels as calcium replacement can be dependent on maintaining normal magnesium levels as well.

   Hungry bone syndrome is a phenomenon that occurs after the PTH stimulus for bone resorption has been taken away and the bones suddenly begin to sequester calcium. The consequence of this sequestration is hypocalcemia. Additionally, phosphorus will be absorbed as well, giving low serum phosphorus levels. PTH levels may be slightly elevated here as they begin to respond to the declining serum calcium concentration. This phenomenon may last days or, sometimes, even weeks. A severe manifestation of this condition occurs in patients with osteitis fibrosa cystica. In addition to the profound hypocalcemia that may occur after parathyroidectomy, these patients may have very high alkaline phosphatase levels.

   Patients treated for a single adenoma are more likely to have hypocalcemia secondary to hungry bone syndrome. This generally presents 2 to 3 days postoperatively. Patients being treated with four-gland exploration with multiple resections are more likely to experience permanent hypocalcemia. This can present within 2 hours of surgery.

   Treatment and prophylaxis for hypocalcemia associated with both problems are similar; in particular, treatment consists of oral calcium, calcitriol, and magnesium when it is also low. It is our practice to give every patient for 5 days after surgery, calcium citrate four times per day and 0.5 mg calcitriol daily. If patients complain of symptoms, we ask them to take double doses. We recommend calcium citrate over calcium carbonate because calcium citrate is better absorbed. Rarely does anyone require intravenous calcium replacement as oral calcium is readily absorbed.
2. *Injury to the recurrent laryngeal nerve.* Unilateral recurrent nerve dysfunction usually results in a hoarse voice and sometimes aspiration when swallowing liquids of thin consistency. If a recurrent nerve is transected during surgery, the ends should be débrided and anastomosed with 6-0 permanent interrupted sutures. This does not restore

vocal cord function but medializes the cord and prevents atrophy. Bilateral injury to the recurrent laryngeal nerve may result in airway obstruction, which often requires tracheostomy.

3. *Bleeding.* Postoperative bleeding can be life threatening in that it can compress the trachea and result in airway obstruction. Any postoperative respiratory distress should be attributed to a neck hematoma until proven otherwise. Most bleeding occurs within 4 hours of operation, and virtually all occurs within 24 hours. Acute airway compromise from hematoma requires that the incision be opened emergently without waiting for reintubation.
4. *Infection.* This complication is exceedingly rare after parathyroidectomy. Any patient with acute pharyngitis or neck cellulitis should not undergo this procedure until the infection resolves.
5. *Seroma.* Most seromas are small and reabsorb spontaneously. Symptomatic seromas can be aspirated. Compression bandages after aspiration are helpful in some cases.
6. *Keloid.* Hypertrophic and keloid scar formation after thyroidectomy is most common in African-American patients and in patients with a history of this problem.

OUTCOME EVALUATION

The patient should have a normal voice and be normocalcemic. The overall complication rate should be less than 2%. Most patients can return to work or full activity in 1 to 2 weeks.

ALTERNATIVE TECHNIQUE

Much has been written and discussed about limiting parathyroid surgery to the exposure and removal of a single parathyroid, with consequent reduced morbidity and improved cosmesis. As experience has been gained with these techniques, we have come to realize that virtually all parathyroid surgery can be performed on an outpatient basis and that the morbidity is independent of the size of the incision or the extent of the exploration. Thus, the advantage of the "limited," "concise," "focused," or "mini" parathyroid exploration may be only to those with cosmetic concerns.

Nonetheless, "mini" parathyroidectomy remains a popular operative method, limiting the necessity for a full four-gland exploration. This uses preoperative ultrasonography and sestamibi scanning to direct a more focused exploration. When both modalities have concordant results suggesting a single abnormal gland, one has a greater than 97% success with a focused parathyroidectomy that avoids bilateral neck dissection. In our experience, we have found it useful to take the time to explore the ipsilateral presumed "normal" parathyroid under these circumstances. On rare occasions, this ipsilateral gland will be abnormal and prompt the appropriate bilateral neck exploration.

Also of utility with this method is intraoperative PTH testing. Because PTH has a half-life of less than 5 minutes, comparison of a predissection PTH level to one obtained 10 minutes after excision of the adenoma should show a 50% or greater drop if all the abnormal parathyroid tissue has been removed. If this does not happen, the surgeon is generally directed to continue exploring the neck. At its inception, this assay received great attention; however, it has become somewhat controversial whether or not it adds much when there is concordance between operative findings and preoperative imaging. Based on our experience, it does not add significantly when preoperative localization studies are concordant. When ultrasonography, sestamibi scanning, and intraoperative PTH testing are combined, patients have an approximately 98% chance of cure. This is equal in success to the results from bilateral neck surgery and four-gland exploration.

Multiple Endocrine Neoplasia Syndromes

The MEN syndromes are an inherited group of disorders characterized by the propensity for patients to develop tumors and diffuse hyperplasia of endocrine tissues. They are inherited in an autosomal dominant fashion. Because these syndromes can present with simultaneous, different endocrine tumors, treatment algorithms will be influenced by the consequences of the various presenting tumors. Additionally, prophylactic operations in these patient populations may be recommended by the high penetrance of endocrine malignancies.

MEN I is characterized by hyperparathyroidism and pituitary and pancreatic neuroendocrine tumors. Ninety percent of patients with this syndrome will have a mutation in the *MENIN* tumor suppressor gene located on chromosome 11q13. All MEN I cases will present with hyperparathyroidism, two thirds of which will be the initial manifestation of this syndrome. Most cases will occur before age 40 and will exhibit multiglandular disease. About 70% of MEN I patients will have neuroendocrine tumors of the pancreas. In this population, the tumors are usually multiple and are generally benign. Gastrinomas are the most common for MEN I patients as opposed to the general population, which has a higher incidence of insulinomas. The most common pituitary tumor is prolactinoma. The workup for these patients should routinely include serum calcium and gastrin levels, pancreatic polypeptide levels, fasting blood glucose, serum prolactin, visual field testing, and head imaging. Because hypercalcemia often exacerbates the symptoms of pancreatic neuroendocrine tumors, it is preferable to treat the hyperparathyroidism in MEN I patients first. All patients should undergo four-gland parathyroidectomy with autotransplantation of a single remnant to prevent permanent hypocalcemia. Supernumerary parathyroids are common in this group.

MEN IIa is characterized by hyperparathyroidism, medullary thyroid cancer, and pheochromocytomas. These patients generally have a mutation in the *ret* proto-oncogene on chromosome 10. This gene codes for a cell membrane receptor tyrosine kinase. Only about half of these patients will have hyperparathyroidism, again involving multiple glands. Around 70% will have pheochromocytomas, and in this patient population, they are often bilateral, multiple, and extra-adrenal. Only rarely are they malignant. Most patients will present with pheochromocytomas in the third or fourth decade of life. All of these patients will develop medullary thyroid carcinoma. Because these tumors present at a younger age than sporadic medullary thyroid carcinoma, it is recommended that patients have prophylactic total thyroidectomies at 2 years of age. All of these patients should undergo *ret* proto-oncogene mutation screening as it is 95% sensitive for this syndrome. Additionally, serum calcium levels should be monitored, pentagastrin-stimulated plasma calcitonin can be used to follow patients for recurrence, and urinary catecholamines and their metabolites, as well as metaiodobenzylguanidine (MIBG) testing, should be considered in patients. In patients with concurrent tumors, pheochromocytomas should be treated first as operative management of other tumors may precipitate hypertensive crisis. Patients with hyperparathyroidism should undergo four-gland parathyroidectomy with single-gland remnant autotransplantation. Some kindreds have uniglandular disease and do not require such extensive surgery.

MEN IIb is characterized by medullary thyroid carcinomas (95%), pheochromocytomas (50%), neuromas (100%), and marfanoid habitus (70%). This syndrome is also associated with the *ret* proto-oncogene mutation. In these patients, medullary thyroid carcinoma presents 15 years earlier than in patients with MEN IIa and is more severe, and metastases are almost always found on presentation. The workup is the same as that for patients with MEN IIa. Again, pheochromocytomas should be treated first. Prophylactic total thyroidectomy should be performed as soon as the diagnosis of MEN IIb is made.

Financial Disclosures: None Reported

Recommended Reading

Chen H, Sokol LJ, Udelsman R. Outpatient minimally invasive parathyroidectomy: a combination of sestamibi-SPECT localization, cervical block anesthesia, and intraoperative parathyroid hormone assay. Surgery 1999;126:1016.

Chertok-Shacham, E: Biomarkers of hypercoagulability and inflammation in primary hyperparathyroidism. Med Sci Monit, 2008;14:CR628–632.

Clark OH. Total thyroidectomy and lymph node dissection for cancer of the thyroid. In: Hyhus LM, Baker RJ, editors. Mastery of surgery. 2nd ed. Boston: Little, Brown and Co; 1992. p. 204.

Clark OH. Total thyroid lobectomy. In: Daly JM, Cady B, Low DW, editors. Atlas of surgical oncology. St. Louis: CV Mosby; 1993. p. 41.

Clark O, Duh QY, Kebebew El. Textbook of endocrine surgery. 2nd ed. Philadelphia (PA): Elsevier Saunders; 2005.

Clark OH: Endocrine surgery of the thyroid and parathyroid glands. Philadelphia (PA): WB Saunders; 2003.

Gawande AA, Monchik JM, Abbruzzese TA, et al. Reassessment of PTH monitoring during parathyroidectomy for primary hyperparathyroidism after two preoperative localization studies. Arch Surg 2006;141:381.

Gerlach C, et al. Increased plasma N-terminal pro-B-type natriuretic peptide and markers of inflammation related to atherosclerosis in patients with primary hyperparathyroidism. Clin Endo 2005;63:493–498.

Gordon LL, Snyder WH, Wians JR, et al. The validity of quick intraoperative hormone assay: an evaluation of seventy two patients based on gross morphology criteria. Surgery 1999;126:1030.

Irvin GL, Molinari AS, Figuero C, et al. Improved success rate in reoperative parathyroidectomy with intraoperative PTH assay. Ann Surg 1999;229:874.

Henry JF, Audiffret J, Denizot A, et al. The nonrecurrent inferior laryngeal nerve: review of 33 cases, including two on the left side. Surgery 1988;104:977.

Tezelman S, Shen W, Shaver JK, et al. Double parathyroid adenomas: clinical and biochemical characteristics before and after parathyroidectomy. Ann Surg 1993;218:300.

Thompson NW, Olsen WR, Hoffman GL. The continuing development of the technique of thyroidectomy. Surgery 1973;73:913.

Wang H. Reporting thyroid fine-needle aspiration: literature review and a proposal. Diagnostic Cytopathology 2005;34:67–76.

Acknowledgment

Figures 1 through 5 Tom Moore

1 BREAST CANCER

*Stephen B. Edge, MD, FACS**

Breast cancer is the most common malignancy in women in the Western world. It is increasingly prevalent in developing countries and leads to the death of hundreds of thousands of women worldwide annually. In the United States, general surgeons treat most breast cancers. It is the responsibility of surgeons to have a thorough understanding of the principles and current practices of breast cancer surgery and care beyond surgery, including the use of imaging and other diagnostic modalities, pathology, radiation, and systemic therapy, so that surgical care is coordinated as a component of comprehensive breast cancer care.

Breast cancer refers primarily to a malignancy of the epithelium of the ductal and lobular epithelial components of the breast. Nonepithelial malignancies of the breast are much less common and include tumors of mesenchymal origin (phylloides tumors, soft tissue sarcomas) and lymphoma.[1,2] The breast is only rarely the site of metastases from other primary malignancies. This chapter addresses only the treatment of epithelial malignancies.

Investigative Studies

HISTORY AND PHYSICAL EXAMINATION

SCORE Most women with breast cancer are asymptomatic at the time of presentation, but a complete history of breast-related symptoms and evaluation for symptoms related to metastatic disease should be performed. Particular attention should be paid to skeletal symptoms and their extent or degree and duration. A prior history of imaging findings and biopsies is important. The history should include the presence of masses or lumps in the breast, any apparent swelling, edema or thickening in the breast tissue or skin, and the presence or absence of discharge from the nipple (character, color, consistency, frequency, and mode of expression—spontaneous or elicited). The patient should be queried regarding any changes in the appearance of the nipple and the areola, the presence of scaling, eczematous changes, or peeling of the skin. The physician should also document factors related to breast cancer risk: age at onset of menarche and menopause, age at first-term pregnancy and hormone use, and a detailed family history, including the type of cancer and age at onset of all first-degree and second-degree relatives with breast cancer and ovarian cancer, on both the maternal and paternal sides of the family. If there is evidence of a syndrome of inherited susceptibility to breast and ovarian cancer or to other inherited syndromes, consideration should be made for referral to a genetic specialist for genetic counseling and possible genetic testing. Finally, a thorough history of medication use should be recorded. In addition to common prescription medication, the patient should be queried regarding the use of supplements and other alternative medicine because of the potential effect on hormone metabolism and bleeding.

Examination of the breast and chest wall begins maneuvers to accentuate skin puckering or retraction, including extending the arms over the head and/or flexing the pectoral muscles with the hands on the patient's hips. Examination of the axilla is best performed in the sitting position. The key to successful examination of the axilla is relaxation of the muscles of the shoulder girdle. This is best accomplished with the examiner supporting the full weight of the arm abducted from the body at about an angle of 60{198} while palpating the axilla with the other hand. Care should be taken to examine the axilla fully underneath the pectoral muscles and along the chest wall toward the latissimus muscle. It is important to examine both axillae. The supraclavicular region should be carefully examined for the presence of enlarged lymph nodes.

The most common technique for examining the breast includes accentuating the skin of the breast by placing the patient's hand behind her head. The surgeon should develop a standard manner of examining the breast so that the entirety of both breasts is fully examined. It is generally best to begin the examination with the breast opposite the breast of concern so that this examination is not forgotten. Most examiners use a process of pushing the breast tissue back against the underlying rib cage starting at the areola and working out in a circular motion extending through the entire breast, recognizing that the breast tissues goes into the axilla. The character and size of any masses identified should be noted. The density and glandularity of the breast should be identified. It is important to compare areas of dense glandular tissue with the contralateral side to identify subtle differences in the size and density of breast tissue. Although the primary examination is performed in the supine position, the patient should be queried as to whether she perceives a palpable lesion and should be asked to reproduce the position where the lesion is best examined. Frequently, patients will identify a lesion in a position other than the supine position, and subtle findings may be identified in this way. After examination of the breast, the skin of the nipple and areola should also be carefully examined, and after warning the patient, the nipple may be compressed to elicit a discharge.

Ultrasonography is an excellent adjunct to physical examination to allow the characterization of palpable lesions as solid or cystic and to help define whether there is a specific lesion identified in areas of dense breast. Surgeons who perform ultrasonography in the office need to be fully familiar with its value and limitations and should undergo appropriate training and certification of their skill. Surgeon-performed

* The author and editors gratefully acknowledge the contributions of the previous authors, Doreen M. Agnese, MD, FACS, Stephen P. Povoski, MD, FACS, and Wiley W. Souba, MD, ScD, FACS, to the development and writing of the original chapter.

ultrasonography may or may not replace ultrasonography performed as part of the diagnostic breast imaging.

IMAGING

Mammography

The majority of breast cancers are detected by screening mammography. Controversy continues over the exact populations that benefit from screening mammography, but most organizations recommend mammography annually beginning at age 40 and at a younger age for women at substantial risk for increased risk of cancer.[3–5]

Concerning findings include new masses, asymmetry, distortion in the architecture of the breast tissue, and the presence of calcifications grouped ("clustered") in an area of breast tissue. When an abnormality is identified, the mammogram becomes a "diagnostic mammogram," and supplemental views are obtained in addition to the standard bilateral craniocaudad and mediolateral oblique screening views. These include accentuated positions, localized "spot" compression, and magnified settings. Any finding should be compared with previous mammograms to determine if it is new. Mammogram findings are assigned a score of 0 to 6 using the Breast Imaging Reporting and Data System (BI-RADS), with BI-RADS 4 and 5 findings requiring biopsy.[6] Mammography detects only 80 to 90% of breast cancers and is less sensitive in women with dense glandular tissue (more common in younger women) and for lobular cancer. Suspicious physical findings (e.g., a lump or discharge) should be evaluated and biopsied even if breast imaging is normal. Mammography also has a relatively low specificity, with about 60 to 70% of all lesions requiring biopsy proving benign.

Ultrasonography

Ultrasonography is an adjunctive imaging tool to define the characteristics of a lesion identified by other imaging modalities. Ultrasonography itself is not a useful screening tool. It primarily defines whether a lesion is cystic or solid. Malignant lesions are solid and tend to have irregular borders and inhomogeneous acoustic shadowing. However, ultrasound features alone are insufficient to define if the lesion is malignant. Ultrasonography may also be used to direct needle biopsy by fine-needle aspiration (FNA), core biopsy, or vacuum-assisted needle biopsy.

Magnetic Resonance Imaging

Magnetic resonance imaging (MRI) may be used in breast cancer screening and evaluation of breast cancers.[7] MRI visualization of breast cancers requires contrast enhancement using intravenous gadolinium. Indications for breast MRI continue to evolve. MRI may detect cancers that are occult on mammography but suffers from a substantial rate of false positive findings, which leads to otherwise unnecessary biopsies and significant patient concern. MRI screening is useful in women at defined increased risk of developing breast cancer. Standard criteria in 2009 are to consider MRI screening for women with a lifetime breast cancer risk of at least 20 to 25%.[8]

The use of MRI in women with a known breast cancer has the dual purpose of screening the remainder of breast tissue and providing additional information on the extent of the known cancer. MRI detects mammographically occult breast cancer in the contralateral breast in as many as 3% of women.[9]

MRI may assist in surgical planning. It is critical to recognize that surgical planning for cancer treatment cannot be based on the MRI finding alone and requires biopsy confirmation of any suspicious findings. Retrospective studies show that the surgical treatment planning is changed by MRI findings in as many as 20% of cases—most commonly, alteration from planned breast conservation to mastectomy. However, every study to date that has examined the question has failed to show any difference in outcomes, including local recurrence in women having presurgical MRI.[10] Use of MRI may, paradoxically, unnecessarily increase the use of mastectomy. Therefore, the use of MRI in treatment planning remains controversial.

MRI may be useful in women with locally advanced breast cancer for whom neoadjuvant chemotherapy is being considered to downsize the tumor to allow breast conservation. In addition, MRI clinical response quantified by changes in enhancement and in reduction in tumor volume may be prognostic of ultimate cancer outcome.

Other Imaging Modalities

Other imaging modalities include sestamibi imaging and positron emission tomography (PET).[11–13] Sestamibi imaging remains investigational. PET scanning is of minimal value in evaluating the primary tumor. Other whole body imaging of the asymptomatic patient with breast cancer is not useful in stage I and II breast cancer unless there are symptoms suggestive of metastatic disease but may be used in those with advanced disease.

Evaluation of Suspicious Findings

A breast lesion suspicious for malignancy requires tissue biopsy. Percutaneous needle biopsy is preferred over surgical excision in all circumstances. Surgical excision as a diagnostic procedure is not a justifiable alternative simply because of "patient choice" and should be performed only when needle biopsy cannot be performed for specific technical reasons, when a needle biopsy is either nondiagnostic, the result is not concordant with the imaging findings (i.e., the needle biopsy is benign, but the lesion is of high suspicion), or in highly select other cases. Technical reasons that may preclude needle biopsy include anatomic location of the lesion on mammography directly opposed to the chest wall or in the far periphery of the breast so that it cannot be visualized on stereotactic imaging devices.

FNA that provides cytology only, used extensively in the past, has largely been supplanted by core biopsy or vacuum-assisted needle biopsy that provides tissue for histologic examination. The specimens also allow performance of tumor marker studies.

Needle biopsy may be directed by direct palpation or image guidance. Lesions that are clearly palpable may be accurately localized for biopsy by palpation in the office without using imaging equipment. However, it is best to use image guidance if there is any question or if the lesion is not palpable. The choice between ultrasound, stereotactic mammographic, or MRI guidance is based on the character of the lesion (i.e., calcifications require mammographic guidance) and the expertise and preference of the provider. In a few cases, surgical excision is required for lesions defined as benign by needle biopsy.

In addition to the "nonconcordant" finding, this includes cases where the biopsy shows the benign lesions atypical hyperplasia (ductal or lobular) or lobular carcinoma in situ. Excision is necessary in these cases because there is a small chance that there is cancer in the tissue immediately surrounding the biopsy-sampled tissue.[14]

Breast Cancer Management

The treatment of breast cancer requires coordination between multiple disciplines.

Surgical care cannot be done in a vacuum and must be integrated with adjuvant therapies, including radiation and systemic therapy. Although it is not mandatory that every breast cancer patient consult with specialists in each relevant discipline prior to surgery, it is incumbent upon the surgeon to ensure that the surgical care is appropriately coordinated in overall breast cancer care.

Breast cancer management addresses two major issues. The first is the treatment of the local disease in the breast itself. This is generally accomplished through surgical resection with or without radiation. The second is the adjuvant systemic therapy (chemotherapy and endocrine therapy) because any woman with invasive cancer has the risk of harboring occult microscopic metastatic disease that will ultimately lead to clinically apparent metastatic disease and death.

Decisions about treatment require accurate information on the extent of the cancer at the time of diagnosis codified using staging systems. The clinically used staging system is the TNM system of the American Joint Committee on Cancer (AJCC).[15] This classifies the size and extent of the primary tumor (T), the involvement of regional lymph nodes (N), the presence or absence of distant metastases (M), and a "stage group" derived from the T, N, and M. The AJCC TNM system was recently revised for cases diagnosed beginning in 2010.

Stage should be documented in the medical record at two distinct points in treatment.

Clinical stage is the initial cancer stage used in treatment planning and includes information gleaned from the history and physical examination and any available imaging studies prior to surgery or the start of systemic or radiation therapy. Pathologic stage is the clinical stage supplemented with the findings from surgical resection. When neoadjuvant therapy is used, the extent of disease after treatment is the posttreatment stage. The degree of response to neoadjuvant therapy may be prognostic. The rules and specifics of the TNM staging system are presented in detail in the *AJCC Cancer Staging Manual* (seventh edition).[15]

Breast cancer management continues to evolve, and no book chapter can remain up to date. Surgeons are urged to remain current with the relevant literature and refer to guidelines in making treatment decisions. The most comprehensive guidelines that are updated at least annually are supplied by the National Comprehensive Cancer Network (NCCN) and are available at www.nccn.org.[16]

Noninvasive Cancer

Cancer that is confined to the lumen of the duct or lobule of the breast and has not penetrated the basement membrane is termed in situ cancer. This generally refers to ductal carcinoma in situ (DCIS) but also encompasses a benign entity called lobular carcinoma in situ (LCIS).

LOBULAR CARCINOMA IN SITU

Small uniform cells confined to the lobule of the breast characterize LCIS. It is generally a clinically and mammographically occult lesion that is identified only incidentally when a biopsy is performed for calcifications or a mass that proves to be some other benign lesion. LCIS is actually not cancer but rather is a benign lesion and does not require cancer treatment per se. The primary issue with LCIS is that it conveys an increased lifelong risk of subsequent invasive cancer quantified at 0.5 to 0.75% per year.[17] In addition, when LCIS is identified on a core-needle biopsy, there is a 10 to 20% chance of DCIS or invasive cancer in the surrounding tissue; therefore, surgical excision is warranted.[18]

Long-term follow-up shows that the large majority of women with LCIS never develop invasive breast cancer. Therefore, ablative surgical therapy and radiation for LCIS are not necessary. Previously, LCIS was considered in and of itself an indication to consider bilateral mastectomy. However, mastectomy is generally not indicated in women with LCIS and should be performed only in the context of risk reduction for those at very high risk related to factors such as inherited susceptibility.[19]

Because women with a diagnosis of LCIS are at increased risk for subsequent invasive cancer, they should be counseled regarding that risk and may benefit from consultation with genetics professionals if they have a family history of breast or ovarian cancer. Women with a biopsy showing LCIS may also consider risk-reducing chemoprevention with one of the selective estrogen receptor modulators (SERM's), tamoxifen or raloxifene. These reduce the risk of subsequent invasive cancer by about 50%, with an acceptable toxicity profile.[20,21] Raloxifene is the preferred agent in postmenopausal women.

DUCTAL CARCINOMA IN SITU

The histologic hallmark of DCIS is the presence of malignant-appearing cells confined to the lumen of the ductal system in the breast. DCIS is most often diagnosed because of the presence of calcifications clustered in one area of the breast. The calcifications suspicious for DCIS are often linear (not round), growing in a ductal distribution. The DCIS may not be confined to the extent of calcifications, and not all DCIS is manifested by calcification. Therefore, the size or extent of DCIS may not be defined by the mammographic appearance. Although DCIS occasionally presents as a mass, the presence of the mass even in the setting of a biopsy showing DCIS most often signifies that the cancer is primarily invasive.

DCIS is generally considered a precursor to invasive cancer.[22] The purpose of treatment of DCIS is to prevent progression to invasive cancer with the sequelae of metastatic disease and death. However, indirect evidence suggests that not all DCIS lesions will progress to invasive cancer. Unfortunately, despite extensive research, there is insufficient evidence to identify which DCIS lesions will progress to invasive cancer and which will remain clinically occult for the duration of a woman's life.[23] Therefore, all women diagnosed with DCIS should undergo appropriate treatment.

DCIS encompasses a spectrum of histologic subtypes. Malignant-appearing cells confined to the breast duct characterize all of these. However, the appearance ranges from bland, uniform cells growing from the wall of the duct or bridging the duct (papillary; cribriform) to cells filling the entire duct (solid). These cells also vary in nuclear morphology, ranging from low-grade, uniform-appearing nuclei to varying size and shape and large nuclei (high grade) and in the presence or absence of central necrosis within the duct. The combination of high nuclear grade and central necrosis is termed "comedo-DCIS" or "comedocarcinoma." It is possible that these subtypes of DCIS are different disease entities with different potential for progression to invasive cancer, but this is poorly understood. The clinical relevance of the DCIS subtypes is that they may have different potential for local recurrence after breast-conserving surgery, which may impact on the utility of radiation as an adjunct to wide excision. The presence of high-grade cells or comedonecrosis is not an indication of metastatic potential and does not itself warrant systemic therapy or lymph node staging.

Treatment

The overall cancer-specific survival for women with DCIS approaches 100% almost irrespective of the subtype of DCIS and the type of treatment [*see Figure 1*].[22] Mastectomy is effective in DCIS, but in most cases, a breast-conserving approach is possible. Recurrence in the skin of the mastectomy site or on the chest wall muscle ("local recurrence") may occur, but the frequency after mastectomy for DCIS is extremely low (1 to 3%).[24] Most women with DCIS may be treated by surgical excision ("lumpectomy" or "wide excision") of the DCIS with some surrounding normal breast tissue to achieve a "negative margin." The choice between breast-conserving surgery (BCS) and mastectomy may be influenced by the size of the area of involvement, the size of the breast, and the location of the DCIS.

There is no specific size above which mastectomy is mandatory. Wide excision ("lumpectomy") with a generous margin of normal breast tissue can be accomplished in most women.

Large-scale randomized clinical trials in North America and Europe have demonstrated the effectiveness of BCT and the role of radiation in DCIS. The National Surgical Adjuvant Breast and Bowel Project (NSABP), the European Organization for Research and Treatment of Cancer (EORTC), and others conducted trials comparing wide excision alone versus wide excision plus radiation therapy.[25–28] Every study demonstrated long-term overall survival approaching 100% irrespective of treatment. However, women treated with BCT had a substantial risk of recurrence in the same breast, and radiation reduced this risk. The rate of local recurrence in the NSABP study was 30% without radiation and about 12% with radiation. The size and histologic characteristics of the DCIS as well as the extent of the margin of resection also affect the risk of local recurrence.

A key factor in breast-conserving surgery for DCIS is obtaining a negative surgical margin. Because the DCIS may extend beyond the area of calcifications seen on mammography, the rate of positive margins on the initial excision for DCIS ranges as high as 20 to 25%. Women who have a positive margin on the initial excision for DCIS must undergo repeat surgery to obtain a negative margin. On occasion, even with such "reexcision," the DCIS extends to the new margin, and some of these women ultimately require mastectomy. The definition of a "negative margin" is an area of controversy.[29,30]

The NSABP studies used the definition of a negative margin as the absence of the ink used to paint the surgical margin on any cancer cells. However, the margin width, measured as the distance from the closest surgical margin to the DCIS, affects the risk of local recurrence, with the lowest rates among women with a full 1 cm margin.[31] The best current evidence is that a margin of at least 2 mm is required to obtain optimal rates of local recurrence.[32]

Substantial research has focused on identification of those women with DCIS who may not require radiation. Some evidence from nonrandomized series suggests that the size of the area of DCIS coupled with the nuclear grade and the width of the resection margin may identify subsets of women with DCIS for whom the risk of local recurrence is so low that radiation is not warranted.[33,34] However, in randomized trials, there are no subsets that can be identified for whom radiation does not reduce the risk of local recurrence. Therefore, the decision to omit radiation therapy with DCIS requires careful counseling of the patient coupled with multidisciplinary input.

The standard radiation treatment is whole-breast radiation therapy to a dose of about 50 Gy potentially coupled with a 15 Gy boost to the site of the surgical excision. Because most local recurrences occur in the breast tissue close to the original DCIS, it is possible that radiation administered only to the affected region of the breast may be as effective as whole-breast radiation therapy. Techniques for administering so-called accelerated partial-breast irradiation therapy allow treatment to be delivered over a much shorter period of time (as short as 5 days), making it an attractive alternative.[35] However, as of 2009, there are no long-term data demonstrating the effectiveness of accelerated partial-breast irradiation in DCIS, and it remains investigational.

The choice between mastectomy and breast conservation may be difficult. It is different for women with DCIS than for those with invasive cancer primarily because those with DCIS do not face the threat of death from metastatic disease. For women with disease treatable by breast conservation, mastectomy remains a reasonable option if selected by the patient. The choice may also be influenced by the risk of developing a subsequent second breast cancer related to family history and biologically defined inherited susceptibility. An initial reaction of "just remove it" is insufficient justification for mastectomy and should be followed by careful counseling and reassurances regarding the long-term outlook for women with DCIS.

Reconstruction of the breast mound is available to most women who require or choose mastectomy for DCIS. Breast reconstruction may be performed at the same time as the mastectomy using implant techniques or tissue transfer using a variety of tissue flaps (see below).

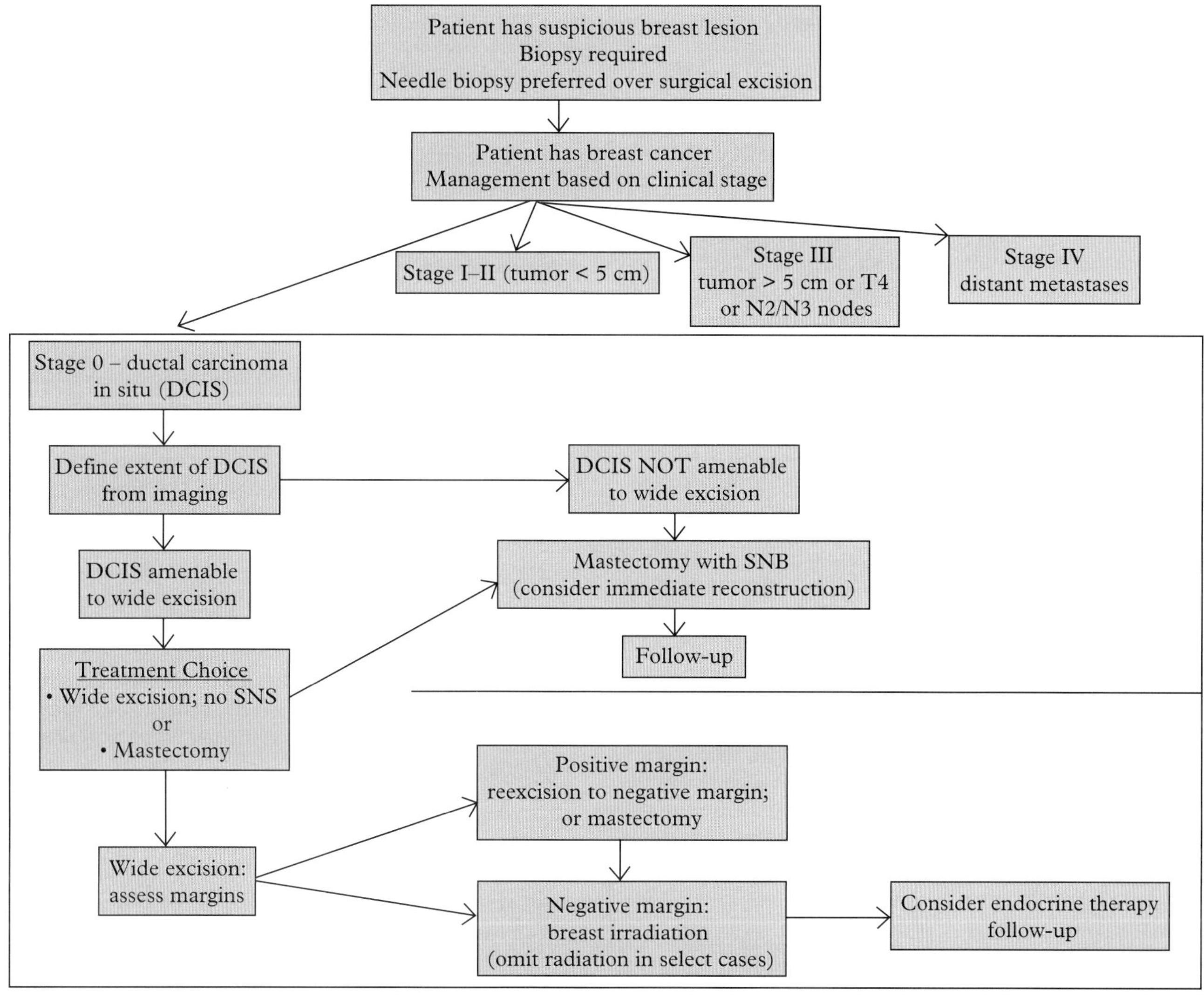

Figure 1 **Guidelines for treatment of ductal carcinoma in situ (DCIS). SNB = sentinel node biopsy.**

An important issue with DCIS is that there is a risk that invasive cancer is identified in the final surgical specimen in 5 to 20% of women for whom needle biopsy showed DCIS. Invasive cancer is more likely in cases where a mass is present on imaging or physical examination. This leads some surgeons to recommend lymph node surgery in all women with DCIS. However, lymph node surgery is unnecessary in the management of DCIS because it has no metastatic potential. For women undergoing breast-conserving treatment, if an invasive cancer is identified in the final surgical specimen, lymph node staging with sentinel node biopsy (SNB) may be performed at a subsequent surgical procedure with the same level of accuracy as if done at the time of excision. Some surgeons advocate SNB in all women with DCIS, making the argument that it is cost-effective compared with a separate SNB procedure for those with invasive cancer, but there are no high-level data to support this statement. In addition, SNB carries some risk of long-term morbidity; careful evaluation on prospective studies demonstrates that women with SNB have about a 6% risk of at least mild lymphedema.[36,37] Therefore, with breast-conserving surgery, SNB should not be performed. Exceptions are the presence of a suspicious mass—indicative of invasive cancer—or when the DCIS is in the axillary tail of the breast, and excision may preclude subsequent SNB because of interruption of lymphatic flow to the axilla. SNB is appropriate when mastectomy is used for DCIS because of the chance that the breast harbors an invasive cancer. Mastectomy may preclude subsequent SNB; therefore, mastectomy without SNB for women with DCIS may commit those women to undergoing a full axillary lymph node dissection if invasive cancer is present.

Women who undergo radiation with DCIS may also benefit from adjuvant endocrine therapy. The NSABP conducted a clinical trial of wide excision plus radiation with or without tamoxifen.[38] Tamoxifen reduced the risk of local recurrence by 40%. A subsequent clinical trial not as yet reported in 2010 addresses whether an aromatase inhibitor is effective and comparable or superior to tamoxifen in reducing the rate of local recurrence in DCIS. The use of endocrine treatment in DCIS must be balanced against the toxicity of the selected drug, recognizing that endocrine therapy is not lifesaving in this situation. There are no data supporting the use of endocrine therapy in women treated for DCIS with mastectomy.

PAGET DISEASE OF THE BREAST

An uncommon presentation of breast cancer is with eczematoid changes directly in the nipple, often with beet red and ulcerated skin in the nipple. This is due to malignant cells with a characteristic "fried egg" appearance occurring in the nipple skin or "Paget cells." This is Paget disease of the nipple. In most cases of Paget disease, there is a cancer in the underlying breast, and the cells in the nipple may represent intraductal spread of the cancer to the nipple, although this process is poorly understood. In most cases, the underlying cancer is relatively close to the nipple and in most cases is DCIS.

Women with these changes in the nipple are often misdiagnosed as having benign skin conditions and are treated with topical agents, including steroids. If such treatments are used and the lesion does not resolve, or if there is any clinical suspicion, a biopsy of the affected skin is needed. If the biopsy shows Paget disease, then the breast should be carefully imaged by mammography supplemented by MRI if the breast is dense to search for primary tumor in the breast. If a breast lesion is found, it, too, should be biopsied.

Treatment is generally based on the type (in situ or invasive) of primary tumor in the breast and treatment of the nipple. This may be accomplished in many cases with removal of the nipple in continuity with the breast cancer, followed by radiation.[39] Mastectomy is still often used but may be reserved for cases with more extensive involvement.[40] Lymph node surgery is warranted only with invasive cancer. Adjuvant systemic therapy is administered by standard guidelines.

Invasive Breast Cancer

The majority of breast cancers are classified as invasive or infiltrating, characterized by the cancer invading through the basement membrane of the duct or lobule. The same properties allow basement membrane invasion may allow the malignant cells to invade surrounding blood vessels or lymphatic channels and raise a possibility of spread to distant sites. Although most have probably not spread as assessed by long-term survival without distant metastases, the treatment issues for invasive breast cancer include not only the local treatment of the breast but also the potential for distant spread and the role for adjuvant systemic drug therapy.

CLASSIFICATION

The majority of breast cancers arise from the ductal component of the terminal ductal lobular unit and are termed invasive ductal cancer. An additional 10 to 15% arise within the lobule and have a characteristic appearance of small cells infiltrating in a linear fashion through the breast stroma, termed invasive lobular cancer. Invasive lobular carcinoma carries the same risk of distant metastases as ductal carcinoma. However, lobular carcinoma may be more insidious because of the infiltrative nature of the disease, which results in a lesion more difficult to detect by mammographic or clinical means.

Certain subtypes may have a different prognosis than typical invasive ductal cancer. These include tubular carcinoma, mucinous carcinoma, medullary carcinoma, and metaplastic carcinoma. Tubular and mucinous carcinomas may have a lower propensity for lymphatic metastases and a generally better prognosis than typical ductal cancers.[41,42]

Medullary cancer was historically considered a cancer with a better prognosis, but the term is overused, and most tumors classified this way are high-grade cancers with a poor prognosis. Standard guidelines do not assign medullary cancer to a good prognosis subgroup.[16] Because of the potential overuse of these subgroup terms, great care should be taken in making treatment decisions based on these subgroups without ensuring with the pathologist that the tumor truly is the special histology.

Inflammatory breast cancer is an infiltrating cancer characterized by skin edema and erythema encompassing over half the breast and associated with an especially high likelihood of subsequent metastases and death. It often correlates with the histologic finding of dermal lymphatics clogged by tumor cells, but the diagnosis of inflammatory cancer is only a clinical diagnosis. Skin biopsy showing dermal lymphatic involvement is not necessary to classify a cancer as inflammatory.[15]

Breast cancers may be better classified by biologic characteristics rather than histologic appearance. At the very least, all breast cancers should be analyzed for expression of the hormone receptors for estrogen and progesterone and the level of expression or amplification of the HER-2/*neu* gene.[16] These provide key prognostic information and "predictive" information about sensitivity to specific drugs to treat breast cancer. It is expected that biologic classification of breast cancers beyond these three receptors will ultimately allow a higher degree of personalization of both local and systemic treatment.[43,44]

The accuracy of testing for estrogen, progesterone, and HER-2 varies, and this variation impacts significantly on patient outcome. To improve this situation, national organizations have established practice standards for laboratories performing this testing.[45,46] Pathology should be reported using structured documentation according to the templates provided by the College of American Pathologists (www.cap.org). Surgeons should be sure that testing for their patients is performed and reported in accordance with these standards.

LOCAL THERAPY OF T1 AND T2 INVASIVE BREAST CANCER

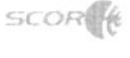

The primary goal of local therapy of breast cancer is eradication of the primary tumor to prevent progression and further dissemination of the disease [*see Figure 2*]. In addition, staging of the regional lymph nodes is performed to provide prognostic information and to guide systemic treatment as well as provide regional control in the common regional nodal basins.

Mastectomy versus Breast-Conserving Surgery

Historically, local treatment of breast cancer meant mastectomy. One can argue that the development of the operation of radical mastectomy was the single most important advance in the treatment of breast cancer. At the time it was developed in the late 1800s, most women presented with breast cancers that were locally advanced and were likely to progress to difficult painful and infected local problems. However, the ability to treat breast cancer effectively led to

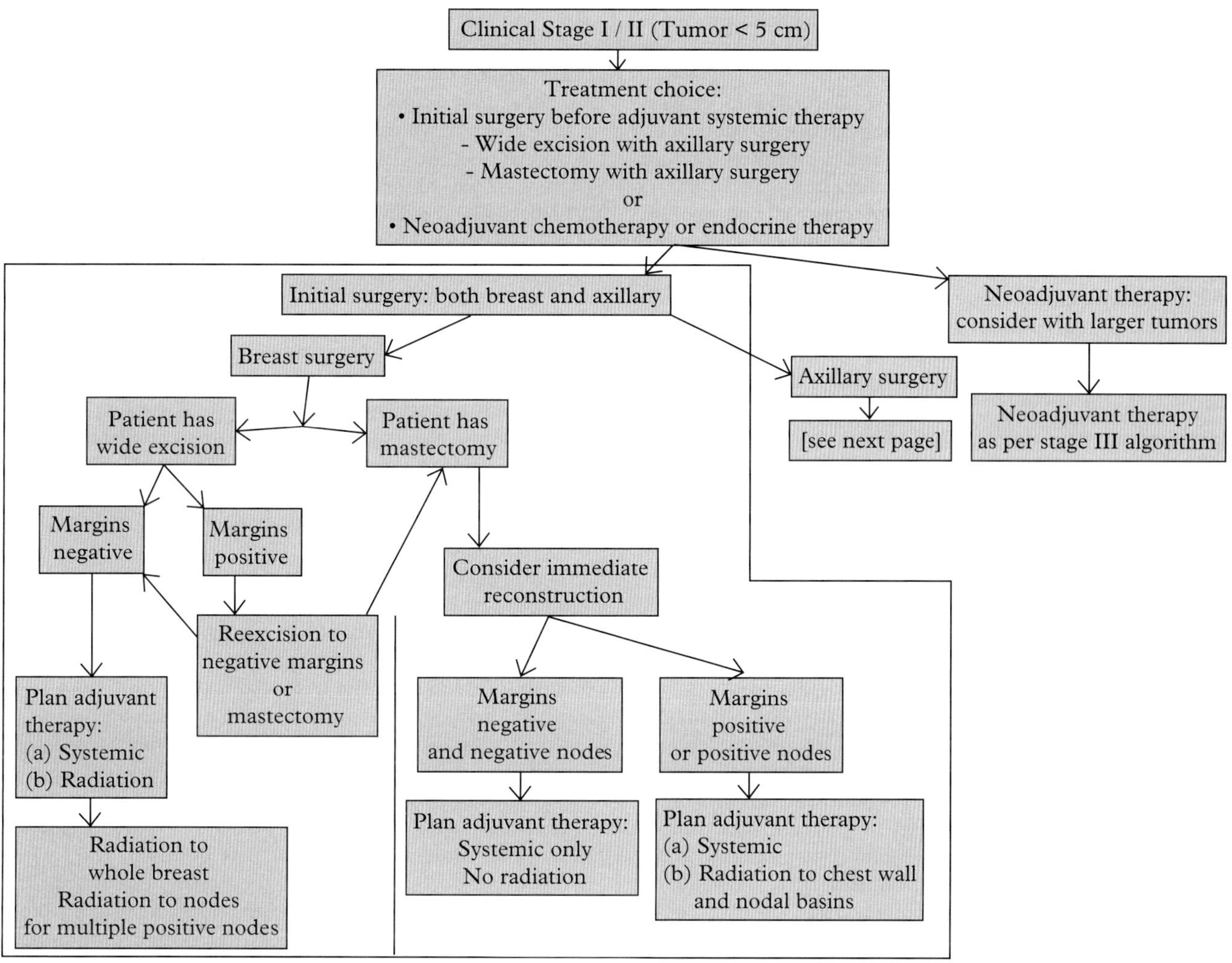

Figure 2 **Overview schema for local therapy for stage I/II breast cancer.**

women presenting with smaller cancers. However, it was not until the 1970s that the so-called "halstedian" thesis, that breast cancers progressed in a stepwise fashion from the breast (local) to lymph nodes (regional) to distant disease (metastases), was proven incorrect. In the 1970s and 1980s, landmark clinical trials demonstrated that breast cancer is a systemic disease with the possibility of disseminated disease even at the smallest primary tumor and that removal of the tumor without mastectomy provided long-term outcome equivalent to mastectomy. The most significant study was the NSABP B-06 trial comparing mastectomy with lumpectomy alone and with lumpectomy plus radiation therapy.[47] Long-term follow-up on this trial demonstrated no difference in overall survival between the three groups. However, with lumpectomy alone, the cancer recurred in the same breast in as many as 40% of women. Radiation reduced this rate of local recurrence to approximately 12%. On the basis of this finding, lumpectomy plus radiation therapy became an accepted standard in the late 1980s and became widely used through the 1990s.

Breast-conserving surgery may be performed in a majority of women with invasive breast cancer. Successful BCT requires obtaining negative margins of resection around the tumor. As with DCIS, major clinical trials testing BCT defined a negative margin as no ink on the tumor. However, in general, a minimum 2 mm margin is optimal. A specific exception may be at the chest wall, where the pectoralis fascia has been taken, and anteriorly at the skin. If a negative margin cannot be obtained with lumpectomy, including with a second or occasionally a third operation for "reexcision," mastectomy is necessary.

Indications for mastectomy include the presence of multicentric disease in the breast—separate cancers in distinct parts of the breast separated by at least 5 cm of normal breast tissue, occurring in 2 to 5% of cases; a very large tumor in relation to the size of the breast that is not amenable to lumpectomy or does not respond sufficiently to neoadjuvant systemic therapy; and previous radiation treatments to the breast, such as with a prior breast cancer or for treatment of other cancers, such as lymphoma. Radiation may not be administered during pregnancy, but with standard sequencing of systemic and radiation after BCT, radiation is usually timed such that it is administered after delivery of the baby; therefore, BCT is possible for women presenting with breast cancer during pregnancy. In addition, mastectomy is indicated after completion of systemic chemotherapy for inflammatory breast cancer because of the likelihood of the microscopic extent of disease both in the skin and within the breast beyond the area of known cancer.

An unusual presentation of breast cancer is with axillary lymph node involvement without the presence of a detectable primary cancer in the breast (occult breast primary tumor). If a woman has suspicious lymph nodes in the axilla, biopsy is warranted. If the histology shows an adenocarcinoma (as opposed to lymphoma or melanoma), the primary source of this metastatic deposit is almost invariably the breast, even if the hormone receptors are negative. Mammography usually shows the primary tumor, but MRI may find some of these cancers not seen on mammography.[48] However, in a few cases, even MRI will be negative, yet the source is invariably the breast. A whole-body search for another source of adenocarcinoma is not indicated. The woman should receive therapy assuming that this is a breast cancer.

In the past, mastectomy was used for all women with an occult breast primary tumor with a positive axillary node. However, recent data show that mastectomy is not necessary.

They should undergo axillary lymph node dissection and then receive adjuvant systemic therapy (chemotherapy and endocrine therapy) as appropriate based on stage and biologic features and then radiation to the breast.[49,50]

Women who have inherited susceptibility with a mutation known in *BRCA1* or *BRCA2* also often choose mastectomy or bilateral mastectomy. The overall survival for women treated with BCT in this situation is the same as for women without inherited susceptibility.[51] However, they are at increased risk for developing a second primary cancer in the same breast, a chance that approaches 50%, especially in women under age 50 at the initial diagnosis.[52]

Radiation in Local Therapy

Mastectomy should be supplemented with radiation when the cancer is over 5 cm in size, when surgical resection margins are close or positive, or when multiple lymph nodes are involved.[53] The "textbook" standard is that radiation is indicated with four or more positive nodes. However, radiation should be considered even when only one to three nodes are involved based on the findings of randomized clinical trials demonstrating improved survival. Unfortunately, a major American clinical trial addressing the use of radiation after mastectomy for women with one to three positive nodes failed to accrue sufficient numbers of patients to provide an answer to this critical question.

The possible need for radiation after mastectomy may affect decisions regarding the cosmetic outcome of immediate breast reconstruction.[54] Immediate reconstruction may complicate radiation dosimetry and uniform dose delivery over the entire field and increase the volume of tissue outside the field, including the lung and heart. In addition, radiation may compromise the cosmetic result of immediate reconstruction through contracture of the scar capsule around an implant and/or contracture of tissues within an autologous tissue flap. The potential need for radiation after mastectomy should be discussed with all women having mastectomy for invasive breast cancer.

Radiation is generally administered in all cases with BCT. Radiation reduces the risk of local recurrence by as much as 70%, and this may improve survival.[55] Subset analysis of large clinical trials and limited clinical trials in women with small cancers failed to identify cancers of sufficiently small size that radiation does not reduce the risk of local recurrence.

One group in whom the omission of radiation is reasonable is women over age 70 with cancers that are hormone receptor positive, 2 cm or smaller, with clinically negative nodes. A clinical trial conducted by Cancer and Leukemia Group B (CALGB) randomized such women to lumpectomy and tamoxifen with or without radiation.[56] There was no difference in long-term survival. Local recurrence occurred in 1% with and 6% without radiation. However, the same number of women in both groups ultimately underwent mastectomy as those who had not received radiation or were most often treated with lumpectomy and radiation. Therefore, omission of radiation is reasonable in this group. A similar trial conducted in Canada for women age 50 and over demonstrated local recurrence rates of about 15% among women between age 50 and 70, lending caution to omitting radiation for younger women.[57]

The standard radiation treatment after breast-conserving surgery is treatment of the entire breast to a dose of about 50 Gy, with an additional boost of radiation to the primary tumor site of about 15 Gy. Radiation treatment takes about 6 weeks of therapy and is well tolerated. Long-term serious sequelae of whole-breast radiation are uncommon.

Recent clinical research has focused on the potential for limiting the extent and time required to deliver radiation to the breast. This research is based on the finding that most recurrences occur within a short distance from the primary tumor site. Only about 15% of new events in the treated breast occur outside the area of the original tumor area and are most likely a new second primary cancer. It is hypothesized that limitation of radiation treatment only to the site of the primary cancer can provide local control equivalent to whole-breast radiation therapy. So-called accelerated partial-breast irradiation (APBI) has one major advantage: because of the technical issues in radiation dosimetry and tissue tolerance, APBI may be delivered in a much shorter time frame—generally two fractions a day over only 5 days. Another purported advantage is that if there is a second disease event in the affected breast, this may be treated by a repeat lumpectomy rather than mastectomy. However, there are no data to support this thesis.

There are a number of techniques to deliver APBI.[58] The technique with the longest-term follow-up, albeit in a limited number of patients, is multicatheter brachytherapy. This technique is cumbersome, unsightly, and seldom used. More recent alternative techniques for delivery of APBI include three-dimensional computed tomography (CT)–directed external beam radiation, brachytherapy using a radiation seed in a balloon catheter placed in the lumpectomy site, and a single intraoperative dose of radiation. These are promising technologies, but there are no long-term data from controlled clinical trials demonstrating the safety and effectiveness of these techniques.[58] Data from noncontrolled series are scant and have very short-term follow-up in a setting where, at the very least, 5-year follow-up is required. Large clinical trials are ongoing, including a study by the NSABP. Therefore, as of 2010, APBI remains investigational and whole-breast radiation therapy remains the standard.[16,59]

Local Recurrence with Mastectomy or Breast-Conserving Surgery

Local recurrence after surgical treatment of breast cancer occurs with both mastectomy and BCT. The risk of local recurrence after lumpectomy is somewhat lower than reported in the NSABP B-06 trial. When performed by experienced surgeons with careful pathologic control, appropriate radiation, and stage-appropriate adjuvant systemic therapy, the rate of local recurrence with BCT is as low as 1 to 5%. Local recurrences are also a significant issue among women treated with mastectomy. This risk is about 2 to 5% for women with negative lymph nodes and ranges as high as 25% for women with multiple positive lymph nodes.[60,61]

Local recurrence is a serious event whether it occurs after BCT or mastectomy. These women have a higher risk of developing distant metastases compared with women with similar-stage cancer who do not suffer local recurrence. It has previously been generally cited that radiation impacts only the risk of local recurrence and not overall survival. However, a meta-analysis of all available data for women treated with BCT and mastectomy demonstrated that radiation therapy not only reduces the risk of local failure but also improves survival.[55] The best estimate is that radiation saves one life for every four local recurrences prevented. Radiation is therefore recommended for women who have a risk of local failure over 10% regardless of the type of primary surgery.

The accepted treatment for local recurrence after BCT is mastectomy. This is because the recurrence may be multifocal and because full-dose radiation cannot be administered safely a second time because of tissue toxicity. Local recurrence after mastectomy is more difficult to treat and carries a more serious prognosis. Treatment usually includes resection of a local recurrence in the skin, muscle, or regional nodes if possible, followed by radiation to the chest wall and regional nodes. The role for additional adjuvant systemic therapy after local recurrence is uncertain, and there are no clinical trial data supporting its use. However, many oncologists will deliver additional systemic treatment based on the type of previous treatment and the nature and extent of the local recurrence.

Selection of Breast-Conserving Surgery versus Mastectomy

The decision between BCT and mastectomy is a complex and difficult one for women with breast cancer. From a technical standpoint, BCT is possible in the large majority of women with breast cancer. More than 90% of women with tumors under 2 cm in size (T1) may undergo BCT given the absolute and relative contraindications to BCT discussed above. However, many other factors in addition to the technical ability to perform BCT affect the decision. Ultimately, the individual patient is the determinant of whether or not she will have mastectomy. Her choice may be influenced by perceptions or values based on personal or family experiences, real or perceived increased risks of recurrent cancer based on family history, and other factors.

Counseling women regarding the choice of surgery is one of the most important tasks for the treating surgeon.[62] Surgeons need to learn the skills of nondirective counseling and must incorporate other professionals and resources into their practice. Careful study of the decision-making process has shown that physicians are not necessarily fully sensitive to their patient's concerns or to their styles of decision making.[63] This has led to the development of decision assistance and support tools and to the recognition of the need for multidisciplinary counseling, especially in more complex situations or those associated with questions surrounding inherited susceptibility and genetics.[64]

One of the key factors in this process is the recognition that breast cancer treatment is not an immediate emergency. There are no data to support the contention that treatment initiated within a few days of diagnosis improves outcome compared with that delayed a reasonable period of time, measured in a number of weeks or even months. Women should be given the opportunity to seek additional counseling, research information on their own, and obtain second opinions if they so desire. Inclusion of professionals of other disciplines, including radiation oncology, plastic surgery, medical oncology, radiology, psychology and social support, nursing, and genetics, may be warranted.

MANAGEMENT OF THE CONTRALATERAL BREAST

Women with breast cancer have a risk of second malignancies and especially the risk of developing a contralateral primary breast cancer. Outside the setting of inherited susceptibility, the chance of developing a contralateral primary breast cancer is about 10% over 20 to 30 years.[47] Given that the average woman is in her 50s or 60s and that most of these contralateral breast cancers will be effectively treated, the risk that a woman with a breast cancer will succumb to a new contralateral breast cancer is far outweighed by both the risk of death from the current breast cancer and the long-term risk of death from other causes during the very long-term follow-up in which second cancers occur. Therefore, treatment addressing the other breast is generally not necessary.

Previously, it was believed that women with invasive lobular cancer had a much higher risk of a contralateral breast cancer compared with ductal cancer. The added risk of contralateral cancer with lobular cancer is relatively small and should have little bearing on treatment decisions.

The issues are different for women with inherited susceptibility, most notably those with mutations in *BRCA1* and *BRCA2*. They are generally younger at breast cancer diagnosis and have a higher risk of developing a second cancer. This risk appears dependent on the age at which they are diagnosed with their first breast cancer: 25 to 50% for those under age 50 at the initial diagnosis and 15 to 20% for those over age 50.[52]

Careful counseling can largely allay a woman's fears of the impact of the risk of a second cancer. However, some women, especially those undergoing mastectomy for the index cancer, may request contralateral mastectomy. Recent observational studies demonstrate that the number of women undergoing prophylactic contralateral mastectomy increased significantly over the last decade. In New York State, about 4% of women treated with mastectomy in 1995 had a contralateral mastectomy compared with 15% in 2005.[65]

LYMPH NODE STAGING IN BREAST CANCER

The presence of metastases in regional lymph nodes is a key prognostic factor used in making treatment decisions, as discussed below [*see Figure 3*]. In addition, removing lymph

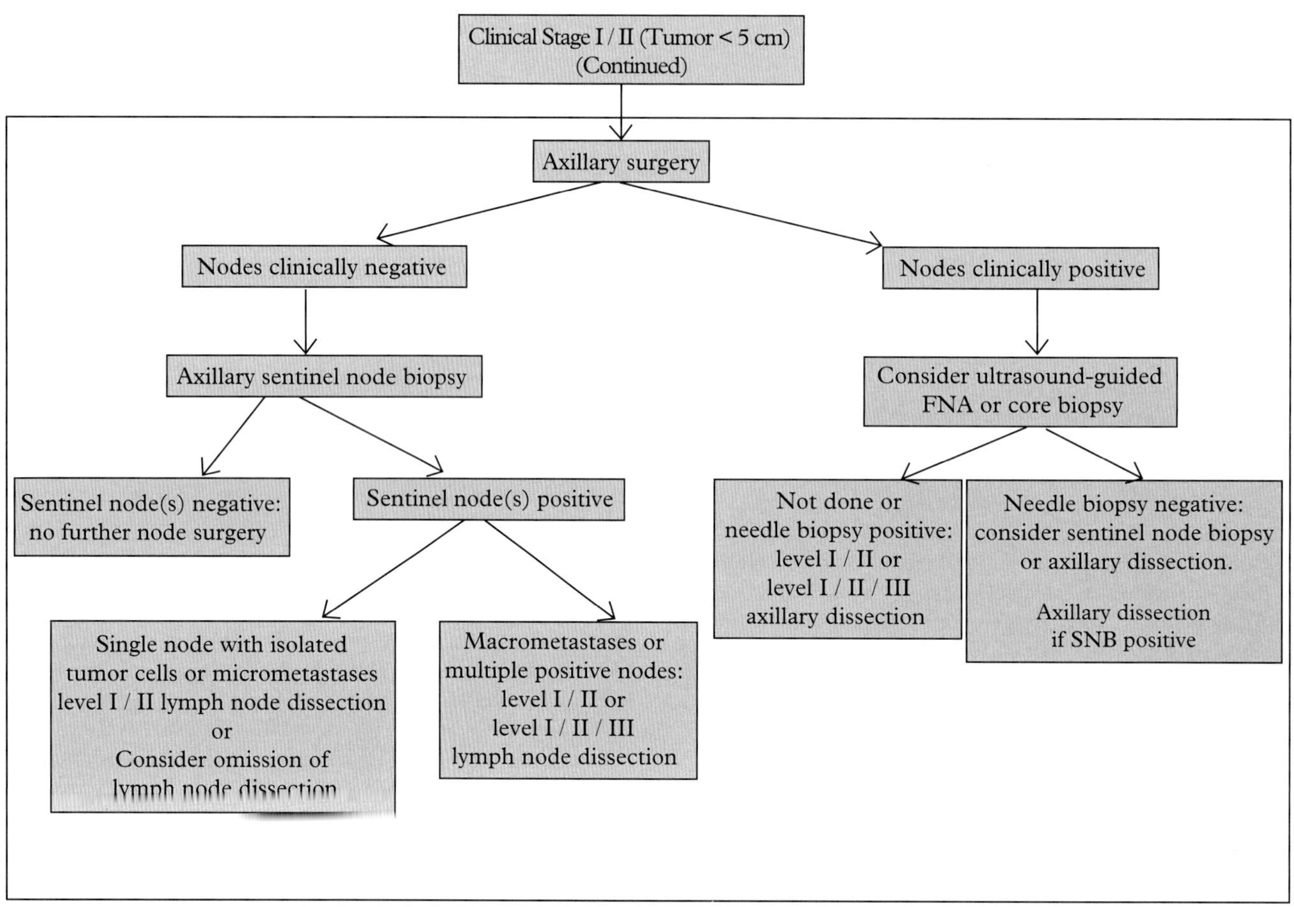

Figure 3 **Axillary surgery management schema. FNA = fine-needle aspiration; SNB = sentinel node biopsy.**

nodes prevents recurrence risk in the regional lymph node basin. However, treatment of lymph nodes does not itself affect survival. Defining the involvement of regional lymph nodes requires surgical resection. No noninvasive test of the regional lymph nodes has proven insufficient sensitivity and specificity to replace surgical resection. Therefore, surgical evaluation of regional nodes remains a key component of breast cancer treatment.[66]

Lymph fluid from the breast drains primarily through the axillary lymph nodes.[67] A small fraction of lymph drainage from the breast is through other pathways, including direct drainage through the supraclavicular nodes and via the internal mammary chain.[68] Because the majority of drainage is through the axilla, and because of potential morbidity of internal mammary lymph node dissection, most surgeons limit surgical evaluation of lymph nodes to the axilla.

The axilla contains an average of 15 to 20 lymph nodes extending under the axillary vein medially toward the thoracic inlet. Until the last decade, evaluating these nodes required dissection of the entire axillary contents. A safe operation, it carries substantial risk of long-term morbidity related to disruption of the lymphatic flow from the arm and permanent swelling, termed lymphedema.[69–71] Lymphedema is a chronic lifelong condition that ranges from minimal effects to disabling swelling. The risk of lymphedema is about 10% with axillary dissection alone and substantially higher when radiation is also required after node dissection.[37,72]

During the 1990s, the hypothesis that lymphatic drainage to the axilla could be mapped using radioactive or large colloidal particle tracers and that the first few lymph nodes identified by these mappings would define the status of the lymph nodes was tested and proven accurate.[73] Termed the sentinel lymph node, the first few lymph nodes can be identified and full axillary lymph node dissection limited only to those women with proven nodal metastases. Morbidity, including the risk of lymphedema, is lower with SNB than with axillary dissection, but lymphedema still may occur.[36]

SNB is appropriate for women with clinically negative nodes. Those with clinically positive nodes are not candidates for SNB and should have full axillary lymph node dissection. If there is a question about nodes, involvement of nodes may be confirmed before surgery using ultrasound-guided needle biopsy (core biopsy or FNA).

SNB is performed by injecting radiolabeled tracer and/or vital dyes that drain to and are trapped in the initial lymph nodes in the chain. The injection is generally in the periareolar skin and under the nipple-areola complex. This identifies an average of three lymph nodes, which are then removed and examined for metastases. SNB is appropriate in virtually all women with invasive breast cancer clinically negative nodes. SNB may be performed in women with local recurrence after previous breast-conserving surgery and radiation, although the accuracy of SNB in this setting has never been tested.

BREAST RECONSTRUCTION

Women treated with mastectomy may consider reconstruction of the breast mound performed either at the time of mastectomy (immediate reconstruction) or at a later time (delayed reconstruction).[74] Immediate reconstruction is reasonable in women with early-stage breast cancer. However, the potential need for postmastectomy radiation must be considered in reconstruction planning.[54] Although satisfactory cosmetic outcomes may be obtained even with radiation to the implant, radiation increases the rate of painful scar contracture. Decisions regarding immediate breast reconstruction should be made in collaboration with the entire multidisciplinary treatment team. Conversely, delayed reconstruction requires that the woman live without the reconstructed breast for a period of 1 to 2 years and may be more difficult to perform because there is less skin remaining from the original mastectomy to be used in reconstruction.

Options for breast reconstruction include prosthetic reconstruction with an implant or "tissue expander implant" generally placed beneath the pectoralis major muscle or transfer of autologous tissue from another region in the body.[74] Implant reconstruction is generally simpler and quicker to perform but may not leave as attractive an aesthetic result. Complications of implant reconstruction include contracture around the implant (which may be exacerbated if radiation is necessary) and infection, resulting in loss of the implant. Autologous tissue reconstruction often leaves a superior cosmetic result but at the cost of more complex surgery, longer recovery, and the potential for complications at the site of the donor tissue. The most common donor sites are the rectus abdominus muscle (so-called transverse rectus abdominus myocutaneous [TRAM] flap), the more superficial fat and skin from the abdominal wall (deep inferior epigastric perforator [DIEP] flap), and the latissimus dorsi muscle flap. These flaps may be used in conjunction with complete sparing of all the skin of the breast that provides for an even better cosmetic result. In general, the nipple and areola are resected with mastectomy, but in select circumstances, such as small tumors located in the periphery of the breast, some surgeons have been experimenting with mastectomy that preserves the nipple.[75–77]

ADJUVANT SYSTEMIC THERAPY

Women with invasive cancer also face the risk of developing distant metastases. These metastases develop from microscopic dissemination of cancer cells prior to diagnosis. Staging studies including CT, PET, and MRI are not insensitive at detecting this microscopic disease. In stage I and stage II cancer, these studies are unnecessary unless there are symptoms such as new skeletal pain or other constitutional symptoms. The chance of identifying metastatic disease is very low, and there is a substantial chance of false positive scans, requiring extensive evaluation and invasive studies.

Therefore, every woman with invasive cancer must consider whether to receive systemic adjuvant therapy to prevent the growth of this microscopic metastatic disease [*see Figure 4*]. The decision depends on both the estimated risk of developing metastatic disease and the degree of benefit that treatment may provide. These risks are estimated by analysis of features about the cancer, including the size of the invasive component of the cancer, the presence or absence of regional lymph node metastases, the grade of the cancer, and the presence or absence of specific biomarkers associated with prognosis and response to treatment. The three clinically used markers are the estrogen receptor, the progesterone receptor, and HER-2/neu protein expression or gene amplification. In making these assessments, it must be recognized that a substantial fraction of women with negative lymph nodes still develop metastatic disease.[15]

Clinical Stage I / II (Tumor < 5 cm)
Adjuvant systemic therapy:

Consider in all cases:
Based on
• Primary tumor characteristics
• Hormone receptor status
• HER-2/*neu* status
• Genomic profiling

Principles of Systemic Therapy
• ER positive: endocrine therapy and consider adding chemotherapy even with negative nodes
• ER negative: consider chemotherapy even with negative nodes
• HER-2/*neu* positive: add trastuzumab to chemotherapy

Figure 4 **Principles of adjuvant systemic therapy. ER = estrogen receptor.**

Treatment entails two major classes of drugs: endocrine drugs, which block the effect of circulating estrogen on breast cancers that express estrogen and progesterone receptors, and systemic cytotoxic chemotherapy. The best available treatments are codified in widely accepted practice guidelines developed and updated annually by the NCCN.[16]

Endocrine therapy is effective only for women whose tumors express hormone receptors. This includes premenopausal women and postmenopausal women as they have low levels of circulating estrogens from non-ovarian sources. There are two primary classes of endocrine drugs: SERMs, of which the primary agent used in breast cancer is tamoxifen, and aromatase inhibitors, which block peripheral synthesis of estrogen and are effective only in postmenopausal women.[78] Recent clinical trials demonstrated that aromatase inhibitors are superior to tamoxifen in preventing the recurrence of breast cancer, with a slightly improved safety profile in postmenopausal women. Aromatase inhibitors are not effective in premenopausal women, for whom tamoxifen remains the drug of choice. These drugs are remarkably safe and effective, with only rare serious side effects.

With only a few exceptions, all women with hormone receptor–positive breast cancers should receive prolonged endocrine therapy. At least 5 years of therapy is warranted.

Ongoing clinical trials are addressing whether prolonged therapy with aromatase inhibitors may be of value.

Women with hormone receptor–positive breast cancers should consider whether to also receive systemic chemotherapy. A large body of evidence from clinical trials shows that survival may be improved by the addition of chemotherapy.[79,80] However, the magnitude of benefit over the benefit of endocrine therapy alone may be small. For otherwise healthy women who have positive lymph nodes, additional chemotherapy may be strongly considered. For those with negative nodes, the benefit varies according to the characteristics of the cancer. Until recently, many women received chemotherapy for a survival advantage as low as 1%. Recently, genomic profiling of cancers through characterization of the expression of multiple genes has allowed identification of women in this situation with a very high and with a very low risk of distant disease and also has to find which patients benefit from chemotherapy.[81,82] The most widely used genomic profiling system in breast cancer in 2009 is OncotypeDx. This profiling is validated for use in women with hormone receptor–positive, lymph node–negative invasive breast cancer.

Endocrine therapy is not effective in women with hormone receptor–negative breast cancer. For these women, the only treatment to reduce the risk of distant metastases is cytotoxic chemotherapy.[79,80] Unless otherwise contraindicated by serious comorbidities, women with cancers over 1 cm and negative hormone receptors should receive chemotherapy.[16] Those with tumors under 1 cm have a lower risk of distant metastases and may derive substantially less benefit from chemotherapy.

Breast cancers that express the HER-2/neu protein have a higher risk of developing distant metastases. However, the monoclonal antibody trastuzumab (Herceptin) directed against HER-2 has proven to be safe and effective when given in combination with chemotherapy. The risk of distance metastatic disease is cut by about half over the benefit of chemotherapy alone when combined with trastuzumab.[83]

The most difficult situation is when estrogen, progesterone, and HER-2/neu are negative. So-called "triple negative cancers" are more common in younger women, those of African American ancestry, and those with inherited susceptibility. There is active ongoing clinical research to define improved approaches in this setting.

Clinical trials over the last three decades have defined the most effective drugs in breast cancer. Chemotherapy drugs are most effective when used in combination with other drugs. The most effective drugs in breast cancer are the anthracyclines, of which the most widely used agent is doxorubicin (Adriamycin), cyclophosphamide (Cytoxan), and the taxanes (paclitaxel and docetaxil). Readers are referred to a large-scale meta-analysis of the value of adjuvant chemotherapy and endocrine therapy and to recent reviews on the subject.[79,80,84]

Decisions regarding adjuvant systemic therapy are complex for both patients and their physicians. To aid these decisions, there are mathematical models that incorporate relevant prognostic factors and provide individualized risk of distant recurrence and benefit from treatment. The most widely used models are Adjuvant! (www.adjuvantonline.com) and CancerMath.net (http://cancer.lifemath.net/).[85–87]

NEOADJUVANT SYSTEMIC THERAPY AND LOCALLY ADVANCED BREAST CANCER

Locally advanced breast cancer is generally defined as any tumor over 5 cm, involving the skin, or with extensive lymph node involvement [*see Figure 5*]. In these cases, surgery may be difficult and even standard mastectomy may not be possible. With the advent of chemotherapy in the 1970s, clinical trials investigated the value of systemic treatments, most notably chemotherapy, prior to surgery. These demonstrated that such "neoadjuvant" presurgical therapy with locally advanced breast cancer often reduced the size and extent of the cancer more than 50%, which often allowed standard surgery. Equally interesting was that 15 to 25% had complete disappearance of cancer clinically and half of these women had no viable tumor identified pathologically (pathologic complete response). Neoadjuvant chemotherapy became the accepted standard treatment for locally advanced and inflammatory breast cancer (stage III).

This finding with locally advanced breast cancer led to studies of presurgical chemotherapy with lower-stage cancer.[88] Large-scale studies, most notably the NSABP B-18 study, demonstrated similar cancer responses with presurgical chemotherapy.[89] Neoadjuvant therapy did not convey any survival advantage over chemotherapy administered postoperatively. However, women treated with presurgical chemotherapy were more likely to have BCT, and the rate of local recurrence after this treatment was equivalent to that of others receiving BCT. The degree of response to neoadjuvant therapy is itself of significant prognostic importance.[89–91] Those women who achieve a major response, especially those who achieve a complete pathologic response in the tumor, are more likely to have long-term survival compared with those who do not.[88] These and other factors have led to an increasing use of neoadjuvant therapy.

Presurgical endocrine therapy may also be of value in select cases.[92,93] A response to neoadjuvant chemotherapy is most likely among women with high-grade and hormone receptor–negative cancers. Those with endocrine receptor–positive cancers may be somewhat less likely to respond. However, these tumors may also respond to presurgical endocrine therapy, with similar benefits in terms of surgical treatment. With endocrine therapy, the time to maximal tumor response is longer than with chemotherapy; it may take 6 months to achieve maximum tumor response prior to surgery.

It is therefore reasonable to administer neoadjuvant therapy to any woman who would otherwise receive chemotherapy for treatment for breast cancer. In general, neoadjuvant therapy is administered to those with larger T2 cancers (those over three or 4 cm in size) and T3 cancers in an effort to allow breast conservation. In addition, neoadjuvant therapy is the treatment of choice for those with cancer that involves the skin or chest wall (T4), with extensive lymph node involvement clinically, or those who have inflammatory cancer. Regardless of the final surgery type and the degree of tumor response, women with locally advanced breast cancer should receive surgery and radiation.[94]

STAGE IV BREAST CANCER

A small fraction of breast cancers have distant metastases (stage IV) at the time of the initial cancer presentation [*see*

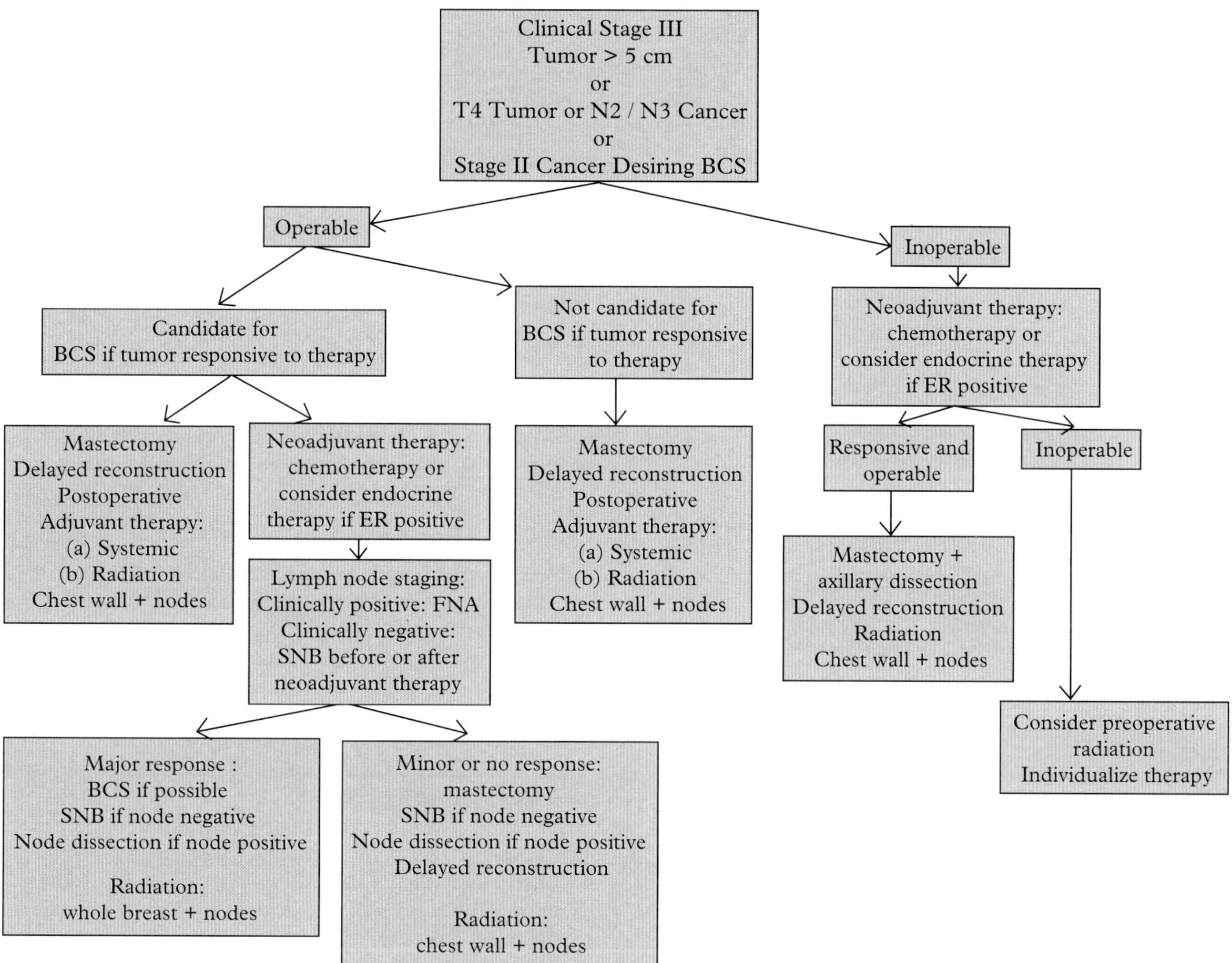

Figure 5 **Schema for treatment of locally advanced breast cancer. BCS = breast-conserving surgery; ER = estrogen receptor; FNA = fine-needle aspiration; SNB = sentinel node biopsy.**

Figure 6]. This disease is generally incurable, and treatment is targeted at preventing disease progression for the longest time possible while maintaining high quality of life. It is generally necessary to obtain tissue from the primary tumor to obtain hormone receptor and HER-2/neu information, as well as to biopsy a metastatic site if there is any doubt regarding whether the metastatic deposit is truly a metastasis.

First-line treatment is generally systemic therapy.[16] In the absence of symptomatic or aggressive visceral disease, those with endocrine-sensitive tumors are best treated with oral endocrine therapy. Many may achieve a major response and have long, progression-free intervals with high quality of life without significant treatment-related toxicity. Those with hormone receptor–negative cancers may begin with systemic chemotherapy.

For those diagnosed with metastases before the primary tumor in the breast is removed, there is generally no reason to do surgery. Systemic treatment often provides a major response in the breast and achieves sufficient local control for the duration of the woman's life. For those women fortunate enough to have prolonged survival but in whom the primary tumor does progress, surgery and/or radiation may be used for local control and preserving quality of life.

There is an interesting literature from population cancer registries suggesting that those women who present with metastatic disease who undergo surgery at the time of diagnosis have longer survival than those who do not have surgery.[95–97] However, this finding is most likely a selection bias in that women with a lower burden of disease are more likely to have undergone surgery before the discovery of the metastatic cancer and are therefore more likely to survive longer. There are no controlled clinical trial data to support either argument.

Breast Cancer in Pregnancy

Breast cancer is uncommon in young women but may occur during the childbearing years. Therefore, breast cancer may occur during pregnancy and, in fact, is the second most common cancer associated with pregnancy. Women in this age group are generally not undergoing routine breast cancer screening, and changes in the breast associated with pregnancy can mask the presence of a mass. Therefore, breast

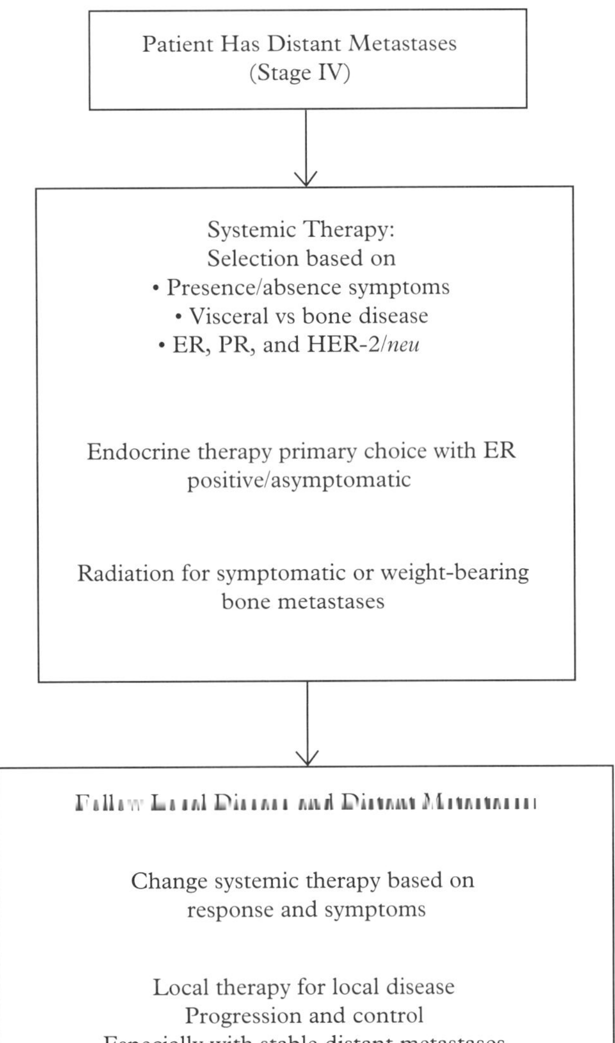

Figure 6 **Schema for treatment of women with cancer with distant metastases at presentation (stage IV). ER = estrogen receptor; PR = progesterone receptor.**

cancer diagnosis is often delayed in this situation. Women with a suspicious breast mass detected during pregnancy should be evaluated aggressively. Imaging can generally be done with judicious use of mammography, ultrasonography, and biopsy performed as in any woman with a suspicious breast lesion.

The principles of treatment are the same as in any woman with breast cancer.[98] The only limitations are that chemotherapy cannot be administered during the first trimester and radiation cannot be administered until after delivery. However, neither of these issues limits aggressive treatment of women with breast cancer during pregnancy. Termination of the pregnancy is not necessary, although some women diagnosed early in pregnancy may choose to do so.

Older texts suggested that mastectomy is the preferred treatment in women with breast cancer during pregnancy. However, the same choices are available to women with cancer during pregnancy because the radiation that is administered is generally delayed until after chemotherapy and therefore is timed to occur after delivery of the child. Therefore, breast conservation can be used safely during pregnancy. Similarly, chemotherapy may be used safely during pregnancy. There are extensive data demonstrating the safety of chemotherapy for both the mother and the fetus. SNB may also be performed during pregnancy using the radioactive tracers. The estimated radiation dose to the fetus is exceedingly low and is considered safe.[99] The vital dyes isosulfan blue and methylene blue have potential teratogenic effects and are contraindicated during pregnancy.

Women who have breast cancer at a young age or during pregnancy may wish to have additional children. Decades ago, they were advised against this because of concern that hormonal changes associated with pregnancy could promote recurrence. This has been proven incorrect. Women may choose to have children after breast cancer treatment with no additional risk of breast cancer recurrence and death.

Breast Cancer in Men

Breast cancer occurs in men with an incidence less than 1% of that of women. No screening for men is warranted, but a mass in the breast should be fully evaluated. Most masses proved to be gynecomastia. Breast cancer in a younger man may be indicative of inherited susceptibility within that family particularly related to *BRCA2*. Careful family history and counseling regarding this risk should be provided.

The treatment of breast cancer in men follows the same principles as in women.[100,101]

Surgery is generally mastectomy because of the tumor is directly under the nipple complex. Wide margins should be obtained. Radiation may be administered if the tumor is larger or involves the skin and/or chest wall. SNB and axillary lymph node dissection should be performed using the same indications as in women. Men should also receive adjuvant systemic therapy using the same criteria as women. Most are hormone receptor positive, and endocrine therapy is effective.

Follow-up after Breast Cancer Treatment

Patients who have been treated for invasive breast cancer are at risk for developing distant metastases, local recurrence, and a contralateral or ipsilateral new breast cancer. Most recurrences occur within the first 5 to 10 years, with the peak at 4 to 6 years. Occasionally, women develop distant metastases many years later.

Women with breast cancer often assume that careful screening is warranted to allow early detection of metastases on the assumption that early detection will provide a better chance of a successful outcome. Unfortunately, there is no such entity as early metastatic cancer. Once breast cancer metastases are established to the extent that they are detectable, there is no therapy that is curative, and treatment is largely palliative, as discussed above related to stage IV breast cancer. Because of this, extensive testing for metastatic disease on a periodic basis does not provide any advantage to a woman with breast cancer.[102] This question has actually been tested in randomized clinical trials of extensive testing versus simple follow-up for local recurrence only combined with evaluation of any symptoms suggestive of metastatic disease.

These studies showed no survival advantage despite detection of metastatic disease, and those recurred an average of 3 months earlier in the screened group.

Screening women for evidence of local recurrence with both invasive and in situ cancer may be of value. This should include mammography of the ipsilateral breast in women treated with breast conservation, contralateral mammography for all women, and a careful history and physical examination. Mammography should be done annually, with the history and physical examination done every 6 to 12 months. The role of breast MRI in breast cancer follow-up is unclear. Women should maintain a primary care provider to be sure that other regular medical care is provided.

CANCER SURVIVORSHIP

In addition to covering medical issues in cancer follow-up, surgeons should provide ongoing resources to help women adjust to the cancer diagnosis, deal with psychological issues, address cancer genetic and family concerns, and identify other long-term sequelae of cancer.[103] Patients should be provided with a written "care plan" for their ongoing care and should be encouraged to seek individual counseling and participate in support groups as they see the need and to gain the value of engagement in the vast array of support and advocacy activities available in most communities.[104]

Financial Disclosures: None Reported

References

1. Telli ML, Horst KC, Guardino AE, et al. Phyllodes tumors of the breast: natural history, diagnosis, and treatment. J Natl Compr Canc Netw 2007;5:324–30.
2. Lum YW, Jacobs L. Primary breast sarcoma. Surg Clin North Am 2008;88:559–70, vi.
3. Smith RA, Cokkinides V, Brawley OW. Cancer screening in the United States, 2009: a review of current American Cancer Society guidelines and issues in cancer screening. CA Cancer J Clin 2009;59: 27–41.
4. Smith RA, Cokkinides V, Eyre HJ. Cancer screening in the United States, 2007: a review of current guidelines, practices, and prospects. CA Cancer J Clin 2007;57: 90–104.
5. Screening for breast cancer: U.S. Preventive Services Task Force recommendation statement. Ann Intern Med 2009;151:716–26, W-236.
6. Eberl MM, Fox CH, Edge SB, et al. BI-RADS classification for management of abnormal mammograms. J Am Board Fam Med 2006;19:161–4.
7. Lehman CD, Smith RA. The role of MRI in breast cancer screening. J Natl Compr Canc Netw 2009;7:1109–15.
8. Saslow D, Boetes C, Burke W, et al. American Cancer Society guidelines for breast screening with MRI as an adjunct to mammography. CA Cancer J Clin 2007;57: 75–89.
9. Brennan ME, Houssami N, Lord S, et al. Magnetic resonance imaging screening of the contralateral breast in women with newly diagnosed breast cancer: systematic review and meta-analysis of incremental cancer detection and impact on surgical management. J Clin Oncol 2009;27: 5640–9.
10. Houssami N, Hayes DF. Review of preoperative magnetic resonance imaging (MRI) in breast cancer: should MRI be performed on all women with newly diagnosed, early stage breast cancer? CA Cancer J Clin 2009; 59:290–302.
11. Singh V, Saunders C, Wylie L, Bourke A. New diagnostic techniques for breast cancer detection. Future Oncol 2008;4:501–13.
12. Lee JH, Rosen EL, Mankoff DA. The role of radiotracer imaging in the diagnosis and management of patients with breast cancer: part 1—overview, detection, and staging. J Nucl Med 2009;50:569–81.
13. Lee JH, Rosen EL, Mankoff DA. The role of radiotracer imaging in the diagnosis and management of patients with breast cancer: part 2—response to therapy, other indications, and future directions. J Nucl Med 2009;50:738–48.
14. Eby PR, Ochsner JE, DeMartini WB, et al. Frequency and upgrade rates of atypical ductal hyperplasia diagnosed at stereotactic vacuum-assisted breast biopsy: 9- versus 11-gauge. AJR Am J Roentgenol 2009;192: 229–34.
15. Edge SB, Byrd DR, Compton CC, et al, editors. AJCC cancer staging manual. 7th ed. New York: Springer; 2010.
16. Carlson RW, Allred DC, Anderson BO, et al. Breast cancer. Clinical practice guidelines in oncology. J Natl Compr Canc Netw 2009;7:122–92.
17. Chuba PJ, Hamre MR, Yap J, et al. Bilateral risk for subsequent breast cancer after lobular carcinoma-in-situ: analysis of surveillance, epidemiology, and end results data. J Clin Oncol 2005;23:5534–41.
18. Karabakhtsian RG, Johnson R, Sumkin J, Dabbs DJ. The clinical significance of lobular neoplasia on breast core biopsy. Am J Surg Pathol 2007;31:717–23.
19. Anderson BO, Calhoun KE, Rosen EL. Evolving concepts in the management of lobular neoplasia. J Natl Compr Canc Netw 2006;4:511–22.
20. Vogel VG. Recent results from clinical trials using SERMs to reduce the risk of breast cancer. Ann N Y Acad Sci 2006;1089: 127–42.
21. Vogel VG. The NSABP Study of Tamoxifen and Raloxifene (STAR) trial. Expert Rev Anticancer Ther 2009;9:51–60.
22. Allegra CJ, Aberle DR, Ganschow P, et al. National Institutes of Health State-of-the-Sciences Conference Statement: Diagnosis and Management of Ductal Carcinoma In Situ September 22–24, 2009. J Natl Cancer Inst 2010;102:161–9.
23. Kuerer HM, Albarracin CT, Yang WT, et al. Ductal carcinoma in situ: state of the science and roadmap to advance the field. J Clin Oncol 2009;27:279–88.
24. Carlson GW, Page A, Johnson E, et al. Local recurrence of ductal carcinoma in situ after skin-sparing mastectomy. J Am Coll Surg 2007;204:1074–8; discussion 1078–80.
25. Fisher B, Dignam J, Wolmark N, et al. Lumpectomy and radiation therapy for the treatment of intraductal breast cancer: findings from National Surgical Adjuvant Breast and Bowel Project B-17. J Clin Oncol 1998; 16:441–52.
26. Bijker N, Meijnen P, Peterse JL, et al. Breast-conserving treatment with or without radiotherapy in ductal carcinoma-in-situ: ten-year results of European Organisation for Research and Treatment of Cancer randomized phase III trial 10853—a study by the EORTC Breast Cancer Cooperative Group and EORTC Radiotherapy Group. J Clin Oncol 2006;24:3381–7.
27. Holmberg L, Garmo H, Granstrand B, et al. Absolute risk reductions for local recurrence after postoperative radiotherapy after sector resection for ductal carcinoma in situ of the breast. J Clin Oncol 2008;26:1247–52.
28. Goodwin A, Parker S, Ghersi D, Wilcken N. Post-operative radiotherapy for ductal carcinoma in situ of the breast—a systematic review of the randomised trials. Breast 2009;18:143–9.
29. Blair SL, Thompson K, Rococco J, et al. Attaining negative margins in breast-conservation operations: is there a consensus among breast surgeons? J Am Coll Surg 2009;209:608–13.
30. Azu M, Abrahamse P, Katz SJ, et al. What is an adequate margin for breast-conserving surgery? Surgeon attitudes and correlates. Ann Surg Oncol 2010;17:558–63.
31. Macdonald HR, Silverstein MJ, Lee LA, et al. Margin width as the sole determinant of local recurrence after breast conservation in patients with ductal carcinoma in situ of the breast. Am J Surg 2006;192:420–2.
32. Dunne C, Burke JP, Morrow M, Kell MR. Effect of margin status on local recurrence after breast conservation and radiation therapy for ductal carcinoma in situ. J Clin Oncol 2009;27:1615–20.
33. Silverstein MJ, Lagios MD, Craig PH, et al. A prognostic index for ductal carcinoma in situ of the breast. Cancer 1996;77: 2267–74.
34. Silverstein MJ, Buchanan C. Ductal carcinoma in situ: USC/Van Nuys Prognostic Index and the impact of margin status. Breast 2003;12:457–71.
35. Keisch M, Vicini F, Beitsch P, et al. American Society of Breast Surgeons MammoSite Radiation Therapy System Registry Trial: ductal carcinoma-in-situ subset analysis—4-year data in 194 treated lesions. Am J Surg 2009;198:505–7.
36. Lucci A, McCall LM, Beitsch PD, et al. Surgical complications associated with sentinel lymph node dissection (SLND) plus axillary lymph node dissection compared with SLND alone in the American College of Surgeons Oncology Group Trial Z0011. J Clin Oncol 2007;25:3657–63.
37. McLaughlin SA, Wright MJ, Morris KT, et al. Prevalence of lymphedema in women with breast cancer 5 years after sentinel lymph node biopsy or axillary dissection: objective measurements. J Clin Oncol 2008; 26:5213–9.

38. Fisher B, Dignam J, Wolmark N, et al. Tamoxifen in treatment of intraductal breast cancer: National Surgical Adjuvant Breast and Bowel Project B-24 randomised controlled trial. Lancet 1999;353:1993–2000.
39. Marshall JK, Griffith KA, Haffty BG, et al. Conservative management of Paget disease of the breast with radiotherapy: 10- and 15-year results. Cancer 2003;97:2142–9.
40. Chen CY, Sun LM, Anderson BO. Paget disease of the breast: changing patterns of incidence, clinical presentation, and treatment in the U.S. Cancer 2006;107:1448–58.
41. Rakha EA, Lee AH, Evans AJ, et al. Tubular carcinoma of the breast: further evidence to support its excellent prognosis. J Clin Oncol 2010;28:99–104.
42. Barkley CR, Ligibel JA, Wong JS, et al. Mucinous breast carcinoma: a large contemporary series. Am J Surg 2008;196:549–51.
43. Cianfrocca M, Gradishar W. New molecular classifications of breast cancer. CA Cancer J Clin 2009;59:303–13.
44. Martin M, Gonzalez Palacios F, Cortes J, et al. Prognostic and predictive factors and genetic analysis of early breast cancer. Clin Transl Oncol 2009;11:634–42.
45. Carlson RW, Moench SJ, Hammond ME, et al. HER2 testing in breast cancer: NCCN Task Force report and recommendations. J Natl Compr Canc Netw 2006;4 Suppl 3:S1–22; quiz S3–4.
46. Wolff AC, Hammond ME, Schwartz JN, et al. American Society of Clinical Oncology/Coll[illegible] Pathologists guideline [illegible] human epidermal growth factor receptor 2 testing in breast cancer. Arch Pathol Lab Med 2007;131:18–43.
47. Fisher B, Anderson S, Bryant J, et al. Twenty-year follow-up of a randomized trial comparing total mastectomy, lumpectomy, and lumpectomy plus irradiation for the treatment of invasive breast cancer. N Engl J Med 2002;347:1233–41.
48. de Bresser J, de Vos B, van der Ent F, Hulsewe K. Breast MRI in clinically and mammographically occult breast cancer presenting with an axillary metastasis: a systematic review. Eur J Surg Oncol 2010;36:114–9.
49. Varadarajan R, Edge SB, Yu J, et al. Prognosis of occult breast carcinoma presenting as isolated axillary nodal metastasis. Oncology 2006;71:456–9.
50. Yang TJ, Yang Q, Haffty BG, Moran MS. Prognosis for mammographically occult, early-stage breast cancer patients treated with breast-conservation therapy. Int J Radiat Oncol Biol Phys 2010;76:79–84.
51. Bordeleau L, Panchal S, Goodwin P. Prognosis of BRCA-associated breast cancer: a summary of evidence. Breast Cancer Res Treat 2010;119:13–24.
52. Graeser MK, Engel C, Rhiem K, et al. Contralateral breast cancer risk in BRCA1 and BRCA2 mutation carriers. J Clin Oncol 2010;27:5887–92.
53. Fernando SA, Edge SB. Evidence and controversies in the use of postmastectomy radiation. J Natl Compr Canc Netw 2007;5:331–8.
54. Kronowitz SJ, Robb GL. Radiation therapy and breast reconstruction: a critical review of the literature. Plast Reconstr Surg 2009;124:395–408.
55. Clarke M, Collins R, Darby S, et al. Effects of radiotherapy and of differences in the extent of surgery for early breast cancer on local recurrence and 15-year survival: an overview of the randomised trials. Lancet 2005;366:2087–106.
56. Hughes KS, Schnaper LA, Berry D, et al. Lumpectomy plus tamoxifen with or without irradiation in women 70 years of age or older with early breast cancer. N Engl J Med 2004;351:971–7.
57. Fyles AW, McCready DR, Manchul LA, et al. Tamoxifen with or without breast irradiation in women 50 years of age or older with early breast cancer. N Engl J Med 2004;351:963–70.
58. Offersen BV, Overgaard M, Kroman N, Overgaard J. Accelerated partial breast irradiation as part of breast conserving therapy of early breast carcinoma: a systematic review. Radiother Oncol 2009;90:1–13.
59. Dirbas FM. Accelerated partial breast irradiation: where do we stand? J Natl Compr Canc Netw 2009;7:215–25.
60. Buchanan CL, Dorn PL, Fey J, et al. Locoregional recurrence after mastectomy: incidence and outcomes. J Am Coll Surg 2006;203:469–74.
61. Nielsen HM, Overgaard M, Grau C, et al. Study of failure pattern among high-risk breast cancer patients with or without postmastectomy radiotherapy in addition to adjuvant systemic therapy: long-term results from the Danish Breast Cancer Cooperative Group DBCG 82 B and C randomized studies. J Clin Oncol 2006;24:2268–75.
62. Morrow M, Jagsi R, Alderman AK, et al. Surgeon recommendations and receipt of mastectomy for treatment of breast cancer. JAMA 2009;302:1551–6.
63. Opatt D, Morrow M, Hawley S, et al. Conflicts in [illegible] for breast cancer surgery. [illegible]
64. Collins ED, Moore CP, Clay KF, et al. Can women with early-stage breast cancer make an informed decision for mastectomy? J Clin Oncol 2009;27:519–25.
65. McLaughlin CC, Lillquist PP, Edge SB. Surveillance of prophylactic mastectomy: trends in use from 1995 through 2005. Cancer 2009;115:5404–12.
66. Quan ML, McCready D. The evolution of lymph node assessment in breast cancer. J Surg Oncol 2009;99:194–8.
67. Estourgie SH, Nieweg OE, Olmos RA, et al. Lymphatic drainage patterns from the breast. Ann Surg 2004;239:232–7.
68. Chen RC, Lin NU, Golshan M, et al. Internal mammary nodes in breast cancer: diagnosis and implications for patient management—a systematic review. J Clin Oncol 2008;26:4981–9.
69. Hayes SC, Janda M, Cornish B, et al. Lymphedema after breast cancer: incidence, risk factors, and effect on upper body function. J Clin Oncol 2008;26:3536–42.
70. Warren AG, Brorson H, Borud LJ, Slavin SA. Lymphedema: a comprehensive review. Ann Plast Surg 2007;59:464–72.
71. Tsai RJ, Dennis LK, Lynch CF, et al. The risk of developing arm lymphedema among breast cancer survivors: a meta-analysis of treatment factors. Ann Surg Oncol 2009;16:1959–72.
72. Hinrichs CS, Watroba NL, Rezaishiraz H, et al. Lymphedema secondary to postmastectomy radiation: incidence and risk factors. Ann Surg Oncol 2004;11:573–80.
73. Lyman GH, Giuliano AE, Somerfield MR, et al. American Society of Clinical Oncology guideline recommendations for sentinel lymph node biopsy in early-stage breast cancer. J Clin Oncol 2005;23:7703–20.
74. Kronowitz SJ, Kuerer HM. Advances and surgical decision-making for breast reconstruction. Cancer 2006;107:893–907.
75. Brachtel EF, Rusby JE, Michaelson JS, et al. Occult nipple involvement in breast cancer: clinicopathologic findings in 316 consecutive mastectomy specimens. J Clin Oncol 2009;27:4948–54.
76. Gerber B, Krause A, Dieterich M, et al. The oncological safety of skin sparing mastectomy with conservation of the nipple-areola complex and autologous reconstruction: an extended follow-up study. Ann Surg 2009;249:461–8.
77. Edge SB. Nipple-sparing mastectomy: how often is the nipple involved? J Clin Oncol 2009;27:4930–2.
78. Zelnak AB, O'Regan R. Adjuvant hormonal therapy for early-stage breast cancer. Cancer Treat Res 2008;141:63–78.
79. Ravdin P. Overview of randomized trials of systemic adjuvant therapy. Cancer Treat Res 2008;141:55–62.
80. McArthur HL, Hudis CA. Advances in adjuvant chemotherapy of early stage breast cancer. Cancer Treat Res 2008;141:37–53.
81. Bao T, Davidson NE. Gene expression profiling of breast cancer. Adv Surg 2008;42:249–60.
82. Marchionni L, Wilson RF, Wolff AC, et al. Systematic review: gene expression profiling assays in early-stage breast cancer. Ann Intern Med 2008;148:358–69.
83. Hudis CA. Trastuzumab—mechanism of action and use in clinical practice. N Engl J Med 2007;357:39–51.
84. Effects of chemotherapy and hormonal therapy for early breast cancer on recurrence and 15-year survival: an overview of the randomised trials. Lancet 2005;365:1687–717.
85. [illegible], Bajdik CD, Ravdin PM, et al. [illegible] validation of the prognostic model ADJUVANT! for early breast cancer. J Clin Oncol 2005;23:2716–25.
86. Mook S, Schmidt MK, Rutgers EJ, et al. Calibration and discriminatory accuracy of prognosis calculation for breast cancer with the online Adjuvant! program: a hospital-based retrospective cohort study. Lancet Oncol 2009;10:1070–6.
87. Chen LL, Nolan ME, Silverstein MJ, et al. The impact of primary tumor size, lymph node status, and other prognostic factors on the risk of cancer death. Cancer 2009;115:5071–83.
88. Kaufmann M, Hortobagyi GN, Goldhirsch A, et al. Recommendations from an international expert panel on the use of neoadjuvant (primary) systemic treatment of operable breast cancer: an update. J Clin Oncol 2006;24:1940–9.
89. Wolmark N, Wang J, Mamounas E, et al. Preoperative chemotherapy in patients with operable breast cancer: nine-year results from National Surgical Adjuvant Breast and Bowel Project B-18. J Natl Cancer Inst Monogr 2001:96–102.
90. Jeruss JS, Mittendorf EA, Tucker SL, et al. Combined use of clinical and pathologic staging variables to define outcomes for breast cancer patients treated with neoadjuvant therapy. J Clin Oncol 2008;26:246–52.
91. Symmans WF, Peintinger F, Hatzis C, et al. Measurement of residual breast cancer burden to predict survival after neoadjuvant chemotherapy. J Clin Oncol 2007;25:4414–22.
92. Wong ZW, Ellis MJ. Neoadjuvant endocrine therapy for breast cancer: an overlooked option? Oncology (Williston Park) 2004;18:411–20; discussion 21, 24, 29 passim.
93. Ma CX, Ellis MJ. Neoadjuvant endocrine therapy for locally advanced breast cancer. Semin Oncol 2006;33:650–6.
94. Bristol IJ, Woodward WA, Strom EA, et al. Locoregional treatment outcomes after multimodality management of inflammatory

breast cancer. Int J Radiat Oncol Biol Phys 2008;72:474–84.

95. Khan SA, Stewart AK, Morrow M. Does aggressive local therapy improve survival in metastatic breast cancer? Surgery 2002;132: 620–6; discussion 6–7.
96. Rapiti E, Verkooijen HM, Vlastos G, et al. Complete excision of primary breast tumor improves survival of patients with metastatic breast cancer at diagnosis. J Clin Oncol 2006;24:2743–9.
97. Hazard HW, Gorla SR, Scholtens D, et al. Surgical resection of the primary tumor, chest wall control, and survival in women with metastatic breast cancer. Cancer 2008; 113:2011–9.
98. Molckovsky A, Madarnas Y. Breast cancer in pregnancy: a literature review. Breast Cancer Res Treat 2008;108:333–8.
99. Spanheimer PM, Graham MM, Sugg SL, et al. Measurement of uterine radiation exposure from lymphoscintigraphy indicates safety of sentinel lymph node biopsy during pregnancy. Ann Surg Oncol 2009;16: 1143–7.
100. Giordano SH. A review of the diagnosis and management of male breast cancer. Oncologist 2005;10:471–9.
101. Pant K, Dutta U. Understanding and management of male breast cancer: a critical review. Med Oncol 2008;25:294–8.
102. Khatcheressian JL, Wolff AC, Smith TJ, et al. American Society of Clinical Oncology 2006 update of the breast cancer follow-up and management guidelines in the adjuvant setting. J Clin Oncol 2006;24:5091–7.
103. Ganz PA. Breast cancer, menopause, and long-term survivorship: critical issues for the 21st century. Am J Med 2005;118 Suppl 12B:136–41.
104. Ganz PA, Hahn EE. Implementing a survivorship care plan for patients with breast cancer. J Clin Oncol 2008;26:759–67.

2 SOFT TISSUE INFECTION

Mark A. Malangoni, MD, FACS, and Christopher R. McHenry, MD, FACS

Approach to the Patient with Soft Tissue Infection

Soft tissue infections are a diverse group of diseases that involve the skin and underlying subcutaneous tissue, fascia, or muscle. Such infections may be localized to a small area or may involve a large portion of the body. They may affect any part of the body, although the lower extremities, the perineum, and the abdominal wall are the most common sites of involvement. Some soft tissue infections are relatively harmless if treated promptly and adequately; others can be life-threatening even when appropriately treated. The symptoms and signs range from subtle or nonspecific indicators (e.g., pain, localized tenderness, and edema without fever) to obvious features (e.g., necrosis, blistering, and crepitus associated with systemic toxicity).

Soft tissue infections were first defined as such more than a century ago. In 1883, Fournier described a gangrenous infection of the scrotum that continues to be associated with his name.[1] In 1924, Meleney documented the pathogenic role of streptococci in soft tissue infection.[2] Shortly thereafter, Brewer and Meleney described progressive polymicrobial postoperative infection of the muscular fascia with necrosis[3] (although the term *necrotizing fasciitis* was not introduced until more than 25 years later[4]). The association between toxic-shock syndrome (TSS) and streptococcal soft tissue infection was delineated as this disease reemerged in the 1980s.[5]

Various classification systems and eponyms are used to describe specific forms of soft tissue infection [*see* Discussion, Etiology and Classification of Soft Tissue Infection, *below*]. In our view, however, it is more important to develop a common approach to the diagnosis and treatment of these conditions than to refine the minor details of classification. For therapeutic purposes, the primary consideration is to distinguish between necrotizing soft tissue infections and nonnecrotizing infections. Nonnecrotizing soft tissue infections involve one or both of the superficial layers of the skin (epidermis and dermis) and the subcutaneous tissue and usually respond to antibiotic therapy alone. Necrotizing soft tissue infections may involve not only the skin, the subcutaneous tissue, and the superficial fascia but also the deep fascia and muscle, and they must be treated with urgent surgical débridement. At times, it is difficult to distinguish between these two categories of infection, especially when obvious clinical signs of necrotizing soft tissue infection are absent.

In this chapter, we review the diagnosis and management of the main soft tissue infections seen by surgeons, including both superficial infections (e.g., pyoderma, animal and human bites, and cellulitis) and necrotizing infections involving superficial and deep tissues [*see Table 1*].

Clinical Evaluation

The diagnosis of soft tissue infection is usually made on the basis of the history and the physical examination. Patients typically seek medical attention because of pain, tenderness, and erythema of recent onset. They should be asked about environmental factors that may have disrupted the normal skin barrier [*see Table 2*], as well as about any host factors that may increase their susceptibility to infection and limit their ability to contain it. It is particularly important that they be questioned about specific clinical scenarios associated with unusual pathogens, such as an animal bite (associated with *Pasteurella multocida*), a human bite (*Eikenella corrodens*), chronic skin diseases (*Staphylococcus aureus*), saltwater exposure or ingestion of raw seafood (*Vibrio vulnificus*), and brackish or freshwater exposure (*Aeromonas hydrophila*).

Physical examination usually reveals erythema, tenderness, and induration. Vesicular lesions and honey-colored crusted plaques are seen in patients with impetigo. Intense, sharply demarcated erythema is characteristic of erysipelas.

Table 1 Common Soft Tissue Infections
Superficial infections
Pyoderma
Impetigo
Erysipelas
Folliculitis
Furuncles and carbuncles
Infections developing in damaged skin
Animal bites
Human bites
Cellulitis
Nonnecrotizing
Necrotizing
Deep necrotizing cutaneous infections
Necrotizing fasciitis
Myonecrosis
Gas gangrene
Metastatic gas gangrene

Table 2 Environmental Factors that Disrupt Skin and Alter Normal Barrier Function
Cuts, lacerations, or contusions
Injections from contaminated needles
Animal, human, or insect bites
Burns
Skin diseases (e.g., atopic dermatitis, tinea pedis, eczema, scabies, or varicella infection)
Decubitus, venous stasis, or ischemic ulcers
Contaminated surgical incisions

A tender, swollen, erythematous papule, often containing a visible hair shaft, is indicative of folliculitis. A single painful, tender, indurated, erythematous skin nodule suggests a furuncle, and the presence of multiple inflammatory nodules with sinus tracts is consistent with a carbuncle. Cellulitis in association with a decubitus ulcer or an ischemic leg ulcer frequently signals a polymicrobial infection with gram-negative organisms. An erythematous linear streak, characteristic of lymphangitis, usually indicates a superficial infection secondary to *Streptococcus pyogenes*; associated lymphadenopathy may be present as well.

Patients with necrotizing soft tissue infections often complain of severe pain that is out of proportion to their physical findings. Compared with patients who have nonnecrotizing infections, they are more likely to have fever, bullae, or blebs [*see Figure 1*]; signs of systemic toxicity; hyponatremia; and leukocytosis with a shift in immature forms. Physical findings characteristic of a necrotizing infection include tenderness beyond the area of erythema, crepitus, cutaneous anesthesia, and cellulitis that is refractory to antibiotic therapy.[6] Tenderness beyond the borders of the erythematous area is an especially important clinical clue that develops as the infection in the deeper cutaneous layers undermines the skin. Early in the course of a necrotizing soft tissue infection, skin changes may be minimal despite extensive necrosis of the deeper cutaneous layers. Bullae, blebs, cutaneous anesthesia, and skin necrosis occur as a result of thrombosis of the nutrient vessels and destruction of the cutaneous nerves of the skin, which typically occur late in the course of infection.

Clinicians should be mindful of certain diagnostic barriers that may delay recognition and treatment of necrotizing soft tissue infections.[7] In particular, these infections have a variable clinical presentation. Although most patients present with an acute, rapidly progressive illness and signs of systemic toxicity, a subset of patients may present with a more indolent, slowly progressive infection. Patients with postoperative necrotizing infections often have a more indolent course. Moreover, in the early stages, underlying necrosis may be masked by normal-appearing overlying skin. As many as 20% of necrotizing soft tissue infections are primary (idiopathic) and occur in previously healthy patients who have no predisposing factors and no known portal of entry for bacterial inoculation. Finally, crepitus is noted in only 30% of patients with necrotizing soft tissue infections. Overall, fewer than 40% of patients exhibit the classic symptoms and signs described.[7,8] Accordingly, it is imperative to maintain a high index of suspicion for this disease in the appropriate setting.

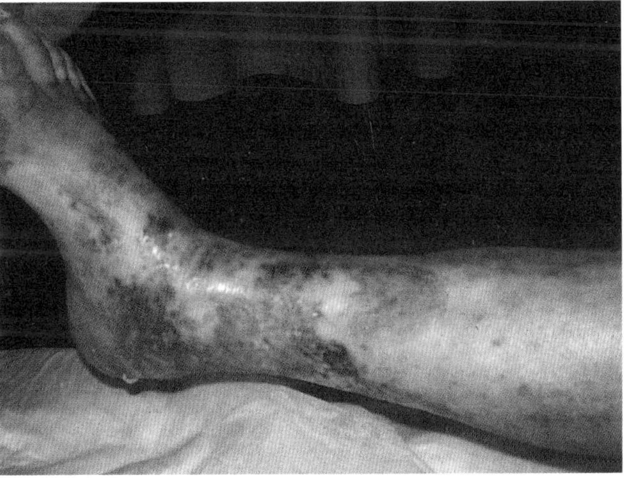

Figure 1 **Lower extremity necrotizing fasciitis is characterized by bullae, blebs, and discolored skin.**

Investigative Studies

Diagnostic studies have a low yield in patients with superficial soft tissue infections. They are rarely necessary and are used only in specific clinical circumstances. Either needle aspiration at the advancing edge of erythema with Gram staining and culture or full-thickness skin biopsy and culture may be helpful when cellulitis is refractory to antibiotic therapy or when an unusual causative organism is suspected. Because of their low yield, blood cultures are obtained only in patients with signs of systemic toxicity, those with buccal or periorbital cellulitis, and those with infection suspected of being secondary to saltwater or freshwater exposure; these clinical situations are associated with a higher likelihood of a positive culture.

When the characteristic clinical features of necrotizing soft tissue infection are absent, diagnosis may be difficult. In this setting, laboratory and imaging studies become important [*see Figure 2*]. In one study, logistic regression analysis showed that an elevated white blood cell (WBC) count (≥ 15,400/µL) and hyponatremia (serum sodium level lower than 135 mmol/L) at the time of hospital admission were highly sensitive for the presence of a necrotizing soft tissue infection; however, the positive predictive value of these findings was only 26%.[9] The absence of these findings in a patient without obvious clinical signs of a necrotizing soft tissue infection had a negative predictive value of 99%. In a prospective observational study, a WBC greater than 15,400/µL and a serum sodium level less than 135 mEq/L were shown to significantly increase the likelihood of a necrotizing soft tissue infection and may aid in more rapid diagnosis in patients without hard clinical signs.[10] A normal serum creatine kinase (CK) level rules out muscle necrosis.

In a 2004 report, one group of investigators described the development and application of the Laboratory Risk Indicator for NECrotizing fasciitis (LRINEC) score.[11] This scoring system assigns points for abnormalities in six independent variables: serum C-reactive protein level (> 150 mg/L), WBC count (> 15,000/µL), hemoglobin level (< 13.5 g/dL), serum sodium level (< 135 mmol/L), serum creatinine level (> 1.6 mg/dL), and serum glucose level (> 180 mg/dL). With a score of 8 or higher, there is a 75% risk of a necrotizing soft tissue infection. The authors of the report recommended that the LRINEC score be used to determine which patients require further diagnostic testing, given that the negative predictive value of this screening tool was 96%. However, this has not been validated in larger prospective studies.

Radiographic studies may be necessary to establish a diagnosis of necrotizing soft tissue infection. A plain x-ray of

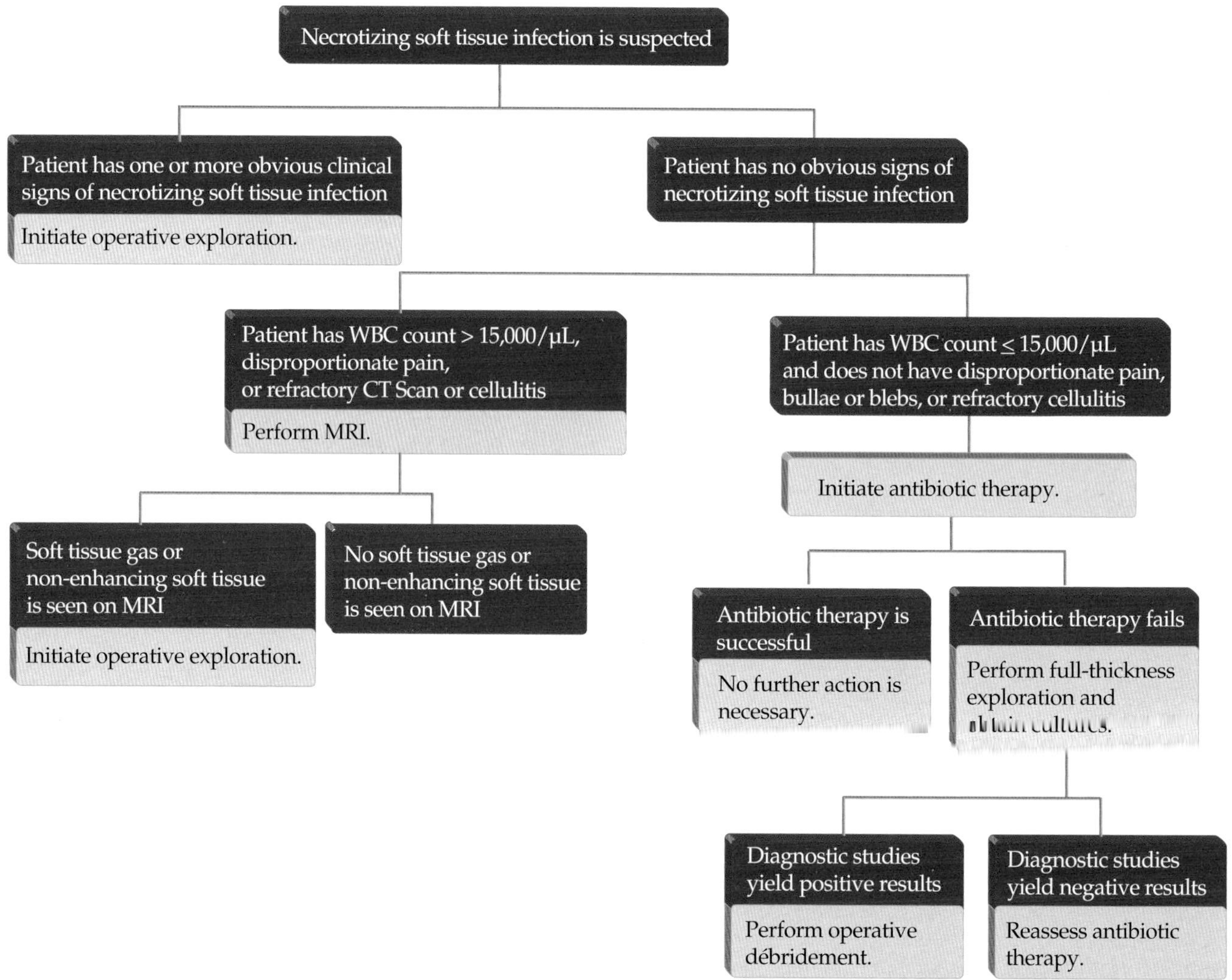

Figure 2 **Algorithm outlining diagnostic evaluation of patients with soft tissue infection.[6] MRI = magnetic resonance imaging; WBC = white blood cell.**

the involved area may demonstrate soft tissue gas but in only 15 to 30% of patients with necrotizing infections [*see Figure 3*].[6] Computed tomography (CT) and magnetic resonance imaging (MRI) are more sensitive in identifying soft tissue gas. The absence of subcutaneous gas does not absolutely rule out a necrotizing soft tissue infection.

MRI can be helpful for documenting deep necrotizing infections [*see Figure 4*]. The presence of soft tissue gas on MRI is diagnostic of a necrotizing soft tissue infection. T_2-weighted images demonstrate thickening and increased signal intensity of the deep fascial planes.[12,13] Increased signal intensity in the subcutaneous tissue and edema of the adjacent muscle are also frequently present. High signal intensity on T_2-weighted images and tissue enhancement after gadolinium administration are indicative of inflamed tissue and may also occur with certain nonnecrotizing soft tissue conditions (e.g., exertional muscle injury, lymphedema, dermatomyositis, polymyositis, eosinophilic fasciitis, and neoplastic disease).[13–17] Low or absent signal intensity on gadolinium-enhanced T_1-weighted images is indicative of necrosis, a finding that is more specific for a necrotizing soft tissue infection.[18–20] The reported sensitivity of MRI for diagnosis of necrotizing soft tissue infection ranges from 89 to 100%, and its specificity ranges from 46 to 86%.[18,20]

MRI is not always immediately available in many institutions and still has a low specificity, overestimating the extent of deep fascial involvement. Advances in CT technology have resulted in improvement in the diagnosis and the exclusion of necrotizing soft tissue infection. It is also more readily available and expeditious. Zacharias and colleagues, using new-generation 16- or 64-section helical scanners, reported a sensitivity for diagnosis of necrotizing soft tissue infection of 100%, a specificity of 81%, a positive predictive value of 76%, and a negative predictive value of 100%.[21] Asymmetrical and diffuse areas of soft tissue inflammation and ischemia, muscle necrosis, and soft tissue gas and fluid collections were the imaging features associated with a necrotizing soft tissue infection. However, only the presence of nonenhancing tissue and gas traversing tissue planes was diagnostic of a necrotizing soft tissue infection.[21] Davis

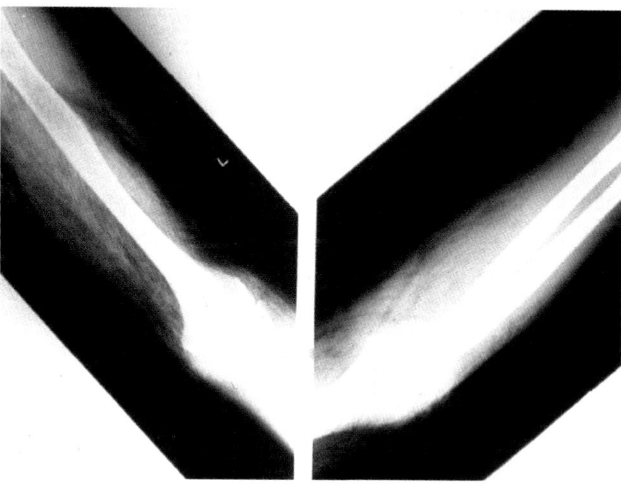

Figure 3 **Upper extremity x-ray of a patient with necrotizing soft tissue infection demonstrating soft tissue gas outlining the muscles.**

pointed out that CT is less likely to identify necrotizing infections involving the skin and subcutaneous tissue because they are less vascular and less likely to contain gas, emphasizing that CT should continue to be used judiciously as an adjunct to clinical judgment.[22]

The finding of nonenhancing soft tissue and soft tissue gas on diagnostic imaging warrants immediate operative exploration and débridement. Because of the high sensitivity of CT and MRI, necrotizing infection is unlikely when there is no involvement of the superficial fascia, subcutaneous tissue, or deeper cutaneous layers. However, the inflammatory changes seen on CT and MRI when necrotizing soft tissue infection is present may also be seen in patients with nonnecrotizing infections, as well as in those with other inflammatory conditions affecting the deep soft tissues. Because of the relatively low specificity of imaging studies, operative exploration and direct tissue examination may be needed to diagnose or rule out soft tissue infection [*see Figure* 2]. This procedure may be performed at the bedside with local anesthesia. The observation of necrotic or infected tissue through the biopsy incision indicates that immediate débridement is needed.

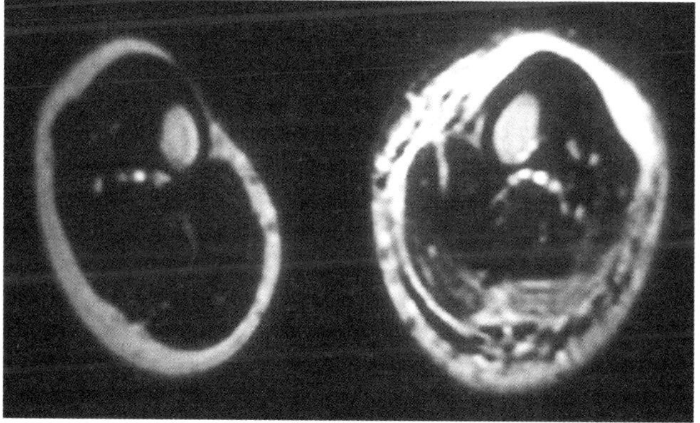

Figure 4 **Lower extremity magnetic resonance image of a patient with necrotizing fasciitis of the left leg demonstrating inflammatory changes typical of necrosis.**

General Management of Nonnecrotizing and Necrotizing Soft Tissue Infection

NONNECROTIZING INFECTION

Antibiotic therapy is the cornerstone of treatment for patients with nonnecrotizing infections. Such patients usually require antibiotics that are effective against group A streptococci or *S. aureus*. The prevalence of community-acquired methicillin-resistant *Staphylococcus aureus* (MRSA) strains has increased significantly. These strains now outnumber methicillin-sensitive strains by a 2 to 1 margin.[23] This development has necessitated a change in the empirical treatment of these infections. Topical, oral, or intravenous (IV) preparations may be employed, depending on the nature and severity of the disease process [*see* Management of Specific Soft Tissue Infections, *below*]. If polymicrobial infection is suspected, broad-spectrum antimicrobial agents should be given, either alone or in combination.

NECROTIZING INFECTION

Management of necrotizing soft tissue infections is predicated on early recognition of symptoms and signs and on emergency operative débridement. Once the diagnosis of necrotizing soft tissue infection is established, patient survival and soft tissue preservation are best achieved by means of prompt operation; precise identification of the causative bacteria and correct assignment of the patient to a specific clinical syndrome are unnecessary. The delay between hospital admission and initial débridement is the most critical factor influencing morbidity and mortality: a number of reports have demonstrated a strong correlation between survival and the interval between onset of symptoms and initial operation.[8,24–26]

The key components of the initial treatment of necrotizing soft tissue infection are (1) resuscitation and correction of fluid and electrolyte disorders, (2) physiologic support of failing organ systems, (3) broad-spectrum antimicrobial therapy, (4) urgent and thorough débridement of necrotic tissue, and (5) supportive care [*see Figure* 5].

Initial Resuscitation and Correction of Fluid and Electrolyte Disorders

Patients with necrotizing soft tissue infections frequently present with tachycardia and hypotension, reflecting depleted intravascular volume and sepsis syndrome. These patients often exhibit extensive extracellular fluid sequestration within the affected area, as well as more generalized sequestration resulting from sepsis. A balanced isotonic electrolyte solution, such as lactated Ringer solution (or 0.9% normal saline, for patients with renal dysfunction), is administered to replace these fluid deficits. The adequacy of intravascular volume repletion is usually assessed by monitoring vital signs and urinary output; however, it sometimes proves necessary to use a central venous catheter to

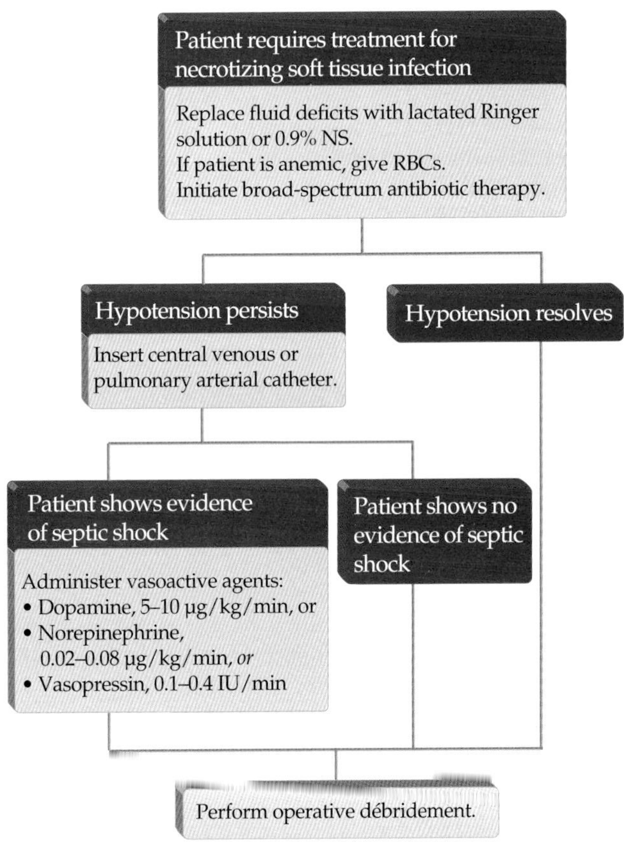

Figure 5 **Algorithm outlining the treatment of necrotizing soft tissue infection. NS = normal saline; RBC = red blood cell.**

monitor central venous or pulmonary arterial pressure in patients with associated myocardial dysfunction, septic shock, chronic pulmonary disease, renal insufficiency, or other severe chronic illnesses.

Mild hyponatremia, commonly seen with necrotizing soft tissues infections, is usually corrected by infusing isotonic fluids. Hypocalcemia, which can result from calcium precipitation in patients with extensive fat necrosis, is usually corrected by administering IV calcium gluconate. Because hypoalbuminemia is also common in these patients, it is important to measure ionized calcium to guide replacement therapy. Hyperglycemia is corrected with insulin, given either via subcutaneous injection or, for patients with more severe abnormalities, via IV infusion. Lactic acidosis generally responds to fluid administration. Renal function is assessed by measuring blood urea nitrogen (BUN) and serum creatinine concentrations. CK levels should be monitored and a qualitative evaluation of urine myoglobin done if muscle necrosis is suspected or renal failure is present. Myoglobinuria and elevated CK levels are suggestive of myonecrosis and should be treated aggressively. Anemia is treated with packed red blood cell transfusions.

Physiologic Support

Patients whose hypotension does not resolve with appropriate intravascular fluid resuscitation often experience septic shock. In these circumstances, low dosages of IV norepinephrine (0.02 to 0.08 μg/kg/min), vasopressin (0.1 to 0.4 IU/min), or dopamine (5 to 10 μg/kg/min) are useful for raising blood pressure, improving myocardial function, and increasing organ and tissue perfusion.

Patients with traumatic wounds or other contaminated sites should receive tetanus toxoid or human tetanus immunoglobulin, depending on their immunization status.

Broad-Spectrum Antimicrobial Therapy

IV antimicrobial therapy is indicated in all patients with necrotizing soft tissue infections [*see Table 3*]. Such therapy is important but is not a substitute for prompt and adequate operative débridement as antibiotics do not penetrate necrotic tissues. Necrotizing soft tissue infections are most often caused by a mixed polymicrobial bacterial flora [*see Table 4*]. Approximately 15 to 20% of necrotizing soft tissue infections is monomicrobial. Although *S. pyogenes* is the bacterium most frequently involved in monomicrobial infections, the microbiology of these infections often cannot be accurately predicted before final identification of organisms on culture. Thus, the empirical antibiotic regimen chosen should be effective against a diverse group of potential pathogens.[26] The proliferation of MRSA strains in the community and health care environments mandates the use of an agent effective against these organisms.[23] Doxycycline or a similar tetracycline should be added whenever *Vibrio* or *Aeromonas* species are suspected.[23]

In addition, because these patients have a high incidence of associated nosocomial infections and even of metastatic infections, it is important to ensure that the dosage is high enough to achieve adequate serum concentrations.[8,23] Once the results of intraoperative culture and antimicrobial sensitivity testing become available, antibiotic therapy is adjusted

Table 3 Intravenous Antibiotic Regimens and Dosages for Adults with Necrotizing Soft Tissue Infection and Normal Renal Function

Piperacillin-tazobactam 3.375 g q. 6 hr *plus*
Clindamycin 600–900 mg q. 6–8 hr *plus*
Ciprofloxacin 400 mg q. 12 hr
Imipenem-cilastatin 500–1,000 mg q. 6 hr
Meropenem 1 g q. 8 hr
For patients allergic to penicillins, use
Linezolid 600 mg q. 12 hr *or*
Vancomycin 30 mg/kg/day in two divided doses *or*
Daptomycin 4 mg/kg q. 24 hr in divided doses *or*
Quinupristin-dalfopristin 7.5 mg/kg q. 12 hr
For infections in which only staphylococci, streptococci, or clostridial species are isolated
Clindamycin 600–900 mg q. 6–8 hr *plus*
Penicillin 2–4 million units q. 4–6 hr
For patients allergic to penicillins, use linezolid 600 mg q. 12 hr *or*
Vancomycin 30 mg/kg/day in two divided doses *or*
Daptomycin 4 mg/kg q. 24 hr in divided doses *or*
Quinupristin-dalfopristin 7.5 mg/kg q. 12 hr
For infections in which *Vibrio* or *Aeromonas* species are isolated or suspected, add
Doxycycline 100 mg q. 12 hr

Table 4 Organisms Commonly Causing Necrotizing Soft Tissue Infection

Organisms
Aerobes
Gram positive
Group A *Streptococcus*
Enterococcus species
Staphylococcus aureus
Bacillus species
Gram negative
Escherichia coli
Pseudomonas aeruginosa
Enterobacter cloacae
Klebsiella species
Serratia species
Acinetobacter calcoaceticus
Vibrio vulnificus
Anaerobes
Bacteroides species
Clostridium species
Peptostreptococcus species
Fusobacterium species

accordingly. This adjustment can be challenging in that all of the pathogens identified must be treated.

IV antimicrobial therapy is continued until operative débridement is complete, there is no further evidence of infection in the involved tissues, and all signs of systemic toxicity have resolved. Topical antiseptic agents (e.g., Dakin solution and Burow solution) may help control local infection that progresses despite adequate débridement and IV antibiotics. Topical application of mycostatin powder may help control progressive fungal infection. When patients are able to resume oral intake, they can often be switched from IV to oral antimicrobial therapy. Antimicrobial therapy should not, however, be prolonged merely because oral agents are available.

Operative Treatment

The most critical factors for reducing mortality from necrotizing soft tissue infections are early recognition and urgent operative débridement.[8,22,24,27] The extent of débridement depends on intraoperative findings and cannot be accurately predicted before operation; this fact should be communicated to patients. Operative intervention helps limit tissue damage by removing necrotic tissue, which serves as a nidus for infection.

Thorough exploration is necessary to confirm the diagnosis of necrotizing soft tissue infection and determine the degree of involvement. Aggressive, widespread débridement of all apparent necrotic, infected tissue is essential; antibiotics will not penetrate dead tissues. The underlying necrosis of subcutaneous tissues, fascia, and muscle typically extends beyond the obvious limits of cutaneous involvement. Operative débridement should therefore be continued until viable tissue is reached. In most instances, the involved tissues are easily separated from their surrounding structures. The presence of "dishwater pus" and noncontracting muscle are additional indicators of necrotizing infection. The presence of arterial bleeding generally indicates that tissues are viable; in the absence of arterial bleeding, tissues are nonviable even if venous bleeding is present. With deep necrotizing infections, débridement of the necrotic fascia and muscle may create large skin flaps that are poorly perfused. It is best to preserve as much viable skin and subcutaneous tissue as possible because these tissues can be essential for later coverage of the wound. Nonviable skin, however, should be resected.

Wound drainage or exudate should be submitted for Gram staining, as well as for aerobic, anaerobic, and fungal cultures and antimicrobial sensitivity testing. Fasciotomy is rarely required. The presence of subcutaneous gas extending beyond areas of nonviable tissue does not necessitate débridement if the surrounding tissues are viable. It is sometimes helpful to perform an exploratory incision over an area beyond the limits of débridement when it is uncertain whether necrosis is undermining viable skin. If no necrotizing infection is found, the incision may be closed primarily.

Reexploration should be routinely performed within 24 to 48 hours to ensure that all necrotic tissue has been débrided. Débridement is repeated as necessary until the infection is controlled. After débridement, the exposed areas should be covered with 0.9% normal saline wet-to-dry dressings. Once the initial infection has been controlled and débridement is no longer necessary, dressing changes can often be performed at the bedside after sufficient analgesics have been given to achieve adequate pain management. Patient-controlled analgesia is frequently useful early in the course of treatment. Propofol or ketamine can be given in the intensive care unit to facilitate pain control during dressing changes. Vacuum-assisted closure devices can be applied to the affected area once the infection is controlled. These devices can reduce the exposed surface area and lessen the need for skin graft coverage. If repeated débridement does not control infection, if there are persistent, fulminant infections of the extremities, or if an extremity remains nonfunctional after débridement has been completed, amputation can be lifesaving. Lower extremity amputation is most often required for patients with clostridial myonecrosis and for diabetic patients with necrotizing infections.[27] In two large series of patients with necrotizing soft tissue infections, the incidence of amputation was approximately 15 to 26%.[8,24]

Patients with necrotizing soft tissue infections involving the perineum and perirectal area may need a diverting colostomy to prevent tissue contamination resulting from fecal incontinence and to control local infection. Overall, this measure is required in fewer than 25% of cases.[8] Orchiectomy is rarely needed for necrotizing soft tissue infections involving the scrotum as the blood supply to the testicles is usually maintained.[1]

Supportive Care

Early nutritional support should be instituted to optimize recovery. Enteral nutritional support should begin once resuscitation is complete, the infection is adequately controlled, the signs of sepsis have resolved, and gastrointestinal function is restored. Because it frequently proves necessary to return the patient to the operating room, enteral feeding tubes should be placed beyond the pylorus so that enteral nutrition can be provided with minimal interruption. Alternatively, parenteral nutrition may be employed. Regardless of the type of nutritional support, appropriate supplementation of essential vitamins and minerals promotes wound healing.

Hyperbaric oxygen has been advocated as adjunctive therapy for extensive necrotizing infections, particularly those caused by clostridia.[28] Hyperbaric oxygen improves oxygen tension in perfused tissues, and its beneficial properties include inhibition of bacterial exotoxin production [*see* Discussion, Pathogenesis of Soft Tissue Infections, *below*], improved leukocyte function, and attainment of tissue oxygen levels that are bactericidal for *Clostridium perfringens* and bacteriostatic for other anaerobic bacteria. Hyperbaric oxygen does not, however, neutralize exotoxin that has already been released.[28] There is little evidence supporting the benefits of hyperbaric oxygen therapy for the treatment of necrotizing soft tissue infections, and most prospective studies fail to demonstrate any benefit from its use. Such therapy has not been demonstrated to improve survival or to bring about earlier resolution of infection and has been associated with barotrauma, pneumothorax, and oxygen toxicity.[29,30] Importantly, operative débridement should not be delayed to accommodate hyperbaric oxygen therapy, and such therapy should not be considered a substitute for complete débridement of infected nonviable tissues.

Intravenous immunoglobulin therapy has been advocated for necrotizing soft tissue infections due to streptococci and staphylococci. Intravenous immunoglobulin provides antibodies that can neutralize circulating exotoxins produced by these organisms and may modulate the systemic inflammatory response induced by cytokine stimulation. The evidence supporting use of intravenous immunoglobulin in this situation remains controversial.[31] If used, it should be given selectively to patients with severe sepsis due to known staphylococcal or streptococcal infections.

Once the localized infection is under control and the patient is recovering, the exposed soft tissues should be covered to minimize insensible fluid loss and to reduce pain. This is most commonly done with split-thickness skin grafting, although other reconstructive procedures (e.g., rotational flaps) can be effective in this setting as well. Exposed tendons, nerves, or bone often should be covered with full-thickness skin to prevent desiccation and preserve limb function. Premature closure of highly contaminated or persistently infected sites usually fails and leads to recurrence of infection and a greater likelihood of death.

When the abdominal or chest wall has been excised to control infection, reconstruction is necessary. Prosthetic mesh is useful for restoring continuity of the abdomen or the chest wall, and overlying moist dressings can help prevent desiccation of underlying viscera. Some have advocated using biologic materials or absorbable mesh for restoration of abdominal wall continuity; however, we prefer to use permanent mesh in most circumstances, especially when omentum is available for interposition between the mesh and the small intestine.[8]

Management of Specific Soft Tissue Infections

Normal skin functions as a protective barrier that prevents microorganisms from causing soft tissue infection. The skin is made up of two layers, the epidermis and the dermis [*see Figure 6*]. The epidermis, the outer avascular epithelial layer, functions as a permeability barrier for the rest of the body. The dermis, the inner layer, contains blood vessels, lymphatic vessels, sweat and sebaceous glands, and hair follicles. The subcutaneous tissue separates the skin from the deep fascia, muscle, and bone. Typically, soft tissue infections result from disruption of the skin by some exogenous factor; less commonly, they result from extension of a subjacent infection or hematogenous spread from a distant site of infection.

SUPERFICIAL INFECTIONS

Superficial infections constitute the majority of soft tissue infections. They primarily involve the epidermis or dermis (pyoderma) or the subcutaneous tissue (cellulitis) and secondarily occur in skin damaged by animal or human bites. Nonnecrotizing superficial soft tissue infections are principally treated with antibiotics. Necrosis is rare but may develop in superficial infections that are inadequately treated or neglected.

Pyoderma

Pyoderma is a general term referring to a bacterial infection of the skin. It may be divided into several subcategories, including impetigo, erysipelas, folliculitis, and furuncles and carbuncles.

Impetigo Impetigo is a highly contagious bacterial infection that is confined to the epidermis and that usually involves the face or the extremities. It is most common in infants and preschool children and is seen more frequently

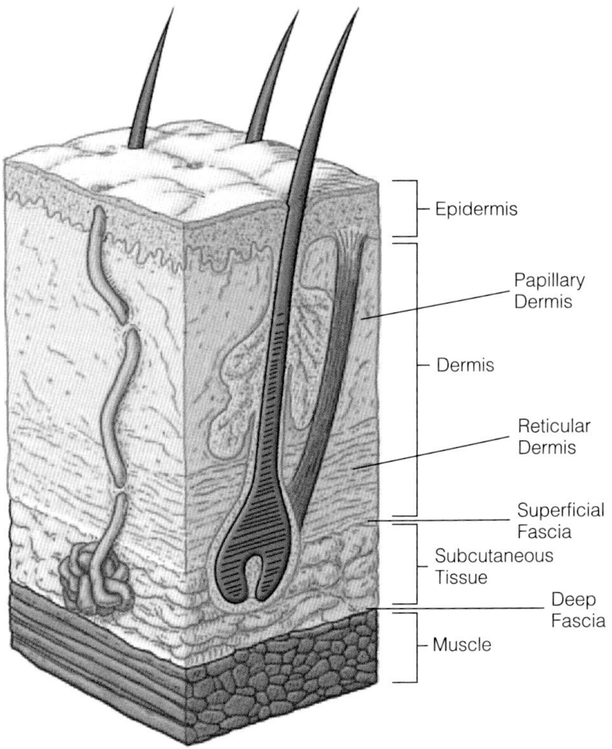

Figure 6 **The normal anatomy of the skin and the deeper cutaneous layers.**[6]

in patients with preexisting skin conditions (e.g., eczema, atopic dermatitis, varicella infection, angular cheilitis, and scabies). Warm and humid weather, crowded living conditions, and poor hygiene can all contribute to the development of impetigo.[32] The dominant pathogen is *S. aureus*, which causes either a bullous or a nonbullous form of the disease; a less common pathogen is *S. pyogenes*, which causes a nonbullous form.[33]

Impetigo usually occurs in areas of skin breakdown, although *S. aureus* may give rise to de novo infection in normal skin. Bullous impetigo is manifested by numerous blisters or bullae that rapidly become pustules and then rupture within 1 to 2 days to form a thick, honey-colored, crusted plaque that remains for days to weeks. Nonbullous impetigo is characterized by erythema and tiny, less prominent vesicles that progress to crusted erosions in the skin. The skin lesions are intensely pruritic, and local spread may occur as a result of scratching and release of infected fluid from the blisters, bullae, or vesicles. Associated regional lymphadenopathy is common. Glomerulonephritis may complicate streptococcal-induced impetigo.[33,34]

The diagnosis is established by Gram stain and culture of the vesicular fluid or the crusted plaque. The skin lesions usually resolve spontaneously within 2 to 3 weeks.[34] Antibiotic therapy accelerates the resolution of these lesions. Mupirocin ointment (2%) is applied topically three times a day until the lesions clear. This agent possesses excellent in vitro activity against both staphylococci and streptococci and achieves high rates of cure in patients with localized disease. Erythromycin and clindamycin ointments are acceptable alternatives [*see Table 5*]. For patients who have disseminated impetigo or impetigo of the scalp or mouth and those in whom topical therapy fails, an oral antibiotic (e.g., dicloxacillin, cephalexin, cefadroxil, erythromycin, or clindamycin) may be used [*see Table 5*]. A 7-day course of oral antibiotic therapy is usually sufficient.[34]

Table 5 Topical and Oral Antibiotic Agents Used for Superficial Soft Tissue Infections*

Mupirocin ointment (2%), applied to affected area t.i.d.†
Erythromycin ointment (2%), applied to affected area b.i.d.†
Clindamycin gel or lotion (1%), applied to affected area b.i.d.†
Gentamicin cream or ointment (0.1%), applied to affected area t.i.d. or q.i.d.
Penicillin V, 250–500 mg q.i.d. (pediatric: 25–50 mg/kg in divided doses q.i.d.)
Amoxicillin, 250–500 mg t.i.d. (pediatric: 20–30 mg/kg/day p.o. in divided doses t.i.d.)
Dicloxacillin, 250–500 mg q.i.d. (pediatric: 12.5–25.0 mg/kg/day in divided doses q.i.d.)
Cephalexin, 250–500 mg q.i.d. (pediatric: 25–100 mg/kg/day in divided doses q.i.d.)
Cefadroxil, 500–1,000 mg b.i.d. (pediatric: 30 mg/kg/day in divided doses b.i.d.)
Erythromycin, 250–500 mg q. 6 hr (pediatric: erythromycin ethyl succinate, 40 mg/kg in divided doses q.i.d.)
Clindamycin, 150–450 mg q.i.d. (pediatric: 20 mg/kg/day in divided doses t.i.d. or q.i.d.)
Trimethoprim-sulfamethoxazole, 160/800 mg b.i.d.
Amoxicillin-clavulanate, 500 mg t.i.d. (pediatric: 40 mg/kg/day in divided doses t.i.d.)
Ciprofloxacin, 500 mg p.o., b.i.d.

*All dosages are for patients with normal renal function.
†Adult dosage and pediatric dosage are the same.

Erysipelas Erysipelas is an acute bacterial infection that principally involves the dermis. It is almost invariably caused by *S. pyogenes*. Most cases are preceded by influenza-like symptoms. Infection extends through the dermal lymphatic vessels and is typically manifested by a tender, pruritic, intensely erythematous, sharply demarcated, and raised plaque. Patients complain of pain, often in conjunction with high fever, increased skin warmth, and leukocytosis. Lymphangitis and lymphadenopathy are sometimes present as well. The leg is the most common site of involvement, but erysipelas may also occur on the face, the arms, and the upper thighs.

The factors predisposing to the development of erysipelas of the extremity include local conditions such as tinea pedis (athlete's foot), leg ulcers, and venous stasis dermatitis.[35] Erysipelas tends to be more common in the presence of associated conditions such as lymphedema, diabetes mellitus, alcoholism, immunocompromise, and obesity[33,35] and is more likely to recur in patients with these associated diseases and in those whose underlying skin conditions are inadequately treated. Erysipelas recurs in 10% of patients within 6 months of their first episode and in 30% within 3 years.[35]

The standard antibiotic treatment for uncomplicated erysipelas is penicillin, which is effective in at least 80% of cases. Oral and intravenous antibiotic regimens are equally efficacious. Amoxicillin appears to work as well as penicillin. Patients with erysipelas of the lower extremity should be placed on bed rest, and the involved leg should be elevated to reduce edema and pain. Once the patient is able to resume normal activities, he or she should be fitted with elastic stockings, which help reduce the occurrence of edema and lower the risk of lymphedema. For patients with tinea pedis, a topical antifungal agent is used to treat the infection and prevent recurrence.

Folliculitis Folliculitis is an infection of the hair follicle that is typically caused by *S. aureus*. It is characterized by a painful, tender, erythematous papule with a central pustule. A shaft of hair is often seen in the center of the pustule. Shaving, plucking, waxing, heat and humidity, the use of corticosteroids or antibiotics, immunosuppression, and occlusion of the skin by clothing, adhesives, or plastics may predispose to folliculitis.[32] Single or multiple lesions may occur in the skin of any hair-bearing area. If the pustule ruptures, superficial erosion often ensues. Infection that principally involves the deeper part of the hair follicle is characterized by a tender, swollen papule without an associated pustule at the skin surface.

In rare cases, folliculitis is caused by pathogens other than *S. aureus*, such as *Pseudomonas aeruginosa*, *Klebsiella* species, *Enterobacter* species, *Proteus* species, yeasts, and fungi. *Pseudomonas* folliculitis usually results from exposure to inadequately chlorinated water in swimming pools, hot tubs, or whirlpools. Patients with this infection have multiple papular or pustular lesions on the back, the buttocks, and the extremities, along with fever and malaise appearing 6 hours to 3 days after exposure.[34,36] Organisms may be cultured either from the pustules or from the infected water. *Klebsiella*, *Enterobacter*, and *Proteus* species can cause folliculitis in patients receiving long-term antibiotic therapy for acne vulgaris.[33] Yeast folliculitis and fungal folliculitis tend to occur in immunocompromised patients.[33]

In most patients, folliculitis resolves spontaneously within 7 to 10 days.[34] Topical therapy with clindamycin, erythromycin, or mupirocin ointments or benzoyl peroxide in combination with warm soaks may accelerate resolution [*see Table 5*]. Isotretinoin can be used to treat gram-negative folliculitis. Gentamicin cream may be helpful in drying out the pustular lesions in patients with *Pseudomonas* folliculitis.

In patients with refractory or disseminated follicular infections, oral antibiotic therapy is indicated. When *S. aureus* is considered the most likely pathogen, trimethoprim-sulfamethoxazole, a tetracycline, or clindamycin should be given, in view of the high prevalence of MRSA[24,37]; an oral quinolone is indicated for the treatment of gram-negative folliculitis [*see Table 5*]. Elimination of predisposing factors is important for reducing the likelihood of recurrence.

Furuncles and carbuncles Furuncles and carbuncles are deeper infections of the hair follicle that extend beyond the follicle to involve the subcutaneous tissue. For both, *S. aureus* is the usual causative organism.

A furuncle, or boil, is a small abscess, manifested as a firm, tender, erythematous nodule that tends to occur in skin areas exposed to friction (e.g., the inner thighs and the axilla). Furuncles also may occur on the face, the neck, the upper back, and the buttocks. Possible predisposing factors include increased friction and perspiration (as seen in obese individuals or athletes), corticosteroid use, diabetes mellitus, and inherited or acquired defects in neutrophil function.[33,34]

Initial treatment consists of applying warm compresses to help promote drainage and administering an oral antimicrobial agent that is effective against *S. aureus* (e.g., dicloxacillin, cephalexin, cefadroxil, erythromycin, or clindamycin for infections presumed to be caused by methicillin-sensitive strains; trimethoprim-sulfamethoxazole, a tetracycline, or clindamycin for suspected MRSA infections) [*see Table 5*]. With time, the furuncle becomes fluctuant, and the pus coalesces at the skin surface. An incision-and-drainage procedure is necessary when these lesions do not drain spontaneously. This procedure should be performed with local anesthesia, and care should be taken to open the abscess cavity completely. Lesions that have drained spontaneously should be examined to confirm that the cavity has been opened sufficiently. Failure to drain these lesions adequately may result in recurrence, as well as in progression to a more serious infection.

A carbuncle is a deep cutaneous infection involving multiple hair follicles that is characterized by destruction of fibrous tissue septa and consequent formation of a series of interconnected abscesses. It is typically manifested by a painful, red, tender, indurated area of skin with multiple sinus tracts. Systemic manifestations (e.g., fever and malaise) are common. Carbuncles occur most frequently on the nape of the neck, the upper part of the back, or the posterior thigh. The thickness of the overlying skin in these areas leads to lateral extension of the infection and loculation. Patients commonly present with relatively large skin lesions that represent a confluence of inflammatory nodules. These lesions are associated with chronic drainage, sinus tracts, and scarring.

An incision-and-drainage procedure is recommended when a fluctuant carbuncle is present. A thorough search for loculated areas should be undertaken to facilitate drainage of deeper accumulations of pus and to ensure adequate treatment. Wide local excision of the involved skin and subcutaneous fat is often necessary to prevent recurrent disease. An oral antistaphylococcal agent should be given. All patients with hair follicle infections should cleanse the site with chlorhexidine or an iodine-containing solution.

Infections Developing in Damaged Skin

Damage to skin as a result of animal or human bites predisposes patients to soft tissue infection. An estimated 50% of all Americans will be bitten by an animal or by another human being during their lifetime.[38] Animal and human bites account for approximately 1% of all emergency department visits.[38] Soft tissue infection is the most common complication of such bites. The risk of infection depends on the type of bite, the site of injury, the time elapsed from the bite until presentation, host factors, and the management of the wound [*see Table 6*].

Most animal and human bites produce minor injuries for which patients do not seek medical attention. The overall risk of infection after a bite is estimated to be 5 to 15%[39]; however, among the subset of patients who seek medical attention, estimated infection rates range from 2 to 20% for dog bites, from 30 to more than 50% for cat bites, and from 10 to 50% for human bites.[40] Most patients with an infected bite can be managed on an outpatient basis with oral antibiotic therapy and elevation of the involved site.

Animal bites In the United States, dog bites account for 80 to 90% of all animal bites and cat bites for 3 to 15%.[40,41] Nondomestic animals are responsible for only 1 to 2% of all animal bites. Patients with infections resulting from animal bites typically present with significant pain, soft tissue swelling, and tenderness; they may also have associated injuries to nerves, tendons, bones, joints, or blood vessels. Bites involving the hand are associated with an increased risk of tenosynovitis, septic arthritis, and abscess formation.[40]

Infections that occur after a dog or cat bite are usually polymicrobial, involving a mixture of aerobes and anaerobes [*see Table 7*]. *P. multocida* is the major pathogen, isolated from 50 to 80% of infections related to cat bites and from 25% of those related to dog bites.[38,40] Infection with *P. multocida* is characterized by the acute onset of severe

Table 6 Risk Factors for Soft Tissue Infection Complicating Animal or Human Bite
Location on the hand or the foot or over a major joint
Immunosuppression
Chronic alcoholism
Location on the scalp or the face of an infant
Diabetes mellitus
Puncture wound
Corticosteroid use
Delay in treatment lasting longer than 12 hr
Preexisting edema in an affected extremity

Table 7 Organisms Most Frequently Isolated from Dog and Cat Bite Wounds

Organisms
Aerobes
Pasteurella multocida
Corynebacterium species
Staphylococcus species
Streptococcus species
Capnocytophaga canimorsus (rare)
Anaerobes
Bacteroides species
Prevotella species
Porphyromonas species
Peptostreptococci
Fusobacterium species
Bacteroides fragilis
Veillonella parvula

pain, tenderness, and swelling, usually within 12 to 18 hours of the bite. In rare cases (usually involving immunocompromised patients), *Capnocytophaga canimorsus* causes soft tissue infection after a dog or cat bite. *C. canimorsus* infection can be quite serious, leading to overwhelming sepsis; the associated mortality is 25 to 30%.[40–42]

Wounds resulting from animal bites should immediately be washed with soap and water. When seen early, dog bites should be copiously irrigated, débrided, and, in most circumstances, closed. Infected wounds, wounds older than 12 hours, cat bites, and bites on the hand should be left open. In all cases of infection related to an animal bite, aerobic and anaerobic cultures should be obtained from the site of infection. Tetanus immune status should be determined, and immunization against tetanus should be provided when appropriate. In cases of bites from nondomestic carnivores (e.g., bats, skunks, raccoons, etc.), wounds should be irrigated with povidone-iodine to reduce the transmission of rabies, and immunization against rabies should be provided.

Antibiotic therapy is recommended for high-risk wounds (e.g., cat bites that are a true puncture, bites to the hand, massive crush injury, late presentation, and poor general health) [*see Table 6*]. A broad-spectrum antibiotic effective against aerobic and anaerobic organisms should be chosen [*see Table 5*]. Amoxicillin-clavulanate is the antibiotic of choice because of its broad spectrum of activity against common pathogens involved in animal bites; trimethoprim-sulfamethoxazole, doxycycline, and ciprofloxacin are also used [*see Table 5*].

Human bites Human bites may be classified as either occlusional bites (in which teeth puncture the skin) or clenched-fist injuries (in which the hand is injured after contact with teeth).[40,42] Occlusional bites carry roughly the same risk of infection as animal bites, except when they occur on the hand. Clenched-fist injuries and all hand injuries are associated with a higher risk of infection. Clenched-fist injuries typically occur at the third metacarpophalangeal joint. Penetration of the metacarpophalangeal joint capsule may occur, with subsequent development of septic arthritis and osteomyelitis.[38]

Human bites result in more infections than animal bites because of the multiple bacteria involved. Soft tissue infections resulting from human bites are polymicrobial, involving a mixture of aerobes and anaerobes. On average, five different microorganisms are isolated from a human bite wound[40]—significantly more than are usually isolated from an animal bite wound. In addition, the concentration of bacteria in the oral cavity is higher in humans than in animals. The anaerobic bacteria isolated from human bite wounds are similar to those that cause infection after dog and cat bites, except that *Bacteroides* species are more common [*see Table 7*]. Unlike the anaerobic pathogens in dog and cat bites, however, those involved in human bite infections often produce β-lactamases.[40] The predominant aerobic organisms in human bite infections are *S. aureus*, *Staphylococcus epidermidis*, α- and β-hemolytic streptococci, *Corynebacterium* species, and *E. corrodens*. *E. corrodens* is a fastidious facultative aerobic gram-negative rod that is cultured from approximately 25% of clenched-fist injuries and frequently causes a chronic indolent infection.[40] It typically is susceptible to amoxicillin-clavulanate, trimethoprim-sulfamethoxazole, doxycycline, and ciprofloxacin. Other pathogens may also be transmitted as a result of contact with blood or saliva, including hepatitis B and C viruses and, possibly, HIV.

Management of human bite wounds is similar to that of animal bite wounds. The wound must be thoroughly irrigated, preferably with povidone-iodine or chlorhexidine, which are both bactericidal and viricidal. Puncture bite wounds should be irrigated with a small catheter to achieve high-pressure irrigation. If the wound appears infected, aerobic and anaerobic cultures are obtained. Devitalized tissue should be débrided, and the wound should be left open, whether infected or not. The injured extremity should be immobilized and elevated.

Because of the high degree of contamination and local tissue damage associated with human bite wounds to the hand, antimicrobial therapy is indicated for all such injuries. A prospective, randomized study of 45 patients with human bites to the hand seen within 24 hours after injury and without evidence of infection, tendon injury, or joint capsule penetration demonstrated that infection developed in 47% of the patients who did not receive antibiotics but in none of those who did.[43] Patients with an uncomplicated human bite to the hand should receive a broad-spectrum oral antimicrobial agent, such as amoxicillin-clavulanate. Alternate regimens for patients with penicillin allergy include clindamycin plus either ciprofloxacin or trimethoprim-sulfamethoxazole or doxycycline. Prophylaxis for 5 to 7 days is preferred, with longer periods required for infected wounds.[44]

Patients with human bite wounds at sites other than the hand who have risk factors for infection [*see Table 6*] should also receive antimicrobial therapy. However, minor bite wounds in patients who have no risk factors for infection do not call for antibiotic therapy. As with animal bite wounds, tetanus immunization status should be determined, and tetanus toxoid, tetanus immunoglobin, or both should be administered as indicated.

Patients with systemic manifestations of infection (e.g., fever or chills); severe cellulitis; compromised immune status; diabetes mellitus; significant bites to the hand; associated joint, nerve, bone, or tendon involvement; or infection refractory to oral antibiotic therapy should be admitted to the hospital for IV antibiotic therapy.[40] Appropriate choices for IV treatment include piperacillin-tazobactam as well as the regimens listed above. Tenosynovitis, joint infections, and associated injuries to deep structures must also be treated if present.

Cellulitis

Cellulitis is an acute bacterial infection of the dermis and the subcutaneous tissue that primarily affects the lower extremities, although it can affect other areas as well (e.g., the periorbital, buccal, and perianal regions; the areas around incisions; and sites of body piercing).[45] The most common causes of cellulitis are (1) soft tissue trauma from injection of illicit drugs, puncture wounds from foreign bodies or bites (animal, human, or insect), or burns; (2) surgical site infection; and (3) secondary infection of preexisting skin lesions (e.g., eczema; tinea pedis; and decubitus, venous stasis, or ischemic ulcers). Less common causes include extension of a subjacent infection (e.g., osteomyelitis) and bacteremia from a remote site of infection. Predisposing factors for the development of cellulitis include lymphatic disruption or lymphedema, interstitial edema, previous irradiation of soft tissue, diabetes mellitus, immunocompromise, and peripheral vascular disease.

Nonnecrotizing The overwhelming majority of patients with cellulitis have a nonnecrotizing form of the disease. Patients typically present for medical attention because of pain and soft tissue erythema and often have constitutional symptoms (e.g., fever, chills, or malaise). Physical examination reveals erythema with advancing borders, increased skin warmth, tenderness, and edema. Lymphangitis may also be present, manifested as an erythematous linear streak that often extends to a draining lymph node basin; associated lymphadenopathy, fever, and leukocytosis with a shift to immature forms may be apparent.

Cellulitis is usually caused by a single aerobic pathogen. The organisms most frequently responsible for cellulitis in otherwise healthy adults are *S. pyogenes* and *S. aureus*. Of the two, *S. pyogenes* is the more common and is the usual pathogen in patients with associated lymphangitis. *S. aureus* is usually present in patients with underlying chronic skin disease. Other microorganisms may cause cellulitis on rare occasions but usually only in specific clinical circumstances. *Haemophilus influenzae* sometimes causes cellulitis in children or adults infected with HIV.[46] *Streptococcus pneumoniae* may cause this condition in patients with diabetes mellitus, alcoholism, nephrotic syndrome, systemic lupus erythematosus, or hematologic malignancies.[47] *P. multocida* may cause cellulitis as a complication of dog or cat bites. *S. epidermidis* is a recognized cause of cellulitis among immunocompromised patients, including those with HIV infection and those receiving organ transplants.[48] *V. vulnificus* occasionally causes cellulitis in patients who have ingested raw seafood or who have experienced minor soft tissue trauma and are exposed to sea water.[45] *A. hydrophila* may cause cellulitis in patients with soft tissue trauma who are exposed to brackish or fresh water, soil, or wood.[45] Cellulitis that complicates decubitus or other nonhealing ulcers is usually a mixed infection that includes gram-negative organisms.

In most situations, cellulitis is treated with empirical antibiotic regimens that include agents effective against *S. pyogenes* and *S. aureus*. MRSA accounts for up to 70% of all *S. aureus* infections acquired in the community and is the most common organism identified in patients presenting to the emergency department with a skin or soft tissue infection.[49,50] Attempts to isolate a causative pathogen are usually unsuccessful; needle aspiration and skin biopsy at an advancing margin of erythema are positive in only 15 and 40% of cases, respectively.[51] Bacteremia is uncommon, and, as a result, blood cultures are positive in only 2 to 4% of patients with cellulitis.[45,52] Blood cultures are obtained selectively when the patient has high fever and chills, preexisting lymphedema, or buccal or periorbital cellulitis or when a saltwater or freshwater source of infection is suspected. In all of these clinical situations, the prevalence of bacteremia is higher.[52] Radiologic examination should be reserved for patients in whom it is difficult to exclude a deep necrotizing infection.

In an otherwise healthy adult, uncomplicated cellulitis without systemic manifestations can be treated with an oral antibiotic on an outpatient basis. Because the vast majority of cellulitides are caused either by *S. pyogenes* or by a penicillinase-producing *S. aureus*, one of the following agents is usually given: dicloxacillin, cephalexin, cefadroxil, erythromycin, or clindamycin. When MRSA infection is suspected, trimethoprim-sulfamethoxazole, a tetracycline, or clindamycin should be administered [*see Table 5*]. The margins of the erythema should be marked with ink to facilitate assessment of the response to treatment. For lower extremity cellulitis, reduced activity and elevation are important ancillary measures. Appropriate analgesic agents should be given.

Patients who are diabetic or immunocompromised and those who have high fever and chills, rapidly spreading cellulitis, or cellulitis that is refractory to oral antibiotic therapy should be admitted to the hospital for IV antibiotic therapy [*see Table 8*]. Nafcillin is the preferred IV agent. Piperacillin-tazobactam should be added if gram-negative organisms are suspected pathogens, as when cellulitis complicates a decubitus or a diabetic foot ulcer. Vancomycin, tigecycline, linezolid, daptomycin, or quinupristin-dalfopristin should be given to patients with MRSA infections and those with serious penicillin allergies.

Necrotizing Necrotizing cellulitis is similar to nonnecrotizing cellulitis in etiology and pathogenesis but is more serious and progressive. Necrosis generally occurs when the infection is neglected or inadequately treated. The microbiology of necrotizing cellulitis is also similar to that of nonnecrotizing cellulitis, except that *C. perfringens* and other clostridial species may be involved when necrosis is present. In addition to antimicrobial therapy [*see Table 8*], urgent operative débridement is indicated. In other respects, necrotizing cellulitis is treated in much the same way as deep necrotizing infections are (see below). In some patients with necrotizing fasciitis, the skin is involved secondarily.

DEEP NECROTIZING INFECTIONS

Infections that involve the soft tissues deep to the skin tend to become apparent after necrosis has developed. It is

Table 8 Suggested Parenteral Antibiotic Regimens for Treatment of Cellulitis in Adults

Agent	IV Dosage
Nafcillin	2 g q. 4 hr
Cefazolin	1–2 g q. 8 hr
Clindamycin	600–900 mg q. 8 hr
Vancomycin	1 g q. 8 hr
Ampicillin-sulbactam	3 g q. 6 hr

IV = intravenous.

possible that deep necrotizing infections begin without necrosis but progress rapidly as a result of intrinsic factors. Alternatively, such infections may develop as a result of delayed recognition attributable to the tissue depth at which the process takes place and the lack of specific early signs and symptoms. The relatively poor blood supply to subcutaneous fat makes this tissue more susceptible to microbial invasion. Contamination of the deep soft tissues occurs either through neglect or inadequate treatment of cutaneous or subcutaneous infections or through hematogenous seeding of microorganisms in an area of injury.

Most deep necrotizing soft tissue infections are polymicrobial and occur on the extremities, the abdomen, and the perineum.[8,25,27] Necrotizing infections that involve only muscle are uncommon; therefore, necrotizing fasciitis can be considered the paradigm for these infectious processes.

The early signs and symptoms of deep necrotizing soft tissue infection are localized pain that is often disproportionate to the physical findings, tenderness, mild edema, and erythema of the overlying skin. These characteristics may be subtle, and this diagnosis may not readily come to mind. Sometimes, there is a history of previous injury to the area of suspected infection, which can lead to confusion about the diagnosis. Early systemic signs include low-grade fever, tachycardia, and mild tachypnea. The more classic findings associated with these infections—skin discoloration, the formation of bullae, and intense erythema—occur much later in the process. It is important to understand this point so that an early diagnosis can be made and appropriate treatment promptly instituted.

Necrotizing Fasciitis

Necrotizing fasciitis is characterized by angiothrombotic microbial invasion and liquefactive necrosis.[6] Progressive necrosis of the superficial fascia develops, and the deep dermis and fascia are infiltrated by polymorphonuclear leukocytes, with thrombosis of nutrient vessels and occasional suppuration of the veins and arteries coursing through the fascia; bacteria then proliferate within the destroyed fascia. Initially, tissue invasion proceeds horizontally, but as the condition progresses, ischemic necrosis of the skin develops, along with gangrene of the subcutaneous fat and dermis (characterized by progressive skin necrosis, the formation of bullae and vesicles, and occasional ulceration [*see Figure 1*]).

Myonecrosis

Myonecrosis is a rapidly progressive life-threatening infection of skeletal muscle that is primarily caused by *Clostridium* species. The classic example of myonecrosis is clostridial gas gangrene, a disease that was common in World War I soldiers who sustained extremity injuries that were contaminated with soil. Delays in definitive treatment and the use of primary closure for these contaminated wounds contributed to the severity and mortality of these infections.[53] Clostridial myonecrosis may also occur as a deep surgical site infection after contaminated operations, particularly those involving the gastrointestinal tract or the biliary tract. Devitalized tissue is a perfect environment for clostridial proliferation. A rare spontaneous form of this disease occurs in patients with colon or hematologic malignancies in whom myonecrosis caused by *Clostridium septicum* develops in the absence of tissue damage. Myonecrosis may also result from the spread of contiguous fascial infections.

Clostridial myonecrosis has a notably short incubation period: severe progressive disease can develop within 24 hours of contamination. This condition is characterized by acute catastrophic pain in the area of infection, with minimal associated physical findings. Systemic signs of toxicity (e.g., confusion, incontinence, and delirium) often precede the physical signs of localized infection. The skin initially is pale and then gradually becomes yellowish or bronze. Blebs, bullae, and skin necrosis do not appear until late in the course of the disease. Edema and tenderness occur early, and the absence of erythema distinguishes clostridial infections from streptococcal infection. A thin serosanguineous discharge is present in involved areas and may emanate from an involved incision. Gram stain reveals gram-positive coccobacilli with few leukocytes.

When clostridial myonecrosis is suspected or confirmed, penicillin G, 2 to 4 million U every 4 hours, should be given immediately; clindamycin, 900 mg every 8 hours, should be added. When *C. septicum* is identified on culture, a search for an occult gastrointestinal tract malignancy should be made. Clostridial myonecrosis is the one soft tissue infection for which hyperbaric oxygen is recommended, although, as yet, there is little evidence that this modality improves outcomes. If hyperbaric oxygen therapy is to be used, it should not be given before operative débridement.

Discussion

Etiology and Classification of Soft Tissue Infection

Soft tissue infection commonly results from inoculation of bacteria through a defect in the epidermal layer of the skin, such as may occur with injury, preexisting skin disease, or vascular compromise. Less commonly, soft tissue infection may be a consequence of extension from a subjacent site of infection (e.g., osteomyelitis) or of hematogenous spread from a distant site (e.g., diverticulitis or *C. septicum* infection in patients with colonic carcinoma). It may also occur de novo in healthy patients with normal-appearing skin, often as a result of invasion of damaged soft tissue by virulent pathogenic organisms.[54]

Conditions that disrupt the skin and alter its normal barrier function [*see Table 2*] predispose patients to bacterial contamination. Host factors may increase susceptibility to infection and limit the patient's ability to contain the bacterial inoculum. Clinically occult infection or inadequate treatment of other conditions may also lead to secondary development of soft tissue infection (as is sometimes seen in patients with perirectal or Bartholin cyst abscesses, strangulated hernias, or panniculitis). Delayed or inadequate treatment of superficial infections (e.g., folliculitis, furuncles, carbuncles, cellulitis, and surgical site infections) may lead to more severe necrotizing infections, particularly when host immunity is otherwise compromised.

Soft tissue infections may be classified as superficial or deep, as nonnecrotizing or necrotizing, as primary (idiopathic) or secondary, and as monomicrobial or polymicrobial. Superficial infections involve the epidermis, dermis, superficial fascia, or subcutaneous tissue, whereas deep infections involve the deep fascia or muscle [*see Figure 6*]. Necrotizing soft tissue infections are distinguished by the presence of extensive, rapidly progressing necrosis and high mortality. Such infections are termed necrotizing cellulitis, necrotizing fasciitis, or myonecrosis according to whether the deepest tissue layer affected by necrosis is subcutaneous tissue, deep fascia, or muscle, respectively.

Primary (idiopathic) soft tissue infections occur in the absence of a known causative factor or portal of entry for bacteria. Such infections are uncommon and are believed to result from hematogenous spread of microorganisms to damaged fat or muscle or bacterial invasion through small unrecognized breaks in the epidermis.[54,55] Soft tissue infection caused by *V. vulnificus* is an example of a primary soft tissue infection: it is attributed to bacteremia developing after the ingestion of contaminated raw seafood. Only 10 to 15% of all necrotizing soft tissue infections are idiopathic; the remaining 85 to 90% are secondary infections, developing as a consequence of some insult to the skin that predisposes to infection. Secondary soft tissue infections may be further categorized as posttraumatic, postoperative, or complications of preexisting skin conditions.

Soft tissue infections are classified as monomicrobial when they are caused by a single organism and as polymicrobial when they are caused by multiple organisms. Most superficial soft tissue infections are caused by a single aerobe, usually *S. pyogenes* or *S. aureus*. Exceptions to this general rule include infections caused by animal or human bites, cellulitis associated with decubitus or other nonhealing ulcers, and infections in immunocompromised patients. These infections are typically polymicrobial, often involving aerobic or facultative gram-negative organisms and anaerobes in addition to aerobic gram-positive bacteria.

Deep necrotizing soft tissue infections are polymicrobial 80 to 85% of the time. They are caused by the synergistic activity of facultative aerobes and anaerobes [*see Figure 7*].[56,57] *S. aureus*, *S. pyogenes*, and enterococci are the most common gram-positive aerobes. *Escherichia coli* is the most common gram-negative enteric organism. *Bacteroides* species and peptostreptococci are the most common anaerobes.[9,30,57] The remaining 15 to 20% of deep necrotizing infections are monomicrobial. Most primary necrotizing soft tissue infections are monomicrobial.[54] These infections are more fulminant and are notable for their acute onset, rapid progression, and systemic toxicity. Their characteristic clinical manifestations are related to exotoxin production by the pathogen involved [*see Table 9 and* Pathogenesis of Soft Tissue Infections, *below*]. *S. pyogenes* is the pathogen in more than half of monomicrobial infections; *S. aureus*, *C. perfringens*, *V. vulnificus*, *A. hydrophila* and *P. aeruginosa* are less common.

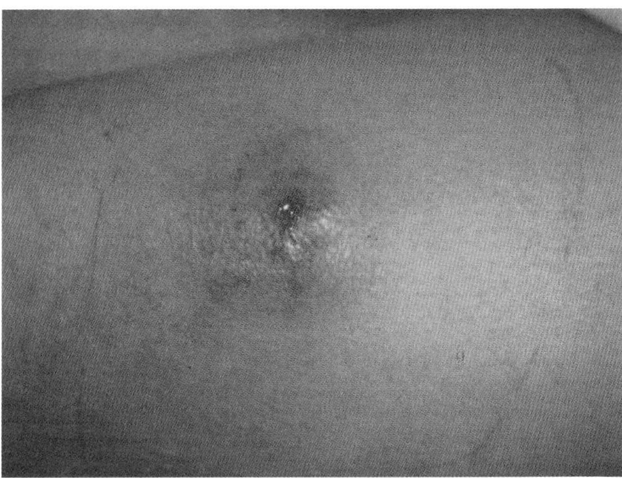

Figure 7 **Meleney ulcer is characterized by central necrosis, erythema, and edema.**

Ludwig angina is a polymicrobial infection involving the submandibular space that can extend into the neck and mediastinum along fascial planes. In 40% of cases, infection extends into the mediastinum, resulting in cervical necrotizing fasciitis, which is associated with a mortality of 40% or more.[58] Ludwig angina and cervical necrotizing fasciitis have several unique features. Ludwig angina has an odontogenic ctiology and is caused by oral anaerobic bacteria, primarily fusobacteria and peptostreptococci.[59,60]

Pathogenesis of Soft Tissue Infections

Soft tissue infections generally induce localized inflammatory changes in the involved tissues, regardless of the species of bacteria involved. As the infection progresses, tissue necrosis occurs as a result of (1) direct cellular injury from

Table 9 Major Exotoxins Associated with Organisms Causing Monomicrobial Necrotizing Soft Tissue Infection

Bacterium	*Exotoxins*
Streptococcus pyogenes	Pyrogenic exotoxins A and B, hemolysin, fibrinolysin, hyaluronidase, streptokinase
Staphylococcus aureus	Hemolysins (intravascular hemolysis and local tumor necrosis), coagulase
Pseudomonas aeruginosa	Collagenase (local tissue damage and necrosis)
Clostridium perfringens	α-Toxin (lecithinase causing tissue necrosis, intravascular hemolysis, hemoglobinemia, and acute renal failure)

bacterial toxins, (2) significant inflammatory edema within a closed tissue compartment, (3) thrombosis of nutrient blood vessels, and (4) tissue ischemia.

The exotoxins produced by gram-positive cocci and some gram-negative bacteria are powerful proteolytic enzymes. *S. pyogenes* produces hemolysins, fibrinolysins, hyaluronidases, and streptolysins that facilitate spread into surrounding tissues. Methicillin-resistant strains of *S. aureus*, in particular the USA300 strain, produce Panton-Valentine leukocidin, which results in leukocyte destruction and tissue necrosis.[24] *S. aureus* and *P. aeruginosa* produce coagulases that result in local tissue damage and necrosis. *C. perfringens* produces numerous exotoxins. The α-toxin, a lecithinase enzyme, is highly lethal: it destroys cell membranes, causes hemolysis, and alters capillary permeability. Other clostridial toxins lyse red blood cells and have direct cardiotoxic effects. These toxins also cause platelet aggregation and fibrin deposition, with resultant vascular thrombosis and necrosis. Production of the α-toxin leads to intravascular leukostasis and inhibits diapedesis of white blood cells into infected tissue. This unique collection of bacterial toxins accounts for the rapid progression of *C. perfringens* infection in a setting of minimal inflammatory changes. Many of the various toxins produced by these bacteria destroy white blood cells directly or inhibit their migration into the area of infection, resulting in a leukocyte-poor "dishwater pus" in the area of necrosis.

That most necrotizing soft tissue infections involve multiple bacterial species strongly suggests that bacterial synergy plays an important role in their pathogenesis. Toxin-induced cellular necrosis establishes an anaerobic environment that facilitates the growth of both facultative and anaerobic bacteria. These anaerobes elaborate additional enzymes and other by-products that facilitate tissue invasion and destruction.

Preexisting local tissue damage frequently serves as a nidus for soft tissue infection. The reduced oxygen tension of this abnormal environment allows pathogens to proliferate. In addition, various patient factors predispose susceptible individuals to these infections. Chronic illnesses can contribute to a diminished immunologic response. Peripheral vascular disease impairs the local blood and oxygen supply. Diabetes mellitus inhibits WBC function. Chronic pulmonary disease can result in systemic hypoxemia. Patients with congestive heart failure or significant coronary artery disease may be unable to increase their cardiac output in response to infection. Malnutrition can result in a lack of nutrients and critical enzymatic cofactors involved in the normal cellular response to infection. Each of these patient factors impairs the host response and thereby increases the likelihood that infection will develop.

Hemolytic streptococci were originally described by Meleney as the cause of a "synergistic gangrene."[2] In the 1920s, Meleney demonstrated that injection of animals with pathogens isolated from patients with infectious gangrene reproduced the characteristics of infection.[2]

Toxic-Shock Syndrome

The current resurgence of necrotizing soft tissue infections attributed to so-called flesh-eating bacteria probably represents an adaptation of group A β-hemolytic streptococci and *S. aureus* to the contemporary environment.[61] TSS is defined as the isolation of *S. pyogenes* or *S. aureus* from a normally sterile body site in conjunction with hypotension and either renal impairment, acute respiratory distress syndrome, abnormal hepatic function, coagulopathy, extensive tissue necrosis, or an erythematous rash.[42] More than 60% of patients with TSS have bacteremia. TSS has been shown to be a major risk factor for mortality among patients with necrotizing soft tissue infections.[62]

Population-based studies in North America and Europe documented a nearly fivefold increase in group A streptococcal infections since the late 1980s.[63] The current incidence of group A streptococcal infections in the population of Ontario, Canada, is estimated to be 1.5 per 100,000.[63] TSS develops in approximately 10 to 15% of these patients and necrotizing fasciitis in about 6%.[64] It is likely that the rise in serious group A streptococcal infections reflects an antigenic shift that has increased the virulence of these organisms.

Soft tissue infections associated with TSS typically involve an extremity. Approximately 70% of patients will progress to necrotizing fasciitis or myositis and will require operative treatment. Only about 50% of patients with streptococcal soft tissue infections have a demonstrable portal of entry for bacteria.[54,65]

Severe pain is the most common initial symptom of TSS. It is of sudden onset and generally precedes tenderness or other physical findings. Fever is another common early sign. About 80% of TSS patients show clinical signs of soft tissue infection (e.g., localized swelling, erythema, and tenderness) [*see Figure 8*]. In approximately 50%, blood pressure is initially normal, but hypotension invariably develops within 4 to 8 hours after presentation.

Hemoglobinuria and an elevated serum creatinine concentration are hallmarks of renal involvement. Even when adequate resuscitation is provided and antibiotics and vasopressors are given, hypotension persists in the overwhelming majority of patients. Renal dysfunction can persist or progress for 48 to 72 hours despite treatment. Hypoalbuminemia is common. Mild leukocytosis is present initially; however, the percentage of immature neutrophils is generally 40% or higher.

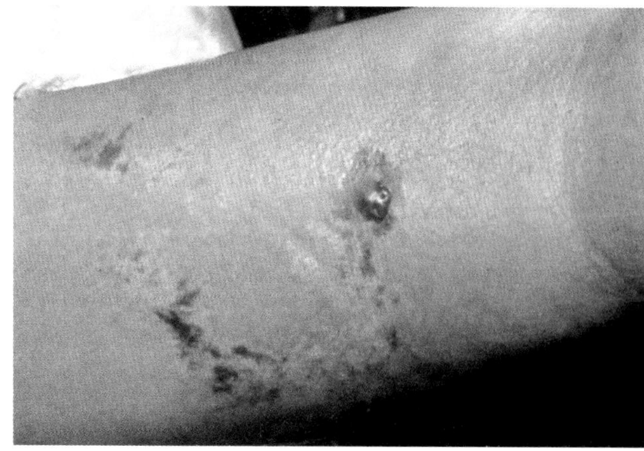

Figure 8 The superficial appearance of streptococcal gangrene of the posterior thigh.

S. pyogenes can be classified into more than 80 different strains, or M types, on the basis of the M proteins expressed. M proteins impede phagocytosis of streptococci and induce vascular leakage by forming complexes with fibrinogen.[66] They also cleave nicotinic acid dinucleotide (NAD), thereby interrupting elemental cellular processes. The M proteins M1 and M3 are associated with the majority of streptococcal necrotizing soft tissue infections.[61] Streptococcal pyrogenic exotoxins (SPEs) are produced by most streptococci that cause severe soft tissue infection and can be transmitted by bacteriophages to different M types. They are the cause of the fever, shock, and tissue injury associated with these infections. SPE-A and SPE-B induce the synthesis of tumor necrosis factor–α (TNF-α), interleukin-1β (IL-1β), and IL-6. Peptidoglycan, lipoteichoic acid, and killed organisms also are capable of inducing TNF-α production.

It has been proposed that M proteins or SPEs act as superantigens. These exotoxins, along with certain staphylococcal toxins (e.g., toxic-shock syndrome toxin–1 [TSST-1] and staphylococcal enterotoxins), can stimulate T cell responses through conventional antigen-presenting cells, as well as through direct binding to the Vβq region of the T cell receptor. Conventional T cell activation through antigen-presenting cells is a multistage process that stimulates a relatively small percentage of T cells and limits the magnitude of the resultant cytokine response. In contrast, superantigens bypass the normal antigen presentation pathway and do not undergo phagocytosis. The superantigen processing pathway can stimulate a polyclonal T cell activation in excess of a thousand times more T cells than the conventional antigen pathway and thus can trigger a massive release of cytokines.

Although *S. pyogenes* is susceptible to penicillin and other β-lactam antibiotics in vitro, clinical treatment failure sometimes occurs when penicillin is used alone against *S. pyogenes* infections.[61] Such failure is a particular problem with more aggressive group A streptococcal infections and may be attributable to the large inoculum size (the so-called Eagle effect). These large inocula reach the stationary growth phase very quickly. Penicillin and other β-lactam antibiotics are ineffective in the stationary growth phase because of the reduced expression of penicillin-binding proteins in this phase. Moreover, toxin production is not inhibited by β-lactam antibiotics during the stationary growth phase. In contrast, antibiotics that inhibit protein synthesis have been associated with improved survival after serious group A streptococcal infections.

Clindamycin has been demonstrated to possess the unique property of suppressing toxin production by *S. aureus*, hemolytic streptococci, and clostridia and should be included in the antibiotic regimen when these organisms are present or suspected as well as for all patients with hypotension, coagulopathy, or organ system failure.[67] Clindamycin inhibits protein synthesis, and its efficacy is unaffected by inoculum size or the stage of bacterial growth. In particular, it suppresses bacterial toxin synthesis and inhibits M-protein synthesis, thus facilitating phagocytosis of *S. pyogenes*. Clindamycin also suppresses synthesis of penicillin-binding proteins and can act synergistically with penicillin. Vancomycin or linezolid should be used for patients who are allergic to clindamycin; however, these agents do not suppress toxin production.

Mortality from necrotizing soft tissue infection has been reported to range from 21 to 29%[9,25,27,30,68]; however, mortality in a recent multi-institutional report was reported to be 12%.[69] Risk factors for mortality include age greater than 50 years, the presence of organ dysfunction at admission, a relatively high percentage of total body surface area involved, hypotension, lactic acidosis, immune compromise, a WBC count greater than 30,000/µL, and, most important, delays in recognition and treatment.[9,25,27,62,69,70] Patients with truncal involvement or positive blood cultures also have a higher mortality.[24,67] A single-institution report of long-term outcomes following necrotizing soft tissue infections demonstrated that 25% of patients who survived at least 30 days during their initial hospitalization for necrotizing soft tissue infection died over a mean follow-up period of 3.3 years.[71] Late causes of death included chronic diseases and malignancies, which provides more evidence for the predisposition of this patient population for this illness as well as evidence for its high mortality.

Financial Disclosures: None Reported

References

1. Eke N. Fournier's gangrene: a review of 1726 cases. Br J Surg 2000;87:718.
2. Meleney FL. Hemolytic streptococcus gangrene. Arch Surg 1924;9:317.
3. Brewer GE, Meleney FL. Progressive gangrenous infection of the skin and subcutaneous tissues, following operation for acute perforative appendicitis. Ann Surg 1926;84:438.
4. Wilson B. Necrotizing fasciitis. Am Surg 1952;18:416.
5. Greenberg RN, Willoughby BG, Kennedy DJ, et al. Hypocalcemia and "toxic" syndrome associated with streptococcal fasciitis. South Med J 1983;76:916.
6. McHenry CR, Compton CN. Soft tissue infections. In: Malangoni MA, Soper NJ, editors. Problems in general surgery. Philadelphia: Lippincott Williams & Wilkins; 2002. p. 7.
7. Anaya DA, Dellinger EP. Necrotizing soft-tissue infection: diagnosis and management. Clin Pract 2007;44:705.
8. McHenry CR, Piotrowski JJ, Petrinic D, et al. Determinants of mortality for necrotizing soft tissue infections. Ann Surg 1995;221:558.
9. Wall DB, Klein SR, Black S, et al. A simple model to help distinguish necrotizing fasciitis from non-necrotizing soft tissue infection. J Am Coll Surg 2000;191:227.
10. Chan T, Yaghoubian A, Rosing D, et al. Low sensitivity of physical examination findings in necrotizing soft tissue infection is improved with laboratory values: a prospective study. Am J Surg 2008;196:926–30.
11. Wong CH, Khin LW, Heng KS, et al. The LRINEC (Laboratory Risk Indicator for Necrotizing Fasciitis) score: a tool for distinguishing necrotizing fasciitis from other soft tissue infections. Crit Care Med 2004;32:1535.
12. Struk DW, Munk PL, Lee MJ, et al. Imaging of soft tissue infections. Radiol Clin North Am 2001;39:277.

13. Loh N, Ch'en IY, Cheung LP, et al. Deep fascial hyperintensity in soft-tissue abnormalities as revealed by T_2-weighted MR imaging. AJR Am J Roentgenol 1997;168:1301.
14. Arslan A, Pierre-Jerome C, Borkine A. Necrotizing fasciitis unreliable MRI findings in the preoperative diagnosis. Eur J Radiol 2000;36:139.
15. DeCiernk LS, Degryse HR, Wouters E, et al. Magnetic resonance imaging in the evaluation of patients with eosinophilic fasciitis. J Rheumatol 1989;16:1270.
16. Haaverstad R, Nilsen, G, Myhre HO, et al. The use of MRI in the investigation of leg edema. Eur J Vasc Surg 1992;6: 124.
17. Duewell S, Hagspiel KD, Zuber J, et al. Swollen lower extremity: role of MR imaging. Radiology 1992;184:227.
18. Hopkins KL, King CP, Bergman G. Gadolinium-DTPA-enhanced magnetic resonance imaging of musculoskeletal infectious processes. Skeletal Radiol 1995;24:325.
19. Schmid MR, Kossman T, Duewell S. Differentiation of necrotizing fasciitis and cellulitis using MR imaging. AJR Am J Roentgenol 1998;170:615.
20. Brothers TE, Tagge DU, Stutley JE, et al. Magnetic resonance imaging differentiates between necrotizing and non-necrotizing fasciitis of the lower extremity. J Am Coll Surg 2000;187:416.
21. Zacharias N, Velmahos GC, Salama A, et al. Diagnosis of necrotizing soft tissue infections by computed tomography. Arch Surg 2010;145:452–5.
22. Davis KA. Computed tomography to exclude necrotizing soft tissue infection. Not quite ready for prime time. Arch Surg 2010;145:455.
23. Miller LG, Perdreau-Remington F, Rieg G, et al. Necrotizing fasciitis caused by community-associated methicillin-resistant *Staphylococcus aureus* in Los Angeles. N Engl J Med 2005;352:1445.
24. Anaya DA, McMahon K, Nathens AB, et al. Predictors of mortality and limb loss in necrotizing soft tissue infections. Arch Surg 2005;140:151–8.
25. Rouse TM, Malangoni MA, Schulte WJ. Necrotizing fasciitis: a preventable disaster. Surgery 1981;92:765.
26. Elliott DC, Kufera JA, Myers RAM. Necrotizing soft tissue infections: risk factors for mortality and strategies for management. Ann Surg 1996;224:672.
27. Ustin JS, Malangoni MA. Necrotizing soft tissue infections. Crit Care Med 2011. [Epub Apr 28]
28. Brown DR, Davis NL, Lepawsky M, et al. A multicenter review of the treatment of major truncal necrotizing infections with and without hyperbaric oxygen therapy. Am J Surg 1994;167:485.
29. Jallali N, Withey S, Butler PE. Hyperbaric oxygen as adjuvant therapy in the management of necrotizing fasciitis. Am J Surg 2005;189:462–6.
30. George ME, Rueth NM, Skarda DE, et al. Hyperbaric oxygen does not improve outcome in patients with necrotizing soft tissue infection. Surg Infect (Larchmt) 2009;10:21–8.
31. Alejandria MM, Lansang MA, Dans LF, et al. Intravenous immunoglobulin for treating sepsis and septic shock. Cochrane Database Syst Rev 2002;(2):CD001090.
32. Trent JT, Federman D, Kirsner RS. Common bacterial skin infections. Ostomy Wound Manage 2001;47:30.
33. Stulberg DL, Penrod MA, Blatny RA. Common bacterial skin infections. Am Fam Phys 2002;66:119
34. Sadick NS. Current aspects of bacterial infections of the skin. Dermatol Clin 1997;15:341.
35. Bonnetblanc JM, Bédane C. Erysipelas: recognition and management. Am J Clin Dermatol 2003;4:157.
36. Shirtcliffe P, Robinson GM. A case of severe Pseudomonas folliculitis from a spa pool. N Z Med J 1998;139:30.
37. Merlino JI, Malangoni MA. Complicated skin and soft-tissue infections: diagnostic approach and empiric treatment options. Cleve Clin J Med 2007;74 Suppl 4:S21–8.
38. Goldstein EJC. Bite wounds and infections. Clin Infect Dis 1992;14:633.
39. Weber DJ, Hansen AR. Infections resulting from animal bites. Infect Dis Clin North Am 1991;5:663.
40. Griego RD, Rosen T, Orengo IF, et al. Dog, cat and human bites: a review. J Am Acad Dermatol 1995;33:1019.
41. Tan JS. Human zoonotic infections transmitted by dogs and cats. Arch Intern Med 1997;157:1933.
42. Presutti RJ. Bite wounds: early treatment and prophylaxis against infectious complications. Postgrad Med 1997;101: 243.
43. Zubowicz VN, Gravier M. Management of early human bites of the hand: a prospective randomized study. Plast Reconstr Surg 1991;88:111.
44. Agency for Healthcare Research and Quality National Guideline Clearinghouse. Management of human bite wounds. Available at: http://www.guideline.gov/content.aspx?id=10860 (accessed July 25, 2011).
45. Swartz MN. Cellulitis. N Engl J Med 2004;350:904.
46. Ginsberg CM, Hurwitz RM. Haemophilus influenzae type B is an unusual organism causing cellulitis in children and patients with HIV infection. Arch Dermatol 1980;4:661.
47. Parada JP, Maslow JN. Clinical syndromes associated with adult pneumococcal cellulitis. Scand J Infect Dis 2000;32: 133.
48. Sadick NS. Bacterial disease of the skin. In: Rakel EE, editor. Conn's current therapy. Philadelphia: WB Saunders; 1997. p. 823.
49. King MD, Humphrey BJ, Yang YF, et al. Emergence of community-acquired methicillin-resistant Staphylococcus aureus. USA 300 clone as the predominant cause of skin and soft tissue infections. Ann Intern Med 2006;144: 309–17.
50. Moran GJ, Krishnadasan A, Gorwitz RJ, et al. Methicillin-resistant S. aureus infections among patients in the emergency department. N Engl J Med 2006;355:666–74.
51. Stevens DL. Streptococcal infections. In: Bennet JC, Plum F, editors. Cecil textbook of medicine. 20th ed. Philadelphia: WB Saunders; 1996. p. 1585.
52. Perl B, Gottehrer NP, Ravek D, et al. Cost-effectiveness of blood cultures for adult patients with cellulitis. Clin Infect Dis 1999;29:1483.
53. Altemeier WA, Fullen WD. Prevention and treatment of gas gangrene. JAMA 1971;217:806.
54. McHenry CR, Brandt CP, Piotrowski JJ, et al. Idiopathic necrotizing fasciitis: recognition, incidence and outcome of therapy. Am Surg 1994;60:490.
55. McHenry CR, Azar T, Ramahi AJ, et al. Monomicrobial necrotizing fasciitis complicating pregnancy and puerperium. Obstet Gynecol 1996;87:823.
56. McHenry CR, Malangoni M. Necrotizing soft tissue infections. In: Fry DE, editor. Surgical infections. Boston: Little, Brown & Co; 1995. p. 161.

57. Giuliano A, Lewis F Jr, Hadley K, et al. Bacteriology of necrotizing fasciitis. Am J Surg 1977;134:52.
58. Mathieu D, Neviere R, Teillon C, et al. Cervical necrotizing fasciitis: clinical manifestations and management. Clin Infect Dis 1995;21:51–6.
59. Boscolo-Rizzo P, Da Mosto MC. Submandibular space infection: a potentially lethal infection. Int J Infect Dis 2009; 13:327–33.
60. Bansal A, Miskoff J, Lis RJ. Otolaryngologic critical care. Crit Care Clin 2003;19:55–72.
61. Stevens DL. Streptococcal toxic-shock syndrome: spectrum of disease, pathogenesis and new concepts in treatment. Emerg Infect Dis 1995;1:69.
62. Golger A, Ching S, Goldsmith CH, et al. Mortality in patients with necrotizing fasciitis. Plast Reconstr Surg 2007; 119:1803.
63. Kaul R, McGeer A, Low DE, et al. Population-based surveillance for group A streptococcal necrotizing fasciitis: clinical features, prognostic indicators and microbiologic analysis of seventy-seven cases. Am J Med 1997;103:18.
64. Davies HD, McGeer A, Schwartz B, et al. Invasive group A streptococcal infections in Ontario, Canada. N Engl J Med 1996;335:547.
65. Bisno AL, Stevens DL. Streptococcal infections of the skin and soft tissues. N Engl J Med 1996;334:240.
66. Herwald H, Cramer H, Orgelin M, et al. M protein, a classical bacterial virulence determinant, forms complexes with fibrinogen that induce vascular leakage. Cell 2004;116:367.
67. Stevens DL, Ma Y, Salmi DB, et al. Impact of antibiotics on expression of virulence associated exotoxin genes in methicillin-sensitive and methicillin-resistant Staphylococcus aureus. J Infect Dis 2007;195:202–11.
68. Bosshardt TL, Henderson VJ, Organ CH. Necrotizing soft-tissue infections. Arch Surg 1996;131:846.
69. Mills MK, Faraklas I, Davis C, et al. Outcomes from treatment of necrotizing soft-tissue infections: results from the National Surgical Quality Improvement Program database. Am J Surg 2010;200:790–7.
70. Yaghoubian A, de Virgilio C, Dauphine C, et al. Use of admission serum lactate and sodium levels to predict mortality in necrotizing soft-tissue infections. Arch Surg 2007;142:840–6.
71. Light TD, Choi KC, Thomsen TA, et al. Long-term outcomes of patients with necrotizing fasciitis. J Burn Care Res 2010; 31:93–9.

Acknowledgment

Figure 6 Tom Moore

3 PRINCIPLES OF WOUND MANAGEMENT AND SOFT TISSUE REPAIR

Jonathan S. Friedstat, MD, Eric G. Halvorson, MD, and Joseph J. Disa, MD, FACS

Difficult Wounds

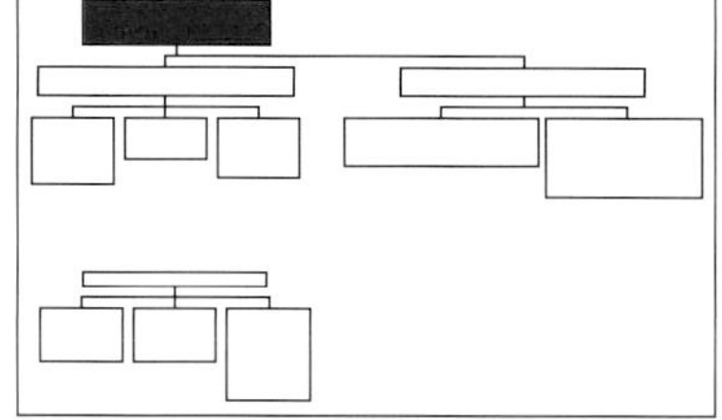

Problem wounds are characterized by one of the following: large size that precludes direct primary closure, gross infection or uncertain bacteriologic status, or threatened loss of critical structures exposed as a result of insufficient soft tissue coverage. Surgically created wounds, which generally pose less of a problem from a bacteriologic standpoint than traumatic wounds, are best managed by an immediate coverage procedure when direct closure is impossible.

Traumatic wounds are more difficult to evaluate than surgical wounds for several reasons. First, the potential for infection is high because of the environment in which the wound is created, the mechanism of injury, and the time that elapses before operative intervention. Second, the mechanism of injury (e.g., crush, avulsion, or gunshot) may extend the zone of injury beyond what is immediately apparent [*see Figure 1*]. Serious postoperative infection may develop in these cases if definitive wound coverage is provided in the absence of adequate débridement. Third, whereas accurate assessment of the chances for recovery of specific structures within the wound is vital for selecting the optimal method of treatment, such assessment is often difficult immediately after injury.

EVALUATION

The initial step in the management of problem wounds is to decide whether the wound is suitable for immediate soft tissue coverage. Wounds that are surgically created during the course of an elective procedure are almost always best treated with primary definitive coverage. Traumatic wounds that present within 1 or 2 hours of injury and have a minimal crush component are also best treated with a primary definitive coverage procedure after thorough débridement (if the patient's hemodynamic status permits).

Injuries with a significant crush component and exposure of critical structures (e.g., nerves, vessels, tendons, or bone) are best treated more aggressively. In these cases, thorough débridement requires considerable surgical experience because the tendency is to débride inadequately. The accuracy with which tissue viability can be assessed varies from one type of tissue to another. For example, skin can be evaluated by its color, the nature of its capillary refill, the quality of its dermal bleeding, or its bleeding response to pinprick. After intravenous fluorescein injection, skin viability can also be assessed qualitatively, with a Wood light, or quantitatively, with a dermofluorometer. Muscle is the most difficult tissue to evaluate. Color, capillary bleeding, and contractile response to stimulation are not always reliable indicators of muscle viability. In severe injuries, they can be misleading. Inadequate débridement may lead to severe consequences resulting from infection. Therefore, serial débridement at 24- to 48-hour intervals is essential for accurately establishing the limits of muscle injury. Efforts should be made during débridement to preserve tissues such as major nerves and blood vessels unless they are severely injured. These structures are vital for function and are of small mass compared with other tissues (e.g., skin, fat, and muscle) at risk for necrosis and subsequent infection.

Wound débridement, therefore, should involve careful analysis of the injury from an anatomic point of view; débridement should not consist of indiscriminate excision of blocks of tissue. Between débridement procedures, the wound should be treated with sterile dressing changes or negative-pressure wound therapy (NPWT) if conditions permit. A definitive soft tissue coverage procedure should then be performed as soon after the initial injury as wound conditions permit. When thorough débridement and definitive coverage can be completed within less than 1 week, the wound will generally heal uneventfully. Inadequate débridement frequently results in the loss of any additional tissue invested to achieve acute soft tissue coverage. The wound becomes grossly infected, and important functional structures within the wound are reexposed.

Infected surgical wounds, neglected wounds, or other complex wounds in which initial wound management fails should be débrided and then treated by open methods. Proper care of these wounds is aimed at converting established gross infection to a much lower level of bacterial contamination, which is then compatible with successful secondary wound closure. For example, advances in the use of NPWT [*see* Initial Treatment, Negative-Pressure Wound Therapy, *below*] have simplified the management of complex lower extremity traumatic wounds, reducing the use of free tissue transfer.[1]

INITIAL TREATMENT

Débridement

Devitalized tissue provides an ideal culture medium for bacteria and isolates them from host defense mechanisms. Surgical débridement must be performed aggressively—and on a serial basis if necessary—to remove all necrotic tissue.

High-Pressure Irrigation

A useful adjunct to débridement is irrigation, which has been shown experimentally to reduce wound infection rates significantly.[2,3] Although many surgeons use high-pressure

Acute reconstruction is indicated

Evaluate and treat open wound. Débride nonviable tissue and use wet-to-dry dressings or negative-pressure wound therapy until infection is cleared and wound is healing.

Select coverage procedure to achieve healed wound.

Wound does not contain exposed bone, cartilage, nerve, or tendon but cannot be closed directly

Apply a skin graft.

Wound is a small defect but is in an area where graft contracture is not desirable (e.g., face, hand, or flexion crease)

Apply full-thickness skin graft; donor sites include the ear, upper eyelid, neck, and groin.

Wound has a large surface area or is a small wound in a noncritical area

Apply split-thickness skin graft.

Wound is clean but in an area prone to contamination

Apply meshed split-thickness skin graft. Reinstitute early dressing changes if infection develops.

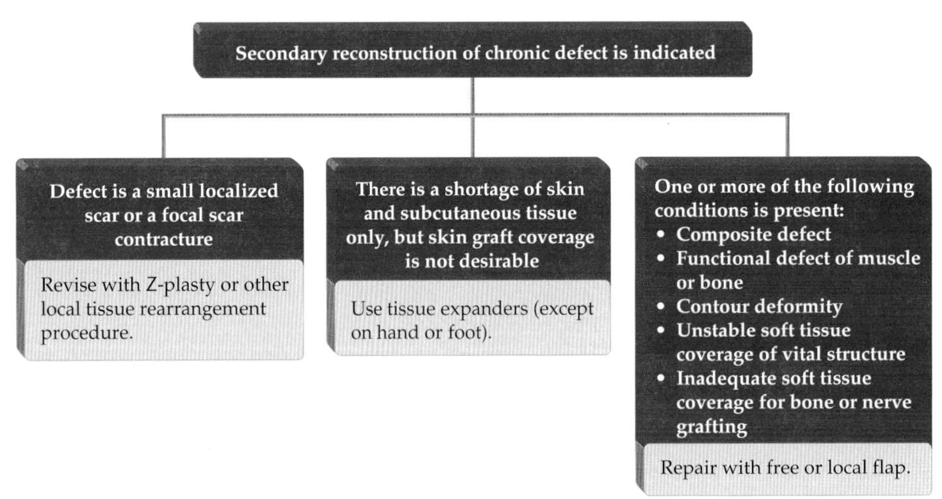

Secondary reconstruction of chronic defect is indicated
Defect is a small localized scar or a focal scar contracture
Revise with Z-plasty or other local tissue rearrangement procedure.
There is a shortage of skin and subcutaneous tissue only, but skin graft coverage is not desirable
Use tissue expanders (except on hand or foot).
One or more of the following conditions is present:
• Composite defect
• Functional defect of muscle or bone
• Contour deformity
• Unstable soft tissue coverage of vital structure
• Inadequate soft tissue coverage for bone or nerve grafting
Repair with free or local flap.

Approach to Surgical Reconstruction

Bone, cartilage, nerve, or tendon is exposed and cannot be covered by direct wound closure

Perform flap coverage procedure.

Local donor site meets needs and is not involved in the primary process

Use local flap.

- *Small or clean wound*: use local skin flap if possible.
- *Large or contaminated wound*: use regional myocutaneous flap.

Local flap is not possible or would not provide appropriate tissue

Use free flap.

- If wound is clean and thin flap is desired, apply skin or fascial free flap.
- If wound is large or contaminated, apply muscle or myocutaneous free flap.

Muscle flaps require coverage with a meshed split-thickness skin graft.

a

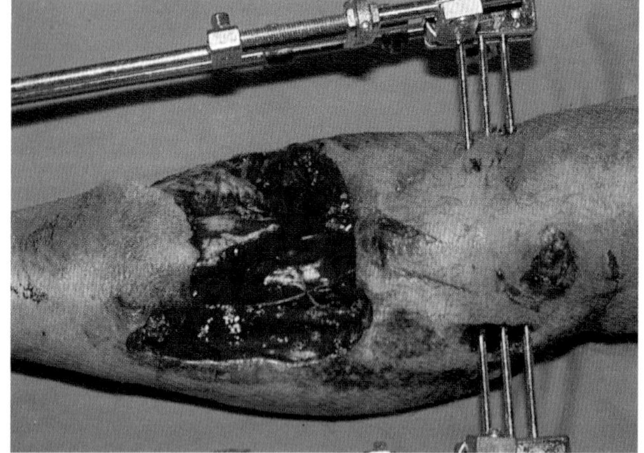

b

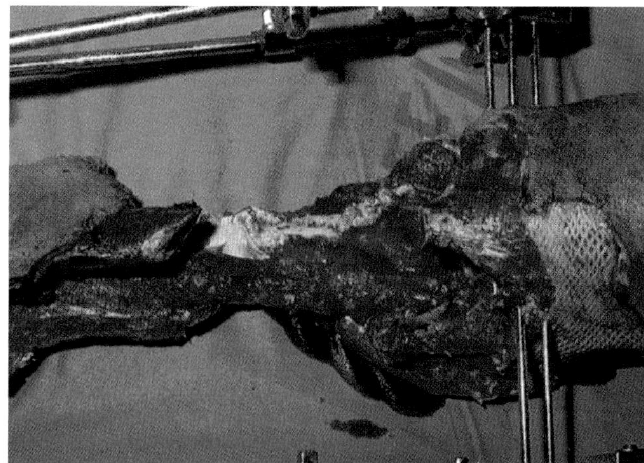

c

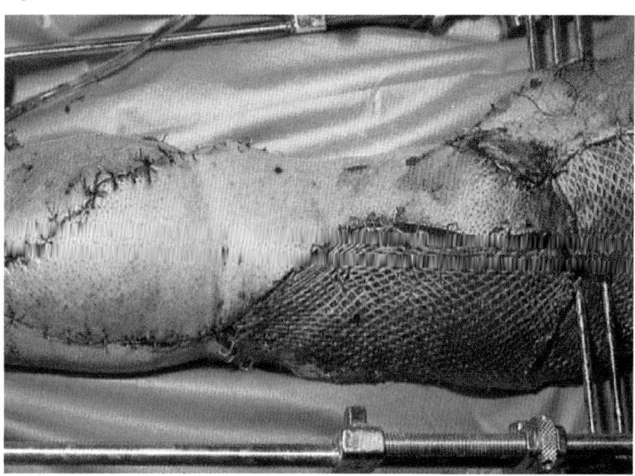

Figure 1 (*a*) A so-called bumper injury of the leg is shown after initial débridement and bony stabilization (2 days after injury). (*b*) After the second débridement, the true extent of devitalization of bone and soft tissue is apparent (4 days after injury). (*c*) A latissimus dorsi free flap has been used to reconstruct the soft tissue defect (5 days after injury).

irrigation, some argue that small particulate materials may get pushed deeper into a wound bed with this technique. High-pressure irrigation is recommended as an adjunct once thorough débridement has been performed manually.

Given that the optimal technique for wound irrigation is debatable, an international, multicenter, randomized, controlled trial is under way aimed at answering this question in the setting of open fractures. The pilot trial compared castile soap versus normal saline at low and high pressure with primary outcomes of unplanned reoperation, infection, wound healing, and nonunion. The researchers found that higher-pressure irrigation was associated with a 28% risk of primary outcomes versus 19% for lower-pressure irrigation.[4]

Quantitative Bacteriology

The degree of bacterial wound contamination can be accurately quantified. The standard technique of quantitative bacteriology requires several days to complete and is therefore of somewhat limited utility in the management of acute wounds. In addition to a count, it provides identification and antibiotic sensitivities of the organism. As an alternative, quantitative bacteriology can be performed by using the rapid slide technique, which provides valuable information about the wound within 20 minutes.[5,6] The level of bacterial contamination has been shown to be a significant predictor of outcome in wound closure by either skin graft or flap coverage techniques. According to the golden period principle of wound closure, a minimum time interval is necessary for bacteria to proliferate to a certain threshold level. Contaminated wounds take a mean time of about 5 hours to reach a bacterial count of 10^5/g of tissue. Attempts to close wounds that have counts higher than 10^5/g of tissue will fail 75 to 100% of the time, whereas attempts to close wounds with lower counts are successful more than 90% of the time.[7] β-Hemolytic streptococci are an exception in that much lower concentrations of these organisms consistently result in failure of wound closure. When a β-hemolytic streptococcus is the dominant isolate, the wound should generally be treated openly until cultures become negative. Good clinical judgment often makes quantitative bacteriology unnecessary, and it is not used frequently. In many modern microbiology laboratories, it is no longer available.

Systemic and Topical Antibiotics

The role of systemic antibiotics in wound management is not clearly defined. Broad-spectrum antibiotics should be given in cases of severe trauma as a prophylactic dose prior to surgery. Certain antibiotics provide broad-spectrum activity when applied topically. Neomycin, 10 mg/mL, or a combination of bacitracin, 50 U/mL, and polymyxin B, 0.05 mg/mL, kills most common wound pathogens. Other solutions that can be considered for their use in wet dressing changes include silver nitrate, sulfamylon (mafenide acetate), acetic acid, and Dakin solution. In the past few years, numerous antibacterial dressings have been developed, including an antibacterial silver-impregnated NPWT sponge. Such dressings may prove useful in the treatment of open, contaminated wounds following adequate débridement; however, discussion of these products is outside the scope of this chapter.

Topical Antiseptics

A variety of topical antiseptics have been used empirically in wound care. In the concentrations usually recommended, however, these solutions can be detrimental to wound healing. Povidone-iodine (1%), hydrogen peroxide (3%), acetic acid (0.25%), and sodium hypochlorite (0.5%) have all been shown to be lethal to fibroblasts, as well as to bacteria. More dilute concentrations of povidone-iodine (0.001%) and sodium hypochlorite (0.005%) are effective against bacteria while being safe for fibroblasts.[8] A number of these agents also inhibit normal white blood cell function in the wound. Therefore, it is best to use these solutions temporarily to treat significant contamination or colonization. Solutions also seen in the treatment of burn patients also cause common side effects; for example, silver nitrate is known to cause hyponatremia and sulfamylon is known to cause metabolic acidosis.

Damp Dressings

Open wounds can be treated with damp dressings, generally consisting of gauze soaked in saline or an acceptable topical antiseptic and then wrung out until just damp. Damp-to-damp dressings prevent desiccation of exposed vital structures or freshly placed skin grafts. Damp-to-dry dressings are useful for assisting in daily wound débridement. These dressings are allowed to dry on the wound; when they are removed, adherent fibrinous debris is removed with the dressing. Damp dressings of either type should be changed at least twice a day.

Small wounds can be expected to close by contraction and secondary epithelialization after appropriate open management with the techniques described. Large wounds will improve with aggressive open care but will then stabilize into a chronic state of wound colonization of varying degrees. A soft tissue coverage procedure may then be necessary to complete closure in these cases.

Negative-Pressure Wound Therapy

In the past 10 years, the vacuum-assisted closure (VAC) device (VAC Dressing System, Kinetic Concepts Inc., San Antonio, TX) has gained widespread acceptance for the treatment of open wounds. Because this device does not accomplish débridement to any significant degree, it should be applied only to a clean wound that has no necrotic debris or infection present. If any significant necrotic tissue remains after sharp débridement, wet-to-dry dressings may be employed until the wound is clean and granulating. Dressing changes are typically carried out every 2 or 3 days; this is a significant advantage given that conventional dressing changes are generally done at least twice daily. Exudate is removed and quantified by the suction device, and more robust wound granulation and contraction can be observed. After treatment with a VAC device, wound closure can be accomplished secondarily with a skin graft, local flaps, or free tissue transfer, depending on the clinical situation. The disadvantages of NPWT include the need for specialized equipment and training and the increased cost.

Nutrition and Wound Healing

Although a complete discussion of the importance of nutrition in wound healing is beyond the scope of this chapter, it is an important consideration in the patient's ability to heal his or her wounds. Some important clues to a patient's nutritional status can be found through the history (e.g., weight loss, new diagnosis of cancer) or physical examination (e.g., temporal wasting). Additional information can be obtained from basic laboratory values, including albumin (which is less reliable in acute trauma and massive fluid shifts and has a prolonged turnover of 3 weeks) and prealbumin, which is best interpreted with a C-reactive protein (CRP). Prealbumin/transthyretin and CRP are inversely related. Therefore, in the setting of high inflammation, CRP will be elevated, and prealbumin will be lower than its actual value. Initial values are helpful to follow as a trend, particularly for patients with long hospital and recovery courses. Early and aggressive nutritional support is imperative, and there are good data supporting improved outcomes, reduced infections, and decreased mortality when enteral feeding is begun quickly [*see Table 1*]. There is a growing body of literature indicating that initiating feeding prior to traditional measures of bowel function restoration (e.g., return of flatus, patient appetite) can be done safely and helps improve patient outcomes, including mortality.[9–11]

SELECTION OF COVERAGE PROCEDURE

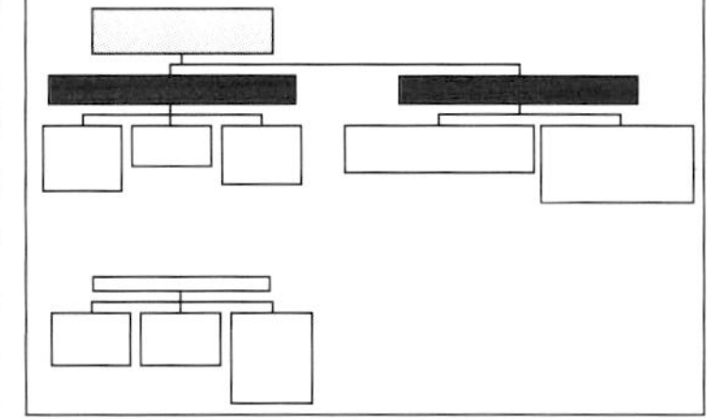

The main goals of coverage procedures in the management of both acute and chronic wounds are (1) to achieve a healed wound and (2) to avoid infection. The treatment of functional problems is generally deferred for secondary reconstruction.

The method of coverage depends on whether vital structures (e.g., vessels, tendons, nerves, and bone) are exposed in the wound. If no vital structures are exposed, skin graft coverage is indicated. Skin grafts can also be used over tendon if the paratenon is intact, over nerve if the epineurium is intact, and over bone if the periosteum is intact. Skin grafts are the most expendable type of soft tissue available for the coverage of open wounds. They allow the wound to heal completely and set the stage for secondary reconstruction, during which more valuable tissue can be used to achieve other goals at minimal risk. When vital structures are exposed in the wound, a flap is preferred because it

Table 1 Indications for Enteral Nutrition (Partial Listing)

Considered routine care in the following:
- Protein-calorie malnutrition with inadequate oral intake of nutrients for the previous 5–7 days
- Normal nutritional status but < 50% of required oral intake of nutrients for the previous 7–10 days
- Severe dysphagia
- Major full-thickness burns
- Low-output enterocutaneous fistulas
- Major trauma

Usually helpful in the following:
- Radiation therapy
- Mild chemotherapy
- Liver failure and severe renal dysfunction
- Massive small bowel resection (> 50%) in combination with administration of total parenteral nutrition

Of limited or undetermined value in the following:
- Intensive chemotherapy
- Immediate postoperative period or poststress period
- Acute enteritis
- > 90% resection of small bowel

Contraindicated in the following:
- Complete mechanical intestinal obstruction
- Abdominal distention
- Ileus or intestinal hypomotility
- Severe diarrhea
- Severe gastrointestinal bleeding
- High-output external fistulas
- Severe, acute pancreatitis
- Shock
- Case of aggressive nutritional support not desired by the patient or legal guardian and respect of such wish being in accordance with hospital policy and existing law
- Prognosis not warranting aggressive nutritional support

provides more substantial soft tissue coverage of the structure. The choice of flap depends on the location of the wound and on its overall size, depth, and topographic configuration (see below).

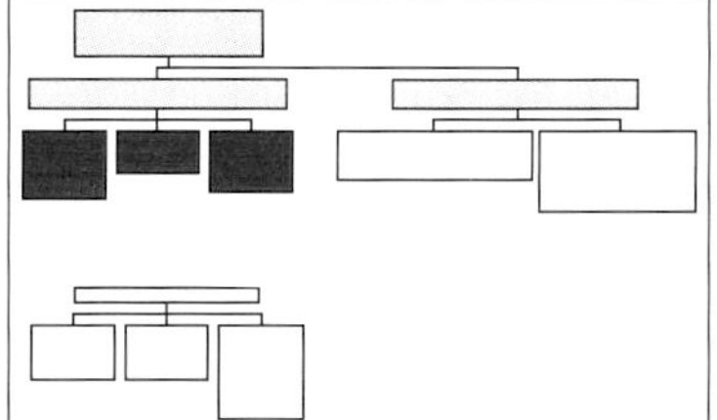

Skin Grafts

Skin grafts may be either partial thickness (i.e., split thickness) or full thickness. Split-thickness grafts are preferred for wounds with a large surface area. Full-thickness grafts are suitable only for small defects because their donor sites must be closed primarily; the most common donor sites for full-thickness grafts are the ears, upper eyelids, neck, and groin. Full-thickness grafts contract less with time than split-thickness grafts and are therefore particularly suitable for wounds of the hands, extremity flexion creases, nose, eyelids, and other areas of the face.

Successful healing of skin grafts requires immobilization of the recipient site to prevent shearing in the plane between the graft and the wound bed. Although complete immobilization is desirable, the required dressings may preclude observation of a wound that is known to be significantly contaminated. In such cases, a meshed split-thickness graft is indicated, and the wound should be treated in an open fashion. A meshed graft can be placed directly over the muscle of a flap and secured over its irregular contour with staples [*see Figure 2*]. Because the graft is meshed, serum can escape between the interstices and there is little risk of separation from the underlying tissue. A meshed graft is also less vulnerable to disruption by shear forces. An additional advantage of a meshed graft is that it permits the wound to be treated with wet dressings if there is still risk of infection. A mesh expansion ratio of 1.5:1 is generally preferred, except when the surface area of the wound is very large and the availability of donor sites is limited.

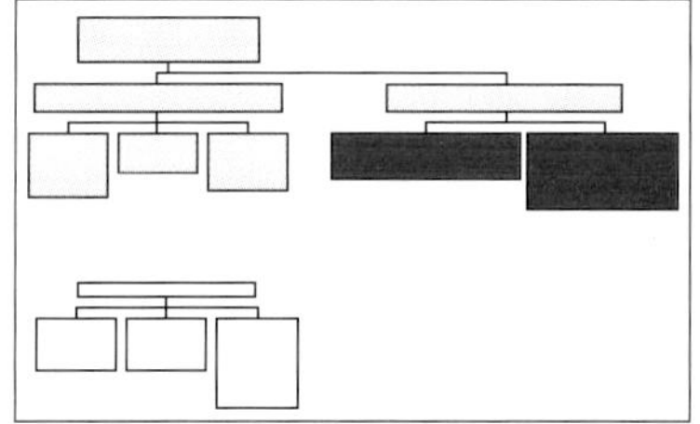

Flaps

Flaps consist of tissues that have a self-contained vascular system. They permit a more substantial transfer of tissue bulk than do skin grafts and may consist of skin and subcutaneous tissue, fascia, muscle, bone, or a combination of several tissue types. Local flaps consist of tissue that is mostly detached from surrounding tissue but retains enough connection to preserve an adequate blood supply to the entire flap. Local flaps are either transposed, rotated, or advanced into adjacent defects for the purpose of reconstruction. Island flaps are local flaps that are based only on their skeletonized axial blood supply. Once created, an island flap is transferred through a subcutaneous tunnel into the defect. The skeletonized pedicle remains in the subcutaneous space, whereas the cutaneous portion of the flap fills the defect. Free flaps, in contrast, are totally detached; their blood supply is reconnected at the recipient site by means of surgically performed microvascular anastomoses between recipient-site blood vessels and the major vessels that supply the flap.

Blood Supply

The earliest flaps in common use were skin flaps that had what is known as a random-pattern type of circulation [*see*

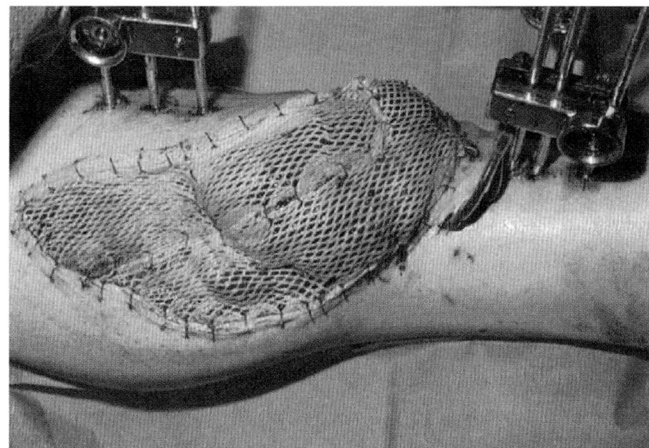

Figure 2 **A meshed (1.5:1 ratio) skin graft has been secured to the irregular contour of a muscle free flap with staples. No additional immobilization of the graft is needed. The interstices of the graft allow free drainage of serous exudate from the muscle.**

Figure 3a], in which blood is supplied by the subdermal-capillary plexus rather than by a named vessel.[12] The precarious nature of the blood supply of such flaps severely limited flap design and resulted in a preoccupation with suitable length-to-width ratios. Greater length-to-width ratios became possible after the empirical discovery that a more vigorous circulation develops in flaps raised in stages (the delay phenomenon).[13] The next flaps to come into common use had an axial-pattern type of circulation, in which a sizable artery coursed directly to a specific cutaneous territory [*see Figure 3b*]. The groin was the first region where this arrangement was carefully described, and it remains a useful source of flaps for selected applications. Because longer flaps can be made in areas where the blood supply has an axial pattern, the length-to-width ratio and the delay phenomenon became less important issues.[14] Identification of an axial-pattern blood supply to a given graft allows so-called islanding of the graft from the donor site except for the vascular connection, which is preserved. Such island flaps have greater mobility than flaps with a less attenuated attachment to the donor site.

A third type of flap was based on the myocutaneous blood supply, a network of vessels that perforate muscles vertically and supply the overlying skin [*see Figure 3c and Figure 3d*]. These vessels are not necessarily the exclusive supply to the skin in a specific region, but they are able to support the skin entirely when other sources of blood supply are eliminated. Investigation of the body musculature showed that there were at least five basic patterns of blood supply to muscle, distinguished by the existence of and balance between primary pedicles and secondary sources of blood supply [*see Figure 4*]. Some muscles can be rotated or transposed as myocutaneous flaps on the basis of either their dominant or their secondary blood supply (e.g., the pectoralis major and the latissimus dorsi). Some muscles have two dominant supplies and can be transposed on

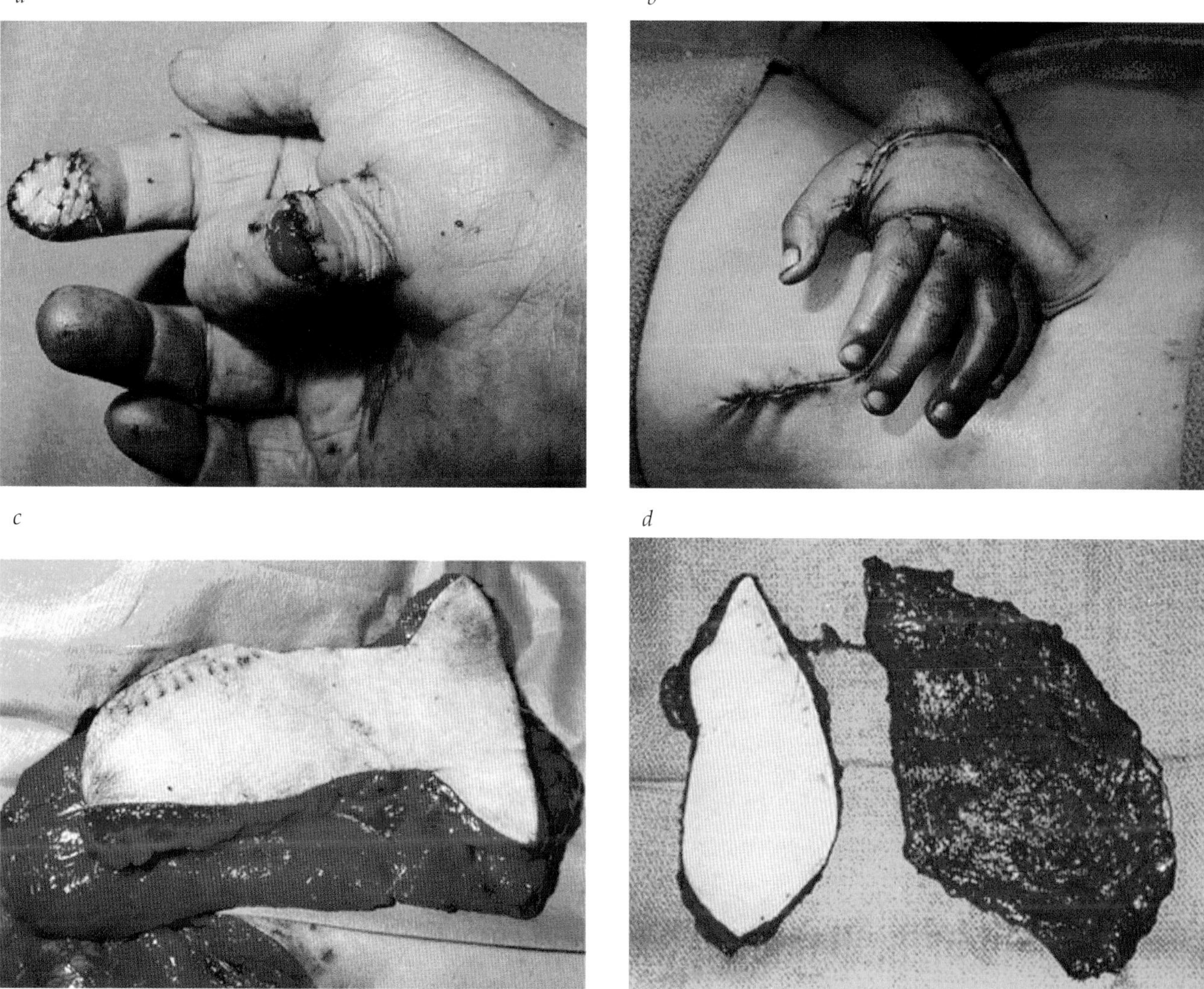

Figure 3 **(*a*) The blood supply of random-pattern skin flaps is limited; only small flaps (e.g., thenar flaps, shown here) are consistently reliable. (*b*) An axial-pattern skin flap. (*c*) The skin and subcutaneous tissue of a myocutaneous flap can exist as a complete island because the blood supply is derived from vertical muscular perforators. (*d*) A large free flap of scapular area skin and the entire latissimus dorsi. The subscapular vessels that connect the two will supply both components of the flap after microvascular anastomoses.**

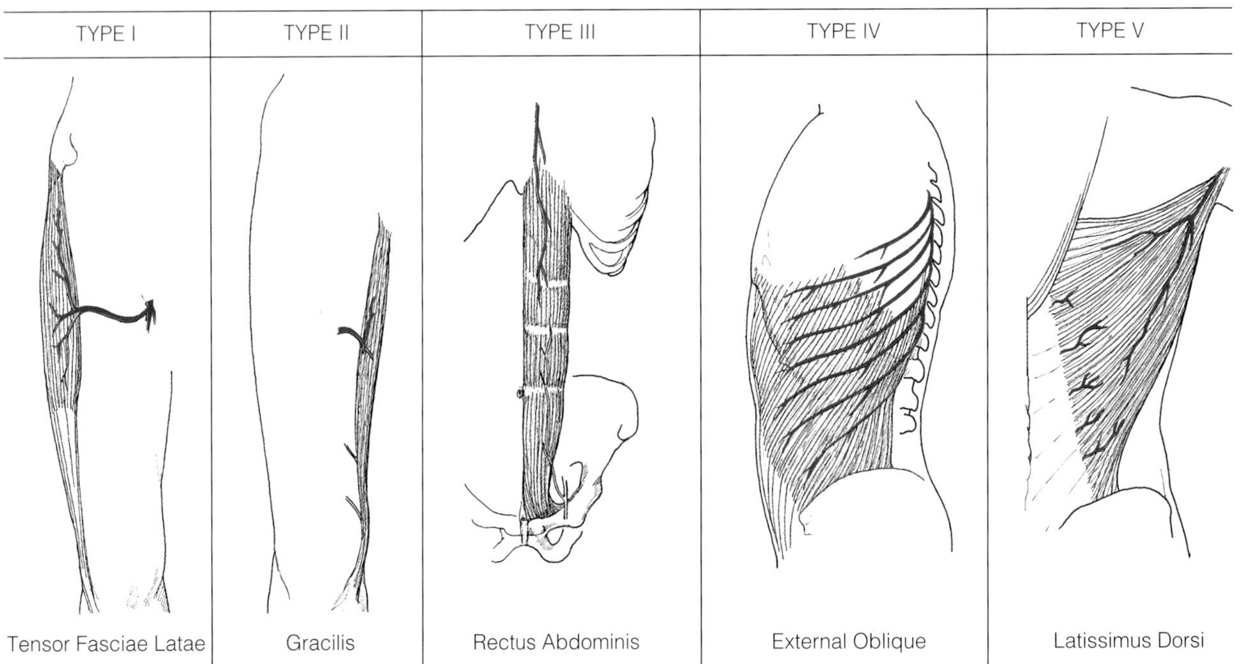

Figure 4 **Schematized are the five basic patterns of blood supply to muscle. Individual muscles are classified on the basis of the dominance, number, and size of the vessels that supply them. Type I is supplied by a single dominant pedicle. Type II is supplied by one dominant vessel and several much smaller vessels. Type III is supplied by two dominant pedicles. Type IV is supplied by multiple vessels of similar size. Type V is supplied by one dominant pedicle and several smaller segmental vascular pedicles.**

either one (e.g., the rectus abdominis). Other muscles do not reliably support skin territories supplied by minor pedicles (e.g., the gracilis).

Other patterns of cutaneous blood supply are now well recognized. Fasciocutaneous flaps with high length-to-width ratios can be reliably raised on the trunk, arms, and legs. The blood supply of deep fascia appears to consist of both a deep and a superficial fascial plexus. These vessels connect both to perforating vessels from the underlying muscles and to the subcutaneous tissue vessels above them.[15] At least three types of fasciocutaneous flaps may be distinguished on the basis of the fascial blood supply to the skin [*see Figure 5*].[16]

In some areas, fascia supplies overlying subcutaneous tissue and skin more directly. Such a blood supply is most evident in the extremities, where direct branches from major vessels course through intermuscular septa to reach the deep fascia and supply the overlying skin and subcutaneous tissue. The forearm is a clinically important donor site because thin septocutaneous flaps fed by the radial artery can be raised as either pedicled or free flaps. Other examples of fasciocutaneous flaps include the lateral arm septocutaneous flap, fed by the profunda brachii artery; the scapular flap, fed by the circumflex scapular artery [*see Figure 3d*]; the fibular osteofasciocutaneous flap, fed by the peroneal artery; and the anterolateral thigh flap, fed by the descending branch of the lateral circumflex femoral artery.

The 21st century has seen the popularization of "perforator" flaps, which are based on musculocutaneous branches (or perforators) of named, axial vessels. In the early years of microsurgery, success was defined by a lack of microvascular thrombosis. As experience was gained and rates of microvascular anastomotic failure decreased, focus was then turned on limiting donor-site morbidity. Several myocutaneous flaps used primarily for their skin and subcutaneous components were modified such that musculocutaneous perforators supplying the overlying fat and skin were dissected through the muscle down to the pedicle origin, thus preserving muscle and function. Common perforator flaps include the deep inferior epigastric perforator flap, or DIEP flap, and the superior and inferior gluteal artery perforator flaps, or SGAP and IGAP flaps. These flaps are commonly performed for breast reconstruction. The anterolateral thigh flap, or ALT flap, is supplied by a musculocutaneous perforator of the descending branch of the lateral circumflex femoral artery roughly two thirds of the time and by a septocutaneous branch one third of the time.

TYPES OF LOCAL FLAPS

Transposition Flaps

A flap that is moved laterally into the primary defect is called a transposition flap. The essential concept in the design of such a flap is to ensure that the flap is long enough to cover the entire defect so that the transfer can be done without tension [*see Figure 6*].

The skin is marked and incised with a scalpel, and dissection is carried through the subcutaneous fat. The flap is retracted with a skin hook, and dissection is performed with blunt scissors until the flap is elevated sufficiently to allow it to be transposed into the defect without tension. The secondary defect is closed primarily; alternatively, depending on the location of the donor area and the degree of skin

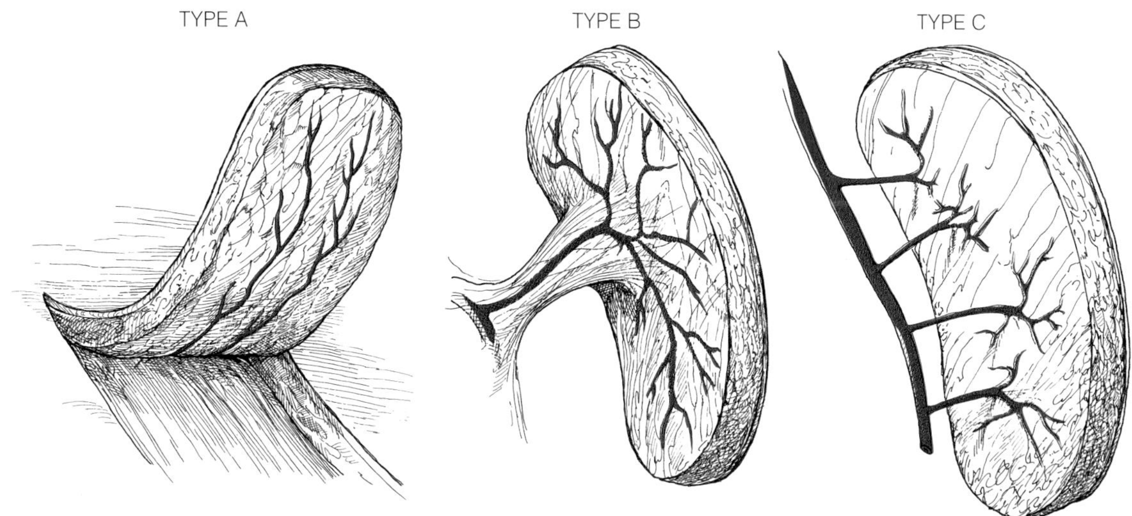

Figure 5 **At least three types of fasciocutaneous flaps exist, categorized by blood supply configuration. Type A is supplied by multiple small, longitudinal vessels coursing with the deep fascia. These flaps must retain a base of a certain width and cannot be raised as islands (e.g., longitudinally oriented flaps of skin and fascia on the lower leg). Type B is supplied by a single major vessel within the fascia (e.g., scapular flap). Type C is supplied by multiple perforating segments from a major vessel coursing through intermuscular septa (e.g., forearm flaps).**

tension present there, a skin graft may be indicated. As with any local flap, wide undermining of the surrounding tissues may be necessary for closure of the defect and the donor site. Closure is then performed in two layers.

Bilobed flap A bilobed flap is a transposition flap consisting of two lobes of skin and subcutaneous tissue based on a common pedicle [*see Figure 7*]. It is often used to correct nasal defects involving the lateral aspect, the ala, or the tip. The keys to a successful bilobed flap are (1) accurate design and (2) wide undermining of the surrounding tissue in the submuscular plane to allow a smooth transposition. The primary lobe is usually at an angle of 45 or less to the defect; the secondary lobe is designed to achieve closure of the donor defect and is substantially smaller than the primary lobe. The angle between the two is 90 to 100 . Both flaps are raised simultaneously in the submuscular plane. Wide undermining of the area (also in the submuscular plane) minimizes tension. The primary lobe of the bilobed flap is transposed into the initial defect, the secondary lobe is transposed into the donor defect left by the primary lobe, and the defect left by the secondary lobe is closed primarily. Closure is accomplished with 5-0 or 6-0 nylon.

Rhomboid flap (Limberg flap) A rhomboid flap is a transposition flap that is designed in a specific geometric fashion [*see Figure 8*]. The initial defect is converted to a rhomboid, with care taken to plan the flap in an area with minimal skin tension. The rhomboid must be an equilateral parallelogram with angles of 60 ; and 120 ; this design allows the surgeon to excise less tissue than would be needed for an elliptical flap. One face of the rhomboid constitutes the first side of the flap (YZ). The short diagonal of the rhomboid is then extended outward for a distance equal to

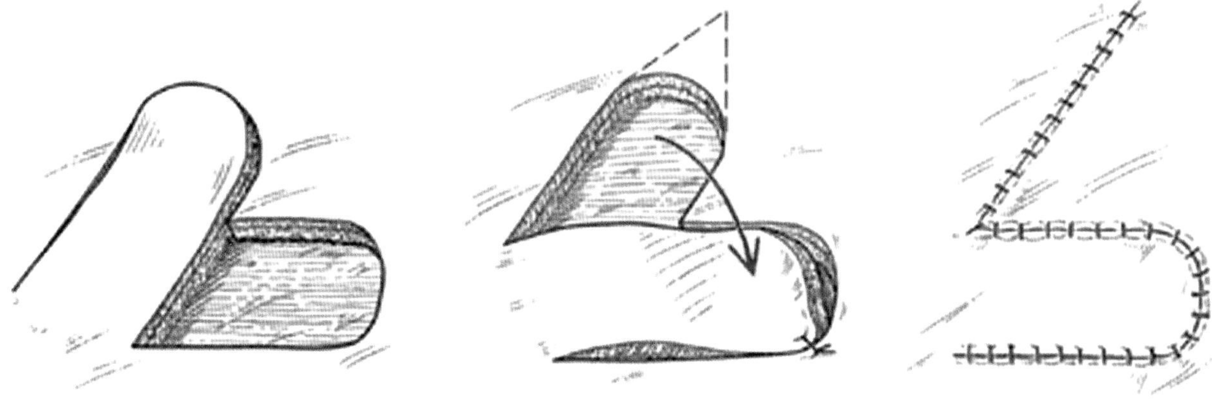

Figure 6 **After excision of the defect, a transposition flap of adequate length is designed and elevated in the subcutaneous plane. The flap is moved laterally into the defect and inset. It may be necessary to excise a dog-ear of excess skin at the tip of the flap harvest site.**

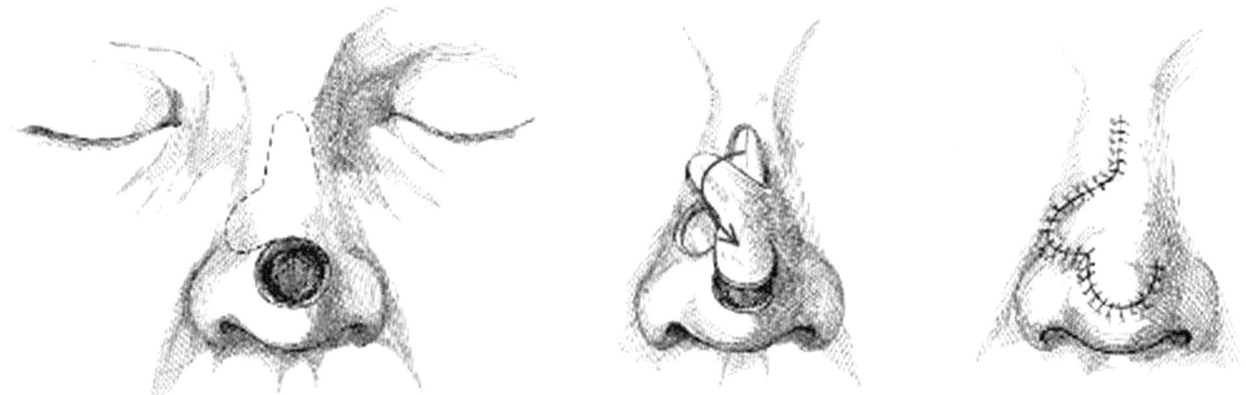

Figure 7 **A flap with two lobes is created, with the first lobe the same size as the defect and the second lobe substantially (50%) smaller than the first. The flap is elevated in the submuscular plane. Wide undermining at this level is necessary for tension-free transposition. The first lobe covers the initial defect, and the second covers the defect from the first. The second lobe is placed in an area of loose skin, and its area of origin is closed primarily.**

its own length. This extension should be oriented along relaxed skin tension lines, perpendicular to the line of maximum extensibility; it constitutes the second side of the flap (XY). Next, a line parallel and equal in length to YZ is drawn from Y to outline the third side of the flap. Correct orientation of the rhomboid is vital for achieving flap repair with minimal tension, particularly with respect to the line of maximum extensibility: it is along this base line that maximum tension results when the donor defect is closed. Once the flap has been correctly designed and elevated, it is transposed into the defect. Closure is done in two layers. Rhomboid flaps work best on flat surfaces (e.g., the upper cheek, the temporal region, and the trunk). Extra attention to flap design is necessary when an attempt is made to close a defect over a convex surface with a rhomboid flap; improper flap design leads to excessive tension and potential flap necrosis.

Rotation Flaps

A flap that is rotated into the defect is called a rotation flap.[17,18] This type of flap is commonly used to repair a defect on the scalp, where large flaps must be designed to overcome the inelasticity of scalp tissue. A rotation flap takes the form of a semicircle, of which the defect occupies a wedge-shaped segment [*see Figure 9*]. The original defect is converted to a triangular shape (ABC). One side of the triangular defect (AC) is extended to a point (D) that will serve as the pivot point for the flap. The distance between A and D should be at least 50% greater than that between A and C. A semicircular line extending from C to D is then defined.

The flap is incised with a scalpel, elevated, and rotated. As with all local skin flaps, wide undermining of the surrounding tissue may be necessary to allow tension-free rotation and wound closure. The flap is secured with a two-layer closure; the secondary defect may be closed primarily. Sometimes a so-called back cut is required to gain adequate rotation. The most common technical error with rotation flaps is improper design: a flap that is too small will not cover the defect adequately.

Advancement Flaps

Advancement flaps are moved directly forward into a defect without either rotation or lateral movement. The

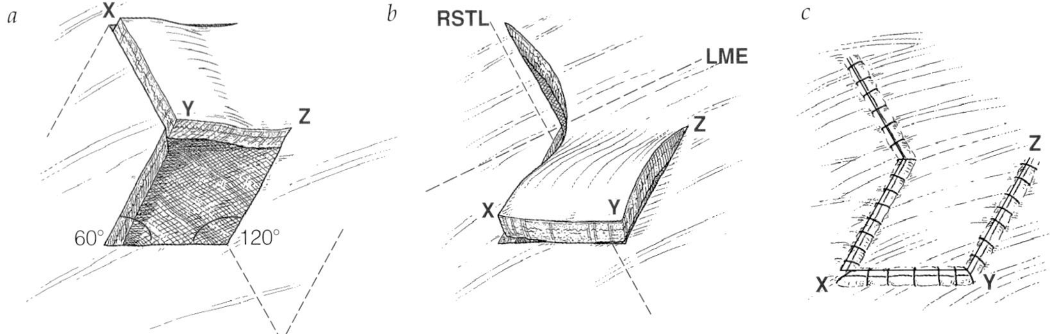

Figure 8 **(*a*) The defect is converted to a rhomboid, with all four sides of equal length and angles of 60 and 120 . An extension XY is made that is the same length as the short diagonal of the rhomboid, and a line of equal length is drawn from X paralleling YZ. (*b*) The flap is oriented so that XY follows the relaxed skin tension lines (RSTL) and YZ the line of maximum extensibility (LME). (*c*) The flap is inset.**

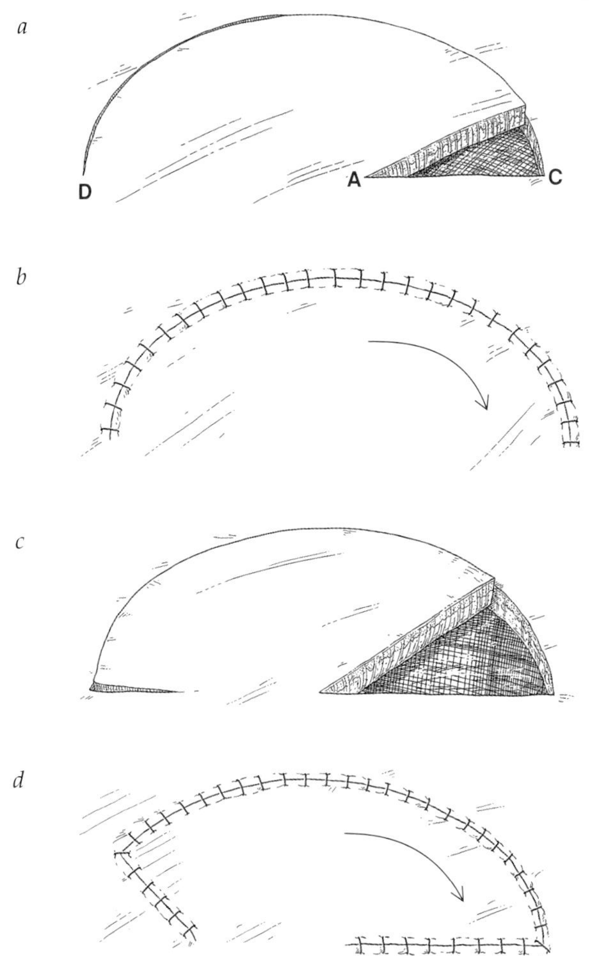

Figure 9 (*a*) The defect is converted into a wedge. One side (AC) is extended to a pivot point D, so that AD is at least 50% longer than AC. A semicircle from C to D is defined. (*b*) The flap is elevated, rotated, and inset. (*c, d*) If there is too much tension, a back cut may be necessary to release the flap and allow rotation. Care is taken not to make the back cut excessively long; to do so could devascularize the flap.

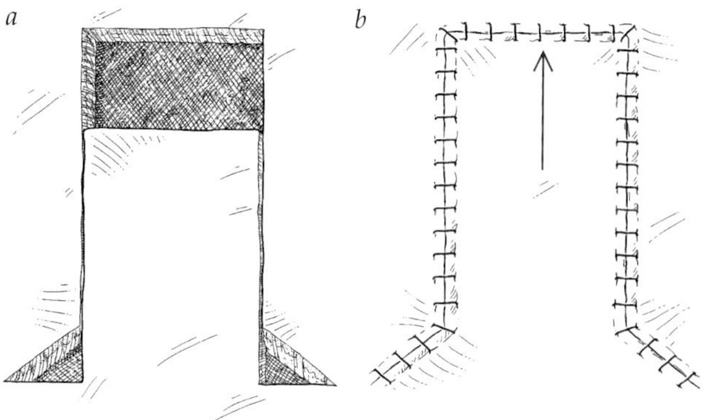

Figure 10 (*a*) A flap whose shape corresponds to that of the defect is elevated in the subcutaneous plane and advanced into the defect. (*b*) Excision of Burow triangles (excess skin at the flap base) may be necessary to permit advancement.

single-pedicle advancement flap is a rectangular or square flap of skin and subcutaneous tissue that is stretched forward. The flap is oriented with respect to the local skin tension, with care taken to plan the advancement in an area where the skin is extensible. A rectangular defect is created, and the flap is elevated in an area of loose skin and advanced to cover the defect [*see Figure 10*]. When closure is performed, some excess skin (dog-ears) at the base of the flap (Burow triangles) may have to be excised.

V-Y advancement flap The V-Y advancement flap is a modification of a basic advancement flap [*see Figure 11*]. The use of a V-Y advancement flap eliminates the need to revise the dog-ears that sometimes result with rotation flaps. When possible, the flap should be oriented in accordance with the line of maximum extensibility. Its length should be 1.5 to 2 times that of the defect in the direction of the closure.

Incisions are made completely through skin. As with other flaps, skin hooks are used to retract the skin flap, and blunt scissors dissection is then performed. The point of the V on the flap is the area where tightness is most frequently encountered; this area may have to be released to facilitate advancement. Care must be taken not to undermine the advancing flap excessively: doing so may impair or interrupt the blood supply to the flap and result in necrosis. Once adequately advanced, the flap is sutured at the advancing edge and at the base of the Y.

Z-Plasty

When reconstruction is indicated for small, localized scars, soft tissue coverage is generally sufficient. With such coverage, there is no threat of breakdown leading to exposure of important structures; instead, the reconstructive problem is generally functional. An example is a flexion crease contracture, which is commonly seen after a burn injury. A local procedure that rearranges the existing tissue can relieve the tension by making more tissue available in one direction, even though the amount of tissue in the area is not actually increased.

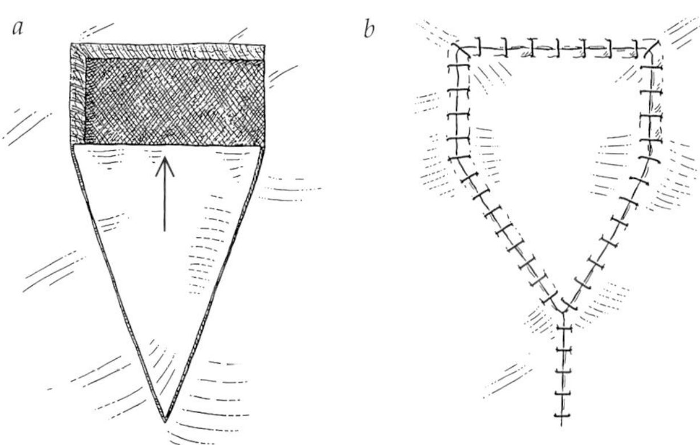

Figure 11 (*a*) A V-shaped flap is created whose length is 1.5 to 2 times that of the defect. With subcutaneous connections to the skin preserved (because these constitute the blood supply to the flap), the flap is advanced into the defect. (*b*) The V incision is converted to a Y as the base is closed primarily.

The Z-plasty [*see Figure 12*] is an example of such tissue rearrangement.[19] Two triangular flaps are designed so that they have in common a central limb aligned in the direction along which additional length is desired. For example, the limb may be placed along the line of a contracture. Two lines, approximately equal in length to the central limb, are drawn from either end of the limb, diverging from it at equal angles varying from 30 to 90 . The degree of lengthening obtained is determined by the size of this angle [*see Table 2*]. In theory, maximal length gain is achieved by using the largest angle possible, but in practice, the maximum usable angle is determined by the limits of skin elasticity. A 60 angle, which is commonly used, will result in a 75% gain in length along the central limb. Triangular flaps are elevated, and the fibrous tissue band responsible for the contracture is divided. The triangular flaps are transposed and inset, yielding increased length in the desired direction, with the original Z rotated 90 and reversed.

Although Z-plasty is conceptually simple, it is not necessarily easy: experience is necessary for the surgeon to realize the limitations of technique and appreciate the subtleties of proper design. Important considerations in the use of Z-plasty include appropriate determination of the length of the central limb and correct orientation of the limbs so that the new central limb formed after transposition is parallel to skin tension lines. Multiple Z-plasties may be useful for some localized scars.

Local flaps versus free flaps The choice between a local flap and a free flap is determined by the amount and the type of tissue needed, as well as by the availability of flaps in the immediate area of the wound [*see Figure 13*]. The availability of local flaps, in turn, is determined by the nature of the regional blood supply. The vascular anatomy of a particular area determines the availability of arterialized skin flaps, fasciocutaneous flaps, myocutaneous flaps, and other forms of composite flaps. Local flaps can be grouped regionally by the types of tissue that they provide.

A local flap is generally preferred over a free flap if the two provide similar tissue, primarily because of the additional effort required to transfer a free flap. A free flap procedure commonly takes twice as long as a local flap procedure.

Free flaps are indicated in areas where local flaps are unavailable (e.g., the distal third of the leg) or when an extremely large flap is needed but cannot be obtained locally. When regional donor sites are affected by the primary process, free tissue transfer allows healthy, well-vascularized tissue to be brought into the compromised area. Moreover, if free tissue is transferred, the size of the wound is not extended, because the donor site is not contiguous but instead is located at a distance from the wound.

If expertise in microvascular surgery is available, free flaps are frequently a first-line choice. Free flaps allow selection of the appropriate type of tissue in the most suitable size and configuration for the specific reconstructive problem. Compared with free flaps, local flaps are inefficient ways of moving tissue because only a small portion of a local flap actually reaches the defect itself. The choice of donor site is greater with free flaps because the limitations imposed by local availability are avoided.

Table 2 Z-Plasty: Incision Angle and Degree of Lengthening Theoretically Possible

Incision Angle (°)	*Theoretical Amount of Lengthening (%)*
30	25
45	50
60	75
75	100
90	120

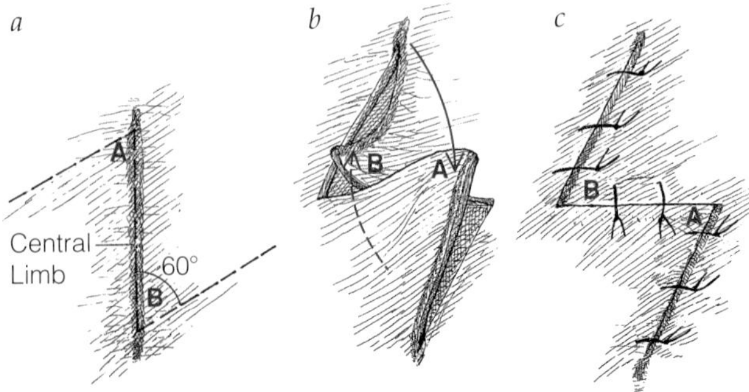

Figure 12 **(*a*) The central limb of the Z is placed along the line of contracture. Incisions diverging from the scar at a 60 angle will yield an increase of approximately 75% in the direction of the central limb. (*b*) The flaps are transposed. (*c*) The length has been increased in the desired direction, and the original Z design has been rotated 90 and reversed.**

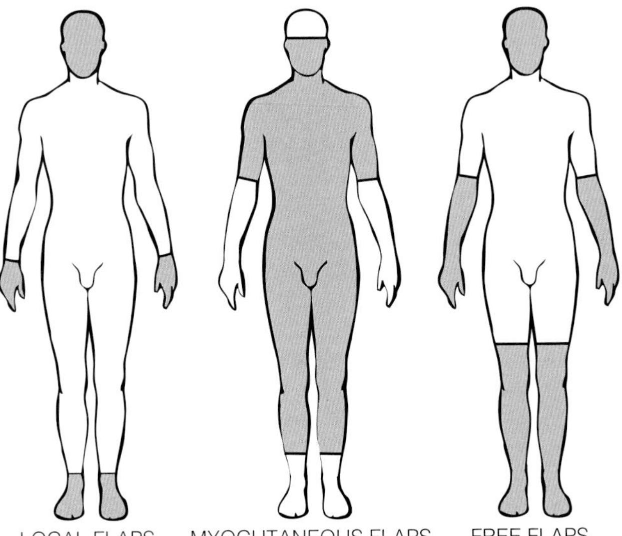

Figure 13 **Defects in the central portion of the body are treated with myocutaneous flaps primarily; defects of the peripheral areas are treated with either local flaps or free flaps. In some areas, several options exist, and the choice is influenced by the size of the defect and the specific tissue requirements.**

REGIONAL ALTERNATIVES IN FLAP SELECTION

Head and Neck

Facial defects of small to moderate size are best treated with local skin flaps [*see Figure 14*]. A variety of flaps are available for reconstruction of limited defects of the eyelids, cheeks, nose, and mouth.[20–22] Small facial defects that do not directly involve the facial features can often be closed with any of several types of flaps that rearrange the existing tissue in the area—for example, a Z-plasty or a Limberg flap. Tissues that are difficult to match (e.g., those of the eyelids or lips) can often be reconstructed with flaps that borrow tissue from their opposite, intact counterparts (e.g., the Abbe lip flap).

For coverage of some large defects in the head and neck region, the trapezius, the latissimus dorsi, and the pectoralis major can be used. Each muscle can be raised with an optional skin island. These flaps are generally too bulky to be used on the face, and their reach is limited when used as pedicled flaps. None of them can cover major portions of the scalp or comfortably reach the upper face.

Latissimus dorsi, scapular, and rectus abdominis free flaps are useful for very large defects of the scalp or upper face. Smaller defects of the scalp are best treated with local scalp flaps.

Other free flaps of a specialized nature are superior for reconstruction of the floor of the mouth and mandible, even though local myocutaneous flaps will reach this area. For example, the forearm free flap based on the radial artery is quite thin and pliable and therefore provides an ideal replacement for the floor of the mouth. Composite free flaps that contain both bone and skin (e.g., those taken from the scapula, the ilium, the radius, and the fibula) provide tissue of the appropriate type and proper configuration for defects of the lower face in which the mandible must be reconstructed along with the intraoral lining, the external skin, or both.

Chest and Back

Most clean defects of the chest and back are amenable to treatment with local myocutaneous flaps because of the wide arc of rotation of muscles located in these areas.[23] In the presence of contamination, open wound management is indicated. Traditionally, this has been accomplished with wet-to-dry dressing changes, which are especially effective for superficial débridement. Currently, these wounds are increasingly being managed with NPWT after all necrotic tissue is débrided. A common example is the wound resulting from the treatment of poststernotomy mediastinitis. After sepsis is eliminated and the wound is granulating, definitive flap closure can be performed.[24,25] Midline sternal wounds can be covered with pectoralis major, rectus abdominis, or omental flaps; lateral chest defects with latissimus dorsi or pectoralis major flaps; and midline back defects with latissimus dorsi or trapezius flaps. To cover midline defects, the pectoralis major, the latissimus dorsi, and the trapezius can be divided from their primary vascular supply and folded over as local flaps based on their medial segmental intercostal secondary blood supply.

Arm and Forearm

Large wounds above the elbow can be covered with a latissimus dorsi myocutaneous flap transposed as a pedicled flap provided that the vascular pedicle of the muscle has not been affected by the injury. Forearm wounds that require flap closure are best treated with free flaps. A rectus abdominis, scapular, anterolateral thigh, or latissimus dorsi muscle flap can be used for large defects of the arm or forearm. Although soft tissue coverage with simultaneous functional forearm muscle replacement can be achieved with a single flap (e.g., a gracilis muscle flap), this is generally reserved as a secondary operation. A skin flap (e.g., a scapular free flap) is preferred as a first stage of reconstruction to achieve wound healing.

Hand

Both free flaps and pedicled skin flaps are useful for soft tissue coverage of hand wounds. A temporalis fascia free flap is particularly thin and is ideal for coverage of exposed tendons on the dorsum of the hand. A lateral arm free flap is ideal for reconstruction of a large defect of the first web space; it has sensory potential because it contains a large sensory nerve. Both of these free flaps are small. Pedicled distant skin flaps from the chest or abdomen are available as an alternative form of coverage for sizable hand defects. However, pedicled skin flaps have major disadvantages: wound care is difficult, edema persists because elevation and movement of the hand are seldom possible while it is attached to the trunk, and a second procedure is needed to divide these flaps.

Digital injuries with exposed tendons can be closed with a variety of cross-finger flaps of skin and subcutaneous tissue raised from either the volar or extensor aspect of an adjacent digit. Because these flaps do not contain a great deal of subcutaneous tissue, they are preferred for coverage of digits proximally, where a thick subcutaneous pad is not essential. A thenar flap is useful for fingertip injuries in which the soft tissue pad of the fingertip is lost and bone is exposed. This flap provides an ideal pulp replacement, as well as better sensory recovery than skin grafts. Fingertip injuries can also be closed with several types of V-Y advancement flaps that can be raised from either the volar surface or the lateral surface of the end of the finger.

Abdomen

Clean defects of the abdominal wall that require flap closure are best treated with local muscle flaps such as the tensor fasciae latae and the rectus femoris from the thigh. The rectus abdominis also can occasionally be transposed to cover an abdominal defect. Each of these flaps is harvested along with skin, although a large tensor fasciae latae flap will probably necessitate skin graft closure of the donor site. The tensor fasciae latae flap has the advantage of including the thickened deep fascia (iliotibial band) of the thigh, which can provide additional strength for abdominal wall closure. Midline defects resulting from previous operation or trauma can often be closed by means of the component separation method. The external oblique fascia is divided lateral to the lateral edge of the rectus sheath, and the bloodless plane between the external and internal oblique muscles is developed. This maneuver mobilizes the recti toward the midline, usually allowing primary closure. Adding a prosthetic mesh reduces the recurrent rate of hernias but is more difficult to manage when exposed or infected.

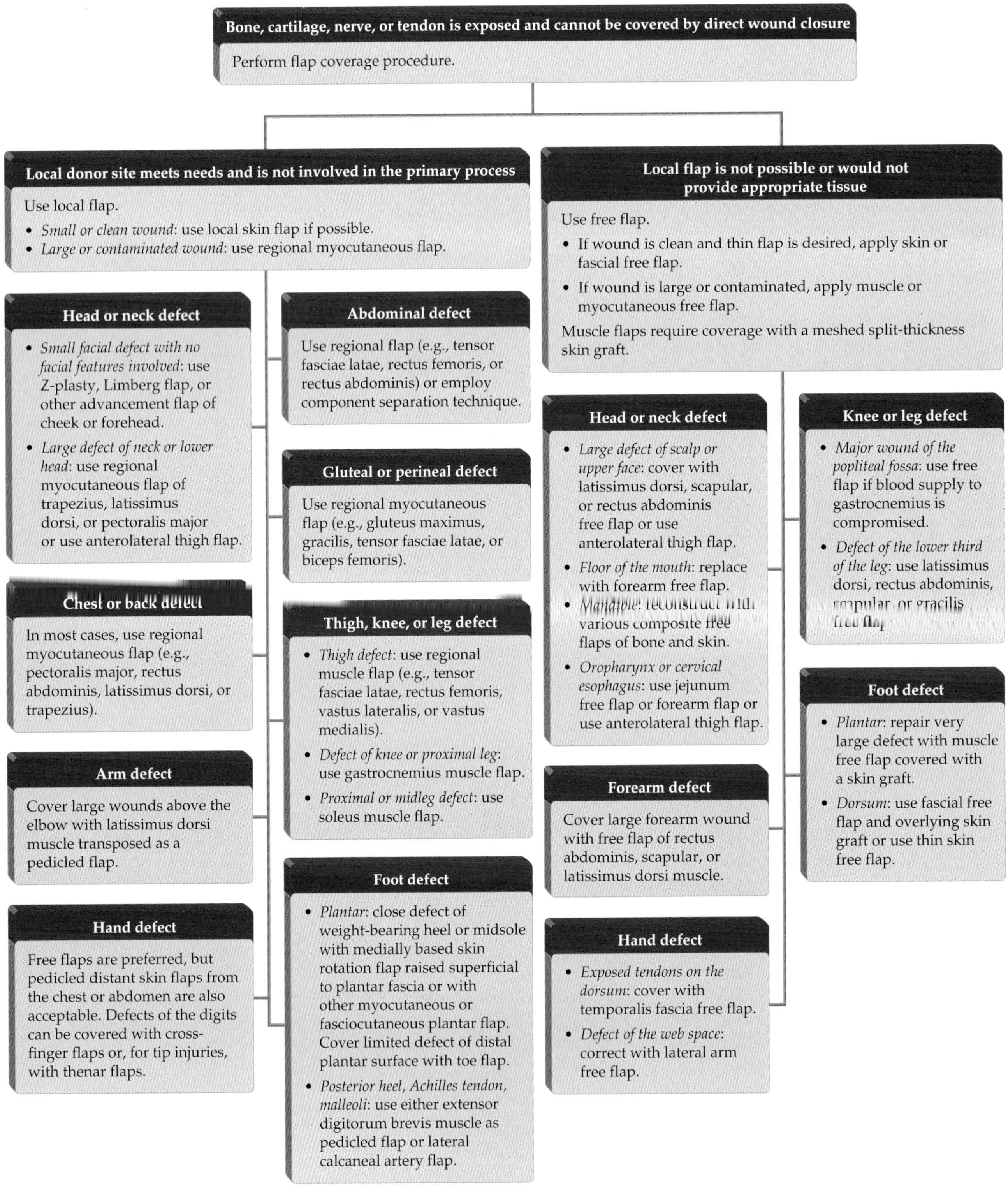

Bone, cartilage, nerve, or tendon is exposed and cannot be covered by direct wound closure

Perform flap coverage procedure.

Local donor site meets needs and is not involved in the primary process

Use local flap.

- *Small or clean wound*: use local skin flap if possible.
- *Large or contaminated wound*: use regional myocutaneous flap.

Head or neck defect

- *Small facial defect with no facial features involved*: use Z-plasty, Limberg flap, or other advancement flap of cheek or forehead.
- *Large defect of neck or lower head*: use regional myocutaneous flap of trapezius, latissimus dorsi, or pectoralis major or use anterolateral thigh flap.

Chest or back defect

In most cases, use regional myocutaneous flap (e.g., pectoralis major, rectus abdominis, latissimus dorsi, or trapezius).

Arm defect

Cover large wounds above the elbow with latissimus dorsi muscle transposed as a pedicled flap.

Hand defect

Free flaps are preferred, but pedicled distant skin flaps from the chest or abdomen are also acceptable. Defects of the digits can be covered with cross-finger flaps or, for tip injuries, with thenar flaps.

Abdominal defect

Use regional flap (e.g., tensor fasciae latae, rectus femoris, or rectus abdominis) or employ component separation technique.

Gluteal or perineal defect

Use regional myocutaneous flap (e.g., gluteus maximus, gracilis, tensor fasciae latae, or biceps femoris).

Thigh, knee, or leg defect

- *Thigh defect*: use regional muscle flap (e.g., tensor fasciae latae, rectus femoris, vastus lateralis, or vastus medialis).
- *Defect of knee or proximal leg*: use gastrocnemius muscle flap.
- *Proximal or midleg defect*: use soleus muscle flap.

Foot defect

- *Plantar*: close defect of weight-bearing heel or midsole with medially based skin rotation flap raised superficial to plantar fascia or with other myocutaneous or fasciocutaneous plantar flap. Cover limited defect of distal plantar surface with toe flap.
- *Posterior heel, Achilles tendon, malleoli*: use either extensor digitorum brevis muscle as pedicled flap or lateral calcaneal artery flap.

Local flap is not possible or would not provide appropriate tissue

Use free flap.

- If wound is clean and thin flap is desired, apply skin or fascial free flap.
- If wound is large or contaminated, apply muscle or myocutaneous free flap.

Muscle flaps require coverage with a meshed split-thickness skin graft.

Head or neck defect

- *Large defect of scalp or upper face*: cover with latissimus dorsi, scapular, or rectus abdominis free flap or use anterolateral thigh flap.
- *Floor of the mouth*: replace with forearm free flap.
- *Mandible*: reconstruct with various composite free flaps of bone and skin.
- *Oropharynx or cervical esophagus*: use jejunum free flap or forearm flap or use anterolateral thigh flap.

Forearm defect

Cover large forearm wound with free flap of rectus abdominis, scapular, or latissimus dorsi muscle.

Hand defect

- *Exposed tendons on the dorsum*: cover with temporalis fascia free flap.
- *Defect of the web space*: correct with lateral arm free flap.

Knee or leg defect

- *Major wound of the popliteal fossa*: use free flap if blood supply to gastrocnemius is compromised.
- *Defect of the lower third of the leg*: use latissimus dorsi, rectus abdominis, scapular, or gracilis free flap.

Foot defect

- *Plantar*: repair very large defect with muscle free flap covered with a skin graft.
- *Dorsum*: use fascial free flap and overlying skin graft or use thin skin free flap.

Figure 14 **Diagnostic algorithm outlining regional alternatives in flap selection.**

As a consequence of the growing realization of the benefits of the open abdomen, increasing numbers of patients treated for abdominal trauma, sepsis, and compartment syndrome are presenting for management and closure. With contaminated wounds, the use of permanent meshes for reconstruction is contraindicated, and definitive flap closure is best delayed. In these difficult situations, the wound must be treated in an open manner, with close attention paid to the unique vulnerability of the intestines to fistula formation. Many treatment options are currently available for the open abdomen. Important considerations for any treatment modality include whether the method controls abdominal contents, whether it avoids promoting fistula formation, whether it achieves skin and fascial closure, whether it removes and quantifies exudate, whether it controls infection, and whether it promotes wound healing. The VAC device performs well with respect to all of these considerations, perhaps because of reverse tissue expansion and full-thickness wound contraction.[26,27] Once all acute problems have been addressed and recovery is well under way, an absorbable mesh is commonly applied, followed by dressing changes or NPWT. To protect the underlying bowel, a layer of nonstick gauze should be applied before dressings or NPWT sponges. Once granulation is achieved, a skin graft can be placed. Chronic hernia formation is the rule and can generally be treated as a stable chronic ventral hernia provided that the wound is closed and free of infection.

Gluteal Area and Perineum

Local muscle flaps with or without skin are indicated for defects in the gluteal area or the perineum. Such flaps are preferable to large, random-pattern advancement skin flaps from the posterior thigh and thoracolumbar rotation skin flaps. The gluteus maximus, for example, can be used as a rotation flap, a V-Y advancement flap, or a turnover flap in the treatment of pressure sores. As a turnover flap, it can be proximally or distally based, or it can be split along its longitudinal axis so that only a portion of it is used. Also useful for covering defects in the gluteal area and the perineum is the myofasciocutaneous gluteal thigh flap, which is a combination of a gluteus muscle flap and a fasciocutaneous flap from the posterior thigh that is supplied by an extension of the inferior gluteal artery. Because of its size and location, the gracilis muscle is well suited for coverage of defects of the perineum. The gracilis and the biceps femoris are generally secondary choices for the treatment of pressure sores over the ischium. The tensor fasciae latae is frequently used for treating open wounds over the greater trochanter. The entire quadriceps can be used to close defects resulting from hemipelvectomy.

Thigh

Flaps are rarely required for soft tissue coverage in the thigh area because critical vital structures are located deep within the thigh and are rarely exposed by injury or by surgical procedures. A number of regional muscle flaps are available for coverage in this region, however, including the tensor fasciae latae, the rectus femoris, the vastus lateralis, and the vastus medialis. An anterior defect that involves exposure of the femoral vessels can be covered with a rectus abdominis myocutaneous flap, a rectus femoris flap divided distally and turned over, or a sartorius flap. The sartorius muscle has a segmental blood supply and will not be reliable if more than one to two segmental pedicles are ligated, which limits its utility for larger defects. A number of smaller local skin flaps that are supplied with blood from the deep fascia can be raised over portions of the thigh. The anterolateral thigh flap is the most commonly employed thigh flap for free tissue transfer.

Knee, Proximal Leg, and Midleg

The two heads of the gastrocnemius can be used either together or independently to cover defects of the knee and the proximal third of the leg. The soleus is useful for coverage of defects of the proximal and middle thirds of the leg. Local flaps should not be used for major leg wounds if the extent of the injury suggests involvement of the muscle donor site. Instead, a free flap should be used to bring healthy tissue into the area. Therefore, free flaps are a first choice, for example, for coverage of major wounds of the popliteal fossa, knee, and proximal leg that involve the sural artery blood supply to the gastrocnemius; they are also highly useful for coverage of defects in the distal third of the leg. Traumatic wounds of the distal lower extremity can also be managed with NPWT. Increased use of this modality has been associated with the performance of fewer free tissue transfers and more delayed local flap procedures for definitive closure.[1]

Skin flaps fed by the fascial blood supply can also be raised over the leg.[28] A number of fasciocutaneous flaps have been described in this area, but they tend to be smaller than muscle flaps and generally less reliable. These flaps are longitudinally oriented over the course of the anterior tibial artery or the peroneal artery. The maximum length at which such fasciocutaneous flaps are safe and their specific applications have not been well established.

Foot

The foot is as complex as the hand and the face in that it is composed of separate regions, each of which has a unique set of alternatives for reconstruction. These regions include the plantar surface; the dorsum; and the posterior (non–weight-bearing) heel, Achilles tendon, and malleoli.

Superficial defects that lie completely within the non–weight-bearing portion of the midsole do not need flap coverage. Defects of the weight-bearing heel and midsole area that are less than 6 cm in diameter can be closed with a medially based skin rotation flap that is raised superficial to the plantar fascia.[29] This flap maintains plantar sensation. Limited defects of the distal plantar surface can be treated with local toe flaps that also maintain sensation. Very large plantar defects are best resurfaced with a muscle free flap (e.g., latissimus dorsi, gracilis, or rectus abdominis) covered with a skin graft or thin fasciocutaneous flaps. Although this type of flap lacks sensation, it appears to provide the most durable form of coverage because it resists shear forces well.[30]

Defects of the dorsum that require flap coverage are best covered either with a fascial free flap (e.g., temporalis fascia) and an overlying skin graft or with a skin free flap that is thin (e.g., from the forearm or the anterolateral thigh). The extensor digitorum brevis can be raised from the dorsum as a pedicled flap fed by the dorsalis pedis artery. This flap, which measures approximately 5 × 6 cm, has an arc of rotation that makes it useful for the coverage of defects of the malleolus or the Achilles tendon area. A narrow transposition skin flap fed by the lateral calcaneal artery is useful for coverage of defects approximately 3 cm in diameter that lie over the Achilles tendon or the non–weight-bearing posterior heel. A distally based reverse sural artery flap transfers skin, subcutaneous fat, and fascia from the proximal posterior calf based on the vasa nervorum of the sural nerve, supplied by a distal branch of the peroneal at the level of the malleolus. This flap can also be used for defects of the ankle; however, it can be prone to venous congestion.

Secondary Reconstruction

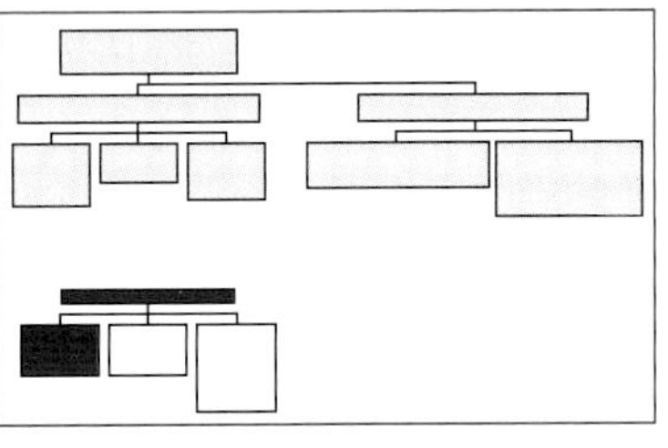

Selection of the proper method for secondary reconstruction requires analysis of the type and extent of tissue deficiency that is present and consideration of the functional goals that are involved. Superficial defects may require replacement or supplementation of only skin and subcutaneous tissue, whereas more complex defects may require replacement of several types of tissue. Specialized tissue, such as vascularized nerve or intestine, may be necessary to provide a functional reconstruction in some cases (see below).

SMALL LOCALIZED SCAR

When reconstruction is indicated for a small localized scar, soft tissue coverage is generally sufficient and poses no threat of breakdown leading to exposure of important structures. Instead, the reconstructive problem is generally functional in nature. An example is a tight scar band across a flexion crease, which is commonly seen after a burn injury. A local procedure that rearranges the existing tissue can relieve the tension by making more tissue available in one direction, although the amount of tissue in the area is not actually increased.

The Z-plasty is an example of such tissue rearrangement. Multiple Z-plasties or other procedures, such as W-plasty, may be useful for some localized scars.

SHORTAGE OF SKIN AND SUBCUTANEOUS TISSUE

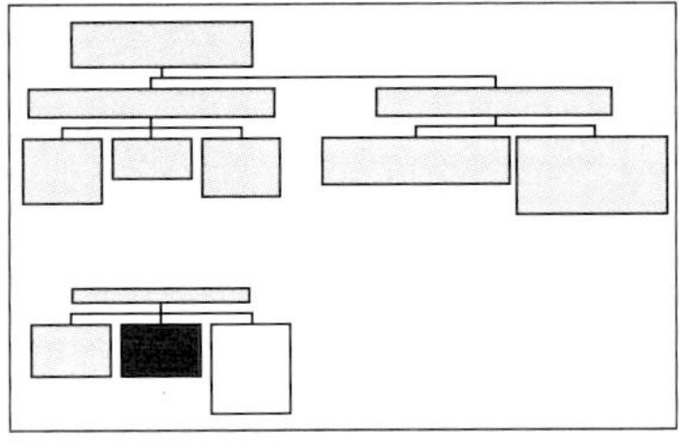

A shortage of skin and subcutaneous tissue may result from excision of a large scar or a large congenital defect (e.g., a nevus). Mastectomy commonly leaves a shortage of skin that prevents creation of a breast mound. In these cases, extra tissue can be created locally with the use of tissue expanders. These devices are inflatable plastic reservoirs of various shapes and volumes that are implanted under the skin. The skin over the expander is stretched during a period of several weeks as the expander is gradually filled by percutaneously injecting saline into an incorporated or remote fill port. The expander is then removed as a second procedure, and the expanded area of skin is advanced to cover the defect. The process of tissue expansion results in thinning of all layers of tissue overlying the expander except for the epidermis, which actually thickens.

A number of important principles govern the use of tissue expanders. The expanders must be placed so as to allow expansion only in normal skin adjacent to the defect, not in the defect itself. To ensure adequate expansion, a sufficiently large expander or multiple expanders must be used. Complications associated with the use of tissue expanders include infection, extrusion, deflation, flipped ports (remote type), and hematoma formation.[31]

Tissue expanders are used in secondary reconstruction only; they play no role in acute wound management. They are not indicated for contour defects (see below), because the tissue they provide is two-dimensional and lacking in bulk. Expanded tissue may not be adequate for coverage of chronically exposed structures (e.g., bone).

The scalp is an ideal location for the use of tissue expanders because no equivalent substitute for this type of hair-bearing tissue exists. Expanders work effectively when implanted over the hard calvarium and are useful in cases of burn alopecia and large nevi involving the scalp. Expanders are also useful for breast reconstruction, for carefully selected large lesions of the face, and for certain scars of the limbs. They are generally not indicated for use in the hands or feet. Although some local flap donor sites (e.g., the forehead) can be expanded before flap transfer, there is a loss of tissue pliability that appears to limit the usefulness of this particular application.

COMPLEX DEFECTS

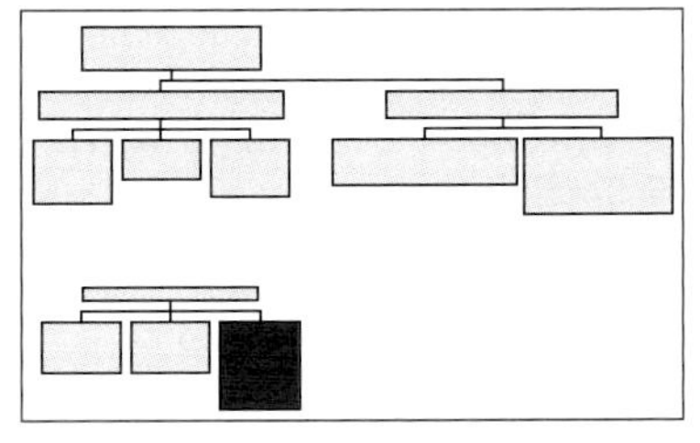

Certain reconstructive problems require substantial amounts of tissue of one or more types or of a very specialized type. Either local or free flaps are used to meet these tissue requirements.

Composite Defect

A composite defect may result from resection of an intraoral carcinoma with loss of the mandible and either the lining of the mouth or external skin. Another example is a crush injury of the leg with loss of soft tissue and a segment of weight-bearing bone. These defects require that a composite flap be brought to the area to meet more than one type of tissue deficiency. Local flaps generally do not provide the necessary types of tissue or permit the freedom of design possible with free flaps. The wide variety of free flap donor sites that exists allows selection of tissue in the appropriate quantity and configuration for a particular defect [*see Figure 15*].

Functional Defect

Functional defects require repair with specialized flaps. Free flaps are frequently used because the specific tissue

a

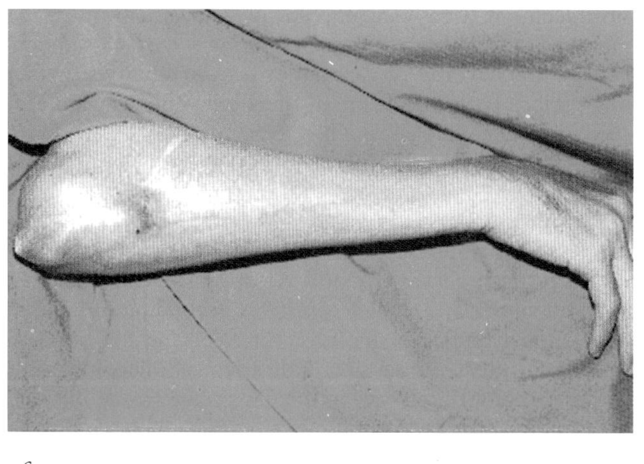

b

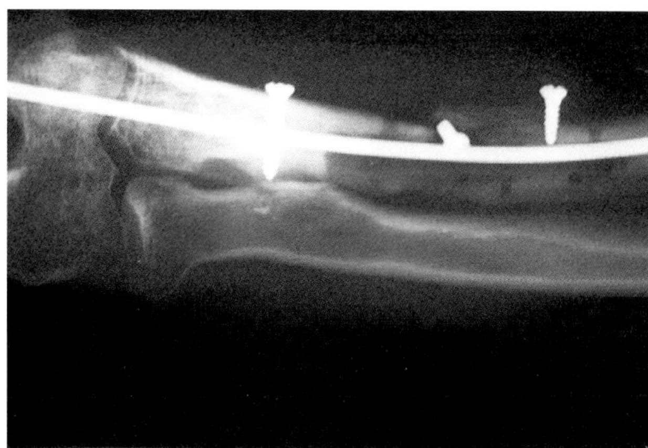

c

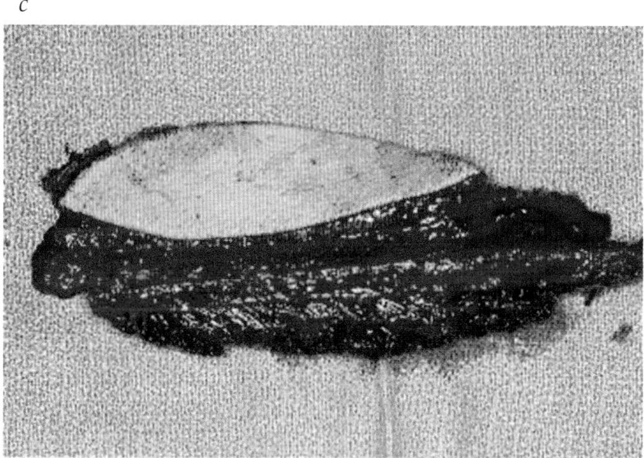

d

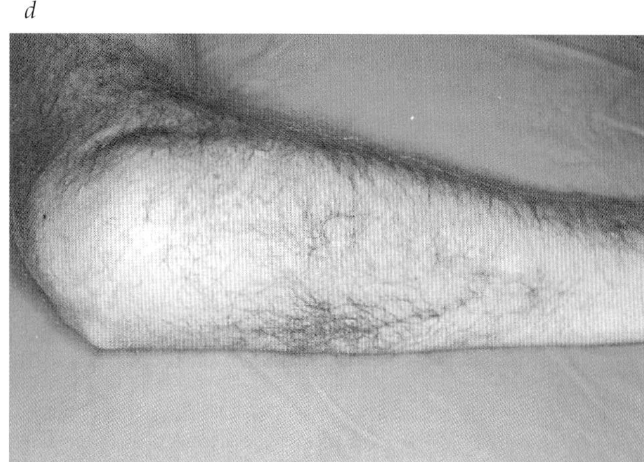

e

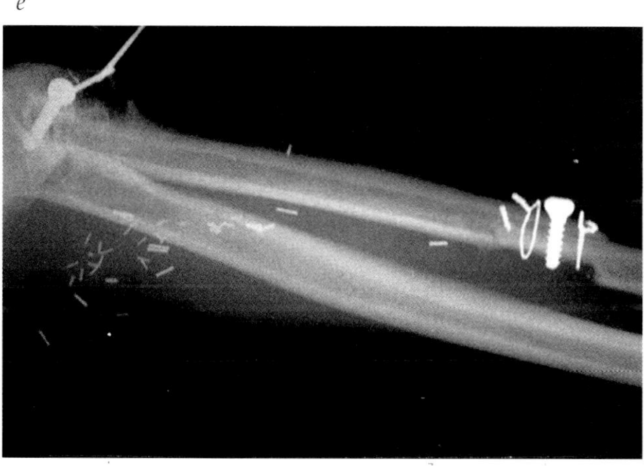

Figure 15 **(*a*) A chronic draining sinus of the ulna with poor overlying soft tissue coverage is shown. Simultaneous replacement of both bone and overlying soft tissue with a composite tissue flap is needed. (*b*) A radiograph shows nonunion of the ulna with orthopedic hardware. (*c*) A fibular free flap provides bone and skin in the appropriate amount and configuration for replacement of the affected tissues in a single stage. (*d*) The segment of ulna and overlying skin has been replaced. (*e*) A radiograph shows the vascularized fibula in place.**

requirements usually cannot be satisfied by a local flap. A functional defect may result, for example, in the cervical esophagus from tumor resection or in the forearm from the Volkmann contracture. A segment of small intestine can repair the esophageal defect; transfer of a vascularized and innervated muscle (e.g., the gracilis) can replace forearm muscle.[32]

Contour Defect

Contour defects, such as those that result from mastectomy or from trauma to the lower extremity, can be reconstructed with either local or free flaps. A mastectomy defect, because of its location on the chest, is suitable for reconstruction with one of several myocutaneous flaps from either the back or the abdomen. A free flap from the abdomen or the gluteal area is another alternative. The best reconstructive solution for a particular person is determined by variables such as body habitus and the size and configuration of the contralateral breast.

A contour defect of the lower extremity is best reconstructed with a large myocutaneous free flap that provides tissue of sufficient quantity and flexibility to allow sculpting into the appropriate shape. An excellent example is the latissimus dorsi free flap, which provides a large volume of thin, pliable muscle, which can be wrapped around orthopedic hardware.

Unstable Soft Tissue Coverage

Marginal soft tissue coverage (e.g., skin grafts) may break down after repeated minor trauma. Bones may become exposed and are then at risk for osteomyelitis. This situation can be avoided by elective replacement of the tissue at risk with a more substantial soft tissue covering. As in acute reconstruction, local flaps are the first choice for lesions of the trunk or the proximal extremities, whereas free flaps are often more appropriate for lesions of the distal extremities.

Soft tissue coverage is sometimes inadequate even in a healed wound. For example, certain procedures (e.g., nerve or bone grafting) require an ideal soft tissue bed to promote adequate graft revascularization. In some cases, it may initially be necessary to replace the existing soft tissue coverage as a first-stage procedure before grafting a bone or nerve gap. A skin or muscle flap is most commonly used in such cases. Muscle flaps tend to provide superior vascularity (e.g., for bone grafts) but are considered inferior for coverage of tendons that need to glide. This problem is most common in areas such as the distal extremities, where native soft tissue coverage is not overly abundant and is easily lost as a consequence of trauma or tumor resection. Free flaps are usually chosen to provide a healthy, well-vascularized soft tissue bed before further functional reconstruction is undertaken.

POSTOPERATIVE CARE AND FLAP MONITORING

Local Flaps

The postoperative care of local flaps is not complex. Flap healing is supported by adequate nutrition and maintenance of a normal hemodynamic state, including normal blood volume. Tension must not be placed on the flap. Tension can develop in flaps on the trunk as a result of changes in patient position or in flaps on the limbs as a result of loss of immobilization. Generally, the tip of any local flap is not only its most valuable portion but also its most vulnerable area. At the tip, the blood supply is the most precarious, and the detrimental effects of tension are magnified. Unfortunately, no pharmacologic agents are of proven benefit in preventing necrosis of a flap with failing circulation. Any flap necrosis that might develop should be minimized by preventing infection of the necrotic tissue. Necrotic tissue must therefore be débrided after the extent of tissue loss becomes clear. Portions of the flap that are undergoing demarcation but do not appear actively infected can be protected by the application of a topical antibiotic (e.g., silver sulfadiazine cream).

Extremities that are recipient sites for flaps, such as those that are recipient sites for skin grafts, should be immobilized and elevated after the operation until satisfactory wound healing has occurred.

Free Flaps

Survival of free flaps, unlike that of local flaps, tends to be an all-or-none phenomenon. Careful postoperative monitoring of flap circulation is essential because flap failure is likely to be the result of a problem at the vascular anastomoses. Flaps are usually monitored for 7 days. However, the most critical time for free flap monitoring is the first 48 hours because the majority of vascular crises usually occur within this period. Early detection and aggressive investigation of such crises generally allow a flap to be salvaged. Maintenance of normal blood volume, treatment of hypothermia, and avoidance of pressors are particularly important in the early postoperative period to prevent vascular spasm.

Free flaps should be monitored on an hourly basis during the early postoperative period. Most free flaps include an exposed skin island, which facilitates evaluation of the flap circulation. The flap is observed for color and for capillary refill—the most important indicators of flap viability. Although color differences in the flap and surrounding skin can be due to the pallor of donor sites (e.g., the abdomen or lateral thigh), traditionally, a pale flap generally indicates arterial insufficiency. In contrast, flaps with venous insufficiency are characteristically blue in color and exhibit rapid capillary refill.

Free flaps exhibit venous engorgement when placed in a dependent position up to several weeks postoperatively. Such engorgement is generally not dangerous, although patients with free flaps below the knee should be gradually mobilized in the same fashion as patients with skin grafts in this location by keeping the lower extremity elevated for at least 10 to 11 days.

Free flaps in the head and neck area require that the patient's head motion be restricted somewhat for the first few days to prevent kinking of the vascular pedicle. It is important that electrocardiographic leads and tracheostomy tube ties not compress the external jugular vein if it was used as a recipient vessel for anastomosis. If central lines are used after operation, they should be placed on the contralateral side of the neck to prevent thrombosis near the microvascular anastomosis.

If a skin island is exposed, Doppler ultrasonography should reveal the presence of a triphasic arterial pulse and its location should be marked with a suture, staple, or permanent ink to facilitate monitoring by nursing staff.

When the flap is buried or when cutaneous signals cannot be found, monitoring becomes more difficult and alternative methods of monitoring are used. One example is the implantable Doppler monitor which is attached to the artery or vein distal to the anastomosis to obtain a continuous Doppler signal.[33] Tissue oximetry has also been developed to monitor flaps with an external skin island.[34] Using this device, a probe is placed on the skin island and attached to a monitor that measures overall tissue oximetry (arterial and venous). A baseline level is reached, and any significant fall below the baseline indicates vascular compromise. The flap can be monitored remotely via the Internet, and when the level falls below a preset point, the machine can notify personnel via a pager. Surface temperature probes can also be used to monitor free flaps that have a skin island. Given that the flap surface temperature is generally about 1.0 to 2.5 C lower than the control temperature, measuring the difference between the flap and surrounding skin can alert providers to potential flap compromise.

Financial Disclosures: None Reported

References

1. Parrett BM, Matros E, Pribaz JJ, et al. Lower extremity trauma: trends in the management of soft-tissue reconstruction of open tibia-fibula fractures. Plast Reconstr Surg 2006; 117:1315.
2. Edlich RF, Jones KC Jr, Buchanan L, et al. A disposable emergency wound treatment kit. J Emerg Med 1992;10:463.
3. Stevenson TR, Thacker JG, Rodeheaver GT, et al. Cleansing the traumatic wound by high pressure syringe irrigation. J Am Coll Emerg Phys 1976;5:17.
4. FLOW Investigators, Petrisor B, Sun X, Bhandari M, et al. Fluid lavage of open wounds (FLOW): a multicenter, blinded, factorial pilot trial comparing alternative irrigating solutions and pressures in patients with open fractures. J Trauma 2011;71:596–606.
5. Hollander JE, Singer AJ, Valentine SM, et al. Risk factors for infection in patients with traumatic lacerations. Acad Emerg Med 2001;8:716.
6. Edlich RF, Rodeheaver GT, Thacker JG. Technical factors in the prevention of wound infection. In: Simmons R, Howard R, editors. Surgical infectious diseases. Norwalk (CT): Appleton-Century-Croft; 1981.
7. Robson MC, Heggers JP. Delayed wound closures based on bacterial counts. J Surg Oncol 1970;2:379.
8. Braunschweig CL, Levy P, Sheean PM, Wang X. Enteral compared with parenteral nutrition: a meta-analysis. Am J Clin Nutr 2001;74:534–42.
9. Codner PA. Enteral nutrition in the critically ill patient. Surg Clin North Am 2012;92:1485–501.
10. Burlew CC, Moore EE, Cuschieri J, et al; WTA Study Group. Who should we feed? Western Trauma Association multi-institutional study of enteral nutrition in the open abdomen after injury. J Trauma Acute Care Surg 2012;73:1380–7.
11. Teepe RG, Koebrugge EJ, Lowik CW, et al. Cytotoxic effects of topical antimicrobial and antiseptic agents on human keratinocytes in vitro. J Trauma 1993;35:8.
12. Daniel RK, Kerrigan CL. Skin flaps: an anatomical and hemodynamic approach. Clin Plast Surg 1979;6:181.
13. Cederna PS, Chang P, Pittet-Cuenod BM, et al. The effect of the delay phenomenon on the vascularity of rabbit abdominal cutaneous island flaps. Plast Reconstr Surg 1997;99:183.
14. Milton SH. Pedicled skin-flaps: the fallacy of the length:width ratio. Br J Surg 1970;57:502.
15. Lamberty BG, Cormack GC. Fasciocutaneous flaps. Clin Plast Surg 1990;17:713.
16. Cormack GC, Lamberty BG. Arterial anatomy of skin flaps. Edinburgh: Churchill Livingstone; 1987.
17. Jackson IT. Local rotational flaps. In: Evans GRD, editor. Operative plastic surgery. New York: McGraw-Hill; 2000.
18. Worthen EF. Scalp flaps and the rotation forehead flap. In: Strauch B, Vasconez LO, Hall-Findlay EJ, editors. Grabb's encyclopedia of flaps. Vol 1. Philadelphia: Lippincott-Raven Publishers; 1998.
19. McGregor IA, McGregor AD. The Z-plasty. In: Fundamental techniques of plastic surgery. Edinburgh: Churchill Livingstone; 1995.
20. Jackson IT. Local flaps in head and neck reconstruction. St. Louis: CV Mosby; 1985.
21. Spinelli HM, Forman DL. Current treatment of post-traumatic deformities: residual orbital, adnexal, and soft-tissue abnormalities. Clin Plast Surg 1997;24:519.
22. Luce EA. Reconstruction of the lower lip. Clin Plast Surg 1995;22:109.
23. Mathes SJ, Nahai F. Reconstructive surgery: principles, anatomy, technique. Vol 1. New York: Churchill Livingstone; 1997.
24. Orgill DP, Austen WG, Butler CE, et al. Guidelines for treatment of complex chest wounds with negative pressure wound therapy. Wounds 2004;16(12 Suppl B):1.
25. Domkowski PW, Smith ML, Gonyon DL Jr, et al. Evaluation of vacuum-assisted closure in the treatment of post-sternotomy mediastinitis. J Thorac Cardiovasc Surg 2003;126:386.
26. Kaplan M, Banwell P, Orgill DP, et al. Guidelines for the management of the open abdomen: recommendations from a multidisciplinary expert advisory panel. Wounds 2005; 17(10 Suppl):1.
27. Miller PR, Thompson JT, Faler B, et al. Late fascial closure in lieu of ventral hernia: the next step in open abdomen management. J Trauma 2002;53:843.
28. Taylor GI, Giantoutsos MP, Morris SF. The neurovascular territories of the skin and muscles: anatomic study and clinical implications. Plast Reconstr Surg 1994;94:1.
29. Hidalgo DA, Shaw WW. Reconstruction of foot injuries. Clin Plast Surg 1986;13:663.
30. May JW Jr, Halls MJ, Simon SR. Free microvascular muscle flaps with skin graft reconstruction of extensive defects of the foot: a clinical and gait analysis study. Plast Reconstr Surg 1985;75:627.
31. Bennett RG, Hirt M. A history of tissue expansion: concepts, controversies, and complications. J Dermatol Surg Oncol 1993;19:1066.
32. Hidalgo DA, Disa JJ, Cordeiro PG. A review of 716 consecutive free flaps for oncologic surgical defects: refinement in donor site selection and technique. Plast Reconstr Surg 1998;102:722.
33. Kind GM, Buntic RF, Buncke GM, et al. The effect of an implantable Doppler probe on the salvage of microvascular tissue transplants. Plast Reconstr Surg 1998;101:1268.
34. Keller A. Noninvasive tissue oximetry for flap monitoring: an initial study. J Reconstr Microsurg 2007;23:189–97.

Acknowledgments

Figures 4, 5, 7, 12, 13 Carol Donner
Figures 6, 8, 9, 10, 11 Tom Moore

4 SURGICAL MANAGEMENT OF MELANOMA AND OTHER SKIN CANCERS

Jennifer A. Wargo, MD, and Kenneth Tanabe, MD

The clinical assessment and management of skin lesions can be challenging as the natural history and prognosis of these lesions are widely variable. Surgeons play a pivotal role in the treatment of these lesions, although initial evaluation of these lesions is often performed by other clinicians. The management of various benign skin lesions is beyond the scope of this review. Evaluation and management of skin cancers are addressed in detail.

The prevalence of malignant skin cancers has increased significantly over the past several years. Approximately 1.2 million cases of nonmelanoma skin cancer are diagnosed per year.[1] More alarming, up to 80,000 cases of melanoma are diagnosed per year,[2] an incidence that has been steadily increasing,[3] with a lifetime risk of 1 in 50 for the development of melanoma.[2] The disturbing increase in the incidence of both nonmelanoma skin cancer and melanoma can largely be attributed to the social attitude toward sun exposure.[4]

Assessment of Skin Lesions

HISTORY AND PHYSICAL EXAMINATION

Obtaining a careful history is critical to the evaluation of skin lesions. Particular attention should be paid to a history of sun exposure and the use of sunscreen. Blistering sunburn in childhood or adolescence is a significant risk factor and is present in virtually all whites who develop melanoma. Patients should also be questioned about any personal or family history of skin cancer as those who report a history of melanoma in a first-degree relative have an eight- to 12-fold risk of developing melanoma.[5] In addition, patients should be questioned regarding immunosuppression and a history of transplantation as these put them at a higher risk for developing skin cancer.

A detailed history regarding when the lesion was first noted as well as changes in the size or appearance of the lesion is important to elucidate. Generally speaking, lesions are nonsuspicious if they remain stable and uniform in their physical characteristics (e.g., size, shape, color, profile, and texture). An example of a nonsuspicious lesion is a simple nevus, which typically becomes apparent at 4 to 5 years of age, darkens with puberty, and fades in the seventh to eighth decades of life. However, pigmented lesions that demonstrate an irregular border or demonstrate a change in size, color, or texture are considered to be suspicious. The "ABCD" guideline for identification of suspicious pigmented lesions is described below in the section on melanoma. Careful attention should also be paid to constitutional symptoms as patients may present with advanced disease with metastases and systemic or focal complaints, such as headaches or visual changes in the case of melanoma metastatic to the brain.

Physical examination should include a complete skin examination and an examination of mucosal membranes. Specific attention should be paid to the presence of ulceration in a skin lesion as this significantly affects the prognosis depending on the histology of the lesion. Also, careful attention should be paid to the potential draining nodal basins as lymph node metastases are known to occur in squamous cell cancer and melanoma.

Nonsuspicious lesions may be safely monitored conservatively with regular self-examination by the patient and regular follow-up with a health care provider. Any change in a lesion constitutes a criterion for biopsy. In addition, lesions that are large in size (1 to 2 cm) should be considered for biopsy.

BIOPSY

Any suspicious lesion should be biopsied. This can be performed by either excisional biopsy if the lesion is small or incisional biopsy if the lesion is large. Excisional biopsy should be performed incorporating a margin of a few millimeters of normal skin surrounding the lesion depending on the clinical characteristics. This may eliminate the need for subsequent reexcision for some types of lesions. For example, dysplastic nevi that have moderate to severe cytologic atypia need to be excised to clear margins. However, no attempt should be made to perform a definitive radical excision until a diagnosis is established by biopsy. Full-thickness excision into the subcutaneous fat should be performed, and margins on the specimen should be marked for orientation. This allows the pathologist to comment on the level of invasion and on margins for possible microscopic involvement with tumor cells. It is preferable to avoid electrocautery to excise the specimen as margins can be distorted significantly by the artifact created by this technique. Shave biopsy for evaluation of pigmented lesions is discouraged as it runs the risk of a positive deep margin, which compromises the ability to determine the true depth of penetration of a melanoma.

Whenever feasible, the long axis of an elliptically shaped excisional biopsy should be oriented along the long axis of the extremity, which facilitates subsequent excision if necessary. If the lesion is benign, no further treatment is warranted. If it proves to be malignant, further excision with an appropriate margin is usually necessary, and staging of the tumor becomes important. The adequacy of margins is discussed under each tumor type.

EXCISION

If a lesion proves to be malignant, complete excision should be performed with adequate margins as dictated by the type of tumor. For large elliptical excisions, the length of the ellipse should be approximately 3.5 to 4 times the width to allow for a cosmetic closure without "dog ears" at the ends. If an area cannot be closed without significant tension, skin grafting may be necessary to achieve a technically acceptable result. Specialized flaps may also be required for very large lesions or for difficult areas, such as on the face.

Specific Types of Skin Cancer

BASAL CELL CARCINOMA

Incidence and Epidemiology

Basal cell carcinoma is the most common malignancy in whites[6] and the most prevalent type of skin cancer. The incidence is widely variable across the globe, with an incidence of 146 per 100,000 in the United States and 726 per 100,000 in Australia.[7] The lifetime risk for whites in the United States of developing a basal cell carcinoma is approximately 30%.[1] Although the metastatic potential of these lesions is very low, the economic and social burden remains quite high.

In general, the vast majority of basal cell carcinomas occur on the head and neck. Basal cell carcinoma develops without a known precursor lesion, although it seems to be most closely related to exposure to ultraviolet radiation. Significant sun exposure during childhood and adolescence confers significant risk for the development of these lesions, although studies have failed to demonstrate a significant correlation between the development of basal cell carcinoma and cumulative exposure to ultraviolet light in adulthood.[8] Several heritable conditions are associated with an increased risk of basal cell carcinoma, including albinism, xeroderma pigmentosum, and Gorlin syndrome. Patients with Gorlin syndrome develop multiple basal cell carcinomas as well as anomalies of the spine and ribs, jaw cysts, pitting of the palms and soles, and calcification of the falx cerebri. Inheritance is autosomal dominant.[9]

Histologic Subtypes of Basal Cell Carcinoma

Several subtypes of basal cell carcinoma exist. Typical patterns seen in more mature lesions include nodular or cystic, superficial, morphoeic, and pigmented. Nodular or cystic basal cell carcinomas typically present as solitary lesions, often on the face, and are usually shiny and red, with central telangiectasias [*see Figure 1a*]. The classic basal cell carcinoma is the nodular type, which is also known as a "rodent ulcer." These lesions are characterized by an indurated edge and an ulcerated center. Superficial basal cell carcinomas are typically found on the trunk and appear as an erythematous patch that is often mistaken for eczema or psoriasis and are typically slow-growing.[9] Perhaps the most pertinent of these lesions is the morphoeic basal cell carcinoma [*see Figure 1b*], which represents the minority of these lesions but has clinical features that are particularly pertinent to the surgeon. These lesions are often larger than they appear clinically and have a more aggressive natural history, which can make complete excision quite challenging.

Treatment

Surgical excision remains the mainstay of treatment for primary basal cell carcinomas. Typically, a surgical margin of 4 mm is recommended when possible.[10] Primary closure can generally be accomplished for small defects and rotation flaps, or skin grafting may be necessary for larger defects. Although present only extraordinarily rarely, lymphatic spread identified in the primary tumor may be an indication for lymphatic mapping.[11]

An important distinction when choosing appropriate means for management is whether or not it is a primary versus a recurrent lesion. Other surgical techniques include cryosurgery, curettage and cautery, and Mohs micrographic surgery. Cryosurgery and curettage should generally be avoided in large or morphoeic tumors or in those in high-risk areas (such as the central face) as surgical margins cannot be assessed. Mohs micrographic surgery is a technique involving excision of serial sections with intraoperative histologic examination of frozen sections to control surgical margins. It is useful in morphoeic or recurrent basal cell carcinomas or those in high-risk sites, where 5-year cure rates approach 95%.[12] It is especially useful in sites in which for cosmetic reasons it is important to minimize the amount of tissue resected.

Nonsurgical modalities available for the treatment of basal cell carcinoma include radiotherapy, photodynamic therapy, and topical agents such as 5-fluorouracil, imiquimod, or intralesional interferon alfa. Radiation therapy is generally reserved for elderly patients with lesions too extensive for excision, with 5-year cure rates approaching 90%.[13] Photodynamic therapy involves the use of δ-aminolevulinic acid in a 20% emulsion that is applied to the lesion followed by exposure to light in the wavelength range of 620 to 640 nm. This treatment is based on the uptake of the porphyrin metabolite by the tumor with subsequent conversion to protoporphyrin IX, which is subject to destruction in the presence of light.[9] Responses to treatment are somewhat lower, with an overall clearance rate of 87% and a lower clearance rate of 53% in nodular basal cell carcinoma.[14] Fluorouracil 5% cream may also be used in the management of multiple basal cell carcinomas of the trunk and limbs. Imiquimod is an immunomodulatory agent that is used in a 5% cream for basal cell carcinomas, with a clearance rate of 70 to 100%.[15] Intralesional interferon alfa has also been used experimentally, with a 67% cure rate in a series of 140 patients treated in this manner.[16]

Patients who have been treated for any skin cancer, including basal cell carcinoma, should perform frequent self-examination to look for suspicious lesions as they are at a greater risk for developing additional skin cancers. Counseling to reduce sun exposure should be undertaken to limit further damage from ultraviolet irradiation. High-risk individuals, such as those with Gorlin syndrome or those who are on immunosuppressive therapy after renal transplantation, are offered oral retinoid treatment in the hope of preventing the development of other nonmelanoma skin cancers.[16]

An interesting advance in the treatment of advanced basal cell carcinoma is the use of inhibitors of the sonic hedgehog pathway. The vast majority of basal cell carcinomas harbor genetic mutations in the hedgehog signaling pathway, which results in constitutive activation and basal cell proliferation.[17] Targeted therapy using small-molecule inhibitors of this pathway is now approved for the treatment

a

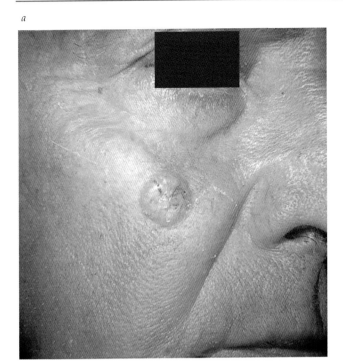

b

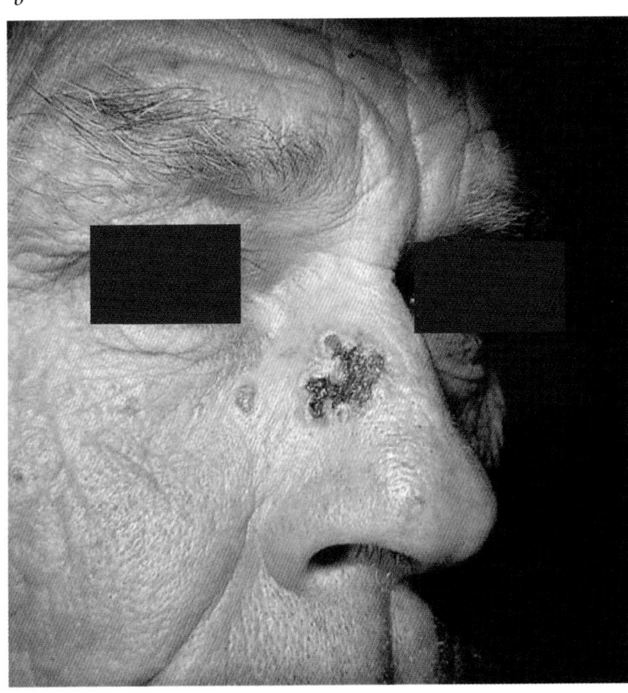

Figure 1 (a) Typical basal cell carcinoma. A pearly luster and telangiectasias are evident in this typical basal cell carcinoma on the cheek of a 43-year-old man. (b) Morpheaform basal cell carcinoma. This sclerosing (morpheaform) basal cell carcinoma on the nose of a 55-year-old man was found to be deeply invasive and exhibited multidirectional growth.

of locally advanced and metastatic basal cell carcinoma.[18] Two recently published trials demonstrated the efficacy of the drug vismodegib (an oral inhibitor of the hedgehog pathway) in treating locally advanced and metastatic basal cell carcinoma[19] and in preventing new lesions or treating existing lesions in individuals with Gorlin syndrome.[20] However, side effects with this therapy are common and are often limiting.[19,20]

SQUAMOUS CELL CARCINOMA

Incidence and Epidemiology

Squamous cell carcinoma of the skin is the second most common form of nonmelanoma skin cancer, with the majority (50 to 60%) of these lesions occurring on the head and neck. It is the most common tumor found in elderly patients, likely representing the results of cumulative doses of sun exposure over the course of their lifetime.

Precursor Lesions

Unlike basal cell carcinomas, squamous cell skin cancers often arise in precursor lesions, such as actinic keratosis.[21] Actinic keratoses, sometimes referred to as solar keratoses, develop in chronically sun-damaged areas of the body. They are generally ill-defined and irregular and may range significantly in size from only a millimeter to a few centimeters. They have a scaly appearance and are often multiple and can range in color from dark brown to flesh-colored. Biopsy may be necessary to rule out the presence of a squamous cell carcinoma. The rate of malignant transformation of actinic keratosis to squamous cell carcinoma is less than 0.1% per year,[22] although lesions should be treated to decrease the chance of progression. Treatment options include cryotherapy, curettage, and topical agents. Surgical excision of actinic keratoses is rarely necessary but may be indicated if there is a high suspicion for a concurrent squamous cell carcinoma.

Intraepithelial squamous cell carcinoma, carcinoma in situ, is thought to be the next step in the progression from actinic keratosis to invasive squamous cell carcinoma. Another term for this lesion is Bowen disease, and lesions are typically located on sun-exposed areas of the head, neck, trunk, or legs. This lesion is referred to as "erythroplasia of Queyrat" when located on the genitalia. When it occurs on non–sun-exposed areas, it may be associated with internal malignancy.[23] These lesions typically appear as erythematous slightly keratotic plaques and are usually larger than lesions of actinic keratosis. These lesions should be excised with a 5 mm to 1 cm margin.

Diagnosis

Squamous cell carcinomas occur on the head and neck in approximately 50% of cases. Whites have nearly a 10% lifetime risk of developing a squamous cell carcinoma. Interestingly, in one series, nearly half of the fatal cases of squamous cell carcinoma occurred in patients in whom the lesion arose on the ear.[24] The mortality associated with squamous cell carcinoma is estimated at 1:100,000.[25]

As noted, squamous cell carcinomas are most often associated with sun exposure, although they may also be seen in a background of old scars, radiation-damaged skin [*see Figure 2a*], or chronic open wounds.[26] Chronic inflammation

a

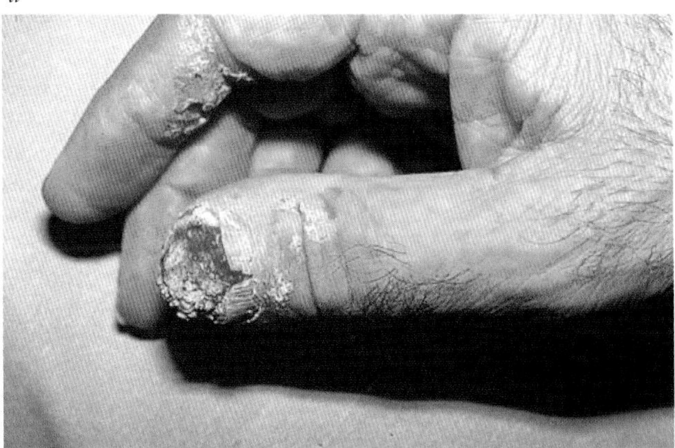

b

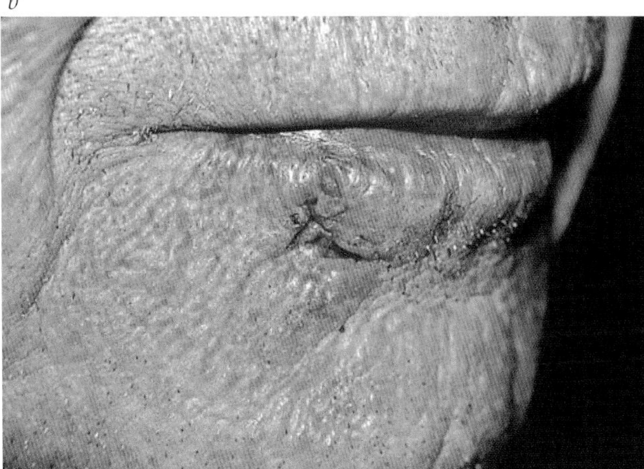

Figure 2 (*a*) **Squamous cell carcinoma related to radiation exposure. This squamous cell carcinoma involving the thumb and index finger of a 72-year-old man, a retired dentist, was related to exposure to occupational hazards; he had subjected these digits to repeated radiation exposure by holding dental x-rays against his patients' teeth. (*b*) Squamous cell carcinoma related to sun exposure. This squamous cell carcinoma on the lip of a 70-year-old man was related to sun exposure; the patient was a nonsmoker.**

and irritation appear to be the common denominators. Marjolin ulcer is a term for squamous cell carcinoma arising in a burn scar or open wound such as osteomyelitis draining sites.

These lesions typically appear as keratotic papules that may ulcerate and may be reddish-brown, pink, or flesh-colored [*see Figure 2b*]. A cutaneous "horn" may be evident if there is extensive hyperkeratosis.[24] Symptoms that may suggest malignant transformation of actinic keratosis include pain, erythema, ulceration, or induration. Histologically, these lesions are characterized by nests of atypical keratinocytes that have invaded into the dermis, which may be well or poorly differentiated.

Once a diagnosis of squamous cell carcinoma is suspected, careful attention should be paid to the draining nodal basins as lymph node metastases are possible. Overall, the risk of metastasis is between 2 and 4% and is higher in larger, poorly differentiated lesions and lesions located on the scalp, nose, ear, lip, and extremities. The most common sites of metastasis are regional lymph nodes, the lungs, and the liver. Recurrence or metastases typically occur within 3 years after treatment of the index lesion.

Treatment

Surgical excision remains the mainstay of treatment for primary squamous cell carcinomas as well, although the recommended margin of excision is generally larger than that for basal cell carcinoma and ranges from 0.5 to 2 cm. Primary closure is often possible for smaller lesions, although larger lesions may require rotation flaps or skin grafting.

Other modalities of therapy for squamous cell carcinoma are similar to those used to treat basal cell carcinoma and include cryosurgery, curettage and cautery, Mohs micrographic surgery, radiotherapy, photodynamic therapy, and topical agents such as 5-fluorouracil, imiquimod, or intralesional interferon alfa. Squamous cell carcinomas that develop from Marjolin ulcer are characterized by aggressive growth after surgical excision.

Patients who have been treated for squamous cell carcinoma should perform frequent self-examinations to look for suspicious lesions as they are at risk for developing other nonmelanoma skin cancers. Counseling to reduce sun exposure should be undertaken to limit further damage from ultraviolet irradiation. High-risk individuals, such as those who are on immunosuppressive therapy after renal transplantation, may be offered oral retinoid treatment in the hope of preventing the development of other nonmelanoma skin cancers.[16]

Sentinel Lymph Node Biopsy in Squamous Cell Carcinoma

The overwhelming majority of squamous cell carcinomas have low metastatic potential and are cured with surgery or ablative therapy alone. However, there is a subpopulation of high-risk patients with significant risk of metastasis. The prognosis is poor for patients with lymph node metastases from squamous cell carcinoma, with 5- and 10-year survival rates of 30% and 16%, respectively.[27] Factors that are associated with a worse prognosis include large lesions (> 2 cm on the trunk and extremities, > 1 cm on the head and neck, and > 0.6 cm on the genitalia, hands, and feet), those with a rapid growth rate, recurrent lesions or those that develop in sites of previous radiotherapy or chronic inflammation, those with histologic features of moderate or poor differentiation and/or perineural invasion, and lesions that occur in high-risk individuals (e.g., patients with heritable disorders such as albinism and xeroderma pigmentosum and patients with immunodeficiency such as transplant patients).[27–30]

Although the utility of sentinel lymph node biopsy (SLNB) is clear in melanoma, its role in staging in clinically node-negative high-risk cutaneous squamous cell carcinoma remains unclear. Several studies have tried to address this, with a recent report showing a positive sentinel node rate of 14.4% in all cutaneous squamous cell carcinomas (including the head and neck and the trunk).[31] Currently, there are no standard of care guidelines for its use in high-risk squamous cell carcinoma, and its use remains investigational in this population.

MELANOMA

Incidence and Epidemiology

Although it is less common than basal cell or squamous cell carcinoma, melanoma is clearly the most deadly of these cancers. Apprxoimately 76,250 cases of melanoma were diagnosed in 2012, with 9,180 deaths.[2] As such, it is one of the fastest-growing cancers in the United States. The lifetime risk is estimated to be 1 in 50 individuals for the development of melanoma.[2] The incidence of melanoma is increasing significantly at a rate of 4.1% per year, faster than any other malignancy. The incidence is slightly higher in men than in women, and the median age at diagnosis is 57 years.[5] An average of 15 years of potential life are lost per death, and the costs attributable to melanoma are $39.2 million to $3.3 billion for morbidity and mortality, respectively.[32]

Melanoma results from the malignant transformation of melanocytes, which are responsible for pigment production. Both genetic and environmental factors are implicated in the development of melanoma. Genetic susceptibility is important, and patients with melanoma often report a family history. Those who report a history of melanoma in a first-degree relative have an eight- to 12-fold risk of developing melanoma.[5] Family members with melanoma tend to be diagnosed at an earlier age and have a higher frequency of multiple primary melanomas. Several genes have been implicated in the pathogenesis of melanoma. *CDKN2A* is a major susceptibility gene, as is *CDK4*. *BRCA2* mutations have been linked to increased risk of melanoma. Melanocortin receptor (*MC1R*) and retinoblastoma (*Rb*) genes are also under investigation. Environmental exposure to ultraviolet radiation also is implicated in the transformation of melanocytes. Patients with xeroderma pigmentosum have an extremely high rate of skin cancers, including melanoma. The risk of developing melanoma is associated with intermittent, intense sun exposure rather than with a cumulative effect, although the exact mechanism behind the pathogenesis remains unknown.

In one study, six risk factors were identified by multivariate analysis to be important in the development of malignant melanoma: a family history of melanoma, a history of three or more blistering sunburns before age 20, the presence of blonde or red hair, the presence of actinic keratosis, a history of 3 or more years of an outdoor summer job as a teenager, and the presence of marked freckling on the upper part of the back. If an individual has one or two of these factors, he or she has a 3.5-fold increased risk of developing melanoma, whereas if an individual has three or more, the increase in risk is 20-fold.

Screening and Diagnosis

The frequency of screening of patients for melanoma should be based on the above risk factors. Routine screening of low-risk patients using a total body skin examination by health care providers is not supported by prospective, randomized clinical trial data. Self-screening, however, is clearly recommended, with excellent educational materials provided by the American Academy of Dermatology and the American Cancer Society. There is an absence of prospective, randomized trial data showing that skin screening by health care providers decreases skin cancer mortality. Nevertheless, physicians should take every opportunity to screen opportunistically as lesions found by physicians are significantly thinner than those detected by patients or their spouse.[33]

Early recognition of melanoma is paramount to its effective treatment. The "ABCD" guideline may be used in the evaluation of pigmented lesions.[34] These lesions often occur on sun-exposed areas of the upper trunk and extremities and are typically asymmetrical with irregular borders and variegated pigmentation [*see Figure 3*]. Occasionally, they lack pigmentation or are associated with significant ulceration. The original "ABCD" has been modified to "ABCDE," with "E" representing evolution of a lesion [*see Table 1*]; pigmented lesions that are new or change over time should be regarded as suspicious. Any lesion suspicious for melanoma should be biopsied.

Histologic Subtypes

Cutaneous melanoma may be further classified into histologic subtypes based on patterns of growth and anatomic location. The significance of these subtypes is less important than the pattern of growth (radial versus vertical growth) and depth of penetration.[35] The most common subtypes

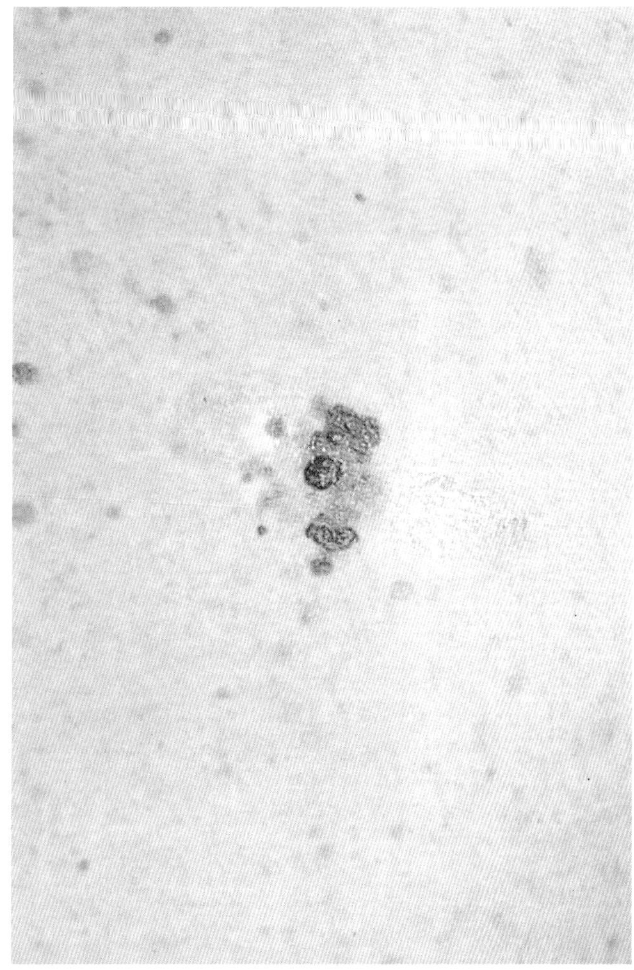

Figure 3 **Typical melanoma. A halo effect caused by loss of pigmentation is visible along the left margin of this melanoma on the upper back of a 33-year-old white woman; irregularities in shape, contour, and pigmentation are also evident.**

Table 1 ABCDE Guidelines for Pigmented Lesions

Asymmetry	Most early lesions grow at an uneven rate, resulting in an asymmetrical pattern
Border irregularity	The uneven growth rate also results in an irregular border
Color variegation	Irregular growth also causes new shades of black, and light and dark brown
Diameter	Lesions with ABC freatures and diameters > 6 mm should be considered suspicious for melanoma
Evolution	Change in a lesion over time

include lentigo maligna melanoma, superficial spreading melanoma, acral lentiginous melanoma, and nodular melanoma. Superficial spreading accounts for over 70% of melanomas. These lesions are most common in white adults and typically occur on the back or legs. Nodular melanomas are the second most common, accounting for between 15 and 30% of all melanomas. These lesions often appear dome shaped and may occur anywhere on the body. They typically invade the dermis early in their natural history owing to an early vertical growth phase. Lentigo maligna melanoma accounts for approximately 5% of all melanomas and is thought to arise in a focus of lentigo maligna, or Hutchinson freckle. These lesions demonstrate a prolonged radial growth phase before developing an invasive component. Acral lentiginous melanomas occur on the hands or feet [*see Figure 4*], often occurring under the nailbed, where the dermis is thinner (e.g., subungual melanoma). A more rare histologic variant is desmoplastic melanoma, which typically occurs in areas of sun damage and tends more often to recur locally. Desmoplastic melanoma has been subclassified into a pure form or as a mixed histologic variant, with the former having a very low incidence of lymph node metastases.[36]

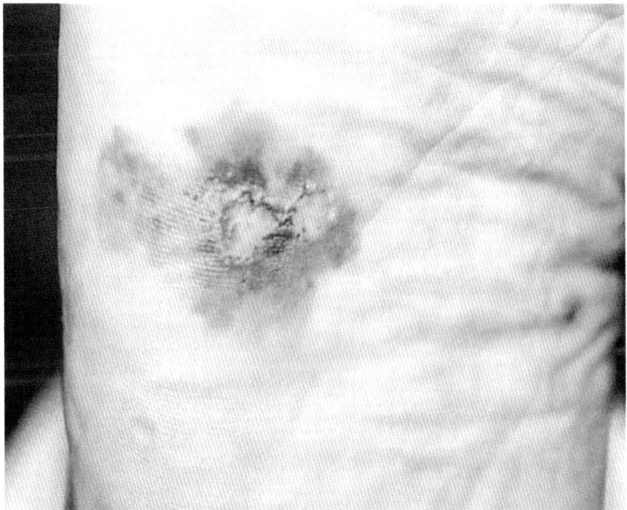

Figure 4 **Acral lentiginous melanoma. This melanoma, on the sole of the foot of a 47-year-old black woman, shows irregularities in shape, contour, and pigmentation.**

Prognostic Factors in Melanoma

An important variable in the prognosis of melanoma is the thickness of the primary tumor as assessed using the Breslow system. Tumor thickness in the Breslow system is measured from the epidermal surface to the deepest point of the tumor with a calibrated ocular micrometer.[37] A historically used microstaging system—the Clark system—categorized the depth of melanoma penetration based on histologically defined layers. However, the value of this microstaging system is considerably less than that of the Breslow system given its absence of prognostic value once other histologic factors are integrated (Breslow thickness, ulceration, mitotic rate), lower reproducibility, and lower concordance of interpretation among expert pathologists. The American Joint Committee on Cancer (AJCC) approved the latest version of the melanoma staging system in 2009, with changes that were validated via analysis of over 30,946 patients with stage I, II, and III melanoma and 7,972 patients with stage IV melanoma[38] [*see Table 2 and Table 3*]. Major changes in this new version include the following: (1) in patients with localized melanoma, tumor thickness, mitotic rate (histologically defined as mitoses/mm^2), and ulceration were the most dominant prognostic factors; (2) the mitotic rate replaces the level of invasion as a primary criterion for defining T1b versus T1a melanomas; and (3) among the 3,307 patients with regional metastases, components that defined the N category were the number of metastatic nodes, tumor burden, and ulceration of the primary melanoma. In patients with more advanced melanoma, all nodal metastases, regardless of the extent of tumor burden, are classified as stage III. Micrometastases detected by immunohistochemistry are specifically included. The two dominant components in defining the M category are the site of distant metastases (nonvisceral versus lung versus all other visceral metastatic sites) and an elevated serum lactate dehydrogenase (LDH) level. Five-year survival rates correlate with stage [*see Figure 5*].[38] Of note, the Clarke microstaging system is no longer a component of the AJCC stage classification of melanoma.

Stage I and II melanoma Those with clinically localized melanoma represent the vast majority of patients, and several prognostic factors have been identified for risk stratification and prognosis in this heterogeneous group. The most important prognostic factors in early-stage melanoma are Breslow tumor thickness (T1 to T4), the presence or absence of ulceration, and the number of mitoses. These have significant implications in prognosis as 5-year survival in stage I to II melanomas falls significantly with increasing thickness and dropped from 80% to 55% in the presence of ulceration in a 2006 analysis.[35] Of late, the mitotic rate in the primary tumor has been identified as an important prognostic factor, possibly even surpassing ulceration in importance in early-stage melanoma.[39–41] Mitotic rate was incorporated into the newest version of the AJCC staging system.[38]

Thin (< 1 mm thick) melanomas in particular have also been studied, with some interesting results. Thin melanomas with ulceration or mitoses greater than or equal to 1/mm^2 are classified as T1b and are associated with a worse prognosis than those without these features. A publication

Table 2 AJCC Staging of Malignant Melanoma

T Classification	*Depth*	*Histologic Features*
T1	≤ 1.0 mm	a: without ulceration and mitoses < 1/mm^2
		b: with ulceration or mitoses ≥ 1/mm^2
T2	1.01–2.0 mm	a: without ulceration
		b: with ulceration
T3	2.01–4.0 mm	a: without ulceration
		b: with ulceration
T4	> 4.0 mm	a: without ulceration
		b: with ulceration
N Classification	*Number of Nodes Involved*	*Histologic Features*
N1	1 lymph node	a: micrometastases
		b: macrometastases
N2	2–3 lymph nodes	a: micrometastases
		b: macrometastases
		c: in-transit metastasis(es), satellite(s) without metastatic nodes
N3	4 or more metastatic lymph nodes, matted lymph nodes, or combinations of in-transit metastasis(es), satellites, or ulcerated melanoma and metastatic lymph node(s)	
M Classification	*Site of Disease*	*LDH Level*
M1	Distant skin, subcutaneous, or lymph node metastases	Normal LDH
M2	Lung metastases	Normal LDH
M3	All other visceral metastases	Normal LDH
	Any distant metastases	Elevated LDH

AJCC = American Joint Committee on Cancer; LDH = lactate dehydrogenase.
Stage 0: Tis, N0, M0; stage IA: T1a, N0, M0; stage IB: T1b, N0, M0; T2a, N0, M0; stage IIA: T2b, N0, M0; T3a, N0, M0; stage IIB: T3b, N0, M0; T4a, N0, M0; stage IIC: T4b, N0, M0; stage IIIA: any T1–4a, N1b, M0; stage IIIB: any T1–4a, N2b, M0; stage IIIC: any T, N2c, M0; any T, N3, M0; stage IV: any T, any N, M1–3.

from the group at the University of Pennsylvania described a prognostic model using four factors based on multivariate analysis: mitotic rate (0 versus ≥ 1 per mm^2), growth phase (radial or vertical), gender, and tumor-infiltrating lymphocytes.[42] They developed an algorithm for risk stratification based on these factors, with minimal- and low-risk patients having a predicted risk of metastasis of less than 4%, whereas those who were considered moderate or high risk had a predicted risk of metastasis of 12% and 30%, respectively.[42]

Intermediate-thickness (1.0 to 4 mm) melanomas have a worse prognosis than T1 melanomas, with 5-year survival rates of 89% for nonulcerated T2 lesions (1 to 2 mm) and 77.4% for ulcerated lesions. Patients with ulcerated T3 lesions (2 to 4 mm) have a predicted 5-year survival of 63%. Thick (> 4 mm) lesions in node-negative patients have an associated 5-year survival of 67.4%, which drops to 45.1% if the lesion is ulcerated.[43]

Stage III melanoma Stage III melanoma is characterized by the presence of nodal metastases (micro- or macrometastases) with or without in-transit/satellite lesions. The presence of lymph node metastases confers a significantly worse prognosis, with less than half of node-positive patients surviving 5 years.[43] The number of involved nodes is also of prognostic significance and is reflected in the AJCC staging system.

In patients with stage III disease, four prognostic factors for survival were identified: number of metastatic lymph nodes, microscopic versus macroscopic tumor deposits in lymph nodes, the presence of in-transit or satellite metastases, and the presence of ulceration in the primary lesion.[38,43]

In-transit and satellite metastases represent dissemination of tumor via lymphatic channels, and the 5-year survival rate in patients with these findings is similar to that of those with lymph node metastases. If these findings are present in association with lymph node metastases (N3), the survival drops significantly.[43]

Stage IV melanoma For stage IV melanoma, the site of distant metastasis and serum LDH seem to have the most value in prognosis, with a far more favorable prognosis in those with cutaneous metastases and a normal serum LDH. On analysis, there is a significant difference in 1-year survival rates between those with cutaneous, subcutaneous, or distant nodal metastases (M1) versus those with lung metastases (M2) versus those with any other visceral metastases or any metastasis with an elevated serum LDH (M3).[38]

Table 3 Anatomic Stage/Prognostic Groups

Stage	Clinical Staging			Pathologic Staging			
0	Tis	N0	M0	0	Tis	N0	M0
IA	T1a	N0	M0	IA	T1a	N0	M0
IB	T1b	N0	M0	IB	T1b	N0	M0
	T2a	N0	M0		T2a	N0	M0
IIA	T2b	N0	M0	IIA	T2b	N0	M0
	T3a	N0	M0		T3a	N0	M0
IIB	T3b	N0	M0	IIB	T3b	N0	M0
	T4a	N0	M0		T4a	N0	M0
IIC	T4b	N0	M0		T4b	N0	M0
III	Any T	≥ N1	M0	IIIA	T1–4a	N1a	M0
					T1–4a	N2a	M0
				IIIB	T1–4b	N1a	M0
					T1–4b	N2a	M0
					T1–4a	N1b	M0
					T1–4a	N2b	M0
					T1–4a	N2c	M0
				IIIC	T1–4b	N1b	M0
					T1–4b	N2b	M0
					T1–4b	N2c	M0
					Any T	N3	M0
IV	Any T	Any N	M1	IV	Any T	Any N	M1

Initial Evaluation

Recommendations for the initial evaluation of patients with melanoma are as follows: for patients with thin melanomas (< 1.0 mm), no routine laboratory or radiologic tests are recommended beyond a careful history and physical examination. SLNB is generally not recommended unless the lesion is between 0.75 and 1.0 mm, high risk based on histologic features (e.g., ulcerated or with > 1 mitoses/mm^2), or inadequately staged (e.g., positive deep margin).[44,45] For patients with melanomas greater than 1.0 mm in thickness, a chest radiograph is considered optional. For patients with stage III disease, chest radiography or computed tomography (CT) of the chest, abdomen, and pelvis without positron emission tomography (PET) may be performed, especially to follow up on any signs or symptoms of metastases. If inguinal lymphadenopathy is apparent, a pelvic CT scan should be obtained to assess iliac lymph nodes.[46] For patients with stage IV disease, a chest radiograph and serum LDH should be obtained. Brain magnetic resonance imaging (MRI) and CT of the chest, abdomen, and pelvis should be performed before embarking on any surgery. Other imaging will be guided by protocol if the patient is enrolled in a clinical trial.[46]

Surgical Treatment of Stage I and II Melanoma

Margins of excision Surgical excision remains the mainstay of treatment for primary melanoma. The width of the recommended surgical margins depends on the thickness of the lesion and has been well defined by a series of prospective, randomized clinical trials. A 0.5 cm margin is adequate for in situ melanoma, whereas margins of 1 cm are suggested for melanomas less than 1.0 mm in thickness. One or 2 cm margins should be obtained for melanomas measuring 1 to 2 mm in depth. Data from a prospective, randomized clinical trial of 1 cm versus 3 cm excision margins for melanomas less than 2 mm in thickness revealed no difference in overall survival between the two assigned treatment arms.[47] However, the arm randomized to the 1 cm margin had a higher incidence of local recurrences, and these were clustered in the group of patients with melanomas between 1 and 2 mm in thickness. Data from the Intergoup prospective, randomized clinical trial comparing 2 cm versus 4 cm margins for melanomas measuring 1 to 4 mm in thickness revealed no reduction in survival or local control rates with use of the narrower (2 cm) surgical margin.[48] Based on these data, for patients with melanomas between 1 and 2 mm in depth, the goal is to achieve 2 cm margins. However, if the morbidity of the operation is increased significantly by use of a 2 cm versus a 1 cm margin (e.g., skin graft or flap required for closure), then a 1 cm margin is considered adequate. Two centimeter margins should be obtained for melanomas less than 2 mm in thickness.[49]

Sentinel lymph node biopsy Another important issue in the surgical management of melanoma is the use of SLNB, which has essentially replaced elective lymph node dissection. Sentinel lymph node (SLN) status is the single

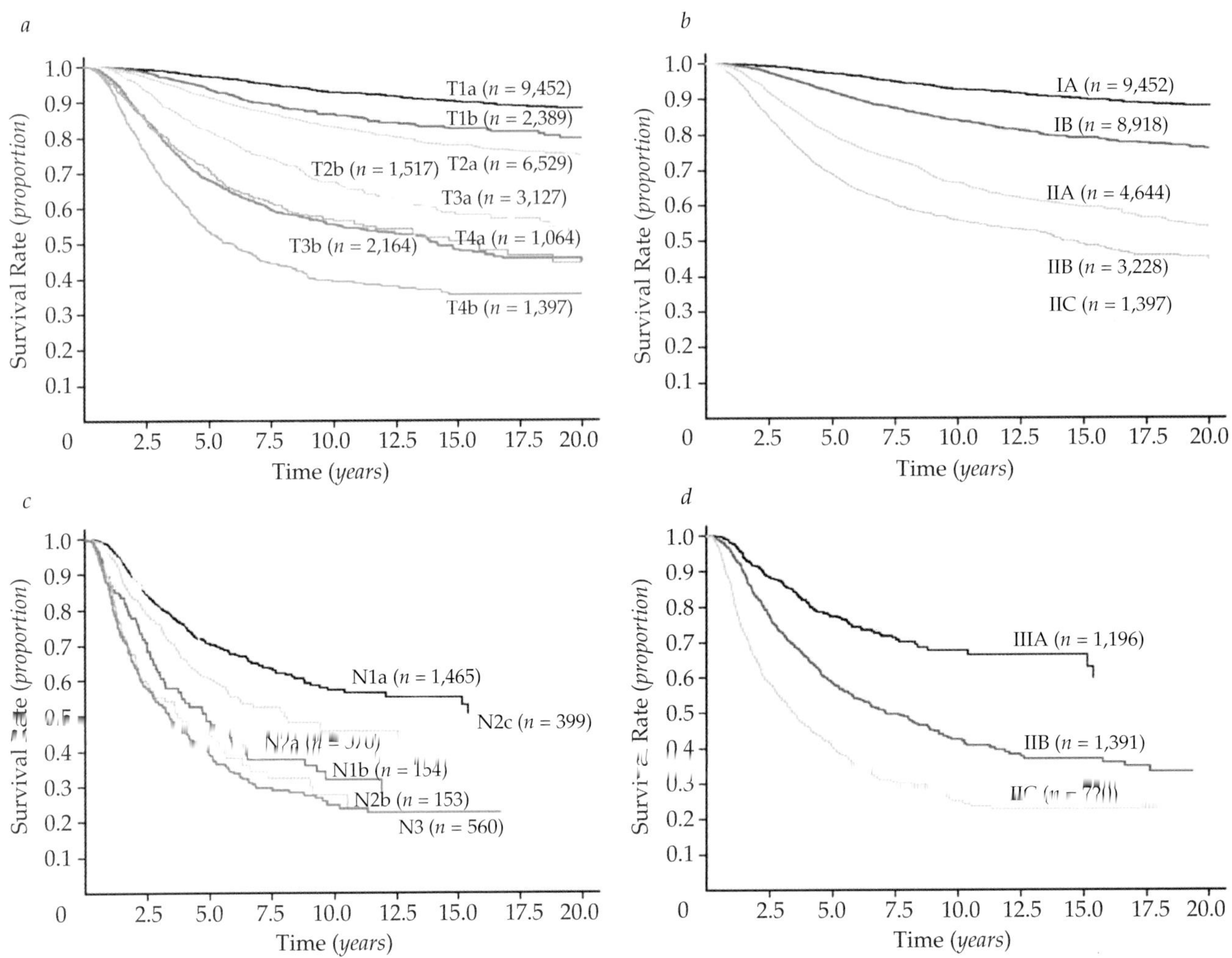

Figure 5 **Survival curves from the American Joint Committee on Cancer (AJCC) Melanoma Staging Database comparing (*a*) the different T categories and (*b*) the stage groupings for stages I and II melanoma. For patients with stage III disease, survival curves are shown comparing (*c*) the different N categories and (*d*) the stage groupings. Adapted from Balch CM, et al.[38]**

most important predictor of survival in patients with melanoma[50–52] and is considered a standard approach in this country. A positive result is defined as the presence of identifiable melanoma cells on either routine hematoxylin-eosin stains and/or by immunohistochemical staining with S-100 or HMB-45. Preoperative lymphatic mapping via lymphoscintigraphy is helpful as some patients have variable drainage basins that cannot be predicted clinically and may even drain to contralateral nodes.[53] The greatest accuracy is achieved when both radioactive colloid and blue dye are used during SLNB.[54] SLNB should not be performed in the setting of clinically positive nodes or in patients who would otherwise not be considered for lymphadenectomy.

SLNB for melanoma is critical for accurate staging and is also important in deciding whether to perform completion lymphadenectomy or offer adjuvant therapy. As mentioned, several studies have demonstrated increased overall survival and disease-free survival in SLN-negative compared with SLN-positive patients.[51,52] One of these studies demonstrated a 3-year disease-free survival of 88.5 versus 55.8% in SLN-negative versus SLN-positive patients, with a 58.6% increase in disease-free survival if the SLNB was negative.[51] The question of whether SLNB impacts survival was addressed in a prospective, randomized clinical trial—the Multicenter Selective Lymphadenectomy Trial (MSLT) I—in which patients with melanomas greater than 1.2 mm in thickness were randomized to either SLNB or observation.[55] Five-year melanoma-specific survival rates were similar in the two groups (87.1 ± 1.3% and 86.6 ± 1.6%, respectively). The 5-year disease-free survival rate for the population was 78.3 ± 1.6% in the SLNB group and 73.1 ± 2.1% in the observation group (hazard ratio [HR] for recurrence 0.74; 95% confidence interval [CI] 0.59 to 0.93; p = .009). The difference in disease-free survival between the groups resulted primarily from regional (nodal) recurrences in the group randomized to nodal observation. Among a subgroup of patients with nodal metastases, the 5-year survival rate was higher among those who underwent immediate lymphadenectomy than among those in whom lymphadenectomy was delayed (72.3 ± 4.6% versus 52.4 ± 5.9%; HR for death 0.51; 95% CI 0.32 to 0.81; p = .004). These data serve to bolster the arguments of proponents of SLNB, who cite improved survival in the subgroup of node-positive patients randomized to SLNB. These data also simultaneously bolster the arguments of opponents of SLNB, who argue that the primary end point of the study was overall survival and that no difference in overall survival was observed between the two arms. It is also important to point out that in node-positive patients, the nodal burden was significantly higher in the observation patients compared with those managed with SLNB.

Surgical Treatment of Stage III Melanoma

Complete (therapeutic) lymph node dissection Full lymphadenectomy is currently recommended for management of the regional lymph node drainage basin in the presence of a positive SLN (termed *completion lymphadenectomy*) and in patients with clinically palpable lymph node metastases (termed *therapeutic lymphadenectomy*). An important factor in considering a completion lymph node dissection following a positive SLNB is the likelihood of finding metastases in the remaining non-SLNs. This was addressed in a recent series of 658 patients in which 90 (14%) were found to have a positive SLN, with 18 (20%) of that group having evidence of metastases in additional non-SLNs.[56] These studies likely underestimate the frequency of melanoma in non-SLNs given that these nodes were analyzed only by routine hematoxylin-eosin staining on a bivalved lymph node. But these studies provide a theoretical rationale for completion lymph node dissection following a positive SLNB. Moreover, as previously discussed, the number of positive nodes impacts the prognosis and is included in the most recent AJCC staging.

The impact of completion lymphadenectomy on overall survival in SLN-positive patients remains a matter of debate and will be addressed further in MSLT-II, which is designed to evaluate the therapeutic value of completion lymph node dissection versus SLNB alone in patients who have metastasis in the SLN.[57] In this trial, patients with melanoma identified in their SLN are randomized to completion lymphadenectomy versus close clinical observation with the use of ultrasonography in the nodal basin.

Despite some controversy regarding the roles of SLNB and completion lymphadenectomy for a positive SLN, there is little debate regarding the value of therapeutic lymph node dissection in patients with clinically palpable nodal disease in the absence of distant metastases. The procedure can result in long-term survival in a subset of patients, reduces morbidity and suffering from uncontrolled tumor burden in a nodal basin, and can be performed with minimal morbidity and good palliation.[55]

Another aspect of lymphadenectomy that is debated is the extent of lymph node dissection required. Morton's group recently reviewed their experience with lymph node dissection prior to the use of SLNB and concluded that the extent of lymph node dissection is more important with a higher tumor burden and less important with a lower tumor burden.[58] Those with micrometastatic disease in an SLN and those with bulky nodal disease are clearly different, and the potential benefits of therapeutic lymph node dissection must be carefully weighed against the morbidity of the procedure.

Isolated limb perfusion Patients with in-transit metastases have an unfavorable prognosis, with a 5-year survival rate of approximately 25 to 30%. Surgical excision is the mainstay of therapy when the size and number of lesions permit. Unlike with primary melanomas, in which appropriate widths of margins are defined, in-transit metastases require only that the surgical margin is "clear." The appropriate surgical margin required for in-transit metastases is simply "margin negative." Limb amputation is almost never indicated.

Another therapeutic option for patients with extensive in-transit metastases in an extremity involves the use of hyperthermic isolated limb perfusion (HILP). This technique was introduced in 1958 and holds the advantage of achieving high regional concentrations of therapeutic agents while minimizing systemic side effects.[59] The arterial supply and venous drainage are isolated and canulated, and an oxygenated extracorporeal circuit is used to circulate chemotherapeutic agents for 1 to 1.5 hours under hyperthermic conditions. A tourniquet is also used to help achieve complete vascular isolation. Melphalan is typically used as a chemotherapeutic agent, and the limb temperature is typically elevated to 39 to 40 C.[60] The use of an extracorporeal circuit and vascular isolation protects the remainder of the body from exposure to melphalan or hyperthermia. In patients who have clinically positive nodes, therapeutic lymph node dissection is performed at the same setting just prior to limb perfusion. Observed responses to isolated limb perfusion can be dramatic. Complete response with melphalan alone is 40 to 60%.[61] However, these responses are often short-lived, with recurrence rates of 50% within 1 to 1.5 years after limb perfusion.[62] Overall 5-year survival after ILP was 32% in a recent series.[62] Recurrences following ILP may be treated with excision, although repeat ILP has also been used with success in patients with extensive disease.[63] Some clinical researchers have championed the addition of biologics such as tumor necrosis factor–α (TNF-α) as this has been shown to increase response rates to 91% in uncontrolled studies.[64] However, a randomized trial did not demonstrate any benefit from the addition of TNF-α.[65]

An alternative type of regional chemotherapy treatment for melanoma that is gaining popularity is isolated limb infusion (ILI), which is conducted under normothermic conditions. The attraction of this approach is that it does not require a surgical incision and therefore may be associated with lower morbidity than HILP. For ILI, the artery and vein of an extremity are accessed percutaneously using catheters, and a pneumatic tourniquet is inflated proximally to isolate the extremity. The blood in an isolated extremity is circulated by hand by means of a syringe "push-pull" technique; thus, the blood and chemotherapy are circulated at a much slower rate than in HILP. In addition, during ILI, the extremity is hypoxic, which leads to marked acidosis. Chemotherapy regimens for ILI typically use melphalan and dactinomycin. The approach was popularized after the original reports suggested a response rate similar to that observed with HILP.[66] But subsequent studies conducted in the United States have been unable to reproduce these results, yielding a rate of complete response of only 30%. Although there are no randomized trials that compare hyperthermic HILP with ILI, the available evidence suggests

receptor tyrosine kinase c-kit occur in approximately 20% of acral lentiginous and mucosal melanomas[95] and may be targeted with imatinib (Gleevac).[96]

Conclusions

The prevalence of malignant lesions of the skin has increased dramatically over the past several years, with nearly 1.2 million cases of nonmelanoma skin cancer diagnosed per year[1] and close to 80,000 cases of melanoma diagnosed per year.[2] The clinical assessment and management of skin lesions are challenging, and surgeons play a pivotal role in the treatment of these lesions. Thus, it is critical for surgeons to have an astute awareness of these lesions, their workup, and their management.

Specific Procedures

The inguinal nodes drain the anterior and inferior abdominal wall, the perineum, the genitalia, the hips, the buttocks, and the thighs. A superficial groin dissection removes the inguinal nodes, whereas a deep groin dissection additionally incorporates the iliac and obturator nodes. Palpable nodes can be marked on the patient before operation.

SUPERFICIAL GROIN DISSECTION

The patient is placed in a supine position on the operating table, with the hip slightly abducted and supported by a pillow and with the hip and knee slightly flexed. A Foley catheter is inserted, and the patient is prepared and draped.

The femoral artery, anterior superior iliac spine, pubic tubercle, and femoral triangle apex are marked, and a diagonally oriented skin incision is planned. The incision courses from the medial to the anterosuperior iliac spine down to the apex of the femoral triangle. An S-shaped incision is used to avoid crossing the thigh flexion crease at a right angle. This incision interferes least with the musculocutaneous and cutaneous vascular territories of the skin, minimizes ischemia to the skin flaps, and avoids a flexion contracture. Flaps are raised to identify the medial border of the sartorius muscle, the lateral border of the adductor longus muscle, and the external oblique fascia on the lower abdominal wall. Fat and nodal tissue are dissected off the external oblique aponeurosis, the spermatic cord, and the inguinal ligament and are reflected inferiorly [*see Figure 6*]. The fat and lymph nodes are then dissected from the femoral triangle starting medially at the lateral edge of the adductor longus and proceeding laterally [*see Figure 7 and Figure 8*]. The femoral vessels are left undisturbed. At the fossa ovalis, the saphenous vein is ligated and divided [*see Figure 9*]. It is also ligated and divided as it exits the femoral triangle distally. The specimen is then dissected free from the femoral nerve, usually sacrificing branches of the lateral femoral cutaneous nerve, thereby resulting in numbness of the anterolateral thigh. Cloquet lymph nodes are located medial to the femoral vein under the inguinal ligament. Following removal of the specimen, these nodes are dissected out and submitted as a separate specimen. If Cloquet nodes contain melanoma, the risk of iliac nodes with melanoma is high, and a deep groin dissection should be performed.

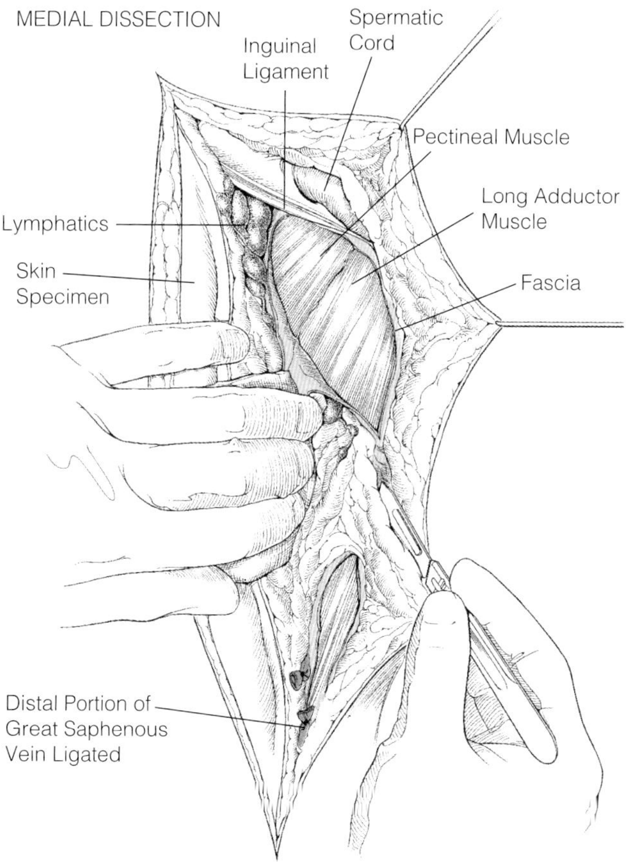

Figure 6 **Superficial groin dissection. In a superficial groin dissection, the incision is deepened to include the deep muscular fascia.**

DEEP GROIN DISSECTION

The iliac region is easily approached through a separate incision in the external oblique fascia, parallel to and above the inguinal ligament. The retroperitoneal space is further exposed by releasing the internal oblique abdominal muscle, the transversus abdominis, and the fascia transversalis. The deep circumflex iliac vessels are ligated, and blunt finger dissection separates the peritoneum from the retroperitoneal fat and nodes. Alternatively, the inguinal ligament may be divided to allow access to the retroperitoneal space, although reconstruction of the inguinal ligament can be challenging.

Retractors are inserted to widen the retroperitoneal space, and the peritoneum and the abdominal viscera are retracted medially. The chain of lymph nodes, areolar tissue, and adventitial tissues along the external iliac vessels is dissected; the dissection proceeds proximally to the origins of the internal iliac vessels (avoiding the ureter) and incorporates the nodes overlying the obturator foramen by removing the internal obturator fascia but carefully avoiding injury to the obturator nerve. The lymph node–bearing specimen is then removed as a unit, oriented, and labeled appropriately with sutures. The inguinal canal is reconstructed to prevent a hernia. The sartorius muscle is detached from the anterior superior iliac spine and the midportion of the inguinal ligament to cover the femoral vessels. The skin and the subcutaneous tissues are then closed in layers over a soft suction drain.

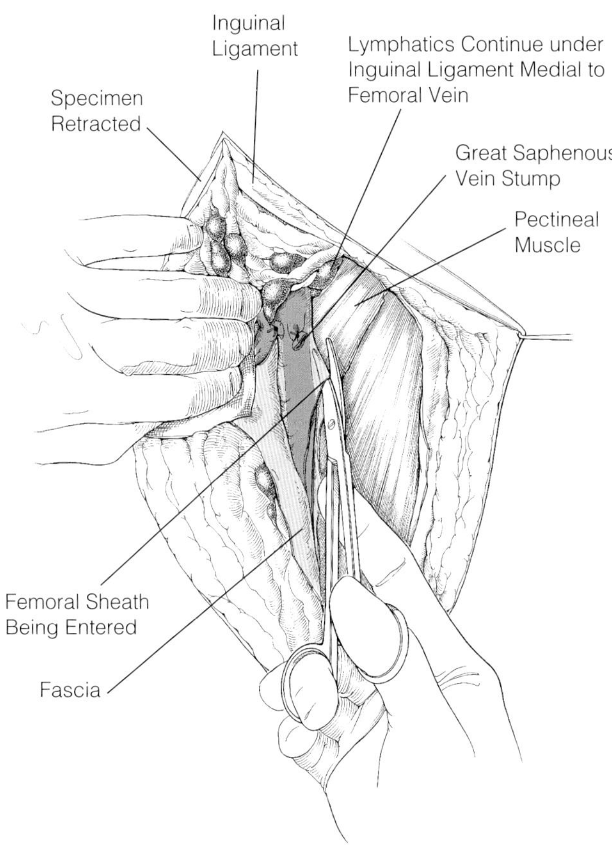

Figure 7 **Removal of investing fascia. As the superficial groin dissection proceeds, the investing fascia overlying the femoral nerve and vessels is removed.**

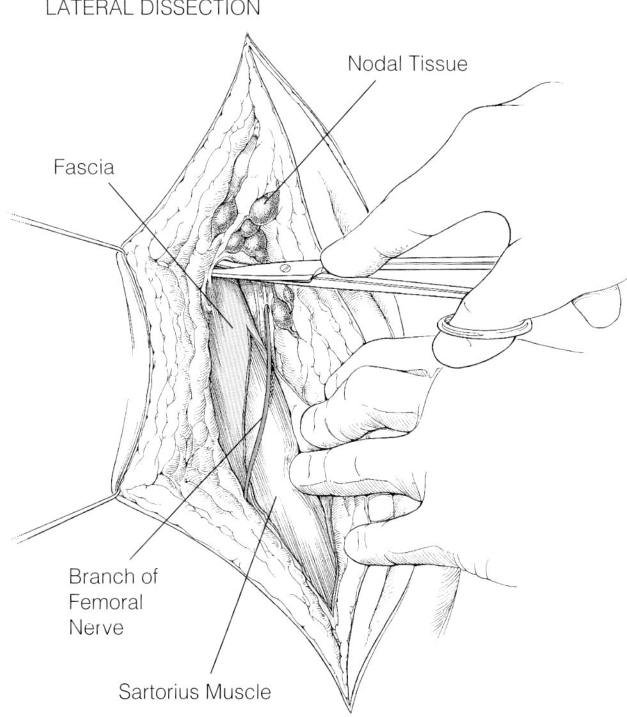

Figure 8 **Continuation of groin dissection on the lateral side. The superficial groin dissection is continued at the same level on the lateral side.**

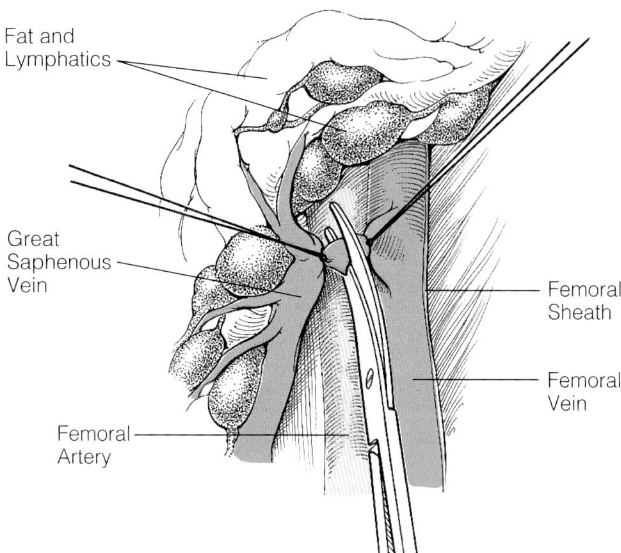

Figure 9 **Ligation and division of the great saphenous vein. The great saphenous vein is ligated and divided.**

Jennifer A. Wargo, MD, has received a speaker fee from DAVA Oncology. Kenneth Tanabe, MD, has no financial disclosures to report.

References

1. Miller DL, Weinstock MA. Nonmelanoma skin cancer in the United States: incidence. J Am Acad Dermatol 1994;30:774–8.
2. Siegel R, Naishadham D, Jemal A. Cancer statistics, 2012. CA Cancer J Clin 2012;62:10–29.
3. Hall HI, Miller DR, Rogers JD, Bewerse B. Update on the incidence and mortality from melanoma in the United States. J Am Acad Dermatol 1999;40:35–42.
4. Urbach F. Incidence of nonmelanoma skin cancer. Dermatol Clin 1991;9:751–5.
5. Rager EL, Bridgeford EP, Ollila DW. Cutaneous melanoma: update on prevention, screening, diagnosis, and treatment. Am Fam Physician 2005;72:269–76.
6. Miller SJ. Etiology and pathogenesis of basal cell carcinoma. Clin Dermatol 1995;13:527–36.
7. Marks R, Staples M, Giles GG. Trends in non-melanocytic skin cancer treated in Australia: the second national survey. Int J Cancer 1993;53:585–90.
8. Vitasa BC, Taylor HR, Strickland PT, et al. Association of nonmelanoma skin cancer and actinic keratosis with cumulative solar ultraviolet exposure in Maryland watermen. Cancer 1990;65:2811–7.
9. Wong CS, Strange RC, Lear JT. Basal cell carcinoma. BMJ 2003;327:794–8.
10. Telfer NR, Colver GB, Bowers PW. Guidelines for the management of basal cell carcinoma. British Association of Dermatologists. Br J Dermatol 1999;141:415–23.
11. Harwood M, Wu H, Tanabe K, Bercovitch L. Metastatic basal cell carcinoma diagnosed by sentinel lymph node biopsy. J Am Acad Dermatol 2005;53:475–8.

12. Rowe DE, Carroll RJ, Day CL Jr. Mohs surgery is the treatment of choice for recurrent (previously treated) basal cell carcinoma. J Dermatol Surg Oncol 1989;15:424–31.
13. Silverman MK, Kopf AW, Gladstein AH, et al. Recurrence rates of treated basal cell carcinomas. Part 4: X-ray therapy. J Dermatol Surg Oncol 1992;18:549–54.
14. Peng Q, Warloe T, Berg K, et al. 5-Aminolevulinic acid-based photodynamic therapy. Clinical research and future challenges. Cancer 1997;79:2282–308.
15. Chimenti S, Peris K, Di Cristofaro S, et al. Use of recombinant interferon alfa-2b in the treatment of basal cell carcinoma. Dermatology 1995;190:214–7.
16. Hodak E, Ginzburg A, David M, Sandbank M. Etretinate treatment of the nevoid basal cell carcinoma syndrome. Therapeutic and chemopreventive effect. Int J Dermatol 1987;26:606–9.
17. Aszterbaum M, Rothman A, Johnson RL, et al. Identification of mutations in the human PATCHED gene in sporadic basal cell carcinomas and in patients with the basal cell nevus syndrome. J Invest Dermatol 1998;110:885–8.
18. Von Hoff DD, LoRusso PM, Rudin CM, et al. Inhibition of the hedgehog pathway in advanced basal-cell carcinoma. N Engl J Med 2009;361:1164–72.
19. Sekulic A, Migden MR, Oro AE, et al. Efficacy and safety of vismodegib in advanced basal-cell carcinoma. N Engl J Med 2012;366:2171–9.
20. Tang JY, Mackay-Wiggan JM, Aszterbaum M, et al. Inhibiting the hedgehog pathway in patients with the basal-cell nevus syndrome. N Engl J Med 2012;366:2180–8.
21. Goldman GD. Squamous cell cancer: a practical approach. Semin Cutan Med Surg 1998;17:80–95.
22. Marks R. Squamous cell carcinoma. Lancet 1996;347:735–8.
23. Miki Y, Kawatsu T, Matsuda K, et al. Cutaneous and pulmonary cancers associated with Bowen's disease. J Am Acad Dermatol 1982;6:26–31.
24. Shelton RM. Skin cancer: a review and atlas for the medical provider. Mt Sinai J Med 2001;68:243–52.
25. Weinstock MA, Bogaars HA, Ashley M, et al. Nonmelanoma skin cancer mortality. A population-based study. Arch Dermatol 1991;127:1194–7.
26. Brownstein MH, Rabinowitz AD. The precursors of cutaneous squamous cell carcinoma. Int J Dermatol 1979;18:1–16.
27. Rowe DE, Carroll RJ, Day CL Jr. Prognostic factors for local recurrence, metastasis, and survival rates in squamous cell carcinoma of the skin, ear, and lip. Implications for treatment modality selection. J Am Acad Dermatol 1992; 26:976–90.
28. North JH Jr, Spellman JE, Driscoll D, et al. Advanced cutaneous squamous cell carcinoma of the trunk and extremity: analysis of prognostic factors. J Surg Oncol 1997;64:212–7.
29. Veness MJ. Time to rethink TNM staging in cutaneous SCC. Lancet Oncol 2008;9:702–3.
30. Mullen JT, Feng L, Xing Y, et al. Invasive squamous cell carcinoma of the skin: defining a high-risk group. Ann Surg Oncol 2006;13:902–9.
31. Kwon S, Dong ZM, Wu PC. Sentinel lymph node biopsy for high-risk cutaneous squamous cell carcinoma: clinical experience and review of literature. World J Surg Oncol 2011; 9:80.
32. Guy GP, Ekwueme DU. Years of potential life lost and indirect costs of melanoma and non-melanoma skin cancer: a systematic review of the literature. Pharmacoeconomics 2011;29:863–74.
33. Schwartz JL, Wang TS, Hamilton TA, et al. Thin primary cutaneous melanomas: associated detection patterns, lesion characteristics, and patient characteristics. Cancer 2002;95: 1562–8.
34. Friedman RJ, Rigel DS, Silverman MK, et al. Malignant melanoma in the 1990s: the continued importance of early detection and the role of physician examination and self-examination of the skin. CA Cancer J Clin 1991;41:201–26.
35. Crowson AN, Magro CM, Mihm MC. Prognosticators of melanoma, the melanoma report, and the sentinel lymph node. Mod Pathol 2006;19 Suppl 2:S71–87.
36. George E, McClain SE, Slingluff CL, et al. Subclassification of desmoplastic melanoma: pure and mixed variants have significantly different capacities for lymph node metastasis. J Cutan Pathol 2009;36:425–32.
37. Breslow A. Thickness, cross-sectional areas and depth of invasion in the prognosis of cutaneous melanoma. Ann Surg 1970;172:902–8.
38. Balch CM, Gershenwald JE, Soong SJ, et al. Final version of 2009 AJCC melanoma staging and classification. J Clin Oncol 2009;27:6199–206.
39. Barnhill RL, Katzen J, Spatz A, et al. The importance of mitotic rate as a prognostic factor for localized cutaneous melanoma. J Cutan Pathol 2005;32:268–73.
40. Francken AB, Shaw HM, Thompson JF, et al. The prognostic importance of tumor mitotic rate confirmed in 1317 patients with primary cutaneous melanoma and long follow-up. Ann Surg Oncol 2004;11:426–33.
41. Thompson JF, Soong SJ, Balch CM, et al. Prognostic significance of mitotic rate in localized primary cutaneous melanoma: an analysis of patients in the multi-institutional American Joint Committee on Cancer melanoma staging database. J Clin Oncol 2011;29:2199–205.
42. Gimotty PA, Guerry D, Ming ME, et al. Thin primary cutaneous malignant melanoma: a prognostic tree for 10-year metastasis is more accurate than American Joint Committee on Cancer staging. J Clin Oncol 2004;22:3668–76.
43. Balch CM, Soong SJ, Gershenwald JE, et al. Prognostic factors analysis of 17,600 melanoma patients: validation of the American Joint Committee on Cancer melanoma staging system. J Clin Oncol 2001;19:3622–34.
44. Coit DG, Andtbacka R, Bichakjian CK, et al. Melanoma. J Natl Compr Cancer Netw 2009;7:250–75.
45. Bichakjian CK, Halpern AC, Johnson TM, et al. Guidelines of care for the management of primary cutaneous melanoma. American Academy of Dermatology. J Am Acad Dermatol 2011;65:1032–47.
46. Johnson TM, Bradford CR, Gruber SB, et al. Staging workup, sentinel node biopsy, and follow-up tests for melanoma: update of current concepts. Arch Dermatol 2004;140: 107–13.
47. Veronesi U, Cascinelli N, Adamus J, et al. Thin stage I primary cutaneous malignant melanoma. Comparison of excision with margins of 1 or 3 cm. N Engl J Med 1988;318: 1159–62.
48. Balch CM, Urist MM, Karakousis CP, et al. Efficacy of 2-cm surgical margins for intermediate-thickness melanomas (1 to 4 mm). Results of a multi-institutional randomized surgical trial. Ann Surg 1993;218:262–7; discussion 7–9.

49. Rigel DS, Carucci JA. Malignant melanoma: prevention, early detection, and treatment in the 21st century. CA Cancer J Clin 2000;50:215–36; quiz 37–40.
50. Gershenwald JE, Colome MI, Lee JE, et al. Patterns of recurrence following a negative sentinel lymph node biopsy in 243 patients with stage I or II melanoma. J Clin Oncol 1998; 16:2253–60.
51. Gershenwald JE, Mansfield PF, Lee JE, Ross MI. Role for lymphatic mapping and sentinel lymph node biopsy in patients with thick (> or = 4 mm) primary melanoma. Ann Surg Oncol 2000;7:160–5.
52. Gershenwald JE, Thompson W, Mansfield PF, et al. Multi-institutional melanoma lymphatic mapping experience: the prognostic value of sentinel lymph node status in 612 stage I or II melanoma patients. J Clin Oncol 1999;17:976–83.
53. Thompson JF, Uren RF. Lymphatic mapping in management of patients with primary cutaneous melanoma. Lancet Oncol 2005;6:877–85.
54. Morton DL. Sentinel node mapping and an International Sentinel Node Society: current issues and future directions. Ann Surg Oncol 2004;11:137S–43S.
55. Hughes TM, A'Hern RP, Thomas JM. Prognosis and surgical management of patients with palpable inguinal lymph node metastases from melanoma. Br J Surg 2000;87: 892–901.
56. Clinical practice guidelines for the management of cutaneous melanoma. Canberra: National Health and Medical Research Council; 1999.
57. Morton DL. Overview and update of the phase III Multicenter Selective Lymphadenectomy Trials (MSLT-I and MSLT-II) in melanoma. Clin Exp Metastasis 2012;29: 699–706.
58. Chan AD, Essner R, Wanek LA, Morton DL. Judging the therapeutic value of lymph node dissections for melanoma. J Am Coll Surg 2000;191:16–22; discussion 3.
59. Benckhuijsen C, Kroon BB, van Geel AN, Wieberdink J. Regional perfusion treatment with melphalan for melanoma in a limb: an evaluation of drug kinetics. Eur J Surg Oncol 1988;14:157–63.
60. Lingam MK, Byrne DS, Aitchison T, et al. A single centre's 10 year experience with isolated limb perfusion in the treatment of recurrent malignant melanoma of the limb. Eur J Cancer 1996;32A:1668–73.
61. Vrouenraets BC, Nieweg OE, Kroon BB. Thirty-five years of isolated limb perfusion for melanoma: indications and results. Br J Surg 1996;83:1319–28.
62. Grunhagen DJ, Brunstein F, Graveland WJ, et al. One hundred consecutive isolated limb perfusions with TNF-alpha and melphalan in melanoma patients with multiple in-transit metastases. Ann Surg 2004;240:939–47; discussion 47–8.
63. Feldman AL, Alexander HR Jr, Bartlett DL, et al. Management of extremity recurrences after complete responses to isolated limb perfusion in patients with melanoma. Ann Surg Oncol 1999;6:562–7.
64. Lejeune F, Lienard D, Eggermont A, et al. Rationale for using TNF alpha and chemotherapy in regional therapy of melanoma. J Cell Biochem 1994;56:52–61.
65. Burmeister BH, Henderson MA, Ainslie J, et al. Adjuvant radiotherapy versus observation alone for patients at risk of lymph-node field relapse after therapeutic lymphadenectomy for melanoma: a randomised trial. Lancet Oncol 2012; 13:589–97.
66. Kroon HM, Lin DY, Kam PC, Thompson JF. Efficacy of repeat isolated limb infusion with melphalan and actinomycin D for recurrent melanoma. Cancer 2009;115: 1932–40.
67. Stevens G, Thompson JF, Firth I, et al. Locally advanced melanoma: results of postoperative hypofractionated radiation therapy. Cancer 2000;88:88–94.
68. Ang KK, Byers RM, Peters LJ, et al. Regional radiotherapy as adjuvant treatment for head and neck malignant melanoma. Preliminary results. Arch Otolaryngol Head Neck Surg 1990;116:169–72.
69. Morris KT, Marquez CM, Holland JM, Vetto JT. Prevention of local recurrence after surgical debulking of nodal and subcutaneous melanoma deposits by hypofractionated radiation. Ann Surg Oncol 2000;7:680–4.
70. Morton DL, Thompson JF, Cochran AJ, et al. Sentinel-node biopsy or nodal observation in melanoma. N Engl J Med 2006;355:1307–17.
71. Kirkwood JM, Strawderman MH, Ernstoff MS, et al. Interferon alfa-2b adjuvant therapy of high-risk resected cutaneous melanoma: the Eastern Cooperative Oncology Group Trial EST 1684. J Clin Oncol 1996;14:7–17.
72. Wheatley K, Ives N, Hancock B, et al. Does adjuvant interferon-alpha for high-risk melanoma provide a worthwhile benefit? A meta-analysis of the randomised trials. Cancer Treat Rev 2003;29:241–52.
73. Eggermont AM, Suciu S, Testori A, et al. Long-term results of the randomized phase III trial EORTC 18991 of adjuvant therapy with pegylated interferon alfa-2b versus observation in resected stage III melanoma. J Clin Oncol 2012;30: 3810–8.
74. Gogas H, Ioannovich J, Dafni U, et al. Prognostic significance of autoimmunity during treatment of melanoma with interferon. N Engl J Med 2006;354:709–18.
75. Morton DL, Foshag LJ, Hoon DS, et al. Prolongation of survival in metastatic melanoma after active specific immunotherapy with a new polyvalent melanoma vaccine. Ann Surg 1992;216:463–82.
76. Butterfield LH, Ribas A, Dissette VB, et al. Determinant spreading associated with clinical response in dendritic cell-based immunotherapy for malignant melanoma. Clin Cancer Res 2003;9:998–1008.
77. Soiffer R, Hodi FS, Haluska F, et al. Vaccination with irradiated, autologous melanoma cells engineered to secrete granulocyte-macrophage colony-stimulating factor by adenoviral-mediated gene transfer augments antitumor immunity in patients with metastatic melanoma. J Clin Oncol 2003;21:3343–50.
78. Rosenberg SA, Yang JC, Restifo NP. Cancer immunotherapy: moving beyond current vaccines. Nat Med 2004;10: 909–15.
79. Wong SL, Coit DG. Role of surgery in patients with stage IV melanoma. Curr Opin Oncol 2004;16:155–60.
80. Cohen GL, Falkson CI. Current treatment options for malignant melanoma. Drugs 1998;55:791–9.
81. Middleton MR, Grob JJ, Aaronson N, et al. Randomized phase III study of temozolomide versus dacarbazine in the treatment of patients with advanced metastatic malignant melanoma. J Clin Oncol 2000;18:158–66.

82. Rosenberg SA, Yang JC, Topalian SL, et al. Treatment of 283 consecutive patients with metastatic melanoma or renal cell cancer using high-dose bolus interleukin 2. JAMA 1994;271: 907–13.
83. Atkins MB, Kunkel L, Sznol M, Rosenberg SA. High-dose recombinant interleukin-2 therapy in patients with metastatic melanoma: long-term survival update. Cancer J Sci Am 2000;6 Suppl 1:S11–4.
84. Dudley ME, Wunderlich J, Nishimura MI, et al. Adoptive transfer of cloned melanoma-reactive T lymphocytes for the treatment of patients with metastatic melanoma. J Immunother 2001;24:363–73.
85. Dudley ME, Wunderlich JR, Robbins PF, et al. Cancer regression and autoimmunity in patients after clonal repopulation with antitumor lymphocytes. Science 2002;298: 850–4.
86. Hughes MS, Yu YY, Dudley ME, et al. Transfer of a TCR gene derived from a patient with a marked antitumor response conveys highly active T-cell effector functions. Hum Gene Ther 2005;16:457–72.
87. Pardoll DM. The blockade of immune checkpoints in cancer immunotherapy. Nat Rev Cancer 2012;12:252–64.
88. Hodi FS, O'Day SJ, McDermott DF, et al. Improved survival with ipilimumab in patients with metastatic melanoma. N Engl J Med 2010;363:711–23.
89. Attia P, Phan GQ, Maker AV, et al. Autoimmunity correlates with tumor regression in patients with metastatic melanoma treated with anti-cytotoxic T-lymphocyte antigen-4. J Clin Oncol 2005;23:6043–53.
90. Topalian SL, Hodi FS, Brahmer JR, et al. Safety, activity, and immune correlates of anti-PD-1 antibody in cancer. N Engl J Med 2012;366:2443–54.
91. Brahmer JR, Tykodi SS, Chow LQ, et al. Safety and activity of anti-PD-L1 antibody in patients with advanced cancer. N Engl J Med 2012;366:2455–65.
92. Davies H, Bignell GR, Cox C, et al. Mutations of the BRAF gene in human cancer. Nature 2002;417:949–54.
93. Chapman PB, Hauschild A, Robert C, et al. Improved survival with vemurafenib in melanoma with BRAF V600E mutation. N Engl J Med 2011;364:2507–16.
94. Flaherty KT, Infante JR, Daud A, et al. Combined BRAF and MEK inhibition in melanoma with BRAF V600 mutations. N Engl J Med 2012;367:1694–703. DOI 10.1056/NEJMoa1210093.
95. Curtin JA, Fridlyand J, Kageshita T, et al. Distinct sets of genetic alterations in melanoma. N Engl J Med 2005;353: 2135–47.
96. Guo J, Si L, Kong Y, et al. Phase II, open-label, single-arm trial of imatinib mesylate in patients with metastatic melanoma harboring c-kit mutation or amplification. J Clin Oncol 2011;29:2904–9.

5 BREAST PROCEDURES

Angela Gucwa, MD, J. Garrett Harper, MD, and D. Scott Lind, MD

The procedures used to diagnose, stage, and treat breast disease are rapidly becoming less invasive and more cosmetically satisfying while remaining oncologically sound. In particular, percutaneous core biopsy has largely replaced excisional breast biopsy for both palpable and nonpalpable breast lesions and has proved to be an equally accurate, less invasive, and less costly means of pathologic diagnosis.[1] Moreover, in clinically appropriate patients, sentinel lymph node biopsy (SLNB) has proved to be an accurate method of staging the axilla that reduces the incidence of many of the complications associated with traditional axillary node dissection.[2] Furthermore, breast conservation has largely supplanted mastectomy for definitive surgical treatment of breast cancer; randomized trials continue to demonstrate equivalent survival rates for the two therapies.[3] Even in those cases where mastectomy is either required or preferred, advances in reconstructive techniques have been made that yield significantly improved outcomes after breast reconstruction.[4] Finally, in an effort to eliminate the need for open surgical treatment of breast cancer, various percutaneous extirpative and ablative local therapies have been developed and are being evaluated for potential use in managing breast cancer in carefully selected patients.[5]

A more minimally invasive approach to breast disease will depend to a substantial extent on the availability of accurate and efficient imaging modalities. Adeptness with such modalities is rapidly becoming an essential part of the general surgeon's skill set. In this chapter, we describe selected standard, novel, and investigational procedures employed in the diagnosis and management of breast disease. The application of these procedures is a dynamic process that is shaped both by technological advances and by physicians' evolving understanding of the biology of breast diseases.

Breast Ultrasonography

Breast ultrasonography can be useful for evaluating palpable breast masses or mammographically indeterminate lesions; for carrying out postoperative and oncologic follow-up; for guiding aspiration and biopsy of lesions; and for facilitating intraoperative tumor localization, margin assessment, placement of catheters for partial-breast irradiation, and investigational tumor-ablating techniques.

In the office, breast ultrasonography has become a useful adjunct to the clinical breast examination, particularly in patients with radiographically dense mammograms. It defines breast lesions more clearly than physical examination does and thus can potentially reduce the number of unnecessary biopsies done for simple cysts or fibroglandular tissue presenting as a palpable nodularity. Whole-breast ultrasonography is not an effective screening tool and therefore should not be a substitute for annual mammography. The American College of Surgeons (ACS) and various surgical subspecialty organizations offer a multitude of courses, at varying skill levels, geared toward training general surgeons in the use of breast ultrasonography.

TECHNIQUE

Most real-time ultrasound imaging is performed with handheld probes generating frequencies between 7.5 and 12 MHz. The procedure is conducted with the patient supine, a pillow behind the shoulder, and the ipsilateral arm extended over the head for maximal spreading of the breast. Sonographic transmission gel is applied between the transducer and the skin to reduce air artifacts, and the transducer is pressed slightly against the skin to improve image quality. The selected breast area is imaged from the nipple outward in a radial pattern.

All lesions should be sonographically characterized with respect to margins, effect on adjacent tissue, internal echo pattern, compressibility, height to width ratio, and presence of shadowing versus posterior enhancement. Classically, simple cysts tend to be oval or lobulated, anechoic, and sharply demarginated; they typically demonstrate posterior enhancement. Benign solid lesions tend to be well circumscribed, hypoechoic, and wider than they are tall; they show homogeneous internal echoes and edge shadowing. Carcinomas are also hypoechoic masses, but they cross tissue planes and therefore tend to be taller than they are wide, with irregular borders; in addition, they can demonstrate heterogeneous interior patterns and broad acoustic shadowing [*see Figure 1*]. A lesion that has a single indeterminate characteristic on ultrasonography or that is clinically suspicious despite appearing benign on ultrasonography is an indication for core or open biopsy. Lesions should be characterized in at least two orthogonal planes, and the image should be saved for future reference.

Ductal Lavage

The majority of breast cancers originate from the epithelium of the mammary ducts. Originally developed to increase the cellular yield after nipple aspiration failed to obtain adequate sampling, ductal lavage is a method of recovering breast duct epithelial cells for cytologic analysis via a microcatheter that is inserted into the duct.[6] Potential applications include

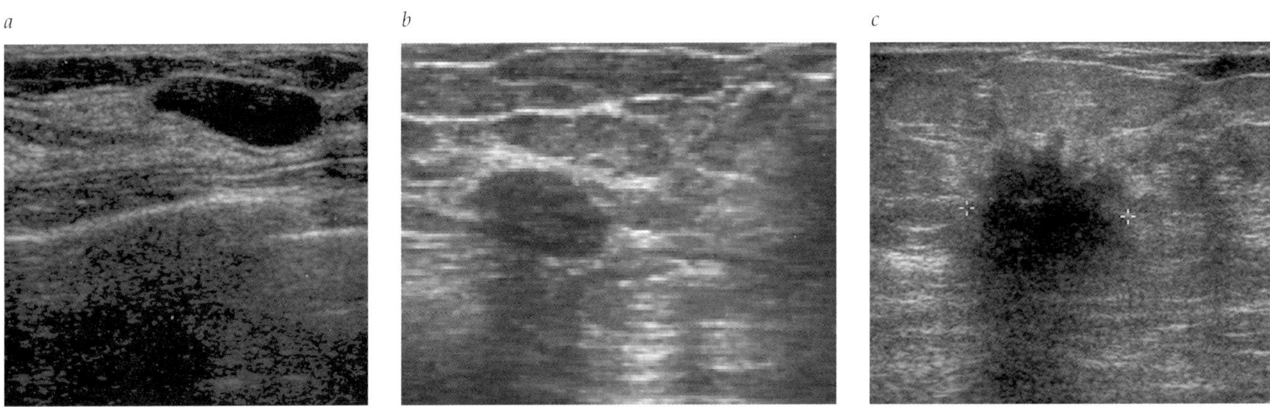

Figure 1 **Breast ultrasonography. Shown are (*a*) a simple cyst that has smooth margins, is anechoic, and shows posterior enhancement; (*b*) a fibroadenoma that has smooth margins, is hypoechoic, and shows posterior shadowing; and (*c*) a mammary carcinoma that has irregular borders, is hypoechoic, and shows irregular posterior shadowing.**

identifying high-risk women, predicting risk with molecular markers, monitoring the effectiveness of chemopreventive agents, and delivering drugs directly into the ducts. At present, however, ductal lavage remains investigational, and its predictive value and clinical utility await further definition.[7]

TECHNIQUE

The breast duct epithelium may be sampled by means of either nipple fluid aspiration or ductal lavage. For the aspiration of nipple fluid, a topical anesthetic is first applied to the nipple, followed by a mild scrub with a dekeratinizing gel. Suction is then applied to the nipple while the breast is gently massaged. Aspirated fluid is sent for analysis. In ductal lavage, the breast and nipple are similarly prepared. The nipple duct orifice that yields fluid spontaneously or as a result of suction is cannulated, the duct is irrigated with saline, and the effluent is collected for cytologic analysis. Cannulation of the duct is possible in the majority of women. Both nipple fluid aspiration and ductal lavage are generally well tolerated. The former is simpler and less expensive, but the latter retrieves more cells.[8]

Ductoscopy

Advances in endoscopic technology have allowed for visualization and biopsy of the mammary ducts, including those in more peripheral locations.[9] Mammary ductoscopy is a procedure in which a 0.9 mm microendoscope is employed to visualize the lining of the ductal system directly. Previous studies have revealed ductoscopy to be safe for use in three main areas: (1) evaluation of patients with pathologic nipple discharge,[10] (2) evaluation of high-risk patients, and (3) evaluation of breast cancer patients to determine the extent of intraductal disease and perhaps reduce the rate of positive margins. This is especially important in those patients with in situ disease and benign radiographic findings.[11] Current research is aimed at the use of ductoscopy-directed biopsy and ablation techniques. Perforation of the mammary duct is the most commonly reported complication; however, this appears to have minimal sequela. At present, this investigational technology is available at only a few centers, and further study will be required to determine its precise role in the evaluation and management of breast disease.

TECHNIQUE

Ductoscopy can be performed either in the office or in the operating room with minimal discomfort. Before the procedure, a nipple block is usually performed with topical lidocaine cream, supplemented (if necessary) by intradermal injection of 1% lidocaine around the nipple-areola complex or intraductal instillation of lidocaine (or both). The breast is massaged to promote expression of nipple aspirate fluid, which facilitates identification of a ductal orifice. The duct is then gently dilated, and the ductoscope is advanced with the help of insufflation under direct visualization. Most ducts with pathologic discharge can readily be identified and dilated sufficiently to allow passage of the ductoscope.[12] Under direct visualization, the ductoscope is advanced using saline insufflation. An outer air channel on the fiberscope permits instillation and collection of saline solution so that cells can be retrieved for ductal lavage.[13] Intraductal lesions can be percutaneously localized under direct endoscopic visualization for subsequent biopsy; alternatively, they may be amenable to endoscopic cytologic brushing or to the newly described technique of intraductal breast biopsy.[12]

The procedure is usually well tolerated. It should be noted that duct excision is still regarded as standard practice for pathologic discharge, regardless of endoscopic findings.

Breast Biopsy

Cytologic or tissue diagnosis of a palpable breast mass may be obtained by means of fine-needle aspiration (FNA) biopsy, core-needle biopsy (CNB), or open incisional or excisional biopsy. Currently, most solid lesions are initially diagnosed by means of CNB, which is less invasive, less costly, and more expeditious than open biopsy while achieving comparable accuracy. In select circumstances, however, FNA biopsy and open biopsy may remain suitable options. All minimally invasive biopsy techniques are facilitated when guided by imaging modalities; such guidance enables the physician to perform a more directed biopsy that targets the lesion precisely while avoiding benign-appearing tissue, necrotic tissue, and adjacent structures (e.g., the chest wall, skin, and axillary vessels). Therefore, even when a lesion is palpable, ultrasound-directed biopsy is preferable to blind biopsy (although not absolutely necessary) and is recommended if the surgeon has a suitable ultrasound device in the office.

The choice of a specific biopsy technique should be individualized on the basis of the clinical and radiographic features of the lesion, the experience of the clinician, and the patient's condition and preference.

FINE-NEEDLE ASPIRATION BIOPSY

FNA biopsy permits the sampling of cells from the breast or the axillary region for cytologic analysis. It is particularly useful for sampling a clinically or sonographically suspicious axillary node and for evaluating cyst fluid that is bloody or that comes from an incompletely collapsed or recurrent cyst. In patients receiving anticoagulants, FNA biopsy is a reasonable alternative to CNB for evaluation of a solid lesion in that there is less potential for hemorrhage if anticoagulation cannot be discontinued. Discrete masses discovered on physical examination may be either cystic or solid. A lesion that is shown by ultrasonography to be a simple cyst need not undergo FNA biopsy unless it is symptomatic.

Technique

The skin of the breast or axilla is prepared, and a local anesthetic is injected superficially via a 25-gauge needle. Although smaller needles may be used, a 21-gauge needle is optimal for FNA biopsy because it can be effectively used both for aspiration of potentially viscous fluid and for procurement of sufficient cellular material from solid masses. To generate adequate suction, a 10 mL or larger syringe should be used. As noted (see above), FNA biopsy ideally is performed under ultrasonographic guidance. If such guidance is unavailable, the lesion is held steady between the thumb and the index finger of the nondominant hand. Before the needle enters the skin, 1 mL of air is introduced into the biopsy syringe. Then, without the application of suction, the needle is advanced into the lesion. Once the needle is in place, strong suction is applied.

If the lesion is cystic, all fluid is aspirated, at which point the mass should disappear. Ultrasonography can confirm the complete collapse of a cyst or help direct the needle to an undrained portion of the cyst. The fluid need not be sent for analysis unless it is bloody or is associated with a residual palpable mass or an incompletely collapsed cyst as seen on ultrasonography. If the fluid is to be sent for analysis, it is injected directly into the pathologic preservative. The patient is reexamined 4 to 8 weeks after successful aspiration. If the same cyst has recurred, aspiration should be repeated and the new aspirate sent for cytologic analysis.

If the lesion is solid, the needle is moved back and forth within the lesion along a 5 to 10 mm tract until tissue is visualized in the hub of the needle. (This oscillation of the needle along the same tract is the most effective way of obtaining a cellular, diagnostic specimen.) Suction is released while the needle is still within the lesion, and the needle is then withdrawn. The contents of the needle are expelled onto prepared glass slides, spread into a thin smear, and fixed according to the preferences of the cytology laboratory. The syringe may be rinsed so that a cellblock can be prepared for further analysis. The lesion should be sampled twice to ensure that a sufficiently cellular sample has been obtained.

Interpretation of Results

Accurate interpretation of FNA requires substantial experience on the part of both the operator and the cytopathologist; only in a few select centers with expert breast cytopathologists has it remained the diagnostic procedure of choice for solid breast masses. Consequently, one must exercise considerable caution about using FNA biopsy rather than CNB as the sole means of confirming a cancer diagnosis before the initiation of definitive operative management or neoadjuvant therapy. FNA biopsy is unable to discriminate carcinoma in situ from invasive carcinoma and therefore is incapable of establishing whether axillary node staging is needed. Furthermore, because of the smaller quantity of tissue extracted, FNA biopsy is a less reliable means of assessing receptor status than CNB is. Finally, in 1 to 2% of cases, FNA biopsy may yield false positive results,[14] potentially leading to an unnecessary cancer operation. For these reasons, it is recommended that malignancies identified by FNA biopsy be confirmed by means of CNB or open biopsy (preferably the former) before definitive therapy is provided.

Cytologic analysis that is diagnostic of a specific benign lesion (e.g., a fibroadenoma) may generally be relied on if it is in concordance with the clinical features of the lesion. However, a negative result from FNA biopsy does not exclude cancer: this procedure fails to diagnose as many as 40% of breast malignancies.[14] Cellular atypia, pathologic discordance, or a nondiagnostic FNA is an indication for tissue diagnosis.

CORE-NEEDLE BIOPSY

As noted (see above), CNB is the diagnostic procedure of choice for breast lesions. Like FNA biopsy, it is easily performed in an outpatient setting. Unlike FNA biopsy, CNB removes a narrow cylinder of tissue that is submitted for pathologic rather than cytologic analysis. Whenever feasible, CNB of both palpable and nonpalpable lesions is performed under ultrasonographic guidance, which permits real-time documentation of the needle's position within the lesion. For lesions not visualized on ultrasonography or for suspicious microcalcifications, stereotactic guidance may be employed instead. A preoperative diagnosis of malignancy obtained via CNB enables the surgeon to perform a single-stage operative procedure. It may also help lower the positive margin rate for patients undergoing breast-conserving therapy (BCT), thereby reducing the need for reexcision and improving the cosmetic outcome.[15]

Various automatic, rotational, and vacuum-assisted devices may be employed to perform CNB; in what follows, we briefly discuss these devices [*see* Technique, *below*]. When CNB is performed with a 14-gauge needle, as is the case with Tru-Cut (Cardinal Health, Dublin, Ohio) devices and spring-loaded guns, up to 30% pathologic upgrading may be seen on subsequent surgical excision.[1] When CNB is done with a larger needle (8 to 11 gauge), as is the case with image-guided vacuum-assisted and rotational devices, a greater volume of tissue is delivered; consequently, less pathologic upgrading is seen.[16] With the vacuum-assisted core biopsy (VACB) devices currently available, it is possible to remove all radiographic evidence of the lesion. It is therefore common practice with all core biopsies to place a titanium clip or another surrogate marker at the biopsy site to facilitate future localization procedures. In addition, a clip should be placed at the biopsy site if the patient has a larger cancer for which neoadjuvant chemotherapy is required; some such lesions exhibit a complete clinical response to chemotherapy and thus are no longer radiographically visible at the time of definitive operative treatment. Two-view postbiopsy mammography should be performed to confirm accurate placement of the clip and adequate sampling of the lesion at the time of biopsy.

Technique

Palpation-guided biopsy In this setting, a manual Tru-Cut–type device or, more commonly, a spring-loaded semiautomatic biopsy gun is used to obtain the specimen. The skin is prepared, and a local anesthetic is infiltrated superficially via a 25-gauge needle. A nick is made in the skin with a No. 11 blade to permit easy entry of the biopsy needle (usually a 14-gauge needle). As with FNA biopsy (see above), the lesion is held steady in the nondominant hand while the biopsy needle is advanced into the periphery of the lesion. Next, the needle is manually advanced through the center of the lesion (if a manual device is used), or the gun is fired (if a spring-loaded device is used). Finally, the needle is withdrawn to retrieve the core. Four to five cores, each from a separate pass, should be obtained to ensure that the lesion is not undersampled. Pressure is applied over the lesion and the biopsy tract for 10 to 15 minutes to ensure adequate hemostasis. The nick in the skin is closed with an adhesive strip (e.g., Steri-Strip, 3M, St. Paul, Minnesota).

Ultrasound-guided biopsy This technique may be employed for both palpable and nonpalpable lesions. The lesion that is to undergo biopsy is centered on the screen of the ultrasound device. A local anesthetic is injected superficially, first along the anticipated biopsy tract and then both anterior and posterior to the lesion; this latter maneuver helps ensure that there is a safe distance between the lesion and the skin or the chest wall. A nick is made in the skin with a No. 11 blade. The biopsy needle is then inserted through the skin, with care taken to keep it in a plane parallel to the footplate of the ultrasound probe as it passes through the breast tissue. The biopsy itself can be either performed in a freehand manner or directed with a needle guide attached to the probe. The ideal final positions of the tip and shaft vary, depending on the particular biopsy device selected for the procedure [*see Figure 2*]. Regardless of which device is used, the tip and shaft of the needle should be visualized throughout the entire approach to and biopsy of the lesion. Prefire and postfire images should be obtained that show the needle in proximity to and within the lesion, respectively. Four to five good cores are required for adequate sampling. Once the biopsy is complete, pressure is applied over the lesion and the biopsy tract, and a Steri-Strip is placed. To facilitate closure of larger entry sites, a single subcuticular stitch may be used.

Brisk bleeding may occur during and immediately after the procedure, but it usually can be controlled by the application of direct pressure. Patients are restricted from engaging in strenuous activity for 24 hours after biopsy. Bruising may result, but it typically resolves within days. Other potential complications include hematoma, fat necrosis, a palpable lump, and infection; however, such events are uncommon. Most patients receiving oral anticoagulants can be switched to a subcutaneous alternative that can be stopped on the morning of the procedure.

Semiautomated gun biopsy When a spring-loaded semiautomatic biopsy gun is used, the tip of the needle should abut the lesion in such a way that the biopsy trough will be in the lesion after the device is fired. Ideally, the repeat passes should sample different portions of the lesion and avoid any necrotic areas that have been visualized.

Vacuum-assisted core biopsy Vacuum-assisted rotational cutting devices employ a 7- to 11-gauge probe with a distal sampling trough and an inner rotating cutter. The sampling trough can be placed either in the center of the lesion or directly under it. The probe is attached to a vacuum system, which draws the target tissue into the trough. Once the tissue has been drawn into the trough, the inner rotating cutter is advanced and cuts a core from it. The tissue core is then delivered by the vacuum system through the barrel of the probe and into a proximal collection chamber. The probe can be rotated up to 360° and can retrieve multiple samples through a single insertion in the skin. The larger tissue volumes obtained with these rotational VACB devices have reduced the incidence of atypical ductal hyperplasia or ductal carcinoma in situ (DCIS) upgrades on subsequent excisional biopsies.[5]

Cryoassisted core biopsy In a cryobiopsy, a thin (19-gauge) solid needle is placed in the middle of the targeted tissue. The tip is then cooled to approximately 10°C, a temperature that freezes the tissue to the needle but does not cause tissue necrosis. An outer rotating cutting cannula (10 gauge) is then advanced over the inner localizing needle. The device is removed from the breast, and the single specimen is removed. As with the semiautomatic biopsy gun, multiple passes into the breast are still required. However, the local anesthetic effect of the cooling process, the ability of the device to spear and stabilize a lesion, and the absence of a firing gun–type action make cryobiopsy advantageous, particularly for a mobile lesion that lies close to the skin or the chest wall.

Stereotactic-guided biopsy Lesions that are visible on mammography—including small solid lesions, asymmetrical densities, and suspicious groups of microcalcifications—can often be targeted and subjected to core biopsy under stereotactic guidance.[17] Stereotaxy refers to the use of three-dimensional coordinates to localize and identify the lesion and determine the precise positioning of the tissue to be sampled.[18] This outpatient procedure commonly makes use of a mounted VACB gun, similar to the handheld VACB device previously described (see above). Stereotactic biopsy is appropriate for lesions that are clearly visible on digital images and identifiable on stereotactic projections. Lesions that lie close to the chest wall or in the subareolar region may not be amenable to stereotactic biopsy and are often best approached via open biopsy with needle localization (see below). Likewise, lesions in thinly compressible breasts may not be amenable to stereotactic biopsy, because firing of the needle may result in a through-and-through injury to the breast. Certain stereotactic systems may not be suitable for patients who are unable to lie prone or are morbidly obese. It should be kept in mind that stereotactic biopsy is a diagnostic procedure and is not intended for therapeutic purposes. On the whole, it is safe, and the complication rate is acceptably low.

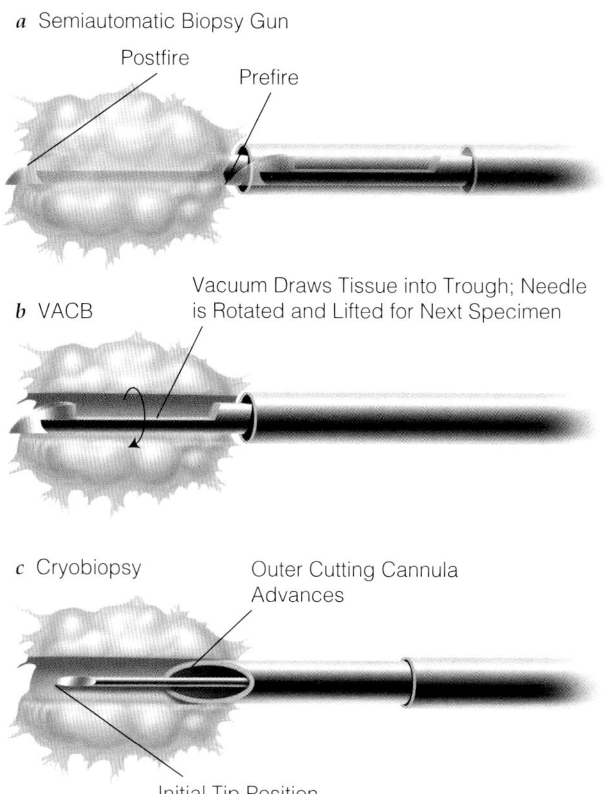

Figure 2 **Core-needle biopsy. The positioning of the needle shaft and tip varies with the particular biopsy device being used. (*a*) For manual or semiautomatic guns that fire through the lesion, the position of the tip before firing should be at the edge of the lesion. Keeping the needle shaft parallel to the chest wall or the skin keeps these structures from being injured when the gun is fired or the core is manually obtained. (*b*) For most vacuum-assisted devices, multiple cores can be obtained through a single placement of the device within the breast. For diagnostic biopsies performed under ultrasonographic or stereotactic guidance, the needle may be placed in the center of the lesion and rotated up to 360° in specified intervals. (*c*) For cryobiopsy, the tip of the needle should be advanced through the center of the lesion toward the far edge of the lesion before firing. This step stabilizes the lesion. The outer cutting and rotating cannula is then fired over the inner needle. VACB = vacuum-assisted core biopsy.**

Depending on the system being employed, the patient either lies prone on the stereotactic table or sits upright. With the breast compressed craniocaudally or mediolaterally, stereotactic digital imaging is then performed to visualize the targeted lesion and calculate its location in three dimensions, and a suitable probe insertion site is identified. The skin is prepared, and a small amount of buffered 1% lidocaine with epinephrine is administered. The skin at the insertion site is punctured with a No. 11 blade, the probe is manually advanced to the prefire site, and the position of the probe is confirmed by means of stereotactic imaging. The device is then fired, repeatedly cutting, rotating, and retrieving samples until the desired amount has been removed. Targeted removal of suspicious microcalcifications is confirmed with specimen mammography.

Once the biopsy is complete, an inert metallic clip is deployed into the biopsy site through the probe for future localization; deployment and positioning are initially confirmed by stereotactic imaging. The biopsy device is then removed, the edges of the skin incision are approximated with Steri-Strips, and a compressive bandage is applied. Typically, 1 g of tissue (equivalent to approximately 10 to 12 samples with an 11-gauge probe) is sufficient for diagnosis. Once the procedure is over and the breast has been released from compression, a two-view mammography should be obtained to verify that the clip was accurately placed and to document that the targeted lesion was adequately sampled.

Magnetic resonance imaging–guided biopsy Contrast-enhanced magnetic resonance imaging (MRI) has been found to be a highly sensitive method for detecting breast cancer, especially those that are nonpalpable or are unable to be viewed using conventional radiographic methods. A stereotactic method similar to the one described above has been developed using a VACB to perform an incisional biopsy under MRI guidance. Similarly, the patient is placed prone and the targeted breast undergoes mediolateral compression. Using MRI, a software program calculates the three-dimensional coordinates for the biopsy device. The VACB gun is used outside the magnet, so MRI compatibility is not required. After several tissue samples are removed, the resulting cavity is directly visualized to ensure precise tissue removal. A metallic marking clip can be placed during the procedure to facilitate future surgical excision if a diagnosis of cancer is determined. The procedure is generally well tolerated. Bleeding and hematoma are the most commonly encountered complications. Compared to conventional stereotactic biopsy, MRI-guided biopsy has a significantly higher cost. MRI-guided biopsy is a promising modality but requires further investigation as there are few long-term studies to determine histopathologic correlation and the false negative rate.[19–21]

Interpretation of Results

CNB is a highly accurate diagnostic tool: the false negative rate is only 1 to 2%,[22] which is comparable to that of open wire-localized biopsy. When pathologic evaluation reveals fibroadenoma, microcalcifications within benign fibrocystic tissue, or other comparably benign pathologic conditions, there is no need for any special follow-up, and routine screening mammography may be resumed. However, when biopsy of the targeted mass lesion fails to yield a mass diagnosis or a biopsy specimen from a group of clustered calcifications is devoid of microcalcifications on pathologic review, the discordant result should be viewed with some suspicion and should be considered an indication for open biopsy. Subsequent excisional biopsy is also indicated when CNB reveals atypical hyperplasia, radial scar, lobular carcinoma in situ (LCIS), or papilloma. The rationale is that the excisional biopsy may result in a pathologic upgrade to cancer. For example, open biopsy after a CNB indicative of atypical ductal hyperplasia may reveal DCIS in approximately 40% of patients when CNB was performed with a 14-gauge automated gun. The use of larger (e.g., 11-gauge) core biopsy devices has reduced the frequency of this finding to approximately 20%,[23] but it has not eliminated the need for excision. False positive results are rare with CNB; therefore, a diagnosis of malignancy may be believed, and a one-stage definitive surgical procedure may then be planned without further biopsy.

Touch Preparation of Cores

For an immediate but preliminary diagnosis, cytologic touch preparation of fresh cores may be performed in the office.[24] The tissue is blotted to remove any gross blood, the core is gently smeared along a glass slide, and the slide is then immediately fixed in 70% ethanol. A layer of cells is left on the surface of the slide for cytologic evaluation, whereas the core is preserved for permanent evaluation. This procedure has a diagnostic accuracy of nearly 90%. Although the false negative rate is approximately 25%, an immediate diagnosis is obtained in 75% of patients.[18] Like all preliminary diagnoses, touch preparation diagnoses should be treated with caution until the final results of histopathologic evaluation are available.

PERCUTANEOUS EXCISIONAL BIOPSY

In some instances, patient preference may dictate complete removal of a mass regardless of its benign appearance. As an alternative to open biopsy (see below), percutaneous excision of small masses may be performed.[25–27] This procedure can be performed in an outpatient setting with the patient under local anesthesia. Some of the devices used for percutaneous excision are vacuum assisted and remove the mass as multiple cores, whereas others deliver large intact samples in a single pass [*see Figure 3*]. Although such approaches clearly show promise for future surgical treatment of breast cancer, these percutaneous devices are currently approved by the US Food and Drug Administration (FDA) only for excision of benign masses. Lesions found to be harboring cancer should undergo subsequent open surgical reexcision. Excision of lesions that are close to the skin or the chest wall or are larger than 2 to 3 cm in diameter may prove technically challenging with percutaneous techniques; open excisional biopsy [*see* Open Biopsy, *below*] may be preferable for such lesions.

OPEN BIOPSY

The vast majority of open breast biopsies are now performed with either local anesthesia alone or local anesthesia with intravenous sedation.

Technique

Various options for incisions are available [*see Figure 4*]. If the pathology is unclear, the incision is placed directly over the lesion to minimize tunneling through breast tissue. The incision should be long to ensure that the mass, together with a small rim of grossly normal tissue, can be excised as a single specimen and be oriented so that it can be included within any future lumpectomy or mastectomy incision should the lesion prove malignant. Resection of overlying skin is not necessary unless the lesion is extremely superficial. Historically, surgeons performing open biopsies have generally employed curvilinear incisions placed within the resting lines of skin tension [*see Figure 4, a and b*]. Currently, however, some surgeons are advocating the use of radial incisions, particularly for medial, lateral, and inferior lesions.[15] If a previous CNB proved the lesion to be benign (e.g., fibroadenoma) but the patient still favors excision, it is acceptable to move the incision to a circumareolar position or another less visible site.

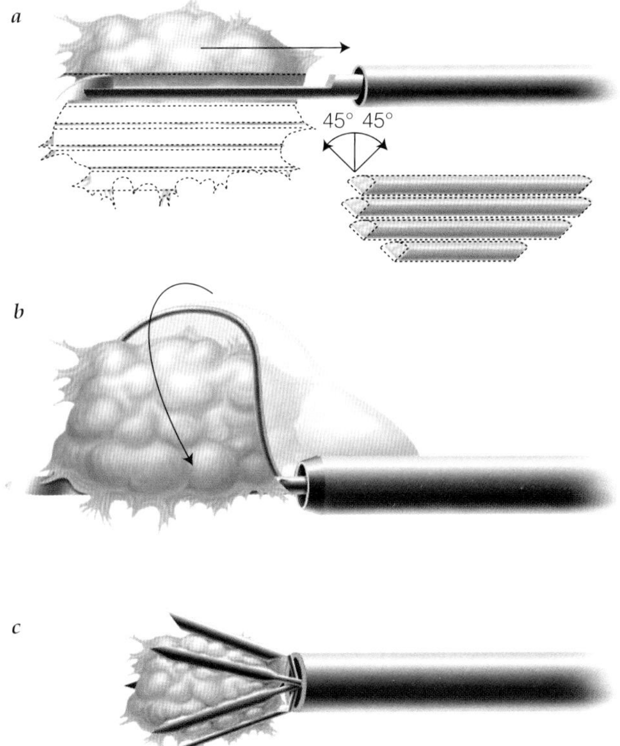

Figure 3 **Percutaneous excisional biopsy. This procedure may be performed by means of several different methods. (*a*) One approach is to employ a vacuum-assisted device, which is placed with the trough under the lesion and the shaft parallel to the posterior aspect of the lesion. The needle is then lifted anteriorly as it is rotated first 45° clockwise, then back to the center position (0°), and finally 45° counterclockwise to remove the entire lesion in multiple cores. (*b*) Another option is to employ an electrosurgical device such as the Ovation (Rubicor Medical, Inc., Redwood City, California), which circumscribes the mass with a cutting wire loop while concurrently deploying a retractable plastic bag that encapsulates the lesion and retracts it through the skin en bloc. (*c*) A third option is to employ a device such as the Intact Breast Lesion Excision System (Intact Medical Corp., Natick, Massachusetts), which circumscribes the mass with a radiofrequency wand and delivers it en bloc.**

For diagnostic biopsies, the surgeon should orient the specimen, and the pathologist should ink all margins. Meticulous hemostasis should be achieved before closure to prevent the formation of hematomas that could complicate subsequent definitive oncologic resection. A cosmetic subcuticular skin closure is preferred.

NEEDLE (WIRE)-LOCALIZATION BREAST BIOPSY

Lesions that are not amenable to stereotactic core biopsy may be excised by means of needle (wire)-localization breast biopsy (NLBB). Such lesions include those that are close to the chest wall or under the nipple, as well as those occurring in a thin breast, where firing the needle may cause it to pass through the opposite side of the breast. Radiographic evidence of a radial scar is also an indication for NLBB: a core pathologic diagnosis of such a scar would ultimately necessitate

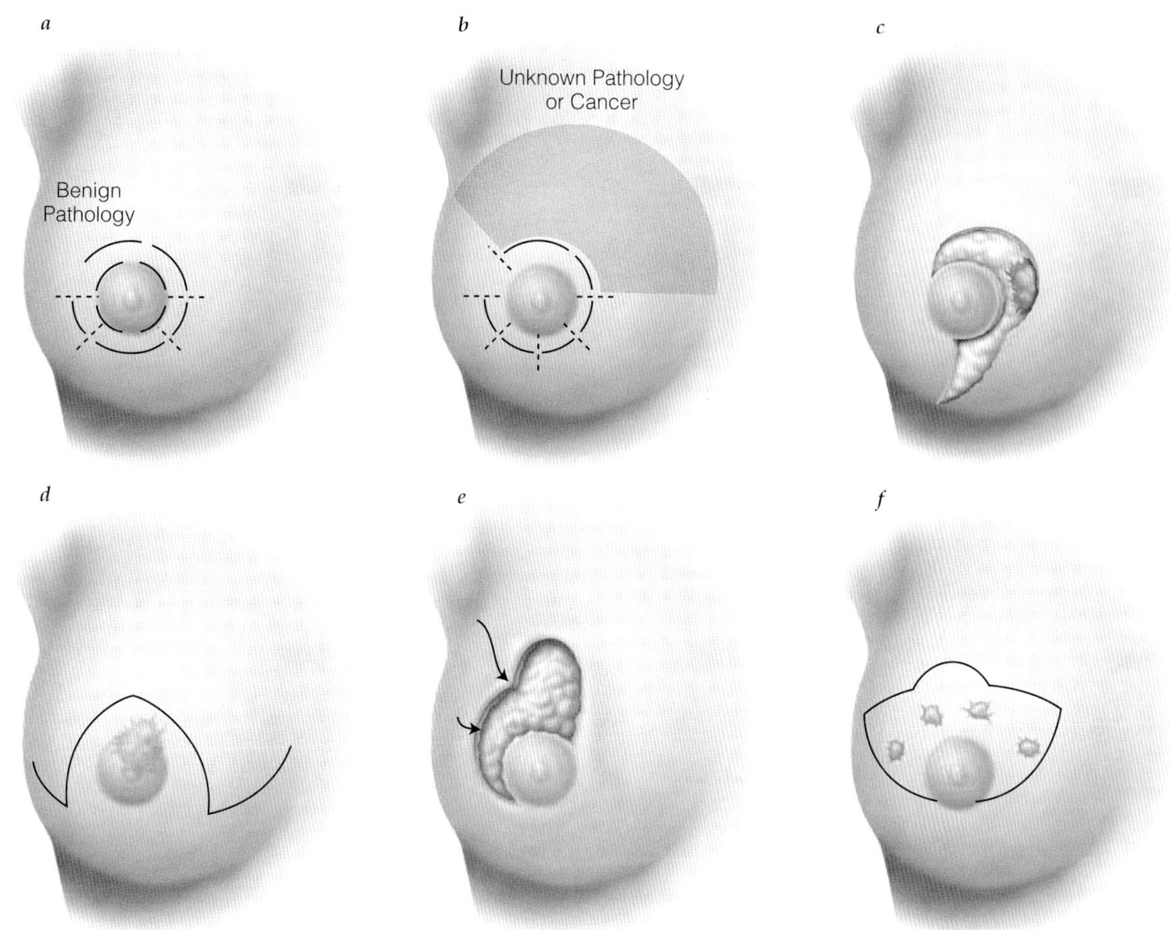

Figure 4 **Open biopsy. (*a*) For biopsy-proven benign masses, a circumareolar incision generally provides excellent cosmesis and a well-hidden scar. If the lesion is too far from the nipple, curvilinear incisions are traditionally employed instead. Alternatively, medial, lateral, and inferior incisions may be placed in a radial fashion. (*b*) For lesions of unknown pathology, incisions should be placed directly over the lesion and should be oriented so that they will be included within a subsequent mastectomy incision if margins prove positive and mastectomy is indicated. As with benign lesions, either curvilinear or radial incisions may be employed. Circumareolar incisions should be avoided in this setting because reexcision to provide clear margins, as is indicated in the case of malignancy, can necessitate excision of a portion of the nipple-areola complex and can commit the surgeon to a mastectomy. In cases where reexcision is indicated, avoidance of incisions in the so-called no man's land may improve cosmesis in that it allows future reconstructive efforts to include advancement of the nipple-areola complex if desired. Various oncoplastic incisions may be employed as alternatives for (*c*) medial, (*d*) central, or (*e, f*) superior lesions.**

open excision. Finally, reexcision is required when stereotactic or ultrasound-guided CNB reveals lesions determined to be high risk on pathologic evaluation (e.g., atypical hyperplasia, LCIS, papilloma, carcinoma, or lesion whose pathologic status is discordant with radiographic findings). In these circumstances, wire localization may be performed on the residual lesion, a clip placed at the time of CNB, or another surrogate marker (see below). To bracket a more extensive area of calcifications, multiple wires may be placed, especially if previous CNB revealed atypia or malignancy in the area.

Technique

The lesion to be excised is localized by inserting a thin needle and a fine wire under mammographic, ultrasonographic, or MR guidance immediately before operation. To facilitate incision placement, images should be sent to the operating room with the wire entry site indicated on them. The incision is placed as directly as possible over the mass to minimize tunneling through breast tissue. With superficial lesions, the wire entry site is usually close to the lesion and thus may be included in the incision. With some deeper lesions, the wire entry site is on the shortest path to the lesion and so may still be included in the incision. Once the incision is made, a block of tissue is excised around and along the wire in such a way as to include the lesion [*see Figure 5, a and b*]. This process is easier and involves less excision of tissue if the localizing wire has a thickened segment several centimeters in length that is placed adjacent to or within the lesion. The wire itself can then be followed into breast tissue until the thick segment is reached, at which point the excision can be extended away from the wire to include the lesion in a fairly small tissue fragment.

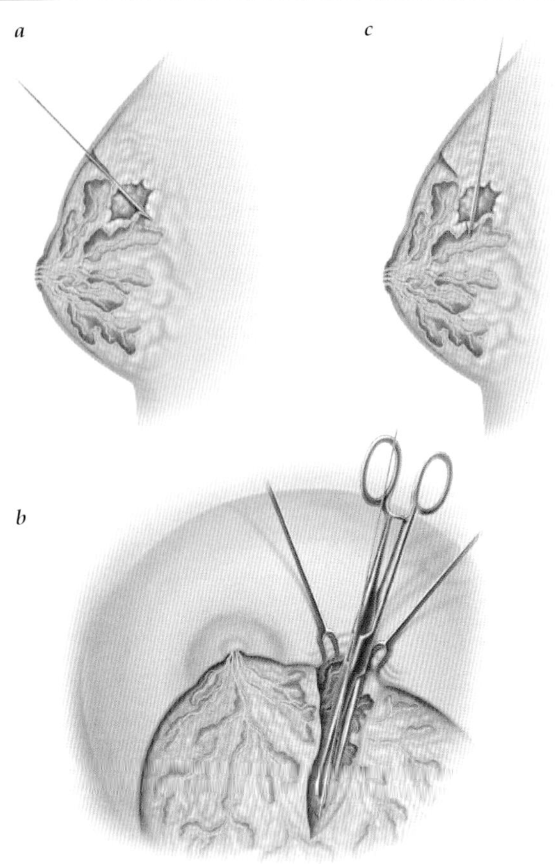

Figure 5 **Needle-localization breast biopsy. (*a*) The mammographic abnormality is localized preoperatively. The relation between the wire, the skin entry site, and the lesion is noted by the surgeon. The skin incision is placed over the expected location of the mammographic abnormality. (*b*) The tissue around the wire is removed en bloc with the wire and sent for specimen mammography. Tunneling and piecemeal removal are to be avoided. (*c*) It is sometimes necessary to insert the localizing wire from a peripheral site to localize a deep or central lesion. The incision should be placed directly over the expected location of the lesion, not over the wire entry site. The dissection is extended into breast tissue to identify the wire a short distance from the lesion. The free end of the wire is pulled into the wound, and the biopsy is performed as previously described.[99]**

With many lesions, the wire entry site is in a fairly peripheral location relative to the position of the lesion, which means that including the wire entry site in the incision would result in excessive tunneling within breast tissue. In such cases, the incision is placed over the expected position of the lesion [*see Figure 5c*], the dissection is extended into breast tissue to identify the wire a few centimeters away from the lesion itself, and the free end of the wire is pulled up into the incision. A generous block of tissue is then excised around the wire. Intraoperative ultrasonography may be useful for identifying the tip of the needle and facilitating excision, particularly in the case of a deep lesion or biopsy site in a large breast.

Radiography should be performed intraoperatively on all wire-localized biopsy specimens to confirm excision of the lesion. If the lesion was missed, another tissue sample may be excised if the surgeon has some idea of the likely location of the missed lesion. If, however, the surgeon suspects that the wire was dislodged before or during the procedure, then the incision should be closed, and repeat localization and biopsy should be performed later. In addition to wire dislocation or transection, wire localization is occasionally associated with vasovagal reactions. Alternatives to wire localization include hematoma ultrasound-guided (HUG) excision (see below), carbon marking,[28] use of methylene blue dye,[29] and placement of radioactive seeds.[30]

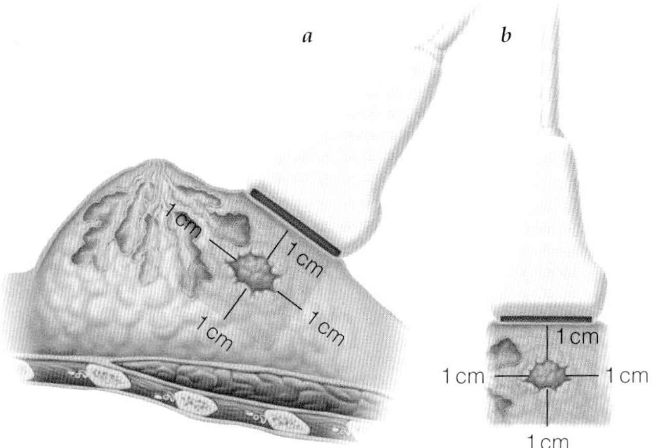

Figure 6 **Hematoma ultrasound-guided excision. (*a*) The hematoma is localized in two planes with intraoperative ultrasonography, and 1 cm margins are marked off around it. Dissection then proceeds down toward the chest wall in a block fashion. Excision of the hematoma is confirmed by ultrasonography of the specimen ex vivo. (*b*) as well as by direct visualization of the hematoma in the gross specimen.[31,32]**

Hematoma ultrasound-guided excision In patients who have undergone CNB, particularly those who have undergone VACB, the hematoma at the biopsy site can often serve as a physiologic marker that accurately guides intraoperative localization [*see Figure 6*].[31,32] This procedure, referred to as HUG excision, renders wire placement unnecessary and can facilitate operative scheduling. The hematoma is localized in two planes using ultrasound guidance and 1 cm margins are marked off around the lesion; dissection is then continued down toward the chest wall in a block fashion. Excision of the hematoma can be confirmed by ultrasonography of the specimen ex vivo, as well as direct visualization of the hematoma in the gross specimen. Another variation of the procedure includes localization of the tumor with MRI and infusion of the patient's own blood into the lesion for future localization and surgical excision.[31]

RADIOISOTOPE-GUIDED OCCULT LESION LOCALIZATION

As widespread mammographic screening programs have been employed, there has been an increase in the detection of nonpalpable breast lesions requiring improved localization techniques for biopsy and/or excision. Radioisotope-guided occult lesion localization (ROLL) is one such modality using an intratumorally injected radiotracer to identify the lesion intraoperatively by use of a gamma probe.[33] Contraindications to the ROLL procedure include patients with a history of albumin allergy attributed to the injection of a colloid into the breast lesion.[34] The ROLL procedure has shown a decrease in the volume of breast tissue excised while preserving surgical margins. Patients have reported less pain and an improved cosmetic result with this procedure.[34–36] Clinical trials have shown adequate excision rates when compared with the needle-localization technique. Combination with the sentinel lymph node (SLN) mapping procedure has been successfully described in the literature.[37–39] Further investigation with randomized clinical trials is currently underway.

Technique

Lesions are identified by image guidance using either ultrasonography or stereotactic mammography, and intratumoral injection of a radionuclide-labeled colloid is performed prior to surgery. The procedure can be performed using local anesthesia with or without sedation. Intraoperatively, a handheld gamma-detecting probe is used to identify the area with the maximum radioactivity, and a small incision is made in the skin overlying this site. Determination of excision volume is made by review of preoperative lymphoscintigraphic imaging and decreased detection of radioactivity in the resection bed. Surgical specimens should undergo radiographic evaluation to confirm removal of the lesion.

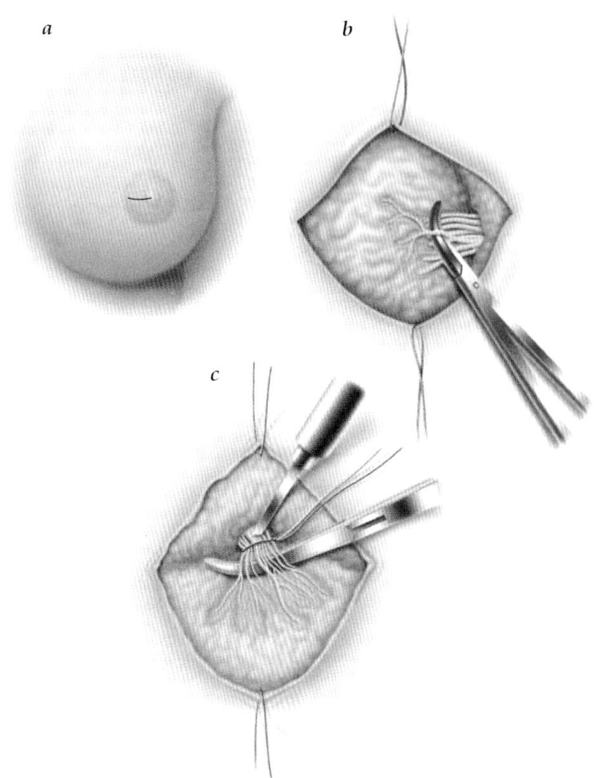

Figure 7 **Terminal duct excision. (*a*) A radial incision is made within the areola. (*b*) The involved duct is identified by means of blunt dissection and removed along with a core of breast tissue. (*c*) If no single duct is identified, the entire subareolar ductal complex is excised from immediately beneath the nipple dermis to a depth of 4 to 5 cm within breast tissue.**[40,42]

Terminal Duct Excision

Terminal duct excision is the procedure of choice in the surgical treatment of pathologic nipple discharge.[40] The goal is to excise the discharging duct with as little additional tissue as possible to maintain cosmesis. To this end, the surgeon should carefully note the precise position of the offending duct at the time of the initial examination. To ensure accurate ductal identification, intraductal injection of methylene blue has been used to aid in visualization of the involved ductal system prior to major duct excision. Other methods used in conjunction with terminal duct excision to limit the volume of tissue removed include ductography and ductoscopy.[41]

OPERATIVE TECHNIQUE

The patient is instructed to refrain from manually expressing her discharge for several days before operation. After local anesthesia (with or without sedation) is administered, the surgeon attempts to express the discharge. If this attempt is successful, the edge of the nipple is grasped with a forceps, and a fine lacrimal duct probe (000 to 0000) is gently inserted into the discharging duct. A radial incision is made within the areola at the same clock position as is occupied by the draining duct [*see Figure 7*]; this incision is preferred to a circumareolar incision because it is believed to preserve more nipple sensation and function.[42] The nipple skin flap is raised, and the duct containing the wire is excised with a margin of surrounding tissue from just below the nipple dermis to a depth of 4 to 5 cm within the breast tissue. The electrocautery should be employed with particular caution in the superficial portions of the dissection to prevent devascularization of the nipple-areola complex. If it is not possible to pass the lacrimal duct probe into the discharging duct or it is unclear which duct has resulted in the pathologic discharge, the entire subareolar duct complex must be excised from immediately beneath the nipple dermis to a depth of 4 to 5 cm within the breast tissue. The breast tissue should be reapproximated beneath the nipple to prevent retraction of the nipple or indentation of the areola.

Minimally Invasive Techniques

The next step in the evolving application of minimally invasive techniques to breast cancer is to determine whether ablative local therapies can safely substitute for standard surgical extirpation. Cryotherapy, interstitial laser therapy, radiofrequency ablation (RFA), microwave ablation, and high-intensity focused ultrasound ablation have all been studied as means of eradicating small breast cancers.[43] In most of these techniques, a probe is placed percutaneously into the breast lesion under imaging guidance, and tumor cell destruction is achieved by means of either heat or cold.

To date, experience with ablative breast therapies has been limited, and long-term follow-up has not been carried out. There is some evidence that patients who have small, well-defined, unifocal cancers without an extensive intraductal component may have greater success with these techniques.[43] Lesions in close proximity to the pectoralis major muscle or the skin should be isolated by injecting normal saline to prevent thermal injury. Most of the time, these minimally invasive techniques are well tolerated and can be performed in an outpatient setting. Additionally, superior cosmesis is achieved by leaving the ablated tissue in situ without loss of tissue volume, thus preventing breast deformity and scarring. However, most of the initial studies of ablative breast therapies involved subsequent surgical excision to obtain histologic evidence of cell death. Unfortunately, when ablative therapies are used alone, the benefits of pathologic assessment of the specimen, including evaluation of margin status, are lost. Limiting factors include the ability of current imaging modalities to detect residual disease, thereby identifying patients who may need subsequent surgical intervention. Clearly, minimally invasive ablative approaches to breast cancer are technically feasible and safe, and they do appear to offer some potential advantages; however, it remains to be determined to what extent they are oncologically appropriate.

CRYOABLATION

Cryotherapy has been successfully used in the treatment of nonresectable liver tumors. It destroys targeted tissue by alternately freezing (–40°C) and thawing the lesion. Intracellular ice formation and osmotic and ischemic injury are believed to contribute to the mechanism of tissue destruction. Because of the natural analgesic effect of cold, cryoablation is generally a well-tolerated procedure that can be performed in an outpatient setting using local anesthesia with minimal need for pain-controlling medications.

Patients with a biopsy-proven fibroadenoma who want their mass removed but desire an alternative to open or percutaneous surgical excision may be candidates for cryoablation. Clinically, resorption of the fibroadenoma increases over time, with 12-month follow-up studies reporting a significant reduction in lesion volume. Despite the occasional residual disease noted when cryoablation is used to treat larger masses, both hospital- and community-based studies have reported that patient satisfaction rates are higher than 90% with this procedure.[44]

The role of cryotherapy in the treatment of primary malignant disease has recently been explored. Immunologic activation from the cryoablative technique may provide an effective tumor-specific response.[45] Early studies reveal the degree of tumor destruction achieved by cryotherapy to be inconsistent.[46–48] Larger clinical trials are currently in the planning stages, and the efficacy of this treatment for selected patient populations remains investigational.

Use of the cryoprobe has also been explored as an alternative to needle localization for excision of nonpalpable lesions prior to BCT. Theoretically, the ability to palpate previously nonpalpable lesions may reduce reexcision rates for positive margins. Pilot studies have shown decreases in resected tissue volume, improved cosmesis, and improved patient satisfaction with a consistently negative margin status.[49] Clearly, the use of cryoablation in this role also requires further examination.

Technique

A 12-gauge cryoprobe is inserted into the center of the lesion under ultrasonographic guidance. To freeze the lesion, inert argon gas is delivered through the tip of the probe in such a way as to create a local temperature of −40°C or lower. An iceball is thereby formed that is well visualized by ultrasonography [see Figure 8]. In a tightly coupled system, helium is then delivered to thaw the lesion. For adequate necrosis to occur, two freeze-thaw cycles must be performed; the exact specifications of these cycles depend on the size of the lesion.

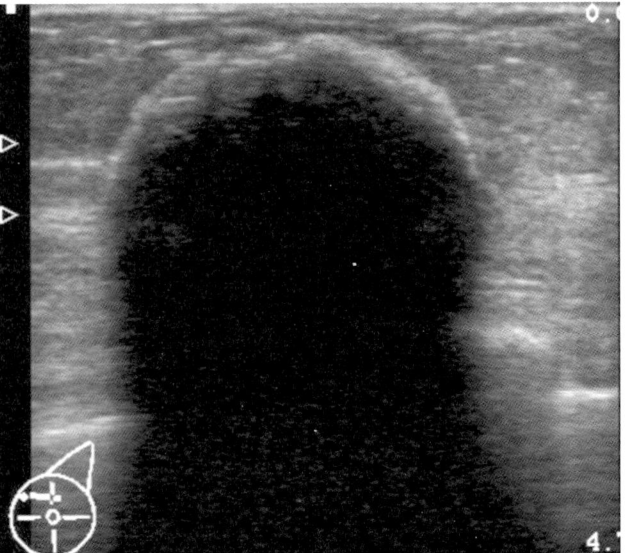

Figure 8 **Cryoablation. The needle is placed through the center of the lesion, and argon gas is delivered to create a local temperature of −40°C. The resulting iceball is well visualized by ultrasonography.**

INTERSTITIAL LASER THERAPY

Interstitial laser therapy causes hyperthermic (80°C to 100°C) cell death and coagulative tissue necrosis by delivering energy through a fiberoptic probe. Precise targeting with the use of an MRI-guided laser or stereotactic mammography is required. Benefits of this treatment include the use of local anesthesia only. One reported complication with significant morbidity included gaseous rupture of the tumor.[46] Small studies employing surgical excision following laser treatment have shown complete ablation to be inconsistent. Smaller tumors were more likely to be completely ablated.[50,51] Complete tumor destruction has been difficult to ensure with this technique. Further investigation and long-term follow-up are required.

Technique

A 16-gauge needle with a thermal sensor is inserted into the center of the tumor using image guidance. The stylet is then replaced with a laser fiber, and the tissue is heated to 80°C to 100°C. For larger lesions, multiple laser fibers may be placed. A thermal sensor needle is placed 1 cm away from the laser needle to monitor peripheral temperatures and ensure an ablative zone of 2.5 to 3.0 cm. Tumor destruction is confirmed by ultrasonography or MRI.[50]

RADIOFREQUENCY ABLATION

Like cryotherapy, RFA has also been extensively used to treat liver tumors. RFA is a minimally invasive thermal ablation technique in which frictional heat is generated by intracellular ions moving in response to alternating current. It is currently the most promising ablative method for small breast cancers; however an accurate treatment algorithm remains to be developed.[50] Complications include superficial skin burning and temporary elevation of body temperature. Early studies with RFA followed by immediate or delayed surgical resection have shown incomplete ablation of tumors.[46] Incomplete ablations were attributed to large tumor size (> 2 cm) and the presence of multifocal disease.[43]

Technique

A large-gauge probe is placed into the center of the tumor using image guidance. A star-shaped set of electrodes is deployed from the tip of the probe to deliver heat at a temperature of 95°C, which is maintained for 15 minutes followed by a period of cooling for 1 minute. Postprocedural MRI may help confirm complete tumor destruction after RFA and other ablative techniques.

MICROWAVE ABLATION

Microwave ablation is an investigational technique similar to RFA causing tumor necrosis by generation of frictional heat using two microwave phased array applicators. Because of the higher water content of cancer tissue (compared to adipose and glandular tissue), agitation of intracellular water molecules causes temperature elevation of the breast lesion, leading to tissue necrosis. Image guidance is usually performed to localize the lesion. Complications have included skin flap necrosis and mild skin burns overlying the treatment area. Pilot studies have shown a reduction in the size of the tumor; however, further prospective trials are needed to investigate the use of microwave ablation as a treatment modality for invasive cancer.[52–55] Current investigations into the added benefit of microwave ablation in conjunction with neoadjuvant chemotherapy are promising.[54]

FOCUSED ULTRASOUND ABLATION

Focus ultrasound ablation (FUS) is a modality used to incur cellular death by thermal injury from an ultrasonic energy source. One of the benefits of FUS is that no implantable device is required, allowing the procedure to be performed through the intact skin. Additionally, larger tumors and lesions with an irregular shape can be ablated using this technique. Image guidance is required to make sure the lesion is adequately ablated including a 2 cm margin, in keeping with the oncologic principles of breast conservation surgery. Short-term follow-up studies ablating smaller tumors have shown contradictory results with FUS regarding complete tumor necrosis. A palpable lump following the procedure is noted by most patients from local tissue edema; however, this is transient and usually resolves within 1 to 2 weeks. Contraindications to FUS include multifocal, deep lesions and tumors in close proximity to the skin and nipple.[54–56]

Surgical Options for Breast Cancer

There are several surgical options for primary treatment of breast cancer. It should be emphasized that for most patients, partial mastectomy (lumpectomy) to microscopically clear margins coupled with axillary staging and radiation therapy yields long-term survival equivalent to that associated with mastectomy and axillary staging. Currently, indications for mastectomy include patient preference, the inability to achieve clean margins without unacceptable deformation of the breast, the presence of disease in multiple quadrants (multicentric disease), previous chest wall irradiation, pregnancy, the presence of severe collagen vascular disease (e.g., scleroderma), and the lack of access to a radiation therapy facility.

Partial Mastectomy

Partial mastectomy—also referred to as wide local excision or lumpectomy—involves excision of all cancerous tissue to microscopically clear margins. Although 1 cm margins are the goal, many surgeons consider 2 mm margins to be adequate for reducing the risk of local recurrence.[57] Hence, reexcision is indicated whenever margins are either positive or too close (< 2 mm). Partial mastectomy is commonly performed with the patient under local anesthesia, with or without sedation. The addition of an axillary staging procedure (a common event) usually necessitates general anesthesia, but in select circumstances, local or epidural anesthesia may suffice.

OPERATIVE TECHNIQUE

An incision is placed directly over the lesion to minimize tunneling through breast tissue; it should be oriented so as to be included within a subsequent mastectomy incision if margins prove positive. As with open biopsy (see above), curvilinear incisions have been the standard, but radial incisions are now being advocated by some surgeons, particularly for upper outer, medial, lateral, and inferior lesions. A radial incision facilitates excision of tumors that extend in a ductal distribution, preserves the contour of the breast, and permits easier reexcision if margins prove positive [*see Figure 4b*]. With current oncoplastic techniques,[58,59] lesions in the central, medial, or superior portions of the breast can be resected with minimal cosmetic deformity [*see Figure 4, c, d, e, and f*]. Resection of a portion of the overlying skin is not necessary unless the lesion is extremely superficial.

To obtain clear margins, a 1 to 1.5 cm margin of normal-appearing tissue should be removed beyond the edge of the palpable tumor or, if excisional biopsy has already been performed, around the biopsy cavity. In the case of nonpalpable lesions diagnosed by means of CNB, wire localization is performed, and 2 to 3 cm of tissue should be excised around the wire to obtain an adequate margin. Intraoperative ultrasonography may reduce the rate of positive margins by allowing visualization of the tumor edge or the previous biopsy site.[60]

The specimen should be oriented by the surgeon and the margins inked by the pathologist; this orientation is useful if reexcision is required to achieve clean margins. Reexcision of any close (< 2 mm) margins may be performed during the same surgical procedure if the specimen margins are assessed immediately by the pathologist. If the specimen was not oriented, the entire biopsy cavity should be reexcised. Surgical clips may be left in the lumpectomy site to help the radiation oncologist plan the radiation boost to the tumor bed or to direct partial-breast irradiation. In the closure of the incision, hemostasis should be meticulous: a hematoma may delay adjuvant therapy. Deep breast tissue should be approximated only if such closure does not result in significant deformity of breast contours. A cosmetic subcuticular closure is preferred. Wearing a support bra during the day and night can reduce shearing of fragile vessels.[15]

ACCELERATED PARTIAL-BREAST IRRADIATION WITH BALLOON CATHETER

Historically, whole-breast irradiation has been the standard treatment to reduce the risk of local recurrence after BCT. Long-term follow-up of patients who have received BCT demonstrates, however, that only 1 to 3% of recurrences within the breast arise at a significant distance from the primary cancer site (i.e., in other breast quadrants); the remainder develop near the original biopsy site.[57,61] These data provide the rationale for the approach known as accelerated partial-breast irradiation (APBI), in which a shortened course of high-dose radiation is delivered to the tissue surrounding the lumpectomy cavity (the region theoretically at greatest risk). Decreasing the volume of tissue receiving radiation therapy allows for patients to undergo a shorter course of therapy (approximately 1 week).[62] Several different APBI techniques have been developed, including placement of interstitial catheters, use of a localized external beam, single-dose intraoperative treatment, implantation of radioactive beads or seeds, and insertion of a balloon catheter into the lumpectomy site. Although long-term follow-up has not been carried out, the short-term results reported for some APBI techniques indicate that in most centers, recurrence rates have been low, with good cosmesis and only mild chronic toxicity.[63]

The technique of APBI can be illustrated by considering the MammoSite Radiation Therapy System (Cytyc Corp., Palo Alto, California), in which a balloon catheter is inserted into the surgical cavity after lumpectomy to provide partial-breast irradiation (see below). Although the catheter may also be inserted at the time of the original operation, it is preferable to wait for final pathologic evaluation to confirm clear margins; if the catheter is inserted and margins are found to be positive, it will have to be replaced (a costly process). The optimal time for insertion of the APBI balloon is within 2 to 3 weeks from the final procedure. Postoperative insertion may be done either percutaneously under ultrasonographic guidance or by means of an open technique. Once the catheter is in place, a radiation source (iridium 192) is delivered into the balloon via a high–dose rate remote afterloader.

Technique

For safe and effective delivery of radiotherapy through the MammoSite balloon catheter, the lumpectomy cavity must be able to conform its shape to that of an ovoid or spherical catheter without significant air pockets, able to accommodate a volume of at least 30 mL (the volume of the smallest available balloon), and able to maintain a minimum distance of 7 mm from the skin with the catheter in place. In addition, if a percutaneous technique is being considered, the surgeon should be comfortable with ultrasonography (which will be employed for initial visualization of the lumpectomy cavity). If the above criteria seem reasonably attainable, one may proceed with a percutaneous approach [*see Figure 9*].

Percutaneous approach A site peripheral to the scar is chosen as the entry site for the balloon catheter, and a local

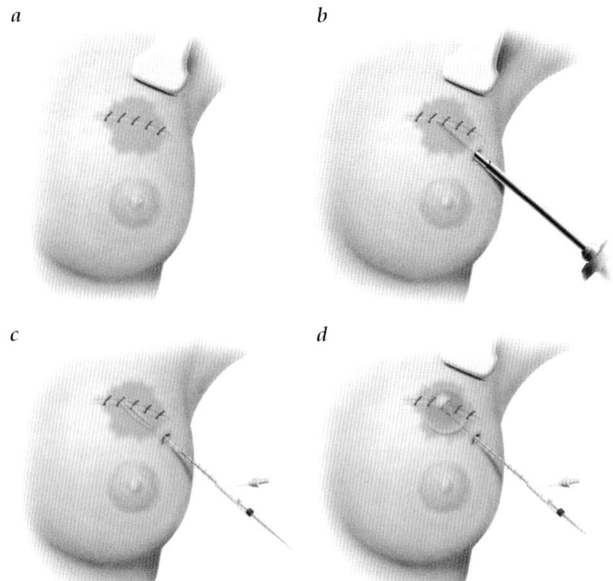

Figure 9 **Accelerated partial-breast irradiation with balloon catheter. (*a*) The lumpectomy cavity is evaluated by means of ultrasonography. (*b*) The trocar is inserted through a separate entry site under ultrasonographic guidance. (*c*) The uninflated balloon catheter is advanced through the trocar path. (*d*) Under ultrasonographic visualization, the balloon is inflated with saline or contrast material. An anterior distance of at least 7 mm between the catheter and the chest wall or skin is confirmed.**

anesthetic is injected along the proposed catheter tract. A trocar (supplied with the insertion kit) is inserted into the cavity via the peripheral entry site and then removed. Removal of the trocar allows for the evacuation of the postlumpectomy seroma and prevents underdosage of tissue around the cavity. The shape of the cavity and skin-to-cavity distance are visualized by means of ultrasonography, and a catheter of appropriate shape (ovoid or spherical) and volume (30 to 65 mL) is advanced through the newly formed tract. Saline is then infiltrated to inflate the catheter balloon to the maximum volume that the cavity can accommodate. A small amount of radiographic contrast may also be infused to aid in visualization. The cavity is then reimaged to confirm that the catheter is an adequate distance (7 mm) from the skin. If the distance is inadequate, the balloon volume is reduced. If it is not possible to keep the catheter at least 7 mm from the skin while maintaining a balloon volume of at least 30 mL, conversion to an open approach is indicated.

Open approach The cavity is reopened through the original skin incision. Occasionally, a thick rind may form around the residual seroma; this rind may be excised to reduce tension and increase the volume of the cavity. If necessary, the anterior skin may be excised in the form of an ellipse to provide improved anterior coverage of the catheter, and the subcutaneous tissue may be pulled together over the catheter and the cavity to help ensure adequate coverage and sufficient distance from the skin. A peripheral site is chosen for insertion of the catheter. After the skin is closed, ultrasonography is employed to confirm that the distance from the skin is adequate. A topical antibiotic is applied at the insertion site; no anchoring stitch is necessary. Correct positioning of the catheter is confirmed by a postplacement treatment-planning computed tomographic (CT) scan that is evaluated by the radiation oncologist.

Mastectomy

The goal of a mastectomy is to remove all breast tissue—including the nipple, the areola, and the pectoral fascia—while leaving viable skin flaps and a smooth chest wall for application of prosthesis. This should be the objective whether the mastectomy is performed for cancer treatment or for prophylaxis. Skin-sparing mastectomy (SSM) performed in conjunction with immediate reconstruction is discussed elsewhere [*see* Breast Reconstruction, *below*]. Proper skin incisions and good exposure are the key components of a well-performed mastectomy. Mastectomy usually calls for general anesthesia, but it may be performed with thoracic epidural anesthesia or local anesthesia in select circumstances.

OPERATIVE TECHNIQUE

The traditional mastectomy incision is an elliptical one that is placed either transversely across the chest wall or at an upward angle toward the axilla. It should be fashioned in such a way as to include the nipple-areola complex and any incision from a previous biopsy [*see Figure 10a*]. Ideally, the upper and lower skin flaps should be of similar length so that there is no redundant skin on either flap. The outline of the incision may be established by using the following five steps:

1. The lateral and medial end points are marked.
2. The breast is pulled firmly downward.
3. To define the path of the upper incision, a straight line is drawn from one end point to the other across the upper surface of the breast.
4. The breast is pulled firmly upward.
5. To define the path of the lower incision, a straight line is drawn from one end point to the other across the lower surface of the breast.

The outlined incision is then checked to confirm that it can be closed without either undue tension or redundant skin. Dog-ears or lateral skin folds can be prevented by extending the incision medially or laterally to remove all the skin that contributes to the forward projection of the breast. The closure should be fairly snug intraoperatively while the arm is extended; significant slack will be created when the arm is returned to the patient's side. The medial and lateral end points of the incision may be adjusted upward or downward to include any previous biopsy incisions.

As noted [*see* Partial Mastectomy, *above*], there is increasing acceptance of the use of radial and oncoplastic incisions for BCT. In a small percentage of women, persistently positive margins may dictate conversion from BCT to mastectomy. In large-breasted women with excess breast skin, traditional elliptical incisions can easily incorporate any previous radial or superior-pole oncoplastic incisions that may have been performed [*see Figure 10b*]. In smaller-breasted women, however, sigmoid, modified Wise, or other oncoplastic mastectomy incisions may be needed to incorporate previous lumpectomy incisions [*see Figure 10c*].

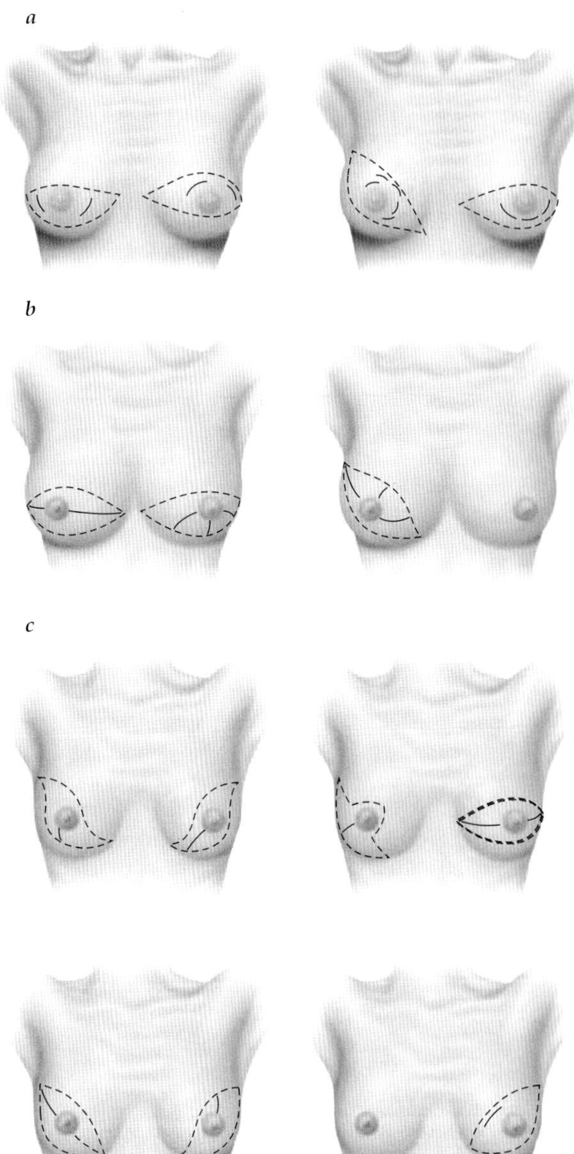

Figure 10 **Mastectomy incisions. (*a*) Elliptical incisions incorporate traditional lumpectomy incisions. (*b*) In large-breasted women with excess breast skin, traditional ellipses can easily incorporate previous radial and superior-pole oncoplastic incisions. (*c*) In smaller-breasted women, sigmoid, modified Wise, or other oncoplastic mastectomy incisions may be needed to incorporate previous radial lumpectomy incisions.**

Once the incision is made, the next step is to create even and viable flaps. In most patients, there is a fairly well-defined avascular plane between subcutaneous fat and breast tissue. This plane is identified by pulling the edges of the incision upward with skin hooks and beginning a flap that is 8 to 10 mm thick. After an initial release of the skin edge, the desired plane is developed by applying firm tension downward on the breast tissue and away from the skin at a 45°

angle. The fine fibrous attachments between breast tissue and subcutaneous fat (Cooper ligaments) are then divided with the electrocautery or a blade, and crossing vessels are coagulated or ligated as they appear. To protect both arterial supply to and venous drainage from the skin flap, one must refrain from excessive ligation or cauterization of vessels on the flap. For most women, flap viability is not an issue. For diabetics, smokers, and other patients with diffuse small vessel disease, however, it is a serious consideration. In such patients, flaps should be no longer than necessary with no excess tension, and extra care should be taken to preserve flap vessels. Patients should be warned that even with these measures, there may be some skin necrosis along the incision. Such necrosis is best treated with gradual débridement of the eschar.

Flaps are raised superiorly to the clavicle, medially to the sternum, inferiorly to the inframammary fold, and laterally to the border of the latissimus dorsi. The pectoral fascia is incised both superiorly and medially. Inferiorly, the fascia of the abdominal muscles is not divided. The pectoralis major, the abdominal muscles, and the anterior serratus muscle form the deep border of the dissection. The pectoral fascia is removed with the breast specimen and may be separated from the muscle with either the electrocautery or a blade.

In a simple mastectomy, the dissection proceeds around the lateral edge of the pectoralis major but stops before entering the axillary fat pad (unless the procedure is being done in conjunction with SLNB). A single closed suction drain is placed through a separate lateral stab wound in such a way that it extends under the lower flap and a short distance upward along the sternal border of the dissection.

A modified radical mastectomy essentially consists of an axillary node dissection added to a simple mastectomy. At the lateral edge of the dissection, the border of the latissimus dorsi is exposed, as is the lateral border of the pectoral muscle. Retraction of these two muscles provides excellent exposure for the axillary dissection [*see* Axillary Dissection, *below*]. Some surgeons prefer to remove the breast from the chest wall first, whereas others leave the breast attached to provide tension for the axillary dissection. On completion of the procedure, two closed suction drains are placed, one in the axilla and another under the lower flap and extending to the midline.

After either a simple or a modified radical mastectomy, the skin is closed and a dressing applied according to the surgeon's preference. Early arm mobilization is encouraged.

SKIN-SPARING MASTECTOMY

SSM, which consists of resection of the nipple-areola complex, any existing biopsy scar, and the breast parenchyma, followed immediately by breast reconstruction, has become an increasingly popular approach for women requiring mastectomy.[64] With this approach, the inframammary fold and contour of the breast are preserved, and a generous skin envelope remains in situ for reconstruction; cosmetic results are thereby optimized. In addition, SSM is oncologically safe and is not associated with an increased incidence of local recurrence.[65] The recurrences that do occur typically develop below the skin flaps and thus are easily detectable; deep recurrences beneath the reconstruction are comparatively uncommon.

The incision for SSM with immediate reconstruction should be planned in collaboration with the plastic surgeon [*see Figure 11*], and the inframammary fold should be marked preoperatively with the patient in a sitting position. Several options are available for SSM. For CNB-diagnosed tumors that are not superficial, a circumareolar incision may be employed, with a lateral extension for exposure if necessary. Different incisions may be used if it proves necessary to incorporate previous incisions or to remove skin anterior to superficial tumors. A separate axillary incision may be useful when axillary dissection or SLNB is being performed. CNB sites generally are not included in the excised skin segment; the surgeon may opt to excise them through a separate skin ellipse. Intraoperatively, flaps are created in a circular fashion to optimize exposure. Although optimal cosmesis is part of the rationale for SSM, cosmetic considerations should never be allowed to compromise the extent of the dissection in any way.

NIPPLE-SPARING MASTECTOMY

Following mastectomy or SSM, many patients report dissatisfaction with the reconstruction of their nipple areolar complex using skin grafting or tattooing. Nipple-sparing mastectomy (NSM) eliminates the need for reconstruction by preservation of the dermis and epidermis of the nipple-areola complex during the initial procedure. Several initial studies have shown NSM to be an oncologically safe procedure in those patients appropriately selected.[66–71] Contraindications to NSM include larger tumors (> 2 cm), centrally located lesions with a small tumor-to-nipple distance, and lymphovascular invasion.[72]

Several types of incisions have been described, including periareolar with lateral extension, transareolar with lateral extension, and inframammary fold incisions. These typically allow for good exposure and dissection of the retroareolar structures.[73] Elevation of the areola off of the breast parenchyma should be performed with sharp dissection to prevent thermal injury to the nipple from electrocautery. The lactiferous ducts are transected at the base of the nipple papilla. Skin flaps are raised in a manner similar to that of SSM or conventional mastectomy. On removal of the subcutaneous breast, the remaining nipple tissue is removed with sharp dissection. A small (2 to 3 mm) rim of peripheral subcutaneous tissue should be preserved behind the nipple to prevent par-

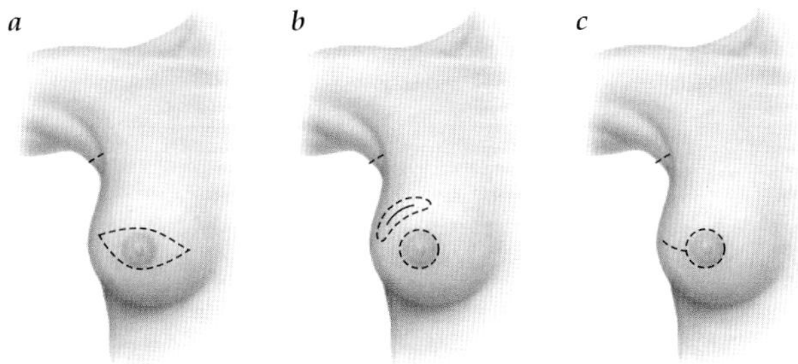

Figure 11 **Shown is (*a*) the recommended placement of the traditional circumareolar incision for skin-sparing mastectomy. (*b*) Separate incisions may be used to excise previous lumpectomy incisions or to gain access to the axilla. (*c*) A lateral extension can provide further exposure for flap development or axillary staging.**

tial or complete nipple necrosis. Pathologic evaluation of the excised lactiferous ducts for tumor involvement is imperative and mandates complete removal of the nipple if in situ or invasive disease is present.

One of the most concerning complications to NSM includes nipple or areolar necrosis, which not only negatively impacts cosmesis but can cause loss of the reconstructed implant. Additional complications include lack of sensation to the nipple, change in nipple pigmentation, and improper nipple positioning following reconstruction.[74] Currently, long-term follow-up to investigate local recurrence rates for NSM is lacking. However, NSM appears to be a good option for those patients undergoing prophylactic mastectomy or those with small, peripheral tumors or in situ disease.

Lymphatic Mapping and SLNB

The pathologic status of the axillary nodes is the single most important prognostic factor for outcome after treatment of breast cancer. The growing recognition of the morbidity of traditional axillary dissection (lymphedema and sensory deficits), together with the increased capability of mammography to detect smaller, potentially node-negative invasive breast cancers, has given rise to the development of SLNB as an axillary staging procedure. SLNB is a minimally invasive means of identifying the first node or nodes draining the breast and hence the first node or nodes to which tumor may spread. In experienced hands, a negative SLNB reliably predicts a tumor-free axilla (false negative rate, 5 to 9%); therefore, when such a result is obtained, no further nodes need to be removed and the patient can be spared the morbidity of a traditional axillary node dissection.[75–77] Surgeons competent in SLNB should be able to identify the SLN with at least 90% accuracy and a false negative rate lower than 5%.[78] It is recommended that surgeons first learning the technique use axillary dissection as a backup for the first 20 procedures to gain experience in identifying the SLN. Currently, axillary dissection is recommended for patients who have a positive SLN; however, prospective, randomized trials are required to determine the extent to which this step is necessary in SLN-positive patients.

The most common method of identifying the SLN involves injection of both a vital blue dye and a radionuclide.[79–82] The radionuclide is first injected into the subareolar lymphatic plexus, either preoperatively or, in some centers, intraoperatively.[80] Because the breast and its overlying skin drain to the same few SLNs,[82] peritumoral, intradermal, and subareolar injections are all acceptable approaches; subareolar injection has the advantage of being expeditious and accurate in cases of multicentric (as well as unicentric) disease.[79] The vital blue dye is then injected, commonly in the subareolar plexus, and the breast is massaged for 5 minutes to stimulate lymphatic flow. Lymph nodes that are "hot" (i.e., radioactive), blue, or both, as well as palpable nodes, are removed for evaluation by frozen-section analysis or touch-print cytology.

SLNB has also been employed in DCIS patients, but, in general, its use should be limited to patients with extensive DCIS who are undergoing mastectomy (in the event of occult invasive disease). Some investigators recommend SLNB for patients with extensive DCIS who are undergoing BCT (in whom CNB may have missed an area of invasion),[83] whereas others caution against this practice.[84,85] Results from the National Surgical Adjuvant Breast and Bowel Project (NSABP) B-27 trial suggest that in patients undergoing neoadjuvant therapy, SLNB may be performed either before or after therapy, with no significant differences in identification and false negative rates[86]; however, this suggestion is not universally accepted.[87] Contraindications to SLNB include the presence of clinically positive axillary nodes, previous axillary surgery, and pregnancy or lactation. Large or locally advanced breast cancers commonly give rise to a positive SLN but are not a contraindication to the procedure in that some patients may still be spared the morbidity of a full axillary dissection.

Axillary Dissection

Before the advent of SLNB, axillary dissection was routinely performed in breast cancer patients. It provided prognostic information that guided subsequent adjuvant therapy, afforded excellent local control, and may have contributed a small overall survival benefit.

Axillary dissection includes resection of level I and level II lymph nodes [*see Figure 12a*].[88] The superior border of the dissection is formed by the axillary vein; the lateral border of the dissection is formed by the latissimus dorsi; the medial border is formed by the pectoral muscles and the anterior serratus muscle; and the inferior border is formed by the tail of the breast. Level II nodes are easily removed by retracting the pectoralis major and the pectoralis minor medially; it is not necessary to divide or remove the pectoralis minor. Level III nodes are not removed unless palpable disease is present.

Axillary dissection, either alone or in conjunction with lumpectomy or mastectomy, usually calls for general anesthesia, but it may be performed with thoracic epidural anesthesia. To facilitate identification and preservation of motor nerves within the axilla, the anesthesiologist should refrain from using neuromuscular blocking agents. In the absence of neuromuscular blockade, any clamping of a motor nerve or too-close approach to a motor nerve with the electrocautery will be signaled by a visible muscle twitch.

STRUCTURES TO BE PRESERVED

A number of vascular structures and nerves passing through the axilla must be preserved during axillary dissection [*see Figure 12b*]. These structures include the axillary vein and artery; the brachial plexus; the long thoracic nerve, which innervates the anterior serratus muscle; the thoracodorsal nerve, artery, and vein, which supply the latissimus dorsi; and the medial pectoral nerve, which innervates the lateral portion of the pectoralis major.

The axillary artery and the brachial plexus should not be exposed during axillary dissection. If they are, the dissection has been carried too far superiorly, and proper orientation at a more inferior position should be established. In some patients, there may be sensory branches of the brachial plexus superficial (and, rarely, inferior) to the axillary vein laterally near the latissimus dorsi; injury to these nerves results in numbness extending to the wrist. To prevent this complication, the axillary vein should initially be identified medially, under the pectoralis major. Medial to the thoracodorsal nerve and adherent to the chest wall is the long thoracic nerve of Bell. The medial pectoral nerve runs from superior to the axillary vein to the undersurface of the pectoralis major, passing through the axillary fat pad and across the level II nodes; it has an accompanying vein whose blue color may be used to identify the nerve. If a submuscular implant reconstruction [*see* Breast Reconstruction, *below*] is planned, preservation of the medial pectoral nerve is especially important to prevent atrophy of the muscle.

The intercostobrachial nerve provides sensation to the posterior portion of the upper arm. Sacrificing this nerve generally leads to numbness over the triceps region. In many women, the intercostobrachial nerve measures 2 mm in diameter and takes a fairly cephalad course near the axillary vein; when this is the case, preservation of the nerve will not interfere with node dissection. Sometimes, however, the nerve is tiny, has multiple branches, and is intermingled with nodal tissue that should be removed; when this is the case, one should not expend a great deal of time on attempting to preserve the nerve. If the intercostobrachial nerve is sacrificed, it should be transected with a knife or scissors rather than with the electrocautery, and the ends should be buried to reduce the likelihood of postoperative causalgia.

OPERATIVE TECHNIQUE

The incision for axillary dissection should be a transverse or curvilinear one made in the lower third of the hair-bearing skin of the axilla. For cosmetic reasons, it should not extend anteriorly onto the pectoralis major; however, it may be extended posteriorly onto the latissimus dorsi as necessary for exposure. Skin flaps are raised to the level of the axillary vein and to a point below the lowest extension of hair-bearing skin, either as an initial maneuver or after the initial identification of key structures.

The key to axillary dissection is obtaining and maintaining proper orientation with respect to the axillary vein, the thoracodorsal bundle, and the long thoracic nerve. After the incision has been made, the dissection is extended down into the true axillary fat pad through the overlying fascial layer. The fat of the axillary fat pad may be distinguished from subcutaneous fat on the basis of its smoother, lipomalike texture. There may be aberrant muscle slips from the latissimus dorsi or the pectoralis major; in addition, there may be an extremely dense fascial encasement around the axillary fat pad. It is important to divide these layers early in the dissection. The borders of the pectoralis major and the latissimus dorsi are then exposed, which clears the medial and lateral borders of the dissection.

The axillary vein and the thoracodorsal bundle are identified next. As discussed (see above), the initial identification of the axillary vein should be made medially, under the pectoralis major, to prevent injury to low-lying branches of the brachial plexus. Sometimes, the axillary vein takes the form of several small branches rather than a single large vessel. If this is the case, all of the small branches should be preserved.

The thoracodorsal bundle may be identified either distally at its junction with the latissimus dorsi or at its junction with the axillary vein. The junction with the latissimus dorsi is

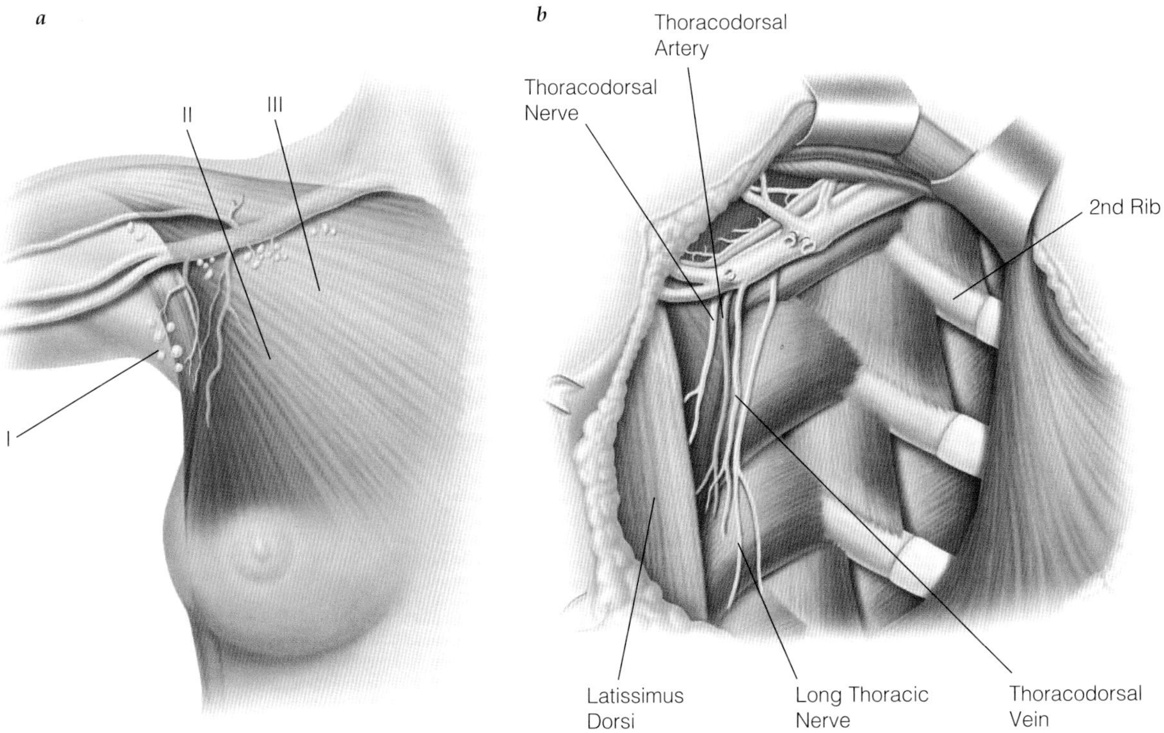

Figure 12 **Axillary dissection.[88] (*a*) Shown are axillary lymph node levels in relation to the axillary vein and the muscles of the axilla (I = low axilla, II = midaxilla, III = apex of axilla). (*b*) Shown is a view of the structures of the axilla after completion of axillary dissection.**

within the axillary fat pad at a point two thirds of the way down the hair-bearing skin of the axilla, or approximately 4 cm below the inferior border of the axillary vein. Occasionally, the thoracodorsal bundle is bifurcated, with separate superior and inferior branches entering the latissimus dorsi; this is particularly likely if the entry point appears very high. If the bundle is bifurcated, both branches should be preserved. The thoracodorsal bundle may be identified at its junction with the latissimus dorsi by spreading within axillary fat parallel to the border of the muscle and looking for the blue of the thoracodorsal vein. Identification is also facilitated by lateral retraction of the latissimus dorsi. The long thoracic nerve lies just medial to the thoracodorsal bundle on the chest wall at this point and at approximately the same anterior-posterior position. It may be identified by spreading tissue just medial to the thoracodorsal bundle and then running the index finger perpendicular to the course of the long thoracic nerve on the chest wall to identify the cordlike nerve as it moves under the finger. Once the nerve is identified, axillary tissue may be swept anteriorly away from the nerve by blunt dissection along the anterior serratus muscle; there are no significant vessels in this area.

The junction of the thoracodorsal bundle with the axillary vein is 1.5 to 2.0 cm medial to the point at which the axillary vein crosses the latissimus dorsi. The thoracodorsal vein enters the posterior surface of the axillary vein, and the nerve and the artery pass posterior to the axillary vein. Generally, one or two scapular veins branch off the axillary vein medial to the junction with the thoracodorsal vein. These are divided during the dissection and should not be confused with the thoracodorsal bundle.

The axillary vein and the thoracodorsal bundle having been identified, the pectoralis major is retracted medially at the level of the axillary vein, and the latissimus dorsi is retracted laterally to place tension on the thoracodorsal bundle. Once this exposure is achieved, the axillary fat and the nodes are cleared away superficial and medial to the thoracodorsal bundle to the level of the axillary vein. Superiorly, dissection proceeds medially along the axillary vein to the point where the fat containing level II nodes crosses the axillary vein. To improve exposure, the fascia overlying the level II extension of the axillary fat pad should be incised to release tension and expose the lipomalike level II fat. As noted [*see* Structures to Be Preserved, *above*], the medial pectoral nerve passes onto the underside of the pectoralis major in this area and should be preserved. One or more small venous branches may pass inferiorly from the medial pectoral bundle; particular attention should be paid to preserving the nerve when ligating these venous branches.

The next step in the dissection is to reflect the axillary fat pad inferiorly by dividing the medial attachments of the axillary fat pad along the anterior serratus muscle. Care must be taken to preserve the long thoracic nerve. Because there are no significant vessels or structures in the tissue anterior to the long thoracic nerve, this tissue may be divided sharply, with small perforating vessels either tied or cauterized. Finally, the axillary fat is freed from the tail of the breast with the electrocautery or a knife.

There is no need to orient the axillary specimen for the pathologist, because treatment is not affected by the anatomic level of node involvement. A closed suction drain is placed through a separate stab wound. (Some practitioners prefer not to place a drain and simply aspirate postoperative seromas as necessary.) A long-acting local anesthetic may be instilled into the axilla—a particularly helpful practice if the dissection was done as an outpatient procedure.

Breast Reconstruction

The vast majority of women undergoing a partial or complete mastectomy are candidates for breast reconstruction and should be offered a plastic surgery consultation before undergoing definitive surgical treatment. Reconstruction is covered by insurance and may be done either at the time of the oncologic surgery (immediate reconstruction) or as a delayed procedure (delayed reconstruction). Despite early concerns and debate, studies show that neither mode of reconstruction interferes with detection of recurrent disease nor does it significantly delay subsequent adjuvant therapy.

REPAIR OF PARTIAL MASTECTOMY DEFECTS (ONCOPLASTY)

Recently, there has been an increase in the proportion of breast cancer patients treated with partial mastectomy followed by radiation therapy, an approach referred to as BCT. This trend is in part attributable to increased mammographic screening that has led to the detection of earlier breast cancers and the use of neoadjuvant chemotherapy, where significant clinical responses can obviate the need for a traditional mastectomy. Alarmingly, 20 to 30% of patients who undergo BCT report having a poor cosmetic result in the treated breast.[89]

The term *oncoplasty* has been used to describe techniques to improve the cosmesis of the breast after oncologic resection. Techniques integral to plastic surgery are often incorporated and include local tissue rearrangement, purse-string defect closure, breast reduction techniques, local pedicled flaps, and lower abdominal flaps.[89,90] The ultimate goal is to obtain a natural-appearing breast with improved cosmesis compared to partial mastectomy alone.

REPAIR OF MASTECTOMY DEFECTS

Options for breast reconstruction continue to evolve and include, but are not limited to, implants with or without tissue expansion, the transverse rectus abdominis myocutaneous (TRAM) flap, the latissimus dorsi myocutaneous flap, and various other free flaps. Patient preference and lifestyle, the availability of suitable autologous tissue, and the demands imposed by additional cancer therapies are variables that can influence the timing and choice of the optimal reconstructive technique [*see Figure 13*].

If the need for postmastectomy radiation therapy is definite or unclear at the time of mastectomy (i.e., final pathology results are not available), a delayed reconstruction may be chosen because of an increased risk of complications related to the reconstructed breast. An expander is typically placed at the time of mastectomy to preserve the breast skin envelope, and the definitive reconstructive plan is formulated once the final pathologic results have become available and the radiation therapy has been completed.[91]

RECONSTRUCTION OPTIONS

Prosthetic Implants

The simplest method of reconstruction is to place a saline- or silicone-filled implant beneath the pectoralis major. However, even after SSM, the pectoralis major is usually so tight that expansion of this muscle and the overlying skin is necessary before an implant that matches the opposite breast can be inserted. A tissue expander is typically placed and serial expansions are performed on an outpatient basis until an appropriate-size breast pocket has been attained. The time required to complete the expansion process usually ranges from 3 to 6 months after mastectomy and is dependent mostly on the desired breast size, the thickness of the mastectomy skin flaps, and the patient's ability to tolerate the expansion.[92] A second operative procedure is then required to exchange the expander for a permanent implant. The nipple-areolar complex is constructed at a later date. AlloDerm (LifeCell Corp., Branchburg, New Jersey) and Flex HD (MTF, Edison, New Jersey) are acellular dermal matrices derived from human cadaver skin that may be sewn to the pectoralis muscle and the inframammary fold to reinforce the lower pole of the breast and enlarge the breast pocket so that it may accommodate a tissue expander or implant.[93] This measure may reduce postoperative pain and improve cosmesis, as well as facilitate immediate implant placement in smaller-breasted women. Porcine-derived dermal matrices are also available and may be used as an alternative to the aforementioned.

The major advantages of implant reconstruction are reduced operative time, faster recuperation, and a reasonably good cosmetic outcome. These advantages must be weighed against the fact that this method is a two-stage approach and that obtaining symmetry with the contralateral native breast can be difficult and often requires a mastopexy (breast lift) with or without an implant augmentation.[94] The cosmetic result may also deteriorate over time as a consequence of capsule formation or implant migration, resulting in replacement of the implant each decade.

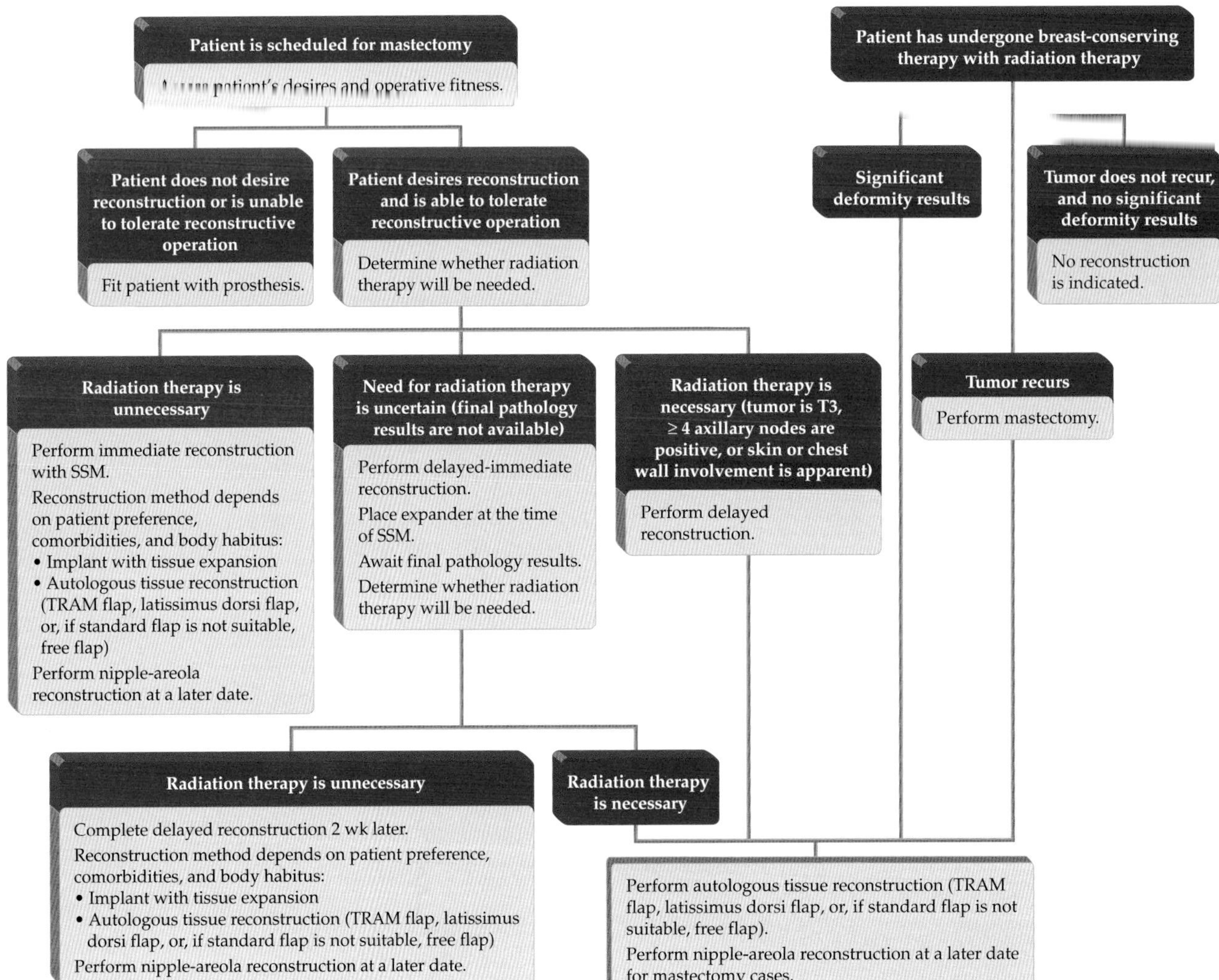

Figure 13 **Algorithm outlining the major steps in breast reconstruction after mastectomy. SSM = skin-sparing mastectomy; TRAM = transverse rectus abdominis myocutaneous.**

Autologous Tissue

An alternative approach to reconstruction that continues to evolve is the transfer of vascularized muscle, skin, fat, or a combination of these from a donor site to the mastectomy defect. The transferred tissue may be relocated either on a vascular pedicle or as a free tissue transfer requiring a microsurgical anastomosis. Although autologous tissue procedures can be lengthy and are associated with a longer recovery period, they often require fewer revision and symmetry procedures.[95] With autologous tissue reconstruction, it is possible to create a natural-appearing breast without the need for a breast implant, often sparing the patient a contralateral breast procedure to obtain symmetry.[94] The most commonly used pedicled myocutaneous flaps are the TRAM flap [*see Figure 14*] and the latissimus dorsi flap [*see Figure 15*]. Recent advances have led to the conception of perforator flaps such as the deep inferior epigastric perforator (DIEP) flap and the superficial inferior epigastric artery (SIEA) flap, which allow for safe and reliable tissue transfer with minimal donor-site morbidity.

The major advantage of autologous tissue reconstruction is that it generally yields a superior cosmetic result and provides variability in breast volume and shape[96]; in addition, the reconstructed breast has a softer, more natural texture than a breast that has undergone implant reconstruction. The main drawbacks are the magnitude of the surgical procedure (involving both a prolonged operating time and longer inpatient hospitalization), the potential need for blood transfusion, and the morbidity related to the donor site. Smokers and patients with significant vascular disease may not be ideal candidates for autologous tissue reconstruction. Partial necrosis of the transferred flap may create firm areas; on rare occasions, complete necrosis and consequent loss of the flap can occur.

Pedicled myocutaneous flaps In a pedicled TRAM flap reconstruction, the contralateral rectus abdominis is transferred along with overlying skin and fat based on the superior epigastric vessels to create a breast mound. This procedure yields a flatter abdominal contour but calls for a long transverse abdominal incision and necessitates repositioning of the umbilicus. The major advantages of TRAM flap reconstruction are that it provides enough tissue to match most contralateral breasts and that it offers the option of performing bilateral TRAM flap procedures in healthy candidates who desire or require bilateral reconstruction. Patients who have undergone abdominal procedures that compromise the TRAM flap's vascular supply are not ideal candidates for TRAM reconstruction. Postoperative discomfort is greater with TRAM flap reconstruction than with other flap reconstructions because of the extent of the abdominal wall dissection and defect.

In a pedicled latissimus dorsi myocutaneous flap reconstruction, the ipsilateral latissimus dorsi is transferred along with overlying skin and fat based on the thoracodorsal vessels to create a breast mound. The operative technique for the latissimus dorsi flap reconstruction is complex, requiring intraoperative changes in patient position (unless the oncologic surgeon is willing to perform the mastectomy with the patient in a lateral decubitus position). Patients who have undergone irradiation of the breast, the chest wall, or the axilla (including irradiation of the thoracodorsal vessels) may not be eligible for this procedure. A major advantage of the latissimus dorsi flap is that its donor site is associated with less postoperative discomfort than the abdominal donor site of the TRAM flap. In addition, transfer of the latissimus dorsi results in substantially less functional impairment than transfer of the rectus abdominis. One major drawback is that in many women, the latissimus dorsi is not bulky enough to

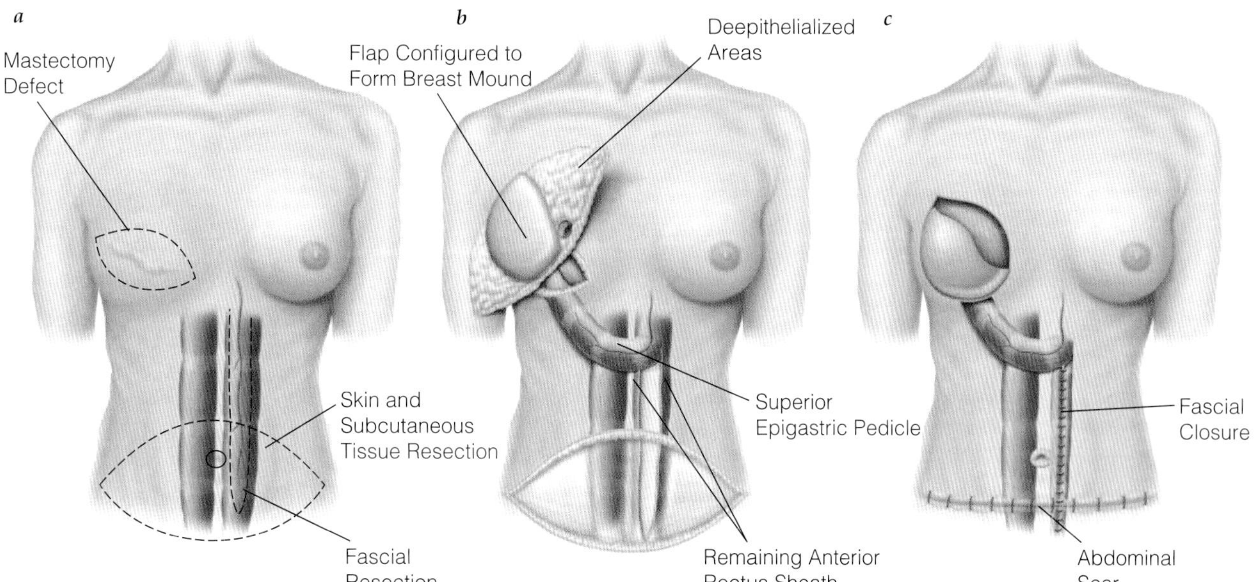

Figure 14 **Breast reconstruction after mastectomy: transverse rectus abdominis myocutaneous (TRAM) flap. (*a*) The infraumbilical flap is designed. The TRAM flap is tunneled subcutaneously into the chest wall cavity. Blood supply to the flap is maintained from the superior epigastric vessels of the rectus abdominis. (*b*) Subcutaneous fat and deepithelialized skin are positioned under the mastectomy flaps as needed to reconstruct the breast mound. (*c*) The fascia of the anterior rectus sheath is approximated to achieve tight closure of the abdominal wall defect and to prevent hernia formation. The umbilicus is sutured into its new position.**

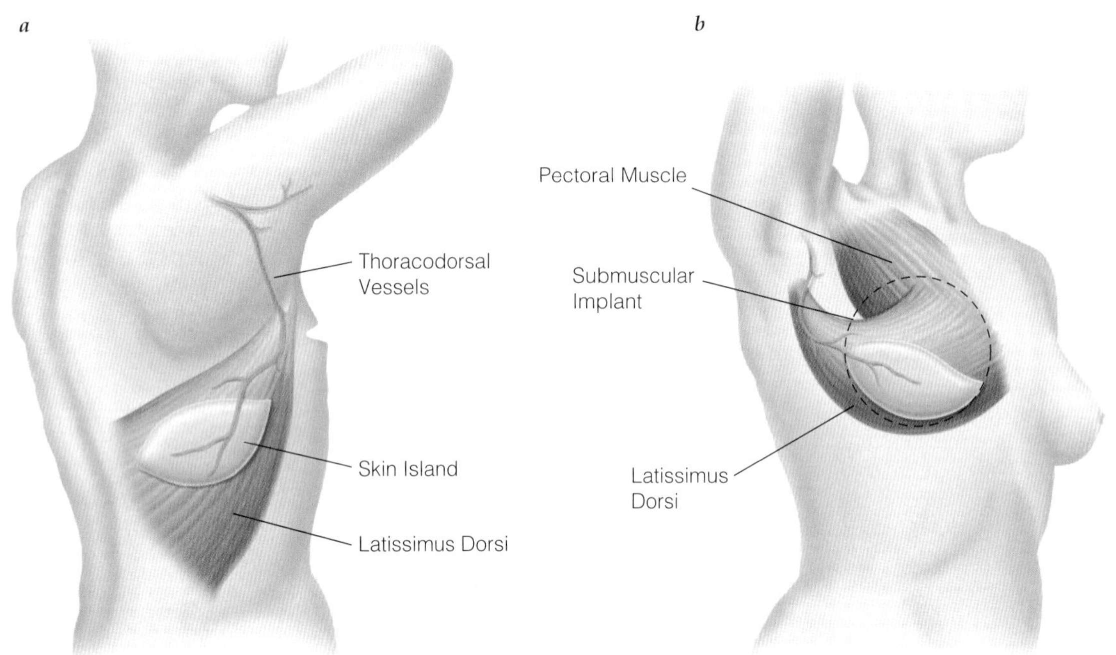

Figure 15 **Breast reconstruction: latissimus dorsi flap Breast reconstruction after mastectomy: latissimus dorsi myocutaneous flap with submuscular implant. With this flap, addition of an implant is often required to provide the reconstructed breast with adequate volume and projection. (*a*) The myocutaneous flap is elevated; it is important to maintain the blood supply to the flap from the thoracodorsal vessels. The flap is tunneled subcutaneously to the mastectomy defect. (*b*) The latissimus dorsi is sutured to the pectoralis major and the skin of the inframammary fold so that the implant is completely covered by muscle.**

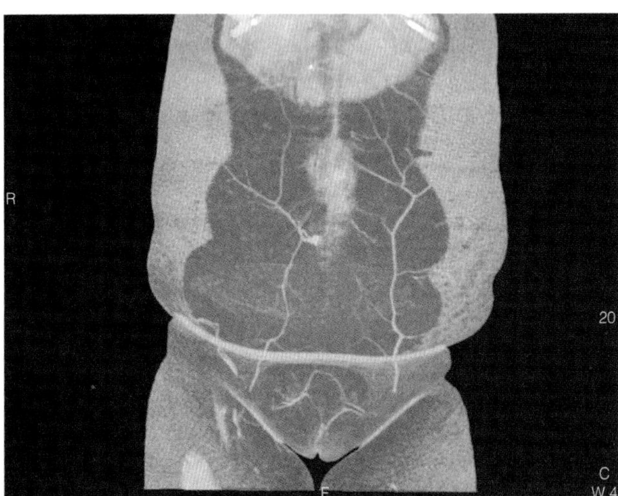

Figure 16 **Pre-operative computed tomographic angiography of the inferior epigastric arterial system, the basis for free transverse rectus abdominis myocutaneous (TRAM), deep inferior epigastric perforator (DIEP), and superficial inferior epigastric artery (SIEA) flaps, used for autologous breast reconstruction.**

provide symmetry with the contralateral breast; consequently, to match the size of the opposite breast, the flap must be supplemented with an implant. Thus, the drawback of the implant's limited life span is added to the drawbacks associated with autologous tissue reconstruction.

Free myocutaneous and perforator flaps Free-flap reconstruction options are used primarily when other autologous and implant reconstruction options are not available, do not provide sufficient tissue volume, or have failed. They are more complex procedures, requiring microvascular anastomoses, and carry a higher risk of total flap loss. Although, historically, the free TRAM flap and the free gluteal artery flap (GAP) have been the most often employed techniques, the introduction of perforator flaps (DIEP, SIEA, superior GAP, inferior GAP) has added options to the reconstructive surgeon's armamentarium. Preoperatively, CT angiography [*see Figure 16*] has replaced duplex ultrasonography as the gold standard for evaluation of donor vessel caliber and patency.[96] Perforator flaps are supplied by blood vessels that perforate through or around overlying muscles to vascularize the overlying skin and fat. During flap harvest, these perforators must be meticulously dissected free from the surrounding muscle, which is preserved intact and left in its natural position. The free tissue flap is then anastomosed to recipient vessels, and the donor site is closed without the need of additional support such as mesh or biologics.[97] Ideally, they provide adequate tissue for reconstruction without the level of donor-site morbidity seen with the free TRAM or other myocutaneous free flaps.[98] The disadvantages of perforator flaps include the considerable technical expertise and long operating time required, as well as the greater potential for flap loss (because these flaps have a more tenuous blood supply than the standard TRAM flap).

Financial Disclosures: None Reported

References

1. Liberman L. Percutaneous image-guided core breast biopsy. Radiol Clin North Am 2002;40:483–500, vi.
2. Shoher A, Lucci A. Emerging patterns of practice in the implementation and application of sentinel lymph node biopsy in breast cancer patients in the United States. J Surg Oncol 2003;83:65–7.
3. Fisher B, Anderson S, Redmond C, et al. Reanalysis and results after 12 years of follow-up in a randomized clinical trial comparing total mastectomy with lumpectomy with or without irradiation in the treatment of breast cancer. N Engl J Med 1995;333:1456–61.
4. Shons AR, Mosiello G. Postmastectomy breast reconstruction: current techniques. Cancer Control 2001;8:419–26.
5. Dowlatshahi K, Francescatti DS, Bloom K, et al. Image-guided surgery of small breast cancers. Am J Surg 2001;182:419–25.
6. Tondre J, Nejad M, Casano A, et al. Technical enhancements to breast ductal lavage. Ann Surg Oncol 2008;15:2734–8.
7. Newman LA, Blake C. Ductal lavage for breast cancer risk assessment. Cancer Control 2002;9:473–9.
8. Dooley WC, Ljung B, Veronesi U, et al. Ductal lavage for detection of cellular atypia in women at high risk for breast cancer. J Natl Cancer Inst 2001;93:1624–32.
9. Kapenhas-Valdes E, Feldman S, Cohen J, et al. Mammary ductoscopy for evaluation of nipple discharge. Ann Surg Oncol 2008;15: 2720–7.
10. Moncrief RM, Nayar R, Diaz LK, et al. A comparison of ductoscopy-guided and conventional surgical excision in women with spontaneous nipple discharge. Ann Surg 2005;241:575–81.
11. Dooley WC. Routine operative breast endoscopy during lumpectomy. Ann Surg Oncol 2003;10:38–42.
12. Escobar PF, Crowe JP, Matsunaga T, et al. The clinical applications of mammary ductoscopy. Am J Surg 2006;191:211–5.
13. Mokbel K, Elkak AE. The evolving role of mammary ductoscopy. Curr Med Res Opin 2002;18:30–2.
14. Stanley MW, Sidawy MK, Sanchez MA, et al. Current issues in breast cytopathology. Am J Clin Pathol 2000;113:(5 Suppl 1): S49–75.
15. Choi JY, Alderman AK, Newman LA. Aesthetic and reconstruction considerations in oncologic breast surgery. J Am Coll Surg 2006;202:943–52.
16. Burbank F. Stereotactic breast biopsy: comparison of 14- and 11-gauge Mammotome probe performance and complication rates. Am Surg 1997;63:988–95.
17. Hoorntje LE, Peeters PH, Mali WP, et al. Vacuum-assisted breast biopsy: a critical review. Eur J Cancer 2003; 39:1676–83.
18. Robinson D, Sundaram M. Stereotactic imaging and breast biopsy. In: Bland KI, Copeland E, editors. The breast: comprehensive management of benign and malignant disorders. Philadelphia: WB Saunders; 2004; p. 686.
19. Kuhl CK, Morakkabati N, Leutner CC, et al. MR imaging–guided large-core (14-gauge) needle biopsy of small lesions visible at breast MR imaging alone. Radiology 2001;220: 31–9.
20. Viehweg P, Heinig A, Amaya B, et al. MR-guided interventional breast procedures considering vacuum biopsy in particular. Eur J Radiol 2002;42:32–9.
21. Orel SG, Rosen M, Mies C, et al. MR imaging-guided 9-gauge vacuum-assisted core-needle breast biopsy: initial experience. Radiology 2006;238:54–61.
22. King TA, Fuhrman GM, Image-guided breast biopsy. Semin Surg Oncol 2001; 20:197–204.
23. Jacobs TW, Connolly JL, Schnitt SJ. Nonmalignant lesions in breast core needle biopsies: to excise or not to excise?. Am J Surg Pathol 2002;26:1095–110.
24. Kass R, Henry-Tillman RS, Nurko J, et al. Touch preparation of breast core needle specimens is a new method for same-day diagnosis. Am J Surg 2003;186:737–41; discussion 742.
25. Bloom K, Fine RE, Lerner AG. Intact specimen capture and collection of image-detected breast lesions via percutaneous radiofrequency device. In: American Society of Breast Surgeons; 2004; Las Vegas (NV).
26. Fine RE, Boyd BA, Whitworth PW, et al. Percutaneous removal of benign breast masses using a vacuum-assisted hand-held device with ultrasound guidance. Am J Surg 2002;184:332–6.
27. Johnson AT, Henry-Tillman RS, Smith LF, et al. Percutaneous excisional breast biopsy. Am J Surg 2002;184:550–4; discussion 554.
28. Mullen DJ, Eisen RN, Newman RD, et al. The use of carbon marking after stereotactic large-core-needle breast biopsy. Radiology 2001;218:255–60.
29. Marx M, Bernstein RM, Wack JP. Xylocaine plus methylene blue vs methylene blue alone for marking breast tissue preoperatively. AJR Am J Roentgenol 1993;160:896.
30. Gray RJ, Salud C, Nguyen K, et al. Randomized prospective evaluation of a novel technique for biopsy or lumpectomy of non-palpable breast lesions: radioactive seed versus wire localization. Ann Surg Oncol 2001;8:711–5.
31. Smith LF, Henry-Tillman R, Harms S, et al. Hematoma-directed ultrasound-guided breast biopsy. Ann Surg 2001; 233:669–75.
32. Smith LF, Henry-Tillman R, Rubio IT, et al. Intraoperative localization after stereotactic breast biopsy without a needle. Am J Surg 2001;182:584–9.
33. van Esser S, Hobbelink M, Van der Ploeg IM, et al. Radio guided occult lesion localization (ROLL) for non-palpable invasive breast cancer. J Surg Oncol 2008;98: 526–9.
34. Medina-Franco H, Abarca-Pérez L, García-Alvarez MN, et al. Radioguided occult lesion localization (ROLL) versus wire-guided lumpectomy for non-palpable breast lesions: a randomized prospective evaluation. J Surg Oncol 2008;97:108–11.
35. Thind CR, Desmond S, Harris O, et al. Radio-guided localization of clinically occult breast lesions (ROLL): a DGH experience. Clin Radiol 2005;60:681–6.
36. Nadeem R, Chagla LS, Harris O, et al. Occult breast lesions: a comparison between radioguided occult lesion localisation (ROLL) vs. wire-guided lumpectomy (WGL). Breast 2005;14:283–9.
37. van Rijk MC, Tanis PJ, Nieweg OE, et al. Sentinel node biopsy and concomitant probe-guided tumor excision of nonpalpable breast cancer. Ann Surg Oncol 2007;14:627–32.
38. Tanis PJ, Deurloo EE, Valdés Olmos RA, et al. Single intralesional tracer dose for radio-guided excision of clinically occult breast cancer and sentinel node. Ann Surg Oncol 2001;8:850–5.
39. Ronka R, Krogerus L, Leppänen E, et al. Radio-guided occult lesion localization in patients undergoing breast-conserving surgery and sentinel node biopsy. Am J Surg 2004;187:491–6.
40. Morrow M. Breast diseases. In: Hellman S, Harris JR, Henderson IC, editors. Breast diseases. Philadelphia: JB Lippincott; 1991.
41. Sharma N, Huston TL, Simmons RM. Intraoperative intraductal injection of methylene blue dye to assist in major duct excision. Am J Surg 2006;191:553–4.
42. Smith J. Ductal exploration for nipple discharge. Contemp Surg 2003;59:518.
43. Simmons RM. Ablative techniques in the treatment of benign and malignant breast disease. J Am Coll Surg 2003;197:334–8.
44. Whitworth PW, Rewcastle JC. Cryoablation and cryolocalization in the management of breast disease. J Surg Oncol 2005;90:1–9.
45. Sabel MS. Cryoablation for breast cancer: no need to turn a cold shoulder. J Surg Oncol 2008;97:485–6.
46. van Esser S, van den Bosch MA, van Diest PJ, et al. Minimally invasive ablative therapies for invasive breast carcinomas: an overview of current literature. World J Surg 2007; 31:2284–92.
47. Sabel MS, Kaufman CS, Whitworth P, et al. Cryoablation of early-stage breast cancer: work-in-progress report of a multi-institutional trial. Ann Surg Oncol 2004;11:542–9.
48. Roubidoux MA, Sabel MS, Bailey JE, et al. Small (< 2.0-cm) breast cancers: mammographic and US findings at US-guided cryoablation—initial experience. Radiology 2004;233:857–67.
49. Tafra L, Fine R, Whitworth P, et al. Prospective randomized study comparing cryo-assisted and needle-wire localization of ultrasound-visible breast tumors. Am J Surg 2006;192: 462–70.
50. Kepple J, Van Zee KJ, Dowlatshahi K, et al. Minimally invasive breast surgery. J Am Coll Surg 2004;199:961–75.
51. Dowlatshahi K, Francescatti DS, Bloom KJ. Laser therapy for small breast cancers. Am J Surg 2002;184:359–63.
52. Fujimoto S, Kobayashi K, Takahashi M, et al. Clinical pilot studies on pre-operative hyperthermic tumour ablation for advanced breast carcinoma using an 8 MHz radiofrequency heating device. Int J Hyperthermia 2003;19:13–22.
53. Gardner RA, Vargas HI, Block JB, et al. Focused microwave phased array thermotherapy for primary breast cancer. Ann Surg Oncol 2002; 9:326–32.
54. Huston TL, Simmons RM. Ablative therapies for the treatment of malignant diseases of the breast. Am J Surg 2005;189:694–701.
55. Kaiser WA, Pfleiderer SO, Baltzer PA. MRI-guided interventions of the breast. J Magn Reson Imaging 2008;27:347–55.
56. Wu F, Wang ZB, Cao YD, et al. "Wide local ablation" of localized breast cancer using high intensity focused ultrasound. J Surg Oncol 2007;96:130–6.
57. Kunos C, Latson L, Overmoyer B, et al. Breast conservation surgery achieving > or =2 mm tumor-free margins results in decreased local-regional recurrence rates. Breast J 2006;12:28–36.
58. Grisotti A. Conservative treatment of breast cancer: reconstructive problems. In: Spear S, editor. Surgery of the breast. Philadelphia: Lippincott Williams & Wilkins; 2006; p. 147.
59. Silverstein M. Ductal carcinoma in situ: basics, treatments controversies, and an oncoplastic approach. In: Spear S, editor. Surgery of the breast. Philadelphia: Lippincott Williams & Wilkins; 2006; p. 92.

60. Smith LF, Rubio IT, Henry-Tillman R, et al. Intraoperative ultrasound-guided breast biopsy. Am J Surg 2000; 180: 419–23.
61. Kuerer HM. The case for accelerated partial-breast irradiation for breast cancer—M.D. Anderson Cancer Center telemedicine symposium. Contemp Surg 2003;59:508.
62. Strauss JB, Dickler A. Accelerated partial breast irradiation utilizing balloon brachytherapy techniques. Radiother Oncol 2009;91: 157–65.
63. Wallner P, Arthur D, Bartelink H, et al. Workshop on partial breast irradiation: state of the art and the science, Bethesda, MD, December 8-10, 2002. J Natl Cancer Inst 2004;96:175–84.
64. Hultman CS, Daiza S. Skin-sparing mastectomy flap complications after breast reconstruction: review of incidence, management, and outcome. Ann Plast Surg 2003;50:249–55; discussion 255.
65. Carlson G. Invasive carcinoma skin sparing mastectomy. In: Wilkins LW, editor. Surgery of the breast. Philadelphia: Lippincott Williams & Wilkins; 2006; p. 140.
66. Benediktsson KP, Perbeck L. Survival in breast cancer after nipple-sparing subcutaneous mastectomy and immediate reconstruction with implants: a prospective trial with 13 years median follow-up in 216 patients. Eur J Surg Oncol 2008;34:143–8.
67. Caruso F, Ferrara M, Castiglione G, et al. Nipple sparing subcutaneous mastectomy: sixty-six months follow-up. Eur J Surg Oncol 2006;32:937–40.
68. Crowe JP Jr, Kim JA, Yetman R, et al. Nipple-sparing mastectomy: [illegible] and results of 54 procedures. Arch Surg 2004; 139:148–50.
69. Gerber B, Krause A, Reimer T, et al. Skin-sparing mastectomy with conservation of the nipple-areola complex and autologous reconstruction is an oncologically safe procedure. Ann Surg 2003; 238:120–7.
70. Petit JY, Veronesi U, Luini A, et al. When mastectomy becomes inevitable: the nipple-sparing approach. Breast 2005;14:527–31.
71. Voltura AM, Tsangaris TN, Rosson GD, et al. Nipple-sparing mastectomy: critical assessment of 51 procedures and implications for selection criteria. Ann Surg Oncol 2008;15:3396–401.
72. Chung AP, Sacchini V. Nipple-sparing mastectomy: where are we now?. Surg Oncol 2008;17:261–6.
73. Sacchini V, Pinotti JA, Barros AC, et al. Nipple-sparing mastectomy for breast cancer and risk reduction: oncologic or technical problem?. J Am Coll Surg 2006;203: 704–14.
74. Sookhan N, Boughey JC, Walsh MF, et al. Nipple-sparing mastectomy—initial experience at a tertiary center. Am J Surg 2008; 196:575–7.
75. Krag D, Weaver D, Ashikaga T, et al. The sentinel node in breast cancer—a multicenter validation study. N Engl J Med 1998;339: 941–6.
76. Sabel MS, Schott AF, Kleer CG, et al. Sentinel node biopsy prior to neoadjuvant chemotherapy. Am J Surg 2003;186:102–5.
77. Turner RR, Ollila DW, Krasne DL, et al. Histopathologic validation of the sentinel lymph node hypothesis for breast carcinoma. Ann Surg 1997;226:271–6; discussion 276–8.
78. Schwartz GF, Guiliano AE, Veronesi U. Proceeding of the consensus conference of the role of sentinel lymph node biopsy in carcinoma or the breast April 19-22, 2001, Philadelphia, PA, USA. Breast J 2002;8: 124–38.
79. Layeeque R, Henry-Tillman R, Korourian S, et al. Subareolar sentinel node biopsy for multiple breast cancers. Am J Surg 2003;186:730–5; discussion 735–6.
80. Layeeque R, Kepple J, Henry-Tillman R, et al. Intraoperative subareolar radioisotope injection for immediate sentinel lymph node biopsy. Ann Surg 2004;239: 841–5; discussion 845–8.
81. Ozmen V, Cabioglu N. Sentinel lymph node biopsy for breast cancer: current controversies. Breast J 2006;12(5 Suppl 2):S134–42.
82. Rubio IT, Klimberg VS. Techniques of sentinel lymph node biopsy. Semin Surg Oncol 2001;20:214–23.
83. Camp R, Feezor R, Kasraeian A, et al. Sentinel lymph node biopsy for ductal carcinoma in situ: an evolving approach at the University of Florida. Breast J 2005;11:394–7.
84. Farkas EA, Stolier AJ, Teng SC, et al. An argument against routine sentinel node mapping for DCIS. Am Surg 2004;70:13–7; discussion 17–8.
85. Lagios MD, Silverstein MJ. Sentinel node biopsy for patients with DCIS: a dangerous and unwarranted direction. Ann Surg Oncol 2001;8:275–7.
86. Mamounas EP, Brown A, Anderson S, et al. Sentinel node biopsy after neoadjuvant chemotherapy in breast cancer: results from National Surgical Adjuvant Breast and Bowel Project Protocol B-27. J Clin Oncol 2005; 23:2694–702.
87. Jones JL, Zabicki K, Christian RL, et al. A comparison of sentinel node biopsy before and after neoadjuvant chemotherapy: timing is important. Am J Surg 2005; 190:517–20.
88. Kinne DW. Primary treatment of breast cancer. In: Hellman S, Harris JR, Henderson IC, editors. Breast diseases. Philadelphia: JB Lippincott; 1991.
89. Kronowitz SJ, Kuerer HM, Buchholz TA, et al. A management algorithm and practical oncoplastic surgical techniques for repairing partial mastectomy defects. Plast Reconstr Surg 2008;122:1631–47.
90. Fitzal F, Mittlboeck M, Trischler H, et al. Breast-conserving therapy for centrally located breast cancer. Ann Surg 2008; 247: 470–6.
91. Kronowitz SJ, Robb GL. Controversies regarding immediate reconstruction: aesthetic risks of radiation. In: Spear S, editor. Surgery of the breast. Philadelphia: Lippincott Williams & Wilkins; 2006; p. 679.
92. Kronowitz SJ, Kuerer HM. Advances and surgical decision-making for breast reconstruction. Cancer 2006;107:893–907.
93. Spear S. Immediate breast reconstruction with tissue expanders and AlloDerm. In: Spear S, editor. Surgery of the breast. Philadelphia: Lippincott Williams & Wilkins; 2006; p. 484.
94. Losken A, Carlson GW, Bostwick J, et al.Trends in unilateral breast reconstruction and management of the contralateral breast: the Emory experience. Plast Reconstr Surg 2002;110:89–97.
95. Kroll SS, Baldwin B. A comparison of outcomes using three different methods of breast reconstruction. Plast Reconstr Surg 1992; 90:455–62.
96. Rozen WM, Ashton MW. Improving outcomes in autologous breast reconstruction. Aesthetic Plast Surg 2008;33:327–35.
97. Granzow JW, Levine JL, Chiu ES, et al. Breast reconstruction with perforator flaps. Plast Reconstr Surg 2007;120:1–12.
98. Craigie JE, Allen RJ, DellaCroce FJ, et al. Autogenous breast reconstruction with the deep inferior epigastric perforator flap. Clin Plast Surg 2003;30:359–69.
99. Urist MM, Bland KI. Indications and techniques for biopsy. In: Bland KI, Copeland EMI, editors. The breast: comprehensive management of benign and malignant diseases. Philadelphia: WB Saunders; 2004; p. 791.

Acknowledgment

The authors wish to acknowledge Rena B. Kass, MD, FACS, and Wiley W. Souba, MD, ScD, FACS, for their contributions to the previous rendition of this chapter on which they have based this update.
Figures 2, 3, 5 to 11, and 13 to 15 Alice Y. Chen.

6 LYMPHATIC MAPPING AND SENTINEL NODE BIOPSY

*David W. Ollila, MD, FACS, Karyn B. Stitzenberg, MD, MPH, and Nancy Klauber-Demore, MD, FACS**

With an estimated 194,280 new cases in the United States in 2009, breast cancer is among the most common malignancies treated by US surgeons.[1] Meanwhile, the incidence of melanoma is rising faster than for all other solid malignancies. In 2009, there were an estimated 68,720 new cases of invasive melanoma in the United States.

Over the past 25 years, significant strides have been made in the management of these two diseases from the standpoint of both surgical and adjuvant therapy. For both diseases, the presence or absence of lymph node metastases is highly predictive of patient outcome and is the most important prognostic factor for disease recurrence and cancer-related mortality. As a result, nodal staging is a critical component of the staging workup and of treatment planning. The focus of this chapter is the role of nodal staging for both diseases.

No patient with tumor-free regional lymph nodes derives any therapeutic benefit from a complete regional lymphadenectomy. For patients with clinically negative nodal basins, the development of intraoperative lymphatic mapping and sentinel node (SN) biopsy has made it possible to map lymphatic pathway from a primary tumor to the initial draining node(s) (i.e., the SN or SNs) in the regional nodal basin. This is the lymph node most likely to harbor metastatic nodal disease, if any exists. It has been demonstrated in both breast cancer and melanoma that the pathologic status of the SN, when performed by an experienced team, is to be concordant with the pathologic status of the entire nodal basin. Integration of these techniques, along with increasingly detailed and sophisticated pathologic examination of the SN, into the surgical treatment of melanoma and breast cancer offers the potential for more conservative nodal basin operations, lower morbidity, and more accurate disease staging.

Lymphatic Mapping and SN Biopsy for Melanoma

RATIONALE

Assessment of Nodal Status

Approximately 20% of melanoma patients have nodal metastases at the time of diagnosis. The presence of lymph node metastases is the single most powerful predictor of recurrence and survival in melanoma patients. Five-year survival is approximately 40% lower in patients who have lymph node metastases than in those who do not.[2] As a result, accurate nodal staging is important for stratifying patients into different risks groups that can be used to direct further therapy.

Elective Lymph Node Dissection

Until the early part of the 1990s, elective lymph node dissection (ELND) was the mainstay of the surgeon's armamentarium for nodal staging of melanoma patients. ELND is the complete surgical removal of the closest nodal basin in patients with clinically negative lymph nodes. In contrast, therapeutic lymph node dissection (TLND) is the complete surgical removal of the draining nodal basin known to have histopathologically confirmed nodal metastases. Three prospective, randomized trials failed to demonstrate better survival in melanoma patients treated with ELND than in patients undergoing wide local excision (WLE) alone as primary surgical therapy.[3–5]

With ELND offering no overall survival advantage, a more accurate method to identify the approximately 20% of melanoma patients who presented with nodal metastasis was needed. In the 1970s, Roth and colleagues were attempting to identify the nodal basin at risk by injecting colloidal gold around a patient's primary melanoma site.[6] This was a very crude technique that identified only the basin at risk and not the specific node at risk. Alternative newer-generation radiopharmaceuticals and improved gamma detection devices were needed.

An alternative method of identifying the node at risk for harboring metastatic disease was first described by Wong and colleagues using a feline model.[7] They demonstrated that a vital blue dye (Lymphazurin, Hirsch Industries, Inc., Richmond, VA) injected into the dermis of the cat would travel via the dermal lymphatics to the regional nodal basin.

The following year, in human melanoma patients, Morton and colleagues demonstrated the feasibility of lymphatic mapping and SN biopsy using vital blue dye injected.[8] These investigators showed that the SN is the first node in the regional lymphatic basin into which the primary melanoma consistently drains (although not necessarily the closest to the primary lesion). They harvested the SN separately from the remainder of the regional nodes and found that the pathologic status of the SN was highly accurate at predicting the pathologic status of the entire nodal basin, which was also surgically removed in all of the patients studied. These findings suggested that melanoma patients could be accurately staged with procedures that were far less extensive than complete regional nodal dissections.

* The authors and editors gratefully acknowledge the contributions of the previous authors, Seth P. Harlow, MD, David N. Krag, MD, FACS, Douglas S. Reintgen, MD, FACS, Frederick L. Moffat Jr, MD, FACS, and Thomas G. Frazier, MD, FACS, to the development and writing of this chapter.

PREOPERATIVE EVALUATION

Selection of Patients

The risk of nodal metastases in any one individual melanoma patient depends on a number of factors, including primary tumor thickness, presence of ulceration, and mitotic rate.[9,10]

SN biopsy is most likely to alter therapy in patients who have a significant risk of nodal metastases but a low risk of systemic disease. As a result, the subgroup of patients with intermediate-thickness melanomas (1.0 to 4.0 mm) is the group most likely to benefit from SN biopsy. In patients with melanomas between 0.76 and 1.0 mm thick, the risk of nodal metastasis is approximately 5 to 6%,[11–16] and a balanced discussion should be held with the patient including other factors such as ulceration, mitotic rate greater than 1, male sex, and axial location.[17] Patients with thin melanomas and multiple risk factors may be at high enough risk to warrant SN biopsy.

On the opposite end of the spectrum are patients with thick melanomas (> 4.0 mm). For these patients, the risk of systemic metastases is as high as 50 to 60%, whereas the risk of nodal metastases ranges from 40 to 50%. ELND was not recommended for such patients in the past because of this high risk of systemic disease. However, even among patients with thick melanomas, survival is better for those with negative nodes than for those with microscopic nodal disease.[18] As a result, patients with thick melanomas and no obvious systemic metastases may benefit from SN biopsy to stage the nodal basin. This is particularly important if the presence of nodal metastases will change the adjuvant treatment plan from observation to active systemic therapy.

The available data suggest that lymphatic mapping is applicable to all primary body sites, including the head and neck (the most technically demanding sites).[19,20] The best results are achieved with a combination mapping approach that employs both a vital blue dye and a radiocolloid. The procedure is associated with slightly higher false negative rates in patients with head and neck melanoma than in those with melanoma of the trunk or extremities (10% versus 1 to 2%). Nevertheless, the false negative rates with head and neck melanoma are still low enough to justify offering lymphatic mapping to patients.

Special Circumstances

The extent of any operation done at the primary site before SN biopsy may affect the success of the biopsy procedure. In patients who have had an appropriate 1 or 2 cm margin resection and then large areas of tissue undermining or have undergone reconstruction with a rotational flap or Z-plasty to close the oncologic resection defect, the normal lymphatic channels may be disrupted. Such disruption may render SN biopsy inaccurate. Nevertheless, there have been reports of SN biopsy being performed successfully after previous WLE.[21] These patients may have more SNs in more regional nodal basins than patients in whom the primary tumor has not been resected with curative intent, but at present, there is no unequivocal evidence that previous WLE of the primary lesion increases the risk of postoperative nodal relapse.[22,23]

Increasingly, surgeons are caring for patients who have undergone previous nodal surgery. Over time, patients develop alternate lymphatic drainage pathways after nodal surgery. Although localization rates tend to be lower under these circumstances, the accuracy of the SN for predicting the status of the nodal basin remains high.[24,25] Preoperative lymphoscintigraphy is critical, even for breast cancer patients, because the altered lymphatic pathways may result in drainage to less common nodal basins. Because development of new drainage pathways takes time, accuracy is related to the amount of time that has elapsed since the first procedure. For patients in whom the previous nodal procedure was performed less than 6 months previously, the reliability of the SN is doubtful.

Breast cancer and melanoma are frequently diagnosed in women of childbearing age, so the safety of lymphatic mapping during pregnancy needs to be discussed. Sentinel lymphadenectomy generally requires general anesthesia, so the risks of surgery during pregnancy need to be considered. In addition, there are potential risks related specifically to the lymphatic mapping. Neither isosulfan blue dye nor methylene blue dye has been tested for safety during pregnancy. In the absence of data, it is recommended that these be avoided. Although radiation is teratogenic, studies suggest that the levels of radiation associated with lymphoscintigraphy are low and safe.[26–28] No adverse events have been documented in reported case series to date.[29,30]

OPERATIVE PLANNING: POSITIONING AND ANESTHESIA

Patients should be prepared to undergo wide excision of the primary melanoma site (if not previously performed) and SN biopsy during the same operative session. Depending on the location of the primary lesion, it may be possible to perform the two procedures with the patient in a single position; however, often the patient must be repositioned during the procedure to afford the surgeon adequate access to the different locations. The choice of anesthesia varies, depending on the size and location of the wide excision and the anatomic depth of the SNs. In very selected cases, local anesthesia may be appropriate, but for most lesions, general or regional anesthesia is preferable.

OPERATIVE TECHNIQUE

Although the technical details of lymphatic mapping and SN biopsy for melanoma vary from institution to institution, the reported results of the different approaches have been very similar. Proper performance of these procedures requires close collaboration between the nuclear medicine physician, the surgeon, and the pathologist, with each member playing a critical role in the process.

Step 1: Injection of Radiolabeled Tracer and Lymphoscintigraphy

On the day of the procedure, the patient reports to the nuclear medicine suite for injection of the radiolabeled tracer and preoperative lymphoscintigraphy. It is crucial to have a mechanism in place by which the location of the primary melanoma site can be reliably communicated to the nuclear radiologist. Some melanoma biopsy sites are difficult to locate, particularly if multiple skin biopsies have already been performed.

A radiolabeled agent is then selected; the most common choices are technetium-99m (^{99m}Tc)–labeled sulfur colloid (TSC) and ^{99m}Tc-labeled antimony trisulfide colloid (T-ATC). The dose of the tracer and the volume of the injectate are largely determined by the location and size of the primary tumor site but generally can be kept to 0.5 mCi or less and 1 mL or less, respectively. Injections are made intradermally around the circumference of the lesion or biopsy site, and dynamic scans are taken 5 to 10 minutes after injection. Although the location of the SN may be marked on the skin by the radiologist to assist the surgeon, this location may vary slightly with changes in patient position and should therefore be confirmed by the surgeon with the gamma probe in the operating room. To allow complete and accurate nodal staging, all regional basins at risk should be marked, along with any in-transit nodes that are identified [*see Figure 1*]. If there is no migration of TSC after approximately 60 to 90 minutes, then a second injection of filtered TSC is performed. If no migration occurs, the nuclear medicine physician communicates this directly with the operating surgeon.

The surgical procedure should be carried out no more than 6 to 8 hours after TSC injection. Activity in the SNs usually reaches its maximum 2 to 6 hours after injection; waiting longer to carry out the procedure may increase the labeling of secondary nodes. There have, however, been several reports of SN procedures being accurately performed 16 to 24 hours after tracer injection.[19] Because TSC is retained in the SN dendritic cells, the SNs can still be easily identified after 6 hours, whereas the radioactivity at the injection site and resultant background interference may be diminished because of the short half-life of technetium (6 hours).

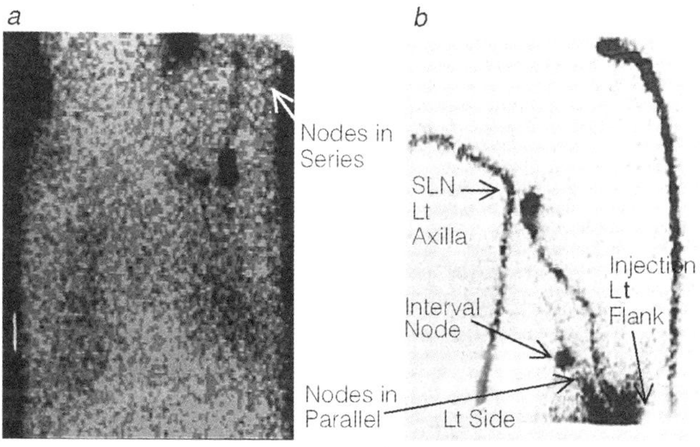

Figure 1 **Lymphatic mapping and sentinel lymph node (SLN) biopsy for melanoma. In-transit nodal areas are identified in 5% of melanoma patients; this is the reason why preoperative lymphoscintigraphy is performed for primary sites on either the upper or the lower extremity. In a patient with a melanoma on the left hand (*a*), the injection site and the left hand are raised above the head, and cutaneous lymphatic flow into an epitrochlear node can be seen. This in-transit node then emits a lymphatic vessel flowing to the left axilla. By definition, the SLN is the first node in the chain that receives primary lymphatic flow. The epitrochlear node and any axillary nodes are nodes in series. Hence, the epitrochlear node is the SLN and thus is the only node that must be harvested. In a patient with a primary melanoma on the left flank (*b*), there are two separate afferent lymphatics, one leading to an SLN in the left axilla and the other leading to an in-transit node on the left flank. These are nodes in parallel in that they both receive primary lymphatic flow from the skin site. Hence, the two nodes are equally at risk for metastatic disease, and both are considered sentinel nodes and must be harvested.**

Step 2: Intraoperative Lymphatic Mapping and Identification of SN

It is our practice to review the lymphoscintigram when the patient arrives in the preoperative holding area. For patients who had either ambiguous drainage or no drainage, we evaluate the patient with the gamma probe before deciding on positioning. Probe evaluation, whether performed in the preoperative holding area or in the operating room, begins by defining the diffusion zone around the primary tumor site, where SN identification is not possible. The area between this diffusion zone and the possible nodal drainage sites is then mapped for possible in-transit nodes by means of a systematic but expeditious evaluation for radioactive "hot spots." The gamma probe is moved in a linear fashion between the diffusion zone and the nodal basin. It is then shifted medial or lateral to the previous line, and the process is repeated until the entire area is evaluated. The location of a radioactive hot spot is confirmed by identifying a discrete location where the radioactive counts are higher than the counts found in the tissue 1 to 2 cm more proximal to the injection site (the background skin count). The counts from the hot spot and the background are recorded. The hot-spot site is marked on the skin to allow more direct dissection to the SN.

Concomitant use of a vital blue dye is favored by many surgeons and is our preferred method. The blue dye is complementary to the radiolabeled tracer; the combination of the two marking agents improves the chances of identifying the SN and facilitates node retrieval. The blue dye is injected into the dermis immediately adjacent to the melanoma. For lesions on an extremity, the dye may be injected along the proximal margin of the lesion or biopsy site; for lesions on other areas, it should be injected circumferentially. The general recommendation is to wait 5 to 10 minutes after injecting the dye before initiating SN retrieval.

To minimize the dissection required for node resection, the incision for the SN biopsy should be made through the hot spot identified by the gamma probe. The incision should also be situated so that it can be incorporated into a longer incision should the finding of a positive SN necessitate performance of a TLND. The gamma probe is placed in a sterile sheath and used again after the incision is made to guide further dissection. If blue dye was used, the surgeon can visually follow the blue lymphatic channels to the blue-stained SN.

An SN is defined as either (1) all radioactive nodes with an ex vivo node to background ratio greater than 10:1, (2) a node that either is blue or clearly has a blue-stained lymphatic vessel entering it, or (3) a firm palpable node. When an SN is removed, the ex vivo radioactivity count in the node is recorded. This count is then used as a reference for determining which, if any, of the remaining nodes in that basin (some of which may be potential SNs) should be removed. In our view, if the radioactivity count in the hottest remaining node in the basin is less than 10% of the ex vivo count in the hottest SN, none of the remaining nodes should be considered SNs.[19,31] Any nodes with radioactivity counts exceeding this 10% threshold, however, should be removed.

Once an SN is identified, it should be dissected out with as little trauma to the surrounding tissues as possible. Lymphatic channels to the node should be identified and either tied or clipped to reduce the risk of postoperative seroma formation. Because the gamma probe can localize SNs with great accuracy, routine dissection of motor nerves is not required; however, knowledge of the likely location of the motor nerves is critical for preventing inadvertent injury to these structures during dissection.

After SN removal, a final count of the SN biopsy bed is taken to document that all significantly radiolabeled nodes have been accounted for and removed. In addition, the tissues are examined for blue-stained lymphatic channels or lymph nodes regardless of radioactivity. (As noted, blue staining confers SN status even if the node is not radioactive.)

Firm tumor-involved nodes with obstructed afferent lymphatics may divert lymph flow to non-SNs, and such diversion is a significant cause of false negative SN biopsy results. Consequently, the final step is to palpate for grossly suspicious nodes. If grossly suspicious nodes are identified after all relevant SNs have been removed, the suspicious nodes should also be removed.

Step 3: Pathologic Evaluation of SN

The optimal extent of pathologic evaluation of SNs in patients with melanoma has been the subject of some debate. SN biopsy allows pathologists to focus their efforts on one node or a small number of nodes, and this focus has led to a process of ultrastaging. Several good methodology articles describing the handling and processing of SN are available in the literature.[32,33] Our current institutional protocol has been published.[34] Briefly, the SN is bivalved and then serially sectioned at 1 to 2 mm section across both halves. The nodal sections are first evaluated with hematoxylin-eosin (H&E) stain. If no obvious metastases are identified, the immunohistochemical stains are applied, S-100 and MART-1. This enables the pathologist to identify tiny (less than 1 mm) deposits of metastatic melanoma.

COMPLICATIONS

Complications of SN biopsy are quite uncommon. Allergic reactions to the blue dyes occur in less than 1% of patients but can range in severity from mild urticaria to anaphylaxis; thus, the surgical team and the anesthesia team should always be prepared for this uncommon but potentially serious problem.[35,36] In experienced hands, motor nerve injury is rare. In a series of 47 patients who had head and neck melanomas with SN drainage to the parotid region, there were no permanent injuries to the facial nerve when the SN was removed without formal nerve dissection.[37] Similar results have been reported for nodes in the posterior triangle of the neck and in the axilla. The incidence of wound complications is quite low (1.7% wound complication rate; 3.0% seroma rate), as is the incidence of postbiopsy lymphedema (0.7%). In the Sunbelt Melanoma Trial, the complication rate in 2,120 patients undergoing SN biopsy was 4.6%, compared with 23.2% in 444 patients undergoing completion lymph node dissection (CLND).[38]

OUTCOME EVALUATION

Ideally, level I evidence from a prospective, randomized, controlled trial would demonstrate that lymphatic mapping and SN biopsy are superior to close nodal observation as the treatment of choice for melanoma patients. The Multicenter Selective Lymphadenectomy Trial (MSLT-1; Donald Morton, principal investigator) was designed to compare WLE and SN biopsy to WLE and close observation in patients with intermediate-thickness melanomas. A detailed description of the trial has been published.[39] Briefly, all patients with intermediate-thickness melanomas eligible for the trial (Breslow thickness 1.2 to 3.5 mm) were randomized in a 60:40 ratio to WLE and SN biopsy or to WLE and watchful waiting. All patients with a tumor-involved SN went on to an immediate TLND. For patients in the watchful waiting arm, a delayed TLND was performed if clinically apparent, pathologically confirmed nodal disease was identified.

After the third interim analysis, the Data Safety Monitoring Board insisted that the data be released to the public because several secondary end points had been met. Most importantly, melanoma-specific survival in patients with nodal disease was improved for patients in the SN biopsy arm compared with watchful waiting. Patients with a tumor-involved SN who underwent immediate LND had a 5-year survival advantage compared with those in the watchful waiting arm who developed a nodal basin metastasis: 72.3% versus 52.4% (hazard ratio 0.51, 95% confidence interval 0.32 to 0.81, $p = .004$).[39] These results continue to hold up after the fourth interim analysis with 10-year survival advantage of 63.2% versus 36.5% ($p < .001$).[40]

To date, the primary end point, improved overall survival, has not been met. Although this has led some critics to advocate abandoning SN biopsy in melanoma patients,[41] several clarifications need to be emphasized. First, no lymph node–negative patient ever derives a survival benefit from undergoing nodal operation, whether ELND or SN biopsy. Given that the incidence of nodal metastases in patients with intermediate-thickness melanoma, as defined by the MSLT-1, would be expected to be around 20%, 80% of patients enrolled on the trial could not possibly derive a survival advantage. These patients who cannot benefit dilute the observed magnitude of effect for those who do benefit. Second, SN biopsy is not proposed as a therapeutic procedure but rather as a highly sophisticated staging procedure. On MSLT-1, the patients with a tumor-involved SN subsequently underwent a directed TLND. The results of MSLT-1 demonstrate a clear survival advantage in performing the TLND early in an association with a tumor-involved SN as opposed to later, when palpable lymphadenopathy is detected.

Lymphatic Mapping and SN Biopsy in Breast Cancer

RATIONALE: ASSESSMENT OF NODAL STATUS

In early breast cancer, as in melanoma, the pathologic status of the regional lymph nodes is the most important predictor of outcome. The presence of regional lymph node metastases in breast cancer reduces 5-year survival by 28 to 40%.[42,43] Prognostic factors related to primary tumor characteristics have consistently been shown to be inferior to nodal status as predictors of overall survival. In addition, axillary lymph node dissection in the setting of breast cancer is superior to observation and at least equivalent to irradiation for regional disease control in clinically node-negative patients.[44] There is some evidence that adequate regional disease control may confer a small survival benefit.[45]

Invasive breast cancer has a relatively high rate of nodal metastasis in clinically node-negative patients. The risk of metastasis is clearly related to the size of the primary tumor, but it is significant (15% or higher) even in patients with early (T1a) lesions.[46,47] The primary nodal drainage basin for the breast is the ipsilateral axilla; however, drainage to extra-axillary sites (e.g., the internal mammary lymph node chain, the supraclavicular nodes, and the intramammary nodes) is also reported. Other potential sites of lymphatic drainage notwithstanding, the recommended surgical procedure for evaluating the regional lymph nodes in clinically node-negative breast cancer patients has been level I and II axillary lymph node dissection (ALND). Such dissections are, however, associated with a significant risk of long-term morbidity, primarily related to the risk of lymphedema in the affected arm. For this reason, SN biopsy was developed and investigated as a possible substitute for standard ALND in the treatment of breast cancer patients with clinically uninvolved axillary lymph nodes.

PREOPERATIVE EVALUATION

Selection of Patients

All clinically node-negative patients with a diagnosis of invasive breast cancer are potential candidates for SN biopsy. Ideal candidates are those patients with unifocal lesions less than 5 cm in greatest dimension who have no history of previous axillary surgery or previous cancer treatment. Performing an SN biopsy after a previous excisional biopsy is technically feasible. Patients who have undergone extensive previous breast procedures (e.g., breast reduction, placement of breast implants, or multiple open biopsies) may have significant alterations in the lymphatic pathways; however, accurate identification of the SN can still be accomplished with proper planning of the injection sites. Patients with multifocal tumors or multicentric breast cancers also require thoughtful planning of the injection sites, although there is some evidence suggesting that using periareolar injection sites may allow the procedure to be performed accurately in patients with multifocal disease.[48] For patients who will be undergoing mastectomy with immediate breast reconstruction, performing SN biopsy as an outpatient procedure prior to the planned mastectomy may facilitate surgical planning depending on the need for postmastectomy radiation or ALND.[49] However, the false negative rate of SN biopsy may be higher in cases with large additive tumor burden.[50]

For patients who present with inflammatory breast carcinoma or who present with palpable adenopathy and pathologically confirmed metastatic nodal disease, there is absolutely no role for SN biopsy at the time of presentation. The role of SN biopsy in patients who present with large breast cancers and are scheduled to receive neoadjuvant chemotherapy is highly controversial. Several recent studies have shown a low false negative rate for patients with T3 tumors who have an SN procedure prior to neoadjuvant chemotherapy,[51–55] as well as those authors advocating the procedure after the neoadjuvant chemotherapy.[56–58] Several good reviews of the controversy are published.[59–61] The remainder of this chapter deals with patients who present with unifocal, T1 or T2, clinically node-negative breast cancer.

OPERATIVE PLANNING: POSITIONING AND ANESTHESIA

Patients should be placed in the supine position, with all potential nodal sites within the operative field. Although SN biopsy may be performed with the patient under local anesthesia, we favor general anesthesia for this procedure, particularly when it is done in conjunction with the breast excision.

OPERATIVE TECHNIQUE

Step 1: Injection of Radiolabeled Tracer and Lymphoscintigraphy

In the United States, the radiocolloid most commonly employed for SN biopsy in breast cancer patients is TSC, which may be used either unfiltered or filtered (< 220 nm) The ^{99m}Tc dose generally ranges from 0.45 to 1.0 mCi, and the injectate volume ranges from 4 to 8 mL. Several routes of tracer injection have been investigated for SN biopsy in breast cancer patients, primarily in response to the difficulties sometimes associated with peritumoral injection (e.g., delayed tracer uptake and wide diffusion zones that can overlap the nodal basins). These routes include intradermal or subdermal injection in the area overlying the tumor, subareolar injection, and periareolar injection. The rationale for the development of these alternatives is that there is significant overlap between the lymphatic vessels of the breast skin and those of the breast parenchyma. Multiple studies have confirmed that the use of these injection routes yields high localization rates and results in accurate removal of SNs that reflect the pathologic nodal status of individual patients. A notable deficiency of these techniques, however, has been the low reported rate of tracer migration to nodes outside the axilla, particularly to the internal mammary lymph node chain. This result is thought to be attributable to a unique set of lymphatic channels deep in the breast parenchyma, separate from the overlying skin, that drain to the internal mammary chain.

The various tracer injection methods have not been directly compared; thus, at present, the optimal route of injection can be inferred only by comparing studies from different institutions. The potential importance of the extra-axillary sites is not entirely clear, but it appears that these sites may be the sole locations of metastatic disease in as many as 20% of the node-positive patients from whom they are removed.[62,63] Most patients in whom SNs are found outside the axilla have additional SNs in the axillary basin.

A thorough literature review on the use of different routes of injection and the associated rates of SN localization by nodal basin, node positivity rates, and false negative rates has been performed. This review included those studies in which a radiolabeled tracer was used for SN identification (either by lymphoscintigraphy or by intraoperative gamma probe localization) and in which the location of the SN basins and the pathologic status of the SNs could be ascertained. The results of previous reviews of almost 9,000 patients indicated that all of the approaches have acceptable SN retrieval rates but that the rates are slightly higher with the more superficial ones (i.e., the dermal, subareolar, and periareolar techniques).[62,64–67] There are, however, significant differences in the locations of the SN basins identified with the different methods: with the superficial injection techniques, drainage is essentially confined to the axillary basin, whereas with the deeper injection techniques, as many as 22% of patients are found to have nodal basins outside the axilla. Approximately 16 to 21% of the extra-axillary SNs will be found to have metastatic disease if removed. The clinical ramifications of these findings are that some patients may be understaged if the extra-axillary sites are not evaluated, and such understaging may affect the recommendations for systemic adjuvant therapy.

Whether the breast cancer is palpable or nonpalpable, we prefer that the injection is guided by ultrasonographic evidence. If an excisional biopsy was previously performed, the tracer should be injected into the breast parenchyma rather than into the biopsy cavity; it will not diffuse out of the cavity. This is also best done under ultrasonographic guidance. In addition, injections should not be made into the retromammary fat or the pectoral fascia, because doing so would lead to wide diffusion of tracer throughout the chest area, which would make nodal identification very difficult.

In breast cancer patients, the timing of SN biopsy after tracer injection is not of critical importance. Good results have been obtained with injection-to-biopsy intervals ranging from 30 minutes to 24 hours. The usual recommendation is to wait 1 to 2 hours.

Step 2: Intraoperative Lymphatic Mapping and Removal of SN

Once the patient is asleep, the vital blue dye (Lymphazurin) is injected either peritumorally, into the parenchyma surrounding an excisional biopsy, intradermally, or subareolarly depending on surgeon preference. The breast is gently massaged for 5 to 10 minutes to enhance transport of the dye to the SNs. Our approach begins by performing a primary survey of the potential nodal sites with the handheld gamma detector. Using one of the commercially available handheld gamma probes, an axillary hot spot is identified, and then a small incision is made. The gamma probe, sterile sheathed, is inserted into the wound and guides the dissection to the radioactive node(s). During the dissection, the surgeon looks for blue-stained lymphatic channels and nodes [*see Figure 2*]. Most of the time, the radiocolloid and the vital blue dye identify the same SNs. The SNs are then carefully removed, and the lymphatic vessels entering them are tied or clipped off whenever possible.

An SN is defined as either (1) all radioactive nodes with an ex vivo node to background ratio greater than 10:1, (2) a node that either is stained blue or clearly has a blue-stained lymphatic vessel entering it, or (3) a firm palpable node. When an SN is removed, the ex vivo radioactivity count in the node is recorded. This count is then used as a reference for determining which, if any, of the remaining nodes in that basin (some of which may be potential SNs) should be removed. In our view, if the radioactivity count in the hottest remaining node in the basin is less than 10% of the ex vivo count in the hottest SN, none of the remaining nodes should be considered SNs, and none should be removed.[67] Any nodes whose radioactivity counts exceed this 10% threshold, however, should be removed.

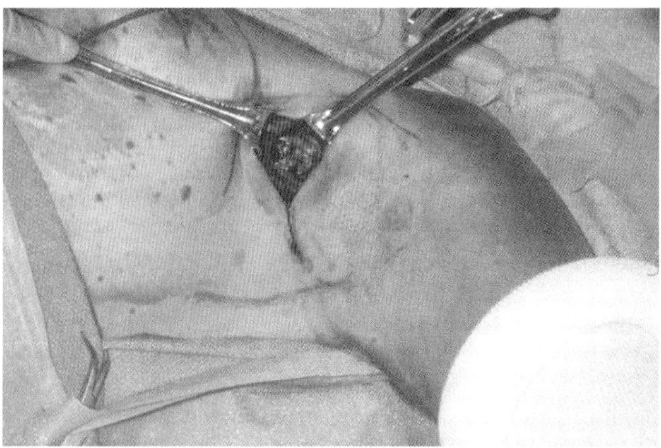

Figure 2 **Lymphatic mapping and sentinel node (SN) biopsy for breast cancer. A small incision is made in the axilla on the basis of the hot-spot location. The SNs identified are both radioactive and stained blue.**

A final count of the SN biopsy bed is then taken to document that all significantly radiolabeled SNs have been accounted for and removed. In addition, the tissues are examined for blue-stained lymphatic channels or lymph nodes regardless of radioactivity; as noted, blue staining confers SN status even if the node is not radioactive. Finally, when it appears that all relevant SNs have been removed, as confirmed by the final bed count, the tissues are palpated for grossly suspicious nodes. Firm tumor-involved nodes with obstructed afferent lymphatics may divert lymph flow to non-SNs, and such diversion is a significant cause of false negative SN biopsy results.

Once an SN is identified, it should be dissected out with as little trauma to the surrounding tissues as possible. Lymphatic channels to the node should be identified and either tied or clipped to reduce the risk of postoperative seroma formation. Because the gamma probe can localize SNs with great accuracy, routine dissection of motor nerves is not required; however, knowledge of the likely location of the motor nerves is critical for preventing inadvertent injury to these structures during dissection.

Step 3: Pathologic Evaluation of SN

Pathologic SN evaluation in breast cancer patients has two main aspects. The first is intraoperative evaluation of the SN when the pathologic status of the node is being used to determine the need for ALND; the second is permanent evaluation of the nodes to determine whether micrometastatic disease is present. Both have conflicting views in the literature.

Two techniques are commonly employed for intraoperative evaluation of SNs: frozen-section analysis and touch-imprint cytology. Frozen-section histopathology is available in most hospitals, and all surgical pathologists have some experience with it. This technique has a drawback, however, in that it sometimes uses up a large portion of the SN, leaving a remnant that is insufficient for permanent paraffin-embedded sections. In addition, the sectioning of radioactive nodes on a cryostat raises radiation safety issues for the pathologists.

Studies of frozen-section techniques of evaluating SNs for metastatic breast cancer report false negative rates of 27 and 32%.[64,68] When 60 frozen sections are made from each SN, the false negative rate can be reduced to about 5%,[64,69] but at the cost of 45 to 60 minutes of operating time and loss of tissues for permanent histopathologic evaluation. Frozen section is far more effective in detecting macrometastatic disease (sensitivity 92%) than micrometastatic disease (sensitivity 17%), and the volume of nodal metastases is highly correlated with tumor size.[70] In comparison, touch-imprint cytology consumes much less time and tissue, is far more accurate (false negative rate 0.8%),[71] and does not contaminate the cryostat. It has also been applied to the evaluation of lumpectomy margins [*see Figure 3*]. The chief limitation of the touch-imprint method is that for optimal results, it requires a pathologist who is highly skilled in the cytologic evaluation of lymph nodes. Some centers use rapid immunohistochemical (IHC) analysis for cytokeratin staining to detect tumor cells in touch-imprint or frozen-section specimens, anticipating that detection of such cells can thereby be improved, particularly in patients with invasive lobular or well-differentiated ductal carcinomas.

The optimal extent of pathologic evaluation of SNs in patients with breast cancer has been the subject of some debate. SN biopsy allows pathologists to focus their efforts on one node or a small number of nodes, and this focus has led to a process of ultrastaging. Several good methodology articles describing the handling and processing of SN are available in the literature.[32,33] Our current institutional protocol has been published previously.[34] Briefly, the SN is bivalved

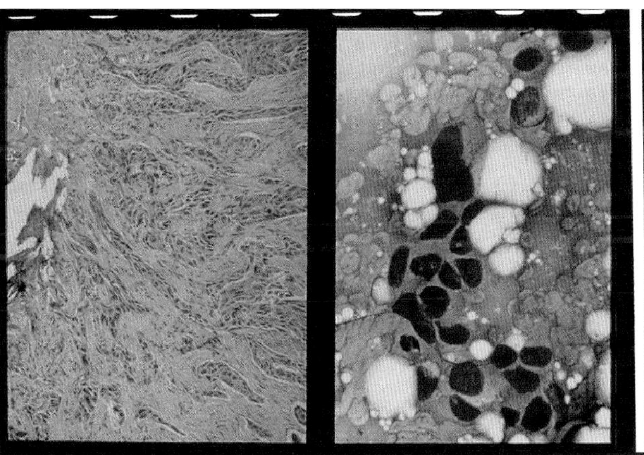

Figure 3 **Lymphatic mapping and sentinel node biopsy for breast cancer. In touch-imprint cytology, slides are touched to tissue from a "hot" specimen, and cells on the section or the margin are exfoliated onto the slide for cytologic preparation. Shown are (*a*) permanent histology of an infiltrating ductal carcinoma extending down to an inked margin and (*b*) a touch preparation demonstrating bizarre malignant cells from the sampling of the margin. The advantages of this technique are that the entire margin can be sampled and that tissue is not lost in the cryostat.**

and then serially sectioned at 1 to 2 mm section across both halves. The nodal sections are first evaluated with H&E stain. In 1999, the College of American Pathologists issued a consensus statement recommending that the staging of SNs be based on routine histologic evaluation of the nodes cut at approximately 2 mm intervals.[72] Routine use of cytokeratin IHC staining should not be adopted as standard until its significance is demonstrated in clinical trials.

COMPLICATIONS

The complications of SN biopsy in breast cancer patients are similar to those seen in melanoma patients.[73] There is a minor (< 1%) risk of allergic reactions to the blue dye.[74] There is a small risk of sensory or motor nerve injury or lymphedema whenever an axillary node procedure is performed; this risk is substantially reduced, although not entirely eliminated, with SN biopsy.[75] With an internal mammary SN biopsy, there is a risk of pneumothorax from unintended opening of the parietal pleura. This risk is very small with careful technique, however, and the problem can almost always be corrected by closing the wound around a rubber catheter inserted through a small stab incision and removing it at the end of a positive pressure breath given by the anesthesiologist. Surgical site infections occur in fewer than 1% of cases, and small seromas occur in about 10%.

OUTCOME EVALUATION

The first report of SN biopsy in breast cancer, published in 1993, described the use of the gamma probe localization technique for SN identification.[76] A second report, published the following year, described the use of the vital blue dye technique for SN identification.[77] Since these initial feasibility reports, many single-center and multicenter studies have been published that achieved remarkably similar results using either or both of these techniques.

The early studies of SN biopsy tended to use either a radiolabeled tracer or a vital blue dye alone. The first trial in which the two agents were used together was published in 1996.[65] This study documented an improvement in SN localization and a 0% false negative rate, albeit in a small series of patients. Subsequent multicenter trials incorporating larger study groups yielded more reliable indications of the applicability of these techniques to the overall surgical community. In one such study, surgeons from 11 centers performed SN biopsies and confirmatory axillary dissection in clinically node-negative patients with invasive breast cancer.[66] The overall success rate for identifying and removing an SN was 93%, the pathologic accuracy rate for predicting the presence of nodal metastases from the SNs removed was 97%, and the pathologic false negative rate was 11.4%. A subsequent multicenter trial, using a combination of blue dye staining and the gamma probe technique in most patients, reported an SN retrieval rate of 88% and a pathologic false negative rate of 7.2%.[67] A third trial, using the gamma probe technique, reported an SN retrieval rate of 87% and a pathologic false negative rate of 13%.[78] A fourth trial, using both blue dye staining and the gamma probe technique, reported an SN retrieval rate of 86% and a pathologic false negative rate of 4%.[79]

To evaluate the true efficacy of a new technology, a prospective trial needs to be performed, and the first one completed was by Veronesi and colleagues.[80] In this trial, 516 evaluable patients were randomly assigned to undergo either SN biopsy with confirmatory axillary dissection (257 patients) or SN biopsy with axillary dissection done only if the biopsy yielded positive results (259 patients). At a median follow-up point of 46 months, no significant survival differences were reported, and there were no regional nodal recurrences in either arm. Admittedly, the study size was small and the follow-up relatively short, but still there was no significance in axillary failure in patients who received only an SN biopsy.

The National Surgical Adjuvant Breast and Bowel Project (NSABP) undertook a trial very similar to that of the Milan group, NSABP B-32. Breast cancer patients with clinically node-negative axillae were randomized to undergo SN biopsy with mandatory ALND or SN biopsy with ALND if the SN revealed metastatic breast cancer.[81] Between 1999 and 2004, 5,611 patients were accrued and randomized. The technical details have been published[81]; previously, the SN identification on the trial was 97% and the false-negative rate was 9.7%, very consistent with some of the early breast SN reports. At the 2010 meeting of the American Society of Clinical Oncology (ASCO 2010), Krag and colleagues stated for the first time that there was no difference in overall survival, disease-free survival, or locoregional recurrences, thus providing level I evidence that the SN biopsy is an accurate and safe alternative to routine ALND in clinically node-negative breast cancer patients.[82]

The American College of Surgeons Oncology Group (ACOSOG) undertook an SN trial designed to evaluate the incidence and prognostic significance of SN and bone marrow micrometastases in patients with early-stage breast cancer. ACOSOG Z0010 was a phase II trial in which all patients enrolled underwent a SN biopsy and bilateral iliac crest bone marrow aspirates. If the SNs were negative by H&E stain, then they were submitted to the central laboratory for IHC stains. From April 1999 through May 2003, 5,539 patients were enrolled. At ASCO 2010, Cote and colleagues presented for the first time the unblinded SN IHC results.[83] There was no difference in overall survival in patients with IHC-detected metastases compared with tumor-free SN (95.1% versus 95.8%, p = .53). Thus, the routine examination of SN with IHC in patients with invasive ductal carcinoma should not be performed.

The advent of the SN has reopened the debate regarding the impact of ALND on overall survival. One of the earliest NSABP studies, B-04, randomized patients to either radical mastectomy, total mastectomy with delayed ALND if necessary, or total mastectomy and radiotherapy.[44] There was no overall survival difference between the three arms of the trial, but the trial was not powered to detect a small survival advantage. Patients receiving an ALND appeared to have improved the locoregional recurrence rate.

The question in the SN era remains: in patients with H&E-detected metastases, what, if anything, should be done to the remainder of the axillary nodes? Two prospective, randomized trials were designed to answer this very important question. The first is the European Organisation for Research and Treatment of Cancer (EORTC) AMAROS (after mapping of the axilla: radiotherapy or surgery) trial in which patients with an H&E-detected SN metastasis were randomized to axillary radiation versus a completion ALND. The trial finished accrual in 2008 but, because of a lower than expected event rate, had to reopen to accrual. The other important trial is ACOSOG Z0011, in which patients with H&E-detected metastases were randomized to completion ALND or observation. At ASCO 2010, Giuliano and colleagues, for the first time, stated that there was no difference in overall survival between the two groups (completion ALND 91.9% versus observation 92.5%) or disease-free survival (82.2% versus 83.8%, p = .13).[84] Thus, in a large phase III trial, albeit underpowered, there is not even a trend toward a survival advantage in patients receiving ALND. Routine ALND following a positive SN adds nothing to the patient's overall survival.

Radiation Exposure Guidelines and Policies

The amount and type of radioactivity injected in the course of lymphatic mapping and SN biopsy are relatively limited. Typically, from 0.1 to 1.0 mCi of ^{99m}Tc is injected. This agent is a pure gamma emitter with a short half life (6 hours); thus, the risks of potentially harmful beta radiation are avoided. The total radiation dose used is quite small—only about 5% of that used in common nuclear scanning techniques (e.g., bone scans). It has been estimated that a maximum of 0.45 Gy could be absorbed at the injection site. Of hospital workers, the surgeon is exposed to the highest levels of radiation. A study from Walter Reed Army Medical Center found that the hands of surgeons performing lymphatic mapping and SN biopsy were exposed to an average of 9.4 ± 3.6 mrem per operation.[85] Therefore, on the basis of skin dosage recommendations set by the Nuclear Regulatory Commission, a surgeon would have to perform more than 5,000 SN procedures a year to incur more than the minimal level of risk.

The low risk notwithstanding, proper handling of radioactive specimens is recommended. All such specimens should be handled as little as possible for at least 24 to 48 hours and should be appropriately labeled. Physicians performing these procedures should develop guidelines for handling and processing specimens in accordance with their institution's radiation safety policies.

Financial Disclosures: None Reported

References

1. National Cancer Institute. Available at: www.cancer.gov.
2. Balch CM, Gershenwald JE, Soong SJ, et al. Multivariate analysis of prognostic factors among 2,313 patients with stage III melanoma: comparison of nodal micrometastases versus macrometastases. J Clin Oncol 2010; 28:2452–9. Epub 2010 Apr 5.
3. Veronesi U, Adamus J, Bandiera DC, et al. Inefficacy of immediate node dissection in stage 1 melanoma of the limbs. N Engl J Med 1977;297:627–30.
4. Sim FH, Taylor WF, Pritchard DJ, Soule EH. Lymphadenectomy in the management of stage I malignant melanoma: a prospective randomized study. Mayo Clin Proc 1986;61: 697–705.
5. Balch CM, Soong SJ, Bartolucci AA, et al. Efficacy of an elective regional lymph node dissection of 1 to 4 mm thick melanomas for patients 60 years of age and younger. Ann Surg 1996;224:255–63; discussion 263–256.
6. Roth JA, Eilber FR, Bennett LR, Morton DL. Radionuclide photoscanning. Usefulness in preoperative evaluation of melanoma patients. Arch Surg 1975;110:1211–2.
7. Wong JH, Cagle LA, Morton DL. Lymphatic drainage of skin to a sentinel lymph node in a feline model. Ann Surg 1991;214:637–41.

8. Morton DL, Wen DR, Wong JH, et al. Technical details of intraoperative lymphatic mapping for early stage melanoma. Arch Surg 1992;127:392–9.
9. AJCC cancer staging manual. 5th ed. New York: Springer; 2010.
10. Balch CM, Gershenwald JE, Soong SJ, et al. Final version of 2009 AJCC melanoma staging and classification. J Clin Oncol 2009;27:6199–206.
11. Stitzenberg KB, Groben PA, Stern SL, et al. Indications for lymphatic mapping and sentinel lymphadenectomy in patients with thin melanoma (Breslow thickness < or =1.0 mm). Ann Surg Oncol 2004;11:900–6.
12. Ranieri JM, Wagner JD, Wenck S, et al. The prognostic importance of sentinel lymph node biopsy in thin melanoma. Ann Surg Oncol 2006;13:927–32.
13. Bleicher RJ, Essner R, Foshag LJ, et al. Role of sentinel lymphadenectomy in thin invasive cutaneous melanomas. J Clin Oncol 2003;21:1326–31.
14. Bedrosian I, Faries MB, Guerry DT, et al. Incidence of sentinel node metastasis in patients with thin primary melanoma (< or = 1 mm) with vertical growth phase. Ann Surg Oncol 2000;7:262–7.
15. Olah J, Gyulai R, Korom I, et al. Tumour regression predicts higher risk of sentinel node involvement in thin cutaneous melanomas. Br J Dermatol 2003;149:662–3.
16. Wong SL, Brady MS, Busam KJ, Coit DG. Results of sentinel lymph node biopsy in patients with thin melanoma. Ann Surg Oncol 2006;13:302–9.
17. Slingluff CL Jr, Vollmer RT, Reintgen DS, Seigler HF. Lethal "thin" malignant melanoma. Identifying patients at risk. Ann Surg 1988;208:150–61.
18. Heaton KM, Sussman JJ, Gershenwald JE, et al. Surgical margins and prognostic factors in patients with thick (>4mm) primary melanoma. Ann Surg Oncol 1998;5:322–8.
19. Byrd D, Nason K, Eary J, et al. Utility of sentinel lymph node dissection in patients with head and neck melanoma [abstract]. Presented at the 54th Annual Cancer Symposium, Society of Surgical Oncology; 2001 Mar 15–18; Washington, DC.
20. Medina-Franco H, Beenken S, Heslin M, et al. Sentinel lymph node biopsy for cutaneous melanoma of the head and neck [abstract]. Presented at the 54th Annual Cancer Symposium of the Society of Surgical Oncology; 2001 Mar 15-18; Washington, DC.
21. Evans HL, Krag DN, Teates CD, et al. Lymphoscintigraphy and sentinel node biopsy accurately stage melanoma in patients presenting after wide local excision. Ann Surg Oncol 2003;10:416–25.
22. Kelemen PR, Essner R, Foshag LJ, Morton DL. Lymphatic mapping and sentinel lymphadenectomy after wide local excision of primary melanoma. J Am Coll Surg 1999;189:247–52.
23. Leong SP, Thelmo MC, Kim RP, et al. Delayed harvesting of sentinel lymph nodes after previous wide local excision of extremity melanoma. Ann Surg Oncol 2003;10:196–200.
24. Cox CE, Furman BT, Kiluk JV, et al. Use of reoperative sentinel lymph node biopsy in breast cancer patients. J Am Coll Surg 2008;207:57–61.
25. Intra M, Trifiro G, Viale G, et al. Second biopsy of axillary sentinel lymph node for reappearing breast cancer after previous sentinel lymph node biopsy. Ann Surg Oncol 2005;12:895–9.
26. Spanheimer PM, Graham MM, Sugg SL, et al. Measurement of uterine radiation exposure from lymphoscintigraphy indicates safety of sentinel lymph node biopsy during pregnancy. Ann Surg Oncol 2009;16:1143–7.
27. Pandit-Taskar N, Dauer LT, Montgomery L, et al. Organ and fetal absorbed dose estimates from 99mTc-sulfur colloid lymphoscintigraphy and sentinel node localization in breast cancer patients. J Nucl Med 2006;47:1202–8.
28. Gentilini O, Cremonesi M, Trifiro G, et al. Safety of sentinel node biopsy in pregnant patients with breast cancer. Ann Oncol 2004;15:1348–51.
29. Khera SY, Kiluk JV, Hasson DM, et al. Pregnancy-associated breast cancer patients can safely undergo lymphatic mapping. Breast J 2008;14:250–4.
30. Mondi MM, Cuenca RE, Ollila DW, et al. Sentinel lymph node biopsy during pregnancy: initial clinical experience. Ann Surg Oncol 2007;14:218–21.
31. Krag DN, Meijer SJ, Weaver DL, et al. Minimal-access surgery for staging of malignant melanoma. Arch Surg 1995;130:654–8; discussion 659–60.
32. Cochran AJ, Starz H, Ohsie SJ, et al. Pathologic reporting and special diagnostic techniques for melanoma. Surg Oncol Clin N Am 2006;15:231–51.
33. Starz H, Siedlecki K, Balda BR. Sentinel lymphonodectomy and s-classification: a successful strategy for better prediction and improvement of outcome of melanoma. Ann Surg Oncol 2004;11(3 Suppl):162S–8S.
34. Stitzenberg KB, Calvo BF, Iacocca MV, et al. Cytokeratin immunohistochemical validation of the sentinel node hypothesis in patients with breast cancer. Am J Clin Pathol 2002;117:729–37.
35. Leong SP, Donegan E, Heffernon W, et al. Adverse reactions to isosulfan blue during selective sentinel lymph node dissection in melanoma. Ann Surg Oncol 2000;7:361–6.
36. Sadiq TS, Burns WW 3rd, Taber DJ, et al. Blue urticaria: a previously unreported adverse event associated with isosulfan blue. Arch Surg 2001;136:1433–5.
37. Ollila DW, Foshag LJ, Essner R, et al. Parotid region lymphatic mapping and sentinel lymphadenectomy for cutaneous melanoma. Ann Surg Oncol 1999;6:150–4.
38. Wrightson WR, Wong SL, Edwards MJ, et al. Complications associated with sentinel lymph node biopsy for melanoma. Ann Surg Oncol 2003;10:676–80.
39. Morton DL, Thompson JF, Cochran AJ, et al. Sentinel-node biopsy or nodal observation in melanoma. N Engl J Med 2006;355:1307–17.
40. Morton DL. MSLT-1: Results of fourth interim analysis. Presented at Sentinel Node Congress; 2008 Feb 19; Sydney, Australia.
41. Rosenberg SA. Why perform sentinel-lymph-node biopsy in patients with melanoma? Nat Clin Pract Oncol 2008;5(1):1.
42. Haagensen CD. Treatment of curable carcinoma of the breast. Int J Radiat Oncol Biol Phys 1977;2:975–80.
43. Bonadonna G. Karnofsky Memorial Lecture. Conceptual and practical advances in the management of breast cancer. J Clin Oncol 1989;7:1380–97.
44. Fisher B, Redmond C, Fisher ER, et al. Ten-year results of a randomized clinical trial comparing radical mastectomy and total mastectomy with or without radiation. N Engl J Med 1985;312:674–81.
45. Orr RK. The impact of prophylactic axillary node dissection on breast cancer survival—a Bayesian meta-analysis. Ann Surg Oncol 1999;6:109–16.
46. Baker LH. Breast Cancer Detection Demonstration Project: five-year summary report. CA Cancer J Clin 1982;32:194–225.
47. Dewar JA, Sarrazin D, Benhamou E, et al. Management of the axilla in conservatively treated breast cancer: 592 patients treated at Institut Gustave-Roussy. Int J Radiat Oncol Biol Phys 1987;13:475–81.
48. Mertz L, Mathelin C, Marin C, et al. [Subareolar injection of 99m-Tc sulfur colloid for sentinel nodes identification in multifocal invasive breast cancer]. Bull Cancer 1999;86:939–45.
49. Klauber-Demore N, Calvo BF, Hultman CS, et al. Staged sentinel lymph node biopsy before mastectomy facilitates surgical planning for breast cancer patients. Am J Surg 2005;190:595–7.
50. Fearmonti RM, Batista LI, Meric-Bernstam F, et al. False negative rate of sentinel lymph node biopsy in multicentric and multifocal breast cancers may be higher in cases with large additive tumor burden. Breast J 2009;15:645–8.
51. Ollila DW, Neuman HB, Sartor C, et al. Lymphatic mapping and sentinel lymphadenectomy prior to neoadjuvant chemotherapy in patients with large breast cancers. Am J Surg 2005;190:371–5.
52. Wong SL, Chao C, Edwards MJ, et al. Accuracy of sentinel lymph node biopsy for patients with T2 and T3 breast cancers. Am Surg 2001;67:522–6; discussion 527–8.
53. Sabel MS, Schott AF, Kleer CG, et al. Sentinel node biopsy prior to neoadjuvant chemotherapy. Am J Surg 2003;186:102–5.
54. Schrenk P, Hochreiner G, Fridrik M, Wayand W. Sentinel node biopsy performed before preoperative chemotherapy for axillary lymph node staging in breast cancer. Breast J 2003;9:282–7.
55. Straver ME, Rutgers EJ, Oldenburg HS, et al. Accurate axillary lymph node dissection is feasible after neoadjuvant chemotherapy. Am J Surg 2009;198:46–50.
56. Hunt KK, Yi M, Mittendorf EA, et al. Sentinel lymph node surgery after neoadjuvant chemotherapy is accurate and reduces the need for axillary dissection in breast cancer patients. Ann Surg 2009 Aug 27. [Epub ahead of print]
57. Tausch C, Konstantiniuk P, Kugler F, et al. Sentinel lymph node biopsy after preoperative chemotherapy for breast cancer: findings from the Austrian Sentinel Node Study Group. Ann Surg Oncol 2008;15:3378–83.
58. Newman EA, Sabel MS, Nees AV, et al. Sentinel lymph node biopsy performed after neoadjuvant chemotherapy is accurate in patients with documented node-positive breast cancer at presentation. Ann Surg Oncol 2007;14:2946–52.
59. Buchholz TA, Lehman CD, Harris JR, et al. Statement of the science concerning locoregional treatments after preoperative chemotherapy for breast cancer: a National Cancer Institute conference. J Clin Oncol 2008;26:791–7.
60. Papa MZ, Zippel D, Kaufman B, et al. Timing of sentinel lymph node biopsy in patients receiving neoadjuvant chemotherapy for breast cancer. J Surg Oncol 2008;98:403–6.
61. van Deurzen CH, Vriens BE, Tjan-Heijnen VC, et al. Accuracy of sentinel node biopsy after neoadjuvant chemotherapy in breast cancer patients: a systematic review. Eur J Cancer 2009;45:3124–30.
62. Tanis PJ, Deurloo EE, Valdes Olmos RA, et al. Single intralesional tracer dose for radio-guided excision of clinically occult breast cancer and sentinel node. Ann Surg Oncol 2001;8:850–5.
63. Tanis PJ, Nieweg OE, Valdes Olmos RA, et al. Impact of non-axillary sentinel node biopsy on staging and treatment of breast cancer patients. Br J Cancer 2002;87:705–10.

64. Veronesi U, Paganelli G, Viale G, et al. Sentinel lymph node biopsy and axillary dissection in breast cancer: results in a large series. J Natl Cancer Inst 1999;91:368–73.
65. Albertini JJ, Lyman GH, Cox C, et al. Lymphatic mapping and sentinel node biopsy in the patient with breast cancer. JAMA 1996;276:1818–22.
66. Krag D, Weaver D, Ashikaga T, et al. The sentinel node in breast cancer—a multicenter validation study. N Engl J Med 1998;339:941–6.
67. McMasters KM, Tuttle TM, Carlson DJ, et al. Sentinel lymph node biopsy for breast cancer: a suitable alternative to routine axillary dissection in multi-institutional practice when optimal technique is used. J Clin Oncol 2000;18:2560–6.
68. Dixon JM, Mamman U, Thomas J. Accuracy of intraoperative frozen-section analysis of axillary nodes. Edinburgh Breast Unit team. Br J Surg 1999;86:392–5.
69. Zurrida S, Mazzarol G, Galimberti V, et al. The problem of the accuracy of intraoperative examination of axillary sentinel nodes in breast cancer. Ann Surg Oncol 2001;8:817–20.
70. Weiser MR, Montgomery LL, Susnik B, et al. Is routine intraoperative frozen-section examination of sentinel lymph nodes in breast cancer worthwhile? Ann Surg Oncol 2000;7:651–5.
71. Rubio IT, Korourian S, Cowan C, et al. Use of touch preps for intraoperative diagnosis of sentinel lymph node metastases in breast cancer. Ann Surg [illegible] 1998;5:680–94.
72. Fitzgibbons PL, Page DL, Weaver D, et al. Prognostic factors in breast cancer. College of American Pathologists Consensus Statement 1999. Arch Pathol Lab Med 2000;124:966–78.
73. Wilke LG, McCall LM, Posther KE, et al. Surgical complications associated with sentinel lymph node biopsy: results from a prospective international cooperative group trial. Ann Surg Oncol 2006;13:491–500.
74. Sadiq TS, Burns WW 3rd, Taber DJ, et al. Blue urticaria: a previously unreported adverse event associated with isosulfan blue. Arch Surg 2001;136:1433–5.
75. Temple LK, Baron R, Cody HS 3rd, et al. Sensory morbidity after sentinel lymph node biopsy and axillary dissection: a prospective study of 233 women. Ann Surg Oncol 2002;9:654–62.
76. Krag DN, Weaver DL, Alex JC, Fairbank JT. Surgical resection and radiolocalization of the sentinel lymph node in breast cancer using a gamma probe. Surg Oncol 1993;2:335–9; discussion 340.
77. Giuliano AE, Kirgan DM, Guenther JM, Morton DL. Lymphatic mapping and sentinel lymphadenectomy for breast cancer. Ann Surg 1994;220:391–8; discussion 398–401.
78. Tafra L, Lannin DR, Swanson MS, et al. Multicenter trial of sentinel node biopsy for breast cancer using both technetium sulfer colloid and isosulfan blue dye. Ann Surg 2001;233:51–9.
79. Shivers S, Cox C, Leight G, et al. Final results of the Department of Defense multicenter breast lymphatic mapping trial. Ann Surg Oncol 2002;9:[illegible]–55.
80. Veronesi U, Paganelli G, Viale G, et al. A randomized comparison of sentinel-node biopsy with routine axillary dissection in breast cancer. N Engl J Med 2003;349:546–53.
81. Krag DN, Anderson SJ, Julian TB, et al. Technical outcomes of sentinel-lymph-node resection and conventional axillary-lymph-node dissection in patients with clinically node-negative breast cancer: results from the NSABP B-32 randomised phase III trial. Lancet Oncol 2007;8:881–8.
82. Krag DN, Anderson SJ, Julian TB, et al. Primary outcome results of NSABP B-32, a randomized phase III clinical trial to compare sentinel node resection (SNR) to conventional axillary dissection (AD) in clinically node-negative breast cancer patients. Presented at American Society of Clinical Oncology Annual Meeting; 2010 March; Chicago, IL.
83. Cote R, Giuliano AE, Hawes D, et al. ACOSOG Z0010: a multicenter prognostic study of sentinel node (SN) and bone marrow (BM) micrometastases in women with clinical T1/T2 N0 M0 breast cancer. Presented at American Society of Clinical Oncology Annual Meeting; 2010 March; Chicago, IL.
84. Giuliano AE, McCall LM, Beitsch PD, et al. ACOSOG Z0011: a randomized trial of axillary node dissection in women with clinical T1-2 N0 M0 breast cancer who have a positive sentinel node. Presented at American Society of Clinical Oncology Annual Meeting; 2010 March; Chicago, IL.
85. Miner TJ, Shriver CD, Flicek PR, et al. Guidelines for the safe use of radioactive materials during localization and resection of the sentinel lymph node. Ann Surg Oncol 1999;6:75–82.

7 EVOLVING MOLECULAR THERAPEUTICS AND THEIR APPLICATIONS TO SURGICAL ONCOLOGY

Melissa Heffler, MD, Vita Golubovskaya, PhD, and Kelli Bullard Dunn, MD, FACS, FACRS

Despite advances in both medical and surgical therapy for cancer, the majority of cancer deaths result from metastasis. Traditionally, chemotherapy has been the mainstay of therapy for systemic disease. However, even the most effective chemotherapeutic agents are rarely curative. Moreover, toxicity is common and can be debilitating and dose limiting. It has proven difficult to find an agent that is toxic to cancer cells but does not in some way damage healthy cells. This treatment paradox has prompted a revolution in drug development. Increasingly, research efforts are focusing on the development of agents that target molecules that are specific to tumor cells. The ability of cancer cells to resist apoptosis, proliferate unchecked, and detach and metastasize results from activation and dysregulation of complex signaling cascades that in normal cells are controlled by intrinsic checkpoints and regulatory processes. Better understanding of these pathways, and of their checks and balances, has led to the development of agents that specifically target these processes in tumor cells. Agents are generally classified based on mechanism of action; however, overlap exists, and class lines are often blurred. The following summary describes historic targeted therapies that have laid the groundwork for current investigations and outlines current breakthroughs that are revolutionizing the way cancer is treated. The ultimate goal of molecular therapeutics is to develop agents that are lethal only to tumor cells, that maintain efficacy without developing resistance, and that possess acceptable toxicities that make them well tolerated by patients.

Tyrosine Kinase Inhibitors

BIOCHEMICAL RATIONALE

Tyrosine kinases (TKs) are enzymatic proteins that catalyze the phosphorylation and activation of other signaling proteins.[1] As their name implies, the target of these kinases is the tyrosine residue on a variety of proteins. TKs have long been known to play a role in cancer progression, and as such, inhibition of TKs has been at the forefront of targeted cancer therapy.

TKs are classified as either receptor or nonreceptor kinases. Fifty-eight membrane-spanning receptor tyrosine kinases (RTKs) have been identified.[2] Structurally, the lipophilic transmembrane domain is flanked by an immunoglobulin-like, ligand-binding extracellular head and an intracellular tyrosine autophosphorylating carboxy-terminal tail. The majority of RTKs function in pairs, and activation induces dimerization [*see Figure 1*].[1,3,4] Dimerization then triggers a phosphorylation cascade involving the cytosolic non-RTKs [*see Figure 2*]. These non-RTKs relay intracellular signals by additional protein phosphorylation.[4] Many processes involved in tumor progression and metastasis, including proliferation, angiogenesis, migration, and cell survival, are influenced by dimerization, autophosphorylation, and the resulting downstream signal cascade.[1,3] Although these processes are necessary for normal cell turnover, mutations can alter the expression or activation of TKs and thereby lead to uncontrolled activation in cancer cells.[5] To date, the 58 RTKs that have been described are classified into over 20 families based on molecular structure and the sequence of the kinase domain.[2,5,6] Of these, approximately 30% have been found to be either mutated or unregulated in cancer.[5] Several RTKs are now known to play important roles in tumorigenesis and have become effective therapeutic targets. For example, c-kit is unregulated in gastrointestinal stromal tumors (GISTs) and acute myelogenous leukemia (AML), HER-2 is elevated in breast cancer, and RET is altered in the multiple endocrine neoplasia (MEN) disorders.[5] These and other RTKs, therefore, provide potential targets for molecular therapeutics.

TYROSINE KINASE INHIBITORS

Delineating the role of TKs in tumorigenic processes such as invasion, angiogenesis, and proliferation prompted the development of several tyrosine kinase inhibitors (TKIs) that target either the receptor or the ligand that promotes the downstream signal cascade.[1] The resulting flood of TKIs has been variably classified by the target receptor or ligand, the signaling pathway affected, or their molecular structure. For the purposes of this review, TKIs are classified based on molecular structure: (1) monoclonal antibodies, (2) small molecule kinase inhibitors, and (3) multitargeted kinase inhibitors [*see Table 1*].

Monoclonal Antibodies

TKIs were first introduced to the anticancer armamentarium with the development of imatinib mesylate for the treatment of chronic myelogenous leukemia (CML), and this monoclonal antibody revolutionized therapy for this disease. The majority of patients with CML possess the t(9;22) translocation mutation (Philadelphia chromosome) that fuses the

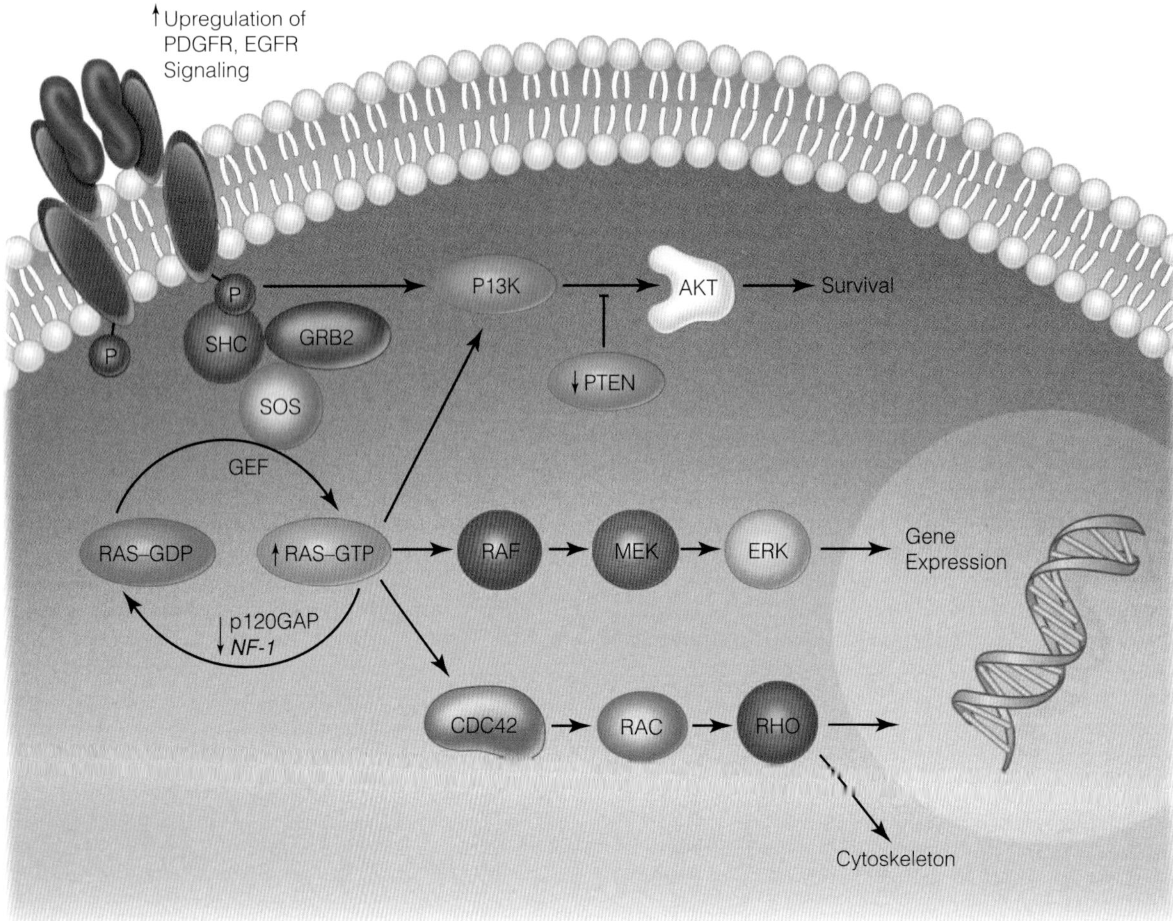

Figure 1 **Activation of a receptor tyrosine kinase induces dimerization and downstream phosphorylation of nonreceptor tyrosine kinases. Major signaling cascades include the RAS/RAF/MAPK pathway, MEK pathway, and PI_3 kinase/AKT pathway. Adapted with permission from Zhu Y, Parada LF. The molecular and genetic basis of neurological tumours. Nat Rev Cancer 2002:2:616–26. EGFR= epidermal growth factor receptor; ERK= extracellular signal-related kinase; GAP= GTPase-activating proteins; GEF= guanosine exchange factors; MEK= mitogen-activated protein kinase; NF1= neurofibromin gene; PDGFR= platelet-derived growth factor receptor; PI3K= phosphotidylinositol-3 kinase.**

Abl TK to the *Bcr* gene on chromosome 22.[1,7] Transcription and translation of this mutation produce two TKs, p190 and p210, both of which are involved in hematopoietic stem cell proliferation and inhibition of apoptosis.[1] Imatinib blocks the adenosine triphosphate (ATP)-binding site on these proteins, hindering activation and downstream signaling. In clinical trials, this early TKI improved long-term survival in CML by prolonging periods of remission and has been an effective treatment modality for both newly diagnosed patients and those who have failed interferon-alfa therapy.[8]

The success of imatinib in the treatment of CML raised the question of whether this agent might be useful for treating solid tumors. The recognition that imatinib also inhibits the c-kit and platelet-derived growth factor receptor (PDGFR) TKs led to trials treating tumors with mutations in these molecules.[9] For example, GISTs are well known to express c-kit, and imatinib has been highly successful in treating these tumors. Currently, there are several clinical trials designed to test the efficacy of imatinib in other solid tumors, including colorectal cancer, ovarian cancer, prostate cancer, and thyroid cancer.[10] Nevertheless, despite successes with this agent, prolonged use of imatinib has resulted in the development of resistant tumors. The most common mechanism of resistance appears to involve mutations in the kinase domain of bcr-abl, which then prevent binding of the drug.[11] As a result, current research is focusing on overcoming this limitation.

Another RTK that has been identified as a target for monoclonal antibody inhibition is epidermal growth factor receptor 2 (EGFR2, ErbB2), also known as human epidermal receptor 2 (HER-2).[12] This RTK can bind a wide array of growth factors, thereby inducing dimerization and stimulating downstream activation of either the RAS/MAPK, PI_3 kinase/Akt/mTOR, or other signaling pathways, which promote cell proliferation and migration and inhibit apoptosis.[12,13] HER-2

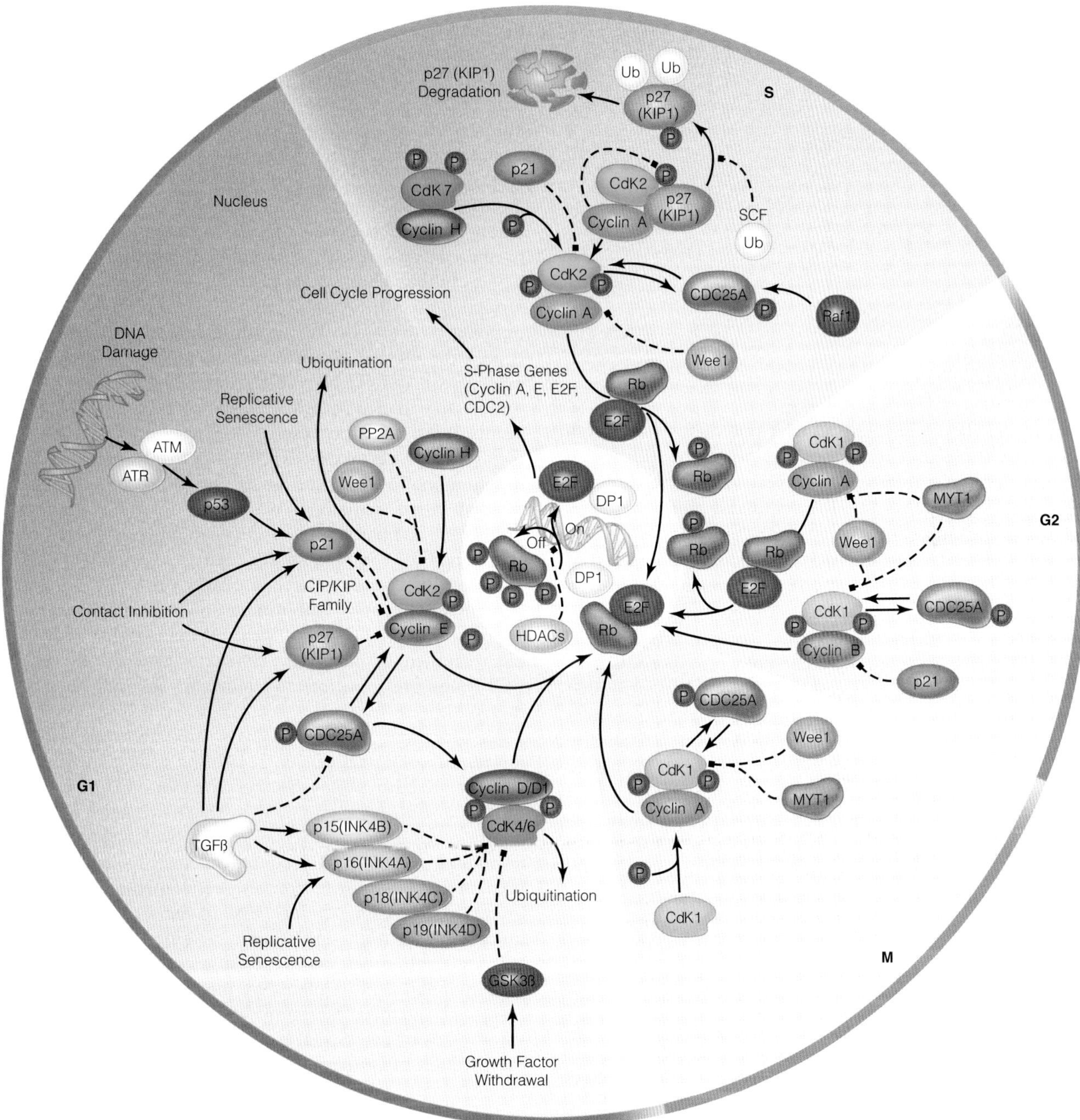

Figure 2 **Regulation of the cell cycle involves a highly complex sequence of events. The interaction of cyclin-dependent kinases (CdKs) and cyclins determines progression through different phases of the cell cycle. Adapted from SABiosciences. Cyclins and cell cycle regulation. Available at: www.sabiosciences.com (accessed October 2010).**

is overexpressed in many malignancies, and between 20 and 30% of advanced breast cancers express this receptor.[12,14] Trastuzumab is a humanized monoclonal antibody that inhibits activation of the HER-2 receptor by binding to the extracellular domain and blunting the activation of downstream signaling.[12] In addition, trastuzumab has been shown to affect breast cancer cells by inducing cell cycle arrest at G_1 via upregulation and translocation of p27 from cytosol to nuclei.[15,16] These findings have led to clinical use of this drug for treating HER-2-positive breast cancer.

Trastuzumab has demonstrated efficacy against both early- and late-stage breast cancer and is currently the standard of care for HER-2-positive tumors.[17,18] This agent was first used as adjuvant therapy for node-positive or advanced node-negative breast cancer with *HER-2* gene amplification. In the National Surgical Adjuvant Breast and Bowel Project (NSABP) B-31 and North Central Cancer Treatment Group (NCCTG) N9831 trials, trastuzumab was studied as a conjugate to the established treatment regimen of doxorubicin and cyclophosphamide plus paclitaxel.[19] The Herceptin

Table 1 Tyrosine Kinase Inhibitors

Monoclonal antibodies
Imitinib
Trastuzumab
Cetuximab
Panitumumab
Small molecule inhibitors
Gefitinib
Erlotinib
Multitargeted inhibitors
Lapatinib
Dasatinib
Sunitinib
Axitinib
Vandetanib

Adjuvant (HERA) and Breast Cancer International Research Group (BCIRG) 006 trials then examined the efficacy of adjuvant trastuzumab for 1 or 2 years following different chemotherapy regimens (HERA) or as an addition to the regimen of anthracycline, cyclophosphamide, and docetaxal (BCIRG 006).[20] In all four trials, both disease-free survival and overall survival were improved in the groups that received trastuzumab. In addition, patients who received trastuzumab developed fewer metastases and had lower mortality compared with patients who received chemotherapy alone. Unfortunately, side effects observed in these studies and attributed to trastuzumab treatment were congestive heart failure and a measurable decline in left ventricular ejection fraction.[19,20] Further investigation revealed that the risk of cardiac failure was greatest in patients who received anthracycline, and although there is evidence that this untoward effect was curtailed with the concomitant administration of epirubicin, it remains a real concern for many patients and physicians.[21] Thus, trastuzumab should not be given with anthracycline, and close monitoring of cardiac function is recommended.

Although trastuzumab has traditionally been administered in conjunction with chemotherapy in advanced HER-2-positive disease, more recent work has focused on using this drug as a single agent in early disease in an effort to delay the use of other, more toxic chemotherapy.[17] In addition, the recent phase III Trastuzumab for Gastric Cancer (ToGA) trial has suggested that trastuzumab may be a reasonable adjunct to capecitabine and cisplatin or 5-fluorouracil (5-FU) and cisplatin for patients with HER-2-positive gastric or gastroesophageal junction cancer. Patients who received trastuzumab experienced 13.8-month median overall survival compared with 11.1 months for those receiving chemotherapy alone, decreasing the rate of death by 26%.[22,23] Trials are also under way to test the efficacy of trastuzumab in combination with other targeted therapies. For example, trastuzumab-DM1 is a combination of the monoclonal antibody and the maytansine derivative DM1, a drug that interferes with microtubule formation. Preclinical studies demonstrate efficacy in lapatinib and trastuzumab-refractory breast cancer cells, and this combination is currently in phase II clinical trials for the treatment of breast cancer.[24,25] Preliminary data show an approximately 40% overall response rate in metastatic disease after 6 months.[26,27]

Like trastuzumab, cetuximab is a monoclonal antibody that targets EGFRs by binding to the extracellular domain.[3,28] The development of this drug began with the identification of a murine monoclonal antibody (called 225) that could bind EGFR and inhibit activation of the intracellular TK domain of the receptor. The downstream effects of 225 included increased apoptosis and cell cycle arrest in G_1.[29] Experimental data were promising; however, concern about the use of a mouse monoclonal antibody in the human population and the potential for antimouse antibody response prompted chimerization of the antibody with human IgG1.[30,31] The resulting chimeric antibody (C225, cetuximab) performed better than the original 225 antibody in inhibiting tumor growth in vivo.[31,32] In addition, early studies demonstrated the efficacy of cetuximab in improving progression-free survival and overall response rate in metastatic colorectal tumors that had developed resistance to chemotherapeutic agents such as irinotecan.[3,33] Moreover, patients with metastatic colorectal cancer refractory to oxaliplatin and fluoropyrimidine (5-FU) experienced prolonged progression-free survival when cetuximab was given in conjunction with irinotecan compared with irinotecan alone. These results established the combination regimen as a standard of care for refractory metastatic colorectal cancer.[3] In 2004, cetuximab either in combination with irinotecan or as a single agent was approved by the Food and Drug Administration (FDA) for the treatment of metastatic colorectal cancers that express EGFR and are refractory to irinotecan- or oxaliplatin-based therapies.[3,34,35]

As cetuximab was increasingly used to treat refractory metastatic colorectal cancer, it became clear that this agent is most effective in a subset of patients.[33,36–38] Specifically, tumors possessing a mutation in the K-*ras* gene responded poorly to cetuximab, whereas tumors with wild-type K-*ras* responded well.[39–41] The consensus that K-*ras* status is a predictive marker for response to cetuximab therapy has led to current recommendations that patients be tested for the mutation prior to the initiation of treatment.[42,43]

In 2001, Shin and colleagues studied the combined effect of cetuximab and cisplatin in patients with recurrent or late-stage squamous carcinoma of the head and neck.[30] In this study, 67% of patients demonstrated a major response with the addition of cetuximab.[30] This drug also showed efficacy in improving the response rates in patients with head and neck cancer when combined with cisplatin, 5-FU, and radiation.[32] As such, in 2006, cetuximab was approved by the FDA for the treatment of squamous cell carcinoma of the head and neck in combination with radiation therapy or as a single agent in cases refractory to platinum-based regimens.[44] Thus, cetuximab has demonstrated efficacy for the treatment of several cancers that in the past have been difficult to treat, and the recognition of optimal applications is growing. Although still under active investigation for more general use, this agent holds promise for treating a variety of cancers.

Another human monoclonal antibody that targets EGFR, panitumumab, has a different mechanism of action. Panitumumab functions by binding to the site of epidermal growth factor and tumor necrosis factor–α (TNF-α) binding on the EFGR.[45] The antibody is then internalized and downregulates EGFR production, induces apoptosis, and inhibits tumor growth and cell cycle progression.[45] Panitumumab has been approved by the FDA for the treatment of EGFR-expressing metastatic colorectal cancer refractory to fluoropyrimidine-, irinotecan-, or oxaliplatin-based therapies.[46] Similar to cetuximab, however, several studies have identified K-*ras* mutation as a predictive marker for panitumumab response and thus recommend that K-*ras* status be identified prior to the initiation of treatment.[43] Recent work also has identified additional markers that have the potential to predict tumor response to monoclonal antibodies, such as cetuximab and panitumumab. For example, *BRAF*, N-*ras*, and PIK3CA have been suggested as potential biomarkers for response to anti-EGFR therapy and hold promise for further personalizing cancer treatment.[47,48]

Finally, other similar agents, such as pertuzumab, an antibody that prevents dimerization of HER-2 receptors, are being developed and tested.[49] In vitro, pertuzumab demonstrated synergy with trastuzumab in inhibiting breast cancer cell growth. A phase I trial demonstrated that this drug was well tolerated and produced promising preliminary clinical results.[49,50]

Small Molecule TKIs

Gefitinib is a small molecule inhibitor that targets the epidermal growth factor receptor 1 (EGFR1/HER-1) by inhibiting autophosphorylation.[27] This small molecule binds the intracellular TK domain of the receptor.[51,52] Gefitinib was originally approved for the treatment of non–small cell lung cancer in 2003. However, in 2005, its use was limited only to patients who had previously benefited from the drug after two clinical trials demonstrated no advantage in patients with non–small cell lung tumors that overexpressed EGFR.[53] As clinical testing has continued, the results with gefitinib treatment have been mixed. Recent data from the North-East Japan Study Group indicated that first-line gefitinib prolonged progression-free survival in patients with metastatic non–small cell lung cancer with EGFR mutation(s) compared with carboplatin and paclitaxel.[54] In contrast, other studies have failed to show any improvement in survival.[55,56] Interestingly, gefitinib appears to reverse drug resistance in breast cancer cells that overexpress Pgp, a multidrug resistance protein, suggesting that this may also be a therapeutic target for this agent.[57]

Erlotinib is another small molecule inhibitor of EGFR autophosphorylation that binds the kinase domain of the receptor and inhibits cell proliferation and cell cycle progression. In preclinical trials, erlotinib effectively inhibited activation of EGFR in colorectal cancer cells, inhibited in vivo growth of squamous cell head and neck cancer cells that overexpress EGFR, and inhibited in vivo growth of non–small cell lung cancer cells.[58–60] In a large randomized, placebo-controlled, double-blind trial studying patients with advanced non–small cell lung cancer (stage IIIB or IV), erlotinib therapy prolonged progression-free and overall survival and was subsequently approved as second-line therapy for treating non–small cell lung cancer in 2004.[61–64] Later, erlotinib was approved in combination with gemcitabine for treating pancreatic cancer (2005) and as maintenance therapy for non–small cell lung cancer (2010).[64]

Multitargeted Inhibitors

Despite the demonstrated efficacy of monoclonal antibodies and small molecule inhibitors of TKIs, the development of resistance has been a concern and, as such, has led to the development of second-generation TKIs that are capable of inhibiting multiple TKs. These molecules are designed to inhibit not only EGFR/HER-2 activation, for example, but also downstream cell signaling molecules such as the src family of kinases and proteins such as c-kit, HER-2, and PDGFR.[65]

Lapatinib is an EGFR and HER-2 inhibitor that has been extensively studied in the treatment of breast cancer. The unique feature of this inhibitor is the extended binding time to EGFR that prolongs its inhibitory effect. As a single agent, only modest clinical benefit was appreciated in phase II trials. However, lapatinib appears to be effective when used in combination with other agents. For example, in patients with metastatic breast cancer who overexpress HER-2, treatment with lapatinib plus capecitabine markedly improved progression-free survival. Also, patients receiving the combination regimen showed 51% reduction in risk of disease progression, decreased incidence of central nervous system (CNS) metastases, and decreased volume of existing CNS metastases.[27] In 2007, lapatinib in combination with capecitabine was approved by the FDA for use in advanced breast cancers that overexpress HER-2. In addition, in 2010, the FDA approved the combination of lapatinib and letrozole in postmenopausal women with advanced breast cancers who overexpress HER-2 and are hormone receptor positive. The combination regimen significantly improved progression-free survival.[66]

Another of the second-generation, multitargeted TKIs, dasatinib, has demonstrated increased inhibitory activity against Bcr-Abl compared with imatinib in vitro and is currently approved for the treatment of CML in patients who have developed resistance to imatinib or are otherwise intolerant of the drug.[8,65] In the SRC/ABL Tyrosine kinase inhibition Activity Research Trials of dasatinib (START-C) trial, 53% of patients who received dasatinib achieved a complete cytogenic response and 62% achieved a major cytogenic response after 24 months.[8,67] Although this investigation involved the initiation of dasatinib treatment after failure of imatinib, there is speculation and early evidence that it may be effective as a first-line agent. Initial studies have suggested that the rate of remission at 24 months was superior with initial treatment of dasatinib when compared with initial treatment with imatinib.[8,68]

Additional multitargeted agents are also under development. For example, neratinib inhibits both EGFR (ErbB1), HER-2 (ErbB2), and HER-4 (ErbB4), and in a phase I study for use against solid tumors, the agent was well tolerated and showed promising clinical activity.[69] A phase II trial of its use against advanced breast cancer supported early findings, and further studies are under way for the treatment of breast cancer and other solid tumors.[10,70]

Another group of TKIs that target multiple receptors is difficult to classify because these agents affect a variety of kinases and downstream signaling cascades. For example, some of these molecules inhibit angiogenesis by blocking the vascular endothelial growth factor receptor (VEGFR) while also inhibiting TKs such as c-kit and HER-2. One such inhibitor is sunitinib, a molecule that inhibits c-kit, PDGFR-α, CSF-1 receptor, and VEGFR-1, -2, and -3.[27] The FDA approved its use in advanced renal cell carcinoma after it demonstrated efficacy by improving progression free survival and overall survival compared with interferon alfa.[71,72] Sunitinib has also been used successfully to treat GISTs that have developed resistance to imatinib and is FDA approved for use in that setting.[71,73,74]

Other clinical trials test sunitinib's efficacy in a variety of settings, and a phase II study using sunitinib for treating thyroid cancer that was resistant to radioactive iodine showed that 3% of patients had a complete response, 29% showed a partial response, and 46% maintained stable disease.[75] In addition, for metastatic breast cancer patients who failed treatment with anthracyclines and taxanes, sunitinib treatment helped some (5%) achieve stable disease.[76] Despite these promising results, toxicity has emerged as a concern with this agent. For example, in the study treating metastatic breast cancer, dose modification was necessary in 56% of patients as a result of adverse effects.[76] Similarly, in a study combining sunitinib with cyclophosphamide and methotrexate, of the 15 patients studied, three developed neutropenia and five developed mucositis.[27] In another phase I dose-escalation study combining sunitinib and capecitabine in patients with solid tumors, five grade 3 adverse effects emerged: abdominal pain, mucosal inflammation, fatigue, neutropenia, and hand-foot syndrome.[77] Similar side effects have been reported in other clinical trials, and one trial was terminated early because of the high incidence of neutropenia, febrile neutropenia, and fatigue.[27] Interestingly, in one study of efficacy against hepatocellular carcinoma, the neutropenia and skin toxicities seemed to correlate with response to therapy, overall survival, and time to tumor progression, suggesting that those toxicities may be a marker for tumor response.[78]

Axitinib is another inhibitor of several RTKs, including all VEGFRs (1, 2, and 3), PDGFR-β, and c-kit.[27] This agent has shown promise in phase I studies and was initially thought to have few severe side effects (hypertension was most common). Phase II studies have suggested a benefit to adding axitinib to docetaxel for patients with metastatic breast cancer and in combination with gemcitabine for treating metastatic pancreatic cancer.[27,79] In the phase II trials, however, toxicity appeared to be greater than suggested in the phase I trials (febrile neutropenia, fatigue, stomatitis, diarrhea, hypertension), and a phase III trial combining the agent with gemcitabine was terminated early because of a lack of improved survival.[27,80] Clinical trials continue to investigate the use of axitinib for the treatment of a variety of solid tumors, including, but not limited to, renal cell carcinoma, hepatocellular carcinoma, colorectal cancer, lung cancer, and melanoma.[10]

Finally, vandetanib is a molecule that inhibits EGFR, the kinase domain of VEGFR2, and ret autophosphorylation that is currently in the early stages of clinical investigation.[27,81–85] Phase I data suggest that although this agent is well tolerated, it provided no clinical benefit for patients with multiple myeloma.[81] Early clinical trials for use against refractory non–small cell lung cancer, however, were more promising, prompting the initiation of phase III investigations for its use in that disease.[83,85] The Ziprasidone Observational Study of Cardiac Outcomes (ZODIAC) trial examined the effect of vandetanib with docetaxel on previously treated non–small cell lung cancer; compared with patients who received docetaxel with placebo, patients who received vandetanib had significantly longer progression-free survival and an improved overall response rate.[86] Early clinical trials in glioblastoma and medullary thyroid cancer also have shown promising results.[87,88] At present, the indications for the use of these agents, both alone and in combination with other drugs, are evolving and await the results of clinical trials.

TKIs are the prototype for targeted therapeutics. These agents have been widely studied, and new and increasingly effective molecules are under development. Interestingly, one consistent theme with TKIs is the ability of biomarkers such as K-*ras* mutation and EGFR overexpression to predict response. This improved understanding of the molecular mechanisms underlying carcinogenesis and tumor response to therapy increasingly is leading to a more individualized approach to cancer treatment.

Angiogenesis Inhibitors

BIOCHEMICAL RATIONALE

Angiogenesis is one of the earliest events in tumor growth.[89] Hypoxic conditions provoke tumor microvascular formation by not only inciting proangiogenic signals but also inhibiting antiangiogenic signals.[90–92] The proangiogenic factors released include, but are not limited to, vascular endothelial growth factors (VEGFA, -B, -C, -D, and -E), basic fibroblast growth factor (bFGF), interleukin-8, placentalike growth factors (PLGF-1 and -2), neurophilins (NRP1 and NRP2), transforming growth factors (TGFs), fibroblast growth factor (FGF), and platelet-derived growth factor (PDGF).[illegible] The effects of these proangiogenic proteins can be classified based on the mechanism by which they stimulate microvascular formation.[89] For example, some stimulate new growth of vasculature from preexisting blood vessels, whereas others induce the formation of de novo vascular channels.[94] VEGFR stimulation activates intracellular phospholipase Cγ (PLC-γ), protein kinase C (PKC) and the MAPK pathway, PI_3 kinase, Akt/PKB (protein kinase B), nuclear factor κB (NF-κB), and endothelial nitric oxide syntheses and inhibits proapoptotic proteins, thereby inducing endothelial cell survival, proliferation, and migration and increasing vasodilation, vascular remodeling, and vessel permeability.[95] In addition, hypoxia-inducible factors (HIFs) are transcription factors that are activated under hypoxic conditions and serve as a major stimulus for angiogenesis.[89]

Folkman's hypothesis suggests that approximately 2 mm^3 is the critical tumor size at which further growth and survival depend on an autonomous vascular network.[96] The resulting neovasculature is tortuous and irregular, and although not efficient enough to satisfy the oxygen needs of the growing tumor, these networks are able to promote growth and metastasis.[89] The most important cell involved in this process is the vascular endothelial cell, and its growth is primarily regulated by VEGF activation of the VEGFR. In normal tissues, VEGFR2 appears to be the major inducer of angiogenesis, whereas the relatively weak signal cascade of VEGFR1 may actually decrease angiogenesis. VEGFR3 is involved in embryologic and postnatal angiogenesis and lymphangiogenesis. In cancer, VEGFR1 and -2 appear to be the receptors most involved in tumor angiogenesis.[3] Both VEGF and VEGFRs have emerged as logical targets for drugs seeking to inhibit angiogenesis.[42,89]

ANGIOGENESIS INHIBITORS

Bevacizumab is the prototypical angiogenesis inhibitor. This anti-VEGFA antibody reduces the amount of effective circulating VEGFA and thereby prevents VEGFR activation.[42] Bevacizumab has shown efficacy in suppressing endothelial cell adhesion and proliferation in vitro and suppressing peritoneal dissemination of gastric cancer in a murine model.[97,98] Clinical efficacy was first demonstrated in colorectal cancer. In stage IV disease, bevacizumab in combination with irinotecan, 5-FU, and folinic acid (leucovorin) (FOLFIRI) induced higher response rates and prolonged progression-free and overall survival compared with traditional chemotherapy.[99] In 2004, bevacizumab was approved by the FDA as a first-line treatment for metastatic colorectal cancer and in 2006 as second-line treatment in combination with oxaliplatin, folinic acid, and 5-FU (FOLFOX4).[100,101] The efficacy of bevacizumab has subsequently been tested in other tumor types, including pancreatic and hepatocellular carcinoma, renal cell carcinoma, neuroendocrine tumors, non–small cell lung cancer, and breast, brain, and ovarian cancers.[10]

Despite early enthusiasm about bevacizumab, additional experience has met with mixed results. The Bevacizumab Regimens' Investigation of Treatment Effects (BRiTE) study, an observational cohort study of 1,953 patients with metastatic colorectal cancer from 248 United State sites between 2004 and 2005, examined the efficacy of bevacizumab combined with chemotherapy as first-line treatment for metastatic colorectal cancer. At 20 months, progression-free survival was observed in 22% of patients who had received bevacizumab, whereas disease progression was seen in 79% of the patients. In addition, 66% of patients died during the study period, and 12% either withdrew from the study or were lost to follow-up.[102] Similarly, in a phase III study by Stathopoulos and colleagues in 2010, median overall survival did not differ between groups that received bevacizumab with chemotherapy (irinotecan, 5-FU, leucovorin) and groups that received chemotherapy alone as the initial treatment for metastatic colorectal cancer.[103] Moreover, in a phase II study of bevacizumab with erlotinib for treating recurrent malignant glioma, progression-free survival was not significantly improved in patients who received bevacizumab.[104] Other early studies, however, have suggested efficacy in the treatment of other types of cancer. In non–small cell lung cancer, the effects on overall survival were inconsistent, but the drug appeared to slow the progression of the disease.[105] In vitro data suggest efficacy in combination with docetaxal for treatment of breast and prostate cancers.[106] In combination therapy with paclitaxel for metastatic breast cancer, bevacizumab improved response rates compared with paclitaxel alone.[107]

To date, the FDA has approved bevacizumab in combination with carboplatin and paclitaxel for the treatment of non–small cell lung cancer and in combination with interferon for the treatment of metastatic renal cell carcinoma.[101,108,109] It has also been approved for use as a second-line single agent for the treatment of glioblastoma.[101] In 2008, bevacizumab was approved as first-line treatment in combination with paclitaxel for metastatic HER-2-negative breast cancer.[101] However, the results of more recent analyses of several clinical trials have failed to show any survival advantage in breast cancer patients who receive bevacizumab compared with chemotherapy alone. As a result, the Oncologic Drugs Advisory Committee of the FDA has recommended withdrawing the approval of bevacizumab as first-line treatment for metastatic breast cancer.[110] The FDA is currently reviewing the data on this drug, and the decision regarding possible revocation of approval is pending.[111]

Toxicity, although not prohibitive, is common, and the most common adverse effects are rash, hepatotoxicity (elevated liver function tests), proteinuria, diarrhea, myelosuppression, fatigue, infection, pain, nausea/vomiting, and hypokalemia.[104,105,107,112] In addition, the BRiTE study found several rare, but more severe, side effects. New onset or worsening hypertension was seen in 22% of patients, and hypertension was implicated in eight serious adverse events. Additional less common but serious adverse events included postoperative wound healing complications (4%), grade 3 to 4 bleeding (2.2%), arterial thromboembolic events (2%), and gastrointestinal perforation (2%). The majority of bleeding events were gastrointestinal. Significant postoperative wound healing complications occurred following major surgery and in patients in whom surgery was undertaken within 2 weeks of the last bevacizumab dose.[102] This observation has led most surgeons to try to avoid operating on patients within 6 to 8 weeks of bevacizumab therapy. Moreover, the FDA has issued a drug warning and safety labeling update concerning these adverse effects.[101]

Aflibercept (VEGF Trap) is a molecule in which the ligand-binding domains of the VEGFR1 and VEGFR2 proteins are fused with human IgG1, forming a decoy receptor that binds all VEGFs and placental growth factor.[27] Preclinical studies have suggested that this agent is well tolerated but have failed to show significant clinical activity. Definitive recommendations about the use of aflibercept await the results of ongoing trials.[27]

Angiogenesis inhibitors have demonstrated efficacy in a variety of disease sites; however, they also have limitations. Of particular concern to surgeons are the risk of increased bleeding and inhibition of wound healing. Nevertheless, antiangiogenic compounds have proven to be useful in well-selected patients.

Cell Cycle Inhibitors

BIOCHEMICAL RATIONALE

Regulation of the cell cycle involves a highly complex sequence of events orchestrated by cyclins and cyclin-dependent kinases (CdKs) [*see Figure 3*]. The interaction of these molecules is regulated by several naturally occurring cyclin-dependent kinase inhibitors (CdKIs) that prevent binding of CdKs to cyclins. Two families of CdKIs have been identified: the INK4/ARF family and the Cip/Kip family. The INK4/ARF family includes p15, p16, p18, and p19, and the Cip/Kip family includes p21, p27, and p57.[113,114] A cell will exit the quiescent phase, G_0, and enter G_1 following the production of cyclin D, which is the result of activation of the Ras/Raf/MAPK signal cascade by mitogens. Progression through the cell cycle is permitted to occur when the CdKIs do not prevent CdK-cyclin interactions. For example, cyclin E–CdK2 complex formation promotes cell entry into

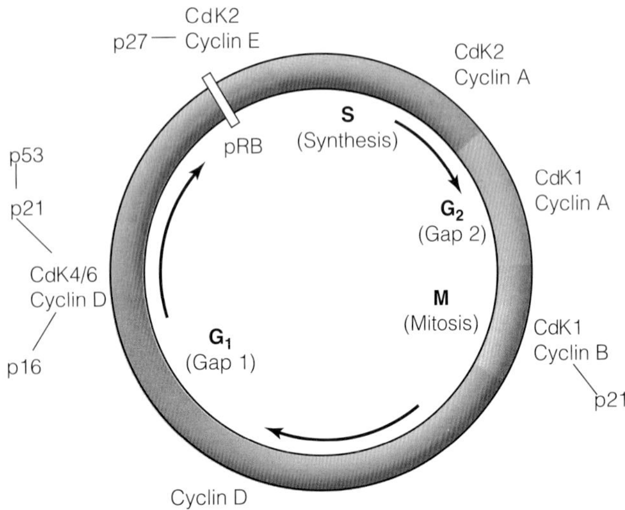

Figure 3 **Progression through each phase of the cell cycle is regulated by cyclin–cyclin-dependent kinase interactions. Adapted from www.sysmex-lifescience.com (accessed October 2010).**

S phase, and cyclin B–CdK1 allows mitosis to occur[115,116] [*see Figure 3*]. Overall, nine CdKs have been described, and these molecules interact with 20 possible cyclins (A to T).[115] Given that cyclins and CdKs play major roles in controlling progression through the cell cycle, they are logically attractive targets for treating cancer. In addition, there is evidence that CdK or cyclin production is disrupted in several malignancies, including melanoma and lung, breast, and colorectal cancers.[115,117,118] Several cell cycle inhibitors are currently under investigation, but clinical results have been mixed, and it has been suggested that these agents may have more utility as chemosensitizers for other agents.[115]

CELL CYCLE INHIBITORS

Currently, CdKIs include flavopiridol, roscovitine, E7070, AZD5438, SNS-032 (BMS-387032), bryostatin-1, PD 0332991, and SCH 727965. Flavopiridol acts on the G_1 and S phases of the cell cycle via inhibition of CdKs 2, 4, 6, and 9 and has demonstrated early success in vitro by inducing arrest of cellular growth and inducing apoptosis in chronic lymphocytic leukemia (CLL) and colorectal cancer cells.[119,120] Currently, flavopiridol is useful for treating recurrent CLL, where it has been shown to induce a clinical response in patients with high-risk genomic features.[121] In addition, when given with cytosine arabinoside and mitoxantrone, flavopiridol induced complete remission in 67% of patients with AML who had poor-risk features (older age, unfavorable genetic mutations, or secondary AML).[122] Phase I trials indicate drug tolerability, and phase II trials continue to test this drug's efficacy in a variety of cancers.[123]

Roscovitine inhibits cyclin E–CdK2, cyclin B–CdK1, cyclin H–CdK7, and cyclin T1–CdK9 and prevents progression through the S, G_2, and M phases of the cell cycle.[115] In vitro studies also indicate that this drug induces apoptosis by activating p53, suppressing NF-κB, and downregulating Mcl-1 (an antiapoptosis protein) in multiple myeloma cells.[124–126] It also inhibits mitosis by decreasing production of promoters of cell division, such as Aurora-A/B, CDC25C, pololike kinase, and WEEL.[127] Preclinical studies have demonstrated the efficacy of this agent in a variety of cancer cell lines. A phase II clinical trial of roscovitine for treating resistant non–small cell lung cancer has recently been completed, and phase I investigation of its clinical safety in treating any solid tumors resistant to standard treatment is under way.[10]

E7070 is a synthetic sulfonamide that inhibits CdK2 and cyclin E, effectively inhibiting progression through G_1 and S phases.[128] In vitro, this agent blocked cell cycle progression in non–small cell lung cancer cells, and in vivo, it not only inhibited tumor growth but also induced regression in models of colon cancer and non–small cell lung cancer.[129,130] Four phase I clinical trials are currently under way evaluating the use of this agent in solid tumors and melanoma. However, the results of phase II trials in other disease sites have been somewhat disappointing. For example, E7070 as a single agent did not show significant response in non–small cell lung cancer.[131] In 2005, Smyth and colleagues reported similar results in metastatic melanoma, with the best response being stable disease in 17% of patients, whereas 58% experienced disease progression.[132] A phase II study in squamous cell head and neck cancer was terminated because of the 15 patients who were treated, none achieved 4 months of progression-free survival.[133] In addition, toxicity was concerning in these trials, prompting some patients to withdraw. Most common problems consisted of gastrointestinal upset (nausea, vomiting, constipation, or diarrhea) and pain at the injection site.[131] However, more severe side effects, such as anemia, thrombocytopenia, bleeding, and one reported death attributable to pulmonary embolus, have also been attributed to E7070 treatment.[132] Since the conclusion of those trials, pharmacokinetic studies have been initiated in an effort to identify the optimal dose of E7070 in combination with other agents in an attempt to minimize toxicity.[134,135]

A number of additional cell cycle inhibitors are currently undergoing early clinical evaluation for the treatment of a variety of malignancies [*see Table 2*]. One such agent is SNS-032, an aminothiazide-based inhibitor that halts cell cycle progression by way of CdK2 and -7 inhibition, and transcription via CdK7 and -9 inhibition.[136,137] Interestingly, the antitumor efficacy of SNS-032 may also result from inhibition of VEGF expression, hindering angiogenesis.[138] Phase I investigations of oral bioavailability in patients with metastatic solid tumors and lymphomas, as well as previously treated CLL and multiple myeloma patients, indicate that oral administration is feasible, and although neutropenia and thrombocytopenia were the most common side effects, the agent was largely well tolerated.[137,139]

Bryostatin-1 is a macrocyclic lactone derived from *Bugula neritina*.[140] This natural antineoplastic agent affects protein kinase C levels, inhibits CdK2, and induces p21.[115,141] Although promising in preclinical investigations, the results of phase II studies have shown inconsistent efficacy as a single agent or in combination with other agents. Some trials, however, did report disease improvement with bryostatin-1 treatment. Most recently, Barr and colleagues demonstrated that combination bryostatin-1 and vincristine induced an overall response rate of 31% with complete remission of disease in two patients with non-Hodgkin lymphoma.[142] Clinical trials continue to test this agent under myriad conditions.[10]

Table 2 Cell Cycle Inhibitors

Cell Cycle Inhibitor	*Mechanism of Action*	*Effects*	*Clinical Trials**
Flavopiridol	Inhibits CdK 2, 4, 6, 9	G_1/S arrest	Phase I/II (hematologic and several solid tumors)
Roscovitine	Inhibits cyclin E/CdK2, cyclin B/CdK1, cyclin H/CdK7, cyclin T1/CdK9; p53 activation, nuclear factor κB, decreases Mcl-1	S/G_2/M arrest	Phase I/II (solid tumors)
E7070	Inhibits CdK2, cyclin E	G_1/S progression	Phase I/II (several solid tumors, melanoma)
SNS-032	Inhibits CdK 2, 7, 9, VEGF	Inhibits progression and transcription, angiogenesis	Phase I (advanced B cell lymphomas, several solid tumors)
Bryostatin-1	Affects protein kinase C, CdK2; induces p21	Cell cycle modulation	Phase I/II (combination therapy for hematologic and several solid tumors)
AZD5438	Inhibits CdK1, 2, 9	Affects all phases of cell cycle	Trials terminated dues to safety concerns

*Adapted from www.clinicaltrials.gov.[10]
CdK = cyclin-dependent kinase; VEGF = vascular endothelial growth factor.

Finally, AZD5438 is one cell cycle inhibitor that exemplifies the difficulty in translating laboratory outcomes to clinical practicality. This agent worked through all phases of the cell cycle by inhibiting CdK1, -2, and -9.[115,143] Preclinical data were promising, but the clinical trials yielded less favorable outcomes. The most recent phase I trial published, studying patient tolerance of AZD5438 for the treatment of recurrent solid malignancies, indicated that weekly dosing was more appropriate than continuous. However, safety concerns prompted manufacturer discontinuation of the agent and thus resulted in early termination of clinical trials.[144]

Cell cycle inhibitors are in the early stages of evaluation, and some have shown promising initial results in combination with other chemotherapies. However, although tumor cells demonstrate accelerated cell turnover and, as such, should be most sensitive to these agents, the nonspecific targeting of the cell cycle can injure normal tissues. Thus, as is the case with angiogenesis inhibitors, toxicity remains a major concern and has limited the clinical applicability of some of these drugs.

Inducers of Apoptosis

BIOCHEMICAL RATIONALE

Apoptosis is the natural process of programmed cell death, and two pathways are involved in this process. The extrinsic pathway is mediated by death receptors such as Fas, TNF, and TRAIL, among others. The intrinsic pathway is mitochondria and apoptosome mediated and can be activated by radiation and chemotherapy. It includes downstream signaling mediated by bcl-2 and the bcl-2 family of antiapoptotic or proapoptotic proteins (e.g., Bid, Bax, Bak), as well as caspases and cytochrome-*c*. These pathways are not mutually exclusive; for example, caspases are known to participate in both intrinsic and extrinsic pathways. Naturally occurring apoptosis proteins interact with the caspases to either inhibit or induce the innate process of programmed cell death.[145,146] Although these molecules balance the proapoptotic/antiapoptotic equilibrium, changes in any number of elements in the signal cascade may disrupt normal apoptosis. For example, a mutation resulting in the loss of antiapoptotic p53 functions can lead to genomic instability and decreased apoptosis. Cancer therapies that target the inappropriate loss of control over apoptosis have been developed to induce the intrinsic and extrinsic pathways either independently or together. Recent work has focused on inhibition of pathways involving the TRAIL receptor, bcl receptors, and inhibitors of apoptosis proteins (AIPs).[147]

APOPTOSIS-INDUCING AGENTS

Apoptosis inducers can be classified based on their mechanism of action. Bortezomib, suberoylanilide hydroxamic acid (SAHA), TLK286, ONYX015, FTI-R115777, and 17AAG target protein kinases, proteosomes, and transcriptional factors. Mapatumumab and lexatumumab target the proapoptotic proteins TRAILR1 and TRAILR2.

Bortezomib is a boronic acid dipeptide and was the first proapoptotic agent used in cancer treatment. Bortezomib promotes apoptosis by inhibiting the 26S proteosome.[148] This proteosome degrades many cellular proteins, including those involved in the cell cycle, transcription, and tumor suppression. Early work suggested that 26S proteosome inhibition promoted apoptosis in multiple myeloma cells and that this molecule stabilized tumor suppressor and cell cycle proteins (p53, p21, and p27).[148] The Assessment of Proteasome Inhibition for Extending Remissions (APEX) trial suggested superior efficacy of bortezomib over dexamethasone for refractory multiple myeloma.[149] Clinical trials also suggest that this agent may effectively augment the antitumor activities of established chemotherapy regimens. For example, the Velcade as Initial Standard Therapy in Multiple Myeloma (VISTA) study was a phase III clinical evaluation of bortezomib in combination with melphalan and prednisone as first-line therapy for multiple myeloma. The addition of bortezomib to the standard melphalan-prednisone regimen slowed time to disease progression, increased the incidence of partial and complete response, and prolonged the duration of response.[150] Further follow-up showed that patients treated with a combination of bortezomib, melphalan, and prednisone had better overall survival at 3 years (69% versus 54%), and 35% reduced risk of death at 26.7 months when compared with patients who received only melphalan and prednisone.[151] The FDA approved bortezomib as a second-line therapy for the treatment of mantle cell lymphoma in 2006 and as first-line therapy for multiple myeloma in 2008.[152]

Several clinical trials have studied the efficacy of bortezomib against solid tumors, such as hepatocellular carcinoma and metastatic rectal cancer.[153–155] Bortezomib has also been proposed as a radiosensitizer in combination with 5-FU for neoadjuvant treatment of locally advanced (stages II and III) rectal cancer. However, in a small study, only one of nine patients treated had a complete pathologic response, arguably equivalent to 5-FU-based strategies alone.[154] At present, there are no indications for use of this agent in solid tumors, despite its efficacy in hematologic malignancies.[156]

SAHA inhibits histone deacetylase, thereby suppressing the expression of genes that can promote tumorigenesis.[157] In vitro and in vivo studies indicated that histone deacetylase inhibitors such as SAHA downregulate TNF-α receptor–1 expression and activation of NF-κB.[158] Several clinical trials have been completed, and in 2006, the agent was approved by the FDA as a third-line treatment option for cutaneous T cell lymphoma.[159] The trials that led to approval demonstrated that patients who had previously failed treatment benefited from treatment with SAHA. Side effects were tolerable, and the most common adverse effects were fatigue (52%), diarrhea (52%), and nausea (40%). More serious effects (pulmonary embolism, deep vein thrombosis, myocardial infarction) occurred in fewer than 10% of patients.[159] Additional clinical investigations are under way, including a phase III trial of SAHA use against advanced mesothelioma.[160]

Several other agents designed to induce apoptosis are under investigation [see Table 3]. TLK286, a modified glutathione analogue, is metabolized by glutathione *S*-transferase (GST) in the tumor cell cytosol, yielding a molecule that is toxic to the cell. Because GST is overexpressed in many resistant tumor cells, TLK286 may be an ideal therapeutic option in these refractory tumors.[161,162] Preliminary data suggest that TLK286 has little efficacy as a single agent, but combination with other agents may be useful.[163–167] A phase III study comparing TLK286 with doxorubicin or topotecan as a third-line treatment for refractory ovarian, fallopian, or primary peritoneal cancer is currently under way.[168]

The adenovirus ONYX015 is an attenuated adenovirus that has also shown antitumor activity, although the mechanism of action remains poorly understood. It was initially thought that the virus selectively invades and replicates in *p53* mutated cells and binds to and inactivates the *p53* gene but has no effect on normal cells.[169,170] However, other studies have suggested that its efficacy results from more complex interactions and not just mutated *p53*.[171,172] In 2004, the agent was approved in China for use against squamous cell head and neck cancer, and in the United States, it has shown promise in phase I and II trials as combination therapy for patients with solid tumors such as advanced sarcoma and recurrent head and neck cancer.[173–175]

Another agent that induces apoptosis is FTI R115777, a methylquinolone farnesyl transferase inhibitor (FTI). Initially thought to inhibit cell growth and induce apoptosis solely by blocking farnesylation of Ras, it now appears that FTI R115777 also induces cell death by disrupting the mitochondrial membrane and inducing caspase-9 activation.[176] Early clinical trials have yielded mixed results. The Children's Oncology Group, however, recently reported that although the pharmacokinetics were more variable in the pediatric population, the agent is well tolerated for the treatment of pediatric hematologic malignancies, and further investigation in solid tumors and neurofibromatosis type 1–related plexiform tumors is warranted.[177,178]

7AAG is an inhibitor of heat shock protein HSP90, a molecule that is frequently overexpressed in tumor cells.[179] This agent has been thoroughly studied in vitro and in vivo

Table 3 Inducers of Apoptosis

Inducer of Apoptosis	*Mechanism of Action*	*Effects*	*Clinical Trials**
Bortezomib	Inhibits 26S proteosome	Decreased degradation of cell cycle and transcription proteins	FDA approved as first-line treatment of multiple myeloma and as second-line treatment of mantle cell lymphoma
Suberoylanilide hydroxamic acid (SAHA)	Inhibits histone deacetylase	Suppress tumorigenic gene expression	FDA approved as third-line treatment of cutaneous T cell lymphoma; phase III (advanced mesothelioma)
TLK286	Formation of a toxic metabolite	Induces apoptosis	Phase III (refractory gynecologic malignancies), combination therapy
ONYX015	Adenovirus; invades and replicates in *p53* mutated cells, inactivates *p53* gene	Lyses *p53* mutated tumor cells	Phase I/II (combination therapy for solid tumors)
FTI-R115777	Blocks farnesylation of Ras, disrupts mitochondrial membrane, induces caspase-9 activation	Inhibit cell growth and induce apoptosis	Phase III (colorectal cancer and AML; no significant improval in progression-free survival or overall survival, respectively); phase I/II (pediatric leukemias, glioma)
17AAG	Inhibits HSP90	Inhibit cell motility and invasion	Phase I/II (multiple myeloma)
Mapatumumab	TRAILR1 agonist	Inhibit TRAIL ligand binding and apoptotic signal cascade	Phase I/II (several solid tumors)
Lexatumumab	TRAILR2 agonist		

*Adapted from www.clinicaltrials.gov.[10]
AML = acute myelogenous leukemia; FDA = Food and Drug Administration.

and affects a variety of cancer cell types by inducing apoptosis, decreasing growth, potentiating the effects of known chemotherapeutic drugs, and sensitizing tumors to radiotherapy.[180] Phase I and II trials suggest a tolerable safety profile and disease stability when administered as a single agent or in combination with bortezomib.[181,182]

Another pathway targeted to induce apoptosis involves TRAILR1 and TRAILR2. TRAILR1 and TRAILR2 are two TRAIL receptors that are believed to be involved in apoptosis via FADD and caspase-8 or -10 recruitment and possibly by activation of other signaling pathways involving NF-κB, MAPK, PI_3 kinase, and Akt. Initiated by TRAIL ligand binding, this process has been linked to tumorigenesis and is a promising target for anticancer therapy. Mapatumumab (HGS-ETR1) and lexatumumab (HGS-ETR2) are two monoclonal antibodies that agonistically bind the TRAILR1 and TRAILR2 receptors, respectively.[147] The role of mapatumumab and lexatumumab in combination with other agents has been supported by the observation of a synergistic effect with either antibody and cisplatin or bortezomib in non–small cell lung cancer cells and malignant mesothelioma cells or with radiotherapy in colorectal cancer cells.[183–185] Clinical trials are under way for both mapatumumab and lexatumumab.[10] Although well tolerated, the clinical response at the dose of mapatumumab administered was not significant.[186] Phase I trials also suggested that lexatumumab is safe and well tolerated and has promising clinical efficacy.[187,188]

Thus, drugs designed to induce apoptosis are showing early promise for the treatment of a variety of cancers. Clinical trials suggest that the side effect profile does not limit use and that these drugs may be most effective as chemo- or radio sensitizers.

Focal Adhesion Kinase Inhibitors

BIOCHEMICAL RATIONALE

Focal adhesion kinase (FAK) is a non-RTK that was identified at adhesion sites between cells and the extracellular environment. The 125 kDa protein is encoded by a gene located on chromosome 8 and houses three domains, the amino-N-terminal domain, the central catalytic domain, and the carboxy-C-terminal domain. FAK activation relies on autophosphorylation of the Y397 site that is found in the N-terminal domain. This is also a binding and activation site for several signaling proteins, such as src, PI_3 kinase, and Grb-7. In addition, this region also binds extracellular matrix and signaling proteins involved in cell motility, invasion, and cytoskeletal changes, as well as EGFR, p53, and other molecules that are critical for carcinogenesis.[189] It is well known that p53 is mutated in many cancers; interestingly, p53 can inhibit FAK expression, and FAK can inhibit p53 expression. In breast cancer cells, p53 mutation is highly correlated with FAK overexpression.[190] Finally, FAK appears to play a key role in motility and migration, invasion, survival, angiogenesis, lymphangiogenesis, and proliferation[189] [*see Figure 4*].

FAK is upregulated in several types of cancer.[189] The potential role of FAK activation in cancer growth and progression has led to the development of several therapeutic agents targeting this molecule. Initial attempts were focused on downregulation of FAK expression. Subsequently, more specific targeted therapeutic approaches have been developed using small molecules designed to inhibit FAK kinase activity and activation or to inhibit protein-protein interactions.

FAK INHIBITORS

Initial attempts at FAK inhibition focused on downregulating FAK expression. Early studies demonstrated that transfection of breast cancer cells with dominant negative C-terminal FAK-CD decreased adhesion, colonization, and in vivo tumor growth.[191] Moreover, cells transfected with FAK-silenced RNA (FAKsiRNA) showed increased rounding, decreased growth, and decreased in vivo tumorigenesis.[191] Combination FAK/src inhibition with adenoviral FAK-CD and the src inhibitor PP2 appeared to have a synergistic effect and functioned by increasing apoptosis.[192] Thus, FAK inhibition via silencing FAK expression seems to decrease tumorigenesis in vitro and in vivo.

Another approach to FAK inhibition involved either activation of p53 or elimination of p53-deficient cells. This indirect approach was studied by introducing retroviruses that express p53 into rapidly dividing p53-deficient cells. A similar tact was applied in the development of AD5CMV-p53, an adenoviral vector encoding p53 that was subsequently used to replenish p53 deficiency in tumor cells. This approach inhibited lung cancer cell growth in vitro and in vivo.[193] Clinically, phase I and II trials suggest that this agent is both safe and effective against esophageal squamous cell carcinoma.[194,195] However, concerns about the safety of a viral vector and about the logistics of production and storage persist.[196]

More recent efforts have focused on the development of small molecules to inhibit FAK activity. The first FAK inhibitor that was developed, TAE226, blocks the ATP-binding site and inhibits FAK phosphorylation at both Y397 and Y861, a site that is involved with VEGF signaling. This molecule showed promise in preclinical in vitro and in vivo trials and most recently was found to inhibit angiogenesis in models of human colon cancer.[197] TAE226 has not yet progressed to clinical evaluation.

In addition to TAE226, several other FAK inhibitors have been developed and are currently in phase I clinical trials. Like TAE226, PF-562,271 blocks the ATP-binding site of FAK and of Pyk2 (protein-rich tyrosine kinase 2), another nonreceptor tyrosine kinase known to bind and activate src.[198,199] PF-562,271 inhibited in vivo breast cancer cell growth and metastasis in a murine model and decreased the in vivo growth of prostate cancer cells and in vitro growth of lung cancer cells.[198,200–202] It also has exhibited synergy with sunitinib in the inhibition of hepatocellular tumor growth in vivo.[203] Phase I clinical trials employing PF-562,271 for treating prostate, pancreatic, and head and neck cancers have recently been completed. Another inhibitor, PF-573,228, works similarly and has been found to inhibit breast cancer cell migration.[200] Interestingly, this agent in combination with tamoxifen decreased proliferation in estrogen receptor–positive breast cancer cells.[204] Other FAK inhibitors include PF-04554878, which is currently in phase I clinical trials for the treatment of advanced nonhematologic malignancies, and GSK2256098, which has completed phase I trials.[10]

PND-1186 is another FAK inhibitor with a different mechanism of action. PND-1186 likely inhibits ATP activity by substituting a pyridine ring for the pyramidine ring found in

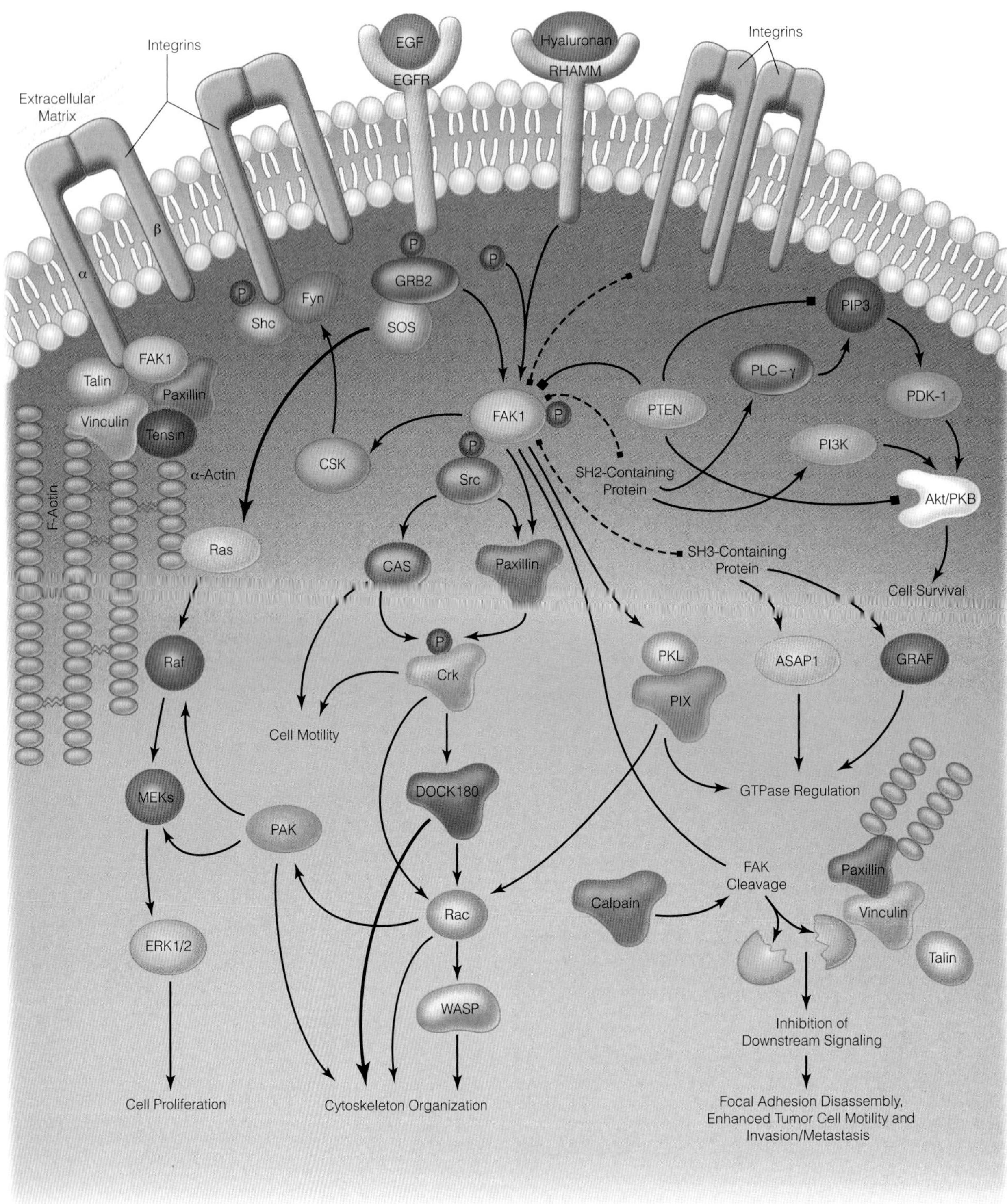

Figure 4 **Focal adhesion kinase (FAK) plays a key role in a signaling cascade that can lead to some of the tumorigenic properties of cancer cells. FAK activation induces cell proliferation, motility, survival, invasion, and metastasis. Adapted from SABiosciences. Retrieved from www.sabiosciences.com (accessed October 2010). EGF = epidermal growth factor; EGFR = epidermal growth factor receptor; PLC-γ = phospholipase Cγ.**

other ATP-binding FAK inhibitors.[205,206] Early studies show that this molecule increases breast cancer cell apoptosis, inhibits in vivo breast cancer cell growth and metastasis, and inhibits ascites and peritoneal seeding in models of ovarian cancer.[205,207]

An obvious concern with any drug is the potential for toxicity. Theoretically, the more specific the drug, the less potential it has to produce untoward effects. Although inhibiting ATP binding prevents FAK activation, this effect is somewhat nonspecific and, as such, raises concern about potential toxicity. Specific inhibition of the Y397 phosphorylation site, without blocking ATP binding, may offer a more specific target for FAK inactivation. Recently, several small molecule inhibitors that directly target the Y397 autophosphorylation site have been developed.[208] One such molecule, 1,2,4,5-benzenetetraamine tetrahydrochloride (Y15), binds specifically to the Y397 site, does not affect ATP binding or Pyk-2, and effectively inhibits FAK activation. In vitro, Y15 increased detachment and inhibited adhesion of breast cancer cells and tumorigenesis in vivo.[208] Additional studies have demonstrated the efficacy of Y15 in inhibiting pancreatic and neuroblastoma tumor growth in vivo.[209–211] In addition, when combined with gemcitabine, these two agents demonstrated synergy in inhibiting pancreatic cancer cell growth.[211] This novel small molecule inhibitor of FAK activation, therefore, holds promise as a potential new therapeutic agent.

FAK inhibition has been a relatively new approach to targeted cancer therapy. This approach is unique, and early studies suggest that FAK inhibition, either alone or in combination with other agents, may provide novel anticancer regimens.

Conclusion

The oncologic arena is changing. As the understanding of the complexities of cell signaling, cell division, apoptosis, and angiogenesis, grows, so does the armamentarium of therapeutic agents against cancer. Some of these agents have been studied extensively and already are used clinically. Others that show promise are at the early stages of development. The objective of studying these molecules is to develop drugs that selectively target malignant cells while sparing normal cells. By doing so, not only can efficacy against cancer be improved, but toxicity can also be minimized. Thus, in addition to more traditional advances in surgical and medical treatment of cancer, targeted therapeutics increasingly will play a role in surgical oncology. This is an exciting area of development with a substantial collection of established regimens and promising new therapies on the horizon.

Dr. Vita Golubovskaya is a co-founder of CureFAKtor Pharmaceuticals.

References

1. Arora A, Scholar EM. Role of tyrosine kinase inhibitors in cancer therapy. J Pharmacol Exp Ther 2005;315:971–9.
2. Robinson D, Yi-Mi Q, Su-Fang L. The protein tyrosine kinase family of the human genome. Oncogene 2000;19:5548–57.
3. Arnold D, Seufferlein T. Targeted treatments in colorectal cancer: state of the art and future perspectives. Gut 2010;59: 838–58.
4. Taniguchi T. Cytokine signaling through nonreceptor tyrosine kinases. Science 1995; 268:251–5.
5. Amit I, Wides, R, Yarden, Y. Evolvable signaling networks of receptor tyrosine kinases: relevance of robustness to malignancy and to cancer therapy. Mol Syst Biol 2007; 3:151.
6. De Bacco F, Fassetta, M, Rasola, A. Receptor tyrosine kinases as targets for cancer therapy. Cancer Ther 2004;2:317–28.
7. Popenoe D, Schaefer-Rego K, Mears JG, et al. Frequent and extensive deletion during the 9,22 translocation in CML. Blood 1986;68:1123–8.
8. Agrawal M, Garg RJ, Cortes J, Quintas-Cardama A. Tyrosine kinase inhibitors: the first decade. Curr Hematol Malig Rep 2010; 5:70–80.
9. Sleijfer S, Seynaeve, C, Wiemer E, Verweij J. Practical aspects of managing gastrointestinal stromal tumors. Clin Colorectal Cancer 2006;6 Suppl 1:S18–23.
10. Clinical Trials.gov. Available at: www.clinicaltrials.gov (accessed October 2010).
11. Lee T, Ma W, Zhang X, et al. BCR-ABL alternative splicing as a common mechanism for imatinib resistance: evidence from molecular dynamics simulations. Mol Cancer Ther 2008;7:3834–41.
12. Hudis C. Trastuzumab—mechanism of action and use in clinical practice. N Engl J Med 2007;357:39–51.
13. Yarden Y, Sliwkowski MX. Untangling the ErbB signaling network. Nat Rev 2001;2: 127–37.
14. Krop I, Muralidhar B, Jones SF, et al. Phase I study of trastuzumab-DM1, and HER2 antibody-drug conjugate, given every 3 weeks to patients with HER2-positive metastatic breast cancer. J Clin Oncol 2010;28:2698–704.
15. Yakes F, Chinraranalab W, Ritter CA, et al. Herceptin-induced inhibition of phosphatidylinositol-3 kinase and Akt is required for antibody-mediated effects of p27, cyclin D1, and antitumor action. Cancer Res 2002;62: 4132–41.
16. Le X, Pruefer F, Bast RC Jr. HER2-targeting antibodies modulate the cyclin-dependent kinase inhibitor p27Kip1 via multiple signaling pathways. Cell Cycle 2005;4:87–95.
17. Chang H. Trastuzumab-based neoadjuvant therapy in patients with HER2-positive breast cancer. Cancer 2010;116:2856–67.
18. Christofanilli M. Novel targeted therapies in inflammatory breast cancer. Cancer 2010; 116:2837–9.
19. Romond E, Perez EA, Bryant J, et al. Trastuzumab plus adjuvant chemotherapy for operable HER2-positive breast cancer. N Engl J Med 2005;353:1673–84.
20. Basegla J, Perez EA, Pienkowski T, Bell R. Adjuvant trastuzumab: a milestone in the treatment of HER-2-positive early breast cancer. Oncologist 2006;11:4–12.
21. Joensuu H, Kellokump-Lehtinin PL, Bono P, et al. Adjuvant docetaxel of vinorelbine with or without trastuzumab for breast cancer. N Engl J Med 2006;354:809–20.
22. Bang Y, VanCutsen E, Feyereislova A, et al. Trastuzumab in combination with chemotherapy versus chemotherapy alone for the treatment of HER2-positive advanced gastric or gastro-oesophageal junction cancer (ToGA): a phase 3, open-label, randomised controlled trial. Lancet 2010; 376:687–97.
23. Breast cancer drug helps patients with gastric cancer. NCI Cancer Bull 2009;6(11).
24. Juntilla T, Li G, Parsons K, et al. Trastuzumab-DM1 (T-DM1) retains all the mechanisms of action of trastuzumab and efficiently inhibits growth of lapatinib insensitive breast cancer. Breast Cancer Res Treat 2010. [Epub ahead of print]
25. Lewis Phillips G, Li G, Dugger DL, et al. Targeting HER2-positive breast cancer with trastuzumab-DM1, an antibody-cytotoxic drug conjugate. Cancer Res 2008;68: 9280–90.
26. Vogel C, Burris HA, Limentani S, et al. A phase II study of trastuzumab-DM1 (T-DM1), a HER2 antibody-drug conjugate (ADC), in patients with HER2+ metastatic breast cancer (MBC): final results [abstract]. J Clin Oncol 2009;27(15S):1017.
27. Alvarez R, Valero V, Hortobagyi GN. Emerging targeted therapies for breast cancer. J Clin Oncol 2010;28:3366–79.
28. Jonker D, O'Callaghan CJ, Karapetis CS, et al. Cetuximab for the treatment of colorectal cancer. N Engl J Med 2007;357: 2040–8.
29. Normanno N, Bianco C, De Luca A, et al. Target-based agents against ErbB receptors and their ligands: a novel approach to cancer treatment. Endocr Relat Cancer 2003;10: 1–21.
30. Shin DM, Donato NJ, Perez-Soler R, et al. Epidermal growth factor receptor-targeted therapy with C225 and cisplatin in patients with head and neck cancer. Clin Cancer Res 2001;7:1204–13.
31. Goldstein N, Prewett M, Zuklys K, et al. Biological efficacy of a chimeric antibody to the epidermal growth factor receptor in a human tumor xenograft model. Clin Cancer Res 1995;1:1311–8.

32. Merlano M, Russi E, Benasso M, et al. Cisplatin-based chemoradiation plus cetuximab in locally advanced head and neck cancer: a phase II clinical study. Ann Oncol 2010. [Epub ahead of print]
33. Cunningham D, Humblet Y, Siena S, et al. Cetuximab monotherapy and cetuximab plus irinotecan in irinotecan-refractory metastatic colorectal cancer. N Engl J Med 2004;351:337–45.
34. US Department of Health and Human Services, US Food and Drug Administration. FDA approves Erbitux for colorectal cancer. 2004. Available at: http://www.fda.gov/NewsEvents/Newsroom/PressAnnouncements/2004/ucm108244.htm (accessed October 2010).
35. US Department of Health & Human Services, US Food and Drug Administration. Cetuximab. 2007. Available at: http://www.fda.gov/AboutFDA/CentersOffices/CDER/ucm129241.htm (accessed October 2010).
36. Van Cutsem E, Nowacki M, Lang I, et al. Randomized phase II study of irinotecan and 5-FU/FA with or without cetuximab in the first-line treatment of patients with metastatic colorectal cancer (mCRC): the CRYSTAL trial [abstract]. J Clin Oncol 2007;25(18 Suppl 4000).
37. Bokemeyer C, Bondarenko I, Makhson A, et al. Cetuximab plus 5-FU/FA/oxaliplatin (FOLFOX-4) versus FOLFOX-4 in the first-line treatment of metastatic colorectal cancer (mCRC): OPUS, a randomized phase II study [abstract]. J Clin Oncol 2007;25(18 Suppl 4035).
38. Saltz L, Meropol NJ, Loehrer PJ Sr, et al. Phase II trial of cetuximab in patients with refractory colorectal cancer that express the epidermal growth factor receptor. J Clin Oncol 2004;22:1201–8.
39. Khambata-Ford S, Garrett CR, Meropol NJ, et al. Expression of epiregulin and amphiregulin and K-ras mutation status predict disease control in metastatic colorectal cancer patients treated with cetuximab. J Clin Oncol 2007;25:2330–7.
40. Tejpar S, Peeters M, Humblet Y, et al. Relationship of efficacy with KRAS status (wild type versus mutant) in patients with irinotecan-refractory metastatic colorectal cancer (mCRC) treated with irinotecan (q2w) and escalating doses of cetuximab (q1w): the EVEREST experience (preliminary data) [abstract]. J Clin Oncol 2008; 265(May 20 Suppl 4001).
41. Bokemeyer C, Bondarenko I, Hartmann JT, et al. KRAS status and efficacy of first-line treatment of patients with metastatic colorectal cancer (mCRC) with FOLFOX with or without cetuximab: the OPUS experience [abstract]. J Clin Oncol 2008;26 (15 Suppl 4000).
42. Winder T, Lenz H-J. Molecular predictive and prognostic markers in colon cancer. Cancer Treat Rev 2010;36:550–6.
43. Allegra C, Jessup JM, Somerfield MR, et al. American Society of Clinical Oncology provisional clinical opinion: testing for KRAS gene mutations in patients with metastatic colorectal carcinoma to predict response to anti-epidermal growth factor receptor monoclonal antibody therapy. J Clin Oncol 2009;27:2091–6.
44. National Cancer Institute. Cetuximab. 2006. Available at: http://www.cancer.gov/cancertopics/druginfo/cetuximab (accessed October 2010).
45. Lynch D, Yang XD. Therapeutic potential of ABX-EGF: a fully human anti-epidermal gorwth factor receptor monoclonal antibody for cancer treatment. Semin Oncol 2002; 29:47–50.
46. Giusti R, Shastri KA, Cohen MH, et al. FDA drug approval summary: panitumumab (Vectibix). Oncologist 2007;12:577–83.
47. DiNicolantonio F, Martini M, Molinari F, et al. Wild-type BRAF is required for response to panitumumab or cetuximab in metastatic colorectal cancer. J Clin Oncol 2008;26:5705–12.
48. De Roock W, Claes B, Bernasconi D, et al. Effects of KRAS, BRAF, NRAS, and PIK-3CA mutations of the efficacy of cetuximab plus chemotherapy in chemotherapy-refractory metastatic colorectal cancer: a retrospective consortium analysis. Lancet Oncol 2010;11:753–62.
49. Agus D, Gordon MS, Taylor C, et al. Phase I clinical study of pertuzumab, a novel HER dimerization inhibitor, in patients with advanced cancer. J Clin Oncol 2005;23: 2534–43.
50. Nahta R, Hung M-C, Esteva FJ. The HER-2-targeting antibodies trastuzumab and pertuzumab synergistically inhibit the survival of breast cancer cells. Cancer Res 2004; 64:2343–6.
51. Normanno N, Tejpar S, Morgillo F, et al. Implications for KRAS status and EGFR-targeted therapies in metastatic CRC. Nat Rev Clin Oncol 2009;6:519–27.
52. Burton A. What went wrong with Iressa? Lancet Oncol 2002;3:708.
53. US Food and Drug Administration. Information for healthcare professionals: gefitinib (marketed Iressa). FDA Alert. Available at: http://www.fda.gov/Drugs/DrugSafety/PostmarketDrugSafetyInformationforPatientsandProviders/DrugSafetyInformationforHealthcareProfessionals/ucm085197.htm (accessed October 2010).
54. Maemondo M, Inoue A, Kobayashi K, et al. Gefitinib or chemotherapy for non-smll-cell lung cancer with mutated EGFR. N Engl J Med 2010;362:2380–8.
55. Ibrahim E. Frontline gefitinib in advanced non-small cell lung cancer: meta-analysis of published randomized trials. Ann Thorac Med 2010;5:153–60.
56. Price K, Azzoli CG, Krug LM, et al. Phase II trial of gefitinib and everolimus in advanced non-small cell lung cancer. J Thorac Oncol 2010;5:1623–9.
57. Kitazaki T, Oka M, Nakamura Y, et al. Gefitinib, an EGFR tyrosine kinase inhibitor, directly inhibits the function of P-glycoprotein in multidrug resistant cancer cells. Lung Cancer 2005;49:337–43.
58. Moyer J, Barbacci EG, Iwata KK, et al. Induction of apoptosis and cell cycle arrest by CP-358,774, an inhibitor of epidermal growth factor receptor tyrosine kinase. Cancer Res 1997;57:4838–48.
59. Pollack VA, Savage DM, Baker DA, et al. Inhibition of epidermal growth factor receptor-associated tyrosine phosphorylation in human carcinomas with CP-358,774: dynamics of receptor inhibition in situ and antitumor effects in athymic mice. J Pharmacol 1999;291:739–49.
60. Higgins B, Kolinsky K, Smith M, et al. Antitumor activity of erlotinib (OSI-774, Tarceva) alone or in combination in human non-small cell lung cancer tumor xenograft models. Anticancer Drugs 2004;15: 503–12.
61. Shepherd F, Pereira JR, Ciuleanu T, et al. Erlotinib in previously treated non-small-cell lung cancer. N Engl J Med 2005; 353:123–32.
62. Cohen M, Johnson JR, Chen Y-F, et al. FDA drug approval summary: erlotinib (Tarceva) tablets. Oncologist 2005;12: 461–6.
63. US Department of Health and Human Services, US Food and Drug Administration. Erlotinib. 2010. Available at: http://www.fda.gov/AboutFDA/CentersOffices/CDER/ucm209058.htm (accessed October 2010).
64. National Cancer Institute. FDA approval for erlotinib hydrochloride. 2004. Available at: http://www.cancer.gov/cancertopics/druginfo/fda-erlotinib-hydrochloride (accessed October 2010).
65. O'Hare T, Walters DK, Stoffregen EP, et al. Combined Abl inhibitor therapy for minimizing drug resistance in chronic myeloid leukemia: Src/Abl inhibitors are compatible with imatinib. Clin Cancer Res 2005;11: 6987–93.
66. National Cancer Institute. FDA approval for lapatinib ditosylate. 2010. Available at: http://www.cancer.gov/cancertopics/druginfo/fda-lapatinib (accessed October 2010).
67. Baccarini M, Kantarjian HM, Apperley JF. Efficacy of dasatinib (Sprycel) in patients with chronic phase chronic myelogenous leukemia resistance to or intolerant of imatinib: updated results of the CA180013 START-C Phase II study [abstract]. Blood 2006;108:53.
68. Cortes J, Kim DW, Martinelli G, et al. Efficacy and safety of dasatinib in imatinib-resistant or -intolerant patients with chronic myeloid leukemia in blast phase. Leukemia 2008;22:2176–83.
69. Wong KK, Fracasso PM, Bukowski RM, et al. A phase I study with neratinib (HKI-272), an irreversible pan ErbB receptor tyrosine kinase inhibitor, in patients with solid tumors. Clin Cancer Res 2009;15: 2552–8.
70. Burstein H, Sun Y, Dirix LY, et al. Neratinib, an irreversible ErbB receptor tyrosine kinase inhibitor, in patients with advanced ErbB2-positive breast cancer. J Clin Oncol 2010;28:1301–7.
71. National Cancer Institute. FDA approval for sunitinib malate. 2006. Available at: http://www.cancer.gov/cancertopics/druginfo/fda-sunitinib-malate (accessed October 2010).
72. Oudard S, Beuselinck B, Decoene J, Albers P. Sunitinib for the treatment of metastatic renal cell carcinoma. Cancer Treat Rev 2010. [Epub ahead of print]
73. Demetri G, van Oosterom AT, Garrett CR, et al. Efficacy and safety of sunitinib in patients with advanced gastrointestinal stromal tumour after failed imatinib; a randomised controlled trial. Lancet 2006; 368:1329–38.
74. Casali PG, Garrett CR, Blackstein ME, et al. Updated results from a phase III trial of sunitinib in GIST patients (pts) for whom imatinib (IM) therapy has failed due to resistance or intolerance [abstract] J Clin Oncol 2006;24(918 Suppl 9513).
75. Carr L, Mankoff D, Goulart BH, et al. Phase II study of sunitinib in FDG-PET positive, differentiated thyroid cancer and metastatic medullary carcinoma of thyroid with functional imaging correlation. Clin Cancer Res 2010. [Epub ahead of print]
76. Burstein H, Elias AD, Rugo HS, et al. Phase II study of sunitinib malate, an oral multitargeted tyrosine kinase inhibitor, in patients with metastatic breast cancer previously treated with and anthracycline and a taxane. J Clin Oncol 2008;26:1810–6.
77. Sweeney C, Chiorean EG, Verschraegen CF, et al. A phase I study of sunitinib plus capecitabine in patients with advanced solid tumors. J Clin Oncol 2010. [Epub ahead of print]
78. Zhu A, Duda DG, Ancukiewicz M, et al. Exploratory analysis of early toxicity of sunitinib in advanced hepatocellular carcinoma patients: kinetics and potential biomarker value. Clin Cancer Res 2010. [Epub ahead of print]

79. Spano J, Chodkiewicz C, Maurel J, et al. Efficacy of gemcitabine plus axitinib compared with gemcitabine alone in patients with advanced pancreatic cancer: an open-label randomised phase II study. Lancet 2008;371:2101–8.
80. Reuters. UPDATE 1-Pfizer pancreatic cancer drug fails, trial halted. 2009. Available at: http://www.reuters.com/article/idINN3039502020090130?rpc=44 (accessed October 2010).
81. Kovacs M, Reece DE, Marcellus D, et al. A phase II study of ZD6474 (Zactima), a selective inhibitor of VEGFR and EGFR tyrosine kinase in patients with relapsed multiple myeloma—NCIC CTG IND.145. Investig New Drugs 2006;24:529–35.
82. Arnold A, Seymour L, Smylie M, et al. Phase II study of vandetanib or placebo in small-cell lung cancer patients after complete or partial response to induction chemotherapy with or without radiation therapy: National Cancer Institute of Canada Clinical Trials Group Study BR.20. J Clin Oncol 2007; 25:4278–84.
83. Heymach J, Johnson BE, Prager D, et al. Randomised, placebo-controlled phase II study of vandetanib plus docetaxel in previously treated non small-cell lung cancer. J Clin Oncol 2007;25:4270–7.
84. Horti J, Widmark A, Stenzi A, et al. A randomized, double-blind, placebo-controlled phase II study of vandetanib plus docetaxel/prednisolone in patients with hormone-refractory prostate cancer. Cancer Biother Radiopharm 2009;24:175–80.
85. Natale R, Bodkin D, Govindan R, et al. Vandetanib versus gefitinib in patients with advanced non-small-cell lung cancer: results from a two-part, double-blind, randomised phase II study. J Clin Oncol 2009;27: 2523–9.
86. Herbst R, Eberhardt WE, Germonpre P, et al. Vandetanib plus docetaxel versus docetaxel as second-line treatment for patients with advanced non-small-cell lung cancer (ZODIAC): a double blind, randomised, phase 3 trial. Lancet Oncol 2010; 11:619–26.
87. Drappatz J, Norden AD, Wong ET, et al. Phase I study of vandetanib with radiotherapy and temozolomide for newly diagnosed glioblastoma. Int J Radiat Oncol Biol Phys 2010;78:85–90.
88. Wells S Jr, Gosnell JE, Gagel RF, et al. Vandetanib for the treatment of patients with locally advanced or metastatic hereditary medullary thyroid cancer. J Clin Oncol 2010;28:767–72.
89. Kesisis G, Broxterman H, Giaccone G. Angiogenesis inhibitors. Drug selectivity and target specificity. Curr Pharm Design 2007;13:2795–809.
90. Rak J, Mitsuhashi Y, Sheehan C, et al. Oncogenes and angiogenesis: differential modes of vascular endothelial growth factor up-regulation in ras-transformed epithelial cells and fibroblasts. Cancer Res 2000; 60:490–8.
91. Fukumura D, Jain RK. Role of nitric oxide in angiogenesis and microcirculation in tumors. Cancer Metastasis Rev 1998;17: 77–89.
92. Dameron K, Volpert OV, Tainsky MA, Bouck N. Control of angiogenesis in fibroblasts by p53 regulation of thrombospondin-1. Science 1994;265: 1582–4.
93. Carmeliet P, Dor Y, Herbert JM, et al. Role of HIF-1alpha in hypoxia-mediated apoptosis, cell proliferation and tumour angiogenesis. Nature 1998;394:485–90.
94. Bergers G, Benjamin LE. Tumorigenesis and the angiogenic switch. Nat Rev Cancer 2003;3:401–10.
95. Gotnik K, Verheul HMW. Anti-angiogenic tyrosine kinase inhibitors: what is their mechanism of action? Angiogenesis 2010; 13:1–14.
96. Folkman J. Tumor angiogenesis: therapeutic implications. N Engl J Med 1971;285: 1182–6.
97. Barzelay A, Lowenstein A, George J, Barak A. Influence of non-toxic doses of bevacizumab and ranibizumab on endothelial functions and inhibition of angiogenesis. Curr Eye Res 2010;35:835–41.
98. Imaizumi T, Aoyagi K, Miyagi M, Shirouzu K. Suppressive effect of bevacizumab on peritoneal dissemination from gastric cancer in a peritoneal metastasis model. Surg Today 2010;40:851–7.
99. Hurwitz H, Fehrenbacher L, Novotny W, et al. Bevacizumab plus irinotecan, fluorouracil, and leukovorin for metastatic colorectal cancer. N Engl J Med 2004;350: 2335–42.
100. Cohen M, Gootenberg J, Keegan Pazdur R. FDA drug approval summary: bevacizumab plus FOLFOX4 as a second-line treatment of colorectal cancer. Oncologist 2007;12: 356–61.
101. National Cancer Institute. FDA approval for bevacizumab. 2009. Available at: http://www.cancer.gov/cancertopics/druginfo/fda-bevacizumab (accessed October 2010).
102. Kozloff M, Yood MU, Berlin J, et al. Clinical outcomes associated with bevacizumab-containing treatment of metastatic colorectal cancer: the BRiTE observational cohort study. Oncologist 2009;14:862–70.
103. Stathopoulos G, Batziou C, Trafalis D, et al. Treatment of colorectal cancer with and without bevacizumab: a phase III study. Oncology 2010;78:376–81.
104. Sathornsumetee S, Desjardins A, Vrendenburgh JJ, et al. Phase II trial of bevacizumab and erlotinib in patients with recurrent malignant glioma. Neurooncology 2010. [Epub ahead of print]
105. Dingemans A, de Langen AJ, van den Boogaart VV, et al. First-line erlotinib and bevacizumab in patients with locally advanced and/or metastatic non-small cell lung cancer: a phase II study including molecular imaging. Ann Oncol 2010. [Epub ahead of print]
106. Ortholan C, Durivault J, Hannoun-Levi JM, et al. Bevacizumab/docetaxal association is more efficient than docetaxal alone in reducing breast and prostate cancer cell growth: a new paradigm for understanding the therapeutic effect of combined treatment. Eur J Cancer 2010. [Epub ahead of print]
107. Kountourakis P, Doufexis D, Maliou S, et al. Bevacizumab combined with two-weekly paclitaxel as first-line therapy for metastatic breast cancer. Anticancer Res 2010;30:2969–72.
108. Cohen M, Gootenberg J, Keegan P, Pazdur R. FDA drug approval summary: bevacizumab (Avastin) plus carboplatin and paclitaxel as first-line treatment of advanced/metastatic recurrent nonsquamous non-small cell lung cancer. Oncologist 2007;12: 713–8.
109. Summers J, Cohen MH, Keegan P, Pazdur R. FDA drug approval summary: bevacizumab plus interferon for advanced renal cell carcinoma. Oncologist 2010;15: 104–11.
110. Medscape Medical News. Will the FDA revoke bevacizumab's approval for breast cancer? 2010. Available at: http://www.medscape.com/viewarticle/725509 (accessed October 2010).
111. Medscape General Surgery. FDA delays decision on breast cancer indication for bevacizumab. 2010. Available at: http://www.medscape.com/viewarticle/728972 (accessed October 2010).
112. Hurvitz S, Allen HJ, Moroose RL, et al. A phase II trial of decetaxel with bevacizumab as first-line therapy for HER2-negative metastatic breast cancer (TORI B01). Clin Breast Cancer 2010;10:307–12.
113. Besson A, Dowdy SF, Roberts JM. CDK inhibitors: cell cycle regulators and beyond. Dev Cell Rev 2008;14:159–69.
114. Humpath.com. Cell-cycle inhibitors. Available at: http://www.humpath.com/cell-cycle-inhibitors (accessed October 2010).
115. Dickson M, Schwartz GK. Development of cell-cycle inhibitors for cancer therapy. Curr Oncol 2009;16:36–43.
116. Cheng T. Cell cycle inhibitors in normal and tumor stem cells. Oncogene 2004; 23:7256–66.
117. Sutherland R, Musgrove, EA. Cyclin E and prognosis in patients with breast cancer. N Engl J Med 2002;347:1546–7.
118. Buckley M, Sweeney KJ, Hamilton JA, et al. Expression and amplification of cyclin genes in human breast cancer. Oncogene 1993; 8:2127–33.
119. Semenov I, Akyuz C, Roginskaya V, et al. Growth inhibition and apoptosis of myeloma cells by the CDK inhibitor flavopiridol. Leuk Res 2002;26:271–80.
120. Ambrosinin G, Seelman SL, Qin LX, Schwartz GK. The cyclin-dependent kinase inhibitor flavopiridol potentiates the effets of topoisomerase I poisons by suppressing Rad51 expression in a p53-dependent manner. Cancer Res 2008;68:2312–20.
121. Lin TS, Ruppert AS, Johnson AJ, et al. Phase II study of flavopiridol in relapsed chronic lymphocytic leukemia demonstrating high response rates in genetically high-risk disease. J Clin Oncol 2009;27:6012–8.
122. Karp J, Blackford A, Smith BD, et al. Clinical activity of sequential flavopiridol, cytosine arabinoside and mitoxantrone for adults with newly diagnosed, poor-risk acute myelogenous leukemia. Leuk Res 2010;34: 877–82.
123. Rathkopf D, Dickson MA, Feldman DR, et al. Phase I study of flavopiridol with oxaliplatin and fluorouracil/leukovorin in advanced solid tumors. Clin Cancer Res 2009;15:7405–11.
124. Dey A, Wong ET, Cheok CF, et al. R-Roscovitine simultaneously targets both the p53 and NF-kappaB pathways and causes potentiation of apoptosis: implications in cancer therapy. Cell Death Differ 2008;15:263–73.
125. Raje N, Kumar S, Hideshima T, et al. Seliciclib (CYC202 of R-roscovitine), a small-molecule cyclin-dependent kinase inhibitor, mediates activity via down-regulation of Mcl-1 in multiple mlyeloma. Blood 2005;106:1042–7.
126. MacCallum D, Melville J, Frame S, et al. Seliclib (CYC202, R-roscovitine) induces cell death in multiple myeloma cell by inhibition of RNA polymerase II-dependent transcription and down-regulation of Mcl-1. Cancer Res 2005;65:5399–407.
127. Whittaker S, Te Poele RH, Chan F, et al. The cyclin-dependent kinase inhibitor seliciclib (R-roscovitine; CYC202) decreases the expression of mitotis control genes and prevents entry into mitosis. Cell Cycle 2007; 6:3114–31.
128. van Kesteren C, Beijnen JH, Schellens JH. E7070: a novel synthetic sulfonamide targeting the cell cycle progression for the treatment of cancer. Anticancer Drugs 2002;13:989–97.
129. Fukuoka K, Usuda J, Iwamoto Y, et al. Mechanisms of action of the novel sulfon-

amide anticancer agent E7070 on cell cycle progression in human non-small cell lung cancer cells. Investig New Drugs 2001;19: 219–27.

130. Ozawa Y, Sugi MH, Nagasu T, et al. E7070, a novel sulphonamide agent with potent antitumor activity in vitro and in vivo. Eur J Cancer 2001;37:2275–82.

131. Talbot D, von Pawel J, Cattell E, et al. A randomized phase II pharmacokinetic and pharmacodynamic study of indisulam as second-line therapy in patients with advanced non-small cell lung cancer. Clin Cancer Res 2007;13:1816–22.

132. Smyth J, Aamdal S, Awada A, et al. Phase II study of E7070 in patients with metastatic melanoma. Ann Oncol 2005;16:158–61.

133. Haddad R, Weinstein LJ, Wieczorek TJ, et al. A phase II clinical and pharmacodynamic study of E707 in patients with metastatic, recurrent, or refractory squamous cell carcinoma of the head and neck: modulation of retinoblastoma protein phosphorylation by a novel chloroindolyl sulfonamide cell cycle inhibitor. Clin Cancer Res 2004; 10:4680–7.

134. Zandvliet A, Schellens JH, Dittrich C, et al. Population pharmacokinetic and pharmacodynamic analysis to support treatment optimization of combination chemotherapy with indisulam and carboplatin. Br J Clin Pharmacol 2008;66:485–97.

135. Dittrich C, Zandvliet AS, Gneist M, et al. A phase I and pharmacokinetic study of indisulam in combination with carboplatin. Br J Clin Pharmacol 2007;96:559–66.

136. [illegible] D, Yinn HY, Kim KS, et al. [illegible] 2-aminothiazole inhibitors of cyclin-dependent kinase-2. N-[5[[[5(1,1-dimethylethyl)2-oxazolyl] methyl]thio]-2-thiazolyl]-4-piperdinecarboxamide (BMS-389032), a highly efficacious and selective antitumor agent. J Med Chem 2004;47:1719–28.

137. Heath EI, Bible K, Martell RE, et al. A phase 1 study of SNS-032 (formerly BMS-387032), a potent inhibitor of cyclin-dependent kinases 2,7 and 9 administered as a single oral dose and weekly infusion in patients with metastatic refractory solid tumors. Investig New Drugs 2008;26:59–65.

138. Ali M, Choy H, Habib AA, Saha D. SNS-032 prevents tumor cell-induced angiogenesis by inhibiting vascular endothelial growth factor. Neoplasia 2007;9:370–81.

139. Tong W, Chen R, Plunkett W, et al. Phase I and pharmacologic study of SNS-032, a potent selective Cdk2,7, and 9 inhibitor in patients with advanced chronic lymphocytic leukemia and multiple myeloma. J Clin Oncol 2010;28:3015–22.

140. Pettit G, Herald CL, Doubeck DL, et al. Isolation and structure of bryostatin 1. J Am Chem Soc 1982;104:6846–8.

141. Asiedu C, Biggs J, Lilly M, Kraft AS. Inhibition of leukemic cell growth by the protein kinase C activator bryostatin 1 correlates with the dephosphorylation of cyclin-dependent kinase 2. Cancer Res 1995;55: 3716–20.

142. Barr P, Lazarus HM, Cooper BW, et al. Phase II study of bryostatin 1 and vincristine for aggressive non-Hodgkin lymphoma relapsing after an autologous stem cell transplant. Am J Hematol 2009;84:484–7.

143. Bythe K, Thomas A, Hughes G, et al. AZD5438, a potent oral inhibitor of cyclin-dependent kinases 1,2, and 9, leads to pharmacodynamic changes and potent antitumor effects in human tumor xenografts. Mol Cancer Ther 2009;8:1856–66.

144. AstraZeneca Clinical trials Website. AZD5438. 2010. Available at: http://www.astrazenecaclinicaltrials.com/other-drug-products/discontinuedproducts/AZD5438/ (accessed October 2010).

145. Danial N, Korsmeyer SJ. Cell death: critical control points. Cell 2004;116:205–19.

146. Gonzalvez F, Ashkenazi A. New insights into apoptosis signaling by Apo2L/TRAIL. Oncogene 2010;29:4753–65.

147. Johnstone R, Frew AJ, Smyth MJ. The TRAIL apoptotic pathway in cancer onset, progression and therapy. Nat Rev Cancer 2008;8:782–98.

148. Richardson P, Hideshima T, Anderson KC. Bortezomib (PS-341): a novel, first-in-class proteosome inhibitor for the treatment of multiple myeloma and other cancers. Cancer Control 2003;10:361–9.

149. Richardson P, Sonneveld P, Schuster MW, et al. Bortezomib or high-dose dexamethasone for relapsed multiple myeloma. N Engl J Med 2005;352:2487–96.

150. San Miguel J, Schlag R, Khuageva NK, et al. Bortezomib plus melphalan and prednisone for the initial treatment of multiple myeloma. N Engl J Med 2008;359:906–17.

151. Mateos MV, Richardson PG, Schlag R, et al. Bortezomib plus melphalan and prednisone compared with melphalan and prednisone in previously untreated multiple myeloma: updated follow-up and impact of subsequent therapy in the phase III VISTA trial. J Clin Oncol 2010;28:2259–66.

152. National Cancer Institute. FDA approval for bortezomib. 2003. Available at: http://www.cancer.gov/cancertopics/druginfo/fda-bortezomib (accessed October 2010).

153. Kim G, Mahony MR, Szydio D, et al. An international multicellular phase II trial of bortezomib in patients with hepatocellular carcinoma. Investig New Drugs 2010. [Epub ahead of print]

154. O'Neil B, Raftery L, Calvo BF, et al. A phase I study of bortezomib in combination with standard 5-fluorouracil and external-beam radiation therapy for the treatment of locally advanced or metastatic rectal cancer. Clin Colorectal Cancer 2010;9:119–25.

155. Messinger Y, Gaynon P, Raetz E, et al. Phase II study of bortezomib combined with chemotherapy in children with relapsed childhood acute lymphoblastic leukemia (ALL): a report from the Therapeutic Advances in Childhood Leukemia (TACL) Consortium. Pediatr Blood Cancer 2010; 55:254–9.

156. Goel S, Hidalgo M, Perez-Soler R. EGFR inhibitor-mediated apoptosis in solid tumors. J Exp Ther Oncol 2007;6:305–20.

157. Richon V, Zhou X, Rifkind RA, Marks PA. Histone deacetylase inhibitors: development of suberoylanilide hydroxamic acid (SAHA) for the treatment of cancers. Blood Cells Mol Dis 2001;27:260–4.

158. Imre G, Gekeler V, Leja A, et al. Histone deacetylase inhibitors suppress the inducibility of nuclear factor-KB by tumor necrosis factor-a receptor-1 down-regulation. Cancer Res 2006;66:5409–18.

159. Mann B, Johnson JR, Cohen MH, et al. FDA approval summary: Vorinostat for treatment of advanced primary cutaneous T-cell lymphoma. Oncologist 2007;12: 1247–52.

160. Paik P, Krug LM. Histone deacetylase inhibitors in malignant pleural mesothelioma: preclinical rationale and clinical trials. J Thorac Oncol 2010;5:275–9.

161. Tew K. Glutathione-associated enzymes in anticancer drug resistance. Cancer Res 1994;54:4313–20.

162. Lewis A, Hayes JD, Wolf R. Glutathione and glutathione-dependent enzymes in ovarian adenocarcinoma cell lines derived from a patient before and after the onset of drug resistance: intrinsic differences and cell cycle effects. Carcinogenesis 1988;9:1283–7.

163. Rosen L, Laxa B, Boulos L, et al. Phase I study of TLK286 (Telcyta) administered weekly in advanced malignancies. Clin Cancer Res 2004;10:3689–98.

164. Rosen L, Brown J, Laxa B, et al. Phase I study of TLK286 (glutathione S-transferase P1-1 activated glutathione analogue) in advanced refractory solid malignancies. Clin Cancer Res 2003;9:1628–38.

165. Kavanagh J, Gershenson DM, Choi H, et al. Multi-institutional phase 2 study of TLK286 (TELCYTA, a glutathione S-transferase P1-1 activated glutathione analog prodrug) in patients with platimun and paclitaxel refractory or resistant ovarian cancer. Int J Gynecol Cancer 2005;15:593–600.

166. Kavanagh J, Levenbeck CF, Ramirez PT, et al. Phase 2 study of canfosfamide in combination with pegylated liposomal doxorubicin in platinum and paclitaxel resistant epithelial ovarian cancer. J Hematol Oncol 2010;11:9.

167. Vergote I, Finkler N, del Campo J, et al. Phase 3 randomised study of canfosfamide (telcyta, TLK286) versus pegylated liposomal doxorubicin or topotecan as third-line therapy in patients with platinum-refractory or -resistant ovarian cancer. Eur J Cancer 2009;45:2324–32.

168. National Cancer Institute. Phase II randomized study of TLK286 versus doxorubicin HCl liposome or topotecan as third-line therapy in patients with platinnum-refractory or -resistant metastatic ovarian epithelial, fallopian tube, or primary peritoneal cancer. 2004. Available at: http://www.cancer.gov/search/ViewClinicalTrials.asp?cdrid=[illegible]version=HealthProfessional&protocol[illegible] (accessed October 2010).

169. Liu X, Gu JF. Targeting gene-virotherapy of cancer. Cell Res 2006;16:25–30.

170. Jiang H, Gomez-Manzano C, Lang F, et al. Oncolytic adenovirus: preclinical and clinical studies in patients with human malignant gliomas. Curr Gene Ther 2009;9:422–7.

171. Garber S, Dix BR, Myers CJ, et al. Evidence that replication of the antitumor adenovirus ONYX-051 is not controlled by the p53 and p14ARF tumor suppressor genes. J Virol 2002;76:12483–90.

172. O'Shea C, Johnson L, Bagus B, et al. Late viral RNA export, rather than p53 inactivation, determines ONYX-015 tumor selectivity. Cancer Cell 2004;6:611–23.

173. Garber K. China approves world's first oncolytic virus therapy for cancer treatment. J Natl Cancer Inst 2006;98:298–300.

174. Galanis E, Okuno SH, Nascimento AG, et al. Phase I-II trial of ONYX-015 in combination with MAP chemotherapy in patients with advanced sarcomas. Gene Ther 2005;12:437–45.

175. Nemunaitis J, Senzer N, Sarmiento S, et al. A phase I trial of intravenous infusion of ONYX-015 and Enbrel in solid tumor patients. Cancer Gene Ther 2007;14: 885–93.

176. Beaupre D, Cepero E, Obeng EA, et al. R115777 induces Ras-independent apoptosis of myeloma cells via multiple intrinsic pathways. Mol Cancer Ther 2004;3: 179–86.

177. Widemann B, Arceci RJ, Jayaprakash N, et al. Phase 1 trial and pharmacokinetic study of the farnesyl transferase inhibitor tipifarnib in children and adolescents with refractory leukemias: a report from the Children's Oncology Group. Pediatr Blood Cancer 2010. [Epub ahead of print]

178. Widemann B, Salzer WL, Arceci RJ, et al. Phase I trial and pharmacokinetic study of the farnesyltransferase inhibitor tipifarnib in children with refractory solid tumors or neurofibromatosis type I and plexiform

neurofibromas. J Clin Oncol 2006;24: 507–16.

179. Ferrarini M, Heltai S, Zocchi MR, Rugarli C. Unusual expression and localization of heat-shock proteins in human tumor cells [abstract]. Int J Cancer 1992;51:613–9.

180. Usmani S, Bona R, Li Z. 17 AAG for HSP90 inhibition in cancer—from bench to bedside. Curr Mol Med 2009;9:654–64.

181. Richardson P, Chanan-Khan AA, Alsina M, et al. Tanespimycin monotherapy in relapsed multiple myeloma: results of a phase 1 dose-escalation study. Br J Haematol 2010;150:438–45.

182. Richardson P, Badros AZ, Jagannath S, et al. Tanespimycin with bortezomib: activity in relapsed/refractory patients with multiple myeloma. Br J Haematol 2010;150: 428–37.

183. Luster T, Carrell JA, McCormick K, et al. Mapatumumab and lexatumumab induce apoptosis in TRAIL-R1 and TRAIL-R2 antibody-resistant NSCLC cell lines when treated in combination with bortezomib. Mol Cancer Ther 2009;8:292–302.

184. Belyanskaya L, Marti TM, Hopkins-Donaldson S, et al. Human agonistic TRAIL receptor antibodies mapatumumab and lexatumumab induce apoptosis in malignant mesothelioma and act synergistically with cisplatin. Mol Cancer 2007;6:66.

185. Marini P, Denzinger S, Schiller D, et al. Combined treatment of colorectal tumours with agonistic TRAIL receptor antibodies HGS-ETR1 and HGS-ETR2 and radiotherapy: enhanced effects in vitro and dose-dependent growth delay in vivo. Oncogene 2006;25:5145–54.

186. Greco F, Bonomi P, Crawford J, et al. Phase 2 study of mapatumumab, a fully human agonistic monoclonal antibody which targets and activates the TRAIL receptor-1, in patients with advanced non-small cell lung cancer. Lung Cancer 2008;61:82–90.

187. Plummer R, Attard G, Pacey S, et al. Phase 1 and pharmacokinetic study of lexatumumab in patients with advanced cancers. Clin Cancer Res 2007;13:6187–94.

188. Wakelee H, Patnaik A, Sikic BI, et al. Phase I and pharmacokinetic study of lexatumumab (HGS-ETR2) given every 2 weeks in patients with advanced solid tumors. Ann Oncol 2010;21:376–81.

189. Golubovskaya VM, Cance WG. Focal adhesion kinase and p53 signaling in cancer cells. Int Rev Cytol 2007;263:103–53.

190. Golubovskaya VM, Conway-Dorsey K, Edmiston SN, et al. FAK overexpression and p53 mutations are highly correlated in human breast cancer. Int J Cancer 2009;125: 1735–8.

191. Golubovskaya VM, Zheng M, Zhang L, Cance WG. The direct effect of focal adhesion kinase (FAK), dominant-negative FAK-CD and FAK siRNA on gene expression and human MCF-7 breast cancer cell tumorigenesis. BMC Cancer 2009;12:280.

192. Golubovskaya VM, Gross S, Kaur AS, et al. Simultaneous inhibition of focal adhesion kinase and SRC enhances detachment and apoptosis in colon cancer cell lines. Mol Cancer Res 2003;1:755–64.

193. Sakai R, Kagawa S, Yamasaki Y, et al. Preclinical evaluation of differentially targeting dual virotherapy for human solid cancer. Mol Cancer Ther 2010;9:1884–93.

194. Wolf J, Bodurka DC, Gano JB, et al. A phase I study of Adp52 (INGN 201; ADVEXIN) for patients with platinum- and paclitaxel-resistant epithelial ovarian cancer. Gynecol Oncol 2004;94:442–8.

195. Shimada H, Matsubara H, Shiratori T, et al. Phase I/II adenoviral p53 gene therapy for chemoradiation resistant advanced esophageal squamous cell carcinoma. Cancer Sci 2006;97:554–61.

196. Yoo GH, Moon J, Leblanc M, et al. A phase 2 trial of surgery with perioperative INGN 201 (Ad5CMV-p53) gene therapy followed by chemoradiotherapy for advanced, resectable squamous cell carcinoma of the oral cavity, oropharynx, hypopharynx, and larynx: report of the Southwest Oncology Group. Arch Otolaryngol Head Neck Surg 2009;135:869–74.

197. Schultze A, Decker S, Otten J, et al. TAE226-mediated inhibition of focal adhesion kinase interferes with tumor angiogenesis and vasculogenesis. Investig New Drugs 2009. [Epub ahead of print]

198. Roberts W, Ung E, Whalen P, et al. Antitumor activity and pharmacology of a selective focal adhesion kinase inhibitor, PF-562,271. Cancer Res 2008;68:1935–44.

199. Dikic I, Tokiwa G, Lev S, et al. A role for Pyk2 and Src in linking G-protein-coupled receptors with MAP kinase activation. Nature 1996;383:547–50.

200. Wendt M, Schiemann WP. Therapeutic targeting of the focal adhesion complex prevents oncogenic TGF-beta signaling and metastasis. Breast Cancer Res 2009;11: R68.

201. Bagi C, Roberts GW, Andresen CJ. Dual focal adhesion kinase/Pyk2 inhibitor has positive effects on bone tumors: implications for bone metastases. Cancer 2008;112: 2313–21.

202. Sun H, Pisle S, Gardner ER, Figg WD. Bioluminescent imaging study: FAK inhibitor, PF-562,271, preclinical study in PC3M-luc-C6 local implant and metastasis xenograft models. Cancer Biol Ther 2010;10(1):38–43.

203. Bagi C, Christensen J, Cohem DP, et al. Sunitinib and PF-562,271 (FAK/Pyk2 inhibitor) effectively block growth and recovery of human hepatocellular carconima in a rat xenograft model. Cancer Biol Ther 2009;8:856–65.

204. Hiscox S, Barnfather P, Hayes E, et al. Inhibition of focal adhesion kinase suppresses the adverse phenotype of endocrine-resistant breast cancer cells and improves endocrine response in endocrine-sensitive cells. Breast Cancer Res Treat 2010. [Epub ahead of print]

205. Tanjoni I, Walsh C, Uryu S, et al. PND-1186 FAK inhibitor selectively promotes tumor cell apoptosis in three-dimensional environments. Cancer Biol Ther 2010;9: 764–77.

206. Schaller M, Frisch SM. PND-1186 FAK inhibitor selectively promotes tumor cell apoptosis in three-dimensional environments. Cancer Biol Ther 2010;9:791–3.

207. Walsh C, Tanjoni I, Uryu S, et al. Oral delivery of PND-1186 FAK inhibitor decreases tumor growth and spontaneous breast to lung metastasis in pre-clinical models. Cancer Biol Ther 2010;9:778–90.

208. Golubovskaya VM, Nyberg C, Zheng M, et al. A small molecule inhibitor, 1,2,4,5-benzenetetraamine tetrahydrochloride, targeting the Y397 site of focal adhesion kinase decreases tumor growth. J Med Chem 2008;51:7405–16.

209. Zheng D, Golubovskaya V, Kurenova E, et al. A novel strategy to inhibit FAK and IGF-1R decreases growth of pancreatic cancer xenografts. Mol Carcinog 2010;49: 200–9.

210. Beierle EA, Ma X, Stewart J, et al. Inhibition of focal adhesion kinase decreases tumor growth in human neuroblastoma. Cell Cycle 2010;9:1005–115.

211. Hochwald S, Nyberg C, Zheng M, et al. A novel small molecule inhibitor of FAK decreases growth of human pancreatic cancer. Cell Cycle 2009;8:2435–43.

8 SOFT TISSUE SARCOMA

Aimee M. Crago, MD, PhD, and Samuel Singer, MD, FACS

The term *soft tissue sarcoma* (STS) defines cancers that develop from mesenchymal cells and their progenitors. STS is rare; the disease is diagnosed in approximately 10,000 individuals yearly in the United States.[1] This represents approximately 1% of adult malignancies and 15% of pediatric malignancies. We now recognize that, as rare as STS is, it actually represents an umbrella diagnosis encompassing over 50 different histologic subtypes of disease. Histologic subtype, in conjunction with tumor location, largely defines the biologic behavior of a given lesion and the associated clinical prognosis [*see Figure 1*]. Approximately half of all STSs occur in the extremities and 15% in the retroperitoneum [*see Figure 2*]. The most common histologic subtype in adults is liposarcoma (24% of extremity STS and 45% of retroperitoneal STS); other common subtypes are malignant fibrous histiocytoma (21% of extremity STS) and leiomyosarcoma (21% of retroperitoneal STS) [*see Figure 3*].

Unfortunately, the complexity created by diverse tumor characteristics means that treatment of STS is similarly complex. This chapter attempts to simplify the principles of STS therapy, defining an algorithm for patient evaluation and treatment while highlighting common indications for diverging from this strategy as dictated by disease subtype and location.

Etiology

SCORE Factors responsible for the development of sporadic STS are poorly understood, and few etiologic relationships have been definitively characterized. The disease is loosely associated with exposure to various herbicides and environmental toxins. The clearest of these connections are associations of vinyl chloride and thorium dioxide (Thorotrast) with hepatic angiosarcoma.[2] Patients who develop chronic lymphedema, often following surgical lymph node dissection, are also at risk for the development of angiosarcoma, a clinical scenario known as Stewart-Treves syndrome.[3]

Exposure to therapeutic and environmental radiation is a factor that clearly puts patients at risk for the development of STS. Radiation-induced sarcomas are defined as those occurring within the prior radiation field and having a pathologic confirmation of sarcoma that is histologically distinct from the primary cancer.[4] In a population-based study of 295,712 patients with solid or hematologic tumors, those treated with radiation therapy had a twofold higher rate of sarcoma development compared with the general population. For patients who received radiation before age 55, the rate was fourfold higher than in the general population.[5] The median interval between radiation administration and development of radiation-associated STS is 10 years. The most common

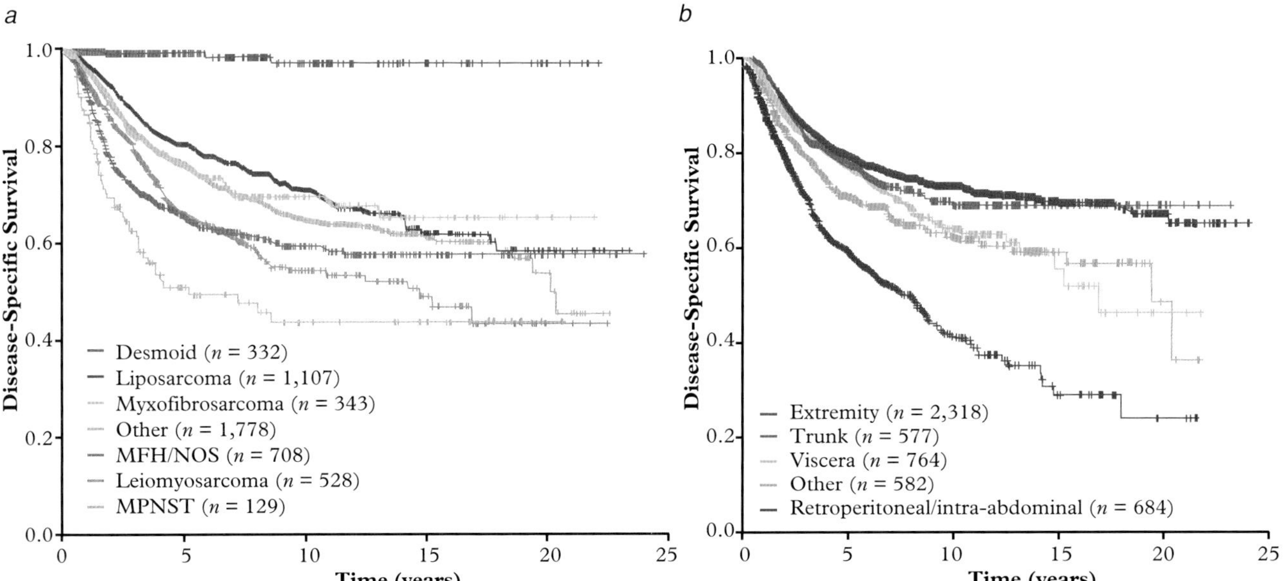

Figure 1 **Disease-specific survival stratified by (*a*) histologic type and (*b*) tumor location. Data are derived from all cases of soft tissue survival evaluated, treated, and followed prospectively at Memorial Sloan-Kettering Cancer Center over a 25-year period. MFH/NOS = malignant fibrous histiocytoma/sarcoma not otherwise specified; MPNST = malignant peripheral nerve sheath tumor.**

The authors and editors gratefully acknowledge the contributions of the previous authors, Eric Kimchi, MD, Herbert Zeh, MD, Yixing Jiang, MD, PhD, and Kevin Staveley-O'Carroll, MD, Phd, FACS, to the development and writing of this chapter.

SCORE Indicates the text is tied to a SCORE learning objective. Please see the HTML version online at www.acssurgery.com.

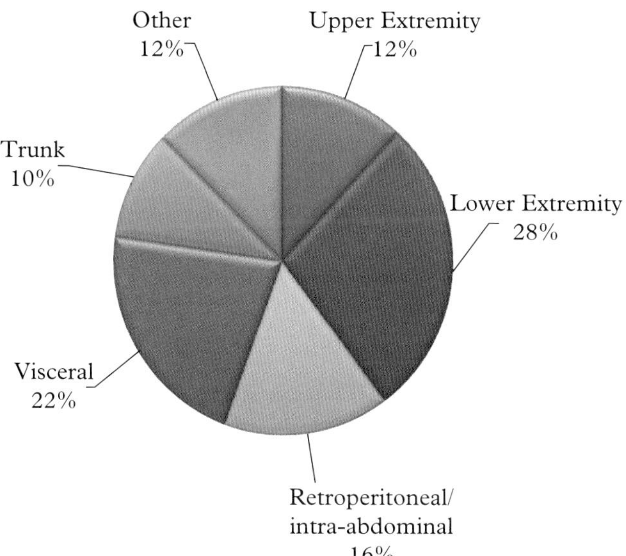

Figure 2 **Anatomic distribution of all cases of soft tissue sarcomas evaluated, treated, and followed prospectively at Memorial Sloan-Kettering Cancer Center over a 25-year period (N = 7,850).**

subtypes of radiation-induced sarcoma are angiosarcoma (27%), high-grade malignant fibrous histiocytoma (26%), and leiomyosarcoma (12%). In retrospective and case-control studies, a sarcoma being radiation associated is an independent risk factor (by multivariate analysis) for disease-specific death.[6]

Although environmental causes for STS are incompletely understood, characteristic molecular changes have been identified in many histologic subtypes of STS. These include chromosome amplifications, point mutations, and gene translocations. In many tumors, these genomic alterations can be used to identify the histologic subtype. For instance, well-differentiated and dedifferentiated liposarcoma cells have characteristic chromosome 12 amplifications that result in increased levels of MDM2 and CDK4 proteins, which can be stained by immunohistochemistry. In myxoid-round cell liposarcomas and synovial sarcomas, gene fusion products (FUS-CHOP and SSX-SYT, respectively) can be detected by polymerase chain reaction. With gastrointestinal stromal tumors (GISTs), genetic characterization (c-kit overexpression) has been used to identify the tumor; in addition, c-kit overexpression is targeted by imatinib in systemic treatment of the disease.

Germline mutations have also been associated with development of STS. Examples include Li-Fraumeni syndrome (*p53* mutation associated with STS and osteosarcoma), neurofibromatosis type 1 (von Recklinghausen disease; *NF1* mutation associated with progression of neurofibromas to malignant peripheral nerve sheath tumors), and Gardner syndrome (*APC* mutation associated with intra-abdominal desmoid tumors). These syndromes can be inherited. Childhood retinoblastoma, Werner syndrome, Gorlin syndrome, Carney triad, and tuberous sclerosis also carry increased risk of STS.

Tumor Staging and Patient Prognosis

T stage for STS is determined not only by tumor size (T1, 5 cm and below; T2, larger than 5 cm) but also whether the lesion is superficial (T1a or T2a) or deep (T1b or T2b) to the muscle fascia. Nodal disease (N1) is rare in STS patients;

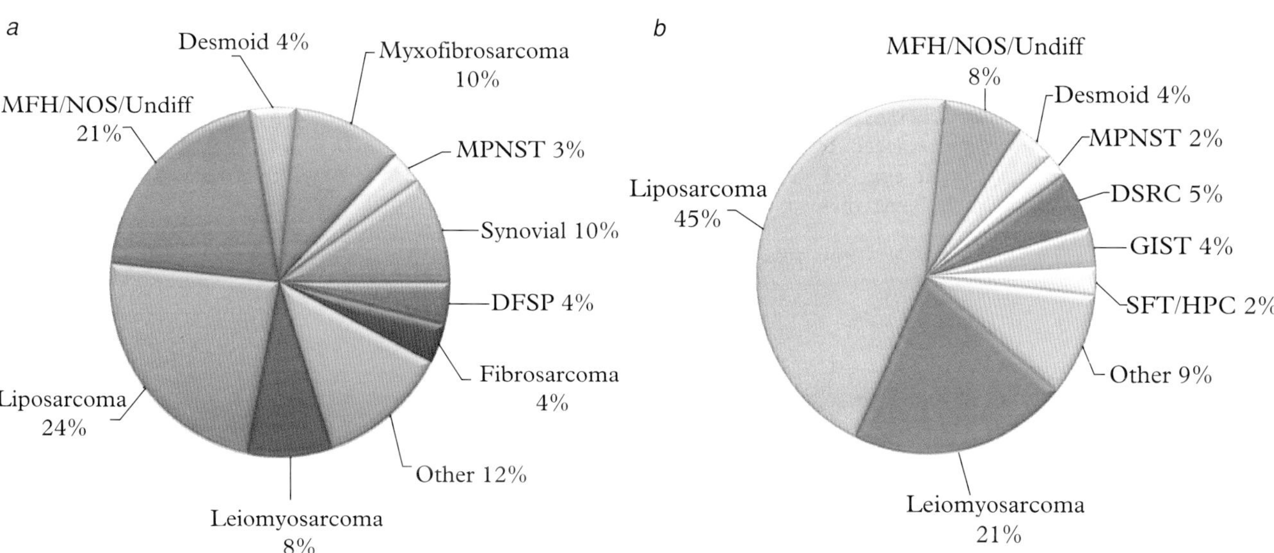

Figure 3 **Histopathologic distribution of (*a*) extremity soft tissue sarcoma (n = 3,123) and (*b*) retroperitoneal/intra-abdominal soft tissue sarcoma (n = 1,241). Data are based on all cases of soft tissue sarcoma evaluated, treated, and followed prospectively at Memorial Sloan-Kettering Cancer Center over a 25-year period. DFSP = dermatofibrosarcoma protuberans; DSRC = desmoplastic small round cell tumor; GIST = gastrointestinal stromal tumor; MFH/NOS/Undiff = malignant fibrous histiocytoma/sarcoma not otherwise specified/undifferentiated pleomorphic sarcoma; MPNST = malignant peripheral nerve sheath tumor; SFT/HPC = solitary fibrous tumor/hemangiopericytoma.**

it does not confer a prognosis as poor as do distant metastases (M1).

The American Joint Committee on Cancer (AJCC) staging system for STS includes not only tumor size and the presence of nodal and metastatic disease, as in adenocarcinomas, but also tumor grade[7]; it is therefore termed TNGM staging. It should be noted, however, that the traditional AJCC grading system, which is based on differentiation (well, moderate, or poor), is not generally applicable to STS. Most sarcoma grading systems incorporate the histology-specific extent of differentiation, mitotic rate, and necrosis. The most widely accepted system, that of the French Federation of Cancer Centers Sarcoma Group (FNLCC), uses these three factors to classify sarcomas as low (G1), intermediate (G2), or high (G3) grade.

TNGM staging classifies STS into four broad stages.[7] Stage I includes all localized, low-grade tumors. Stage II is localized intermediate-grade tumors or high-grade, localized tumors that are small and/or superficial. Stage III disease represents large (> 5 cm), high-grade tumors. Stage III disease also includes STS associated with nodal metastases independent of grade and size. Stage IV disease represents all disease associated with distant metastases.

Outcomes based on TNGM staging are shown in Figure 4. Although stage is a strong prognostic factor, there is a significant degree of variability among patients within each of the localized disease stages (stage I, II, or III) as relates to outcome after surgical resection of the primary tumor. One reason for this limitation may be that the AJCC system does not incorporate multiple prognostic factors important in STS. For example, tumor histology is of significant import; malignant peripheral nerve sheath tumors are associated with poorer disease-specific survival than are myxofibrosarcomas [*see Figure 1a*]. Given these facts, a prognostic nomogram has been developed from retrospective data collected from 2,163 patients treated at Memorial Sloan-Kettering Cancer Center [*see Figure 5*] and validated using a prospectively enrolled cohort of 929 patients treated at the University of California, Los Angeles.[8,9] Tumor size, histologic subtype, and site of disease are all used to improve prediction of patient outcome. Prognostic accuracy is further enhanced by the fact that variables such as size and patient age can be considered continuous variables rather than being divided into a few categories, as they are in staging systems and risk category systems. A Web-based version of the STS nomogram is available for general reference (http://www.mskcc.org/mskcc/html/6181.cfm).

Evaluation and Treatment of Soft Tissue Sarcoma

Surgical excision of STS is the mainstay of our current treatment algorithm. A multidisciplinary approach to the disease is, however, essential, because of the complexity involved in histology-based treatment. The risks and benefits of radiation and chemotherapy as well as adjuvant and neoadjuvant approaches should be carefully weighed when determining the overall treatment plan for a patient with STS. Prevalence of histologic subtypes, treatment-related morbidities, and patterns of recurrence are very different for primary STS of the extremity or superficial trunk versus the abdomen or retroperitoneum. The sections below separately describe extremity and truncal STS and abdominal and retroperitoneal STS.

EXTREMITY AND SUPERFICIAL TRUNCAL STS

Diagnosis and Evaluation

Patients with STS of the extremity and superficial trunk most commonly present with a palpable mass sometimes brought to their attention by a minor trauma in the region. After a careful history and physical examination, a magnetic resonance imaging (MRI) or computed tomographic (CT) scan is indicated for all but small (< 2 cm), superficial lesions, which can be evaluated by excisional biopsy. Cross-sectional imaging provides the size and location of the lesion and identifies involvement of adjacent structures. CT is readily available and less expensive, although MRI can provide better soft tissue definition in the extremity. Histologic subtype, which dictates appropriate treatment, is not, in most instances, well defined by CT or MRI. The exception to this rule is well-differentiated liposarcoma (atypical lipomatous tumors). On cross-sectional imaging, these lesions resemble normal fat in their signal intensity, appear encapsulated, and are associated with thick, internal septations.[10] For tumors located deep to the investing fascia, imaging findings are almost pathognomonic for this subtype, and further workup is not warranted. These lesions should be completely excised with, when possible, a margin of normal muscle or fascial tissue to minimize the risk of local recurrence.

If the STS does not appear consistent with an atypical lipomatous mass, biopsy is indicated prior to defining a treatment plan. Performed improperly, the biopsy of an extremity mass can result in significant oncologic and cosmetic consequences when definitive excision is performed. For this reason, the principles of STS biopsy should be part of the core procedural knowledge for all general surgeons. Although incisional biopsy had been the standard method of diagnosis, core biopsy provides adequate tissue for evaluation in almost all cases and often leads to accurate diagnosis of histologic type and grade.[11] When performing a core biopsy for suspected STS, the surgeon or radiologist should first consider where the surgical incision will be placed. The biopsy site will be excised at the time of surgery and should, therefore, be placed directly adjacent to the planned surgical incision. If multiple cores are taken, they should be angled serially toward a different region of the tumor but always obtained through a single biopsy site.

In the event that core biopsy is insufficient for diagnosis or the lesion is too small to biopsy in this manner, incisional or excisional biopsy is performed. Again, careful planning of the biopsy is essential. The biopsy incision should always be oriented longitudinally along the limb. This is because the definitive surgery for excision of an STS will require resection of the biopsy incision with circumferential margins between 1 and 2 cm (depending on the histologic subtype of the STS). If a biopsy scar is oriented transversely, the diameter of the surgical specimen must increase dramatically to obtain adequate surgical margins. This often means that primary closure of the defect is impossible, and a skin graft or muscle flap is essential to cover the surgical bed.

All STS patients with high-grade disease should undergo a CT scan of the chest to evaluate for pulmonary metastases.

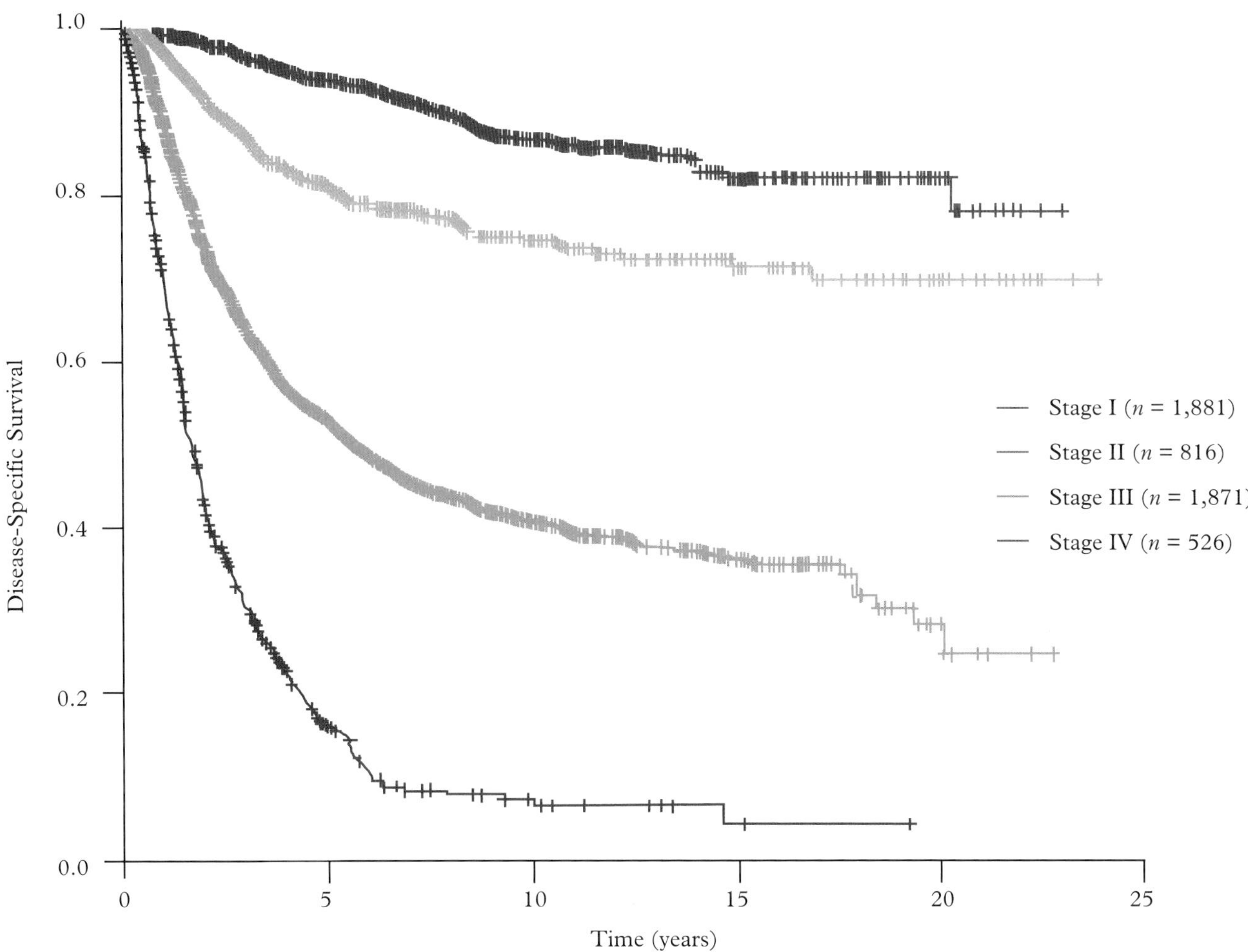

Figure 4 **Disease-specific survival according to American Joint Committee on Cancer TNGM stage based on all cases of soft tissue survival evaluated, treated, and followed prospectively at Memorial Sloan-Kettering Cancer Center over a 25-year period.**

For those with low-grade disease, the risk of metastasis is minimal and chest x-ray is generally adequate and cost-effective. Many STSs are not fluorodeoxyglucose avid; therefore, positron emission tomography (PET) has poor sensitivity for use in the staging of these diseases.

After a pathologic diagnosis of STS has been obtained, the histologic subtype and grade have been identified, and the patient has been assessed for distal metastases, a multidisciplinary treatment plan can be defined. In most cases of localized disease, the primary treatment will be resection or, much less commonly, radiation (discussed below in the context of adjuvant radiation).

Surgical Planning

An algorithm for the treatment of extremity STS is shown in Figure 6.

Prior to 1981, the standard surgical approach to STS of the extremity was amputation. A randomized, controlled trial, coordinated at the National Cancer Institute, defined a role for limb-sparing surgery. The trial followed 43 patients with high-grade tumors treated with amputation or limb-sparing resection with adjuvant radiation. Five years after resection, patients undergoing limb-sparing surgery clearly had a higher incidence of local recurrence, but their disease-free and overall survival rates were no different from those who underwent amputation. Patients experiencing a local recurrence were, in large part, salvaged with additional surgery.[12] Limb-sparing surgery is, therefore, currently considered the standard of care in STS surgery.

Resections should be carefully planned preoperatively to consider functional outcomes and risks of recurrent local disease and distal progression. Importantly, although many extremity lesions are associated with what appears on inspection to be a well-defined pseudocapsule, microscopic disease extends beyond this layer. Therefore, during limb-sparing procedures, a wide margin (1 to 2 cm) of normal tissue should be resected with the specimen to reduce the risk of local recurrence. When the tumor abuts a fascial plane of an adjacent muscle, this layer should be resected with the tumor. When the tumor is superficial, the underlying muscle fascia should always be resected.

When treating extremity STS, the surgeon should consider the relationship between the tumor and nearby neurovascular structures. This will allow him or her to inform the patient about sensory and motor deficits that may be expected after a limb-sparing procedure. It is also vital for surgical planning;

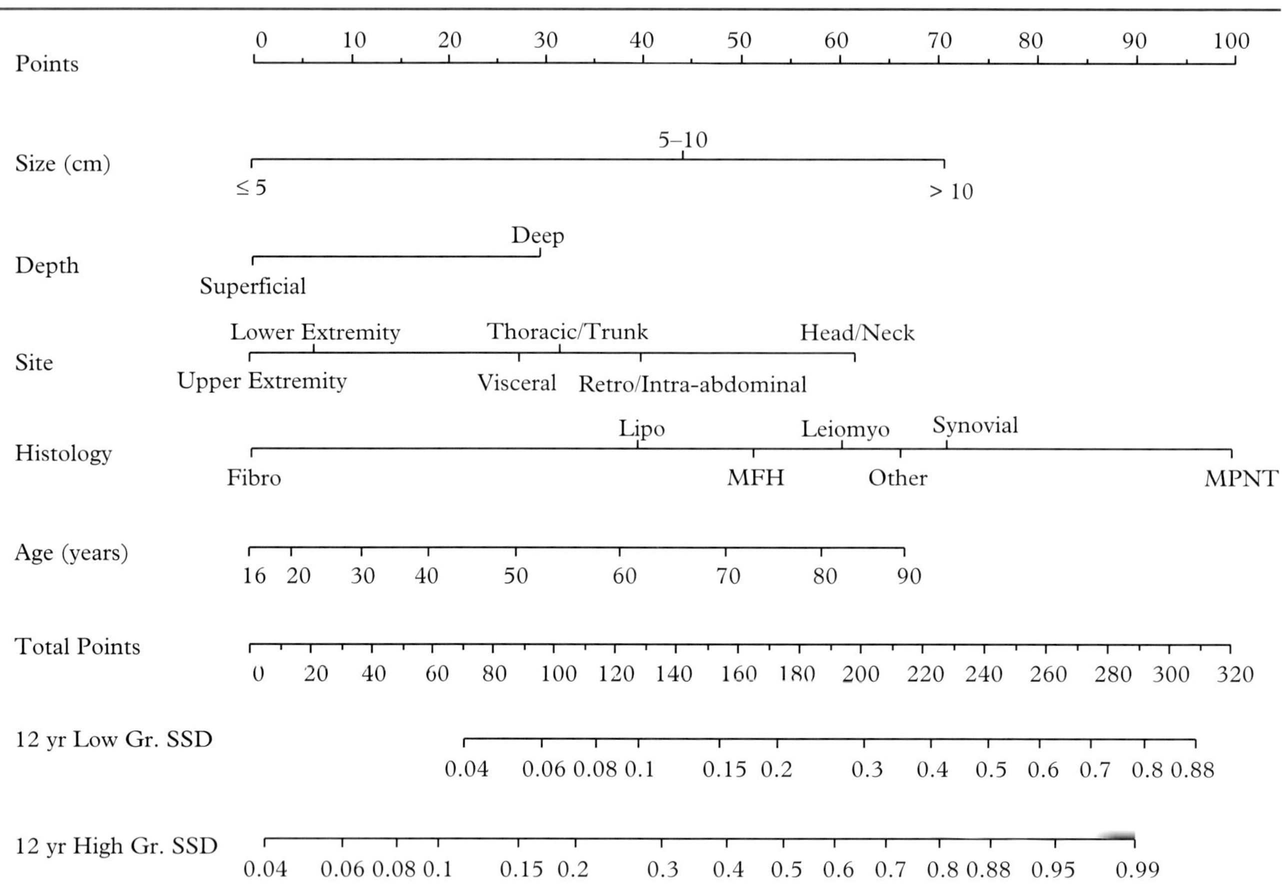

Instructions for Physician: Locate the patient's tumor size on the Size axis. Draw a line straight upward to the **Points** axis to determine how many points toward sarcoma-specific death the patient receives for his tumor size. Repeat this process for the other axes, each time drawing straight upward to the **Points** axis. Sum the points achieved for each predictor and locate this sum on the **Total Points** axis. Draw a line straight down to either the Low Grade or High Grade axis to find the patient's probability of dying from sarcoma within 12 years assuming he or she does not die of another cause first.

Instruction to Patient: "If we had 100 patients exactly like you, we would expect between <predicted percentage from nomogram - 8%> and <predicted percentage + 8%> to die of sarcoma within 12 years if they did not die of another cause first, and death from sarcoma after 12 years is still possible."

Figure 5 **Positive nomogram for prediction of sarcoma-specific death (SSD) at 12 years postresection for patients with soft tissue sarcoma. Fibro = fibrosarcoma; GR = grade; Leiomyo = leiomyosarcoma; Lipo = liposarcoma; MFH = malignant fibrous histiocytoma; MPNT = malignant peripheral nerve sheath tumor.**

nerves, veins, and arteries often limit the extent of the resection to be performed. Whenever possible, vascular structures are skeletonized and major nerves salvaged by resecting perineurium. This will preserve limb function, and if a high-risk lesion is removed with an R1 margin, adjuvant radiation is an option for reducing rates of local recurrence (see below). To avoid amputation when major neurovascular structures are encased by a high-grade tumor, the surgeon may consider advanced maneuvers such as arterial bypass or resection of the sciatic nerve.[13] Venous reconstruction is rarely indicated and when performed is often not successful; compression garments are used to control postoperative symptoms.

Preoperative diagnoses of dermatofibrosarcoma protuberans (DFSP) and myxofibrosarcoma are of particular concern in planning local resection. These lesions often have microscopic tentacles that extend laterally from the lesion.[14–16] DFSP should be resected en bloc with margins of 2 cm, including the underlying fascia, but underlying muscle rarely needs to be removed as this subtype generally does not penetrate the fascia. Myxofibrosarcoma, however, often penetrates fascia and invades muscle and is often multifocal with skip areas. Therefore, excision should be not only wide laterally but also deep with significant surrounding muscle; again, margins of 2 cm should be resected en bloc with the tumor. With either of these subtypes, more conservative resection leads to a high risk of local recurrence. Although recurrence of DFSP in the surgical bed is a difficult local problem, it is almost never associated with distant spread (unless there is histologic evidence of sarcomatous degeneration). Local recurrence of myxofibrosarcoma, however, is potentially more dangerous as it is associated with a high-grade phenotype in as many as 54% of cases. High-grade

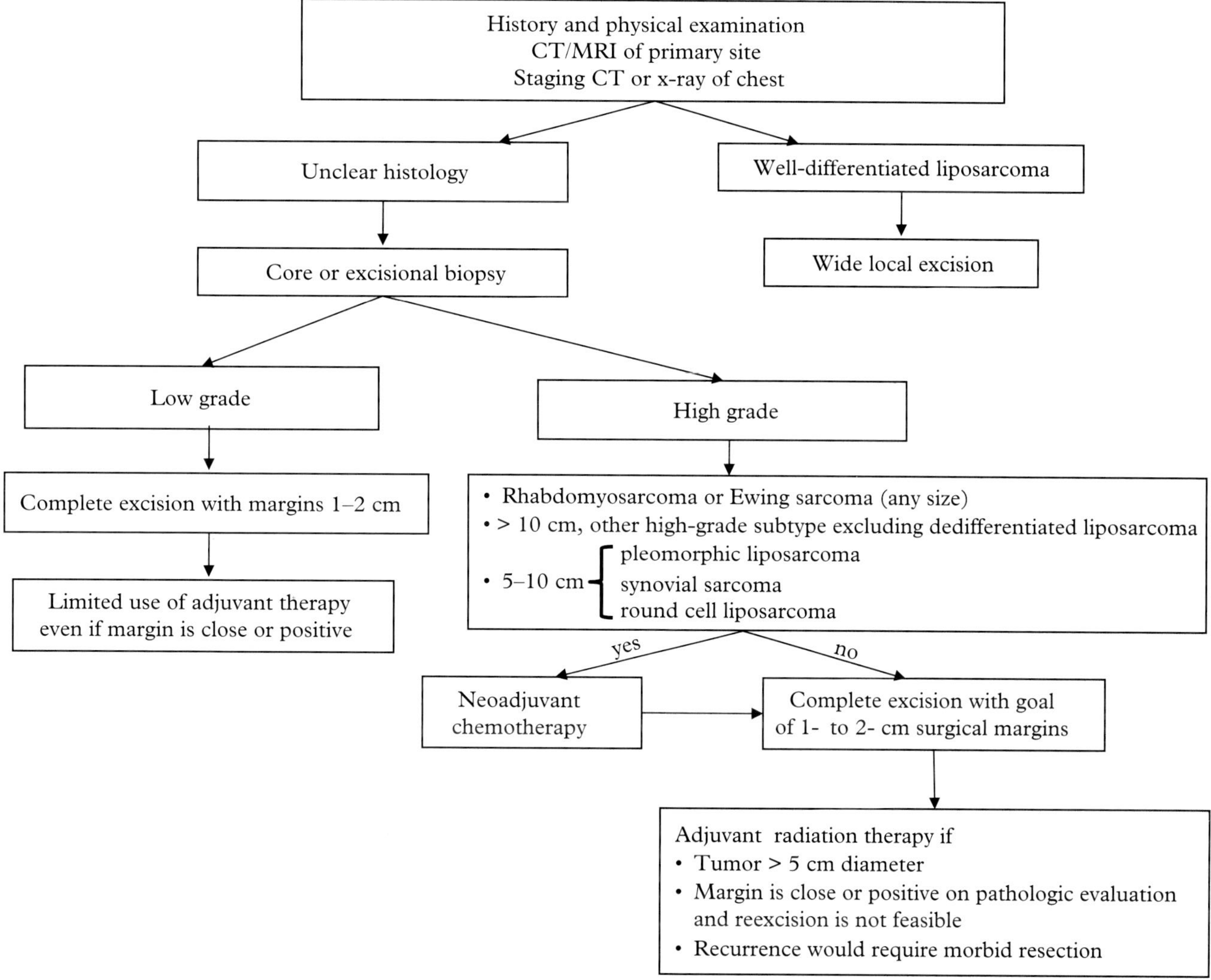

Figure 6 **A treatment algorithm for soft tissue sarcoma of the extremity. CT = computed tomography; MRI = magnetic resonance imaging.**

recurrence of myxofibrosarcoma places the patient at significant risk for metastatic disease.[15,16] Therefore, every attempt should be made to resect myxofibrosarcomas with negative margins, even when they appear as low-grade lesions. Multiple procedures may be required to adequately remove all disease, and reconstruction will often require tissue flaps or a skin graft.

Lymph node metastases are rare in STS and generally occur in the context of epithelioid or clear cell variants of STS.[17] In these cases, sentinel lymph node biopsy has been reported and can give prognostic information as a positive biopsy defines stage III disease. However, this procedure has not been associated with a therapeutic benefit, and no survival advantage has been reported in patients undergoing completion lymph node dissection.[18] For these reasons, the role of sentinel lymph node biopsy in management of STS remains debatable.

Radiation in Extremity STS

Radiation therapy after limb-sparing surgery for STS appears to increase local control but not survival. This conclusion comes from three large randomized, controlled trials. In the first trial, 141 patients with STS of the extremity treated with surgery and chemotherapy were randomized to receive postoperative radiation or no radiation.[19] In the context of both high- and low-grade tumors, the addition of adjuvant radiation significantly reduced the risk of local recurrence (risk at 9 years of 33% versus 4% for low-grade tumors and 19% versus 0% for high-grade tumors). However, radiation afforded no benefit in terms of overall survival. Similarly, brachytherapy applied after complete resection of STS in the extremity and superficial trunk improved local control but did not alter disease-specific survival.[20] Moreover, local benefit of brachytherapy was restricted to patients who presented with high-grade tumors. Because radiation therapy can have long-term complications such as joint fibrosis and secondary malignancies, the potential risk versus benefit of radiation therapy must be carefully weighed for each patient. Radiation therapy is routinely prescribed for high-risk lesions (> 5 cm and high-grade or recurrent tumors that were not previously treated with radiation) with close margins. Given the fact that no trial has shown radiation to improve overall or disease-specific survival, it is reasonable to defer adjuvant therapy when the tumor is low grade or the margin is wide, particularly if a local recurrence could be excised without amputation or major functional impairment.

The decision to prescribe radiation therapy is further complicated in that the modality can be administered either preoperatively or postoperatively. A randomized trial compared these strategies by assigning 190 patients with extremity STS to either adjuvant radiation (66 Gy) or neoadjuvant radiation (50 Gy).[21] This study showed no difference in local control. It did show an increased rate of wound complications in patients treated with radiation prior to resection (35% versus 17%). This difference was most pronounced in patients with STS of the lower extremity. Conversely, patients receiving therapy after resection had a higher risk of long-term fibrotic complications (e.g., joint stiffness), presumably related to the higher dose of radiation.[22] Therefore, preoperative radiation therapy can be an excellent choice for patients with tumors adjacent to a joint or tumors located in the upper extremity that are likely to have close or positive margins. In all other settings, the role of radiation therapy is determined from the final assessment of tumor histology, and margin status following resection determines the contribution radiation may play in the multimodality treatment of extremity STS.

Neoadjuvant Chemotherapy

No prospective study has definitively shown a benefit to administration of adjuvant chemotherapy in STS patients. However, three groups of patients should receive neoadjuvant therapy [*see Figure 6*] because of the high risk of metastasis and/or predicted chemosensitivity of a tumor subtype. The first group includes patients with rhabdomyosarcoma or Ewing sarcoma. Regardless of tumor size, these patients have a high risk of metastasis and are always treated with chemotherapy prior to surgery. The second group encompasses patients with high-grade tumors that are larger than 10 cm. Retrospective studies have demonstrated that neoadjuvant chemotherapy is associated with improved disease-specific survival among these patients.[23] Specifically, neoadjuvant chemotherapy is considered in patients without significant comorbidities and with large, high-grade, round cell liposarcoma, pleomorphic liposarcoma, synovial sarcoma, malignant peripheral nerve sheath tumor, or leiomyosarcoma. However, dedifferentiated liposarcomas, even when they are large and high grade, have a low risk of distant metastasis and are rarely chemosensitive, so initial treatment is surgery when the lesions are resectable.

The third group considered for neoadjuvant chemotherapy includes patients with moderate-size tumors (5 to 10 cm) representing relatively chemosensitive histologies that have a propensity to metastasize. Round cell liposarcoma, pleomorphic liposarcoma, and synovial sarcoma are the most common histologic subtypes treated in this manner.[24–26]

RETROPERITONEAL AND VISCERAL SARCOMAS

Retroperitoneal Disease

The retroperitoneum is the second most common site of STS, although retroperitoneal lesions are significantly less common than those of the extremity [*see Figure 2*]. Patients typically present with a palpable mass or a mass found incidentally on imaging acquired for an unrelated symptom. Patients may have pain and/or symptoms of lower extremity neural compromise. This is particularly true for those with large retroperitoneal tumors, which often remain undetected until they reach sizes greater than 10 cm in diameter. Rarely, patients with retroperitoneal tumors are diagnosed because of paraneoplastic syndromes, such as hypoglycemia related to leiomyosarcoma or solitary fibrous tumor.

A preoperative biopsy is usually needed only if there is suspicion of carcinoma, lymphoma, or germ cell tumor or if the mass appears to be not completely resectable; in other circumstances, biopsy rarely alters the therapeutic plan. Regardless of histologic subtype, the goal of operative intervention is complete gross resection, which can be achieved in 80% of patients. The major hindrance to tumor resectability is involvement of the great or visceral vessels. Retroperitoneal lesions can encase the aorta, vena cava, celiac axis, or porta. In these cases, attempt at resection will leave gross tumor in the surgical bed, and when an R2 resection is anticipated, surgery should be considered only as palliative therapy. Debulking has not been demonstrated to provide survival benefit, and patients with a grossly positive margin have outcomes that are similar to those of patients undergoing no operative intervention [*see Figure 7*].

Involvement of adjacent organs such as the spleen, pancreas, and bowel does not preclude surgical resection. STS associated with these findings can be managed by en bloc resection to achieve R0 or R1 resection. It should be noted that resection of these organs (excluding the kidney) with STS does increase the morbidity associated with surgery.[27,28] If the retroperitoneal lesion involves the kidney, adequate resection can often be achieved by removing only the renal capsule with the tumor. This is possible as retroperitoneal tumors rarely invade the renal parenchyma. Involvement of the kidney hilum, however, will require a nephrectomy to obtain adequate margins.

Visceral Disease

The principles that govern surgical resection of visceral sarcomas are similar to those noted above for retroperitoneal tumors. In all instances, a negative resection margin is the goal of operative intervention. The most common subtype of STS in the viscera is GIST; patients present with gastrointestinal bleeding or bowel obstruction. These tumors are generally well circumscribed and can be removed with a 1 cm gross margin; anatomic resection has not been shown to improve outcomes. For example, in most cases, a gastric GIST can be removed with only a small (1 cm) margin of surrounding tissue, preserving the main body of the stomach. Even with large tumors, this approach allows for preservation of visceral organs and minimizes the complexity of reconstruction.

Adjuvant Therapy in Retroperitoneal and Visceral STS

Retroperitoneal lesions are almost exclusively liposarcoma, leiomyosarcoma, or malignant peripheral nerve sheath tumors. These tumors have low rates of response to chemotherapy, and adjuvant chemotherapy has never been demonstrated to improve survival in this patient population. Radiation therapy, however, is more debatable. Several small, retrospective studies have suggested that its use is associated with reduced

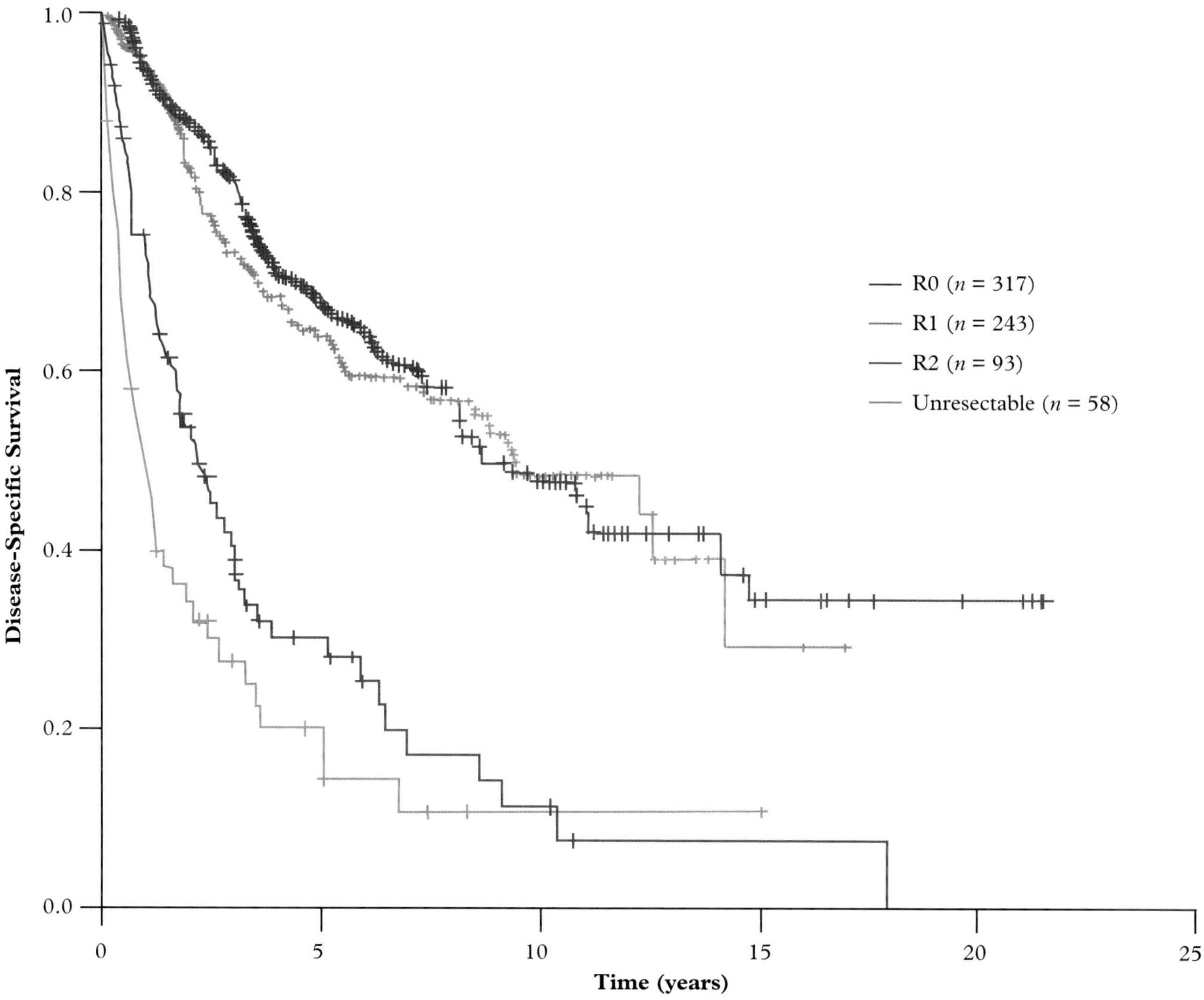

Figure 7 **Disease-specific survival according to extent of resection among patients with retroperitoneal soft tissue sarcoma treated at Memorial Sloan-Kettering Cancer Center over a 25-year period. Outcomes were similar for patients undergoing incomplete gross resection (R2; *n* = 93) and for patients with disease judged unresectable at exploration (*n* = 58).**

risks of local recurrence following surgical resection.[29] Nevertheless, no difference in overall survival has been implied, and selection bias and significant differences in surgical management between institutions remain confounding factors when interpreting the literature. We do understand that adjuvant radiation administered after resection of a retroperitoneal lesion is associated with significant morbidity. Radiation enteritis occurs in up to 60% of patients and can lead to chronic malnutrition, enteric fistulization, and bowel obstruction.[30] Given this drawback of adjuvant radiation therapy, neoadjuvant radiation should be considered if surgical resection is likely to result in positive margins and radiation is to be prescribed. The neoadjuvant approach limits the morbidity of treatment because it can target the radiotherapy to the region at highest risk for microscopic residual disease while limiting the dose to surrounding viscera.

GISTs present a unique case for application of adjuvant treatment because many of them are sensitive to imatinib. This drug targets the c-kit receptor and is a cytostatic reagent. The effect of adjuvant imatinib therapy in high-risk GIST (at least 3 cm in diameter) has been examined in a randomized, controlled trial.[31] In patients treated with adjuvant imatinib, recurrence-free survival at 1 year was increased from 83 to 98%. For this reason, the drug is generally administered in the adjuvant setting to high-risk patients. Imatinib is also of use in the neoadjuvant setting.[32] It can be prescribed in attempt to reduce the size of the tumor and minimize the morbidity of resection when surgical resection of a lesion will prove morbid. Examples of these cases include lesions located at the gastroesophageal junction or rectal lesions. Imatinib can be prescribed in attempt to reduce the size of the tumor and minimize the morbidity or resection.

RECURRENT AND METASTATIC DISEASE

Following surgical resection of STS, the tumor bed is evaluated by cross-sectional imaging every 4 to 6 months,

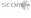

depending on the grade of the tumor. Local recurrence is observed in approximately 10 to 30% of patients with extremity STS and 50% of patients with retroperitoneal lesions.[33] At the time of recurrence, patients should again be staged to rule out metastatic disease.

In the context of extremity recurrence, local resectability is determined as above. Important considerations are the postoperative morbidity of limb-sparing surgery and the ability to spare the neurovascular bundle. The surgeon should excise not only gross tumor and a margin of normal tissue but also the prior surgical incision, drain site, and resected specimen bed. Adjuvant or neoadjuvant radiation or chemotherapy may be considered if the patient was not previously treated with these modalities. Local recurrence is associated with poor prognosis when lesions are high grade, recurrences are greater than 5 cm in diameter, and the recurrence-free interval is short (less than 16 months).[34] Patients whose disease recurs with these features have an increased risk of disease-associated death and should be considered for neoadjuvant chemotherapy or enrolment in clinical trials.

As in the extremity, retroperitoneal recurrence presents a difficult problem and is associated with a poor prognosis. If the lesion is isolated, surgical resection can again be used in an attempt to achieve a cure, and its goal should be negative margins. Neoadjuvant radiation therapy can be considered. As in extremity recurrence, poor prognostic features include large size of tumor recurrence and short disease-free interval, and patients with these features should be considered for neoadjuvant trials. In addition, retroperitoneal liposarcoma patients with local recurrence growth rates exceeding 1 cm per month have an extremely poor prognosis even after aggressive attempts to completely excise all measurable disease. In a retrospective analysis of such patients, surgical resection was not associated with increased survival. Thus, patients with liposarcoma growth rates greater than 1 cm per month should be considered for systemic treatment with novel targeted therapies or conventional chemotherapy.[35]

Indications for Metastasectomy

In patients with high-grade STS, surveillance of the surgical bed is accompanied by cross-sectional imaging of the lung, the most common site of metastatic disease (44%). In most patients, metastases are treated with chemotherapy. The choice of agents is dependent on disease histology and is beyond the scope of this review. Resection, however, is often recommended when disease at the primary site is well controlled and the patient presents with isolated pulmonary metastases. Patients most likely to benefit from metastasectomy include those with metachronous disease and long disease-free intervals, those with slowly growing metastases, and those with a limited number of lesions (one to three). Patients with metastatic disease have an overall survival of less than 20% at 5 years, but long-term survival is observed in patients carefully selected for metastasectomy.[36,37] In these patients, surgery alone may be sufficient for cure as no additional increase in survival has been associated with perioperative chemotherapy.[38]

DESMOID FIBROMATOSIS

Desmoid tumors are rare neoplasms that develop from mesenchymal stem cells.[39] The estimated incidence is only 1,000 cases per year in the United States. Standard management of the disease has included wide resection in the past. Such procedures may be associated with significant morbidity; they can result in short bowel syndrome, incisional hernia, or functional impairment of a limb. Desmoids do not metastasize, however, and this has led to a significant shift in treatment algorithms. Current management strategies do not focus solely on complete eradication of local disease but also on improving functional outcomes for patients with desmoid tumors.

Data supporting current treatment recommendations have been collected only over the last two decades. Large retrospective series showed no difference in the rates of local recurrence following R1 versus R0 resection. This fact was the first that suggested clinicians could adopt a function-preserving approach when planning surgical resection.[40] Subsequently, in the context of recurrent, nonoperable desmoids, it was observed that the growth of tumors was actually self-limited in some cases. An initial period of observation was, therefore, proposed to be a safe treatment option in patients with recurrent disease.[41] The clear benefit thought to be associated with early surgical resection was questioned.

Most recently, an analysis of 142 patients with primary or recurrent desmoid was reported by Fiore and colleagues.[42] This study examined cases in which a frontline, nonoperative approach was employed. Eighty-three of these patients did not receive surgery, radiation, or medical treatment at presentation. They were instead followed with serial imaging every 3 to 6 months. The 5-year progression-free survival in this cohort was 49%. For patients who progressed, surgical resection was considered. If resection would result in significant functional impairment or was not technically feasible, a course of medical management with targeted therapies or cytotoxic therapy was prescribed in the neoadjuvant setting or for long-term maintenance. Sorafenib, tamoxifen, cyclooxygenase-2 inhibitors, imatinib mesylate (Gleevec), and anthracyclines (Doxil) are currently employed for this purpose.[43] No patient with progressive disease was noted in the study by Fiore and colleagues to have unexpected complications or a poor outcome that could be attributed to an initial period of observation. Given these data, many large sarcoma referral centers now uniformly recommend an initial period of observation before undertaking major surgery in the context of desmoid fibromatosis.

Radiation following resection of desmoids has been advocated in both the adjuvant and neoadjuvant settings. Although several analyses have demonstrated an association between radiation and reduced local recurrence after surgery, no difference in overall survival has been observed.[44,45] The long-term complications associated with radiation in a patient population, which is generally diagnosed during their second through fourth decade of life, limit its utility. In the context of a disease that has no metastatic potential, this modality is, therefore, almost always reserved for intractable cases that are symptomatic and have failed all other therapeutic options.

Financial Disclosures: None Reported

References

1. Jemal A, Siegel R, Ward E, et al. Cancer statistics, 2009. CA Cancer J Clin 2009;59: 225–49.
2. Brady J, Liberatore F, Harper P, et al. Angiosarcoma of the liver: an epidemiologic survey. J Natl Cancer Inst 1977;59:1383–5.
3. Stewart FW, Treves N. Lymphangiosarcoma in postmastectomy lymphedema; a report of six cases in elephantiasis chirurgica. Cancer 1948;1:64–81.
4. Cahan WG, Woodard HQ, Higinbotham NL, et al. Sarcoma arising in irradiated bone; report of 11 cases. Cancer 1948;1:3–29.
5. Virtanen A, Pukkala E, Auvinen A. Incidence of bone and soft tissue sarcoma after radiotherapy: a cohort study of 295,712 Finnish cancer patients. Int J Cancer 2006;118: 1017–21.
6. Gladdy RA, Qin LX, Moraco N, et al. Do radiation-associated soft tissue sarcomas have the same prognosis as sporadic soft tissue sarcomas? J Clin Oncol 2010;28:2064–9.
7. American Joint Committee on Cancer. AJCC cancer staging handbook. 6th ed. New York: Springer; 2002.
8. Kattan MW, Leung DH, Brennan MF. Postoperative nomogram for 12-year sarcoma-specific death. J Clin Oncol 2002;20:791–6.
9. Eilber FC, Brennan MF, Eilber FR, et al. Validation of the postoperative nomogram for 12-year sarcoma-specific mortality. Cancer 2004;101:2270–5.
10. Jelinek JS, Kransdorf MJ, Shmookler BM, et al. Liposarcoma of the extremities: MR and CT findings in the histologic subtypes. Radiology 1993;186:455–9.
11. Heslin MJ, Lewis JJ, Woodruff JM, Brennan MF. Core needle biopsy for diagnosis of extremity soft tissue sarcoma. Ann Surg Oncol 1997;4:425–31.
12. Rosenberg SA, Tepper J, Glatstein E, et al. The treatment of soft-tissue sarcomas of the extremities: prospective randomized evaluations of (1) limb-sparing surgery plus radiation therapy compared with amputation and (2) the role of adjuvant chemotherapy. Ann Surg 1982;196:305–15.
13. Brooks AD, Gold JS, Graham D, et al. Resection of the sciatic, peroneal, or tibial nerves: assessment of functional status. Ann Surg Oncol 2002;9:41–7.
14. Farma JM, Ammori JB, Zager JS, et al. Dermatofibrosarcoma protuberans: how wide should we resect? Ann Surg Oncol 2010;17: 2112–8.
15. Mentzel T, Calonje E, Wadden C, et al. Myxofibrosarcoma. Clinicopathologic analysis of 75 cases with emphasis on the low-grade variant. Am J Surg Pathol 1996;20:391–405.
16. Huang HY, Lal P, Qin J, et al. Low-grade myxofibrosarcoma: a clinicopathologic analysis of 49 cases treated at a single institution with simultaneous assessment of the efficacy of 3-tier and 4-tier grading systems. Hum Pathol 2004;35:612–21.
17. Fong Y, Coit DG, Woodruff JM, Brennan MF. Lymph node metastasis from soft tissue sarcoma in adults. Analysis of data from a prospective database of 1772 sarcoma patients. Ann Surg 1993;217:72–7.
18. Maduekwe UN, Hornicek FJ, Springfield DS, et al. Role of sentinel lymph node biopsy in the staging of synovial, epithelioid, and clear cell sarcomas. Ann Surg Oncol 2009; 16:1356–63.
19. Yang JC, Chang AE, Baker AR, et al. Randomized prospective study of the benefit of adjuvant radiation therapy in the treatment of soft tissue sarcomas of the extremity. J Clin Oncol 1998;16:197–203.
20. Pisters PW, Pollock RE, Lewis VO, et al. Long-term results of prospective trial of surgery alone with selective use of radiation for patients with T1 extremity and trunk soft tissue sarcomas. Ann Surg 2007;246:675–81; discussion 81–2.
21. O'Sullivan B, Davis AM, Turcotte R, et al. Preoperative versus postoperative radiotherapy in soft-tissue sarcoma of the limbs: a randomised trial. Lancet 2002;359:2235–41.
22. Davis AM, O'Sullivan B, Turcotte R, et al. Late radiation morbidity following randomization to preoperative versus postoperative radiotherapy in extremity soft tissue sarcoma. Radiother Oncol 2005;75:48–53.
23. Grobmyer SR, Maki RG, Demetri GD, et al. Neo-adjuvant chemotherapy for primary high-grade extremity soft tissue sarcoma. Ann Oncol 2004;15:1667–72.
24. Esnaola NF, Rubin BP, Baldini EH, et al. Response to chemotherapy and predictors of survival in adult rhabdomyosarcoma. Ann Surg 2001;234:215–23.
25. Canter RJ, Qin LX, Maki RG, et al. A synovial sarcoma-specific preoperative nomogram supports a survival benefit to ifosfamide-based chemotherapy and improves risk stratification for patients. Clin Cancer Res 2008;14:8191–7.
26. Eilber FC, Eilber FR, Eckardt J, et al. The impact of chemotherapy on the survival of patients with high-grade primary extremity liposarcoma. Ann Surg 2004;240:686–95; discussion 95–7.
27. Singer S, Antonescu CR, Riedel E, Brennan MF. Histologic subtype and margin of resection predict pattern of recurrence and survival for retroperitoneal liposarcoma. Ann Surg 2003;238:358–70; discussion 70–1.
28. Lewis JJ, Leung D, Woodruff JM, Brennan MF. Retroperitoneal soft-tissue sarcoma: analysis of 500 patients treated and followed at a single institution. Ann Surg 1998;228: 355–65.
29. Pawlik TM, Pisters PW, Mikula L, et al. Long-term results of two prospective trials of preoperative external beam radiotherapy for localized intermediate- or high-grade retroperitoneal soft tissue sarcoma. Ann Surg Oncol 2006;13:508–17.
30. Kinsella TJ, Sindelar WF, Lack E, et al. Preliminary results of a randomized study of adjuvant radiation therapy in resectable adult retroperitoneal soft tissue sarcomas. J Clin Oncol 1988;6:18–25.
31. Dematteo RP, Ballman KV, Antonescu CR, et al. Adjuvant imatinib mesylate after resection of localised, primary gastrointestinal stromal tumour: a randomised, double-blind, placebo-controlled trial. Lancet 2009;373: 1097–104.
32. Gold JS, Dematteo RP. Neoadjuvant therapy for gastrointestinal stromal tumor (GIST): racing against resistance. Ann Surg Oncol 2007;14:1247–8.
33. Singer S, Corson JM, Demetri GD, et al. Prognostic factors predictive of survival for truncal and retroperitoneal soft-tissue sarcoma. Ann Surg 1995;221:185–95.
34. Eilber FC, Brennan MF, Riedel E, et al. Prognostic factors for survival in patients with locally recurrent extremity soft tissue sarcomas. Ann Surg Oncol 2005;12:228–36.
35. Park JO, Qin LX, Prete FP, et al. Predicting outcome by growth rate of locally recurrent retroperitoneal liposarcoma: the one centimeter per month rule. Ann Surg 2009;250: 977–82.
36. Temple LK, Brennan MF. The role of pulmonary metastasectomy in soft tissue sarcoma. Semin Thorac Cardiovasc Surg 2002;14:35–44.
37. Billingsley KG, Burt ME, Jara E, et al. Pulmonary metastases from soft tissue sarcoma: analysis of patterns of diseases and postmetastasis survival. Ann Surg 1999;229: 602–10; discussion 10–2.
38. Canter RJ, Qin LX, Downey RJ, et al. Perioperative chemotherapy in patients undergoing pulmonary resection for metastatic soft-tissue sarcoma of the extremity: a retrospective analysis. Cancer 2007;110:2050–60.
39. Wu C, Nik-Amini S, Nadesan P, et al. Aggressive fibromatosis (desmoid tumor) is derived from mesenchymal progenitor cells. Cancer Res 2010;70:7690–8.
40. Merchant NB, Lewis JJ, Woodruff JM, et al. Extremity and trunk desmoid tumors: a multifactorial analysis of outcome. Cancer 1999;86:2045–52.
41. Phillips SR, A'Hern R, Thomas JM. Aggressive fibromatosis of the abdominal wall, limbs and limb girdles. Br J Surg 2004;91:1624–9.
42. Fiore M, Rimareix F, Mariani L, et al. Desmoid-type fibromatosis: a front-line conservative approach to select patients for surgical treatment. Ann Surg Oncol 2009;16: 2587–93.
43. de Camargo VP, Keohan ML, D'Adamo DR, et al. Clinical outcomes of systemic therapy for patients with deep fibromatosis (desmoid tumor). Cancer 2010;116:2258–65.
44. Francis WP, Zippel D, Mack LA, et al. Desmoids: a revelation in biology and treatment. Ann Surg Oncol 2009;16:1650–4.
45. Ballo MT, Zagars GK, Pollack A, et al. Desmoid tumor: prognostic factors and outcome after surgery, radiation therapy, or combined surgery and radiation therapy. J Clin Oncol 1999;17:158–67.

9 BENIGN BREAST DISEASE

*Helen Cappuccino, MD, FACS, Ermelinda Bonaccio, MD, and Swati Kulkarni, MD, FACS**

Clinicians should have an understanding of the evaluation and management of breast disorders. One in two women will consult a health care provider for a breast-related complaint during her lifetime.[1] The fundamental task facing a physician who is evaluating a patient with a breast concern is to determine whether the abnormality is benign or malignant. Even though most breast complaints do not result in a diagnosis of cancer, any woman presenting with a breast complaint should receive a comprehensive evaluation. In this chapter, we focus on the evaluation and management of benign breast conditions.

Screening Recommendations

In the absence of a specific breast complaint, breast cancer can be detected by screening. The three main methods of breast cancer screening are breast self-examination (BSE), clinical breast examination (CBE), and screening mammography.[2] American Cancer Society (ACS) screening guidelines for women aged 40 years and older specify that mammography and CBE should be included as part of an annual health examination.[3] In addition, health care providers should tell women about the benefits and limitations of BSE, stressing the importance of promptly reporting any new breast symptoms. There is currently no role for routine screening ultrasonography or screening magnetic resonance imaging (MRI) in the general population.

BREAST SELF-EXAMINATION

In BSE, the patient inspects and palpates both breasts and axillae. One might assume that instruction in BSE would improve breast cancer detection. However there is no conclusive evidence that BSE is of significant value in this regard. Many self-detected tumors are found incidentally, not during BSE. Furthermore, the best technique for BSE and optimal frequency has not been established. The ASC recommends counseling patients on the benefits and limitations of BSE as a part of the breast cancer screening process that also includes mammography and CBE.[3]

CLINICAL BREAST EXAMINATION

In CBE, a qualified health care professional carries out a complete examination of the breasts and axillae. As with BSE, there is little evidence indicating that annual or semiannual CBE increases breast cancer detection rates.[4] Nevertheless, it is prudent for the clinician to include CBE as part of the physical examination performed on every female patient.

SCREENING MAMMOGRAPHY

Screening mammography refers to the imaging of asymptomatic women to detect early, clinically occult breast cancers. Mammography is the only breast imaging modality proven to reduce mortality from breast cancer. The Swedish Two-County Trial updated their data in 2000 and demonstrated a 32% reduction in breast cancer mortality in women invited to screening.[5] Based on the findings from these trials, women should begin annual screening mammography at age 40. There are subgroups of women at high risk for breast carcinoma who may benefit from screening at a younger age, although no randomized controlled trials support these recommendations.[6] Currently, there is no accepted upper age limit for mammographic screening; however, the presence of significant comorbidities reducing life expectancy to less than 10 years should be considered when ordering a screening mammogram in women over the age of 70.

Digital mammography is becoming more common in many centers. Results from a large prospective multicenter trial comparing digital to conventional film mammography demonstrated no significant difference in cancer detection rates.[7] However, digital mammography was found to be more sensitive than film in three subgroups: women less than 50 years of age, women with radiographically dense breasts, and women who were pre- or perimenopausal.[8]

Evaluating Breast Complaints and Masses

HISTORY

Evaluation of a woman with a breast complaint should include a thorough history, a physical examination, and appropriate diagnostic studies. A complete history of the current complaint should include onset, duration, and progression of symptoms. Precipitating and ameliorating factors should be noted, as should the relationship of palpable abnormalities, pain, and tenderness to the menstrual cycle. Recent history of trauma to the breast, prior infections, fine-needle aspirations (FNAs), core biopsies, and surgical biopsies should also be recorded. Medical records, including operative reports and corresponding pathology and radiographic reports, should be reviewed carefully. The treating clinician should obtain and review prior breast imaging as part of the patient's history. SCORE

Symptoms or complaints involving the breast should be evaluated in the context of historical breast cancer risk data. Historical risk data include (1) history of the duration and type of hormone use (oral contraceptives and hormone replacement therapy); (2) reproductive history (age at menarche, age at menopause, age at first live birth, number of gestations and completed pregnancies); and (3) complete family history of all malignancies on both the maternal and SCORE

* The authors and editors gratefully acknowledge the contributions of the previous authors, Doreen M. Agnese, MD, FACS, Stephen P. Povoski, MD, FACS, and Wiley W. Souba, MD, ScD, FACS, to the development and writing of this chapter.

SCORE Indicates the text is tied to a SCORE learning objective. Please see the HTML version online at www.acssurgery.com.

the paternal side, including the age at diagnosis. The remainder of the patient's general history should be evaluated with a focus on significant medical problems that may impact surgical planning. Medications and supplements that may contain estrogen-like substances and social history (especially tobacco, alcohol, work, exercise, and even sexual history as it pertains to breast stimulation) can be relevant.

PHYSICAL EXAMINATION

The breasts should be thoroughly examined in the upright and supine positions. Breast asymmetry and overall appearance of the skin, nipples, and areola should be observed with the patient upright. Any erythema, induration, peau d'orange, nipple retraction, and ulceration should be noted. Occult skin retraction can be demonstrated by having the woman raise her hands above her head and then place them against her hips. Bimanual examination of the breast tissue can facilitate identification of masses in women with dense breast tissue. In the supine position, turning the patient to either side to disperse breast tissue facilitates a more thorough examination for women with larger breasts. For the ptotic breast, palpation of the breast tissue between the thumb and index finger of the same hand may be useful. Location, mobility, and characteristics of masses and thickening should be noted, including size, firmness, presence of smooth or irregular borders, overlying skin changes, consistency, and areas of tenderness. Drawings or digital images can be made to document physical findings. All tissue between the clavicle and costal margins should be palpated, from the lateral sternal border to the posterior axillary line. Patients should also be checked for nipple discharge. Axillary, clavicular, and cervical lymph node basins should also be palpated in the upright and supine positions. The presence of adenopathy, including the size, consistency (hard versus soft), number, laterality, location, and mobility of the lymph nodes, should be documented.

DIAGNOSTIC STUDIES

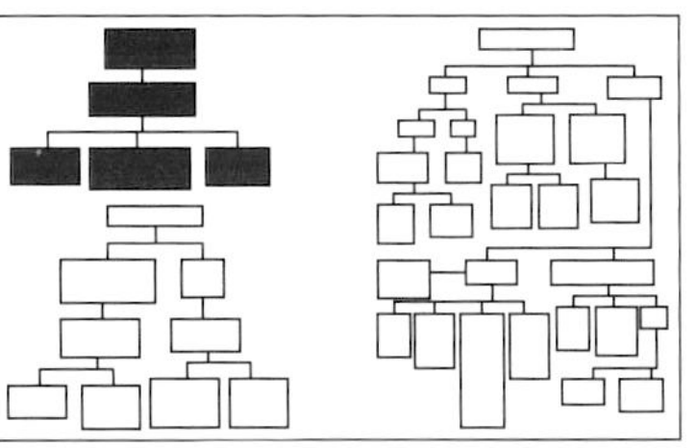

Diagnostic Mammography and Targeted Ultrasonography

As mentioned previously, screening mammography refers to imaging of an asymptomatic woman. Diagnostic mammography, on the other hand, refers to imaging a woman with either a clinical complaint (a palpable lump, thickening, focal pain, discharge) or an abnormal screening mammogram. The initial workup of an abnormal screening mammogram involves additional mammographic imaging directed by a radiologist, which determines if the perceived abnormality is a real lesion. Spot and rolled views (with or without magnification) can sometimes demonstrate that the perceived abnormality was actually only the result of overlapping glandular tissue and there is no underlying lesion. The diagnostic mammogram report would then be given a final assessment 1 (negative), and the patient should return to annual screening mammography.

When an abnormality is detected and the patient needs additional mammographic and/or sonographic imaging, the initial screening mammogram in these patients is given a final assessment 0 [*see Table 1*]. Women with a Breast Imaging Reporting and Data System (BI-RADS) 1 or 2 should continue to undergo routine annual mammography.[8] Women with a BI-RADS 3 should undergo short-term follow–up, which typically involves an ipsilateral mammogram in 6 months followed by a bilateral study at 12 and 24 months. A finding in this category should have a less than 2% risk of malignancy based on morphologic and distribution features.[9,10] Any interval progression at follow-up should prompt a biopsy. Patients with a BI-RADS category 4 or 5 lesion require a tissue diagnosis. As an adjunct to diagnostic mammography, high-frequency breast ultrasonography is often used in the diagnostic workup of a mass and can distinguish between a solid and a cystic lesion. If a solid mass is visualized sonographically, ultrasound-guided core-needle biopsy (CNB) can be performed for pathologic diagnosis.

PERCUTANEOUS CORE BIOPSY

Breast biopsies should be performed percutaneously whenever possible, using stereotactic, ultrasound, or MRI guidance. CNB with an automated gun or vacuum-assisted device has been confirmed in multiple studies to be a reliable alternative to surgical excision.[11,12] Stereotactic (mammographic) guidance is typically used to biopsy indeterminate or suspicious calcifications as well as masses or densities that are sonographically occult. Ultrasound guidance is used to biopsy masses that can be visualized sonographically and is the most cost-effective type of image-guided core biopsy.[13] MRI guided CNB is reserved for lesions that are occult to conventional imaging. The benefit of CNB over FNA is that it provides tissue for histologic rather than cytologic evaluation.

With any image-guided approach, it is important to confirm that the pathologic results are concordant with the imaging findings. Treatment decisions should be based on both pathologic findings and the appearance of the abnormality on diagnostic imaging. Discordant imaging and pathologic findings should prompt a surgical biopsy.

OTHER IMAGING MODALITIES

Magnetic Resonance Imaging

MRI is an imaging modality that uses strong magnetic fields to create a cross-sectional image. Breast MRI requires a specific coil and peripheral intravenous injection of a gadolinium-based contrast medium. Contrast-enhanced breast MRI has been shown to have a high sensitivity for detection of invasive breast cancer and can find both invasive and in situ carcinomas that are occult to conventional imaging. In practice, use of breast MRI is predominantly limited to women diagnosed with breast carcinoma and women at increased risk of developing breast cancer.

At present, there is no indication for the use of positron emission tomographic scans in the diagnostic workup of breast diseases outside a clinical trial. A number of new modalities are being investigated, such as positron emission mammography, breast-specific gamma imaging, tomosynthesis, and coned-beam computed tomography. Although some of these modalities are approved by the Food and Drug Administration (FDA), they are not currently standard practice.

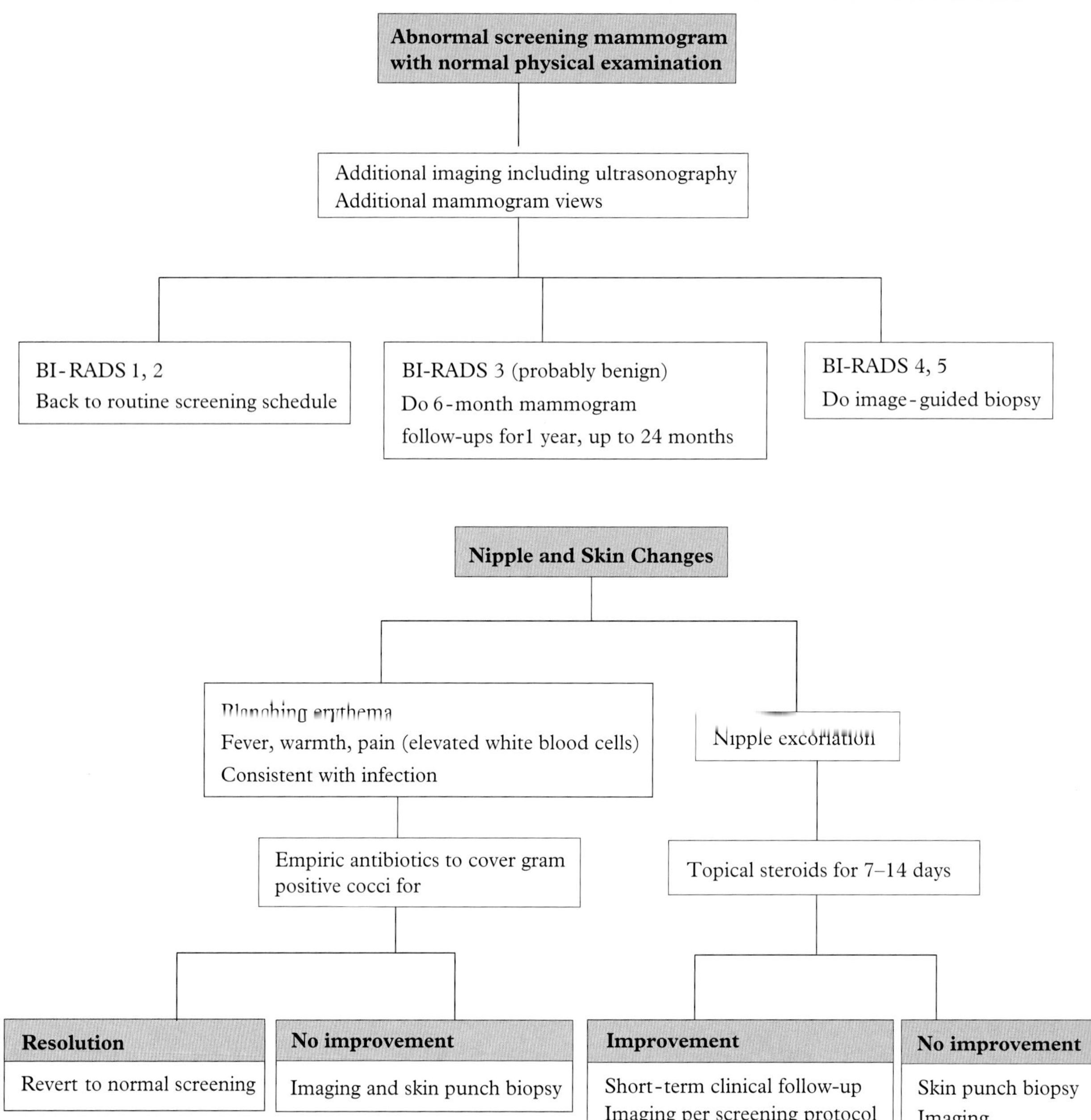
Abnormal screening mammogram with normal physical examination
Additional imaging including ultrasonography
Additional mammogram views
BI-RADS 1, 2
Back to routine screening schedule
BI-RADS 3 (probably benign)
Do 6-month mammogram
follow-ups for1 year, up to 24 months
BI-RADS 4, 5
Do image-guided biopsy
Nipple and Skin Changes
Blanching erythema
Fever, warmth, pain (elevated white blood cells)
Consistent with infection
Nipple excoriation
Empiric antibiotics to cover gram positive cocci for
Topical steroids for 7–14 days
Resolution
Revert to normal screening
No improvement
Imaging and skin punch biopsy
Improvement
Short-term clinical follow-up
Imaging per screening protocol
No improvement
Skin punch biopsy
Imaging

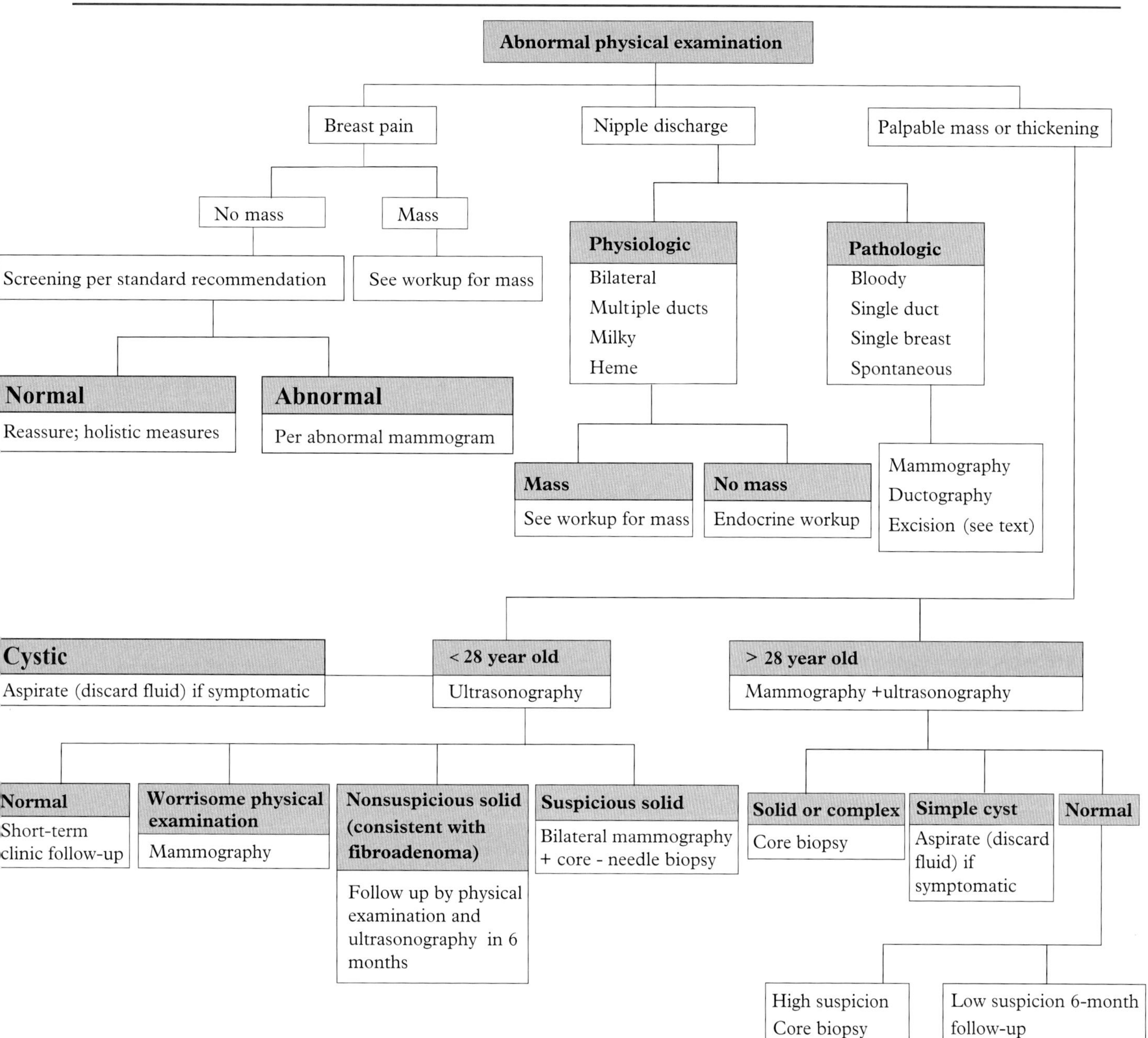
Abnormal physical examination
Breast pain
Nipple discharge
Palpable mass or thickening
No mass
Mass
Screening per standard recommendation
See workup for mass
Normal
Reassure; holistic measures
Abnormal
Per abnormal mammogram
Physiologic
Bilateral
Multiple ducts
Milky
Heme
Pathologic
Bloody
Single duct
Single breast
Spontaneous
Mass
See workup for mass
No mass
Endocrine workup
Mammography
Ductography
Excision (see text)
Cystic
Aspirate (discard fluid) if symptomatic
< 28 year old
Ultrasonography
> 28 year old
Mammography +ultrasonography
Normal
Short-term clinic follow-up
Worrisome physical examination
Mammography
Nonsuspicious solid (consistent with fibroadenoma)
Follow up by physical examination and ultrasonography in 6 months
Suspicious solid
Bilateral mammography + core - needle biopsy
Solid or complex
Core biopsy
Simple cyst
Aspirate (discard fluid) if symptomatic
Normal
High suspicion Core biopsy
Low suspicion 6-month follow-up

Table 1 American College of Radiology Breast Imaging Reporting and Data System (BI-RADS)

Category	Assessment	Description/Recommendation
0	Additional imaging evaluation required	Additional imaging recommended
1	Negative finding	Nothing to comment on; routine screening recommended
2	Benign finding	Negative mammogram, but interpreter may wish to describe a finding; routine screening recommended
3	Probably benign finding	Very high probability of benignity; short-interval follow-up suggested to establish stability
4	Suspicious abnormality	Probability of malignancy; biopsy should be considered
5	Abnormality highly suggestive of malignancy	High probability of cancer; appropriate action should be taken

The report generated after the diagnostic workup is completed will have a final assessment of 1 to 5. The Breast Imaging Reporting and Data System (BI-RADS) lexicon was developed to standardize mammographic reports.[6] It defines the final assessment categories, which informs the referring physician about the likelihood of malignancy.

General Management of Clinical Findings in the Breast

PALPABLE MASS

A dominant breast mass is defined as a discrete lump that is distinctly different from the surrounding breast tissue. Overall, approximately 10% of dominant breast masses are malignant. The workup and management of a discrete breast mass are governed by the age of the patient, the patient's family and medical history, the physical characteristics of the palpable lesion, and findings on diagnostic imaging.

SOLID MASSES

The likelihood of malignancy is greater when the patient is 40 years of age or older and when the mass is solid, hard, immobile and has irregular borders. Appropriate imaging studies, including mammography and ultrasonography should be done. In women over 30 years of age or with a significant family history of breast cancer, contralateral mammography is indicated to rule out synchronous lesions. If the mass is clinically suspicious, CNB or surgical biopsy should be performed for tissue diagnosis even in the setting of negative imaging.

CYSTIC MASSES

Cysts are a common cause of dominant breast masses, particularly in premenopausal women. They can be differentiated from solid lesions by means of ultrasonography. Sonographically, simple cysts tend to be oval, lobulated, and anechoic, with well-defined borders. Complex cysts with indistinct walls or solid components are more likely to be associated with carcinoma; therefore, imaging-guided aspiration, biopsy, or both should be performed. For asymptomatic simple cysts, no further intervention is required. For symptomatic cysts, FNA is appropriate. If the mass does not disappear completely after aspiration, then biopsy of any residual solid component should be performed. Clear fluid should not be sent for cytologic analysis because of the high likelihood of a false positive result. Bloody fluid obtained from a cyst aspiration should be sent for cytologic examination.

VAGUE THICKENING OR NODULARITY

Normal breast texture is often heterogeneous, particularly in premenopausal women. Vague thickening or tender or nontender areas of nodularity are frequently detected by the patient or the clinician. It is important to distinguish this vague breast thickening or nodularity from a discrete or dominant breast mass. In clinical practice, the first step in evaluating a nodular area is to compare it with the corresponding area of the opposite breast. Symmetrical tender nodularity—for example, in the upper outer quadrant of both breasts—is rarely pathologic. These areas often represent fibrocystic changes that may resolve with time and thus should be followed clinically. Asymmetrical areas of vague thickening in premenopausal women should be reexamined after one or two menstrual cycles. If the asymmetry persists, the patient should undergo mammography if she is 35 years of age or older and has not undergone a mammogram within the last 6 months. If the mass is clinically suspicious, a surgical biopsy for adequate sampling should be performed even in the setting of negative imaging.

Management of Specific Benign Breast Complaints

MASTALGIA

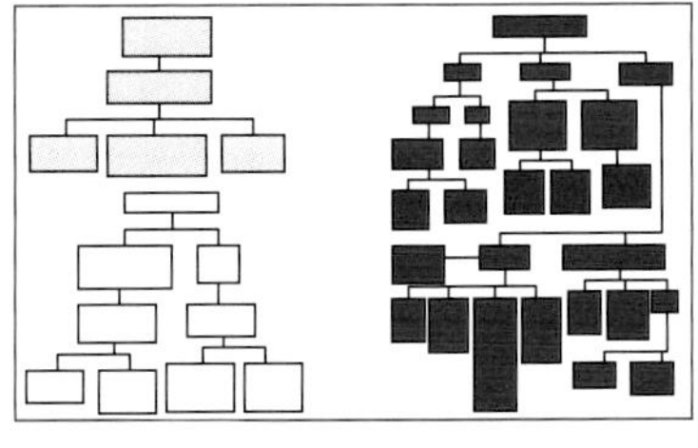

One of the most common complaints for which a woman seeks a doctor's opinion is mastalgia. Mastalgia (breast pain) can be cyclical or noncyclical and may be idiopathic. Often it is related to other common processes that occur in the breast, such as fibrocystic change or infection. Two thirds of women will complain about mastalgia during the course of their lives.[14] Its cause is poorly understood. A history of the onset and course of the pain are important, especially as it relates to a woman's menstrual cycle. Although rarely a presenting complaint of breast cancer, mastalgia often causes considerable concern for patients. Mastalgia resolves spontaneously in 20 to 30% of cases but can recur in up to 60% of women. Some studies suggest a relationship with caffeine intake, premenstrual syndrome, and serum hormone levels.[15] Frequently, after a complete history and physical examination to rule out a malignancy, the clinician is left treating mastalgia of unknown etiology. Many women respond well to reassurance[14,16] and simple interventions, such as wearing a properly fitted bra and reducing caffeine intake. Commonly used remedies, including evening primrose oil, vitamin E, and vitamin B_6, have limited evidence supporting their use to relieve symptoms.[17,18] If simple interventions are not successful, consideration can be given to pharmacologic agents including nonsteroidal antiinflammatory drugs (NSAIDs), danazol, bromocriptine, and tamoxifen.[15,18,19] In extreme and otherwise nonresponsive cases, surgical excision of the tender area can be used.[20]

FIBROCYSTIC CHANGE

Fibrocystic change is often referred to by the misnomer fibrocystic disease. It is a common finding in women who are menstruating, occurring almost exclusively between the ages of 30 and 50. Fibrocystic change is characterized by lumpy or "cobblestone" breasts with ridges of tissue appreciated on palpation. The change is considered a normal variant. If a dominant mass is found in a woman with fibrocystic breasts, diagnostic imaging and biopsy should be undertaken to rule out malignancy. Symptoms generally improve with oral contraceptive use and abate with menopause. Treatment is geared toward symptomatic relief using the agents listed above for mastalgia and reassuring the patient that there is no worrisome etiology or increased risk of developing breast cancer.

NIPPLE DISCHARGE: PAPILLOMAS, DUCTAL ECTASIA, AND GALACTORRHEA

Nipple discharge is the third most common breast complaint after mastalgia and breast mass.[21] In the majority of cases, the discharge is caused by noncancerous processes, including (1) physiologic discharge, (2) ductal ectasia, and (3) intraductal papilloma. However, malignancy should be ruled out as part of the workup for nonphysiologic discharge.[21] For women presenting with this concern, the clinician should elicit a history that includes the characteristics of the discharge. The initial question to the patient should be whether the discharge is spontaneous or self-induced. If self-induced, the patient should be counseled to stop eliciting the discharge. If spontaneous, the characteristics are important in determining the cause, including whether it is unilateral or bilateral, milky, bloody, clear, posttraumatic, or cyclical. The history should also include questions pertaining to symptoms associated with an endocrine disorder (hypothyroidism) or to an intracranial etiology such as a pituitary tumor (amenorrhea, visual disturbances, and headache). A history of recent medication changes should also be taken because numerous medications are associated with galactorrhea (H_2 receptor antagonists, antihypertensives, antidepressants, and antidopaminergic agents).[21]

To understand physiologic nipple discharge, an understanding of breast physiology is critical. During pregnancy, high circulating levels of estrogen result in development of the breast into a predominantly glandular structure. With parturition, estrogen production decreases, resulting in prolactin secretion and increased secretory activity, whereas oxytocin results in "letting down" or ejection of milk into the ducts. A suckling infant or similar stimuli (i.e., sexual breast stimulation, postthoracotomy syndrome)[22] may result in oxytocin release. Any of these conditions can result in physiologic discharge, which is usually milky and bilateral. Pregnancy can result in galactorrhea from the second trimester to as late as 2 years postpartum. Elevated thyroid-stimulating hormone (TSH) levels can also be associated with elevated prolactin levels.

Nipple discharge characterized as nonbloody but darker green or brown is associated with ductal ectasia, a benign condition characterized by dilated ducts resulting from obstruction with keratin plugs, and subsequent inflammation and secretions. Ductal ectasia can arise in one or multiple ducts. Dilated ducts are visualized on ultrasonography and on ductography. The characteristics of the discharge from ductal ectasia can be similar to those seen with papillomas and ductal carcinoma in situ (DCIS) and are therefore included in the differential diagnosis of pathologic nipple discharge.

Bloody nipple discharge can appear as bright red, rusty, brown, or green and is considered pathologic. It is characteristically unilateral and emanates from a single duct. Although the most common etiology of this remains a solitary intraductal papilloma, DCIS and invasive breast cancer can also present with pathologic discharge. Of patients presenting with such a discharge, 17% have malignancy, 65% have papillomas, and the remainder have other benign lesions.[23]

A thorough physical examination that includes a search for signs of an endocrine disturbance should be conducted (e.g., thyromegaly, visual field defects). As part of the breast evaluation, if nipple discharge is not apparent, the clinician should gently squeeze the nipple to determine whether the discharge is coming from a single duct or multiple ducts and whether the discharge is bilateral. The breast should be evaluated for the presence of a discrete mass that may be associated with an underlying carcinoma.

Historical and physical findings suggestive of an endocrine disorder should prompt the clinician to order TSH and prolactin levels. An MRI of the brain should be ordered to rule out a prolactin-secreting tumor of the pituitary if prolactin levels are elevated. In women of childbearing age, a pregnancy test should also be ordered as part of the workup of galactorrhea. Women with medication-induced bilateral discharge should be counseled about the etiology and reassured.

For patients who are found to have pathologic discharge, the diagnostic workup should begin with bilateral diagnostic mammography. If imaging reveals a focal lesion or microcalcifications, tissue diagnosis should be obtained. Ductography may be able to identify an intraductal lesion and guide surgical planning. Ductography involves cannulating the discharging duct with a small catheter and then injecting a small amount of radiographic contrast medium. Magnified mammographic views are then obtained, and lesions within the duct are identified as either a filling defect or an abrupt cutoff. More recently, ductoscopy, which uses a flexible or rigid fibroscopic ductoscope to cannulate the nipple, can be used to isolate areas of pathology for excision. In skilled hands, it can be combined with (brush) cytology for improved accuracy.[24,25]

The role of cytologic analysis remains controversial. FNA is also unreliable in evaluating patients with drainage and/or papillomatous disease[26] (and many feel that even CNB of endoductal lesions remains inadequate for definitive diagnosis of these lesions).[27–30] Therefore, surgical excision is recommended given the incidence of concomitant premalignant and malignant disease in the setting of pathologic nipple discharge.[27,31] When the location of the intraductal pathology is identified prior to surgical resection, a more limited resection (i.e., single duct excision) of the disease is possible.[32] If the duct is peripheral in the breast, the duct can be localized via needle localization. When possible, single duct excision is preferred because it preserves nipple sensation and the ability to breastfeed. In cases where the focal pathology cannot be isolated preoperatively, or in the case of multiduct involvement, a major duct excision is more appropriate. This involves removing all of the central lactiferous ducts and sinuses, preventing further discharge. Both procedures can be done on an outpatient basis and require only local anesthesia and intravenous sedation.

FIBROEPITHELIAL LESIONS: FIBROADENOMA AND PHYLLODES TUMOR

Fibroepithelial lesions encompass a spectrum of breast abnormalities ranging from the fibroadenoma (FA) to the phyllodes tumor (PT). FAs are the most common benign breast lesions and occur most frequently in the second and third decades of life. Their natural history is one of stability or slow growth. Patients will often give a history of a solitary nontender nodule. Physical examination will usually demonstrate a well-defined solitary, rubbery, and mobile nodule. Ultrasonography is particularly useful in younger women and demonstrates a well defined oval or round hypoechoic mass with discrete margins. Mammography should be obtained (in addition to ultrasonography) in women over 35 years of age and typically demonstrates a well-defined radiopaque mass with smooth borders. If the history, physical examination, and imaging are consistent with an FA, careful clinical follow-up is reasonable with ultrasonography and CBE at 6-month intervals to assess the stability of the lesion. When the diagnosis is uncertain, CNB should be performed. For women who request excision of a benign FA, enucleation of the lesion is adequate. Conversely, if the lesion increases in size during clinical follow-up, surgical excision is recommended to rule out a PT.

PTs are unusual, representing only 0.3 to .5% of breast neoplasms.[33] They have the same clinical appearance and imaging characteristics as FAs, but unlike FAs, they are characterized by a clinical history of rapid growth and have larger dimensions. With increased screening, more PTs are being discovered mammographically. Given that these lesions do not have any features on imaging that would be helpful in differentiating them from FAs, CNB is recommended. However, it can be difficult to differentiate between FA and PT on CNB. A pathologic diagnosis of a fibroepithelial lesion on CNB necessitates excision to rule out a PT. Tumors are classified histologically as low, intermediate, or high grade. Although most PTs have minimal metastatic potential, they have a proclivity for local recurrence and should be excised with at least a 1 cm margin. Local recurrence has been correlated with excision margins but not with tumor grade or size.[34] The most common site of metastasis from malignant PT is the lungs.

ATYPICAL DUCTAL HYPERPLASIA, RADIAL SCAR, LOBULAR NEOPLASIA, AND LOBULAR CARCINOMA IN SITU

During the course of a patient's workup for a suspicious physical finding or image-detected abnormality, CNB or FNA may be performed. A pathologic diagnosis demonstrating atypia (on FNA), atypical ductal hyperplasia (ADH), atypical lobular hyperplasia (ALH), lobular carcinoma in situ (LCIS), or radial scar requires formal surgical excision with needle localization to rule out the presence of invasive carcinoma or DCIS. CNB of these lesions understages findings related to these diagnoses in up to 30% of cases.[35–39] These lesions may be an independent risk factor for the development of carcinoma[38] [*see* Evaluation of Patients at High Risk for Breast Cancer, *below*].

FAT NECROSIS

Fat necrosis can masquerade as breast cancer. It often presents as a firm, irregular mass within breast tissue, which is occasionally tender. The patient's history is helpful in providing clues to this diagnosis and will often include a history of trauma, reduction mammoplasty, or prior breast surgery. Large cavity size, postoperative hematoma, or infection, as well as adjuvant radiation, can increase the likelihood of fat necrosis. A compromise to the surrounding parenchymal blood supply is thought to be the underlying factor in its development. Diagnostic mammography and ultrasonography can aid in the diagnosis. Loss of speculation, compressibility, oil cysts, and the presence of eggshell calcifications are suggestive of a benign etiology. Review of prior films is necessary to determine the stability of the lesion.[40] Ultrasonography or stereotactic CNB is appropriate if there is doubt about the diagnosis and will reveal chronic inflammatory cells, lymphocytes, histiocytes, fat necrosis, and saponification. Should the physician opt for short-term clinical follow-up (1 to 2 months) instead of biopsy, it is important to have a patient who will be compliant with keeping follow-up visits.[41]

GALACTOCELE

In the pregnant patient with complaints of a mass or tenderness, the clinician should bear in mind the hormonally stimulated status of the breast, resulting in increased tenderness. However, any mass or thickening in the breast requires prompt evaluation in the pregnant patient. Malignancy should always be ruled out, particularly in older, childbearing-age women. A galactocele, which is a collection of milk within an obstructed, dilated duct, can form during pregnancy, lactation, or recent postlactation. A patient may complain of a tender nodule within the breast tissue. A mammogram will demonstrate a well-circumscribed mixed-density lesion, and ultrasonography will reveal a corresponding partially cystic mass. Simple aspiration can be both diagnostic and therapeutic, providing relief. Malignancy should always be in the differential, particularly in older women of childbearing years.

MONDOR DISEASE

Mondor disease is thrombophlebitis of the superficial veins of the breast. It is characterized by the finding of a tender and often inflamed cord palpated on the patient's breast. After a thorough history and physical examination of the patient's breasts, treatment should consist of NSAIDs, analgesics, and antibiotics. If there is evidence of infection, or should the condition fail to improve, surgical excision is appropriate for definitive management and diagnosis.[42]

GYNECOMASTIA

Gynecomastia, or a breast mass in male breast tissue, is usually a benign condition in adolescent males and presents as discoid, subareolar, rubbery thickening of the breast tissue. In the absence of any other findings, such as testicular pathology, or a history of ingestion or use of substances associated with gynecomastia, these patients should be reassured and reexamined. In the case of especially prominent, large, or symptomatic gynecomastia, surgical excision is reasonable. In the mature male population, a physical examination and history are vitally important. Soft, diffuse enlargement is a result of medication in 20 to 25% of cases.[43] Gynecomastia can also be due to hormonal, physiologic, or idiopathic factors and can usually be managed nonoperatively and with serial examinations. Many medications resulting in gynecomastia are felt to do so by elevating prolactin levels comparatively. If the gynecomastia is attributable to medication, switching the patient off the medication will often result in regression over the course of a few months. For men who would like to avoid surgery, some success has been noted in treating gynecomastia with tamoxifen, raloxifene, and aromatase inhibitors.[44,45] However, a finding of a solitary hard mass, especially with findings of adenopathy and skin changes, requires aggressive workup, including mammogram and tissue diagnosis, usually with CNB.

SKIN AND NIPPLE CHANGES

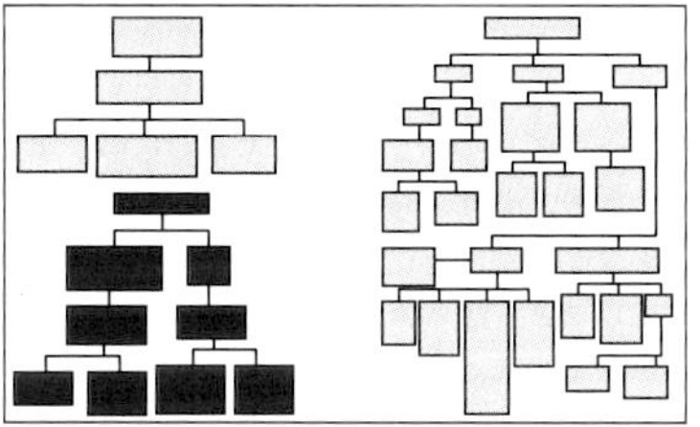

Common breast skin and nipple changes include bacterial infections (mastitis, cellulitis, with or without underlying abscess), fungal infections, and dermatitis. In lactating women, mastitis is generally the result of poor hygiene. Women will often give a history of an abrasion or crack in the nipple. Symptoms typically include erythema, tenderness, and swelling of the breast. *Staphylococcus aureus* is the most common organism identified. Treatment involves continued breastfeeding and antibiotics. The choice of antibiotics should take into consideration the safety of the breastfeeding infant.[46] Nonresolution of the infection with a course of appropriate antibiotics should prompt the surgeon to consider the presence of an underlying abscess or an antibiotic-resistant organism. Fluid from an abscess should be sent for Gram stain and culture to ensure the appropriate choice of antibiotic. If the symptoms persist in the absence of the above causes, inflammatory breast cancer should be considered, followed by appropriate imaging, punch biopsy of the skin, and percutaneous biopsy of any underlying lesion.

In nonlactating women, cellulitis of the breast typically occurs in the lower half of the breast and is more commonly found in women who are overweight, have large, pendulous breasts, or have poor personal hygiene. Breast abscesses are more frequently seen in women with a history of diabetes, rheumatoid arthritis, chronic steroid use, chronic granulomatous lobular mastitis, and trauma.[46] Treatment includes antibiotics and identification of an underlying abscess followed by aspiration or drainage. Aspiration should always precede drainage. Intravenous antibiotics should be considered for women with elevated temperature and white blood cell count. Other skin conditions in the breast include sebaceous cysts and hidradenitis suppurativa. Appropriate antibiotics should be given, and surgical excision is often required for resolution of the symptoms. Fungal (candidal) infections involving the breast are a common complaint in women with large, pendulous breasts. The lower breast and inframammary crease are common locations for the characteristic erythematous moist patches. Treatment includes keeping the area clean and dry and topical antifungal powders or creams.

In nonlactating women, benign processes involving the nipple are often the result of trauma or damage to the nipple or subareolar ducts. Smoking is associated with periductal mastitis, which can present with pain, inflammation, nipple retraction, and discharge. Appropriate antibiotics and abscess aspiration or drainage are the recommended treatments. Trauma, dry skin, or dermatitis can lead to excoriation of the nipple. Allergic or atopic dermatitis frequently occurs as a result of allergies to clothing, dyes, perfumes, and detergents. Treatment is symptomatic, with removal of the offending agent and a course of topical steroids. Short-term clinical follow-up (1 to 2 weeks) is essential to ensure resolution of the symptoms. Breast cancer, including Paget disease of the nipple, can present with these symptoms, and it is vital that the surgeon make an accurate diagnosis. If there is no improvement of the symptoms in 2 weeks, punch biopsy of the nipple should be done.

Evaluation of Patients at High Risk for Breast Cancer

Significant morbidity and cost are associated with breast cancer treatment. Approximately one third of women diagnosed with breast cancer will succumb to the disease. This has led to efforts to provide primary prevention to high-risk women. A number of factors have been identified that increase breast cancer risk [*see Table 2*].[47] These risk factors include

***Table 2* Magnitude of Known Breast Cancer Risk Factors**

Relative risk < 2
Early menarche
Late menopause
Nulliparity
Age > 35 first birth
Hormone replacement therapy
Obesity
Alcohol use
Proliferative breast disease
Prior breast biopsies
Relative risk 2–4
One first-degree relative with breast cancer
Radiation exposure
Prior breast cancer
Mammographic density
Relative risk > 4
Two first-degree relatives with breast cancer
Gene mutation
Lobular carcinoma in situ
Ductal carcinoma in situ
Atypical hyperplasia

Adapted from: Morrow M, Jordan VC. Managing breast cancer risk. 1st edition. Hamilton, ON: BC Decker Inc; 2003. p. 302.

(1) mutations in genes that confer a predisposition to breast cancer[48]; (2) hormonal and reproductive factors[47,49–51]; (3) environmental factors, including diet and lifestyle characteristics of developed Western nations[52]; (4) prior radiation to the chest wall as a teenager or young adult[53]; (5) a history of prior breast cancer, radial scar, or other premalignant lesions[37,54,55]; and (6) increased mammographic density.[56] Recognition of factors that increase breast cancer risk facilitates appropriate screening and clinical management of individual patients. It must be recognized, however, that most women have none of the known risk factors for breast cancer, and the absence of these risk factors should never prevent full evaluation or biopsy of a suspicious breast lesion.

Approximately 10% of all breast cancers are hereditary.[57] Hereditary breast cancer is characterized by early age of onset, bilateral disease and disease in other organ sites. Therefore, an accurate and complete family history, including all malignancies, is essential for quantifying a woman's genetic predisposition to breast cancer. Questions about breast cancer in family members should go back several generations, with age at diagnosis recorded if available. Any personal history of cancer should be recorded, with particular attention paid to breast, ovarian, and endometrial cancers.

BRCA1 and *BRCA2* account for the majority of hereditary breast cancers. The lifetime risk of breast cancer in these individuals can be as high as 85%. Mutations in these genes are associated with other malignancies, most notably ovarian, pancreatic, and prostate cancer. Specific founder mutations in *BRCA1* and *BRCA2* occur within certain ethnic groups (e.g., Ashkenazi Jews).[57] Surgeons should also be aware of mutations in other genes that are commonly associated with an increased risk of breast cancer, including mutations in *p53* (Li-Fraumeni syndrome), mutations in the *PTEN* gene (Cowden syndrome), and hereditary diffuse gastric cancer syndrome (*CHD1*). Tests that detect mutations in these genes are commercially available. Clinicians should consult a licensed genetic counselor to determine appropriate candidates for testing.

Genetic testing has significantly improved our ability to define breast cancer risk for the subset of women who have a mutation. For women without a known genetic predisposition, the Gail[58] and Claus models[59] are two tools that can screen women who may be at increased risk and would therefore benefit from enhanced surveillance and chemoprevention. It should be noted that these mathematical models define population-based risk, not individual risk.

Histologic markers of risk include both ductal and lobular atypia, radial scar, and lobular carcinoma in situ (LCIS). Atypia and radial scar confer a fourfold increased risk of developing breast cancer.[60,61] LCIS is associated with an increased lifetime risk of subsequent carcinoma between 20 and 25%. Pleomorphic LCIS, a pathologically distinct entity of LCIS, appears to be associated more frequently with invasive cancer.[62,63] At present, women with these high-risk lesions should be offered screening and chemoprevention.

Currently, there are three options for women to manage their risk: (1) enhanced surveillance, (2) chemoprevention, and (3) prophylactic mastectomy. For women with LCIS or a family history of breast carcinoma, surveillance should include twice-yearly CBE. Mammography should be performed annually after the diagnosis of LCIS or atypical hyperplasia. Women with a family history of breast cancer should have screening mammography performed annually, beginning 10 years before the earliest age at which cancer was diagnosed in a first-degree relative.[64] For women with known genetic mutations and other women from families with an autosomal dominant pattern of breast cancer transmission, annual mammographic screening should begin at age 25.[64] There are several prospective nonrandomized trials which were designed to assess the benefit for adding yearly screening breast MRI for women at high risk for breast cancer.[65–69] These studies demonstrated that breast MRI is more sensitive than mammography. The ACS recently published recommendations for the use of screening breast MRI as an adjunct to mammography. Annual screening with breast MRI is recommended for the following: (1) *BRCA* mutation carriers; (2) first-degree relatives of a *BRCA* mutation carrier who have never been tested; (3) women with a lifetime risk of 20 to 25% based on risk models that are predominantly dependent on family history; (4) women with a history of radiation to the chest between the ages of 10 and 20 years; (5) women with Li-Fraumeni syndrome (mutations in the *p53* gene) and their first-degree relatives; and (6) women with Cowden and Bannayan-Riley-Ruvalcaba syndromes (mutations in the *PTEN* gene) and first-degree relatives.[70]

It is important to remember that although the sensitivity of breast MRI for cancer is high, the specificity is relatively low and can result in high recall and biopsy rates.[70] Breast MRI should be used as an adjunct to mammography and not a replacement. Mammography and MRI can be done simultaneously or alternating with each other at 6-month intervals to coincide with the CBE. Given the specificity of breast MRI and the fact that many enhancing lesions seen on breast MRI are occult to conventional imaging modalities, it is essential that any facility performing screening breast MRI should have the capability for MRI-guided breast biopsy.

Chemopreventive strategies are designed either to block the initiation of the carcinogenic process or to prevent (or reverse) the progression of the premalignant cells to an invasive cancer.[71] Only tamoxifen and raloxifene are currently FDA approved for chemoprevention in breast cancer. Both are selective estrogen receptor modulators (SERMs). Large multicenter randomized trials demonstrated the efficacy of these agents in the primary prevention setting for women at increased risk of breast cancer based on a Gail score of 1.67 or a personal history of ADH or LCIS. The overall risk of invasive breast cancer was reduced by 50% after treatment for 5 years and limited to estrogen receptor (ER)-positive breast cancers in these high-risk women. Raloxifene is currently approved only for postmenopausal women and has the added benefit of treating postmenopausal osteoporosis. It is noteworthy, however, that raloxifene was not found to prevent noninvasive breast cancers in this trial.[72]

The hot flashes, deep vein thrombosis, and endometrial cancer associated with tamoxifen have made it an unattractive option for many women. This has generated interest in identifying other chemopreventive agents. Aromatase inhibitors, which are used to treat ER-positive breast cancers in postmenopausal women, reduce the risk of contralateral cancers and may have a role to play in chemoprevention. In addition, gonadotropin-releasing hormone agonists, monoterpenes, lignans, retinoids, rexinoids, vitamin D derivatives, and inhibitors of tyrosine kinase are all undergoing evaluation in clinical or preclinical studies with a view to assessing their potential chemopreventive activity. Whether any of these compounds will play a clinically useful role in preventing breast cancer remains to be seen.

For those women at significant risk of breast cancer attributable to genetic predisposition, bilateral prophylactic mastectomy can be considered. High-risk women who underwent this procedure, compared with those who did not, had their breast cancer risk reduced by at least 90%.[73] Oopherectomy also confers up to a 50% breast cancer risk reduction in premenopausal women.[74] The benefits of prophylactic mastectomy must be weighed against the irreversibility and the psychosocial consequences of the procedure.

Research involving high-risk women is challenging because of the large numbers of women who must be recruited and followed for many years and because of the cost associated with such an undertaking. Improved risk assessment tools that can aid in improved risk stratification are under active investigation.[75] Current trials are focused on identifying and using intermediate biomarkers of breast cancer risk to test potential chemopreventive agents.

Financial Disclosures: None Reported

References

1. Seltzer MH. Breast complaints, biopsies, and cancer correlated with age in 10,000 consecutive new surgical referrals. Breast J 2004;10: 111–7.
2. Vahabi M. Breast cancer screening methods: a review of the evidence. Health Care Women Int 2003;24:773–93.
3. Smith RA, Saslow D, Sawyer KA et al. American Cancer Society guidelines for breast cancer screening: update 2003. CA Cancer J Clin 2003;53:141–69.
4. Jatoi I. Screening clinical breast examination. Surg Clin North Am 2003;83:789–801.
5. Tabar I, Vitak B, Chen HH, et al. The Swedish Two-County Trial twenty years later. Up-dated mortality results and new insights from long-term follow-up. Radiologic Clinic North Am 2000;38:625–51.
6. Bevers TB, Anderson BO, Bonaccio E, et al. NCCN clinical practice guidelines in oncology: breast cancer screening and diagnosis. J Natl Compr Canc Netw 2009;7:1060–96.
7. Pisano ED, Gatsonis C, Hendrick E, et al. Diagnostic performance of digital versus film mammography for breast-cancer screening. N Engl J Med 2005;353:1773–83.
8. American College of Radiology (ACR). ACR BI-RADS – Mammography. In: ACR Breast Imaging Reporting and Data System, Breast Imaging Atlas. 4th edition. Reston, VA: American College of Radiology; 2003.
9. Sickles AE. Periodic mammographic follow up of probably benign lesions: results in 3184 consecutive cases. Radiology 1991;179: 463–8.
10. Varas X, Leborgne F, Leborbne JH. Nonpalpable, probably benign lesions: role of follow-up mammography. Radiology 1992; 184:409–14.
11. Schueller G, Jaromi S, Ponhold L, et al. US-guided 14-gauge core-needle breast biopsy: results of a validation study in 1352 cases. Radiology 2008;248:406–13.
12. Brenner RJ, Bassett LW, Fajardo LL, et al. Stereotactic core-needle breast biopsy: a multi-institutional prospective trial. Radiology 2001;218:866–72.
13. Liberman L, Feng TL, Dershaw DD, et al. US-guided core breast biopsy: use and cost-effectiveness. Radiology 1998;208: 717–23.
14. Olawaiye A, Withiam-Leitch M, Danakas G, Kahn K. Mastalgia: a review of management. J Reprod Med 2005;50:933–9.
15. Norlock FE. Benign breast pain in women: a practical approach to evaluation and treatment. J Am Med Womens Assoc 2002;57: 85–90.
16. Bundred NJ. Breast pain. Clin Evid (Online). 2007. Available at: http://www.clinicalevidence.com (accessed April 5, 2010).
17. Neilann KH, Johanna WL. Potential mechanisms of diet therapy for fibrocystic breast conditions show inadequate evidence of effectiveness. J Am Diet Assoc 2000;100: 1368–80.
18. Qureshi S, Sultan N. Topical nonsteroidal anti-inflammatory drugs versus oil of evening primrose in the treatment of mastalgia. Surgeon 2005;3:7–10.
19. Rosolowich V, Saettler E, Szuck B, et al. Mastalgia. J Obstet Gynaecol Can 2006;28: 49–71.
20. Pain JA, Cahill CJ. Management of cyclical mastalgia. Br J Clin Pract 1990;44:454–6.
21. Hussain AN, Policarpio C, Vincent MT. Evaluating nipple discharge. Obstet Gynecol Surv 2006;61:278–83.
22. Morley JE, Dawson M, Hodgkinson H, Kalk WJ. Galactorrhea and hyperprolactinemia associated with chest wall injury. J Clin Endocrinol Metab 1977;45:931–5.
23. Cabioglu N, Hunt KK, Singletary SE, et al. Surgical decision making and factors determining a diagnosis of breast carcinoma in women presenting with nipple discharge. J Am Coll Surg 2003;196:354–64.
24. Beechey-Newman N, Kulkarni D, Kothari A, et al. Breast duct microendoscopy in nipple discharge: microbrush improves cytology. Surg Endosc 2005;19:1648–51.
25. Liu GY, Lu JS, Shen KW, et al. Fiberoptic ductoscopy combined with cytology testing in the patients of spontaneous nipple discharge. Breast Cancer Res Treat 2008;108:271–7.
26. Saad RS, Kanbour-Shakir A, Syed A, Kanbour A. Sclerosing papillary lesion of the breast: a diagnostic pitfall for malignancy in fine needle aspiration biopsy. Diagn Cytopathol 2006;34:114–8.
27. Rizzo M, Lund M, Oprea G, et al. Surgical follow-up and clinical presentation of 142 breast papillary lesions diagnosed by ultrasound-guided core-needle biopsy. Ann Surg Oncol 2008;15:1040–7.
28. Ueng SH, Mezzetti T, Tavassoli FA. Papillary neoplasms of the breast: a review. Arch Pathol Lab Med 2009;133:893–907.
29. Mercado CL, Hamele-Bena D, Oken SM, et al. Papillary lesions of the breast at percutaneous core-needle biopsy. Radiology 2006; 238:801–8.
30. Jaffer S, Nagi C, Bleiweiss IJ. Excision is indicated for intraductal papilloma of the breast diagnosed on core needle biopsy. Cancer 2009;115:2837–43.
31. Brookes MJ, Bourke AG. Radiological appearances of papillary breast lesions. Clin Radiol 2008;63:1265–73.
32. Van Zee KJ, Ortega PG, Minnard E, Cohen MA. Preoperative galactography increases the diagnostic yield of major duct excision for nipple discharge. Cancer 1998;82:1874–80.
33. Roa JC, Tapia O, Carrasco P, et al. Prognostic factors of phyllodes tumor of the breast. Pathol Int 2006;56:309–14.
34. Mangi AA, Smith BL, Gadd MA, et al. Surgical management of phyllodes tumors. Arch Surg 1999;134:487–93.
35. Brem RF, Behrndt VS, Sanow L, Gatewood OM. Atypical ductal hyperplasia: histologic underestimation of carcinoma in tissue harvested from impalpable breast lesions using 11-gauge stereotactically guided directional vacuum-assisted biopsy. AJR Am J Roentgenol 1999;172:1405–7.
36. Harvey JM, Sterrett GF, Frost FA. Atypical ductal hyperplasia and atypia of uncertain significance in core biopsies from mammographically detected lesions: correlation with excision diagnosis. Pathology 2002;34: 410–6.
37. Jacobs TW, Byrne C, Colditz G, et al. Radial scars in benign breast-biopsy specimens and the risk of breast cancer. N Engl J Med 1999;340:430–6.
38. Kennedy M, Masterson AV, Kerin M, Flanagan F. Pathology and clinical relevance of radial scars: a review. J Clin Pathol 2003; 56:721–4.
39. Youk JH, Kim EK, Kim MJ. Atypical ductal hyperplasia diagnosed at sonographically guided 14-gauge core needle biopsy of breast mass. AJR Am J Roentgenol 2009;192: 1135–41.
40. Stavros AT, Parker SH, Rapp LC. Breast ultrasound. Philadelphia: Lippincott Williams & Wilkins; 2004.
41. Hughes LE, Mansel RE, Webster DJT. Benign disorders and diseases of the breast: concepts and clinical management. 2nd ed. Philadelphia: WB Saunders; 2004.
42. Catania S, Zurrida S, Veronesi P, et al. Mondor's disease and breast cancer. Cancer 1992;69:2267–70.
43. Caocci G, Atzeni S, Orru N, et al. Gynecomastia in a male after dasatinib treatment for chronic myeloid leukemia. Leukemia 2008; 22:2127–8.
44. Shulman DI, Francis GL, Palmert MR, Eugster EA, for the Lawson Wilkins Pediatric Endocrine Society Drug and Therapeutics C. Use of aromatase inhibitors in children and adolescents with disorders of growth and adolescent development. Pediatrics 2008;121: e975–83.
45. Fradet Y, Egerdie B, Andersen M, et al. Tamoxifen as prophylaxis for prevention of gynaecomastia and breast pain associated with bicalutamide 150 mg monotherapy in patients with prostate cancer: a randomised, placebo-controlled, dose-response study. Eur Urol 2007;52:106–14.

46. Dixon JM. ABC of breast diseases: breast infection. BMJ 1994;309:946–9.
47. Henderson IC. Risk factors for breast cancer development. Cancer 1993;71 Suppl 6: 2127–40.
48. Slattery ML, Kerber RA. A comprehensive evaluation of family history and breast cancer risk: The Utah Population Database. JAMA 1993;270:1563–8.
49. Squitieri R, Tartter PI, Ahmed S, et al. Carcinoma of the breast in postmenopausal hormone user and nonuser control groups. J Am Coll Surg 1994;178:167–70.
50. Newcomb PA, Storer BE, Longnecker MP, et al. Lactation and a reduced risk of premenopausal breast cancer. N Engl J Med 1994;330:81–7.
51. Colditz GA, Stampfer MJ, Willett WC, et al. Prospective study of estrogen replacement therapy and risk of breast cancer in postmenopausal women. JAMA 1990;264:2648–53.
52. Cummings SR, Tice JA, Bauer S, et al. Prevention of breast cancer in postmenopausal women: approaches to estimating and reducing risk. J Natl Cancer Inst 2009;101: 384–8.
53. Travis LB, Hill D, Dores GM, et al. Cumulative absolute breast cancer risk for young women treated for Hodgkin lymphoma. J Natl Cancer Inst 2005;97:1428–37.
54. Frykberg ER, Bland KI. Management of in situ and minimally invasive breast carcinoma. World J Surg 1994;18:45–57.
55. Page DL, Jensen RA. Evaluation and management of high risk and premalignant lesions of the [illegible]. World J Surg 1994;18:32–8.
56. Martin L, Boyd N. Mammographic density. Potential mechanisms of breast cancer risk associated with mammographic density: hypotheses based on epidemiological evidence. Breast Cancer Res 2008;10:201.
57. Quan ML, Petrek JA. Clinical implications of hereditary breast cancer. Adv Surg 2003;37: 197–212.
58. Gail MH, Brinton LA, Byar DP, et al. Projecting individualized probabilities of developing breast cancer for white females who are being examined annually. J Natl Cancer Inst 1989;81:1879–86.
59. Claus EB, Risch N, Thompson WD. Autosomal dominant inheritance of early-onset breast cancer. Implications for risk prediction. Cancer 1994;73:643–51.
60. Page DL, Dupont WD, Rogers LW, Rados MS. Atypical hyperplastic lesions of the female breast. A long-term follow-up study. Cancer 1985;55:2698–708.
61. Simpson P, Gale T, Fulford L, et al. The diagnosis and management of pre-invasive breast disease: pathology of atypical lobular hyperplasia and lobular carcinoma in situ. Breast Cancer Res 2003;5:258–62.
62. Sneige N, Wang J, Baker BA, et al. Clinical, histopathologic, and biologic features of pleomorphic lobular (ductal-lobular) carcinoma in situ of the breast: a report of 24 cases. Mod Pathol 2002;15:1044–50.
63. Fadare OMD, Dadmanesh FMD, Alvarado-Cabrero IMD, et al. Lobular intraepithelial neoplasia [lobular carcinoma in situ] with comedo-type necrosis: a clinicopathologic study of 18 cases. Am J Surg Pathol 2006;30: 1445–53.
64. Dershaw DD. Mammographic screening of the high-risk woman. Am J Surg 2000;180: 288–9.
65. Warner E, Plewes DB, Hill KA, et al. Surveillance of BRCA1 and BRCA2 mutation carriers with magnetic resonance imaging, ultrasound, mammography, and clinical breast examination. JAMA 2004;292: 1317–25.
66. Leach MO, Boggis CR, Dixon AK, et al. Screening with magnetic resonance imaging and mammography of a UK population at high familial risk of breast cancer: a prospective multicentre cohort study (MARIBS) [published erratum appears in Lancet 2005; 365(9474):1848]. Lancet 2005;365(9473): 1769–78.
67. Kriege M, Brekelmans CTM, Boetes C, et al. Efficacy of MRI and mammography for breast-cancer screening in women with a familial or genetic predisposition. N Engl J Med 2004;351:427–37.
68. Kuhl CK, Schrading S, Leutner CC, et al. Mammography, breast ultrasound, and breast magnetic resonance imaging for surveillance of women at high familial risk for breast cancer. J Clin Oncol 2005;23:8469–76.
69. Lehman CD, Blume JD, Weatherall P, et al. Screening women at high risk for breast cancer with mammography and magnetic resonance imaging. Cancer 2005;103: 1898–905.
70. Saslow D, Boetes C, Burke W, et al. American Cancer Society guidelines for breast screening with MRI as an adjunct to mammography. CA Cancer J Clin 2007;57: 75–89.
71. Zujewski J. Selective estrogen receptor modulators (SERMs) and retinoids in breast cancer chemoprevention. Environ Mol Mutagen 2002;39:264–70.
72. Vogel VG, Costantino JP, Wickerham DL, et al. Effects of tamoxifen vs raloxifene on the risk of developing invasive breast cancer and other disease outcomes: the NSABP Study of Tamoxifen and Raloxifene (STAR) P-2 trial. JAMA 2006;295:2727–41.
73. Hartmann LC, Schaid DJ, Woods JE, et al. Efficacy of bilateral prophylactic mastectomy in women with a family history of breast cancer. N Engl J Med 1999;340:77–84.
74. Rebbeck TR, Kauff ND, Domchek SM. Meta-analysis of risk reduction estimates associated with risk-reducing salpingo-oophorectomy in BRCA1 or BRCA2 mutation carriers. J Natl Cancer Inst 2009;101: 80–7.
75. Fabian CJ, Kimler BF, Mayo MS, Khan SA. Breast-tissue sampling for risk assessment and prevention. Endocr Relat Cancer 2005; 12:185–213.

1 DYSPHAGIA

*P. James Villeneuve, MDCM, PhD, FRCSC, and R. Sudhir Sundaresan, MD, FRCSC, FACS**

The term *dysphagia*, derived from the Greek *dys-* (with difficulty) and *-phagia* (to eat), describes difficulty in the transfer of food or liquid boluses from the mouth to the stomach. Dysphagia is a common complaint, with at least 35% of patients above the age of 50 complaining of weekly dysphagia and up to 60% of nursing home residents suffering feeding difficulties as a result of dysphagia.[1,2]

There are two forms of dysphagia. Oropharyneal dysphagia results from a functional impairment in the initiation of swallowing, including the oral and pharyngeal phases [*see Sidebar* Normal Swallowing Mechanism], and often results from systemic neurologic or myopathic syndromes [*see Table 1*]. Esophageal dysphagia relates to intrinsic functional (motor) and anatomic abnormalities of the esophagus that result in swallowing difficulties [*see Table 2*].[1,3]

This chapter outlines the basic physiology of the swallowing mechanism and proposes an evaluative and diagnostic approach to difficulties with swallowing. The technical details of specific procedures employed in the definitive treatment of certain causes of dysphagia are described in later chapters of this volume.

Evaluation

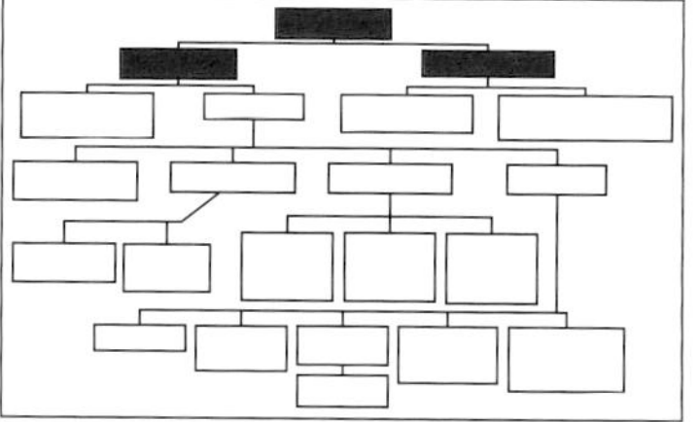

A systematic approach to the patient with dysphagia is mandatory. A thorough history and complete physical examination allow for an accurate assessment of likely etiologies. Confounding diagnoses, such as angina pectoris, thyroid goiter, and pharyngitis, should be eliminated.

IMPORTANT ELEMENTS TO ELICIT ON HISTORY

Timing of Dysphagia

Immediate coughing, choking, or regurgitation suggests oropharyngeal causes for dysphagia. A sensation of food "sticking" or getting "caught" or the delayed regurgitation of food suggests esophageal causes of dysphagia.[2] Patients reporting the constant presence of symptoms not associated with swallowing difficulties may have globus sensation, which is a benign, nonpainful fullness in the neck or throat.[4]

Painful Swallowing

Odynophagia is not typically associated with dysphagia; its presence should prompt consideration of infectious or inflammatory etiologies. Exposure and ingestion of caustic substances must be sought out as an expedient assessment of severity and consideration of immediate surgery must be made.

Location

Patients will self-localize symptoms to the cervical, retrosternal, or epigastric regions. Studies have demonstrated accurate localization, by patient history, to within 4 cm of the culprit lesion in up to 74% of cases.[5] Accuracy seems best for proximal lesions.

Solid or Liquid

Intolerance to both liquids and solids suggests a functional or neuromuscular cause of dysphagia. Difficulties with solid food only strongly implicates a mechanical or anatomic causes of dysphagia[6]; a progression from purely solid food dysphagia to both solid and liquid dysphagia suggests narrowing attributable to an evolving mechanical obstruction.

Onset and Progression

The temporal pattern of symptom onset and duration also gives valuable information as to possible causes for dysphagia. Intermittent, nonprogressive symptoms suggest an intrinsic motor dysfunction (such as diffuse esophageal spasm) or a mechanical cause such as a web or ring. If the symptoms have been present for a short period of time or are rapidly progressive, a malignant etiology must be ruled out.

Associated Symptoms

A history of anorexia or weight loss suggests an underlying malignancy. Passive regurgitation of food particles may arise from achalasia or a cricopharyngeal diverticulum. Retrosternal chest pain, once cardiac etiologies have been eliminated, may be present in cases of esophageal spasm or gastroesophageal reflux. However, dysphagia secondary to peptic strictures and adenocarcinoma are without symptoms of gastroesophageal reflux disease (GERD) in up to 25 to 35% of cases.[7] Medication lists must be examined to rule out culprit medications (alendronate, doxycycline, nonsteroidal antiinflammatory drugs [NSAIDs], and mycophenolate mofetil [MMF]) that may cause drug-induced esophageal injury.[8]

PHYSICAL EXAMINATION

The esophagus is a deep-seated structure that does not lend itself to direct physical assessment. Although a thorough physical examination should follow a complete history, information gathered is useful only in inferring potential diagnoses. A detailed and accurate history is the mainstay of clinical assessment in patients who present with dysphagia.

The head and neck are examined for the size of the thyroid gland, as well as for the presence of any lymphadenopathy or masses. A careful examination of cranial nerves may

* The authors and editors gratefully acknowledge the contributions of the previous author, Ahmad S. Ashrafi, MD, FRCSC, to the development and writing of this chapter.

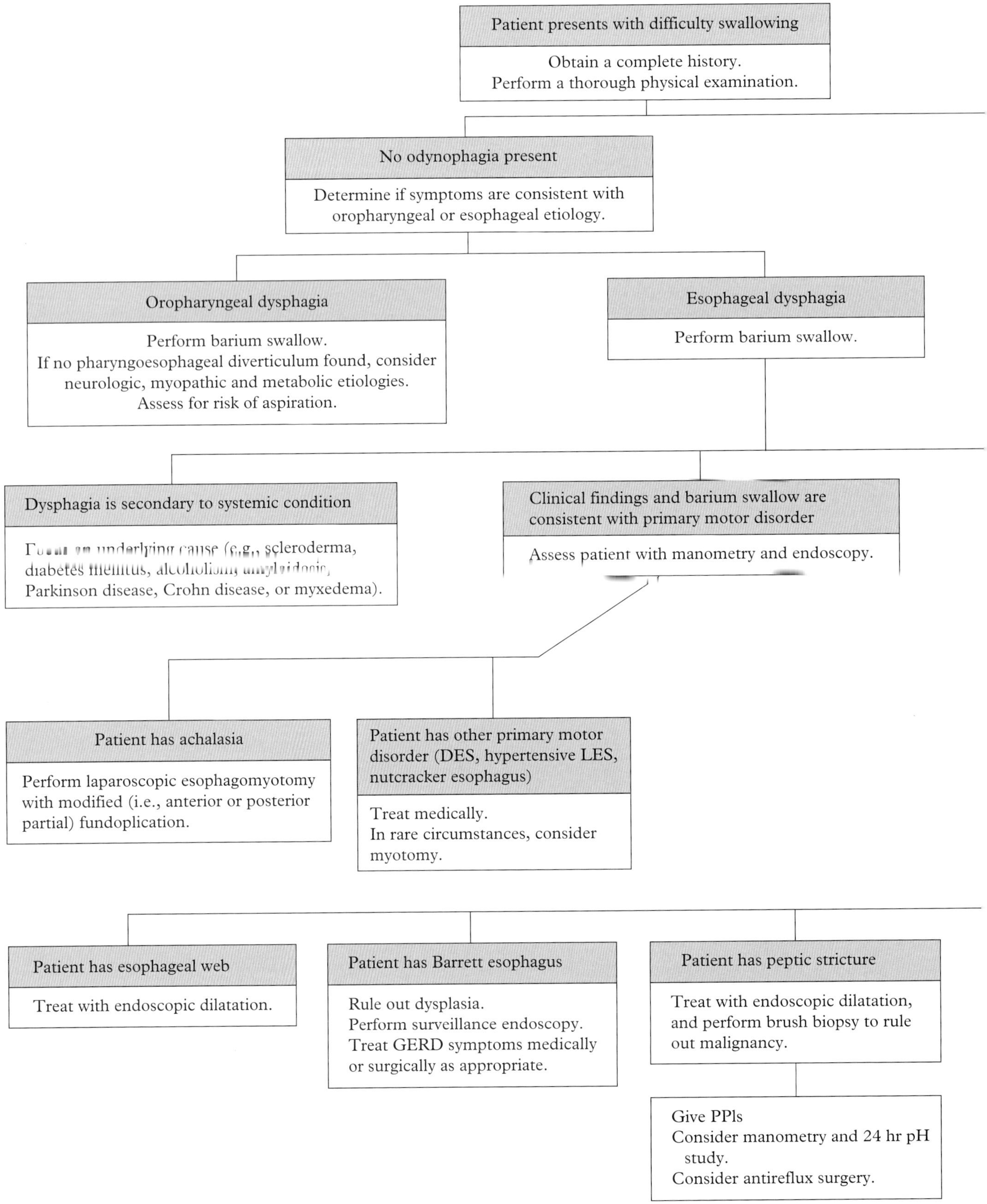

Patient presents with difficulty swallowing

Obtain a complete history.
Perform a thorough physical examination.

No odynophagia present

Determine if symptoms are consistent with oropharyngeal or esophageal etiology.

Oropharyngeal dysphagia

Perform barium swallow.
If no pharyngoesophageal diverticulum found, consider neurologic, myopathic and metabolic etiologies.
Assess for risk of aspiration.

Esophageal dysphagia

Perform barium swallow.

Dysphagia is secondary to systemic condition

Focus on underlying cause (e.g., scleroderma, diabetes mellitus, alcoholism, amyloidosis, Parkinson disease, Crohn disease, or myxedema).

Clinical findings and barium swallow are consistent with primary motor disorder

Assess patient with manometry and endoscopy.

Patient has achalasia

Perform laparoscopic esophagomyotomy with modified (i.e., anterior or posterior partial) fundoplication.

Patient has other primary motor disorder (DES, hypertensive LES, nutcracker esophagus)

Treat medically.
In rare circumstances, consider myotomy.

Patient has esophageal web

Treat with endoscopic dilatation.

Patient has Barrett esophagus

Rule out dysplasia.
Perform surveillance endoscopy.
Treat GERD symptoms medically or surgically as appropriate.

Patient has peptic stricture

Treat with endoscopic dilatation, and perform brush biopsy to rule out malignancy.

Give PPIs
Consider manometry and 24 hr pH study.
Consider antireflux surgery.

DES = diffuse esophageal spasm; LES = lower esophageal sphincter; GERD = gastroesophageal reflux disease; PPI = proton pump inhibitor; NPO = nil per os; CT = computed tomography; PET = positron emission tomography; EUS = endoscopic ultrasound.

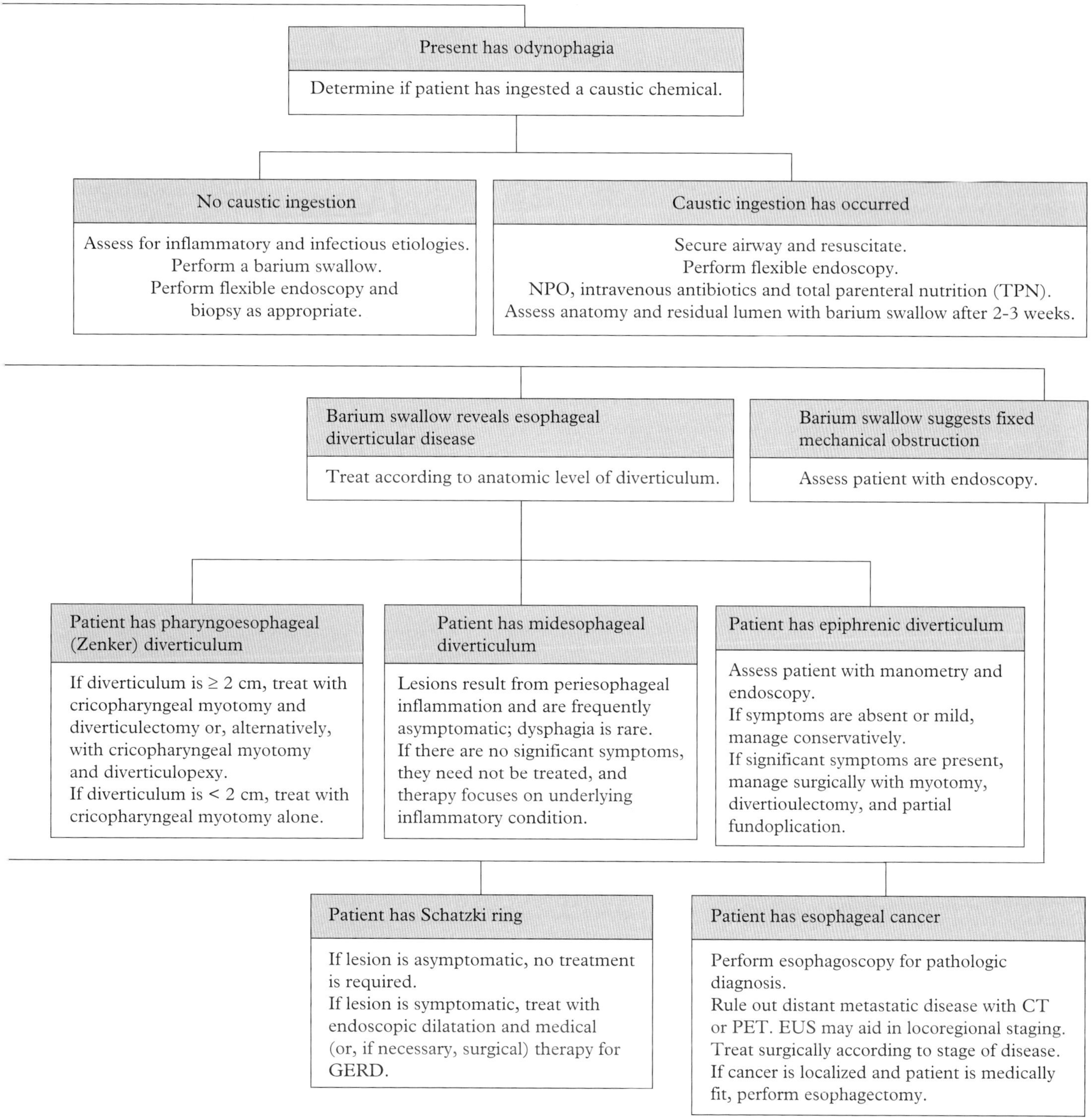

Present has odynophagia

Determine if patient has ingested a caustic chemical.

No caustic ingestion

Assess for inflammatory and infectious etiologies.
Perform a barium swallow.
Perform flexible endoscopy and biopsy as appropriate.

Caustic ingestion has occurred

Secure airway and resuscitate.
Perform flexible endoscopy.
NPO, intravenous antibiotics and total parenteral nutrition (TPN).
Assess anatomy and residual lumen with barium swallow after 2-3 weeks.

Barium swallow reveals esophageal diverticular disease

Treat according to anatomic level of diverticulum.

Patient has pharyngoesophageal (Zenker) diverticulum

If diverticulum is ≥ 2 cm, treat with cricopharyngeal myotomy and diverticulectomy or, alternatively, with cricopharyngeal myotomy and diverticulopexy.
If diverticulum is < 2 cm, treat with cricopharyngeal myotomy alone.

Patient has midesophageal diverticulum

Lesions result from periesophageal inflammation and are frequently asymptomatic; dysphagia is rare.
If there are no significant symptoms, they need not be treated, and therapy focuses on underlying inflammatory condition.

Patient has epiphrenic diverticulum

Assess patient with manometry and endoscopy.
If symptoms are absent or mild, manage conservatively.
If significant symptoms are present, manage surgically with myotomy, divertioulectomy, and partial fundoplication.

Barium swallow suggests fixed mechanical obstruction

Assess patient with endoscopy.

Patient has Schatzki ring

If lesion is asymptomatic, no treatment is required.
If lesion is symptomatic, treat with endoscopic dilatation and medical (or, if necessary, surgical) therapy for GERD.

Patient has esophageal cancer

Perform esophagoscopy for pathologic diagnosis.
Rule out distant metastatic disease with CT or PET. EUS may aid in locoregional staging.
Treat surgically according to stage of disease.
If cancer is localized and patient is medically fit, perform esophagectomy.

Normal Swallowing Mechanism adapted from Matsuo and Palmer[25]

Swallowing was previously described using a three-phase sequential model, whereby the position of the food bolus was used to identify the oral, pharyngeal, and esophageal phases. Later reports expanded this into a four-stage model by dividing the oral phase into preparatory and propulsive stages. These early models accurately depicted liquid swallows but were inadequate to model solid food boluses. The process model accounts for swallowing of solid foods by expanding the oral phase into stage I, transport, food processing, and stage II, transport. The pharyngeal and esophageal phases are common to both liquid and solid transport.

Oral Phases of Liquid Swallowing

Preparatory	Liquid is held against hard palate by tongue and sealed posteriorly by contact between tongue and soft palate
Propulsive	Sequential contact between tongue and hard palate coupled with relaxation of seal between posterior tongue and soft palate squeezes liquid into pharynx

Oral Phases of Solid Swallowing

Stage I transport	Food is positioned against occlusive tooth surfaces by tongue movement.
Oral food processing	Coordinated movements of the jaw, in concert with the tongue, cheek, soft palate, and hyoid bone movement. This results in masticated, moistened food that is optimal for further swallowing.
Stage II transport	Food bolus is positioned on the tongue surface. Sequential contact between the tongue and hard palate coupled with relaxation of seal between posterior tongue and soft palate propels food into the pharynx.

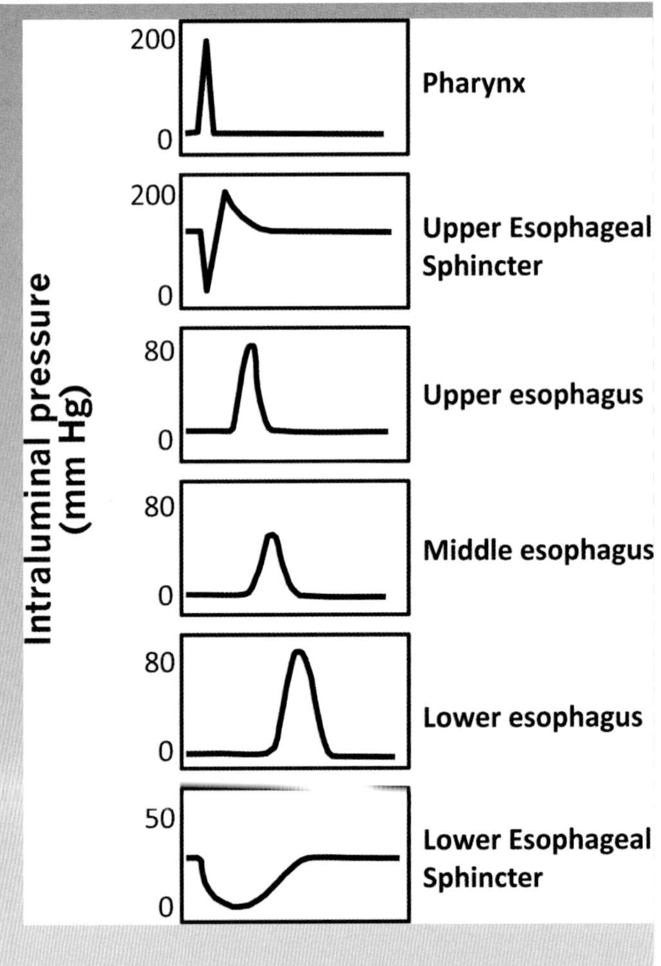

Pharyngeal Phase

This rapid phase must achieve airway protection while facilitating passage of boluses through the upper esophageal sphincter (UES) to the esophagus proper. Airway protection is achieved by concerted closure of the vocal cords and laryngeal movement (anteriorly and superiorly) with concomitant tilting of the epiglottis to seal the laryngeal vestibule. Food propulsion follows: the soft palate rises to block retrograde passage into the nasopharynx. Pharyngeal constrictors sequentially contract from cranial to caudal, shortening the pharynx and propelling the food bolus downward. This "pharyngeal pump" can generate pressures of up to 200 mm Hg. The UES has a resting pressure of between 16 and 118 mm Hg and is closed at rest. Active opening of the UES is achieved by relaxation of the cricopharyngeus, traction by the strap muscles, and distending pressure of the descending food bolus.

Esophageal Phase

Both the UES and the lower esophageal sphincter (LES) remain closed at rest to prevent reflux. Autonomic efferent signals mediate peristalsis; an initial wave of relaxation preceding the food bolus is followed by a wave of contraction, resulting in transit through the esophagus into the stomach. *Primary* esophageal peristalsis is triggered by voluntary swallowing but autonomously propagates at 2 to 5 cm/s through the striated muscles of the upper third of the esophagus, slowing as peristalsis passes into the smooth muscles of the lower esophagus. Secondary esophageal peristalsis is involuntary and arises in response to esophageal distention or irritation. It is thought that these waves of peristalsis serve to keep the esophagus clear. Tertiary esophageal waves can arise normally between swallows but are often nonpropulsive.

The sidebar figure demonstrates normal waveforms and propagation of peristalsis in swallowing. It is evident that coordination between the different anatomic levels of the esophagus is required for effective swallowing. The high-pressure contraction in the pharynx is coordinated with full relaxation of the UES. This allows transfer of swallowed material into the esophagus proper, where peristaltic pressures of up to 80 mm Hg are noted. Orderly progression of moderate-amplitude waves through the esophageal body occurs. The LES relaxes early in response to swallowing and slowly regains its resting pressure of 10 to 25 mm Hg in concert with distal esophageal transport.

demonstrate deficits contributing to oropharyngeal dysphagia, and corresponding neurologic assessment may reveal signs of a cerebrovascular accident (CVA), myasthenia gravis, or Parkinson disease. The chest and abdomen are examined for the presence of subcutaneous nodules or masses that may indicate underlying malignancy. Dermatologic rashes may indicate a paraneoplastic syndrome or a primary autoimmune disorder. Murmurs or thrills on cardiac auscultation may represent atrial enlargement (secondary to mitral valvular stenosis), causing extrinsic esophageal compression. Refer to *Table 1* and *Table 2* for specific causes of oropharyngeal and esophageal dysphagia.

Table 1 Etiologies of Oropharyngeal Dysphagia

Systemic conditions
Cerebrovascular accident
Myasthenia gravis
Intrinsic motor disorders
Cricopharyngeal (Zenker) diverticulum
Fixed mechanical obstruction
Oropharyngeal cancer
Webs
Previous surgical/radiation treatment

DIAGNOSTIC TESTS

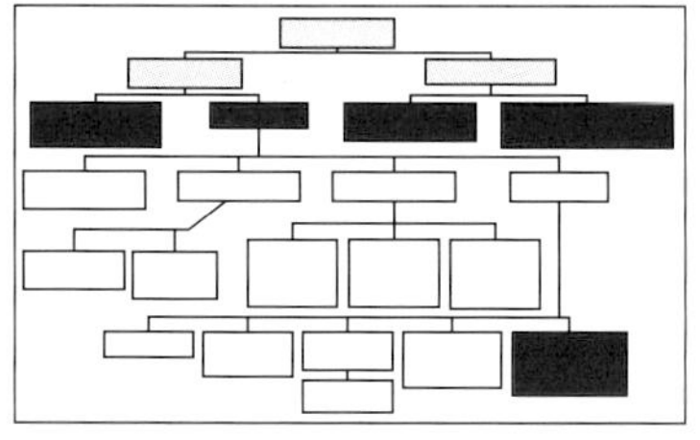

Many diagnostic tests can be used to assess dysphagia, including endoscopic, radiologic, and manometric modalities. The application of these should be predicated by the history.

In cases of suspected or confirmed caustic ingestion, the first test is emergent upper flexible endoscopy to assess the anatomic extent of damage and to grade the injury.[9] In all other cases of dysphagia, the barium swallow is the ideal first test as it is readily available, cost-effective, and rapidly performed. Information can be gained from the barium study regarding anatomic relations, esophageal transit patterns, and the presence or absence of mass lesions and diverticulae. The safety and diagnostic yield of subsequent upper endoscopy are enhanced.

Upper endoscopy allows for a visual assessment of mucosa; diagnostic and therapeutic maneuvers such as biopsies, brushings, and dilatations can be performed.

Endoscopic ultrasonography (EUS) is an emerging diagnostic modality that allows for assessment of the esophageal wall and surrounding tissues. This permits the characterization of esophageal masses (depth of invasion, T stage) and an assessment of adjacent lymphadenopathy (N stage), and guides endoscopic fine-needle aspiration biopsies. EUS-guided biopsies have excellent predictive value in the assessment of lymph node involvement in cases of esophageal carcinoma.[10]

Table 2 Etiologies of Esophageal Dysphagia

Systemic conditions
Scleroderma
Diabetes mellitus
Intrinsic motor disorders
Secondary to GERD
Achalasia
Esophageal spasms
Fixed mechanical obstruction
Webs
Neoplasms
Extrinsic compression
Inflammatory
Eosinophilic esophagitis
HSV/CMV/*Candida*

CMV = cytomegalovirus; GERD = gastroesophageal reflux disease; HSV = herpes simplex virus.

When reflux disease is suspected, extended pH monitoring is invaluable in assessing the presence and severity of GERD. Motility disorders are best diagnosed using manometric techniques.

In cases where extrinsic compression is suspected or demonstrated, cross-sectional imaging using computed tomography (CT) or magnetic resonance imaging (MRI) may be useful in identification of malignant masses or vascular anomalies (aberrant subclavian vessels, aortic aneurysms, or Kommerell diverticulae).[11,12] Dysphagia lusoria is a rare entity in which dysphagia results from extrinsic vascular compression of the esophagus from an aberrant right subclavian artery, which arises from the thoracic aorta and typically courses posterior to the esophagus [*see Figure 1*].

The assessment of esophageal cancer also requires cross-sectional imaging with CT and fluorodeoxyglucose–positron emission tomography (PET). The use of PET is highly sensitive for the detection of unsuspected metastatic lesions in patients deemed candidates for curative resection on the basis of CT alone.[13]

Management of Esophageal Dysphagia

MOTOR DISORDERS

Motility disorders affect the smooth muscle of the distal esophagus and the lower esophageal sphincter (LES). Symptoms typically include dysphagia to solids and liquids; noncardiac chest pain may also be present.

Achalasia

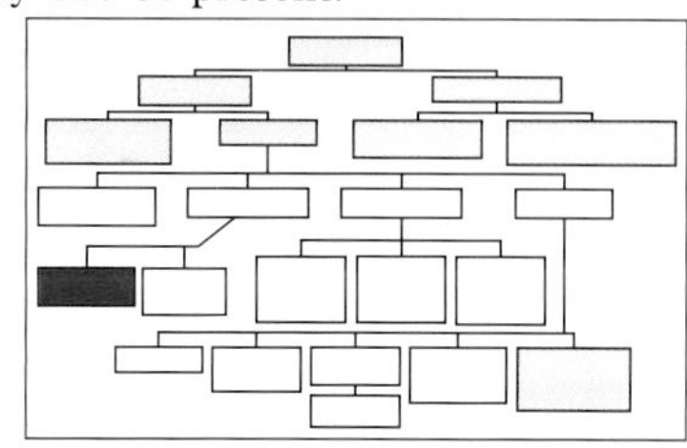

Ninety-eight percent of all cases of achalasia are idiopathic. The disease is thought to result from a loss of inhibitory neurons in the Auerbach plexus, altering neural input to the LES and preventing normal relaxation.[14] Achalasia affects females and males equally at a rate of 1 per 100,000 individuals per year. The usual presentation is between 20 and 50 years, but it has been described in all age groups. The disease is slowly progressive, and presentation is typically at advanced stages. Symptoms include progressive dysphagia to both solids and liquids, accompanied by regurgitation of food particles, chest pain, and weight loss. GERD-like symptoms were present in up to 48% of patients in a study of 32 patients[15]; these symptoms are a consequence of stasis esophagitis (secondarily to fermentation of retained food) rather than reflux of gastric acid.

Plain x-rays may reveal an air-fluid level in the distal esophagus, and a barium swallow will demonstrate a dilated and atonic esophagus with the pathognomonic "bird's-beak" narrowing of the gastroesophageal junction (GEJ) [*see Figure 2*]. Long-standing achalasia may manifest with an extremely dilated and tortuous esophagus (often described as a sigmoid esophagus) [*see Figure 3*]. Manometric findings of aperistalsis and failure of LES relaxation are key in establishing the diagnosis. Resting LES pressures may be normal or elevated. Endoscopic assessment is required to visually assess mucosal appearance to rule out cancer.

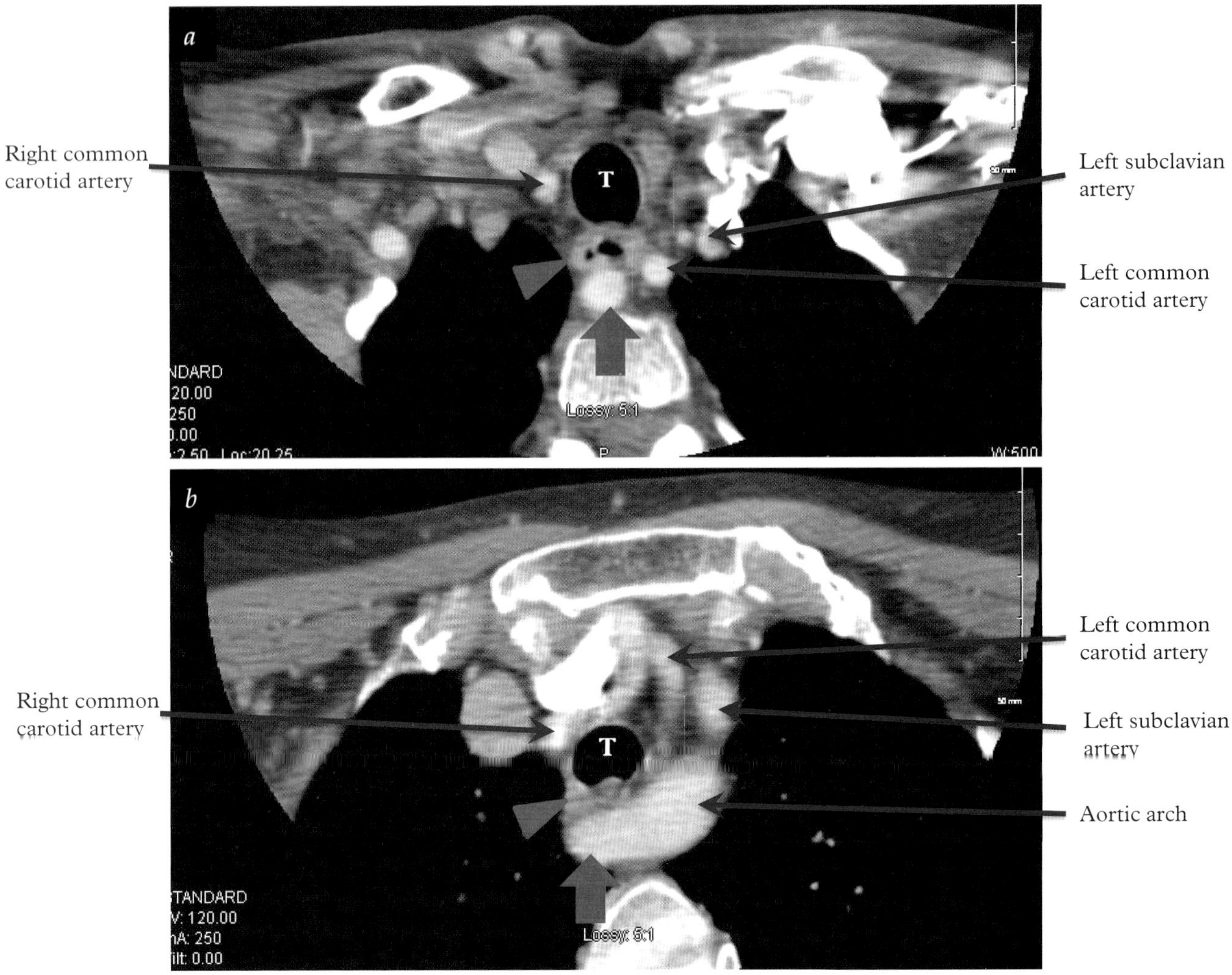

a

Right common carotid artery

T

Left subclavian artery

Left common carotid artery

b

Left common carotid artery

Right common carotid artery

T

Left subclavian artery

Aortic arch

Figure 1 **Dysphagia lusoria. Contrast-enhanced CT scan of the upper chest at the level of the clavicular heads (*a*) and near the carina (*b*) demonstrating the retroesophageal course of the right subclavian artery (*arrow*) causing compression of the esophagus (*arrowhead*) against the trachea (T) and right carotid artery. One can appreciate the idea of a "vascular ring" in such cases causing esophageal compression.**

Treatment modalities for achalasia must achieve enhanced LES compliance and lower resting LES pressures. Medical management with calcium channel blockers or nitrates has no meaningful benefit. Endoscopic management includes endoscopically injected botulinum toxin, or balloon dilatation, to mechanically disrupt the lower esophageal muscle fibers. Recurrent dysphagia (up to 50%) has been noted in some studies at 5 years after balloon dilatation, with a 5% periprocedural risk of esopheageal rupture.[16] In comparison, a laparoscopically performed Heller esophagomyotomy with partial anterior (Dor) fundoplication is considered to be the standard of care in terms of both durable outcomes (90 to 95% resolution of dysphagia) and low complication rates.[14]

Long-standing achalasia is a risk factor for esophageal squamous cell carcinoma, and tumors of the GEJ may present with symptoms similar to those of achalasia.

Dysmotility Syndromes

Motility disorders can be considered within a spectrum that includes diffuse esophageal spasm (DES), nutcracker esophagus, and hypertensive LES. These disorders are traditionally considered separate entities; however, the manometric findings and the mainstays of medical treatment are similar.

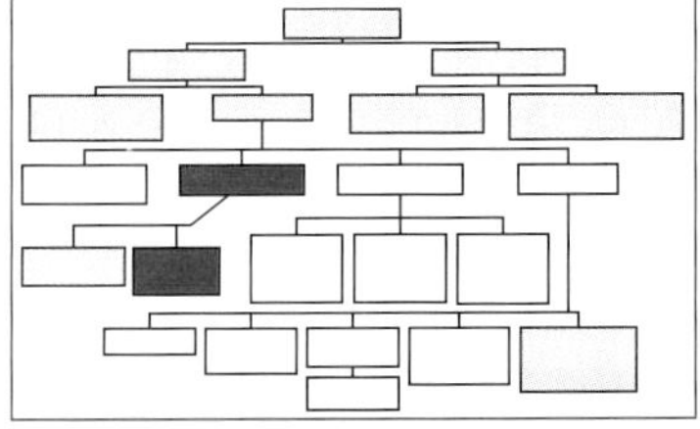

DES is a dysmotility syndrome of unknown etiology. It is characterized in 50% of patients by intermittent dysphagia to solids and liquids. Up to 5% of patients with unexplained chest pain are found to have DES on manometric testing.[7] Evidence for DES on manometry includes periodic prolonged, multipeaked, high-amplitude contractions in more than one in five wet swallows, with observation of normal peristalsis in intervening periods. Incomplete LES relaxation or hypertensive LES may also be observed. Figure 4 demonstrates the classic corkscrew appearance that is observed in some cases of DES.

Nutcracker esophagus presents more commonly with chest pain rather than dysphagia. Manometry also forms the

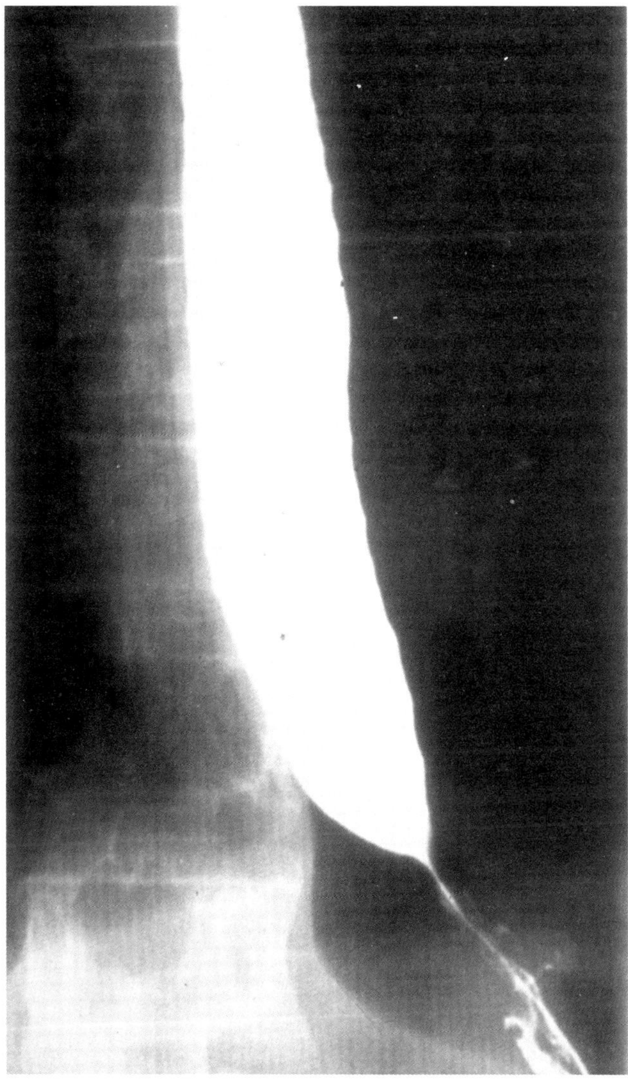

Figure 2 **Achalasia. Barium swallow demonstrates the proximal dilatation and classic "bird's beak" narrowing at the esophagogastric junction, consistent with achalasia, in a 22-year-old woman being evaluated for dysphagia.**

mainstay of diagnosis: a normal peristaltic pattern is noted, with extremely increased pressure amplitudes of more than 180 mm Hg. In contrast to DES, normal peristalsis is not observed within trains of high-pressure waves. Barium swallow is of normal appearance.

Hypertensive LES may be found in isolation but often coexists with other dysmotility syndromes. Resting pressures at the LES by manometry are found to be 45 mm Hg or greater.

Treatment for DES, nutcracker esophagus, and hypertensive LES is based on smooth muscle relaxation using nitrates such as isosorbide dinitrate or calcium channel blockers such as diltiazem. Balloon dilatation may be effective for isolated hypertensive LES.

Esophageal Diverticulae

Diverticulae are classified according to the degree to which the esophageal wall is involved in the outpouching: true

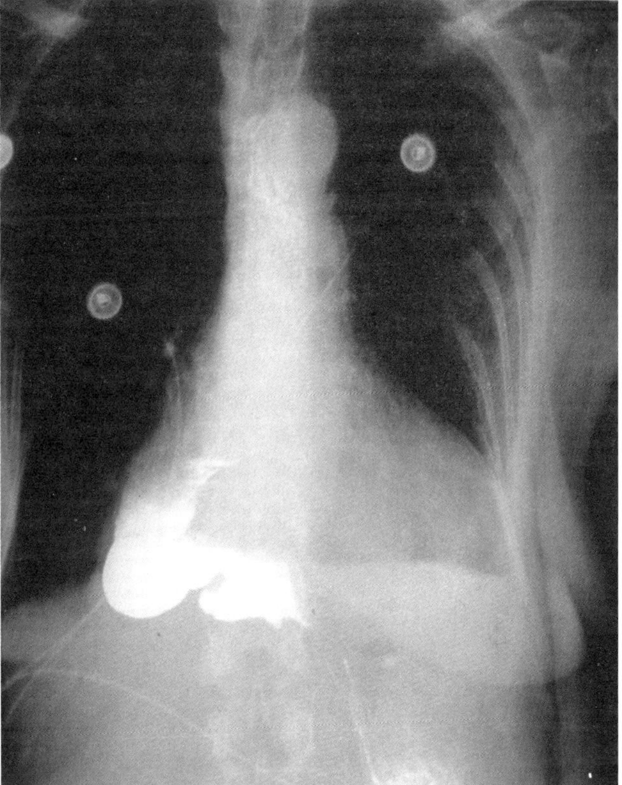

Figure 3 **Sigmoid esophagus. Barium study demonstrates dilated esophagus with right-sided deviation and tortuous course of the distal esophagus. Treatment most often involves resection of diseased esophagus with conduit interposition.**

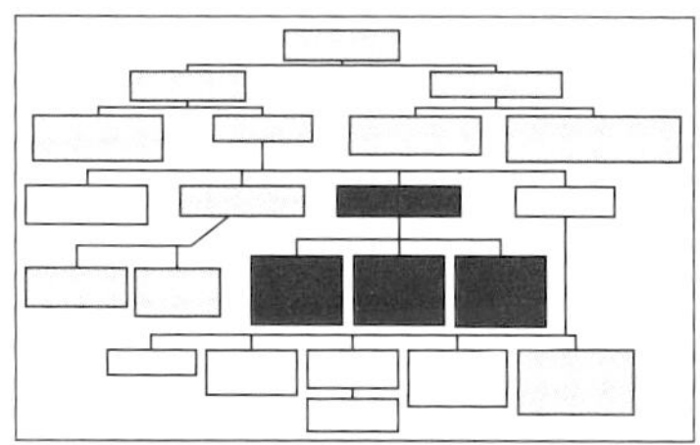

diverticulae involve all layers of the esophageal wall, whereas false diverticulae involve only the mucosal layer. Both types of diverticulae can also be classified by the mechanism underlying their formation: True diverticulae usually form in the midesophagus and are most often related to extrinsic traction from extramural inflammation in adjacent mediastinal lymph nodes. These are also referred to as traction diverticulae. False diverticulae relate to dysmotility and consist of the mucosa being extruded through external muscular layers above a high-pressure zone and are thus pulsion-type diverticulae.

Intramural pseudodiverticulosis is a rare cause of dysphagia characterized by multiple outpouchings of the esophageal wall; these outpouchings represent the dilatation of submucosal glands.[17] Although a benign condition, complications related to infection, inflammation, perforation, stricture, and bleeding have been reported. The mainstay of treatment is reduction of inflammation and dilatation of strictures as necessary.

Pharyngoesophageal diverticulae (Zenker diverticulum) are the most common diverticulae observed. These pulsion-type false diverticulae arise in the Killian triangle and are located just superior to the cricopharyngeus muscle. The

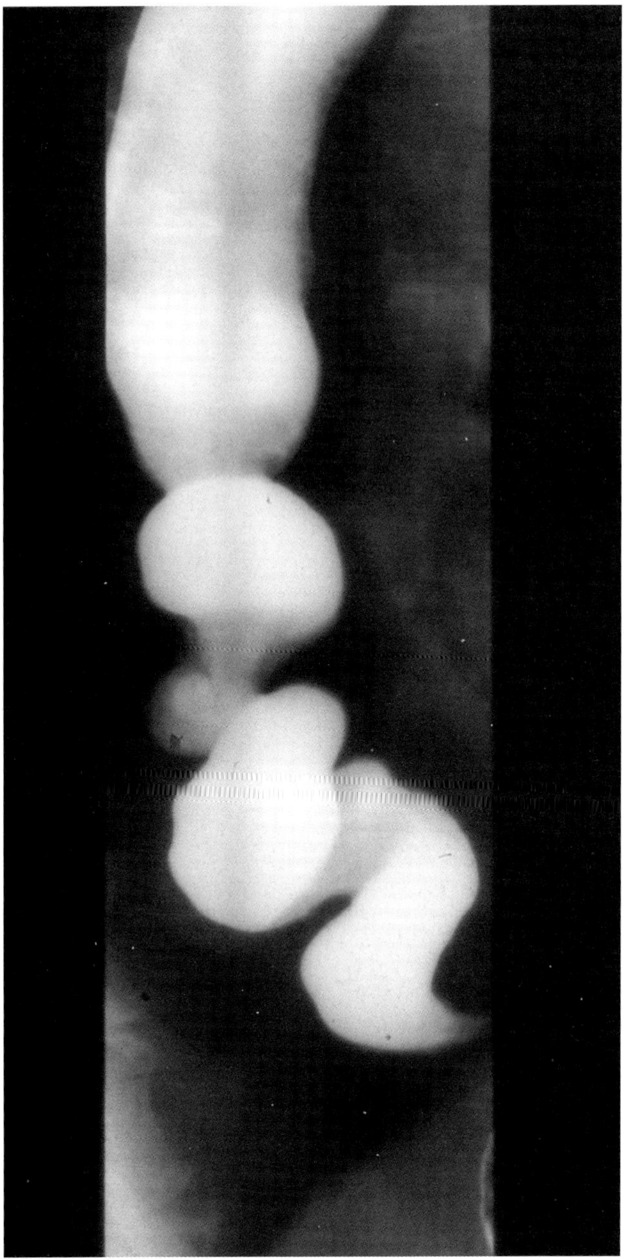

Figure 4 **Diffuse esophageal spasm. The classic corkscrew appearance of the esophagus is evident in this barium study in a middle-aged patient presenting with dysphagia and intermittent chest pain.**

basis for the formation of a Zenker diverticulum is pharyngo-cricopharyngeal dyscoordination. When the cricopharyngeal sphincter fails to immediately and fully relax during swallowing, the pharyngeal pump mechanism produces extremely high pressures. As a result of these high pressures, progressive bulging of the mucosa occurs in the posterior midline through a potential gap between the pharyngeal constrictors and the cricopharyngeus muscles (the Killian space). There has been a long-standing appreciation of an association between the pathologic severity of gastroesophageal reflux and the development of Zenker diverticulae: it is thought that repeated exposure of the proximal esophagus and pharynx to low pH refluxate results in cricopharyngeal spasm and loss of normal coordination.

Symptoms of a cricopharyngeal diverticulum include dysphagia, halitosis, throat discomfort, a palpable mass, and regurgitation of undigested food. Some patients may suffer from recurrent aspiration pneumonia and in severe cases may develop lung abscesses.

The first diagnostic test should be a barium swallow [*see Figure 5*], which will delineate the size and position of the diverticulum. Initial assessment by endoscopic means is not recommended as there is a sizable risk of perforating the pouch with the endoscope.

Treatment is surgical and must include the division of the cricopharyngeus muscle. Smaller pouches may be treated by myotomy alone, whereas those larger than 2 cm should

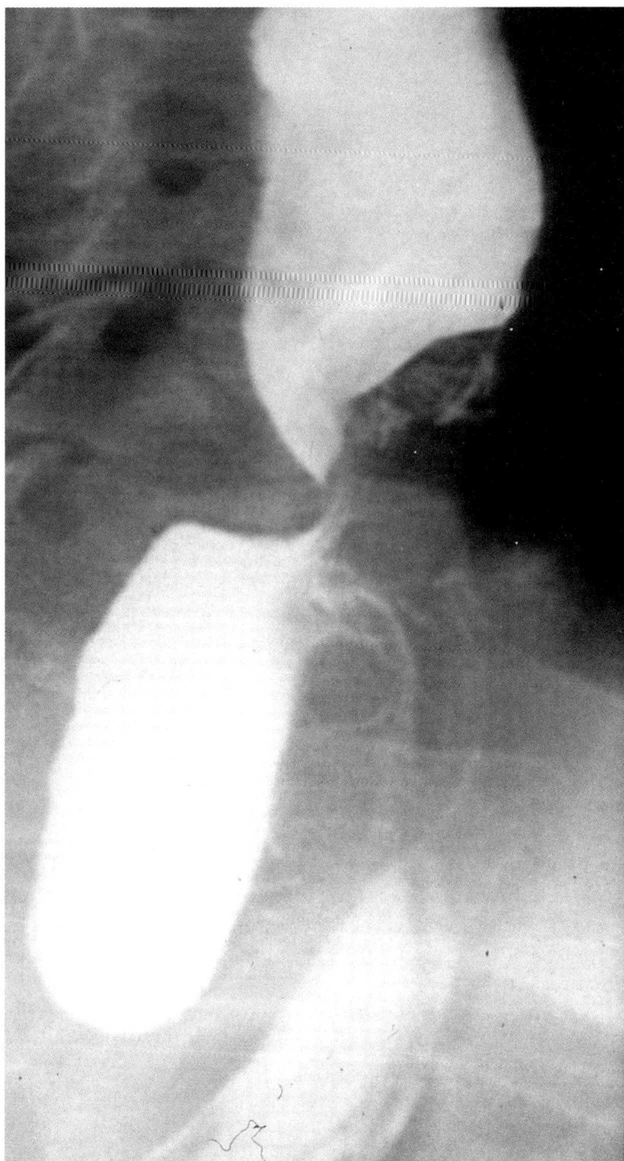

Figure 5 **Pharyngoesophageal diverticulum. A large Zenker diverticulum is shown in an elderly patient who presented with dysphagia, recurrent pneumonia, and regurgitation.**

be excised.[18] Endoscopic (transoral) approaches to diverticulostomy have also been described.[19]

Midesophageal diverticulae are not typically associated with dysphagia. These true diverticulae are formed by traction from extraesophageal inflammation, most often granulomatous disease in subcarinal lymph nodes. Midesophageal diverticulae are usually asymptomatic, and treatment is focused on the underlying inflammatory process.

Epiphrenic diverticulae arise in the distal esophagus. These pulsion-type diverticulae are associated with underlying esophageal dysmotility[20,21] and are also occasionally an isolated finding [*see Figure 6*]. In the absence of symptoms, expectant management is appropriate. When dysphagia is present, surgical management is necessary. The surgical approach, understood to incorporate "triple therapy," must include (1) excision of the diverticulum, (2) an esophageal myotomy, and (3) an antireflux procedure.[22,23]

Secondary Motor Disorders

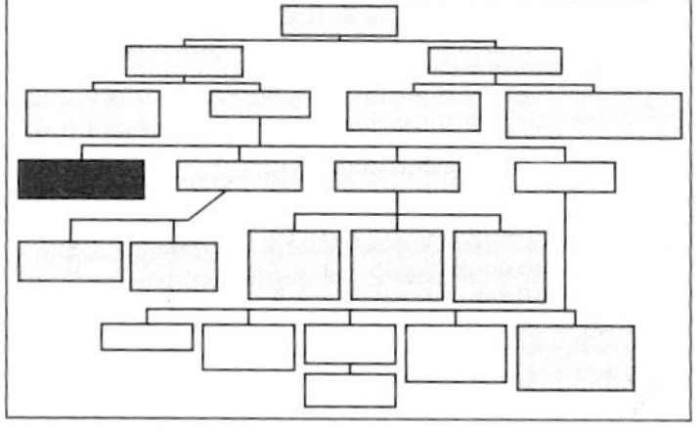

In secondary dysmotility syndromes, the esophageal symptoms are a manifestation of a generalized systemic process. The etiology is thought to be progressive neuropathy and subsequent fibrosis. Common diseases associated with secondary dysmotility include rheumatologic syndromes, such as scleroderma, and diabetes mellitus.

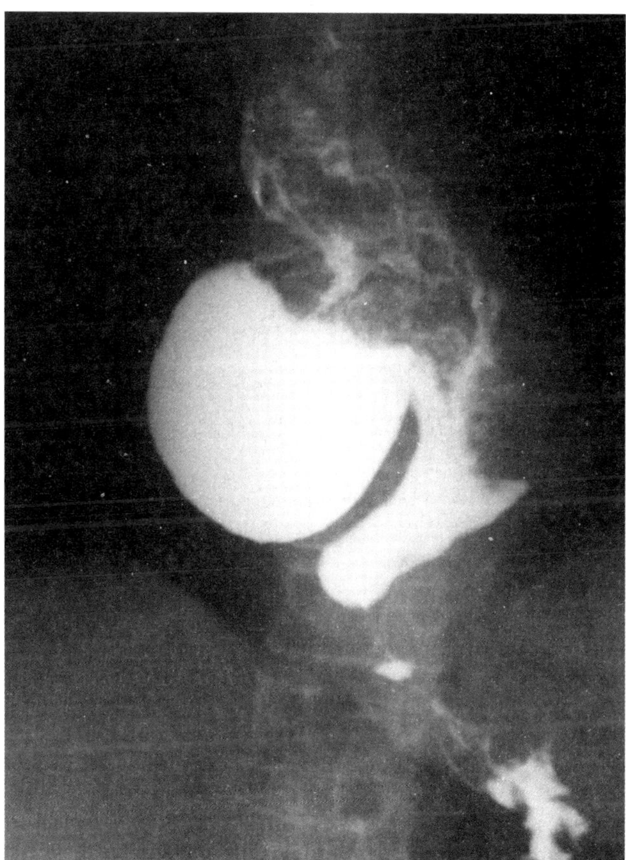

Figure 6 **Giant epiphrenic diverticulum. Barium swallow shows an epiphrenic diverticulum in an elderly female with progressive dysphagia and weight loss; cancer was initially suspected.**

MECHANICAL OBSTRUCTION

Webs

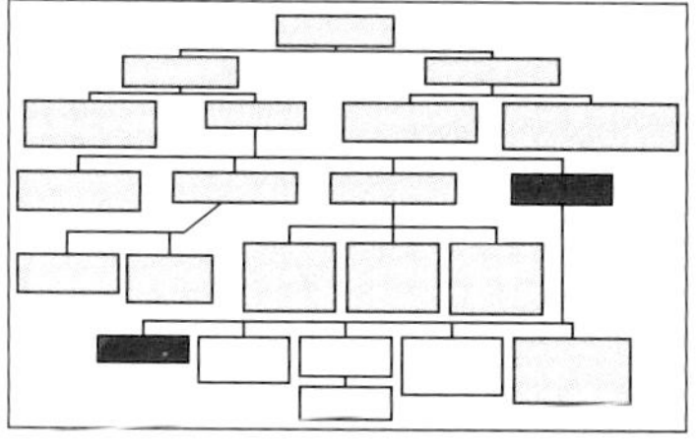

A web is a thin mucosal fold that protrudes into the esophageal lumen. Congenital webs are rare and usually restricted to the pediatric population. These are located in the middle and lower thirds of the esophagus.[7] Acquired webs are normally located in the postcricoid cervical esophagus and are mostly asymptomatic. Etiologies for acquired webs include iron deficiency anemias (Plummer-Vinson and Paterson-Kelly syndromes) and dermatologic diseases. Webs are twice as common in female patients.

Dysphagia occurs intermittently with solids, and when symptoms arise, the orifice of the web is found to be less than 1.3 cm. Diagnosis is by barium swallow, and treatment involves mechanical dilatation using Savary bougies or endoscopic balloons. Underlying anemias and dermatologic conditions should also undergo assessment and appropriate treatment.

Rings

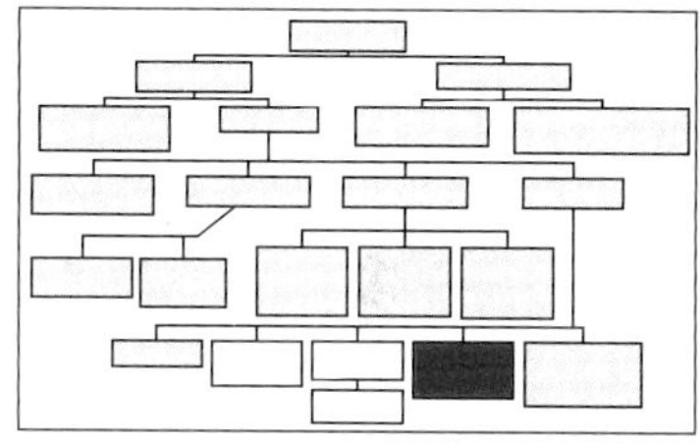

Esophageal rings are typically located in the lower third of the esophagus. Two types are typically described: muscular rings and mucosal or Schatzki rings.

Muscular rings are rarely associated with dysphagia and are often found incidentally in children undergoing barium swallow for other reasons. Schatzki rings are located at the Z-line (squamocolumnar junction) and are almost always seen in patients with GERD [*see Figure 7*]; consequently, the upper surface of a Schatzki ring is covered by squamous epithelium, whereas the lower surface is covered by columnar epithelium. Associations with eosinophilic esophagitis and GERD have been proposed. Diagnosis and treatment are as for esophageal webs.

Peptic Stricture

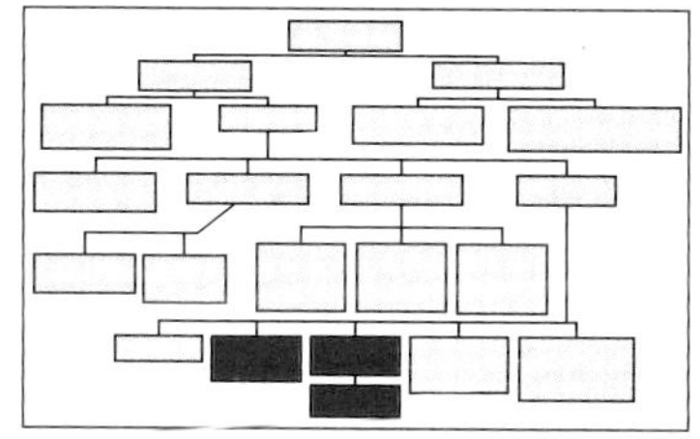

Peptic stricture was previously found in up to 10% of patients with GERD and represents the end stage of reflux-associated ulcerative esophagitis [*see Figure 8*]. The incidence of peptic strictures has been drastically reduced with the increased use of effective antireflux medications, chiefly the proton-pump inhibitors (PPIs).

Symptoms are described as progressive in nature and involve initial solid food dysphagia, progressing to liquid dysphagia. A history of reflux symptoms will also be elicited.

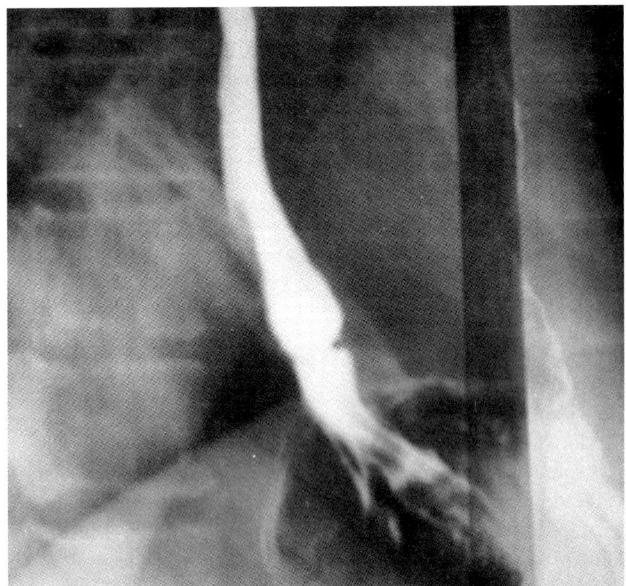

Figure 7 **Schatzki ring. Barium swallow demonstrates a ring in a middle-aged man with severe gastroesophageal reflux disease symptoms and recent-onset dysphagia.**

Initial assessment is by barium swallow. Peptic strictures are short segment, circumferential, and located at the squamocolumnar junction. A high index of suspicion for concomitant Barrett esophagus or frank cancer at the site of stricture must be kept. Treatment of isolated peptic strictures includes acid suppression and endoscopic dilatation. In the past, peptic strictures were usually an indication for surgical correction; however, recent clinical experience with careful repeated dilatations combined with effective acid suppression

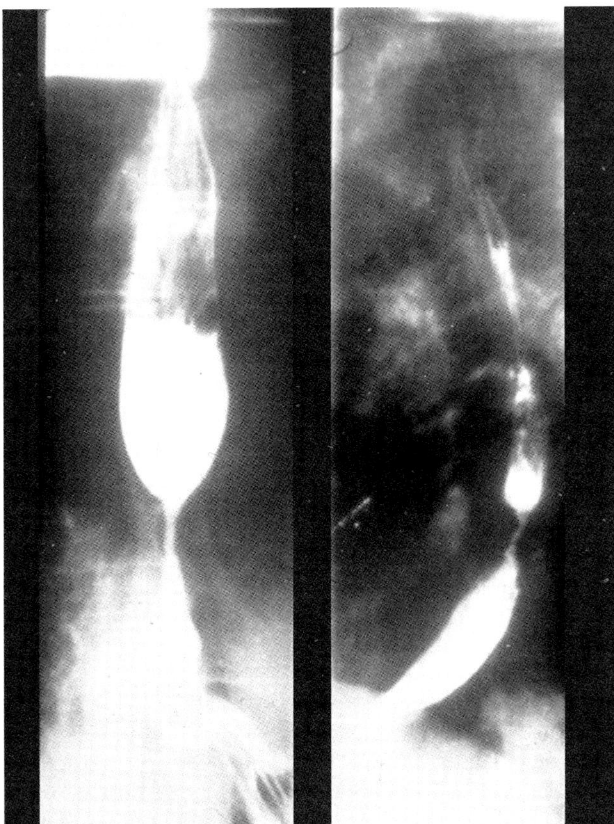

Figure 8 **Severe ulcerative esophagitis. Shown is the appearance of severe ulcerative esophagitis, annular stricture, and evidence of esophageal shortening. The caliber of the narrowed segment suggests a benign etiology.**

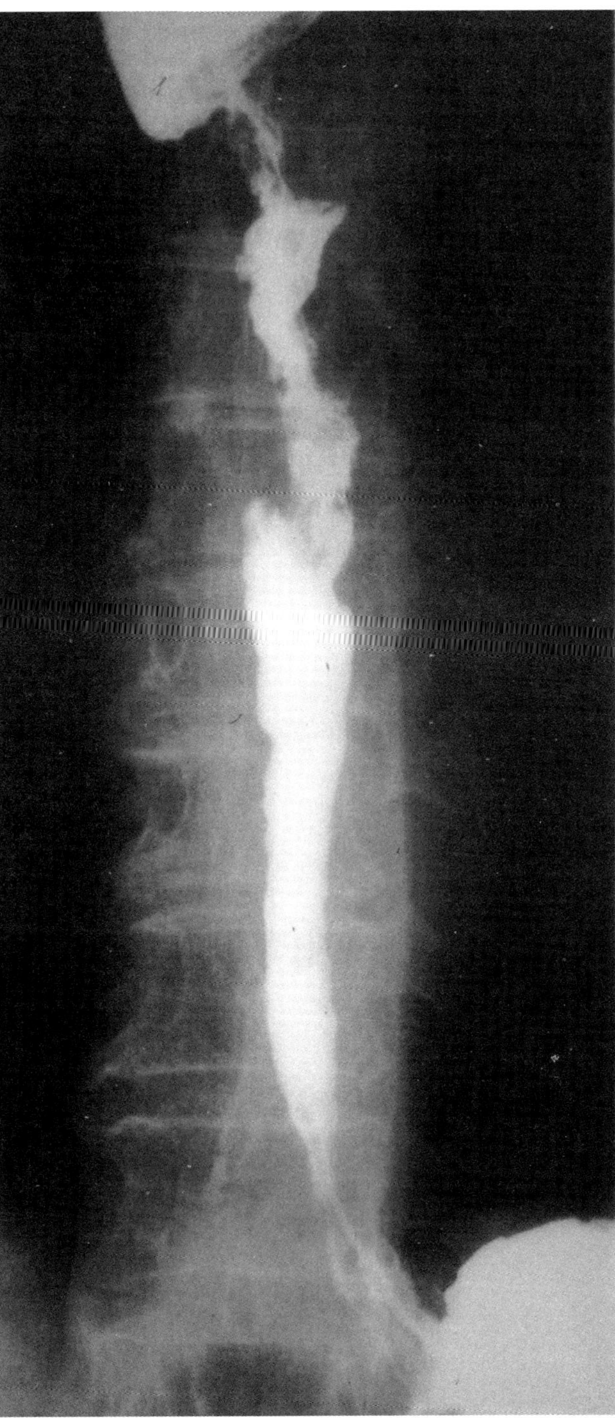

Figure 9 **Midesophageal squamous cell carcinoma. Shown is the classic appearance of a midesophageal squamous cell carcinoma. Mucosal irregularity is apparent within the lesion, along with proximal dilatation and shouldering at the upper and lower borders. Bronchoscopy confirmed anterior penetration of tumor into the airway mucosa.**

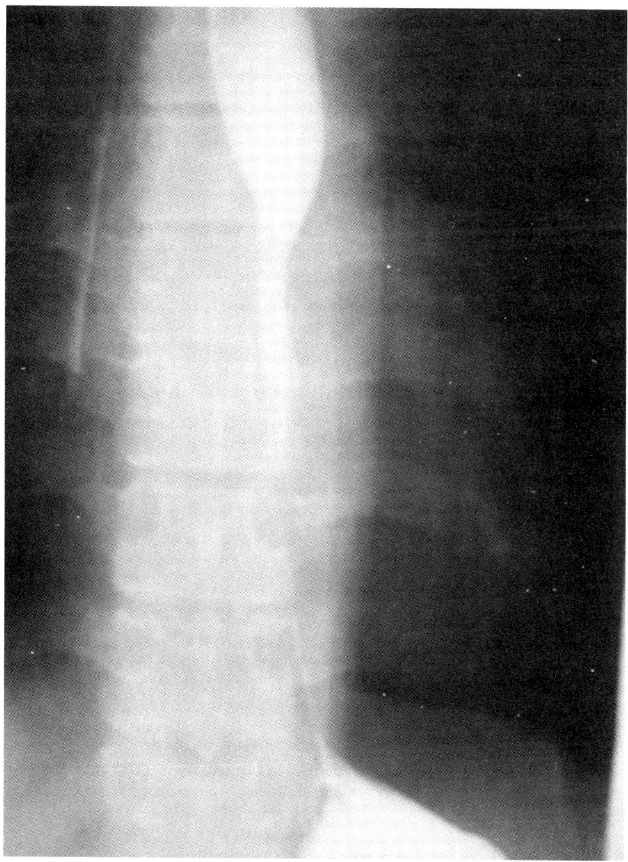

Figure 10 **Caustic ingestion. Barium swallow from a 22-year-old patient after ingestion of toilet cleaner showing a long, stringlike lumen spanning the midesophagus to the stomach. Dilatation was impossible, and esophageal resection with colonic interposition was performed.**

therapy (using PPIs) has rendered surgical treatment an uncommon occurrence.

Cancer

Dysphagia is the presenting complaint in the majority of patients with esophageal cancer. The temporal course is usually short and rapidly progressive. Weight loss is a prominent feature. Locally advanced cancers causing airway fistulization may present with aspiration (swallow-cough sequence) [*see Figure 9*]. Evaluation and staging should proceed as per established guidelines.

ODYNOPHAGIC SYNDROMES

Caustic Ingestion

Caustic agents are found in many household cleaning products. Ingestion is typically accidental but may be related to a suicide attempt. The pH of the offending agent (less than 2 or greater than 12), the volume ingested, and the total contact time with the esophageal muscosa are the determinants of the severity of the esophageal injury.[8] Immediate flexible endoscopy is required to assess the degree and severity of the injury.[9] Frank perforation or instability mandates immediate surgical exploration and resection. Sites most commonly affected include the distal esophagus and stomach; there is relative sparing of the upper pharynx and esophagus because of rapid transit through these regions.

Injuries will mature into strictures, which require serial assessment by barium studies starting 4 weeks after the initial injury [*see Figure 10*]. Repeated dilatations are typically required, although these procedures are technically challenging and sometimes dangerous as a result of the intense fibrosis, which virtually obliterates the esophageal lumen. A large majority of these patients do not have satisfactory results with dilatation as a result of an inability to

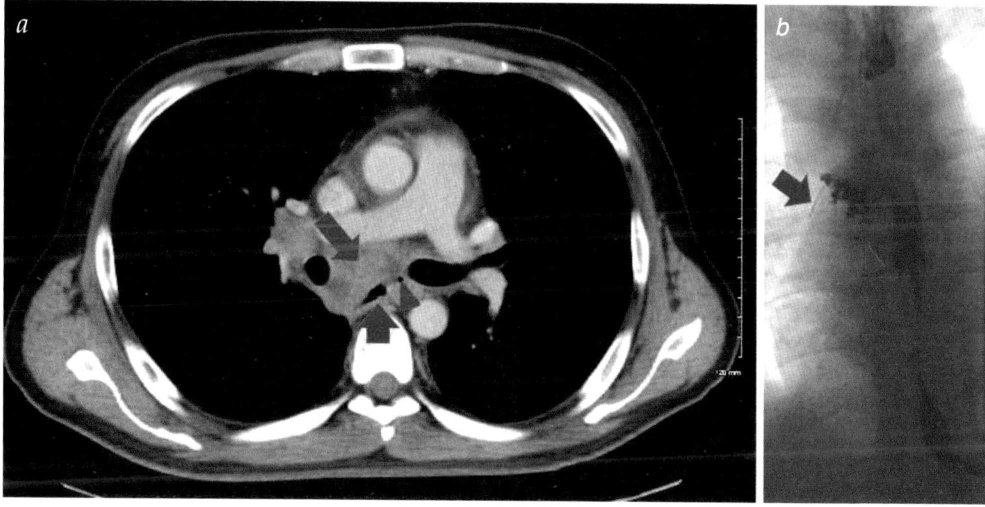

Figure 11 **Dysphagia and odynophagia secondary to tuberculous lymphadenitis in the neck and mediastinum arising in an immunocompromised patient with chronic HIV infection. (*a*) Computed tomography image showing extensive necrotizing inflammation in the mediastinal lymph nodes (*long arrow*), air within the esophagus (*arrowhead*), and a collection of extraluminal air in the mediastinum (*short arrow*). (*b*) Contrast swallow study using water-soluble contrast, showing extravasation of contrast into the mediastinum (*arrowhead*) and fistulization between the esophagus and the right bronchial tree (*arrow*). Esophagoscopy showed extensive destruction of the esophagus by the mediastinal infection and multiple small fistulae into the airway. A covered self-expanding esophageal stent was inserted to block the fistula, followed by aggressive antituberculous therapy. The fistula healed, and the patient continues to do well clinically.**

establish an esophageal lumen or an inability to maintain an adequate lumen despite repeated dilatations. Resection and reconstruction using colonic interposition become necessary.

Eosinophilic Esophagitis

This rare inflammatory condition is characterized by eosinophilic infiltrates isolated to the esophagus.[24] Intermittent dysphagia to solid food and pain are commonly noted, and associated manometric abnormalities (hypercontractility) are found in up to 60% of patients. Barium studies and endoscopy are often normal in appearance. Glucocorticoids and leukotriene antagonists represent currently accepted treatment.[7]

Infections

Infectious causes of dysphagia associated with odynophagia include intrinsic infections such as esophageal candidiasis, herpetic infections, and cytomegaloviral illness. Treatment is based on the infectious agent involved. Rarely, extrinsic infection of the esophagus (originating in neighboring necrotizing mediastinal lymph nodes) can occur, causing dysphagia, odynophagia, and other potentially disastrous complications [*see Figure 11*].

Conclusion

Evaluation of the patient presenting with dysphagia represents a challenge for the surgeon. A careful history is key in determining likely etiologies. The barium swallow should be the first diagnostic test to be considered, with endoscopy to follow. Esophageal manometry represents the gold standard for diagnosing benign, functional (motor) disorders. Treatment is varied and depends on the etiology of the dysphagia.

Financial Disclosures: None Reported

References

1. Cook IJ, Kahrilas PJ. AGA technical review on management of oropharyngeal dysphagia. Gastroenterology 1999;116:455–78.
2. Saud B, Szyjkowski RD. A diagnostic approach to dysphagia. Clin Fam Pract 2004; 6:525–46.
3. Spechler SJ. AGA technical review on treatment of patients with dysphagia [illegible] by benign disorders of the distal esophagus. Gastroenterology 1999;117:233–54.
4. Allescher HD. Globus sensation and hyperdynamic upper esophageal sphincter: another piece in the puzzle? Gastroenterology 2009; 137:1847–9.
5. Wilcox CM, Alexander LN, Clark WS. Localization of an obstructing esophageal lesion. Is the patient accurate? Dig Dis Sci 1995;40:2192–6.
6. Rice T. Dilation of peptic esophageal strictures. In: Patterson G, Cooper J, Deslauriers J, et al, editors. Pearson's thoracic & esophageal surgery. Vol 2. Philadelphia: Churchill Livingstone Elsevier; 2008. p. 251–60.
7. Lawal A, Shaker R. Esophageal dysphagia. Phys Med Rehabil Clin N Am 2008;19:729–45, viii.
8. Pace F, Antinori S, Repici A. What is new in esophageal injury (infection, drug-induced, caustic, stricture, perforation)? Curr Opin Gastroenterol 2009;25:372–9.
9. Cheng HT, Cheng CL, Lin CH, et al. Caustic ingestion in adults: the role of endoscopic classification in predicting outcome. BMC Gastroenterol 2008;8:31.
10. Peng HQ, Greenwald BD, Tavora FR, et al. Evaluation of performance of EUS-FNA in preoperative lymph node staging of cancers of esophagus, lung, and pancreas. Diagn Cytopathol 2008;36:290–6.
11. Sitzman TJ, Mell MW, Acher CW. Adult-onset dysphagia lusoria from an uncommon vascular ring: a case report and review of the literature. Vasc Endovasc Surg 2009;[illegible]: 100–2.
12. Wu JY, Chen HY, Shu CC, Yu CJ. Kommerell diverticulum, right-sided aorta, and left aberrant subclavian artery in a patient with dysphagia. J Thorac Cardiovasc Surg 2009 Mar 25. [Epub ahead of print].
13. Flanagan FL, Dehdashti F, Siegel BA, et al. Staging of esophageal cancer with 18F-fluorodeoxyglucose positron emission tomography. AJR Am J Roentgenol 1997;168: 417–24.
14. Williams VA, Peters JH. Achalasia of the esophagus: a surgical disease. J Am Coll. Surg 2009;208:151–62.
15. Spechler SJ, Souza RF, Rosenberg SJ, et al. Heartburn in patients with achalasia. Gut 1995;37:305–8.
16. West RL, Hirsch DP, Bartelsman JF, et al. Long term results of pneumatic dilation in achalasia followed for more than 5 years. Am J Gastroenterol 2002;97:1346–51.
17. Van LW, Urbain D, Reynaert H. Esophageal intramural pseudodiverticulosis. Clin Gastroenterol Hepatol 2007;5:A22.
18. Lerut A, Luketich JD, Bizekis C. Esophageal diverticulae. In: Patterson G, Cooper J, Deslauriers J, et al, editors. Pearson's thoracic & esophageal surgery. Vol 2. Philadelphia: Churchill Livingstone Elsevier; 2008. p. 702–13.
19. Hillel AT, Flint PW. Evolution of endoscopic surgical therapy for Zenker's diverticulum. Laryngoscope 2009;119:39–44.
20. D'Journo XB, Ferraro P, Martin J, et al. Lower oesophageal sphincter dysfunction is part of the functional abnormality in epiphrenic diverticulum. Br J Surg 2009;96: 892–900.
21. Rice TW, Goldblum JR, Yearsley MM, et al. Myenteric plexus abnormalities associated with epiphrenic diverticula. Eur J Cardiothorac Surg 2009;35:22–7.
22. Kilic A, Schuchert MJ, Awais O, et al. Surgical management of epiphrenic diverticula in the minimally invasive era. J Soc Laparoendosc Surg 2009;13:160–4.
23. Varghese TK Jr, Marshall B, Chang AC, et al. Surgical treatment of epiphrenic diverticula: a 30-year experience. Ann Thorac Surg 2007;84:1801–9.
24. Rothenberg ME. Biology and treatment of eosinophilic esophagitis. Gastroenterology 2009;137:1238–49.
25 Matsuo K, Palmer JB. Anatomy and physiology of feeding and swallowing: normal and abnormal. Phys Med Rehabil Clin N Am 2008;19:691–707, vii.

2 COUGH AND HEMOPTYSIS

Shahriyour Andaz, MD, FACS, FRCS, and Svetlana Danovich, DO, PhD

Cough is one of the most common symptoms in patients seeking medical attention from the office-based physician.[1] In the United States, it accounts for approximately 30 to 50 million physician visits each year, and more than $1 billion is spent annually on its workup and treatment.[2] Despite its massive burden on health care resources, cough is often dismissed as an unimportant irritation rather than a symptom of major socioeconomic importance.[3] Hemoptysis, however, may not be as common a presenting complaint, and even mild hemoptysis is distressing to many patients and physicians and calls for prompt attention and diagnosis. It may range in severity from mild blood streaking in sputum to massive hemorrhage that, if left untreated, can lead to shock and rapid death from blood loss and asphyxiation. Every case of hemoptysis warrants a thorough clinical evaluation. Cough and hemoptysis can result from a wide variety of conditions, ranging from fairly non–life-threatening causes (e.g., bronchitis) to life-threatening ones (e.g., lung cancer). Because both cough and hemoptysis may be signs of urgent or life-threatening disease, patients who present with either or both of these symptoms should undergo a thorough, methodical workup consisting of a detailed history, a careful physical examination, and appropriate diagnostic studies.

Cough

DEFINITION

Cough is a forceful release of air from the lungs that can be heard. Coughing protects the respiratory system by clearing it of irritants and secretions. Although people can cough voluntarily, a cough is usually a reflex triggered when an irritant stimulates one or more of the cough receptors found at different points in the respiratory system.

Cough is a reflex defense mechanism that consists of an acute rapid inspiratory phase followed by an equally rapid and forceful expiratory phase against a closed glottis. Rapid opening of the glottis and brisk forceful expulsion result in the clearance of inhaled pathogens, aeroallergens, irritants, particulate matter, secretions, and aspirate.[4] Impaired cough reflexes significantly increase the risk of pulmonary infection from retained secretions. Cough helps maintain airway function and lung capacity for gas exchange.[5,6]

The cough reflex is initiated by the irritation of cough receptors that exist not only in the epithelium of the upper and lower respiratory tract but also in the pericardium, lower esophagus, stomach, and diaphragm.[7,8] These receptors can be triggered by chemical and mechanical stimuli such as foreign bodies, irritant particles, fumes, and extrinsic pressure from masses (e.g., lung cancer), edema from pulmonary parenchymal infection (e.g., pneumonia or abscess), or pulmonary parenchymal fibrosis resulting from any of a variety of interstitial lung diseases (e.g., idiopathic pulmonary fibrosis or sarcoidosis).

The airway sensory receptors are either primarily mechanically sensitive (low-threshold mechanoreceptors) or primarily chemically sensitive (chemosensors or, alternatively, nociceptors). Mechanoreceptors are of two types: rapidly adapting receptors (RARs) and slowly adapting receptors (SARs). They are sensitive to many mechanical stimuli, including changes in lung volume, airway smooth muscle constriction, and airway wall edema. As their names suggest, RARs display rapid adaptation (i.e., a rapid reduction in the number of action potentials) during sustained lung inflations, whereas SARs adapt slowly to this stimulus. RARs and SARs have different mechanical activation profiles. Thus, RARs may be activated during both inflation and deflation of the lungs (including lung collapse). SARs, on the other hand, display activity during tidal inspirations, peaking just prior to the initiation of expiration. Even though the RARs and SARs are not chemosensitive, they do get activated secondary to airway smooth muscle contraction, mucous secretion, or edema formation caused by bradykinin and capsaicin.

Chemically sensitive airway afferent fibers become recruited during airway inflammation or irritation. They are typically activated by a wide range of chemicals, including capsaicin, bradykinin, adenosine, and prostaglandin E_2. Chemosensors are stereotypically defined by their responsiveness to the irritant chemical capsaicin and, hence, the expression of the capsaicin receptor. The transient receptor potential cation channel, subfamily V, member 1 (TRPV1), also known as the capsaicin receptor, is a protein that, in humans, is encoded by the *TRPV1* gene. This protein is a member of the TRPV group of the transient receptor potential family of ion channels. TRPV1 is a nonselective cation channel that may be activated by a wide variety of exogenous and endogenous physical and chemical stimuli. The best known activators of TRPV1 are heat greater than 43°C and capsaicin, the pungent compound in hot chili peppers. Airway chemosensors are sometimes thought of as high-threshold mechanosensors. Within this group are fibers that are not readily excited by mechanical stimulation (e.g., bronchoconstriction, lung inflations, light touch) but can be activated using severe mechanical manipulations (e.g., lung hyperinflation, forceful punctate stimuli) and one or more chemical stimuli (e.g., capsaicin, bradykinin, adenosine).[9–12]

Afferent fibers from cough receptors in the airways converge via the vagus nerve on brainstem sites in the nucleus tractus solitarus. The nucleus tractus solitarius is connected to respiratory-related neurons in the central respiratory generator that coordinate the efferent cough response.[13] Sensation of the cough reflex can also arise in the brainstem neurons. Higher cortical centers can also voluntarily inhibit or produce cough.[14,15]

CLINICAL EVALUATION

Guidelines from the American College of Chest Physicians distinguish three categories of cough based on duration:

- Acute cough, lasting less than 3 weeks
- Subacute cough, lasting between 3 and 8 weeks
- Chronic cough, lasting more than 8 weeks[16]

Cough can be the first indication of serious pulmonary or extrapulmonary pathologic conditions; the differential diagnosis of cough includes infectious, inflammatory, and neoplastic conditions and many pulmonary disorders [*see Table 1*]. The most common cause of acute, transient cough is the common cold. The most prevailing genesis in a series of 184 patients with subacute cough (lasting 3 to 8 weeks) was postinfectious cough (48%), postnasal drip (33%), and cough-variant asthma (16%).[4] The most frequent etiology of chronic cough includes asthma, postnasal drip, sinusitis, chronic bronchitis, and reflux disease. The etiology of chronic cough can be multifactorial. For example, in a study of 88 consecutive unselected immunocompetent patients referred to pulmonary outpatient clinic for evaluation of chronic cough, 39% had a single cause of cough, 42% had two causes, and 17% had three causes. The most common causes of chronic cough were gastroesophageal reflux disease (GERD) (71.6%), postnasal drip syndrome (67%), asthma (23.9%), and bronchiectasis (8%). When considering only patients with cough for at least 3 weeks, who are nonsmokers and not on angiotensin-converting enzyme (ACE) inhibitors, with normal or nearly normal and stable chest radiographs, 99.4% will have GERD, postnasal drip syndrome, and/or asthma.[17]

Table 1 Differential Diagnosis of Cough
Acute infections
Acute bronchitis
Viral and bacterial pneumonias
Pertussis
Chronic infections
Bronchiectasis
Tuberculosis
Cystic fibrosis
Airway diseases
Asthma
Chronic postnasal drip
Chronic bronchitis
Parenchymal diseases
Emphysema
Chronic interstitial lung fibrosis
Sarcoidosis
Tumors
Primary lung carcinoma
Benign airway tumors
Mediastinal tumors
Cardiovascular diseases
Congestive heart failure
Pulmonary embolism
Other diseases
GERD
Recurrent aspiration
Endobronchial stents
Drugs
ACE inhibitors

ACE = angiotensin-converting enzyme; GERD = gastroesophageal reflux disease.

The cause of cough can be determined from a comprehensive history and physical examination. In fact, some studies estimated that the cause of cough is found in up to 80% of cases from the history and physical examination alone.[17,18] The initial approach to the diagnosis of cough is a careful and detailed review of the history of the patient's cough, especially its features, including time of occurrence, frequency, duration, precipitating or aggravating factors, whether it is productive or nonproductive, and the color of the expectorant.[19] In the study of 71 immunocompetent patients with chronic cough productive greater than 30 mL of sputum/day, all patients underwent careful evaluation, including chest radiography, and other tests being selectively administered, including sinus x-rays, allergy evaluation, pre- and post-bronchodilator spirometry, methacholine challenge, barium swallow, sputum culture, sputum cytology, fiberoptic bronchoscopy, and studies of cardiac function. A specific cause of chronic cough was determined in 97%: postnasal drainage syndrome (40%), asthma (24%), GERD (15%), acute and chronic bronchitis (11%), bronchiectasis (4%), and left ventricular failure (3%).[4]

MANAGEMENT

Acute Cough

Pneumonia (bacterial, viral, and aspiration) can present with fever, cough, and shortness of breath. Patients may also complain of pleuritic chest pain. Diagnosis is often made on a chest x-ray, sputum, and blood cultures, and treatment is directed toward the causative organism.

Asthmatic patients can develop cough in response to various provoking factors (allergens, cold, and exercise) and may not always be associated with airflow obstruction, wheezing, or dyspnea. The cough is often nocturnal, and the diagnosis is supported by bronchial hyperresponsiveness using a bronchial challenge test using nebulized methacholine or histamine and spirometry flow rates.[20] Cough can be the first sign of worsening of asthma; physicians should look for a fall in early-morning peak flows [*see Figure 1*].

Chronic Cough

Chronic bronchitis Chronic bronchitis accounts for about 10% of cases of chronic cough.[21] The typical patient is a smoker experiencing productive cough. There is a wide spectrum of the disease, from mild early-morning sputum production to a chronic variety in patients with severe disabling chronic obstructive airway diseases.[22–28] In a smoker, a chronic cough is not a particularly worrisome symptom; however, if the character of the cough or the quality of the sputum changes, further workup is indicated to look for a possible superimposed infection or neoplasm.[27] Any degree of hemoptysis in a former smoker should be taken seriously, especially if it is not associated with an infection. A chest x-ray may not be diagnostic, and evaluation with chest computed tomography (CT) and/or bronchoscopy may be indicated.[27,28] Treatment consists of cessation of smoking, antibiotics, bronchodilators, and oral or inhaled steroids [*see Figure 2*].

Postnasal drip Postnasal drip, also known as upper airway cough syndrome, occurs when excessive mucus is produced by the nasal membrane. The excess mucus

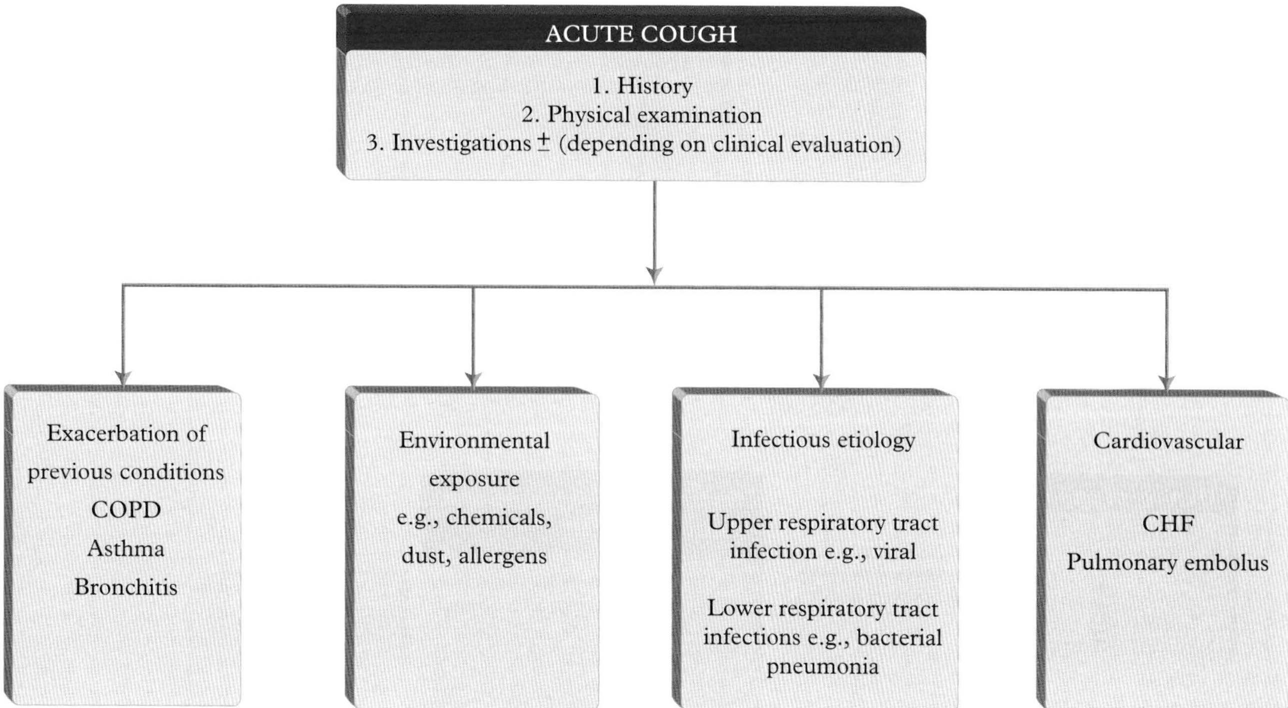

Figure 1 **Acute cough algorithm for the management of patients over 15 years of age with cough lasting less than 3 weeks. CHF = congestive heart failure; COPD = chronic obstructive pulmonary disease.**

accumulates in the back of the nose and trickles down the throat. It is characterized by a sensation of nasal secretions of a drip at the back of the throat, often accompanied by the frequent need to clear the throat, and is associated with nasal discharge or nasal stiffness. Nasal secretions irritate the larynx and trachea, leading to activation of the cough reflex arc.[29] Postnasal drip occurs during the day or night and may be worse at night. Generally, the diagnosis is made on the basis of the history and the symptom complex. The symptoms may be vague at times, and the diagnosis is confirmed only when the patient responds to empirical therapy. In recalcitrant cases, an otolaryngologic examination may be required to exclude sinus disorders. Physical examination may reveal nasal edema, mucopurulent secretions, and the typical cobblestone appearance of the posterior pharyngeal wall.[29] CT scanning of the sinuses may be required if the diagnosis is uncertain. Steroid nasal sprays, antihistamines, and nasal irrigations with saline are useful for ameliorating symptoms.

Medications Cough is a well-recognized complication of ACE inhibitor therapy.[30] ACE inhibitors are prescribed for the treatment of hypertension and heart failure; 2 to 33% of patients report a dry cough.[31] The cough can arise within a few hours of taking the drug but can also become apparent after only a few weeks or months; it improves within days or weeks of withdrawal of the drug but can take longer to resolve completely. ACE inhibitor cough can be caused by the accumulation of bradykinin and prostaglandin, which directly sensitize cough receptors. Cough may also result from nonselective beta-blocker therapy or may develop as a consequence of idiosyncratic reactions to a variety of drugs and herbal remedies.

Reflux disease GERD is commonly implicated as a cause of chronic cough. In fact, it may be the only symptom in GERD.[32] Typically, symptoms of acid reflux, other than cough, are heartburn, chest pain, a sour taste, and regurgitation. Reflux of gastric contents to the larynx can cause reflux laryngitis with thickening, redness, and edema of the posterior larynx.[33–35] The diagnosis is difficult to make if the typical symptoms of reflux and heartburn are absent. As awareness of reflux-induced asthma and cough grows, more patients are being evaluated with barium studies and esophageal pH monitoring, which often provide the correct diagnosis when clinical evaluation cannot.

Tumors In smokers, a change in the nature of cough or hemoptysis should alert the physician to an underlying carcinoma.[27] There may be associated weight loss and weakness. Malignant central tumors tend to be squamous cell carcinoma or small cell cancers and can have associated mediastinal lymphadenopathy detected as hilar or mediastinal fullness on a chest x-ray and confirmed on CT scans. Carcinoid tumors, for the most part, tend to be central endobronchial lesions, causing obstruction to the lumen of the bronchus, and appear as smooth, round, fleshy, and highly vascular lesions on bronchoscopy. Not uncommonly, patients with a carcinoid tumor of the airway will have been treated with inhalers and steroids for years because of the presumptive diagnosis of asthma. Patients with malignant fistulas between the airway and the esophagus either from the cancers eroding the lumens or as a result of breakdown after radiotherapy present with copious secretions and foul breath. These patients usually have advanced disease and are best palliated with covered stents in the trachea and/or the esophagus.

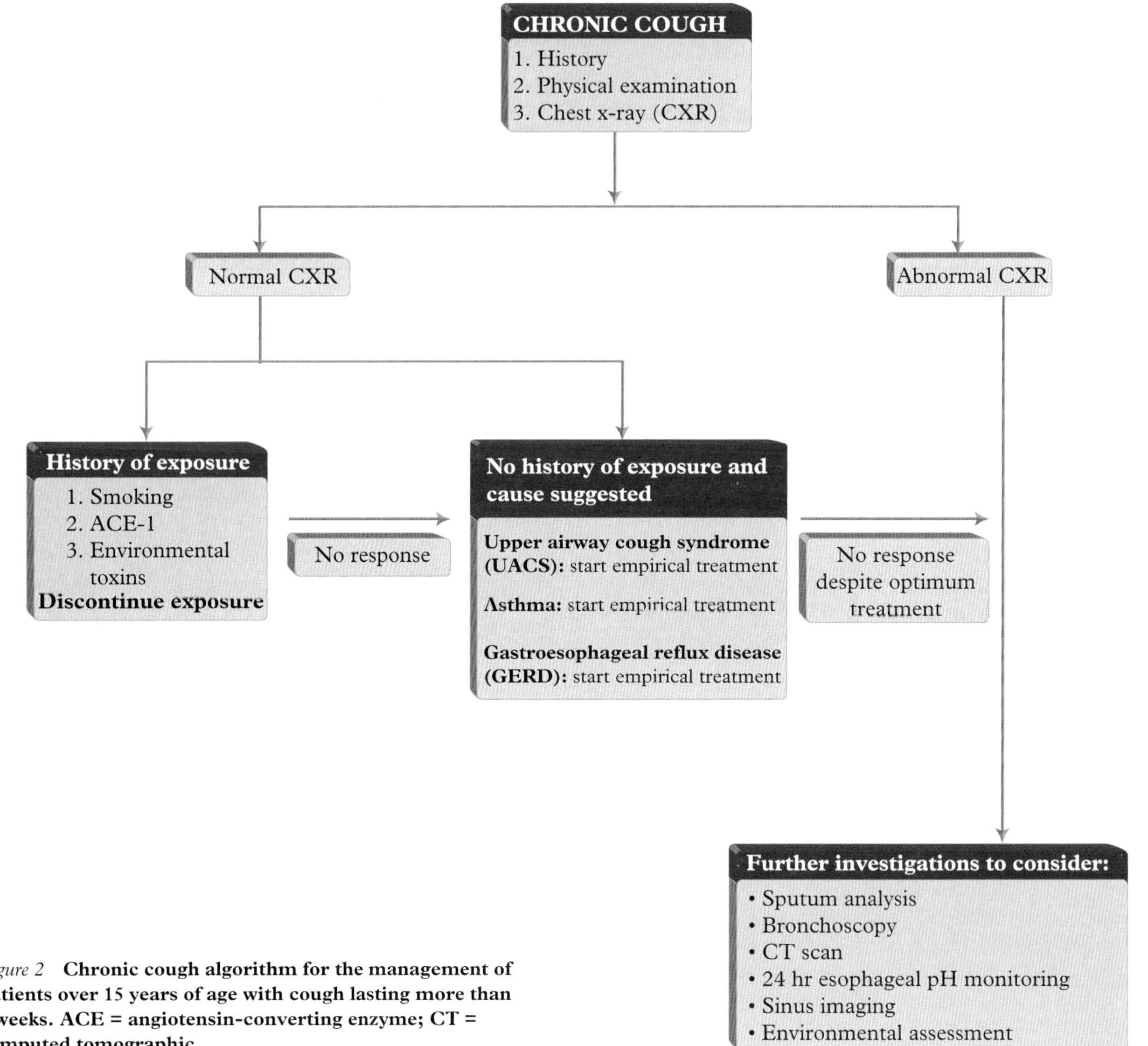

Figure 2 **Chronic cough algorithm for the management of patients over 15 years of age with cough lasting more than 8 weeks. ACE = angiotensin-converting enzyme; CT = computed tomographic.**

Other conditions associated with cough Bronchiectasis cough is associated with extensive secretions from overproduction, together with reduced clearance, of airway secretions[36] The patient produces mucoid or mucopurulent sputum, sometimes accompanied by fever, hemoptysis, and weight loss.[36] Cough can be the only presenting symptom. Bronchiectasis can be associated with postnasal drip and rhinosinusitis, asthma, GERD, and chronic bronchitis.[37] Bronchiectasis can lead to clubbing of the fingers. Common pathogens cultured from sputum include *Haemophilus influenzae*, *Staphylococcus aureus*, and *Pseudomonas aeruginosa*.[37] Patients with immotile cilia syndrome (Kartagener syndrome) will have other hallmarks of disease, such as situs inversus, sinusitis, and recurrent otitis.[38] Diagnosis is made by the delay (over 12 minutes) in the patient's ability to taste the saccharine placed on the anterior nares. Treatment is directed at the recurrent infections in the sinuses, ears, and chest.

A chronic cough may also be a consequence of congestive heart failure (CHF) (from any cause), although this is not a common occurrence. Mild CHF with symptoms of orthopnea at night may be associated with coughing. The diagnosis is made on the basis of a history of orthopnea and associated cardiac risk factors or valvular disease, followed by cardiac echocardiography. Occasionally, the presence of a small unrecognized tracheobronchial foreign body can lead to chronic irritation of the bronchial epithelium and then to a persistent cough; this presentation is more common in children than in adults.[39] The diagnosis is usually made by performing bronchoscopy in a patient who is believed to be harboring a foreign body on the basis of chest imaging.

Eosinophilic bronchitis is a rare cause of chronic cough that may be suspected in patients with no other clearly explainable diagnosis.[40,41] Patients typically have a history of atopy, and the diagnosis is made on the basis of clinical suspicion and the results of bronchial epithelial biopsy. Steroids are the mainstay of treatment. Chronic cough can be a prominent symptom of occupational exposure in glass workers exposed to low-molecular-weight irritants, hydrochloric acid, and organic oils.[42,43]

In the occasional patient, a chronic cough may be of psychogenic origin. Such a cough classically occurs during the daytime and is absent when the patient is asleep. This is described as short and explosive and usually has been triggered by a precipitating upper respiratory tract infection that leads to a "sensation of a trickle in the throat" and has subsequently persisted. It can be socially disruptive. The mainstay of treatment is creating an awareness in the patient and encouraging voluntary suppression of the cough and attempts at increasing the time interval between coughs.[44,45]

Hemoptysis

DEFINITION

Hemoptysis is defined as expectoration of blood originating from the lower airways (tracheobronchial or pulmonary parenchymal). Hemoptysis can be traces or massive, potentially resulting in asphyxia by flooding the airways. By definition, a loss of over 600 mL over 24 hours is considered massive. However, even as little as 150 mL of rapid blood loss in a patient with compromised pulmonary functions can be disastrous because the total dead space of the airway is 150 mL.

HISTORY

Hemoptysis dates back to 400 BC, when Hippocrates described hemoptysis in patients with advanced phthisis (Latin, from Greek, from *phthinein*, to waste away). Greek physicians recognized hemoptysis as being caused by underlying tuberculosis. In 1938, Eloesser suggested lobectomy for hemoptysis.[46] In 1941, Pitkin performed the first pneumonectomy in a patient with bronchiectasis,[47] and in 1973, Remy and colleagues reported the first case of bronchial arterial embolization.[48]

SURGICAL ANATOMY

There are two major sources of independent arterial inflow to the lungs: an anatomically consistent pulmonary circuit with the inflow through the pulmonary artery and return via the pulmonary veins and a highly variable and complex bronchial arterial system originating from the arch of the aorta, intercostals, or other arterial branches that supply the esophagus, mediastinal lymph glands, and spinal artery.

A bronchial artery greater than 2 mm is considered pathologic, and the bronchial arteries play the dominant role in hemoptysis as these vessels are subjected to higher systemic pressures.[49] As a rule, the blood seen in the sputum is derived from either the pulmonary arteries or the bronchial arteries; only rarely does it come from the pulmonary veins.[50–52] Although the bronchial arteries provide less blood flow than the pulmonary arteries do, they supply the bulk of the blood received by the airways and, accordingly, are the source of the blood in most cases of hemoptysis.

ETIOLOGY

Inflammatory processes, including bronchitis, bronchiectasis, tuberculosis, fungal infections, lung abscess, and cystic fibrosis, account for 60 to 70% of cases of hemotypsis, with tumors being responsible for 23%.[53,54] In 7 to 34% of patients with hemoptysis, no identifiable cause can be found after careful evaluation.[55] Acute or chronic bronchitis leads to airway inflammation and is usually minor. Bronchiectasis [*see Figure 3*] results in the destruction of the cartilage and is associated with proliferation of bronchial arteries in the smaller bronchi (third and fourth generation), resulting in massive hemoptysis.[36] Hemoptysis in tuberculosis results from the development of false aneurysms (Rasmussen aneurysm) of the bronchial or pulmonary artery as they traverse the walls of a tuberculous cavity or occasionally from a broncholith (calcified lymph gland) eroding through the bronchus. Broncholithiasis is also seen in histoplasmosis infections.

Various benign and malignant primary epithelial and soft tissue tumors have been associated with hemoptysis. The majority of primary airway tumors are malignant, with squamous cell carcinoma and adenoid cystic carcinoma being the primary malignancies most frequently seen in the trachea.[56–62] In the case of primary lung cancers, massive hemorrhage is rare. Terminal bleeding in primary lung cancer is usually associated with a cavitary squamous cell cancer and involves major vessels adjacent to the main tracheobronchial airways.[63,64] Endobronchial carcinoid tumors are highly vascular and appear as smooth, cherry red endobronchial tumors seen on bronchoscopy. Care must be taken when performing a biopsy of endobronchial tumors such as a carcinoid tumor as serious hemorrhage can result. Tumors arising from adjacent structures such as the esophagus and thyroid can erode the tracheobronchial tree, resulting in hemoptysis.

Trauma from penetrating injuries and iatrogenic injuries caused by the Swan-Ganz catheter and transbronchial biopsies can result in hemorrhage. Granulation tissue in a tracheobronchial stent placed for malignant tracheobronchial

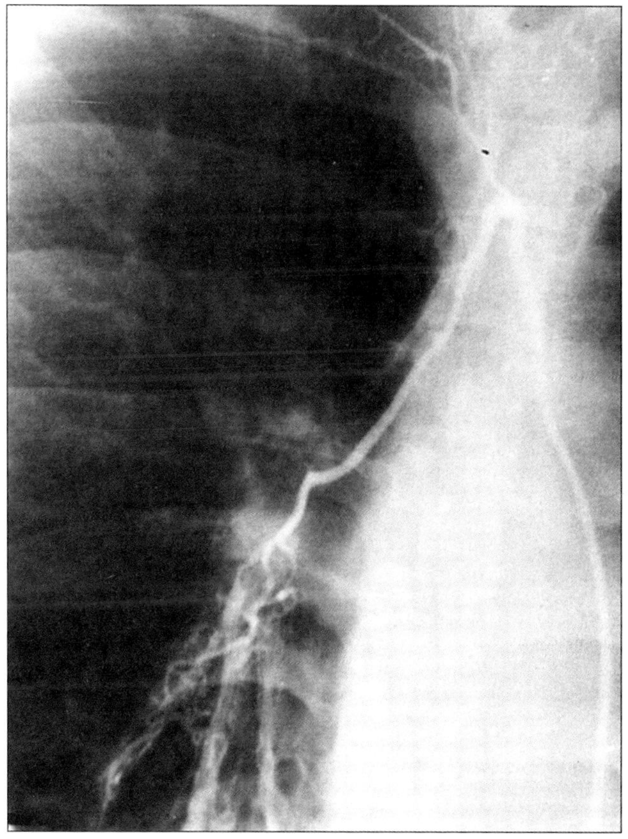

Figure 3 **Bronchial angiogram in bronchiectasis.**

disease can bleed, requiring bronchoscopy and fulguration. Massive hemoptysis from a tracheostomy should alert the physician to the possibility of a tracheoinnominate fistula.

Mitral stenosis results in pulmonary congestion leading to hemoptysis. Other cardiovascular causes include pulmonary infarction, septic emboli,[63] and congenital diseases resulting in pulmonary hypertension, for example, Eisenmenger complex and primary pulmonary hypertension. Arteriovenous fistulas are a rare cause of massive hemoptysis.[65] Patients with Rendu-Osler-Weber syndrome may have telangiectasis of the skin or superficial mucous membranes.

DIAGNOSIS

History and Physical Examination

Taking a detailed history is essential to differentiate true hemoptysis from other sources of hemorrhage, such as the upper airways or blood being aspirated from the gastrointestinal (GI) tract. A history of coughing must be obtained. A history of spitting, epistaxis or nausea, vomiting, heartburn, and abdominal pain may differentiate other sources of the bleeding, that is, the upper airway or the GI tract. The physician must determine the duration and quantify the bleeding (e.g., a teaspoon, a cupful), the presence of clots, and other respiratory symptoms, such as shortness of breath, chronic cough, and chest pain. Direct observation is sometimes the first way to quantify the bleeding. Obtaining a history of previous cardiac or pulmonary diseases, smoking, and medications, including blood thinners such as aspirin, clopidogrel, or warfarin, is vital. Clinical evaluation may reveal clubbing in patients with chronic disease such as bronchiectasis, calf tenderness, or swelling in deep vein thrombosis, and the presence of telangiectasias, suggesting hereditary telangiectasia, may help narrow the differential diagnosis [*see Table 2*].

Investigations

Noninvasive investigations Routine chest x-rays are insensitive. Chest CT with contrast can often identify the cause of hemoptysis, especially for parenchymal lesions. CT scanners capable of three-dimensional helical reconstruction are especially useful in this regard. The coagulation profile should be determined and, if abnormal, corrected aggressively.

Endoscopy: diagnostic and therapeutic The key is to determine the side and site of bleeding, and bronchoscopy is particularly effective if performed within 48 hours of presentation.[50–52] Bronchoscopy should preferably be carried out in a dedicated suite or the operating room by an experienced bronchoscopist with access to a variety of methods to arrest the hemorrhage using balloon catheters, endobronchial lasers, or endobronchial fulguration. Flexible bronchoscopy can be used for diagnostic purposes when the bleeding is minimal; however, in patients with massive hemoptysis, a rigid bronchoscope will allow not only rapid evacuation of active bleeding but also the use of other modalities to stop the hemorrhage. Selective ventilation with a double-lumen endotracheal tube may be used to temporize a critical situation.

Angiography: diagnostic and therapeutic Failure to identify the source of hemorrhage at bronchoscopy should prompt systematic bilateral angiography of the bronchial, nonbronchial, and pulmonary vascular bed. Direct evidence of extravasation of blood into the bronchi or the lung parenchyma occurs only during active hemorrhage. On occasion, the source of bleeding is a systemic vessel from the subcalvian, intercostal, or phrenic vessels.[66] Most often, we rely on indirect evidence of the bleeding vessel, as suggested by vascular hypertrophy and tortuosity [*see Figure 4*], and aneurysm formation and collateral circulation [*see Figure 5 and Figure 6*]. Bleeding from the pulmonary vasculature resulting in hemoptysis is seen in less than 10% of patients with massive hemoptysis, especially in patients with arteriovenous malformations, lung abscess, and Rasmussen aneurysm seen in tuberculosis.[66] Bronchial arteriography and embolization should be considered in patients in whom resection is contraindicated [*see Table 3*]. Embolization can result in dramatic relief of hemorrhage. Unfortunately, the majority of patients with massive hemoptysis do not survive, dying of suffocation, and the goal of the treating physician should be to identify and treat these patients before they experience their final bleeding.

Table 2 **Differential Diagnosis of Hemoptysis**
Tracheobronchial disease
Acute or chronic bronchitis
Bronchiectasis
Neoplasms
Foreign bodies
Trauma
Tracheoinnominate fistula
Parenchymal disease
Infection
Interstitial lung disease
Pulmonary embolism
Pulmonary arteriovenous malformations
Miscellaneous conditions
Mitral valve disease
Coagulopathy

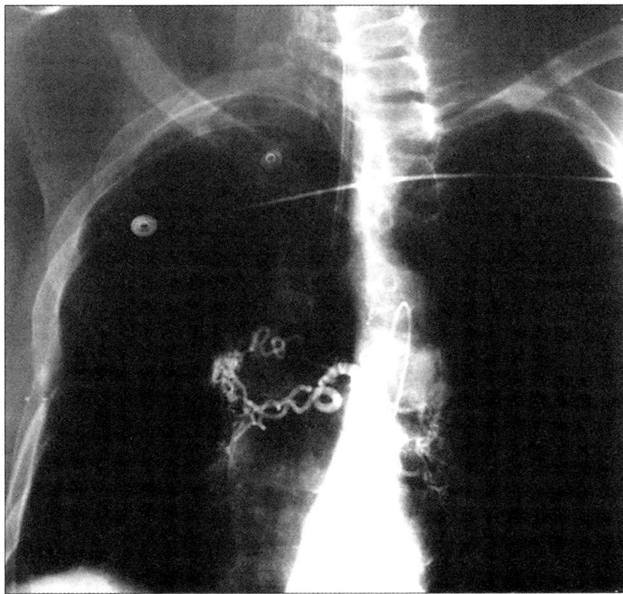

Figure 4 **Bronchial arteriogram showing tortuosity.**

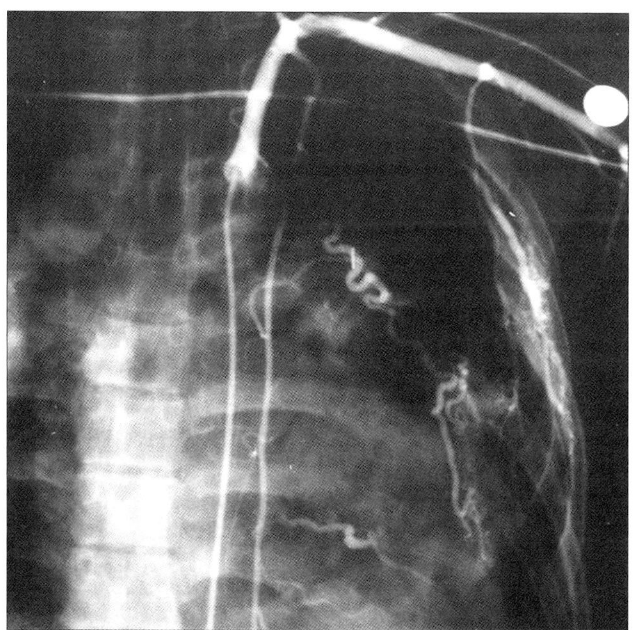

Figure 5 **Collateral circulation from the subclavian artery.**

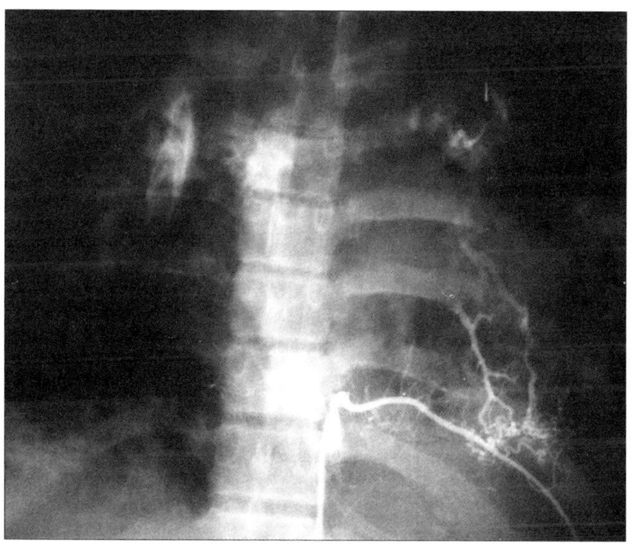

Figure 6 **Collateral channels from phrenic artery.**

MANAGEMENT

Medical

As with any potentially serious condition, evaluation of the "ABCs" (i.e., airway, breathing, and circulation) is the initial step. The overall goals of management of the patient with hemoptysis are threefold: aspiration prevention, bleeding cessation, and treatment of the underlying cause. Any patient with significant hemoptysis should be admitted to a monitored unit and evaluated promptly. Initial medical management consists of sedatives, cough suppressants, supplemental oxygen, and bed rest with dependent positioning of the pathologic side. Most cases of minor hemoptysis usually settle down with conservative measures. Patients with massive hemoptysis are, however, best monitored in intensive care units. Interventional techniques described earlier using bronchoscopy (flexible or rigid) and arteriography with embolization as required are used in stabilizing the patient.

Table 3 **Contraindications to Surgical Resection**
FEV_1 < 40% of predicted
Unable to localize site at bronchoscopy
Unresectable cancer
Metastatic disease
Coagulopathy
Systemic disorder
Bilateral lung involvement

FEV_1 = forced expiratory volume in 1 second.

Surgical

Surgery is best performed once the acute situation is under control and the site has been identified. There should be no medical contraindications, and the patient must have adequate pulmonary reserve. Pulmonary resection is the most effective method for controlling and preventing recurrent bleeding in most patients. Emergency surgery has a significantly higher morbidity and mortality than elective surgery. Surgical resection prior to hospital discharge must be considered in patients with massive hemoptysis even if the bleeding is stabilized as the recurrence rate is high (> 30%).[67] Surgical procedures depend on the pathology and pulmonary reserve. For benign disease and in patients with poor reserve, a limited resection may be appropriate, whereas in patients with malignant disease and with better pulmonary functions, a more radical approach with a lobectomy or even a pneumonectomy may be necessary.

SUMMARY

Hemoptysis must always be taken seriously. Death from massive hemoptysis occurs from asphyxiation. Every attempt must be made to localize the site of bleeding. Whenever possible, attempts must be made to control massive hemorrhage by interventional techniques. Elective resection has less morbidity and mortality than emergency surgery.

Financial Disclosures: None Reported

References

1. Schappert SM. National Ambulatory Medical Care Survey: 1991 summary. 13th ed. Atlanta (GA): Centers for Disease Control and Prevention; 1995.
2. Irwin RS, Boulet LP, Cloutier MM, et al. Managing cough as a defense mechanism and as a symptom: a consensus panel report of the American College of Chest Physicians. Chest 1998;114:133S.
3. Coultas DB, Mapel D, Gagnon R, Lydick E. The health impact of undiagnosed airflow obstruction in a national sample of United States adults. Am J Respir Crit Care Med 2001;64:372–7.

4. McCool FD. Global physiology and pathophysiology of cough. Chest 2006;129:1142.
5. Korpas J, Tomori Z. Cough and other respiratory reflexes. In: Herzog H, ed. Progress in respiratory research. Vol 12. Basel (Switzerland): Karger; 1979. p. 94–105.
6. Widdicombe JG. Reflex control of breathing. In: Widdicombe JG, editor. MTP in Rev Sci. Respiratory physiology. London: Butterworths; 1974. p. 286–91.
7. Widdicombe JG. Afferent receptors in the airways and cough. Respir Physiol 1998;114: 5–15.
8. Canning BJ, Mori N, Mazzone SB. Vagal afferent nerves regulating the cough reflex. Respir Physiol Neurobiol 2006;152:223–42.
9. Groneberg DA, Niimi A, Dinh QT, et al. Increased expression of transient receptor potential vanilloid-1 in airway nerves of chronic cough. Am J Respir Crit Care Med 2004;170:1276–80.
10. Canning BJ, Mazzone SB, Meeker SN, et al. Identification of the tracheal and laryngeal afferent neurons mediating cough in anaesthetized guinea-pigs. J Physiol 2004;557: 543–58.
11. Undem BJ, Chuaychoo B, Lee MG, et al. Subtypes of vagal afferent C-fibers in guinea-pig lungs. J Physiol 2004;556:905–17.
12. Baluk P, Nadel JA, McDonald DM. Substance-P-immunoreactive sensory axons in the rat respiratory tract: a quantitative study of their distribution and role in neurogenic inflammation. J Comp Neurol 1992; 319:586–98.
13. Shannon R, Baekey DM, Morris KF, Lindsey BG. Ventrolateral medullary respiratory network and a model of cough motor pattern generation. J Appl Physiol 1998;84:2020–35.
14. Widdicombe J, Eccles R, Fontana G. Supramedullary influences on cough. Respir Physiol Neurobiol 2006;152:320–8.
15. Hutchings HA, Morris S, Eccles R, Jawad MSM. Voluntary suppression of cough induced by inhalation of capsaicin in healthy volunteers. Respir Med 1993;87:379–82.
16. Irwin RS, Baumann MH, Bolser DC, et al. Diagnosis and management of cough executive summary: ACCP evidence-based clinical practice guidelines. Chest 2006;129:1S.
17. Irwin RS, Corrao WM, Pratter MR. Chronic persistent cough in the adult: the spectrum and frequency of causes and successful outcome of specific therapy. Am Rev Respir Dis 1981;123:413.
18. Parks DP, Ahrens RC, Humphries CT, et al. Chronic cough in childhood: approach to diagnosis and treatment. J Pediatr 1989; 115:856.
19. Pratter MR, Bartter T, Akers S, et al. An algorithmic approach to chronic cough. Ann Intern Med 1993;119:977.
20. Corrao WM, Braman SS, Irwin RS. Chronic cough as the sole presenting manifestation of bronchial asthma. N Engl J Med 1979; 300:633–7.
21. Kohno S, Ishida T, Uchida Y, et al. The Japanese. Respiratory Society guidelines for management of cough. Respirology 2006; 11 Suppl 4:S135–86.
22. Braman SS. Postinfectious cough: ACCP evidence-based clinical practice guidelines. Chest 2006;129:138S.
23. Irwin RS, Madison JM. The persistently troublesome cough. Am J Respir Crit Care Med 2002;165:1469–74.
24. Page C, Reynolds SM, Mackenzie AJ, et al. Mechanisms of acute cough. Pulm Pharmacol Ther 2004;17:389.
25. McGarvey LP, Nishino T. Acute and chronic cough. Pulm Pharmacol Ther 2004;17:351.
26. Pratter MR, Bartter T, Akers S, et al. An algorithmic approach to chronic cough. Ann Intern Med 1993;119:977.
27. Ebihara S, Ebihara T, Okazaki T, et al. Cigarette smoking, cough reflex, and respiratory tract infection. Arch Intern Med 2005;165: 814.
28. Hamilton W, Sharp D. Diagnosis of lung cancer in primary care: a structured review. Fam Pract 2004;21:605.
29. Morice AH. Post-nasal drip syndrome—a symptom to be sniffed at? Pulm Pharmacol Ther 2004;17:343.
30. Israili ZH, Hall WD. Cough and angioneurotic edema associated with angiotensin-converting enzyme inhibitor therapy. A review of the literature and pathophysiology. Ann Intern Med 1992;117:234–42.
31. Berkin KE, Ball SG. Cough and angiotensin converting enzyme inhibition. BMJ 1988;296: 1279.
32. Ahmed T, Vaezi MF. The role of pH monitoring in extraesophageal gastroesophageal reflux disease. Gastrointest Endosc Clin N Am 2005;15:319.
33. Bocskei C, Viczian M, Bocskei R, et al. The influence of gastroesophageal reflux disease and its treatment on asthmatic cough. Lung 2005;183:53.
34. Ciprandi G, Buscaglia S, Catrullo A, et al. Loratadine in the treatment of cough associated with allergic rhinoconjunctivitis. Ann Allergy Asthma Immunol 1995;75:115.
35. Leggett JJ, Johnston BT, Mills M, et al. Prevalence of gastroesophageal reflux in difficult asthma: relationship to asthma outcome. Chest 2005;127:1227.
36. Barker AF. Bronchiectasis. N Engl J Med 2002;346:1383.
37. Morrissey BM, Evans SJ. Severe bronchiectasis. Clin Rev Allergy Immunol 2003;25:233.
38. Sturgess JM,Turner JAP. The immotile cilia syndrome. In: Chernick V, Kending EL Jr, editors. Kendig's disorders of the respiratory tract in children. 5th ed. Philadelphia: WB Saunders; 1990. p. 675.
39. Saquib Mallick M, Rauf Khan A, Al-Bassam A. Late presentation of tracheobronchial foreign body aspiration in children. J Trop Pediatr 2005;51:145.
40. Gibson PG, Fujimura M, Niimi A. Eosinophilic bronchitis: clinical manifestations and implications for treatment. Thorax 2002;57: 178.
41. Birring SS, Berry M, Brightling CE, et al. Eosinophilic bronchitis: clinical features, management and pathogenesis. Am J Respir Med 2003;2:169.
42. Lee SY, Cho JY, Shim JJ, Kim HK. Airway inflammation as an assessment of chronic nonproductive cough. Chest 2001;120:1114.
43. Morice AH, Committee Members. The diagnosis and management of chronic cough. Eur Respir J 2004;24:481.
44. McGarvey LP, Ing AJ. Idiopathic cough, prevalence and underlying mechanisms. Pulm Pharmacol Ther 2004;17:435.
45. Shuper A, Mukamel M, Mimouni M, et al. Psychogenic cough. Arch Dis Cild 1983;58: 745.
46. Eloesser L. Observation on sources of pulmonary hemorrhage and attempts at its control. J Thorac Surg 1938;7:671.
47. Pitkin CE. Repeated severe hemoptysis necessitating pneumonectomy. Ann Otol Rhinol Laryngol 1941;50:914.
48. Remy J, Voisin C, Dupis C. Traitement, par embolization, des hemoptysis graves ou repeaters liees a une hypervascularization systemique. Presse Med 1973;2:2060.
49. Furuse M, Saito K, Kunieda E. Bronchial arteries: CT demonstration with arteriograhic correlation. Radiology 1987;162:393.
50. Corder R. Hemoptysis. Emerg Med Clin North Am 2003;21:421.
51. Hirshberg B, Biran I, Glazer M, et al. Hemoptysis: etiology, evaluation, and outcome in a tertiary referral hospital. Chest 1997;112:440.
52. Thompson AB, Teschler H, Rennard SI. Pathogenesis, evaluation, and therapy for massive hemoptysis. Clin Chest Med 1992; 13:69.
53. Harrison TR, Braunwald E. Hemoptysis. In: Harrison's principles of internal medicine. 15th ed. New York: McGraw-Hill; 2001. p. 203–6.
54. Reisz G, Stevens D, Boutwell C, Nair V. The causes of hemoptysis revisited. A review of the etiologies of hemoptysis between 1986 and 1995. Mo Med 1997;94:633–5.
55. Herth F, Ernst A, Becker HD. Long-term outcome and lung cancer incidence in patients with hemoptysis of unknown origin. Chest 2001;120:1592–4.
56. Gaissert HA. Primary tracheal tumors. Chest Surg Clin N Am 2003;13:247.
57. Meyers BF, Mathisen DJ. Management of tracheal neoplasms. Oncologist 1997;2:245.
58. Compeau CG, Keshavjee S. Management of tracheal neoplasms. Oncologist 1996;1:347.
59. Ampil FL. Primary malignant tracheal neoplasms: case reports and literature radiotherapy review. J Surg Oncol 1986;33:20.
60. Gaissert HA, Mathisen DJ, Moncure AC, et al. Survival and function after sleeve lobectomy for lung cancer. J Thorac Cardiovasc Surg 1996;111:948.
61. Pearson FG, Todd TR, Cooper JD. Experience with primary neoplasms of the trachea and carina. J Thorac Cardiovasc Surg 1984; 88:511.
62. Litzky L. Epithelial and soft tissue tumors of the tracheobronchial tree. Chest Surg Clin N Am 2003;13:1.
63. Thompson AB, Tessler H, Rennard SI. Pathogenesis, evaluation, and therapy for massive hemoptysis. Clin Chest Med 1992; 13:69.
64. Miller RR, McGregor DH. Hemorrhage from carcinoma of the lung. Cancer 1980;46:200.
65. Conlan AA, Hurwitz SS, Krige L. Massive hemoptysis: diagnostic and therapeutic implications. Surg Annu 1985;17:337.
66. Cahil BC, Ingbar DH. Massive hemoptysis: assessment and management. Clin Chest Med 1994;15:147.
67. Kim KJ, Yoo JH, Sung NC, et al. The factors related to recurrence after transcatheter arterial embolization for the treatment of hemoptysis. Korean J Intern Med 1997;12:45–51.

3 CHEST WALL MASS

Michael E. Friscia, MD, and John C. Kucharczuk, MD

Chest wall masses are relatively uncommon in clinical practice. Together they encompass a variety of different processes, which may be benign or malignant. Unfortunately, few surgeons have a working knowledge of the etiology, evaluation, treatment, and prognosis of patients with primary or secondary chest wall masses. Often unfamiliarity leads to inappropriate diagnostic studies, delays in treatment, and frustration for the patient and surgeon alike. The intent of this chapter is to review the clinical presentation and diagnostic procedures required to evaluate and treat a patient presenting with a chest wall mass. We begin with the formulation of a clinical algorithm to streamline the evaluation, diagnosis, and treatment of patients with chest wall masses and conclude with a review of the specific causes of chest wall masses.

The chest wall contains a number of distinct tissues, including skin, fat, muscle, bone, cartilage, lymphatics, blood vessels, and fascia. Each of these component tissues has the capability of producing either a benign or a malignant primary chest wall mass. The chest wall is also in intimate proximity to a number of organs, which may cause a mass by extension of a malignancy or infection. These include the breast, the lung, the mediastinum, and the pleura. Additionally, because of the large surface area of the chest wall, it can be the site of metastasis from distant malignancies, including carcinomas and sarcomas. The primary framework for classification of chest wall masses is shown in Table 1.

Clinical Evaluation

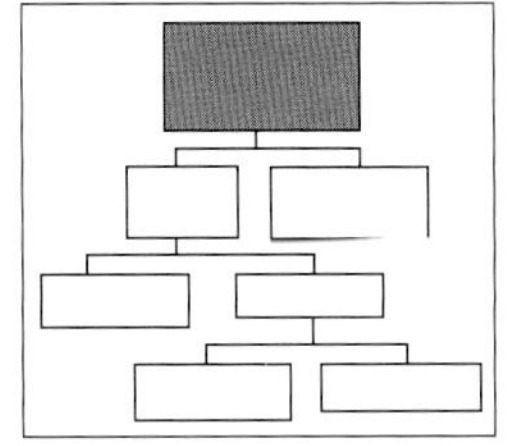

The initial evaluation of these patients begins with a careful history noting the symptoms associated with the mass and the history of its growth. A personal history of malignancy should raise concern for a metastatic lesion. A complete physical examination is performed to evaluate other sites of disease and delineate comorbid medical conditions that will impact the patient's candidacy for resection. Previous radiographs, if available, are reviewed to determine the rapidity of the growth. If the mass is palpable, its size and characteristics (hard versus soft, fixed versus mobile) are noted.

A computed tomographic (CT) scan of the chest is required if chest wall involvement of an intrathoracic lesion is suspected. For primary chest wall masses, magnetic resonance imaging (MRI) can be useful for further characterization. An MRI allows delineation of tissue planes and the relationships to major neurovascular structures.[1] Chest radiography is often performed initially but is of little use.

Table 1 Framework for Classification of Primary and Secondary Chest Wall Masses

Primary masses of the chest wall
Benign masses
Infectious masses
Soft tissue neoplasms
Bone and cartilage neoplasms
Malignant masses
Soft tissue malignant neoplasms
Bone and cartilage malignant neoplasms
Secondary masses of the chest wall
Tumor invasion from contiguous organs
Metastasis from distant organs

The next step is to decide whether to pursue a tissue diagnosis prior to proceeding with definitive therapy. For lesions less than 3 cm, whether suspected of being benign or malignant, excisional biopsy is performed for diagnosis and treatment. For lesions greater than 3 cm that can produce significant morbidity with resection, a preoperative tissue diagnosis is obtained.

Fine-needle aspirations (FNAs) are technically simple and can be performed in the office at the initial patient evaluation but are best used when metastasis is suspected. Lack of histology and tissue architecture severely limits the use of FNA in distinguishing benign from malignant primary chest wall tumors. In these cases, a core-needle biopsy or incisional biopsy is performed. Both techniques provide tissue for histology, and both must be performed so that the biopsy track will be completely excised at the time of definitive surgery. Given the easy access to most chest wall masses, many patients will tolerate a core-needle biopsy in the office, which can expedite the diagnostic process.[2]

Benign Primary Masses of the Chest Wall

INFECTIOUS MASSES OF THE CHEST WALL

Sternal Infections

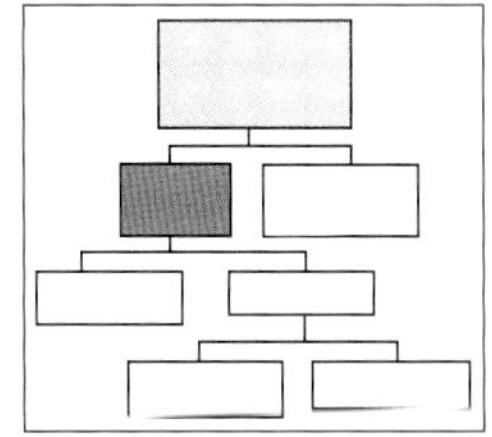

Primary sternal osteomyelitis is rare but may be seen in intravenous drug abusers. Much more common is osteomyelitis following median sternotomy. Approximately 1 to 3% of median sternotomies for cardiac surgery are complicated by sternal

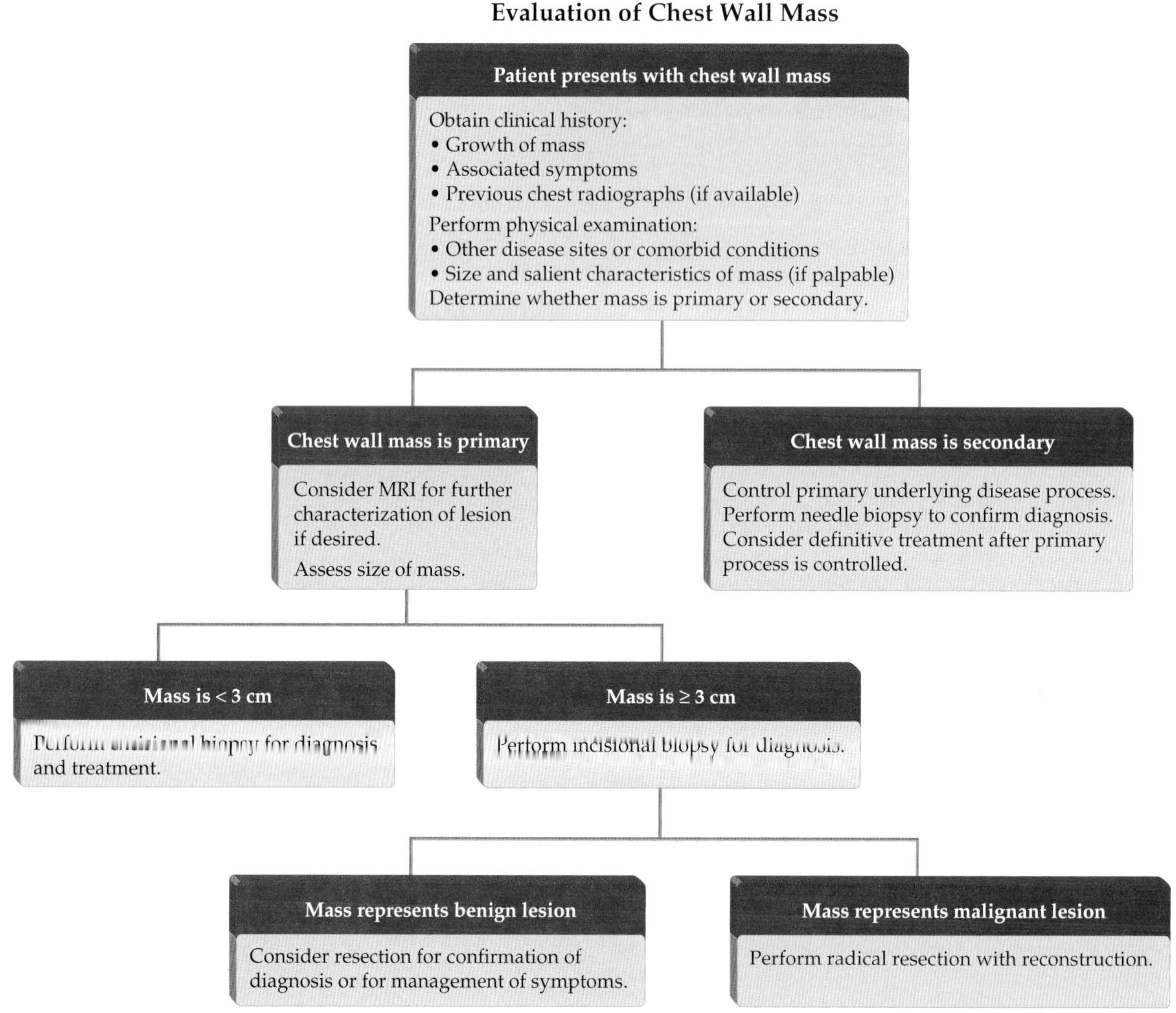

wound infection.[2] The risk factors for this complication include diabetes, use of bilateral internal mammary arteries, and reoperation.[3] These patients present with pain, drainage, and systemic signs of infection. Most of these infections have deep extension into the mediastinum as well as sternal osteomyelitis. When sternal osteomyelitis is suspected, a CT scan of the chest can help determine the extent of mediastinal soilage, but, generally, the patient is taken directly to the operating room for exploration and sternal débridement. Aggressive surgical débridement of the bone and cartilage with flap closure is associated with the best clinical outcomes.[4]

Special mention must be made of the patient who presents after sternotomy with a pulsating sternal mass. These patients have a pseudoaneursym of the underlying aorta and are at risk for exsanguination. They should undergo an emergent CT angiogram or aortogram to confirm the diagnosis. They must then be taken directly to the operating room, where they are placed on cardiopulmonary bypass through femoral cannulation and are cooled to hypothermia prior to opening the sternum as repair may require circulatory arrest.

Evaluation of Chest Wall Mass
Patient presents with chest wall mass
Obtain clinical history:
• Growth of mass
• Associated symptoms
• Previous chest radiographs (if available)
Perform physical examination:
• Other disease sites or comorbid conditions
• Size and salient characteristics of mass (if palpable)
Determine whether mass is primary or secondary.
Chest wall mass is primary
Consider MRI for further characterization of lesion if desired.
Assess size of mass.
Chest wall mass is secondary
Control primary underlying disease process.
Perform needle biopsy to confirm diagnosis.
Consider definitive treatment after primary process is controlled.
Mass is < 3 cm
biopsy for diagnosis
and treatment.
Mass is ≥ 3 cm
Perform incisional biopsy for diagnosis.
Mass represents benign lesion
Consider resection for confirmation of diagnosis or for management of symptoms.
Mass represents malignant lesion
Perform radical resection with reconstruction.

Sternoclavicular Joint Infections

Sternoclavicular joint infections present as painful palpable masses overlying the sternoclavicular joint, as shown in Figure 1. These infections are often associated with intravenous drug abuse, infected indwelling subclavian catheters, and trauma. The majority of patients have some underlying risk factor, including diabetes, hepatic or renal insufficiency, or a history of systemic sepsis. The diagnosis is made by a combination of history, physical examination, and MRI of the chest with attention to the sternoclavicular joint. The typical findings include a collection around the joint and abnormal signal intensity in the bone and cartilage [*see Figure 2*]. Treatment consists of wide resection of the sternoclavicular joint, including the proximal third of the clavicle as well as débridement of the manubrium.[5] The proximal portion of the first or second ribs can be involved and also requires resection. Immediate reconstruction is performed by rotation of a pectoralis muscle flap into the resection cavity. Postoperatively, the patients are treated with 6 weeks of intravenous antibiotics. Most require intensive postoperative physical therapy to restore strength, function, and mobility in the upper extremity.

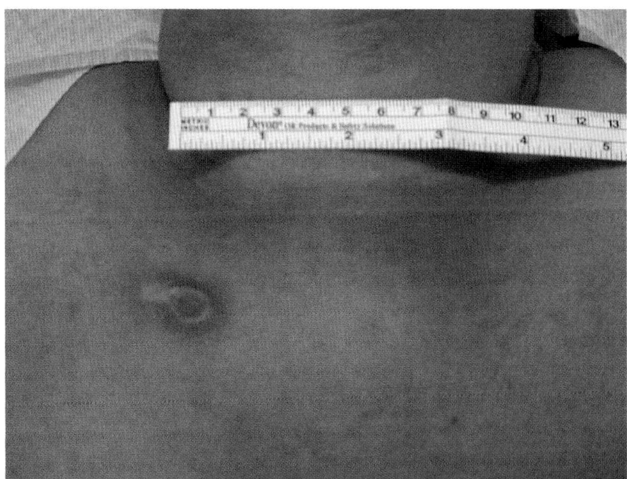

Figure 1 **Sternoclavicular joint infections present as painful palpable masses overlying the joint.**

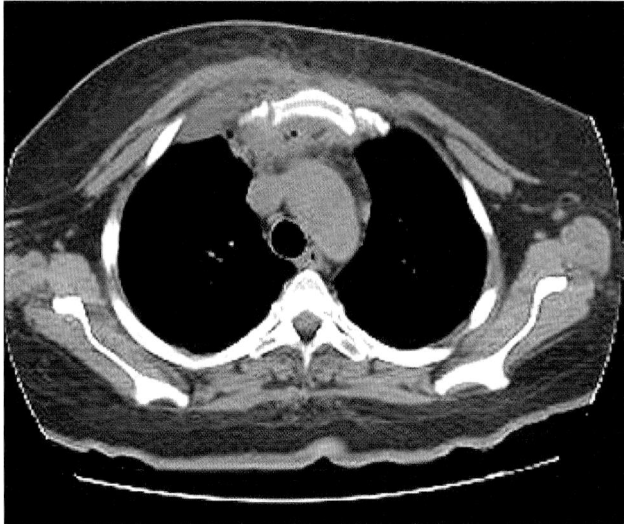

Figure 2 **A computed tomographic (CT) scan shows the typical appearance of sternoclavicular joint infection, including fluid collection around the joint and tissue stranding.**

Osteomyelitis of the Rib

Osteomyelitis of a rib presents as a painful, swollen mass overlying an infected segment of rib. Often a draining sinus tract is present. The diagnosis is made on a clinical basis. A CT scan of the chest is obtained to rule out underlying intrathoracic pathology such as an empyema. Treatment is resection of the infected bone with soft tissue coverage of the defect. Care is taken to avoid contamination of the underlying pleural cavity during rib resection. In children, the diagnosis can be facilitated by the use of ultrasonography, which demonstrates obliteration of the intermuscular planes adjacent to the infected rib and pericostal edema.[6] As with adults, the range of pathologic organisms recovered can be quite wide.

BENIGN NEOPLASMS OF THE CHEST WALL

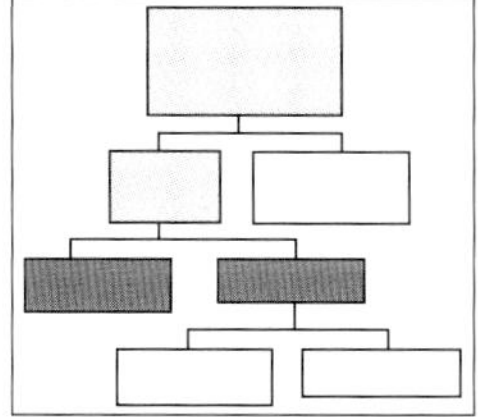

The benign neoplasms of the chest wall are shown in Table 2.

Benign soft tissue neoplasms of the chest wall usually present as slowly growing, painless masses. Often plain radiographs and a CT scan of the chest are obtained, although they are not always necessary. On examination, benign soft tissue lesions are usually soft and mobile. The CT scan shows a homogeneous mass without necrosis, infiltration of associated soft tissue, or destruction of associated bone. Small (< 3 cm) soft tissue lesions are completely removed by excisional biopsy for definitive diagnosis and treatment. Larger lesions (> 3 cm) are approached with a core-needle biopsy first to rule out a malignant soft tissue neoplasm. If the lesion is confirmed to be benign, it is resected with close negative margins to minimize the size of the surgical defect. If it is determined to be malignant, an aggressive wide excision is performed with immediate reconstruction.

Desmoid tumors deserve special mention in that they are borderline neoplasms.[7] These tumors generally arise in the muscle and fascia around the shoulder. Although they appear histologically benign, they can infiltrate adjacent structures and have a high tendency for local recurrence, which can make surgical treatment for recurrence morbid and disfiguring. For these reasons, desmoid tumors are best treated with radical surgical excision. The largest current series demonstrates that a positive surgical margin is associated with an 89% recurrence rate, whereas with a negative margin, recurrence is less than 20%.[8]

Benign Bone and Cartilage Neoplasms

Osteochondroma is a benign cartilaginous neoplasm that can occur in any bone that undergoes enchondral bone formation. Essentially, these tumors are hamartomas of the growth plate. The knee is the most common site of occurrence. In the

Table 2 **Benign Neoplasms of the Chest Wall by Site of Origin**
Benign soft tissue neoplasms
Lipoma
Fibroma
Hemangioma
Granuloma
Neurofibroma
Elastoma
Desmoid
Benign bone and cartilage neoplasms
Osteochondroma
Chondroma
Fibrous dysplasia
Eosinophilic granuloma

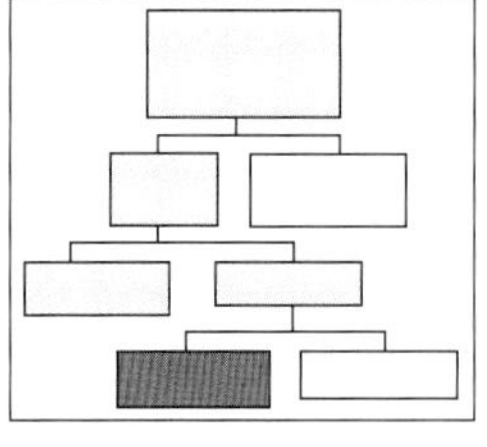

chest, they arise in the metaphyseal regions of the anterior ribs. Most are asymptomatic and found on a screening chest radiograph where an eccentric growth pattern is noted at the costochondral junction. The diagnosis is made from a characteristic pattern of stippled calcification within the tumor on plain x-ray. In children, they are followed unless causing pain or increasing in size; in postpubescent and adult patients, they are resected to confirm the diagnosis and rule out malignancy.

Chondromas are the next most common benign neoplasm of the chest wall. They occur along the costochondral junctions between the anterior ribs and the sternum. Unfortunately, the distinction between chondroma and chondrosarcoma cannot be made on clinical or radiographic grounds; therefore, excision is required for diagnosis. This results in a significant surgical defect, which usually requires complex reconstruction, including prosthetic material to provide rigid structure and soft tissue coverage.

Fibrous dysplasia is a benign cystic lesion of the medullary cavity of the rib that usually presents as a painless lesion incidentally found on a screening chest x-ray. Medullary replacement by fibrous tissue creates a radiolucent appearance on an x-ray. These lesions are treated conservatively and simply followed. Local resection is indicated if pain develops or the lesion enlarges on serial x-rays.

Malignant Primary Masses of the Chest Wall

Malignant soft tissue lesions of the chest wall constitute a large number of diverse pathologies. The primary malignant masses of the chest wall are listed in Table 3.

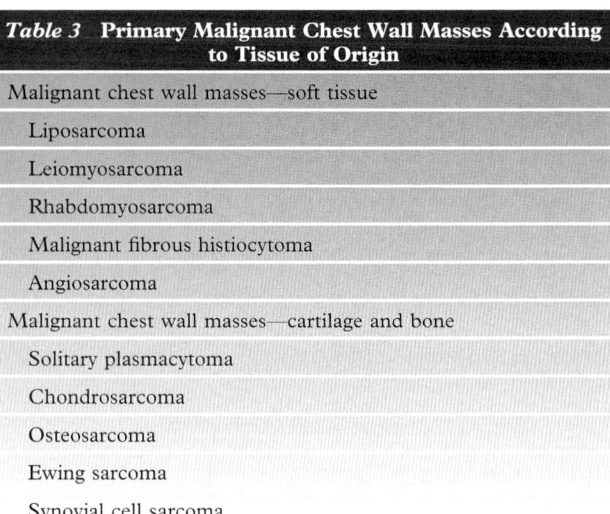

Table 3 **Primary Malignant Chest Wall Masses According to Tissue of Origin**

Malignant chest wall masses—soft tissue
Liposarcoma
Leiomyosarcoma
Rhabdomyosarcoma
Malignant fibrous histiocytoma
Angiosarcoma
Malignant chest wall masses—cartilage and bone
Solitary plasmacytoma
Chondrosarcoma
Osteosarcoma
Ewing sarcoma
Synovial cell sarcoma

SOFT TISSUE

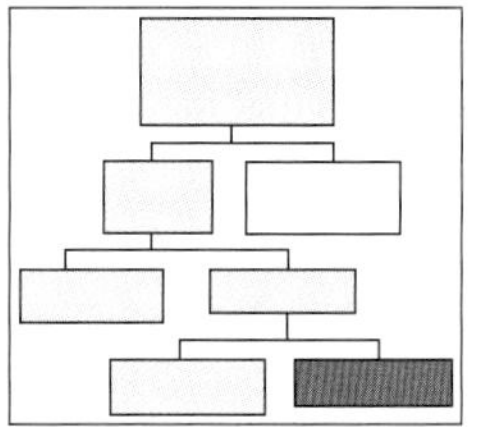

Sarcomas are the most common primary malignant neoplasm of the chest wall. On examination, sarcomas of the chest wall can be quite sizable, as shown in Figure 3. They are painless in half of the patients. The clinical finding is a hard, fixed mass. No calcifications are visible on a CT scan of the chest, but bony invasion is common. The treatment is wide surgical excision. Gordon and colleagues reported the largest surgical series of patients with soft tissue sarcomas of the chest wall in 1991.[9] The study included 149 patients who had undergone resection at the Memorial Sloan-Kettering Cancer Center in New York. The 5-year survival rate was 66%. Unfortunately, the study also included 32 patients who had desmoid tumors, which are not histologically classified as sarcomas or as malignant. A large retrospective study containing 55 surgically treated patients with soft tissue sarcomas of the chest wall was reported from a single institution in Brazil in 2005.[10] In this series, fibrosarcoma accounted for nearly 53% of the cases. With wide surgical resection, the authors reported disease-free survival rates of 75% at 5 years and 64% at 10 years. The histologic grade of the tumor and the type of surgical resection were found to be independent prognostic factors for disease-free survival. This is consistent with other studies that suggest that age, gender, symptoms, and size do not significantly impact survival.[11] The French Sarcoma Group published its retrospective series of soft tissue sarcomas of the trunk wall in 2009, which included 283 patients with chest wall sarcomas treated primarily with surgery.[12] Overall survival at 5 and 10 years was 57% and 52%, respectively. Interestingly, 22% of patients in this study had a previous history of radiation therapy, which adversely affected survival.

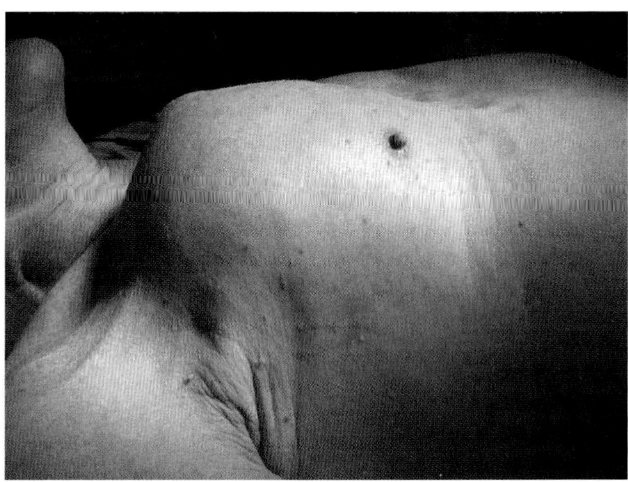

Figure 3 **Shown is the appearance of a chest wall sarcoma on physical examination. Such lesions can be quite large.**

Currently, no good data are available to recommend neoadjuvant treatment, which has become routine in the treatment of soft tissue sarcomas of the extremities. A single-institution, multidisciplinary experience with primary chest wall sarcomas was reported from The University of Texas M.D. Anderson Cancer Center in 2001.[13] The retrospective review included patients with sarcomas of soft tissue, cartilage, and bone origin, as well as desmoid tumors. The cumulative 5-year survival was 64%, which is to be expected from surgery alone.

CARTILAGE AND BONE

Solitary plasmacytoma represents an uncommon chest wall mass caused by a localized collection of monoclonal plasma cells. Histologically, the plasma cells are identical to those seen in patients with multiple myeloma; however, unlike patients with multiple myeloma, they are confined to a single site. Patients generally present with pain and often have pathologic rib fractures. With soft tissue involvement, a palpable mass becomes evident. Tissue is required to make the diagnosis either by FNA, core-needle, or small incisional biopsy. The specimen should be sent for flow cytometry, which confirms the clonal nature of the cells.[14] Definitive local radiotherapy is the treatment of choice for solitary bone plasmacytoma.[15] Although local control is achieved in over 90% of patients with radiation alone, about 50% of patient progress to multiple myeloma within 2 years and require systemic treatment.[16]

Chondrosarcoma is the most common primary malignant tumor of the chest wall. Chondrosarcomas are found along the anterior sternal border or the costochondral arches and are more common in males than in females. The primary symptom leading to evaluation is pain. The best imaging modality is CT; however, there are no distinguishing radiographic characteristics to provide a definitive diagnosis, and core or incisional biopsy is required.[17] Complete surgical resection with adequate surgical margins and immediate reconstruction is the treatment of choice. The Scandinavian Sarcoma Group published the largest series of patients with chest wall chondrosarcoma.[18] Ninety-seven patients were treated with surgery; wide excision was associated with a 92% 10-year survival and a 4% local recurrence rate, compared with a 47% 10-year survival and a 73% local recurrence rate when margins were positive.

Ewing sarcoma is an aggressive primary malignant bone tumor that presents in children and adolescents with a painful, enlarging mass often associated with fever and malaise. Ewing sarcoma was initially distinguished from osteosarcoma because of its sensitivity to radiation. Although the cellular origin of Ewing sarcoma remains unclear, there appears to be a spectrum of tumors that share the same genetic translocation and are referred to as the Ewing family of tumors.[19] The initial role of surgery in primary chest wall Ewing sarcoma is to obtain tissue for diagnosis. With smaller rib lesions, this may be in the form of an excisional biopsy. Therapeutically, these tumors are best approached with multimodality treatment, including preoperative chemotherapy followed by complete resection of residual disease.[20] A review of three multi-institutional trials from the Pediatric Oncology Group in 2003 suggested that the likelihood of a complete resection is improved with neoadjuvant chemotherapy followed by wide resection in patients with Ewing sarcoma and closely related primitive neuroectodermal tumors of the chest wall.[21] If the resection is complete and the pathologic margins are negative, no radiation therapy is given. The avoidance of radiation therapy may be particularly important in children and adolescents because of the risk (10 to 30%) of developing a radiation-induced malignancy over their lifetime.[22] Askin tumors are a small round cell tumor of the thoracopulmonary region and are members of the Ewing family of tumors. They are best managed by diagnostic biopsy and preoperative chemotherapy followed by complete surgical resection.[23]

Synovial sarcomas are rare but may arise on the trunk, where they present as a palpable chest wall mass. Despite the name, these lesions do not arise from synovial cells or joint cavities. They were originally named based on the appearance under light microscopy; however, these tumors are now known to arise from pluripotential mesenchymal cells.[24] The most important prognostic factor is tumor size.[25] Limited data suggest that although there may be an objective response to neoadjuvant chemotherapy, there is no detectable benefit on survival.[26] The current recommendation is aggressive surgical resection. Patients with very large tumors or positive surgical margins receive postoperative adjuvant treatment.

Secondary Masses of the Chest Wall

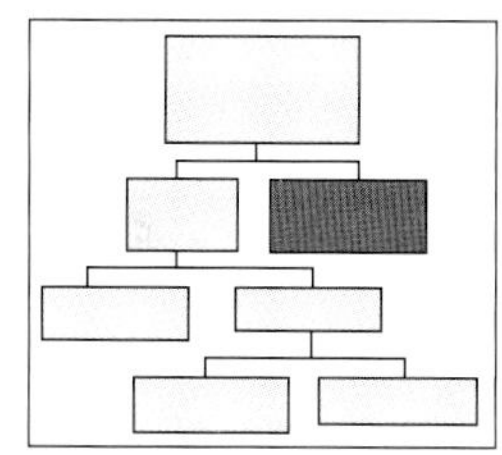

Secondary chest wall masses arise as direct extensions of a malignancy from a contiguous organ. Breast and lung cancer are the most common. The initial evaluation centers on staging the underlying disease. For example, a patient with a chest wall mass attributable to direct invasion of a primary lung cancer should undergo a staging workup to determine the extent of disease. If the patient is deemed an appropriate candidate for resection and is medically operable, he or she should undergo pulmonary resection with en bloc chest wall resection.[27] Following resection, the patient should be referred for adjuvant chemotherapy. The intent is cure, and the outcomes are stage specific.

Unfortunately, most women presenting with a chest wall mass from breast cancer have a local recurrence. Resection with reconstruction can be performed in this situation, but the benefit remains unclear. The Memorial Sloan-Kettering Cancer Center reported on 38 women who underwent extensive chest wall resection for recurrent breast cancer with a 0% operative mortality rate, but the 5-year survival rate was only 18%, and by 5 years, 87% of the patients had local recurrence.[28] Currently, chest wall resection of locally recurrent breast cancer must be considered on a case-by-case basis.

A large necrotic ulcer of the chest wall presenting after radiation therapy to the chest wall for previous malignancy should raise the suspicion for osteoradionecrosis. This is a locally destructive lesion characterized by infection and necrosis. The first step is to perform biopsies of the area to ensure that the lesion does not represent tumor recurrence. The preferred treatment is wide excision to healthy tissue and local or free flap coverage of the soft tissue defect, avoiding the use of prosthetic material whenever possible. Close collaboration with a plastic and reconstructive surgeon is critical to operative planning and success.[29]

Conclusions

Chest wall masses are relatively unusual in clinical practice. Most surgeons have limited experience in diagnosis and treatment. In general, it is important to move quickly to establish a tissue diagnosis as a physical examination and a radiographic study often cannot distinguish a benign from a malignant chest wall mass. The very unusual tumors will often require consultation with a highly specialized pathologist to make the diagnosis and an oncologist to assist in treatment planning to optimize patient outcome.

Financial Disclosures: None Reported

References

1. Fortier M, Mayo JR, Swensen SJ, et al. MR imaging of chest wall lesions. Radiographics 1994;14:597–606.
2. Toumpoulis IK, Anagnostopoulos CE, DeRose JJ, Swistel DG. The impact of deep sternal wound infection on long-term survival after coronary artery bypass grafting. Chest 2005;127:464–71.
3. Ridderstolpe L, Gill H, Granfeldt H, et al. Superficial and deep sternal wound complications: incidence, risk factors and mortality. Eur J Cardiothorac Surg 2001;20:1168–75.
4. DeFeo M, Gregorio R, Della Corte A, et al. Deep sternal wound infection: the role of early debridement surgery. Eur J Cardiothorac Surg 2001;19:811–6.
5. Song HK, Guy TS, Kaiser LR, Shrager JB. Current presentation and optimal surgical management of sternoclavicular joint infections. Ann Thorac Surg 2002;73:427–31.
6. Bar-Ziv J, Barki Y, Maroko A, Mares AJ. Rib osteomyelitis in children. Early radiologic and ultrasonic findings. Pediatr Radiol 1985;15:315–8.
7. Hayry P, Reitamo JJ, Totterman S, et al. The desmoid tumor. Analysis of factors possibly contributing to the etiology and growth behavior. Am J Clin Pathol 1982;77:674–80.
8. Abbas AE, Deschamps C, Cassivi SD, et al. Chest wall desmoid tumors: results of surgical intervention. Ann Thorac Surg 2004;78:1219–23.
9. Gordon MS, Hadju SI, Bains MS, et al. Soft tissue sarcomas of the chest wall. J Thorac Cardiovasc Surg 1991;101:843–54.
10. Gross JL, Younes RN, Haddad FJ, et al. Soft-tissue sarcomas of the chest wall: prognostic factors. Chest 2005;127:902–8.
11. King Rm, Pairolero PC, Trastek VF, et al. Primary chest wall tumors: factors affecting survival. Ann Thorac Surg 1986;41:597–601.
12. Salas S, Bui B, Stoeckle E, et al. Soft tissue sarcomas of the trunk wall (STS-TW): a study of 343 patients from the French Sarcoma Group (FSG) database. Ann Oncol 2009;20:1127–35.
13. Walsh GL, Davis BM, Swisher SG, et al. A single-institutional, multidisciplinary approach to primary sarcomas involving the chest wall requiring full-thickness resections. J Thorac Cardiovasc Surg 2001;121:48–68.
14. Jennings CD, Foon KA. Recent advances in flow cytometry: application to the diagnosis of hematologic malignancy. Blood 1997;90:2863–92.
15. Dimopoulos MA, Moulopouls LA, Maniatis A, Alexanian R. Solitary plasmacytoma of bone and asymptomatic multiple myeloma. Blood 2000;96:2037–44.
16. Liebross RH, Ha CS, Cox JD, et al. Solitary bone plasmacytoma: outcome and prognostic factors following radiotherapy. Int J Radiat Oncol Biol Phys 1998;41:1063–7.
17. Murphey MD, Flemming DJ, Boyea SR, et al. Enchondroma versus chondrosarcoma in the appendicular skeleton: differentiating features. Radiographics 1998;5:1213–37.
18. Widhe B, Bauer HC; Scandinavian Sarcoma Group. Surgical treatment is decisive for outcome in chondrosarcoma of the chest wall: a population-based Scandinavian Sarcoma Group study of 106 patients. J Thorac Cardiovasc Surg 2009;137:610–4.
19. Delattre O, Zucman J, Melot T, et al. The Ewing family of tumors—a subgroup of small-round-cell tumors defined by specific chimeric transcripts. N Engl J Med 1994;331:294–9.
20. Saenz NC, Hass DJ, Meyer P, et al. Pediatric chest wall Ewing's sarcoma. J Pediatr Surg 2000;35:550–5.
21. Shamberger RC, LaQuaglia MP, Gebhardt MC, et al. Ewing sarcoma/primitive neuroectodermal tumor of the chest wall: impact of initial versus delayed resection on tumor margins, survival and use of radiation therapy. Ann Surg 2003;238:563–8.
22. Paulussen M, Ahresn S, Lehnert M, et al. Second malignancies after Ewing tumor treatment in 690 patients from a cooperative German/Austrian/Dutch study. Ann Oncol 2001;12:1619–30.
23. Veronesi G, Spaggiari L, De Pas T, et al. Preoperative chemotherapy is essential for conservative surgery of Askin tumors. J Thorac Cardiovasc Surg 2003;125:429–9.
24. Miettinen M, Virtanen I. Synovial sarcoma: a misnomer. Am J Pathol 1984;117:18–25.
25. Deshmukh R, Mankin H, Singer S. Synovial [illegible] the importance of size and location for survival. Clin Orthop Relat Res 2004;419:155–61.
26. Singer S, Baldini EH, Demetri GD, et al. Synovial sarcoma: prognostic significane of tumor size, margin of resection and mitotic activity for survival. J Clin Oncol 1996;14:1201–8.
27. Burkhart HM, Allen MS, Nichols FC, et al. Results of en bloc resection for bronchogenic carcinoma with chest wall invasions. J Thorac Cardiovasc Surg 2002;123:670–5.
28. Downey RJ, Rusch V, Hsu FI, et al. Chest wall resection for locally recurrent breast cancer: is it worthwhile? J Thorac Cardiovasc Surg 2000;119:420–8.
29. Granick MS, Larson DL, Solomon MP. Radiation-related wounds of the chest wall. Clin Plast Surg 1993;20:559–71.

4 PLEURAL EFFUSION

Michael A. Maddaus, MD, FACS, and Rafael S. Andrade, MD, FACS

Approach to the Patient with a Pleural Effusion

Pleural effusion is a common problem in surgical practice. It results from perturbations of normal pleural fluid transport, which are produced by three main mechanisms: abnormalities in Starling equilibrium, increased capillary and mesothelial permeability, and interference with lymphatic drainage. These mechanisms are associated with a variety of different causes [*see Table 1*].[1,2] Often more than one mechanism is involved. An inflammatory effusion, for instance, is marked by increases in capillary and mesothelial permeability, which lead to elevated intrapleural oncotic pressure.

Pleural effusion is classified as either transudative or exudative, depending on the chemical composition of the fluid. A transudate is an ultrafiltrate of serum and has a low total protein content ($\leq$ 3 g/dL); an exudate is the result of increased permeability and has a high total protein content. Increased pleural permeability results from complex inflammatory mediator interactions between the mesothelium (whose cells play an active role in inflammation, phagocytosis, leukocyte migration, tissue repair, antigen presentation, coagulation, and fibrinolysis[3,4]) and the capillary endothelium. The distinction between transudative and exudative pleural effusion is clinically significant in that the two types of effusion have different causes [*see Table 2*].[1,4]

Table 1 Pathophysiologic Mechanisms of Pleural Effusion

Mechanism	Specific Alteration	Cause
Abnormality in Starling equilibrium	Increased capillary and lymphatic hydrostatic pressure	Increased venous pressure (e.g., biventricular heart failure, renal failure)
	Decreased capillary oncotic pressure	Hypoproteinemia (e.g., nephrotic syndrome)
	Decreased intrapleural hydrostatic pressure	Ex vacuo effusion (e.g., atelectasis)
	Increased intrapleural oncotic pressure	Inflammation (e.g., infection, cancer, autoimmune disease)
Increase in capillary and mesothelial permeability	Increased filtration	Inflammation (e.g., infection, cancer, autoimmune disease)
Interference with lymphatic drainage	Obstruction	Cancer, structural abnormalities

Table 2 Causes of Transudative and Exudative Pleural Effusion

Type of Effusion	Cause
Transudative	Congestive heart failure Cirrhosis Nephrotic syndrome Acute atelectasis Renal failure Peritoneal dialysis Postoperative state Myxedema Postpartum state
Exudative	Pneumonia Malignancy Infection Esophageal perforation Hemothorax Chylothorax Pseudochylothorax Connective tissue diseases Drug-induced pleuritis Pancreatitis Uremia Postmyocardial infarction (Dressler syndrome) Chronic atelectasis Radiation therapy Asbestos esposure Meigs syndrome Ovarian hyperstimulation
Transudative or exudative	Pulmonary embolus

Clinical Evaluation

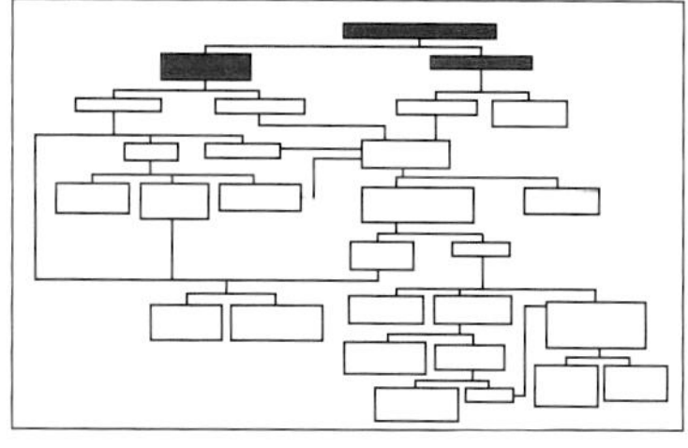

A complete history, physical examination, and clinical acuity are the initial tools used for diagnosing pleural effusion. Important facts from a patient's history (e.g., respiratory symptoms, pain, extrathoracic symptoms, duration of symptoms, previous medical conditions, and risk factors for cardiopulmonary diseases or cancer) can raise the index of suspicion for an effusion and provide guidance regarding possible causes. Careful physical examination of the chest can detect an effusion, and many physical signs may provide clues to the cause. Physical signs that are particularly useful for diagnostic purposes include jugular venous distention and tachycardia (suggestive of congestive heart failure); lymphadenopathy, digital clubbing, and localized bone tenderness (suggestive of lung cancer); and ascites (suggestive of ovarian tumors or cirrhosis).

Approach to the Patient with a Pleural Effusion

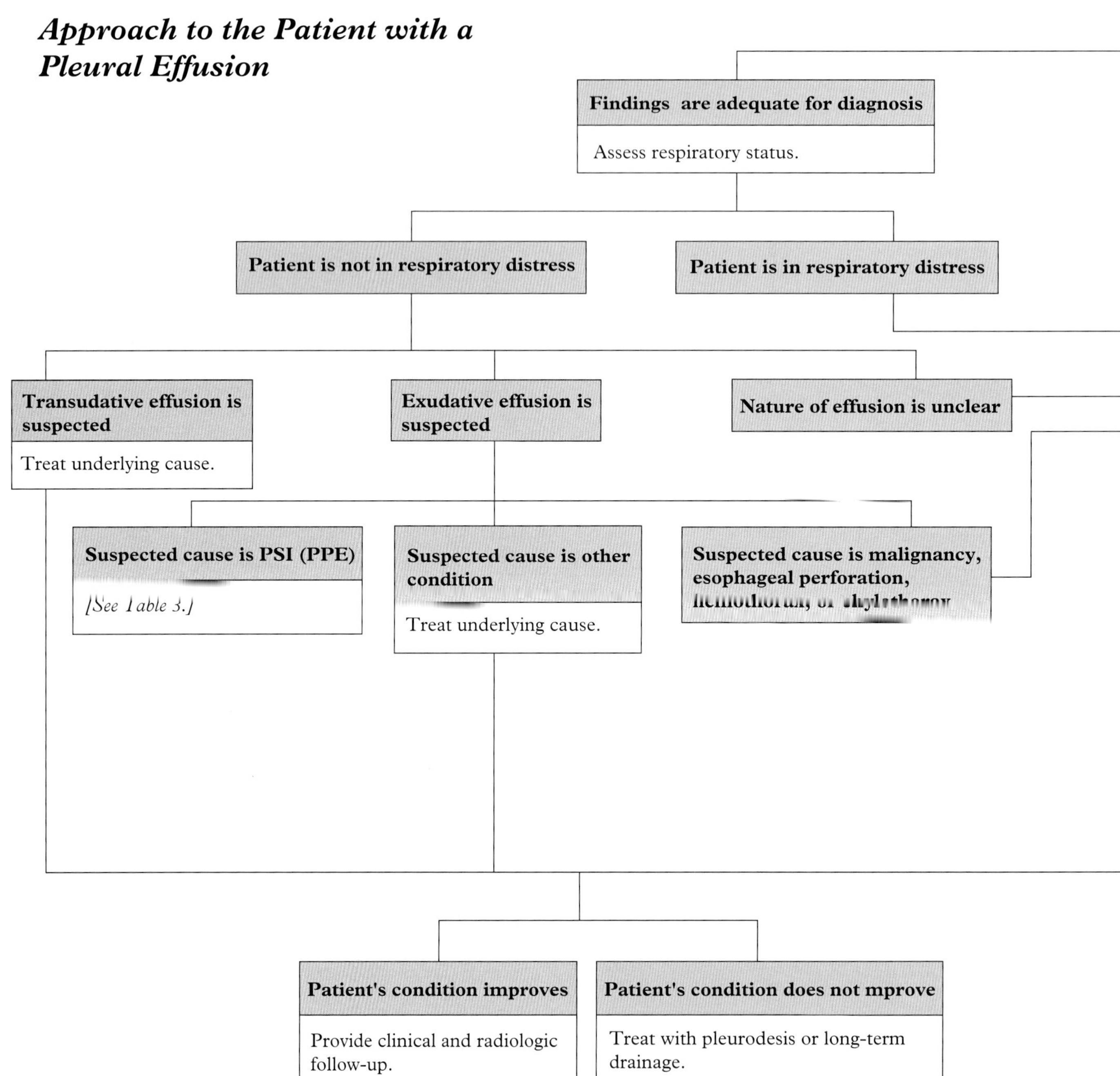

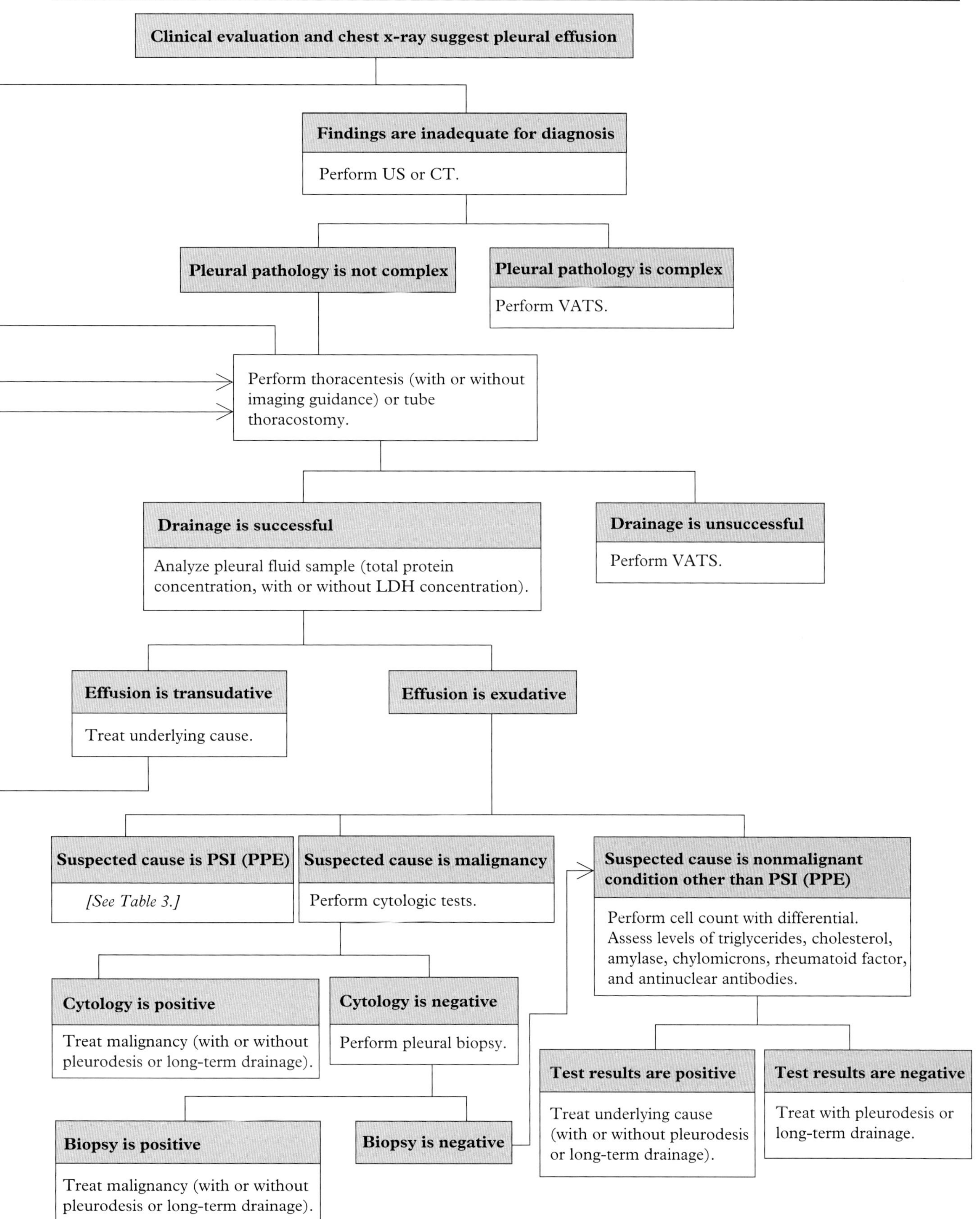
Clinical evaluation and chest x-ray suggest pleural effusion
Findings are inadequate for diagnosis
Perform US or CT.
Pleural pathology is not complex
Pleural pathology is complex
Perform VATS.
Perform thoracentesis (with or without imaging guidance) or tube thoracostomy.
Drainage is successful
Analyze pleural fluid sample (total protein concentration, with or without LDH concentration).
Drainage is unsuccessful
Perform VATS.
Effusion is transudative
Treat underlying cause.
Effusion is exudative
Suspected cause is PSI (PPE)
[See Table 3.]
Suspected cause is malignancy
Perform cytologic tests.
Suspected cause is nonmalignant condition other than PSI (PPE)
Perform cell count with differential. Assess levels of triglycerides, cholesterol, amylase, chylomicrons, rheumatoid factor, and antinuclear antibodies.
Cytology is positive
Treat malignancy (with or without pleurodesis or long-term drainage).
Cytology is negative
Perform pleural biopsy.
Test results are positive
Treat underlying cause (with or without pleurodesis or long-term drainage).
Test results are negative
Treat with pleurodesis or long-term drainage.
Biopsy is positive
Treat malignancy (with or without pleurodesis or long-term drainage).
Biopsy is negative

Pleural effusion can occur in a wide variety of clinical situations, however, and it often evades clinical detection by history and physical examination. Consequently, imaging tests are indispensable in the workup of a patient with a possible pleural effusion. Pleural fluid analysis, pleural biopsy, and thoracoscopy may also be required for evaluation.

Investigative Studies

IMAGING

Chest Radiography

To be detectable on a standard upright posteroanterior chest radiograph, an effusion must have a volume greater than 150 mL. If the volume is 150 to 500 mL, the lateral costophrenic angle will be blunted; if the volume is greater than 500 mL, a meniscus will be created.[5,6] A lateral decubitus chest radiograph can detect minute effusions (< 50 mL), and as a general rule, a layering effusion that is at least 1 cm thick is accessible to thoracentesis.[6,7] A loculated effusion may appear as a so-called pseudotumor on a chest radiograph and typically will not layer freely on a lateral decubitus radiograph. Subtle changes on an upright chest radiograph (e.g., accentuation of a fissure, elevation of a hemidiaphragm or increased separation between the lung and subdiaphragmatic gas [*see Figure 1*]) may also signal an effusion. Additional findings on a standard chest radiograph (e.g., laterality, the size of the cardiac silhouette, the position of the mediastinum, pulmonary parenchymal changes, pleural calcifications, and osseous abnormalities) may point to a specific cause.

Supine chest radiographs are less sensitive than other chest radiographs. With these images, suspicion of an effusion is triggered by increased homogeneous density of the lower hemithorax, loss of normal diaphragmatic silhouette, blunting of the lateral costophrenic angle, or apical capping [*see Figure 2*].[8]

Ultrasonography

Chest ultrasonograms are more reliable for detecting and localizing small (5 to 100 mL) or loculated pleural effusions than chest radiographs are.[5,9,10] Ultrasonography is particularly helpful for guiding thoracentesis for small-volume effusions and for assessing pleural effusions in critically ill patients.[6,11]

Computed Tomography of Chest

Computed tomography (CT) of the chest is a very sensitive tool for evaluating pleural effusion. Free-flowing fluid causes a sickle-shaped opacity in the most dependent portion of the thorax, and even small effusions are readily detected [*see Figure 3*]. CT may also reveal clues to the cause of the effusion, such as a fluid-fluid level (suggestive of acute hemorrhage), pleural thickening and enhancement (suggestive of pleural space infection [PSI] [*see Figure 4*]), calcified pleural plaques (suggestive of asbestosis), and diffuse irregular nodularity and pleural thickening (suggestive of pleural metastases or mesothelioma). CT is especially useful for characterizing loculated effusions, for differentiating pleural thickening or pleural masses from pleural effusions, for distinguishing between effusion and lung abscess, and for guiding and monitoring closed drainage of effusions.[6,10,12,13]

Magnetic Resonance Imaging

Magnetic resonance imaging (MRI) of the chest provides no useful information beyond what can be obtained with CT.

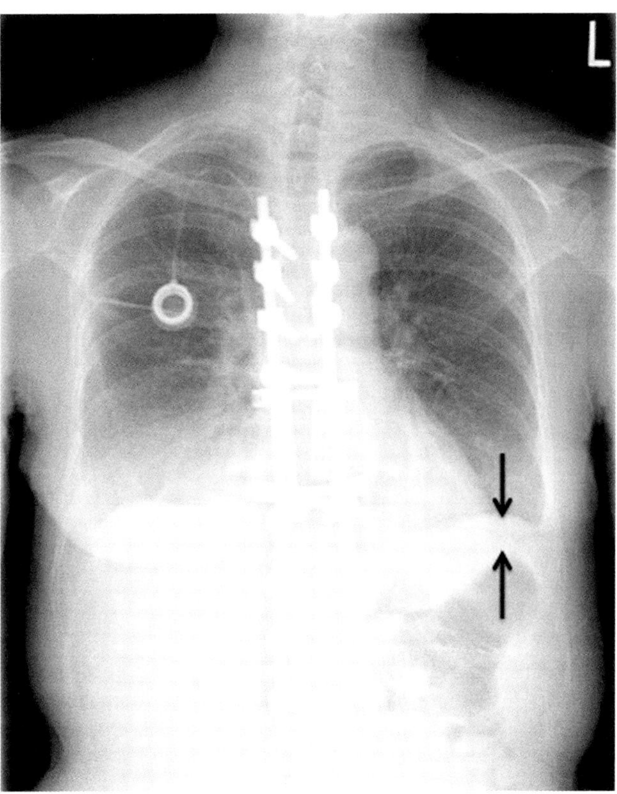

Figure 1 **Posteroanterior chest radiograph of a patient with bilateral pleural effusion reveals increased separation between the left lung and subdiaphragmatic gas (*arrows*).**

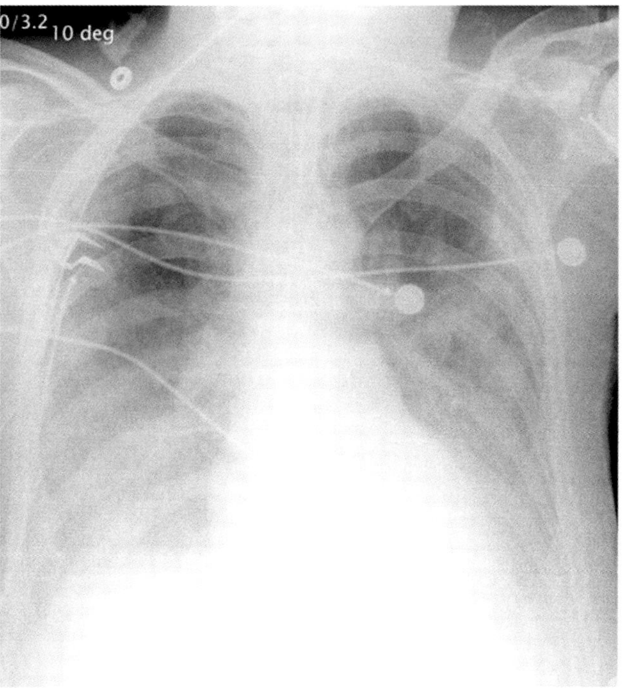

Figure 2 **Supine chest radiograph of a patient with bilateral pleural effusion shows increased homogeneous density of the lower hemithoraces.**

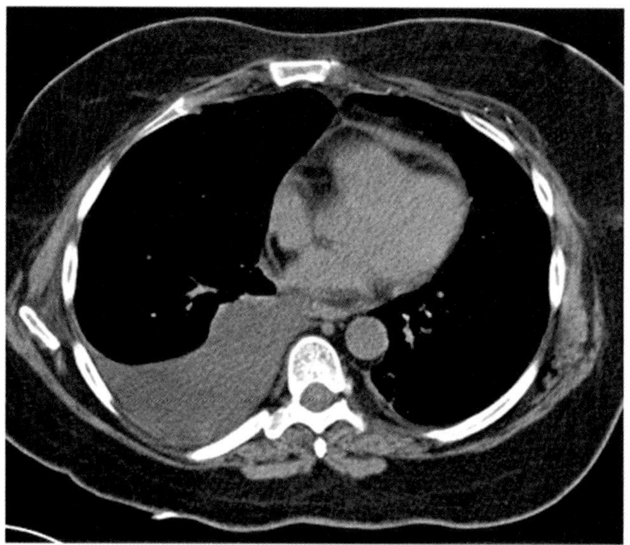

Figure 3 **Computed tomographic scan of the chest shows a free-flowing, sickle-shaped, right-sided effusion.**

MRI is neither efficient nor cost-effective in standard evaluation of pleural effusion.[12,14]

THORACENTESIS

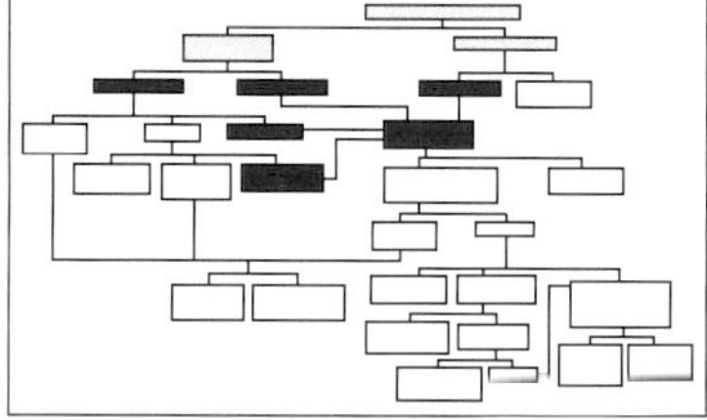

If the cause of a pleural effusion cannot be explained by the clinical circumstances (e.g., congestive heart failure or a recent surgical procedure), diagnostic thoracentesis [*see Sidebar* Techniques for Bedside Thoracentesis and Tube Thoracostomy] is indicated. Thoracentesis may also have therapeutic value in that drainage of fluid may relieve dyspnea. Absolute contraindications to thoracentesis include a lack of cooperation on the patient's part, clinical instability with hemodynamic or respiratory compromise, severe coagulopathy, and high-pressure ventilation. Relative contraindications to thoracentesis include a nonlayering effusion, loculations, and previous thoracic trauma, chest tube placement, or surgery.

A large effusion can be drained without any special imaging guidance other than an upright posteroanterior and lateral chest radiograph. Thoracentesis for a small or loculated effusion is best done with ultrasound guidance; success rates are as high as 97%.[15]

The incidence of complications associated with thoracentesis varies, depending on the experience of the operator and on the use of imaging guidance. Pneumothorax occurs in 3 to 20% of patients, of whom approximately 20% require tube thoracostomy [*see Sidebar* Techniques for Bedside Thoracentesis and Tube Thoracostomy]. Patients commonly experience pain and cough with lung reexpansion during drainage. Reexpansion pulmonary edema is an uncommon complication that can occur with rapid drainage of a large-volume effusion. It is common practice to drain no more than 1 to 1.5 L at a time, even though no evidence supports this practice. Experimental data suggest that active aspiration of fluid can cause high negative intrapleural pressures, potentially precipitating edema formation; gravity drainage may be preferable to minimize the chance of edema. Additional potential complications include so-called dry tap, vasovagal reaction, hemorrhage, hypovolemia, and PSI.[10,16–18]

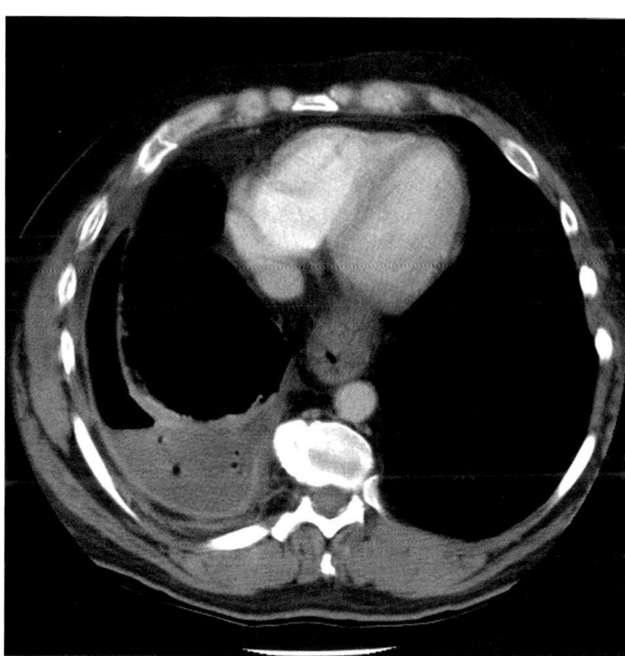

Figure 4 **Chest computed tomographic scan of a patient with right-side empyema shows a loculated effusion. The pleura is enhanced with intravenous contrast.**

PLEURAL FLUID ANALYSIS

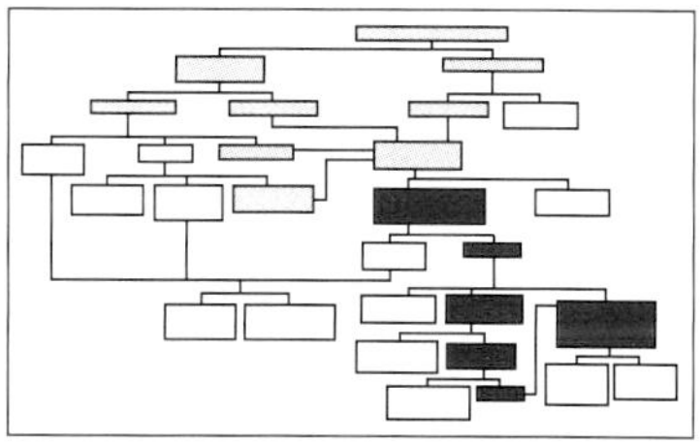

Assessment of a pleural fluid sample is guided, to some extent, by the clinical context in which the pleural effusion occurs. When the cause of the effusion is unknown, evaluation of a pleural fluid sample typically includes measurement of total protein and lactate dehydrogenase (LDH) concentrations, a cell count with differential, cause-specific testing, and microbiologic and cytologic analysis.

Biochemical Analysis of Pleural Fluid

A total protein concentration higher than 3 g/dL is sometimes used as the main criterion for distinguishing a transudate from an exudate; however, the use of this criterion may result in misclassification of as many as 15% of effusions. According to Light and colleagues' criteria,[19] which have a sensitivity of 99% and a specificity of 98% for identifying exudates, an effusion is an exudate if one of the following three findings is present:

1. A pleural fluid–to–serum protein ratio higher than 0.5
2. A pleural fluid–to–serum LDH ratio higher than 0.6
3. A pleural fluid LDH concentration higher than two thirds of the upper limit of the serum reference range

Techniques of Bedside Thoracentesis and Tube Thoracostomy

Bedside Thoracentesis

Bedside thoracentesis should be performed on a bed or an examination table (as a safeguard if hypotension develops). The patient should be upright and seated (provided that he or she is awake and cooperative), with the arms leaning comfortably on a bedside table and the back facing the surgeon.

The proper intercostal space for catheter insertion is determined through physical examination and radiologic evaluation of the effusion; generally, the ninth or 10th intercostal space in the midscapular line is a good choice. The area is prepared and anesthetized with 1% lidocaine, 3 to 5 mg/kg, with care taken not to injure the intercostal bundle. To confirm that the catheter is in the correct location, we recommend drawing a small amount of pleural fluid at the time of local anesthetic infiltration. Several thoracentesis kits with one-way valves are available. Fluid should be allowed to drain by gravity; however, to minimize the risk of reexpansion pulmonary edema, drainage should not exceed 1.5 L. Frequently, a dry cough and pleuritic pain develop as drainage approaches its end. To minimize anxiety, the patient should be warned about this possibility in advance. After the completion of thoracentesis, a chest radiograph should be obtained.

Bedside Tube Thoracostomy

Bedside tube thoracostomy should be performed with the patient supine. The side on which the thoracostomy will be created should be elevated, and the patient's ipsilateral arm should be abducted. Supplemental oxygen should be supplied. Monitoring must include, at the least, continuous oxygen saturation plethysmography and intermittent measurement of blood pressure and heart rate. Tube thoracostomy is potentially very painful; accordingly, in a nonemergency situation, every effort should be made to minimize pain and anxiety. We usually administer intravenous ketorolac about 30 to 60 minutes before the procedure. During preparation for chest tube placement, narcotics and sedatives should be administered intravenously; additional doses should then be administered at the beginning of and during the procedure.

The ideal location for chest tube placement is determined by clinical and radiographic examination. The area is prepared and draped widely, and a local anesthetic is used at a near-maximum dosage, with care taken to anesthetize skin, subcutaneous tissue, muscle, and periosteum. A 1.5 cm skin incision is made, a soft tissue tunnel is created with blunt instrument and finger dissection, the upper edge of the rib is identified clearly, and additional local anesthetic is applied to the periosteum and the intercostal muscles. The subcutaneous tunnel should generally be directed posteriorly so that the chest tube will sit along the posterior chest wall and will not be trapped in a fissure. The intercostal muscle is pierced bluntly, and digital examination of the pleural space is performed to confirm that an intrapleural location has been reached and to search for abnormalities such as adhesions or tumor implants. The chest tube is then directed to the desired location with the aid of a clamp. As with thoracentesis, fluid should be allowed to drain by gravity, but drainage should not exceed 1.5 L. If the effusion exceeds 1.5 L, the chest tube should be clamped and the remaining fluid allowed to drain intermittently in 200 mL aliquots every 2 hours. Immediately after completion of the procedure, a chest radiograph should be obtained to verify lung expansion and confirm the position of the chest tube. When chest tube output falls below 200 mL/day and reexpansion of the lung is verified, pleurodesis should be performed. We recommend that patient-controlled analgesia be employed while the chest tube remains in place.

The size of the chest tube is determined by the suspected cause and by the radiologic characteristics of the effusion. For a free-flowing transudative effusion, a small (20 to 24 French) chest tube or even a pigtail catheter usually suffices; for a thick exudative effusion or a hemothorax, a tube as large as 40 French may be required.

A 1997 meta-analysis of the diagnostic value of tests used to distinguish transudates from exudates did not find any test or combination of tests to be clearly superior.[20] The choice of a test for this purpose is therefore a matter of individual preference. If only one test is to be performed, measurement of the total protein concentration is the most practical choice in view of its accuracy and availability.

Assessment of pleural fluid pH and glucose levels may be used adjunctively for risk stratification in patients with PSI, but the clinical utility of these measurements is not well established (see below).[21]

There are numerous substances whose concentrations can be measured to help determine the specific cause of a pleural effusion, such as triglycerides, chylomicrons, and cholesterol (to help diagnose chylothorax); amylase (to help diagnose esophageal perforation or pancreatitis); rheumatoid factor (to help diagnose rheumatoid effusion); antinuclear antibodies (to help diagnose lupus pleuritis); carcinoembryonic antigen (to help diagnose malignancy); and adenosine deaminase (to help diagnose tuberculous pleurisy).[3,22–25]

Cell Counts

Analysis of the number and type of white blood cells (WBCs) present in pleural fluid is often diagnostically useful. Pleural effusions can be categorized according to the type of WBC that is predominant. Generally, pleural fluid neutrophilia points to acute inflammation (e.g., from PSI or pulmonary infarction) as the underlying cause; however, the presence of a neutrophilic effusion does not exclude malignancy. Pleural fluid lymphocytosis, in which lymphocytes account for more than 50% of WBCs, most frequently is indicative of malignancy (occurring in 50% of malignant effusions), tuberculosis (occurring in 15 to 20% of tuberculous effusions), or chylothorax.[26] Pleural fluid eosinophilia, in which eosinophils account for more than 10% of WBCs, can be caused by a wide variety of benign and malignant conditions—even, in some cases, by the mere presence of air or blood in the pleural space. Approximately one third of eosinophilic effusions are idiopathic. As a rule, the presence of mesothelial cells is of little diagnostic value; the exception to this rule is that if such cells account for more than 5% of WBCs, a tuberculous effusion is unlikely.[23,27]

Microbiologic Tests

If a PSI is suspected, Gram staining and standard bacterial cultures are indicated. If tuberculous pleurisy is a possibility, acid-fast stains and mycobacterial cultures should be performed. Fungal, viral, and parasitic PSIs are uncommon; accordingly, special stains and cultures for these conditions are indicated only if dictated by a specific clinical setting.[28]

Cytologic Tests

Cytologic testing of pleural fluid is routinely performed whenever the cause of an effusion is unclear. The diagnostic yield for malignancy varies depending on the stage of the disease, but it generally is in the range of 50 to 60% (higher in patients with bulky pleural tumors). Repeat cytologic testing may increase the yield to more than 70%,[10,29] and testing of three or more samples may increase the yield to 90%.[30]

PLEURAL BIOPSY

In approximately 25% of patients with exudative effusion, the cause remains unknown after clinical evaluation, imaging, and pleural fluid analysis. The next step in the evaluation of such patients is pleural biopsy.

Percutaneous pleural biopsy is an infrequently used tool that has a diagnostic yield of 57% for carcinoma. Its low yield for malignant effusion can be explained by the uneven distribution of pleural metastases. For tuberculous pleurisy, however, the diagnostic yield of percutaneous pleural biopsy is 75%, and the yield rises to 90% when this procedure is combined with pleural fluid culture. In about 10 to 20% of patients with exudative pleural effusion, laboratory analysis of pleural fluid and percutaneous biopsy fail to produce a specific diagnosis.[18] The contraindications and complications associated with percutaneous pleural biopsy are similar to those associated with thoracentesis.[31]

Video-assisted thoracoscopic surgery (VATS) is also employed for pleural biopsy; its diagnostic yield in this setting is 92% for malignancy and nearly 100% for tuberculous pleurisy. VATS is a therapeutic procedure as well, allowing the surgeon to perform pleurodesis, decortication, or pleurectomy if necessary. VATS pleural biopsy is typically performed with the patient under general anesthesia, but if the patient is highly debilitated, it can be done with regional and local anesthesia.[32] Procedure-specific complications include hypoxemia, hemorrhage, prolonged air leakage, subcutaneous emphysema, and empyema, each of which occurs at a rate of about 2%. The mortality associated with diagnostic thoracoscopy ranges from 0.01 to 0.09%.[29,31] When VATS is performed to remove a suspected malignant lesion, a protective plastic device is required to minimize the possibility of tumor seeding. Incisional tumor seeding after a VATS biopsy is rare but can occur at any time after the procedure (reported range 2 weeks to 29 months).[33]

If mesothelioma is suspected, pleural biopsy (through a 5 cm incision) is the preferred diagnostic procedure. Ideally, the biopsy incision should be placed at the location of a potential thoracotomy incision so that future excision of the biopsy scar can be accomplished in a manner that minimizes the risk of local tumor recurrence.[34]

Management

PLEURAL EFFUSION IN THE INTENSIVE CARE UNIT

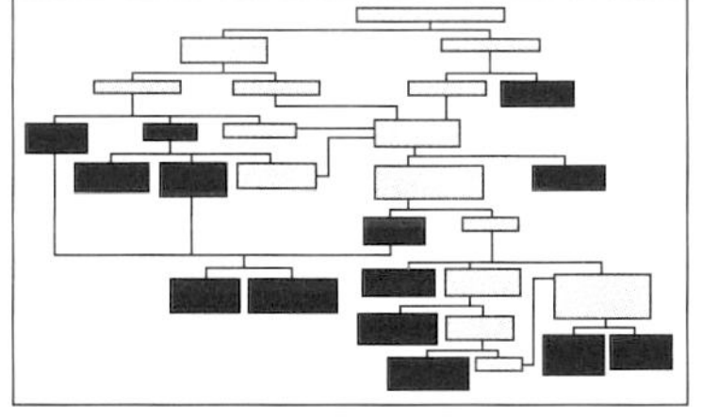

Pleural effusion develops in as many as 60% of intensive care unit (ICU) patients evaluated with ultrasonography.[11] When pleural effusion occurs in the ICU, drainage should be liberally employed to optimize the patient's hemodynamic and respiratory status and to detect PSI early. Thoracentesis can be done in critically ill ventilator-dependent patients with the help of bedside ultrasonography. Chest tube thoracostomy does not require ultrasonographic guidance and may be a safer choice for patients on high-pressure ventilation.

MALIGNANT PLEURAL EFFUSION

Pleural effusion is associated with malignancy in 30 to 65% of patients, and approximately 75% of patients with malignant effusion have lung or breast cancer.[35] The principal aim of therapy is to relieve dyspnea and to limit the number of procedures and hospital days that patients with a limited life expectancy must endure.

Drainage can be achieved by means of thoracentesis, chest tube placement, or VATS. Thoracentesis is a valuable option for initial patient evaluation, particularly in the office setting. Because malignant pleural effusion recurs rapidly unless patients undergo effective systemic or local treatment, repeat thoracentesis is generally not recommended for anything other than urgent relief of symptoms. Chest tubes are placed primarily with the intention of performing bedside pleurodesis.

Small-bore subcutaneously tunneled catheters may be employed for long-term management of malignant pleural effusions. Long-term drainage is preferable in patients with a very short life expectancy ($\leq$ 3 months), patients who have a poor performance status, and patients with a trapped lung.[36] Two options are available: the Pleurx catheter (Denver Biomedical, Golden, Colorado) [*see Figure 5*] and the Tenckhoff peritoneal dialysis catheter. With either device, the procedure is essentially the same: the catheter is inserted with the patient under local or general anesthesia, the patient is discharged on the day of or the day after insertion, and the pleural fluid is drained either according to a schedule or on an as-needed basis. Small-bore tunneled catheters are comfortable, but patients may object to having a permanent catheter or to undergoing home-based procedures. In 20 to 70% of patients with a permanent catheter, pleurodesis develops within 4 to 6 weeks. Patients with malignant pleural effusions secondary to breast or gynecologic cancers are more likely to develop pleurodesis (about 70%) than patients with lung cancer (about 40%).[37] Catheter removal is easily done in the office setting with local anesthetic. Technical failures and infection

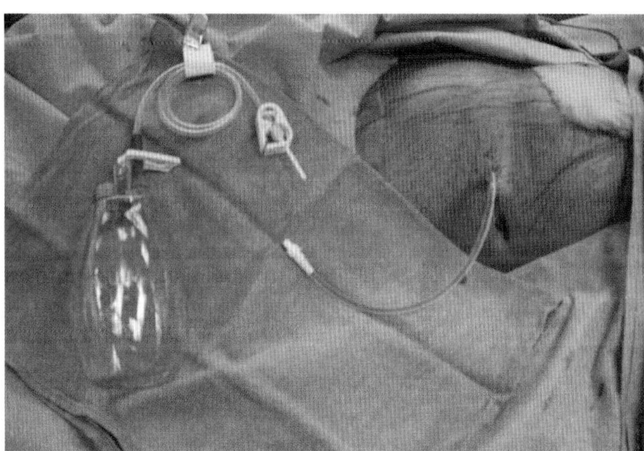

Figure 5 **Shown is a Pleurx catheter after placement and subcutaneous tunneling. The vacuum container is not connected.**

may occur in as many as 20% of patients with permanent catheters, but very few patients require operative management.[38–41]

Pleuroperitoneal shunting has been advocated as an alternative for long-term management of malignant pleural effusions. However, experience with this mode of drainage is limited and the potential for technical complications is high.[42,43]

Recurrence of malignant pleural effusion is best prevented by using sclerosants to induce pleurodesis. The sclerosant may be instilled either via a bedside tube thoracostomy or thoracoscopically; a median hospitalization of 6.5 days is required.[38] Of the various sclerosants available, talc is the most efficacious, with an overall success rate of 80 to 96%.[44–46] The ideal talc dose has not been determined; the usual dose is 4 or 5 g. Talc pleurodesis with a 5 g dose has generally proved efficient and safe. For obvious reasons, simultaneous bilateral talc instillation should be avoided.[44] A phase III intergroup study (Cancer and Leukemia Group B 9334) that compared bedside talc slurry pleurodesis versus thoracoscopic talc insufflation pleurodesis found no difference in outcome at 30 days; however, subgroup analysis revealed that thoracoscopic talc insufflation pleurodesis was superior in patients with primary lung cancer or breast cancer.[47] Thoracoscopically guided talc pleurodesis can be performed with an operative mortality of less than 1%.[48,49]

Pain and fever are frequent side effects of talc pleurodesis, but the main concern is the possible development of acute lung injury (ALI) and respiratory failure. Respiratory failure is reported to occur in approximately 1 to 4% of patients. The cause of respiratory failure secondary to talc pleurodesis is not clear and is probably related to multiple factors (e.g., talc dose, talc absorption, underlying lung disease, reexpansion pulmonary edema, systemic inflammatory response, tumor burden, and lymphatic obstruction). There is no definitive evidence that the talc dose is correlated with the incidence of ALI; respiratory failure has been reported even with a 2 g talc dose.[44,50–54] Moreover, a recent multicenter prospective cohort study reported a 0% incidence of acute respiratory distress syndrome in 558 patients undergoing talc pleurodesis (4 g dose).[55]

Iodopovidone (10%; 20 mL) is a very effective and inexpensive alternative for chemical pleurodesis that is of value in the setting of limited financial resources.[56,57]

Treatment of malignant pleural effusion must be individualized. The key factors governing the choice of treatment approach are the (1) patient's performance status, (2) prognosis, (3) patient's choice, (4) ability of the lung to reexpand, and (5) pleural tumor bulk. Patients who have poor performance status (e.g., those with advanced tumors or significant comorbid conditions) or a very poor short-term prognosis should undergo the least invasive treatment—namely, drainage only. Patients who have better functional status and are expected to survive longer should preferably undergo thoracoscopically guided talc pleurodesis, but it is not unreasonable for a patient to elect to have long-term drainage in this scenario. Pleural tumor bulk is important in that bulky pleural lesions will interfere with pleurodesis. The lung's ability to reexpand after drainage of a malignant effusion is significant because if the lung is atelectatic as a result of airway obstruction or trapped as a result of pleural seeding, no agent will be able to induce pleurodesis, and the best treatment will be long-term drainage. Table 3 summarizes practical guidelines for the definitive management of malignant pleural effusion.

PLEURAL SPACE INFECTION

PSI can be caused by a variety of factors, including pneumonia, trauma, and intrathoracic procedures. It has a wide clinical spectrum, ranging from a small parapneumonic effusion (PPE) to a pus-filled pleural space (empyema) with respiratory compromise and sepsis. (The terms PSI and PPE are often used interchangeably.) PSI can be classified according to its pathophysiologic stage (exudative, fibrinopurulent, or organizing) or its anatomic appearance (nonloculated versus loculated or noncomplicated versus complicated). The term empyema is commonly reserved for the most advanced stage of PSI.[58]

The pathophysiology of PSI or PPE can be divided into three stages. The exudative stage is characterized by the development of an exudative effusion secondary to increased pleural permeability; the pleural space is often sterile initially, but if it is left untreated, bacterial infection is likely to ensue. The fibrinopurulent stage is marked by the progressive deposition of fibrin and the increasing presence of WBCs; gradual angioblastic and fibroblastic proliferation leads to extensive fibrin deposits, and the effusion becomes loculated (complicated). The organizing stage starts as early as 1 week after infection, with increasing collagen deposition and lung entrapment; after 3 or 4 weeks, the organized collagen has formed a peel. The pleural fluid is grossly purulent. Eventually, dense fibrosis, contraction, and lung entrapment develop.[59,60]

In most patients, PSI is caused by bacteria. The most common pathogens are *Staphylococcus aureus*, *Streptococcus pneumoniae*, enteric gram-negative bacilli, and anaerobes. Approximately 30 to 40% of cultures are polymicrobial. In a subgroup of patients, there is sterile pus in the pleural space as a consequence of either previous antimicrobial therapy or bacterial autolysis. The pathogens identified vary according to the cause of PSI. For instance, *S. aureus* and *S. pneumoniae* predominate in PPE, *S. aureus* in postthoracotomy PSI, mixed oropharyngeal organisms in PSI resulting from esophageal perforation,[28] and acid-fast bacteria in tuberculous empyema.[61]

Parapneumonic Effusion

PPE occurs in as many as 57% of patients hospitalized with pneumonia, and pneumonia accounts for 42 to 73%

Table 3 Practical Guidelines for Definitive Management of Malignant Pleural Effusion

Patient Characteristics	Chemical Pleurodesis	Long-Term Drainage
Performance status		
Good	Yes	Yes
Poor	No	Yes
Life expectancy		
> 6 mo	Yes	Yes
3–6 mo	Individualize	Yes
< 3 mo	No	Yes
Bulky pleural implants	Individualize	Yes
Trapped lung	No	Yes

of cases of PSI. In most cases, early PPE is effectively treated by timely antibiotic therapy aimed at the underlying pneumonia.[21,28]

In 2000, a panel convened by the Health and Science Policy Committee of the American College of Chest Physicians (ACCP) reviewed the available literature with the aim of developing an evidence-based clinical practice guideline for the treatment of PPE.[21] The panel formulated a clear and relatively simple classification system that used pleural anatomy and bacteriology to stratify patients according to the risk of a poor outcome [*see Table 4*]. It then made therapeutic recommendations on the basis of this classification. Some authors have used pleural fluid chemistry test results (e.g., pH and glucose concentration) as additional criteria for categorizing PPE; for example, a pleural fluid pH lower than 7.20 or a glucose level lower than 60 mg/dL has been considered suggestive of moderate risk. To date, however, the clinical utility and decision thresholds of pH and glucose values have not been well defined. Accordingly, the panel omitted pleural fluid chemistry from its guidelines.

The ACCP Health and Science Policy Committee evaluated six primary management approaches: no drainage, therapeutic thoracentesis, tube thoracostomy, fibrinolytic therapy, VATS, and open surgery. Overall, pooled outcomes favored patients treated with fibrinolytics, VATS, and open surgery. However, the success of an approach is related to the patient's risk category. The recommendations for drainage in relation to risk category are general guidelines, based on level C and D evidence (with level C referring to historically controlled series and case series and level D to expert opinion). With these recommendations (and their limitations) in mind, treatment should be tailored to the specific situation of each patient.

Category 1 and 2 PPE PPE in categories 1 (very low risk) and 2 (low risk) can be treated with antibiotic therapy directed at the underlying pneumonia. Some patients with category 2 PPE may require drainage for relief of dyspnea through either thoracentesis or tube thoracostomy.

Category 3 and 4 PPE Drainage options for category 3 (moderate risk) and 4 (high risk) PPE include tube thoracostomy alone, tube thoracostomy with intrapleural fibrinolytic therapy, VATS drainage, and open surgical drainage. These various approaches are not mutually exclusive: in some cases, patient outcomes may be optimized by a combination of treatment modalities.[62]

Tube thoracostomy alone may be appropriate for category 3 patients with free-flowing effusion. With loculated effusion, however, the key to successful therapy is breaking down the fibrin septations. Evidence from three small randomized, controlled trials suggested that intrapleural fibrinolytic therapy has an advantage over tube thoracostomy alone for patients with category 3 or 4 PPE; a large trial is being conducted to address this specific issue.[59] To date, only one randomized study, including 20 patients with category 3 or 4 PPE, has compared VATS with fibrinolytic therapy. The primary treatment success rate was significantly higher in the VATS treatment group, the duration of chest tube drainage was less, and the total hospital stay was shorter.[63] VATS allows not only adequate drainage and visualization of the pleural space but also decortication of the lung if required; however, if decortication cannot be thoroughly accomplished by means of VATS and satisfactory lung expansion cannot be achieved, a thoracotomy should be performed.[64,65]

The principles of PPE treatment can be applied to PSI from any cause, but in view of the paucity of reliable data, caution should be exercised.

Posttraumatic PSI

PSI occurs in about 1 to 5% of patients who have sustained blunt or penetrating thoracic injury. The incidence of PSI in the setting of trauma increases with the number of chest tubes placed and with the duration of chest tube drainage. The effect of an undrained hemothorax on the risk of PSI has not been completely defined, and prophylactic antibiotics have not been shown to reduce the incidence of PSI.[58]

As noted (see above), the general guidelines for the treatment of PPE apply to the treatment of posttraumatic PSI.

Iatrogenic PSI

Iatrogenic PSI develops when a preexisting pleural effusion is inoculated with bacteria during an invasive procedure (e.g., thoracentesis or tube thoracostomy). The presence of fluid in the pleural space appears to be a prerequisite for infection.[58]

A bronchopleural fistula (BPF) is by definition a PSI and therefore has a similarly broad spectrum of clinical presentation. The overall incidence of BPF after lobar resection is approximately 1%; it is somewhat higher after resections for inflammatory diseases than after resections for cancer. The incidence of BPF after pneumonectomy varies depending on the side on which the pneumonectomy was done, the indications for surgery, the extent of preoperative irradiation,

Table 4 **Categorization of Parapneumonic Effusion by Risk of Poor Outcome**

Pleural Space Anatomy	Pleural Fluid Bacteriology	Category	Risk of Poor Outcome	Drainage
Minimal free-flowing effusion (< 10 mm on lateral decubitus x-ray)	Culture and Gram stain results unknown	1	Very low	No
Small to moderate free-flowing effusion (> 10 mm but < 50% hemithorax)	Negative culture and Gram stain	2	Low	No
Large free-flowing effusion (> 50% hemithorax), loculated effusion, or effusion with thickened parietal pleura (as seen on contrast-enhanced CT)	Positive culture or Gram stain	3	Moderate	Yes
	Pus	4	High	Yes

CT = computed tomography.

and the comorbid conditions present. In a report encompassing 464 pneumonectomies for cancer, the incidence of BPF was 8.6% after right pneumonectomy and 2.3% after left pneumonectomy.[66,67]

Almost every PSI after a lung resection is synonymous with BPF, and operative management is generally required.

Tuberculous PSI

Pleural effusion is common in patients with clinically evident pulmonary tuberculosis. Most cases of tuberculous effusion are secondary to hypersensitivity and resolve spontaneously. Tuberculous empyema is relatively rare; it is typically the result of active pleural infection by acid-fast bacteria.[61]

Tuberculous PSI is also treated in accordance with the general treatment guidelines for bacterial PSI. Chronic tuberculous PSI may present specific problems, such as drug resistance and impaired ability (or even inability) to reexpand the lung. Surgical procedures performed to manage chronic tuberculous empyema include VATS, standard open decortication, thoracoplasty, parietal wall collapse, open drainage, myoplasty, and omentopexy.[61]

CHYLOTHORAX AND PSEUDOCHYLOTHORAX

Chylothorax is the presence of chyle in the pleural space as a consequence of blockage of or damage to the thoracic duct or one of its tributaries. The rate at which chyle flows through the thoracic duct can be higher than 100 mL/hr; thus, large amounts of chyle can leak into the pleural space.[68] The principal causes of chylothorax are surgical trauma and malignancy (70 to 80% are caused by non-Hodgkin lymphoma).[49,68,69] Congenital chylothorax is more often attributable to malformation of the thoracic duct than to birth trauma.[24]

The diagnosis of chylothorax is made by measuring triglyceride levels in pleural fluid. Levels higher than 110 mg/dL are highly suggestive of chylothorax, levels between 50 and 100 mg/dL are equivocal, and levels lower than 50 mg/dL rule out chylothorax.[24] A pleura-to-serum triglyceride ratio higher than 1 can be a useful indicator[70]; the presence of chylomicrons is synonymous with chylothorax.[25]

Treatment of chylothorax depends on its cause and severity. Postoperative chylothorax may be treated initially with conservative measures (e.g., with a nihil per os [NPO] regimen, total parenteral nutrition, and administration of octreotide). However, drainage totaling more than 500 mL/day is considered to predict failure of conservative management. Thoracic duct ligation is the surgical treatment of choice and can often be performed thoracoscopically. To help identify the leak intraoperatively, it may be helpful to administer 100 to 200 mL of heavy cream or olive oil orally 2 to 3 hours before operation.[71,72] Early surgical intervention is important because the ongoing loss of lymph has significant effects on fluid homeostasis, nutrition, and immunocompetence (secondary to lymphocyte loss). In the early postligation period, medical management should be continued to allow any small leaks to seal. An alternative to surgical ligation that has evoked some interest is transabdominal percutaneous embolization of the thoracic duct. This technique requires significant expertise.[73]

Lymphoma-related chylothorax is caused principally by obstruction and usually develops on the left side [*see Figure 6*]. In a stiff and infiltrated duct, minor triggers (e.g., a Valsalva maneuver) can lead to duct rupture. Although patients with chylothorax often have extensive disease, supradiaphragmatic disease is not always present. Lymphoma-related chylothorax is best managed with thoracentesis and with therapy directed at the underlying cause. If first-line therapy fails, thoracoscopic talc pleurodesis is recommended; a small series reported 100% resolution of lymphoma-related chylothorax with thoracoscopic talc pleurodesis. If the chylothorax does not respond to any of these approaches, it may respond to thoracic duct ligation or pleuroperitoneal shunting. Chylothorax in the presence of lymphoma-related chylous ascites is a difficult problem that is generally refractory to most forms of therapy (although pleurodesis is occasionally successful).[49,68,69,74,75]

Pseudochylothorax is a rare disorder associated with the formation of persistent exudates that last for months or years. The most common cause is tuberculosis; the second most common cause is rheumatoid arthritis. Biochemical analysis of pleural fluid from patients with pseudochylothorax reveals very high cholesterol levels (> 200 mg/dL) and the presence of cholesterol crystals. Treatment is generally conservative.[24,25]

IDIOPATHIC PERSISTENT PLEURAL EFFUSION

In a small percentage of patients, the cause of pleural effusion remains unknown despite extensive diagnostic evaluation. Eventually, most cases of idiopathic effusion turn out to be caused most frequently by tuberculosis and other granulomatous diseases, malignancy, and pulmonary embolism; less common causes include constrictive pericarditis, subphrenic abscess, connective tissue diseases, drug-induced pleuritis, peritoneal dialysis, and cirrhosis.[23] In the management of persistent benign or idiopathic effusion, talc pleurodesis has a high success rate and minimal long-term implications.[76,77] A chronic drainage catheter (i.e., Pleurx) can be used for refractory pleural effusion in patients with congestive heart failure; however, prolonged use (> 4 months) can lead to empyema.[78]

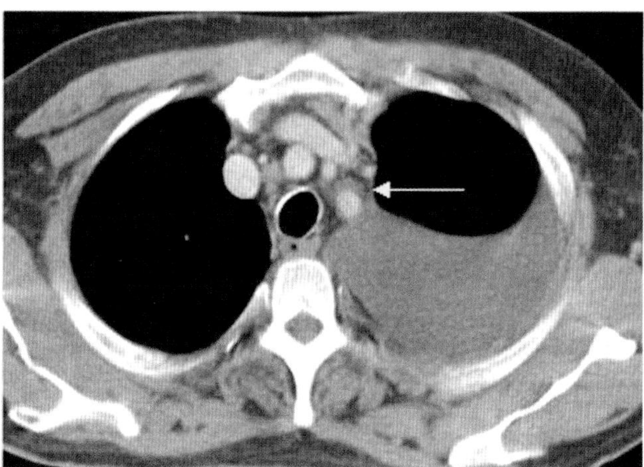

Figure 6 **Chest computed tomographic scan shows left-side chylothorax secondary to lymphoma. Subtle mediastinal lymphadenopathy obstructing the thoracic duct (*arrow*) is apparent.**

Hence, in the setting of a benign, refractory pleural effusion, a chronic drainage catheter should be considered only as a last resort.

Pleura: Basic Facts

PLEURAL ANATOMY

The pleura is a continuous membrane that covers the parietal and visceral surfaces of the thorax. In adults, it has an estimated surface area of 2,000 cm^2.[79] Light microscopy shows the pleura to have five layers: (1) a mesothelial cell layer; (2) a mesothelial connective tissue layer with basal lamina; (3) a superficial elastic layer; (4) a loose connective tissue layer with adipose tissue, blood vessels, nerves, and lymphatic vessels; and (5) a deep fibroelastic layer. The parietal pleura establishes a pleurolymphatic communication on the diaphragm to allow clearance of large (> 1,000 nm) particles and cells from the normal pleural space. The structure of this pleurolymphatic communication consists of stomata 2 to 12 μm in diameter, which overlie bulblike lymphatic channels (lacunae) separated by a layer of loose connective tissue (the membrana cribriformis).

Electron microscopy reveals microvilli on the mesothelial cell surface of the pleura. The main function of these microvilli is to enmesh glycoproteins rich in hyaluronic acid for purposes of lubrication. The structure of the intercellular junction in the mesothelial cells of the pleura is similar to that in the endothelial cells of the venules, which suggests that the pleural mesothelial cell layer may be as leaky as the venular endothelium.[3,4,80]

PLEURAL FLUID PHYSIOLOGY

The amount of pleural fluid in an adult is 1 to 10 mL and forms a 10 μm thick layer.[1,3,79,80] Fluid exchange across the pleural surface depends on three mechanisms: (1) passive filtration following Starling equilibrium, (2) active solute transport, and (3) lymphatic clearance. In the normal pleura, Starling equilibrium favors the flow of fluid in a parietal-to-visceral direction.[79] The rate at which fluid traverses the pleura ranges from 20 to 160 mL/day in adults; maximal lymphatic clearance is believed to be approximately 700 mL/day.[2,79,81–84]

The chemical composition of normal pleural fluid is similar to that of interstitial fluid. The protein concentration is typically 1 to 2 g/dL. The concentration of high-molecular-weight proteins (e.g., LDH) is approximately half that seen in serum. Cell counts in normal pleural fluid range from 1,400 to 4,500 cells/μL; macrophages account for the majority of the cells.[3,80]

Financial Disclosures: None Reported

References

1. Tran AC, Lapworth RL. Biochemical analysis of pleural fluid: what should we measure? Ann Clin Biochem 2001;38:311–22.
2. Jaker SA. Pleural anatomy, physiology and diagnostic procedures. In: Baum GL, Crapo JD, Celli BR, et al, editors. Textbook of pulmonary diseases. 6th ed. Vol 1. New York: Lippincott-Raven; 1998. p. 255.
3. Antony VB, Mohammed KA. Pathophysiology of pleural space infections. Semin Respir Infect 1999;14:9–17.
4. Mutsaers S. Mesothelial cells: their structure, function and role in serosal repair. Respirology 2002;7:171–91.
5. Rubins JB, Colice GL. Evaluating pleural effusions: how should you go about finding the cause? Postgrad Med 1999;105:39–42.
6. Levin DL, Klein JS. Imaging techniques for pleural space infections. Semin Respir Infect 1999;14:31–8.
7. Moskowitz H, Platt RT, Schachar R, et al. Roentgen visualization of minute pleural effusion—an experimental study to determine the minimum amount of pleural fluid visible on a radiograph. Radiology 1973;109:33–5.
8. Woodring JH. Recognition of pleural effusion on supine radiographs: how much fluid is required? AJR Am J Roentgenol 1984;142: 59–64.
9. Eibenberger KL, Dock WI, Ammann ME, et al. Quantification of pleural effusions: sonography versus radiography. Radiology 1994;191:681–4.
10. Bartter T, Santarelli R, Akers SM, et al. The evaluation of pleural effusion. Chest 1994; 106:1209–14.
11. Azoulay E. Pleural effusions in the intensive care unit. Curr Opin Pulm Med 2003;9:291–7.
12. McLoud TC. CT and MR in pleural disease. Clin Chest Med 1998;19:261–76.
13. Stark DD, Federle MP, Goodman PC, et al. Differentiating lung abscess and empyema: radiography and computed tomography. AJR Am J Roentgenol 1983;141:163–7.
14. Rusch VW. Mesothelioma and less common pleural tumors. In: Pearson FG, Cooper JD, Deslauriers J, et al, editors. Thoracic surgery. New York: Churchill Livingstone; 2002. p. 1241.
15. Tsai TH, Yang PC. Ultrasound in the diagnosis and management of pleural disease. Curr Opin Pulm Med 2003;9:282–90.
16. Light RW, Jenkinson SG, Minh VD, et al. Observations on pleural fluid pressures as fluid is withdrawn during thoracentesis. Am Rev Respir Dis 1980;121:799–804.
17. Grogan DR, Irwin RS, Channick R, et al. Complications associated with thoracentesis: a prospective, randomized study comparing three different methods. Arch Intern Med 1990;150:873–7.
18. American Thoracic Society. Guidelines for thoracentesis and needle biopsy of the pleura. Am Rev Respir Dis 1989;140:257–8.
19. Light R, Macgregor MI, Luchsinger PC, et al. Pleural effusions: the diagnostic separation of transudates and exudates. Ann Intern Med 1972;77:507–13.
20. Heffern JE, Brown LK, Barbier CA. Diagnostic value of tests that discriminate between exudative and transudative pleural effusion. Chest 1997;111:970–80.
21. Colice GL, Curtis A, Deslauriers J, et al. Medical and surgical treatment of parapneumonic effusions: an evidence-based guideline. Chest 2000;118:1158–71.
22. Banales JL, Pineda PR, Fitzgerald JM, et al. Adenoside deaminase in the diagnosis of tuberculous pleural effusions: a report of 218 patients and review of the literature. Chest 1991;99:355–7.
23. Ansari T, Idyll S. Management of undiagnosed persistent pleural effusions. Clin Chest Med 1998;19:407–17.
24. Hillerdal G. Chylothorax and pseudochylothorax. Eur Respir J 1997;10:1157–62.
25. Garcia-Zamalloa A, Ruiz-Irastorza G, Aguayo FJ, et al. Pseudochylothorax: report of 2 cases and review of the literature. Medicine (Baltimore) 1999;78:200–7.
26. O'Callaghan AM, Meade GM. Chylothorax in lymphoma: mechanisms and management. Ann Oncol 1995;6:603–7.
27. Kalomenidis I, Light RW. Eosinophilic pleural effusions. Curr Opin Pulm Med 2003; 9:254–80.
28. Everts RJ, Relle B. Pleural space infections: microbiology and antimicrobial therapy. Semin Respir Infect 1999;14:18–40.
29. Boutin C, Astoul P. Diagnostic thoracoscopy. Clin Chest Med 1998;19:295–309.
30. Light RW, Erozan YS, Ball WC Jr, et al. Cells in pleural fluid: their value in differential diagnosis. Arch Intern Med 1973;132:854–60.
31. Sahn SA. State of the Art. The pleura. Am Rev Respir Dis 1988;138:184–234.
32. Rusch VW, Mountain C. Thoracoscopy under regional anesthesia for the diagnosis and management of pleural disease. Am J Surg 1987;154:274–8.
33. Downey RJ, McCormack P, LoCicero J 3rd, et al. Dissemination of malignant tumors after video-assisted thoracic surgery: a report of twenty-one cases. J Thorac Cardiovasc Surg 1996;111:954–60.
34. Boutin C, Rey F, Viallat JR. Prevention of malignant seeding after invasive diagnostic procedures in patients with pleural mesothelioma. A randomized trial of local radiotherapy. Chest. 1995;108:754–8.
35. Moghissi K. The malignant pleural effusion tissue diagnosis and treatment. In: Deslauriers J, Lacquet LK, editors. Thoracic surgery: surgical management of pleural diseases. Vol 6. St Louis: Mosby; 1990. p. 397.
36. Efthymiou CE, Masudi T, Thorpe JAC, Papagiannopoulos K. Malignant pleural

effusion in the presence of trapped lung. Five-year experience of PleurX tunneled catheters. Interact Cardiovasc Thorac Surg 2009; 9:961–4.
37. Warren WH, Kim AW, Liptay MJ. Identification of clinical factors predicting Pleurx catheter removal in patients treated for malignant pleural effusion. Eur J Cardiothorac Surg 2008;33:89–94.
38. Pollak J. Malignant pleural effusions: treatment with tunneled long-term drainage catheters. Curr Opin Pulm Med 2002;8:302–7.
39. Robinson R., Fullerton DA, Albert JD, et al. Use of pleural Tenckhoff catheter to palliate malignant pleural effusion. Ann Thorac Surg 1994;57:286–8.
40. Musani A, Haas AR, Seijo L, et al. Outpatient management of malignant pleural effusions with small-bore, tunneled pleural catheter. Respiration 2004;71:559–66.
41. Pollak JS, Burdge CM, Rosenblatt M, et al. Treatment of malignant pleural effusions with tunneled long-term drainage catheters. J Vasc Interv Radiol 2001;2:201–8.
42. Little A, Kadowaki MH, Ferguson MK, et al. Pleuro-peritoneal shunting: alternative therapy for pleural effusions. Ann Surg 1988; 208:443–50.
43. Genc O, Petrou M, Ladas G, et al. The long-term morbidity of pleuroperitoneal shunts in the management of recurrent malignant effusions. Eur J Cardiothorac Surg 2000; 18:143–6.
44. Sahn SA. Talc should be used for pleurodesis. Am J Respir Crit Care Med 2000; 162:2023–4.
45. Shaw P, Agarwal R. Pleurodesis for malignant pleural effusions. Cochrane Database Syst Rev 2004;(1):CD002916.
46. Tan C, Sedrakyan A, Browne J, et al. The evidence on the effectiveness of management for malignant pleural effusion: a systematic review. Eur J Cardiothorac Surg 2006; 29:829–38.
47. Dresler C, Olak J, Herndon JE 2nd, et al. Phase III intergroup study of talc poudrage vs talc slurry sclerosis for malignant pleural effusion. Chest 2005;127:909–15.
48. Cardillo G, Facciolo F, Carbone L, et al. Long-term follow-up of video-assisted talc pleurodesis in malignant recurrent pleural effusions. Eur J Cardiothorac Surg 2002;21: 302–5.
49. Mares DC, Mathu PN. Medical thoracoscopic talc pleurodesis for chylothorax due to lymphoma: a case series. Chest 1998;114: 731–5.
50. de Campos M, Ribas J. Thoracoscopy talc poudrage. Chest 2001;119:801–6.
51. Prevost A, Costa B, Elamarti R, et al. Long-term effect and tolerance of talc slurry for control of malignant pleural effusions. Oncol Rep 2001;8:1327–31.
52. Webb WR. Iodized talc pleurodesis for the treatment of pleural effusions. J Thorac Cardiovasc Surg 1992;103:881–5.
53. Kennedy L, Rusch VW, Strange C, et al. Pleurodesis using talc slurry. Chest 1994; 106:342–6.
54. Montes JF, Ferrer J, Villarino MA, et al. Influence of talc dose on extrapleural talc dissemination after talc pleurodesis. Am J Respir Crit Care Med 2003;168:348–55.
55. Janssen JP, Collier G, Astoul P, et al. Safety of pleurodesis with talc poudrage in malignant pleural effusion: a prospective cohort study. Lancet 2007;369:1535–9.
56. Olivares-Torres CA, Laniado-Laborin R, Chavez-Garcia C, et al. Iodopovidone pleurodesis for recurrent pleural effusions. Chest 2002;122:581–3.
57. Das SK, Saha SK, Das A, et al. A study of comparison of efficacy and safety of talc and povidone iodine for pleurodesis of malignant pleural effusions. J Indian Med Assoc 2008; 106:589–90.
58. Strange C, Sahn S. The definitions and epidemiology of pleural space infection. Semin Respir Infect 1999;14:3–8.
59. Cameron R, Davies HR. Intra-pleural fibrinolytic therapy versus conservative management in the treatment of parapneumonic effusions and empyema. Cochrane Database Syst Rev 2004;(2):CD002312.
60. McLaughlin JS, Krasna MJ. Parapneumonic empyema. In: LoCicero J III, Ponn RB, Shields TW, editors. General thoracic surgery. 5th ed. New York: Lippincott Williams & Wilkins; 2000. p. 699.
61. Sahn SA, Iseman M. Tuberculous empyema. Semin Respir Infect 1999;14:82–7.
62. Lim TK, Chin NK. Empirical treatment with fibrinolysis and early surgery reduces the duration of hospitalization in pleural sepsis. Eur Respir J 1999;13:514–8.
63. Wait MA. A randomized trial of empyema therapy. Chest 1997;111:1548–51.
64. Landreneau R. Thoracoscopy for empyema and hemothorax. Chest 1995;109:18–24.
65. Luh SP, Chou MC, Wang LS, et al. Video-assisted thoracoscopic surgery in the treatment of complicated parapneumonic effusions or empyemas: outcome of 234 patients. Chest 2005;127:1427–32.
66. Shields TW, Ponn RB. Complications of pulmonary resection. In: LoCicero J III, Ponn RB, Shields TW, editors. General thoracic surgery. 5th ed. New York: Lippincott Williams & Wilkins; 2000. p. 481.
67. Asamura H, Naruke T, Tsuchiya R, et al. Bronchopleural fistulas associated with lung cancer operations: univariate and multivariate analysis of risk factors, management and outcome. J Thorac Cardiovasc Surg 1992; 104:1456–64.
68. Johnstone DW. Postoperative chylothorax. Chest Surg Clin N Am 2002;12:597–603.
69. Simpson L. Chylothorax in adults: pathophysiology and management. In: Deslauriers J, Lacquet LK, editors. Thoracic surgery: surgical management of pleural diseases. Vol 6. St. Louis: Mosby; 1990. p. 366.
70. Romero S. Nontraumatic chylothorax. Curr Opin Pulm Med 2000;6:287–91.
71. Peillon C, D'Hont C, Melki J, et al. Usefulness of video thoracoscopy in the management of spontaneous and post operation chylothorax. Surg Endosc 1999;13:1106–9.
72. Haniuda M, Nishimura H, Kobayashi O, et al. Management of chylothorax after pulmonary resection. J Am Coll Surg 1995; 180:537–40.
73. Cope C. Management of chylothorax via percutaneous embolization. Curr Opin Pulm Med 2004;10:311–4.
74. Pratap U, Slavik Z, Ofoe VD, et al. Octreotide to treat postoperative chylothorax after cardiac operations in children. Ann Thorac Surg 2001;72:1740–2.
75. Gabbieri D, Bavutti L, Zaca F, et al. Conservative treatment of postoperative chylothorax with octreotide. Ital Heart J 2004;5:479–82.
76. Lange P, Mortensen J, Groth S. Lung function 22–35 years after treatment of idiopathic spontaneous pneumothorax with talc poudrage or simple drainage. Thorax 1988; 43:559–61.
77. Glazer M, Berkman N, Lafair JS, et al. Successful talc slurry pleurodesis in patients with nonmalignant pleural effusion: report of 16 cases and review of the literature. Chest 2000;117:1404–9.
78. Herlihy JP, Loyalka P, Gnananandh J, et al. PleurX catheter for the management of refractory pleural effusions in congestive heart failure. Tex Heart Inst J 2009;36:38–43.
79. Jones JSP. The pleura in health and disease. Lung 2002;179:397–413.
80. Wang NS. Anatomy of the pleura. Clin Chest Med 1998;19:229–40.
81. Agostoni E, Zocchi L. Mechanical coupling and liquid exchanges in the pleural space. Clin Chest Med 1988;19:241–60.
82. Kinasewitz GT, Fishman AP. Influence of alterations in Starling forces on visceral pleural fluid movement. J Appl Physiol 1981;51: 671–7.
83. Miserocchi G. Physiology and pathophysiology of pleural fluid turnover. Eur Respir J 1997;10:219–25.
84. Pistolesi M, Miniati M, Giunti C. Pleural liquid and solute exchange. Am Rev Respir Dis 1989;140:825–47.

5 SOLITARY PULMONARY NODULE

*Taine T.V. Pechet, MD, FACS**

Assessment of a Solitary Pulmonary Nodule

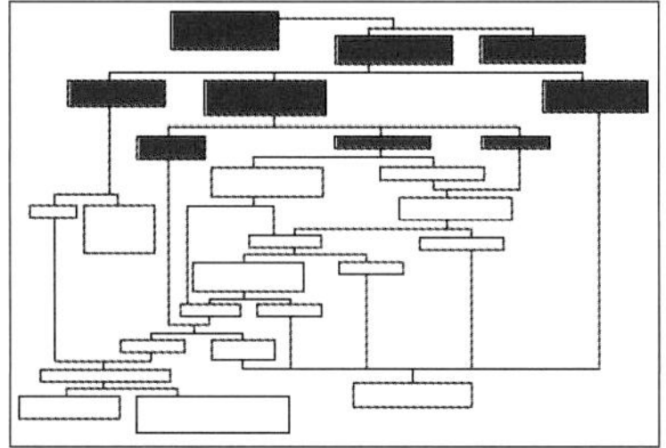

The solitary pulmonary nodule (SPN) is a common finding that is observed in more than 150,000 persons each year in the United States.[1] An SPN is defined as a single radiographically visible pulmonary lesion that is less than 3 cm in diameter, is completely surrounded by pulmonary parenchyma, and is not associated with atelectasis or adenopathy.[2] Any pulmonary lesion larger than 3 cm is considered a mass and as such has a greater likelihood of being malignant.[3,4] SPNs are detected on routine chest radiography at a rate of 1 in 500 x-rays, but with the growing use of computed tomographic (CT) scanning, they are now being diagnosed with increasing frequency.

The differential diagnosis of an SPN is broad and includes vascular diseases, infections, inflammatory conditions, congenital abnormalities, benign tumors, and malignancies [*see Table 1*]. Although most SPNs are benign, as many as one third represent primary malignancies, and nearly one quarter may be solitary metastases.[1,5,6] Various approaches have been developed to aid in the characterization and identification of SPNs. Certain clinical characteristics—such as greater age, history of tobacco use, and previous history of cancer—have been shown to increase the likelihood that the SPN is malignant.[7] Some authors have attempted to use the Bayes theorem, logistic regression models, or neural network analysis to predict the likelihood of malignancy.[7–9] Such methods are highly sensitive and specific, but they are cumbersome and of limited clinical applicability.

Clinical Evaluation

Once an SPN has been identified, it is necessary to determine whether the lesion is benign or malignant and what further investigations should be pursued. Evaluation should generally be governed by the dictum "malignant until proven otherwise." The basis for an initial assumption of malignancy is the observation that the overall 5-year survival rate is low (10 to 15%) once a diagnosis of lung cancer is established.[10] Appropriate evaluation involves careful assessment of the patient's history and risk factors for malignancy in conjunction with the results of radiographic studies [*see* Investigative Studies, *below*] to develop an individualized care plan.

Table 1 Differential Diagnosis of Solitary Pulmonary Nodule

Behavior	Category	Disease
Benign	Vascular disease	Arteriovenous malformations Pulmonary artery aneurysm
	Infection	*Mycobacterium avium* complex infection Aspergilloma Histoplasmosis Echinococcosis Blastomycosis Cryptococcosis Coccidioidomycosis Ascariasis Dirofilariasis
	Inflammatory condition	Rheumatoid nodule Sarcoidosis Wegener granulomatosis
	Congenital abnormality	Foregut duplication cyst
	Other	Rounded atelectasis Pulmonary amyloidosis
	Benign tumor	Hamartoma Lipoma Fibroma
Malignant	Primary lung cancer	Non–small cell lung cancer Squamous cell carcinoma Adenocarcinoma Large cell cancer Bronchoalveolar carcinoma Small cell lung cancer Carcinoid Lymphoma
	Metastatic cancer	Colon cancer Testicular cancer Melanoma Sarcoma Breast cancer

FACTORS INFLUENCING PROBABILITY OF MALIGNANCY

A number of factors influence the probability that an SPN is malignant. Those most strongly associated with lung cancer are age, smoking history, and occupational history. Pulmonary function test results indicative of a severe obstructive ventilatory impairment are also associated with an increased likelihood of malignancy.[11] In addition, the presence of endemic granulomatous disease has been shown to increase the probability that an SPN is harboring cancer.[7]

The radiographic appearance of an SPN, particularly on a CT scan, also influences the probability of malignancy

* The authors and editors gratefully acknowledge the contributions of the previous author, Shamus Carr, MD, to the development and writing of this chapter.

Assessment of a Solitary Pulmonary Nodule

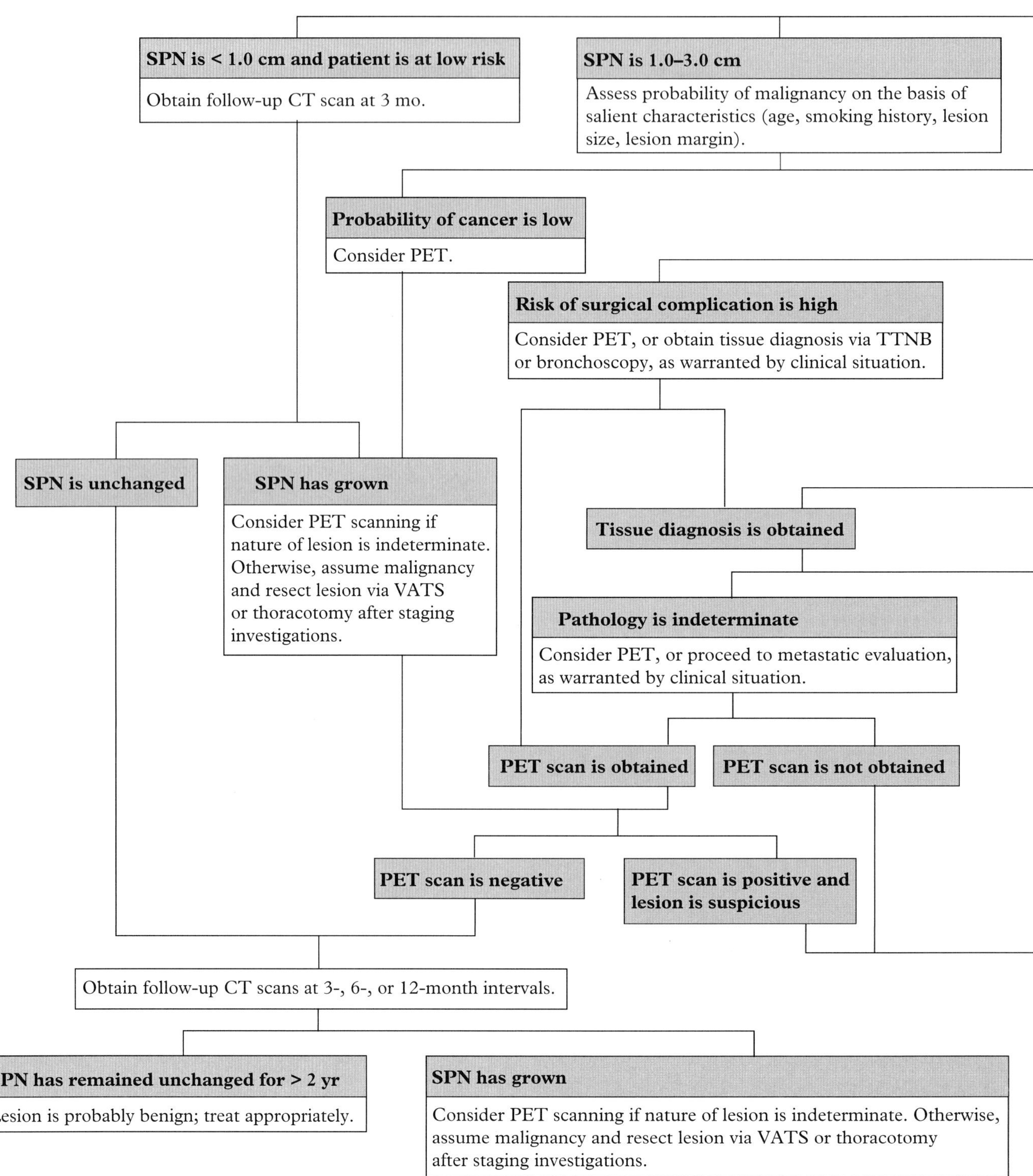
SPN is seen on chest x-ray or CT scan
Obtain history and perform thorough physical examination.
Review previous diagnostic images (if available).
SPN is < 1.0 cm and patient is at low risk
Obtain follow-up CT scan at 3 mo.
SPN is 1.0–3.0 cm
Assess probability of malignancy on the basis of salient characteristics (age, smoking history, lesion size, lesion margin).
Probability of cancer is low
Consider PET.
Risk of surgical complication is high
Consider PET, or obtain tissue diagnosis via TTNB or bronchoscopy, as warranted by clinical situation.
SPN is unchanged
SPN has grown
Consider PET scanning if nature of lesion is indeterminate. Otherwise, assume malignancy and resect lesion via VATS or thoracotomy after staging investigations.
Tissue diagnosis is obtained
Pathology is indeterminate
Consider PET, or proceed to metastatic evaluation, as warranted by clinical situation.
PET scan is obtained
PET scan is not obtained
PET scan is negative
PET scan is positive and lesion is suspicious
Obtain follow-up CT scans at 3-, 6-, or 12-month intervals.
SPN has remained unchanged for > 2 yr
Lesion is probably benign; treat appropriately.
SPN has grown
Consider PET scanning if nature of lesion is indeterminate. Otherwise, assume malignancy and resect lesion via VATS or thoracotomy after staging investigations.

SPN = solitary pulmonary nodule; CT = computed tomography; PET = positron emission tomography; VATS = video assisted thoracic surgery; TTNB = trans-thoracic needle biopsy.

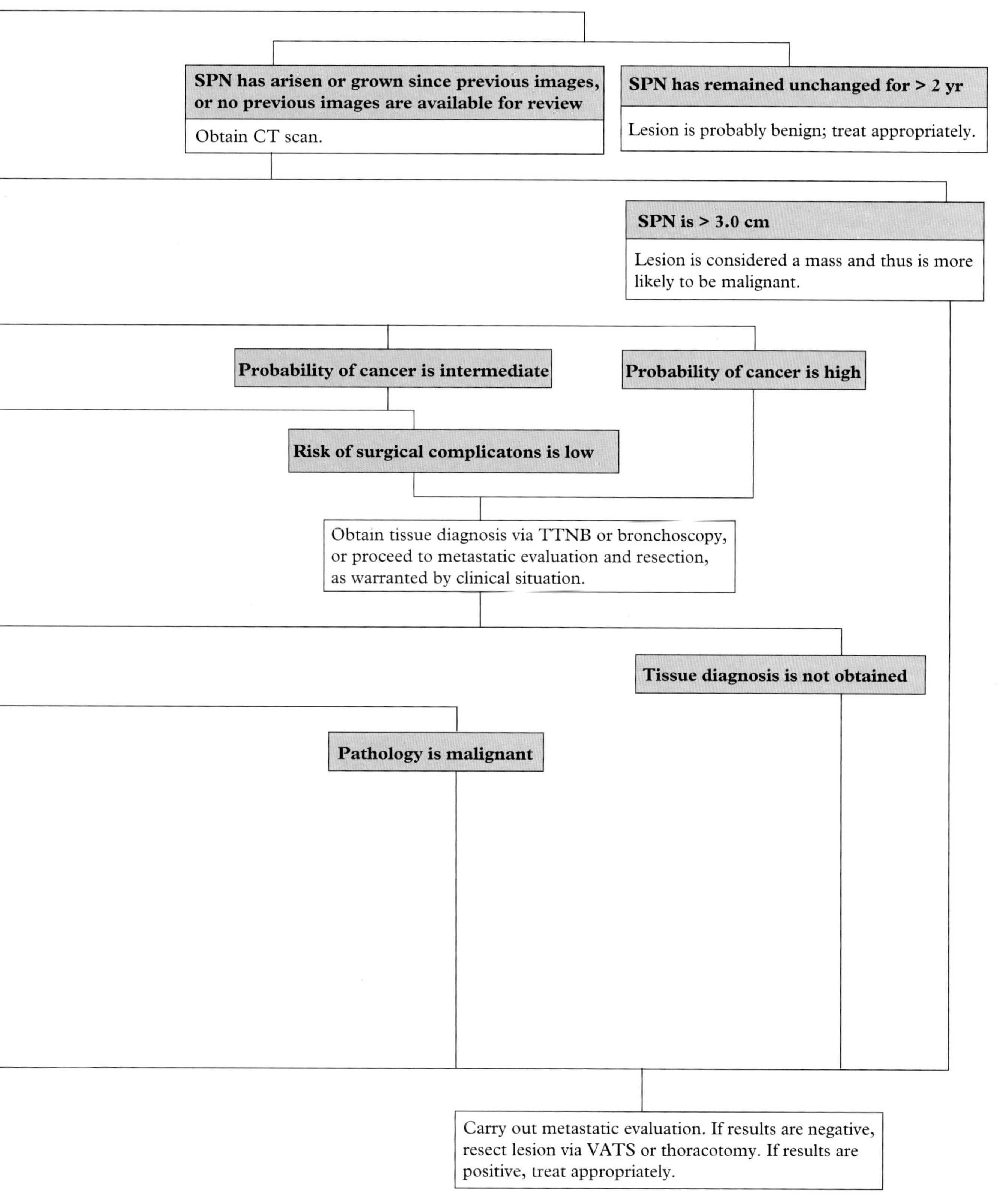
SPN has arisen or grown since previous images, or no previous images are available for review
Obtain CT scan.
SPN has remained unchanged for > 2 yr
Lesion is probably benign; treat appropriately.
SPN is > 3.0 cm
Lesion is considered a mass and thus is more likely to be malignant.
Probability of cancer is intermediate
Probability of cancer is high
Risk of surgical complicatons is low
Obtain tissue diagnosis via TTNB or bronchoscopy, or proceed to metastatic evaluation and resection, as warranted by clinical situation.
Tissue diagnosis is not obtained
Pathology is malignant
Carry out metastatic evaluation. If results are negative, resect lesion via VATS or thoracotomy. If results are positive, treat appropriately.

[*see* Investigative Studies, Imaging, Computed Tomography, *below*]. The size, contour, internal characteristics, and growth rate of the nodule are all potentially significant indicators of malignant disease [*see Table 2*].

Age

Lung cancer is rare before the age of 40 years, but its incidence steadily increases from that point until the age of 80.[5] Above the age of 70, the likelihood that an SPN is malignant increases.[8] After the age of 80, the incidence of malignancy in an SPN seems to level off or even decrease.[12]

Environmental Exposures

The link between cigarette smoking and lung cancer has been well established since the 1950s, and the incidence of lung cancer in smokers is directly correlated with the number of pack-years of smoking.[13] The surgeon general's report from 2004 states that "the evidence is sufficient to infer a causal relationship between smoking and lung cancer."[14] There is also ample evidence of a causal relationship between environmental tobacco exposure, termed "secondhand smoke," and lung cancer.[15]

Radon exposure is the second leading cause of lung cancer in America, and cigarette smoking further increases the risks associated with radon exposure.[16] Asbestos exposure in combination with cigarette smoking also places patients at significantly increased risk for lung cancer. Patients with a history of workplace exposure to a radioactive substance (e.g., uranium or plutonium) are at increased risk for lung cancer, but this association is not as well documented as the association of lung cancer with tobacco use. Miners of heavy metals (e.g., nickel, cadmium, and silica) are also at increased risk, and a variety of other environmental toxins, from diesel exhaust through vinyl, have been associated with the development of lung cancer.[15] There is some evidence to suggest that patients with idiopathic pulmonary fibrosis and pneumoconiosis are at increased risk for bronchoalveolar cell carcinoma.[17]

Table 2 Factors Affecting Malignant Probability of Solitary Pulmonary Nodule[8]

Factor	Likelihood Ratio for Malignancy
Spiculated margins on CT scan	5.54
Age > 70 yr	4.16
Lesion size 2.1–3.0 cm	3.67
Doubling time < 465 days	3.40
History of smoking	2.27
Age 50–69 yr	1.90
Lesion size 1.1–2.0 cm	0.74
Lesion size < 1 cm	0.52
Smooth margins on CT scan	0.30
No history of smoking	0.19
Doubling time > 465 days	0.01

CT = computed tomographic.

Investigative Studies

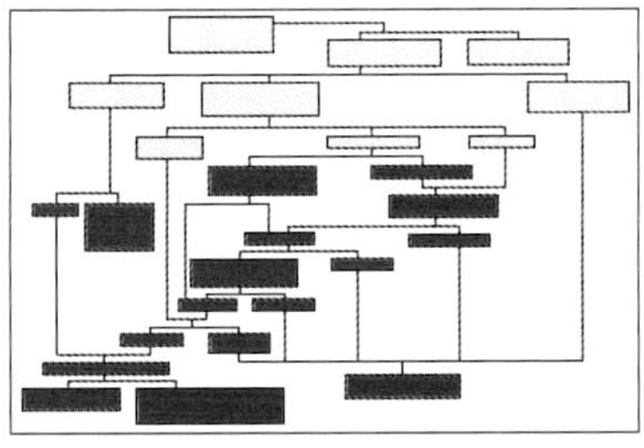

IMAGING

Chest Radiography (X-Ray)

Whereas the prevalence of lung cancer is low in comparison with that of breast or prostate cancer, the mortality for lung cancer exceeds that for breast, prostate, and colon cancer combined. As noted [*see* Clinical Evaluation, *above*], the overall 5-year survival rate for lung cancer patients is poor, in part because lung cancer is frequently diagnosed at a more advanced stage than other forms of cancer. Several trials performed before the advent of CT scanning evaluated chest radiography for early screening of lung cancer but were unable to demonstrate that such screening yielded better survival.[18–20] One explanation for these disappointing results may be that fewer than 10% of lung cancers are stage I at presentation.[18]

Although chest radiography is ineffective as a screening tool for early-stage lung cancer, it remains a valuable investigative tool in the evaluation of SPNs. If an SPN's appearance on chest x-rays has not changed for more than 2 years, the SPN will be benign in more than 90% of cases. In such cases, only yearly follow-up is typically required; additional diagnostic tests are usually unnecessary.[21,22] Therefore, an effort should always be made to obtain old chest radiographs if they are known to exist.

Computed Tomography

The advent of CT scanning has led to an increase in the number of SPNs detected.[23] But, of course, it has also led to an increase in the number of benign SPNs found. Advocates of CT scanning for assessment of SPNs base their argument on two central points. First, as many as 83% of CT-detected stage I malignancies are not visible on chest x-ray.[24] Second, non–small cell lung cancer (NSCLC) is the malignancy most commonly identified, and the survival rate for stage I NSCLC is relatively high in comparison with more advanced disease stages. In patients whose SPN proves to be NSCLC, the 5-year survival rate is 67% for stage IA disease. This figure falls rapidly as the disease stage rises: the 5-year survival rate is 55% for stage IIA NSCLC and only 10% for stage IIIA NSCLC with mediastinal nodal metastasis.[25]

Numerous studies have evaluated the use of screening CT both in the general population and in at-risk groups consisting of older patients with a smoking history.[24,26,27] The greatest drawback to screening CT is the high false positive rate: nodules are identified on 23 to 66% of all CT scans, depending on the thickness of the slices,[12,24] and nearly 98% of these nodules are eventually determined to be benign. Sequential CT scanning is often required to determine whether an SPN is benign or malignant. In 10 to 15% of patients, however, this determination cannot be made even when two CT scans are compared. Such patients may be assessed with other imaging modalities (e.g., positron emission tomography [PET]) or may be referred for transthoracic needle biopsy (TTNB) or other invasive diagnostic tests.

Controversy exists in both the literature and in clinical practice around the optimal intervals for follow-up CT scanning after initial identification of an SPN. In the literature, the recommended interval between initial CT scanning and repeat CT scanning has ranged from 1 month to 1 year.[12,24,27] These varying recommendations are based on what is considered the doubling time for an SPN. In a study from 2000 that included 13 patients with a known diagnosis and lesions less than 10 mm in diameter at initial evaluation, volumetric growth rates were measured to establish the doubling times of the nodules.[10] The doubling times ranged from 51 days to more than 1 year. For malignant lesions, the average doubling time was less than 177 days, whereas for benign lesions, it was more than 396 days. New volumetric modeling methods have been developed that may be capable of detecting conformational changes over much shorter intervals, but they remain infrequently used.[28] Because the doubling time is considerably shorter for malignant lesions than for benign lesions, a repeat CT scan should typically be performed for most lesions 3 months after the initial study. If the lesion is visibly larger on the repeat scan, it is likely malignant, and diagnostic evaluation should progress toward presumed resection. If, however, the lesion has neither regressed nor progressed, a follow-up CT scan closer to 12 months is warranted; the precise timing remains controversial and should be determined on the basis of individual patient and SPN characteristics. The Fleischner Society Statement from the Radiological Society of North America provides commonly cited guidelines for the radiographic evaluation of nodules, with recommendations divided into size categories and recommendations that range from 3 to 12 months.[29]

The morphologic characteristics of an SPN visualized on a CT scan can be extremely helpful in characterizing the probability of malignancy [*see* Differential Diagnosis, *below*]. Size, margin appearance, cavitation, and attenuation are important criteria. Air bronchograms, ground-glass opacity, and adjacent vascular distortion patterns can also help suggest malignancy. Although an SPN with a spiculated margin is perhaps most suspicious for malignancy, one fifth of lung cancers may have well-defined margins.[30,31] Within areas of ground-glass opacity, characteristic changes, such as the development of nodularity and solid attenuation, have been identified that increase the probability of malignancy.[32–34] Other CT characteristics may point more toward a benign condition. For example, although cavitation may occur in either benign or malignant lesions, SPNs with walls thinner than 4 mm are much more likely to be benign, whereas those with walls thicker than 16 mm are more likely to be malignant.[35] Intranodular fat is a reliable indicator of a hamartoma, a benign lesion, and is seen in as many as 50% of hamartomas.[36] In addition, calcification is most commonly associated with hamartomas and other benign nodules. Unfortunately, between one third and two thirds of benign lesions visualized are not calcified, and as many as 6% of malignant lesions are calcified.[31,37,38] Finally, increased enhancement (measured in Hounsfield units [HU]) after injection with intravenous contrast is strongly suggestive of malignancy and has been included in the American College of Chest Physicians (ACCP) consensus recommendations.[39] Lesions that enhance by less than 15 HU are most likely benign (positive predictive value 99%), whereas lesions that enhance by more than 20 HU are typically malignant (sensitivity 98%; specificity 73%).[40] Lesions that enhance by 15 to 20 HU should be considered indeterminate.

Because most SPNs are benign and because the risk of misdiagnosing a malignant lesion is so great, it is important to make use of all of the data obtained from CT scanning in the effort to make cost-effective, logical decisions regarding further evaluation or treatment. Careful evaluation of the size, contours, and internal characteristics of an SPN on successive CT scans, balanced by the patient's risk profile, including age, smoking history, and environmental exposures, provides the framework for developing an individualized evaluation strategy

Positron Emission Tomography

PET is an imaging modality that employs radiolabeled isotopes of fluorine, carbon, or oxygen; the most commonly used isotope is ^{18}F-fluorodeoxyglucose (FDG). The rationale for FDG-PET scanning in the evaluation of SPNs is based on the higher metabolic rate of most malignancies and the preferential trapping of FDG in malignant cells.[41] However, increased FDG activity can also occur in benign SPNs,[42,43] especially those arising from active granulomatous diseases[44,45] or inflammatory processes.[46] These benign diseases can produce false positive PET scans and thereby reduce the sensitivity of the test. Conversely, some malignancies—bronchoalveolar carcinoma and carcinoid tumors, in particular—have low metabolic activity and commonly produce false negative PET scans.[47–51] Thus, a negative PET scan is not a particularly helpful result, and it is necessary to follow the lesion with serial CT scans. Accuracy calculations for PET scanning vary widely, with some of the highest sensitivity and specificity figures reported in an early meta-analysis identifying sensitivity of 96% and specificity of 77%.[52] More recent pooled sensitivity and specificity figures were 87% and 83%, with specificity ranging from 40 to 100%.[39]

Efforts have been made to improve the sensitivity and specificity of PET scanning in the diagnosis of SPNs. One such effort involves the use of the standardized uptake value (SUV), which is a numerical indication of the activity concentration in a lesion, normalized for the injected dose.[53] In many studies, an SPN is considered malignant when its SUV is higher than 2.5. Because of the methodology used to calculate SUV, however, small tumors (< 1.0 cm) may have an SUV lower than 2.5 and still be malignant. Their small volume causes their true activity concentration to be underestimated, with the result that their SUV drops below the threshold value for malignancy. In one prospective study of patients with SPNs, the overall sensitivity of FDG-PET scanning was 79% and the overall specificity was 65%.[54] When the SPN was smaller than 1.0 cm, however, all of the scans were negative, even though 40% of the nodules were malignant. Another effort involves recent technology combining PET and CT scans. CT-PET fusion imaging is clinically available in many locales, and combination imaging has been found to be particularly important for staging.[55,56]

In cases where the SPN is larger than 8 mm and no previous radiographs or CT scans are available for comparison, PET scanning can provide information that may facilitate the decision whether to follow the lesion closely or to proceed with tissue acquisition. ACCP consensus recommendations include the use of PET scanning in select lesions greater than 8 mm identified in patients with low to moderate pretest probability of malignancy.[39] Cost analysis is also an important criterion in considering PET scanning. One study that examined the cost-effectiveness of PET in the evaluation of SPNs concluded that it was cost-effective for patients who had an intermediate pretest probability of a malignant SPN and who were at high risk for surgical complications.[57] In all other groups, PET was not cost-effective, and CT led to similar outcomes (in terms of quality-adjusted life-years) and to lower costs.

BIOPSY

If an SPN displays characteristics suggestive of malignancy, a tissue diagnosis should be obtained. In many cases, the appropriate form of tissue acquisition will be excisional biopsy by wedge resection, often followed by anatomic lung resection. Traditionally, excisional biopsy was performed, accepting the morbidity associated with thoracotomy. Especially for peripheral lesions, however, video-assisted thoracic surgery (VATS) has now supplanted thoracotomy as the procedure of choice. However, several alternative biopsy techniques may be performed in place of resection, including TTNB and bronchoscopy.

Transthoracic Needle Biopsy

Lesions that are between 1.0 and 3.0 cm in diameter should be considered for TTNB. The diagnostic yield of this procedure for SPNs is excellent, reaching 95% in some studies. The reported sensitivity ranges from 80 to 95% and the specificity ranges from 50 to 88%.[58–60] A study of 222 patients who underwent TTNB for an SPN reported a positive predictive value of 98.6% and a negative predictive value of 96.6%[61]; however, several other studies reported false negative rates ranging from 3 to 29%.[58,62] The complication rate associated with TTNB is relatively high—potentially as high as 30% and rarely lower than 10%, in even the most experienced hands.[59,63] Most commonly, a pneumothorax results; however, chest tube placement is required only if the patient becomes symptomatic, a situation that occurs in approximately 50% of cases. In the absence of symptoms, observation with serial chest x-rays is generally appropriate. If no increase in the size of the pneumothorax is observed, the patient can be discharged with the expectation that the pneumothorax will resolve.

For lesions smaller than 1.0 cm, the risk-to-benefit ratio of TTNB rises to the point where other techniques are typically preferred. The utility of TTNB depends primarily on the characteristics of the SPN—in particular, its location. Nodules that are central or close to the diaphragm or the pericardium are less well suited to this technique than those at other sites.

Bronchoscopy

Bronchoscopy has a well-established role in the evaluation of central SPNs, which are amenable to direct visualization and biopsy. Most SPNs, however, are not central. Various adjunctive measures, including transbronchial needle biopsy and cytology brushings, are employed to improve the yield of bronchoscopy. For SPNs between 2.0 and 3.0 cm in diameter, the diagnostic yield of bronchoscopy ranges from 20 to 80%, depending on the size of the lesion, the incidence of malignancy in the study population, and the proximity of the lesion to the bronchial tree.[64,65] For SPNs smaller than 1.5 cm, the yield drops to 10%.[66] Even though bronchoscopy has a low complication rate (about 5%), its low diagnostic yield for malignancy limits its utility in the evaluation of SPNs.

New technology has allowed the application of guidance techniques to the field of bronchoscopy. Ultrasound transducers affixed to the tip of a bronchoscope, endobronchial ultrasonography (EBUS), has become an important tool in mediastinal staging, with EBUS-transbronchial needle aspiration (EBUS-TBNA) sensitivities in the range of 92% and specificities of 98% reported.[67] Electromagnetic navigational bronchoscopy (ENB) uses three-dimensional CT reconstructions to provide guidance for bronchoscopic sampling of peripheral lesions. The diagnostic yield for peripheral lesions is in the range of 70%,[68] and experience within the community is growing. ENB is a technique that can provide tissue from central nodules as well as an alternative to TTNB or VATS for peripheral lesions, and offers the ability to place a fiducial marker for subsequent radiation therapy guidance.

Excisional Biopsy

The decision to proceed to excisional lung biopsy (open or VATS) must be carefully considered. The risk-to-benefit ratio of excisional biopsy for an individual patient is determined by clinical characteristics affecting perioperative morbidity and mortality, as well as by the expected risk of malignancy in the SPN.

Resection is the reference standard for tissue acquisition. The morbidity associated with VATS is less than that associated with thoracotomy; accordingly, when VATS lung biopsy is technically feasible, it is preferable to open lung biopsy. The overall morbidity is lower than 1% for VATS wedge resection, compared with 3 to 7% for the equivalent open procedure. Patients who have undergone VATS resection experience less pain, have shorter hospital stays, and recover sooner than those who have undergone open biopsy.[69–71]

A technical consideration that must be contemplated when VATS is planned is possible conversion to thoracotomy. The conversion rate for VATS to thoracotomy has been reported to be as high as 33%, but there is evidence to suggest that this rate can be significantly reduced with careful patient selection and increasing experience in minimally invasive techniques.[72,73] For example, modern experience with VATS techniques has demonstrated a low conversion rate of 2.5% in a series of 1,100 patients undergoing the more complex VATS lobectomy procedure.[74]

Peripheral SPNs more than 1.0 cm in diameter are the lesions best suited to VATS excision. As SPNs become smaller and more central, they become harder to identify, and the rate of conversion to thoracotomy or the need to perform an anatomic resection increases. A wide variety of techniques have been employed to improve the identification of SPNs for VATS, ranging from dye staining through guide-wire localization. One of the more recent developments has been the use of technetium-labeled microalbumin combined with a gamma probe to successfully resect 96% of lesions using thoracoscopic techniques.[75] Despite demonstrated cost-effectiveness,[76] however, none of these techniques have achieved wide acceptance, and most surgeons rely on digital palpation combined with radiographic guidance.

Differential Diagnosis

MALIGNANT LESIONS

Non–Small Cell Lung Cancer

As noted, NSCLC is the malignancy most frequently identified in an SPN. Most lung cancer patients are asymptomatic, and those who are symptomatic usually have advanced disease, including mediastinal lymph node involvement. Arterial invasion has also been shown to have an adverse effect on survival in patients with early-stage NSCLC.[77] The most common sites of metastases are the lymph nodes, the brain, the bones, and the adrenal glands. Accordingly, it is essential to perform a metastatic evaluation that focuses on these areas before proceeding with resection.

Adenocarcinoma and squamous cell carcinoma remain the most common types of NSCLC, but bronchoalveolar carcinoma is a well-differentiated subtype that has a prolonged doubling time. Because of its slow growth rate, it may be missed by PET scan.[49] Bronchoalveolar carcinoma may present as an SPN, particularly with a ground-glass appearance, as airspace disease, or as multiple nodules.

Small Cell Lung Cancer

Small cell carcinoma accounts for approximately 20% of lung cancers. Typically, it presents as a central mass in association with significant nodal disease, often accompanied by distant metastases.[78] Small cell carcinoma typically has a very short doubling time. Paraneoplastic syndromes are more common with small cell lung cancer than with NSCLC.

Pulmonary Carcinoid Tumor

Pulmonary carcinoid tumors are uncommon neuroendocrine neoplasms that account for 1 to 2% of lung cancers.[79] They are classified as either typical or atypical, depending on their histology, but represent a spectrum of neuroendocrine tumors.[80] Either type of carcinoid may present as an SPN, usually in the fifth or sixth decade of life. Typical carcinoid tumors have a very long doubling time—up to 80 months—and thus may be mistaken for benign lesions.[81] Atypical carcinoid tumors have a much shorter doubling time and are more likely to show an increase in size on serial CT scans. Typical carcinoid tumors have an extremely low incidence of recurrence and are not usually associated with nodal metastasis.

Metastatic Malignancies

Metastases to the lung frequently appear as smooth, round, well-demarcated lesions. They often are multiple, tend to be found in the better vascularized lower lung zones, and rarely are associated with mediastinal adenopathy. Most pulmonary metastases derive from the lungs, the colon, the testicles, the breasts, melanomas, or sarcomas. Treatment tends to be palliative, based on the diagnosis of the primary tumor, but it may be curative in cases of metastatic sarcoma or testicular carcinoma. In patients with these cancers, limited wedge resection of a metastasis to the lung has been shown to confer a survival advantage; this measure may also be beneficial for patients with metastatic head and neck cancer and, occasionally, for those with metastatic melanoma.[82] Recent reports with modern chemotherapeutic strategies and resection have suggested that prolonged survival is possible in colorectal cancer metastatic to the lung, with 5-year survival of 67%.[83] Improved outcomes are thought to be more likely in colorectal cancer patients with less than two pulmonary metastases.[84]

BENIGN LESIONS

Pulmonary Hamartoma

Pulmonary hamartomas are the most common benign pulmonary tumors and the third most common cause of SPNs overall. Most (90%) arise in the periphery of the lung, but endobronchial hamartomas are seen as well. Because they are most common in the periphery, hamartomas are usually asymptomatic. When a potential hamartoma appears as an SPN on a chest x-ray, CT scanning is warranted for further evaluation.

Certain typical CT findings suggest that the SPN is likely to be a hamartoma. One such finding is a particular pattern of calcification. Calcification is more common in benign lesions than in malignant tumors. Four patterns of calcification are considered benign: central, diffuse, laminated, and "popcornlike." The first three patterns are most commonly associated with an infectious condition (e.g., histoplasmosis or tuberculosis). The popcornlike pattern, however, indicates that the lesion is probably a hamartoma. Unfortunately, calcification is present in only about 50% of benign lesions, and only about 50% of hamartomas are calcified.[31] It is important to remember that pulmonary carcinoid tumors and metastases to the lung (especially those from osteosarcomas, chondrosarcomas, or synovial cell sarcomas) may also have calcifications. Another reliable marker of a hamartoma is the finding of fat within the lesion on a CT scan; however, fewer than 50% of hamartomas demonstrate this characteristic. PET scanning, particularly the correlation between PET and CT findings on PET-CT, has been suggested as a useful diagnostic tool.[85]

Inflammatory Nodules

Sarcoidosis is known as the great mimicker, but it rarely presents as an SPN.[86] Most commonly, it presents as hilar and mediastinal lymphadenopathy and diffuse parenchymal involvement. When it does present as an SPN, it is almost invariably a solid lesion, hardly ever a cavitary one. The incidence of sarcoidosis is highest in African-American women between 20 and 40 years of age. If sarcoidosis is suspected during the evaluation of an SPN, an elevated angiotensin-converting enzyme level supports the diagnosis, but a normal level does not exclude it. If a biopsy is performed, the presence of noncaseating granulomas on pathologic evaluation helps establish the diagnosis. If a diagnosis of sarcoidosis is suspected, PET scanning has been suggested as an effective method to identify extrathoracic sites of disease to target for pathologic confirmation.[87]

Pulmonary rheumatoid nodules are present in fewer than 1% of patients with rheumatoid arthritis.[88] They are usually associated with rheumatoid nodules in other parts of the body but may precede any systemic manifestations of the disease. Pulmonary rheumatoid nodules, although generally asymptomatic in themselves, arise from underlying rheumatoid activity. When the underlying disease is active, the nodules may grow, simulating malignancy. An elevated serum rheumatoid factor level is typical and helps confirm the diagnosis.

Wegener granulomatosis is a necrotizing vasculitis that affects both the upper and the lower respiratory tract, as well as the kidneys. It presents with an SPN in approximately 20% of patients.[89] If vasculitis is suspected during evaluation of an SPN, laboratory studies should include testing for cytoplasmic antineutrophil cytoplasmic antibodies (c-ANCAs); a positive result on this test is highly suggestive of Wegener granulomatosis. Treatment includes the cytotoxic drug cyclophosphamide, either alone or in combination with corticosteroids.

Infectious Nodules

An SPN can also represent an infectious granuloma caused by tuberculosis, atypical mycobacterial diseases, histoplasmosis, coccidioidomycosis, or aspergillosis. Such granulomas frequently have a cavitary appearance on CT scans. Occasionally, a chest x-ray taken with the patient in different positions shows shifting of the position of the cavity's contents or a crescent of air around the mass (the Monod sign).[90] This radiographic finding is characteristic of a mycetoma, usually aspergilloma. Depending on the circumstances—in particular, on whether there has been significant hemoptysis and whether pulmonary function is reasonably well preserved—many of these lesions are best treated with resection. Others are best diagnosed by noninvasive techniques and treated with antimicrobial therapy.

Pulmonary dirofilariasis is a rare but well-attested cause of SPNs that is the consequence of infestation of human lungs by the canine heartworm *Dirofilaria immitis*. This organism is transmitted to humans in larval form by mosquitoes that have ingested blood from affected dogs.[91] Because humans are not suitable hosts for this organism, the larvae die and embolize to the lungs, where they initiate a granulomatous response. Typically, these lesions are pleura based, and the diagnosis is made at the time of resection.[92] Once the diagnosis is made, no further therapy is required.

Echinococcosis is a hydatid disease caused by the tapeworm *Echinococcus granulosus*. It is endemic to certain areas of the world where sheep and cattle are raised. Normally, it is ingested incidentally; the parasite penetrates the bowel wall and travels to the lungs in 10 to 30% of cases.[93,94] A complete blood count usually demonstrates peripheral eosinophilia. If echinococcosis is suspected, a hemagglutination test, which has a sensitivity of 66 to 100% and a specificity of 98 to 99% for *Echinococcus*, should be performed. TTNB should not be performed because there is a risk that cyst rupture triggers an anaphylactic reaction to the highly antigenic contents. Patients may be treated with anthelmintic agents, but the incidence of persistent or recurrent disease is high. Accordingly, surgical resection should be considered.

OTHER CONSIDERATIONS

Pulmonary amyloidosis may present in either a diffuse or a nodular form. The prognosis is most favorable when it presents as an asymptomatic SPN. Typically, the nodule is well defined and between 2 and 4 cm in diameter. Unless the patient exhibits systemic manifestations of amyloidosis, the diagnosis can be confirmed only by biopsy of the nodule.[42]

Rounded atelectasis usually presents as a pleura-based nodular density that occurs secondary to pleural scarring and thickening. An effort should be made to look for associated pleural plaques resulting from asbestos exposure. The CT scan usually demonstrates an SPN with a "comet tail." Biopsy is not required unless mesothelioma is strongly suspected or the SPN is seen to have grown on successive CT scans.

Management

The ACCP attempted to provide evidence-based guidelines to direct the evaluation of patients with SPNs 8 to 10 mm in diameter in their 2007 consensus statement.[39] Unfortunately, few, if any, randomized controlled trials exist to direct management. Most clinicians rely on a combination of single-institution studies, a few prospective trials, and clinical acumen to assess a given patient's risk profile to inform decisions on invasive and noninvasive testing. The initial step in decision making is to confirm that the lesion is, in fact, new, and to compare current chest x-rays or CT scans with any previous images that are available. An SPN whose size has been stable for 2 years on diagnostic images will be benign 90 to 95% of the time. If no previous images are available for comparison, the patient should undergo a clinical evaluation to determine their risk profile. This evaluation must be individualized according to the characteristics of the patient and the lesion. On the basis of the patient's age, exposure and smoking history, the size of the SPN, and the characteristics of the lesion's borders, an SPN for which no previous diagnostic images are available can be initially classified as having a low, intermediate, or high probability of cancer [*see Table 3*].[7,95,96] This classification governs the subsequent workup. Whereas a patient with a high-probability SPN needs a complete evaluation progressing toward resection with minimal delay, the same strategy would not be cost-effective for a patient with a low-probability SPN. It is important not to subject a patient with a high-probability SPN to studies that will not change clinical management or outcome: doing so will delay diagnosis and treatment unnecessarily.

At this point in the evaluation, if the nature of the SPN is still indeterminate and the lesion is larger than 1 cm, there may be a role for PET or PET-CT scanning. If PET scanning yields negative results, the SPN is likely benign, and follow-up CT scanning is appropriate. If PET scanning yields positive results and the patient is at high surgical risk, TTNB, bronchoscopy, or guided bronchoscopy may be performed to

Table 3 Initial Assessment of Probability of Cancer in Solitary Pulmonary Nodule

Characteristics of Patient or Lesion	Probability of Cancer		
	Low	Intermediate	High
Patient age (yr)	< 40	40–60	> 60
Patient smoking history	Never smoked	< 20 pack-yr	≥ 20 pack-yr
Lesion size (cm)	< 1.0	1.1–2.2	≥ 2.3
Lesion margin	Smooth	Scalloped	Spiculated

establish a diagnosis. If, however, the patient is at reasonable surgical risk, proceeding directly to VATS resection (and, potentially, to lobectomy) offers the best chance of cure for a probable carcinoma.

For patients with SPNs smaller than 1.0 cm, the optimal approach may be to perform serial CT scanning at an initial 3-month interval for a minimum of 2 years. The rationale for this approach is based on the difficulty of identifying these lesions with VATS, the low likelihood of establishing a diagnosis with TTNB, and the possibility that the lesion may be benign. If the lesion has grown visibly between scans, it is probably malignant, and proceeding with resection for diagnosis and treatment is appropriate. The likelihood that nodal metastases will develop in a closely followed SPN smaller than 1.0 cm is low.[73] If the SPN proves to be malignant, scanning at 3-month intervals is unlikely to alter the eventual outcome. Society guidelines continue to be refined in an effort to provide helpful recommendations.

Financial Disclosures: None Reported

References

1. Leef JL 3rd, Klein JS. The solitary pulmonary nodule. Radiol Clin North Am 2002;40: 123–43, ix.
2. Tuddenham WJ. Glossary of terms for thoracic radiology: recommendations of the Nomenclature Committee of the Fleischner Society. AJR Am J Roentgenol 1984;143: 509–17.
3. Lillington GA. Management of the solitary pulmonary nodule. Hosp Pract (Off Ed) 1993;28(5):41–8.
4. Midthun DE, Swensen SJ, Jett JR. Approach to the solitary pulmonary nodule. Mayo Clin Proc 1993;68:378–85.
5. Jemal A, Murray T, Ward E, et al. Cancer statistics, 2005. CA Cancer J Clin 2005;55: 10–30.
6. Swanson SJ, Jaklitsch MT, Mentzer SJ, et al. Management of the solitary pulmonary nodule: role of thoracoscopy in diagnosis and therapy. Chest 1999;116(6 Suppl):523S–4S.
7. Swensen SJ, Silverstein MD, Ilstrup DM, et al. The probability of malignancy in solitary pulmonary nodules. Application to small radiologically indeterminate nodules. Arch Intern Med 1997;157:849–55.
8. Gurney JW. Determining the likelihood of malignancy in solitary pulmonary nodules with Bayesian analysis. Part I. Theory. Radiology 1993;186:405–13.
9. Henschke CI, Yankelevitz DF, Mateescu I, et al. Neural networks for the analysis of small pulmonary nodules. Clin Imaging 1997;21: 390–9.
10. Yankelevitz DF, Henschke CI. Small solitary pulmonary nodules. Radiol Clin North Am 2000;38:471–8.
11. Kishi K, Gurney JW, Schroeder DR, et al. The correlation of emphysema or airway obstruction with the risk of lung cancer: a matched case-controlled study. Eur Respir J 2002;19:1093–8.
12. Libby DM, Smith JP, Altorki NK, et al. Managing the small pulmonary nodule discovered by CT. Chest 2004;125:1522–9.
13. Wynder EL, Graham EA. Tobacco smoking as a possible etiologic factor in bronchiogenic carcinoma; a study of 684 proved cases. J Am Med Assoc 1950;143:329–36.
14. The 2004 United States Surgeon General's Report: the health consequences of smoking. N S W Public Health Bull 2004;15:107.
15. Moritsugu KP. The 2006 Report of the Surgeon General: the health consequences of involuntary exposure to tobacco smoke. Am J Prev Med 2007;32:542–3.
16. Pawel DJ, Puskin JS. The U.S. Environmental Protection Agency's assessment of risks from indoor radon. Health Phys 2004;87: 68–74.
17. Pairon JC, Brochard P, Jaurand MC, Bignon J. Silica and lung cancer: a controversial issue. Eur Respir J 1991;4:730–44.
18. Melamed MR, Flehinger BJ, Zaman MB, et al. Screening for early lung cancer. Results of the Memorial Sloan-Kettering study in New York. Chest 1984;86:44–53.
19. Kubik A, Haerting J. Survival and mortality in a randomized study of lung cancer detection. Neoplasma 1990;37:467–75.
20. Kubik A, Parkin DM, Khlat M, et al. Lack of benefit from semi-annual screening for cancer of the lung: follow-up report of a randomized controlled trial on a population of high-risk males in Czechoslovakia. Int J Cancer 1990; 45:26–33.
21. Lillington GA. Management of solitary pulmonary nodules. Dis Mon 1991;37: 271–318.
22. Yankelevitz DF, Henschke CI. Does 2-year stability imply that pulmonary nodules are benign? AJR Am J Roentgenol 1997;168: 325–8.
23. Diederich S, Lenzen H, Windmann R, et al. Pulmonary nodules: experimental and clinical studies at low-dose CT. Radiology 1999; 213:289–98.
24. Henschke CI, Naidich DP, Yankelevitz DF, et al. Early lung cancer action project: initial findings on repeat screenings. Cancer 2001; 92:153–9.
25. Mountain CF. Revisions in the International System for Staging Lung Cancer. Chest 1997; 111:1710–7.
26. Sone S, Li F, Yang ZG, et al. Results of three-year mass screening programme for lung cancer using mobile low-dose spiral computed tomography scanner. Br J Cancer 2001;84: 25–32.
27. Swensen SJ, Jett JR, Sloan JA, et al. Screening for lung cancer with low-dose spiral computed tomography. Am J Respir Crit Care Med 2002;165:508–13.
28. Winer-Muram HT, Jennings SG, Tarver RD, et al. Volumetric growth rate of stage I lung cancer prior to treatment: serial CT scanning. Radiology 2002;223:798–805.
29. MacMahon H, Austin JH, Gamsu G, et al. Guidelines for management of small pulmonary nodules detected on CT scans: a statement from the Fleischner Society. Radiology 2005;237:395–400.
30. Erasmus JJ, Connolly JE, McAdams HP, Roggli VL. Solitary pulmonary nodules: part I. Morphologic evaluation for differentiation of benign and malignant lesions. Radiographics 2000;20:43–58.
31. Siegelman SS, Khouri NF, Leo FP, et al. Solitary pulmonary nodules: CT assessment. Radiology 1986;160:307–12.
32. Park CM, Goo JM, Lee HJ, et al. Nodular ground-glass opacity at thin-section CT: histologic correlation and evaluation of change at follow-up. Radiographics 2007;27: 391–408.
33. Oda S, Awai K, Liu D, et al. Ground-glass opacities on thin-section helical CT: differentiation between bronchioloalveolar carcinoma and atypical adenomatous hyperplasia. AJR Am J Roentgenol 2008;190:1363–8.
34. Suzuki K, Asamura H, Kusumoto M, et al. "Early" peripheral lung cancer: prognostic significance of ground glass opacity on thin-section computed tomographic scan. Ann Thorac Surg 2002;74:1635–9.
35. Woodring JH, Fried AM. Significance of wall thickness in solitary cavities of the lung: a follow-up study. AJR Am J Roentgenol 1983;140:473–4.
36. Weisbrod GL, Towers MJ, Chamberlain DW, et al. Thin-walled cystic lesions in bronchioalveolar carcinoma. Radiology 1992;185: 401–5.
37. Ledor K, Fish B, Chaise L, Ledor S. CT diagnosis of pulmonary hamartomas. J Comput Tomogr 1981;5:343–4.
38. Mahoney MC, Shipley RT, Corcoran HL, Dickson BA. CT demonstration of calcification in carcinoma of the lung. AJR Am J Roentgenol 1990;154:255–8.
39. Gould MK, Fletcher J, Iannettoni MD, et al. Evaluation of patients with pulmonary nodules: when is it lung cancer?: ACCP evidence-based clinical practice guidelines (2nd edition). Chest 2007;132(3 Suppl): 108S–30S.
40. Swensen SJ, Viggiano RW, Midthun DE, et al. Lung nodule enhancement at CT: multicenter study. Radiology 2000;214: 73–80.
41. Wahl RL, Hutchins GD, Buchsbaum DJ, et al. 18F-2-deoxy-2-fluoro-D-glucose uptake into human tumor xenografts. Feasibility studies for cancer imaging with positron-emission tomography. Cancer 1991;67: 1544–50.
42. Ollenberger GP, Knight S, Tauro AJ. False-positive FDG positron emission tomography in pulmonary amyloidosis. Clin Nucl Med 2004;29:657–8.
43. Alavi A, Gupta N, Alberini JL, et al. Positron emission tomography imaging in nonmalignant thoracic disorders. Semin Nucl Med 2002;32:293–321.
44. El-Haddad G, Zhuang H, Gupta N, Alavi A. Evolving role of positron emission tomography in the management of patients with inflammatory and other benign disorders. Semin Nucl Med 2004;34:313–29.
45. Zhuang H, Yu JQ, Alavi A. Applications of fluorodeoxyglucose-PET imaging in the detection of infection and inflammation and other benign disorders. Radiol Clin North Am 2005;43:121–34.
46. Croft DR, Trapp J, Kernstine K, et al. FDG-PET imaging and the diagnosis of non-small cell lung cancer in a region of high histoplasmosis prevalence. Lung Cancer 2002;36: 297–301.
47. Higashi K, Ueda Y, Seki H, et al. Fluorine-18-FDG PET imaging is negative in bronchioloalveolar lung carcinoma. J Nucl Med 1998;39:1016–20.
48. Yap CS, Schiepers C, Fishbein MC, et al. FDG-PET imaging in lung cancer: how

sensitive is it for bronchioloalveolar carcinoma? Eur J Nucl Med Mol Imaging 2002;29: 1166–73.
49. Heyneman LE, Patz EF. PET imaging in patients with bronchioloalveolar cell carcinoma. Lung Cancer 2002;38:261–6.
50. Erasmus JJ, McAdams HP, Patz EF Jr, et al. Evaluation of primary pulmonary carcinoid tumors using FDG PET. AJR Am J Roentgenol 1998;170:1369–73.
51. Marom EM, Sarvis S, Herndon JE 2nd, Patz EF Jr. T1 lung cancers: sensitivity of diagnosis with fluorodeoxyglucose PET. Radiology 2002;223:453–9.
52. Gould MK, Maclean CC, Kuschner WG, et al. Accuracy of positron emission tomography for diagnosis of pulmonary nodules and mass lesions: a meta-analysis. JAMA 2001; 285:914–24.
53. Vansteenkiste J, Fischer BM, Dooms C, Mortensen J. Positron-emission tomography in prognostic and therapeutic assessment of lung cancer: systematic review. Lancet Oncol 2004;5:531–40.
54. Nomori H, Watanabe K, Ohtsuka T, et al. Evaluation of F-18 fluorodeoxyglucose (FDG) PET scanning for pulmonary nodules less than 3 cm in diameter, with special reference to the CT images. Lung Cancer 2004; 45:19–27.
55. Shim SS, Lee KS, Kim BT, et al. Non-small cell lung cancer: prospective comparison of integrated FDG PET/CT and CT alone for preoperative staging. Radiology 2005;236: 1011–9.
56. Fischer B, Lassen U, Mortensen J, et al. Preoperative staging of lung cancer with combined PET-CT. N Engl J Med 2009;361: 32–9.
57. Gould MK, Sanders GD, Barnett PG, et al. Cost-effectiveness of alternative management strategies for patients with solitary pulmonary nodules. Ann Intern Med 2003;138:724–35.
58. Levine MS, Weiss JM, Harrell JH, et al. Transthoracic needle aspiration biopsy following negative fiberoptic bronchoscopy in solitary pulmonary nodules. Chest 1988;93: 1152–5.
59. Lacasse Y, Wong E, Guyatt GH, Cook DJ. Transthoracic needle aspiration biopsy for the diagnosis of localised pulmonary lesions: a meta-analysis. Thorax 1999;54:884–93.
60. Larscheid RC, Thorpe PE, Scott WJ. Percutaneous transthoracic needle aspiration biopsy: a comprehensive review of its current role in the diagnosis and treatment of lung tumors. Chest 1998;114:704–9.
61. Conces DJ Jr, Schwenk GR Jr, Doering PR, Glant MD. Thoracic needle biopsy. Improved results utilizing a team approach. Chest 1987;91:813–6.
62. Yung RC. Tissue diagnosis of suspected lung cancer: selecting between bronchoscopy, transthoracic needle aspiration, and resectional biopsy. Respir Care Clin N Am 2003;9: 51–76.
63. Geraghty PR, Kee ST, McFarlane G, et al. CT-guided transthoracic needle aspiration biopsy of pulmonary nodules: needle size and pneumothorax rate. Radiology 2003;229: 475–81.
64. Wallace JM, Deutsch AL. Flexible fiberoptic bronchoscopy and percutaneous needle lung aspiration for evaluating the solitary pulmonary nodule. Chest 1982;81:665–71.
65. Cortese DA, McDougall JC. Bronchoscopic biopsy and brushing with fluoroscopic guidance in nodular metastatic lung cancer. Chest 1981;79:610–1.
66. Swensen SJ, Jett JR, Payne WS, et al. An integrated approach to evaluation of the solitary pulmonary nodule. Mayo Clin Proc 1990;65:173–86.
67. Yasufuku K, Nakajima T, Motoori K, et al. Comparison of endobronchial ultrasound, positron emission tomography, and CT for lymph node staging of lung cancer. Chest 2006;130:710–8.
68. Eberhardt R, Anantham D, Herth F, et al. Electromagnetic navigation diagnostic bronchoscopy in peripheral lung lesions. Chest 2007;131:1800–5.
69. Davies AL. The current role of video-assisted thoracic surgery (VATS) in the overall practice of thoracic surgery. A review of 207 cases. Int Surg 1997;82:229–31.
70. Asamura H. Thoracoscopic procedures for intrathoracic diseases: the present status. Respirology 1999;4:9–17.
71. Flores RM, Park BJ, Dycoco J, et al. Lobectomy by video-assisted thoracic surgery (VATS) versus thoracotomy for lung cancer. J Thorac Cardiovasc Surg 2009;138:11–8.
72. Allen MS, Deschamps C, Jones DM, et al. Video-assisted thoracic surgical procedures: the Mayo experience. Mayo Clin Proc 1996; 71:351–9.
73. Hazelrigg SR, Magee MJ, Cetindag IB. Video-assisted thoracic surgery for diagnosis of the solitary lung nodule. Chest Surg Clin N Am 1998;8:763–74, vii.
74. McKenna RJ Jr, Houck W, Fuller CB. Video-assisted thoracic surgery lobectomy: experience with 1,100 cases. Ann Thorac Surg 2006;81:421–5; discussion 425–6.
75. Stiles BM, Altes TA, Jones DR, et al. Clinical experience with radiotracer-guided thoracoscopic biopsy of small, indeterminate lung nodules. Ann Thorac Surg 2006;82:1191–6; discussion 1196–7.
76. Grogan EL, Stukenborg GJ, Nagji AS, et al. Radiotracer-guided thoracoscopic resection is a cost-effective technique for the evaluation of subcentimeter pulmonary nodules. Ann Thorac Surg 2008;86:934–40; discussion 934–40.
77. Pechet TT, Carr SR, Collins JE, et al. Arterial invasion predicts early mortality in stage I non-small cell lung cancer. Ann Thorac Surg 2004;78:1748–53.
78. Chute CG, Greenberg ER, Baron J, et al. Presenting conditions of 1539 population-based lung cancer patients by cell type and stage in New Hampshire and Vermont. Cancer 1985;56:2107–11.
79. Harpole DH Jr, Feldman JM, Buchanan S, et al. Bronchial carcinoid tumors: a retrospective analysis of 126 patients. Ann Thorac Surg 1992;54:50–4; discussion 54–5.
80. McMullan DM, Wood DE. Pulmonary carcinoid tumors. Semin Thorac Cardiovasc Surg 2003;15:289–300.
81. DeCaro LF, Paladugu R, Benfield JR, et al. Typical and atypical carcinoids within the pulmonary APUD tumor spectrum. J Thorac Cardiovasc Surg 1983;86:528–36.
82. Greelish JP, Friedberg JS. Secondary pulmonary malignancy. Surg Clin North Am 2000;80:633–57.
83. Watanabe K, Nagai K, Kobayashi A, et al. Factors influencing survival after complete resection of pulmonary metastases from colorectal cancer. Br J Surg 2009;96: 1058–65.
84. Onaitis MW, Petersen RP, Haney JC, et al. Prognostic factors for recurrence after pulmonary resection of colorectal cancer metastases. Ann Thorac Surg 2009;87: 1684–8.
85. De Cicco C, Bellomi M, Bartolomei M, et al. Imaging of lung hamartomas by multidetector computed tomography and positron emission tomography. Ann Thorac Surg 2008; 86:1769–72.
86. Gotway MB, Tchao NK, Leung JW, et al. Sarcoidosis presenting as an enlarging solitary pulmonary nodule. J Thorac Imaging 2001; 16:117–22.
87. Iannuzzi MC, Rybicki BA, Teirstein AS. Sarcoidosis. N Engl J Med 2007;357: 2153–65.
88. Voulgari PV, Tsifetaki N, Metafratzi ZM, et al. A single pulmonary rheumatoid nodule masquerading as malignancy. Clin Rheumatol 2005;24:556–9.
89. Elrifai AM, Bailes JE, Shih SR, et al. Rewarming, ultraprofound hypothermia and cardiopulmonary bypass. J Extra Corpor Technol 1993;24:107–12.
90. Suen HC, Mathisen DJ, Grillo HC, et al. Surgical management and radiological characteristics of bronchogenic cysts. Ann Thorac Surg 1993;55:476–81.
91. Echeverri A, Long RF, Check W, Burnett CM. Pulmonary dirofilariasis. Ann Thorac Surg 1999;67:201–2.
92. Asimacopoulos PJ, Katras A, Christie B. Pulmonary dirofilariasis. The largest single-hospital experience. Chest 1992;102:851–5.
93. Morar R, Feldman C. Pulmonary echinococcosis. Eur Respir J 2003;21:1069–77.
94. Gottstein B, Reichen J. Hydatid lung disease (echinococcosis/hydatidosis). Clin Chest Med 2002;23:397–408, ix.
95. Cummings SR, Lillington GA, Richard RJ. Estimating the probability of malignancy in solitary pulmonary nodules. A Bayesian approach. Am Rev Respir Dis 1986;134: 449–52.
96. Henschke CI, Yankelevitz D, Westcott J, et al. Work-up of the solitary pulmonary nodule. American College of Radiology. ACR appropriateness criteria. Radiology 2000;215 Suppl:607–9.

6 PARALYZED DIAPHRAGM

*Matthew O. Hubbard, MD, Raymond P. Onders, MD, FACS, and Philip A. Linden, MD, FACS**

Diaphragmatic dysfunction may be unilateral or bilateral, with symptoms ranging from dyspnea only on extreme exertion to ventilator dependence. The etiology, treatment, and prognosis are quite different in unilateral and bilateral paralysis. A paralyzed hemidiaphragm may occur in isolation or as part of a systemic disease, whereas bilateral diaphragmatic paralysis usually occurs as result of a traumatic or neuromuscular degenerative process. The symptoms related to a paralyzed diaphragm are explained by both the loss of muscular action of the diaphragm in respiration and the loss of anatomic domain between the thorax and abdomen.

Unilateral dysfunction usually results from transection, bruising, stretching, or manipulation of one of the phrenic nerves. A paralyzed hemidiaphragm may restrict a patient's vital capacity by almost 20% in a seated position and up to 40% in a supine position. Compression of the lower lobe of the lung may result in ventilation-perfusion mismatch. A small but significant reduction in the arterial oxygenation may be seen, although hypercarbia is usually not present.[1] These alterations are usually well tolerated in a young, healthy patient, with the sole symptom being dyspnea on exertion. A patient at the extremes of life (early childhood or late adulthood) or suffering from underlying lung diseases, obesity, or other systemic disorders may be more adversely affected by unilateral diaphragmatic paralysis.

Bilateral dysfunction may be attributable to central nervous system disorders (central hypoventilation resulting in diminished central triggering of the diaphragms), diffuse nerve dysfunction (disorders such as amyotrophic lateral sclerosis [ALS]), or spinal cord injury (SCI) above C5. Bilateral paralysis causes more severe respiratory symptoms than unilateral paralysis. Vital capacity can be reduced 45 to 50% from predicted in patients with bilateral paralysis.[2] Arterial hypoxemia can be seen as a result of ventilation-perfusion mismatches at the lung bases, and hypercarbia may result from a decrease in tidal volume and minute ventilation. Assisted ventilation (either noninvasive or invasive) is usually required.

Clinical Evaluation

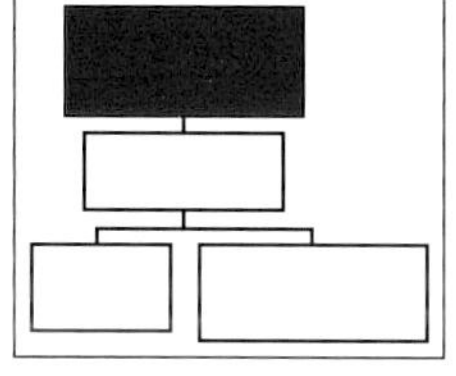

HISTORY

In adults with a paralyzed hemidiaphragm, the most common complaint is typically dyspnea on exertion. Often there are no symptoms at rest.

Bilateral diaphragmatic paralysis results in more severe symptoms than unilateral paralysis, resulting in profound respiratory compromise. Patients depend on accessory muscles of inspiration more, may experience dyspnea in the supine position and related sleep disturbances with daytime fatigue, and may suffer from chronic respiratory failure.

Infants and young children depend on the diaphragm to achieve adequate vital capacities because they have a more compliant chest wall, weaker accessory muscles of respiration, and a more mobile mediastinum than adults. Unilateral paralysis may cause severe respiratory compromise requiring mechanical ventilation; bilateral diaphragmatic paralysis almost always requires prompt ventilator support.

COMMON CAUSES OF DIAPHRAGMATIC PARALYSIS

The most common causes of diaphragmatic paralysis are listed in Table 1. The most common causes of unilateral paralysis are neoplastic invasion, idiopathic, and iatrogenic.

Malignancies account for roughly one third of cases of diaphragm paralysis. Neoplasms of bronchogenic origin are most common, although malignancies of the mediastinum, including thymomas, lymphomas, and germ cell tumors, can also result in interruption of the phrenic nerve input to the diaphragm. The phrenic nerve can be damaged by either direct mediastinal invasion of a tumor or metastasis of a tumor to the mediastinal lymph nodes with subsequent lymph node enlargement. Overall, only about 10% of patients with unexplained diaphragmatic paralysis will regain function of the diaphragm.[3]

Phrenic nerve damage can occur during thoracic and cervical surgery as well as during cervical vein catheter insertion and has even been described as a result of cervical chiropractic manipulation. Injury to the phrenic nerve during cardiac surgery has fallen dramatically with the transition from topical ice slushes to cooling jackets but still may occur as a result of stretching, compression, or sectioning. The use of cautery during high dissection of the internal mammary artery near the first rib may also injure the nerve. Patients with an elevated hemidiaphragm on chest radiographs at the time of discharge after cardiac surgery have a 20% chance at 1 year

Table 1 **General Causes of Unilateral and Bilateral Diaphragmatic Paralysis**
Neoplasm invasion
Phrenic nerve injury: surgical section or stretching, cooling, chiropractic cervical manipulation, cervical venipuncture, birth trauma, cervical disk surgery, blunt or penetrating chest trauma
Neuritis: brachial neuritis, herpes zoster infection, mononeuritis multiplex, paraneoplastic neuritis
CNS or spinal cord disorders: neuralgic amyotrophy, stroke, multiple sclerosis, rhizotomy, infantile spinomuscular atrophy, Arnold-Chiari malformation, syringomelia
Nerve compression: cervical spondylosis, mediastinal lymph node enlargement, substernal goiter
Miscellaneous: diabetes mellitus, carbon monoxide poisoning, upper abdominal surgery, liver transplantation

CNS = central nervous system.

* The authors and editors gratefully acknowledge the contributions of the previous authors, Bryan F. Mayers, MD, FACS, and Benjamin D. Kozower, MD, to the development and writing of this chapter.

Evaluation of Elevated Hemidiaphragm

Patient presents with elevated hemidiaphragm on chest x-ray

Obtain clinical history:
- Previous operations (iatrogenic phrenic nerve injury)
- Malignancy involving phrenic nerve
- Respiratory symptoms (exertional dyspnea, cough, difficulty in sleeping)
- GI symptoms (dysphagia, dyspepsia)
- Cardiac symptoms (dysrhythmia)

Perform physical examination:
- Auscultation for decreased breath sounds
- Percussion to assess diaphragmatic excursion

Order investigative studies:
- Inspiratory and expiratory chest x-ray (to confirm elevated hemidiaphragm)
- Fluoroscopy and sniff test (to distinguish diaphragmatic paralysis from weakness)
- Cervical phrenic nerve stimulation (to clarify diagnosis in patients on mechanical ventilation when sniff test is inconclusive—rarely necessary)

Patient is asymptomatic or has only mild symptoms

Treat conservatively:
- Physical therapy
- Pulmonary rehabilitation
- Weight loss
- Consider enrollment in trial of unilateral diaphragmatic pacing

Patient has significant symptoms (e.g., dyspnea, recurrent pneumonia, chronic bronchitis, chest pain, poor exercise tolerance, cardiac dysrhythmia, or functional gastric disorder)

Order further tests as required:
- Pulmonary (pulmonary function tests)
- Cardiac (ECG, echocardiography)
- GI (gastric motility study)

Treat surgically with diaphragmatic plication (open or thoracoscopic).

of continued diaphragmatic dysfunction. Injury can occur during dissection of mediastinal vessels during lobectomy. Typically, this is more common on the right than the left (the phrenic nerve courses closer to the hilum on the right than on the left) and may be more commonly injured after upper lobectomies than lower (the nerve courses closer to the superior pulmonary vein than the inferior vein). The phrenic nerve is at risk during a supraclavicular (or scalene) lymph node biopsy as it courses directly anterior to the anterior scalene muscle. The phrenic nerve is also at risk during thymectomy as perithymic tissue often extends bilaterally near both phrenic nerves. If one nerve is invaded by a thymoma, it should be resected en bloc with the thymoma provided that the other nerve is healthy and can be spared. Cautery should generally be avoided within 1 cm of the phrenic nerve. Typically, morbidity surrounding injuries to the phrenic nerves is minimal. Exceptions to this, however, are in pediatric patients undergoing open heart surgery, patients post–lung transplantation, and those adult patients with preexisting respiratory compromise. This may result in a failure to wean from mechanical ventilation after surgery.

PHYSICAL EXAMINATION

At rest, adult patients with a paralyzed diaphragm may appear asymptomatic or have the nonspecific complaints discussed above. On physical examination, diminished breath sounds are heard on the affected base, with decreased excursion of the diaphragm noted on percussion. Paradoxical inward motion of the ipsilateral abdominal wall may also be seen.[4]

A patient with bilateral diaphragmatic paralysis is much more likely to become symptomatic, complaining of the symptoms above, and is also subject to the neurologic or neuromuscular complaints related to the underlying etiology. Physical examination almost always reveals significant use of accessory inspiratory muscle use. Tachycardia and tachypnea are usually present. Characteristically, paradoxical inward movement of the abdominal wall is seen with inspiration.[4]

Investigative Studies

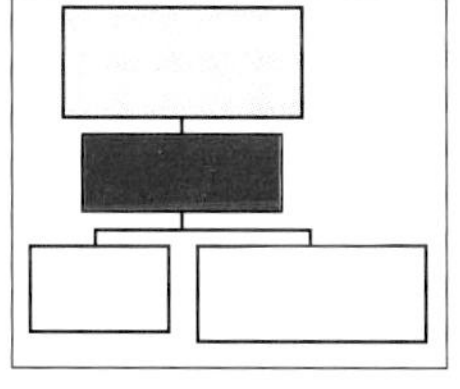

Diaphragmatic paralysis is usually discovered following an inspiratory chest radiograph, which may demonstrate an elevated diaphragmatic dome with sharpened and deepened costovertebral and costophrenic sulci [*see Figure 1*]. With left-sided paralysis, the stomach may rotate with the greater curvature facing cephalad and showing two fluid levels corresponding to the inverted fundus and body.[4]

Fluoroscopy or ultrasonography can be used for functional evaluation of the diaphragm in patients with suspected paralysis. Elevation of the diaphragm above the normal range, paradoxical movement with inspiration (especially while sniffing, the "sniff test"), and a mediastinal swing during respiration may all be seen. All of these findings may also be seen in other respiratory ailments and require a good deal of judgment to evaluate. The "sniff test," rapidly inhaling with a closed mouth, should show a paradoxical upward motion of the diaphragm of at least 2 cm to be considered a positive test for paralysis. This test may be unobtainable in patients with severe weakness or on mechanical ventilation.[5]

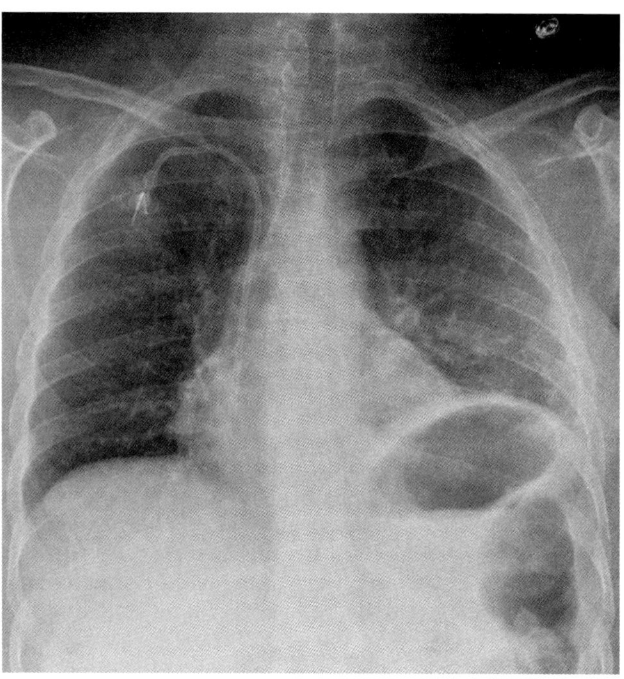

Figure 1 **Chest radiograph showing left diaphragmatic paralysis in a breast cancer patient with malignant adenopathy involving the left phrenic nerve near the left main pulmonary artery.**

Ultrasound evaluation can also be used to evaluate suspected diaphragmatic paralysis and may be slightly more sensitive than fluoroscopy.[6] Using ultrasonography, a paralyzed diaphragm fails to increase in thickness during inspiration compared with a normally functioning diaphragm. This was seen in single patients comparing paralytic hemidiaphragms with the contralateral leaflets and also comparing experimental and control patients. Rarely, equivocal noninvasive testing may be augmented with phrenic nerve stimulation with electromyographic measurement of nerve latency; this may be helpful with patients being supported by mechanical ventilation.[7]

Management

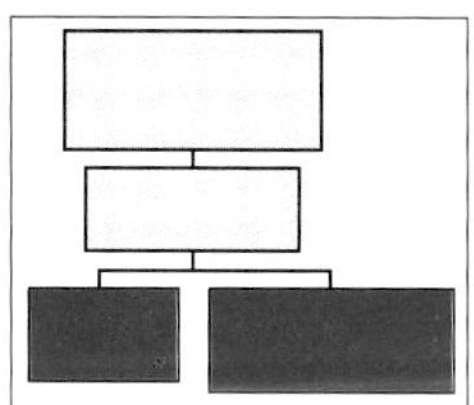

CONSERVATIVE VERSUS SURGICAL TREATMENT

Surgical treatment of diaphragmatic paralysis should be reserved for patients with moderate to severe symptoms of respiratory compromise. Adult patients with mild symptoms, such as dyspnea on exertion, would benefit from conservative treatment focusing on physical therapy, pulmonary rehabilitation, and weight loss.

The standard treatment of diaphragmatic paralysis is plication of the affected diaphragm, first performed by Bisgard in 1947 to treat congenital eventration of the diaphragm in an infant with respiratory distress. Several descriptions of plication of the diaphragm exist in the literature for diaphragmatic paralysis and eventration, varying in suture placement and surgical approach. Developments in phrenic nerve repair and diaphragm pacing (DP) have emerged in recent years.

PLICATION OF THE DIAPHRAGM

A posterolateral incision at the seventh or eighth intercostal space provides access to the thoracic cavity for a plication procedure. Four to six parallel rows of nonabsorbable suture with pledgets should be placed in an anteroposterior orientation within the central tendon of the diaphragm. Ideally, these sutures should not strike the phrenic vessels and nerve branches. The phrenic vessels often course under the diaphragm and are not visible from above [*see Figure 2*].

Thoracoscopic approaches to diaphragmatic plication have been described. One study of 25 patients undergoing video-assisted thoracoscopic diaphragm plication showed that forced vital capacity (FVC), forced expiratory volume at 1 second (FEV_1), functional residual capacity (FRC), and total lung capacity (TLC) improved by 17%, 21.4%, 20.3%, and 16.1%, respectively, at 6 months.[8] Symptomatic dyspnea also improved, and 17 patients were able to return to work.

Radial plication of the muscular portion of the diaphragm, avoiding the mediastinal pleura, has been described through a transabdominal and transthoracic approach.[9] This procedure allows for protection of the phrenic nerve branches and vessels. This has also been described through a thoracoscopic approach in children and adults: a three-port technique using anterior and posterior thoracic ports at the sixth and eighth interspaces, respectively, for plication, and a subcostal port used for grasping and displacing the central tendon of the diaphragm through the abdomen.[10]

A study of plication in 17 patients (16 men, one woman), with an average age of 54 years, showed subjective improvement in dyspnea score, as well as objective improvement in FVC, TLC, and FRC, as well as arterial oxygenation, at 6 months.[11] These results were maintained in the six patients who were followed for more than 5 years. A different study of 15 patients with a mean follow-up of 10 years after plication showed continued improvement in FVC, FEV_1, FRC, and TLC by 11.8%, 15.4%, 26%, and 13.3%, respectively.[12]

Infants and children who suffer from diaphragmatic paralysis are much more susceptible to respiratory compromise. These children are much more likely to require mechanical ventilation and to be exposed to the complications therein. Diaphragmatic plication has been shown to be an effective means to wean children from mechanical ventilation.[13]

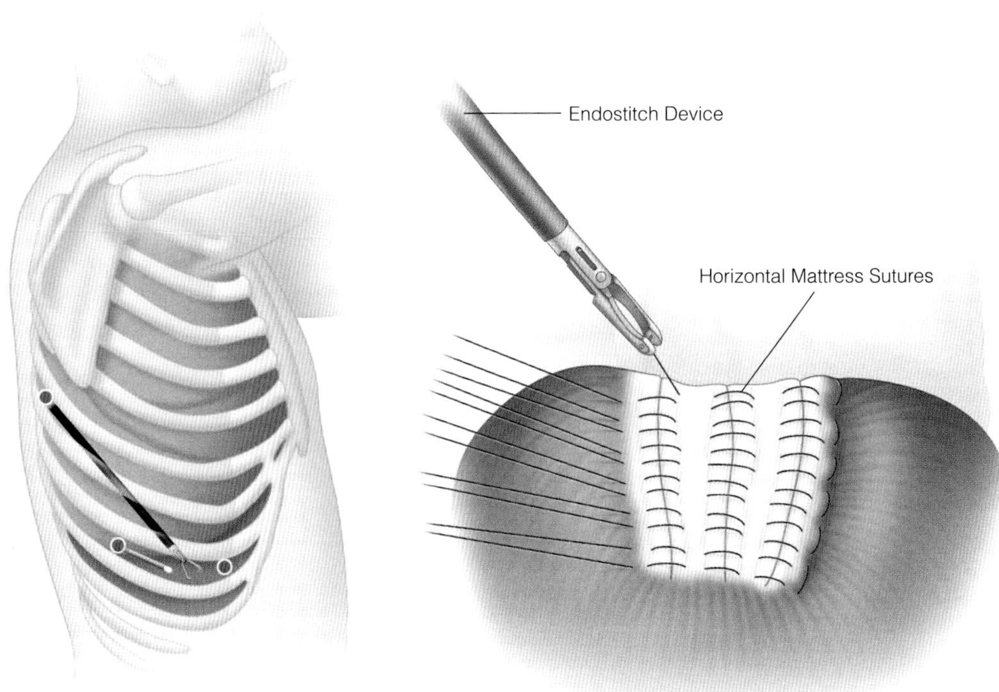

Figure 2 **Several parallel rows of sutures are placed in the muscular portion and central tendon of the diaphragm and tied with the aid of a knot pusher. A pledget should be placed at the ends of the suture if the diaphragm is thinned.**

REPAIR OF PHRENIC NERVE INJURY

Some cases of diaphragmatic paralysis result from traumatic or iatrogenic severing of the phrenic nerve. Case reports of direct repair of the phrenic nerve using microsurgery techniques have been described in adults and children by end-to-end anastomosis and sural nerve graft techniques; an improvement in diaphragmatic function occurred as early as 6 months after surgery.[14] Repair of the phrenic nerve can be performed for simple transection, whereas sural nerve grafting is used for replacement of phrenic nerve segments that were resected en bloc with tumor. There are no reports of nerve repair in large numbers of patients.

DIAPHRAGMATIC PACING

Indications for Diaphragm Pacing

Direct phrenic nerve pacing and intramuscular DP systems were designed to replace or delay the need for patients requiring long-term positive pressure mechanical ventilation via tracheostomies. In the 1980s, Mortimer and colleagues showed that the diaphragm could be directly stimulated at the motor point (area of phrenic nerve insertion) of the diaphragm to provide ventilation.[15]

The initial clinical indications for phrenic nerve or DP have been cervical SCIs and congenital central hypoventilation syndromes. SCI involves the disruption of the signal pathway from the respiratory center in the brain to the respiratory nerves (primarily the phrenic nerves), whereas central hypoventilation syndromes generally involve a decreased respiratory drive. Central hypoventilation is a rare diagnosis, affecting one in 50,000 live births; these children require permanent nighttime positive pressure ventilation unless phrenic nerve pacing is possible.

Of 11,000 new SCIs each year in the United States, slightly more than half are affected by quadriplegia, with only 4% requiring long-term mechanical ventilation. In a prospective worldwide trial of DP in this group, 50 patients were implanted.[16] The average age was 36 years (range 18 to 74 years), and the time from injury to implantation was 5.6 years (range 0.3 to 27 years). Ninety-eight percent of the patients had DP-stimulated tidal volumes above 5 to 7 cc/kg for 4 or more continuous hours, with 50% using DP for continuous 24-hour ventilation. Age and time from injury directly affect the conditioning time needed to achieve independent ventilation, with younger and more recently injured patients weaning from the ventilator faster.[17] In a long-term analysis of 24 patients, 60% reported fewer secretions, and 95% reported greater freedom and independence. This multicenter trial led to approval by the Food and Drug Administration in June 2008.

DP is used in patients with ALS (Lou Gehrig disease), where respiratory insufficiency is the major cause of mortality. There is a significant risk of impending respiratory failure and death when FVC falls below 25 to 30%.[18] In this group of patients, the goal is to delay the need for mechanical ventilation by implanting the DP and stimulating the muscle to maintain diaphragm strength prior to end-stage weakness.

The results of a multicenter prospective trial comparing noninvasive ventilation with DP combined with noninvasive ventilation in 145 subjects with ALS showed a decreased respiratory decline and improved survival with pacing.[19] After conditioning the diaphragm with the DP, the rate of decline in FVC fell from 2.62% per month to 1.25% per month. Respiratory compliance increased 18% from improving posterior lobe ventilation.

The use of DP for the treatment of ventilator dependence following iatrogenic diaphragmatic paralysis is currently under sporadic investigation

Surgical Technique of Laparoscopic Diaphragm Pacing

For DP to be effective, the phrenic nerve must be intact and able to provide intramuscular conduction pathways. Unfortunately, many patients with tetraplegia have sustained injury to the phrenic motor neurons in the spinal cord and/or phrenic rootlets. Prior to implantation, an assessment of phrenic nerve function should be performed. In patients with ALS or central hypoventilation, fluoroscopy of the diaphragm can also be done to see that volitional diaphragm movement is intact, commonly referred to as a sniff test.

Paralytic agents cannot be used during the pacer insertion procedure as the diaphragm has to be stimulated during the operation. The surgery is described in four phases: exposure, mapping, implantation, and routing. The exposure consists of the setup for the standard laparoscopy with the initial port supraumbilical for adequate visualization of the diaphragm. Two lateral subcostal 5 mm ports are placed for the mapping probe for each side, and these are used initially to completely divide the falciform ligament, which allows easier visualization of the medial aspect of the right diaphragm and easier exit of the pacing electrodes through a 12 mm epigastric port. The epigastric port is used for the diaphragm implant instrument.

Mapping involves finding the point on the abdominal side of the diaphragm where stimulation causes the greatest diaphragm excursion. The mapping instrument has flexible tubing inside a rigid cannula that connects to the operating room suction. The working part of the mapping instrument has a circular electrode that can be stimulated when temporarily attached to the diaphragm by the suction [*see Figure 3*]. Stimulation is applied in either a twitch or burst mode from the clinical station through a connecting cable. Mapping allows qualitative and quantitative data to be obtained. Quantitatively, changes in abdominal pressures are measured. Qualitatively, observation of the diaphragm contraction is performed. The stronger the stimulated contraction, the closer the mapping probe is to the motor point of the diaphragm. The primary electrode site is identified at the location of maximal pressure change in each hemidiaphragm. A secondary electrode site is identified as either a backup to the primary site or at a location in each hemidiaphragm that recruits another region (e.g., anterior, lateral, or posterior) of the diaphragm at a similar magnitude. On the right diaphragm, the motor point is just lateral to the central tendon, and on the left diaphragm, the motor point tends to be much more lateral because the phrenic nerve travels on the lateral aspect of the pericardium and enters the diaphragm more laterally.

Once the primary and secondary electrode sites are identified in each hemidiaphragm, the implantation phase begins.

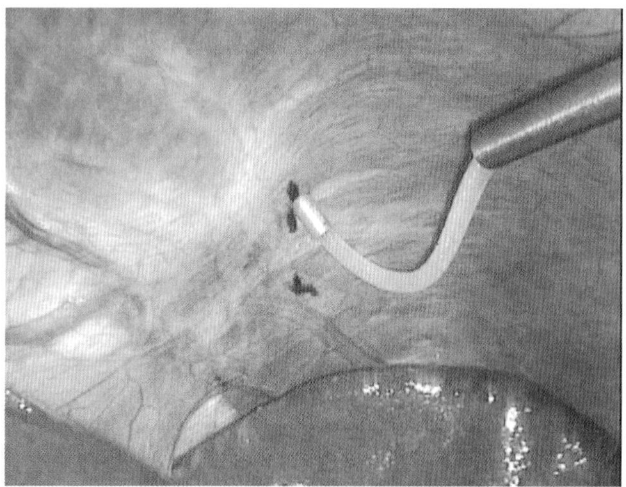

Figure 3 **A laparoscopic mapping probe is being held onto the left diaphragm with suction and receives electrical stimuli from an external clinical station. The blue marks were placed at the locations of the strongest contractions.**

An intramuscular electrode is introduced into the abdominal cavity with the electrode delivery instrument. The implant instrument needle is inserted into the diaphragm at an angle so that the electrode lead travels parallel to the plane of the diaphragm prior to exit, and the delivery instrument is withdrawn [*see Figure 4*]. The electrode is then tested to ensure that the desired response to twitch stimuli is achieved, and if the response is not adequate, the electrode may be withdrawn and another implanted. Once all four electrodes are implanted, they are brought out through the epigastric port, keeping the right and left sides separated. Excess electrode length is kept in the abdomen on top of the liver. The electrodes will be tunneled subcutaneously to an area in the upper chest or abdomen at a site deemed appropriate by the surgeon and patient's caregivers. An additional indifferent electrode will be placed subcutaneously through a separate percutaneous exit site.

Electrode evaluation is performed by adjusting individual stimulus parameters (amplitude, pulse width, rate, and frequency) so that a comfortable level of stimulation can be identified for the diaphragm conditioning sessions. The DP system will be set to provide a tidal volume that provides 15% above the basal needs (5 to 7 cc/kg) and that the patient can easily tolerate. For SCI patients and for ALS patients, the highest setting that causes no discomfort will be used.

ALS patients begin conditioning by pacing five 30-minute sessions a day. Continuous positive airway pressure (CPAP) or noninvasive ventilation may still be needed to maintain an upper airway and can be used in conjunction with the DP system. A weaning program for SCI patients is begun where the DP unit is turned on and the ventilator is turned off. The patients are placed back on the ventilator when they feel uncomfortable or if their tidal volumes start dropping because of diaphragm fatigue. Initially, patients may tolerate only 15 minutes of DP. If the DP system is implanted early after an SCI, the patient can be rapidly transitioned from the mechanical ventilator to DP. Figure 5 shows the system attached to a pediatric patient for whom weaning will be started the day of surgery. The diaphragm can recover quite rapidly from training, so patients and their caregivers can repeat a session every hour. The length of time it takes to go more than 4 continuous hours depends on the amount of time the patient and caregivers devote to this process.

The future application for temporary use in the intensive care unit (ICU) has some excellent theoretical possibilities, but well-designed trials will need to be done to identify the actual role of DP in the ICU.

Dr. Raymond P. Onders has received research grants from Synapse Biomedical Inc, Oberlin, OH.

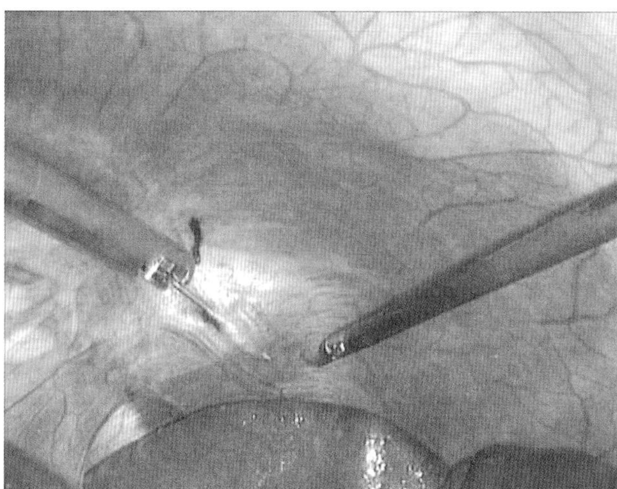

Figure 4 **The electrode implant device houses the electrode in the needle and is placed into the diaphragm tangentially. Countertraction can be applied by a second instrument to help deploy the electrode, which has a small barb on the end of it.**

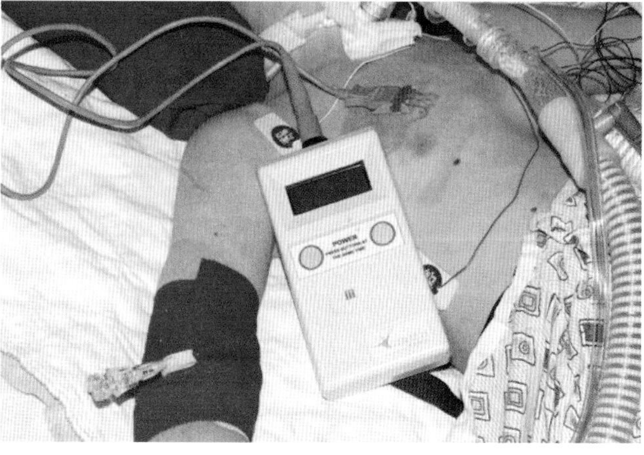

Figure 5 **The diaphragm pacing system has already been programmed for conditioning and is attached via percutaneously placed diaphragm electrodes in this spinal cord–injured child for early conditioning and weaning from the ventilator.**

References

1. Clague HW, Hall DR. Effect of posture on lung volume: airway closure and gas exchange in hemidiaphragmatic paralysis. Thorax 1970;34:523–6.
2. Molho M, Katz I, Schwartz E, et al. Familial bilateral paralysis of the diaphragm. Chest 1987;91:466–7.
3. Piehler JM, Pairolero PC, Gracey DR, et al. Unexplained diaphragmatic paralysis: a harbinger of malignant disease? J Thorac Cardiovasc Surg 1982;84:861–4.
4. Fraser RS, Muller NL, Colman N, Pare PD, editors. The diaphragm. In: Diagnosis of diseases of the chest. 4th ed. Philadelphia: W.B. Saunders Company; 1999. p. 2987–3010.
5. Alexander C. Diaphragm movements and the diagnosis of diaphragmatic paralysis. Clin Radiol 1966;17:79–83.
6. Houston JG, Fleet M, Cowan MD, et al. Comparison of ultrasound with fluoroscopy in the assessment of suspected hemidiaphragmatic movement abnormality. Clin Radiol 1995;50:95–8.
7. Wilcox P, Baile EM, Hards J, et al. Phrenic nerve function and its relationship to atelectasis after coronary artery bypass surgery. Chest 1988;93:693–8.
8. Freeman RK, Wozniak TC, Fitzgerald EB. Functional and physiological results of video-assisted thoracoscopic diaphragm plication in adult patients with unilateral diaphragm paralysis. Ann Thorac Surg 2006;81:1853–7.
9. Shoemaker R, Palmer G, Brown JW, et al. Aggressive treatment of acquired phrenic nerve paralysis in infants and small children. Ann Thorac Surg 1981;32:250–9.
10. Wiener DC, Jaklitsch MT. Surgery of the diaphragm: a deductive approach. In: Selke FW, del Nido PJ, Swanson SJ, editors. Sabiston & Spencer surgery of the chest. 7th ed. Philadelphia: Elsevier Saunders; 2005. p. 501–15.
11. Graham DR, Kaplan D, Evans CC, et al. Diaphragmatic plication for unilateral diaphragmatic paralysis: a 10-year experience. Ann Thorac Surg 1990;49:248–51.
12. Higgs SM, Hussain A, Jackson M, et al. Long term results of diaphragmatic plication for unilateral diaphragm paralysis. Eur J Cardiothorac Surg 2002;21:294–7.
13. Simansky DA, Paley M, Refaely Y, et al. Diaphragm plication following phrenic nerve injury: a comparison of paediatric and adult patients. Thorax 2002;57:613–6.
14. Merav AD, Attai LA, Condit DD. Successful repair of a transected phrenic nerve with restoration of diaphragmatic function. Chest 1983;84:642–4.
15. Peterson DK, Nochomovitz ML, DiMarco AF, Mortimer JT. Intramuscular electrical activation of the phrenic nerve. IEEE Trans Biomed Eng 1986;33:342–51.
16. Onders RP, Elmo M, Khansarinia S, et al. Complete worldwide operative experience in laparoscopic diaphragm pacing: results and differences in spinal cord injured patients and amyotrophic lateral sclerosis patients. Surg Endosc 2009;23:1433–40. [Epub 2008 Dec 6].
17. Onders RP, Elmo MJ, Ignagni AR. Diaphragm pacing stimulation system for tetraplegia in individuals injured during childhood or adolescence. J Spinal Cord Med 2007;30:25–9.
18. Benditt JO. Respiratory complications of amyotrophic lateral sclerosis. Semin Respir Crit Care Med 2002;23:239–47.
19. Onders R, Katirji B, So Y, et al. Multicenter study results of motor point stimulation for condidtioning the diaphragm of patients with amyotrophic lateral sclerosis/motor neuron disease: preliminary trend toward slowed respiratory decline and improved survival. Amyotroph Lateral Scler 2009;10:60–1.

7 OPEN ESOPHAGEAL PROCEDURES

Cameron D. Wright, MD, FACS

The remarkable developments in diagnosis, imaging, and surgical treatment of esophageal diseases over the past 15 years have resulted in markedly better patient outcomes, and the morbidity and mortality associated with surgery of the esophagus have been substantially reduced. In particular, the operative techniques employed to treat esophageal disease have advanced considerably as a result of the successful introduction of minimally invasive approaches to the esophagus. For a number of diseases (e.g., achalasia and routine antireflux surgery), minimally invasive procedures have proved to be as effective as their open counterparts while causing less postoperative morbidity. The growing stature of minimally invasive approaches does not, however, diminish the importance of the equivalent open approaches. In this chapter, we describe common open operations performed to excise Zenker diverticulum, to manage complex gastroesophageal reflux disease (GERD), and to resect esophageal and proximal gastric tumors.

General Preoperative Considerations

METHODS OF PATIENT ASSESSMENT

The functional results achieved with esophageal procedures become more predictable when the approach to preoperative patient evaluation is precise and reproducible. The ciné barium swallow remains the most cost-effective method for initial evaluation of esophageal anatomy and function. It should be employed before endoscopy because the results may direct the endoscopist's attention to particular areas of concern. In addition, endoscopic examination alone is often insufficient for assessing esophageal motility disorders or defining the complex anatomy of a paraesophageal hiatal hernia.

Endoscopic ultrasonography (EUS) is an extension of the visual mucosal examination. The information it can provide about the extension of mass lesions beyond the confines of the esophageal wall is helpful in planning surgical resection. In addition, EUS can differentiate benign stromal tumors from cystic or malignant neoplasms on the basis of characteristic echogenicity patterns. EUS-FNA (fine-needle aspiration) is used to confirm suspected nodal metastases seen during the EUS examination. The combination of EUS and computed tomography (CT) permits highly precise anatomic assessment of esophageal neoplasms, definition of the extent of local invasion, and identification of regional metastases.

Functional imaging with photodynamic or vital staining allows accurate diagnosis of dysplastic or malignant mucosal lesions in their earliest stages. Positron emission tomography (PET) yields similar results by localizing metabolically active tissue regionally or at distant sites. The combination of morphologic data from high-resolution CT and functional data from PET is particularly effective for identifying occult metastases that would preclude curative resection for esophageal cancer.

Esophageal manometry, 24-hour esophageal pH testing, and nuclear studies for assessment of esophageal and gastric transit provide functional data that can facilitate the diagnosis and treatment of GERD, achalasia, and other disorders of the esophagus. They are useful complements to standard investigations (e.g., ciné barium swallow and endoscopy).

Complete preoperative investigation of all patients, even those with classic histories and physical findings, is mandatory. The data from anatomic and functional testing allow the surgeon to plan the operation more appropriately and effectively (e.g., deciding on the need for esophageal lengthening in patients with paraesophageal hernias or choosing between a complete and a partial fundoplication in patients with hernias associated with varying degrees of esophageal dysmotility).

OPTIMIZATION OF PATIENT HEALTH STATUS

Patients with obstructing esophageal diseases are often elderly, debilitated, and malnourished. Although months of insufficient nutrition cannot be corrected in the space of a few hours, anemia, dehydration, and electrolyte abnormalities can be mitigated by means of intravenous support and appropriate laboratory monitoring. If esophageal obstruction prevents oral intake, endoscopic dilation of the stricture, accompanied by either nasogastric intubation or percutaneous endoscopic gastrostomy (PEG), is often indicated; the patient should then be able to resume at least a liquid diet. Caution should be used when addressing esophageal obstruction in preoperative patients before induction therapy is given. Most surgeons prefer not to have a PEG tube placed in the stomach for fear of compromising its blood supply when an esophagectomy is planned. Alternative options include a nasogastric tube, a jejunostomy tube, or total parenteral nutrition. If weight loss has exceeded 10%, enteral nutrition, comprising at least 2,000 kcal/day of a high-protein liquid diet, should be administered for at least 10 days before the operation. Cardiovascular, renal, hepatic, and respiratory function should be documented and optimized. If the patient is aspirating, the esophagus should be evacuated and the patient should be given nothing by mouth until after the operation. Aspiration pneumonia should always be corrected preoperatively.

Cricopharyngeal Myotomy and Excision of Zenker Diverticulum

PREOPERATIVE EVALUATION

Patients who are candidates for cricopharyngeal myotomy usually present with difficulty initiating swallowing, cervical dysphagia, and a history of pulmonary aspiration. These symptoms of cricopharyngeal dysfunction may or may not be associated with a Zenker diverticulum. Ciné contrast studies may reveal poor pharyngeal contractility, pulmonary or nasal aspiration, abnormalities of the upper esophageal sphincter, pharyngeal pouches, or other structural abnormalities in the distal esophagus. Barium is the usual contrast agent as it is inert if aspirated.

Zenker diverticulum is a pulsion diverticulum that arises adjacent to the inferior pharyngeal constrictor, between the oblique fibers of the posterior pharyngeal constrictors and the cricopharyngeus muscle. This mucosal outpouching results from a transient incomplete opening of the upper esophageal sphincter. The diverticulum ultimately enlarges, drapes over the cricopharyngeus, and dissects behind the esophagus into the prevertebral space. The pouch usually deviates to one side or the other; accordingly, the side on which the deviation occurs must be determined by means of a barium swallow so that the appropriate operative approach can be selected. Esophageal motility studies (not usually performed) may show either incomplete upper esophageal relaxation on swallowing or poor coordination of the upper esophageal relaxation phase with pharyngeal contractions. Upper gastrointestinal (GI) endoscopy is performed preoperatively to exclude the presence of a pharyngeal or esophageal carcinoma and to assess the upper GI anatomy. If there is evidence of GERD, proton pump inhibitors (PPIs) are given.

In symptomatic patients (e.g., those with dysphagia, nocturnal cough, or recurrent pneumonia from aspiration), surgical therapy is indicated regardless of whether a pouch is present or how large it may be. Such treatment involves correcting the underlying cricopharyngeal muscle dysfunction with a cricopharyngeal myotomy. If there is a diverticulum larger than 2 cm, it should be excised in addition to the cricopharyngeal myotomy. Alternatively, the diverticulum may be managed via endoscopic obliteration of the common wall between the pharyngeal pouch and the esophagus with either a stapler or a laser. Cricopharyngeal incoordination may be temporarily relieved by injecting botulinum toxin into the cricopharyngeus.

OPERATIVE PLANNING

The patient is placed on a clear fluid diet for 2 days before the operation. With the patient under general anesthesia, the trachea is intubated with a single-lumen endotracheal tube. Cricoid pressure is applied to prevent aspiration of diverticular contents. A soft roll is placed behind the shoulders to extend the neck. The patient is placed in a 20° reverse Trendelenburg position, and the legs are wrapped with pneumatic calf compressors to prevent deep vein thrombosis (DVT). With the endotracheal tube placed to the side of the mouth, a preliminary flexible esophagogastroscopy is performed to empty the diverticulum of all food and to examine the esophagus and the stomach. The scope is then brought back up into the oropharynx and moved into the pouch. The location of the diverticulum (on the left or the right side) is confirmed by turning off the room lights and noting which side is transilluminated by the gastroscope.

OPERATIVE TECHNIQUE

Step 1: Incision and Dissection of Pharyngeal Pouch

The patient lies with the head turned away from the side on which the incision is made (usually the left). The cricoid cartilage is palpated and marked. A 6 cm skin incision is made, either obliquely along the sternocleidomastoid muscle [*see Figure 1*] or transversely in a skin crease at the level of the cricoid. The platysma is divided in the same line. Self-retaining retractors are inserted. The anterior border of the sternocleidomastoid muscle is incised throughout its length. The omohyoid muscle and the sternohyoid and sternothyroid muscles are retracted [*see Figure 2*]. The sternocleidomastoid muscle is retracted laterally to expose the carotid sheath and the internal jugular vein. The middle thyroid vein is ligated and divided, and the thyroid gland and the trachea are retracted medially by the assistant's finger to minimize the risk of injury to the underlying recurrent laryngeal nerve. There is no need to encircle the esophagus or to dissect in the tracheoesophageal groove. The deep cervical fascia is divided. The inferior thyroid artery is divided as laterally as possible. The carotid sheath is retracted laterally, and dissection is carried down to the prevertebral fascia [*see Figure 2*]. The endoscope placed in the diverticulum is palpated, and the pouch is dissected away from the cervical esophagus up as far as the pharyngoesophageal junction. The flexible endoscope is then removed from the pouch and advanced into the thoracic esophagus so that it can be used as a stent for the cricopharyngeal myotomy. Dissection of the pharyngeal pouch is then completed.

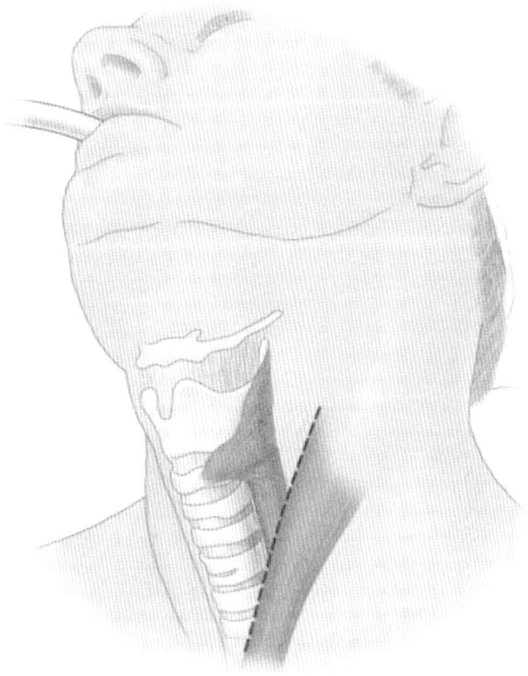

Figure 1 **Cricopharyngeal myotomy and excision of Zenker diverticulum. A soft roll is placed behind the shoulders to extend the neck. The head is turned to the side opposite the incision. The cricoid cartilage is palpated and marked. The skin is incised obliquely along the sternocleidomastoid muscle, as shown, or transversely in a skin crease at the level of the cricoid.**

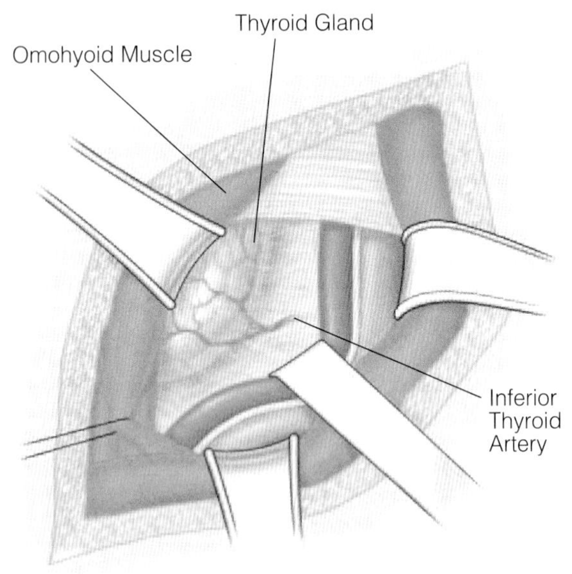

Figure 2 **Cricopharyngeal myotomy and excision of Zenker diverticulum. The sternocleidomastoid is incised along the anterior border so as to expose the omohyoid muscle and the sternohyoid and sternothyroid muscles, which are retracted. The thyroid gland and the trachea are retracted medially by the assistant's finger, and the inferior thyroid artery is ligated and divided laterally to avoid injury to the recurrent laryngeal nerve.**

Step 2: Myotomy

The esophageal myotomy is started approximately 1 cm below the cricopharyngeus on the posterolateral esophageal wall [*see Figure 3a*]. The esophageal muscle is divided down to the mucosa, which is recognizable from its bluish coloration with the submucosal plexus overlying it. The esophageal muscle is dissected away from the mucosa with a right-angle dissector and divided with either a knife, scissors, or a low-intensity diathermy unit. The myotomy is then continued proximally through the cricopharyngeus and up into the muscular wall of the hypopharynx for 1 to 2 cm if no diverticulum is present. The hypopharynx is distinguished by a pronounced submucosal venous plexus. The muscle is then swept off the mucosa for 120°.

Step 3: Freeing or Excision of Diverticulum

If there is a diverticulum less than 2 cm in diameter, the cricopharyngeus is transected and the muscularis around the diverticulum is freed. The myotomy is extended onto the hypopharynx for 1 to 2 cm. The diverticulum is then suspended to the back wall of the pharynx to prevent food from easily entering it. It should not be sutured to the prevertebral fascia, because the passage of sutures through the diverticulum can contaminate the fascia or intervertebral disk, leading to an increased risk of infection.

If the diverticulum is more than 2 cm in diameter, it is excised with a linear stapler loaded with 2.5 mm staples, which is placed at the base of the sac and pressed firmly against the esophagoscope [*see Figure 3b*]. Particular care must be taken at this point so as not to injure the recurrent laryngeal nerve. The stapler is fired, and the diverticulum is excised. The staple line is cleaned with an antiseptic solution, and the incision is filled with saline. The esophagus is insufflated with air to determine whether mucosal leakage has occurred, and the esophagoscope is removed; any mucosal leaks found are closed with fine absorbable sutures. In the absence of a stapler, the best way of excising the sac is to make a series of short incisions through the neck of the sac with scissors, suturing the edges after each cut with absorbable monofilament sutures (the so-called cut-and-sew technique). The esophagoscope ensures that the esophageal lumen is not narrowed. If an esophagoscope is not used, then a Maloney dilator (50 to 54 French) is used to ensure that excessive esophagus is not removed.

Step 4: Drainage and Closure

Once hemostasis has been achieved, a short vacuum drain is placed through the skin into the retroesophageal space. The platysma is repaired with absorbable sutures, and the skin is closed with a subcuticular absorbable suture. Nasogastric intubation is unnecessary. Prokinetic agents and PPIs are administered to prevent gastroesophageal reflux. A water-soluble contrast study can be done the day after the operation. If the results are normal, the patient is started on a liquid diet, the drain is removed, and the patient is discharged on liquids for 1 week.

COMPLICATIONS

The main complications associated with cricopharyngeal myotomy are recurrent laryngeal nerve trauma (occurring in 1% of cases), fistulas (1%), hematoma formation, infection (2%), aspiration, and recurrence (4%). Hematomas and infections must be drained promptly. Fistulas usually close once the prevertebral space is drained and the associated infection is controlled. Aspiration is the most serious complication after cricopharyngeal myotomy. Gastroesophageal reflux may contribute to oropharnygeal dysphagia. Division of the upper esophageal sphincter in a patient with an incompetent esophagogastric junction may lead to massive tracheobronchial aspiration. Therefore, documented severe gastroesophageal reflux, gastroesophageal regurgitation, and severe distal esophagitis may be relative contraindications to cricopharyngeal myotomy until the lower esophageal sphincter defect has been remedied with an antireflux operation.

OUTCOME EVALUATION

Of patients with a Zenker diverticulum, at least 90% experience excellent results from surgical treatment. Of patients without a Zenker diverticulum, one third experience excellent results, another third show moderate improvement, and the remaining third show no improvement.[1] Patients with poor pharyngeal contractility in conjunction with normal upper esophageal sphincter function show little improvement with cricopharyngeal myotomy. Patients with oropharyngeal dysphagia secondary to neurologic involvement who have intact voluntary deglutination, adequate pulsion of the tongue, and normal phonation may show improvement with cricopharyngeal myotomy. Appropriate selection of patients for cricopharyngeal myotomy leads to better surgical outcomes.

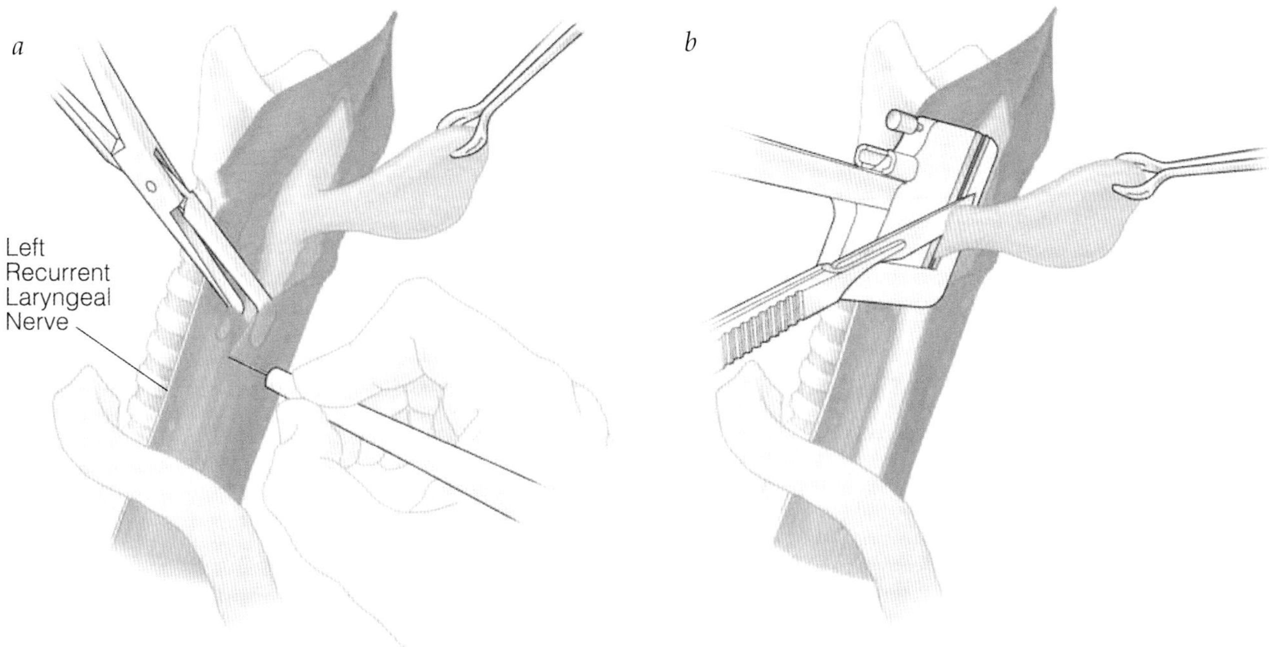

Figure 3 **Cricopharyngeal myotomy and excision of Zenker diverticulum. (*a*) The diverticulum is dissected away from the esophagus, and an esophageal myotomy is started approximately 3 cm below the cricopharyngeus. The myotomy is continued proximally through the cricopharyngeus, and the muscle around the diverticulum is freed. (*b*) A linear stapler is placed at the base of the sac and pressed firmly against the esophagoscope. The stapler is fired, and the diverticulum is excised.**

Transthoracic Hiatal Hernia Repair

Unlike most operations on the esophagus, which are extirpative procedures, hiatal hernia repair with fundoplication is a reconstructive procedure, the aim of which is to restore a high-pressure zone at the esophagogastric junction that prevents reflux but also permits comfortable swallowing. Currently, this repair is usually accomplished via minimally invasive approaches. The degree of tension on the hiatal repair sutures, the length of the esophagus, the quality of the crural tissue itself, and the caliber of the esophageal hiatus after repair all must be assessed. In certain patients, laparoscopic reconstruction of a competent gastroesophageal high-pressure zone may be very difficult and may demand a degree of skill not yet achievable by laparoscopy. The most common indications for transthoracic hiatus hernia repair are a failed previous repair and a hostile abdomen.

The long-term success of antireflux surgery, whether done via the transthoracic approach or by means of laparoscopy, depends on three factors: (1) a tension-free repair that maintains a 4 cm long segment of esophagus in the intra-abdominal position, (2) durable approximation of the diaphragmatic crura, and (3) correct matching of the fundoplication technique according to the peristaltic function of the esophagus. The transthoracic approach should be considered whenever the standard abdominal approaches to hiatal hernia repair carry an increased risk of failure or complication—for example, in patients who have a foreshortened esophagus associated with a massive hernia and an incarcerated intrathoracic stomach, patients with severe peptic strictures of the esophagus, patients in whom the hiatal hernia coexists with an esophageal motility disorder or morbid obesity, and patients who have undergone multiple previous abdominal operations. The transthoracic repair is particularly useful when a previous open abdominal procedure has failed. In this situation, the reasons for such failure, whether technical or tissue related, should be assessed so that a compensatory strategy can be devised.

PREOPERATIVE EVALUATION

Symptomatic Evaluation

All patients being considered for fundoplication to treat GERD must undergo a comprehensive evaluation to determine whether there is indeed an anatomic substrate for their symptoms and what the most appropriate form of repair is. Specifically, a history of heartburn and effortless regurgitation should be sought. Dysphagia and odynophagia are not typically associated with hiatal hernia unless there is a significant paraesophageal component. Persistent dysphagia may reflect the presence of a stricture or a neoplasm. Reflux-induced esophageal spasm may present with occasional episodes of cervical dysphagia, but the transient nature of the symptoms easily differentiates this condition from dysphagia caused by a fixed obstruction. Chest pain that radiates toward the back after meals and is relieved by nonbilious vomiting may indicate the presence of an incarcerated intrathoracic stomach that is hindering the emptying of the paraesophageal component. Atypical chest pain from cholelithiasis, peptic ulcer, or coronary artery disease may confound the diagnosis.

Imaging

Radiographic investigation should begin with a ciné barium swallow, which will yield valuable information regarding the length of the esophagus, its peristaltic function, and the integrity of the mucosal surface. The gastric views can be used for qualitative assessment of distal emptying. Any paraesophageal component will be clearly demonstrated, along with any associated organoaxial volvulus. A simple barium swallow often yields the most useful information for managing the complex problem of recurrent hiatal hernia and a slipped Nissen fundoplication.

Next, esophagogastroscopy should be performed to examine the mucosa for the presence of esophagitis, Barrett mucosa, stricture, or malignancy. The locations of any lesions observed, along with the position of the squamocolumnar junction, should be carefully documented in terms of their distance from the incisors. All strictures must undergo cup or brush biopsy to rule out an occult malignancy. The presence of severe esophagitis raises the possibility of acquired shortening of the esophagus secondary to transmural inflammation and contraction scarring. Every effort should be made to measure the length of the esophagus accurately.

Dilation

If a stricture is found during esophagoscopy, a decision must be made about whether to attempt esophageal dilation. This procedure carries the risk of perforation and should be performed only after careful consideration. If the stricture is diagnosed at the time of the initial endoscopic examination, it is advisable to perform only the brush biopsy at this point, deferring dilation to a subsequent visit. Delaying dilation gives the surgeon time to reassess the anatomy depicted on the barium swallow, to decide whether wire-guided dilation is necessitated by angulation of the esophagus, to obtain informed consent, to assemble the requisite equipment, and to plan sedation for what is often an uncomfortable procedure. If a malignancy is suspected at the time of the initial endoscopic examination, dilation should be avoided. In this situation, repair is impossible; thus, if iatrogenic perforation of a malignant stricture occurs, the surgeon will have to attempt emergency resection in an inadequately prepared patient in whom proper staging is unlikely to have been completed.

The standard flexible adult esophagoscope is approximately 32 French in caliber. In advancing the scope into the stricture, only very gentle pressure should be necessary. As a rule, a mild stricture that is not associated with steep angulation of the esophagus will readily accept passage of the endoscope and will be amenable to subsequent blind dilation with Hurst-Maloney bougies.

After successful passage, the scope is removed, and sequential insertion of progressively larger dilators (starting at 32 French) into the stricture is attempted. The weight of the dilator alone should be sufficient to effect its passage, with little or no forward force applied. Although the patient will be able to swallow comfortably only after satisfactory passage of a dilator at least 48 French in caliber, it is essential never to try to force passage. To this end, the surgeon must take careful note of the subtle signs of increasing resistance transmitted through the dilator. Sequential dilation should be stopped whenever significant resistance is encountered or blood streaks appear on the dilator. Sudden pain during dilation is an ominous sign and calls for immediate investigation with a swallow study using a water-soluble contrast agent (e.g., Gastrografin, Schering AG, Berlin, Germany). Subcutaneous emphysema in the neck or mediastinal air on a plain chest radiograph may also indicate an injury to the esophagus. Perforation must be definitively ruled out before the patient can be discharged.

Highly stenotic strictures that do not allow the passage of a standard adult endoscope may be associated with a distorted and a steeply angulated esophagus. In such cases, the use of a pediatric endoscope may permit directed placement of a guide wire through the stricture; fluoroscopy is a useful adjunct for this purpose. A series of progressively larger Savary-Gillard dilators may then be passed over the guide wire to enlarge the lumen and allow subsequent endoscopic biopsy. As a rule, less tactile feedback is available during wire-guided dilation than during passage of standard Maloney-Hurst bougies. Increased pressure is required to pass the Savary-Gillard dilators because of the resistance caused by the wire passing through the dilator itself. It is essential that the wire be well lubricated and not be allowed to dislodge proximally between the sequential insertions of progressively larger dilators. The caveats that apply to blind dilation also apply to wire-guided dilation.

Patients whose esophagus can be dilated to 48 French and who are candidates for antireflux surgery may undergo subsequent intraoperative dilation to 54 to 60 French. Patients who cannot be dilated to 48 French and fail to achieve comfortable swallowing should be classified as having a nondilatable stricture and should be considered for transhiatal esophagectomy [*see* Resection of Esophagus and Proximal Stomach, *below*].

Functional Evaluation

Esophageal manometry permits quantitative assessment of peristalsis, a capability that is critically important for determining which type of fundoplication is most suitable for reconstructing a nonoccluding high-pressure zone at the esophagogastric junction. Stationary pH tests measure the capacity of the esophagus to clear acid, its sensitivity to instilled acid, the relation of reflux episodes to body position, and the correlation between changes in esophageal pH and the subjective symptoms of heartburn. Ambulatory 24-hour pH testing allows further quantification of reflux episodes with respect to duration, frequency, and association with patient symptoms.

OPERATIVE PLANNING

The transthoracic hiatus hernia repair may be completed with either a partial fundoplication (as in the 240° Belsey Mark IV procedure) or a complete fundoplication (as in the 360° Nissen procedure). Acquired shortening of the esophagus may necessitate lengthening of the esophagus by means of a Collis gastroplasty, in which the portion of the gastric cardia along the lesser curvature and directly contiguous to the distal esophagus is fashioned into a tube [*see* Operative Technique, Step 6a, *below*].

A thoracic epidural catheter is placed for regional analgesia. General anesthesia is administered, and flexible esophagoscopy is performed by the operating team. Insufflation should be done with as little air as is practical, particularly in the case of large paraesophageal hernias. The extent of the pathologic condition is documented, and the absence of malignancy is verified. The stomach is decompressed with suction, and the endoscope is removed. A nasogastric tube is placed while the patient is supine.

Tracheal intubation is performed with a double-lumen endotracheal tube. A Foley catheter is placed. Subcutaneous heparin is administered for DVT prophylaxis, and pneumatic calf compression devices are applied. Antibiotic prophylaxis is provided.

The patient is positioned for a left thoracotomy. The table is flexed to distract the ribs. The right leg is bent at the hip and knee while the left leg is kept straight. Pillows are placed between the legs, and all pressure points are padded. The arms are positioned so that the humeri are at right angles to the chest and the elbows are bent 90°.

OPERATIVE TECHNIQUE

Step 1: Incision and Entry into Chest

A standard left posterolateral thoracotomy is performed. The latissimus dorsi is divided. The serratus fascia is incised, but the muscle itself can generally be preserved. For most patients, the sixth interspace is the most appropriate incision site for exposing the hiatus. The seventh interspace can also be used, particularly if the patient is tall or has a hyperextended chest as a result of chronic pulmonary disease. The paraspinal muscles are elevated away from the posterior aspect of the adjacent ribs, and a 1 cm segment of the rib below the selected interspace is resected to facilitate exposure. The chest is then entered, and the lung and the pleural space are thoroughly inspected. The leaves of the retractor are spread slowly over the course of the next several minutes so as not to cause iatrogenic rib fractures.

Step 2: Mobilization of Esophagus and Excision of Hernia Sac

The inferior pulmonary ligament is divided with the electrocautery to the level of the inferior pulmonary vein [*see Figure 4*]. The mediastinal pleura overlying the esophagus is longitudinally incised to expose the esophagus from the level of the carina to the diaphragm. Particular care is taken to avoid injury to the vagi. Vessels supplying the esophagus and arising from the adjacent aorta are cauterized and divided. A few larger vessels may have to be ligated with 2-0 silk. The esophagus is encircled just below the inferior pulmonary vein with a wide Penrose drain [*see Figure 4*]. The two vagi are mobilized and carried with the esophagus. (The right vagus is located along the right anterior border of the descending aorta and can easily be missed.)

The esophagus is then elevated, and mobilization is circumferentially completed in the direction of the diaphragm, starting from the level of the carina. In cases of giant paraesophageal hernia or reoperation for a failed repair, the stomach will have a large intrathoracic component. Dissection continues inferiorly to separate the sac from the pericardium anteriorly and the aorta posteriorly. The right pleura is closely approximated to the esophagus for 2 to 5 cm above the diaphragm; in the presence of a substantial hiatal hernia and its sac, it may be difficult to identify. The right pleura should be gently dissected away from the sac without entry into the right chest. This can generally be done with a small sponge on a stick. If a tear occurs, it should be closed with absorbable suture material to prevent accumulation of blood and fluid on the right side during the operation.

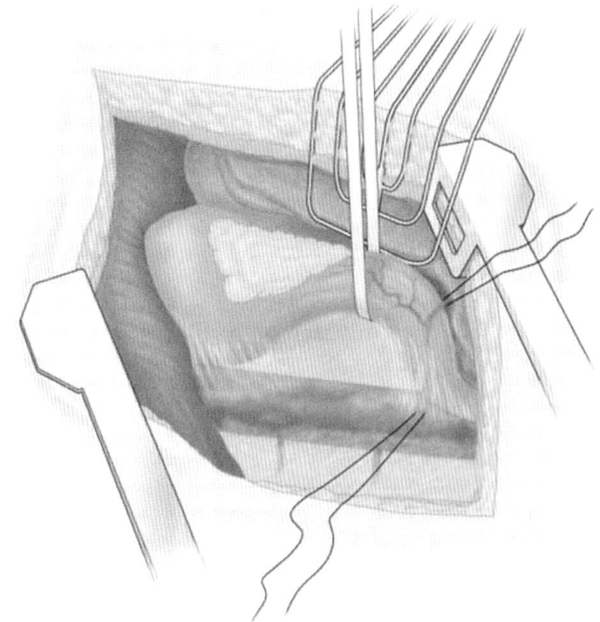

Figure 4 **Transthoracic hiatal hernia repair. The lung is retracted, and the inferior pulmonary ligament is divided to the level of the inferior pulmonary vein. The mediastinal pleura overlying the esophagus is incised to expose the esophagus from the level of the carina to the diaphragm. The esophagus and both vagi are encircled just below the inferior pulmonary vein with a Penrose drain. Vessels supplying the esophagus and arising from the adjacent aorta are ligated and divided.**

Dissection is continued inferiorly to expose the right and left crura. The left crus is generally more robust and is certain to be easily seen with this exposure. Its medial fibers may be attenuated and may blend into the hernia sac superiorly. The sac should be incised 1 cm above the muscle fibers because the muscle alone will not hold sutures well for the subsequent repair. Skeletonization of the crural muscle must be avoided; it is the fibroconnective tissue that provides the most tensile strength. The hernia sac is dissected away from the left crus in an anterior-to-posterior direction. The right crus is generally less robust than the left. In the case of a previous failed repair, the right crus may be very difficult to see, being obscured from the operator's view by the intrathoracic stomach. Dissection of the right crus is best accomplished in a posterior-to-anterior direction.

Once the sac is circumferentially freed from the crura, dissection proceeds cephalad along the esophagus. To minimize the risk of vagal injury, the sac should be incised parallel to the esophagus.

Step 3: Division of Phrenoesophageal Membrane and Gastrohepatic Ligament

The esophagus is retracted anteriorly to expose the posteriorly located phrenoesophageal membrane, which is then divided to yield entry into the lesser sac. The remainder of the phrenoesophageal membrane is elevated with a right-angle clamp as it courses anteriorly, yielding a view of the spleen below. The esophagus and the stomach are thus completely mobilized from the left crus. The esophageal branch of the left phrenic artery, visible near the left vagus, is divided near the crus.

The uppermost portion of the gastrohepatic ligament is found along the undersurface of the right crus. It is divided with the electrocautery. The Belsey artery, a communicating branch between the left gastric artery and the inferior phrenic artery, lies in this area and may have to be ligated directly. It is vital to divide the gastrohepatic ligament down to the level of the left gastric artery. The caudate lobe of the liver must be clearly visible beneath the right crus. This opening is essential for subsequent passage of the fundoplication wrap behind the esophagus.

Step 4: Mobilization of the Stomach

The highest short gastric arteries are ligated between ties to permit mobilization of the fundus. Excessive traction must be avoided to prevent splenic injury. Three or four vessels are usually divided. The esophagogastric junction is elevated well into the chest, and any organoaxial rotation of the stomach is released as the short gastric vessels are divided. It is crucial that ligation be limited to the vessels along the greater curvature. Inadvertent ligation of the vessels along the lesser curvature can easily occur, especially if there was a previous operation. Loss of blood supply from the branches of the left gastric artery along the lesser curvature will lead to ischemia of the Collis gastroplasty tube and will predispose to either leakage at the staple line or subsequent stricture formation.

In the case of a redo repair, the previous fundoplication often will have slipped down onto the cardia or even onto the body of the stomach. Generally, the inner aspect of the previous fundoplication can be freed from the esophagus without any difficulty; rarely will any major dissection have been done in this area during the original operation. The vagi will be found within the wrap and should be specifically visualized. Because of scarring, it may be difficult to see the point at which the previous fundoplication attaches to itself. Not uncommonly, a serosal tear develops on the fundus as the wrap is undone. Any areas of concern can be reinforced with a simple stitch of 4-0 silk. Mobilization is complete when the fundus is restored to its original anatomic position and the greater curvature can be followed down to the left gastroepiploic artery.

Step 5: Closure of Crura

Because the right crus is often quite attenuated, it is crucial to incorporate an adequate amount of tissue into the repair. An Allis or Babcock clamp is placed at the apex of the hiatus and into the central tendon so that both crura can be placed under tension. The esophagus is retracted anteriorly, and a No. 1 silk suture is passed through the most posterior aspect of the left crus, with care taken to avoid the adjacent spleen [*see Figure 5*]. A notched spoon retractor is placed through the hiatus and into the abdomen behind the left crus. The spleen is thus protected while the suture is brought through the left crus.

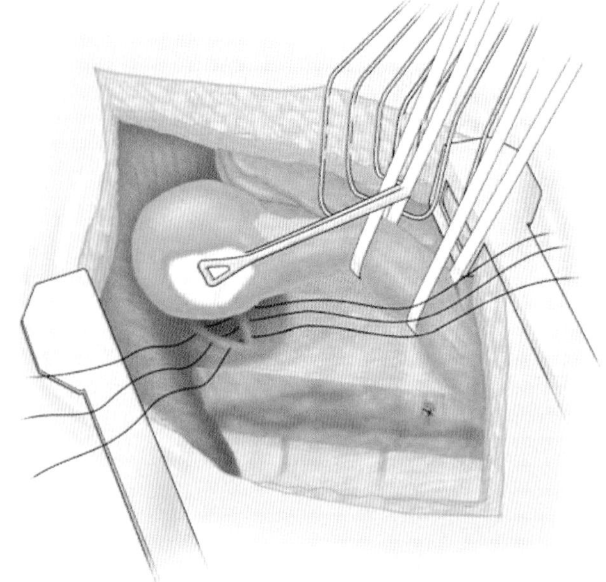

Figure 5 **Transthoracic hiatal hernia repair. The esophagogastric junction is mobilized by dividing the phrenoesophageal ligament and some short gastric vessels. No. 1 silk sutures are passed through the exterior aspect of the right crus (with care taken to avoid the adjacent inferior vena cava) and through the left crus.**

Next, the suture is brought out through the right crus, with care taken to prevent injury to the aorta or entry through the right pleura. Three to five crural repair stitches are then placed at 1 cm intervals, from posterior to anterior. The sutures should be staggered slightly so that the needle entry points are not all in a straight line; this measure helps prevent longitudinal shredding of the muscle fibers when the sutures are placed under tension. The sutures are held together with hemostats but left untied at this point in the operation.

Placement of traction on the last suture should close the defect while still allowing easy passage of one finger along the esophagus. The final decision on whether to tie this last suture or to cut it out is made later, after construction of the fundoplication. It is better to err on the side of an overly narrow opening: removing a suture is easier than having to place an extra one at a time when exposure is less than optimal.

Step 6: Assessment of Esophageal Length and Removal of Anterior Fat Pad

After placement of the crural stitches, an assessment of the esophageal length is made. Ideally, the stomach can easily be reduced into the abdomen without placing tension on the thoracic esophagus. When esophageal foreshortening is found, a Collis gastroplasty is performed [*see* Step 6a, *below*].

If an esophageal stricture is present, the assistant performs dilation by passing a tapered bougie orally while the surgeon supports the esophagus. The anteriorly located esophageal fat pad is removed in anticipation of the gastroplasty, with care taken not to injure the vagi located on either side [*see Figure 6*].

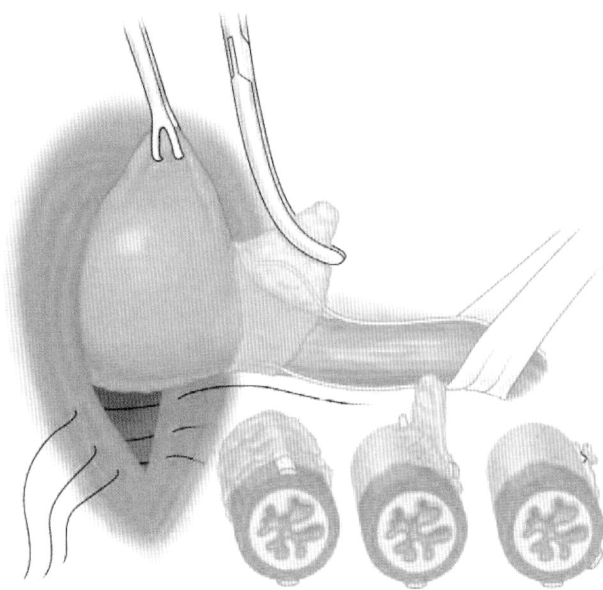

Figure 6 **Transthoracic hiatal hernia repair. The anterior fat pad is removed from the esophagus with sharp dissection, with care taken to avoid injury to the vagi.**

Step 6a: Collis Gastroplasty

In a Collis gastroplasty for a short esophagus, a stapler is used to form a 4 to 5 cm neoesophagus out of the proximal stomach, thereby effectively lengthening the esophagus and transposing the esophagogastric junction more distally. A large-caliber Maloney bougie (54 French for women, 56 French for men) is placed in the esophagus to prevent narrowing of the lumen as the stapler is fired. The bougie is advanced well into the stomach so that its widest portion rests at the esophagogastric junction. The bougie is held against the lesser curvature, and the fundus is retracted away at a right angle to the esophagus with a Babcock clamp. A 60 mm gastrointestinal anastomosis (GIA) stapler loaded with 3.5 mm staples is applied immediately alongside the bougie on the greater curvature side [*see Figure 7a*] and fired, simultaneously cutting and stapling the cardia. The staple line is oversewn with nonabsorbable 4-0 monofilament suture material on both sides [*see Figure 7b*]. Two metal clips are placed to mark the distal extent of the gastroplasty tube, denoting the new esophagogastric junction.

Step 7: Fundoplication and Reduction of Wrap into Abdomen

The fundus is passed posteriorly behind the esophagus and brought up against the anterior stomach, with care taken to avoid torsion of the fundal wrap. The fundus is then wrapped either over the lower 2 cm of the esophagus, if no gastroplasty was done, or over a 2 cm length of the gastroplasty tube while the bougie is in place. The seromuscular layer of the fundus is approximated to that of the esophagus or the gastroplasty tube and that of the adjacent anterior stomach with two interrupted 2-0 silk sutures [*see Figure 8*]. When tied, the wrap should still be loose enough to accommodate a finger alongside the esophagus. The fundoplication sutures are again oversewn with a continuous seromuscular nonabsorbable monofilament suture. Two clips are placed at the superior aspect of the wrap. These, along with the previously placed clips, help confirm both the length and the location of the wrap on chest x-ray.

Once the fundoplication is complete, the dilator is removed and the wrap is reduced into the abdomen. Two mattress sutures of 2-0 polypropylene are placed to secure the top of the fundoplication to the underside of the diaphragm. The crural sutures are then sequentially tied, from the most posterior one to the most anterior. When the final suture is tied, one finger should still be able to pass through the hiatus alongside the esophagus.

Step 8: Drainage and Closure

A nasogastric tube is passed into the stomach and secured. Hemostasis is verified, and a single thoracostomy tube is placed. The wound is closed in layers. A chest x-ray is performed to verify the position of the tubes and the location of the clips marking the wrap. The patient is then extubated in the operating room (OR) and transported to the recovery area.

POSTOPERATIVE CARE

Patients typically remain in the hospital for about 5 days. The nasogastric tube is left on low suction and removed on postoperative day 3. Patients then begin liquid oral intake, advancing to a full-fluid diet as tolerated. Early ambulation is encouraged to prevent respiratory complications. Judicious use of analgesics and antiemetics minimizes nausea and vomiting. The thoracostomy tube is removed as drainage subsides. The epidural and Foley catheters are generally removed later the same day. A barium swallow is performed on postoperative day 5 to verify the position of the wrap, to ensure that there is no significant esophageal obstruction, and to provide a qualitative impression of gastric emptying. Gastroparesis secondary to vagal nerve dysfunction may be apparent.

Once patients can tolerate a soft solid diet, they are discharged home with instructions about the gradual resumption of a normal diet at home. Large meals and carbonated beverages should be avoided in the early postoperative period.

COMPLICATIONS

The root causes of the complications arising after transthoracic hiatal hernia repair are often technical; thus, the best prevention, in most cases, is meticulous surgical technique. Mobilization of the stomach with ligation of short gastric vessels may result in injury to the spleen. Injury to the vagi predisposes to gastric dysfunction, early satiety, and so-called gas-bloat syndrome. Poor crural approximation increases the chances that the repair will fail. Dehiscence allows upward migration of the wrap into the chest or the development of a paraesophageal hernia. The gastroplasty may leak at the staple line. Overzealous dissection along the lesser curvature can devascularize the cardia and cause ischemic stenosis of the gastroplasty tube. Torsion of the fundus results in perforation and sepsis. Excessive distraction of the ribs can lead to pain and splinting with subsequent atelectasis or pneumonia. Inadequate mobilization of the fundus may place

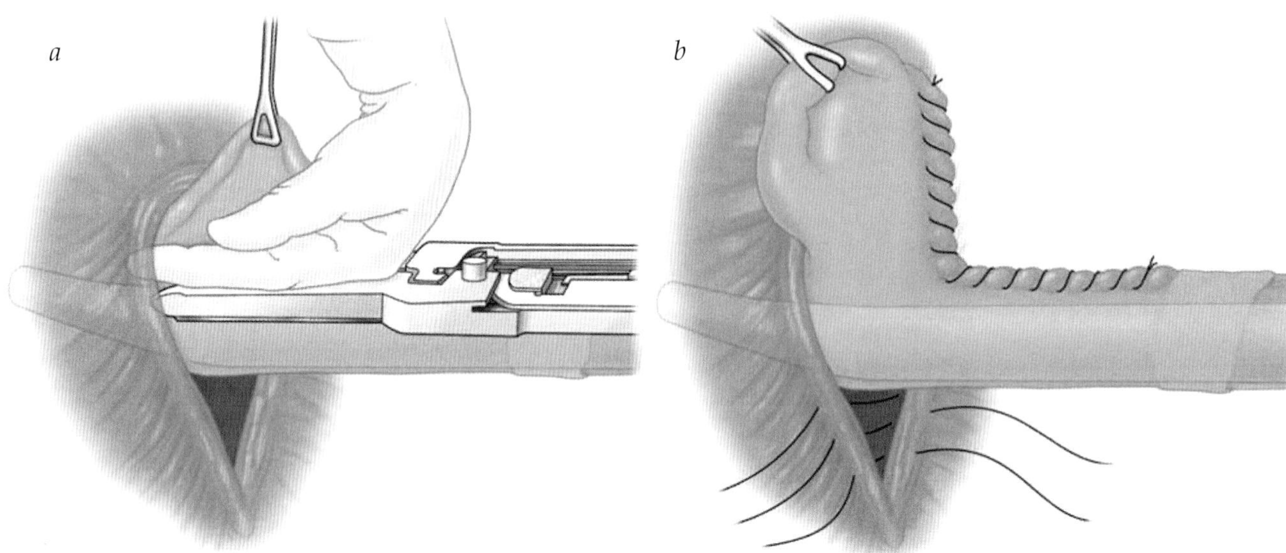

Figure 7 **Transthoracic hiatal hernia repair. (*a*) If esophageal foreshortening is present, a Collis gastroplasty is performed. A 54 French Maloney bougie is inserted through the esophagogastric junction. A 4 to 5 cm neoesophagus is formed with a 60 mm gastrointestinal anastomosis stapler loaded with 3.5 mm staples. (*b*) Both the fundal staple line and the lesser curvature staple line are oversewn with nonabsorbable monofilament suture.**

excessive tension in the wrap and promote later disruption and recurrent reflux. A slipped Nissen can result when the wrap is inadequately fixed to the esophagus or the gastroplasty tube and the stomach telescopes through the intact fundoplication to assume an hourglass configuration. This event leads to varying degrees of heartburn, regurgitation, and dysphagia because the proximal pouch tends to empty

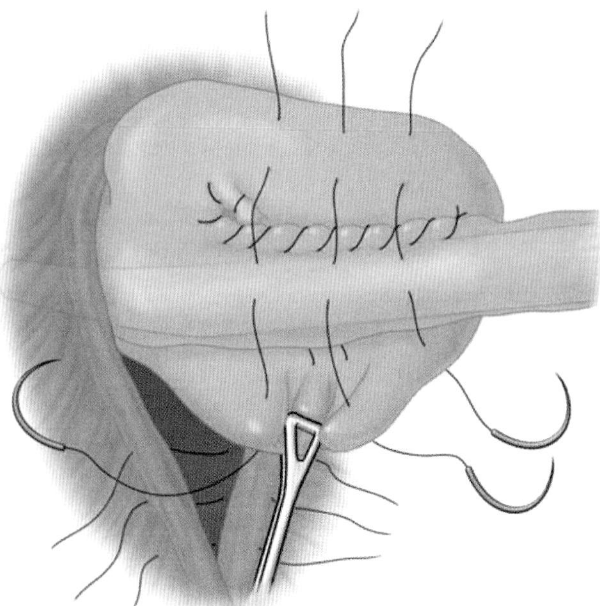

Figure 8 **Transthoracic hiatal hernia repair. The fundus is passed behind the esophagus and sewn to the neoesophagus and the anterior stomach over a 2 cm length with interrupted 2-0 silk sutures.**

slowly and remain distended after meals. A wrap that is too tight or too long results in persistent dysphagia.

Recurrent heartburn and regurgitation call for evaluation with contrast studies and esophagoscopy. The barium swallow is the most useful test for assessing whether the repair has failed. If there is an anatomic condition that is responsible for recurrent symptoms (e.g., slipping of the fundoplication or disruption of the crural repair), reoperation is usually necessary; continued medical treatment of symptoms related to a structural failure invariably proves to be of little use. A barium swallow may also identify gastroparesis secondary to vagal nerve injury. Nuclear transit studies for gastric emptying will help confirm this diagnosis. Dysphagia that is not related to recurrent reflux, ulceration, or stricture usually responds to dilation; reoperation is not required if the barium swallow shows contrast flowing through the esophagus and an intact wrap beneath the diaphragm. Given that patients with long-standing reflux are at higher risk for Barrett dysplasia and esophageal adenocarcinoma, it is important to perform endoscopy to rule out malignancy.

OUTCOME EVALUATION

Transthoracic hiatal hernia repair yields good to excellent results in more than 85% of patients undergoing a primary repair. Approximately 75% of patients who have previously undergone hiatal hernia repair experience symptomatic improvement.[2]

Resection of Esophagus and Proximal Stomach

In the remainder of the chapter, we describe the standard open techniques for resection of the esophagus and the esophagogastric junction. The technique of esophagectomy is largely surgeon dependent, with often strong preferences expressed for a particular operative approach. There is a paucity of definitive evidence as to which technique is superior. Transhiatal esophagectomy is commonly performed to treat end-stage benign esophageal disease and carcinomas of the cardia and the lower esophagus. Esophageal resection through a combined laparotomy–right thoracotomy approach (Ivor Lewis esophagectomy) is ideal for cancers of the middle esophagus but is also used by many for lower third cancers. A three-hole esophagectomy (also known as a McKeown esophagectomy) is sometimes preferred for its excellent exposure of all lymph node stations. The gastric conduit may be anastomosed to the cervical esophagus either high in the right chest (as in an Ivor Lewis esophagectomy) or in the neck (as in a transhiatal esophagectomy or three-hole esophagectomy). The left thoracoabdominal approach is less commonly used but may be indicated for resection of the distal esophagus and the proximal stomach in the case of a bulky tumor that is locally aggressive. Although the traditional anastomosis of the gastric conduit is in the left chest, it may also be placed in the neck.

PREOPERATIVE EVALUATION

Thorough preoperative preparation is essential for a good postoperative outcome. Smoking cessation and a graded regimen of home exercise will help minimize postoperative complications and encourage early mobilization. Schematic diagrams have proved useful for educating patients and shaping their expectations about quality of life and ability to swallow after esophagectomy. Illustrations, by emphasizing the anatomic relations, greatly facilitate discussion of potential complications (e.g., hoarseness from recurrent laryngeal nerve injury, pneumothorax, anastomotic leakage, mediastinal bleeding, and splenic injury).

Potential postoperative problems (e.g., reflux, regurgitation, early satiety, dumping, and dysphagia) must be discussed before operation. Such discussion is particularly relevant for patients undergoing esophagectomy for early-stage malignant tumors or for high-grade dysplasia in Barrett mucosa. These patients generally have no esophageal obstruction and may be completely asymptomatic; accordingly, their expectations about postoperative function may be quite different from those of patients with profound dysphagia secondary to near-complete esophageal occlusion. Support groups in which patients with upcoming operations can contact patients who have already undergone treatment have proved to be highly beneficial to all parties. Realistic expectations improve the chances of a satisfactory outcome.

Evaluation of Operative Risk

Preoperative assessment should include a thorough review of the patient's cardiopulmonary reserve and an estimate of the level of operative risk. Spirometry, arterial blood gas analysis, and exercise stress testing should be considered. Even when a transhiatal esophagectomy is planned, patients should be assessed with an eye to whether they can tolerate a laparotomy and a thoracotomy, in case the latter is made necessary by findings that become apparent only at the time of operation. Thoracic epidural analgesia should be administered for pain control. If a transthoracic approach is taken, a double-lumen endotracheal tube should be placed for separate lung ventilation before beginning the chest portion of the resection.

Imaging

Esophagoscopy with biopsy and contrast-enhanced CT of the chest and the upper abdomen are required before esophagectomy. If performed, the esophagogram identifies the location of the tumor and may indicate whether it extends into the proximal stomach. Esophagoscopy allows direct assessment of the mucosa, precise localization of the tumor, and collection of tissue for histologic study. Retroflexion views of the stomach, after distention with air, are particularly important if proximal gastric invasion is suspected, in which case distal esophagectomy and total gastrectomy with reconstruction of alimentary continuity by means of intestinal interposition may be required. In cases of midesophageal cancer, bronchoscopy is mandatory to rule out airway involvement. The carina and the proximal left mainstem bronchus are the sites most at risk for local invasion.

Contrast-enhanced CT scans of the chest and abdomen are standard. Thoracic and abdominal CT scans yield information on the extent of any celiac or mediastinal adenopathy, the degree of esophageal thickening, and the possibility of invasion of the adjacent aorta or tracheobronchial tree. The lung parenchyma is assessed for metastatic nodules, as are the liver and the adrenal glands. When the distal extent of tumor cannot be defined as a result of near-complete obstruction on endoscopy, a prone abdominal CT scan can help differentiate a tumor at the gastric cardia from a collapsed but normal stomach. If the obstruction is not complete, the stomach can be distended with air (through either the ingestion of effervescent granules or the passage of a small-bore nasogastric tube) to improve visualization. A prone CT scan also yields improved imaging of the gastrohepatic and celiac lymph nodes by allowing the stomach to fall away from these adjacent structures. Metastatic cancer in the celiac lymph nodes portends a poor prognosis.

PET is useful for the detection of occult distant metastases that preclude curative resection. Suspicious areas should undergo needle biopsy or laparoscopic or thoracoscopic assessment. Similarly, pleural effusions must be tapped for cytologic evaluation. Invasion of mediastinal structures and the presence of distant metastases are contraindications to esophagectomy.

At present, EUS, although quite sensitive for detection of paraesophageal adenopathy, is incapable of accurately differentiating reactive lymph nodes from nodes invaded by malignancy. EUS-FNA of suspicious lymph nodes should be done if possible. This is often not possible because of intervening tumor in the wall of the esophagus. CT and PET have limitations; thus, locoregional involvement may not be recognized before resection is attempted. In patients who are marginal candidates for surgical treatment and in whom metastatic disease is suspected, laparoscopy has been advocated for histologic evaluation of small superficial liver nodules, peritoneal abnormalities, and celiac nodes. Although this approach adds to the cost of investigation, it can save the patient from having to undergo a major operation for what would later prove to be an incurable condition.

Neoadjuvant Therapy

Patients with esophageal cancer who are candidates for resection may benefit from neoadjuvant chemotherapy and concurrent radiation therapy. In particular, patients with good performance status and locally advanced disease should be considered for such therapy. To date, no randomized trials have conclusively demonstrated a survival benefit with this approach, but several series have documented a 20 to 30% rate of complete response with no viable tumor found at the time of resection. After chemoradiation, patients are restaged with a CT. PET after treatment may yield spurious results in that inflammatory conditions can mimic the increased tracer uptake seen in malignant tissue. Microscopic disease cannot be assessed, and scarring from radiation may further confound the situation by preventing tracer uptake in areas that actually harbor malignancy.

If there are no contraindications to surgical treatment, resection is scheduled 4 to 6 weeks after the completion of neoadjuvant therapy. This interval allows time for patients to return to their baseline activity level and for any induced hematologic abnormalities to be corrected. Previous chemoradiation therapy does not make transhiatal esophagectomy significantly more difficult or complicated. Many tumors are downstaged and less bulky at the time of resection. In centers with experience in this approach, the rates of bleeding and anastomotic leakage remain low.

OPERATIVE PLANNING

Transhiatal Esophagectomy

In transhiatal esophagectomy, the stomach is mobilized through an upper midline laparotomy, the esophagus is mobilized from adjacent mediastinal structures via dissection through the hiatus without the use of a thoracotomy, and the stomach is transposed through the posterior mediastinum and anastomosed to the cervical esophagus at the level of the clavicles. The main advantages of this approach are (1) a proximal surgical margin that is well away from the tumor site, (2) an extrathoracic esophagogastric anastomosis that is easily accessible in the event of complications, and (3) reduced overall operative trauma. Single-center studies throughout the world have shown transhiatal esophagectomy to be safe and well tolerated, even in patients who may have significantly reduced cardiopulmonary reserve. Long-term survival is equivalent to that reported after transthoracic esophagectomy.

Although transhiatal esophagectomy has been used for resection of tumors at any location in the esophagus, it is best suited for resection of tumors in the lower esophagus and at the esophagogastric junction. It should also be considered for certain advanced nonmalignant conditions of the esophagus. Nondilatable strictures of the esophagus may occur as an end-stage complication of gastroesophageal reflux. Intractable reflux after failed hiatal hernia repair may not be amenable to further attempts at reconstruction of the esophagogastric junction and thus may call for esophagectomy. Because of the high cervical anastomosis, transhiatal esophagectomy is less likely to predispose to postoperative reflux and recurrent stricture formation than transthoracic esophagectomy would be. Achalasia may result in a sigmoid megaesophagus and dysphagia that cannot be managed without removal of the esophagus. Transhiatal esophagectomy permits complete removal of the thoracic esophagus and, in the majority of patients, restoration of comfortable swallowing without the need for a thoracotomy.

Generally, patients are admitted to the hospital on the day of the operation. Thoracic epidural analgesia is administered, both intraoperatively and postoperatively, and appropriate antibiotic prophylaxis is provided. Heparin, 5,000 U subcutaneously, is given before induction, and pneumatic calf compression devices are applied. A radial artery catheter is placed to permit continuous monitoring of blood pressure. Central venous access is rarely required. General anesthesia is administered via an uncut single-lumen endotracheal tube. Flexible esophagoscopy is performed (if it was not previously performed by the surgical team). A nasogastric tube is placed before final positioning and draping.

The patient is placed in the supine position with a small rolled sheet between the shoulders. The arms are secured to the sides, and the head is rotated to the right with the neck extended. The neck, the chest, and the abdomen are prepared as a single sterile field. The drapes are placed so as to expose the patient from the left ear to the pubis. The operative field is extended laterally to the anterior axillary lines to permit placement of thoracostomy tubes as needed. A self-retaining table-mounted retractor is used to facilitate upward and lateral traction along the costal margin.

Ivor Lewis Esophagectomy

At many institutions, Ivor Lewis esophagectomy is preferred because it provides excellent direct exposure for dissection of the intrathoracic esophagus in that it combines a right thoracotomy with a laparotomy. This procedure should be especially considered when there is concern regarding the extent of esophageal fixation within the mediastinum. One advantage of Ivor Lewis esophagectomy is that an extensive local lymphadenectomy can easily be performed through the right thoracotomy. Any attachments to mediastinal structures can be freed under direct vision. Whether any regional lymph node dissection is necessary is highly controversial; no significant survival advantage has yet been demonstrated. Long-term survival after Ivor Lewis resection is equivalent to that after transhiatal esophagectomy.[3]

The main disadvantages of the Ivor Lewis procedure are (1) the physiologic impact of the two major access incisions employed (a right thoracotomy and a midline laparotomy) and (2) the location of the anastomosis (in the chest). Incision-related pain may hinder deep breathing and the clearing of bronchial secretions, resulting in atelectasis and pneumonia. The use of thoracic epidural catheters for pain management has greatly improved pain-related respiratory complications. Complications of the intrathoracic anastomosis may be hard to manage. Although the anastomotic leakage rate associated with Ivor Lewis esophagectomy has typically been 5% or lower—and thus substantially lower than the rate cited for the cervical anastomosis after transhiatal esophagectomy—intrathoracic leaks are much more dangerous and difficult to handle than intracervical leaks. In many cases, drainage of the leak will be incomplete and empyema will result. Reoperation may prove necessary to manage mediastinitis.

Three-Hole Esophagectomy

Three-hole esophagectomy is performed when the surgeon desires direct exposure to all phases of dissection, extensive lymph node clearance, and an anastomosis in the neck. The right chest is opened first, and the intrathoracic esophagus and the regional lymph nodes are dissected and mobilized free. The patient is then turned supine for the abdominal and neck phase, very similar to a transhiatal esophagectomy.

Left Thoracoabdominal Esophagogastrectomy

The left thoracoabdominal approach is indicated for large gastroesophageal junction tumors and resection of the distal esophagus and the proximal stomach when removal of the stomach necessitates the use of an intestinal substitute to restore swallowing. This approach can also be used for very obese patients to obtain optimal exposure. If the proximal stomach must be resected for adequate resection margins to be obtained, then the distal stomach may be anastomosed to the esophagus in the left chest. This operation can be associated with significant esophagitis from bile reflux. Consequently, many surgeons prefer to resect the entire stomach and the distal esophagus and then to restore swallowing with a Roux-en-Y jejunal interposition anastomosed to the residual thoracic esophagus. Alternatively, some surgeons use this approach for most cancers and routinely place the anastomosis in the left neck. Similar to other transthoracic approaches, the use of a thoracic epidural catheter for pain control ameliorates pain-related respiratory complications.

OPERATIVE TECHNIQUE

Transhiatal Esophagectomy

Transhiatal esophagectomy is best understood as consisting of three components: abdominal, mediastinal, and cervical. The abdominal portion involves mobilization of the stomach, pyloromyotomy (if performed), and placement of a temporary feeding jejunostomy.

Step 1: incision and entry into peritoneum A midline laparotomy is performed from the tip of the xiphoid to the umbilicus. The peritoneum is opened to the left of the midline so that the falciform and the preperitoneal fat may be retracted en bloc to the right. Body wall retractors are placed at 45° angles from the midline to elevate and distract both costal margins. The retractors are placed so as to lift up the costal margin gently and open the wound. The abdomen is then inspected for metastases.

Step 2: division of gastrohepatic ligament and mobilization of distal esophagus The left lobe of the liver is mobilized by dividing the triangular ligament and then folded to the right and held in this position with a moist laparotomy pad and a deep-bladed self-retaining retractor. Next, the gastrohepatic ligament is divided. Occasionally, there is an aberrant left hepatic artery arising from the left gastric artery [*see Figure 9*]. The peritoneum over the right crus is incised, and the hiatus is palpated; the extent and mobility of any tumor may then be assessed. The peritoneum over the left crus is similarly divided, and the esophagus is encircled with a 2.5 cm Penrose drain. Traction is applied to draw the esophagogastric junction upward and to the right; this measure facilitates exposure of the short gastric arteries coursing to the fundus and the cardia.

Step 3: mobilization of stomach The greater curvature of the stomach is inspected, and the right gastroepiploic artery is palpated. The lesser sac is generally entered near the midpoint of the greater curvature. The transition zone between the right gastroepiploic arcade and the short gastric arteries is usually devoid of blood vessels.

Dissection then proceeds along the greater curvature toward the pylorus. The omentum is mobilized from the right gastroepiploic artery. Vessels are ligated between 2-0 silk ties, and great care is exercised to avoid placing excessive traction on the arterial arcade. A 1 cm margin is always maintained between the line of dissection and the right gastroepiploic artery. Venous injuries, in particular, can occur with injudicious handling of tissue. The ultrasonic scalpel is particularly efficient and effective for mobilization of the stomach; again, this instrument must be applied well away from the gastroepiploic arcade. Dissection is continued rightward to the level of the pylorus. It should be noted that the location of the gastroepiploic artery in this area may vary; often it is at some unexpected distance from the stomach wall. Posterior adhesions between the stomach and the pancreas are lysed so that the lesser sac can be completely opened.

The assistant's left hand is then placed into the lesser sac to retract the stomach gently to the right and place the short gastric vessels on tension. The Penrose drain previously placed around the esophagus facilitates exposure by retracting the cardia to the right. Dissection along the greater curvature proceeds cephalad. The vessels are divided well away from the wall of the stomach to prevent injury to the fundus. Clamps should never be placed on the stomach. A high short gastric artery is typically encountered just adjacent to the left crus. Precise technique is required to prevent injury to the spleen. The Penrose drain [*see* Step 2, *above*] is exposed as the peritoneum is opened over the left crus. Mobilization of the proximal stomach and liberation of the distal esophagus are thereby completed.

Once the stomach has been completely mobilized along the greater curvature, it is elevated and rotated to the right [*see Figure 10*]; the left gastric artery and associated nodal tissues can then be visualized via the lesser sac. The superior edge of the pancreas is visible, and the remaining posterior attachments of the stomach are divided along the hiatus and the left crus. These may be quite extensive if there has been a history of pancreatitis or preoperative radiation therapy.

If the operation is being done for malignant disease, a final determination of resectability can be made at this point. Tumor fixation to the aorta or the retroperitoneum can be assessed. Celiac and para-aortic lymph nodes can be palpated and, if necessary, sent for biopsy. The left gastric artery and vein are then ligated proximally, either through the lesser sac or directly through the divided gastrohepatic ligament. All nodal tissue is dissected free in anticipation of subsequent removal en bloc with the specimen.

Step 4: mobilization of duodenum and pyloromyotomy The duodenum is mobilized with a Kocher maneuver. Careful attention to the superior extent of this dissection is critical. Adhesions to either the porta hepatis or the gallbladder must be divided to ensure that the pylorus is sufficiently freed for later migration to the diaphragmatic hiatus.

Gastric drainage can be provided by a pyloromyotomy and is performed by most surgeons. The pyloromyotomy is begun 1 to 2 cm on the gastric side of the pylorus. The serosa and

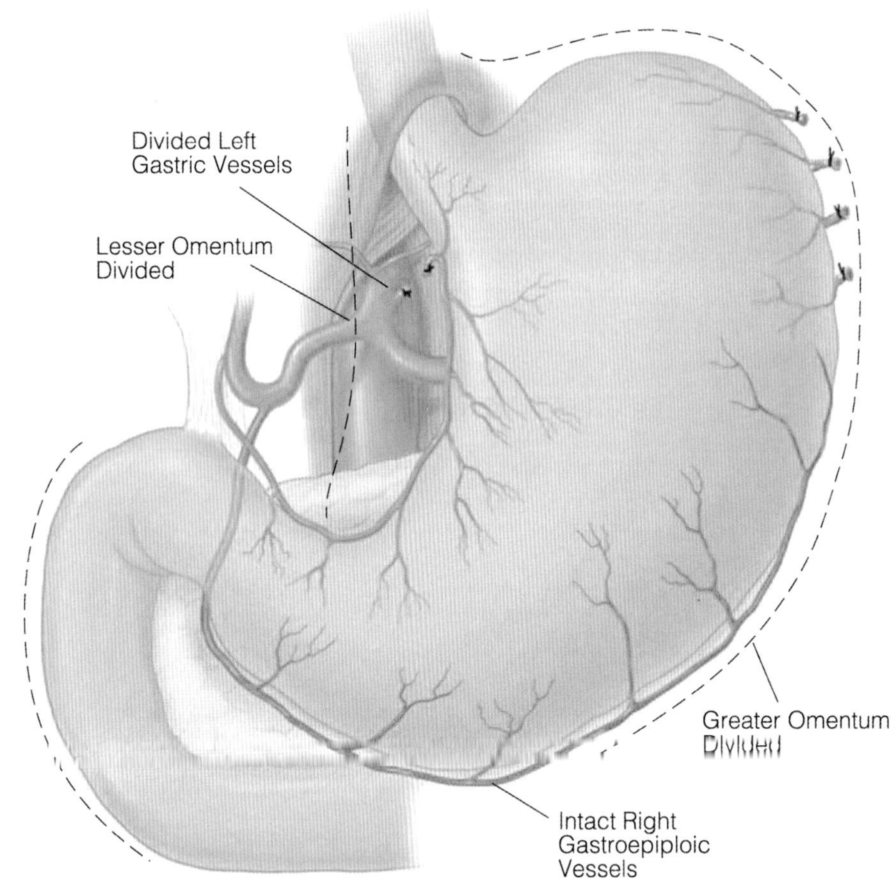

Figure 9 **Transhiatal esophagectomy. The duodenum is mobilized, and the gastrohepatic and gastrocolic omenta are divided.**

the muscle are divided with a small scalpel to expose the submucosa; generally, these layers of the stomach are robust, making the proper plane easy to find.

Dissection is extended toward the duodenum with the aid of a fine-tipped right-angle or tonsil clamp. The duodenal submucosa, recognizable by its fatty deposits and yellow coloration, is exposed for approximately 0.5 cm. The duodenal submucosa is usually much more superficial than expected, and accidental entry into the duodenum often occurs just past the left edge of the circular muscle of the pylorus. Should entry into the lumen occur, a simple repair using interrupted fine monofilament (4-0 or 5-0 polypropylene) sutures to close the mucosa is performed. Small metal clips are applied to the knots of the traction sutures before removal of the ends; these clips serve to indicate the level of the pyloromyotomy on subsequent radiographic studies. A tag of omentum can be easily sutured over the myotomy site for an added layer of security. My own preference is not to perform a pyloromyotomy primarily to reduce the possibility of postoperative bile reflux, which is very problematic to treat. In addition, I remain unconvinced that pyloromyotomy helps gastric drainage that much. With the availability of balloon dilation, it is now simple to enhance emptying postoperatively if needed. Many studies have confirmed that not performing a pyloromyotomy is safe.

Step 5: feeding jejunostomy Placement of a standard Weitzel jejunal feeding tube approximately 30 cm from the ligament of Treitz completes the abdominal portion of the transhiatal esophagectomy.

Step 6: exposure and encirclement of cervical esophagus The cervical esophagus is exposed through a 6 to 8 cm incision along the anterior edge of the left sternocleidomastoid muscle [*see Figure 1*] that is centered over the level of the cricoid cartilage. The platysma is divided to expose the omohyoid, which is divided at its tendon. The strap muscles are divided low in the neck at their origin on the back of the manubrium. The esophagus and its indwelling nasogastric tube can be palpated.

The carotid sheath is retracted laterally, and blunt dissection is employed to reach the prevertebral fascia. The inferior thyroid artery is ligated laterally; the recurrent laryngeal nerve is visible just deep and medial to this vessel. No retractor other than the surgeon's finger should be applied medially: traction injury to the recurrent laryngeal nerve will result in both vocal cord palsy and uncoordinated swallowing with aspiration. In particular, metal retractors must not be used in this area. The tracheoesophageal groove is incised close to the esophageal wall while gentle finger traction is applied cephalad to elevate the thyroid cartilage toward the right. This measure usually suffices to define the location of the nerve.

The esophagus is then encircled by passing a right-angle clamp posteriorly from left to right while the surgeon's finger remains in the tracheoesophageal groove. The tip of the

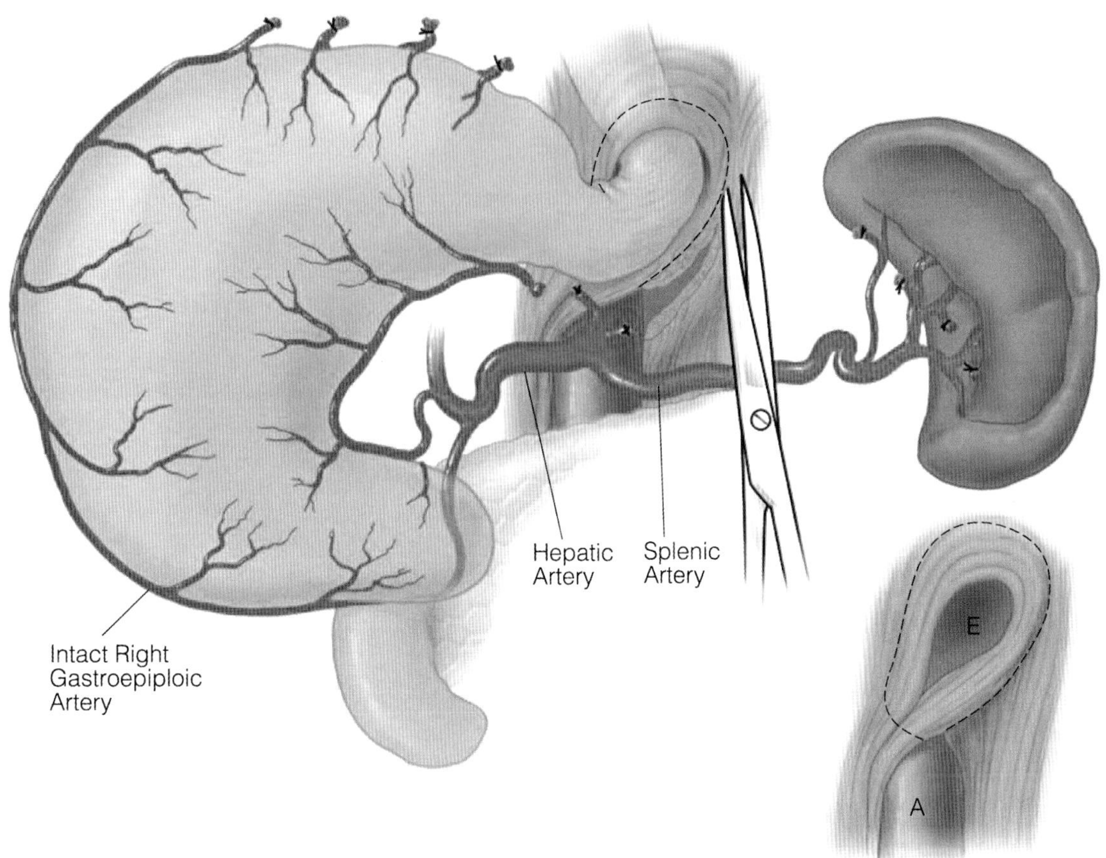

Figure 10 **Transhiatal esophagectomy. After the stomach has been completely mobilized along the greater curvature, it is elevated and rotated to the right. The left gastric vessels are suture-ligated and divided. A 1 cm margin of the diaphragmatic crura is taken in continuity with the esophagogastric junction, providing ample clearance of the tumor and improved exposure of the lower mediastinum. *A* denotes the aorta, *E* denotes the esophageal hiatus.**

clamp is brought into the pulp of the fingertip. The medially located recurrent laryngeal nerve and the membranous trachea are thereby protected from injury. The clamp is brought around, and a narrow Penrose drain is passed around the esophagus [*see Figure 11*]. Blunt finger dissection is employed to develop the anterior and posterior planes around the esophagus at the level of the thoracic inlet.

Step 7: mediastinal dissection Some authors describe this portion of the procedure as a blunt dissection, but, in fact, the vast majority of the mediastinal mobilization is done under direct vision. Narrow, long-handled, handheld, curved Harrington retractors are placed into the hiatus and lifted up to expose the distal esophagus. Caudal traction is placed on the esophagus, allowing excellent visualization of the hiatus and the distal esophagus. Long right-angle clamps are used to expose these attachments. Vascularity in this area is often minimal, and hemostasis can easily be achieved with either the electrocautery, ultrasonic scalpel, metal clips, or ties. The left crus can be divided to facilitate exposure. Paraesophageal lymph nodes are removed either en bloc or as separate specimens. Dissection is continued cephalad with the electrocautery and a long-handled right-angle clamp. The two vagi are divided, and the periesophageal adhesions are lysed. Mobilization of the distal esophagus under direct vision is thus completed up to the level of the carina.

Three specific maneuvers are now carried out. First, the plane posterior to the esophagus is developed [*see Figure 12*]. The surgeon's right hand is advanced palm upward into the hiatus, with the fingers closely applied to the esophagus. The volar aspects of the fingers run along the prevertebral fascia, elevating the esophagus off the spine. A moist sponge stick is placed through the cervical incision, also posterior to the esophagus. The sponge is advanced toward the right hand, which is positioned within the mediastinum. As the sponge is advanced into the right palm, the posterior plane is completed.

Second, the anterior plane is developed [*see Figure 13*]. This is often much more difficult than developing the posterior plane because the left mainstem bronchus may be quite close to the esophagus. Again, the surgeon's right hand is placed through the hiatus, but it is now palm down and anterior to the esophagus. The fingertips enter the space between the esophagus and the left mainstem bronchus. The hand is gently advanced, and the airway is displaced anteriorly. A blunt curved suction handle is employed from above as a

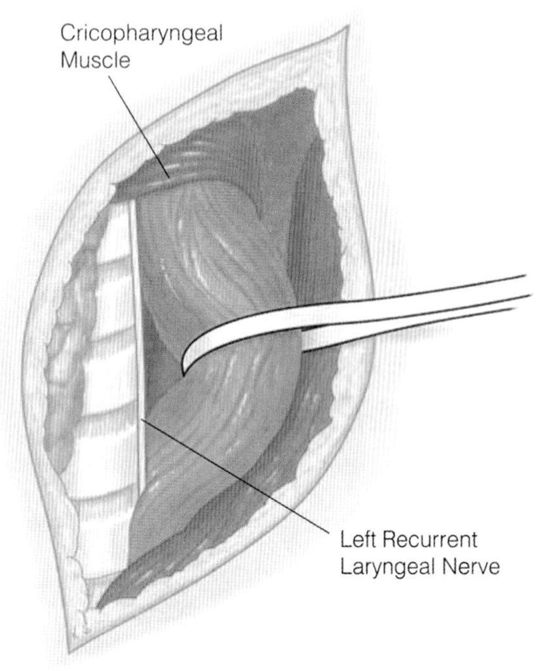

Figure 11 **Transhiatal esophagectomy. Once the cervical esophagus is exposed through an incision along the left sternocleidomastoid muscle, strap muscles are divided and retracted, and the cervical esophagus is dissected away from the left and right recurrent laryngeal nerves.**

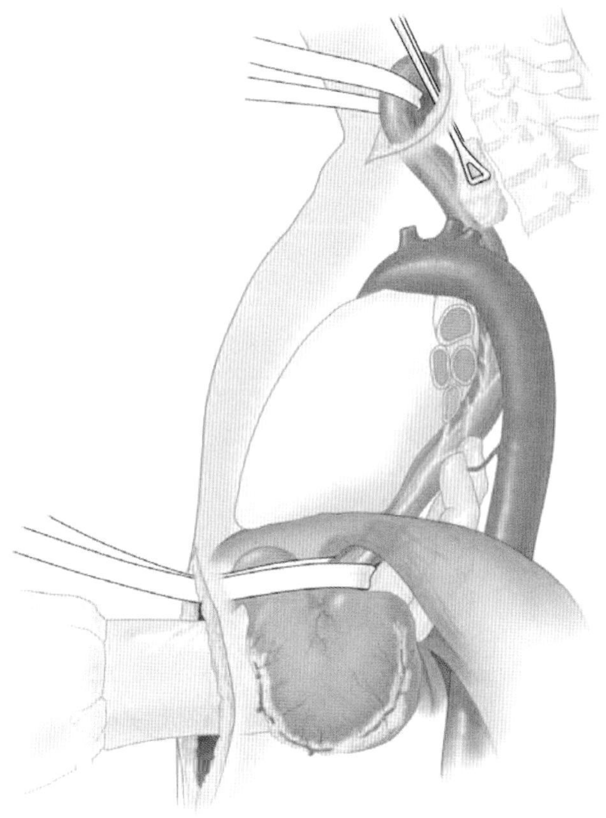

Figure 12 **Transhiatal esophagectomy. The plane posterior to the esophagus is developed by placing the surgeon's right hand into the hiatus along the prevertebral fascia. A moist sponge stick is placed through the cervical incision posterior to the esophagus, and the posterior plane is completed.**

substitute finger. It is advanced along the anterior aspect of the esophagus through the cervical incision. The right hand guides the tip of the suction handle beneath the bronchus. Lateral displacement of the handle allows further mobilization of the bronchus away from the esophagus. Completion of the anterior and posterior planes usually results in a highly mobile esophagus.

Third, the lateral attachments of the upper and middle esophagus are divided. Upward traction is applied with the Penrose drain previously placed around the cervical esophagus, allowing further dissection at the level of the thoracic inlet. Lateral attachments are pushed caudally into the mediastinum, and traction applied to the esophagus from below allows these attachments to be visualized inferiorly through the hiatus and then isolated with long right-angle clamps and divided with the electrocautery. Caution must be exercised so as not to injure the azygos vein. Dissection on the right side must therefore be kept close to the esophagus. Once the last lateral attachment is divided, the esophagus is completely free and can be advanced into the cervical wound.

Close monitoring of arterial blood pressure is maintained throughout. Transient hypotension may occur as a result of mediastinal compression and temporary impairment of cardiac venous return as the surgeon's hand or retractors are passed through the hiatus. Vasopressors are never required for management: simple repositioning of the retractors or removal of the dissecting hand usually results in prompt restoration of normal blood pressure. Placement of the patient in a slight Trendelenburg position is often helpful.

Step 8: proximal transection of esophagus and delivery into abdomen The nasogastric tube is retracted to the level of the cricopharyngeus, and the esophagus is divided with a cutting stapler 5 to 6 cm distal to the muscle. The esophagus is then removed via the abdomen [*see Figure 14*]. Retractors are placed in the hiatus, and the mediastinum is inspected for hemostasis. Both pleurae are inspected. The lungs are inflated so that it can be determined which pleural space requires thoracostomy drainage. The mediastinum is packed with dry laparotomy pads from below. A narrow pack is placed into the thoracic inlet from above. Chest tubes are then placed as required along the inframammary crease in the anterior axillary line. The drainage from these tubes should be closely monitored throughout the rest of the operation to ensure that any bleeding from the mediastinal dissection does not go unnoticed.

Step 9: excision of specimen and formation of gastric tube The gastric fundus is grasped, and gentle tension is applied along the length of the stomach. The esophagus is held at right angles to the body of the stomach, and the fat in the gastrohepatic ligament is elevated off the lesser curvature; all lymph nodes are thus mobilized. A point approximately midway along the lesser curvature is selected. The blood vessels traversing this area from the right gastric artery are

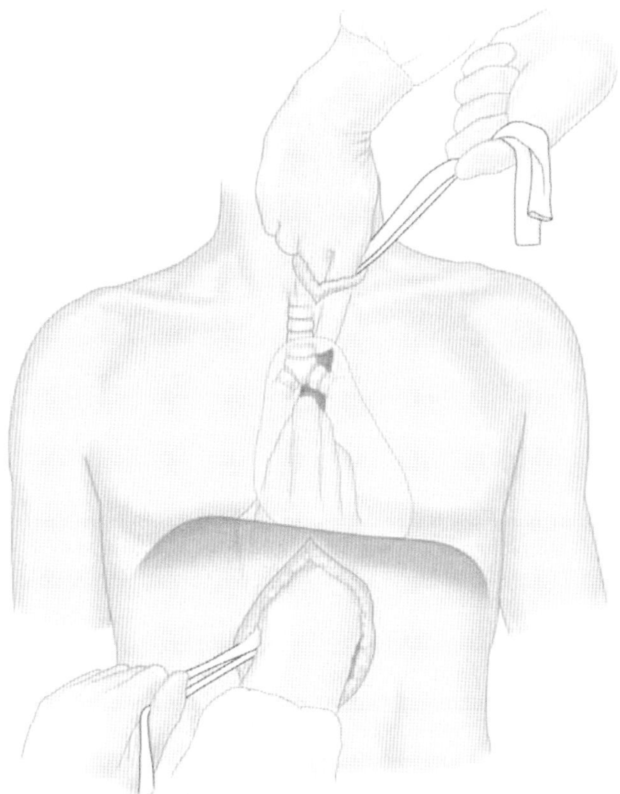

Figure 13 **Transhiatal esophagectomy. The anterior plane is developed by placing the surgeon's right hand through the hiatus anterior to the esophagus. The fingertips enter the space between the esophagus and the left mainstem bronchus, to be met by a blunt suction handle passed downward through the cervical incision. The lateral attachments of the esophagus are divided from above downward as far as the aortic arch.**

ligated to expose the lesser curvature. The distal resection margin is then marked; it should be 4 to 6 cm from the esophagogastric junction, extending from the selected point on the lesser curvature to a point medial to the fundus. A 60 mm GIA stapler loaded with 3.5 or 4.8 (depending on the thickness of the stomach) mm staples is then used to transect the proximal stomach, proceeding from the lesser curvature toward the fundus [*see Figure 15*]. Resection of the cardia along with the adjacent portion of the lesser curvature effectively converts a J-shaped stomach into a straight tube and harvests many left gastric territory lymph nodes.

For maximizing the length of the gastric tube, several technical points are critical. Tension must be maintained on the stomach as the stapler is serially applied. The stapler should be simply placed on the stomach and fired: no attempt should be made to telescope tissue into the jaws because to do so would effectively reconstitute the curve of the stomach and diminish its upward reach. Typically, five or six staple loads are required.

The specimen is removed, and frozen-section examination is done on the distal margin. The completed staple line is then oversewn with a continuous Lembert suture of 4-0 polypropylene. Once again, tension is maintained along the stomach to prevent any foreshortening of the lesser curvature. The use of two separate sutures, each reinforcing half of the staple line, is helpful in this regard. Alternatively, interrupted 4-0 sutures can be used.

Step 10: advancement of stomach into chest or neck The mediastinal packs are removed, and hemostasis is verified in the chest. The stomach is inspected as well. The ends of any short gastric vessels that were divided with the

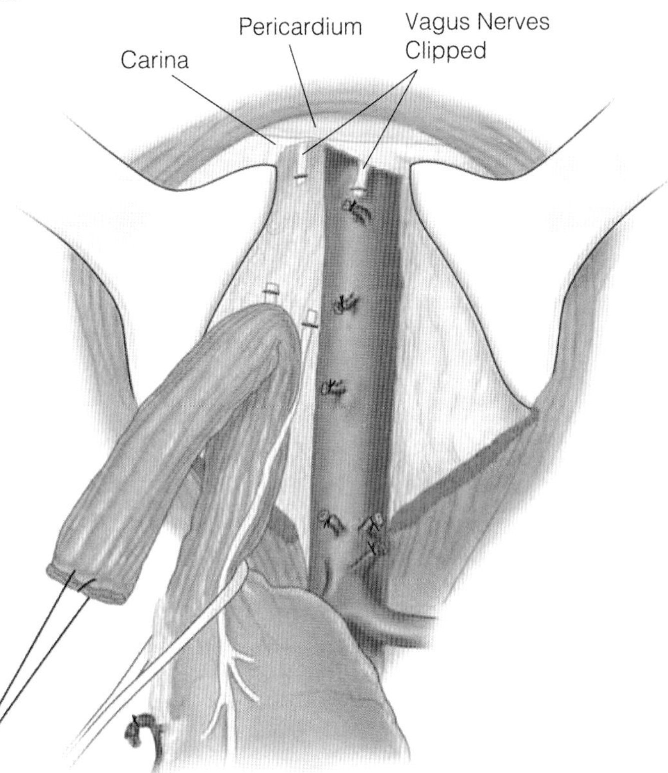

Figure 14 **Transhiatal esophagectomy. The esophagus is divided in the neck and delivered into the abdomen. Retractors are placed in the hiatus, and any vessels entering into the esophagus are clipped and divided. The vagi are also clipped and divided.**

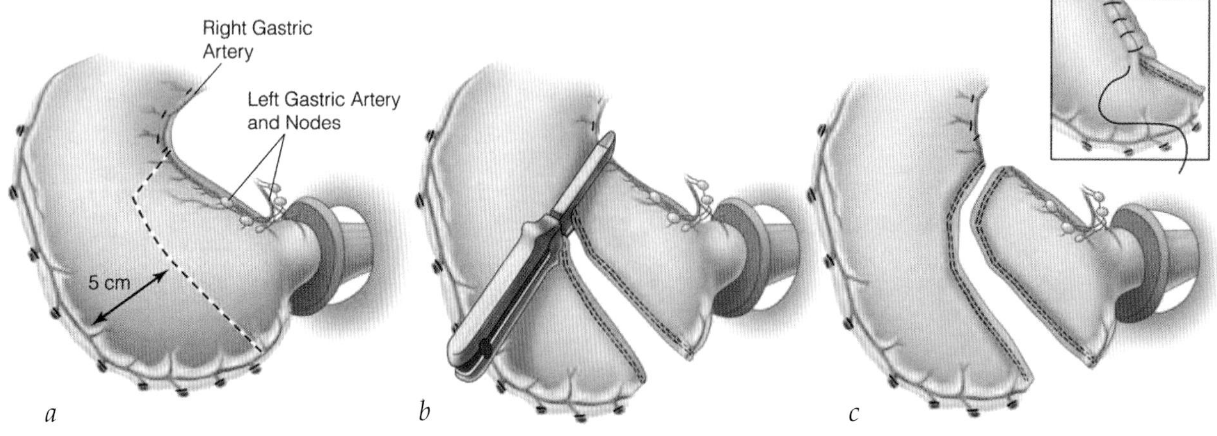

Figure 15 **Transhiatal esophagectomy. A gastric tube is formed by stapling along the lesser curvature of the stomach from the junction of the right and left gastric vessels to the top of the fundus. This staple line is oversewn with either an interrupted or a continuous fine suture, with care taken not to foreshorten the gastric tube. The gastric tube is made at least 5 cm wide to avoid undo ischemia.**

ultrasonic scalpel are now tied so that subsequent manipulation does not precipitate bleeding. The stomach is oriented so that the greater curvature is to the patient's left. There must be no torsion. The anterior surface of the fundal tip should be marked with ink so that proper orientation of the stomach can be confirmed after its passage into the neck. The stomach can usually be advanced through the posterior mediastinum without any traction sutures or clamps. The surgeon's hand is placed palm down on the anterior surface of the stomach, with the fingertips about 5 cm proximal to the tip of the fundus. The hand is then gently advanced through the chest, pushing the stomach ahead of itself. The tip of the fundus is gently grasped with a Babcock clamp as it appears in the neck. To prevent trauma at this most distant aspect of the gastric tube, the clamp should not be ratcheted closed.

No attempt should be made to pull the stomach up into the neck: the position of the fundus is simply maintained as the surgeon's hand is removed from the mediastinum. Further length in the neck can usually be gained by gently readvancing the hand along the anterior aspect of the stomach. This measure uniformly distributes tension along the tube and ensures proper torsion-free orientation in the chest. The stomach is pushed up into the neck rather than drawn up by the clamp.

A useful alternative approach for positioning the gastric tube involves passing a large-bore Foley catheter through the mediastinum from the neck incision. The balloon is inflated, and a 50 cm section of a narrow plastic laparoscopic camera bag is tied onto the catheter just above the balloon. The gastric tube is positioned within the bag, and suction is applied through the catheter, creating an atraumatic seal between the stomach and the surrounding plastic bag. As the bag is drawn upward through the neck with gentle traction on the Foley catheter, the stomach advances through the mediastinum. The stomach is not secured to the prevertebral fascia in any way.

The feeding jejunal tube is brought out the left midabdomen through a separate stab incision. The hiatus is inspected for hemostasis, as is the splenic hilum. It may be necessary to reconstitute the hiatus with one or two simple sutures of 1-0 silk placed through the crura. These sutures must be placed with care to ensure that injury to the gastroepiploic arcade does not occur at this late point in the procedure. The hiatus is narrowed, but not so much that three fingers cannot be easily passed alongside the gastric conduit. This reconstitution will help prevent herniation of other abdominal contents alongside the gastric conduit. The liver is returned to its anatomic position, thus also preventing any subsequent herniation of bowel into the chest. The pylorus is generally found at the level of the diaphragm. The laparotomy is then closed in the usual fashion. The viability of the fundus in the neck incision is checked periodically as the abdominal portion of the procedure is completed.

Step 11: cervical esophagogastric anastomosis The construction of the esophagogastric anastomosis is the most important part of the entire operation: any anastomotic complication will greatly compromise the patient's ability to swallow comfortably. Accordingly, meticulous technique is essential.

A seromuscular traction suture of 4-0 polyglactin is placed through the anterior stomach at the level of the clavicle and drawn upward, thus elevating the fundus into the neck wound and greatly facilitating the anastomosis.

The site of the anterior gastrotomy is then carefully selected: it should be midway between the oversewn lesser curvature staple line and the greater curvature of the fundus (marked by the ligated ends of the short gastric vessels). The staple line on the cervical esophagus is removed, and the anterior aspect of the esophagus is grasped with a fine-toothed forceps at the level of the planned gastrotomy. A straight DeBakey forceps is then applied across the full width of the esophagus to act as a guide for division. The esophagus is cut with a new scalpel blade at a 45° angle so that the anterior wall is slightly longer than the posterior wall; the anterior wall then forms the hood of the anastomosis. The fine-toothed forceps is used to maintain orientation of the esophagus throughout. Two full-thickness stay sutures of 4-0 polyglactin are placed, one at the midpoint of the anterior cut edge of the esophagus and one at the corresponding location posteriorly. The posterior stitch is placed from inside the lumen, and the needle is left on the suture for later use.

A small gastrotomy is then performed with a needle-tipped electrocautery using cutting current. The incision is obliquely oriented, with the cephalad extent proceeding slightly medially. The needle from the stay suture previously placed on the posterior wall of the esophagus is then passed the full thickness of the cephalad aspect of the gastrotomy [*see Figure 16a*]. Traction on this untied suture brings the esophagus toward the stomach. A 45 mm endoscopic stapler loaded with 3.5 mm staples is used to form the back wall of the anastomosis. The thicker portion of the device (the cartridge) is advanced cephalad into the esophagus, with the narrower portion (the anvil) in the gastric lumen [*see Figure 16b*]. The tip of the stapler should be aimed toward the patient's right ear. Tension is applied to the stay suture holding the esophagus and stomach together so as to bring tissue into the jaws of the device. The portion of the fundus extending beyond the stapler is then rotated medially to ensure that the new staple line is well away from the one previously placed along the lesser curvature. This is a crucial point: crossing of the two staple lines may create an ischemic area that can give rise to a large leak in the postoperative period.

The stapler is then closed, holding the esophagus and stomach together, but not yet fired. The position of the nasogastric tube should be maintained just at the level of the cricopharyngeus during the construction of the anastomosis. This positioning keeps the tube out of the operative field and protects it from being entrapped by the jaws of the stapler; it also facilitates subsequent passage of the tube into the gastric conduit once the posterior wall of the anastomosis is complete. Two suspension sutures are placed on either side of the closed stapler, one toward the tip and the other near the heel of the jaws. These four sutures alleviate any potential tension on the staple line by approximating the muscular layer of the esophagus to the seromuscular layer of the stomach. The suspension sutures are tied, and the stapler is fired, thereby completing the posterior portion of the anastomosis [*see Figure 16c*].

The anterior portion of the anastomosis is closed in two layers. The inner layer consists of a continuous 4-0 polydioxanone suture placed as full-thickness inverting stitches, and the second layer consists of interrupted seromuscular Lembert sutures [*see Figure 17*]. The lateral and medial corners of the anastomosis, where the staple line meets the handsewn portion, merit extra attention. These corners are quite fragile, and excessive traction may result in dehiscence progressing cephalad along the staple line in a zipperlike fashion. The inner layer should therefore be started at each corner, incorporating the last 5 mm of the staple line. Once several stitches have been placed from the two corners, the nasogastric tube can be passed through the anastomosis. The nasogastric tube is properly positioned when the most distal black marker is at the nares. The inner layer is then completed as the two sutures are tied at the midpoint.

Step 12: drainage, closure, and completion x-ray The incision is irrigated. The strap muscles are not reapproximated but are merely attached loosely to the underside of the

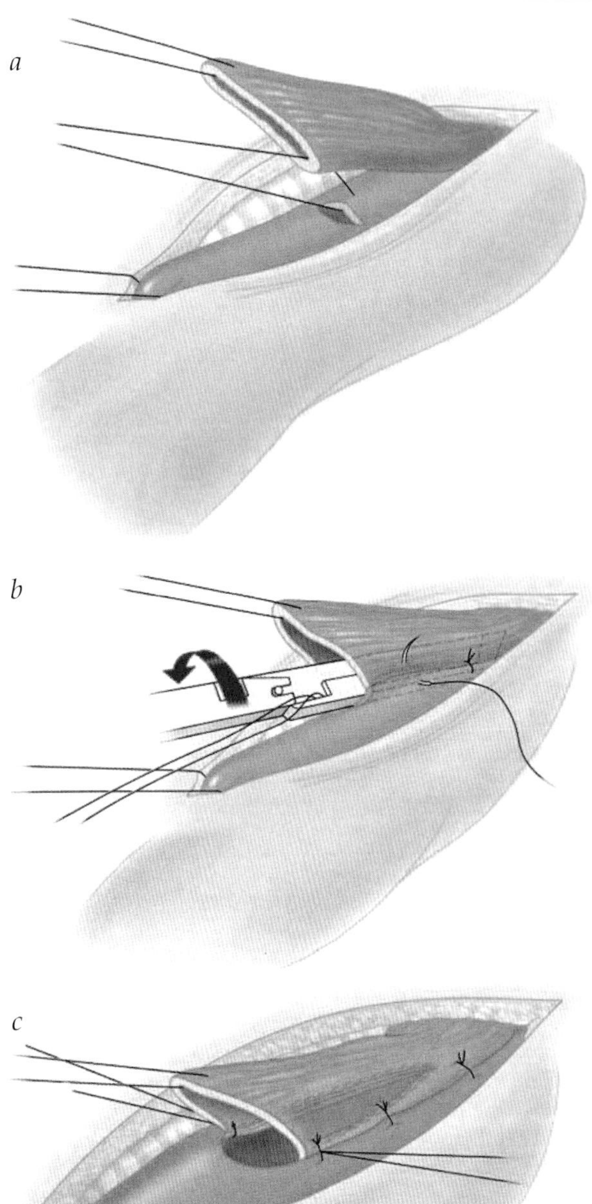

Figure 16 **Transhiatal esophagectomy. (*a*) After the proximal end of the stomach tube is delivered into the neck, the esophagus is cut at a 45° angle so that the anterior wall is longer than the posterior wall. A gastrotomy is placed between the oversewn lesser curvature staple line and the greater curvature of the fundus. A full-thickness suture is placed through all layers of the esophagus and all layers of the gastrotomy. (*b*) An endoscopic gastrointestinal anastomosis stapler is used to form the back wall of the anastomosis. The thicker portion of the device (the cartridge) is advanced cephalad into the esophagus, with the narrower portion (the anvil) in the gastric lumen. The tip of the stapler should be aimed toward the patient's right ear. The staple line must be well away from the lesser curvature staple line. Two suspension sutures are placed on either side of the closed stapler, one toward the tip and the other near the heel of the jaws. (*c*) The stapler is fired to complete the posterior portion of the anastomosis.**

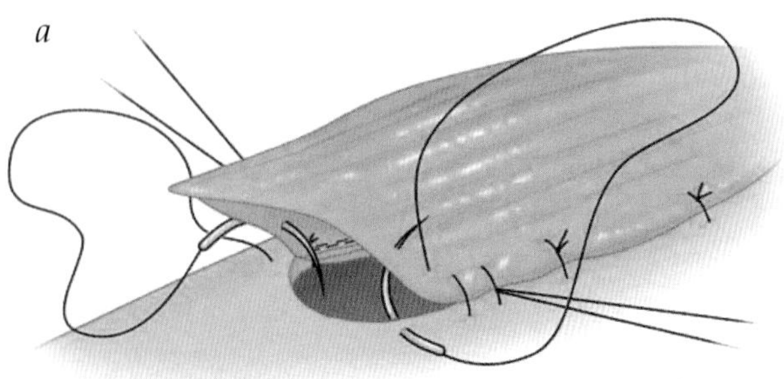

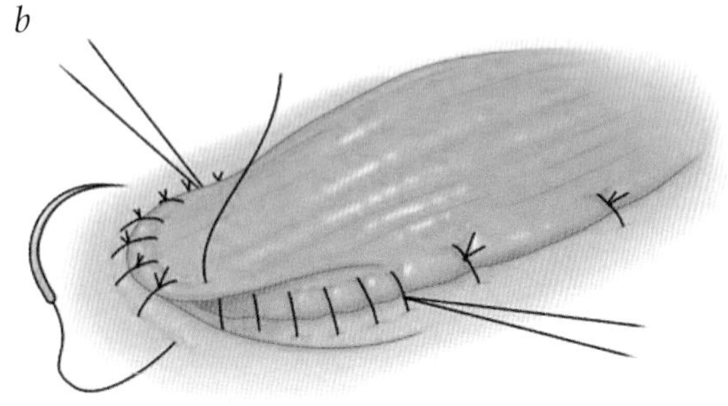

Figure 17 **Transhiatal esophagectomy. The anterior portion of the anastomosis is completed with (*a*) an inner layer consisting of a continuous 4-0 polydioxanone suture and (*b*) an outer layer consisting of interrupted sutures.**

sternocleidomastoid muscle with two interrupted 4-0 polyglactin sutures. The platysma is reconstituted with interrupted 4-0 polyglactin sutures. The nasogastric tube is secured.

A chest x-ray is obtained in the OR to verify the position of the drains and the absence of any abnormal collections in the chest. Patients are extubated in the OR and transported to the anesthetic recovery area. Extubation should be carried out only when the health care team is confident that subsequent reintubation is unlikely to be necessary. Emergency reintubation after a cervical anastomosis is hazardous in that vigorous neck extension may threaten the suture line. Once patients are awake and alert, which is usually 3 to 4 hours after the operation, they are taken to the general ward. As a rule, admission to an intensive care unit is not required unless there are substantial comorbidities or intraoperative concerns. To prevent excessive traction on the anastomosis, the neck should be maintained in a flexed position with two pillows placed behind the head.

In certain patients, a stapled anastomosis may be impractical. In patients with a bull-neck habitus, for example, a partial sternal split may be required for adequate exposure of the cervical esophagus, and a handsewn true end-to-end anastomosis (EEA) may be necessary. In addition, patients who have previously undergone antireflux surgery may have a relatively short gastric tube that will necessitate an end-to-end reconstruction.

Patients should, if possible, begin walking the morning after the operation. An incentive spirometer should be constantly within arm's length of the patient, and hourly use of this device should be encouraged. The nasogastric tube is removed on postoperative day 3, and the patient is allowed ice chips in the mouth. The thoracic epidural catheter is removed the afternoon after the chest tube is removed. The diet is gradually advanced so that a soft diet is begun on postoperative day 5 or 6. A barium swallow is performed on postoperative day 6 in preparation for hospital discharge on day 7 or 8.

Ivor Lewis Esophagectomy

Steps 1 through 5 Esophagoscopy is performed to confirm the location of the tumor. Steps 1 through 5 of an Ivor Lewis esophagectomy are virtually identical to the first five steps (i.e., the abdominal portion) of a transhiatal esophagectomy. Once complete mobilization of the stomach is verified, the pylorus is manually advanced to the level of the diaphragm to ensure that it is not being tethered by the duodenum or the greater omentum. Although it is possible to form the gastric tube in the chest, it is easier to do in the abdomen. Similar to step 9 in a transhiatal esophagectomy, a 5 to 6 cm wide gastric tube is created. The proximal divided stomach is sewn to a large Penrose drain. The other end of the drain is sutured to the tip of the gastric tube so that it can be pulled into the chest when needed. A jejunostomy is performed, and the laparotomy is closed.

Step 6: exposure and mobilization of esophagus The patient is shifted to the left lateral decubitus position and redraped. Single-lung ventilation is instituted, and the chest is entered through a right fifth interspace thoracotomy. The inferior pulmonary ligament is divided, and the lung is retracted cephalad. The esophagus is mobilized from the level of the diaphragm to a point above the azygos vein [*see Figure 18*], which can be divided with a vascular stapler. I prefer not to divide the vein as the azygos helps keep the stomach conduit in the midline for comfortable swallowing. The pleura overlying the esophagus is divided to the level of the thoracic inlet, superior to the azygos vein. The esophagus is encircled with a Penrose drain in the retrotracheal region. The pleura is then divided to the level of the diaphragm, with care taken to stay close to the right bronchus and the pericardium and avoid injury to the thoracic duct. The soft tissue between the esophagus and the aorta posteriorly and between the esophagus and the trachea or the pericardium anteriorly is dissected free and maintained en bloc with the esophagus. Periesophageal and subcarinal nodes are thereby mobilized [*see Figure 18b*].

Step 7: excision and removal of specimen The hiatus is incised, and the abdomen is entered. The stomach is drawn up into the chest, with care taken not to place excessive traction on the gastroepiploic pedicle. The esophagus is divided proximally at least 5 cm away from any grossly evident tumor, typically just below the thoracic inlet. The esophageal specimen is removed from the operative field, and proximal and distal margins are sent for frozen-section examination. [*see Figure 19*]. The stomach is positioned in the posterior mediastinum with care to avoid any twisting.

Step 8: intrathoracic esophagogastric anastomosis The site of the esophagogastric anastomosis should be about 2 to 4 cm above the azygos vein. Several interrupted sutures are used to secure the transposed stomach to the adjacent pleura. The staple line on the esophagus is removed, and a

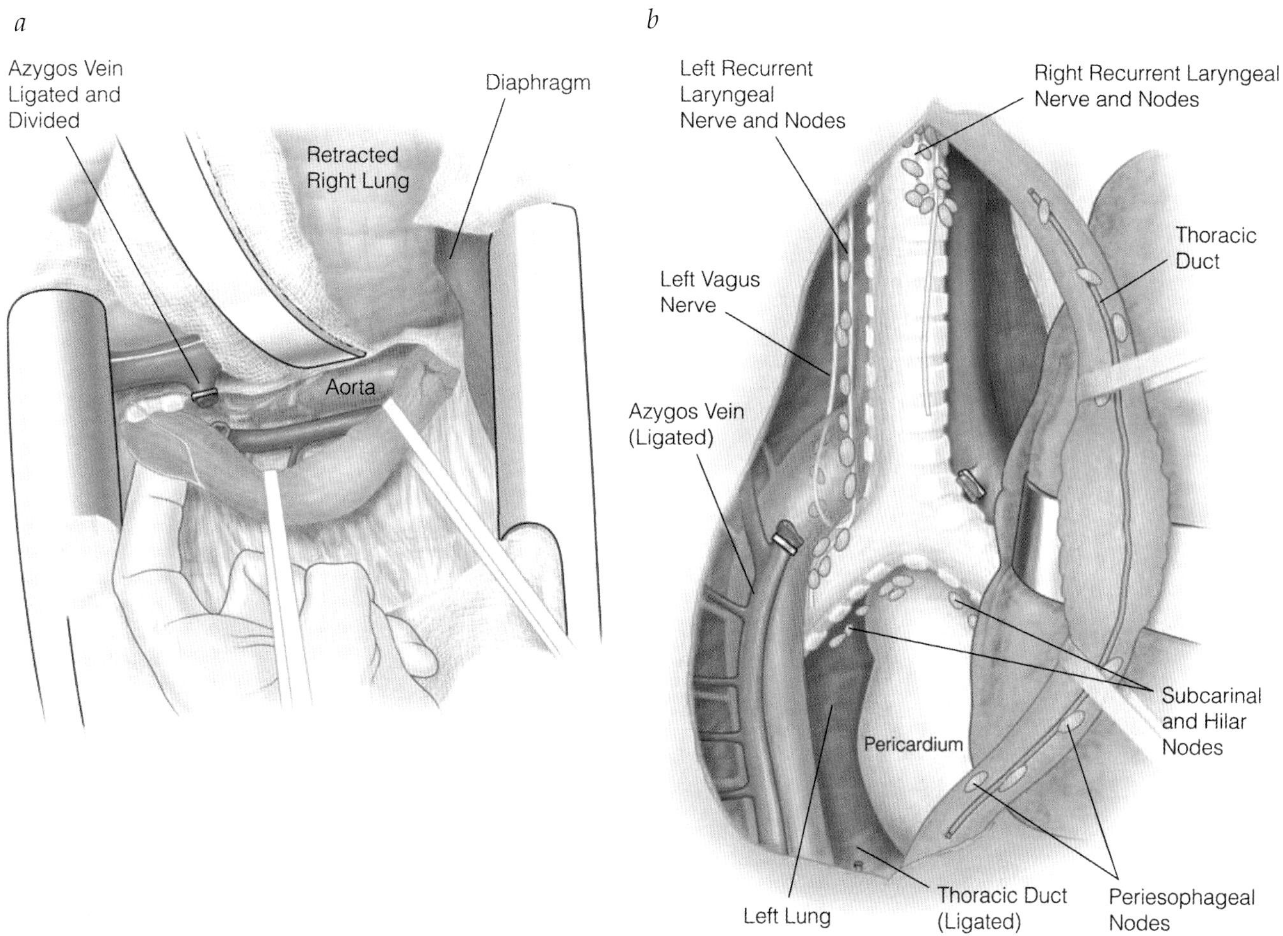

Figure 18 **Ivor Lewis esophagectomy. (*a*) The lung is retracted, and the azygos vein is stapled and divided. The esophagus and the vagi are mobilized from the level of the diaphragm to the thoracic inlet. (*b*) Dissection en bloc via right thoracotomy of the thoracic duct, the azygos vein, the ipsilateral pleura, and all periesophageal tissue in the mediastinum. The specimen includes the lower and middle mediastinal, subcarinal, and right-side paratracheal lymph nodes.**

gastrotomy is performed in preparation for a side-to-side functional EEA [*see Figure 20*]. With the aid of full-thickness traction sutures, the esophagus is positioned along the surface of the stomach and well away from the oversewn staple line defining the gastric resection margin. The posterior aspect of the anastomosis is completed with an endoscopic GIA stapler as described earlier [*see* Transhiatal Esophagectomy, Step 11, *above, and Figure 16 and Figure 17*]. A nasogastric tube is passed, and the anterior wall is completed in two layers. The first layer consists of a full-thickness continuous 3-0 polydioxanone suture; the second consists of interrupted absorbable sutures approximating the seromuscular layer of the stomach to the muscular layer of the esophagus.

Two alternative methods of anastomosis are sometimes used: (1) a totally handsewn end-to-side anastomosis and (2) a totally stapled EEA. I prefer a handsewn anastomosis, although it is no longer in vogue. An outer layer of interrupted 4-0 silk is used followed by a mucosal layer of interrupted inverting 4-0 silk [*see Figure 20*]. The stapled circular technique involves opening the previously placed gastric staple line and advancing the handle of an EEA stapler through the stomach. The proximal esophagus is dilated sufficiently to accommodate at least a 25 mm head. The anvil is placed into the distal esophagus and secured with a purse-string suture. The tip of the stapler is brought out through the apical wall of the stomach and attached to the anvil. The stapler is then fired to create the EEA, and the gastrotomy is closed. The advantages of this technique are its relative simplicity and the theoretical security of a completely stapled anastomosis; the main potential disadvantage is the risk of postoperative dysphagia resulting from an overly narrow anastomotic ring.

After completion of the anastomosis, the stomach is inspected for any potential redundancy or torsion in the chest. To prevent torsion, the stomach is anchored to the pericardium and pleura with nonabsorbable sutures. The diaphragmatic hiatus is then inspected: it should allow easy passage of two fingers into the abdomen alongside the transposed stomach. Interrupted sutures may be used to approximate the edge of the crura to the adjacent stomach wall, thereby preventing any later herniation of abdominal contents into the pleural space.

a

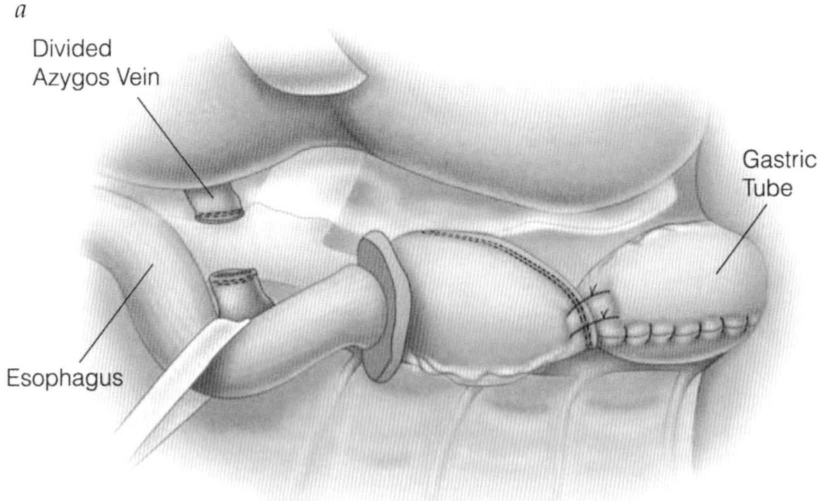

b

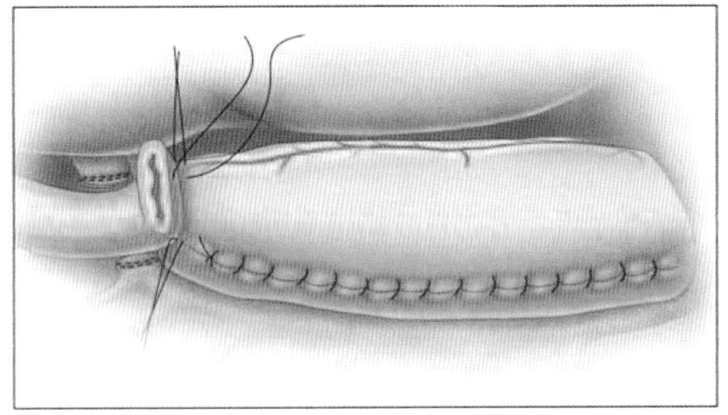

Figure 19 **Ivor Lewis esophagectomy. (*a*) After full mobilization of the esophagus, the gastric conduit (sutured to the divided proximal stomach) is pulled up into the chest. (*b*) An open anastomosis is begun at or above the level of the azygos vein.**

Step 9: drainage and closure A chest tube is placed. The tip of the chest drain is positioned alongside the stomach at the level of the anastomosis. Fine gut sutures secured to the adjacent parietal pleura will help maintain the position of the tube. The thoracotomy is then closed in the standard fashion.

Patients should begin walking on postoperative day 1. The nasogastric tube is generally removed on postoperative day 3. Oral intake is not begun at this point; feeding is accomplished via the temporary jejunostomy. A barium contrast study is performed approximately 5 to 7 days after the operation. If there is no anastomotic leakage, oral intake is initiated and advanced as tolerated. The chest tube and epidural catheter are removed, usually on day 4. Patients are generally discharged from the hospital by postoperative days 8 to 10.

Three-Hole Esophagectomy

Step 1: thoracotomy phase Esophagoscopy is performed to confirm the location of the tumor. A double-lumen endotracheal tube is placed. The first step is a right thoracotomy and mobilization of the esophagus and the regional lymph nodes, similar to step 6 of an Ivor Lewis esophagectomy. The chest is closed after esophageal mobilizaton is performed.

Step 2: abdominal and cervical phase The patient is turned back to the supine position. The double-lumen endotracheal tube is replaced by a standard single-lumen tube. Thereafter, the operation proceeds exactly like a transhiatal esophagectomy with steps 1 through 12. The mediastinal phase is, of course, much easier because all of the dissection was done in the thoracotomy phase of the operation.

Patients should begin walking on postoperative day 1. The nasogastric tube is generally removed on postoperative day 3. Oral intake is not begun at this point; feeding is accomplished via the temporary jejunostomy. A barium contrast study is performed approximately 5 to 7 days after the operation. If there is no anastomotic leakage, oral intake is initiated and advanced as tolerated. The chest tube and epidural catheter are removed, usually on day 4. Patients are generally discharged from the hospital by postoperative days 8 to 10.

Left Thoracoabdominal Esophagogastrectomy

Step 1: incision and entry into peritoneum The patient is placed in the right lateral position, with the hips rotated backward about 30°. An exploratory laparotomy is performed through an oblique incision extending from the tip of the sixth costal cartilage to a point about halfway between the sternum and the umbilicus. The peritoneal cavity is carefully examined to rule out peritoneal and hepatic metastases. The region of the cardia is palpated, and the mobility of the tumor is assessed. If there is minor involvement of the crura or the

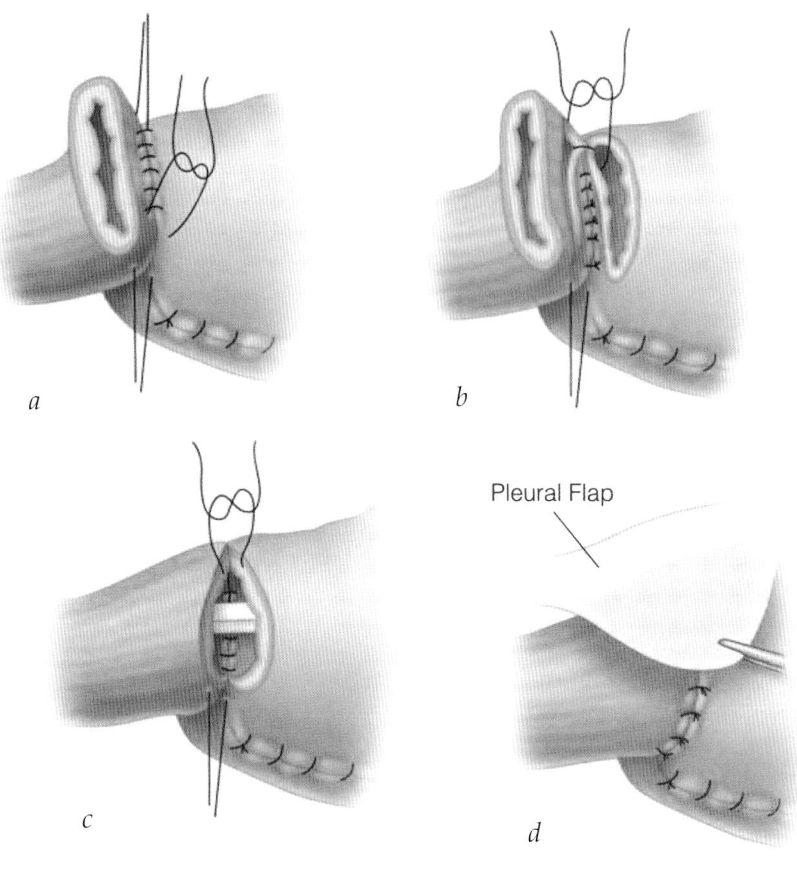

Figure 20 **Ivor Lewis esophagectomy. The two-layer anastomosis is performed with fine 4-0 sutures in an interrupted fashion. It is important to locate the gastrostomy away from the turned-in lesser curve suture line to avoid ischemia. (*a*) Posterior layer. (*b*) Posterior inner mucosal layer. (*c*) Anterior mucosal layer. (*d*) After the anterior seromuscular layer is done, local pleura is used to cover the anastomosis to buttress it and to keep the conduit in the middle of the mediastinum. The anastomosis can also be completed as in a transhiatal esophagectomy or with an end-to-end anastomosis [*see Figure 16 and Figure 17*].**

tail of the pancreas, resection may still be possible; however, if the tumor is firmly fixed or there are peritoneal or hepatic metastases, resection should be abandoned. A feeding jejunostomy, an esophageal stent, or both may be inserted to improve swallowing and allow nutrition.

Step 2: assessment of gastric involvement and incision of diaphragm The extent to which the tumor involves the stomach determines whether a total gastrectomy or a proximal gastrectomy is indicated along with the distal esophagectomy. If no metastases are found, the incision is extended and the chest is opened with a left posterolateral incision through the sixth interspace. If the thoracic component of the tumor appears to be resectable, the costal margin is divided. It is advisable to remove a 1 to 2 cm segment of the costal margin to facilitate repair of the diaphragm at the end of the operation and reduce postoperative costal margin pain. The diaphragm is incised radially. Alternatively, a circumferential incision may be made about 2 cm from the costal margin to reduce the risk of postoperative diaphragmatic paralysis.

Step 3: division of pulmonary ligament and mobilization of esophagus and stomach The pulmonary ligament is divided, and the mediastinal pleura is incised over the esophagus as far as the aortic arch. The esophagus is mobilized above the tumor and is retracted by a Penrose drain. The esophageal vessels are carefully dissected, ligated, and divided. The tumor is mobilized; the plane of the dissection is kept close to the aorta on the left, and, if necessary, the right parietal pleura is taken in continuity with the lesion. About 1 cm of the crura is taken in continuity with the tumor to provide good local clearance. The stomach is then mobilized in much the same way as in a transhiatal esophagectomy [*see Figure 9*].

Step 4: assessment of pancreatic involvement and hepatic viability The lesser sac is opened through the greater omentum so that it can be determined whether the primary tumor involves the distal pancreas. If so, it is reasonable to resect the distal pancreas, the spleen, or both in continuity with the stomach; if not, the short gastric vessels are ligated and divided, with the spleen preserved. The lesser omentum is detached from the right side of the esophagus and the hilum of the liver and then divided down to the area of the pylorus, with the right gastric artery and vein preserved. There is often a hepatic branch from the left gastric artery running through the gastrohepatic omentum. If this hepatic branch is of significant size, a soft vascular clamp should be placed on the artery for 20 minutes so that the viability of the liver can be assessed. If the liver is viable, the artery is suture-ligated and divided.

Step 5: division of greater omentum and short gastric vessels The greater omentum is divided, with care taken to preserve the right gastroepiploic artery and vein. These two vessels are suture-ligated and divided well away from the stomach. Ligation and division of the short gastric vessels allow complete mobilization of the greater curvature of the stomach. Dissection is extended downward as far as the pylorus. The stomach is turned upward, and the left gastric vessels are exposed through the lesser sac [*see Figure 10*]. The lymph nodes along the celiac axis and the left gastric artery are swept up into the specimen, and the gastric vessels are either suture-ligated or stapled and divided.

Step 6: choice of partial or total gastrectomy At this time, the surgeon determines whether the whole stomach must be resected to remove the gastric part of the cancer or whether a partial (i.e., proximal) gastrectomy will suffice.

If the surgeon decides that resection of the proximal stomach will remove all of the tumor while leaving at least 5 cm of tumor-free stomach, a proximal esophagogastrectomy is performed [*see Figure 21*]. A gastric tube is fashioned with a linear stapler [*see* Transhiatal Esophagectomy, Step 9, *above, and Figure 15*]. The staple line is oversewn with inverting 3-0 or 4-0 sutures. Because the vagus nerves are divided and gastric stasis may result, a pyloromyotomy may be performed, much as in a transhiatal esophagectomy.

The proximal gastric resection margin is covered with a sponge and turned upward over the costal margin. The stomach tube is then brought up through the hiatus and into the thorax behind the proximal esophageal resection margin [*see Figure 21*]. The margin should be at least 10 cm from the proximal end of the esophagogastric cancer. If the esophageal resection margin is not adequate, the stomach tube is mobilized and brought to the left neck and then anastomosed to the cervical esophagus through a left neck incision; alternatively, the left colon is interposed between the gastric stump and the cervical esophagus. If the resection margin is adequate, the tip of the stomach tube is anastomosed to the esophagus by any of the previously described techniques [*see Figure 22*].

The anastomosis is then performed with the stapling technique previously described for transhiatal esophagectomy [*see Figure 16 and Figure 17*]. A nasogastric tube is passed down into the gastric remnant. The tube is sewn to the pericardium and the endothoracic fascia to prevent torsion or herniation into the pleural space.

Total gastrectomy with Roux-en-Y esophagojejunostomy If the surgeon decides that a total gastrectomy is necessary, the right gastroepiploic and right gastric vessels are suture-ligated and divided distal to the pylorus. The duodenum is divided just distal to the pylorus with a linear stapler. The staple line is inverted with interrupted 3-0 nonabsorbable sutures and covered with omentum to prevent duodenal stump blowout.

The esophagus is then mobilized up to the level of the inferior pulmonary vein. Two retaining sutures are placed in the esophageal wall. A monofilament nylon purse-string suture is placed around the circumference of the proximal esophagus in preparation for stapling. The resected specimen is sent to the pathologist for examination of the margins.

A jejunal interposition is then fashioned by using the Roux-en-Y technique. One or two jejunal arteriovenous arcades are divided to mobilize enough jejunum to allow anastomosis to the thoracic esophagus [*see Figure 23*]. A 25 or 28 mm EEA stapler is passed through the jejunum into the

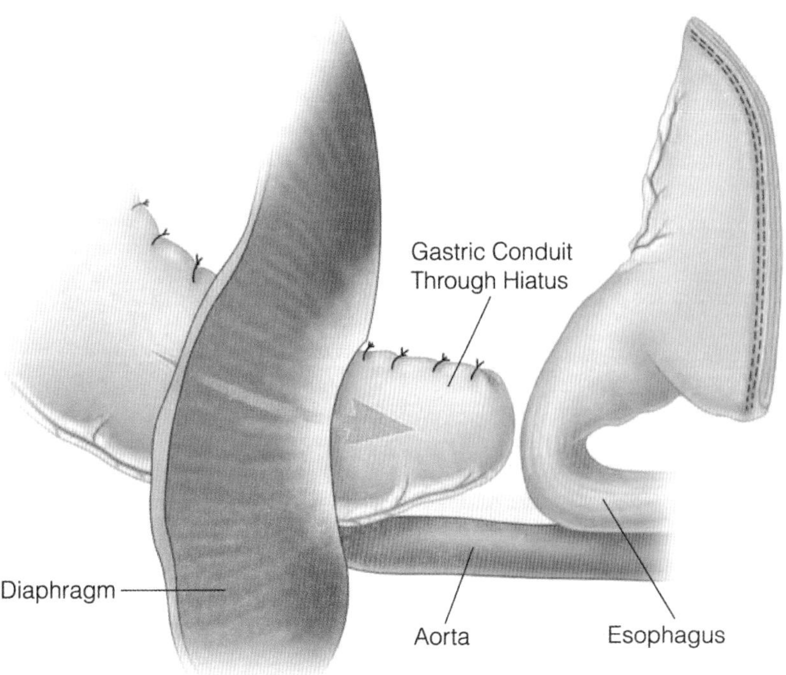

Figure 21 **Left thoracoabdominal esophagogastrectomy. The diaphragm is incised radially sparing major branches of the phrenic nerve. The pulmonary ligament is divided, and the esophagus is mobilized above the tumor and retracted with a Penrose drain. The esophageal vessels are ligated and divided. The tumor and the esophagus are mobilized off the aorta down to the hiatus; 1 cm of the diaphragmatic crura is taken in continuity with the tumor to provide local clearance. The stomach is then mobilized in much the same way as in a transhiatal esophagectomy and brought through the diaphragmatic hiatus [*see Figure 9*].**

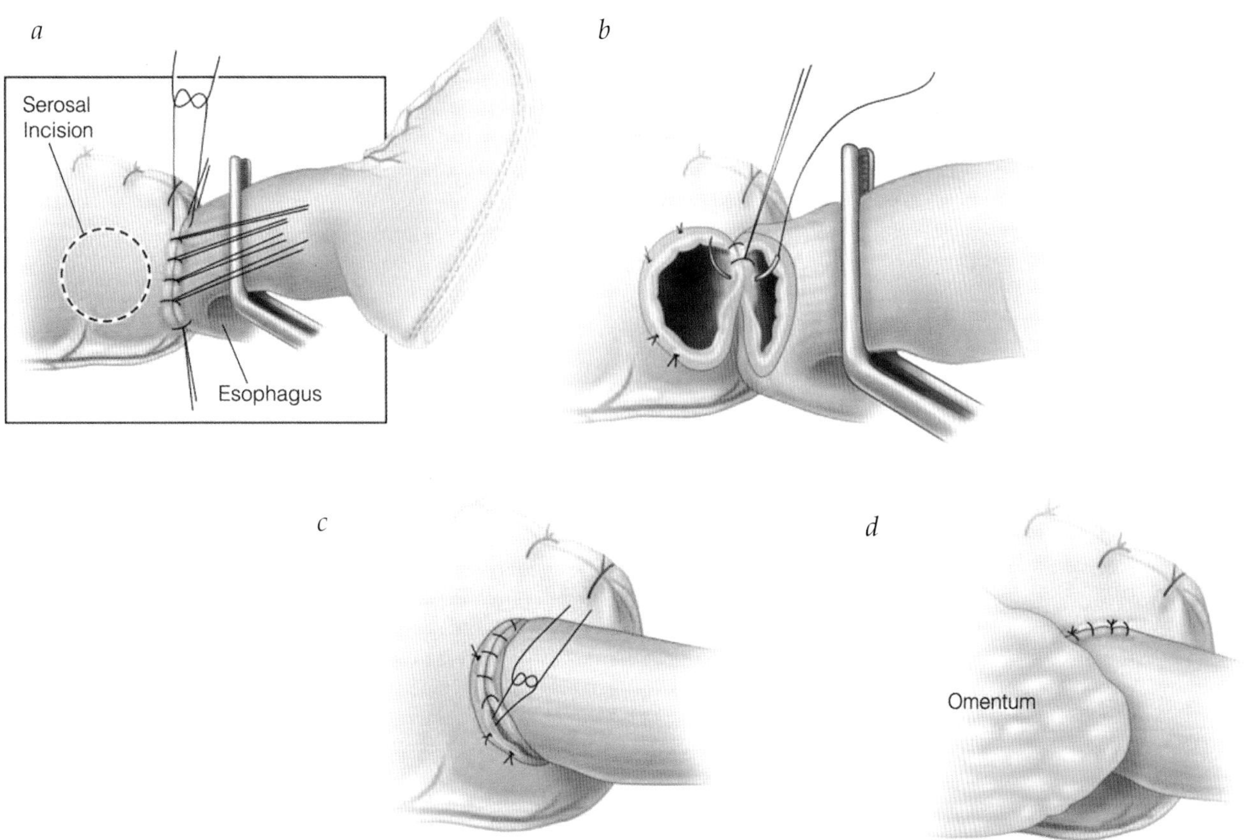

Figure 22 **Left thoracoabdominal esophagogastrectomy: proximal esophagogastrectomy with esophagogastrostomy. The esophagus is sewn to the tip of the stomach tube, halfway between the lesser curvature suture line and the greater curvature. (*a*) The Sweet anastomosis developed at the Massachusetts General Hospital. The outer posterior layer is performed with fine 4-0 silk sutures. A serosal "button" is inscribed with a scalpel down to the level of the submucosal vascular plexus. Fine 4-0 silk sutures are used to ligate these vessels so they do not obscure the anastomosis while it is being performed. (*b*) The gasric button is excised, and the inner posterior layer is anastomosed with interrupted 4-0 silks. This is continued anteriorly as well. (*c*) The outer anterior layer is performed also with interrupted 4-0 silks. (*d*) A tag of omentum from the high greater curve is sutured over the anastomosis to buttress it. Alternatively, an anastomosis can be fashioned with the stapling technique used in transhiatal esophagectomy or with an end-to-end anastomosis [*see Figure 16 and Figure 17*].**

esophagus, fired, and removed. The jejunum is anchored to the pericardium and the proximal esophagus. The duodenal loop is anastomosed to the jejunum at least 45 to 50 cm distal to the esophagojejunal anastomosis to minimize bile reflux [*see Figure 23*]. The blind end of the jejunal loop is then stapled closed.

After careful irrigation of the chest, the first step in the closure is to repair the diaphragm around the hiatus. The gastric or jejunal interposition is sewn to the crura with interrupted nonabsorbable sutures. The remainder of the diaphragm is closed with interrupted nonabsorbable 0 mattress sutures. A chest tube is placed into the pleural space close to but not touching the anastomosis. The final sutures in the peripheral part of the diaphragm are placed but are not tied until the ribs are brought together with pericostal sutures. The left lung is reexpanded. The costal cartilages are not approximated but are left to float free. If the ends of the costal margin are abutting, another 2 cm of costal cartilage should be removed to reduce postoperative pain. Thoracic and abdominal skin layers are closed with a continuous absorbable suture. The skin and the subcutaneous tissue are closed in the usual fashion.

POSTOPERATIVE CARE

As a rule, patients are not routinely admitted to the intensive care unit after esophagectomy; however, individual practices depend on the distribution of skilled nursing and physiotherapy personnel. Early ambulation is the mainstay of postoperative care. As a rule, patients are able to walk slowly, with assistance, on postoperative day 1. Patient-controlled epidural analgesia is particularly useful in facilitating good pulmonary toilet and minimizing the risk of atelectasis or pneumonia.

The nasogastric tube is removed on postoperative day 3 or 4; jejunostomy tube feedings are gradually started at the same time. Once bowel function normalizes, patients are allowed small sips of liquids. Chest tubes are removed as pleural drainage subsides. By postoperative day 6, most patients have progressed to a soft solid diet. Dietary education is provided, focusing primarily on eating smaller and more frequent meals,

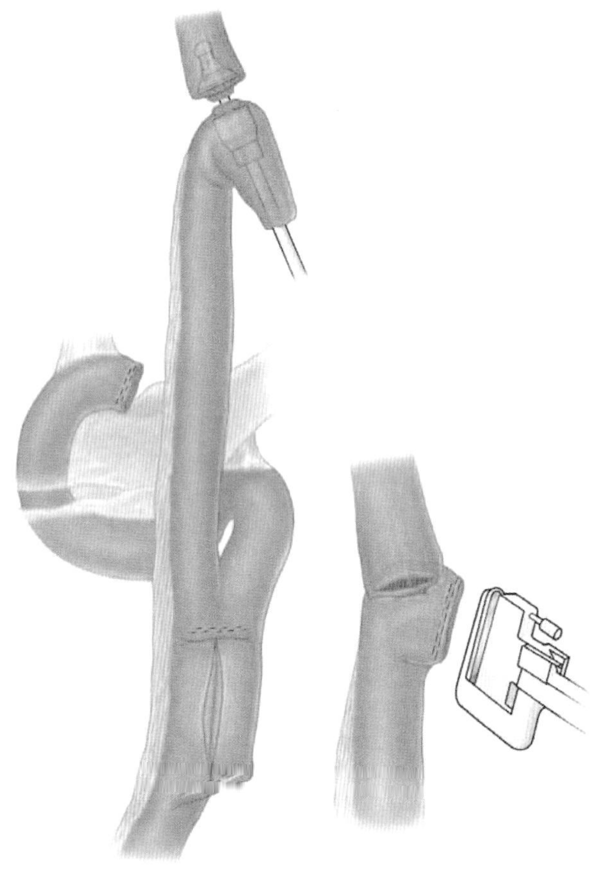

Figure 23 **Left thoracoabdominal esophagogastrectomy: total gastrectomy with Roux-en-Y esophagojejunostomy. A jejunal interposition is fashioned with the Roux-en-Y technique. One or two jejunal arteriovenous arcades are divided to mobilize enough jejunum for anastomosis to the thoracic esophagus. A 25 or 28 mm end-to-end anastomosis stapler is passed through the jejunum into the esophagus. The jejunum is anchored to the pericardium and the proximal esophagus. The duodenal loop is anastomosed to the jejunum at least 45 to 50 cm distal to the esophagojejunal anastomosis. The blind end of the jejunal loop is then stapled closed.**

avoiding bulky foods (e.g., meat and bread) in the early postoperative period, and taking measures to minimize postprandial dumping. Patients are also taught how to care for their temporary feeding jejunostomy. Consumption of caffeine and carbonated beverages is usually limited during the first few weeks after discharge.

A barium swallow is performed on postoperative day 7 to verify the integrity of the anastomosis and gastric emptying. Patients are usually discharged on postoperative day 7 or 8. The feeding jejunostomy is left in place until the first postoperative evaluation, which usually takes place 2 to 3 weeks after the operation. The feeding tube is removed during that visit if oral intake and weight are stable.

COMPLICATIONS OF ESOPHAGECTOMY

Pulmonary Impairment

Atelectasis and pneumonia should be considered preventable complications of esophagectomy. Patients with recognized preoperative impairment of pulmonary reserve should be considered for transhiatal esophagectomy. Existing pulmonary function can be optimized through incentive spirometry, use of bronchodilators, and physical rehabilitation. Chronic nocturnal aspiration from esophageal obstruction should be watched for in the postoperative patient; the head of the bed should be elevated 30° to 45° as a preventive measure. Effective pain control is essential to prevent postoperative atelectasis. Routine use of patient-controlled thoracic epidural analgesia should be considered. Deep breathing, early ambulation, and chest physiotherapy encourage the clearing of bronchial secretions. Certain patients will require nasotracheal aspiration or bronchoscopy for pulmonary toilet.

Tracheobronchial Injury

On rare occasions, lacerations of the membranous trachea or the left mainstem bronchus occur during esophagectomy. When such injuries occur during transthoracic resection, management is relatively simple, thanks to the already excellent operative exposure. Direct suture repair and tissue reinforcement with adjacent pleura or a pedicle of intercostal muscle provide safe closure in almost all cases. When tracheobronchial injuries occur during transhiatal esophagectomy, they are less obvious but no less urgent. This rare complication arises during mediastinal dissection. Typically, the anesthetic team notes a loss of ventilatory volume, and the surgeon may detect the smell of inhalational agents in the operative field. Bronchoscopy should be promptly performed to identify the site of the injury. The uncut endotracheal tube is then advanced over the bronchoscope and past the site of the laceration to restore proper ventilation. High tracheal injuries can usually be repaired by extending the cervical incision and adding a partial sternotomy. Injury to the carina or the left mainstem bronchus must be repaired via a right thoracotomy.

Bleeding

Hemorrhage should be rare during esophagectomy. In routine situations, blood loss should amount to less than 500 mL. The blood supply to the esophagus consists of small branches coming from the aorta, which are easily controlled and generally constrict even if left untied. Splenic injuries sometimes occur during mobilization of the stomach. The resultant hemorrhage can be immediate or delayed; blood loss may be significant, and splenectomy is usually required. Precise dissection around the left gastric artery is vital: the bleeding vessels may retract, and attempts at control may result in injury to the celiac artery or its hepatic branches. Similarly, peripancreatic vessels may be difficult to control if inadvertently injured during the Kocher maneuver.

Bleeding that arises during the mediastinal stage of the transhiatal esophagectomy generally subsides with packing if it derives from periesophageal arterial branches. Brisk loss of dark blood usually signifies injury to the azygos vein. The first step in addressing such injuries is to pack the mediastinum quickly so as to allow the anesthetic team to stabilize the patient and restore volume. Chest tubes are immediately placed to allow detection of any free hemorrhage into the pleural space. Precise localization of the bleeding site may then follow. Injury to the azygos vein may be addressed via an upper sternal split; however, when the exposure is poor, the surgeon should not hesitate to proceed to a full sternotomy. Bleeding from the subcarinal area is usually bright red and may involve bronchial arteries or small periesophageal vessels arising from the aorta, both of which can usually be controlled through the hiatus with a long-handled pistol-grip clip applier or electrocautery.

Laryngeal Nerve Injury

Injury to the recurrent laryngeal nerve is a major potential complication of transhiatal esophagectomy. Traction neuropraxia may be temporary and require no specific treatment. Permanent injury will lead to hoarseness and impaired protection of the airway during deglutition. Pneumonia from aspiration is a major problem. Meticulous protection of the nerve during the cervical stage should minimize the incidence of this complication. If laryngeal nerve injury becomes apparent in the postoperative period, early medialization of the affected cord should be performed by an otolaryngologist to enhance the ability of the patient to cough and to prevent aspiration.

Of particular concern is the risk of bilateral nerve injury after a transthoracic esophagectomy with a cervical esophagogastric anastomosis (i.e., a so-called three-hole esophagectomy). Any dissection of the upper esophagus performed through the right chest should be done as close to the esophagus as possible to avoid placing traction on the right recurrent laryngeal nerve; the subsequent left cervical dissection may put the left recurrent laryngeal nerve at risk for damage. Bilateral paralysis of the vocal cords is very poorly tolerated and has a devastating impact on quality of life.

Chylothorax

Thoracic duct injuries typically present by postoperative day 3 or 4. Dyspnea and pleural effusion may be noted if thoracostomy tubes are not in place. Thoracentesis yields an opaque, milky fluid. In patients who already have a chest drain in place, there is typically a high volume of serous drainage in the first 2 postoperative days. As enteral nutrition is established and dietary fat is reintroduced, the fluid assumes a characteristic milky appearance. In most cases, the gross appearance is diagnostic, and there is rarely a need to confirm the diagnosis by measuring the triglyceride level. A thoracostomy drain is placed to monitor the volume of the chyle leak if one is not present. Chest x-rays should be obtained to verify complete drainage of the pleural space and full expansion of the lung.

Patients with chylothorax should be converted to fat-free enteral nutrition. Persistent drainage exceeding 500 mL per day is an indication for early operation and ligation of the thoracic duct; high-volume chyle leaks are unlikely to close spontaneously. Prolonged loss of chyle causes significant electrolyte, nutritional, and immunologic derangements that may prove fatal if allowed to progress. Accordingly, patients with persistent chyle leakage should undergo operation within 1 week of diagnosis. A feeding tube is placed in the duodenum before operation if a jejunostomy tube is not already in place. Jejunal feeding with 35% cream at a rate of 60 to 80 mL/hr is maintained for at least 4 hours before operation. Feeding is continued even during the procedure: the enteral fat stimulates a brisk flow of chyle and greatly facilitates visualization of any thoracic duct injury.

Right-side chyle leaks are approached via either a thoracotomy or video-assisted thoracoscopy. The magnification and excellent illumination associated with thoracoscopy are partially counterbalanced by the constraints imposed by port placement and limited tissue retraction. The inferior pulmonary ligament is divided, and the posterior mediastinum is inspected for extravasation of milky fluid. Any visible sources of chyle leakage can be controlled with clips or suture ligatures. In some cases, mass ligation of the thoracic duct at the level of the diaphragm, incorporating all of the soft tissue between the aorta and the azygos vein, may be required.

Left-side leaks can be difficult to manage. The subcarinal area is typically involved; this is the level at which the thoracic duct crosses over from the right. Exploration should begin on the left side. If the leak cannot be visualized, a right-side approach may be necessary to control the thoracic duct as it first enters the chest.

Anastomotic Leakage

The consequences of anastomotic complications after esophagectomy vary considerably in severity, depending on their location and cause. The cervical anastomotic leaks that may develop after transhiatal esophagectomy are generally simple to treat. Leaks in the early postoperative period are usually related to technical factors (e.g., excessive tension across the anastomosis). A nonviable stomach may not give rise to obvious signs; thus, any possibility of ischemia in the transposed stomach must be addressed promptly. Tachycardia, confusion, leukocytosis, cervical wound drainage, and neck tenderness may or may not be present.

The morbidity of an open cervical wound is not high—it is certainly lower than that of an untreated leak. Accordingly, any clinical suspicion of a leak should prompt a diagnostic contrast swallow study using dilute barium. Large leaks are manifested as persistent collections of contrast material outside the esophagus. Although such leaks rarely extend into the pleural space, any fluid in the chest must be drained so that its nature can be determined. The neck wound is opened by removing the sutures and performing gentle digital exploration of the prevertebral space behind the esophagus as the finger is advanced into the mediastinum; this is usually done at the bedside and requires little, if any, patient sedation.

Saline-moistened gauze packing is changed three or four times a day. Prolonged or copious cervical drainage may call for supplemental deep wound aspiration with a Yankauer suction handle. Administering water orally during aspiration facilitates removal of any necrotic debris. A fetid, malodorous breath associated with sanguineous discharge from the nasogastric tube and purulent fluid in the opened neck incision are ominous signs that should prompt early esophagoscopy. Diffuse mucosal ischemia may indicate the presence of a nonviable stomach; reoperation with completion gastrectomy and proximal esophagostomy is required to treat this rare catastrophic complication.

Generally, leaks that occur more than 7 days after operation are small and are related to some degree of late ischemic disruption along the anastomosis. They can usually be managed by opening the cervical wound at the bedside and packing the site with gauze. Oral diet is advanced as tolerated. It may be noted that the volume of the leak is markedly greater or less depending on the position of the head during swallowing. Accordingly, before discharge, patients are taught how to temporarily adjust their swallowing and how to manage their dressing changes. Applying gentle pressure to the neck wound and turning the head to the left may help the patient ingest liquids with minimal soiling of the open neck incision. Dysphagia, even with an opened neck incision, should be treated by passing tapered esophageal dilators orally between 2 and 4 weeks after surgery. When a bougie at least 48 French in caliber can be passed through the anastomosis, the patient can usually swallow comfortably. The size of the leak often decreases after dilation as food is allowed to proceed preferentially into the stomach. To maximize the diameter of the anastomosis and reduce the likelihood of a symptomatic stricture, subsequent dilations should be scheduled at 2-week intervals for the next few months.

When a routine predischarge barium swallow after transhiatal esophagectomy raises the possibility of an anastomotic leak in an asymptomatic patient, the question arises of whether the wound should be opened at all. For small, contained leaks associated with preferential flow of contrast material into the stomach, observation alone may suffice in selected cases. Patients must be closely watched for fever or other signs of major infection. Given the quite low morbidity of cervical wound exploration, the surgeon should not hesitate to drain the neck if the patient's condition changes.

The incidence of anastomotic leakage is low after Ivor Lewis resection, but the consequences are significant. Leaks presenting early in the postoperative period are usually related to technical problems and are difficult to manage; those presenting later are generally related to some degree of ischemic tissue loss. Patients who have received radiation therapy or are nutritionally depleted may be especially vulnerable to problems with anastomotic healing. A contrast swallow with dilute barium is the best method of evaluating the anastomosis. Leaks may be manifested either as a free flow of contrast into the pleural space or as a contained fluid collection.

Small leaks that drain immediately into properly placed thoracostomy tubes can usually be managed by giving antibiotics and withholding oral intake. Local control of infection generally results in spontaneous healing. Anastomotic disruptions that are large or are associated with a major pleural collection typically necessitate open drainage with decortication; percutaneous drainage may be considered as a preliminary approach in selected patients. Persistent soiling of the mediastinum and the pleural space is fatal if untreated.

Early esophagoscopy is strongly advised to evaluate the viability of the gastric remnant. Ischemic necrosis of the stomach necessitates reexploration, decortication, takedown of the anastomosis, gastric débridement, return of any viable stomach into the abdomen, closure of the hiatus, and proximal diversion with a cervical esophagostomy. Repair or revision of the anastomosis in an infected field is certain to fail and should never be considered. In certain cases, diversion via a cervical esophagostomy and a completion gastrectomy may be required.

Late Complications

At every postoperative visit, symptoms of reflux, regurgitation, dumping, poor gastric emptying, and dysphagia must be specifically sought: these are the major quality-of-life issues for postesophagectomy patients.[4] Reflux and regurgitation may complicate any form of alimentary reconstruction after esophagectomy, although cervical anastomoses are less likely to be associated with symptomatic reflux than intrathoracic anastomoses are. Reflux symptoms generally respond to dietary modifications, such as smaller and more frequent meals. Regurgitation is usually related to the supine position and thus tends to be worse at night; elevating the bed and avoiding late meals may suffice for symptom control. Dumping is exacerbated by foods with high fat or sugar content. Dysphagia may be related to narrowing at the anastomosis or, in rare instances, to poor emptying of the transposed stomach. Anastomotic strictures are most commonly encountered as a sequel to a postoperative leak. There may be excessive scarring at the anastomosis, associated with local distortion or angulation. Specific tests for gastric atony include nuclear medicine gastric emptying studies using radiolabeled food. A simple barium swallow may indicate an incomplete pyloromyotomy as a cause of poor gastric emptying; balloon dilation often corrects this problem.

Any form of anastomotic leak will increase the incidence of late stricture. Dysphagia may be treated by means of progressive dilation with Maloney bougies. This procedure is performed in the outpatient clinic and often does not require sedation or any other special patient preparation. Complications are rare if due care is exercised during the procedure. As noted [*see* Transthoracic Hiatal Hernia Repair, Preoperative Evaluation, Dilation, *above*], it is essential that the caliber of the dilators be increased gradually and that little or no force be applied in advancing them. The appearance of blood on a withdrawn dilator signals a breach of the mucosa; further dilation should be done cautiously lest a transmural injury results. Comfortable swallowing, of liquids at least, is usually achieved after the successful passage of a 48 French bougie. It is preferable, however, to advance dilation until at least a 54 French bougie can be passed with ease. For late strictures that are particularly difficult to dilate, endoscopic examination and histologic evaluation may be required to rule out a recurrent tumor. CT of the chest should also be performed whenever there is unexplained weight loss or fatigue late after esophagectomy.

The Savary system of wire-guided dilators has been particularly helpful in the management of tight or eccentric strictures. Patients are generally treated in the endoscopy suite. Temporary sedation with intravenous fentanyl and midazolam is required. Fluoroscopy can be used to confirm proper placement of a flexible-tip wire across the stricture. Serial wire-guided dilation can then be performed with confidence and increased patient safety.

OUTCOME EVALUATION

Transhiatal Esophagectomy

A 2001 study from the University of Michigan presented data on 1,085 patients who underwent transhiatal esophagectomy without thoracotomy, of whom 74% had carcinoma and 26% had nonmalignant disease.[5] Transhiatal esophagectomy was completed in 98.6% of the patients; the remaining 1.4% were converted to a transthoracic esophagectomy as a result of either thoracic esophageal fixation or bleeding.

Previous chemotherapy or radiation therapy did not preclude performance of a transhiatal esophagectomy. Nine patients experienced inordinate intraoperative blood loss; three died as a result. The overall hospital mortality was 4%. The overall 5-year survival rate for patients undergoing transhiatal esophagectomy is approximately 20% for adenocarcinoma of the cardia and the esophagus and 30% for squamous cell carcinoma of the esophagus.

The stapled anastomosis described earlier [*see* Operative Technique, Transhiatal Esophagectomy, Step 8, *above*] reflects numerous refinements introduced at the University of Michigan. The endoscopic GIA stapler has a low-profile head that is ideally suited to the tight confines of the neck, enabling the surgeon to fashion a widely patent side-to-side functional EEA with three rows of staples along the back wall. The rate of anastomotic stricture is markedly lower with this anastomosis than with a totally handsewn anastomosis. As regards postoperative function, stomach interposition through the posterior mediastinum after transhiatal esophagectomy is associated with low rates of aspiration and regurgitation. Esophageal reflux and esophagitis—commonly seen with intrathoracic esophagogastric anastomoses—are usually not clinically significant problems with this approach. Patients are advised to elevate the head of their bed and to continue taking acid blockers for about 3 months after the operation. Approximately one third will require esophageal dilation for dysphagia after the operation. Some 7 to 10% experience postvagotomy dumping symptoms, which, in most cases, can be controlled by simply avoiding high-carbohydrate foods and dairy products.

Ivor Lewis Esophagectomy

Ivor Lewis esophagectomy is associated with anastomotic leakage rates and operative mortalities of less than 3%.[3,6] Approximately 5% of patients will require anastomotic dilation. Again, patients are advised to elevate the head of the bed and to continue taking acid blockers if they have any reflux symptoms. In some patients, the gastric interposition rotates into the right posterolateral thoracic gutter, resulting in postprandial gastric tension and rendering them more susceptible to aspiration. Compared to transhiatal esophagectomy, extended transthoracic esophagectomy is associated with higher pulmonary morbidity but no difference in operative mortality or in 5-year survival. A post hoc subset analysis did suggest a survival advantage of transthoracic resection with one to eight positive lymph nodes.[7,8]

Three-Hole Esophagectomy

Three-hole esophagectomy is also associated with low anastomotic leak rates and mortality similar to Ivor Lewis esophagectomy.[9] Again, patients are advised to elevate the head of the bed and to continue taking acid blockers if they have any reflux symptoms. In some patients, the gastric interposition rotates into the right posterolateral thoracic gutter, resulting in postprandial gastric tension and rendering them more susceptible to aspiration. A special note should be made that cervical leaks with a three-hole esophagectomy can be more problematic than with a transhiatal esophagectomy presumably because of the wide opening of the mediastinum resulting in a greater tendency of leaks to track down into the mediastinum.

Left Thoracoabdominal Esophagogastrectomy

Left thoracoabdominal esophagogastrectomy is also associated with anastomotic leakage rates and operative mortalities of less than 3%.[3,10] Approximately 5% of patients will require esophageal dilation. Reconstructions involving anastomosis of the distal stomach to the esophagus are associated with a higher incidence of bile gastritis and esophagitis. Of all the operations we have described, this one results in the lowest postoperative quality of life. Accordingly, most surgeons prefer to carry out a total gastrectomy. Swallowing is restored with a Roux-en-Y jejunal interposition.

Financial Disclosures: None Reported

References

1. Crescenzo DG, Trastek VF, Allen MS, et al. Zenker's diverticulum in the elderly: is operation justified? Ann Thorac Surg 1998;66:347.
2. Stirling MC, Orringer MB. Continued assessment of the combined Collis-Nissen operation. Ann Thorac Surg 1989;47:224.
3. Mathiesen DJ, Grillo HC, Wilkens EW Jr. Transthoracic esophagectomy: a safe approach to carcinoma of the esophagus. Ann Thorac Surg 1988;45:137.
4. Finley RJ, Lamy A, Clifton J, et al. Gastrointestinal function following esophagectomy for malignancy. Am J Surg 1995;169:471.
5. Orringer MB, Marshall B, Iannettoni MD. Transhiatal esophagectomy for treatment of benign and malignant esophageal disease. World J Surg 2001;25:196.
6. Visbal AL, Allen MS, Miller DL, et al. Ivor Lewis esophagogastrectomy for esophageal cancer. Ann Thorac Surg 2001;71:1803.
7. Hulscher JBF, van Sandick JW, de Boer AG, et al. Extended transthoracic resection compared with limited transhiatal resection for adenocarcinoma of the esophagus. N Engl J Med 2002;347:1662.
8. Omloo JMT, Lagarde SM, Hulscher JBF, et al. Extended transthoracic resection compared with limited transhiatal resection for adenocarcinoma of the mid/distal esophagus. Five year survival of a randomized clinical trial. Ann Surg 2007;246:992.
9. Swanson SJ, Battirel HF, Bueno R, et al. Transthoracic esophagectomy with radical mediastinal and abdominal lymph node dissection and cervical esophagastrostomy for esophageal carcinoma. Ann Thorac Surg 2001;72:1918.
10. Akiyama H, Miyazono H, Tsurumaru M, et al. Thoracoabdominal approach for carcinoma of the cardia of the stomach. Am J Surg 1979;137:345.

Acknowledgments

The authors and editors gratefully acknowledge the contributions of the previous authors, John Yee, MD, FRCSC, and Richard J. Finley, MD, FACS, FRCSC, to the development and writing of this chapter.

Figures 1 through 23 Tom Moore

8 MINIMALLY INVASIVE ESOPHAGEAL PROCEDURES

*Daniel C. Wiener, MD, and Jon O. Wee, MD, FACS**

In this chapter, we focus on minimally invasive surgical approaches to the treatment of the following benign esophageal disorders: gastroesophageal reflux disease (GERD), achalasia, and paraesophageal hernias. These minimally invasive procedures have continued to evolve over the past two decades, thanks to better instrumentation and improved surgical expertise. With greater experience and longer follow-up, it has become possible to analyze techniques and their results more rigorously. In most instances, laparoscopy has replaced open procedures as the standard of care. Nevertheless, equipoise remains in the literature regarding the benefits of surgery compared with alternative treatment strategies such as medications in the case of GERD or endoscopic procedures in the case of achalasia. As technologies such as transoral incisionless endoscopic fundoplication continue to evolve, the standards of care will continue to be challenged. The chapter is organized by surgical procedure, all of which are derivatives of the laparoscopic Nissen fundoplication described below.

Laparoscopic Nissen Fundoplication

GERD is defined as "a condition which develops when the reflux of stomach contents causes troublesome symptoms and/or complications."[1] Complications include esophagitis, stricture, or Barrett esophagus. GERD is quite prevalent, with up to 20% of adults in Western society experiencing symptoms of heartburn and/or reflux at some point in their lives,[2] and is the most frequent first-listed digestive system condition at ambulatory care visits every year in the United States.[3] Proton pump inhibitors (PPIs) are the third largest-selling drug class, generating more than $13.6 billion in sales in 2009.[4] Although there is an ongoing debate regarding the benefit of surgery versus medical management, a 2010 Cochrane systematic review of randomized, controlled trials reported improved outcome with laparoscopic fundoplication in the short to medium term.[5] There is also a growing body of literature categorizing the adverse effects of long-term use of PPIs, ranging from increased risk of *Clostridium difficile* to osteoporotic fractures.[6] According to Society of American Gastrointestinal and Endoscopic Surgeons (SAGES) guidelines published in 2010, indications for surgery include (1) failure of medical management, (2) patient preference, (3) complications of GERD (Barrett esophagus, peptic stricture), and (4) extraesophageal manifestations (asthma, hoarseness, cough, chest pain, aspiration).[7]

* The authors and editors gratefully acknowledge the contributions of the previous authors, Francesco Palazzo, MD, Piero M. Fisichella, MD, and Marco G. Patti, MD, FACS, to the development and writing of this chapter.

Here we present a standard approach to patients referred for surgical management of GERD. We briefly mention some of the controversies in both evaluation and surgical technique with the understanding that these issues are covered in more depth elsewhere in the literature.

PREOPERATIVE EVALUATION

Patients who are potential candidates for a laparoscopic fundoplication often undergo a battery of preoperative testing that includes the following: (1) symptomatic evaluation, (2) an upper gastrointestinal (GI) series, (3) endoscopy, (4) esophageal manometry, and (5) ambulatory pH monitoring. Below we discuss the relative merits of these studies.

Symptomatic Evaluation

Clinical symptoms of GERD are classically divided into typical (heartburn, regurgitation, and dysphagia) and atypical (cough, asthma, chest pain, dental erosions, and hoarseness). This is a significant distinction that has implications for the likelihood of success of the procedure. Specifically, there is a 95% success rate in controlling typical symptoms compared with a 53% success rate with atypical symptoms.[8]

Some physicians assert that the diagnosis can be made reliably from the clinical history,[9] so a complaint of heartburn should lead to the presumption that acid reflux is present; however, testing of this diagnostic strategy demonstrates that symptoms are far less sensitive and specific than is usually believed.[10] For instance, a study from the University of California, San Francisco (UCSF), found that of 822 consecutive patients referred for esophageal function tests with a clinical diagnosis of GERD (based on symptoms and endoscopic findings), only 70% had abnormal reflux on pH monitoring.[11] Heartburn and regurgitation were no more frequent in patients who had genuine reflux than in those who did not; thus, symptomatic evaluation, by itself, could not distinguish between the two groups.

The response to PPIs is a good predictor of abnormal reflux. In the UCSF study cited above, 75% of patients with GERD reported a good or excellent response to PPIs, compared with only 26% of patients without GERD.[11] Similarly, a study involving multivariate analysis of factors predicting outcome after laparoscopic fundoplication identified a clinical response to acid suppression therapy as one of three factors predictive of a successful outcome, the other two being an abnormal 24-hour pH score and the presence of a typical primary symptom (e.g., heartburn).[12] Given the unreliability of clinical history, a more definitive workup to confirm a diagnosis of GERD needs to be performed prior to proceeding with surgical intervention.

Upper GI Series

An upper GI series is useful for diagnosing and characterizing an existing hiatal hernia. The size of the hiatal hernia helps predict how difficult it will be to reduce the esophagogastric junction below the diaphragm, a critical component of a successful antireflux procedure. In addition, large hiatal hernias are associated with more severe disturbances of esophageal peristalsis and esophageal acid clearance.[13] Esophagograms are also useful for determining the location, shape, and size of a stricture.

Endoscopy

Endoscopy is helpful to assess the mucosal damage caused by reflux, although mucosal changes are absent in about 50% of GERD patients.[11] That said, there are major interobserver variations with esophageal endoscopy, particularly for low-grade esophagitis.[14] In one study, for instance, 60 (24%) of 247 patients with negative results on pH monitoring had been diagnosed as having grade I or II esophagitis.[11] Endoscopy can be helpful in identifying a hiatal hernia and is most valuable for detecting the presence of Barrett esophagus and excluding gastric and duodenal pathologic conditions.

Esophageal Manometry

Esophageal manometry provides useful information about the motor function of the esophagus by determining the length and resting pressure of the lower esophageal sphincter (LES) and assessing the quality (i.e., the amplitude and propagation) of esophageal peristalsis. In addition, it allows proper placement of the pH probe for ambulatory pH monitoring (5 cm above the upper border of the LES).

The notion of tailoring the type of fundoplication to the patient based on esophageal function is quite controversial and revolves around the issue of balancing postoperative dysphagia with effective antireflux control. Whereas short-term results of randomized, controlled trials comparing total versus partial fundoplication demonstrate less dysphagia and equivalent efficacy with partial wraps, retrospective studies with longer-term follow-up maintain superior results with total fundoplication.[7]

Ambulatory pH Monitoring

Ambulatory pH monitoring is the most reliable test for the diagnosis of GERD, with a sensitivity and specificity of about 92%.[15] It is of key importance in the workup for the following reasons:

1. It determines whether abnormal reflux is present. In the UCSF study mentioned earlier, pH monitoring yielded normal results in 30% of patients with a clinical diagnosis of GERD, thereby obviating the continuation of inappropriate and expensive drugs (e.g., PPIs) or the performance of a fundoplication.[11] In addition, pH monitoring prompted further investigation that in a number of cases pointed to other diseases (e.g., cholelithiasis and irritable bowel syndrome).
2. It establishes a temporal correlation between symptoms and episodes of reflux. Such a correlation is particularly important when atypical GERD symptoms (e.g., cough and chest pain) are present because 50% of these patients experience no heartburn and 50% do not have esophagitis on endoscopy.[16]
3. It allows staging on the basis of disease severity. Specifically, esophageal manometry and pH monitoring identify a subgroup of patients characterized by worse esophageal motor function (manifested by a defective LES or by abnormal esophageal peristalsis), more acid reflux in the distal and proximal esophagus, and slower acid clearance. These patients more frequently have Barrett metaplasia and experience respiratory symptoms; thus, they might benefit from early antireflux surgery.[17]
4. It provides baseline data that may prove useful postoperatively if symptoms do not respond to the procedure.

Combined multichannel intraluminal impedance and pH testing (MII-pH) has the ability to detect episodes of reflux, regardless of the pH of the refluxate, by identifying changes induced by the presence of a bolus in the esophagus; the episodes are then simply classified as acid or nonacid on the basis of concomitantly recorded pH values. Studies of healthy persons have demonstrated that MII-pH possesses increased sensitivity and specificity in detecting and characterizing gastroesophageal reflux, and the results have been shown to be highly reproducible.[18] Evaluation of bolus transit time can also provide a real-time evaluation of esophageal function. Impedance has also been demonstrated to be useful in the workup of patients with GERD refractory to PPIs and patients with respiratory symptoms of unknown origin.[19]

OPERATIVE TECHNIQUE

The patient is placed under general anesthesia and intubated with a single-lumen endotracheal tube. Abdominal wall relaxation is ensured by the administration of a nondepolarizing muscle relaxant, the action of which is rapidly reversed at the end of the operation. Adequate muscle relaxation is essential because increased abdominal wall compliance allows increased pneumoperitoneum, which yields better exposure. An orogastric tube is inserted at the beginning of the operation to keep the stomach decompressed. A Foley catheter is used routinely.

The patient is placed in a steep reverse Trendelenburg position. The surgeon stands off to the right side of the patient. To prevent the patient from sliding as a result of the steep position used during the operation, foot boards should be secured at the end of the table. Because increased abdominal pressure from pneumoperitoneum and the reverse Trendelenburg position decrease venous return, pneumatic compression stockings are always used as prophylaxis against deep vein thrombosis.

The equipment required for a laparoscopic Nissen fundoplication includes five trocars, a 30 or 45 laparoscope, an instrument for coagulation (Harmonic scalpel [Ethicon Inc, Somerville, NJ], LigaSure Vessel Sealing System [Covidien, Mansfield, MA], vascular clips, and hook cautery), and various other grasping instruments [*see Table 1*].

A total fundoplication is our procedure of choice. A partial fundoplication [*see* Laparoscopic Partial Fundoplication (Anterior/Posterior), *below*] can be performed in certain settings.[20,21] The operation may be divided into nine key steps as follows.

Table 1 Equipment for Laparoscopic Esophageal Procedures

Equipment
Five trocars (5–10 mm depending on camera, suture equipment)
30 scope
Graspers and needle holder
Babcock clamp
L-shaped hook cautery with suction-irrigation capacity
Scissors
Laparoscopic clip applier
LigaSure* or Harmonic scalpel†
Fan retractor
Endo Stitch device‡
2-0 silk sutures
56 French esophageal bougie

*Valleylab, Boulder, CO
†Ethicon Endo-Surgery, San Diego, CA.
‡Autosuture, Norwalk, CT.

Step 1: Placement of Trocars

Five trocars are used for the operation [*see Figure 1*]. Port A is a 10 mm port placed slightly (2 to 3 cm) to the right of the midline, approximately one third the distance from the umbilicus to the xiphoid via an open technique. This is the camera port. Port B is 5 mm and is placed in the right lateral subcostal region just caudal to the inferior edge of the right lobe of the liver. It is used for the liver retractor to provide upward retraction on the left lobe of the liver exposing the esophageal hiatus. Port C is another 5 mm incision in the mid right subcostal region and serves the operating surgeon's left hand. Port D is 10 mm and is located adjacent to Port A to the right of the midline. This port services the operating surgeon's right hand. These ports are used for insertion of the graspers, energy source, and suturing instruments. Port E is a 5 mm assistant port in the lateral left subcostal region and is used primarily for retraction and exposure.

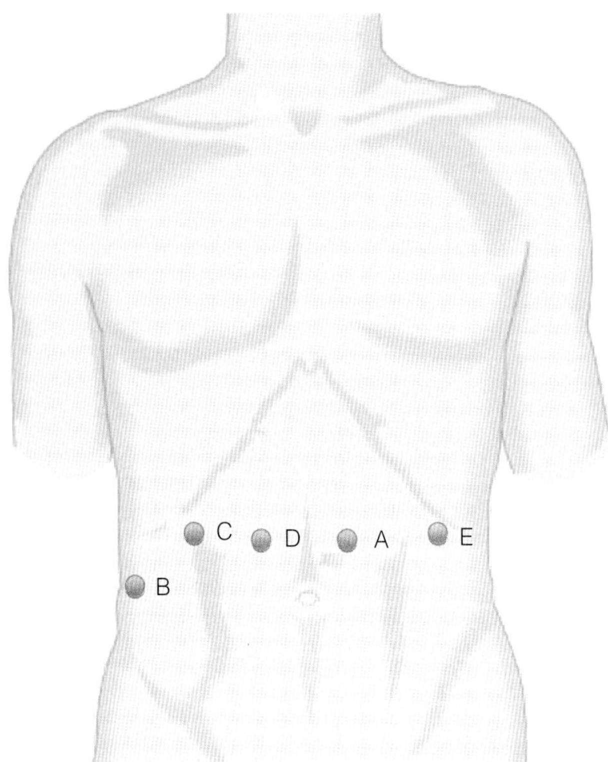

Figure 1 **Laparoscopic Nissen fundoplication. Illustrated is the recommended placement of the trocars.**

Troubleshooting If the ports are placed too low in the abdomen, the operation is made more difficult. If port B is too low, the fan retractor will not retract the left lateral section of the liver well, and the esophagogastric junction will not be properly exposed. If port A is too low, visualization of the hiatus will be difficult. If ports C and D are too low, the dissection at the beginning of the procedure and the suturing at the end are problematic. This becomes increasingly important when a large hiatal hernia is present. Port A must be placed with caution. We routinely use the open approach and a Hasson trocar. Maintaining the proper distance between ports is important to avoid clashing with the trocar or instrument of the adjacent port. Generally keeping four fingerbreadths between ports provides reasonable working space. Finally, if a trocar is not in the ideal position, it is better to insert another one than to operate through an inconveniently placed port.

If the surgeon spears the epigastric vessels with a trocar, bleeding will occur, in which case, we prefer to ligate the vessel under laparoscopic guidance. We favor the Carter-Thomason CloseSure System (Inlet Medical, Inc., Eden Prairie, MN) to ligate the vessel securely with 0 absorbable suture. Once hemostasis is obtained, the surgeon can simply reposition the trocar away from the vessels or leave the trocar in place and reinspect at the end of the case.

Step 2: Division of Gastrohepatic Ligament; Identification of Right Crus of Diaphragm and Posterior Vagus Nerve

Once the ports are in place, the gastrohepatic ligament is divided. Dissection begins above the caudate lobe (segments 1 and 9) of the liver, where this ligament usually is very thin, and continues toward the diaphragm until the right crus is identified. The crus is then separated from the right side of the esophagus by blunt dissection, and the posterior vagus nerve is identified. The dissection continues inferiorly along the right crus toward the junction with the left crus.

Troubleshooting An accessory left hepatic artery originating from the left gastric artery is frequently encountered in the gastrohepatic ligament. If this vessel creates problems of exposure, it may be divided; in our experience, doing so has not caused problems. In dissecting the right crus from the esophagus, the electrocautery should be used with particular caution. Because the monopolar current tends to spread laterally, the posterior vagus nerve may sustain damage simply from being in proximity to the device, even when there is no direct contact. A better alternative is to use a bipolar instrument or Harmonic scalpel.

Step 3: Division of Peritoneum and Phrenoesophageal Membrane above Esophagus; Identification of Left Crus of Diaphragm and Anterior Vagus Nerve

The peritoneum and the phrenoesophageal membrane above the esophagus are divided, and the anterior vagus nerve is identified. The left crus of the diaphragm is dissected downward toward the junction with the right crus.

Troubleshooting Care must be taken not to damage the anterior vagus nerve or the esophageal wall. To this end, the nerve should be left attached to the esophageal wall, and the peritoneum and the phrenoesophageal membrane should be lifted from the wall by blunt dissection before they are divided.

Step 4: Division of Short Gastric Vessels

The Harmonic scalpel or laparoscopic LigaSure Vessel Sealing System is introduced. Gentle retraction of the stomach to the right and the omentum to the left affords exposure to the vessels. The spleen side of the vessel is sometimes clipped while the stomach side is divided.

Troubleshooting There are two problems to watch for during this part of the procedure: (1) bleeding, either from the short gastric vessels or from the spleen, and (2) damage to the gastric wall.

Bleeding from the short gastric vessels is usually caused by excessive traction or by division of a vessel that is not completely coagulated. It is important to orient the Harmonic scalpel or LigaSure Vessel Sealing System perpendicular to the vessel being divided as vessels approached obliquely are often inadequately coagulated. The highest short gastrics are often quite short and have close approximation to both the spleen and the stomach. It is often better to dissect from inferior to superior along the greater curvature of the stomach to get as much length and mobility as possible on the attachments between the stomach and spleen. Clipping the spleen site of the vessel before dividing can help decrease bleeding. Damage to the gastric wall can be caused by a burn from the electrocautery used to dissect between vessels or by traction applied with the graspers or the Babcock clamp.

Step 5: Mobilization of the Esophagus and Fat Pad

With gentle inferior retraction on the stomach, dissect up into the hiatus for several centimeters while mobilizing the esophagus. With the esophagus elevated, divide the attachments to the aorta posteriorly. Once the esophagus is mobilized, carefully dissect the anterior fat pad off of the stomach and follow this circumferentially around the gastroesophageal junction (GEJ) until a window is created posteriorly. Dissection must be close to the esophagus to avoid injury to both the anterior and posterior vagal nerves. Once the fat pad is fully mobilized, the GEJ can be identified. Esophageal length must be determined. If the GEJ is less than 2 to 3 cm from the hiatus, additional esophageal mobilization can be performed higher in the hiatus to get additional abdominal esophageal length. Dissection can be performed to above the level of the inferior pulmonary veins.

Troubleshooting During the hiatal mobilization, be careful not to dissect too close to the aorta. Elevate the esophagus and divide the attachments in the midline. Also be aware of the anterior vagal nerve as it moves anteriorly and to the left as you move proximally along the esophagus.

During the mobilization of the fat pad, stay close to the esophagus, moving left to right. It should remain attached superiorly and inferiorly. There are small arterial branches from the fat pad to the esophagus that may bleed as you mobilize. Follow the wall of the eosophagus until a window is created posteriorly to the left side.

If there is not adequate esophageal length (GEJ 2 to 3 cm from the hiatus) even with additional esophageal mobilization, a wedge (Collis) gastroplasty should be considered [*see* Laparoscopic Paraesophageal Hernia Repair, *below, for a description*].

Step 6: Wrapping of Gastric Fundus around Lower Esophagus

Graspers are used to grab the cardia of the stomach in the line of the short gastrics through the posterior window created within the fat pad and posterior to the esophagus. The gastric fundus is gently pulled under the esophagus with the graspers. A bougie is placed through the oropharynx and guided into the esophagus and stomach until it lies on the lesser curvature. The size of the bougie is typically 54 to 56 French. The bougie must be inserted enough for the thickest portion to be at the area of the wrap. The left and right sides of the fundus are wrapped within the fat pad at and above the level of the GEJ. Three 2-0 sutures are used to secure the two ends of the wrap to each other as well as the esophagus in the midline.

Troubleshooting The wrap should measure no more than 2 to 2.5 cm. Care must be used when placing the bougie. Any resistance must be carefully examined as misplacement of the bougie can result in perforation. You should be able to place an instrument easily between the wrap and the esophagus laterally. If not, the wrap may be too tight.

Step 7: Closure of Crura

The diaphragmatic crura are closed with interrupted 0-0 sutures on an Endo Stitch device (Autosuture, Norwalk, CT); the sutures are tied intracorporeally. Exposure is provided by retracting the esophagus upward and toward the patient's abdominal wall. Typically, this is done with gentle upward retraction of a closed grasper placed posterior to the esophagus. The first stitch should be placed just above the junction of the two pillars. Additional stitches are placed 1 cm apart, and a space of about 1 cm is left between the uppermost stitch and the esophagus.

Troubleshooting Care must be taken not to spear the esophageal wall with the needle. So as not to limit the space available for suturing, the bougie is not placed inside the esophagus during this part of the procedure. Additional care must be taken when tying the crural sutures. The tendency is to blindly push the needle driver or Endo Stitch device into the left upper quadrant posterior to the esophagus when tightening the square knot, which poses the risk of splenic injury.

Step 8: Final Inspection, Removal of Instruments and Ports from Abdomen, and Closure of Port Sites

After hemostasis is obtained, the instruments and the ports are removed from the abdomen under direct vision.

We usually close the initial 10 mm trocar site with 0 absorbable suture material using the Carter-Thomason CloseSure System.

Troubleshooting If any areas of oozing were observed, they should be irrigated and dried with sponges rolled into a cigarettelike shape before the ports are removed. In addition, if some grounds for concern remain, the oozing areas should be examined after the pneumoperitoneum is decreased to 7 to 8 mm Hg to abolish the tamponading effect exerted by the high intra-abdominal pressure.

All ports should be removed from the abdomen under direct vision so that any bleeding from the abdominal wall can be readily detected. Such bleeding is easily controlled, either from inside or from outside.

COMPLICATIONS

A feared complication of laparoscopic Nissen fundoplication is esophageal or gastric perforation, which may result either from traction applied with the clamp or a grasper to the esophagus or the stomach (particularly when the stomach is pulled under the esophagus) or from inadvertent electrocautery burns during any part of the dissection. A leak will manifest itself during the first 48 hours. Peritoneal signs will be noted if the spillage is limited to the abdomen; shortness of breath and a pleural effusion will be noted if spillage also occurs in the chest. The site of the leak can be confirmed by a contrast study with barium or a water-soluble contrast agent. If a perforation is detected intraoperatively, it may be closed laparoscopically. If there is a delayed recognition of the leak postoperatively, management is dependent on the location and extent of the leak.

Almost every patient experiences some degree of dysphagia postoperatively. This problem usually resolves after 4 to 6 weeks. Diet is advanced slowly postoperatively starting with a liquid diet and slowly progressing to soft solids followed by a regular diet. If, however, dysphagia persists beyond this period, one or more of the following causes is responsible:

1. A wrap that is too tight or too long (i.e., > 2.5 cm)[22]
2. Lateral torsion with a corkscrew effect. If the wrap rotates to the right (because of tension from intact short gastric vessels or because the fundus is small), a corkscrew effect is created.
3. A wrap made with the body of the stomach rather than the fundus. The relaxation of the LES and the gastric fundus is controlled by vasoactive intestinal polypeptide and nitric oxide[23,24]; after fundoplication, the two structures relax simultaneously with swallowing. If part of the body of the stomach rather than the fundus is used for the wrap, it will not relax as the LES does on arrival of the food bolus.

If the wrap slips into the chest, a recurrent hernia, the patient may experience dysphagia and regurgitation. The diagnosis is confirmed by means of a barium swallow. Paraesophageal hernia may occur if the crura have not been closed or if the closure is too loose. Closure of the crura is not only essential for preventing paraesophageal hernia but also is important from a physiologic point of view in that it acts synergistically with the LES against stress reflux.

POSTOPERATIVE CARE

Postoperative care has become fairly standardized at our institution. Patients remain nihil per os (NPO) on postoperative day 0 and are advanced to clear liquid diet on posteroperative day 1. A nutritionist consultation provides post–Nissen fundoplication dietary instructions. Patients are advanced to full liquids by postoperative day 2 whether they are have been discharged or remain in the hospital. They continue with full liquids for 2 weeks until seen back in the clinic for a routine follow-up. At the time of this visit, a detailed history is obtained to assess for dysphagia and the patient's diet is typically advanced to a regular diet, with some exceptions. Carbonated beverages are prohibited to minimize bloating. As mentioned above, bread and meat are discouraged for the next 2 to 4 weeks. It is important to discuss these postoperative dietary restrictions ahead of time so that patients have realistic expectations. Furthermore, all patients should be alerted to the likelihood of experiencing mild dysphagia in the initial postoperative period as well as some bloating, both of which resolve with time.

Laparoscopic Partial Fundoplication (Anterior/Posterior)

PREOPERATIVE EVALUATION AND OPERATIVE PLANNING

As mentioned in the above section, there is considerable controversy regarding the utility of partial fundoplication in antireflux surgery. Specifically, questions regarding the efficacy and longevity of partial wraps have been raised by retrospective studies. Although these concerns are not supported by more recent randomized, controlled trials, there is limited long-term follow-up to settle this controversy. In general, the partial fundoplication operation is reserved for patients with severe esophageal dysmotility due to concerns of increased dysphagia with a complete fundoplication [*see* Outcome Evaluation, *below*]. In addition, laparoscopic partial fundoplication is often performed after laparoscopic Heller myotomy for achalasia [*see* Laparoscopic Heller Myotomy with Partial Fundoplication, *below*].[25] Either an anterior or a posterior fundoplication is typically performed in conjunction with a Heller myotomy. The Dor fundoplication is an anterior 180 wrap. Its advantages are that (1) it does not require posterior dissection and the creation of a window between the esophagus, the stomach, and the left pillar of the crus and (2) it covers the exposed esophageal mucosa after completion of the myotomy. Its main disadvantage is that achieving the proper geometry can be difficult, and a wrong configuration can lead to dysphagia even after a properly performed myotomy.[26] The advantages of the posterior fundoplication are that (1) it theoretically keeps the edges of the myotomy well separated in the context of a Heller myotomy and (2) it might be more effective than a Dor procedure in preventing reflux. Its main disadvantages are that (1) it requires more dissection for the creation of a posterior window and (2) it leaves the esophageal mucosa exposed, again in the context of a Heller myotomy. Although there is variation in technique, the basic principles of partial posterior and anterior plications are described below.

OPERATIVE TECHNIQUE

Posterior Fundoplication: Steps 1 through 5, 7

These steps in a posterior fundoplication are identical to the steps in a Nissen fundoplication.

Step 6: Wrapping the Gastric Fundus around the Lower Esophagus

As the name implies, the partial wraps do not extend around the esophageal circumference. For the posterior approach, the gastric fundus is delivered under the esophagus. Eighty to 120 of the anterior esophagus is left uncovered, and each of the two sides of the wrap (right and left) is separately affixed to the esophagus and the corresponding crura [*see Figure 2*]. The gastric fundus is grasped and delivered posteriorly. With the fundus now posterior to the esophagus, a suture is placed securing the superior left portion of the wrap to the esophagus and left crus. Additionally, another suture is placed securing the right portion of the fundus to the right side of the esophagus and the right crus. Once secured, 2-0 Ethibond sutures (Ethicon) are then used to approximate seromuscular layers of the esophageal wall to the gastric fundus on both the left and right sides. Care is taken to avoid full-thickness bites on the esophagus.

Anterior Fundoplication: Steps 1 through 5, 7

The steps in a posterior fundoplication are identical to these first steps in a Nissen fundoplication.

Step 6: Wrapping the Gastric Fundus around the Lower Esophagus

The gastric fundus is mobilized. Two rows of sutures are placed. The first row (on the left side) comprises three stitches: the uppermost stitch incorporates the gastric fundus, the esophageal wall, and the left pillar of the crus [*see Figure 3*], and the other two incorporate only the gastric fundus and the left side of the esophageal wall [*see Figure 4*]. The gastric fundus is then folded over the myotomy, and the second row (also comprising three stitches) is placed on the right side between the fundus and the right side of the esophageal wall, with only the uppermost stitch incorporating the right pillar of the crus [*see Figure 5 and Figure 6*]. Finally, two additional stitches are placed between the anterior rim of the hiatus and the superior aspect of the fundoplication [*see Figure 7*]. These stitches remove any tension from the second row of sutures.

Troubleshooting Efforts must be made to ensure that the fundoplication does not become a cause of postoperative dysphagia. Accordingly, we always take down the short gastric vessels, even though some authorities suggest that this step can be omitted.[27,28] In addition, the gastric fundus rather than

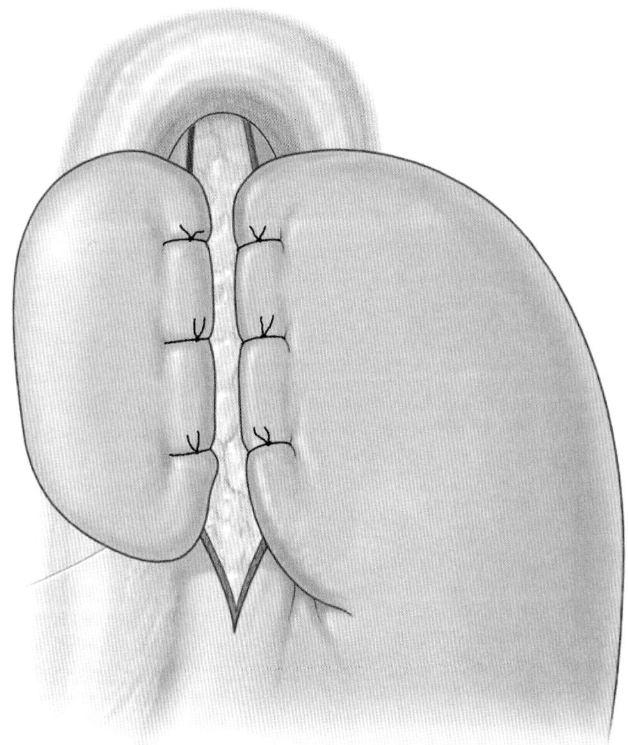

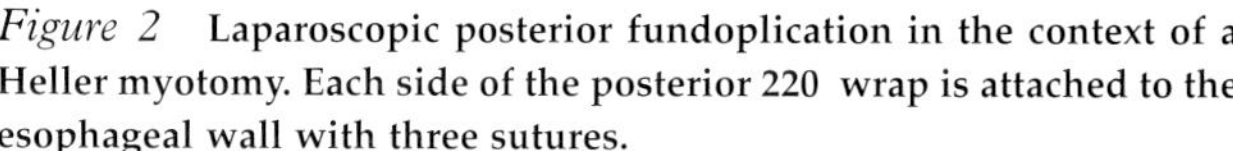

Figure 2 Laparoscopic posterior fundoplication in the context of a Heller myotomy. Each side of the posterior 220 wrap is attached to the esophageal wall with three sutures.

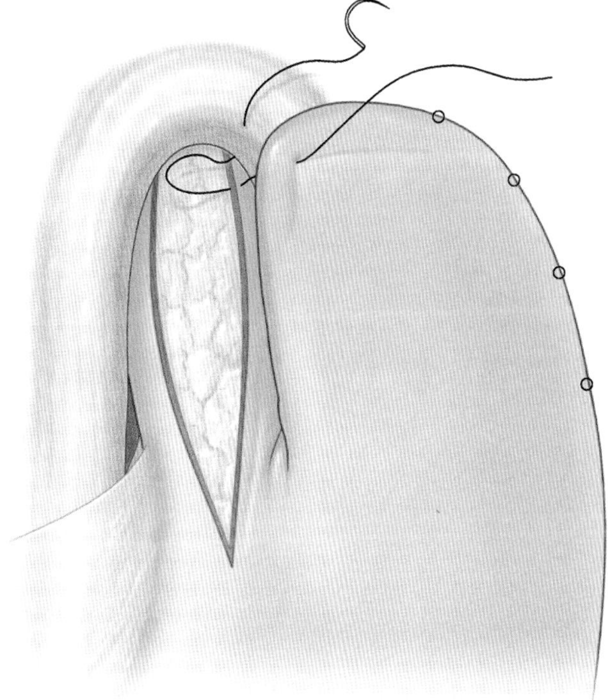

Figure 3 Laparoscopic anterior partial fundoplication in the context of a Heller myotomy. The uppermost stitch in the first row incorporates the fundus, the esophageal wall, and the left pillar of the crus.

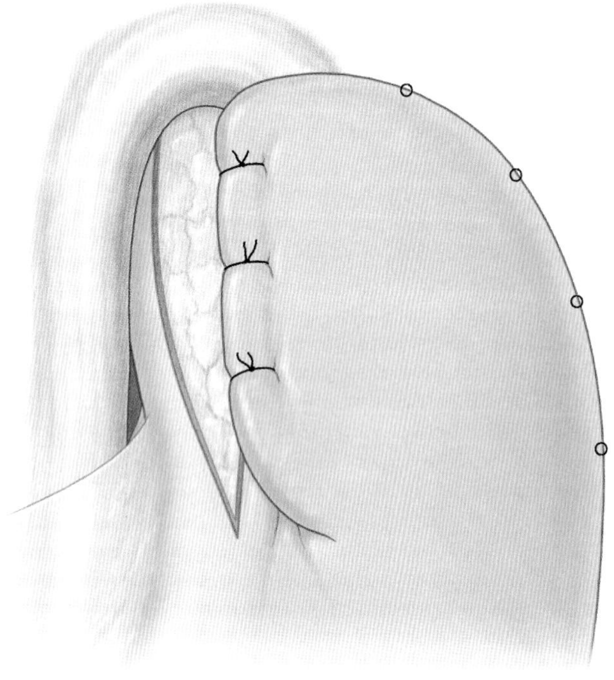

Figure 4 Laparoscopic anterior partial fundoplication in the context of a Heller myotomy. The second and third stitches in the first row incorporate only the fundus and the left side of the esophageal wall.

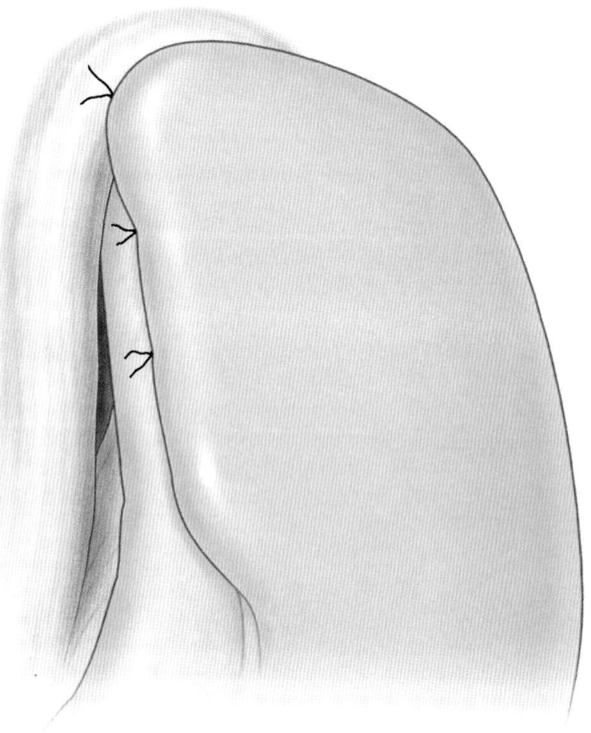

Figure 6 Laparoscopic anterior partial fundoplication in the context of a Heller myotomy. The second and third stitches in the second row incorporate only the fundus and the right side of the esophageal wall.

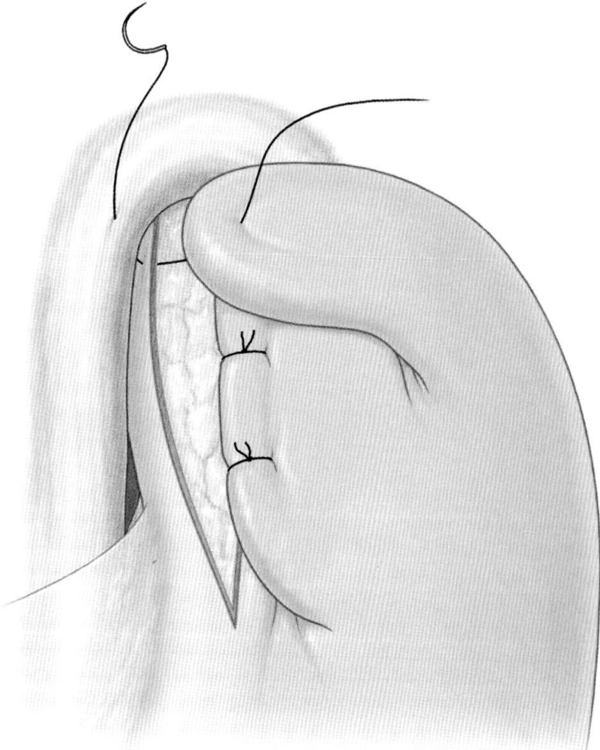

Figure 5 Laparoscopic anterior partial fundoplication in the context of a Heller myotomy. The uppermost stitch in the second row incorporates the fundus, the esophageal wall, and the right crus.

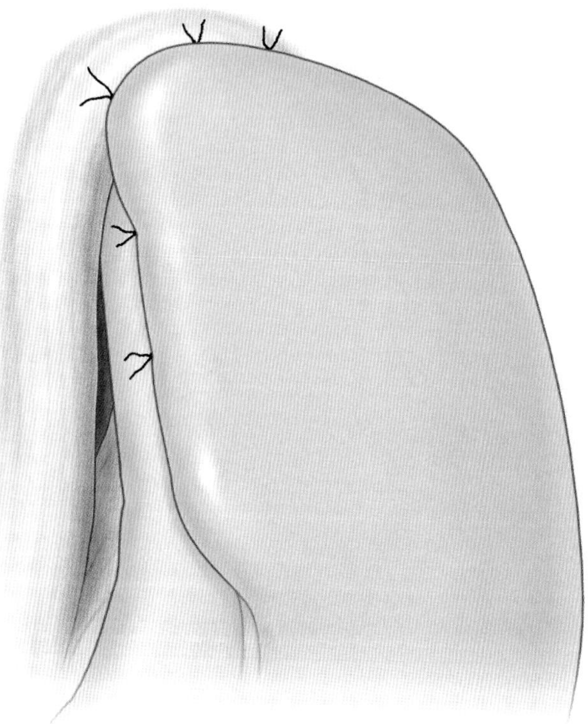

Figure 7 Laparoscopic anterior partial fundoplication in the context of a Heller myotomy. Two final stitches are placed between the superior portion of the wrap and the anterior rim of the hiatus.

the body of the stomach should be used for the wrap. Some argue that only the uppermost stitch of the right row of sutures should incorporate the right pillar of the crus.[29]

POSTOPERATIVE CARE

Postoperative care is the same as for Nissen fundoplication.

OUTCOME EVALUATION

The initial results of laparoscopic fundoplication obtained in the early 1990s indicated that the operation was effective in controlling reflux but that postoperative dysphagia occurred more often than had been anticipated.[30] Many experts thought that this problem could be avoided by tailoring the fundoplication to the strength of esophageal peristalsis as measured by esophageal manometry.[30] Accordingly, partial fundoplication (240) was recommended for patients with impaired peristalsis, and total fundoplication (360) was recommended for those with normal peristalsis. The short-term results of this tailored approach were promising.[30] Gradually, however, it became evident that a partial fundoplication was not as durable as a total fundoplication[31] and that a total fundoplication was not associated with a higher incidence of postoperative dysphagia even in patients with weak peristalsis.[32,33]

These findings suggest that the initial problems with postoperative dysphagia were primarily attributable to unknown technical factors that were largely eliminated from the procedure as surgeons garnered more experience with it. As a result, total fundoplication is currently considered the procedure of choice for patients with GERD, regardless of the strength of their esophageal peristalsis.

In a 2007 study, pre- and postoperative manometric results were reviewed in 71 patients who underwent laparoscopic fundoplication. Not only did LES pressure increase after the procedure, but distal esophageal amplitude also increased in patients with abnormal preoperative motility, with normalization of peristalsis occurring in the majority of patients.[34]

A 2001 report found that 62% of fundoplication patients were using antireflux medications 10 years after the operation, a finding that raised concerns about long-term durability of the procedure.[35] This study has been criticized on the grounds that many of the patients were taking PPIs for reasons other than reflux symptoms and that the reflux status was not assessed by pH monitoring. A 2006 study aimed at critically assessing 10-year outcomes reported the results from 100 consecutive patients after complete and partial fundoplication.[36] In this series, the rate of symptomatic control of reflux symptoms at 5 and 10 years was 90%, with fewer than 10% of patients using antacid medications at 10 years; only one patient required reintervention for persistent dysphagia. Similar results were documented in subsequent studies,[37,38] confirming laparoscopic Nissen fundoplication as an effective long-term treatment for GERD.

Laparoscopic Heller Myotomy with Partial Fundoplication

Achalasia is an esophageal motor disorder characterized by manometric findings. Specifically, this disease is defined by failure of LES relaxation and impaired or absent esophageal body contractions. Patients typically present with progressive dysphagia, chest pain, and/or regurgitation of undigested food matter. Surgical and endoscopic treatment strategies focus on alleviating dysphagia by disrupting the LES, facilitating the passage of food into the stomach.

Minimally invasive surgical procedures for other primary esophageal motility disorders (diffuse esophageal spasm, nutcracker esophagus, and hypertensive LES) are controversial. We will thus focus on laparoscopic Heller myotomy with partial fundoplication for achalasia, which has supplanted left thoracoscopic myotomy as the procedure of choice.[39–42]

PREOPERATIVE EVALUATION

All candidates for a laparoscopic Heller myotomy should undergo a thorough and careful evaluation to establish the diagnosis and characterize the disease.[43]

An upper GI series is useful. A characteristic so-called bird's beak is usually seen in patients with achalasia. A dilated, sigmoid esophagus may be present in patients with long-standing disease, whereas a corkscrew esophagus is often seen in patients with diffuse esophageal spasm. Endoscopy is performed to rule out a tumor of the esophagogastric junction and gastroduodenal pathologic conditions.

Esophageal manometry is the key test for establishing the diagnosis of esophageal achalasia. The classic manometric findings are (1) absence of esophageal peristalsis and (2) an LES that fails to relax appropriately in response to swallowing.

Ambulatory pH monitoring should always be done in patients who have undergone pneumatic dilatation to rule out abnormal gastroesophageal reflux. In addition, pH monitoring should be performed postoperatively to detect abnormal reflux, which, if present, should be treated with acid-reducing medications.[43] A prospective randomized trial of Heller myotomy noted that approximately 50% of patients had acid reflux following the procedure. The addition of the Dor fundoplication decreased that rate to 9%.[44]

In patients older than 60 years who have experienced the recent onset of dysphagia and excessive weight loss, secondary achalasia or pseudoachalasia from cancer of the esophagogastric junction should be ruled out. Endoscopic ultrasonography or computed tomography (CT) can help establish the diagnosis.[28]

OPERATIVE PLANNING

Patient preparation (i.e., anesthesia, positioning, and instrumentation) is identical to that for laparoscopic fundoplication except for the preoperative diet. Patients are required to transition to a full liquid diet 3 days preoperatively followed by a clear liquid diet for 24 hours preoperatively. Otherwise, large food particles may be found in the esophagus at the time of surgery, even in patients who have been NPO for 24 hours. Surgery is not advised unless the esophagus is clean. Hence, an on-table endoscopy is important.

OPERATIVE TECHNIQUE

Many of the steps in a laparoscopic Heller myotomy are the same as the corresponding steps in a laparoscopic fundoplication. The ensuing description focuses on those steps that differ significantly.

Steps 1 through 5

The steps of a laparoscopic Heller myotomy are essentially identical to the first steps of a laparoscopic fundoplication. Steps 6 and 7, however, are necessary only if a posterior partial fundoplication is to be performed. Care must be taken not to narrow the esophageal hiatus too much and push the esophagus too far anteriorly.

Step 7: Intraoperative Endoscopy

At the beginning of a surgeon's experience with laparoscopic Heller myotomy, intraoperative endoscopy is an important and helpful step; however, once the surgeon has gained adequate experience with this procedure and has become familiar with the relevant anatomy from a laparoscopic perspective, it may be omitted.

Troubleshooting The most worrisome complication during intraoperative endoscopy is perforation of the esophagus. This complication can be prevented by having the procedure done by an experienced endoscopist who is familiar with achalasia. If a perforation is identified, immediate laparoscopic closure of the perforation is an effective treatment.

Step 8: Initiation of Myotomy and Entry into Submucosal Plane at Single Point

The myotomy is performed at the 11 o'clock position [*see Figure 8 and Figure 9*]. The myotomy is started about 3 cm

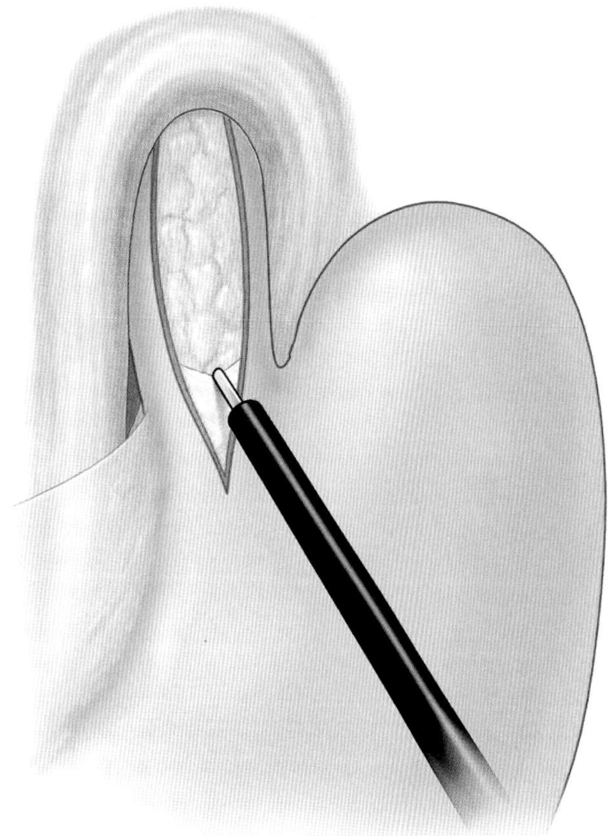

Figure 8 **Laparoscopic Heller myotomy. The myotomy is extended proximally and distally.**

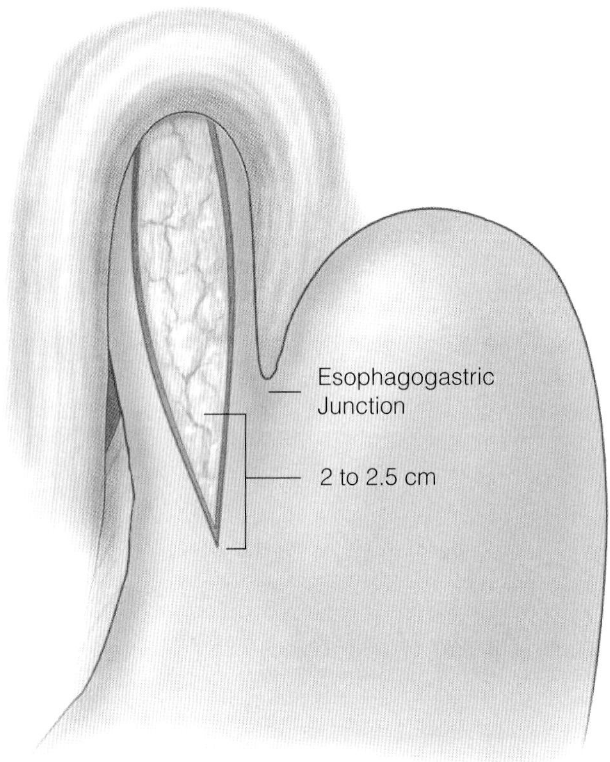

Figure 9 **Laparoscopic Heller myotomy with partial fundoplication. The myotomy is approximately 8 cm long, extending distally for about 2 to 2.5 cm onto the gastric wall and proximally for about 6 cm above the esophagogastric junction.**

proximal to the esophagogastric junction. Before it is extended upward and downward, the proper submucosal plane should be reached at a single point; in this way, the likelihood of subsequent mucosal perforation can be reduced.

Troubleshooting The myotomy should not be started close to the esophagogastric junction, because at this level, the layers are often poorly defined, particularly if multiple dilatations or injections of botulinum toxin have been performed. At the preferred starting point, about 3 cm above the esophagogastric junction, the esophageal wall is usually normal. As a rule, we do not open the entire longitudinal layer first and then the circular layer; we find it easier and safer to try to reach the submucosal plane at a single point and then move upward and downward from there. In the course of the myotomy, there is always some bleeding from the cut muscle fibers, particularly if the esophagus is dilated and the wall is very thick. After the source of the bleeding is identified, gentle pressure is often all that is needed for hemostasis. The electrocautery is unnecessary and sometimes dangerous. The most troublesome bleeding comes from the submucosal veins encountered at the esophagogastric junction (which are usually large). A sponge introduced through one of the ports facilitates the application of direct pressure.

Step 9: Proximal and Distal Extension of Myotomy

Once the mucosa has been exposed, the myotomy can safely be extended. Distally, it is extended for about 2 to 2.5 cm onto the gastric wall; proximally, it is extended for about 6 cm above the esophagogastric junction. Thus, the total length of the myotomy is typically about 8 to 8.5 cm. A plane can be creased between the mucosa and the circular muscular layer. Gentle dissection and division with scissors or energy devices such as the Harmonic scalpel are performed.

Troubleshooting The course of the anterior vagus nerve must be identified before the myotomy is started. This nerve often crosses the line of the myotomy. It must be lifted away from the esophageal wall, and the muscle layers must then be cut under it. Previous balloon dilations and/or treatment with botulinum toxin occasionally results in fibrosis with scarring and loss of the normal anatomic planes; this occurs more frequently at the level of the esophagogastric junction.

If a perforation seems possible or likely, it should be carefully investigated, as described earlier [*see* Step 7: Intraoperative Endoscopy, *above*]. Any perforation found should be repaired immediately, with interrupted sutures employed for a small perforation and a continuous suture for a larger one. When a perforation has occurred, an anterior fundoplication is usually chosen in preference to a posterior one because the stomach will offer further protection against a leak.

Step 10: Anterior or Posterior Partial Fundoplication

Once the myotomy has been created, we proceed with either an anterior or posterior plication. Please refer to the section on partial fundoplication for details.

Step 11: Final Inspection and Removal of Instruments and Ports from Abdomen

Step 11 of a laparoscopic Heller myotomy is identical to step 8 of a laparoscopic Nissen fundoplication.

COMPLICATIONS

Delayed esophageal leakage, usually resulting from a burn to the esophageal mucosa, may occur during the first 24 to 36 hours after operation. The characteristic signs and symptoms are chest pain, fever, and a pleural effusion on the chest x-ray. The diagnosis is confirmed by an esophagogram. Treatment options depend on the time of diagnosis and on the size and location of the leak. Early, small leaks can be repaired directly. If the damage to the esophagus is too extensive to permit repair, treat as you would an esophageal perforation, which may include diversion and drainage.

Dysphagia may either persist after the operation or recur after a symptom-free interval. In either case, a complete workup is necessary, and treatment is individualized on the basis of the specific cause of dysphagia. Reoperation may be indicated [*see* Reoperation for Esophageal Achalasia, *below*].

Abnormal gastroesophageal reflux occurs in 7 to 20% of patients after operation.[39,40] Because most patients are asymptomatic, it is essential to try to evaluate all patients postoperatively with manometry and prolonged pH monitoring. Reflux should be treated with acid-reducing medications.

POSTOPERATIVE CARE

We routinely obtain an esophagogram before initiating feeding. Diet progression is the same as that for a Nissen fundoplication. Patients are counseled to avoid strenuous activity for 4 to 6 weeks to decrease strain at the hiatus.

OUTCOME EVALUATION

The results obtained to date with laparoscopic Heller myotomy and partial fundoplication are excellent and are generally comparable to those obtained with the corresponding open surgical procedure: dysphagia is alleviated or eliminated in more than 90% of patients.[26,39,42] These results have been confirmed in long-term follow-up outcome studies. One report from the University of Padua found that at a minimum of 6 years after surgical intervention, 85% of myotomy patients were satisfied.[45]

A randomized, controlled trial published in the *New England Journal of Medicine* in 2011 examined pneumatic dilation versus laparoscopic Heller myotomy and found no significant difference at 2 years in either subjective or objective measures.[46] That said, several retrospective longer-term studies strongly favor a surgical approach. In a 2008 report describing the UCSF experience with 113 patients treated for achalasia with laparoscopic Heller myotomy and Dor fundoplication, surgeons found that at a median follow-up of 45 months (range 7 months to 12.5 years), 80% experienced complete relief of dysphagia after the operation.[47] The remaining 20% required endoscopic dilatation, which was successful in 50% of the cases. Many studies have demonstrated inferior outcomes in patients who have had endoscopic therapies prior to surgical intervension.[48] Hence, gastroenterologists typically refer these patients for surgical treatment before any other therapy has been instituted, reserving endoscopic dilatation for cases where operative treatment has failed.[49] With the recent randomized, controlled trial, one wonders if this practice pattern will change. Overall, combined treatment yields a success rate of about 90%.

Historically, the presence of a sigmoid-shaped esophagus has been considered a contraindication to performing a myotomy to treat long-standing achalasia, making esophagectomy the only option. In the study just mentioned, the UCSF group subdivided the patients according to the degree of esophageal dilatation and observed the responses to surgery in the various groups.[47] Even in those cases where the esophageal diameter exceeded 6 cm and the esophagus was sigmoid, the outcomes of laparoscopic myotomy were not significantly different.[47]

Laparoscopic Paraesophageal Hernia Repair

A hiatal hernia is defined as displacement of abdominal cavity contents through the esophageal hiatus of the diaphragm into the chest. The prevalence of hiatal hernias is difficult to estimate given that the majority of patients are asymptomatic. Quoted ranges vary widely from 20 to 100%.[50] Hiatal hernias are classified into four types based on their anatomic configuration [*see Figure 10*]. True paraesophageal hernias (types II, III, and IV) comprise only 5 to 14% of all hiatal hernias.[51] The majority of patients with paraesophageal hernias are asymptomatic, and their hernias are found incidentally with a retrocardiac gastric bubble on an

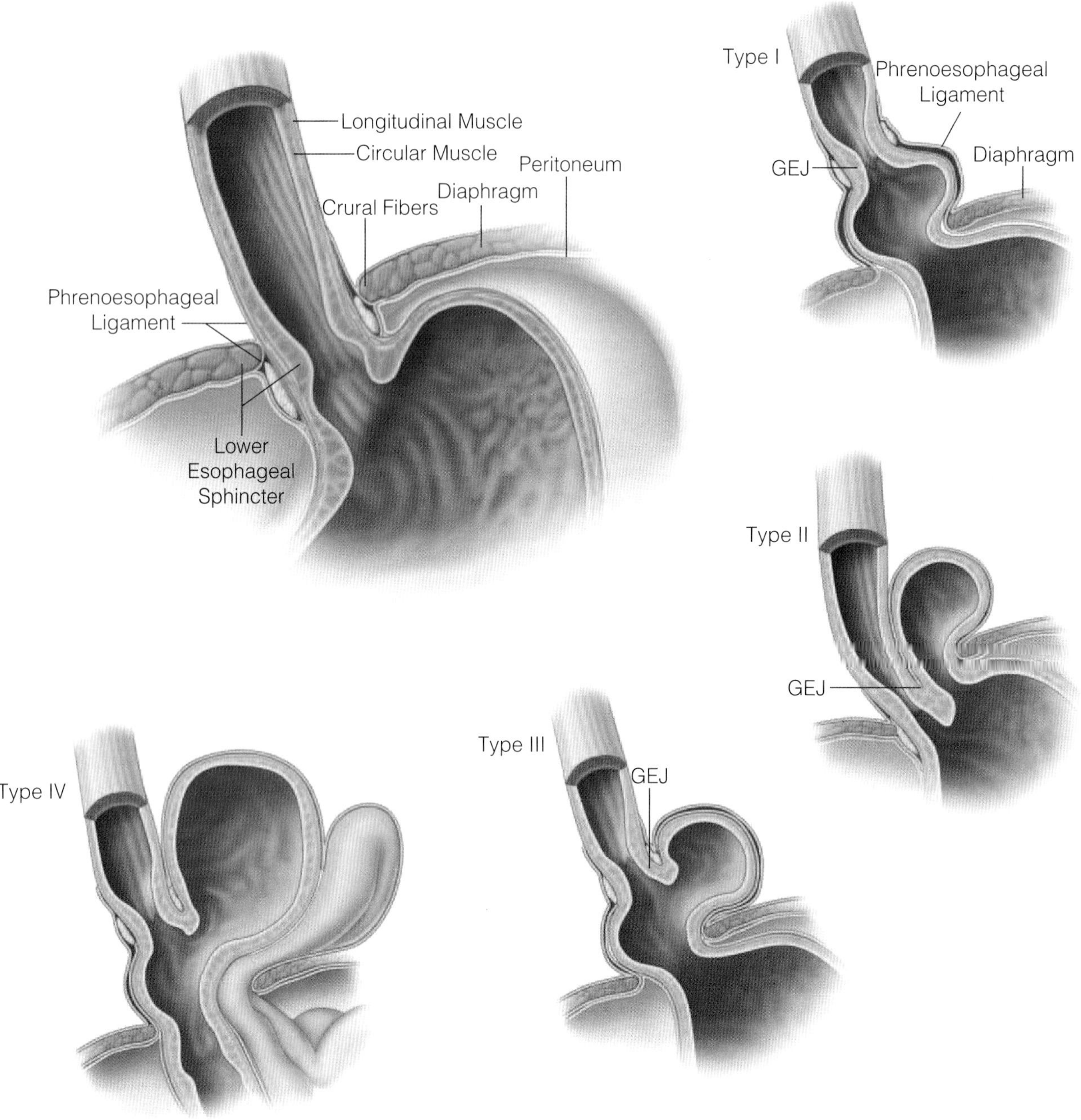

Figure 10 **Types of hiatal hernias. GEJ = gastroesophageal junction.**

upright chest x-ray or herniated GEJ seen on a chest or abdominal CT scan. In a recently published series of giant paraesophageal hernia repairs, the most common symptom in this surgical population was heartburn (66%), followed by chest and abdominal pain (59%), regurgitation (54%), and dysphagia (43%).[52]

Whether or not all paraesophageal hernias ought to be repaired is the subject of debate. Skinner and Belsey's initial report in 1967 detailing six of 21 patients treated medically dying from complications of their paraesophageal hernias prompted a widespread belief that all paraesophageal hernias need surgical repair.[53] A series published in 1993 by Allen and colleagues followed 23 patients for a median of 78 months and described only three cases of gastric strangulation in 735 patient-years, with only one mortality.[54] Clearly, for patients who are symptomatic, surgical repair is indicated as there is no medical treatment for this mechanical problem. For asymptomatic patients, clinical judgment needs to be used. Most patients who are reasonable surgical candidates should consider repair given the natural history of disease with progressive enlargement of the hernia and the increasing likelihood of symptoms over time.

PREOPERATIVE EVALUATION

Preoperative evaluation should include a contrast study of the upper GI tract, typically an upper GI series with barium. This study helps characterize the anatomy, assess rotation, and evaluate for strictures. Esophagogastroduodenoscopy is helpful to assess for evidence of esophagitis and gastric ulcers, although it may be challenging to get beyond the hiatus. The utility of pH probe and manometry is questioned in certain institutions given the inherent abnormality of the anatomy.

OPERATIVE TECHNIQUE

Step 1: Port Placement

The port placements for paraesophageal hernia repair are similar to those for a Nissen fundoplication (see above).

Troubleshooting Depending on the size of the hernia and the anatomy of the patient, ports may need to be placed more cranial, closer to the costal margin, to comfortably reach the intrathoracic portion of the hernia.

Step 2: Complete Dissection of the Hernia Sac

The repair starts with reduction of the hernia sac. The sac is grasped within the mediastinum and everted by retracting it caudally into the abdomen. The sac is then incised with an ultrasonic scalpel or cautery, thereby exposing a loose connective tissue plane between the sac and the mediastinal structures and pleura. The dissection allows for complete reduction of the hernia sac and its contents into the abdomen with restoration of proper anatomy. Depending on the duration and extent of the hernia, there may be significant lengthening of the short gastric arteries and thinning of the ligamentous attachments of the stomach. Once reduced and delivered into the abdomen, the sac is incised at the hiatus, completing the sac mobilization and allowing for sac excision.

Troubleshooting Depending on the size of the hernia and the hiatus, it can be challenging to reduce contents into the abdomen. Forceful retraction should be avoided as this can lead to unrecognized perforations. Nasogastric decompression is essential. It is imperative that all attempts be made to preserve the peritoneal lining over the crura as this provides integrity to the crural closure later in the procedure.

Step 3: Esophageal Mobilization

Esophageal mobilization within the mediastinum is routinely performed and can be achieved up to the level of the inferior pulmonary veins. Vagal nerves must be identified and preserved.

Troubleshooting Arterial supply to this portion of the esophagus is directly off the aorta. These branches need to be identified, ligated, and divided. Care must be taken to avoid inadvertent thermal energy transfer to the esophagus or aorta for obvious reasons. In general, it is best to leave some length on the aortic side of the vessel so that it can be grasped and clipped in the event of bleeding.

Step 4: Assessment of Esophageal Length

We routinely mobilize the gastric fat pad to allow visualization of the GEJ and determination of intra-abdominal esophageal length in the absence of retraction or tension. The goal is to achieve at least 2 cm of tension-free intra-abdominal esophagus. If a tension-free adequate segment of intra-abdominal esophagus is not achievable with mobilization, we perform a wedge gastroplasty to create a neoesophagus.

Troubleshooting The issue of the foreshortened esophagus and its management is controversial. Some contend that mediastinal mobilization of the intrathoracic esophagus via a laparoscopic approach is sufficient to allow for a tension-free fundoplication. Others are convinced that one of the main reasons for high rates of recurrence is an underappreciation of the shortened esophagus and the resultant tension on the repair of the esophageal hiatus. The reality probably can be found somewhere in between. As is evident from Luketich and colleagues' series, the use of the wedge gastroplasty decreased with time as technical skill improved, allowing for more extensive mediastinal mobilization of the intrathoracic esophagus.[52]

The steps involved a laparoscopic wedge gastroplasty are as follows: a Maloney dilator is carefully inserted and used to calibrate the gastroplasty. Typical sizes range from 48 to 58 French. Multiple firings of a roticulating endostapler (Covidien, 45 mm cartridge length, 3.5 mm staple thickness) are used to staple from the greater curve toward the dilator and then cranially along the dilator to the left of the GEJ at the angle of His. The goal is to create a 2.5 cm neoesophagus, which becomes the part of the "esophagus" that is incorporated within the wrap. Placing the wrap around this distal "esophagus" buttresses the staple lines and allows for a tension-free repair.

Step 5: Fundoplication

An antireflux procedure (a floppy Nissen fundoplication in most cases) is routinely performed [*see* Step 6, Laparoscopic Nissen Fundoplication, *above*].

Step 6: Crural Closure

As described above for the Nissen fundoplication, the crura are reapproximated without tension using a nonabsorbable Ethibond suture. Because of the presence of a hernia, the size of the hiatus is likely to be quite large, but the muscle is often quite lax. If the crura are denuded of overlying peritoneum from dissection of the hernia sac or are unable to hold sutures because of significant attenuation, or cannot be reapproximated without tension, we will typically reinforce the closure with a biologic absorbable mesh.

Troubleshooting We use biologic mesh and a Protack device (Covidien) to secure the mesh. The mesh is configured in a U shape, with the broad base of the U overlying the sutures reapproximating the crura posterior to the esophagus. The limbs of the U are positioned along side the hiatus. Malpositioned, bulky mesh may be partially responsible for dysphagia, although this is controversial in the literature.

COMPLICATIONS

Mortality in the laparoscopic era is 1 to 2% and has been associated with advanced age and the urgency of the operation.[52] Elective repair of paraesophageal hernia has been found to have a 0.5% mortality in contrast to a 7.5% mortality for urgent repair. Major morbidity rates in a single academic institution are reported at 20%. These adverse outcomes included pneumonia, congestive heart failure, pulmonary embolism, postoperative leak, perioperative hernia recurrence, need for reintubation, acute renal failure, cerebrovascular accident, and myocardial infarction. It is worthwhile noting that the majority of perioperative leaks were in patients who underwent gastroplasty.[52]

POSTOPERATIVE CARE

We routinely obtain an esophagogram before initiating feeding. Diet progression is the same as that for a Nissen fundoplication. Patients are counseled to avoid strenuous activity for 4 to 6 weeks to decrease strain at the hiatus. Every attempt is made to minimize nausea and wretching in the postoperative period.

OUTCOME EVALUATION

There is considerable variability in reporting of recurrences after laparoscopic paraesophageal hernia repair. Short-term recurrence rates range from 12.0 to 42%.[55–57] Variation seems to depend on whether one measures radiographic or symptomatic recurrence as there is significant discordance between the two. In Luketich and colleagues' largest series published in 2010, recurrent hiatal hernia was identified in 70 of 445 patients who underwent postoperative upper GI studies more than 3 months postoperatively (14.5%).[52] Radiographic recurrence and significant symptoms leading to reoperation, however, were limited to 21 of 662 patients (3.2%). Interestingly, Luketich and colleagues found no association between radiographic recurrence and recurrent symptoms. In a smaller study from the University of Minnesota looking specifically at patients with giant or recurrent hiatal hernia who underwent wedge gastroplasty, there was a 98% satisfaction rate with the surgical outcome in the 51 of 61 patients who completed the GERD-HRQOL survey, with only 25% of patients reporting antacid medication use of any sort. More than 80% of respondents experienced resolution of symptoms such as heartburn, regurgiation, chest pain, abdominal pain, and respiratory symptoms. Only two of 42 patients had a small asymptomatic recurrence seen on a contrast study at the 2-year follow-up.[58]

Reoperation for GERD

Currently, an increasing number of patients are being seen for evaluation and treatment of foregut symptoms after laparoscopic antireflux surgery. These patients are treated as follows:

PREOPERATIVE EVALUATION

Some degree of dysphagia, bloating, and abdominal discomfort is common during the first 6 to 8 weeks after a fundoplication. If these symptoms persist or heartburn and regurgitation occur, a thorough evaluation (with barium swallow, endoscopy, esophageal manometry, and pH monitoring) is carried out with the aim of answering the following three questions:

1. Are the symptoms attributable to persistent gastroesophageal reflux?
2. Are the symptoms attributable to the fundoplication itself?
3. Can the cause of the failure of the first operation be identified and corrected by a second operation?

Many patients report heartburn after a fundoplication. It is often assumed that this symptom must be the result of a failed operation and that acid-reducing medications should be restarted. In most cases, however, this assumption is mistaken: postoperative pH monitoring yields abnormal results in only about 20% of patients.[59] The value of manometry lies in its ability to document the changes caused by the operation at the level of the LES and the esophageal body. The pH monitoring assesses the reflux status and determines whether there is a correlation between symptoms and actual episodes of reflux. If abnormal reflux is present, the therapeutic choice is between medical therapy and a second operation.

Other patients complain of dysphagia arising de novo after the operation. This symptom is usually attributable to the operation itself and may occur in the absence of abnormal reflux. In addition to manometry and pH monitoring, a barium swallow is essential to define the anatomy of the esophagogastric junction. A study from the University of Washington found that the anatomic configurations observed could be divided into three main types: (1) type I hernia, in which the esophagogastric junction was above the diaphragm (subdivided into type IA, with both the esophagogastric junction and the wrap above the diaphragm, and type IB, with only the esophagogastric junction above the diaphragm); (2) type II hernia, a paraesophageal configuration; and (3) type III hernia, in which the esophagogastric junction was below the diaphragm and there was no evidence of hernia but in which the body of the stomach rather than the fundus was used for the wrap.[20] In 10% of patients, however, the cause of the failure could not be identified preoperatively.[60]

Some patients present with a mix of postprandial bloating, nausea, and diarrhea. These symptoms may be the result of damage to the vagus nerves. Radionuclide evaluation of gastric emptying often helps quantify the problem.

OPERATIVE PLANNING

Patient preparation (i.e., anesthesia, positioning, and instrumentation) for a reoperation for reflux is identical to that for the initial laparoscopic fundoplication.

OPERATIVE TECHNIQUE

We routinely attempt a second antireflux operation laparoscopically. To provide a stepwise technical description that would be suitable for all reoperations for reflux is impossible because the optimal procedure depends on the original approach (open versus laparoscopic), the severity of the adhesions, and the specific technique used for the first operation (total or partial fundoplication). The key goals of reoperation for reflux are as follows:

1. To dissect the wrap and the esophagus away from the crura. This is the most difficult part of the operation. The major complications seen during this part of the procedure are damage to the vagus nerves and perforation of the esophagus and the gastric fundus.
2. To take down the previous repair. The earlier repair must be completely undone and the gastric fundus returned to its natural position. If the short gastric vessels were not taken down during the first procedure, they must be taken down during the second.
3. To dissect the esophagus in the posterior mediastinum so as to have enough esophageal length below the diaphragm and avoid placing tension on the repair.
4. To reconstruct the cardia. The same steps are followed as for a first-time repair. If, after extensive esophageal mobilization, the esophagogastric junction remains above the diaphragm (short esophagus), esophageal lengthening can be accomplished by adding a thoracoscopic Collis gastroplasty to the fundoplication. To date, however, we have never found this step to be necessary.

COMPLICATIONS

Because the risk of gastric or esophageal perforation or damage to the vagus nerves is much higher during a second antireflux operation, the surgeon must proceed with extreme care, making sure to identify structures completely before dividing them. Most perforations are recognized and repaired intraoperatively. Leaks manifest themselves during the first 48 hours. Peritoneal signs are noted if the spillage is limited to the abdomen; shortness of breath and a pleural effusion are noted if spillage also occurs in the chest. The site of the leak should always be confirmed by means of a contrast study with barium or a water-soluble agent. Perforation is best handled with laparotomy and direct repair of the leak.

OUTCOME EVALUATION

Whereas the success rate is around 80 to 90% for a first antireflux operation, it falls to 70 to 80% for a second such operation and falls an additional 10 to 15% for each redo. In our view, a second operation should be attempted by an expert team only if medical management fails to control heartburn or dilatation has not relieved dysphagia.

Reoperation for Esophageal Achalasia

Laparoscopic Heller myotomy improves swallowing in more than 90% of patients. What causes the relatively few failures reported is still incompletely understood. Typically, a failed Heller myotomy is signaled either by persistent dysphagia or by recurrent dysphagia that develops after a variable symptom-free interval following the original operation.

A complete workup (routinely including barium swallow, endoscopy, manometry, and pH monitoring) is required before treatment is planned. Such errors typically fall into one of the following three categories:

1. A myotomy that is too short either distally or proximally. If the myotomy is too short distally, a barium swallow shows persistent distal esophageal narrowing and manometry shows a residual high-pressure zone. If the myotomy is too short proximally, it will be apparent from the barium swallow.
2. A constricting Dor fundoplication. Often manometry and pH monitoring yield normal results, but a barium swallow shows slow passage of contrast media from the esophagus into the stomach. In one study from UCSF, problems with Dor fundoplications occurred in four (4%) of 102 patients.[28] Analysis of the video records of the first operations showed that in three of the four patients, all the stitches in the right suture row had incorporated the esophagus, the right pillar of the crus, and the stomach, thereby constricting the myotomy. In one patient, the short gastric vessels had not been taken down, and the body of the stomach rather than the fundus had been used for the fundoplication.
3. Transmural scarring caused by previous treatment. In patients treated with intrasphincteric injection of botulinum toxin, transmural fibrosis can sometimes be found at the level of the esophagogastric junction. This unwelcome finding makes the myotomy more difficult and the results less reliable.

There are two treatment options for persistent or recurrent dysphagia after Heller myotomy: (1) pneumatic dilatation and (2) a second operation tailored to the results of preoperative evaluation. In a 2002 study, pneumatic dilatation was successfully used to treat seven of 10 patients who experienced dysphagia postoperatively; of the remaining three patients, two required a second operation and one refused any treatment.[27]

Reoperation for achalasia is technically challenging. It is of paramount importance to avoid perforating the exposed esophageal mucosa during the dissection. A small hole can be repaired, but a larger laceration might necessitate an esophagectomy. This option should always be discussed with the patient before the operation. Several reports have stressed the feasibility of laparoscopic reoperation after a failed myotomy.[61]

Overall, about 10 to 20% of patients experience some degree of dysphagia after a Heller myotomy. Pneumatic dilatation, a second myotomy, or both should always be tried before an esophagectomy is considered.

Financial Disclosures: None Reported

References

1. Kahrilas PJ, Shaheen NJ, Vaezi MF, et al. American Gastroenterological Association Medical Position Statement on the management of gastroesophageal reflux disease. Gastroenterology 2008;135:1383–1391, 1391.e1-5.
2. Dent J, El-Serag HB, Wallander MA, Johansson S. Epidemiology of gastro-oesophageal reflux disease: a systematic review. Gut 2005;54:710–7.
3. Everhart JE, Ruhl CE. Burden of digestive diseases in the United States part I: overall and upper gastrointestinal diseases. Gastroenterology 2009;136:376–86.
4. IMS Health National Sales Perspectives. Top Therapeutic Classes by U.S. Sales. 2009. Available at: http://www.imshealth.com/ims/Global/Content/Corporate/Press

%20Room/Top-line%20Market%20Data/2009%20Top-line%20Market%20Data/Top%20Therapy%20Classes%20by%20U.S.Sales.pdf

5. Wileman SM, McCann S, Grant AM, et al. Medical versus surgical management for gastro-oesophageal reflux disease (GORD) in adults. Cochrane Database Syst Rev 2010;(3):CD003243.
6. Ito T, Jensen R. Association of long-term proton pump inhibitor therapy with bone fractures and effects on absorption of calcium, vitamin B_{12}, iron, and magnesium. Curr Gastroenterol Rep 2010;12:448–57.
7. Stefanidis D, Hope WW, Kohn GP, et al. Guidelines for surgical treatment of gastroesophageal reflux disease. Surg Endosc 2010;24:2647–69.
8. So JB, Zeitels SM, Rattner DW. Outcomes of atypical symptoms attributed to gastroesophageal reflux treated by laparoscopic fundoplication. Surgery 1998;124:28–32.
9. Sonnenberg A, Delco F, El-Serag HB. Empirical therapy versus diagnostic tests in gastroesophageal reflux disease: a medical decision analysis. Dig Dis Sci 1998;43:1001–8.
10. Johnsson F, Joelsson B, Gudmundsson K, Greiff L. Symptoms and endoscopic findings in the diagnosis of gastroesophageal reflux disease. Scand J Gastroenterol 1987;22:714–8.
11. Patti MG, Diener U, Tamburini A, et al. Role of esophageal function tests in diagnosis of gastroesophageal reflux disease. Dig Dis Sci 2001;46:597–602.
12. Campos GM, Peters JH, DeMeester TR, et al. Multivariate analysis of factors predicting outcome after laparoscopic Nissen fundoplication. J Gastrointest Surg 1999;3:292–300.
13. Patti MG, Goldberg HI, Arcerito M, et al. Hiatal hernia size affects lower esophageal sphincter function, esophageal acid exposure, and the degree of mucosal injury. Am J Surg 1996;171:182–6.
14. Bytzer P, Havelund T, Hansen JM. Interobserver variation in the endoscopic diagnosis of reflux esophagitis. Scand J Gastroenterol 1993;28:119–25.
15. Fuchs KH, DeMeester TR, Albertucci M. Specificity and sensitivity of objective diagnosis of gastroesophageal reflux disease. Surgery 1987;102:575–80.
16. Patti MG, Arcerito M, Tamburini A, et al. Effect of laparoscopic fundoplication on gastroesophageal reflux disease-induced respiratory symptoms. J Gastrointest Surg 2000;4:143–9.
17. Diener U, Patti MG, Molena D, et al. Esophageal dysmotility and gastroesophageal reflux disease. J Gastrointest Surg 2001;5:260–5.
18. Mainie I, Tutuian R, Shay S, et al. Acid and non-acid reflux in patients with persistent symptoms despite acid suppressive therapy: a multicentre study using combined ambulatory impedance-pH monitoring. Gut 2006;55:1398–402.
19. Hirano I, Richter JE, Practice Parameters Committee of the American College of Gastroenterology. ACG practice guidelines: esophageal reflux testing. Am J Gastroenterol 2007;102:668–85.
20. Horgan S, Pohl D, Bogetti D, et al. Failed antireflux surgery: what have we learned from reoperations? Arch Surg 1999;134:809–15; discussion 815–7.
21. Patti MG, Robinson T, Galvani C, et al. Total fundoplication is superior to partial fundoplication even when esophageal peristalsis is weak. J Am Coll Surg 2004;198:863 –9; discussion 869–70.
22. Patterson EJ, Herron DM, Hansen PD, et al. Effect of an esophageal bougie on the incidence of dysphagia following Nissen fundoplication: a prospective, blinded, randomized clinical trial. Arch Surg 2000;135:1055 –61; discussion 1061–2.
23. Guelrud M, Rossiter A, Souney PF, et al. The effect of vasoactive intestinal polypeptide on the lower esophageal sphincter in achalasia. Gastroenterology 1992;103:377–82.
24. Tottrup A, Svane D, Forman A. Nitric oxide mediating NANC inhibition in opossum lower esophageal sphincter. Am J Physiol 1991;260:G385–9.
25. Champion JK, Delisle N, Hunt T. Laparoscopic esophagomyotomy with posterior partial fundoplication for primary esophageal motility disorders. Surg Endosc 2000;14:746–9.
26. Patti MG, Molena D, Fisichella PM, et al. Laparoscopic Heller myotomy and Dor fundoplication for achalasia: analysis of successes and failures. Arch Surg 2001;136:870–7.
27. Zaninotto G, Costantini M, Portale G, et al. Etiology, diagnosis, and treatment of failures after laparoscopic Heller myotomy for achalasia. Ann Surg 2002;235:186–92.
28. Moonka R, Patti MG, Feo CV, et al. Clinical presentation and evaluation of malignant pseudoachalasia. J Gastrointest Surg 1999;3:456–61.
29. Watson DI, Liu JF, Devitt PG, et al. Outcome of laparoscopic anterior 180 degree partial fundoplication for gastroesophageal reflux disease. J Gastrointest Surg 2000;4:486–92.
30. Patti MG, Arcerito M, Feo CV, et al. An analysis of operations for gastroesophageal reflux disease: identifying the important technical elements. Arch Surg 1998;133:600–6; discussion 606–7.
31. Horvath KD, Jobe BA, Herron DM, Swanstrom LL. Laparoscopic Toupet fundoplication is an inadequate procedure for patients with severe reflux disease. J Gastrointest Surg 1999;3:583–91.
32. Oleynikov D, Eubanks TR, Oelschlager BK, Pellegrini CA. Total fundoplication is the operation of choice for patients with gastroesophageal reflux and defective peristalsis. Surg Endosc 2002;16:909–13.
33. Novitsky YW, Wong J, Kercher KW, et al. Severely disordered esophageal peristalsis is not a contraindication to laparoscopic Nissen fundoplication. Surg Endosc 2007;21:950–4.
34. Herbella FA, Tedesco P, Nipomnick I, et al. Effect of partial and total laparoscopic fundoplication on esophageal body motility. Surg Endosc 2007;21:285–8.
35. Spechler SJ, Lee E, Ahnen D, et al. Long-term outcome of medical and surgical therapies for gastroesophageal reflux disease: follow-up of a randomized controlled trial. JAMA 2001;285:2331–8.
36. Dallemagne B, Weerts J, Markiewicz S, et al. Clinical results of laparoscopic fundoplication at ten years after surgery. Surg Endosc 2006;20:159–65.
37. Morgenthal CB, Shane MD, Stival A, et al. The durability of laparoscopic Nissen fundoplication: 11-year outcomes. J Gastrointest Surg 2007;11:693–700.
38. Kelly JJ, Watson DI, Chin KF, et al. Laparoscopic Nissen fundoplication: clinical outcomes at 10 years. J Am Coll Surg 2007;205:570–5.

39. Patti MG, Pellegrini CA, Horgan S, et al. Minimally invasive surgery for achalasia: an 8-year experience with 168 patients. Ann Surg 1999;230:587 –93; discussion 593–4.
40. Zaninotto G, Costantini M, Molena D, et al. Treatment of esophageal achalasia with laparoscopic Heller myotomy and Dor partial anterior fundoplication: prospective evaluation of 100 consecutive patients. J Gastrointest Surg 2000; 4:282–9.
41. Ackroyd R, Watson DI, Devitt PG, Jamieson GG. Laparoscopic cardiomyotomy and anterior partial fundoplication for achalasia. Surg Endosc 2001;15:683–6.
42. Finley RJ, Clifton JC, Stewart KC, et al. Laparoscopic Heller myotomy improves esophageal emptying and the symptoms of achalasia. Arch Surg 2001;136:892–6.
43. Patti MG, Diener U, Molena D. Esophageal achalasia: preoperative assessment and postoperative follow-up. J Gastrointest Surg 2001;5:11–2.
44. Richards WO, Torquati A, Holzman MD, et al. Heller myotomy versus Heller myotomy with Dor fundoplication for achalasia: a prospective randomized double-blind clinical trial. Ann Surg 2004;240:405–12; discussion 412–5.
45. Costantini M, Zaninotto G, Guirroli E, et al. The laparoscopic Heller-Dor operation remains an effective treatment for esophageal achalasia at a minimum 6-year follow-up. Surg Endosc 2005;19:345–51.
46. Boeckxstaens GE, Annese V, Varannes SBD, et al. Pneumatic dilation versus laparoscopic Heller's myotomy for idiopathic achalasia. N Engl J Med 2012;364:1807–16.
47. Sweet MP, Nipomnick I, Gasper WJ, et al. The outcome of laparoscopic Heller myotomy for achalasia is not influenced by the degree of esophageal dilatation. J Gastrointest Surg 2008;12:159–65.
48. Smith CD, Stival A, Howell DL, Swafford V. Endoscopic therapy for achalasia before Heller myotomy results in worse outcomes than heller myotomy alone. Ann Surg 2006;243:579–84; discussion 584–6.
49. Patti MG, Fisichella PM, Perretta S, et al. Impact of minimally invasive surgery on the treatment of esophageal achalasia: a decade of change. J Am Coll Surg 2003;196:698–703; discussion 703–5.
50. Kahrilas PJ, Pandolfino JE. Hiatus hernia in the esophagus. In: Costell DO, Richter JE, editors. Philadelphia: 2004. p. 389–407.
51. Hashemi M, Sillin LF, Peters JH. Current concepts in the management of paraesophageal hiatal hernia. J Clin Gastroenterol 1999;29(1):8–13.
52. Luketich JD, Nason KS, Christie NA, et al. Outcomes after a decade of laparoscopic giant paraesophageal hernia repair. J Thorac Cardiovasc Surg 2010;139:395–404, 404.e1.
53. Skinner DB, Belsey RH. Surgical management of esophageal reflux and hiatus hernia. Long-term results with 1,030 patients. J Thorac Cardiovasc Surg 1967;53(1):33–54.
54. Allen MS, Trastek VF, Deschamps C, Pairolero PC. Intrathoracic stomach. Presentation and results of operation. J Thorac Cardiovasc Surg 1993;105:253–8; discussion 258–9.
55. Dahlberg PS, Deschamps C, Miller DL, et al. Laparoscopic repair of large paraesophageal hiatal hernia. Ann Thorac Surg 2001;72:1125–9.
56. Hashemi M, Peters JH, DeMeester TR, et al. Laparoscopic repair of large type III hiatal hernia: objective followup reveals high recurrence rate. J Am Coll Surg 2000;190:553–60; discussion 560–1.
57. Lin E, Swafford V, Chadalavada R, et al. Disparity between symptomatic and physiologic outcomes following esophageal lengthening procedures for antireflux surgery. J Gastrointest Surg 2004;8:31–9; discussion 38–9.
58. Whitson BA, Hoang CD, Boettcher AK, et al. Wedge gastroplasty and reinforced crural repair: important components of laparoscopic giant or recurrent hiatal hernia repair. J Thorac Cardiovasc Surg 2006;132:1196–1202.e3.
59. Lord RV, Kaminski A, Oberg S, et al. Absence of gastroesophageal reflux disease in a majority of patients taking acid suppression medications after Nissen fundoplication. J Gastrointest Surg 2002;6:3–9; discussion 10.
60. Patti MG, Gorodner MV, Galvani C, et al. Spectrum of esophageal motility disorders: implications for diagnosis and treatment. Arch Surg 2005;140:442–8; discussion 448–9.
61. Iqbal A, Tierney B, Haider M, et al. Laparoscopic reoperation for failed Heller myotomy. Dis Esophagus 2006; 19:193–9.

Acknowledgment

Figures 1 through 10 Tom Moore

9 CHEST WALL PROCEDURES

Bryon J. Boulton, MD, and Seth D. Force, MD

Chest wall procedures are an important component of any thoracic surgeon's practice. The approach to these procedures is somewhat different from the approach to esophageal or pulmonary resections and requires specific knowledge of thoracic musculoskeletal anatomy, as well as of the different types of autologous and artificial grafts available for chest wall reconstruction. Broadly, chest wall procedures may be divided into those performed to treat congenital chest wall disease and those done to treat acquired disease. In what follows, we describe the major surgical techniques in both categories and review the pitfalls that may accompany them.

Procedures for Congenital Chest Wall Disease

Congenital chest wall defects arise from abnormal development of the sternum, the costal cartilages, and the ribs. Such defects include pectus excavatum (funnel chest), pectus carinatum (pigeon chest), cleft sternum, and Poland syndrome (absence of the breast and the underlying pectoralis muscle and ribs). Of these, pectus excavatum is by far the most common, accounting for more than 90% of all congenital chest wall procedures; accordingly, the ensuing discussion focuses on the surgical aspects of pectus excavatum repair.

REPAIR OF PECTUS EXCAVATUM

Preoperative Evaluation

Because pectus excavatum occurs in varying degrees of severity, patients may seek surgical treatment for any of a number of different reasons, such as shortness of breath, early fatigue with exercise, or simple dissatisfaction with their appearance. Thus, one of the most important tasks for surgeons treating pectus excavatum is determining which patients are candidates for operative management. In an attempt to facilitate this determination, the Congenital Heart Surgery Nomenclature and Database Project has developed a classification system for pectus excavatum, in which a deformity less than 2 cm in depth is classified as mild, a deformity 2 to 3 cm in depth is classified as moderate, and a deformity greater than 3 cm in depth is classified as severe.[1] A computed tomography (CT)–based index has also been devised, in which the transverse chest diameter is divided by the anteroposterior diameter; an index greater than 3.2 is considered indicative of severe disease.[2]

These classification attempts notwithstanding, the precise indications for surgery remain unclear. Many studies have attempted to show that the depressed sternum leads to pulmonary compromise, but, for the most part, these studies have had small sample sizes and have employed differing measures of lung function, both of which have made accurate comparisons difficult. In one study that included 25 US Air Force personnel with symptomatic pectus excavatum, lung volumes were comparable to those in normal persons, but there was a significant difference in maximum voluntary ventilation.[3] In a study that compared 37 patients who had undergone surgical repair of pectus excavatum both with normal persons and with persons who had uncorrected deformities, no differences in physical working capacity among the three groups were noted.[4] Other studies have reported improvements in exercise tolerance and regional ventilation and perfusion after surgical repair of pectus excavatum.[5,6] On the other hand, some investigators have reported decreases in pulmonary function in symptomatic patients after corrective surgery. One group attributed this result to overly aggressive resection in very young patients that led to growth restriction of the chest wall; accordingly, they recommended delaying surgical repair until 6 to 8 years of age.[7]

Severe pectus excavatum has also been reported to cause cardiac dysfunction secondary to sternal compression of the right ventricle. Several early studies found stroke volume and cardiac output to be lower in exercising upright patients than in supine patients.[8,9] However, improvement in cardiac function after pectus excavatum repair has not been universally documented. In one study, first-pass radionuclide angiocardiography failed to show any improvements in left ventricular function after repair of pectus excavatum.[10] At present, there is no consensus on the cardiopulmonary benefits of pectus excavatum repair, and the major reasons for surgical treatment are still patient discomfort and dissatisfaction with appearance.

Operative Technique

A number of different procedures have been employed to treat pectus excavatum, but, for present purposes, we focus on (1) the Ravitch procedure (and variations thereof) and (2) the Nuss procedure. For historical reasons, the turnover technique, originally described by Judet and Judet[11] and later employed by Wada and colleagues,[12] warrants a brief mention. Wada and colleagues' series included 199 patients whose deformities were corrected with a version of this technique; good results were achieved in 63% of patients, and there were only three instances of partial sternal necrosis. Today, however, the turnover technique is rarely used because of the good results that can be achieved with techniques that do not carry a risk of sternal necrosis. It is usually reserved for extreme cases of pectus excavatum, which often include deformities of the sternum in addition to abnormalities of the costal cartilages.

Ravitch procedure Repair of pectus excavatum is based on the principle that the deformity is secondary to abnormal growth of the costal cartilages. Accordingly, correction involves (1) resection of the abnormal cartilages, (2) a transverse anterior sternal osteotomy to allow anterior displacement of the sternum, and (3) sternal fixation to prevent posterior displacement after the repair. Most of the variations in the Ravitch procedure have to do with the use of different sternal fixation techniques.

Step 1: initial incision and exposure Either a midline incision or a bilateral inframammary incision is made [*see Figure 1a, b*]; the latter incision yields superior cosmetic results, especially in female patients, but necessitates the elevation of large subcutaneous skin flaps to the level of the angle of Louis or the sternal notch superiorly and to the xiphoid process inferiorly. The pectoralis muscles are then mobilized from the chest wall, beginning medially and proceeding laterally until the costal cartilages are exposed [*see Figure 1c*].

Step 2: resection of abnormal cartilages For each abnormal costal cartilage, the anterior perichondrium is scored with the electrocautery along the length of the cartilage, and the cartilage is dissected from the perichondrium with a periosteal elevator [*see Figure 2a*]. The posterior plane between the cartilage and the perichondrium is then developed in one area, and the cartilage is divided with a scalpel between the jaws of a right-angle clamp [*see Figure 2b*]. The cut end of the cartilage is grasped with a clamp, and the rest of the cartilage is dissected from the perichondrium. Once the correct plane is established, the dissection can be facilitated by gently pushing the perichondrium off the cartilage with a finger. The entire cartilage should be removed from the sternum to the rib, with every attempt made to maintain the integrity of the perichondrium. During this part of the procedure, the xiphoid process is also detached from the sternum. The extent of cartilage removal depends on the individual defect present but usually includes the third rib.

Step 3: sternal osteotomy An osteotomy is made in the upper anterior table of the sternum with either a periosteal elevator or a small reticulating bone saw [*see Figure 3a*], and the posterior table of the sternum is fractured. The sternum can then be angled anteriorly. When the desired angle is reached, the osteotomy is closed with three interrupted nonabsorbable sutures or with microplates and screws [*see Figure 3b,* c]. At this point, rotational sternal defects can be corrected by making anterior and posterior lateral osteotomies on either side of the sternum and then closing the osteotomies with sutures or microplates.

Step 4: sternal fixation Sternal fixation can be accomplished by any of several means. Posterior sternal support can be achieved by placing a Kirschner wire or retrosternal bar that is secured to the periosteum of the rib and left in place for approximately 3 months after operation [*see Figure 4*]. Alternatively, the sternum can be supported with a piece of polypropylene mesh or with two polypropylene sutures sutured to the xiphoid process and then brought around the right and left second ribs.[13]

Step 5: closure and drainage The pectoralis muscles are reapproximated in the midline, closed suction drains are placed in the subcutaneous flaps, and the subcutaneous layer and the skin are closed. To prevent seroma formation, one closed suction drain may be placed posterior to the pectoralis muscles and another between the pectoralis muscles and the subcutaneous layer; the right pleural space may then be

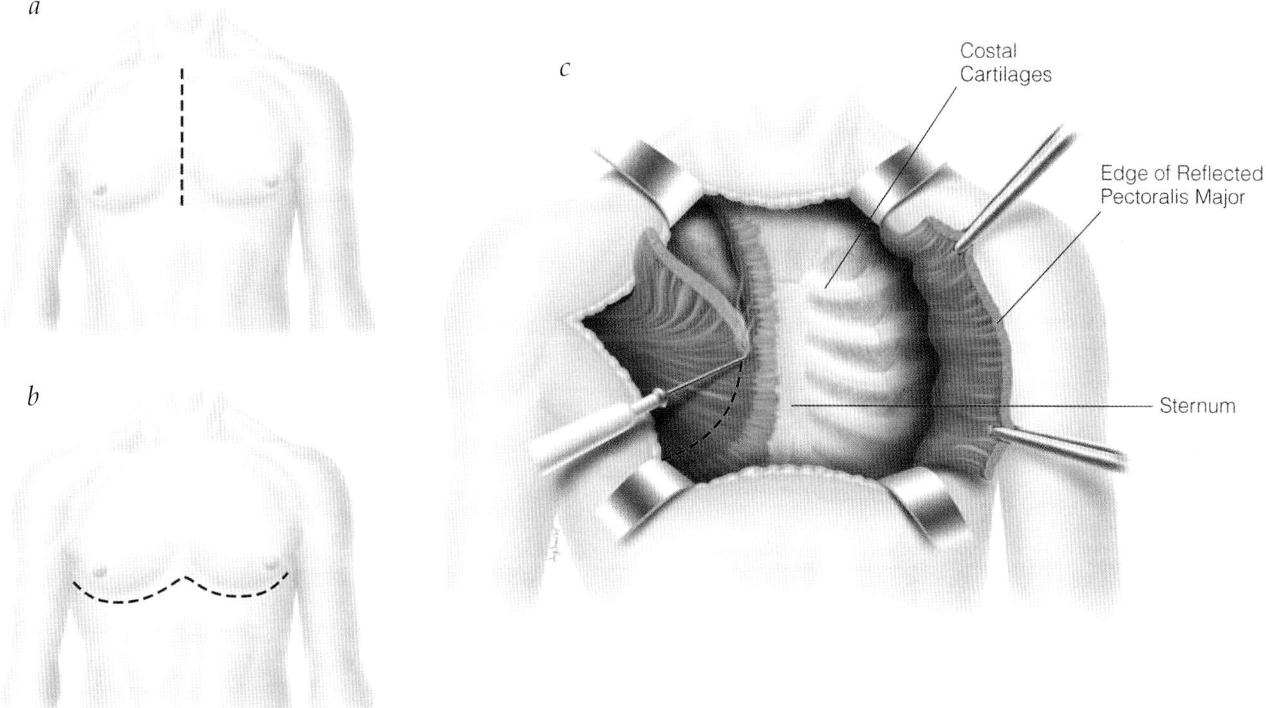

Figure 1 **Repair of pectus excavatum: Ravitch procedure. The procedure begins with a midline incision (*a*) or a bilateral inframammary incision (*b*). The pectoralis muscles are then dissected off the chest wall (*c*).**

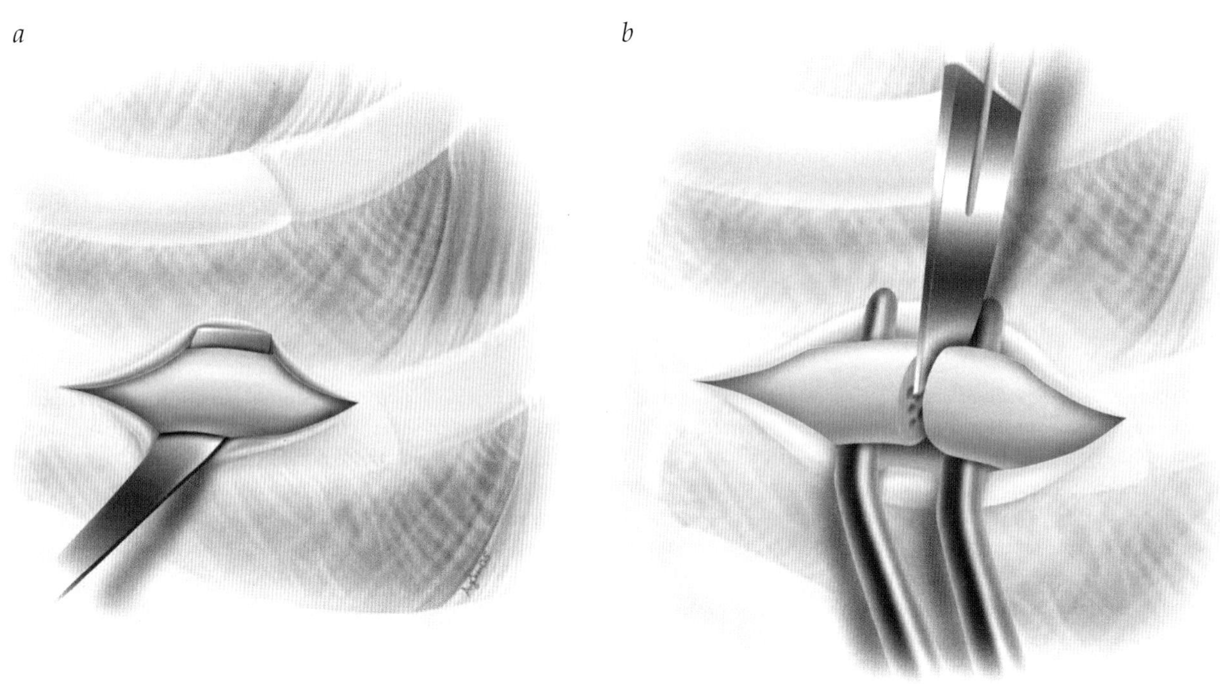

Figure 2 **Repair of pectus excavatum: Ravitch procedure. (*a*) The anterior perichondrium is opened, and the abnormal cartilage is dissected free with a periosteal elevator. (*b*) The cartilage is divided.**

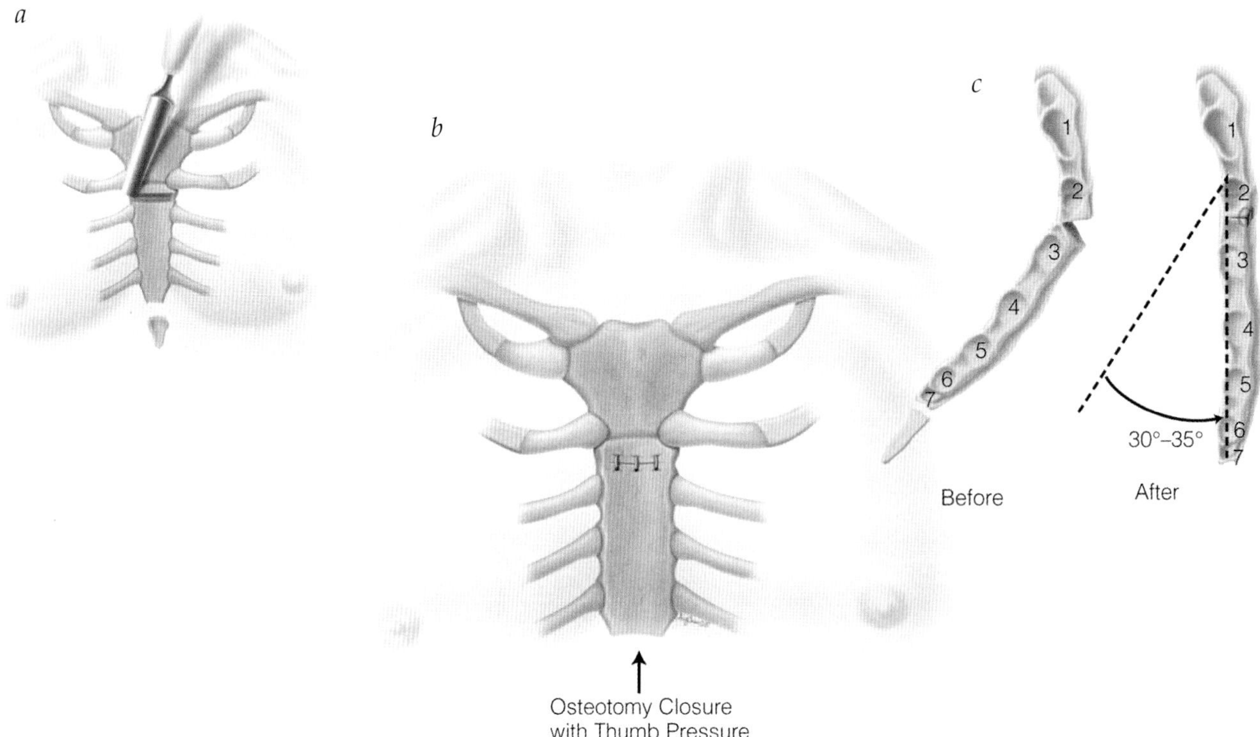

Figure 3 **Repair of pectus excavatum: Ravitch procedure. (*a*) An osteotomy is made in the upper sternum. (*b*) The sternum is angled anteriorly; when the desired angle is reached, the osteotomy is closed. (*c*) Shown is a lateral view of the sternal angle before and after correction.**

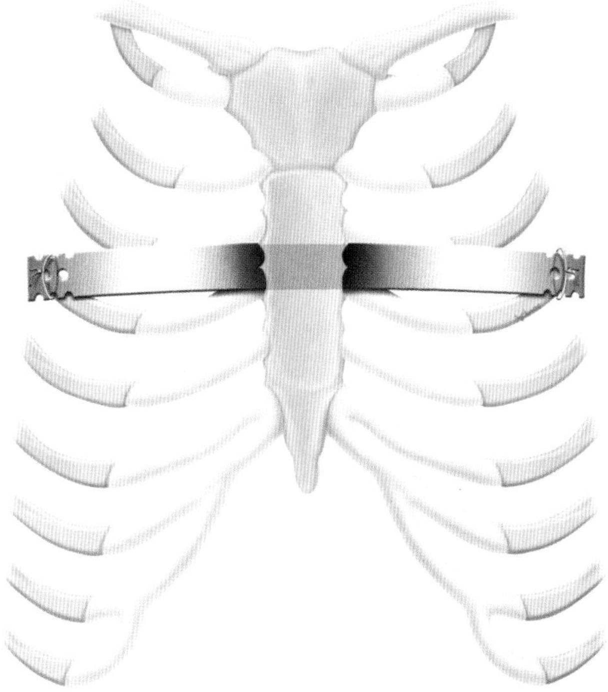

Figure 4 **Repair of pectus excavatum: Ravitch procedure. Sternal fixation is accomplished through placement of a retrosternal bar.**

opened anteriorly and a right pleural tube placed through a separate incision.[14]

Nuss procedure Minimally invasive repair of pectus excavatum, also referred to as the Nuss procedure, has gained popularity over the past decade.

Step 1: configuration of bar The patient is placed in the supine position with the arms abducted, and marks are made on either side of the chest at spots that correspond to the deepest point of the defect. The bar that will be used for the repair is shortened to a length equivalent to the measured distance between the two midaxillary lines minus 1 cm. A complex series of bends are then placed in the bar to match its contours to those of the patient's deformity.

Step 2: initial incisions and creation of intrathoracic tunnel Incisions are made in the right and left midaxillary lines at the level of the marks, and a subcutaneous flap is raised from each incision and extended to the defect. A Crawford vascular clamp or a Lorenz pectus introducer is then placed through the right intercostal space under thoracoscopic visualization and advanced along the posterior sternum and out the corresponding left intercostal space [*see Figure 5*].

Step 3: placement and fixation of bar An umbilical tape is pulled through the anterior mediastinum and attached to the bar, which is then gently pulled, with the concave side up, through the intercostal space. A Lorenz pectus bar rotator is employed to flip the bar over, and the ends of the bar are positioned in the subcutaneous space [*see Figure 6*]. Occasionally, for proper alignment, the bar may have to be removed and rebent, or stabilizers may have to be placed alongside it.

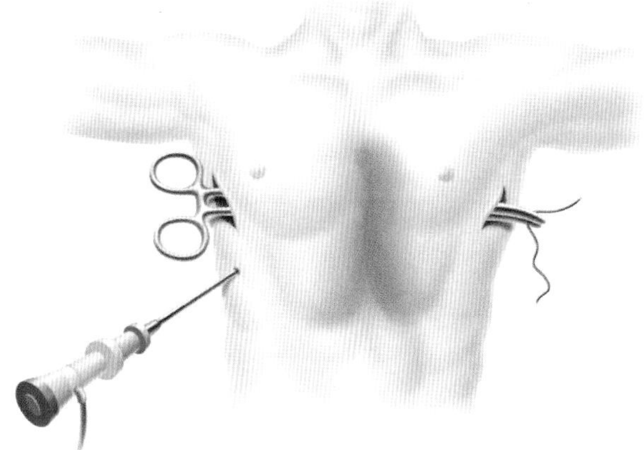

Figure 5 **Repair of pectus excavatum: Nuss procedure. Incisions are made on either side of the chest. A Crawford vascular clamp is inserted through the right intercostal space and advanced along the sternum and out the left intercostal space.**

When the bar is correctly positioned, it is sutured to the chest wall musculature with an absorbable suture on one end and a permanent suture on the other.

The bar is usually left in place for 2 years. Excellent results have been reported.[15] Significant complications include bar displacement necessitating reoperation (9.2% of procedures), pneumothorax (4.8%), infection (2%), and pleural effusion (2%). Rare complications include cardiac injury, thoracic outlet syndrome (TOS), pericarditis, and sternal erosion caused by the bar.

Outcome Evaluation

In general, the results of pectus excavatum repair are good, and the overall complication rate is low. In one study, 90% of 76 patients operated on over a 30-year period experienced excellent outcomes, and only one patient required reoperation for a recurrent defect.[14] The incidence of complications (pleural effusions, pneumonia, and wound seromas) was 14%.[14] In another study, no operative deaths occurred in more than 800 repairs, and only a few cases of serious infections and bleeding were reported.[16] Other investigators have reported rare complications arising from the migration of sternal support bars and wires.[17]

REPAIR OF PECTUS CARINATUM

Operative Technique

Surgical repair of pectus carinatum resembles surgical repair of pectus excavatum in several respects. The same skin incision is employed, and the pectoralis major muscles are elevated in a similar manner. Subperichondrial resection of the abnormal cartilages is then carried out, usually extending to the second costal cartilage. Next, a generous V-shaped osteotomy is made in the upper portion of the sternum at the point of maximal protrusion, which is usually near the insertion of the second cartilage. Occasionally, a second osteotomy is required near the caudal end of the sternum to facilitate elevation of the manubrium and depression of the sternum.

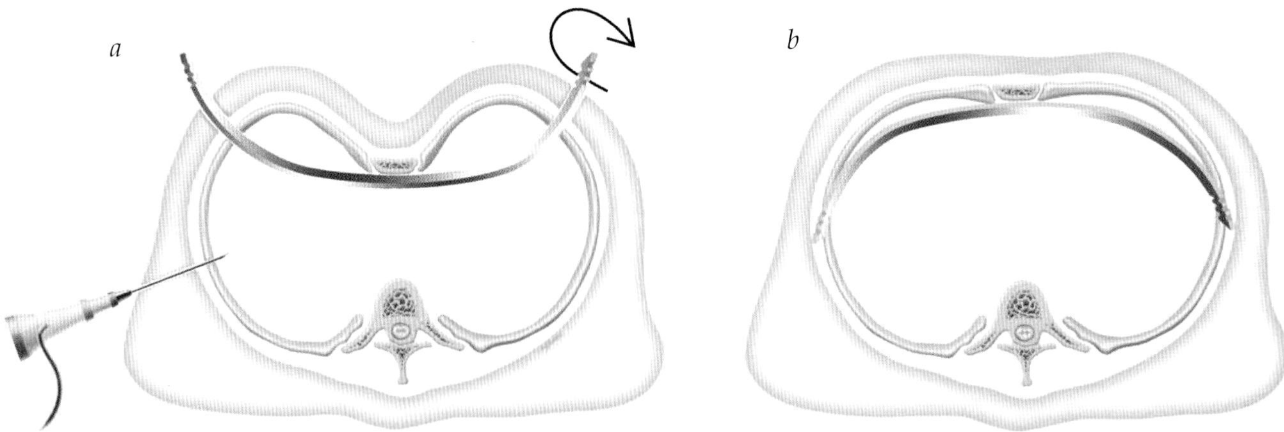

Figure 6 **Repair of pectus excavatum: Nuss procedure. (*a*) The pectus bar is pulled into the tunnel opened by the vascular retractor and then flipped to provide the desired chest contour. (*b*)The ends of the bar are then sutured to the chest wall musculature.**

Finally, the osteotomy is closed with nonabsorbable monofilament sutures, drains are placed, and soft tissue is closed as in a pectus excavatum repair.

Outcome Evaluation

The results of pectus carinatum repair are generally comparable to those of pectus excavatum repair. Most patients experience good outcomes, and operative morbidity is low.

Procedures for Acquired Chest Wall Disease

TRANSAXILLARY FIRST RIB RESECTION FOR THORACIC OUTLET SYNDROME

Preoperative Evaluation

TOS results from compression of the subclavian blood vessels or the brachial plexus as these structures exit the bony thorax. Symptoms may be primarily vascular (e.g., arm swelling or loss of pulse) or neurogenic (e.g., pain and paresthesias). The workup for TOS includes a detailed physical examination, as well as imaging and nerve conduction studies.

Operative Planning

Surgical treatment of TOS typically involves resection of the first rib, which widens the thoracic outlet and relieves the neurovascular impingement. First rib resection can be accomplished via several different approaches, including posterior, supraclavicular, infraclavicular, transthoracic, and transaxillary. I focus here on the transaxillary approach, which provides good exposure of the first rib and allows the surgeon to avoid the subclavian blood vessels and the brachial plexus. Regardless of the specific surgical approach followed, any surgeon embarking on a first rib resection must have a detailed knowledge of the thoracic outlet to keep from injuring the neurovascular structures in the area.

Operative Technique

The patient is placed in the lateral decubitus position, and the affected arm is kept at a 90° angle either by an arm holder or, alternatively, by an assistant. Care must be taken not to hyperabduct or hyperextend the shoulder. The arm, the axilla, and the chest are prepared and draped into the sterile field.

Step 1: initial incision and exposure An incision is made just below the axillary hair line and extended from the pectoralis major to the latissimus dorsi [*see Figure 7*]. The subcutaneous tissue is incised down to the chest wall with the electrocautery, with care taken to stay perpendicular to the axis of the chest. Dissection is then begun along the chest wall and carried toward the first rib. The intercostal brachial

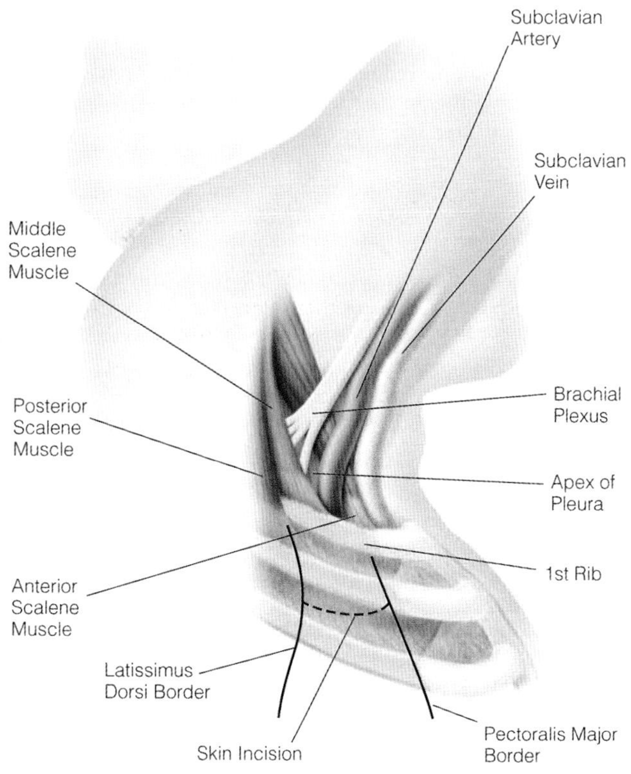

Figure 7 **Transaxillary first rib resection. Shown are the transaxillary incision and the thoracic outlet anatomy.**

nerve is identified where it exits between the first and second ribs. This nerve should be spared: dividing it leads to numbness of the upper inner biceps region.

Step 2: dissection and division of anterior portion of first rib When the first rib is encountered, it is dissected from the periosteum with a periosteal elevator. Dissection is continued anteriorly along the rib until just past the subclavian vein, at which point a right-angle clamp can be passed around the rib in the subperiosteal plane. A Gigli saw or a first rib cutter is then used to divide the anterior portion of the rib [*see Figure 8a*].

Next, the first rib is retracted inferiorly to permit visualization of the anterior scalene muscle, which is then divided at its attachment to the rib. To prevent thermal injury to the phrenic nerve, a scalpel rather than an electrocautery is used to divide the muscle [*see Figure 8b*]. Care should also be taken not to injure the subclavian vein and artery, which lie anterior and posterior to the anterior scalene muscle, respectively. As an alternative, the anterior scalene muscle may be divided before the anterior portion of the rib is cut.

Step 3: dissection and division of posterior portion of first rib The subperiosteal dissection is continued posteriorly, freeing the first rib from the pleura, the subclavian vessels, and the brachial plexus. The posterior portion of the rib is then divided with a first rib cutter as close as possible to the articulation of the rib with the transverse process. Every effort should be made to keep from injuring the C8 and T1 nerve roots.

Step 4: closure The incision is closed without drainage. If the pleura was inadvertently entered, air may be aspirated from the chest with a red rubber tube, which is removed before the subcutaneous tissue is closed. One authority recommends further neurolysis of the C7 to T1 nerve roots and the middle and lower trunks of the brachial plexus, as well as resection of the anterior and middle scalene muscles up into the neck.[18]

Complications

Surgical complications include injuries to the subclavian vein and artery (leading to massive blood loss), the brachial plexus, the phrenic nerve, the long thoracic nerve, and the thoracic duct.

Outcome Evaluation

The long-term results of first rib resection appear to be independent of the exposure technique employed. Good results, defined as relief of major symptoms, have been reported in as many of 90% of patients in the first year and in as many as 70% of patients 5 to 10 years after operation. Considerable debate continues over the preferred surgical approach. but, to date, no studies have shown any one approach to have significant advantages over any of the others.

CHEST WALL RESECTION

Chest wall resection has become a critical component of the thoracic surgeon's armamentarium. It may be performed to treat either benign conditions (e.g., osteoradionecrosis, osteomyelitis, and benign neoplasms) or malignant disease.

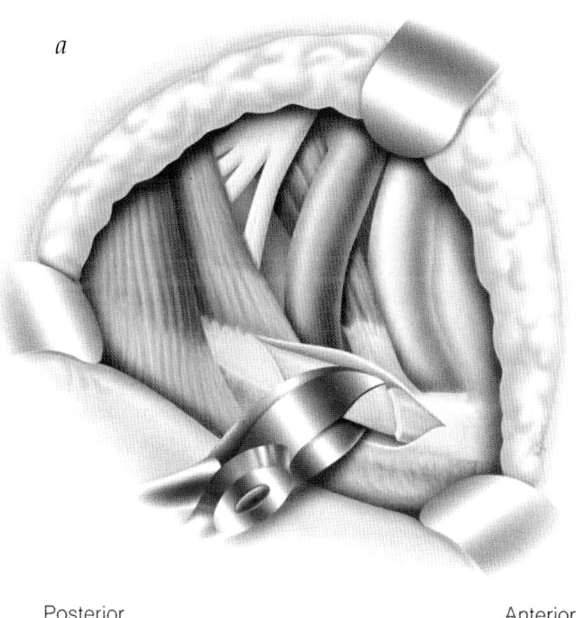

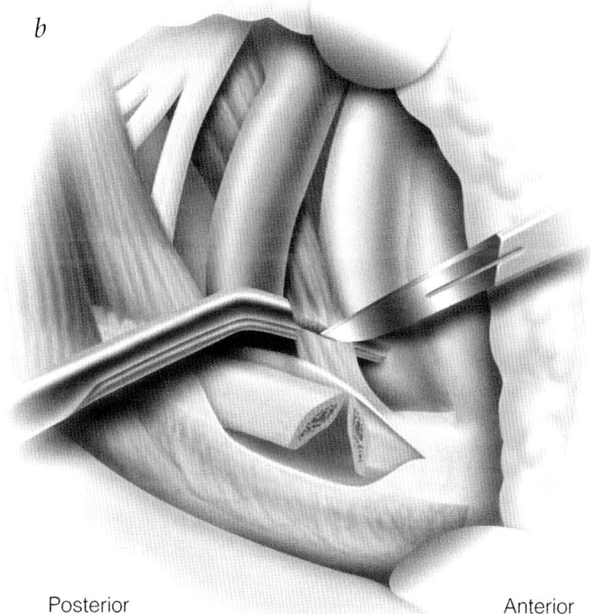

Figure 8 **Transaxillary first rib resection. (*a*) The anterior portion of the first rib is cut. (*b*) The anterior scalene muscle is then divided.**

Preoperative Evaluation

Preoperative imaging studies may include chest x-ray, chest CT [*see Figure 9*], and magnetic resonance imaging if vertebral involvement is suspected. The other preoperative tests ordered are much the same as those required for any other large thoracic procedure, including pulmonary function testing, nutritional assessment, and cardiac stress testing in patients who are older or have a history of cardiac disease.

Operative Planning

Operative planning for chest wall resection should include establishing the extent of the resection, weighing options for chest wall stabilization, and deciding on the method of tissue coverage to be employed. A multidisciplinary approach, involving the participation of a neurosurgeon and a plastic surgeon, may be required.

The technique of chest wall resection is essentially the same for benign conditions as for malignant ones and is mainly dependent on the location of the lesion. For malignant tumors of the chest wall, a 5 cm margin, or at least resection of one uninvolved rib above and below the tumor, is required. Additionally, any involved skin and any biopsy site must be resected along with the chest wall specimen. For infection or osteoradionecrosis, the resection must include all nonviable skin and underlying bone; if it does not, skin and muscle flaps may not heal properly. Any destroyed lung tissue may also have to be resected along with the chest wall specimen. In addition, recurrent cancer must be ruled out before the operation can proceed. A particular challenge is posed by breast cancer patients who have already had muscle flaps for breast reconstruction; in these patients, tissues other than muscle (e.g., omentum) may be required for tissue coverage after chest wall resection.

Standard Chest Wall Resection

In cases in which a concomitant lung resection is required, the chest wall resection is usually performed first; this measure renders the lung more mobile and facilitates the pulmonary resection. The lateral decubitus position is the best choice for most combined lung–chest wall procedures, whereas the supine position is preferable for isolated anterior chest wall procedures. If a larger chest wall resection is expected, every attempt should be made to spare major muscle groups so that these muscles can be used later to cover any prosthetic material used in reconstruction.

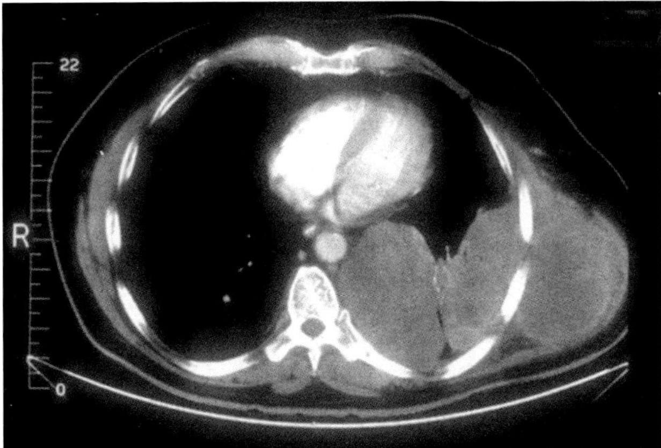

Figure 9 **Chest computed tomographic scan reveals a large pulmonary and chest wall mass.**

Operative technique

Step 1: initial incision and exposure The usual incision is a standard posterolateral thoracotomy incision through the fifth interspace.

Step 2: determination of extent of required chest wall resection As soon as the pleura is opened, the surgeon should palpate the tumor to evaluate the extent of chest wall involvement, which determines the extent of the resection. Removal of uninvolved ribs may make reconstruction of the chest wall more complicated. For example, posterior resections that do not require removal of the fifth rib are protected by the scapula, so reconstruction is unnecessary. If the fifth rib is removed, however, the tip of the scapula will tend to become stuck under the sixth rib with shoulder movement; this is very uncomfortable for the patient, and chest wall reconstruction will therefore be required at the time of resection.

At this point, the surgeon should also rule out diffuse pleural disease before proceeding with resection. In some cases, the tumor can be removed by means of extrapleural dissection, without any need for chest wall resection. If there is any suspicion of chest wall involvement, however, chest wall resection is mandatory because leaving any tumor behind guarantees a recurrence.

The extent of the chest wall resection is marked with the electrocautery on the outside of the thoracic cavity. At least one grossly uninvolved rib should be included both above and below the tumor.

Step 3: completion of anterior boundary of resection Initially, the periosteum over the lowest rib to be resected is scored, and a periosteal elevator is used to separate the intercostal bundle from the rib. Alternatively, the intercostal bundle can be doubly ligated and divided at the anterior resection margin. Once the intercostal vessels are cleared from the lowest rib, the electrocautery is used to divide the pleura below the rib toward the anterior boundary of the resection. The rib is then divided with a rib cutter, with care taken to ensure a margin of at least 5 cm from the tumor [*see Figure 10*]. Next, the intercostal bundle of the next higher rib is ligated and divided, the intercostal muscle is divided with the electrocautery, and the rib is cut with a rib cutter in the same manner as the previous rib. This process is repeated until the anterior boundary of resection is completed. A subperiosteal plane is then developed over the highest rib to be resected, the adjacent intercostal bundle is separated from the rib, and the parietal pleura is divided with the electrocautery.

Step 4: completion of posterior boundary of resection If the tumor margin does not involve the vertebrae, the posterior portion of the chest wall resection is identical to the anterior portion [*see* Step 3, *above*]. If, however, the tumor appears to encroach on the head of the rib or the transverse process, it will be necessary to disarticulate the rib from the transverse process or, in the latter situation, remove the transverse process entirely.

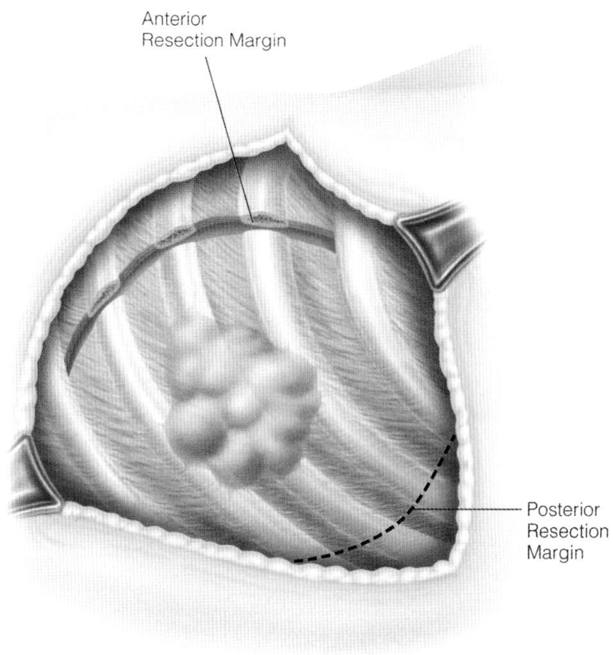

Figure 10 **Chest wall resection. The anterior and posterior margins of the required resection are determined. The anterior margin is completed first.**

Disarticulation of the rib from the transverse process is performed by dissecting the paraspinal ligament and erector spinae muscles away from the spine with the electrocautery, thereby exposing the joint between the head of the rib and the transverse process. The ligaments attaching the rib to the transverse process are then incised with the electrocautery, and an osteotome is inserted into the joint, which is then levered anteriorly and posteriorly to disarticulate the rib from the transverse process [*see Figure 11*]. The intercostal neurovascular bundle must be ligated and divided at this point:

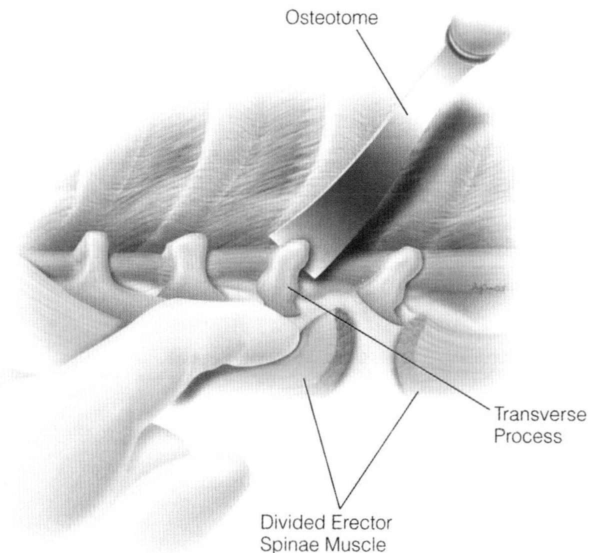

Figure 11 **Chest wall resection. Depicted is disarticulation of the rib from the transverse process.**

failure to do so will result in bleeding and possibly in leakage of cerebrospinal fluid (CSF). If bleeding occurs, it can be controlled with bipolar electrocauterization and temporary packing with a hemostatic agent. The hemostatic agent must not be left in place permanently, because it may expand or result in a neural foramen hematoma, and either of these events can lead to spinal cord compression and significant neurologic injury. If at any time the surgeon feels uncomfortable about ongoing intercostal bleeding or a possible CSF leak, intraoperative neurosurgical consultation should be obtained. In cases in which the tumor involves the transverse process, this structure must be removed from the vertebral body with an osteotome and a mallet or with a first rib cutter. If the tumor has invaded the vertebral body and resection is still being considered, neurosurgical consultation should be obtained. Generally, if the tumor involves more than one quarter of the vertebral body or extends into multiple vertebral levels, it is considered unresectable.

Step 5: lung resection (if required) Once the posterior chest wall margin has been completed, the lung resection (if required) is performed. The entire lung–chest wall specimen is then submitted for pathologic examination, and histopathologic margins are obtained both on the lung and on the chest wall. If the chest wall margins are positive, the involved area must be trimmed back and a new margin submitted.

Step 6: chest wall reconstruction Chest wall reconstruction is required for all anterior defects and for posterior defects that involve any rib lower than the fourth rib. Reconstruction can be performed either with polypropylene or Gore-Tex (W. L. Gore and Associates, Flagstaff, Arizona) mesh or with a polypropylene-methylmethacrylate sandwich. The latter is employed when rigid reconstruction is warranted (as in anterior reconstruction); it not only provides added protection of pleural and mediastinal structures but also creates a better cosmetic effect by recreating the shape of the chest wall.

To create the polypropylene-methylmethacrylate sandwich, two pieces of polypropylene mesh are cut to the size of the defect. A thin layer of methylmethacrylate cement is spread on one of the mesh pieces, and the other piece is then applied over the methylmethacrylate layer. As this sandwich begins to harden, it is molded to the contours of the chest wall, with care taken to protect the patient's skin against injury from the heat given off by the hardening cement. When the sandwich is sufficiently hardened, it is sewn to the ribs with 0 polypropylene sutures [*see Figure 12a*]. The sutures may be passed around the uppermost and lowermost ribs and may be placed directly through the anterior and posterior margins [*see Figure 12b*]. If rib disarticulation was required to complete the posterior margin, holes may be drilled in the transverse processes and the sutures passed through these holes; alternatively, the sandwich may be sutured to the paraspinal ligament.

If polypropylene or Gore-Tex mesh is used without cement, it should be cut to a size smaller than that of the defect. Thus, the mesh will effectively be stretched when it is sutured to the chest wall, and any laxity in the reconstruction will thereby be alleviated.

Step 7: closure and drainage The serratus anterior and the latissimus dorsi are closed in the standard fashion, as

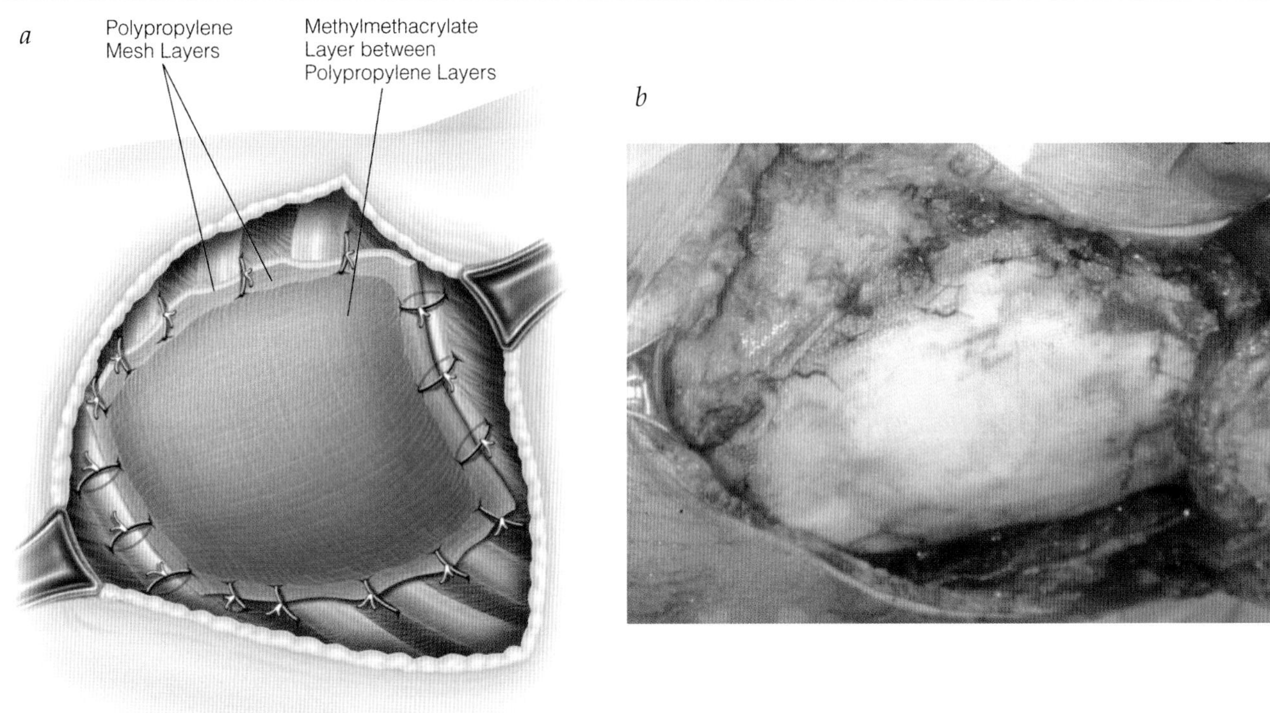

Figure 12 **Chest wall resection. (*a*) A polypropylene-methylmethacrylate sandwich is created by spreading a layer of methylmethacrylate cement between two pieces of polypropylene mesh. When sufficiently hardened, the sandwich is sutured to the ribs. (*b*) Photograph shows a polypropylene-methylmethacrylate sandwich sutured in place.**

are the subcutaneous and skin layers. With the exception of pleural tubes, drains are not routinely used. Special attention should be paid to postoperative analgesia: patients who have undergone extensive resections often experience considerable pain and are therefore prone to atelectasis and pneumonia. Epidural analgesia should be employed routinely in such cases.

Troubleshooting If chest wall infection is a possibility (as with osteoradionecrosis or osteomyelitis), alternative reconstructive techniques are required to obviate concerns about superinfection resulting from the use of synthetic material. In particular, radiation injury may involve all layers of the chest wall, necessitating very large resections [*see Figure 13a*]. Muscle or omental flaps with split-thickness skin grafts may be required for coverage; thus, preoperative consultation with an experienced plastic surgeon is advisable. A particular concern is what to use to reconstruct the chest wall. Various tissues (e.g., fascia lata and ribs) have been employed, but an easier substitute that works quite well is an absorbable synthetic mesh (e.g., Vicryl). The mesh is sewn to the ribs as previously described [*see* Step 6, *above*], and the tissue flap is placed on top of the mesh, followed by a skin graft [*see Figure 13b, c*]. Alternatively, some authors recommend the use of muscle or myocutaneous flaps without rigid chest wall reconstruction after resection, particularly in infected fields.[19]

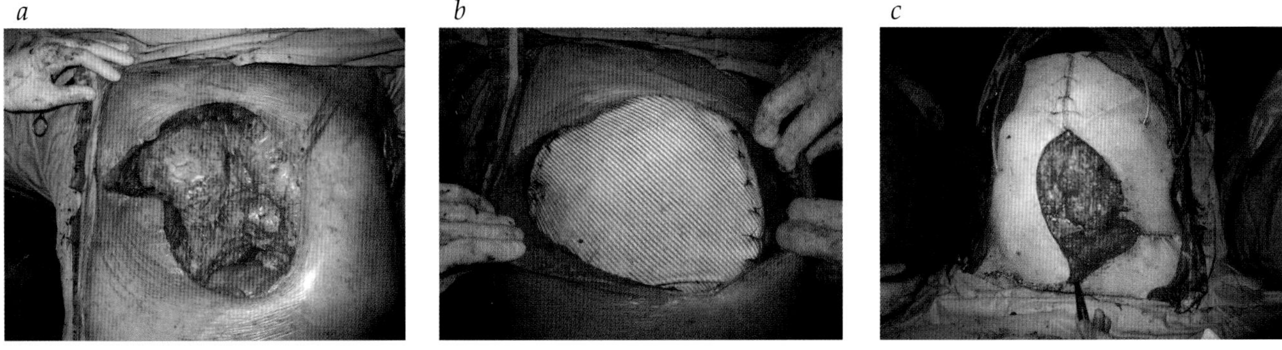

Figure 13 **Chest wall resection. The presence of osteoradionecrosis may necessitate very large resections and resulting defects (*a*). Such defects may be covered with absorbable mesh (*b*), followed by an omental flap (*c*) or a muscle flap.**

Outcome evaluation The results achieved after major chest wall resection have generally been excellent. One study reviewed 200 patients who underwent resection and reconstruction over a 25-year period.[20] The reconstructions ranged from relatively straightforward two-rib resections to more complex forequarter amputations. The indications for resection were lung cancer (38%), osteoradionecrosis (29%), chest wall tumor (27%), and osteomyelitis (16%). Immediate reconstruction was performed in 98% of patients. The major muscle flaps used were latissimus dorsi (20%), rectus abdominis (17%), pectoralis major (16%), and serratus anterior (9%). Free flaps were used in only 9% of cases, and split-thickness skin grafts were required in 12% of patients. Reconstruction was performed with Prolene mesh (25%), Marlex mesh (11%), Vicryl mesh (6%), or a polypropylene-methylmethacrylate sandwich (6%). Operative mortality was 7%, and major morbidity occurred in 24% of patients. Most of the morbidity was accounted for by pneumonia (14%) and acute respiratory distress syndrome (6%).

Manubrial and Clavicular Resection

Resection of the manubrium or the clavicle may be necessary if these structures become infected or involved with tumors. Clavicular and manubrial resections follow the same operative approach as other chest wall resections. Specifically, attention must be paid to how much bone to resect, how to reconstruct the defect, and how to provide tissue coverage.

Resection of sternoclavicular joint for infection Clavicular resections are rarely performed but may be required to treat tumors, vascular compression from healed fractures, or infection. Occasionally, infections involve the sternoclavicular joint (SCJ). Patients with osteomyelitis of this joint are often immunosuppressed and may have had an indwelling subclavian vein catheter that became infected. In a study of seven patients who underwent SCJ resection for infection, five of six patients initially treated with antibiotics and simple drainage experienced recurrences, whereas six of six patients treated with resection of the joint and pectoralis muscle advancement flaps were cured. None of the patients experienced problems with arm mobility in the course of long-term follow-up.[21]

An incision is made that extends along the distal clavicle and curves down onto the manubrium. The soft tissue is divided with the electrocautery down to the clavicle and the manubrium. The muscular attachments of the pectoralis major and the sternocleidomastoid muscle are dissected off the clavicle and the manubrium with a periosteal elevator. Dissection in the subperiosteal plane is then continued circumferentially around the distal clavicle, with special care taken to keep from injuring the subclavian vessels that lie deep to the clavicle. A Gigli saw is passed around the clavicle with a right-angle clamp and used to divide the distal clavicle. The distal cut end of the clavicle is grasped with a penetrating towel clamp and bluntly dissected away from the deep tissue toward the manubrium. Any pockets of infection encountered should be cultured, drained, and débrided.

At this point, a large separation in the SCJ, caused by the infection, should be apparent. Resection of a small portion of the manubrium is usually required to remove all of the infected bone. Once the tissue deep to the manubrium has been dissected, a small band retractor is placed beneath the manubrium, and an oscillating sternal saw is used to resect the lateral portion of the manubrium, adjacent to the SCJ. Alternatively, a rongeur may be used to débride infected bone from the manubrium. All tissue should be sent for culture.

Severe infections may necessitate more extensive resection of bone or soft tissue, but if the infection is caught early, simple resection of the SCJ is generally curative. In more extensive resections, muscle flap coverage may be required, but in simple SCJ resections, good results can be obtained by using only deep closed suction drainage, followed by multilayer closure of the wound. To prevent any recurrent osteomyelitis, antibiotics should be continued for several weeks after resection.

Resection of manubrium for cancer Manubrial resections may be required for rare cases of primary or metastatic cancers.

Because of the relative paucity of tissue overlying the manubrium, cancers in this area may involve the dermis. In such cases, it may be necessary to resect skin along with the specimen. Alternatively, if the skin is not involved, an upper midline incision may be employed. The incision is carried down circumferentially to the chest wall, with care taken to maintain a 2 to 3 cm margin from the tumor. The clavicles and ribs are divided in the same fashion as for chest wall and clavicular resections [*see Figure 14a*]. Associated structures (e.g., the thymus) can be resected along with the manubrium; these tumors rarely involve the innominate vein.

A polypropylene-methylmethacrylate sandwich is useful for reconstruction of this area of the chest wall [*see Figure 14b*]. The patch is secured to the remaining ribs and clavicles with 0 polypropylene sutures. Coverage is then provided with a pectoralis major advancement flap or, if skin was excised, a pedicled pectoralis myocutaneous flap. A pleural drain may be placed if either pleural space was entered, but this measure is not routinely employed.

Open Chest Drainage (Eloesser Flap)

Open drainage procedures are usually included in discussions of treatment of empyema, but they really represent a type of chest wall resection. Open drainage techniques for empyema were first described in the late 1800s by Poulet and subsequently by Schede. Graham, who headed the Army Empyema Commission during World War I, is credited with the observation that ensuring pleural-pleural symphysis was the key to preventing the often fatal complication of pneumothorax.[22] Indications for open chest drainage include postpneumonectomy empyema or bronchopleural fistula, long-standing empyema in a patient who cannot undergo decortication, and chronic bronchopleural fistula in a high-risk patient.

Operative technique The technique currently employed by most thoracic surgeons follows Symbas's modification of Eloesser's open drainage technique.[23] This procedure has come to be known as the Eloesser flap. Preoperative chest CT is essential for identifying the exact location of the empyema, which determines the placement of the incision.

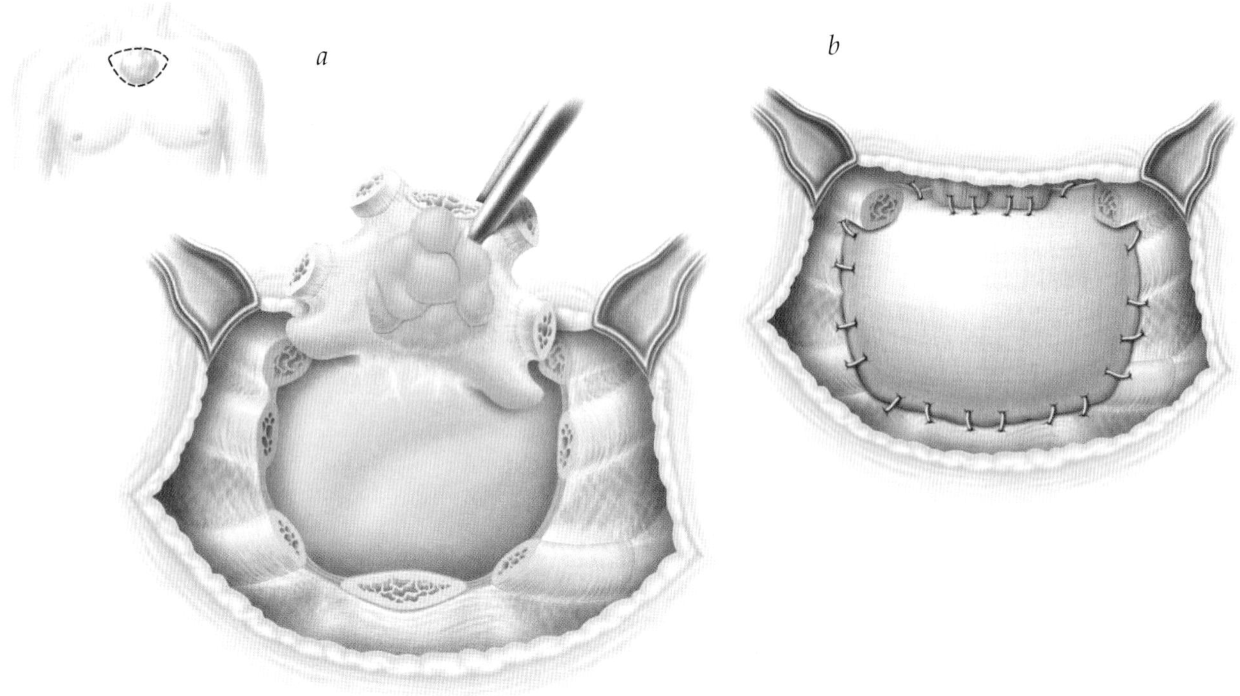

Figure 14 **Manubrial resection and reconstruction. (*a*) The clavicles and ribs are divided as in clavicular and other chest wall resections. (*b*) A polypropylene-methylmethacrylate sandwich may be used to reconstruct the chest wall.**

Step 1: initial incision and exposure The patient is placed in the decubitus position, and a 6 to 8 cm incision is made over the area corresponding to the most dependent area of the infected cavity. Symbas employed a U-shaped incision; however, a simple linear incision can also be used with good results. The subcutaneous tissue and muscle are then divided down to the chest wall with the electrocautery.

Step 2: resection of ribs and creation of thoracostomy The pleural space is opened with the electrocautery, any pus present is drained, and the chest cavity is manually and visually explored. Next, 6 to 8 cm segments of two or three adjacent ribs are resected according to the same principles employed for other chest wall resections. The resulting thoracostomy is large enough to permit drainage and packing. The skin overlying this thoracostomy is then marsupialized to the thickened parietal pleura with absorbable sutures [*see Figure 15*]. If the pleura does not possess sufficient integrity to hold the sutures, they can be placed through the periosteum of the ribs.

Step 3: packing and drainage The wound is irrigated with normal saline and packed with saline-moistened gauze. Postoperatively, a chest x-ray should be obtained to rule out pneumothorax, and twice- to thrice-daily packing is initiated. Packing is continued on an outpatient basis, and the wound is monitored. The wound will begin to close over the next several weeks. If the empyema or bronchopleural fistula has not healed by the time the wound starts closing, the thoracostomy will have to be revised. In some cases, this can be

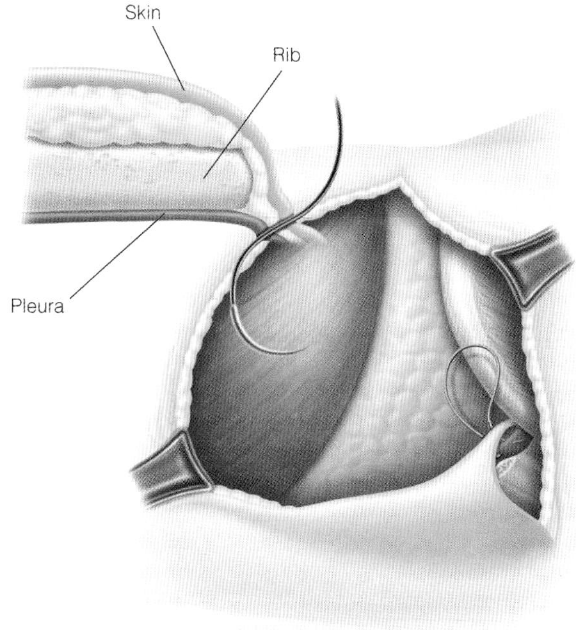

Figure 15 **Open chest drainage (Eloesser flap). Once the ribs have been resected, the skin overlying the thoracostomy is marsupialized to the parietal pleura to permit packing and open pleural drainage.**

accomplished merely by manually dilating the opening in the operating room; in others, the entire thoracostomy must be revised. In either case, the goal is to maintain a large enough opening to allow adequate packing.

Step 4: closure of thoracostomy Once the lung and the pleural space have healed, the thoracostomy is closed. The procedure for closing the thoracostomy depends on the size and nature of the remaining defect [*see Figure 16a*]. For small defects, simple closure of the skin will suffice. For larger defects or residual spaces in the pleura, however, muscle flap closure will be required [*see Figure 16b*]. Improvements in radiographic techniques and greater emphasis on early intervention for empyemas have significantly reduced the need for open chest drainage; however, this technique can still be valuable in the appropriate clinical situation.

PROCEDURES FOR CHEST WALL FRACTURES/TRAUMA

A recent survey of American trauma, orthopedic, and thoracic surgeons found that the majority of polled surgeons had not performed a repair on sternal or rib fractures, nor was there a consensus of surveyed surgeons with agreed upon surgical indications. Also, a large majority were unaware of any published randomized trials addressing rib or sternal fractures.[24] Although rib and sternal fracture repairs have been performed for many years, the operative indications remain somewhat controversial. However, there is increasing consensus that operative fixation of these fractures is underused; therefore, basic repair techniques are discussed below.[25]

Repair of Rib Fractures

Although there are a number of potential indications for operative repair for rib fractures, two recent randomized trials demonstrate that patients with flail chest can benefit from operative repair in selected scenarios. Flail chest can be defined as three or more consecutive ribs fractured in two or more locations, clinically creating a segment of the chest wall that visibly demonstrates paradoxical motion with respiratory variations. In both of these trials, the operative group demonstrated a reduced number of ventilator days, intensive care unit length of stay, and lower incidence of pneumonia. One of the trials reported that more of the operative group returned to work at the 6-month follow-up compared to the nonoperative group.[26,27] Retrospective reviews and nonrandomized cohort studies demonstrate that patients with severe flail segments without underlying pulmonary contusion are offered the greatest advantage in surgical repair of rib fractures.[28] Opponents to surgical correction of rib fractures suggest that the nonoperative groups were not managed with modern strategies, including epidural anesthesia and chest physiotherapy.[29] It is not, however, within the scope of this chapter to argue the merits of the literature surrounding the subject matter but simply to delineate some of the techniques. Other indications include chest wall defect and pulmonary hernia.

Operative planning In preoperative planning, it is useful to define the location and characteristics of all the rib fractures with a CT scan, and three-dimensional reconstruction may provide the surgeon with added information to the fracture geometry. As the main complications of the procedure are infectious in etiology, removal of chest tubes if possible, prior to the operation, is encouraged. The use of an epidural catheter for pre- and postoperative pain management should be considered. Many different techniques have been described, including variations of intramedullary fixation, plate attachment, or wiring, but the most commonly

a

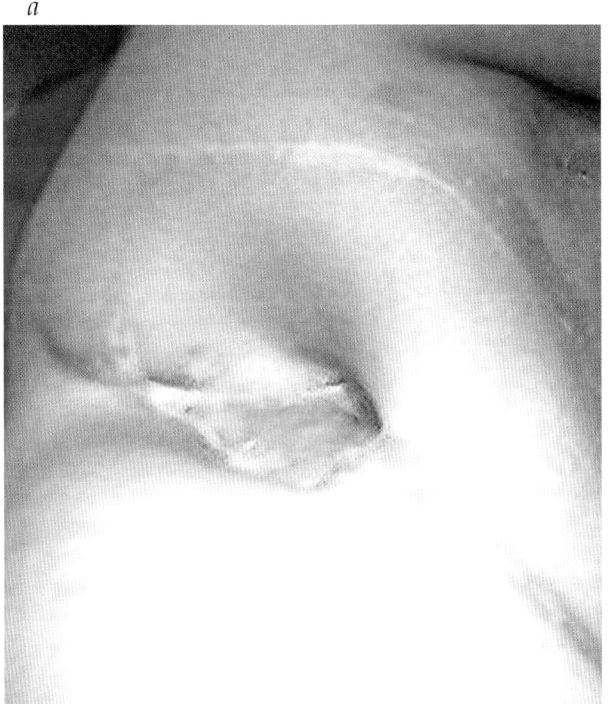

b

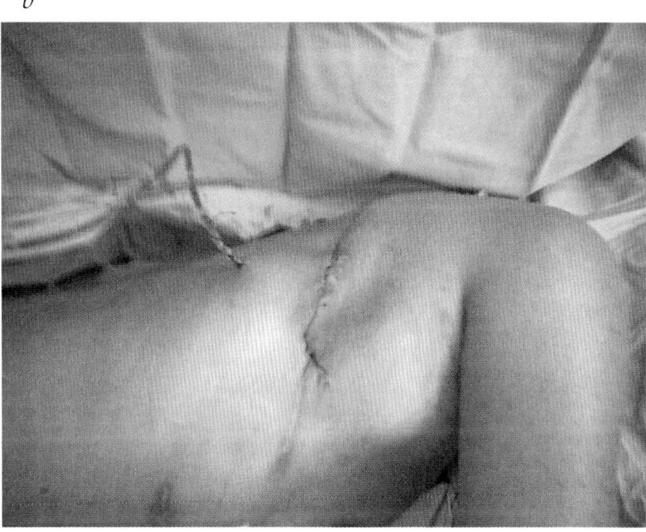

Figure 16 **Open chest drainage (Eloesser flap). (*a*) Photograph shows a right Eloesser flap 8 months after creation. (*b*) Photograph shows an Eloesser flap that was closed with a muscle flap.**

employed technique is anterior plating with bicortical screw fixation.

Operative technique The patient is intubated with a single-lumen endotracheal tube or a double-lumen tube if single-lung ventilation is preferred, but this is not mandatory. The patient is placed in standard lateral decubitus positioning for a posterior lateral thoracotomy. A muscle-sparing thoracotomy incision is used if possible, and the scapulothoracic bursa is incised, giving access to the thoracic cage. This allows for fracture site localization, easily accessing ribs 3 to 9. Soft tissue immediately overlying the fractures is removed with a periosteal elevator, and the ribs are realigned with the use of bone forceps. Plates of the surgeon's selection are secured to the ribs with bicortical screw placement. Careful attention is placed to ensure that the screws are of the appropriate length to prevent screw tips from entering the pleural space. For stabilization of the chest wall, not all the fractured ribs need to be fixed. Depending on the surgeon's comfort, single-lung ventilation can be used, and by inserting a thoracoscope inferior to the fractures, the pleural space can be visualized and monitored during screw placement. Assuming that satisfactory fixation has been accomplished, the pneumothorax can be evacuated on lung reexpansion, and no chest tube would be required.

Complications Postoperative complications are primarily infectious in etiology and include superficial wound infections and empyemas. A postoperative pneumothorax should always be evaluated for on standard postoperative chest x-ray and if there is any respiratory deterioration, even if the pleural space was not entered during the procedure. Other, less frequent complications include fixation failures, chronic pain, reactive pleural effusions, and wound hematomas.

Repair of Sternal Fractures

The diagnosis of sternal fractures is usually suspected because of pain in the precordial area with tenderness and instability on palpation. There is evidence of increased diagnosis of sternal fracture in the trauma literature as a result of the increased use of CT scanning in this patient population. However, because of the prevalence of median sternotomies in cardiac procedures, more operations for sternal fixation are performed for postoperative chronic sternal nonunion than acute fracture. Sternal fracture nonunion is commonly defined as persistent instability after 6 weeks of nonoperative management and is the most common operative indication. Other indications include fractures that create paradoxical motion with respirations altering respiratory mechanics, and a multitude of anterior plating systems are available for the surgeon to use; other techniques include placement of sternal wires through the fracture fragments.

Operative planning In the preoperative planning of surgical repair, a CT scan with three-dimensional reconstruction provides added geometric insight to the fracture pattern. In an attempt to reduce postoperative infectious complications, mediastinal or chest tubes should be removed if in place. Also, one should consider the use of an epidural catheter for postoperative pain management.

Operative technique The sternum is exposed using a previous surgical incision if present or through a longitudinal or transverse incision depending on the need for exposure. If sternal wires are in place, they are removed, and the fibrous tissue and soft tissue are removed with electrocautery and the periosteal elevator. If there is a fibrous union, this is removed as well. Once all fractures are identified, they are reduced using bone forceps. Plates are selected to allow for at least three screws to be seated on either side of the fracture. Careful attention is placed ensuring that the screws do not penetrate the inner table of the sternum. The pectus muscles are reapproximated and a drain placed to prevent seroma or hematoma formation. The drain is removed on postoperative day 1 or 2 depending on the output.

Complications Postoperative complications have a low incidence for sternal fixation procedures and are similar to rib fixation, including superficial wound infections, wound hematomas and seromas, fixation failures, chronic pain, pleural effusions, and empyemas.

Financial Disclosures: None Reported

References

1. Backer CL, Mavroudis C. Congenital heart surgery nomenclature and database project: vascular rings, tracheal stenosis, pectus excavatum. Ann Thorac Surg 2000;69(4 Suppl):S308.
2. Haller JA, Kramer SS, Lietman SA. Use of CT scans in selection of patients for pectus excavatum surgery: a preliminary report. J Pediatr Surg 1987;22:904.
3. Weg JG, Krumholz RA, Harkleroad LE. Pulmonary dysfunction in pectus excavatum. Am Rev Respir Dis 1967;96:936.
4. Gyllensward A, Irnell L, Michaelsson M, et al. Pectus excavatum: a clinical study with long term postoperative follow-up. Acta Paediatr 1975;255 Suppl:2.
5. Cahill JL, Lees GM, Robertson HT. A summary of preoperative and postoperative cardiorespiratory performance in patients undergoing pectus excavatum and carinatum repair. J Pediatr Surg 1984;19:430.
6. Blickman JG, Rosen PR, Welch KJ, et al. Pectus excavatum in children: pulmonary scintigraphy before and after corrective surgery. Radiology 1985;156:781.
7. Haller JA, Colombani PM, Humphries CT, et al. Chest wall constriction after too extensive and too early operations for pectus excavatum. Ann Thorac Surg 1996;61:1618.
8. Bevegard S. Postural circulatory changes at rest and during exercise in patients with funnel chest, with special reference to the influence on the stroke volume. Acta Physiol Scand 1960;49:279.
9. Gattiker H, Buhlmann A. Cardiopulmonary function and exercise tolerance in supine and sitting position in patients with pectus excavatum. Helv Med Acta 1967;33:122.
10. Peterson RJ, Young WG Jr, Godwin JD, et al. Noninvasive assessment of exercise cardiac function before and after pectus excavatum repair. J Thorac Cardiovasc Surg 1985;90: 251.
11. Judet J, Judet R. Sternum en entonnoir par resection et retournement. Mem Acad Chir 1956;82:250.
12. Wada J, Ikeda K, Ishida T, et al. Results of 271 funnel chest operations. Ann Thorac Surg 1970;10:526.
13. Robicsek F, Cook JW, Daugherty HK, et al. Pectus carinatum. J Thorac Cardiovasc Surg 1979;78:52.
14. Mansour KA, Thourani VH, Odessey EA, et al. Thirty-year experience with repair of pectus deformities in adults. Ann Thorac Surg 2003;76:391.
15. Hebra A. Minimally invasive pectus surgery. Chest Surg Clin N Am 2000;10:329.
16. Robicsek F. Surgical treatment of pectus excavatum. Chest Surg Clin N Am 2000;10: 277.
17. Stefani A, Morandi U, Lodi R. Migration of pectus excavatum correction metal support into the abdomen. Eur J Cardiothorac Surg 1998;14:434.
18. Urschel HC. The transaxillary approach for treatment of thoracic outlet syndrome. Chest Surg Clin N Am 1999;9:771.
19. Arnold PG, Pairolero PC. Use of pectoralis major muscle flaps to repair defects of

anterior chest wall. Plast Reconstr Surg 1979;63:105.
20. Mansour KA, Thourani VH, Losken A, et al. Chest wall resections and reconstruction: a 25-year experience. Ann Thorac Surg 2002; 73:1720.
21. Song HK, Guy TS, Kaiser LR, et al. Current presentation and optimal surgical management of sternoclavicular joint infections. Ann Thorac Surg 2002;73:427.
22. Somers J, Faber LP. Historical developments in the management of empyema. Chest Surg Clin N Am 1996;6:404.
23. Symbas PN, Nugent JT, Abbott OA, et al. Nontuberculous pleural empyema in adults. Ann Thorac Surg 1971;12:69.
24. Mayberry JC, Ham LB, Schipper PH, et al. Surveyed opinion of American trauma, orthopedic, and thoracic surgeons on rib and sternal fracture repair. J Trauma 2009;66:875.
25. Richardson JD, Franklin GA, Heffley S, et al. Operative fixation of chest wall fractures: an underused procedure? Am Surg 2007;73: 591.
26. Tanaka H, Yukioka T, Yamaguti Y, et al. Surgical stabilization of internal pneumatic stabilization? A prospective randomized study of management of severe flail chest patients. J Trauma 2002;52:727.
27. Granetzny A, Abd El-Aal M, Emam E, et al. Surgical versus conservative treatment of flail chest. Evaluation of the pulmonary status. Int Cardiovasc Thorac Surg 2005;4:583.
28. Nirula R, Diaz JJ Jr, Trunky DD, et al. Rib fracture repair: indications, technical issues, and future directions. World J Surg 2009;33: 14.
29. EAST Practice Management Workgroup for Pulmonary Contusion-Flail Chest 2006. Available at: http://www.east.org/tpg/pulmcontflailchest.pdf (accessed October 30, 2009).

Acknowledgment

Figures 1 through 8, 10 through 12, 14, and 15 Alice Y. Chen

10 VIDEO-ASSISTED THORACIC SURGERY

Marcelo C. DaSilva, MD, and Scott J. Swanson, MD⋆

Although Sir Francis Richard Cruise has been credited with performing the first thoracoscopy for evacuation of empyema in 1865,[1] Hans Christian Jacobaeus coined the term "thoracoscopy" in an article published in 1910.[2] In the latter report, Jacobaeus described the use of a cystoscope to examine the chest cavity and to lyse adhesions, allowing the lungs to collapse for the treatment of tuberculosis.[3] With the introduction of streptomycin, which revolutionized the treatment of tuberculosis, thoracoscopy was relegated to the occasional case report. It was not until the introduction of laparoscopic procedures in the 1980s that surgeons started to apply this technology to the thoracic cavity. In 1992, Lewis and colleagues reported 100 consecutive patients who underwent video-assisted thoracoscopic surgery, including three lobectomies with anatomic hilar dissection.[4] From these early studies, minimally invasive video-assisted thoracic surgery (VATS) has emerged as a safe and reliable technique. It has, in many instances, supplanted standard thoracic procedures. Approximately 20% of all lobectomies now are performed thoracoscopically in the United States.[5]

Historical Background

The first single institution prospective randomized trial comparing VATS to the muscle-sparing open technique for lobectomy was published by Kirby and colleagues in 1995.[6] Sixty-one patients undergoing lobectomy for stage I non–small cell lung cancer (NSCLC) were randomized to VATS or open thoracotomy. There was no significant difference in operating time, intraoperative complications, estimated blood loss, chest tube drainage, length of stay, or postthoracotomy pain between the groups, although it was a small study and many VATS patients had a minithoracotomy. In the early 1990s, the National Institute of Cancer funded an intergroup consortium of thoracic surgeons to investigate the efficacy of thoracoscopy and VATS in the diagnosis, staging, and treatment of intrathoracic malignancies. Cancer and Leukemia Group B (CALGB) 9335 was the first multicenter, clinical research phase II trial to look at the feasibility of treating patients with poor cardiopulmonary reserve and T1 peripheral NSCLC by VATS wedge resection or radiotherapy.[7] This clinical trial concluded that VATS wedge resection in high-risk patients is safe and feasible. The CALGB 9380 phase II clinical trial was designed to determine the feasibility, morbidity, and mortality for thoracoscopic and/or laparoscopic staging of esophageal cancer.[8] One hundred seventeen patients were accrued; 82 patients (70%) met the entry criteria for thoracoscopy. Of those, 57% had positive nodes and 43% had all negative nodes. Node-negative status was confirmed on final pathology in 12 (75%) of 16 patients who underwent surgery, whereas three patients had node-positive status in the specimen (19% false negative rate). The authors concluded that thoracoscopic and/or laparoscopic staging lung and esophageal cancer was feasible and doubled the number of positive lymph nodes identified by conventional surgery.

The first multicenter prospective trial to examine standardized VATS lobectomy was CALGB 39802.[9] One hundred twenty-eight patients were enrolled for VATS lobectomy as defined by one access incision (4 to 8 cm), two 5 mm port incisions, and no retractor use or rib spreading. The perioperative morbidity was 7.4% and 30-day mortality was 2.7%, both comparable to standards of open thoracotomy in patients with small (≤3 cm) peripheral NSCLC. In 1998, CALGB 39803 answered the question of restaging patients with histologic documented stage IIIA NSCLC with VATS on the basis of involved N2 nodes from mediastinoscopy prior to induction therapy.[10] Seventy patients were accrued in 10 institutions. Of those, 47 patients (67%) had radiation therapy and 68 (97%) had chemotherapy. The number of incisions ranged from one to four, with a median of three incisions. VATS restaging criteria were met in 40 patients (57%): four had pleural carcinomatosis, 17 had persistent N2 disease, and 19 had three negative nodal stations. In addition, 13 (18.6%) patients in the VATS group had no evidence of persistent N2 disease attributable to unanticipated obliteration of nodal tissue. VATS was unsuccessful in 17 (24%) patients as a result of adhesions or fibrosis and tumor bulk preventing nodal access. Of the 53 patients who completed VATS restaging, 21 provided cancer tissue and 31 had histologic tissue obtained during thoracotomy; N2 downstaging occurred in 32 patients (46%). The sensitivity of VATS was 75%, the specificity was 100%, and the negative predictive value was 75.8%. No deaths occurred, but one airway injury was directly attributed to VATS. The authors concluded that VATS was feasible and provided pathologic assessment of ipsilateral nodes in treated IIIA (N2) NSCLC.

Eastern Cooperative Oncology Group (ECOG) 2202 was the first multi-institutional phase II trial to assess the feasibility of minimally invasive esophagectomy (MIE) in a multi-institutional setting.[11] Of 106 patients enrolled in this study, 99 underwent MIE. Anastomotic leak (7.8%) and pneumonia (4.9%) were the major complications, whereas the mortality rate was 2% (2 of 106), with a mean follow-up

⋆ The authors and editors gratefully acknowledge the contributions of the previous authors, Raja M. Flores, MD, Bernard Park, MD, and Valerie W. Rusch, MD, FACS, to the development and writing of this chapter.

of 19 months, and the estimated 3-year survival rate for the cohort was 50% (95% confidence interval 35 to 655). The authors concluded that MIE was safe and feasible, with low perioperative mortality and morbidity and with oncologic outcomes similar to those of open esophagectomy.

The era of VATS is sufficiently mature that enough data have accrued to compare the efficacy of VATS with that of open procedures. In this regard, anatomic pulmonary resection by VATS has led to significant reductions in morbidity, mortality, and hospital length of stay, allowing patients a more expeditious return to regular activities. VATS has been used in the treatment of both benign and malignant diseases of the chest. Furthermore, VATS may be used in selected patients with early-stage lung cancer without breaching oncologic surgical principles.

DEFINITION

The terms "VATS" and "thoracoscopic" refer to totally thoracoscopic approaches, where visualization is dependent on video monitors, and rib spreading is avoided by using a thoracoscope, video monitors, and one to four small (1 to 2 cm) incisions.[12]

INDICATIONS AND CONTRAINDICATIONS

The indications for VATS are the same as for conventional approaches to thoracic surgery. However, tumor size greater than 6 cm, inability to tolerate single-lung ventilation, and previous thoracotomy with obliteration of the pleural space [*see Table 1*] are considered relative contraindications. The individual experience of the surgeon and the complexity of the operation also influence the procedures that can be performed by VATS.

Table 1 Indications and Relative Contraindications for VATS Procedures

Diagnostic indications
- All biopsies: nodules, interstitial lung disease
- Pulmonary infection in the immunosuppressed patient
- Nodal staging of a primary thoracic tumor
- Staging a primary extrathoracic tumor
- Trauma: lung laceration, hemothorax diaphragmatic injury

Therapeutic indications
- Lung
  - Spontaneous pneumothorax
  - Bullous disease/lung volume reduction
  - Persistent parenchymal airleak
  - Pleural effusion
  - Pleural disease: empyema, fibrothorax, decortication
  - Anatomic resection
    - Lobectomy
    - Segmentectomy
    - Pneumonectomy
- Esophageal
  - Benign
  - Malignant
- Mediastinal
  - VATS thymectomy for thymoma
  - Nodal dissection
  - Pericardial window
  - Cysts
- Chest wall
  - Rib resection
    - Sarcoma
    - First rib for thoracic outlet syndrome
- Other
  - Metastatectomy
  - Sympathectomy for hyperhidrosis
  - Ligation of thoracic duct
  - Repair/plication of the diaphragm

Relative contraindications to VATS pulmonary resection
- Intolerance of single-lung ventilation
- Tumor size > 6 cm
- Anticipated sleeve resection
- Hilar lymphadenopathy
- Chest wall or mediastinal involvement
- Neoadjuvant radiation therapy or chemotherapy

VATS = video-assisted thoracic surgery.

PREOPERATIVE EVALUATION

The preoperative evaluation of patients undergoing VATS is similar to that of those undergoing open thoracotomy procedures. The risks related to surgical resection include perioperative morbidity and mortality and long-term functional disability. Individual patient circumstances increase or decrease the risks from standard thoracotomy resection and VATS [*see Figure 1*]. In addition, a discussion of the balance between the risks and benefits of surgical resection by the surgeon and the patient should also include nonstandard treatment options, such as sublobar resections, conventional radiotherapy, stereotactic radiotherapy, and radiofrequency ablation.

A thorough physical examination, past medical history, social history including tobacco smoking and exposure to arsenic and asbestos, radiologic studies (chest x-rays, computed tomographic [CT] scan, positron emission tomographic [PET]-CT scan, magnetic resonance imaging [MRI]), and pulmonary function tests are part of the preoperative preparation. Although thoracoscopic procedures tend to be less stressful than open thoracotomy, with fewer cardiopulmonary complications (e.g., atrial fibrillation or myocardial infarction),[13] it is important to recognize that risk assessment is a complex process, and the surgeon should focus on determining the individual patient's resectability and operability. Resectability refers to the amount of lung tissue and tumor that can be safely removed without developing respiratory insufficiency. It depends directly on the amount of pulmonary reserve of the patient. Operability, on the other hand, refers to the ability of a patient to survive the proposed procedure and its perioperative complications. It depends on the patient's comorbid conditions. However, neither the operability of an individual patient nor the resectability of a tumor should influence the decision concerning the role of a complete resection on survival.[14]

Pulmonary function testing includes pulmonary spirometry, pulmonary hemodynamic response testing, and exercise testing. Pulmonary spirometry is affected by height, age, weight, sex, race, and posture, as well as arterial oxygenation and diffusion capacity. Although pulmonary spirometry and arterial oxygenation help predict mortality, they are not good predictors of postoperative complications. Diffusion capacity of the lung for carbon monoxide (DLCO) is a more sensitive predictor of postoperative complications. DLCO measures the partial pressure difference between inspired and expired carbon monoxide. It relies on the strong affinity and large absorption capacity of erythrocytes for carbon monoxide and thus demonstrates gas uptake by the capillaries that is less dependent on cardiac output.[15] Thus, value is decreased in

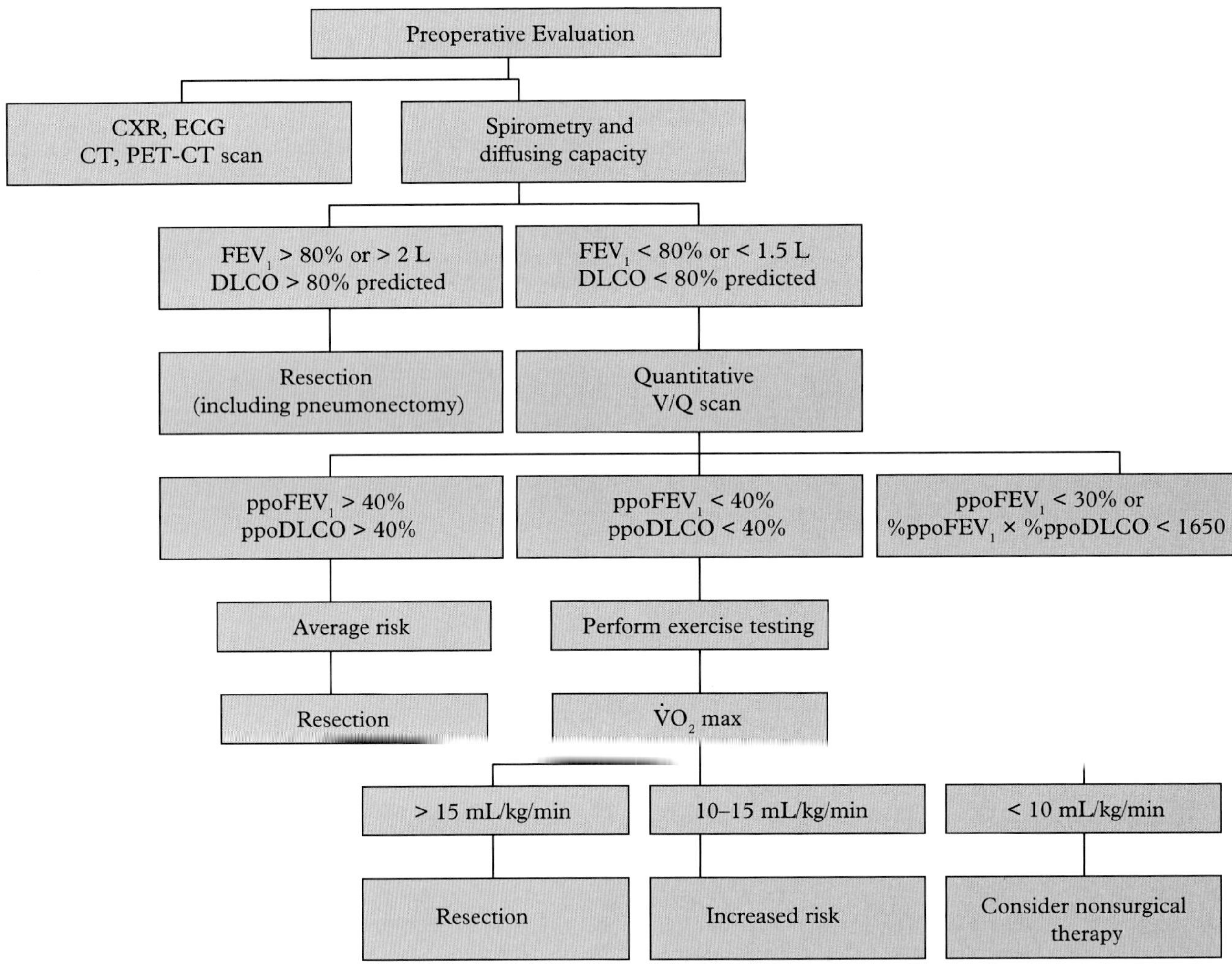

Figure 1 **Preoperative evaluation. CXR = chest x-ray; CT = computed tomographic; ECG = electrocardiogram; DLCO = diffusing capacity for carbon monoxide; FEV_1 = forced expiratory volume in 1 second; PET = positron emission tomographic; ppo = postoperative; $\dot{V}O_2$ max = maximum oxygen consumption; V/Q = ventilation-perfusion.**

patients with emphysema, chronic pulmonary hypertension, and interstitial lung disease. DLCO is an important and independent predictor of postoperative complications after major lung resection, even in patients without COPD.[16,17]

Quantitative ventilation/perfusion (V/Q) scan, along with pulmonary spirometry, is useful for predicting postoperative lung function. A calculated predictive postoperative forced expiratory volume in 1 second (ppoFEV_1 of less than 40% is associated with a 50% mortality rate. The absolute minimum ppoFEV_1 in patients undergoing lobectomy is 800 mL. Pulmonary hemodynamic response testing includes the measurement of pulmonary artery pressure and pulmonary vascular resistance. It is an invasive test and requires right heart catheterization. Systolic pulmonary artery pressure greater than 35 mm Hg is associated with a 10-fold decrease in survival rate, and pulmonary vascular resistance greater than 190 dyne is associated with a 90% mortality rate. Maximum exercise testing is concerned with the amount of arterial desaturation that occurs during exercise. Patients with a maximum oxygen consumption ($\dot{V}O_2$ max) less than 15 mL/kg/min are considered high risk, whereas those with a $\dot{V}O_2$ max of 16 to 20 mL/kg/min could probably undergo surgery.

Flexible bronchoscopy is generally indicated in patients with hemoptysis, wheezing, and evidence of bronchial obstruction. In patients with lung cancer, bronchoscopy is always performed to assess endobronchial invasion. If a mass is found beneath the mucosa or intraparenchyma, endobronchial ultrasonography and electromagnetic navigational bronchoscopy are potential diagnostic tools, but their discussion is beyond the scope of this chapter. Bronchoscopy is also useful for the diagnosis of infectious diseases, such as tuberculosis, fungus, *Pneumocystis* pneumonia, and cytomegalovirus, prior to a thoracoscopic procedure. Finally, a multidisciplinary discussion with medical and radiation oncologists is especially useful in patients who are marginal surgical candidates and serves as a basis for discussing the proposed surgical procedure and treatment options with the patient and appropriate family or surrogates.

The goal of the preoperative evaluation is to identify those patients who can tolerate a thoracic surgical procedure. By integrating the concept of operability and resectability while achieving a complete surgical resection, along with a thorough preoperative evaluation, the surgeon will be able to identify a group of patients who would benefit from VATS.

Operative Planning

ANESTHESIA AND MONITORING

VATS is performed under general anesthesia with single-lung ventilation. A double-lumen endotracheal tube is generally used, but an endobronchial blocker may also be employed to collapse the lung. Alternatively, limited operations such as diagnostic pleuroscopy and pleural biopsy, insertion of pleural drainage catheters, or procedures performed on pneumonectomy patients can be safely done with a single-lumen endotracheal tube and intermittent lung ventilation. The degree of intraoperative monitoring needed depends on the extent of the planned procedure and on the patient's general medical condition. Standard monitoring techniques are used to measure the patient's oxygenation, ventilation, circulation, and temperature.[18] Whenever indicated, a peripheral arterial line, central venous pressure and pulmonary artery (PA) catheters, and transesophageal echocardiography may be used. A Foley catheter is inserted at the beginning of the procedure to monitor urine output. Depending on the pulmonary reserve of the patient, extent of the procedure, and postoperative pain, epidural catheters can provide excellent pain relief, but they are not commonly used for thoracoscopic procedures because of the time required for insertion and frequent side effects, such as hypotension and urinary retention. Alternatively, recent studies have demonstrated the safety and efficacy of continuous infusion pumps delivering local anesthetic through a catheter in the extrapleural pocket during thoracotomy,[19] as well as patient-controlled analgesia for perioperative pain management.

POSITIONING OF THE PATIENT AND PORT PLACEMENT

The general technique for VATS is neither simple nor uniform. Absolute understanding of thoracic anatomy and video orientation is critical. Thoracoscopy is made difficult by paradoxical motion when the camera and instruments are facing each other. Preparation and positioning are the same for all major VATS procedures. The surgeon stands facing the patient, who is placed in the full lateral decubitus position, elevated on pontoons [*see Figure 2*] designed to protect pressure points. Flexing the operating table to open the intercostal spaces (ICSs) for maneuvering instruments can be used but is not mandatory.

Port placement involves triangulation of the target with trocar ports [*see Figure 3*]. Alignment of the thoracoscope and positioning of the video monitors in the operating room are of paramount importance. The thoracoscope is usually placed in the seventh or eighth ICS over the mid-to-anterior axillary line [*see Figure 4*]. Additional 1 cm incisions, usually two, are placed along the line of the standard posterolateral thoracotomy incision approximately on the fifth ICS, one at the anterior axillary line and one at the posterior axillary line. The incisions are placed such that a triangular configuration is achieved. This setup facilitates the most efficient use of the instruments by the surgeon and the assistant. In females, the skin incision can be made in the inframammary fold for

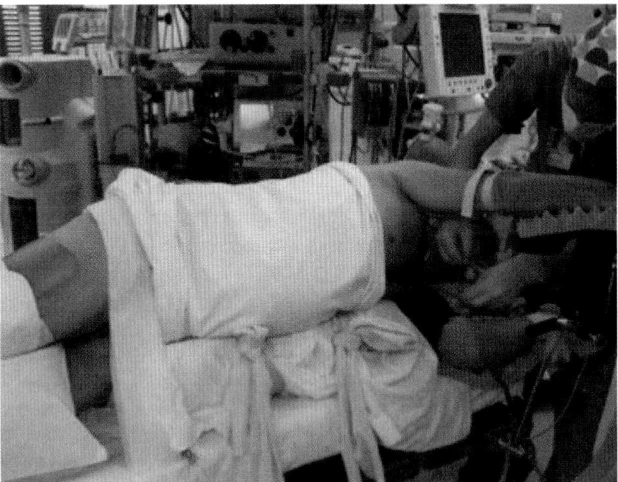

Figure 2 **Proper patient position in the operating room, with the patient propped on pontoons.**

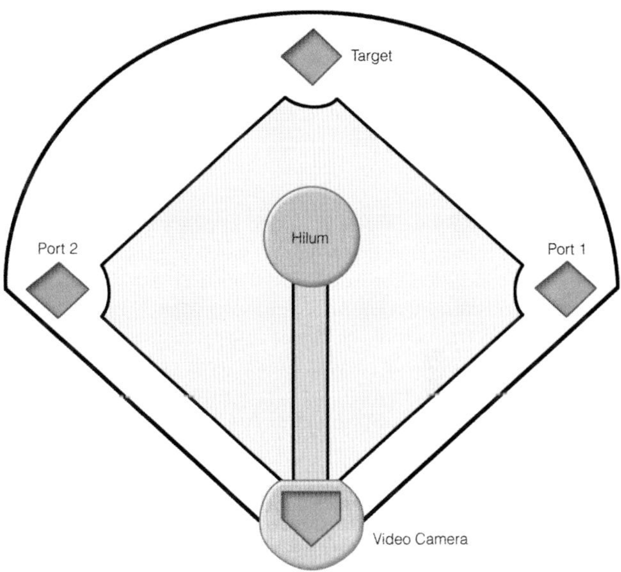

Figure 3 **Triangulation technique for port placement in relation to intrathoracic structures and targets.**

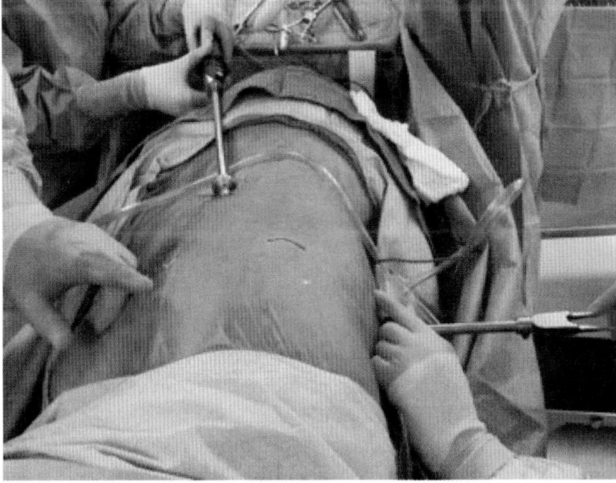

Figure 4 **Thoracoscope and trocar placement.**

cosmesis. These incision sites may vary according to the proposed procedure, the location of the pathology, patient body habitus, and previous scars. Alternatively, a ring forceps or endo-Kittner (Ethicon Endo-Surgery, Cincinnati, OH) can be used to inspect the chest cavity and expose the hilum to determine the proper position for the other incisions. The so-called access incision should be placed so as to provide direct access to the hilum. A soft tissue retractor may be used to provide adequate exposure. Intraoperative conversion to a standard thoracotomy will be necessary in approximately 5 to 20% of patients undergoing VATS depending on the level of experience for several reasons, including extensive pleural adhesions and pulmonary lesions that cannot be located thoracoscopically or that necessitate a more extensive resection than can be accomplished by VATS.

INSTRUMENTATION

The equipment used for VATS comprises (1) a video camera and tower; (2) monitors, usually two at 45° from the midline; (3) thoracoscopes and ports; (4) staplers; (5) thoracic instruments (e.g., lung clamps and retractors) that have been modified for endoscopic use; (6) various devices for tissue cauterization; and (7) a suction irrigation device [*see Figure 5*]. A basic open thoracotomy tray and instruments should be available in the event of conversion to open thoracotomy [*see Table 2*].

Video Equipment

The basic components of all video systems used for thoracoscopy are similar: a large-screen video monitor, a xenon light source, a video recorder, and a printer for still photography. A second video monitor, either mounted on a cart or hanging from the ceiling, is connected by cable to the main monitor and is placed across from it at the head of the operating table. Alternatively, a single monitor can be placed at the head of the operating table. A CO_2 insufflator is used for the combined thoracoscopic/laparoscopic procedures, such as in MIE.

Thoracoscopes and Thoracoports

Both rigid and flexible thoracoscopes can be used for VATS. Depending on individual surgeon preference, level of expertise, and comfort zone, a 5 or 10 mm 0° or 30° rigid telescope with a forward-viewing scope or a 5 or 10 mm flexible scope can be used. The rigid thoracoscope has an excellent resolution. Placing the video camera at the distal end of a flexible thoracoscope, as in the electronic videothoracoscope (EVE-L, Fujinon, Wayne, NJ), yields better visualization of some relatively inaccessible areas in the chest. The disadvantages of the flexible thoracoscope include increased expense and complexity and reduced resolution compared with rigid systems.[20] For most VATS procedures, a 10 mm 30° rigid telescope is used. This thoracoscope allows better orientation and visualization around structures such as the pulmonary artery and bronchus. Thoracoports are shorter and have a corkscrew configuration on the outside that stabilizes them within the chest wall. The trocar is simply a blunt-tipped obturator that facilitates passage of the cannula through the chest wall. A long laparoscopic trocar may be used in morbidly obese patients. Thoracoports are available in several sizes (5, 10.5, 12, and 15 mm in diameter) to accommodate various instruments.

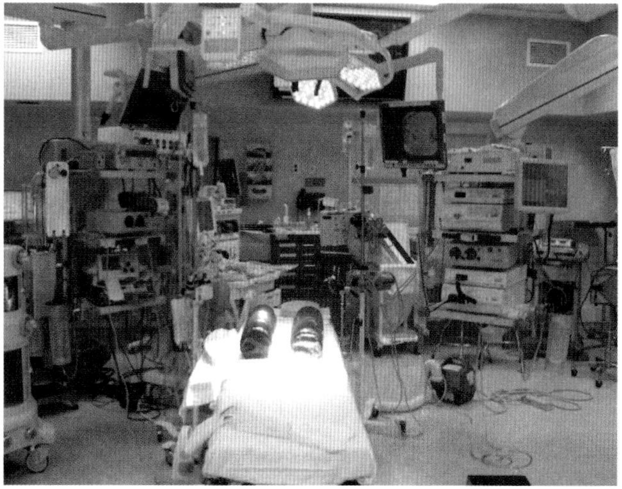

Figure 5 **Video and monitors.**

***Table 2* Basic Instruments and Equipment Used for VATS Procedures**

Standard open thoracotomy set
Standard thoracoscopic instruments set
- Thoracoscope, rigid or flexible
  - 0°, 30°, and 45°
  - 5 or 10 mm (diameter)
- Endoscopic staplers*
  - Echelon ENDOPATH 45 and 60 mm
  - Echelon ENDOPATH ETS 35 or 45 mm
- Thoracoscopic endo-Kittner†
- ENDOPATH 5 mm babcocks, graspers, curved dissector and scissors*
- EnSeal (bipolar coagulation, mechanical transection of tissue allows simultaneous sealing and transection of blood vessels up to 7 mm)*
- Harmonic shears (for lymph node dissection only, cut /coagulate vessels up to 5 mm in diameter)*
- Specimen retrieval bags
  - ENDOPOUCH Retriver 224 mL retrival bag, polyurethane*
  - Endo-Catch Gold (10 mm specimen pouch)‡
  - Endo-Catch II (15 mm specimen pouch)‡
- Endoscopic, surgical irrigation and suction systems

* VATS = video-assisted thoracic surgery. Ethicon Endo-Surgery, Cincinnati, OH
† Aspen Surgical, Caledonia, MI
‡ Covidien, Norwalk, CT

Staplers

Endoscopic gastrointestinal anastomosis (Endo-GIA) staplers have revolutionized the surgeon's ability to perform minimally invasive pulmonary resections. Furthermore, tissue reinforcements that buttress the staple line with prosthetic materials (Gore-Tex [W.L. Gore & Associates, Newark, DE] or bovine pericardium) are highly reliable and provide excellent hemostasis as well as closure of air leaks reducing postoperative air leakage. The vascular stapler cartridge with six rows of 2.0 or 2.5 mm staples is designed for division of thin vascular tissue such as the pulmonary vessels. Some surgeons are reluctant to use it on hilar vessels because if the stapler fails mechanically (e.g., cuts without applying both staple lines properly), life-threatening hemorrhage can ensue.[21] Endoscopic staplers that do not cut (transverse anastomosis [TA] staplers) are also available. Some advocate using two applications of the endovascular stapling device to minimize the risk of transecting the vessel as a consequence of a stapling misfire. In this approach, the stapler is first fired proximally with the knife removed, leaving six rows of staples in place. Next, the stapler is fired again more distally with the cutting mechanism intact to transect the vessel, leaving a total of nine rows of staples on the patient side and three rows of staples on the specimen side.

Instruments

Various types of Pennington and Duval clamps are available. Sponge sticks modified by the introduction of various curves and a line of lung clamps are used for retracting lungs, dissecting hilar structures, and holding lymph nodes. The vein retractor and the fan retractor, which can be opened and closed like a fan by turning a knob on the end, can also be used during VATS. Vein retractors are best suited for gentle retraction of hilar or mediastinal structures (e.g., vessels, bronchi, esophagus, or lymph nodes), whereas the fan retractor can be used to hold the whole lung during MIE.

In major VATS procedures (e.g., VATS lobectomy), the soft tissues of the access incision may be retracted by means of a cerebellar (or Weitlaner [Miltex, Inc, York, PA]) retractor. This allows the surgeon to dissect and encircle hilar vascular structures by using two instruments through the same incision. A Harken clamp (Scanlan, Saint Paul, MN) is useful in that it is long enough to reach behind a vascular structure, pass a silk suture to the tip of the instrument, and tie it to an endoleader to guide the stapler across these delicate arterial branches.[22] A long Allis forceps is an excellent instrument for holding and retracting lymph nodes during a mediastinal lymph node dissection. Although biopsy forceps have been specifically created for laparoscopy and thoracoscopy, those used for mediastinoscopy are, in fact, well suited for thoracoscopy. Various curved and right-angle dissecting clamps, needle holders, and scissors have been developed. In addition, standard thoracotomy instruments can be inserted through a minithoracotomy incision and used just as they would be in an open procedure.

Devices for Tissue Cauterization

The standard disposable electrocautery device (Bovie Medical Corporation, Clearwater, FL) with a long tip extension, or the Harmonic Scalpel (Ethicon Endo-Surgery, Cincinnati, OH), the LigaSure vessel sealing system (Covidien, Valleylab, Boulder, CO) and the argon beam electrocoagulator handpiece are narrow enough to pass through a thoracoport. These instruments can be used for dissection and cauterization during VATS. The argon beam electrocoagulator (ConMed Corporation, Utica, NY) is a noncontact form of electrocautery that provides hemostasis on raw surfaces (e.g., denuded pulmonary parenchyma or the chest wall after pleurectomy) and helps seal air leaks from the surface of the lung. Instrumentation for videothoracoscopy continues to evolve. Nevertheless, it may still be necessary to combine disposable and nondisposable instruments from different manufacturers and to use instruments originally designed for other procedures. It is best to maintain a single standard tray that includes the basic instruments required for most operations and to add instruments as needed.

Basic Operative Technique

At our institution, VATS is conducted under general anesthesia using a double-lumen endotracheal tube and single-lung ventilation. The patient is placed in the full lateral decubitus position, but depending on the location of the target, the patient can be tilted 5° forward or backward. Ventilation to the lung being operated on is stopped as soon as the patient is rotated into the lateral decubitus position, to ensure that the lung will be thoroughly collapsed by the time the videothoracoscope is inserted into the pleural space. The incisions are made on the superior aspect of the ribs to avoid injury to the neurovascular bundle. A standard thoracoscopy is performed with three 10 mm incisions: a camera port is placed in the anterior axillary line in the seventh or eighth ICS; an anterior or access port is placed between the latissimus dorsi and the pectoralis major muscles in the fourth or fifth ICS, and a posterior or working port is placed adjacent to the scapula in the fifth or sixth ICS. Alternatively, a 5 mm incision can be used for a 5 mm camera, and one working port ranging from 3 to 10 mm can be used. It is important to orient the instruments and the thoracoscope such that they face the target within a 180° arc; this positioning prevents mirror imaging and helps the surgery team develop a three-dimensional spatial anatomic orientation in the chest. The incisions should also be placed widely distant from each other so that the instruments do not crowd one another. Should it become necessary to convert to a thoracotomy, the two upper incisions can be incorporated into the thoracotomy incision and the lower incision can be used as a chest tube site. When a patient is being operated on for an apical lesion, the camera port can be placed at the fifth or sixth ICS, and the two instrument ports may also be moved higher, toward the axilla, and the other higher on the posterior chest wall at approximately the third ICS. Also, a fourth port may be helpful for the introduction of additional instruments or to palpate the lesion, depending on its location. An infant Finochietto (Medicon, Bedford, VA) or a Weitlaner retractor is used to keep the soft tissues from falling into the wound without spreading the ribs. These are the basic steps on which modification of the technique will occur depending on the pathology, the location of the target being removed, and the surgeon's skills.

VATS Procedures for Pleural Disease

OPERATIVE TECHNIQUE

One or two 10 mm incisions are made for the videothoracoscope and instruments. The videothoracoscope is inserted through either a 5 or 10 mm thoracoport at the seventh or eighth ICS in the midaxillary line. In cases of pleurodesis, either by mechanical or talc poudrage, the incisions are used for placement of chest tubes, with a right-angle tube inserted over the diaphragm through the lower incision and a straight tube advanced up to the apex of the pleural space through the upper incision. Alternatively, a small 19 French Silastic flexible drain (Blake drain, Ethicon, Somerville, NJ) can be placed in the chest cavity as well, but it has to be looped around the base of the lung and over the diaphragmatic surface and guided posteriorly along the parietal pleura with its tip up in the apex.[23] Special attention must be paid to the placement of the incision in patients with suspected malignant mesothelioma because of the propensity of this tumor to implant in incisions and needle tracks. Once the videothoracoscope has been inserted, pleural fluid is drained with

Yankauer suction tip (Cardinal Health, Dublin, OH) and is sent for cytology, microbiology, and chemistry. Inspection of the cavity is performed, and multiple pleural biopsies are obtained. Fibrinous debris can be removed by irrigating the pleural space with a pulsating water irrigation system. This technique is particularly useful for the débridement and drainage of loculated fibrinopurulent empyema. Talc poudrage for the treatment of malignant pleural effusion can be accomplished by delivering 2 to 6 g of talc in the pleural cavity with a pneumatic atomizer using 10 L of high-flow O_2.[24] At the end of the procedure, an intercostal nerve block is performed under the direct vision of the thoracoscope.

TROUBLESHOOTING

In patients with loculated effusion, the thoracoport placement must sometimes be modified. The preoperative chest CT scan should help ensure that the ports are placed in areas where the lung is not adherent to the chest wall. In some cases, the pleural space is obliterated by adhesions or tumor. This event occurs most frequently in patients who have had severe inflammatory disease (e.g., pneumonia, empyema, or tuberculosis) or extensive pleural malignancy (e.g., locally advanced malignant mesothelioma). In these circumstances, the anterior thoracoport incision can be extended to a length of 5 to 6 cm, the underlying rib section can be resected, and the parietal pleura can undergo biopsy. If thoracotomy is subsequently warranted for therapeutic reasons (e.g., for pleurectomy, decortication, or extrapleural pneumonectomy for mesothelioma), this small incision can be incorporated into the thoracotomy incision.

VATS Pulmonary Wedge Resection

VATS pulmonary wedge resection has become a standard approach to diagnosing small, indeterminate pulmonary nodules and pulmonary infiltrates of uncertain origin, particularly in immunocompromised patients in whom transbronchial biopsy is neither safe nor appropriate. The role of VATS wedge resection is less well defined in the management of primary lung cancers but may be indicated in patients with marginal lung function who otherwise would not tolerate a lobectomy. Although no prospective studies have been performed to clearly assess the benefit of pulmonary metastasectomy, there is an abundance of retrospective data to indicate a long-term survival benefit from complete pulmonary resection. The general criteria in selecting patients for pulmonary metastasectomy include the following: (1) the primary neoplasm must be completely controlled or imminently controllable; (2) metastatic lesions must be limited to the lung without evidence of other distant organ involvement; (3) all metastases must be resectable with adequate pulmonary reserve; and (4) nonavailability of another effective therapy. In cases that meet these resection criteria, long-term survival rates have been reported to be in the range of 30 and 58% for patients with soft tissue and osteogenic sarcomas, respectively. Similar cure rates have been reported with the resection of isolated pulmonary metastases from colon cancer (30.5%), renal cell carcinoma (52.4%), head and neck cancers (48%), and germ cell tumors (59%). Although some melanoma patients with a solitary metastasis may benefit from pulmonary metastasectomy, most patients with this disease do not survive long-term despite aggressive resection of the metastasis.[25] Improved survival in patients with pulmonary metastases appears to be directly linked to the ability to remove all macroscopic tumor. The biology of pulmonary metastases may favor VATS resection based on the following arguments: (1) metastases have been present prior to treatment of the primary lesion and in that sense have been "missed" for a significant period of time already; (2) as noted above, multiple resections do not adversely affect the overall outcome of patients with metachronously detected metastases; (3) patients with unresectable disease who have a recurrence will not be subject to a larger operation, i.e., thoracotomy; (4) VATS resection may be less stressful for patients and therefore result in less immunosuppression, resulting in a more favorable disease course; and (5) VATS may permit patients to return to their regular work or family schedules significantly earlier than an open approach. Other considerations include quality of life and cost of treatment. Historical data, tumor biology, and recent advances in radiologic and surgical techniques support the use of video-assisted surgery in the resection of pulmonary metastases, following the paramount principle of removing all lesions found on a high-resolution CT scan.

Anecdotal reports of port-site recurrence also have raised concerns about VATS as a treatment method in patients with malignancies. However, a 2001 study of 410 patients from a prospective VATS database found only one case of port-site recurrence.[26] The authors concluded that the incidence of such recurrences could be kept low if surgical oncologic principles are respected. These principles include (1) reserving VATS for lesions that can be widely excised; (2) conversion to an open thoracotomy for definitive or extensive operations; and (3) meticulous technique for extraction of specimens from the pleural space, with small specimens removed directly through a thoracoport and larger specimens removed in an endo-bag.

OPERATIVE TECHNIQUE

Once general anesthesia has been induced and a double-lumen endotracheal tube inserted, the patient is placed in the full lateral decubitus position. Small subpleural pulmonary nodules are most easily identified in a fully atelectatic lung because they protrude from the surrounding collapsed pulmonary parenchyma. Most pulmonary wedge resections are performed as true videothoracoscopic procedures using just three port incisions placed in a triangulated manner [*see Figure 4*]. The pulmonary nodules to be removed are grasped with an endoscopic lung clamp (Pennington, ring forceps, or Duval) inserted through one instrument port, and wedge resection is done with repeated applications of an endoscopic stapler inserted through the opposite port. An endoscopic lung compression clamp is a linear clamp that can be placed deep to the lesion to ensure a 1 cm margin from the lesion to the staple line [*see Figure 6*]. As the resection is performed, it is often helpful to introduce the stapler through each of two instrument ports to obtain the correct angle for application to the lung. To prevent tumor implantation in the chest wall, all specimens are placed in a disposable endo-bag and brought out through a slightly enlarged anterior thoracoport incision. At the end of the procedure, intercostal nerve blocks are performed under direct vision of the thoracoscope, and a single chest tube is inserted through the inferior port after the videothoracoscope is withdrawn.

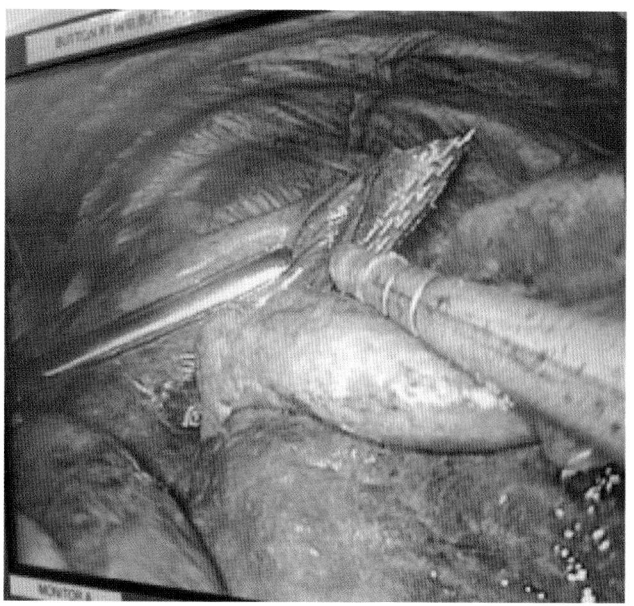

Figure 6 **Wedge resection, lung compression clamp.**

TROUBLESHOOTING

Several techniques may be used to locate pulmonary nodules that are either too deep or too small to be easily visible on simple inspection of the lung. All of these should be used in conjunction with a high-quality preoperative chest CT scan to identify the lung segment in which the nodule is located. Thoracoscopic examination of the lung nodule can be performed by gently running an endo-Kittner or a ring forceps on the surface of the lung as a surrogate to digital palpation. With experience, one can "feel" a bump and grasp the visceral pleura adjacent to the location. The nodule can be brought up toward the examining finger placed through one of the ports. Alternatively, under prior CT guidance preoperatively, a needle may be inserted into the nodule for intraoperative localization, much like a breast needle localization procedure. Localization is accomplished by injecting methylene blue or by inserting a barbed mammography localization needle, which is then cut off at the skin exit site and later retrieved thoracoscopically. Needle localization techniques are effective, but they also are costly and time-consuming and need to be coordinated with the radiology team and surgeons. Finally, if careful endoscopic examination of the lung fails to reveal the location of a nodule, an access incision is added to the videothoracoscopy. Each lobe of the lung is sequentially rotated up to this non–rib-spreading utility thoracotomy for direct digital palpation. This technique almost always permits identification of a nodule when other techniques fail.

Pulmonary nodules located on the broad surface of the lung may not be amenable to a wedge resection with an endoscopic stapler. Such nodules can be removed by means of electrocauterization, just as in an open thoracotomy. An extension is placed on the handle of the electrocautery device, which is then introduced into the pleural space through either a port or an access incision. Another approach is to resect the pulmonary nodule with a laser in either contact or noncontact mode. To minimize bleeding and air leakage, raw pulmonary surfaces can be cauterized with either the neodymium: yttrium-aluminum-garnet (Nd:YAG) laser or the argon beam coagulator. Numerous types of absorbable sealant patches or materials are also available to control air leaks from areas of raw pulmonary parenchyma.

Occasionally, after a wedge resection, it is necessary to suture together the pleural edges over an area of raw pulmonary parenchyma. The suturing can be done directly through a non–rib-spreading access incision or through port sites. In the latter case, the ports are removed and a 3-0 polypropylene suture is passed through the anterior port site with a standard needle holder. A second needle holder is introduced via the posterior port site and used in place of a forceps to pick up and reposition the needle as it is passed through the lung. The surgeon and the first assistant work together to oversew the lung, in contrast to the normal practice for an open procedure, in which the surgeon uses a needle holder and a forceps to place the sutures.

VATS Procedures for Spontaneous Pneumothorax and Bullous Disease

OPERATIVE TECHNIQUE

VATS is now frequently performed for the management of recurrent spontaneous pneumothorax and for bullous disease. The approach is similar to that followed in a wedge resection, with three or four port sites being used. The videothoracoscope is inserted at the fifth ICS in the midaxillary line, and two other port sites are added at the fourth ICS in the anterior and posterior axillary lines. In patients with spontaneous pneumothorax, the responsible bulla (which is usually apical in location) is identified, and wedge resection is done with a tissue-reinforced endoscopic stapler. Bullae can be excised by applying the stapler across the base of the area of bullous disease. They also can be ablated with the argon beam coagulator or the Nd:YAG laser and then suture-plicated if necessary.

TROUBLESHOOTING

The placement of port incisions should be determined by the location of the bullae. Because bullous disease is generally apical, port sites are correspondingly higher than for the average wedge resection (i.e., at the fourth and sixth ICSs rather than at the fifth or sixth and eighth ICSs). The precise placement should, however, be determined by determining the exact location of the disease site(s) on the preoperative CT scans. The main problem after resection for bullous disease is prolonged air leak from the staple line. This problem can be minimized by applying commercially available sleeves made of bovine pericardium or with tissue-reinforced staplers and by performing pleurodesis. Mechanical pleurodesis is done with a small gauze sponge passed through a port site. Some surgeons scarify the pleura by cauterizing it with the argon beam coagulator or the Nd:YAG laser, but this is not as effective as mechanical pleurodesis. Chemical pleurodesis by talc poudrage should be reserved for older patients with emphysema and bullous disease and avoided in young patients with spontaneous pneumothorax, who might require a thoracotomy later in life. Another option in younger patients is a limited apical pleurectomy. Special angulated instruments and blunt dissectors have been designed for this procedure; however, a parietal pleurectomy is also easily performed with combinations of standard blunt and sharp instruments.

VATS Lung Volume Reduction Surgery

OPERATIVE TECHNIQUE

VATS may also be applied to the performance of lung volume reduction surgery (LVRS). If unilateral LVRS is planned, the patient is placed in the lateral decubitus position, and port placement is similar to that for a patient undergoing a wedge resection of the upper lobe. Most patients undergoing LVRS, however, benefit from bilateral LVRS. For this procedure, the patient is placed in the standard supine bilateral lung transplantation position, with shoulder rolls placed vertically in an inverted U fashion behind the back and with the arms positioned above the head. The camera port is placed in the anterior axillary line at the sixth ICS. A lung compression clamp is placed on the area that will be resected. A tissue-reinforced stapler is then inserted into the chest and fired sequentially until the desired area is excised [*see Figure 7*].

TROUBLESHOOTING

A major cause of morbidity and mortality with this procedure is the occurrence of air leaks, which sometimes are large enough to compromise ventilation significantly. Thus once LVRS has been done on one side, the lung is reexpanded and any air leaks are carefully assessed. If the leak is small, the other side is operated on in the same setting; if the leak is large, the contralateral procedure is postponed to a later date. The use of fibrin glue or another commercially available pneumostatic sealant along the staple line should be considered to minimize postoperative air leakage.

VATS Lobectomy and Pneumonectomy

Although VATS lobectomy is much less frequently performed than VATS pulmonary wedge resection, standard techniques have been developed.[27] VATS pneumonectomy is performed with less frequency. There are emerging data using VATS, but this approach is experimental at this point in time. These tumors are usually larger and centrally located, making it difficult to assess for the option of a sleeve lobectomy. Therefore, this operation is best performed through an open thoracotomy. However, these operations are done as VATS procedures using an access incision, which facilitates insertion of standard thoracotomy instruments, extraction of the resected specimen from the pleural space, and performance of the technically complex aspects of the procedure, including dissection of the hilar vessels and the mediastinal lymph nodes.

Two approaches to lobectomy have been developed. One involves sequential anatomic ligation of the hilar structures, much as in a standard anatomic lobectomy, and the other involves mass ligation of the pulmonary vessels and the bronchus. The latter is not considered an anatomic lobectomy; therefore, we do not endorse its practice. Both approaches require at least two port incisions in addition to the access incision. The sequential anatomic ligation approach has been well described and follows sound surgical oncologic principles. Accordingly, it is our preferred method of performing VATS lobectomy. In an effort to standardize the approach, we define a VATS lobectomy as an anatomic dissection that is performed entirely under thoracoscopic visualization, proceeds in an anterior to posterior fashion, and uses a 4 cm utility incision, two thoracoscopy ports (one for the camera and one for retraction), and no rib spreading. Avoiding rib spreading is the key element in VATS lobectomy to prevent postoperative pain and trauma to the intercostal nerve bundles, which are responsible for the postthoracotomy pain syndrome. A metastatic survey is performed in all patients undergoing VATS lobectomy for malignant disease. The chest is inspected for metastatic pleural and pericardial implants and effusion, chest wall invasion, adhesions, enlarged lymph nodes, and anatomic variations. Radical lymph node dissection includes evaluation of lymph node levels 2, 4, 7, 8, and 9 on the right side. On the left side, it should also include lymph node levels 5 and 6.

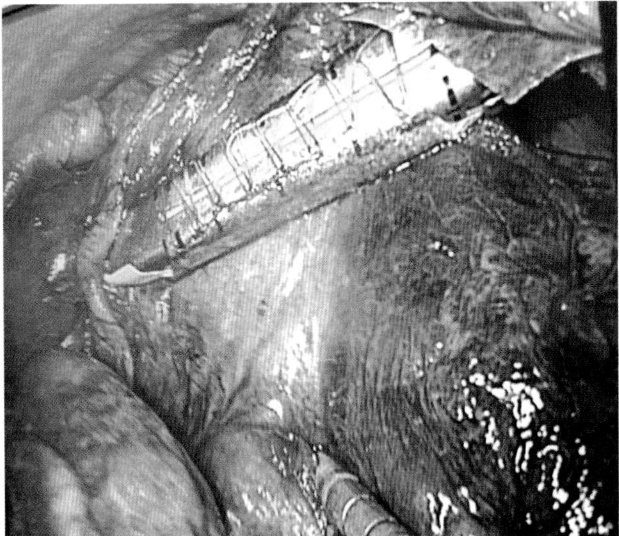

Figure 7 **Tissue-reinforced stapler is inserted into the chest.**

OPERATIVE TECHNIQUE

Lobectomy (Sequential Anatomic Ligation)

Correct positioning and port placement are essential for a successful VATS lobectomy. The first port placed is the camera port. It is usually placed through the seventh or eighth ICS and should provide visualization of the anterior and posterior hilum and align with the major fissure in a caudal-cephalic orientation. Whether the port is in the anterior, middle, or posterior axillary line depends on the level of the diaphragm as seen from a review of the preoperative chest x-ray or CT scan, on the location of the target, and on the side of the procedure.

The anterior or utility port (< 4 cm) should be placed right over the hilum. The hilum and the fissures will be dissected through this port. The port usually is created anterior to the latissimus dorsi in the fourth ICS for upper lobectomies and in the fifth ICS for lower lobectomies. A soft tissue retractor may be used to keep the subcutaneous tissue and muscle away from the incision. The third (posterior) port is usually placed where the edge of the lower lobe touches the diaphragm under the vision of the thoracoscope either inferior or posterior to the scapular tip. This port usually is used for retracting the lung. A ring forceps is placed through the posterior port, and the upper lobe is retracted laterally to permit visualization of the superior pulmonary vein. Table 3 shows the general operative steps for VATS lobectomy.[28]

Right-Side Resections

Right upper lobectomy The initial dissection is carried out at the anterior hilum. The phrenic nerve is identified, and the mediastinal pleura is opened posterior to it. This plane is developed anteriorly, superiorly, and then posteriorly between the lung and the azygos vein. If any level 10 lymph nodes are found at this location, they are sampled and sent for frozen section. This dissection can, for the most part, be accomplished with blunt dissection using two endo-Kittners. Next, the lung is retracted anteriorly and the posterior hilum is opened to expose the right mainstem bronchus. Further dissection is carried out to expose the bifurcation of the upper lobe bronchus and the bronchus intermedius. The superior pulmonary vein is dissected from the overlying pleura via the access incision with long Pearson or Metzenbaum scissors and DeBakey forceps, similar to an open lobectomy. A Harken clamp is passed behind the superior pulmonary vein after clear identification of the middle lobe vein. The superior pulmonary vein is encircled with an oiled 2-0 silk suture, which is then tied to the endoleader.[29] A lung clamp is placed through the utility incision, and the upper lobe is retracted posteriorly. An endovascular stapler is placed through the posterior port and, guided by the endoleader, is passed behind the superior pulmonary vein and deployed [*see Figure 8*].

Once the pulmonary vein has been divided, the truncus anterior of the pulmonary artery and its variable apical branches are exposed. A Harken clamp is passed around the anterior and apical pulmonary arterial branches, and an oiled 2-0 silk suture followed by the endoleader is passed around these vessels and brought out through the utility incision. The endovascular stapler is passed though the posterior port and used to transect the vessels. Transection of the truncus artery and its branch exposes the right upper lobe bronchus [*see Figure 9*]. Dissection is performed to separate the ongoing pulmonary artery from the bronchus. An endoscopic 4.8 mm GIA stapler is placed through the posterior port and closed but not fired until the lung is inflated, demonstrating that the middle lobe bronchus is patent. Once the upper lobe bronchus has been divided [*see Figure 10*], the fissure is completed with the stapler. The upper lobe is then placed in a large surgical tissue endo-bag and removed via the utility incision.

Table 3 Operative Steps for VATS Lobectomy

Step 1	Positioning and incision/thoracoscopic port placement
Step 2	Lung mobilization
Step 3	Isolation and division of pulmonary arterial and venous branches
Step 4	Fissure completion
Step 5	Bronchial division
Step 6	Lymph node dissection
Step 7	Closure

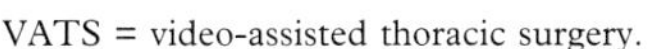
VATS = video-assisted thoracic surgery.

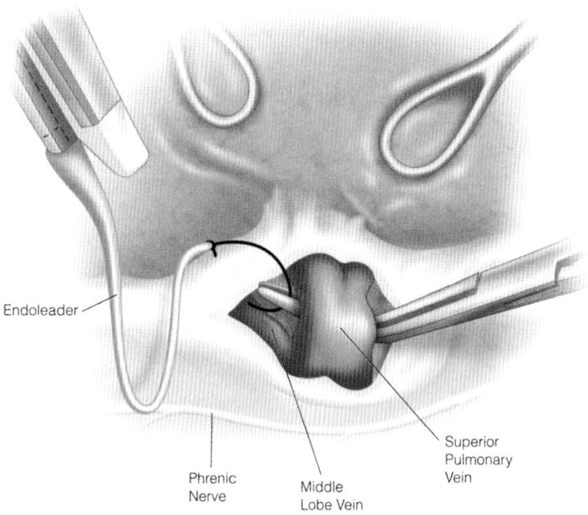

Figure 8 **The endoleader looped around the superior pulmonary vein.**

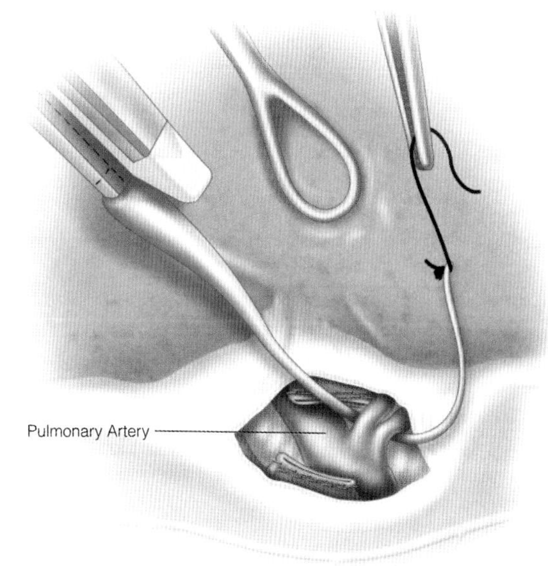

Figure 9 **The endoleader looped around the truncus anterior and its branch.**

Certain basic surgical concepts—dissection of hilar structures, passage of a monofilament suture around the structure, and transection with a stapler—are similar for all lobectomies. However, the order in which structures are transected and the ports through which staplers are passed differ.

Right middle lobectomy The camera port is placed in the seventh ICS in the midaxillary line. The anterior or access port is placed in the fifth ICS. The posterior or working port is placed either at the scapula tip or posterior to it in the sixth or seventh ICS. The right middle lobe is retracted laterally, and the middle lobe vein is exposed by dissecting it on the anterior hilum. Once the middle lobe vein is dissected free, it is divided using the same maneuvers as described earlier

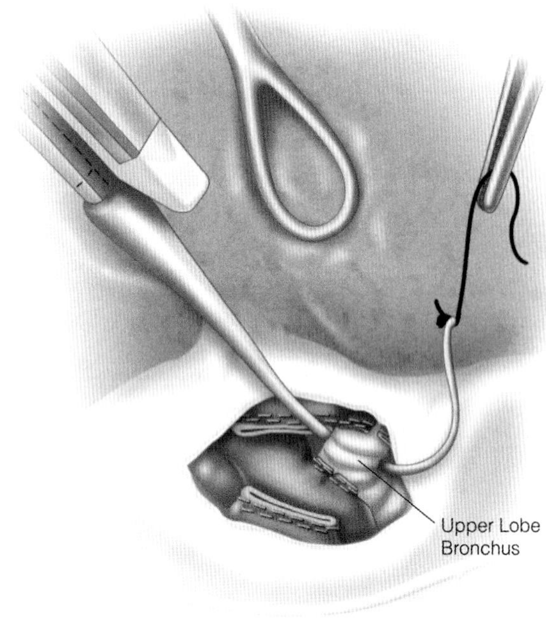

Figure 10 **Division of the upper lobe bronchus.**

using the endovascular stapler. The middle lobe bronchus is exposed and divided before the artery because it lies anterior to the pulmonary artery to the middle lobe. Caution should be exercised while dissecting around the middle bronchus so as not to injure the arterial branches to the middle lobe. Maciejewski described two arterial branches of the pulmonary artery to the middle lobe in 57% of the patients and a single artery penetrating the middle lobe in 43% of patients.[30] The length of arteries can be up to 30 mm and the diameter up to 10.6 mm. The pulmonary artery branches are dissected free, isolated, and divided with the endovascular stapler. The fissure is completed, and the middle lobe is removed in a specimen endo-bag through the access port.

Right lower lobectomy The camera port is inserted in the seventh ICS in the posterior axillary line. The posterior port is placed either at the tip of the scapula or immediately behind it. The access port is placed directly over the fissure between the middle and lower lobe at the level of the inferior pulmonary vein. Ring forceps are used to retract the middle lobe medially and the lower lobe posteriorly. Next, the lower lobe is retracted superiorly and the inferior pulmonary ligament is taken down with either electrocautery device (Bovie) or Harmonic shears (Ethicon Endo-Surgery, Cincinnati, OH). Level 9 lymph nodes are taken during this step of the operation. Next, the posterior mediastinal pleura is opened at the level of the inferior pulmonary vein and the dissection continues posteriorly between the posterior hilum and the esophagus. If a level 8 lymph node is found at this location, it is removed as well. This dissection is carried out to the level of the azygos vein. The lung is then retracted anteriorly toward the anterior mediastinum. Next, level 7 (subcarinal) lymph nodes are dissected with two endo-Kittner dissectors and removed. At this point, most of the pleura along the hilum has been opened posteriorly and the inferior pulmonary vein dissected. Next, the apex of the lung is gently grasped with a ringed forceps and retracted toward the diaphragm. This maneuver exposes the paratracheal lymph nodes. The pulmonary artery is then identified just under the surface of the pleura at the fissure. The visceral pleura overlying it is opened. A tunnel of visceral pleura is created over the pulmonary artery by gently pulling the visceral pleura toward the chest wall and dissecting it with endo-Kittners. This maneuver allows for identification of the middle lobe bronchus. Once this tunnel is developed, the fissure is completed posteriorly with the endo-stapler. At this point, the lower lobe pulmonary artery is visualized. A Harken clamp is passed under the artery, and the artery is dissected. The flat tip of a 35 mm vascular load stapler (white load) is passed under the pulmonary artery to the lower lobe and the basilar trunk is transected. The lung is retracted upwards and toward the anterior mediastinum. The inferior pulmonary vein is then transected with the same technique as for the pulmonary artery. The vascular stapler is brought in from the access incision toward the back while lifting the lung up with the ring forceps through the posterior port. The lung is then pulled upwards, the lower lobe bronchus is dissected out, and the stapler is applied but not fired. The anesthesiologist should then inflate the middle lobe. Bronchoscopy is also performed, and the orifice to the middle lobe is visualized. Only after these maneuvers have been performed is the bronchus to the lower lobe transected. The lobe is placed in the endo-bag and brought out through the access port incision.

Left-Side Resections

Left upper lobectomy The left upper lobectomy is technically the most challenging approach because of the anatomic variability in the pulmonary artery branches as well as a common pulmonary vein trunk that drains to the back of the left atrium. Maciejewski reported that in most cases of his series, there were four, and, in a few cases, up to seven, branches of the pulmonary artery to the upper lobe, measuring 30 mm in length and 12 mm in diameter.[31] In about 50% of the cases, the branches were divided in (a) apicoanterior trunk, (b) lingular, and (c) one or two subsegmental branches. In 25% of the cases, almost all segmental branches penetrated into the lobe separately. In 20% of the cases, a single apicoposterior trunk or independent segmental or subsegmental branches were present. Only in 5% of the cases did the branches include the apicoposteroanterior trunk and the remaining segmental and subsegmental branches.

Although port placement is similar to that for right upper lobectomy, the camera port is placed more posteriorly through a seventh or sixth ICS in the anterior axillary line, to avoid obstruction of the camera view by the heart and the pericardial fat pad. Once all ports have been placed, dissection of the anteroposterior window lymph nodes is carried out. This provides information about metastatic nodal spread. It also opens up the space around the artery and vein. The posterior port is placed just behind the tip of the scapula. The lung is retracted posteriorly, the hilum is opened anteriorly, and the superior pulmonary vein is dissected free. Caution must be exercised during this phase of the dissection to avoid injuring the back wall of the vein while it is being dissected off the airway. The upper lobe is retracted posteriorly and the lower lobe is retracted somewhat anteriorly, toward the pericardium, splaying out the fissure. The pulmonary artery is usually found in the fissure, where it is visualized as a white, shiny structure. Dissection of the pulmonary artery creates a space on the top of the artery, a so-called vascular tunnel that allows one to complete the fissure with a stapler, thereby avoiding problems with air leak. A ringed forceps is placed through the fourth ICS to access the incision anteriorly. The lung is now moved anteriorly. The endo-Kittners are placed through the posterior port to dissect the lymph nodes located above the pulmonary artery as it traverses into the fissure. The first apical branch of the pulmonary artery is dissected free and transected with an endoscopic GIA vascular stapler introduced via the posterior port. The anterior aspect of the fissure is opened with one or two applications of an endoscopic GIA stapler introduced via the access incision. The bifurcation of the left upper and left lower lobe bronchi is identified, and the left upper lobe bronchus is transected with an endoscopic GIA stapler with 4.8 mm staples introduced via the posterior port. A ringed forceps is used to retract the stump of the bronchus laterally, which facilitates exposure of several branches of the pulmonary artery, including the lingular artery. These branches are transected individually via the posterior port. The fissure is completed with an endoscopic GIA stapler with 4.8 mm staples through the posterior port and dividing it. The lobe is placed in the endo-bag and brought out through the access port incision. A 24 French chest tube is placed toward the apex of the lung.

Left lower lobectomy The camera port is placed in the eighth ICS in the posterior axillary line to provide exposure to the posterior hilum and to avoid crowding of the instruments. The access port is placed anteriorly in the fifth ICS. The posterior working port is usually posterior to the scapular tip in the sixth or seventh ICS. First, the lung is retracted superiorly and the inferior pulmonary ligament is identified and level 9 lymph nodes are sampled. The left lower lobe is held superiorly with a ring forceps through the posterior port, with the ligament under tension. A long-tipped electrocautery device, or ultrasonic scalpel, divides the ligament at the base of the inferior pulmonary vein. Next, the inferior pulmonary vein is completely dissected. Once the inferior pulmonary vein has been dissected free, an endoscopic GIA vascular stapler is placed via the utility incision to transect the vessel. The interlobar pulmonary artery is isolated within the fissure. The branches of the pulmonary artery to the left lower lobe are of three types: trunk, segmental, and subsegmental. In 70% of the cases, the branches penetrating the basal segments showed a treelike configuration; in 3% of the cases, the segments had a bushlike configuration; and in 27% of the cases, the branches had an intermediate anatomic configuration.[32] The basilar trunk and the artery to the superior segment are identified, dissected, and divided with the endovascular stapler. The superior segmental artery is divided first and the basilar trunk next. This strategy avoids injury to the superior segmental branch with the stapler used to divide the basilar branches. Finally, the bronchus to the lower lobe is dissected and divided with an endo GIA 4.8 mm stapler through the access incision. Attention must be paid to avoid impingement on the lingular bronchus. In cases of incomplete fissure, the fissure between the lingula and lower lobe should be opened prior to dissection of the pulmonary artery to facilitate subsequent arterial exposure.

Pneumonectomy

This operation is best performed through an open thoracotomy.

VATS Mediastinal Lymph Node Dissection

OPERATIVE TECHNIQUE

For biopsy of the aortopulmonary window nodes or anterior mediastinal masses, VATS mediastinal lymph node dissection is often performed as an alternative to a Chamberlain procedure and is thought by some surgeons to provide better exposure and a superior cosmetic result. The thoracoscope is inserted at the fifth or sixth ICS in the posterior axillary line. Instruments for retracting the lung inferiorly are introduced via a port at the seventh ICS in the midaxillary line. Instruments for dissecting nodes are introduced through ports placed at the fourth ICS in the anterior axillary line and in the auscultatory triangle. The lymph nodes are dissected free with graspers (e.g., curved sponge sticks or polyp forceps), scissors, the electrocautery device, and endoscopic hemostatic clips. A similar approach can be used for biopsy of other mediastinal nodes, including the paratracheal and periesophageal nodes. Dissection of level 4 and level 2 nodes on the right is facilitated by transection of the azygos vein. It is more difficult to do a complete en bloc subcarinal lymph node dissection on the left than on the right with this method, although nodal sampling of this region by means of VATS is certainly feasible, especially when an access incision is used.

TROUBLESHOOTING

Care should be taken not to injure the phrenic nerve as it courses along the superior vena cava on the right and across the anterior aspect of the aortopulmonary window on the left. The vagus nerve should be visualized and the origin of the recurrent laryngeal nerve avoided during dissection. The recurrent laryngeal nerve is easily injured on the left side, where it passes around the ligamentum arteriosum before traveling under the aortic arch; however, it can also be injured on the right side if mediastinal lymph node dissection is carried too high superiorly along the origin of the innominate artery.

It is unwise to perform a VATS mediastinal lymph node dissection after induction chemotherapy or chemoradiotherapy because the lymph nodes will often be densely adherent to surrounding structures. This is especially true on the right side, where the superior mediastinal lymph nodes usually adhere densely to the superior vena cava, the azygos vein, and the right main pulmonary artery. A thoracotomy, with extensive exposure and sharp dissection, is usually required for a safe and complete mediastinal lymphadenectomy.

All lymphatic branches should be ligated during node biopsy or dissection to prevent a chyle leak. There are often large lymphatic branches in the distal right paratracheal area. In addition, the thoracic duct can be injured if periesophageal or posterior mediastinal lymph nodes are being removed.

VATS Esophagectomy

OPERATIVE TECHNIQUE

Transthoracic Approach

The most widely accepted method of performing a thoracoscopic and laparoscopic esophagectomy is the technique developed by Luketich and colleagues.[33] All patients undergo bronchoscopy and on-the-table esophagogastroduodenoscopy (EGD) to make a final assessment of the location of the tumor and the suitability of the gastric conduit for reconstruction. If the EGD, endoscopic ultrasonography, or CT scan findings suggest gastric extension, T4 local extension, or possible metastases, we perform a staging laparoscopy, a thoracoscopy, or both. Patients are intubated with a double-lumen tube and placed in the left lateral decubitus position. The surgeon stands on the right and the assistant on the left. Four thoracoscopic ports are used [*see Figure 11*]. A 10 mm camera port is placed at the seventh to eighth ICS, just anterior to the midaxillary line. A 5 mm port is placed at the eighth or ninth ICS, posterior to the posterior axillary line, for the Harmonic shears. A 10 mm port is placed in the anterior axillary line at the fourth ICS; this port is used to pass a fan-shaped retractor to retract the lung anteriorly and allow exposure of the esophagus. The last 5 mm port is placed just posterior to the scapula tip; it is used to place instruments for retraction and countertraction. In most patients, a single retracting suture (G-Endostitch, US Surgical, Norwalk, CT) is placed near the central tendon of the diaphragm and brought out through the inferior anterior chest wall through a 1 mm skin incision, providing downward traction on the diaphragm and allowing exposure of the distal esophagus.

The intrathoracic esophagus is exposed by dividing the inferior pulmonary ligament. The mediastinal pleura overlying the esophagus is opened, and dissection is carried out cephalad toward the azygos vein. The azygos vein is divided with an endoscopic stapler [*see Figure 12*]. Care is taken to preserve the mediastinal pleura above the azygos vein. This maneuver helps to maintain the gastric tube in the posterior mediastinum. By keeping the mediastinal pleura intact near the thoracic inlet, it may help to seal the plane around the gastric tube, preventing downward extension of a cervical leak into the chest. Circumferential mobilization of the esophagus is performed up to the level of 1 to 2 cm above the carina, including all surrounding lymph nodes; periesophageal tissue and fat; the plane along the pericardium, aorta, and contralateral mediastinal pleura up to but not including the thoracic duct; and the azygos vein laterally. Esophageal branches of the aorta are cut with a Harmonic scalpel. No effort is made to find the thoracic duct. A Penrose drain is placed around the esophagus to facilitate traction and exposure [*see Figure 12*].

The entire intrathoracic esophagus is mobilized from the thoracic inlet to the diaphragmatic reflection. As the dissection proceeds toward the thoracic inlet, care is taken to stay near the esophagus to avoid trauma to the posterior membranous trachea and the recurrent laryngeal nerves. Once the esophagus is completely mobilized in the chest, a single 28 French chest tube is inserted through the most anterior and inferior port and the lung is inflated to search for any air leaks from the trachea and proximal bronchus. The thoracic ports are closed, and the patient is turned to the supine position. The surgeon remains on the patient's right; the patient is positioned in the steep reverse Trendelenburg position.

Five abdominal ports (four 5 mm and one 11 mm) are used for the dissection [*see Figure 13*]. The gastrohepatic ligament is divided. The right and left crura of the diaphragm are dissected; division of the phrenoesophageal membrane is avoided at this stage of the operation because this may cause loss of the pneumoperitoneum into the chest cavity and lead

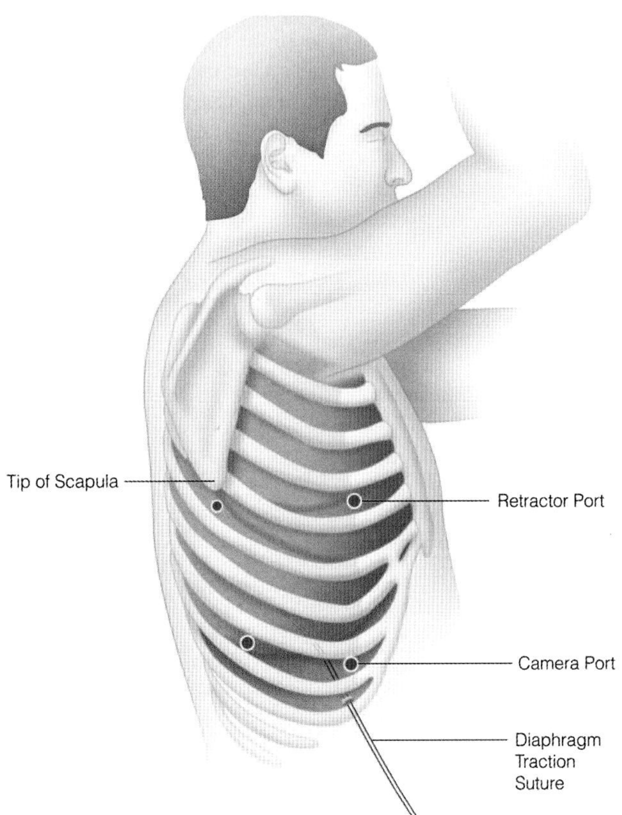

Figure 11 **Thoracic port placement for minimally invasive esophagectomy.**

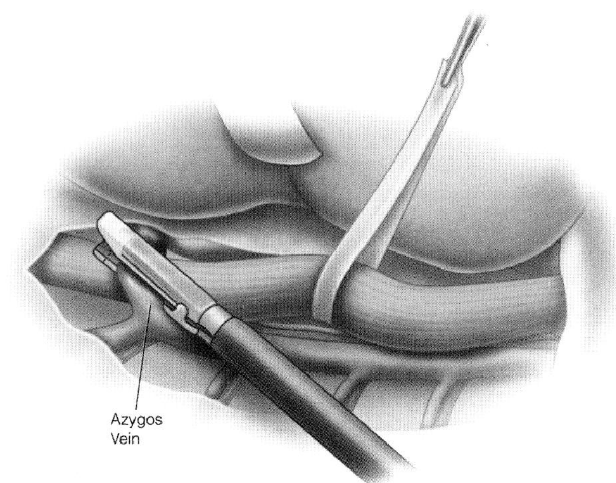

Figure 12 **Stapling of the azygos vein.**

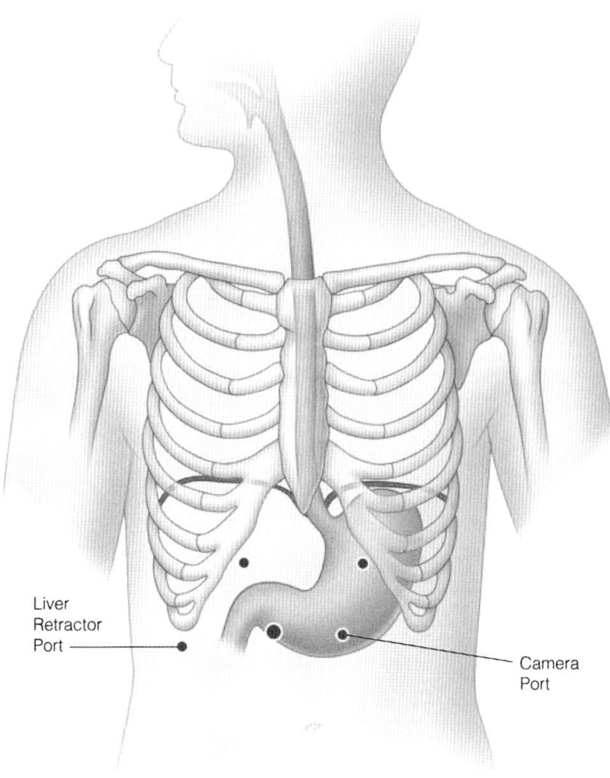

Figure 13 **Abdominal port placement.**

to technical difficulties. The stomach is mobilized by dividing the short gastric vessels using the Harmonic scalpel. The gastrocolic omentum is divided, with care taken to preserve the right gastroepiploic arcade [*see Figure 14*]. The stomach is

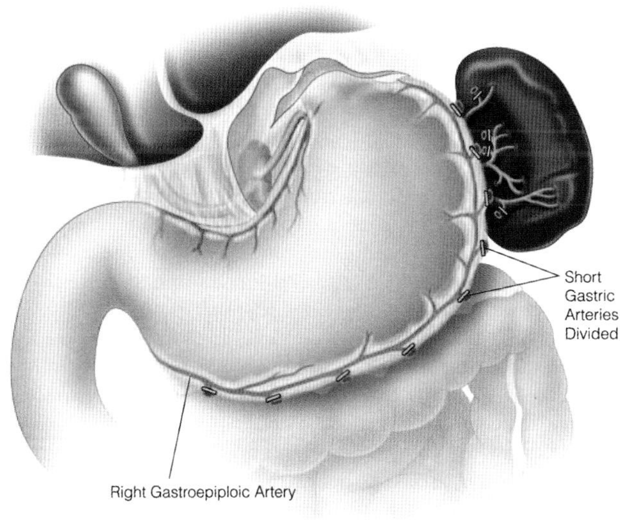

Figure 14 **Division of the gastrocolic omentum along the greater curvature of the stomach and dissection of the hiatus.**

retracted superiorly, and the left gastric vessels are identified. The left gastric artery and vein can be divided from the retrogastric or lessor curve view, depending on the anatomy, using the Endo-GIA stapler.

PYLOROPLASTY

The Harmonic scalpel is used to open the pylorus, and the Endo Stitch (2.0, US Surgical) is used to close the pylorus transversely [*see Figure 15*]. A gastric tube is then constructed by dividing the stomach starting at the lesser curvature and preserving the right gastric vessels with the 4.8 mm stapler (Endo-GIA II, US Surgical) [*see Figure 16*]. There is some variability in the construction of the gastric tube based on the characteristics of the tumor. It may be necessary to construct a slightly more narrow tube or to resect some of the proximal stomach in tumors with significant gastric extension. If gastric extension of the tumor is significant, the resection of the stomach is larger and an intrathoracic anastomosis is performed. Currently, we prefer a gastric tube of 5 to 6 cm in diameter. Extreme caution must be used when manipulating the gastric tube during mobilization and stapling to avoid trauma. The most cephalad portion of the gastric tube is then attached to the esophageal and gastric specimen using two 2-0 endo-sutures. An additional superficial stitch may be placed on the anterior proximal gastric tube to facilitate orientation and prevent twisting as the tube is brought up into the neck [*see Figure 17*]. A feeding jejunostomy tube is done laparoscopically. First, a proximal limb of jejunum (25 cm distal to the ligament of Treitz) is attached to the anterior abdominal wall in the left lateral quadrant with the endo-stitch. An additional 10 mm port in the right lower quadrant may be inserted to facilitate suturing of the jejunum

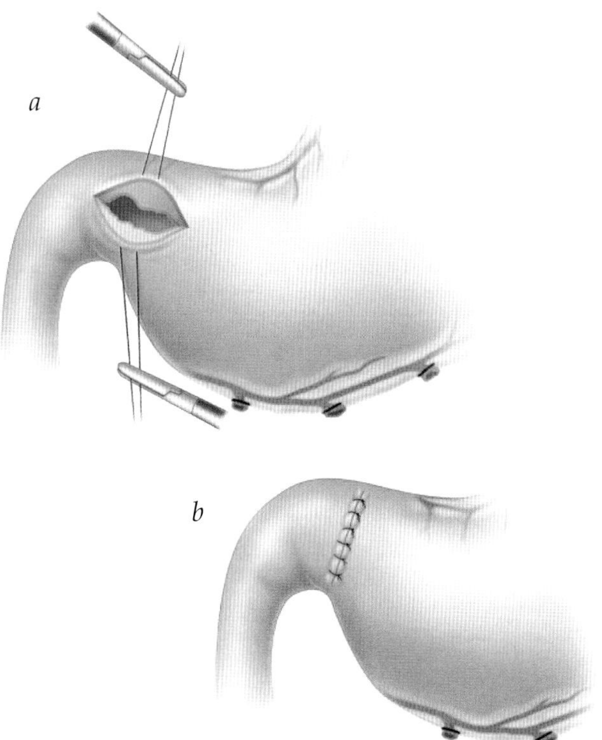

Figure 15 **Pyloroplasty. (*a*) Pyloroplasty is performed using Harmonic shears. (*b*) Transverse closure of the pyloroplasty with endo-stitch technique.**

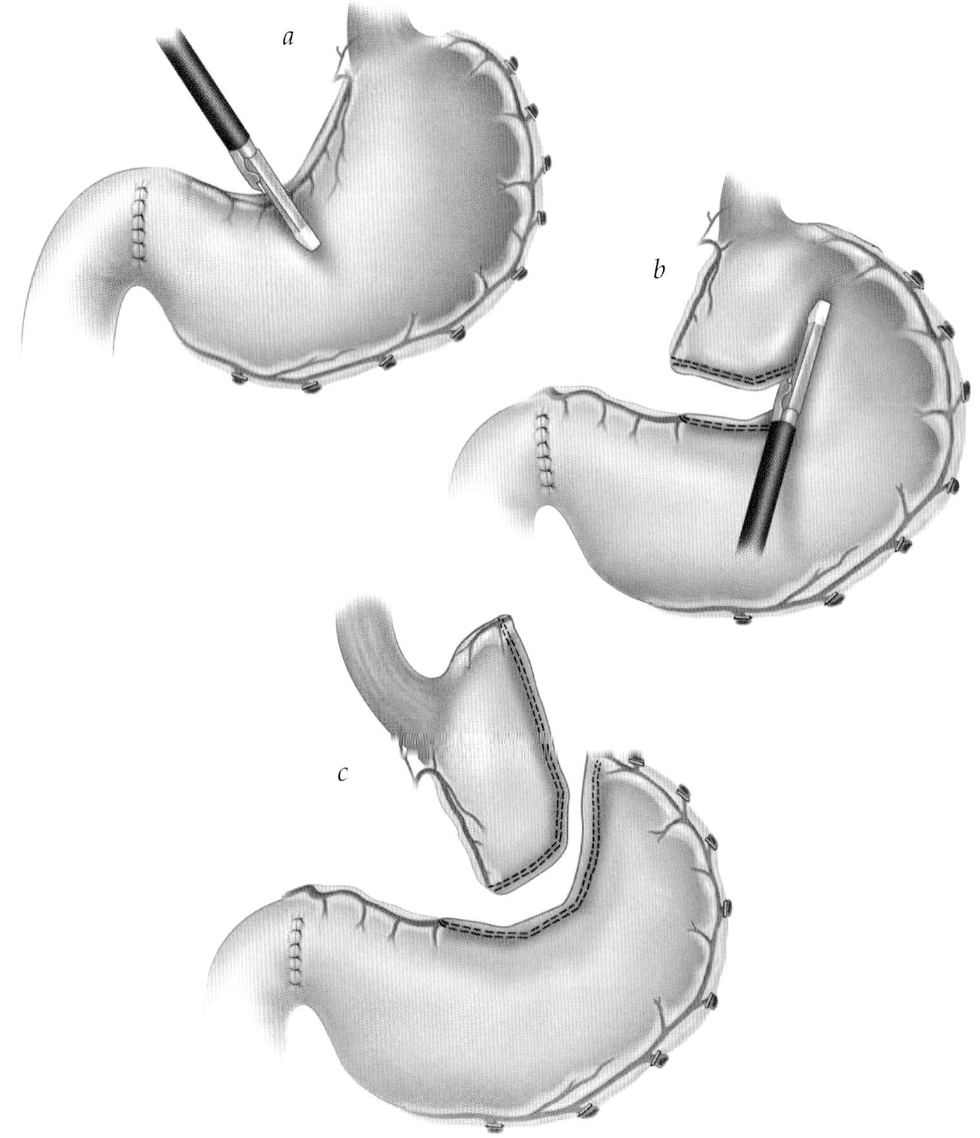

Figure 16 **Creation of a gastric tube. (*a*) The gastric tube is created by dividing the stomach starting at the distal lesser curve, preserving the right gastric vessels. (*b*) A 5 to 6 cm in diameter gastric tube is preferred. (*c*) Division of the gastric tube is from the esophagus.**

to the anterior abdominal wall. A needle catheter (Compact Biosystems, Minneapolis, MN) is placed percutaneously into the peritoneal cavity. Under direct laparoscopic vision, the guide wire and catheter are directed into the loop of jejunum that has been tacked to the anterior abdominal wall. The entry site of the needle catheter J tube is tacked completely to the anterior abdominal wall for a distance of several centimeters.

The last step in the abdominal operation is the dissection of the phrenoesophageal membrane, which was delayed earlier to minimize the risk of losing the pneumoperitoneum into the mediastinum. The right and left crura are partially divided to permit easy passage of the gastric specimen and tube through the hiatus and to prevent later gastric outlet obstruction.

Next, a 4 to 6 cm horizontal neck incision is made [*see Figure 18*]. The cervical esophagus is exposed. Careful dissection is performed inferiorly until the thoracic dissection plane is encountered. This is generally quite easy because the VATS dissection is continued well into the thoracic inlet. In addition, we leave the Penrose drain around the esophagus during the thoracic dissection and push the drain into the periesophageal plane at the thoracic inlet so that it is easily visualized during the neck dissection. This maneuver allows the surgeon to pull the Penrose drain out through the neck to facilitate the neck dissection. The esophagogastric specimen is pulled out of the neck incision and the cervical esophagus is divided high (1 to 2 cm below the cricopharyngeal muscle). The specimen is removed from the field. An anastomosis is performed between the cervical esophagus and gastric tube using a GIA stapler [*see Figure 19*]. Next, the surgeon returns to the laparoscopic view and gently pulls downward on the pyloroantral area to retrieve any excess gastric tube that may have been pulled up into the chest during the neck

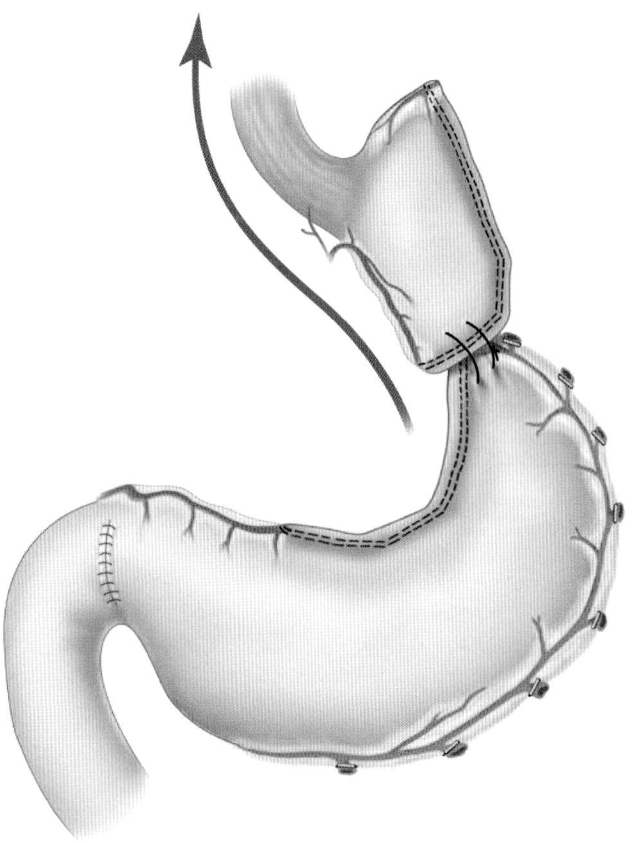

Figure 17 **Pulling up the gastric tube for cervical anastomosis.**

anastomosis and mobilization. The laparoscopic pull is performed gently and only until the assistant at the neck observes the tube beginning to be pulled down at the level of the anastomosis. The esophagogastric cervical anastomosis is placed high in the neck, just below the level of the cricopharyngeus, to ensure adequate removal of any islands of Barrett and to ensure that any anastomotic leaks will be more likely to drain out via the neck. Three tacking sutures are placed: one between the left crus and stomach just anterior to the greater curve arcade; the second on the right side of the gastric tube just above the right gastric vessels to the right crus; and the third suture anteriorly between the stomach and the diaphragm.

TROUBLESHOOTING

The technical problems associated with VATS esophagectomy are similar to those associated with open thoracic esophagectomy, including thoracic duct injury, recurrent nerve palsy, bleeding from the intercostal vessels, and anastomotic leakage. These problems are best prevented by obtaining good visualization of the superior and posterior mediastinum, which can be achieved by using a 30° angled thoracoscope. The most common reason for conversion to thoracotomy is the presence of a locally advanced tumor that necessitates extensive dissection for safe mobilization away from adjacent mediastinal structures.

To date, comparison of the results of VATS esophagectomy with those of open esophagectomy has not shown VATS to yield a significant decrease in major complications, especially postoperative respiratory insufficiency and cardiac arrhythmias. As a result, most centers still prefer the standard open transhiatal or transthoracic approaches to esophagectomy. VATS may also be used in the management of postoperative chylothorax. The thoracic duct can be ligated thoracoscopically, although it is sometimes difficult to identify and ligate the primary site of a postoperative lymphatic leak without reopening the thoracotomy.

VATS Pericardial Window

OPERATIVE TECHNIQUE

Some surgeons create a pericardial window by means of VATS as an alternative to taking the subxiphoid approach or the left anterior thoracotomy approach. A double-lumen endotracheal tube is inserted with the patient under general anesthesia, and the patient is rotated into the right lateral decubitus position. Three access sites are used, with the thoracoscope inserted at the seventh ICS in the posterior axillary line and the instruments introduced through two ports, one at the tip of the scapula and the other at the sixth ICS in the axillary line. The pericardium is retracted with a grasper forceps, and scissors are used to resect 8 to 10 cm^2 areas of pericardium both anterior and posterior to the phrenic nerve. If indicated, talc pleurodesis can be performed to control an associated pleural effusion. One or two chest tubes are then inserted through the port-site incisions.

TROUBLESHOOTING

When a pericardial effusion causes cardiac tamponade, a subxiphoid approach is preferable to VATS for creating a pericardial window because it is safer to perform in a hemodynamically unstable patient. A VATS pericardial window is also inadvisable in patients with constrictive physiology or with intrapericardial adhesions discovered at the time of operation. Conversion to an open procedure with formal pericardiectomy is advisable under these circumstances.

VATS Procedures for Mediastinal Masses

A 1998 multicenter trial aimed at defining the role of VATS in the management of mediastinal tumors suggested that VATS can be used safely to diagnose and resect most middle and posterior mediastinal masses, especially in view of the typically benign nature of these tumors.[34]

VATS thymectomy has been used to treat myasthenia gravis and thymoma. To date, only anecdotal experience has been reported, and no studies examining long-term outcomes have been published. Although a VATS approach to myasthenia gravis may appear attractive at first, it is not the least invasive approach to the thymus. Transcervical thymectomy is a minimally invasive approach to the thymus that does not require a chest incision, does not violate the pleural space, and allows most patients to be discharged home the next day. There is still a degree of controversy as to whether complete thymic resection, including all ectopic thymic tissue, is necessary to obtain clinical remission in patients with myasthenia gravis. For patients with a thymic mass, we prefer a transsternal approach. It is imperative to maintain oncologic surgical principles; accordingly, en bloc resection is emphasized so that pleural seeding is avoided and the risk of incomplete

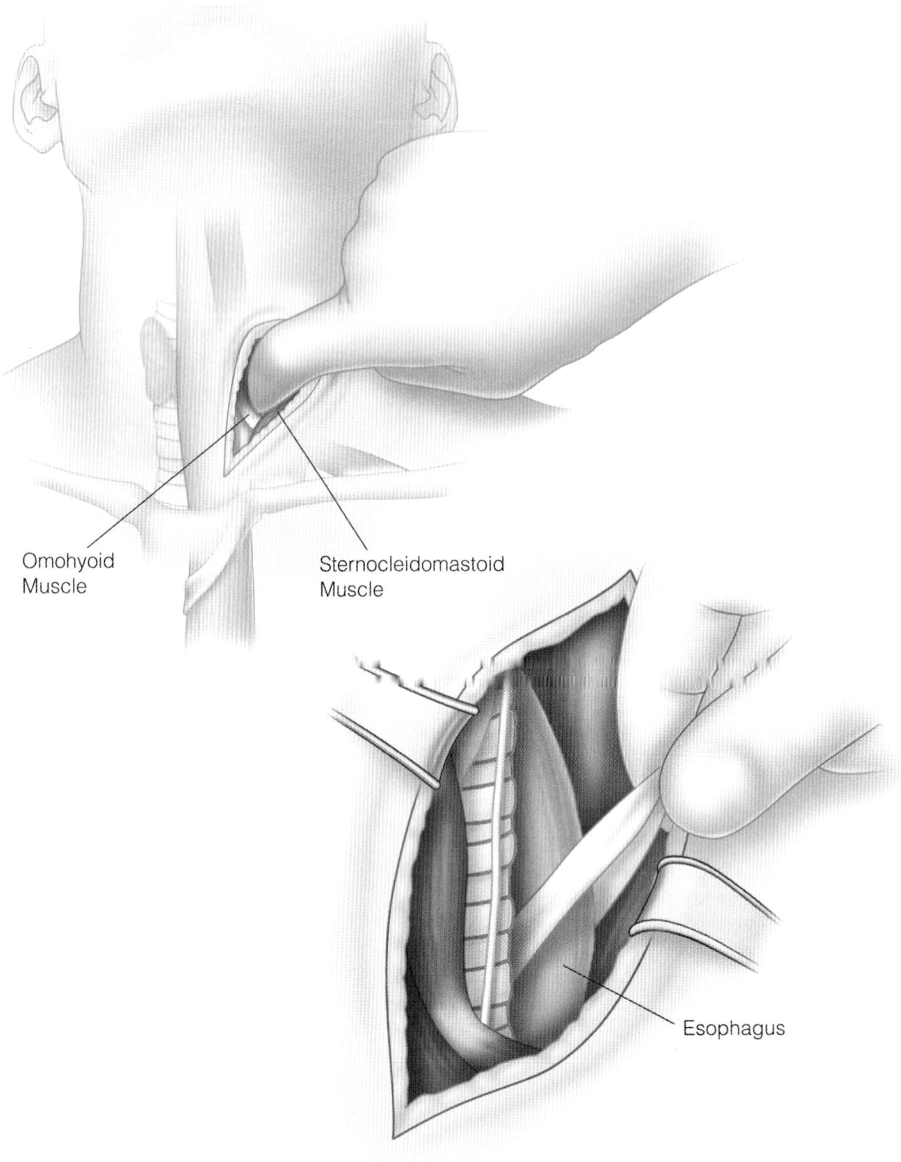

Figure 18 **Neck incision.**

resection is minimized. For patients with myasthenia gravis who do not have a thymoma, however, there is a need for prospective studies comparing VATS with other surgical approaches to thymectomy.

OPERATIVE TECHNIQUE

VATS has been used to resect masses in all of the mediastinal compartments. VATS resection is an ideal approach to posterior neurogenic tumors that do not extend into the neural foramen or the spinal canal. With the patient in the lateral decubitus position, the operating table is rotated anteriorly so that the lung falls away from the paravertebral region. The port sites are placed anteriorly: the thoracoscope is inserted at the fifth ICS in the midaxillary line, a lung retractor is inserted at the sixth ICS in the anterior axillary line, and dissecting instruments are inserted at the second and fourth ICSs at the anterior axillary line. The mass is manipulated with a grasper to expose the posteriorly located pedicle, which is then dissected, ligated, and divided with the scissors, clip appliers, and electrocautery device.

For removal of anterior mediastinal masses, the port sites are placed in more posterior locations. The thoracoscope

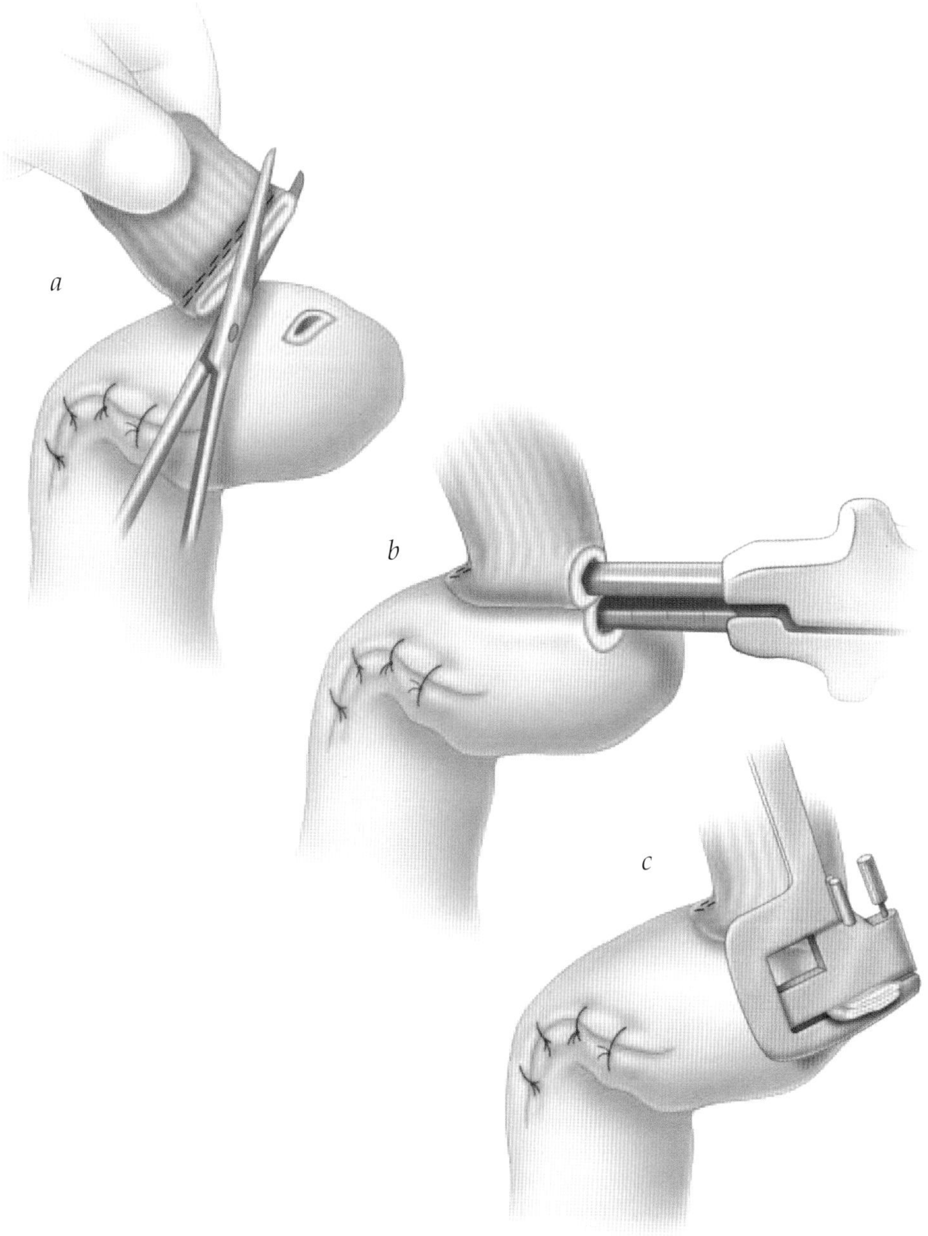

Figure 19 **Cervical anastomosis. (*a*) The cervical esophagus is divided high (1 to 2 cm below the cricopharyngeal muscle). (*b*) A side-to-side esophagogastric cervical anastomosis is performed using a gastrointestinal anastomosis (GIA) stapler. (*c*) Closure of the anastomosis by a 45 mm transverse anastomosis stapler.**

is introduced at the fifth ICS at the midaxillary or posterior axillary line, and instruments are inserted through two ports, one at the second ICS at the midaxillary line and the other at the fifth or sixth ICS at the anterior axillary line. The mass is retracted with a grasper and dissected free with a combination of sharp and blunt dissection, clip appliers, and the electrocautery device. A similar technique is used to resect middle mediastinal masses, most of which are pericardial or bronchogenic cysts. The access sites should be chosen according to the location of the mass on the preoperative CT scan. Generally, however, the triangulated site placement used for pulmonary wedge resections provides more suitable exposure than the site placement used for anterior or posterior mediastinal masses.

TROUBLESHOOTING

The placement of the thoracoports and the positioning of the operating team for the resection of posterior mediastinal tumors or for thoracic discectomy differ significantly from the usual practice in most other VATS procedures. In place of the standard arrangement of trocars in an inverted triangle, the viewing port is placed in the posterior axillary line and the operating ports in the anterior axillary line. The thoracic surgeon and the neurosurgeon both stand on the anterior side of the patient, each viewing a monitor on the opposite side. In addition, a 30° scope is essential for visualizing the intervertebral disk space.

Removal of dumbbell neurogenic tumors can be accomplished thoracoscopically if immediately preceded by posterior surgical removal of the spinal component of the tumor via laminectomy and intervertebral foraminotomy. Preoperative MRI is crucial for defining the extent of the tumor within the spinal canal. Resection of posterior mediastinal tumors is sometimes associated with significant bleeding from intercostal or spinal arteries. If such bleeding occurs, there should be no hesitation in converting to a thoracotomy. Ideally, anterior mediastinal cysts should be resected in toto to prevent recurrence. However, if the cysts are firmly adherent to vital mediastinal structures, partial excision with cauterization of the endothelial lining may be safer.

VATS Management of Thoracic Trauma

The major contraindication to thoracoscopy in thoracic trauma is hemodynamic instability. For major life-threatening injuries involving the great vessels and the mediastinum, thoracotomy is required to obtain expeditious control of injured structures. However, hemodynamically stable patients with certain thoracic problems (e.g., diaphragmatic injury; slow, continued intrathoracic bleeding; persistent air leakage; and empyema) may be diagnosed and often treated by means of VATS.[35,36]

In the assessment of a trauma patient with a potential diaphragmatic injury, it is important not to ignore the high incidence of associated intra-abdominal injury. If intra-abdominal injury has been ruled out and there is concern about the presence of a diaphragmatic tear, thoracoscopic assessment of the diaphragm is justified. Such assessment allows a more thorough evaluation of the entire diaphragm than the laparoscopic approach, which is limited by the liver on the right side. In the largest series published to date, 60 of 171 patients who underwent thoracoscopy for penetrating chest injuries had diaphragmatic injuries that necessitated repair.[37]

When a patient has an ongoing intrathoracic problem (e.g., persistent bleeding or a large air leak 24 to 48 hours after a traumatic injury), VATS should be considered before a thoracotomy is done because most problems encountered at this time (e.g., chest wall bleeding and laceration of the lung parenchyma) can be managed endoscopically, without the need for a thoracotomy.

TROUBLESHOOTING

The main pitfall in thoracoscopic evaluation of the diaphragm is failure to assess the abdomen appropriately and consequent failure to recognize an occult intra-abdominal injury. When laparoscopy is performed in a patient with a diaphragmatic injury, insufflation of CO_2 may cause a tension pneumothorax to develop on the side of the diaphragmatic injury. Accordingly, whenever diaphragmatic injury is a possibility, the chest should be included in the operative field to allow chest tube insertion if required. Because thoracoscopy does not require CO_2 insufflation, it is safer in such situations.

VATS Sympathectomy and Splanchnicectomy

Thoracic sympathectomy is known to be the most effective treatment for upper limb hyperhidrosis, and VATS is now an accepted approach to this operation. The main indication for splanchnicectomy is intractable abdominal pain from unresectable malignancies (e.g., pancreatic or gastric carcinoma) and chronic pancreatitis. The effects of celiac ganglion blocks are transient, and surgical manipulation of this area is usually very difficult because of the primary disease process, previous operations, or both. In the past, thoracotomy was generally considered too invasive an approach to splanchnic denervation in these patients. Currently, however, because of the less invasive nature of thoracoscopy and the quicker recovery time associated with it, thoracoscopic splanchnicectomy is an attractive therapeutic option.

OPERATIVE TECHNIQUE

Sympathectomy

VATS sympathectomy is performed with the patient under general anesthesia and a double lumen tube in place. Several techniques have been described. Initially, the common practice was to use three port sites: one for the thoracoscope at the third ICS in the midaxillary line, one at the third ICS in the anterior axillary line, and one at the tip of the scapula. Currently, the procedure is most often performed with two incisions: one at the fifth ICS at the border of the pectoralis and one at the fourth ICS in the anterior axillary line. The pleura is incised and divided from T2 to T5, and the sympathetic chain is dissected free with scissors and excised. For complete control of upper limb hyperhidrosis, VATS must be done bilaterally.[38,39]

A 1998 study reviewed the long-term results in 630 patients who had undergone thoracoscopic sympathectomy for hyperhidrosis (median follow-up 15 years).[40] Of these patients, 68% were fully satisfied and 26% were only partially satisfied but nevertheless would agree again to the operation. Hyperhidrosis was cured permanently in 93%. Compensatory sweating and gustatory sweating occurred in 67% and 47% of cases, respectively. Overall, patients were well satisfied with the results and considered the compensatory sweating less of a problem than the original hyperhidrosis.

Splanchnicectomy

The technical aspects of VATS splanchnicectomy are quite simple: sound knowledge of the splanchnic anatomy and a basic set of thoracoscopic instruments are all that is needed. Single-lung ventilation is required. Three thoracoports are placed. A silk stitch is placed in the central tendon of the diaphragm and pulled through the most anterior and inferior port to allow better visualization of the splanchnic nerves. The camera is also placed through this port. An endoscopic grasper and an endoscopic scissors with an electrocautery attachment are used to remove the nerve segment from T5 to T9. The greater and lesser splanchnic nerves are resected. The least splanchnic nerve is rarely visualized.

TROUBLESHOOTING

Care should be taken to identify the first and second ribs. Division of the sympathetic trunk at the level of the first rib causes Horner syndrome and does not reduce palmar hyperhidrosis. Division of the rami communicantes rather than the main sympathetic trunk reduces the incidence of undesirable side effects, especially compensatory hyperhidrosis of the trunk, but its overall success rate in controlling upper limb hyperhidrosis is lower. Abolition of only the T2 and T3 ganglia may control palmar hyperhidrosis without being as likely to result in unacceptable compensatory truncal sweating. Some have advocated limited T3 sympathectomy for primary hyperhidrosis to prevent compensatory sweating.[41] Target areas for axillary sweating also include T4 and T5. In addition, an accessory sympathetic nerve fiber that runs lateral to the sympathetic chain (known as the nerve of Kuntz) should be sought and, if identified, divided. Compensatory hyperhidrosis of the inner thighs is a common complication. Neuralgia is frequent after VATS sympathectomy. Some authors advocate a 2-day postoperative course of dexamethasone to reduce the incidence of this problem.[42]

Miscellaneous VATS Procedures

Several other procedures have been performed by VATS, including ligation of the thoracic duct[43] and resection of the adrenal gland.[44] For adrenal resection, three incisions are placed at the ninth or 10th ICS, extending from the anterior axillary line to the posterior axillary line. A fan retractor is inserted through a radial incision in the diaphragm and used to retract the perirenal fat. The adrenal gland is dissected free and removed, and the associated vessels are clipped or cauterized.

Cost Considerations

It is hard to estimate the cost-effectiveness of VATS procedures because the instrumentation, the types of procedures performed, and the surgical expertise with these operations are all still evolving. Initially, VATS procedures proved expensive for several reasons (e.g., the cost of purchasing video and endoscopic equipment, the cost of disposable instrumentation, and the need for long operating times as surgeons and nursing staff gained experience with the procedures). Soon after VATS was introduced, a study from the Mayo Clinic compared the cost of performing VATS pulmonary wedge resections with that of the same operation done by thoracotomy.[45] The VATS approach was associated with substantially shorter hospital stays but also with increased operating room costs; hence, the use of VATS did not result in any significant overall savings. Since that study, however, as some VATS procedures (e.g., pulmonary wedge resection) have become standard operations and more reusable instrumentation has become available, the cost of VATS has undoubtedly decreased. Whether other, more complex VATS procedures (e.g., thoracoscopic esophagectomy) are cost-effective remains to be determined.

Within this context, the Society of Thoracic Surgeons (STS) and the American Association for Thoracic Surgery (AATS) formed a joint committee to establish standards and guidelines for training and certification in VATS.[46] As a result of the educational efforts of this committee, many surgeons were trained within a short time, and VATS was quickly incorporated into thoracic surgical practice and residency training. The important considerations with respect to the training and practice of VATS have been well articulated.[46,47]

VATS is not minor surgery: it is a minimally invasive, complex intrathoracic procedure that should be performed only by persons who are familiar with intrathoracic anatomy and pathology and are fully competent to manage complications and make intraoperative decisions in such a way as to ensure safe outcomes for thoracic surgical patients. The complications encountered during thoracoscopic operations are potentially immediately life-threatening, whereas those encountered during other endoscopic procedures usually are not. For that reason, VATS procedures should not be performed by anyone—surgeon or nonsurgeon—who lacks the training and experience to perform immediate thoracotomy and repair of intrathoracic injuries.

Conclusion

Since its reintroduction into clinical practice in the early 1990s, VATS has been investigated in a scholarly and academically rigorous manner. It represents a paradigm for the evaluation of surgical innovation, leading to safe and effective application in patients. This chapter describes the most common video-assisted thoracic procedures performed in the current practice of thoracic surgery.

Financial Disclosures: None Reported

References

1. Hoksch B, Birken-Bertsch H, Muller JM. Thoracoscopy before Jacobaeus. Ann Thorac Surg 2002;74:1288–90.
2. Jacobaeus HC. Ueber die Moglichkeit die Zystoskopie bei Untersuchung sero ser Hohlungen anzuwenden. Munch Med Wochenschr 1910;57:2090–2.
3. Yim APC, Izzat MB, Lee TW. Thoracoscopic surgery for pulmonary tuberculosis. World J Surg 1999;23:1114–7.
4. Lewis RJ, Caccavale RJ, Sisler GE, Mackenzie JW. One hundred consecutive patients undergoing video-assisted thoracic operations. Ann Thorac Surg 1992;54:421–6.
5. Boffa DJ, Allen MS, Grab JD, et al. Data from the Society of Thoracic Surgeons General Thoracic Surgery database: the surgical management of primary lung tumors. J Thorac Cardiovasc Surg 2008;135:247–54. [Epub 2007 Dec 21]
6. Kirby TJ, Mack MJ, Landreneau RJ, Rice TW. Lobectomy-video assisted thoracic surgery versus muscle sparing thoracotomy: a randomized trial. J Thorac Cardiovasc Surg 1995;109:997–1002.
7. Shennib HAF, Landreneau R, Mulder DS, Mack M. Video-assisted thoracoscopic wedge resection of T1 lung cancer in high-risk patients. Ann Surg 1993;218:555 60.
8. Krasna MJ, Reed CE, Nedzwiecki D, et al. CALGB 9380: a prospective trial of the feasibility of thoracoscopy/laparoscopy in staging esophageal cancer. Ann Thorac Surg 2001; 71:1073–9.
9. Swanson SJ, Herndon JE II, D'Amico TA, et al. Video-assisted thoracic surgery lobectomy: report of CALGB 39802—a prospective, multi-institution feasibility study. J Clin Oncol 2007;25:4993–7.
10. Jaklitsch MT, Gu L, Harpole DH, et al. Prospective phase II trial of pre-resection thoracoscopic (VATS) restaging following neoadjuvant therapy for IIIA (N2) non-small cell lung cancer (NSCLC): results of

CALGB 39803. J Clin Oncol 2005;23(16S Suppl):7065.
11. Luketich J, Pennathur A, Catalano PJ, et al. Results of a phase II multicenter study of minimally invasive esophagectomy (Eastern Cooperative Oncology Group Study E2202). J Clin Oncol 2009;27(15S Suppl):4516.
12. Burfeind WR Jr, D'Amico TA. Thoracoscopic lobectomy. In: Cox JL, Patterson GA, editors. Operative techniques in thoracic and cardiovascular surgery. Vol 9. New York: W.B. Saunders; 2004. p. 98–114.
13. Colice GL, Shafazand S, Griffin JP, et al. Physiologic evaluation of the patient with lung cancer being considered for resectional surgery. Chest 2007;132:161S–77S.
14. Kutlu CA, Olgac G. How does definition of 'complete resection' conduct surgical management of non-small cell lung cancer? Interact Cardiovasc Thorac Surg 2006;5: 643–5.
15. Sue DY, Oren A, Hansen JE, Wasserman K. Diffusing capacity for carbon monoxide as a predictor of gas exchange during exercise. N Engl J Med 1987;316:1301–6.
16. Ferguson MK, Gaissert HA, Grab JD, Sheng S. Pulmonary complications after lung resection in the absence of chronic obstructive pulmonary disease: the predictive role of diffusing capacity. J Thorac Cardiovasc Surg 2009;138:1297–302.
17. Ferguson MK, Vigneswaran WT. Diffusing capacity predicts postoperative morbidity after major lung resection in patients without obstructive pulmonary disease. Ann Thorac Surg 2008;85:1158–65.
18. American Society of Anesthesiologists. Standards for Basic Anesthesia Monitoring. 1998 Directory of Members. Park Ridge: ASA. 1998. p. 438.
19. Detterbeck FC. Efficacy of methods of intercostal nerve blockade for pain relief after thoracotomy. Ann Thorac Surg 2005;80: 1550–9.
20. Allen MS, Trastek VF, Daly RC, et al. Equipment for thoracoscopy. Ann Thorac Surg 1993;56:620–3.
21. Yim APC, Ho JKS. Malfunctioning of vascular staple cutter during thoracoscopic lobectomy. J Thorac Cardiovasc Surg 1995; 109:1252.
22. Nicastri DG, Yun J, Swanson SJ. VATS lobectomy. In: Sugarbaker SJ, Bueno R, Krasna MJ, et al, editors. Adult chest surgery: concepts and procedures. New York: McGraw-Hill; 2009. p. 541–51.
23. Nakamura H, Taniguchi Y, Miwa K, et al. The 19Fr Blake drain versus the 28Fr conventional drain after a lobectomy for lung cancer. Thorac Cardiovasc Surg 2009;57: 107–9. [Epub 2009 Feb 24]
24. Stefani A, Natali P, Casali C, Morandi U. Talc poudrage versus talc slurry in the treatment of malignant pleural effusion: a prospective comparative study. Eur J Cardiothorac Surg 2006;30:827–32.
25. Sonett JR. Pulmonary metastases: biologic and historical justification for VATS. Eur J Cardiothorac Surg 1999;16:13–6.
26. Parekh K, Rusch V, Bains M, et al. VATS port site recurrence: a technique dependent problem. Ann Surg Oncol 2001;8:175.
27. Weiser TD, Swanson SJ. Surgical pitfalls: prevention and management. In: Evans SRT, editor. Lobar resections. 1st ed. Philadelphia: W.B. Saunders; 2009. p. 671.
28. Demmy TL, James TA, Swanson SJ, et al. Troubleshooting video-assisted thoracic surgery lobectomy. Ann Thorac Surg 2005; 79:1744–53.
29. Grondin SC, Sugarbaker DJ. Pleuropneumonectomy in the treatment of malignant pleural mesothelioma. Chest 1999; 116 Suppl: 450–4S.
30. Maciejewski R. Branches of the right pulmonary artery to the middle lobe of the right lung. Folia Morphol (Warsz) 1991;50: 187–92.
31. Maciejewski R. Branches of the left pulmonary artery vascularizing the left upper pulmonary lobe. Acta Anat (Basel) 1990;138: 224–9.
32. Maciejewski R. Branches of the left pulmonary artery supplying the basal segments of the lung. Acta Anat (Basel) 1991;140:284–6.
33. Luketich JD, Alvelo-Rivera M, Buenaventura PO, et al. Minimally invasive esophagectomy outcomes in 222 patients. Ann Surg 2003;238: 486–95.
34. Demmy TL, Krasna MJ, Detterbeck FC, et al. Multicenter VATS experience with mediastinal tumors. Ann Thorac Surg 1998; 66:187.
35. Lang-Lazdunski L, Mouroux J, Pons F, et al. Role of videothoracoscopy in chest trauma. Ann Thorac Surg 1997;63:327.
36. Spann JC, Nwariaku FE, Wait M. Evaluation of video-assisted thoracoscopic surgery in the diagnosis of diaphragmatic injuries. Am J Surg 1995;170:628.
37. Freeman RK, Al-Dossari G, Hutcheson KA, et al. Indications for using video-assisted thoracoscopic surgery to diagnose diaphragmatic injuries after penetrating chest trauma. Ann Thorac Surg 2001;72:342.
38. Dumont P, Denoyer A, Robin P. Long-term results of thoracoscopic sympathectomy for hyperhidrosis. Ann Thorac Surg 2004;78: 1801.
39. Krasna MJ, Demmy TL, McKenna RJ, et al. Thoracoscopic sympathectomy: the U.S. experience. Eur J Surg Suppl 1998;580:19.
40. Zacherl J, Huber ER, Imhof M, et al. Long-term results of 630 thoracoscopic sympathicotomies for primary hyperhidrosis: the Vienna experience. Eur J Surg Suppl 1998; 580:43.
41. Yoon do H, Ha Y, Park YG, et al. Thoracoscopic limited T-3 sympathicotomy for primary hyperhidrosis: prevention for compensatory hyperhidrosis. J Neurosurg Spine 2003;99:39.
42. Wong C-W. Transthoracic video endoscopic electrocautery of sympathetic ganglia for hyperhidrosis palmaris: special reference to localization of the first and second ribs. Surg Neurol 1997;47:224.
43. Shirai T, Amano J, Takabe K. Thoracoscopic diagnosis and treatment of chylothorax after pneumonectomy. Ann Thorac Surg 1991;52: 306.
44. Mack MJ, Aronoff RJ, Acuff TE, et al. Thoracoscopic transdiaphragmatic approach for adrenal biopsy. Ann Thorac Surg 1993; 55:772.
45. Allen MS, Deschamps C, Lee RE, et al. Video-assisted thoracoscopic stapled wedge excision for indeterminate pulmonary nodules. J Thorac Cardiovasc Surg 1993;106: 1048.
46. McKneally MF, Lewis RJ, Anderson RP, et al. Statement of the AATS/STS Joint Committee on Thoracoscopy and Video Assisted Thoracic Surgery. J Thorac Cardiovasc Surg 1992;104:1.
47. Thoracoscopy forum, continuing dialogue. Chest 1992;102:1915.

Acknowledgments

Figures 8–19 Christine Kenney

11 MEDIASTINAL PROCEDURES

Joseph B. Shrager, MD, FACS, and Vivek Patel, MBBS

Procedures for Lesions of the Anterior Mediastinum

More than half of all mediastinal masses arise from the anterior compartment. Most primary malignancies of the mediastinum also develop in the anterior mediastinum. Because of the narrowness of the space that makes up the thoracic inlet, as well as the presence of the trachea and esophagus traversing this region, anterior mediastinal masses become symptomatic earlier than their counterparts in other anatomic spaces of the mediastinum. Whereas adults with masses of the middle or posterior mediastinum usually report no significant symptoms, more than 50% of patients with anterior mediastinal masses present with chest pain, fever, cough, dyspnea, dysphagia, or vascular obstruction. Thymic neoplasms and lymphoma, the two most common masses in the anterior mediastinum, may have systemic manifestations (e.g., weakness associated with myasthenia gravis [MG] or symptoms associated with International Working Formulation [IWF] group B lymphoma).

In what follows, we focus on surgical approaches to the diagnosis and treatment of the more common neoplasms of the anterior mediastinum, including thymic tumors, lymphomas, and germ cell tumors. Embryologic anomalies and neoplasms arising from normal structures in this region broaden the differential diagnosis [*see Table 1*]. Finally, we address thymectomy for MG, a procedure that is frequently performed even in the absence of neoplastic disease.

PREOPERATIVE EVALUATION

In a patient with an anterior mediastinal mass, it is frequently possible to make a strong provisional diagnosis of the tumor type on the basis of clinical evaluation and diagnostic imaging.[1] As noted (see above), the presence of systemic manifestations may be helpful. Physical examination must include examination of peripheral lymph node groups and testes. Computed tomography (CT) yields valuable information about the anatomic location of the tumor, its characteristics (i.e., fatty, solid, or cystic), and its degree of invasiveness (if any) [*see Figure 1*]. Occasionally, magnetic resonance imaging (MRI) provides useful additional information about the obliteration of normal tissue planes. Positron emission tomography (PET) generally demonstrates strong fluorodeoxyglucose (FDG) uptake in lymphoma; thus, PET and CT may be useful in guiding sites for biopsy in that disease. Several small trials have been conducted evaluating the utility of PET in the evaluation of thymoma.[2] Uptake of FDG appears to be greater in thymoma than in thymic hyperplasia, and thymic carcinomas appear to have the highest FDG uptake. The reproducibility and thus diagnostic utility of this finding, though, have yet to be clearly elucidated.

Lymphoma is the most likely diagnosis in persons younger than 40 years, and the presence of IWF group B symptoms further raises the level of suspicion. The presence of palpable remote adenopathy or an elevated serum lactate dehydrogenase level is also suggestive.[3] When peripheral nodes are palpable, the diagnosis may be most easily obtained by excising one of them. Patients with suspected lymphoma who have an isolated anterior mediastinal mass should undergo core-needle biopsy or a Chamberlain procedure (anterior mediastinotomy), depending on the pathologists' level of comfort with classifying lymphoma on the basis of small specimens at one's institution. Resection of lymphoma is not indicated; it may be avoided by performing a diagnostic biopsy whenever lymphoma is suspected.

Unlike lymphomas, thymic neoplasms are uncommon before the fourth decade of life. Thymoma [*see Figure 1a*] may be associated with any of several paraneoplastic syndromes. MG occurs in conjunction with a pathologic condition of the thymus—either thymoma or thymic hyperplasia—in 80 to 90% of cases. Thymoma may also be associated with pure red cell aplasia, agammaglobulinemia, systemic lupus erythematosus, and various autoimmune disorders. The presence of any of these associated syndromes essentially clinches the diagnosis of thymoma. Autoantibodies to the acetylcholine receptor (anti-AChR antibodies) should be measured: their presence is diagnostic of MG, and they are found in nearly 60% of patients who have thymoma without neurologic symptoms.[4] Once the diagnosis of thymoma has been made, the goal is to proceed to direct resection without preliminary biopsy; these tumors have a predilection for local recurrence once the capsule has been violated.

The majority of germ cell tumors, whether malignant or benign, are diagnosed in the second or third decade of life. Benign teratomas are usually well encapsulated, with frequent recapitulation of one or more tissue elements seen on radiography.[5] The appearance of the lesions on CT is often diagnostic [*see Figure 1b*]. Surgical extirpation is the mainstay of treatment for these mature germ cell tumors, and biopsy is not indicated. Malignant germ cell tumors, on the other hand, are treated with primary chemotherapy, radiotherapy, or both; when suspected, these patients should undergo biopsy rather than being taken directly to resection. Characteristic serum tumor markers, including β–human chorionic gonadotropin (β-hCG) and α-fetoprotein (AFP), are elaborated by most malignant germ cell neoplasms but are not found in benign germ cell tumors.[6] Elevation of the AFP level beyond 500 ng/mL is considered diagnostic of a nonseminomatous component in a malignant germ cell tumor and is usually associated with a concomitant increase in serum β-hCG levels.[7] In the absence of any marked elevation in the AFP or β-hCG level, percutaneous needle biopsy usually suffices to establish the diagnosis.

OPERATIVE PLANNING

Biopsy versus Resection

Clearly, the decision whether to perform a biopsy of an anterior mediastinal mass is not a simple one. Routine biopsy

Table 1 Differential Diagnosis of Anterior Mediastinal Mass

Neoplastic conditions
Thyroid
Substernal goiter
Ectopic thyroid tissue
Thymus
Thymic hyperplasia
Thymoma
Thymic carcinoma
Thymic carcinoid
Thymic small cell carcinoma
Thymic cyst
Thymolipoma
Teratoma
Mature teratoma
Immature teratoma
Teratoma with malignant component
Lymphoma
Ectopic parathyroid with adenoma
Germ cell tumors
Seminoma
Nonseminoma
Yolk sac tumor
Embryonal carcinoma
Choriocarcinoma
Hemangioma
Lipoma
Liposarcoma
Fibroma
Fibrosarcoma
Cervicomediastinal hygroma
Infectious conditions
Acute descending necrotizing mediastinitis
Subacute mediastinitis
Vascular conditions
Aneurysm of aortic arch with projection in anterior mediastinum
Innominate vein aneurysm
Superior vena cava aneurysm
Dilation of superior vena cava (with anomalous pulmonary venous return)
Persistent left superior vena cava

a

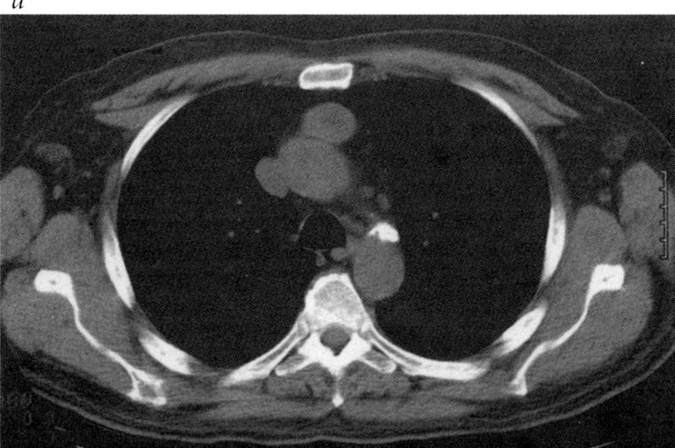

b

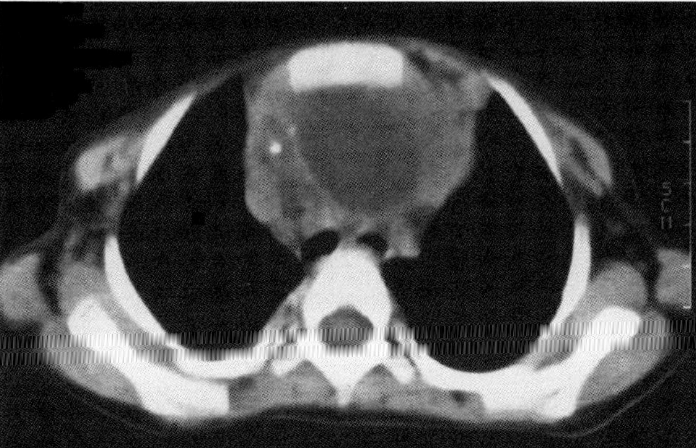

Figure 1 **(*a*) Computed tomography (CT) scan shows a well-encapsulated anterior mediastinal mass—a thymoma. (*b*) CT scan shows a benign teratoma of the anterior mediastinum; calcification and varying tissue densities may be seen.**

should be avoided, not only because of the cost and the unnecessary morbidity but also because of the risk that biopsy may spread thymoma. The choice to proceed with biopsy should be made according to which tumor type is believed to be most likely on the basis of the diagnostic workup.

Well-encapsulated lesions that are believed not to represent lymphoma are resected, without a preceding biopsy, for both diagnosis and treatment. Neoplasms that commonly fall into this category include noninvasive thymomas, mature teratomas, mesenchymal tumors, and, occasionally, benign cysts. Most patients with MG should be offered thymectomy whether they have a thymic mass or not.

When lymphoma is suspected, biopsy is required. The technique employed should be minimally invasive while still permitting the acquisition of a sufficient tissue sample. CT-guided core-needle biopsy may be attempted, but, frequently, this technique does not provide enough tissue for the analyses required to classify the tumor.[8,9] Thus, the Chamberlain procedure (anterior mediastinotomy) is recommended in these situations.

For locally invasive or frankly unresectable anterior mediastinal masses other than those felt likely to represent lymphoma, biopsy is also preferable to immediate attempt at resection. Such lesions may represent aggressive thymomas that may benefit from neoadjuvant treatment, malignant germ cell tumors, or other rare disease processes. Once the decision has been made to proceed with biopsy rather than resection, selection of a biopsy approach is based on anatomic considerations and patient factors.

BIOPSY OF ANTERIOR MEDIASTINAL MASS

Chamberlain Approach

Anterior parasternal mediastinotomy (the Chamberlain procedure) is favored by most surgeons for biopsy of lesions in the anterior mediastinum and the aortopulmonary window. It is usually done under general anesthesia, although local anesthesia may be used instead, and it does not require single-lung ventilation. This operation affords good exposure and allows generous biopsy specimens to be taken, and it can be performed as an outpatient procedure.

Operative technique *Step 1: initial incision* A 5 cm transverse incision is made over the second costal cartilage on the side to be operated on (the second cartilage is identified by its continuity with the sternal angle). The pectoralis major is separated in a direction parallel to the direction of its fibers,

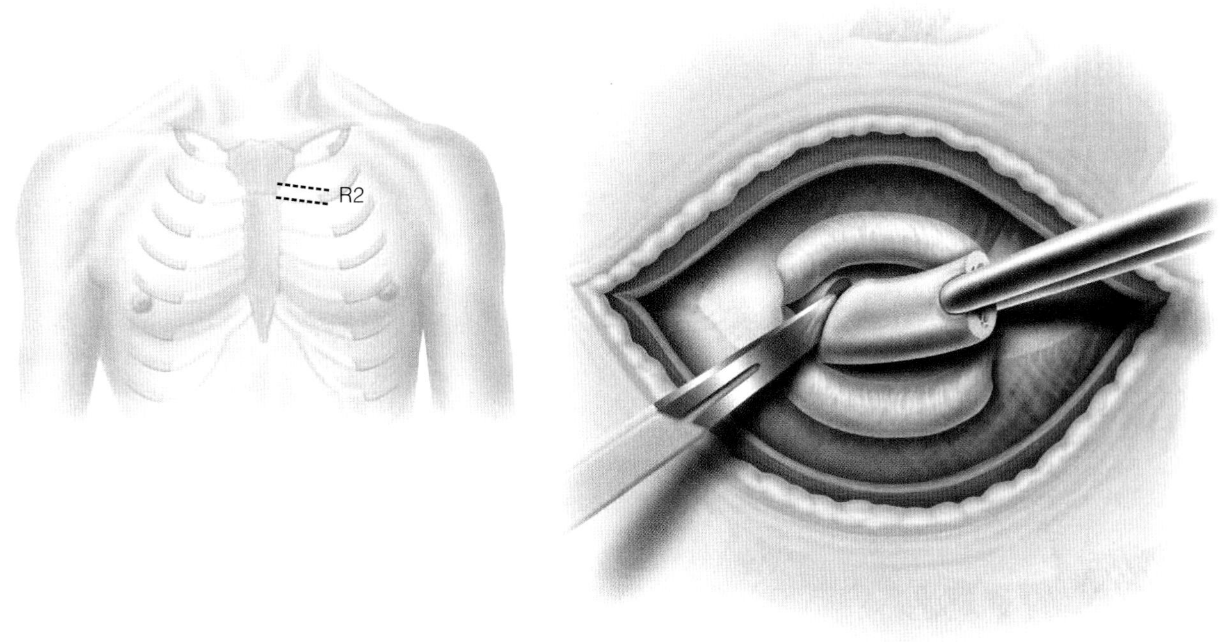

Figure 2 **Biopsy of anterior mediastinal mass: Chamberlain approach. Depicted are incision and subperichondrial resection of the second costal cartilage.**

and the cartilage is resected in a subperichondrial plane [*see Figure 2*]. Leaving perichondrium behind facilitates postoperative regrowth of the cartilage.

Step 2: dissection and exposure The posterior perichondrium is incised, and the parietal pleura is bluntly dissected laterally with a peanut sponge; this affords entry into the mediastinal fat and direct access to the tumor mass. Almost invariably, the internal mammary vessels can be mobilized medially and preserved, but, if necessary, they may be ligated to improve exposure.

Step 3: biopsy A generous wedge-shaped portion of the mass is excised with a scalpel. Frozen-section examination is then performed to confirm that diagnostic tissue has been obtained. It is important to remember to request that flow cytometry be performed on the specimen.

Step 4: closure The posterior perichondrium is reapproximated, followed by the pectoralis major, the subcutaneous fat, and the skin.

Troubleshooting If the pleura was entered, a red rubber catheter is used to evacuate the pleural space as the lung is inflated with a large positive pressure breath, and the catheter is withdrawn through the layers of closure. A small postoperative pneumothorax is almost always attributable to residual air rather than to an ongoing air leak.

Sometimes the tumors are fairly vascular and bleed moderately after biopsy is performed. This bleeding can always be controlled with electrocauterization. We often leave an absorbable hemostatic agent in place as well.

Transcervical Approach

As an alternative to the Chamberlain procedure, a mass of the anterior mediastinum may be approached for biopsy through a cervical incision, exactly as in a transcervical thymectomy [*see* Resection of Anterior Mediastinal Mass, Transcervical Approach, *below*]. The use of a Cooper thymectomy retractor (Pilling Company, Fort Washington, Pennsylvania), which elevates the sternum, affords excellent exposure of the anterior mediastinum and sometimes allows direct examination to ascertain the invasiveness of an otherwise uncertain mass. In most cases, general anesthesia is required, but transcervical biopsy can be performed as an outpatient procedure. We have used this technique occasionally and have achieved results comparable to those of anterior mediastinotomy.[10] Proper performance of this procedure does, however, require a level of experience with the technique that is not widely available.

Video-Assisted Thoracic Surgery

Video-assisted thoracic surgery (VATS) has been applied to diagnostic biopsy of anterior mediastinal masses, but VATS biopsy procedures are not widely employed for this purpose. The necessity of single-lung ventilation adds a level of complexity to the procedure beyond what is required for the

Chamberlain procedure or the transcervical approach. Furthermore, intercostal incisions are frequently more painful than transcervical incisions or the incision for an anterior mediastinotomy. VATS does have certain advantages that may be of value in individual cases, such as the capacity to provide simultaneous access to other compartments of the mediastinum and the ability to evaluate the pleural space for evidence of tumor dissemination. Robot-assisted thoracoscopic procedures for anterior mediastinal masses have also been described,[11] but their availability does not eliminate the major objection to transpleural approaches to mediastinal masses—namely, the possibility of spreading a disease that had been contained within the mediastinum into the pleural space.

RESECTION OF ANTERIOR MEDIASTINAL MASS

Operative Planning

The most frequent indications for resection (as opposed to biopsy) of an anterior mediastinal mass are (1) thymoma and (2) thymectomy for MG. The principles underlying thymoma resection can be applied to resection of other, rarer anterior mediastinal masses such as thymic carcinoma, thymolipoma, and germ cell tumors. The first successful resection of a thymic mass for MG was described in 1939.[12] Since the introduction of transcervical thymectomy (TCT), there has been ongoing debate regarding the optimal method for thymectomy in patients with nonthymomatous MG. There is little debate, however, regarding the optimal approach to resection of anterior mediastinal malignancies.

For all primary invasive masses of the anterior mediastinum—including invasive thymomas, malignant germ cell tumors (after systemic treatment), thymic carcinomas, and other, less common malignancies—the most important prognostic factor is complete resection. Accordingly, the operative approach must be selected with an eye to providing optimal exposure. There is little doubt that a full median sternotomy is ideal in this regard. However, a less than full sternotomy is a reasonable choice for small (< 3 cm) noninvasive thymomas or other noninvasive mediastinal tumors (e.g., mature teratomas), particularly when the diagnosis of thymoma is in doubt before operation. In such situations, we usually begin with TCT,[13,14] but we do not hesitate to convert to a sternotomy if unexpected invasion is identified. Some surgeons have employed a partial upper sternotomy in these settings; however, this approach limits exposure, and we do not believe that it actually reduces morbidity in comparison with a full sternotomy. Video thoracoscopic (VATS) and even robotic thymectomy have now been described by a number of groups employing several technical variations and with apparently good results. These approaches have, like TCT, been applied generally to patients with MG without thymoma or those with small, noninvasive thymomas. Studies with longer follow-up reporting myasthenia remission rates and thymoma cure rates will be required before these VATS and robotic approaches can be considered to have a proven role in the management of these diseases.

En bloc resection of malignancies is mandatory, and resection of adjacent serosal membranes (including pleura or pericardium) is required if there is any suggestion of attachment during the operation. Resection of adjacent lung parenchyma is not uncommon, and resection of the great vessels has been performed with both technical success and good long-term survival. All great vessels resected must be reconstructed, with the exception of the innominate vein, which may be ligated with little deleterious effect. Every effort should be made to preserve the phrenic nerves: damage to even one of these nerves can be disastrous in an already weakened myasthenia patient. In a patient with a malignancy, however, one phrenic nerve may be sacrificed if tumor invasion necessitates this step, provided that the patient's preoperative respiratory status is acceptable and curative resection is likely.

In cases of thymectomy for advanced MG, every effort must be made to optimize the patient's condition preoperatively. To this end, a multidisciplinary approach that includes a neurologist and, possibly, a pulmonologist is necessary. If the disease does not stabilize with medication (e.g., pyridostigmine, low-dose steroids, or intravenous γ-globulin), preoperative plasmapheresis may be required. Patients with moderate or greater generalized weakness despite optimization of medication should certainly undergo plasmapheresis. The question of which MG patients should be offered thymectomy is, at best, difficult to answer. Most studies have found the impact of thymectomy to be greater if it is performed in patients with less severe and shorter-duration disease. Accordingly, our practice is to offer TCT sooner in the course of the disease rather than later; however, we will perform the procedure at any stage, from ocular only disease to severe, generalized weakness. Because TCT is associated with minimal morbidity, requires only a small incision, and can generally be done as an outpatient procedure, it is a very attractive option for patients with milder disease. At the same time, it is also more easily tolerated by patients with severe disease than is a median sternotomy.

An approach to thymectomy for MG that is favored by a few surgeons is so-called maximal transsternal-transcervical thymic resection, which combines a median sternotomy with an additional neck incision to provide wide access to all areas where thymic tissue has been identified. The rationale for such extensive exposure is the observation that thymic tissue may reside in several extrathymic locations. Proponents of the maximal approach argue that if thymectomy for MG is to provide optimal benefit, it should include removal of all of this extraglandular thymic tissue. This approach has never been compared to TCT in a randomized trial, but, in our view, most of the available data suggest that remission rates after maximal transsternal-transcervical thymic resection are not remarkably different from those after TCT, which is much less invasive. Because we do not personally perform the maximally invasive procedure, we do not describe it in this chapter.

Median Sternotomy Approach

As noted (see above), the standard approach to masses of the anterior mediastinum is via a median sternotomy. Resection of a thymoma of the anterior mediastinum is performed as follows.

Operative technique *Step 1: initial incision and exposure* The patient is placed in the supine position and intubated with a double-lumen endotracheal tube. The skin incision typically extends from 2 cm below the jugular notch to the xiphisternal junction; however, depending on the extent of the expected pathologic condition, the incision may be shortened further and the full sternum divided by reaching beneath skin flaps. Finger dissection is performed beneath the sternum to rule out tumor invasion into the posterior sternal table. If the posterior sternal table is clear, the sternum is divided, hemostasis is achieved, and the edges are separated with a sternal retractor.

Step 2: determination of resectability The anterior mediastinum is inspected, the mass is visually identified, and an initial assessment of resectability is undertaken.

Step 3: mobilization of inferior poles of thymus Dissection of the thymus begins at the caudad aspect, with the inferior poles and surrounding mediastinal fat mobilized first from the underlying pericardium and diaphragm by electrocautery dissection. It is difficult to determine by visual means precisely where thymic tissue merges into simple mediastinal fat; accordingly, to ensure complete resection of the thymus, all fatty tissue between the phrenic nerves and down to the level of the diaphragm is removed with the specimen. The mediastinal pleura, to which this fatty and thymic tissue tends to be adherent, is also taken with the specimen [*see Figure 3*]. This is done by first opening the mediastinal pleura along the entire length of the chest, approximately 1 cm posterior to the sternum.

Step 4: continuation of dissection cephalad From within the pleural space, the phrenic nerves are identified and followed along their entire path up to the point where they course beneath the innominate vein. Sharp dissection is carried close to the nerves, dividing the mediastinal pleura again along this more posterior line, to secure an adequate tumor margin and ensure removal of all thymic tissue that is progressively mobilized medially. It is advisable to clip small vessels near the nerves before dividing them so as to prevent irritating bleeding, which can be difficult to control without compromising the nerve.

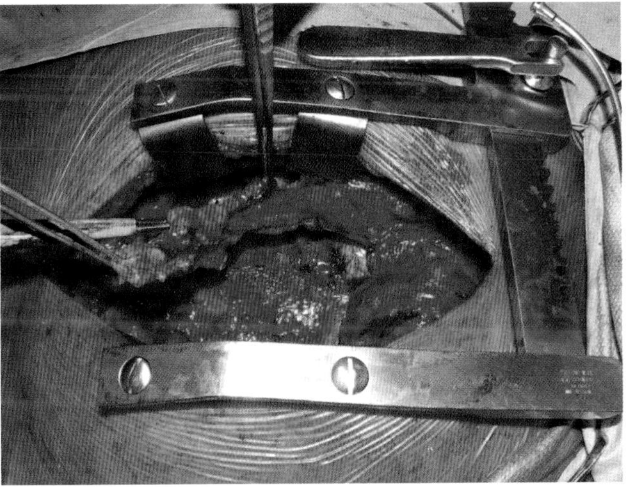

Figure 3 **Resection of anterior mediastinal mass: median sternotomy approach. Intraoperative photograph shows dissection of the right inferior thymic pole and associated mediastinal fat.**

The small arteries supplying the thymus, which are most often not even clearly seen arising laterally via branches from the internal mammary vessels, are coagulated or ligated and divided as they are encountered. Care must be taken to stay away from the phrenic nerves while controlling the arterial blood supply.

Step 5: mobilization of superior poles of thymus Dissection is then continued in the neck, where the two cervical extensions are isolated by means of gentle traction and blunt dissection and followed until they trail off into the thyrothymic ligament. This ligament is clamped, divided, and ligated superiorly at a point where only a small blood vessel is present and no visible glandular tissue remains.

Step 6: dissection of thymus from innominate vein The cervical poles are followed down over the innominate vein. Sharp dissection is continued onto the surface of the vein, and the two to five veins draining the gland into the innominate vein are ligated and divided [*see Figure 4*].

Step 7: removal of specimen Once the body of the thymus has been freed from the innominate vein, the H-shaped gland and the associated mass are removed [*see Figure 5*]. If the

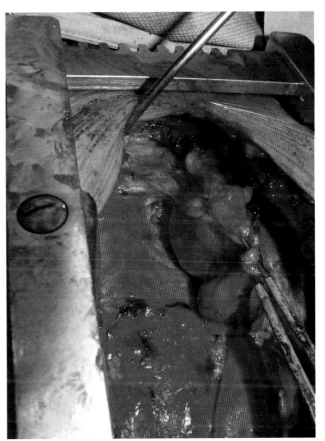

Figure 4 **Resection of anterior mediastinal mass: median sternotomy approach. View from feet shows the thymus and tumor mobilized off the innominate vein. The entire right thymus (both the upper and the lower pole) has been fully mobilized.**

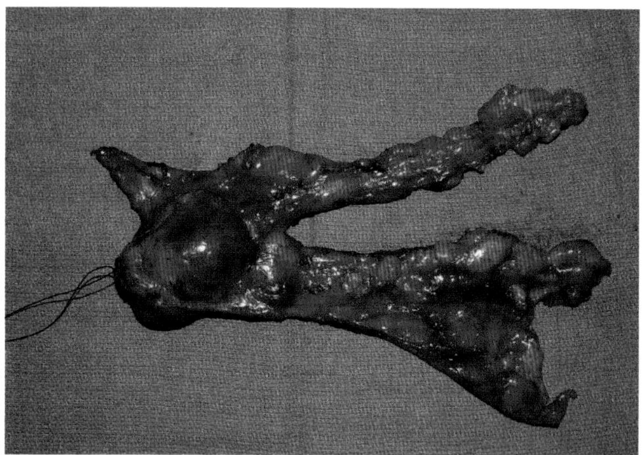

Figure 5 **Resection of anterior mediastinal mass: median sternotomy approach. Shown is the resected thymoma specimen.**

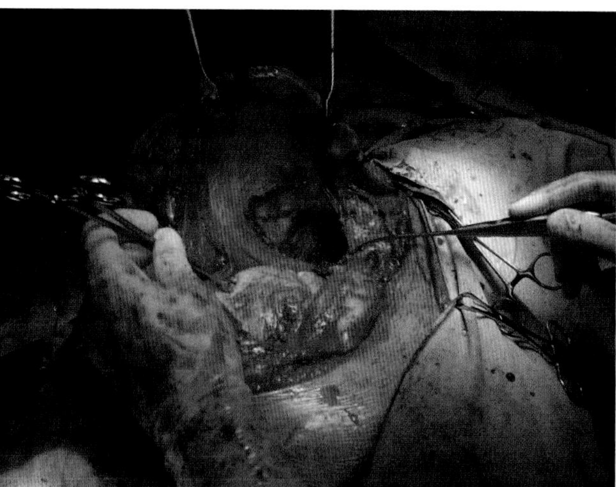

Figure 6 **Resection of anterior mediastinal mass: median sternotomy approach. Hemiclamshell incision provides exposure to masses located at the thoracic apex.**

clean plane between the mass and the underlying pericardium—a plane normally composed of fine, filmy adhesions—is at all compromised, one should not hesitate to resect a portion of the pericardium en bloc with the specimen, with care taken to maintain a gross margin of at least 2 cm at all times.

Step 8: closure Two pleural drains that traverse the mediastinum and reach the apex of each hemithorax are placed, and the sternum and the soft tissues are reapproximated in layers.

Troubleshooting If invasion of great vessels is considered a possibility before the start of the operation, the groin should be prepared and draped into the field to provide access for cardiopulmonary bypass if needed. Giant anterior mediastinal masses may necessitate extension of a partial median sternotomy incision into an ipsilateral intercostal space (usually the fourth space). Such extension may be achieved by making an ipsilateral incision in the neck along the anterior border of the sternocleidomastoid muscle and making a submammary skin incision continuous with the incision over the sternum (a hemiclamshell incision) [*see Figure 6*].

Transcervical Approach

Although the transcervical approach to thymic resection was the first one used in the early 1900s, it fell into disuse during the middle of the 20th century, when the median sternotomy approach became feasible. During the past 20 years, however, there has been a resurgence of interest in TCT. Today, TCT is used primarily for thymectomy in the setting of MG, although, as noted (see above), a transcervical approach can be useful for biopsy or resection of other anterior mediastinal processes as well. Proponents of TCT have published data establishing that complete remission rates from MG after so-called extended TCT using the sternum-lifting Cooper retractor[15] are very similar to remission rates after the more invasive approaches.[14,16,17] Because TCT is an outpatient procedure, hospital stay and operative recovery are certainly dramatically shorter than after thymectomy by sternotomy.

TCT should be employed very cautiously in cases in which a neoplasm is suspected or proved on the basis of preoperative studies or is identified during the course of intraoperative exploration. Because thymoma is often an indolent tumor, with recurrence developing many years after resection, long-term follow-up studies are required before TCT can be firmly recommended for treatment of even small thymomas. On the other hand, it is likely that surgeons who have extensive experience with TCT can safely resect small (< 3 cm) thymomas via this approach without risking tumor spillage or incomplete resection.

Operative technique *Step 1: initial incision and exposure* The patient is placed on the operating table in the supine position, with the head supported by a foam doughnut and an inflatable bag placed horizontally beneath the scapulae. The bag is inflated until the cervical spine is maximally extended. It is important that the top of the patient's head be all the way up to the edge of the table so that the surgeon can easily reach all areas of the mediastinum from a seated position at the head.

A 5 to 6 cm curvilinear incision is made about 2 cm superior to the jugular notch and extending about 1 cm above each clavicular head [*see Figure 7*]. Electrocautery dissection is continued through the platysma, and subplatysmal flaps are elevated. The strap muscles are separated in the midline, and the interclavicular ligament is divided. Separating a small portion of the attachment of each sternocleidomastoid muscle from the corresponding clavicular head allows the sternum to be elevated somewhat higher, thereby improving exposure.

Step 2: mobilization of superior poles of thymus The superior poles of the thymus are located (usually on the left side first) by means of gentle blunt dissection beneath the strap muscles. After one pole is identified, it is divided between ties at its superior extent. Its medial edge is then followed down to where it meets the medial edge of the opposite superior pole, and this opposite pole can then be similarly traced upward

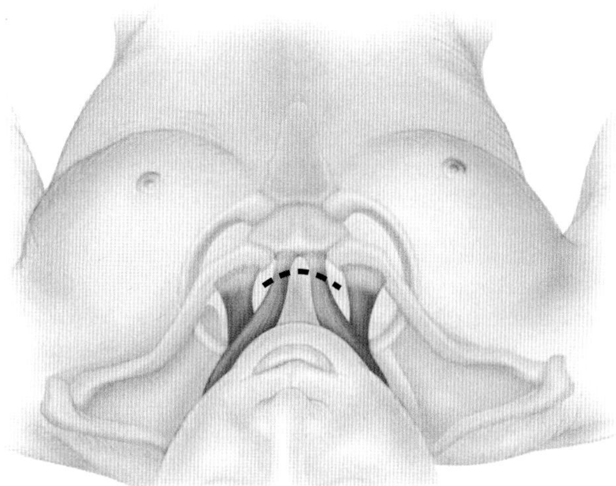

Figure 7 **Resection of anterior mediastinal mass: transcervical approach. Shown is the location of the skin incision for transcervical thymectomy in relation to the sternal notch and the heads of the clavicles.**

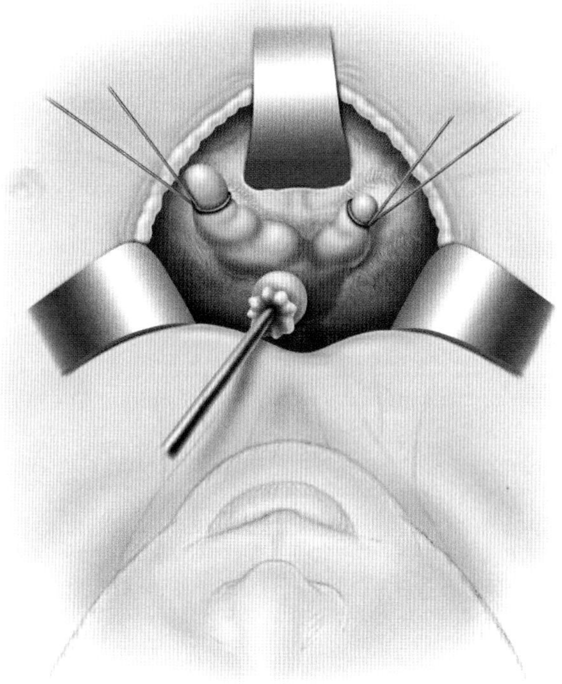

Figure 8 **Resection of anterior mediastinal mass: transcervical approach. A Cooper thymectomy retractor is placed beneath the sternum, and retraction on the upper poles of the thymus is maintained with silk sutures.**

into the neck, ligated, and divided. A very important part of the procedure is the placement of 0 silk ligatures around an area containing strong tissue within each superior pole. These ligatures are left long and clamped. The surgeon or an assistant places traction on them during the remaining course of the dissection to manipulate and progressively mobilize the gland [*see Figure 8*].

Step 3: continuation of dissection downward into superior mediastinum As traction is being placed on the upper poles, sharp and blunt dissection, staying outside the well-defined capsule of the gland, is extended downward into the superior mediastinum to the level of the innominate vein. The procedure becomes much more difficult if the capsule is violated.

Step 4: elevation of sternum Finger dissection is performed in the substernal plane, and the arm of a Cooper thymectomy retractor is placed into the retromanubrial space to elevate the sternum. The retracting arm is placed under upward tension as the inflatable bag beneath the shoulders is deflated. This step leaves most patients actually hanging from the retractor, thereby opening up a sizable space that allows good visualization and ready passage of dissecting instruments into the anterior mediastinum. Army-Navy retractors are placed in each of the two upper corners of the incision, and their distal ends are tied to the siderails of the table with Penrose drains to provide countertraction and to hold the skin incision open.

Step 5: dissection of venous tributaries to innominate vein With the superior poles gently pulled upward by an assistant (and at times looped over the Cooper retractor), the inferior surface of the gland is dissected until the innominate vein is encountered. The venous tributaries draining the thymus into the innominate vein are isolated sharply, ligated with fine silk sutures, and divided.

Step 6: dissection of posterior aspect of thymus Once the thymus is freed from the innominate vein, dissection of the posterior aspect of the gland must be continued directly on the surface of the pericardium. This posterior dissection is carried as far down as possible, primarily in a blunt fashion. Most of the time, the surgeon holds one ring clamp containing a sponge dissector in each hand while an assistant holds the upper poles. Occasionally, the surgeon holds the sutures attached to the upper poles in one hand while employing the sponge dissector in the other hand.

Step 7: removal of specimen When the posterior dissection has been extended as far as possible toward the diaphragm, further mobilization of the thymus is typically accomplished by working the glandular tissue laterally, first off the pleura on one side, then off the sternum anteriorly, and finally off the pleura on the opposite side. In this way, the entire gland is ultimately removed between the phrenic nerves and down to the diaphragm. During this final mobilization, the surgeon periodically asks to have ventilation held temporarily so that the pleura can fall back and thus permit improved visualization. Small feeding vessels from the mammary are doubly clipped and divided as they are encountered.

Often the final stages of blunt dissection may be facilitated by placing a ring clamp on the body of the gland to allow slightly more vigorous retraction than can be achieved by using the upper poles alone. If any suspicious residual tissue is seen in the mediastinum at this point, it can be removed piecemeal; however, this is an unusual occurrence.

Step 8: closure After inspection of the surgical field for hemostasis, the strap muscles and the platysma are closed over a red rubber catheter, to which suction may be applied. The catheter is subsequently removed, and the skin is closed.

Troubleshooting In the course of preoperative evaluation before TCT, it is important to be sure that the patient is able to extend the neck to a reasonable degree. TCT is simplest in young persons who are capable of good extension; it can be difficult or impossible in persons with cervical spine disease that hinders extension.

During the procedure itself, it is important that the branches of the innominate vein be tied rather than clipped; the space anterior to the vein becomes the avenue through which dissecting instruments are passed into and out of the mediastinum, and these instruments often rub against the vein fairly vigorously.

When working laterally, one must take care not to injure the phrenic nerves, and one certainly should not use the electrocautery while working at the lateral extremes of the dissection. If the pleural space is entered while one is working laterally, a red rubber catheter [*see* Operative Technique, Step 8, *above*] is advanced well into that pleural space, and suction in the form of several large positive-pressure breaths is applied before the catheter is removed.

If a thymoma is encountered during TCT, continuation via this approach may be considered. In our view, most noninvasive thymic lesions less than 3 cm in diameter can be safely and completely resected via the transcervical approach. In addition, it generally is not difficult to resect a portion of the anterior pericardium as well if a tumor or the thymus is adherent to it. However, because the evidence currently available does not conclusively establish that TCT is equivalent to resection via sternotomy for thymoma, some surgeons prefer to convert to a sternotomy if a suspicious mass is discovered during transcervical exploration. Certainly, if any difficulty is encountered that might lead to an incomplete thymectomy or incomplete removal of a thymoma, the incision should be extended.

Approximately 90% of patients are able to go home on the same day as their procedure. The most common cause for hospital admission is a pneumothorax that must be monitored or drained. Occasionally, a seroma develops at the site of the incision, but it almost always resolves either spontaneously or after a single percutaneous drainage procedure in the office.

VATS/Robotic Thymectomy

Although we do not have personal experience with VATS or robotic thymectomy and will therefore not include a discussion on its technique, an increasing number of published reports suggest that these are safe and effective alternatives to transsternal and transcervical approaches. Since the first sporadic case reports of VATS thymectomy in the early 1990s, the popularity of this procedure has increased, likely because of the increased availability of VATS instrumentation, surgeon familiarity with VATS techniques, and increased awareness of minimally invasive strategies. Proponents of VATS thymectomy cite decreased postoperative pain, decreased length of stay, improved cosmesis, and less morbidity than sternotomy as reasons in support of VATS thymectomy. Most case series report complete stable remission rates from MG[18,19] comparable to transsternal and transcervical approaches. The data in this area, however, are not nearly as mature as those in support of TCT or sternotomy for thymectomy.

The drawbacks of VATS thymectomy depend on the particular technical approach that is chosen, which include unilateral, bilateral, and substernal approaches. As with any minimally invasive technique, detractors have pointed out that there may be an inability to provide complete clearance of all thymic tissue. It has been suggested that a unilateral VATS approach may provide inadequate access to the portion of the gland approaching the contralateral phrenic nerve. Aside from the question of the completeness of thymectomy, any transthoracic, minimally invasive approach may create a small risk of transpleural seeding in patients with thymoma. Given that "drop metastasis" to the pleural surfaces is the typical mode of spread of thymoma, there is substantial concern that a transpleural, thoracoscopic approach may facilitate this mode of spread.

Procedures for Lesions of the Middle Mediastinum

The majority of masses found in the middle mediastinum in adults are malignant, representing either lymphoma or lymph node metastases from primary lung carcinoma. Accordingly, the procedures performed in this anatomic area primarily involve biopsy for staging or diagnosis rather than curative or palliative resection. On infrequent occasions, however, benign or primary malignant lesions of the middle mediastinum occur for which resection is appropriate. In what follows, we briefly discuss resection of such lesions; for the most part, the principles are the same as those underlying resection of masses in the posterior mediastinum [*see* Procedures for Lesions of the Posterior Mediastinum, *below*].

Of particular surgical interest in the middle mediastinum are benign cysts, which may arise from the pleura, the pericardium, the airways, or the esophagus. Bronchogenic cysts, which typically develop in proximity to the carina, are probably the middle mediastinal cysts most commonly encountered in clinical practice, with pericardial cysts running a close second. On rare occasions, ectopic remnants from cervical structures (e.g., the parathyroid and thyroid glands) are encountered in this compartment.[20]

PREOPERATIVE EVALUATION

CT generally provides an accurate preoperative diagnosis of a benign middle mediastinal cyst, as well as information regarding abutment of adjacent structures, the consistency of the mass, and potential invasiveness. MRI may be helpful if there is concern that a cyst might actually represent an aberrant vascular structure or an aneurysm, if the simple nature of the cyst is in doubt, or if clearer delineation of suspected invasion of surrounding structures is required. Radionuclide scans (e.g., with technetium-99m or radioactive iodine) may be useful if the differential diagnosis includes a parathyroid or thyroid mass. Cystic structures adjacent to the airways and the esophagus are evaluated by means of bronchoscopy, esophagoscopy, barium esophagography, or some combination of these imaging modalities to rule out communication with the lumina.

OPERATIVE PLANNING

Middle mediastinal cysts that are symptomatic should be treated surgically. However, simple cysts of the middle mediastinum that are asymptomatic and meet all radiographic criteria for benignity may be followed. This conservative approach is often more appropriate for asymptomatic middle mediastinal cysts than for asymptomatic posterior mediastinal cysts in that complete cyst resection (at least for bronchogenic cysts) tends to be more complex in the middle mediastinum than in the posterior mediastinum, given the closer proximity to vital structures and the deeper placement within soft tissue. Complete resection of pericardial cysts, on the other hand, typically is easily accomplished by means of VATS; therefore, such cysts are probably best resected when discovered, even if they are asymptomatic. VATS resection of subcarinal bronchogenic cysts is feasible and has been described in published reports.[21] It is our experience, however, that larger and more chronic cysts in this location may be difficult to remove completely by a VATS approach.

Thus, for a symptomatic, large, or chronic subcarinal bronchogenic cyst (a not uncommon occurrence), one is left to choose between (1) thoracotomy for complete resection and (2) some other approach for incomplete resection. Because this area is easily accessible by means of mediastinoscopy, and because we believe that mediastinoscopy is simpler and causes less morbidity than VATS, we prefer partial resection via mediastinoscopy as the initial approach to these lesions.[22] If cysts treated in this manner recur with associated symptoms, one can always perform thoracotomy for complete resection at that time, and little will have been lost in the meantime.

MEDIASTINOSCOPIC PARTIAL RESECTION OF SUBCARINAL BRONCHOGENIC CYST

Operative Technique

Step 1: mediastinoscopy and pretracheal dissection A standard cervical mediastinoscopy is performed, with dissection in the pretracheal plane down to the level of the carina.

Step 2: freeing of cyst from surrounding tissues With the cyst wall kept intact, as much of the wall as can safely be exposed is visualized by bluntly dissecting it away from the undersurface of the carina and the mainstem bronchi. Next, the mass is dissected away from the soft tissues anterior and posterior to it; obviously, this must be done with caution, given that the right main pulmonary artery and the esophagus are located nearby (anteriorly and posteriorly, respectively).

Step 3: aspiration of cyst contents and excision of exposed cyst wall The contents of the cyst are aspirated for cytologic and microbiologic examination, and the exposed portion of cyst wall is excised. Typically, approximately 50% of the cyst wall can be removed in this fashion. Some of the remaining cyst wall may be cauterized; this too must be done with caution, given the proximity of the adjacent vital structures.

Procedures for Lesions of the Posterior Mediastinum

The majority of posterior mediastinal masses occurring in adults are benign. These lesions may be usefully classified according to their radiologic appearance—that is, as either cystic or solid. Cystic masses in this region typically are bronchogenic cysts or esophageal duplication cysts, whereas solid masses most frequently are benign neurogenic tumors (e.g., schwannomas, neurofibromas, or ganglioneuromas). Esophageal leiomyomas (benign intramuscular tumors within the esophageal wall) are often grouped with these posterior mediastinal lesions and are managed in a similar fashion. In many cases, posterior mediastinal masses come to light as asymptomatic radiographic abnormalities; however, they may also be associated with signs of infection (in the case of infected cysts), dysphagia, chest pain, or respiratory complaints. At present, because of the growing availability of less morbid, minimally invasive approaches to posterior mediastinal masses, most authors recommend resection even when the lesion is asymptomatic. Although this recommendation remains somewhat controversial, we agree with it.

OPERATIVE PLANNING

VATS versus Thoracotomy

Resection of posterior mediastinal masses may be accomplished by means of either VATS or thoracotomy. The procedure is essentially the same with either approach, and the goal is complete resection. With some exceptions, VATS is considered preferable to thoracotomy in this setting; generally, VATS results in less postoperative pain and quicker functional recovery.[23,24] Some surgeons argue that a VATS approach may be more likely to leave a patient with microscopic residual disease. In our experience and that of others, however, recurrences of these lesions are very rare after VATS excision.[25,26] Given the low recurrence rate and the fact that these masses are almost always benign, we believe that the risk-benefit ratio favors VATS in most cases.

There are, however, several circumstances in which thoracotomy is indicated from the outset [*see Table 2*]. A suggestion of malignancy (in particular, invasion of surrounding structures) on preoperative radiography mandates exploration and resection by thoracotomy; in this situation, the potential consequences of positive margins justify the more aggressive approach. The presence of active infection within a cyst is a relative indication for thoracotomy in that it can cause disruption of normal tissue planes and thereby render VATS dissection more hazardous. Masses larger than approximately 6 cm also call for an open approach: such lesions are typically more difficult to mobilize safely from underlying structures than smaller lesions are, they are more likely to be malignant, and their removal between the ribs is likely to necessitate rib spreading, which may negate some of the benefit of true VATS.

Table 2 **Indications for Planned Thoracotomy Approach to Middle or Posterior Mediastinal Mass**

Suggestion of malignancy on preoperative radiography
Presence of inflammation or infection, blurring tissue planes
Large mass (> 5–6 cm)
Esophageal duplication cyst believed to communicate with esophageal lumen on the basis of preoperative computed tomography, barium esophagography, or esophagoscopy
Esophageal lesions without evidence of overlying normal esophageal mucosa on preoperative esophagoscopy or endoscopic ultrasonography
Previous ipsilateral thoracotomy with adhesions
Tumor located at apex of the chest, which may necessitate thoracosternotomy

When a cyst is arising from or abutting the esophagus, the possibility of a communication between the cyst and the esophageal lumen should be investigated preoperatively. Such a communication may be suggested on CT scans by the presence of an air-fluid level. To rule out this phenomenon, we perform barium esophagography during the preoperative workup, followed by intraoperative esophagoscopy at the commencement of the operation. If a communication is identified or cannot be ruled out, thoracotomy is performed. After excision of an esophageal duplication cyst with a communication, reapproximation of the esophageal mucosa is a paramount consideration; in our view, this is best done through an open approach.

In cases of suspected leiomyoma of the esophagus, preoperative investigation should be done to confirm the presence of intact overlying mucosa, which is virtually pathognomonic of this disease. Esophagoscopy is done to assess the mucosa; if the mucosa is intact, the possibility of malignancy is essentially ruled out. Simultaneously, endoscopic ultrasonography may be performed to establish the depth to which the esophageal wall is involved. With a preoperative diagnosis of probable leiomyoma, VATS is the approach of choice in our practice.

So-called dumbbell neurogenic tumors (tumors that invade the neural foramen) are special cases. Any solid mass in the costovertebral sulcus should be evaluated by means of MRI to determine whether it is invading the neural foramen if the absence of invasion was not clearly established by CT. Although invasion of the neural foramen by tumor is not in itself an indication for thoracotomy, it does necessitate a combined anterior-posterior approach with neurosurgical involvement for the intraspinal portion of the procedure. Several versions of such an approach have been described.[27–29] We prefer to perform the posterior neurosurgical resection of the intraspinal component (laminectomy and intervertebral foraminotomy) first and then to reposition the patient and carry out the remainder of the procedure (generally via VATS).[30]

Although VATS is often an excellent approach to posterior mediastinal lesions, it must be emphasized that one should never hesitate to convert a VATS procedure to a thoracotomy if required. Accordingly, informed consent to undergo thoracotomy should be sought before operation from all patients being treated for posterior mediastinal lesions, even when VATS is the intended approach.

VATS RESECTION OF NEUROGENIC TUMOR OF POSTERIOR MEDIASTINUM

Operative Technique

Resection of a solid neurogenic tumor of the posterior mediastinum that does not invade the neural foramen [*see Figure 9*] proceeds as follows.

Step 1: intubation and endoscopy The patient is intubated with a double-lumen endotracheal tube to allow single-lung ventilation. Preoperative bronchoscopy (for cystic lesions) or esophagoscopy (for lesions abutting the esophagus) is performed as indicated (see above).

Step 2: patient positioning and placement of ports The patient is placed in the lateral thoracotomy position and stabilized with bean bags so that the operating table can safely be tilted as much as 45° to either side. With this degree of tilt, the lung tends to fall away from the field of vision; thus, there usually is no need to place an additional port for a lung retractor.

The port for the scope is placed through an incision in the midaxillary line at the level of the mass; if it is placed much more anteriorly than the midaxillary line, the surgeon's view of posterior lesions may be obscured by the lung. The two working ports are placed through separate incisions in the posterior axillary line, made as far cephalad and caudad as possible. Sometimes placement of an alternative upper working port posterior to the scapula is advantageous [*see Figure 10*]. The main working instruments are an endoscopic scissors-cautery, a ring clamp, an endoscopic peanut dissector, a Maryland dissector, a long right-angle clamp, and an endoscopic clip applier.

Step 3: incision of pleura The parietal pleura is incised around the mass, with a margin of approximately 2 cm circumferentially. The pleura is tented up with the aid of

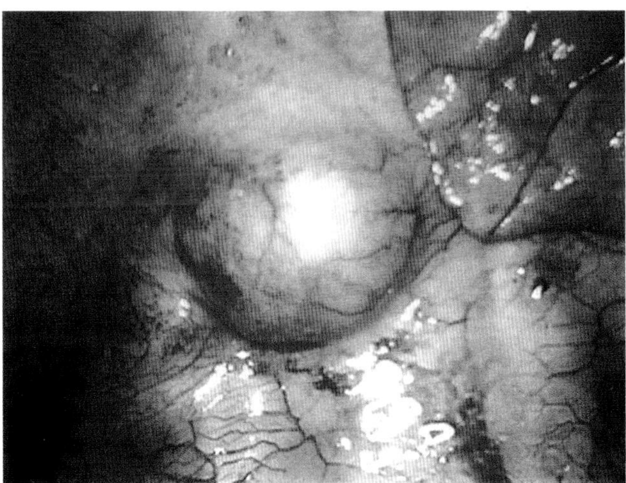

Figure 9 **Resection of neurogenic tumor of posterior mediastinum. Intraoperative photograph shows a solid neurogenic tumor of the costovertebral sulcus.**

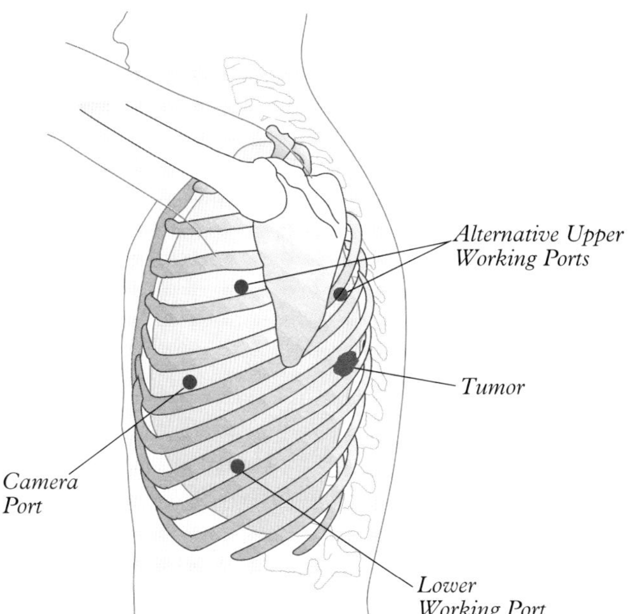

Figure 10 **Resection of neurogenic tumor of posterior mediastinum. Shown is typical port placement for video thorascopic resection of a posterior mediastinal mass.**

the right-angle clamp or the Maryland dissector to separate it from the underlying structures [*see Figure 11*]. This separation allows the use of the electrocautery, which provides hemostasis while protecting the underlying esophagus, vagus and intercostal nerves, and azygos vein. This dissection and all subsequent work are facilitated by placing gentle traction on the mass with a sponge stick or, for smaller masses, by grasping the entire mass within a ring clamp.

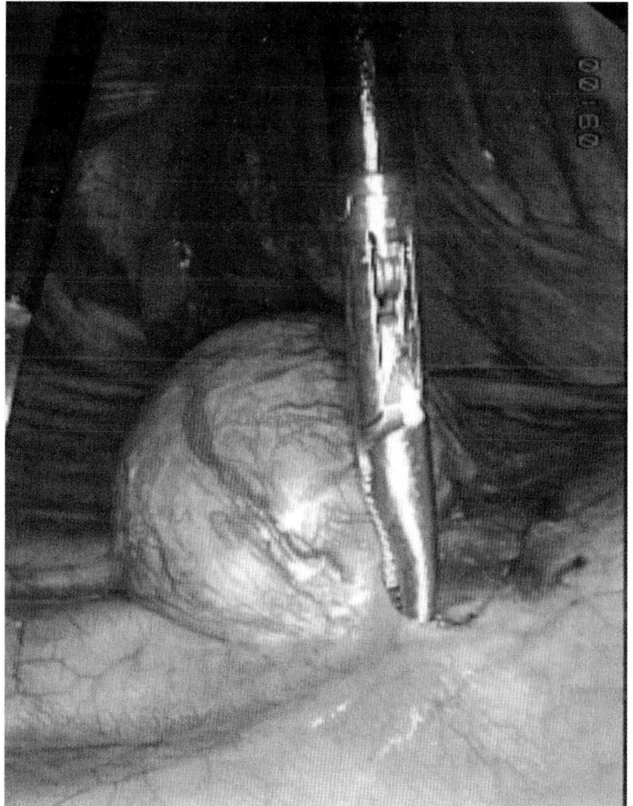

Figure 11 **Resection of neurogenic tumor of posterior mediastinum. Shown is circumferential incision of the pleura around a neurogenic mass.**

Step 4: dissection of soft tissue attachments Once the pleura has been incised circumferentially, the soft tissue attachments are further dissected bluntly with the endoscopic peanut dissector. Attachments that are relatively thick or vascular are best controlled by double-clipping and division. If the tumor originates from an intercostal nerve, gentle dissection is done beneath the tumor to identify the intercostal bundle that is the source of the lesion.

Step 5: division of source intercostal bundle The source intercostal bundle lateral to the tumor is mobilized, doubly clipped, and divided. Once this has been accomplished, blunt dissection is performed until the nerve root emerging from the neural foramen and the associated intercostal vessels are the last remaining attachments. If the tumor originates from the sympathetic chain, the chain is clipped above and below the tumor, and the intercostal bundle is spared if possible.

Step 6: removal of specimen The remaining stalk is doubly clipped and divided [*see Figure 12*], and the mass is removed in an endoscopic bagging device.

Step 7: drainage A 24 French chest tube is positioned posteriorly at the apex.

Troubleshooting

Care must be taken to ensure that only very gentle traction is exerted on a mass adjacent to the neural foramen. Overzealous traction can cause tearing of the nerve root proximal to the extraspinal extent of the dura, and this tearing can lead to a cerebrospinal fluid (CSF) leak, which most often becomes evident only postoperatively (in the form of persistent clear

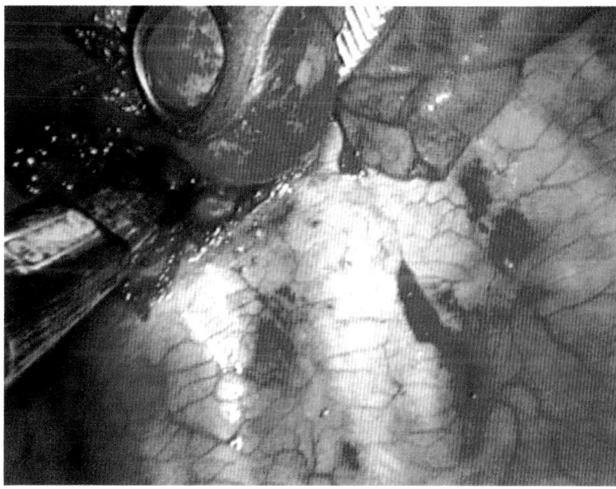

Figure 12 **Resection of neurogenic tumor of posterior mediastinum. The final remaining intercostal stalk is divided.**

chest tube output). The diagnosis of CSF leakage can be confirmed by measuring the β_2-transferrin level in the fluid. If CSF leakage is confirmed, reoperation with a neurosurgeon is mandatory; the leak is repaired and buttressed with vascularized tissue.

After resection of a tumor at the costoverterbral sulcus, regular neurologic examinations of the lower extremities are indicated. Tamponade with hemostatic agents should never be employed for bleeding at the neural foramen: doing so can result in an intraspinal hematoma with subsequent cord compression. Careful use of the electrocautery at the bony margins of the foramen or watchful waiting is preferable. If hemostasis cannot be achieved with these measures, a neurosurgical consultation should be obtained. In the event of oozing from the vicinity of a foramen that is not easily controlled, there should be no hesitation in converting a VATS procedure to an open procedure.

In a minority of patients, clipping and division of an intercostal nerve result in intercostal neuralgia after the procedure; the possibility that this may occur must be discussed with the patient preoperatively. Many patients who undergo division of a lower thoracic intercostal nerve that supplies an upper abdominal dermatome notice postoperative bulging of the ipsilateral abdomen in the area supplied by that nerve.

RESECTION OF BENIGN CYST OF POSTERIOR MEDIASTINUM

Resection of a benign cystic mass of the posterior mediastinum closely resembles resection of a neurogenic tumor [*see* Resection of Neurogenic Tumor of Posterior Mediastinum, *above*]; the differences are relatively minor [*see* Troubleshooting, *below*].

Troubleshooting

In the initial stages of dissection of a benign cyst of the posterior mediastinum, care should be taken not to rupture the cyst; initial mobilization from surrounding structures is easier when the cyst wall is under tension [*see Figure 13*]. If the area of the cyst wall that directly abuts the mediastinum is found to be too adherent to underlying structures to be removed safely, we intentionally rupture the cyst and then remove as much of the cyst wall as possible. As much as 35% of the cyst wall may be left in place. In such cases, we ablate the residual intact cyst wall with the electrocautery to destroy any potential secretory tissue. In our estimation, if more than approximately 35% of the cyst must be left in place, conversion to thoracotomy should be considered.

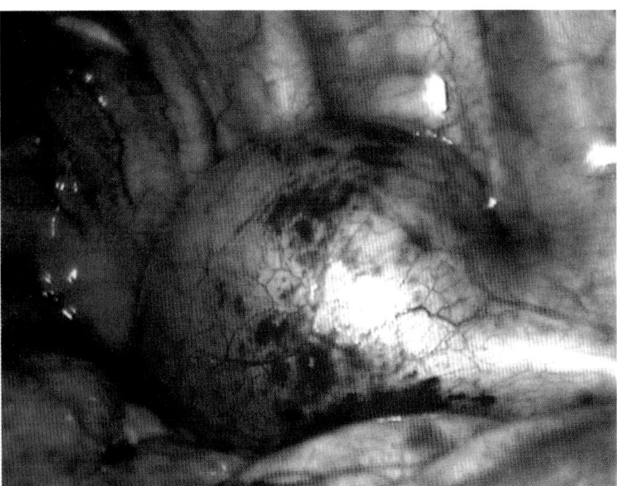

Figure 13 **Resection of benign cyst of posterior mediastinum. Intraoperative photograph shows a fluid-filled posterior mediastinal cyst. The tenseness of the cyst wall facilitates initial dissection.**

RESECTION OF ESOPHAGEAL LEIOMYOMA

Operative Technique

In addition to the steps described for resection of a neurogenic mass, there are several special maneuvers that facilitate resection of esophageal intramural masses, such as leiomyomata [*see Figure 14a*] and duplication cysts:

1. The pleura is incised longitudinally with the electrocautery after it is tented up away from the esophagus, the vagus nerve, and the azygos vein with a right-angle clamp or a Maryland dissector [*see Figure 14b*].
2. In some cases, exposure is facilitated by dividing the azygos vein with an endoscopic stapler [*see Figure 14c*].
3. The longitudinal esophageal muscle fibers that overlie the mass are separated bluntly or with the electrocautery in the line of the fibers. These fibers are often markedly attenuated as a result of the expansion of the mass [*see Figure 14d*].
4. Blunt dissection with an endoscopic peanut dissector allows careful, progressive mobilization of the mass, first from the muscle layer and then from the underlying mucosa. Gentle traction on the mass facilitates exposure at this point in the procedure [*see Figure 14e*]. A suture may be placed into the tumor to facilitate this retraction. Having an assistant place the endoscope within the esophageal lumen to distend and illuminate the mucosa also may be helpful at this stage. Once the mass has been completely resected, it is sent for pathologic examination [*see Figure 14f*].
5. The esophagus is distended by insufflating air from above while the distal esophagus is occluded with a sponge stick. The air-filled esophagus is then submerged in saline, and the area of the resection is examined for air leakage.

Troubleshooting

The muscular defect in the esophageal wall must be closed after resection to ensure that an esophageal diverticulum will not develop. Such closure may be accomplished by means of thoracoscopic suturing.

Frequently, duplication cysts are more adherent to the underlying esophageal mucosa than leiomyomata are, and transillumination of the esophageal wall helps define the plane at which blunt dissection should be performed. Where the cyst wall becomes difficult to separate from the mucosa, a small amount of the wall may be left in place if, in the surgeon's judgment, attempting to remove all of it might lead to a breach in the mucosa.

Financial Disclosures: None Reported

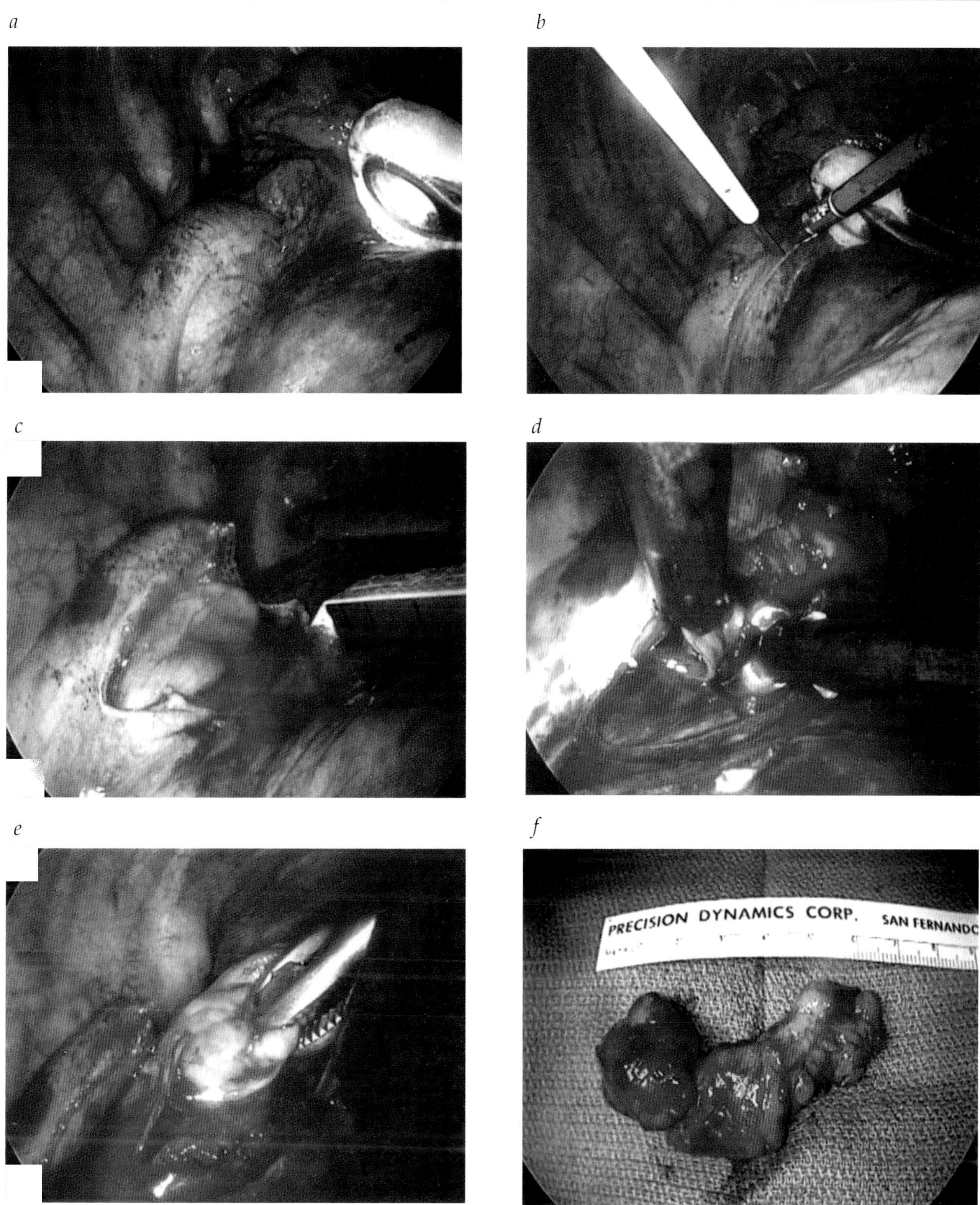

Figure 14 **Resection of esophageal leiomyoma. (*a*) Shown is an esophageal leiomyoma beneath the azygos vein. (*b*) The mediastinal pleura overlying the leiomyoma is incised. (*c*) The azygos vein is divided with an endoscopic stapler. (*d*) The muscle fibers overlying the mass are divided. (*e*) Gentle traction is applied to facilitate blunt dissection. (*f*) Shown is a completely resected horseshoe-shaped esophageal leiomyoma.**

References

1. Hoerbelt R, Keunecke L, Grimm H. The value of a noninvasive diagnostic approach to mediastinal masses. Ann Thorac Surg 2003; 75:1086.
2. Kumar A, Regmi SK, Dutta R, et al. Characterization of thymic masses using 18F-FDG PET CT. Ann Nucl Med 2009 July 8. [Epub ahead of print]
3. Koduri P. The diagnostic approach to mediastinal masses. Ann Thorac Surg 2004;78: 1888.
4. Vernino S, Lennon VA. Autoantibody profiles and neurological correlations of thymoma. Clin Cancer Res 2004;10:7270.
5. Drevelegas A, Palladas P, Scordalaki A. Mediastinal germ cell tumors: a radiopathological review. Eur Radiol 2001;11: 1925.
6. Schneider DT, Calaminus G, Reinhard H, et al. Primary germ cell tumors in children and adolescents: results of the German cooperative protocols MEKEI 83/86, 89 and 96. J Clin Oncol 2000;18:832.
7. Wood DE. Mediastinal germ cell tumors. Semin Thorac Cardiovasc Surg 2000;12: 278.
8. Watanabe M, Takagi K, Aoki T. A comparison of biopsy through a parasternal anterior mediastinotomy under local anesthesia and percutaneous needle biopsy for malignant anterior mediastinal tumors. Surg Today 1998;28:1022.
9. Powers CN, Silverman JF, Geisinger KR, et al. Fine-needle aspiration biopsy of the anterior mediastinum: a multi-institutional analysis. Am J Clin Pathol 1996;105:168.
10. Deeb ME, Brinster CJ, Kucharzuk J, et al. Expanded indication for transcervical thymectomy in the management of anterior mediastinal masses. Ann Thorac Surg 2001; 72:208.
11. Savitt MA, Gao G, Furnary AP, et al. Application of robotic-assisted techniques to the surgical evaluation and treatment of the anterior mediastinum. Ann Thorac Surg 2005; 79:450.
12. Blalock A, Masoj MF, Riven SS. Myasthenia gravis and tumors of the thymic region. Ann Surg 1939;110:544.
13. Shrager JB, Deeb ME, Mick R, et al. Transcervical thymectomy for myasthenia gravis achieves results comparable to thymectomy by sternotomy. Ann Thorac Surg 2002; 74:320.
14. Shrager JB, Nathan D, Brinster CJ, et al. Outcomes following 151 extended transcervical thymectomies for myasthenia gravis. Ann Thorac Surg 2006;82:1863–9.
15. Cooper JD, Al-Jilaihawa AN, Pearson FG, et al. An improved technique to facilitate transcervical thymectomy for myasthenia gravis. Ann Thorac Surg 1988;45:242.
16. Bril V, Kojic J, Ilse WK, et al. Long-term clinical outcome after transcervical thymectomy for myasthenia gravis. Ann Thorac Surg 1998;65:1520.
17. Calhoun RF, Ritter JH, Guthrie TJ, et al. Results of transcervical thymectomy for myasthenia gravis in 100 consecutive patients. Ann Surg 1999;230:555.
18. Meyer DM, Herbert MA, Sobhani NC, et al. Comparative clinical outcomes of thymectomy for myasthenia gravis performed by extended transsternal and minimally invasive approaches. Ann Thorac Surg 2009;87: 385–90.
19. Rückert JC, Ismail M, Swierzy M, et al. Thoracoscopic thymectomy with the da Vinci robotic system for myasthenia gravis. Ann N Y Acad Sci 2008;1132:329–35.
20. Nwariaku F, Snyder WH, Burkey SH, et al. Infra-manubrial parathyroid glands in patients with primary hyperparathyroidism: alternatives to sternotomy. World J Surg 2005 March 22. [Epub ahead of print]
21. Demmy TL, Krasna MJ, Detterbeck FC, et al. Multicenter VATS experience with mediastinal tumors. Ann Thorac Surg 1998; 66:187.
22. Smythe WR, Bavaria JE, Kaiser LR. Mediastinoscopic subtotal removal of mediastinal cysts. Chest 1998;114:1794.
23. Santambrogio L, Nosotti M, Bellaviti N, et al. Videothoracoscopy versus thoracotomy for the diagnosis of the intermediate solitary pulmonary nodule. Ann Thorac Surg 1995; 59:868.
24. Nagahiro I, Andou A, Aoe M, et al. Pulmonary function, postoperative pain, and serum cytokine level after lobectomy: a comparison of VATS and conventional procedure. Ann Thorac Surg 2001;72:362.
25. Martinod E, Pons F, Azorin J, et al. Thoracoscopic excision of mediastinal bronchogenic cysts: results in 20 cases. Ann Thorac Surg 2000;69:1525.
26. Zambudio AR, Lanzas JT, Calvo MJ, et al. Non-neoplastic mediastinal cysts. Eur J Cardiothorac Surg 2002;22:712.
27. Shadmehr MB, Gaissert HA, Wain JC, et al. The surgical approach to “dumbbell tumors” of the mediastinum. Ann Thorac Surg 2003; 76:1650.
28. Osada H, Aoki H, Yokote K, et al. Dumbbell neurogenic tumor of the mediastinum: a report of three cases undergoing single-staged complete removal without thoracotomy. Jpn J Surg 1991;21:224.
29. Rzyman W, Skokowski J, Wilimski R, et al. One step removal of dumb-bell tumors by postero-lateral thoracotomy and extended foraminectomy. Eur J Cardiothorac Surg 2004;25:509.
30. Vallières E, Findlay JM, Fraser RE. Combined microneurosurgical and thorascopic removal of neurogenic dumbbell tumors. Ann Thorac Surg 1995;59:469.

Acknowledgments

Figure 1b Photo courtesy of Wallace T. Miller Sr, MD, University of Pennsylvania School of Medicine
Figures 2, 7, and 8 Alice Y. Chen
Figure 10 Tom Moore

12 PERICARDIAL PROCEDURES

Dawn Emick, MD, and Thomas A. D'Amico, MD

Surgical procedures are performed on the pericardium either for diagnostic purposes or for relief of the hemodynamic consequences of pericardial disease. The pericardial processes for which surgical intervention is required can be divided into two broad categories: pericardial effusion and constrictive pericarditis. Pericardial effusion can either be acute or chronic, and the management of effusion depends largely on the rapidity of fluid accumulation and the risk of cardiac tamponade. The decisions that must be made regarding the selection of patients, the timing of surgery, and the choice of technique or approach often pose substantial challenges to the surgeon. Accordingly, a thorough knowledge of the anatomy, physiology, and pathophysiology of the pericardium is essential for successful management of pericardial disease processes.

Anatomic and Physiologic Considerations

ANATOMY

Like the pleura, the pericardium consists of two layers. The inner layer, the visceral pericardium (or epicardium), is a monolayer of mesothelial cells that is adherent to the heart. The outer layer, the parietal pericardium, is a tough fibrous structure composed of dense bundles of collagen fibers with occasional elastic fibers. The fibrous structure of this layer renders the pericardial sac relatively noncompliant, and this noncompliance plays a significant role in pericardial function and pathophysiology.

The pericardium surrounds the heart and the great vessels [*see Figure 1*]. Its parietal and visceral surfaces meet superiorly at the ascending aorta and the superior vena cava. From that point, the pericardium continues down the right border of the heart and over the anterior surface of the pulmonary veins to the inferior vena cava. After crossing the inferior vena cava, the inferior pericardium is densely adherent to the diaphragm. Just past the apex of the heart, it turns superiorly again and runs over the pulmonary veins back to the aorta.

Anteriorly, there are normally no connections between the visceral and parietal layers of the pericardium. Posteriorly, the pattern of pericardial reflections around the pulmonary veins and the venae cavae creates two sinuses. The oblique pericardial sinus is the space in the center of the pulmonary veins, directly behind the left atrium. The transverse pericardial sinus is bordered anteriorly by the aorta and the main pulmonary artery and posteriorly by the dome of the left atrium and the superior vena cava.

NORMAL PHYSIOLOGY

The pericardium is normally filled with 15 to 50 mL of serous fluid, which serves as lubrication to facilitate the motion of the heart within this structure. By virtue of its relative noncompliance, the pericardium exerts an influence on cardiac hemodynamics. This influence can easily be seen in the normal inspiratory variation in systemic arterial pressure. Under normal circumstances, intrapericardial pressure is slightly less than 0 mm Hg, becoming more negative during inspiration and less negative during expiration. Negative intrathoracic pressure during inspiration augments right ventricular filling. Because the pericardium does not allow significant acute right ventricular dilation, the ventricular cavity enlarges by shifting the septum toward the left ventricle. In addition, the noncompliance of the pericardium prevents the free wall of the left ventricle from distending to recapture its normal cavitary volume. Thus, the volume ejected from the left ventricle is slightly decreased, resulting in lower systemic arterial pressure. Normally, this effect is exceedingly small. However, it becomes more pronounced when the pericardium is filled with fluid: ventricular distention is restricted even further, and paradoxical pulse becomes clinically apparent.

PATHOPHYSIOLOGY

Although the pericardium is resistant to rapid distention, it is capable of distending over time. If filled slowly, it can expand to contain significant amounts of fluid (sometimes more than 1 L) before hemodynamic consequences develop. In the setting of an acute pericardial effusion (e.g., from trauma), however, devastating hemodynamic consequences may occur with only 100 to 200 mL of blood in the pericardium. When the elastic capacity of the pericardium is exceeded, even small increases in volume cause large increases in intrapericardial pressure and, if untreated, can lead to rapidly fatal cardiac tamponade. Although large, chronic effusions accumulate slowly over time, there is still a point at which the pericardium can no longer accommodate more volume, and tamponade can develop quickly. In a series of 28 patients with large idiopathic pericardial effusions, nearly 30% developed cardiac tamponade unexpectedly.[1] Thus, drainage of large effusions even without signs of tamponade may be appropriate, particularly if there is evidence of right-sided diastolic collapse. A number of different processes can result in the accumulation of fluid in the pericardial space [*see Table 1*].

Constrictive pericarditis is defined as a chronic fibrous thickening of the pericardium that causes cardiac compression sufficient to prevent normal diastolic filling. It can best be thought of as the chronic sequela of acute pericarditis or of any situation resulting in pericardial irritation and adhesion formation. Almost any cause of acute pericarditis can result in pericardial constriction [*see Table 2*]. In many patients, there is no clear antecedent event, and the cause of the constrictive pericarditis cannot be determined with certainty.

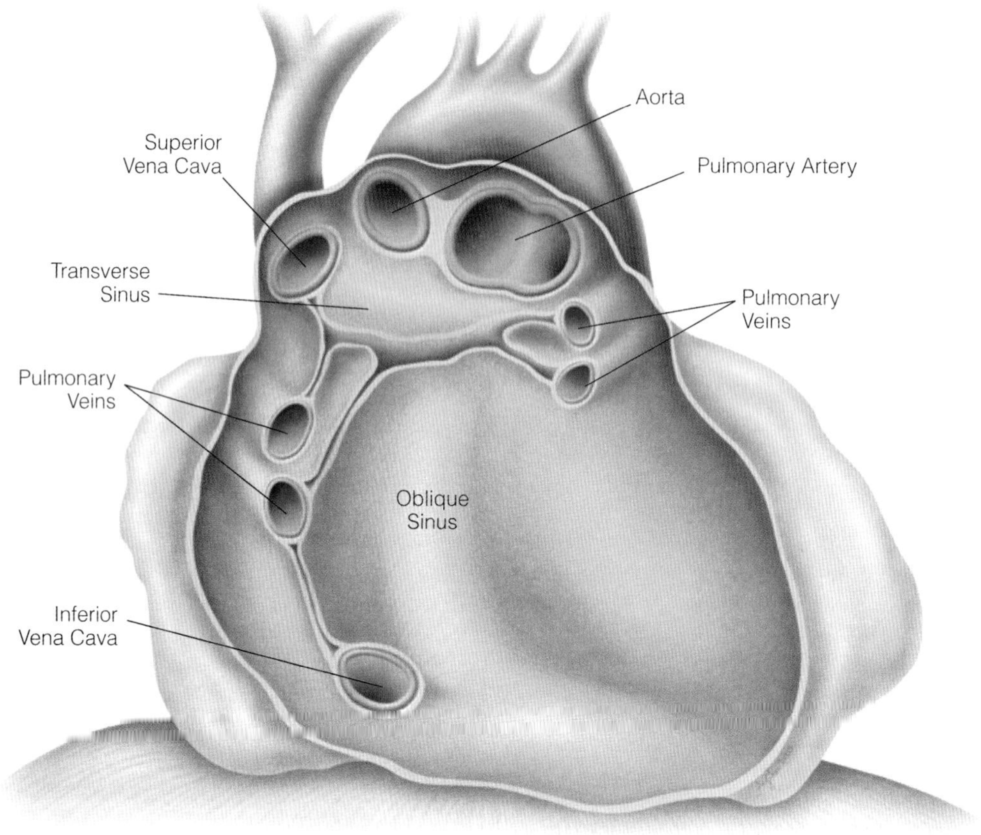

Figure 1 **Shown is a view of the pericardium with the heart removed.**

Pathologic examination typically demonstrates end-stage fibrosis, and these cases are presumed to be viral in origin. Historically, mycobacterial tuberculosis has been the most common infectious cause of constrictive pericarditis, and it is still the dominant infectious cause in many developing countries today.[2,3] In the United States, tuberculosis is the cause of constrictive pericarditis in approximately 6% of patients who undergo pericardiectomy.[4] Constrictive pericarditis also occurs after instrumentation of the pericardium and is seen occasionally (in 0.2 to 0.3% of cases) after cardiac surgery.[5,6] It also may develop after iatrogenic cardiac perforation in the course of catheterization or pacemaker

Table 1 **Common Causes of Pericardial Effusion**
Malignancy
Trauma
Uremia
Infection (viral, bacterial, fungal, tubercular)
Autoimmune processes
Cardiac surgery (postoperative complication)
Myocardial infarction
Iatrogenesis (intracardiac procedures)
Aortic dissection
Radiation
Idiopathic origin

Table 2 **Causes of Constrictive Pericarditis**
Common Causes
Unknown
Infection
Tuberculosis
Viral infection (coxsackievirus B)
Bacterial infection
Fungal infection (histoplasmosis, coccidioidomycosis)
Parasitic infection (amebiasis, echinococcosis)
Cardiac surgery or pacemaker insertion
Penetrating, nonpenetrating, or iatrogenic trauma
Radiation therapy
Connective tissue disorders (rheumatoid arthritis, systemic lupus erythematosus, scleroderma)
Renal failure
Neoplasm
Metastatic disease (breast, lung, lymphatic system, skin)
Primary mesothelioma
Drugs (procainamide, methysergide, hydralazine)
Uncommon Causes
Myocardial infarction
Asbestosis
Amyloidosis
Sarcoidosis
Dermatomyositis
Actinomycosis
Lassa fever
Whipple disease
Mulibrey nanism

placement and after blunt or penetrating trauma—essentially, after any process resulting in an incompletely drained hemopericardium.[7,8]

The pericardium may harbor metastatic disease or locally advanced disease (e.g., mesothelioma), which may lead to pericardial constriction.[9,10] Connective tissue disorders (e.g., rheumatoid arthritis and lupus) can cause recurrent acute pericarditis and pericardial effusions, eventually resulting in constrictive pericarditis. A similar situation may arise in patients receiving radiation therapy and patients with renal failure.

The stiffening and thickening of the pericardium have three major physiologic effects. First, the thicker pericardium isolates the heart from changes in intrathoracic pressure. Normally, the pulmonary veins (which are intrathoracic structures) and the cardiac chambers experience the same changes in intrathoracic pressure. In the presence of pericardial constriction, however, the negative intrathoracic pressure generated during inspiration cannot be transmitted to the heart. This isolation of the heart results in decreased flow through the pulmonary veins during inspiration and reduced left-side filling.

Second, the ventricles become interdependent. Because total pericardial volume does not change, the inspiratory decrease in left ventricular filling seen with constriction must be accompanied by an increase in right ventricular filling, with a resultant septal shift toward the left ventricle. During expiration, the opposite occurs: left ventricular filling increases and right ventricular filling decreases, and there is a septal shift toward the right ventricle.

Third, the encasement of the heart impairs the diastolic filling of all cardiac chambers. Elevated atrial pressure causes rapid initial filling of the ventricle (with as much as 75% of the ventricle filled during the first 25% of diastole), but by the middle of diastole, filling abruptly decreases as a result of the rigid pericardium. Because of this limit to diastolic filling, increasing the heart rate becomes the most effective method of increasing cardiac output.[11]

Other uncommon but potentially significant pericardial diseases include congenital defects and cysts. In one study, congenital defects of the pericardium were found in 1 of 10,000 autopsies.[12] Most commonly, these included partial or total absence of pericardium on the left (70%), right (17%), or total bilateral (rare), and 30% had other associated anatomic anomalies. Most patients with complete absence or large defects are asymptomatic; partial left-sided defects can be complicated by herniation of the heart through the defect and possible strangulation leading to chest pain, shortness of breath, syncope, or sudden death. Surgical pericardioplasty may be indicated in patients with imminent strangulation. Pericardial cysts may be congenital, inflammatory, or echinococcal in origin. Regardless of origin, most cysts are asymptomatic and detected incidentally. Patients with symptoms from compression on the heart are candidates for percutaneous aspiration and ethanol sclerosis, with the addition of pretreatment with albendazole for echinococcal cysts.[13] Patients with symptomatic inflammatory or congenital cysts who do not respond to aspiration and sclerosis may be candidates for video-assisted thoracotomy or surgical excision.

Pericardial Drainage Procedures for Pericardial Effusion

Pericardial effusion fluid may be transudate, exudate, pyopericardium, or hemopericardium. Regardless of the origin of the fluid accumulation, once the pericardium has reached the limits of its elasticity, the only way in which it can increase its volume is by reducing the volume occupied by the heart within it. Increases in pericardial pressure result in progressive cardiac compression and reductions in intracardiac volumes and myocardial diastolic compliance. This effect is most pronounced in the chambers with the lowest normal intracavitary pressures—namely, the right atrium and the right ventricle.[14] Changes in systemic cardiac output occur as a result of right heart compression, which leads to diminished right ventricular stroke volume, reduced pulmonary blood flow, and decreased left ventricular filling. In the early stages of pericardial effusion, various compensatory changes act to preserve cardiac output. Such changes include an increased ejection fraction, tachycardia, increased intravascular volume via renal conservation of salt and water, increased peripheral vascular resistance, and time-dependent pericardial stretch.[15,16]

PREOPERATIVE EVALUATION

The presenting symptoms of pericardial effusion may be nonspecific and related to the underlying disorder (e.g., fever, chest pressure, and fatigue). Fluid accumulation that is substantial enough to have hemodynamic consequences is defined as cardiac tamponade. Patients with early tamponade may have dyspnea, tachycardia, mild hypotension, decreased urine output, and paradoxical pulse. As tamponade progresses, patients may manifest signs of end-organ hypoperfusion (e.g., mental status changes, renal insufficiency, and shock). The classic physical findings known as the Beck triad (i.e., jugular venous distention, systemic hypotension, and distant heart sounds) are more common with acute tamponade (such as results from trauma) than with slow-developing tamponade (such as results from medical processes). In patients with slow-developing tamponade, systemic fluid retention is observed, often manifested by peripheral edema or ascites.

Most commonly, pericardial effusion is diagnosed when a patient exhibits new symptoms in the context of an underlying disorder associated with pericardial effusion (e.g., renal failure or malignancy). Chest x-rays may reveal a globular heart or an increasing cardiac silhouette on serial films. Currently, echocardiography is the most commonly employed and most useful modality for the diagnosis of pericardial effusion: it reliably determines the presence, location, and relative volume of fluid accumulations. The size of effusions can be graded based on echocardiographic findings. Grade I effusions are small (echo-free space in diastole <10 mm), grade II effusions are moderate (10 to 20 mm), grade III are large (≥ 20 mm), and grade IV are very large (>20 mm and compression of the heart).[17] In many cases, echocardiography can identify early tamponade, often before symptoms develop. A variety of echocardiographic findings are helpful in diagnosing hemodynamically significant effusions, the most useful being right atrial collapse and right ventricular collapse. Right atrial collapse during late diastole tends to occur early in the development of tamponade because of the normally low right atrial filling pressures. Right ventricular free wall collapse during early diastole suggests progression of tamponade. Other useful signs are loss of the normal inspiratory collapse of the inferior vena cava and an increase in right ventricular diameter with a reciprocal decrease in left ventricular diameter during inspiration.

In patients who are undergoing invasive hemodynamic monitoring (e.g., those who have just undergone cardiac surgery), hemodynamic findings suggestive of tamponade include elevation of right atrial pressure and equalization of right atrial pressure and pulmonary capillary wedge pressure. It is important to remember, however, that localized tamponade can occur (especially in the postoperative period) without these changes. A common cause is localized clot in the oblique pericardial sinus behind the left atrium, which causes reduced left atrial compliance. Transesophageal echocardiography here may be particularly useful, but it is important to have a high degree of suspicion in these cases as thrombosis does not have the typical echolucent area on echocardiography.

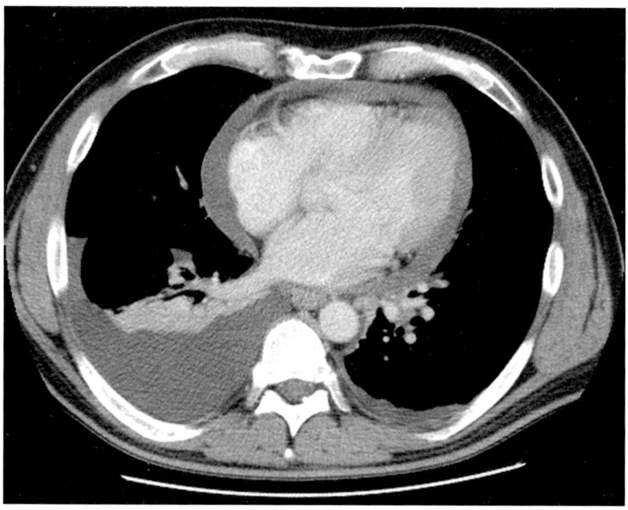

Figure 2 **Computed tomography demonstrates right pleural and pericardial effusions, for which a right thoracoscopic approach is ideal.**

OPERATIVE PLANNING

Choice of Procedure

Three procedures are commonly performed for surgical diagnosis and treatment of pericardial effusion: pericardiocentesis, subxiphoid pericardiostomy (pericardial window), and thoracoscopic pericardiostomy (via either the right or the left pleural space). The choice of a surgical approach to the pericardial space depends on the clinical condition of the patient, the presence or absence of associated pleural effusion or other thoracic process, and the underlying diagnosis (if known). Patients with tamponade may decompensate rapidly during the vasodilatation and positive pressure ventilation associated with general anesthesia. Accordingly, careful consideration must be given to the type of anesthesia employed for pericardial drainage procedures.

Pericardiocentesis is routinely done with local anesthesia only and may be the best choice in an acutely unstable patient with tamponade. If this option is chosen, however, the choice must be made with the understanding that pericardiocentesis, because of its high recurrence rate and its limited diagnostic capacity, is unlikely to constitute definitive therapy. Subxiphoid pericardiostomy is generally done with initial local anesthesia followed by induction of general anesthesia, and most patients with tamponade can undergo this procedure. The subxiphoid approach provides the hemodynamic benefits of pericardiocentesis, offers the enhanced diagnostic capability of pericardial biopsy, and has a low recurrence rate. Consequently, it is the procedure of choice for patients with tamponade who are stable enough to be transported to the operating suite. Thoracoscopic pericardiostomy has the advantage of enabling simultaneous treatment of pleural processes, which are commonly present in these patients [*see Figure 2*]. Ipsilateral pleural and pericardial spaces can be fully explored, pleural effusions can be drained, loculations can be divided, and biopsy specimens can be obtained as needed. The thoracoscopic approach can be especially useful in the case of a known loculated effusion that is limited to one area of the pericardium, in that a pericardial window can be created via either pleural space. This approach also allows resection of a larger segment of pericardium, which may improve the diagnostic yield and reduce the likelihood of recurrent effusion. The major limitation of thoracoscopic pericardiostomy is the need for lung isolation and lateral positioning, which should not be attempted in patients with evidence of tamponade. By weighing the relative risks and benefits of these three procedures, the surgeon can choose the optimal approach for each patient.

PERICARDIOCENTESIS

Operative Technique

Pericardiocentesis is performed either at the bedside in an urgent situation or, preferably, under echocardiographic or fluoroscopic guidance in a catheterization laboratory. The basic technique is simple.

Step 1: placement of needle A local anesthetic is infiltrated along the left side of the xiphoid. An 18-gauge spinal needle attached to a three-way stopcock and syringe is then advanced into the pericardial space and directed cephalad toward the left shoulder at a 45° angle until fluid is aspirated [*see Figure 3*]; if air is aspirated, the needle is withdrawn and redirected more medially. Once fluid is aspirated freely, it is inspected. If the fluid is bloody, 5 mL is withdrawn and placed on a sponge. If the fluid on the sponge clots, it is fresh blood, probably from a cardiac injury occurring during the procedure or from intracardiac positioning of the needle; blood that has been in the pericardium for even a short time becomes defibrinated and will not clot.[18]

Troubleshooting The inherent danger of cardiac injury during pericardiocentesis should be obvious. The risk is highest with small or loculated effusions and patients with coagulation abnormalities. The possibility of cardiac aspiration or injury can be minimized, although not eliminated, by means of various safety measures. Of historical interest, the simplest of these measures was to attach an electrocardiographic (ECG) lead to the needle and employ continuous ECG monitoring. If the needle contacts the epicardium, ST

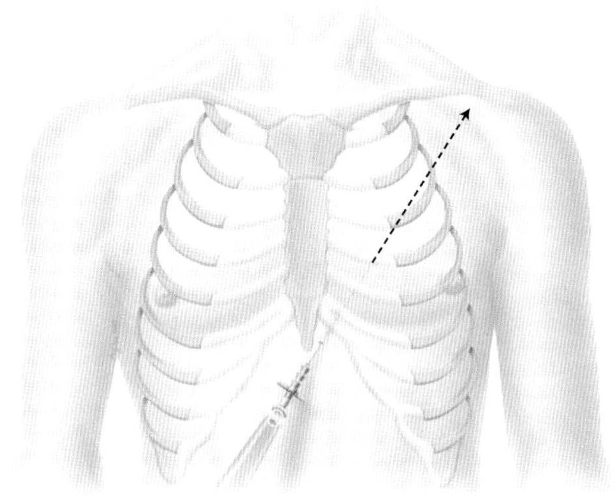

Figure 3 **Pericardiocentesis. The needle is angled toward the left shoulder at an angle of 45°.**

segment elevation will be observed, in which case, the needle is withdrawn until the ST elevation disappears. This is not considered to be an adequate safeguard anymore, and most experts recommend direct visualization using fluoroscopic or echocardiographic guidance. Fluoroscopy or echocardiography is essential in cases of loculated effusions to help direct aspiration. Simultaneous cardiac catheterization has also been used to locate the right coronary artery and the atrioventricular groove.

Step 2: placement of drainage catheter and aspiration of fluid Once the needle is within the pericardial space, a guide wire is placed through it, and a small-bore drainage catheter is advanced into the effusion by means of a modified Seldinger technique. Fluid is aspirated and sent for laboratory evaluation (including cell count, chemistry, culture, and cytology). The catheter is then connected to a closed drainage system for 24 to 72 hours; this may help reduce recurrence.

Complications

The most serious complications of pericardiocentesis are laceration and/or rupture of the myocardium and coronary vessels. Thankfully, these are rare (< 1% when fluoroscopy is used).[19] More common complications of pericardiocentesis include arrhythmias, pneumothorax, air embolism, puncture of the abdominal cavity or abdominal organs, misdiagnosis, and recurrence of pericardial effusion. In every patient undergoing pericardiocentesis, pneumothorax must be ruled out by means of chest x-ray at the completion of the procedure or, if respiratory or hemodynamic changes develop intraoperatively, during the procedure. Cardiac injuries range from minor needle lacerations to the epicardium, which are self-limited in patients with normal coagulation parameters, to potentially fatal injuries to the myocardium or coronary vessels that can lead to acute cardiac tamponade. Incorrect diagnoses based on pericardiocentesis are not uncommon. Although a diagnosis can be confirmed by positive results from fluid culture or cytology, negative results from cytology do not rule out malignant effusion. Cytologic analysis of pericardial fluid is diagnostic in only 55 to 85% of patients.[20] Further diagnostic maneuvers often must be undertaken, usually involving subxiphoid or thoracoscopic approaches with pericardial biopsy. Recurrence of pericardial effusion after pericardiocentesis is extremely common. In a review that included 139 patients with malignant pericardial effusions who were treated with pericardiocentesis, successful fluid removal with symptomatic relief was achieved in 97.1% of cases.[21] Of the 139 patients, 2.9% experienced complications (e.g., pneumothorax and ventricular laceration) and one (0.7%) died. In all, 45 of the patients received no further therapy, and in 25 (55%) of the 45, recurrent effusions developed that necessitated reintervention.

Several techniques for preventing recurrent pericardial effusion have been tried. Instillation of a sclerosing agent (e.g., tetracycline, thiotepa, or bleomycin) into the pericardium to promote fusion of the two layers of the pericardium has been shown to increase the success rate of pericardiocentesis by as much as 85%.[22-24] Placement of an indwelling catheter (see above) also has been shown to improve the success rate.[21,25] Several authors have described creating a pericardial window percutaneously by means of balloon dilation of the tract created by pericardiocentesis, which theoretically allows fluid to drain into the pleural space or the subcutaneous tissues, where it can be absorbed.[26,27] However, it is unclear how long a window created in this fashion will remain patent. Although pericardiocentesis provides initial symptomatic relief in most patients, the observation that 15 to 45% of patients require a further procedure for diagnosis and as many as 55% require reintervention for recurrence has led some authorities to question its benefit.

SUBXIPHOID PERICARDIOSTOMY (PERICARDIAL WINDOW)

Operative Technique

Subxiphoid pericardiostomy may be performed either to diagnose pericardial effusion or to manage tamponade. For diagnosis, the procedure is usually done with general anesthesia. In an unstable patient with significant tamponade, who would be at risk for hemodynamic collapse with general anesthesia, the procedure may be performed with the patient under local anesthesia and mild sedation and breathing spontaneously. If there is any question of tamponade, the patient is prepared and draped while awake, and anesthesia is induced only when the surgeon is ready to begin. In all patients, the entire chest should be prepared in case a left anterior thoracotomy or median sternotomy is required. Ideally, the patient is sedated and the airway controlled while spontaneous respiration is maintained to minimize hemodynamic effects. If necessary, a local anesthetic may be infiltrated and the incision made before induction of anesthesia.

Step 1: initial incision and exposure of pericardium A small vertical incision is made from the xiphisternal junction downward to a point slightly below the tip of the xiphoid process [*see Figure 4a*]. The upper extent of the linea alba is divided, with care taken not to enter the peritoneum. Peritoneal openings are easily repaired but can make the

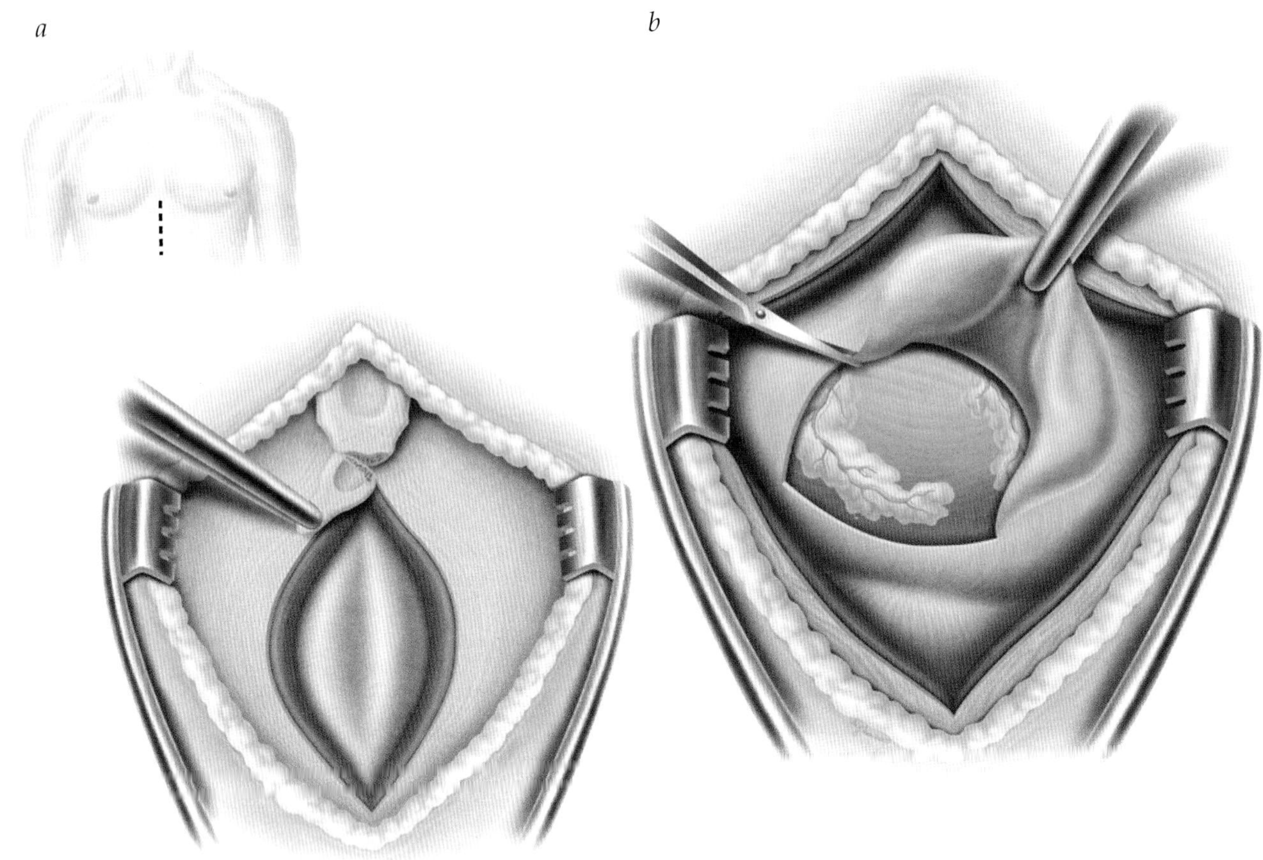

Figure 4 **Subxiphoid pericardiostomy. (*a*) A small vertical incision is made from the xiphisternal junction down to a point just below the tip of the xiphoid, the upper extent of the linea alba is divided, and the xiphoid is removed. (*b*) The pericardium is opened, and the edge of the opening is grasped and elevated. A pericardial specimen several square centimeters in size is then resected to create the pericardial window.**

procedure technically more difficult in that abdominal contents tend to impede visualization, especially in spontaneously breathing patients. Positioning patients with feet down in a reverse Trendelenburg position prior to the procedure may allow the abdominal organs to fall toward the pelvis and out of the way. The soft tissue attachments to the xiphoid are divided, the veins running along either side of the xiphoid are controlled, and the xiphoid process is removed.

The tissue plane behind the lower sternum is developed by means of blunt dissection. This maneuver exposes the retrosternal space to allow visualization of the pericardium. To enhance exposure, the sternum is retracted upward by an assistant. The anterior pericardial surface is then exposed by sweeping away the remaining mediastinal fat. If necessary, the confluence of the pericardium and the diaphragm may be retracted caudally to improve exposure.

Step 2: opening of pericardium The location of the pericardial incision can be confirmed by palpating cardiac motion through the exposed pericardium. The pericardium is then opened with a scalpel; shallow strokes should be employed to reduce the chances of injuring underlying myocardium that may be adherent to the pericardium. Upon entry into the pericardium, there is an initial outrush of fluid. A sanguineous effusion can be difficult to differentiate from cardiac injury; therefore, the patient's hemodynamics should be carefully monitored during this time. When the pressure placed on the heart by an effusion is released, blood pressure will usually rise and heart rate fall; however, if the heart has been accidentally injured, the opposite will occur. Once hemodynamic stability is achieved, administration of a diuretic (e.g., furosemide) should be considered to reduce the risk of pulmonary edema developing as a result of systemic fluid retention.

Step 3: creation of pericardial window Pericardial fluid is collected for microbiologic and cytologic analysis and for any additional testing suggested by the clinical scenario. The pericardial space is gently explored with the fingers, and all remaining fluid is evacuated. The edge of the pericardial opening is grasped with a clamp and elevated [*see Figure 4b*]. A pericardial specimen several square centimeters in size—or as large as can safely be managed—is resected and sent for pathologic and microbiologic analysis.

Step 4: drainage and closure A separate stab incision for drain placement is made below and to one side of the lowermost aspect of the skin incision. Bringing the drainage tube out through a separate incision helps prevent incisional complications (e.g., infection and hernia). A 24 to 28 French chest tube (either straight or right-angle) is tunneled through the fascia at the entry site so that it lies beneath the divided linea alba in the preperitoneal space. The tube is then directed through the pericardial window and into the pericardial space and secured at skin level. The fascia at the linea alba is closed with interrupted sutures to provide secure closure and prevent late hernia; the skin and subcutaneous tissue are closed in the standard fashion. The chest tube is connected to a drainage system with a water seal. Pericardial drainage is maintained for several days postoperatively until the output falls below 100 mL/day. This period allows time for apposition and adhesion formation between the visceral pericardium and the parietal pericardium.

Although some fluid may initially drain into the subcutaneous tissues and be absorbed, the name pericardial window is something of a misnomer. The surgically created window in the pericardium is unlikely to remain patent over the long term, and, in fact, obliteration of the pericardial space has been shown to be the mechanism responsible for the success of this procedure.[28,29]

Complications

Complications from subxiphoid pericardiostomy are rare; bleeding, infection, incisional hernia, anesthetic complications, and cardiac injury have been reported. In a study that included 155 patients who underwent subxiphoid pericardiostomy over a 5-year period, not a single death was attributable to the operative procedure itself.[23] The 30-day mortality was high but was related to the underlying disease process: 33% in patients with malignant effusions and 5% in those with benign effusions. Recurrent pericardial effusion necessitating additional procedures occurred in four patients (2.5%). In a study that compared 94 patients who underwent subxiphoid pericardiostomy with 23 patients who underwent pericardiocentesis, the rate of recurrent effusion that necessitated reintervention was 1.1% after the subxiphoid window procedure but 30.4% after pericardiocentesis.[30] In this series, the rate of major complications after the pericardial window procedure was 1.1% (one patient with bleeding that necessitated reexploration), compared with a major complication rate of 17% after pericardiocentesis (including a mortality of 4%).

Several studies have shown that the most important predictor of long-term outcome is the underlying disease process. In one, the median survival time was 800 days for patients with benign disease, 105 days for patients with known cancer but negative results from pericardial cytology and pathology, and only 56 days for patients with malignant effusions.[28] It appears, however, that cancer patients with hematologic malignancies and pericardial effusion survive significantly longer than patients with other malignancies. In another study, the mean survival time after drainage of pericardial effusion was 20 months for patients with hematologic malignancies, compared with 5 months for patients with any other malignancies.[31] The investigators suggested that this finding may be related to the relative responsiveness of hematologic cancers to systemic chemotherapy. Patients with HIV disease have been shown to have universally dismal outcomes after they present with pericardial effusion. In this population, surgical pericardial drainage generally is not diagnostically revealing and is of little therapeutic value. Several authors have questioned whether pericardial drainage should even be offered to these patients.[32]

THORACOSCOPIC PERICARDIOSTOMY

Operative Technique

Thoracoscopic pericardiostomy is a safe and effective approach to the diagnosis and management of pericardial effusion, especially in patients with a unilateral pleural disease process that can be simultaneously addressed in the course of the procedure. Thoracoscopic pericardial drainage necessitates single-lung ventilation and thus is unsuitable for unstable patients, especially those with tamponade. Such ventilation can be accomplished by means of either a dual-lumen endotracheal tube or a bronchial blocker placed through a standard endotracheal tube.

Once the tube is in place, the patient is turned to the appropriate lateral decubitus position. The side of approach is chosen on the basis of the location of a loculated effusion or the site of any coexisting pathologic condition (e.g., a pleural effusion, pleural nodules or thickening, or pulmonary nodule). If the disease process or processes present do not dictate a particular side of approach, the right side is preferred. It is often easier to operate on the right side because there is more working room within the pleural space; however, operating on the left side usually allows the surgeon to create a larger pericardial window. If tamponade is present in a patient for whom the thoracoscopic approach is desired, pericardiocentesis may be performed before induction of general anesthesia.[33]

Step 1: placement of ports and entry into pleural space An initial camera port is placed in the posterior axillary line at the eighth intercostal space [*see Figure 5*]. The pleural space is entered and explored, and any effusion present is drained. Pleural fluid is sent separately for culture and cytologic analysis. To prevent inadvertent entry into the pericardium, which is often distended, a second incision is created anteriorly at the fifth intercostal space under camera visualization.

Step 2: opening of pericardium On the left side, the phrenic nerve, which runs midway between the hilum and the anterior chest wall, is carefully identified, and an initial pericardial incision is made approximately 1 cm anterior to this nerve. Care must be taken to place this first incision in an area that is free of cardiac adhesions. When grasped, the pericardium should tent outward slightly. Often cardiac motion is visible through the pericardium.

Step 3: creation of pericardial window A pericardial window several square centimeters in area is removed. A similar window may be created posterior to the phrenic nerve—again, with care taken to stay at least 1 cm away from the nerve. The pericardial space is inspected, and any loculations are opened. The procedure is similar when performed on the right side, except that the phrenic nerve on the right runs much closer to the hilum; accordingly, instead of two pericardial windows (anterior and posterior to the nerve), only a single, larger pericardial window is created (anterior to the nerve).

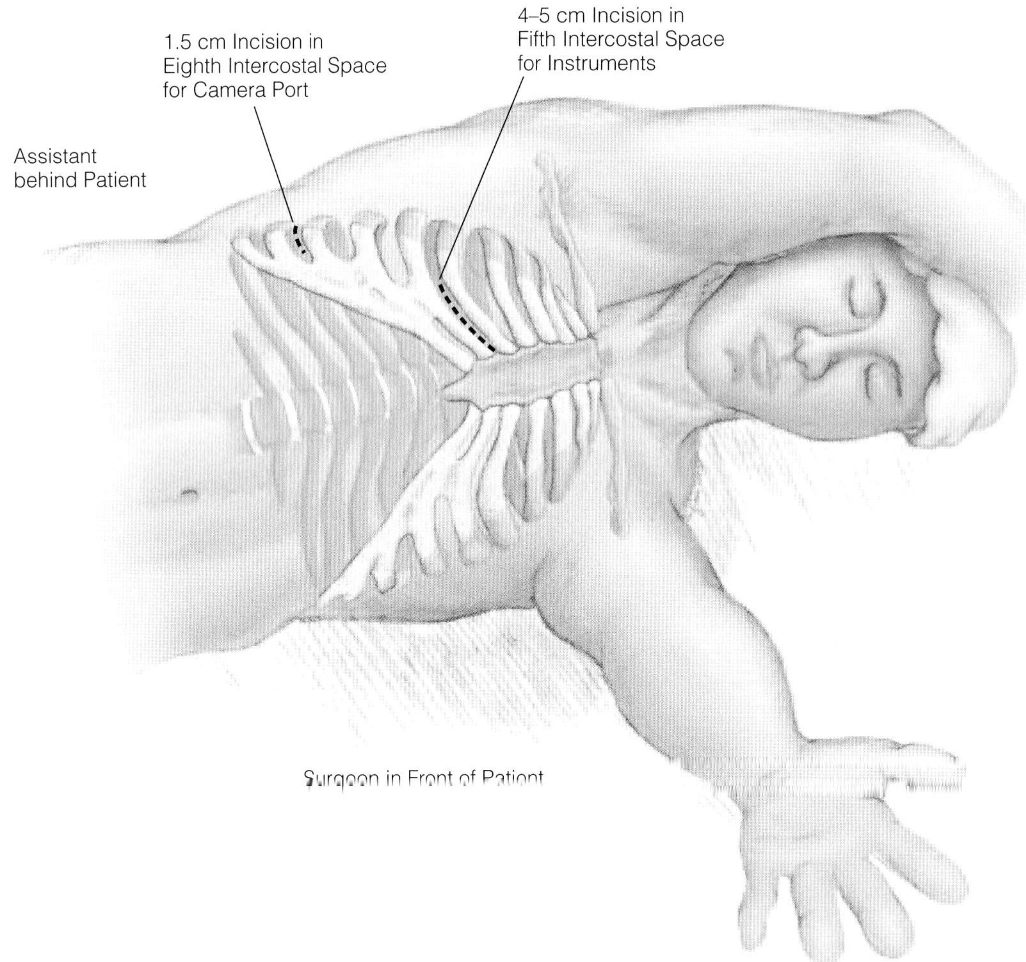

Figure 5 **Thoracoscopic pericardiostomy. Shown are the appropriate patient positioning and the proper placement of ports and instruments.**

In patients who can tolerate general anesthesia, a pericardial window can be created thoracoscopically with excellent diagnostic yield and relief of symptoms.[34] The thoracoscopic approach allows directed access and can be useful in treating effusions that recur after subxiphoid pericardiostomy.[35]

Complications

Complications from thoracoscopic pericardiostomy occur more frequently than from the subxiphoid approach. Reported complications include bleeding, infection, and cardiac injury similar to the subxiphoid approach, but compared to the subxiphoid approach, patients who undergo thoracoscopic procedures have longer anesthesia times and require single-lung ventilation, which increases the incidence of anesthesia-related complications. Patients who undergo thoracoscopic procedures require pleural tubes in the immediate postoperative period, and various complications related to chest tubes (e.g., recurrent pneumothorax, trapped lung) may occur. One recent study compared subxiphoid to videothoracoscopic pericardial window procedures in 71 patients.[36] In this retrospective review, 56 patients underwent subxiphoid pericardiostomy and 15 underwent the procedure thoracoscopically. Nonpericardial procedures were performed in 10 of 15 thoracoscopic procedures (67%) and only 18 of 56 (32%) of the subxiphoid approach. Anesthesia time (117 ± 32 vs 81 ± 26 minutes) and minor procedural morbidity (27% versus 2%) were higher for the thoracoscopic approach, but long-term control of the effusion seemed to be improved in the thoracoscopic approach. Equal percentages of patients had recurrence of their effusions (≈ 10%), but time to recurrence was much longer for the thoracoscopic procedures (36 versus 11 months).

Pericardiectomy for Constrictive Pericarditis

Constrictive pericarditis appears to be about three times as common in males as in females, and it may occur at any point in life from childhood to the ninth decade.[37] The symptoms of constrictive pericarditis usually develop progressively over a period of years but may develop within weeks to months after a defined inciting event (e.g., mediastinal irradiation or cardiac surgery). Signs and symptoms are related to pulmonary venous congestion (e.g., exertional dyspnea) and systemic venous congestion (e.g., elevated jugular venous pressure, hepatomegaly, ascites, and peripheral edema).

PREOPERATIVE EVALUATION

The physiologic effects of the thickened pericardium form the basis for the diagnosis of constrictive pericarditis and, more important, for the differentiation of constrictive pericarditis from restrictive cardiomyopathy, which often presents a similar picture. Echocardiography can be employed to rule out other causes of right-side failure. Specific findings that suggest pericardial constriction include septal bounce (a respiratory phase–related septal shift) and decreased transmitral flow velocity during inspiration. Computed tomography and magnetic resonance imaging may demonstrate thickened, often calcified, pericardium; however, the degree of pericardial thickening does not necessarily correlate with the presence of hemodynamic effects.

Cardiac catheterization may demonstrate increases in and equalization of end-diastolic pressure in all four cardiac chambers, a dip-and-plateau pattern (the square-root sign) in the ventricular pressure curves as a result of rapid early filling and limited late filling, and rapid x and y descents in the atrial pressure curves. The most useful information obtainable through cardiac catheterization has to do with the respiratory variation of ventricular pressure. In a patient with a normal heart or a patient with restrictive cardiomyopathy, inspiration causes a decrease in both right ventricular pressure and left ventricular pressure as a consequence of decreased intrathoracic pressure. In a patient with constrictive pericarditis, because of the interdependence of the ventricles, inspiration causes a decrease in left ventricular pressure but an increase in right ventricular pressure.[38]

OPERATIVE PLANNING

Choice of Approach

Pericardiectomy may be performed via either a median sternotomy or a left anterolateral thoracotomy, with equivalent results. Median sternotomy provides better access to the right atrium and the great vessels, as well as easier access for cannulation if cardiopulmonary bypass is required; left anterolateral thoracotomy allows more complete release of the left ventricle. With either approach, the patient should undergo full monitoring, including radial artery catheterization and central venous catheterization, with consideration given to placement of a pulmonary arterial catheter if there is significant hemodynamic compromise. Because significant blood loss can occur when densely adherent pericardium is resected, large-bore intravenous access should be available as well.

OPERATIVE TECHNIQUE

Median Sternotomy

Step 1: initial incision and exposure The patient is placed in the supine position, and the skin incision is carried down to the level of the sternum. If there is no history of previous pericardial procedures and it is possible to develop the plane behind the sternum bluntly at the superior and inferior aspects, a standard sternotomy saw can be used for the median sternotomy. If, however, there are likely to be adhesions between the sternum and the pericardium or the heart (as in the case of constrictive pericarditis after coronary artery bypass grafting), a careful reoperative sternotomy should be performed with an oscillating saw. Access to the femoral vessels should be available within the sterile field; placement of a femoral arterial line will facilitate percutaneous cannulation in the event that the heart is injured during sternal reentry.

After the sternum is opened, all adhesions are dissected away from the sternum, with care taken to stay as close to the posterior surface of the sternum as possible. Both pleural spaces are opened, and the left and right phrenic nerves are identified.

Step 2: dissection and resection of pericardium The phrenic nerves define the limits of pericardial resection bilaterally. Small loculated spaces are often present within the pericardium, especially near the great vessels and the diaphragm, and provide good starting places for pericardiectomy. Once an initial flap is raised, it is used to provide retraction to facilitate further dissection. Careful attention must be paid to the coronary artery anatomy: coronary arteries and bypass grafts are vulnerable to injury. If the pericardium is densely adherent in the region of a coronary artery, small islands of pericardium may be left on the heart. Areas of calcification can be addressed with the use of bone-cutting instruments; however, if an island of calcification appears to extend into the myocardium, it should not be removed.

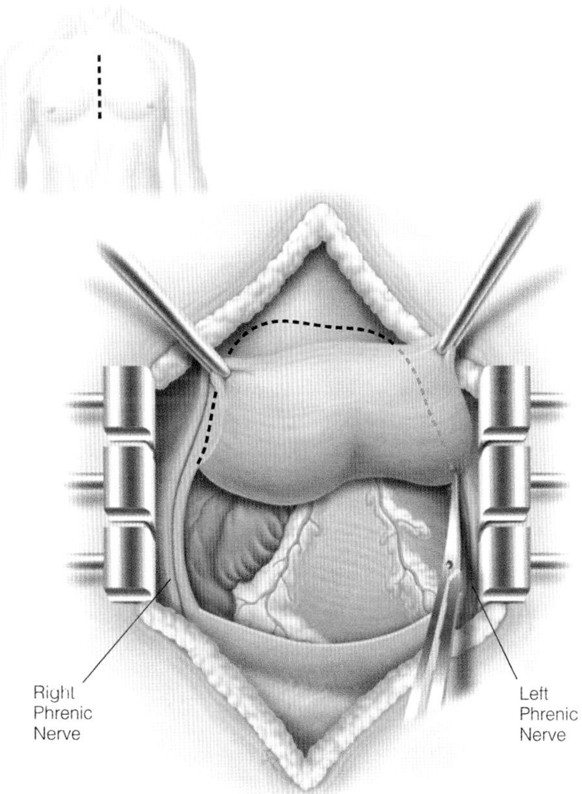

Figure 6 **Pericardiectomy: median sternotomy approach. The pericardium is resected from the left phrenic nerve to the right phrenic nerve.**

Epicardium can also be involved in the disease process and should be resected or scored until no further restriction to ventricular filling remains. The heart should be dissected free of the left pulmonary veins all the way over to the right pulmonary veins (including the origins of the venae cavae). The pericardium is resected from the left phrenic nerve to the right phrenic nerve [*see Figure 6*].

Cardiopulmonary bypass can make dissection easier, but in view of the greater risk of bleeding and the increased transfusion requirements, it is best avoided if possible. Cardiopulmonary bypass does facilitate repair of cardiac injuries during sternal reentry or dissection and should be used if cardiac procedures are to be performed concomitantly.

Step 3: drainage and closure After completion of the pericardiectomy, mediastinal and pleural drains are placed, and the sternum is closed in the usual fashion.

Left Anterolateral Thoracotomy

Step 1: initial incision and exposure The patient is placed in the supine position, with a roll under the left side of the torso to elevate the left side 45°. It is often difficult to establish cardiopulmonary bypass through the chest via this approach; therefore, the femoral vessels should be available within the sterile field so that femorofemoral bypass can be instituted if necessary. A curvilinear submammary incision is created, and the chest is entered at the fifth interspace. For improved exposure, the internal thoracic vessels may be divided and the intercostal muscles divided posteriorly. The left phrenic nerve is carefully identified.

Step 2: dissection and resection of pericardium As with the median sternotomy approach, loculated spaces are often present near the great vessels and the diaphragm, and these vessels provide good starting places for dissection. The entire pericardium is dissected free over the left ventricle, and an island of pericardium is left attached to the phrenic nerve along its length [*see Figure 7*]. The pericardium is resected from the pulmonary veins to a point just posterior to the phrenic nerve. Resection resumes anterior to the nerve and continues across the anterior aspect of the heart as far as possible, ideally to the right atrioventricular groove. The same precautions should be taken around the coronary vessels as are taken with the median sternotomy approach.

Step 3: drainage and closure After completion of the pericardiectomy, mediastinal and pleural drains are placed, and the thoracotomy is closed in the usual fashion.

OUTCOME EVALUATION

There is no proven difference between the two approaches to pericardiectomy with respect to outcome. Accordingly, the choice between them is based on whether one option affords better access to the areas believed to be most involved

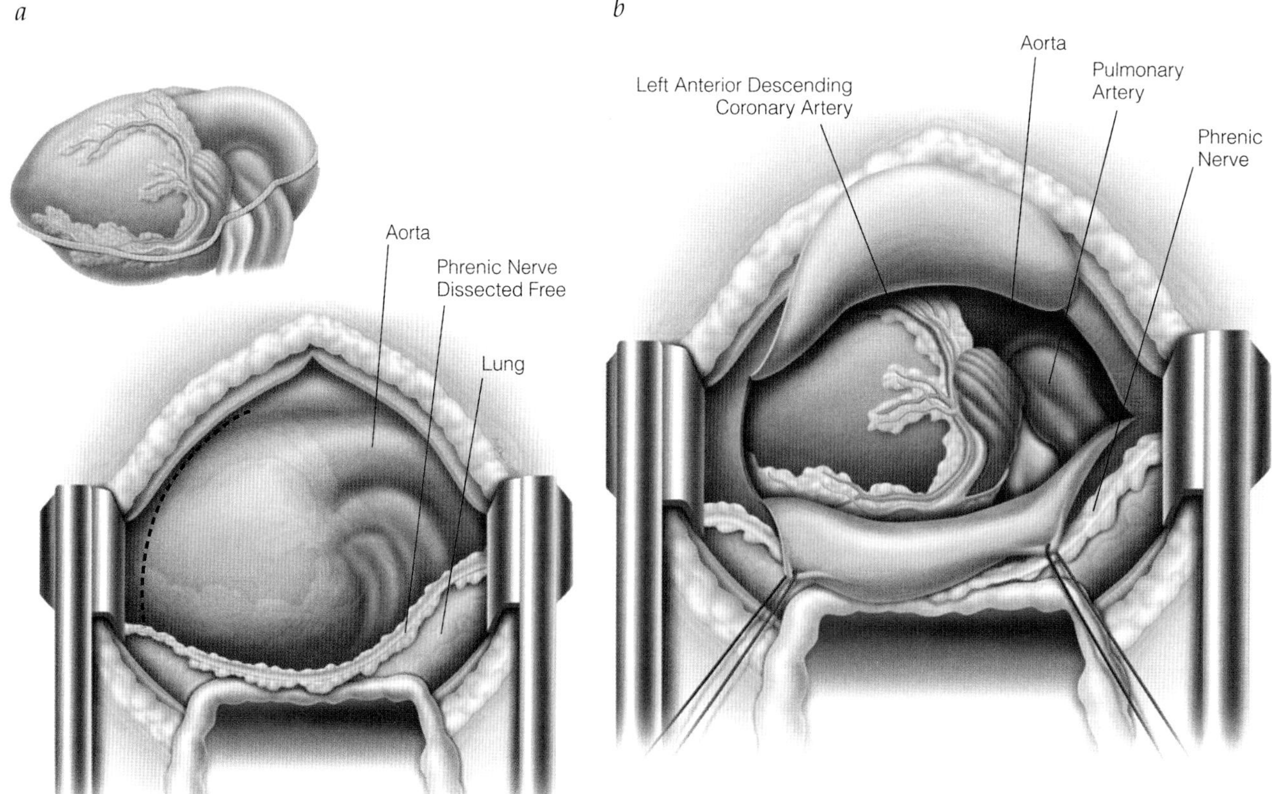

Figure 7 **Pericardiectomy: left anterolateral thoracotomy approach. (*a*) The left phrenic nerve is identified. (*b*) The entire pericardium is dissected free over the left ventricle, with an island of pericardium left attached to the phrenic nerve along its length. Care must be taken to avoid injuring coronary vessels.**

(e.g., a median sternotomy is more effective for releasing the right side of the heart) and whether the surgeon is more comfortable with one approach or the other.

The underlying cause of constrictive pericarditis is a significant predictor of long-term survival. In a study of 163 patients who underwent pericardiectomy, 7-year survival rates were highest in patients with idiopathic constrictive pericarditis (88%), somewhat lower in patients with postoperative constriction (66%), and lowest in patients with radiation-induced constriction (27%).[39] Predictors of decreased survival included previous radiation therapy, renal dysfunction, pulmonary hypertension, and abnormal left ventricular systolic function. Perioperative mortality was 6% overall but 21% in patients who had received radiation therapy and 8% in postsurgical patients. The slightly higher mortality recorded in postoperative patients may reflect underlying cardiac dysfunction, as well as the vulnerability of previous bypass grafts to injury. The poor outcomes after pericardiectomy for radiation-induced constriction indicate that constriction is not the sole factor responsible for cardiac failure in this situation. Although cardiac failure has been attributed to myocardial atrophy caused by prolonged constriction, the excellent outcomes reported after pericardiectomy for idiopathic constrictive pericarditis suggest that constriction is rarely the only cause of cardiac failure.

Another study reported similar findings, with radiation-induced constriction leading to significantly decreased 10-year survival after pericardiectomy.[37] The authors also noted that patients who underwent pericardiectomy for radiation-induced constriction had demonstrably worse late functional status. Fifteen of 17 long-term survivors with a history of previous radiation therapy showed New York Heart Association class III or IV symptoms, whereas only 31 of 112 patients without a history of radiation therapy had major symptoms of heart failure.

Financial Disclosures: None Reported

References

1. Sagrista-Sauleda J, Angel J, Permanyer-Miralda G, Soler-Soler J. Long-term follow-up of idiopathic chronic pericardial effusion. N Engl J Med 1999;341:2054.
2. Fowler NO. Tuberculous pericarditis. JAMA 1991;266:95.
3. Butany J, El Demellawy D, Collins MJ, et al. Constrictive pericarditis: case presentation and a review of the literature. Can J Cardiol 2004;20:1137.
4. Tuna IC, Danielson GK. Surgical management of pericardial diseases. Cardiol Clin 1990;84:683.
5. Cimino JJ, Kogan AD. Constrictive pericarditis after cardiac surgery: report of three cases and review of the literature. Am Heart J 1989;118:1292.
6. Matsuyama K, Matsumoto M, Sugita T, et al. Clinical characteristics of patients with constrictive pericarditis after coronary bypass surgery. Jpn Circ J 2001;65:480.
7. Swallow RA, Thomas RD. Pericardial constriction after a stab wound to the chest. Heart 2004;90:276.
8. Isaacs D, Stark P, Nichols C, et al. Post traumatic pericardial calcification. J Thorac Imaging 2003;18:250.
9. Eren NT, Akar AR. Primary pericardial mesothelioma. Curr Treat Options Oncol 2002;3:369.
10. Quinn DW, Qureshi F, Mitchell IM. Pericardial mesothelioma: the diagnostic dilemma of misleading images. Ann Thorac Surg 2000; 69:1926.
11. Myers RBH, Spodick DH. Constrictive pericarditis: clinical and pathophysiologic characteristics. Am Heart J 1999;138:219.
12. Cottrill CM, Tamaren J, Hall B. Sternal defects associated with congenital pericardial and cardiac defects. Cardiol Young 1998; 8:100.
13. Simeunovic D, Seferovic PM, Ristic AD, et al. Pericardial cysts: incidence, clinical presentations and treatment. In: Seferovic PM, Spodick DH, Maisch B, editors. Pericardiology: contemporary answers to continuing challenges. Belgrade: Science; 2000. p. 203–9.
14. Fowler NO, Gabel M. The hemodynamic effects of cardiac tamponade: mainly the result of atrial, not ventricular, compression. Circulation 1985;71:154.
15. Ameli S, Shah PK. Cardiac tamponade: pathophysiology, diagnosis and management. Cardiol Clin 1991;9:665.
16. Spodick DH. Pathophysiology of cardiac tamponade. Chest 1998;113:1372.
17. Maisch B, Seferovid PM, Ristic AD, et al, for the Task Force on the Diagnosis and Management of Pericardial Diseases of the European Society of Cardiology. Guidelines on the diagnosis and management of pericardial diseases: executive summary. Eur Heart J 2004;25:587.
18. Nkere UU, Whawell SA, Thompson EM, et al. Changes in pericardial morphology and fibrinolytic activity during cardiopulmonary bypass. J Thorac Cardiovasc Surg 1993; 106:339.
19. Duvernow O, Borowiex J, Helmius G, et al. Complications of percutaneous pericardiocentesis under fluoroscopic guidance. Acta Radiol 1992;33:309.
20. Posner MR, Cohen GI, Skarin AT. Pericardial disease in patients with cancer. Am J Med 1981;71:407.
21. Vaitkus PT, Herrmann HC, LeWinter MM. Treatment of malignant pericardial effusion. JAMA 1994;272:59.
22. Shepherd FA, Morgan C, Evans WK, et al. Medical management of malignant pericardial effusion by tetracycline sclerosis. Am J Cardiol 1987;60:1161.
23. Davis S, Rambotti P, Grignani F. Intrapericardial tetracycline sclerosis in the treatment of malignant pericardial effusion. J Clin Oncol 1984;2:631.
24. Girardi LN, Ginsberg RJ, Burt ME. Pericardiocentesis and intrapericardial sclerosis: effective therapy for malignant pericardial effusions. Ann Thorac Surg 1997;64:1422.
25. Kopecky SL, Callahan JA, Tajik AJ, et al. Percutaneous pericardial catheter drainage: report of 42 consecutive cases. Am J Cardiol 1986;58:633.
26. del Barrio LG, Morales JH, Delgado C, et al. Percutaneous balloon pericardial window for patients with symptomatic pericardial window. Cardiovasc Intervent Radiol 2002; 25:360.
27. DiSegni E, Lavee J, Kaplinsky E, et al. Percutaneous balloon pericardiostomy for treatment of cardiac tamponade. Eur Heart J 1995;16:184.
28. Moores DWO, Allen KB, Faber LP, et al. Sub-xiphoid pericardial drainage for pericardial tamponade. J Thorac Cardiovasc Surg 1995;109:546.
29. Sugimoto JT, Little AG, Ferguson MF, et al. Pericardial window: mechanism of efficacy. Ann Thorac Surg 1990;50:442.
30. Allen KB, Faber LP, Warren WH, et al. Pericardial effusion: subxiphoid pericardiostomy versus percutaneous catheter drainage. Ann Thorac Surg 1999;67:437.
31. Dosios T, Theaskos N, Angouras D, et al. Risk factors affecting the survival of patients with pericardial effusion submitted to subxiphoid pericardiostomy. Chest 2003;124:242.
32. Flum DR, McGinn JT, Tyras DH. The role of the 'pericardial window' in AIDS. Chest 1995;107:1522.
33. Burfeind WR, D'Amico TA. VATS for mediastinal and pericardial diseases. In: Soper NL, Swanstrom LL, Eubanks WS, editors. Mastery of endoscopic and laparoscopic surgery. 2nd ed. Philadelphia: Lippincott Williams & Wilkins; 2005. p. 550–58.
34. Nataf P, Cocoub P, Regan M, et al. Video-thoracoscopic pericardial window in the diagnosis and treatment of pericardial effusions. Am J Cardiol 1998;82:124.
35. Campione A, Cacchiarelli M, Ghiribelli, et al. Which treatment in pericardial effusion? J Cardiovasc Surg 2002;43:735.
36. O'Brien PKH, Kucharczuk JC, Marshall MB, et al. Comparative study of subxiphoid versus video-thoracoscopic pericardial "window." Ann Thorac Surg 2005;80:2013.
37. Ling LH, Oh JK, Schaff HV, et al. Constrictive pericarditis in the modern era: evolving clinical spectrum and impact on outcome after pericardiectomy. Circulation 1999;100: 1380.
38. Nishimura RA. Constrictive pericarditis in the modern era: a diagnostic dilemma. Heart 2001;86:619.
39. Bertog SC, Thambidorai SK, Parakh K, et al. Constrictive pericarditis: etiology and cause-specific survival after pericardiectomy. J Am Coll Cardiol 2004;43:1445.

Acknowledgment

The authors wish to acknowledge Shari L. Meyerson, MD, for contributions to the previous rendition of this chapter on which we have based this update.

Figures 1 and 3 through 7 Alice Y. Chen.

13 DECORTICATION AND PLEURECTOMY

Eric S. Lambright, MD

The pleural space is a potential cavity between the lung and the chest wall—more specifically, between the visceral and parietal pleura. The pleura typically is less than 1 mm thick in the normal, healthy patient. However, a variety of pathologic processes can occur that alter the transport of cell and fluid within the pleural space. The processes compromising the pleural space can lead severe clinical symptoms and resultant patient compromise. By definition, a fibrothorax is characterized by the presence of abnormal fibrous tissue within the pleural space, with resultant entrapment of the underlying pulmonary parenchyma. A variety of terminology is commonly used to describe this process, including "trapped lung," restrictive pleurisy, or encased lung.

Decortication refers to the process of peeling this restrictive fibrous layer or peel from the lung and literally means stripping the "rind" from the lung. The goal of therapy is to improve patient symptoms and control any ongoing intrapleural process. Typically, surgical interventions are required. The technical goals of the operation are complete lung expansion and resolution of the pleural space pathology. If achieved, this will result in improved pulmonary function and chest wall mechanics. This translates into symptom relief for the patient. We review the common causes, physiology, and diagnosis of fibrothorax; management and indications for decortication; technical aspects of the operation, management of residual pleural space issues; and the expected outcomes.

Pleural space complications remain a clinical challenge. The therapeutic options are extremely broad, and several disciplines, including pulmonary medicine, radiology, infectious disease, and surgery, are involved in the care of the patient. Unfortunately, comparative data as to optimal therapy are lacking, and clinical judgment is typically the driver of care decisions. As such, a multidisciplinary approach is a key factor to ensuring optimal patient outcomes.

Causes and Pathophysiology of Fibrothorax

Any insult to the pleura can result in an inflammatory response with fibrin deposition and resultant fibrothorax.[1] Blood and infection (bacterial and mycobacterium) remain the common causes of fibrothorax [*see Table 1*]. Classically, empyemas evolve over a 4- to 6-week period, which is indicative of pleural space disease progression. The initial exudative phase is characterized by thin exudative fibrin fluid. This progresses to the fibropurulent phase, with a heavy fibrin deposit over the pleural surface and development of loculations and fibrinous debris within the thoracic cavity. The organization phase (3 to 5 weeks) results in a thick fibrous peel that imprisons the lung and prevents expansion. As described by Wachsmuth and Schautz, the fully developed peel consists of three layers: (1) a loosely organized vascular tissue nearest the parietal pleura; (2) a layer of fibrous connective tissue, which is relatively avascular and acellular; and (3) an inner layer consisting of necrotic tissues and fibrinoid masses.[2] Typically, small hemothoraces will reabsorb through an intact lymphatic system. Drummond and Craig found that if the hemothorax is larger, there is continued bleeding, or bacteria is present, the clot will ultimately organize, with resultant peel formation.[3]

Table 1 Common Causes of Fibrothorax
Chronic bacterial empyema
Retained hemothorax—traumatic/iatrogenic
Pleural effusive disease
Parapneumonic
Transudative
Chylous
Pancreatic
Sequelae of *Mycobacterium tuberculosis* infection
Chronic pneumothorax

Pathophysiology and Diagnosis: Preoperative Considerations

The physiologic consequences of a fibrothorax culminate in pulmonary restriction, including a decrease in lung volumes, diffusion capacity, and expiratory flows. Movement of the chest is impaired.[4] The clinical presentation of the patient who has fibrothorax depends on the underlying cause and the presence of underlying parenchymal disease. Typically, dyspnea on exertion is the most common presenting symptom. Cough, fever, pleuritic chest discomfort, malaise, night sweats, weight loss, or chest pressure may also be present. In obtaining the clinical history, one should define the chronicity of the illness and attempt to identify other underlying disease processes that may confound the pulmonary disease process. Physical examination is relatively nonspecific but typically reveals decreased breath sounds and decreased chest wall excursion.

Radiographic evaluation is the mainstay of diagnosis [*see Figures 1 and 2*]. Chest computed tomography (CT) is a required test. Malignancy must also be included in the differential diagnosis of fibrothorax and ruled out as management options are quite different. CT can assess the extent and thickness of pleural involvement and identify associated parenchymal disease. Parenchymal abnormalities such as fibrosis, bronchiectasis, and malignancy may be seen on CT imaging. Such factors would greatly impact surgical decision making. Physiologic assessment with spirometry and diffusing capacity are mandatory to define the degree of pulmonary dysfunction and assist with perioperative risk stratification. The results of pulmonary function testing may be quite abnormal preoperatively. Often pulmonary function tests are more impaired than would otherwise be anticipated by radiographic studies. Marked abnormalities

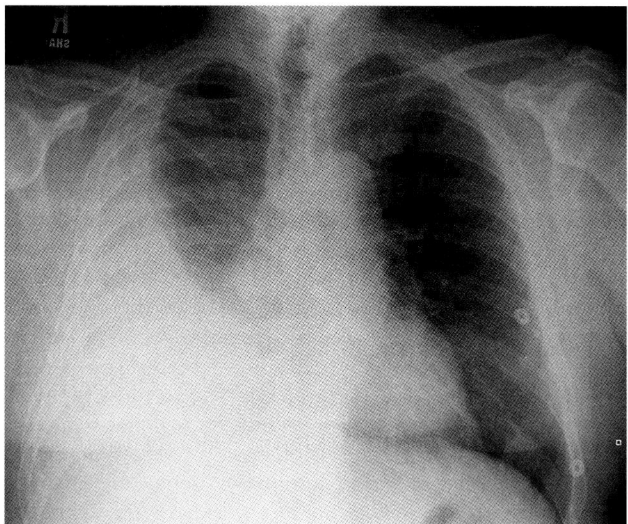

Figure 1 **Chest x-ray in a patient with a 4-month history of dyspnea and cough associated with intermittent fever and night sweats. Treatments included three courses of antibiotics and bronchodilator therapy.**

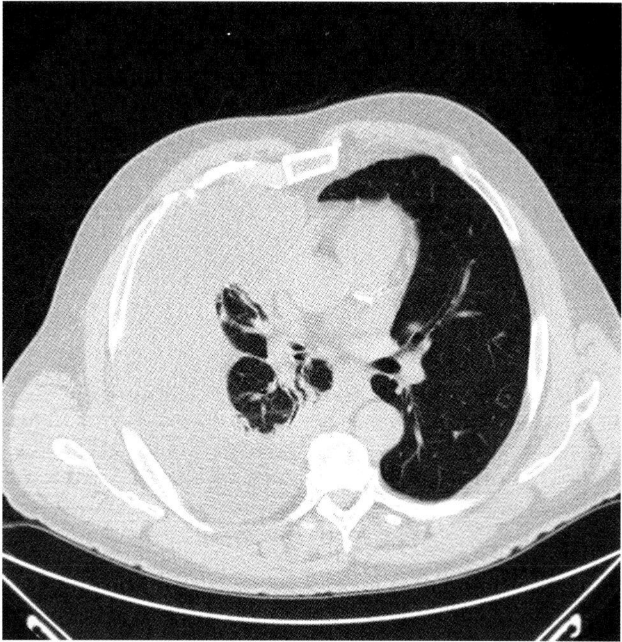

Figure 2 **Chest computed tomographic scan on the same patient documenting a large pleural effusion, pleural thickening, and atelectasis.**

in physiologic testing should not be used as absolute contraindications for surgical intervention as improvement would be anticipated. Preoperative radiographic and physiologic testing is used to provide an assessment of the expected realistic improvement in dyspnea, pulmonary reexpansion, and parenchyma function following decortication. Surgical judgment ultimately plays a key role.

The clinician must also keep in mind the possibility of a malignant pleural process. If malignancy is a concern, this diagnosis should be excluded prior to proceeding with recommended surgical therapy. If cancer is present, palliative interventions such as pleurodesis or small bore indwelling catheter placement would be more appropriate. Cytologic evaluation of the pleural fluid can typically establish the diagnosis of metastatic pleural involvement. However, pleural fluid cytology is often less helpful in providing the diagnosis of mesothelioma, a primary pleural malignancy. If the presentation of a chronic pleural process is atypical and the etiology is poorly defined, one must maintain a high degree of suspicion for malignancy. Appropriate initial pleural biopsies can be helpful to rule out underlying malignancy prior to proceeding with decortication. If malignancy is defined, therapeutic alternatives such as pleurodesis or placement of an indwelling small bore pleural catheter may be optimal.

Surgical Management

Fibrothorax is a potentially preventable disease process. As it is a manifestation of a chronic problem, intervention at an earlier stage of the disease may prevent this challenging complication. With regard to traumatic hemothorax, Pomerantz argued that early and complete drainage can prevent fibrothorax complications.[5] Observation studies have consistently demonstrated that early evacuation of clotted hemothorax decreased morbidity and mortality and prevented empyema.[6,7] Additionally, when parapneumonic effusions are thin, simple aspiration or chest tube drainage may suffice. The fibropurulent stage of loculated empyema or clotted hemothorax can often be successfully managed with thoracoscopic intervention with débridement of the intrathoracic material and irrigation, thus allowing for pulmonary reexpansion prior to the establishment of a restrictive peel.[8] These factors again reinforce the need for optimal multidisciplinary care of the patient at a time in the clinical course when morbidities of the required interventions may be less.

The indications for decortication of fibrothorax are symptoms that compromise quality of life and/or an ongoing pleural process that has systemic manifestations. Timing of the operation is an important consideration. Often pleuropulmonary processes are self-limiting, and symptoms will resolve with time. Decortication should be considered if pleural thickening has been present for a chronic period (> 4 to 6 weeks), respiratory symptoms remain disabling, and there is radiographic evidence of a reversible entrapment of the lung. Decortication is often necessary when lesser interventions have not achieved control of the pleural space infection or allowed for lung reexpansion. For tuberculosus empyema, treatment remains primarily medical. Decortication is reserved for persistent pleural effusion despite long-term medical therapy.

The surgical care for the patient with fibrothorax is multifactorial. In addition to the technical aspects of pleural space management, other factors must be considered. Often patients will have been ill for a prolonged period. Attention to the basic surgical principles of optimizing nutrition, improved control of chronic medical diseases such as diabetes or heart disease, and defining appropriate antimicrobial therapy is required to ensure the best possible patient outcomes.

A major challenge for the thoracic surgeon is a pleural space infection with underlying parenchymal disease or airway stenosis.[9,10] When there is severe underlying parenchymal disease, decortication attempts will fail and are futile. The lung parenchyma will not reexpand, and surgical intervention on the diseased lung will only aggravate the underlying process. Pleuropneumonectomy may be the only option. Decortication may be precluded by invasive uncontrolled pulmonary infection, contralateral pulmonary disease, or a chronically debilitated state with significant or prohibitive operative risk. Again, medical optimization may be required as an initial step. However, the challenge is often that the underlying pleural infectious process remains unresolved despite optimal medical management and necessitates surgical intervention in the medically fragile patient. Optimally, nutritional status should be normalized, which may require a period of forced feedings, and any systemic sepsis should be controlled with appropriate antibiotic therapy.

Conduct of Operation and Technical Considerations

The complications of pleural cavity infections and fibrosis are essentially a problem of residual intrapleural space. The lung does not adequately expand to fill the hemithorax. As such, the residual space becomes or remains infected. This is often a difficult challenge for the thoracic surgeon. Surgical judgment is required to ensure optimal outcomes. Several issues must be considered related to surgical decortication and include the following: timing of intervention with relation to a chronicity of the process, the quality of the underlying pulmonary parenchyma, the expected ability of lung reexpansion and possible need to address any residual space issues, and the physiologic status of the patient. The goal of any decortication procedure is to remove the peel from the visceral pleura of the lung so as to allow the lung to reexpand and, as importantly, to ensure obliteration of any potential residual space [*see Figure 3*].

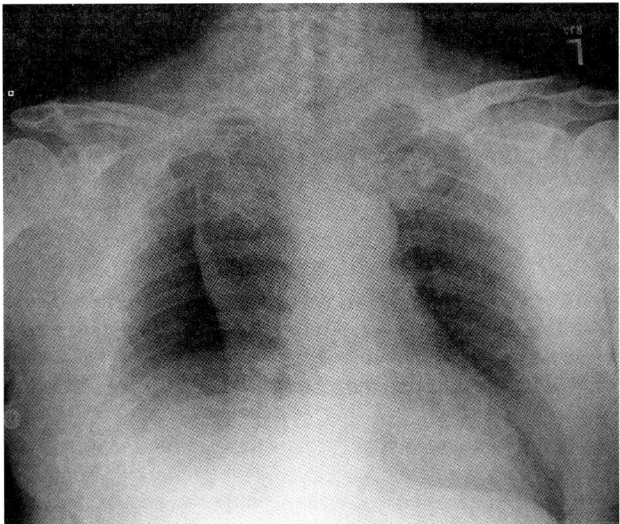

Figure 3 **Chest x-ray following thoracentesis revealing a large hydropneumothorax consistent with fibrothorax.**

Realistically, there are few absolute contraindications to pulmonary decortication. Patient operability status is critical, as with any recommended surgical procedure. In the extremely frail patient, less invasive interventions, such as chest tube thoracostomy, rib resection, or open window thoracostomy, may provide a better patient-centered outcome. An ongoing need for positive pressure ventilation is also a relative contraindication for pulmonary decortication. In general, decortication is not required for a small, well-defined residual cavity and is usually reserved for a diffuse pleural process. An accurate assessment of the chronicity of the pleural space process is required as well. In earlier pleural space infectious processes, where the peel is less organized, a thoracoscopic approach with cleansing of the pleural space, removal of the pleural debris, and deloculation may prove adequate. Thoracoscopic management to decorticate a chronic process remains debated. However, outcomes appear to be similar as experience with the techniques continues to improve.[11]

For open decortication, the surgeon must start with bronchoscopy to evaluate for endobronchial obstruction, which may prevent satisfactory lung expansion. Unexpected findings may include malignancy, bronchial stenosis, or broncholith. Initial thoracoscopic exploration may be warranted if malignancy remains a clinical concern. The chest is entered in the appropriate predetermined interspace, often the fifth or sixth interspace, through a standard posterolateral thoracotomy. Alternatively, a vertical axillary thoracotomy incision may be a reasonable option. Regardless of the approach, the latissimus dorsi and serratus anterior muscles should be spared as either or both could potentially be used as a transposition muscle flap should pleural space challenges persist. A rib is often resected in a subperiostial fashion to facilitate exposure as the chest is often rigid and contracted from the underlying inflammatory process. This rib removal facilitates exposure and may be helpful to initially define an extrapleural plane for the initiation of parietal pleurectomy. In chronic (> 6 weeks) conditions, the parietal and visceral pleura are often partially fused, and one would then proceed with planned pleurectomy. When present, adhesions between the visceral and parietal pleura are lysed with a combination of sharp and electrocautery dissection.

The key to a technically successful decortication is to define the correct plane between the parietal peel and the visceral pleura.[12] If the pleural resection is inadequate, lung expansion is compromised; thus, the clinical results of the operation would be suboptimal. When the pleurectomy is too deep, there is parenchymal injury with resultant bleeding and air leakage. These factors may result in a prolonged postoperative recovery. Gentle hand ventilation on the operative lung or the addition of continuous positive airway pressure (CPAP) is helpful to provide appropriate countertension from the underlying lung parenchyma. Incision of the pleural peel is made sharply over a broad area, and the appropriate plane is identified. The pleural peel is grasped with hemostats, and, working over a broad area, the surgeon then proceeds with blunt and sharp dissection of the peel from the visceral pleura. A sponge ball or "peanut" dissector can be helpful with this. Care must be taken to protect the underlying fragile pulmonary parenchyma as inadvertent injury may result in prolonged and unnecessary air leaks. The integrity of the underlying pulmonary parenchyma is far less than the fibrotic feel and will be significantly injured if dissection is too aggressive. Patience is required as quite often the operation becomes very tedious. To ensure an optimal surgical outcome, all portions of the lung encased by the peel should be addressed, which often requires following the peel into the fissure, down onto the diaphragm, and into the posterior and anterior sulci. At times, entrance into the chest through an additional interspace is required to ensure an optimal technical result. The surgeon should not hesitate to proceed with this counterincision through an additional interspace should the additional exposure be deemed necessary [*see Table 2*].[12]

The peel should be sent for appropriate pathologic and microbiologic evaluation. The lung is tested to ensure complete reexpansion. Large parenchymal air leaks can be oversewn, but this is often unnecessary and risks additional lung injury. One may consider use of commercially available pulmonary parenchymal sealants for control of parenchymal air leaks. Chest tubes are placed for wide drainage of the chest: one tube along the diaphragm, one anterior, and one posterior toward the apex. Provided that there was satisfactory parenchyma reexpansion, any pulmonary air leaks will promptly resolve with simple drainage once positive pressure is discontinued. Hemostasis must be ensured as residual hemothorax in the setting of a pleural space infection is a nidus for ongoing infection challenges.

The role for parietal pleurectomy remains unclear. Opinions differ, but objective data regarding the optimal approach are sparse. The mechanics of the thoracic cage improve with parietal pleurectomy.[13] However, parietal pleurectomy adds to the risk of bleeding, prolongs the procedure, and places intrathoracic vital structures (phrenic and vagus nerves, esophagus, brachial plexus, vascular structures) at risk. Additionally, the pleural process may resolve once the underlying issues are addressed. A compromise approach with partial parietal pleurectomy with care in the dissection near the vital mediastinal structures may be technically optimal.

Table 2 Conduct of Pulmonary Decortication

Conduct of Pulmonary Decortication
Preoperative evaluation
Chest computed tomography
Complete pulmonary function testing
Nutritional assessment
Control of systemic illness with appropriate antibiotics
Optimal management of chronic medical comorbidities
Operative planning
Lateral decubitus for thoracotomy
General anesthesia with double-lumen endotracheal tube
Operative technique
Bronchoscopy
Thoracotomy (muscle sparing recommended)
Rib resection (define extrapleural plane)
Lysis of adhesions between visceral and parietal pleura
Débridement of intrapleural debris
Identification of appropriate decortication plane
Complete decortication (into fissure and onto the diaphragmatic surface)
Partial parietal pleurectomy
Assessment of pulmonary parenchyma and reexpansion
Wide chest tube drainage

Management of chest tubes postoperatively is dictated by the culture results, intraoperative findings, and clinical status of the patient [*see Figure 4*]. Residual space concerns may be managed by open tube thoracostomy, open window thoracostomy, or placement of a muscle flap. Rarely, thoracoplasty must be considered to obliterate any residual space infection.

Results

Morbidity and mortality following decortication depend on the severity of the underlying illness and perioperative complications. Mayo reported mortality of less than 8%.[14] Complications are often infection related, with perioperative sepsis syndrome, or technically related, including bronchopleural fistula, hemorrhage, or persisting air leaks. Additional surgical intervention may be required to address these. As with all operations in the chest, attention to detail with meticulous surgical technique is required to lessen the rates of these postoperative challenges [*see Table 3*].

Functional improvement following decortication is mostly dependent on the extent of underlying lung parenchymal disease.[15–17] Complete lung reexpansion and obliteration of the pleural space should be achieved if the lung is otherwise normal. Decortication is usually followed by measurable improvement in lung volumes, although, typically, they do not return to normal.[15,18] Changes in the chest with mediastinal shift and diaphragm elevation, with a resultant decrease in the size of the thorax, may account for these findings. The relation of the chronicity of the pleural process is unclear in terms of expected functional improvement. Some authors suggest that a shorter duration of pleural disease prior to treatment is associated with improved outcomes.[19,20] Others have not observed this.[15] Failure to achieve improvement following decortication is most related to surgical judgment related to patient selection and surgical technique, with resultant perioperative complications.

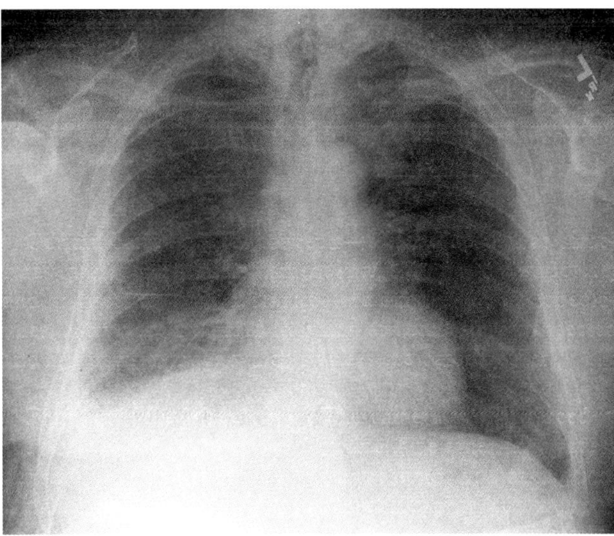

Figure 4 Postoperative chest x-ray on the sixth postoperative day in the same patient following decortication documenting complete reexpansion of the lung.

Table 3 Causes of Failed Decortication
Underlying pulmonary disease
Active tuberculosis or invasive pulmonary infection
Bronchial stenosis
Chronicity of lung collapse
Technical considerations
Residual space
Incomplete decortication
Air leakage
Postoperative hemothorax

Although there are no specific studies related to failure following decortication, technical challenges are probably the most common cause of failure, with the main problem being inadequate obliteration of the pleural space. A confounding technical challenge can be the inability to define the plane of dissection between the peel and the visceral pleura. If visceral pleurectomy is performed, air-leak and postoperative hemorrhage may compromise pulmonary function. The phrenic nerve must also be protected throughout the operation. This is typically not an issue as the mediastinal pleura is not typically involved in the inflammatory process. Incomplete parietal pleurectomy or inability to free the diaphragm may also compromise results.

Complete reexpansion of the lung following decortication will typically be achieved in the appropriately selected patient. However, the surgeon must recognize a residual pleural space issue following otherwise technically satisfactory successful decortication. This space must be obliterated, or failure is predictable. Options to address the residual space problem include thoracoplasty or tissue transposition. The latissimus dorsi muscle and the abdominal omentum provide satisfactory bulk for space obliteration.[21,22] The omentum is most helpful for issues in the inferior hemithorax, whereas the latissimus is better for the superior hemithorax. The surgeon must keep these facts in mind at the time of thoracotomy and should preferentially consider a muscle-sparing thoracotomy approach.

The use of thoracoscopy to definitively address fibrothorax continues to evolve [*see Figure 5*]. Thoracoscopy appears to have a clear clinical advantage over open thoracotomy in managing the earlier stages of empyema and clotted hemothorax.[8] There is a growing experience with the use of thoracoscopic techniques for the management of fibrothorax.[11,23,24] As with any minimally invasive operative, the technical goals of the operation must not be compromised. Complete lung expansion and avoidance of pulmonary parenchymal injury are critical. Common themes in the literature[11,23,24] related to thoracoscopic decortication and improved outcomes correlate with increased technical experience and the timeliness of appropriate surgical intervention. These observations suggest that appropriate use of centers with experience and expertise with these procedures may be optimal for clinical care.

Summary

Fibrothorax can be a challenging surgical problem. The successful management of the patient with fibrothorax requires adherence to basic surgical tenets: appropriate

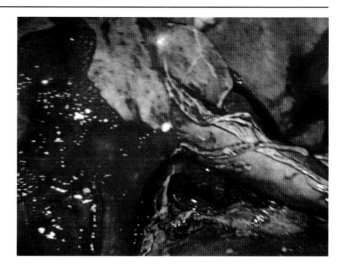

Figure 5 **Thoracoscopic appearance of the lung with fibrin peel. The lung did not expand, even with positive pressure ventilation to 35 cm water pressure. Decortication was required.**

patient selection for surgery, preoperative optimization, exacting attention to the technical aspects of the procedure, and timely interventions for perioperative events. Failure to achieve improvement in patient symptoms or physiologic status following decortication may result from inattention to any of these important details and render the patient in an even more physiologically compromised state. Insights into these important factors with attention to the technical aspects of decortication have been provided. The combined expertise of the pulmonary medicine team, radiology, and the surgical team is typically needed to ensure optimal patient-centered outcomes.

Financial Disclosures: None Reported

References

1. Samson PC. Some surgical considerations in pulmonary decortication. Am J Surg 1955;89:364.
2. Wachsmuth W, Schautz R. Untersuchungen uber die Lungen-Pleura-Grenzschicht beider extrapleuralen Dekortikation. Chirurg 1961;22:237.
3. Drummond DS, Craig RH. Traumatic hemothorax: complications and management. Am Surg 1967;33:404.
4. Bollinger CT, de Kock MA. Influence of a fibrothorax on the flow volume curve. Respiration 1988;54:197.
5. Pomerantz M. Discussion of Wilson JM, et al. Traumatic hemothorax: is decortication necessary? J Thorac Cardiovasc Surg 1979;77:494.
6. Milfield DJ, Mattox KL, Beall AC. Early evacuation of clotted hemothorax. Am J Surg 1978;136:686.
7. Beall AC, Crawford HW, DeBakey ME. Considerations in the management of acute traumatic hemothorax. J Thorac Cardiovasc Surg 1966;52:353.
8. Deslauriers J, Mehran RJ. Role of thoracoscopy in the diagnosis and management of pleural disease. Semin Thorac Cardiovasc Surg 1993;5:284.

9. Savage T, Flemin JA. Decortication of the lung in tuberculous disease. Thorax 1955;10:293.
10. Magdeleinat P, Icard P, Pouzet B, et al. Indications actuelles et resultats des decortications pulmonaries pour pleurisies purulentes non tuberculeuses. Ann Chir 1999;53:41.
11. Tong BC, Hanna J, Toloza EM, et al. Outcomes of video-assisted thoracoscopic decortication. Ann Thor Surg 2010;89:220.
12. Kaiser LR. Pleurectomy and decortication. In: Atlas of general thoracic surgery. Philadelphia: Mosby-Year Book; 1997.
13. Waterman DH, Domm SE, Roger WK. A clinical evaluation of decortication. J Thorac Cardiovasc Surg 1957;33:1.
14. Mayo P. Early thoracotomy and decortication for nontuberculous empyema in adults with and without underlying disease. A twenty-five year review. Am Surg 1985;51:230.
15. Patton WE, Watson TR, Gaensler EA. Pulmonary function before and at intervals after surgical decortication of the lun. Surg Gynecol Obstet 1952;95:477.
16. Siebens AA, Storey CF, Newman MM, et al. The physiological effects of fibrothorax and the functional results of surgical treatment. J Thorac Surg 1956;32:53.
17. Barker WL, Neuhaus H, Langston HT. Ventilatory improvement following decortication in pulmonary tuberculosis. Ann Thor Surg 1965;1:532.
18. LeMense GF, Strange CH, Sahn S. Empyema thoracis: therapeutic management and outcome. Chest 1994;107:1532.
19. Carroll D, McClement J, Himmelstein A, Cournand A. Pulmonary function following decortication of the lung. Am Rev Tuberc 1951;63:231.
20. Morton JR, Boushy SF, Guinn GA. Physiological evaluation of results of pulmonary decortication. Ann Thorac Surg 1970;4:321.
21. Marshall MD, Kaiser LR, Kucharczuk JC. Simple technique for maximal thoracic muscle harvest. Ann Thorac Surg 2004;4:1465.
22. Shrager JB, Wain JC, Wright CD, et al. Omentum is highly effective in the management of complex cardiothoracic surgical problems. J Thorac Cardiovasc Surg 2003;125:526.
23. Waller DA, Rengarajan A. Thoracoscopic decortication: a role for video-assisted surgery in chronic postpneumonic pleural empyema. Ann Thor Surg 2001;71:1813.
24. Manunga J, Olak J. Is thoracoscopic decortication sufficient for the treatment of empyema? Am Surgeon 2010;76:1050.

14 PULMONARY RESECTION

Min P. Kim, MD, and Ara Vaporciyan, MD, FACS

Anatomic resections of the lung (including pneumonectomy and lobectomy) are the standard operative techniques employed to treat both neoplastic and nonneoplastic diseases of the lung. In neoplastic disease of the lung the disease process can be divided between primary and metastatic lung cancers. In patients with primary lung cancer, the staging of the patient is critical to provide best therapy for the patient. There is no role of pulmonary resection for patients with metastatic disease or stage IV disease. In terms of the nodal stations, pulmonary resection maybe offered in patients with N1 disease or metastatic cancer to ipsilateral hilar lymph nodes (level 10, 11, 12, 13, 14). There is controversy about the role of pulmonary resection in patients with N2 disease or metastatic cancer to ipsilateral mediastinal lymph nodes (on right: level 2R, 4R, 7 and on left: level 2L, 4L, 5, 6, 7). The options include either induction chemotherapy followed by surgery then consolidative radiation to the mediastinum, induction chemoradiotherapy followed by surgery, or chemoradiation therapy without surgery. The final option is most commonly chosen when multiple N2 lymph nodes are involved, the nodal disease is bulky and deemed unresectable, or when the surgical risk is felt to be too high (for example when a right pneumonectomy is required). Finally, there is no role for pulmonary resection in patients with N3 disease or metastatic cancer to contralateral mediastinal lymph nodes. In patients with no nodal or metastatic disease, pulmonary resection is a primary therapy. Any surgeon who intends to operate on the pulmonary system must be keenly aware of the anatomy of the pulmonary vasculature and the bronchi and the relation between the two. There is no substitute for this degree of familiarity. Detailed discussions are available in existing anatomy textbooks. In what follows, we describe several of the more common techniques employed for anatomic resections of the lung.

Preoperative Evaluation

Detailed discussion of the physiologic evaluation of the patient and of the indications for lobectomy or pneumonectomy is beyond the scope of this chapter. In general, the patient must have sufficient pulmonary reserve to tolerate the planned resection. A common contraindication for surgery is an estimated postresectional forced expiratory volume in 1 second (FEV_1) and carbon monoxide diffusion capacity (DLCO) of less than 35 to 40%. The choice of what volume of lung to resect for lung cancer should be a balance between achieving an adequate oncologic outcome and preservation of pulmonary function. When wedge resection was compared with lobectomy for tumors smaller than 3 cm there was a higher local recurrence rate after a wedge resection compared with a lobectomy. Based on these data the current recommendation is to perform a lobectomy if the patient's pulmonary status will tolerate that volume of resection. A minimally invasive lobectomy can be substituted for an open lobectomy although the presence of hilar nodal involvement by tumor or granulomatous disease is a relative contraindication to this procedure. For metastatic tumors and diagnostic resections of pulmonary nodules a wedge resection, if feasible, is considered adequate. In addition, it is essential to carry out a thorough evaluation of all other systems, especially the cardiac system. In patients who have received preoperative chemotherapy, the hematologic and renal systems should receive particular attention.

Operative Planning

ANESTHESIA

Although pulmonary resections can be performed with bilateral lung ventilation, careful hilar dissection is greatly facilitated by using unilateral lung ventilation. The advent of double-lumen endotracheal tubes and bronchial blockers has made it possible to isolate the ipsilateral lung and has made it easier for surgeons to carry out complex hilar dissections with the required precision. In patients with centrally located tumors, care must be taken with tube placement: inadvertent trauma to an endobronchial tumor during placement of a double-lumen tube can lead to significant bleeding and compromise of the airway. Bronchoscopic confirmation of tube position is recommended after the patient has been positioned.

Requirements for monitoring and intravenous access are determined by the patient's preoperative status and by the complexity of the resection. In most cases, the standard practice is to place a radial arterial catheter, two large-bore peripheral intravenous catheters, and a Foley catheter, with more invasive monitoring employed if mandated by the patient's clinical condition. Thoracic epidural catheters are also commonly employed for postoperative pain control. If carefully placed by an experienced anesthesiologist, these catheters can remain in place for as long as 7 days or until the chest tubes are removed.

PATIENT POSITIONING

Patients are routinely placed in the lateral decubitus position, with the table flexed just cephalad to the superior iliac crest. This positioning allows sufficient access for most incisions. If an anterior thoracotomy or a sternotomy is planned, the patient may be placed in the supine position, with a pillow placed in such a way as to elevate the area of the thorax that will be operated on.

When the patient is in the lateral decubitus position, several measures should be adopted to guard against injury. Adequate padding should be employed to prevent the development of pressure points on the contralateral lower extremity. A low axillary roll should be used to prevent injury to the contralateral brachial plexus and shoulder girdle. Finally, adequate padding should be placed beneath the head to keep the cervical spine in a neutral position.

GENERAL TECHNICAL CONSIDERATIONS

Incisions

Posterior lateral thoracotomy remains the standard incision for anatomic pulmonary resections; however, safe and complete resections can also be performed through a variety of smaller incisions, including posterior muscle-sparing, anterior muscle-sparing, and axillary thoracotomies. In most cases, the thorax is entered at the fifth intercostal space, an approach that affords excellent exposure of the hilar structures. The anterior muscle-sparing thoracotomy is generally placed at the fourth intercostal space because of the more caudal positioning of the anterior aspects of the ribs. Although a sternotomy may be employed to gain access to the upper lobes, it does not provide good exposure of the lower lobes and the bronchi.

Thoracoscopic lobectomy [*see 5:10 Video-Assisted Thoracic Surgery*] is being performed with increasing frequency, especially for early-stage lesions. This procedure employs two or three 1 cm ports and a utility thoracotomy (frequently in the axillary position) for instrumentation and removal of the specimen. Rib spreading is not necessary, because visualization is achieved via the thoracoscope. The various thoracoscopic lobar resections are generally similar with regard to isolation and division of the hilar vessels and bronchi. Complete nodal dissections are also performed thoracoscopically. The main advantages of this approach seem to be reduced postoperative pain and earlier return to normal activity, but to date, no randomized trials have shown these advantages to be significant. Because of the technical challenges posed by thoracoscopic pulmonary resections, surgeons should have a complete mastery of the hilar anatomy before attempting these procedures.

Special Intraoperative Issues

Upon entry into the thoracic cavity, all benign-appearing filmy adhesions should be mobilized. Any malignant-appearing, broad-based, or dense adhesions should be noted, and a decision whether to perform an extrapleural dissection or a chest wall resection should be made on the basis of the depth of involvement and the preoperative imaging studies. If there is reason to believe that the chest wall or the parietal pleura may be involved, a more aggressive approach may be required to achieve a complete resection. These techniques are beyond the scope of this chapter.

Once the lung is freed of all adhesions, the inferior pulmonary ligament is divided and the lung rendered completely atelectatic. The entire lung and the parietal pleura are inspected and palpated. In patients with malignant disease, biopsies of any suspicious nodules are performed. The presence or absence of pleural fluid should be noted; if fluid is present, it should be aspirated and sent for immediate cytologic analysis.

Frequently, the fissures are incomplete as a consequence of congenital absence, inflammatory disease, or a neoplasm. If the adhesions within the fissure are filmy, they may be divided sharply or with the electrocautery while the lung is being ventilated. If the adhesions are more densely adherent, the fissures may have to be completed with staplers. During resection for malignancy, any evidence of tumor extension across a fissure or of hilar nodal involvement should be noted. A decision is then made regarding the extent of the required resection. If there is only minor extension, wedge resection of a portion of the additional lobe is indicated. If, however, the involvement is significant, segmentectomy, bilobectomy, or pneumonectomy may be indicated. Often we develop the fissures during ventilation until a dense or incomplete region is encountered, at which point we complete the remainder of the fissure with staples. For this approach to work, the vascular and bronchial anatomy must already have been completely delineated. If the vascular structures cannot be identified in the fissure because the fissure is fused, the pulmonary artery branches will have to be approached from the anterior and posterior hilum.

Traditionally, during a lobectomy, the arterial branches are divided first, followed by the venous branches. However, if conditions exist that limit exposure (e.g., a centrally placed tumor or significant inflammation and scarring), the surgeon should start with the structures that provide the most accessible targets. Veins may be ligated first. Proponents of this approach believe that it may limit the escape of circulating tumor cells (an event that rarely, if ever, occurs); opponents claim that initial vein ligation may lead to venous congestion and retention of blood that is subsequently lost with the specimen, although peribronchial venous channels will frequently prevent this result. The bronchus may also be ligated first. However, two points should be kept in mind if this is done. First, the distal limb of the bronchus (the specimen side) should be oversewn to prevent drainage of mucus into the chest. Second, after division of the bronchus, the lobe is much more mobile; therefore, to prevent avulsion of the pulmonary artery branches, care should be taken not to employ excessive torsion or traction.

The techniques used for dissection, ligation, and division of pulmonary arteries and their branches differ from those used for other vessels. Pulmonary vessels are low-pressure, high-flow, thin-walled, fragile structures. Accordingly, for rapid and safe dissection, a perivascular plane, known as the plane of Leriche, should be sought. This plane may be absent in the presence of long-standing granulomatous or tuberculous disease, after major chemotherapy, after thoracic radiotherapy, and in cases of reoperation. In these situations, proximal control of the main pulmonary artery and the two pulmonary veins may be necessary before the more peripheral arterial dissection can be started. Before any pulmonary vessel is divided, it should be controlled either with two separate suture ligatures proximal to the line of division or with vascular staples; stapling devices are especially useful for larger vessels.

Exposure of the bronchus should not involve stripping the bronchial surface of its adventitia. Aggressive dissection may compromise the vascular supply and lead to impaired healing and bronchial dehiscence. Overlying nodal tissues should be cleared, and major bronchial arteries should be clipped just proximal to the point of division. Bronchial closure has been greatly facilitated by the use of automatic staplers. Because the bronchus is frequently the last structure to be divided before removal of the specimen, we often apply staples only to the proximal side of the bronchus and divide the bronchus distal to the staple line. Once the stapler is applied, every effort should be made to minimize its movement during firing so as to prevent injury to the remaining proximal bronchial segment. With the stapler applied but not yet fired, the remaining lung should be ventilated to determine whether there is any impairment of ventilation secondary to placement of the stapler too close to a proximal lobar bronchus. Only when the absence of ventilatory impairment has been confirmed should the stapler be fired. When bronchial length is limited, one may perform suture closure of the bronchial stump rather than attempt to force a stapler around the bronchus. Whenever there is a high risk of bronchial stump dehiscence (e.g., after chemotherapy, radiotherapy, or chemoradiotherapy; in patients for whom adjuvant therapy is planned; or after right pneumonectomy), a vascularized rotational tissue flap (e.g., from the pericardium, the pericardial fat pad, or intercostal muscle) should be used to reinforce the bronchial closure.

Closure and Drainage

Once the bronchial closure is complete, the next step is to test its adequacy. The bronchial stump is submerged under normal saline, and the lung is inflated to a tracheal pressure of 45 cm H_2O. Any area of hilar dissection and divided fissures should be evaluated in a similar fashion. Significant parenchymal air leaks should be repaired with interrupted fine sutures (e.g., 4-0 polypropylene). If the air leak is from a diffuse raw surface, especially after upper lobectomy, construction of a pleural tent should be considered. Any air leak from the bronchial stump should be assessed very carefully. A simple repair with fine absorbable sutures may suffice, or the entire closure may have to be redone. Strong consideration should be given to reinforcing the stump with vascularized tissue (see above).

The chest is usually drained with two chest tubes that are positioned anteriorly and posteriorly and exit through separate stab incisions in the chest wall. If an epidural or a paravertebral catheter is being employed for postoperative pain management, the chest tubes should exit through an intercostal space that is no more than two spaces below the intercostal space used for entry into the chest. Failure to follow this recommendation is likely to result in pain originating from the chest tube site that will not be adequately addressed postoperatively and will lead to a significant increase in discomfort.

After a pneumonectomy, the chest tubes can be omitted. If this option is chosen, a needle should be used to aspirate 1,000 to 1,200 mL of air from the hemithorax operated on after closure of the skin. If a chest tube is used, a balanced drainage system is employed without suction. At most institutions, suction is employed postoperatively for all other resections (i.e., lobectomy, segmentectomy, and wedge resection); however, careful use of water seal in selected patients (i.e., those with small air leaks whose lungs do not collapse while on water seal) may allow earlier withdrawal of the tube.

Operative Technique

INITIAL STEPS

After making a posterior lateral thoracotomy and exposing the chest cavity through the fifth intercostal space, the inferior pulmonary ligament is taken down and the hilum is mobilized. A lung grasper is used to provide tension on the lower lobe, and the inferior pulmonary ligament is taken down using a cautery or bluntly to the inferior pulmonary vein. One needs to be very careful not to injure the pulmonary vein. After this is done, the lung is freed of any filmy pleural attachments. Dense attachments may indicate chest wall involvement and should be approached as such.

RIGHT LUNG

Right Hilar Dissection

In the right thoracic cavity, it is important to identify the inferior pulmonary vein draining the right lower lobe, superior pulmonary vein draining the right upper and right middle lobe, the main pulmonary artery, and the truncus anterior branch of the pulmonary artery. In addition, the right main bronchus and the right upper-lobe takeoff and the right bronchus intermedius should be identified. Then the lung is rotated posteriorly, and the pleura is incised posterior to the course of the phrenic nerve, which usually passes close to the base of the superior pulmonary vein. The phrenic nerve is carefully and gently mobilized anteriorly, avoiding the use of cautery. This will expose the superior pulmonary vein and inferior pulmonary vein. The right upper lobe is then rotated more inferiorly to provide a better view of the superior aspect of the hilum. This step allows complete exposure of the truncus anterior branch of the pulmonary artery. Finally, the lung is rotated anteriorly, and the right main bronchus as well as the right upper-lobe bronchus and the bronchus intermedius are exposed.

Right Upper Lobectomy

Pulmonary arteries: truncus anterior and posterior ascending Two branches of the pulmonary artery go into the right upper lobe: the truncus anterior and posterior ascending arteries. The truncus anterior is the first branch coming off the main pulmonary artery and, most of the time, is a large branch that immediately bifurcates to two arteries; however, at times two truncus anterior arteries may be coming off the pulmonary artery. It is imperative that dissection be performed with care. Once the vessel is exposed, it is either suture-ligated and divided or transected with an endovascular stapler.

It is very important to accurately identify all the vessels to prevent inadvertent ligation of the wrong artery. To expose the posterior ascending pulmonary artery, the dissection begins within the interlobar fissure, and the pulmonary artery is exposed at the junction of the major and minor fissures [*see Figure 1*]. In many cases, the artery is partially obscured by a level 11 interlobar lymph node, which should be removed. Also

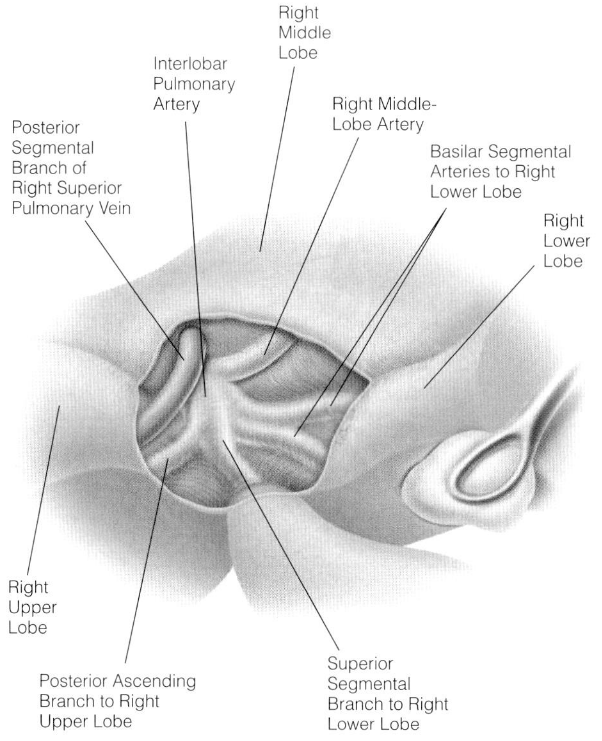

Figure 1 **Right upper lobectomy. Shown is the surgeon's view of the right interlobar fissure. The fissures have been completed, and the segmental arteries to the upper, middle, and lower lobes have been identified. The posterior ascending branch to the upper lobe most commonly varies with respect to size and origin. This vessel may be absent or diminutive and may arise from the superior segmental branch to the lower lobe. The posterior segmental vein draining into the superior pulmonary vein (not seen) is clearly visualized in the right upper lobe, lateral to the pulmonary artery branches.**

present is the posterior segmental branch of the superior pulmonary vein, which traverses the fissure in a posterior-to-anterior direction. The pulmonary artery lies medial and inferior to this venous branch. Once the pulmonary artery is identified, the branches within the fissure are exposed, including the posterior ascending artery to the right upper lobe. The posterior ascending artery typically comes off the main pulmonary artery opposite to the right middle-lobe pulmonary artery. However, at times there may be no posterior ascending artery or there may be two posterior ascending arteries, or the posterior ascending artery may originate as a branch of the superior segment artery to the right lower lobe. Distal to the posterior ascending artery is the superior segmental artery to the right lower lobe and the basilar branches to the right lower lobe. If the exposure is adequate, the posterior ascending branch can be ligated and divided.

Fissure between the right lower lobe and the right upper lobe If additional length is required to expose the posterior ascending artery, the fissure between the superior segment of the lower lobe and the posterior segment of the upper lobe can be completed. This is accomplished by opening the pleura in the posterior hilum along the lateral edge of the bronchus intermedius. A level 11 lymph node will be encountered between the right upper-lobe bronchus and the bronchus intermedius. Removal of this interlobar node (sometimes referred to as the "sump node") will expose the posterior ascending branch of the pulmonary artery. A right-angle clamp can be passed from the interlobar fissure between the superior segmental branch of the pulmonary artery and the posterior ascending pulmonary artery to the opening between the right upper-lobe bronchus and the bronchus intermedius. A silk can be placed through this opening, which will guide in separation of the right upper lobe and the right lower lobe. The fissure can be completed with gastrointestinal anastomosis (GIA) staplers. The posterior ascending artery can be ligated and divided after completion of the fissure.

Pulmonary vein: right upper-lobe branch of the superior pulmonary vein The superior pulmonary vein is dissected, and the apical, anterior, and posterior branches are encircled [*see Figure 2*]. Care is taken to preserve the middle-lobe branches. Both the right upper lobe and the middle lobe often drain into the superior pulmonary vein. However, at times the right middle lobe may drain into the inferior pulmonary vein or into both the superior and the inferior pulmonary vein. The right middle-lobe pulmonary vein branch has to be clearly identified prior to taking the right upper-lobe pulmonary vein branches. The branches draining the upper lobe are then ligated and divided or controlled with a vascular stapler. Division of the veins before division of the arterial supply will not cause the lobe to become engorged. Instead, through collateral venous drainage to the middle lobe or via bronchial venous channels, blood will be shunted away from the upper lobe.

Fissure between the right upper lobe and the right middle lobe After the division of the right upper-lobe pulmonary veins, the interlobar (or truncus posterior) branch of the right pulmonary artery will be visible as it courses posterior to the superior pulmonary vein branches. Dissection continues along the lateral surface of the interlobar artery. Once the branches to the middle-lobe artery are identified, the dissection should reach the region previously dissected within the fissure. A right-angle clamp can be used to pass a silk along this opening and keep the right middle pulmonary artery and vein with the right middle lobe. The fissure between the middle lobe and the upper lobe can now be completed through serial application of GIA staplers.

Right upper-lobe bronchus The upper lobe is retracted superiorly and posteriorly, and the interlobar artery is gently retracted anteriorly. The bronchus to the right upper lobe is circumferentially exposed, and all nodal tissue surrounding the right upper-lobe bronchus is swept distally so that it can be included with the specimen. Every effort is made to avoid devascularizing the bronchus. Once an adequate length of the right upper-lobe bronchus is exposed, the lung is rotated anteriorly to allow visualization of the course of the bronchus intermedius. The bronchus is ligated with a transverse anastomosis (TA)–30 stapler loaded with 4.8 mm staples. Care is taken to achieve close apposition of the anterior wall to the posterior membranous wall of the bronchus. With the stapler applied but not fired, the right lung is ventilated to confirm that the bronchus intermedius has not been compromised. The stapler is fired, the bronchus is divided, and the specimen is removed.

To prevent middle-lobe syndrome resulting from torsion of the narrow hilum of the middle lobe after an upper lobectomy, the middle lobe should be secured to the lower lobe. Once the lungs are reexpanded, a small portion of the lower lobe and a comparable portion of the middle lobe are grasped along the major fissure. A single application (or, at most, two applications) of a TA stapler should suffice to secure the lobes to each other at this site and thus prevent middle-lobe torsion.

Right Middle Lobectomy

Pulmonary arteries: one or two right middle-lobe pulmonary arteries The initial steps in a right middle lobectomy are similar to those in a right upper lobectomy. The pulmonary artery and its branches are identified within the fissure. The middle-lobe artery is identified [*see Figure 1*]. Not infrequently, there are two middle-lobe arteries. When this is the case, the most proximal branch is commonly located across from the posterior ascending branch to the right upper lobe. Once the anatomy has been confirmed, the arterial branches to the middle lobe can be individually ligated and divided. If additional exposure is needed before ligation, the fissures can be completed to yield added exposure of a proximal middle-lobe artery.

Pulmonary vein: right middle-lobe branch of the superior pulmonary vein Once the arteries are divided (or if additional exposure is required), the lung is rotated posteriorly to expose the superior pulmonary vein [*see Figure 2*]. The branches to the middle lobe are carefully identified, doubly ligated, and divided. The posterior segmental branch of the superior pulmonary vein should now be easily identifiable, originating just cephalad to the middle-lobe vein and coursing posteriorly (lateral to the interlobar artery) to drain the posterior segment of the right upper lobe. As noted (see above), this venous branch is easily identified during dissection of the interlobar artery within the fissure.

Fissure between the right upper and middle lobes and fissure between the right middle and lower lobes To complete the fissure between the upper and middle lobes, dissection continues along the caudal and lateral surface of the posterior segmental venous branch until the previously performed dissection of the interlobar artery within the fissure is reached. The fissure is then completed through serial application of GIA staplers. When the fissure is complete, the surgeon has a clear view of the posterior segmental branch of the superior pulmonary vein and the interlobar branch of the pulmonary artery coursing posterior and medial to the veins. If the proximal arterial branch to the middle lobe could not be safely ligated from the fissure before, it should be easily accessible now. The fissure between the right middle and lower lobes can be completed using serial application of the GIA staplers by keeping the right middle lobe and the right middle-lobe bronchus to one side and the right lower lobe

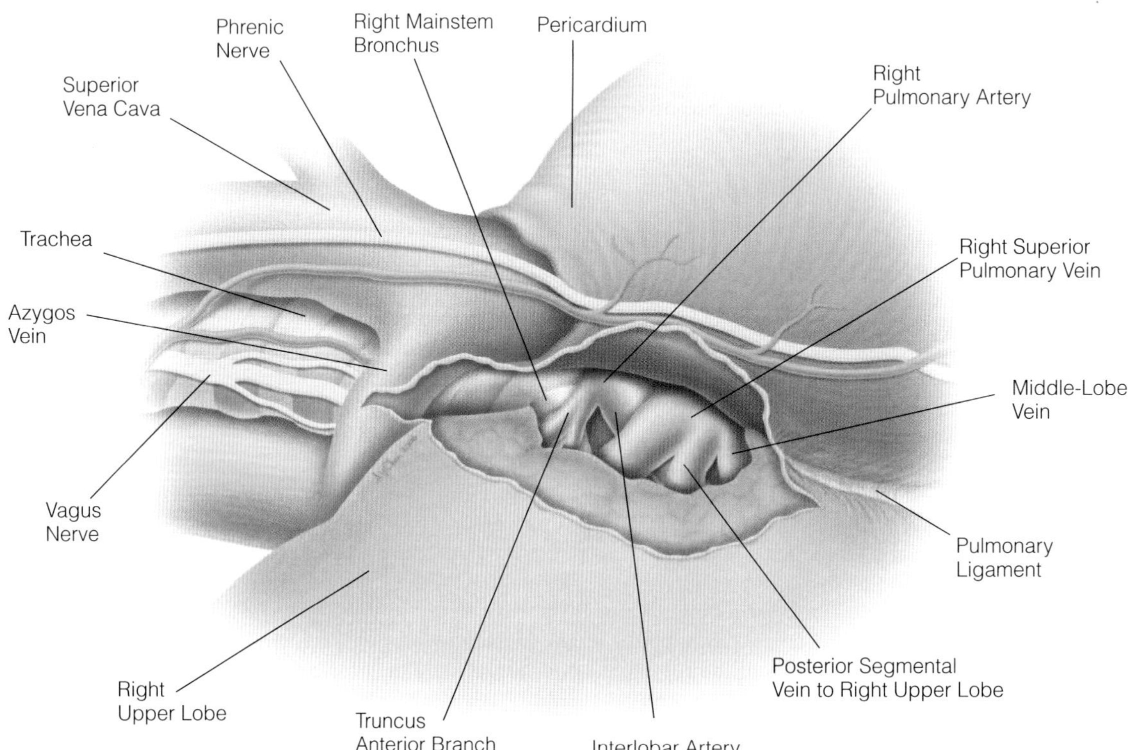

Figure 2 **Right upper lobectomy. Shown is the surgeon's view of the anterior right hilum. The apical venous branches of the superior pulmonary vein obscure the interlobar pulmonary artery and, to a lesser degree, the truncus anterior branch. Division of these venous branches during upper lobectomy improves exposure of the truncus anterior. The splitting of the main pulmonary artery into its two main branches may occur more proximally, and care should be taken to identify both branches before either one is divided. Another significant possible variation is a branch of the middle-lobe vein that arises from the intrapericardial portion of the superior pulmonary vein.**

with the basilar branches of the pulmonary artery and the right lower-lobe bronchus to the other side.

Right middle-lobe bronchus The middle lobe is then rotated superiorly and posteriorly to expose the right middle-lobe bronchus [*see Figure 3*], which usually arises anterior and inferior to the right middle-lobe branches of the pulmonary artery. The basilar artery branches to the right lower lobe are gently mobilized posteriorly to expose the bronchus intermedius and the origin of the right middle-lobe bronchus. Peribronchial lymph nodes located in this region should be dissected and removed, with care taken not to injure the bronchial arterial branches. Once the bronchus is free, it is either divided and ligated with an automatic stapler or transected and oversewn as previously described (see above).

Right Lower Lobectomy

Pulmonary artery: superior segmental branch and basilar branches Once again, the pulmonary artery is exposed within the oblique fissure. The pulmonary branches to the superior segment and the basilar segments of the right lower lobe are identified [*see Figure 1*]. Most of the time, there is one branch to the superior segment of the right lower lobe; however, at times there are two branches, and, rarely, there is a common branch that gives rise to the posterior ascending branch of the right upper lobe and the superior segmental branch of the right lower lobe. Careful identification of the pulmonary artery is important. All branches within the fissure are identified, including the middle-lobe artery and the posterior ascending branch to the right upper lobe. The superior segmental artery is encircled and doubly ligated, with care taken not to injure the posterior ascending branch if it arises from or close to the origin of the superior segmental branch. The basilar segmental branches are then encircled and doubly ligated, with the same care taken not to injure the middle-lobe branch. Both vessels are then divided.

Fissure between the right upper lobe and right lower lobe The fissure between the superior segment of the lower lobe and the posterior segment of the upper lobe is frequently incomplete. If necessary, it is completed as previously described [*see* Right Upper Lobectomy, *above*]. The pleura is incised along the bronchus intermedius, and the lymph node (sump node) just distal to the takeoff of the right upper-lobe bronchus is removed so that the previously dissected pulmonary artery is exposed. Serial application of GIA staplers is employed to complete the fissure.

Fissure between the right middle lobe and right lower lobe The fissure between the middle and lower lobes may also have to be completed (although, in many cases, it is congenitally complete). The pleura is incised within the anterior hilum to allow identification of the superior and inferior pulmonary veins. The basilar segmental bronchi and the middle-lobe bronchus should be exposed. Removal of lymphoid tissue allows easy application of a GIA stapler to complete the fissure.

Pulmonary vein: inferior pulmonary vein The inferior pulmonary vein is then encircled as it exits the pericardium [*see Figure 4*]. This step is facilitated by dissecting the superior edge of the inferior pulmonary vein with the lung rotated first anteriorly and then posteriorly. Once encircled, the pulmonary vein can easily be ligated and divided with a vascular stapler. An infrequent anatomic variant is a vein draining the posterior segment of the right upper lobe into the inferior pulmonary vein. Although an effort can be made to save this branch, there is adequate collateral venous drainage within the right upper lobe to allow this branch to be sacrificed without consequences.

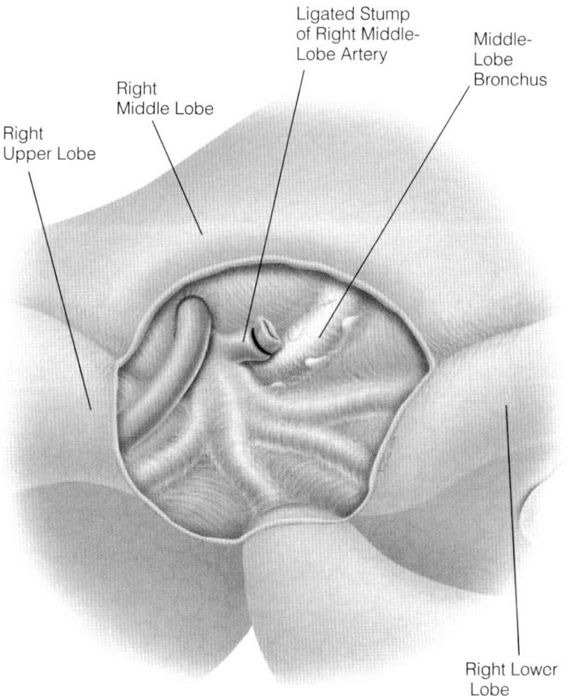

Figure 3 **Right middle lobectomy. Shown is the surgeon's view of the right middle-lobe bronchus. Gentle retraction of the basilar segmental artery to the lower lobe posteriorly allows clear visualization of the origin of the middle-lobe bronchus.**

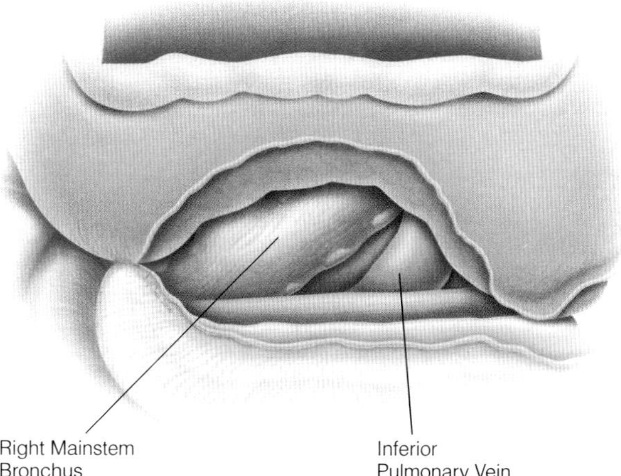

Figure 4 **Right lower lobectomy. Shown is the surgeon's view of the right inferior pulmonary vein. For encirclement of this vein, dissection may also have to be performed on its anterior surface. The branch to the superior segment can be seen overlying the origin of the superior segmental bronchus.**

Right lower-lobe bronchus Division of the lower-lobe bronchus is best accomplished through the fissure; this approach facilitates identification of the middle-lobe bronchus and helps prevent inadvertent damage to or compromise of the origin of this structure. Level 11 and 12 lymph nodes are cleared distally along the bronchi to expose the origin of the superior segmental bronchus [*see Figure 5*]. In some patients, there is adequate length to permit oblique placement of a stapler for control of all of the lower-lobe segmental bronchi without compromise of the middle-lobe bronchus. If this step is not possible, separate ligation and division of the superior segmental bronchus and of all the basilar bronchi as a unit should be performed.

The lung is rotated anteriorly, and the bronchus intermedius is dissected distally until the origin of the superior segmental bronchus is identified from this side. The branch of the inferior pulmonary vein draining the superior segment will be encountered and should be mobilized distally to allow adequate exposure of the superior segmental bronchus origin. This bronchus can now be encircled, ligated, and divided with a stapler or divided and oversewn.

Next, the basilar segmental bronchi are encircled at a point where closure will not affect airflow to the middle-lobe bronchus. Appropriate placement is confirmed by asking the anesthesiologist to ventilate the right lung while the stapler or clamp is applied to the base of the basilar bronchi. If placement is adequate, the basilar segmental bronchi are ligated and divided.

Right Pneumonectomy

Pulmonary artery: right main trunk With the pleura incised circumferentially around the hilum, the lung is rotated inferiorly and posteriorly [*see Figure 2*]. The main trunk of the right pulmonary artery is exposed as it exits the pericardium posterior to the vena cava. Care is taken not to dissect distally on the vessel and not to encircle only the truncus anterior branch by mistake. Ligation and division of the right pulmonary artery can be accomplished in several different ways; either dividing the vessel between clamps and oversewing it with 3-0 nonabsorbable suture material or using vascular staplers is acceptable.

Pulmonary vein: superior and inferior pulmonary vein Next, attention is directed toward the superior pulmonary vein. The vessel is mobilized on its superior and inferior aspects with blunt and sharp dissection, encircled with blunt dissection, and ligated and divided with either clamps or a vascular stapler. With the lung retracted superiorly, the inferior pulmonary vein is dissected as in a right lower lobectomy [*see Figure 4*]. Once isolated, this vein is also ligated and divided as previously described (see above).

Right mainstem bronchus With the lung retracted anteriorly, attention is directed toward the right mainstem bronchus. The subcarinal lymph nodes are mobilized, and the bronchial artery on the posterior medial aspect of the right mainstem bronchus is controlled. The remaining peribronchial tissues are then mobilized distally with blunt and sharp dissection. To avoid leaving a long bronchial stump, exposure of the bronchus to within 1 cm of the carina is advisable.

The bronchus can be closed with a TA stapler loaded with 4.8 mm staples. The staples should be oriented so as to allow good approximation of the anterior and posterior membranous walls. If suture closure is selected instead, the bronchus is divided with the clamp placed on the distal bronchus to prevent spillage. The open end of the bronchus is then closed with nonabsorbable simple sutures, with the cartilaginous wall

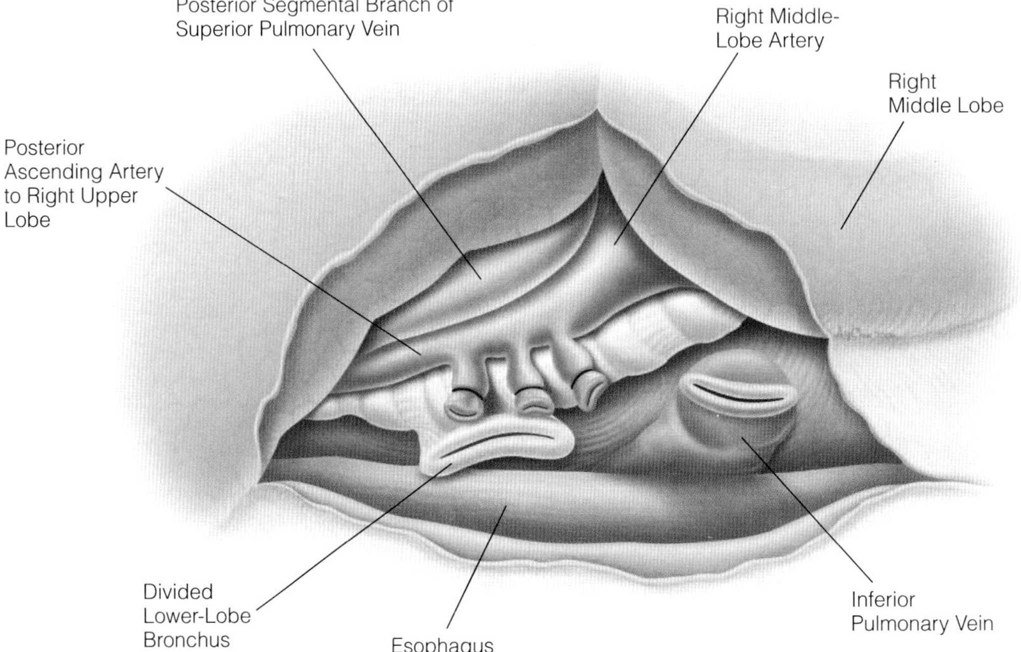

Figure 5 **Right lower lobectomy. Shown is the surgeon's view of the right fissure after division of the lower-lobe vessels. The decision whether to divide the bronchi separately or to transect them with a single oblique application of the stapler depends on the proximity of the middle-lobe bronchus to the superior segmental and basilar bronchi.**

approximated to the membranous wall. To guard against necrosis of the bronchus, care should be taken not to tie the sutures too tightly. Coverage of the pneumonectomy stump with viable tissue is preferred, especially if the patient has received or will receive chemotherapy, radiation therapy, or both. The ideal choice for this purpose is either a rotated intercostal muscle flap or a pericardial fat pad rotational flap. The flap is secured with carefully placed 4-0 polypropylene sutures.

In the preceding description, the artery is divided first, followed by the individual veins and, finally, by the bronchus; however, the steps of this operation can be carried out in any order. The position of the tumor may make the approach we describe difficult. For example, an anteriorly placed tumor may hinder exposure of the anterior hilum. In this situation, the bronchus can be divided first, and the pulmonary artery can be approached from the posterior hilum. As another example, if the tumor is very proximal, the pericardium can be entered via a U-shaped incision along the anterior, caudal, and posterior hilum. The pulmonary veins can then be divided en masse as they originate from the left atrium, and the pulmonary artery can be divided as it courses posterior to the ascending aorta.

LEFT LUNG

Left Hilar Dissection

In the left chest cavity, it is important to identify the inferior pulmonary vein, pulmonary artery, bronchus, and superior pulmonary artery. Retract the lung anteriorly and take down the mediastinal pleura to expose the inferior pulmonary vein and continue superiorly to expose the left main bronchus and the pulmonary artery. With the lung retracted inferiorly, dissection continues proximally along the pulmonary artery. The pleura is incised under the arch of the aorta to expose the left main pulmonary artery. A variable number of small vessels and vagal branches to the lung are encountered that must be ligated and divided. Care is taken not to injure the recurrent laryngeal nerve as it branches from the vagus and travels under the arch just distal to the ligamentum arteriosum. With the lung now retracted posteriorly, the mediastinal pleura is opened parallel to and posterior to the course of the phrenic nerve [*see Figure 6*]. This will expose the main trunk of the left pulmonary artery and the superior pulmonary vein.

Left Upper Lobectomy

Pulmonary artery: apicoanterior, posterior, and lingular The interlobar fissure is developed with a combination of sharp and electrocautery dissection. The posterior aspect of the fissure, between the apicoposterior segment of the left upper lobe and the superior segment of the left lower lobe, is completed (with a linear stapler if necessary) to expose the proximal portion of the pulmonary artery. The left upper lobe is then retracted anteriorly and superiorly to expose the pulmonary arteries supplying the lobe [*see Figure 7*]. The left upper-lobe pulmonary artery anatomy is most variable among the lobes. The most common anatomy is three branches from the pulmonary artery: apicoanterior, posterior, and lingular branches. However, not infrequently, multiple posterior apical branches are encountered; in fact, as many as seven vessels supplying the left upper lobe may be identified. Typically, the posterior segmental branch frequently arises directly opposite the superior segmental branch to the lower lobe, as well as a more distally situated lingular branch. These vessels should be identified, individually ligated, and divided.

Next, the whole lung is retracted inferiorly to expose the aortic arch. A large arterial branch supplying the apicoposterior aspect of the upper lobe is usually encountered. Although the superior and posterior aspects of this artery are easily dissected, the anterior aspect is frequently obscured by an apical branch of the superior pulmonary vein; division of this venous branch may improve exposure and facilitate control of the artery. Once the artery is encircled, it is ligated and divided. To prevent avulsion of this vessel from the main pulmonary artery, care must be taken not to exert excessive traction on the lung.

Pulmonary vein: superior pulmonary vein The superior pulmonary vein can then be identified easily. If the apical branch was not previously ligated, the surgeon should make every effort not to damage the pulmonary artery branches that lie posterior to this portion of the vein. The majority of the superior pulmonary vein lies anterior to the left upper-lobe bronchus. Once this vein is encircled, it is ligated and divided.

Left upper-lobe bronchus Attention is then redirected toward the fissure, and the peribronchial nodal tissue surrounding the left upper-lobe bronchus is swept distally with blunt and sharp dissection. The fissure between the lingula and the lower lobe is completed with serial application of GIA staplers [*see Figure 8*]. The left upper-lobe bronchus is encircled and either clamped or controlled with a TA stapler. To prevent inadver-

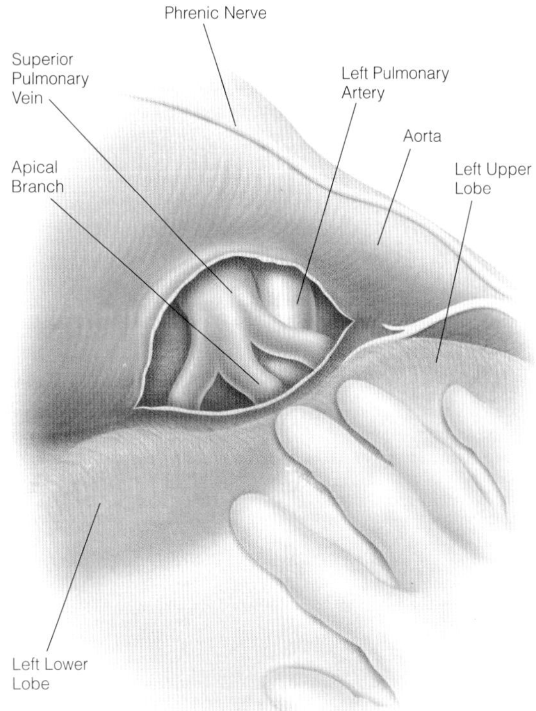

Figure 6 **Left upper lobectomy. Shown is the surgeon's view of the anterior left hilum. The apical branches of the superior pulmonary vein course anterior to the apicoposterior branches of the pulmonary artery. If additional vessel length is needed because of the presence of a central tumor, the pericardium may be entered and the vein divided at that location.**

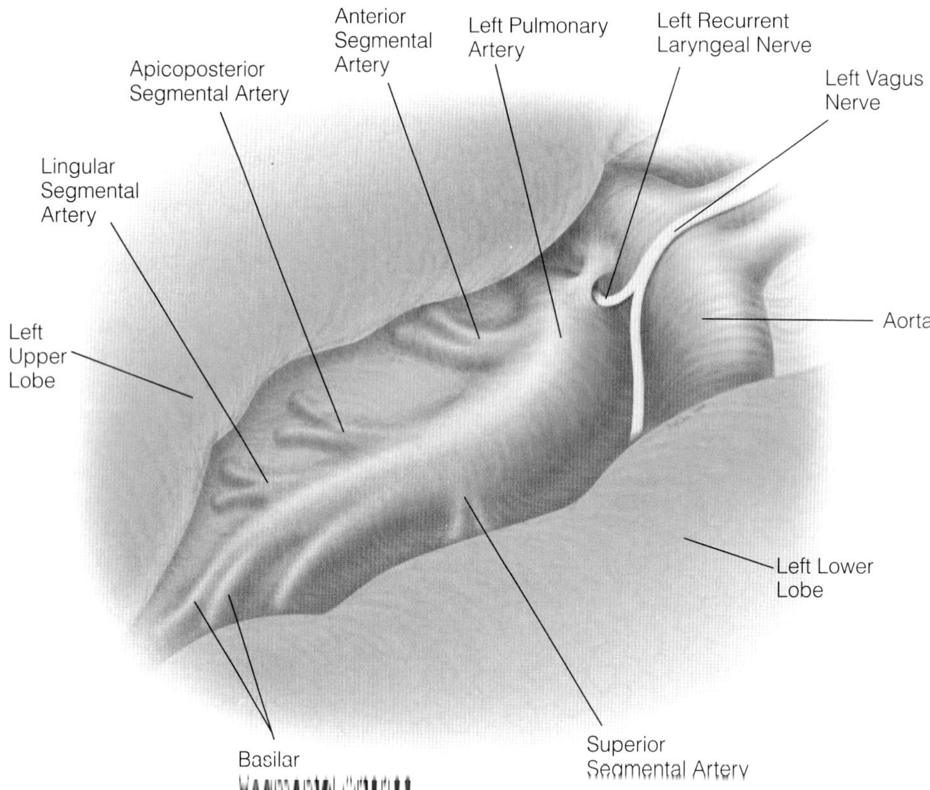

Figure 7 **Left upper lobectomy. Shown is the surgeon's view of the left interlobar fissure. The recurrent laryngeal nerve can be seen coursing lateral to the ligamentum arteriosum. The arterial branches supplying the left upper lobe between the apicoposterior segmental branch and the lingular branch can vary substantially in number and size. Another frequently encountered variation is a distal lingular branch that arises from a basilar segmental branch.**

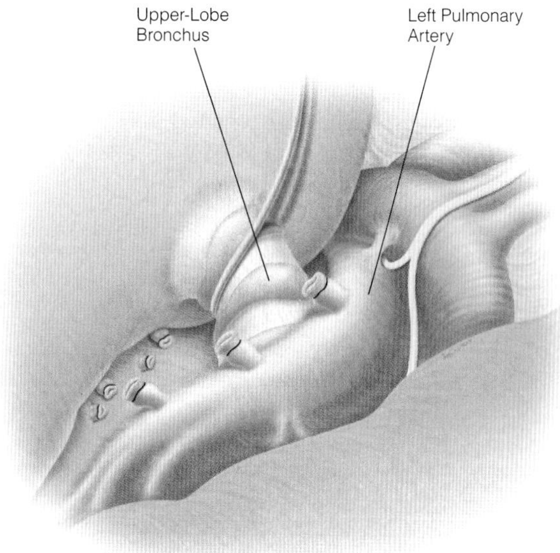

Figure 8 **Left upper lobectomy. Shown is the surgeon's view of the left fissure after division of the upper-lobe arteries. Care should be taken not to injure the pulmonary artery inadvertently when applying a stapler.**

tent injury, the pulmonary artery branches to the lower lobe should be gently retracted posteriorly during stapler placement. With the stapler applied (or the clamp in place), the anesthesiologist ventilates the left lung to verify that air is flowing freely to the entire left lower lobe. Once unobstructed airflow is confirmed, the stapler is fired and the bronchus is divided.

Left Lower Lobectomy

Pulmonary artery: superior segmental and basilar As in a left upper lobectomy, dissection begins within the interlobar fissure. The pulmonary artery is identified, and the branches to the upper and lower lobes are dissected [*see Figure 7*]. The superior segmental artery is encircled first and is ligated and divided; not uncommonly, there are actually two separate superior segmental arteries. The basilar segmental arteries are then encircled distal to the origin of the lingular artery. These vessels are also ligated and divided, with care taken not to encroach on the blood flow to the lingula.

Pulmonary vein: inferior pulmonary vein The lung is rotated superiorly to expose the inferior pulmonary vein. As in a right lower lobectomy, the vein is encircled by dissecting first on its anterior surface with the lung rotated posteriorly, then on its posterior surface with the lung rotated anteriorly [*see Figure 9*]. Once the vein is encircled, it is ligated and divided.

Left lower-lobe bronchus Attention is then redirected toward the interlobar fissure, and the left lower-lobe bronchus

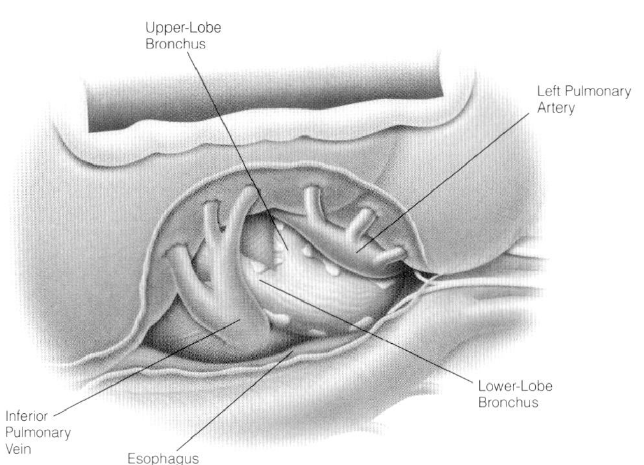

Figure 9 **Left lower lobectomy. Shown is the surgeon's view of the left inferior pulmonary vein. The left side, unlike the right side, affords only limited access to the subcarinal space. However, the length of the inferior pulmonary vein outside the pericardium is greater on the left side than on the right.**

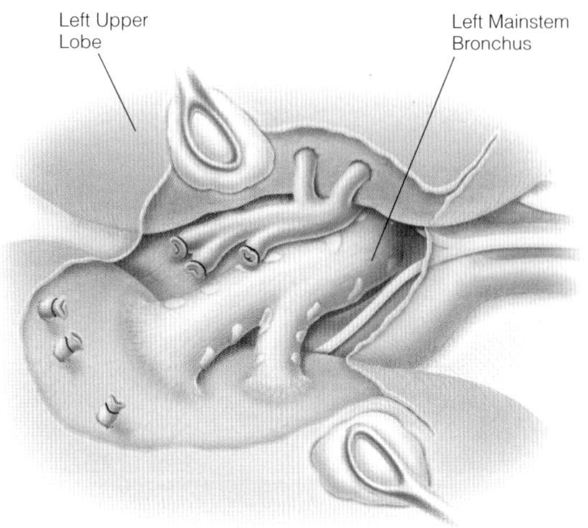

Figure 10 **Left lower lobectomy. Shown is the surgeon's view of the left fissure after division of the lower-lobe vessels. In this procedure, a single oblique transection of the entire left lower-lobe bronchus can be employed without any concern that a proximal bronchus will be compromised; this step would not be feasible in a right lower lobectomy, in that the right middle-lobe bronchus arises from the bronchus intermedius.**

is identified [*see Figure 10*]. The origin of the bronchus is cleared by sweeping nodal tissue distally with blunt and sharp dissection. The upper-lobe branches of the pulmonary artery are gently retracted superiorly to allow placement of a TA stapler on the bronchus. With the stapler applied, the anesthesiologist ventilates the left lung to confirm the adequacy of airflow to the upper lobe. The stapler is fired, and the bronchus is divided distal to the staple line.

Left Pneumonectomy

Pulmonary artery: left main pulmonary artery The initial steps of a left pneumonectomy are similar to those of a left upper lobectomy. The lung is retracted caudally, and the pleura is incised along the course of the aortic arch [*see Figure 7*]. The superior and posterior surfaces of the pulmonary artery are dissected as it enters the thorax under the aortic arch. Once the perivascular space is entered, the entire vessel can usually be encircled with blunt dissection. If the superior pulmonary vein's apical branch limits access to the anterior surface of the pulmonary artery, the branch may be ligated and divided first to improve exposure of the artery; alternatively, the superior pulmonary vein itself may be ligated and divided first to facilitate arterial exposure (see below).

Once the pulmonary artery is encircled, the vessel can be ligated and divided. Our preferred method is to use an endovascular GIA stapler, the advantages of which include its rapidity of use, its consistently reproducible results, and its ability to control the vessel along a broad surface. Mass ligation is not advisable, because the risk of dislocation of the tie is too great. When the length of exposed artery is too short or a stapler cannot be placed safely, the surgeon may apply vascular clamps to the proximal and distal portions of the vessel instead. Once the vessel is divided, the proximal end may be oversewn with a continuous polypropylene suture.

If additional vessel length is required because of the presence of a proximal tumor, the ligamentum arteriosum may be divided. The recurrent laryngeal nerve should be identified and preserved. In dividing the left pulmonary artery proximal to the ligamentum arteriosum, care should be taken not to narrow the main pulmonary artery and thereby reduce right-side blood flow. For maximal safety, systemic blood pressures and oxygenation should be evaluated for 15 to 20 seconds after application of the clamp or stapler but before ligation.

Pulmonary vein: superior and inferior pulmonary vein With the lung retracted posteriorly, the pleura is incised posterior to the course of the phrenic nerve, and the superior pulmonary vein is identified [*see Figure 6*]. The vein is encircled with blunt dissection, then ligated and divided. As noted (see above), the apical branch usually travels across the apical branch of the pulmonary artery, and care should be taken not to injure this vessel during dissection.

The lung is then retracted superiorly to expose the inferior pulmonary vein. Dissection is performed on the anterior and posterior aspects of the inferior pulmonary vein, and blunt dissection is used to achieve complete encirclement of the vein [*see Figure 9*], which is ligated and divided.

Left main bronchus Next, the lung is retracted anteriorly and superiorly. Complete dissection of the subcarinal lymph nodes is performed, facilitated by division of one or two pulmonary branches of the left vagus nerve and both bronchial arteries. Gentle traction is applied in conjunction with blunt dissection to allow encirclement of the proximal left mainstem bronchus [*see Figure 11*]. An effort should be made to encircle the bronchus within 1 cm of the carina. A TA stapler is then passed around the left mainstem bronchus and applied at this point. If excessive traction is required to achieve this placement, the bronchial stump can be left slightly longer: 1 to 1.5 cm, as measured from the carina. The stapler is fired, and the bronchus is divided distal to the staple line.

Frequently, the position of the bronchial stump under the aortic arch and deep within the mediastinum renders coverage of the stump unnecessary. If the surgeon is concerned about

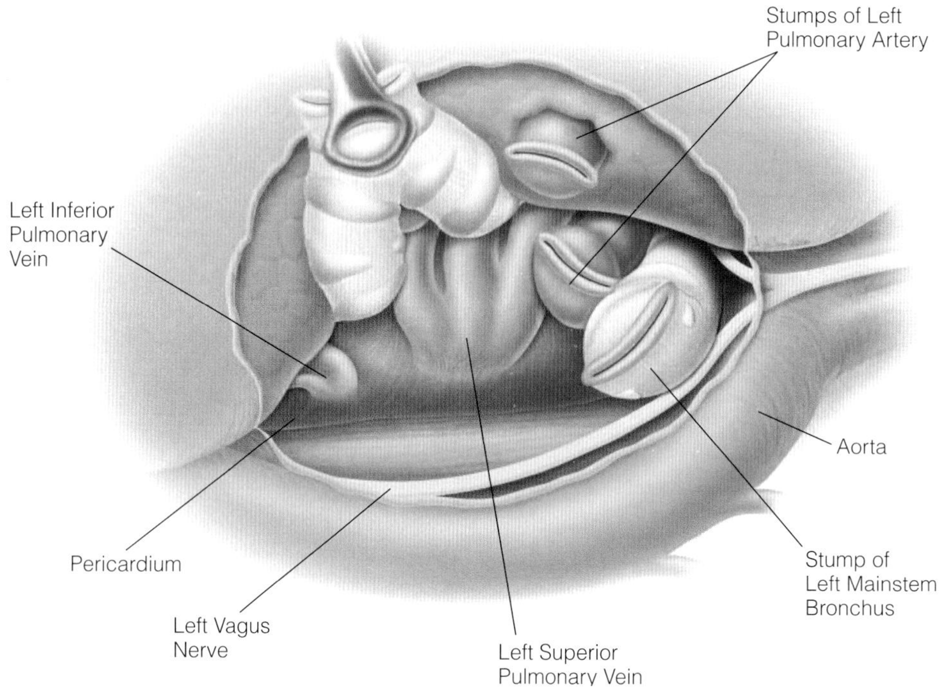

Figure 11 **Left pneumonectomy. Shown is the surgeon's view of the posterior left hilum. The carina is located deep under the aortic arch. A left-side double-lumen tube or bronchial blocker may have to be withdrawn to afford better exposure of the proximal left mainstem bronchus. The orientation of the superior pulmonary vein and the pulmonary artery (anterior and superior to the bronchus, respectively) should be noted.**

possible stump dehiscence (e.g., in a patient who has undergone high-dose preoperative radiotherapy), coverage with a flap from the pericardial fat pad or intercostal muscle is appropriate.

Postoperative Management

A key to successful postoperative management after pulmonary resection is pain control, pulmonary toilet and chest tube management. Thoracic epidural can provide great pain relief after the operation. If this modality is not available or not efficacious, patient controlled analgesia with or without continuous local anesthetic to the thoracotomy incision can be a good alternative. Although adequate pain control is one of the key elements of good pulmonary toilet it is not sufficient by itself. Patient education should begin preoperatively with clear explanation of the goals of pulmonary toilet and the methods used to achieve this. This includes coughing, deep breathing, usually assisted with an incentive spirometer, ambulation, bronchodilators, and, if necessary, nasotracheal suctioning or even flexible bronchoscopy. An x-ray is obtained after the operation to evaluate for appropriate lung expansion, shift of the mediastinum and the diaphragm. After a lobectomy or any lesser resection, the chest tube is usually placed on suction at –20 cm H_2O then transitioned to a water seal once there is a minimal air leak. Although there are wide variations in chest tube management most surgeons will remove the tube when the air leak has resolved and the output is less then 300–400 cc in 24 hours. Patients are then transitioned to oral pain medication and discharged home.

Min P. Kim, MD, owns stock, stock options, or bonds in ATSI, General Electric, and Johnson & Johnson Inc.

Selected Reading

Fell SC, Kirby TJ. Technical aspects of lobectomy. In: Shields TW, LoCicero J, Ponn RB, et al, editors. General thoracic surgery. 6th ed. Philadelphia: Lippincott Williams & Wilkins; 2005. p. 433.

Hood RM. Techniques in general thoracic surgery. 2nd ed. Philadelphia: Lea & Febiger; 1993.

Kirby TJ, Fell SC. Pneumonectomy and its modifications. In: Shields TW, LoCicero J, Ponn RB, et al, editors. General thoracic surgery. 6th ed. Philadelphia: Lippincott Williams & Wilkins; 2005. p. 470.

Martini N, Ginsberg RJ. Lobectomy. In: Pearson FG, Cooper JD, Deslauriers J, et al, editors. Thoracic surgery. 2nd ed. Philadelphia: Churchill Livingstone; 2002. p. 981.

Nesbitt JC, Wind GG. Thoracic surgical oncology. In: Exposures and techniques. 1st ed. Philadelphia: Lippincott Williams & Wilkins; 2003. p. 320.

Waters PF. Pneumonectomy. In: Pearson FG, Cooper JD, Deslauriers J, et al, editors. Thoracic surgery. 2nd ed. Philadelphia: Churchill Livingstone; 2002. p. 974.

Acknowledgment

Figures 1, 2, and 3 through 11 Alice Y. Chen.

15 DIAPHRAGMATIC PROCEDURES

Ayesha S. Bryant, MSPH, MD, and Robert James Cerfolio, MD, FACS, FCCP

Although the diaphragm is sometimes thought of as little more than a partition between the thoracic organs and the abdominal organs, it is, in fact, a dynamic anatomic structure that plays a pivotal role in the physiology of respiratory mechanics. For example, paralysis of just one hemidiaphragm can lead to the loss of 50% of a patient's vital capacity.[1] Like any other anatomic structure, the diaphragm may be affected by either benign or malignant conditions. Overall, benign diseases of the diaphragm (e.g., paralysis) are far more common than malignant ones. With either type of condition, however, the development of a safe surgical treatment strategy depends on a solid knowledge of diaphragmatic anatomy and physiology. Accordingly, we begin with a brief review of the embryology and anatomy of the diaphragm. We then describe the main procedures performed to treat the more common congenital diseases (e.g., congenital diaphragmatic hernia [CDH]) and acquired pathologic conditions (e.g., paralysis and tumor) that affect this structure.

Anatomic Considerations

DEVELOPMENTAL ANATOMY

The diaphragm is a modified half-dome of musculofibrous tissue that lies between the chest and the abdomen and serves to separate these two compartments. It is formed from four embryologic components: (1) the septum transversum, (2) two pleuroperitoneal folds, (3) cervical myotomes, and (4) the dorsal mesentery. Development of the diaphragm begins during week 3 of gestation and is complete by week 8. Failure of the pleuroperitoneal folds to develop, with subsequent muscle migration, results in congenital defects.

CLASSICAL ANATOMY

The diaphragmatic musculature originates from the lower six ribs on each side, from the posterior xiphoid process, and from the external and internal arcuate ligaments. A number of different structures traverse the diaphragm, including three distinct apertures (foramina) that allow the passage of the vena cava, the esophagus, and the aorta [*see Figure 1*]. The aortic aperture is the lowest and most posterior of the diaphragmatic foramina, lying at the level of the 12th thoracic vertebra. Besides the aorta, the thoracic duct and, sometimes, the azygos and hemiazygos veins also pass through this aperture. The esophageal aperture is the middle foramen; it is surrounded by diaphragmatic muscle and lies at the level of the 10th thoracic vertebra. The vena caval aperture is the highest of the three foramina, lying level with the disk space between T8 and T9.

VASCULAR SUPPLY

The diaphragm is supplied by the right and left phrenic arteries, the intercostal arteries, and the musculophrenic branches of the internal thoracic arteries. Some blood is supplied by small branches of the pericardiophrenic arteries that run with the phrenic nerve, mainly where the nerves penetrate the diaphragm. Venous drainage occurs via the inferior vena cava and the azygos vein on the right and via the suprarenal and renal veins and the hemiazygos vein on the left.

INNERVATION

The diaphragm receives its muscular neurologic impulse from the phrenic nerve, which arises primarily from the fourth cervical ramus but also has contributions from the third and fifth rami. The phrenic nerve originates around the level of the scalenus anterior and runs inferiorly through the neck and thorax before reaching its terminal point, the diaphragm. Because the phrenic nerve follows such a long course before reaching its final destination, a number of processes can disrupt the transmission of neurologic impulses through the nerve at various points and thereby cause diaphragmatic paralysis.

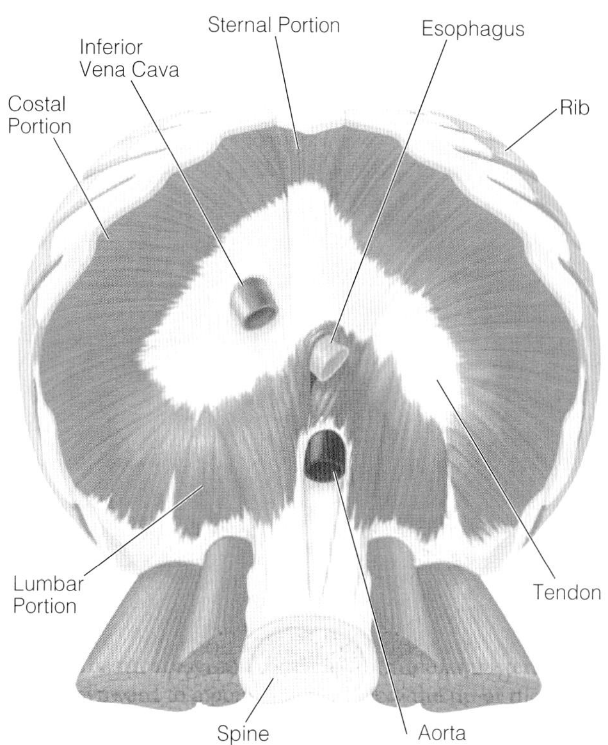

Figure 1 **Shown is an inferior view of the diaphragm.**

Procedures for CDH

REPAIR OF BOCHDALEK HERNIA

Bochdalek hernia, named after the Czech anatomist Vincent Alexander Bochdalek, is the most common form of CDH and is also the most common surgical emergency in neonates.[1] It involves an opening on the left side of the diaphragm. The stomach and intestines usually herniate into the thoracic cavity. The usual presenting symptoms are severe respiratory distress and a scaphoid abdomen. The primary pathologic condition is the presence of posterolateral defects of the diaphragm, which result either in maldevelopment of the pleuroperitoneal folds or in improper or absent migration of the diaphragmatic musculature.

Bochdalek hernias occur in approximately one of every 2,500 live births and are twice as common in male neonates as in female neonates. Mortality ranges from 45 to 50%. The bulk of the morbidity and mortality of CDH is attributable to the resultant hypoplasia of the lung on the affected side and to various associated abnormalities (e.g., malrotation of the gut, neural tube defects, and cardiovascular anomalies).

Preoperative Evaluation

Prenatal ultrasound examination accurately diagnoses CDH in 40 to 90% of cases.[2] In most instances, the examination is performed to rule out polyhydramnios. It is noteworthy that polyhydramnios is present in as many as 80% of pregnant women whose fetuses have CDH.[3] In neonates with CDH, besides the upper gastrointestinal tract, parts of the colon, the spleen, the kidneys, and the pancreas may herniate, and the abnormal position of these organs can be identified by means of ultrasonography. Malrotation and malfixation of the small bowel should be ruled out. Once the diagnosis is confirmed, additional radiographic, echocardiographic, and ultrasonographic studies should be performed to rule out associated anomalies.

Operative Technique

As a rule, neonates with Bochdalek hernias are taken to the operating room immediately after birth. Some studies, however, have shown that delayed surgical repair yields improved survival rates.[4]

For left-side hernias, a transabdominal subcostal approach is generally preferred, whereas for right-side hernias, a transthoracic approach may be more useful. The herniated organs are returned to the peritoneal cavity. The lung is inspected, but no attempt to expand the hypoplastic lung should be made. If any extralobar pulmonary sequestration is present (as is occasionally the case), it should be excised. Most of the defects may be closed primarily with interrupted nonabsorbable sutures; particularly large defects may be closed with a prosthetic patch. The left pleural space is drained with a chest tube, which should be placed on water seal.

Some surgeons have attempted surgical correction of severe Bochdalek hernias in the prenatal period. The safety and feasibility of this therapeutic approach continue to be debated. Prenatal correction of these hernias poses a risk to both the mother and the fetus, with possibly fatal results for both.[5]

REPAIR OF MORGAGNI HERNIA

Morgagni hernias, named after the Italian anatomist and pathologist Giovanni Battista Morgagni, are related to maldevelopment of the embryologic septum transversum and to failed fusion of the sternal and costal fibrotendinous elements of the diaphragm.[6] The Morgagni hernia involves an opening on the right side of the diaphragm. The liver and intestines usually herniate into the thoracic cavity. These hernias are generally asymptomatic[7] and are usually detected as incidental findings on radiographs. Accordingly, the average age at diagnosis is typically greater for Morgagni hernia than for Bochdalek hernia: in one report, the mean age at which the former was diagnosed was 45 years.[8] Morgagni hernias are most commonly seen on the right side. The hernia sac usually contains omentum, but it may also contain part of the transverse colon or, less commonly, parts of the stomach, the liver, or the small bowel; almost any upper abdominal structure may herniate in this setting.

Preoperative Evaluation

On chest radiography, a Morgagni hernia appears as a mass at the right cardiophrenic angle [*see Figure 2*]. Computed tomography (CT) of the chest and abdomen, liver scintigraphy, and multiplanar magnetic resonance imaging (MRI) are occasionally helpful in the diagnostic process.

Operative Technique

Morgagni hernias can be repaired via a subcostal, a paramedian, or a midline incision. We prefer to use an upper midline abdominal incision. Once the peritoneal cavity is entered, the hernia sac is identified just posterior to the xiphoid and the posterior sternal border and then opened. The herniated abdominal viscera are restored to their normal abdominal anatomic positions, and the sac is ligated. The entire hernia sac is defined, resected, and closed. The diaphragmatic defect may be repaired in several different ways, depending on its size and position. Because there is weak tissue in the area of the defect, we generally use a prosthetic patch for the repair. Either polypropylene mesh (e.g., Marlex; C. R. Bard, Inc., Murray Hill, New Jersey) or polytetrafluoroethylene (PTFE) mesh (e.g., Gore-Tex; W. L. Gore and Associates, Newark, Delaware) may be used for this purpose. We prefer PTFE because it may cause fewer adhesions to the underlying abdominal structure, which may be an important consideration if further abdominal surgery subsequently proves necessary. The prosthetic patch is sewn to the midline abdominal fascia, with wide bites taken to prevent an abdominal incisional hernia. The rest of the patch is sewn to the thickened investing fascia that made up the edges of the hernia sac. As noted, the frequently marginal quality of this tissue is the reason why a patch repair is almost always required.

Repair of a Morgagni hernia via a thoracic incision follows the same basic principles. The hernia sac is entered, the visceral contents are mobilized and reduced into the abdomen, the sac is resected, and the diaphragm is repaired. Again, the closure should be completed without tension. If the defect cannot be closed with horizontal mattress sutures, a prosthetic patch should be used.

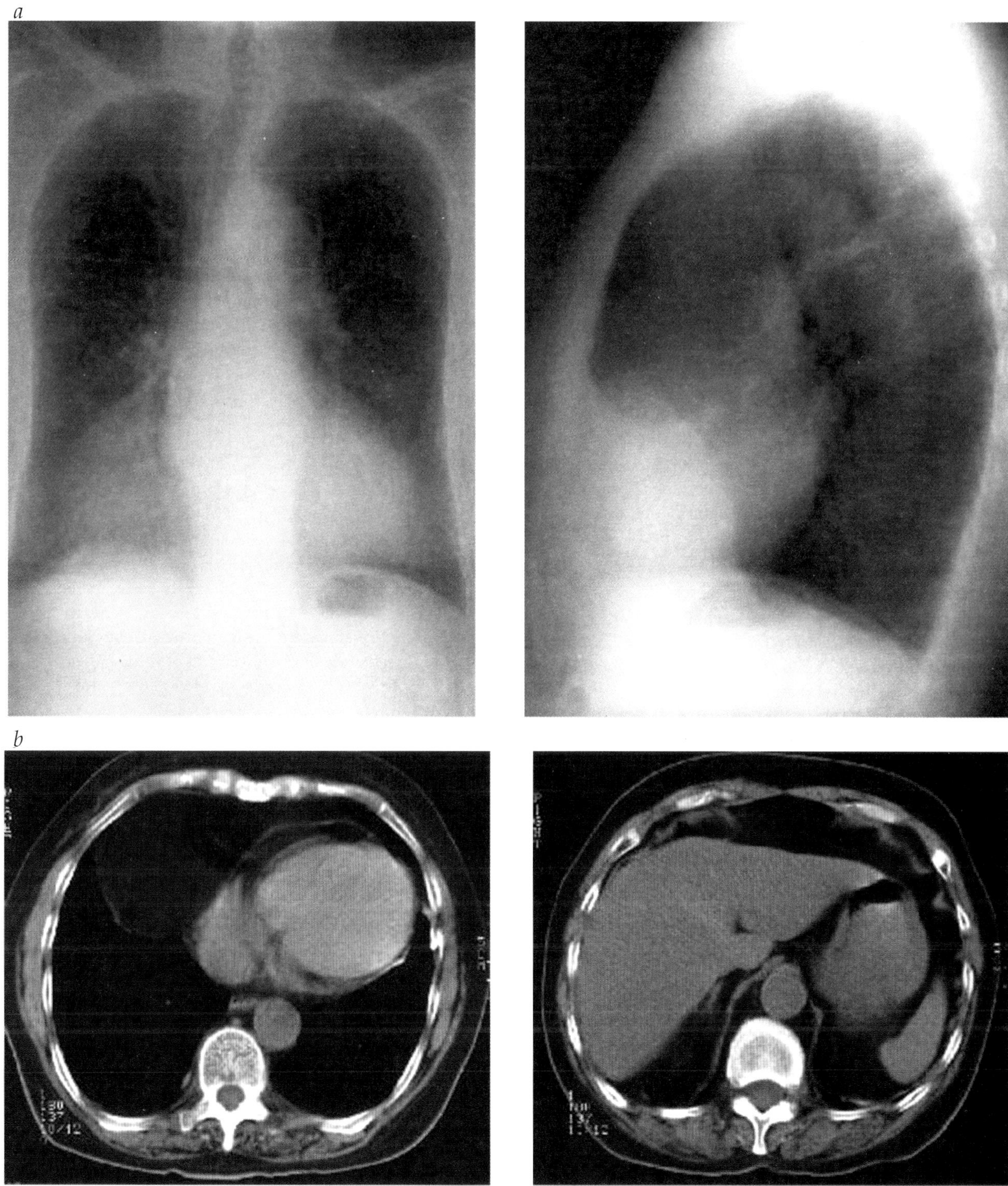

Figure 2 **Repair of Morgagni hernia. The differential diagnosis of a cardiophrenic-angle mass includes pericardial fat, a lipoma, a pericardial cyst, a Morgagni hernia, and a thymoma. Shown are (*a*) chest x-rays and (*b*) chest computed tomographic scans from a 33-year-old man with an incidental finding of a Morgagni hernia.**

Complications

The potential complications of surgical treatment of Morgagni hernia depend to an extent on the type of procedure undertaken to repair the defect. Laparoscopy may result in failure to reduce the contents of the hernia sac, which necessitates conversion to an open procedure. Laparotomy has been associated with postoperative pleural effusion,[9] wound infection,[10] deep vein thrombosis,[11] and pulmonary embolism.[12] Thoracotomy has been associated with pneumonia, sepsis, and bowel obstruction in the postoperative period.[13]

Outcome Evaluation

Most patients do not have any significant postoperative limitations after repair of a Morgagni hernia, nor are such hernias likely to recur. In one study, 16 patients who underwent transthoracic repair of a Morgagni hernia were followed for 5.7 years; no recurrences or symptoms related to the operation were reported.[14]

Procedures for Diaphragmatic Paralysis

The diaphragm is the most important of the respiratory muscles: diaphragmatic contraction decreases intrapleural pressure during inspiration, expands the rib cage, and thereby facilitates the movement of gases into the lungs. Accordingly, paralysis of the diaphragm can have a major adverse effect on respiratory function. Diaphragmatic paralysis may involve either the whole diaphragm (bilateral paralysis) or only one leaflet or hemidiaphragm (unilateral paralysis). The possible causes of diaphragmatic paralysis are numerous [*see Table 1*]; the most common causes are phrenic nerve trauma related to a surgical procedure (e.g., stretching, crushing, or transection) and invasion by a malignant neoplasm.

DIAPHRAGMATIC PLICATION FOR UNILATERAL PARALYSIS

Preoperative Evaluation

With unilateral diaphragmatic paralysis, the paralyzed hemidiaphragm paradoxically moves upward on inspiration and downward on expiration, passively following changes in intrapleural and intra-abdominal pressure. Patients with a paralyzed hemidiaphragm who are otherwise healthy usually have no symptoms at rest but experience dyspnea during exertion and show a decrease in exercise performance. Physical examination may reveal dullness to percussion and an absence of breath sounds over the lower chest on the involved side.

In most cases, the diagnosis of hemidiaphragmatic paralysis is suspected on the basis of incidental findings on a chest x-ray. Typically, the roentgenogram reveals an elevated hemidiaphragm, diminished lung volume, and basilar atelectasis. Fluoroscopy may also be performed. The diagnosis is confirmed by performing a fluoroscopic sniff test, in which paradoxical elevation of the paralyzed diaphragm is observed with sniffing.[15] The sniff test is the gold standard for the diagnosis of this condition. In certain patients, a chest CT scan may be indicated for evaluating the potential cause of the paralysis. If an obvious cause is not apparent from the history or a previous evaluation, CT scanning of the chest should be performed to ensure that no pathologic process is compressing or invading the phrenic nerve. Similarly, MRI of the neck or the spine may be indicated in certain patients to look for conditions that might be causing the diaphragmatic paralysis.

Two other tests that are also (albeit less commonly) used for the diagnosis of unilateral diaphragmatic paralysis are electromyography and transdiaphragmatic pressure assessment. In the first, the phrenic nerve is electrically stimulated in the neck in an effort to distinguish between neuropathic and myopathic causes of paralysis. In the second, transdiaphragmatic pressures are measured by placing a thin walled balloon transnasally at the lower end of the esophagus in such a way as to reflect changes in pleural pressure; a second balloon manometer is then placed in the stomach in such a way as to reflect changes in intra-abdominal pressure. The difference between the two pressures is the transdiaphragmatic pressure. Measurement of transdiaphragmatic pressure can help differentiate diaphragmatic paralysis from other causes of respiratory failure.

Yet another test involves measurement of maximal inspiratory pressures. Patients with diaphragmatic dysfunction and paralysis show a decrease in their maximal inspiratory pressures. These patients cannot generate high negative inspiratory pressures; thus, their maximal inspiratory pressures will be less negative than −60 cm H_2O.

Operative Planning

Surgical treatment of hemidiaphragmatic paralysis is reserved for symptomatic patients who, after a follow-up period of at least 6 months, have persistent shortness of breath with exertion that is sufficiently pronounced to interfere with lifestyle. For a patient to be considered for operation, the sniff test should show significant paradoxical motion.

The basic principle of the surgical procedure is to "reef" (i.e., reduce the surface area of) the redundant floppy diaphragm by plicating it. This measure lowers the resting position of the hemidiaphragm and thus affords the lung the opportunity to expand fully. The effective result is an increase in the functional vital capacity of the ipsilateral lung. The results of plication have been shown to be better in children compared to adults. Plication is of limited benefit in weaning ventilated adults; however, it still results in lifetime improvement in nonventilated adults.[16] A couple of studies have found

Table 1 Common Causes of Diaphragmatic Paralysis
Neurologic conditions
Spinal cord transection
Multiple sclerosis
Amyotrophic lateral sclerosis
Cervical spondylosis
Poliomyelitis
Guillain-Barré syndrome
Phrenic nerve dysfunction
Compression by tumor
Cardiac surgery cold injury
Blunt trauma
Idiopathic phrenic neuropathy
Diabetes mellitus
Postviral phrenic neuropathy (herpes zoster)
Radiation therapy
Cervical chiropractic manipulation
Myopathic conditions
Limb-girdle dystrophy
Hyperthyroidism/hypothyroidism
Malnutrition
Acid maltase deficiency
Connective tissue disease
Systemic lupus erythematosus
Dermatomyositis
Mixed connective tissue disease
Amyloidosis
Idiopathic myopathy
Muscular dystrophy
Multiple siclerosis

that plication of the diaphragm led to long-term improvements in pulmonary function test results, as well as reduced dyspnea.[17,18]

Operative Technique

Diaphragmatic plication may be performed with either sutures or staples; we prefer sutures for this procedure. The chest is entered through a thoracotomy in the seventh or eighth intercostal space. Horizontal mattress sutures buttressed with Teflon pledgets are then placed in a lateral-to-medial direction [*see Figure 3*]. We typically use monofilament nonabsorbable sutures that pass easily through the muscle and can be tightened without dragging through tissue. To distribute the tension, multiple sutures must be placed; this is especially important on the right side, where the diaphragm must be pulled down against the upward force exerted by the presence of the right hemiliver. When the sutures are tied, the hemidiaphragm should be almost back to its normal anatomic location. Care must be taken to ensure that the repair is not under undue tension: excessive tension is likely to result in early dehiscence. Occasionally, a prosthetic patch may be used to buttress the repair further, but in the majority of cases, this measure should be unnecessary. If the choice is made to use staples rather than sutures, care must be taken to ensure that the underlying abdominal contents are not caught in the staple line.

Diaphragmatic plication can also be performed via video-assisted thoracoscopic approach. Some studies have shown that the minimally invasive approach reduces the risk and the recovery time when compared to a thoracotomy.[19]

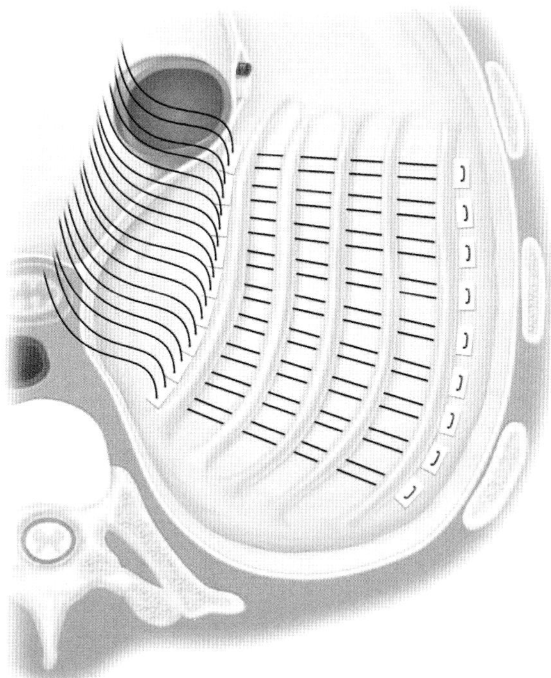

Figure 3 **Diaphragmatic plication. Shown is suture plication of the right hemidiaphragm. Placement of sutures buttressed with pledgets extends anteriorly to the level of the vena cava.**

DIAPHRAGMATIC PACING FOR BILATERAL PARALYSIS

Preoperative Evaluation

In patients with bilateral diaphragmatic paralysis, the respiratory accessory muscles assume all the work of breathing by contracting more intensely. Both hemidiaphragms move upward on inspiration, concomitant with inward (rather than the normal outward) movement of the abdominal wall.[20] Patients typically present with severe respiratory failure or with dyspnea (sometimes misinterpreted as a sign of heart failure) that worsens in the supine position, and they generally exhibit tachypnea and rapid, shallow breathing when in the recumbent position. Increased expenditure of effort in the struggle to breathe may fatigue the accessory muscles and lead to ventilatory failure. Patients also report anxiety, insomnia, morning headache, excessive daytime somnolence, confusion, fatigue, poor sleep habits, and signs of cor pulmonale.[21]

During physical examination, auscultation of the chest reveals limitation of diaphragmatic excursion and bilateral lower-chest dullness with absent breath sounds. The finding that establishes the diagnosis is a paradoxical inward movement of the abdomen with inspiration. As with unilateral diaphragmatic paralysis, however, it is more common for the diagnosis to be suspected on the basis of a chest roentgenogram that shows bilateral diaphragmatic elevation and then confirmed by means of the sniff test.

Operative Planning

Treatment depends on the cause and severity of the diaphragmatic paralysis. Most patients are treated with ventilatory support, but some are treated with bilateral plication or with pacing (as shown in Figure 4). Plication for bilateral paralysis is performed in the same way as plication for unilateral paralysis [*see* Diaphragmatic Plication for Unilateral Paralysis, *above*], except that both hemidiaphragms are lowered.

There are patients who have suffered high cervical injuries and are either quadriplegic or have loss of the C3, C4, and C5 anterior horn cells in the nerve roots. These patients are on ventilators for life and usually nonambulatory. To date, two pacing devices have been approved by the Food and Drug Administration: the Mark IV Breathing Pacemaker System (Avery Biomedical Devices, Commack, New York) uses an electrode that is placed on the skeletonized phrenic nerve, and the NeuRx (Synapse Biomedical, Cleveland, Ohio) uses electrodes placed directly in the diaphragm fibers either video-assisted thoracoscopically or laparoscopically. Both are connected to a small receiving electrode unit placed under the skin. A battery-powered external transmitting box connected to an antenna is taped over the surface of the skin, just above the subcutaneous receiver. This transmitting box permits adjustment of pulse duration, pulse train duration, respiratory rate, pulse frequency, and current amplitude. In most patients, the only parameters that the clinician adjusts are current amplitude and respiratory rate.

Implantation of a diaphragmatic pacer requires experience on the part of the surgeon—not so much because of any particular technical demands imposed by the implantation itself but because of the procedures for diaphragm training that must be carried out in the postoperative period.

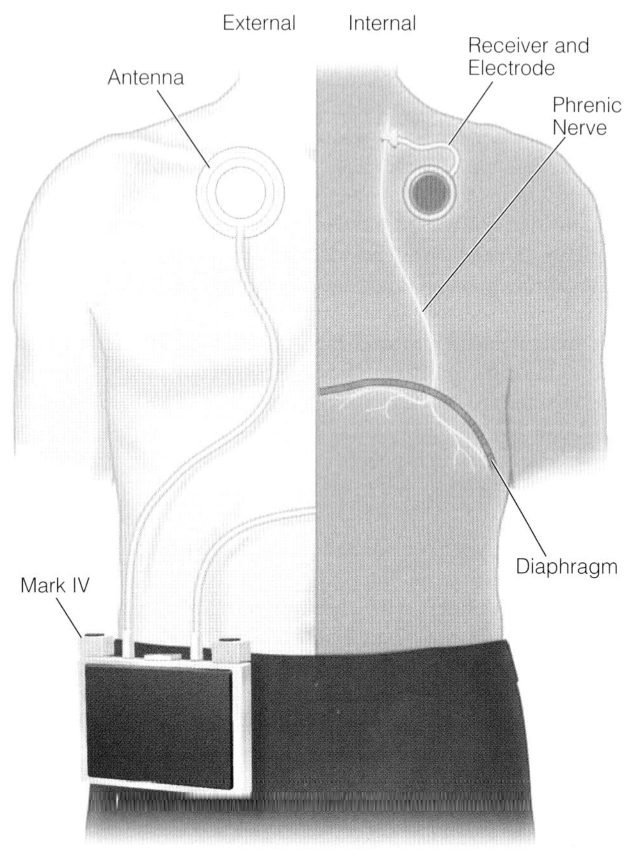

Figure 4 **Diaphragmatic pacing. Shown are internal and external pacer connections.**

Surgical implantation of a diaphragmatic pacer can be done via either a cervical approach or a thoracic approach. The primary advantage of the cervical approach is that it avoids the morbidity associated with bilateral thoracotomies, which may not be well tolerated in patients who have marginal pulmonary function or a history of severe pulmonary contusions. However, there are other ways of avoiding this morbidity, either laparoscopically, by video-assisted thoracoscopic surgery (VATS), or with a small muscle-sparing, rib-sparing, nerve-sparing thoracotomy.[22] One disadvantage of the cervical approach is that in a small percentage of patients, the current amplitude necessary to stimulate the phrenic nerve results in transmission of the current through the soft tissues. The transmitted current stimulates the functioning portions of the brachial plexus, causing rhythmic jerking motions of the upper extremities. Another disadvantage is that a number of accessory nerve branches arise distal to the neck.

One advantage of the thoracic approach is that inadvertent stimulation of portions of the brachial plexus (as sometimes occurs with the cervical approach) may be avoided. Another advantage is that there is some neuroanatomic evidence that a small branch of the phrenic nerve joins the main nerve trunk only after it enters the chest cavity; thus, the thoracic approach may stimulate a larger portion of the phrenic nerve than the cervical approach would. The disadvantage of the thoracic approach is the preconceived notion that entry into the chest is associated with a higher morbidity than entry into the neck.

Operative Technique

Cervical placement In the neck, the phrenic nerve runs between the scalenus anterior and the scalenus medius. A transverse skin incision is made in the midportion of the neck, just lateral to the sternocleidomastoid muscle, and the borders of the two scalene muscles are dissected. The scalene muscles are then divided, and the phrenic nerve is identified lying in a layer of fascia just anterior to the anterior surface of the scalenus medius. Identification of this nerve is often facilitated by the use of a handheld nerve stimulator. Intraoperative fluoroscopy allows observation of diaphragmatic contraction in response to phrenic nerve stimulation, which confirms that pacing is successful.

Once the phrenic nerve is identified, it is carefully dissected free of its investing fascia, and the Y-shaped electrode is placed under it and secured with sutures. Care must be taken to ensure that the nerve is not injured during this step. The connecting wire from the electrode is then tunneled subcutaneously to a subcutaneous pocket that is created just below the ipsilateral clavicle. The connections are made and sealed, and the small incisions are closed.

Thoracic placement In the thoracic approach, the chest is entered through a high thoracotomy (usually over the fourth interspace), and the proximal phrenic nerve is identified. On the right side, the nerve lies along the mediastinum, situated just anterior to the vena cava and coursing along the pericardial surface. On the left side, it lies on the pericardium for most of its length. The proximal nerve is freed of its fibrous investments, and the electrode is placed under it and secured with sutures. The electrode is connected to the receiver, which is placed in a subcutaneous pocket.

As noted (see above), there are alternative approaches to pacer implantation that avoid the cervical approach but also do not involve standard thoracotomies. For example, there is limited (but growing) experience with thoracoscopic placement of phrenic nerve pacing leads.[23] In addition, laparoscopic implantation of intramuscular pacing electrodes onto the inferior aspect of the diaphragm has been reported.[24]

Taking into account all the advantages and disadvantages of each approach to pacer implantation, we generally prefer the thoracic approach, either via VATS or via a thoracotomy.[23,25] The evolution of less invasive surgical techniques may allow the thoracic approach to be employed in patients who are unable to tolerate thoracotomy.

Complications

Besides the usual complications associated with any thoracic procedure (i.e., infection, bleeding, atrial fibrillation, and pneumonia), several specific complications are associated with diaphragmatic pacing. The most common of these are dislodgment of the pacer electrode, transmission of pacer impulses to the brachial plexus with resultant rhythmic jerking of the upper extremity (seen with cervical placement of the electrode), and hardware malfunction.

Outcome Evaluation

Retrospective analysis of the collective experience at a single center between 1981 and 1987 suggested that long-term pacing did not lead to progressive diaphragmatic dysfunction.[26] Six of the 12 patients in this cohort continued to undergo diaphragmatic pacing on a full-time basis for a median period of more than 14 years. Pacing was well tolerated in this group; the reasons for discontinuance included intercurrent medical illness and lack of social support. Concerns have been raised that prolonged diaphragmatic pacing might damage the phrenic nerve. In the series cited, however, the ability to pace the phrenic nerve was not lost in any of the patients, and the mean threshold currents for pacing did not change significantly over time.

Resection of Diaphragmatic Tumors

Primary tumors of the diaphragm are extremely rare. Benign tumors (e.g., lipomas and cystic masses) are more common than malignant tumors, which mostly are sarcomas of fibrous or muscular origin. Thoracic and abdominal tumors (e.g., bronchogenic carcinomas, pleural malignancies, and chest wall malignancies) may involve the diaphragm secondarily through direct extension. Malignant pleural mesothelioma represents a different scenario and is not discussed here. Schwannomas, chondromas, pheochromocytomas, and endometriomas have all been reported. Bilateral occurrence, calcification, sharp margins, and flattened contours are indicative of a malignant process, such as pleural metastases, mesothelioma, or a primary diaphragmatic tumor.

The most common indication for diaphragmatic resection is mesothelioma. This remains true even though mesothelioma is relatively uncommon in comparison with bronchogenic malignancy and even though few patients with mesothelioma are actually candidates for resection. Again, resection of a mesothelioma is not addressed here. The ensuing operative description focuses on diaphragmatic resection to treat either a lung cancer invading the diaphragm or a primary diaphragmatic tumor [*see Figure 5*].

OPERATIVE TECHNIQUE

Once the decision is made to resect a tumor involving the diaphragm, the key considerations are (1) the surgical approach to be taken and (2) the placement of the incision in the diaphragm. We prefer a skin incision that is lower and slightly more anterior than a normal posterolateral thoracotomy; such an incision allows easy entry over the top of the seventh rib. After entry into the chest, the lung, the pericardium, and the pleural surface are carefully visualized and palpated to search for any signs of metastatic disease.

Next, the incision in the diaphragm is planned. Ideally, the incision should be made anterior or lateral to the tumor so that a hand can be placed easily into the peritoneal cavity [*see Figure 5a*]. Intra-abdominal palpation confirms that the tumor

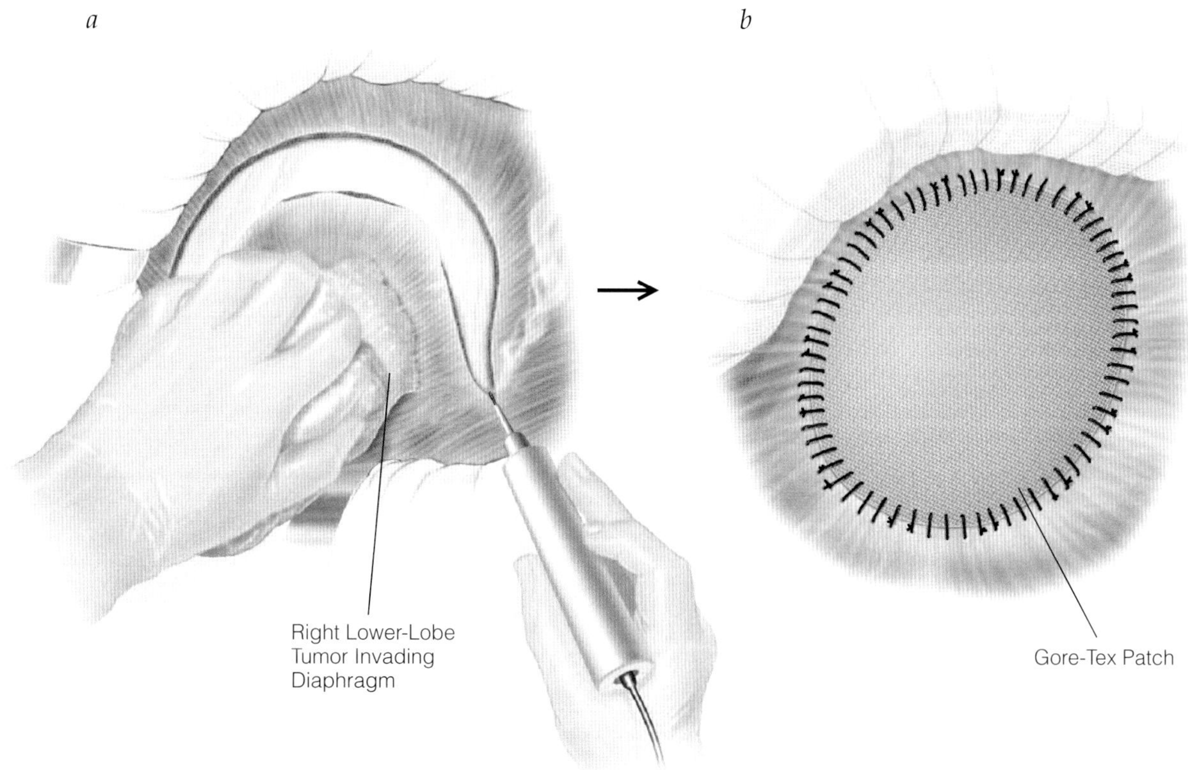

Figure 5 **Resection of diaphragmatic tumor. The patient has a right lower-lobe bronchogenic malignancy with erosion into the right hemidiaphragm. (*a*) The tumor is resected en bloc with the diaphragmatic fibers; the electrocautery is used to achieve clear surgical margins and hemostasis. (*b*) The defect in the right hemidiaphragm is closed with a mesh patch.**

has not extended into underlying structures. This information is almost always gleaned from the preoperative CT scan, but if any uncertainty remains after the scan, diagnostic laparoscopy may be performed before the thoracotomy to look for possible tumor extension.

The tumor is then resected with 2 to 4 cm margins. The large arteries that course through the diaphragmatic fibers are ligated. It is our practice also to place a few silk sutures (stay stitches) in the edges of the defect; this prevents the edges from retracting, helps keep the defect as small as possible, and keeps abdominal contents from interfering with the resection. In addition, we place clips on the edges for guidance purposes in case adjuvant radiotherapy is delivered after the operation. If adequate margins are obtained, which is usually relatively easy in a diaphragmatic resection, postoperative radiotherapy should be unnecessary. If, however, the tumor abuts vital structures (e.g., the suprahepatic vena cava), postoperative radiotherapy may have a useful role to play.

Once the entire tumor has been resected and clear margins have been confirmed by frozen-section examination, the diaphragm is reconstructed. Primary repair is rarely indicated because in most cases, the defect is too large and the tension on the repair would be too great. Moreover, the tissue in the anterior aspect of the diaphragm is thin and is likely to tear under tension. Accordingly, repair with a prosthetic patch is the usual choice. Infection of such a patch is exceedingly rare, and with the exception of the cost, there is little downside to the use of prosthetic material in this setting. As in the repair of a CDH, we prefer PTFE mesh [*see Figure 5b*] to polypropylene mesh because it is less likely to adhere to underlying abdominal structures.

The mesh patch is sewn to the edges of the defect (preferably with nonabsorbable suture material, such as 0 polypropylene), starting at the most anterior and inferior portions of the opening and continuing toward the surgeon [*see Figure 5*]. The inferior half of the repair is done with a continuous suture. The repair is completed with two or three sutures, which are tied circumferentially. To prevent paradoxical motion, the diaphragm must not be too redundant or floppy. It should remain in the normal anatomic position so that the remaining lung can expand completely. In general, however, it is best to keep the repair taut so as to optimize pulmonary mechanics after the procedure.

Dr. Cerfolio is a speaker and consultant for Ethicon, Millicore, Medela, and Atrium. He is a consultant for Neomend, and Closure (J&J). He is a speaker for E Plus Health Care, OSI Pharmaceuticals, Oncotech, Covidien, and Precision.

References

1. Kirks DR, Caron KH. Gastrointestinal tract. In: Kirs DR, editor. Practical pediatric imaging. 2nd ed. Boston: Little, Brown & Co, 1991; p. 709–904.
2. Lewis DA, Reickert C, Bowerman R, Hirschi RB. Prenatal ultrasonography frequently fails to diagnose congenital diaphragmatic hernia. J Pediatr Surg 1997;32:352–6.
3. Adzick NS, Harrison MR, Glick PL, et al. Diaphragmatic hernia in the fetus: prenatal diagnosis and outcome in 94 cases. J Pediatr Surg 1985;20:357.
4. Breaux CW Jr, Rouse TM, Cain WS, et al. Improvement in survival of patients with congenital diaphragmatic hernia utilizing a strategy of delayed repair after medical and/or extracorporeal membrane oxygenation stabilization. J Pediatr Surg 1991;26:333.
5. Wenstrom KD, Weiner CP, Hanson JW. A five year statewide experience with congenital diaphragmatic hernia. Am J Obstet Gynecol 1991;165:838.
6. Panicek DM, Benson CB, Gottlieb RH, et al. The diaphragm: anatomic, pathologic, and radiologic considerations. Radiographics 1988;8:385.
7. Fraser RS, Pare JAP, Fraser RG, et al. Synopsis of diseases of the chest. 2nd ed. Philadelphia: WB Saunders Co; 1984.
8. Minneci PC, Deans KJ, Kim P, et al. Foramen of Morgagni hernia: changes in diagnosis and treatment. Ann Thorac Surg 2004;77: 1956.
9. Jani PG. Morgagni hernia: case report. East Afr Med J 2001;78:559.
10. Ngaage DL, Young RA, Cowen ME. An unusual combination of diaphragmatic hernias in a patient presenting with the clinical features of restrictive pulmonary disease: report of a case. Surg Today 2001;31:1079.
11. Missen AJB. Foramen of Morgagni hernia. Proc R Soc Med 1973;66:654.
12. Dawson RE, Jansing CW. Case report: foramen of Morgagni hernias. J Kentucky Med Assoc 1997;75:325.
13. Lev-Chelouche D, Ravid A, Michowitz M, et al. Morgagni hernia: unique presentations in elderly patients. J Clin Gastroenterol 1999; 28:81.
14. Kiliç D, Nadir A, Döner E, et al. Transthoracic approach in surgical management of Morgagni hernia. Eur J Cardiothorac Surg 2001;20:1016.
15. Miller JM, Moxham J, Green M. The maximal sniff in the assessment of diaphragm function in man. Clin Sci (Colch) 1985;69: 91.
16. Simansky DA, Paley M, Rafaely Y, Yellin A. Diaphragm plication following phrenic nerve injury: a comparison of paediatric and adult patients. Thorax 2002;57:613–6.
17. Higgs SM, Hussain A, Jackson M, et al. Long term results of diaphragmatic plication for unilateral diaphragm paralysis. Eur J Cardiothorac Surg 2002;21:294.
18. Versteegh MI, Braun J, Voigt PG, et al. Diaphragm plication in adult patients with diaphragm paralysis leads to long-term improvement of pulmonary function and level of dyspnea. Eur J Cardiothorac Surg 2007; 32:449–56.
19. Freeman RK, Wozniak TC, Fitzgerald EB. Functional and physiologic results of video-assisted thoracoscopic diaphragm plication in adult patients with unilateral diaphragm paralysis. Ann Thorac Surg 2006;81:1853–7.
20. Higgenbottam T, Allen D, Loh L, et al. Abdominal wall movement in normals and patients with hemidiaphragmatic and bilateral diaphragmatic palsy. Thorax 1977;32:589.
21. Piehler JM, Pairolero PC, Gracey DR, et al. Unexplained diaphragmatic paralysis: a harbinger of malignant disease? J Thorac Cardiovasc Surg 1982;84:861.
22. Cerfolio RJ, Bryant AS, Patel B, et al. Intercostal muscle flap decreases the pain of thoracotomy: a prospective randomized trial. J Thorac Cardiovasc Surg 2005;130:987.
23. Morgan JA, Morales DL, John R, et al. Endoscopic, robotically assisted implantation of phrenic pacemakers. J Thorac Cardiovasc Surg 2003;126:582.
24. DiMarco AF, Onders RP, Kowalski KE, et al. Phrenic nerve pacing in a tetraplegic patient via intramuscular diaphragm electrodes. Am J Respir Crit Care Med 2002;166:1604.
25. Cerfolio RJ, Price TN, Bryant AS, et al. Intracostal sutures decrease the pain of thoracotomy. Ann Thorac Surg 2003;76: 407.
26. Elefteriades JA, Quin JA, Hogan JF, et al. Long-term follow-up of pacing of the conditioned diaphragm in quadriplegia. Pacing Clin Electrophysiol 2002;25:897.

Acknowledgment

Figures 1 and 3 through 5 Tom Moore

16 THORACIC DIAGNOSTIC AND STAGING PROCEDURES

Farzaneh Banki, MD and Larry R. Kaiser, MD, FACS

Thoracic diagnostic and staging procedures can be divided into those that involve the lungs, pleural space, mediastinum, and esophagus. Surgeons must be familiar with the TNM staging system for each major thoracic disease to decide on appropriate treatment. A general principle is to proceed with the diagnostic modality that will potentially yield or rule out the highest stage. As an example, in a patient with presumed non–small cell lung cancer and a pleural effusion, there is no reason to proceed with mediastinoscopy to assess lymph node involvement prior to interrogating the pleural space with video-assisted thoracoscopy (VATS). In this chapter, we review the diagnostic and staging procedures that relate to the most common thoracic malignancies that occur in the thoracic cavity that have relevance to the general surgeon.

Clinical Diagnosis and Staging

The diagnosis and staging of intrathoracic disease have major implications for treatment planning, especially in light of recent advances in both neoadjuvant and adjuvant treatment regimens in both lung cancer and esophageal cancer. These two malignancies account for the majority of the pathology seen within the chest cavity and treated by thoracic surgeons. TNM staging for both lung cancer and esophageal cancer recently has undergone revision as noted in the seventh edition of the American Joint Committee on Cancer (AJCC) cancer staging manual, effective since January 2010.[1] It is mandatory for every surgeon who treats these diseases to be intimately familiar with the staging classification as mentioned in the latest edition of this manual. The surgeon needs to be familiar with clinical staging based on preoperative imaging studies and pathologic staging that result from either preoperative invasive staging techniques or the findings that are generated by the pathologist who reviews the histology of the material obtained at the time of definitive resection. Optimal surgical resection that results in definitive information detailing the final clinical stage includes complete removal of the primary tumor as well as, ideally, a systematic dissection or, at minimum, sampling of the regional lymph nodes. Any procedure that is not this inclusive results in partial information that makes a decision regarding postoperative treatment significantly more difficult and may result in a poorer outcome for the patient.

Clinical staging of intrathoracic disease, specifically intrathoracic malignancies, relies on imaging modalities that range from plain chest radiography to positron emission tomography (PET). Most commonly, patients with intrathoracic complaints obtain a chest radiograph that may or may not delineate the relevant pathology. Computed tomographic (CT) scans of the chest most commonly performed following the injection of intravenous contrast are the mainstay of thoracic imaging procedures. These scans are the most sensitive for defining parenchymal lung lesions and can detect lesions down to a size of several millimeters.

The appearance of a parenchymal lung nodule does not necessarily indicate malignancy. The only definitive information that can be obtained regarding a lung nodule seen on a CT scan is its size. There are no specific defining characteristics that are accurate in delineating a benign from a malignant nodule. If previous CT scans are available for comparison, an increase in the size of a nodule points toward malignancy but, again, is not definitive. The presence of a new nodule on a CT scan may mandate nothing more than a repeat scan in 3 months to assess whether the nodule is changing in size. An increase in the size of a nodule should mandate further diagnostic procedures to define the nodule. The size increase alone may be an indication for resection or, depending on the clinical setting, may mandate a needle aspiration biopsy to obtain material for cytologic analysis. However, one must be aware that only a positive result is helpful, as with any diagnostic test. A "negative" biopsy is of no use because a sampling error may account for the negative result and we are still faced with a nodule that has increased in size. Thus, prior to obtaining a needle aspiration biopsy, the surgeon should know how the information will be used. One recognizes intuitively that if the biopsy is positive for malignancy and there is no evidence of locally advanced or distant disease, the patient is a candidate for resection unless that option is precluded because of other underlying medical problems. But if operation is also indicated in the presence of a negative result on biopsy, one has to think seriously as to whether the risk of a needle biopsy is warranted.

CT scans are also excellent for demonstrating enlargement of mediastinal and hilar lymph nodes, but, once again, an increase in size alone does not necessarily translate into malignancy. By convention, we define mediastinal lymph nodes larger than 1 cm on short axis as pathologic, although some prefer to use 1.5 cm as the definition for pathologic.[2] Many surgeons have used CT scans to identify those patients without pathologic lymph nodes as defined by size criteria so that certain patients may proceed to resection without the need for invasive mediastinal staging. It has been reported that only 3 to 16% of patients with mediastinal lymph nodes less than 1 cm in size on a CT scan are found to have tumor involvement at mediastinoscopy.[3,4] Sensitivity and specificity will vary depending on what size criteria for positivity one chooses to use. A meta-analysis looking at CT scans in assessing mediastinal lymph node involvement in bronchogenic carcinoma found an overall sensitivity and specificity of

79% and 78%, respectively.[5] McLoud and colleagues reported even lower sensitivity and specificity of 64% and 62%, respectively.[6] The bottom line here is that the presence of enlarged lymph nodes should prompt additional staging studies, including ^{18}F-fluorodeoxyglucose (^{18}F-FDG) PET and most likely mediastinoscopy to document the presence or absence of malignancy before deciding that a patient is not an operative candidate.[7]

PET is highly sensitive in the detection of mediastinal lymph node involvement in patients with bronchogenic carcinoma, with a lower limit of detection reported at 4 mm.[8] It has been estimated to have a sensitivity as high as 91 to 96% and a specificity as high as 86 to 93% in staging of mediastinal lymph nodes.[9–13] PET has also been found to be quite useful in differentiating benign from malignant parenchymal lung nodules. A nodule with positive ^{18}F-FDG uptake on PET has a better than 90% likelihood of being malignant. Figure 1a demonstrates a right upper lobe nodule seen on a CT scan, whereas Figure 1b shows the same nodule on a PET scan. Increased metabolic activity is suggestive of malignancy, as seen in the hilar lymph node. The use of combined PET-CT is growing, and several studies suggest that the use of integrated PET-CT improves anatomic localization of lymph nodes compared with PET alone.[11] This study provides both the anatomic localization and size information when looking at the mediastinal lymph nodes, as well as the metabolic information obtained from the PET scan, which provides additional information useful in determining benign from malignant tumors. The same applies to parenchymal lesions.

Diagnostic and Staging Procedures for the Lungs, Pleura, and Mediastinum

BRONCHOSCOPY

Bronchoscopy is the standard diagnostic modality used for the assessment of disease that involves the airway, lungs, and pleura. The use of the fiberoptic bronchoscope has, for the most part, supplanted the use of rigid bronchoscopy for all but lesions thought to involve the trachea or proximal mainstem bronchi. It is safe, although sad, to say that rigid bronchoscopy is a dying art except for the few thoracic surgeons and interventional bronchoscopists who continue to use it for certain indications. Flexible bronchoscopes allow for visualization of the entire tracheobronchial tree out to the level of subsegmental bronchi, and lesions may be sampled via the working channel of the instrument. Techniques for sampling include brushings, washings, and use of a flexible biopsy forceps to obtain tissue samples. The procedure may easily be performed with the patient awake and lightly sedated with the instrument passed either via the nares or through the mouth using topical anesthetic to attenuate the gag reflex. Use of an endotracheal tube is not required to place the bronchoscope but may be used to secure the airway if necessary.

Once the instrument is passed, the vocal cords are visualized and traversed, with inspection then carried out of the entire airway. Topical anesthetic may be injected through the instrument as needed to prevent the patient from coughing. Orientation is secured by visualizing the origin of the right upper lobe bronchus, which is the most proximal orifice

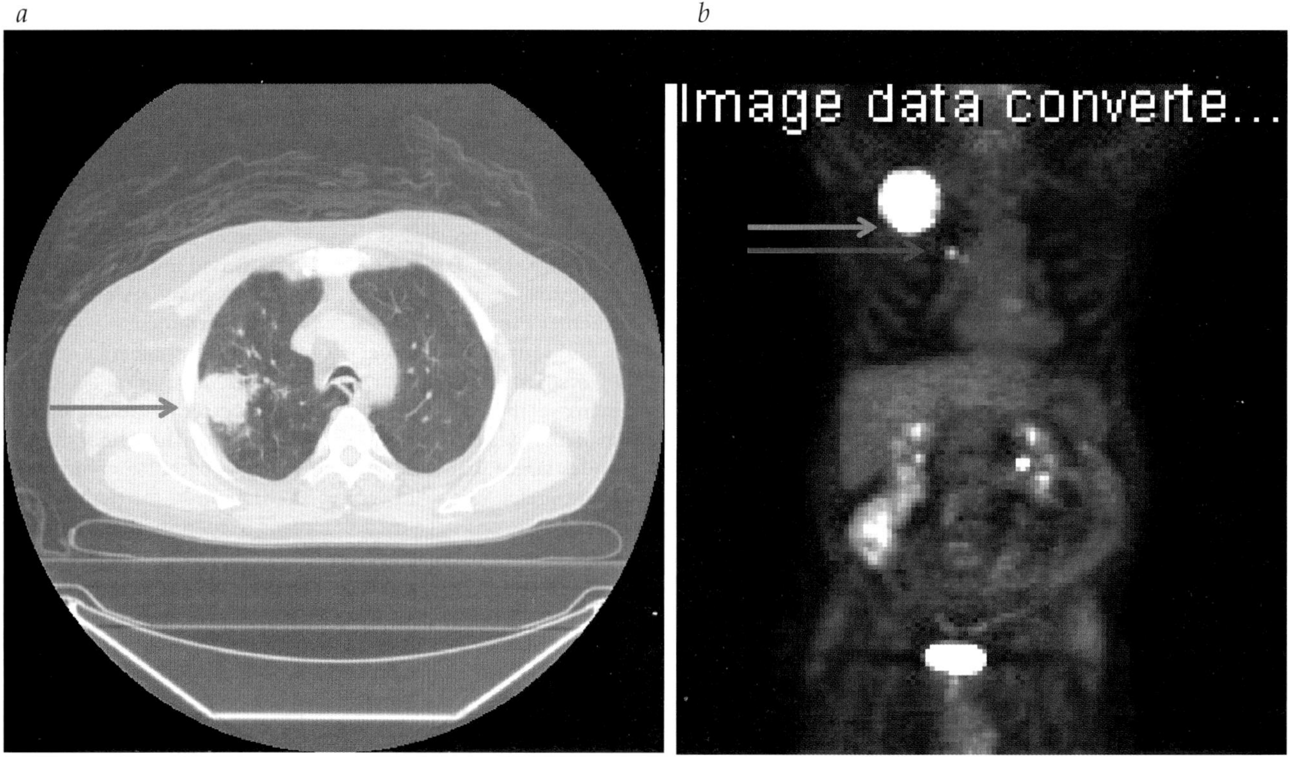

Figure 1 **(*a*) Right upper lobe non–small cell lung cancer on a computed tomographic scan. (*b*) Positron emission tomographic scan. The *blue arrows* indicate the primary tumor, and the *red arrow* indicates the hilar lymph node.**

visualized when one proceeds beyond the carina and takes off at an acute angle [*see Figure 2*]. Proceeding down the right mainstem bronchus, the bronchus intermedius is entered distal to the right upper lobe takeoff, and the origin of the middle lobe and lower lobe bronchus can be seen. The takeoff of the superior segment of the lower lobe is visualized heading posteriorly. Next, the left main bronchus is entered and both upper and lower lobe bronchi are interrogated. Any endobronchial lesions seen may be sampled with the cup biopsy forceps. Parenchymal lesions may also be sampled via a transbronchial approach using fluoroscopy for precise localization of the biopsy forceps. Special alligator forceps are passed distally into the airway via the appropriate segmental bronchus, and either a discrete lesion or diffusely involved parenchyma may be sampled. Bleeding, if encountered, usually only requires saline lavage and tamponade with the bronchoscope. Occasionally, epinephrine in saline is used to control bleeding after a transbronchial lung biopsy.

Transbronchial Needle Aspiration

Transbronchial needle aspiration (TBNA) is another diagnostic technique that may be used to assess regional lymph nodes and is performed via the flexible bronchoscope. A needle catheter is passed through the working channel of the instrument and guided to the area of the tracheobronchial tree adjacent to the mediastinal lymph node of interest. The needle catheter is advanced through the tracheal or carinal wall into the mediastinal lymph node, and a syringe is connected to aspirate cellular material. Several passes may be necessary until an adequate specimen is confirmed by the cytopathologist, who, ideally, is present. On-site cytopathologic examination of needle aspiration specimens significantly improves the yield of TBNA.

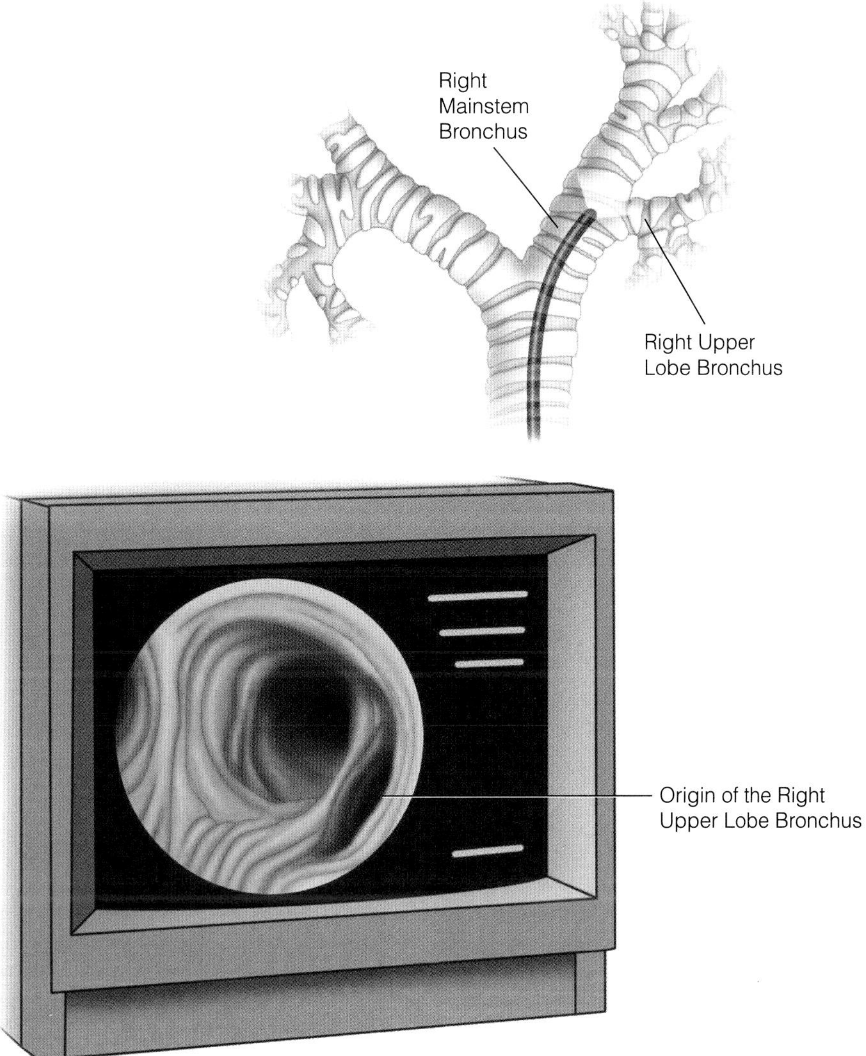

Figure 2 **Diagrammatic representation of the right mainstem bronchus and the origin of the right upper lobe bronchus. Note the position of the upper lobe takeoff. This is the point of orientation for bronchoscopy. Reproduced with permission from Kaiser LR et al.[25]**

TBNA is used most frequently to assess subcarinal lymph nodes. Paratracheal lymph nodes may also be sampled with TBNA, but these are somewhat more difficult to access mainly because of the technical difficulty of sufficiently angulating the bronchoscope containing the needle catheter.[14] It has been reported that it is feasible to obtain adequate specimens via TBNA in approximately 80 to 90% of cases.[15] Results achieved for lymph nodes less than 1 to 1.5 cm may be substantially reduced but may improve up to 90% for nodes of greater than 1.5 cm.[16–18]

Endobronchial Ultrasound-Guided Needle Aspiration

Endobronchial ultrasound-guided needle aspiration (EBUS-NA) is a procedure similar to conventional TBNA that also uses local anesthesia and sedation. However, the patient is intubated because of the larger external diameter of the EBUS-NA bronchoscope. EBUS-NA is a relatively new technique for mediastinal staging and employs a bronchoscope with a convex ultrasound probe that allows for real-time ultrasound-guided TBNA [*see Figure 3*]. EBUS-NA can be used to sample the highest mediastinal, upper and lower paratracheal, and subcarinal lymph nodes, as well as hilar lymph nodes. The overall reported sensitivity is 90%, with values ranging from 79 to 95%. The average reported false negative rate is 24% but varies significantly among reported series.[19–21]

Rigid Bronchoscopy

Rigid bronchoscopy, when indicated, is performed with the patient anesthetized and in the supine position. The head should be placed in the "sniffing" position, and using the operator's thumb as a fulcrum, the instrument tip is used to elevate the epiglottis. Once the vocal cords are visualized, the instrument is turned so as to facilitate passage into the airway. The rigid instrument cannot be passed beyond the lobar level and is directed by turning the head. Rigid forceps may be used for sampling proximal lesions, and larger specimens may be obtained than can be using the flexible instrument. The rigid bronchoscope may also be used as a therapeutic tool to remove foreign bodies, dilate strictures, or debulk tumor that may be occluding proximal airways. It remains a very useful tool for those who have the expertise to use it.

MEDIASTINOSCOPY

This procedure remains the gold standard for assessing the status of the mediastinal lymph nodes whether for patients with a parenchymal lung lesion or for those who simply present with mediastinal adenopathy of unknown etiology. The CT scan of the chest is used to identify enlarged mediastinal lymph nodes, and the PET scan may be highly suggestive or even "definitive" that these nodes may harbor malignancy, but until there is histologic proof from tissue obtained, some doubt remains. Even with a positive PET scan, at least a 10 to 20% chance of a false positive result attributable mainly to inflammatory disease remains.

In 2007, Detterbeck and colleagues published evidence-based clinical practice guidelines for invasive mediastinal staging of lung cancer that concluded the following[14]:

1. In patients with discrete mediastinal nodal enlargement, staging by CT or PET scan is not sufficiently accurate. The sensitivity of various techniques is similar in this setting, although the false negative rate of needle techniques is higher than that for mediastinoscopy.
2. In patients with a stage II or central tumor, invasive staging of the mediastinal nodes is necessary.

a

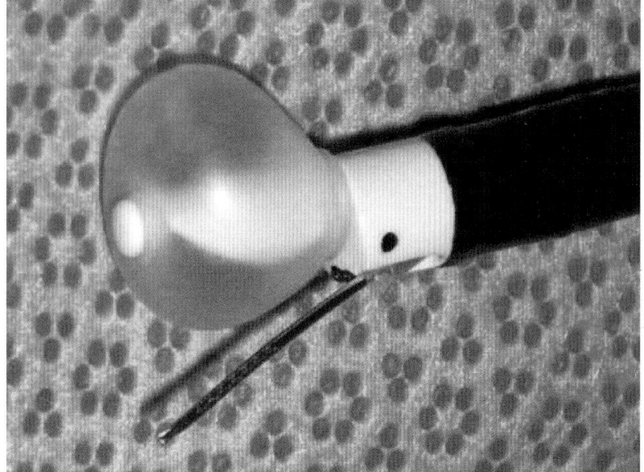

b

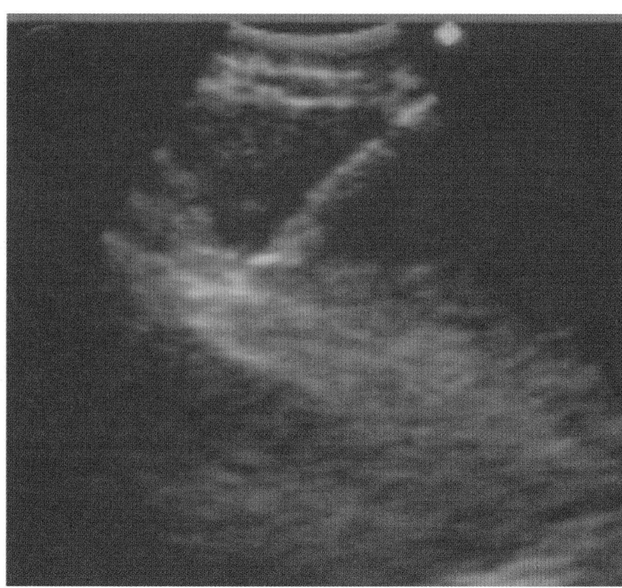

Figure 3 **(*a*) Endobronchial ultrasound probe with the inflated balloon. (*b*) Ultrasound image with the tip of the needle in the mediastinal lymph node. Reproduced with permission from Yasufuku K et al.[20]**

3. Mediastinoscopy is generally preferable because of the higher false negative rates of needle techniques in the setting of normal-sized lymph nodes.
4. Patients with a peripheral clinical stage I non–small cell lung cancer do not usually need invasive confirmation of mediastinal nodes unless a PET scan finding is positive in the nodes.
5. The staging of patients with left upper lobe tumors should include an assessment of the aortopulmonary window lymph nodes.

Mediastinoscopy is performed with the patient under general anesthesia and positioned supine with the neck hyperextended. A small cervical incision is made approximately 2 cm above the sternal notch, and the strap muscles are separated in the midline. The pretracheal fascia is incised, and the mediastinal plane is defined with finger dissection [*see Figure 4*]. In most patients, the carina may be palpated with the back of the finger at the distal extent of the defined plane. The innominate artery is palpated anteriorly, as is the arch of the aorta. Thus, the mediastinoscope is passed in a plane with the trachea immediately posterior and the brachiocephalic vessels immediately anterior. Both the right and left upper and lower paratracheal nodal locations may be accessed, as well as the subcarinal space. The mediastinoscope is passed posterior to the right main pulmonary artery as the artery traverses the carina. Recognizing the major vascular structures that are within the field, the operator can see the potential for causing havoc if he or she is not intimately familiar with the performance of this diagnostic procedure [*see Figure 5*]. Mediastinoscopy is not for the occasional operator; it is a difficult procedure to teach and difficult to perform well. The advent of the video-assisted mediastinoscope has helped advance the teaching of the technique.

It is difficult to overestimate the value of this procedure and the significance of the information in guiding therapy, especially for patients with non–small cell lung cancer. The presence of ipsilateral nodal, or N2, disease portends a somewhat dismal prognosis but also indicates the need for multimodality therapy to achieve optimal results. If at the time of mediastinoscopy, contralateral nodal, or N3, disease is found, this rules out the possibility of surgical resection adding anything to the overall outcome and the patient is, in most circumstances, considered inoperable. The finding of contralateral nodal disease is most common with tumors that arise in the left lower lobe.

This points out the importance of performing a complete and thorough examination of the mediastinum with appropriate specimens taken. This includes sampling the right upper and lower paratracheal locations (levels 2 and 4), left lower paratracheal locatoin (level 4; it is unusual to find upper paratracheal nodes on the left, likely because of the position of the aortic arch), and the subcarinal space (level 7) [*see Figure 6*]. Finding left level 4 lymph nodes can be challenging, especially for the inexperienced operator, and exploration in this location puts the left recurrent nerve at risk. Complete sampling is not required if contralateral nodal disease is identified first or for those patients who present simply with mediastinal adenopathy but without a lung lesion where the differential diagnosis includes malignancy, sarcoidosis, and other inflammatory or infectious disease. In the latter situations, a single sample from the most easily accessible location suffices, but adequate tissue for diagnosis must be confirmed by the pathologist on frozen section at the time of the procedure prior to terminating the operation.

The possibility of a major injury to the azygos vein, innominate artery, or pulmonary artery is very real if the surgeon should inadvertently attempt to obtain a specimen from what appears to be a lymph node but is actually a vessel. Often the azygos vein looks very much like an enlarged lymph node, but palpation with the suction or cautery gives the tactile sense of something other than a solid structure. The development of this tactile sense often comes only with significant experience with this procedure. Injury to a vessel may also occur if a lymph node is adherent, unbeknownst to the surgeon, who encounters significant bleeding after sampling a node.

Anyone performing this procedure should know how to manage a potentially lethal complication should a major vascular injury occur. The initial maneuver should be to tamponade the bleeding either with a finger or preferably by packing. Vaginal packing should be on the field just for such use. Only if the bleeding appears minimal should any attempt be made to control it through the mediastinoscopy with clips or electrocautery. Bleeding is common following sampling of the subcarinal space and is easily controlled with minimal packing. When the bleeding is such that the field becomes dark, it is time to pack the mediastinum and prepare for median sternotomy. Once the bleeding has been stopped by packing, the anesthesiologist should have blood in the room and fluids given to optimize perfusion while preparations are made for median sternotomy. The sternotomy approach allows access to any potential bleeding site and because the patient already is supine obviates the need to turn the patient to the lateral decubitus position. The azygos vein is also accessible and can be controlled via this approach as well.

Also vulnerable to injury during mediastinoscopy, as discussed above, is the left recurrent laryngeal nerve. This can be injured with electrocautery if used too close to the nerve or by the biopsy forceps. Unfortunately, this is an all too common complication that results in significant morbidity. The hoarseness or breathy voice that results is one issue, but the major one is the possibility of aspiration on swallowing that can result because of the incomplete glottic closure that is a consequence of the left vocal cord being in the abducted position.

PARASTERNAL MEDIASTINOTOMY

This procedure is related to mediastinoscopy but usually does not require the use of a mediastinoscope. Originally referred to as a Chamberlain procedure, this technique was formerly used most commonly to sample enlarged lymph nodes (level 5) located in the aortopulmonary window on the left side. Currently, most surgeons employ VATS to sample that area if indicated to make a treatment decision. This procedure is most commonly used to obtain tissue from an anterior mediastinal mass to establish a diagnosis. The most common lesion to occur in this location is a lymphoma, either Hodgkin disease or non-Hodgkin lymphoma. Adequate tissue is necessary not only to establish a diagnosis but also to aid in typing the lymphoma. As mentioned above, the procedure most commonly is performed on the left side but may also be

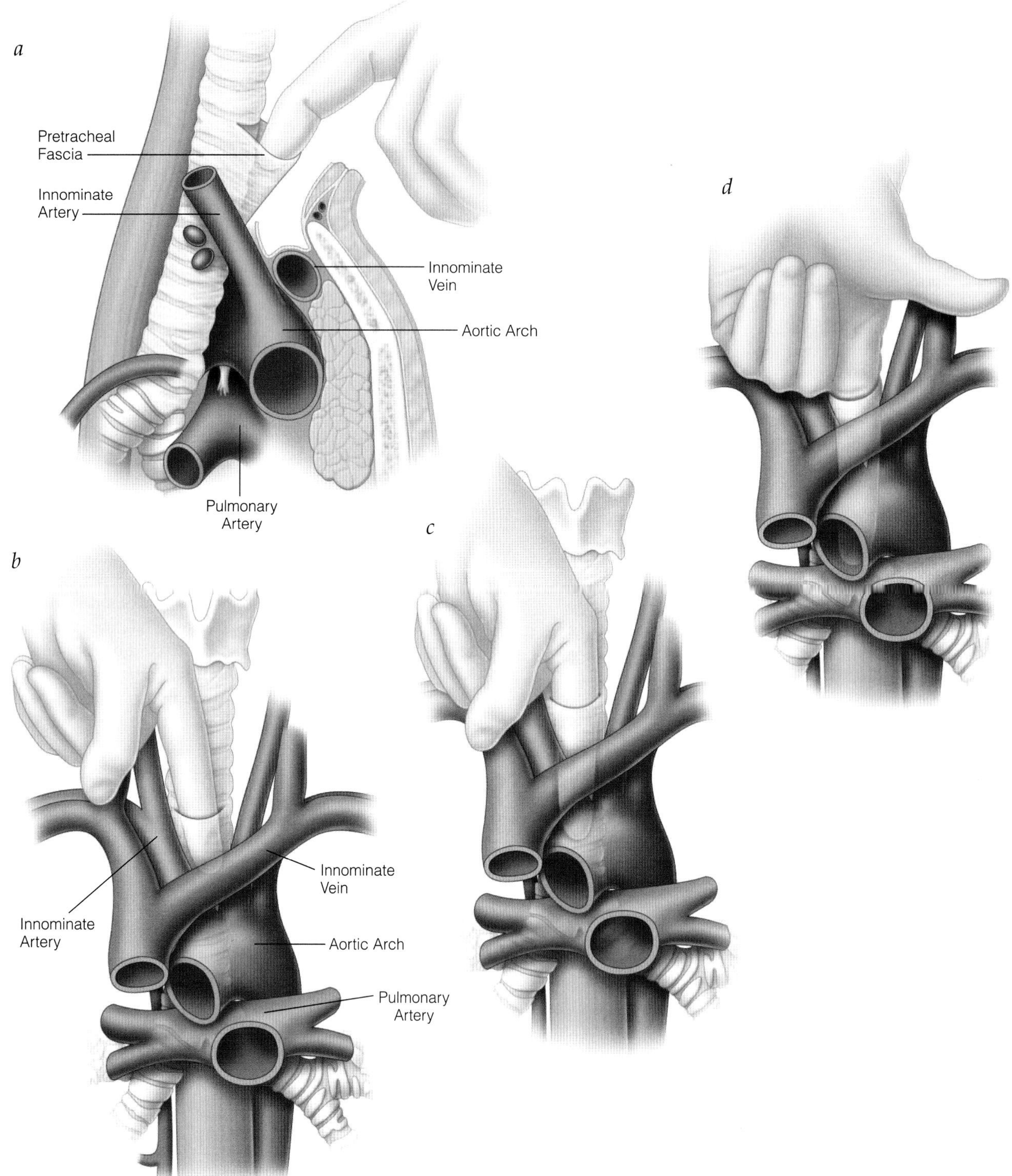

Figure 4 **Development of the mediastinal plane prior to introducing the mediastinoscope. (*a, b*) Oblique and anterior views of the finger entering the pretracheal space after the fascia has been incised. The finger goes along the anterior aspect of the trachea, and the innominate artery is palpated anteriorly. (*c*) The finger is passed beyond the innominate artery, and both the right and left paratracheal areas are palpated. (*d*) The finger now is at the level of the carina, which, in most cases, can be palpated. The mediastinal space is now ready for insertion of the mediastinoscope. Reproduced with permission from Kaiser LR et al.[25]**

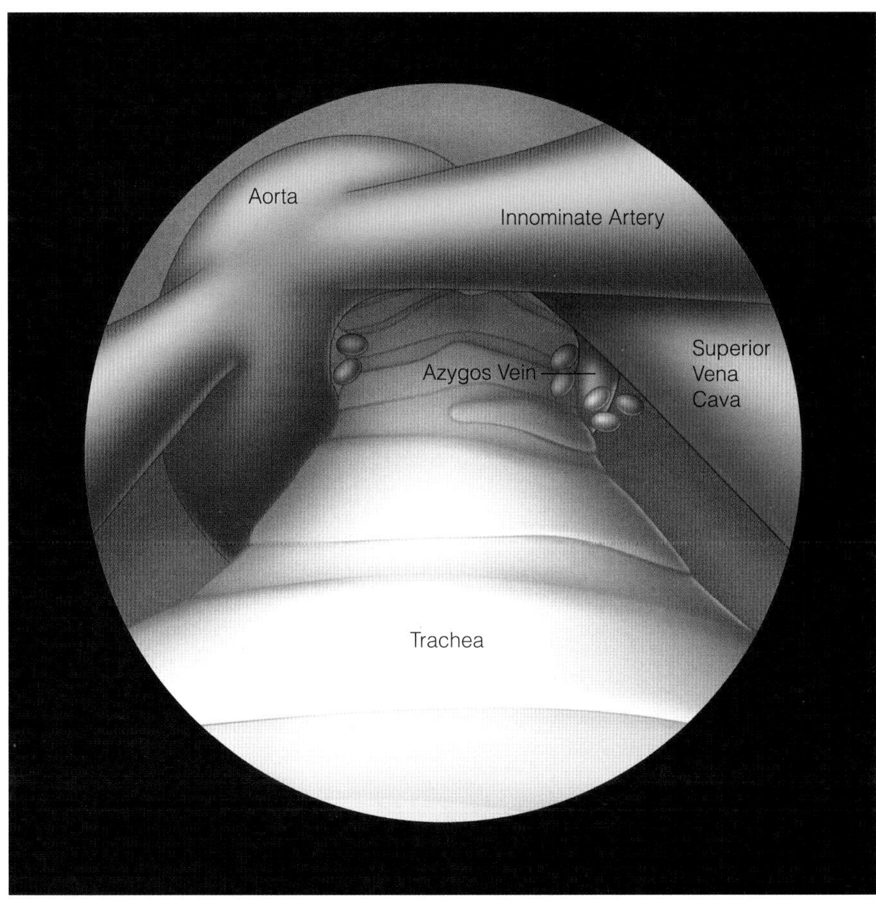

Figure 5 **Schematic representation of blood vessels in the superior mediastinum also showing the location of lymph nodes at the tracheobronchial angle. The mediastinoscope is inserted into this space, anterior to the trachea and posterior to the innominate artery. The trachea is always the reference point for location during the conduct of the procedure. Reproduced with permission from Mentzer SJ.[26]**

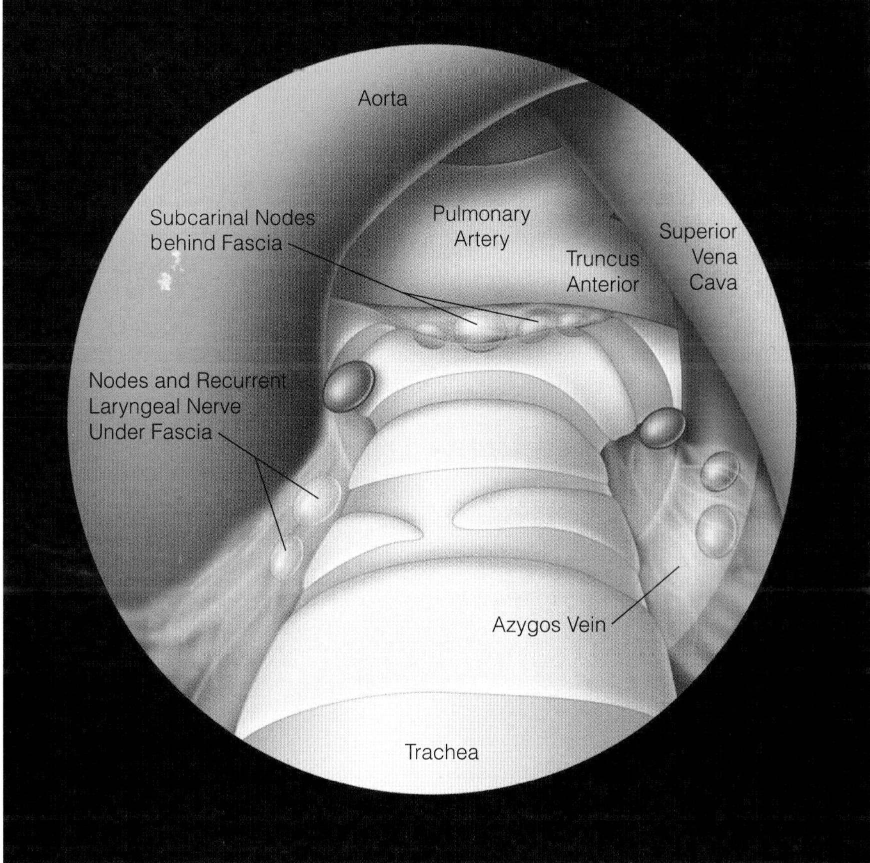

Figure 6 **View as seen through the mediastinoscope of the carina and subcarinal space. Note the location of the right main pulmonary artery as it traverses the carina and its proximity to the subcarinal space. Note also the location of the azygos vein. Reproduced with permission from Mentzer SJ.[26]**

carried out on the right side depending on the location of the anterior mediastinal mass.

A small incision is made over the second rib cartilage immediately adjacent to the sternum [*see Figure 7*]. Resecting the second costal cartilage in a subperichondrial plane facilitates entry into the mediastinum without breaching the pleural reflection. Some surgeons choose not to resect the costal cartilage and either attempt to stay out of the pleural space or routinely enter it. In any case, care must be taken to avoid the internal thoracic artery pedicle, which usually may

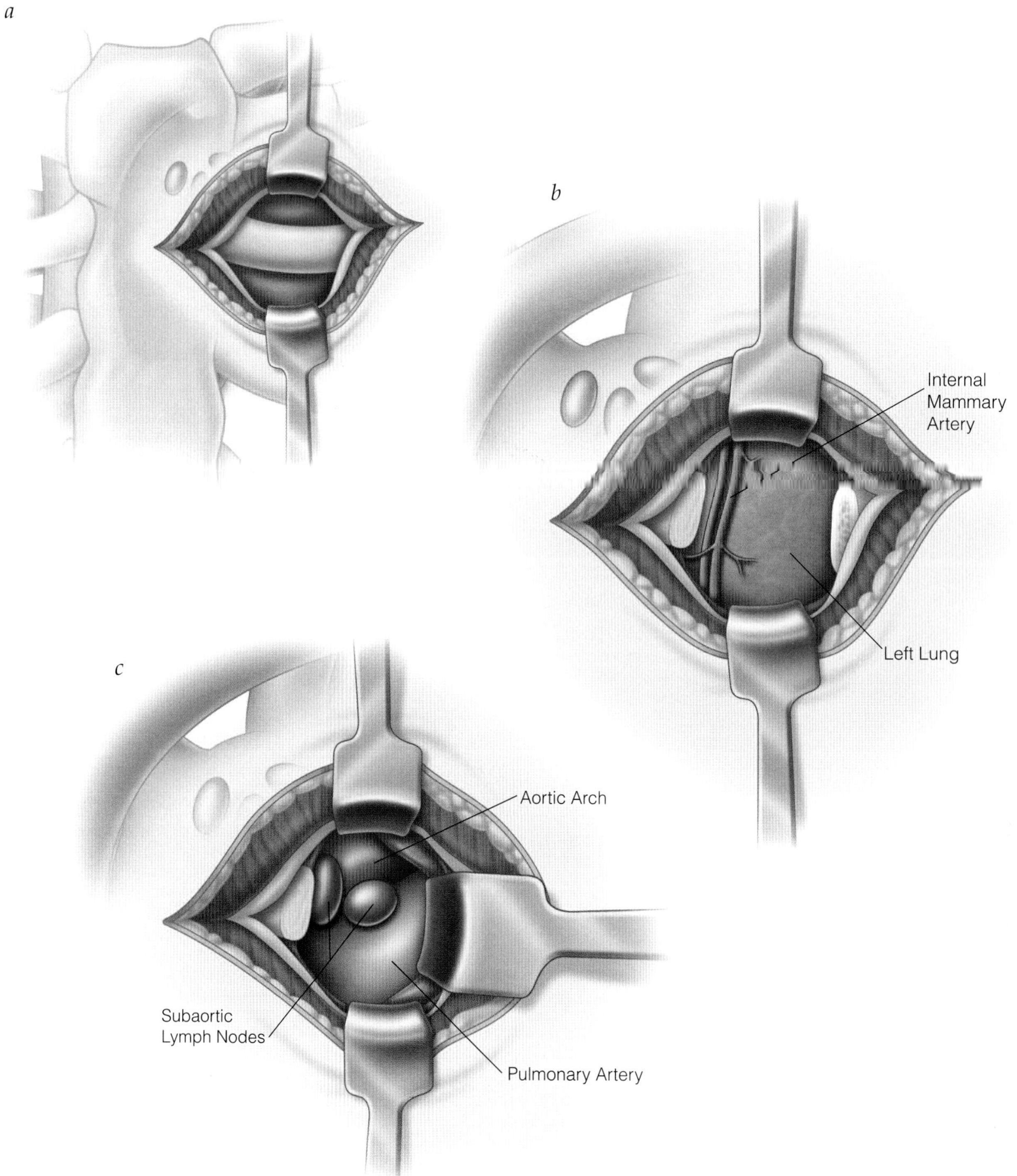

Figure 7 **Diagrammatic representation of a left anterior mediastinotomy. (*a*) An incision is made immediately adjacent to the sternum over the left second costal cartilage. (*b*) The second costal cartilage is removed, allowing access to the mediastinum without entering the pleural space, or the pleura may be incised. Note the location of the internal mammary vessels. (*c*) Enlarged lymph nodes in the aortopulmonary window. Reproduced with permission from Kaiser LR et al.[25]**

be identified and reflected out of the way. The endothoracic fascia is incised, the pleural reflection is swept laterally, and the mass is encountered. Multiple samples of the mass may be taken with a biopsy forceps, and frozen section will determine if adequate material has been obtained. If the pleural space is entered, simply placing a red rubber catheter prior to closure and removing it just prior to skin closure following a Valsalva maneuver removes any air from the pleural space. Given that there is no ongoing air leak from lung parenchyma, this is all that is required. Some have warned of the possibility of "seeding" the pleural space when sampling what turns out to be a thymoma, but staying out of the pleural space renders that concern moot.

VIDEO-ASSISTED THORACIC SURGERY

There are multiple uses for VATS procedures in the diagnosis and staging of intrathoracic pathology. As mentioned above, its use for mediastinal staging, for the most part, is confined to accessing the aortopulmonary window to sample the level 5 lymph nodes, if indicated [*see Figure 8*]. By far the most common use is to assess the pleural space, especially when a pleural effusion is present and there is a question of pleural involvement. Not all pleural effusions indicate pleural space involvement by tumor. In a patient who presents with a pleural effusion for which there is no plausible explanation, thoracentesis is first performed. If positive, the patient is staged M1a and no further invasive diagnostic or staging procedure is necessary. If negative and the patient has a parenchymal lung lesion, a VATS procedure may be performed to visually examine the parietal and visceral pleural surfaces and sample any abnormal areas seen. Not all malignancies that involve the pleura will shed cells; thus, false negative thoracenteses are not uncommon, especially with certain histologies. If the VATS procedure fails to detect any pleural involvement, then resection can proceed assuming that there is no other evidence of metastatic disease.

In addition to the diagnosis of pleural involvement, VATS has been used routinely to resect parenchymal nodules for diagnosis prior to proceeding with resection. A wedge excision of a pulmonary nodule confirms the diagnosis prior to proceeding with lobectomy, and resection may then be carried out completely via VATS or open thoracotomy. Finding a benign nodule saves the patient a lobectomy and the attendant morbidity. In addition, VATS has been particularly useful in obtaining lung parenchyma in those patients with diffuse interstitial lung disease where a diagnosis guides therapy. For interstitial disease, samples are taken from at least two locations, ideally in different lobes, to fully assess the process. Most commonly, VATS is performed with three incisions placed in a triangulated fashion, which allows for the scope to be placed in one port, leaving the other two for instrument placement. Thus, the lung parenchyma may be grasped via one port and an endoscopic stapler placed in the other to perform the excision. The presence of diagnostic material should be confirmed by the pathologist prior to terminating the procedure.

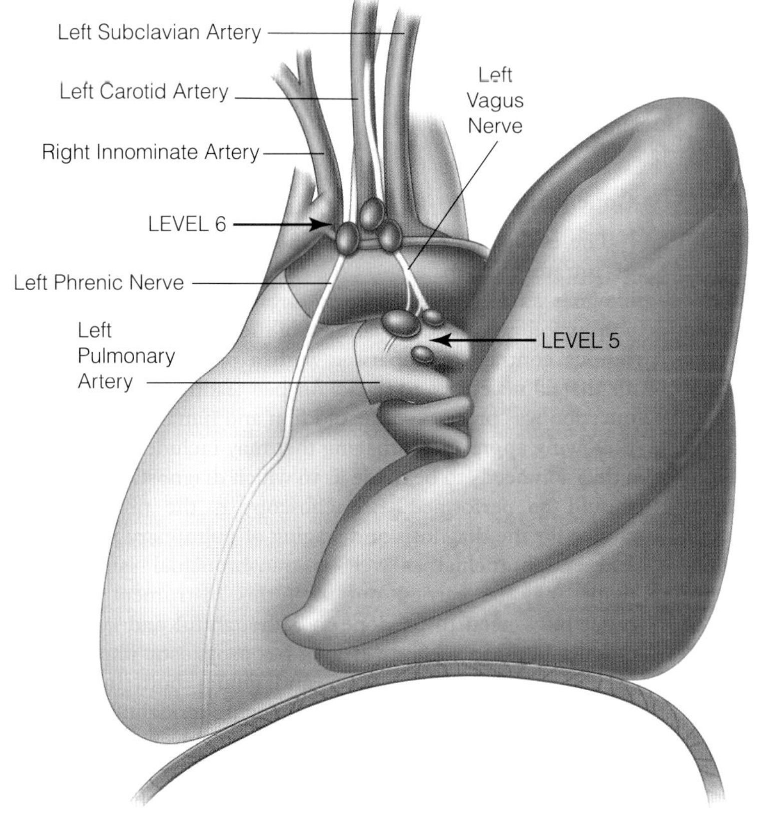

Figure 8 **Video-assisted thoracoscopic view of the aortopulmonary window. The third and seventh intercostal space access ports are placed. The lung is reflected posteriorly. The phrenic nerve is traced to the level 6 lymph nodes at the base of the innominate artery. The *arrows* show the level 5 aortopulmonary window and level 6 para-aortic lymph nodes. Reproduced with permission from Mentzer SJ.**[26]

17 THORACIC OUTLET SYNDROME

Mark W. Fugate, MD, and Julie A. Freischlag, MD

Thoracic outlet syndrome (TOS) is a condition caused by compression of the neurovascular structures leading to the arm passing through the thoracic outlet. The incidence of TOS is reported as 0.3 to 2% in the general population.[1] There are three distinct types of TOS: neurogenic (95%), venous (4%), and arterial (1%). Treatment algorithms depend on the type of TOS. Arterial and venous TOS often present urgently with arterial or venous thrombosis, which is fairly easily identified by thorough history taking and a physical examination. Diagnosis is also aided by duplex ultrasonography. Restoration of arterial or venous flow can often be readily accomplished by thrombolysis. More important, however, is the diagnosis of the underlying structural component involved in the development of symptoms. Although statistically the most common, neurogenic TOS is often the most difficult to diagnose and treat. There are good data indicating that appropriately selected patients benefit from surgical therapy for neurogenic TOS as well. To prevent recurrence of symptoms, patients must undergo first rib resection and anterior scalenectomy, as well as resection of any rudimentary or cervical ribs. Regardless of the type of TOS encountered, proper therapy requires a thorough diagnostic evaluation and multidimodal treatment.

History

Historically, TOS has been a controversial syndrome in terms of its causes, diagnosis, and management. Galen first described a cervical rib in human cadaver dissections.[2] As his work had fallen out of favor during the Dark Ages, Vesalius, who revived much of Galen's work, again described the cervical rib among human cadavers.[2] In 1821, Sir Astley Cooper observed that a subclavian artery occlusion was caused by compression from a cervical rib, which came to be known as cervical rib syndrome.[3] In 1927, the first rib was implicated in neurogenic TOS.[4] In 1935, Ochsner and colleagues described the scalenus anticus syndrome, and an association was first made with trauma.[5] Compression of the subclavian artery and vein was termed costoclavicular syndrome in 1943.[6] The term thoracic outlet syndrome was first introduced in 1956 by Peet and colleagues, who also described a therapeutic exercise regimen in the management of the syndrome.[7] This was an important contribution as physical therapy continues to be one of the mainstays of therapy for neurogenic TOS.

As the views of the anatomic causes of TOS evolved over the years, so did the surgical approaches to its management. In 1861, Coote completed the first successful cervical rib resection for relief of arterial compression.[8] Murphy performed a first rib resection in 1910 for neurogenic TOS.[9] Adson and Coffey performed the first scalenectomy in 1927, without first rib resection.[10] Later, it was realized that the division of the muscle alone led to recurrent symptoms. The posterior approach to first rib resection was described by Clagett in 1962,[11] and the transaxillary approach to first rib resection was described by Roos in 1966.[12] Other surgical approaches include supraclavicular as well as combined techniques using transaxillary first rib resection and transcervical scalenectomy.[1,13]

Anatomy and Predisposing Factors

TOS is divided into three distinct subtypes: neurogenic, venous, and arterial. Symptoms are produced relative to which of the neurovascular structures is compressed in the thoracic outlet [*see Table 1*]. In this regard, the scalene triangle is the most important anatomic space in the thoracic outlet. The anterior and middle scalene muscles comprise the sides of the scalene triangle, with the first rib forming the base of the triangle. The anterior and middle scalene both arise from the lower cervical spine. Through this relatively small space pass the subclavian artery and vein, as well as the five nerve roots of the brachial plexus. These muscles can potentially scar and/or hypertrophy with repetitive motion or trauma, further contributing to compression of the neurovascular structures. The subclavius muscle, which is found between the clavicle and the first rib, also may compress the subclavian vein, contributing to venous TOS. This muscle is frequently found to be hypertrophied in patients presenting with effort thrombosis.[14]

A combination of congenital anatomic predispositions and acquired extrinsic factors results in the spectrum of symptoms associated with TOS. Cervical ribs, which are congenital, can predispose to all three types of TOS. They have an incidence of approximately 1% in the general population with 50% bilaterality.[15,16] Although most cervical ribs are asymptomatic, they occur in up to 11% of patients undergoing surgical decompression for TOS.[17,18] A long C7 transverse process or bifid first rib may also predispose to TOS, but these are even less common. Particularly in neurogenic TOS, congenital fibromuscular bands often are observed—in more than 80% of patients, according to some authors.[19] These congenital bands and ligaments have been categorized into nine different types by Roos.[20] Anatomic variation in the size and insertion points of the scalene muscles has also been implicated.

In addition to these predisposing anatomic factors, trauma and repetitive motion also play a role in the development of TOS. Some authors have reported that up to 80% of TOS patients have a history of trauma to the neck or shoulder area.[21] Repetitive motion attributable to athletic activity (e.g., swimming or weight lifting) or occupational environment (e.g., poor posture and/or prolonged computer use) also may contribute to the development of TOS.

Table 1 Thoracic Outlet Syndrome: Types and Characteristics

Characteristic	Neurogenic Most Common Form of TOS	Venous Subclavian Vein Thrombosis	Arterial Subclavian Artery Thrombosis
Sex	Female (3.5:1)	Male	Female/male equally
Age (yr)	20–40	20–30	20–30
Risk factors	Repetitive movements Previous trauma	Strenuous work Athletics	Vigorous arm activity
Symptoms	Pain down arm, forearm, ring finger, and little finger Paresthesias (pain, numbness) at night Arm/hand weakness Arm/hand swelling Loss of dexterity Cold intolerance Headache	Pain in affected arm often associated with strenuous work Arm/hand swelling Veins of shoulder and chest appear more visible Hand/arm appears blue in color	Pain Claudication Hand appears white in color Hand/arm cool Decreased pulse
Laboratory studies	None	Hypercoagulable studies	Hypercoagulable studies
Imaging studies	Chest x-ray	Chest x-ray Duplex ultrasonography Venography	Chest x-ray Duplex ultrasonography Arteriography
Other studies	Nerve conduction study	Nerve conduction study	Nerve conduction study
Consultations	Vascular surgeon Physical therapy (PT) Pain management	Vascular surgeon Hematologist	Vascular surgeon Hematologist
Treatment	Physical therapy (PT) Lidocaine bocks Botulinum toxin blocks* Surgical intervention† Postoperative PT	Anticoagulant Surgical intervention Venography/venoplasty Postoperative PT	Anticoagulant Surgical intervention Arteriography/arterioplasty Postoperative PT
Prognosis	Good	Good	Good
Recovery time	Longer period of time (time needed is dependent on duration of symptoms prior to treatment and commitment to PT)	Quick	Quick

TOS = thoracic outlet syndrome.
*Brand of botulinum toxin type A manufactured by Allergan (Irvine, CA).
†Not all neurogenic TOS patients need or are candidates for surgery.

Preoperative Evaluation

NEUROGENIC THORACIC OUTLET SYNDROME

Symptoms attributable to neurogenic TOS are caused by compression of the roots of the brachial plexus and are much the same as those experienced with nerve compression in other parts of the body. Pain, paresthesias, and weakness in the pattern of the affected nerve roots are common. Pain and/or point tenderness in the anterior or posterior shoulder region, as well as the neck and occipital or mastoid region, is also a common finding. Headaches may also be present. On physical examination, there is often tenderness over the scalene muscles and/or the supraclavicular fossa on the involved side. Radiation of pain or paresthesias in the symptomatic arm can often be reproduced by deep palpation of the scalene muscles or other provocative maneuvers, such as abducting the arms to 90° in external rotation. With the arms in the same position, the patient can be asked to repeatedly open and close the hands for several minutes, the so-called Roos stress test. Reproduction of the patient's symptoms with this maneuver may be an indication of neurogenic TOS. During the Adson maneuver, the arm on the affected side is abducted and the head is rotated toward the same side. Disappearance of the radial pulse is a nonspecific finding, but reproduction of the patient's symptoms may again be an indication of neurogenic TOS. Decreased grip strength and mild to moderate sensory abnormalities in the affected hand are common findings. Atrophy of the intrinsic muscles of the hand is a late and uncommon finding. A chest x-ray to rule out bony abnormalities is mandatory. Magnetic resonance imaging, nerve conduction studies, and electromyography can be helpful. However, as there is no definitive diagnostic test for neurogenic TOS, the diagnosis is typically clinical. Prior to considering surgery for neurogenic TOS, nerve conduction studies should be obtained as they are the best objective test for this condition.

VENOUS THORACIC OUTLET SYNDROME

The most common presentation of venous TOS is acute effort thrombosis of the axillosubclavian vein, also known as Paget-Schroetter syndrome. This is characterized by the sudden onset of swelling, pain, and discoloration of the affected upper extremity. Edema is nonpitting and involves the entire arm. Additionally, superficial veins of the upper arm, shoulder, and chest wall may be distended and visible. Typically, these patients are young and healthy and often quite athletic. Swimmers, weight lifters, and volleyball players are particularly common. Again, the diagnosis is typically clinical but can be confirmed with duplex ultrasonography. If ultrasonography is for some reason unavailable or equivocal, contrast venography will confirm the diagnosis. Again, chest x-ray to rule out bony abnormalities should be performed.

ARTERIAL THORACIC OUTLET SYNDROME

Symptoms attributable to arterial TOS are commonly the result of thromboemboli from intimal lesions or post-stenotic arterial aneurysms. Patients present with varying degrees of arm or hand ischemia. Ischemia may manifest with many signs and symptoms, including weakness, paresthesias, pain and pallor, and diminished pulses distally, especially with activity or positional changes. A positive Adson test aids in the diagnosis but is not pathognomonic. Chest x-ray is extremely important in the diagnosis as cervical ribs are often present in cases of arterial TOS. Duplex ultrasonography is also essential to assess the presence and degree of arterial stenosis and to detect subclavian artery aneurysm.[22] Arteriography is not mandatory but can be quite useful in identifying arterial lesions caused by extrinsic compression or post-stenotic aneurysms.

Treatment

NEUROGENIC THORACIC OUTLET SYNDROME

Initial therapy for neurogenic TOS is always conservative. This consists of two broad categories, lifestyle modification and physical therapy. Lifestyle modification includes posture training for proper posture when walking, sitting, and standing, which promotes relaxation of the neck muscles and may help decompress the thoracic outlet. It also includes modification of daily activities, including minimization of repetitive motion, overhead work, and weight lifting, if applicable. Exercises directed toward improved range of motion and flexibility also may provide symptomatic improvement. Physical therapy is TOS specific [*see Table 2*] and consists of three sessions per week for 8 weeks before surgery is considered. If the patient proceeds to surgical treatment, physical therapy is also used postoperatively for the same frequency and duration to include increased range of motion, strengthening exercises, and soft tissue or scar tissue massage.

If lifestyle modification and physical therapy are unsuccessful, a computed tomography (CT)-guided anterior scalene block is performed with local anesthetic. The block causes relaxation of the anterior scalene muscle, allowing the first rib to drop, which should relieve tension on the brachial plexus. Symptomatic relief as the result of a scalene muscle block is a reasonable procedure to give some indication as to whether a first rib resection and anterior scalenectomy will be beneficial. CT-guided scalene muscle block is used by some investigators for diagnosing neurogenic TOS.[23] We have also found that CT-guided botulinum toxin type A (Botox, Allergan, Irvine, CA) injections provide symptomatic relief for at least 1 month and often up to 3 months.[24] These treatments may be used as a bridge to surgery or as an adjunct to nonoperative treatment with physical therapy. We do not offer more

Table 2 Thoracic Outlet Syndrome: Specific Physical Therapy Protocol

Weeks 1–3
Manual therapy:
Soft tissue mobilization (STM) of scar when closed
STM of anterior thorax, intercostal spaces, diaphragm
Joint mobilization of sternoclavicular (SC) and costosternal joints and acromioclavicular joint (AC)
Positioning and mobility of the ribs
Mobilization of the thoracic and cervical spine
Usually thoracic extension and cervical flexion
Focus of occiput-atlantis (OA) flexion
Brachial plexus and peripheral neural mobility
Teasing stretch or pain sensation—with caution to avoid exacerbating symptoms
Therapeutic exercise and neuromuscular reeducation:
Diaphragmatic breathing
OA flexion
Gentle scapular posterior depression exercises
Use prolonged holds > 45″ to retain position and movement with gentle manual resistance
Gentle neural mobility
Posture training:
Activity restriction education, patient self-care education
Sleep position and transfers
Lifting and reaching related to activities of daily living (ADL)
Weeks 4–6 (build-off gains made in weeks 1–3)
Manual therapy:
STM to pectoralis, serratus anterior, and latissimus dorsi
STM to neck and along track of brachial plexus (neck to hand)
Gentle mobility of glenohumeral joint and AC joint separation
Focus on inferior glide of humeral head and mobility of the posterior rotator cuff
Therapeutic exercise and neuromuscular reeducation:
Continue with prolonged holds of OA flexion with manual and self-progressive resistance exercise
Continue with prolonged holds of scapular posterior depression
Add mild resistance with Thera-Band or weights
Train scapular stability in prone or elbow position before progressing to quadruped
Supine shoulder flexion exercises with wand
Add gentle manual resistance in flexion when patient can perform full flexion without scapular substitution, thoracic extension, or sternum elevation
Posture training
Focus on sitting posture and assumption of work position while holding proper posture
Weeks 7–8
Manual therapy:
Moderate to aggressive glenohumeral mobilizations (specifically Mulligan glenohumeral mobilizations with movement)
Continue neural mobilization until patient can reach full tension position without complaints of pain/stretch symptoms
Address other limitations in soft tissue and joint mobility as needed
Therapeutic exercise and neuromuscular reeducation:
Scapular posterior depression exercises against resistance as tolerated
Still focus on prolonged hold of postural muscles
Plank exercises maintaining scapular neutral position
Add weight shifts, walking out with a Thera-Ball, and pushups from the knees
Independent maintenance of neural mobility
Progress to resisted exercises of shoulder flexion against gravity if patient is able to perform without scapular substitution
Perform exercises until fatigue or substitution
Posture training:
Lifting crates/boxes with full squat while maintaining scapular neutral position
Mimic work-related activities

than two injections because the muscle and surrounding tissues tend to scar and the long-term effects of repeated botulinum toxin injections are not known.

Surgical treatment consists of first rib resection and anterior scalenectomy, and our favored approach is transaxillary (see below). When neurogenic TOS patients are appropriately selected for surgical intervention, we have shown good outcomes in terms of quality-of-life improvements.[25]

VENOUS THORACIC OUTLET SYNDROME

Traditionally, treatment of secondary axillosubclavian vein thrombosis has consisted of conservative measures: systemic anticoagulation with rest and elevation of the affected extremity. However, in primary axillosubclavian vein thrombosis, conservative treatment alone leaves most patients with residual symptoms attributable to venous outflow obstruction. As most of these patients are young and active, more aggressive therapy is required. Once the diagnosis of thrombosis as a result of venous TOS is suspected, the patient should undergo contrast venography. Once thrombosis is confirmed, catheter-directed thrombolysis should be performed. Once the thrombosis has been cleared, venography should be repeated to confirm extrinsic compression of the subclavian vein. Compression and narrowing of the vein at the costoclavicular junction are almost universally present in cases of venous TOS. Angioplasty and stenting should not be performed in the initial setting until the patient has undergone thoracic outlet decompression via first rib resection and anterior scalenectomy. This can be performed days to weeks after the initial thrombolysis. Again, our preferred approach is transaxillary. To avoid bleeding complications, no anticoagulation is given until 3 days after surgery. Therapeutic low-molecular-weight heparin injections are given until 2 weeks later, when repeat venography is performed. At this time, residual stenotic areas can be percutaneous and dilated effectively as extrinsic compression has been relieved. If the vein has remained patent and no intervention is required, anticoagulation is discontinued. If the vein has rethrombosed, repeat thrombolysis may be performed and anticoagulation continued with warfarin, with an international normalized ratio of 2 to 3. The patient is followed long term with duplex ultrasonography monthly, and anticoagulation is continued as long as areas of increased velocities in the subclavian vein are visualized during arm abduction, up to 6 months. In our series of more than 80 patients with venous thrombosis secondary to venous TOS, we found that after 6 months, all remained patent. Therefore, we do not anticoagulate beyond this time.

The final important consideration is a thorough hypercoagulable workup. We have observed an increased frequency of hypercoagulable disorders in patients with Paget-Schroetter syndrome. Therefore, we now perform a hypercoagulable workup in all our venous TOS patients, as well as in arterial thrombosis patients. If the patient presents acutely, these laboratory values will be assessed initially. If the patient presents from another institution where he or she has already undergone thrombolysis and is being maintained on warfarin therapy, the hypercoagulable evaluation is done 6 months after discontinuation of warfarin. These laboratory tests include protein C and S levels, factor V Leiden mutation, prothrombin gene mutation 20210, antithrombin III level, antiphospholipid antibodies (lupus anticoagulant and anticardiolipin antibodies), homocysteine levels, and methylene tetrahydrofolate reductase (MTHFR) 677T variant. If the patient is confirmed to have a hypercoagulable disorder, then he or she is continued on lifelong anticoagulation.

ARTERIAL THORACIC OUTLET SYNDROME

The timing and sequence of therapy for arterial TOS depend on the degree and acuteness of ischemia. The majority of patients with arterial TOS present chronic ischemic symptoms and a nonthreatened limb. In this situation, the proximal embolic source is eliminated first. This is typically accomplished by direct arterial reconstruction, preferably with an autologous vein. This can be undertaken at the same time of resection of the commonly found cervical or rudimentary rib, depending on the surgical approach. In arterial TOS, a transaxillary approach may be employed for rib resection and scalenectomy, but arterial reconstruction is not possible from this approach. This typically requires a supraclavicular approach. If the patient presents with acute and limb-threatening ischemia, distal thromboemboli must be cleared first, either surgically or via thrombolysis, before rib resection and arterial reconstruction.

TRANSAXILLARY APPROACH TO FIRST RIB RESECTION AND ANTERIOR SCALENECTOMY

A detailed description of the multiple approaches to thoracic outlet decompression is beyond the scope of this chapter. Our preferred approach is transaxillary because it allows for safe exposure and excellent visualization of the major structures through a cosmetically acceptable, low-morbidity incision. First and cervical ribs, as well as rudimentary ribs, are all readily removed via this approach. The vast majority of patients are easily treated through transaxillary thoracic outlet decompression. As previously mentioned, direct arterial reconstruction is the only task not amenable to this technique.

The patient undergoes general anesthesia with a short-acting neuromuscular blockade such as succinylcholine, allowing for safer dissection around the brachial plexus, as well as easier identification of the long thoracic nerve. The patient is placed in the lateral decubitus position and prepared from the neck to beyond the nipples. An adjustable arm support, the Machleder retractor [*see Figure 1*], is attached to the operating room table and allows for elevation of the arm. This elevation is vital for adequate exposure of the axilla during dissection. Prior to placement on the retractor, the arm is well padded to prevent injury to the median and ulnar nerves at the elbow. The skin incision is made at the lower border of the axillary hair line between the latissimus dorsi and pectoralis major muscles. Dissection with cautery proceeds down to the flimsy areolar tissue superficial to the chest wall. Gentle blunt dissection is then used in an anterior and cephalad direction. Manual palpation is used to identify the first rib as it approaches the clavicle. A self-retaining retractor is then placed and the Machleder retractor is elevated to facilitate exposure in the axilla. The soft tissue overlying the subclavian vessels and the scalene muscles is swept away with a Kittner blunt dissector. Frequently, a small branch of the subclavian artery must be ligated and divided to fully mobilize the artery. The first rib is identified and the

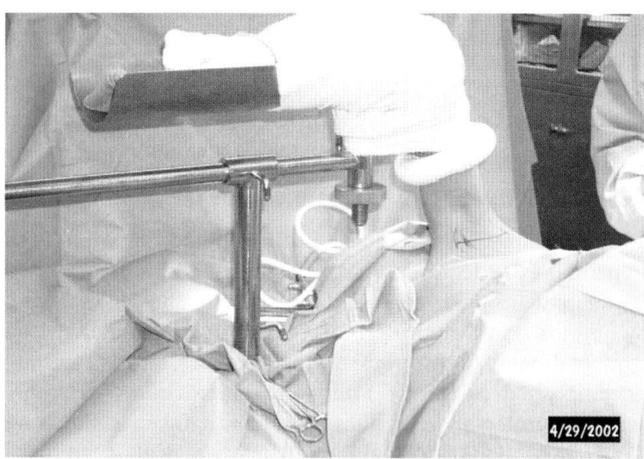

Figure 1 **Machleder retractor used for positioning during transaxillary first rib resection. The patient is placed in a decubitus position with the nonoperative side down. Ample sterile towels are used for padding, and the arm is secured in the retractor with a combination of gauze and elastic wraps.**

intercostal muscle attachments are bluntly cleared from the lower edge using a Kittner blunt dissector followed by a flat periosteal elevator [*see Figure 2*]. The first rib is separated from the underlying pleura by gently sliding a small periosteal elevator beneath the first rib. The pleura is pushed away from the rib, and this mobilization extends from behind the brachial plexus posteriorly to in front of the subclavian vein anteriorly. The subclavius muscle, which has a crescent-shaped ligamentous attachment on the first rib adjacent to the subclavian vein, is sharply divided with scissors, taking care not to injure the subclavian vein. Division of the subclavius muscle provides greater anterior mobilization of the first rib, allowing for more anterior resection, which is of particular importance in venous TOS. The scalene medius fibers are dissected bluntly using a periosteal elevator. Sharp dissection is avoided because of the adjacent course of the long thoracic nerve. The anterior scalene muscle must be clearly visualized between the subclavian artery and vein. A right-angle clamp is then placed behind the anterior scalene muscle, lifting it away from the adjacent artery. The muscle is divided sharply with scissors, leaving as much length as possible attached to the rib [*see Figure 3*]. This maneuver is performed with care and may need to be repeated multiple times to divide the muscle safely. A bone cutter is then placed anteriorly and the first rib is divided adjacent to the subclavian vein. The posterior division of the rib occurs once the remainder of the rib is mobilized. This allows for optimal visualization of the brachial plexus to prevent injury when cutting the rib posteriorly. The rib cutter is gently applied to the rib just anterior to the brachial plexus. The nerve must be visualized prior to making any cut [*see Figure 4*]. The rib is divided and removed. The rib is always cut in front of the nerve so that posterior nerve roots are not unintentionally damaged. The remainder of the rib anteriorly and posteriorly is trimmed with a rongeur. The nerve root is pushed away and protected with a Roos retractor as the posterior remnant of the rib is rongeured. The bone edges should be fairly uniform, and there should be no impingement on the neurovascular structures [*see Figure 5*]. Saline is then instilled into the axillary cavity, and the patient is given several positive pressure ventilations to check for tears in the parietal pleura. If a pneumothorax is present, a 12 French chest tube is placed in the second intercostal space through a separate stab incision. This is applied to 20 cm of water suction after the arm is lowered and the wound is closed in two layers.

Outcomes

The most common complication of transaxillary thoracic outlet decompression is pneumothorax, occurring in approximately 10% of patients. Fortunately, this is easily dealt with intraoperatively by placement of a small chest tube, which is

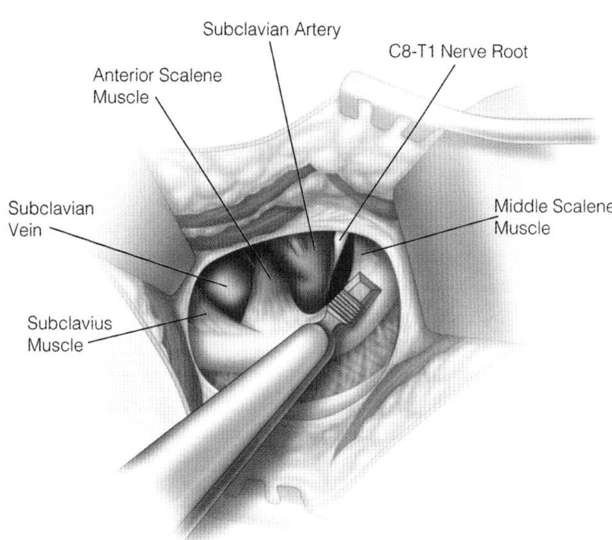

Figure 2 **Gentle dissection of the first rib with a periosteal elevator.**

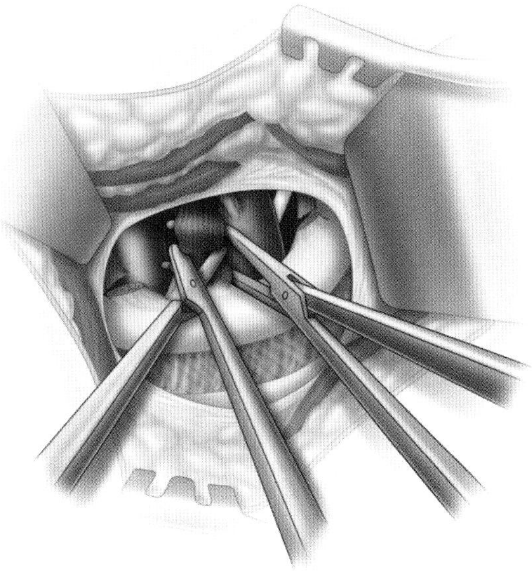

Figure 3 **Anterior scalene muscle isolated by a right-angle clamp prior to dissection.**

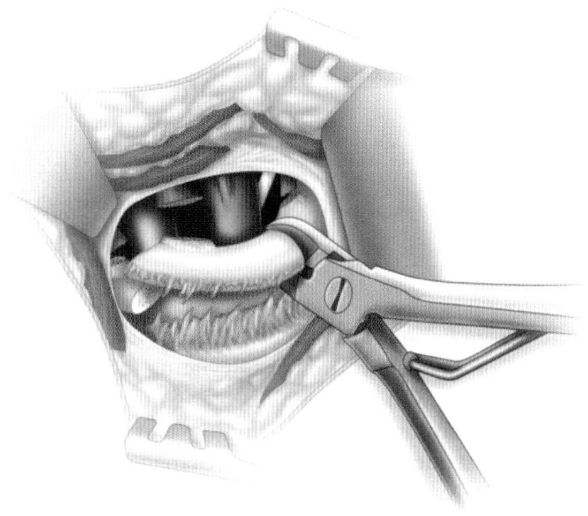

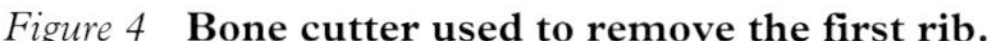

Figure 4 **Bone cutter used to remove the first rib.**

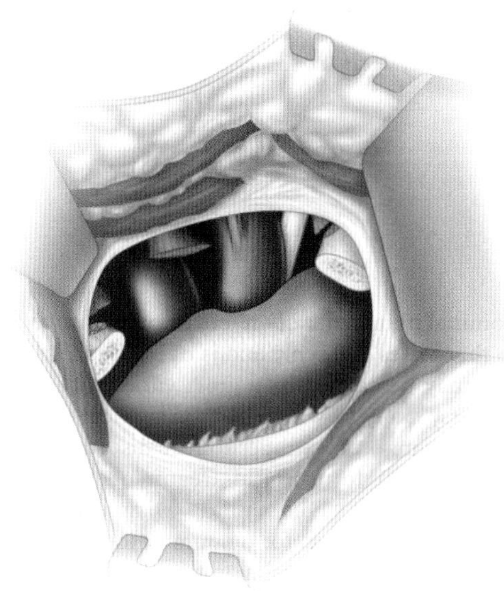

Figure 5 **Anatomic space immediately prior to closure. The neurovascular structures are no longer restricted following rib resection.**

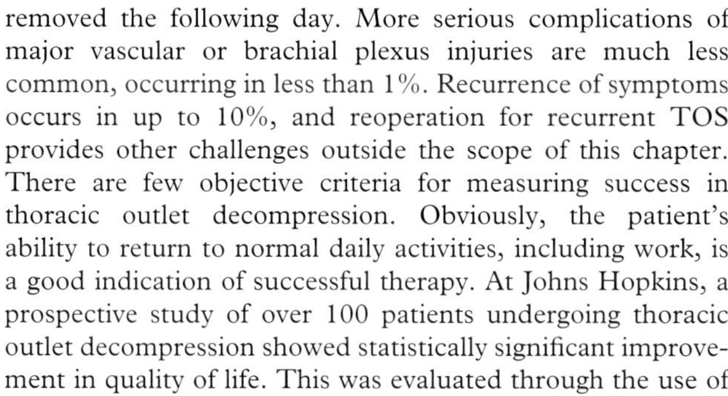

removed the following day. More serious complications of major vascular or brachial plexus injuries are much less common, occurring in less than 1%. Recurrence of symptoms occurs in up to 10%, and reoperation for recurrent TOS provides other challenges outside the scope of this chapter. There are few objective criteria for measuring success in thoracic outlet decompression. Obviously, the patient's ability to return to normal daily activities, including work, is a good indication of successful therapy. At Johns Hopkins, a prospective study of over 100 patients undergoing thoracic outlet decompression showed statistically significant improvement in quality of life. This was evaluated through the use of a novel survey instrument.[25] The majority of patients in this study were able to return to work or activity within 6 months. Ultimately, successful outcomes depend on thorough diagnostic evaluation, carefully selected and often multimodal therapy, and long-term follow-up.

Financial Disclosures: None Reported

References

1. Atasoy E. Thoracic outlet compression syndrome. Orthop Clin North Am 1996;27:265–303.
2. Atasoy E. History of thoracic outlet syndrome. Hand Clin 2004;20:15–6.
3. Cooper A. An exostosis. In: Cooper A, Cooper B, Travers B, editors. Surgical essays. 3rd ed. London: Longman; 1821. p. 128.
4. Bramwell E, Dykes HB. Rib pressure and the brachial plexus. Edinburgh Med J 1927;27:65.
5. Ochsner A, Gage M, Debakey M. Scalenus anticus syndrome. Am J Surg 1935;28:669–95.
6. Falconer MA, Weddell G. Costoclavicular compression of the subclavian artery and vein. Lancet 1943;2:539–43.
7. Peet RM, Henriksen JD, Anderson TD, Martin GM. Thoracic outlet syndrome: evaluation of a therapeutic exercise program. Mayo Clin Proc 1956;31:281–7.
8. Coote H. Exostosis of the left transverse process of the seventh cervical vertebra surrounded by blood vessels and nerves: successful removal. Lancet 1861;1:360–1.
9. Murphy T. Brachial neuritis caused by pressure of first rib. Aust Med J 1910;15:582–5.
10. Adson JW, Coffey JR. Cervical rib: a method of anterior approach for relief of symptoms by division of the scalenus anticus. Ann Surg 1927;85:839–57.
11. Clagett OT. Presidential address: research and prosearch. J Thorac Cardiovasc Surg 1962;44:153–66.
12. Roos DB. Transaxillary approach to first rib resection to relieve thoracic outlet syndrome. Ann Surg 1966;163:354–8.
13. Gol A, Patrick DW, McNeel DP. Relief of costoclavicular syndrome by infraclavicular removal of first rib: technical note. J Neurosurg 1968;28:81–4.
14. Caparrelli DJ, Freischlag JA. Thoracic outlet syndromes. In: Cameron JC, editor. Current surgical therapy. 9th ed. Philadelphia: Elsevier Mosby; 2007. p. 878–84.
15. Leffert RD. Thoracic outlet syndromes. Hand Clin 1992;8:285–97.
16. Adson WA. Surgical treatment for symptoms produced by cervical ribs and the scalenus anticus muscle. Surg Gynecol Obstet 1947;85:687–700.
17. Novak CB, Mackinnon SE. Thoracic outlet syndrome. Orthop Clin North Am 1996;27:747–62.
18. Oates SD, Daley RA. Thoracic outlet syndrome. Hand Clin 1996;12:705–18.
19. Thomas GI, Jones TW, Stavney LS, Manhas DR. The middle scalene muscle and its contribution to the thoracic outlet syndrome. J Am Dent Assoc 1993;145:589–92.
20. Roos DB. Congenital anomalies associated with thoracic outlet syndrome: anatomy, symptoms, diagnosis and treatment. Am J Surg 1976;132:771–8.
21. Sanders RJ, Pearce WH. The treatment of thoracic outlet syndrome: a comparison of different operations. J Vasc Surg 1989;10:626–34.
22. Caparrelli DJ, Tabulov DM, Freischlag JA. Image of the month. Subclavian artery aneurysm secondary to cervical rib. Arch Surg 2006;141:513.
23. Jordan SE, Machleder HI. Diagnosis of thoracic outlet syndrome using electrophysiologically guided anterior scalene blocks. Ann Vasc Surg 1998;12:260–4.
24. Jordan SE, Ahn SS, Freischlag JA, et al. Selective botulinum chemodenervation of the scalene muscles for treatment of neurogenic thoracic outlet syndrome. Ann Vasc Surg 2000;14:365–9.
25. Chang DC, Rotellini-Coltvet LA, Mukherjee D, et al. Surgical intervention for thoracic outlet syndrome improves patient's quality of life. J Vasc Surg 2009;49:630–7.

Acknowledgments

Figures 2–5 Christine Kenney

perforated viscus, or a ruptured ectopic pregnancy; a near loss of consciousness or stamina associated with sudden-onset pain should heighten the level of concern for such a catastrophe. Rapidly progressive pain that becomes intensely focused in a well-defined area within a period of a few minutes to an hour or two suggests a condition such as acute cholecystitis or pancreatitis. Pain that has a gradual onset over several hours, usually beginning as slight or vague discomfort and slowly progressing to steady and more localized pain, suggests a subacute process and is characteristic of processes that lead to peritoneal inflammation. Numerous disorders may be associated with this mode of onset, including acute appendicitis, diverticulitis, pelvic inflammatory disease (PID), and intestinal obstruction.

Pain can be either intermittent or continuous. Intermittent or cramping pain (colic) is pain that occurs for a short period (a few minutes), followed by longer periods (a few minutes to one half-hour) of complete remission during which there is no pain at all. Intermittent pain is characteristic of obstruction of a hollow viscus and results from vigorous peristalsis in the wall of the viscus proximal to the site of obstruction. This pain is perceived as deep in the abdomen and is poorly localized. The patient is restless, may writhe about incessantly in an effort to find a comfortable position, and often presses on the abdominal wall in an attempt to alleviate the pain. Whereas the intermittent pain associated with intestinal obstruction (typically described as gripping and mounting) is usually severe but bearable, the pain associated with obstruction of small conduits (e.g., the biliary tract, the ureters, and the uterine tubes) often becomes unbearable. Obstruction of the gallbladder or the bile ducts gives rise to a type of pain often referred to as biliary colic; however, this term is a misnomer in that biliary pain is usually constant because of the lack of a strong muscular coat in the biliary tree and the absence of regular peristalsis.

Continuous or constant pain is pain that is present for hours or days without any period of complete relief; it is more common than intermittent pain. Continuous pain is usually indicative of a process that will lead, or has already led, to peritoneal inflammation or ischemia. It may be of steady intensity throughout, or it may be associated with intermittent pain. For example, the typical colicky pain associated with simple intestinal obstruction changes when strangulation occurs, becoming continuous pain that persists between episodes or waves of cramping pain.

Certain types of pain are generally held to be typical of certain pathologic states. For example, the pain of a perforated ulcer is often described as burning, that of a dissecting aneurysm as tearing, and that of bowel obstruction as gripping. One may imagine that the first type of pain is explained by the efflux of acid, the second by the sudden expansion of the retroperitoneum, and the third by the churning of hyperperistalsis. Colorful as these images may be, in most cases, the pain begins in a nondescript way. It is only by carefully following the patient's description of the evolution and time course of the pain that such images may be formed with confidence.

For several reasons—atypical pain patterns, dual innervation by visceral and somatic afferents, normal variations in organ position, and widely diverse underlying pathologic states—the location of abdominal pain is only a rough guide to diagnosis. It is nevertheless true that in most disorders, the pain tends to occur in characteristic locations, such as the right upper quadrant (cholecystitis), the right lower quadrant (appendicitis), the epigastrium (pancreatitis), or the left lower quadrant (sigmoid diverticulitis) [*see Figure 2*]. It is important to determine the location of the pain at onset because this may differ from the location at the time of presentation (so-called shifting pain). In fact, the chronological sequence of events in the patient's history is often more important for diagnosis than the location of the pain alone. For example, the classic pain of appendicitis begins in the periumbilical region and settles in the right lower quadrant. Another example is the pain from a perforated ulcer which can shift to the right lower quadrant as escaping gastroduodenal content tracks down the right gutter.

It is also important to take into account radiation or referral of the pain, which tends to occur in characteristic patterns [*see Figure 3*]. For example, biliary pain is referred to the right subscapular area, and the boring pain of pancreatitis typically radiates straight through to the back. Obstruction of the small intestine and the proximal colon is referred to the umbilicus, and obstruction distal to the splenic flexure is often referred to the suprapubic area. Spasm in the ureter often radiates to the suprapubic area and into the groin. The more severe the pain is, the more likely it is to be associated with referral to other areas.

The intensity or severity of the pain is related to the magnitude of the underlying insult. It is important to distinguish between the intensity of the pain and the patient's reaction to it because there appear to be significant individual differences with respect to tolerance of and reaction to pain. Pain that is intense enough to awaken the patient from sleep usually indicates a significant underlying organic cause. Past episodes of pain and factors that aggravate or relieve the pain often provide useful diagnostic clues. For example, pain caused by peritonitis tends to be exacerbated by motion, deep breathing, coughing, or sneezing, and patients with peritonitis tend to lie quietly in bed and avoid any movement. The typical pain of acute pancreatitis is exacerbated by lying down and relieved by sitting up. Pain that is relieved by eating or taking antacids suggests duodenal ulcer disease, whereas diffuse abdominal pain that appears 30 minutes to 1 hour after meals suggests intestinal angina.

Associated gastrointestinal symptoms (e.g., nausea, vomiting, anorexia, diarrhea, and constipation) often accompany abdominal pain; however, these symptoms are nonspecific and therefore may not be of great value in the differential diagnosis. Vomiting in particular is common: when sufficiently stimulated by pain impulses traveling via secondary visceral afferent fibers, the medullary vomiting centers activate efferent fibers and cause reflex vomiting. Once again, the chronology of events is important in that pain often precedes vomiting in patients with conditions necessitating operation, whereas the opposite is usually the case in patients with medical (i.e., nonsurgical) conditions.[5,12] This is particularly true for adult patients with acute appendicitis, in whom pain almost always precedes vomiting by several hours. In children, vomiting is commonly observed closer to the onset of the pain, although it is rarely the initial symptom.

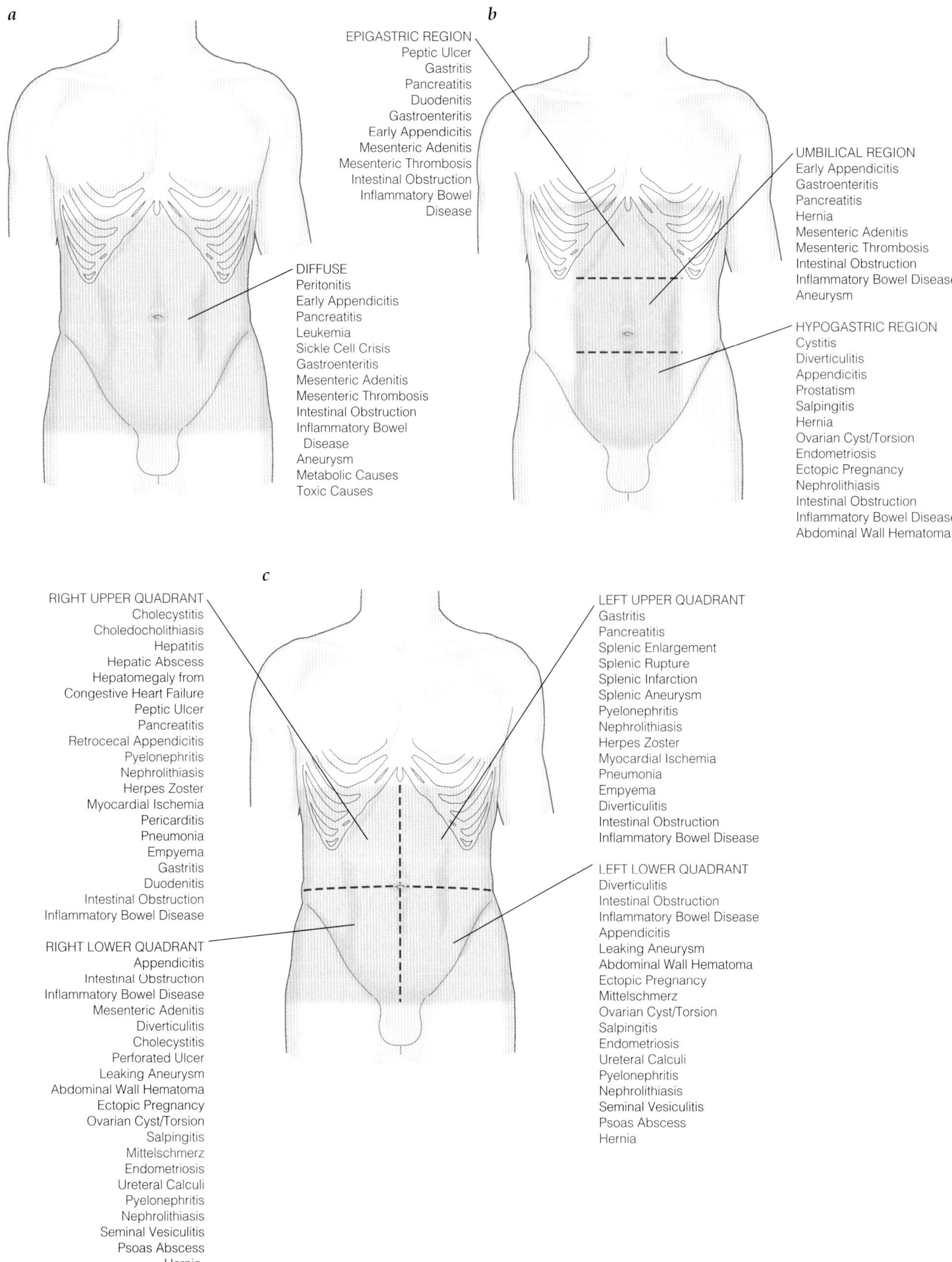

Figure 2 **In most disorders that give rise to acute abdominal pain, the pain tends to occur in specific locations. (*a*) Diffuse pain suggests a certain set of diagnostic possibilities. (*b*) Differing groups of disorders give rise to abdominal pain in the epigastric, umbilical, and hypogastric regions. (*c*) Disorders that give rise to acute abdominal pain may be grouped according to the quadrant of the abdomen in which pain tends to occur.**

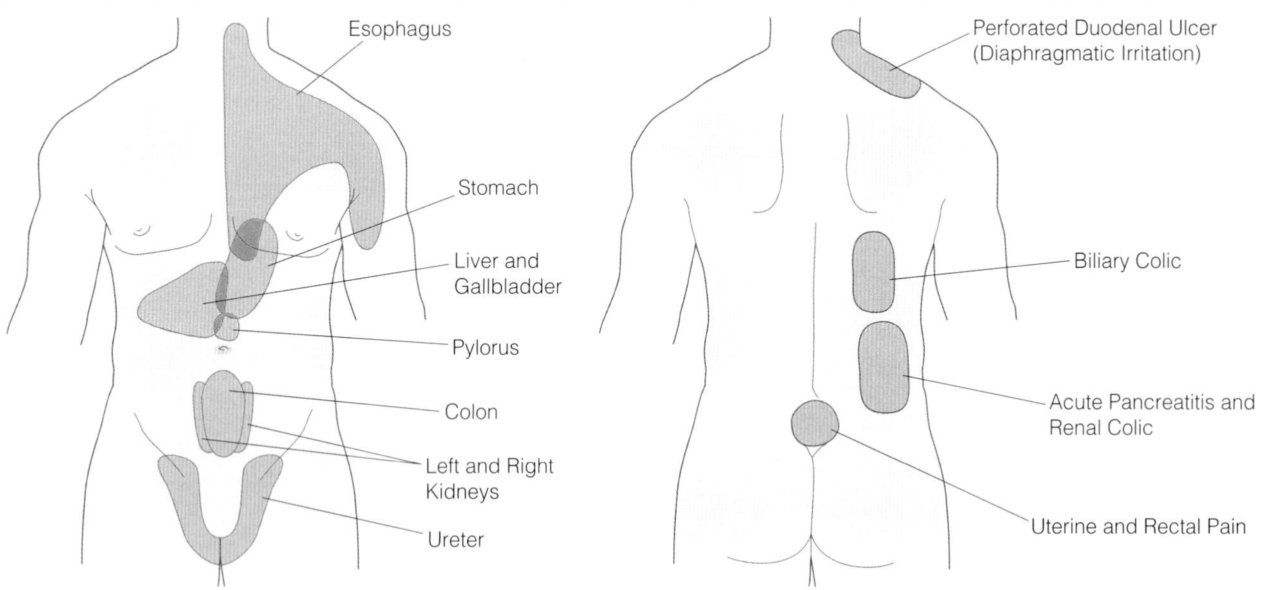

Figure 3 **Pain of abdominal origin tends to be referred in characteristic patterns.[80] The more severe the pain is, the more likely it is to be referred. Shown are anterior (*left*) and posterior (*right*) areas of referred pain.**

Similarly, constipation may result from a reflex paralytic ileus when sufficiently stimulated visceral afferent fibers activate efferent sympathetic fibers (splanchnic nerves) to reduce intestinal peristalsis. Diarrhea is characteristic of gastroenteritis but may also accompany incomplete intestinal or colonic obstruction. More significant is a history of obstipation because if it can be definitely established that a patient with acute abdominal pain has not passed gas or stool for 24 to 48 hours, it is certain that some degree of intestinal obstruction is present. Other associated symptoms that should be noted include jaundice, melena, hematochezia, hematemesis, and hematuria. These symptoms are much more specific than the ones just discussed and can be extremely valuable in the differential diagnosis. Most conditions that cause acute abdominal pain of surgical significance are associated with some degree of fever if they are allowed to continue long enough. Fever suggests an inflammatory process; however, it is usually low grade and often absent altogether, particularly in elderly and immunocompromised patients. The combination of a high fever with chills and rigors indicates bacteremia, and concomitant changes in mental status (e.g., agitation, disorientation, and lethargy) suggest impending septic shock.

A history of trauma (even if the patient considers the traumatic event trivial) should be actively sought in all cases of unexplained acute abdominal pain; such a history may not be readily volunteered (as is often the case with trauma resulting from domestic violence). The history may be particularly relevant in a patient taking anticoagulants and presenting with acute onset of abdominal pain accompanied by tenderness but no clear signs of inflammation. Hematoma within the rectus muscle sheath can easily be mistaken for appendicitis or other lower abdominal illnesses; hematoma elsewhere can produce symptoms of obstruction or acute bleeding into the peritoneum and the retroperitoneum. In female patients, it is essential to obtain a detailed gynecologic history that includes the timing of symptoms within the menstrual cycle, the date of the last menses, previous and current use of contraception, any abnormal vaginal bleeding or discharge, an obstetric history, and any risk factors for ectopic pregnancy (e.g., PID, use of an intrauterine device, or previous ectopic or tubal surgery). Pregnancy should be excluded in all women of childbearing age with abdominal pain.

A complete history of previous medical conditions must be obtained because associated diseases of the cardiac, pulmonary, and renal systems may give rise to acute abdominal symptoms and may also significantly affect the morbidity and mortality associated with surgical intervention. The use of regular and as needed medications must also be obtained. Weight changes, past illnesses, recent travel, and environmental exposure to toxins or infectious agents used should also be investigated. A history of previous abdominal operations should be obtained but should not be relied on too heavily in the absence of operative reports. A careful family history is important for detection of hereditary disorders that may cause acute abdominal pain. A detailed social history should also be obtained that includes any history of tobacco, alcohol, or illicit drug use, as well as a sexual history.

TENTATIVE DIFFERENTIAL DIAGNOSIS

Once the history has been obtained, the examiner should generate a tentative differential diagnosis and carry out the physical examination in search of specific signs or findings that either rule out or confirm the diagnostic possibilities.

Given the diversity of conditions that can cause acute abdominal pain [see Table 1 and Table 2], there is no substitute for general awareness of the most common causes of acute abdominal pain and the influence of age, gender, and geography on the likelihood of any of these potential causes. Although acute abdominal pain is the most common surgical emergency and most non–trauma-related surgical admissions (and 1% of all hospital admissions) are accounted for by patients complaining of abdominal pain, little information is available regarding the clinical spectrum of disease in these patients.[13] Nevertheless, detailed epidemiologic information can be an invaluable asset in the diagnosis and treatment of acute abdominal pain. Now that patients from different parts of the world are increasingly being seen in North American

Table 1 Intraperitoneal Causes of Acute Abdominal Pain

Inflammatory	Mechanical (obstruction, acute distention)
Peritoneal	Hollow visceral
Chemical and nonbacterial peritonitis	Intestinal obstruction
Perforated peptic ulcer/biliary tree, pancreatitis, ruptured ovarian cyst, mittelschmerz	Adhesions, hernias, neoplasms, volvulus
Bacterial peritonitis	Intussusception, gallstone ileus, foreign bodies
Primary peritonitis	Bezoars, parasites
Pneumococcal, streptococcal, tuberculous	Biliary obstruction
Spontaneous bacterial peritonitis	Calculi, neoplasms, choledochal cyst, hemobilia
Perforated hollow viscus	Solid visceral
Esophagus, stomach, duodenum, small intestine, bile duct, gallbladder, colon, urinary bladder	Acute splenomegaly
Hollow visceral	Acute heptomegaly (congestive heart failure, Budd-Chiari syndrome)
Appendicitis	Mesenteric
Cholecystitis	Omental torsion
Peptic ulcer	Pelvic
Gastroenteritis	Ovarian cyst
Gastritis	Torsion or degeneration of fibroid
Duodenitis	Ectopic pregnancy
Inflammatory bowel disease	Hemoperitoneum
Meckel diverticulitis	Ruptured hepatic neoplasm
Colitis (bacterial, amebic)	Spontaneous splenic rupture
Diverticulitis	Ruptured mesentery
Solid visceral	Ruptured uterus
Pancreatitis	Ruptured graafian follicle
Hepatitis	Ruptured ectopic pregnancy
Pancreatic abscess	Ruptured aortic or visceral aneurysm
Hepatic abscess	Ischemic
Splenic abscess	Mesenteric thrombosis
Mesenteric	Hepatic infarction (toxemia, purpura)
Lymphadenitis (bacterial, viral)	Splenic infarction
Epiploic appendagitis	Omental ischemia
Pelvic	Strangulated hernia
Pelvic inflammatory disease (salpingitis)	Neoplastic
Tubo-ovarian abscess	Primary or metastatic intraperitoneal neoplasms
Endometritis	Traumatic
	Blunt trauma
	Penetrating trauma
	Iatrogenic trauma
	Domestic violence
	Miscellaneous
	Endometriosis

Adapted from McFadden DW et al.[81]

Table 2 **Extraperitoneal Causes of Acute Abdominal Pain**

Genitourinary	Neurogenic
Pyelonephritis	Herpes zoster
Perinephric abscess	Tabes dorsalis
Renal infarct	Nerve root compression
Nephrolithiasis	Spinal cord tumors
Ureteral obstruction (lithiasis, tumor)	Osteomyelitis of the spine
Acute cycstitis	Abdominal epilepsy
Prostatitis	Abdominal migraine
Seminal vesiculitis	Multiple sclerosis
Epididymitis	Inflammatory
Orchitis	Schönlein-Henoch purpura
Testicular torsion	Systemic lupus erythematosus
Dysmenorrhea	Polyarteritis nodosa
Threatened abortion	Dermatomyositis
Pulmonary	Scleroderma
Pneumonia	Infectious
Empyema	Bacterial
Pulmonary embolus	Parasitic (malaria)
Pulmonary infarction	Viral (measles, mumps, infectious mononucleosis)
Pneumothorax	Rickettsial (Rocky Mountain spotted fever)
Cardiac	Hematologic
Myocardial ischemia	Sickle cell crisis
Myocardial infarction	Acute leukemia
Acute rheumatic fever	Acute hemolytic states
Acute pericarditis	Coagulopathies
Metabolic	Pernicious anemia
Acute intermittent porphyria	Other dyscrasias
Familial Mediterranean fever	Vascular
Hypolipoproteinemia	Vasculitis
Hemochromatosis	Periarteritis
Hereditary angioneurotic edema	Toxins
Endocrine	Bacterial toxins (tetanus, *Staphylococcus*)
Diabetic ketoacidosis	Insect venom (black widow spider)
Hyperparathyroidism (hypercalcemia)	Animal venom
Acute adrenal insufficiency (Addisonian crisis)	Heavy metals (lead, arsenic, mercury)
Hyperthyroidism or hypothyroidism	Poisonous mushrooms
Musculoskeletal	Drugs
Rectus sheath hematoma	Withdrawal from narcotics
Arthritis/diskitis of thoracolumbar spine	Retroperitoneal
Psychogenic	Retroperitoneal hemorrhage (spontaneous adrenal hemorrhage)
Hypochondriasis	Psoas abscess
Somatization disorders	
Factitious	
Munchausen syndrome	
Malingering	

emergency rooms, it is important to consider endemic diseases, including tuberculosis,[14,15] parasitic diseases,[16–18] bezoars from unusual dietary habits,[19,20] and unusual malignancies.[21,22]

The value of detailed epidemiologic knowledge notwithstanding, it is worthwhile to keep in mind the truism that common things are common. Regarding which things are common, the most extensive information currently available comes from the ongoing survey begun in 1977 by the Research Committee of the OMGE. As of the last progress report on this survey, which was published in 1988, more than 200 physicians at 26 centers in 17 countries had accumulated data on 10,320 patients with acute abdominal pain [*see Table 3*].[23] The most common diagnosis in these patients was nonspecific abdominal pain (NSAP)—that is, the retrospective diagnosis of exclusion in which no cause for the pain can be identified.[24,25] NSAP accounted for 34% of all patients seen; the four most common diagnoses accounted for more than 75%. The most common surgical diagnosis in the OMGE survey was acute appendicitis, followed by acute cholecystitis, small bowel obstruction, and gynecologic disorders. Relatively few patients had perforated peptic ulcer, a finding that confirms the current downward trend in the incidence of this condition. Cancer was found to be a significant cause of acute abdominal pain. There was little variation in the geographic distribution of surgical causes of acute abdominal pain (i.e., conditions necessitating operation) among developed countries. In patients who required surgery, the most common causes were acute appendicitis (42.6%), acute cholecystitis (14.7%), small bowel obstruction (6.2%), perforated peptic ulcer (3.7%), and acute pancreatitis (4.5%).[23] The OMGE survey's finding that NSAP was the most common diagnosis in patients with acute abdominal pain has been confirmed by several srudies[12,13,25]; the finding that acute appendicitis, cholecystitis, and intestinal obstruction were the three most common diagnoses in patients with acute abdominal pain who require operation has also been amply confirmed [*see Table 3*].[1,12,13]

The data described so far provide a comprehensive picture of the most likely diagnoses for patients with acute abdominal pain in many centers around the world; however, this picture does not take into account the effect of age on the relative likelihood of the various potential diagnoses. It is well known that the disease spectrum of acute abdominal pain is different in different age groups, especially in the very old[4,26,27] and the very young.[28–30] In the OMGE survey, well over 90% of cases of acute abdominal pain in children were diagnosed as having acute appendicitis (32%) or NSAP (62%).[28] Similar age-related differences in the spectrum of disease have been confirmed by other studies,[16] as have various gender-related differences.

This variation in the disease spectrum is readily apparent when the 10,320 patients from the OMGE survey are segregated by age [*see Table 4*]. In patients 50 years of age

***Table 3* Frequency of Specific Diagnoses in Patients with Acute Abdominal Pain**

Diagnosis	Frequency in Individual Studies (% of Patients)					
	OMGE[23] (*N* = 10,320)	Wilson et al[82] (*N* = 1,196)	Irvin[13] (*N* = 1,190)	Brewer et al[12] (*N* = 1,000)	de Dombal[1] (*N* = 552)	Hawthorn[83] (*N* = 496)
Nonspecific abdominal pain	34.0	45.6	34.9	41.3	50.5	36.0
Acute appendicitis	28.1	15.6	16.8	4.3	26.3	14.9
Acute cholecystitis	9.7	5.8	5.1	2.5	7.6	5.9
Small bowel obstruction	4.1	2.6	14.8	2.5	3.6	8.6
Acute gynecologic disease	4.0	4.0	1.1	8.5	—	—
Acute pancreatitis	2.9	1.3	2.4	—	2.9	2.1
Urologic disorders	2.9	4.7	5.9	11.4	—	12.8
Perforated peptic ulcer	2.5	2.3	2.5	2.0	3.1	—
Cancer	1.5	—	3.0	—	—	—
Diverticular disease	1.5	1.1	3.9	—	2.0	3.0
Dyspepsia	1.4	7.6	1.4	1.4	—	—
Gastroenteritis	—	—	0.3	6.9	—	5.1
Inflammatory bowel disease	—	—	0.8	—	—	2.1
Mesenteric adenitis	—	3.6	—	—	—	1.5
Gastritis	—	2.1	—	1.4	—	—
Constipation	—	2.4	—	2.3	—	—
Amebic hepatic abscess	1.2	—	1.9	—	—	—
Miscellaneous	6.3	1.3	5.2	15.5	4.0	8.0

OMGE = World Organization of Gastroenterology.

Table 5 (continued) **Common Abdominal Signs and Findings Noted on Physical Examination**

Sign or Finding	Description	Associated Clinical Condition(s)
Cullen sign	Periumbilical darkening of skin from blood	Hemoperitoneum (especially in ruptured ectopic pregnancy)
Cutaneous hyperesthesia	Increased abdominal wall sensation to light touch	Parietal peritoneal inflammation secondary to inflammatory intra-abdominal pathology
Dance sign	Slight retraction in area of right iliac fossa	Intussusception
Danforth sign	Shoulder pain on inspiration	Hemoperitoneum (especially in ruptured ectopic pregnancy)
Direct abdominal wall tenderness	—	Localized inflammation of abdominal wall, peritoneum, or an intra-abdominal viscus
Fothergill sign	Abdominal wall mass that does not cross midline and remains palpable when rectus muscle is tense	Rectus muscle hematoma
Grey Turner sign	Local areas of discoloration around umbilicus and flanks	Acute hemorrhagic pancreatitis
Iliopsoas sign	Elevation and extension of leg against pressure of examiner's hand causes pain	Appendicitis (retrocecal) or an inflammatory mass in contact with psoas
Kehr sign	Left shoulder pain when patient is supine or in the Trendelenburg position (pain may occur spontaneously or after application of pressure to left subcostal region)	Hemoperitoneum (especially ruptured spleen)
Kustner sign	Palpable mass anterior to uterus	Dermoid cyst of ovary
Mannkopf sign	Acceleration of pulse when a painful point is pressed on by examiner	Absent in factitious abdominal pain
McClintock sign	Heart rate > 100 beats/min 1 hr postpartum	Postpartum hemorrhage
Murphy sign	Palpation of right upper abdominal quadrant during deep inspiration results in inspiratory arrest	Acute cholecystitis
Obturator sign	Flexion of right thigh at right angles to trunk and external rotation of same leg in supine position result in hypogastric pain	Appendicitis (pelvic appendix); pelvic abscess; an inflammatory mass in contact with muscle
Puddle sign	Alteration in intensity of transmitted sound in intra-abdominal cavity secondary to percussion when patient is positioned on all fours and stethoscope is gradually moved toward flank opposite percussion	Free peritoneal fluid
Ransohoff sign	Yellow pigmentation in umbilical region	Ruptured common bile duct
Rovsing sign	Pain referred to the McBurney point on application of pressure to descending colon	Acute appendicitis
Subcutaneous crepitance	Palpable crepitus in abdominal wall	Subcutaneous emphysema or gas gangrene
Summer sign	Increased abdominal muscle tone on exceedingly gentle palpation of right or left iliac fossa	Early appendicitis; nephrolithiasis; ureterolithiasis; ovarian torsion
Ten Horn sign	Pain caused by gentle traction on right spermatic cord	Acute appendicitis
Toma sign	Right-sided tympany and left-sided dullness in supine position as a result of peritoneal inflammation and subsequent mesenteric contraction of intestine to right side of abdominal cavity	Inflammatory ascites

Adapted from Hickey MS et al.[6]

deeply palpated), which is associated with acute cholecystitis. These signs are indicative of localized peritoneal inflammation. Similarly, specific maneuvers can elicit signs of localized peritoneal irritation. The psoas sign is elicited by placing the patient in the left lateral decubitus position and extending the right leg. In settings where appendicitis is suspected, pain on extension of the right leg indicates that the psoas is irritated and thus that the inflamed appendix is in a retrocecal position. The obturator sign is elicited by raising the flexed right leg and rotating the thigh internally. In settings where appendicitis is suspected, pain on rotation of the right thigh indicates that the obturator is irritated and thus that the inflamed appendix is in a pelvic position. The Kehr sign is elicited when the patient is placed in the Trendelenburg position. Pain in the shoulder indicates irritation of the diaphragm by a noxious fluid (e.g., gastric contents from a perforated ulcer, pus from a ruptured appendix, or free blood from a fallopian tube pregnancy). Another useful maneuver is the Carnett test, in which the patient elevates his or her head off the bed, thus tensing the abdominal muscles. When the pain is caused by abdominal wall conditions (e.g., rectal sheath hematoma), tenderness to palpation persists, but when the pain is caused by intraperitoneal conditions, tenderness to palpation decreases or disappears (the Carnett sign).

Rectal, genital, and (in women) pelvic examinations are essential to the evaluation of all patients with acute abdominal pain. The rectal examination should include evaluation of sphincter tone, tenderness (localized versus diffuse), and prostate size and tenderness, as well as a search for the presence of hemorrhoids, masses, fecal impaction, foreign bodies, and gross or occult blood. The genital examination should search for adenopathy, masses, discoloration, edema, and crepitus. The pelvic examination in women should check for vaginal discharge or bleeding, cervical discharge or bleeding, cervical mobility and tenderness, uterine tenderness, uterine size, and adnexal tenderness or masses. Although a carefully performed pelvic examination can be invaluable in differentiating nonsurgical conditions (e.g., pelvic inflammatory disease and tubo-ovarian abscess) from conditions necessitating prompt operation (e.g., acute appendicitis), the possibility that a surgical condition is present should not be prematurely dismissed solely on the basis of a finding of tenderness on a pelvic or rectal examination.

Investigative Studies

Laboratory tests and imaging studies rarely, if ever, establish a definitive diagnosis by themselves; however, if used in the correct clinical setting, they can confirm or exclude specific diagnoses suggested by the history and the physical examination.

LABORATORY TESTS

In all patients except those in extremis, a complete blood count, blood chemistries, and a urinalysis are routinely obtained before a decision to operate. The hematocrit is important in that it allows the surgeon to detect significant changes in plasma volume (e.g., dehydration caused by vomiting, diarrhea, or fluid loss into the peritoneum or the intestinal lumen), preexisting anemia, or bleeding. An elevated white blood cell (WBC) count is indicative of an inflammatory process and is a particularly helpful finding if associated with a marked left shift; however, the presence or absence of leukocytosis should never be the single deciding factor as to whether the patient should undergo an operation. A low WBC count may be a feature of viral infections, gastroenteritis, or NSAP. Other tests, such as C-reactive protein assay, may be useful for increasing confidence in the diagnosis of an acute inflammatory condition. An important consideration in the use of any such test is that derangements develop over time, becoming more likely as the illness progresses; thus, serial examinations might be more useful than a single test result obtained at an arbitrary point. Indeed, for the diagnosis of acute appendicitis, serial observations of the leukocyte count and the C-reactive protein level have been shown to possess greater predictive value than single observations.[33]

Serum electrolyte, blood urea nitrogen, and creatinine concentrations are useful in determining the nature and extent of fluid losses. Blood glucose and other blood chemistries may also be helpful. Liver function tests (serum bilirubin, alkaline phosphatase, and transaminase levels) are mandatory when abdominal pain is suspected of being hepatobiliary in origin. Similarly, amylase and lipase determinations are mandatory when pancreatitis is suspected, although it must be remembered that amylase levels may be low or normal in patients with pancreatitis and may be markedly elevated in patients with other conditions (e.g., intestinal obstruction, mesenteric thrombosis, and perforated ulcer).

Urinalysis may reveal red blood cells (RBCs) (suggestive of renal or ureteral calculi), WBCs (suggestive of urinary tract infection or inflammatory processes adjacent to the ureters, such as retrocecal appendicitis), increased specific gravity (suggestive of dehydration), glucose, ketones (suggestive of diabetes), or bilirubin (suggestive of hepatitis). A pregnancy test should be obtained in any woman of childbearing age who is experiencing acute abdominal pain.

Electrocardiography is mandatory in elderly patients and in patients with a history of cardiomyopathy, dysrhythmia, or ischemic heart disease. Abdominal pain may be a manifestation of myocardial disease, and the physiologic stress of acute abdominal pain can increase myocardial oxygen demands and induce ischemia in patients with coronary artery disease.

IMAGING

Until relatively recently, initial radiologic evaluation of the patient with acute abdominal pain included plain films of the abdomen in the supine and standing positions and chest radiographs.[34] Currently, CT scanning (when available) is generally considered more likely to be helpful in most situations.[35,36] Still, some situations remain in which plain films may be a more useful and safe form of investigation—as, for example, when a strangulating obstruction is thought to be the most likely diagnosis and plain films are used for rapid confirmation. If the diagnosis of strangulating obstruction is in doubt, however, CT scanning—particularly with the newer generations of scanning instruments—is useful for making a definitive diagnosis and for identifying clinically unsuspected strangulation.[37–39]

When performed in the correct clinical setting, imaging studies may confirm diagnoses such as pneumonia (signaled by pulmonary infiltrates); intestinal obstruction (air-fluid levels and dilated loops of bowel); intestinal perforation (pneumoperitoneum); biliary, renal, or ureteral calculi (abnormal calcifications); appendicitis (fecalith); incarcerated hernia (bowel protruding beyond the confines of the peritoneal cavity); mesenteric infarction (air in the portal vein); chronic pancreatitis (pancreatic calcifications); acute pancreatitis (the so-called colon cutoff sign); visceral aneurysms (calcified rim); retroperitoneal hematoma or abscess (obliteration of the psoas shadow); and ischemic colitis (so-called thumbprinting on the colonic wall).

Although in most settings, CT is the preferred modality for primary evaluation of acute abdominal pain, there are certain settings in which US should be considered. When gallstones are considered a likely diagnosis, US is more apt to be diagnostic than CT is, given that about 85% of gallstones are not detectable by x-rays. In disorders of the female genitourinary tract, US is also quite sensitive and specific for diagnoses such as ovarian cyst, fallopian tube pregnancy, and intrauterine pregnancy. Although there are reassuring reports that the risks of radiation from CT scanning can be managed in children and pregnant women with abdominal pain,[40,41] theoretical concerns remain regarding the teratogenicity of the radiation dose.[42] Accordingly, it would seem prudent to consider US the preferred initial imaging test for such patients. In these circumstances, CT is employed only if the diagnosis remains unresolved and if the potential delay in diagnosis (from not obtaining a CT scan) is likely to cause harm.

Working or Presumed Diagnosis

The tentative differential diagnosis developed on the basis of the clinical history is refined on the basis of the physical examination and the investigative studies performed, and a working or presumed diagnosis is generated. Once a working diagnosis has been established, subsequent management depends on the accepted treatment for the particular condition believed to be present. In general, the course of management follows four basic pathways [*see* Management: Surgical versus Nonsurgical Treatment, *below*], depending on whether the patient (1) has an acute surgical condition that necessitates immediate laparotomy, (2) is believed to have an underlying surgical condition that does not necessitate immediate laparotomy but does call for urgent or early operation, (3) has an uncertain diagnosis that does not necessitate immediate or urgent laparotomy and that may prove to be nonsurgical, or (4) is believed to have an underlying nonsurgical condition.

It must be emphasized that the patient must be constantly reevaluated (preferably by the same examiner) even after the working diagnosis has been established. If the patient does not respond to treatment as expected, the working diagnosis must be reconsidered, and the possibility that another condition exists must be immediately entertained and investigated by returning to the differential diagnosis.

Management: Surgical versus Nonsurgical Treatment

ACUTE SURGICAL ABDOMEN

A thorough but expeditious approach to patients with acute abdominal pain is essential because in some patients, action must be taken immediately and there is not enough time for an exhaustive evaluation. As outlined (see above), such an approach should include a brief initial assessment, a complete clinical history, a thorough physical examination, and targeted laboratory and imaging studies. These steps can usually be completed in less than 1 hour and should be insisted on in the evaluation of most patients. In most cases, it is wise to resist the temptation to rush to the operating room with an incompletely evaluated, unprepared, and unstable patient. Sometimes, the anxiety of the patient or the impatience of the health care providers requesting the surgeon's consultation creates an unwarranted feeling of urgency. Often, however, the anxiety or impatience is on the part of the surgeon and, if indulged, may be a cause of subsequent regret.

Very few abdominal crises mandate immediate operation, and even with these conditions, it is still necessary to spend a few minutes on assessing the seriousness of the problem and establishing a probable diagnosis. Among the most common of the abdominal catastrophes that necessitate immediate operation are ruptured AAAs or visceral aneurysms, ruptured ectopic pregnancies, and spontaneous hepatic or splenic ruptures. The relative rarity of such conditions notwithstanding, it must always be remembered that patients with acute abdominal pain may have a progressive underlying intra-abdominal disorder causing the acute pain and that unnecessary delays in diagnosis and treatment can adversely affect outcome, often with catastrophic consequences.

SUBACUTE SURGICAL ABDOMEN

When immediate operation is not called for, the physician must decide whether urgent laparotomy or nonurgent but early operation is necessary. Urgent laparotomy implies operation within 4 hours of the patient's arrival; thus, there is usually sufficient time for adequate resuscitation, with proper rehydration and restoration of vital organ function, before the procedure. Indications for urgent laparotomy may be encountered during the physical examination, may be revealed by the basic laboratory and radiologic studies, or may not become apparent until other investigative studies are performed. Involuntary guarding or rigidity during the physical examination, particularly if spreading, is a strong indication for urgent laparotomy. Other indications include increasing severe localized tenderness, progressive tense distention, physical signs of sepsis (e.g., high fever, tachycardia, hypotension, and mental status changes), and physical signs of ischemia (e.g., fever and tachycardia). Basic laboratory and radiologic indications for urgent laparotomy include pneumoperitoneum, massive or progressive intestinal distention, signs of sepsis (e.g., marked or rising leukocytosis, increasing glucose intolerance, and acidosis), and signs of continued hemorrhage (e.g., a falling hematocrit). Additional findings that constitute indications for urgent laparotomy include free extravasation of radiologic contrast material, mesenteric occlusion on angiography, endoscopically uncontrollable bleeding, and positive results from peritoneal lavage (i.e., the presence of blood, pus, bile, urine, or gastrointestinal contents). Acute appendicitis, perforated hollow viscera, and strangulated hernias are examples of common conditions that necessitate urgent laparotomy.

If early operation is contemplated, it may still be prudent to obtain additional studies to obtain information related to the site of the lesion or to associated anatomic pitfalls. In deciding whether to order such studies, it is important to consider not only whether the additional information obtained will increase confidence in the diagnosis but also whether the extra time, expense, and discomfort involved will be justified by the quality and usefulness of the information.[43] During a short, defined period of resuscitation, it may be possible to employ CT scanning to identify the location of the inflamed appendix in difficult (i.e., retrocecal or pelvic) locations. Knowing the location of the appendix and its morphology can be helpful in directing the incision in an open operation or determining the most expeditious exposure in a laparoscopic procedure. CT scanning may also be used to identify an atypical site of a visceral perforation (e.g., the proximal stomach, the distal or posterior wall of the duodenum, or the transverse colon), thereby guiding placement of the incision and obviating needless dissection of tissue planes. In the setting of distal bowel obstruction, an expeditious Gastrografin (Bracco Diagnostics, Princeton, NJ) enema or CT scan may alert the surgeon to the possibility of an otherwise undetectable malignancy (e.g., cecal carcinoma causing distal bowel obstruction). In cases in which ischemic bowel is suspected, the site of vascular blockage can be localized by using a CT angiogram imaging protocol. In each of these examples, the information gained may permit the surgeon to plan the operation, to optimize time spent under anesthesia, and to minimize postoperative discomfort after laparotomy.

The use of preoperative imaging has become increasingly important as an operative planning tool, particularly when laparoscopic approaches are contemplated for management of acute abdominal emergencies. In the 1990s and the first few years of the 21st century, a number of trials were performed to determine whether laparoscopy or open operation should be the approach of choice when the primary clinical diagnosis is acute appendicitis. This topic has been reviewed extensively in the literature[44–46] and in a 2004 update of a Cochrane meta-analysis.[47] In some environments, the answer to this question remains unclear.[48,49] In many settings, however, the current consensus is that uncomplicated appendicitis can be treated laparoscopically, with a clear expectation of less postoperative pain, a shorter hospital stay, and an earlier return to work and regular activities. These advantages, although significant, do not indicate that a laparoscopic approach is to be preferred in all or most clinical settings or that it is necessarily more cost-effective than an open approach.[47] Laparoscopic appendectomy requires a high level of organization with respect to operating room resources, and this level of organization may be difficult to achieve in institutions where the procedure is not performed regularly (particularly in the middle of the night). In addition, it is not clear whether patients with appendicitis that is complicated by a well-established abscess or bowel obstruction benefit from laparoscopic approaches.

Anatomic considerations also enter into the decision whether to perform the procedure laparoscopically. For instance, it can be very difficult to separate a perforated retrocecal appendix from adherent colon in a safe manner. In many cases, it is prudent not to persist in attempting to extract the appendix without a standard open incision, excellent exposure, and controlled technique. The importance of anatomic considerations underscores the usefulness of preoperative CT in identifying pathologic anatomy, associated abnormalities, and potential pitfalls for either open or laparoscopic approaches.

The advantages of laparoscopy in the management of other abdominal emergencies are less clear-cut. It is important that the surgeon determine not only whether the particular clinical scenario is amenable to a laparoscopic approach but also whether the experience of the entire team and that of the institution as a whole are sufficient for what may be an advanced procedure performed in an acute situation. With this caveat in mind, various investigators have demonstrated that laparoscopy can be employed safely and with good clinical results in selected patients with perforated peptic ulcers.[50–54] Two prospective, randomized, controlled trials comparing open repair of perforated peptic ulcers with laparoscopic repair found that the latter was safe and reliable and was associated with shorter operating times, less postoperative pain, fewer chest complications, shorter postoperative hospital stays, and earlier return to normal daily activities than the former.[52,54]

ACUTE ABDOMINAL PAIN REQUIRING OBSERVATION

It is widely recognized that of all patients admitted for acute abdominal pain, only a minority require immediate or urgent operation.[2,12] It is therefore both cost-effective and prudent to adopt a system of evaluation that allows for thought and investigation before definitive treatment in all patients with acute abdominal pain except those identified early on as needing immediate or urgent laparotomy. The traditional wisdom has been that spending time on observation opens the door for complications (e.g., perforating appendicitis, intestinal perforation associated with bowel obstruction, or strangulation of an incarcerated hernia). However, clinical trials evaluating active in-hospital observation of patients with acute abdominal pain of uncertain origin have demonstrated that such observation is safe, is not accompanied by an increased incidence of complications, and results in fewer negative laparotomies.[55] Many institutions now employ CT scanning liberally in patients with uncertain diagnoses; this practice should greatly minimize the incidence of diagnostic failures or delays in patients with acute conditions necessitating surgical intervention.[32]

The initial resuscitation and assessment are followed by appropriate imaging studies and serial observation. Specific monitoring measures are chosen (e.g., examination of the abdomen, measurement of urine output, a WBC count, and repeat CT scans), and end points of therapy should be identified. Active observation allows the surgeon to identify most of the patients whose acute abdominal pain is caused by NSAP or by various specific nonsurgical conditions. It must be emphasized that active observation involves more than simply admitting the patient to the hospital and passively watching for obvious problems: it implies an active process of thoughtful, discriminating, and meticulous reevaluation (preferably by the same examiner) at intervals ranging from minutes to a few hours, complemented by appropriately timed additional investigative studies.

A major point of contention in the management of patients with acute abdominal pain is the use of narcotic analgesics during the observation period. The main argument for withholding pain medication is that it may obscure the evolution of specific findings that would lead to the decision to operate. The main argument for giving narcotic analgesics is that in a controlled setting where patients are being observed by experienced clinicians, outcomes are not compromised and patients are more comfortable.[56] It has also been suggested that providing early pain relief may allow the more critical clinical signs to be more clearly identified[57] and that severe pain persisting despite adequate doses of narcotics suggests a serious condition for which operative intervention is likely to be necessary.

In my view, the decision whether to provide or withhold narcotic analgesia must be individualized.[58] The current consensus is that for most patients undergoing evaluation and observation for acute abdominal pain, it is safe to provide medication in doses that would “take the edge off” the pain without rendering the patient unable to cooperate during the observation period. It may be especially desirable to provide medication in a manner that allows the patient to be comfortable while lying in the CT scanner. In these cases, the goal of pain relief is to make it easier to obtain accurate information that will facilitate and expedite the diagnosis and the development of a treatment plan. Given the high diagnostic yield and accuracy of the new generation of CT scanners, it is generally safe to provide pain medication while obtaining the diagnosis.

On occasion, however, reflex administration of pain medication solely with the aim of relieving pain may be undesirable or even harmful. For example, in situations for which advanced imaging is unavailable, physical examination may be so crucial to decision making that any risk of obscuring important physical findings is deemed unacceptable; therefore, pain medication should be withheld. In addition, narcotic analgesia should be used cautiously in patients with acute intestinal obstruction when strangulation is a concern.[59] These patients present with abdominal pain that is out of proportion to the physical findings, a syndrome whose differential diagnosis includes acute intestinal ischemia, pancreatitis, ruptured aortic aneurysm, ureteral colic, and various medical causes (e.g., sickle cell crisis and porphyria). A period of resuscitation and evaluation, in conjunction with advanced imaging studies (e.g., CT), may then yield a tentative diagnosis of intestinal obstruction caused by adhesions (e.g., if the patient has a history of abdominal surgery and no evidence of herniation or obturation) without evidence of bowel ischemia. In this setting, the decision whether to admit the patient for observation rather than immediate operation depends on the extent to which the surgeon is confident that the obstruction is not a "closed loop."[59] However, within a relatively short period (perhaps 4 to 24 hours), the surgeon must determine whether any indications for operation will arise, and the main parameters for observation include the WBC count, the urine output, and the development of peritoneal findings. In such cases, it may well be prudent to withhold pain medication until there is a high level of confidence that the timing of surgery will not be delayed.

A final point is that over the course of a 24- to 48-hour observation period, the patient's condition may neither deteriorate nor improve, and supplemental investigation may be considered. Diagnostic laparoscopy has been recommended in cases in which surgical disease is suspected but its probability is not high enough to warrant open laparotomy.[60,61] It is particularly valuable in young women of childbearing age, in whom gynecologic disorders frequently mimic acute appendicitis.[62–64] A 1998 report showed that diagnostic laparoscopy had the same diagnostic yield as open laparotomy in 55 patients with acute abdomen; 34 (62%) of these patients were safely managed with laparoscopy alone, with no increase in morbidity and with a shorter average hospital stay.[63] Diagnostic laparoscopy has also been shown to be useful for assessing acute abdominal pain in acutely ill patients in the intensive care unit.[60,65]

In patients with AIDS,[66,67] a number of unusual diagnoses may be related to or coincident with an episode of abdominal pain. The differential diagnosis includes lymphoma, Kaposi sarcoma, tuberculosis and variants thereof, and opportunistic bacterial, fungal, and viral (especially cytomegaloviral) infections. Laparoscopy has been used for the purposes of diagnosis, biopsy, and treatment in patients with an established AIDS diagnosis who manifest acute abdominal pain syndrome.[66,67] The complication rate and mortality associated with surgery are related to the underlying illness, and outcomes have improved steadily over the years.[68] It is important to note that patients who are infected with HIV but have no clinical manifestations of AIDS are evaluated and managed in the same fashion as patients without HIV infection when they present with acute abdominal pain. The differential diagnosis and the outcomes are essentially no different, unless there are reasons to think that the new onset of pain in an HIV-infected patient is a manifestation of AIDS.[58,68]

Subacute or Chronic Relapsing Abdominal Pain: Role of Outpatient Evaluation and Management

For every patient who requires hospitalization for acute abdominal pain, at least two or three others have self-limiting conditions for which neither operation nor hospitalization is necessary. Much or all of the evaluation of such patients, as well as any treatment that may be needed, can now be completed in the outpatient department. To treat acute abdominal pain cost-effectively and efficiently, the surgeon must be able not only to identify patients who need immediate or urgent laparotomy or laparoscopy but also to reliably identify those whose condition does not present a serious risk and who therefore can be managed without hospitalization. The reliability and intelligence of the patient, the proximity and availability of medical facilities, and the availability of responsible adults to observe and assist the patient at home are factors that should be carefully considered before the decision is made to evaluate or treat individuals with acute abdominal pain as outpatients.

SUSPECTED NONSURGICAL ABDOMEN

Numerous disorders cause acute abdominal pain but do not call for surgical intervention. These nonsurgical conditions are often extremely difficult to differentiate from surgical conditions that present with almost indistinguishable characteristics.[2] For example, the acute abdominal pain of lead poisoning or acute porphyria is difficult to differentiate from the intermittent pain of intestinal obstruction in that marked hyperperistalsis is the hallmark of both. As another example, the pain of acute hypolipoproteinemia may be accompanied by pancreatitis, which, if not recognized, can lead to unnecessary laparotomy. Similarly, acute and prostrating abdominal pain accompanied by rigidity of the abdominal wall and a low hematocrit may lead to unnecessary urgent laparotomy in patients with sickle cell anemia crises. To further complicate the clinical picture, cholelithiasis is also often found in patients with sickle cell anemia.

In addition to numerous extraperitoneal disorders [*see Table 2*], nonsurgical causes of acute abdominal pain include a wide variety of intraperitoneal disorders, such as acute gastroenteritis (from enteric bacterial, viral, parasitic, or fungal infection), acute gastritis, acute duodenitis, hepatitis, mesenteric adenitis, salpingitis, Fitz-Hugh–Curtis syndrome, mittelschmerz, ovarian cyst, endometritis, endometriosis, threatened abortion, spontaneous bacterial peritonitis, and tuberculous peritonitis. As noted (see above), acute abdominal pain in immunosuppressed patients or patients with AIDS is now encountered with increasing frequency and can be caused by a number of unusual conditions (e.g., cytomegalovirus enterocolitis, opportunistic infections, lymphoma, and Kaposi sarcoma), as well as by the more usual ones.

Although such disorders typically are not treated by operative means, operation is sometimes required when the diagnosis is uncertain or when a surgical illness cannot be excluded with confidence. In such cases, laparoscopy can be very helpful, permitting relatively complete and systematic exploration without involving the potential morbidity or the longer postoperative recovery and rehabilitation period associated with open exploration.[69–72] From the surgeon's point of view, an optimal outcome for laparoscopic exploration in these settings is one in which a diagnosis is established by means of visualization, with or without biopsy, and in which symptoms improve as a consequence of a therapy directed by the laparoscopic findings. Overall, candidate lesions—including appendiceal pathology (e.g., chronic appendicitis or carcinoid tumor), adhesions, hernias, endometriosis, mesenteric lymphadenopathy—are identified in about 50% of cases, with pelvic adhesions being the most common finding. From the patient's point of view, however, establishing a precise diagnosis may not be particularly critical, and symptomatic improvement, by itself, may suffice to render the outcome successful. Indeed, a number of reports have emphasized that laparoscopy often leads to improvement in symptoms even if no lesion is identified or treated.[69,70] This point may be illustrated by considering pelvic adhesions.

Given the frequency with which laparoscopic exploration identifies pelvic adhesions, adhesiolysis might be expected to alleviate abdominal pain in many cases. However, it is unclear whether adhesiolysis is therapeutically beneficial when there is no firm evidence that the adhesions are contributing to the pain syndrome. In one prospective, randomized trial, 100 patients with laparoscopically identified adhesions were randomly allocated to either a group that underwent adhesiolysis or one that did not.[73] Both groups reported substantial pain relief and a significantly improved quality of life, but there were no differences in outcome between them, which suggested that the benefit of laparoscopy could not be attributed to adhesiolysis. Longer-term studies also failed to support the hypothesis that pelvic adhesions are responsible for chronic pelvic pain.[74] However, in a study conducted concurrently with the aforementioned randomized trial, 224 consecutive patients underwent laparoscopically assisted adhesiolysis, and 74% of the 224 obtained short-term relief.[75] Factors that contributed to a successful outcome were gender, age, and adhesions severe enough to have led to inadvertent enterotomy and a consequent need for open exploration. It may, therefore, be possible to identify specific subgroups that would benefit from the addition of adhesiolysis to exploratory laparoscopy.

A similar issue arises with respect to pathologic conditions of the appendix—namely, whether appendectomy should be performed when no other source of the abdominal pain can be identified. Early enthusiasm for appendectomy in patients with chronic right lower quadrant pain was sparked by observations of acute or chronic inflammation in specimens that seemed visibly normal.[76,77] In subsequent reports, however, this enthusiasm was tempered by the recognition that these pathologic findings were not very prevalent and that appendectomy did not always reduce the pain.[78,79] No randomized trial of appendectomy for chronic abdominal pain has been performed in a clearly defined patient group, as has been done for adhesiolysis.[73]

At present, the surgeon can only use his or her best judgment as to the likelihood that a given episode of abdominal pain may originate from a set of visible adhesions or a visually normal appendix. It should be remembered that unnecessary or potentially meddlesome interventions are always best avoided; however, it should also be remembered that failure to alleviate chronic relapsing abdominal pain will lead to a program of chronic pain management, including long-term management with potentially addictive and enervating agents. Thus, if adhesiolysis or appendectomy can be performed with the expectation of low morbidity and without conversion to laparotomy, it seems reasonable to perform these procedures during laparoscopy if no other source of pain can be identified.

Financial Disclosures: None Reported

References

1. de Dombal FT. Diagnosis of acute abdominal pain. 2nd ed. London: Churchill Livingstone; 1991.
2. Purcell TB. Nonsurgical and extraperitoneal causes of abdominal pain. Emerg Med Clin North Am 1989;7:721.
3. Silen W. Cope's early diagnosis of the acute abdomen. 20th ed. New York: Oxford University Press; 2000.
4. Marco CA, Schoenfeld CW, Keyl PM, et al. Abdominal pain in geriatric emergency patients: variables associated with adverse outcomes. Acad Emerg Med 1998;5:1163.
5. Flasar MH, Goldberg E. Acute abdominal pain. Med Clin North Am 2006;90:481.
6. Hickey MS, Kiernan GJ, Weaver KE. Evaluation of abdominal pain. Emerg Med Clin North Am 1989;7:437.
7. Adams ID, Chan M, Clifford PC, et al. Computer aided diagnosis of acute abdominal pain: a multicentre study. Br Med J 1986;293:800.
8. de Dombal FT, Dallos V, McAdam WA. Can computer aided teaching packages improve clinical care in patients with acute abdominal pain? BMJ 1991;302:1495.
9. Korner H, Sondenaa K, Soreide JA, et al. Structured data collection improves the diagnosis of acute appendicitis. Br J Surg 1998;85:341.
10. American College of Emergency Physicians. Clinical policy for the initial approach to patients presenting with a chief complaint of nontraumatic acute abdominal pain. Ann Emerg Med 1994;23:906.
11. de Dombal FT. Surgical decision making in practice: acute abdominal pain. Oxford: Butterworth-Heinemann; 1993. p. 65.
12. Brewer RJ, Golden GT, Hitch DC, et al. Abdominal pain: an analysis of 1,000 consecutive cases in a university hospital emergency room. Am J Surg 1976;131:219.
13. Irvin TT. Abdominal pain: a surgical audit of 1190 emergency admissions. Br J Surg 1989;76:1121.
14. Di Placido R, Pietroletti R, Leardi S, et al. Primary gastroduodenal tuberculous infection presenting as pyloric outlet obstruction. Am J Gastroenterol 1996;91:807.
15. Padussis, J, Loffredo B, McAneny D. Minimally invasive management of obstructive gastroduodenal tuberculosis. Am Surg 2005;71:698.
16. Petro M, Iavu K, Minocha A. Unusual endoscopic and microscopic view of *Enterobius vermicularis*: a case report with a review of the literature. South Med J 2005;98:927.
17. Ross AG, Bartley PB, Sleigh AC, et al. Schistosomiasis. N Engl J Med 2002;346:1212.
18. Akgun Y. Intestinal obstruction caused by *Ascaris lumbricoides*. Dis Colon Rectum 1996;39:1159.
19. Krausz MM, Moriel EZ, Ayalon A, et al. Surgical aspects of gastrointestinal persimmon phytobezoar treatment. Am J Surg 1986;152:526.
20. Lee JF, Leow CK, Lai PB, et al. Food bolus intestinal obstruction in a Chinese population. Aust N Z J Surg 1997;67:866.
21. Parente F, Anderloni A, Greco S, et al. Ileocecal Burkitt's lymphoma. Gastroenterology 2004;127:368.
22. Qiu DC, Hubbard AE, Zhong B, et al. A matched, case-control study of the association between *Schistosoma japonicum* and liver and colon cancers, in rural China. Ann Trop Med Parasitol 2005;99:47.
23. de Dombal FT. The OMGE acute abdominal pain survey. Progress report, 1986. Scand J Gastroenterol 1988;144 Suppl:35.
24. Jess P, Bjerregaard B, Brynitz S, et al. Prognosis of acute nonspecific abdominal pain: a prospective study. Am J Surg 1982;144:338.
25. Lukens TW, Emerman C, Effron D. The natural history and clinical findings in undifferentiated abdominal pain. Ann Emerg Med 1993;22:690.
26. Martinez JP, Mattu A. Abdominal pain in the elderly. Emerg Med Clin North Am 2006;24:371.
27. Telfer S, Fenyo G, Holt PR, et al. Acute abdominal pain in patients over 50 years of age. Scand J Gastroenterol 1988;144 Suppl:47.
28. Dickson JAS, Jones A, Telfer S, et al. Acute abdominal pain in children. Progress report, 1986. Scand J Gastroenterol 1988;144 Suppl:43.

29. Scholer SJ, Pituch K, Orr DP, et al. Clinical outcomes of children with acute abdominal pain. Pediatrics 1996;98:680.
30. Malaty HM, Abudayyeh S, O'Malley KJ, et al. Development of a multidimensional measure for recurrent abdominal pain in children: population-based studies in three settings. Pediatrics 2005;115:e210.
31. Gill BD, Jenkins JR. Cost-effective evaluation and management of the acute abdomen. Surg Clin North Am 1996;76:71.
32. Rao PM, Rhea JT, Novelline RA, et al. Effect of computed tomography of the appendix on treatment of patients and use of hospital resources. N Engl J Med 1998;338:141.
33. Thompson MM, Underwood MJ, Dookeran KA, et al. Role of sequential leucocyte counts and C-reactive protein measurements in acute appendicitis. Br J Surg 1992;79:822.
34. Plewa MC. Emergency abdominal radiography. Emerg Med Clin North Am 1991;9:827.
35. Ahn SH, Mayo-Smith WW, Murphy BL, et al. Acute nontraumatic abdominal pain in adult patients: abdominal radiography compared with CT evaluation. Radiology 2002;225:159.
36. MacKersie AB, Lane MJ, Gerhardt RT, et al. Nontraumatic acute abdominal pain: unenhanced helical CT compared with three-view acute abdominal series. Radiology 2005;237:114.
37. Balthazar EJ, Liebeskind ME, Macari M. Intestinal ischemia in patients in whom small bowel obstruction is suspected: evaluation of accuracy, limitations, and clinical implications of CT in diagnosis. Radiology 1997;205:519.
38. Zalcman M, Sy M, Donckier V, et al. Helical CT signs in the diagnosis of intestinal ischemia in small-bowel obstruction. AJR Am J Roentgenol 2000;175:1601.
39. Mallo RD, Salem L, Lalani T, et al. Computed tomography diagnosis of ischemia and complete obstruction in small bowel obstruction: a systematic review. J Gastrointest Surg 2005;9:690.
40. Wagner LK, Huda W. When a pregnant woman with suspected appendicitis is referred for a CT scan, what should a radiologist do to minimize potential radiation risks? Pediatr Radiol 2004;34:589.
41. Fefferman NR, Bomsztyk E, Yim AM, et al. Appendicitis in children: low-dose CT with a phantom-based simulation technique—initial observations. Radiology 2005;237:641.
42. Hurwitz LM, Yoshizumi T, Reiman RE, et al. Radiation dose to the fetus from body MDCT during early gestation. AJR Am J Roentgenol 2006;186:871.
43. Ng CS, Watson CJ, Palmer CR, et al. Evaluation of early abdominopelvic computed tomography in patients with acute abdominal pain of unknown cause: prospective randomised study. BMJ 2002;325:1387.
44. Garbutt JM, Soper NJ, Shannon WD, et al. Meta-analysis of randomized controlled trials comparing laparoscopic and open appendectomy. Surg Laparosc Endosc 1999;9:17.
45. Sauerland S, Lefering R, Holthausen U, et al. Laparoscopic vs conventional appendectomy— a meta-analysis of randomised controlled trials. Langenbecks Arch Surg 1998;383: 289.
46. Guller U, Hervey S, Purves H, et al. Laparoscopic versus open appendectomy: outcomes comparison based on a large administrative database. Ann Surg 2004;239:43.
47. Sauerland S, Lefering R, Neugebauer EA. Laparoscopic versus open surgery for suspected appendicitis. Cochrane Database Syst Rev 2004:(4)CD001546.
48. Katkhouda N, Mason RJ, Towfigh S, et al. Laparoscopic versus open appendectomy: a prospective randomized double-blind study. Ann Surg 2005;242:439.
49. Moberg AC, Berndsen F, Palmquist I, et al. Randomized clinical trial of laparoscopic versus open appendicectomy for confirmed appendicitis. Br J Surg 2005;92:298.
50. Fritts LL, Orlando R. Laparoscopic appendectomy: a safety and cost analysis. Arch Surg 1993;128:521.
51. Hansen JB, Smithers BM, Schache D, et al. Laparoscopic versus open appendectomy: prospective randomized trial. World J Surg 1996;20:17.
52. Lau WY, Leung KL, Kwong KH, et al. A randomized study comparing laparoscopic versus open repair of perforated peptic ulcer using suture or sutureless technique. Ann Surg 1996;224:131.
53. Matsuda M, Nishiyama M, Hanai T, et al. Laparoscopic omental patch repair for the perforated peptic ulcer. Ann Surg 1995;221:236.
54. Siu WT, Leong HT, Law BK, et al. Laparoscopic repair for perforated peptic ulcer: a randomized controlled trial. Ann Surg 2002;235:313.
55. Thomson HJ, Jones PF. Active observation in acute abdominal pain. Am J Surg 1986;152:522.
56. McHale PM, LoVecchio F. Narcotic analgesia in the acute abdomen—a review of prospective trials. Eur J Emerg Med 2001;8:131.
57. Attard AR, Corlett MJ, Kidner NJ, et al. Safety of early pain relief for acute abdominal pain. BMJ 1992;305:554.
58. Soybel DI. Appendix. In: Norton JA, Barie PS, Bollinger RR, editors. Surgery: basic science and clinical evidence. New York: Springer; 2000. p. 647.
59. Saund M, Soybel DI. Ileus and bowel obstruction. In: Mulholland MW, Lillemoe KD, Doherty GM, editors. Greenfield's surgery: scientific principles and practice. 4th ed. Philadelphia: Lippincott Williams & Wilkins; 2006. p. 767.
60. Majewski W. Diagnostic laparoscopy for the acute abdomen and trauma. Surg Endosc 2000;14:930.
61. Golash V, Willson PD. Early laparoscopy as a routine procedure in the management of acute abdominal pain: a review of 1,320 patients. Surg Endosc 2005;19:882.
62. Taylor EW, Kennedy CA, Dunham RH, et al. Diagnostic laparoscopy in women with acute abdominal pain. Surg Laparosc Endosc 1995;5:125.
63. Chung RS, Diaz JJ, Chari V. Efficacy of routine laparoscopy for the acute abdomen. Surg Endosc 1998;12:219.
64. Ou CS, Rowbotham R. Laparoscopic diagnosis and treatment of nontraumatic acute abdominal pain in women. J Laparoendosc Adv Surg Tech A 2000;10:41.
65. Orlando R, Crowell KL. Laparoscopy in the critically ill. Surg Endosc 1997;11:1072.
66. Box JC, Duncan T, Ramshaw B, et al. Laparoscopy in the evaluation and treatment of patients with AIDS and acute abdominal complaints. Surg Endosc 1997;11:1026.
67. Endres JC, Salky BA. Laparoscopy in AIDS. Gastrointest Endosc Clin N Am 1998;8:975.
68. Saltzman DJ, Williams RA, Gelfand DV, et al. The surgeon and AIDS: twenty years later. Arch Surg 2005;140:961.
69. Klingensmith ME, Soybel DI, Brooks DC. Laparoscopy for chronic abdominal pain. Surg Endosc 1996;10:1085.
70. Onders RP, Mittendorf EA. Utility of laparoscopy in chronic abdominal pain. Surgery 2003;134:549.
71. Paajanen H, Julkunen K, Waris H. Laparoscopy in chronic abdominal pain: a prospective nonrandomized long-term follow-up study. J Clin Gastroenterol 2005;39:110.
72. Salky BA, Edye MB. The role of laparoscopy in the diagnosis and treatment of abdominal pain syndromes. Surg Endosc 1998;12:911.
73. Swank DJ, Swank-Bordewijk SC, Hop WC, et al. Laparoscopic adhesiolysis in patients with chronic abdominal pain: a blinded randomised controlled multi-centre trial. Lancet 2003;361:1247.
74. Dunker MS, Bemelman WA, Vijn A, et al. Long-term outcomes and quality of life after laparoscopic adhesiolysis for chronic abdominal pain. J Am Assoc Gynecol Laparosc 2004;11:36.
75. Swank DJ, Van Erp WF, Repelaer Van Driel OJ, et al. A prospective analysis of predictive factors on the results of laparoscopic adhesiolysis in patients with chronic abdominal pain. Surg Laparosc Endosc Percutan Tech 2003;13:88.
76. Chao K, Farrell S, Kerdemelidis P, et al. Diagnostic laparoscopy for chronic right iliac fossa pain: a pilot study. Aust N Z J Surg 1997;67:789.
77. Greason KL, Rappold JF, Liberman MA. Incidental laparoscopic app[illegible] acute right lower quadrant abdominal pain. Its time has come. Surg Endosc 1998;12:223.
78. Teh SH, O'Ceallaigh S, Mckeon JG, et al. Should an appendix that looks 'normal' be removed at diagnostic laparoscopy for acute right iliac fossa pain? Eur J Surg 2000;166:388.
79. van den Broek WT, Bijnen AB, de Ruiter P, et al. A normal appendix found during diagnostic laparoscopy should not be removed. Br J Surg 2001;88:251.
80. Cheung LY, Ballinger WF. Manifestations and diagnosis of gastrointestinal diseases. In: Hardy JD, editor. Hardy's textbook of surgery. Philadelphia: Lippincott; 1983. p. 445.
81. McFadden DW, Zinner MJ. Manifestations of gastrointestinal disease. In: Schwartz SI, Shires GT, Spencer FC, editors. Principles of surgery. 6th ed. New York: McGraw-Hill; 1994. p. 1015.
82. Wilson DH, Wilson PD, Walmsley RG, et al. Diagnosis of acute abdominal pain in the accident and emergency department. Br J Surg 1977;64:249.
83. Hawthorn IE. Abdominal pain as a cause of acute admission to hospital. J R Coll Surg Edinb 1992;37:389.

Acknowledgments

Figures 2 and 3 Tom Moore.

The majority of this chapter is based on previous iterations written for *ACS Surgery*. The author wishes to thank the previous authors, specifically Drs. Delcore, Cheung, and Soybel.

2 ABDOMINAL MASS

Wilbur B. Bowne, MD, and Michael E. Zenilman, MD, FACS

Evaluation of an Abdominal Mass

Abdominal masses are commonly addressed by surgeons, as well as by members of many clinical subspecialties. In terms of clinical importance, abdominal masses cover a broad spectrum: some have few or no apparent consequences, others significantly impair quality of life, and still others represent severe conditions that are associated with poor outcomes and high mortalities. For each patient, therefore, it is essential to formulate a management approach that is tailored to the particular clinical situation. Effective decision-making in this regard involves establishing the correct diagnosis, introducing an effective treatment plan, eliminating risks and complicating factors, initiating preventive measures, and determining the prognosis.

The history of the abdominal mass in the medical literature is ancient, dating back to the Egyptians. The varied differential diagnosis of such masses was discussed in the Papyrus Ebers (ca. 1500 B.C.).[1] Egyptian medical scholars kept detailed notes chronicling conditions encountered and describing methods of abdominal examination that were based on studies of basic anatomy and embalming practices. Centuries later, in his *Book of Prognostics*, the Greek physician Hippocrates (ca. 400 B.C.) discussed the prognostic significance of various types of abdominal masses:

> The state of the hypochondrium is best when it is free from pain, soft, and of equal size on the right side and the left. But if inflamed, or painful, or distended; or when the right and left sides are of disproportionate sizes; all of these appearances are to be dreaded. A swelling in the hypochondrium, that is hard and painful, is very bad.... Such swellings at the commencement of disease prognosticate speedy death. Such swellings as are soft, free from pain, and yield to the finger, occasion more protracted crises, and are less dangerous than others.[2]

Along with the basic methods of clinical evaluation known since antiquity, the modern surgeon has an armamentarium of sophisticated diagnostic studies that aid in the detection, diagnosis, and appropriate treatment of abdominal masses.

In this chapter, we begin with essential definitions and anatomic considerations and then outline our fundamental approach to evaluating patients with an abdominal mass, which integrates the clinical history, the physical examination, and various investigative studies. In particular, we address current developments in investigative techniques, including radiographic and molecular imaging studies that facilitate anatomic evaluation, diagnosis, and determination of the biologic significance of the abdominal mass; we also address minimally invasive diagnostic interventions. Throughout, we emphasize an algorithmic, evidence-based approach to detection and evaluation of abdominal masses. Specific perioperative and operative strategies for addressing particular diagnoses are outlined in other chapters.

Clinical Evaluation

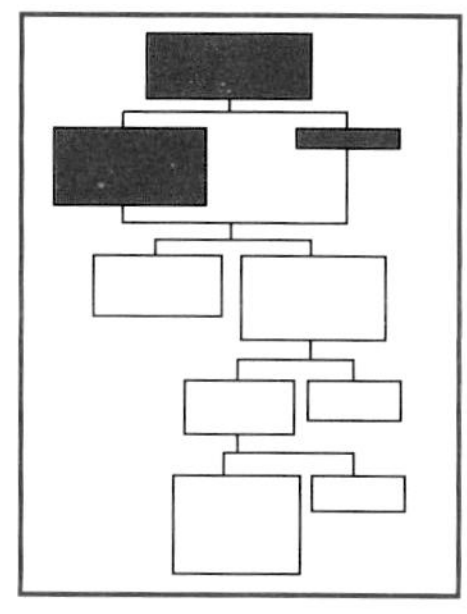

In general, the term abdominal mass refers to a palpable mass that lies anterior to the paraspinous muscles in a region bordered by the costal margins, the iliac crests, and the pubic symphysis. One method of description divides the abdomen into nine areas: epigastric, umbilical, suprapubic, right hypochondriac, left hypochondriac, right lumbar, left lumbar, right inguinal, and left inguinal.[3] Our preferred method divides the abdominal cavity into four quadrants—right upper, right lower, left upper, and left lower—and makes specific reference to the epigastrium and the hypogastrium as necessary. This method of description also includes masses discovered within the retroperitoneum and the abdominal wall. For practical purposes, the abdominal wall begins from the diaphragm superiorly and continues inferiorly to the pelvic cavity through the pelvic inlet. The anterior, posterior, and lateral boundaries of the abdominal wall should be familiar to surgeons. Further anatomic detail is available in other sources.[4,5]

A sound understanding of the normal anatomy in each abdominal quadrant is essential for the evaluation of the abdominal mass. Particular abnormalities tend to be associated with particular regions or quadrants of the abdomen, and these associations should be considered first in the differential diagnosis. Commonly, an abnormal enlargement or mass in the abdomen comes to the clinician's attention in one of three ways: it is detected and reported by the patient, it is discovered by the clinician on physical examination, or it is noticed as an unrelated incidental finding on a radiographic study. Subsequent clinical decision making is then influenced by whether the lesion is intra-abdominal, pelvic, retroperitoneal, or situated within the abdominal wall. In certain cases, a prompt diagnosis can be made after the physical examination, with no further investigation required; obesity, ascites, pregnancy, hernias, infection or abscess, cysts, and lipomas are examples of conditions that can generally be diagnosed at this point.

Evaluation of an Abdominal Mass

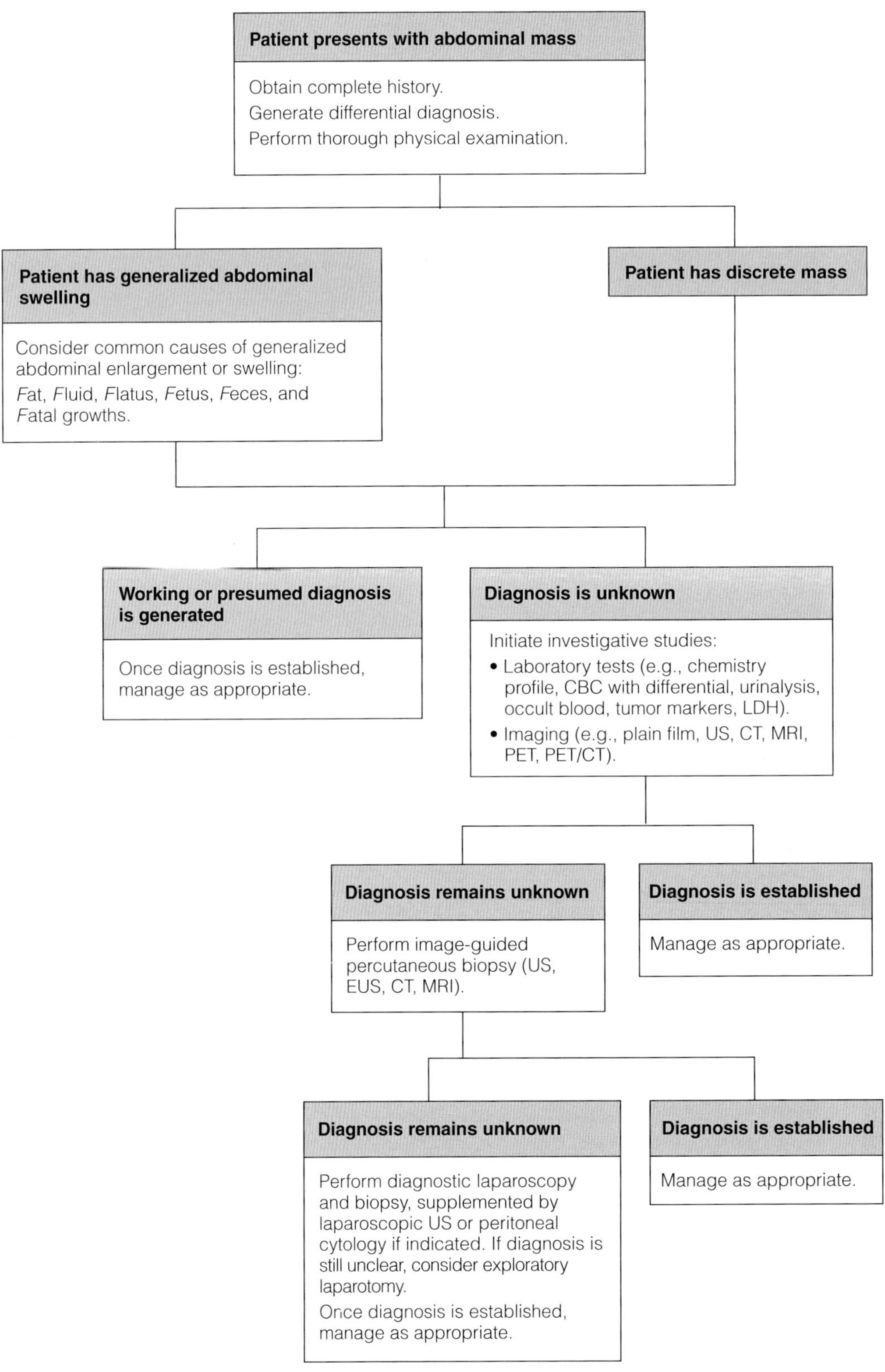

Patient presents with abdominal mass
Obtain complete history.
Generate differential diagnosis.
Perform thorough physical examination.
Patient has generalized abdominal swelling
Consider common causes of generalized abdominal enlargement or swelling:
*F*at, *F*luid, *F*latus, *F*etus, *F*eces, and *F*atal growths.
Patient has discrete mass
Working or presumed diagnosis is generated
Once diagnosis is established, manage as appropriate.
Diagnosis is unknown
Initiate investigative studies:
• Laboratory tests (e.g., chemistry profile, CBC with differential, urinalysis, occult blood, tumor markers, LDH).
• Imaging (e.g., plain film, US, CT, MRI, PET, PET/CT).
Diagnosis remains unknown
Perform image-guided percutaneous biopsy (US, EUS, CT, MRI).
Diagnosis is established
Manage as appropriate.
Diagnosis remains unknown
Perform diagnostic laparoscopy and biopsy, supplemented by laparoscopic US or peritoneal cytology if indicated. If diagnosis is still unclear, consider exploratory laparotomy.
Once diagnosis is established, manage as appropriate.
Diagnosis is established
Manage as appropriate.

Of the various factors that go into making the diagnosis and implementing therapy, clinical experience is undoubtedly paramount. Nevertheless, even the most experienced physicians are subject to some degree of clinical inaccuracy. A randomized study from 1981 found that even when experienced clinicians were certain about the presence of a mass, there was still an appreciable (22%) chance that further investigation would not reveal any abnormality.[6] The evaluation of abdominal masses continues to pose many clinical challenges for the surgeon. There is no magical formula for mastering the necessary diagnostic skills; the closest thing to such a formula is an approach that combines knowledge and application of fundamental anatomic principles with continuous development and appropriate utilization of new diagnostic modalities. For accurate assessment of the origin and character of the abdominal mass, it is essential to possess a thorough understanding of the normal anatomy, the anatomic variations that may be observed, and the distortions that may be caused by the various potential disease processes. As has been said of many professions besides surgery, "You must know the territory." Ultimately, whether a correct diagnosis calls for further intervention or for referral to colleagues with complementary technical expertise depends on the experience of the practitioner.

Fundamental to the successful diagnosis of any abdominal mass are a detailed medical and surgical history and a meticulous physical examination (see below).

HISTORY

Establishing a solid surgeon-patient relationship is vital for building patient trust and confidence, particularly during a period of great uncertainty and vulnerability in the patient's life. Accordingly, our philosophy in dealing with an abdominal mass is to evaluate the patient first and then consider radiographic and laboratory studies if the initial assessment does not yield a diagnosis. A careful and methodical clinical history should be taken that includes all factors pertaining to the lesion. Information about the lesion's mode of onset, duration, character, chronology, and location should be obtained, as well as confirmation of the presence or absence of associated symptoms.

Interviewing strategies for collecting clinical data may vary from surgeon to surgeon.[7] For example, some prefer to conduct a clinical history while sitting rather than standing because this posture tends to suggest the absence of undue haste and the presence of appropriate concern and empathy. A focused, comprehensive interview usually provides all the information necessary for making the correct diagnosis. Our practice is to start by asking nondirective questions—for example, "When did you first notice the mass on your left side?" or "How long did you experience this pain in your abdomen?" It is important to allow patients to describe the history in their own words. It is also important to avoid questions with a built-in degree of bias—for example, "Didn't you know the mass was on your left side?" or "The pain must have been there for some time?" Such questions can lead to biased answers that may misrepresent the chronology or the true natural history of the disease. In most cases, we then proceed to ask questions designed to elicit more specific information (e.g., previous operations, previous medical conditions or therapies, family medical history, or recent travel). It is sometimes necessary to fill in the details by asking direct questions about particular points not already mentioned by the patient. For example, an inquiry regarding gastrointestinal symptoms associated with the abdominal mass may be either nonspecific (e.g., concerned with nausea, vomiting, diarrhea, or constipation) or specific (e.g., concerned with jaundice, melena, hematochezia, hematemesis, hematuria, or changes in stool caliber). Non-GI symptoms (including urologic, gynecologic or obstetric, vascular, and endocrinologic symptoms) should not be overlooked. A history of surgery, trauma, or neoadjuvant or adjuvant cancer therapy may be diagnostically important.[8] For instance, the presence of an abdominal mass representing recurrent cancer raises important clinical questions concerning the advisability of additional therapy or palliative measures, which may carry significant morbidity and mortality.[9–12]

DIFFERENTIAL DIAGNOSIS

For practical purposes, the differential diagnosis for an abdominal mass is divided into categories corresponding to the anatomic divisions of the abdomen (i.e., the four quadrants, the epigastrium, and the hypogastrium) [*see Figure 1*]. The challenge for the modern surgeon is how to narrow down the diagnostic possibilities while avoiding needlessly extensive and expensive evaluations. To accomplish this goal with efficiency, the surgeon must draw both on his or her own reservoir of fundamental knowledge and on the available patient data (e.g., age, gender, associated symptoms, and comorbidities).

After obtaining a thorough clinical history, the surgeon should be able to generate a differential diagnosis. The physical examination may then help confirm or rule out diagnostic possibilities. For example, the presence or absence of pain or tenderness may distinguish an inflammatory or nonneoplastic process from a neoplastic one (e.g., cholecystitis from Courvoisier gallbladder or, perhaps, diverticulitis from carcinoma of the colon). Likewise, the acuteness of the condition may help eliminate diagnostic possibilities, as when an incarcerated abdominal wall hernia is distinguished from a lipomatous mass. So too may the nature of the process, as when a pulsatile mass such as an aneurysm is distinguished from a nonpulsatile one such as a hematoma or a cyst.

Masses of the abdominal wall commonly are subcutaneous lipomas, and care should be taken to differentiate them from neoplastic lesions such as desmoid tumors,[13] dermatofibrosarcoma protuberans (DFSP),[14] and other related[15] or nonrelated tumors.[16,17] When an abdominal mass is associated with uncommon or unexpected findings, the surgeon must be alert to the possibility of an uncommon or unexpected disease process.[18,19] It remains true, however, that knowledge of the most common disease processes associated with region-specific abdominal masses, combined with familiarity with the characteristic signs and symptoms, is the foundation of the clinical assessment of such masses.

PHYSICAL EXAMINATION

The physical examination plays an essential role in the evaluation and workup of an abdominal mass. Current investigative studies are also important in this setting, but all too often, clinicians become overly reliant on various imaging modalities, sometimes overlooking the importance of a careful

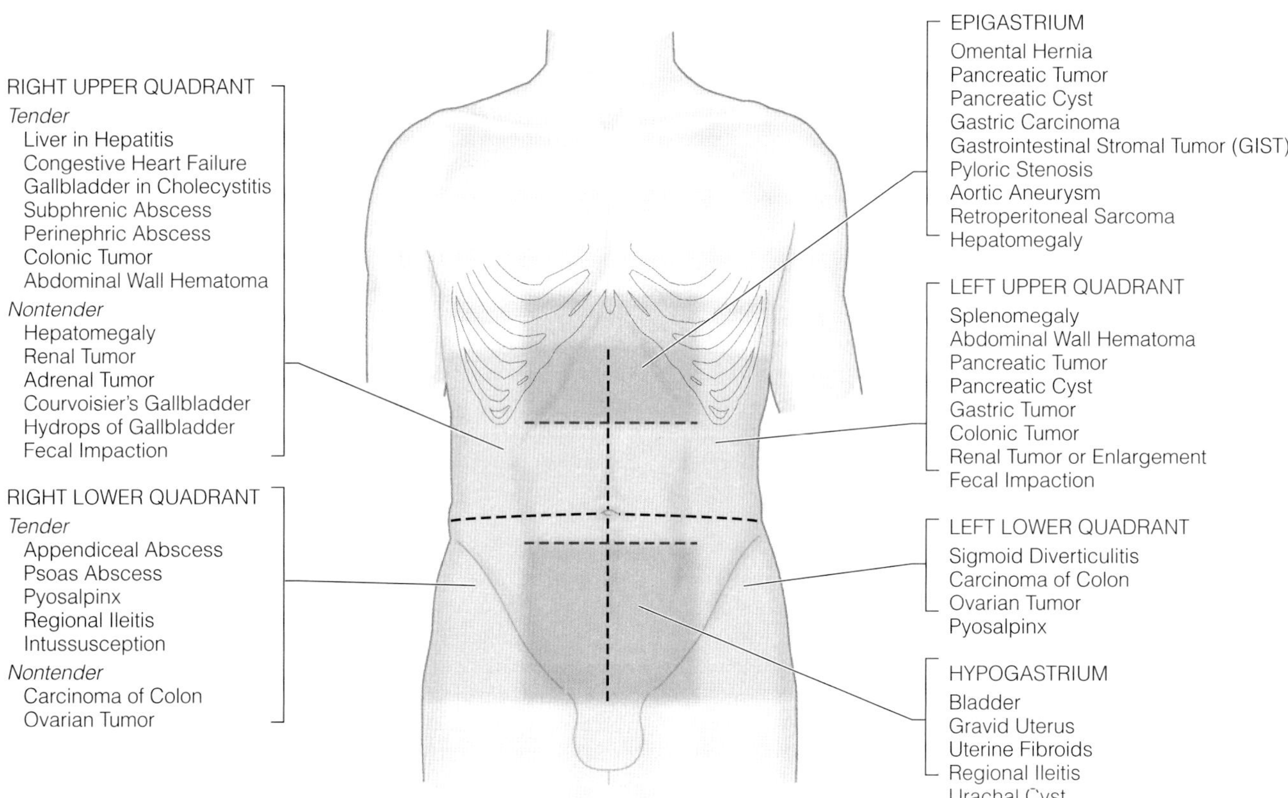

Figure 1 **Schema represents differential diagnosis of an abdominal mass by quadrant or region. Fundamental knowledge of normal anatomy and clinical presentations is the basis for distinguishing the various disease processes. Abdominal wall hernia is considered a possibility in every region or quadrant.**

and thorough examination. Such overreliance can increase the chances of missing subtle physical findings—such as an enlarged lymph node, subcutaneous irregularity, or referred pain—that could have a significant effect on the management of the abdominal mass. Our practice in examining patients with an abdominal mass is to follow an organized, systematic approach consisting of inspection, auscultation, percussion, and palpation, in that order. More detailed discussions of these specific maneuvers are available elsewhere.[20]

The physical examination has three main objectives. First, the examiner must evaluate the patient's condition as it directly or indirectly relates to the mass (e.g., by noting associated systemic illness, pain, malaise, or cachexia). Second, the examiner must assess the acuteness of the patient's condition (e.g., by determining whether a left upper quadrant mass is likely to be a ruptured spleen or simply a long-standing mass in the abdominal wall), which will dictate whether the next step is immediate treatment or further evaluation. Third, the examiner must carefully examine each abdominal quadrant, assessing both normal and abnormal anatomic relations as possible sources of the presumed mass.

How to distinguish a normal abdominal mass or swelling from an abnormal one remains a common challenge for the surgeon. Physical findings on examination are sometimes variable and can be affected by factors such as obesity, body habitus, associated medical conditions, and the patient's ability to cooperate. For example, the normal aorta is often palpable within the epigastrium and may be slightly tender; in elderly, asthenic patients, the normal aorta may be mistaken for an aneurysm. Likewise, the cecum and the descending colon, both of which are usually palpable in thin patients (especially when they contain feces), sometimes masquerade as a cancerous mass; subsequent disimpaction causes such "masses" to resolve. Obesity may preclude evaluation of a potential abdominal mass: it can be difficult to identify discrete palpable masses amid the often remarkable adiposity present within the abdominal wall and the surrounding structures. Ascites may also obscure abdominal masses, making examination more problematic. Transient gaseous distention or intestinal bloating occasionally presents a similar problem, but it usually resolves spontaneously, except in cases of intestinal obstruction. Either gastric dilatation or intestinal obstruction may lead to abdominal distention that is severe enough to necessitate nasogastric decompression. Not uncommonly, in women of childbearing age, a lower abdominal mass may represent a gravid uterus. In such cases, a gynecologic examination must be conducted and a pregnancy test performed before further studies are ordered. The multiplicity of potential benign causes notwithstanding, the possibility of a neoplasm (single or multiple) clearly remains a matter of considerable concern in the evaluation of any patient with abdominal distention. A convenient method of recalling the main causes of generalized enlargement or distention of the abdomen is to use the so-called "six Fs" mnemonic device: *F*at, *F*luid, *F*latus, *F*etus, *F*eces, and *F*atal growths.[21-23]

Palpable or discrete masses should always be localized with respect to the previously described landmarks (see above), and they should, if possible, be described in terms of size, shape, consistency, contour, presence or absence of tenderness, pulsatility, and fixation. Knowledge of the location of the mass in the abdomen shortens the list of structures or organs to be considered and may give insight into the nature and extent of the pathologic process. Frequently, however, the mass's location can only be vaguely outlined, particularly when fluid is present, when the abdomen is tender or tense, or when the patient is obese. Gastric neoplasms, pancreatic neoplasms, colonic neoplasms, sarcomas, pancreatic cysts, and distended gallbladders may be palpable, typically at advanced stages of disease. Recognition of such masses can be facilitated by repeating the abdominal examination after analgesics have been administered or after the patient has been anesthetized in preparation for a procedure.

Working or Presumed Diagnosis

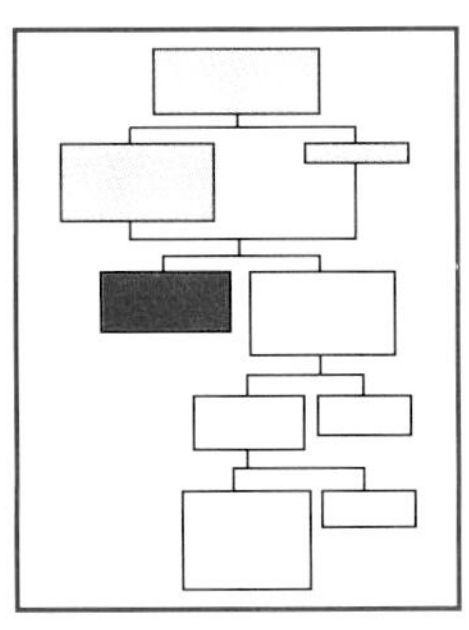

Once a thorough clinical history has been obtained and a careful physical examination conducted, it is usually possible to generate a working diagnosis. Once the working diagnosis has been established, subsequent management is considered in light of its appropriateness for the presumed condition. Sometimes, however, the diagnosis remains unknown even after a comprehensive clinical history and physical examination; in such cases, further studies are required. A wide range of laboratory and imaging studies are now available for establishing the diagnosis. If these studies do not resolve the diagnostic uncertainty, additional procedures, including image-guided percutaneous biopsy, diagnostic laparoscopy, and exploratory laparotomy, may be employed as necessary.

Investigative Studies

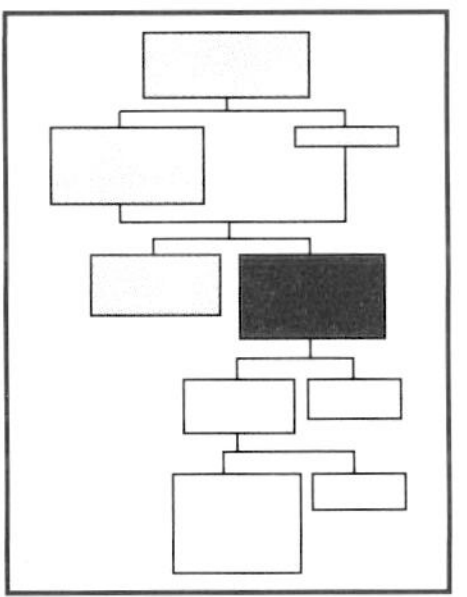

Surgeons are in a unique position to care for patients presenting with an abdominal mass and should guide the collaborative management effort and the choice of appropriate investigative studies. It is therefore essential that surgeons be familiar with every available method for efficient and cost-effective diagnosis of an abdominal mass. For any given situation, the selection of investigative studies should be based on the preferences of the patient, the knowledge and judgment of the surgeon, and the capabilities of the institution. In this way, surgeons who practice outside large, specialized referral centers will still be able to provide integral leadership for most disease management efforts arising from the diagnosis of an abdominal mass.

LABORATORY STUDIES

The diagnostic workup of an abdominal mass usually includes laboratory evaluation. If the cause of the mass remains unknown, preliminary laboratory analysis should include a chemistry profile (electrolyte, blood urea nitrogen [BUN], and creatinine concentrations, as well as liver function tests), a complete blood count (CBC) with differential, and urinalysis. An abnormal laboratory value sometimes plays an important role in establishing the identity or pathogenesis of an abdominal mass. For example, an elevated alkaline phosphatase or liver transaminase level may suggest metastasis to the liver. Likewise, an elevated serum amylase concentration may be suggestive of a pancreatic pseudocyst rather than a cystic neoplasm or an adenocarcinoma; however, an elevated total serum bilirubin level (i.e., > 10 mg/dl) may be more suggestive of a malignant process secondary to adenocarcinoma of the pancreatic head or cholangiocarcinoma. Routine testing for occult blood in the stool should not be overlooked. Tumor markers (e.g., carcinoembryonic antigen [CEA], the cancer antigens CA 19-9 and CA 125, and α-fetoprotein [AFP]) may also help differentiate between benign disease processes and malignant ones, distinguish high-level disease from low-level disease, and, in some cases, establish a disease diagnosis (e.g., elevated AFP levels in patients with hepatocellular carcinoma). Similarly, an elevated serum lactate dehydrogenase (LDH) level may prove invaluable in the staging and prognosis of certain diseases (e.g., melanoma) connected with an abdominal mass.[24] Furthermore, the ability to distinguish between functional abdominal masses and nonfunctional ones (e.g., adrenal tumors) also has important implications for evaluation and management.

In some cases, when the type of mass remains unknown, needless and expensive laboratory analysis can and should be avoided if it appears that other studies may prove more beneficial.

IMAGING

Diagnostic radiology is a dynamic specialty that has undergone rapid change in conjunction with the ongoing evolution of imaging technology. Not only has the number of imaging modalities increased, but each modality continues to be improved and refined for use in evaluating abdominal masses. In particular, advances in cross-sectional imaging techniques, such as ultrasonography (US), computed tomography, magnetic resonance imaging, and positron emission tomography (PET), have made it possible to assess these lesions more precisely. Consequently, whenever the surgeon is confronted with the scenario of a clinically suspected or palpable abdominal mass, accurate diagnostic imaging is of paramount importance. The appropriate use of different imaging modalities in the evaluation of the palpable abdominal mass is well described by the American College of Radiology guidelines,[25,26] which are updated every 6 years.

The use of noninvasive US and CT as first-line procedures for the evaluation of palpable masses has received considerable clinical attention.[6,27–30] Investigators have found both US and CT to be excellent for affirming or excluding a clinically suspected abdominal mass, with sensitivity and specificity values exceeding 95%. This finding is particularly noteworthy because in only 16% to 38% of patients referred for a suspected abdominal mass will the diagnosis be corroborated by an imaging study.[31] Both US and CT are also capable of visualizing the organ from which the mass arises: US successfully determines the organ of origin approximately 88% to 91% of the time, and CT does so approximately 93% of the time. Prediction of the pathologic diagnosis of an abdominal mass, however, remains a challenge for both modalities. US correctly predicts the pathologic diagnosis in 77% to 81% of cases, whereas CT suggests the diagnosis in 88% of cases. Further advancements in cross-sectional imaging (e.g., multidetector CT [MDCT] with three-dimensional reconstruction and magnetic resonance angiography [MRA]) and the addition of molecular and functional imaging modalities (e.g., PET) will undoubtedly improve the predictive abilities of CT and US. At any rate, the current state of imaging technology affords clinicians the ability to distinguish benign from malignant processes, to assess tumor biology, and to detect lesions that impose a minimal disease burden. As a consequence, clinicians are more likely to detect clinically occult disease or discover it incidentally.

Employing an integrative assessment approach (which includes clinical history, physical examination, and investigative studies) should lead to more targeted, efficient, and cost-effective strategies for evaluating abdominal masses. For example, the surgeon can correlate the clinical location of the abdominal mass with pertinent findings from the history and laboratory studies to determine which imaging modality is the most expeditious and cost-effective for a given circumstance. Each imaging modality has unique strengths and weaknesses.

Plain Abdominal Radiographs

By definition, a plain film is a radiograph made without the use of an artificially introduced contrast substance.[32] Commonly employed for initial surveillance of the abdomen, the plain film still has an important place within the investigative armamentarium. Otherwise known as a KUB (kidney-ureter-bladder) study, this low-cost technique may reveal nonspecific or indirect evidence of an abdominal mass, such as variations in the size and density of an organ or displacement of normal structures or fat planes. Furthermore, the radiolucency of air within the bowel may also prove helpful for recognizing worrisome displacement of viscera as a result of a large abdominal mass. Occasionally, a simple plain radiograph can assist the surgeon in making a specific diagnosis, such as calcified aortic aneurysm, acute gastric distention, fecal impaction, porcelain gallbladder, and certain malignancies [*see Figure 2*].

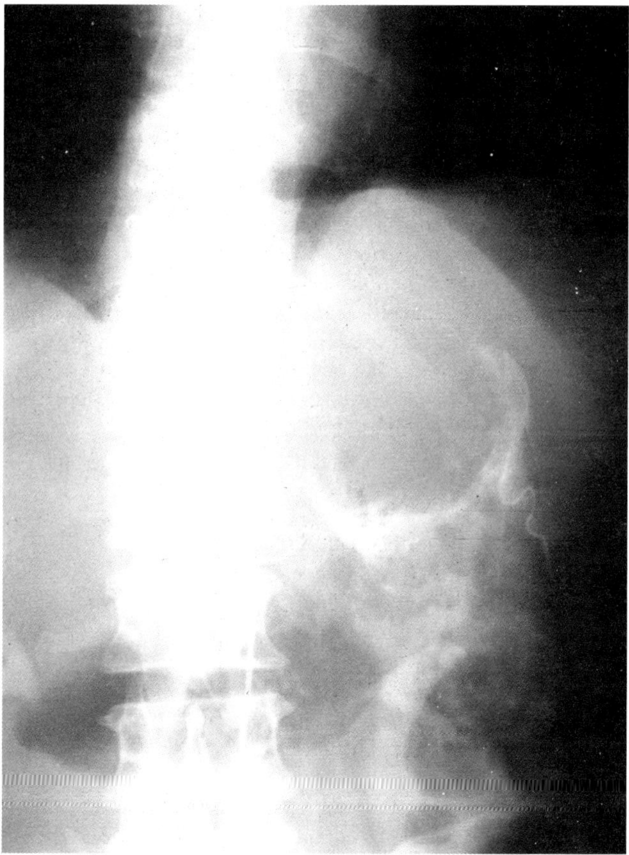

Figure 2 **Plain abdominal radiograph shows a 10 cm functional left adrenocortical carcinoma. Calcifications creating a rim enhancement are easily identified. The diagnosis was confirmed by means of laboratory analysis and abdominal CT.**

Conventional Gastrointestinal Imaging

As a consequence of the technical advances in cross-sectional imaging and endoscopy, conventional GI contrast studies are now largely relegated to more adjunctive roles in the evaluation of abdominal masses. In the upper and middle portions of the abdomen, we occasionally use upper GI studies, small bowel follow-through (SBFT), or enteroclysis to evaluate inflammatory masses (e.g., lesions arising from Crohn disease), masses that are inaccessible to endoscopy, or unusual masses with uncertain diagnoses. For such lesions, we employ single- or double-contrast barium protocols to ensure that significant pathology is not missed; however, these studies are notoriously insensitive and do not provide an opportunity for tissue diagnosis. In the lower portion of the abdomen, barium studies still play a significant role in the evaluation of masses whose history includes GI symptoms (e.g., anemia and weight loss) suggestive of a colonic neoplasm, as well as for evaluating inflammatory masses arising from diverticular disease. In certain cases, we employ a single-contrast barium enema for masses that are causing near-complete obstruction; this study is also helpful for assessing the remaining large bowel for synchronous disease. For small lesions (masses < 1 cm), we typically favor a double-contrast barium enema.

Currently, in the evaluation of an abdominal mass, barium studies are used mainly to complement colonoscopy and CT. Novel approaches (e.g., CT virtual colonoscopy), in conjunction with advances in cross-sectional imaging, may eventually render conventional GI imaging unnecessary.

Ultrasonography

Compared with other modalities, US has several advantages in the evaluation of suspected abdominal masses, including widespread availability, speed of use, the absence of ionizing radiation, low cost, and the ability to document the size, consistency (solid or cystic), and origin of a mass with real-time images.[27,33] When directed at solving a specific clinical problem, US generally provides more diagnostic information. Moreover, the necessary equipment can easily be transported to the patient's bedside or another clinical setting; thus, no patient preparation is required, and only minimal patient cooperation is needed.

We consider US indispensable in the assessment of abdominal masses. At the same time, we acknowledge that one disadvantage of US is the extent to which the quality of the results depends on the technical proficiency and diligence of the operator or technician (though this disadvantage can actually become an advantage when personnel are well trained and experienced). In the hands of an inexperienced operator, US may yield inconclusive or untrustworthy results that contribute to delayed diagnosis or even misdiagnosis. In an effort to help minimize this problem, we encourage the surgeons at our institution (who are trained in US) to perform their own studies in the clinic and the operating room. This approach further expedites recognition of disease [*see Figure 3*], positively influences management, and facilitates operative decision making regarding abdominal masses [*see Figure 4*].

Another disadvantage of US is its inability to visualize the entire abdominal cavity as a consequence of the acoustic barriers presented by gas-containing structures (e.g., the bowel) and the absorptive interfaces (acoustic shadowing) provided by soft tissue and bone. For optimal visualization of abdominal masses, US should be performed through "acoustic windows" that allow adequate transmission of sound. Accordingly, US is most effective as a tool for evaluating masses in those regions of the abdomen where an acoustic window exists (e.g., the right and left upper quadrants and the pelvis). Fortunately, the shortcomings of US can be compensated for by employing other cross-sectional imaging modalities.

Computed Tomography

At present, helical (spiral) CT is the most efficient and cost-effective imaging modality for the evaluation of abdominal masses.[6,27,34,35] Unlike US, CT provides cross-sectional images with excellent spatial resolution and exquisite density discrimination that are unaffected by bowel gas, bone, or excessive abdominal fat. CT routinely visualizes the abdominal wall, the viscera, the mesentery, and the retroperitoneum, clearly defining important tissue planes and delineating the relations between the abdominal mass and adjacent structures [*see Figure 5*]. Such data are essential for guiding diagnostic procedures, determining whether operative management is indicated, and selecting the optimal operative approach. Although modalities such as MRI, PET, and endoscopic ultrasonography (EUS) have advantages over CT in one area or another, CT continues to be superior overall for assessing abdominal masses and remains our preferred imaging method for this purpose.

The use of contrast during the acquisition of CT scans is vital. Opacification of the bowel enables the examiner to distinguish the abdominal mass from surrounding viscera or other adjacent structures. Contrast-enhanced scans also allow delineation of the relevant vascular anatomy; in fact, CT angiography has now relegated conventional angiography to a minimal role in the evaluation of certain abdominal masses.[36,37] Triple-phase or multiphase scanning that includes noncontrast images is now recommended. Such scans achieve

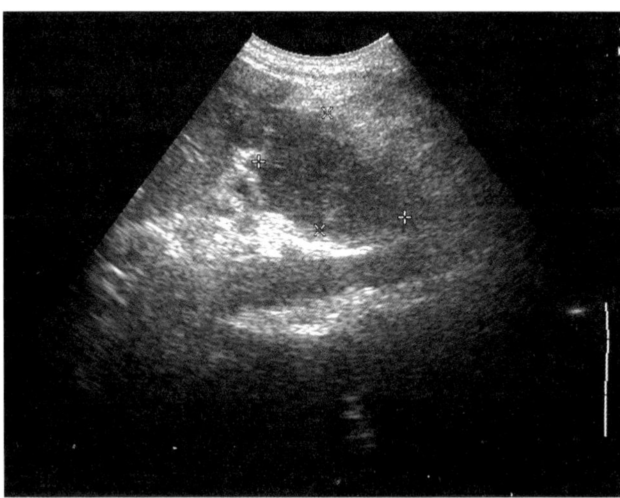

Figure 3 **Sagittal ultrasonogram of the pancreas demonstrates a large mass in the pancreatic head of a 71-year-old patient referred for "gallstones" after experiencing a 10 lb weight loss. The mass lies anterior to the inferior vena cava.**

a

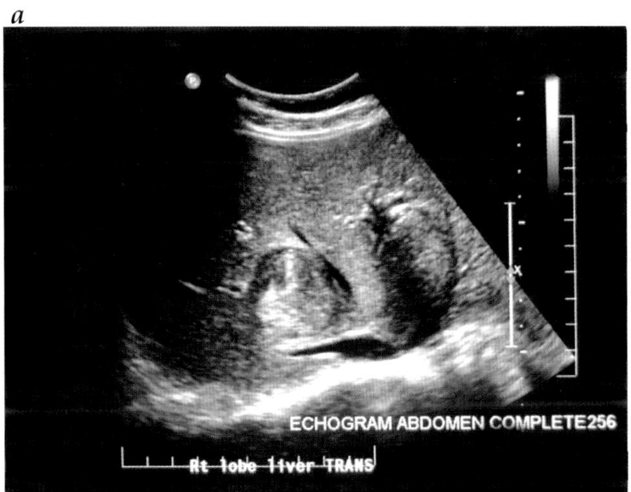

b

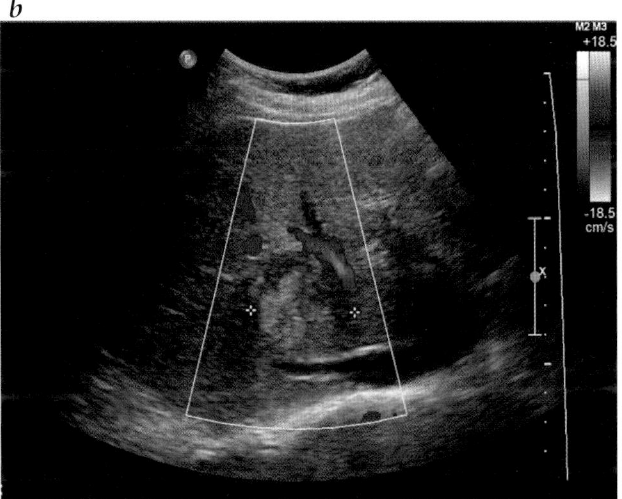

Figure 4 **(*a*) Transverse ultrasonogram of the liver of a 72-year-old cirrhotic patient with a hepatitis C infection shows a 4.0 × 3.5 cm hepatoma, nestled between the right and middle hepatic veins and closely apposed to the inferior vena cava. (*b*) Color Doppler ultrasonogram from the same patient displays blood flow in the middle hepatic vein and the surrounding liver parenchyma. Blood flow toward the transducer is usually displayed in shades of red, whereas blood flow away from the transducer is displayed in shades of blue. Color Doppler ultrasonography allows evaluation of the patency and flow characteristics of the hepatic circulation as it relates to the mass.**

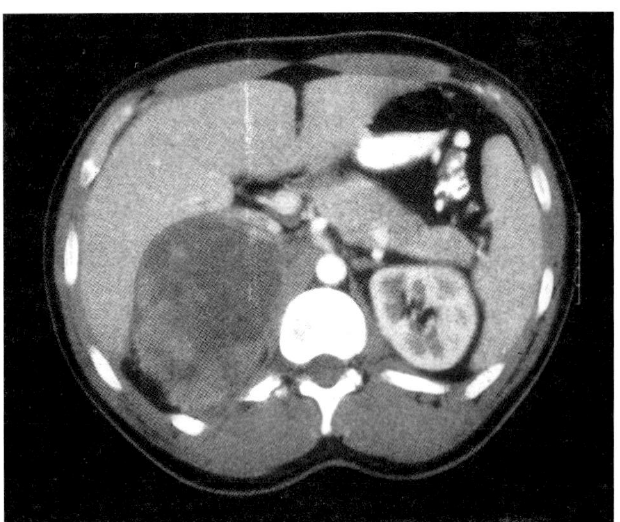

Figure 5 **CT scan of a 65-year-old man with a large retroperitoneal leiyomyosarcoma clearly demonstrates close association of this mass with the right hemiliver, as well as displacement of the inferior vena cava.**

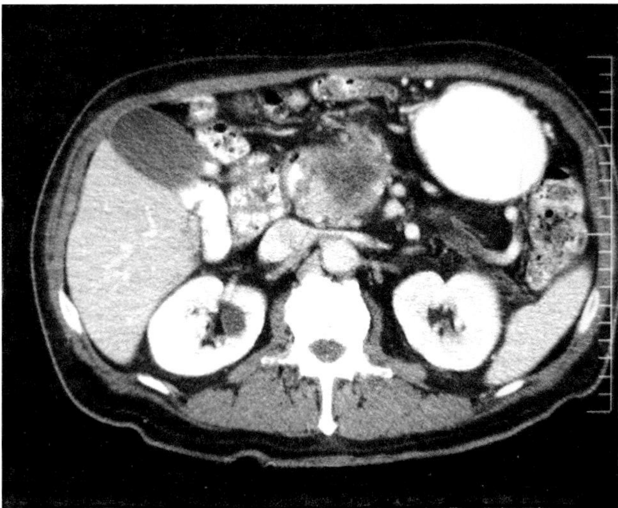

Figure 6 **CT angiography performed to evaluate vascular invasion in a 58-year-old patient with a pancreatic mass demonstrates nearly complete encasement of the superior mesenteric vein. The superior mesenteric artery is not involved with the mass.**

optimal definition and characterization of liver and pancreatic masses. This achievement is of significant clinical value: state-of-the-art CT imaging of malignant pancreatic masses, as well as of other malignancies, has the potential to improve outcome not only by correctly detecting the mass but also by accurately assessing the extent of disease, thereby helping determine which patients may benefit from surgical management or neoadjuvant therapy [*see Figure 6*].

The advent of MDCT technology offers the possibility of even better imaging of abdominal masses than standard contrast CT provides. MDCT scanners can image specific organs or masses with 1 mm slices in less than 20 seconds, and the resultant data can be displayed not only as an axial image but also in a three-dimensional representation that includes detailed vascular mapping.[35] Studies suggest that MDCT may be the most useful modality for preoperative assessment of the resectability of pancreatic and other abdominal masses.[36] MDCT has a sensitivity of 90% and a specificity of 99%, respectively, and it is not observer dependent.

Currently, although MRI (see below) offers unique tissue contrast and inherent multiplanar capabilities for imaging abdominal masses, CT has several advantages—high resolution, short scan times, and fast patient throughput—that make it a more widely preferred imaging modality for this purpose.

Magnetic Resonance Imaging

Since its introduction in the mid-1980s, MRI has become one of radiology's great success stories (though, because it still is not as widely available as US or CT, its cost-effectiveness has yet to be determined). Few would dispute the enormous impact MRI has had on our ability to diagnose pathologic conditions of the brain, the spine, and the musculoskeletal system. Whereas MRI has clear advantages over CT in these areas of the body, this is not the case in the abdomen. Nevertheless, there are situations in which MRI is a better choice than CT for evaluating an abdominal mass. An example is a case in which the use of iodinated contrast material is contraindicated. The extracellular gadolinium chelates used in MRI are very safe and can be given to patients with mild to moderate azotemia without causing renal impairment. MRI has unique characteristics that can be effectively employed to distinguish normal from pathologic tissue in a patient with an abdominal mass.[38]

Detailed information about the principles and practices of abdominal MRI is beyond the scope of this chapter and is readily available elsewhere.[39] A brief technical summary may, however, be worthwhile. The abdomen and its contents are subjected to a momentary radiofrequency pulse, then allowed to return to a state of equilibrium. During the return to equilibrium, the nuclei within each specific tissue will emit specific radiofrequency signals. The strength and type of the emitted signal determine the image intensity. The way in which the different tissues are visually rendered depends on (1) the longitudinal relaxation time (T_1) and the transverse relaxation time (T_2) of the nuclei in the tissues and (2) the method of image weighting employed. By convention, tissues with short T_1 values (such as solid structures) appear bright on T_1-weighted images, whereas structures with long T_2 values (e.g., fluid-containing tissues) appear bright on T_2-weighted images. The tissue contrast and multiplanar capabilities of MRI allow surgeons and radiologists to distinguish not only obvious but also subtle differences between abdominal masses and normal anatomy. For example, T_1-weighted images may be valuable for detecting abdominal masses that contain fluid (e.g., cystic masses or masses containing necrotic tissue), whereas T_2-weighted images may be useful for characterizing these masses as either benign or malignant [*see Figure 7*]. Similarly, magnetic resonance cholangiopancreatography (MRCP) uses T_2-weighted images to distinguish masses with different signal intensities in the pancreas, the liver, and the biliary tract.[40]

Positron Emission Tomography

In 1930, Warburg reported that cancer cells show higher rates of glycolysis than normal cells do.[41] This discovery has

a

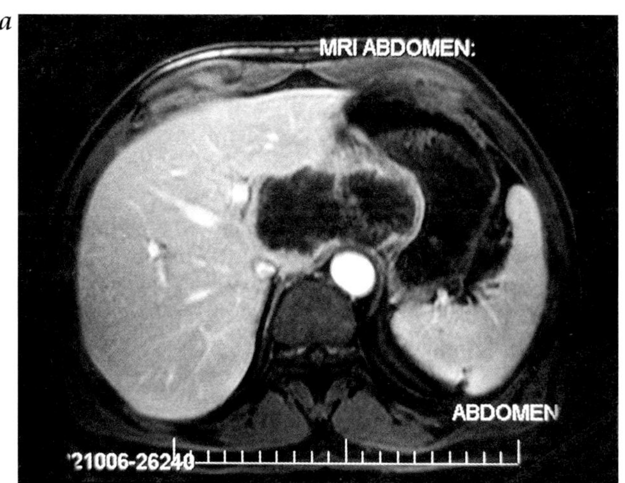

b

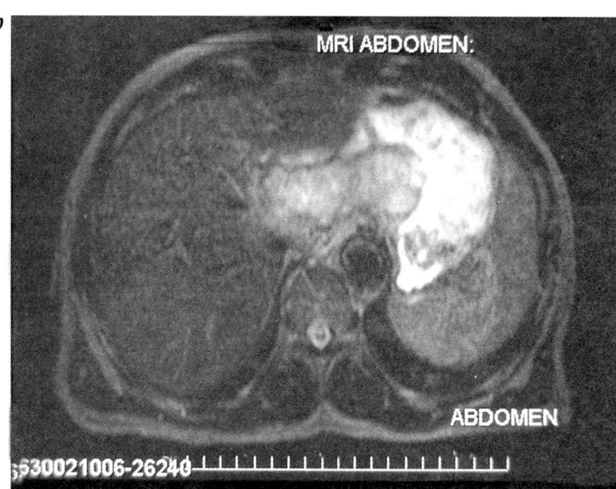

Figure 7 **(*a*) Gadolinium-enhanced, T_1-weighted MRI shows a large mass that appears dark and well-circumscribed in comparison with the normal-appearing enhanced liver and spleen. This abnormal mass clearly contains some fluid. The fluid-filled stomach also appears dark. (*b*) T_2-weighted MRI of the same patient details subtle inhomogeneities characteristic of a malignant mass (less organized appearance with an enhanced necrotic component). Subsequent biopsy showed this mass to be a poorly differentiated adenocarcinoma from recurrent colon cancer.**

stood the test of time and now serves as the theoretical rationale for the use of ^{18}F-fluorodeoxyglucose (^{18}FDG) PET imaging to assess abdominal masses caused by cancer. Briefly, ^{18}FDG is a glucose analogue that crosses the cell membrane by sharing the glucose transporter molecules used by glucose. Like glucose, it undergoes phosphorylation by the enzyme hexokinase. The resulting molecule, ^{18}FDG-6-phosphate, is polar and is unable to cross cell membranes or serve as a substrate for metabolism. The net effect is that ^{18}FDG both accumulates in and is retained by cancer cells.

Figure 8 **^{18}FDG PET scan demonstrates a large metabolically active non-Hodgkin lymphoma giving rise to an abdominal mass.**

The molecular information obtained from PET, as measured by standard uptake values (SUV), allows identification of hypermetabolic (^{18}FDG-avid) abdominal masses (typically arising from lymphomas, melanomas, or certain GI malignancies [*see Figure 8*]).[12] PET may also prove to be an important surrogate modality for distinguishing malignant abdominal masses from benign ones.[43] When PET is used alone, it has the disadvantage of being unable to provide sufficient anatomic information to guide biopsy or further therapy. When PET is used with CT in PET/CT fusion imaging, however, the functional advantages of PET and the structural advantages of CT combine to enhance the detection rate for abdominal masses.[42] If a mass is anatomically evident but metabolically inactive, it will be detected by CT. If it shows increased glycolysis but few or no CT abnormalities, it will be detected by PET. The apparent advantages of PET/CT notwithstanding, prospective, randomized validation is necessary before the widespread application of this approach to the evaluation of abdominal masses can be justified. At present, the use of PET/CT is mostly restricted to large tertiary referral centers.

BIOPSY

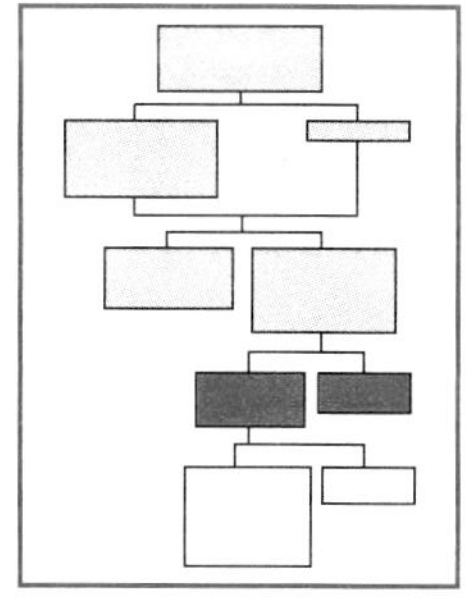

In many cases, the pathologist is the surgeon's greatest teacher. Despite the surgeon's most strenuous efforts, the biology of the disease or lesion will inevitably dictate the outcome. Nowhere is this statement more true than in the evaluation of the abdominal mass, and its truth becomes increasingly evident as ongoing refinements in molecular diagnosis permit ever more sophisticated discrimination among different tumor types and their respective behaviors.[44] Aside from the treatment of lymphoma, in which the surgeon is frequently called on to provide technical assistance in obtaining tissue for diagnosis, the decision whether to perform a biopsy (as well as when and how to do so) rests on the surgeon's understanding of the probable disease. For example, surgeons who treat pancreatic cancer usually proceed to surgery without biopsy if the evidence for malignancy is strong. In other cases, biopsy is performed to confirm what is already suspected on the basis of clinical and radiographic findings. Moreover, establishing the type of tumor or mass present has important implications for the use of neoadjuvant or adjuvant therapy, as well as for the planning of the surgical approach. We view the biopsy of an abdominal mass as the first stage of surgery. This procedure, though seemingly innocuous, has the potential to contaminate tissue planes and must therefore be performed carefully. Accordingly, in order to make the appropriate choice when confronted with an abdominal mass, the surgeon must possess a thorough understanding of the various methods of obtaining an accurate and safe biopsy. Factors related to the size and location of the abdominal mass, as well as factors related to institutional preference and experience, may influence the choice of biopsy technique.

Image-Guided Percutaneous Biopsy

The value of image-guided percutaneous biopsy in the evaluation of the abdominal mass is well established.[45,46] In practice, the procedure begins with identification of the mass by means of a cross-sectional imaging modality such as US, CT, or MRI. Often, three-dimensional imaging reconstructions are generated to detail the relations of the abdominal mass to the surrounding anatomy. Once the mass is identified, decisions are made regarding the safest approach and the most appropriate technique. The biopsy needle is then inserted percutaneously under the guidance of US, CT, or MRI. The choice among the different modalities depends on several factors, including the size and location of the mass, the surgeon's judgment regarding which method is best in the circumstances, and the availability of the various modalities at a particular institution. The most important consideration, however, is the personal preference and experience of the radiologist performing the biopsy. We favor either US or CT, both of which yield good results.

In general, we prefer US-guided biopsy for large, superficial, and cystic masses. This technique is also appropriate for lesions lying at moderate depths in thin to average-size persons. In some cases, US can be employed to guide biopsy of small, deep, and solid abdominal masses; however, US-guided biopsy of these deep-seated masses (as well as of masses in obese patients) often proves difficult because of inadequate visualization resulting from sound attenuation in the soft tissues. Similarly, lesions located within or behind bone or gas-filled bowel cannot be easily visualized (a consequence of the nearly complete reflection of sound from bone or air interfaces).

US possesses several strengths as a guidance modality for percutaneous biopsy. It is readily available, inexpensive, and portable, and it provides guidance in multiple transverse, longitudinal, or oblique planes. Moreover, it offers real-time visualization of the needle tip as it passes through tissue planes into the target area,[47] thereby allowing the surgeon to place the needle precisely and to avoid important intervening structures. In addition, color flow Doppler imaging can help prevent complications of needle placement by identifying the blood vessels involved with the mass, as well as any vessels lying within the needle path. Because of its real-time capabilities, US guidance has the potential to allow quicker, more accurate, and less expensive biopsies than CT guidance does.[48] In theory, any mass that is well visualized with US should be amenable to US-guided biopsy. In practice, however, this modality remains best suited for superficial to moderately deep abdominal masses and for patients with a thin to average body habitus.

The utility of US notwithstanding, CT remains indispensable at our institution as a guidance method for percutaneous biopsy of most regions in the body. It is particularly useful when an abdominal mass is in a location that is inaccessible to US as a result of bowel gas or body habitus. In the abdomen, CT provides excellent spatial resolution of all structures between the skin and the mass, regardless of body habitus or lesion depth, and it provides an accurate image of the needle tip. We favor CT guidance for abdominal masses that are located deep in the abdomen or in the retroperitoneum. The only limitation of CT in this setting is that it does not offer continuous visualization of the needle during insertion and biopsy. In most cases, however, CT guidance can reliably establish the direction and depth of the needle [*see Figure 9*].

Numerous different needles, covering a broad spectrum of calibers, lengths, and tip designs, are commercially available for use in percutaneous image-guided fine-needle aspiration (FNA) biopsy. For convenience, these needles can be grouped into two main size categories: small caliber (20 to 25 gauge) and large caliber (14 to 19 gauge). Small-caliber needles are used primarily for cytologic analysis but may also be employed to obtain small pieces of tissue for histologic analysis. The flexible shaft of small-caliber needles allows them to be passed with minimal risk of tissue or organ laceration or of damage from tearing. Such needles are often used to confirm tumor

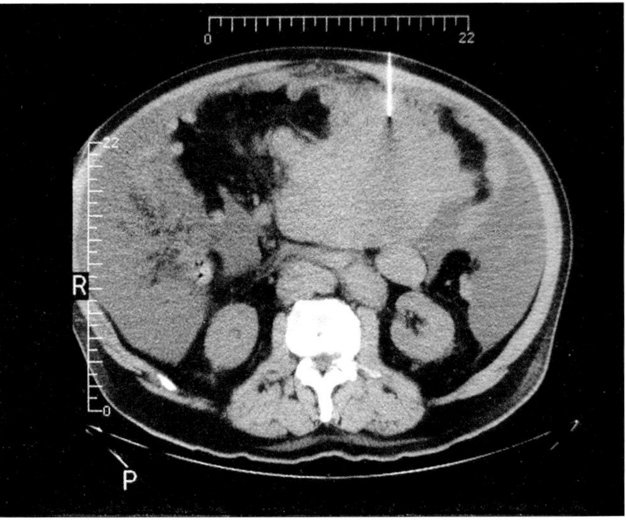

Figure 9 **In a percutaneous biopsy of a large abdominal mass, CT guidance is a reliable means of determining the direction and depth of the needle.**

recurrence or metastasis in patients with a pathologically confirmed primary malignancy. Large-caliber needles are typically used to obtain greater amounts of material for histologic or cytologic analysis.[49] In practice, the choice of a biopsy needle is often influenced by whether the suspected pathology is benign or malignant. For example, large-caliber needles may be necessary to obtain a sufficiently large histologic specimen when certain types of malignancies (e.g., lymphoma) are suspected. When an inflammatory mass is suspected and material is needed for culture, however, a small-caliber needle may be preferred.

Additional considerations for image-guided biopsy include the accuracy, safety, and potential complications of the proposed technique. These considerations are essential for an evidence-based approach to diagnosis of an abdominal mass.

The reported accuracy of US-guided biopsy ranges from 66% to 97%. The location, size, and histologic origin of the abdominal mass appear to influence the diagnostic accuracy of the procedure.[47] In a series that included 126 consecutive small (< 3 cm) solid masses distributed among various anatomic locations and histologic types, US-guided biopsies showed an overall accuracy of 91%.[47] Biopsy results improved as the size of the mass increased: accuracy rose from 79% in masses 1 cm or less in diameter to 98% in masses 2 to 3 cm in diameter. The accuracy of US-guided biopsy in the liver, where most of the biopsies were performed, exceeded 96%. Another study found US-guided biopsy to be 91% accurate for abdominal masses less than 2.5 cm in diameter.[50] Two organ-specific reviews concluded that US-guided biopsy of hepatic masses had an accuracy of 94%[51] and that US-guided biopsy of pancreatic masses had an accuracy of 95%.[52]

The reported accuracy of CT-guided biopsy ranges from 80% to 100%. As with US-guided biopsy, the size, location, and histologic origin of the mass influence the results.[53–55] In a study of 200 consecutive CT-guided needle biopsies, the overall accuracy for all sites biopsied was 95%. The reported organ-specific accuracy was as follows: kidneys, 100%; liver, 99%; retroperitoneum, 87.5%; and pancreas, 82%.[56] In a prospective study of 1,000 consecutive CT-guided biopsies, the reported sensitivity was 91.8% and the specificity 98.9%.[55] At our institution, as well as others, CT-guided biopsy is now considered a reliable tool for the diagnosis and classification of malignant abdominal lymphomas.[57]

The safety of image guided percutaneous biopsy is well documented. Several large multi-institutional reviews reported major complication rates ranging from 0.05% to 0.18% and mortalities ranging from 0.008% to 0.031%.[58–60] A large prospective study of 3,393 biopsies (1,825 US-guided; 1,568 CT-guided) documented an overall mortality of 0.06%, a major complication rate of 0.34% (0.3% with US; 0.5% with CT), and a minor complication rate of 2.9% (2.4% with US; 3.3% with CT).[47] Procedure-related morbidity and mortality appear to be largely unaffected by whether a small-caliber or a large-caliber biopsy needle is used. A review of 11,700 patients who underwent percutaneous abdominal biopsy with 20- to 23-gauge needles found an overall complication rate of only 0.05% and an overall mortality of only 0.008%.[58] A single-institution review of 8,000 US-guided needle biopsies performed with both small- and large-caliber needles reported equivalent results: a major complication rate of 0.187% and a mortality of 0.038%.[61] Of the rare major complications that occur, hemorrhage is the most frequently reported; pneumothorax, pancreatitis, bile leakage, peritonitis, and needle track seeding may also develop.

Needle-track seeding remains an important theoretical consideration when an abdominal mass appears likely to be malignant. According to some investigators, percutaneous needle biopsy has the potential to seed between 103 to 104 tumor cells into the needle track.[62,63] Nevertheless, tumor dissemination after percutaneous biopsy remains exceedingly rare: with fewer than 100 cases reported in the world literature, it has an estimated frequency of 0.005%,[64–66] mostly occurring after biopsy of pancreatic, hepatic, or retroperitoneal masses. Poorly planned biopsies of malignant abdominal masses have the potential to exert adverse effects on subsequent surgery and to compromise local tumor control; fortunately, such negative consequences remain rare.

EUS-Guided Imaging and Biopsy

EUS provides unique imaging information because it involves the close apposition of a high-frequency ultrasound transducer, called an echoendoscope (whereby image resolution is directly related to frequency), to the structures being studied. As a result, it can delineate abdominal masses and associated structures with greater anatomic detail than standard transcutaneous ultrasonography can. In general, EUS-guided biopsy is well suited for abdominal masses that are too small for visualization by means of other cross-sectional imaging modalities or that are inaccessible to percutaneous biopsy.[67] The most frequently used EUS device is the radial echoendoscope, which creates a 360° tomographic image perpendicular to the scope. The circumferential view obtained with this instrument facilitates orientation and therefore is more efficient for diagnostic imaging. Alternatively, the linear-array echoendoscope, which generates an image parallel to the shaft of the scope, may be used. This instrument produces high-quality gray-scale images, as well as color and duplex images. EUS-guided biopsy with a linear scanning system offers clear and consistent visualization of the biopsy needle along its entire path in real time, with excellent delineation of intervening tissues and without any interference from intestinal gas.

EUS has proved to be superior to other cross-sectional imaging modalities for detection and staging of pancreatic, gastric, and esophageal masses.[68–71] For instance, in a patient with a pancreatic mass, EUS not only identifies the size of the mass and the peripancreatic lymph nodes but also delineates the relations of these structures to major blood vessels. EUS has also proved to be helpful in selecting patients for various neoadjuvant protocols. Furthermore, the availability of high-frequency catheter-based intraductal ultrasonography (IDUS) now enables surgeons to visualize masses within the biliary tree and obtain biopsy specimens from them.[72]

Advantages notwithstanding, EUS technology has several important limitations. As with all forms of ultrasonography, a substantial period is required before the operator achieves proficiency. EUS is highly operator dependent; when it is done by an inexperienced operator, the potential exists for serious misinterpretations. For example, if an operator obtains only one view of a mass in the head of the pancreas, the mass may appear to be invading vascular structures when it is not actually doing so. In the evaluation of pancreatic

3 JAUNDICE

Prosanto Chaudhury, MD, CM, MSc (Oxon), FRCSC, FACS, Alan Barkun, MD, MSc, FRCPC, Jeffrey Barkun, MD, MSc, FRCSC

Approach to the Jaundiced Patient

The term "jaundice" refers to the yellowish discoloration of skin, sclerae, and mucous membranes that results from excessive deposition of bilirubin in tissues. It usually is unmistakable but, on occasion, may manifest itself subtly. Jaundice develops when serum bilirubin levels rise above 34.2 mmol/L (2 mg/dL)[1]; however, the appearance of jaundice also depends on whether it is conjugated or unconjugated bilirubin that is elevated and on how long the episode of jaundice lasts.

In what follows, we outline a problem-based approach to the jaundiced patient that involves assessing the incremental information provided by successive clinical and laboratory investigations, as well as the information obtained by means of modern imaging modalities. We also propose a classification of jaundice that stresses the therapeutic options most pertinent to surgeons. We have not attempted a detailed review of bilirubin metabolism and the various pediatric disorders that cause jaundice; such issues are beyond the scope of this chapter. Finally, we emphasize that modern decision making in the approach to the jaundiced patient includes not only careful evaluation of anatomic issues but also close attention to patient morbidity and quality-of-life concerns, as well as a focus on working up the patient in a cost-effective fashion. For optimal treatment, in our view, an integrated approach that involves the surgeon, the gastroenterologist, and the radiologist is essential.

Clinical Evaluation and Investigative Studies

HISTORY AND PHYSICAL EXAMINATION

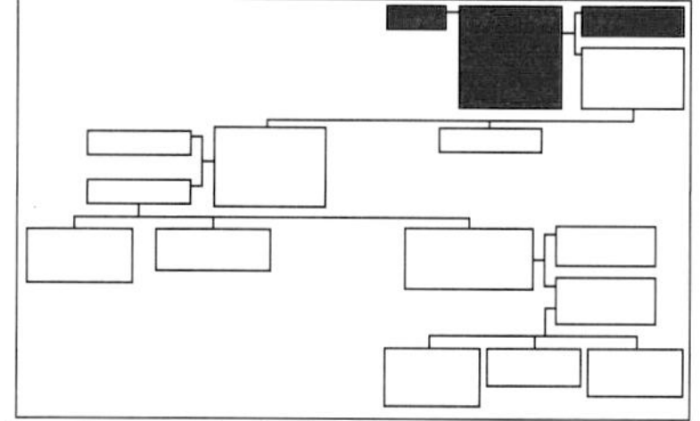

When a patient presents with a skin discoloration suggestive of jaundice, the first step is to confirm that icterus is indeed present. To this end, the mucous membranes of the mouth, the palms, the soles, and the sclerae should be examined in natural light. Because such areas are protected from the sun, photodegradation of bile is minimized; thus, the yellowish discoloration of elastic tissues may be more easily detected. Occasionally, deposition of a yellowish pigment on skin may mimic jaundice but may, in fact, be related to the consumption of large quantities of food containing lycopene or carotene or drugs such as rifampin or quinacrine. In these cases, the skin is usually the only site of coloration, and careful inspection of sclerae and mucous membranes generally reveals no icteric pigmentation. In certain cultures, long-term application of tea bags to the eyes may lead to a brownish discoloration of the sclerae that can mimic jaundice (M. Jabbari, personal communication, 1994).

DIRECT VERSUS INDIRECT HYPERBILIRUBINEMIA

Once the presence of jaundice has been confirmed, further clinical assessment determines whether the hyperbilirubinemia is predominantly direct or indirect. This distinction is based on the division of bilirubin into conjugated and unconjugated fractions, which are also known, respectively, as direct and indirect fractions on the basis of their behavior in the van den Bergh (diazo) reaction.[2] If the patient has normal-colored urine and stools, unconjugated bilirubin [*see Sidebar* Unconjugated (Indirect) Bilirubin] is predominant [*see Table 1*]. If the patient has dark urine, pale stools, or any other signs or

Unconjugated (Indirect) Bilirubin

The breakdown of heme leads to the production of unconjugated bilirubin, which is water insoluble, is tightly bound to albumin, and does not pass into the urine. Excessive production of unconjugated bilirubin typically follows an episode of hemolysis. In the absence of concomitant liver disease or biliary obstruction, the liver can usually handle the extra bilirubin, and only a modest rise in serum levels is observed. There is a substantial increase in bile pigment excretion, leading to large quantities of stercobilinogen in the stool. A patient with hemolysis may therefore be slightly jaundiced with normal-colored urine and stools. Blood tests reveal that 60 to 85% of bilirubin is indirect.[127]

Possible causes of indirect hyperbilirubinemia include a variety of disorders that result in significant hemolysis or ineffective erythropoiesis. The diagnosis of indirect hyperbilirubinemia attributable to hemolysis is confirmed by an elevated serum lactate dehydrogenase (LDH) level, a decreased serum haptoglobin level, and evidence of hemolysis on microscopic examination of the blood smear.

Disorders associated with defects in hepatic bilirubin uptake or conjugation can also produce unconjugated hyperbilirubinemia. The most common of these, Gilbert syndrome, is a benign condition affecting up to 7% of the general population.[128,129] It is not a single disease but a heterogeneous group of disorders, all of which are characterized by a homozygosity for a defect in the promoter controlling the transcription of the UDP glucuronyl transferase I gene.[130] The consequent impairment of bilirubin glucuronidation presents as a mild unconjugated hyperbilirubinemia. The elevated bilirubin level is usually detected on routine blood testing, and affected patients may report that their skin turns yellow when they are fatigued or at stressful times (e.g., after missing meals, after vomiting, or in the presence of an infection). Other causes of an unconjugated hyperbilirubinemia are beyond the scope of this chapter.

Table 1 Causes of Unconjugated Hyperbilirubinemia

Causes
Increased RBC breakdown
Acute hemolysis
Chronic hemolytic disorders
Large hematoma resorption, multiple blood transfusions
Gilbert syndrome
Decreased hepatic bilirubin conjugation
Gilbert syndrome
Crigler-Najjar syndrome types I and II
Familial unconjugated hyperbilirubinemia

RBC = red blood cell.

symptoms of a cholestatic syndrome (see below), the serum bilirubin fractionation usually indicates that conjugated bilirubin is predominant. Rarely, the clinical picture may be secondary to a massive increase in both direct and indirect bilirubin production after the latter has overcome the ability of the hepatocytes to secrete conjugated bilirubin.

It is nearly always possible to distinguish between direct and indirect hyperbilirubinemia on clinical grounds alone.[3] Our emphasis here is on direct hyperbilirubinemia, which is the type that is more relevant to general surgeons.

Cholestatic Syndrome

The term "cholestasis" refers to decreased delivery of bilirubin into the intestine (and subsequent accumulation in the hepatocytes and in blood), irrespective of the underlying cause. When cholestasis is mild, it may not be associated with clinical jaundice. As it worsens, a conjugated hyperbilirubinemia develops that presents as jaundice. The conjugated hyperbilirubinemia may derive either from a defect in hepatocellular function (hepatic jaundice, also referred to as nonobstructive or medical jaundice) or from a blockage somewhere in the biliary tree (posthepatic jaundice, also referred to as obstructive or surgical jaundice). In this chapter, we refer to hepatic and posthepatic causes of jaundice, reserving the term cholestasis for the specific clinical syndrome that is attributable to a chronic lack of delivery of bile into the intestine. This syndrome is characterized by signs and symptoms that are related either to the conjugated hyperbilirubinemia or to chronic malabsorption of fat-soluble vitamins (i.e., vitamins A, D, E, and K): jaundice, dark urine, pale stools, pruritus, bruising, steatorrhea, night blindness, osteomalacia, and neuromuscular weakness.[4]

HEPATIC VERSUS POSTHEPATIC JAUNDICE

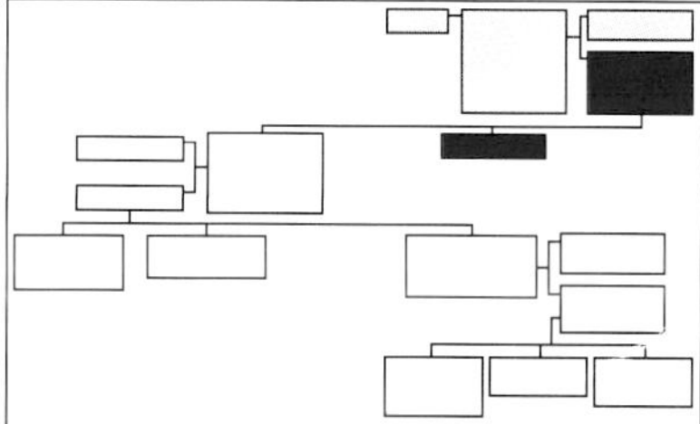

Once the presence of direct hyperbilirubinemia is confirmed, the next step is to determine whether the jaundice is hepatic or posthepatic. A number of authors have studied the reliability of clinical assessment for making this determination.[5-16] The sensitivities of history, physical examination, and blood tests alone range from 70 to 95%,[5-10] whereas the specificities are approximately 75%.[9,10] The overall accuracy of clinical assessment of hepatic and posthepatic causes of jaundice ranges from 87 to 97%.[7,11] Clinically, hepatic jaundice is most often signaled by acute hepatitis, a history of alcohol abuse, or physical findings reflecting cirrhosis or portal hypertension[12]; posthepatic jaundice is most often signaled by abdominal pain, rigors, itching, or a palpable liver more than 2 cm below the costal margin.[13]

By using discriminant analysis in a pediatric patient population, two investigators were able to isolate three biochemical tests that differentiated between biliary atresia and intrahepatic cholestasis with an accuracy of 95%: total serum bilirubin concentration, alkaline phosphatase level, and γ-glutamyltranspeptidase level.[14] Serum transaminase levels added no independent information of significance to the model. Another multivariate analysis model demonstrated that patients with posthepatic jaundice were younger, had a longer history of jaundice, were more likely to present with fever, and had greater elevations of serum protein concentrations and shorter coagulation times than patients with hepatic jaundice.[15] This model, however, despite its 96% sensitivity (greater than that of any single radiologic diagnostic modality), could not accurately predict the level of a biliary obstruction. Other investigators have reported similar findings,[7,11,12] and most agree that strategies that omit ultrasonography are clearly inferior.[16]

In summary, a clinical approach supported by simple biochemical evaluation displays good predictive ability to distinguish hepatic from posthepatic jaundice; however, a clinical approach alone does not accurately identify the level of biliary obstruction in a patient with posthepatic jaundice.

The remainder of this chapter focuses primarily on management of posthepatic jaundice; hepatic jaundice is less often seen and dealt with by general surgeons [*see Table 2 and Sidebar* Hepatic Jaundice].

IMAGING

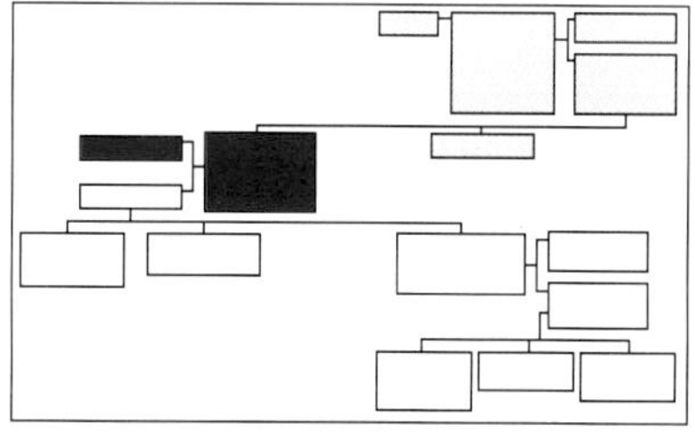

Once the history has been obtained and bedside and laboratory assessments have been completed, the next step is imaging, the goals of which are (1) to confirm the presence of an extrahepatic obstruction (i.e., to verify that the jaundice is indeed posthepatic rather than hepatic), (2) to determine the level of the obstruction, (3) to identify the specific cause of the obstruc-

Table 2 Causes of Hepatic Jaundice[131]

Causes
Hepatitis
Viral
Autoimmune
Alcoholic
Drugs and hormones
Diseases of intrahepatic bile ducts
Liver infiltration and storage disorders
Systemic infections
Total parenteral nutrition
Postoperative intrahepatic cholestasis
Cholestasis of pregnancy
Benign recurrent intrahepatic cholestasis
Infantile cholestatic syndromes
Inherited metabolic defects
No identifiable cause (idiopathic hepatic jaundice)

Hepatic Jaundice

Hepatic jaundice may be either acute or chronic and may be caused by a variety of conditions [*see Table 2*].

Acute hepatic jaundice may arise de novo or in the setting of ongoing liver disease. Historical clues may suggest a particular cause, such as medications or viral hepatitis. Physical examination usually reveals little. In the presence of preexisting chronic liver disease, bedside stigmata (e.g., ascites, spider nevi, caput medusae, palmar erythema, gynecomastia, or Dupuytren contracture) may be present. Although specific therapies exist for certain clinical problems (e.g., acetylcysteine for acetaminophen ingestion and penicillin plus silibinin for *Amanita phalloides* poisoning), treatment in most cases remains supportive. Patients in whom encephalopathy develops within 2 to 8 weeks of the onset of jaundice are usually classified as having fulminant hepatic failure. Evidence of encephalopathy, renal failure, or a severe coagulopathy is predictive of poor outcome in this setting.[126] The most common causes of fulminant hepatic failure are viral hepatitis and drug toxicity. The mortality from fulminant hepatic failure remains high even though liver transplantation has favorably affected the prognosis.[127]

In cases of chronic hepatic jaundice, the patient may have chronic hepatitis or cholestasis, with or without cirrhosis. The cause usually is determined on the basis of the history in conjunction with the results of serology, biochemistry, viral DNA analysis, and, occasionally, histology. Causes include viral infection, drug-induced chronic hepatitis, autoimmune liver disease, genetic disorders (e.g., Wilson disease and α_1-antitrypsin deficiency), chronic cholestatic disorders, alcoholic liver disease, and steatohepatitis.[128] Physical examination reveals the stigmata of chronic liver disease and occasionally suggests a specific cause (e.g., Kayser-Fleischer rings on slit-lamp examination in Wilson disease). Treatment, once again, is usually supportive, depending on the clinical presentation; whether more specific therapy is needed and what form it takes depend on the cause of liver disease. Although physiologic tests have been developed to quantify hepatic reserve, the most widely used and best-validated prognostic index remains the Child-Pugh classification (see below), which correlates with individual survival and has been shown to predict operative risk.[129] Liver transplantation is the treatment of choice in most cases of end-stage liver disease.

The Child-Pugh Classification[129] *Numerical Score (points)*			
Variable	1	2	3
Encephalopathy	Nil (0)	Slight to moderate (1, 2)	Moderate to severe (3–5)
Ascites	Nil	Slight	Moderate to severe
Bilirubin, mg/dL (mmol/L*)	< 2 (< 34)	2–3 (34–51)	> 3 (> 51)
Albumin, g/dL (g/L*)	> 3.5 (> 35)	2.8–3.5 (28–35)	< 2.8 (< 28)
Prothrombin index	> 70%	40–70%	< 40%

Modified Child-Pugh risk grade (depending on total score): 5 or 6 points, grade A; 7 to 9 points, grade B; 10 to 15 points, grade C.
*Système International d'Unités, or SI units.
The Model for End-Stage Liver Disease (MELD) score is now used to prioritize the allocation of organs for liver transplantation by the United Network for Organ Sharing.[130] This score is based on the serum bilirubin and creatinine concentrations, the international normalized ratio (INR), and the presence of hepatocellular carcinoma; it does not make use of some of the more subjective components of the Child-Pugh score (e.g., ascites and encephalopathy).

tion, and (4) to provide complementary information relating to the underlying diagnosis (e.g., staging information in cases of malignancy).

Of the many imaging methods available today, the gold standard for defining the level of a biliary obstruction before operation in a jaundiced patient remains direct cholangiography, which can be performed either via endoscopic retrograde cholangiopancreatography (ERCP) or via percutaneous transhepatic cholangiography (PTC). Unlike other imaging modalities, direct cholangiography poses significant risks to the patient: there is a 4 to 7% incidence of pancreatitis or cholangitis after ERCP,[17,18] and there is a 4% incidence of bile leakage, cholangitis, or bleeding after PTC.[19] There are also several risks that are particular to the manipulation of an obstructed biliary system (see below). For these reasons, the role of ERCP and PTC is increasingly a therapeutic one: therefore, it is important to gather as much imaging information as possible on the likely cause of the jaundice before performing either investigation.[20] We have found the following approach to be an efficacious, cost-effective,[21] and safe way of obtaining such information in a patient with presumed posthepatic jaundice.

The presence of ductal dilatation of the intrahepatic or extrahepatic biliary system confirms that a posthepatic cause is responsible for the jaundice. Ultrasonography detects ductal dilatation with an accuracy of 95%, although the results are to some extent operator dependent.[22] If ultrasonography does not reveal bile duct dilatation, it is unlikely that an obstructing lesion is present. In some cases, even though ductal dilatation is absent, other ultrasonographic findings may still point to a specific hepatic cause of jaundice (e.g., cirrhosis or infiltration of the liver by tumor).

There are a few specific instances in which ultrasonography may fail to detect a posthepatic cause of jaundice. For instance, very early in the course of an obstructive process, not enough time may have elapsed for biliary dilatation to occur. In this setting, a hepatoiminodiacetic acid (HIDA) scan has often helped identify bile duct blockage.[23] The yield from this test is highest when the serum bilirubin level is lower than 100 mmol/L.[1] Occasionally, the intrahepatic biliary tree is unable to dilate; possible causes of such inability include extensive hepatic fibrosis, cirrhosis, sclerosing cholangitis, and liver transplantation. If one of these diagnoses is suspected, ERCP, magnetic resonance cholangiopancreatography (MRCP), or PTC will eventually be required to confirm the diagnosis of biliary obstruction. Occasionally, the biliary tree dilatation may be intermittent; possible causes of this condition include choledocholithiasis and some biliary tumors. In a patient with gallstones, transient liver test abnormalities by themselves may suggest an intermediate to high likelihood of common bile duct (CBD) stones, even if there is no biliary ductal dilatation.[24,25] If one of these diagnoses is suspected, ultrasonography may be repeated after a short period of observation (when clinically applicable); biliary ductal dilatation then generally becomes apparent. If all of these unusual clinical situations have been ruled out, a hepatic cause for the jaundice should be sought [*see Table 2*] and a liver biopsy considered.[26,27]

Besides being able to identify the presence of extrahepatic ductal obstruction with a high degree of reliability, ultrasonography can accurately determine the level of the obstruction in 90% of cases.[28] For example, a dilated gallbladder suggests that the obstruction is probably located in the middle third or the distal third of the CBD.

Some centers prefer computed tomography (CT) to ultrasonography as the initial imaging modality,[29] but we, like a number of other authors,[30] find ultrasonography to be the most expedient, least invasive, and most economical imaging method for differentiating between hepatic and posthepatic causes of jaundice, as well as for suggesting the level of obstruction.[31] Traditional imaging techniques, such as oral or intravenous (IV) cholangiography, have a negligible role to play in this setting because of their very poor accuracy and safety, especially in jaundiced patients.

MRCP [*see Figure 1*] and endoscopic ultrasonography (EUS) have been used to visualize the biliary and pancreatic trees in various populations of patients with obstructive jaundice.[32–36] Compared with direct cholangiography, both appear to be excellent at diagnosing biliary obstruction and establishing its location and nature.[37,38] MRCP exhibits more modest detection rates when diagnosing small CBD stones.[39,40] Spiral (helical) CT scanning is also useful in diagnosing biliary obstruction and determining its cause, although concomitant oral or IV cholangiography is required to detect choledocholithiasis.[41–43]

In addition to their ability to detect choledocholithiasis, spiral CT, EUS, and MRCP in combination with abdominal magnetic resonance imaging (MRI) (e.g., of the pancreas) are very useful in diagnosing and staging biliopancreatic tumors.[44–46] Cytology specimens are readily obtained via fine-needle aspiration (FNA) during CT or EUS.[45]

It is our current practice to employ these modalities as second-line tests after the initial abdominal ultrasonographic examination. To obtain a diagnosis, we favor EUS for periampullary pathologic conditions and MRI with MRCP for more proximal diseases of the biliary tree.

In making the choice among the various available second-line tests, local expertise and cost-effectiveness become important considerations. Unfortunately, the reports on cost-effectiveness published to date have suffered either from limited assumptions (when the methodology involved decision modeling) or from the lack of an effectiveness-type design (when the methodology involved allocation of patients).

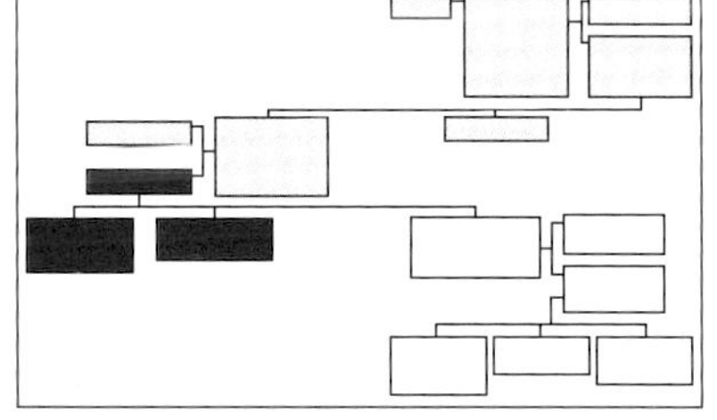

Workup and Management of Posthepatic Jaundice

Once ultrasonography has confirmed that ductal obstruction is present, there are three possible clinical scenarios: suspected cholangitis, suspected choledocholithiasis without cholangitis, and a suspected lesion other than choledocholithiasis. The direction of the subsequent workup depends on which of the three appears most likely

a

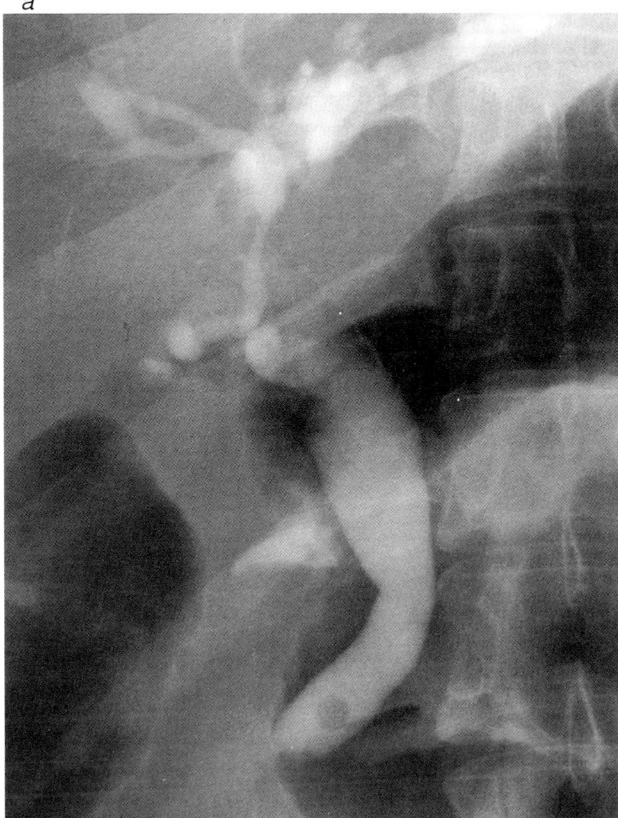

b

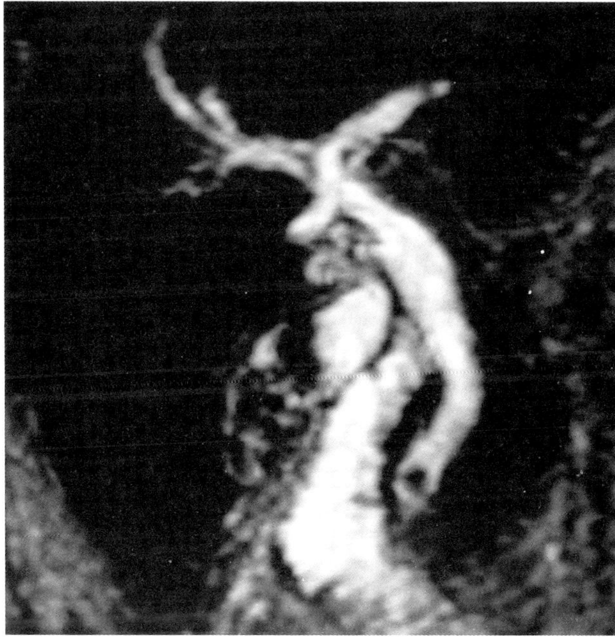

Figure 1 **Endoscopic retrograde cholangiopancreatography (*a*) and corresponding magnetic resonance cholangiopancreatography (*b*) demonstrate the presence of a stone in the distal common bile duct.**

SUSPECTED CHOLANGITIS

If a jaundiced patient exhibits a clinical picture compatible with acute suppurative cholangitis (Charcot triad),[47,48] the most likely diagnosis is choledocholithiasis. After appropriate resuscitation, correction of any coagulopathies present, and administration of antibiotics, ERCP is indicated for diagnosis and treatment.[49] If ERCP is unavailable or is not feasible (e.g., because of previous Roux-en-Y reconstruction), transhepatic drainage or surgery may be necessary. It is important to emphasize here that the mainstay of treatment of severe cholangitis is not just the administration of appropriate antibiotics but rather the establishment of adequate biliary drainage.

SUSPECTED CHOLEDOCHOLITHIASIS WITHOUT CHOLANGITIS

Choledocholithiasis is the most common cause of biliary obstruction.[12,13] It should be strongly suspected if the jaundice is episodic or painful or if ultrasonography has demonstrated the presence of gallstones or bile duct stones. Patients with suspected choledocholithiasis should be referred for laparoscopic cholecystectomy with either preoperative ERCP, intraoperative cholangiography, or intraoperative ultrasonography.[50] We favor preoperative ERCP in this setting of jaundice because its diagnostic yield is high,[51] it allows confirmation of the diagnosis preoperatively (thus obviating intraoperative cholangiography), and it is capable of clearing the CBD of stones in 95% of cases. Decision analyses appear to confirm the utility of this strategy when laparoscopic CBD exploration is not an option.[52–56] Many authors, however, favor a fully laparoscopic approach, in which choledocholithiasis is detected in the operating room by means of intraoperative cholangiography[57,58] or ultrasonography[59–61] and laparoscopic biliary clearance is performed when choledocholithiasis is confirmed. Given that both the ERCP approach and the fully laparoscopic approach have advantages and limitations, the optimal approach in a particular setting should be dictated by local expertise.

SUSPECTED LESION OTHER THAN CHOLEDOCHOLITHIASIS

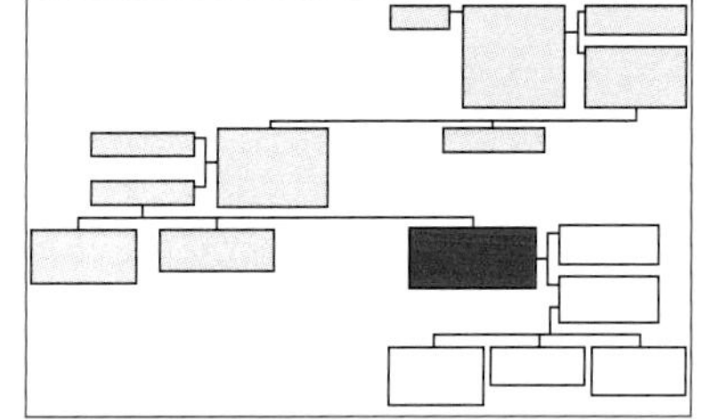

If no gallstones are identified, if the clinical presentation is less acute (e.g., constant abdominal or back pain), or if there are associated constitutional symptoms (e.g., weight loss, fatigue, and long-standing anorexia), the presence of a lesion other than choledocholithiasis should be suspected. In such cases, another imaging modality besides the ultrasonography already performed must be considered before the decision is made to proceed to cholangiography or operation.

Possible causes of posthepatic obstruction (other than choledocholithiasis) may be classified into three categories, depending on the location of the obstructing lesion (as suggested by the pattern of gallbladder and biliary tree dilatation on the ultrasonogram): the upper third of the biliary tree, the middle third, or the lower (distal) third [*see Table 3*]. Once it has been determined that choledocholithiasis is unlikely, the most common cause of such obstruction is pancreatic cancer.[12,13] In adults, many of the other possible causes also involve malignant processes. Consequently, the next step in the workup of the patient is typically the assessment of resectability and operability.

***Table 3* Causes of Posthepatic Jaundice**

Upper-third obstruction
Polycystic liver disease
Caroli disease
Hepatocellular carcinoma
Oriental cholangiohepatitis
Hepatic arterial thrombosis (e.g., after liver transplantation or chemotherapy)
Hemobilia (e.g., after biliary manipulation)
Iatrogenic bile duct injury (e.g., after laparoscopic cholecystectomy)
Cholangiocarcinoma (Klatskin tumor)
Sclerosing cholangitis
Papillomas of the bile duct
Middle-third obstruction
Cholangiocarcinoma
Sclerosing cholangitis
Papillomas of the bile duct
Gallbladder cancer
Choledochal cyst
Intrabiliary parasites
Mirizzi syndrome
Extrinsic nodal compression (e.g., from breast cancer or lymphoma)
Iatrogenic bile duct injury (e.g., after open cholecystectomy)
Cystic fibrosis
Benign idiopathic bile duct stricture
Lower-third obstruction
Cholangiocarcinoma
Sclerosing cholangitis
Papillomas of the bile duct
Pancreatic tumors
Ampullary tumors
Chronic pancreatitis
Sphincter of Oddi dysfunction
Papillary stenosis
Duodenal diverticula
Penetrating duodenal ulcer
Retroduodenal adenopathy (e.g., lymphoma, carcinoid)

Diagnosis and Assessment of Resectability

Assessment of the resectability of a tumor usually hinges on whether the superior mesenteric vein, the portal vein, the superior mesenteric artery, and the porta hepatis are free of tumor and on whether there is evidence of significant local adenopathy or extrapancreatic extension of tumor. Unfortunately, the majority of lesions will be clearly unresectable, either because of tumor extension or because of the presence of hepatic or peritoneal metastases.

Many imaging modalities are currently used to determine resectability, and several of these have been established as effective alternatives to direct cholangiography because they involve little, if any, morbidity. Their accuracy varies according to the underlying pathology and the expertise of the user. They have been studied mostly with respect to the staging and diagnosis of pancreatic, periampullary, and biliary hilar cancers.

For determining resectability and staging lesions before operation, we rely mainly on spiral CT. The advent and widespread availability of multidetector CT have made this modality the dominant second-line imaging method in cases of suspected pancreatic masses. For optimal evaluation of the pancreas, a fine-cut dual-phase (arterial phase and portal venous phase) scan should be obtained. Oral administration of water allows better evaluation of the duodenum and the ampulla.[62,63] At present, spiral CT is considered to be superior for the diagnosis and staging of lesions such as pancreatic cancer.[44,64,65] It exhibits a high negative predictive value and has a false positive rate of less than 10%; its sensitivity is optimal for pancreatic lesions larger than 1.5 cm in diameter. Ascites, liver metastases, lymph nodes larger than 2 cm in diameter, and invasion into adjacent organs are all signs of advanced disease.[66] On the basis of these criteria, spiral CT can predict that a lesion will not be resectable with an accuracy approaching 95%; however, as many as 33% of tumors that appear to be resectable on CT are found to be unresectable at operation.[65]

MRI-based staging, along with MRCP, can further dictate the subsequent choice of therapy.[66–69] MRI may be particularly useful for following up patients in whom clip artifacts interfere with a CT image.[66] It also appears to be successful in detecting cholangiocarcinoma spreading along the proximal biliary tree.[70] Given the renewed interest in biliary contrast media and the availability of software optimized for multidetector scanners, CT cholangiography may soon rival MRCP for evaluation of the biliary tree in cases of suspected malignancy.[71]

Only in a few very rare instances is traditional angiography used to assess resectability or stage a hepatobiliary or pancreatic neoplasm. Increasingly, it is being replaced by CT angiography or duplex Doppler ultrasonography, which can confirm the presence of flow in the hepatic arterial or portal venous systems and occasionally can demonstrate invasion of these vessels by tumor.[72] Magnetic resonance angiography (MRA) has also been used, with excellent results. As yet, none of these noninvasive modalities have been shown to be clearly superior to any of the others.[73]

EUS is a highly sensitive method of imaging the pancreas and the duodenum.[45,74,75] In two large studies, it was found to be superior to CT and standard ultrasonography in staging pancreatic and ampullary cancers.[76,77] Subsequent studies indicated that whereas EUS is superior to CT for detection and staging, it provides similar information regarding nodal status and overall assessment of resectability.[62,78] From a cost-minimization point of view, the optimal strategy is to begin with a dual-phase CT scan and to follow up with EUS only in cases in which further information or a tissue diagnosis is required.[79,80] In another large series, EUS was reported to be more accurate than CT in the comparative staging of pancreatic and ampullary cancers. It has also been found useful for identifying small (< 2 cm) pancreatic tumors, which may be suspected in a patient who has an obstruction of the distal third of the bile duct and whose CT scan is normal.[75] Furthermore, EUS is currently the dominant technique for staging ampullary tumors.[81]

In patients with a suspected pancreatic tumor, direct FNA of the lesion at the time of EUS has become the gold-standard method for obtaining a tissue diagnosis. In the case of potentially resectable lesions, however, this measure adds very little to the decision-making process. The limited data currently available suggest that assays of tumor markers in serum and pancreatic fluid are useful, particularly for cystic lesions of the pancreas.[82]

At this point in the evaluation, patients can be referred either for cholangiography (ERCP or MRCP) to clarify a still unclear diagnosis or for biliary decompression (see below). MRI of the pancreas with MRCP continues to improve rapidly. It is a noninvasive modality that evaluates the pancreas, vasculature, and pancreatobiliary ductal system in a single examination, with the additional benefit of avoiding ionizing radiation and iodinated contrast agents.[83] MRCP remains our test of choice for evaluation of middle- and upper-third lesions in cases in which decompression is not required.

In the event that none of these modalities point to a diagnosis, the use of ^{18}F-fluorodeoxyglucose (FDG) positron emission tomography (PET) may be considered to help differentiate benign pancreatic conditions from malignant ones.[84,85] Besides facilitating diagnosis, FDG-PET provides information regarding occult metastases and can be useful in detecting recurrent disease. Experience with FDG-PET is growing rapidly as this imaging modality becomes more readily accessible.

When a biliary stricture is detected at cholangiography, brush cytology or biopsy is mandatory. Biliary cytology, however, has been disappointing, particularly at ERCP: diagnostic accuracy ranges from 40 to 85%,[86,87] mostly because the negative predictive value is poor. Accuracy improves with multiple sampling and when a biliary rather than a pancreatic malignancy is detected. In addition, biopsy tends to be more accurate than brush cytology.[86]

Nonoperative Management: Drainage and Cholangiography

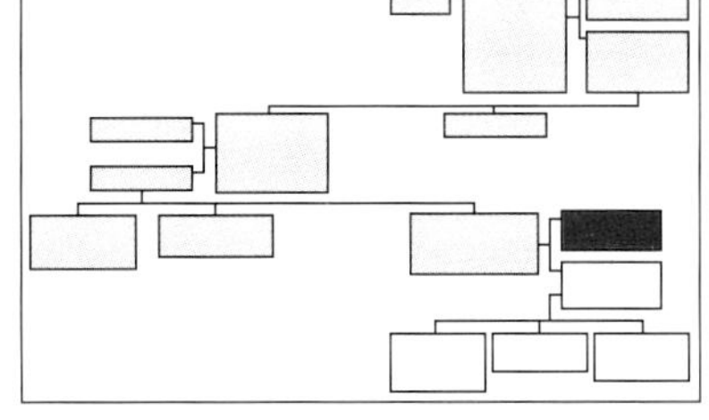

In the majority of patients with malignant obstructions, treatment is palliative rather than curative. It is therefore especially important to recognize and minimize the iatrogenic risks related to the manipulation of an obstructed biliary system; this is why staging and cholangiography are currently being performed with EUS and MRCP.

Cholangiography and decompression of obstructed biliary system As a rule, we favor ERCP, although PTC may be preferable for obstructions near the hepatic duct bifurcation. Whichever imaging modality is used, the following four principles apply:

1. In the absence of preexisting or concomitant hepatocellular dysfunction, drainage of one half of the liver is generally sufficient for resolution of jaundice.[88]
2. Because of its external diameter, a transhepatic drain, once inserted, does not necessarily permit equal drainage of all segments of the liver, particularly if there are a number of intrahepatic ductal stenoses. Accordingly, some patients with conditions such as sclerosing cholangitis or a growing tumor may experience persistent sepsis from an infected

excluded liver segment even when the prosthesis is patent [*see Figure 2*]. An excluded segment may even be responsible for severe persistent pruritus.

3. Any attempt at opacifying an obstructed biliary tree introduces a significant risk of subsequent cholangitis, even when appropriate antibiotic prophylaxis is provided. Accordingly, when one elects to perform direct cholangiography, there should be a plan for biliary drainage either at the time of ERCP or PTC or soon thereafter.
4. Even though jaundice is believed to be associated with multiple adverse systemic effects (e.g., renal failure, sepsis, and impaired wound healing),[89,90] routine preoperative drainage of an obstructed biliary system does not benefit patients who will soon undergo resection.[91,92] A growing body of evidence suggests that in patients with either pancreatic[93,94] or hepatic[95] malignancies, routine preoperative direct cholangiography with decompression is associated with a higher incidence of postoperative complications when tumor resection is ultimately carried out.

When direct cholangiography is ordered, it should be thought of as more than just a diagnostic test: it is the ideal setting for cytology, biopsy, or even drainage of the obstructed bile duct via a sphincterotomy, a nasobiliary tube, or a catheter or stent. Accordingly, it is essential that the surgeon, the gastroenterologist, and the radiologist discuss the possible need for drainage well before it is required. Early, open communication among all members of the treating team is a hallmark of the modern management of biliary obstruction.

Palliation in patients with advanced malignant disease

When a patient has advanced malignant disease, drainage of the biliary system for palliation is not routinely indicated, because the risk of complications related to the procedure may outweigh the potential benefit. Indeed, the best treatment for a patient with asymptomatic obstructive jaundice and liver metastases may be supportive care alone.[96] Biliary decompression is indicated if cholangitis or severe pruritus interferes with quality of life.

We, like others,[21] consider a stent placed with ERCP to be the palliative modality of choice for advanced disease, although upper-third lesions may be managed most easily through the initial placement of an internal or external catheter at the time of PTC. Metal expandable stents remain patent longer than large conventional plastic stents[97,98] and are becoming the standard of care.[99,100] Whether plastic biliary stents should be replaced prophylactically or only after obstruction has occurred remains controversial; however, results from a randomized, controlled trial (RCT) favor the former approach.[101] In another RCT, the use of prophylactic ciprofloxacin did not prolong stent patency but did reduce the incidence of cholangitis and improve quality-of-life scores.[102]

RCTs suggest that surgical biliary bypass should be reserved for patients who are expected to survive for 6 months or longer because bypass is associated with more prolonged palliation at the cost of greater initial morbidity.[103]

The role of prophylactic gastric drainage at the time of operative biliary drainage remains controversial,[104,105] although two RCTs demonstrated a reduced incidence of subsequent clinical gastric outlet obstruction when this measure was employed. Jaundiced patients with unresectable lesions who also present with duodenal or jejunal obstruction should be referred for gastrojejunostomy at the time of biliary bypass surgery. There is evidence to suggest that when a pancreatic malignancy is present, intraoperative celiac ganglion injection should be performed for either prophylactic or therapeutic pain control.[106]

Operative Management at Specific Sites: Bypass and Resection

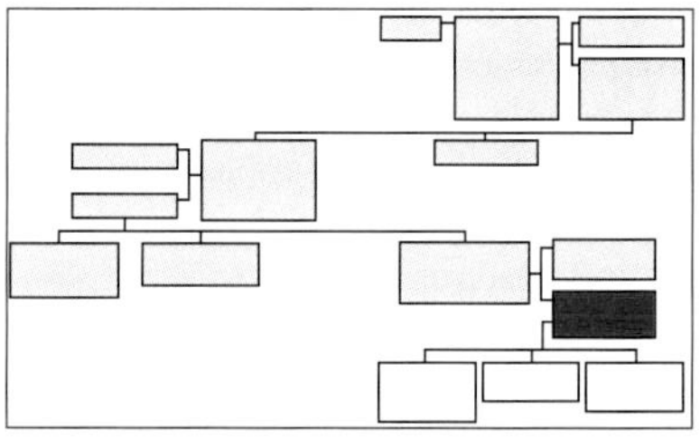

Surgical treatment of tumors causing biliary obstruction is determined primarily by the level of the biliary obstruction.

a

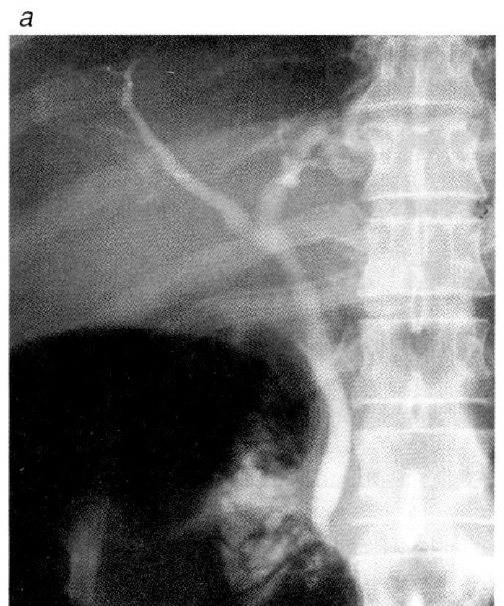

b

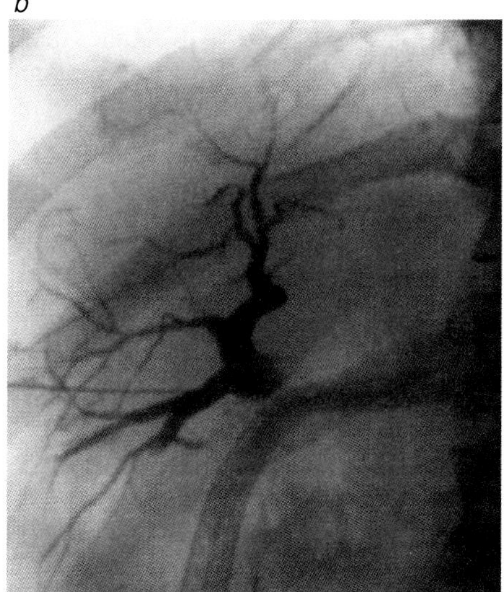

c

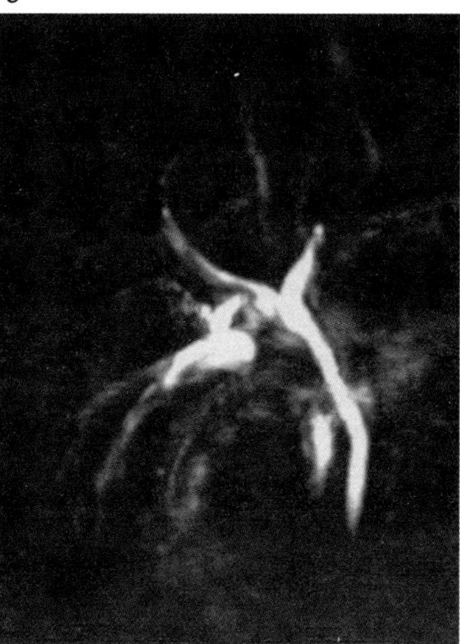

Figure 2 **(*a*) Endoscopic retrograde cholangiopancreatography demonstrates missing liver segments. (*b*) Transhepatic cholangiography of segment 6 reveals the excluded liver ductal system. (*c*) Magnetic resonance cholangiopancreatography shows the excluded liver segments, as well as the biliary system, which still communicates with the common hepatic duct.**

Current evidence indicates that modern surgical approaches are resulting in lower postoperative morbidity and, possibly, improved 5-year survival[107]; however, the prognosis is still uniformly poor, except for patients with ampullary tumors. In fact, the surgical procedure rarely proves curative, even after meticulous preoperative patient selection.

At one time, there was considerable enthusiasm for routine use of staging laparoscopy; at present, however, selective use is recommended.[108] The benefits of staging laparoscopy include more accurate assessment of resectability and prevention of the prolonged hospital stay and convalescence associated with an unnecessary laparotomy. Laparoscopy is used mostly to detect peritoneal carcinomatosis, liver metastases, malignant ascites, and gross hilar adenopathy.[109,110] The main limitation of laparoscopy in this setting appears to be that it does not accurately detect the spread of tumors to lymph nodes or the vascular system.[111] In several studies, a combined approach that included both laparoscopy and laparoscopic ultrasonography was associated with shorter hospital stays and lower costs.[108,110–112]

In what follows, only the general principles of resection or bypass at each level of obstruction are discussed; operative technical details are addressed elsewhere. Our preferred method of biliary anastomosis, for either reconstruction or bypass, involves the fashioning of a Roux-en-Y loop, followed by a mucosa-to-mucosa anastomosis. In all cases, a cholecystectomy is performed to facilitate access to the biliary tree.

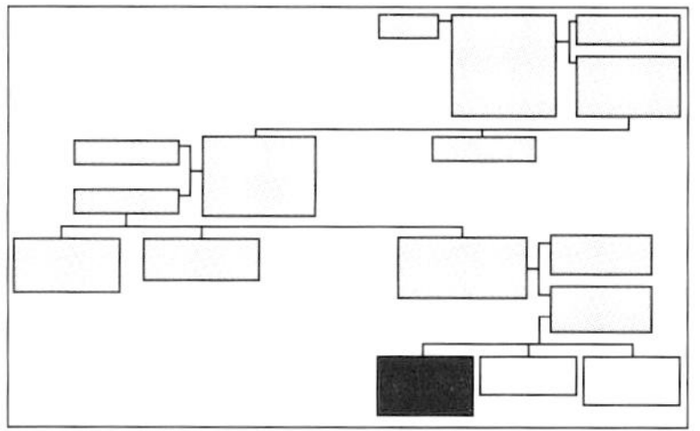

Upper-third obstruction

Palliation Because the left hepatic duct has a long extrahepatic segment that makes it more accessible, the preferred bypass technique for an obstructing upper-third lesion is a left (or segment 3) hepaticojejunostomy. This operation has superseded the Longmire procedure because it does not involve formal resection of liver parenchyma. Laparoscopic bypass techniques that make use of segment 3 have been developed, but their performance has yet to be formally assessed, and they cannot yet be incorporated into a management algorithm.[113,114]

Resection for cure The hilar plate is taken down to lengthen the hepatic duct segment available for subsequent anastomosis. Often a formal hepatectomy or segmentectomy is required to ensure an adequate proximal margin of resection. If the resection must be carried out proximal to the hepatic duct bifurcation, several cholangiojejunostomies will have to be done to anastomose individual hepatic biliary branches. Frozen-section examination of the proximal and distal resection margins is important because of the propensity of tumors such as cholangiocarcinoma to spread in a submucosal or perineural plane.

The results of aggressive hilar tumor resections that included as much liver tissue as was necessary to obtain a negative margin appear to justify this approach.[115] In cases of left hepatic involvement, resection of the caudate lobe (segments 1 and 9) is indicated as well.[116,117]

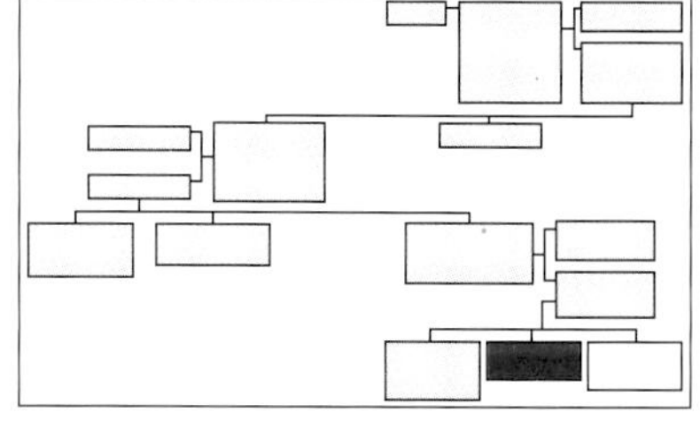

Middle-third obstruction

Palliation Surgical bypass of middle-third lesions is technically simpler because a hepaticojejunostomy can often be performed distal to the hepatic duct bifurcation, which means that exposure of the hilar plate or the intrahepatic ducts is unnecessary.

Resection for cure Discrete tumors in this part of the bile duct, although uncommon, are usually quite amenable to resection along with the lymphatic chains in the porta hepatis. Resection of an early gallbladder cancer may, on occasion, necessitate the concomitant resection of segment 5, although the value of resecting this segment prophylactically has not been conclusively demonstrated.[118] Sometimes jaundice from a suspected middle-third lesion is, in fact, caused by a case of Mirizzi syndrome [*see Figure 3*]. In such cases, a gallstone is responsible for extrinsic obstruction of the CBD, either by causing inflammation of the gallbladder wall or via direct impingement. Proper treatment of this syndrome may involve hepaticojejunostomy in addition to cholecystectomy if a cholecystocholedochal fistula is present.[119]

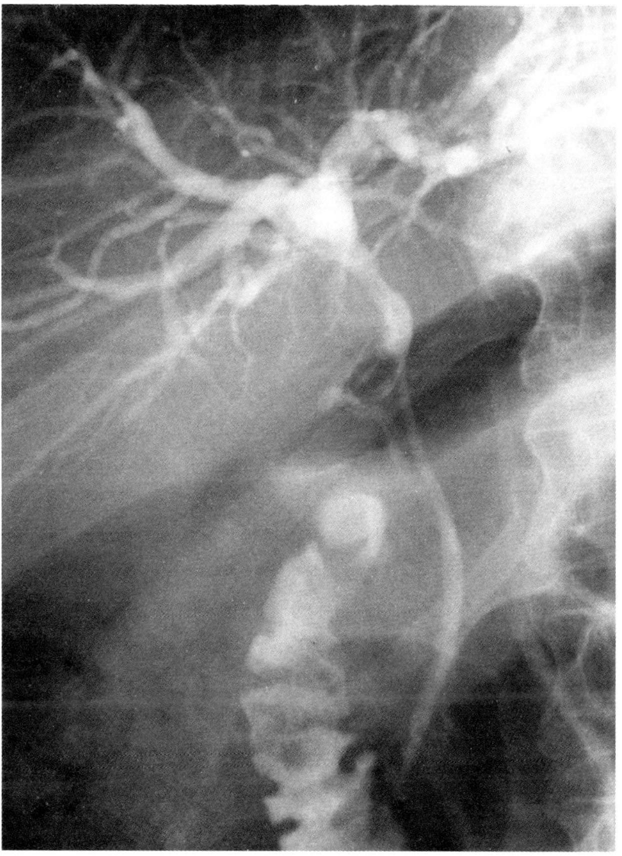

Figure 3 **Endoscopic retrograde cholangiopancreatography demonstrates extrinsic compression of the common hepatic duct by a stone in the Hartmann pouch. A biliary stent has been inserted for drainage.**

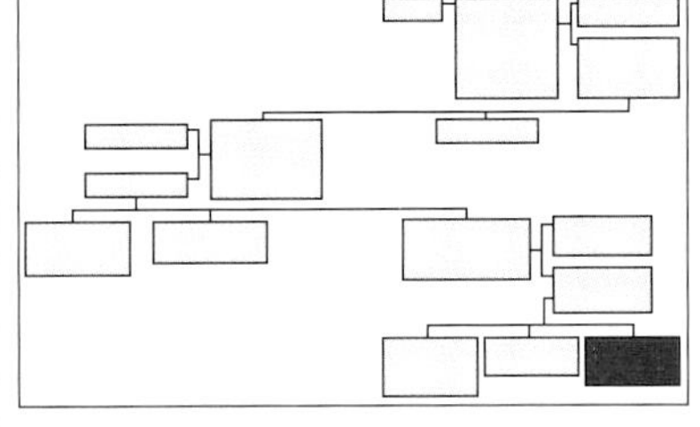

Lower-third obstruction

Palliation The preferred bypass technique for lower-third lesions is a Roux-en-Y choledochojejunostomy. Cholecystojejunostomy carries a higher risk of complications and subsequent development of jaundice[120]; this remains true even when it is performed laparoscopically. Occasionally, it may be done as a temporizing measure before a more definitive procedure in the context of an upcoming transfer to a specialized center.

Resection for cure Occasionally, an impacted CBD stone at the duodenal ampulla mimics a tumor and is not clearly identified preoperatively. Because of the growing use of EUS and MRCP, such a situation is increasingly uncommon. Resection of a lower-third lesion usually involves a pancreaticoduodenectomy, although transduodenal ampullary resection may be an acceptable alternative for a small adenoma of the ampulla; local duodenal resection without removal of the head of the pancreas has also been described.[121] For optimal results, pancreaticoduodenectomy is best performed in specialized centers.[122]

It has been suggested that postoperative adjuvant therapy may improve the prognosis after resection of a pancreatic adenocarcinoma,[illegible] but this debate falls outside the scope of our discussion.

Postoperative Jaundice

A clinical scenario of particular pertinence to surgeons that we have not yet addressed is the development of jaundice in the postoperative setting.

Jaundice develops in approximately 1% of all surgical patients after operation.[123] When jaundice occurs after a hepatobiliary procedure, it may be attributable to specific biliary causes, such as retained CBD stones, postoperative biliary leakage (through reabsorption of bile leaking into the peritoneum) [*see Figure 4*], injury to the CBD, and the subsequent development of biliary strictures. In most instances, however, the jaundice derives from a combination of disease processes, and only rarely is invasive testing or active treatment required.[124]

A diagnostic approach similar to the one outlined earlier (see above) is applicable to postoperative jaundice. However, as the possible causes of postoperative jaundice vary depending on the time interval between the operation and the development of jaundice, the following diagnostic approach may also be useful:

- Jaundice may develop within 48 hours of the operation; this is most often the result of the breakdown of red blood cells, occurring in the context of multiple blood transfusions (particularly with stored blood), the resorption of a large hematoma, or a transfusion reaction. Hemolysis may also develop in a patient with a known underlying hemolytic anemia and may be precipitated by the administration of specific drugs (e.g., sulfa drugs in a patient who has glucose-6-phosphate dehydrogenase deficiency).[125] Cardiopulmonary bypass or the insertion of a prosthetic valve may be associated with the development of early postoperative jaundice as well. Gilbert syndrome [*see Sidebar* Hepatic Jaundice] may first manifest itself early in the postoperative period. Occasionally, a mild conjugated hyperbilirubinemia may be related to Dubin-Johnson syndrome, which is an inherited disorder of bilirubin metabolism. This condition is usually self-limited and is characterized by the presence of a melaninlike pigment in the liver.
- Intraoperative hypotension or hypoxemia or the early development of heart failure can lead to conjugated hyperbilirubinemia within 5 to 10 days after operation. The hyperbilirubinemia may be associated with other end-organ damage (e.g., acute tubular necrosis). In fact, any impairment of renal function causes a decrease in bilirubin excretion and can be responsible for a mild hyperbilirubinemia.
- Jaundice may develop 7 to 10 days after operation in association with a medication-induced hepatitis attributable to an anesthetic agent. This syndrome has an estimated incidence of 1 in 10,000 after an initial exposure.[125] More commonly, the jaundice is related to the administration of antibiotics or other medications used in the perioperative setting.[125]

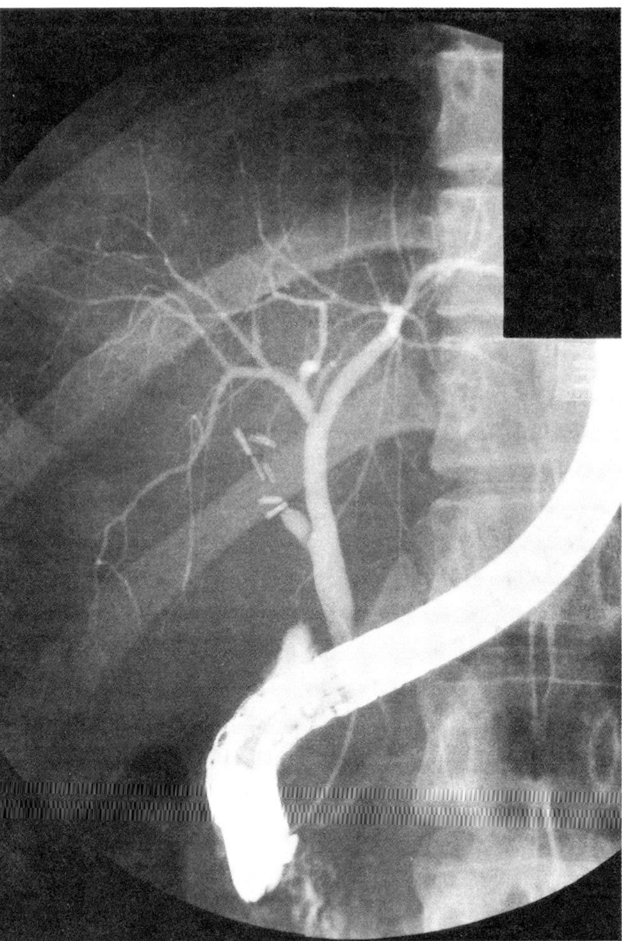

Figure 4 **Jaundice has occurred after laparoscopic cholecystectomy as a result of bile leakage from a distal biliary tributary. A stent has been inserted to decrease bile duct luminal pressure and foster spontaneous resolution.**

- After the first week, jaundice associated with intrahepatic cholestasis is often a manifestation of a septic response and usually presents in the setting of overt infection, particularly in patients with multiple organ dysfunction syndrome. Gram-negative sepsis from an intra-abdominal source is typical; if it persists, the outcome is likely to be poor. Jaundice may occur in as many as 30% of patients receiving total parenteral nutrition (TPN). It may be attributable to steatosis, particularly with formulas containing large amounts of carbohydrates. In addition, decreased export of bilirubin from the hepatocytes may lead to cholestasis, the severity of which appears to be related to the duration of TPN administration. Acalculous cholecystitis or even ductal obstruction may develop as a result of sludge in the gallbladder and the CBD. An elevated postoperative bilirubin level at any time may also result from unsuspected hepatic or posthepatic causes (e.g., occult cirrhosis, choledocholithiasis, or cholecystitis). A rare cause of postoperative jaundice is the development of thyrotoxicosis. Another entity to consider (as a diagnosis of exclusion) is so-called benign postoperative cholestasis, a primarily cholestatic, self-limited process with no clearly demonstrable cause that typically arises within 2 to 10 days after operation. Benign postoperative cholestasis may be attributable to a combination of mechanisms, including an increased pigment load, impaired liver function resulting from hypoxemia and hypotension, and decreased renal bilirubin excretion caused by varying degrees of tubular necrosis.[126] The predominantly conjugated hyperbilirubinemia may reach 40 mg/dL and remain elevated for as long as 3 weeks.[125]
- In the late postoperative period, the development of non-A, non-B, non-C viral hepatitis after transfusion of blood products will usually occur within 5 to 12 weeks of operation.

Financial Disclosures: None Reported

References

1. Schiff L. Jaundice: a clinical approach. In: Schiff L, Schiff ER, editors. Diseases of the liver. 7th ed. Philadelphia: JB Lippincott; 1993. p. 334.
2. Scharschmidt BF, Gollan JL. Current concepts of bilirubin metabolism and hereditary hyperbilirubinemia. In: Popper H, Schaffner F, editors. Progress in liver diseases. New York: Grune & Stratton; 1979. p. 187.
3. Frank BB. Clinical evaluation of jaundice: a guideline of the Patient Care Committee of the American Gastroenterological Association. JAMA 1989;262:3031.
4. Schiff ER, Sorrell MF, Maddrey WC, editors. Schiff's diseases of the liver. 8th ed. Philadelphia: Lippincott-Raven; 1999. p. 119.
5. Lindberg G, Björkman A, Helmers C. A description of diagnostic strategies in jaundice. Scand J Gastroenterol 1983;18:257.
6. Lumeng L, Snodgrass PJ, Swonder JW. Final report of a blinded prospective study comparing current non-invasive approaches in the differential diagnosis of medical and surgical jaundice. Gastroenterology 1980;78:1312.
7. Martin W, Apostolakos PC, Roazen H. Clinical versus actuarial prediction in the differential diagnosis of jaundice. Am J Med Sci 1960,240:571.
8. Matzen P, Malchow-Möller A, Hilden J, et al. Differential diagnosis of jaundice: a pocket diagnostic chart. Liver 1984;4:360.
9. O'Connor K, Snodgrass PJ, Swonder JE, et al. A blinded prospective study comparing four current non-invasive approaches in the differential diagnosis of medical versus surgical jaundice. Gastroenterology 1983; 84:1498.
10. Schenker S, Balint J, Schiff L. Differential diagnosis of jaundice: report of a prospective study of 61 proved cases. Am J Dig Dis 1962;7:449.
11. Theodossi A, Spiegelhalter D, Portmann B, et al. The value of clinical, biochemical, ultrasound and liver biopsy data in assessing patients with liver disease. Liver 1983;3: 315.
12. Pasanen PA, Pikkarainen P, Alhava E, et al. The value of clinical assessment in the diagnosis of icterus and cholestasis. Ital J Gastroenterol Hepatol 1992;24:313.
13. Theodossi A. The value of symptoms and signs in the assessment of jaundiced patients. Clin Gastroenterol 1985;14:545.
14. Fung KP, Lau SP. Differentiation between extrahepatic and intrahepatic cholestasis by discriminant analysis. J Paediatr Child Health 1990;26:132.
15. Pasanen PA, Pikkarainen P, Alhava E, et al. Evaluation of a computer-based diagnostic score system in the diagnosis of jaundice and cholestasis. Scand J Gastroenterol 1993;28: 732.
16. Malchow-Möller A, Gronvall S, Hilden J, et al. Ultrasound examination in jaundiced patients: is computer-assisted preclassification helpful? J Hepatol 1991;12:321.
17. Loperfido S, Angelini G, Benedetti G, et al. Major early complications from diagnostic and therapeutic ERCP: a prospective multicenter study. Gastrointest Endosc 1998; 48:1.
18. Freeman ML, DiSario JA, Nelson DB, et al. Risk factors for post-ERCP pancreatitis: a prospective, multicenter study. Gastrointest Endosc 2001;54:425.
19. Lillemoe KD. Surgical treatment of biliary tract infections. Am Surg 2000;66:138.
20. NIH state-of-the-science statement on endoscopic retrograde cholangiopancreatography (ERCP) for diagnosis and therapy. NIH Consens State Sci Statements 2002; 19:1.
21. Rossi LR, Traverso W, Pimentel F. Malignant obstructive jaundice: evaluation and management. Surg Clin North Am 1996;76: 63.
22. Taylor KJW, Rosenfield A. Grey-scale ultrasonography in the differential diagnosis of jaundice. Arch Surg 1977;112:820.
23. Kaplun L, Weissman HS, Rosenblatt RR, et al. The early diagnosis of common bile duct obstruction using cholescintigraphy. JAMA 1985;254:2431.
24. Abboud PA, Malet PF, Berlin JA, et al. Predictors of common bile duct stones prior to cholecystectomy: a meta-analysis. Gastrointest Endosc 1996;44:450.
25. Roston AD, Jacobson IM. Evaluation of the pattern of liver tests and yield of cholangiography in symptomatic choledocholithiasis: a prospective study. Gastrointest Endosc 1997;45:394.
26. Richter JM, Silverstein MD, Schapiro R. Suspected obstructive jaundice: a decision analysis of diagnostic strategies. Ann Intern Med 1983;99:46.
27. Bravo AA, Sheth SG, Chopra S. Liver biopsy. N Engl J Med 2001;344:495.
28. Blackbourne LH, Earnhardt RC, Sistrom CL, et al. The sensitivity and role of ultrasound in the evaluation of biliary obstruction. Am Surg 1994;60:683.
29. Sherlock S. Ultrasound (US), computerized axial tomography (CT) and magnetic resonance imaging (MRI). Dis Liver Biliary System 1989;5:70.
30. Cosgrove DO. Ultrasound in surgery of the liver and biliary tract. In: Blumhart LH, editor. Surgery of the liver and biliary tract. 2nd ed, vol 1. New York: Churchill Livingstone; 1994. p. 189.
31. Lindsell DRM. Ultrasound imaging of pancreas and biliary tract. Lancet 1990; 335:390.
32. Gillams A, Gardener J, Richards R, et al. Three-dimensional computed tomography cholangiography: a new technique for biliary tract imaging. Br J Radiol 1994;67:445.
33. Low RN, Sigeti JS, Francis IR, et al. Evaluation of malignant biliary obstruction: efficacy of fast multiplanar spoiled gradient-recalled MR imaging vs spin-echo MR imaging, CT, and cholangiography. AJR Am J Roentgenol 1994;162:315.
34. Amouyal P, Amouyal G, Levy P, et al. Diagnosis of choledocholithiasis by endoscopic ultrasonography. Gastroenterology 1994; 106:1062.
35. Guibaud L, Bret PM, Reinhold C, et al. Bile duct obstruction and choledocholithiasis: diagnosis with MR cholangiography. Radiology 1995;197:109.
36. Ishizaki Y, Wakayama T, Okada Y, et al. MR cholangiography for evaluation of obstructed jaundice. Am J Gastroenterol 1993;88:2072.
37. Bardou M, Romagnuolo J, Barkun AN, et al. Magnetic resonance cholangiopancreatography: a meta-analysis of test performance in suspected biliary disease. Ann Intern Med 2002;139:547.
38. Mallery S, Van Dam J. Current status of diagnostic and therapeutic endoscopic ultrasonography. Radiol Clin North Am 2001; 39:449.
39. Sugiyama M, Atomi Y, Hachiya J. Magnetic resonance cholangiography using half

Fourier acquisition for diagnosing choledocholithiasis. Am J Gastroenterol 1998;93:1886.

40. Jendresen MB, Thorboll JE, Adamsen S, et al. Preoperative routine magnetic resonance cholangiopancreatography before laparoscopic cholecystectomy: a prospective study. Eur J Surg 2002;168:690.
41. Soto JA, Alvarez O, Munera F, et al. Diagnosing bile duct stones: comparison of unenhanced helical CT, oral contrast-enhanced CT cholangiography, and MR cholangiography. AJR Am J Roentgenol 2000;175:1127.
42. Soto JA, Velez SM, Guzman J. Choledocholithiasis: diagnosis with oral-contrast-enhanced CT cholangiography. AJR Am J Roentgenol 1999;172:943.
43. Stabile Ianora AA, Memeo M, Scardapane A, et al. Oral contrast enhanced three-dimensional helical-CT cholangiography: clinical applications. Eur Radiol 2003;13:867.
44. Freeny PC. Computed tomography in the diagnosis and staging of cholangiocarcinoma and pancreatic carcinoma. Ann Oncol 1999;10 Suppl 4:12.
45. Hawes RH, Xiong Q, Waxman I, et al. A multispecialty approach to the diagnosis and management of pancreatic cancer. Am J Gastroenterol 2000;95:17.
46. Megibow AJ, Lavelle MT, Rofsky NM. MR imaging of the pancreas. Surg Clin North Am 2001;81:307.
47. Charcot JM. Leçons sur les maladies du fore des voices biliarcs et des veins faites à [illegible] Bournesville et sevestre; 1877.
48. Reynolds BM, Dargan EL. Acute obstructive cholangitis: a distinct clinical syndrome. Ann Surg 1959;150:299–303.
49. Lai EC, Mok FP, Tan ES, et al. Endoscopic biliary drainage for severe acute cholangitis. N Engl J Med 1992;326:1582.
50. Siperstein AE, Pearl J, Macho J, et al. Comparison of laparoscopic ultrasonography and fluorocholangiography in 300 patients undergoing laparoscopic cholecystectomy. Surg Endosc 1999;13:967.
51. Barkun JS, Fried GM, Barkun AN, et al. Cholecystectomy without operative cholangiography: implications for bile duct injury and common bile duct stones. Ann Surg 1993;218:371.
52. Sahai AV, Mauldin PD, Marsi V, et al. Bile duct stones and laparoscopic cholecystectomy: a decision analysis to assess the roles of intraoperative cholangiography, EUS, and ERCP. Gastrointest Endosc 1999;49(3 Pt 1):334.
53. Abraham N, Barkun AN, Barkun JS, et al. What is the optimal management of patients with suspected choledocholithiasis in the era of laparoscopic cholecystectomy? A decision analysis. Gastroenterology 1999;116:G0012.
54. Tse F, Barkun JS, Barkun AN. The elective evaluation of patients with suspected choledocholithiasis undergoing laparoscopic cholecystectomy. Gastrointest Endosc 2004;60:437.
55. Erickson RA, Carlson B. The role of endoscopic retrograde cholangiopancreatography in patients with laparoscopic cholecystectomies. Gastroenterology 1995;109:252.
56. Urbach DR, Khajanchee YS, Jobe BA, et al. Cost-effective management of common bile duct stones: a decision analysis of the use of endoscopic retrograde cholangiopancreatography (ERCP), intraoperative cholangiography, and laparoscopic bile duct exploration. Surg Endosc 2001;15:4.
57. Memon MA, Hassaballa H, Memon MI. Laparoscopic common bile duct exploration: the past, the present, and the future. Am J Surg 2000;179:309.
58. Crawford DL, Phillips EH. Laparoscopic common bile duct exploration. World J Surg 1999;23:343.
59. Falcone RA Jr, Fegelman EJ, Nussbaum MS, et al. A prospective comparison of laparoscopic ultrasound vs intraoperative cholangiogram during laparoscopic cholecystectomy. Surg Endosc 1999;13:784.
60. Thompson DM, Arregui ME, Tetik C, et al. A comparison of laparoscopic ultrasound with digital fluorocholangiography for detecting choledocholithiasis during laparoscopic cholecystectomy. Surg Endosc 1998;12:929.
61. Wu JS, Dunnegan DL, Soper NJ. The utility of intracorporeal ultrasonography for screening of the bile duct during laparoscopic cholecystectomy. J Gastrointest Surg 1998;2:50.
62. Stroszczynski C, Hunerbein M. Malignant biliary obstruction: value of imaging findings. Abdom Imaging 2005;30:314.
63. Legmann P, Vignaux O, Dousset B, et al. Pancreatic tumors: comparison of dual-phase helical CT and endoscopic sonography. AJR Am J Roentgenol 1998;170:1315.
64. Freeny PC, Traverso LW, Ryan JA. Diagnosis and staging of pancreatic adenocarcinoma with dynamic computed tomography. Am J Surg 1993;165:600.
65. Moosa AR, Gamagami RA. Diagnosis and staging of pancreatic neoplasms. Surg Clin North Am 1995;75:871.
66. [illegible] H, et al. Pancreatic carcinoma: CT vs MR imaging in the evaluation of resectability. Radiology 1995;195:327.
67. Hann LE, Winston CB, Brown KT, et al. Diagnostic imaging approaches and relationship to hepatobiliary cancer staging and therapy. Semin Surg Oncol 2000;19:94.
68. Zidi SH, Prat F, Le Guen O, et al. Performance characteristics of magnetic resonance cholangiography in the staging of malignant hilar strictures. Gut 2000;46:103.
69. Kim MJ, Mitchell DG, Ito K, et al. Biliary dilatation: differentiation of benign from malignant causes—value of adding conventional MR imaging to MR cholangiopancreatography. Radiology 2000;214:173.
70. Georgopoulos SK, Schwartz LH, Jarnagin WR, et al. Comparison of magnetic resonance and endoscopic retrograde cholangiopancreatography in malignant pancreaticobiliary obstruction. Arch Surg 1999;134:1002.
71. McNulty N, Francis I, Platt J, et al. Multidetector row helical CT of the pancreas: effect of contrast-enhanced multiphasic imaging on enhancement of the pancreas, peripancreatic vasculature, and pancreatic adenocarcinoma. Radiology 2001;220:97.
72. Smits NJ, Reeders JW. Current applicability of duplex Doppler ultrasonography in pancreatic head and biliary malignancies. Baillieres Clin Gastroenterol 1995;9:153.
73. Arslan A, Buanes T, Geitung JT. Pancreatic carcinoma: MR, MR angiography and dynamic helical CT in the evaluation of vascular invasion. Eur J Radiol 2001;38:151.
74. Giovannini M, Seitz JF. Endoscopic ultrasonography with a linear-type echoendoscope in the evaluation of 94 patients with pancreatobiliary disease. Endoscopy 1994;26:579.
75. Snady H, Cooperman A, Siegel J. Endoscopic ultrasonography compared with computed tomography and E.R.C.P. in patients with obstructive jaundice or small peri-pancreatic mass. Gastrointest Endosc 1992;38:27.
76. Nakaizumi A, Uehara H, Iishi H, et al. Endoscopic ultrasonography in diagnosis and staging of pancreatic cancer. Dig Dis Sci 1995;40:696.
77. Bakkevold KE, Arnesjo B, Kambestad B. Carcinoma of the pancreas and papilla of Vater—assessment of resectability and factors influencing resectability in stage I carcinomas: a prospective multicentre trial in 472 patients. Eur J Surg Oncol 1992;18:494.
78. DeWitt J, Devereaux B, Chiswell M, et al. Comparison of endoscopic ultrasonography and multidetector computed tomography for detecting and staging pancreatic cancer. Ann Intern Med 2004;141:753.
79. Soriano A, Castells A, Ayuso C, et al. Preoperative staging and tumor resectability assessment of pancreatic cancer: prospective study comparing endoscopic ultrasonography, helical computed tomography, magnetic resonance imaging and angiography. Am J Gastroenterol 2004;99:492.
80. Agarwal B, Abu-Hamda E, Molke KL, et al. Endoscopic ultrasound-guided fine needle aspiration and multidetector spiral CT in the diagnosis of pancreatic cancer. Am J Gastroenterol 2004;99:844.
81. Cannon ME, Carpenter SL, Elta GH, et al. EUS compared with CT, magnetic resonance imaging, and angiography and the influence of biliary stenting on staging accuracy of ampullary neoplasms. Gastrointest Endosc 1999;50:27.
82. Brugge WR, Lauwers GY, Sahani D, et al. Current concepts: cystic neoplasms of the pancreas. N Engl J Med 2004;351:1218.
83. Keppke AL, Miller FH. Magnetic resonance imaging of the pancreas: the [illegible] Semin Ultrasound CT MR 2005;26:132.
84. Delbeke D, Pinson CW. Pancreatic tumors: role of imaging in the diagnosis, staging and treatment. J Hepatobiliary Pancreat Surg 2004;11:4.
85. Heinrich S, Goerres G, Schafer M, et al. Positron emission tomography/computed tomography influences in the management of resectable pancreatic cancer and its cost-effectiveness. Ann Surg 2005;242:235.
86. Davidson BR. Progress in determining the nature of biliary strictures. Gut 1993;34:725.
87. Hawes RH. Endoscopy and non-calculus biliary obstruction. In: Cotton PB, Tytgat GNJ, Williams CB, editors. Annuals of gastrointestinal endoscopy, 8th ed. London, England: Current Science; 1995. p 101.
88. Baer HU, Rhyner M, Stain SC, et al. The effect of communication between the right and left liver on the outcome of surgical drainage from jaundice due to malignant obstruction at the hilus of the liver. HPB Surg 1994;8:27.
89. Rege RV. Adverse effects of biliary obstruction: implications for treatment of patients with obstructive jaundice. AJR Am J Roentgenol 1995;164:287.
90. Grande L, Garcia-Valdecasas JC, Fuster J, et al. Obstructive jaundice and wound healing. Br J Surg 1990;77:440.
91. Pitt HA, Gomes AS, Lois JF. Does preoperative percutaneous biliary drainage reduce operative risk or increase hospital cost? Ann Surg 1985;201:545.
92. McPherson GA, Benjamin IS, Hodgson HJ, et al. Preoperative percutaneous transhepatic biliary drainage: results of a controlled trial. Br J Surg 1984;71:371.
93. Povoski SP, Karpeh MS Jr, Conlon KC, et al. Preoperative biliary drainage: impact on intraoperative bile cultures and infectious morbidity and mortality after pancreaticoduodenectomy. J Gastrointest Surg 1999;3:496.

94. Sohn TA, Yeo CJ, Cameron JL, et al. Do preoperative biliary stents increase postpancreaticoduodenectomy complications? J Gastrointest Surg 2000;4:258.
95. Jarnagin WR, Bodniewicz J, Dougherty E, et al. A prospective analysis of staging laparoscopy in patients with primary and secondary hepatobiliary malignancies. J Gastrointest Surg 2000;4:34.
96. Abraham N, Barkun J, Barkun AN, et al. Clinical risk factors of plastic biliary stent obstruction: a prospective trial. Am J Gastroenterol 2000;95:2471.
97. Knyrim K, Wagner HJ, Pausch J, et al. A prospective, randomized controlled trial of metal stents for malignant obstruction of the common bile duct. Endoscopy 1993; 25:207.
98. Davids P, Groen A, Rauws E, et al. Randomized trial of self-expanding metal stents versus polyethylene stents for distal malignant biliary obstruction. Lancet 1992;340: 1488.
99. Moss, AC, Morris E, MacMathuna P. Palliative biliary stents for obstructing pancreatic carcinoma. Cochrane Database Syst Rev 2006;(2):CD004200.
100. Weber A, Mittermeyer T, Wagenpfeil S, et al. Self-expanding metal stents versus polyethylene stents for palliative treatment in patients with advanced pancreatic cancer. Pancreas 2009;38:e7–11.
101. Isayama H, Komatsu Y, Tsujino T, et al. A prospective randomised study of "covered" versus "uncovered" diamond stents for the management of distal malignant biliary obstruction. Gut 2004;53:729–34.
102. Prat F, Chapat O, Ducot B, et al. A randomized trial of endoscopic drainage methods for inoperable malignant strictures of the common bile duct. Gastrointest Endosc 1998;47:1.
103. Chan G, Barkun J, Barkun AN, et al. The role of ciprofloxacin in prolonging polyethylene biliary stent patency: a multicenter, double-blinded effectiveness study. J Gastrointest Surg 2005;9:481.
104. Smith AC, Dowsett JF, Russell RC, et al. Randomized trial of endoscopic stenting vs surgical bypass in malignant low bile duct obstruction. Lancet 1994;344:1655.
105. Lillemoe KD, Sauter P, Pitt HA, et al. Current status of surgical palliation of periampullary carcinoma. Surg Gynecol Obstet 1993;176:1.
106. Van Heek NT, De Castro SM, Van Eijck CH, et al. Need for a prophylactic gastrojejunostomy for unresectable periampullary cancer: a prospective randomized multicenter trial with special focus on assessment of quality of life. Ann Surg 2003; 238:894.
107. Lillemoe KD, Cameron JL, Kaufman HS, et al. Chemical splanchnicectomy in patients with unresectable pancreatic cancer: a prospective randomized trial. Ann Surg 1993; 217:447.
108. Lillemoe KD, Cameron JL, Yeo CJ, et al. Pancreaticoduodenectomy: does it have a role in the palliation of pancreatic cancer? Ann Surg 1996;223:718.
109. D'Angelica M, Fong Y, Weber S, et al. The role of staging laparoscopy in hepatobiliary malignancy: prospective analysis of 401 cases. Ann Surg Oncol 2003;10:183.
110. Conlon KC, Dougherty E, Klimstra DS, et al. The value of minimal access surgery in the staging of patients with potentially resectable pancreatic malignancy. Ann Surg 1996;223:134.
111. John TG, Greig JD, Carter DC, et al. Carcinoma of the pancreatic head and periampullary region: tumor staging with laparoscopy and laparoscopic ultrasonography. Ann Surg 1995;221:156.
112. Jarnagin WR, Bodniewicz J, Dougherty E, et al. A prospective analysis of staging laparoscopy in patients with primary and secondary hepatobiliary malignancies. J Gastrointest Surg 2000;4:34.
113. Hunerbein M, Rau B, Schlag PM. Laparoscopic ultrasound for staging of upper gastrointestinal tumours. Eur J Surg Oncol 1995;21:50.
114. Scott-Conner CE. Laparoscopic biliary bypass for inoperable pancreatic cancer. Semin Laparosc Surg 1998;5:185.
115. Date RS, Siriwardena AK. Current status of laparoscopic biliary bypass in the management of non-resectable peri-ampullary cancer. Pancreatology 2005;5:325.
116. Chamberlain RS, Blumgart LH. Hilar cholangiocarcinoma: a review and commentary. Ann Surg Oncol 2000;7:55.
117. Ogura Y, Kawarada Y. Surgical strategies for carcinoma of the hepatic duct confluence. Br J Surg 1998;85:20.
118. Jarnagin W, Shoup M. Surgical management of cholangiocarcinoma. Semin Liver Dis 2004;24:189.
119. Bartlett D. Gallbladder cancer. Semin Surg Oncol 2000;19:145.
120. Baer HU, Matthews JB, Schweizer WP, et al. Management of the Mirizzi syndrome and the surgical implications of cholecystocholedochal fistula. Br J Surg 1990;77:743.
121. Sarfeh MG, Rypins EB, Jakowatz JG, et al. A prospective, randomized clinical investigation of cholecystoenterostomy and choledochoenterostomy. Am J Surg 1988;155: 411.
122. Kalady MF, Clary BM, Tyler DS, Pappas TN. Pancreas-preserving duodenectomy in the management of duodenal familial adenomatous polyposis. J Gastrointest Surg 2002;6:82.
123. Lieberman MD, Kilburn H, Lindsey M, et al. Relation of perioperative deaths to hospital volume among patients undergoing pancreatic resection for malignancy. Ann Surg 1995;222:638.
124. Lamont JT, Isselbacher KJ. Current concepts of postoperative hepatic dysfunction. Conn Med 1975;39:461.
125. Matlof DS, Kaplan MM. Postoperative jaundice. Orthop Clin North Am 1978;9: 799.
126. Moody FG, Potts JR III. Postoperative jaundice. In: Schiff L, Schiff ER, editors. Diseases of the liver. 7th ed. Philadelphia: JB Lippincott; 1993. p. 370.
127. Watson CJ. Prognosis and treatment of hepatic insufficiency. Ann Intern Med 1959; 31:405.
128. Sherlock S. Jaundice. In: Sherlock S, editor. Diseases of the liver and biliary system, 8th ed. Oxford: Blackwell Scientific Publications; 1989. p. 230.
129. Gollan JL, Keefe EB, Scharschmidt BF. Cholestasis and hyperbilirubinemia. In: Gitnick G, editor. Current hepatology, Vol I. Boston: Houghton Mifflin; 1980. p. 277.
130. Bosma PJ, Chowdhury JR, Bakker C, et al. The genetic basis of the reduced expression of bilirubin UCP-glucuronosyltransferase 1 in Gilbert's syndrome. N Engl J Med 1995; 333:1171.
131. Fallon MB, Anderson JM, Boyer JL. Intrahepatic cholestasis. In: Schiff L, Schiff ER, editors. Diseases of the liver, 7th ed. Philadelphia: JB Lippincott Co; 1993. p. 343.

Acknowledgment

Figure 2c From *MRI of the Abdomen and Pelvis: A Text-Atlas*, by R.C. Semelka, S. M. Asher, and C. Reinhold. John Wiley and Sons, New York, 1997. Used with permission.

4 INTESTINAL OBSTRUCTION

Phillip A. Bilderback, MD, Ryan K. Smith, BA, and W. Scott Helton, MD, FACS

Intestinal obstruction is a common medical problem and accounts for a large percentage of surgical admissions for acute abdominal pain.[1] It develops when air and secretions are prevented from passing aborally as a result of either intrinsic or extrinsic compression (i.e., mechanical obstruction) or gastrointestinal (GI) paralysis (i.e., nonmechanical obstruction in the form of ileus or pseudo-obstruction). Small intestinal ileus is the most common form of intestinal obstruction; it occurs after most abdominal operations and is a common response to acute extra-abdominal medical conditions and intra-abdominal inflammatory conditions [*see Table 1*].[2] Acute colonic pseudo-obstruction occurs most frequently in the postoperative period or in response to another acute medical illness. Mechanical small bowel obstruction (SBO) is somewhat less common; such obstruction is secondary to intra-abdominal adhesions, hernias, or cancer in about 90% of cases [*see Table 2*]. Mechanical colonic obstruction accounts for only 10 to 15% of all cases of mechanical obstruction and most often develops in response to obstructing carcinoma, diverticulitis, or volvulus [*see Table 3*].

There are several different methods of classifying mechanical obstruction: acute versus chronic, partial versus complete, simple versus closed loop, and gangrenous versus nongangrenous. The importance of these classifications is that the natural history of the condition, its response to treatment, and the associated morbidity and mortality all vary according to which type of obstruction is present.

When chyme and/or gas can traverse the point of obstruction, obstruction is partial; when this is not the case, obstruction is complete. When the bowel is occluded at a single point along the intestinal tract, leading to intestinal dilatation, hypersecretion, and bacterial overgrowth proximal to the obstruction and decompression distal to the obstruction, simple obstruction is present. A closed-loop obstruction occurs when a segment of bowel is obstructed along its course by a single constrictive lesion that occludes both the proximal and the distal end of the intestinal loop and traps the bowel's mesentery. When the blood supply to a closed loop segment of bowel becomes compromised, leading to ischemia and eventually to bowel wall necrosis and perforation, strangulation is present. The most common causes of simple obstruction are intra-abdominal adhesions, tumors, and strictures; the most common causes of closed-loop obstruction are hernias, adhesions, and volvulus.

Table 1 Causes of Ileus

- Intra-abdominal causes
  - Intraperitoneal problems
    - Peritonitis or abscess
    - Inflammatory condition
      - Mechanical: operation, foreign body
      - Chemical: gastric juice, bile, blood
      - Autoimmune: serositis, vasculitis
    - Intestinal ischemia: arterial or venous, sickle cell disease
  - Retroperitoneal problems
    - Pancreatitis
    - Retroperitoneal hematoma
    - Spine fracture
    - Aortic operation
    - Renal colic
    - Pyelonephritis
    - Metastasis
- Extra-abdominal causes
  - Thoracic problems
    - Myocardial infarction
    - Pneumonia
    - Congestive heart failure
    - Rib fractures
  - Metabolic abnormalities
    - Electrolyte imbalance (e.g., hypokalemia)
    - Sepsis
    - Lead poisoning
    - Porphyria
    - Hypothyroidism
    - Hypoparathyroidism
    - Uremia
  - Medicines
    - Opiates
    - Anticholinergics
    - Alpha agonists
    - Antihistamines
    - Catecholamines
  - Spinal cord injury or operations
  - Head, thoracic, or retroperitoneal trauma
  - Chemotherapy, radiation therapy

Table 2 Causes of Small Bowel Obstruction in Adults

- Extrinsic causes
  - Adhesions*
  - Hernias (external, internal [paraduodenal], incisional)*
  - Metastatic cancer*
  - Volvulus
  - Intra-abdominal abscess
  - Intra-abdominal hematoma
  - Pancreatic pseudocyst
  - Intra-abdominal drains
  - Tight fascial opening at stoma
- Intraluminal causes
  - Tumors*
  - Gallstones
  - Foreign body
  - Worms
  - Bezoars
- Intramural abnormalities
  - Tumors
  - Strictures
  - Hematoma
  - Intussusception [*see Figure 4*]
  - Regional enteritis
  - Radiation enteritis

*Approximately 90% of all small bowel obstructions are secondary to adhesions, hernias, or tumors.

Table 3 Causes of Colonic Obstruction

Causes
Common causes
Cancer (primary, anastomotic, metastatic)
Volvulus
Diverticulitis
Pseudo-obstruction
Hernia
Anastomotic stricture
Unusual causes
Intussusception
Fecal impaction
Strictures (from one of the following)
Inflammatory bowel disease
Endometriosis
Radiation therapy
Ischemia
Foreign body
Extrinsic compression by a mass
Pancreatic pseudocyst
Hematoma
Metastasis
Primary tumors

One of the most difficult tasks in general surgery is deciding when to operate on a patient with intestinal obstruction; however, new methods for detecting ischemic bowel and determining when obstruction will be amenable to nonoperative therapy are emerging. The purpose of the following discussion is to outline a safe, efficient, and cost-effective stepwise approach to making this difficult decision and optimizing the management of patients with this problem [*see Figure 1*]. Absolutes are few and far between: treatment must always be highly individualized. Consequently, the following recommendations are intended only as guidelines, not as surgical dicta.

Clinical Evaluation

HISTORY AND CLINICAL SETTING

When a patient complains of acute obstipation, abdominal pain and distention, nausea, and vomiting, the probability that either mechanical bowel obstruction or ileus is present is very high.[3] Mechanical obstruction can often be distinguished from ileus or pseudo-obstruction on the basis of the location, character, and severity of abdominal pain as well as the setting within which the symptoms occur. Pain from mechanical obstruction is usually located in the middle of the abdomen, whereas pain from ileus and pseudo-obstruction is diffuse. Pain from ileus is usually mild, and pain from obstruction is typically more severe. In general, pain increases in severity and depth over time as obstruction progresses; however, in mechanical obstruction, pain severity may decrease over time as a result of bowel fatigue and atony. The periodicity of pain can help localize the level of obstruction: pain from proximal intestinal obstruction has a short periodicity (3 to 4 minutes), and distal small bowel or colonic pain has longer intervals (15 to 20 minutes) between episodes of nausea, cramping, and vomiting.

Abdominal distention, nausea, and vomiting usually develop after pain has already been felt for some time. The patient should be asked what degree of abdominal distention is present and whether there has been a sudden or rapid change. Distention developing over many weeks suggests a chronic process or progressive partial obstruction. Massive abdominal distention coupled with minimal crampy pain, nausea, and vomiting suggests long-standing intermittent mechanical obstruction or some form of chronic intestinal pseudo-obstruction. The combination of a gradual change in bowel habits, progressive abdominal distention, early satiety, mild, crampy pain after meals, and weight loss also suggests chronic partial mechanical bowel obstruction. If the patient has undergone evaluation for similar symptoms before, any previous abdominal radiographs or contrast studies should be reviewed. The patient should be asked when flatus was last passed: failure to pass flatus may signal a transition from partial to complete bowel obstruction. Patients with an intestinal stoma (ileostomy or colostomy) who present with signs and symptoms of obstruction often report abdominal distention and pain after a sudden change in stomal output of stool, liquid, or air.

The patient should also be asked about (1) previous episodes of bowel obstruction, (2) previous abdominal or pelvic operations, (3) a history of malignancy, and (4) a history of intra-abdominal inflammation (e.g., inflammatory bowel disease, cholecystitis, pancreatitis, pelvic inflammatory disease, or abdominal trauma). The presence of various factors provides clues as to the etiology of the obstruction. If the patient has experienced episodes of obstruction before, one should ask about the etiology and the response to treatment. If the patient has ever undergone an abdominal operation, one should try to obtain and read the operative report, which can provide a great deal of helpful information (e.g., description of adhesions, assessment of their severity, and evaluation of intra-abdominal pathology and anatomy). If abdominal cancer was present, one should find out what operation was performed and attempt to determine the likelihood of intra-abdominal recurrence. Obstructive symptoms without a history of previous surgery or identified hernias should raise the suspicion for cancer. Symptoms that come and go suddenly over several days in a patient older than 65 years should increase the index of suspicion for gallstone ileus.[4]

The clinical setting often provides clues to the cause and type of bowel obstruction. In hospitalized patients, there is likely to be an associated medical condition or metabolic derangement that led to obstruction. A thorough review of the patient's medical history and hospital course should be undertaken to identify precipitating events that could have led to intestinal obstipation. One should ask the patient about any previous abdominal irradiation and should note and take into account all medications the patient is taking, especially anticoagulants and agents with anticholinergic side effects. Patients who are receiving chemotherapy or have undergone abdominal radiation therapy are prone to ileus. Severe infection, fluid and electrolyte imbalances, narcotic and anticholinergic medications, and intra-abdominal inflammation of any origin may be implicated. Acute massive abdominal distention in a hospitalized patient usually results from acute gastric atony, small bowel ileus, or acute colonic pseudo-obstruction. Excessive anticoagulation can lead to retroperitoneal, intra-abdominal, or intramural hematoma that can cause mechanical obstruction or ileus. Finally, there are specific problems that tend to arise in the

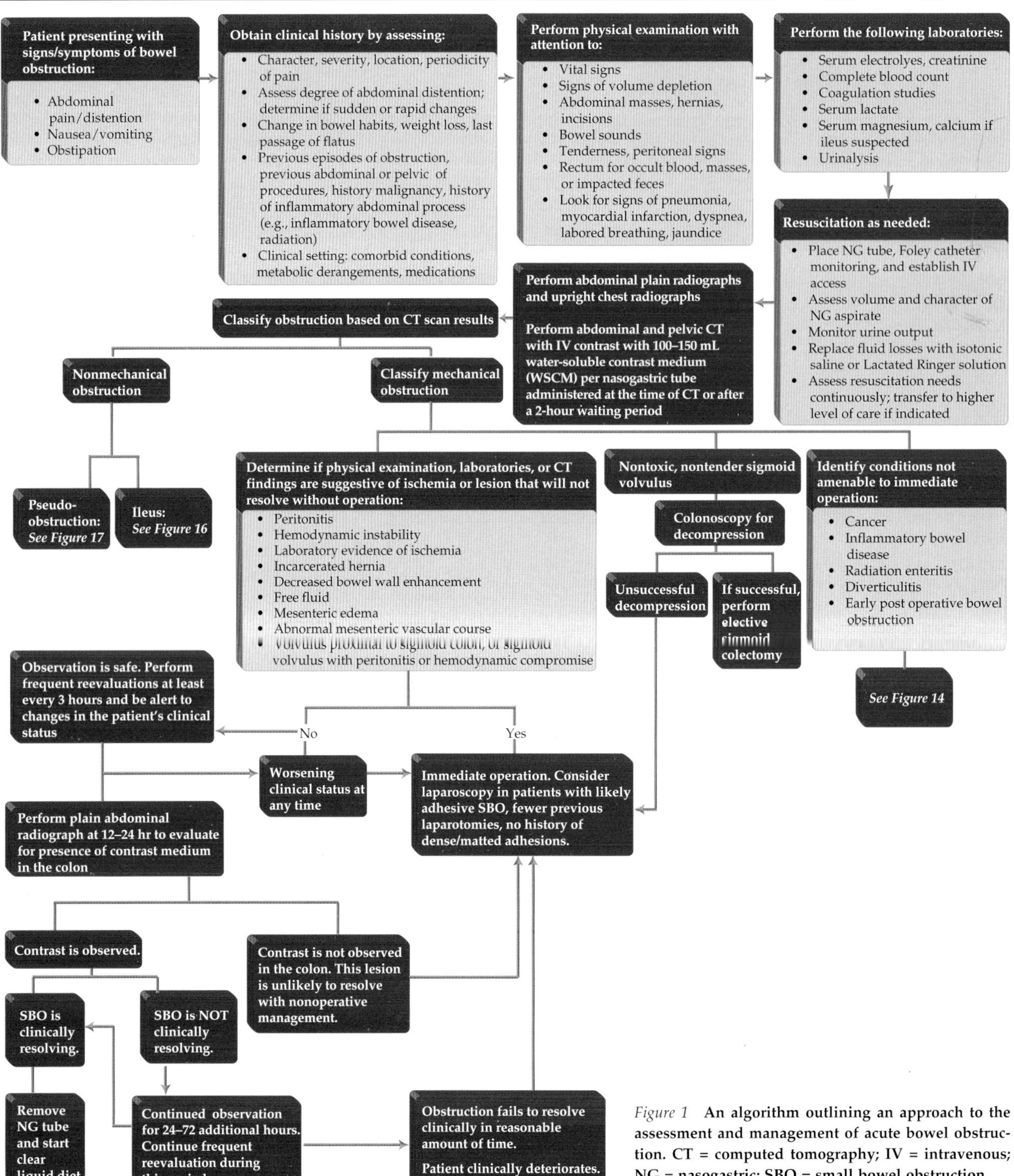

Patient presenting with signs/symptoms of bowel obstruction:
• Abdominal pain/distention
• Nausea/vomiting
• Obstipation
Obtain clinical history by assessing:
• Character, severity, location, periodicity of pain
• Assess degree of abdominal distention; determine if sudden or rapid changes
• Change in bowel habits, weight loss, last passage of flatus
• Previous episodes of obstruction, previous abdominal or pelvic of procedures, history malignancy, history of inflammatory abdominal process (e.g., inflammatory bowel disease, radiation)
• Clinical setting: comorbid conditions, metabolic derangements, medications
Perform physical examination with attention to:
• Vital signs
• Signs of volume depletion
• Abdominal masses, hernias, incisions
• Bowel sounds
• Tenderness, peritoneal signs
• Rectum for occult blood, masses, or impacted feces
• Look for signs of pneumonia, myocardial infarction, dyspnea, labored breathing, jaundice
Perform the following laboratories:
• Serum electrolyes, creatinine
• Complete blood count
• Coagulation studies
• Serum lactate
• Serum magnesium, calcium if ileus suspected
• Urinalysis
Resuscitation as needed:
• Place NG tube, Foley catheter monitoring, and establish IV access
• Assess volume and character of NG aspirate
• Monitor urine output
• Replace fluid losses with isotonic saline or Lactated Ringer solution
• Assess resuscitation needs continuously; transfer to higher level of care if indicated
Perform abdominal plain radiographs and upright chest radiographs
Perform abdominal and pelvic CT with IV contrast with 100–150 mL water-soluble contrast medium (WSCM) per nasogastric tube administered at the time of CT or after a 2-hour waiting period
Classify obstruction based on CT scan results
Nonmechanical obstruction
Classify mechanical obstruction
Pseudo-obstruction: See Figure 17
Ileus: See Figure 16
Determine if physical examination, laboratories, or CT findings are suggestive of ischemia or lesion that will not resolve without operation:
• Peritonitis
• Hemodynamic instability
• Laboratory evidence of ischemia
• Incarcerated hernia
• Decreased bowel wall enhancement
• Free fluid
• Mesenteric edema
• Abnormal mesenteric vascular course
• Volvulus proximal to sigmoid colon, or sigmoid volvulus with peritonitis or hemodynamic compromise
Nontoxic, nontender sigmoid volvulus
Colonoscopy for decompression
Unsuccessful decompression
If successful, perform elective sigmoid colectomy
Identify conditions not amenable to immediate operation:
• Cancer
• Inflammatory bowel disease
• Radiation enteritis
• Diverticulitis
• Early post operative bowel obstruction
See Figure 14
No
Yes
Observation is safe. Perform frequent reevaluations at least every 3 hours and be alert to changes in the patient's clinical status
Worsening clinical status at any time
Immediate operation. Consider laparoscopy in patients with likely adhesive SBO, fewer previous laparotomies, no history of dense/matted adhesions.
Perform plain abdominal radiograph at 12–24 hr to evaluate for presence of contrast medium in the colon
Contrast is observed.
Contrast is not observed in the colon. This lesion is unlikely to resolve with nonoperative management.
SBO is clinically resolving.
SBO is NOT clinically resolving.
Remove NG tube and start clear liquid diet
Continued observation for 24–72 additional hours. Continue frequent reevaluation during this period.
Obstruction fails to resolve clinically in reasonable amount of time.
Patient clinically deteriorates.

Figure 1 **An algorithm outlining an approach to the assessment and management of acute bowel obstruction. CT = computed tomography; IV = intravenous; NG = nasogastric; SBO = small bowel obstruction.**

postoperative period; these are discussed more fully elsewhere [*see* Urgent Operation, Early Postoperative Technical Complications; *and* No Operation, Early Postoperative Obstruction, *below*].

PHYSICAL EXAMINATION AND RESUSCITATION

The initial steps in the physical examination are (1) developing a sense of the patient's illness and course and (2) assessing the patient's vital signs, hydration status, and cardiopulmonary system. A nasogastric (NG) tube, a Foley catheter, and an intravenous (IV) line should be placed immediately while the physical examination is in progress. The volume and character of the gastric aspirate and urine are noted. A clear, gastric effluent is suggestive of gastric outlet obstruction. A bilious, nonfeculent aspirate is a typical sign of middle to proximal SBO or colonic obstruction with a competent ileocecal valve. A feculent aspirate is a typical sign of distal, high-grade SBO. Volume replacement, if necessary, is initiated with isotonic saline or lactated Ringer solution. Adequate resuscitation is critical prior to taking the patient to the operating room; measurement and repletion of electrolytes that may have occurred from prolonged periods of vomiting should also be undertaken.

Fever or tachycardia may be present, suggesting that the obstruction may be a manifestation of an intra-abdominal abscess, or they may indicate perforation, especially if peritonitis is noted. Signs of pneumonia or myocardial infarction should be sought: these conditions, like intestinal obstruction, can have upper abdominal pain, distention, nausea, and vomiting as presenting symptoms. Dyspnea and labored breathing may occur secondary to severe abdominal distention or pain, in which case, immediate relief should be provided by placing the patient in the lateral decubitus position and offering narcotics as soon as the initial physical examination is performed. Jaundice raises the possibility of gallstone ileus or metastatic cancer.

Examination of the abdomen proceeds in an orderly manner from observation to auscultation to palpation and percussion. The patient is placed in the supine position with the legs flexed at the hip to decrease tension on the rectus muscles. The degree of abdominal distention observed varies, depending on the level of obstruction: proximal obstructions may cause little or no distention. Abdominal scars should be noted. Abdominal asymmetry or a protruding mass suggests an underlying malignancy, an abscess, or closed-loop obstruction. The abdominal wall should be observed for evidence of peristaltic waves, which are indicative of acute SBO.

Auscultation should be performed for at least 3 to 4 minutes to determine the presence and quality of bowel sounds. High-pitched bowel tones, tingles, and rushes are suggestive of an obstructive process, especially when temporally associated with waves of crampy pain, nausea, or vomiting. The absence of bowel tones is typical of intestinal paralysis but may also indicate intestinal fatigue from long-standing obstruction, closed-loop obstruction, or pseudo-obstruction.

Approximately 70% of patients with bowel obstruction have symmetrical tenderness, whereas fewer than 50% have rebound tenderness, guarding, or rigidity.[3] Traditional teaching is that localized tenderness and guarding indicate underlying strangulated bowel; however, prospective studies have demonstrated that these physical findings are neither specific nor sensitive for detecting underlying strangulation[5] or even obstruction.[3] Nevertheless, most surgeons still believe that guarding, rebound tenderness, and localized tenderness reflect underlying strangulation and therefore are indications for operation. Patients with ileus tend to have generalized abdominal tenderness that cannot be distinguished from the tenderness of mechanical obstruction. Gentle percussion is performed over all quadrants of the abdomen to search for areas of dullness (suggestive of an underlying mass), tympany (suggestive of underlying distended bowel), and peritoneal irritation. A thorough search is made for inguinal, femoral, umbilical, and incisional hernias. The rectum is examined for masses, fecal impaction, and occult blood. If the patient has an ileostomy or a colostomy, the stoma is examined digitally to make sure that there is no obstruction at the level of the fascia.

It is important to note that no constellation of signs, symptoms, or physical examination findings can reliably presume the diagnosis of bowel obstruction 100% of the time, and a low threshold should be maintained to initiate further workup with laboratory and imaging studies when clinical suspicion exists.[6]

Investigative Studies

IMAGING

In general, one should obtain a chest x-ray in all patients with bowel obstruction to exclude subdiaphragmatic free air. In most cases, supine, upright, or lateral decubitus films of the abdomen can distinguish the type of obstruction present (mechanical or nonmechanical, partial or complete) and establish the general location of the obstruction (stomach, small bowel, or colon). A useful technique for evaluating abdominal radiographs is to look systematically for intestinal gas along the normal route of the GI tract, beginning at the stomach, continuing through the small bowel, and, finally, following the course of the colon to the rectum. The following questions should be kept in mind as this is done:

- Are there abnormally dilated loops of bowel, signs of small bowel dilatation, or air-fluid levels?
- Are air-fluid levels and bowel loops in the same place on supine and upright films?
- Is there gas throughout the entire length of the colon (suggestive of ileus or partial mechanical obstruction)?
- Is there a paucity of distal colonic gas or an abrupt cutoff of colonic gas with proximal colonic distention and air-fluid levels (suggestive of complete or near-complete colonic obstruction)?
- Is there evidence of strangulation (e.g., thickened small bowel loops, mucosal thumb printing, pneumatosis cystoides intestinalis, or free peritoneal air)?
- Is there massive distention of the colon, especially of the cecum or sigmoid (suggestive of either volvulus or pseudo-obstruction)?
- Are there any biliary or renal calculi, and is there any air in the biliary tree (suggestive of gallstone ileus[6] or a renal stone that could be causing ileus)?

It is important to be able to distinguish between small and large bowel gas. Gas in a distended small bowel outlines the valvulae conniventes, which traverse the entire diameter of the bowel lumen [*see Figure 2*]. Gas in a distended colon, on the other hand, outlines the colonic haustral markings, which cross only part of the bowel lumen and typically interdigitate [*see Figure 3 and Figure 4*]. Distended small bowel loops usually occupy the central abdomen [*see Figure 2*], whereas distended large bowel loops are typically seen around the periphery [*see Figure 3*]. In patients with ileus, distention usually extends uniformly throughout the stomach, the small bowel, and the colon [*see Figure 4*], and air-fluid levels may be found in the colon and the small intestine.

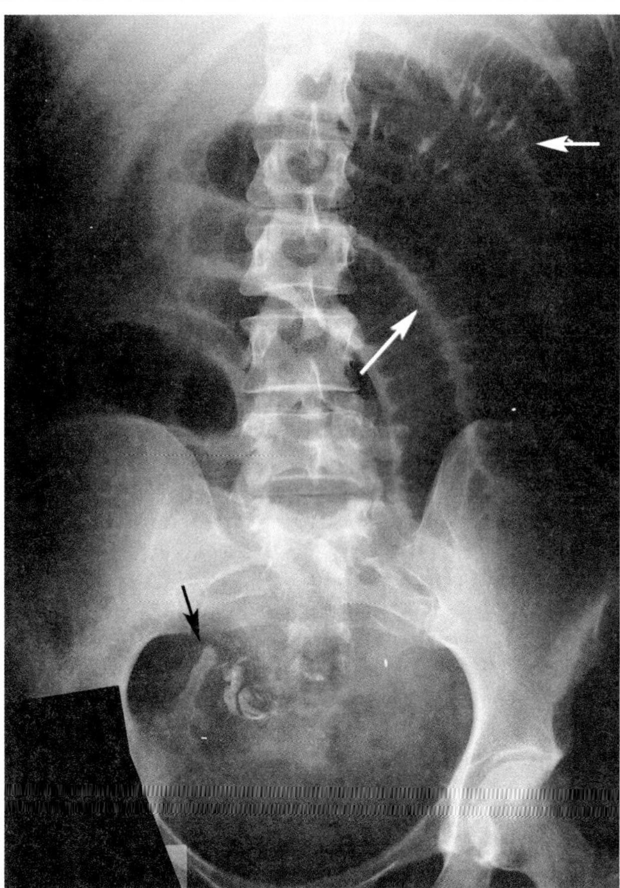

Figure 2 **Supine radiograph from a patient with complete small bowel obstruction shows distended small bowel loops in the central abdomen with prominent valvulae conniventes (*small white arrow*). The bowel wall between the loops is thickened and edematous (*large white arrow*). No air is seen in the colon or the rectum. Note the presence of an isolated small bowel loop in the right lower quadrant (*black arrow*), which is seen fixed in the same location on upright films, as shown in Figure 5.**

Patients with gastric outlet obstruction or gastric atony typically have a giant gastric bubble if no nasogastric tube has been placed, with little or no air in the small bowel or the colon. Patients with mechanical SBO usually have multiple air-fluid levels, with distended bowel loops of varying sizes arranged in an inverted U configuration [*see Figure 5*]. A dilated loop of small bowel appearing in the same location on supine and upright films suggests obstruction of a fixed segment of bowel by an adhesion or an internal hernia [*see Figure 2 and Figure 5*]. SBO is often accompanied by a paucity of gas in the colon. The complete absence of colonic gas is strongly suggestive of complete SBO; however, the presence of colonic gas does not exclude complete SBO in that there may have been unevacuated gas distal to a point of complete obstruction before the radiograph was taken. On the other hand, if repeat radiographs demonstrate decreased or absent colonic or rectal gas in a patient with SBO who previously had more colonic or rectal gas, it is probable that partial obstruction has become complete, and an operation may be indicated. High-grade obstruction of the colon with an incompetent ileocecal valve may manifest itself as distended small bowel loops with air-fluid levels, thereby mimicking SBO. Hence, it is sometimes necessary to perform a barium enema to exclude colonic obstruction.

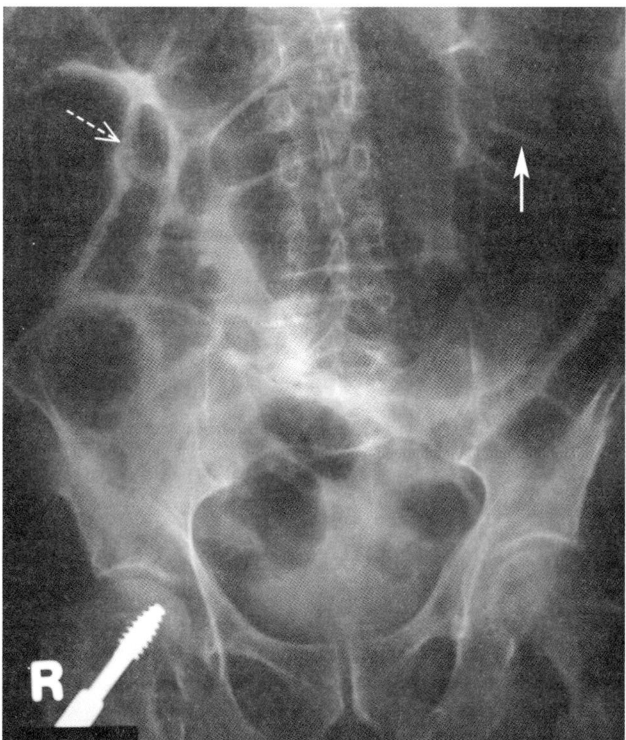

Figure 3 **Radiograph from a patient with acute [illegible] pseudo-obstruction shows a dilated colon with haustral markings (*white arrow*) and edematous small bowel loops (*dotted white arrow*). Air extends down to the distal sigmoid. This picture is also consistent with rectal obstruction, which could have been excluded by rigid sigmoidoscopy.**

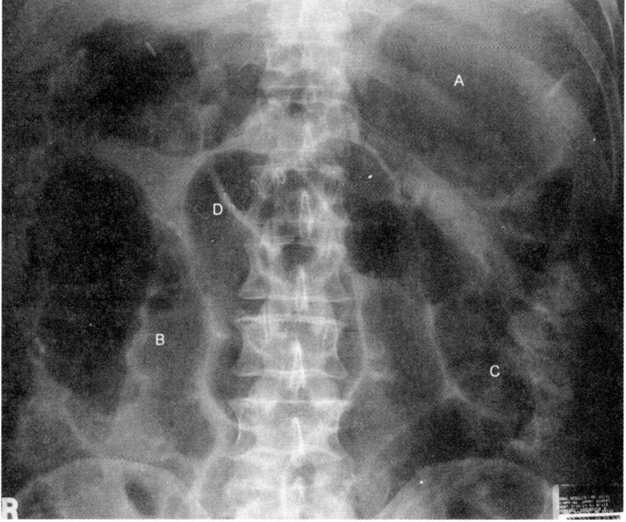

Figure 4 **Radiograph from a patient with postoperative ileus shows massive gastric distention (A), distended small bowel loops (B), air throughout the colon, mild dilatation of the sigmoid colon (C) with air mixed with stool, and a haustral fold in the apex of the sigmoid colon (D).**

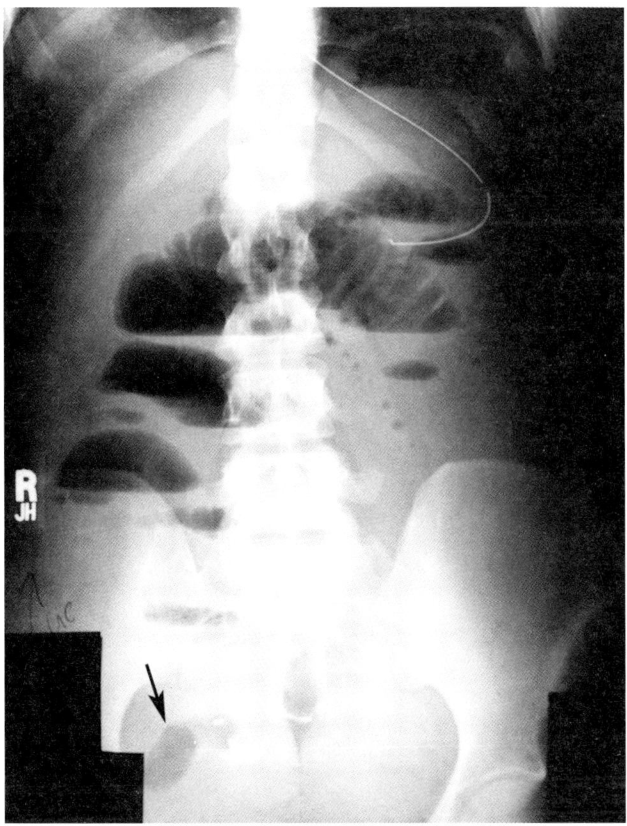

Figure 5 **Upright radiograph from the same patient as the supine radiograph in Figure 2 shows multiple air-fluid levels of varying size arranged in inverted Us. In the right lower pelvis, a loop of small bowel is seen in exactly the same location as on the supine abdominal film (*black arrow*), a finding suggestive of adhesive obstruction.**

Massive gaseous distention of the colon is usually secondary to distal colonic or rectal obstruction, volvulus, or pseudo-obstruction [*see Figure 2, Figure 6, Figure 7, and Figure 8*]. There are well-defined radiographic criteria that are highly sensitive and specific for sigmoid volvulus.[7] If there is any uncertainty regarding the presence, type, or level of colonic obstruction, immediate sigmoidoscopy followed by barium enema is diagnostic.

LABORATORY TESTS

Serum electrolyte concentrations, hematocrit, serum creatinine concentration, coagulation profile (prothrombin time [or international normalized ratio] and platelet count), and serum lactate are helpful in determining the severity of volume depletion, identifying ischemia, and guiding resuscitative efforts. If ileus is suspected, serum magnesium and calcium levels should be measured, and urinalysis should be done to check for hematuria.

Determination of Need for Operation and Classification of Obstruction

The combination of a thorough history, a carefully performed physical examination, and correctly interpreted abdominal radiographs usually allows an experienced surgeon to identify the type of bowel obstruction present and to decide whether a patient requires immediate, urgent, or delayed operation [*see Table 4*] or can safely be treated initially with nonoperative measures. On the other hand, even experienced surgeons have difficulty in properly identifying the cause and in deciding when to operate on a patient with intestinal obstruction. Given the importance of establishing a timely and accurate diagnosis on patient outcomes and costs of care, it is strongly recommended that all patients suspected of having intestinal obstruction be admitted to a surgical service; failure to do so can increase patient morbidity and mortality.[8] An exception to this guideline may be patients admitted to a hospitalist service but with early surgical consultation, frequent reevaluation, and good interservice communication.

It is particularly important and useful to stratify patients into those with mechanical obstruction and those with nonmechanical obstruction. In patients with mechanical bowel obstruction, an effort should be made to determine whether the obstruction is partial or complete and whether it is accompanied by ischemia. This can be accomplished early in most cases using the aid of computed tomography (CT) with IV contrast and use of a water-soluble contrast medium (WSCM) challenge [*see* Adjunctive Tests, Ultrasonography, Fast Magnetic Resonance Imaging, and Computed Tomography; *and* Mechanical Obstruction, Immediate Operation, CT-based scoring systems, *and* Urgent Operation, Water-soluble contrast medium challenge, *below*]. Strong consideration for immediate operation may be given to patients with high-grade to complete obstruction and/or clinical or radiologic signs of ischemia; conversely, patients with partial bowel obstruction, especially from adhesions, rarely require an emergent operation. Finally, an effort should be made to establish the level and cause of obstruction because these factors often help guide therapy and affect the probability of success in response to specific therapeutic intervention. Patients with nonmechanical obstruction, which derives from ileus or pseudo-obstruction [*see* Ileus *and* Pseudo-obstruction, *below*], do not require immediate, or often any, operation.

ADJUNCTIVE TESTS

Sigmoidoscopy

When one is uncertain whether or not an obstruction is mechanical on the basis of the information at hand, additional diagnostic measures are immediately indicated. When large amounts of colonic air extend down to the rectum, a digital rectal examination and flexible or rigid sigmoidoscopy will readily exclude a rectal or distal sigmoid obstruction. Care must be exercised to avoid insufflating large amounts of air during endoscopy: excessive insufflation can cause overdistention of the colon above the level of the possible obstruction, which can be counterproductive and harmful. If sigmoidoscopy yields normal findings but partial colonic obstruction seems to be the correct diagnosis, a water-soluble contrast enema should be administered.[9]

Barium studies may be harmful in patients with acute obstruction when they are performed before the nature of the obstruction (complete or partial) is determined. Abdominal ultrasonography, although not as definitive as a contrast examination, is also able to diagnose suspected colonic obstruction in 85% of patients.[10]

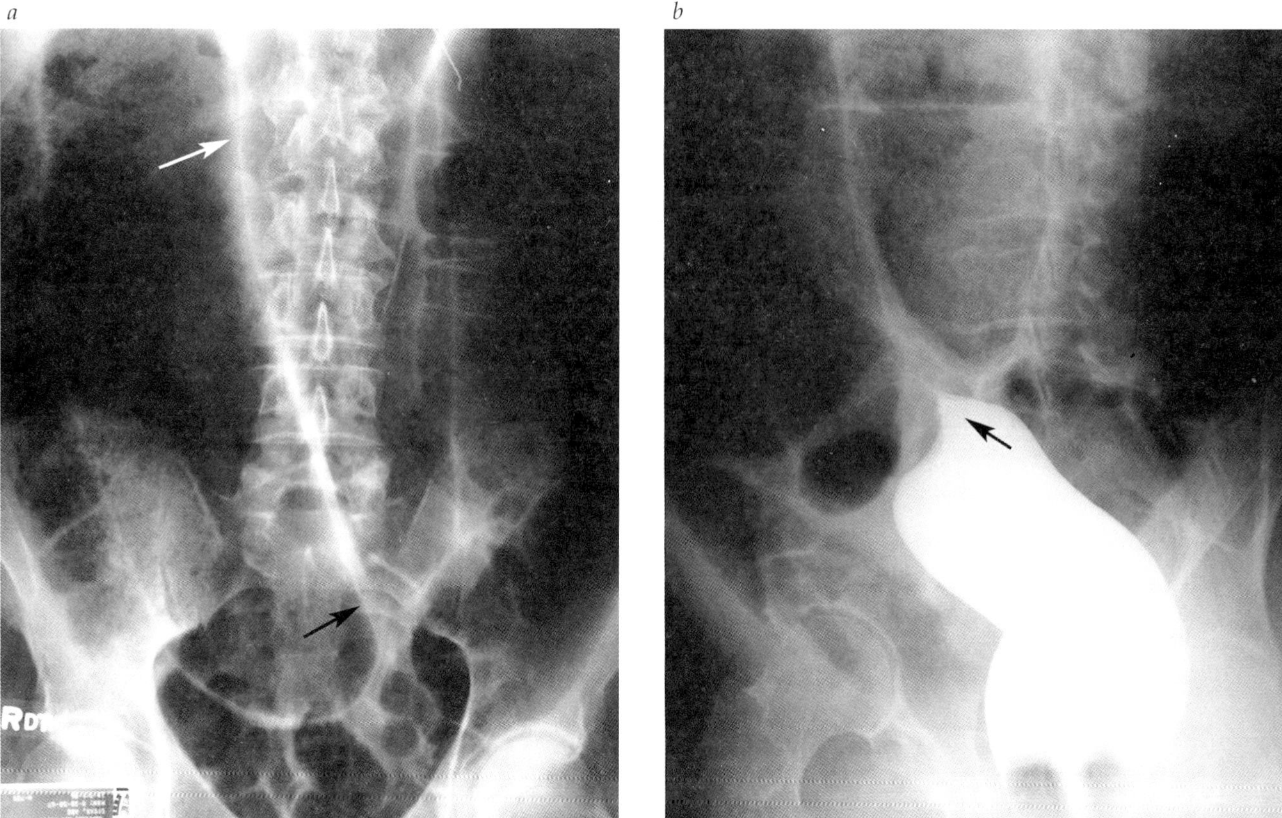

Figure 6 (*a*) Radiograph from a patient with massive sigmoid volvulus shows a distended ahaustral sigmoid loop (*white arrow*), inferior convergence of the walls of the sigmoid loop to the left of the midline, and approximation of the medial walls of the sigmoid loop as a summation line (*black arrow*). (*b*) Barium enema of the colon shows a tapered obstruction at the rectosigmoid junction with a typical bird's beak deformity (*black arrow*).

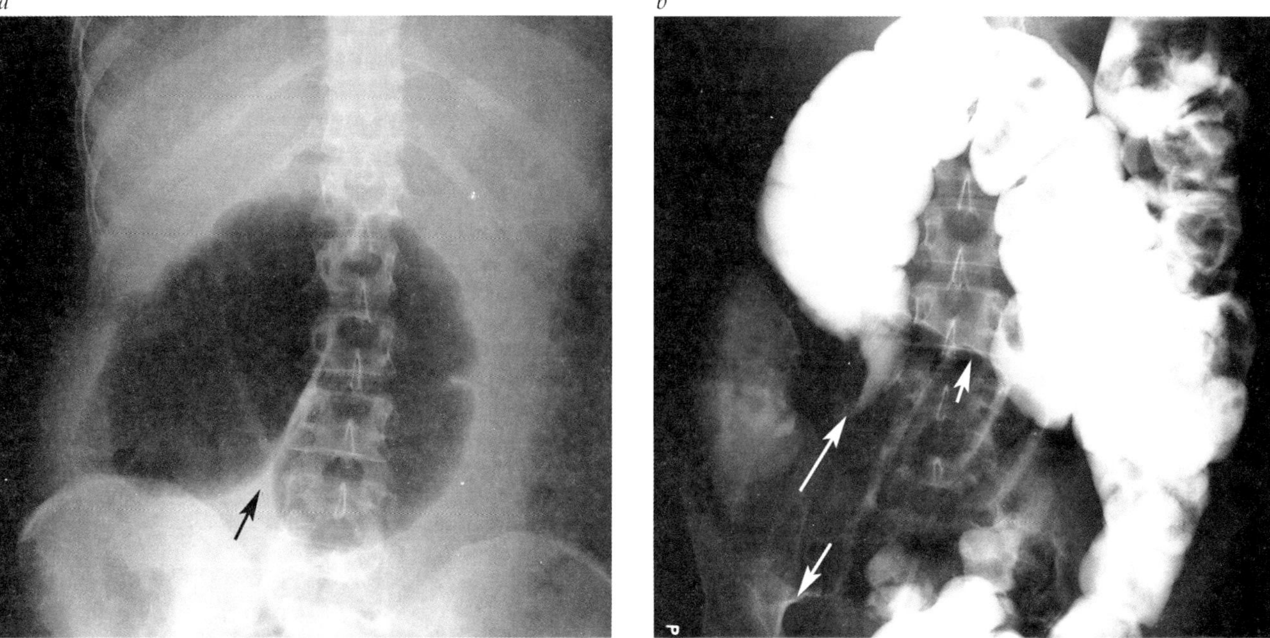

Figure 7 (*a*) Radiograph from a patient with cecal volvulus shows a dilated cecum with no air distally in the colorectum. Convergence of the medial walls of the loop (*black arrow*) points to the right, a typical finding in cecal volvulus. (*b*) Barium examination demonstrates a bird's beak deformity tapering at the point of volvulus (*large white arrow*). Note walls of dilated cecum (*small white arrows*).

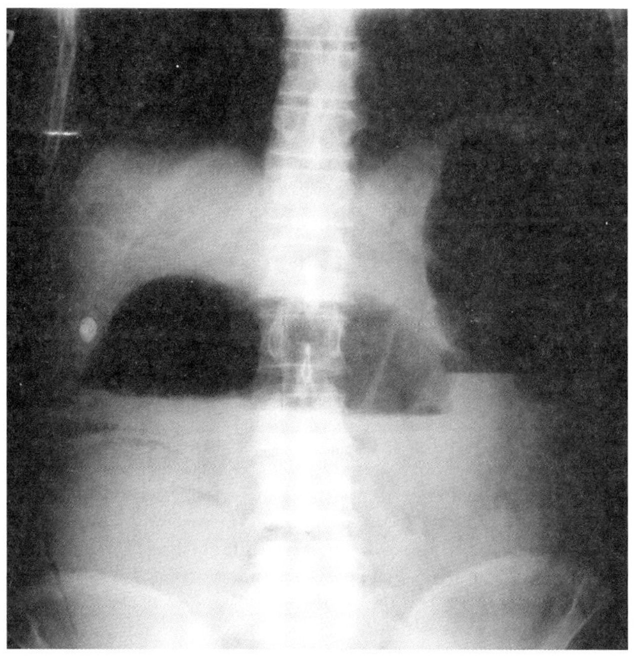

Figure 8 **Radiograph from a patient with complete colonic obstruction from an obstructing carcinoma in the descending left colon with proximal air-fluid levels. The absence of air distally in the rectum or the sigmoid is suggestive of complete obstruction. The ileocecal valve is competent; thus, there is no small bowel air.**

Ultrasonography, Fast Magnetic Resonance Imaging, and Computed Tomography

Abdominal radiographs can be entirely normal in patients with complete, closed-loop, or strangulation obstruction.[11] Controversy exists over the role of abdominal radiography in the diagnosis of bowel obstruction, and studies of its diagnostic accuracy have been mixed.[12] A recent study, however, found that abdominal radiographs were accurate in detecting acute SBO using three patterns of air-fluid levels and that senior radiologists were more accurate than less experienced readers.[13]

Therefore, if the patient's clinical profile and the results of physical examination are consistent with intestinal obstruction despite normal abdominal radiographs, abdominal ultrasonography, CT, or fast magnetic resonance imaging (MRI) should be performed immediately.[12] All three modalities are highly sensitive and specific for intestinal obstruction when performed properly and interpreted by experienced clinicians. Ultrasonography, MRI, and CT are all capable of detecting the cause of the obstruction, as well as the presence of closed-loop or strangulation obstruction.[12,14]

Sonographic criteria have been established for small bowel and colonic obstruction[10,15,16]: (1) simultaneous observation of distended and collapsed bowel segments; (2) free peritoneal fluid; (3) inspissated intestinal contents; (4) paradoxical pendulating peristalsis; (5) highly reflective fluid within the bowel lumen; (6) bowel wall edema between serosa and mucosa; and (7) a fixed mass of aperistaltic, fluid-filled, dilated intestinal loops. Ultrasonography is well suited to critically ill patients: because it can be performed at the bedside, the risk associated with transport to the radiology suite is avoided. Recent prospective trials have also shown bedside ultrasonography to have superior diagnostic accuracy to abdominal plain films when performed by emergency department physicians, radiologists, and residents after appropriate training.[17,18] Given that ultrasonography is relatively inexpensive, is easy and quick to perform, and often can provide a great deal of information about the location, nature, and severity of the obstruction, it is often used in regions outside the United States.[14] However, concerns over interobserver variability, sonographer inexperience, obesity, impaired imaging relative to overlying bowel gas, and the ready availability of CT imaging have made ultrasonography an uncommon choice in the United States.

Fast MRI with T_2-weighted (spin-spin relaxation time) images is an accurate modality to establish the location and cause of bowel obstruction.[19] Because of its higher cost, decreased availability, longer study time, and lack of convincing incremental diagnostic gain compared with CT, MRI should not be used routinely for evaluating suspected high-grade SBO. It remains a useful option in children or pregnant patients.[12]

The American College of Radiology recommends that patients with suspected complete or high-grade SBO and equivocal plain abdominal films undergo CT with IV contrast routinely.[12] CT has several advantages over a small bowel contrast examination in this setting: (1) it can ascertain the level of obstruction, (2) it can assess the severity of the obstruction and determine its cause, and (3) it can detect closed-loop obstruction and signs of ischemia [*see Figure 9, Figure 10, Figure 11, Figure 12, and Figure 13*]. Furthermore, several scoring systems and models have been developed that use a combination of clinical and CT findings to detect ischemia and help predict the need for operative intervention [*see* Mechanical Obstruction, Immediate Operation,

Table 4 Guidelines for Operative and Nonoperative Therapy

Situations suggesting emergent operation
- Incarcerated, strangulated hernias
- Peritonitis
- Pneumatosis cystoides intestinalis
- Pneumoperitoneum
- Suspected or proven intestinal strangulation
- Closed-loop obstruction
- Nonsigmoid colonic volvulus
- Sigmoid volvulus associated with toxicity or peritoneal signs

Situations necessitating urgent operation
- Failure of water-soluble contrast medium to reach the colon within 24 hours
- Progressive bowel obstruction at any time after nonoperative measures are started
- Failure to improve with conservative therapy within 36–48 hr
- Early postoperative technical complications

Situations in which delayed operation is usually safe
- Immediate postoperative obstruction
- Sigmoid volvulus successfully decompressed by sigmoidoscopy
- Acute exacerbation of Crohn disease, diverticulitis, or radiation enteritis
- Chronic, recurrent partial obstruction
- Paraduodenal hernia
- Gastric outlet obstruction
- Postoperative adhesions
- Resolved partial colonic obstruction

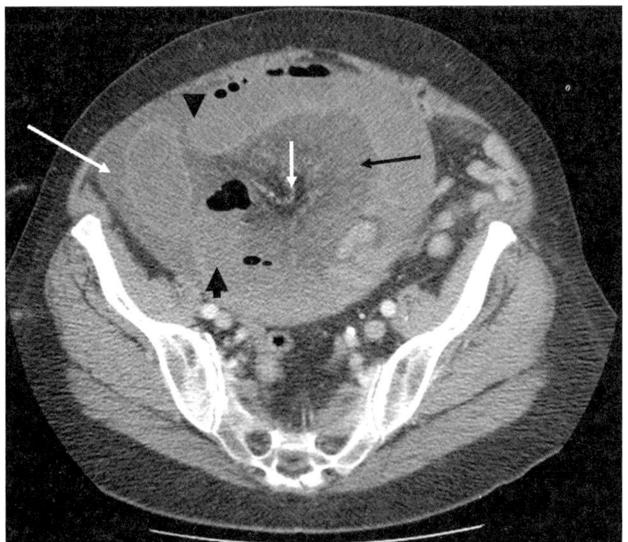

Figure 9 **Axial intravenous contrast–enhanced computed tomographic scan demonstrating the classic appearance of a closed-loop obstruction (*between black arrowheads*). There is a swirling appearance of the mesenteric vessels, also known as the "whirl sign" (*short white arrow*), accompanied by mesenteric edema (*black arrow*) and free intraperitoneal fluid (*long white arrow*). This patient was markedly tender and acidotic and had a leukocytosis. She was taken for laparotomy and found to have a small section of ischemic small bowel that was resected.**

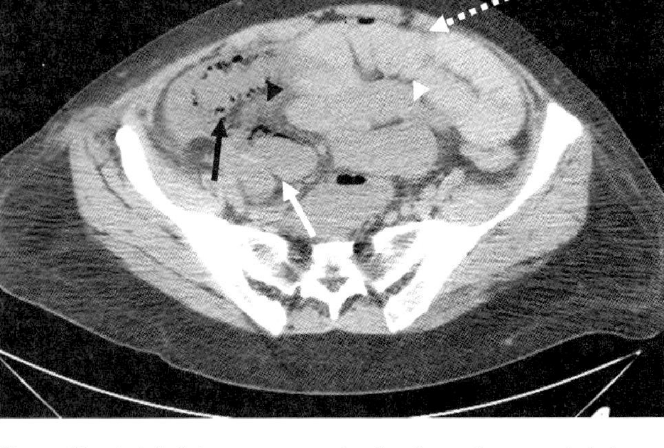

Figure 11 **Axial intravenous contrast–enhanced computed tomographic scan demonstrating ischemic bowel obstruction. There is mesenteric edema (*black arrowhead*) and, importantly, pneumatosis intestinalis (*black arrow*), which can be distinguished from air within the bowel lumen given its appearance in antidependent bowel in a supine patient. A transition point from distended to decompressed bowel is demonstrated (*white arrowhead*). Note the normal mucosal enhancement (*broken white arrow*) compared to the decreased enhancement in the section of ischemic bowel (*white arrowhead*). These findings, combined with tachycardia and leukocytosis, prompted an early exploration.**

Strangulation and Closed-Loop Obstruction, CT-based scoring systems, *below*]. CT can also detect inflammatory or neoplastic processes both outside and inside the peritoneal cavity and can visualize small amounts of intraperitoneal air or pneumatosis cystoides intestinalis not seen on conventional films [*see Figure 11*]. Prospective studies have demonstrated that the accuracy of CT in diagnosing bowel obstruction is higher than 95% and that its sensitivity and specificity are each higher than 94%.[20] CT distinguishes colonic mechanical obstruction from pseudo-obstruction more accurately than conventional films do and thus is the preferred modality in many cases.[12]

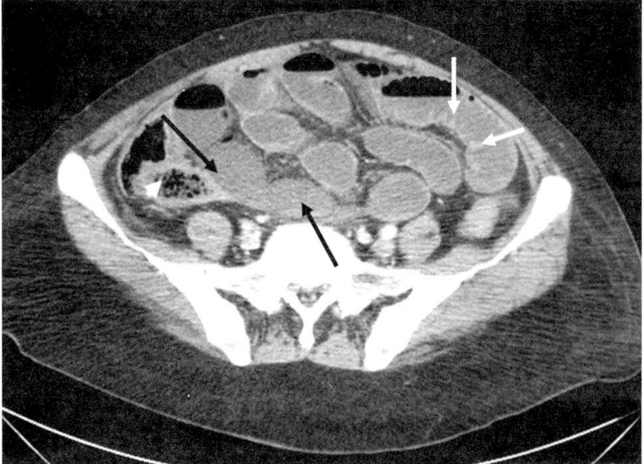

Figure 10 **Axial intravenous contrast–enhanced computed tomographic scan demonstrating decreased bowel wall enhancement in a patient with ischemia secondary to adhesive small bowel obstruction. Note the mucosal detail in the normal bowel (*white arrows*), where the mucosal folds can clearly be seen. This is in contrast to the loss of detail in the areas of ischemia (*black arrows*). There is air in the colon (*white arrowhead*), a finding indicative of partial obstruction; however, because of evidence of ischemia, this patient was taken for laparotomy and found to have strangulated obstruction.**

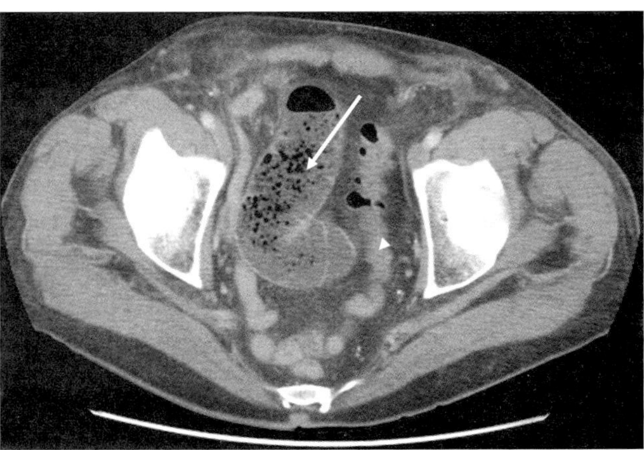

Figure 12 **Axial intravenous contrast–enhanced computed tomographic scan of a patient with small bowel obstruction secondary to an incarcerated femoral hernia demonstrating "fecalization" of small bowel contents within an obstructed segment (*white arrow*). Note the dilated small bowel adjacent to a loop of decompressed bowel (*white arrowhead*). Although small bowel fecalization is thought to indicate a more indolent course and suggests that nonoperative management may be successful, because this lesion would not resolve on its own, the patient was taken for early laparotomy.**

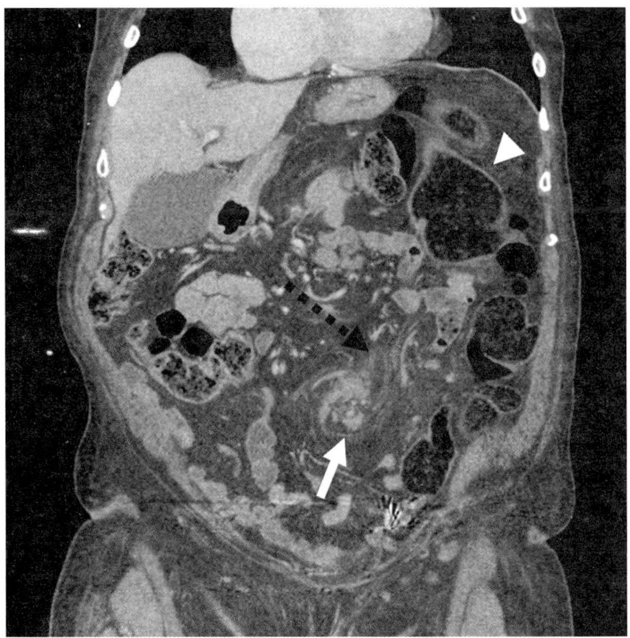

Figure 13 **Coronal section of an intravenous contrast–enhanced computed tomographic scan in a patient with sigmoid volvulus. Note the swirling mesentery ("whirl sign") (*white arrow*) with associated mesenteric edema (*dashed black arrow*) and marked colonic dilatation in the left upper quadrant (*white arrowhead*). This patient underwent prompt colonoscopic decompression of his volvulus and subsequent elective sigmoid colectomy.**

Contrast Studies

Enteroclysis (direct injection of contrast into the small bowel using a long intestinal tube) was previously considered the most sensitive method of distinguishing between ileus and partial mechanical SBO. Fluoroscopic enteroclysis has become unnecessary in the vast majority of cases of acute SBO with the advent of newer imaging techniques. However, because of its ability to challenge the distensibility of the bowel wall, enteroclysis has continued utility in cases of subclinical, low-grade, or intermittent obstruction.[21] CT and magnetic resonance enteroclysis is now possible, and the use of cross-sectional imaging overcomes the limitations of radiographic enteroclysis, including overlapping bowel loops and the requirement for a skilled fluoroscopist.[12] Furthermore, cross-sectional imaging detects a greater number of abnormalities both inside and outside the intestinal tract.[14] Because enteroclysis challenges the distensibility of the bowel, it is more sensitive than small bowel follow-through or CT enterography in detecting low-grade or partial SBO.[14,21] If partial obstruction is identified in either the small or the large bowel, the patient is treated accordingly. If (1) mechanical obstruction is not identified and (2) a point of obstruction, as evidenced by the finding of both dilated and decompressed intestinal loops, cannot be identified through abdominal ultrasonography, CT, or fast MRI, then the diagnosis is almost certainly ileus, in which case, one's attention is directed toward identifying and correcting the underlying precipitating cause [*see Table 1 and* Mechanical Obstruction, No Operation, Adhesive Partial Small Bowel Obstruction, *below*]

Mechanical Obstruction

MALIGNANT BOWEL OBSTRUCTION

Malignant bowel obstruction (MBO) is a serious complication and most commonly affects patients with abdominal and pelvic tumors. Some patients will present with advanced disease for which curative surgical intervention is not feasible. For those patients, palliative efforts should focus on controlling GI symptoms and restoring or preserving quality of life. Etiologies for MBO include extrinsic occlusion of the lumen, malignant infiltration of mesentery and intestinal muscle and serosal surfaces, and intraluminal obstruction. Avoidance of operation in patients with extrinsic obstruction due to carcinomatosis is desirable, and resolution may be obtained by medical or endoscopic means. Intestinal immobility secondary to opioids, certain antiemetics, and secondary adrenal insufficiency may all play a role in MBO.

Early and intensive pharmacologic treatment with a combination of antisecretory drugs, analgesics, and antiemetics has been shown to be effective in controlling GI symptoms and even reverse functional MBO [*see Figure 14*].[22,23] Three prospective, randomized clinical trials demonstrated that octreotide significantly attenuated the severity of nausea and vomiting and the degree of subjective discomfort in patients with inoperable obstruction and permitted the discontinuance of NG tube decompression.[24] One of these studies also demonstrated that octreotide significantly reduced the degree of fatigue and anorexia experienced.[24] Malignant obstruction has been treated safely on an outpatient basis with octreotide, metoclopramide, morphine, and dexamethasone.[25] Long-acting preparations of octreotide may aid in the development of protocols designed to keep patients at home as long as possible.[23] Therefore, patients with terminal illness should be offered hospice care or home visiting nurse services with continuous octreotide infusion, IV rehydration, and decompression.[22–24] Attention must always be paid to quality of life issues and to the patient's interest in pursuing nonoperative forms of palliation. For many terminally ill or incurable patients with bowel obstruction, the most humane and sensible treatment comprises institution of comfort measures, including continuous morphine infusion, rehydration, and administration of antisecretory agents.[22–24]

Self-expanding metallic stents

Many patients with gastric, duodenal, or colorectal MBO may be successfully treated by endoscopic deployment of self-expanding metallic stents (SEMSs) as a means of palliation or as a bridge surgery.[26,27] Malignant obstruction of the gastric outlet or duodenum is a frequent late complication of gastric, duodenal, or pancreatic cancer and has been traditionally managed with surgical gastrojejunostomy. Two systematic reviews have found that placement of a SEMS for malignant gastroduodenal obstruction leads to faster resumption of oral intake, decreased length of hospital stay, lower incidence of delayed gastric emptying, and similar complication rates when compared with gastroenterostomy.[28,29] In a multicenter, randomized trial comparing the two approaches, more rapid symptom improvement was noted in the stenting group, but longer-lasting results were achieved with gastrojejunostomy, with decreased need for reintervention.[30] In general, for patients with shorter life

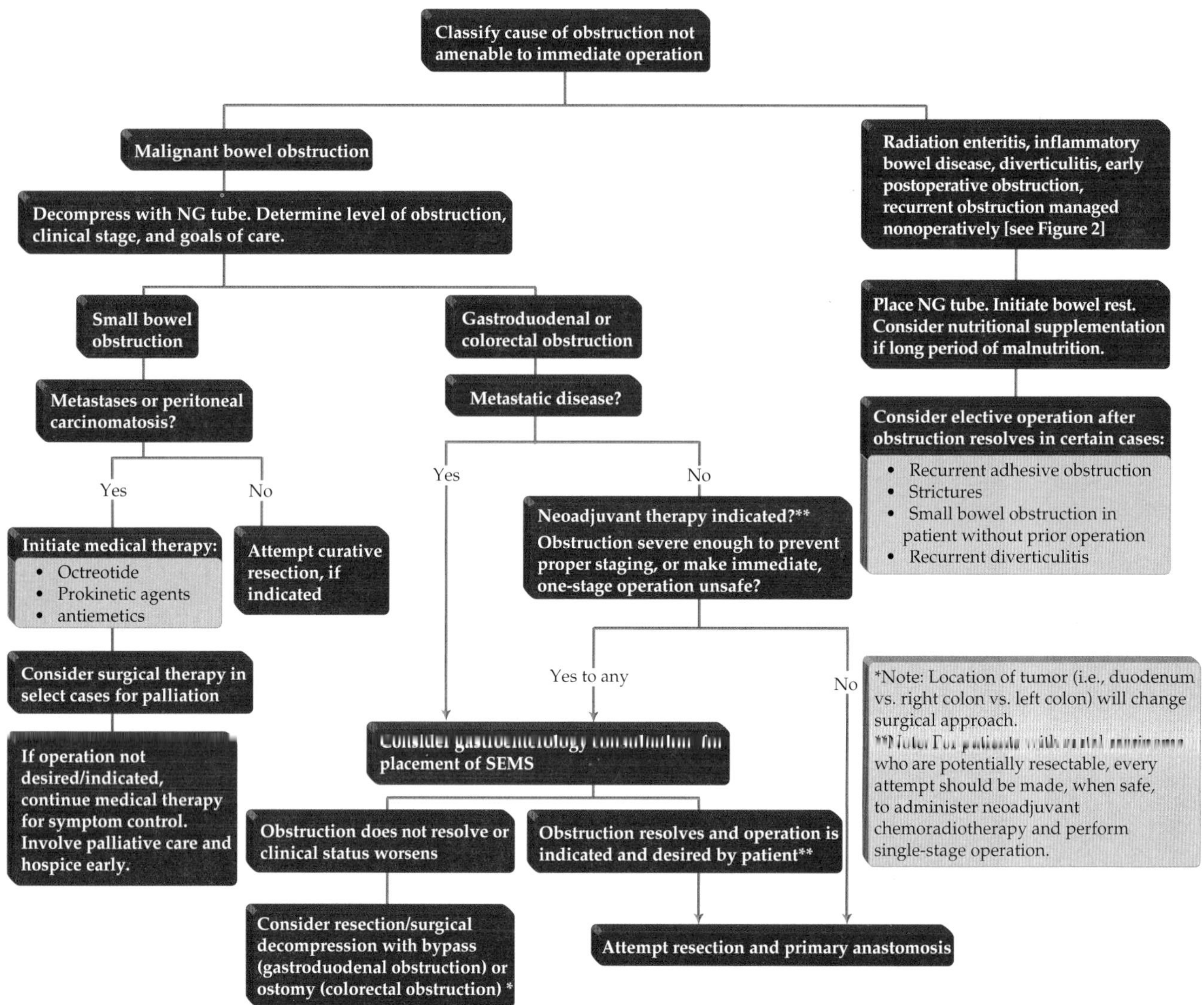

Figure 14 **An algorithm outlining an approach to the management of patients with obstructions not amenable to immediate operation. NG = nasogastric; SEMS = self-expanding metallic stent.**

expectancies (i.e., less than 2 months), SEMS is the preferred palliative therapy and is cost-effective.[29–32] Long-term gastric or enteric decompression may also be achieved with percutaneous endoscopic gastrostomy or jejunostomy.

In the case of malignant colorectal obstruction, a robust body of evidence is mounting for the safety, efficacy, and cost-effectiveness of SEMS as palliative therapy alone or as a bridge to surgery in the case of resectable disease.[26,27] For palliation, high technical and clinical success rates have been observed with prompt colonic decompression following stent placement in more than 90% of cases.[33–38] The most common observed complications were stent migration (5 to 22%), early or late perforation (4 to 8%), and reobstruction (7 to 30%).[27,33–36] Three randomized, controlled trials have compared palliative stenting versus palliative surgery revealing shorter time with resumption of oral intake and shorter hospital stay,[39,40] but unacceptably high perforation rates in the SEMS group caused an early closure of one study.[41] Systematic reviews have suggested that SEMS placement is safe and effective in achieving relief of obstruction, decreasing hospital stay, and improving quality of life with similar or fewer complications when compared with surgery.[33,37] SEMSs do appear to be more prone to reobstruction; however, placement of a second stent will relieve reobstruction in most cases.[35] Balloon dilation of malignant strictures prior to stenting has been associated with increased risk of perforation and should be avoided.[37]

Malignant colorectal obstruction often presents acutely with significant metabolic derangements secondary to dehydration. Bowel may be distended and friable, making operating conditions hazardous.[37,38,42] Most often these lesions are left-sided, and historical treatment has been a Hartmann procedure with creation of an end-colostomy. These emergency procedures are associated with high morbidity and mortality, and many of these colostomies will not be reversed.[38,42] Placement of a SEMS provides an opportunity for patient stabilization, completion of a proper staging workup, and the opportunity to pursue an elective resection and often primary anastomosis.[38,42,43] Placement of a SEMS followed by surgery leads to higher rates of primary anastomosis, lower rates of colostomy, shorter hospital stays, and possibly fewer complications.[33,37,38] Three randomized, controlled trials address the use of SEMSs as a bridge to surgery, with mixed results[42–44]; however, two of the three trials were plagued by lower than average technical and clinical success rates for SEMS deployment.[43,44] In a well-designed randomized, controlled trial, Cheung and colleagues found that SEMS placement followed by elective laparoscopic colonic resection resulted in significantly lower blood loss, pain scores, incidence of anastomotic leak, and wound infection than those treated with emergency open surgery.[42] Sixty-six percent of patients in the SEMS group underwent successful one-stage operation versus 38% with emergency surgery.[42] Another surgical approach is segmental colectomy and primary anastomosis with intraoperative colonic irrigation; however, a recent systematic review failed to find an advantage over manual colonic decompression.[45] Further study of endoscopic and surgical management of acute malignant colorectal obstruction is warranted as prospective, randomized, controlled trials have been conflicting.[26]

IMMEDIATE OPERATION

Traditional teaching has been that all patients with complete bowel obstruction, whether of the small or large intestine, should undergo immediate operation unless extraordinary circumstances (e.g., diffuse carcinomatosis, terminal illness, radiation enteritis, or sigmoid volvulus that responds to sigmoidoscopic decompression) are present. The fear is that if one attempts to manage complete intestinal obstruction nonoperatively, one risks delaying definitive treatment of patients with intestinal ischemia and subjecting them to significantly increased morbidity and mortality should perforation or severe infection develop.[5,46] However, in the absence of findings suggestive of ischemia or strangulation, high-grade to complete SBO will resolve without surgery in 37 to 46% of cases.[47,48] Rocha and colleagues reported that in a cohort of patients initially managed nonoperatively but progressing to surgery in an average time of 68 hours, there was no difference in mortality or requirement for bowel resection at the time of operation compared with the immediate surgery group.[47] Consensus guidelines now suggest that a trial of nonoperative management in patients with likely adhesive SBO is appropriate, with the knowledge that high-grade to complete obstruction carries a higher risk of failure of nonoperative management and a shorter time to recurrence [*see* No Operation, *below*].[49]

Immediate operation should be strongly considered when bowel obstruction is associated with peritonitis and/or collective clinical and radiographic signs of bowel ischemia. Immediate operation remains unequivocally indicated for patients with incarcerated, strangulated hernias, suspected or confirmed strangulation, sigmoid volvulus accompanied by systemic toxicity or peritoneal irritation, colonic volvulus proximal to the sigmoid colon, or sigmoid volvulus that cannot be reduced endoscopically. These conditions will not resolve without operation and are associated with increased morbidity, mortality, and cost if diagnosis and treatment are delayed. The only time one would not operate immediately on any patient with one of these diagnoses is when the patient requires cardiopulmonary stabilization or additional resuscitation or refuses operation. Whenever there is any doubt as to the presence of any of these conditions, additional diagnostic tests (e.g., IV contrast–enhanced CT scan) are indicated to confirm or exclude them.

Strangulation and Closed-Loop Obstruction

Morbidity and mortality from intestinal obstruction vary significantly and depend primarily on the presence of strangulation and subsequent infarction. Strangulation obstruction occurs in approximately 10% of all patients with small intestinal obstruction. It carries a mortality of 10 to 37%, whereas simple obstruction carries a mortality of less than 5%.[5,50] Early recognition and immediate operative treatment of strangulation obstruction are the only current means of decreasing this mortality. Strangulation obstruction occurs most frequently in patients with incarcerated hernias [*see Figure 12*], closed-loop obstruction [*see Figure 9*], or volvulus [*see Figure 13*]; hence, identification of any of these specific causes of obstruction is an important and clear indication for immediate operation.

Surgeons often base the decision of whether to operate on patients with bowel obstruction on the presence or absence of the so-called "classic signs" of strangulation obstruction—continuous abdominal pain, fever, tachycardia, peritoneal signs, and leukocytosis—and on their clinical experience. Unfortunately, these classic signs, even in conjunction with abdominal x-rays and clinical judgment, are incapable of reliably detecting closed-loop or gangrenous bowel obstruction.[5,46] In fact, one prospective clinical trial concluded that the five classic signs of strangulation obstruction and experienced clinical judgment were neither sensitive, specific, nor predictive of strangulation: in more than 50% of the patients who had intestinal strangulation, the condition was not recognized preoperatively.[5] Such findings suggest that early nonoperative recognition of intestinal strangulation is not feasible without advanced imaging (CT, ultrasonography, or fast MRI).

Many investigators have examined the role of CT alone [*see Table 5*] or in conjunction with clinical findings [*see Table 6*] for the diagnosis of ischemia and strangulation.[51–56] A systematic review of 11 studies (seven prospective trials and four retrospective studies) demonstrated a positive predictive value of 79% and a negative predictive value of 93% of CT to detect ischemia, suggesting that CT scanning can reliably diagnose ischemic bowel.[57] However, there were no standard criteria among the studies included for the diagnosis of strangulation. Reduced bowel wall enhancement on IV contrast–enhanced CT has been identified by multiple reports as an independent predictor of ischemia (odds ratio 4.87 to 143) [*see Figure 10*].[53–56,58] Using maximal attenuation of a region of interest can detect subtle differences in enhancement and improve the diagnostic accuracy

Table 5 Independent Predictors of Ischemia on Computed Tomographic Scan

Free fluid volume > 500 cc on computed tomographic scan
Mesenteric edema
Lack of a "small bowel feces sign"
Abnormal swirling course of mesenteric vessels (also known as "whirl sign")
Reduced bowel wall enhancement

Table 6 Clinicoradiologic Scoring Systems Using Computed Tomographic Scan

Reference	*Study Type*	*Criteria*	*Results*
Jones et al[51]	Retrospective chart review	Free air = 5 points Transition point = 3 points Complete obstruction = 3 points Closed-loop = 3 points Free fluid = 3 points Partial obstruction = 2 points Signs of worsening vs. resolution on repeat CT imaging = 3–5 points	Score of 8 or higher is 75% accurate in predicting the need for operative exploration
Schwenter et al[55]	Prospective trial	One point each for: History of pain lasting ≥ 4 days Guarding on exam C-reactive protein ≥ 75 mg/L Leukocyte count ≥ 10 x 10^9/L Free abdominal fluid identified on CT with volume ≥ 500 mL Decreased bowel wall enhancement	Score 3 = 67% sensitive, 90.8% specific to predict ischemic bowel Score ≥ 4 = 100% specific, 38.7% sensitive to predict ischemic bowel
Zielinski et al[52]	Prospective trial	One point each for: Mesenteric edema Lack of a "small bowel feces sign" Clinical finding of obstipation	Score 3 = 46% sensitive and 82% specific to predict the presence of strangulation obstruction Negative predictive value of 91% when all three criteria absent

CT = computed tomography

of this sign; however, this novel technique is currently not widely used in clinical practice.[54] Using multivariate logistic regression models, free fluid volume greater than 500 cc on a CT scan [*see Figure 9*], mesenteric edema [*see Figure 9 and Figure 13*], lack of a "small bowel feces sign" [*see Figure 12*], and an abnormal vascular course of mesenteric vessels (also known as the "whirl sign") [*see Figure 9 and Figure 13*] have all been identified as independent predictors of bowel ischemia.[52,55,56,58–60]

CT-based scoring systems To assist in operative decision making, a great deal of effort has gone into the development of scoring systems that combine various historical, examination, laboratory, and radiologic findings to diagnose ischemia and/or predict the need for operative exploration [*see Table 6*]. Although sensitivity in predicting the need for operation and the presence of strangulation with these models is low, such approaches may provide a means for objective early diagnosis of patients with ischemia and reduce delays in operation for at-risk patients. Taken together, there is a growing body of evidence that CT scan with IV contrast, when appropriately combined with clinical features, can reliably assist in identifying patients with ischemia who will benefit from early laparotomy.

Incarcerated or Strangulated Hernias

A hernia that is incarcerated, tender, erythematous, warm, or edematous is an indication for immediate operation. Primary or incisional hernias may not be palpable in obese patients, in which case, advanced imaging should be performed [*see Figure 12*].

Nonsigmoid Volvulus and Sigmoid Volvulus with Systemic Toxicity or Peritoneal Signs

All intestinal volvuli are closed-loop obstructions and thus carry a high risk of intestinal strangulation, infarction, and perforation. Patients typically present with acute, colicky abdominal pain, massive distention, nausea, and vomiting. Sigmoid volvulus is the most common form of colonic volvulus, followed by cecal volvulus. Abdominal radiographs are fairly diagnostic for colonic volvulus [*see Figure 6, Figure 7, and Figure 13*]. In contrast, small bowel volvulus may not be visualized on plain radiographs, because the closed loop fills completely with fluid and no air-fluid level can be seen. Small bowel volvulus is readily detected by ultrasonography or CT; one or both of these procedures should be performed in patients presenting with signs and symptoms of bowel obstruction and normal abdominal radiographs [*see Figure 9*]. Small bowel or cecal volvulus is an indication for immediate operation.

If one observes signs of systemic toxicity, a bloody rectal discharge, fever, leukocytosis, or peritoneal irritation in a patient with sigmoid volvulus, the patient should undergo immediate operation; if all of these signs are absent, the patient should undergo sigmoidoscopy. When there are no signs of peritonitis or generalized toxicity, sigmoidoscopic decompression is safe and effective in more than 95% of patients with sigmoid volvulus.[61] If mucosal gangrene or a bloody effluent is noted at the time of sigmoidoscopy, immediate operative intervention is necessary even in the absence of any clinical signs or symptoms of strangulation. After sigmoidoscopy, the patient can undergo elective bowel preparation and a single-stage sigmoid resection before being discharged from the hospital. If, however, clinical toxicity, a bloody rectal discharge, fever, or peritoneal irritation arises at any time after sigmoidoscopic decompression while the patient is being prepared for an elective procedure, immediate operation is indicated.

Patients with volvulus proximal to the sigmoid colon should undergo immediate operation regardless of whether peritoneal irritation is present. The incidence of strangulation infarction is high in such patients, and nonoperative therapy often fails. If the diagnosis of nonsigmoid colonic volvulus is in doubt, a barium enema is indicated to exclude colonic pseudo-obstruction.

Fecal Impaction

Complete colonic obstruction secondary to fecal impaction in the rectum can sometimes be successfully relieved through disimpaction at the bedside; however, this can be difficult and extremely uncomfortable for the patient. The most expeditious and successful method of relieving the obstruction is to disimpact the patient while he or she is under general or spinal anesthesia. In one study, the pulsed-irrigated enhanced-evacuation procedure, which can be performed at the bedside, successfully resolved fecal impaction in approximately 75% of geriatric patients.[62] In another study, administration of a polyethylene glycol 3350 solution over 3 days successfully resolved intestinal obstruction from fecal impaction in 75% of pediatric patients.[63]

URGENT OPERATION

Failure of Water-Soluble Contrast Medium Challenge at 24 Hours

It is usually safe to manage partial bowel obstruction initially by nonoperative means: a nihil per os (NPO) regimen, NG tube decompression, and analgesics. Such therapy is successful in most cases, especially if the cause of obstruction is postoperative adhesions, but there is always the risk that strangulation obstruction already exists but is undetected. Routine CT with IV contrast in all patients undergoing nonoperative management is indicated to decrease this possibility. Furthermore, there is the risk that while the patient is being observed, partial obstruction will progress to complete, unresolving obstruction, or strangulation and perforation will develop. Repeated examination of the abdomen by the same clinician is the most sensitive way of detecting progressive obstruction and clinical deterioration. Examinations should be performed no less frequently than every 3 hours. If abdominal pain, tenderness, or distention increases or the gastric aspirate changes from nonfeculent to feculent, abdominal exploration is usually indicated. It is therefore crucial to be alert to such changes in the patient's condition.

Water-soluble contrast medium challenge Level 1a evidence now exists supporting the use of WSCM (also known as Gastrografin or ditrizoate meglumine) as a diagnostic and therapeutic tool in the management of patients with adhesive SBO. WSCM administered orally or via a NG tube that arrives in the colon within 4 to 24 hours of administration can predict the resolution of SBO with 96% sensitivity and 98% specificity and should be used routinely to aid in determining which patients are unlikely to resolve with nonoperative management [*see Figure 15*].[64] There are no reported complications related directly to the administration of WSCM and no difference in overall complication rates. Importantly, these studies excluded all patients with clinical signs of ischemia or strangulation (peritonitis, fever, tachycardia, and leukocytosis), patients who had surgery within 4 to 6 weeks of the obstructive episode, those with nonreducible hernia, and patients with abdominal or pelvic malignancy. A rational approach to a patient presenting with likely adhesive SBO would begin with the history, physical examination, NG tube placement and decompression, and appropriate laboratory and radiologic examinations, including IV contrast–enhanced CT, to exclude patients with likely

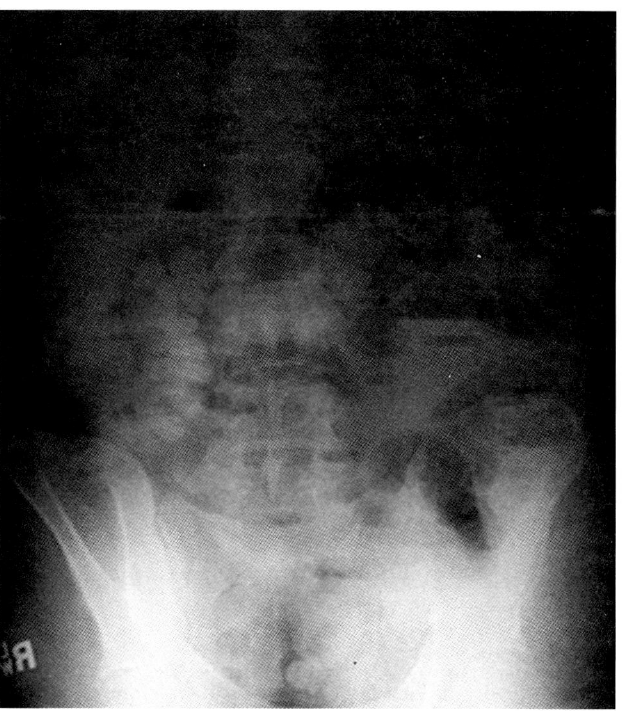

Figure 15 **The presence of contrast in the colon within 4 to 24 hours of administration is highly sensitive and specific for predicting resolution with nonoperative management.**

ischemia or strangulation [*see* Immediate Operation, Strangulation and Closed-Loop Obstruction, CT-based scoring systems, *above*]. At the time of initial CT, or after a short waiting period (i.e., 1 to 2 hours) to allow for adequate decompression, a WSCM meal of 50 to 150 mL should be administered via a NG tube, which is clamped for 4 hours. If there is no sign of strangulation by either clinical or CT findings, a waiting period of 24 hours with close clinical follow-up should begin. If at 24 hours no contrast is visible within the colon on an upright abdominal plain film, the patient should progress to operative intervention as the obstruction is unlikely to resolve. Level 1a evidence also indicates that WSCM may accelerate resolution of partial SBO[64] [*see* No Operation, Adhesive Partial Small Bowel Obstruction, *below*].

Early Postoperative Technical Complications

When normal bowel function initially returns after an abdominal operation but then is replaced by a clinical picture suggestive of early postoperative mechanical obstruction, the explanation may be a technical complication of the operation (e.g., phlegmon, abscess, intussusception, a narrow anastomosis, an internal hernia, or obstruction at the level of a stoma). An early, aggressive diagnostic workup should be performed to identify or exclude these problems because they are unlikely to respond to NG decompression or other forms of conservative management. It is critical to know exactly what was done within the abdomen in the course of the operation. To this end, one should try to speak directly with the operating surgeon rather than attempt to deduce the needed information from the operative report.

If the patient had peritonitis or a colonic anastomosis at the initial operation, one should order a CT scan to look for an intra-abdominal abscess. An abscess or a phlegmon at the site of an anastomosis is usually secondary to anastomotic leakage and is an indication for reoperation or endoscopic stenting in some cases. CT can also identify intra-abdominal hematomas, which should be evacuated through early reoperation. In patients recovering from a proctectomy, herniation of the small bowel through a defect in the pelvic floor is a common cause of intestinal obstruction. Oral contrast studies can help identify patients with an internal hernia, intussusception, or anastomotic obstruction and should be performed after the CT scan. A retrograde barium examination by gravity drainage should be performed in patients thought to have a problem related to a stoma or an intestinal anastomosis. High-pressure contrast examination should be avoided to reduce trauma to the anastomosis. When none of the above factors appear to be the cause of the postoperative obstruction, it is reasonable for the surgeon to assume that the obstruction is secondary to postoperative adhesions, which are best treated conservatively (see below).

NO OPERATION

In selected patients, nonoperative management of partial bowel obstruction is highly successful and carries an acceptably low morbidity and mortality. Nonoperative management is most often successful in patients with obstruction secondary to intra-abdominal adhesions, occurring in the immediate postoperative period, or deriving from an inflammatory condition (e.g., inflammatory bowel disease, radiation enteritis, or diverticulitis).

Adhesive Partial Small Bowel Obstruction

Adhesions are the major cause of bowel obstruction. Obstruction resulting from adhesions can occur as early as 1 month or as late as 20 years after operation.[65] Adhesive partial SBO is treated initially with NG tube decompression, IV rehydration, and analgesia.

Some studies suggest that the nature of the previous abdominal operation or the type of adhesions present may influence the probability that the obstruction will respond to medical therapy.[66,67] Operations associated with a lower likelihood of response to medical therapy include those performed through a midline incision; those involving the aorta, colon, rectum, appendix, or pelvic adnexa; and those done to relieve previous carcinomatous obstruction. Matted adhesions, which are more common in patients who have undergone midline incisions or colorectal procedures, are less amenable to conservative management than a simple adhesive band.[66] In the context of this kind of operative history, strong consideration should be given to surgical intervention if the obstruction does not resolve within 24 hours—unless comorbid medical conditions tip the risk-benefit balance in the direction of nonoperative therapy.

When operative adhesiolysis is performed, the mortality is 5% for all comers[68]; however, it may be as high as 30% for patients with strangulation or necrotic bowel necessitating intestinal resection.[65] In view of this substantial difference in mortality, it is extremely important to determine which patients have ischemic bowel at presentation. Given the high reliability of IV contrast–enhanced CT for the detection of ischemia [*see* Immediate Operation, Strangulation and Closed-Loop Obstruction, CT-based scoring systems, *above*], it should be performed routinely in all patients to be given a trial of nonoperative management.[57,58]

After exclusion of patients with contraindications to nonoperative management on clinical or radiologic grounds, the key factor in determining whether to continue with nonoperative management is WSCM challenge followed by a period of close observation [*see* Urgent Operation, Failure of Water-Soluble Contrast Medium Challenge at 24 Hours, Water-soluble contrast medium challenge, *above*]. During this observation period, the overall clinical picture (vital signs, laboratory values, abdominal examination findings, nature of NG aspirate) should be continuously evaluated, ideally by the same examiner. Analgesics can be safely administered, and repeat abdominal examinations should be performed at 3-hour intervals when the influence of narcotics has waned. Repeat abdominal x-rays should be obtained no later than 24 hours after WSCM administration. If contrast is visible in the colon within 24 hours on an upright abdominal radiograph, then nonoperative management is likely to succeed and should be continued [*see Figure 15*].[64] There is heterogeneity among published reports regarding the time interval prior to follow-up abdominal radiograph, and shorter intervals than 24 hours may be appropriate.[64] If abdominal pain and/or distention are increasing, or the gastric aspirate changes from bilious to feculent, strong consideration should be given to operation. Importantly, WSCM administration has been shown to decrease the time to resolution of SBO by almost 20 hours and to reduce hospital length of stay by nearly 2 days when compared with standard therapy.[64]

By quickly identifying patients who are unlikely to resolve nonoperatively and accelerating the resolution of partial SBO, administration of WSCM can shorten the expected hospital stay and thereby reduce the cost of care. Thus, intragastric administration of WSCM is the logical first step in managing suspected partial SBO from adhesions or postoperative ileus. Even if bowel function does not return within 24 hours but a partial obstruction is demonstrated, continued observation is safe, and resolution without operation is still highly probable.[49,64] Eventually, there will be a point beyond which continued observation is no longer cost-effective in comparison with operative adhesiolysis (especially laparoscopic adhesiolysis). In the first prospectively validated model for managing bowel obstruction, drainage of more than 500 mL from the NG tube at day 3, when combined with an age over 65 and the presence of ascites on CT, demonstrated a positive predictive value of 72% for requiring operation. Drainage volume of gastric aspirate, particularly on hospital day 3, appears to be another important factor to consider when deciding if a patient should progress to operative therapy.[69] Additional prospective trials are necessary to determine the appropriate time interval before operative treatment is pursued.

Experimental studies in animals suggest that there may be some benefit from administration of somatostatin analogues in patients undergoing nonoperative treatment of bowel obstruction as a result of the potent effects these substances exert on intestinal sodium, chloride, and water absorption.[70] In one study, animals with either complete or closed-loop partial SBO were given either long-acting somatostatin or saline; the treatment group had significantly less intestinal distention, less infarction, and longer survival than the control group.[70,71] In a prospective, randomized clinical trial evaluating the use of somatostatin in patients who had complete SBO without clinical or radiologic evidence of strangulation, the treatment group was less likely to need operation, had less proximal intestinal distention, and exhibited decreased mucosal necrosis proximal to the point of obstruction.[72] These results have not been replicated in further studies.

Laparoscopic adhesiolysis A recent systematic review of over 2,000 cases has confirmed that laparoscopic adhesiolysis for acute SBO is both feasible and safe.[73] Laparoscopic or laparoscopy-assisted lysis of adhesions relieves bowel obstruction in more than 70% of patients and is associated with lower morbidity, earlier return of bowel function, and a shorter hospital stay than open operative lysis. An average conversion rate of 29% was observed; the majority of conversions were related to dense adhesions, bowel ischemia requiring resection, or iatrogenic bowel injury. The overall enterostomy rate was 6.6%, with the majority recognized at the time of operation.[73] To minimize the risk of bowel injury at the beginning of the operation, the first trocar is inserted under direct vision and the incision is placed well away from any previous scars.[74] Meticulous, atraumatic handling of edematous bowel, avoidance of electrocautery, and a low threshold for early conversion are critical to minimize the risk of perforation.[75,76] In spite of its demonstrated safety and efficacy, current opinion still demonstrates a reluctance to embrace laparoscopic lysis of adhesions.[77] In 2002, a study examining the Nationwide Inpatient Sample revealed that only 11.4% of over 6,000 randomly selected operations for SBO were attempted laparoscopically[78] [*see Video 1, online version only*].

There are no prospective, randomized, controlled clinical trials comparing laparoscopic adhesiolysis with open adhesiolysis.[79] Two retrospective, matched-pair, intention-to-treat analyses have demonstrated lower morbidity (16 to 19% versus 40 to 45%) and reduced hospital stay (7 to 11 days versus 13 to 18 days, in respective studies).[76,80] A 45 to 52% rate of conversion either for completion of adhesiolysis, resection of necrotic bowel, or management of complications was observed. Large, retrospective series suggest that conversion rates may be much lower (15 to 30%) with conservative patient selection.[73,78] It is important to note that laparoscopic operations converted to open operations have essentially the same morbidity, cost, and length of stay as primary open operations; however, early conversions in response to dense adhesions or poor visibility carry significantly less morbidity than reactive conversions in response to an iatrogenic injury.[73] In the report by Wullstein and Gross, intraoperative perforations were more common overall in the laparoscopic group than in the open group, but this difference was largely eliminated when patients from the laparoscopic group who underwent conversion to open lysis were not considered.[80] In the other retrospective controlled trial, Khaikin and colleages reported no intraoperative perforations in the laparoscopic group, which they attributed to meticulous operative technique and a low threshold for conversion.[76]

There is conflicting evidence regarding indications for attempted laparoscopic adhesiolysis. Patients with two or more previous laparotomies had a higher incidence of intraoperative complications and an increased rate of conversion than those with fewer laparotomies in one study[80]; on the other hand, a systematic review found that the number of previous laparotomies was not associated with unsuccessful laparoscopic adhesiolysis in multiple studies.[73] Appendectomy was the only previous operation predictive of laparoscopic success. Bowel dilatation greater than 4 cm on preoperative imaging may be associated with conversion, but reports are conflicting. Consistently, a documented history of dense adhesions has been associated with a higher rate of conversion. Primary laparotomy may still be an appropriate choice for such patients as well as those with complex pathology, for example, a history of malignancy or inflammatory bowel disease. When laparoscopic adhesiolysis fails to identify and relieve an obvious point of obstruction or when adhesiolysis is inadequate or unsafe, conversion to an open approach is indicated. Conversion should not be viewed as failure but rather as sound surgical judgment. At present, the laparoscopic approach appears best suited to those patients who have undergone fewer previous operations, especially if they have undergone appendectomy only, as well as those in whom the probable cause of obstruction is from one to several adhesive bands.[73] One must be vigilant in monitoring for signs or symptoms of a missed enterotomy in patients treated laparoscopically as these injuries may present in a delayed fashion and prompt recognition is key to reducing the morbidity associated with this complication.

By reducing the number of days spent in the hospital when compared with open surgery, laparoscopic lysis of adhesions stands to significantly decrease the cost associated with adhesive SBO. Few studies have examined cost directly, but Khaikin and colleagues demonstrated a reduction in total hospital charges of over $30,000 with a totally laparoscopic approach compared with an open approach.[76] Importantly, these cost benefits disappeared when patients who underwent conversion to open lysis of adhesions were considered with the laparoscopic group. Another important potential cost benefit of laparoscopic adhesiolysis is that it results in fewer intra-abdominal adhesions than open laparotomy[81,82] and thus may reduce the risk of recurrent bowel obstruction. No studies comparing recurrence rates after laparoscopic versus open adhesiolysis have yet been performed.

Early Postoperative Obstruction

Early postoperative mechanical SBO is not uncommon: it occurs in approximately 10% of patients undergoing abdominal procedures.[83] Postoperative bowel obstruction is often difficult to diagnose because it gives rise to many of the same signs and symptoms as postoperative ileus: obstipation, distention, nausea, vomiting, abdominal pain, and altered bowel sounds. In most cases, there are radiographic signs indicative of small bowel obstruction rather than ileus; however, in some cases, abdominal x-rays fail to diagnose the obstruction.[84] Traditionally, when plain radiographs are equivocal, an upper GI barium study with follow-through views is the next test performed to distinguish ileus from partial or complete SBO[85]; however, such studies may yield the wrong diagnosis in as many as 30% of cases.[84] A water-soluble contrast study may prove useful in this scenario, although its previously described accuracy in determining which cases of SBO will require operation was not tested in the setting of recent operation. WSCM may also have therapeutic benefits in the treatment of ileus [*see* Nonmechanical Obstruction, Ileus, *below*].

Early postoperative obstruction is caused by adhesions in about 90% of patients.[84,86] When there are no signs of toxicity and no acute abdominal signs, such obstruction can usually be managed safely with NG decompression.[84,86] As many as 87% of patients respond to NG suction within 2 weeks. About 70% of the patients who respond to nonoperative treatment do so within 1 week, and an additional 25% respond during the following 7 days. If postoperative obstruction does not resolve in the first 2 weeks, it is unlikely to do so with continued nonoperative therapy, and reoperation is probably indicated[84,86]; about 25% of patients whose postoperative obstruction was initially treated nonoperatively eventually require reoperation. An exception to this guideline arises in patients known to have severe dense adhesions (sometimes referred to as obliterative peritonitis) in response to multiple sequential laparotomies. These patients may have a combination of mechanical obstruction and diffuse small bowel and colonic ileus. The risk of closed-loop obstruction, volvulus, or strangulation in this group of patients is low. Repeat laparotomies and attempts to lyse adhesions may lead to complications, the development of enterocutaneous fistulas, or exacerbation of the adhesions. Often the best approach to managing these patients is observation for prolonged periods (i.e., months). Total parenteral nutrition (TPN) is indicated.

Because the risk of intestinal strangulation in patients with postoperative adhesive obstruction is extremely low (< 1%),[84] one can generally treat these patients nonoperatively for longer periods. In fact, the conservative approach is often the wise one: reoperation may do more harm than good (e.g., by causing enterotomies and inducing denser adhesions). The traditional indications for operation in patients with early postoperative obstruction include (1) deteriorating clinical status, (2) worsening obstructive symptoms, and (3) failure to respond to nonoperative management within 2 weeks. With the rising cost of hospitalization, it might, in fact, be more cost-effective to reoperate on patients who have persistent obstruction after 7 days. This speculation would have to be tested by a well-organized cost-benefit study conducted in a prospective fashion.

Some physicians have maintained that long intestinal tubes are beneficial in the management of postoperative bowel obstruction.[87] However, there is no convincing evidence that long intestinal tubes are any better for resolving bowel obstruction than conventional NG tubes. In fact, some authorities have reported that the use of such tubes increases morbidity.[50] One prospective, randomized clinical trial that addressed this issue found no differences between the two types of tube with respect to the percentage of patients who were able to avoid operation, the incidence of complications, the time between admission and operation, or the duration of postoperative ileus.[88]

Inflammatory Conditions

Partial bowel obstruction secondary to inflammatory bowel disease, radiation enteritis, or diverticulitis usually resolves with nonoperative therapy. Bowel obstruction accompanying an acute exacerbation of Crohn disease usually resolves with NG suction, IV antibiotics, and antiinflammatory agents. If, however, CT detects an intra-abdominal abscess, there is evidence of a chronic stricture, or the patient exhibits persistent obstructive symptoms, an operation may be necessary. Similarly, bowel obstruction arising from acute enteritis caused by radiation exposure or chemotherapy usually resolves with supportive care. Chronic radiation-induced strictures are problematic; astute clinical judgment must be exercised to determine when operative treatment is the best option.

Patients with acute diverticulitis typically present with a history of altered bowel movements, fever, leukocytosis, localized pain, tenderness, and guarding in the left lower quadrant of the abdomen. Approximately 20% of patients with colonic diverticulitis also present with signs and symptoms of partial colonic obstruction. A CT scan should be obtained early in all patients with diverticulitis to ascertain whether there is a pericolic abscess that could be drained percutaneously.[89] Partial colonic obstruction in these patients usually resolves with antibiotic therapy, an NPO regimen, and NG decompression. If obstructive symptoms persist for more than 7 days or if obstructive symptoms from a documented stricture recur, operation is indicated.

ELECTIVE OPERATION

Nontoxic, Nontender Sigmoid Volvulus

Patients with nontoxic, nontender sigmoid volvulus whose bowel obstruction is initially treated successfully with sigmoidoscopic decompression are at risk for recurrent colonic obstruction. Accordingly, these patients should undergo elective sigmoid resection after complete bowel preparation during their index admission [*see Figure 14*].

Recurrent Adhesive or Stricture-Related Partial Small Bowel Obstruction

Many patients whose adhesive bowel obstruction resolves experience no further obstructive episodes. If a patient does present with recurrent obstruction from presumed adhesions, either a contrast examination of the bowel or CT is indicated to determine whether there is a surgically correctable point of stenosis. A strong argument can be made that non–high-risk patients should undergo elective operation after presenting with their second episode of mechanical obstruction. Similarly, patients with recurrent obstruction from strictures of any sort should undergo elective operation given that these lesions are unlikely to resolve [*see Figure 14*].

Partial Colonic Obstruction

The most common causes of partial colonic obstruction are colon cancer, strictures, and diverticulitis. Cancer and strictures usually must be managed surgically because they generally go on to cause obstruction later. Strictures from ischemia or endometriosis usually call for elective colonic resection. Inflammatory strictures from diverticulitis may resolve; however, if obstructive symptoms persist or if barium enema examination continues to yield evidence of colonic narrowing, elective resection is warranted.

When abdominal x-rays suggest distal colonic obstruction, digital examination and rigid sigmoidoscopy are performed to exclude fecal impaction, tumors, strictures, and sigmoid volvulus. If obstruction is proximal to the sigmoidoscope, barium contrast examination is indicated. If barium examination does not demonstrate mechanical obstruction, a presumptive diagnosis of colonic pseudo-obstruction is made.

The morbidity and mortality associated with elective colorectal procedures are significantly lower than those associated with emergency colonic surgery. Furthermore, immediate operation for left-sided colonic obstruction almost always necessitates the creation of a diverting colostomy. If a colostomy takedown subsequently proves necessary, the overall cost of caring for the patient will be significantly higher than it would have been had a single-stage procedure been performed. For these reasons, one should initially treat partial colonic obstruction with NG suction, enemas, and IV rehydration in the hope that the obstruction will resolve and that the patient thus can undergo mechanical and antibiotic bowel preparation and a single-stage procedure comprising resection and primary anastomosis. Placement of SEMSs has a growing role as both a bridge to a single-stage resection and a primary palliative intervention [*see Figure 14 and* Mechanical Obstruction, Malignant Bowel Obstruction, Self-expanding metallic stents, *above*].

Bowel Obstruction without Previous Abdominal Operation

When partial SBO develops and resolves in a patient who has not previously undergone an abdominal operation, a diagnostic workup should be performed to identify the cause of the obstruction. Incarcerated inguinal, femoral, and umbilical hernias should be ruled out. There may be an underlying condition that is likely to cause recurrent obstruction (e.g., an internal hernia, malrotation, or malignancy). The first diagnostic test to be ordered should be a CT scan, followed by an upper GI barium study with follow-through views and a barium enema.[90] If a pathologic lesion is identified, elective operation is indicated [*see Figure 14*]. An argument can be made that no additional diagnostic tests should be performed in these patients and that diagnostic laparoscopy should be performed instead to enable laparoscopic surgery in case a cause of obstruction is identified that can be treated with a minimally invasive procedure. If no cause of obstruction is found at laparoscopy, open laparotomy is performed.

Paraduodenal hernia, a congenital defect resulting from intestinal malrotation, is probably more common than was once thought. It accounts for approximately 50% of internal hernias. Patients with paraduodenal hernia may present with a catastrophic closed-loop obstruction; more often, however, they exhibit mild, nonspecific GI symptoms such as nausea, vomiting, esophageal reflux, and abdominal pain. Duodenogastric reflux and prominent bile gastritis in the absence of a previous operation or diabetic gastroparesis are indirect signs of a paraduodenal hernia. The diagnosis is established by means of either an upper GI contrast study with small bowel follow-through or CT scanning. When a paraduodenal hernia is identified, operative treatment is indicated. Such treatment is usually successful in alleviating symptoms and preventing strangulation obstruction.

Nonmechanical Obstruction

ILEUS

Ileus, or intestinal paralysis, is most common after abdominal operations but can also occur in response to any acute medical condition or metabolic derangement [*see Table 1*]. The pathophysiologic mechanisms that cause ileus are incompletely understood but appear to involve disruption of normal neurohumoral responses that result in elevated sympathetic nerve activity. Moreover, immunohistochemistry in rats has shown an increase in inflammatory mediators such as macrophages, mast cells, dendritic cells, and T cells as a result of surgical manipulation of the bowel, which, in addition to the sympathetic nervous system stimulation, leads to decreased circular muscle contractile activity. The intensity of the paralysis is directly proportional to the degree of trauma (e.g., physical manipulation, incision).[91]

Ileus may be classified into two broad categories: postoperative ileus and ileus without antecedent abdominal operation [*see Figure 16*]. Postoperative ileus is manifested by atony of the stomach, small intestine, and colon and usually resolves spontaneously within a few days as normal bowel motility returns. Typically, the small bowel regains its motility within 24 hours of operation, followed 3 to 4 days later by the stomach and colon. Initial therapy of ileus is directed at identifying and correcting the presumed cause. If the patient experiences abdominal distention, abdominal pain, nausea, or vomiting, then NG decompression, placement of a Foley catheter, and IV rehydration are indicated. When ileus develops in patients who have not recently undergone an operation, a thorough history, a careful physical examination, and well-chosen laboratory tests are necessary to identify the possible causes. Serum electrolytes, including calcium and magnesium, should be routinely measured.

Perioperative measures to reduce postoperative ileus include early postoperative mobilization, avoidance of NG tube insertion when appropriate, prokinetic administration, early enteral feeding, judicious use of IV fluids, and minimization of narcotics (often with the assistance of thoracic epidural analgesia).[92] Institution of these measures can be aided with the use of enhanced recovery protocols. Additionally, gum chewing has emerged as an effective perioperative intervention to alleviate ileus. A form of "sham feeding," gum chewing improves intestinal motility through cephalic-vagal stimulation. A systematic review and meta-analysis demonstrated that gum chewing reduced length of stay by 1.1 days and shortened the time to first flatus by 14 hours when compared with control.[93] As well, the adoption of gum chewing for patients with postoperative paralytic ileus, as an alternative to early feeding, eliminates the common complications associated with enteric feeding of recovering bowel, such as nausea and vomiting. Additionally, gum chewing can be tolerated sooner than even small amounts of food. Gum chewing appears to be a useful adjunct for reducing the duration of postoperative ileus to reduce cost and improve outcomes.[93]

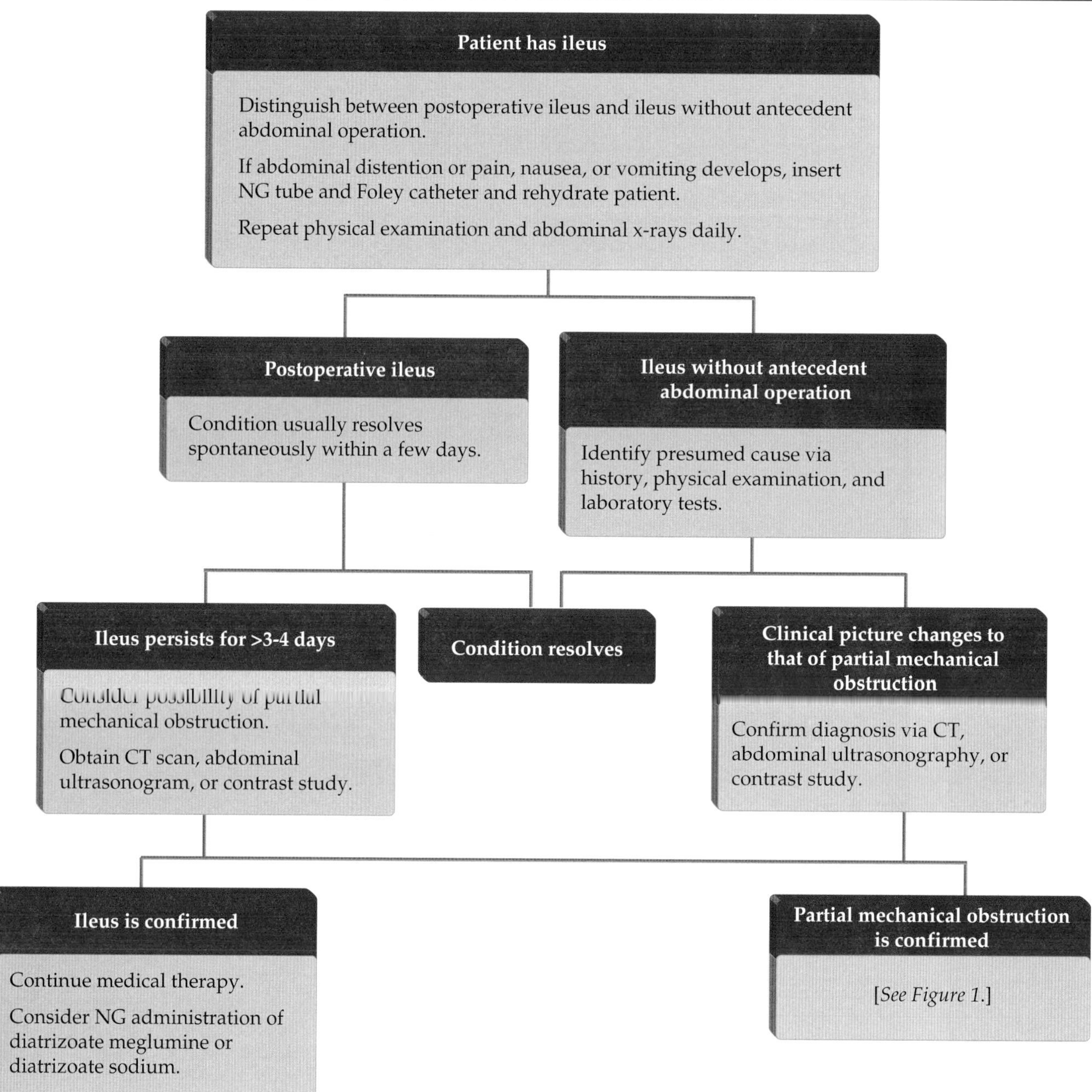

Figure 16 **An algorithm outlining an approach to the management of ileus. CT = computed tomography; IV = intravenous; NG = nasogastric; PO = by mouth; WSCM = water-soluble contrast medium.**

When ileus persists for what is, in one's best clinical judgment, an inordinate length of time for the operation performed (typically, longer than 3 to 4 days), the possibility of partial mechanical obstruction or other surgical complication must be considered. Prolonged operative ileus (defined as no flatus for > 6 days) was independently associated with male gender, chronic obstructive pulmonary disease, and placement of an ileostomy in a study of colorectal surgery patients.[94] If an abscess is suspected, an abdominal CT scan should be obtained. Abdominal ultrasonography has been reported to distinguish postoperative ileus from mechanical obstruction reliably.[16] A small bowel contrast examination with barium identifies partial mechanical SBO in about 75% of patients.[95] CT distinguishes ileus from obstruction in about 80% of patients.

Intragastric administration of a water-soluble contrast agent has shown great potential in the treatment of ileus. In one study, administration of 120 mL of WSCM via an NG tube to 40 adults with postoperative ileus led to restored intestinal motility within 6 hours in all 40, allowing them to resume oral alimentation within 24 hours.[96] A phase IV prospective, randomized clinical trial is currently under way to study the efficacy of WSCM on postsurgical ileus.[97] Also in the expanding repertoire of pharmacologic modalities is a prokinetic ghrelin agonist, TZP-101 (ulimorelin). This agent, when administered beginning 1 hour after operation and continued daily until the first bowel movement, was independently, prospectively associated with accelerated return of GI function and an increased proportion of patients recovering bowel function within 72 hours.[98] Alvimopan, a selective mu-opioid receptor antagonist, is well tolerated and has been shown to accelerate GI recovery and the time to writing of the discharge order (by 16 hours over placebo).[99] Further investigation into pharmacologic treatment and prevention is likely to yield synergistic, cost-saving strategies to prevent and reduce the severity and duration of postoperative ileus.

PSEUDO-OBSTRUCTION

Pseudo-obstruction [*see Figure 17*] can exist in the small bowel or colon and can be either acute or chronic. Acute colonic pseudo-obstruction, also known as Ogilvie syndrome, is the most common form. Colonic pseudo-obstruction occurs most commonly in hospitalized patients in the postoperative period or in response to a nonsurgical acute illness (e.g., pneumonia, myocardial infarction, hypoxia, shock, intestinal ischemia, or electrolyte imbalance). The pathophysiologic mechanisms underlying idiopathic pseudo-obstruction appear to be related to an imbalance in the parasympathetic and sympathetic influences on colonic motility.

The presenting symptoms of acute colonic pseudo-obstruction are massive dilatation of the colon seen on a plain abdominal radiograph (with the cecum more dilated than the distal colon), crampy pain, nausea, and vomiting.[100] If peritoneal irritation or systemic toxicity is present, immediate laparotomy is indicated; if not, treatment begins with conservative methods and proceeds in a stepwise fashion.

Conservative modalities include NG decompression, placement of a rectal tube, tap-water enemas, correction of any underlying metabolic disturbances, and avoidance of narcotic and anticholinergic medications. With conservative management, acute colonic pseudo-obstruction resolves within 4 days in more than 80% of cases.[101] In unalleviated cases, colonoscopy was previously the method of choice for decompression.[102] However, it is now recommended that acute colonic pseudo-obstruction that does not resolve within 24 to 48 hours be treated pharmacologically.[103] IV administration of 2.5 mg neostigmine, an acetylcholinesterase inhibitor, over 2 to 3 minutes, leads to prompt resolution of acute colonic pseudo-obstruction within minutes in nearly all cases.[104,105] Although other prokinetic agents (IV erythromycin, cisapride, metoclopramide) are reportedly effective, neostigmine has emerged as the only option backed by a randomized, controlled trial.[103,105] When using neostigmine, serious GI, cardiovascular, and respiratory side effects can occur, including bronchospasm, bradycardia, and hypotension, potentially leading to syncope. Therefore, the patient's vital signs and electrocardiogram should be monitored, with medical support immediately available during the infusion. Now that this previously difficult and potentially lethal problem can readily be treated pharmacologically, colonoscopic decompression and surgical intervention should be reserved for cases in which pharmacologic measures fail.

Chronic intestinal pseudo-obstruction is a rare acquired disorder that is caused by various diseases involving GI smooth muscle, the enteric nervous system, or the extrinsic autonomic nerve supply to the gut.[106] These disorders are treated with an NPO regimen, home TPN, and octreotide. Patients with chronic intestinal pseudo-obstruction should be followed closely for the development of nutritional deficiencies. Surgical approaches are sometimes helpful, but often the condition is progressive, such that removal of a defunctional segment of bowel may not provide long-term relief. Bowel transplantation has been attempted, with varying degrees of success.[106]

Recurrence and Prevention of Small Bowel Obstruction

The largest series to date of over 32,000 patients with adhesive SBO indicated that nonoperative therapy leads to resolution of obstruction in approximately three quarters of patients; however, resolution was followed by recurrence of obstruction within 5 years of the index admission in approximately 20% of cases.[68] Of note, patients initially managed nonoperatively have a slightly higher recurrence rate requiring readmission than those managed operatively during their index admission (20% versus 16%) and a shorter median time to recurrence (194 days versus 354 days).[68] Even high-grade to complete obstructions may be managed nonoperatively, but there is an increased incidence of recurrent obstruction requiring hospitalization when compared with operative management (24% versus 9%), with nearly half of all recurrences in the nonoperative group occurring within 2 years.[47] However, approximately one fifth of all patients undergoing initial laparotomy for SBO will have recurrence within 10 years.[107] Because of the significant risk of SBO posed by adhesions and the considerable risk of recurrence with both operative and nonoperative therapy, a great deal of effort has gone into adhesion prevention.

Multiple Cochrane reviews have examined the evidence on adhesion prevention with placement of bioresorbable membranes beneath fascial closures (typically composed of sodium hyaluronate and carboxymethylcellulose, i.e., Seprafilm, or oxidized regenerated cellulose, i.e., Interceed)[108,109] and instillation of fluid agents (solutions containing dextran, icodextrin, and hyaluronic acid)[108,110] in both gynecologic[109,110] and nongynecologic surgery.[108] Although products containing hyaluronic acid and cellulose significantly reduced the severity and density of postoperative adhesions, longer-term studies are required to determine whether the use of these products will result in fewer adhesion-related admissions. In the only prospective long-term study, the incidence of obstruction-related readmissions following the Hartmann procedure was not statistically different between groups in which Seprafilm was placed versus those without it (0 versus 2). Unfortunately, the study only enrolled 35 patients for long-term follow-up and was underpowered to detect such a difference.[111] Therefore, a well-designed, appropriately powered, long-term, prospective examination of adhesion prevention and its relation to real-world prevention of adhesive bowel obstruction is still required. Also, logic would dictate that smaller incisions needed for laparoscopic surgery would result in fewer adhesions to the abdominal wall and reduce the risk of subsequent bowel obstruction; however, no study examining adhesion-related readmissions following laparoscopic versus open procedures of a similar type has been conducted.

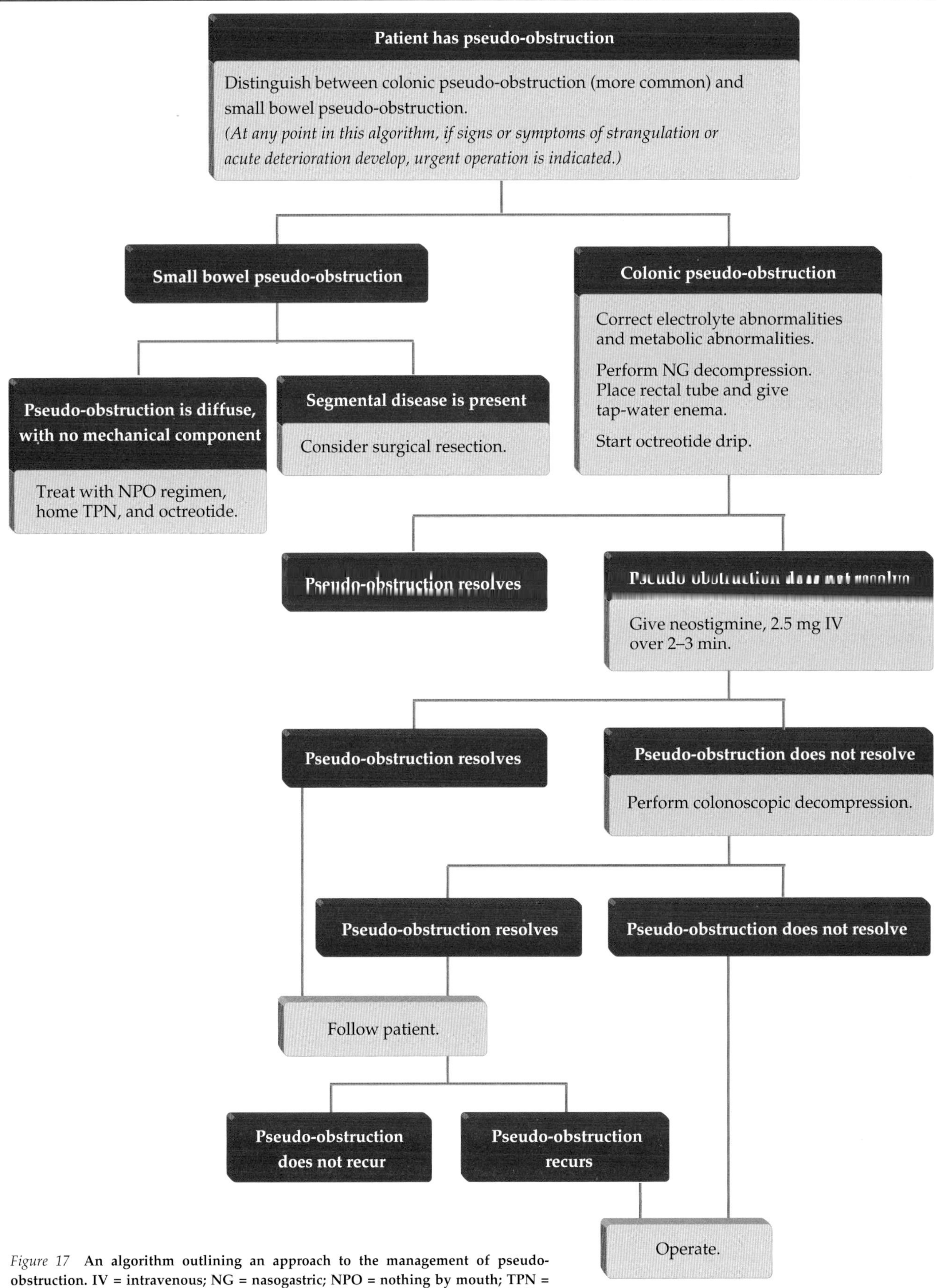

Figure 17 An algorithm outlining an approach to the management of pseudo-obstruction. IV = intravenous; NG = nasogastric; NPO = nothing by mouth; TPN = total parenteral nutrition.

Cost Considerations

Cost considerations are exerting an ever-growing influence on surgical care in general and on the decision whether to operate in particular. A large percentage of the high total cost of caring for patients with ileus or mechanical intestinal obstruction is accounted for by the cost associated with hospitalization or the need for laparotomy. Bed stay for these admissions represents the equivalent of almost one surgical bed per year and at least 2 days of operating room time.[112]

Strategies for reducing the overall cost of managing patients with bowel obstruction have taken several forms: the development of diagnostic and therapeutic methods that lead to more rapid diagnosis and resolution of ileus and partial SBO; the development of techniques for rapid identification of patients with complete or closed-loop obstruction and early reversible strangulation, which should permit earlier operative intervention and thereby reduce the incidence of complications; the development of therapeutic approaches that prevent postoperative ileus, including the use of selective postoperative inhibition of GI opioid receptors,[113] the use of a well-defined postoperative care program, including continuous thoracic epidural analgesia and enforced early mobilization and enteral nutrition,[92] gum chewing,[93] and avoiding positive salt and water balance[114]; and the development of proven methods for preventing intra-abdominal adhesions, which can significantly reduce the overall incidence of adhesive bowel obstruction.

From a management viewpoint, if a specific diagnostic test, medication, or approach (e.g., laparoscopy) costs less than a day of hospitalization does, it immediately becomes cost-effective if it reduces complications and shortens length of stay by 1 day. Intragastric administration of a water-soluble contrast agent to diagnose and relieve small bowel ileus or partial adhesive obstruction is an example of an innovative, cost-effective diagnostic and therapeutic strategy with the support of high-level evidence. CT has emerged as an effective aid for earlier definitive management decisions and to prevent unrecognized gangrenous obstruction. Laparoscopic adhesiolysis is safe and leads to earlier hospital discharge. On the basis of the collective experience reported in a substantial number of studies (see above), a logical proposal for cost-effective management of patients with bowel obstruction is to perform abdominal CT immediately after initial resuscitation and then to perform laparoscopic surgery on those patients in whom the contrast agent does not arrive in the right colon within 24 hours [*see Figure 1*]. However, prospective, randomized clinical trials are needed to evaluate the cost-effectiveness of this and other newer management strategies.

W. Scott Helton has received speaker and contractual fees from Covidien, and speaker fees from Life Call.

Phillip A. Bilderback and Ryan K. Smith have no commercial relationships with the products and services discussed in this chapter.

References

1. Irvin TT. Abdominal pain: a surgical audit of 1190 emergency admissions. Br J Surg 1989;76:1121–5.
2. Luckey A, Livingston E, Tache Y. Mechanisms and treatment of postoperative ileus. Arch Surg 2003;138:206–14.
3. Eskelinen M, Ikonen J, Lipponen P. Contributions of history-taking, physical examination, and computer assistance to diagnosis of acute small-bowel obstruction. A prospective study of 1333 patients with acute abdominal pain. Scand J Gastroenterol 1994;29:715–21.
4. Reisner RM, Cohen JR. Gallstone ileus: a review of 1001 reported cases. Am Surg 1994;60:441–6.
5. Sarr MG, Bulkley GB, Zuidema GD. Preoperative recognition of intestinal strangulation obstruction. Prospective evaluation of diagnostic capability. Am J Surg 1983;145:176–82.
6. Jang TB, Schindler D, Kaji AH. Predictive value of signs and symptoms for small bowel obstruction in patients with prior surgery. Emerg Med J 2012;29:769–70.
7. Burrell HC, Baker DM, Wardrop P, Evans AJ. Significant plain film findings in sigmoid volvulus. Clin Radiol 1994;49:317–9.
8. Oyasiji T, Angelo S, Kyriakides TC, Helton SW. Small bowel obstruction: outcome and cost implications of admitting service. Am Surg 2010;76:687–91.
9. Fataar S, Schulman A. Small-bowel obstruction masking synchronous large-bowel obstruction: a need for emergency barium enema. AJR Am J Roentgenol 1983;140:1159–62.
10. Lim JH, Ko YT, Lee DH, et al. Determining the site and causes of colonic obstruction with sonography. AJR Am J Roentgenol 1994;163:1113–7.
11. Gough IR. Strangulating adhesive small bowel obstruction with normal radiographs. Br J Surg 1978;65:431–4.
12. Small WC, Rose TA, Rosen MP, et al. American College of Radiology appropriateness criteria: suspected small bowel obstruction. Available at: http://www.acr.org/Secondary-MainMenuCategories/quality_safety/app_criteria/pdf/ExpertPanelonGastrointestinalImaging/SuspectedSmall-BowelObstructionDoc15.aspx (accessed September 25, 2011).
13. Thompson WM, Kilani RK, Smith BB, et al. Accuracy of abdominal radiography in acute small-bowel obstruction: does reviewer experience matter? AJR Am J Roentgenol 2007;188:W233–8.
14. Maglinte DD, Howard TJ, Lillemoe KD, et al. Small-bowel obstruction: state-of-the-art imaging and its role in clinical management. Clin Gastroenterol Hepatol 2008;6:130–9.
15. Meiser G, Meissner K. Intermittent incomplete intestinal obstruction: a frequently mistaken entity. Ultrasonographic diagnosis and management. Surg Endosc 1989;3:46–50.
16. Meiser G, Meissner K. Ileus and intestinal obstruction—ultrasonographic findings as a guideline to therapy. Hepatogastroenterology 1987;34:194–9.
17. Unluer EE, Yavasi O, Eroglu O, et al. Ultrasonography by emergency medicine and radiology residents for the diagnosis of small bowel obstruction. Eur J Emerg Med 2010;17:260–4.
18. Jang TB, Schindler D, Kaji AH. Bedside ultrasonography for the detection of small bowel obstruction in the emergency department. Emerg Med J 2011;28:676–8.
19. Beall DP, Fortman BJ, Lawler BC, Regan F. Imaging bowel obstruction: a comparison between fast magnetic resonance imaging and helical computed tomography. Clin Radiol 2002;57:719–24.

20. Megibow AJ. Bowel obstruction. Evaluation with CT. Radiol Clin North Am 1994;32:861–70.
21. Kohli MD, Maglinte DD. CT enteroclysis in incomplete small bowel obstruction. Abdom Imaging 2009;34:321–7.
22. Mercadante S, Casuccio A, Mangione S. Medical treatment for inoperable malignant bowel obstruction: a qualitative systematic review. J Pain Symptom Manage 2007;33:217–23.
23. O'Connor B, Creedon B. Pharmacological treatment of bowel obstruction in cancer patients. Expert Opin Pharmacother 2011;12:2205–14.
24. Mercadante S, Porzio G. Octreotide for malignant bowel obstruction: twenty years after. Crit Rev Oncol Hematol 2012;83:388–92.
25. Porzio G, Aielli F, Verna L, et al. Can malignant bowel obstruction in advanced cancer patients be treated at home? Support Care Cancer 2011;19:431–3.
26. Ansaloni L, Andersson RE, Bazzoli F, et al. Guidelines in the management of obstructing cancer of the left colon: consensus conference of the World Society of Emergency Surgery (WSES) and Peritoneum and Surgery (PnS) Society. World J Emerg Surg 2010;5:29.
27. Manes G, de BM, Fuccio L, et al. Endoscopic palliation in patients with incurable malignant colorectal obstruction by means of self-expanding metal stent: analysis of results and predictors of outcomes in a large multicenter series. Arch Surg 2011;146:1157–62.
28. Hosono S, Ohtani H, Arimoto Y, Kanamiya Y. Endoscopic stenting versus surgical gastroenterostomy for palliation of malignant gastroduodenal obstruction: a meta-analysis. J Gastroenterol 2007;42:283–90.
29. Jeurnink SM, van Eijck CH, Steyerberg EW, et al. Stent versus gastrojejunostomy for the palliation of gastric outlet obstruction: a systematic review. BMC Gastroenterol 2007;7:18.
30. Jeurnink SM, Steyerberg EW, van Hooft JE, et al. Surgical gastrojejunostomy or endoscopic stent placement for the palliation of malignant gastric outlet obstruction (SUSTENT study): a multicenter randomized trial. Gastrointest Endosc 2010;71:490–9.
31. Jeurnink SM, Polinder S, Steyerberg EW, et al. Cost comparison of gastrojejunostomy versus duodenal stent placement for malignant gastric outlet obstruction. J Gastroenterol 2010;45:537–43.
32. Piesman M, Kozarek RA, Brandabur JJ, et al. Improved oral intake after palliative duodenal stenting for malignant obstruction: a prospective multicenter clinical trial. Am J Gastroenterol 2009;104:2404–11.
33. Sebastian S, Johnston S, Geoghegan T, et al. Pooled analysis of the efficacy and safety of self-expanding metal stenting in malignant colorectal obstruction. Am J Gastroenterol 2004;99:2051–7.
34. Fernandez-Esparrach G, Bordas JM, Giraldez MD, et al. Severe complications limit long-term clinical success of self-expanding metal stents in patients with obstructive colorectal cancer. Am J Gastroenterol 2010;105:1087–93.
35. Lee HJ, Hong SP, Cheon JH, et al. Long-term outcome of palliative therapy for malignant colorectal obstruction in patients with unresectable metastatic colorectal cancers: endoscopic stenting versus surgery. Gastrointest Endosc 2011;73:535–42.
36. Small AJ, Coelho-Prabhu N, Baron TH. Endoscopic placement of self-expandable metal stents for malignant colonic obstruction: long-term outcomes and complication factors. Gastrointest Endosc 2010;71:560–72.
37. Watt AM, Faragher IG, Griffin TT, et al. Self-expanding metallic stents for relieving malignant colorectal obstruction: a systematic review. Ann Surg 2007;246:24–30.
38. Zhang Y, Shi J, Shi B, et al. Self-expanding metallic stent as a bridge to surgery versus emergency surgery for obstructive colorectal cancer: a meta-analysis. Surg Endosc 2012;26:110–9.
39. Fiori E, Lamazza A, De Cesare A, et al. Palliative management of malignant rectosigmoidal obstruction. Colostomy vs. endoscopic stenting. A randomized prospective trial. Anticancer Res 2004;24:265–8.
40. Xinopoulos D, Dimitroulopoulos D, Theodosopoulos T, et al. Stenting or stoma creation for patients with inoperable malignant colonic obstructions? Results of a study and cost-effectiveness analysis. Surg Endosc 2004;18:421–6.
41. van Hooft JE, Fockens P, Marinelli AW, et al. Early closure of a multicenter randomized clinical trial of endoscopic stenting versus surgery for stage IV left-sided colorectal cancer. Endoscopy 2008;40:184–91.
42. Cheung HY, Chung CC, Tsang WW, et al. Endolaparoscopic approach vs conventional open surgery in the treatment of obstructing left-sided colon cancer: a randomized controlled trial. Arch Surg 2009;144:1127–32.
43. van Hooft JE, Bemelman WA, Oldenburg B, et al. Colonic stenting versus emergency surgery for acute left-sided malignant colonic obstruction: a multicentre randomised trial. Lancet Oncol 2011;12:344–52.
44. Pirlet IA, Slim K, Kwiatkowski F, et al. Emergency preoperative stenting versus surgery for acute left-sided malignant colonic obstruction: a multicenter randomized controlled trial. Surg Endosc 2011;25:1814–21.
45. Kam MH, Tang CL, Chan E, et al. Systematic review of intraoperative colonic irrigation vs. manual decompression in obstructed left-sided colorectal emergencies. Int J Colorectal Dis 2009;24:1031–7.
46. Silen W, Hein MF, Goldman L. Strangulation obstruction of the small intestine. Arch Surg 1962;85:121–9.
47. Rocha FG, Theman TA, Matros E, et al. Nonoperative management of patients with a diagnosis of high-grade small bowel obstruction by computed tomography. Arch Surg 2009;144:1000–4.
48. Fevang BT, Jensen D, Svanes K, Viste A. Early operation or conservative management of patients with small bowel obstruction? Eur J Surg 2002;168:475–81.
49. Catena F, Di Saverio S, Kelly MD, et al. Bologna guidelines for diagnosis and management of adhesive small bowel obstruction (ASBO): 2010 evidence-based guidelines of the World Society of Emergency Surgery. World J Emerg Surg 2011;6:5.
50. Sosa J, Gardner B. Management of patients diagnosed as acute intestinal obstruction secondary to adhesions. Am Surg 1993;59:125–8.
51. Jones K, Mangram AJ, Lebron RA, et al. Can a computed tomography scoring system predict the need for surgery in small-bowel obstruction? Am J Surg 2007;194:780–3.

52. Zielinski MD, Eiken PW, Heller SF, et al. Prospective, observational validation of a multivariate small-bowel obstruction model to predict the need for operative intervention. J Am Coll Surg 2011;212:1068–76.
53. Sheedy SP, Earnest F, Fletcher JG, et al. CT of small-bowel ischemia associated with obstruction in emergency department patients: diagnostic performance evaluation. Radiology 2006;241:729–36.
54. Jang KM, Min K, Kim MJ, et al. Diagnostic performance of CT in the detection of intestinal ischemia associated with small-bowel obstruction using maximal attenuation of region of interest. AJR Am J Roentgenol 2010;194:957–63.
55. Schwenter F, Poletti PA, Platon A, et al. Clinicoradiological score for predicting the risk of strangulated small bowel obstruction. Br J Surg 2010;97:1119–25.
56. Zalcman M, Sy M, Donckier V, et al. Helical CT signs in the diagnosis of intestinal ischemia in small-bowel obstruction. AJR Am J Roentgenol 2000;175:1601–7.
57. Mallo RD, Salem L, Lalani T, Flum DR. Computed tomography diagnosis of ischemia and complete obstruction in small bowel obstruction: a systematic review. J Gastrointest Surg 2005;9:690–4.
58. Jancelewicz T, Vu LT, Shawo AE, et al. Predicting strangulated small bowel obstruction: an old problem revisited. J Gastrointest Surg 2009;13:93–9.
59. Duda JB, Bhatt S, Dogra VS. Utility of CT whirl sign in guiding management of small-bowel obstruction. AJR Am J Roentgenol 2008;191:743–7.
60. Hwang JY, Lee JK, Lee JE, Baek SY. Value of multidetector CT in decision making regarding surgery in patients with small-bowel obstruction due to adhesion. Eur Radiol 2009; 19:2425–31.
61. Mangiante EC, Croce MA, Fabian TC, et al. Sigmoid volvulus. A four-decade experience. Am Surg 1989;55:41–4.
62. Gilger MA, Wagner ML, Barrish JO, et al. New treatment for rectal impaction in children: an efficacy, comfort, and safety trial of the pulsed-irrigation enhanced-evacuation procedure. J Pediatr Gastroenterol Nutr 1994;18:92–5.
63. Youssef NN, Peters JM, Henderson W, et al. Dose response of PEG 3350 for the treatment of childhood fecal impaction. J Pediatr 2002;141:410–4.
64. Branco BC, Barmparas G, Schnuriger B, et al. Systematic review and meta-analysis of the diagnostic and therapeutic role of water-soluble contrast agent in adhesive small bowel obstruction. Br J Surg 2010;97:470–8.
65. Ellis H. The clinical significance of adhesions: focus on intestinal obstruction. Eur J Surg Suppl 1997;(577):5–9.
66. Miller G, Boman J, Shrier I, Gordon PH. Natural history of patients with adhesive small bowel obstruction. Br J Surg 2000;87:1240–7.
67. Ellis H, Moran BJ, Thompson JN, et al. Adhesion-related hospital readmissions after abdominal and pelvic surgery: a retrospective cohort study. Lancet 1999;353:1476–80.
68. Foster NM, McGory ML, Zingmond DS, Ko CY. Small bowel obstruction: a population-based appraisal. J Am Coll Surg 2006;203:170–6.
69. Komatsu I, Tokuda Y, Shimada G, et al. Development of a simple model for predicting need for surgery in patients who initially undergo conservative management for adhesive small bowel obstruction. Am J Surg 2010;200:215–23.
70. Mulvihill SJ, Pappas TN, Fonkalsrud EW, Debas HT. The effect of somatostatin on experimental intestinal obstruction. Ann Surg 1988;207:169–73.
71. Gittes GK, Nelson MT, Debas HT, Mulvihill SJ. Improvement in survival of mice with proximal small bowel obstruction treated with octreotide. Am J Surg 1992;163: 231–3.
72. Bastounis E, Hadjinikolaou L, Ioannou N, et al. Somatostatin as adjuvant therapy in the management of obstructive ileus. Hepatogastroenterology 1989;36:538–9.
73. O'Connor DB, Winter DC. The role of laparoscopy in the management of acute small-bowel obstruction: a review of over 2,000 cases. Surg Endosc 2012;26:12–7.
74. Tierris I, Mavrantonis C, Stratoulias C, et al. Laparoscopy for acute small bowel obstruction: indication or contraindication? Surg Endosc 2011;25:531–5.
75. Ghosheh B, Salameh JR. Laparoscopic approach to acute small bowel obstruction: review of 1061 cases. Surg Endosc 2007;21:1945–9.
76. Khaikin M, Schneidereit N, Cera S, et al. Laparoscopic vs. open surgery for acute adhesive small-bowel obstruction: patients' outcome and cost-effectiveness. Surg Endosc 2007;21:742–6.
77. Oyasiji T, Helton SW. Survey of opinions on operative management of adhesive small bowel obstruction: laparoscopy versus laparotomy in the state of Connecticut. Surg Endosc 2011;25:2516–21.
78. Mancini GJ, Petroski GF, Lin WC, et al. Nationwide impact of laparoscopic lysis of adhesions in the management of intestinal obstruction in the US. J Am Coll Surg 2008;207: 520–6.
79. Cirocchi R, Abraha I, Farinella E, et al. Laparoscopic versus open surgery in small bowel obstruction. Cochrane Database Syst Rev 2010;(2):CD007511.
80. Wullstein C, Gross E. Laparoscopic compared with conventional treatment of acute adhesive small bowel obstruction. Br J Surg 2003;90:1147–51.
81. Garrard CL, Clements RH, Nanney L, et al. Adhesion formation is reduced after laparoscopic surgery. Surg Endosc 1999;13:10–3.
82. Tittel A, Treutner KH, Titkova S, et al. Comparison of adhesion reformation after laparoscopic and conventional adhesiolysis in an animal model. Langenbecks Arch Surg 2001;386:141–5.
83. Ellozy SH, Harris MT, Bauer JJ, et al. Early postoperative small-bowel obstruction: a prospective evaluation in 242 consecutive abdominal operations. Dis Colon Rectum 2002;45:1214–7.
84. Pickleman J, Lee RM. The management of patients with suspected early postoperative small bowel obstruction. Ann Surg 1989;210:216–9.
85. Brolin RE. The role of gastrointestinal tube decompression in the treatment of mechanical intestinal obstruction. Am Surg 1983;49:131–7.
86. Stewart RM, Page CP, Brender J, et al. The incidence and risk of early postoperative small bowel obstruction. A cohort study. Am J Surg 1987;154:643–7.
87. Gowen GF. Long tube decompression is successful in 90% of patients with adhesive small bowel obstruction. Am J Surg 2003;185:512–5.

88. Fleshner PR, Siegman MG, Slater GI, et al. A prospective, randomized trial of short versus long tubes in adhesive small-bowel obstruction. Am J Surg 1995;170:366–70.
89. Hulnick DH, Megibow AJ, Balthazar EJ, et al. Computed tomography in the evaluation of diverticulitis. Radiology 1984;152:491–5.
90. Stelmach WS, Cass AJ. Small bowel obstructions: the case for investigation for occult large bowel carcinoma. Aust N Z J Surg 1989;59:181–3.
91. Kalff JC, Schraut WH, Simmons RL, Bauer AJ. Surgical manipulation of the gut elicits an intestinal muscularis inflammatory response resulting in postsurgical ileus. Ann Surg 1998;228:652–63.
92. Lassen K, Soop M, Nygren J, et al. Consensus review of optimal perioperative care in colorectal surgery: Enhanced Recovery After Surgery (ERAS) Group recommendations. Arch Surg 2009;144:961–9.
93. Noble EJ, Harris R, Hosie KB, et al. Gum chewing reduces postoperative ileus? A systematic review and meta-analysis. Int J Surg 2009;7:100–5.
94. Millan M, Biondo S, Fraccalvieri D, et al. Risk factors for prolonged postoperative ileus after colorectal cancer surgery. World J Surg 2012;36:179–85.
95. Brolin RE. Partial small bowel obstruction. Surgery 1984; 95:145–9.
96. Watkins DT, Robertson CL. Water-soluble radiocontrast material in the treatment of postoperative ileus. Am J Obstet Gynecol 1985;152:450–5.
97. Biondo S. Study of the effect of water soluble oral contrast (Gastrografin) on postoperative ileus after colorectal surgery. Available at: http://clinicaltrials.gov/ct2/show/NCT01440712 (Accessed September 25, 2012).
98. Bochicchio G, Charlton P, Pezzullo JC, et al. Ghrelin agonist TZP-101/ulimorelin accelerates gastrointestinal recovery independently of opioid use and surgery type: covariate analysis of phase 2 data. World J Surg 2012;36: 39–45.
99. Delaney CP, Wolff BG, Viscusi ER, et al. Alvimopan, for postoperative ileus following bowel resection: a pooled analysis of phase III studies. Ann Surg 2007;245:355–63.
100. Vanek VW, Al-Salti M. Acute pseudo-obstruction of the colon (Ogilvie's syndrome). An analysis of 400 cases. Dis Colon Rectum 1986;29:203–10.
101. Sloyer AF, Panella VS, Demas BE, et al. Ogilvie's syndrome. Successful management without colonoscopy. Dig Dis Sci 1988;33:1391–6.
102. Nakhgevany KB. Colonoscopic decompression of the colon in patients with Ogilvie's syndrome. Am J Surg 1984;148:317–20.
103. De Giorgio R, Knowles CH. Acute colonic pseudo-obstruction. Br J Surg 2009;96:229–39.
104. Hutchinson R, Griffiths C. Acute colonic pseudo-obstruction: a pharmacological approach. Ann R Coll Surg Engl 1992;74:364–7.
105. Ponec RJ, Saunders MD, Kimmey MB. Neostigmine for the treatment of acute colonic pseudo-obstruction. N Engl J Med 1999;341:137–41.
106. De Giorgio R, Cogliandro RF, Barbara G, et al. Chronic intestinal pseudo-obstruction: clinical features, diagnosis, and therapy. Gastroenterol Clin North Am 2011;40:787–807.
107. Fevang BT, Fevang J, Lie SA, et al. Long-term prognosis after operation for adhesive small bowel obstruction. Ann Surg 2004;240:193–201.
108. Kumar S, Wong PF, Leaper DJ. Intra-peritoneal prophylactic agents for preventing adhesions and adhesive intestinal obstruction after non-gynaecological abdominal surgery. Cochrane Database Syst Rev 2009;(1):CD005080.
109. Ahmad G, Duffy JM, Farquhar C, et al. Barrier agents for adhesion prevention after gynaecological surgery. Cochrane Database Syst Rev 2008;(2):CD000475.
110. Metwally M, Watson A, Lilford R, Vandekerckhove P. Fluid and pharmacological agents for adhesion prevention after gynaecological surgery. Cochrane Database Syst Rev 2006;(2):CD001298.
111. van der Wal JB, Iordens GI, Vrijland WW, et al. Adhesion prevention during laparotomy: long-term follow-up of a randomized clinical trial. Ann Surg 2011;253:1118–21.
112. Menzies D, Parker M, Hoare R, Knight A. Small bowel obstruction due to postoperative adhesions: treatment patterns and associated costs in 110 hospital admissions. Ann R Coll Surg Engl 2001;83:40–6.
113. Taguchi A, Sharma N, Saleem RM, et al. Selective postoperative inhibition of gastrointestinal opioid receptors. N Engl J Med 2001;345:935–40.
114. Lobo DN, Bostock KA, Neal KR, et al. Effect of salt and water balance on recovery of gastrointestinal function after elective colonic resection: a randomised controlled trial. Lancet 2002;359:1812–8.

Acknowledgments

Figures 8, 9, 10, 11, 12 Lawrence Holder, MD
Figure 15 Marcia Krammerer

5 GASTROINTESTINAL BLEEDING

Ezra N. Teitelbaum, MD, and Eric S. Hungness, MD, FACS

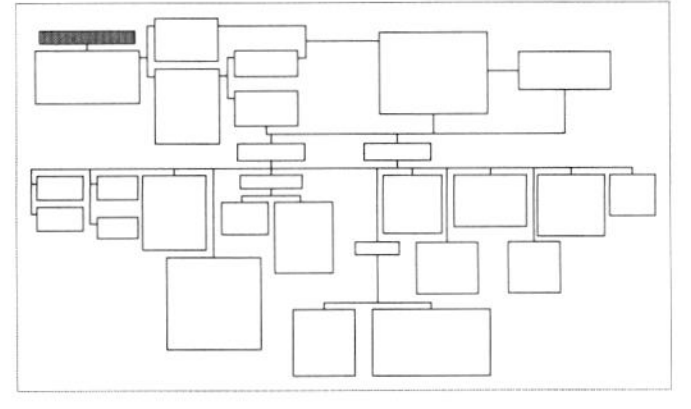

Despite recent advances in therapeutic endoscopy and the widespread use of antisecretory medications, upper gastrointestinal bleeding (UGIB), defined as bleeding that occurs proximal to the ligament of Treitz, continues to be one of the more common reasons for surgical consultation. It also remains a significant source of mortality for both emergency admissions (11%) and inpatients (33%).[1] The most common causes of UGIB are esophageal and gastric varices, Mallory-Weiss tears, acute hemorrhagic gastritis, gastric and duodenal ulcers, and neoplasms.[1] Less common causes include various other gastrointestinal (GI) conditions and certain hepatobiliary and pancreatic disorders.

Lower gastrointestinal bleeding (LGIB), defined as abnormal hemorrhage into the lumen of the bowel from a source distal to the ligament of Treitz, usually derives from the colon; however, the small bowel is identified as the source of bleeding in as many as one third of cases.[2] In as many as 11% of patients presenting with hematochezia, brisk UGIB is identified as the source.[3] The most common causes of LGIB are colonic, with diverticular disease being the most common and accounting for 30 to 40% of all cases.[4] Arteriovenous malformations (AVMs), although extensively described in the literature, are considerably less common causes, accounting for 1 to 4% of cases.[5] Other less common causes include inflammatory bowel disease (IBD), benign and malignant neoplasms, ischemia, infectious colitis, benign anorectal disease, coagulopathy, use of nonsteroidal antiinflammatory drugs (NSAIDs), radiation proctitis, AIDS, and small bowel disorders.

Presentation and Initial Management

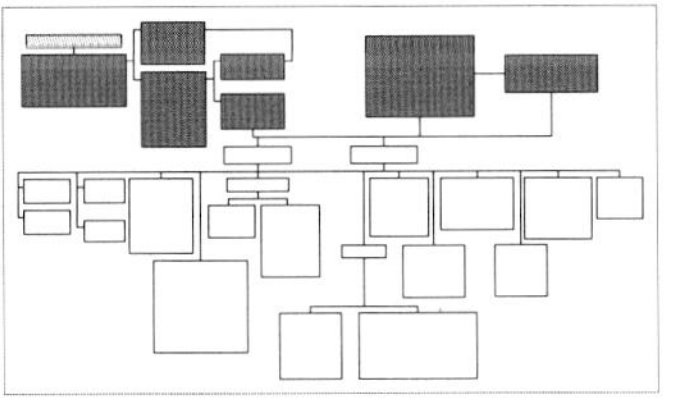

Gastrointestinal bleeding (GIB) may present as severe bleeding with hematemesis (UGIB), hematochezia (UGIB or LGIB), and/or symptoms of hypotension or severe anemia (syncope, light-headedness, dyspnea, chest pain). UGIB may be gradual, presenting with melena, or occult, presenting with symptoms of chronic anemia (fatigue, dyspnea). The initial steps in the evaluation of patients with GIB are based on the perceived rate of bleeding and the degree of hemodynamic stability. Hemodynamically stable patients who show no evidence of active bleeding or comorbidities may be treated on an outpatient basis,[6] whereas patients who show evidence of serious bleeding should be managed aggressively and hospitalized.

In the acute setting, the airway, breathing, and circulation should be rapidly assessed, and the examiner should note whether the patient has a history of or currently exhibits hematemesis, melena, or hematochezia. Blood should be sent to the blood bank for typing/crossmatching, complete blood count, blood chemistries (including tests of liver function and renal function), and measurement of the prothrombin time and the partial thromboplastin time. If UGIB is suspected, the patient should be given an intravenous (IV) proton pump inhibitor (PPI) empirically (e.g., omeprazole 80 mg bolus dose followed by a 8 mg/hr continuous infusion in high-risk patients) as preendoscopy PPI administration has been shown to decrease the need for endoscopic therapy for bleeding peptic ulcers.[7,8]

If the patient is stable and shows no evidence of recent or active hemorrhage, the surgeon may proceed with the workup. If the patient is unstable or shows evidence of recent or active bleeding, short, large-bore IV lines should be placed before the workup is begun to ensure that immediate IV access is possible should the patient subsequently become unstable. He or she should be taken to an intensive care unit and resuscitated immediately. Resuscitation of an unstable patient is begun by establishing a secure airway and ensuring adequate ventilation.[9] Oxygen should be given, with a low threshold for endotracheal intubation. Much as in trauma resuscitation, either short, large-bore, peripheral IV lines or a single-lumen 8 French catheter in the femoral vein should then be placed, through which lactated Ringer solution or 0.9% normal saline should be infused at a rate high enough to maintain tissue perfusion. A urinary catheter should be inserted and urine output monitored. Blood products should be given as necessary, and any coagulopathies should be corrected. Transfusion should aim at maintaining both a hemoglobin level of 7 g/dL or greater and adequate end-organ perfusion (as measured by urine output, mental status, etc.). It is all too easy to forget these basic steps in a desire to evaluate and manage massive GI hemorrhage.

Every effort should be made to resuscitate and stabilize the patient sufficiently to allow clinical evaluation and diagnostic testing to help determine the cause of the bleeding and direct subsequent care. Only if the patient remains unstable and continues to bleed despite maximal supportive measures should he or she be taken to the operating room (OR) for intraoperative diagnosis.

Clinical Evaluation

Only after the initial measures to protect the airway and stabilize the patient have been completed should an attempt be made to establish the cause of the bleeding. The history should focus on known causes of GIB (e.g., previous GIB, peptic ulcer disease, diverticulosis, AVM, esophageal varices, liver disease, alcohol abuse, and IBD) and on the possible use of medications that interfere with coagulation (e.g.,

Assessment and Management of Gastrointestinal Bleeding

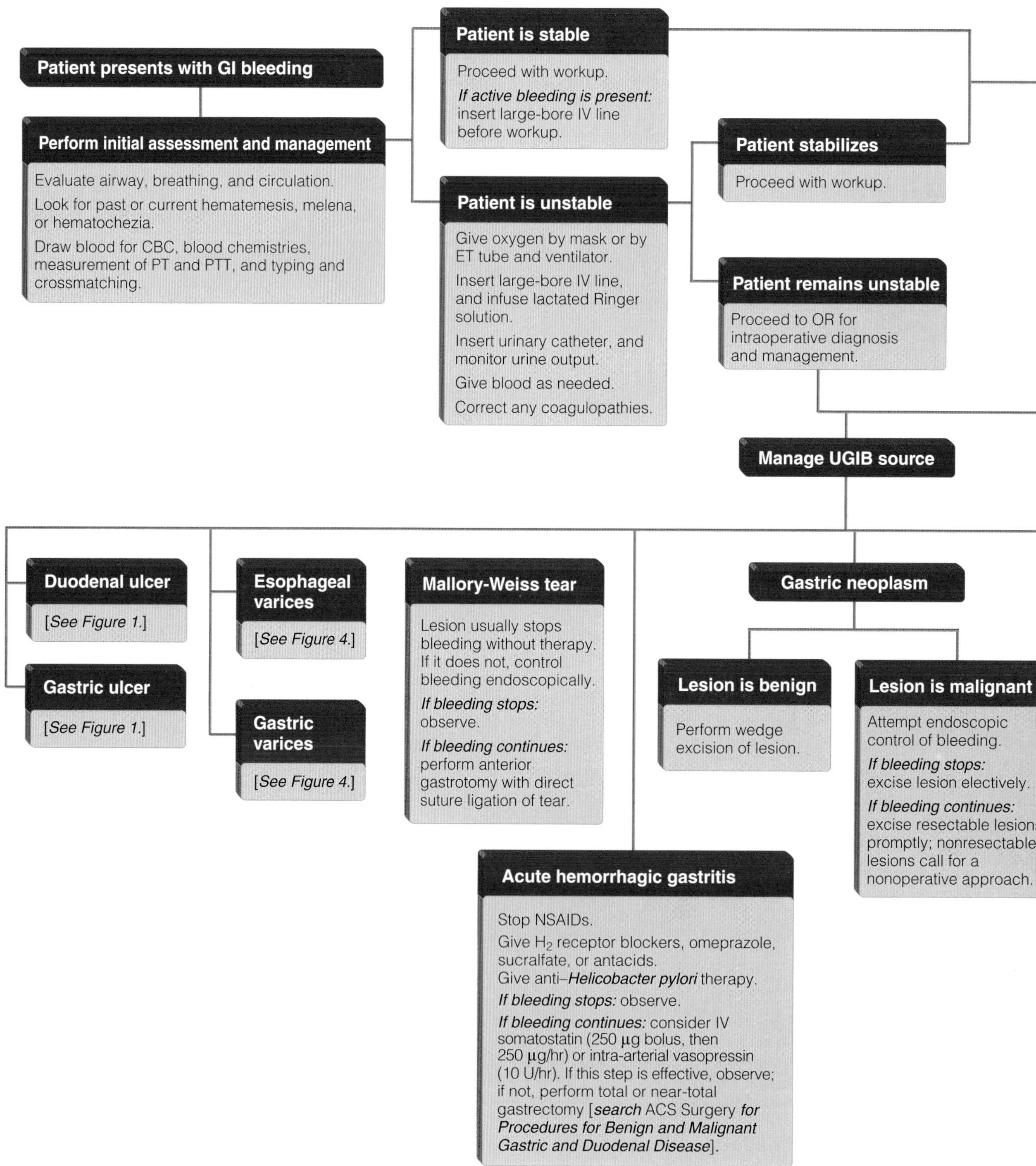

Patient presents with GI bleeding
Perform initial assessment and management
Evaluate airway, breathing, and circulation.
Look for past or current hematemesis, melena, or hematochezia.
Draw blood for CBC, blood chemistries, measurement of PT and PTT, and typing and crossmatching.
Patient is stable
Proceed with workup.
If active bleeding is present: insert large-bore IV line before workup.
Patient is unstable
Give oxygen by mask or by ET tube and ventilator.
Insert large-bore IV line, and infuse lactated Ringer solution.
Insert urinary catheter, and monitor urine output.
Give blood as needed.
Correct any coagulopathies.
Patient stabilizes
Proceed with workup.
Patient remains unstable
Proceed to OR for intraoperative diagnosis and management.
Manage UGIB source
Duodenal ulcer
[See Figure 1.]
Gastric ulcer
[See Figure 1.]
Esophageal varices
[See Figure 4.]
Gastric varices
[See Figure 4.]
Mallory-Weiss tear
Lesion usually stops bleeding without therapy. If it does not, control bleeding endoscopically.
If bleeding stops: observe.
If bleeding continues: perform anterior gastrotomy with direct suture ligation of tear.
Gastric neoplasm
Lesion is benign
Perform wedge excision of lesion.
Lesion is malignant
Attempt endoscopic control of bleeding.
If bleeding stops: excise lesion electively.
If bleeding continues: excise resectable lesions promptly; nonresectable lesions call for a nonoperative approach.
Acute hemorrhagic gastritis
Stop NSAIDs.
Give H_2 receptor blockers, omeprazole, sucralfate, or antacids.
Give anti–Helicobacter pylori therapy.
If bleeding stops: observe.
If bleeding continues: consider IV somatostatin (250 μg bolus, then 250 μg/hr) or intra-arterial vasopressin (10 U/hr). If this step is effective, observe; if not, perform total or near-total gastrectomy [search ACS Surgery for Procedures for Benign and Malignant Gastric and Duodenal Disease].

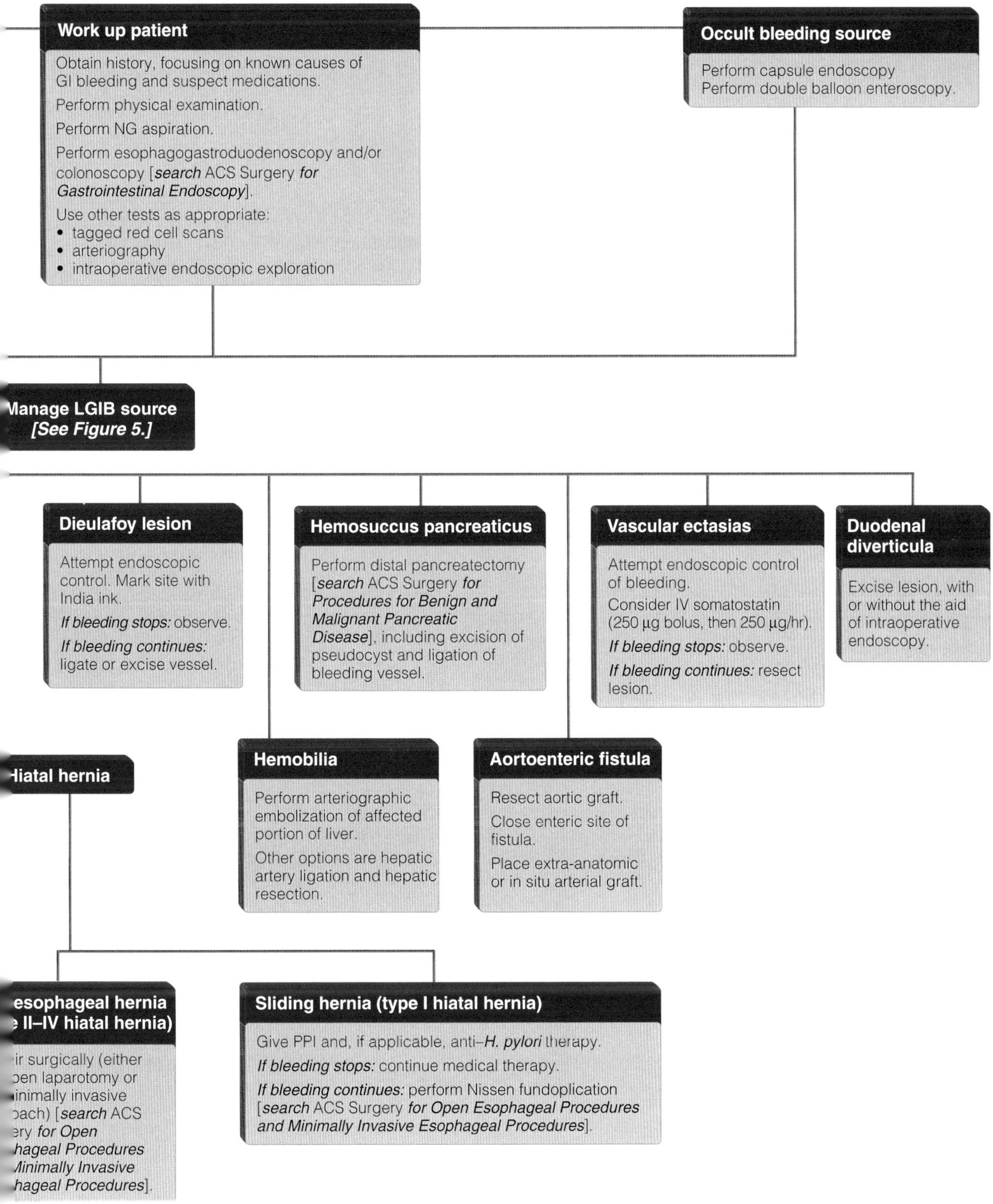

Work up patient

Obtain history, focusing on known causes of GI bleeding and suspect medications.

Perform physical examination.

Perform NG aspiration.

Perform esophagogastroduodenoscopy and/or colonoscopy [*search* ACS Surgery *for Gastrointestinal Endoscopy*].

Use other tests as appropriate:
- tagged red cell scans
- arteriography
- intraoperative endoscopic exploration

Occult bleeding source

Perform capsule endoscopy
Perform double balloon enteroscopy.

lanage LGIB source
[See Figure 5.]

Dieulafoy lesion

Attempt endoscopic control. Mark site with India ink.

If bleeding stops: observe.

If bleeding continues: ligate or excise vessel.

Hemosuccus pancreaticus

Perform distal pancreatectomy [*search* ACS Surgery *for Procedures for Benign and Malignant Pancreatic Disease*], including excision of pseudocyst and ligation of bleeding vessel.

Vascular ectasias

Attempt endoscopic control of bleeding.

Consider IV somatostatin (250 μg bolus, then 250 μg/hr).

If bleeding stops: observe.

If bleeding continues: resect lesion.

Duodenal diverticula

Excise lesion, with or without the aid of intraoperative endoscopy.

Hemobilia

Perform arteriographic embolization of affected portion of liver.

Other options are hepatic artery ligation and hepatic resection.

Aortoenteric fistula

Resect aortic graft.

Close enteric site of fistula.

Place extra-anatomic or in situ arterial graft.

liatal hernia

esophageal hernia
e II–IV hiatal hernia)

ir surgically (either
pen laparotomy or
inimally invasive
pach) [*search* ACS
ery *for Open*
hageal Procedures
linimally Invasive
hageal Procedures].

Sliding hernia (type I hiatal hernia)

Give PPI and, if applicable, anti–*H. pylori* therapy.

If bleeding stops: continue medical therapy.

If bleeding continues: perform Nissen fundoplication [*search* ACS Surgery *for Open Esophageal Procedures and Minimally Invasive Esophageal Procedures*].

warfarin, aspirin, clopidogrel, dabigatran, and NSAIDs) or alter hemodynamics (e.g., beta blockers and antihypertensive agents). Of particular importance in taking the history is to ascertain the nature and duration of the bleeding, including stool color, frequency, and volume. The patient should also be asked about any associated symptoms of potential significance (e.g., abdominal pain, changes in bowel habits, fever, urgency, tenesmus, or weight loss). Knowledge of the patient's cardiac history is useful to assess the patient's ability to withstand varying degrees of anemia.

The physical examination is seldom of much help in determining the exact site of bleeding, but determination of postural vital signs can accurately estimate intravascular volume status. A drop in the orthostatic blood pressure greater than 10 mm Hg or an increase in the pulse rate greater than 10 beats/min indicates that more than 800 mL of blood (> 15% of the total circulating blood volume) has been lost. Marked tachycardia and tachypnea in association with hypotension and depressed mental status indicate that more than 1,500 mL of blood (> 30% of the total circulating blood volume) has been lost. A complete abdominal examination, including digital rectal examination and anoscopy, should be performed as it may reveal jaundice, ascites, or other signs of hepatic disease; a tumor mass; or a bruit from an abdominal vascular lesion.

A nasogastric (NG) tube should be placed for gastric lavage. If lavage yields positive results (i.e., the aspirate contains gross blood or so-called coffee grounds), UGIB is confirmed and esophagogastroduodenoscopy (EGD) is indicated. An aspirate that contains no blood and copious amounts of bile is strongly suggestive of LGIB, and the workup proceeds accordingly. The choice is less clear-cut with a clear aspirate. In the absence of bile, such an aspirate cannot rule out a duodenal source for the bleeding. Accordingly, there is some degree of latitude for clinical judgment: depending on the overall clinical picture, the surgeon may choose either to perform EGD to rule out a duodenal bleeding source or to proceed with colonoscopy on the assumption that the source of the bleeding is in the lower GI tract.

Several clinical prediction scores have been developed to risk-stratify patients presenting with UGIB and can help guide the sequence of diagnostic tests and subsequent management. The two most commonly used are the Blatchford score[10] and the Rockall score.[11] The Blatchford score predicts the need for clinical intervention (blood transfusion, endoscopic, or operative treatment) based on clinical variables obtained on presentation (blood urea, hemoglobin, pulse, blood pressure, presenting symptoms, and comorbidities) [*see Table 1*]. It has an area under the receiver operating characteristic (ROC) curve of 0.92 and a sensitivity of 99% (for a score ≥ 1), so it is best used as an initial screening tool to alert emergency department personnel of patients who may have serious UGIB and therefore need more urgent diagnostic evaluation. The Rockall score incorporates clinical and EGD findings (age, level of shock, comorbidities, endoscopic diagnosis, and the presence of stigmata of recent hemorrhage) to predict hospital mortality and the risk of rebleeding [*see Table 2*]. As such, it is used after the initial EGD evaluation and may help predict patients who will go on to need a surgical intervention.

Separate risk stratification scores also exist for LGIB. Strate and colleagues developed and validated a prediction model based on the presence of seven clinical variables (heart rate ≥ 100 beats/min, systolic blood pressure ≤ 115 mm Hg, syncope, a nontender abdomen, rectal bleeding in the first 4 hours of evaluation, aspirin use, and more than two medical comorbidities) to predict the risk of need for blood transfusion, surgical intervention, and mortality.[12] In this study, patients with four of more of these risk factors were determined to be at high likelihood for severe bleeding, and therefore in general patients meeting this criterion should be triaged to receive emergent intervention.

UGIB Investigative Tests

ESOPHAGOGASTRODUODENOSCOPY

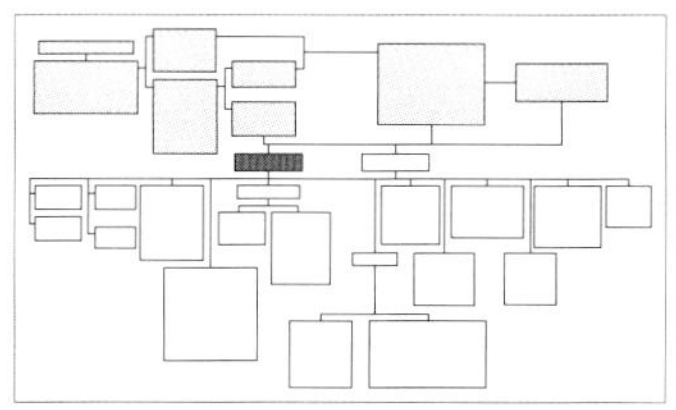

EGD almost always reveals the source of UGIB; its utility and accuracy have been well documented in the literature.[13] Performance of this procedure requires considerable skill: identification of bleeding sites in a blood filled stomach is far from easy. Hematemesis is an indication for emergency EGD, usually within 1 hour of presentation. If the rate of bleeding is high, saline lavage may be performed to clear the stomach of blood and clots. If the rate of bleeding is moderate or low, as is often the case in patients with melena, urgent EGD is indicated. In these cases, EGD should be performed within 24 hours of presentation, and several studies have shown that EGD within 12 hours results in shorter hospital stays and possibly decreased rates of rebleeding and mortality in high-risk patients.[14–16] Erythromycin can be given prior to endoscopy to facilitate gastric emptying as pretreatment has been shown to decrease the need for multiple endoscopic evaluations.[17]

EGD is not only an excellent diagnostic tool but also a valuable therapeutic modality. Indeed, most UGIB may be controlled endoscopically, although the degree of success to be expected in individual cases varies according to the expertise of the endoscopist and the specific cause of the bleeding. Therapeutic endoscopic maneuvers include injection, thermal coagulation, and mechanical occlusion of bleeding sites (clip application or variceal banding). The choice of therapy depends on the cause, the site, and the rate of bleeding.

OTHER UGIB IMAGING

Tagged red blood cell (RBC) scans may confirm the presence of an active bleeding site; however, scans are fairly nonspecific with respect to determining the anatomic location of the bleeding.[18] Arteriography may demonstrate that a lesion is present, but it cannot reliably identify a bleeding site unless the bleeding is brisk (> 1 mL/min). Occasionally, arteriography reveals the cause of the bleeding even if the bleeding has stopped. Angiography may also be considered a therapeutic modality for high-risk surgical patients. These tests, in conjunction with EGD, should allow the surgeon to establish the cause of UGIB more than 90% of the time.

Table 1 Blatchford Prediction Score for Upper Gastrointestinal Bleeding[10]

	Score					
Variable	*0*	*1*	*2*	*3*	*4*	*6*
Blood urea (mmol/L)	< 6.5		6.5–8	8–10	10–25	> 25
Hemoglobin (g/dL) for men	> 13	12–13		10–12		< 10
Hemoglobin for women	> 12	10–12				< 10
Systolic BP	> 109	100–109	90–99	< 90		
Other markers		Pulse ≥ 100 beats/min, presentation with melena	Presentation with syncope, hepatic disease, cardiac failure			

BP = blood pressure.

LGIB Investigative Tests

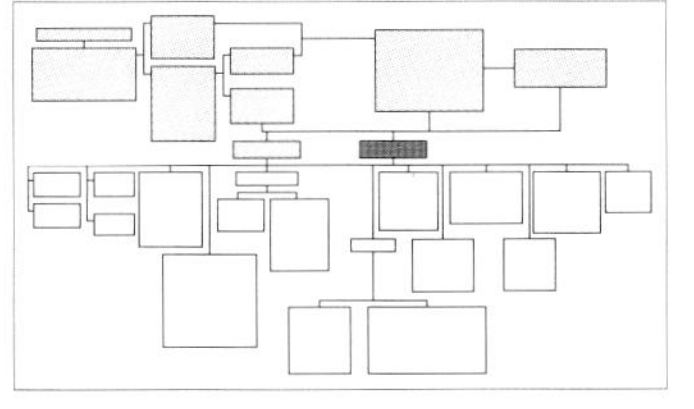

A number of diagnostic techniques are available for determining the source of LGIB, including colonoscopy radionuclide scanning, computed tomography (CT), and angiography (in the form of selective mesenteric arteriography), as well as enteroscopy and capsule endoscopy (CE) to localized small bowel etiologies. The goal of these tests is to locate the site of bleeding accurately so that definitive therapy can be properly directed as the potential source ranges from the ligament of Treitz to the anus. The diagnostic test chosen for a specific patient depends on several factors, including the hemodynamic stability of the patient, the bleeding rate, patient comorbidities, therapeutic options, and local expertise available. Unlike radionuclide and CT scanning, arteriography and colonoscopy provide a therapeutic option. Arteriography has a lower diagnostic yield and a higher complication rate than colonoscopy does; therefore, it is reasonable to attempt colonoscopy first and to reserve angiography for patients in whom the volume of bleeding is such that colonoscopy would be neither safe nor accurate.[19]

COLONOSCOPY

Several large series that evaluated the diagnostic utility of colonoscopy in patients with LGIB found this modality to be moderately to highly accurate, with overall diagnostic yields ranging from 53 to 97%.[3,20,21] In studies reporting morbidity, colonoscopy was safe, with an average complication rate of 0.5%. Colonoscopy has both a higher diagnostic yield and a lower complication rate than arteriography in this setting.[3,21] A randomized, controlled trial in 2005 demonstrated that early colonoscopy (< 8 hours from presentation) was better able to localize and identify the source of LGIB than standard care (elective colonoscopy or radionuclide scanning followed by angiography in patients with ongoing bleeding).[22] An argument has been made that colonoscopy should be considered the procedure of choice for structural evaluation of LGIB and that arteriography should be reserved for patients with massive, ongoing bleeding in whom endoscopy is not feasible or colonoscopy fails to reveal the source of the hemorrhage.[23]

As with EGD, early colonoscopy (within 12 hours) results in higher diagnostic yields and increased opportunity for endoscopic intervention. One study showed that a therapeutic intervention was successful in 29% of colonoscopies performed within 12 hours, 13% of those between 12 and 24 hours, 4% in those between 24 and 48 hours, and none

Table 2 Rockall Prediction Score for Upper Gastrointestinal Bleeding[11]

	Score			
Variable	*0*	*1*	*2*	*3*
Age (yr)	< 60	60–79	≥ 80	
Shock	Systolic BP ≥ 100 mm Hg and pulse < 100 beats/min	Systolic BP ≥ 100 mm Hg and pulse ≥ 100 beats/min	Systolic BP < 100 mm Hg	
Comorbidites	No major comorbidities		Heart failure, ischemic heart disease, other major comorbidity	Renal failure, liver failure, metastatic cancer
Diagnosis	Mallory-Weiss tear, no lesion identified, and no stigmata of recent hemorrhage	All other diagnoses	Upper GI malignancy	
Stigmata of recent hemorrhage	None or dark spot only		Blood in upper GI tract, adherent clot, visible or spurting vessel	

BP = blood pressure; GI = gastrointestinal.

performed later than 48 hours after presentation.[24] The merits of colonic preparation have been extensively debated in the literature.[3,25] Although no firm conclusion has been reached, adequate colonic preparation may improve both the diagnostic yield and the safety of colonoscopy. Given the absence of any definitive data suggesting that bowel preparation either reactivates or increases bleeding, one should consider administering an oral bowel preparation after the patient has been adequately resuscitated.

If the entire colon has been adequately visualized and no source for the bleeding has been identified, the ileum should be intubated; fresh blood in this region suggests a possible small bowel source. If no active bleeding is observed in the ileum, upper GI endoscopy should be performed to rule out a UGIB site.

When colonoscopy identifies a bleeding source, endoscopic treatment may be an option. Endoscopic modalities used to treat LGIB include use of thermal contact probes, laser photocoagulation, electrocauterization, injection of vasoconstrictors, application of metallic clips, and injection sclerotherapy. The choice of a specific modality often depends on the nature of the offending lesion and on the expertise and resources available locally. A 1995 survey of members of the American College of Gastroenterology found that endoscopic therapy was used in 27% of patients presenting with LGIB.[26]

RADIONUCLIDE SCANNING

Radionuclide scanning is highly sensitive for lower LGIB, capable of detecting bleeding at rates as slow as 0.1 to 0.4 mL/min.[27] The patient's RBCs are labeled with technetium-99m (^{99m}Tc), which can be detected on images as long as 24 to 48 hours after injection [*see Figure 1*]. The high sensitivity of ^{99m}Tc-labeled RBC scanning (80 to 98%) is well attested, but there is considerable disagreement in the literature with regard to its specificity in identifying the anatomic site of bleeding.[28,29] For example, a 1997 study found radiolabeled RBC scanning to be 97% accurate for localizing bleeding in 37 patients undergoing surgical resection,[29] whereas a 1990 study reported a 42% rate of incorrect resection when surgical therapy was based solely on this modality.[28] In 2005, one group retrospectively reviewed 127 bleeding scans in an effort to identify factors that might predict a positive scan.[30] The investigators found that tagged RBC scans were 48% accurate in localizing bleeding sites later confirmed by endoscopy, surgery, or pathologic evaluation. Multivariate analysis demonstrated that both the number of units of blood transfused in the 24 hours preceding the scan and the lowest recorded hematocrit differed significantly between patients with positive scans and those with negative scans. However, the clinical significance of a positive scan was unclear in this study in that the rate of endoscopy was not significantly different between patients who had positive scans and those who did not. For this reason, an anatomically selective colon resection for LGIB should not be performed based on localization obtained through radionuclide scanning alone.

Given that radionuclide scanning has no therapeutic intervention capabilities, its best use is in patients with non–life-threatening LGIB as a prelude and a guide to mesenteric angiography after active hemorrhage has been confirmed. However, one should keep in mind that many interventional radiologists may be reluctant to perform an angiography without first confirming bleeding with a positive radionuclide study.

Radionuclide scanning is also useful for diagnosing a Meckel diverticulum, a rare cause of LGIB. Patients are injected with ^{99m}Tc pertechnetate, which is taken up by the ectopic gastric mucosa. Although studies in the pediatric population have demonstrated high diagnostic accuracy, the sensitivity of the scan is only 60 to 70% in the adult population.[31]

MESENTERIC ANGIOGRAPHY

Selective mesenteric arteriography is somewhat less sensitive than radionuclide scanning for lower GI hemorrhage: bleeding must be occurring at a rate of at least 0.05 to 1 mL/min to be detectable with this test.[32,33] The procedure involves percutaneous placement of a transfemoral arterial catheter for evaluation of the superior mesenteric, inferior mesenteric, and celiac arteries. A positive test result is defined as extravasation of contrast into the lumen of the bowel. The probability of a positive study increases with the severity of bleeding. A systolic blood pressure less than 90 mm Hg and the need for five or more units of blood transfusion result in an 85% positive predictive value for bleeding localization.[34]

In several large series, the overall diagnostic yield of arteriography ranged from 27 to 67%.[illegible] The complication rate for arteriography performed for LGIB ranges from 2 to 4%.[2,37] Reported complications include contrast allergy, renal failure due to contrast nephropathy, bleeding and/or pseudoaneurysm formation at the arterial puncture site, and embolism from a dislodged thrombus.[23] Diagnostic use of angiography in patients with LGIB can often be followed by angiographic therapy. The two main angiographic treatment options are intra-arterial injection of vasopressin and transcatheter embolization.

Vasopressin acts to control bleeding by causing arteriolar vasoconstriction and bowel wall contraction. Once the bleeding site has been localized angiographically, the catheter is positioned in the main trunk of the vessel. Infusion of vasopressin is initiated at a rate of 0.2 U/min and can be increased to a rate of 0.4 U/min. Within 20 to 30 minutes, angiography is performed again to determine whether the bleeding has ceased. If the bleeding is under control, the catheter is left in place and vasopressin is continuously infused for 6 to 12 hours. If the bleeding continues to be controlled, infusion is continued for an additional 6 to 12 hours at 50% of the previous rate. Finally, vasopressin infusion is replaced by continuous saline infusion, and if bleeding does not recur, the catheter is removed.[38]

The vasoconstrictive action of vasopressin can have deleterious systemic side effects, including myocardial ischemia, peripheral ischemia, hypertension, dysrhythmias, mesenteric thrombosis, intestinal infarction, and death. Occasionally, simultaneous IV administration of nitroglycerin is necessary to counteract these systemic effects. The reported success rate of vasopressin in controlling LGIB ranges from 60 to 100%, and the incidence of major complications ranges from 10 to 20%.[39-41] Rebleeding rates as high as 50% have been reported.[39,40]

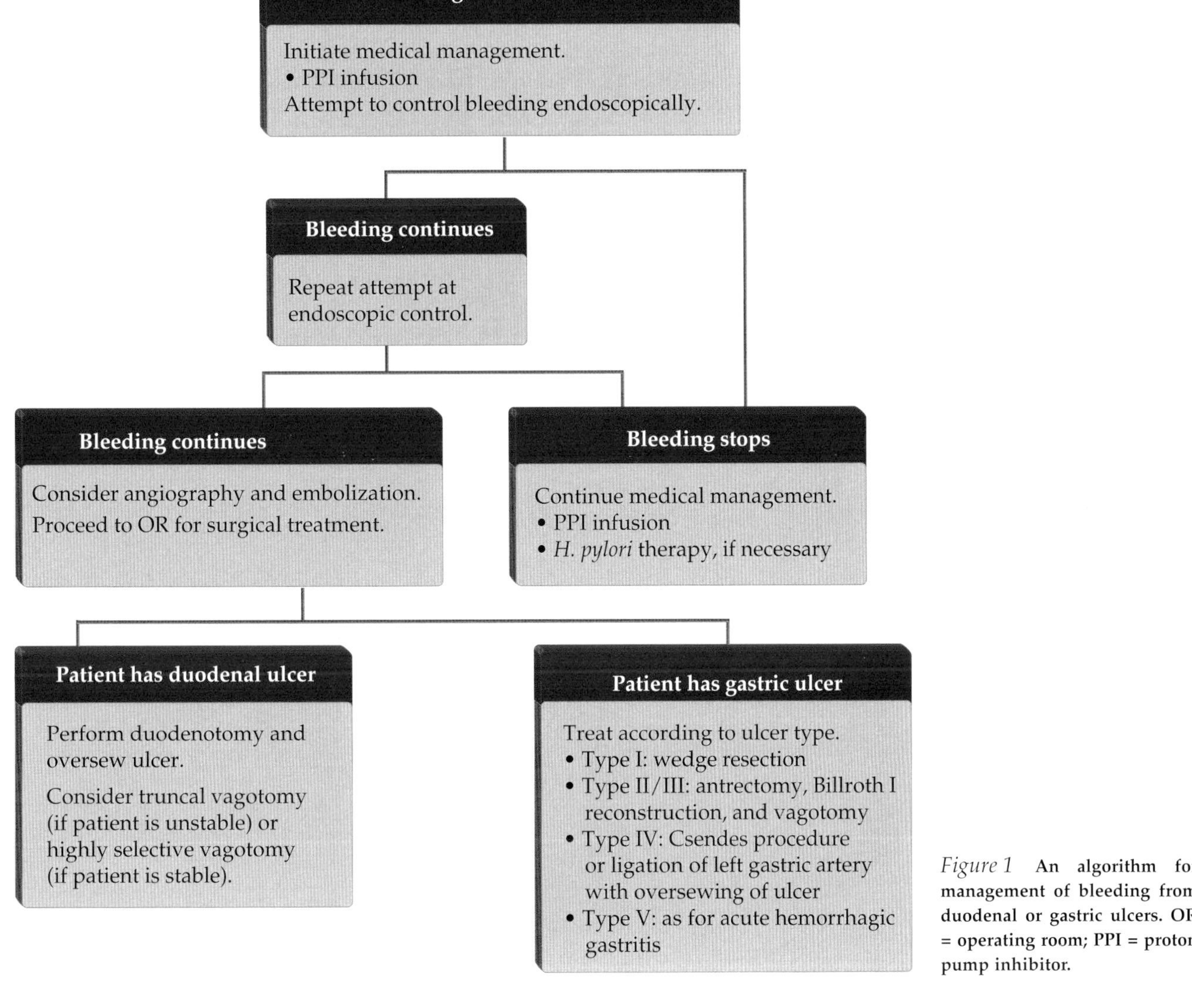

Figure 1 **An algorithm for management of bleeding from duodenal or gastric ulcers. OR = operating room; PPI = proton pump inhibitor.**

Recently, transcatheter embolization has largely replaced vasopressin infusion due to the above-mentioned complications and high rebleeding rates. In this technique, a catheter is superselectively placed into the identified bleeding vessel and an embolizing agent (e.g., a gelatin sponge, a microcoil, polyvinyl alcohol particles, or a balloon) is injected. Several small series found this technique to be 90 to 100% successful at stopping bleeding.[41-43] Equally impressive was the finding that the rebleeding rates in these series were 0%. The complication rates of this procedure are generally reasonable as well; however, intestinal infarction has been reported.[44,45]

The use of small microcatheters and the ability to superselectively embolize individual vessels have reduced the potential for ischemic perforation. It is possible that as more experience is gained with these techniques, superselective embolization may entirely replace catheter-directed vasoconstrictive therapy, thus obviating the potential deleterious systemic effects of vasopressin administration. Some researchers have suggested that with the exception of cases of diffuse bleeding lesions or cases whose demands exceed the technical limitations of superselective catheterization, embolization therapy should be the first choice for angiographic treatment of LGIB.[45,46]

If embolization is not possible, once the bleeding vessel has been localized angiographically, the area must be marked so that it can be successfully identified intraoperatively; this is commonly accomplished by infusing methylene blue into the bleeding artery or leaving a transfemoral catheter to the offending vessel in place [*see Figure 2*].[37] In a minority of patients, obscure bleeding persists despite negative findings from endoscopy, mesenteric arteriography, and radiolabeled RBC scanning. This obscure bleeding presents a considerable diagnostic challenge, which some investigators have proposed addressing by means of so-called provocative angiography.[47] Provocative angiography involves the use of short-acting anticoagulant agents (unfractionated heparin, vasodilators, thrombolytics, or combinations thereof) in association with angiography. Once the bleeding point has

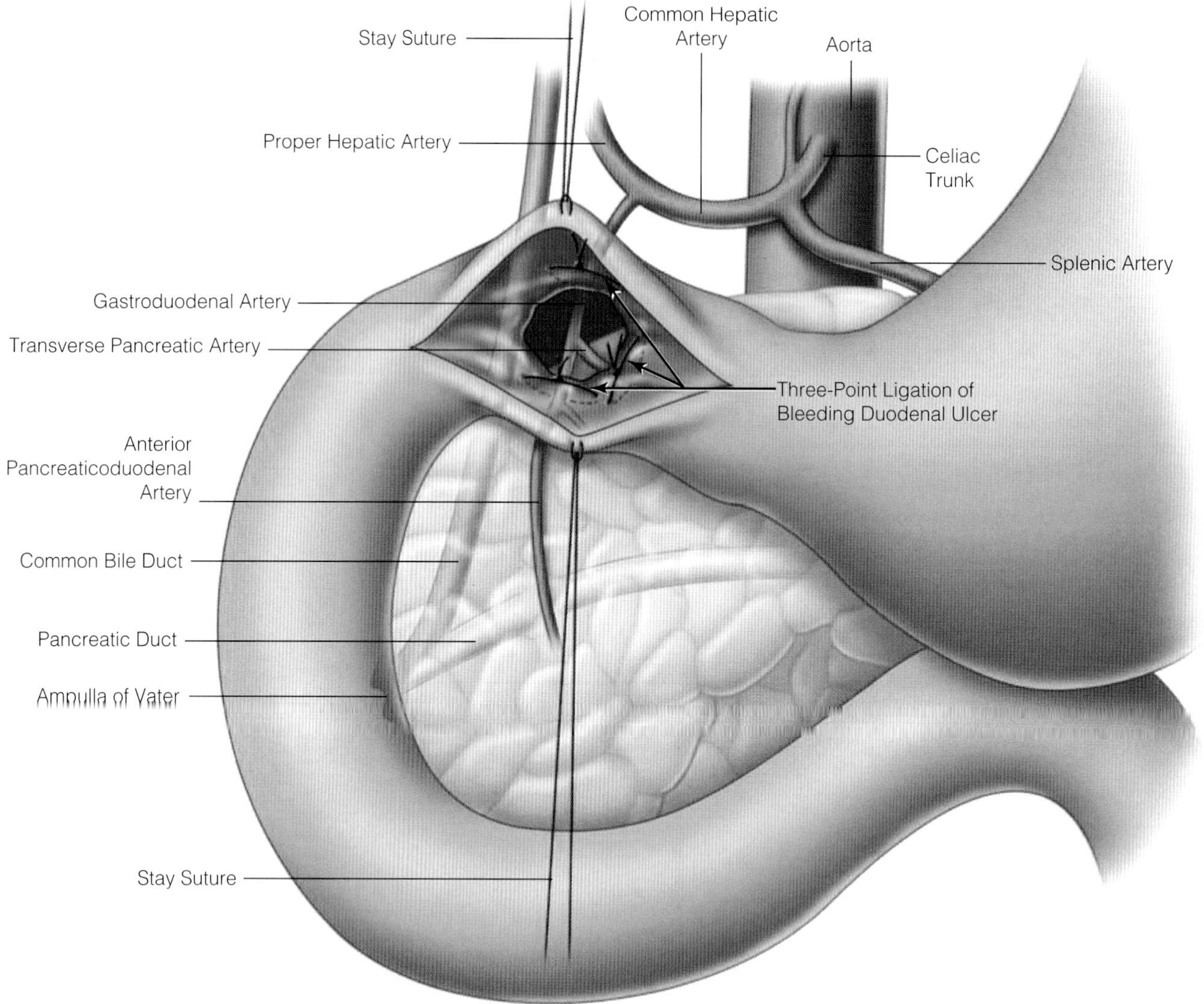

Figure 2 **Technique for duodenotomy and three-point ligation of a bleeding duodenal ulcer.**

been localized (in up to 89% of cases in a recent study),[48] superselective embolization can be attempted or methylene blue is injected and the patient is immediately brought to the OR for surgical treatment.

COMPUTED TOMOGRAPHY

With the ongoing improvements in high-speed abdominal CT scanning, interest has been growing in the evaluation of GIB with CT angiography.[49] Helical CT scanners can provide direct or indirect evidence of the source of GIB. Typical findings that can facilitate localization of bleeding sites include spontaneous hyperdensity of the peribowel fat, contrast enhancement of the bowel wall, vascular extravasation of the contrast medium, thickening of the bowel wall, polyps, tumors, and vascular dilatation.

CT evaluation of GIB has several noteworthy advantages: the scanners typically are readily available, mobilization of special teams or units is not required, the scans can be completed rapidly in the emergency department, and bowel preparation is unnecessary. In one experimental study, CT scanners were able to detect arterial bleeding at rates as low as 0.07 mL/min, which suggests that CT scanning is more sensitive than angiography for this purpose.[50] In addition, CT scans are noninvasive and carry little morbidity. Unfortunately, like radionuclide scanning, CT has no therapeutic capability.

A 2003 study of 19 patients with GI hemorrhage compared triphasic helical CT evaluation with colonoscopy and surgery for localization of bleeding sites.[50] In this series, five patients had small bowel bleeding sites and 14 patients had colonic sites. Helical CT scanning correctly identified four of the five small bowel lesions and 11 of the 14 colonic lesions. A 2012 study of CT evaluation in 114 patients demonstrated a sensitivity of 80% in patients with severe bleeding and 64% in those with mild bleeding.[51] Additionally, CT was able to identify both upper and lower sources of bleeding. This ability to rapidly distinguish between UGIB and LGIB may be of particular value in patients with severe hematochezia when NG lavage is inconclusive. These findings, although preliminary, suggest that CT is a potentially valuable evaluation method in certain cases of GIB. Perhaps CT scanning can eventually replace radionuclide scanning, which is often inaccurate. One potential drawback to the use of CT in this setting is the excessive dye load if angiography is employed as well. Additionally, a specific CT protocol employing timed angiography is required, and the surgeon should discuss this with the radiologist and CT technician prior to performing the study to ensure optimal sensitivity.

CT ENTEROGRAPHY

A novel method for evaluating occult GIB with a suspected origin in the small bowel is CT enterography. As opposed to CT scanning to evaluate for acute bleeding in the upper GI tract or colon, patients undergoing CT enterography are given oral contrast after fasting for 4 hours. Multiphase CT is then performed with additional IV contrast, and timed images are taken at arterial, enteric (50 seconds after injection), and delayed (90 seconds after injection) phases. A 2011 study of 58 patients with occult GIB found CT enterography to be superior to CE in localizing the bleeding source, with sensitivities of 100% and 33%, respectively.[52] This method may be an attractive option in the future as this test can be performed much more quickly than CE, although it requires a specific CT protocol and CT technicians and radiologists who are experienced in the technique.

ENTEROSCOPY

When other tests fail to locate a bleeding source, enteroscopy may be helpful to localize the LGIB. This procedure can be carried out in several ways. It can be performed purely endoscopically with a pediatric colonoscope. Termed "push" endoscopy, this approach generally requires a high level of skill on the part of the endoscopist in that the lack of retroperitoneal attachments of the small intestine makes endoscopic navigation extremely challenging. In most cases, only the proximal 150 cm of the small intestine can be evaluated in this way. Depending on the indication and on the technique employed, the diagnostic yield from push enteroscopy has ranged from 13 to 78%.[53] Typically, yields are highest (40 to 60%) in patients with significant GI hemorrhage.

Recently, double-balloon enteroscopy (DBE) has evolved as an effective method of identifying and endoscopically treating occult LGIB. Using this technique, the entire length of the small intestine can be examined in up to 50% of cases using combined antegrade (transoral) and retrograde (transanal) insertion by milking the bowel in a push/pull technique between two balloons.[54] A recent study demonstrated that 66% of occult bleeding sources were identified using DBE. DBE should be considered the first choice in stable patients with occult active bleeding.

CAPSULE ENDOSCOPY

Another option for stable patients with occult GIB is CE, in which a miniature camera is swallowed and intermittent images are taken along the entire length of the GI tract as the capsule advances. Recent studies, including a prospective, blinded trial and several meta-analyses, have demonstrated that the diagnostic yield of CE is similar to that of DBE, although CE does not allow for therapeutic intervention.[54–56] Because it is less invasive, however, CE should be considered the first choice in stable patients in whom occult bleeding has stopped.

Failure of Nonoperative Intervention

If nonoperative measures, including endoscopy and angiography with embolization, fail and the patient continues to bleed despite maximal supportive measures, should he or she be taken to the OR for intraoperative diagnosis and management? If UGIB is the etiology, the abdomen should be opened through an upper midline incision, and an anterior duodenotomy should be performed at the duodenal bulb. If inspection does not reveal the source of the bleeding or if bleeding is from a duodenal ulcer, the duodenotomy can be extended proximally, or a separate gastrotomy can be performed, to examine the stomach. Bleeding from the proximal stomach may be difficult to verify, but it should be actively sought if no other bleeding site is identified. Intraoperative endoscopy should be considered in this situation.

For LGIB, intraoperative options for bleeding site localization include colonoscopy (to allow for this option, patients should always be placed in the lithotomy position), EGD, and transoral passage of a pediatric colonoscope for enteroscopy with simultaneous intraperitoneal assistance for small bowel manipulation. If the bleeding site is identified, directed segmental resection is the procedure of choice: it is associated with rebleeding rates less than 10% and low mortality rates ranging from 0 to 13%.[44] Blind segmental colectomy without accurate localization of the bleeding lesion should never be performed as it is associated with rebleeding rates as high as 75% and mortality rates as high as 50%.[57] If the bleeding site still cannot be accurately localized, subtotal colectomy (with end ileostomy if the patient remains hemodynamically unstable) is the procedure of choice. This procedure is associated with high morbidity,[58] which underscores the importance of accurate preoperative localization of bleeding before surgical intervention.

Discussion and Management of Specific Sources of UGIB

DUODENAL ULCER

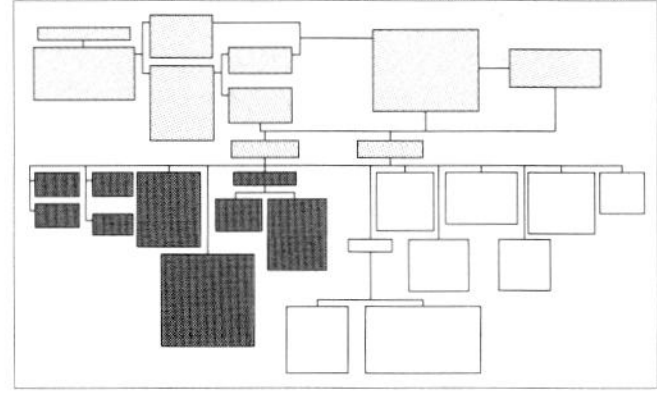

The development of effective medical regimens for controlling uncomplicated duodenal ulcers has led to a drastic reduction in the number of elective surgical procedures performed for this purpose. Nevertheless, the incidence of bleeding from duodenal ulcers that is severe enough to necessitate emergency endoscopic or operative intervention has not decreased over the past decade.[59]

Once EGD has demonstrated that a duodenal ulcer is the source of the bleeding, the first question that must be addressed is whether active bleeding is present. If it is, an attempt should be made to control the hemorrhage endoscopically [*see Figure 1*]. Because ongoing blood loss eventually leads to coagulopathy, the surgeon must exercise good judgment in deciding how long to pursue endoscopic treatment before concluding that such treatment has failed and that surgical treatment is necessary. In general, substantial bleeding (six units or more) or bleeding that is not controlled endoscopically is an indication for surgical intervention. Likewise, ongoing hemorrhage in a hemodynamically unstable patient (especially an elderly one) calls for immediate surgical therapy. An ulcer should be inspected for stigmata of recent hemorrhage. These include (in descending order of risk of further bleeding) active pulsatile bleeding, active oozing, presence of a visible vessel, an adherent clot, a flat, pigmented spot, and a clean-based ulcer [*see Table 3*].[60]

If bleeding is controlled endoscopically, then if not already initiated, PPI therapy, such as pantoprazole, should be given intravenously, either in a bolus twice daily or by continuous infusion.[61] Normal gastric mucosa should be biopsied on initial EGD to pathologically evaluate for *Helicobacter* pylori infection. If *H. pylori* is present, appropriate antibiotic therapy (e.g., a 7 to 14-day course of amoxicillin 1 g p.o., b.i.d.; omeprazole, 20 mg p.o., b.i.d.; and clarithromycin, 500 mg p.o., b.i.d.) should be given as such therapy has been shown to reduce rebleeding rates after antacid medication has been stopped.[62] Food need not be withheld unless the likelihood of rebleeding is high because resumption of oral feeding does not appear to affect rebleeding rates.[63] If bleeding recurs despite medical and endoscopic therapy, a second attempt at endoscopic control should be made. Repeat endoscopic treatment reduces the need for surgery without increasing the risk of death and is associated with fewer complications than is surgery.[64]

If endoscopy fails to control bleeding or bleeding recurs after initial endoscopic therapy, angiographic embolization can be considered a therapeutic alternative to surgery. A systematic review of studies evaluating embolization therapy for nonvariceal UGIB found a mean 84% technical success rate and a 67% clinical success rate.[65] A comparison of angiographic embolization with surgical intervention for UGIB after failed endoscopic therapy found a lower rate of bleeding recurrence after surgery (13% versus 34%) but a higher rate of complications (68% versus 41%).[66] Based on this evidence, embolization may be best targeted toward patients at higher risk for complications after surgical intervention.

Table 3 Forrest Classification for Stigmata of Recent Hemorrhage Used to Evaluate Bleeding Ulcers and Prevalence Data for Each Class from Enestvedt et al[60]

Stigmata of Recent Hemorrhage	*Forrest Classification*	*Prevalence (%)*
Active bleeding		
Active spurting	IA	12 (spurting and oozing combined)
Active oozing	IB	
Recent hemorrhage		
Nonbleeding vessel	IIA	8
Adherent clot	IIB	8
Flat pigmented spot	IIC	16
No signs of hemorrhage		
Clean-based ulcer	III	55

In patients whose UGIB cannot be controlled via other means, surgical management may be accomplished either laparoscopically or via an open approach, although laparoscopy should not be attempted in hemodynamically unstable patients [*search ACS Surgery for more information*]. The latter begins with an upper midline incision. The duodenum is mobilized using a Kocher maneuver, and an anterior longitudinal duodenotomy is performed at the duodenal bulb as the most common source of bleeding is the gastroduodenal artery (GDA), which lies behind the posterior wall of the first portion of the duodenum. The GDA is ligated with nonabsorbable sutures at sites proximal and distal (i.e., superior and inferior) to the bleeding point. A third stitch is placed medial to the bleeding vessel to prevent back-bleeding from the transverse pancreatic artery [*see Figure 2*]. Pains must be taken to avoid injury to the common bile duct during the placement of these sutures, and cannulation of the duct through the ampulla of Vater may be helpful in identifying its course. The duodenotomy is then closed. If a truncal vagotomy is to be performed, the duodenotomy should extend through the pylorus and be closed transversely to perform a pyloroplasty.

A decision is then made whether to perform an acid-reducing procedure. Options are a truncal vagotomy with or without an antrectomy and Billroth I or II reconstruction. The recommendation for truncal vagotomy is based on data from studies done before PPIs and *H. pylori* therapy came into use. Subsequent studies and a 2004 Cochrane review that evaluated rebleeding rates with current medical regimens demonstrated much lower rebleeding rates.[67] Furthermore, it seems probable that long-term PPI therapy (the medical equivalent of vagotomy), in conjunction with eradication of *H. pylori* and avoidance of NSAIDs, should reduce rebleeding rates significantly. Studies from the United States[59] and the United Kingdom[68] have shown that a vagotomy is performed less than 50% of the time during surgical treatment of an acute bleeding duodenal ulcer. Therefore, although there are no prospective, randomized studies to support it, one may consider an alternative treatment approach in patients who have not been receiving ulcer therapy before the bleeding began—namely, ligation of the bleeding vessel, postoperative administration of PPIs, and *H. pylori* therapy. This approach avoids the complications associated with truncal vagotomy.

Another option for preventing postvagotomy symptoms when operating on stable patients for bleeding duodenal ulcer is to perform a highly selective vagotomy (HSV). This procedure is considered preferable to truncal vagotomy because of the decreased incidence of gastric atony, alkaline reflux gastritis, dumping, and diarrhea; however, HSV is associated with a higher recurrence rate than is truncal vagotomy and takes significantly longer to perform.[69]

GASTRIC ULCER

Gastric ulcers are classified according to their location and to the role (if any) that gastric acid hypersecretion plays in their development. Type I ulcers are located on the lesser curvature and are not associated with acid secretion. Type II ulcers are associated with high acid secretion and are located on the lesser curvature, occurring in synchrony with duodenal ulcers. Type III ulcers are also associated with acid hypersecretion but occur in the prepyloric region. Type IV ulcers are not associated with acid secretion and are located in the cardia near the esophagogastric junction [*see Figure 3*]. Type V ulcers are diffuse and are related to the use of medications (e.g., NSAIDs) [*see* Acute Hemorrhagic Gastritis, *below*].

Bleeding is less common than with duodenal ulcers, but initial management of a bleeding gastric ulcer is the same as that of a duodenal ulcer (i.e., endoscopic control) [*see Figure 1*]. To prevent aggravation of the bleeding, early biopsy generally is not recommended; repeat endoscopy and biopsy are done at a later date. The indications for emergency surgical intervention for gastric ulcers are the same as those for duodenal ulcers.

Bleeding gastric ulcers that necessitate operative intervention should be treated with resection. For type I ulcers, wedge resection is typically performed. For type II and III ulcers, the usual approach consists of antrectomy with Billroth I reconstruction and truncal vagotomy. Type IV ulcers can pose a technical challenge as a consequence of their close proximity to the esophagogastric junction. A distal gastrectomy with a tongue-shaped extension upward along the lesser curvature to incorporate the ulcer, followed by a Roux-en-Y reconstruction (the Csendes procedure), is often required.[70] Another option is ligation of the left gastric artery followed by oversewing of the ulcer. If the bleeding ulcer is not resected, a biopsy of the ulcer should be performed to rule out malignancy, taking care to avoid further exacerbating bleeding as a result of the biopsy.

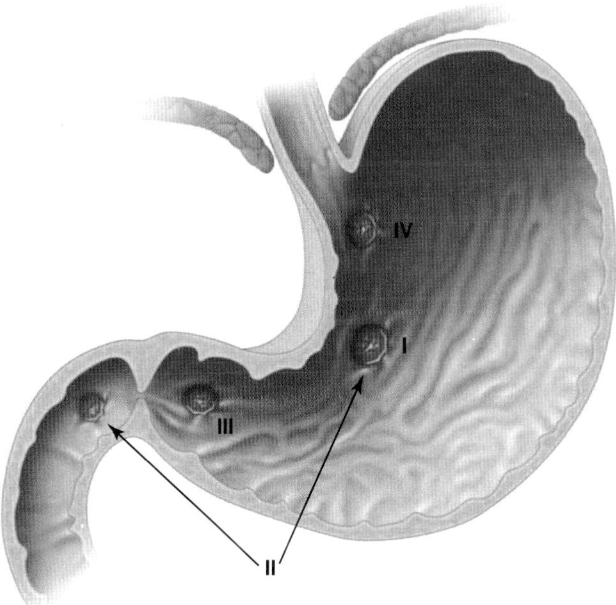

Figure 3 **Anatomic locations of gastric ulcers according to the modified Johnson classification. Type I lies along the lesser curvature. Type II are multiple ulcers, one in the gastric body and one or more in the duodenum. Type III is a prepyloric ulcer. Type IV is a proximal ulcer. Type V (not shown) is an ulcer due to nonsteroidal antiinflammatory drug use, which can occur in any anatomic location.**

ESOPHAGEAL VARICES

The value of endoscopy in the diagnosis and management of variceal bleeding cannot be overemphasized. Even in patients with known varices, the site of bleeding is frequently nonvariceal; endoscopy is therefore essential.[71] If bleeding varices are identified, rubber banding or intravariceal sclerotherapy with a sclerosing agent (1.5% sodium tetradecyl sulfate, ethanolamine, sodium morrhuate, or absolute alcohol) is performed [*see Figure 4*].[72] If these measures do not control the hemorrhage, balloon tamponade is indicated.[73] Successful balloon tamponade is followed by endoscopic variceal injection or variceal banding.

IV somatostatin should be administered in conjunction with the above-mentioned steps. Vasopressin may also be given; however, it causes diffuse vasoconstriction, and nitroglycerin may be required to alleviate cardiac side effects. Somatostatin has proved superior to placebo in controlling variceal hemorrhage when used in conjunction with endoscopic sclerotherapy.[74] It is as effective as vasopressin while giving rise to fewer side effects. Octreotide, a synthetic analogue of somatostatin, shares many of the properties of somatostatin but perhaps not all. Both agents decrease secretion of gastric acid and pepsin; however, the decreased gastric blood flow observed with somatostatin administration has not been reported with octreotide administration. Nevertheless, most clinicians in the United States elect to use octreotide (25 to 50 μg/hr) in place of IV somatostatin because the former tends to be more widely available.

Cirrhotic patients presenting with acute variceal bleeding should also be given prophylactic antibiotics (e.g., ceftriaxone 1 g IV, q.d. for 7 days). Antibiotic administration has been shown to decrease rates of infection, including spontaneous bacterial peritonitis, and may even decrease overall mortality.[75] Human recombinant activated factor VII (rHuFVIIa) has gained recent attention for use in patients with massive hemorrhage and coagulopathy, including patients with esophageal variceal bleeding due to liver failure. However, a 2012 Cochrane meta-analysis of randomized trials comparing rHuFVIIa with conventional treatment failed to show an advantage in terms of mortality or other clinical outcomes.[76] Based on the existing evidence, rHuFVIIa should not be used in patients with bleeding esophageal varices outside an investigational setting.

After the acute variceal bleeding has been controlled, any remaining varices should be subjected to injection sclerotherapy or banding at 2-week intervals until they too are obliterated.

The main indications for surgical intervention in patients with bleeding esophageal varices are uncontrolled hemorrhage and/or persistent rebleeding despite endoscopic and medical therapy. When such intervention is considered, it is essential to determine whether the patient is a transplant candidate. If so, operation should be avoided and bleeding managed by decompressing the portal venous system with a transjugular intrahepatic portosystemic shunt (TIPS). A TIPS significantly reduces rebleeding rates but poses a risk of encephalopathy.[77]

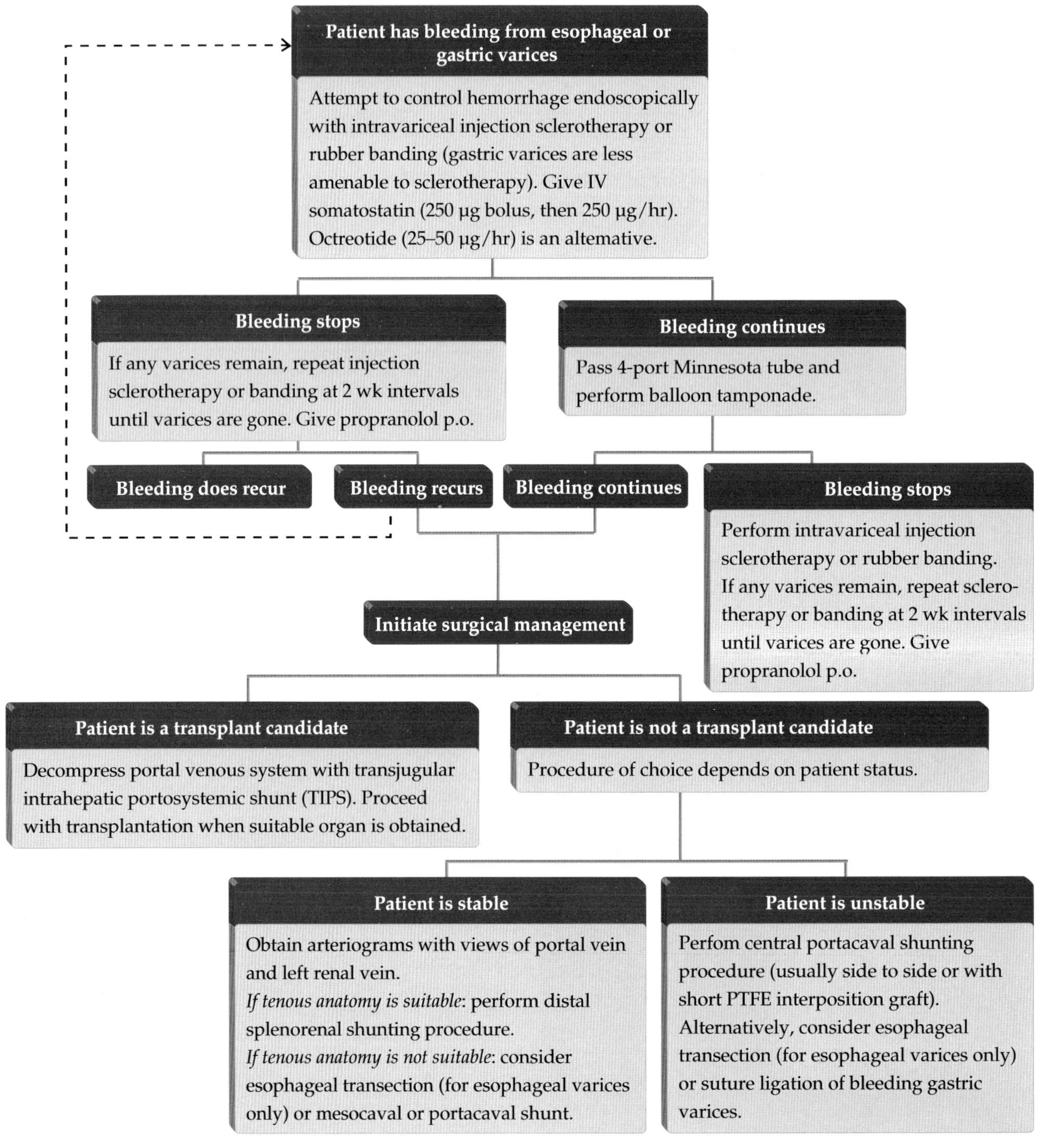

Figure 4 **An algorithm for management of bleeding from esophageal or gastric varices. IV = intravenous; PTFE = polytetrafluoroethylene.**

If the patient is not a transplant candidate and is not actively bleeding, a distal splenorenal shunt (DSRS) is preferable.[78] In the emergency setting, a central portacaval shunt may be placed. Esophageal transection is also a reasonable choice. This procedure is associated with a lower incidence of encephalopathy than a portacaval shunting procedure; however, it is associated with higher rates of rebleeding (particularly late rebleeding) and can be difficult to perform when active bleeding is present. Suture ligation of the bleeding varices with devascularization (the Sugiura procedure) should also be considered.

In general, the prognosis is related to the underlying liver disease. For example, patients with varices that are secondary to chronic extrahepatic portal venous or splenic venous occlusion generally have a much better prognosis than those whose portal hypertension is secondary to hepatic parenchymal causes. The severity of the cirrhosis also determines short-term and long-term survival and may influence the decision whether to perform a shunting procedure.

Several prospective, randomized trials have shown that propranolol (40 mg b.i.d., p.o.) decreases the incidence of first-time variceal bleeding and the incidence of recurrent variceal bleeding.[79,80] However, propranolol should not be used during active bleeding but rather should be started only after bleeding stops.

GASTRIC VARICES

Gastric varices due to portal hypertension are managed in much the same way as esophageal varices [*see Figure 4*], although they are less amenable to sclerotherapy.[81] Other endoscopic treatments (e.g., ligation or sclerotherapy plus ligation) and interventional radiologic treatments (e.g., TIPS or intravascular balloon occlusion) should be considered before surgical management (i.e., DSRS, portosystemic shunting, or suture ligation with gastric devascularization). If the patient is a suitable candidate, liver transplantation may be performed as an alternative to shunting. Occasionally, UGIB can be due to gastric varices secondary to left-sided, or sinistral, portal hypertension. This is usually the result of pancreatic pathology (pancreatitis, pseudocyst, neoplasm) causing splenic vein thrombosis and selective left-sided portal hypertension. Clinical suspicion should be high when varices are present only in the gastric fundus in a patient without liver disease. Treatment in these patients consists of splenectomy, which is usually curative; the procedure may be performed laparoscopically if the patient is hemodynamically stable.[82]

MALLORY-WEISS TEARS

Mallory-Weiss tears are linear mucosal tears at the esophagogastric junction that are usually caused by vomiting. Any patient who presents with vomiting that initially is not bloody but later turns so should be suspected of having a Mallory-Weiss tear. As a rule, these lesions stop bleeding without therapy. If bleeding is substantial or persistent, however, endoscopic injection, clipping, banding, or coagulation may be necessary.[83,84] In rare instances, the tear will have to be oversewn at operation. This is accomplished via an anterior gastrotomy and direct suture ligation of the tear.

ACUTE HEMORRHAGIC GASTRITIS

Bleeding from gastritis is virtually always managed medically with H_2 blockers, PPIs, sucralfate, or antacids (either alone or in combination), along with antibiotics if *H. pylori* is present.[85] Somatostatin may be beneficial. Sometimes administration of vasopressin via the left gastric artery is needed to control bleeding. In rare cases, total or near-total gastrectomy is required; however, the mortality associated with this operation in this setting is high. Stress ulcer prophylaxis in severely ill or traumatized patients is essential to prevent this problem.[86] The gastric pH should be kept as close to neutral as possible. If the gastritis is relatively mild, a biopsy specimen should be obtained and tested for *H. pylori*. Treatment consists of acid reduction and *H. pylori* therapy.

NEOPLASMS

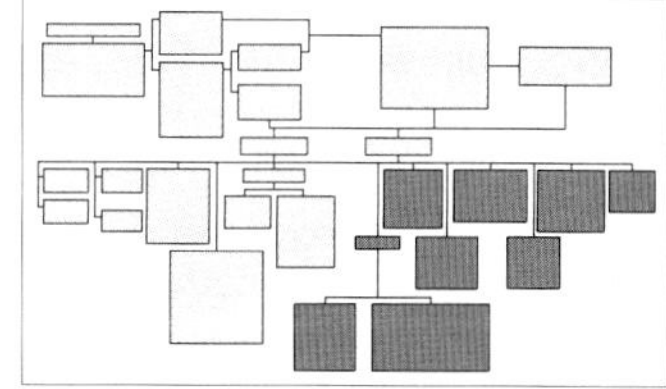

Benign tumors of the upper GI tract (e.g., gastrointestinal stromal tumors [GISTs], hamartomas, and hemangiomas) occasionally bleed. Wedge excision of the offending lesion is the procedure of choice. GISTs (previously classified as leiomyomas or leiomyosarcomas) run the gamut from benign to highly aggressive. They typically present as a submucosal mass that may cause bleeding as a result of mucosal ulceration. The bleeding may be treated with wedge excision of the tumor, which can be challenging when the GIST is located in the gastric cardia. Such excision can often be accomplished laparoscopically or even through a laparoscopic intragastric approach.[87] A combined intragastric laparoscopic approach using a flexible endoscope for visualization and specimen retrieval may be helpful in reducing the number and size of laparoscopic trocars required.[88] Bleeding from malignant neoplasms, whether early stage or late stage, generally can be controlled initially by endoscopic means; however, rebleeding rates are high.[89] If the lesion is resectable, it should be excised promptly once the patient is stable (provided that it has been appropriately staged). If disease is advanced, however, surgical options are limited, and a nonoperative approach, although necessarily imperfect, is preferable.

HIATAL HERNIA

Not infrequently, the source of chronic enteric blood loss is a hiatal hernia. Major bleeding is rare in this condition but may occur as a result of linear erosions at the level of the diaphragm (Cameron lesions),[90] gastritis within the hernia, or torsion of a paraesophageal hernia. Endoscopy is generally diagnostic, although the sources of chronic blood loss are not always obvious. Recognition that the bleeding derives from a Cameron lesion should incline the surgeon toward operative intervention; this lesion is usually mechanically induced and therefore tends to be less responsive to antacid therapy.

Chronic bleeding from a type I hiatal hernia should be treated initially with a PPI. *H. pylori* therapy should be added if biopsy shows this organism to be present. Operative management (i.e., laparoscopic Nissen fundoplication) should be considered for fit patients who have complications associated with their hiatal hernia and for all symptomatic patients with type II, III, or IV hiatal hernias (laparoscopic paraesophageal hernia repair).[91]

DIEULAFOY LESION

A Dieulafoy lesion is the rupturing of a 1 to 3 mm bleeding vessel through the GI mucosa without surrounding ulceration. This lesion is most commonly found high on the lesser curvature of the stomach, but it can also occur anywhere throughout the GI tract. Histologic studies have not revealed any intrinsic abnormalities either of the mucosa or of the vessel.

Initial treatment consists of either endoscopically based coagulation of the bleeding vessel with a heater probe or mechanical control with clips or rubber bands; local injection of epinephrine may help control acute hemorrhage while this is being done. In skilled hands, endoscopic therapy has a 95% success rate, and long-term control is excellent. If endoscopic therapy fails, surgical options, including ligation or excision of the vessel involved, come into play.[92] Having the endoscopist mark the site with India ink is helpful for localization.

HEMOBILIA

Hemobilia should be suspected in all patients who present with the classic triad of epigastric and right upper quadrant pain, GIB, and jaundice; however, only about 40% of patients with hemobilia present with the entire triad. Hemobilia should also be suspected in any patient who had previous liver trauma, percutaneous transhepatic cholangiography, TIPS, or other liver instrumentation. Endoscopy demonstrating blood coming from the ampulla of Vater points to a source in the biliary tree or the pancreas (hemosuccus pancreaticus).

Arteriography may provide the definitive diagnosis: a bleeding tumor, a ruptured artery from trauma, or another cause. Arteriographic embolization of the affected portion of the liver is the preferred treatment option; hepatic artery ligation (selective if possible) or hepatic resection may be required.

HEMOSUCCUS PANCREATICUS

Bleeding into the pancreatic duct, generally from erosion of a pancreatic pseudocyst into the splenic artery, is signaled by upper abdominal pain followed by hematochezia.[93] If endoscopy is performed when hematochezia is present, the bleeding site may not be seen; however, if endoscopy is performed when pain is first noted, blood may be seen coming from the ampulla of Vater. The combination of significant GIB, abdominal pain, a history of alcohol abuse or pancreatitis, and hyperamylasemia should suggest the diagnosis. If there are no pancreatitis-related indications for surgery, angiographic embolization can be definitive treatment.[94] If there are pancreatitis-related indications for operation, angiographic embolization may allow an elective operative procedure based on the structural changes observed in the pancreas. If embolization fails, pancreatic resection is usually required, often on an emergency basis.

AORTOENTERIC FISTULA

Aortoenteric fistulas may occur spontaneously as a result of rupture of an aortic aneurysm or perforation of a duodenal lesion (primary); more often, they arise after aortic surgery (secondary).[95] The most common cause is a graft infection, resulting in graft erosion into the posterior aspect of the third section of the duodenum. A common initial manifestation of an aortoenteric fistula is small herald or "sentinel" bleeding that is followed a few days later by a massive hemorrhage. Patients often present with the triad of GI hemorrhage, a pulsatile mass, and infection; however, not all of these symptoms are invariably present. A high index of suspicion facilitates diagnosis. Endoscopy may [illegible] graft eroding into the enteric lumen, but this is an uncommon finding. CT scanning is the procedure of choice for diagnosis. The finding of air around the aorta or the aortic

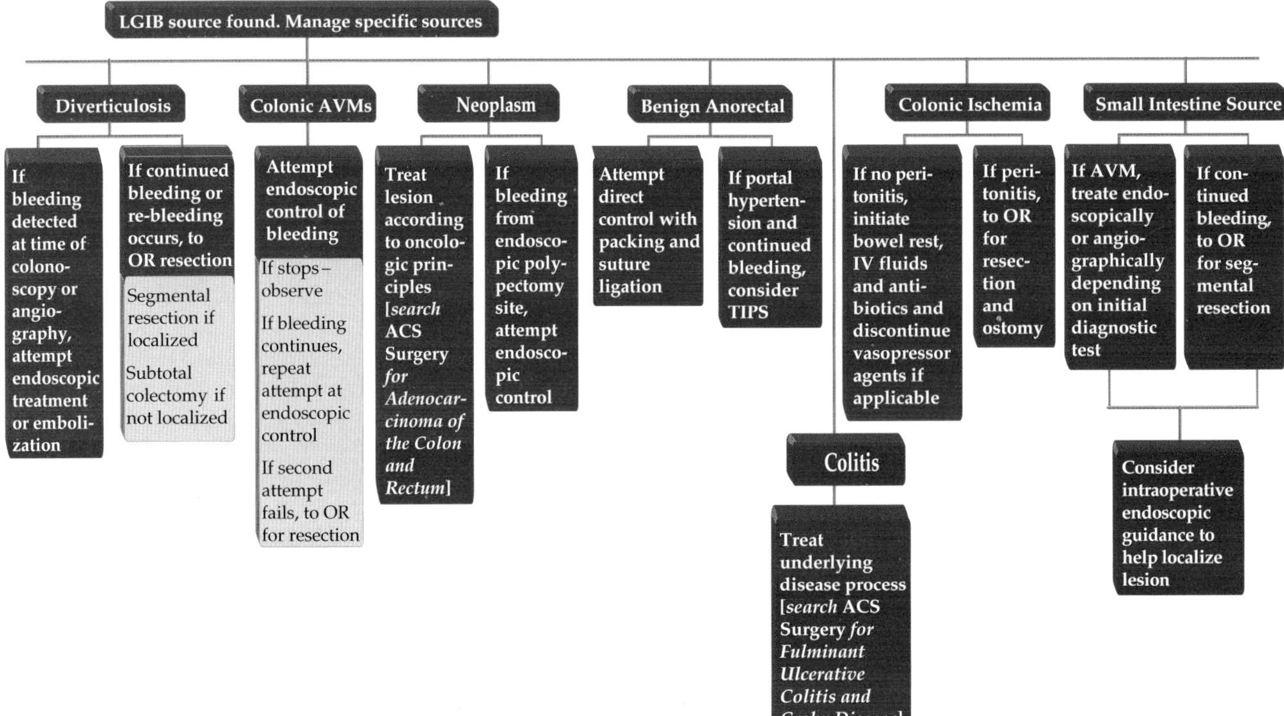

Figure 5 **An algorithm for management of lower gastrointestinal bleeding (LGIB). AVM = arteriovenous malformation; IV = intravenous; OR = operating room; TIPS = transjugular intrahepatic portosystemic shunt.**

graft is diagnostic and is an indication for emergency exploration. The preferred surgical treatment is extra-abdominal bypass (e.g., axillary-femorofemoral bypass) with subsequent excision of the graft and closure of the aorta proximally and aorta or common iliac arteries distally. Some authorities, however, advocate resection of the graft with in situ graft replacement.[96] Some now advocate endovascular stent repair for high-risk patients without evidence of infection.[97]

VASCULAR ECTASIAS

Vascular ectasias (also referred to as vascular dysplasia, angiodysplasia, angiomata, telangiectasia, and AVMs) may bleed briskly. As a rule, gastric lesions can be readily identified and the bleeding controlled by endoscopic means.[98] Lesions that continue to bleed, either acutely or chronically, despite endoscopic measures should be excised. Some patients have multiple and extensive lesions that necessitate resection of large portions of the stomach. Pharmacotherapy and hormone therapy have been tried; the results have been mixed.

DUODENAL DIVERTICULA

Duodenal diverticula are rare causes of UGIB. Accurate identification of a bleeding site within a given diverticulum is difficult, but an attempt should be made to accomplish this by means of per oral enteroscopy or video-CE. Excision is the preferred treatment and is accomplished by means of segmental resection.[99] Great care must be taken in the treatment of duodenal diverticula in the region of the ampulla of Vater to ensure that the pancreatic duct and the bile ducts are not injured during excision.

Discussion and Management of Specific Sources of LGIB

DIVERTICULOSIS

The vast majority of colonic diverticula are actually false diverticula (pseudodiverticula) that contain only serosa and mucosa. They occur at weak points in the colonic wall where the vasa recta penetrate the muscularis to supply the mucosa; as the diverticulum expands, these vessels are displaced. A 1976 anatomic study of colonic specimens from patients with diverticular bleeding used angiography to demonstrate that in all cases, the vasa recta overlying the diverticulum ruptured into the lumen of the diverticulum, not into the peritoneum.[100]

It has been estimated that approximately 17% of patients with colonic diverticulosis experience bleeding, which may range from minor to severe and life-threatening. Endoscopic treatment of diverticular hemorrhage can be difficult because of the high bleeding rate and the location of the bleeding point within the diverticulum. In 2000, one group of investigators reported their experience with endoscopic therapy for severe hematochezia and diverticulosis in a prospective series of 121 patients.[101] In this series, none of the patients treated endoscopically with epinephrine injections, bipolar coagulation, or both required surgery and none experienced recurrent bleeding episodes. A 2001 study from another group, however, reported high rates of recurrent bleeding episodes in both the early and the late posttreatment periods.[102] In the absence of prospective, randomized trials, it is difficult to draw definitive conclusions about the utility of endoscopic therapy in treating diverticular hemorrhage.

Fortunately, most diverticular hemorrhages stop spontaneously. In one series, surgery was unlikely to be necessary if fewer than four units of packed RBCs were transfused in a 24-hour period, whereas 60% of patients receiving more than four units of packed RBCs in a 24-hour period required surgical intervention.[103] Semielective surgical therapy is usually offered after a second diverticular bleeding episode because once a second such episode has occurred, the risk that a third will follow exceeds 50%. In a series of 83 conservatively managed cases of diverticular disease, the predicted yearly recurrence rates were 9% at 1 year, 10% at 2 years, 19% at 3 years, and 25% at 4 years.[104]

In general, patients who require more than four units of blood in a 24-hour period to remain hemodynamically stable, who have not stopped bleeding after 72 hours, or who experience rebleeding within 1 week after an initial episode should undergo surgery.

COLONIC AVMS

The term *arteriovenous malformation* includes vascular ectasias, angiomas, and angiodysplasias. AVMs are ectatic blood vessels seen in the mucosa and submucosa of the GI tract. They are degenerative lesions of the GI tract, occurring more frequently with advancing age. In patients older than 50 years, the incidence of colonic AVMs is estimated to range from 2 to 30%.[105]

Colonic AVMs are believed to derive from chronic colonic wall muscle contraction, which leads to chronic partial obstruction of the submucosal veins, causing the vessels to become dilated and tortuous. This process eventually renders the precapillary sphincters incompetent, resulting in direct arteriovenous communication. Colonic AVMs are most commonly found in the cecum. They have been associated with several systemic diseases, including atherosclerotic cardiovascular disease, aortic stenosis, chronic renal disease, collagen vascular disease, von Willebrand disease, chronic obstructive pulmonary disease, and cirrhosis of the liver; to date, however, no definite causal relation to any of these conditions has been established.[4]

The diagnosis of a colonic AVM is made at the time of angiography or colonoscopy. During angiography, visualization of ectatic, slow-emptying veins, vascular tufts, or early-filling veins establishes the diagnosis.[90] During endoscopy, angiodysplasias appear as red, flat lesions about 2 to 10 mm in diameter, sometimes accompanied by a feeding vessel.

Typically, the bleeding caused by colonic AVMs is chronic, slow, and intermittent. Although these lesions can cause severe lower GI hemorrhage, they are a relatively uncommon cause. The bleeding stops spontaneously in 85 to 90% of cases[106] but recurs in 25 to 85%.[107] Accordingly, definitive surgical or colonoscopic treatment should be rendered once the lesion has been identified.

Colonic AVMs are usually amenable to endoscopic treatment. That these lesions are frequently found in the right colon makes perforation a concern; this complication is reported in approximately 2% of patients. Good success rates have been reported with both injection and thermal methods.[108] In one series, endoscopic fulguration was successful in 87% of patients, and no rebleeding episodes occurred over a 1- to 7-year follow-up period.[108] Bleeding from multiple telangiectatic lesions in the distal colon resulting from radiation injury can be treated with thermal contact probes, lasers, or noncontact devices such as the argon plasma coagulator.

NEOPLASIA

Significant GIB from colorectal neoplasia accounts for 7 to 33% of cases of severe lower GI hemorrhage.[3,25] Such bleeding is believed to result from erosions on the luminal surface. Adenomatous polyps are implicated in 5 to 11% of cases of acute LGIB.[109]

LGIB, either immediate or delayed, is the most common reported complication after endoscopic polypectomy, occurring in 0.2 to 6% of cases.[3,104] Immediate postpolypectomy bleeding is believed to result from incomplete coagulation of the stalk before transection. Delayed bleeding has been reported as long as 15 days after polypectomy and is thought to be secondary to sloughing of the coagulum; it is less common than immediate bleeding, occurring in only 0.3% of cases.[110] Postpolypectomy hemorrhage can often be successfully treated by endoscopic means. Methods used include simple resnaring of the stalk while pressure is maintained[94]; electrocauterization, with or without epinephrine injection; endoscopic band ligation; and placement of metallic clips.

BENIGN ANORECTAL DISEASE

Hemorrhoids, ulcer or fissure disease, and fistula in ano must not be overlooked as causes of GI hemorrhage: in one review comprising almost 18,000 cases of LGIB, 11% were attributable to anorectal pathology. It is therefore imperative to perform a digital rectal examination and anoscopy in all patients with LGIB. However, identification of a benign anorectal lesion does not eliminate the possibility of a more proximal cause of hemorrhage. Patients with hemorrhoids identified on physical examination should therefore still undergo thorough endoscopic evaluation of the colon to rule out other pathologic conditions. For patients whose bleeding is attributable to benign anorectal causes, endoscopic therapy may include epinephrine injection, sclerosant injection, or band ligation of internal hemorrhoids.[111]

Portal hypertension, congestive heart failure, and splenic vein thrombosis can cause colonic or anorectal varices, which can result in massive lower GI hemorrhage. The reported incidence of anorectal varices in patients with portal hypertension ranges from 78 to 89%.[112] If local measures fail to control hemorrhage, some form of portosystemic shunting is indicated.

COLITIS

The broad term *colitis* includes IBD, infectious colitis, radiation colitis, and idiopathic ulcers. IBD, in turn, includes Crohn disease and ulcerative colitis. Patients with IBD usually present with bloody diarrhea that is not life-threatening; however, 6 to 10% of patients with ulcerative colitis have LGIB severe enough to necessitate emergency surgical resection, and 0.6 to 1.3% of patients with Crohn disease have acute life-threatening LGIB.[113] In one review, 50% of patients with intestinal hemorrhage from IBD experienced spontaneous cessation of bleeding.[113] Approximately 35% of patients whose bleeding stops without intervention will have another bleeding episode. Because of this high recurrence rate, semielective surgery is recommended after the first episode of severe GIB secondary to IBD.

Colitis caused by various infectious agents (e.g., typhi, *Escherichia coli* O157:H7, *Clostridium difficile*, and cytomegalovirus) can result in severe LGIB, but this is a relatively rare occurrence.

Increasing use of radiation therapy to treat pelvic malignancies has led to a corresponding increase in the incidence of chronic radiation proctitis. Radiation therapy damages bowel mucosa, resulting in the formation of vascular ectasias that are prone to bleeding. From 1 to 5% of cases of acute LGIB from radiation-induced proctocolitis are severe enough to necessitate hospitalization.[86] In a survey of patients with prostate cancer who underwent pelvic irradiation, 5% of the patients reported hematochezia daily.[114] Initial therapy for clinically significant hematochezia related to radiation proctitis should include some form of endoscopic treatment (e.g., argon-beam coagulation). Surgery should be reserved for unstoppable hemorrhage or other major complications, such as fistulas and strictures.

COAGULOPATHY

LGIB or UGIB can be a presenting symptom for both patients with iatrogenic coagulopathy from heparin or warfarin therapy and patients with a hematologic coagulopathy from thrombocytopenia. It is unclear, however, whether severe coagulopathy leads to spontaneous hemorrhage or whether it predisposes to bleeding from an existing lesion.[115] In an early series of leukemic patients with thrombocytopenia and severe GI hemorrhage, 50% of bleeding patients had platelet counts lower than 20,000/µL without any identifiable mucosal lesions; furthermore, when the platelet count rose above 20,000/µL, the incidence of bleeding decreased to 0.8%.[115] The investigator concluded that severe thrombocytopenia led to spontaneous GI hemorrhage. Other investigators subsequently challenged this conclusion, arguing that spontaneous bleeding from coagulopathy is, in fact, rare. In one report, the distribution of pathologic lesions in patients with GIB who were taking heparin or warfarin was essentially equivalent to that in the general population.[116] Regardless of what the precise relation between coagulopathy and GI hemorrhage may be, a thorough investigation for an anatomic lesion is imperative in the workup of patients with LGIB even in the face of coagulopathy or thrombocytopenia.

COLONIC ISCHEMIA

Acute LGIB can also be a presenting symptom of colonic ischemia. In several large series, colonic ischemia accounted for 3 to 9% of cases of acute lower GI hemorrhage.[104,109] Other vascular diseases reported as potential causes are polyarteritis nodosa, granulomatosis with polyangiitis, and rheumatoid vasculitis. The resultant vasculitis can cause ulceration, necrosis, and, ultimately, hemorrhage.

More than 80% of patients with colonic ischemia respond to bowel rest, IV fluids, and antibiotics and do not require surgical intervention.[117] When exploration is indicated because of peritonitis or recalcitrant disease, all questionable bowel should be resected with stoma creation unless a second-look operation is planned.

SMALL INTESTINAL SOURCES

Small intestinal sources account for 0.7 to 9% of cases of acute LGIB.[3,104] About 70 to 80% of cases of small bowel hemorrhage are attributable to AVMs; other, less common causes are jejunoileal diverticula, Meckel diverticulum, neoplasia, regional enteritis, and aortoenteric fistulas. Accurate localization of a bleeding site in the small intestine can be highly challenging: the length and the free intraperitoneal position of the small bowel make endoscopic examination difficult, and the nature of the overlying loops makes angiographic localization imprecise. For these reasons, the small intestine is usually left for last in the attempt to localize the source of LGIB and is examined only after sources in the colon, upper GI tract, and anorectum have been ruled out.

AIDS

The etiology of LGIB in patients with AIDS differs from that in the general population. In AIDS patients, LGIB is caused predominantly by conditions related to the underlying HIV infection. Cytomegalovirus colitis is the most common cause of such bleeding in this population, occurring in 39% of cases. AIDS patients with hemorrhoids or anal fissures often experience significant bleeding as a result of HIV-induced thrombocytopenia. A 1998 study reported that in 23% of AIDS patients hospitalized for LGIB, benign anorectal disease was the cause.[118] Other significant causes of lower GI hemorrhage in this population are colonic histoplasmosis, Kaposi sarcoma of the colon, and bacterial colitis.[118]

NSAIDS

Although the association between NSAID use and UGIB is well known, current data suggest that NSAIDs have a toxic effect on colonic mucosa as well. An epidemiologic study estimated the incidence of NSAID-associated large bowel bleeding to be seven in 100,000.[119] A retrospective review found that patients who had experienced LGIB were twice as likely to have taken NSAIDs as those who had not.[120] NSAIDs have also been linked to diverticular hemorrhage. The exact mechanism of NSAID-induced colonic injury is unknown.

Summary

Despite recent advances in diagnostic and therapeutic capabilities, in-hospital mortality rates have remained significant in patients presenting with both upper and lower GIB. Starting with the initial evaluation in the emergency department, these patients should be managed with the same sense of clinical urgency that is now standard for severely injured trauma patients and patients with sepsis. Such prompt diagnostic and resuscitative efforts can stabilize patients early in their clinical course and save them from unnecessarily invasive interventions further on. Although the widespread use of PPI therapy and advances in less invasive procedures such as flexible endoscopy and angiography have decreased the volume of surgery for peptic ulcers and other causes of GIB, there will always be a role for surgery for bleeding that is refractory to other therapies. The surgical techniques for management of such critically ill patients remain an essential component of any general surgery training program.

Financial Disclosures: None Reported

References

1. Rockall TA, Logan RF, Devlin HB, et al. Incidence of and mortality from acute upper gastrointestinal haemorrhage in the United Kingdom. Steering Committee and members of the National Audit of Acute Upper Gastrointestinal Haemorrhage. BMJ 1995;311:222.
2. Koval G, Benner KG, Rosch J, et al. Aggressive angiographic diagnosis in acute lower gastrointestinal hemorrhage. Dig Dis Sci 1987;32:248.
3. Jensen DM, Machicado GA. Diagnosis and treatment of severe hematochezia: the role of urgent colonoscopy after purge. Gastroenterology 1988;95:1569.
4. Foutch PG, Rex DX, Lieberman DA. Prevalence and natural history of colonic angiodysplasia among healthy asymptomatic people. Am J Gastroenterol 1995;90:564.
5. Krevsky B. Detection and treatment of angiodysplasia. Gastrointest Endosc Clin North Am 1997;7:509–24.
6. Cebollero-Santamaria F, Smith J, Gioe S, et al. Selective outpatient management of upper gastrointestinal bleeding in the elderly. Am J Gastroenterol 1999;94:1242.
7. Lau JY, Leung WK, Wu JC, et al. Omeprazole before endoscopy in patients with gastrointestinal bleeding. N Engl J Med 2007;356:1631–40.
8. Sreedharan A, Martin J, Leontiadis GI, et al. Proton pump inhibitor treatment initiated prior to endoscopic diagnosis in upper gastrointestinal bleeding. Cochrane Database Syst Rev 2010;(7):CD005415.
9. Liebler JM, Benner K, Putnam T, et al. Respiratory complications in critically ill medical patients with acute upper gastrointestinal bleeding. Crit Care Med 1991;19:1152.
10. Blatchford O, Murray WR, Blatchford M. A risk score to predict need for treatment for upper-gastrointestinal haemorrhage. Lancet 2000;356:1318–21.
11. Rockall TA, Logan RF, Devlin HB, Northfield TC. Risk assessment after acute upper gastrointestinal haemorrhage. Gut 1996;38:316–21.
12. Strate LL, Saltzman JR, Ookubo R, et al. Validation of a clinical prediction rule for severe acute lower intestinal bleeding. Am J Gastroenterol 2005;100:1821–7.
13. Savides TJ, Jensen DM. Therapeutic endoscopy for nonvariceal upper gastrointestinal bleeding. Gastroenterol Clin North Am 2000;29:465.
14. Jairath V, Kahan BC, Logan RF, et al. Outcomes following acute nonvariceal upper gastrointestinal bleeding in relation to time to endoscopy: results from a nationwide study. Endoscopy 2012;44:723–30.
15. Lim LG, Ho KY, Chan YH, et al. Urgent endoscopy is associated with lower mortality in high-risk but not low-risk nonvariceal upper gastrointestinal bleeding. Endoscopy 2011;43:300–6.

16. Bjorkman DJ, Zaman A, Fennerty MB, et al. Urgent vs. elective endoscopy for acute non-variceal upper-GI bleeding: an effectiveness study. Gastrointest Endosc 2004;60: 1–8.
17. Barkun AN, Bardou M, Martel M, et al. Prokinetics in acute upper GI bleeding: a meta-analysis. Gastrointest Endosc 2010;72:1138–45.
18. Jacobson AR, Cerqueira MD. Prognostic significance of late imaging results in technetium-99m-labeled red blood cell-gastrointestinal bleeding studies with early negative images. J Nucl Med 1992;33:202.
19. Dempsey DT, Burke DR, Reilly RS, et al. Angiography in poor-risk patients with massive nonvariceal upper gastrointestinal bleeding. Am J Surg 1990;159:282.
20. Richter JM, Christensen MR, Kaplan LM, et al. Effectiveness of current technology in the diagnosis and management of lower gastrointestinal hemorrhage. Gastrointest Endosc 1995;41:93.
21. Ohyama T, Sakurai Y, Ito M, et al. Analysis of urgent colonoscopy for lower gastrointestinal tract bleeding. Digestion 2000;61:189.
22. Green BT, Rockey DC, Portwood G, et al. Urgent colonoscopy for evaluation and management of acute lower gastrointestinal hemorrhage: a randomized controlled trial. Am J Gastroenterol 2005;100:2395–402.
23. Zuccaro G Jr. Management of the adult patient with acute lower gastrointestinal bleeding. American College of Gastroenterology Practice Parameters Committee. Am J Gastroenterol 1998;93:1202.
24. Strate LL, Syngal S. Timing of colonoscopy: impact on length of hospital stay in patients with acute lower intestinal bleeding. Am J Gastroenterol 2003;98:317–22.
25. Caos A, Benner KG, Manier J, et al. Colonoscopy after Golytely preparation in acute rectal bleeding. J Clin Gastroenterol 1986;8:46.
26. Peura DA, Lanza FL, Gostout CJ, et al. The American College of Gastroenterology. Bleeding Registry: preliminary findings. Am J Gastroenterol 1997;92:924.
27. Mariani G, Pauwels EK, AlSharif A, et al. Radionuclide evaluation of the lower-gastrointestinal tract. Nucl Med 2008;49:776–87.
28. Hunter JM, Pezim ME. Limited value of technetium 99m-labeled red cell scintigraphy in localization of lower gastrointestinal bleeding. Am J Surg 1990;159:504.
29. Ng DA, Opelka FG, Beck DE, et al. Predictive value of technetium Tc 99m-labeled red blood cell scintigraphy for positive angiogram in massive lower gastrointestinal hemorrhage. Dis Colon Rectum 1997;40:471.
30. Olds GD, Cooper GS, Chak A, et al. The yield of bleeding scans in acute lower gastrointestinal hemorrhage. J Clin Gastroenterol 2005;39:273.
31. Lin S, Suhocki PV, Ludg KA, Shetzline MA. Gastrointestinal bleeding in adult patients with Meckel's diverticulum: the role of -technetium 99m pertechnetate scan. South Med J 2002;95:1338–41.
32. Nusbaum M, Baum S. Radiographic demonstration of unknown sites of gastrointestinal bleeding. Surg Forum 1963;14:374–5.
33. Baum S, Athanasoulis CA, Waltman AC. Angiographic diagnosis and control of large-bowel bleeding. Dis Colon Rectum 1974;17:447.
34. Pennoyer WP, Vignati PV, Cohen JL. Mesenteric angiography for lower gastrointestinal hemorrhage: are there predictors for a positive study? Dis Colon Rectum 1997;40: 1014–8.
35. Pennoyer WP, Vignati PV, Cohen JL. Management of angiogram positive lower gastrointestinal hemorrhage: long term follow-up of non-operative treatments. Int J Colorectal Dis 1996;11:279.
36. Rantis PC Jr, Harford FJ, Wagner RH, et al. Technetium-labelled red blood cell scintigraphy: is it useful in acute lower gastrointestinal bleeding? Int J Colorectal Dis 1995;10:210.
37. Athanasoulis CA, Moncure AC, Greenfield AJ, et al. Intraoperative localization of small bowel bleeding sites with combined use of angiographic methods and methylene blue injection. Surgery 1980;87:77.
38. Rahn NH 3rd, Tishler JM, Han SY, et al. Diagnostic and interventional angiography in acute gastrointestinal hemorrhage. Radiology 1982;143:361.
39. Clark RA, Colley DP, Eggers FM. Acute arterial gastrointestinal hemorrhage: efficacy of transcatheter control. AJR Am J Roentgenol 1981;136:1185.
40. Browder W, Cerise EJ, Litwin MS. Impact of emergency angiography in massive lower-gastrointestinal bleeding. Ann Surg 1986;204:530.
41. Matolo NM, Link DP. Selective embolization for control of gastrointestinal hemorrhage. Am J Surg 1979;138:840.
42. Peck DJ, McLoughlin RF, Hughson MN, et al. Percutaneous embolotherapy of lower gastrointestinal hemorrhage. J Vasc Interv Radiol 1998;9:747.
43. Gady JS, Reynolds H, Blum A. Selective arterial embolization for control of lower gastrointestinal bleeding: recommendations for a clinical management pathway. Curr Surg 2003;60:344.
44. Leitman IM, Paull DE, Shires GT 3rd. Evaluation and management of massive lower gastrointestinal hemorrhage. Ann Surg 1989;209:175.
45. Funaki B. Microcatheter embolization of lower gastrointestinal hemorrhage: an old idea whose time has come. Cardiovasc Intervent Radiol 2004;27:591.
46. Darcy M. Treatment of lower gastrointestinal bleeding: vasopressin infusion versus embolization. J Vasc Interv Radiol 2003;14:535.
47. Bloomfeld RS, Smith TP, Schneider AM, et al. Provocative angiography in patients with gastrointestinal hemorrhage of obscure origin. Am J Gastroenterol 2000;95:2807.
48. Shetzline MA, Suhocki P, Dash R, et al. Provocative angiography in obscure gastrointestinal bleeding. South Med J 2000;93:1205.
49. Yamaguchi T, Yoshikawa K. Enhanced CT for initial localization of active lower-gastrointestinal bleeding. Abdom Imaging 2003;28:634.
50. Ernst O, Bulois P, Saint-Drenant S, et al. Helical CT in acute lower gastrointestinal bleeding. Eur Radiol 2003;13: 114.
51. Sun H, Jin Z, Li X, et al. Detection and localization of active gastrointestinal bleeding with multidetector row computed tomography angiography: a 5-year prospective study in one medical center. J Clin Gastroenterol 2012;46:31–41.
52. Huprich JE, Fletcher JG, Fidler JL, et al. Prospective blinded comparison of wireless capsule endoscopy and

multiphase CT enterography in obscure gastrointestinal bleeding. Radiology 2011;260:744–51.
53. Lin S, Branch MS, Shetzline M. The importance of indication in the diagnostic value of push enteroscopy. Endoscopy 2003;35:315.
54. Kamesa N, Higuchi K, Masatsugu S, et al. A prospective single-blind trial comparing wireless capsule endoscopy and double--balloon enteroscopy in patients with obscure gastrointestinal bleeding. J Gastroenterol 2008;43:434–40.
55. Pasha SF, Leighton JA, Das A, et al. Double-balloon enteroscopy and capsule endoscopy have comparable diagnostic yield in small-bowel disease: a meta analysis. Clin Gastroenterol Hepatol 2008;6:671–6.
56. Chen X, Ran ZH, Tong JL. A meta-analysis of the yield of capsule endoscopy compared to double-balloon enteroscopy in patients with small bowel diseases. World J Gastroenterol 2007;13:4372–8.
57. Eaton AC. Emergency surgery for acute colonic haemorrhage—a retrospective study. Br J Surg 1981;68:109.
58. Setya V, Singer JA, Minken SL. Subtotal colectomy as a last resort for unrelenting, unlocalized, lower gastrointestinal hemorrhage: experience with 12 cases. Am Surg 1992;58: 295.
59. Reuben BC, Stoddard G, Glasgow R, et al. Trends and predictors for vagotomy when performing oversew of acute bleeding duodenal ulcer in the United States. J Gastrointest Surg 2007;11:22.
60. Enestvedt BK, Gralnek IM, Mattek N, et al. An evaluation of endoscopic indications and findings related to nonvariceal upper-GI hemorrhage in a large multicenter consortium. Gastrointest Endosc 2008;67:422–9.
61. Barkun AN, Cockeram AW, Plourde V, et al. Review article: acid suppression in non-variceal acute upper gastrointestinal bleeding. Aliment Pharmacol Ther 1999;13:1565.
62. Graham DY, Hepps KS, Ramirez FC, et al. Treatment of Helicobacter pylori reduces the rate of rebleeding in peptic ulcer disease. Scand J Gastroenterol 1993;28:939.
63. Laine L, Cohen H, Brodhead J, et al. Prospective evaluation of immediate versus delayed refeeding and prognostic value of endoscopy in patients with upper gastrointestinal hemorrhage. Gastroenterology 1992;102: 314.
64. Lau JY, Sung JJ, Lam YH, et al. Endoscopic retreatment compared with surgery in patients with recurrent bleeding after initial endoscopic control of bleeding ulcers. N Engl J Med 1999;340:751.
65. Mirsadraee S, Tirukonda P, Nicholson A, et. al. Embolization for non-variceal upper gastrointestinal tract haemorrhage: a systematic review. Clin Radiol 2011;66:500–9.
66. Wong TC, Wong KT, Chiu PW, et al. A comparison of angiographic embolization with surgery after failed endoscopic hemostasis to bleeding peptic ulcers. Gastrointest Endosc 2011;73:900–8.
67. Gisbert JP, Khorrami S, Carballo F, et al. H. pylori eradication therapy vs. antisecretory non-eradication therapy (with or without long-term maintenance antisecretory therapy) for the prevention of recurrent bleeding from peptic ulcer. Cochrane Database Syst Rev 2004;(2):CD004062.
68. Gilliam AD, Speake WJ, Lobo DN, et al. Current practice of emergency vagotomy and Helicobacter pylori eradication for complicated peptic ulcer in the United Kingdom. Br J Surg 2003;90:88.
69. Chan VM, Reznick RK, O'Rourke K, et al. Meta-analysis of highly selective vagotomy versus truncal vagotomy and pyloroplasty in the surgical treatment of uncomplicated duodenal ulcer. Can J Surg 1994;37:457.
70. Csendes A, Braghetto I, Calvo F, et al. Surgical treatment of high gastric ulcer. Am J Surg 1985;149:765.
71. Cook DJ, Guyatt GH, Salena BJ, et al. Endoscopic therapy for acute nonvariceal upper gastrointestinal hemorrhage: a meta-analysis. Gastroenterology 1992;102:139.
72. Hartigan PM, Gebhard RL, Gregory PB. Sclerotherapy for actively bleeding esophageal varices in male alcoholics with cirrhosis. Gastrointest Endosc 1997;46:1.
73. Panes J, Teres J, Bosch J, et al. Efficacy of balloon tamponade in treatment of bleeding gastric and esophageal varices: results in 151 consecutive episodes. Dig Dis Sci 1988;33:454.
74. Avgerinos A, Nevens F, Raptis S, et al. Early administration of somatostatin and efficacy of sclerotherapy in acute oesophageal variceal bleeds: the European Acute Bleeding Oesophageal Variceal Episodes (ABOVE) randomised trial. Lancet 1997;350:1495.
75. Chavez-Tapia NC, Barrientos-Gutierrez T, Tellez-Avila FI, et al. Antibiotic prophylaxis for cirrhotic patients with upper gastrointestinal bleeding. Cochrane Database Syst Rev 2010;(9):CD002907.
76. Marti-Carvajal AJ, Karakitsiou DE, Salanti G. Human recombinant activated factor VII for upper gastrointestinal bleeding in patients with liver diseases. Cochrane Database Syst Rev 2012;(3):CD004887.
77. Khan S, Tudur Smith C, Williamson P, et al. Portosystemic shunts versus endoscopic therapy for variceal rebleeding in patients with cirrhosis. Cochrane Database Syst Rev 2006;(4):CD000553.
78. Warren WD, Henderson JM, Millikan WJ, et al. Distal splenorenal shunt versus endoscopic sclerotherapy for long-term management of variceal bleeding: preliminary report of a prospective, randomized trial. Ann Surg 1986;203:454.
79. Conn HO, Grace ND, Bosch J, et al. Propranolol in the prevention of the first hemorrhage from esophagogastric varices: a multicenter, randomized clinical trial. Hepatology 1991;13:902.
80. Groszmann RJ, Bosch J, Grace ND, et al. Hemodynamic events in a prospective randomized trial of propranolol versus placebo in the prevention of a first variceal hemorrhage. Gastroenterology 1990;99:1401.
81. Ryan BM, Stockbrugger RW, Ryan JM. A pathophysiologic, gastroenterologic, and radiologic approach to the management of gastric varices. Gastroenterology 2004;126: 1175.
82. Jaroszewski DE, Schlinkert RT, Gray RJ. Laparoscopic splenectomy for the treatment of gastric varices secondary to sinistral portal hypertension. Surg Endosc 2000;14:87.
83. Huang SP, Wang HP, Lee YC, et al. Endoscopic hemoclip placement and epinephrine injection for Mallory-Weiss syndrome with active bleeding. Gastrointest Endosc 2002; 55:842.
84. Park CH, Min SW, Sohn YH, et al. A prospective, randomized trial of endoscopic band ligation vs. epinephrine injection for actively bleeding Mallory-Weiss syndrome. Gastrointest Endosc 2004;60:22.

85. Metz CA, Livingston DH, Smith JS, et al. Impact of multiple risk factors and ranitidine prophylaxis on the development of stress-related upper gastrointestinal bleeding: a prospective, multicenter, double-blind, randomized trial. Crit Care Med 1993;21:1844.
86. Tryba M. Prophylaxis of stress ulcer bleeding: a meta-analysis. J Clin Gastroenterol 1991;13 Suppl 2:S44.
87. Kimata M, Kubota T, Otani Y, et al. Gastrointestinal stromal tumors treated by laparoscopic surgery: report of three cases. Surg Today 2000;30:177.
88. Wilhelm D, von Delius S, Burian M, et al. Simultaneous use of laparoscopy and endoscopy for minimally invasive resection of gastric subepithelial masses—analysis of 93 interventions. World J Surg 2008;32:1021–8.
89. Loftus EV, Alexander GL, Ahlquist DA, et al. Endoscopic treatment of major bleeding from advanced gastroduodenal malignant lesions. Mayo Clin Proc 1994;69:736.
90. Cameron AJ, Higgins JA. Linear gastric erosion: a lesion associated with large diaphragmatic hernia and chronic blood loss anemia. Gastroenterology 1986;91:338.
91. Stylopoulos N, Gazelle GS, Rattner DW. Paraesophageal hernias: operation or observation? Ann Surg 2002;236:492.
92. Norton ID, Petersen BT, Sorbi D, et al. Management and long-term prognosis of Dieulafoy lesion. Gastrointest Endosc 1999;50:762.
93. Stabile BE. Hemorrhagic complications of pancreatitis and pancreatic pseudocyst. In: Beger HG, Warshaw AL, Buchler MW, et al, editors. The pancreas: a clinical textbook. Oxford: Blackwell Scientific Publications; 1998. p. 606–13.
94. Sakorafas GH, Sarr MG, Farley DR. Hemosuccus pancreaticus complicating chronic pancreatitis: an obscure cause of upper gastrointestinal bleeding. Langenbecks Arch Surg 2000;385:124.
95. Lemos DW, Raffetto JD, Moore TC, et al. Primary aortoduodenal fistula: a case report and review of the literature. J Vasc Surg 2003;37:686.
96. Walker WE, Cooley DA, Duncan JM, et al. The management of aortoduodenal fistula by in situ replacement of the infected abdominal aortic graft. Ann Surg 1986;205:727.
97. Kotsis T, Lioupis C, Tzanis A, et al. Endovascular repair of a bleeding secondary aortoenteric fistula with acute leg ischemia: a case report and review of the literature. J Vasc Interv Radiol 2006;17:563.
98. Weiner FR, Simon DM. Gastric vascular ectases. Gastrointest Endosc Clin North Am 1996;6:681.
99. Mathis KL, Farley DR. Operative management of symptomatic duodenal diverticula. Am J Surg 2007;193:305.
100. Meyers MA, Alonso DR, Gray GF, et al. Pathogenesis of bleeding colonic diverticulosis. Gastroenterology 1976;71:577.
101. Jensen DM, Machicado GA, Jutabha R, et al. Urgent colonoscopy for the diagnosis and treatment of severe diverticular hemorrhage. N Engl J Med 2000;342:78.
102. Bloomfeld RS, Rockey DC, Shetzline MA. Endoscopic therapy of acute diverticular hemorrhage. Am J Gastroenterol 2001;96:2367.
103. McGuire HH Jr. Bleeding colonic diverticula: a reappraisal of natural history and management. Ann Surg 1994;220:653.
104. Longstreth GF. Epidemiology and outcome of patients hospitalized with acute lower gastrointestinal hemorrhage: a population-based study. Am J Gastroenterol 1997;92:419.
105. Zuckerman G, Benitez J. A prospective study of bidirectional endoscopy (colonoscopy and upper endoscopy) in the evaluation of patients with occult gastrointestinal bleeding. Am J Gastroenterol 1992;87:62.
106. Boley SJ, Sprayregen S, Sammartano RJ, et al. The pathophysiologic basis for the -angiographic signs of vascular ectasias of the colon. Radiology 1977;125:615.
107. Helmrich GA, Stallworth JR, Brown JJ. Angiodysplasia: characterization, diagnosis, and advances in treatment. South Med J 1990;83:1450.
108. Santos JC Jr, Aprilli F, Guimaraes AS, et al. Angiodysplasia of the colon: endoscopic diagnosis and treatment. Br J Surg 1998;75:256.
109. Peura DA, Lanza FL, Gostout CJ, et al. The American College of Gastroenterology. Bleeding Registry: preliminary findings. Am J Gastroenterol 1997;92:924.
110. Habr-Gama A, Waye JD. Complications and hazards of gastrointestinal endoscopy. World J Surg 1989;13:193.
111. Trowers EA, Ganga U, Rizk R, et al. Endoscopic hemorrhoidal ligation: preliminary clinical experience. Gastrointest Endosc 1998;48:49.
112. Chawla Y, Dilawari JB. Anorectal varices—their frequency in cirrhotic and non-cirrhotic portal hypertension. Gut 1991;32:309.
113. Robert JR, Sachar DB, Greenstein AJ. Severe gastrointestinal hemorrhage in Crohn's disease. Ann Surg 1991;213:207.
114. Crook J, Esche B, Futter N. Effect of pelvic radiotherapy for prostate cancer on bowel, bladder, and sexual function: the patient's perspective. Urology 1996;47:387.
115. Gaydos LA, Freireich EJ, Mantel N. The quantitative relation between platelet count and hemorrhage in patients with acute leukemia. N Engl J Med 1962;266:905.
116. Mittal R, Spero JA, Lewis JH, et al. Patterns of gastrointestinal hemorrhage in hemophilia. Gastroenterology 1985;88:515.
117. Theodoropoulou A, Koutroubakis IE. Ischemic colitis: clinical practive in diagnosis and treatment. World J Gastroenterol 2008;14:7302–8.
118. Chalasani N, Wilcox CM. Etiology and outcome of lower gastrointestinal bleeding in patients with AIDS. Am J Gastroenterol 1998;93:175.
119. Davies NM. Toxicity of nonsteroidal anti-inflammatory drugs in the large intestine. Dis Colon Rectum 1995;38:1311.
120. Holt S, Rigoglioso V, Sidhu M, et al. Nonsteroidal antiinflammatory drugs and lower gastrointestinal bleeding. Dig Dis Sci 1993;38:1619.

Acknowledgments

Figures 2 and 3 Christine Kenney

6 SURGICAL TREATMENT OF OBESITY AND METABOLIC SYNDROME

*Robert B. Dorman, MD, PhD, and Sayeed Ikramuddin, MD, FACS**

Why the Need for Bariatric Surgery?

Obesity is associated with increased morbidity and an increased incidence of comorbid illness. Failure of sustained weight loss following dietary therapy and the proven long-term success of weight loss surgery have driven the increasing popularity of bariatric operations in the United States. Emerging data regarding the improvements in metabolic disorders following bariatric surgery, such as type 2 diabetes mellitus (T2DM), are not explained simply by weight loss alone. The complex hormonal and molecular signaling changes encountered following many weight loss procedures today have resulted in increased popularity of the term "metabolic surgery" to describe the field more completely.

Definition of Obesity, Current Indications for Surgery, and the Metabolic Syndrome

Obesity is divided into three classes, with class I, II, and III obesity defined as a body mass index (BMI) of 30 to 34.9 kg/m², 35 to 39.9 kg/m², and 40 kg/m² or greater, respectively.[1] Morbid obesity encompasses those within class III or patients who are more than 100 pounds above ideal body weight. The National Institutes of Health Consensus Statement drafted in 1991 still dictates the criteria for who should undergo bariatric surgery.[2] Patients can undergo bariatric surgery if they have a BMI greater than or equal to 40 kg/m² or a BMI between 35 and 39 kg/m² if an additional major comorbidity is present. Major comorbidities include T2DM, hypertension, and obstructive sleep apnea (OSA). Since the release of this statement, the profound effects of bariatric surgery on metabolic diseases such as T2DM have been thoroughly documented[3–5]; also, several studies are currently under way to investigate the effects of various bariatric operations on T2DM in patients with a BMI less than 35 kg/m².

Metabolic syndrome involves the presence of multiple metabolic risk factors for the development of cardiovascular disease and T2DM. Specifically, hypertension, dyslipidemia, glucose intolerance, and central obesity cluster together to form metabolic syndrome.[6] To be officially diagnosed with metabolic syndrome, one must meet three of the five criteria presented in Table 1.[7] The diagnosis of metabolic syndrome carries increased mortality,[8,9] and weight loss is an effective method to manage this disease to reduce both cardiovascular risk and mortality. The impacts of bariatric surgery on all aspects of the metabolic syndrome are discussed separately in this chapter.

Medical Management of Obesity

Either alone or in combination, the global epidemic of obesity has not been well managed using behavior modification, dietary management, exercise, or pharmaceutical interventions. Medical management of obesity is clearly the mainstay and initial focus of treatment of both obesity and obesity-related comorbid illnesses. The impact of modest weight loss has been clearly shown. Lifestyle modification has also been shown to produce a robust 8.6% weight loss in the Look-AHEAD study at 1 year; however, by 4 years, there was significant weight regain.[10] However, this is a remarkably intense program that may be difficult to implement in clinical reality. Caloric restriction in addition to lifestyle modification produces even more significant weight loss, as much as 15.5% of total body weight[11]; however, a number of these studies demonstrate rapid regain of weight. Long-term follow-up in these studies has been a significant challenge.

Surgical Procedures: An Overview

Bariatric surgery has changed dramatically in the last several years. Over the last two decades, jejunoileal bypass and vertical banded gastroplasty have become obsolete. The Roux-en-Y gastric bypass (RYGB) has become the "gold standard." The quick rise of the adjustable gastric band (AGB) has been overcome by the introduction of vertical sleeve gastrectomy (VSG). The biliopancreatic diversion with duodenal switch (DS) has maintained a small but constant presence.

Procedures can be grouped into either restrictive, malabsorptive, or a combination of both. An example of a purely restrictive procedure would be the AGB. The VSG is also theoretically a purely restrictive procedure; however, there may be a hunger suppression effect following the VSG that far exceeds its restrictive value, possibly modulated through the hormone ghrelin.[12] The RYGB and DS work via restrictive mechanisms but also add a component of malabsorption. With the RYGB, the total intestinal bypass is typically no more than 250 cm but will involve most of the stomach and the entire duodenum, which will have a significant impact on iron, vitamin B_{12}, and calcium absorption. Given that folic acid is absorbed throughout the entire gastrointestinal tract, its absorption will be affected differentially. With the DS, the stomach and a small portion of ileum are in continuity, making vitamin B_{12} absorption less of a concern. Iron absorption following DS may be marginally improved compared with the RYGB given the small amount

* The authors and editors gratefully acknowledge the contributions of the previous authors, Eric DeMaria, MD, FACS, and Christopher Myers, MD, to the development and writing of this chapter.

Table 1 Diagnosis of Metabolic Syndrome

Measure	*Categorical Cut Points*
Elevated waist circumference	Population- and country-specific definitions
Elevated triglycerides (drug treatment for elevated triglycerides is an alternate indicator)	≥ 150 mg/dL (1.7 mmol/L)
Reduced HDL-C (drug treatment for reduced HDL-C is an alternate indicator)	< 40 mg/dL (1.0 mmol/L) in males; < 50 mg/dL (1.3 mmol/L) in females
Elevated blood pressure (antihypertensive drug treatment in a patient with a history of hypertension is an alternate indicator)	Systolic ≥ 130 and/or diastolic ≥ 85 mm Hg
Elevated fasting glucose (drug treatment of elevated fasting glucose is an alternate indicator)	≥ 100 mg/dL

Adapted from Alberti KGMM, Eckel RH, Grundy SM.[7]
HDL-C = high-density lipoprotein cholesterol.

of duodenum in continuity with the stomach. The presence of duodenum distal to the stomach may confer some protection against marginal ulceration.

OPEN PROCEDURES

In 2004, the number of laparoscopic gastric bypass operations exceeded that of open procedures according to a national audit of bariatric surgery performed at academic centers.[13] Open procedures are associated with larger incisions, greater postoperative pain, a greater number of wound-related complications, and a higher incidence of both readmission (2.6% versus 4.7%) and mortality (0.1% versus 0.3%) at 30 days.[14–16] In addition, laparoscopic procedures achieve comparable weight loss. However, open procedures have a role in select patients with previous intra-abdominal operations, particularly in patients undergoing revision bariatric surgery.

Preoperative Preparation

WEIGHT LOSS

The role of preoperative weight loss in perioperative outcomes has been a significant area of consideration in bariatric surgery over the past few years. Indeed, a major impetus for preoperative weight loss has come from insurance companies, presumably to ensure that patients have made adequate attempts at weight loss. This, however, has fallen out of favor. Rather, the focus has been more on demonstrating compliance preoperatively. Preoperative weight loss may be a means to ensure patient compliance with dietary regimens.

An emerging rationale is to improve perioperative safety by reducing the size of the liver. Liver size has been demonstrated in a number of studies to be impacted greatly by weight loss preoperatively, which can facilitate the laparoscopic approach.[17,18] Preoperative weight loss has other advantages, such as improving OSA, hyperglycemia, and other weight-related comorbid illnesses that can adversely affect the patient in the perioperative period. Whether long-term weight loss outcomes are impacted by preoperative weight loss is unclear.[19]

NUTRITION

The role of the nutritionist/dietitian in the bariatric surgery process has evolved significantly over recent years. Historically, it primarily included involvement in the immediate postoperative period alone. However, with the dramatic rise in the number of surgical procedures being performed and an increased awareness of possible nutritional complications, the role of the nutritionist or dietitian has become a vital component of both the pre- and the post-operative process. Nutritional assessment and the ongoing management of nutritional needs in surgical weight loss have both been shown to be an important correlate with long-term success.[20]

A comprehensive nutritional assessment should be completed preoperatively on all patients who are considering weight loss surgery. This assessment process is often initiated several months prior to surgery and may involve multiple visits with a dietitian or other qualified health professional. It is essential to determine any preexisting nutritional deficiencies and necessary diet interventions to assist with weight management or loss prior to surgery and to develop a plan for behavior modification in dietary intake postoperatively. The preoperative nutritional assessment should include weight history, medical history, laboratory values, psychological history, current dietary intake, eating behavior, current level of physical activity, and psychosocial components that may affect compliance postoperatively. A list of all recommended laboratory tests for patients undergoing bariatric surgery is provided in Table 2.

The dietitian must also prepare patients for surgery via education. Extensive counseling to ensure understanding of the planned procedure, guidelines for progression of diet consistency, postoperative dietary restrictions, and potential nutritional complications is critical. Patients must understand that weight loss surgery is only a tool and that modification of lifestyle is paramount to both successful weight loss and maintenance.

OBSTRUCTIVE SLEEP APNEA

OSA is a potentially fatal complication of morbid obesity. A diagnosis of OSA should be suspected when there is a history of loud snoring, frequent nocturnal awakening with

Table 2 Preoperative Laboratory Assessment for All Bariatric Patients

Lipid panel*
Comprehensive metabolic panel†
Complete blood count including platelets
Copper
Ferritin
Folic acid
Magnesium
Phosphorus
Parathyroid hormone
Vitamin A
Vitamin B_1
Vitamin B_6
Vitamin B_{12}
25-Hydroxyvitamin D (D_2 and D_3)
Zinc
Glycosylated hemoglobin‡
Random urine microalbumin‡

*Cholesterol, triglycerides, high-density lipoprotein with reflex to low-density lipoprotein when triglycerides are greater than 400 mg/dL.
†Sodium, potassium, chloride, carbon dioxide, creatinine, blood urea nitrogen, glucose, calcium, albumin, alkaline phosphatase, alanine aminotransferase, aspartate aminotransferase, total bilirubin, total protein.
‡Only if there is a preoperative history of diabetes or borderline diabetes.

air hunger, or daytime somnolence. The incidence of OSA is markedly higher in the obese population compared with the nonobese population and may be as high as 78%.[21,22] The pathogenesis of OSA is likely multifactorial and related, but not limited, to tongue volume; excessive fat deposits in the uvula, pharynx, and hypopharynx; increased airway length; a lower end-expiratory volume (often observed in obesity); and a larger neck circumference.[23] If OSA is suspected, then the patient should undergo preoperative polysomnography to confirm the diagnosis, and continuous positive airway pressure (CPAP) treatment should be initiated if indicated. In patients who are unable to tolerate CPAP, preoperative weight loss requires enhanced emphasis.

ANESTHESIA

Morbidly obese patients are at significant risk for complications from anesthesia, and obese patients with respiratory insufficiency are particularly prone to complications. An obese patient often has a short, fat neck and a heavy chest wall, which makes both intubation and ventilation a challenge.

A volume ventilator is required during operation on obese patients. Placing the patient in the reverse Trendelenburg position can expand total lung volume and facilitate ventilation.[24] The reverse Trendelenburg position increases lower extremity venous pressure and therefore mandates the use of intermittent sequential venous compression boots.

CARDIAC DISEASE

Morbidly obese patients are at significant risk for coronary artery disease as a result of an increased incidence of systemic hypertension, hypercholesterolemia, and diabetes. Because of this increased risk of cardiac dysfunction, preoperative electrocardiography should be performed on all obese patients 30 years of age or older.

Morbidly obese patients often have systemic hypertension, which can aggravate left ventricular dysfunction; however, mild left ventricular dysfunction can be documented in many morbidly obese patients in the absence of systemic hypertension. Circulating blood volume, plasma volume, and cardiac output increase in proportion to body weight.[25] Significant weight loss corrects pulmonary hypertension and the left ventricular dysfunction associated with respiratory insufficiency.[26,27]

PSYCHOLOGICAL ASSESSMENT

Clearly, obesity is associated with significant psychological burden, as are the comorbidities associated with obesity, particularly T2DM. The spectrum of preoperative psychological evaluation is an unclear one in terms of its true benefit to improving outcomes in patients. The mainstay of focus for preoperative evaluations is to demonstrate if (1) the patient has psychological stability, (2) there is an adequate support group, (3) the patient understands that lifestyle modifications are necessary to be successful, and (4) the patient understands the procedure and its risks and potential benefits. Therefore, the psychological evaluation should evaluate for all of these parameters.[28] Another important adjunct to the psychological evaluation is a detailed substance abuse history, which is typically not revealed during a routine history and physical examination by the bariatric surgeon. Another area that is stressed during the psychological assessment is any recent history of psychological instability such as psychiatric admissions or suicide attempts. Whether a Minnesota Multiphasic Personality Inventory (MMPI)[29] is necessary for this is not completely clear, and a number of inventories and questionnaires have not demonstrated a significant impact in outcomes following bariatric surgery, although this area remains controversial at best.

GASTROINTESTINAL EVALUATION

By and large, the RYGB is a remarkably effective operation for the treatment of gastroesophageal reflux disease (GERD), whether it is alkaline or acid based. Hiatal hernias can be fixed concomitantly, and even dysphagia, due to the significant impact on GERD, can be improved following the RYGB. With the AGB, the data are far less clear, but it may improve GERD, with overall improvements in Demeester scores postoperatively.[30,31] The presence of a hiatal hernia may complicate placement of the band, although this has not been demonstratively confirmed. Operations such as VSG and the DS may, at least temporarily, negatively impact the symptoms of GERD in patients due to their strong restrictive nature.[32]

A number of things need to be confirmed prior to the bariatric operation. Any patients with dysphagia, stricture, premalignant disease, or Barrett esophagus changes need to be carefully screened and evaluated before surgery. Patients with ulcer diathesis need to be screened for *Helicobacter pylori*, and this can be evaluated either through direct biopsy, stool analysis, or a breath test. Whether this should be a standard of care in all patients is unclear, but, certainly, patients with a known history of epigastric abdominal pain, a history of ulcer disease, or a history of gastritis should be screened and have this excluded; otherwise, it is not mandatory.

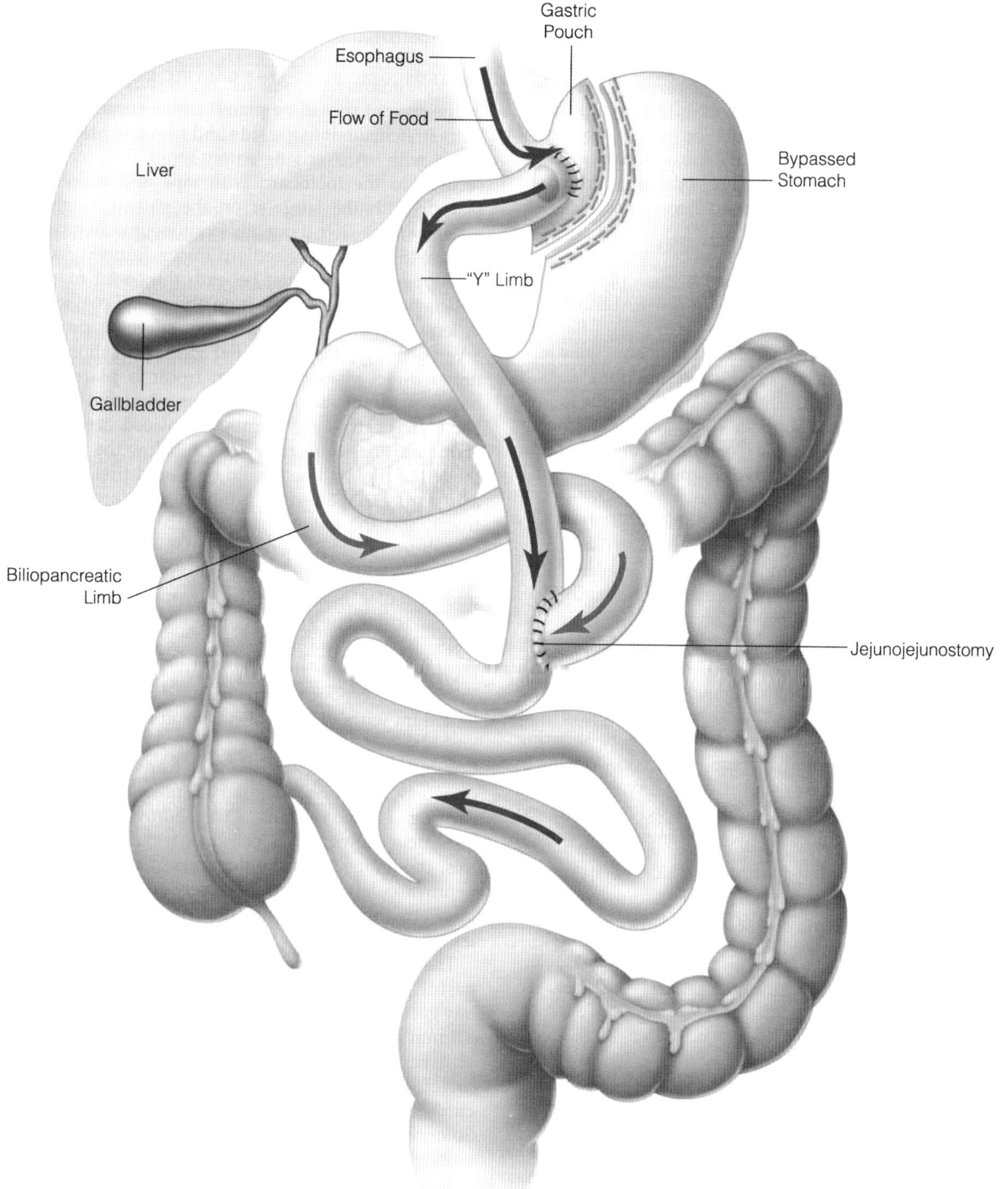

Figure 2 **Final anatomy following a Roux-en-Y gastric bypass.**

Return the operating room table to the reverse Trendelenberg position and place the back row of sutures along the gastrojejunostomy using an Endostitch suturing device (Covidien, Norwalk, CT) with 3-0 braided nylon [*see Figure 5*]. The posterior row should be a running seromuscular suture that begins at the angle of His on the gastric pouch and along the start of the mesentery on the Roux limb. The gastrotomy is made at the right, inferior portion of the gastric pouch using a Harmonic scalpel; an enterotomy is created at the corresponding point on the Roux limb. The goal is to create a gastrojejunostomy no larger than 2 cm in diameter; this is accomplished by placing a linear staple with a 3.5 mm staple cartridge into the pouch and the Roux limb no more than 2.0 cm [*see Figure 6*].

The assistant then moves to the head of the bed to place a 30 French endoscope into the pouch and into the Roux limb.

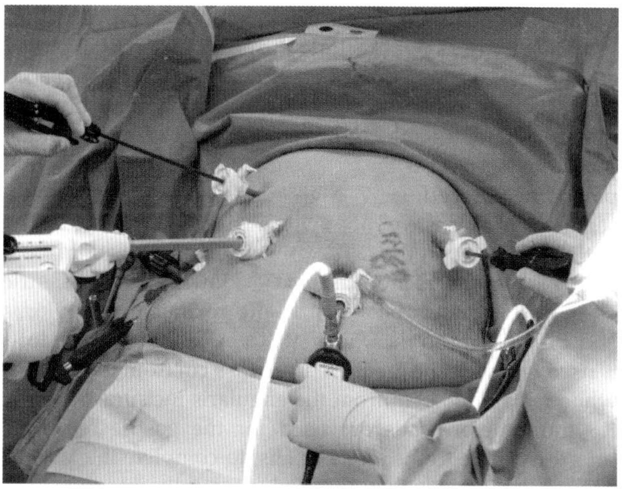

Figure 3 Final port placement for a Roux-en-Y gastric bypass. A 5 mm trocar is placed at the left upper quadrant (the site of Veress needle insufflations); an 11 mm trocar is placed 15 cm below the xiphoid just to the left of the midline; one 5 mm trocar is placed subcostally on the right at the midclavicular line; a 12 mm port is placed medial to the midclavicular line and just superior to the camera port; and a 5 mm trocar is placed in the patient's right flank to assist with liver retraction.

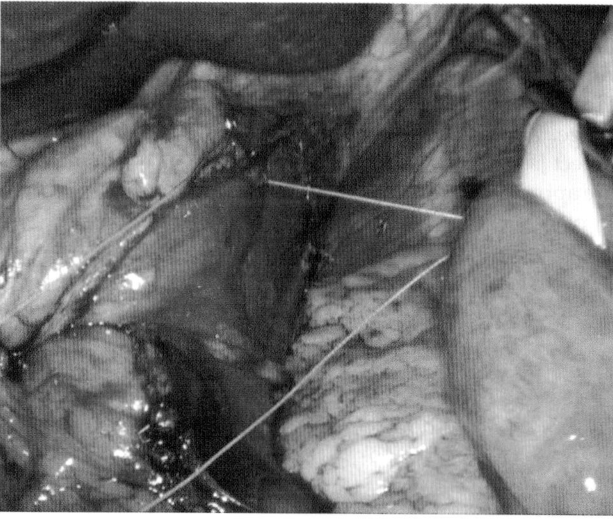

Figure 5 The first stitch creating the back wall of the gastrojejunostomy anastomosis. The Penrose drain is seen looped through the jejunum on the right. A running suture is started near the angle of His on the gastric pouch.

The defect is closed in two layers over the endoscope using an Endostitch. The jejunum is divided to the left of the anastomosis using a "white" staple load, and the Penrose drain is removed from the abdomen. The anastomosis should be tested for leak by placing a bowel clamp approximately 5 cm distal to the newly formed anastomosis and insufflating air through the endoscope while submerging the anastomosis in normal saline irrigation fluid. Defects should be oversewn if identified and the submersion process repeated.

We make a 150 cm Roux limb that is measured out from the gastrojejunostomy. The use of 150 cm is principally to avoid alkaline reflux. Weight loss differences beyond 2 years are not significantly different with shorter Roux limbs.[40]

The biliopancreatic limb is sutured to the Roux limb at the 150 cm point along their antimesenteric borders to form the back wall of the anastomosis. It is very important that extra caution be taken to be certain that the mesenteries are appropriately aligned to prevent twisting of the bowel. A functional side-to-side anastomosis is formed by making enterotomies in both the Roux limb and the biliopancreatic limb with a Harmonic scalpel. A 6 cm linear endostapler loaded with a white cartridge is inserted to its full length into each limb and fired. The heal of the anastomosis is secured with a single suture. The common enterotomy is closed with one additional white staple load using a 6 cm linear endostapler.

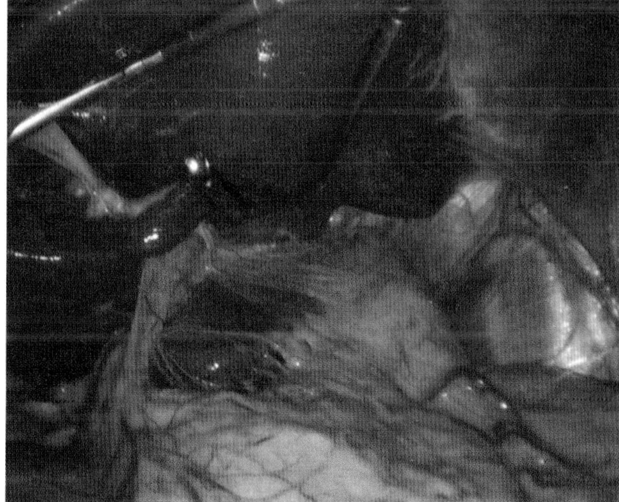

Figure 4 A laparoscopic view demonstrating the liver retractor in place elevating the left lobe of the liver anteriorly.

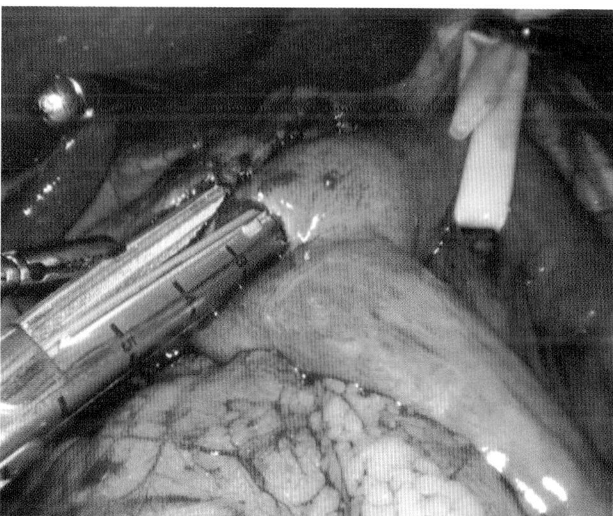

Figure 6 Creation of the gastrojejunostomy is performed using a linear endostapler with a 3.5 mm cartridge. The gastrojejunostomy should be about 2 cm in size.

effect are glucagonlike peptide–1 (GLP-1) and gastrointestinal inhibitory peptide (GIP). GLP-1 is secreted by the L cells, which are the neuroendocrine cells located in the ileum and colon. In response to a mixed meal, GLP-1 will augment the effect of insulin by impairing hepatic gluconeogenesis, increasing insulin secretion, attenuating the effect of pancreatic glucagon secretion, slowing gastric emptying, and directly impacting the hypothalamus to reduce hunger.[53,54] GIP is another widely recognized factor of insulin secretion, but its clinical implications in this setting are not well understood.

Although postprandial hyperglycemia may be addressed with more robust insulin secretion, patients following a gastric bypass, compared with the VSG or an AGB, demonstrate a more marked reduction in glucose levels very early after surgery. The mechanisms for this are quite unclear and poorly explored. Glucose and insulin dynamics are improved dramatically in a way that is consistent between the gastric bypass and equivalent caloric reduction. Although these studies are not well controlled, they certainly raise the interest for further investigation into this area. Thus, the importance of caloric restriction in this setting cannot be underemphasized. Also, following gastric bypass, patients have a marked reduction in hunger that may also contribute.[55]

Another putative factor is the hormone ghrelin, the "hunger hormone." Ghrelin is a 28–amino acid peptide that is secreted by the stomach and pancreas. Its exact function is unclear, but in its active form, ghrelin will induce hunger in humans. Ghrelin has a cyclical behavior that rises before and is reduced by ingestion of a mixed meal. The reduction in ghrelin is profound following both the gastric bypass and the VSG.[56] Long-term results are contradictory regarding ghrelin secretion patterns following gastric bypass procedures.[57]

Clearly, the most robust long-term results for T2DM improvement come from the most malabsorptive procedures. Although these have been demonstrated to have the most weight loss in comparative trials, it appears that the DS may have an augmented effect on reduction of HbA_{1C}, one of the key parameters for the control and management of T2DM. By its very nature, this operation involves malabsorption, and as such, it may be that malabsorption of certain types of fat known to increase insulin resistance, particularly ceramides, may impact insulin signaling at the level of muscle. It is important to understand that of the multiple tissue determinants of insulin resistance, which include fat, liver, and muscle, not to mention reduced glucose responsiveness at the level of the pancreas, muscle is the most important determinant of whole body insulin resistance. It is curious that regarding the most sophisticated studies, insulin resistance is not reduced early after bariatric surgery and that these changes are not seen until 6 months later. Tissue-specific measurements of insulin resistance after bariatric surgery comparing different operations or dietary interventions have not been thoroughly investigated.

IMPACT ON GERD

The effect of bariatric surgery on GERD is an important consideration in procedural selection. Of the four procedures considered primary, the gastric bypass, the VSG, the AGB, and the DS, relatively little is known about direct comparisons of the various operations to impact on GERD. Considering the band, patients tend to have initial improvement in GERD. Long-term GERD appears to be a potentially significant comorbid illness, potentially due to overtightening, particularly associated with nocturnal reflux. There have been no good studies evaluating concomitant repair of hiatal hernias as there tends to be a dichotomous approach to repair of these either to anterior plication of the cura or dissection posteriorly. The latter tends to be performed less commonly. It was accepted to be the definitive way to repair a hiatal hernia, principally because of concerns over slippage of the band, but this has never been substantiated. The VSG is an operation that clearly worsens GERD, at least initially, based on a number of studies.[58,59]

The RYGB demonstrates significant improvement in GERD, and although it is controversial, if a traditional antireflux surgery such as the Nissen fundoplication is compromised in its outcome on a morbidly obese patient, it is clear that the RYGB improves many other comorbid conditions beyond GERD. Although there are no clear head-to-head comparisons in assessing pH studies before and after the AGB and RYGB, there appears to be no significant change in the Demeester score following banding; however, a significant reduction in the Demeester score following the RYGB has been reported.[60] In comparing the RYGB with the DS, we expect there to be a similar increase in GERD following DS, at least initially, putatively related to the difficulty of passage of food through the narrow sleeve. Typically in a DS, the sleeve is a little larger, and alkaline contents will be diverted; however, in a study by Prachand and colleagues, it appears that GERD is significantly more prevalent in patients with a BMI greater than 50 kg/m^2 who undergo DS versus the gastric bypass.[61]

OUTCOMES ON SURVIVAL

Two long-term studies have examined long-term survival following bariatric surgery. The Swedish Obesity Study is a large prospective analysis comparing bariatric surgery with no surgery in morbidly obese patients.[43] With nearly 11 years of average follow-up, the Swedish Obesity Study found a significant mortality benefit for patients who underwent bariatric surgery with a mortality rate of 5% compared with 6.3% for obese patients who did not undergo weight loss surgery. Interestingly, there was also a significant decrease in mortality related to cardiovascular events and cancer among the surgery group. A study performed by Adams and colleagues examined mortality as well.[62] This study also found a significant survival advantage for obese patients who underwent weight loss surgery compared with those who did not. Other large-scale studies have not been able to show a significant survival advantage when the follow-up is less than 7 years.[63] Also of significance, death related to accidents and suicide is reported to be significantly greater among patients who undergo bariatric procedures.

OUTCOMES ON CANCER

Specifically addressing cancer-related deaths, Adams and colleagues at 7 years found a 60% reduction in cancer-related deaths among patients who underwent RYGB compared with matched BMI patients who did not undergo surgery.[62] With 11 years of average follow-up in the Swedish Obesity Study, the risk of death from cancer was significantly greater among patients who underwent surgery (1.4%) compared with those who did not (2.3%).[43] An additional study by Adams and colleagues reported that patients who underwent gastric bypass had a significantly lower incidence of cancer compared with obese, nonsurgical controls (hazard ratio0.76; 95% CI 0.65 to 0.89).[64] This study also found that patients who underwent gastric bypass had a reduction in cancer-related mortality of 46% compared with nonoperative controls.

Complications

MORTALITY AND READMISSION RATE

One of the greatest achievements in bariatric surgery over the past 20 years is the dramatic improvement in perioperative mortality rates. Recent publications place the 30-day mortality rate at 0.15%.[65,66] Readmission, however, continues to be a concern, especially in the era of payers imposing penalties on institutions for readmissions. At 1 year, readmission rates have been reported as high as 11.6% following gastric bypass, 6.7% following AGB, and 14.8% following DS.[49] Overall complication rates for the procedures at 1 year were 15.1%, 10%, and 40.7% for the gastric bypass, gastric band, and DS, respectively. These high complication rates associated with the DS preclude it from being the preferred procedure for weight loss despite its superior effect on metabolic diseases such as dyslipidemia and T2DM.

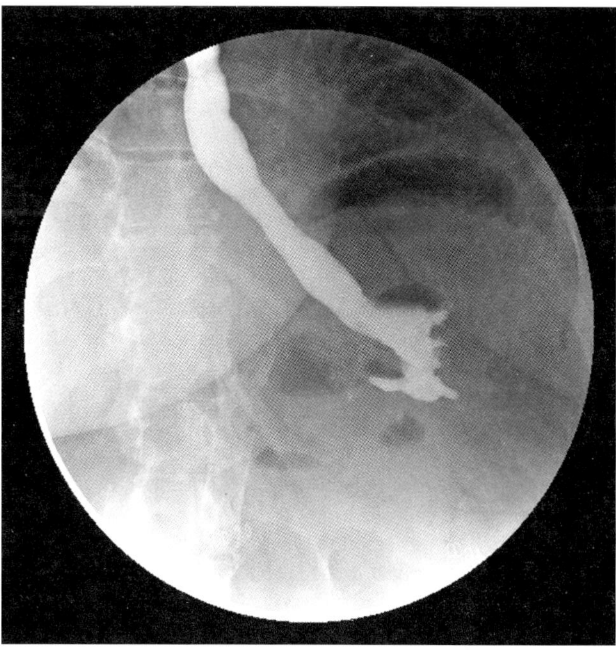

Figure 11 **An upper gastrointestinal study obtained as part of our routine postoperative workup on postoperative day 1, which shows clear extravasation of contrast out of the gastrointestinal lumen at the site of the gastrojejunal anastomosis.**

GASTROINTESTINAL LEAK

One of the most feared complications is a gastrointestinal leak occurring either at an anastomosis or a staple line [*see Figure 11*]. We recommend a routine upper gastrointestinal swallow study on all laparoscopic RYGB patients on the morning of postoperative day 1 prior to instituting a clear liquid diet. Increasing abdominal pain, peritoneal signs, and tachycardia should all raise suspicion for a leak. Early exploration is paramount to reduce the serious sequelae that can result from such an insult.

STRICTURE

Stricture formation can occur in up to 7% of patients following RYGB.[67,68] It is heralded by a discrete inability to progress in terms of dietary intake. The definitive diagnosis is made by performing an upper endoscopy, which should be as soon as possible to the time of presenting symptoms. Classically, the time of presentation is about 3 weeks after surgery but can be found later. Our standard approach to management of this is dilatation with a 12 mm 36 French balloon up to six atmospheres for 5 minutes. In many cases, fluoroscopic guidance is not necessary except with very tight strictures, in which case, a guide wire may be necessary to pass through the stricture. Upper gastrointestinal swallow evaluations have very little role in the acute management of these patients.

GASTRIC REMNANT DISTENTION

A surgical emergency in patients following RYGB that can occur is acute gastric remnant distention. Distention of the remnant can lead to gastric perforation or perforation of jejunojejunostomy. Presenting symptoms can include a bloated sensation, left shoulder pain, hiccups, and, if severe, shock. The diagnosis can be confirmed by a plain upright abdominal film, which may reveal a dilated stomach. If the stomach is fluid filled, CT may be necessary for diagnosis. Urgent percutaneous decompression performed by an interventional radiologist is appropriate, but if this option is not available, then the patient will require an emergent laparotomy with gastrostomy tube placement. At the time of exploration, the integrity of the jejunojejunostomy should be evaluated.

MARGINAL ULCER

Marginal ulceration is a common problem following RYGB, perhaps more so than any of the other bariatric procedures. Common causes for marginal ulceration include excessive use of nonsteroidal antiinflammatory agents, smoking, and possibly stress. It is difficult to control; however, removal of these risk factors is absolutely necessary. Placement of the patient on proton pump inhibitors is essential to control, as well as coating agents such as sucralfate. It is imperative that these be controlled as they certainly can progress to perforation anteriorly and chronic pain posteriorly. In many cases, admission to the hospital for intravenous proton inhibitors may be necessary with frequent endoscopies for monitoring.

INTERNAL HERNIA

The RYGB places patients at risk for internal hernia that can lead to bowel strangulation. Internal hernias can occur at locations where mesenteric defects are created, including the jejunojejunostomy, the transverse mesocolon if a retrocolic Roux limb is brought up to the gastric pouch, and through the Petersen defect, which is located posterior to the Roux limb between the Roux mesentery and the transverse mesocolon. Patients can present with periumbilical pain that is usually colicky in nature. Caution should be exercised with imaging at upper gastrointestinal contrast studies, and abdominal CT scans can be normal. Exploration is safest in these patients with recurring cramping and periumbilical pain. These defects should be closed at the time of primary operation to prevent the occurrence of internal hernia. The current internal hernia rate following laparoscopic gastric bypass is between 1 and 3%.[69]

DUMPING SYNDROME

Dumping syndrome is common after gastric bypass surgery and can be seen following sleeve gastrectomy. Sweating, flushing, weakness, tachycardia, palpitations, nausea, abdominal cramps, and loose stools are all signs and symptoms associated with dumping syndrome. Following RYGB, as many as 70% of patients will have some dumping symptoms, but less than 5% will have severe symptoms. Due to the loss of pylorus following RYGB, hyperosmotic food enters the jejunum more readily, resulting in fluid shifts and release of vasoactive substances such as serotonin. One to 3 hours after a meal, reactive hypoglycemia occurs and is generated by an exaggerated and prolonged insulin secretion. Most of these issues can be successfully treated with dietary advice, which includes small, frequent, dry meals with a low glycemic index and high protein. Medications are rarely needed to control symptoms, and most often symptoms improve over time.

GASTRIC BAND

There are three principal complications of the AGB that must be evaluated: slippage, erosion, and concentric dilatation. Slippage is the most common complication of the AGB and occurs in anywhere from 1 to 20% of cases.[70–72] In many instances, this is heralded by signs and symptoms of difficulty swallowing and left upper quadrant pain. In these patients, it is important to obtain a flat plate of the abdomen and upper gastrointestinal study, which can demonstrate a change in angulation of the band. There are two types of slippage: anterior and posterior. Since the advent of the pars flaccida approach, the patient is less likely to have posterior slippage. Anterior slippage, however, is quite common, and there are no bona fide techniques that have been studied to reduce their occurrence. Chronic slippage can result in excessive weight loss, which often complicates the care of patients, such that they would like to keep their band longer; however, it must be removed to facilitate appropriate esophageal emptying. Acute obstruction without relief from removal of the fluid of the band necessitates emergent surgery with reduction of the stomach and removal of the band. This must not be delayed to prevent gastric strangulation and perforation.

Erosion of the band into the stomach occurs less frequently, perhaps in 1 in 100 cases [*see Figure 12*]. Risk factors for erosion are unclear and can sometimes occur early, which may be related to a subclinical perforation. Late perforation is due to the buckle eroding into the stomach; therefore, it is advised to angulate and turn the buckle away from the greater curvature during implantation.

More worrisome long-term complications include concentric dilatation and esophageal dilatation. Indeed, concentric dilatation may be a precursor to esophageal dilatation. In effect, concentric dilatations represent equal dilatation of the pouch of the stomach as opposed to slippage, which is an asymmetrical dilatation. This is often the case in a patient who has excess fluid in the band, but it is a very difficult clinical entity to deal with as there is no clear point of slippage. Thus, it is necessary to remove the fluid from the band, reinitiate careful eating habits, and observe if this process continues. If the size of the pouch exceeds the edges of the band fluoroscopically, then the band will need to be removed. If the patient is otherwise well, conversion to a RYGB may be considered. Similarly, with esophageal dilatation, the fluid in the band should be removed and reimaging performed to ensure a return to normal anatomy. If a return to normal anatomy does not occur, the band should be removed. Further, bariatric surgery should not be performed until the esophagus has returned to normal as visualized via endoscopy and fluoroscopic imaging.

VERTICAL SLEEVE GASTRECTOMY

Complications of VSG principally include nausea and vomiting, which will resolve with time; esophageal reflux disease, which, in rare cases, can be incapacitating; and leakage. Management of a leak from the VSG represents a unique clinical problem, principally in that the leak is potentiated by a relative distal obstruction, usually between the angularis incisura and the staple line. It is imperative that this relative obstruction be managed using either stents or indwelling tubes such as a T tube, which goes percutaneously through the leak and past the angularis incisura. Management of these leaks can be quite challenging, and adequate drainage of the abscess and adequate nutrition are essential for the healing process.

Failure of Bariatric Surgery and Revision

Failure of bariatric procedures is one of the most vexing problems that the bariatric surgeon has to manage. Failure can be defined in a number of ways, such as less than 30% excess weight loss or not achieving a BMI less than 35 kg/m^2.[73] Multiple additional definitions exist that are relative to the preoperative BMI. Perhaps the single most understood preoperative factor that is related to failure long term is the preoperative BMI.[40,74] Superobese patients, with a BMI greater than 50 kg/m^2, tend to do the worst and as a result are more likely suited for the most malabsorptive procedure (i.e., the DS) based on weight criteria alone. Revision surgery is clearly associated with more complications, and outcomes in terms of weight loss are mixed.[75–79] It is important to note that preoperative consideration for such procedures needs to be discussed thoroughly as these procedures carry a higher postoperative morbidity risk.

The approach to revisions is determined by either the presence of complications, the failure of weight loss, or both. Approaches for the different operations are varied; with

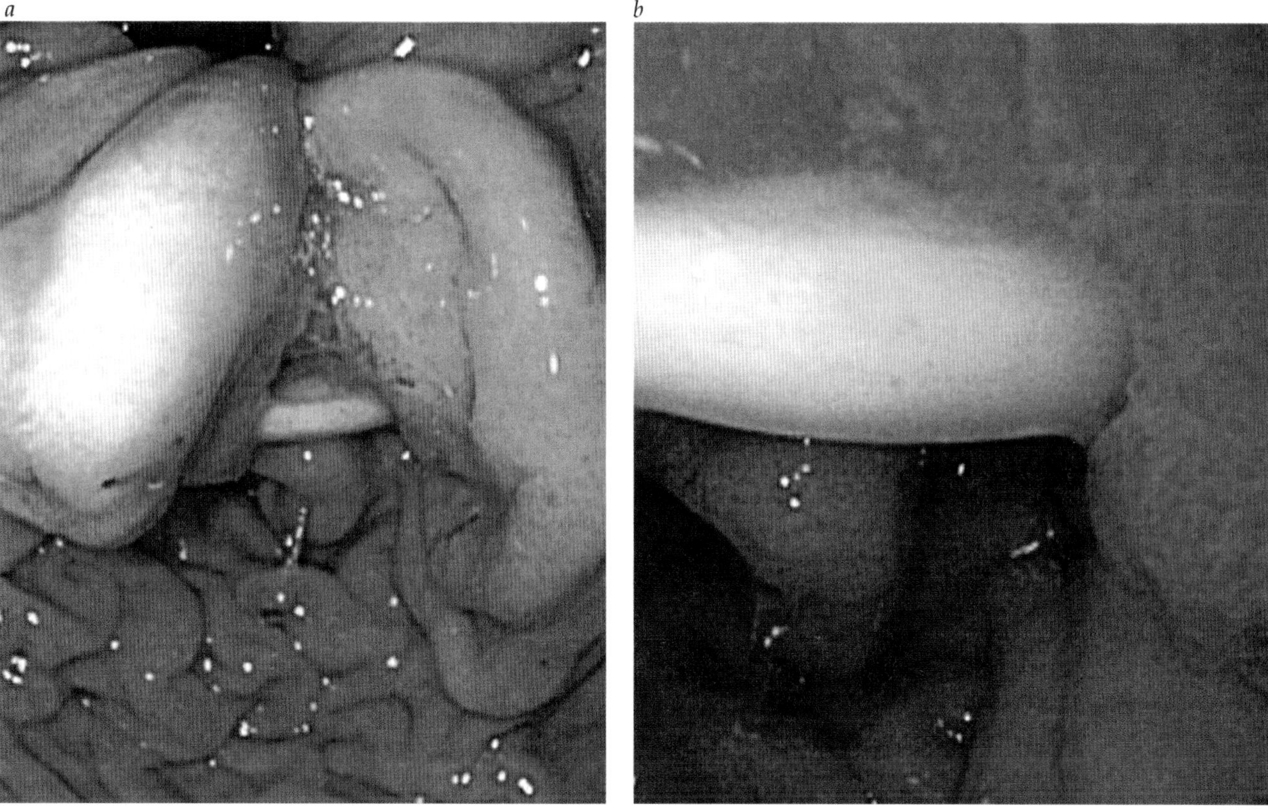

Figure 12 **Two photographs (*a* and *b*) from the same patient of an adjustable gastric band that has eroded into the stomach.**

banding, for example, management is rather straightforward. Patients who have had slippages, outright failure, or technical problems with the band are best suited to having a conversion to either RYGB or DS. Although studies of outcomes are relatively small, evidence points to excellent outcomes with either of these operations[80–82]; the choice of revision procedure should be based on both comorbid illnesses and preoperative weight.

Failure of the RYGB, on the other hand, is a far more vexing problem. Different options include revision of the RYGB in its entirety, which carries a high risk without clear clinical benefit.[83] In the case of a large gastric pouch (i.e., greater than three times normal) or gastrogastric fistula, revision might be considered, especially with the presence of concomitant complications such as ulceration. Another option is conversion to a long-limb RYGB. This operation has been performed extensively in the past, but the outcome in terms of protein malnutrition is significant.[84] Notably, malnutrition can occur in the absence of significant weight loss, which can make the clinical picture confusing.[85,86] A much more palatable option for those patients who have recurrent T2DM following gastric bypass is conversion to a DS if they still have the ability to secrete adequate levels of insulin. The prospect of this is certainly daunting and should be carried out only in specialized centers, but it may produce long-term demonstrable improvement in T2DM.[87] In any event, this decision should be thoroughly discussed with the patient who has demonstrated the ability to follow up in clinic preoperatively before these considerations have been made. Although appealing, a simple reduction in the stomach pouch size, unless extremely large (greater than three times normal size), using endoscopic techniques or other methods has demonstrated no benefit long term and at this point should be considered experimental. The current climate of medical care is to perform one weight loss procedure per lifetime. As such, the goal is to avoid revision procedures in their entirety by choosing the right procedures for the right patient at the outset.

Evaluation of Old Procedures

Often a surgeon will see patients following either a jejunoileal bypass or vertical banded gastroplasty presenting for complications or for simple failure of weight loss. In the case of the jejunoileal bypass, these patients tend to be considerably older as this operation has not been performed routinely for many years in the United States; however, these patients can suffer significant problems, with arthralgias, skin rashes, hepatic and renal failure, and bacterial overgrowth issues. In these cases, it is routine to either reverse these operations or convert to another bariatric procedure. In patients who are suffering from significant metabolic compromises, reversal is the best option; however, it must be stressed that these patients may have significant differences in bowel caliber, which can make these very technically difficult. For vertical banded gastroplasty, many of these patients will present with complications, such as GERD, with loss of tooth enamel and maladaptive eating. Some patients

adults with type 2 diabetes mellitus and body mass index <35 kg/m(2). Surgery 2011;150:684.
52. Creutzfeldt W, Ebert R. New developments in the incretin concept. Diabetologia 1985;28:565.
53. Nauck MA. Incretin-based therapies for type 2 diabetes mellitus: properties, functions, and clinical implications. Am J Med 2011;124:S3.
54. Drucker DJ, Nauck MA. The incretin system: glucagon-like peptide-1 receptor agonists and dipeptidyl peptidase-4 inhibitors in type 2 diabetes. Lancet 2006;368:1696.
55. le Roux CW, Aylwin SJ, Batterham RL, et al. Gut hormone profiles following bariatric surgery favor an anorectic state, facilitate weight loss, and improve metabolic parameters. Ann Surg 2006;243:108.
56. Lee WJ, Chen CY, Chong K, et al. Changes in postprandial gut hormones after metabolic surgery: a comparison of gastric bypass and sleeve gastrectomy. Surg Obes Relat Dis 2011;7:683–90.
57. Martins C, Kjelstrup L, Mostad IL, et al. Impact of sustained weight loss achieved through Roux-en-Y gastric bypass or a lifestyle intervention on ghrelin, obestatin, and ghrelin/obestastin ratio in morbidly obese patients. Obes Surg 2011; 21:751.
58. Carter PR, Leblanc KA, Hausmann MG, et al. Association between gastroesophageal reflux disease and laparoscopic sleeve gastrectomy. Surg Obes Relat Dis 2011;7:569.
59. Himpens J, Dobbeleir J, Peeters G. Long term results of laparoscopic sleeve gastrectomy for obesity. Ann Surg 2010; 252:319.
60. Patterson EJ, Davis DG, Khajanchee Y, Swanstrom LL. Comparison of objective outcomes following laparoscopic Nissen fundoplication versus laparoscopic gastric bypass in the morbidly obese with heartburn. Surg Endosc 2003;17; 1561–5.
61. Prachand VN, Ward M, Alverdy JC. Duodenal switch provides superior resolution of metabolic comorbidities independent of weight loss in the super-obese (BMI > or = 50 kg/m2) compared with gastric bypass. J Gastrointest Surg 2010;14:211.
62. Adams TD, Gress RE, Smith SC, et al. Long-term mortality after gastric bypass surgery. N Engl J Med 2007;357:753.
63. Maciejewski ML, Livingston EH, Smith VA, et al. Survival among high-risk patients after bariatric surgery. JAMA 2011;305:2419.
64. Adams TD, Stroup AM, Gress RE, et al. Cancer incidence and mortality after gastric bypass surgery. Obesity 2009;17: 796.
65. Longitudinal Assessment of Bariatric Surgery Consortium. Perioperative safety in the longitudinal assessment of bariatric surgery. N Engl J Med 2009;361:445.
66. Dorman RB, Abraham A, Al-Refaie WB, et al. Bariatric surgery outcomes in the elderly: an ACS NSQIP study. J Gastrointest Surg 2012;16(1):35–44.
67. Takata MC, Ciovica R, Cello JP, et al. Predictors, treatment, and outcomes of gastrojejunostomy stricture after gastric bypass for morbid obesity. Obes Surg 2007;17:878.
68. Carrodeguas L, Szomstein S, Zundel N, et al. Gastrojejunal anastomotic strictures following laparoscopic RYGB surgery: analysis of 1291 patients. Surg Obes Relat Dis 2006;2: 92.
69. Higa KD, Ho T, Boone KB. Internal hernias after laparoscopic Roux-en-Y gastric bypass: incidence, treatment and prevention. Obes Surg 2003;13:350.
70. Stroh C, Hohmann U, Schramm H, et al. Fourteen-year long-term results after gastric banding. J Obes 2011;2011: 128451.
71. Suter M, Calmes JM, Paroz A, et al. A 10-year experience with laparoscopic gastric banding for morbid obesity: high long-term complication and failure rates. Obes Surg 2006;16: 829.
72. Egan RJ, Monkhouse SJ, Meredith HE, et al. The reporting of gastric band slip and related complications; a review of the literature. Obes Surg 2011;21:1280.
73. Biron S, Hould FS, Label S, et al. Twenty years of biliopancreatic diversion: what is the goal of the surgery? Obes Surg 2004;14:160.
74. Chevallier JM, Paita M, Rodde-Dunet MH, et al. Predictive factors of outcome after gastric banding: a nationwide survey on the role of center activity and patients' behavior. Ann Surg 2007;246:1034.
75. Sanchez H, Cabrera A, Cabrera K, et al. Laparoscopic Roux-en-Y gastric bypass as a revision procedure after restrictive bariatric surgery. Obes Surg 2008;18:1539.
76. Weiss HG, Kirchmayr W, Klaus A, et al. Surgical revision after failure of laparoscopic adjustable gastric banding. Br J Surg 2004;91:235.
77. Gagné DJ, Dovec E, Urbandt JE. Laparoscopic revision of vertical banded gastroplasty to Roux-en-Y gastric bypass: outcome of 105 patients. Surg Obes Relat Dis 2011;7:493.
78. Fronza JS, Prystowsky JB, Hungness ES, et al. Revisional bariatric sugery at a single institution. Am J Surg 2010;200: 651.
79. Parikh M, Heacock L, Gagner M. Laparoscopic "gastrojejunal sleeve reduction" as a revision procedure for weight loss failure after Roux-en-Y gastric bypass. Obes Surg 2011; 21:650.
80. Ardestani A, Lautz DB, Tavakkolizadeh A. Band revision versus Roux-en-Y gastric bypass conversion as a salvage operation after laparoscopic adjustable gastric banding. Surg Obes Relat Dis 2011;7:33.
81. Moore R, Perugini R, Czerniach D, et al. Early results of conversion of laparoscopic adjustable gastric band to Roux-en-Y gastric bypass. Surg Obes Relat Dis 2009;5:439.
82. Topart P, Becouarn G, Ritz P. Biliopancreatic diversion with dudodenal switch or gastric bypass for failed gastric banding: retrospective study from two institutions with preliminary results. Surg Obes Relat Dis 2007;3:521.
83. Griffen WO Jr, Bivins BA, Bell RM, et al. Gastric bypass for morbid obesity. World J Surg 1981;5:817.
84. Sugerman HJ, Kellum JM, DeMaria EJ. Conversion of proximal to distal gastric bypass for failed gastric bypass for superobesity. J Gastrointest Surg 1997;1:517.
85. Rawlins ML, Teel D II, Hedgcorth K, et al. Revision of Roux-en-Y gastric bypass to distal bypass for failed weight loss. Surg Obes Relat Dis 2011;7:45.
86. Kellum JM, Chikunguwo SM, Maher JW, et al. Long-term results of malabsorptive distal Roux-en-Y gastric bypass in superobese patients. Surg Obes Relat Dis 2011;7:189.
87. Parikh M, Pomp A, Gagner M. Laparoscopic conversion of failed gastric bypass to duodenal switch: technical considerations and preliminary outcomes. Surg Obes Relat Dis 2007;3:611.

88. Institute of Medicine (US) and National Research Council (US) Committee to Reexamine IOM Pregnancy Weight Guidelines. Weight gain during pregnancy: reexamining the guidelines. Washington, DC: National Academic Press; 2009.
89. Maggard MA, Yermilov I, Li Z, et al. Pregnancy and fertility following bariatric surgery: a systematic review. JAMA 2008;300:2286.
90. Patel JA, Patel NA, Shinde T, et al. Endoscopic retrograde cholangiopancreatography after laparoscopic Roux-en-Y gastric bypass: a case series and review of the literature. Am Surg 2008;74:689.

Acknowledgments

Figures 1, 2, 8, and 9 Christine Kenney

7 TUMORS OF THE STOMACH, DUODENUM, AND SMALL BOWEL

Karl Y. Bilimoria, MD, MS, Mark S. Talamonti, MD, FACS, and Jeffrey D. Wayne, MD, FACS

Gastric Adenocarcinoma

The incidence of gastric carcinoma exhibits significant geographic variability. The disease is most common in Japan and China, and high rates of occurrence have also been reported in Central and South America, eastern Europe, and parts of the Middle East.[1] In most of the more developed nations, however, gastric carcinoma is relatively uncommon. The overall incidence of this condition has decreased in the past few decades, but gastric carcinoma remains the second leading cause of cancer death worldwide. The reported reductions in gastric cancer mortality appear to be linked to better refrigeration and a concomitant decrease in the intake of salted, pickled, smoked, and chemically preserved foods. An inverse association with the consumption of fresh fruits and vegetables has also been noted.[2]

Gastric cancer occurs 1.5 to 2.5 times more frequently in males than in females. It is rarely diagnosed before the age of 40, and its incidence peaks in the seventh decade of life. African Americans, Hispanic Americans, and Native Americans are two times more likely to have gastric cancer than white Americans are.[3]

In the United States in particular, the incidence of stomach cancer has fallen substantially over the past 70 years.[4] Whereas this disease was once a leading cause of cancer-related death in the United States, it now ranks 13th among major causes. Unfortunately, the decline in incidence has not translated into an improvement in the 5-year survival rate.[5] Across all races, the 5-year relative survival was 23% for the period extending from 1992 to 1999.[3] This result is probably related to the advanced stage at which most patients present. A 2000 study from the National Cancer Data Base found that 55% of patients with gastric cancer presented with locally advanced or metastatic disease.[6] Resection rates ranged from 40 to 60%, and 5-year survival rates after resection with curative intent were directly related to stage at presentation. For stage IA disease, the survival rate was 78%; for stage IB, 58%; for stage II, 34%; for stage IIIA, 20%; for stage IIIB, 8%; and for stage IV, 7%.

Another relevant change in the epidemiology of gastric cancer is a shift in the distribution of primary lesion sites within the stomach. In the first quarter of the 20th century, two thirds of gastric cancers were located in the antrum and the prepyloric area and only 10% arose in the cardia or the esophagogastric junction. Since the 1970s, however, adenocarcinoma of the proximal stomach has become increasingly common. In one study, the incidence of adenocarcinoma of the gastric cardia rose from 29.1 to 52.2% in the period between 1984 and 1993.[7] In another study, which included 18,365 gastric cancer patients from Commission on Cancer–approved hospitals, 31% of tumors were found to be in the proximal stomach, compared with only 26% in the distal third.[8] In the United States, carcinoma of the cardia occurs primarily in whites, with a male-to-female ratio of approximately 2:1. Cancer of the cardia appears to be distinct from adenocarcinoma of the distal esophagus, which frequently arises in the setting of Barrett esophagus.[9] Associations have also been reported between cancer of the gastric cardia and infection with *Helicobacter pylori* or Epstein-Barr virus.[10,11]

CLASSIFICATION

Adenocarcinoma of the stomach may be divided into two histologic subtypes, intestinal and diffuse.[12] Each subtype has unique pathologic, epidemiologic, etiologic, and prognostic [illegible] in the distal stomach (often after a long precancerous phase), is more common in elderly patients, and has been closely associated with atrophic gastritis and diets high in nitrates and nitrose compounds.[13] The characteristic histologic finding is cohesive neoplastic cells that form glandlike tubular structures. The diffuse subtype occurs more frequently in younger patients and has no identifiable precursor lesion. It may develop in any part of the stomach but shows a predilection for the cardia. Cell cohesion is absent; thus, individual cancer cells infiltrate and thicken the stomach wall without forming a discrete ulcer or mass.

In general, the prognosis for the diffuse subtype is worse than that for the intestinal subtype. Whereas intestinal lesions are seen more frequently in regions with a high incidence of gastric cancer, the incidence of diffuse lesions is constant among various populations throughout the world.[14] Accordingly, the overall decline in gastric cancer over the past century has been attributed to a decline in intestinal lesions and to a decline in the incidence of *H. pylori* infection (see below).

RISK FACTORS

Historical studies of specimens obtained during operation or at autopsy suggest that gastric carcinoma, especially of the intestinal subtype, frequently develops in the presence of chronic atrophic gastritis and associated intestinal metaplasia. It has generally been assumed that adenocarcinoma of the distal stomach progresses from chronic gastritis to metaplasia through the teratogenic influence of environmental factors. The most commonly studied environmental factors are the nitrates and nitrose compounds present in high levels in salted, smoked, or pickled foods consumed in areas where gastric cancer is endemic.[15] To date, however, no prospective studies have conclusively demonstrated that modern refrigeration practices and the subsequent decline in the salting, smoking, and pickling of food have been responsible for the relative decline in intestinal gastric cancer. Furthermore, the intestinal subtype may arise in the absence of metaplasia. Finally, the emergence of chronic infection with *H. pylori* as the dominant risk factor for gastric adenocarcinoma has challenged the paradigm of the atrophic gastritis–intestinal metaplasia–gastric cancer sequence.

Epidemiologic studies across various populations worldwide have consistently demonstrated a strong association between *H. pylori* infection and gastric cancer.[16] Prospective serologic studies have confirmed that persons with evidence of such infection are three to six times more likely to have gastric cancer than persons who are seronegative.[17] Still, only a very small fraction of infected persons develop gastric cancer. It has been estimated that more than half of the world's inhabitants may be infected with *H. pylori*—a number that dwarfs the actual incidence of gastric cancer. What is clear is that *H. pylori* infection of the gastric mucosa leads to a state of chronic active inflammation that lasts for decades. This inflammatory process appears to be modulated by multiple forces, including genetic and environmental factors.[18] Inherited traits may confer susceptibility or resistance to carcinogenesis. Indeed, first-degree relatives of gastric cancer patients have a two to three times higher relative risk of contracting the disease.[19] Gastric irritants may act as promoters, and antioxidants may have a protective effect (which may be part of the reason for the reduced risk of gastric cancer associated with diets rich in fruits and vegetables).[20]

Unlike intestinal cancers, diffuse cancers appear not to be associated with *H. pylori* infection. Diffuse adenocarcinoma of the stomach is more common in young patients and has no known precursor lesion.[9] The incidence of genetically associated diffuse cancers is estimated to be in the range of 5 to 10%.[19] Familial cases of diffuse gastric cancer occur at an average age of 38 years and are inherited in an autosomal dominant fashion with 70% penetrance.[21] Patients with blood group A have a 16 to 20% increased risk of gastric cancer.[22]

CLINICAL EVALUATION

In high-risk areas (e.g., Japan), mass screening programs have been successful in identifying early gastric cancer, which is generally amenable to surgical cure.[23] In fact, in some Japanese studies, as many as 40% of newly diagnosed patients had early gastric cancer. Unfortunately, in Western countries, the disease is almost always diagnosed relatively late, when it is locally advanced or metastatic. When it is superficial, gastric cancer typically produces no symptoms. As it progresses, however, a constellation of vague, nonspecific symptoms may develop, including anorexia, fatigue, weight loss, and epigastric discomfort. Dysphagia, early satiety, vomiting, and hematemesis also are seen, albeit rarely; when present, they often indicate advanced disease. Indeed, early gastric cancer has no characteristic physical findings, and many patients are not diagnosed until they present with jaundice, ascites, or a palpable mass, all of which signal incurable disease. Although rare, certain physical examination findings are indicative of metastases, including the Virchow node (left supraclavicular lymph node), Sister Mary Joseph nodule (periumbilical metastasis), Irish node (axillary lymph node), and Blumer shelf (metastases palpable on a rectal examination in the rectouterine or rectovesical space).

INVESTIGATIVE STUDIES

Until comparatively recently, an upper gastrointestinal (GI) series was often the first diagnostic test ordered to evaluate symptoms related to the upper GI tract. However, even with double-contrast techniques, which allow improved visualization of mucosal detail, false negative rates as high as 25% were reported, especially with small lesions (i.e., 5 to 10 mm).[24] Accordingly, in most large series, fiberoptic endoscopy with biopsy has replaced contrast radiography as the primary diagnostic technique.[25] Upper GI endoscopy with biopsy has been reported to have a diagnostic accuracy of 95%.[20] However, false negatives have been reported, especially in the context of inadequate biopsies. Thus, it is recommended that at least four biopsies be taken from the region of any atypical findings.[26]

STAGING

Two major classification systems are available for staging gastric cancer. The first is the one used in Japan, where gastric cancer is staged according to the general rules for gastric study in surgery and pathology published by the Japanese Research Society for Gastric Cancer (JRSGC).[27] This elaborate system focuses on the anatomic involvement of specifically numbered lymph node stations. The second system is the one generally used in Western countries—namely, the familiar tumor-node-metastasis (TNM) system developed by the American Joint Committee on Cancer (AJCC) and the International Union Against Cancer (UICC) [*see Table 1 and Table 2*].[28] The AJCC/UICC staging system is based on a gastric cancer database and classifies lesions according to the depth to which the primary tumor penetrates the gastric wall, the extent of lymph node involvement, and the presence or absence of distant metastases.

The primary goal in the evaluation of gastric cancer patients is to stratify them into two clinical stage groups: those with locoregional disease (AJCC stages I to III) and those with systemic disease (AJCC stage IV).[29] The National Comprehensive Cancer Network (NCCN) has developed consensus guidelines for the clinical evaluation and staging of patients with possible gastric cancer. These guidelines are accessible to any practitioner via the Internet (http://www.nccn.org/) and are updated annually. Multidisciplinary evaluation is recommended for all patients. A careful history is obtained and a thorough physical examination is performed, with special attention paid to performance status and to comorbid conditions that might preclude operative intervention. Initial laboratory studies include a complete blood cell count with a platelet count; determination of serum electrolyte, blood urea nitrogen, creatinine, and glucose concentrations; and a liver function panel. Chest radiography is performed, along with computed tomography (CT) of the abdomen and pelvis.

Whereas CT is invaluable for detecting ascites, bulky adenopathy, and significant visceral metastases, its overall accuracy in staging tumors is modest: only 70% for advanced lesions and 44% for early lesions.[30] CT assesses lymph node involvement primarily on the basis of node size. Thus, its sensitivity for N1 and N2 disease is low, ranging from 24 to 43%; however, its specificity is high, approaching 100%.

Table 1 American Joint Committee on Cancer TNM Clinical Classification of Gastric Carcinoma, 7th Edition[96]

Primary tumor (T)	TX	Primary tumor cannot be assessed
	T0	No evidence of primary tumor
	Tis	Carcinoma in situ: intraepithelial tumor without invasion of lamina propria
	T1	Tumor invades lamina propria, muscularis mucosae, or submucosa T1a: Tumor invades lamina propria or muscularis mucosae T1b: Tumor invades submucosa
	T2	Tumor invades muscularis propria
	T3	Tumor penetrates subserosal connective tissue without invasion of visceral peritoneum or adjacent structures
	T4a	Tumor invades serosa (visceral peritoneum)
	T4b	Tumor invades adjacent structures
Regional lymph nodes (N)	NX	Regional lymph node(s) cannot be assessed
	N0	No regional lymph node metastasis
	N1	Metastasis in 1–2 regional lymph nodes
	N2	Metastasis in 3–6 regional lymph nodes
	N3	Metastasis in 7 or more regional lymph nodes N3a: Metastasis in 7–15 regional lymph nodes N3b: Metastasis in 16 or more regional lymph nodes
Distant metastasis (M)	M0	No distant metastasis
	M1	Distant metastasis

Technical advances, such as spiral (helical) CT with intravenous contrast plus appropriate gastric distention with 600 to 800 mL of water (a negative contrast agent), have allowed modest improvements in overall staging with CT [*see Figure 1*]. Although improving, CT is still limited in its ability to evaluate peritoneal disease and liver metastases smaller than 5 mm.[31]

Given the limitations of CT, in the absence of obvious metastatic disease, locoregional staging with endoscopic ultrasonography (EUS) is vital for accurately assessing tumor penetration through the gastric wall (T stage) and ascertaining whether regional nodes (N stage) or even mediastinal or para-aortic lymph nodes may be involved [*see Figure 2*]. EUS is unique among imaging modalities in its ability to image the gastric wall as a five-layer structure, with each layer correlating with an actual histologic layer.[32] The overall accuracy of EUS in determining the extent of infiltration ranges from 67 to [illegible]%.[33] EUS features that suggest lymph node metastasis include a rounded shape, hypoechoic patterns, and a size larger than 1 cm. In one study comparing preoperative findings from EUS with pathologic findings at operation, EUS was 100% sensitive for N0 disease and 66.7% sensitive for N1 disease.[34] EUS also allows identification and aspiration of small-volume ascites. If cytologic study of the ascitic fluid so obtained confirms the presence of malignant cells, the patient is considered to have metastatic disease and therefore is not eligible for curative-intent surgery. For all of these reasons, EUS is now widely accepted as superior to conventional CT in the regional staging of gastric cancer.[9]

Table 2 American Joint Committee on Cancer Staging of Gastric Carcinoma, 7th Edition[96]

Stage	Tumor	Node	Metastasis
0	Tis	N0	M0
IA	T1	N0	M0
IB	T1 T2	N1 N0	M0 M0
IIA	T1 T2 T3	N2 N1 N0	M0 M0 M0
IIB	T1 T2 T3 T4a	N3 N2 N1 N0	
IIIA	T2 T3 T4a	N3 N2 N1	M0 M0 M0
IIIB	T3 T4a T4b T4b	N3 N2 N1 N0	M0
IIIC	T4a T4b T4b	N3 N2 N3	
IV	Any T	Any N	M1

The ultimate goal of any staging evaluation is to ensure that patients with metastatic disease are not treated with nontherapeutic laparotomy or other local therapies (e.g., radiation therapy), which are generally ineffective against advanced disease. Even small-volume metastatic disease identified on the surface of the liver or the peritoneum at laparotomy is associated with poor survival: in one study, patients with such disease had a life expectancy of only 6 to 9 months.[35] In these situations, there is little to be gained from attempts at palliative resection.

Staging laparoscopy has proved to be highly relevant to the evaluation of patients with gastric cancer. In a study from the Memorial Sloan-Kettering Cancer Center (MSKCC), the investigators performed laparoscopic exploration on 110 of 111 patients with newly diagnosed gastric cancer.[36] Of these 110 patients, 94% were accurately staged, with a sensitivity of 84% and a specificity of 100%, and 37% were found to have subclinical metastatic disease. Hospital stay was substantially shorter in the 24 patients who underwent diagnostic laparoscopy with biopsy only (average 1.4 days) than in comparable patients who underwent exploratory laparotomy

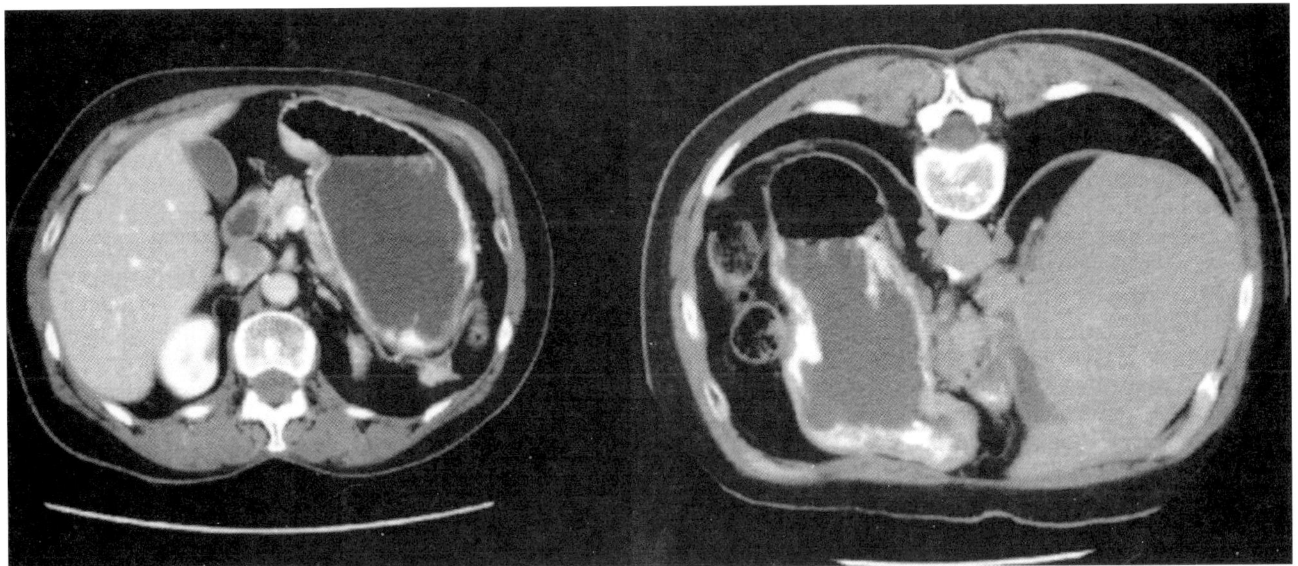

Figure 1 **Shown is a computed tomographic scan of a patient with advanced gastric carcinoma. Water (a negative contrast agent) has been used to distend the stomach. The images were acquired with the patient in the prone position to allow the stomach to fall away from the retroperitoneum and to define the interface between the stomach and pancreas.**

without resection (average 6.5 days). Finally, at the time the data were reported, none of the patients who underwent laparoscopy had required palliative surgery. Subsequent single-institution series confirmed the utility of staging laparoscopy, reporting accuracy rates ranging from 95 to 97% and occult M1 disease rates approaching 30%.[37,38] Taken as a whole, the data are compelling and have led the NCCN to encourage laparoscopic staging strongly, either before or at the time of the planned resection.[39]

MANAGEMENT

Surgical Therapy

Surgical resection remains the only potentially curative therapy for localized gastric cancer [*see Figure 3*]. Cure requires removal of all gross and microscopic disease. More specifically, a margin-negative (R0) resection entails wide local excision of the primary tumor with en bloc removal of all associated lymphatic vessels and any local or regional

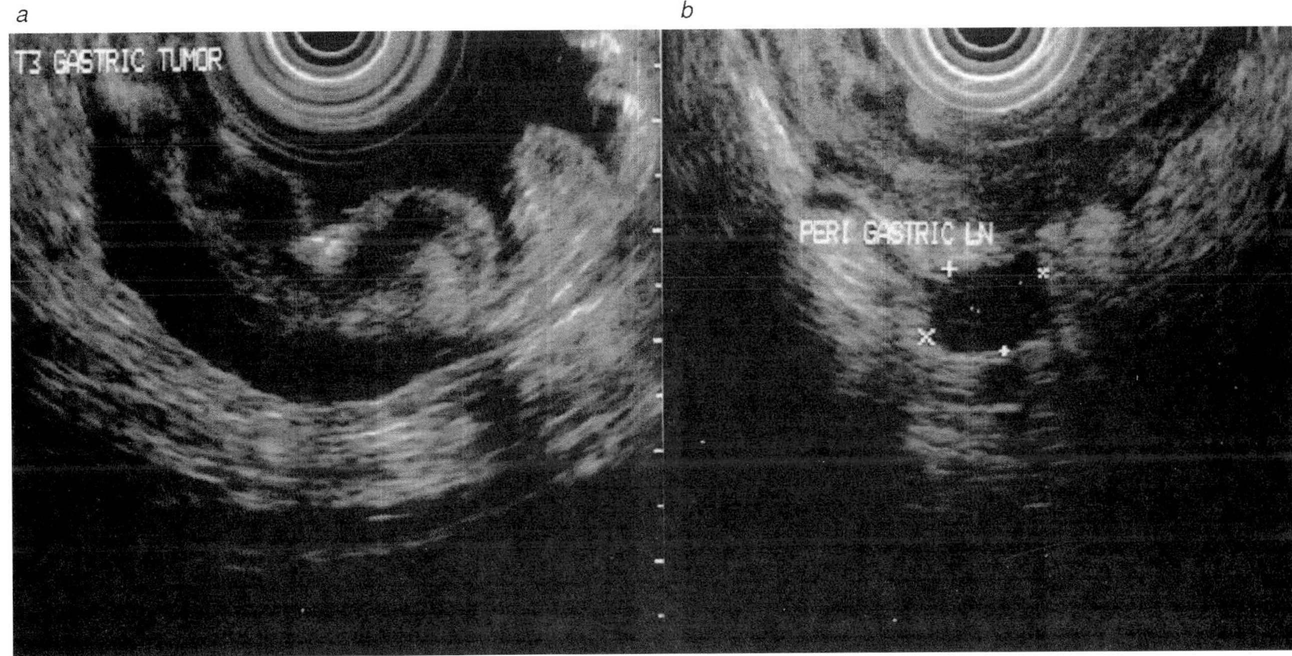

Figure 2 **(*a*) Shown is an endoscopic ultrasonographic (EUS) image of a T3 gastric neoplasm. (*b*) EUS reveals the presence of suspicious perigastric (N1) nodes, later confirmed as malignant at operation.**

common hepatic artery, the left gastric artery, the celiac axis, and the splenic artery. A D3 lymph node dissection adds resection of nodes in the hepatoduodenal ligament and the root of the mesentery. Finally, a D4 resection calls for a D3 dissection plus resection of the retroperitoneal para-aortic and paracolic lymph nodes.[55] The JRSGC defines a curative operation as a gastric resection that includes lymph nodes one level beyond the level of pathologic nodal involvement. Thus, in Japan, a D2 lymph node dissection is considered the standard resection for even relatively early cancers, and numerous studies have cited the benefits of D3 and even D4 lymphadenectomy for advanced carcinoma.[56–58]

Western surgeons have been reluctant to embrace radical lymphadenectomy, arguing that it has yet to demonstrate an unequivocal survival advantage in any prospective, randomized trial from a Western institution or cooperative group. Detractors further argue that the survival advantage associated with more radical procedures simply reflects stage migration, a higher incidence of early gastric cancers, and differences in tumor biology and body habitus between Japanese and Western populations and point to the increases in operating time and morbidity that often accompany extended gastric resections. One retrospective review of the tumor registries of over 2,000 hospitals in the United States found that D2 lymph node dissection had no survival advantage over D1 lymph node dissection in terms of either the median survival time or the 5-year survival rate.[59]

Two prospective trials from Western Europe examined this issue further in an effort to evaluate the safety and efficacy of ELND. In the Dutch Gastric Cancer Group trial, 711 patients were randomly assigned to undergo either D1 or D2 lymphadenectomy as part of a potentially curative gastrectomy for biopsy-proven adenocarcinoma.[60] This trial was unique in its use of extensive quality control measures, which included instruction and operative supervision by an expert gastric cancer surgeon from Japan (who also assisted with the processing and pathologic examination of the surgical specimens). Patients without evidence of disseminated metastases underwent either total gastrectomy or, if 5 cm proximal margins could be obtained, distal gastrectomy. In this study, a D2 lymph node dissection entailed distal pancreatectomy and splenectomy. Both morbidity and mortality were significantly higher in the D2 group than in the D1 group, and D2 dissection conferred no demonstrable survival advantage at a median follow-up of 72 months.

In a trial from the Medical Research Council in the United Kingdom, 400 patients with stage I to IIB disease were randomly assigned to undergo either a D1 or a D2 lymph node dissection.[61] There was no significant difference in overall 5-year survival between the two arms, but multivariable analysis demonstrated that clinical stages II and III, advanced age, male sex, and removal of the pancreas and the spleen were independently associated with poor outcome. The authors concluded that the classic Japanese D2 dissection offered no survival advantage over D1 dissection. However, they hypothesized that D2 dissection with preservation of the distal pancreas and the spleen might lead to decreased morbidity and mortality within the extended resection group and thus potentially to superior outcomes.

Further support for this hypothesis was provided by two nonrandomized trials from specialized centers. The Italian Gastric Cancer Study Group (IGCSG) completed a phase II multicenter trial designed to evaluate the safety and efficacy of pancreas-preserving D2 lymph node dissection.[62] Quality control measures included supervision by a surgeon who had studied the technique of D2 lymph node dissection at the National Cancer Center Hospital in Tokyo. At a median follow-up time of 4.38 years, the overall morbidity rate for D2 dissection in the 191 patients enrolled was 20.9% and the in-hospital mortality was 3.1%. The 5-year survival rate among eligible patients was 55%. In a prospective series of 125 patients undergoing standardized D2 lymph node dissection at a single Western center, the investigators reported a mortality of 1.37% and an overall morbidity rate of 33.5%.[63] As in the IGCSG study, distal pancreatectomy was avoided in all cases, except when direct extension was suspected on the basis of macroscopic findings (5.5% of cases). Overall 5- and 10-year survival rates for this highly selected cohort were 52.3% and 40%, respectively. These studies suggest that D2 lymph node dissection may be safely performed in Western centers when accompanied by careful selection of patients, strict standardization of technique, and a strategy of pancreatic preservation.

Current AJCC guidelines state that pathologic examination of at least 15 lymph nodes is required for adequate staging.[28] Specifically, examination of at least 15 nodes is required to confidently deem a patient free of nodal metastases. However, multiple studies have demonstrated inadequate nodal assessment that is somewhat related to hospital type.[64] In an effort to confirm the benefit of this staging system, investigators from the MSKCC reviewed their experience with 1,038 patients who underwent R0 resection for gastric cancer.[65] The location of positive lymph nodes (within 3 cm of the primary tumor versus more than 3 cm away) did not significantly affect median survival; however, the number of positive lymph nodes had a profound effect on survival. Furthermore, in cases in which at least 15 nodes were examined (27% of the total), the median survival for patients with metastasis in one to six regional lymph nodes, metastasis in seven to 15 regional lymph nodes, and metastasis in more than 15 regional lymph nodes was significantly longer than the median survival reported in cases in which 14 or fewer nodes were resected with the specimens. These findings are consistent with published data from our own institution (Northwestern University Feinberg School of Medicine), which indicate that the number of positive lymph nodes is a highly significant predictor of survival.[66] In our series of 110 patients, those with seven or more positive lymph nodes had a median disease-free survival (DFS) of 17.6 months, whereas those with six or fewer positive nodes had a median DFS of 44 months. Data from other centers support this view as well.

It is our current practice to perform a D2 lymph node dissection with resection of all perigastric lymph nodes along the greater and lesser curvatures of the stomach, as well as those along the common hepatic artery, the left gastric artery, the celiac axis, and the splenic artery. We make every attempt to preserve the tail of the pancreas and spleen, with multivisceral resection reserved for cases of overt direct extension of malignant disease in the absence of disseminated metastasis. This strategy should provide adequate staging in terms of the AJCC guidelines, minimize morbidity, and possibly confer a survival advantage on certain patient subgroups, as suggested by the results of the trials mentioned.

Role of splenectomy Routine splenectomy has been proposed as a means of facilitating clearance of metastatic nodes along the splenic artery and in the splenic hilum, but there is little evidence to support this practice in the treatment of proximal gastric cancers. Indeed, numerous studies have documented the deleterious effect of splenectomy when it is performed as part of an extended gastric resection.

In a retrospective study of 392 patients who underwent curative gastrectomy at a high-volume cancer center, the impact of splenectomy on survival and postoperative morbidity was evaluated.[67] Splenectomy was not predictive of death on multivariable analysis, but complications were far more frequent in patients who underwent splenectomy as part of surgical treatment than in those who did not (45% versus 21%). Specifically, the incidence of infectious complications was far higher in the splenectomy group than in the nonsplenectomy group (75% versus 47%).

In a review of data from an American College of Surgeons Pattern of Care Study, the investigators reported that the operative mortality was 9.8% in patients who underwent splenectomy during gastric resection, compared with 8.6% for those who did not.[68] More significantly, the 5-year observed survival rate was 20.9% in the splenectomy group, compared with 31% in the nonsplenectomy group.

In a randomized, prospective trial, early and late results of total gastrectomy alone were compared with those of total gastrectomy plus splenectomy in patients being treated for cancers of the upper third of the stomach.[69] All patients underwent a D2 lymph node dissection. The operative mortalities and the 5-year survival rates were similar in the two groups, but the splenectomy group had more infectious complications. Specifically, the splenectomy group had higher incidences of pulmonary complications, postoperative fever higher than 38°C (100.4°F), and subphrenic abscess formation. We agree with the conclusions of the authors of this study: routine splenectomy does not increase survival and should be reserved for situations in which the gastric tumor directly invades the splenic hilum or there is evidence of gross nodal metastases along the splenic artery.

Nonsurgical Therapy

Adjuvant therapy As noted (see above), the majority of patients who present with gastric carcinoma and undergo potentially curative surgical treatment will experience locoregional failure, distant metastasis, or both and will succumb to their disease. Accordingly, numerous adjuvant approaches—including chemotherapy, radiotherapy, chemoradiation, immunochemotherapy, and intraperitoneal chemotherapy—have been tried in gastric cancer patients with the aim of improving overall survival and DFS. The results, for the most part, have been disappointing.

The results from prospective, randomized, controlled trials of adjuvant radiation therapy in this setting have failed to establish a survival benefit. In a multi-institutional trial from 1994, patients were randomly assigned to undergo surgery alone, surgery plus adjuvant radiation, or surgery plus adjuvant multiagent chemotherapy.[70] There was no significant benefit to either adjuvant regimen: overall 5-year survival was 20% for surgery alone, compared with 12% for surgery plus radiation therapy and 19% for surgery plus chemotherapy.

The results from trials of chemotherapy alone have been equally unsatisfactory. Because of the established inefficacy of single-agent 5-fluorouracil (5-FU) therapy, combination chemotherapy regimens have been employed. Such regimens have included nitrosourea compounds, mitomycin C, anthracyclines, and members of the cisplatin family.[23] In a meta-analysis of 13 trials comparing adjuvant chemotherapy with observation in non-Asian countries, the odds ratio for death in the treated group was 0.8, corresponding to a relative risk of 0.94.[71] This result did not, however, reflect a statistically significant improvement. Most oncologists have now abandoned the use of chemotherapy by itself in the adjuvant setting.

In an effort to derive greater therapeutic benefit than can be achieved with either radiation therapy or chemotherapy alone, combination chemoradiation therapy has been used in the adjuvant setting. In Intergroup Trial 0116, 556 patients who had undergone R0 resection of adenocarcinoma of the stomach or the esophagogastric junction were randomly assigned to treatment with either surgery alone or surgery plus postoperative chemoradiotherapy.[72] Patients with tumors ranging from stage IB to stage IVM0 were included; the majority had T3 tumors and node-positive disease. The therapeutic regimen consisted of 5-FU and leucovorin therapy administered concomitantly with 45 Gy of external-beam irradiation over a period of 5 weeks. Median overall survival in the surgery-only group was 27 months, compared with 36 months in the surgery-chemoradiation group. In addition, the 3-year survival rate was 41% in the surgery-only group, compared with 50% in the chemoradiotherapy group. The hazard ratio for death in the surgery-only group compared with the chemotherapy group was 1.35.

In the United States, the results of Intergroup Trial 0116 have led to the acceptance of combined chemoradiation therapy as standard adjuvant therapy for patients who have undergone curative-intent resection of gastric cancer. Nonetheless, numerous criticisms of this trial have been expressed. Specifically, a review of the operative and pathology reports of 453 of the patients revealed a lack of surgical standardization.[73] When the extent of lymphadenectomy was categorized, the majority (54.2%) of the patients were found to have undergone a D0 resection; 38.1% underwent a D1 resection, and only 7.5% underwent a D2 or D3 lymph node dissection. These findings suggest that the main effect of the chemoradiation therapy may have been simply to compensate for inadequate surgery. This suggestion is supported by the observation that the number of patients with local and regional recurrences was higher in the surgery-only group (178 versus 101), whereas the number of patients with distant failure was slightly higher in the adjuvant therapy arm (40 versus 32). Furthermore, when the Maruyama Index of Unresected Discasc (a computer model developed for accurate prediction of nodal station involvement in gastric cancer) was applied to the 556 patients eligible for the Intergroup trial, the median Maruyama Index was 70.[74] This value was far above the level considered to represent optimal surgical therapy (i.e., Maruyama Index < 5) and led the authors to conclude that the vast majority of patients in the trial had been surgically undertreated.

Currently, physicians, especially in Europe, generally avoid adjuvant therapy after R0 resection of gastric cancer, except under the auspices of a clinical trial.[9] The Radiation Therapy Oncology Group has initiated a phase II trial of adjuvant chemoradiotherapy using 45 Gy of external beam radiation therapy with cisplatin and paclitaxel, with or without 5-FU. If promising results are found, a phase III trial will follow. It is hoped that ongoing trials will shed further light on this complex management issue.

Neoadjuvant therapy As a response to the disappointing results of adjuvant therapy and the inability of many patients to regain adequate performance status after radical gastric surgery to undergo systemic therapy, neoadjuvant protocols have been proposed.[75] The theoretical benefits of a neoadjuvant treatment strategy include treatment-induced tumor downstaging, which may enhance resectability, and early administration of systemic therapy, which allows almost all patients to receive and complete the prescribed treatment. Furthermore, because treatment is administered when measurable disease is present, the response to therapy may be assessed and continued only in patients who are likely to benefit. Finally, patients found to have rapidly progressive disease during preoperative chemotherapy may be spared having to undergo a nontherapeutic gastrectomy.[76]

In a report of three phase II trials from the M.D. Anderson Cancer Center encompassing 83 patients who received neoadjuvant chemotherapy before planned surgical resection, the clinical response rates ranged from 24 to 38%, with three patients (4%) exhibiting a complete pathologic response.[76] Sixty-one patients (73%) were able to undergo a curative-intent resection, and the response to chemotherapy was the only significant predictor of survival on multivariable analysis.

Preoperative chemoradiation therapy has also been shown to be feasible in phase II trials. In a 2001 trial that included 23 patients, 96% of the study population received combined modality therapy.[75] Nineteen patients (83%) were able to undergo surgical resection with D2 lymphadenectomy; four patients (17%) had progressive disease and did not undergo resection. Morbidity and death rates were acceptable (32% and 5%, respectively), and 11% of patients exhibited complete pathologic responses. Overall, 63% of patients showed pathologic evidence of a significant treatment effect.

Newer neoadjuvant strategies employ multiagent induction chemotherapy followed by chemoradiotherapy and planned gastric resection in patients with locally advanced but potentially resectable gastric cancer.[73] Based on the results of the Intergroup Trial 0116, the Medical Research Council Adjuvant Gastric Infusional Chemotherapy (MAGIC) trial was developed to determine whether neoadjuvant epirubicin, cisplatin, and infused fluorouracil (ECF) resulted in improved outcomes compared with surgery alone.[77] Postoperative morbidity and mortality were comparable between the two groups, but overall survival (5-year survival 36% versus 23%; hazard ratio 0.75) and progression-free survival (hazard ratio 0.66) were improved in patients who received neoadjuvant ECF. Thus, the NCCN now recommends neoadjuvant therapy for locally advanced (T3 or node positive based on EUS) gastric cancer.

FOLLOW-UP AND MANAGEMENT OF RECURRENT DISEASE

Even after gross resection of all disease with microscopically negative margins (R0 resection), recurrence of gastric carcinoma is common. Adenocarcinoma of the stomach may spread through direct extension, via lymphatic channels to regional and distant lymph nodes, or via the bloodstream to distant sites. Furthermore, once tumors have penetrated the serosa (T3), peritoneal metastasis becomes a possibility. Through autopsy series and clinical studies, certain definite patterns of locoregional failure and distant metastasis have been established. Locoregional recurrences are common in the gastric bed and the adjacent lymph nodes. Clinical and reoperative evaluation have documented recurrent disease at the anastomosis, in the retroperitoneum, or in the regional lymph nodes in 3 to 69% of patients; the incidence of recurrence may vary, depending on whether the patients had received adjuvant therapy.[23] One autopsy series documented a locoregional recurrence rate of 94% in patients treated with surgery alone. The peritoneum is ultimately involved in 17 to 50% of all patients. The most common sites of visceral metastases are the liver and the lungs.

In view of the high recurrence rates, all patients who have undergone resection should be seen for routine surveillance examinations. Currently, the NCCN recommends that a complete history and physical examination be conducted every 3 to 6 months for 1 to 3 years, every 6 months for 3 to 5 years, and then annually thereafter.[39] A complete blood [illegible] (e.g., CT), and endoscopy should be done if clinically indicated, usually in response to new symptoms. In addition, long-term vitamin B_{12} supplementation should be initiated for patients who have undergone a proximal or subtotal gastrectomy.

Nonadenocarcinomatous Gastric Malignancies

GASTRIC LYMPHOMA

Gastric lymphoma is the second most common malignancy of the stomach, accounting for 2 to 9% of gastric tumors in the United States. Lymphomas of the stomach are of the non-Hodgkin type. The stomach is the most common site of extranodal involvement of non-Hodgkin lymphoma (NHL) and accounts for nearly 50% of all such cases.[78]

Clinical Evaluation

The presenting symptoms of gastric lymphoma, like those of gastric adenocarcinoma, are nonspecific and include loss of appetite, weight loss, vomiting, and bleeding. B symptoms (e.g., fever and night sweats) are relatively rare: in one multicenter trial concerned with primary gastric lymphoma, they occurred in fewer than 12% of patients enrolled.[79] Risk factors for gastric lymphoma include *H. pylori* infection, immunosuppression after solid-organ transplantation, celiac disease, inflammatory bowel disease, and HIV infection.[80]

Investigative Studies

The diagnosis is most frequently established by means of endoscopy with biopsy. Staging studies include a comprehensive blood count, a lactate dehydrogenase level, and a comprehensive chemistry panel; CT of the chest, abdomen, and pelvis; and, often, a bone marrow biopsy. All pathology slides should be reviewed by an experienced hematopathologist.[81]

Staging and Prognosis

Numerous staging systems have been employed to stage NHL of the GI tract. Of these, the one most commonly applied is a modification of the Ann Arbor staging system for lymphoma.[80] For surgeons, the most important determination is often whether the NHL (1) is confined to the stomach and the perigastric nodes (stage I and II disease), (2) involves other intra-abdominal nodes and organs (stage III), or (3) extends outside the abdomen (stage IV).[82]

Management

Over the past decade, the management of patients with gastric lymphoma has undergone significant changes. Generally, there has been a shift away from surgical management, even in relatively localized cases (stages I and II).[83] This shift is the result not only of the documented success of chemotherapy alone for more advanced cases (stages III and IV) but also of a better understanding of the etiology of gastric lymphoma.[84] Approximately 45% of all gastric lymphomas are low-grade mucosa-associated lymphoid tissue (MALT) lymphomas.[79] The gastric mucosa is normally devoid of lymphoid tissue. It is hypothesized that MALT develops in the stomach in response to chronic *H. pylori* infection.[85]

Nonsurgical therapy Low-grade MALT lymphoma usually presents as stage I or II disease and has an indolent course. Since 1993, when regression of low-grade MALT lymphoma after eradication of *H. pylori* was first reported, numerous trials have documented the efficacy of anti–*H. pylori* therapy, with complete remission rates ranging from 50 to 100%.[79] In the German MALT Lymphoma Study, the complete remission rate was 81%; 9% of patients exhibited partial responses, and 10% showed no response.[86] Low-grade lymphomas that are more advanced or do not regress with antibiotic therapy may be treated with combinations of *H. pylori* eradication, radiation, and/or combination chemotherapy.[87] For localized persistent disease, modest doses of radiation, on the order of 30 Gy, may be employed. When chemotherapy is required, multiagent regimens, such as cyclophosphamide-vincristine (Oncovin)-prednisolone (COP), are often used.

Approximately 55% of gastric lymphomas are high-grade lesions, which can occur with or without a low-grade MALT component.[79] These lymphomas are treated with chemotherapy and radiation therapy according to the extent of the disease. The cyclophosphamide-doxorubicin-vincristine (Oncovin)-prednisolone (CHOP) regimen is the one most frequently employed. In some studies, the anti-CD20 monoclonal antibody rituximab has been either added to standard therapy or used alone, with encouraging results.[88]

Surgical therapy Surgical resection, once thought to be essential for the diagnosis, staging, and treatment of early-stage gastric lymphoma, now is used mainly in patients who experience bleeding or perforation. In the German Multicenter Study Group trial, 185 patients with stage I or II gastric lymphoma were treated either with gastrectomy followed by radiation or (in the case of high-grade lesions) chemotherapy plus radiation or with chemotherapy and radiotherapy alone.[79] There was no significant difference in survival between the group receiving surgical treatment and the group receiving nonoperative therapy: overall 5-year survival rates were 82.5 and 84%, respectively. There were no perforations and only one hemorrhage (in a patient treated with chemotherapy alone). Similarly, in a single-institution, prospective, randomized trial comparing chemotherapy alone with chemotherapy plus surgery for stage I and II lymphoma, there were no instances of perforation and only three instances of GI bleeding in the chemotherapy group, compared with two bleeding episodes in the surgery plus chemotherapy group.[83]

Currently, patients with early-stage high-grade gastric lymphomas are treated primarily with chemotherapy or radiation therapy; only rarely do they require surgical intervention for complications encountered during therapy. Patients with locally advanced (stage III) or disseminated (stage IV) gastric lymphoma are clearly best treated with chemotherapy, with or without radiation. Occasionally, surgery is indicated in such patients to treat residual disease confined to the stomach or to palliate bleeding or obstruction that does not resolve with nonoperative therapy. Primary surgical therapy is to be avoided in these patients because of the significant risk of complications and the delay in initiating systemic therapy.

GASTROINTESTINAL STROMAL TUMOR

Gastrointestinal stromal tumor (GIST), although relatively rare in absolute terms, is the most common sarcoma of the GI tract,[89] with approximately 6,000 cases reported each year in the United States alone. The stomach is the most common site of involvement, accounting for 60 to 70% of cases[90]; the small intestine (25%), the rectum (5%), the esophagus (2%), and a variety of other locations account for the remainder. On the basis of their appearance on light microscopy, GISTs were once thought to be of smooth muscle origin, and most were classified as leiomyosarcomas.[91] Thus, extended gastric resection, often including contiguous organs, was advised. Recurrence developed after R0 resection in approximately 50% of cases.[92] With the advent of immunohistochemistry and electron microscopy, it became clear that GIST has both smooth muscle and neural elements, and the cell of origin is now believed to be a precursor of the interstitial cells of Cajal, an intestinal pacemaker cell.[93] The diagnosis of GIST is secured by immunohistochemical staining for the tyrosine kinase receptor KIT (CD 117), which highlights the presence of interstitial cells of Cajal. More than 95% of GISTs exhibit unequivocal staining for KIT.[90] Approximately two thirds of GISTs also express CD34. Histologically, these tumors may exhibit a spindle cell pattern, an epithelioid pattern, or a mixed subtype.

Clinical Evaluation

The median age of incidence is 63 years, and tumors are generally between 0.5 and 44 cm in diameter at the time of diagnosis (median diameter 6 cm).[90] Mass-related symptoms (e.g., abdominal pain, bloating, and early satiety) may be present. Melena or anemia from overlying mucosal ulceration may be present as well. A small subset of patients have peritonitis as a consequence of tumor rupture and subsequent hemorrhage. Finally, many GISTs are discovered incidentally during operation, abdominal imaging, or endoscopy

Investigative Studies

When a GIST is suspected, abdominal and pelvic imaging with either CT or magnetic resonance imaging (MRI) is indicated. Chest imaging is performed as well. Endoscopy, with or without EUS, may occasionally help with surgical planning, but because of the infrequency of mucosal involvement, it is rarely diagnostic.[94] Surgical consultation should be obtained to determine whether the lesion can be resected. If the tumor is resectable, biopsy should not be performed, because of the risk of tumor rupture and intra-abdominal dissemination. Biopsy may be required, however, if the patient has widespread disease or may be enrolling in a trial of neoadjuvant therapy. In such cases, biopsy may be performed percutaneously or at the time of EUS.

Staging and Prognosis

Although the majority of gastric GISTs have a benign course, a wide spectrum of biologic behavior has been observed. Of the prognostic factors examined to date, tumor size and mitotic rate appear to be the most valuable. If the tumor is less than 2 cm in diameter and the mitotic count is lower than five per high-power field (HPF), the risk of an aggressive disease course is considered to be very low. Conversely, if the tumor is larger than 10 cm, if the mitotic count is higher than 10/HPF, or if the tumor is larger than 5 cm with a mitotic count higher than 5/HPF, the risk of aggressive clinical behavior is considered to be high. For all other tumors, the risk of aggressive disease is considered to be intermediate.[90] The site of the primary tumor has also been shown to be important, with gastric GISTs having a better prognosis compared with small bowel GISTs of comparable size and mitotic rate.[95] In addition, the most recent version of the AJCC Cancer Staging Manual (7th Edition) has an added staging system for GISTs (*Table 3 and Table 4*).[96]

Management

Surgical therapy The role of surgery in the treatment of a GIST is to resect the tumor with grossly negative margins and an intact pseudocapsule. Lymph node involvement is rare with GISTs; thus, no effort is made to perform ELND. The tumor must be handled with care to prevent intra-abdominal rupture. Formal gastric resection is rarely required: as a rule, it is indicated only for lesions in close proximity to the pylorus or the esophagogastric junction. The NCCN has guidelines updated annually specifically for the management of GISTs.[97]

Table 3 American Joint Committee on Cancer TNM Clinical Classification of Gastrointestinal Stromal Tumors, 7th Edition[96]

Primary tumor (T)	TX	Primary tumor cannot be assessed
	T0	No evidence of primary tumor
	Tis	Carcinoma in situ
	T1	Tumor 2 cm or less
	T2	Tumor 2–5 cm
	T3	Tumor 5–10 cm
	T4	Tumor > 10 cm in greatest diameter
Regional lymph nodes (N)	NX	Regional lymph node(s) cannot be assessed
	N0	No regional lymph node metastasis
	N1	Regional lymph node metastasis
Distant metastasis (M)	M0	No distant metastasis
	M1	Distant metastasis

Table 4 American Joint Committee on Cancer Staging of Gastric and Small Bowel GISTs, 7th Edition[96]

Stage	Tumor	Node	Metastasis	Mitotic Rate
Gastric				
IA	T1, T2	N0	M0	Low
IB	T3	N0	M0	Low
II	T1 T3 T4	N0	M0	High High Low
IIIA	T3	N1	M0	High
IIIB	T4	N0	M0	High
IV	Any T	N1	M1	Any rate
Small intestine				
I	T1, T2	N0	M0	Low
II	T3	N0	M0	Low
IIIA	T1 T4	N0	M0	High Low
IIIB	T2 T3 T4	N0	M0	High High High
IV	Any T	N1 Any N	M0 M1	Any rate

GIST = gastrointestinal stromal tumor

Nonsurgical therapy If the tumor has metastasized or has advanced locally to the point where surgical therapy would result in excessive morbidity, the patient is treated with the tyrosine kinase inhibitor imatinib mesylate. Imatinib is a selective inhibitor of a family of protein kinases that includes the KIT receptor tyrosine kinase, which is expressed in the majority of GISTs. Originally indicated for the treatment of chronic myelocytic leukemia, imatinib was approved for the treatment of KIT-positive GIST in 2002, when phase II clinical trials documented sustained objective responses in a majority of patients with advanced unresectable or metastatic GIST.[98] Patients with borderline resectable lesions should be treated with imatinib until they exhibit a maximal response as documented by CT and positron emission tomography (PET); surgery may then be undertaken to resect any residual foci of disease. Similarly, although patients with metastatic disease are unlikely to manifest a complete response to imatinib therapy, they should be periodically reevaluated and considered for resection should surgical treatment become technically feasible.[94]

In 2009, the results of the American College of Surgeons Oncology Group (ACOSOG) phase III trial (Z9001) were reported. After resection of intermediate-risk GIST, patients were randomized to treatment with 1 year of imatinib (400 mg/day) versus placebo. Adjuvant imatinib was well tolerated. After a median follow-up of 19.7 months, patients treated with imatinib had a considerably better recurrence-free survival compared with the placebo group (98% versus 83%, $p < .0001$; hazard ratio 0.35). After resection of a

GIST, adjuvant imatinib is recommended for patients with moderate-to-high risk of recurrence.

GASTRIC CARCINOID

Gastric carcinoid tumors are rare, but this incidence is increasing. These tumors now account for approximately 10% of all GI carcinoids and 2% of all gastric tumors.[99–101] The median age at diagnosis is 64, and the tumors are somewhat more common in women than in men.

Clinical Evaluation and Investigative Studies

Gastric carcinoid tumors are often discovered during endoscopic examination of patients experiencing chronic abdominal pain; patients may also complain of vomiting and diarrhea. These tumors are rarely associated with symptoms of the carcinoid syndrome. Diagnosis is usually confirmed by endoscopic biopsy, and EUS is helpful in determining the extent of gastric wall penetration and the degree of regional lymph node involvement.

Gastric carcinoid tumors have been divided into three types, primarily on the basis of their association (or lack thereof) with hypergastrinemia. Type I tumors are associated with chronic atrophic gastritis, are generally small (< 1 cm), and are often multiple and polypoid. They grow slowly and only rarely metastasize to regional nodes or distant sites. Type II tumors are associated with the Zollinger-Ellison syndrome and multiple endocrine neoplasia type I and, like type I tumors, are usually small and multiple. They also grow slowly but are more likely to metastasize than type I gastric carcinoids are. Type III (sporadic) gastric carcinoid tumors are the most biologically aggressive type. They are often large (> 1 cm) at the time of diagnosis and are not associated with hypergastrinemia. Type III lesions frequently metastasize to regional nodes (54%) or the liver (24%).[99]

Management

For patients with small, solitary type I tumors, endoscopic polypectomy or open resection via gastrotomy (local excision) is the procedure of choice. For patients with multiple or recurrent tumors, antrectomy is indicated to remove the source of the hypergastrinemia. For patients with type II lesions, treatment is similar to that for patients with type I lesions, with the extent of gastric resection determined by the size and number of lesions. For patients with type III lesions, however, either distal or total gastrectomy with ELND is required.[102] All patients undergoing a less than total gastrectomy should be followed with serial endoscopy at regular intervals.[103]

Small Bowel Malignancies

Malignant tumors of the small intestine are rare, accounting for fewer than 5% of all GI tract malignancies. In the United States, approximately 6,000 new cases of small bowel cancer are reported each year.[3] The majority of small bowel malignancies are carcinoid tumors, adenocarcinomas, or lymphomas,[104] although GISTs are being noted with increasing frequency in the small intestine. Although adenocarcinomas had traditionally been the most common tumor of the small bowel, a recent report from our group has shown that the incidence of carcinoid tumors has increased over the past 20 years and carcinoids are now the most common tumor of the small intestine.[105] Treatment of lymphomas, carcinoid tumors, and GISTs in the small bowel is nearly identical to treatment of the same lesions in the stomach [*see* Nonadenocarcinomatous Gastric Malignancies, *above*] and thus are not covered further in this chapter. Our focus here is on the presentation, diagnosis, and treatment of adenocarcinoma of the small bowel (*Table 5 and Table 6*).

CLINICAL EVALUATION

Between 46 and 55% of small bowel adenocarcinomas occur in the duodenum and approximately 13% occur in the ileum.[97,98,104–106] Patients frequently present with nausea, vomiting, abdominal pain, weight loss, and GI bleeding; occasionally, they present with iron deficiency anemia or a positive fecal occult blood test result. In rare cases, small bowel obstruction, often with the tumor serving as a lead point for intussusception, is the first manifestation of the disease.[106]

INVESTIGATIVE STUDIES

When an adenocarcinoma is located in the duodenum, the diagnosis is often made by means of esophagogastroduodenoscopy (EGD). Lesions within the first 100 cm of the small bowel may be evaluated with push enteroscopy. When the adenocarcinoma is situated elsewhere in the small bowel, it is localized with small bowel radiographs. Some authors consider enteroclysis to be superior to the more commonly used small bowel follow-through in this setting in that enteroclysis is better able to demonstrate fine mucosal detail.[107] In experienced hands, enteroclysis may therefore be more sensitive.[108] Some lesions are identified when CT or MRI is performed to evaluate complaints of abdominal pain. Furthermore, abdominal imaging may yield complementary staging information (e.g., the presence of regional adenopathy or metastatic disease). One new method for the identification of small bowel tumors is wireless capsule endoscopy.[109] This minimally invasive technique may be particularly useful in identifying small lesions in the distal jejunum and ileum that cannot be identified radiographically.

MANAGEMENT

Aggressive surgical resection remains the cornerstone of therapy for adenocarcinoma of the small intestine.[110] For periampullary lesions, pancreaticoduodenectomy is typically required to achieve a margin-negative resection. For lesions in the distal duodenum, a segmental sleeve resection with a duodenojejunostomy is appropriate. For lesions in the jejunum or the ileum, segmental resection may be performed with a wide mesenteric resection to encompass potentially involved regional lymph nodes. Contiguous organs are resected en bloc as necessary.[99]

Because the presenting signs and symptoms are often vague and nonspecific, diagnosis is often delayed. In one series, only six (11%) of the 53 patients were suspected of having a small bowel tumor at admission.[110] In a retrospective review of patients with small bowel tumors treated at our institution, the mean duration of symptoms before surgical management was 110 months, and more than 50% of the patients were found to have stage III or IV disease.[111] In our work with the National Cancer Data Base, we found that only 24% of patients presented with metastatic disease.[105]

Table 5 American Joint Committee of Cancer TNM Clinical Classification of Small Bowel Carcinoma, 7th Edition[96]

Primary tumor (T)	TX	Primary tumor cannot be assessed
	T0	No evidence of primary tumor
	Tis	Carcinoma in situ
	T1a	Tumor invades lamina propria
	T1b	Tumor invades submucosa
	T2	Tumor invades muscularis propria
	T3	Tumor penetrates the muscularis propria into the subserosa or into the nonperitonealized perimuscular tissue (mesentery or retroperitoneum) with extension of 2 cm or less
	T4	Tumor perforates the visceral perioneum or directly invades other organs or structures (includes other loops of small intestine, mesentery, or retroperitoneum > 2 cm and abdominal wall by way of serosa; for duodenum only, invasion of pancreas or bile duct)
Regional lymph nodes (N)	NX	Regional lymph node(s) cannot be assessed
	N0	No regional lymph node metastasis
	N1	Metastasis in 1–3 regional lymph nodes
	N2	Metastasis in 4 or more regional lymph nodes
Distant metastasis (M)	M0	No distant metastasis
	M1	Distant metastasis

Table 6 American Joint Committee on Cancer Staging of Small Bowel Carcinoma, 7th Edition[96]

Stage	Tumor	Node	Metastasis
0	Tis	N0	M0
I	T1, T2	N0	M0
IIA	T3	N0	M0
IIB	T4	N0	M0
IIIA	Any T	N1	M0
IIIB	Any T	N2	M0
IV	Any T	Any N	M1

The 5-year survival rate continues to be low (24 to 37%).[105,111–113] Significant predictors of good overall survival include location in the jejunum, complete (R0) resection, low-grade tumors, and low AJCC tumor stage.[105,111–113] The available evidence indicates that all patients with small bowel neoplasms should be offered an oncologically sound surgical resection. In one series, curative (R0) resection was accomplished in 71% of cases.[113] No prospective data are available regarding adjuvant therapy, but the treatments and results for colon adenocarcinoma are often extrapolated to small bowel adenocarcinomas.

Financial Disclosures: None Reported

References

1. Roder DM. The epidemiology of gastric cancer. Gastric Cancer 2002;5 Suppl 1:5–11.
2. Neugut AI, Hayek M, Howe G. Epidemiology of gastric cancer. Semin Oncol 1996;23: 281–91.
3. Jemal A, Siegel R, Ward E, et al. Cancer statistics, 2009. CA Cancer J Clin 2009;59: 225–49.
4. Alberts SR, Cervantes A, van de Velde CJ. Gastric cancer: epidemiology, pathology and treatment. Ann Oncol 2003;14 Suppl 2: ii31–6.
5. United States cancer statistics: 1999–2001 incidence and mortality. Washington, DC: Department of Health and Human Services, Centers for Disease Control and Prevention, and National Cancer Institute; 2004.
6. Hundahl SA, Phillips JL, Menck HR. The National Cancer Data Base Report on poor survival of U.S. gastric carcinoma patients treated with gastrectomy: Fifth Edition American Joint Committee on Cancer staging, proximal disease, and the "different disease" hypothesis. Cancer 2000;88: 921–32.
7. Wayman J, Forman D, Griffin SM. Monitoring the changing pattern of esophagogastric cancer: data from a UK regional cancer registry. Cancer Causes Control 2001;12:943–9.
8. Wanebo HJ, Kennedy BJ, Chmiel J, et al. Cancer of the stomach. A patient care study by the American College of Surgeons. Ann Surg 1993;218:583–92.
9. Hohenberger P, Gretschel S. Gastric cancer. Lancet 2003;362:305–15.
10. Corvalan A, Koriyama C, Akiba S, et al. Epstein-Barr virus in gastric carcinoma is associated with location in the cardia and with a diffuse histology: a study in one area of Chile. Int J Cancer 2001;94:527–30.
11. Fukayama M, Chong JM, Uozaki H. Pathology and molecular pathology of Epstein-Barr virus-associated gastric carcinoma. Curr Top Microbiol Immunol 2001; 258:91–102.
12. Lauren P. The two histological main types of gastric carcinoma: diffuse and so-called intestinal-type carcinoma. an attempt at a histo-clinical classification. Acta Pathol Microbiol Scand 1965;64:31–49.
13. Ogimoto I, Shibata A, Fukuda K. World Cancer Research Fund/American Institute of Cancer Research 1997 recommendations: applicability to digestive tract cancer in Japan. Cancer Causes Control 2000;11: 9–23.
14. Plummer M, Franceschi S, Munoz N. Epidemiology of gastric cancer. IARC Sci Publ 2004;157:311–26.
15. Hansson LE, Nyren O, Bergstrom R, et al. Nutrients and gastric cancer risk. A population-based case-control study in Sweden. Int J Cancer 1994;57:638–44.
16. Helicobacter and Cancer Collaborative Group. Gastric cancer and Helicobacter pylori: a combined analysis of 12 case control studies nested within prospective cohorts. Gut 2001;49:347–53.
17. Correa P. Bacterial infections as a cause of cancer. J Natl Cancer Inst 2003;95(7):E3.
18. Peek RM Jr, Blaser MJ. Helicobacter pylori and gastrointestinal tract adenocarcinomas. Nat Rev Cancer 2002;2(1):28–37.
19. La Vecchia C, Negri E, Franceschi S, Gentile A. Family history and the risk of stomach and colorectal cancer. Cancer 1992;70:50–5.
20. Fuchs CS, Mayer RJ. Gastric carcinoma. N Engl J Med 1995;333:32–41.
21. Lin J, Beerm DG. Molecular biology of upper gastrointestinal malignancies. Semin Oncol 2004;31:476–86.
22. Ebert MP, Malfertheiner P. Review article: Pathogenesis of sporadic and familial gastric cancer—implications for clinical management and cancer prevention. Aliment Pharmacol Ther 2002;16:1059–66.
23. Karpeh MS, Kelsen DP, Tepper JE. Cancer of the stomach. 6th ed. Philadelphia: Lippincott Williams & Wilkins; 2001.
24. Oohara T, Aono G, Ukawa S, et al. Clinical diagnosis of minute gastric cancer less than 5 mm in diameter. Cancer 1984;53:162–5.
25. Grise K, McFadden D. Gastric cancer: three decades of surgical management. Am Surg 1998;64:930–3.
26. Yalmarthi S, Witherspoon P, McCole D. Missed diagnosis in patients with upper

gastrointestinal cancers. Endoscopy 2004; 36:874.

27. Nio Y, Tsubono M, Kawabata K, et al. Comparison of survival curves of gastric cancer patients after surgery according to the UICC stage classification and the General Rules for Gastric Cancer Study by the Japanese Research Society for Gastric Cancer. Ann Surg 1993;218:47–53.
28. Edge SB, Byrd DR, Compton CC, et al. Stomach. 6th ed. New York: Springer, 2002.
29. Abdalla EK, Pisters PW. Staging and preoperative evaluation of upper gastrointestinal malignancies. Semin Oncol 2004;31: 513–29.
30. Takao M, Fukuda T, Iwanaga S, et al. Gastric cancer: evaluation of triphasic spiral CT and radiologic-pathologic correlation. J Comput Assist Tomogr 1998;22:288–94.
31. Davies J, Chalmers AG, Sue-Ling HM, et al. Spiral computed tomography and operative staging of gastric carcinoma: a comparison with histopathological staging. Gut 1997;41:314–9.
32. Pollack BJ, Chak A, Sivak MV Jr. Endoscopic ultrasonography. Semin Oncol 1996; 23:336–46.
33. Messmann H, Schlottmann K. Role of endoscopy in the staging of esophageal and gastric cancer. Semin Surg Oncol 2001;20: 78–81.
34. De Manzoni G, Di Leo M, Bonfiglio P. Experience of endoscopic ultrasound in staging adenocarcinoma of the cardia. Eur J Surg Oncol 1999;25:595.
35. Macdonald JS, Gohmann JJ. Chemotherapy of advanced gastric cancer: present status, future prospects. Semin Oncol 1988;15 (3 Suppl 4):42–9.
36. Burke EC, Karpeh MS, Conlon KC, Brennan MF. Laparoscopy in the management of gastric adenocarcinoma. Ann Surg 1997; 225:262–7.
37. Feussner H, Omote K, Fink U, et al. Pretherapeutic laparoscopic staging in advanced gastric carcinoma. Endoscopy 1999;31:342–7.
38. Charukhchyan SA, Lucas GW. Laparoscopy and lesser sac endoscopy in gastric carcinoma operability assessment. Am Surg 1998; 64:160–4.
39. National Comprehensive Cancer Network. Gastric cancer. Practice guidelines in oncology. Version 1. 2010. Available at www.nccn.org (accessed March 1, 2010).
40. Strong VE, Devaud N, Allen PJ, et al. Laparoscopic versus open subtotal gastrectomy for adenocarcinoma: a case-control study. Ann Surg Oncol 2009;16:1507–13.
41. Huscher CG, Mingoli A, Sgarzini G, et al. Laparoscopic versus open subtotal gastrectomy for distal gastric cancer: five-year results of a randomized prospective trial. Ann Surg 2005;241:232–7.
42. Siewert JR, Bottcher K, Stein HJ, Roder JD. Relevant prognostic factors in gastric cancer: ten-year results of the German Gastric Cancer Study. Ann Surg 1998;228:449–61.
43. Hallissey MT, Jewkes AJ, Dunn JA, et al. Resection-line involvement in gastric cancer: a continuing problem. Br J Surg 1993; 80:1418–20.
44. Jakl RJ, Miholic J, Koller R, et al. Prognostic factors in adenocarcinoma of the cardia. Am J Surg 1995;169:316–9.
45. Kooby DA, Coit DG. Controversies in the surgical management of gastric cancer. J Natl Compr Canc Netw 2003;1:115–24.
46. Kattan MW, Karpeh MS, Mazumdar M, Brennan MF. Postoperative nomogram for disease-specific survival after an R0 resection for gastric carcinoma. J Clin Oncol 2003;21:3647–50.
47. Gouzi JL, Huguier M, Fagniez PL, et al. Total versus subtotal gastrectomy for adenocarcinoma of the gastric antrum. A French prospective controlled study. Ann Surg 1989;209:162–6.
48. Robertson CS, Chung SC, Woods SD, et al. A prospective randomized trial comparing R1 subtotal gastrectomy with R3 total gastrectomy for antral cancer. Ann Surg 1994;220:176–82.
49. Bozzetti F, Marubini E, Bonfanti G, et al. Subtotal versus total gastrectomy for gastric cancer: five-year survival rates in a multicenter randomized Italian trial. Italian Gastrointestinal Tumor Study Group. Ann Surg 1999;230:170–8.
50. Spechler SJ. The role of gastric carditis in metaplasia and neoplasia at the gastroesophageal junction. Gastroenterology 1999;117: 218–28.
51. Devesa SS, Blot WJ, Fraumeni JF Jr. Changing patterns in the incidence of esophageal and gastric carcinoma in the United States. Cancer 1998;83:2049–53.
52. Rudiger Siewert J, Feith M, Werner M, Stein HJ. Adenocarcinoma of the esophagogastric junction: results of surgical therapy based on anatomical/topographic classification in 1,002 consecutive patients. Ann Surg 2000;232:353–61.
53. Harrison LE, Karpeh MS, Brennan MF. Total gastrectomy is not necessary for proximal gastric cancer. Surgery 1998;123: 127–30.
54. Kajitani T. The general rules for the gastric cancer study in surgery and pathology. Part I. Clinical classification. Jpn J Surg 1981; 11:127–39.
55. Association JGC. Japanese classification of gastric carcinoma. 2nd English ed. Gastric Cancer 1998;1:11.
56. Baba M, Hokita S, Natsugoe S, et al. Para-aortic lymphadenectomy in patients with advanced carcinoma of the upper-third of the stomach. Hepatogastroenterology 2000; 47:893–6.
57. Isozaki H, Okajima K, Fujii K, et al. Effectiveness of paraaortic lymph node dissection for advanced gastric cancer. Hepatogastroenterology 1999;46:549–54.
58. Maeta M, Yamashiro H, Saito H, et al. A prospective pilot study of extended (D3) and superextended para-aortic lymphadenectomy (D4) in patients with T3 or T4 gastric cancer managed by total gastrectomy. Surgery 1999;125:325–31.
59. Wanebo HJ, Kennedy BJ, Winchester DP, et al. Gastric carcinoma: does lymph node dissection alter survival? J Am Coll Surg 1996;183:616–24.
60. Bonenkamp JJ, Hermans J, Sasako M, et al. Extended lymph-node dissection for gastric cancer. N Engl J Med 1999;340:908–14.
61. Cuschieri A, Weeden S, Fielding J, et al. Patient survival after D1 and D2 resections for gastric cancer: long-term results of the MRC randomized surgical trial. Surgical Co-operative Group. Br J Cancer 1999;79: 1522–30.
62. Degiuli M, Sasako M, Ponti A, Calvo F. Survival results of a multicentre phase II study to evaluate D2 gastrectomy for gastric cancer. Br J Cancer 2004;90:1727–32.
63. Roukos DH, Lorenz M, Encke A. Evidence of survival benefit of extended (D2) lymphadenectomy in western patients with gastric cancer based on a new concept: a prospective long-term follow-up study. Surgery 1998;123:573–8.
64. Bilimoria KY, Talamonti MS, Wayne JD, et al. Effect of hospital type and volume on lymph node evaluation for gastric and pancreatic cancer. Arch Surg 2008;143: 671–8; discussion 678.
65. Karpeh MS, Leon L, Klimstra D, Brennan MF. Lymph node staging in gastric cancer: is location more important than number? An analysis of 1,038 patients. Ann Surg 2000; 232:362–71.
66. Talamonti MS, Kim SP, Yao KA, et al. Surgical outcomes of patients with gastric carcinoma: the importance of primary tumor location and microvessel invasion. Surgery 2003;134:720–7; discussion 727–9.
67. Brady MS, Rogatko A, Dent LL, Shiu MH. Effect of splenectomy on morbidity and survival following curative gastrectomy for carcinoma. Arch Surg 1991;126:359–64.
68. Wanebo HJ, Kennedy BJ, Winchester DP, et al. Role of splenectomy in gastric cancer surgery: adverse effect of elective splenectomy on longterm survival. J Am Coll Surg 1997;185:177–84.
69. Csendes A, Burdiles P, Rojas J, et al. A prospective randomized study comparing D2 total gastrectomy versus D2 total gastrectomy plus splenectomy in 187 patients with gastric carcinoma. Surgery 2002;131: 401–7.
70. Hallissey MT, Dunn JA, Ward LC, Allum WH. The second British Stomach Cancer Group trial of adjuvant radiotherapy or chemotherapy in resectable gastric cancer: five-year follow-up. Lancet 1994;343:1309–12.
71. Earle CC, Maroun JA. Adjuvant chemotherapy after curative resection for gastric cancer in non-Asian patients: revisiting a meta-analysis of randomised trials. Eur J Cancer 1999;35:1059–64.
72. Macdonald JS, Smalley SR, Benedetti J, et al. Chemoradiotherapy after surgery compared with surgery alone for adenocarcinoma of the stomach or gastroesophageal junction. N Engl J Med 2001;345:725–30.
73. Estes NC, MacDonald JS, Touijer K, et al. Inadequate documentation and resection for gastric cancer in the United States: a preliminary report. Am Surg 1998;64: 680–5.
74. Hundahl SA, Macdonald JS, Benedetti J, Fitzsimmons T. Surgical treatment variation in a prospective, randomized trial of chemoradiotherapy in gastric cancer: the effect of undertreatment. Ann Surg Oncol 2002;9:278–86.
75. Lowy AM, Feig BW, Janjan N, et al. A pilot study of preoperative chemoradiotherapy for resectable gastric cancer. Ann Surg Oncol 2001;8:519–24.
76. Lowy AM, Mansfield PF, Leach SD, et al. Response to neoadjuvant chemotherapy best predicts survival after curative resection of gastric cancer. Ann Surg 1999;229: 303–8.
77. Cunningham D, Allum WH, Stenning SP, et al. Perioperative chemotherapy versus surgery alone for resectable gastroesophageal cancer. N Engl J Med 2006;355: 11–20.
78. Gurney KA, Cartwright RA, Gilman EA. Descriptive epidemiology of gastrointestinal non-Hodgkin's lymphoma in a population-based registry. Br J Cancer 1999;79:1929–34.
79. Koch P, del Valle F, Berdel WE, et al. Primary gastrointestinal non-Hodgkin's lymphoma: II. Combined surgical and conservative or conservative management only in localized gastric lymphoma—results of the prospective German Multicenter Study GIT NHL 01/92. J Clin Oncol 2001;19: 3874–83.
80. Crump M, Gospodarowicz M, Shepherd FA. Lymphoma of the gastrointestinal tract. Semin Oncol 1999;26:324–37.

81. National Comprehensive Cancer Network. Non-Hodgkin's lymphoma. Practice guidelines in oncology. Version 1. 2005. Available at www.nccn.org (accessed March 1, 2010).
82. Talamonti MS. Gastric cancer. Philadelphia: Lippincott Williams & Wilkins; 1998.
83. Yoon SS, Coit DG, Portlock CS, Karpeh MS. The diminishing role of surgery in the treatment of gastric lymphoma. Ann Surg 2004;240:28–37.
84. Parsonnet J, Hansen S, Rodriguez L, et al. Helicobacter pylori infection and gastric lymphoma. N Engl J Med 1994;330: 1267–71.
85. Isaacson PG. Recent developments in our understanding of gastric lymphomas. Am J Surg Pathol 1996;20 Suppl 1:S17.
86. Stolte M, Bayerdorffer E, Morgner A, et al. Helicobacter and gastric MALT lymphoma. Gut 2002;50 Suppl 3:III19–24.
87. Schechter NR, Yahalom J. Low-grade MALT lymphoma of the stomach: a review of treatment options. Int J Radiat Oncol Biol Phys 2000;46:1093–103.
88. Martinelli G, Laszlo D, Ferreri AJ, et al. Clinical activity of rituximab in gastric marginal zone non-Hodgkin's lymphoma resistant to or not eligible for anti-Helicobacter pylori therapy. J Clin Oncol 2005;23:1979–83.
89. Nilsson B, Bumming P, Meis-Kindblom JM, et al. Gastrointestinal stromal tumors: the incidence, prevalence, clinical course, and prognostication in the preimatinib mesylate era—a population-based study in western Sweden. Cancer 2005;103:821–9.
90. Miettinen M, Sobin LH, Lasota J. Gastrointestinal stromal tumors of the stomach: a clinicopathologic, immunohistochemical, and molecular genetic study of 1765 cases with long-term follow-up. Am J Surg Pathol 2005;29:52–68.
91. Ng EH, Pollock RE, Munsell MF, et al. Prognostic factors influencing survival in gastrointestinal leiomyosarcomas. Implications for surgical management and staging. Ann Surg 1992;215:68–77.
92. Conlon KC, Casper ES, Brennan MF. Primary gastrointestinal sarcomas: analysis of prognostic variables. Ann Surg Oncol 1995;2:26–31.
93. Corless CL, Fletcher JA, Heinrich MC. Biology of gastrointestinal stromal tumors. J Clin Oncol 2004;22:3813–25.
94. National Comprehensive Cancer Network. Soft tissue sarcoma. Practice guidelines in oncology. Version 1. 2009. Available at www.nccn.org (accessed March 1, 2010).
95. Miettinen M, Lasota J. Gastrointestinal stromal tumors: pathology and prognosis at different sites. Semin Diagn Pathol 2006; 23:70–83.
96. Edge SB, Byrd DR, Compton CC, et al, editors. AJCC cancer staging manual. 7th ed. New York; Springer, 2010.
97. Demetri GD, Benjamin RS, Blanke CD, et al. NCCN Task Force report: management of patients with gastrointestinal stromal tumor (GIST)—update of the NCCN clinical practice guidelines. J Natl Compr Canc Netw 2007;5 Suppl 2:S1–29; quiz S30.
98. Demetri GD, von Mehren M, Blanke CD, et al. Efficacy and safety of imatinib mesylate in advanced gastrointestinal stromal tumors. N Engl J Med 2002;347:472–80.
99. Gilligan CJ, Lawton GP, Tang LH, et al. Gastric carcinoid tumors: the biology and therapy of an enigmatic and controversial lesion. Am J Gastroenterol 1995;90:338–52.
100. Maggard MA, O'Connell JB, Ko CY. Updated population-based review of carcinoid tumors. Ann Surg 2004;240:117–22.
101. Modlin IM, Lye KD, Kidd M. A 50-year analysis of 562 gastric carcinoids: small tumor or larger problem? Am J Gastroenterol 2004;99:23–32.
102. Schindl M, Kaserer K, Niederle B. Treatment of gastric neuroendocrine tumors: the necessity of a type-adapted treatment. Arch Surg 2001;136:49–54.
103. Modlin IM, Cornelius E, Lawton GP. Use of an isotopic somatostatin receptor probe to image gut endocrine tumors. Arch Surg 1995;130:367–73; discussion 373–4.
104. Frost DB, Mercado PD, Tyrell JS. Small bowel cancer: a 30-year review. Ann Surg Oncol 1994;1:290–5.
105. Bilimoria KY, Bentrem DJ, Wayne JD, et al. Small bowel cancer in the United States: changes in epidemiology, treatment, and survival over the last 20 years. Ann Surg 2009;249:63–71.
106. Torres M, Matta E, Chinea B, et al. Malignant tumors of the small intestine. J Clin Gastroenterol 2003;37:372–80.
107. Zuckerman GR, Prakash C, Askin MP, Lewis BS. AGA technical review on the evaluation and management of occult and obscure gastrointestinal bleeding. Gastroenterology 2000;118:201–21.
108. Lewis BS. Small intestinal bleeding. Gastroenterol Clin North Am 2000;29:67–95, vi.
109. de Mascarenhas-Saravina MN, de Silva Araujo Lopes LM. Small bowel tumors diagnosed by wireless capsule endoscopy: report of five cases. Endoscopy 2003;35: 865.
110. Lambert P, Minghini A, Pincus W, et al. Treatment and prognosis of primary malignant small bowel tumors. Am Surg 1996;62: 709–15.
111. Talamonti MS, Goetz LH, Rao S, Joehl RJ. Primary cancers of the small bowel: analysis of prognostic factors and results of surgical management. Arch Surg 2002;137:564–70; discussion 570–1.
112. Dabaja BS, Suki D, Pro B, et al. Adenocarcinoma of the small bowel: presentation, prognostic factors, and outcome of 217 patients. Cancer 2004;101:518–26.
113. Ito H, Perez A, Brooks DC, et al. Surgical treatment of small bowel cancer: a 20-year single institution experience. J Gastrointest Surg 2003;7:925–30.

8 TUMORS OF THE PANCREAS, BILIARY TRACT, AND LIVER

Steven M. Strasberg, MD, FACS, FRCS(C), FRCS(Ed), and David C. Linehan, MD, FACS

Several different types of tumors affect the pancreas, the biliary tree, and the liver. Each year, hundreds of articles are published regarding pancreatic, biliary, and hepatic cancers. Accordingly, this chapter concentrates on essential principles. In particular, it focuses on common malignant tumors, addressing benign tumors and uncommon tumors only insofar as they are important in differential diagnosis.

When a patient presents with an apparent cancer of the pancreas, the biliary tree, or the liver, the surgeon must attempt to answer the following three important questions:

1. What is the diagnosis?
2. What is the surgical stage of the disease—that is, is the tumor resectable?
3. What is the operative rationale that will encompass the disease and produce a margin-free resection (and, for pancreatobiliary cancers, an N1 resection)?

These questions form the underpinning for the process of investigation and management. In what follows, we describe our approach to each of the cancers in these terms.

Pancreatic Cancer

DUCTAL ADENOCARCINOMA

Ductal Adenocarcinoma of the Head of the Pancreas

Adenocarcinoma of the pancreatic head is one of the most common gastrointestinal malignancies and, because of its aggressive nature, one of the hardest cancers to cure. The safety of surgical procedures for cancers of the pancreas has improved dramatically, but 5-year actual survival rates of patients who have undergone resection are still low (about 15%).[1] Cancer of the head of the pancreas is the prototypical tumor that causes painless jaundice; however, other cancers that obstruct the bile ducts also cause jaundice, including extrahepatic bile duct cancer, ampullary malignancy, duodenal cancer, and gallbladder cancer. Some of the following discussion is generalized to determining the diagnosis in patients presenting with obstructive jaundice [*see 6:3 Jaundice*].

Clinical evaluation *History* The classic presentation of cancer of the head of the pancreas is unremitting jaundice, usually accompanied by dark urine, light stool, and pruritus. Darkening of the urine or pruritus is often the first symptom, and scleral icterus frequently is first noted by family members or coworkers. The pruritus is often severe. The jaundice sometimes is painless but more frequently is associated with epigastric pain, which is often mild. Severe acute pain is more often associated with other conditions that may cause jaundice (e.g., choledocholithiasis and pancreatitis). Back pain suggests that the tumor has invaded tissues outside the pancreas and is unresectable. Significant weight loss (> 10% of body weight) is common even when the pancreatic cancer is resectable.

In some patients, the presenting symptom is steatorrhea or diarrhea from obstruction of the pancreatic duct, weight loss, pain, or a combination of these rather than jaundice. Steatorrhea or diarrhea in the absence of jaundice is usually the result of a tumor in the uncinate process that obstructs the pancreatic duct but not the bile duct. Often these symptoms are overlooked until the tumor extends and causes jaundice. About 5% of patients have a history of diabetes of recent onset. Migratory thrombophlebitis (Trousseau sign) is uncommon and usually signifies metastatic disease. Pancreatobiliary malignancies cause biliary obstruction, but such obstruction is not commonly associated with biliary tract infection unless instruments have been employed in the biliary tree. Therefore, other diagnoses should be suspected in patients presenting with cholangitis who have not undergone biliary tract instrumentation. Patients with pancreatic cancer may also present with acute pancreatitis as the first manifestation. Vomiting and gastrointestinal (GI) bleeding are uncommon presenting symptoms and suggest the presence of advanced tumors that are obstructing or eroding the duodenum.

Physical examination Examination reveals scleral icterus. In some cases, the distended gallbladder may be palpable. In advanced cases, signs of metastatic disease (e.g., hepatomegaly and ascites) may be detected.

Investigative studies *Laboratory tests* Liver function tests (LFTs) are of limited value in diagnosis. The serum bilirubin level is elevated in jaundiced patients, with the direct fraction exceeding 50%. The serum alkaline phosphatase level is almost always elevated when the bile duct is obstructed, and levels three to five times normal are common. Aminotransferase levels usually are moderately elevated as well. Very high aminotransferase levels suggest a hepatocellular cause of jaundice, usually viral, although impaction of a stone in the bile duct can cause transient rises in serum aspartate aminotransferase to levels higher than 1,000 IU/mL. By themselves, LFTs cannot effectively distinguish among jaundice arising from a hepatocellular cause (e.g., viral hepatitis or drug-induced cholestasis), jaundice resulting from a disease of microscopic bile ducts (e.g., primary biliary cirrhosis), or jaundice caused by any of the malignancies that obstruct the major bile ducts. To make this distinction, radiologic imaging tests are required [*see* Imaging, *below*].

Serum concentrations of the tumor marker CA 19-9 are often elevated in patients with pancreatic or biliary adenocarcinomas.[2] The upper limit of the normal range is 37 U/mL. Concentrations higher than 100 U/mL are highly suggestive of malignancy, but elevations between 37 and 100 U/mL are less specific. Serum levels generally reflect the extent of the tumor: small tumors (1 cm in diameter) are rarely associated with levels higher than 100 U/mL, whereas very high concentrations (> 1,000 U/mL) suggest metastatic disease. High levels may also accompany cholangitis, but these levels should subside to normal with relief of obstruction or infection, when malignancy is absent. Measurement of CA 19-9 concentrations may be employed to detect recurrences. In patients who have elevated CA 19-9 levels that return to normal after tumor resection; a second rise in the CA 19-9 level in the follow-up period is indicative of recurrence.

Imaging Several different diagnostic imaging tests may be used in jaundiced patients, including computed tomography (CT), magnetic resonance imaging (MRI), endoscopic retrograde cholangiopancreatography (ERCP), endoscopic ultrasonography (EUS), and transabdominal ultrasonography. The technical advances in imaging achieved over the past few years are remarkable. CT and MRI can now provide high-quality images of blood vessels and ducts and their anatomic relation to tumors. These images can even be projected in three dimensions if desired, although, to date, no high level studies have shown an advantage for this type of display.

Selection of appropriate imaging tests in a jaundiced patient is influenced by patient characteristics and by the symptoms observed. For instance, the type and order of investigations appropriate for an older patient presenting with obstructive jaundice, who is likely to have a malignancy, differ from those appropriate for a young woman with severe pain, who is more likely to have choledocholithiasis. The best initial imaging test in a patient in whom malignancy is suspected is either a fine-cut (3 mm between slices) three-phase (no-contrast phase, arterial phase, and venous phase) helical (spiral) CT scan or a high-quality MRI scan. Although MRI has the advantage of being able to provide a cholangiogram (i.e., magnetic resonance cholangiopancreatography [MRCP]), small and medium-sized radiologic facilities currently tend to be more skilled at CT than at MRI; this difference should be taken into account when the first test is ordered. High-quality MRI scanners and the very latest generation of CT scanners are capable of providing cholangiograms and angiograms, as well as axial images.

The typical pancreatic cancer appears as an area of reduced attenuation (darker zone) in the pancreatic head [*see Figure 1*], associated with upstream dilatation of bile ducts and the gallbladder. Often the pancreatic duct is also obstructed. As a result, the pancreatic duct may be dilated in the tail, body, and neck of the pancreas, with dilatation terminating sharply at the edge of the tumor. Pancreatic duct dilatation is often accompanied by atrophy of the body and the tail of the pancreas [*see Figure 2*].

When a jaundiced patient is discovered to have a typical-appearing localized cancer of the pancreatic head on CT scanning, no further diagnostic tests are needed, and operative management should be the next step. Tissue diagnosis is unnecessary. Negative biopsy results rarely change the therapeutic approach, and in that they may be falsely negative, they are

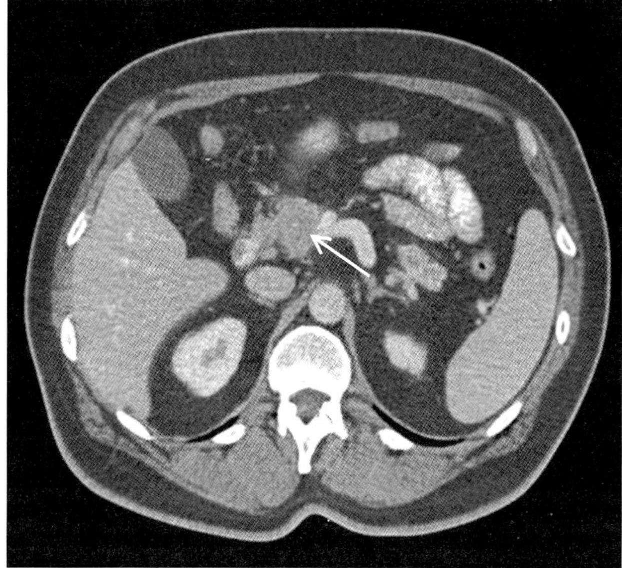

Figure 1 **Shown is a typical hypoattenuating cancer of the pancreatic head. The tumor (*arrow*) is invading the right side of the portosplenic confluence, as evidenced by the "beaking" of the vein at that point.**

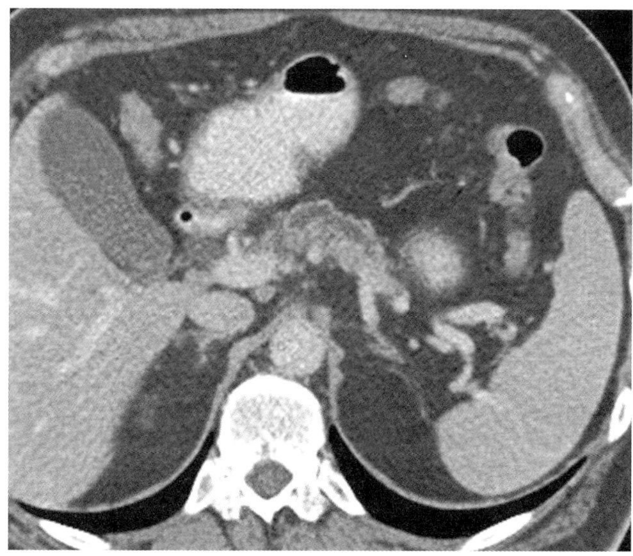

Figure 2 **In the same patient as in Figure 1, pancreatic duct dilation is apparent in the body of the pancreas, with atrophy of the parenchyma.**

potentially misleading. Furthermore, omitting biopsy eliminates the small risk of tumor implantation in the needle tract. Selection of axial imaging as the first test often renders diagnostic ERCP, which is a more invasive test, unnecessary as well. Cholangiography also is not required for staging pancreatic head tumors [*see* Surgical Staging, *below*]. The advantages of starting with axial imaging in jaundiced patients with suspected cancer are discussed in greater detail elsewhere [*see* Biliary Tract Cancer, Extrahepatic Cholangiocarcinoma, Upper Duct Cholangiocarcinoma, Investigative Studies, *below*].

Additional diagnostic imaging for atypical CT or MRI findings In many patients with adenocarcinoma of the pancreatic head, the typical CT findings described above are absent and additional diagnostic imaging is required. Such patients may be categorized into two groups: those with an *atypical mass* and those with *no mass* on axial imaging. In either case, before ordering additional tests, it is appropriate to determine whether the CT scan is of adequate quality. The scan may have been performed without contrast, the arterial and venous phases may not have been captured appropriately, or the slice thickness may have been too great for precise visualization of the head of the pancreas. Small adenocarcinomas may be missed when the venous phase is poorly timed, especially if slice thickness is 5 mm or greater, and masses that initially appear atypical may exhibit a typical appearance when the CT scan is optimized. Neuroendocrine cancers commonly display arterial-phase enhancement, which will be missed if the scan is mistimed. In our experience, about 40% of referred patients who underwent CT scanning before arrival require a so-called pancreas protocol CT scan (i.e., a fine-cut three-phase helical scan) when they are first seen; in many of these cases, the second CT scan yields important diagnostic findings.

When no mass is present in a jaundiced patient with a periampullary tumor or another focal obstructing process (e.g., pancreatitis), the CT scan usually shows bile duct dilatation extending down to the intrapancreatic portion of the duct. The dilatation may terminate anywhere from the upper border of the pancreas to the duodenum, depending on the site of the tumor and the nature of the process obstructing the bile duct. In these conditions, ERCP is a good choice as the second test.

ERCP provides an endoscopic view of the duodenum that allows identification and biopsy of ampullary and duodenal tumors, which may be blocking the bile duct and producing jaundice. It confirms the presence of a bile duct stricture and displays its form, which is helpful in diagnosis. Focal strictures, especially those with shoulders, suggest malignancy. Long, tapering strictures limited to the intrapancreatic portion of the bile duct suggest chronic pancreatitis. Concomitant narrowing of the pancreatic duct in the head of the pancreas (the double-duct sign) suggests the presence of a small pancreatic cancer that is not visible on the CT scan. Longer or multiple pancreatic strictures suggest chronic pancreatitis. A single focal bile duct stricture in the absence of pancreatic duct abnormalities is the hallmark of cancer of the lower bile duct. Infiltrating cancers of the bile duct may cause more than one stricture along the bile duct, but when more than one stricture is present, other diagnoses (e.g., primary sclerosing cholangitis) should be considered. Both pancreatic and bile ducts may be assessed with brush cytology. This test has a 45 to 50% sensitivity for cancer[3]; therefore, only a positive test result is significant.

ERCP findings in a patient with no mass must be evaluated in the light of findings from other investigations. Patients with the classic double-duct sign or single focal shouldered bile duct strictures are likely to have small pancreatic or bile duct tumors. Further diagnostic support is usually not needed before laparotomy, although such support may be reassuring when the CA 19-9 concentration is lower than 100 U/mL. When doubt persists, EUS often helps resolve it. EUS may identify a small mass that was not seen on the CT scan, and biopsies may then be done. Occasionally, EUS reveals enlarged lymph nodes, which may also undergo biopsy. However, negative EUS-guided biopsy results in patients who present with painless jaundice do not exclude malignancy. When such patients have an identifiable mass on EUS and a presentation in keeping with the diagnosis of cancer, pancreaticoduodenectomy is recommended, even if EUS-guided biopsy yields negative results. If a nonoperative approach is taken, short-term follow-up at 4 to 6 weeks with repeat imaging and biopsy is mandatory. If the findings persist, laparotomy is advisable.

Occasionally, preoperative testing reveals no mass, but a mass is subsequently discovered by intraoperative palpation or intraoperative ultrasonography (IOUS). A mass palpated in the head of a pancreas that is otherwise normal or near normal in texture in the remainder of the gland is highly suggestive of malignancy and constitutes sufficient justification for resection. The same is true of a mass detected by IOUS if the mass has characteristics of malignancy (i.e., is hypoechoic). If the IOUS findings are inconclusive, biopsy with frozen-section examination is a reasonable approach. In many such cases, the whole pancreas is diffusely firm or hard, and IOUS demonstrates a diffuse change in the normal texture of the gland. When the pancreas is diffusely firm and no localized process is seen on IOUS, biopsies should be directed toward the stent in the bile duct at the point where the bile duct narrows (as seen on ultrasonography).

The ultimate diagnostic test is pancreaticoduodenectomy. If there is a strong suspicion of cancer before laparotomy or the findings at laparotomy are strongly suggestive, this procedure should be performed without preliminary biopsy. When this approach is followed, a small number of patients with suspected malignant disease will be found to have benign disease; this possibility should be explained to patients who do not undergo confirmatory tissue diagnosis before operation. Because of the limited negative predictive value of currently available tests, pancreaticoduodenectomy is sometimes still required to make a definitive diagnosis.

The finding of an atypical pancreatic head mass on a CT scan poses an additional challenge. Atypical masses may take different forms. In some cases, they exhibit attenuation that differs only slightly from that of the surrounding pancreas; in others, they have a ground-glass appearance. They may extend into the body and tail of the pancreas, or they may be localized to the head. With atypical masses, the most common problem is how to differentiate focal pancreatitis from adenocarcinoma. This differentiation can be very difficult. Pancreatitis may be present without antecedent acute attacks; without a history of alcoholism, gallstones, or hyperlipidemia; without diabetes or steatorrhea; and without calcifications in the gland. Cancer appears to be more common in patients who have had chronic pancreatitis, and the diseases may coexist. Therefore, one cannot feel confident that cancer is absent simply because chronic pancreatitis is present. Cancer should be suspected in patients with an established diagnosis of chronic pancreatitis who undergo a rapid change in status (e.g., weight loss). Diabetes is common in patients with chronic pancreatitis, but it may also be the first sign of pancreatic cancer in patients without chronic pancreatitis. Chronic pancreatitis can cause painless jaundice. A rare immune form of chronic pancreatitis, known as lymphoplasmacytic sclerosing pancreatitis, has been recognized that is particularly hard to differentiate from cancer.[4] However, in these patients, the serum IgG4 level is characteristically elevated.

EUS is becoming increasingly important in the management of patients with atypical pancreatic head masses.[5] When jaundice is present, EUS with or without ERCP is our usual approach; when it is absent, EUS alone is performed. EUS-guided biopsy is superior to CT-guided transabdominal biopsy in that access to the head of the pancreas is easier and the chance of needle tracking is reduced (because the biopsy is taken through the duodenal wall, which is resected if a Whipple procedure is done).

At the conclusion of all of the preceding investigations, it still may not be clear whether a malignancy is present. Clinical judgment must be exercised in deciding whether to operate or to repeat investigative studies after an interval of 2 to 3 months. Operation is favored in patients who are jaundiced, who have less pain, who have elevated CA 19-9 levels, and whose mass is suspicious for cancer. Elevation of the CA 19-9 concentration beyond 100 U/mL should be regarded as a very important finding. When EUS is inconclusive, ultrasound-guided diagnostic laparoscopy may be performed to obtain core tissue biopsies from several areas of the mass. This technique is especially useful when chronic pancreatitis is strongly suspected[6] in that the multiple long core biopsies obtainable with this procedure provide a greater degree of assurance against false negative findings for cancer. Even this test, however, is not 100% accurate. The penultimate diagnostic test is laparotomy with mobilization of the pancreatic head and IOUS-guided transduodenal core biopsies of the mass. The ideal outcome with this approach is to perform pancreaticoduodenectomy in all patients who actually have cancer while reducing to a reasonable minimum resection in patients with benign disease, who in most cases are better served by biliary bypass. Fortunately, today, because of improved axial imaging and EUS, a definitive preoperative diagnosis is usually available.

Surgical staging The term "staging" is currently used to denote the process by which the surgeon determines whether a tumor is resectable. We prefer to use the term "surgical staging" for this process so as to distinguish it from those staging classifications that define the life history and prognosis of tumors and provide the basis for comparison of results—namely, the TNM classifications developed by the American Joint Committee on Cancer (AJCC). These latter systems are also of great importance to the surgeon dealing with pancreatic tumors.

Surgical staging is started preoperatively and completed intraoperatively. Preoperative staging tests determine operability—that is, whether the tumor appears resectable after preoperative testing. However, the final decision regarding resectability is made only during the operation, on the basis of intraoperative staging. A tumor of the head of the pancreas is deemed unresectable when it is determined to have extended beyond the boundaries of a pancreaticoduodenectomy. Common reasons for unresectability include (1) vascular invasion (i.e., invasion of the superior mesenteric vein, the portal vein, the superior mesenteric artery, or, less commonly, the hepatic artery); (2) lymph node metastases that fall outside the scope of a pancreaticoduodenectomy (e.g., metastases to para-aortic and celiac lymph nodes); (3) hepatic metastases; (4) peritoneal metastases; and (5) extra-abdominal metastases (usually pulmonary). Limited vascular invasion of the superior mesenteric vein and the portal vein may be overcome by resection and reconstruction and thus is only a relative contraindication to resection. This is especially true when the tumor is small and has arisen in the vicinity of the veins. In a series from our institution (Washington University in St. Louis), about 27% of resections done for pancreatic cancer involved resection of these veins.[7] Recently, the term "borderline" has been introduced to describe tumors that are unresectable by standard criteria but that can be encompassed by extending the zone of resection.[8] Usually, such tumors are first treated with chemoradiation. Attempts are also being made to downsize more advanced pancreatic tumors to a resectable state by chemotherapy and radiation. To date, no long-term studies have evaluated either approach. However, given the aggressive nature of this tumor, it is likely that chemotherapy and radiation will effectively downsize tumors in only a small number of patients, at least until much more effective chemotherapeutic agents are available.

The tests used to establish the diagnosis and those used to accomplish surgical staging go hand in hand. Abdominal CT scans, abdominal MRI, thoracic CT scans, and chest radiographs are obtained to detect hepatic metastases, vascular invasion, and pulmonary metastases. To assess vascular invasion, fine-cut three-phase helical CT scans or MRI scans are required. These tests may also detect enlarged lymph nodes, but it should be remembered that nodes may be enlarged for reasons other than cancer. Sometimes intraperitoneal fluid collections or peritoneal or omental nodules are identified; fluid may be sent for cytologic analysis, and omental nodules may undergo ultrasound-guided biopsy. Invasion of the mesentery, the mesocolon, or retroperitoneal tissues may also be detected by CT scanning. In the view of some surgeons, such invasion may render the tumor unresectable, but in our experience, this is rarely the case in the absence of concomitant vascular invasion: the resection may still be accomplished with clear margins by resecting the portion of the mesocolon or the mesentery that is locally invaded.

EUS may be used to guide biopsy of suspicious lymph nodes when these lie outside the planned resection zone. It has also been employed to assess vascular invasion, but in our experience, it has no advantage over CT in this regard; moreover, it is more operator dependent than CT. Staging laparoscopy is particularly effective at finding small hepatic and peritoneal nodules. About 20% of patients thought to have resectable pancreatic adenocarcinoma of the head of the pancreas before staging laparoscopy are found to have liver or peritoneal metastases at laparoscopy.[9] Staging is completed intraoperatively by carefully inspecting the intra-abdominal contents, including the lesser sac, mobilizing the head of the pancreas, performing biopsies of suspicious nodules or nodes outside the planned resection zone, and attempting dissection of the superior mesenteric vein or the portal vein. Formal clinicopathologic staging according to the AJCC's TNM system is useful for establishing the prognosis and planning additional treatment [*see Table 1 and Table 2*].

All authorities agree that axial imaging of the abdomen and chest (or roentgenography of the chest) is standard practice for staging pancreatic cancer; however, not all agree on the value of other staging tests. Many authorities advocate omission of staging laparoscopy or EUS-guided biopsy of nodes on the grounds that patients are better served by palliative surgery than by endoscopic stenting of the bile duct. There is no advantage in knowing preoperatively whether small liver metastases or celiac node metastases are present if laparotomy is to be undertaken anyway. Trials examining whether better palliation is offered by surgical bypass or endoscopic stenting report conflicting results; on balance, surgical bypass is still a very good treatment for localized unresectable tumors in younger patients without serious comorbidities. We no longer perform staging laparoscopy in patients with adenocarcinoma of the pancreas except in patients who are suspected to have liver or peritoneal metastases on axial imaging. Finally, ^{18}F-fluorodeoxyglucose positron emission tomography (FDG-PET) may be useful in staging pancreatic cancer. Given that inflammation is frequently confused with cancer, the major role of this modality will probably be in the detection of distant metastases.

Management *Preoperative preparation* All jaundiced patients should receive vitamin K, a fat-soluble vitamin whose absorption is reduced by biliary or pancreatic duct obstruction. Routine preoperative bile duct decompression is unnecessary, except when jaundice has been prolonged or operative treatment will be delayed (e.g., for correction of cardiac or other comorbid conditions). Several studies have shown that surgical outcome is not improved by routine preoperative decompression in jaundiced patients. In fact, stent placement may increase the incidence of postoperative infection.[10]

Rationale for pancreaticoduodenectomy The technical details of pancreaticoduodenectomy are discussed more fully elsewhere [*see 6:23 Procedures for Benign and Malignant Pancreatic Disease*]. Therapeutic decision making necessarily includes consideration of the extent of the procedure. The operative goal is to remove the tumor with clear margins, as well as the N1 regional lymph nodes. Attempts have been made to improve results by extending the operation, either through more extensive lymph node dissections[11] or through resections of superior mesenteric, hepatic, or celiac arteries.[12] Four randomized trials have now shown no advantage for extended lymph node dissection. Resection of celiac or superior mesenteric arteries has also not been successful in improving overall survival. The lesson seems to be that invasion of additional lymph node regions (N2) or the superior mesenteric or celiac arteries signals an aggressive tumor biology that is unlikely to be overcome by wider resections. Except for resection of the portal vein or the superior mesenteric vein and perhaps short segments of the hepatic artery to address invasion of these structures by otherwise favorable tumors, extended resections are generally unsuccessful. Even these recommended vascular resections are probably best restricted to tumors that have arisen close to the particular vessels and involved them while still small; resections of large adenocarcinomas that have grown over time to involve long stretches of the veins are best avoided. These comments do not apply to tumors that initially might have required resection of the celiac or superior mesenteric arteries but that have been downsized by chemotherapy of chemoradiation so that they can be resected without such vascular resections.

There is also continuing controversy regarding the respective merits of the standard version of the operation and its pylorus-preserving variant. There is no evidence that the two procedures differ with respect to overall survival. Pylorus preservation is associated with gastric-emptying problems in the postoperative period, but, overall, it may be associated with slightly less postoperative GI dysfunction.[13] We employ pylorus preservation selectively in older, thinner patients, with the aim of minimizing disruption of GI function.

Adjuvant therapy is often given in resected patients; however, there is controversy regarding the role of chemotherapy

Table 1 American Joint Committee on Cancer TNM Clinical Classification of Pancreatic Cancer[1]

Primary tumor (T)	TX	Primary tumor cannot be assessed
	T0	No evidence of primary tumor
	Tis	Carcinoma in situ
	T1	Tumor limited to pancreas, ≤ 2 cm in greatest dimension
	T2	Tumor limited to pancreas, > 2 cm in greatest dimension
	T3	Tumor extends beyond pancreas but without involvement of celiac axis or SMA
	T4	Tumor involves celiac axis or SMA
Regional lymph nodes (N)	NX	Regional lymph nodes cannot be assessed
	N0	No regional lymph node metastasis
	N1	Regional lymph node metastasis
Distant metastasis (M)	MX	Distant metastasis cannot be assessed
	M0	No distant metastasis
	M1	No distant metastasis

SMA = superior mesenteric artery.

Table 2 American Joint Committee on Cancer Staging System for Pancreatic Cancer

Stage	T	N	M
0	Tis	N0	M0
IA	T1	N0	M0
IB	T2	N0	M0
IIA	T3	N0	M0
IIB	T1, T2, T3	N1	M0
III	T4	Any N	M0
IV	Any T	Any N	M1

versus chemoradiation. Randomized trials have shown that chemotherapy is beneficial and have questioned the role of radiotherapy. The latter may be helpful when an R1 resection has been performed.

Adenocarcinoma of Body and Tail of the Pancreas

Adenocarcinoma of the body and tail of the pancreas is less common than adenocarcinoma of the head. Because it does not produce jaundice, it tends to be recognized relatively late. Accordingly, patients are often in an advanced stage of disease at presentation. Tumors of the midbody tend to invade posteriorly to involve the superior mesenteric artery or the celiac axis, even when these lesions are only 2 to 3 cm in diameter. As a result, tumors of the tail are more likely to be resectable than tumors of the midbody when they are discovered. Many resectable tumors are discovered incidentally; by the time the tumors give rise to symptoms, they are frequently unresectable.

Clinical evaluation Symptoms are nonspecific, consisting of abdominal and back pain (which is usually relieved by sitting up and leaning forward), weight loss, and diabetes of recent onset.

Investigative studies The CA 19-9 concentration may be elevated. CT usually shows a lucent (hypoattenuating) mass [*see Figure 3*], often with extension outside the pancreas and dilatation of the distal pancreatic duct, when the tumor is proximal to the tail of the gland. EUS is very useful for assessing indeterminate lesions.

Surgical staging Surgical staging of cancers of the body and the tail is similar to that of cancers of the pancreatic head and is based primarily on CT scanning of the abdomen and the thorax. Unresectability by reason of local invasion is usually attributable to the involvement of the superior mesenteric artery, hepatic artery, or the celiac artery and less commonly to the involvement of the portal vein, the superior mesenteric vein, or the aorta. Another indicator of unresectability is enlarged para-aortic nodes. Invasion of the spleen, the stomach, the left adrenal gland, the mesocolon, the colon, the retroperitoneum, or even the left kidney is not a contraindication to resection provided that clear margins may be expected.[14] Staging laparoscopy is of great value: between 20 and 50% of patients with these tumors are found to have unresectable tumors with this modality, usually due to small liver or peritoneal implants.[15] Cancer of the body and the tail differs from cancer of the head in that there is no effective palliation and therefore no rationale for laparotomy if the lesion is unresectable. Celiac nerve block, which is very helpful in reducing the use of narcotics for pain control, may also be performed laparoscopically or endoscopically.

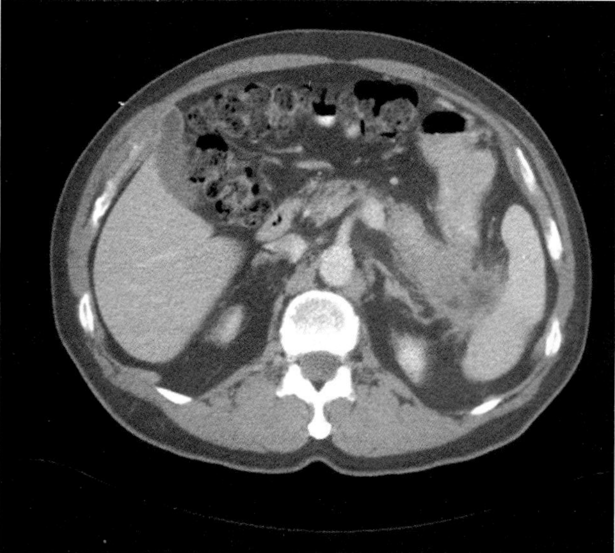

Figure 3 **Shown is a typical hypoattenuating cancer of the tail of the pancreas with invasion of the hilum of the spleen and the splenic flexure of the colon. Peritumoral stranding suggests inflammation or invasion of peripancreatic fat.**

Management *Rationale for radical antegrade modular pancreatosplenectomy* Logically, the goal of resection of tumors of the body and tail should be the same as that of resection of tumors of the head—namely, excision of the tumor with clear margins, along with the N1 lymph nodes. In practice, this goal generally is not achieved by the traditional retrograde distal pancreatectomy, in which the spleen is taken first and which is not based on the lymph node drainage of the pancreas. Lymph node counts have been low with the traditional procedure, and positive posterior margin rates have been high. As an alternative, we have developed a technique referred to as radical antegrade modular pancreatosplenectomy (RAMPS), which accomplishes the desired goals by performing the resection in an antegrade manner from right to left and which is based on the established lymph node drainage of the gland [*see Figure 4*].[16] Negative tangential margin rates of 90% have been achieved with this approach. RAMPS also allows early control of the vasculature.

Mucinous Adenocarcinoma

Mucin-producing cancers are special variants of adenocarcinoma of the pancreas that often arise in preexisting lesions. The two main types of premalignant lesions are mucinous cystic neoplasm (MCN) and intraductal papillary mucinous neoplasm (IPMN) (also referred to as intraductal papillary mucinous tumor).[17] A complete discussion of pancreatic cyst disease is beyond the scope of this chapter. Accordingly, we briefly address such disease as it relates to cancer of the pancreas, omitting discussion of less common cystic malignancies of the pancreas.

Mucinous cystic neoplasm MCN occurs most often in middle-aged women, typically in the body or tail of the pancreas. MCNs are unilocular or septated cysts whose diameter ranges from subcentimeter size to 15 cm or larger. Occasionally, calcium is present in the wall. Excrescences may be present on the inner wall; if so, malignancy is more likely. Most symptomatic MCNs are between 4 and 7 cm in diameter.

Clinical evaluation and investigative studies Patients with MCNs typically present with left-sided abdominal pain, often in the flank and the back. These lesions also are frequently discovered incidentally. Pancreatitis is rare and jaundice is uncommon, even when the lesions are situated in the head of the pancreas. MCNs must be differentiated from pseudocysts and from serous cystadenomas (SCAs), which are benign cysts. Differentiation between MCNs and pseudocysts is based on the history, imaging studies, and cyst fluid analysis. The diagnosis of pseudocyst is supported by a history of pancreatitis,

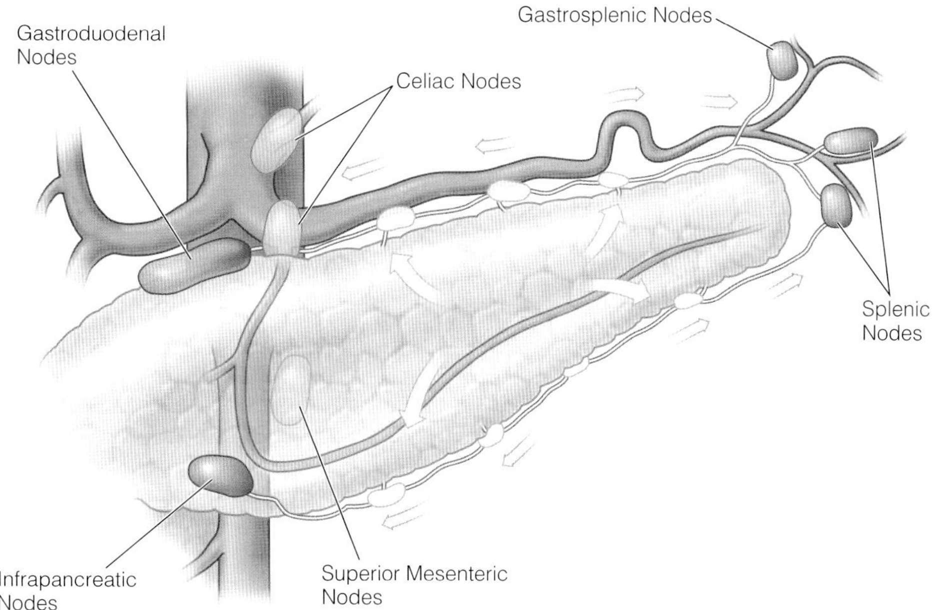

Figure 4 **Illustrated is the pattern of lymphatic drainage of the pancreas. The darker nodes are N1 nodes for the body and tail of the pancreas. The lighter nodes on the aorta to the left side of the celiac artery and the superior mesenteric artery are N1 for the central part of the pancreas and N2 for other regions.**

a thick-walled, uncalcified cyst with associated radiologic signs of pancreatitis and often cholelithiasis, as well as cyst fluid containing high levels of amylase and lipase and a relatively low level of carcinoembryonic antigen (CEA) (< 500 ng/mL).

SCAs have the same clinical presentation as MCNs. SCAs are more frequently polycystic than MCNs, but this difference is not a certain means of discriminating between the two. In a minority (25%) of cases, SCAs have a pathognomonic central calcification with radiating arms ringed by multiple grape-sized cysts. When the individual cysts are tiny (honeycomb pattern), there are many cyst walls within the lesion, and then SCAs may be mistaken for solid tumors. Unlike pseudocysts and IPMNs, neither MCNs nor SCAs communicate with the pancreatic duct, although they may compress it. Measurement of the CEA level in cyst fluid is a good means of distinguishing MCN from SCA. SCAs have very low levels of CEA, with the cutoff being 5 ng/mL.[18] The cyst fluid obtained from MCNs is often mucinous, and cytologic assessment may show mucin-producing cells; typically, the fluid is high in CEA. The CA 19-9 concentration may also be used to distinguish MCNs from SCAs, but it is not as reliable as the CEA concentration for this purpose.[18]

Surgical staging Surgical staging is required when investigations suggest that MCNs are malignant. Essentially, the same methods are used as for any pancreatic adenocarcinoma (see above). Malignancy is suggested by a solid intracystic or extramural component. Sometimes a mucinous tumor is frankly malignant with a large or dominant solid component. Such a tumor is better termed a mucinous cystadenocarcinoma, and it should be evaluated and treated from the outset in the same manner as other adenocarcinomas of the pancreas.

Management In symptomatic patients, preoperative differentiation between MCNs and SCAs is unnecessary because resection is the treatment for both. In asymptomatic patients, MCNs more than 4 cm in diameter should be excised because of the possibility of malignant degeneration.[19] MCNs associated with internal excrescenses or associated with a local solid mass should be removed independent of the size of the cyst.[19] The standard procedure has been open distal pancreatectomy with splenectomy, although lesser procedures, such as spleen-sparing distal pancreatectomy, central pancreatectomy, and enucleation, have all been used as well. Recently, laparoscopic distal pancreatectomy with or without sparing of the spleen has emerged as the procedure of choice because of the advantages of reduced postoperative pain and shortened length of stay.[20] These procedures appear to be reasonable choices provided that there is no suggestion of invasive malignancy on imaging (i.e., that there are no excrescences on the inner lining and that the surrounding pancreas appears normal). In these cases, a more formal resection that obeys oncologic goals such as a RAMPS procedure should be employed. Enucleation may be associated with a higher incidence of postoperative fistula. If invasive cancer is not detected in the resected specimen, the chances that the malignancy will recur are small; in fact, we have never seen such a recurrence.

The 4 cm cutoff for surgical treatment of MCNs in asymptomatic patients[19] without other signs associated with malignant degeneration is reasonable, but recommendations could change based on additional studies of natural history. Furthermore, it is still possible that malignant degeneration could occur in smaller cysts, although the probability is low. Many cysts smaller than 2 cm are found in the course of axial imaging performed for other reasons. Such cysts are difficult to diagnose because of the small volume of cyst fluid present, and the benefit to be gained from performing a large number of pancreatectomies for these small cysts is questionable, even when they are diagnosable as MCNs. Occasionally, MCNs or symptomatic SCAs are located in the head of the pancreas and require pancreaticoduodenectomy. Some authorities feel that very large asymptomatic SCAs should also be excised because of rare instances of malignant degeneration.

Intraductal papillary mucinous neoplasm IPMN begins as a metaplastic change in the cells lining the pancreatic ducts altering from a low cuboidal serous type of cell to a mucin-producing type. These cells are prone to progresss to dysplasia and eventual malignant transformation. Overall, IPMNs appear to undergo malignant transformation more frequently than MCNs. There are two recognized types of IPMN, which may occur either separately or together.[19,21] The more common type affects the main pancreatic duct [*see Figure 5*] and is called "main duct IPMN." In this type, the main pancreatic duct becomes dilated and filled with mucin. As the disease progresses toward malignancy, papillary processes may project into the lumen. The less common type, called "side-branch IPMN," affects the smaller ducts and presents as multiple (usually small) pancreatic cysts. In either type of IPMN, the disease may be either diffuse or focal; when it is focal, the head of the pancreas is the site of disease in the majority (60%) of cases. About 20% of IPMN patients have a malignancy at the time of diagnosis, although the cancer may not be evident until the specimen is examined pathologically.

Clinical evaluation and investigative studies[19,21] IPMN occurs predominantly in males and usually affects patients in their sixties. Pain (usually attributable to pancreatitis arising as a result of mucous obstruction of the pancreatic duct) is a common presenting symptom. Another common presentation is pancreatic insufficiency with diabetes or steatorrhea. Accordingly, it is not surprising that, formerly, many IPMN patients were diagnosed as having chronic pancreatitis. IPMN may also be discovered incidentally or may present as a cancer with signs and symptoms similar to those of other pancreatic cancers, depending on the part of the gland in which they arise. On rare occasions, cholangitis from obstruction of the common channel by mucus is the presenting problem.

The diagnosis is made on the basis of the presentation and the findings from axial imaging and ERCP. The characteristic ERCP findings are a dilated papillary orifice ("fish mouth") with mucus bulging from the orifice and a dilated pancreatic duct when contrast is injected. Sometimes, mucus prevents complete filling of the duct with dye. In this situation, CT scans or MRI with MRCP may be quite useful for detecting ductal dilatation and atrophy of the pancreas. MRCP is best at detecting excrescences projecting from the wall of the duct into the lumen. These signal progression of the disease toward neoplasia. In side-branch IPMN, ERCP (and often MRCP) typically demonstrates communication between the cysts and the main duct, which is often normal in size; this finding is not present in MCN or SCA and is very useful for distinguishing side-branch IPMN from these other types of cysts.

Management Knowledge of this entity is evolving, and recommendations are the current ones.[19,21–23]

Large duct IPMN As this entity is highly premalignant, resection is indicated once the diagnosis is made. Pancreatoduodenectomy is usually required as the disease affects the duct in the head of the pancreas in most cases. Although the duct in the body and tail of the gland may be dilated, this does not mean that it is involved in dysplastic changes as dilation may be secondary to obstruction caused by the viscous mucus in the proximal duct.[21] Therefore, the decision of whether to perform a complete pancreatectomy is made at the time of pancreatoduodenectomy, based on frozen section of the transected pancreatic neck. In most cases, the frozen section will show normal ductal epithelium or only mild or moderate dysplasia. Such patients do not require more pancreas to be resected. Occasionally, carcinoma, carcinoma in situ, or severe dysplasia is found, necessitating the resection of part or all of the remaining pancreas.[21]

Small duct IPMN This entity is less likely to degenerate into malignancy, and the probability of malignant degeneration is related to size.[22] Current indications for resection are cysts exceeding 3 cm in diameter or smaller cysts that are

a

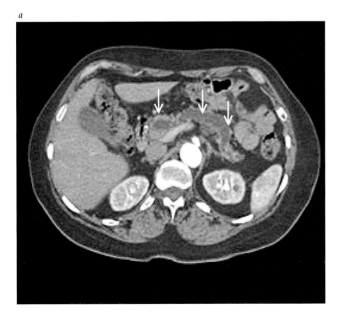

b

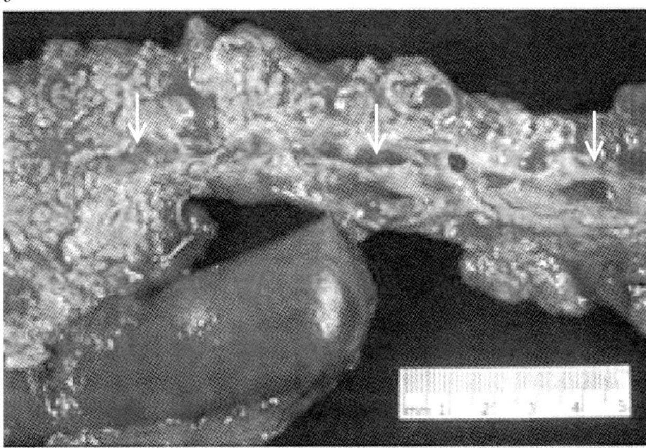

Figure 5 **(*a*) Computed tomographic scan of a patient with main duct intraductal papillary mucinous neoplasm involving the entire length of the pancreatic duct (*arrows*) reveals substantial distention of the duct. (*b*) Shown is a cross section through the resected specimen.**

associated with symptoms, internal excrescences, pericyst solid tumor, or pancreatic duct obstruction manifested as a dilation of the duct distal to the cyst.

With either type of IPMN, lifelong follow-up with axial imaging is needed.[21] This problem should be thought of as a field defect in the pancreas. Large duct and small duct IPMNs may coexist, and pancreatic intraepithelial neoplasia (PanIN) lesions (dyslastic lesions of the duct) may coexist with IPMN.

Most patients who require total pancreatectomy tolerate the procedure well when they are enrolled in a program keyed to this operation. Frank mucinous cancers may appear in patients with IPMN as well; they should be managed in much the same fashion as other adenocarcinomas, with the additional requirement that the resection should encompass the entire IPMN-bearing portion of the pancreas. The mucinous cancers associated with IPMN have a better prognosis than ductal adenocarcinomas do.[21,23]

NEUROENDOCRINE CANCERS

Neuroendocrine cancers account for fewer than 5% of surgically treated pancreatic malignancies. Some of these cancers are functional tumors, which produce hormones that lead to paraneoplastic syndromes. Examples include insulinoma, gastrinoma, glucagonoma, and vasoactive intestinal polypeptide–secreting tumor (VIPoma), all of which are associated with characteristic clinical syndromes. These syndromes are often produced while the tumors are still small. A detailed discussion of functional neuroendocrine tumors is beyond the scope of this chapter.

Other neuroendocrine tumors are nonfunctional and, as a result, reach a larger size before giving rise to symptoms. These lesions present with symptoms caused by mass effect and must be differentiated from ductal adenocarcinomas. Nonfunctional neuroendocrine cancers are relatively slow growing tumors that tend to push rather than invade structures but are capable of metastasizing to lymph nodes, as well as to the liver and other organs. Pain is the most common presenting symptom. Jaundice, pancreatitis, and systemic symptoms (e.g., weight loss) are less common with these tumors than with adenocarcinoma of the pancreas. Because of the propensity of neuroendocrine tumors to deflect rather than invade the bile duct, jaundice may be absent even when tumors are located in the head of the gland.

Diagnosis, surgical staging, and treatment rationale are essentially the same for neuroendocrine cancers as for ductal adenocarcinomas. On CT scans, these lesions characteristically show enhancement in the arterial phase and are seen to push on bile ducts and vascular structures rather than encase them. Complete resection by means of pancreatoduodenectomy or distal pancreatectomy [*see 6:23 Procedures for Benign and Malignant Pancreatic Disease*] is indicated. Given the slow growth rate of neuroendocrine cancers and their relatively favorable prognosis (a 50 to 60% 5-year survival rate), removal of the primary lesion and any hepatic secondary lesions is justified if all tumor tissue can be removed with clear margins.

Biliary Tract Cancer

Cancers of the biliary tract (cholangiocarcinomas) may arise at any level of the biliary tree from the smallest, most peripheral intrahepatic bile duct to the termination of the common bile duct. The lesions may be subdivided into intrahepatic and extrahepatic cholangiocarcinomas. The former are described below under "Liver Tumors." Cholangiocarcinomas may grow in one of three phenotypic forms, a mass, a stricture, or an intraluminal polyp or excrescence, although combinations of these forms in different parts of the tumor may be present. The formal designations are "mass forming" (MF), periductal infiltrating (PI), and intraductal growth (IG). The type of growth pattern may affect the clinical presentation.

EXTRAHEPATIC CHOLANGIOCARCINOMA

Extrahepatic cholangiocarcinoma (CCA) may be subdivided into lower duct CCA and upper duct CCA, with the former arising in the intrapancreatic or retroduodenal portion of the bile duct and the latter arising above it. In practice, most upper duct CCAs (also referred to as hilar CCAs or Klatskin tumors) arise just below the union of the right and left hepatic ducts, at the union of the ducts, or in the main right or left hepatic ducts. Cancer of the midportion of the bile duct at the usual insertion point of the cystic duct is more likely to be an extension of a gallbladder cancer than a primary CCA. AJCC staging criteria for these tumors are useful for establishing the prognosis and planning further treatment [*see Table 3 and Table 4*].

Table 3 American Joint Committee on Cancer TNM Clinical Classification of Extrahepatic Bile Duct Cancer

Primary tumor (T)	TX	Primary tumor cannot be assessed
	T0	No evidence of primary tumor
	Tis	Carcinoma in situ
	T1	Tumor confined to bile duct histologically
	T2	Tumor invades beyond wall of bile duct
	T3	Tumor invades liver, gallbladder, pancreas, or unilateral branches of portal vein or hepatic artery
	T4	Tumor invades any of the following: main portal vein or branches bilaterally, common hepatic artery, or other adjacent structures (e.g., colon, stomach, duodenum, or abdominal wall)
Regional lymph nodes (N)	NX	Regional lymph nodes cannot be assessed
	N0	No regional lymph node metastasis
	N1	Regional lymph node metastasis
Distant metastasis (M)	MX	Distant metastases cannot be assessed
	M0	No distant metastasis
	M1	Distant metastasis

Table 4 American Joint Committee on Cancer Staging System for Extrahepatic Bile Duct Cancer

Stage	T	N	M
0	Tis	N0	M0
IA	T1	N0	M0
IB	T2	N0	M0
IIA	T3	N0	M0
IIB	T1, T2, T3	N1	M0
III	T4	Any N	M0
IV	Any T	Any N	M1

Lower Duct Cholangiocarcinoma

Clinical evaluation and investigative studies Much of what the surgeon needs to know about lower duct CCA has already been addressed elsewhere [*see* Pancreatic Cancer, Adenocarcinoma of the Head of the Pancreas, *above*]. By far the most common presentation is painless jaundice with its constellation of associated symptoms (especially pruritus). Laboratory tests reveal the characteristic pattern of obstructive jaundice. A serum CA 19-9 concentration higher than 100 U/mL facilitates the diagnosis. Axial imaging reveals dilation of the intrahepatic bile ducts, the gallbladder (in most cases), and the extrahepatic bile ducts down to the level of the pancreatic head, where the dilatation terminates abruptly. Usually, no mass is visible. ERCP or MRCP shows a focal stricture, and ERCP brushings are positive in about 50% of cases. EUS may be helpful in that it is more sensitive for small tumors than CT. Needle biopsy is directed toward the mass or, if no mass is visible, toward the narrowest segment of the bile duct. A negative biopsy result does not rule out a small bile duct cancer. "Spyglass" cholangioscopy, in which a small endoscope is directed into the biliary tree along a catheter placed by duodenoscopy, facilitates direct biopsy of the bile duct wall and lesions that project into the lumen.

The differential diagnosis includes other potential causes of focal strictures of the bile duct.[24] The most common cause of a benign stricture of the intrapancreatic bile duct is pancreatitis, which may be diffuse or focal. Other causes of benign stricture include iatrogenic injury, choledocholithiasis, sclerosing cholangitis, and benign inflammatory pseudotumors [*see* Upper Duct Cholangiocarcinoma, Investigative Studies, Imaging, *below*]. Iatrogenic injuries rarely involve the intrapancreatic portion of the bile duct, although such injuries can occur in this area as a consequence of forceful instrumentation. Sclerosing cholangitis may affect this section of the bile duct but usually affects other areas of the biliary tree as well. The diagnostic steps for differentiating benign neoplasms from malignant tumors are essentially the same for lower duct CCA as for pancreatic cancer. As noted, resection may be required to make the diagnosis. In any patient presenting with jaundice and a focal stricture of the bile duct, lower duct CCA should be strongly suspected. Mass-forming bile duct cancers may also arise in the lower bile duct, but, for obvious reasons, they are difficult to differentiate from pancreatic adenocarcinomas. Perhaps in the future genetic profiling will permit this to be done. The surgical workup and management are identical.

Surgical staging Surgical staging of lower duct CCAs is usually straightforward. These tumors are usually remote from major vascular structures and thus are not subject to the same local staging considerations as adenocarcinomas of the pancreatic head are. The exception is a tumor that extends to the top of the retroduodenal portion of the bile duct. At this point, the bile duct is apposed to the portal vein and the hepatic artery, and these structures may be invaded by bile duct tumors in this location.

Management The treatment for resectable lesions is pancreaticoduodenectomy, and the rationale for the extent of the resection is the same as for adenocarcinoma of the head of the pancreas.

Upper Duct Cholangiocarcinoma

Upper duct (or hilar) CCA is a sporadically occurring tumor that may also be seen in patients with primary sclerosing cholangitis, ulcerative colitis, or parasitic infestation. It is characteristically slow growing and locally invasive, and it metastasizes more readily to lymph nodes than systemically, although intrahepatic and peritoneal metastases are not uncommon. Most hilar CCAs are cicatrizing diffusely infiltrating cancers (PI tumors), but some form masses (MF type), and others present as papillary ingrowths (IG type). These tumors are also subdivided by the upper level of the tumor in the biliary tree according to the Bismuth classification [*see Figure 6*].[25]

When the CCA originates in one of the hepatic ducts, that duct may be obstructed for a considerable period before the tumor causes jaundice by growing into the other hepatic duct or the common bile duct. Such prolonged unilateral obstruction before the onset of the presenting symptom of jaundice may result in atrophy of the obstructed side of the liver, which may affect subsequent management. For example, because the disease is more advanced on the obstructed side, the atrophied half of the liver will be removed in almost all cases in which resection is indicated. In addition, when one side of the liver undergoes atrophy, the other side undergoes hypertrophy. These changes may lead to rotation of the liver, which, in turn, may cause the structures in the hepatoduodenal ligament to be rotated out of their normal anatomic location. For instance, if hypertrophy of the left hemiliver develops, the hepatic artery may come to lie directly in front of the bile duct.

Clinical evaluation The usual presentation of hilar CCA consists of painless jaundice with its accompanying symptoms (especially pruritus), although some pain may be present. Cholangitis before instrumentation of the bile duct is uncommon. In patients who present in the late stages of the disease, general manifestations of cancer (e.g., malaise, weight loss, or ascites) may be noted. In patients with primary sclerosing cholangitis, the presence of CCA is often suggested by a rapid deterioration in the patient's general condition. It is not unusual for patients with hilar CCA to have undergone a cholecystectomy in the recent past; the symptoms of pain and jaundice may be mistaken for symptoms of gallbladder disease in patients who happen also to have gallstones.

Investigative studies *Laboratory tests* Laboratory testing follows the pattern previously described for obstructive jaundice [*see* Pancreatic Cancer, *above*]. Again, the most helpful diagnostic laboratory test is the serum CA 19-9 concentration: levels higher than 100 U/mL are strongly suggestive of cancer.

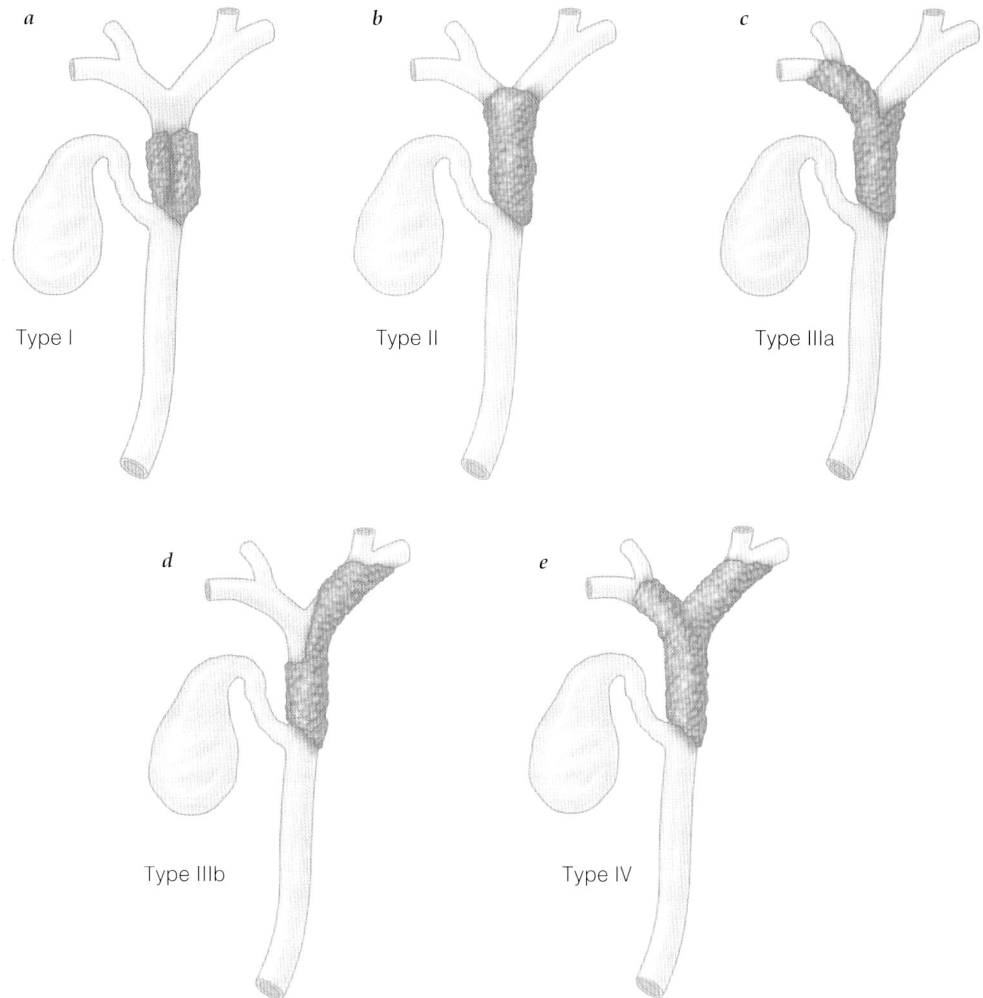

Figure 6 **Depicted is the Bismuth classification of hilar cholangiocarcinoma (*a* through *e*).**

Imaging Earlier [*see* Pancreatic Cancer, Ductal Adenocarcinoma, Adenocarcinoma of the Head of the Pancreas, *above*], the point was made that it is preferable to employ axial imaging rather than ERCP as the first imaging test in the jaundiced patient because doing so will often render ERCP, an invasive test, unnecessary. This point carries even more force in the setting of hilar CCA. Injection of dye above the malignant stricture is an integral part of ERCP. Once the dye has been injected, stents must be placed to prevent post-ERCP cholangitis. This process may involve insertion of bilateral stents, including a stent in the atrophic hemiliver. Bilateral stenting is disadvantageous because the aim is to encourage atrophy of the hemiliver to be resected and hypertrophy of the hemiliver to be retained, and insertion of a stent in the atrophic side negates that aim. Starting with CT or MRI rather than with ERCP allows detection of any hilar CCA present simultaneously with detection of atrophy. At this point, the patient can be evaluated by a multidisciplinary team with expertise in this disease, and a decision can be made regarding which side of the biliary tree to decompress (if either). Whether stents should be employed in treating hilar CCA is debatable, but if a stent is inserted, only the side to be retained should be intubated. MRCP now provides resolution that is close to that obtained with direct cholangiography [*see Figure 7*].

ERCP does have one significant advantage in that it allows brushings to be obtained. Standard brushing techniques at this high level in the biliary tree are even less sensitive than those at lower levels, but spyglass technology (see above) has opened this area of the biliary tree to direct biopsy on a routine basis. EUS has been employed to obtain diagnostic tissue, with some degree of success; however, because the biopsy needle passes through the peritoneal cavity, concerns have been expressed regarding possible tumor seeding. Such seeding has not been an issue with lower duct cancers, because the biopsy tract is entirely within the future resection specimen. In many cases, a tissue diagnosis cannot be obtained preoperatively, and the diagnosis is based on the presence of a focal hilar stricture that causes jaundice.

Focal strictures of the upper bile ducts are strongly suggestive of cancer, but CCAs must also be differentiated from benign inflammatory tumors (also referred to as hepatic inflammatory pseudotumors and benign fibrosing disease).[26] These inflammatory masses mimic upper duct CCAs but

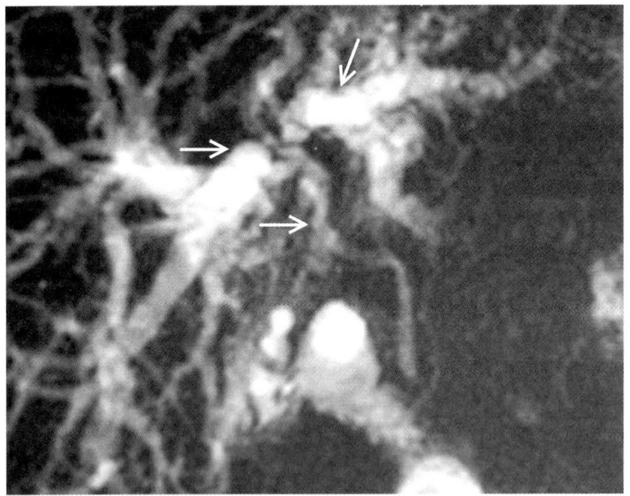

Figure 7 **Shown is Bismuth type II cholangiocarcinoma. The right and left hepatic ducts are dilated (*upper arrows*), whereas the common hepatic duct is normal sized.**

consist of chronic inflammatory cells and fibrous material. One distinguishing characteristic is that they do not involve blood vesels. Even today, they are very difficult to distinguish from cancers before pathologic examination of a resected specimen. Benign inflammatory tumors appear to occur most frequently in extrahepatic upper ducts, but they also occur intrahepatically and, less commonly, in lower ducts.

Gallbladder cancer may invade the porta hepatis and appear as a CCA, especially on ERCP. Gallstones are usually present. Axial imaging usually shows thickening of the gallbladder wall or the presence of a mass involving the infundibulum. Mirizzi syndrome is another cause of a focal stricture of the middle or upper bile duct. This syndrome results from compression of the bile duct by a large gallstone in the infundibulum and is usually associated with severe inflammation of the gallbladder and the characteristic signs and symptoms of acute cholecystitis. The duct is typically bowed to the left rather than focally narrowed, as in cancer. Iatrogenic causes should be considered if the patient has had a cholecystectomy. On occasion, a stricture appears years after the operation. In these cases, the probable cause of the stricture is ischemic injury to the bile duct. The presence of clips close to or indenting the duct is a clue that such injury is a possibility. Choledocholithiasis may also cause strictures, especially if cholangitis has occurred. Strictures are also frequent with recurrent pyogenic (oriental) cholangitis. Other rare tumors of the bile duct (e.g., neuroendocrine tumors) may mimic cholangiocarcinoma.

Surgical staging Often the first axial imaging test reveals only the presence of intrahepatic bile duct dilatation, which stops abruptly as the ducts merge in the hepatic hilum. This finding, however, leads to MRI or CT aimed at providing high-quality cholangiograms and angiograms of the hepatic arteries and the portal veins. Surgical staging of hilar CCA, unlike that of lower duct CCA, requires exact knowledge of the macroscopic upper extent of the tumor in the bile duct. Furthermore, invasion of hepatic arteries and portal veins is common and frequently affects resectability. Thus, surgical staging also requires accurate determination of the extent of hepatic arterial or portal venous invasion and assessment of the degree of atrophy.

Bismuth type IV tumors are not resectable, except by liver transplantation. Type I through III tumors are resectable provided that the main portal vein and the proper hepatic artery, as well as the portal vein and the hepatic artery to the side of the liver to be retained, are not invaded by tumor and that the side to be retained is not atrophic. Involvement of the main portal vein or the hepatic artery is a relative rather than an absolute contraindication; lesser degrees of involvement can be handled by means of vascular resection and reconstruction in specialized centers. Unusual combinations of events may preclude resection (e.g., atrophy on one side of the liver and invasion of the hepatic artery supplying the other side, or invasion of the portal vein to one side and the bile duct on the other side to the level of the secondary biliary branches).

MRI (with MRCP and magnetic resonance angiography [MRA]) or CT with the latest generation of scanners can provide complete information regarding the extent of bile duct involvement and the degree of vascular invasion. Doppler ultrasonography is also excellent for evaluating vascular invasion. In our experience, the combination of these two investigations usually provides more usful staging information than either individually. Both are dependent on highly experienced radiologists. ERCP may be used for additional assessment of the extent of the tumor on the side to be retained if a stent on that side is deemed necessary. The use of percutaneous cholangiography is controversial, the main concern being the risk of tumor seeding along the tube, into the peritoneal cavity, and onto the surface of the liver or the abdominal wall. Nevertheless, this procedure is used extensively in Japan, where surgeons have considerable experience with selective decompression of parts of the liver as a preoperative strategy.[27]

Assessment of distant metastases is achieved by means of axial imaging of the chest and the abdomen. Staging laparoscopy identifies 10 to 15% of cancers that are unresectable because of peritoneal or liver metastases. FDG-PET identifies about 15% of patients with distant metastases. At present, neither of these tests is routinely employed in this setting. Staging laparoscopy has provided a good yield of unresectable cases in some studies but not in others.

Management *Preoperative preparation* Unlike cancers of the lower bile duct, cancers of the upper bile duct usually necessitate major liver resection [*see 6:21 Procedures for Benign and Malignant Biliary Tract Disease*]. Consequently, it has been argued that the risk of postoperative hepatic failure may be lowered by preoperative decompression, especially decompression of the side to be retained, which has the dual purpose of allowing that side to recover function and of actually encouraging hypertrophy. On the other hand, stents may introduce bacteria and cause cholangitis. As noted (see above), selective percutaneous decompression is an accepted strategy in Japan; often multiple stents are inserted.[28]

A reasonable strategy is to proceed to operation if (1) the patient is relatively young (< 70 years), (2) there are no serious comorbid conditions, (3) the jaundice has been present for less than 4 weeks, (4) the serum bilirubin concentration is lower than 10 mg/dL, (5) the future remnant liver will include more than 35% of the total liver mass, and (6) the patient has not undergone biliary instrumentation (which always contaminates the obstructed biliary tract). In all other cases, we routinely decompress the side of the liver to be retained and wait until the serum bilirubin concentration falls to 3 mg/dL. When the future remnant liver will include less than 30 to 35% of the total liver mass, portal vein embolization (PVE) of the side to be resected may be performed to induce hypertrophy of the remnant. Because resection for hilar CCA is a major procedure in a somewhat compromised liver, it is contraindicated in patients who are in poor general condition or who have major organ dysfunction.

Rationale for surgery Patients with upper duct CCA are candidates for resection if they have no distant metastases (including intrahepatic metastases) and if the tumor can be removed in its entirety by means of bile duct resection [*see 6:21 Procedures for Benign and Malignant Biliary Tract Disease*] combined with liver resection [*see 6:22 Hepatic Resection*]. The goal of resection of upper duct CCA is to achieve clear resection margins by removing the tumor, the portal and celiac lymph nodes, the side of the liver in which the ductal involvement is greater (via hemihepatectomy or trisectionectomy), and the caudate lobe. (The caudate lobe is resected because cholangiocarcinomas tend to invade along the short caudate bile ducts, which enter the posterior surfaces of the main right and left bile ducts at the bifurcation of the common hepatic duct.) Recently, some surgeons have extended the portal dissection to include the portal vein when the right side of the liver is to be resected. This provides a wide resection zone and removes an area that is frequently involved by microscopic tumor.[28]

Liver transplantation has been used successfully to manage Bismuth type IV tumors and is usually performed after neoadjuvant chemoradiation therapy and staging laparotomy in highly selected patients.[29] Liver transplantation for Bismuth tumors of lesser Bismuth grades is highly controversial.

Table 5 American Joint Committee on Cancer TNM Clinical Classification of Gallbladder Cancer

Primary tumor (T)	TX	Primary tumor cannot be assessed
	T0	No evidence of primary tumor
	Tis	Carcinoma in situ
	T1	Tumor invades lamina propria or muscle layer
	T1a	Tumor invades lamina propria
	T1b	Tumor invades muscle layer
	T2	Tumor invades perimuscular connective tissue; no extension beyond serosa into liver
	T3	Tumor perforates serosa (visceral peritoneum) and/or directly invades one adjacent organ or structure such as the stomach, duodenum, colon, pancreas, omentum, or extrahepatic bile ducts
	T4	Tumor extends > 2 cm into liver or invades two or more adjacent organs (e.g., duodenum, colon, pancreas, omentum, or extrahepatic bile ducts)
Regional lymph nodes (N)	NX	Regional lymph nodes cannot be assessed
	N0	No regional lymph node metastasis
	N1	Regional lymph node metastasis
Distant metastasis (M)	MX	Distant metastasis cannot be assessed
	M0	No distant metastasis
	M1	Distant metastasis

Gallbladder Cancer

The incidence of gallbladder cancer in the United States is about 9,000 cases a year. This cancer almost always arises in patients with preexisting gallstones and is most often seen in elderly patients. Like ductal adenocarcinoma of the pancreas, it is highly malignant and tends to spread at an early stage to lymph nodes, to peritoneal surfaces, and to areas of the liver distant from the gallbladder fossa. AJCC staging criteria are helpful for planning management of this cancer [*see Table 5 and Table 6*].

Clinical Evaluation

Gallbladder cancer is discovered either incidentally during performance of cholecystectomy for symptomatic cholelithiasis or when the tumor causes symptoms related to invasion of the bile duct or to the effects of metastatic disease. In early stages of the disease in which the tumor is confined to the wall of the gallbladder, the symptoms are usually those of the associated stones—that is, the patient has biliary colic, and the cancer is silent. In later stages of disease, jaundice, weight loss, a palpable right upper quadrant mass, hepatomegaly, or ascites may develop. Jaundice occurs in about 50% of patients. It is a poor prognostic sign because it signifies extension of the tumor beyond the gallbladder and obstruction of the extrahepatic bile ducts. Consequently, most gallbladder cancer patients with jaundice have unresectable tumors. Because the signs and symptoms of gallbladder cancer are nonspecific, delays in diagnosis are common. As a result, most gallbladder cancers are not diagnosed until they have reached stage III or IV; thus, most of these aggressive tumors are unresectable at presentation, even when the patient is not jaundiced.

Investigative Studies

Laboratory tests In stages I and II, LFTs usually yield normal results. In later stages, laboratory test abnormalities may be noted that are not diagnostic but are consistent with bile duct obstruction. Elevated alkaline phosphatase and bilirubin levels are common. An elevation in the serum CA 19-9 concentration is the most helpful diagnostic indicator.

Table 6 American Joint Committee on Cancer Staging System for Gallbladder Cancer

Stage	T	N	M
0	Tis	N0	M0
IA	T1	N0	M0
IB	T2	N0	M0
IIA	T3	N0	M0
IIB	T1, T2, T3	N1	M0
III	T4	Any N	M0
IVB	Any T	Any N	M1

Imaging Because gallbladder cancer is most curable in its early stages and because the symptoms in those stages are those of cholelithiasis, it is important for surgeons to be aware of subtle signs of gallbladder cancer that are occasionally present on sonograms. These signs include asymmetrical thickening of the gallbladder wall, thickening of the wall in a patient without a history of biliary colic, a mass projecting into the lumen, multiple masses or a fixed mass in the gallbladder, calcification of the gallbladder wall (so-called porcelain gallbladder), and an extracholecystic mass. Displacement of a stone to one side of the gallbladder should also be viewed with suspicion.

In later stages of disease, CT scans usually show a gallbladder mass with or without invasion of the liver or other adjacent organs. Obstruction of the bile duct produces the usual features associated with obstructive jaundice. Percutaneous CT-guided biopsy is a useful technique for confirming the diagnosis in patients with unresectable tumors.

Porcelain gallbladder is a premalignant condition, although there is some evidence that the incidence of cancer depends on the pattern of calcification: selective mucosal calcification apparently carries a significant risk of cancer, whereas diffuse intramural calcification does not.[30] It seems reasonable to resect only tumors with the former pattern, but whenever there is a question about the pattern of calcification, one should err on the side of resection.

Surgical Staging

Staging of gallbladder cancer requires knowledge of the extent of direct invasion into the liver and other adjacent organs and tissues (especially the bile duct, the portal veins, and the hepatic arteries). As in hilar CCA, this information may be obtained by means of MRCP and MRA or CT with the latest generation of scanners. Staging laparoscopy is very helpful in managing gallbladder cancer. As many as 50% of patients with this disease are found to have peritoneal or liver metastases on staging laparoscopy,[8] and as with carcinoma of the body of the pancreas, no useful palliative measures can be undertaken at laparotomy.

Management

Rationale for surgery When early-stage gallbladder cancer is suspected on the basis of diagnostic imaging, open cholecystectomy, rather than laparoscopic cholecystectomy, is probably the procedure of choice [*see 6:20 Cholecystectomy and Common Bile Duct Exploration and 6:21 Procedures for Benign and Malignant Biliary Tract Disease*]. Intraoperatively, if there is no evidence of spread outside the gallbladder, we recommend performing an extraserosal cholecystectomy, in which the fibrous liver plate is excised along with the gallbladder so that bare liver is exposed. It is possible to perform an extraserosal resection laparoscopically; however, in our opinion, this should not be attempted, because gallbladder perforation and bile spillage are more common with the laparoscopic version of the procedure. The negative consequences of tumor implantation or incomplete excision far outweigh any benefit that a minimally invasive approach might confer.

The excised specimen should be inked and a frozen section obtained. If there is gallbladder cancer in the specimen but the resection margins are clear and the tumor is a T1 lesion (i.e., has not penetrated the muscularis), the procedure is considered complete in that lymph node metastases are uncommon with T1 tumors (incidence < 10%). However, lymph node metastases are present in 50% of patients with T2 lesions (i.e., tumors that have invaded the muscularis). Therefore, if margins are positive or the tumor is a T2 lesion, resection of segments 4b and 5 of the liver and dissection of the portal and celiac lymph nodes are recommended. Resection of the extrahepatic bile duct and hepaticojejunostomy may be needed in some cases to obtain a complete node clearance, but this is being done less frequently as experience with portal node clearance has been obtained. If it is already clear at the commencement of the operation that the tumor is T2, one should proceed directly to liver, lymph node, and bile duct resection.

In more advanced stages of disease (T3 and T4), the aim is still excision with clear margins and resection of portal and celiac lymph nodes. To obtain clear local margins with these tumors, in addition to what is required for T2 tumors, more extensive hepatic resections—up to a trisectionectomy (resection of segments 4 through 8) [*see* Liver Cancer, Anatomic Considerations, *below*][31]—may be necessary, as well as resection of adjacent organs.

Incidentally discovered gallbladder cancer Gallbladder cancer may be an incidental finding at laparoscopic cholecystectomy, as it has been at open cholecystectomy. The incidence of this finding ranges from 0.3 to 1.0%. A concern that has arisen in the current era, in which the laparoscopic approach to cholecystectomy is dominant, is the risk of port-site implantation of tumor. Port-site implantation is the result of contact between the malignancy and the tissues surrounding the port site at the time of gallbladder extraction. Therefore, when evidence of gallbladder wall thickening is noted intraoperatively, the gallbladder should be extracted in a sac. The gallbladder should be inspected at the time of extraction, and any questionable areas should undergo biopsy.

If a gallbladder cancer is discovered at the time of operation, it should be treated without delay according to the principles stated earlier (i.e., depending on whether the margins on the excised gallbladder are clear and on the T stage of the tumor). From an oncologic viewpoint, it would seem ideal to resect the tissue around all trocar port sites. From a technical viewpoint, however, it would be very difficult and impractical to excise the full thickness of the abdominal wall circumferentially around four port sites, especially because the tract of the port site often is not at a 90° angle to the abdominal wall. If the gallbladder was extracted through a port site without having been placed into a bag, it is reasonable to attempt excision of that one port site.

Sometimes cancer is suspected, but frozen-section examination is inconclusive, and the definitive diagnosis of cancer is not made until the early postoperative period. More often, cancer is not suspected intraoperatively, and the diagnosis is made only when permanent sections of the gallbladder are examined. In these situations, patients with completely excised T1 lesions require no further therapy, and patients with higher-stage lesions should undergo reoperation in accordance with the principles outlined earlier (see above). Other appropriate reasons for not performing the additional surgery at the time of the cholecystectomy are (1) the desire to discuss the management scheme with the patient and (2) a lack of experience with the procedure for T2 tumors. Not infrequently, patients are referred to hepatic-pancreatic-biliary centers 10 to 14 days after surgery, which is an inopportune time for reoperation, especially if the first procedure was difficult. Surgery may then be delayed for 3 to 4 weeks. We restage patients with abdominal CT scans when they are referred with this diagnosis, and it is not unusual to find hepatic metastases when this is done. The survival rate is much higher after radical resection than after cholecystectomy, even when cholecystectomy was the first procedure.[32]

Gallbladder polyps Benign gallbladder poyps may be adenomas or more commonly a focal form of cholesterolosis. Multiple polyps are most often due to cholesterolosis. Gallbladder polyps are discovered incidentally on ultrasonograms or CT scans or are diagnosed when they cause biliary colic. They may be malignant but are rarely so when less than 1 cm in diameter, especially when they are multiple. Most gallbladder polyps are less than 0.5 cm in diameter; these are almost always benign cholesterol polyps and may be followed if they are not giving rise to symptoms. Single polyps between 0.5 and 1 cm in diameter should probably be removed by means of cholecystectomy. Multiple asymptomatic polyps in this size range should be followed because they are more likely to be due to cholesterolosis. About one quarter of all single gallbladder polyps more than 1 cm in diameter are malignant, and such polyps should be treated as malignant as a matter of policy. Almost all polyps more than 1.8 cm in diameter are malignant.[33] Gallbladder sludge and stones may be mistaken for polyps. They are differentiated by using Doppler ultrasonography to determine if the lesion has internal blood flow. If internal blood flow is absent, the lesion is unlikely to be a polyp.

Liver Cancer

ANATOMIC CONSIDERATIONS

A long-standing problem in discussing any surgical liver disease, especially liver cancer, has been the confusing terminology applied to liver anatomy and the various hepatic resections. Fortunately, a lucid and cogent terminology has emerged that is sanctioned by both the International Hepato-Pancreato-Biliary Association (IHPBA) and the American Hepato-Pancreato-Biliary Association (AHPBA).[31] This terminology has been widely adopted around the world and translated into many languages. It may be briefly summarized as follows.

The fundamental principle is that the anatomic divisions of the liver are based on vascular and biliary anatomy rather than on surface markings [*see Figure 8*]. This is an important point because surgical resection is a process of isolating specific liver volumes serviced by specific vascular and biliary

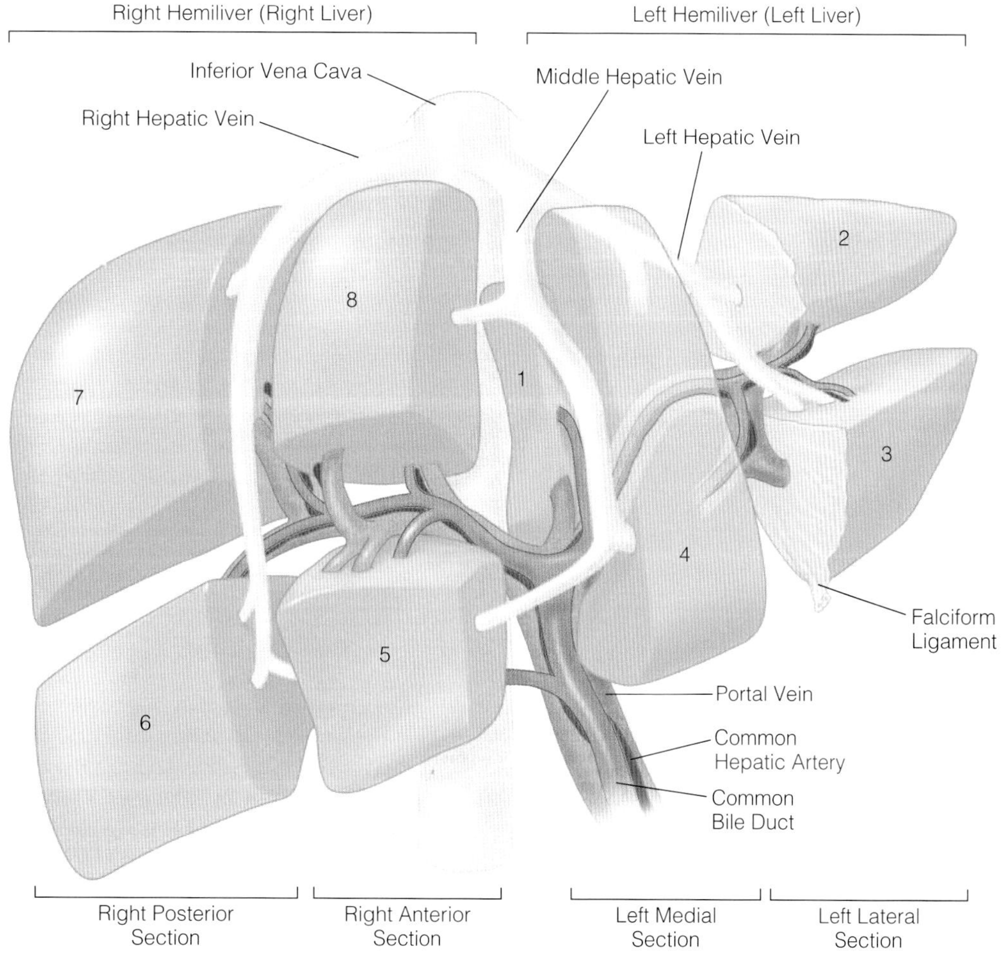

Figure 8 **Illustrated are the anatomic divisions of the liver according to IHPBA/AHPBA-sanctioned terminology, including first-order divisions (hemilivers), second-order divisions (sections), and third-order divisions (segments).**

nodules, which typically do not show washout. Multifocality is also common in HCC, unlike other hepatic neoplasms. Routine biopsy is not indicated in patients with a characteristic mass, those who have a mass and an elevated AFP level, or those who are symptomatic and require treatment for pain. HCC may be very well differentiated and difficult to distinguish from hepatic adenoma and focal nodular hyperplasia on biopsy. It may also be hard to distinguish from cirrhotic nodules. Biopsy is associated with a small risk of bleeding or tumor seeding.

Surgical staging Staging of sporadic HCC requires axial imaging of the abdomen and imaging of the chest. FDG-PET scanning is only marginally useful: HCCs are typically well differentiated, and, as a result, only 50% of the tumors are visualized. Staging laparoscopy is helpful: additional tumors are found in about 15% of patients.[34]

Staging also requires evaluation of the extent of liver disease. The Child-Pugh classification is used to determine operability. With few exceptions, resection is limited to Child-Pugh class A patients with near-normal bilirubin levels (< 1.5 mg/dL), a normal or marginally raised prothrombin time, and no or minimal portal hypertension. The extent of resection must be tailored to the severity of the liver disease. For instance, resection of more than two segments is limited to patients with normal liver function. Too extensive resection puts the patients at risk for liver failure in the postoperative period. In Japan and China, indocyanine green clearance is used in Child-Pugh class A patients to determine the possible extent of resection.

Management *Rationale for surgery* The rationale for surgery is clear in patients without liver disease or in Child-Pugh class B or C patients with chronic liver disease. The rationale for surgery in Child-Pugh class A patients, however, remains controversial.

Partial liver resection [*see 6:22 Hepatic Resection*] is the procedure of choice for sporadic HCC in patients with normal livers. In Child-Pugh class B or C patients with chronic liver disease, liver resection can be hazardous, and orthotopic liver transplantation (OLT) is the procedure of choice. To justify the use of donor organs, however, it is necessary to select patients with HCC so that the long-term outcome of OLT for HCC is similar to that of OLT for benign conditions. To achieve this goal, OLT is restricted to patients with a single tumor less than 5 cm in diameter or to patients with as many as three tumors, none of which are more than 3 cm in diameter (the Milan criteria). These criteria have been shown to be associated with OLT outcomes comparable to those for benign conditions.[35]

In Child-Pugh class A patients with liver disease, hepatic resection and OLT are options if the Milan criteria are met. The optimal therapeutic approach in this situation has been the subject of considerable debate, with proponents arguing for one of two strategies—namely, (1) primary OLT or (2) resection followed by OLT if HCC recurs,[36,37] provided that the patients still meet the criteria for OLT (so-called salvage OLT). A complete discussion of this controversy is beyond the scope of this chapter. Currently, it would seem that the best strategy in patients who meet the criteria for OLT is to perform resection followed by transplanation if disease recurs.[36,37] There is a trend toward liberalizing the OLT criteria to include single tumors 6 or 7 cm in diameter, especially if the source of the organ is a living donor.

When OLT is to be performed, it is important that the waiting time be short; these tumors progress over a timescale of a few months, and when viewed on an intention-to-treat basis, the results of OLT deteriorate significantly if the waiting time is long.[38] In the United States, this concern has been dealt with by the introduction of the Model for End-stage Liver Disease (MELD) scoring system, which gives priority to recipients with HCC. It is common in the United States—and even more usual in countries with longer waiting times—to inhibit the growth of the HCC with various bridging-to-transplantation strategies during the waiting period for OLT. Such strategies include systemic chemotherapy, local treatments (e.g., radiofrequency [RF] ablation and alcohol injection), transarterial chemoembolization (TACE), and even resection of the HCC (so-called bridge resection). TACE may also be used to downsize tumors so that they meet transplant criteria.

In patients with nondiseased livers, the extent of resection depends on the size and position of the tumor. As much as 75% of the liver may be safely excised when normal liver function is present. The size of the future hepatic remnant may be determined by means of imaging. PVE of the side of the liver to be resected may be performed preoperatively to increase the size of the future remnant. It may also be used for this purpose in patients with liver disease. In these patients, PVE functions as a test of the liver's ability to regenerate. Failure to respond to PVE is itself a contraindication to surgery in patients with chronic liver disease.

As a rule, liver resections for HCC should be anatomic [*see 6:22 Hepatic Resection*]. Recurrence rates are higher with nonanatomic resections because HCCs grow along portal veins and metastasize locally within segments, sections, or hemilivers, depending on how far they reach back along the portal veins. When a nonanatomic resection is performed, the resection margings should be 2 cm or greater. When HCC reaches the main portal vein, resection is generally contraindicated; the results are very poor in this situation.

Intrahepatic Cholangiocarcinoma

Clinical evaluation Intrahepatic CCAs arise from intrahepatic bile ducts. The three phenotypic types, MF, PI, and IG, are described above. The MF type is by far the most common. Intrahepatic CCA tumor usually occurs in normal livers. The presentation is similar to that of sporadic HCC.

Investigative studies The appearance of intrahepatic CCA on CT is suggestive of a secondary tumor [*see Figure 10*]. Unlike HCC, diagnosis of intrahepatic CCA often requires biopsy, which reveals an adenocarcinoma that is indistinguishable from a hepatic metastasis. Special stains may be helpful in differentiating this tumor from a true secondary malignancy, but the differentiation is rarely certain. An elevated CA 19-9 concentration is strongly suggestive of this diagnosis if it is higher than 100 U/mL. To make the diagnosis of intrahepatic CCA, primary tumors in other sites must be excluded by means of axial imaging of the chest, the abdomen, and the pelvis; upper and lower GI endoscopy; and mammography. FDG-PET scanning is another helpful method by which an extrahepatic primary tumor may be identified.

Surgical staging FDG-PET scanning appears to be a promising staging tool for identifying portal lymph node and distant metastases when the primary tumor is actually an intrahepatic CCA. Portal lymph node metastases are a relative contraindication to resection in patients with MF tumors; the results of resection in this situation are poor. Left-side tumors

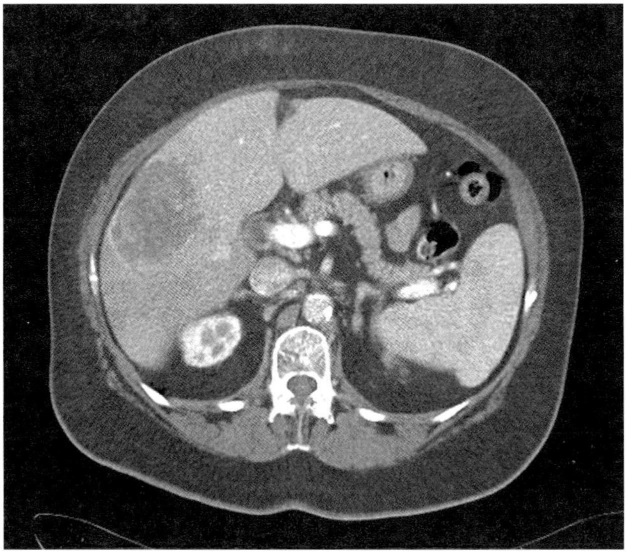

Figure 10 **Computed tomographic scan shows a mass-forming intrahepatic cholangiocarcinoma.**

may metastasize to lymph nodes at the cardia of the stomach and along the lesser curvature or to the mediastinum.

Management The considerations related to resection for intrahepatic CCA are similar to those for sporadic HCC (see above). Liver transplantation generally is not performed for this tumor, because of the typically poor results.

SECONDARY CANCERS

Colorectal Metastases

Clinical evaluation and investigative studies About 50% of the 150,000 patients who are diagnosed with colorectal cancer annually in the United States either have or will have liver metastases. About 10% of patients with these colorectal metastases (CRMs) are eligible for liver resection. CRMs may be diagnosed either at the time of treatment of the primary colorectal cancer (synchronous tumors) or at a later stage (metachronous tumors).

Synchronous tumors are diagnosed by means of either preoperative CT scanning [*see Figure 11*] or intraoperative palpation. LFTs may show elevations (especially of the serum alkaline phosphatase level), but these results are not specific. CEA levels are not helpful as long as the primary tumor is in place. Metachronous tumors are most often diagnosed in the course of a postcolectomy surveillance program, either by imaging the liver with CT or FDG-PET scans or by detecting a rise in the CEA level. When synchronous metastases are discovered preoperatively, a FDG-PET scan should be done to complete the staging.

Surgical staging In about 25% of patients, FDG-PET scans change management as a result of detecting unsuspected extrahepatic or intrahepatic disease. Sometimes it demonstrates that apparent metastases are actually benign lesions. Second primary tumors are not uncommon in patients with metachronous lesions; accordingly, such patients should also be staged by means of colonoscopy, if this procedure was not done in the preceding 6 months, as well as FDG-PET scanning. Staging laparoscopy adds little to staging if an FDG-PET scan has been done.

Intraoperative staging consists of careful palpation of intra-abdominal structures, including hepatic and portal venous lymph nodes. In patients with metachronous lesions, however, palpation of the entire abdomen may be limited by adhesions from previous operations. IOUS of the liver may also detect unsuspected lesions, although this is less likely if the patient has already been staged by means of FDG-PET.

The main value of FDG-PET in this setting is its ability to discover unsuspected extrahepatic disease. In so doing, it helps eliminate futile hepatic resections. If a patient

a

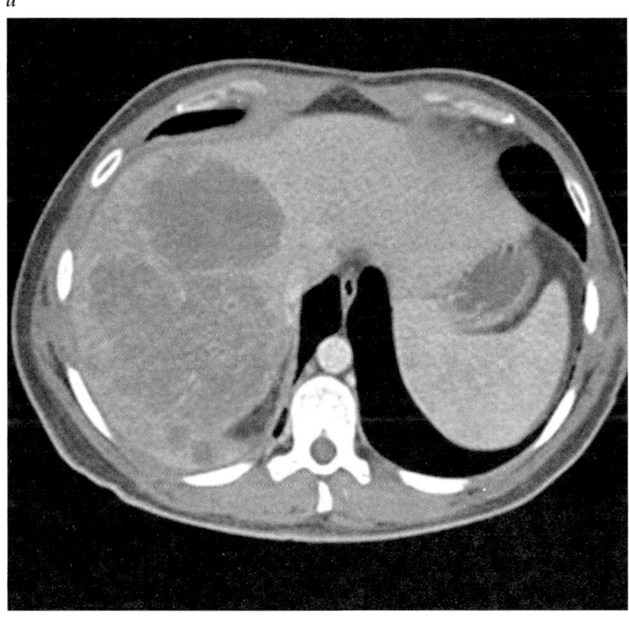

b

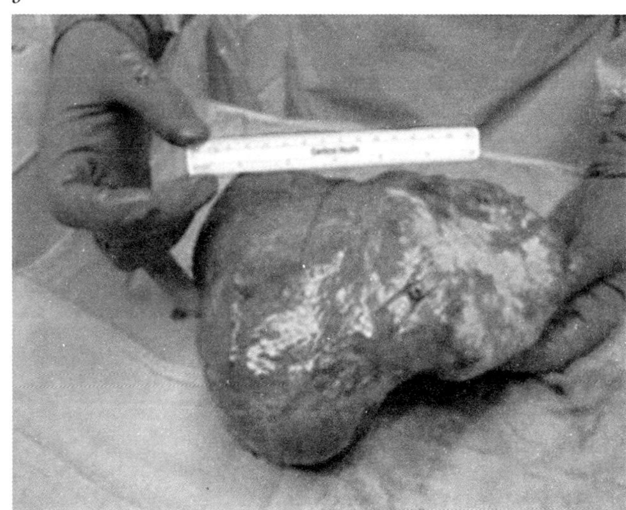

Figure 11 **Colorectal metastasis. (*a*) Computed tomography shows a single large tumor in right hemiliver; (*b*) is the resected specimen.**

with extrahepatic disease is treated with hepatic resection, a "recurrence" is inevitable. Elimination of pointless resections has a positive effect on survival: a 2004 study from our institution found that the overall 5-year survival rate after FDG-PET was about 60%, compared with 40% after conventional imaging.[39] Furthermore, after FDG-PET scanning has been done, the most important prognostic factors determining long-term outcome are the grade of the primary colorectal tumor and whether the primary tumor had metastasized to lymph nodes.[40] FDG-PET–scanned patients with poorly differentiated primary tumors do poorly in terms of overall survival after hepatic resection.[39] In recent years, standard PET scanners have been replaced with CT-PET scanners, which fuse the images and provide superior diagnosis and staging. For planning surgical extirpation, however, the level of detail provided by high-quality contrast-enhanced CT or MRI is also required.

Management *Rationale for surgery* The classic criteria that determined eligibility for resection are (1) that the primary tumor has been or can be completely resected, (2) that (with uncommon exceptions) there is no extrahepatic tumor (other than the primary tumor), and (3) that it is possible to resect all tumors in the liver while leaving enough of a hepatic remnant to ensure that hepatic failure does not develop postoperatively. The considerations governing the extent of the resection and the use of PVE are similar to those for sporadic HCC.

Treatment of multiple tumors is much more common with CRMs than with HCC. However, nonanatomic resections are as effective as anatomic resections as long as the resection margin is microscopically clear. The traditional view has been that resection margins of 1 cm are mandatory and lesser margins lead to poorer results. This view has been challenged in several studies that claim that margins as narrow as 1 mm are satisfactory and are probably as effective as traditional margins provided that they are free of microscopic and gross cancer. This issue must be considered to still be unsettled, and, certainly, 1 cm margins should be the goal whenever feasible. When close margins are expected, transection of the liver with a saline-linked RF ablation device may be useful in that this device leaves a margin of devitalized tissue in the patient and in the specimen.[41] When the margin is very close, it may be extended by painting the cut surface of the hepatic remnant with the RF device.

Synchronous resection of the primary tumor and the liver metastases has proved to be safe[42] and is desired by many patients. The decision to proceed with hepatic resection should not be made until resection of the primary tumor has been completed and it has been determined that the margins are clear and the patient is stable. Some patients with a small number of lung lesions in addition to liver lesions have been cured by resection.

The classic criteria for resection have been challenged and extended by new surgical approaches and the advent of much improved chemotherapy, including oxaliplatin and irinotecan, as well as the targeted monoclonal antibodies bevacizumab and cetuximab. These agents have demonstrated the ability to downsize colorectal tumors both in the liver and at extrahepatic sites. Thus, many formerly unresectable patients can now have liver resection after downsizing with chemotherapy. It is generally agreed that the best time for surgery is when the size and the position of tumors are such that liver resection can be done safely.[43] Continuing chemotherapy until maximal effect is undesirable because irinotecan has been associated with the development of steatohepatitis[44] and oxaliplatin with endotheliolitis.[45] These injuries can make liver resection hazardous. Furthermore, continued downsizing may make tumors difficult to locate. This is important because although tumors may show a complete radiologic response on CT and FDG-PET scans, this is infrequently associated with a complete pathologic response. The ability to resect multiple large tumors from the liver has been enhanced by PVE and two-stage hepatectomy. In this approach, one side of the liver is cleared of tumor and the portal vein on the other side is occluded. At a second stage, the atrophied side containing the bulk of the disease (usually the right hemiliver) is excised.

Extrahepatic disease in patients with hepatic metastases Good results have been obtained in patients with recurrent disease in the primary colorectal site and liver metastases, as well as liver and lung metastases.[46] With the advent of the new chemotherapy, it may be warranted to extend this approach to patients with liver and portal lymph node metastases but not with positive lymph nodes in the celiac or para-aortic regions.[47] Peritoneal metastases have been treated successfully by resection combined with hyperthermic intraperitoneal chemotherapy. Whether this approach combined with liver resection would be effective in patients with liver and peritoneal metastases is uncertain. Its application seems warranted in selected well followed cases.

Ablation of colorectal metastases In situ destruction of tumors with cryotherapy or RF ablation may expand the surgeon's ability to eradicate CRMs localized to the liver.[48] RF ablation has largely supplanted cryotherapy in this context as a result of its lower incidence of complications and greater ease of use. Ablation may be used either as an adjunct to operative management or as the sole treatment when there are many metastases (but usually < 10). The efficacy of RF ablation as an adjunct to surgery remains to be determined. It is doubtful, however, that using this modality alone to eradicate multiple lesions will improve overall survival significantly because the tumor biology in such cases is likely to be that of an aggressive tumor. Recent data suggest that the preceeding statement is correct.[49] FDG-PET scans should be performed in all such patients; the likelihood of discovering extrahepatic tumors increases as the number of hepatic tumors increases.[39]

RF ablation is not recommended for treatment of resectable metastases: it is not approved for this purpose, and using it in this way would mean substituting an unproven therapy of unknown efficacy for a proven therapy of known value. Again, based on recent publications, it is highly likely that RF ablation results in poorer long-term survival than liver resection.[48] If a consenting patient with resectable metastases nevertheless insists on this less invasive therapy, the surgeon should document that the preceding considerations have been explained. RF ablation may be applied by means of open, laparoscopic, or percutaneous methods. There is good reason to believe that targeting ability is degraded as one moves to less invasive methods. This consideration should also be explained to patients, although, undoubtedly, there are some patients who, because of comorbid conditions, are candidates only for percutaneous or laparoscopic approaches.

Neuroendocrine Metastases

Neuroendocrine metastases are characteristically slow growing. Some are functional, especially if they arise from the ileum; metastatic liver disease from this source may produce carcinoid syndrome. ^{111}In-pentetreotide imaging (OctreoScan, Mallinckrodt Inc., Hazelwood, Missouri) provides staging information comparable to that provided by FDG-PET in patients with CRMs.

The aims of surgical treatment are (1) to eradicate the cancer and (2) to reduce hormonal symptoms. The considerations regarding tumor eradication for neuroendocrine metastases are similar to those for CRMs—that is, resection should be performed if all cancer can be removed and no extrahepatic cancer is detectable. In highly symptomatic patients in whom conservative therapy with octreotide has failed, debulking the tumor by means of either chemoembolization or surgery may provide relief. The former is more suitable for patients with multiple small, diffuse metastases, whereas the latter is preferred for patients with large localized tumors. RF ablation may also be employed, either combined with surgical treatment or alone; this is an excellent use of this procedure in that the aim is cytoreduction rather than eradication. Debulking tumors in asymptomatic patients with the intention of extending survival is controversial. It is not recommended when more than 10% of the tumor wil remain.

Noncolorectal, Non-neuroendocrine Metastases

Occasionally, liver metastases from other primary sites behave like CRMs in that they are localized to part of the liver in the absence of extrahepatic disease. Such patients can be managed according to the same approach employed for CRMs, although the outcome is somewhat less satisfactory. Tumors that have been treated in this way with acceptable results include breast cancers, renal cell cancers, gastric cancers, acinar cell cancers of the pancreas, and ovarian cancers. Liver resection for more aggressive malignancies (e.g., metastases from gallbladder cancer and pancreatic ductal adenocarcinomas) can be expected to yield very poor results.

INCIDENTALLY DISCOVERED ASYMPTOMATIC HEPATIC MASS

Now that transaxial imaging of the abdomen is commonly performed for a variety of complaints, the problem of the incidentally discovered asymptomatic hepatic mass is being encountered with increased frequency. Generally, cysts are easily distinguished from solid tumors; the main diagnostic issue is differentiation of the various solid lesions.

The differential diagnosis of the benign solid hepatic mass includes hepatic adenoma, focal nodular hyperplasia (FNH), focal fatty infiltration, cavernous hemangioma, and other rare neoplasms (e.g., mesenchymal hamartoma and teratoma)—all of which must be distinguished not only from one another but also from malignant tumors. In the past, several diagnostic tests (e.g., ultrasonography, CT, sulfur colloid scanning, and angiography) were used to differentiate these neoplasms. Currently, our usual practice is to perform MRI with gadolinium contrast enhancement, which generally allows accurate differentiation among benign tumors with a single test. Cavernous hemangiomas are usually easy to distinguish because they have a characteristic appearance on MRI (hypointense on T_1-weighted images, very intense on T_2-weighted images, and filling in from the periphery with gadolinium injection); if they are asymptomatic, they need not be resected. It is important to distinguish asymptomatic FNHs from hepatic adenomas: whereas resection is recommended for adenomas because of their potential for hemorrhage or malignant degeneration, asymptomatic FNHs can safely be observed. An FNH is nearly isointense on T_1- and T_2-weighted images; it shows slightly more enhancement than normal liver parenchyma in the early phase after contrast injection and then becomes isointense. A central scar is often, but not always, seen. Conversely, a hepatic adenoma exhibits strong early-phase enhancement with contrast administration and tends to be hyperintense on T_1-weighted images.

Given that a symptomatic hepatic mass is usually treated with resection, preoperative biopsy for tissue diagnosis is rarely necessary or desirable. Modern noninvasive radiologic tests, in conjunction with a careful patient history, are often quite accurate in predicting histologic diagnosis. Biopsy of hepatic lesions should not be performed indiscriminately, because there is a small risk of complications or tumor tracking and because biopsy results often do not change management. As a rule, biopsies should be performed when definitive surgical intervention is not planned and when pathologic confirmation is necessary for institution of nonsurgical therapy.

Steven M. Strasberg is a consultant for Salient Surgical Technologies and for Valleylab Inc.

David C. Linehan has no financial disclosures.

References

1. Cleary SP, Gryfe R, Guindi M, et al. Prognostic factors in resected pancreatic adenocarcinoma: analysis of actual 5-year survivors. J Am Coll Surg 2004;198:722.
2. Patel AH, Harnois DM, Klee GG, et al. The utility of CA 19-9 in the diagnoses of cholangiocarcinoma in patients without primary sclerosing cholangitis. Am J Gastroenterol 2000;95:204.
3. Logrono R, Wong JY. Reporting the presence of significant epithelial atypia in pancreaticobiliary brush cytology specimens lacking evidence of obvious carcinoma: impact on performance measures. Acta Cytol 2004; 48:613.
4. Hardacre JM, Iacobuzio-Donahue CA, Sohn TA, et al. Results of pancreaticoduodenectomy for lymphoplasmacytic sclerosing pancreatitis. Ann Surg 2003;237:853.
5. Kahl S, Malfertheiner P. Role of endoscopic ultrasound in the diagnosis of patients with solid pancreatic masses. Dig Dis 2004;22:26.
6. Strasberg SM, Middleton WD, Teefey SA, et al. Management of diagnostic dilemmas of the pancreas by ultrasonographically guided laparoscopic biopsy. Surgery 1999;126:736.
7. Strasberg SM, Drebin JA, Mokadam NA, et al. Prospective trial of a blood supply–based technique of pancreaticojejunostomy: effect on anastomotic failure in the Whipple procedure. J Am Coll Surg 2002;194:746.
8. Varadhachary GR, Tamm EP, Abbruzzese JL, et al. Borderline resectable pancreatic cancer: definitions, management, and role of preoperative therapy. Ann Surg Oncol 2006; 13:1035–46.
9. Vollmer CM, Drebin JA, Middleton WD, et al. Utility of staging laparoscopy in subsets of peripancreatic and biliary malignancies. Ann Surg 2002;235:1.
10. Povoski SP, Karpeh MS Jr, Conlon KC, et al. Preoperative biliary drainage: impact on intraoperative bile cultures and infectious morbidity and mortality after pancreaticoduodenectomy. J Gastrointest Surg 1999; 3:496.
11. Pedrazzoli S, DiCarlo V, Dionigi R, et al. Standard versus extended lymphadenectomy associated with pancreatoduodenectomy in the surgical treatment of adenocarcinoma of the head of the pancreas: a multicenter, prospective, randomized study. Lymphadenectomy Study Group. Ann Surg 1998; 228:508.
12. Sindelar WF. Clinical experience with regional pancreatectomy for adenocarcinoma of the pancreas. Arch Surg 1989;124:127.

PHARMACOLOGIC THERAPY

The pharmacologic agents that decrease splanchnic blood flow are vasopressin and its analogues, somatostatin and its analogues, and nonselective beta-adrenergic blockers. Vasopressin and somatostatin and their analogues are given parenterally and are used only in the acute situation. Vasopressin, a splanchnic vasoconstrictor, can control acute bleeding in nearly half of patients but is not currently used because of an increased risk of cardiovascular ischemia. The semisynthetic analogue of vasopressin, terlipressin, has been used extensively in Europe because of its superior safety profile but is not currently available in the United States. The agent most commonly used within the United States is the somatostatin analogue octreotide because of its safety profile. Octreotide reduces portal pressure by decreasing portal blood flow through arteriolar splanchnic vasoconstriction. Octreotide is administered intravenously as a bolus of 50 μg followed by a continuous infusion at the rate of 50 μg/hr.

Nonselective beta-adrenergic agents are the preferred treatment for long-term use in decreasing portal pressure. A nonselective beta blocker is essential because blockade of beta$_1$-adrenergic receptors in the heart decreases cardiac output, whereas blockade of beta$_2$-adrenergic receptors results in a decrease in portal blood flow. Of the two nonselective beta blockers, nadolol is preferred to propranolol because it is excreted predominantly by the kidney and has lower lipid solubility, which is associated with a lower risk of central nervous system side effects. The initial starting dose of nadolol is 20 mg daily and that of propranolol is 40 mg daily as a long-acting preparation. The dose of the agents is titrated upward every 3 to 5 days until a target heart rate of 55 to 60 beats per minute is reached or a decrease in resting heart rate by 25% is achieved. Recently, carvedilol, a nonselective beta blocker with additional alpha blocking activity, has been introduced for the prevention of variceal bleeding. The effect of alpha blockade is to decrease intrahepatic vascular resistance. Thus, carvedilol causes further decrease in portal pressure than do nonselective beta-blockers alone.[15] Carvedilol is currently recommended in patients with portal hypertension who, in addition, have coronary artery disease or systemic hypertension but, in future, may be recommended for the majority of patients with portal hypertension. Nitrates act by causing venous dilatation and decreased portal blood flow because of the resulting reflex splanchnic vasoconstriction. Nitrates are seldom used within the United States because of the inability of most patients to tolerate the medication for prolonged periods because of headaches.

ENDOSCOPIC THERAPY

Endoscopic therapy is the only modality that can be used to prevent variceal bleeding, control variceal bleeding, and prevent variceal rebleeding. The preferred endoscopic technique is variceal ligation [*see Figure 4*]. Multiband devices are available that can apply several bands without withdrawal of the endoscope. The procedure involves suctioning of the varix into the device at the end of the endoscope. A band is then deployed around the varix, which strangulates the vessel and causes thrombosis. Banding the varices is

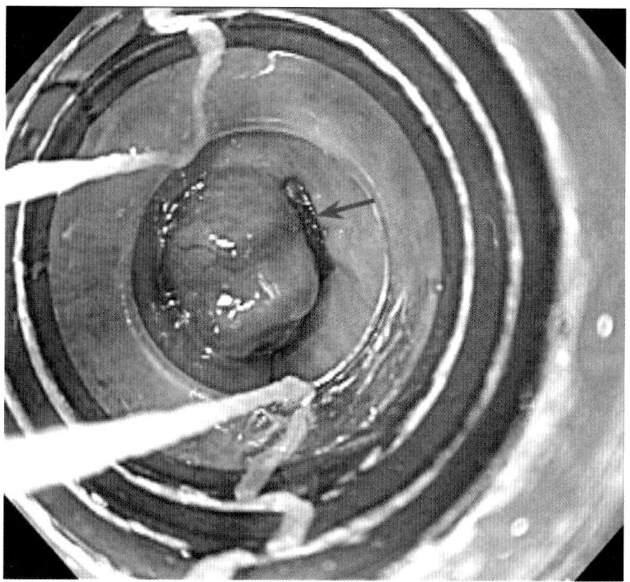

Figure 4 **Endoscopic image of esophageal varix following ligation. The *arrow* points to the band ligating the varix.**

started at the gastroesophageal junction and, moving more proximally in a spiral fashion, at approximately 2 cm intervals. Care should be taken to avoid applying the bands at the same level because of the risk of triggering esophageal strictures. Complications of variceal ligation include esophageal ulceration and esophageal strictures. Pulmonary aspiration may also occur. Gastric varices and ectopic varices may be treated using cyanoacrylate glue, which obturates the varices. These glues are used off label in the United States.

TRANSJUGULAR INTRAHEPATIC PORTOSYSTEMIC SHUNTS

A transjugular intrahepatic portosystemic shunt (TIPS) functions effectively as a side-to-side portocaval shunt [*see Figure 5*]. The technique involves creating a communication in the intrahepatic portion of the liver between the hepatic vein and a portal vein. Because TIPS functions like a side-to-side portocaval shunt, it may be used to treat not only acute or recurrent variceal bleeding but also refractory ascites, Budd-Chiari syndrome, and hepatic hydrothorax. The TIPS placement is usually performed with the patient under sedation. A platelet count of more than 50 × 10^3/μL and an INR less than 2 are usually recommended. The hepatic vein is cannulated through a transjugular approach by an interventional radiologist. Using a Rosch needle, the portal vein is cannulated through the intervening liver from the hepatic vein. The tract is dilated over a guide wire, and an expandable metal stent is placed across the tract to reduce the portocaval pressure gradient to below 12 mm Hg. The stent may be balloon dilated to reduce the pressure so that the target pressure of less than 12 mm Hg is reached. A coated stent is preferred nowadays. The uncoated portion anchors the stent to the portal vein, whereas the polytetrafluoroethylene-coated portion lines the tract within the liver. Shunt stenosis is reduced when coated stents are used. TIPS can be placed successfully in over 95% of patients and is associated with a procedure-related mortality of approximately 1%.[16]

a

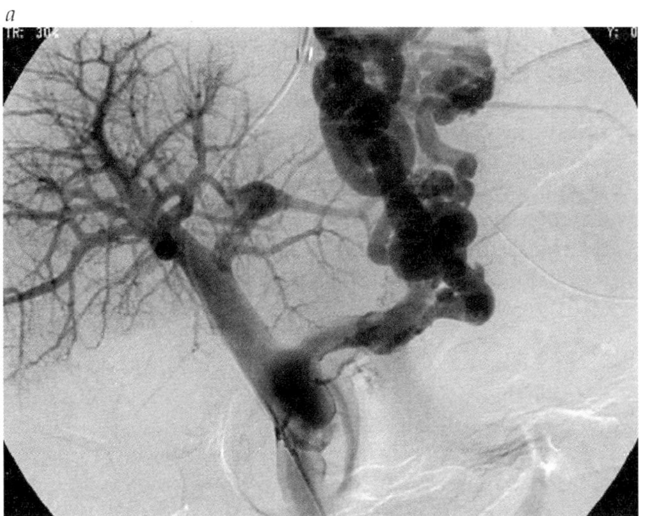

b

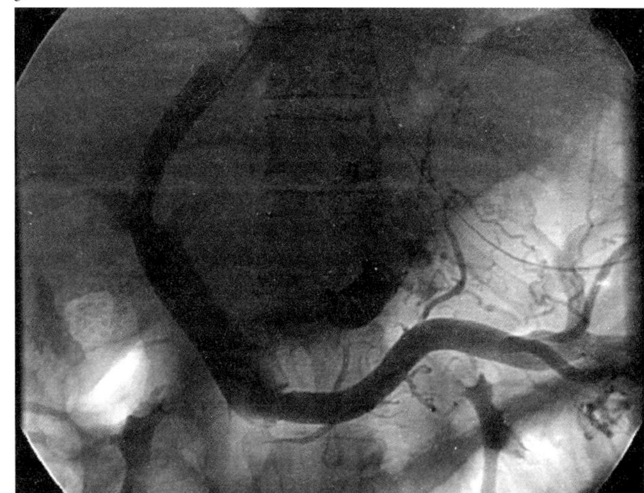

Figure 5 **Transjugular intrahepatic portosystemic shunt (TIPS). (*a*) Portogram demonstrating gastroesophageal varices and portal perfusion of the liver. (*b*) Portogram following creation of TIPS. Note the absence of portal hypertension.**

Complications may occur early or late. Intra-abdominal bleeding is the most serious immediate complication. Long-term complications are related to shunt stenosis. Survival of patients following placement of a TIPS may be determined using the MELD score.[17] Follow-up ultrasonography at 6-month intervals is recommended as surveillance for shunt patency. The patency of TIPS can usually be maintained through repeated radiographic intervention.

Surgery for Portal Hypertension

Surgical treatment for portal hypertension includes portosystemic shunts, nonshunt procedures, and liver transplantation. Surgical procedures are used infrequently for patients with portal hypertension from cirrhosis because of the efficacy of both TIPS and liver transplantation. In fact, all patients with cirrhosis and variceal bleeding should be evaluated for liver transplantation, but patients with a MELD score less than 15 are not likely to have a survival benefit with liver transplantation. Portal hypertensive bleeding should be managed preferably by nonoperative alternatives as a bridge to transplantation, and only failure of nonoperative management should prompt consideration of operative intervention. When a surgical procedure is being considered, the choice of nontransplant procedure is dependent on the presence or absence of underlying liver disease, the patency of the portal venous system, the acuity of the variceal hemorrhage and its response to nonoperative therapy, and candidacy for liver transplantation. Patients who are CTP class A are the best candidates for nontransplant operations for portal hypertension from cirrhosis. However, patients with portal hypertension and variceal bleeding from portal vein thrombosis should be evaluated for nontransplant operative procedures.

NONSHUNT SURGICAL PROCEDURES

Nonshunt procedures include esophageal transection and gastroesophageal devascularization. Gastroesophageal devascularization is generally reserved for patients with extensive portal venous thrombosis in whom the absence of a suitable patent branch of the portal vein precludes portosystemic shunting.

Esophageal Transection

Esophageal transection involves division and anastomosis of the esophagus, usually by stapling, to disrupt esophageal varices. Often splenectomy is performed to further reduce portal blood flow. The Suguira procedure has been the primary transection procedure employed and is usually coupled with selective vagotomy. Importantly, this operation attempts to maintain patency of paraesophageal collaterals to permit the development of additional portoazygos collaterals, thus diverting the hypertensive portal blood flow from the esophagogastric junction. Esophageal transection has reportedly been safe and highly effective in controlling variceal bleeding and is associated with a lower risk of encephalopathy than that for portosystemic shunts in the East but not in the West. Patient selection and modifications in the originally described technique likely account for the differences in outcome. Esophageal transection typically has been undertaken when patients continued to bleed from esophageal varices despite two endoscopic sessions within a 24-hour period. With the increasing use of emergency TIPS to control acute variceal bleeding, esophageal transection is seldom used.

Devascularization Procedures

Devascularization procedures are performed to prevent recurrent variceal bleeding in patients with CTP class A in whom a portosystemic shunt is precluded, either surgically or radiologically. Typically, these procedures are employed in patients with extensive splenic and portal venous thrombosis. As originally described by Sugiura, a combined thoracotomy and laparotomy approach was required, but, subsequently, the operation has been carried out through an abdominal approach combined with a splenectomy.[18] Total devascularization of the greater curvature of the stomach and the upper two thirds of the lesser curvature of the stomach and circumferential devascularization of the lower 7.5 cm of the esophagus are required [*see Figure 6*]. The rate of recurrent bleeding following this procedure depends a great deal on the extent of devascularization and may be as high as 40% if devascularization is incomplete.

PORTOSYSTEMIC SHUNTS

Surgical portosystemic shunts are divided into selective shunts, partial shunts, and total portosystemic shunts.

Selective Shunts

Selective shunts isolate and decompress only a portion of the portal venous system, that is, only the gastroesophageal junction, proximal stomach, and spleen. The most widely used selective shunt is the distal splenorenal shunt or Warren shunt [*see Figure 7*]. Portal hypertensive blood flow is maintained to the liver through the uninterrupted superior mesenteric and portal veins, and hepatic sinusoidal pressure remains elevated; therefore, selective shunts are ineffective in treating ascites. The distal splenorenal shunt is constructed by anastomosing the distal end of the splenic vein from the preserved spleen to the side of the left renal vein. The right and left gastric and right epiploic veins and greater curve perforating branches to the gastroepoploic vein are ligated, but the short gastric veins are preserved to decompress the gastroesophageal junction through the shunt. Additionally, all pancreatic branches to the splenic vein from the splenic hilus to the portal vein are divided to prevent the late loss of selectivity of this shunt. In expert hands, the distal splenorenal shunt can prevent variceal bleeding in more than 90% of patients with low operative mortality and morbidity and a low risk of hepatic encephalopathy, approximately 25% have two episodes of hepatic encephalopathy requiring hospitalization, and approximately 50% have one episode at 5 years.

Partial Portosystemic Shunts

A partial portosystemic shunt is actually a type of side-to-side portocaval shunt, but the shunt is calibrated by the size of the synthetic interposition graft placed between the portal vein and the inferior vena cava. Shunt diameters of 8 mm usually reduce the portal pressure to less than 12 mm Hg and maintain most antegrade portal blood flow to the liver. Construction of a partial shunt is technically simpler than construction of a distal splenorenal shunt. Although partial shunts are nonselective because they do not selectively decompress an isolated portion of the portal system, their efficacy in terms of reduction of variceal bleeding and the rate of encephalopathy is similar to that seen with a distal splenorenal shunt.

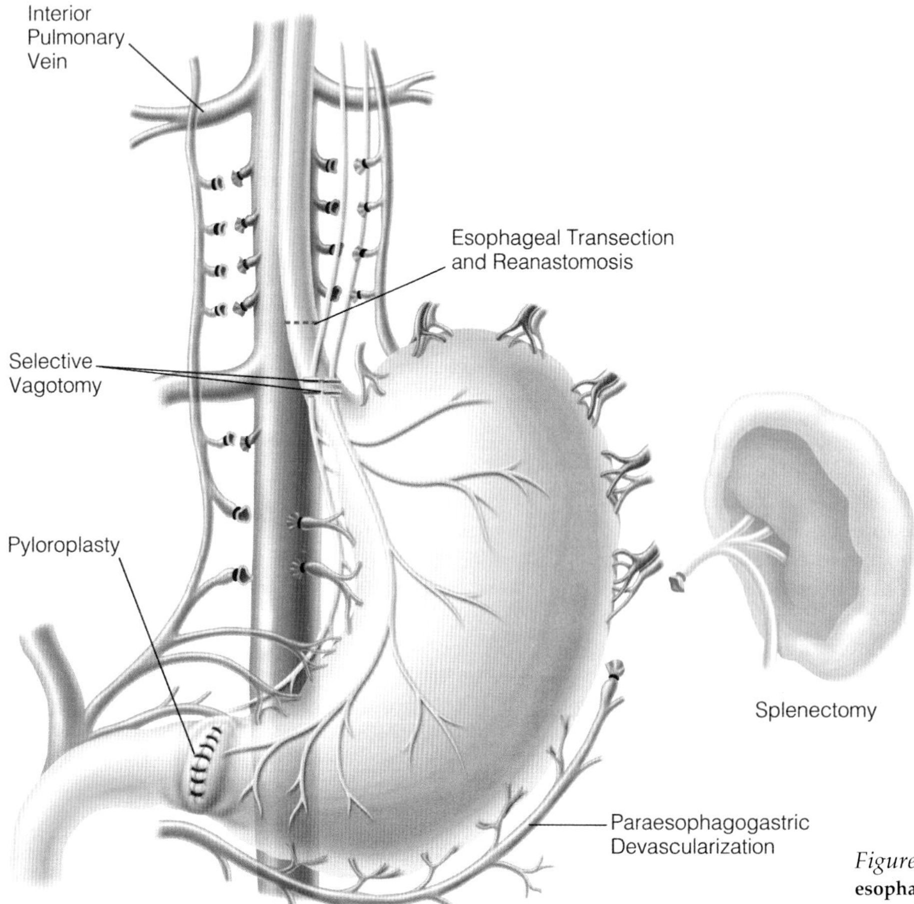

Figure 6 **By extensively devascularizing the esophagogastric junction, this procedure may provide means of interrupting esophagogastric varices without portosystemic shunting.**

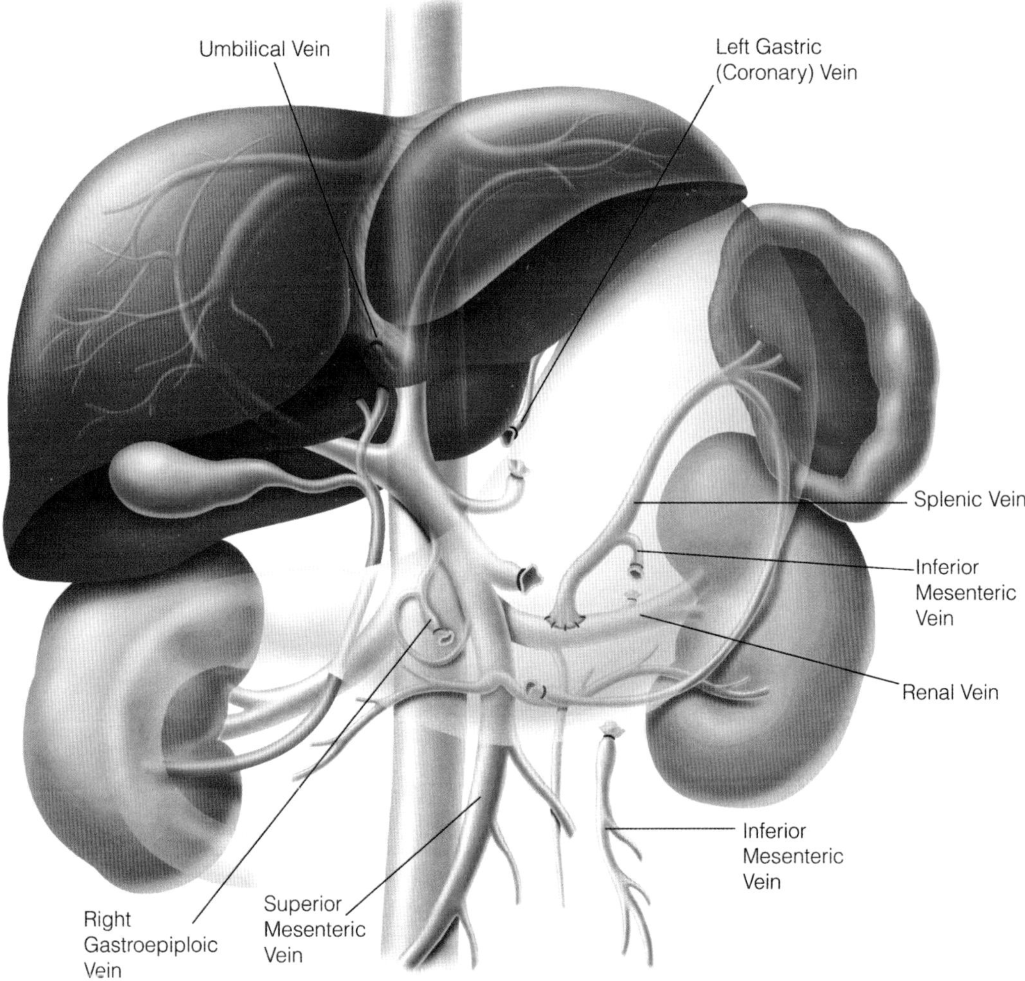

Figure 7 **The distal splenorenal shunt (DSRS) diverts portal flow from the spleen and short gastric veins into the left renal vein. The DSRS provides selective shunting by preserving portal flow from the mesenteric circulation. Potential sites of collateralization (e.g., the left gastric vein, the gastroepiploic vein, and the umbilical vein) are routinely interrupted to preserve hepatopedal portal flow.**

Nonselective Portosystemic Shunts

Nonselective shunts effectively decompress the entire portal venous system and divert portal blood flow from the liver to a significant degree. Nonselective portosystemic shunts include the end-to-side and side-to-side portocaval shunts, the central splenorenal shunt [*see Figure 8a*]), and the mesocaval shunt [*see Figure 8b*]). The end-to-side portocaval shunt [*see Figure 8c*]), which was an excellent procedure for preventing variceal bleeding but which could not be used to treat ascites because hepatic sinusoidal pressure was maintained, is no longer used. Nowadays, the side-to-side portocaval shunt is used predominantly [*see Figure 8d*]). Any portocaval shunt more than 12 mm in diameter results in almost total shunting of portal blood flow. These shunts are very effective in controlling bleeding and ascites because the hepatic sinusoids are decompressed, but hepatic encephalopathy occurs in about 40% of patients followed long term. Moreover, these shunts may be associated with increased morbidity and intraoperative transfusion requirements in those patients who undergo liver transplantation.

Management of Specific Causes of Portal Hypertension–Related Bleeding

ESOPHAGEAL VARICES

Treatment of esophageal variceal bleeding is classified as either (a) primary prophylaxis to prevent the first bleeding [*see Figure 9*]; (b) control of acute variceal bleeding [*see Figure 10*]; or (c) secondary prophylaxis to prevent rebleeding in patients in whom the initial bleeding is controlled [*see Figure 11*].[19]

Primary Prophylaxis

Either nonselective beta blockers or endoscopic variceal ligation should be considered in patients with large varices. In patients with CTP class C cirrhosis, small varices should also be considered for treatment with a beta blocker. The benefit of primary prophylaxis is greatest in patients with large varices, with the prevention of variceal bleeding in approximately one of 10 patients treated. Either nadolol or a long-acting preparation of propranolol may be used. In

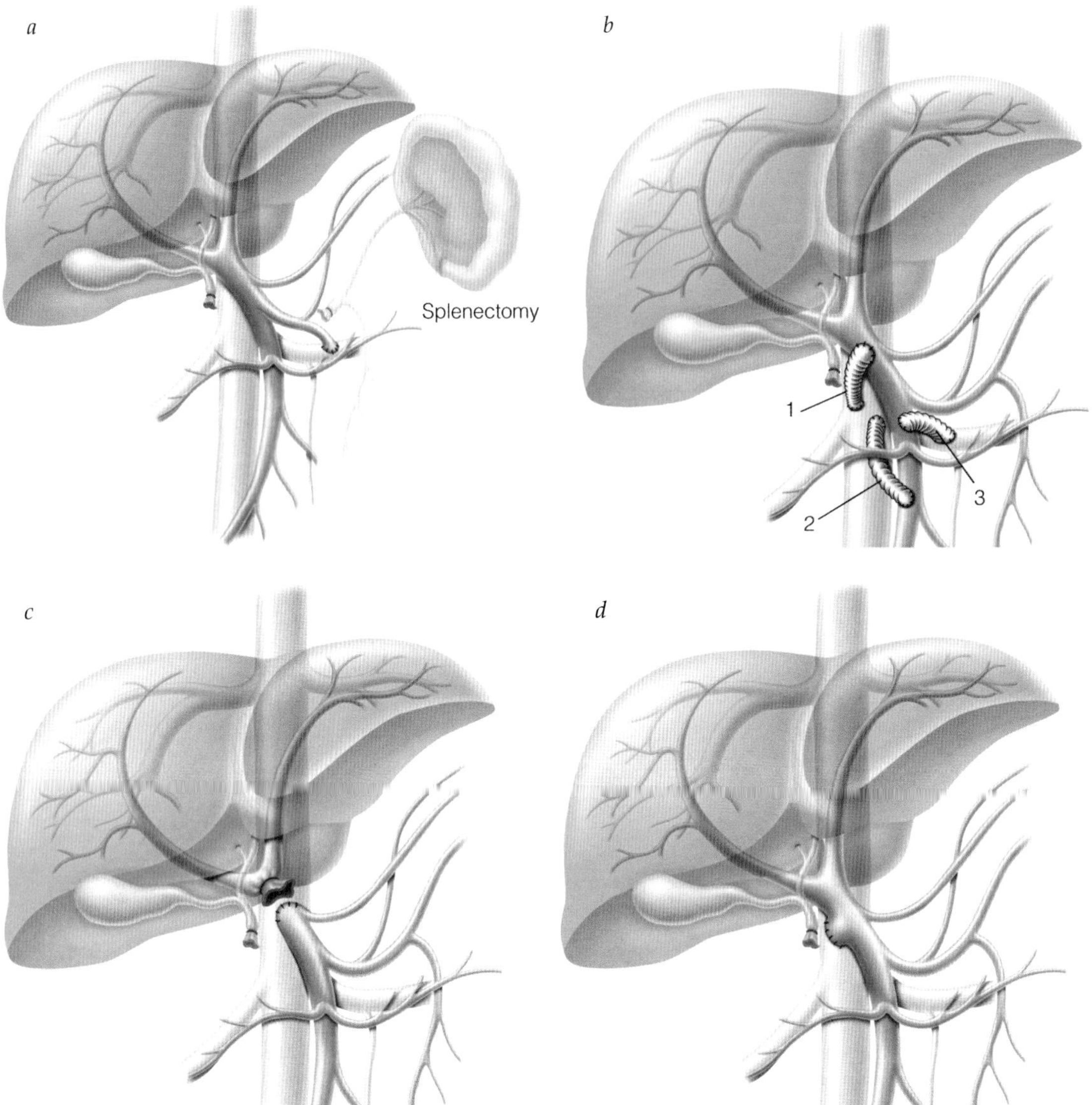

Figure 8 **Nonselective portosystemic shunts either immediately or eventually divert all portal blood flow from the liver into the systemic venous circulation. Shown are the four main variants: (*a*) conventional (proximal) splenorenal shunt, (*b*) interposition shunt (portacaval [1], mesocaval [2], and mesorenal [3]), (*c*) end-to-side portacaval shunt, and (*d*) side-to-side portacaval shunt.**

approximately 15% of patients, the drug is discontinued because of side effects. The physiologic goal of treatment with beta blockers is a resting heart rate of between 55 and 60 beats per minute, provided that the systolic blood pressure is more than 90 mm Hg. If patients are started on pharmacologic treatment, follow-up endoscopy is not required unless gastrointestinal bleeding occurs.

Endoscopic variceal ligation is an alternative treatment. Variceal ligation is associated with a lower risk of bleeding and bleeding-related mortality than therapy with beta blockers, but overall mortality is similar. Complications of variceal ligation include esophageal ulcers and strictures, which may be severe but are infrequent with careful technique. Beta blockers are cheaper and convenient to use and may also reduce the risk of bleeding from gastric varices and portal hypertensive gastropathy, but side effects such as fatigue, erectile dysfunction, and cold extremities are more frequent. Moreover, in patients with refractory ascites on beta blockers, long-term survival may be reduced.[20] Therefore, the choice of therapy should be individualized.

Control of Acute Esophageal Variceal Bleeding

The aims of treatment in a patient with active esophageal variceal bleeding are resuscitation of the patient, control of hemorrhage, and prevention of complications such as infections and liver-specific conditions such as ascites and hepatic encephalopathy. Two large-caliber intravenous access catheters should be inserted as the patient is evaluated. Red blood cells are transfused with the goal of maintaining the hematocrit around 25%, and coagulopathy is corrected as indicated. There are no data to guide the use of platelets and fresh frozen plasma during an episode of

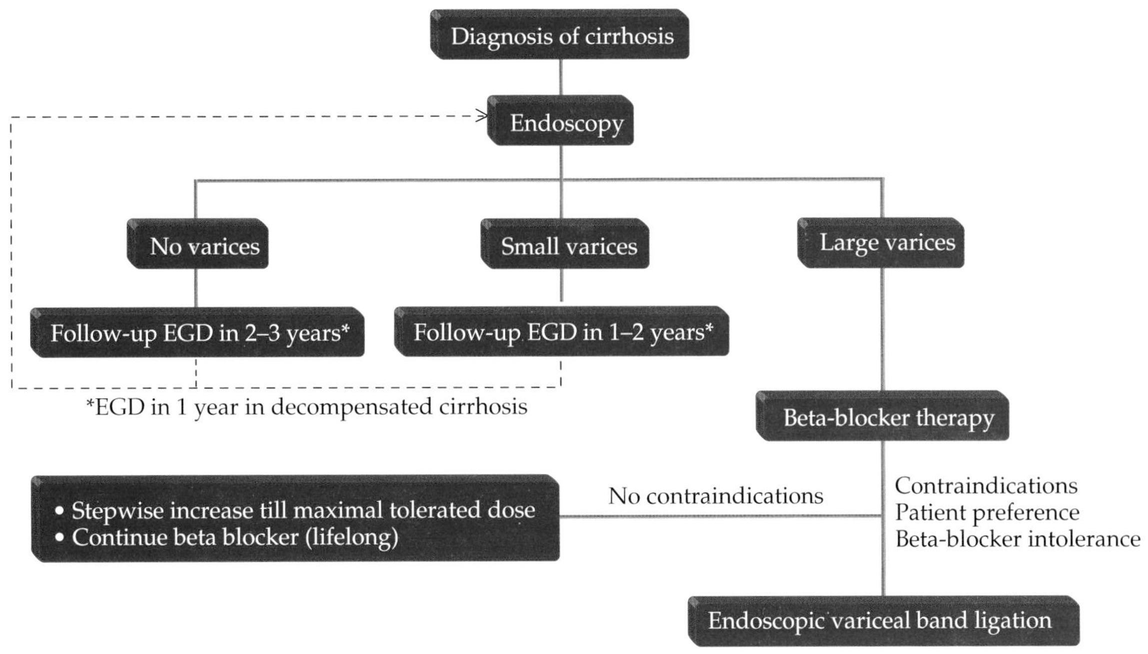

Figure 9 **Esophageal variceal bleeding: primary prophylaxis. EGD = esophagogastroduodenoscopy.**

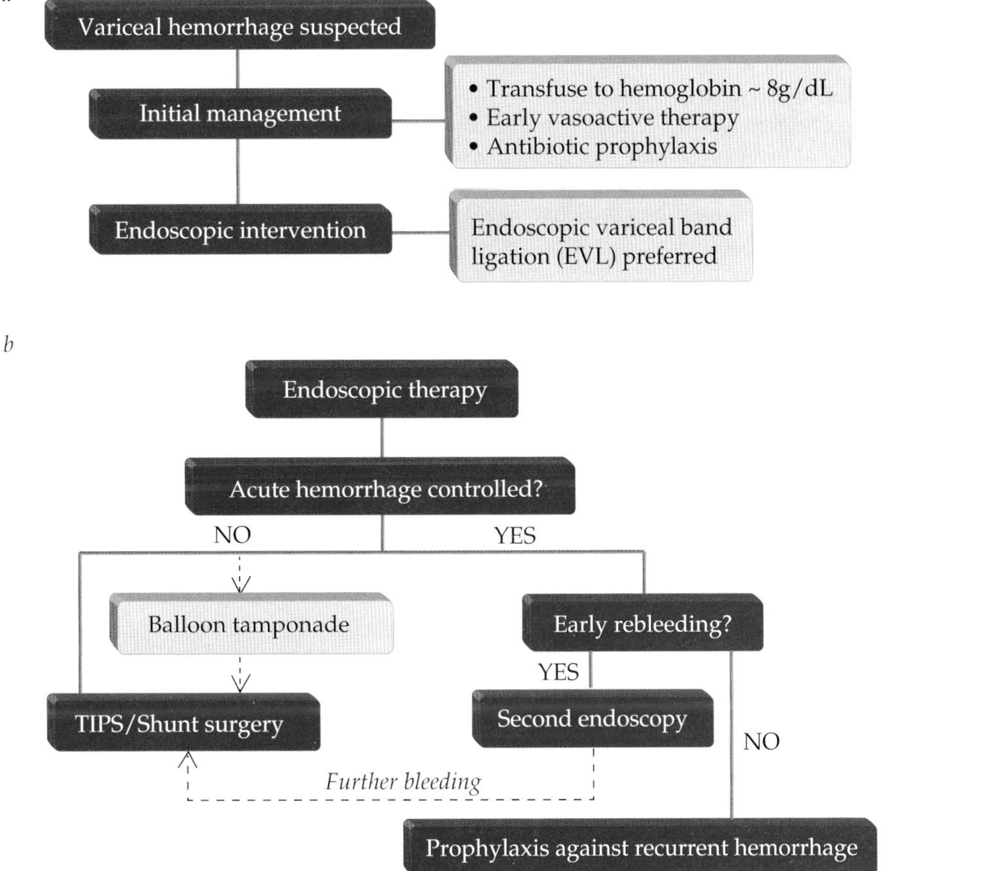

Figure 10 **Management of acute variceal bleeding: (*a*) initial management; (*b*) subsequent management. Early transjugular intrahepatic portosystemic shunt (TIPS) (within 24 to 72 hours) is recommended in patients with Child-Turcotte-Pugh class C or active bleeding at endoscopy.**

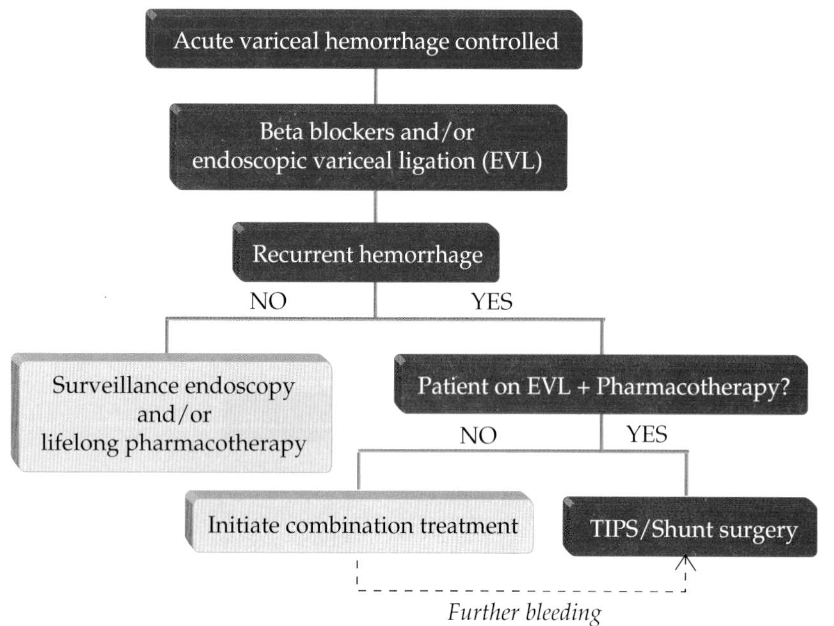

Figure 11 **Esophageal variceal bleeding: secondary prophylaxis. TIPS = transjugular intrahepatic portosystemic shunt.**

variceal bleeding.[19] Endotracheal intubation is advisable in the presence of active bleeding. Antibiotics should be administered to all patients to prevent bacteremia. Norfloxacin 400 mg orally twice daily, intravenous ciprofloxacin 400 mg every 12 hours, ceftriaxone 1 g every 24 hours, or levofloxacin 500 mg every 24 hours for 7 days is recommended. Pharmacologic therapy with vasoactive agents should be started as early as possible. Within the United States, the vasoactive agent most commonly used is octreotide. Endoscopic treatment is undertaken as soon as the patient is hemodynamically stable and the vasoactive agent has been infused for at least 30 minutes. Esophageal variceal bleeding is confirmed if active bleeding is seen from the varices or a white fibrin plug or red blood clot is noted over a varix. Esophageal varices are considered the site of bleeding if blood is seen in the stomach and no other bleeding source is identified.

Acute variceal bleeding cannot be controlled by endoscopic variceal ligation and pharmacotherapy in approximately 10% of patients. When two endoscopic sessions within a 24-hour period fail to control variceal bleeding, TIPS should be considered. Balloon tamponade with either a Minnesota tube or a Sengstaken-Blakemore tube may be used to control bleeding until TIPS is undertaken. The Minnesota tube has a suction port in the esophagus that decreases the risk of aspiration. Both have a gastric balloon and an esophageal balloon, but most operators prefer to inflate only the gastric balloon because inflating the esophageal balloon increases the risk of esophageal necrosis. Under no account should the gastric balloon be kept inflated for greater than 12 to 24 hours and the esophageal balloon for greater than 6 hours. Endotracheal intubation greatly reduces the risk of pulmonary aspiration. Patients with CTP class C and a MELD score of 11 to 13, patients with CTP class B with active bleeding at endoscopy, and patients with a MELD score greater than 18 who require transfusion of more than 4 units of red cells to maintain a hematocrit greater than 25% are patients considered at high risk for early rebleeding. Early TIPS (within 24 to 72 hours of control of bleeding) should be considered in these patients.[21] Emergency surgical shunts have largely been abandoned.

Secondary Prophylaxis

All patients who have had even a single episode of esophageal variceal bleeding should receive prophylactic therapy to reduce the risk of recurrent bleeding from esophageal varices. In the absence of secondary prophylaxis, nearly 80% of these patients will have recurrent variceal bleeding at 2 years. Pharmacologic therapy with nonselective beta blockers, endoscopic therapy, and portosystemic shunts (both surgical and TIPS) either alone or in combination have been used for secondary prophylaxis.[22]

The preferred initial treatment to prevent variceal rebleeding is a combination of endoscopic variceal ligation and a nonselective beta blocker. Isosorbide mononitrate is seldom used in the United States as patients typically are intolerant of this medication after beta blockade. Endoscopic variceal ligation alone is carried out in patients who are intolerant of beta blockers. Following control of the acute variceal bleeding with variceal ligation, the next session of endoscopic variceal ligation is carried out at 7 to 14 days. Subsequent sessions are repeated every 3 to 4 weeks until esophageal varices are ablated. If patients have recurrent bleeding after endoscopic variceal ligation alone, beta blockers are added. Conversely, if patients are initially started on nonselective beta blockers alone and have recurrent bleeding, endoscopic variceal ligation is added. For those patients with recurrent bleeding after a combination of endoscopic variceal ligation and beta blocker therapy, an evaluation for a portosystemic shunt is recommended. TIPS is the preferred modality in patients with Child-Pugh class B and C cirrhosis. Even in patients with Child-Pugh class A cirrhosis, the TIPS procedure may be as effective as a distal splenorenal shunt,[23] but the choice of therapy depends on local expertise.

GASTRIC VARICES

The two classes of gastric varices are GOVs and isolated gastric varices (IGVs). Type 1 gastroesophageal varices (GOV1) extend below the gastroesophageal junction along the lesser curvature of the stomach and are in continuity with esophageal varices; type 2 gastroesophageal varices (GOV2) extend into the cardia and fundus of the stomach and are also in continuity with the esophageal varices [*see Figure 12*]. GOV1 varices comprise approximately 70% of all gastric varices and are treated endoscopically similar to esophageal varices. Varices in the stomach in the absence of esophageal varices are called isolated gastric varices. Type 1 isolated gastric varices (IGV1) are in the fundus, whereas varices that occur elsewhere in the stomach in the absence of esophageal varices are termed IGV2. Although splenic vein thrombosis usually causes IGV1, the most common cause of fundic varices overall is probably cirrhosis. Gastric varices occur in association with advanced portal hypertension, and bleeding is more common in patients with GOV2 and IGV1. Gastric varices that bleed tend to be larger than esophageal varices and are likely to bleed only when their diameter is greater than 1 cm.

Primary Prophylaxis

No large studies have evaluated pharmacologic or endoscopic treatment for primary prophylaxis of gastric variceal hemorrhage, although a recent small study suggests that obturation of the gastric varices with cyano-acrylate glue might be beneficial. In patients with large gastric varices, pharmacologic treatment with nonselective beta blockers may be started to prevent variceal bleeding. Endoscopic therapy is not currently recommended as primary prophylaxis for gastric variceal bleeding.

Control of Bleeding

The principles of treatment for patients with gastrointestinal bleeding from gastric varices again include volume resuscitation, antibiotic prophylaxis, and a vasoactive agent such as octreotide [*see Figure 13*].[24] Endoscopic treatment is performed only after endotracheal intubation because these patients typically have large-volume bleeding. A diagnosis of gastric variceal hemorrhage is sometimes difficult because blood pools in the fundus of the stomach, obscuring visualization of the varices. Gastric variceal hemorrhage is suspected whenever bleeding is noted from a gastric varix; if blood is found in the stomach and gastric varices with a white nipple sign are noted; if active bleeding is seen at either the gastroesophageal junction or in the gastric fundus; or if blood is seen in the stomach and gastric varices are noted in the absence of other lesions in the esophagus and stomach.

The preferred endoscopic treatment for fundal gastric variceal bleeding is injection of cyanoacrylate polymers, usually N-butyl-2-cyanoacrylate in the United States.[25] These cyanoacrylate tissue adhesives are not licensed for use in the United States for variceal injection. Varices are obliterated when the cyanoacrylate adhesives harden on contact with blood. Cyanoacrylate glue injection is superior to both endoscopic variceal ligation and alcohol sclerotherapy in the treatment of gastric fundal varices. Pulmonary and cerebral emboli have been reported, especially in patients with spontaneous large portosystemic shunts or intrapulmonary shunts, and may even be associated with mortality.

If endoscopic and pharmacologic therapies have failed to control gastric variceal hemorrhage, TIPS is performed. A Linton-Nachlas tube with a 600 mL volume gastric balloon may be used temporarily to tamponade bleeding from gastric varices in patients requiring TIPS. The Minnesota tube and the Sengstaken-Blakemore tube with only 250 mL gastric balloons may not be as effective.

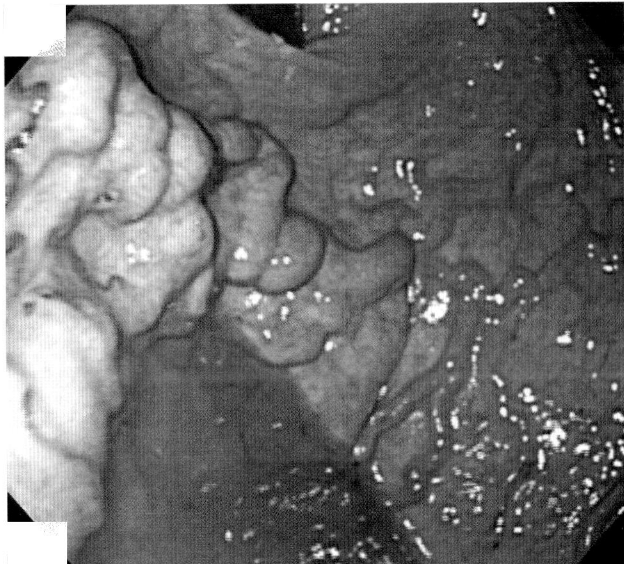

Figure 12 Endoscopic image of gastric varix (*arrow*) in continuity with esophageal varices.

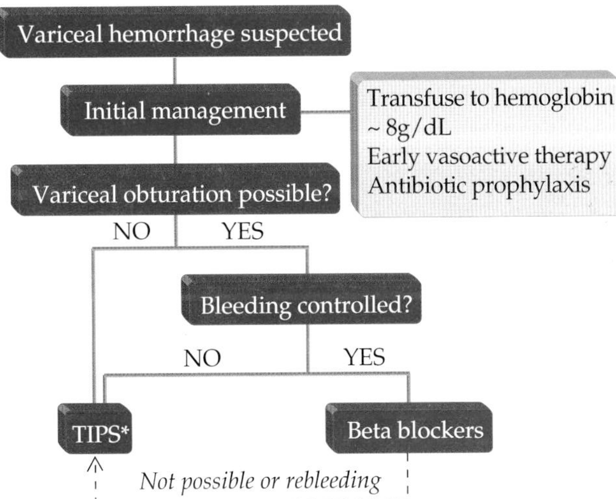

Figure 13 In patients with acute gastric variceal bleeding, initial management consists of transfusion to a hemoglobin of 8 g/dL, pharmacotherapy with vasoactive agents, and antibiotic prophylaxis. Endoscopic treatment is carried out, but if acute hemorrhage is not controlled, transjugular intrahepatic portosystemic shunt (TIPS) is recommended. If the acute hemorrhage is controlled and cyanoacrylate is available, obliteration of the gastric varices is attempted with cyanoacrylate. If cyanoacrylate is not available, then TIPS is recommended. *A surgical shunt may be considered in patients with Child-Turcotte-Pugh class A cirrhosis.

Secondary Prophylaxis

No control trials have determined the preferred therapy for the prevention of recurrent gastric variceal bleeding. Cyanoacrylate glue injection for secondary prophylaxis has been used, with excellent results. Alternatively, transvenous obliteration of gastric varices can also be undertaken in patients with demonstrable spontaneous splenorenal shunts by interventional radiologists. This technique requires considerable radiologic skill and is currently popular only in some centers in the Far East. TIPS is effective in preventing gastric variceal rebleeding in patients with cirrhosis. However, TIPS does not always result in a decrease in the size of gastric varices even when the HVPG is less than 12 mm Hg; therefore, the target HVPG in these patients is not clear.

ECTOPIC VARICES

Varices that occur at a site other than the gastroesophageal junction and stomach are termed ectopic varices.[26] Ectopic varices account for fewer than 5% of all variceal-related bleeding. Depending on the site of rupture of the varices, clinical manifestations include melena, hematemesis, hemobilia, hematuria, and retroperitoneal or intraperitoneal bleeding. Ectopic varices occur in patients with both extrahepatic portal vein obstruction and cirrhosis.

The most common site of ectopic varices is the duodenum. The site of gastrointestinal stomas, particularly in patients with inflammatory bowel disease and primary sclerosing cholangitis who have had an ileostomy following proctocolectomy, is the next most frequent. Peristomal varices present as a bluish halo surrounding the stoma. Anorectal varices are noted in about 10 to 40% of patients with cirrhosis who undergo colonoscopy.

In patients with suspected ectopic variceal bleeding, vasoactive drugs may be used initially to control bleeding. If the ectopic varices are visualized endoscopically, as in the duodenum or colon and rectum [*see Figure 14*], they are treated with band ligation or glue injection. Colonic varices may require application of hemostatic clips. Stomal varices are initially treated with local compression, but, subsequently, patients require either ultrasound-guided variceal sclerotherapy, transhepatic embolization of the stomal varices, or TIPS.

Ectopic varices that present as intraperitoneal hemorrhage are associated with a poor outcome because the diagnosis is often made late and patients may require a laparotomy.

PORTAL HYPERTENSIVE GASTROPATHY AND GASTRIC VASCULAR ECTASIA

Portal hypertensive gastropathy is common in patients with cirrhosis and is characterized by a cobblestone appearance of the gastric mucosa on endoscopy. If red spots are superimposed on the cobblestone appearance, the patients are said to have severe portal hypertensive gastropathy [*see Figure 15*]. Gastric vascular ectasia is an entity in which there are ectatic vessels in the absence of a background mosaic pattern [*see Figure 16*]. When these vascular aggregates occur in the antrum of the stomach arranged in a linear pattern, the term *watermelon stomach* is used. If the aggregates are more widely dispersed, the term used is *gastric antral vascular ectasia*. Portal hypertensive gastropathy responds to beta blockers or TIPS. However, vascular ectasia may require thermoablative therapy and, occasionally, antrectomy. TIPS does not reduce the risk of bleeding from gastric vascular ectasia.[27]

ASCITES

The initiating event in the formation of ascites is sinusoidal portal hypertension. The resulting splanchnic vasodilatation results in a decrease in the effective arterial blood volume. As a means of increasing the circulating intravascular volume, there is activation of the renin-angiotensin-aldosterone system, vasopressin, and the sympathetic

a

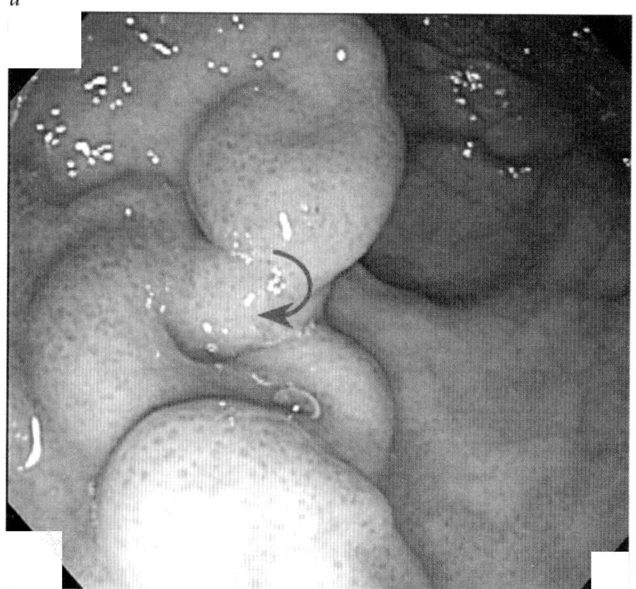

b

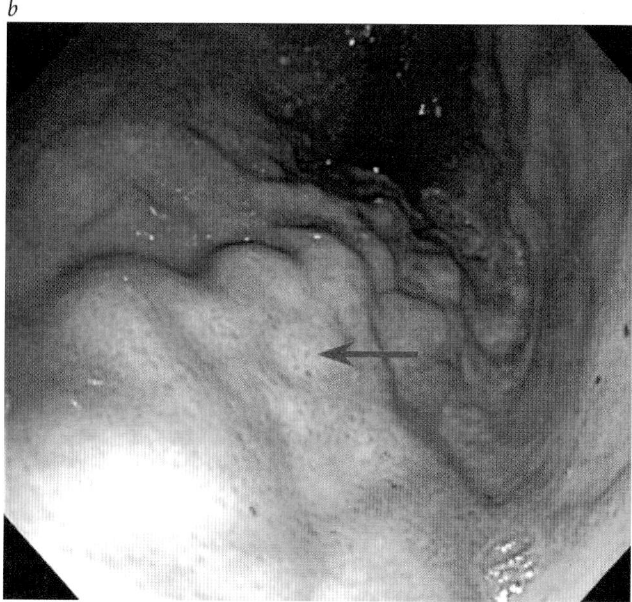

Figure 14 **(*a*) Colonic varix (*arrow*). (*b*) Rectal varix (*arrow*) seen on retroflexion of the colonoscope in the rectum.**

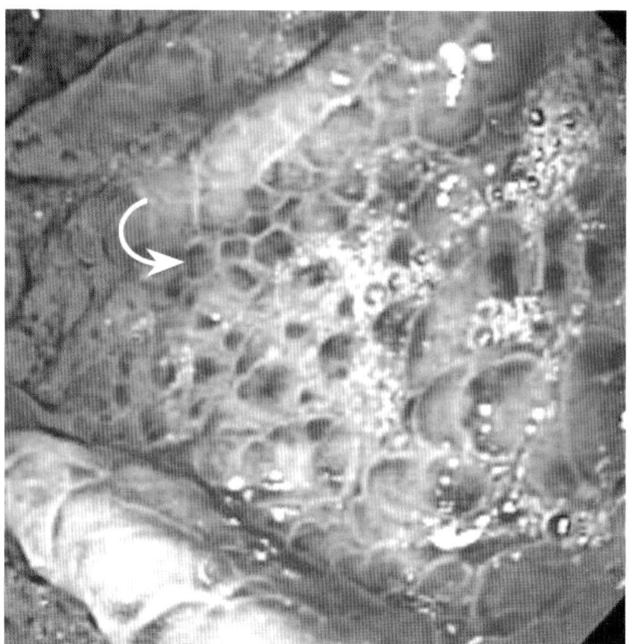

Figure 15 **Endoscopic image of severe portal hypertensive gastropathy. Note the cobblestone appearance (*arrow*) with red signs on the cobblestone.**

nervous system. The net result of these actions is renal retention of sodium and water and renal vasoconstriction. The excess fluid is compartmentalized into the peritoneal space because of portal hypertension. As cirrhosis progresses, there is further splanchnic vasodilatation and renal vasoconstriction. Ultimately, refractory ascites and hyponatremia, both of which are associated with decreased survival, occur. When renal vasoconstriction occurs and the serum creatinine is greater than 2.5 mg/dL, the condition is termed type 1 hepatorenal syndrome, which is associated with a median

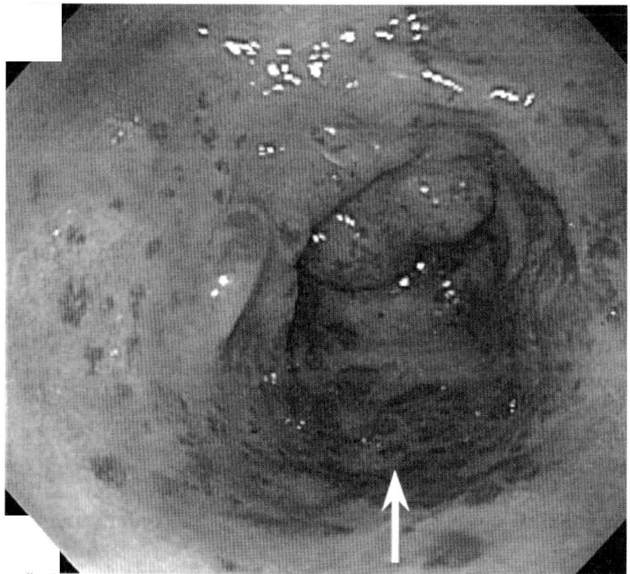

Figure 16 **Gastric vascular ectasia (*arrow*), which are ectatic vessels seen in the absence of background mosaic pattern.**

survival of only 2 weeks without treatment. When the serum creatinine rises above 1.5 mg/dL, patients are said to have type 2 hepatorenal syndrome, the major manifestation of which is refractory ascites. The median survival in patients with refractory ascites is 6 months. Another manifestation associated with increased renal retention of sodium and water is hepatic hydrothorax, that is, pleural effusions in the presence of ascites.

Treatment of ascites is aimed toward maintaining a negative sodium balance.[28] Specifically, renal sodium losses should exceed sodium intake because extrarenal losses of sodium via perspiration and stooling are more limited and difficult to control. Patients with ascites are typically placed on a 2 g sodium restricted diet (88 mEq of sodium). Spironolactone is the preferred diuretic because it is an aldosterone antagonist. The maximum dose of spironolactone is 400 mg per day. Spironolactone alone can achieve adequate renal sodium losses in 60 to 70% of patients. Furosemide is added in escalating doses if sodium restriction and spironolactone alone do not result in a daily weight loss of more than 500 g per day. The goal of treatment with diuretics is to achieve a daily weight loss of 500 g per day in the absence of lower limb edema and 1 kg a day in the presence of edema. The dose of diuretics is increased every 3 to 5 days if weight loss is less than 200 g per day.

If, in spite of sodium restriction and diuretics, a weight loss of more than 200 g per day is not achieved, the patient has refractory ascites. Most of these patients have diuretic-intractable ascites; that is, ascites persists because further increases in the dose of diuretics are associated with complications such as hyponatremia, renal insufficiency, and hepatic encephalopathy. Patients in whom ascites cannot be adequately immobilized in spite of 400 mg of spironolactone and 160 mg of furosemide per day have diuretic resistance ascites.

When ascites is refractory to diuretic treatment, large-volume paracentesis is recommended. Albumin is infused in a dose of 6 to 8 g per liter of ascitic fluid removed to prevent renal dysfunction and rapid reaccumulation of ascites. If more than two to three large-volume paracenteses are required every month in spite of optimal sodium restriction and maximal diuretics, TIPS is performed [*see Figure 17*]. TIPS results in better control of ascites in more than 80% of patients but is associated with an increased risk of hepatic encephalopathy and no change in overall survival. A peritoneovenous shunt should be considered in patients with refractory ascites in whom venous anatomy precludes TIPS. Peritoneovenous shunts are avoided in patients who are candidates for liver transplantation because of the risk of procedure-related mortality and, potentially, peritoneal fibrosis around the catheter. Peritoneovenous shunts are associated with frequent shunt occlusion and disseminated intravascular coagulation. The Denver shunt is the only peritoneovenous shunt currently on the market.

SPONTANEOUS BACTERIAL PERITONITIS

Spontaneous bacterial peritonitis (SBP) is caused by infection of ascites in the absence of a perforated viscus. SBP is suspected clinically in patients with ascites who develop fever and, sometimes, abdominal tenderness with associated other complicating factors. Symptomatic fistulas, such as those associated with obstruction or those associated with disabling symptoms (e.g., rectovaginal fistulas or enterocutaneous fistulas [*see Figure 2*]), may have to be treated surgically. Ileosigmoid fistulas, which effectively bypass the entire colon, may be associated with profound and refractory diarrhea (i.e., > 20 bowel movements/day) and may also have to be treated operatively.

Abscess Formation

Abscesses are particularly common with ileocolic Crohn disease. If they cannot be controlled by means of computed tomography (CT)-guided drainage, surgical therapy may be indicated.

Cancer or Dysplasia

The risk of colorectal cancer is approximately three times higher in patients with Crohn disease than in the general population.[15–17] Screening recommendations for patient's with long-standing Crohn colitis are similar to those for ulcerative colitis.[18] In Crohn disease, cancer may also arise in long-standing fistula tracts.

Failure to Grow

In children, failure to grow and develop normally is one of the main indications that medical therapy for Crohn disease has been unsuccessful. Timely surgical therapy will permit normal development. On occasion, when bone age lags significantly behind chronological age, treatment with recombinant human growth hormone is required.

Special Considerations

PREGNANCY

Persons who have Crohn disease may be less fertile than healthy age-matched persons. One possible explanation for this difference is that feeling ill may result in reduced sexual desire or decreased sexual activity. Another is that pelvic inflammation caused by Crohn disease or by scarring and adhesion formation resulting from surgery may impair fertility. To reduce the chances of the latter, hyaluronic acid sheets may be placed around the tubes and ovaries; alternatively, the ovaries may be tacked to the undersurface of the anterior abdominal wall with absorbable sutures and thereby prevented from entering the pelvis and being trapped in scar tissue.

There is no evidence that pregnancy exacerbates Crohn disease; however, there are some specific concerns that apply to pregnant patients with this condition. Because patients with Crohn disease often have bowel movements that are more liquid, they have a particular need for a well-functioning anal sphincter. If there is any chance of an obstetrics-related injury (e.g., from a large baby in a primagravida or from a breech presentation), a cesarean section is advisable to minimize the risk of sphincter trauma. The same is true in the presence of severe perianal Crohn disease. During pregnancy, prednisone and 5-aminosalicylic acid (5-ASA) medications are safe, whereas drugs such as metronidazole are not.[19] If imaging studies are needed, magnetic resonance imaging and ultrasonography are the modalities of choice.

MARKING OF STOMA SITES AND CHOICE OF INCISION

When a patient with Crohn disease is expected to need an ileostomy, it is extremely important to mark the site preoperatively. What looks flat when the patient is on the operating table may not be flat when he or she is upright. The patient must be asked to sit and lean over to confirm that the marked stoma site is in an area without folds, creases, or previous incisions. Stoma appliances do not adhere well to areas of previous scarring, and these should be avoided whenever possible.

Patients with Crohn disease do not react to intra-abdominal infection in a typical fashion. It is not unusual to find unsuspected abscesses that were not revealed by preoperative CT scans and other imaging studies. If there is even a remote chance of an unsuspected abscess (particularly in cases of obstructing ileocolic Crohn disease), the possibility of a temporary stoma should be raised with the patient and the proposed stoma site marked preoperatively.

A key point is the necessity of planning for the future. Many patients with Crohn disease will eventually require a stoma. Operating through a midline abdominal incision preserves all four quadrants for possible future stoma sites (if needed). Similarly, when surgery is performed laparoscopically, specimen retrieval sites should be kept away from potential stoma sites.

LAPAROSCOPY

Laparoscopic surgical techniques have gained acceptance in the treatment of Crohn disease. In performing a laparoscopic operation for Crohn disease, it is essential to adhere to the same technical standards that apply to corresponding open procedures. Careful intraoperative exploration of the abdomen is important in that many patients have multifocal disease. Without such exploration, patients may experience persistent postoperative symptoms as a consequence of persistent proximal pathologic states that were not addressed. As with other treatment modalities, there are some circumstances in which laparoscopy is particularly useful and others in which it should not be used. For example, a laparoscopic approach may not be suitable for fixed mesenteric abscesses associated with complex fistulae.

Ileocolic resection for Crohn disease also lends itself particularly well to a laparoscopically assisted approach; compared with open resection, laparoscopic resection has been reported to result in shorter hospital stays and reduced costs.[20,21] The ileocolic vessels originate centrally, and they lie only over the retroperitoneum. Once the lateral peritoneal attachments are divided, the colon and the small bowel mesentery can be exteriorized, and the mesentery can be divided and the anastomosis performed extracorporeally.

Many studies have shown that even fistulizing Crohn disease can be safely addressed laparoscopically, depending on the skill of the surgeon. A hand-assisted approach is often useful with cases of dense fixation, in which fistulas are common and finger dissection may facilitate definition of the anatomy. If in doubt, one should not hesitate to convert to an open procedure. Typically, most areas that feel fibrotic or contain fibrotic adhesions are actually areas of fistulizing disease and should be treated as such until proved otherwise. In one study, patients with recurrent disease, those older than 40 years, and those with an abdominal mass were more likely to require conversion to an open procedure.[22]

Surgical Management of Crohn Disease at Specific Sites

ESOPHAGEAL, GASTRIC, AND DUODENAL DISEASE

Crohn disease of the upper alimentary tract can be difficult to diagnose, largely because it is relatively uncommon. Obstructing strictures as a result of Crohn disease in this area are unusual; the unsuspected finding of noncaseating granulomas in biopsies of erythematous areas in a patient with Crohn disease in other locations is diagnostic.

Occasionally, a patient with Crohn disease of the distal esophagus requires dilatations, but this is uncommon. Surgical treatment for Crohn disease of the upper alimentary tract is almost exclusively reserved for disease affecting the duodenum. Diagnosis of duodenal Crohn disease can be difficult and requires a certain amount of suspicion. Frequently, the diagnosis is not made until relatively late because diagnostic imaging tends to focus on endoscopy and because the degree of duodenal obstruction is often not evident except on barium studies. The rigidity and luminal narrowing of the second portion of the duodenum are typically much more readily apparent on contrast studies than on endoscopy. Duodenal Crohn disease can lead to gastric outlet obstruction. In children, it can be mistaken for annular pancreas.

When duodenal Crohn disease does not respond to medical therapy, gastrojejunostomy with vagotomy is the preferred surgical treatment.[23,24] Failure to perform a vagotomy may result in marginal ulcer formation and obstruction. Some surgeons have performed duodenal strictureplasty to treat duodenal Crohn disease. The results have been conflicting[25,26]; the feasibility of this operative approach is limited by the pliability of the duodenum. Many patients experience prompt and full recovery of normal gastric emptying after operation, but some patients with long standing gastric outlet obstruction continue to experience impaired emptying. The latter may benefit from administration of a prokinetic agent (e.g., metoclopramide or erythromycin).

JEJUNOILEAL DISEASE

Short Bowel Syndrome

Although Crohn disease of the small bowel is not common and accounts for a relatively small proportion of all cases, disease in this area is associated with one of the highest overall recurrence rates. Resection of large portions of the small bowel can result in short bowel syndrome. For this reason, before proceeding with any type of small bowel or ileocolic resection, one should measure the length of the existing small bowel to determine the patient's "bowel resource." One naturally would more readily perform a resection in a patient who has 400 cm of normal small bowel than in one who has only 200 cm.

Resection versus Strictureplasty

The major advance in the surgical treatment of Crohn disease over the past quarter-century has been the technique of small bowel strictureplasty, first proposed by Lee and subsequently popularized by Williams, Fazio, and others.[25] Currently, the two most prevalent strictureplasty techniques are Heineke-Mikulicz strictureplasty [*see Figure 3*] and Finney strictureplasty [*see Figure 4*]. The former is best suited for strictures up to 5 to 7 cm long [*see Figure 5*] and the latter for strictures up to 10 to 15 cm long. The side-to-side strictureplasty described by Michelassi and colleagues[27] is suitable for longer areas of stricture; however, this technique involves longer suture lines and is mainly considered for patients who already have, or are at high risk for, short bowel syndrome.

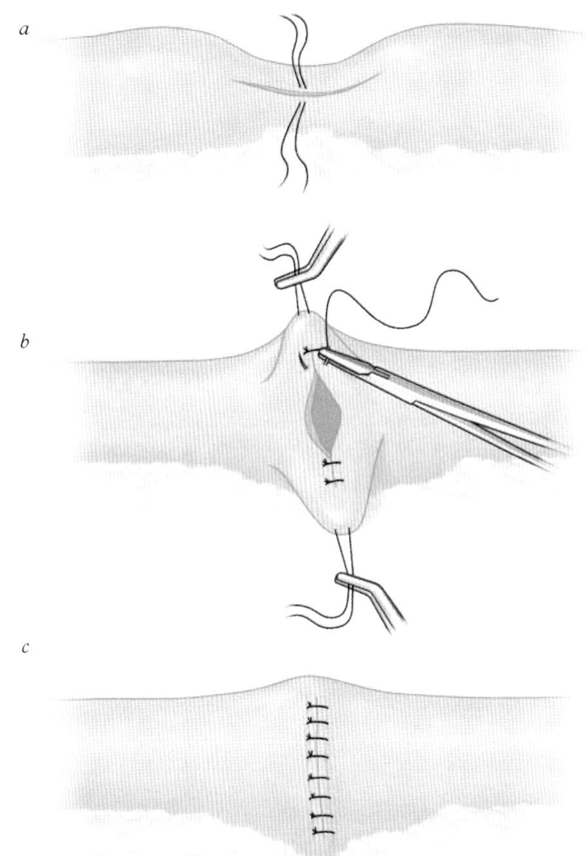

Figure 3 **Heineke-Mikulicz strictureplasty. Stay sutures are placed parallel to each other on the antimesenteric border of the bowel over the area of the stricture. (*a*) The antimesenteric border of the bowel is then opened with the electrocautery over the area of the stricture, and the opening is extended for approximately 1 to 2 cm on either side of the stricture. (*b*, *c*) Traction is placed on the stay sutures, and the original longitudinal enterotomy is closed in a horizontal fashion in one or two layers.**

The short, isolated strictures characteristic of diffuse jejunoileal Crohn disease are more frequently described in patients with long-standing Crohn disease. It has been postulated that over time, Crohn disease progresses from an edematous condition to a more fibrotic, stricturing condition.[28] The fibrotic strictures characteristic of the later stage of the disease are amenable to treatment with strictureplasty. Patients with these short fibrotic strictures typically have obstructive symptoms and often are unable to tolerate solid food, experiencing dramatic weight loss as a result. Although strictureplasty leaves active disease in situ, it usually leads to prompt resolution of obstructive symptoms, regaining of lost body weight, and restoration of normal nutritional status

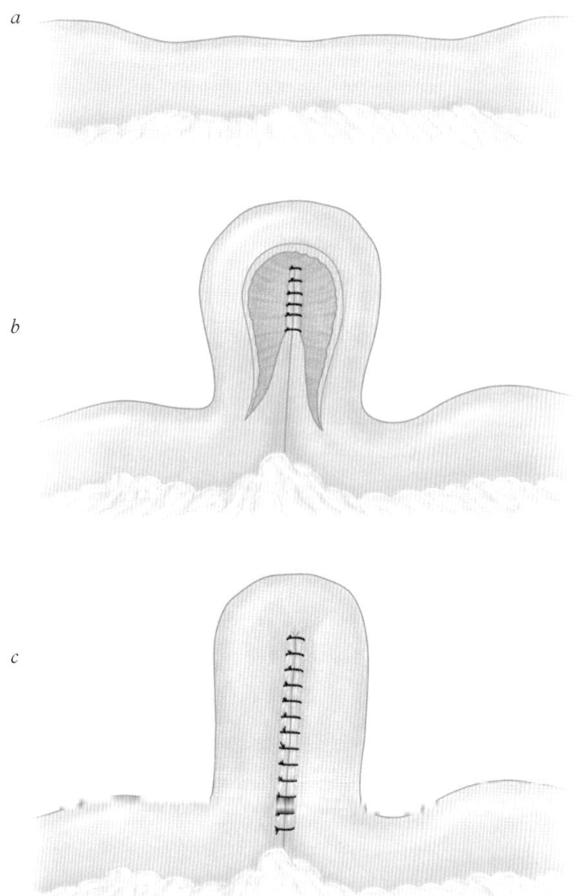

Figure 4 **Finney strictureplasty. (*a*) This procedure is suitable for longer areas of stricture (up to 10 to 15 cm). (*b*) The strictured bowel is bent into the shape of an inverted U. Stay sutures are placed at the apex of the U, which is at the midpoint of the stricture, and at the far ends, which lie 1 to 2 cm proximal and distal to the stricture. A longitudinal enterotomy is made on the antimesenteric border of the bowel with the electrocautery. A side-to-side anastomosis is then performed, with the posterior wall done first. (*c*) Shown is the completed anastomosis.**

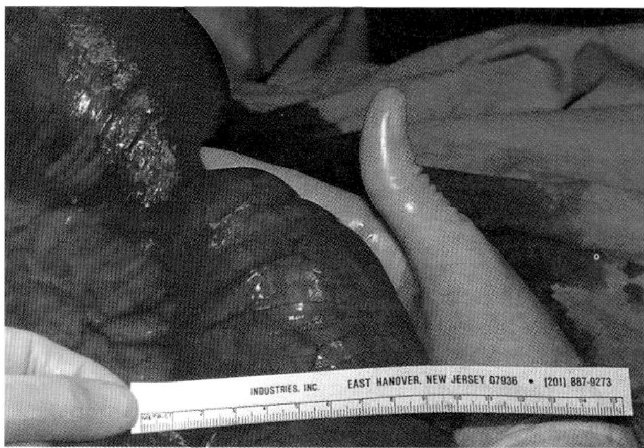

Figure 5 **Shown is a short fibrotic stricture that is ideally suited to treatment with Heineke-Mikulicz strictureplasty.**

A significant concern with strictureplasty is the possibility that small bowel adenocarcinoma may develop; several cases have been reported.[29,30] I have treated a patient in whom a poorly differentiated jejunal adenocarcinoma developed at the site of a strictureplasty that had been performed 10 years earlier. Accordingly, many surgeons advocate routine biopsy of the active ulcer on the mesenteric side of the bowel at the time of strictureplasty [*see Figure 6*]. Another concern has to do with the number of strictureplasties that can safely be performed in a single patient in the course of a single operation. As many as 19 strictureplasties have been performed during one procedure without increased morbidity.[31]

Strictureplasty can be performed with either a single-layer or a double-layer anastomosis. It should not be performed in the presence of an abscess, a phlegmon, or a fistula, and like any other anastomosis, it should not be performed proximal to an existing obstruction that is not treated at the time of operation.

Areas of small bowel Crohn disease that are too long to be treated with strictureplasty can be treated with segmental resection. The area to be resected should be as short as possible. There is no need to obtain frozen-section margins to determine the extent of resection; doing so leads to

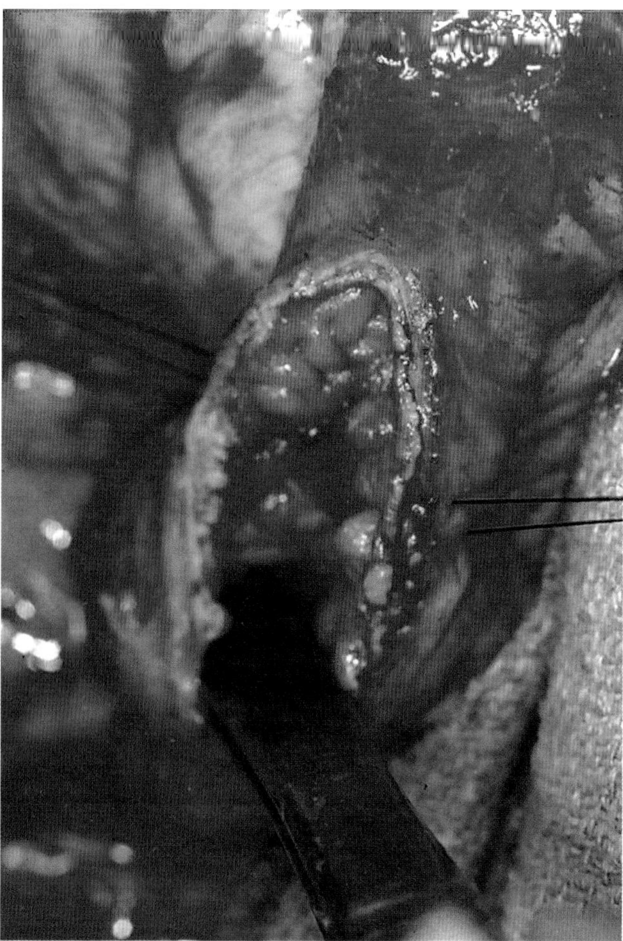

Figure 6 **A large ulcer is nearly always present on the mesenteric luminal border of small bowel strictures.**

unnecessary loss of small bowel length.[32] The resection should extend into palpably normal areas of small bowel. The easiest way of determining the area to be resected is to feel the mesenteric margin of the bowel until palpably normal tissue is reached. Because Crohn disease is generally more severe on the mesenteric side of the bowel, palpation in this area gives the most accurate impression of the intraluminal character of the bowel. Because it is not uncommon for patients to have multifocal Crohn disease, the entire small bowel should always be inspected at the time of operation. Operating on one area of disease while failing to treat a more proximal lesion is clearly not in the patient's interest.

Because of the high rate of recurrence in patients with isolated small bowel disease, postoperative chemoprophylaxis should be strongly considered. In these patients, I prefer to use a more potent agent, such as an antimetabolite, rather than a 5-ASA agent.

ILEOCOLIC DISEASE

Approximately half of those diagnosed with Crohn disease have ileocolic disease. Ileocolic resection is, in fact, the operation most frequently performed to treat Crohn disease. Currently, there is a trend toward more aggressive medical management of Crohn disease; at the same time, surgeons are seeing more complicated disease at the time of operation. These developments have implications for management. In the large Crohn's Therapy, Resource, Evaluation, and Assessment Tool (TREAT) Registry, prednisone therapy was associated with increased mortality with medical treatment, and narcotic use and therapy were both associated with serious infections with medical therapy, in this case most often infliximab.[14] These are both often given for amelioration of symptoms in patients with obstructing ileocolic disease. An easy ileocolic resection is an experience that a patient generally tolerates well and recovers from very quickly; however, delaying operative management with years of aggressive medical therapy can lead to more complicated disease associated with enteroenteric fistulas, which can be difficult to treat. Ileosigmoid fistulas are among the most common fistulas associated with ileocolic Crohn disease, along with fistulas between the terminal ileum and the ascending colon and fistulas between the terminal ileum and adjacent loops of small bowel.

Disease recurrence is common after ileocolic resection. Colonoscopy is the most accurate modality for postoperative surveillance and the easiest to use; it is more sensitive than either small bowel follow-through or air-contrast barium enema. For this reason, I favor an end-to-end anastomosis after ileocolic resection. In the event of recurrent disease, an end-to-side, side-to-end, or side-to-side anastomosis may be difficult to intubate. There is some evidence in the literature to suggest that the postoperative recurrence rate may be lower with a wider anastomosis.[33] The anastomosis can be performed in either one or two layers. If the bowel is thicker, a handsewn anastomosis is preferred to a stapled one.

The incidence of reoperation for recurrent disease after ileocolic resection is high and increases with the number of resections.[34] Postoperative chemoprophylaxis with mesalamine can significantly reduce the recurrence rate.[35] Patients who smoke should be strongly encouraged to stop: the rate and severity of recurrence are increased in smokers.[26]

Special Circumstances

Ileocolic Crohn disease is often associated with intra-abdominal abscesses or fistulas. If an associated abscess is known to be present, CT-guided drainage should be done preoperatively so that a single-stage procedure can then be performed. If an unsuspected abscess is identified at the time of operation, the safest approach is to proceed with bowel resection, perform the posterior wall of the anastomosis, and exteriorize the anastomosis as a loop ileostomy. This loop ileostomy can then be safely closed, often without a formal laparotomy, 8 weeks after operation if there are no signs of ongoing sepsis. If the abscess or the terminal ileal loop is adherent to the sigmoid colon, an ileosigmoid fistula may be present. The decision whether to resect the sigmoid colon is dictated by the appearance and feel of the sigmoid in the involved areas. If only a portion of the anterior colon wall is involved, that portion can be excised in a wedgelike fashion and the excision site closed primarily. If the entire circumference of the sigmoid colon at that point is indurated and woody feeling, a short segmental resection with anastomosis is the best option.

COLONIC DISEASE

Colonic involvement is present in 29 to 44% of patients with Crohn disease.[36] One of the challenges in treating colonic Crohn disease is obtaining the correct diagnosis. Whereas Crohn disease of the small bowel is fairly easy to diagnose, colonic disease often is not. Because granulomas are not present in most cases of colonic Crohn disease and because this condition can look very similar to ulcerative colitis both endoscopically and macroscopically, differentiation between Crohn colitis and ulcerative colitis can be difficult in the absence of small bowel or anal disease. Colonic Crohn disease appears to be more frequently associated with cutaneous manifestations (e.g., pyoderma gangrenosum) [*see Figure 7*].

Indications for Surgical Treatment

The main indications for operative management of colonic Crohn disease are stricture [*see Figure 8*], malignancy, side effects of medical therapy, and failure of medical therapy. In children, failure to recognize and treat this condition promptly may result in growth retardation. It is important to monitor both bone age and insulinlike growth factor–1 levels. If these are abnormal, timely institution of human growth hormone therapy, operative management of inflammatory bowel disease, or both may still permit normal growth and development.

Side effects of medical therapy can be substantial. They may include such varied complications as aseptic necrosis of the femoral head and cataract formation (both related to steroid use), as well as an increased incidence of opportunistic infections (from immunosuppression secondary to antimetabolite or biologic therapy).[37]

Failure of medical therapy can refer to continuing severe disease activity or, at worst, to so-called toxic megacolon. The term *toxic megacolon* is actually a misnomer in that not all patients with this condition actually have a true megacolon [*see Figure 9a*]. In common usage, the term *toxic megacolon* refers to any condition associated with colitis that is severe enough to result in sloughing of the colonic mucosa; such

a

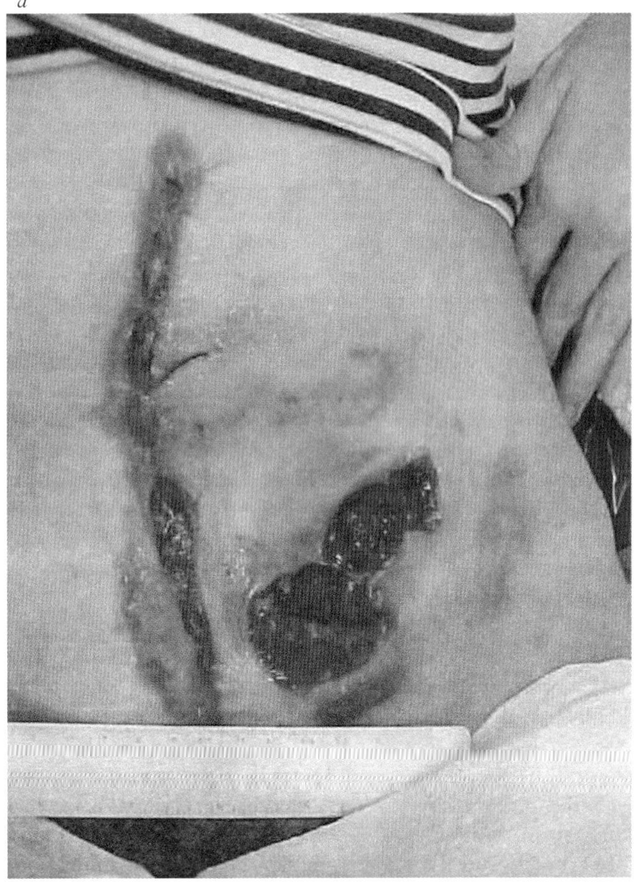

b

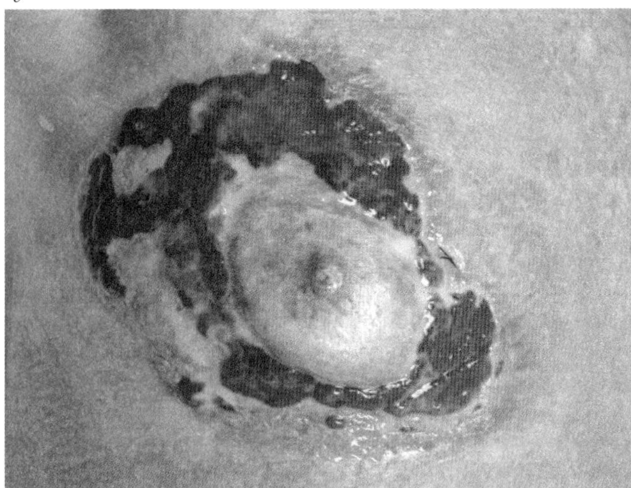

Figure 7 **(*a*) Shown is pyoderma gangrenosum affecting the peristomal and incisional area 6 months after creation of a loop ileostomy in a 16-year-old girl who had undergone colectomy with ileal pouch-anal anastomosis for a presumed initial diagnosis of ulcerative colitis. (*b*) Shown is peristomal gangrenosum of the breast in an otherwise asymptomatic patient with Crohn colitis and perianal Crohn disease who had a diverting loop ileostomy.**

sloughing permits endotoxins to enter the circulatory system and evoke a septic response. The signs and symptoms of toxic megacolon include those characteristic of sepsis-leukocytosis, fever, tachycardia, and hypoalbuminemia. These patients are very ill and often manifest ileus, which is an ominous development that frequently signals impending perforation. Emergency surgical intervention is required. At operation, the colon is often distended, and when the specimen is opened, the colon may appear almost autolytic [*see Figure 9b*]. In this state, the bowel frequently does not hold staples well; accordingly, it is often helpful to sew the distal Hartmann stump between the left and right halves of the anterior inferior rectus fascia at the lower abdominal incision and then to close the skin over it.[38] Thus, if the staple line is disrupted, the result is essentially a surgical site infection that can be opened and drained rather than the pelvic abscess [*see Figure 9c*] that could develop if the rectal stump were located deep within the pelvis.

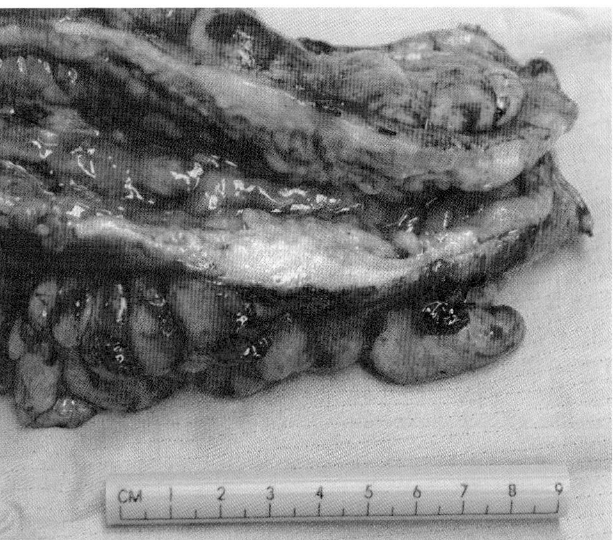

Figure 8 **Shown is a sigmoid colon stricture secondary to Crohn disease that caused obstructing symptoms refractory to medical therapy.**

Types of Disease

Segmental disease In a 2003 review of 92 consecutive cases of patients with Crohn colitis, the number of patients with segmental colonic Crohn disease and the number of those with pancolonic disease were nearly equal.[36] Approximately 63% of those with segmental colitis had other disease involvement as well (e.g., jejunoileal, ileocolic, or perianal), compared with only 12% of those with pancolitis. The recurrence rate, however, was higher in patients with segmental colitis than in those with pancolitis. In addition, the risk of recurrence was higher in patients who had granulomatous disease than in those who did not.

Pancolonic disease In cases of pancolonic Crohn disease with associated perianal, jejunoileal, or ileocolic

a

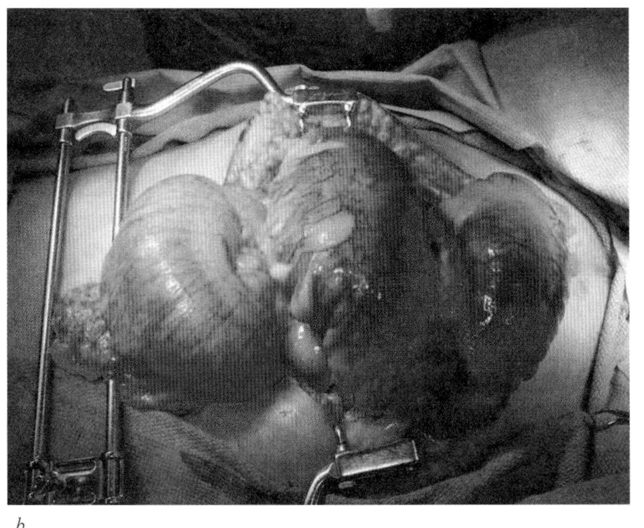

b

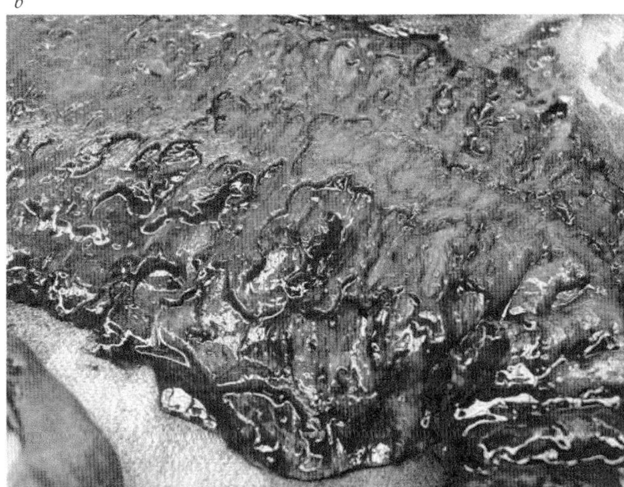

c

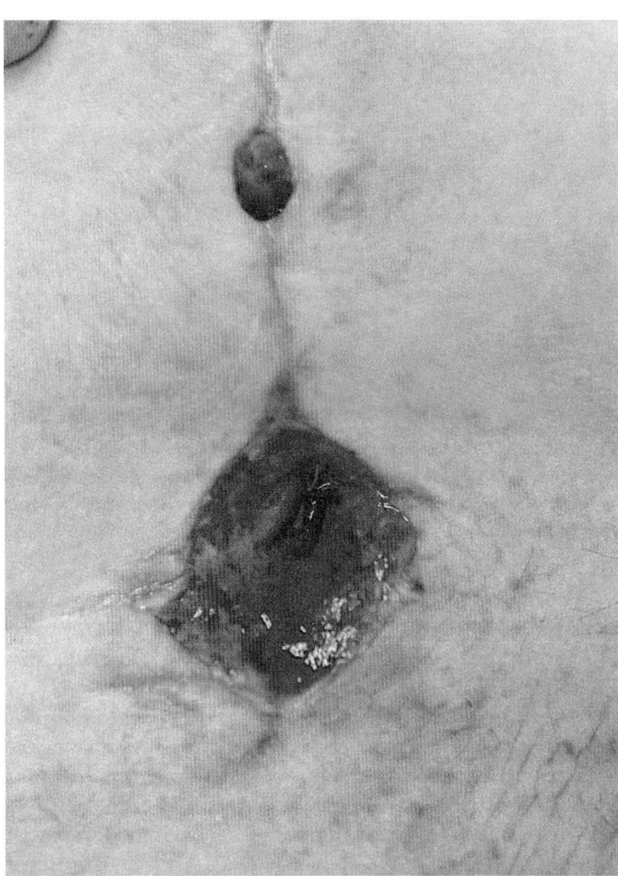

Figure 9 **(*a*) Shown is toxic megacolon in a 17-year-old girl with Crohn colitis. The colon is massively distended and near perforation at the time of operation. (*b*) When the specimen is opened, it is apparent that large segments of the mucosa have sloughed off, leaving denuded muscle wall. (*c*) The distal rectosigmoid is incorporated between the left and right halves of the anterior inferior rectus fascia at the lower abdominal incision and placed underneath the skin, which is then closed over it. Thus, in the event of disruption of the distal stump, the contents drain harmlessly through the wound rather than resulting in a pelvic abscess.**

involvement, diagnosis is not difficult. However, most patients with Crohn pancolitis do not have other sites of disease involvement, nor do they have granulomas.[36] Consequently, differentiation of Crohn pancolitis from ulcerative colitis can be very difficult. Many patients with Crohn disease have been subjected to colectomy with ileal pouch-anal anastomosis (IPAA) because they were initially presumed to have ulcerative colitis.

Operative Procedures

Total proctocolectomy with end ileostomy The traditional procedure for colonic Crohn disease is total proctocolectomy with end ileostomy, which is associated with an 8 to 15% rate of recurrence in the small bowel proximal to the stoma.[39–41] This operation remains the best choice in patients with severe rectal and anal Crohn disease (e.g., those with so-called watering-can perineum [*see Figure 10a*]) and carries the lowest risk of disease recurrence. In contrast to the approach taken in patients with rectal cancer, which involves excising the external anal sphincter and a large portion of the levator muscles, the approach taken in those with colonic Crohn disease is intersphincteric, with dissection performed in the plane between the internal and external anal sphincters to reduce the size of the perineal wound and facilitate healing [*see Figure 10b*]. Even with the intersphincteric approach, delayed healing of the perineal wound is common, occurring in as many as 30% of patients.

Subtotal colectomy with ileorectal or ileosigmoid anastomosis Because many patients with Crohn disease are young, surgeons have long been interested in operations that do not involve an ileostomy. In the absence of significant

a

b

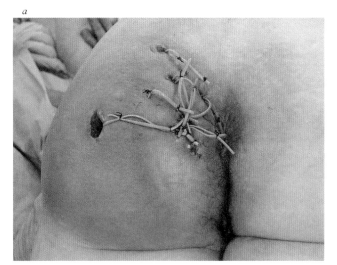

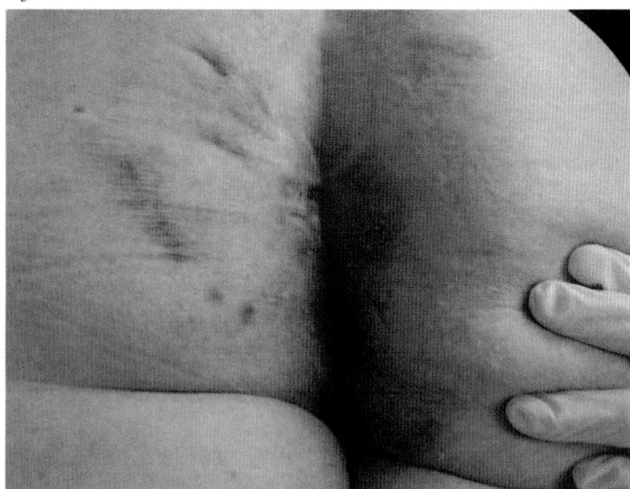

Figure 10 **(*a*) Vessel loops can be used as setons for drainage of abscesses caused by perianal Crohn disease. They can be left in as long as necessary and help prevent recurrent abscess formation. (*b*) Same patient 6 months following total proctocolectomy.**

rectal and anal disease, subtotal colectomy with ileorectal or ileosigmoid anastomosis is an option. Unfortunately, this operation is associated with high recurrence rates (up to 70%)[41]; however, with the advent of more effective immunosuppressive and biologic therapy, it is hoped that these rates can be reduced. As much palpably normal distal rectum and colon as possible should be spared. The anastomosis can be stapled, although if the bowel wall is thickened, many surgeons would feel more secure with a handsewn anastomosis in either one or two layers.

Segmental resection Currently, more surgeons are advocating colon-sparing procedures for Crohn disease. Although this is a relatively new approach, there have already been some reports documenting the safety of segmental resection in cases of limited disease.[43] In patients with colonic strictures resulting in obstruction, segmental resection into palpably normal areas of the bowel yields prompt resolution of symptoms. Because the colon performs an important water-absorbing function, many patients with a limited amount of small bowel can still live without intravenous supplementation if a significant segment of the colon is left in situ. However, patients with segmental Crohn disease appear to have a higher recurrence rate than those with pancolitis, as do patients with granulomas.[36] Surgical treatment of Crohn disease continues to undergo reevaluation and reassessment of results on the basis of the availability of newer medical therapies.

Colectomy with IPAA Although colectomy with IPAA is usually not an operation that one would knowingly perform in a patient with Crohn disease, every year many such patients undergo this procedure as treatment of colonic inflammatory bowel disease that initially is incorrectly presumed to be ulcerative colitis but later is diagnosed as Crohn disease (on the basis of either final pathologic analysis of the resected specimen or the disease's clinical behavior). Generally speaking, in the absence of fistulizing disease, most of these patients are able to maintain their pouch, but they require medical therapy for disease control.[36,44–47] Some surgeons, after very careful patient counseling regarding the real risks of fistulizing disease and other adverse sequelae, will consider IPAA for select patients with Crohn colitis with no evidence of other sites of involvement.[48]

ANAL DISEASE

Types of Disease

With stenosis For patients with anal strictures that are not regularly dilated, the outlook is poor. Such strictures pose functional obstructions and typically lead to continuing problems with fistulas and suppurative disease. They frequently become more and more fibrotic over time and often extend proximally. Most of these patients eventually require fecal diversion. Management generally involves self-dilation, which can often be done with Hegar dilators. If the stenosis is not dealt with, all other treatment of the Crohn disease is doomed to failure; obstruction at the level of the anal canal inevitably results in the persistence of anorectal disease.

Without stenosis Anal Crohn disease without stenosis is much easier to treat medically. Long-term oral metronidazole therapy is often helpful; other medications (e.g., anti–tumor necrosis factor antibody) may be useful as well. Broad fissures are usually asymptomatic. Surgical treatment should be avoided unless the lesions are causing symptoms. Because they tend to have more liquidy bowel movements, patients with Crohn disease need an optimally functioning anal sphincter; hence, fistulotomies, which divide portions of the sphincter, should be avoided if at all possible. Placement of setons through fistula tracts can often prevent abscess formation, provide drainage, and thereby prevent perianal pain while minimizing sphincter trauma. Silk sutures, vessel loops, or Penrose drains also can be used as setons [*see*

Figure 10]. Although some have reported good results with a collagen fistula plug for Crohn disease,[49] others, including the author, have not had similarly favorable experiences.[50,51] Rectovaginal fistulas pose a particular challenge. In the presence of active Crohn disease, advancement flap repair of such fistulas has a low success rate.[52] Laparoscopically assisted loop ileostomy improves the success rate, but, unfortunately, the fistulas may recur when intestinal continuity is reestablished.

CHEMOPROPHYLAXIS

In 1995, a prospective, randomized study showed that patients who underwent ileocolic resection and were given mesalamine postoperatively had a significant reduction in both the symptomatic and the endoscopic rate of recurrence.[35] Not all of the work done since then has confirmed these results, but several studies and a meta-analysis have indicated that mesalamine does reduce the postoperative recurrence rate of Crohn disease.[53] Many patients undergoing surgical treatment of Crohn disease are advised to take some type of postoperative preventive medical therapy, either a 5-ASA derivative (e.g., mesalamine) or a stronger immunosuppressive agent (e.g., 6-mercaptopurine or azathioprine). Better studies are required to document the efficacy of the latter agents in preventing recurrence. It is hoped that chemoprophylaxis will reduce the anticipated recurrence rates by 30 to 40%.

SURVEILLANCE

At present, there are no clear guidelines for surveillance after operative treatment of Crohn disease. In my opinion, however, given the increased risk of colorectal cancer in this setting, patients with Crohn disease who retain some colon should undergo colonoscopy every 2 years, not only to detect any development of colonic neoplasia but also to identify any recurrence of disease in a timely manner. If recurrent Crohn disease is detected, appropriate medical therapy should be promptly instituted, with the aim of avoiding subsequent operation if possible.

BEHAVIORAL MODIFICATION

Exposure to cigarette smoke is known to exacerbate the symptoms of Crohn disease. Smoking has been reported to affect the overall severity of the disease, with smokers having a 34% higher recurrence rate and a higher rate of reoperation than nonsmokers.[54–56] A 1999 study of 141 Crohn disease patients who had undergone ileocolic resection, of whom 79 were nonsmokers and the remainder were smokers, found that the respective 5- and 10-year recurrence-free rates were 65% and 45% in smokers and 81% and 64% in nonsmokers. The recurrence rates were higher in heavy smokers ($\geq$15 cigarettes/day) than in moderate smokers.[57]

Dr. Galandiuk is principal investigator of the University of Louisville site clinical trial registry study on HUMIRA®, which is sponsored by Abbott Pharmaceutical, Inc.

References

1. Farmer RG, Hawk WA, Turnbull RB Jr. Clinical patterns in Crohn's disease: a statistical study of 615 cases. Gastroenterology 1975;68:627
2. Gasche C, Scholmerich J, Brynskov J, et al. A simple classification of Crohn's disease: report of the Working Party for the World Congresses of Gastroenterology, Vienna 1998. Inflamm Bowel Dis 2000;6:8
3. Michelassi F, Balestracci T, Chappell R, et al. Primary and recurrent Crohn's disease: experience with 1379 patients. Ann Surg 1991; 214:230.
4. Bodger K. Cost of illness of Crohn's disease. Pharmacoeconomics 2002;20:639
5. Feagan BG, Vreeland MG, Larson LR, et al. Annual cost of care for Crohn's disease: a payor perspective. Am J Gastroenterol 2000; 95:1955.
6. Colombel JF, Loftus EV Jr, Tremaine WJ, et al. The safety profile of infliximab in patients with Crohn's disease: the Mayo Clinic experience in 500 patients. Gastroenterology 2004; 126:19.
7. Ljung T, Karlen P, Schmidt D, et al. Infliximab in inflammatory bowel disease: clinical outcome in a population based cohort from Stockholm County. Gut 2004;53:849.
8. Appau KA, Fazio VW, Shen B, et al. Use of infliximab within 3 months of ileocolonic resection is associated with adverse postoperative outcomes in Crohn's patients. J Gastrointest Surg 2008;12:1738–44.
9. Mor IJ, Vogel JD, da Luz Moreira A, et al. Infliximab in ulcerative colitis is associated with an increased risk of postoperative complications after restorative proctolectomy. Dis Colon Rectum 2008;51:1202–7.
10. Selvasekar CR, Cima RR, Larson DW, et al. Effect of infliximab on short-term complications in patients undergoing operation for chronic ulcerative colitis. J Am Coll Surg 2007;204:956–63.
11. Crohn BB, Ginzburg L, Oppenheimer GO. Landmark article Oct 15, 1932. Regional ileitis: a pathological and clinical entity. JAMA 1984;251:73.
12. Fazio VW, Marchetti F, Church M, et al. Effect of resection margins on the recurrence of Crohn's disease in the small bowel: a randomized controlled trial. Ann Surg 1996; 224:563.
13. Galandiuk S, O'Neill M, McDonald P, et al. A century of home parenteral nutrition for Crohn's disease. Am J Surg 1990;159:540.
14. Lichtenstein GR, Feagan BG, Cohen RD, et al. Serious infections and mortality in association with therapies for Crohn's disease: TREAT therapy. Clin Gastroenterol Hepatol 2006;4:621–30.
15. Greenstein AJ. Cancer in inflammatory bowel disease. Mt Sinai J Med 2000;67:227.
16. Rhodes JM, Campbell BJ. Inflammation and colorectal cancer: IBD-associated and sporadic cancer compared. Trends Mol Med 2002;8:10.
17. Gillen CD, Walmsley RS, Prior P, et al. Ulcerative colitis and Crohn's disease: a comparison of the colorectal cancer risk in extensive colitis. Gut 1994;35:1590.
18. Itzkowitz SH, Present DH, for the Crohn's and Colitis Foundation of American Colon Cancer in IBD Study Group. Consensus Conference: colorectal cancer screening and surveillance in inflammatory bowel disease. Inflamm Bowel Dis 2005;11:314–21.
19. Mahadevan U, Kane S. American Gastroenterological Association Institute technical review on the use of gastrointestinal medications in pregnancy. Gastroenterology 2006; 131:283–311.
20. Milsom JW, Hammerhofer KA, Bohm B, et al. Prospective, randomized trial comparing laparoscopic vs. conventional surgery for refractory ileocolic Crohn's disease. Dis Colon Rectum 2001;44:1.
21. Young-Fadok TM, Hall Long K, McConnell EJ, et al. Advantages of laparoscopic resection for ileocolic Crohn's disease: improved outcomes and reduced costs. Surg Endosc 2001; 15:450.
22. Moorthy K, Shaul T, Foley RJ. Factors that predict conversion in patients undergoing laparoscopic surgery for Crohn's disease. Am J Surg 2004;187:47.
23. Murray JJ, Schoetz DJ Jr, Nugent FW, et al. Surgical management of Crohn's disease involving the duodenum. Am J Surg 1984; 147:58.
24. Ross TM, Fazio VW, Farmer RG. Long-term results of surgical treatment for Crohn's disease of the duodenum. Ann Surg 1983; 197:399.
25. Worsey MJ, Hull T, Ryland L, et al. Strictureplasty is an effective option in the operative management of duodenal Crohn's disease. Dis Colon Rectum 1999;42:596.
26. Yamamoto T, Bain IM, Connolly AB, et al. Outcome of strictureplasty for duodenal Crohn's disease. Br J Surg 1999;86:259.
27. Michelassi F, Hurst RD, Melis M, et al. Side-to-side isoperistaltic strictureplasty in extensive Crohn's disease: a prospective longitudinal study. Ann Surg 2000;232:401.
28. Marshak RH, Wolf BS. Chronic ulcerative granulomatous jejunitis and ileojejunitis. AJR Am J Roentgenol 1953;70:93.
29. Jaskowiak NT, Michelassi F. Adenocarcinoma at a strictureplasty site in Crohn's disease: report of a case. Dis Colon Rectum 2001;44: 284.

30. Marchetti F, Fazio VW, Ozuner G. Adenocarcinoma arising from a strictureplasty site in Crohn's disease: report of a case. Dis Colon Rectum 1996;39:1315.
31. Dietz OW, Laureti S, Strong SA, et al. Safety and long-term efficacy of strictureplasty in 314 patients with obstructing small bowel Crohn's disease. J Am Coll Surg 2001; 192:330.
32. Hamilton SR, Reese J, Pennington L, et al. The role of resection margin frozen section in the surgical management of Crohn's disease. Surg Gynecol Obstet 1985;160:57.
33. Munoz-Juarez M, Yamamoto T, Wolff BG, et al. Wide-lumen stapled anastomosis vs. conventional end-to-end anastomosis in the treatment of Crohn's disease. Dis Colon Rectum 2001;44:20.
34. Greenstein AJ, Sachar DB, Pasternack BS, et al. Reoperation and recurrence in Crohn's colitis and ileocolitis: crude and cumulative rates. N Engl J Med 1975;293:685.
35. McLeod RS, Wolff BG, Steinhart AH, et al. Prophylactic mesalamine treatment decreases postoperative recurrence of Crohn's disease. Gastroenterology 1995;109:404.
36. Morpurgo E, Petras R, Kimberling J, et al. Characterization and clinical behavior of Crohn's disease initially presenting predominantly as colitis. Dis Colon Rectum 2003;46: 918.
37. Davis B, Galandiuk S. Invasive histoplasmosis activated by maintenance imfliximab initially mimicking an invasive squamous cell carcinoma then invasive nectrotizing infection: case report. Nat Clin Pract Gastro- [illegible]
38. Hull T, Fazio VW. Surgery for toxic megacolon. In: Nyhus LM, Baker RJ, Frischer JE, editors. Mastery of surgery. 3rd ed. Boston: Little Brown & Co; 1996. p. 1437.
39. Goligher JC. The outcome of excisional operations for primary and recurrent Crohn's disease of the large intestine. Surg Gynecol Obstet 1979;148:1.
40. Ritchie JK, Lockhart-Mummery HE. Non-restorative surgery in the treatment of Crohn's disease of the large bowel. Gut 1973;14:263.
41. Goligher JC. The long-term results of excisional surgery for primary and recurrent Crohn's disease of the large intestine. Dis Colon Rectum 1985;28:51.
42. Goligher JC. Surgical treatment of Crohn's disease affecting mainly or entirely the large bowel. World J Surg 1988;12:186.
43. Allan A, Andrews H, Hilton CJ, et al. Segmental colonic resection is an appropriate operation for short skip lesions due to Crohn's disease in the colon. World J Surg 1989;13: 611.
44. Hyman NH, Fazio VW, Tuckson WB, et al. Consequences of ileal pouch-anal anastomosis for Crohn's colitis. Dis Colon Rectum 1991; 34:653.
45. Galandiuk S, Scott NA, Dozois RR, et al. Ileal pouch-anal anastomosis. Reoperation for pouch related complications. Ann Surg 1990;212:446.
46. Panis Y, Poupard B, Nemeth J, et al. Ileal pouch/anal anastomosis for Crohn's disease. Lancet 1996;347:854.
47. Ricart E, Panaccione R, Loftus EV, et al. Successful management of Crohn's disease of the ileoanal pouch with infliximab. Gastroen- [illegible]
48. Joyce MR, Fazio VW. Can ileal pouch anal anastomosis be used in Crohn's disease? Adv Surg 2009;43:111–37.
49. O'Connor L, Champagne BJ, Ferguson MA, et al. Efficacy of anal fistula plug in closure of Crohn's anorectal fistulas. Dis Colon Rectum 2006;49:1569–73.
50. Ky AJ, Sylla P, Steinhagen R, et al. Collagen fistula plug for the treatment of anal fistulas. Dis Colon Rectum 2008;51:838–43.
51. Christoforidis D, Pieh MC, Madoff RD, Mellgren AF. Treatment of trassphincteric anal fistulas by endorectal advancement flap or collagen fistula plug: a comparative stuy. Dis Colon Rectum 2009;52:18–22.
52. Sonoda T, Hull T, Piedmonte MR, et al. Outcomes of primary repair of anorectal and rectovaginal fistulas using the endorectal advancement flap. Dis Colon Rectum 2002; 45:1622.
53. Achkar JP, Hanauer SB. Medical therapy to reduce postoperative Crohn's disease recurrence. Am J Gastroenterol 2000;95:1139.
54. Duffy LC, Zielezny MA, Marshall JR, et al. Cigarette smoking and risk of clinical relapse in patients with Crohn's disease. Am J Prev Med 1990;6:161.
55. Sutherland LR, Ramcharan S, Bryant H, et al. Effect of cigarette smoking on recurrence of Crohn's disease. Gastroenterology 1990;98:1123.
56. Cottone M, Rosselli M, Orlando A, et al. Smoking habits and recurrence in Crohn's disease. Gastroenterology 1994;106:643.
57. Yamamoto T, Keighley MR. The association of cigarette smoking with a high risk of recurrence after ileocolonic resection for ileocecal [illegible]

11 DIVERTICULITIS

John P. Welch, MD, FACS, Jeffrey L. Cohen, MD, FACS, FASCRS, and Rafal Barczak, MD

Diverticula are small (0.5 to 1.0 cm in diameter) outpouchings of the colon that occur in rows at sites of vascular penetration between the single mesenteric taenia and one of the antimesenteric taeniae. At the sites of most diverticula, the muscular layer is absent [*see Figure 1*]. Technically, such lesions are really pseudodiverticula; true diverticula (which are much less common than pseudodiverticula) involve all layers of the bowel wall. Nevertheless, both pseudodiverticula and true diverticula are generally referred to as diverticula.

The sigmoid colon is the most common site of diverticula: in 90% of patients with diverticulosis, the sigmoid colon is involved.[1] If a diverticulum becomes inflamed as a result of obstruction by feces or hardened mucus or of mucosal erosion, a localized perforation (microperforation) may occur—a process known as diverticulitis. The incidence of diverticulitis has been estimated to be about 10 to 25% in patients with colonic diverticula.[1] Limited prospective data suggest that the risk of developing diverticulitis is low in patients with symptomatic diverticulosis.[2] Both diverticulosis and variants of diverticulitis may be subsumed under the more encompassing term *diverticular disease*.

The incidence of diverticular disease increases with age. Diverticula are quite common in elderly patients, being present in more than 80% of patients older than 85 years. Consequently, as the population of the United States continues to age, the overall risk of diverticular complications continues to increase. Before the 20th century, diverticular disease was rare in the United States. By 1996, however, 131,000 patients were being admitted to hospitals with diverticulitis each year.[3]

A diet containing refined carbohydrates and low-fiber substances, such as is currently widespread in many developed countries (especially in the West), has been associated with the emergence of this disease entity. A low-residue diet facilitates the development of constipation, which can lead to increased intraluminal pressure in the large bowel. In addition, elevated elastin levels are commonly noted at colon wall sites containing diverticula,[4] and this change causes shortening of the taeniae.[1] High-pressure zones or areas of segmentation may develop [*see Figure 2*], usually in the sigmoid colon, and diverticula begin to protrude at these locations.[5] If microperforation of a thin-walled diverticulum takes place, local or, uncommonly, widespread contamination with fecal organisms may ensue. The pericolic tissue (typically, the mesentery and the pericolic fat) thus becomes inflamed, whereas the mucosa tends to remain otherwise normal.

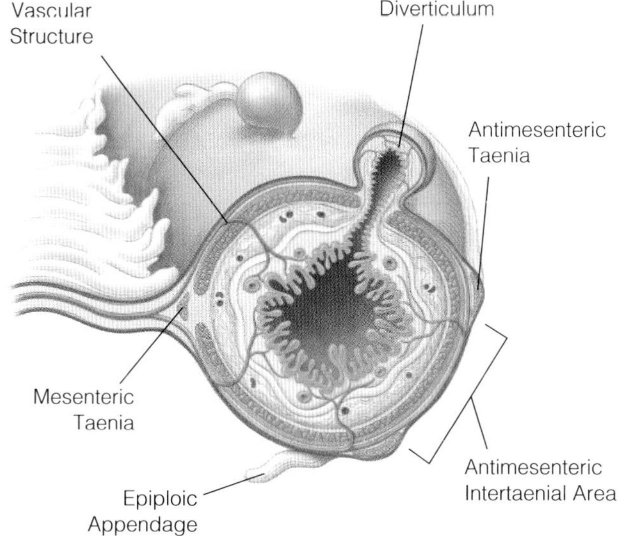

Figure 1 **Illustrated are anatomic findings in a segment of colon containing diverticula. Diverticula are located at sites where blood vessels enter the colonic wall.[87]**

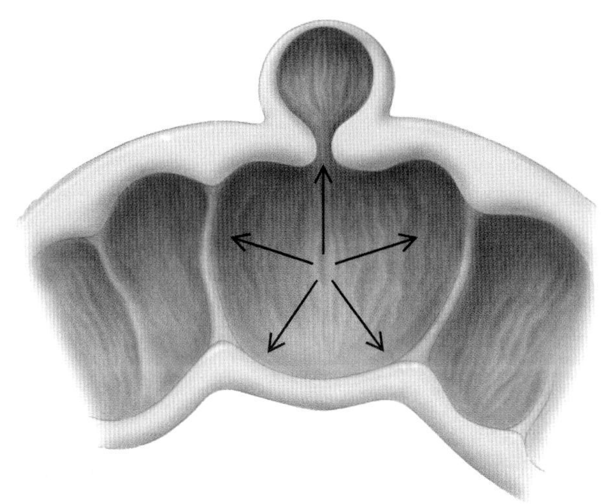

Figure 2 **Depicted is a schematic representation of the process termed segmentation in the colon. It has been theorized that high-pressure compartments lead to the development of diverticula.[88]**

Several factors appear to promote the development of diverticular disease and its complications, including decreased physical activity,[6] obesity,[7] intake of nonsteroidal antiinflammatory drugs (NSAIDs),[8] smoking,[9] and constipation from any cause (e.g., diet or medications). The well-known Western afflictions cholelithiasis, diverticulosis, and hiatal hernia frequently occur together (the Saint triad). Obesity has been associated with the intake of low-fiber diets,[10] and growing numbers of young, obese patients with diverticulitis are being seen by physicians. Consumption of nuts, corn, or popcorn does not increase the incidence of diverticulitis or diverticular bleeding.[11]

Clinical Evaluation

HISTORY

Uncomplicated (Simple) Diverticulitis

The classic symptoms of uncomplicated acute diverticulitis are left lower quadrant abdominal pain, a low-grade fever, irregular bowel habits, and, possibly, urinary symptoms if the affected colon is adjacent to the bladder. If the sigmoid colon is highly redundant, pain may be greatest in the right lower quadrant. Diarrhea or constipation may occur, together with rectal urgency.

The differential diagnosis includes gynecologic and urinary disorders, perforated colon carcinoma, Crohn disease, ischemic colitis, and, sometimes, appendicitis. Chronic diarrhea, multiple areas of colon involvement, perianal disease, perineal or cutaneous fistulas, or extraintestinal signs are suggestive of Crohn disease. Rectal bleeding should raise the possibility of inflammatory bowel disease, ischemia, or carcinoma; such bleeding is uncommon with diverticulitis alone. Given the prevalence of diverticula, it is not surprising that colon carcinoma may coexist with diverticular disease [*see Figure 3*].

Complicated Diverticulitis

Some cases of diverticulitis are classified as complicated, meaning that the disease process has progressed to obstruction, abscess or fistula formation, or free perforation [*see Figure 4*]. Complicated diverticulitis may be particularly challenging to manage,[12] especially because patients may have no known history of diverticular disease. Lower gastrointestinal (GI) bleeding is also a complication of diverticular disease in 30 to 50% of cases; in fact, diverticula are the most common colonic cause of lower GI bleeding. When diverticular hemorrhage occurs [*see 6:5 Gastrointestinal Bleeding*], it is usually associated with diverticulosis rather than with diverticulitis. Approximately 50% of diverticular bleeding originates in the right colon, despite the low incidence of diverticula in this

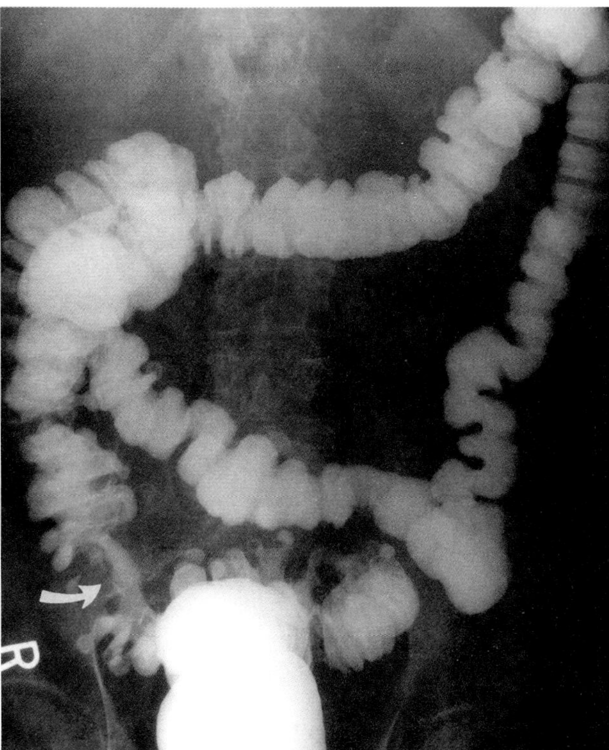

Figure 3 **Barium enema shows a napkin-ring carcinoma (*arrow*) in the middle of multiple diverticula in a redundant sigmoid colon.**

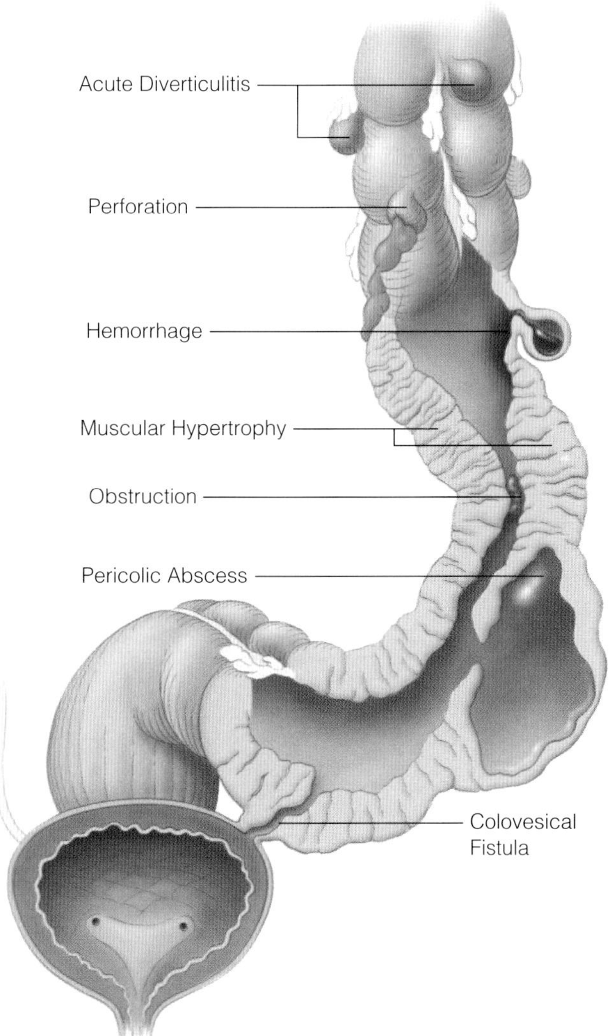

Figure 4 **Shown are major complications of diverticular disease of the sigmoid colon.[89]**

segment of the colon. Patients tend to be elderly and to have cardiovascular disease and hypertension. Regular intake of NSAIDs may increase the risk of this complication. Although patients may lose 1 to 2 units of blood, the bleeding usually ceases spontaneously,[13] and expeditious operative treatment generally is not necessary.

The most common form of complicated diverticulitis involves the development of a pericolic abscess, typically signaled by high fever, chills, and lassitude. Such abscesses may be small and localized or may extend to more distant sites (e.g., the pelvis). They may be categorized according to the Hinchey classification of diverticular perforations,[14] in which stage I refers to a localized pericolic abscess and stage II to a larger mesenteric abscess spreading toward the pelvis [*see Figure 5*]. On rare occasions, an abscess forms in the retroperitoneal tissues, subsequently extending to distant sites such as the thigh or the flank. The location of the abscess can be defined precisely by means of computed tomography (CT) with contrast.

Some abscesses rupture into adjacent tissues or viscera, resulting in the formation of fistulas. The fistulas most commonly seen in this setting (50 to 65% of cases) are colovesical fistulas. This complication is less common in women because of the protection afforded by the uterus. Symptoms of colovesical fistulas tend to involve the urinary tract (e.g., pneumaturia, hematuria, and urinary frequency). Fecaluria is diagnostic of colovesical or enterovesical fistulas. Colovaginal fistulas (which account for 25% of all diverticular fistulas) are usually seen in women who have undergone hysterectomies. The diseased colon is adherent to the vaginal cuff. Most commonly, patients complain of a foul vaginal discharge; however, some patients present with stool emanating from the vagina.

About 10% of colon obstructions are attributable to diverticulitis. Acute diverticulitis can cause colonic edema and a functional obstruction that usually resolves with antibiotic infusion and bowel rest. Stricture formation is more common, usually occurring as a consequence of recurrent attacks of diverticulitis. Circumferential pericolic fibrosis is noted, and marked angulation of the pelvic colon with adherence to the pelvic sidewall may be seen. Patients complain of constipation and narrowed stools. Colonoscopy can be difficult and potentially dangerous in this setting. Differentiating a diverticular stricture from carcinoma may be impossible by any means short of resection.

The term *malignant diverticulitis* has been employed to describe an extreme form of sigmoid diverticulitis that is characterized by an extensive phlegmon and inflammatory

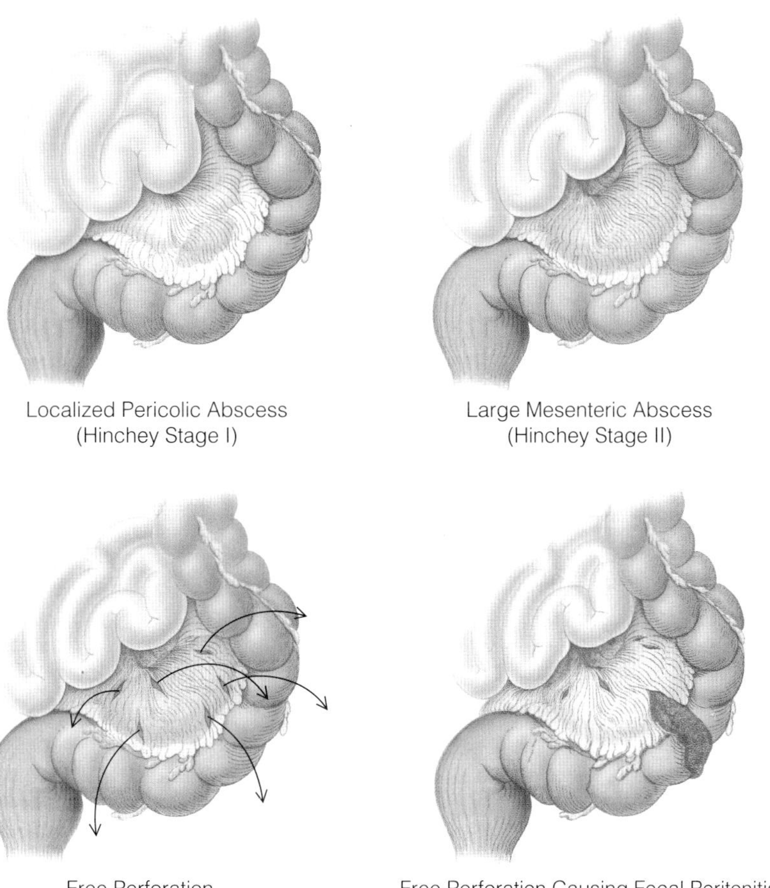

Figure 5 **The Hinchey classification divides diverticular perforations into four stages. Mortality increases significantly in stages III and IV.**[18]

reaction extending below the peritoneal reflection, with a tendency toward obstruction and fistula formation.[15] Malignant diverticulitis is seen in fewer than 5% of patients older than 50 years who are operated on for diverticulitis.[15] The process is reminiscent of Crohn disease, and CT scans demonstrate extensive inflammation. In this setting, a staged resection might be preferable to attempting a primary resection through the pelvic phlegmon. The degree of pelvic inflammation may subside significantly after diversion.[15]

A dangerous but rare complication of acute diverticulitis (occurring in 1 to 2% of cases) is free perforation,[16] which includes both perforation of a diverticular abscess throughout the abdomen leading to generalized peritonitis (purulent peritonitis; Hinchey stage III) and free spillage of stool thorough an open diverticulum into the peritoneal cavity (fecal peritonitis; Hinchey stage IV). The incidence of free perforations may be increasing, at least in the southwestern United States.[17] The overall mortality in this group is between 20 and 30%, that for purulent peritonitis is approximately 13%, and that for fecal peritonitis is about 43%.[16]

PHYSICAL EXAMINATION

Uncomplicated Diverticulitis

Physical examination reveals localized left lower quadrant abdominal tenderness with variable degrees of guarding and rebound tenderness. A mass is occasionally felt. The stool may contain traces of blood, but gross bleeding is unusual. Localized inflammation of the perforated diverticulum and the adjacent mesentery is present, and a phlegmon may be seen as well. Depending on the severity of the physical findings, patients may be managed either as inpatients or outpatients.

Complicated Diverticulitis

In a patient with a pericolic abscess, a mass may be detectable on abdominal, rectal, or pelvic examination. In a patient with a colovaginal fistula, a site of granulation tissue and drainage is seen at the apex of the vaginal cuff. In a patient with obstruction, there may be marked abdominal distention, usually of slow onset; abdominal tenderness may or may not be present, but if tears develop in the cecal taeniae, right lower quadrant tenderness is typically seen. In a patient with a free perforation, there is marked abdominal tenderness, usually commencing suddenly in the left lower quadrant and spreading within hours to the remainder of the abdomen. Hypotension and oliguria may develop later. Patients with rectal bleeding usually have no complaints of abdominal pain or tenderness, and they may be hypovolemic and hypotensive, depending on the rapidity of the bleeding.

Investigative Studies

IMAGING

The most useful diagnostic imaging study in the setting of suspected diverticulitis is a CT scan with oral and rectal contrast.[18] Localized thickening of the bowel wall or inflammation of the adjacent pericolic fat is suggestive of diverticulitis; extraluminal air or fluid collections are sometimes seen together with diverticula [*see Figure 6*]. The most frequent findings (seen in 70 to 100% of cases) are bowel wall thickening, fat stranding, and diverticula.[19] In some cases, small abscesses in the mesocolon or bowel wall are not detected.

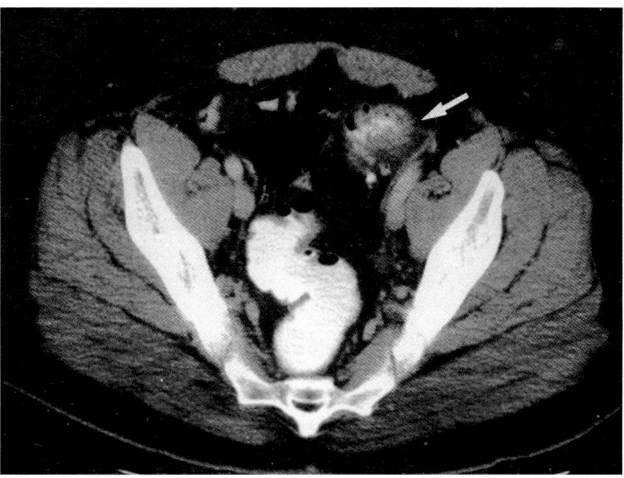

Figure 6 **Computed tomographic scan shows thickening of the sigmoid colon (*arrow*) caused by acute diverticulitis.**

The diagnosis of carcinoma cannot be excluded definitively when there is thickening of the bowel wall [*see Figure 7*]. Limited studies show that magnetic resonance imaging has high sensitivity and specificity for acute diverticulitis, and this technique does not expose the patient to ionizing radiation.[20]

Although CT has [illegible] in the evaluation of diverticulitis,[19] the latter may be more useful in differentiating carcinoma from diverticulitis. A contrast study can also be complementary when the CT scan raises the suspicion of carcinoma.[18] When diverticulitis is suspected, water-soluble contrast material should be used instead of barium because of the complications that follow extravasation of barium [*see Figure 8 and Figure 9*]. Furthermore, in the acute setting, only the left colon should be evaluated. Carcinoma is suggested by an abrupt transition to an abnormal mucosa over a relatively short segment; diverticulitis is usually characterized by a gradual transition into diseased colon over a longer segment, with the mucosa remaining intact. If the contrast study reveals extravasation of contrast outlining an abscess cavity [*see Figure 9*], an intramural sinus tract, or a fistula, diverticulitis is likely.[1]

Colonoscopy is avoided when acute diverticulitis is suspected because of the risk of perforation. It may, however, be done 6 to 8 weeks after the process subsides to rule out other disorders (e.g., colon cancer) [*see Figure 10*]. When a patient does not respond to therapy, gentle flexible sigmoidoscopy may detect a carcinoma or some other abnormality.[21,22] If diverticular disease is advanced, the endoscopic procedure may be difficult; the diverticular segment must be fully traversed for the examiner to be able to exclude a neoplasm with confidence. When major lower GI bleeding occurs, colonoscopy is done to search for polyps, carcinoma, or a site of diverticular bleeding. In the case of massive bleeding, selective arteriography is useful for localizing the source, and superselective embolization frequently quells the hemorrhage. The actual risk of bowel ischemia is low when superselective techniques are employed. Bleeding at the time of arteriography may be facilitated by the infusion of heparin or urokinase; however, this is a risky approach that should be taken only

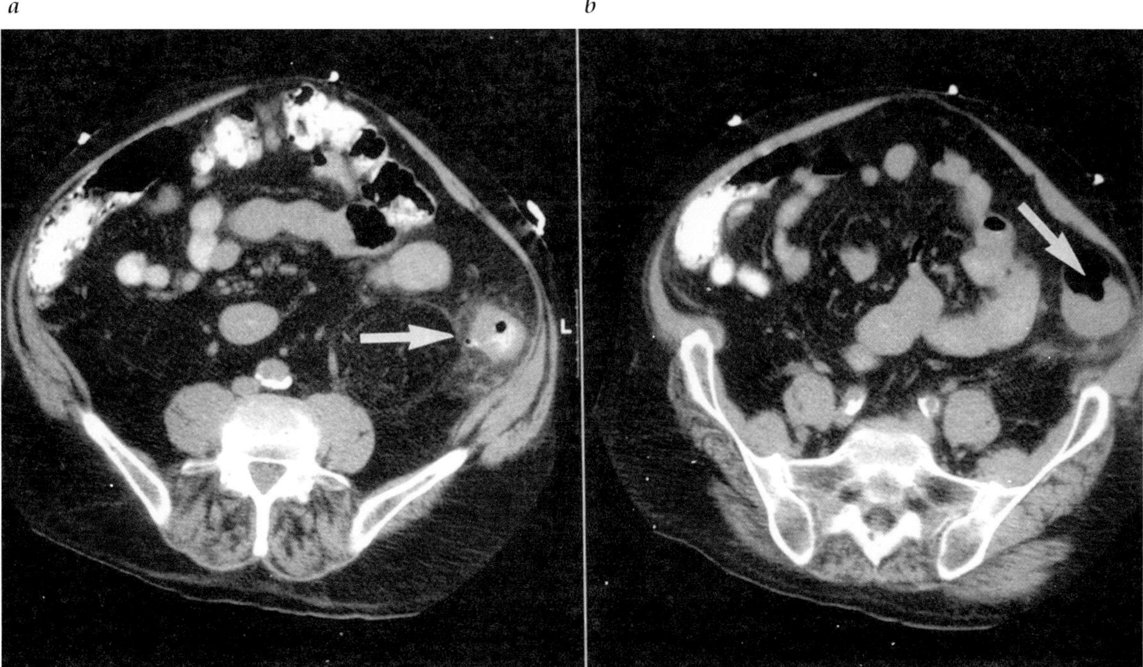

Figure 7 **(*a*) Computed tomographic (CT) scan shows a thickened left colonic wall and diverticulum (*arrow*). Diverticulitis was considered the most likely diagnosis. (*b*) CT scan through an adjacent plane shows deformity of the mucosa, suggesting a possible apple-core lesion (*arrow*). Subsequent endoscopy revealed a carcinoma that was obstructing the colon almost completely.**

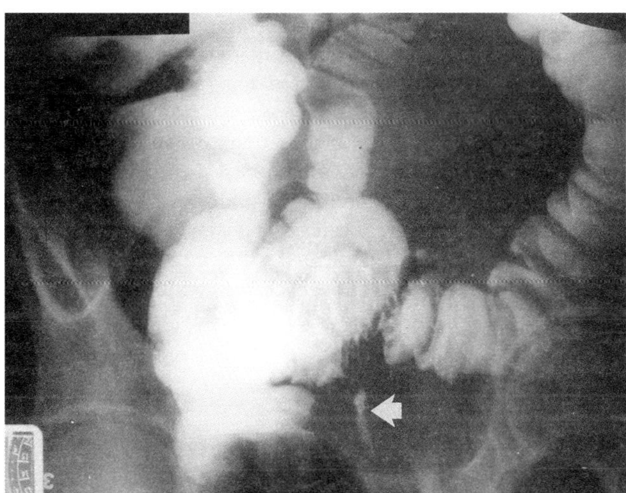

Figure 8 **Contrast study shows local extravasation from the sigmoid colon (*arrow*); a diverticulum is visible.**

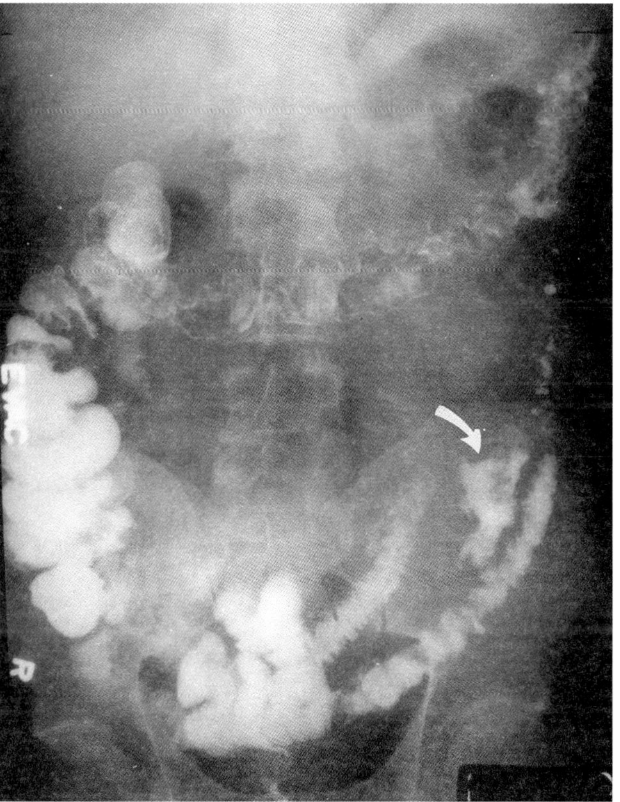

Figure 9 **Shown is extravasation into an abscess cavity (*arrow*) from diverticulitis at the sigmoid colon–descending colon junction in a postevacuation film.**

when other attempts at localization have failed and recurrent bouts of bleeding have occurred.

When a colovesical fistula occurs, contrast CT with narrow cuts in the pelvis can be very helpful. The classic findings are sigmoid diverticula, thickening of the bladder and the colon, air in the bladder, opacification of the fistula tract and the bladder, and, possibly, an abscess [*see Figure 11*]. Cystoscopy is less specific, showing possible edema or erythema at the site of the fistula. A contrast enema helps rule out malignant

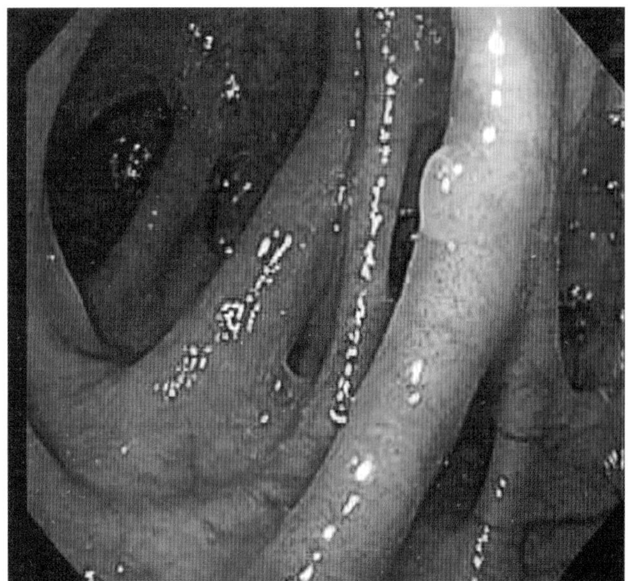

Figure 10 **Colonoscopic view of several sigmoid diverticula reveals no evidence of active diverticulitis (e.g., edema or narrowing).**

disease. The diagnostic tests that are most useful for detecting colovaginal fistulas are contrast CT and vaginography via a Foley catheter. Charcoal ingestion helps confirm the presence of colovesical or colovaginal fistulas. On rare occasions, colocutaneous fistulas may develop, causing erythema and breakdown of the skin. Colouterine fistulas may occur as well; these are also quite rare.

Management

MEDICAL

Uncomplicated diverticulitis is usually managed on an outpatient basis by instituting a liquid or low-residue diet and administering an oral antibiotic combination that covers anaerobes and gram-negative organisms (e.g., ciprofloxacin with metronidazole or clindamycin) over a period of 7 to 10 days. Provided that symptoms and signs have subsided, the colon may be evaluated more fully several weeks later with a contrast study or colonoscopy if the diagnosis of diverticular disease has not already been established. If symptoms worsen, hospitalization should be considered. Over the long term, patients should be maintained on a high-fiber diet, although it may take months for the diet to have an effect on symptoms. Limited trials suggest that other substances such as probiotics and antiinflammatory agents such as mesalazine may help prevent recurrent attacks.[23,24]

If more significant physical findings and symptoms of toxicity develop, hospitalization is warranted [*see Figure 12*]. Patients are placed on a nihil per os (NPO) regimen, and intravenous fluids and antibiotics are administered (e.g., a third-generation cephalosporin with metronidazole) until abdominal pain and tenderness have resolved and bowel function has returned. As a rule, resolution occurs within several days. If there is clinical evidence of intestinal obstruction or ileus, a nasogastric tube is placed. In most cases, ileus-related symptoms resolve with antibiotic treatment. CT scans are useful for establishing the correct diagnosis in the emergency department[25]; furthermore, the severity of diverticulitis on CT scans predicts the risk of subsequent medical failure. Following the sedimentation rate may be helpful in assessing the effectiveness of treatment. Most patients recover with conservative management alone. By observing early trends in the leukocyte count and the maximum temperature in patients with acute diverticulitis, one can predict whether they will recover quickly as expected or if they will likely require prolonged intravenous antibiotics and/or an operation.[26] It has been estimated that 15 to 30% of patients admitted with acute diverticulitis will require surgical treatment during the same admission.[1]

If fever and leukocytosis persist despite antibiotic therapy, the presence of an abscess should be suspected. Small (< 5 cm) abscesses may respond to antibiotic infusion and bowel rest. Larger abscesses that are localized and isolated may be accessible to percutaneous drainage [*see Figure 13*].[27] Generally, this technique is reserved for abscesses greater than 5 cm in

a

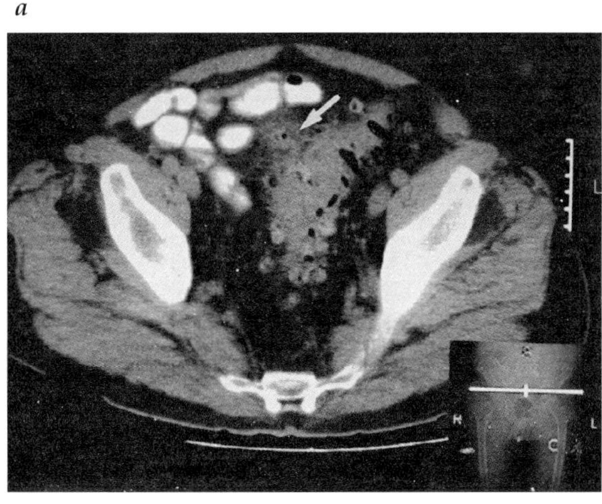

b

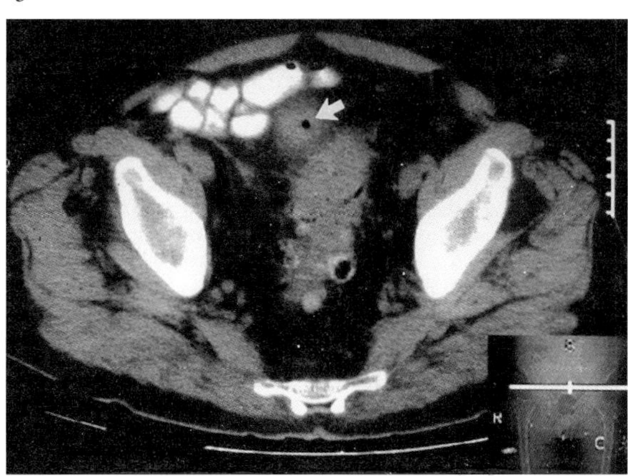

Figure 11 **(*a*) Computed tomographic (CT) scan in a patient with a colovesical fistula shows air in the thickened tract (*arrow*) adjacent to the sigmoid colon. (*b*) CT scan through an adjacent plane shows air in the bladder (*arrow*) as a result of the fistula. No contrast is present in the bladder.**

diameter in low-risk patients who are not immunocompromised. It often leads to resolution of sepsis and the resulting symptoms and signs (e.g., abdominal pain and tenderness and leukocytosis), usually within 72 hours, thereby facilitating subsequent elective surgical resection of the colon. In addition, percutaneous drainage offers cost advantages in that it reduces the number of operative procedures required and shortens hospital stay.[28] Patients with severe comorbidities at times can be managed with drainage alone.[29]

Access to a pelvic collection may be difficult to obtain, and the drainage procedure typically must be done with the patient in a prone or lateral position. If the catheter drainage amounts to more than 500 mL/day after the first 24 hours, a fistula should be suspected. Before the catheter is removed, a CT scan is done with injection of contrast material through the tube to determine whether the cavity has collapsed. If this approach fails (as it usually does in patients with multiple or multiloculated abscesses), an expeditious operation may be necessary.[17] An initial surgical procedure is required in about 20% of cases.

SURGICAL

Overall, approximately 20% of patients with diverticulitis require surgical treatment.[30] Most surgical procedures are reserved for patients who experience recurrent episodes of acute diverticulitis that necessitate treatment (inpatient or outpatient) or who have complicated diverticulitis. The most common indication for elective resection is recurrent attacks—that is, several episodes of acute diverticulitis documented by studies such as CT. Rerecurrences may be more common than recurrences.[31] In 2000, a task force of the American Society of Colon and Rectal Surgeons recommended sigmoid resection after two attacks of diverticulitis.[32] A subsequent cost analysis using a Markov model suggested that cost savings could be achieved if resection was done after three attacks.[33] There is a growing tendency to question arbitrary guidelines for surgical management of recurrent attacks, with the exception of certain groups, such as immunocompromised patients.[34,35] Current practice guidelines state that the recommendation to perform elective sigmoid resection after recovery from uncomplicated acute diverticulitis should be made on a case-by-case basis. The decision-making process should be influenced by the age and medical condition of the patient, the frequency and severity of attacks, and the presence of symptoms after the acute attack. Elective resection is generally recommended after an episode of complicated diverticulitis.[36] Efforts are made to time surgical treatment so that it takes place during a quiescent period 8 to 10 weeks after the last attack. Barium enema or colonoscopy may be employed to evaluate the diverticular disease and rule out carcinoma. The bowel can then be prepared mechanically and with antibiotics (e.g., oral neomycin and metronidazole on the day before operation).

Elective resection is a common sequel to successful percutaneous drainage of a pelvic abscess in an otherwise healthy, well-nourished patient.[37] The timing of surgery may be guided by the extent of the inflammatory changes (as documented by CT scanning) and the patient's clinical course. Most patients can be operated upon within 6 weeks. Elective resection is the preferred approach to diverticular fistulas as well. Colovesical fistulas are usually resected because of the risk of urinary sepsis and the concern that a malignancy might be overlooked. Preferably, the operation is done when the acute inflammation has subsided.

Elective resection is done via either the open route or, increasingly, the laparoscopic route.[38] The learning curve for laparoscopic colectomy is 20 to 50 cases.[39] Obese patients with severe colonic inflammation are poorer candidates for laparoscopic resection.[38] In our institution, the development of hand-assisted procedures has widened the opportunities for using minimally invasive surgery [*see 6:30 Procedures for Diverticular Disease*], allowing all types of diverticular resections to be performed more safely.[40,41] Hand-assisted laparoscopic sigmoidectomy for diverticular disease is associated with lower conversion rates and shorter operative times when compared with purely laparoscopic surgery.[42] In addition, the hand-assisted approach affords a better opportunity to complete complicated cases in a minimally invasive fashion.[2,43] Minimally invasive procedures have several advantages over conventional procedures: decreased intraoperative trauma, fewer postoperative adhesions, reduced postoperative pain, shorter duration of ileus, quicker discharge from the hospital, and earlier return to work.[44] Such procedures can be done safely in obese patients,[44] and the conversion rate is now low.[39,44,45] The technical details of the procedures are addressed elsewhere [*see 6:30 Procedures for Diverticular Disease*].

Some patients with complicated diverticulitis require emergency resection because of free perforation and widespread peritonitis. In such patients, the American Society of Anesthesiologists (ASA) physical status score and the degree of preoperative organ failure may be significant predictors of outcome.[46] Unfavorable systemic factors (e.g., hypotension, renal failure, diabetes, malnutrition, immune compromise, and ascites) play a vital role in determining patient outcome,[46] as does the severity of the peritonitis (i.e., extent, contents, and speed of development). One of the unfortunate limitations of the Hinchey classification is that it does not take comorbidities into account. Because the bowel is not prepared before operation, the surgeon may feel uncomfortable doing an anastomosis. On-table lavage may be considered if contamination is minimal, but it adds to the time spent under anesthesia during an emergency procedure.

As a general rule, resection and immediate anastomosis (open or laparoscopic)[45] are suitable for Hinchey stage I and perhaps stage II diverticular perforations, whereas resection with diversion (the Hartmann procedure) is the gold standard for stage III and especially stage IV.[47] This recommendation is based on the finding that an anastomosis involving the left colon is risky when performed under emergency conditions.[48] The once-popular three-stage procedures are now of historical interest only. There are some reports of successful outcomes for type III and type IV cases after extensive abdominal lavage and two-layer anastomoses[49] or after on-table lavage of the colonic contents to allow primary anastomosis.[50] There have been a number of recent reports of laparoscopic peritoneal lavage and intraperitoneal drainage for the treatment of purulent peritonitis (Hinchey III) scenarios. Morbidity has been low, and a delayed laparoscopic sigmoid resection has been possible.[51,52] Grading of comorbidities with classification systems such as APACHE II or the Mannheim peritonitis index can facilitate decision making with respect to the question of anastomosis versus diversion.[53,54] The surgeon's decision must be individualized on the basis of each patient's

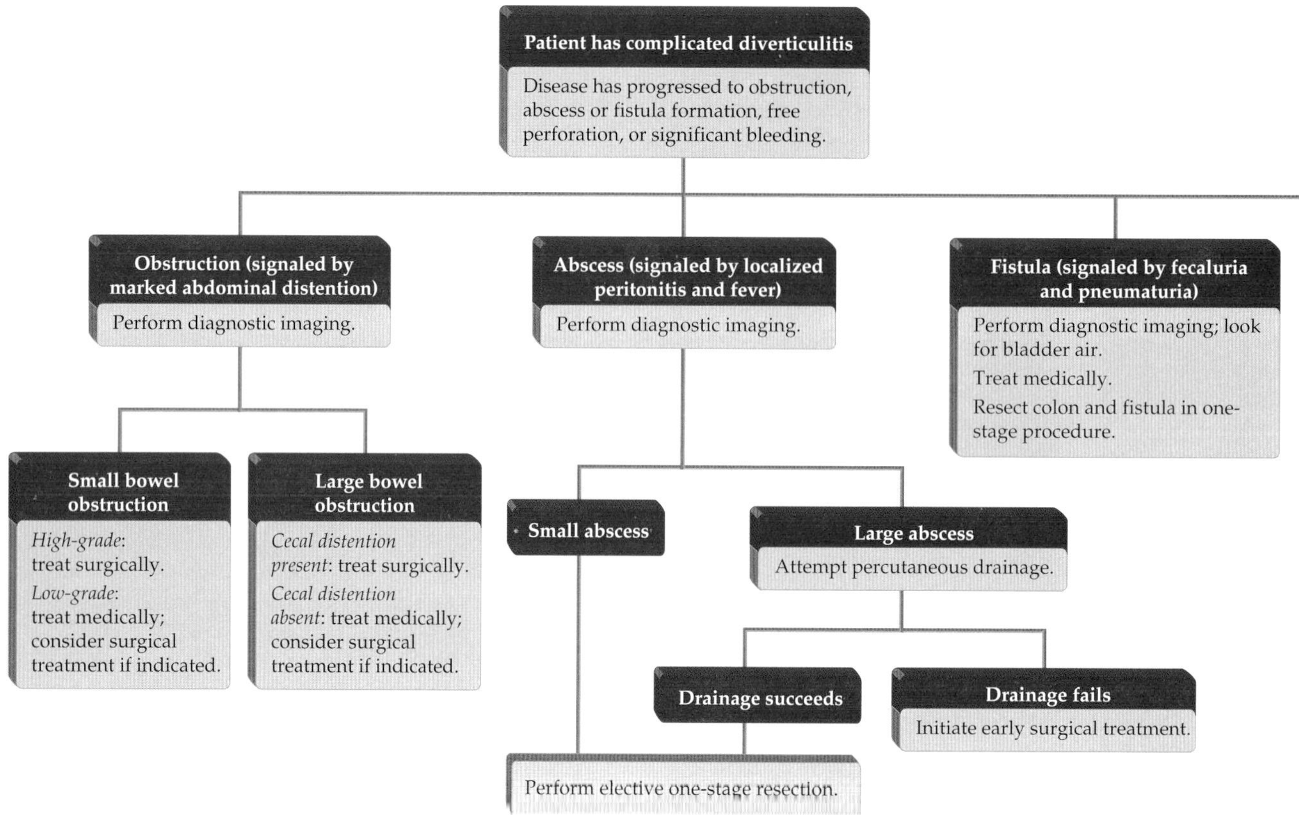

Figure 12 **Algorithm outlining treatment options for complicated diverticulitis. GI = gastrointestinal; RBC = red blood cell.**

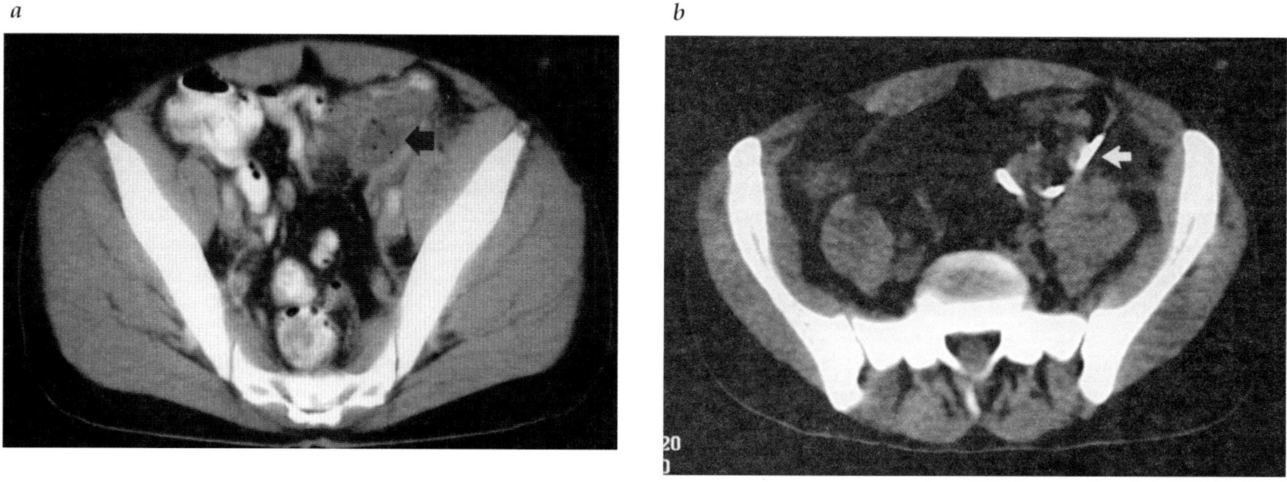

Figure 13 **(*a*) Computed tomographic scan shows a pericolic abscess (*arrow*) caused by a contained perforation arising from sigmoid diverticulitis. (*b*) A pigtail catheter (*arrow*) has been placed into the abscess cavity by the interventional radiologist.**

condition and needs. The literature on this topic is confusing in that most of the published reports are small and retrospective, with only limited classification of disease severity.

Currently, surgeons encountering acute diverticulitis are more likely to do one-stage resections, as opposed to Hartmann procedures, than they once were.[46,55,56] The advantage of the one-stage approach is that the colostomy takedown, frequent postoperative complications,[57] and attendant 4% mortality are avoided.[58] Furthermore, at least 30% of patients who undergo a Hartmann procedure never return for colostomy closure. A primary anastomosis can be protected with a proximal ileostomy as well.[47,59] Transverse colostomy and loop ileostomy

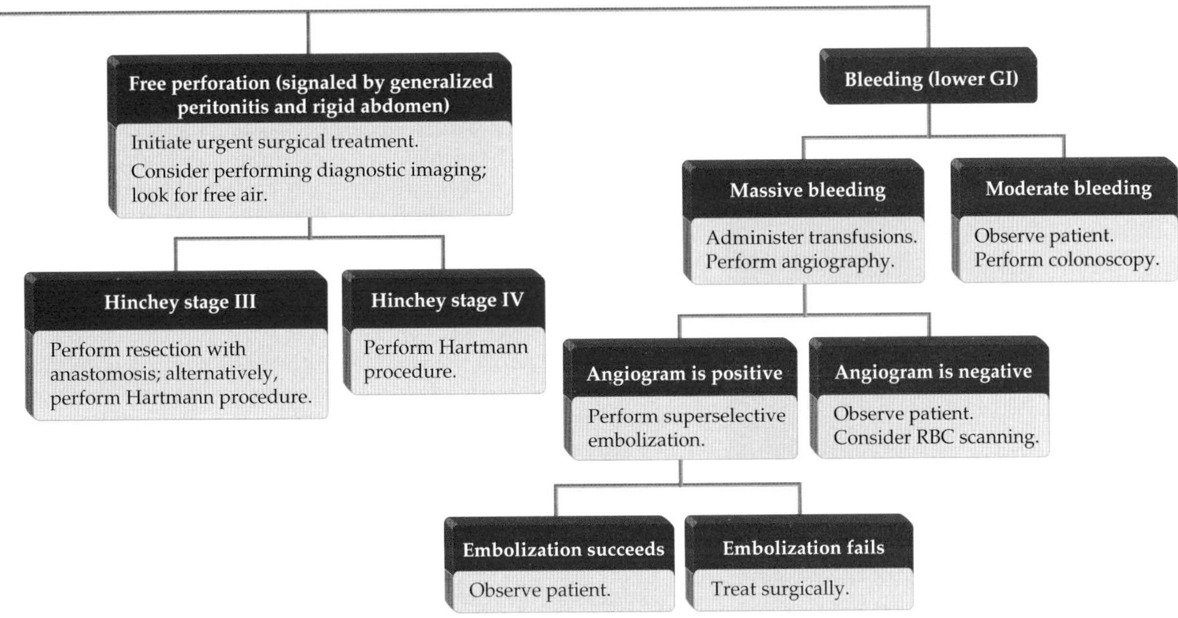

appear to be equally safe, although skin changes may be more problematic after a colostomy,[60] and an ileostomy closure tends to be less complex than a colostomy closure. On-table lavage may also be used as an adjunct to anastomosis.

The risk of complications inherent in operations on the colon should always be kept in mind, especially in the relatively few patients undergoing emergency procedures.[61,62] In this setting, the bowel is unprepared and systemic sepsis may be present. Potential complications include ureteral injuries; anastomotic leakage, anastomotic stricture, and postoperative intra-abdominal abscesses; perioperative bleeding involving the mesentery, adhesions, the splenic capsule, or the presacral venous plexus; postoperative small bowel obstruction; stomal complications; wound infection, wound dehiscence, and abdominal compartment syndrome; acute respiratory distress syndrome; and multiple organ dysfunction syndrome. Even after successful operations, some patients continue to have abdominal pain attributable to factors such as irritable bowel syndrome.[63,64]

Large bowel obstruction secondary to diverticulitis can lead to considerable morbidity and may necessitate surgical intervention.[59] The obstruction is usually partial [*see Figure 14 and Figure 15*], allowing preparation of the bowel in many cases. High-grade obstruction represents a complex problem. If the cecum is dilated to a diameter of 10 cm or greater and there is tenderness in the right lower quadrant, expeditious surgery is necessary because of the risk of cecal necrosis and perforation. High-grade obstruction with fecal loading of the colon is usually managed by performing a Hartmann procedure, although on-table lavage may be considered.[17] A survey of GI surgeons in the United States indicated that 50% would opt for a one-stage procedure in low-risk patients with obstruction, whereas 94% would opt for a staged procedure in high-risk patients.[65]

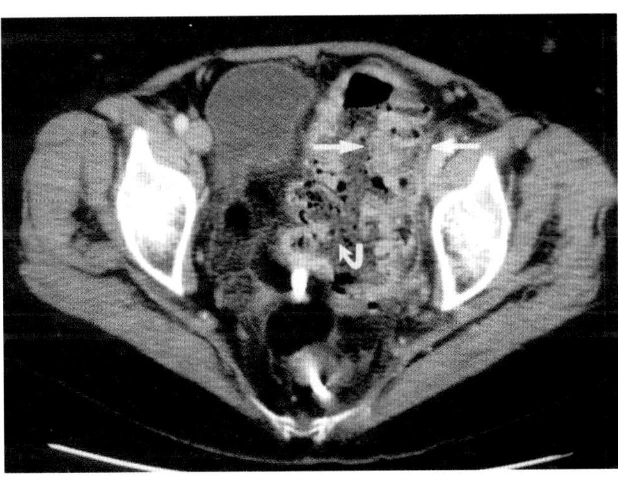

Figure 14 **Computed tomographic scan shows marked thickening of the sigmoid wall (*arrows*) in a patient with diverticular disease who presented with symptoms of intractable constipation. No contrast is present in the lumen (*curved arrow*).**

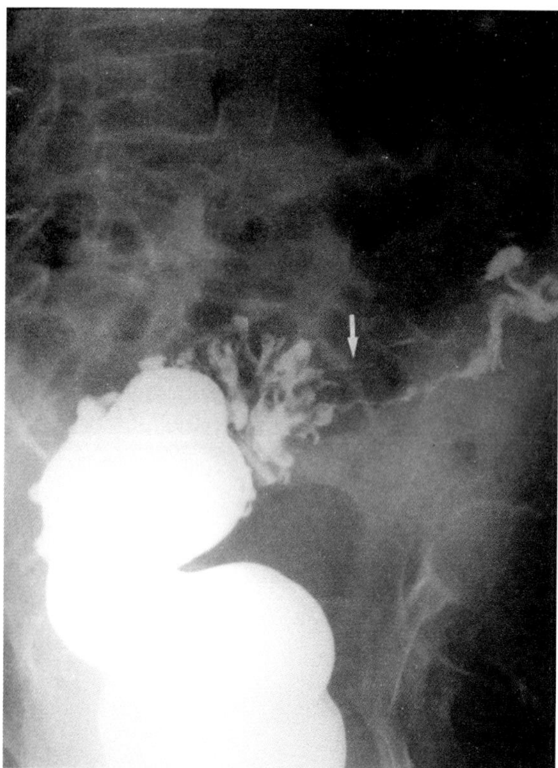

Figure 15 **Contrast study shows high grade retrograde obstruction, multiple diverticula, and a long proximal sigmoid stricture. A tiny extraluminal tract (possibly intramural) from a diverticulum (*arrow*) is seen.**

Small bowel obstruction may also complicate the clinical picture. Mechanical small bowel obstruction may occur as a consequence of adherence of the small bowel to a focus of diverticulitis, especially in the presence of a large pericolic abscess. Whereas small bowel obstruction tends to cause periumbilical crampy abdominal pain and vomiting, these characteristic manifestations may be obscured in part by pain attributed to diverticulitis. The concern in this situation is that ischemic small bowel may be ignored, with potentially disastrous consequences. Diarrhea should trigger the suspicion of colonic disease, and formation of a fistula into the small bowel should raise the possibility of Crohn disease. CT scanning often helps the surgeon differentiate between primary and secondary small bowel obstruction, but, ultimately, exploratory surgery may be required for both diagnosis and treatment.

Lower GI bleeding caused by diverticular disease rarely calls for emergency resection because the bleeding is self-limited in most patients (80 to 90%). Furthermore, active diverticulitis is rare when active bleeding is the presenting symptom. Attempts are made to establish the active bleeding site by means of colonoscopy,[66] tagged red blood cell nuclear scans, or angiography; barium contrast studies have no role to play in this situation. Emergency resection is indicated if the bleeding is life-threatening and if colonic angiography and attempted superselective embolization prove unsuccessful. In an unstable patient, total abdominal colectomy is necessary if the site of bleeding is unknown, although identification of the bleeding site with intraoperative colonoscopy has been reported. In a stable patient with ongoing bleeding, repeat angiography at a later time is appropriate, or so-called pharmacoangiography (infusion of heparin) can be employed in an attempt to induce bleeding.

Special Types of Diverticulitis

CECAL DIVERTICULITIS

In the United States, diverticulitis rarely involves the cecum or the right colon. Right-side diverticula occur in only 15% of patients in Western countries, compared with 75% in Singapore.[1] The incidence of cecal diverticulitis appears to be related to the number of diverticula present.[67] A classification system has been proposed that divides cecal diverticulitis into four grades [*see Figure 16*] to facilitate comparisons between different clinical series and to help surgeons formulate treatment plans in the operating room.[67] Some cecal diverticula are true diverticula, containing all layers of the bowel wall, but the majority are pseudodiverticula. Diverticulitis of the hepatic flexure and the transverse colon is even less common and can present with symptoms suggesting appendicitis.[68]

Patients with right-side disease tend to be younger and to have less generalized peritonitis than patients with left-side diverticulitis.[67,68] Because they typically present with right lower quadrant pain, fever, and leukocytosis, acute appendicitis is usually suspected. CT scans are helpful for differentiating cecal diverticulitis from appendicitis or colon cancer [*see Figure 17*].[69] If cecal diverticulitis is suspected (as in a patient who has previously undergone appendectomy or in a patient with known right-side diverticulosis who has experienced similar attacks in the past), medical management with observation and antibiotics is generally the favored strategy, just as with simple sigmoid diverticulitis. In Japan, where right-side diverticulitis is more common, medical treatment has been successfully used for recurrent attacks of uncomplicated right-side diverticulitis.[70] After a few weeks, colonoscopy should be performed to rule out a colonic neoplasm.

If the patient has significant peritonitis or the diagnosis is unclear, laparoscopy or laparotomy is indicated. It is important that one or the other be done because the mortality associated with delayed treatment of perforated cecal diverticulitis is high. In our institution, laparoscopy is usually employed; if the diagnosis is unclear, laparotomy is recommended. When inflammation is localized and minimal, colectomy is unnecessary, and incidental appendectomy should be considered if the cecum is uninvolved at the base of the appendix.[71] If desired, the diverticulum may be removed as well.

Diverticulectomy should be done only if (1) carcinoma can be ruled out, (2) the resection margins are free of inflammation, (3) the ileocecal valve and the blood supply of the bowel are not compromised, and (4) perforation, gangrene, and abscess are absent.[67] Localized diverticulectomy, in general, should be reserved for grade I and grade II disease.[67] Sometimes, the ostium of the inflamed diverticulum is palpable if the cecum is mobilized surgically. On-table cecoscopy through the appendiceal stump has also been helpful in establishing the diagnosis in the operating room.[71] Grade III and IV cecal diverticulitis may be difficult to differentiate from carcinoma; resection is favored for these lesions. An anastomosis may be created if contamination is limited, but, generally, primary resection, ileostomy, and a mucous fistula are favored for treatment of grade IV disease.

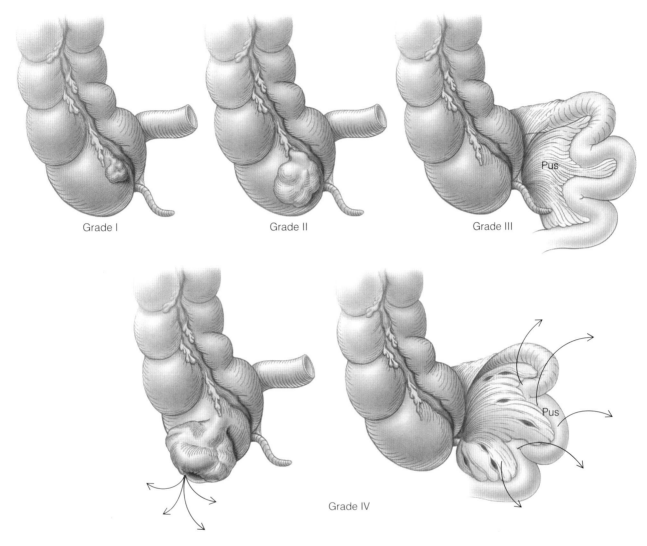

Figure 16 **Illustrated is a proposed classification of pathologic types of cecal diverticulitis. Grade I is a specific inflamed diverticulum; grade II is a cecal mass; grade III is characterized by a localized abscess or fistula; and grade IV represents a free perforation or a ruptured abscess with peritonitis.**[59]

DIVERTICULITIS IN YOUNG PATIENTS

Diverticulitis in patients younger than 40 years has been a focus of considerable attention in the literature, although this group represents only about 2 to 5% of the patients in large series.[32] The incidence of diverticulitis in young patients may be increasing, and obese Latino men appear to be at particular risk.[72] This predominance in males reflects a tendency to underdiagnose acute diverticulitis in young women.[73] Some authors have asserted that diverticulitis is particularly virulent in young patients; however, current data tend not to support this concept, suggesting that patients with mild diverticulitis are misdiagnosed when hospitalized or are treated as outpatients. The high rate of early operation in young patients probably reflects misdiagnosis of diverticulitis as acute appendicitis rather than the development of particularly severe forms of diverticulitis.[72] Patients found to have uncomplicated acute diverticulitis may, if desired, undergo incidental appendectomy in conjunction with medical treatment of diverticulitis.

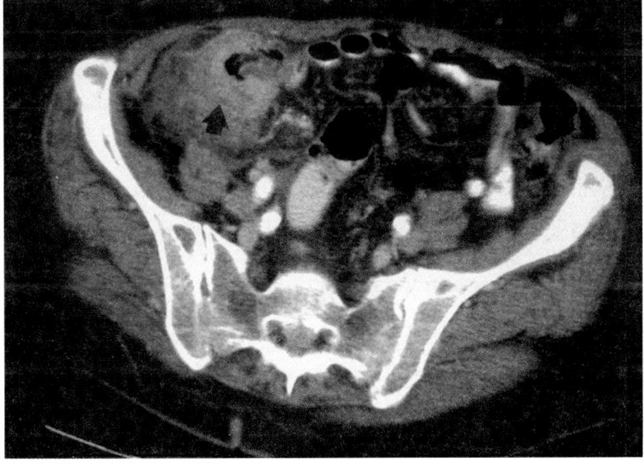

Figure 17 **Computed tomographic scan shows inflammation in the pericecal area (*arrow*) and cecal edema, which could represent cecal diverticulitis. Because the appendix is not clearly visualized, appendicitis cannot be ruled out.**

Unlike elderly patients, hospitalized young patients with diverticulitis tend to have few comorbidities other than obesity. Furthermore, young patients hospitalized for diverticulitis tend to have relatively advanced disease, perhaps as a consequence of delayed diagnosis, whereas elderly patients hospitalized with an admitting diagnosis of diverticulitis tend to exhibit a wider spectrum of disease severity. Young patients appear not to have a higher rate of recurrent diverticulitis than older patients do; thus, aggressive resection is not necessary at the time of the first attack.[72] However, a finding of advanced diverticulitis on CT scans is a predictor of subsequent disease complications in this population.[74]

In general, diverticulitis should be approached in the same fashion in younger patients as in older patients.[74] The pathophysiology of the disease is probably identical. As in the elderly, elective resection is recommended after recurrent attacks, not after a single attack; with follow-up, the majority of patients hospitalized with acute diverticulitis do not require operation.[34,74–76]

Table 1 Unusual Extra-Abdominal Presentations of Diverticulitis[90]

Dermatologic	**Pyoderma gangrenosum**
Urinary	Ureteral obstruction Coloureteral fistula
Soft tissue	Thigh abscess Necrotizing fasciitis
Orthopedic	Osteomyelitis Arthritis
Gynecologic	Colouterine fistula Ovarian tumor/abscess
Genital	Epididymitis Pneumoscrotum
Neurologic	Coloepidural fistula
Vascular	Femoral vein thrombosis Mesenteric vein thrombosis Pylephlebitis Colovenous fistula
Perineal	Fournier gangrene Complex anal fistula

DIVERTICULITIS IN IMMUNOCOMPROMISED PATIENTS

In view of their known predisposition to infection, immunocompromised patients (e.g., chronic alcoholics, transplant patients, and persons with metastatic tumors who are receiving chemotherapy) with diverticulitis are at particular risk.[77] There is no evidence that the incidence of diverticulitis is higher in this population than in the general population, but it is clear that immunocompromised patients have higher rates of operation once diverticulitis develops and that their postoperative mortality is higher.[78] Corticosteroid intake causes a number of significant problems, such as thinning of the colonic wall, lessening of the physical findings with diverticulitis, and an attenuated inflammatory response.

Any immunocompromised patient with abdominal pain should be evaluated aggressively. Contrast-enhanced CT is the imaging study of choice. The risk of perforation is increased in this setting, as is the risk of postoperative complications such as wound dehiscence. For an immunocompromised patient who has recovered from an episode of symptomatic diverticulitis, elective surgical treatment is recommended. A renal transplant patient with asymptomatic diverticulosis, however, need not undergo prophylactic colectomy. Pretransplantation colonic screening of patients older than 50 years does not reliably predict posttransplantation colonic complications.[79]

ATYPICAL PRESENTATIONS

Diverticulitis may give rise to various unusual manifestations involving multiple organ systems [*see Table 1*]. Not surprisingly, immunocompromised patients are at particular risk.

Retroperitoneal abscesses can track into anatomic planes (e.g., along the psoas muscle) or through the obturator foramen to areas such as the neck, the thigh, the knee, the groin, and the genitalia. CT scanning is essential to outline the extent of such abscesses. Contrast enemas show the diverticula along with a sinus tract into the abscess cavity. Cultures of the abscess demonstrate the presence of colonic organisms such as *Bacteroides fragilis*. Definitive treatment consists of wide abscess drainage and colon resection. Without aggressive surgical management, mortality is high.

The protean manifestations of diverticulitis also include pylephlebitis (which causes liver abscesses), arthritis, and skin changes. Diverticulitis has, in fact, replaced appendicitis as the most common source of liver abscesses of portal origin. Simple abscesses may be drained percutaneously if they are not too large, and multiple loculated abscesses may be managed with open drainage. The main risk factors for mortality from liver abscesses are immunosuppression, underlying malignancy, the presence of multiple organisms, and liver dysfunction. If the decision is made to perform a colectomy, the procedure may be done after drainage of the liver abscess or simultaneously with drainage during an open procedure.

GIANT DIVERTICULA

An anatomic curiosity sometimes encountered in patients with diverticular disease is a giant diverticulum, also termed a giant gas cyst or a pneumocyst of the colon.[80] These lesions, which may reach diameters of 40 cm, are believed to develop as a consequence of a ball-valve mechanism created by intermittent occlusion of the neck by fecal material that traps air in the diverticulum. Most giant diverticula are minimally symptomatic, causing only mild abdominal pain, and perforation is rare. A mobile mass may be palpable, and the gas-filled cyst can be seen on plain abdominal films. As many as two thirds of giant diverticula are opacified during a barium enema and can thereby be differentiated from other abnormalities (e.g., a mesenteric cyst, emphysematous cholecystitis, or a colon duplication) [*see Figure 18*]. The cyst tends to adhere densely to adjacent structures (e.g., the bladder and the small bowel). The treatment of choice is resection of the colon and the cyst; performing diverticulectomy alone can lead to the development of a colocutaneous fistula.

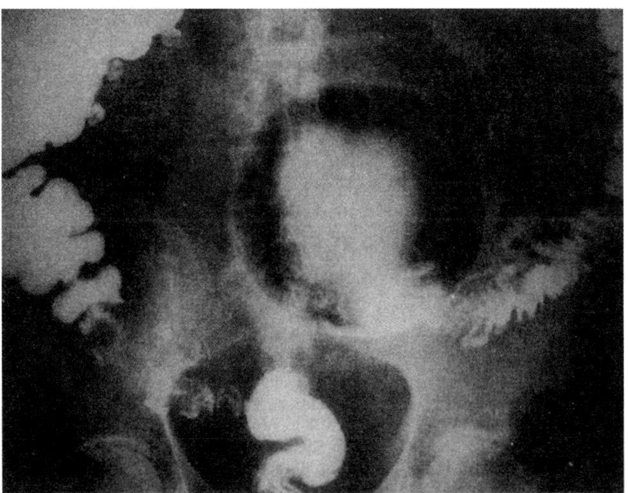

Figure 18 **Giant sigmoid diverticulum opacified during a barium enema examination.**[80]

RECURRENT DIVERTICULITIS AFTER RESECTION

Recurrent diverticulitis is rare after a colectomy for diverticulitis, occurring in 1 to 10% of patients.[81] As many as 3% of patients who have undergone resection for diverticulitis will require repeat resection. The differential diagnosis includes Crohn disease, irritable bowel syndrome, carcinoma, and ischemic colitis. CT and colonoscopy should be carried out. Particular care should be taken to review pathologic specimens for evidence of Crohn disease.

The only significant determinant of recurrent diverticulitis is the level of the anastomosis; the high pressure in the sigmoid colon distal to the anastomosis appears to be responsible. In one study, the risk of recurrence was four times greater in patients with a colosigmoid anastomosis than in those with a colorectal anastomosis.[82] Reoperation requires a dissection that commences in noninflamed tissue. Dissection may be particularly difficult near the pelvic sidewall because of fibrosis; ureteral stenting may facilitate identification of the ureters.

SUBACUTE AND ATYPICAL DIVERTICULITIS

A small number of patients experience recurrent episodes of left lower quadrant abdominal pain that are not accompanied by the classic findings of acute diverticulitis (e.g., fever and leukocytosis). The inflammatory changes associated with diverticula in this subgroup have been referred to as atypical, subacute, or smoldering diverticulitis.[83,84] In this setting, there is not always a direct association between endoscopic and clinical findings; endoscopic evidence of diverticular inflammation has been seen in asymptomatic patients.[85] It has been suggested that there is a relation between diverticular disease and colitis.[86] Patients with chronic lower abdominal pain should undergo imaging studies and endoscopic evaluation, and other disorders (e.g., irritable bowel syndrome, inflammatory bowel disease, drug-induced symptoms, and bowel ischemia) should be excluded. In most cases of atypical diverticulitis, endoscopic findings are normal.[84] In carefully selected patients, colectomy often eliminates the abdominal pain, and many of these patients are eventually found to have histologic signs of acute and chronic mucosal inflammation.[84]

Financial Disclosures: None Reported

References

1. Stollman NH, Raskin JB. Diverticular disease of the colon. J Clin Gastroenterol 1999;29:241.
2. Salem TA, Mohillo RG, O'Dwyer PJ. Prospective, five-year follow-up study of patients with symptomatic uncomplicated diverticular disease. Dis Colon Rectum 2007;50:1460.
3. Munson KD, Hensien MA, Jacob LN, et al. Diverticulitis: a comprehensive follow-up. Dis Colon Rectum 1996;39:318.
4. Whiteway J, Morson BC. Elastosis in diverticular disease of the sigmoid colon. Gut 1985;26:258.
5. Heise CP. Epidemiology and pathogenesis of diverticular disease. J Gastrointest Surg 2008; 12:1309.
6. Alsoori WH, Giovannucci EL, Rimm EB, et al. Prospective study of physical activity and the risk of symptomatic diverticular disease in men. Gut 1995;36:276.
7. Strate LL, Liu YL, Aldoori WH, et al. Obesity increases the risks of diverticulitis and diverticular bleeding. Gastroenterology 2009; 136:115.
8. Goh H, Bourne R. Non-steroidal anti-inflammatory drugs and perforated diverticular disease: a case-control study. Ann R Coll Surg Engl 2002;84:93.
9. Papagrigorladis S. Macey L, Bourantas N, et al. Smoking may be associated with complications in diverticular disease. Br J Surg 1999;86:923.
10. Pereira MA, Ludwig DS. Dietary fiber and body weight regulation: observations and mechanisms. Pediatr Clin North Am 2001; 48:969.
11. Strate LL, Liu YL, Syngal S, et al. Nut, corn, and popcorn consumption and the incidence of diverticular disease. JAMA 2008;300:907.
12. McConnell EJ, Tessier DJ, Wolff BG. Population-based incidence of complicated diverticular disease of the sigmoid colon based on gender and age. Dis Colon Rectum 2003;46:1110.
13. McGuire HH. Bleeding colonic diverticula: a reappraisal of natural history and management. Ann Surg 1994;220:653.
14. Hinchey GC, Schall GH, Richards MB. Treatment of perforated diverticulitis of the colon. Adv Surg 1978;12:85.
15. Morgenstern L. "Malignant" diverticulitis: a clinical entity. Arch Surg 1979;114:1112.
16. Sanford MB, Ryan JA Jr. The proper surgical treatment of perforated sigmoid diverticulitis with generalized peritonitis. In: Welch JP, Cohen JL, Sardella WV, et al, editors. Diverticular disease: management of the difficult surgical case. Baltimore: Williams & Wilkins; 1998. p. 223.
17. Schwesinger WH, Page CP, Gaskill HV III, et al. Operative management of diverticular emergencies: strategies and outcomes. Arch Surg 2000;135:558.
18. Ambrosetti P, Jenny A, Becker C, et al. Acute left colonic diverticulitis-compared performance of computed tomography and water-soluble contrast enema: prospective evaluation of 420 patients. Dis Colon Rectum 2000;43:1363.
19. Kircher MF, Rhea JT, Kihiczak D, et al. Frequency, sensitivity, and specificity of individual signs of diverticulitis on thin-section helical CT with colonic contrast material: experience with 312 cases. AJR Am J Roentgenol 2002; 178:1313.
20. Heverhagen JT, Sitter H, Zielke A, et al. Prospective evaluation of the value of magnetic resonance imaging in suspected acute sigmoid diverticulitis. Dis Colon Rectum 2008;51:1810.
21. Lahat A, Yanai H, Sakhnini E, et al. Role of colonoscopy in patients with persistent acute diverticulitis. World J Gastroenterol 2008; 14:2763.
22. Aydin HN, Remzi FH. Diverticulitis: when and how to operate? Dig Liver Dis 2004;36:435.
23. Di Mario F, Comparato G, Fanigliulo L, et al. Use of mesalazine in diverticular disease. J Clin Gastroenterol 2006;40 Suppl 3:155.

12 FULMINANT ULCERATIVE COLITIS

Roger Hurst, MD, Sharon L. Stein, MD, and Fabrizio Michelassi, MD

Fulminant ulcerative colitis is a potentially life-threatening disorder that requires expert management to allow for optimal outcomes. Once associated with very high mortality,[1] the medical and surgical treatment of fulminate ulcerative colitis has greatly improved such that mortality from fulminant ulcerative colitis currently is less than 3%.[2,3] Optimal management necessitates coordination between medical and surgical therapy; hence, multidisciplinary strategies are required.

Disease Definition

The most commonly applied classification for the severity of ulcerative colitis was described by Truelove and Witts, who identified clinical parameters to categorize mild, moderate, and severe colitis.[4] The Truelove Witts classification, however, does not specify a unique category for fulminant disease. Hanauer modified this classification scheme to include the designation of fulminant colitis [*see Table 1*].[5] There is, however, no universally agreed-upon distinction between severe and fulminant ulcerative colitis.[6] Some authors use the terms "severe" and "fulminant" interchangeably, whereas others, concerned over the lack of a clear definition, recommend that the term "fulminant ulcerative colitis" be avoided.[7] This recommendation aside, the term "fulminant ulcerative colitis" is an established component of the medical vernacular even if the term itself is not clearly defined.[8–10] Fulminant ulcerative colitis is certainly a severe condition associated with systemic deterioration related to progressive ulcerative colitis. Most would agree that a flare of ulcerative colitis can be considered fulminant if it is associated with one or more of the following: high fever, tachycardia, profound anemia requiring transfusion, dehydration, low urine output, abdominal tenderness with distention, and profound leukocytosis with left shift, severe malaise, or prostration. Patients with these symptoms should be hospitalized for aggressive resuscitation while clinical assessment and treatment are initiated.[11]

Table 1 **Criteria for Evaluating the Severity of Ulcerative Colitis**

Variable	Mild Disease	Severe Disease	Fulminant Disease
Stools (no./day)	< 4	> 6	> 10
Blood in stool	Intermittent	Frequent	Continuous
Temperature (°C)	Normal	> 37.5	> 37.5
Pulse (beats/min)	Normal	> 90	> 90
Hemoglobin	Normal	< 75% of normal value	Transfusion required
Erythrocyte sedimentation rate (mm/hr)	□ 30	> 30	> 30
Colonic features on radiography	—	Air, edematous wall, thumb printing	Dilatation
Clinical signs	—	Abdominal tenderness	Abdominal distention and tenderness

Clinical Assessment

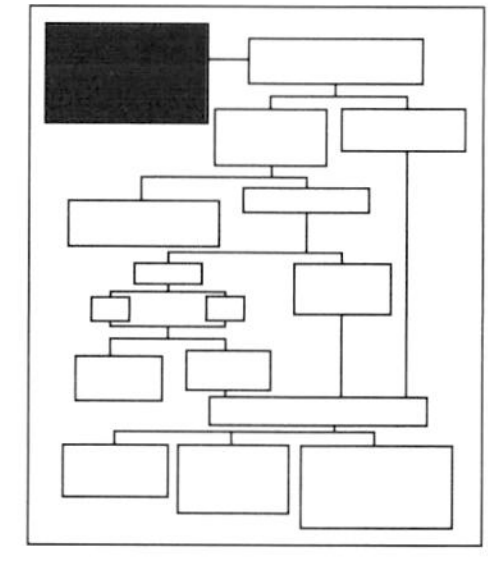

Patients admitted with severe or fulminant ulcerative colitis require a complete history and physical examination. Fulminant ulcerative colitis is rarely the initial presentation of ulcerative colitis, and most patients will have a prior diagnosis. The abdominal examination should focus on signs of peritoneal irritation that may suggest perforation or abscess formation. Any patients admitted with severe ulcerative colitis may have already received substantial doses of corticosteroids, which can mask the physical findings of peritonitis. Initial laboratory studies should include a complete blood count with differential, a coagulation profile, and a complete metabolic profile with assessment of nutritional parameters such as the serum albumin. Abdominal films and an upright chest x-ray should be obtained to assess for colonic distention indicating toxic megacolon and to assess for the presence of pneumoperitoneum indicating perforation. Infectious agents should be ruled out by multiple stool specimens sent for *Clostridium difficile*, cytomegalovirus, and *Escherichia coli* O157:H7.[12,13] It is important to identify the presence of opportunistic infections, particularly *C. difficile*, even in patients with an established diagnosis of ulcerative colitis, as superinfection with *C. difficile* in ulcerative colitis patients is common. Assessment with endoscopic

Management of Fulminant Ulcerative Colitis

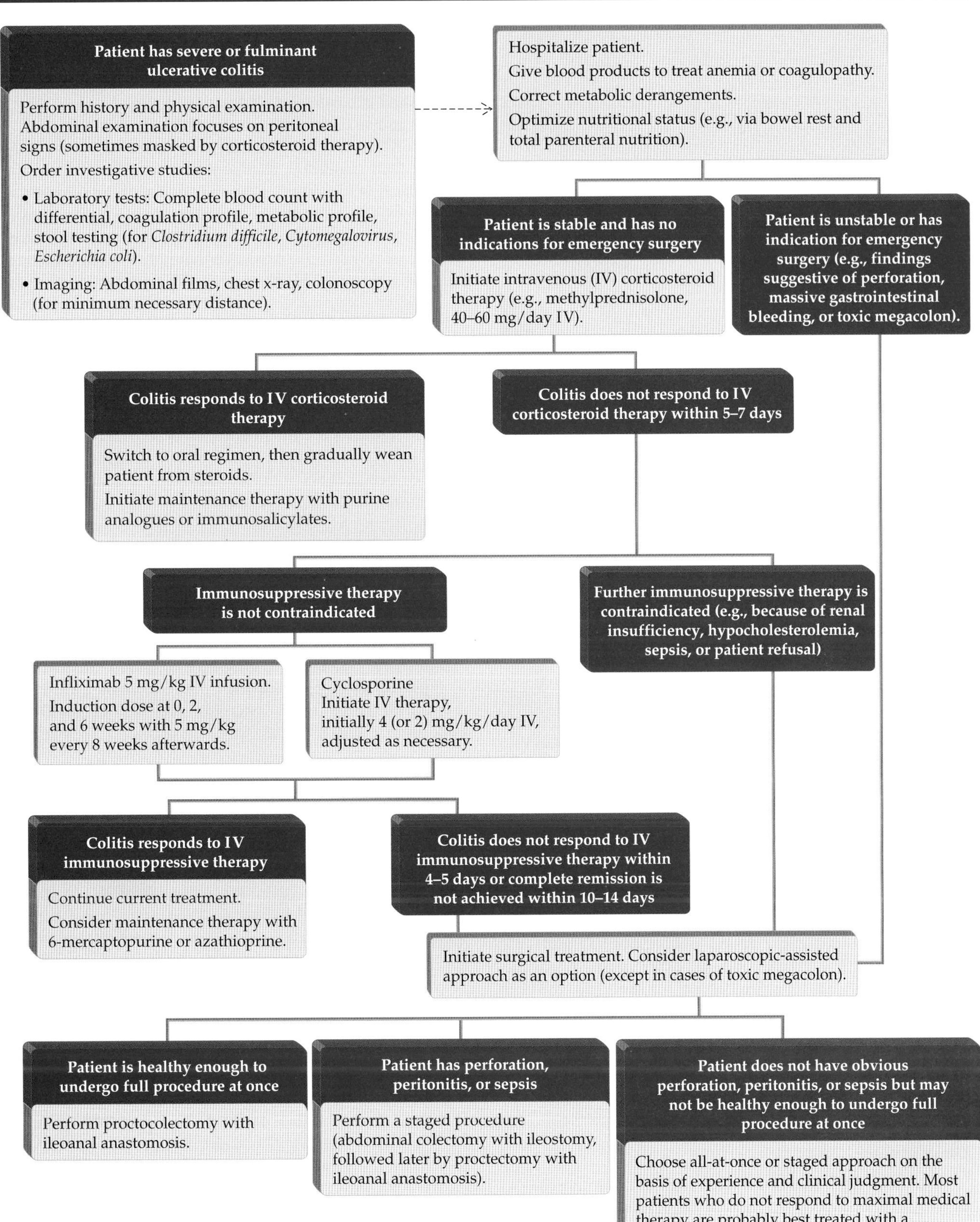

Patient has severe or fulminant ulcerative colitis
Perform history and physical examination. Abdominal examination focuses on peritoneal signs (sometimes masked by corticosteroid therapy).
Order investigative studies:
• Laboratory tests: Complete blood count with differential, coagulation profile, metabolic profile, stool testing (for *Clostridium difficile*, *Cytomegalovirus*, *Escherichia coli*).
• Imaging: Abdominal films, chest x-ray, colonoscopy (for minimum necessary distance).
Hospitalize patient.
Give blood products to treat anemia or coagulopathy.
Correct metabolic derangements.
Optimize nutritional status (e.g., via bowel rest and total parenteral nutrition).
Patient is stable and has no indications for emergency surgery
Initiate intravenous (IV) corticosteroid therapy (e.g., methylprednisolone, 40–60 mg/day IV).
Patient is unstable or has indication for emergency surgery (e.g., findings suggestive of perforation, massive gastrointestinal bleeding, or toxic megacolon).
Colitis responds to IV corticosteroid therapy
Switch to oral regimen, then gradually wean patient from steroids.
Initiate maintenance therapy with purine analogues or immunosalicylates.
Colitis does not respond to IV corticosteroid therapy within 5–7 days
Immunosuppressive therapy is not contraindicated
Further immunosuppressive therapy is contraindicated (e.g., because of renal insufficiency, hypocholesterolemia, sepsis, or patient refusal)
Infliximab 5 mg/kg IV infusion. Induction dose at 0, 2, and 6 weeks with 5 mg/kg every 8 weeks afterwards.
Cyclosporine
Initiate IV therapy, initially 4 (or 2) mg/kg/day IV, adjusted as necessary.
Colitis responds to IV immunosuppressive therapy
Continue current treatment.
Consider maintenance therapy with 6-mercaptopurine or azathioprine.
Colitis does not respond to IV immunosuppressive therapy within 4–5 days or complete remission is not achieved within 10–14 days
Initiate surgical treatment. Consider laparoscopic-assisted approach as an option (except in cases of toxic megacolon).
Patient is healthy enough to undergo full procedure at once
Perform proctocolectomy with ileoanal anastomosis.
Patient has perforation, peritonitis, or sepsis
Perform a staged procedure (abdominal colectomy with ileostomy, followed later by proctectomy with ileoanal anastomosis).
Patient does not have obvious perforation, peritonitis, or sepsis but may not be healthy enough to undergo full procedure at once
Choose all-at-once or staged approach on the basis of experience and clinical judgment. Most patients who do not respond to maximal medical therapy are probably best treated with a staged procedure.

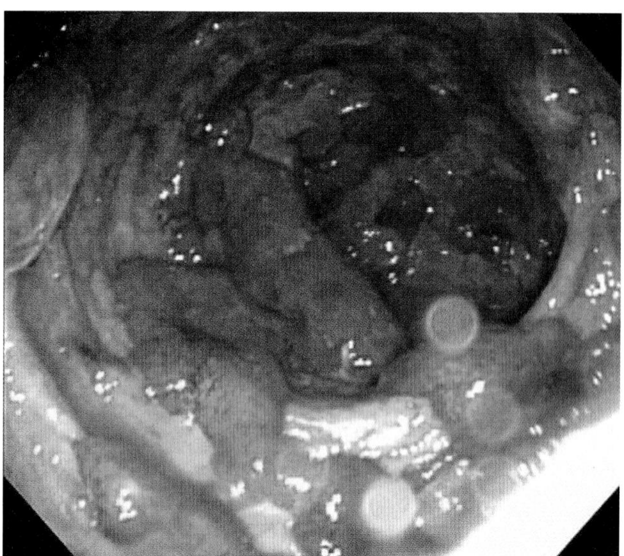

Figure 1 **Sigmoidoscopy demonstrating deep ulcerations in a patient suffering from fulminant ulcerative colitis.**

examination of the colon and rectum in the face of fulminant ulcerative colitis is controversial.[14–16] Colonoscopy with biopsy can provide useful diagnostic information. Reports indicate that in experienced hands, colonoscopy can be performed in patients with severe colitis with little risk.[14,15] In general, however, it is recommended that endoscopic examination be limited to the minimum distance necessary to confirm severe colitis. If an endoscopic examination is to be performed, it is important to minimize the amount of air insufflation as overdistention of the colon may lead to perforation or the development of megacolon. Typical endoscopic findings in fulminant ulcerative colitis are severe inflammation, ulcerations, and mucosal sloughing. Colitis typically is worst in the rectum and continues proximally in a contiguous fashion. Occasionally, the distal rectum may be spared secondary to the use of topical medications such as steroid suppositories. Although these findings help differentiate ulcerative colitis from Crohn disease and indeterminate colitis, the differentiation is probably not important in the setting of fulminant disease, where maximal medical therapy or surgical treatment with subtotal colectomy will be the same regardless of diagnosis. Beyond the diagnostic information, endoscopy can provide useful prognostic information. Carbonell and colleagues noted that the presence of deep extensive colonic ulcerations indicates a low probability for successful medical treatment of fulminant ulcerative colitis, with less than 10% of patients with deep ulcers responding to medical treatment.[14] Such an endoscopic finding thus may assist in the decision to proceed with early surgery if medical therapy does not show rapid and significant improvement [*see Figure 1*].

General Care

All patients with fulminant ulcerative colitis require hospitalization. Blood products should be administered to treat significant anemia or coagulopathy. Metabolic derangements should be corrected.[17] Patients with perforation or massive lower gastrointestinal hemorrhage need emergent operative treatment. More stable patients are initially managed with medical therapy. Narcotics, antidiarrheal agents, and other anticholinergic medications should be avoided as they can precipitate toxic dilation of the colon. Bowel rest typically reduces the volume of diarrhea, but it is not yet clearly established if bowel rest affects the clinical course of the fulminant colitis.[18,19] McIntyre and colleagues reported no significant change in outcome in patients with acute flares of ulcerative colitis managed with total parenteral nutrition (TPN) and bowel rest compared to patients taking enteral nutrition.[19] This study, however, involved varying degrees of severity of colitis such that only a small number of patients with fulminant ulcerative colitis appear to have been included in the study. Conversely, Mikkola and Jarvinen reported a potential clinical advantage to bowel rest and TPN in patients suffering from fulminant ulcerative colitis.[18] The most common approach is to initially place these patients on bowel rest with hyperalimentation. Oral feedings are initiated once symptoms of the fulminant attack begin to improve. Whether patients are maintained on bowel rest or given oral feeds, each patient should always receive adequate nutritional support; hence, TPN should be maintained until the patient is tolerating full enteral feedings.

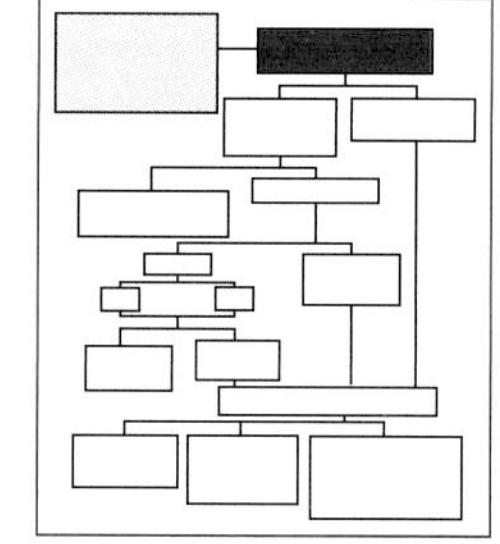

Medical Therapy

The main standard medical therapy for fulminant ulcerative colitis involves the induction of remission with intravenous (IV) corticosteroids or biologics followed by long-term maintenance treatment in the form of purine analogues or biologics for those patients who achieve remission. Cases that are unresponsive to IV steroids are considered for IV cyclosporine and, more recently, infliximab.

STEROIDS

Steroid treatment has been the frontline therapy for acute flares of ulcerative colitis for almost 50 years. Response rates for cases of fulminant ulcerative colitis fall in the range of 50 to 60% when steroids are given over a 5- to 10-day course of treatment.[20,21] Methylprednisolone in a dose of 40 to 60 mg per day, given as a continuous IV infusion, is a common regimen.[5,22–24] The duration of treatment to allow for response from IV steroid therapy has been controversial. Truelove and Witts in 1955 recommended urgent surgery after 5 days if the patient has not responded to IV steroid therapy.[4] This 5-day rule has been widely adopted, but experience suggests that courses up to 7 to 10 days can be safely administered under careful observation to allow for further time for response.[12] Patients who respond to IV steroid therapy are converted to oral steroids, typically prednisone. Corticosteroids, however, should never be used as a long-term maintenance therapy.[5,25] The toxic effects of corticosteroids are related to both the dose and duration of treatment. Severe complications, including diabetes, osteoporosis, mood

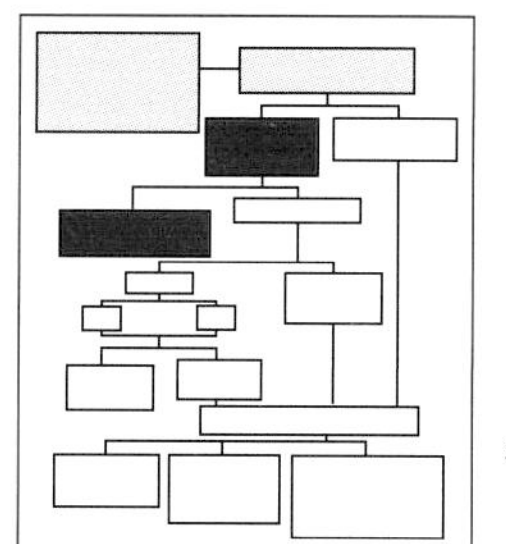

disturbances, and weight gain, are common with extended use of even modest doses of steroids. Patients should be slowly but completely weaned from steroid therapy. Because recurrence of symptomatic colitis occurs in between 40 and 50% of initial responders to IV therapy, maintenance therapy with either purine analogues, immunosalicylates, or biologics should be administered.[5,20] Unfortunately, dependency on corticosteroids is often encountered in patients with ulcerative colitis. In these cases, the dose of steroids cannot be tapered without an increase in disease activity and symptoms. When such patients cannot be taken off steroids within 3 to 6 months, then surgical treatment is indicated.

CYCLOSPORINE

Nonresponders to IV steroid treatment, once universally referred for surgery, may be treated with IV cyclosporine. Cyclosporine is an immunosuppressant macrolide that suppresses the production of interleukin-2 by activated T cells through a calcineurin-dependent pathway.[26] Originally applied as a means of preventing tissue rejection following transplantation, cyclosporine has become the standard for the treatment of steroid-refractory severe ulcerative colitis. The first report of the use of cyclosporine for the treatment of ulcerative colitis was by Gupta and colleagues in 1984.[27] It was not until 10 years later that a randomized placebo-controlled trial of cyclosporine for steroid-refractory ulcerative colitis by Lichtiger and colleagues demonstrated the effectiveness of this agent.[28] This revealed a response rate of 82% with 4 mg/kg of cyclosporine in patients with steroid-refractory ulcerative colitis compared to zero response with continued IV steroid therapy alone. Since this initial report, response rates of 56 to 91% have been reported in the medical literature, confirming cyclosporine as a major advance in the treatment of severe and fulminate ulcerative colitis.[29–31] Dosing and monitoring of cyclosporine are complicated and cumbersome for both physicians and patients, limiting its use. In addition, recurrence of disease after initial remission with cyclosporine is high, with as many as 60% of patients developing recurrent disease.[32] Recurrence rates can be substantially lowered with maintenance therapy with mercaptopurine or azathioprine. With appropriate maintenance therapy, early recurrence of symptoms after successful IV cyclosporine treatment have been recorded as low as 22%.[30,33] Even if disease activity recurs and surgery is necessary, cyclosporine therapy can allow for elective surgical management when the patient is in better general health. This is a clear advantage as urgent surgery for ulcerative colitis carries a much higher risk for complications when compared with surgery performed in a more elective setting.[18,34,35]

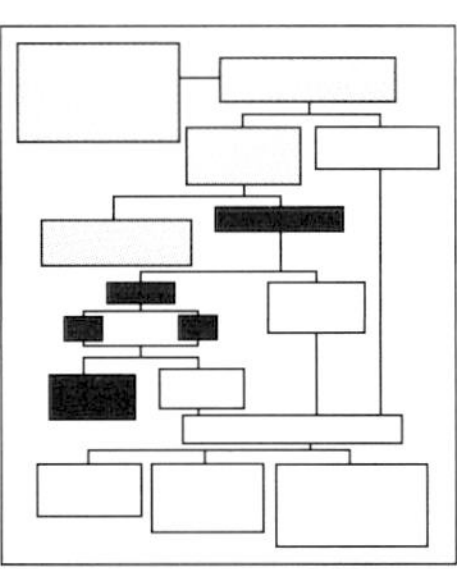

Major side effects associated with cyclosporine treatment include renal insufficiency, opportunistic infections, and seizures. The risk for seizures appears to be highest in patients with hypocholesterolemia. As such, patients with significant (less than 100 mg/dL) hypocholesterolemia should not receive cyclosporine treatment. Hypomagnesemia is commonly seen in patients with fulminant ulcerative colitis undergoing cyclosporine treatment; hence, serum magnesium levels should be closely followed.

Dosing regimens for cyclosporine vary, but patients are typically started on 4 mg/kg per day of IV cyclosporine, with the dose then adjusted to achieve a whole blood level between 150 and 400 ng/mL as measured by high-performance liquid chromatography or radioimmunoassay.[36,37] Higher levels up to 800 ng/mL in whole blood have been cited as acceptable by some investigators.[28] If the patient does not show any improvement within 4 to 5 days or if complete remission is not achieved by 10 to 14 days, surgery is then advised.[12] Most of the side effects from cyclosporine are dose dependent, and some studies have shown that an initial dose of 2 mg/kg per day of IV cyclosporine can also be effective in achieving a remission.[38–40]

INFLIXIMAB

Infliximab is a chimeric monoclonal antibody directed against human tumor necrosis factor (TNF). Infliximab has been used to treat Crohn disease for over 10 years. It was not until 2005, however, that infliximab was approved for use in patients with ulcerative colitis. Potential adverse effects from infliximab include activation of tuberculosis, infusion reactions, hypersensitivity reactions, the development of lymphoma, and infectious complications.[41] Additionally, recent accumulating data suggest that infliximab may significantly increase the risk for postoperative infection and healing complications following surgery for ulcerative colitis.[42,43]

The use of infliximab therapy in the setting of fulminant colitis is controversial. Whereas the data supporting infliximab in the treatment of moderate to moderately severe disease are convincing, the data demonstrating safety and efficacy in the setting of fulminant colitis are limited. Based on the current data, some experts have supported the initiation of infliximab treatment in patients with fulminant colitis who have failed IV steroid therapy.[44] On the other hand, others have advocated the avoidance of infliximab therapy in patients with fulminant colitis.[41] With wider use of anti-TNF therapy for ulcerative colitis, a greater percentage of patients admitted to the hospital with fulminant colitis are likely to already be on infliximab therapy; hence, the decision whether or not to initiate therapy is often moot. Because of the risk of severe complications, infliximab therapy should not be given in combination with cyclosporine therapy.[45]

Because of the increased risk for anastomotic leak and pelvic sepsis in patients undergoing the ileoanal procedure while on anti-TNF therapy, patients with fulminant or severe ulcerative colitis should have a staged abdominal colectomy prior to the ileoanal procedure if they are being treated with infliximab. The negative effect of infliximab on wound healing and infection is prolonged and appears to persist beyond 3 to 4 months after the last dose given.[42,43]

The prolongation of medical therapy in patients with severe disease who have already received high doses of corticosteroids has caused concerns that those patients who fail both steroid and subsequent cyclosporine or infliximab therapy may be at high risk for perioperative morbidity and mortality. Current experience, however, has not identified an increased risk for perioperative complications in patients who fail to respond to cyclosporine therapy and thus does not appear to compromise surgical results.[46] Yet recent data on infliximab in ulcerative colitis do demonstrate a trend toward increased number and severity of septic complications.[42,43,46]

Surgical Therapy

INDICATIONS FOR SURGERY

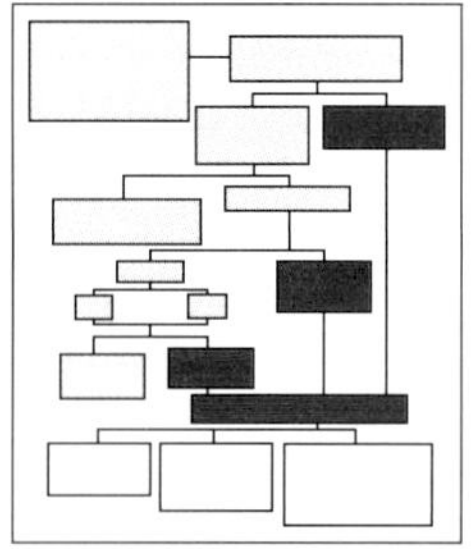

The indications for surgery in a patient suffering from fulminant ulcerative colitis are listed in Table 2. When the options for appropriate medical treatment have been exhausted, surgery will, of course, be required. Because most patients suffering from fulminant ulcerative colitis will respond to aggressive medical therapy, an attempt at medical treatment is warranted in almost all cases. Care must be exercised, however, not to overtreat the patient with fulminant ulcerative colitis who is unresponsive or shows minimal response to medical treatment. The immunosuppressive effects of high-dose corticosteroids and IV cyclosporine or infliximab, along with the debilitation of prolonged severe disease, can place the patient at high risk for perioperative complications. If the patient fails to show significant improvement with IV steroids in 5 to 7 days, then the patient should be started on IV cyclosporine or infliximab or referred for surgery.[12] For patients who fail to show improvement on second-line medications within 4 days or fail to achieve remission of major symptoms by 2 weeks, surgery should be undertaken. If symptoms progress during the course of IV therapy or if no sign of improvement occurs, then the patient should be considered for early surgery. Additionally, patients known to have deep longitudinal ulcerations may also be referred for early surgery, given that these patients are more likely to fail IV medical therapy. The decision when best to abandon medical therapy in favor of surgery for patients with fulminant ulcerative colitis is difficult and requires experience and special expertise. Thus, patients with fulminant ulcerative colitis are best managed in a center specializing in inflammatory bowel disease.

Patients with perforation or severe bleeding require urgent surgery.[47] Debilitation from disease and immunosuppression from intensive medical therapy can mask the signs and symptoms of sepsis and peritonitis associated with perforation. When perforation occurs, the risk for perioperative mortality is up to 10 times greater compared to cases of fulminant colitis without perforation.[48] For these reasons, patients with high fever, marked leukocytosis, and persistent tachycardia should be referred for early surgery, independent of other indications of perforation or peritonitis.

Toxic megacolon is an uncommon complication of severe ulcerative colitis. Associated with impending colonic perforation, toxic megacolon requires aggressive management. Two specific parameters are required to confer the diagnosis of toxic megacolon.[49] First, there must be colonic dilatation. Second, the patient should appear "toxic." Patients with mild symptoms of ulcerative colitis can experience colonic dilatation, perhaps associated with a colonic ileus. This is distinctly different from patients with fulminant ulcerative colitis, some degree of generalized toxicity, and colonic dilatation. Patients with fulminant ulcerative colitis should have an abdominal x-ray to assess for colonic dilatation [*see Figure 2*]. Additionally, patients with fulminant ulcerative colitis who develop abdominal distention or have a sudden decrease in the number of bowel movements without signs of significant clinical improvement should also be assessed radiographically for colonic dilatation.

As noted, patients with toxic megacolon should be treated aggressively. Individuals who are otherwise stable may undergo a brief trial of conservative management consisting of eliminating narcotics and anticholinergic agents. Changing the patient's position from side to side, supine to prone, and into the knee-elbow prone position is thought to assist in the expulsion of colonic gas.[50] Patients should be kept NPO, and broad-spectrum IV antibiotics are advocated. Attempts at endoscopic decompression are to be avoided, and blind placement of rectal tubes is ineffective and may be harmful. Patients with

Table 2 **Indications for Operation**
Perforation
Peritonitis
Progressive signs of sepsis
Failure to respond to medical treatment
Inability of tolerate medical treatment
Severe hemorrhage
Toxic megacolon

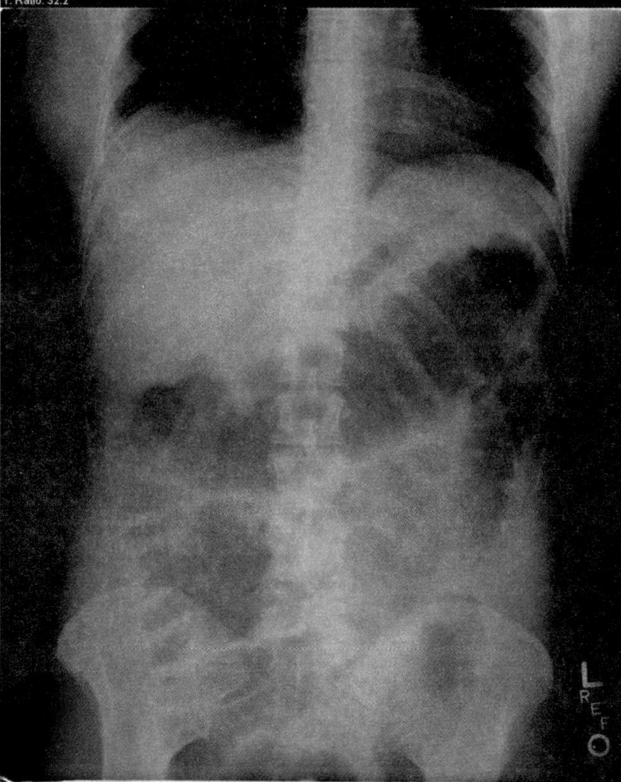

Figure 2 **Abdominal radiograph of a patient with toxic megacolon. Printed with permission of University of Chicago Department of Surgery Archives.**

toxic megacolon who do not rapidly respond to conservative management and those who show signs of peritonitis are otherwise unstable and should undergo urgent surgery.[51]

PREPARATION FOR SURGERY

Patients with fulminant ulcerative colitis who are stable but not responding to medical therapy may have time to prepare for surgery. Patients who are not NPO should be maintained on clear liquids and then kept NPO for 6 to 8 hours prior to surgery. Usually, these patients do not require any form of bowel preparation as they have multiple bloody, liquid bowel movements and will require an emergent colectomy with diversion. If used, bowel preparations may be limited to a rectal washout at the time of surgery. If time allows, patients should be provided with a consultation with an experienced enterostomal therapist and an optimal site for the ostomy should be marked on the abdomen. Prophylactic antibiotics should be given prior to the creation of the surgical incision, and appropriate stress-dose steroids should also be administered.

SURGICAL STRATEGIES

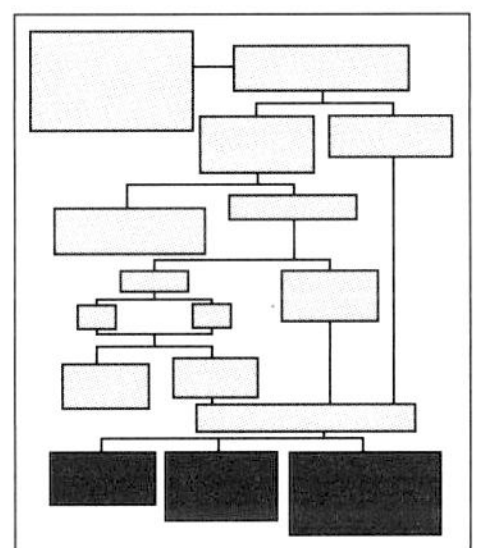

The operative strategies for the treatment of fulminant ulcerative colitis are controversial. Ultimately, almost all patients will end up with a restorative proctocolectomy and an ileoanal anastomosis. Most patients with fulminant ulcerative colitis, however, will have the final surgical goal achieved in multiple steps. The safety of performing an extensive resection with a prolonged and delicate reconstructive procedure in an acutely ill patient is questionable. It has thus been the practice of many to first perform a total abdominal colectomy with an ileostomy, leaving the rectum as a stapled stump or a mucous fistula.[47,48] This approach allows the patient to recover from the acute illness, to wean off the immunosuppressive agents, and to improve the nutritional status. Although the remaining rectal stump will be affected by ulcerative colitis, the activity of disease is greatly diminished with the fecal diversion, and almost all patients can be completely weaned from steroids and other immunosuppressive medications. A subsequent restorative proctectomy with ileoanal anastomosis can then be performed in a more controlled situation.

The benefits of undergoing a staged procedure may be multiple; some studies have demonstrated a reduced risk of anastomotic leak, but findings are not universal. Ziv and colleagues reported excellent long-term results and acceptable short-term morbidity in 12 patients undergoing immediate restorative proctocolectomy with ileal pouch-anal anastomosis.[52] The authors used a liberal definition for fulminant colitis that included patients who may not have been as acutely ill and represent an extraordinarily small proportion of the total number of ileoanal procedures performed at their institution. Harms and colleagues reported on 20 patients undergoing restorative proctocolectomy with ileal pouch-anal anastomosis for the urgent treatment of ulcerative colitis and also reported excellent long-term results and exceptional perioperative morbidity.[53] However, Heyvaert and colleagues reported on 12 patients also undergoing urgent restorative proctocolectomy with ileoanal procedure for ulcerative colitis and noted a 41% anastomotic leak rate compared to an 11% leak rate in patients undergoing ileoanal anastomosis under more controlled conditions.[54] Based on these results, Heyvaert and colleagues counseled against ileoanal anastomosis in the urgent setting. Fukushima and colleagues also noted a higher risk for anastomotic leak (36%) in patients undergoing urgent restorative proctocolectomy with ileoanal anastomosis.[55] This group likewise advised against performing an ileoanal anastomosis in the urgent setting.

Precise parameters under which it is best to stage the procedure with an initial abdominal colectomy have not been clearly defined. It is universally accepted that patients with perforation, peritonitis, or sepsis require a staged procedure. Any patient with suspicion of Crohn colitis or indeterminate colitis should undergo subtotal colectomy to allow for further diagnostic evaluation prior to creation of ileal pouch-anal anastomosis. Beyond this, there is no clear consensus. The available studies addressing this issue unfortunately involve a small number of patients, do not clearly define what is meant by "fulminant" colitis, or do not directly compare results between the two alternative strategies of staged colectomy versus immediate ileoanal anastomosis. Clearly, there is a small subset of patients with symptoms severe enough to require hospitalization who are healthy enough to safely undergo a primary ileoanal anastomosis. On the other end of the spectrum, severely ill patients, that is, most patients with fulminant colitis, should have a staged procedure. Because specific criteria to quantify the risk have not been defined, the decision to stage or not to stage ultimately rests with the clinical judgment of the experienced surgeon. It has been the author's experience, however, that a large majority of patients who fit the criteria of fulminant colitis as noted in Table 1 and have failed maximal medical therapy are best managed with a staged approach.

If the procedure is staged and the proctectomy delayed, there are several advantages to the patient in terms of having time to fully consider lifestyle and reproductive options. Living with an ileostomy for 2 to 4 months ensures that the patient understands the relationship between the timing and quality of oral intake and the frequency and consistency of ileostomy output. This knowledge is extremely helpful to the patient in affecting the frequency, timing, and consistency of bowel movements after completion of all stages associated with a restorative proctectomy and ileoanal pouch procedure. Further, it gives the patient confidence that life with an ileostomy is manageable, a notion that may be important if complications of an ileoanal procedure escalate to the point of considering reversal.

All patients who undergo proctectomy face the risk of decreased fertility and sexual function postoperatively, and consideration of timing of surgery is appropriate. If the rectum is acutely inflamed, dissection may be more difficult and injuries to pelvic nerves and formation of adhesions and abscesses may be greater. As a large percentage of the population with ulcerative colitis are in their reproductive prime, preoperative consideration of issues is appropriate.

In males, erectile dysfunction appears to be altered after damage to the parasympathetic nerves, whereas ejaculatory dysfunction results from sympathetic nerve injury. It is estimated that between 0 and 10% of males experience some degree of sexual dysfunction postoperatively.[56,57] Although studies demonstrate that dysfunction may be transient and relieved with pharmaceutical agents such as sildenafil, this is a significant consideration for males in the peak of their reproductive years.[58] Subtotal colectomy has not been associated with decreased function; therefore, males in need of an urgent procedure may defer the proctectomy to a later time and consider cryopreservation prior to the removal of the rectum.

In women, causes of sexual dysfunction are more difficult to determine, but infertility rates are significantly elevated following proctocolectomy. Fecundity rates, or the percentage of women who become pregnant per unit time, are reduced to one third of baseline populations after proctectomy for ulcerative colitis.[59,60] Adhesions and occlusion of fallopian tubes have been noted in a large number of postoperative patients obstructing normal ovulation and fertilization.[61,62] Although it would be simple to blame surgery alone, patients requiring ileal pouch-anal anastomosis for familial adenomatous polyposis do not experience this radical decrease in fertility postopertively.[63] Although in vitro fertilization has been highly successful in this group, consideration of postponement of proctectomy for family planning may be reasonable in these patients.[64]

SURGICAL TECHNIQUE

Surgical exploration can be performed with a midline or transverse incision. The abdomen should be carefully examined with particular attention given to the small intestine looking for signs of Crohn disease. The colon often shows the changes of colitis with serosal hyperemia, corkscrew vessels, and edema [*see Figure 3*]. Colectomy can be performed in the standard fashion with mesenteric division occurring at a convenient distance from the bowel. Wide mesenteric resection is not necessary.

If a staged colectomy is performed, an ileostomy is created in the standard fashion at the site selected as least inconvenient for the patient preoperatively, and the rectum is left behind either stapled or brought up to the abdominal wall as a mucous fistula. When stapled, it is important that the stump be of the appropriate length. Too short of a pouch can lead to a very difficult proctectomy at the next stage of the procedure sequence. Too long of a stump can run the risk of complications related to persistent disease in the rectum, including bleeding, discharge, and tenesmus. In most cases, the rectum can be safely stapled at the level of the sacral promontory [*see Figure 4*]. When performing the colectomy, the sigmoid branches of the inferior mesenteric artery are divided, whereas the terminal branches of the inferior mesenteric artery are preserved. This will ensure a good blood supply to the remaining rectal stump and aid in the healing of the stapled closure. Preservation of the terminal branches of the inferior mesenteric artery and the superior rectal artery also simplifies the subsequent proctectomy by keeping the pelvic sympathetic nerves free of surrounding scar tissue and by providing a key anatomic landmark that will assist in the location of the appropriate presacral dissection plane at the time of the proctectomy. To staple the proximal rectum safely, the mesenteric and pericolonic fat are removed from the bowel wall. Approximately 2 cm of bowel is prepared in such a manner, and the bowel is then closed with a transverse anastomosis stapler (TIA stapler) using 4.8 mm staples. The bowel is then divided proximal to the staple line. It is important to closely examine the staple line to ensure that the staples are formed properly into two rows of well-formed "B's." The staple line should also be examined to make sure that individual staples are not cutting into the muscularis propria of the bowel. To provide extra assurance against dehiscence, the staple line can be oversewn with interrupted Lembert sutures [*see Figure 4*]. If used, these sutures should be carefully placed so that the anterior and posterior serosal surfaces are approximated without undue tension. In a well-constructed rectal pouch, placement of pelvic drains is not necessary and can be harmful as their placement close to the suture line may promote dehiscence.

In some cases, the colon at the level of the sacral promontory will be affected by deep ulcerations and severe inflammation such that the closure of the rectum at this level may be at high risk for dehiscence [*see Figure 5*]. If the severity of the disease precludes safe closure of the rectal stump, then creation of a mucous fistula should be considered. The mucous fistula does require a longer segment of bowel and thus is

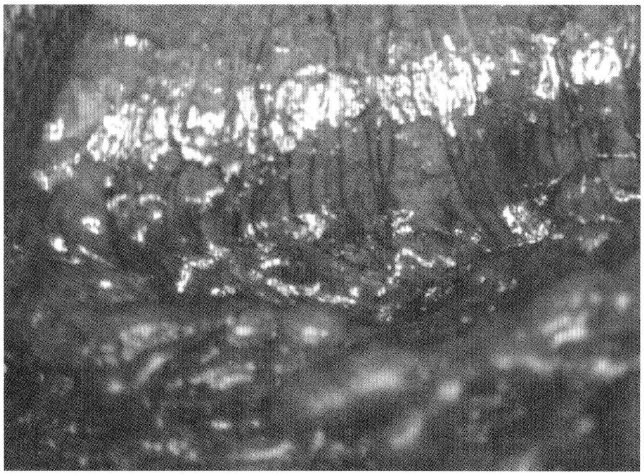

Figure 3 **Intraoperative photograph of colon affected by fulminant ulcerative colitis. Changes on the serosal aspect are typically subtle. Serosal hyperemia with small "corkscrew" vessels is present.**

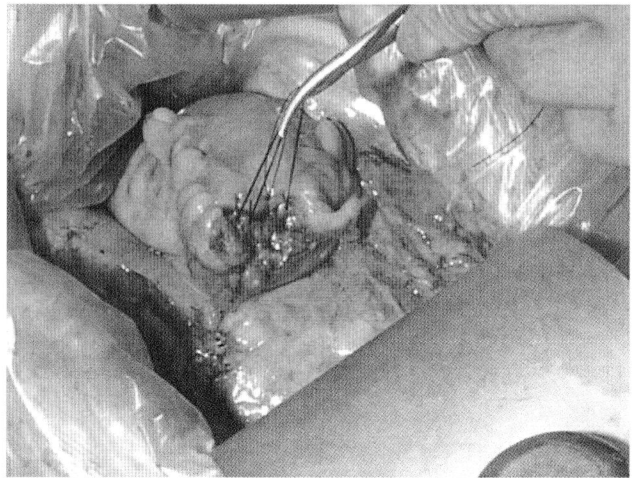

Figure 4 **Hartmann pouch constructed at the level of the sacral promontory. The transverse anastomosis stapler line is reinforced with interrupted silk Lembert sutures.**

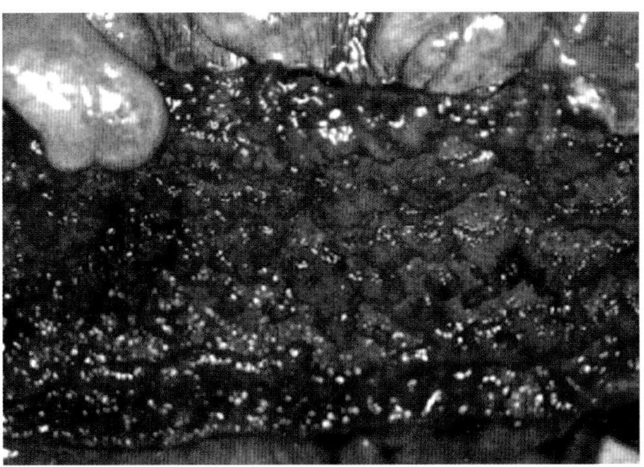

Figure 5 **Surgical specimen showing severe ulceration and inflammation seen with fulminate ulcerative colitis.**

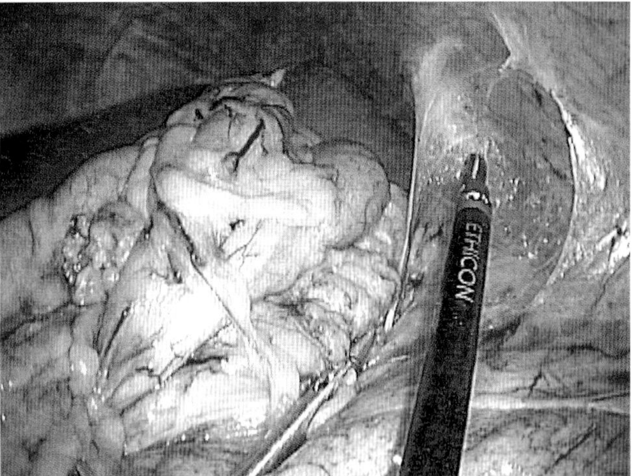

Figure 6 **Laparoscopic colectomy for fulminant ulcerative colitis. Mobilization of the splenic flexure.**

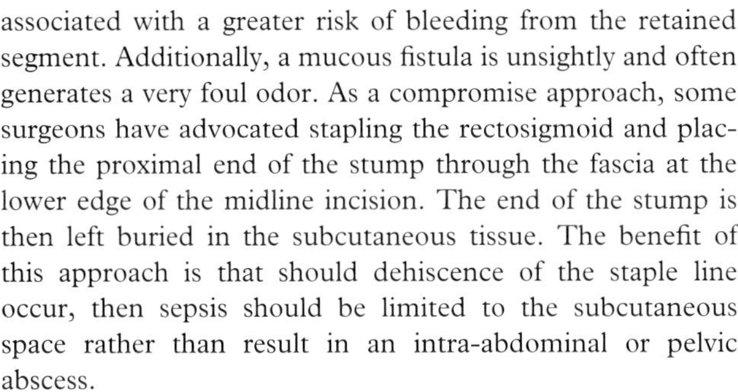

associated with a greater risk of bleeding from the retained segment. Additionally, a mucous fistula is unsightly and often generates a very foul odor. As a compromise approach, some surgeons have advocated stapling the rectosigmoid and placing the proximal end of the stump through the fascia at the lower edge of the midline incision. The end of the stump is then left buried in the subcutaneous tissue. The benefit of this approach is that should dehiscence of the staple line occur, then sepsis should be limited to the subcutaneous space rather than result in an intra-abdominal or pelvic abscess.

If attempts to fashion a secure rectal closure fail, and the remaining rectal stump is too short to bring out as a mucous fistula, then two options remain: an additional inch or two of proximal rectum can be resected and closure of the rectal stump performed lower, sometimes just below the peritoneal reflection. In this situation, closed suction drains should be placed in the deep pelvis and, if possible, the peritoneum closed over the rectal stump. Such a short rectal stump, however, will make finding it during subsequent completion restorative proctectomy and ileoanal anastomosis more difficult. Alternatively, a large Malecott drain, inserted through the lower abdominal wall, can be placed in the proximal rectum and the opening of the rectum can be synched around it with a purse-string suture. In this case, as well as in any case where the closure of the rectal stump seems precarious, transanal placement of a rectal tube to drain rectal secretions and blood may be beneficial in reducing the risk of intra-abdominal spillage of rectal contents or of dehiscence of the stapled rectal stump.

LAPAROSCOPY

Experience with laparoscopic-assisted approaches has demonstrated that abdominal colectomy can be performed safely in patients suffering from ulcerative colitis using these minimally invasive approaches.[65–67] Mobilization of the colon and division of the mesentery can be accomplished laparoscopically with the specimen being removed through a small Pfannenstiel incision [*see Figure 6*]. An end ileostomy is also fashioned with the aid of inspection through the Pfannenstiel incision. Alternatively, the Pfannenstiel incision can be made early on in the procedure and used as a hand assist port and the colon removed using a hand-assisted laparoscopic approach. The clinical advantages of a laparoscopic-assisted approach in the management of fulminate ulcerative colitis have not been fully defined. However, increasing experience with this approach indicates that laparoscopic-assisted colectomy is a safe and reasonable alternative that may well result in shorter hospital stays, decreased postoperative pain, decreased complication rates, and possible reduced adhesions.[68,69] The laparoscopic-assisted approach thus appears to be a reasonable option for most patients suffering from fulminant ulcerative colitis.

Patients suffering from toxic megacolon, however, should be managed with an open surgical approach as the laparoscopic instruments used to grasp the bowel are likely to cause perforation in the severely thinned walls of the dilated colon.

Summary

The optimal management of fulminate ulcerative colitis is challenging. Most patients will respond to medical therapy such that long-term control of disease can be achieved or at least surgery can be undertaken at later, safer, elective conditions. Surgical strategies must be tailored to account for each individual patient's overall physical condition, with most patients who fail medical therapy requiring an abdominalcolectomy as the first step in a staged surgical approach.

Financial Disclosures: None Reported

13 HEREDITARY COLORECTAL CANCER AND POLYPOSIS SYNDROMES

*Jose G. Guillem, MD, MPH, FACS, and John B. Ammori, MD**

The majority of cases of inherited colorectal cancer (CRC) are accounted for by two syndromes: Lynch syndrome and familial adenomatous polyposis (FAP). In both, the predisposition to disease is a germline mutation transmitted in an autosomal dominant fashion. Although the two syndromes are similar in some respects, differences in their phenotypic expression and in the certainty of disease development mandate distinctly different surgical approaches, including the timing and extent of prophylactic procedures in carefully selected patients. In the management of FAP, the role of prophylactic surgery is clearly defined, although the optimal procedure for an individual patient depends on a number of factors. In the management of Lynch syndrome, the indications for prophylactic procedures are emerging.

In addition to classic FAP, attenuated familial adenomatous polyposis (AFAP) and *MUTYH*-associated polyposis (MAP) are two other adenomatous polyposis syndromes being seen with increasing frequency because of increasing genetic testing. AFAP retains autosomal dominant inheritance, whereas MAP is autosomal recessive with increased risk, also described in heterozygote carriers. Given the variability in phenotypes with these syndromes, the role of prophylactic colectomy has to be carefully determined on a case-by-case basis.

Two less common polyposis syndromes, Peutz-Jeghers syndrome (PJS) and juvenile polyposis syndrome (JPS), are also inherited in an autosomal dominant fashion and are associated with a significant risk of CRC. Carefully selected persons affected by these syndromes may also benefit from prophylactic surgical procedures. Current evidence supports a role for prophylactic surgery in JPS but not in PJS.

Recently, hyperplastic polyposis syndrome (HPPS) has been suspected to have a familial basis. There is active ongoing investigation into determining the exact genetic profile, screening, and treatment for this syndrome.

Finally, there are other, less common, inherited hamartomatous polyposis syndromes, such as Cowden disease and Ruvalcaba-Myhre-Smith syndrome. At present, these syndromes appear to be associated with a low risk of CRC, which may not be different from that of the general population; accordingly, the role for prophylactic surgery remains uncertain.[1,2]

Familial Adenomatous Polyposis

FAP is caused by a mutation in the tumor suppressor gene *APC*, located at 5q21. Nearly 80% of FAP patients belong to known FAP kindreds; 10 to 30% have new mutations.[1] More than 300 distinct mutations have been identified within the *APC* gene locus in persons manifesting the FAP phenotype. More than half of the known germline mutations associated with classic FAP phenotype are concentrated in the 5′ region of exon 15.[1] Genotype-phenotype correlative studies have revealed a wide range of phenotypic heterogeneity, ranging from the relatively mild presentation associated with attenuated FAP (discussed below) to the severe presentation associated with mutations downstream of codon 1250, particularly those in codon 1309.

CLINICAL EVALUATION

FAP, which accounts for less than 1% of the annual CRC burden, is characterized by the presence of more than 100 adenomatous polyps of the colorectum, virtually 100% penetrance, and a nearly 100% risk of CRC by the age of 40 if prophylactic colectomy is not performed.[1,3] Extracolonic manifestations are common and include desmoid tumors, osteomas, odontomas, sebaceous and epidermoid cysts, hepatoblastomas, thyroid tumors, congenital hypertrophy of the retinal pigmented epithelium (CHRPE), and periampullary neoplasms.[1]

INVESTIGATIVE FINDINGS

Pathologic Findings

Polyps develop by the age of 20 years in 75% of cases and are typically less than 1 cm in size. In severe FAP, they may carpet the entire surface of the colorectal epithelium. Adenomas may be either pedunculated or sessile and may have tubular, villous, or tubulovillous histology. Microscopic evaluation may reveal innumerable microadenomas within grossly normal-appearing colorectal mucosa. Foci of carcinoma in situ and invasive carcinoma may be found within larger polyps, and the incidence of invasive cancer is proportional to the extent of polyposis. Unlike CRC in the setting of Lynch syndrome, CRC in the setting of FAP is more commonly located on the left side.[1]

Screening and Surveillance

Screening (genetic testing or annual or biennial flexible sigmoidoscopy) for at-risk family members should begin at 10 to 12 years of age [*see Table 1*]. In families with a demonstrated *APC* mutation, informative genetic testing can be carried out with the protein truncation test [*see Table 2*]. This test, which detects foreshortened proteins resulting from truncated *APC* mutations, is approximately 80% sensitive; however, the test results are commonly misinterpreted, even by physicians.[4,5] Patients with the FAP phenotype and a negative protein truncation test should undergo *APC* gene sequencing. It is essential to first determine if the test is informative for that particular family. This is done by confirming that the test is abnormal in a family member

* The authors and editors gratefully acknowledge the contributions of the previous author, Harvey G. Moore, MD, to the development and writing of this chapter.

Table 1 Genetic Basic, Clinicopathologic Features, Diagnosis, Surveillance, and Surgical Management of Hereditary CRC and Polyposis Syndromes

Syndrome	*Genetic Basis*	*Diagnosis*	*GI Manifestations*	*Extracolonic Manifestations*	*Pathologic Features*	*CRC Screening and Surveillance*	*Surgical Management*
FAP	*APC*, 5q21 (> 90%)	≥ 100 adenomatous polyps of colorectum *or* *APC* mutation	Adenomatous polyps of colon and rectum 100% risk of colorectal cancer by age 40 without colectomy	Desmoids Osteomas Odontomas Sebaceous and epidermoid cysts CHRPE Periampullary neoplasms	Tubular, villous, or tubulovillous histology	Consider genetic counseling/ testing Carry out early surveillance with sigmoidoscopy (at age 10–12 yr)[165,166] For at-risk, untested individuals, perform FS every 1–2 yr	If polyposis is confirmed, colectomy is indicated Options include the following: TAC with ileostomy, TAC/IRA, TPC with IPAA
Attenuated FAP	*APC*, 5′ or 3′ end	10–99 adenomatous polyps of colorectum *and* *APC* mutation	Adenomatous polyps of colon and rectum	Desmoids Osteomas Periampullary neoplasms	Tubular, villous, or tubulovillous histology	Consider genetic counseling/ testing If patient is mutation positive or is untested but meets criteria, perform colonoscopy at 20–25 yr (or 10 yr earlier than youngest affected individual), then every 1–2 yr, then annually after age 40	Options include the following: TAC with ileostomy, TAC/IRA, TPC with IPAA
MYH-associated polyposis	Biallelic *MYH* mutation	*MYH*	Adenomatous polyps of colon and rectum 80% risk of CRC by age 70 without colectomy	Desmoids Osteomas Odontomas Sebaceous and epidermoid cysts CHRPE Periampullary neoplasms Breast cancer	Tubular, villous, tubulovillous, or sessile serrated adenomas or hyperplastic polyps	Consider genetic counseling/ testing Biennial colonoscopy beginning at age 18–20 yr	Options include the following: TAC with ileostomy, TAC/IRA, TPC with IPAA
Lynch syndrome	MMR genes: *MLH1* and *MSH2* (80–90%), *MSH6* (10%), *PMS2*	MMR mutation demonstrated *or* Family meets Amsterdam II criteria[86,87]	Possibly few or no colorectal polyps Right-sided tumor (60–70%) MSI-high tumor (80–90%) Synchronous/ metachronous tumors 80% lifetime risk of CRC	Associated tumors of endometrium, small bowel, ureter, or renal pelvis	Adenocarcinoma, frequently mucinous or signet-ring cell histology Solid or cribriform growth pattern Tumor-infiltrating or peritumoral lymphocytes	Consider genetic counseling/ testing If patient is mutation positive or is untested but meets criteria, perform colonoscopy at 20–25 yr (or 10 yr earlier than youngest affected individual), then every 1–2 yr, then annually after age 40[165,166]	Affected patient with identified mutation or meeting Amsterdam criteria: colon cancer or advanced adenoma: perform TAC/ IRA with annual rectal surveillance or segmental colectomy with annual colonoscopy Unaffected patient with identified mutation or meeting Amsterdam criteria: colonoscopy every 1–2 yr

Table 1 Continued

Syndrome	Genetic Basis	Diagnosis	GI Manifestations	Extracolonic Manifestations	Pathologic Features	CRC Screening and Surveillance	Surgical Management
PJS	*LTKB1/ STK11, 19p13.3* (18–63%)	Hamartomas of GI tract *and* At least 2 of the following: small bowel disease, mucocutaneous melanin, family history of PJS	Hamartomatous polyps throughout entire GI tract (small intestine, 90%; colon, 50%) Relative risk of CRC = 84	Mucocutaneous pigmentation (perioral and buccal areas, 95%)	Hyperplasia of smooth muscle of muscularis mucosa Arborization Pseudoinvasion	Consider genetic counseling/ testing Perform colonoscopy starting at age 18, then every 2–3 yr[151]	Perform operative or laparoscopically assisted polypectomy or segmental colectomy for polyps > 1.5 cm that are not amenable to endoscopic removal Perform segmental bowel resection for invasive cancers In the setting of laparotomy, perform intraoperative endoscopy (peroral or via enterotomy) Prophylactic colectomy has no role[154]
JPS	*SMAD4/ DPC4*, 18q21.1 (50%), *BM-PR1A*, 10q22.3	≥ 3 juvenile polyps of colon and juvenile polyps throughout GI tract *or* Any number of polyps with family history of JPS	Multiple hamartomatous polyps throughout gastroduodenum 15% risk of CRC by age 35, 68% risk by age 65	Tumors of stomach, pancreas, duodenum	50–200 polyps Cystic, mucus-filled spaces with epithelial lining Attenuated smooth muscle layer Focal epithelial hyperplasia and dysplasia	Consider genetic counseling/ testing Perform colonoscopy in middle to late teenage years, with EGD and SBS; if results are negative, repeat in 3 yr, then every 3 yr if results remain negative; if results are positive, perform biopsy of polyps and intestinal mucosa	Disease is local and no significant symptoms are present: manage endoscopically, with colonoscopic surveillance every 1–3 yr Disease is diffuse or significant symptoms are present: perform TAC/IRA with rectal surveillance every 1–3 yr
HPS						Consider genetic counseling/ testing	

CHRPE = congenital hypertrophy of retinal pigment epithelium; CRC = colorectal cancer; EGD = esophagogastroduodenoscopy; FAP = familial adenomatous polyposis; FS = flexible sigmoidoscopy; GI = gastrointestinal; IPAA = ileal-pouch-anal anastomosis; JPS = juvenile polyposis syndrome; MMR = mismatch repair; MSI = microsatellite instability; PJS = Peutz-Jeghers syndrome; SBS = small bowel series; TAC/IRA = total abdominal colectomy with ileorectal anastomosis; TPC = total proctocolectomy.

demonstrating the FAP phenotype. Subsequent family members who have a normal genetic analysis may then be discharged from further screening with a nearly 100% certainty that the mutation is absent. However, they should still undergo CRC screening starting at the age of 50 years, as is recommended for average-risk persons. When an *APC* mutation has not previously been identified in the family of an affected person, the patient should be tested first to identify the causative mutation. In families in which the protein truncation test and *APC* gene sequencing fail to provide conclusive information on carrier status, at-risk individuals should continue with the recommended endoscopic surveillance program. Other options for detecting *APC* mutations include linkage analysis and single-stranded confirmation polymorphism.[1]

Genetic counseling is an essential component of the evaluation of patients for FAP. Patients who have a positive genotype or who have adenomatous polyps on sigmoidoscopy should undergo full colonoscopy to establish the extent of polyposis.

Table 2 Availability of Commercial Genetic Testing for Inherited CRC Syndromes

Test	*Approximate Time Frame*	*Approximate Cost*	*Clinical Availability (in United States)*
Protein truncation test (*APC*)	4–6 wk	$1,100; if mutation known, $600	Mayo Clinic, Rochester, MN; (800) 533-1710 Washington University, St. Louis, MO; (314) 454-7601
DNA sequencing, germline *APC*	3 wk	$1,500; if mutation known, $400	Baylor College of Medicine, Houston, TX; (800) 411-GENE Huntington Medical Research Institute, Pasadena, CA; (626) 795-4343 Myriad Inc., Salt Lake City, UT; (800) 469-7423 University of Pennsylvania, Philadelphia, PA; (215) 573-9161
MSI analysis	2–4 wk	$1,150	ARUP Laboratories, Salt Lake City, UT; (800) 583-2787 Baylor College of Medicine, Houston, TX; (800) 411-GENE Mayo Clinic, Rochester, MN; (800) 533-1710 Memorial Sloan-Kettering Cancer Center, New York, NY; (212) 639-5170 Ohio State University, Columbus, OH; (614) 293-7774
IHC MMR (*MLH1, MSH2, PMS2, MSH6*)	2–3 wk	$1,100	Memorial Sloan-Kettering Cancer Center, New York, NY; (212) 639-5170
DNA sequencing, germline MMR mutation (*MLH1, MSH2, MSH6*)	3 wk	$2,950	Baylor College of Medicine, Houston, TX; (800) 411-GENE Huntington Medical Research Institute, Pasadena, CA; (626) 795-4343 Myriad Inc., Salt Lake City, UT; (800) 469-7423 Quest Diagnostics, Inc., San Juan Capistrano, CA; (949) 728-4279 University of Pennsylvania, Philadelphia, PA; (215) 573-9161
MSH6 rearrangement	3 wk	$1,800	Quest Diagnostics, Inc., San Juan Capistrano, CA; (949) 728-4279
PMS2 sequencing and deletion/duplication	4–5 wk	$1,400	ARUP Laboratories, Salt Lake City, UT; (800) 583-2787
MYH	4 wk	$325	Myriad Inc., Salt Lake City, UT; (800) 469-7423 Mayo Clinic, Rochester, MN; (800) 533-1710
MLH1 hypermethylation/ *BRAF*	4–6 wk	$660	Mayo Clinic, Rochester, MN; (800) 533-1710
LKB1/STK11 testing	6–12 wk	$1,176–1,400; if mutation known, $200–350	Ohio State University, Columbus, OH; (614) 293-7774 GeneDx Inc., Gaithersburg, MD; (301) 519-2100
SMAD4/BMPR1A testing	2 mo	$1,234–1,260; if mutation known, $200	Ohio State University, Columbus, OH; (614) 293-7774

CRC = colorectal cancer; IHC = immunohistochemical; MMR = mismatch repair; MSI = microsatellite instability.

MANAGEMENT

Medical Therapy

A number of nonsteroidal antiinflammatory drugs, including sulindac and its metabolite exisulind, have been shown to reduce the number and size of polyps in FAP patients.[6–10] However, long-term use of chemopreventive agents for primary treatment of FAP is not recommended.[11] In a randomized, placebo-controlled, double-blind study of genotype-positive, phenotype-negative patients, the use of sulindac had no effect on the subsequent development of colorectal polyposis.[12] A randomized, placebo-controlled, double-blind study studying a selective cyclooxygenase-2 (COX-2) inhibitor, celecoxib, found a 28% reduction in polyp load at 6 months using a relatively high dose of 800 mg/day.[8] There is no clear advantage in the long term. Furthermore, the development of rectal cancer has been reported in patients whose rectal polyps were effectively controlled with sulindac.[6] Finally, these medications necessitate continued compliance and may be associated with significant side effects.[10] Chemopreventive agents may be useful for reducing polyp load and facilitating endoscopic management of polyps in patients who have an ileorectal anastomosis, are at high risk for polyp development, and refuse proctectomy. In such cases, however, it is still necessary to perform careful surveillance of the residual rectum or the ileoanal pouch every 6 to 12 months.[11]

Surgical Therapy

The timing of surgical treatment depends to some degree on the extent of polyposis in that the risk of CRC is partially dependent on the number of polyps present.[13] Practically speaking, the best time is usually the summer between high school and college. However, in carefully selected cases of mild polyposis, it may be beneficial to delay surgery until after college, particularly to reduce the rate of development of desmoids.[14] Patients with severe polyposis, dysplasia, adenomas larger than 5 mm, and significant symptoms should undergo surgery as soon after diagnosis as is practical.[11] One may consider delaying prophylactic colectomy in very carefully selected asymptomatic patients with small adenomas who have a strong family history of aggressive abdominal desmoids because the risk of desmoid-related complications may outweigh the risk of developing CRC.

There are three basic surgical options for treating FAP: (1) total proctocolectomy (TPC) with permanent ileostomy, (2) total abdominal colectomy with ileorectal anastomosis (TAC/IRA), and (3) proctocolectomy with ileal-pouch-anal anastomosis (IPAA). The optimal procedure for a given patient is determined on a number of factors, including endoscopic and *APC* mutation status, differences in postoperative functional outcome, preoperative anal sphincter status, and patient preference.

TPC TPC with permanent ileostomy is rarely chosen as a primary procedure. More commonly, it is considered an option for patients in whom a proctectomy is required but an IPAA is contraindicated (e.g., those with rectal tumors involving the anal sphincters or those with poor baseline sphincter function) or for patients in whom an IPAA is not technically feasible (e.g., those with desmoid disease and foreshortening of the small bowel mesentery). Occasionally, however, TPC is chosen as a primary procedure in patients whose lifestyle would be compromised by frequent bowel movements.

IPAA versus IRA The choice between IPAA and TAC/IRA is generally more challenging. The main considerations to be taken into account are the risk of rectal cancer development if the rectum is left in site and the differences in functional outcome (and associated quality of life) between procedures.

It has been estimated that the risk of rectal cancer after a TAC/IRA may be as high as 4 to 8% at 10 years and 26 to 32% at 25 years.[15,16] The true risk, however, may be somewhat lower. Most of the studies from which these figures were derived were completed before IPAA became available; thus, patients and physicians may have been more likely to choose IRA even in the setting of more extensive rectal disease, given that TPC with permanent ileostomy was the only other option at the time. The magnitude of risk in an individual patient is related to the overall extent of colorectal polyposis. TAC/IRA may be an option for patients with fewer than 1,000 colorectal polyps and fewer than 20 rectal adenomas because these patients appear to be at relatively low risk for rectal cancer.[11,13,17] Ideally, patients with severe rectal adenomas (> 20 adenomas) or colonic (> 1,000 adenomas) polyposis, an adenoma larger than 3 cm, or an adenoma with severe dysplasia should be treated with IPAA.[11,13]

The risk of secondary rectal excision as a consequence of uncontrollable rectal polyposis or rectal cancer may be estimated on the basis of the specific location of the causative *APC* mutation.[17–19] In a study of 87 FAP patients with an identified *APC* mutation who underwent TAC/IRA, those with a mutation located downstream from codon 1250 had an approximately threefold higher incidence of secondary rectal resection than those with a mutation located upstream of codon 1250.[16] Furthermore, patients with a mutation located between codons 1250 and 1464 had a 6.2-fold higher risk of rectal cancer than those with a mutation before codon 1250 or after codon 1464.[15]

A more recent study examined genotype-phenotype correlations as a potential guide to select patients with FAP for either TAC/IRA or IPAA.[20] A total of 475 patients who underwent TAC/IRA from four national European polyposis registries were examined. Attenuated phenotypes (discussed later in this chapter) were at codons 1 to 157, 312 to 412, and 1596 to 2843; intermediate phenotypes at 158 to 311, 413 to 1249, and 1465 to 1595; and severe phenotype at codon 1250 to 1464. Cumulative risk of secondary proctectomy in the 20 years following TAC/IRA were 10%, 39%, and 61% in the attenuated, intermediate, and severe genotype groups, respectively. Cumulative risks of rectal cancer after TAC/IRA were 3.7%, 9.3%, and 8.3%. These data should be considered when counseling patients regarding surgical options; however, given the phenotypic variability that occurs even among family members, at this time, the choice of surgical procedure should be made based on the clinical phenotype of the patient's disease rather than the patient's genotype.

The risk of polyp and cancer development after index surgery is not limited to patients undergoing TAC/IRA. In patients undergoing IPAA, the pouch-anal anastomosis may be either handsewn after complete anal mucosectomy or stapled to a 1 to 2 cm anal transition zone. Neoplasia may occur at the site of the anastomosis, and the incidence appears to be higher after stapled anastomosis (28 to 31%) than after mucosectomy and handsewn anastomosis (10 to 14%).[21,22] Function, however, may be better after stapled anastomosis.[21] In the case of anal transition zone neoplasia after stapled anastomosis, transanal mucosectomy can sometimes be performed, followed by advancement of the pouch to the dentate line. Of additional concern is the development of adenomatous polyps in the ileal pouch itself, which occurs in 35 to 42% of patients at 7 to 10 years.[23–25]

With respect to postoperative bowel function and associated quality of life, IPAA has been associated with a higher frequency of both daytime and nocturnal bowel movements, a higher incidence of passive incontinence and incidental stooling, and higher postoperative morbidity than TAC/IRA.[26] Accordingly, some authors recommend TAC/IRA for patients with mild rectal polyposis. Other authors, however, have found the two approaches to be equivalent in terms of functional results and quality of life and therefore recommend IPAA for most patients because of the risk of rectal cancer associated with TAC/IRA.[27,28]

Regardless of which procedure is performed, however, lifetime surveillance of the rectal remnant (after TAC/IRA) or the ileal pouch (after IPAA) is required.[11] Endoscopic surveillance of the bowel at intervals of 6 months to 1 year after index surgery is recommended.[4,11] After TAC/IRA, small (< 5 mm) adenomas may be safely observed, with biopsy performed to rule out severe dysplasia. If adenomas increase in number, the frequency of surveillance should be increased, and polyps larger than 5 mm should be removed. When fulguration and polypectomy are repeated over a period of many years, subsequent polypectomy may become difficult, rectal compliance may be reduced, and flat cancers may be hard to identify against a background of scar tissue. The development of severe dysplasia or a villous adenoma larger than 1 cm is considered an indication for proctectomy.[11]

Extracolonic Disease

After TAC/IRA and regular surveillance, the risk of death appears to be three times higher for FAP patients than for age- and sex-matched control populations.[29] The main causes of death after IRA are desmoid disease and upper gastrointestinal (GI) malignancy.

Desmoid disease Desmoids are histologically benign tumors that arise from fibroaponeurotic tissue and occur in 12 to 17% of FAP patients.[11,30,31] Unlike those in the general population, desmoids in FAP patients tend to be intra-abdominal (up to 80% of cases) and mainly occur after abdominal surgical procedures.[30,31] Females who undergo colectomy younger than age 18 are twice as likely to develop intra-abdominal desmoids compared with females operated on after age 18.[14] Patients with *APC* mutations located between codons 1310 and 2011 are at increased risk for these tumors.[18] To avoid the occurrence of desmoids and the possibility of fertility issues, some authors suggest that selected young nulliparous women may benefit from delaying surgery, undergoing laparoscopic surgery, or undergoing TAC/IRA instead of TPC with IPAA.[32,33] Desmoids often involve the small bowel mesentery (> 50% of cases), making complete resection difficult or impossible.[30,31] Not uncommonly, patients present with small bowel obstruction. Morbidity after attempted resection, which often involves the removal of a significant length of small bowel, is substantial. The recurrence rate after attempted resection is also high, and the recurrent disease is often more aggressive than the initial desmoid.[30,31]

Intra-abdominal desmoid formation may be more common after TAC/IRA than after IPAA, and the disease may be more severe after TAC/IRA as well.[18,31,33] When desmoid tumors involve the small bowel mesentery, the mesentery may become foreshortened and thereby render IPAA impracticable, especially in patients undergoing a subsequent completion proctectomy after an initial TAC/IRA.[11] This possibility should be considered when making the choice between TAC/IRA and IPAA as the initial procedure for FAP.

Medical therapy When desmoid tumors are clinically inert, they may be treated with sulindac.[11] Tamoxifen or other antiestrogens may be added for slow-growing or mildly symptomatic tumors.[11,34–36] More aggressive desmoid tumors may be treated with chemotherapy. Vinblastine and methotrexate achieve some degree of response in 40 to 50% of patients.[37] For more rapidly growing desmoids, an antisarcoma agent, such as doxorubicin and dacarbazine, may be administered.[38,39] Radiation therapy may also be effective but can result in substantial small bowel morbidity.

Surgical therapy Surgical treatment of intra-abdominal desmoid tumors is challenging because the natural history is variable and uncertain. Therefore, although surgery should be considered in all cases, it should be reserved for small, well-defined lesions with clear margins.[11] When intra-abdominal desmoids involve the bowel mesentery, they should be treated according to their initial presentation and rate of growth. In patients with desmoid lesions that are refractory to all medical treatments and call for surgical treatment with extensive small bowel resection, small bowel transplantation may be feasible in selected cases.[40] In contradistinction, abdominal wall desmoids that are symptomatic and appear amenable to a complete removal with negative margins should be resected.

Periampullary neoplasms In approximately 80 to 90% of persons with FAP, duodenal adenomas, periampullary adenomas, or both will develop.[41] Of these patients, 14 to 50% will eventually exhibit advanced polyposis, and as many as 6% will eventually have invasive cancer.[1,42–46] Although the risk of periampullary or duodenal cancer in FAP patients is relatively low, it is still several hundred times higher than that in the general population. Among FAP patients, those with *APC* mutations between codons 976 and 1067 appear to have the highest incidence of duodenal adenoma.

Surveillance should begin with side-viewing esophagogastroduodenoscopy (EGD) and biopsy of suspicious polyps either at the age of 20 years or at the time of prophylactic colectomy, whichever is earlier.[11] The purpose of screening is not to remove all disease but to watch for the development of high-grade dysplasia. Duodenal polyposis can be staged using the Spigelman classification [see *Table 3*].[47] The surveillance interval is determined by Spigelman stage: stage 0 or 1, every 5 years; stage 2, every 3 years; stage 3, every 1 to 2 years; stage 4, surgery is recommended.[36] Small tubular adenomas without high-grade dysplasia may be biopsied and observed; adenomas that are larger than 1 cm or that exhibit high-grade dysplasia, villous changes, or ulceration should be removed. Surgical options include endosocopic removal and transduodenal excision, but both approaches have drawbacks: endoscopic ablation generally requires multiple settings, and recurrence is high after either procedure.[42,48] Endoscopic ablation is a reasonable initial approach for most patients without invasive cancer and is an attractive alternative for patients who are unfit for duodenal resection. For patients with persistent or recurrent high-grade dysplasia in the papilla or duodenal adenomas and for patients with Spigelman stage IV disease, pancreas-preserving duodenectomy or pancreaticoduodenectomy is recommended, depending on local expertise.[11,36] The results reported for duodenal resection in patients with malignant lesions are encouraging, with good local control and low morbidity.[42,49,50]

Attenuated Familial Adenomatous Polyposis

An attenuated form of FAP (AFAP) has been described that is associated with fewer adenomas and later development of CRC compared with classic FAP. It is associated

Table 3 Spigelman Classification for Staging Duodenal Polyposis

	Points		
	1	*2*	*3*
Polyp number	1–4	5–20	> 20
Polyp size (mm)	1–4	5–10	> 10
Histology	Tubular	Tubulovillous	Villous
Dysplasia	Mild	Moderate	Severe

No polyp, stage 0; 1 to 4 points, stage 1; 5 to 6 points, stage 2; 7 to 8 points, stage 3; 9 to 12 points, stage 4 with germline mutations at the 5′ and 3′ ends of the *APC* gene, usually codons 78 to 167 and codons 1581 to 2843.[51]

CLINICAL EVALUATION

The AFAP phenotype occurs in less than 10% of FAP patients. The clinical criteria for AFAP are no family members with more than 100 adenomas before the age of 30 years and (1) at least two patients with 10 to 99 adenomas at age over 30 years or (2) one patient with 10 to 99 adenomas at age over 30 years and a first-degree relative with CRC with few adenomas.[52]

INVESTIGATIVE STUDIES

Pathologic Findings

Polyps are typically diagnosed at a mean age of 44 years, with cancers diagnosed at a mean age of 54 to 58 years.[52–54] The youngest reported case of CRC in the setting of AFAP is 24 years.[52] As in classic FAP, adenomas may be either pedunculated or sessile and may have tubular, villous, or tubulovillous histology. However, there is a higher propensity for sessile polyps in AFAP compared with classic FAP. Some authors have reported a predominance of right-sided CRC in the setting of AFAP, whereas others report a more uniform distribution.[54,55] Extracolonic manifestation, such as desmoids, osteomas, and periampullary tumors, occurs in AFAP.[56,57] CHRPE, however, has not been reported in AFAP.

Screening and Surveillance

The cumulative risk of CRC by age 80 has been estimated to be 69%.[54] Given that CRC tends to be right-sided and appears approximately 10 years later than in classic FAP, screening (genetic testing or annual or biennial colonoscopy) for at-risk family members should begin at 18 to 20 years of age. Like classic FAP, AFAP is associated with duodenal polyposis. As such, the duodenum should be surveyed in the same manner as in classic FAP. As in all genetic syndromes, genetic counseling is an essential component of the evaluation of the AFAP patient.

MANAGEMENT

Surgical Therapy

Given that polyposis has a later onset and the risk of CRC is less well established in AFAP, some authors question whether prophylactic colectomy is necessary in all AFAP patients.[53,58–60] In patients with few adenomas, repeated colonoscopic polypectomies may be preferable to surgery.[53,59,60] Colectomy should be considered for those patients whose colonic polyps cannot be controlled endoscopically.[53,58] However, because there is clearly an increased risk of CRC, some authors support prophylactic colectomy.[13,17,19,61,62] One author recommends colectomy at age 20 to 25 as the gold standard.[13] Most recommend TAC/IRA, as opposed to IPAA, in AFAP patients due to the tendency for rectal sparing.[63] One study that examined four national polyposis registries reported a 10% cumulative risk of secondary proctectomy and 3.7% cumulative risk of rectal cancer in 58 AFAP patients following TAC/IRA.[20]

***MYH*-Associated Polyposis**

In 2002, mutY human homologue (MYH)-associated polyposis (MAP) was documented in three siblings with multiple colorectal adenomas and carcinomas.[64] MAP is an autosomal recessive disorder caused by biallelic mutation in the *MYH* gene. MYH is a base excision repair gene that, when absent, leads to a high proportion of somatic G:C to T:A tranversions.[64] Over 80 germline *MYH* mutations have been identified.[65] The most common *MYH* mutations are Y165C and G396D, which are found in 1 to 2% of North Americans and northern Europeans.[66–70] These transversions are found in the *APC* and *KRAS* genes in adenomas of MAP patients.[64,71,72]

CLINICAL EVALUATION

The number of polyps in MAP is highly variable, ranging from a few adenomas to hundreds of adenomas, making it sometimes difficult to distinguish between AFAP and classic FAP. MAP has been diagnosed in over 7% of patients with polyposis (greater than 100 adenomas) and lack of an *APC* mutation.[73] Polyps may be found throughout the colon, but, as in AFAP, there is a slight propensity to CRC proximal to the splenic flexure.[74] It has been suggested that approximately 30% of MAP patients with CRC do not develop polyposis.[75,76] The mean age at CRC diagnosis is between the late forties and early fifties, which is later than classic FAP but similar to AFAP. Synchronous cancers occur in up to 24% of patients.[77] The estimated cumulative risk of CRC in biallelic *MYH* mutation carriers is 80% by age 70.[78] Additionally, there is a twofold increased risk of CRC for heterozygous carriers of *MYH* mutations compared with the general population.[79]

The extracolonic manifestations typical in FAP are also seen in MAP. Duodenal polyps occur in nearly one third of MAP patients, and an increased risk of duodenal adenocarcinoma has been reported.[74] Interestingly, a Dutch registry study reported an increased risk of breast cancer, which occurred in 18% of female patients.[74]

INVESTIGATIVE STUDIES

Pathologic Findings

As in classic FAP, adenomas may be either pedunculated or sessile and may have tubular, villous, or tubulovillous histology. Unlike FAP, patients with MAP may also have hyperplastic polyps (HPs) and sessile serrated adenomas (SSAs), whereas others may have no polyps.[75,76,80] Adenomas are microsatellite stable. Deficiency in *MYH* leads to G:C to T:A transversions in the *APC* and *KRAS* genes. In one study of 17 MAP patients with multiple adenomas, eight were also found to have HPs and SSAs. Three of eight patients with HPs met the criteria for HPPS. *KRAS* mutations were detected in 70% of the HPs and SSAs of MAP patients compared with 17% of controls. *KRAS* mutations were also identified in 23% of adenomas. *APC* mutations with G:C to T:A transversions were observed in 41% of adenomas in MAP patients and not in controls. No *APC* mutations were identified in HPs and SSAs.[80]

The genotype of *MYH* mutations can predict phenotype. Patients with a homozygous G396D mutation are diagnosed with CRC at a mean age of 46 years. Patients with a compound heterozygous mutation (G396D/Y179C) are diagnosed with CRC at a mean age of 52 years, whereas those with a homozygous Y179C mutation have a mean age of 58 years at CRC diagnosis. This information is important when counseling patients with known mutations.

Screening and Surveillance

Given that CRC tends to be right-sided, the European guidelines from the Mallorca group recommend biennial colonoscopy beginning between ages 18 and 20 years. Upper GI endoscopy is advised starting from between 25 and 30 years of age. The recommended screening interval is determined by the Spigelman classification.[36]

MANAGEMENT

Surgical Therapy

Most MAP patients present with an attenuated phenotype and relative sparing of the rectum.[74,81] It is sometimes possible to control these patients with endoscopic polypectomies. If surgery is necessary and the rectum is spared, TAC/IRA is recommended. If rectal polyposis is severe, total proctocolectomy with IPAA is advised.[36] The rectal stump should be examined by yearly surveillance endoscopy.

Lynch syndrome

Lynch syndrome was initially described as an inherited form of CRC. The name *hereditary nonpolyposis colorectal cancer* (HNPCC) syndrome was used to clarify to physicians the nature of the disease. However, over time, there has been recognition that Lynch syndrome is associated with an increased risk of other cancers in addition to CRC. Therefore, the name Lynch syndrome was reintroduced at an international meeting in Bethesda, Maryland, in 2004.[82] Currently, the Lynch syndrome diagnosis is reserved purely for those with a documented mutation in one of the DNA mismatch repair (MMR) genes (*MLH1, MSH2, MSH6, PMS2*).[83,84] A heterodimer of *MSH2/MSH6* recognizes DNA mismatches and recruits other components of the mismatch machinery, such as the MLH1/PMS2 heterodimer. Two genes (*MLH1, MSH2*) are responsible for as many as 80 to 90% of causative germline MMR mutations. A significant percentage of cases may be attributable to large germline deletions that are difficult to detect by means of direct sequencing. It appears that genomic deletions may account for as many as 7% of Lynch syndrome cases defined on the basis of clinical criteria.[85]

CLINICAL EVALUATION

Lynch syndrome is characterized by early-onset CRC, a predominance of lesions proximal to the splenic flexure (60 to 70% of cases), benign and malignant extracolonic tumors, and a predilection for synchronous and metachronous colorectal tumors.[3] Microsatellite instability (MSI), reflecting an accumulation of mutations within regions of repetitive nucleotides called microsatellites, occurs due to a deficiency in the DNA repair secondary to a mutation in the MMR genes. MSI is noted in approximately 80 to 90% of Lynch syndrome–related tumors.[3] The lifetime risk of CRC in Lynch syndrome is approximately 80%.[1,16,86] Endometrial cancer occurs in 43%, gastric cancer in 19%, urinary tract cancer in 18%, and ovarian cancer in 9%.[87]

Deciding who to test for a diagnosis of Lynch syndrome is much more challenging than establishing a clinical diagnosis of FAP in that it requires a careful and detailed family history. The Amsterdam II criteria [*see Table 4*] require that there be three relatives (of which one must be a first-degree relative of the other two) with a Lynch syndrome–related cancer (of the colorectum, endometrium, small bowel, ureter, or renal pelvis), that two or more successive generations be involved, and that at least one relative have a CRC diagnosed before the age of 50.[88,89] Finally, FAP should be excluded.

The Muir-Torre variant of Lynch syndrome is associated with dermatologic manifestations in addition to the other common tumors. This rare variant is most often associated with *MSH2* mutations.[90] Typical skin tumors include sebaceous adenomas and carcinomas, keratoacanthomas, and basal cell carcinomas with sebaceous differentiation.[91]

INVESTIGATIVE STUDIES

Pathologic Findings

Adenomas in Lynch syndrome patients show high-grade dysplasia and villous changes more frequently than adenomas in sporadic CRC patients.[1] Adenomas may also appear at an earlier age and are often larger than those found in the general population. Other pathologic features reported to be more common in Lynch syndrome–related cancers include a mucinous or poorly differentiated histology, a solid or cribriform growth pattern, signet-ring cell tumors, and the presence of tumor-infiltrating and peritumoral lymphocytes. Lynch syndrome–related CRCs have also been shown to have a lower rate of lymph node involvement.[92]

Given that antibodies for MMR proteins are available, immunohistochemical (IHC) testing is becoming more routinely reported as part of the pathology report. Studies assessing the addition of MMR IHC staining have found that approximately 20% of specimens will detect loss of MMR proteins.[93,94] Loss of MMR proteins in tissue can be followed by germline mutation testing. Some tumors show loss of *MSH2* and *MSH6* staining without evidence of germline *MSH2* or *MSH6* mutation. This can be explained by mutations in genes upstream to *MSH2*, such as the epithelial cell adhesion molecule gene (*EpCAM*), also known as *TACSTD1*. Deletions in the last exons of the *EpCAM* gene can lead to *EpCAM/MSH2* fusion transcripts causing the Lynch phenotype in 6.3 to 19% of families without MMR gene mutation.[95–97] Thus, patients who show loss of *MSH2* and/or *MSH6* on IHC without germline mutation should undergo *EpCAM* testing.

Table 4 Clinical Criteria for Diagnosis of Lynch Syndrome

Amsterdam II Criteria	Three or more relatives with a Lynch syndrome-associated cancer (in colorectum, endometrium, small bowel, ureter, or renal pelvis). One first-degree relative of the other two. Two or more successive generations. One CRC diagnosed at age < 50 yr. FAP excluded.

CRC = colorectal cancer; FAP = familial adenomatous polyposis.

Approximately 15 to 20% of sporadic CRC will have MSI. This may occur by epigenetic silencing of the *MLH1* gene by hypermethylation of its promoter region.[98–100] Loss of MLH1 protein by IHC may be seen. *MLH1* hypermethylation is exceedingly rare in sporadic microsatellite stable (MSS) CRC and in Lynch syndrome, in which there is a germline mutation.[98,99] Furthermore, sporadic MSI CRC with MLH1 hypermethylation also shows a high level of a characteristic *BRAF* V600E mutation, in contrast to Lynch syndrome CRC and sporadic MSS CRC.[98,100] Therefore, in selected cases, where there is a loss of MLH1 on IHC testing but a low clinical suspicion for Lynch syndrome, upfront *BRAF* mutation testing can be performed to rule out Lynch syndrome.[101,102]

A founder mutation has been recognized in the Askenazi Jewish population. The mutation is a mutation in a single amplicon, A636P, of the *MSH2* gene.[103] Testing for this single amplicon is rapid, relatively inexpensive, and suggested for Ashkenazi Jewish patients meeting the revised Bethesda criteria because the test result can be obtained in a timely fashion to help decide between segmental versus a TAC.[104]

Screening and Surveillance

CRC patients who have a pedigree suggestive of Lynch syndrome should be offered screening by MSI testing or four-marker IHC panel for loss of MMR protein expression. MSI testing will yield positive results (i.e., an MSI-high tumor) in 80 to 90% of patients belonging to families that meet the Amsterdam criteria.[87] Patients with *MSH6* mutations can test falsely as MSS when using a panel of two mononucleotide and three dinucleotide repeats, but a pentaplex panel comprising five mononucleotide repeats for MSI detection more efficiently discriminates the MSI status of tumors with an *MSH6* defect.[105] IHC for loss of MMR proteins and MSI testing are comparable in sensitivity, but IHC testing is less expensive and can help target a specific mutation for germline testing. Patients with MSI-high tumors or loss of MMR proteins on IHC should undergo testing for germline MMR mutations [*see Table 2*]. However, if there is absence of *MLH1* on IHC testing, *BRAF* mutation testing can be performed prior to germline testing. If there is absence of MLH2 and *MSH6* on IHC testing but no germline mutation is identified, testing can be performed for deletion in the *EpCAM* gene. If tumor tissue is not available, initial germline testing may be considered. As in FAP, a mutation in an affected individual must first be established for testing in at-risk individuals to be informative.[4]

Recommended surveillance in Lynch syndrome includes colonoscopy, initially every 1 to 2 years beginning at the age of 20 to 25 and then annually after age 40.[106,107] Given the increasing evidence of an accelerated adenoma-carcinoma sequence in Lynch syndrome, annual colonoscopy should be strongly considered, especially in families with early-age onset of CRC.[3] Some have recommended that female patients undergo annual transvaginal ultrasonography and measurement of CA 125 levels starting at 25 to 35 years of age, as well as annual endometrial aspiration.[106] Annual EGD is recommended for patients belonging to kindreds with a history of gastric cancer. Finally, ultrasonography and urine cytology every 1 to 2 years may be considered to screen for urinary tract malignancy, although the yield appears to be limited.

MANAGEMENT

Surgical Therapy

Although the development of CRC in persons with Lynch syndrome is not a certainty, the 80% lifetime risk, the 45% rate of metachronous tumors, and the possibility of an accelerated adenoma-carcinoma sequence mandate consideration of prophylactic surgical options.[1,3] Patients who have Lynch syndrome and who have a colon cancer or more than one advanced adenoma should be offered either (1) prophylactic TAC/IRA and yearly flexible sigmoidoscopy or (2) segmental colectomy with yearly colonoscopy.[1,108,109] The first option, however, is open only to patients with normal rectal and anal sphincter function. Although the risk of metachronous colon cancers may be higher after partial colectomy than after TAC/IRA, intensive colonoscopic surveillance and polypectomy may minimize the number of metachronous cancers in the remaining colon.[88,110] Careful surveillance is also necessary after TAC/IRA, given that the risk of metachronous rectal cancer after total colectomy is approximately 12% at 10 to 12 years.[111] However, because of increased risk of metachronous high-risk polyp/carcinoma development and subsequent laparotomy in patients with prior segmental resections, TAC/IRA is our preferred approach and has emerged as the treatment of choice for the index cancer.[112,113]

Lynch syndrome patients with an index rectal cancer that is amenable to a sphincter-preserving resection should be offered either (1) total proctocolectomy with IPAA or (2) low anterior resection (LAR) with primary reconstruction.[11,108] The rationale for total proctocolectomy is based on the 17 to 45% rate of metachronous cancer in the remaining colon associated with an index rectal cancer in Lynch syndrome patients.[114] The decision between the two procedures depends in part on the patient's willingness to undergo intensive surveillance of the retained proximal colon, as well as on the level of bowel function.

Mutation-positive patients with a normal colon and rectum may also be offered prophylactic colectomy in selected cases.[106,115] This approach is supported by the similarity of lifetime cancer risk between patients with germline *APC* mutations and those with MMR mutations, as well as by the observation that TAC/IRA yields less functional disturbance than a prophylactic procedure often recommended for FAP (total proctocolectomy with IPAA).[106,115] An alternative strategy in these patients is to carry out colonoscopic surveillance every 1 to 2 years. This strategy has proven to be cost-effective and to reduce both the rate of CRC development and overall mortality.[88,116–118] There is a risk that CRC may develop in the intervals between colonoscopies. However, when the surveillance interval is shorter than 2 years, tumors generally tend to be found in the early stages, when they are curable.[88,116,118]

A study using a decision analysis model suggested that prophylactic TAC at the age of 25 might offer a survival benefit of 1.8 years when compared with colonoscopic surveillance. The benefit of prophylactic colectomy decreased when surgery was delayed until later in life and became negligible when it was performed at the time of cancer development. However, surveillance provided a greater benefit with respect to quality of life (measured in quality-adjusted life-years).[117] On the basis of this evidence, some surgeons recommended that prophylactic colectomy be performed only in highly selected situations (e.g., when colonoscopic surveillance is not technically possible or when a patient refuses to undergo regular surveillance). Thus, the decision between prophylactic surgery and surveillance for gene-positive unaffected patients is based on many factors, including the penetrance of disease in a family, the age at cancer onset in family members, functional and quality of life considerations, and the likelihood of patient compliance with surveillance.

Extracolonic Disease

Management of extracolonic cancers in Lynch syndrome patients is less well defined. Female patients with a family history of uterine cancer should be offered prophylactic total abdominal hysterectomy (TAH) if their childbearing is complete or if they are undergoing abdominal surgery for other conditions.[11] This recommendation is based on the high (43%) rate of endometrial cancer in mutation-positive persons and on the inefficacy of screening demonstrated in some studies.[89,119] In addition to having a higher incidence of MSS CRC, patients with *MSH6* mutations have a particularly high risk of developing endometrial cancer (71% by the age of 70, with a mean age at diagnosis of 54 years).[120] Oophorectomy should be added to TAH because of the high (9%) incidence of ovarian cancer in Lynch syndrome patients and the frequent coexistence of endometrial cancer with ovarian cancer.[89,121] The optimal timing for prophylactic TAH is unclear. However, given that endometrial cancer has been reported in Lynch syndrome patients before the age of 35, it seems reasonable to begin surveillance at the age of 25 and delay prophylactic surgery until childbearing is complete.[11]

Familial Colorectal Cancer Syndrome Type X

The term *familial colorectal cancer type X* (FCCTX) was coined to describe families meeting the Amsterdam criteria or with an apparent autosomal dominant CRC predisposition who do not have a mutation in the MMR genes. As many as 45% of all families meeting Amsterdam criteria qualify for this syndrome.[122] These families have an increased risk of CRC compared with the general population, but the risk is not as high as that for families with Lynch syndrome.[122] In contrast to Lynch syndrome, CRC in patients with FCCTX is MSS, occurs more commonly on the left side, and presents about 10 years later (mid to late fifties).[123–125] These families do not have other Lynch syndrome–associated tumors.

CLINICAL EVALUATION

The clinical evaluation in a patient presenting with adenoma or nonpolyposis carcinoma and an apparent familial CRC syndrome should proceed as for Lynch syndrome, namely, tissue IHC testing for loss of MMR protein or MSI testing. Patients with loss of an MMR protein or with an MSI tumor should undergo confirmatory germline testing in blood. If these do not confirm a mutation, *APC* and *MYH* gene testing is performed.

INVESTIGATIVE STUDIES

Pathologic Findings

Adenomas and CRC tend to be left-sided. Patients present with less synchronous or metachronous tumors compared with Lynch syndrome patients. A slower progression from adenoma to carcinoma is suggested because there are more adenomas and a greater adenoma/carcinoma ratio than in Lynch syndrome patients.

Screening and Surveillance

FCCTX patients should be screened with colonoscopy beginning 10 years prior to the age at the earliest CRC diagnosis in the family. The frequency of subsequent colonoscopy is determined by the initial findings but should be no longer than 5 years.

MANAGEMENT

Segmental colectomy should be offered for CRC diagnosis. Annual surveillance colonoscopy is performed. The time between colonoscopies can be lengthened if the examination is normal.

Hyperplastic Polyposis Syndrome

HPs are sessile polyps of the colon marked by lengthening and cystic dilation of mucosal glands. HPs are the most common benign colorectal polyp, most commonly located in the distal colon.[126] They have long been thought to be clinically innocuous. More recent data suggest an association of hyperplasic polyposis and CRC.[127] The World Health Organization definition of HPPS includes one of the following: (1) at least five HPs proximal to the sigmoid colon, two of which are greater than 1 cm in diameter, or (2) more than 30 HPs at any site in the colon, or (3) any number of HPs in a patient who has a first-degree relative with HPPS.[128] There have been conflicting data regarding the development of CRC in HPPS by the serrated neoplasia pathway.[129,130] Thus far, no germline mutation has been identified, but multiple factors suggest a hereditary etiology, including familial clustering.[131]

CLINICAL EVALUATION

The number of polyps is variable and may exceed 100 but typically ranges from 40 to 100 polyps.[130,132] CRC develops at a median age between 48 and 55 years but has been diagnosed as early as 11 years of age.[130,133,134] Polyps are distributed throughout the entire colon; however, there appears to be a predilection for right-sided colon cancers.[126]

INVESTIGATIVE STUDIES

Pathologic Findings

No germline mutation has been identified for HPPS. Patients have acquired somatic mutations in either *BRAF* or *KRAS* in HPs, but not in both.[130] Unlike HPs with *KRAS* mutations, HPs with *BRAF* mutations are associated with a high level of DNA methylation in CpG islands.[135] MSI status is variable, but most HPs are microsatellite stable.[130,136] The increased risk of CRC is proposed through the SSA pathway. Dysplastic polyps that are larger than 1 cm are at highest risk for malignant transformation.[131]

Screening and Surveillance

There is no identified germline mutation for testing. There are no specific screening guidelines, although yearly colonoscopy should be performed once the diagnosis is made.

MANAGEMENT

There are no consensus guidelines for the management of HPSS. A logical approach would be to manage these patients in a manner similar to that for Lynch syndrome. Patients who have a colon cancer or more than one advanced adenoma should be offered either (1) prophylactic TAC/IRA and yearly flexible sigmoidoscopy or (2) segmental colectomy with yearly colonoscopy.

Conundrum of Oligopolyposis

In practice, one may encounter a patient who has several adenomatous polyps but without a known genetic syndrome identified. In such a patient, a genetic syndrome should be suspected and a rational workup performed. Initial testing includes *APC* gene testing and MSI testing or IHC for loss of MMR proteins. Patients with loss of MMR protein or MSI tumors should undergo MMR gene testing. If these do not confirm a mutation, *MYH* gene testing is performed.

Treatment should be based on the genetic syndrome, if found. Often, however, no known genetic defect is identified. In these cases, management is determined by the disease phenotype. If there is oligopolyposis, as defined by 5 to 100 polyps without cancer, yearly surveillance colonoscopy with endoscopic treatment as required is an option that would need to be carefully considered on a case-by-case basis. If cancer is identified, segmental colectomy with yearly colonoscopy is recommended. Alternatively, total colectomy with IRA and yearly flexible sigmoidoscopy is an option to be considered, particularly for patients with a strong family history and no indentifiable gene mutation. Similarly for a diagnosis of rectal cancer, segmental resection with yearly colonoscopy is the preferred approach, whereas total proctocolectomy with IPAA is a less often required option. Surgical treatment should be tailored to best address the patient's phenotype.

Peutz-Jeghers Syndrome

Like FAP and Lynch syndrome, PJS follows an autosomal dominant pattern of inheritance with variable penetrance. It is caused in part by mutations in the gene *LKB1/STK11*, which maps to the telomeric region of chromosome 19p13.3. This gene, which codes for a multifunctional serine-threonine kinase, is thought to function as a tumor suppressor gene.[137–140] Germline mutations in *LKB1/STK11* can be demonstrated in 18 to 63% of PJS patients, which suggests the existence of additional PJS loci.[140–143] Genetic testing for PJS can be accomplished through direct sequencing of the *LKB1/STK11* gene [*see Table 2*]; however, such testing is not widely available. In families with an established mutation, genetic testing of at-risk individuals is informative, with a reported accuracy of 95%.[144]

CLINICAL EVALUATION

PJS is a hereditary polyposis syndrome characterized by hamartomas of the GI tract, as well as by mucocutaneous melanin pigmentation. Hamartomatous polyps may occur throughout the GI tract but are most frequently found in the small intestine (90%). Other common sites of hamartomas in PJS are the large intestine (50%) and the stomach; less common sites are the renal pelvis, bile ducts, urinary bladder, lungs, and nasopharynx.[1,145,146] Mucocutaneous pigmentation generally appears during infancy. The perioral and buccal areas are involved in 95% of cases. The periorbital and facial areas, genital region, and acral areas (including the hands and feet) may be involved.[1] The average age at diagnosis of PJS is 22 years in men and 26 years in women.

In as many as 86% of cases, the initial presentation of PJS is small bowel obstruction secondary to intussusception of hamartomas. Other presentations include acute or chronic GI bleeding, biliary and gastric outlet obstruction, and anal protrusion of polyps. The diagnosis of PJS is established by the presence of histologically confirmed hamartomas of the GI tract plus two of the following three criteria: (1) small bowel polyposis, (2) mucocutaneous melanin pigmentation, and (3) a family history of PJS.[147]

Patients with PJS are at significantly increased risk for both intestinal and extraintestinal malignancies. A meta-analysis found that in comparison with the general population, PJS patients were at a 15.2 relative risk for the development of any malignancy.[148] The relative risks for the development of specific cancers were as follows: small bowel, 520; gastric, 213; pancreatic, 132; colorectal, 84; esophageal, 57; ovarian, 27; lung, 17; endometrial, 16; and breast, 15. The cumulative risk for the development of any cancer between the ages of 15 and 64 was 93%.[148] Although the relative risk for the development of CRC was high in this study, the reported magnitude of risk in the individual studies included in the meta-analysis varied considerably.[148] Given that other studies also report a wide range of CRC incidence in these patients, the true incidence of CRC in PJS patients remains unclear.[1] Other cancers associated with PJS are cholangiocarcinomas, testicular neoplasms, and duodenal tumors.[1]

INVESTIGATIVE STUDIES

Pathologic Findings

The polyps seen in PJS are hamartomas characterized by hypertrophy or hyperplasia of the smooth muscle of the muscularis mucosa. Smooth muscle extends into the superficial epithelial layer of the bowel wall in a treelike fashion (a process referred to as arborization). Epithelial cells may become entrapped within the muscle layer, and this "pseudoinvasion" can be mistaken for malignant transformation. Therefore, to diagnose a malignancy in a PJS polyp, cellular atypia or an elevated mitotic rate must be documented.[149] Sporadic PJS polyps do occur, generally secondary to somatic *LKB1/STK11* mutations in one or both alleles, and are histologically identical to their hereditary counterparts.

These sporadic polyps appear not to be associated with an increased risk of GI cancer.[150]

Histologically, areas of cutaneous pigmentation reveal an increased number of melanocytes at the dermal-epidermal junction, with elevated melanin levels in the basal cells. These lesions do not appear to have any malignant potential.

Screening and Surveillance

Clinical screening of asymptomatic persons is facilitated by the appearance of perioral hyperpigmentation during early childhood. Once the diagnosis of PJS is made, patients generally enter a surveillance program. Recommended surveillance for GI disease includes annual serum hemoglobin measurement and EGD and small bowel series every 2 to 3 years, beginning at the age of 8. Colonoscopy is added at age 18. Sigmoidoscopy is usually not employed for surveillance, because the rectum may be spared in some patients with more proximal disease. Upper endoscopic ultrasonography is recommended every 1 to 2 years, whereas computed tomography and/or CA 19-9 may be offered as options. Boys may be offered ultrasonography of the testicles every 2 years until age 12. Women should undergo annual pelvic examinations and Papanicolaou smears beginning at age 21. Starting at age 25, annual transvaginal ultrasonography and serum CA 125, as well as semiannual clinical breast examinations with annual mammography (magnetic resonance imaging may be offered as an alternative), are recommended.[151] The frequency of surveillance examinations may be modified in individual circumstances.

MANAGEMENT

Medical Therapy

COX-2 is known to be overexpressed in the hamartomatous tissue of PJS patients, and there is a correlation between the expression of the COX-2 protein and expression of the *LKB1/STK11* protein in PJS polyps and cancers.[152,153] These findings suggest that COX-2 may be a potential target for chemoprevention of PJS.

Surgical Therapy

Indications for surgical management of PJS include the presence of polyps larger than 1.5 cm that cannot be removed endoscopically, incomplete removal of polyps with adenomatous changes, the development of polyp-associated complications (e.g., obstruction, intussusception, and bleeding), and the management of malignant disease.[154]

Endoscopic polypectomy is generally employed as initial therapy when it is technically feasible. For some polyps, however, operative polypectomy performed through an enterotomy is required. Segmental resection should be avoided. In the context of a laparotomy, intraoperative endoscopy (either peroral or via an enterotomy) allows direct visualization of the remainder of the small bowel and endoscopic clearance of any synchronous polyps. This procedure significantly reduces the need for subsequent laparotomy. The St. Mark's Hospital group in London found that none of 25 patients who underwent enteroscopy during laparotomy required subsequent laparotomy within a 4-year period, whereas 17% of historical control patients who did not undergo intraoperative enteroscopy required repeat laparotomy within a 1-year period.[155]

Laparoscopy-assisted polypectomy and laparoscopic management of small bowel intussusception are additional surgical options.

Given the risk of CRC development in PJS patients, careful colonoscopic surveillance is clearly warranted. However, the role of prophylactic colectomy in patients who are at risk or are mutation positive is unclear. Because the true risk of CRC in these patients is unknown and genetic testing for PJS is not widely available, no recommendations can be made at present regarding the role of prophylactic colectomy in the PJS population.[154]

Juvenile Polyposis Syndrome

Initial evidence suggested that mutations in the *PTEN* gene were responsible for JPS; however, subsequent evidence implicated *SMAD4/DPC4* at 18q21.1 as a more common case, accounting for as many as 50% of familial cases.[156–159] Mutations in *BMPR1A* at 10q22-q23 have also been reported to cause JPS but display variable penetrance [*see Table 2*].[160,161] Clonal genetic alterations are detected in stromal rather than epithelial cells, which suggests that the genetic changes in juvenile polyps originate in the nonepithelial component of the polyps.

CLINICAL EVALUATION

Like PJS, JPS is characterized by the development of multiple hamartomas throughout the GI tract. Isolated juvenile polyps are common in children and are found in approximately 1% of persons younger than 21 years. Juvenile polyposis, however, is much less common. A family history of juvenile polyposis is present in 20 to 50% of JPS patients.[1] Although JPS is an autosomal dominant disorder, its variable penetrance results in a less obvious pattern of inheritance than is seen with FAP or Lynch syndrome.

JPS affects both sexes equally and generally manifests itself during the first or second decade of life (mean age at diagnosis 18.5 years).[1] Common presenting symptoms include chronic anemia, acute GI bleeding, prolapse of rectal polyps, protein-losing enteropathy, and intussusception with or without obstruction.[1]

Extracolonic manifestations of JPS include gastroduodenal and small bowel polyps, malrotation of the midgut, and mesenteric lymphangiomas. Extraintestinal manifestations include clubbing, hypertrophic pulmonary osteoarthropathy, hydrocephalus and macrocephaly, alopecia, cleft lip and palate abnormalities, supernumerary teeth, porphyria, congenital cardiac and arteriovenous malformations, psorias, vitellointestinal duct abnormalities, renal structural abnormalities, and bifid uterus and vagina. JPS is also part of the phenotype for Ruvalcaba-Myhre-Smith syndrome and Gorlin syndrome. Cowden disease, which is characterized by hamartomatous polyposis and is associated with breast and thyroid cancer, may be a phenotypic variant of JPS.[1,161]

The diagnostic criteria for JPS are as follows: (1) the presence of three or more juvenile polyps of the colon; (2) the presence of three or more juvenile polyps throughout the entire GI tract; or (3) the presence of any number of polyps in a patient with a known family history of JPS [*see*

Table 1].[162] The clinical presentation of JPS can be divided into three main clinical variants: (1) JPS of infancy, which is a non–sex-linked recessive condition characterized by failure to thrive, susceptibility to infections, protein-losing enteropathy, bleeding, diarrhea, rectal prolapse, intussusception, and death by the age of 2 years in severe cases; (2) generalized JPS, which occurs in the first decade of life and is characterized by juvenile polyps throughout the GI tract; and (3) JPS of the colon, the most common presentation, which is characterized by colonic polyposis only.[1]

Patients with JPS appear to be at increased risk for GI malignancies, especially CRC. One study estimated the risk of CRC to be 15% by age 35 and 68% by age 65.[163] In another study, GI malignancies (mostly CRC) were diagnosed in 17% of JPS patients at a mean age of 33 years.[164] Associated gastric, pancreatic, duodenal cancers have also been reported. CRCs are thought to arise from malignant transformation of dysplastic polyps.[1] Adenocarcinomas occur, on average, 15 years after diagnosis of JPS and generally are poorly differentiated or mucinous tumors with a poor prognosis.[1]

INVESTIGATIVE STUDIES

Pathologic Findings

The number of polyps seen in JPS patients varies but typically ranges from 50 to 200. The polyps are usually smaller than 1.5 cm but can be as large as 3 cm. Grossly, they appear as red-brown, smooth, pedunculated lesions with lobulated or spherical heads and superficial ulceration; the cut surface demonstrates cystic spaces corresponding to mucus-filled glands. Histologically, polyps are characterized by an inflammatory infiltration of the lamina propria, an attenuated smooth muscle layer, and cystically dilated mucus-filled glands lined by columnar epithelium. Focal epithelial hyperplasia and dysplasia may be present.

Screening and Surveillance

Initial evaluation of the proband and the first-degree relatives, which ideally would be done in the middle to late teenage years, should include colonoscopy, EGD, and a small bowel series. If the initial evaluation yields negative results, a repeat evaluation should be performed in 3 years and then every 3 years thereafter as long as the results remain negative. If disease is encountered, random biopsies of polyps and intervening mucosa should be performed to detect adenomatous and dysplastic changes. Management depends on the presence of symptoms and on the extent and severity of polyposis. When polyposis is mild, endoscopic management may be feasible. Continued annual surveillance after endoscopic management is required; the surveillance interval may be lengthened to 3 years if subsequent evaluations reveal no disease.[1,162]

MANAGEMENT

When polyposis is severe or significant symptoms are apparent, prophylactic colectomy with IRA may be considered for suitable surgical candidates. Although rectal polyposis can generally be managed with rigid or flexible proctoscopy, IPAA may be considered if the polyposis is extensive. Continued annual surveillance of the rectal remnant (after IRA) or the ileal pouch (after IPAA) is required. Surveillance intervals may be increased to 3 years if subsequent evaluations find no evidence of disease.[1,162]

Financial Disclosures: None Reported

References

1. Guillem JG, Smith AJ, Calle JP, Ruo L. Gastrointestinal polyposis syndromes. Curr Probl Surg 1999;36:217–323.
2. Pilarski R. Cowden syndrome: a critical review of the clinical literature. J Genet Couns 2009;18:13–27.
3. Lynch HT, de la Chapelle A. Hereditary colorectal cancer. N Engl J Med 2003;348:919–32.
4. Giardiello FM, Brensinger JD, Petersen GM. AGA technical review on hereditary colorectal cancer and genetic testing. Gastroenterology 2001;121:198–213.
5. Giardiello FM, Brensinger JD, Petersen GM, et al. The use and interpretation of commercial APC gene testing for familial adenomatous polyposis. N Engl J Med 1997;336: 823–7.
6. Cruz-Correa M, Hylind LM, Romans KE, et al. Long-term treatment with sulindac in familial adenomatous polyposis: a prospective cohort study. Gastroenterology 2002;122: 641–5.
7. Giardiello FM, Hamilton SR, Krush AJ, et al. Treatment of colonic and rectal adenomas with sulindac in familial adenomatous polyposis. N Engl J Med 1993;328:1313–6.
8. Steinbach G, Lynch PM, Phillips RK, et al. The effect of celecoxib, a cyclooxygenase-2 inhibitor, in familial adenomatous polyposis. N Engl J Med 2000;342:1946–52.
9. van Stolk R, Stoner G, Hayton WL, et al. Phase I trial of exisulind (sulindac sulfone, FGN-1) as a chemopreventive agent in patients with familial adenomatous polyposis. Clin Cancer Res 2000;6:78–89.
10. Winde G, Schmid KW, Schlegel W, et al. Complete reversion and prevention of rectal adenomas in colectomized patients with familial adenomatous polyposis by rectal low-dose sulindac maintenance treatment. Advantages of a low-dose nonsteroidal anti-inflammatory drug regimen in reversing adenomas exceeding 33 months. Dis Colon Rectum 1995;38:813–30.
11. Church J, Simmang C. Practice parameters for the treatment of patients with dominantly inherited colorectal cancer (familial adenomatous polyposis and hereditary nonpolyposis colorectal cancer). Dis Colon Rectum 2003;46:1001–12.
12. Giardiello FM, Yang VW, Hylind LM, et al. Primary chemoprevention of familial adenomatous polyposis with sulindac. N Engl J Med 2002;346:1054–9.
13. Debinski HS, Love S, Spigelman AD, Phillips RK. Colorectal polyp counts and cancer risk in familial adenomatous polyposis. Gastroenterology 1996;110:1028–30.
14. Durno C, Monga N, Bapat B, et al. Does early colectomy increase desmoid risk in familial adenomatous polyposis? Clin Gastroenterol Hepatol 2007;5:1190–4.
15. Bertario L, Russo A, Radice P, et al. Genotype and phenotype factors as determinants for rectal stump cancer in patients with familial adenomatous polyposis. Hereditary Colorectal Tumors Registry. Ann Surg 2000;231: 538–43.

16. Vasen HF, van der Luijt RB, Slors JF, et al. Molecular genetic tests as a guide to surgical management of familial adenomatous polyposis. Lancet 1996;348:433–5.
17. Bulow C, Vasen H, Jarvinen H, et al. Ileorectal anastomosis is appropriate for a subset of patients with familial adenomatous polyposis. Gastroenterology 2000;119:1454–60.
18. Bertario L, Russo A, Sala P, et al. Multiple approach to the exploration of genotype-phenotype correlations in familial adenomatous polyposis. J Clin Oncol 2003;21:1698–707.
19. Wu JS, Paul P, McGannon EA, Church JM. APC genotype, polyp number, and surgical options in familial adenomatous polyposis. Ann Surg 1998;227:57–62.
20. Nieuwenhuis MH, Bulow S, Bjork J, et al. Genotype predicting phenotype in familial adenomatous polyposis: a practical application to the choice of surgery. Dis Colon Rectum 2009;52:1259–63.
21. Remzi FH, Church JM, Bast J, et al. Mucosectomy vs. stapled ileal pouch-anal anastomosis in patients with familial adenomatous polyposis: functional outcome and neoplasia control. Dis Colon Rectum 2001;44:1590–6.
22. van Duijvendijk P, Vasen HF, Bertario L, et al. Cumulative risk of developing polyps or malignancy at the ileal pouch-anal anastomosis in patients with familial adenomatous polyposis. J Gastrointest Surg 1999;3:325–30.
23. Parc YR, Olschwang S, Desaint B, et al. Familial adenomatous polyposis: prevalence of adenomas in the ileal pouch after restorative proctocolectomy. Ann Surg 2001;233: 360–4.
24. Thompson-Fawcett MW, Marcus VA, Redston M, et al. Adenomatous polyps develop commonly in the ileal pouch of patients with familial adenomatous polyposis. Dis Colon Rectum 2001;44:347–53.
25. Wu JS, McGannon EA, Church JM. Incidence of neoplastic polyps in the ileal pouch of patients with familial adenomatous polyposis after restorative proctocolectomy. Dis Colon Rectum 1998;41:552–6; discussion 6–7.
26. van Duijvendijk P, Slors JF, Taat CW, et al. Functional outcome after colectomy and ileorectal anastomosis compared with proctocolectomy and ileal pouch-anal anastomosis in familial adenomatous polyposis. Ann Surg 1999;230: 648–54.
27. Kartheuser AH, Parc R, Penna CP, et al. Ileal pouch-anal anastomosis as the first choice operation in patients with familial adenomatous polyposis: a ten-year experience. Surgery 1996;119:615–23.
28. Van Duijvendijk P, Slors JF, Taat CW, et al. Quality of life after total colectomy with ileorectal anastomosis or proctocolectomy and ileal pouch-anal anastomosis for familial adenomatous polyposis. Br J Surg 2000;87:590–6.
29. Nugent KP, Spigelman AD, Phillips RK. Life expectancy after colectomy and ileorectal anastomosis for familial adenomatous polyposis. Dis Colon Rectum 1993;36: 1059–62.
30. Clark SK, Neale KF, Landgrebe JC, Phillips RK. Desmoid tumours complicating familial adenomatous polyposis. Br J Surg 1999;86:1185–9.
31. Soravia C, Berk T, McLeod RS, Cohen Z. Desmoid disease in patients with familial adenomatous polyposis. Dis Colon Rectum 2000;43:363–9.
32. Elayi E, Manilich E, Church J. Polishing the crystal ball: knowing genotype improves ability to predict desmoid disease in patients with familial adenomatous polyposis. Dis Colon Rectum 2009;52:1762–6.
33. Heiskanen I, Jarvinen HJ. Occurrence of desmoid tumours in familial adenomatous polyposis and results of treatment. Int J Colorectal Dis 1996;11:157–62.
34. Bus PJ, Verspaget HW, van Krieken JH, et al. Treatment of mesenteric desmoid tumours with the anti-oestrogenic agent toremifene: case histories and an overview of the literature. Eur J Gastroenterol Hepatol 1999;11:1179–83.
35. Tsukada K, Church JM, Jagelman DG, et al. Noncytotoxic drug therapy for intra-abdominal desmoid tumor in patients with familial adenomatous polyposis. Dis Colon Rectum 1992;35:29–33.
36. Vasen HF, Moslein G, Alonso A, et al. Guidelines for the clinical management of familial adenomatous polyposis (FAP). Gut 2008;57:704–13.
37. Skapek SX, Hawk BJ, Hoffer FA, et al. Combination chemotherapy using vinblastine and methotrexate for the treatment of progressive desmoid tumor in children. J Clin Oncol 1998;16:3021–7.
38. Lynch HT, Fitzgibbons R Jr, Chong S, et al. Use of doxorubicin and dacarbazine for the management of unresectable intra-abdominal desmoid tumors in Gardner's syndrome. Dis Colon Rectum 1994;37:260–7.
39. Poritz LS, Blackstein M, Berk T, et al. Extended follow-up of patients treated with cytotoxic chemotherapy for intra-abdominal desmoid tumors. Dis Colon Rectum 2001;44: 1268–73.
40. Chatzipetrou MA, Tzakis AG, Pinna AD, et al. Intestinal transplantation for the treatment of desmoid tumors associated with familial adenomatous polyposis. Surgery 2001;129:277–81.
41. Wallace MH, Phillips RK. Upper gastrointestinal disease in patients with familial adenomatous polyposis. Br J Surg 1998;85:742–50.
42. Alarcon FJ, Burke CA, Church JM, van Stolk RU. Familial adenomatous polyposis: efficacy of endoscopic and surgical treatment for advanced duodenal adenomas. Dis Colon Rectum 1999;42:1533–6.
43. Bjork J, Akerbrant H, Iselius L, et al. Periampullary adenomas and adenocarcinomas in familial adenomatous polyposis: cumulative risks and APC gene mutations. Gastroenterology 2001;121:1127–35.
44. Groves CJ, Saunders BP, Spigelman AD, Phillips RK. Duodenal cancer in patients with familial adenomatous polyposis (FAP): results of a 10 year prospective study. Gut 2002;50:636–41.
45. Saurin JC, Gutknecht C, Napoleon B, et al. Surveillance of duodenal adenomas in familial adenomatous polyposis reveals high cumulative risk of advanced disease. J Clin Oncol 2004;22:493–8.
46. Vasen HF, Bulow S, Myrhoj T, et al. Decision analysis in the management of duodenal adenomatosis in familial adenomatous polyposis. Gut 1997;40:716–9.
47. Spigelman AD, Williams CB, Talbot IC, et al. Upper gastrointestinal cancer in patients with familial adenomatous polyposis. Lancet 1989;2:783–5.
48. Soravia C, Berk T, Haber G, et al. Management of advanced duodenal polyposis in familial adenomatous polyposis. J Gastrointest Surg 1997;1:474–8.

116. Jarvinen HJ, Aarnio M, Mustonen H, et al. Controlled 15-year trial on screening for colorectal cancer in families with hereditary nonpolyposis colorectal cancer. Gastroenterology 2000;118:829–34.
117. Syngal S, Weeks JC, Schrag D, et al. Benefits of colonoscopic surveillance and prophylactic colectomy in patients with hereditary nonpolyposis colorectal cancer mutations. Ann Intern Med 1998;129:787–96.
118. Vasen HF, van Ballegooijen M, Buskens E, et al. A cost-effectiveness analysis of colorectal screening of hereditary nonpolyposis colorectal carcinoma gene carriers. Cancer 1998;82:1632–7.
119. Dove-Edwin I, Boks D, Goff S, et al. The outcome of endometrial carcinoma surveillance by ultrasound scan in women at risk of hereditary nonpolyposis colorectal carcinoma and familial colorectal carcinoma. Cancer 2002; 94:1708–12.
120. Hendriks YM, Wagner A, Morreau H, et al. Cancer risk in hereditary nonpolyposis colorectal cancer due to MSH6 mutations: impact on counseling and surveillance. Gastroenterology 2004;127:17–25.
121. Watson P, Butzow R, Lynch HT, et al. The clinical features of ovarian cancer in hereditary nonpolyposis colorectal cancer. Gynecol Oncol 2001;82:223–8.
122. Lindor NM, Rabe K, Petersen GM, et al. Lower cancer incidence in Amsterdam-I criteria families without mismatch repair deficiency: familial colorectal cancer type X. JAMA 2005;293:1979–85.
123. Dove-Edwin I, de Jong AE, Adams J, et al. Prospective results of surveillance colonoscopy in dominant familial colorectal cancer with and without Lynch syndrome. Gastroenterology 2006;130:1995–2000.
124. Mueller-Koch Y, Vogelsang H, Kopp R, et al. Hereditary non-polyposis colorectal cancer: clinical and molecular evidence for a new entity of hereditary colorectal cancer. Gut 2005;54:1733–40.
125. Valle L, Perea J, Carbonell P, et al. Clinicopathologic and pedigree differences in Amsterdam I-positive hereditary nonpolyposis colorectal cancer families according to tumor microsatellite instability status. J Clin Oncol 2007;25: 781–6.
126. Hyman NH, Anderson P, Blasyk H. Hyperplastic polyposis and the risk of colorectal cancer. Dis Colon Rectum 2004;47:2101–4.
127. Jass JR, Whitehall VL, Young J, Leggett BA. Emerging concepts in colorectal neoplasia. Gastroenterology 2002;123: 862–76.
128. Burt RW, Jass JR. Hyperplastic polyposis. In: Hamilton SR, Aaltonen LA, editors. World Health Organization classification of tumors. Pathology and genetics. Tumors of the digestive system. Berlin: Springer-Verlag; 2000.
129. Goldstein NS, Bhanot P, Odish E, Hunter S. Hyperplastic-like colon polyps that preceded microsatellite-unstable adenocarcinomas. Am J Clin Pathol 2003;119:778–96.
130. Carvajal-Carmona LG, Howarth KM, Lockett M, et al. Molecular classification and genetic pathways in hyperplastic polyposis syndrome. J Pathol 2007;212:378–85.
131. Jass JR. Gastrointestinal polyposes: clinical, pathological and molecular features. Gastroenterol Clin North Am 2007;36:927–46, viii.
132. Lage P, Cravo M, Sousa R, et al. Management of Portuguese patients with hyperplastic polyposis and screening of at-risk first-degree relatives: a contribution for future guidelines based on a clinical study. Am J Gastroenterol 2004;99:1779–84.
133. Bengoechea O, Martinez-Penuela JM, Larrinaga B, et al. Hyperplastic polyposis of the colorectum and adenocarcinoma in a 24-year-old man. Am J Surg Pathol 1987;11: 323–7.
134. Keljo DJ, Weinberg AG, Winick N, Tomlinson G. Rectal cancer in an 11-year-old girl with hyperplastic polyposis. J Pediatr Gastroenterol Nutr 1999;28:327–32.
135. Yang S, Farraye FA, Mack C, et al. BRAF and KRAS mutations in hyperplastic polyps and serrated adenomas of the colorectum: relationship to histology and CpG island methylation status. Am J Surg Pathol 2004;28:1452–9.
136. Young J, Barker MA, Simms LA, et al. Evidence for BRAF mutation and variable levels of microsatellite instability in a syndrome of familial colorectal cancer. Clin Gastroenterol Hepatol 2005;3:254–63.
137. Amos CI, Bali D, Thiel TJ, et al. Fine mapping of a genetic locus for Peutz-Jeghers syndrome on chromosome 19p. Cancer Res 1997;57:3653–6.
138. Hemminki A, Markie D, Tomlinson I, et al. A serine/threonine kinase gene defective in Peutz-Jeghers syndrome. Nature 1998;391:184–7.
139. Jenne DE, Reimann H, Nezu J, et al. Peutz-Jeghers syndrome is caused by mutations in a novel serine threonine kinase. Nat Genet 1998;18:38–43.
140. Lim W, Hearle N, Shah B, et al. Further observations on LKB1/STK11 status and cancer risk in Peutz-Jeghers syndrome. Br J Cancer 2003;89:308–13.
141. Boardman LA, Couch FJ, Burgart LJ, et al. Genetic heterogeneity in Peutz-Jeghers syndrome. Hum Mutat 2000;16: 23–30.
142. Jiang CY, Esufali S, Berk T, et al. STK11/LKB1 germline mutations are not identified in most Peutz-Jeghers syndrome patients. Clin Genet 1999;56:136–41.
143. Westerman AM, Entius MM, Boor PP, et al. Novel mutations in the LKB1/STK11 gene in Dutch Peutz-Jeghers families. Hum Mutat 1999;13:476–81.
144. Burt RW. Colon cancer screening. Gastroenterology 2000; 119:837–53.
145. Corredor J, Wambach J, Barnard J. Gastrointestinal polyps in children: advances in molecular genetics, diagnosis, and management. J Pediatr 2001;138:621–8.
146. Keller JJ, Westerman AM, de Rooij FW, et al. Molecular genetic evidence of an association between nasal polyposis and the Peutz-Jeghers syndrome. Ann Intern Med 2002;136: 855–6.
147. Aaltonen LA. Hereditary intestinal cancer. Semin Cancer Biol 2000;10:289–98.
148. Giardiello FM, Brensinger JD, Tersmette AC, et al. Very high risk of cancer in familial Peutz-Jeghers syndrome. Gastroenterology 2000;119:1447–53.
149. Westerman AM, van Velthuysen ML, Bac DJ, et al. Malignancy in Peutz-Jeghers syndrome? The pitfall of pseudo-invasion. J Clin Gastroenterol 1997;25:387–90.
150. Oncel M, Remzi FH, Church JM, et al. Course and follow-up of solitary Peutz-Jeghers polyps: a case series. Int J Colorectal Dis 2003;18:33–5.

151. Giardiello FM, Trimbath JD. Peutz-Jeghers syndrome and management recommendations. Clin Gastroenterol Hepatol 2006;4:408–15.

152. McGarrity TJ, Peiffer LP, Amos CI, et al. Overexpression of cyclooxygenase 2 in hamartomatous polyps of Peutz-Jeghers syndrome. Am J Gastroenterol 2003;98:671–8.

153. Wei C, Amos CI, Rashid A, et al. Correlation of staining for LKB1 and COX-2 in hamartomatous polyps and carcinomas from patients with Peutz-Jeghers syndrome. J Histochem Cytochem 2003;51:1665–72.

154. Chessin DB, Markowitz AJ, Guillem JG. Peutz-Jeghers syndrome. Cancer de Colon, Reto Anus. In: Mauro Rossi B, Nakagawa WT, Ferreira FO, et al., editors. Sao Paulo, Brazil: Lemar and Temedd; 2004.

155. Edwards DP, Khosraviani K, Stafferton R, Phillips RK. Long-term results of polyp clearance by intraoperative enteroscopy in the Peutz-Jeghers syndrome. Dis Colon Rectum 2003;46:48–50.

156. Howe JR, Roth S, Ringold JC, et al. Mutations in the SMAD4/DPC4 gene in juvenile polyposis. Science 1998;280:1086–8.

157. Huang SC, Chen CR, Lavine JE, et al. Genetic heterogeneity in familial juvenile polyposis. Cancer Res 2000;60:6882–5.

158. Kim IJ, Ku JL, Yoon KA, et al. Germline mutations of the DPC4 gene in Korean juvenile polyposis patients. Int J Cancer 2000;86:529–32.

159. Woodford-Richens K, Williamson J, Bevan S, et al. Allelic loss at SMAD4 in polyps from juvenile polyposis patients and use of fluorescence in situ hybridization to demonstrate clonal origin of the epithelium. Cancer Res 2000;60: 2477–82.

160. Sayed MG, Ahmed AF, Ringold JR, et al. Germline SMAD4 or BMPR1A mutations and phenotype of juvenile polyposis. Ann Surg Oncol 2002;9:901–6.

161. Zhou XP, Woodford-Richens K, Lehtonen R, et al. Germline mutations in BMPR1A/ALK3 cause a subset of cases of juvenile polyposis syndrome and of Cowden and Bannayan-Riley-Ruvalcaba syndromes. Am J Hum Genet 2001; 69:704–11.

162. Wirtzfeld DA, Petrelli NJ, Rodriguez-Bigas MA. Hamartomatous polyposis syndromes: molecular genetics, neoplastic risk, and surveillance recommendations. Ann Surg Oncol 2001;8:319–27.

163. Desai DC, Neale KF, Talbot IC, et al. Juvenile polyposis. Br J Surg 1995;82:14–7.

164. Coburn MC, Pricolo VE, DeLuca FG, Bland KI. Malignant potential in intestinal juvenile polyposis syndromes. Ann Surg Oncol 1995;2:386–91.

165. Smith RA, Cokkinides V, Eyre HJ. American Cancer Society guidelines for the early detection of cancer, 2003. CA Cancer J Clin 2003;53:27–43.

166. Winawer S, Fletcher R, Rex D, et al. Colorectal cancer screening and surveillance: clinical guidelines and rationale—update based on new evidence. Gastroenterology 2003;124:544–60.

14 ADENOCARCINOMA OF THE COLON AND RECTUM

Bruce M. Brenner, MD, FACS, and David M. Ota, MD, FACS

Colorectal cancer (CRC) remains a major public health problem throughout the world. In the United States, CRC is the third most frequently diagnosed cancer in both men and women and the second most common fatal cancer (behind lung cancer).[1] During 2008, there were an estimated 108,000 cases of colon cancer and 41,000 cases of rectal cancer in the United States, resulting in 50,000 total deaths.[1] The cost of treating CRC in the United States is believed to be between 5.5 and 6.5 billion dollars a year.[2] Worldwide, the risk of death from CRC is highest in developed countries and especially low in Asia and Africa.[3]

Data from the Surveillance, Epidemiology, and End Results (SEER) program and the National Center for Health Statistics indicate that the overall incidence of and mortality from CRC have been continuously decreasing in the United States since the 1980s among both men and women.[4] They remain generally higher among men than women. Overall, the incidence of and mortality from CRC are highest among African Americans, somewhat lower among European Americans, and lowest among Asian and Hispanic Americans [*see Table 1*].[4] Most CRCs still occur in the distal colon (beyond the splenic flexure), but the incidence of proximal adenocarcinomas relative to that of distal adenocarcinomas has been increasing over the past 30 years [*see Figure 1*].[5] The cause of this shift is not known.

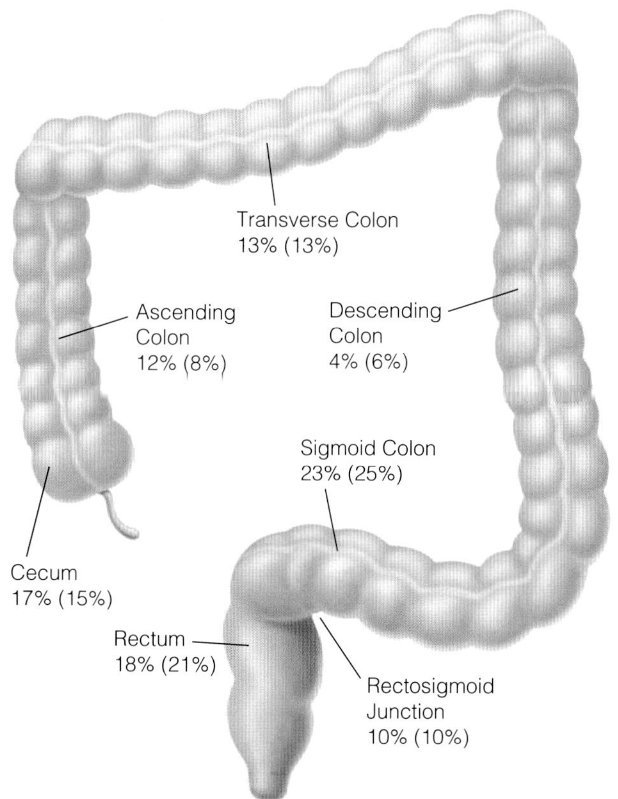

Figure 1 **Shown are the relative frequencies of colorectal cancer for various anatomic subsites of the colon in 1996. For comparative purposes, figures for 1976 are provided in parentheses.**

Genetics

The development of CRC involves a progression from normal mucosa through adenoma to carcinoma.[6] A genetic model of colorectal carcinogenesis was first proposed in the early 1990s that describes a sequence of key mutations driving

Table 1 Incidence and Mortality of Colorectal Cancer by Race and Sex[4]

Race	Incidence* and APC		Mortality* and APC	
	Male	Female	Male	Female
White	60.6 (−2.2)	44 (−1.8)	22.7 (−2.7)	15.3 (−2.6)
African American	69.4 (−1.0)	52.4 (−1.0)	31.8 (−1.6)	22.4 (−1.9)
Asian/Pacific Islander	45.5 (−2.2)	33.6 (−1.4)	14.4 (−2.1)	10.2 (−2.1)
Hispanic	51.5 (−1.0)	36.2 (−1.2)	16.5 (−2.0)	10.9 (−0.9)

*No./100,000.
APC = annual percentage change.

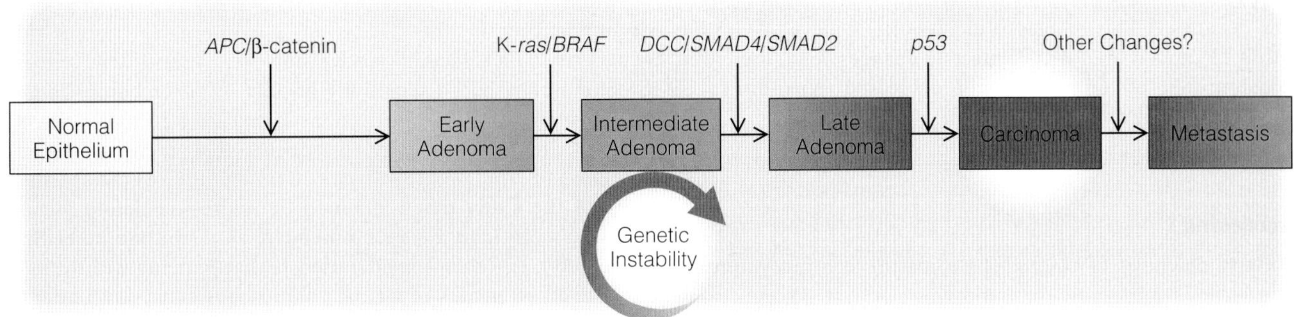

Figure 2 **Diagram illustrates genetic model of colorectal tumorigenesis.**[8]

the process of colorectal carcinogenesis [*see Figure 2*].[7] This progression was recently reevaluated using large-scale genetic sequencing of multiple lesions from an individual patient.[8] Using this "comparative lesion sequencing" approach, it is estimated that it takes approximately 17 years for a large adenoma to progress to invasive malignancy but less than 2 additional years to develop the capacity to metastasize.

The process of colorectal carcinogenesis may involve the accumulation of mutations in both tumor suppressor genes and proto-oncogenes, as well as epigenetic phenomena such as DNA hypermethylation or hypomethylation.[9] The onset of genomic instability increases the mutation rate and accelerates this progression. Inactivation of the adenomatous polyposis coli (*APC*) gene on chromosome 5q is thought to be one of the earliest mutations in sporadic cancers and is seen as a germline mutation in patients with familial polyposis. Mutations in other tumor suppressor genes play an important role in this pathway as well, including mutations in *DCC*, *SMAD2*, and *SMAD4* on chromosome 18q and *p53* on chromosome 17p; these events are thought to occur at a later stage of tumor progression. Mutations in the K-*ras* and *BRAF* oncogenes occur at an intermediate stage. The accumulation of additional mutations (as yet poorly defined) allows metastases to develop.

Microsatellite instability (MSI) is an alternative pathway to genomic instability and subsequent colorectal carcinogenesis. This phenomenon arises from defects in mismatch repair genes, which cause significantly increased mutation rates in comparison with those in normal cells. MSI in hereditary nonpolyposis colorectal cancer (HNPCC) [*see* Risk Factors, *below*] is most commonly attributable to germline mutations in the *hMLH1* and *hMSH2* genes.[10] MSI in sporadic CRC is most frequently associated with hypermethylation of the promoter region of the *hMLH1* gene,[11] which leads to inactivation of the gene and loss of expression of the hMLH1 protein.

Risk Factors

A number of risk factors for CRC have been described, including a family history of cancer or adenomatous polyps, familial CRC syndromes, inflammatory bowel disease (both ulcerative colitis and Crohn's disease), and dietary and lifestyle factors.[12,13] The vast majority of CRCs worldwide are sporadic—that is, they are not associated with known genetic syndromes. In the United States, no more than 5% of CRCs are associated with known genetic syndromes.

In a meta-analysis of studies addressing CRC risk and family history, the relative risk of CRC in those with an affected first-degree relative was 2.25; this figure rose to 4.25 if more than one relative was involved and to 3.87 if CRC was diagnosed before the age of 45.[14] The National Polyp Study found that the relative risk of CRC was 1.78 in first-degree relatives of patients with adenomatous polyps.[15] In another study, the relative risk of CRC was 1.74 in first-degree relatives of patients with adenomatous polyps and was especially high (4.36) in those diagnosed with polyps at or before the age of 50.[16]

The most common of the genetic syndromes known to be associated with CRC is HNPCC, which accounts for the majority of patients with familial CRC. MSI is the characteristic finding of HNPCC, although it is also present in approximately 15% of all sporadic CRCs. HNPCC can be diagnosed clinically on the basis of what are known as the Amsterdam Criteria.[17] Polyposis syndromes (e.g., familial polyposis and juvenile polyposis) account for the remainder of patients with familial CRC syndromes.

As determined by a 2001 meta-analysis, the lifetime risk of CRC for patients with ulcerative colitis is 3.7%, which increases to 5.4% for patients with pancolitis and rises further with greater duration of disease.[18] Despite the common misconception, Crohn's disease may be associated with a similarly increased risk of CRC.[19]

Numerous lifestyle and dietary factors have been put forward as potential causes of increased CRC risk. Lower levels of physical activity and increased body mass are associated with an increased risk of CRC in both men and women.[20] The Western-style diet, which is high in calories and fat and low in fiber, is associated with high rates of CRC. There is evidence that increased dietary intake of calcium may confer some protection against the development of CRC and adenomatous polyps. The Calcium Polyp Prevention Study, a large randomized trial done in the United States, reported a small but statistically significant reduction in the incidence of recurrent colorectal adenomas with dietary calcium supplementation.[21] To date, the evidence from randomized trials has not shown dietary fiber supplementation to have a similar effect. In Japan, where the incidence of CRC has traditionally been low, CRC has become considerably more common in the past few decades.[22] This increased incidence is believed to be the result of post–World War II lifestyle changes (e.g., increased consumption of animal fat and decreased expenditure of energy) that mirror Western habits.

Screening

Early diagnosis of colorectal neoplasms at a presymptomatic stage is important for improving survival. Polypectomy has consistently been shown to decrease the subsequent development of CRC: the National Polyp Study found that the incidence of CRC in patients who underwent colonoscopic polypectomy was as much as 90% less than would otherwise have been expected.[23] Identifying patients with early-stage disease that has not yet metastasized can prevent many CRC-related deaths. Detection of adenomatous polyps prior to the development of invasive cancer has become the focus of screening recommendations. Early detection of and screening for CRC have become important components of routine care and public health programs both in the United States and abroad. The benefits of screening for CRC are especially substantial in patients who are at high risk for CRC (e.g., those with affected first-degree relatives), but even average-risk patients derive significant benefit.

There is no ideal method of screening for CRC that is applicable to all patients. Physical examination is generally not helpful in making the diagnosis; various investigative tests are used instead. In patients at increased or high risk for CRC, colonoscopy is the only recommended screening modality. For average-risk patients, current recommendations divide these tests into those that detect both cancers and premalignant adenomas and those that primarily detect cancer and possibly advanced adenomas.[24] Recommended modalities for CRC screening that are also effective in detecting adenomas include colonoscopy, flexible sigmoidoscopy, double-contrast barium enema (DCBE), and virtual colonoscopy (computed tomographic [CT] colonography). Those that are predominantly effective in detecting cancers and some large adenomas include fecal occult blood testing (FOBT) with guaiac-based or immunochemical tests and stool DNA testing.

Only a limited number of randomized trials have evaluated the above screening modalities. Sigmoidoscopy has been shown to decrease both CRC incidence and mortality, but only in case-control studies,[25] and colonoscopy detects many CRCs in asymptomatic patients that would not be detected by this procedure.[26] FOBT is the sole modality that has consistently been shown to decrease CRC mortality in randomized trials.[27,28] Few studies directly compare different types of FOBT, but fecal immunochemical tests appear to have a higher sensitivity than guaiac-based tests. The specificity may be slightly lower, however, resulting in more patients requiring follow-up colonoscopy.

Virtual colonoscopy, which uses high-resolution CT scanning to image the colon, has been evaluated in at least two multicenter trials in the United States, with varying results.[29,30] One of the studies reported a sensitivity and a specificity of 89% and 80%, respectively, for polyps larger than 6 mm and up to 94% and 96%, respectively, for polyps larger than 10 mm.[29] The sensitivities were equivalent to those of optical colonoscopy in this group of asymptomatic average-risk patients. The second study, however, found that virtual colonoscopy had a sensitivity of only 39% for lesions larger than 6 mm and 55% for lesions larger than 10 mm.[30] Given these divergent findings, it appears that there are issues related to equipment, software, training, and overall sensitivity of the study that remain to be addressed before virtual colonoscopy can be recommended as a routine screening modality. Another consideration is that patients with lesions detected by means of virtual colonoscopy must still undergo optical colonoscopy for treatment or tissue diagnosis.

Fecal DNA assays have been developed to test for mutations in multiple genes known to be involved in colorectal neoplasia and are currently being evaluated in clinical trials.[31] A study comparing fecal DNA testing with a commercially available multigene panel to guaiac-based testing in asymptomatic patients showed both to have a poor sensitivity in detecting cancers and advanced adenomas detected by screening colonoscopy.[32] DNA testing was significantly better, but still only detected 52% of cancers and 18% of advanced adenomas.

Colonoscopy has been consistently shown to be a safe and effective method of CRC screening in asymptomatic, average-risk patients. CT colonography has replaced barium enema as the radiologic screening test of choice but has not been clearly demonstrated to be equivalent to colonoscopy. FOBT and DNA testing are less sensitive and specific than colonoscopy in addition to being relatively ineffective in detecting premalignant polyps. These other modalities may be useful in patients who are unable or unwilling to comply with endoscopic screening.

Many groups have advocated CRC screening, and published guidelines are available from several organizations, including a collaborative guideline published by the American Cancer Society, the US Preventive Services Task Force, and the American College of Radiology.[33] Others include the American College of Gastroenterology[34] and the National Comprehensive Cancer Network (NCCN).[35] All of these guidelines recommend that screening begin at age 50 for average-risk patients with colonoscopy at 10-year intervals. The recommended screening options in patients unwilling or unable to undergo colonoscopy are fairly consistent among the various organizations and include (1) FOBT yearly, (2) flexible sigmoidoscopy every 5 years, (3) yearly FOBT and flexible sigmoidoscopy every 5 years, (4) DCBE every 5 years, and (5) CT colonography every 5 years. In high-risk patients (e.g., those with a family history of CRC), screening may begin at an earlier age—generally at age 40 or 10 years younger than the age of the affected first-degree relative and with shorter, 5-year intervals. There are also specific intensive screening and follow-up regimens for patients with known or suspected familial cancer syndromes.

Clinical Evaluation

As a consequence of the use of screening modalities, patients with CRC are often asymptomatic at diagnosis. Some CRC patients present with occult gastrointestinal bleeding and anemia. Many patients do not exhibit symptoms until relatively late in the course of the disease. The duration of symptoms, however, is not necessarily associated with the stage of the tumor.[36]

The most common symptoms of CRC are bleeding per rectum, abdominal or back pain, and changes in bowel habits or stool caliber. Other symptoms are fatigue, anorexia, weight loss, nausea, and vomiting. Some patients present with acute bowel obstruction or perforation.

Staging and Prognosis

Accurate staging of CRC is extremely important for determining patient prognosis and assessing the need for adjuvant therapy. Traditionally, staging of CRC has been based on modifications of the Dukes classification, which was initially developed as a prognostic tool for rectal cancer in the 1930s.[37] Since this classification was first implemented, it has undergone multiple modifications, of which the most widely used is the modified Astler-Coller system, initially introduced in the 1950s.[38] Currently, the TNM classification, developed by the American Joint Committee on Cancer (AJCC) and the International Union against Cancer (UICC), is the preferred staging system [*see Table 2 and Table 3*].[39] This system takes into account the depth of penetration into the bowel wall (T) [*see Figure 3*], the presence and number of involved mesenteric nodes (N), and the presence of distant metastases (M).

CLINICAL STAGING

Clinical staging is based on the history and the physical examination, endoscopic findings, and biopsy results. If colonoscopy cannot be completed, an air-contrast barium enema study should be performed to evaluate the remainder of the colon. Additional staging information may be obtained by means of imaging studies (e.g., roentgenography, CT, magnetic resonance imaging [MRI], and positron emission tomography [PET]). A chest x-ray is routinely obtained to rule out metastases and prepare for operation.

There is some debate regarding the utility of preoperative CT scans in the management of primary colon cancer. The rationale for obtaining these scans includes evaluation of potential metastatic disease and assessment of the local extent of disease. In a 2002 study of preoperative CT in patients with intraperitoneal colon cancer, however, the results of the imaging changed management in only 19% of patients, and CT had a sensitivity of only 78% for all metastatic disease.[40] Nonetheless, many surgeons routinely perform staging CT in

Table 2 American Joint Committee on Cancer TNM Clinical Classification of Colorectal Cancer

Primary tumor (T)	
T0	No evidence of primary tumor
Tis	Carcinoma in situ, intraepithelial or invasion of lamina propria
T1	Tumor invades submucosa
T2	Tumor invades muscularis propria
T3	Tumor invades through muscularis propria
T4	Tumor invades other organs or perforates visceral peritoneum
Regional lymph nodes (N)	
N0	No regional lymph node metastases
N1	Metastases in 1 to 3 regional lymph nodes
N2	Metastases in 4 or more regional lymph nodes
Distant metastasis (M)	
M0	No distant metastasis
M1	Distant metastasis

Table 3 American Joint Committee on Cancer Staging of Colorectal Cancer[39]

Stage	T	N	M
0	Tis	N0	M0
I	T1, T2	N0	M0
IIA	T3	N0	M0
IIB	T4	N0	M0
IIIA	T1, T2	N1	M0
IIIB	T3, T4	N1	M0
IIIC	Any T	N2	M0
IV	Any T	Any N	M1

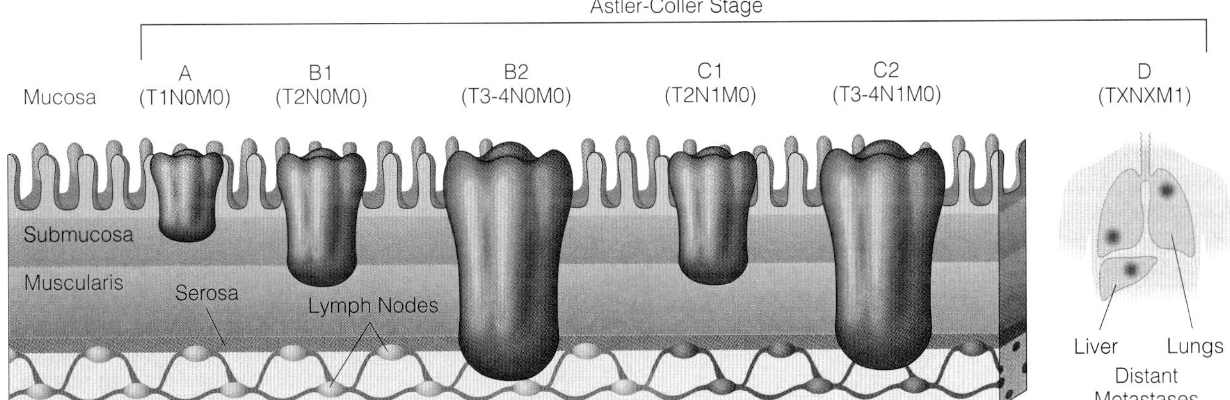

Figure 3 **Classification of colorectal cancer takes into account the depth of tumor penetration and involvement of lymph nodes.**

patients with primary colon cancer. PET is a sensitive study, but its routine use for staging primary CRC is not generally recommended. PET may be considered for high-risk patients in whom the detection of metastases would change initial management.[41]

In cases of rectal cancer, locoregional staging may significantly affect therapeutic decision making. Such staging includes determination of the depth of invasion of the rectal wall and the degree of regional node involvement. Modalities commonly used include CT, MRI, and endoscopic ultrasonography (EUS). In a 2004 meta-analysis that examined the relative utility of each of these studies in rectal cancer staging, EUS proved to be the most accurate technique for evaluating muscularis propria involvement and perirectal tissue invasion.[42] The various techniques were equally accurate in assessing lymph node involvement, with none of them being highly sensitive.

PATHOLOGIC STAGING

Definitive pathologic staging is carried out after surgical exploration and examination of the resected specimen. The final stage of the cancer is then determined on the basis of the TNM system [*see Table 2 and Table 3*]. Survival is correlated with the stage of the tumor [*see Figure 4 and Figure 5*]. In the current (sixth) edition of the AJCC staging system, stage II is subdivided into stages IIA and IIB, and stage III is subdivided into stages IIIA, IIIB, and IIIC on the basis of the extent of wall penetration and the number of nodes involved.[39] These changes were implemented as a result of studies demonstrating differences in survival among these subgroups [*see Figure 6*].[43]

Numerous other criteria have been evaluated as additional prognostic factors in CRC. The degree of lymphatic invasion and the extent of vascular invasion are important adjuncts to the TNM staging system and are incorporated in the current schema.[39] Certain histologic types, including signet-ring and mucinous carcinomas, are associated with poor outcomes. The preoperative serum carcinoembryonic antigen (CEA) level may be an independent prognostic factor that is predictive of resectability and the presence of distant metastases.[44]

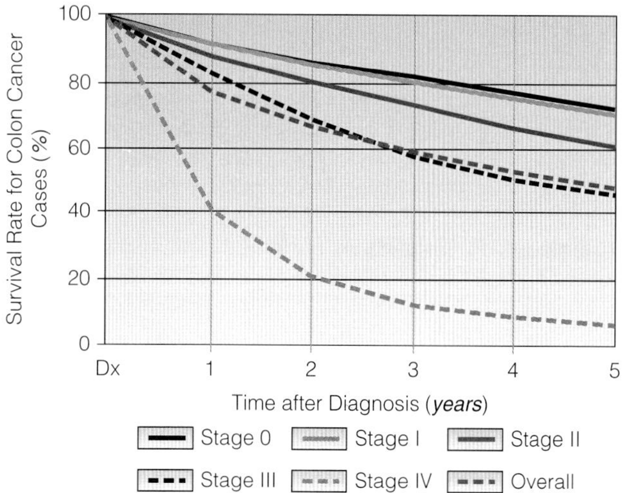

Figure 4 **Shown are 5-year survival rates for cases of colon cancer diagnosed in 1,735 US hospitals in 1995 and 1996.**

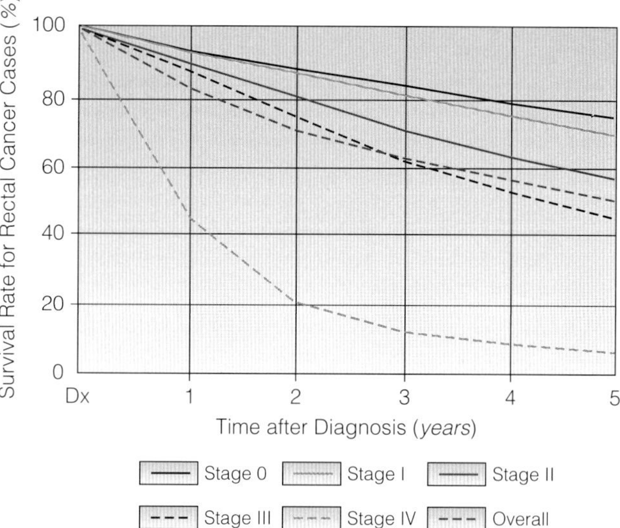

Figure 5 **Shown are 5-year survival rates for cases of rectal cancer diagnosed in 1,683 US hospitals in 1995 and 1996.**

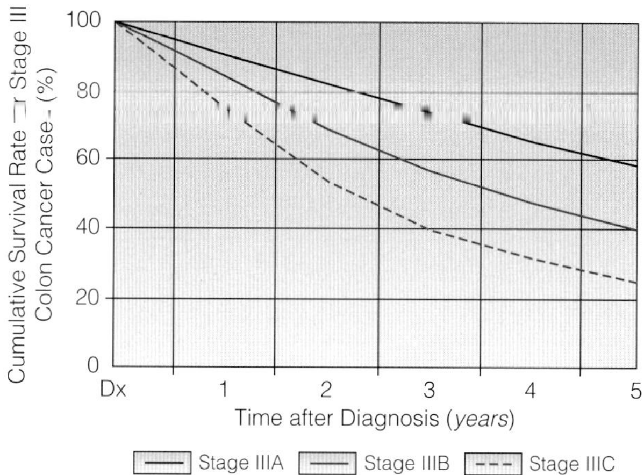

Figure 6 **Shown are 5-year survival rates for cases of stage III colon cancer diagnosed between 1987 and 1993, stratified according to stage III subgroups established by the 6th edition of the *AJCC Staging Manual*.[39]**

MOLECULAR MARKERS

Various molecular markers have been investigated with respect to prognosis and response to therapy in CRC patients. Unfortunately, there are conflicting data on the prognostic impact and clinical utility of most of these markers. As noted [*see* Risk Factors, *above*], MSI is seen in as many as 15% of patients with sporadic CRC. Patients with MSI typically have proximal, poorly differentiated tumors with mucinous or signet-ring components, but they usually exhibit improved overall survival.[45] These patients may be less sensitive to 5-fluorouracil (5-FU)–based chemotherapy.[46]

The long arm of chromosome 18 (18q) harbors at least three candidate tumor suppressor genes, including *DCC*, *SMAD2*, and *SMAD4*. Deletions of chromosome 18q in CRC patients are associated with decreased survival. One study found that patients with stage II cancers and 18q allelic loss had a prognosis similar to that of patients with stage III disease.[47] In addition, *p53* mutations and overexpression are associated with poor outcomes in CRC.[48] Thymidylate synthase is an enzyme active in DNA synthesis that is targeted by 5-FU and similar chemotherapeutic agents. Overexpression of this enzyme is associated with a poor prognosis but also with improved sensitivity to 5-FU–based chemotherapy.[49]

All of these molecular alterations, as well as others (e.g., K-*ras* mutations and 5q deletions), are commonly observed in CRC patients, but further study is required to establish their real prognostic significance.

Management of Colon Cancer

SURGICAL THERAPY

Surgery with curative intent remains the mainstay of therapy for colon cancer [*see Figure 7*]. Complete R0 resection (leaving no gross or microscopic disease) with wide margins along the bowel wall, coupled with regional lymphadenectomy, is the standard of care. The major arterial vessels supplying the segment of the colon containing the tumor should be excised at their origins. A minimum margin of 5 cm of normal bowel on each side of the tumor is considered adequate.

Extent of Resection

The standard extent of resection for various colon cancers has been defined. For tumors of the cecum and the ascending colon, a right hemicolectomy that includes the right branch of the middle colic artery at its origin should be performed. For tumors of the hepatic flexure, an extended right colectomy that includes the entire middle colic artery is indicated. For tumors of the transverse colon, an extended right or left colectomy or a transverse colectomy may be performed. For tumors of the splenic flexure region, a left hemicolectomy is performed, and for sigmoid tumors, a sigmoid colectomy is performed.

In patients who have small or flat tumors or who are undergoing resection after a polypectomy, intraoperative identification of the tumor may be difficult. This is especially true with laparoscopic procedures, in which the bowel often cannot be palpated. If the lesion is in the cecum, the ileocecal valve and the appendiceal orifice are visualized endoscopically, and localization of the tumor is simple. If the lesion is at another location, endoscopic measurements of the distance from the anus or estimates of the location of the tumor may be inaccurate. Endoscopic tattooing, a process in which an agent is injected into the bowel wall submucosally at or near the site of the lesion, has been employed to facilitate intraoperative identification of the tumor site. India ink is the agent most commonly used for this purpose and generally yields excellent results.[50] As an alternative, many institutions use a commercially available sterile suspension of carbon particles, which is also very safe and effective.[51] Intraoperative endoscopy is another option for locating these lesions.

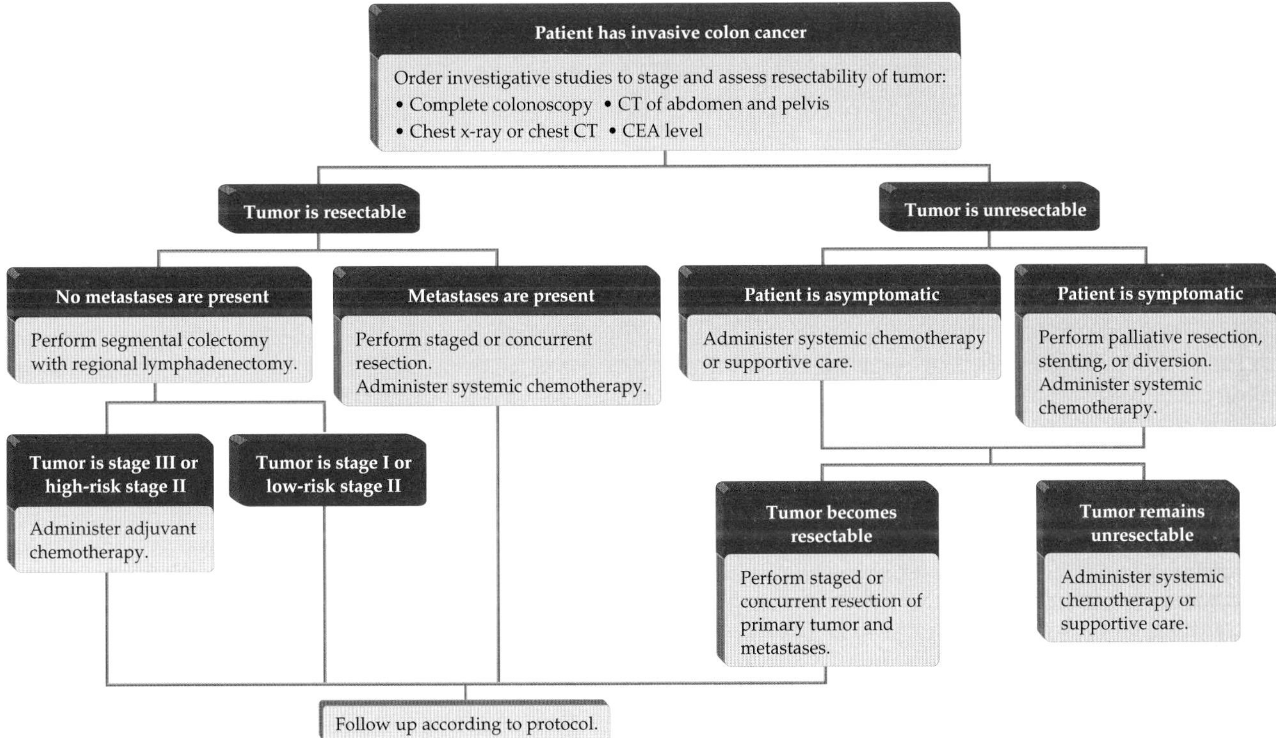

Figure 7 **Algorithm outlines treatment of colon cancer. CEA = carcinoembryonic antigen; CT = computed tomography.**

Surgical Staging

The selection of patients for adjuvant therapy relies heavily on accurate staging. A significant percentage of patients with early-stage node-negative disease present with recurrences or metastases; such a presentation implies that the patients had occult metastatic disease at the time of operation. Surgical resection of CRC should include division of the appropriate mesenteric vessels at their origins, along with resection of the regional nodes. Optimal staging of CRC patients, especially with regard to nodal status, remains controversial. One area of debate is the number of nodes that must be examined to confirm node negativity. This number depends both on the surgeon's technique (i.e., how many nodes were resected) and on the pathologist's efforts to harvest nodes from the specimen. Most groups recommend analysis of at least 12 nodes to confirm node negativity.[52]

Because of the importance of nodal status, ultrastaging of harvested nodes with techniques such as serial sectioning, immunohistochemistry (IHC), and reverse transcriptase polymerase chain reaction (RT-PCR) has been proposed as a means of detecting micrometastases. All of these techniques may result in upstaging of patients who are node negative on standard pathologic analysis, which involves only bivalving the nodes and examining a limited number of sections. The prognostic impact of micrometastases that are detected only by IHC or RT-PCR and are not verified by hematoxylin-eosin staining remains unclear. It is impractical to perform these assays on all nodes harvested; accordingly, the use of lymphatic mapping to identify sentinel lymph nodes (SLNs) has been proposed as a means of selecting a small number of nodes for further analysis.

SLN biopsy in the setting of CRC remains investigational. Lymphatic mapping may be done with either in vivo or ex vivo injection of tracer dye. The dye rapidly diffuses through the lymphatic vessels, and SLNs can be identified and marked in the mesocolon within minutes. This procedure has been shown to be feasible in a number of studies[53]; however, its sensitivity and false negative rates have been variable. In a 2004 multicenter trial, SLN biopsy with serial sectioning had a false negative rate of 54% in patients with node-positive colon cancer.[54] In a large single-institution trial, both SLNs and non-SLNs were studied with serial sectioning and IHC in patients who were node negative on routine pathologic analysis[55]; 19.5% of patients were upstaged by the combination of serial sectioning and IHC of SLNs. These results imply that the main role of this technique may be in upstaging patients who are node negative on routine pathologic analysis. Further study is required before the use of SLN techniques in the context of CRC becomes standard clinical practice.

Occult metastatic disease may also be present in the peritoneal cavity or systemically in the blood or bone marrow at the time of operation. The presence of tumor cells in the peritoneum may be detected by performing cytologic analysis of washings done at the time of operation. In one study, disseminated tumor cells were identified in peritoneal washings or blood in 25% of patients, and their presence was found to be an independent prognostic factor for survival.[56] In another study, patients with positive peritoneal washings had significantly higher rates of local recurrence and peritoneal carcinomatosis but manifested no differences in survival.[57] Again, further study is required before these assays can be routinely used for staging CRC.

Laparoscopic versus Open Colectomy

At present, open colectomy remains the most widely used treatment of resectable colon cancer. Initially, there were concerns about port-site recurrences,[58] but current data suggest that these concerns are unfounded.[59] With respect to comparative cost, data from a subset of patients in the European COlon cancer Laparoscopic or Open Resection (COLOR) trial demonstrated that although the total cost to society from laparoscopic colectomy is similar to that from open colectomy, the costs to the health care system are significantly higher with the former.[60] The Clinical Outcomes of Surgical Therapy (COST) study group, a large, randomized, multicenter trial conducted in the United States, found that laparoscopic-assisted colectomy conferred only minimal (although statistically significant) short-term quality-of-life benefits when compared with open colectomy.[61,62] Cancer-specific outcomes (e.g., recurrence rates, wound recurrences, and overall survival rates) were similar at 3 years with the two approaches, leading to the conclusion that laparoscopic colectomy is an acceptable alternative to open colectomy.[62] This finding was confirmed at 7 years of median follow-up with no difference demonstrated in disease-free or overall survival.[63] The COLOR trial could not rule out a small difference in disease-free survival at 3 years in favor of open colectomy, but the authors concluded that this is "clinically acceptable."[64] The CLASSIC trial from the United Kingdom showed equivalent disease-free and overall survival at 3 years of follow-up.[65] Based on these and other studies, laparoscopic colectomy has become accepted as equivalent to open colectomy for the treatment of colon cancer.

Special Situations

Obstructing and perforated cancers Obstructing and perforated colon cancers are associated with a poor prognosis and with increased surgical morbidity (as a consequence of the need for emergency surgery). Perforation can occur either via direct erosion of the tumor through the wall of the colon or secondary to obstruction with resultant bowel distention proximal to the tumor. Patients with perforated colon cancer are managed with emergency laparotomy, washout, and resection of the primary lesion to prevent further soilage. A diverting stoma is usually indicated, with either a Hartmann pouch or a mucous fistula constructed distally. Select patients may be managed by means of primary anastomosis, with or without a proximal diverting colostomy or ileostomy.

Obstructing right-side cancers (up to the splenic flexure) can usually be treated with resection and primary anastomosis. The traditional emergency treatment of obstructing left-side colon cancers is a diverting colostomy, with or without resection of the lesion. In many such cases, the stoma is never taken down. Some surgeons advocate emergency treatment of these lesions with total abdominal colectomy and ileorectal anastomosis as a means of improving outcomes.[66] Another treatment option is primary resection and anastomosis, with or without on-table intestinal lavage. Yet another option for managing obstructing left-side colon and rectal cancers is the use of colorectal stents with the aim of avoiding emergency surgery. Stents can serve as a bridge to definitive resection by decompressing the colon and thereby allowing subsequent bowel preparation. In patients with advanced disease, stents may also be employed for palliation as an alternative to surgical resection or a diverting stoma.

Synchronous primary colorectal cancers The incidence of synchronous CRCs is reported to range from 3 to 5%[67,68] but may be as high as 11%.[69] Stage for stage, there appear to be no differences in survival between synchronous cancers and single primary cancers.[70,71] Synchronous adenomatous polyps are present in as many as 35% of patients undergoing surgical treatment of CRC.[68,71] In one study, the presence of synchronous lesions made the surgical procedure more extensive than was initially planned for resection of the primary tumor in 11% of patients.[68]

Most synchronous polyps are identified on preoperative colonoscopy, and the colon can often be cleared of these lesions before operation. Management of adenomas not amenable to endoscopic resection and management of synchronous cancers are more challenging. Each primary cancer must be managed surgically according to sound oncologic principles. One option is to perform multiple segmental resections with multiple anastomoses. Another is to perform an extended resection that encompasses all of the lesions or even total abdominal colectomy if needed. The presence of a rectal cancer and a second synchronous lesion makes surgical treatment even more challenging, especially if sphincter preservation and a low rectal or coloanal anastomosis are contemplated.

ADJUVANT THERAPY

Significant progress in systemic adjuvant therapy for patients undergoing resection of a colorectal adenocarcinoma has been made in the past 20 to 30 years, primarily through a series of phase III randomized trials and the development of new drugs. The evolution of adjuvant therapies is likely to continue for the foreseeable future, and surgeons will play a pivotal role as the primary entrance point for standard adjuvant therapy and new phase III randomized trials. Surgeons' awareness of past accomplishments, current study findings, and future phase III trials is crucial for improving the survival of potentially cured patients.

The 5-year survival rate after resection of colon cancer is inversely correlated with the pathologic stage [*see Figure 4*]. The diminishing 5-year survival rates for stage II and III colon cancer became the basis of several phase III randomized trials designed to test the hypothesis that postoperative systemic adjuvant chemotherapy would significantly improve survival in patients with resected but high-risk cancers. Multi-institutional, cooperative cancer group trials were necessary to obtain populations large enough to test this hypothesis. The North Central Cancer Treatment Group (NCCTG) initiated a randomized trial of postoperative systemic adjuvant 5-FU plus levamisole for Dukes stage B and C (AJCC stage II and III) colon carcinomas.[72] Patients were randomly assigned to receive either levamisole alone or 5-FU plus levamisole. Overall survival was significantly improved in stage C patients treated with 5-FU plus levamisole. This was the first randomized trial to demonstrate the efficacy of systemic adjuvant therapy.

The NCCTG trial led to second-generation trials of adjuvant therapy for patients with resected colon cancers. In one such study, patients with high-risk stage II or stage III colon cancer were randomly assigned to receive either 5-FU plus leucovorin and levamisole or 5-FU plus levamisole.[73] Survival rates after 12 months of adjuvant chemotherapy were no better than those after 6 months of chemotherapy; however, 5-FU plus levamisole proved to be inferior to 5-FU plus leucovorin and levamisole with respect to survival.

National Surgical Adjuvant Breast and Bowel Project (NSABP) protocol C-04 randomly assigned Dukes stage B and C colon cancer patients to receive (1) postoperative 5-FU plus leucovorin, (2) 5-FU plus levamisole, or (3) 5-FU plus leucovorin and levamisole.[74] A slight improvement in 5-year disease-free survival was noted with 5-FU plus leucovorin, but overall 5-year survival did not differ significantly among the three treatment arms. Accordingly, 5-FU plus leucovorin became the standard adjuvant regimen.

Intergroup Trial 0089 randomly assigned patients with high-risk stage II and III disease to receive either 5-FU plus high-dose leucovorin or 5-FU plus low-dose leucovorin. The investigators concluded that (1) the high-dose and low-dose regimens were equivalent, (2) a regimen consisting of four cycles of 5-FU with high-dose weekly leucovorin was equivalent to the low-dose leucovorin Mayo Clinic regimen, and (3) the addition of levamisole to the 5-FU plus leucovorin regimen did not improve survival.

These clinical trials established 5-FU plus leucovorin as standard therapy for patients with high-risk stage II and stage III colon cancer. A new series of studies has now provided data regarding newer agents such as oxaliplatin, irinotecan, bevacizumab, and cetuximab. The MOSAIC trial, a large multinational trial,[75] and the NSABP C-07 trial[76] both demonstrated improved outcomes with the addition of oxaliplatin to 5-FU–based regimens. In the MOSAIC trial, the addition of oxaliplatin resulted in a 5.9% increase in disease-free survival at 5 years.[77] There was also a statistically significant 4.6% improvement in overall survival seen in stage III patients with a 6-year median follow-up. Oxaliplatin is now considered a standard component of adjuvant therapy protocols for CRC. Irinotecan has not been shown to improve survival in the adjuvant setting and is associated with increased toxicity[78] and is therefore not generally used. Addition of targeted agents such as bevacizumab, which is a vascular endothelial growth factor antibody, and cetuximab, which is an epidermal growth factor receptor antibody, is currently being studied in trials.

Routine use of systemic adjuvant therapy for stage II colon cancer remains controversial. Patients with stage II colon cancers, including those at high risk (e.g., those who present with large bowel obstruction or perforation), are typically included in adjuvant chemotherapy trials. A meta-analysis of stage II patients included in NSABP colon cancer trials demonstrated that adjuvant chemotherapy did confer a survival benefit at this disease stage.[79] This study was criticized, however, for having included patients from trials that lacked a surgery-only arm, as well as from trials that employed outmoded chemotherapeutic regimens.[80] Another meta-analysis, which included only trials that compared 5-FU plus leucovorin with observation after curative resection in stage II patients, found no statistically significant survival benefit with chemotherapy.[81] A 2004 meta-analysis formulated recommendations on this controversial topic and provided a Web-based tool for calculating risk.[82] This report included data from seven randomized trials that compared surgery alone with surgery plus chemotherapy. Patients with node-negative disease derived a much lower reduction in risk and no statistically significant improvement in overall survival. The authors concluded that the use of postoperative adjuvant chemotherapy for stage II colon cancer patients should be individualized on the basis of the estimated prognosis and the potential treatment benefit. In the MOSAIC trial, there was no long-term overall survival benefit in stage II patients receiving oxaliplatin compared to 5-FU and leucovorin alone.[77]

In summary, postoperative systemic adjuvant therapy is the standard of care in patients with stage III disease. In stage II colon cancer patients who have undergone complete surgical resection, the relative risk of recurrence is small enough that adjuvant chemotherapy yields relatively little benefit in terms of survival. There is, however, a subgroup of patients who have recognized prognostic factors that significantly reduce survival and in whom adjuvant therapy is therefore more likely to be beneficial. These risk factors include (1) bowel obstruction, (2) colonic perforation, (3) high-grade or lymphovascular invasion, and (4) the presence of fewer than 12 lymph nodes in the resected specimen. Additional risk factors such as chromosome 18 deletions and MSI continue to be evaluated.

Management of Rectal Cancer

Rectal cancer presents special management issues with respect to local recurrence after surgical resection. With cancer of the intraperitoneal colon, local recurrence is rare. With rectal cancer, however, surgical treatment alone results in recurrence rates of 16.2% after low anterior resection (LAR) and 19.3% after abdominoperineal resection (APR).[83] Higher stages are associated with higher recurrence rates: 8.5% for Dukes stage A, 16.3% for stage B, and 26% for stage C.[83] Multimodality management, including adjuvant radiation therapy or chemotherapy (or both) in combination with appropriate operative therapy, can reduce local recurrence rates significantly.

SURGICAL THERAPY

Extent of Resection

Sphincter preservation has become a major goal in the multimodality treatment of rectal cancer. Surgical procedures are chosen and performed with this goal firmly in mind.

Radical resection Traditionally, tumors of the rectum have been treated with either LAR or APR [*see Figure 8*]; in numerous series, APR rates of 60% or higher have been reported. Surgical techniques such as stapled or handsewn coloanal anastomoses, when combined with total mesorectal excision (TME), have led to excellent cancer-related outcomes without the need for permanent colostomy. The use of preoperative chemoradiation therapy for tumor downstaging may also reduce the need for APR.[84]

The morbidity associated with radical rectal resection can be substantial. Anastomotic leakage rates vary widely, ranging from less than 10% to more than 30% after resection with anastomosis. Leaks can lead to substantial morbidity and mortality and can necessitate reoperation. Such concerns have prompted the use of temporary diverting ileostomies or colostomies in patients with low rectal anastomoses. Defunctioning stomas may be overused, however, thereby increasing the cost of care in low-risk patients.[85] Preoperative chemoradiation therapy has not been shown to increase anastomotic leakage rates. Urinary and sexual dysfunction are also fairly common after radical resection of rectal cancer. Autonomic nerve preservation in conjunction with TME may improve the functional results of these procedures.[86] The use of local resection techniques (see below) is another means of reducing surgical morbidity and mortality in rectal cancer patients.

Local excision Local excision—including transanal, transsphincteric, and transcoccygeal techniques, as well as transanal endoscopic microsurgery (TEM)—is another option for curative resection of low rectal cancers with preservation of sphincter function. These procedures were initially implemented for local control in patients who were medically unfit for or unwilling to undergo major resections. Transsphincteric and transcoccygeal resections have been associated with an increased incidence of complications, including fecal fistulas and incontinence, and have largely been abandoned now that other, better techniques are available.

Local excision with curative intent is generally reserved for the treatment of early-stage (T1-2N0) lesions and remains controversial even in these patients. Selection of patients for these procedures is critical and is based on preoperative staging and on the probability of harboring nodal metastases, which increases with the T stage. EUS and endorectal coil MRI have become an important staging procedure in these patients, both for assessing the depth of tissue invasion and for detecting the presence of nodal disease. CT is generally performed to rule out distant metastases. Palliative procedures (e.g., fulguration and endocavitary irradiation) may also be considered in patients who are unfit for major surgery.

Several criteria have been established to identify patients who may be candidates for transanal excision (TAE) (NCCN guidelines).[87] According to guidelines published by the NCCN, the lesion must be no more than 3 cm in diameter, must encompass no more than 30% of the circumference of the rectum, and must be less than 8 cm from the anal verge. With the advent of TEM, these criteria have been expanded to include patients with higher lesions. Poorly differentiated tumors and the presence of lymphovascular invasion may also be associated with increased nodal involvement and higher recurrence rates. At least two prospective trials have reported their results with TAE.[88,89] Local recurrence rates ranged from 5 to 7% for T1 lesions treated with surgery alone. The results were not as promising for T2 lesions: local recurrence rates ranged from 14 to 16%, even when adjuvant radiation or chemoradiation therapy was provided. Long-term follow-up data were recently published for one of these studies, showing local recurrence rates of 8 and 18% for T1 and T2 lesions, respectively, with a median follow-up of 7 years.[90] In a recent nationwide cohort study using National Cancer Data Base

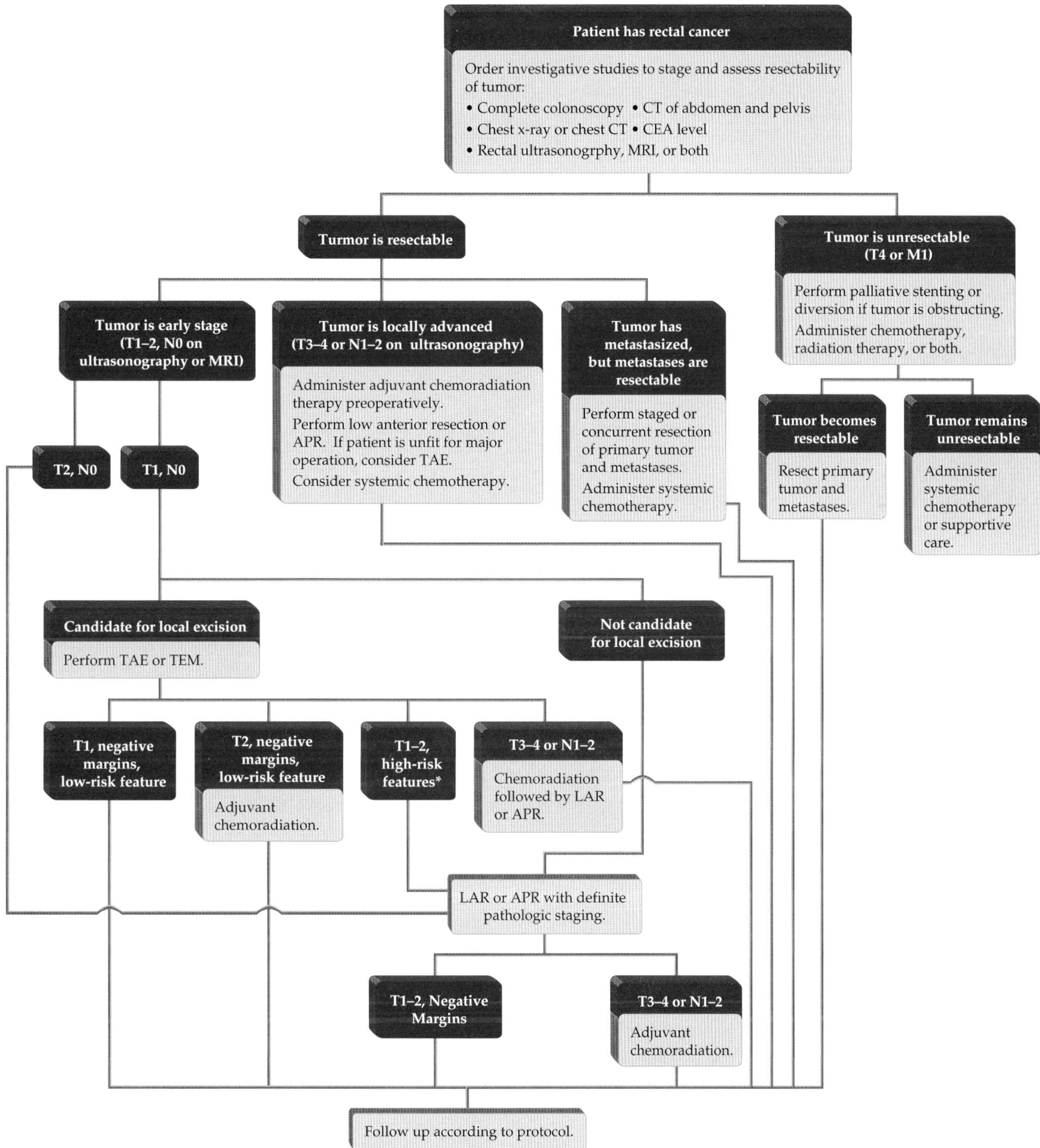

Figure 8 **Algorithm outlines treatment of rectal cancer. APR = abdominoperineal resection; CEA = carcinoembryonic antigen; CT = computed tomography; LAR = low anterior resection; MRI = magnetic resonance imaging; TAE = transanal excision; TEM = transanal endoscopic microsurgery. *High-risk features include a positive margin, lymphovascular invasion, and poorly differentiated or mucinous histopathology.**

data, local excision resulted in significantly higher local recurrence rates than radical surgery for both T1 (12.5 versus 6.9%) and T2 (22.1 versus 15.1%) tumors.[91] Five-year overall survival rates were not significantly different, however.

The use of local excision in patients with more locally advanced disease is even more controversial. Such patients are at considerably greater risk for nodal metastases and thus for local recurrence even after adequate resection of the primary lesion. Traditionally, local excision in patients with locally advanced disease has been associated with unacceptably high recurrence rates. Some authors advocate combining chemoradiation therapy with local excision to manage these patients. In a 2004 retrospective series, the results of local excision were comparable to those of radical resection in T3 patients who had a good response to preoperative chemoradiation therapy and who refused or were medically unfit for major surgery.[92] The role of local excision in these patients remains poorly defined.

Patients undergoing local resection must receive careful follow-up, including digital examination, measurement of CEA levels, proctoscopy, and, possibly, transanal ultrasonography. A subset of these patients with local-only recurrences who are medically fit for surgery may be candidates for resection. At present, few good data are available on the results of salvage surgery for local recurrence after local excision of rectal cancer, but it is unlikely that outcomes are equivalent to those of initial radical resection.[93]

Importance of Radial and Distal Resection Margins

There has been a great deal of debate about what constitutes an adequate margin of resection in surgical treatment of rectal cancer. With respect to distal margins, 2 to 5 cm has traditionally been considered to be the minimum necessary for curative resection. Growing interest in sphincter preservation has led investigators to consider smaller distal margins (i.e., < 2 cm). Studies have shown that clear margins smaller than 2 cm are not associated with higher local recurrence rates or reduced survival.[94] Subsequent reports have suggested that even smaller histologically negative margins (i.e., < 1 cm) may be adequate in patients receiving adjuvant chemoradiation therapy.[95,96]

The importance of radial margin involvement after rectal cancer resection was not recognized until comparatively recently.[97] Radial margins are assessed by means of serial slicing and evaluation of multiple coronal sections of the tumor and the mesorectum.[97] Involvement of radial margins is a predictor of both local recurrence and survival after potentially curative rectal cancer surgery[98] and may be associated with an increased risk of distant metastases.[99] Radial margins smaller than 2 mm are associated with increased local recurrence rates.[99] Adjuvant radiation therapy does not compensate for the adverse impact of positive margins on local recurrence rates.[100]

ADJUVANT AND NEOADJUVANT THERAPY

Adjuvant therapy for rectal cancer has focused on both locoregional control of disease and treatment of systemic disease. Several large studies have evaluated local recurrence of disease after surgical resection alone. Local failure rates of 30 to 40% for T2N0 disease and 50 to 70% for node-positive disease strongly suggested that postoperative adjuvant therapy was needed.[101–103] In distinct contrast to these data, however, other series in which TME was performed reported extremely low local recurrence rates with surgery alone.[104,105]

A series of randomized trials were conducted to assess adjuvant therapy for rectal cancer. Initial studies reported a decrease in local recurrence rates with postoperative radiation therapy.[106,107] In a multi-institutional trial conducted by the NCCTG, the combination of 5-FU with radiation therapy led to improvements in local control rates and in survival.[108] These results were confirmed in large intergroup trials, the results of which indicated that continuous infusion of 5-FU during radiation therapy resulted in significantly better disease-free survival and overall survival than bolus infusion of 5-FU.

Simultaneously with the ongoing development of postoperative locoregional adjuvant therapy for rectal cancer, interest in preoperative (neoadjuvant) therapy has been growing. Preoperative radiation therapy has been associated with excellent local control of disease, sphincter preservation, and acceptable postoperative recovery. There is evidence that rectal adenocarcinoma is sensitive to preoperative radiation therapy, with or without 5-FU. Pathologic complete response rates of 10 to 20% have been noted in resected rectal specimens[109]; pathologic complete response is associated with improved outcomes.[110]

Perhaps the strongest reason to consider preoperative therapy for rectal cancer is its potential for inducing significant tumor regression before surgical resection. Such regression makes clear radial and distal margins easier to obtain. Moreover, tumor regression with preoperative therapy may result in higher sphincter preservation rates. In many published series, the APR rate in rectal cancer patients is between 40 and 60%; more aggressive preoperative efforts to induce regression may give surgeons a better chance to achieve sphincter preservation without compromising local control of disease.[109] One advantage of the postoperative approach is that the disease is more accurately staged before adjuvant therapy begins; thus, patients with early-stage disease are less likely to be overtreated. Data continue to accumulate on the relative merits of preoperative versus postoperative adjuvant treatment of rectal cancer.

Two Swedish studies considered the role of preoperative radiation therapy in treating rectal cancer. The first demonstrated that a short course of preoperative radiation therapy (2.5 Gy in five fractions) was comparable to high-dose postoperative radiation therapy (60 Gy over a period of 8 weeks). The local recurrence rate was significantly lower with the short-course preoperative regimen (12% versus 21%), and there was no overall survival difference between the two regimens.[111] In the second trial, patients received either a short course of preoperative radiation therapy or surgery alone.[112] The local recurrence rate at a median follow-up of 13 years was 9% for preoperative therapy plus surgery compared with 26% for surgery alone. The combined regimen also resulted in significantly better overall survival (38% versus 30%).

The relative benefits of preoperative versus postoperative radiation therapy have been elucidated by the findings from more recent trials. A 2004 German trial randomly assigned patients to receive either preoperative or postoperative 5-FU plus radiation followed by systemic 5-FU therapy.[84] This study was limited to patients with locally advanced disease, including those who had T3 or T4 disease or were node positive on ultrasonography. TME was performed in all patients and was done 6 weeks after treatment in patients receiving preoperative chemoradiation therapy. The primary end point of this study was overall survival; secondary end points included disease-free survival, local and distant control of disease, sphincter preservation, toxicity of adjuvant therapy, surgical complications, and quality of life. There was no difference between the preoperative group and the postoperative group with respect to 5-year survival, but the local recurrence rate was significantly lower with the former (6% versus 13%), as were both the short-term and the long-term toxicity of adjuvant therapy.

Although, overall, the rates of complete (R0) resection and sphincter preservation were similar in the two groups, the APR rate was significantly lower in patients determined by the surgeon to require APR before randomization.

A large multinational trial of preoperative radiation versus selective postoperative chemoradiation demonstrated a significantly decreased local recurrence rate and improved disease-free survival in the preoperative radiation group.[113] Overall survival was not significantly different. A French trial studied the benefits of adding chemotherapy to preoperative radiation.[114] The addition of 5-FU–based chemotherapy at any point in the patients' treatment resulted in a significant improvement in local recurrence but no difference in survival.

The use of adjuvant 5-FU–based chemotherapy and radiation, particularly in the preoperative setting, in the treatment of rectal cancer has demonstrated clear benefit in multiple trials. Studies are currently in progress, including the NSABP R-04, to evaluate the benefits of additional chemotherapeutic agents in combination with preoperative radiation.

Special Considerations

SYNCHRONOUS METASTATIC (STAGE IV) DISEASE

As many as 20% of CRC patients have metastatic disease at the time of initial presentation. The need for surgical intervention in this group of patients is not well defined. Clearly, surgical resection or diversion is indicated in patients who present with significant bleeding, perforation, or obstruction. In asymptomatic patients with unresectable metastatic disease, the role of surgical resection of the primary lesion remains controversial. In patients with resectable metastatic disease (e.g., isolated liver or lung metastases), curative resection may be undertaken.

In a retrospective review of patients presenting with unresectable stage IV CRC, there was no difference in survival between those who were initially managed surgically and those who were initially managed nonoperatively.[115] In the surgical group, the morbidity was 30% and the mortality was 5%. Only 9% of the nonoperative patients subsequently required surgical intervention for bowel obstruction. In another retrospective series, patients managed surgically had significantly better overall survival than those managed nonoperatively but had a lesser tumor burden[116]; 29% of the nonoperative patients eventually required surgery for bowel obstruction. When prognostic factors were evaluated in the surgical arm of this series, the only factor associated with improved outcomes was a less than 25% extent of liver involvement. On the basis of these and other studies, asymptomatic patients with unresectable metastatic CRC should be managed selectively: those with limited tumor burdens may benefit from surgical treatment, whereas those with more extensive disease (especially extensive liver involvement) may initially be managed nonoperatively.

Management of patients with synchronous resectable isolated liver metastases continues to evolve. Many studies have documented improved survival after liver resection in patients with metastatic disease that is confined to the liver. Patients presenting with synchronous lesions have a worse prognosis than those presenting with metachronous lesions.[117] Many of these patients have been managed with staged resections of the primary cancers and the liver metastases. Several groups have reported that such combined procedures do not substantially increase surgical morbidity and mortality or compromise cancer survival.[118,119] These combined procedures should be done only in carefully selected patients at specialized centers with significant experience in resection of both CRC and liver tumors.

PERITONEAL CARCINOMATOSIS

Peritoneal carcinomatosis develops in approximately 13% of all CRC patients.[120] The survival rate of patients who present with peritoneal carcinomatosis from CRC is dismal. In patients with stage IV CRC, the presence of carcinomatosis is associated with a significant reduction in survival (from 18.1 months to 6.7 months).[121] Treatment has traditionally included systemic chemotherapy, with surgery reserved for palliation of symptoms such as bowel obstruction. Newer chemotherapy regimens that include agents such as oxaliplatin may improve survival, but they certainly are not curative.

Peritoneal carcinomatosis is often associated with hematogenous metastases, but in some 25% of patients, the peritoneal cavity is the only site of disease. Several groups have advocated the use of cytoreductive surgery and hyperthermic intraperitoneal chemotherapy (HIPEC) as a means of improving survival in these patients.[122] This treatment, however, is associated with significant morbidity and mortality.[123] A randomized trial from the Netherlands that compared cytoreduction surgery plus HIPEC with systemic chemotherapy plus palliative surgery found that patients in the former group exhibited a statistically significant improvement in median survival (22.3 months versus 12.6 months).[124] At 8 years of follow-up, a significant improvement in median disease-specific survival was maintained.[125] Cytoreductive surgery plus HIPEC seems to be a viable option for the treatment of peritoneal carcinomatosis. Patient selection for these aggressive procedures remains a major issue given the substantial morbidity and mortality associated with them.

Follow-Up and Management of Recurrent CRC

The goal of any CRC follow-up regimen should be to detect any recurrences or metachronous lesions that are potentially curable. In a large, multicenter trial, the incidence of second primary CRCs in patients with resected stage II and III lesions was found to be 1.5% at 5 years.[126] Between 40 and 50% of patients experience relapses after potentially curative resection of CRC. Detection and treatment of recurrent disease before symptom development may improve survival. The time to recurrence is critical in that as many as 80% of recurrences occur within the first 2 years and as many as 90% within the first 4 years. Patterns of recurrence should also be taken into account—for example, the markedly increased risk of local recurrence in rectal cancer patients compared with that in colon cancer patients. Even when recurrent CRC is detected, only a small percentage of patients are candidates for reoperation, and resection in these patients may not improve overall survival. Systemic therapy may improve survival in some patients who have unresectable recurrent lesions.

Various modalities are available for follow-up after surgical treatment of CRC. The history and the physical examination continue to be useful in that a significant percentage of patients present with symptomatic recurrences. Measurement of serum CEA levels has proved effective in detecting asymptomatic recurrences. More recent studies have shown a survival benefit for CT scanning as part of routine follow-up in patients at a high risk of recurrence. One study that evaluated routine CEA measurement and CT scanning of the chest, abdomen, and pelvis for follow-up of stage II and III CRC demonstrated that both modalities were able to identify asymptomatic patients with resectable disease.[127] Colonoscopy is valuable for detecting metachronous cancers and polyps. Other studies, such as liver function tests (LFTs), complete blood count (CBC), and chest x-ray, have not been consistently shown to detect asymptomatic resectable recurrences.

Some authorities advocate so-called intensive follow-up. However, this term lacks a standard definition, and such follow-up has not been conclusively shown to be beneficial. In a meta-analysis that compared an intensive follow-up regimen (including history, physical examination, and CEA measurement) with no follow-up, the former detected more candidates for curative re-resection and led to improvements in both overall survival and survival of patients with recurrences.[128] Three other meta-analyses have been published that assessed the value of intensive follow-up of CRC patients.[129–131] These meta-analyses included only randomized, controlled trials, and all documented a survival advantage with intensive follow-up. Some caution is required in interpreting these results, however, because the meta-analyses included trials with vastly different follow-up regimens in their baseline and intensive groups.

At present, the ideal follow-up regimen for CRC patients remains to be determined. Intensive follow-up regimens obviously are more costly. Patients with stage I disease are at very low risk for recurrence and therefore do not generally require intensive follow-up.[132] Patients with stage II and III disease are at significantly higher risk for recurrence and therefore need more specific cancer-related follow-up, but how intensive such a follow-up regimen should be is still a matter of debate.

Several organizations, including the American Society of Clinical Oncology[133] and the American Society of Colon and Rectal Surgeons,[134] have developed algorithms for postoperative surveillance of CRC patients. Their recommendations generally apply to patients with stage II or III disease (and sometimes patients with T2 lesions) who are candidates for resection of recurrent disease. The recommendations vary somewhat among groups, but the following are generally agreed on:

1. Measurement of CEA levels every 2 to 3 months for 2 years, then every 3 to 6 months for 3 years, then annually
2. Clinical examination every 3 to 6 months for 3 years, then annually
3. Colonoscopy perioperatively, then every 3 to 5 years if the patient remains free of polyps and cancer (some guidelines also recommend colonoscopy 1 year after primary therapy)
4. CT of the chest and abdomen for 3 years; pelvic CT should also be done in patients with rectal cancer

Other imaging studies (e.g., PET and chest x-ray) are not routinely recommended, nor are other blood tests (e.g., CBC and LFTs).

A complete review of the treatment of recurrent CRC is beyond the scope of this chapter. The primary aim of postoperative surveillance is the detection of treatable recurrences or metastatic disease. The most common sites of metastasis in CRC patients are the liver and the peritoneal cavity. Surgery is the only potentially curative therapy for recurrent CRC. Only a select group of patients with isolated peritoneal, liver, or lung metastases are candidates for surgical resection. As noted [*see* Special Considerations, Peritoneal Carcinomatosis, *above*], cytoreductive surgery and HIPEC improve survival in patients with peritoneal carcinomatosis and may lead to long-term survival in a very select group of patients.

Numerous studies have addressed the treatment of patients with isolated liver metastases from CRC. Resection of isolated hepatic metastases has been reported to yield 5-year survival rates higher than 30%, with acceptable surgical morbidity and mortality. Investigators from the Memorial Sloan-Kettering Cancer Center developed a staging system known as the clinical score in an attempt to predict which patients are likely to benefit from aggressive surgical resection.[135] This system used five factors that were found to be independent predictors of poor outcome: (1) node-positive primary disease, (2) a disease-free interval shorter than 12 months, (3) the presence of more than one hepatic tumor, (4) a maximum hepatic tumor size exceeding 5 cm, and (5) a CEA level higher than 200 ng/mL. Patients who met no more than two of these criteria generally had good outcomes, whereas those who met three or more were recommended for inclusion in adjuvant therapy trials.

PET scanning has also been used to detect occult metastatic disease and thus to aid in the selection of patients for surgical resection. In one series, a 5-year overall survival of 58% was reported after resection of CRC liver metastases in patients screened with PET.[136] When combined with the clinical risk score, PET was found to be helpful only in patients with a score of 1 or higher.[137]

Modalities for treating unresectable disease confined to the liver include cryotherapy, radiofrequency (RF) ablation, microwave ablation, hepatic artery infusion of chemotherapeutic agents, and hepatic perfusion. Of these, RF ablation is the one most commonly employed. It may be performed via an open approach, percutaneously, or laparoscopically; it may also be combined with resection and with local or systemic chemotherapy. The survival benefit (if any) associated with use of these modalities has not been well established.

Patients with isolated lung metastases from CRC may also benefit from surgical resection. Because there are relatively few of these patients, treatment of such metastases has not been studied as well as treatment of liver metastases. Some series have reported 5-year survival rates higher than 40% after complete resection. Patient selection remains a major issue. Several prognostic factors that may predict poor outcomes have been identified, including (1) a maximum tumor size greater than 3.75 cm, (2) a serum CEA level higher than 5 ng/mL, and (3) pulmonary or mediastinal lymph node involvement.[138,139] Patients with both pulmonary and hepatic metastases may also be considered for surgical resection.

Pelvic recurrences of rectal cancer present another difficult management issue. These tumors may cause significant pain and disability, and if they are not treated, survival is measured in months. Radiation and chemotherapy provide symptomatic relief and yield a modest increase in survival. Surgery may provide excellent palliation and is potentially curative in patients who do not have distant metastases.

Multimodality therapy has been advocated as a means of improving the chances of cure. In one study, a 37% 5-year survival rate was reported in patients who underwent multimodality therapy, including resection with negative margins.[140] A subgroup of patients in whom complete resection was impossible underwent intraoperative radiation therapy; the 5-year survival in this subgroup was 21%. Several predictors of poor outcomes were identified, including incomplete resection, multiple points of tumor fixation, and symptomatic pain. In another series, hydronephrosis was associated with the presence of unresectable disease.[141] Selection of appropriate patients for curative surgery remains a major issue in the management of locally recurrent rectal cancer.

Chemotherapy is the mainstay of palliative treatment for patients with CRC and unresectable recurrent or metastatic disease. Combinations of 5-FU and leucovorin with newer agents such as irinotecan, oxaliplatin, and bevacizumab define the current standard. Patients in whom these regimens fail may be considered for treatment with other agents such as cetuximab or other targeted therapies.

Financial Disclosures: None Reported

References

1. Jemal A, Siegel R, Ward E, et al. Cancer statistics, 2008. CA Cancer J Clin 2008;58:71.
2. Redaelli A, Cranor CW, Okano GJ, et al. Screening, prevention and socioeconomic costs associated with the treatment of colorectal cancer. Pharmacoeconomics 2003; 21:1213.
3. Pisani P, Parkin DM, Bray F, et al. Estimates of the worldwide mortality from 25 cancers in 1990. Int J Cancer 1999;83:18.
4. Jemal A, Thun MJ, Ries LA, et al. Annual report to the nation on the status of cancer, 1975–2005, featuring trends in lung cancer, tobacco use, and tobacco control. J Natl Cancer Inst 2008;100:1672.
5. Hawk ET, Limburg PJ, Viner JL. Epidemiology and prevention of colorectal cancer. Surg Clin North Am 2002;82:905.
6. Muto T, Bussey HJ, Morson BC, The evolution of cancer of the colon and rectum. Cancer 1975;36:2251.
7. Fearon ER, Vogelstein B. A genetic model for colorectal tumorigenesis. Cell 1990;61:759.
8. Jones S, Chen WD, Parmigiani G, et al. Comparative lesion sequencing provides insights into tumor evolution. Proc Natl Acad Sci U S A 2008;105:4283.
9. Rodriguez-Bigas MA, Stoler DL, Bertario L, et al. Colorectal cancer: how does it start? How does it metastasize? Surg Oncol Clin N Am 2000;9:643.
10. Chung DC, Rustgi AK. The hereditary nonpolyposis colorectal cancer syndrome: genetics and clinical implications. Ann Intern Med 2003;138:560.
11. Herman JG, Umar A, Polyak K, et al. Incidence and functional consequences of hMLH1 promoter hypermethylation in colorectal carcinoma. Proc Natl Acad Sci U S A 1998;95:6870.
12. Slattery ML, Levin TR, Ma K, et al. Family history and colorectal cancer: predictors of risk. Cancer Causes Control 2003;14:879.
13. Le Marchand L, Zhao LP, Quiaoit F, et al. Family history and risk of colorectal cancer in the multiethnic population of Hawaii. Am J Epidemiol 1996;144:1122.
14. Johns LE, Houlston RS. A systematic review and meta-analysis of familial colorectal cancer risk. Am J Gastroenterol 2001;96:2992.
15. Winawer SJ, Zauber AG, Gerdes H, et al. Risk of colorectal cancer in the families of patients with adenomatous polyps. National Polyp Study Workgroup. N Engl J Med 1996; 334:82.
16. Ahsan H, Neugut AI, Garbowski GC, et al. Family history of colorectal adenomatous polyps and increased risk for colorectal cancer. Ann Intern Med 1998;28:900.
17. Park JG, Vasen HF, Park YJ, et al. Suspected HNPCC and Amsterdam criteria II: evaluation of mutation detection rate, an international collaborative study. Int J Colorectal Dis 2002;17:109.
18. Eaden JA, Abrams KR, Mayberry JF. The risk of colorectal cancer in ulcerative colitis: a meta-analysis. Gut 2001;48:526.
19. Bernstein CN, Blanchard JF, Kliewer E, et al. Cancer risk in patients with inflammatory bowel disease: a population-based study. Cancer 2001;91:854.
20. Le Marchand L, Wilkens LR, Kolonel LN, et al. Associations of sedentary lifestyle, obesity, smoking, alcohol use, and diabetes with the risk of colorectal cancer. Cancer Res 1997;57:4787.
21. Baron JA, Beach M, Mandel JS, et al. Calcium supplements for the prevention of colorectal adenomas. Calcium Polyp Prevention Study Group. N Engl J Med 1999;340:101.
22. Yiu HY, Whittemore AS, Shibata A. Increasing colorectal cancer incidence rates in Japan. Int J Cancer 2004;109:777.
23. Winawer SJ, Zauber AG, Ho MN, et al. Prevention of colorectal cancer by colonoscopic polypectomy. The National Polyp Study Workgroup. N Engl J Med 1993;329:1977.
24. Levin B, Lieberman DA, McFarland B, et al. Screening and surveillance for the early detection of colorectal cancer and adenomatous polyps, 2008: a joint guideline from the American Cancer Society, the US Multi-Society Task Force on Colorectal Cancer, and the American College of Radiology. CA Cancer J Clin 2008;58:130.
25. Walsh JM, Terdiman JP. Colorectal cancer screening: scientific review. JAMA 2003;289: 1288.
26. Imperiale TF, Wagner DR, Lin CY, et al. Risk of advanced proximal neoplasms in asymptomatic adults according to the distal colorectal findings. N Engl J Med 2000; 343:169.
27. Mandel JS, Bond JH, Church TR, et al. Reducing mortality from colorectal cancer by screening for fecal occult blood. Minnesota Colon Cancer Control Study. N Engl J Med 1993;328:1365.
28. Hewitson P, Glasziou P, Watson E, et al. Cochrane systematic review of colorectal cancer screening using the fecal occult blood test (hemoccult): an update. Am J Gastroenterol 2008;103:1541.
29. Pickhardt PJ, Choi JR, Hwang I, et al. Computed tomographic virtual colonoscopy to screen for colorectal neoplasia in asymptomatic adults. N Engl J Med 2003;349:2191.
30. Cotton PB, Durkalski VL, Pineau BC, et al. Computed tomographic colonography (virtual colonoscopy): a multicenter comparison with standard colonoscopy for detection of colorectal neoplasia. JAMA 2004;291:1713.
31. Deenadayalu VP, Rex DK. Fecal-based DNA assays: a new, noninvasive approach to colorectal cancer screening. Cleve Clin J Med 2004;71:497.
32. Imperiale TF, Ransohoff DF, Itzkowitz SH, et al. Fecal DNA versus fecal occult blood for colorectal-cancer screening in an average-risk population. N Engl J Med 2004;351: 2704–14.
33. Levin B, Lieberman DA, McFarland B, et al. Screening and surveillance for the early detection of colorectal cancer and adenomatous polyps, 2008: a joint guideline from the American Cancer Society, the US Multi-Society Task Force on Colorectal Cancer, and the American College of Radiology. CA Cancer J Clin 2008;58:130–60.
34. Rex DK, Johnson DA, Anderson JC, et al. American College of Gastroenterology guidelines for colorectal cancer screening 2009. Am J Gastroenterol 2009;104: 739–50.
35. Levin B, Barthel JS, Burt RW, et al. Colorectal cancer screening clinical practice guidelines. J Natl Compr Canc Netw 2006;4: 384–420.
36. Majumdar SR, Fletcher RH, Evans AT. How does colorectal cancer present? Symptoms, duration, and clues to location. Am J Gastroenterol 1999;94:3039.
37. Dukes C, The classification of cancer of the rectum. J Pathol Bacteriol 1932;34:323.
38. Astler VB, Coller FA, The prognostic significance of direct extension of carcinoma of the colon and rectum. Ann Surg 1954; 139:846.
39. Greene F, Page DL, Fleming ID, et al, editors. AJCC cancer staging manual. 6th ed. New York: Springer Verlag New York; 2002.
40. Barton JB, Langdale LA, Cummins JS, et al. The utility of routine preoperative computed tomography scanning in the management of veterans with colon cancer. Am J Surg 2002;183:499.
41. Delbeke D, Martin WH. PET and PET-CT for evaluation of colorectal carcinoma. Semin Nucl Med 2004;34:209.
42. Bipat S, Glas AS, Slors FJ, et al. Rectal cancer: local staging and assessment of lymph node involvement with endoluminal US,

CT, and MR imaging—a meta-analysis. Radiology 2004;232:773.
43. Greene FL, Stewart AK, Norton HJ. A new TNM staging strategy for node-positive (stage III) colon cancer: an analysis of 50,042 patients. Ann Surg 2002;236:416.
44. Marchena J, Acosta MA, Garcia-Anguiano F, et al. Use of the preoperative levels of CEA in patients with colorectal cancer. Hepatogastroenterology 2003;50:1017.
45. Lawes DA, SenGupta S, Boulos PB. The clinical importance and prognostic implications of microsatellite instability in sporadic cancer. Eur J Surg Oncol 2003;29:201.
46. Carethers JM, Smith EJ, Behling CA, et al. Use of 5-fluorouracil and survival in patients with micro-satellite-unstable colorectal cancer. Gastroenterology 2004;126:394.
47. Jen J, Kim H, Piantadosi S, et al. Allelic loss of chromosome 18q and prognosis in colorectal cancer. N Engl J Med 1994; 331:213.
48. Petersen S, Thames HD, Nieder C, et al. The results of colorectal cancer treatment by p53 status: treatment-specific overview. Dis Colon Rectum 2001;44:322.
49. Edler D, Glimelius B, Hallstrom M, et al. Thymidylate synthase expression in colorectal cancer: a prognostic and predictive marker of benefit from adjuvant fluorouracil-based chemotherapy. J Clin Oncol 2002;20:1721.
50. Botoman VA, Pietro M, Thirlby RC. Localization of colonic lesions with endoscopic tattoo. Dis Colon Rectum 1994;37:775.
51. Askin MP, Waye JD, Fiedler L, Harpaz N. Tattoo of colonic neoplasms in 113 patients with a new sterile carbon compound. Gastrointest Endosc 2002;56:339.
52. Nelson H, Petrelli N, Carlin A, et al. Guidelines 2000 for colon and rectal cancer surgery. J Natl Cancer Inst 2001;93:583.
53. Saha S, Dan AG, Bilchik AJ, et al. Historical review of lymphatic mapping in gastrointestinal malignancies. Ann Surg Oncol 2004:11 (3 Suppl):245S.
54. Bertagnolli M, Miedema B, Redston M, et al. Sentinel node staging of resectable colon cancer: results of a multicenter study. Ann Surg 2004;240:624.
55. Wong JH, Johnson DS, Namiki T, et al. Validation of ex vivo lymphatic mapping in hematoxylin-eosin node-negative carcinoma of the colon and rectum. Ann Surg Oncol 2004;11:772.
56. Bosch B, Guller U, Schnider A, et al. Perioperative detection of disseminated tumour cells is an independent prognostic factor in patients with colorectal cancer. Br J Surg 2003;90:882.
57. Kanellos I, Demetriades H, Zintzaras E, et al. Incidence and prognostic value of positive peritoneal cytology in colorectal cancer. Dis Colon Rectum 2003;46:535.
58. Wexner SD, Cohen SM. Port site metastases after laparoscopic colorectal surgery for cure of malignancy. Br J Surg 1995;82:295.
59. Zmora O, Weiss EG. Trocar site recurrence in laparoscopic surgery for colorectal cancer. Myth or real concern? Surg Oncol Clin N Am 2001;10:625.
60. Janson M, Bjorholt I, Carlsson P, et al. Randomized clinical trial of the costs of open and laparoscopic surgery for colonic cancer. Br J Surg 2004;91:409.
61. Weeks JC, Nelson H, Gelber S, et al. Short-term quality-of-life outcomes following laparoscopic-assisted colectomy vs open colectomy for colon cancer: a randomized trial. JAMA 2002;287:321.
62. A comparison of laparoscopically assisted and open colectomy for colon cancer. N Engl J Med 2004;350:2050.
63. Fleshman J, Sargent DJ, Green E, et al. Laparoscopic colectomy for cancer is not inferior to open surgery based on 5-year data from the COST Study Group trial. Ann Surg 2007;246:655–62.
64. Colon Cancer Laparoscopic or Open Resection Study Group. Survival after laparoscopic surgery versus open surgery for colon cancer: long-term outcome of a randomised clinical trial. Lancet Oncol 2009;10:44–52.
65. Jayne DG, Guillou PJ, Thorpe H, et al. Randomized trial of laparoscopic-assisted resection of colorectal carcinoma: 3-year results of the UK MRC CLASICC Trial Group. J Clin Oncol 2007;25:3061–8.
66. Arnaud JP, Bergamaschi R, Emergency subtotal/total colectomy with anastomosis for acutely obstructed carcinoma of the left colon. Dis Colon Rectum 1994;37:685.
67. Fante R, Roncucci L, Di Gregorio C, et al. Frequency and clinical features of multiple tumors of the large bowel in the general population and in patients with hereditary colorectal carcinoma. Cancer 1996;77:2013.
68. Arenas RB, Fichera A, Mhoon D, et al. Incidence and therapeutic implications of synchronous colonic pathology in colorectal adenocarcinoma. Surgery 1997;122:706.
69. Cunliffe WJ, Hasleton PS, Tweedle DE, et al. Incidence of synchronous and metachronous colorectal carcinoma. Br J Surg 1984;71:941.
70. Passman MA, Pommier RF, Vetto JT. Synchronous colon primaries have the same prognosis as solitary colon cancers. Dis Colon Rectum 1996;39:329.
71. Chen HS, Sheen-Chen SM. Synchronous and "early" [illegible] carcinoma: analysis of prognosis and current trends. Dis Colon Rectum 2000;43:1093.
72. Moertel CG, Fleming TR, Macdonald JS, et al. Fluorouracil plus levamisole as effective adjuvant therapy after resection of stage III colon carcinoma: a final report. Ann Intern Med 1995;122:321.
73. O'Connell MJ, Laurie JA, Kahn M, et al. Prospectively randomized trial of postoperative adjuvant chemotherapy in patients with high-risk colon cancer. J Clin Oncol 1998; 16:295.
74. Wolmark N, Rockette H, Mamounas E, et al. Clinical trial to assess the relative efficacy of fluorouracil and leucovorin, fluorouracil and levamisole, and fluorouracil, leucovorin, and levamisole in patients with Dukes' B and C carcinoma of the colon: results from National Surgical Adjuvant Breast and Bowel Project C-04. J Clin Oncol 1999;17:3553.
75. Andre T, Boni C, Mounedji-Boudiaf L, et al. Oxaliplatin, fluorouracil, and leucovorin as adjuvant treatment for colon cancer. N Engl J Med 2004;350:2343.
76. Kuebler JP, Wieand HS, O'Connell MJ, et al. Oxaliplatin combined with weekly bolus fluorouracil and leucovorin as surgical adjuvant chemotherapy for stage II and III colon cancer: results from NSABP C-07. J Clin Oncol 2007;25:2198–204.
77. André T, Boni C, Navarro M, et al. Improved overall survival with oxaliplatin, fluorouracil, and leucovorin as adjuvant treatment in stage II or III colon cancer in the MOSAIC trial. J Clin Oncol 2009;27: 3109–16. [Epub 2009 May 18]
78. Saltz LB, Niedzwiecki D, Hollis D, et al. Irinotecan fluorouracil plus leucovorin is not superior to fluorouracil plus leucovorin alone as adjuvant treatment for stage III colon cancer: results of CALGB 89803. J Clin Oncol 2007;25:3456–61.
79. Mamounas E, Wieand S, Wolmark N, et al. Comparative efficacy of adjuvant chemotherapy in patients with Dukes' B versus Dukes' C colon cancer: results from four National Surgical Adjuvant Breast and Bowel Project adjuvant studies (C-01, C-02, C-03, and C-04). J Clin Oncol 1999;17: 1349.
80. Pignon JP, Ducreux M, Rougier P. More patients needed in stage II colon cancer trials. J Clin Oncol 2000;18:235.
81. Efficacy of adjuvant fluorouracil and folinic acid in B2 colon cancer. International Multicentre Pooled Analysis of B2 Colon Cancer Trials (IMPACT B2) Investigators. J Clin Oncol 1999;17:1356.
82. Gill S, Loprinzi CL, Sargent DJ, et al. Pooled analysis of fluorouracil-based adjuvant therapy for stage II and III colon cancer: who benefits and by how much? J Clin Oncol 2004;15:1797.
83. McCall JL, Cox MR, Wattchow DA. Analysis of local recurrence rates after surgery alone for rectal cancer. Int J Colorectal Dis 1995;10:126.
84. Sauer R, Becker H, Hohenberger W, et al. Preoperative versus postoperative chemoradiotherapy for rectal cancer. N Engl J Med 2004;351:1731.
85. Koperna T. Cost-effectiveness of defunctioning stomas in low anterior resections for rectal cancer: a call for benchmarking. Arch Surg 2003;138:1334.
86. Havenga K, Enker WE. Autonomic nerve preserving total mesorectal excision. Surg Clin North Am 2002;82:1009.
87. Moore HG, Guillem JG. Local therapy for rectal cancer. Surg Clin North Am 2002; [illegible].
88. Steele GD Jr, Herndon JE, Bleday R, et al. Sphincter-sparing treatment for distal rectal adenocarcinoma. Ann Surg Oncol 1999; 6:433.
89. Russell AH, Harris J, Rosenberg PJ, et al. Anal sphincter conservation for patients with adenocarcinoma of the distal rectum: long-term results of Radiation Therapy Oncology Group protocol 89-02. Int J Radiat Oncol Biol Phys 2000;46:313.
90. Greenberg JA, Shibata D, Herndon JE, 2nd, et al. Local excision of distal rectal cancer: an update of cancer and leukemia group B 8984. Dis Colon Rectum 2008;51:1185–91.
91. You YN, Baxter NN, Stewart A, Nelson H. Is the increasing rate of local excision for stage I rectal cancer in the United States justified?: a nationwide cohort study from the National Cancer Database. Ann Surg 2007; 245:726–33.
92. Bonnen M, Crane C, Vauthey JN, et al. Long-term results using local excision after preoperative chemoradiation among selected T3 rectal cancer patients. Int J Radiat Oncol Biol Phys 2004;60:1098.
93. Friel CM, Cromwell JW, Marra C, et al. Salvage radical surgery after failed local excision for early rectal cancer. Dis Colon Rectum 2002;45:875.
94. Pollett WG, Nicholls RJ. The relationship between the extent of distal clearance and survival and local recurrence rates after curative anterior resection for carcinoma of the rectum. Ann Surg 1983;198:159.
95. Kuvshinoff B, Maghfoor I, Miedema B, et al. Distal margin requirements after preoperative chemoradiotherapy for distal rectal carcinomas: are < or = 1 cm distal margins sufficient? Ann Surg Oncol 2001;8:163.
96. Andreola S, Leo E, Belli F, et al. Adenocarcinoma of the lower third of the rectum surgically treated with a <10-MM distal clearance: preliminary results in 35 N0 patients. Ann Surg Oncol 2001;8:611.
97. Quirke P, Durdey P, Dixon MF, et al. Local recurrence of rectal adenocarcinoma due to

inadequate surgical resection. Histopathological study of lateral tumour spread and surgical excision. Lancet 1986;2:996.

98. Wibe A, Rendedal PR, Svensson E, et al. Prognostic significance of the circumferential resection margin following total mesorectal excision for rectal cancer. Br J Surg 2002; 89:327.
99. Nagtegaal ID, Marijnen CA, Kranenbarg EK, et al. Circumferential margin involvement is still an important predictor of local recurrence in rectal carcinoma: not one millimeter but two millimeters is the limit. Am J Surg Pathol 2002;26:350.
100. Marijnen CA, Nagtegaal ID, Kapiteijn E, et al. Radiotherapy does not compensate for positive resection margins in rectal cancer patients: report of a multicenter randomized trial. Int J Radiat Oncol Biol Phys 2003; 55:1311.
101. Rich T, Gunderson LL, Lew R, et al. Patterns of recurrence of rectal cancer after potentially curative surgery. Cancer 1983; 52:1317.
102. Pilipshen SJ, Heilweil M, Quan SH, et al. Patterns of pelvic recurrence following definitive resections of rectal cancer. Cancer 1984;53:1354.
103. Mendenhall WM, Million RR, Pfaff WW. Patterns of recurrence in adenocarcinoma of the rectum and rectosigmoid treated with surgery alone: implications in treatment planning with adjuvant radiation therapy. Int J Radiat Oncol Biol Phys 1983;9:977.
104. Zaheer S, Pemberton JH, Farouk R, et al. Surgical treatment of adenocarcinoma of the rectum. Ann Surg 1998;227:800.
105. Cecil TD, Sexton R, Moran BJ, et al. Total mesorectal excision results in low local recurrence rates in lymph node-positive rectal cancer. Dis Colon Rectum 2004; 47:1145.
106. Prolongation of the disease-free interval in surgically treated rectal carcinoma. Gastrointestinal Tumor Study Group. N Engl J Med 1985;312:1465.
107. Wolmark N, Wieand HS, Hyams DM, et al. Randomized trial of postoperative adjuvant chemotherapy with or without radiotherapy for carcinoma of the rectum: National Surgical Adjuvant Breast and Bowel Project Protocol R-02. J Natl Cancer Inst 2000;92:388.
108. O'Connell MJ, Martenson JA, Wieand HS, et al. Improving adjuvant therapy for rectal cancer by combining protracted-infusion fluorouracil with radiation therapy after curative surgery. N Engl J Med 1994; 331:502.
109. Ota DM, Jacobs L, Kuvshinoff B. Rectal cancer: the sphincter-sparing approach. Surg Clin North Am 2002;82:983.
110. Garcia-Aguilar J, Hernandez de Anda E, Sirivongs P, et al. A pathologic complete response to preoperative chemoradiation is associated with lower local recurrence and improved survival in rectal cancer patients treated by mesorectal excision. Dis Colon Rectum 2003;46:298.
111. Pahlman L, Glimelius B. Pre- or postoperative radiotherapy in rectal and rectosigmoid carcinoma. Report from a randomized multicenter trial. Ann Surg 1990;211:187.
112. Folkesson J, Birgisson H, Pahlman L, et al. Swedish Rectal Cancer Trial: long lasting benefits from radiotherapy on survival and local recurrence rate. J Clin Oncol 2005;23: 5644–50.
113. Sebag-Montefiore D, Stephens RJ, Steele R, et al. Preoperative radiotherapy versus selective postoperative chemoradiotherapy in patients with rectal cancer (MRC CR07 and NCIC-CTG C016): a multicentre, randomised trial. Lancet 2009;373:811–20.
114. Bosset JF, Collette L, Calais G, et al. Chemotherapy with preoperative radiotherapy in rectal cancer. N Engl J Med 2006;355: 1114–23.
115. Scoggins CR, Meszoely IM, Blanke CD, et al. Nonoperative management of primary colorectal cancer in patients with stage IV disease. Ann Surg Oncol 1999;6:651.
116. Ruo L, Gougoutas C, Paty PB, et al. Elective bowel resection for incurable stage IV colorectal cancer: prognostic variables for asymptomatic patients. J Am Coll Surg 2003;196:722.
117. Scheele J, Stangl R, Altendorf-Hofmann A, et al. Indicators of prognosis after hepatic resection for colorectal secondaries. Surgery 1991;110:13.
118. Martin R, Paty P, Fong Y, et al. Simultaneous liver and colorectal resections are safe for synchronous colorectal liver metastasis. J Am Coll Surg 2003;197:233.
119. Chua HK, Sondenaa K, Tsiotos GG, et al. Concurrent vs. staged colectomy and hepatectomy for primary colorectal cancer with synchronous hepatic metastases. Dis Colon Rectum 2004;47:1310.
120. Jayne DG, Fook S, Loi C, et al. Peritoneal carcinomatosis from colorectal cancer. Br J Surg 2002;89:1545.
121. Rosen SA, Buell JF, Yoshida A, et al. Initial presentation with stage IV colorectal cancer: how aggressive should we be? Arch Surg 2000;135:530.
122. Elias DM, Pocard M, Treatment and prevention of peritoneal carcinomatosis from colorectal cancer. Surg Oncol Clin N Am 2003;12:543.
123. Stephens AD, Alderman R, Chang D, et al. Morbidity and mortality analysis of 200 treatments with cytoreductive surgery and hyperthermic intraoperative intraperitoneal chemotherapy using the coliseum technique. Ann Surg Oncol 1999;6:790.
124. Verwaal VJ, van Ruth S, de Bree E, et al. Randomized trial of cytoreduction and hyperthermic intraperitoneal chemotherapy versus systemic chemotherapy and palliative surgery in patients with peritoneal carcinomatosis of colorectal cancer. J Clin Oncol 2003;21:3737.
125. Verwaal VJ, Bruin S, Boot H, et al. 8-year follow-up of randomized trial: cytoreduction and hyperthermic intraperitoneal chemotherapy versus systemic chemotherapy in patients with peritoneal carcinomatosis of colorectal cancer. Ann Surg Oncol 2008;15:2426–32.
126. Green RJ, Metlay JP, Propert K, et al. Surveillance for second primary colorectal cancer after adjuvant chemotherapy: an analysis of Intergroup 0089. Ann Intern Med 2002; 136:261.
127. Chau I, Allen MJ, Cunningham D, et al. The value of routine serum carcino-embryonic antigen measurement and computed tomography in the surveillance of patients after adjuvant chemotherapy for colorectal cancer. J Clin Oncol 2004;22:1420.
128. Rosen M, Chan L, Beart RW, Jr, et al. Follow-up of colorectal cancer: a meta-analysis. Dis Colon Rectum 1998;41:1116.
129. Renehan AG, Egger M, Saunders MP, et al. Impact on survival of intensive follow up after curative resection for colorectal cancer: systematic review and meta-analysis of randomised trials. BMJ 2002;324:813.
130. Jeffery GM, Hickey BE, Hider P, Follow-up strategies for patients treated for non-metastatic colorectal cancer. Cochrane Database Syst Rev 2002;(1):CD002200.
131. Figueredo A, Rumble RB, Maroun J, et al. Follow-up of patients with curatively resected colorectal cancer: a practice guideline. BMC Cancer 2003;3:26.
132. Wichmann MW, Muller C, Hornung HM, et al. Results of long-term follow-up after curative resection of Dukes A colorectal cancer. World J Surg 2002;26:732.
133. Benson AB 3rd, Desch CE, Flynn PJ, et al. 2000 update of American Society of Clinical Oncology colorectal cancer surveillance guidelines. J Clin Oncol 2000;18: 3586.
134. Anthony T, Simmang C, Hyman N, et al. Practice parameters for the surveillance and follow-up of patients with colon and rectal cancer. Dis Colon Rectum 2004;47:807.
135. Fong Y, Fortner J, Sun RL, et al. Clinical score for predicting recurrence after hepatic resection for metastatic colorectal cancer: analysis of 1001 consecutive cases. Ann Surg 1999;230:309.
136. Fernandez FG, Drebin JA, Linehan DC, et al. Five-year survival after resection of hepatic metastases from colorectal cancer in patients screened by positron emission tomography with F-18 fluorodeoxyglucose (FDG-PET). Ann Surg 2004;240:438.
137. Schussler-Fiorenza CM, Mahvi DM, Niederhuber J, et al. Clinical risk score correlates with yield of PET scan in patients with colorectal hepatic metastases. J Gastrointest Surg 2004;8:150.
138. Pfannschmidt J, Muley T, Hoffmann H, et al. Prognostic factors and survival after complete resection of pulmonary metastases from colorectal carcinoma: experiences in 167 patients. J Thorac Cardiovasc Surg 2003;126:732.
139. Vogelsang H, Haas S, Hierholzer C, et al. Factors influencing survival after resection of pulmonary metastases from colorectal cancer. Br J Surg 2004;91:1066.
140. Hahnloser D, Nelson H, Gunderson LL, et al. Curative potential of multimodality therapy for locally recurrent rectal cancer. Ann Surg 2003;237:502.
141. Cheng C, Rodriguez-Bigas MA, Petrelli N. Is there a role for curative surgery for pelvic recurrence from rectal carcinoma in the presence of hydronephrosis? Am J Surg 2001;182:274.

Acknowledgment

Figure 1 Alice Y. Chen.

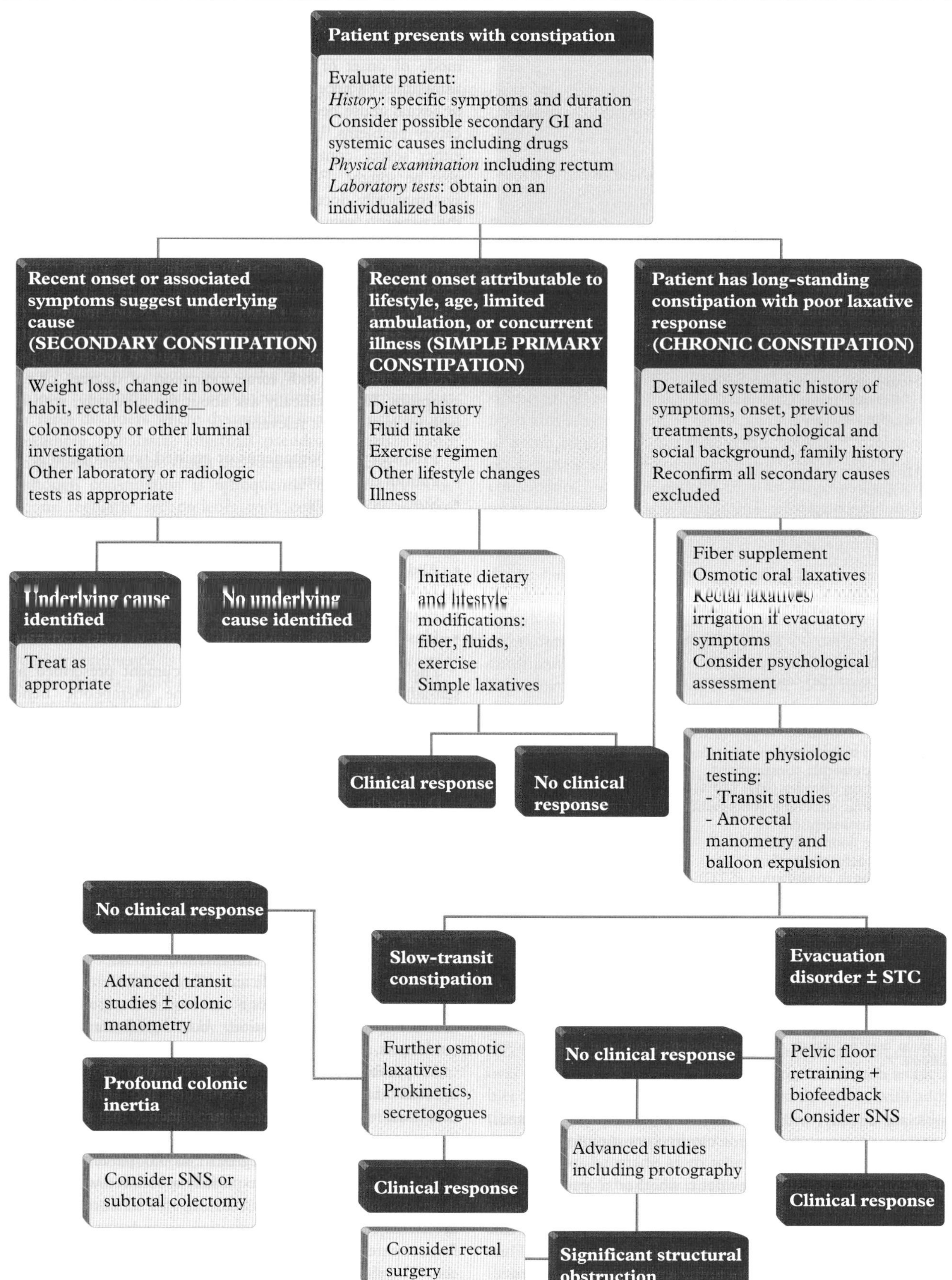

Figure 1 **Algorithm outlining the workup and management of constipation. GI = gastrointestinal; SNS = sacral nerve stimulation; STC = slow-transit constipation.**

squeezing, and ascertain obvious sphincter defects. Furthermore, an effort should be made to look for any anterior defect in the rectovaginal septum leading to a rectocele (your digit will appear within a pouch visible in the posterior vagina). On removing the digit from the anus, it is sometimes possible to appreciate the presence of an intra-anal intussusception or mucosal prolapse that "drags" out with the examining digit.[17] It is unlikely that a digital examination can give useful information on paradoxical puborectalis contraction (dyssynergia), although the experienced examiner can sometimes have the impression of pelvic floor contraction during straining. The finding of a rectal mass warrants further investigation. Anoscopy and proctoscopy should be performed if there is any history of rectal bleeding and may indicate fissure or internal piles.

INVESTIGATIVE STUDIES

In general, diagnostic studies can be divided into those conducted to rule out an underlying cause of secondary constipation (e.g., partially obstructing colon cancer, metabolic or endocrine cause) and those used to diagnose specific anorectal or colonic physiologic abnormalities associated with chronic idiopathic constipation.

Investigations for Secondary Causes of Chronic Constipation

Although the findings from the history or physical examination may indicate a possible secondary cause of constipation, making further investigation mandatory (e.g., for a change in bowel habit), it is also typical practice in patients with chronic constipation to exclude certain secondary causes by investigation even though the diagnostic utility of such investigations is acknowledged to be low (the most common undiagnosed systemic disease is hypothyroidism). Thus, serum calcium concentrations, thyroid function tests, hemoglobin concentrations, glucose levels, serum electrolyte levels, and creatinine concentrations are usually performed. The approach taken to structural investigation of the colon when patients have no suspected intraluminal pathology varies internationally and on the basis of available resources. In the United States, for patients older than 50 years, the baseline risk of colorectal cancer is sufficiently high that screening colonoscopy is recommended even in the absence of alarming symptoms. These older patients should therefore undergo routine colonoscopy, and many authors recommend that patients younger than 50 years undergo routine flexible sigmoidoscopy. Routine biopsies have no benefit however. In Europe, this approach is being increasingly adopted. At some stage, it is worth assessing the rectum and colon so that subsequent management (which may be protracted or unsuccessful) can start with a baseline of reassurance that no organic disease is present. Barium enema can still be a useful investigation in this instance because it yields more information on colonic diameter (for rarer cases of megacolon) and the distribution and severity of diverticular disease, which may coexist and be responsible in part for symptomatology.

Investigations for Primary (Idiopathic) Chronic Constipation

In patients with chronic constipation in whom basic laxatives have failed, further specialist investigative tests are usually warranted. These tests are conducted to provide information on the underlying pathophysiologic abnormalities of the colon and/or anorectum on the basis that the results will guide further management. Most opinion leaders agree that such tests are of value, although opinions differ on how rigorous such investigations should be and when in the algorithm they should be performed. Although there is a general lack of evidence that targeted management strategies are superior to empirical stepwise treatments in earlier pharmacologic and behavioral interventions, it is at least generally agreed that such tests are mandatory if surgery is considered.[18,19] Finally, it should be noted that all are dependent on adequate normative data (sex and age relevant), the expertise of the investigator, and correct interpretation in the context of the clinical information.

These investigations also vary in their availability and complexity internationally. Table 2 lists standard and advanced tests. An additional, often-neglected investigation that can be performed and reviewed immediately in the ambulatory setting is plain abdominal radiography. This is particularly useful as a screening tool for determining whether the symptoms volunteered by patients correlate with a colon loaded with feces and may be shown to the patient to aid discussion.

The mainstay for the rapid evaluation of colonic transit is the radiopaque marker study. Although variations in technique exist in terms of the number of markers, the interval to radiography and definition of slow transit (in the United Kingdom, typically 50 markers, 100 hours, and > 20% remaining),[20] the basic premise is that a number of markers (small pieces of plastic tubing, prepackaged in gelatin capsules) are ingested, and an abdominal x-ray (which includes the pelvis) is taken at an interval. The patient abstains from laxatives for the duration of the study. In patients with significant numbers of retained markers (based on control data), slow transit is diagnosed [*see Figure 2a*]. Alternatively, transit can be measured by radioscintigraphy[21,22] [*see Figure 2b*] or a wireless motility capsule[23] [*see Figure 2c*]. These techniques are valid but not yet widely available. On the basis of radiopaque marker studies, approximately 40% of patients with chronic constipation will have delayed transit.[18,24] Abnormal transit may be demonstrated either throughout the colon or within a limited portion thereof (most commonly, the sigmoid and the rectum).[21] In the latter, it is unresolved whether such markers represent a primary disturbance of rectosigmoid motility or are retained secondary to a primary problem of evacuation,[25] which is also present in more than half of the slow-transit constipation (STC) group.

Figure 3 schematically shows the normal process of defecation [*see Figure 3, a–c*] and the three most common causes of evacuation disorder (ED) [*see Figure 3, d–f*). Pelvic floor studies are valuable for determining the presence and pathophysiology of ED and are best conducted in a pelvic floor laboratory with a specific interest in anorectal function. The balloon expulsion test can be performed in the office as an initial screening measure. A balloon filled with 50 mL of water is attached to tubing and placed in the rectum. Patients with an evacuation disorder are then defined as those who cannot expel the balloon from the rectum in 1 minute while sitting on a commode. It should be kept in mind, however, that as many as 12% of patients with normal pelvic floor function will have difficulty with balloon expulsion in this setting.[24] Furthermore, the literature has become confused by constipation). In many centers, the ability of the patient to sense rectal balloon distention is also determined because loss of the urge to defecate may be caused by blunted rectal sensation (rectal hyposensation).[28] In patients with suspected puborectalis dyssynergia, manometry can be employed during straining to demonstrate either failure to relax to enable expulsion or paradoxical contraction.[24,29] Similar findings during straining can also (if required) be documented by means of electromyography (EMG) with a sponge electrode in the anal canal.[29]

MANAGEMENT

Chronic Idiopathic Constipation

Figure 1 illustrates that many treatments can be initiated without prior physiologic testing. Following detailed history taking, the patient's past drug use will be documented and can guide further therapy. The evidence base for an exact protocol of laxative use is poor,[30] with only polyethylene glycol (PEG)-based osmotic laxatives having been rigorously subjected to trials in the modern randomized, controlled trial age.[31] Nevertheless, stool softeners (e.g., docusate), stimulant laxatives (e.g., senna and bisacodyl), and osmotic laxatives (e.g., PEG, lactulose, and magnesium salts) may be used alone or in combination with good effect. Bulking agents often cause further abdominal pain and bloating in patients with chronic constipation. Furthermore, attempts to prescribe such products (such as encouraging further dietary fiber intake, exercise, and fluids) will in general be met with hostility by patients who have exhausted such measures many years before and lead to an erosion of trust. In the absence of evidence, we make the following practical suggestions:

- Reassure the patient that modern laxatives do not damage the bowel.
- Try to stop all current laxatives, that is, do something definite (this is referred to as "switching" in the psychiatric literature).
- Consider use of rectal laxatives (±oral purgatives) in patients with defecatory symptoms; these have often not been tried.
- Consider laxative dose titration (e.g., magnesium salts).
- Prescribe and monitor the chosen therapy at a fixed interval, for example, 3 months.
- Warn of side effects but emphasize the need for compliance.
- Rotate the laxative type at regular intervals to avoid tolerance.

Other drugs acting on secretion and motility are discussed under Slow-Transit Constipation (see below) but may equally be employed for patients with chronic constipation that has not been further physiologically defined. Similarly, there is some evidence that behavioral treatments may benefit all patients with chronic constipation[32] rather than just those with pelvic floor dyssynergia. However, for clarity and better understanding, further discussion of these has been separated by subtypes of chronic constipation.

Slow-Transit Constipation

Medical treatment Patients with STC are primarily treated by addressing the transit disturbance of the colon (although ED commonly coexists). In this group, the mainstay of therapy is the use of osmotic and stimulant laxatives (alone or in combination) to effect changes in transit[33,34] with benefit proven in controlled trials.[35] A theoretical problem with all classic laxative therapies is their bioavailability in the colon. All require transport to the colon for site of action, and some require metabolism via the enteral flora to produce active products, for example, hydrolysis of stimulant laxatives. Furthermore, laxatives are often poorly tolerated because of pain (mainly stimulant) or unpredictable diarrhea with or without incontinence (mainly osmotic). Given the burden of disease, much investment has been made to find newer classes of drug to treat chronic constipation. To date, two classes of drug are being developed: colonic prokinetics, based on activity at serotonin receptor subtype 4 (5-HT_4 agonists), and intestinal secretagogues.

The main development in the 5-HT_4 agonist class is prucalopride. This drug has much greater selectivity to the 5-HT_4 receptor than the now withdrawn 5-HT_4 agonists such as tegaserod and cisapride. In particular, it has no proven effect on QTc interval caused by activation of the cardiac conducting system channels that led to arrhythmias with less selective drugs. Prucalopride has been the subject of three rigorously conducted phase III pivotal trials with pooled data available on over 2,000 patients.[5] Abundant cross-species data (including humans) show that prucalopride leads to increases in propagated colonic contractile activity, leading to coordinated mass movements and spontaneous defecation.[36] It has an acceptable side-effect profile and is currently licensed in Europe for women with chronic constipation; it has some effect in approximately 50% of patients.[5] In particular, it has a significant advantage over laxatives in terms of reducing rather than increasing abdominal pain and bloating.

Two drugs, lubiprostone (a chloride channel activator) and linaclotide (a guanylate cyclase C receptor activator), accelerate colonic transit in humans by mediating luminal secretion. Lubiprostone has a phase III portfolio and is approved by the Food and Drug Administration (FDA) for chronic constipation but is reported to cause problematic nausea in approximately 20% of patients.[37] Linaclotide is at an earlier developmental stage and has proved effective in phase II trials.[38]

Surgical treatment Until very recently, colonic excision was the only popularized form of surgery to address STC. It is a fact that colectomy has a "finality" that separates it not only from medical treatments but also from most other invasive interventions for constipation. The results of colectomy have been extensively reviewed previously,[19,39] with overall success rates varying between 40 and 100%. It is probable that colectomy peaked in popularity in the mid-1990s but has seen a gradual decline in application since publications of more modest longer-term results became available and the potential for serious complications and poor functional outcomes was realized.[40] Nevertheless, most would agree that colectomy continues to have a limited role as a treatment option for highly selected patients with proven STC (probably < 5% chronic constipation) who have failed all nonsurgical interventions and in whom symptoms are sufficiently severe to contemplate major surgery. Such surgery should be undertaken only in specialized centers where the techniques required for selection are available. Subtotal colectomy with ileorectal anastomosis has the best results, leading to a median stool frequency of three (range one to five) per day. Unfortunately, surgery may not satisfactorily alleviate other symptoms (e.g., abdominal discomfort or bloating),[41] and patients should be made aware of this possibility before operation. Overall, the majority of well-selected patients are satisfied with the results of surgical treatment[42,43]; however, long-term postoperative complications, particularly small bowel obstruction, are common. In addition, patients may manifest symptoms of a more global GI dysmotility disorder in the long term.

The role of sacral nerve stimulation (SNS) is being critically evaluated following the very recent publication of a multicenter European trial showing the beneficial effect of SNS in 39 of 62 (63%) chronic constipation patients who predominantly had STC[44] and other studies with less encouraging results.[45] Mechanistically, SNS increases pancolonic anterograde propogated sequences in patients with STC.[46] Controlled studies are required particularly because SNS is not cheap. However, the attraction of this minimally invasive treatment and possibility of pretesting patients prior to stimulator implantation make it a promising tool for patients who might otherwise progress to colectomy.[39]

A stoma may be used as a definitive procedure, as a guide to further treatment, or as salvage from previously failed or complicated surgical intervention. There are few published data to support an evidence-based use; however, an ileostomy may be employed as a guide to colectomy, with subsequent resection avoided if the ileostomy output is unsatisfactorily high or symptoms such as pain and bloating are untouched by diversion.[47] As a definitive procedure, both colostomy and ileostomy have been described for a diversity of disorders characterized by constipation, including spinal cord injury, megacolon, and ED. There is little evidence in adults to guide the choice of ileostomy or colostomy[48]; however, some report high complication rates of ileostomy,[49] and STC may be unsatisfactorily treated by colostomy.

The Malone anterograde continent enema technique may also be an option for refractory STC but has been employed more frequently in patients with severe ED [*see* Evacuation Disorder, *below*].

Evacuation Disorder

Patients with evidence of ED can be subdivided broadly into those with an obvious structural cause, such as a large rectocele or intussusception, and those in whom no such cause is found but in whom defecation is still ineffective. Depending on the definition and methods used to diagnose, 20 to 75% of the latter will be found to have puborectalis dyssynergia[24,29]—the term used to describe paradoxical or noncontraction of the pelvic floor during straining. The evidence base for ED management is fraught with semantic differences; however, a few key management strategies have general agreement:

- All patients may benefit from nurse-led bowel retraining and rectal laxatives and/or anal irrigation.
- Patients with large rectoceles in whom clinical (the patient can successfully effect evacuation by digital pressure in the vagina) and radiologic findings concur should have these repaired by one of the numerous transvaginal, transperineal, or transanal approaches.[50,51] However, the optimal operation for rectocele remains a matter of debate.
- Patients with proven or suspected puborectalis dyssynergia should undergo behavioral retraining incorporating biofeedback.

Behavioral therapy The predominant behavioral treatment is biofeedback. This (usually nurse-led) therapy retrains the patient to appropriately contract her abdominal and relax her pelvic floor muscles during defecation, with the patient receiving feedback of anal and pelvic floor muscle activity as recorded by surface EMG, anal pressure sensors, or digital examination by the therapist. Several controlled trials and meta-analyses provide data on biofeedback outcomes in comparison with sham or alternative treatments.[18] Opinions vary on which patient groups most benefit, with some favorable[32] and some unfavorable[52] results for patients with STC. However, most would agree that this treatment is best targeted at those with ED, particularly those with proven puborectalis dyssynergia. The results range from approximately 70 to 90% success rates in adults with ED,[52–54] with a recent meta-analysis of three randomized, controlled trials giving an odds ratio of success over placebo of 3.7 (95% CI 2.1 to 6.3).[55] Training may have to be reinforced at intervals but is generally sustained in the longer term.

Anorectal surgery The repair of large rectoceles has been noted above and can be performed by urogynecologists who are more familiar with approaches that avoid the rectal lumen.[51] Much more contentious are the numerous surgical approaches for smaller rectoceles, intussuscepta, or both (these frequently coexist). An "industry" of operations that either hitch, reinforce, or excise rectal tissue have been described.[39] All are beset with the following problems in relation to the treatment of ED:

1. Anatomic abnormalities such as rectocele and intussusception are detectable in significant proportions (at least 40%) of asymptomatic subjects.[56]
2. Such abnormalities often belie a complex multifactorial problem with several contributing etiologies that cannot be corrected by surgery alone.[57,58]
3. Promising early success in case series (e.g., 90%[59]) often becomes less encouraging in the longer term (approximately 50%).[60,61]
4. There are no bona fide data from randomized, controlled trials for any procedure.[39]
5. Although many procedures have generally low morbidity, none are without the risk of serious complications in at least a minority of patients.[62]

Two procedures require specific mention as a result of their current popularity.

Laparoscopic ventral rectopexy was first described for full-thickness rectal prolapse[63] but has been applied to the treatment of intussusception since 2008.[64] The rectum is mobilized anteriorly to the pelvic floor and a mesh is sutured to the ventral rectum, posterior vagina, and vaginal fornix and secured to the sacral promontory. Excellent short-term results have recently been published for this procedure[65]; however,

a

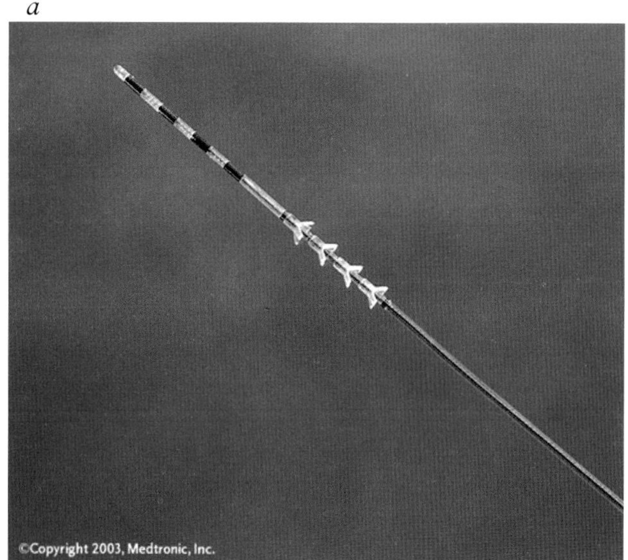

b

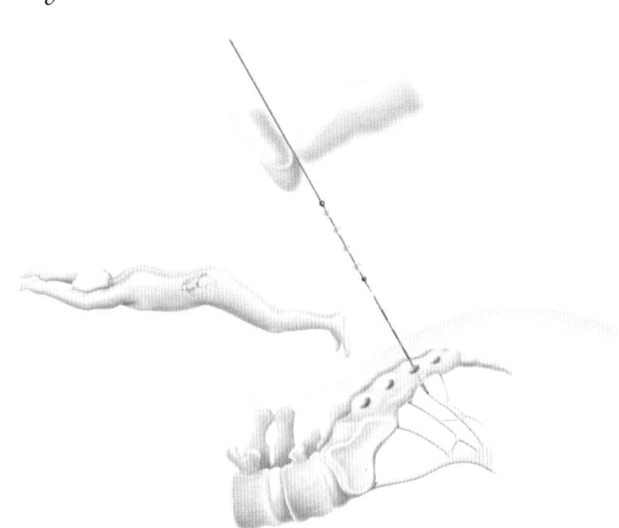

c

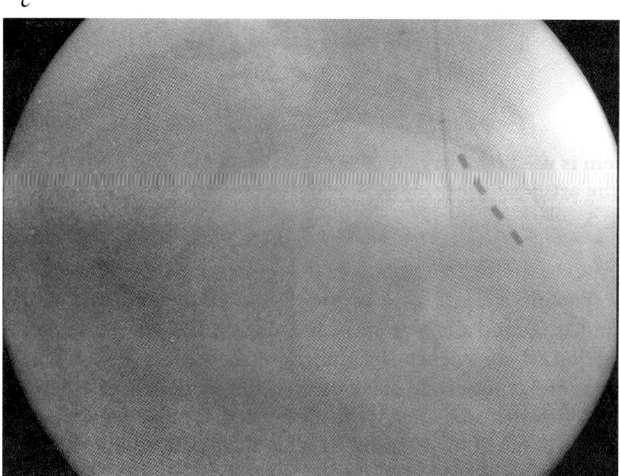

Figure 9 **Sacral nerve stimulation. (*a*) A lead containing four electrodes is used. (*b*) The sacral foramina are identified; in most cases, S3 is the optimal choice for stimulation. (*c*) Shown is the quadripolar lead in position.**

choice for patients with refractory incontinence. If SNS fails, more aggressive treatments may still be tried at a later time.

Colostomy

Although creation of a colostomy does not restore continence, it does provide a degree of bowel control in a manner that allows patients to resume their normal activities without fear of accidents. Surprisingly few data are available regarding colostomy for incontinence; however, one questionnaire study of patients who underwent colostomy for incontinence reported extremely high levels of patient satisfaction and marked improvements in subjective quality of life.[116] In most cases, a simple end sigmoid colostomy with a Hartmann pouch is the appropriate procedure and can often be performed with relatively little operative trauma by using a laparoscopic or minilaparotomy technique. Patients should receive preoperative counseling from an enterostomal therapist, and the optimal stoma site should be marked before the procedure is initiated.

Financial Disclosures: None Reported

References

1. Stewart WF, Liberman JN, Sandler RS, et al. Epidemiology of Constipation (EPOC) study in the United States: relation of clinical subtypes to sociodemographic features. Am J Gastroenterol 1999;94:3530–40.
2. McCrea GL, Miaskowski C, Stotts NA, et al. Review article: self-report measures to evaluate constipation. Aliment Pharmacol Ther 2008;27:638–48.
3. Cook IJ, Talley NJ, Benninga MA, et al. Chronic constipation: overview and challenges. Neurogastroenterol Motil 2009;21 Suppl 2:1–8.
4. Talley NJ. Definitions, epidemiology, and impact of chronic constipation. Rev Gastroenterol Disord 2004;4 Suppl 2:S3–10.
5. Camilleri M, Kerstens R, Rykx A, Vandeplassche L. A placebo-controlled trial of prucalopride for severe chronic constipation. N Engl J Med 2008;358:2344–54.
6. Drossman DA. The functional gastrointestinal disorders and the Rome III process. Gastroenterology 2006;130:1377–90.
7. Probert CS, Emmett PM, Cripps HA, Heaton KW. Evidence for the ambiguity of the term constipation: the role of irritable bowel syndrome. Gut 1994;35:1455–8.

8. Pare P, Ferrazzi S, Thompson WG, et al. An epidemiological survey of constipation in Canada: definitions, rates, demographics, and predictors of health care seeking. Am J Gastroenterol 2001;96:3130–7.
9. Mertz H, Naliboff B, Mayer EA. Symptoms and physiology in severe chronic constipation. Am J Gastroenterol 1999;94:131–8.
10. Knowles CH, Scott SM, Rayner C, et al. Idiopathic slow-transit constipation: an almost exclusively female disorder. Dis Colon Rectum 2003;46:1716–7.
11. Preston DM, Lennard-Jones JE. Severe chronic constipation of young women: 'idiopathic slow transit constipation.' Gut 1986; 27:41–8.
12. Roe AM, Bartolo DC, Mortensen NJ. Slow transit constipation. Comparison between patients with or without previous hysterectomy. Dig Dis Sci 1988;33:1159–63.
13. Leroi AM, Berkelmans I, Denis P, et al. Anismus as a marker of sexual abuse. Consequences of abuse on anorectal motility. Dig Dis Sci 1995;40:1411–6.
14. Agachan F, Chen T, Pfeifer J, et al. A constipation scoring system to simplify evaluation and management of constipated patients. Dis Colon Rectum 1996;39:681–5.
15. Knowles CH, Eccersley AJ, Scott SM, et al. Linear discriminant analysis of symptoms in patients with chronic constipation: validation of a new scoring system (KESS). Dis Colon Rectum 2000;43:1419–26.
16. Lunniss PJ, Gladman MA, Hetzer FH, et al. Risk factors in acquired faecal incontinence. J R Soc Med 2004;97:111–6.
17. Karlbom U, Lundin E, Graf W, Pahlman L. Anorectal physiology in relation to clinical subgroups of patients with severe constipation. Colorectal Dis 2004;6:343–9.
18. Camilleri M, Bharucha AE. Behavioural and new pharmacological treatments for constipation: getting the balance right. Gut 2010; 59:1288–96.
19. Knowles CH, Scott M, Lunniss PJ. Outcome of colectomy for slow transit constipation. Ann Surg 1999;230:627–38.
20. Dinning PG, Smith TK, Scott SM. Pathophysiology of colonic causes of chronic constipation. Neurogastroenterol Motil 2009;21 Suppl 2:20–30.
21. Roberts JP, Newell MS, Deeks JJ, et al. Oral [111In]DTPA scintigraphic assessment of colonic transit in constipated subjects. Dig Dis Sci 1993;38:1032–9.
22. Scott SM, Knowles CH, Newell M, et al. Scintigraphic assessment of colonic transit in women with slow-transit constipation arising de novo and following pelvic surgery or childbirth. Br J Surg 2001;88:405–11.
23. Rao SS, Kuo B, McCallum RW, et al. Investigation of colonic and whole-gut transit with wireless motility capsule and radiopaque markers in constipation. Clin Gastroenterol Hepatol 2009;7:537–44.
24. Rao SS, Ozturk R, Laine L. Clinical utility of diagnostic tests for constipation in adults: a systematic review. Am J Gastroenterol 2005;100:1605–15.
25. Zarate N, Knowles CH, Newell M, et al. In patients with slow transit constipation, the pattern of colonic transit delay does not differentiate between those with and without impaired rectal evacuation. Am J Gastroenterol 2008;103:427–34.
26. Rao SS. Constipation: evaluation and treatment of colonic and anorectal motility disorders. Gastrointest Endosc Clin N Am 2009;19:117–39, vii.
27. Jorge JM, Habr-Gama A, Wexner SD. Clinical applications and techniques of cinedefecography. Am J Surg 2001;182:93–101.
28. Gladman MA, Lunniss PJ, Scott SM, Swash M. Rectal hyposensitivity. Am J Gastroenterol 2006;101:1140–51.
29. Scott SM, Gladman MA. Manometric, sensorimotor, and neurophysiologic evaluation of anorectal function. Gastroenterol Clin North Am 2008;37:511–38, vii.
30. Emmanuel AV, Tack J, Quigley EM, Talley NJ. Pharmacological management of constipation. Neurogastroenterol Motil 2009;21 Suppl 2:41–54.
31. Corazziari E, Badiali D, Bazzocchi G, et al. Long term efficacy, safety, and tolerabilitity of low daily doses of isosmotic polyethylene glycol electrolyte balanced solution (PMF-100) in the treatment of functional chronic constipation. Gut 2000;46:522–6.
32. Chiotakakou-Faliakou E, Kamm MA, Roy AJ, et al. Biofeedback provides long-term benefit for patients with intractable, slow and normal transit constipation. Gut 1998; 42:517–21.
33. Skoog SM, Bharucha AE, Camilleri M, et al. Effects of an osmotically active agent on colonic transit. Neurogastroenterol Motil 2006;18:300–6.
34. Manabe N, Cremonini F, Camilleri M, et al. Effects of bisacodyl on ascending colon emptying and overall colonic transit in healthy volunteers. Aliment Pharmacol Ther 2009;30:930–6.
35. Kienzle-Horn S, Vix JM, Schuijt C, et al. Efficacy and safety of bisacodyl in the acute treatment of constipation: a double-blind, randomized, placebo-controlled study. Aliment Pharmacol Ther 2006;23:1479–88.
36. Bouras EP, Camilleri M, Burton DD, et al. Prucalopride accelerates gastrointestinal and colonic transit in patients with constipation without a rectal evacuation disorder. Gastroenterology 2001;120:354–60.
37. Johanson JF, Drossman DA, Panas R, et al. Clinical trial: phase 2 study of lubiprostone for irritable bowel syndrome with constipation. Aliment Pharmacol Ther 2008;27:685–96.
38. Lembo AJ, Kurtz CB, Macdougall JE, et al. Efficacy of linaclotide for patients with chronic constipation. Gastroenterology 2010; 138:886–95.
39. Knowles CH, Dinning PG, Pescatori M, et al. Surgical management of constipation. Neurogastroenterol Motil 2009;21 Suppl 2:62–71.
40. Kamm MA. The surgical treatment of severe idiopathic constipation. Int J Colorectal Dis 1987;2:229–35.
41. Platell C, Scache D, Mumme G, Stitz R. A long-term follow-up of patients undergoing colectomy for chronic idiopathic constipation. Aust N Z J Surg 1996;66:525–9.
42. FitzHarris GP, Garcia-Aguilar J, Parker SC, et al. Quality of life after subtotal colectomy for slow-transit constipation: both quality and quantity count. Dis Colon Rectum 2003;46:433–40.
43. Nyam DC, Pemberton JH, Ilstrup DM, Rath DM. Long-term results of surgery for chronic constipation. Dis Colon Rectum 1997;40:273–9.
44. Kamm MA, Dudding TC, Melenhorst J, et al. Sacral nerve stimulation for intractable constipation. Gut 2010;59:333–40.
45. Vitton V, Roman S, Damon H, et al. Sacral nerve stimulation and constipation: still a long way to go. Dis Colon Rectum 2009;52: 752–3; author reply 3–4.
46. Dinning PG, Fuentealba SE, Kennedy ML, et al. Sacral nerve stimulation induces pan-colonic propagating pressure waves and increases defecation frequency in patients with slow-transit constipation. Colorectal Dis 2007;9:123–32.
47. Wong SW, Lubowski DZ. Slow-transit constipation: evaluation and treatment. Aust N Z J Surg 2007;77:320–8.
48. Gladman MA, Knowles CH. Surgical treatment of patients with constipation and fecal incontinence. Gastroenterol Clin North Am 2008;37:605–25, viii.
49. Scarpa M, Barollo M, Keighley MR. Ileostomy for constipation: long-term postoperative outcome. Colorectal Dis 2005;7: 224–7.
50. Heriot AG, Skull A, Kumar D. Functional and physiological outcome following transanal repair of rectocele. Br J Surg 2004;91: 1340–4.
51. Altman D, Zetterstrom J, Lopez A, et al. Functional and anatomic outcome after transvaginal rectocele repair using collagen mesh: a prospective study. Dis Colon Rectum 2005;48:1233–41; discussion 41–2; author reply 42.
52. Chiarioni G, Salandini L, Whitehead WE. Biofeedback benefits only patients with outlet dysfunction, not patients with isolated slow transit constipation. Gastroenterology 2005;129:86–97.
53. Rao SS, Seaton K, Miller M, et al. Randomized controlled trial of biofeedback, sham feedback, and standard therapy for dyssynergic defecation. Clin Gastroenterol Hepatol 2007;5:331–8.
54. Heymen S, Scarlett Y, Jones K, et al. Randomized, controlled trial shows biofeedback to be superior to alternative treatments for patients with pelvic floor dyssynergia-type constipation. Dis Colon Rectum 2007; 50:428–41.
55. Enck P, Van der Voort IR, Klosterhalfen S. Biofeedback therapy in fecal incontinence and constipation. Neurogastroenterol Motil 2009;21:1133–41.
56. Shorvon PJ, McHugh S, Diamant NE, et al. Defecography in normal volunteers: results and implications. Gut 1989;30:1737–49.
57. Thompson JR, Chen AH, Pettit PD, Bridges MD. Incidence of occult rectal prolapse in patients with clinical rectoceles and defecatory dysfunction. Am J Obstet Gynecol 2002;187:1494–9.
58. Pescatori M, Spyrou M, Pulvirenti d'Urso A. A prospective evaluation of occult disorders in obstructed defecation using the 'iceberg diagram.' Colorectal Dis 2007;9: 452–6.
59. Christiansen J, Zhu BW, Rasmussen OO, Sorensen M. Internal rectal intussusception: results of surgical repair. Dis Colon Rectum 1992;35:1026–8; discussion 8–9.
60. Pescatori M, Aigner F. Stapled transanal rectal mucosectomy ten years after. Tech Coloproctol 2007;11:1–6.
61. Roman H, Michot F. Long-term outcomes of transanal rectocele repair. Dis Colon Rectum 2005;48:510–7.
62. Gagliardi G, Pescatori M, Altomare DF, et al. Results, outcome predictors, and complications after stapled transanal rectal resection for obstructed defecation. Dis Colon Rectum 2008;51:186–95.
63. D'Hoore A, Cadoni R, Penninckx F. Long-term outcome of laparoscopic ventral rectopexy for total rectal prolapse. Br J Surg 2004;91:1500–5.
64. van den Esschert JW, van Geloven AA, Vermulst N, et al. Laparoscopic ventral rectopexy for obstructed defecation syndrome. Surg Endosc 2008;22:2728–32.
65. Collinson R, Wijffels N, Cunningham C, Lindsey I. Laparoscopic ventral rectopexy for internal rectal prolapse: short-term functional results. Colorectal Dis 2010;12:97–104.

66. Boccasanta P, Venturi M, Calabro G, et al. Stapled transanal rectal resection in solitary rectal ulcer associated with prolapse of the rectum: a prospective study. Dis Colon Rectum 2008;51:348–54.
67. Hirst GR, Arumugam PJ, Watkins AJ, et al. Antegrade continence enema in the treatment of obstructed defaecation with or without faecal incontinence. Tech Coloproctol 2005;9:217–21.
68. Lees NP, Hodson P, Hill J, et al. Long-term results of the antegrade continent enema procedure for constipation in adults. Colorectal Dis 2004;6:362–8.
69. Uludag O, Morren GL, Dejong CH, Baeten CG. Effect of sacral neuromodulation on the rectum. Br J Surg 2005;92:1017–23.
70. Nelson R, Furner S, Jesudason V. Fecal incontinence in Wisconsin nursing homes: prevalence and associations. Dis Colon Rectum 1998;41:1226–9.
71. Johanson JF, Lafferty J. Epidemiology of fecal incontinence: the silent affliction. Am J Gastroenterol 1996;91:33–6.
72. Snooks SJ, Swash M, Setchell M, Henry MM. Injury to innervation of pelvic floor sphincter musculature. Lancet 1984;2:546–50.
73. Wrenn K. Fecal impaction. N Engl J Med 1989;321:658–62.
74. Garcia-Aguilar J, Belmonte C, Wong WD, et al. Open vs. closed sphincterotomy for chronic anal fissure: long-term results. Dis Colon Rectum 1996;39:440–3.
75. Garcia-Aguilar J, Belmonte C, Wong WD, et al. Anal fistula surgery. Factors associated with recurrence and incontinence. Dis [illegible]
76. MacIntyre IM, Balfour TW. Results of the Lord non-operative treatment for haemorrhoids. Lancet 1972;1:1094–5.
77. Sultan AH, Kamm MA, Talbot IC, et al. Anal endosonography for identifying external sphincter defects confirmed histologically. Br J Surg 1994;81:463–5.
78. Gilliland R, Altomare DF, Moreira H Jr, et al. Pudendal neuropathy is predictive of failure following anterior overlapping sphincteroplasty. Dis Colon Rectum 1998; 41:1516–22.
79. Buie WD, Lowry AC, Rothenberger DA, Madoff RD. Clinical rather than laboratory assessment predicts continence after anterior sphincteroplasty. Dis Colon Rectum 2001; 44:1255–60.
80. Heymen S, Jones KR, Ringel Y, et al. Biofeedback treatment of fecal incontinence: a critical review. Dis Colon Rectum 2001; 44:728–36.
81. Norton C, Kamm MA. Anal sphincter biofeedback and pelvic floor exercises for faecal incontinence in adults—a systematic review. Aliment Pharmacol Ther 2001;15: 1147–54.
82. Norton C, Chelvanayagam S, Wilson-Barnett J, et al. Randomized controlled trial of biofeedback for fecal incontinence. Gastroenterology 2003;125:1320–9.
83. Heymen S, Scarlett Y, Jones K, et al. Randomized controlled trial shows biofeedback to be superior to pelvic floor exercises for fecal incontinence. Dis Colon Rectum 2009;52:1730–7.
84. Pinta TM, Kylanpaa ML, Salmi TK, et al. Primary sphincter repair: are the results of the operation good enough? Dis Colon Rectum 2004;47:18–23.
85. Pemberton JH. Spincter and pelvic floor reconstruction. In: Keighley MR, Pemberton JH, Fazio VW, Parc RF, editors. Atlas of colorectal surgery. Edinburgh: Churchill Livingstone; 1996. p. 131–44.
86. Engel AF, Kamm MA, Sultan AH, et al. Anterior anal sphincter repair in patients with obstetric trauma. Br J Surg 1994;81: 1231–4.
87. Karoui S, Leroi AM, Koning E, et al. Results of sphincteroplasty in 86 patients with anal incontinence. Dis Colon Rectum 2000;43:813–20.
88. Halverson AL, Hull TL. Long-term outcome of overlapping anal sphincter repair. Dis Colon Rectum 2002;45:345–8.
89. Malouf AJ, Norton CS, Engel AF, et al. Long-term results of overlapping anterior anal-sphincter repair for obstetric trauma. Lancet 2000;355:260–5.
90. Bravo Gutierrez A, Madoff RD, Lowry AC, et al. Long-term results of anterior sphincteroplasty. Dis Colon Rectum 2004; 47:727–31; discussion 31–2.
91. Pinedo G, Vaizey CJ, Nicholls RJ, et al. Results of repeat anal sphincter repair. Br J Surg 1999;86:66–9.
92. Jensen LL, Lowry AC. Biofeedback improves functional outcome after sphincteroplasty. Dis Colon Rectum 1997;40:197–200.
[illegible] RJ. Long-term results of postanal repair for neurogenic faecal incontinence. Br J Surg 1994;81:140–4.
94. van Tets WF, Kuijpers JH. Pelvic floor procedures produce no consistent changes in anatomy or physiology. Dis Colon Rectum 1998;41:365–9.
95. Kumar D, Benson MJ, Bland JE. Glutaraldehyde cross-linked collagen in the treatment of faecal incontinence. Br J Surg 1998;85:978–9.
96. Kenefick NJ, Vaizey CJ, Malouf AJ, et al. Injectable silicone biomaterial for faecal incontinence due to internal anal sphincter dysfunction. Gut 2002;51:225–8.
97. Siproudhis L, Morcet J, Laine F. Elastomer implants in faecal incontinence: a blind, randomized placebo-controlled study. Aliment Pharmacol Ther 2007;25:1125–32.
98. Luo C, Samaranayake CB, Plank LD, Bissett IP. Systematic review on the efficacy and safety of injectable bulking agents for passive faecal incontinence. Colorectal Dis 2001;12:296–303.
99. Devesa JM, Madrid JM, Gallego BR, et al. Bilateral gluteoplasty for fecal incontinence. Dis Colon Rectum 1997;40:883–8.
100. Faucheron JL, Hannoun L, Thome C, Parc R. Is fecal continence improved by nonstimulated gracilis muscle transposition? Dis Colon Rectum 1994;37:979–83.
101. Baeten C, Spaans F, Fluks A. An implanted neuromuscular stimulator for fecal continence following previously implanted gracilis muscle: report of a case. Dis Colon Rectum 1988;31:134–7.
102. Konsten J, Baeten CGMI, Havenith MG, Soeters PB. Morphology of dynamic graciloplasty compared with the anal sphincter. Dis Colon Rectum 1993;36:559–63.
103. Rongen MJ, Uludag O, El Naggar K, et al. Long-term follow-up of dynamic graciloplasty for fecal incontinence. Dis Colon Rectum 2003;46:716–21.
104. Mander BJ, Wexner SD, Williams NS, et al. Preliminary results of a multicentre trial of the electrically stimulated gracilis neoanal sphincter. Br J Surg 1999;86:1543–8.
105. Baeten CG, Bailey HR, Bakka A, et al. Safety and efficacy of dynamic graciloplasty for fecal incontinence: report of a prospective, multicenter trial. Dynamic Graciloplasty Therapy Study Group. Dis Colon Rectum 2000;43:743–51.
106. Madoff RD, Rosen HR, Baeten CG, et al. Safety and efficacy of dynamic muscle plasty for anal incontinence: lessons from a prospective, multicenter trial. Gastroenterology 1999;116:549–56.
107. Lehur PA, Roig JV, Duinslaeger M. Artificial anal sphincter: prospective clinical and manometric evaluation. Dis Colon Rectum 2000;43:1100–6.
108. Parker SC, Spencer MP, Madoff RD, et al. Artificial bowel sphincter: long-term experience at a single institution. Dis Colon Rectum 2003;46:722–9.
109. Malouf AJ, Vaizey CJ, Kamm MA, Nicholls RJ. Reassessing artificial bowel sphincters. Lancet 2000;355:2219–20.
110. Siegel SW. Management of voiding dysfunction with an implantable neuroprosthesis. Urol Clin North Am 1992;19:163–70.
111. Matzel KE, Stadelmaier U, Hohenfellner M, Hohenberger W. Chronic sacral spinal nerve stimulation for fecal incontinence: long- term results with foramen and cuff electrodes. Dis Colon Rectum 2001;44:59–66.
112. Rosen HR, Urbarz C, Holzer B, et al. Sacral nerve stimulation as a treatment for fecal incontinence. Gastroenterology 2001;121: 536–41.
113. Kenefick NJ, Vaizey CJ, Cohen RC, et al. Medium-term results of permanent sacral nerve stimulation for faecal incontinence. Br J Surg 2002;89:896–901.
114. Matzel KE, Kamm MA, Stosser M, et al. Sacral spinal nerve stimulation for faecal incontinence: multicentre study. Lancet 2004;363:1270–6.
115. Wexner SD, Coller JA, Devroede G, et al. Sacral nerve stimulation for fecal incontinence: results of a 120-patient prospective multicenter study. Ann Surg 2010;251: 441–9.
116. Norton C. Patients' views of a colostomy for faecal incontinence. Neurourol Urodyn 2003;22:403–4.

Acknowledgment

Figures 3, 7, 8, and 9 Alice Y. Chen

16 BENIGN AND MALIGNANT RECTAL, ANAL, AND PERINEAL PROBLEMS

David E. Beck, MD, FACS, FASCRS

Problems of the rectum, anus, and perineum are common, and an understanding of the anatomy is essential to properly diagnose and treat anorectal conditions.[1] As shown in Figure 1, the dentate line divides the rectal mucosa above (generally insensate and lined with columnar mucosa) and the anoderm below (highly sensitive because of somatic enervation provided by the inferior hemorrhoidal nerve and lined with modified squamous mucosa). The anal canal is surrounded by two muscles. The internal anal sphincter, innervated by the autonomic nervous system, maintains the resting anal tone and is under involuntary control. The external sphincter, innervated by somatic nerve fibers, generates the voluntary anal squeeze and is most important in maintaining anal continence. The area surrounding the anorectum is divided into four spaces, which are particularly important when evaluating perirectal abscesses and fistulas.

This chapter briefly reviews the evaluation and management of benign and malignant conditions of the anus and rectum, as well as retrorectal tumors. Rectal cancer is covered in another chapter of this text.

Benign Conditions

HEMORRHOIDS

Hemorrhoids are fibromuscular cushions that line the anal canal and are classically found in three locations: right anterior, right posterior, and left lateral.[2,3] Smaller secondary cushions may occasionally lie between these main cushions. Contrary to popular belief, hemorrhoids are not related to the superior hemorrhoidal artery and vein, to the portal vein, or to portal hypertension.[4] Hemorrhoids are part of normal

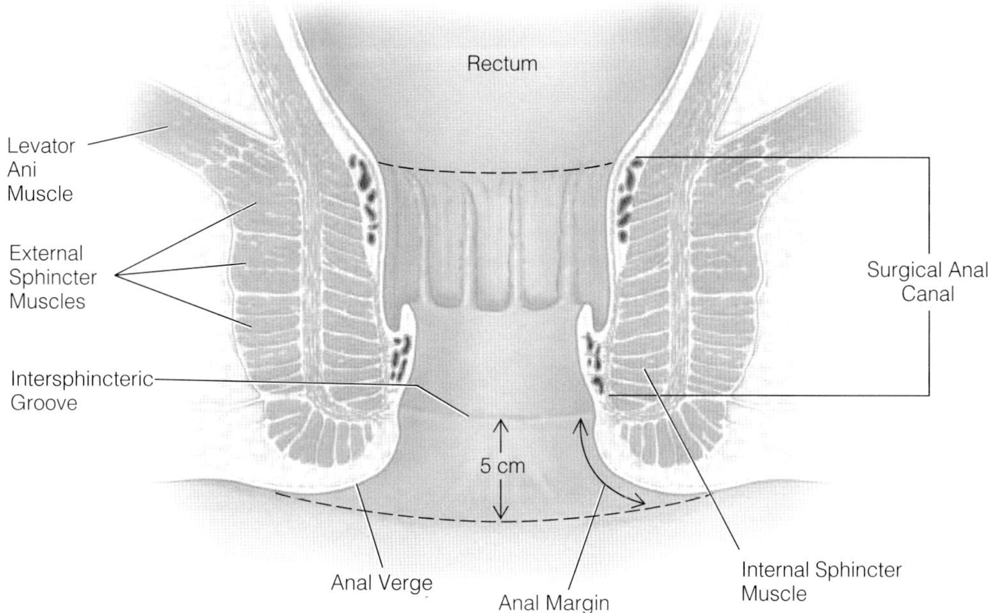

Figure 1 **Depicted is the anatomy of the anal canal.**[53]

anatomy and become engorged during straining or performance of the Valsalva maneuver as a component of the normal mechanism of fecal continence. Hemorrhoidal engorgement most likely completes the occlusion of the anal canal and prevents the stool loss associated with nondefecatory straining. However, when the term "hemorrhoid" is used in the medical literature, it almost exclusively refers to pathologic hemorrhoids, and it will be used as such in the following paragraphs.

Hemorrhoids are divided into internal and external components. Internal hemorrhoids are found proximal to the dentate line, whereas external hemorrhoids occur distally [*see Figure 2*]. External hemorrhoids are redundant folds of perianal skin generally related to previous anal swelling; they remain asymptomatic unless they are thrombosed and are treated entirely differently from internal hemorrhoids.

Internal Hemorrhoids

Evaluation Internal hemorrhoidal disease is demonstrated by two main symptoms: painless bleeding and protrusion.[4] Pain is rarely associated with internal hemorrhoids because they originate above the dentate line in insensate rectal mucosa. The most popular etiologic theory states that hemorrhoids result from chronic straining at defecation (upright posture and heavy lifting may also contribute). This straining not only causes hemorrhoidal engorgement but also creates forces that decrease the fixation between the hemorrhoids and the anal muscular wall. Continued straining causes further engorgement and bleeding, as well as hemorrhoidal prolapse. Internal hemorrhoids are categorized into four grades based on clinical findings and symptoms: 1, bleeding without prolapse; 2, prolapse that spontaneously reduces; 3, prolapse requiring manual reduction; and 4, irreducible prolapse.

Questioning often reveals a long history of constipation and straining at defecation. Patients with internal hemorrhoids are commonly extensive bathroom readers, spending many hours in the bathroom each week. Symptoms start with painless bleeding and may progress to anal protrusion. Hemorrhoidal prolapse must be distinguished from true full-thickness rectal prolapse. The physical examination begins with visual inspection and may reveal prolapsing hemorrhoidal tissue as a rosette of three distinct pink-purple hemorrhoidal groups. If prolapse is not present, anoscopy reveals redundant anorectal mucosa just proximal to the dentate line in the classic locations.

Surgical treatment of hemorrhoids in a patient whose main disease process is Crohn disease, a pelvic floor abnormality, or fissure disease invariably yields imperfect results. It is especially important to recognize anal pain and spasm and fissure in ano because in patients with this problem, excision of the hemorrhoids without concomitant management of the fissure leads to increased postoperative pain and poor wound healing. Not uncommonly, patients are treated for hemorrhoids when the true primary condition is fissure disease.

Treatment Treatment for symptomatic internal hemorrhoids varies from simple reassurance to operative hemorrhoidectomy [*see Table 1*]. Treatments are classified into three categories: (1) dietary and lifestyle modification; (2) nonoperative or office procedures; and (3) operative hemorrhoidectomy. All patients with grade 1 or 2 hemorrhoids and most patients with grade 3 hemorrhoids should be

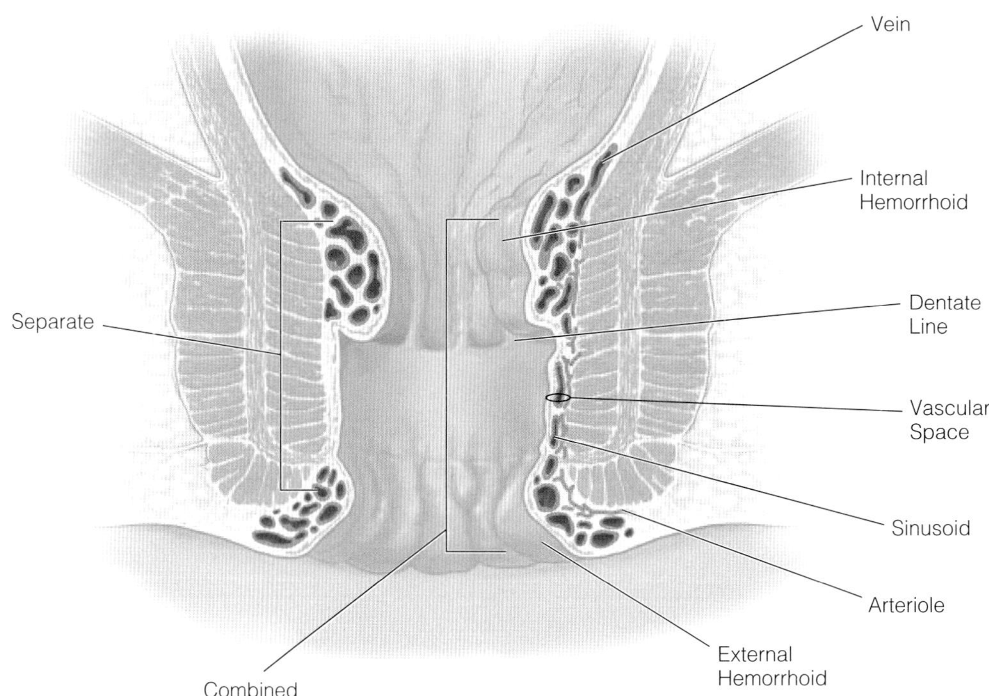

Figure 2 **Separate external and internal hemorrhoids are seen on the left and a combined internal-external hemorrhoidal complex is seen on the right.**

Table 1 Treatment Alternatives for Hemorrhoids

Treatment	Internal (Grade)				External
	1	2	3	4	
Diet modification	X				
Sclerotherapy	X	X			
Infrared coagulation	X	X	(X)		
Rubber band ligation	(X)	X	X		
Stapled anoplasty (PPH)		X	X		
Excisional hemorrhoidectomy		(X)	X	X	X

PPH = procedure for prolapsing hemorrhoids; (X) = selected patients.

treated initially with efforts to correct their constipation. Recommendations should include a high-fiber diet; liberal water intake (six to eight 8-ounce glasses of water daily); fiber supplements such as psyllium, methylcellulose, calcium polycarbophyl, or gum; or stool modifiers such as polyethylene glycol. Sitz baths are recommended for their soothing effect and ability to relax the anal sphincter muscles. Topical creams may reduce some associated symptoms but do not affect the hemorrhoids themselves. Suppositories are avoided as they deliver medication to the rectum and not the anus. Patients are instructed to avoid prolonged trips to the bathroom, and reading should be performed only when sitting atop the toilet lid. If these initial measures are not effective, a number of nonoperative therapies are available. Current recommended options include rubber band ligation, infrared photocoagulation, and sclerotherapy.

Rubber band ligation is currently the most common method in use for the outpatient treatment for hemorrhoids.[5] One to three bands are applied. Complications of hemorrhoid banding include bleeding, pain, thrombosis, and life-threatening perineal sepsis.[5,6] The cardinal signs of perineal sepsis are significant pain, fever, and difficulty urinating. Patients developing any of these symptoms require urgent evaluation and treatment with broad-spectrum antibiotics and selective débridement of any anal necrotic tissue.

Hemorrhoidal banding is successful in two thirds to three quarters of all individuals with first- and second-degree hemorrhoids.[2] Repeated banding may be necessary to resolve all symptoms. Rarely, individuals fail to respond whatsoever or cannot tolerate banding. Some of these patients will respond to infrared coagulation, whereas others may require formal hemorrhoidectomy.

The infrared photocoagulator generates infrared radiation, which coagulates tissue protein and evaporates water from cells.[7] The amount of destruction depends on the intensity and the duration of application. An anoscopic examination is performed, and the infrared coagulator is applied to the apex of each hemorrhoid at the top of the anal canal [*see Figure 3*]. A duration of 1 to 1.5 seconds is used to treat each hemorrhoid bundle three to four times. The infrared coagulator was designed to decrease blood flow to the region and is less

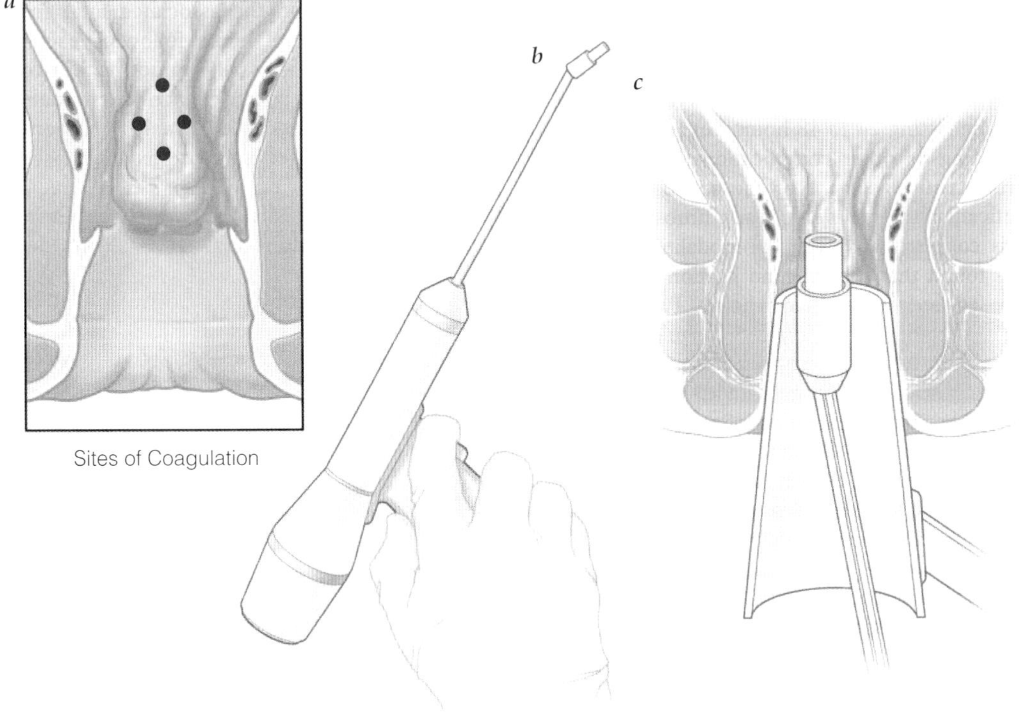

Figure 3 **The infrared coagulator is applied to each hemorrhoid bundle three or four times for 1 to 1.5 seconds at a time.[4]**

ANORECTAL ABSCESS

Anorectal abscesses are the result of local, walled-off infections of a cryptogenic origin.[18,19] That is, they begin as infections in the anal glands that surround the anal canal and empty into the anal crypts at the dentate line. The ducts leading to and from these glands are thought to become obstructed as a result of feces or trauma, and a secondary infection develops that follows the path of least resistance, resulting in an anorectal abscess.

Abscesses are characterized as perianal, ischiorectal, supralevator, or intersphincteric [*see Figure 8*]. Perianal abscesses are the most common; together with ischiorectal abscesses, they account for more than 90% of perianal infections. Perianal abscesses occur in the perianal space immediately adjacent to the anal verge. Ischiorectal abscesses are larger and often more complex than their perianal counterparts, and they usually present as a tender buttock mass. Supralevator abscesses occur above the levator ani muscles, present with poorly localized pain, and are exceedingly rare. Intersphincteric or intermuscular abscesses occur in the plane between the internal and external sphincters, high within the anal canal. The location of an abscess is important as it dictates subsequent therapy.[20]

Regardless of their location, anorectal abscesses are associated with constant perianal pain. Accompanying symptoms may include fever, chills, and malaise. In rare cases, systemic toxicity may be evident. History reveals a gradual onset of rectal pain that progressively increased until the time of presentation. Occasionally, spontaneous drainage decompresses the abscess, and the patient presents with a purulent discharge.

Again, visual inspection of the perineum often clinches the diagnosis. A fluctuant, erythematous, tender area identifies the abscess. In the rare case of a supralevator or intersphincteric abscess, there may be no external manifestations, and a tender mass on digital examination above the anal canal, adjacent to the rectal ampulla (supralevator abscess), or within the anal canal (intersphincteric abscess) provides the clue to diagnosis.

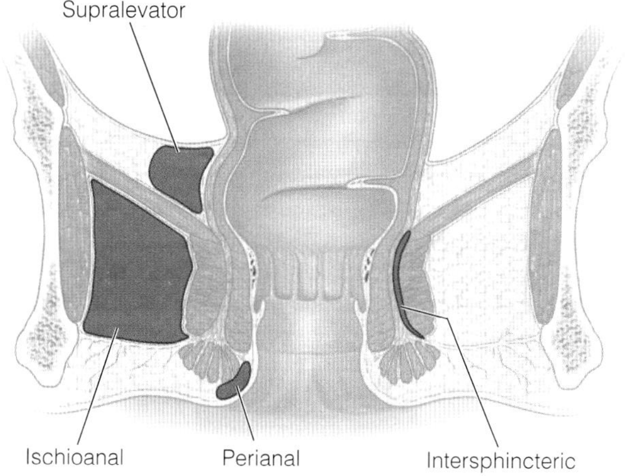

Figure 8 **Anorectal abscesses are classified according to the space in which they develop.**

The treatment for anorectal abscesses is adequate drainage performed either in the office, the emergency room, or the operating room.[18] Most abscesses can be drained in the office, but recurrent or complex abscesses, abscesses in immunosuppressed hosts (including some diabetics), and intersphincteric or supralevator abscesses are more appropriately drained in the operating room.

Adequate drainage is essential and may be established in several ways. One method is to place a catheter (such as a 10 to 16 French de Pezzer catheter) through a small stab incision.[18] This allows the pus to drain through the catheter as the cavity closes down. After the cavity closes down, the catheter is removed, and the small remaining cavity heals. The incision for the catheter is placed over the fluctuant area, as close to the anal canal as possible. This results in a shorter fistula tract if the abscess does not heal completely. A second drainage option involves creating a larger elliptical incision.[20] Unroofing the abscess cavity allows it to heal without the need for packing. A small incision should be avoided as it requires painful packing to keep the skin open until the abscess cavity heals.

The most difficult and potentially quite serious abscess to diagnose and manage is a deep postanal space abscess. Deep postanal space abscesses are caused by fistulization from the posterior anal canal, usually in the bed of a chronic posterior fissure. The patient is impressively uncomfortable and febrile, but there is no apparent sign of a problem perianally. A simple digital examination pushing posteriorly toward the coccyx and deep postanal space is extremely uncomfortable and leads one to suspect the diagnosis. The patient should be taken to the operating room and anesthetized. The deep postanal space is often felt on digital examination to be bulging. The diagnosis is confirmed by aspirating this space with an 18-gauge needle. Once the diagnosis is confirmed, then an incision is made in the perianal skin posterior to the anal verge and deepened into the space. The space is adequately drained. In selected patients, a cutting seton is placed from the primary site in the posterior anal canal directly into the deep postanal space abscess. Any horseshoeing is dealt with using counterincisions.

Following adequate drainage, antibiotics are rarely needed. Patients should be discharged with fiber supplements (stool softeners), pain medication, and instructions for sitz baths two to three times daily.

FISTULA IN ANO

An anal fistula is a communication from the anal canal to the perianal skin. The fistula usually begins in a crypt at the dentate line and follows a course between the internal and external sphincters (the most common location), resulting in an ischiorectal abscess, or above the sphincters, leading to a supralevator abscess.[18,20] Following acute drainage of an abscess, one of three things may occur if a fistula is present: (1) the fistula will heal spontaneously, and the patient will experience no further symptoms; (2) the abscess may heal only to recur in the future; or (3) the abscess may heal, leaving a chronic draining anal fistula or fistula in ano. Only the third scenario is discussed here.

Following drainage of one or more abscesses, a fistula is usually associated with chronic serosanguineous to

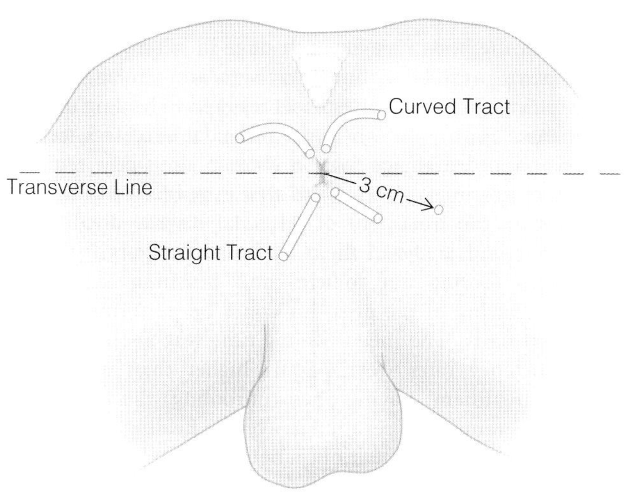

Figure 9 **Goodsall's rule. An external opening seen posterior to a line drawn transversely across the perineum will originate from an internal opening in the posterior medline. An anterior opening will originate in the nearest crypt (for fistulas within 23 cm of the anus).**[4]

seropurulent drainage. As long as the fistula remains open and draining, patients report little pain. But should the fistula close externally, an anorectal abscess may develop. Physical examination reveals a 2 to 3 mm opening in the perianal skin, with surrounding induration. Often a fistula tract may be palpated as a firm cord running between the external opening and the anal canal. The relationship of the external opening to the internal opening is suggested by Goodsale's rule [*see Figure 9*]. Fistulas are classified according to their relation to the anal sphincters [*see Figure 10*].[21]

Essentially, all chronic fistulas require surgical treatment. The most common option consists of unroofing the entire fistula tract (fistulotomy) and leaving the wound open to heal secondarily. Fistulas that course through significant amounts of sphincter muscle, are anterior in women, or are associated with inflammatory bowel disease or weakened sphincter muscles cannot be opened entirely because incontinence will result. These fistulas may be partially opened, leaving the anal musculature intact, which is encircled with a seton.[20] A seton is a nonabsorbable suture (e.g., 0 silk) or elastic suture (Silastic vessel loop) that is inserted into the fistulous tract, and the ends of the suture or elastic are tied with multiple knots to

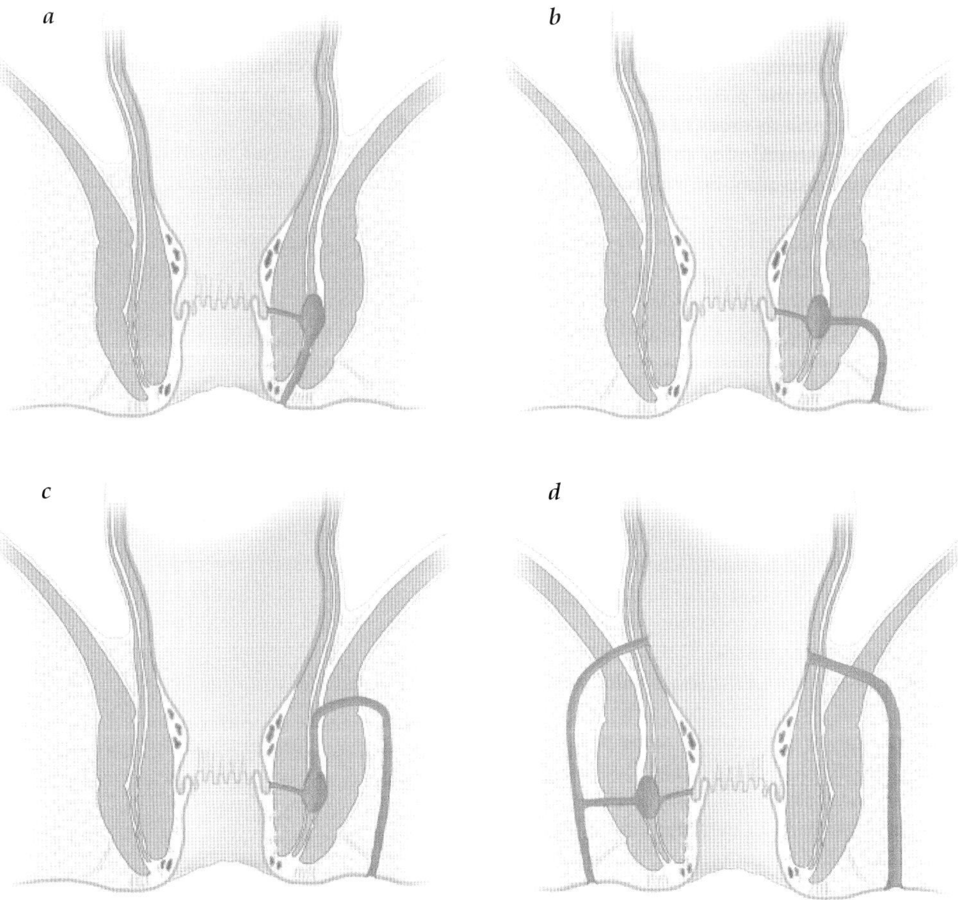

Figure 10 **Fistula in ano is classified on the basis of its relation to the anal sphincter muscles. Shown are (*a*) intersphincteric fistula, (*b*) transsphincteric fistula, (*c*) suprasphincteric fistula, and (*d*) extrasphincteric fistula.**

An endoscopic evaluation of the distal colon and rectum will reveal the lesions described above. The differential diagnosis of both CCF and SRUS includes polyps, endometriosis, inflammatory granulomas, infectious disorders, drug-induced colitidies, or mucus-producing adenocarcinoma. Differentiation among these entities is possible with an adequate biopsy.

Treatment is directed at reducing symptoms or preventing some of the proposed etiologic mechanisms. Conservative therapy (high-fiber diet, lifestyle changes, and biofeedback) will reduce symptoms in most patients and should be tried first. Patients without rectal intussusception are offered biofeedback to retrain their bowel function. Pharmacologic therapy (antiinflammatory enemas or suppositories) has had limited success but is reasonable to try before embarking on surgery. If symptoms persist, a localized resection may be considered in selected patients. Patients with prolapse are considered for perineal procedures (mucosal or perineal proctectomy) and abdominal procedures (fixation or resection and rectopexy). Patients without prolapse may be offered excision, which varies from a transanal excision to a major resection with coloanal pull-through. Surgeons have been understandably hesitant to offer surgical therapy for this benign condition, and the results are often unsatisfactory.[35,36]

Malignant Conditions

Anal neoplasms are uncommon, with an incidence one twentieth that of rectal adenocarcinoma or 1.5 to 4% of large bowel cancers.[28] Current statistics indicate that this incidence is increasing, and the management of these tumors has recently undergone significant changes.

ANATOMY

For clinical purposes, the anus can be divided into two areas: the anal canal and the anal margin [*see Figure 1*]. The anal canal runs from the anorectal junction (top of the anal sphincter muscles) to the intersphincteric groove (approximately 2 cm distal to the dentate line). Thus, it corresponds to the internal sphincter. The lining of this portion of the anus is formed by transitional epithelium, which contains elements of both columnar and squamous epithelium above the dentate line and squamous epithelium distal to the dentate line.

The anal margin runs from the intersphincteric groove to approximately 5 cm on the perineum. This area is covered by nonkeratinizing squamous epithelium, which changes to keratinizing squamous epithelium at the anal margin's outer border with the perineal skin.

ANAL CANAL

Epidermoid Carcinoma

Epidermoid carcinomas are the most common forms of anal canal neoplasms.[37] On histologic review of these neoplasms, 70% are found to be squamous cell neoplasms, 25% are basaloid neoplasms, and 5% are mucoepidermoid. Clinically, the different histologic types act in a similar manner.

The lymphatic drainage of the anus follows the arterial vessels. Thus, metastatic anal disease can spread in three different directions. Superiorly, this includes the pararectal and superior hemorrhoidal nodes; laterally, the internal iliac nodes; and inferiorly, the inguinal and external iliac nodes. For prognostic purposes, anal canal cancers have been grouped into four stages: stage 1 tumors are confined to the sphincteric mechanism, stage 2 have extended into the perirectal fat, stage 3 have involved lymph nodes, and stage 4 have distant metastases. Other staging systems have been described, and the TNM system has been adopted by the American Joint Committee on Cancer [*see Table 2*]. Unfortunately, lymph node involvement is difficult to determine in the absence of surgical specimens.

Diagnosis Patients with anal cancer usually present with bleeding per rectum and pain. The bleeding is red and usually more constant than that associated with hemorrhoids.[38] The pain is less severe than with an acute fissure and more constant. An occasional patient will also complain of an ulcerated or mass lesion of the anus. Additional questions help evaluate these symptoms and exclude other differential diagnoses.

The physical examination is helpful in making the diagnosis and is essential to determine the clinical stage of disease. Anal cancers are within reach of the examining finger and are hard, irregular, and usually ulcerated [*see Figure 13*]. The exact location and size of the lesion must be documented. This includes the vertical and horizontal diameters of the lesion and the height above the anal verge. The anatomic location (e.g., anterior versus posterior and right or left) should also be noted. An assessment of the lesion's fixity, relation to other structures, and status of the sphincteric muscles completes the perineal examination. In addition to an evaluation of the lesion, the patient should be examined for the presence of inguinal adenopathy.

Direct visualization of the anus and rectum is essential to exclude other lesions and allows biopsy of the lesion to confirm the clinical diagnosis. Anoscopy provides good exposure and is the least expensive method to examine the anal canal. After identification, the lesion should undergo biopsy. Several specimens should be obtained from the edges of the lesion. A local anesthetic is usually not required.

Table 2 Tumor Node Metastasis (TNM) Staging System for Anal Cancer

Stage	Description
T1	Carcinoma < 2 cm in diameter
T2	> 2 and < 5 cm in diameter
T3	> 5 cm in diameter
T4	Invading adjacent organ
N0	No regional node involvement
N1	Metastasis in perirectal lymph nodes
N2	Metastasis in unilateral iliac or inguinal nodes
N3	Metastasis in bilateral iliac or inguinal nodes
M0	No distant metastasis
M1	Distant metastasis

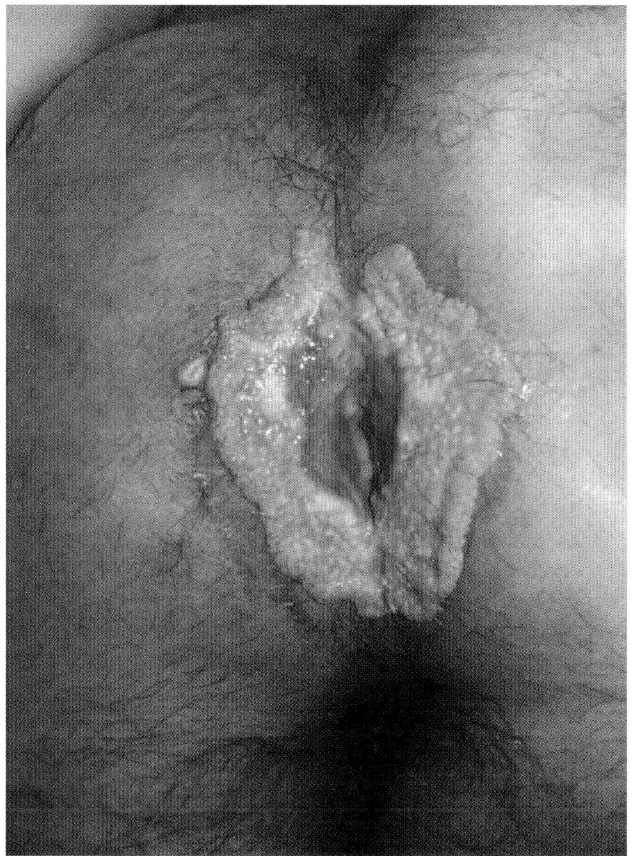

Figure 13 **Anal cancer.**

To assist in clinical staging, several modalities are currently available. Anorectal ultrasonography is being used with increased frequency and is helpful in assessing the depth of anal tumors and in identifying the presence and characteristics of lymph nodes. The difficulty remains with the identification of suspicious nodes. The quality of the examination depends on the operator, and further widespread experience is necessary.

Computed tomographic (CT) scans help assess the extent of the primary tumor and the presence of enlarged lymph nodes. A scan can determine the size and location of lymph nodes but, again, cannot accurately determine if the nodes contain tumor. This study can also evaluate the liver to exclude the presence of large hepatic metastases (greater than 1 cm). Magnetic resonance imaging (MRI) is also being used to stage anal cancer.

Treatment Anal cancer is currently treated by surgery and chemoradiotherapy. Surgical options include transanal excision and abdominoperineal resection (APR). For early lesions, local excision (transanal excision) is a valid consideration but must be limited to lesions that are well differentiated, less than 2 cm in diameter, and located in the distal anal canal. The procedure is similar to that described for early rectal cancers. Using this procedure in selected patients, the reported 5-year survival has ranged from 45 to 100%.[39,40] An APR performed for anal cancer is similar to that described for rectal cancer, with the exception that a slightly wider margin of perineal skin is removed. This procedure is used in patients who cannot undergo chemoradiotherapy or fail this therapy. The 5-year survival rate after this form of treatment averaged 50%, with a published range of 30 to 70%, and local recurrence ranged from 11 to 40%.[39,41]

Inadequate results from surgery or radiotherapy alone led Nigro at Wayne State University to propose initial chemotherapy (5-fluorouracil [5-FU], mitomycin C) and radiotherapy followed by APR.[37] Subsequent experience demonstrated that chemoradiotherapy was curative in most patients, and the subsequent APR has been abandoned unless the tumor persists or recurs.

The reported experience with multimodality treatment for anal carcinoma continues to expand.[37,42] The radiotherapy entails 30 to 60 Gy (given over 3 to 5 weeks) using apposed fields. Chemotherapy is given at the same time as the radiotherapy according to the following scheme: 5-FU (1,000 mg/m^2/day) on days 1 to 5 and days 31 to 35 and mitomycin C (15 mg/m^2) on day 1. Using an anoscope, the lesion site is inspected 4 to 6 weeks after the radiotherapy is completed, and a biopsy is performed on any abnormalities. Some providers will allow additional time after therapy to confirm complete clinical regression of the tumor before embarking on additional therapy. An APR, local excision, or additional chemoradiotherapy is offered to patients with residual disease following combined therapy.

Melanoma

Anorectal melanomas are rare; they account for 1% of all melanomas and 0.25 to 1% of anorectal tumors.[43] The mean age at occurrence is in the fifth decade; females are affected more frequently than males. The most frequent presenting symptom is bleeding, followed by an anal mass or pain. The lesions are usually elevated, and 34 to 75% will be pigmented.

These tumors are locally invasive and have a high metastatic potential. Because many patients present late, the reported 5-year survival rates range from 0 to 12%. The prognosis is related to tumor size, thickness, and clinical stage. Evaluation should include a biopsy and a search for metastatic disease (by CT of the abdomen, pelvis, and chest; liver function tests; chest x-ray evaluation; and bone scans). Special stains or electron microscopy may be required to confirm the diagnostic biopsy.

Surgery provides the only hope for cure. However, the small chance for cure and limited experience have led to controversy about the appropriate procedure. An APR has significant morbidity and mortality. Local excision has less associated morbidity. Reports have shown little difference in the mean survival rates following either procedure. Prophylactic lymphadenectomy is not indicated for clinically negative nodes but is helpful for clinically suspicious nodes. Radiotherapy and chemotherapy have demonstrated little benefit in this disease.

ANAL MARGIN

Premalignant Lesions

Premalignant lesions of the anal margin are uncommon and include Bowen disease and Paget disease. Bowen disease is an intraepithelial squamous cell carcinoma, and a few hundred produce devastating neurologic morbidity. The most common malignant neurogenic lesions are neuroblastomas, schwannomas, and ependymomas, whereas benign tumors include neurilemomas and ganglioneuromas. Osseous tumors can derive from cartilage, bone, or fibrous tissue. They behave similarly to bony tumors in other anatomic locations, with sarcomas having a predilection for hematogenous spread to the lungs.

Miscellaneous

Carcinoid tumors of the retrorectal space are rare but have been described. Most represent direct extension or metastatic spread from rectal carcinoids. Retrorectal carcinoid tumors may also arise from the glandular cells present in rectal duplication or tailgut cysts.[51] These lesions are potentially malignant and should be treated by local excision, typically using a perineal approach.

CLINICAL PRESENTATION

Retrorectal tumors are frequently asymptomatic, and they are often found incidentally during evaluation for unrelated physical complaints. Furthermore, even patients with symptoms directly referable to a retrorectal tumor may be initially misdiagnosed as having fistulae in ano; pilonidal cysts; perianal abscesses; psychogenic, posttraumatic, or postpartum pain; or proctalgia fugax. Patients may initially complain of constipation, paradoxical diarrhea, and frequent urge to defecate as the tumor causes compression of the adjacent rectum or pain (either pelvic discomfort or sciatic symptoms). Malignant tumors that invade the sacral plexus or nerve roots can lead to bowel and bladder incontinence or urinary retention.

In most cases, these lesions are palpable on digital rectal examination.[52] The presence of a postanal skin dimple is suggestive of a developmental cyst. Most retrorectal tumors will feel soft and compressible, whereas teratomas may contain abnormal calcifications that are palpable. A tender mass is suggestive of either an infected developmental cyst or a primary perirectal abscess with supralevator extension.

All patients with suspected retrorectal tumors should undergo complete colonoscopy. The rectal mucosa overlying a retrorectal tumor will appear normal, and larger lesions will demonstrate extraluminal compression of the rectum.

EVALUATION

Plain radiographs of the pelvis are typically normal unless a malignant tumor has produced bony destruction of the sacrum or rare, benign, bone-based lesions such as aneurysmal bone cysts, giant cell tumors, and osteochondromas are present. Teeth or small bone fragments may be visible in presacral teratomas. The "scimitar sign" (a concave sacral deformity suggestive of the curved sword) is characteristic of anterior sacral meningocele. Normal transrectal ultrasonography (TRUS) performed by an experienced surgeon effectively rules out a retrorectal tumor.

CT or MRI is the standard for the preoperative evaluation of retrorectal tumors. Either modality will demonstrate whether the lesion is cystic or solid and the extent of the lesion, but radiologists have difficulty in differentiating benign from malignant lesions.[50] Sixty percent of solid tumors are malignant, whereas 90% of cystic lesions are benign. Thus, although certain characteristics on imaging may be suggestive of a benign pathology, imaging alone cannot obviate the need for surgical resection.

TREATMENT

In appropriate surgical candidates, all retrorectal tumors should be resected, even if asymptomatic.[48] A multidisciplinary approach involving colorectal surgeons, neurosurgeons, and possibly orthopedists is important. In general, preservation of at least unilateral S3 nerve roots typically allows normal bowel and bladder function following sacral resection.[51] The surgical approach is based on preoperative imaging and expected extent of resection.

Biopsy of a retrorectal tumor prior to surgical resection should be avoided. Transrectal biopsy can lead to superinfection of cystic lesions, produce rapidly fatal meningitis in patients with anterior sacral meningocele, and seed needle tracts.[48]

Perhaps the only indication for biopsy is to make a diagnosis in the patient who is not a candidate for surgery but may benefit from palliative radiation or chemotherapy.

Abdominal- or Perineal-Only Approaches

The perineal-only approach is typically reserved for smaller retrorectal tumors that lie mostly caudal to the S4 level, which are typically palpable on digital rectal examination. An abdominal-only approach may be used for high retrorectal tumors that do not involve the sacrum and lie above S4; however, most large lesions are best treated with a combined abdominoperineal approach, as discussed below.

For the perineal approach, the patient is placed in the prone jackknife position with the buttocks retracted laterally with tape. Either a transperineal or parasacral incision may be used. After the incision is made and muscular attachments to the coccyx and lower sacrum are divided, the coccyx can be dislocated and resected to facilitate further exposure and resection.

Once the coccyx has been disarticulated, the presacral space is readily accessible, and dissection of the tumor from the posterior wall of the rectum can proceed. Alternatively, further sacral disarticulation can be performed as needed. Extensive involvement of the rectal wall can necessitate en bloc proctectomy. Following tumor excision, a closed suction drain is placed in the retrorectal space and the muscles are reapproximated. For large tumors, closure of the pelvic floor with a gluteal flap (often in conjunction with a plastic surgeon) can aid in filling the residual tissue defect.

Combined Abdominoperineal Approach

For the combined approach, the procedure begins with the patient in either the supine or the modified lithotomy position, and the abdomen is opened using a low midline incision. The sigmoid colon is mobilized medially, and the inferior mesenteric artery is identified. Both ureters and the hypogastrtic nerves are also identified, swept laterally, and preserved. The retrorectal space is entered by incising the peritoneum in the posterior midline at the sacral promontory. The areolar plane between the mesorectal fascia and presacral fascia is then sharply dissected, proceeding caudally until the tumor is encountered. The middle sacral vessels can be ligated, as can branches from the hypogastric arteries, to gain vascular control of the tumor and reduce bleeding during the deeper portions of the pelvic dissection and the subsequent perineal phase of the operation. The upper aspect of the tumor is then carefully dissected from the surrounding structures, typically, the presacral fascia posteriorly, the levators laterally, and the posterior wall of the rectum anteriorly. If the tumor is adherent to the rectum, an en bloc proctectomy should be performed, with most patients able to undergo restoration of intestinal continuity by coloanal or low-colorectal anastomosis. Once vision becomes limited in the deep pelvis and accurate planes of dissection can no longer be defined, the abdomen is closed, and the patient is either repositioned in the prone jack-knife position or left in the modified lithotomy position for the perineal phase of the operation, which then proceeds as previously described. If en bloc proctectomy has been necessary and the resection completed in the prone jackknife position, the patient can be returned to the modified lithotomy position for creation of the anastomosis.

Adjuvant Therapy

The rarity and heterogeneity of retrorectal tumors make it difficult to demonstrate the efficacy of adjuvant treatment. Radiation therapy may have a role in palliation of unresectable presacral tumors.

Financial Disclosures: None Reported

References

1. Beck DE. Hemorrhoids, anal fissure, and anorectal abscess and fistula. In: Rakel RE, editor. Conn's current therapy. Philadelphia: W.B. Saunders; 1997. p. 482–5.
2. Beck DE. Hemorrhoidal disease. In: Beck DE, Wexner SD, editors. Fundamentals of anorectal surgery. 2nd ed. London: W.B. Saunders; 1998. p. 237–53.
3. Thomsson WHE. The nature of haemorrhoids. Br J Surg 1975;62:542–52.
4. Beck DE. Hemorrhoids. In: Beck DE, editor. Handbook of colorectal surgery. 2nd ed. New York: Marcel Dekker; 2003. p. 325–44.
5. Larach SW, Cataldo PA, Beck DE. Nonoperative treatment of hemorrhoidal disease. In: Hicks TC, Beck DE, Opelka FG, Timmcke AE, editors. Complications of colon & rectal surgery. Baltimore: Williams & Wilkins; 1996. p. 173–80.
6. Scarpa FJ, Hillis W, Sabetta JR. Pelvic cellulitis: a life-threatening complication of hemorrhoidal banding. Surgery 1988;103:383–5.
7. Neiger S. Hemorrhoids in everyday practice. Proctology 1979;2:22–8.
8. MacRae HM, McLeod RS. Comparison of hemorrhoidal treatment modalities. A meta-analysis. Dis Colon Rectum 1995;38;687–94.
9. Cataldo PA. Hemorrhoids. Clin Colon Rectal Surg 2001;14:203–14.
10. Ferguson JA, Mazier WP, Ganchrow MI, Friend WG. The closed technique of hemorrhoidectomy. Surgery 1971;70:480–4.
11. Singer M, Abcarian H. Stapled hemorrhoidopexy. Clin Colon Rectal Surg 2004;17:131–42.
12. Beck DE, Timmcke AE. Pruritus ani and fissure-in-ano. In: Beck DE, editor. Handbook of colorectal surgery. 2nd ed. New York: Marcel Dekker; 2003. p. 367–90.
13. Schouten WR, Briel JW, Auwerda JJ. Relationship between anal pressure and anodermal blood flow. The vascular pathogenesis of anal fissures. Dis Colon Rectum 1994;37:664–9.
14. Eisenhammer S. The evaluation of the internal anal sphincterotomy operation with special reference to anal fissure. Surg Gynecol Obstet 1959;109:583–90.
15. Wiley KS, Chinn BT. Anal fissures. Clin Colon Rectal Surg 2001;14:193–201.
16. Richard CS, Gregoire R, Plewes EA, et al. Internal sphincterotomy is superior to topical nitroglycerin in the treatment of chronic anal fissure. Dis Colon Rectum 2000;43:1048–58.
17. Minguez M, Melo F, Espi A, et al. Therapeutic effects of different doses of botulinum toxin in chronic anal fissure. Dis Colon Rectum 1999;42:1016–21.
18. Beck DE, Vasilevsky CA. Anorectal abscess and fistula-in-ano. In: Beck DE, editor. Handbook of colorectal surgery. 2nd ed. New York: Marcel Dekker; 2003. p. 345–65.
19. Parks AG. Pathogenesis and treatment of fistula-in-ano. Br Med J 1961;1:463–9.
20. Luchtefeld MA. Anorectal abscess and fistula-in-ano. Clin Colon Rectal Surg 2001;14:221–32.
21. Parks AG, Gordon PH, Hardcastle JD. A classification of fistula-in-ano. Br J Surg 1976;63:1–12.
22. Lewis P, Bartolo DCC. Treatment of trans-sphincteric fistulae by full thickness anorectal advancement flap. Br J Surg 1990;77:1187–9.
23. Vasilevsky CA, Gordon PH. Benign anorectal: abscess and fistula. In: Wolff BG, Fleshman JW, Beck DE, et al, editors. ASCRS textbook of colorectal surgery. New York: Springer-Verlag; 2007. p. 192–214.
24. Beck DE, Karulf RE. Pilonidal disease. In: Beck DE, editor. Handbook of colorectal surgery. 2nd ed. New York: Marcel Dekker; 2003. p. 391–403.
25. Beck DE. Operative procedures for pilonidal disease. Oper Techn Gen Surg Anorectal Surg 2001;3:124–31.
26. Allen-Marsh TG. Pilonidal sinus: finding the right tract for treatment. Br J Surg 1990;77:123–32.
27. Armstrong JH, Barcia PJ. Pilonidal sinus disease: the conservative approach. Arch Surg 1994;129:914–9.
28. Bascom JU. Repeat pilonidal operations. Am J Surg 1987;154:118–22.
29. Mitchel KM, Beck DE. Hidradenitis suppurativa. Surg Clin North Am 2002;82:1187–97.
30. Waters GS, Nelson H. Perianal hidradenitis suppurativa. In: Beck DE, Wexner SD, editors. Fundamentals of anorectal surgery. 2nd ed. London: W.B. Saunders; 1998. p. 233–6.
31. Singer M, Cintron JR. Hidradenitis suppurativa. Clin Colon Rectal Surg 2001;14:233–42.
32. Hicks TC, Stamos MJ. Pruritis ani: diagnosis and treatment. In: Beck DE, Wexner SD, editors. Fundamentals of anorectal surgery. 2nd ed. London: W.B. Saunders; 1998. p. 198–208.
33. Madoff RD. Rectal prolapse and intussusception. In: Beck DE, Wexner SD, editors. Fundamentals of anorectal surgery. 2nd ed. London: W.B. Saunders; 1998. p. 99–114.
34. Beck DE. Surgical therapy for colitis cysticia profunda and solitary rectal ulcer syndrome. Curr Treat Options Gastroenterol 2002; 5:231–7.
35. Keighley MRB, Williams NS. Solitary rectal ulcer syndrome. In: Keighley MRB, Williams NS, editors. Surgery of the anus, rectum, and colon. London: W.B. Saunders; 1993. p. 720–38.
36. Localio SA, Eng K, Coppa GF. Anorectal presacral and sacral tumors: anatomy, physiology, and management. Philadelphia: W.B. Saunders; 1987. p. 46–67.
37. Beck DE, Karulf RE. Combination therapy for epidermoid carcinoma of the anal canal. Dis Colon Rectum 1994;37:1118–25.
38. Beck DE. Malignancy of the colon, rectum and anus. In: Beck DE, editor. Handbook of colorectal surgery. 2nd ed. New York: Marcel Dekker; 2003. p. 447–82.
39. Frost DB, Richards PC, Montague ED, et al. Epidermoid cancer of the anorectum. Cancer 1984;53:1285–93.
40. Gordon PH. Current status—perianal and anal canal neoplasms. Dis Colon Rectum 1990;33:799–808.
41. Nivatvongs S. Perianal and anal canal neoplasms. In: Gordon PH, Nivatvongs S, editors. Principles and practice of surgery for the colon, rectum, and anus. St. Louis: Quality Medical Publishing; 1992. p. 401–17.
42. Nguyen W, Mitchell K, Hawkins T, et al. Risk factors associated with requiring a stoma for management of anal cancer. Dis Colon Rectum 2004;47:843–6.
43. McNamara MJ. Melanoma and basal cell cancer. In: Fazio VW, editor. Current therapy in colon and rectal surgery. Philadelphia: BC Decker; 1990. p. 62–3.
44. Glasgow SC, Dietz DW. Retrorectal tumors. Clin Colon Rectal Surg 2006;19:61–8.
45. Beck DE. Paget's disease and Bowen's disease of the anus. Semin Colon Rectal Surg 1995;6:143–9.
46. Beck DE, Timmcke AE. Anal margin lesions. Clin Colon Rectal Surg 2002;15:277–84.
47. Lev-Chelouche D, Gutman M, Goldman G, et al. Presacral tumors: a practical classification and treatment of a unique and

NARROW-BAND IMAGING

Most endoscopes now have the ability to switch the bandwidth of projected light just by pressing a button on the scope handle. Narrow-band imaging (NBI) can differentiate squamous from nonsquamous epithelium to help identify Barrett esophagus [*see Figure 1 and Figure 2*]. The use of white light as well as NBI has also enabled endoscopists to provide an immediate assessment of small colonic and gastric lesions without histopathologic evaluation.[3]

OPTICAL COHERENCE TOMOGRAPHY

This technique uses reflection of near-infrared light to produce real-time two-dimensional cross-sectional images of the gastrointestinal tract. A small probe similar to an endoscope ultrasound probe that does not require tissue contact is passed through the scope. Optical coherence tomography produces a high-resolution image of the layers of the gastrointestinal tract. Although not yet in widespread use, investigation into the accurate identification of diseases such as Barrett esophagus is ongoing.

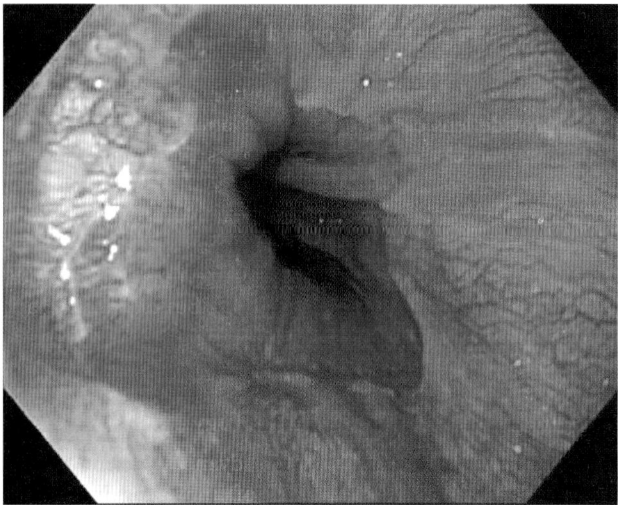

Figure 1 **The squamocolumnar junction seen with routine white light.**

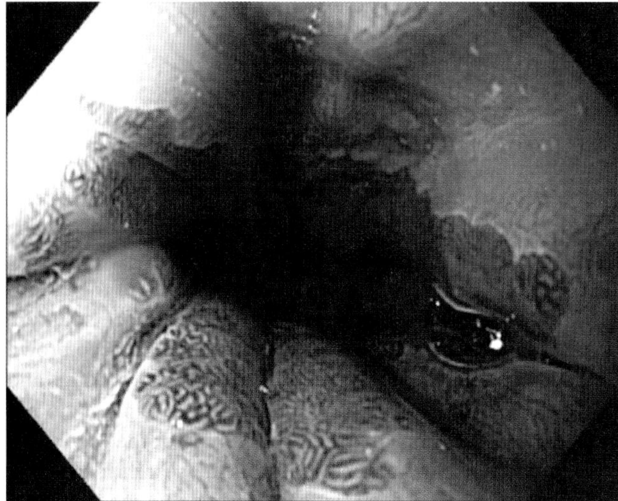

Figure 2 **The squamocolumnar junction as seen with narrow-band imaging.**

Basic Upper Endoscopy

INDICATIONS

Upper endoscopy, or esophagogastroduodenoscopy (EGD), is indicated when a patient has abnormal findings on traditional gastrointestinal x-ray series or one of the "alarm symptoms," such as weight loss, early satiety, hematemesis, dysphagia, odynophagia, epigastric pain that does not respond to medical therapy, persistent heartburn, suspected foreign body, or iron deficiency anemia. It is also indicated for surveillance of patients at high risk for malignancy and for sampling of gastrointestinal tissue or fluid. Unsedated transnasal endoscopy with slim endoscopes can also be performed in patients with suspected esophageal or gastric pathology. Biopsies can be performed, but no therapeutic interventions can be provided because of the limitation of the biopsy channel.

CONTRAINDICATIONS

Contraindications to EGD include underlying patient comorbidity and inability to tolerate conscious sedation. Recent surgery or anastomosis is not a contraindication to an EGD, and the risks and benefits of any procedure must be weighed before proceeding.

ASSESSMENT AND MONITORING

Following initial patient evaluation, including American Society of Anesthesiologists classification and Malampati scoring to assess risk for airway compromise, the patient is placed in a left-side-down decubitus position. One prepares for the examination by ensuring the patient's hemodynamic stability, having the patient fast for 6 to 8 hours beforehand, and then proceeding with the delivery of medications to provide conscious sedation, which generally involves applying a topical anesthetic to the posterior pharynx and administering a narcotic and a benzodiazepine intravenously. Monitoring of arterial blood pressure and oxygen saturation throughout the procedure is now standard practice.

TECHNIQUE OF UPPER ENDOSCOPY

With the patient in the left lateral decubitus position, a topical anesthetic may be applied to the posterior pharynx and an intravenous sedative administered. The forward-viewing panendoscope—a small-caliber instrument that is long enough to permit examination of the foregut from the mouth to the third portion of the duodenum—is employed. The endoscope is held in the left hand regardless of the individual physician's hand dominance. The internal upward and downward deflection knob is controlled by the left thumb while the air, water, and suction knobs are controlled by the left index and middle fingers. The smaller left/right knob then is usually manipulated by the right hand.

The endoscope should be introduced under direct visualization rather than using two-handed techniques, which increase the risk for both the patient and the physician. The instrument is advanced slowly until the epiglottis and vocal cords are visualized [*see Figure 3*]; it is then angled posteriorly

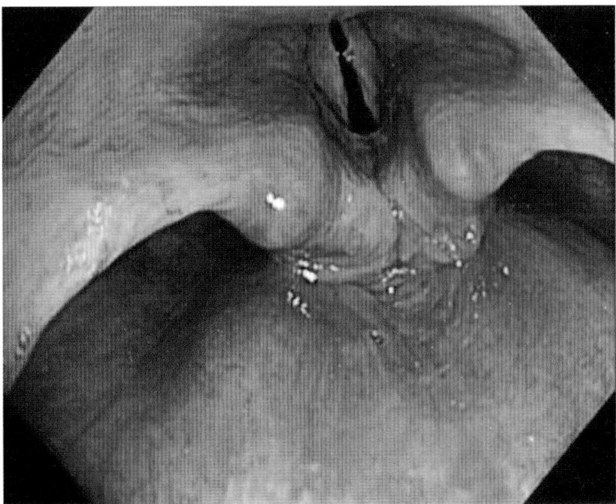

Figure 3 **Normal appearance of the vocal cords and arytenoid cartilages.**

to the esophageal introitus and gently advanced as the patient is asked to swallow. Insufflation of air is begun to distend the esophagus, which appears as a long, round tube. Frequent peristaltic waves are seen; these are normal. Mucosal surfaces must be closely inspected for signs of ulceration, stricture, tumor, or Barrett (columnar) epithelium, which manifests itself as orange patches in otherwise pale salmon-pink esophageal (squamous) mucosa. When abnormalities are noted, biopsy, brushing for cytologic evaluation, or both should be performed [*see Figure 4*]. As the endoscope is advanced, insufflation is continued, and the curve of the lumen is followed to the left as the esophagus traverses the diaphragm to enter the stomach. If the lumen is not fully visualized, the endoscope is withdrawn and the examination resumes. The distance from the incisors to the esophagogastric junction must be identified and recorded. The diaphragmatic incursion is next identified as it "pinches" on the esophageal lumen. Increased length between these two markers is classic for sliding or type I hiatal hernia, as is the presence of gastric folds above this pinched area. The pinching may be better visualized when the patient sniffs.

When the stomach is entered, the tip of the endoscope is elevated so as to center it within the gastric lumen. It should be noted that with the patient lying in the left lateral decubitus position, the stomach is also on its side, with the greater curvature at 6 o'clock, the lesser curvature at 12 o'clock, the posterior wall at 3 o'clock, and the anterior wall at 9 o'clock. Air should be insufflated to distend the stomach fully and permit careful inspection of all mucosal surfaces [*see Figure 5 and Figure 6*].

After the stomach has been viewed, the instrument is advanced under direct vision through the pylorus and into the duodenal bulb. Insufflation of air should continue as the scope is pressed against the pylorus to facilitate passage of the instrument [*see Figure 7*]. The scope tends to pop into the duodenal bulb rather than slide smoothly; it should be pulled

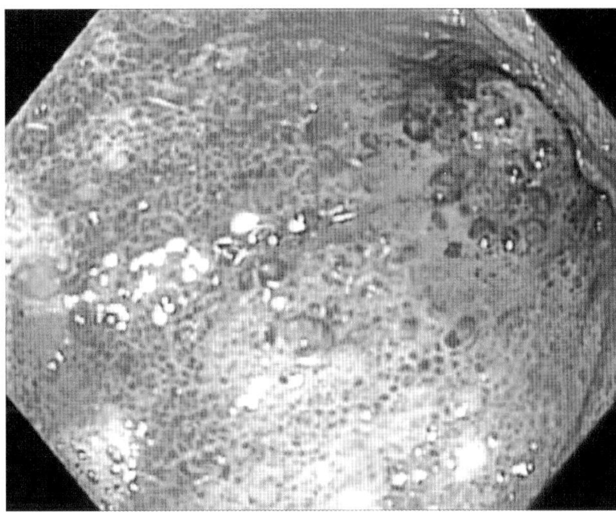

Figure 5 **Esophagogastroduodenoscopy revealing linitis plastica of the stomach.**

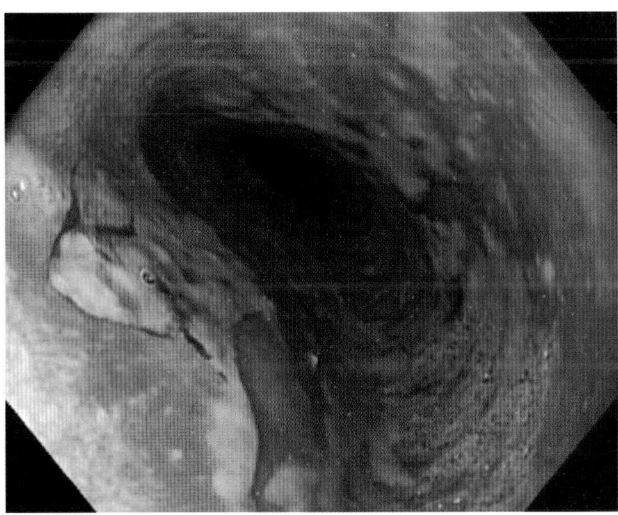

Figure 4 **Evidence of severe *Candida* esophagitis.**

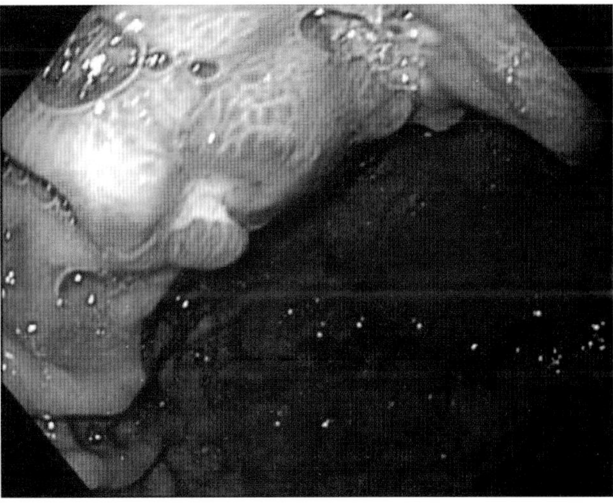

Figure 6 **Esophagogastroduodenoscopy revealing a small, nonbleeding, gastric ulcer.**

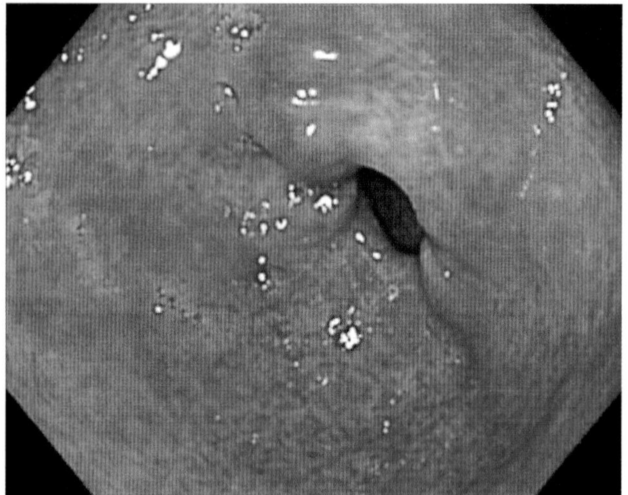

Figure 7 **Normal-appearing pylorus and antrum.**

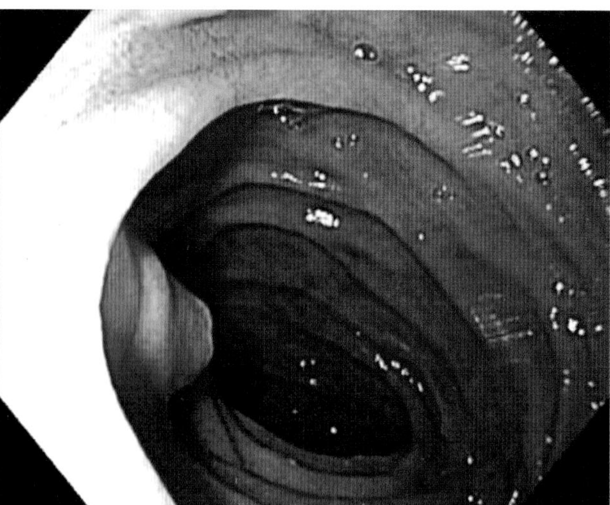

Figure 9 **Normal appearance of the second portion of the duodenum. The major papilla is seen at the 9 o'clock position, along the medial wall of the duodenum.**

back slightly to allow one to observe the mucosal surfaces of the bulb before moving ahead. Unlike the rest of the small bowel, the duodenal bulb has no semicircular folds [*see Figure 8*]. The tip of the scope must be rotated slightly to permit examination of the walls of the bulb. It is advisable to pull the instrument back into the stomach while observing the walls of the bulb and the pyloric channel for lesions; several such withdrawals may be required for full assessment of this area.

Once the duodenal bulb has been examined, the endoscope is advanced just past the bulb to the point where the first duodenal folds are observed. Here, the duodenum turns sharply to the rear and downward as it becomes retroperitoneal. Advancement of the scope into the second portion of the duodenum is one of the few endoscopic maneuvers that cannot be accomplished under direct vision [*see Figure 9*]. Because of the sharp angle of the turn, one will experience a moment of so-called "red-out" as the tip of the endoscope touches the mucosa during the turn. To ensure that the

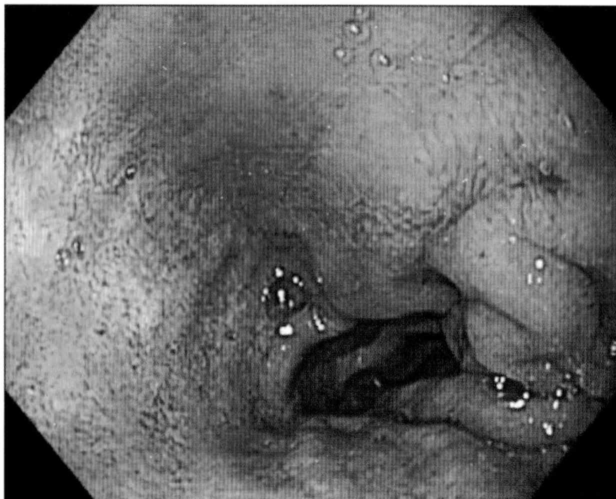

Figure 8 **Normal appearance of the duodenal bulb.**

turn is accomplished safely, the instrument is advanced as far through the bulb as is possible under direct vision. The control handle of the scope is then rotated approximately 90° to the right as the tip of the scope is turned to the right and angled first upward and then downward. As the second portion of the duodenum appears, the scope is rotated back to its neutral position. When done correctly, the turn is actually quite easy. It should never be forced: if the instrument does not proceed easily into the descending duodenum, the scope should be pulled back and the attempt repeated. Pushing against resistance may result in perforation.

Entering the descending duodenum causes the scope to form a large loop in the stomach. Therefore, once the second portion of the duodenum is successfully entered, the shaft of the instrument is pulled back. Paradoxically, as this movement straightens the gastric loop, it also advances the tip of the instrument deeper into the duodenum. Further advancement of the instrument under direct vision often permits entry into the third or even the fourth portion of the duodenum. Once the distal limit of intubation is reached, the scope is withdrawn and the luminal surfaces are carefully examined. Rotating the scope with small right-left movements of the controls and side-to-side movements of the control handle itself will help demonstrate the more subtle details of duodenal anatomy. The endoscope is then withdrawn back into the gastric lumen and full upward deflection is performed as the scope is inserted. This allows a retroflex view of the cardia and fundus [*see Figure 10*]. Often the upper gastrointestinal tract is inspected more completely while the instrument is being withdrawn than while it is being advanced.

COMPLICATIONS OF DIAGNOSTIC EGD

Complications of diagnostic EGD are divided between those related to the actual performance of the procedure and those related to the delivery of conscious sedation. Perforation secondary to EGD can occur related to scope tip or elbow trauma, or barotrauma, which is the insufflation of air. In the cervical esophagus, anatomic alterations such as Zenker

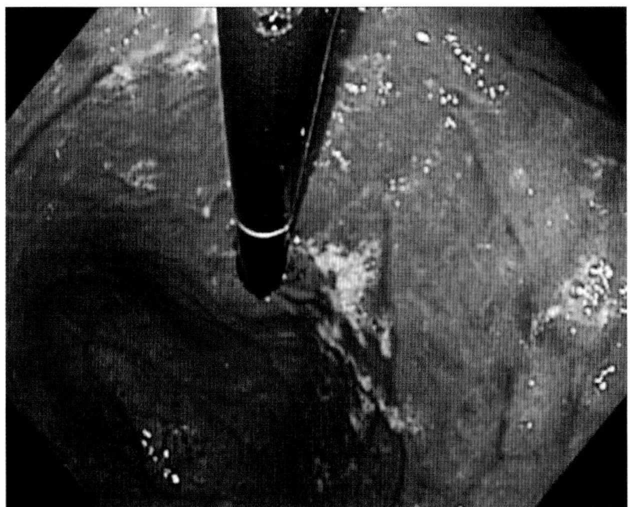

Figure 10 **Retroflex view of the gastric fundus. The angularis is seen at the 2 o'clock position along the lesser curvature.**

diverticulum, vertebral osteophytes, and cervical ribs can contribute to the occurrence of perforation. Cervical esophageal perforation can usually be managed conservatively with observation and antibiotics but rarely requires cervical drainage of abscess formation. Perforation of the mid- or distal esophagus is very rare with diagnostic EGD. In the stomach and duodenum, perforation is also very rare. Other rare complications include bleeding and infection.

The delivery of conscious sedation can lead to cardiac and pulmonary complications. The presence of an endoscope across the upper esophageal sphincter can increase the risk for airway compromise and aspiration. Cardiac events such as arrhythmias and hypotension are usually the result of primary respiratory compromise such as hypoventilation and resultant hypoxia.[4] Oxygen saturation is closely monitored throughout the procedure, and if there is a noticeable drop, jaw thrust, increased supplemental oxygen, and verbal communication can all be used to improve the patient's respiratory status. If this is not effective, the procedure should be aborted immediately with scope removal and consideration given to delivery of reversal agents. Appropriate drugs must always be readily available to reverse sedative effects, and a suction apparatus must be ready for use at all times.

Therapeutic Esophagogastroduodenoscopy

ENDOSCOPIC TISSUE SAMPLING

Sampling of tissue is most frequently obtained by passage of a spiked forceps via the endoscope's biopsy channel. Multiple biopsies should usually be obtained. For ulcers, one should biopsy the edge of the lesion in at least four quadrants. Standard biopsy techniques are quite superficial; however, if deeper biopsies are desired, these can be obtained by using either a jumbo forceps or the practice of repetitive biopsies at the same site, which will lead to a deeper sampling. Tissue and lesions can also be sampled by the use of brush cytology.

ENDOSCOPIC TECHNIQUES FOR MANAGEMENT OF BLEEDING

Endoscopy plays a direct role in the evaluation and treatment of upper gastrointestinal bleeding (UGIB). The timing for endoscopy should be based on each individual clinical scenario, understanding that EGD has both a diagnostic and a therapeutic potential. Prior to EGD, the patient must be stabilized with transfusion of blood products for correction of anemia and coagulopathy as needed, and endotracheal intubation for airway protection if warranted. Techniques of providing endoscopic hemostasis can be divided into thermal and nonthermal categories. It is also possible to treat bleeding with combined modalities such as coagulation and injection or clipping and injection. Given the relatively high success rates of controlling UGIB by endoscopic means, it is appropriate to pursue EGD initially before considering surgical or interventional radiology options.[5]

Thermal Endoscopic Tools

Thermal therapies control hemorrhage by inducing tissue coagulation, collagen contraction, and vessel shrinkage. Thermal energy tools are divided between contact and noncontact categories. These techniques overall are easy to use, although perforation may occur with an extensive delivery of energy in areas of thinner viscus walls, such as the duodenum or cecum.

Contact thermal tools Contact or coaptive techniques involve the use of probes passed via the biopsy channel, which allow for pressure tamponade of the bleeding point with simultaneous application of thermal energy for coagulation. The firmer one applies the device to the tissue, the greater the depth of energy penetration. The heat generated, which can reach several thousand degrees, is sufficient to cause full-thickness tissue damage, so care is required when using this modality.

Noncontact thermal tools Energy delivered to the mucosal without direct contact is referred to as a noncontact thermal tool. Argon plasma coagulation (APC) is an example of this technique in which thermal energy is applied to tissue via ionized argon gas. The energy is actually "sprayed" rather than delivered via direct contact. APC is particularly well suited for settings where large mucosal areas require treatment, such as gastric antral vascular ectasia (GAVE), or where the risk of deeper thermal injury leading to perforation is of heightened concern, for example, in the duodenum or cecum[6] [*see Figure 11 and Figure 12*].

NONTHERMAL ENDOSCOPIC HEMOSTASIS TOOLS

Injection Sclerotherapy

The delivery of hemostatic agents is performed by passage of a needle catheter system via the biopsy channel of the endoscope. The 5 mm needle can be advanced into the adjacent tissues and withdrawn as needed. The sclerosant agent is routinely injected submucosally at three or four sites surrounding a bleeding. The amount injected varies with different agents, and it must be remembered that systemic absorption will occur. The affect of hemostasis occurs secondary to direct tamponade and to vasoconstriction. Dilute

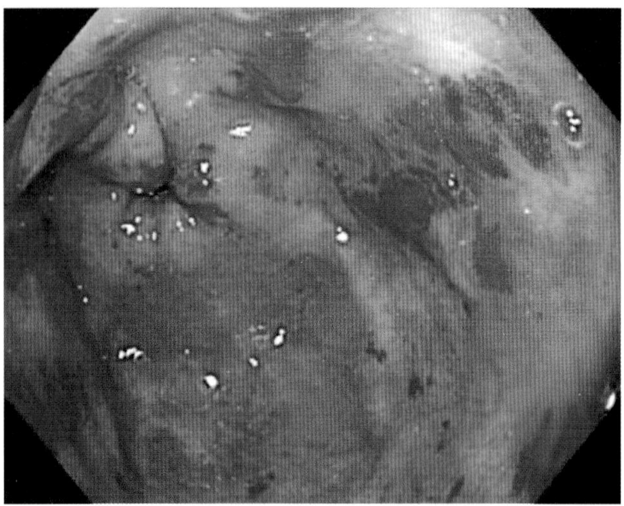

Figure 11 **Esophagogastroduodenoscopy revealing gastric antral vascular ectasia.**

1:10,000 epinephrine solution is the most commonly used agent and should be limited to less than 10 cc total volume. For esophageal varices, injections are begun just above the gastroesophageal junction. Sclerosants can be injected either directly into the varix or alongside it, intravariceal or paravariceal.

Endoscopic Band Placement

Endoscopic rubber band ligating devices can be used with most standard endoscopes and provide an alternative for management of variceal and nonvariceal bleeding. This technique is based on the ability to suction tissue into a cap placed at the tip of the endoscope and then, with the turning of a control knob, fire a small, tightly constricting rubber band. Applications for endoscopic banding include treatment of internal hemorrhoids, Dieulafoy ulcers, esophageal and gastric varices, and mucosal neoplasia in conjunction with endoscopic mucosal resection.[7]

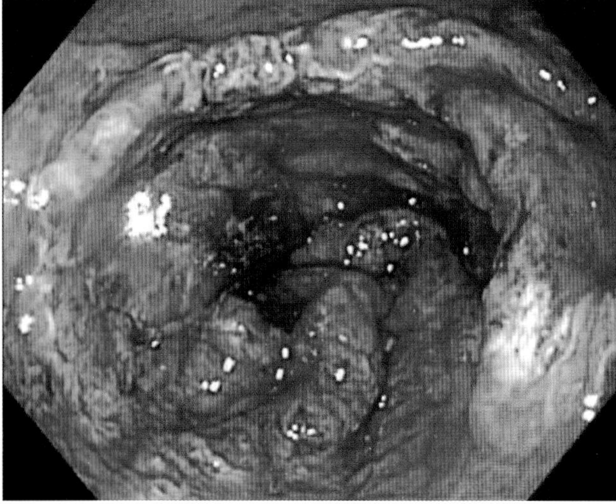

Figure 12 **Appearance of gastric antral vascular ectasia following treatment with argon plasma coagulation.**

Endoscopic Clip Placement

Endoscopic clip placement is an effective method to control bleeding and can be used safely at multiple sites throughout the gastrointestinal tract in conjunction with other endoscopic therapies. The clips are created with different characteristics but routinely provide only a very superficial tissue approximation. The clips will usually slough off within 2 weeks and pass spontaneously through the gastrointestinal tract.[8]

Endoscopic Loop Placement

Pretied endoscopic loops can also be applied through a standard endoscope biopsy channel and can be used for ligation of pedunculated structures before or after endoscopic resection. These single-application devices are similar to laparoscopic endoloops, although they are nylon sutures, and instead of an actual slip knot, a plastic cinching device holds the loop in place once deployed.

ENDOSCOPIC DILATION TECHNIQUES

Endoscopic dilation can be performed for any enteral stricture that can be reached by endoscopic means. Stenoses and anastomotic strictures secondary to ischemia, inflammation, radiation, and neoplasm are all amenable to endoscopic dilation. The use of fluoroscopy as an adjunct to endoscopic dilation is believed to decrease the risk of perforation, although this has not been fully proven in randomized prospective trials. The two most common dilators available are the guide wire–driven type, which applies both axial and radial forces, and the balloon type, which applies only radial forces. Fluoroscopic guidance allows the endoscopist to gauge several components of the procedure. First, it ensures the positioning of the balloon or the guide wire in the viscus lumen. Second, if contrast is injected in the balloon as the dilating fluid, expansion of the balloon can be fully appreciated. This is termed "waist ablation" and refers to the full dilation of the balloon at the site of the stricture [*see Figure 13 and Figure 14*]. Fluoroscopy also can monitor the position of the guide wire as Savary-type dilators are advanced over the wire in a trolley system fashion. Long, complex strictures may be less responsive to endoscopic dilation, and many strictures may also require repeat treatments. Aggressive biopsying of the mucosa after dilation is necessary in cases of unclear etiology. Complications secondary to endoscopic dilation include bleeding, perforation, mucosal tears, and recurrent structuring.

ENDOSCOPIC ENTERAL STENT PLACEMENT

Endoscopic stents can be used for the treatment of. strictures, leaks, fistulae, and obstructing neoplasms. The delivery system is dependent on the type of stent and the location for deployment. Endoscopic stent deployment is either through-the-scope (TTS) or wire guided using fluoroscopic guidance. TTS stents are delivered through the endoscope channel, are routinely a 10 French system, and require a therapeutic scope. Non-TTS stents are limited to the esophagus, including the esophagogastric junction or the rectosigmoid region. In patients following gastric resection, these systems can also traverse a gastrojejunal anastomosis.

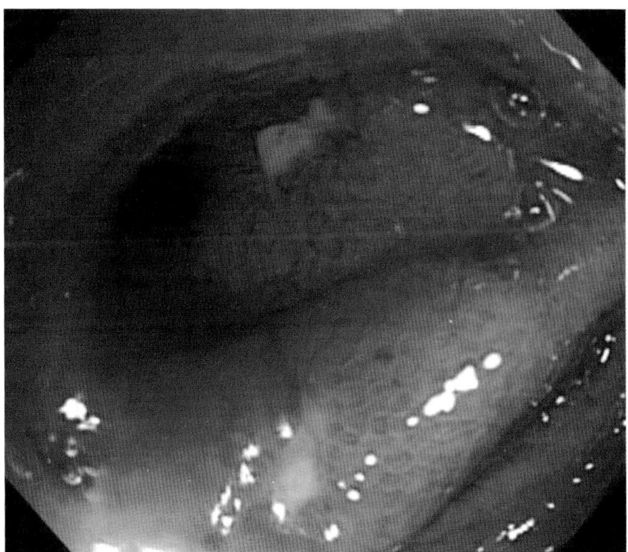

Figure 13 **Enteroscopy revealing small bowel stricture secondary to inflammatory bowel disease.**

The characteristics of endoscopic stents are quite diverse, including different lengths, widths, and morphologies. In addition, stents can be uncovered, partially covered, or fully covered. Covered endoscopic stents have been created for the sole purpose of temporarily bridging esophageal and proximal anastomotic leaks and fistulae.[9] These stents are considered removable as there is minimal tissue ingrowth, which occurs usually at the proximal and distal ends. The greatest problem with these stents is the high risk of migration. Bleeding, perforation, and obstruction are far less common complications.

Uncovered enteral stents, using TTS deployment systems, are not intended for removal and can be placed for temporary relief of benign and malignant strictures throughout the gastrointestinal tract.[10] They are associated with tissue ingrowth and occasional occlusion if they are left in place, but they have a lower rate of migration. In unresectable disease states, palliation of obstruction with enteral stents can provide an alternative to surgical bypass procedures.

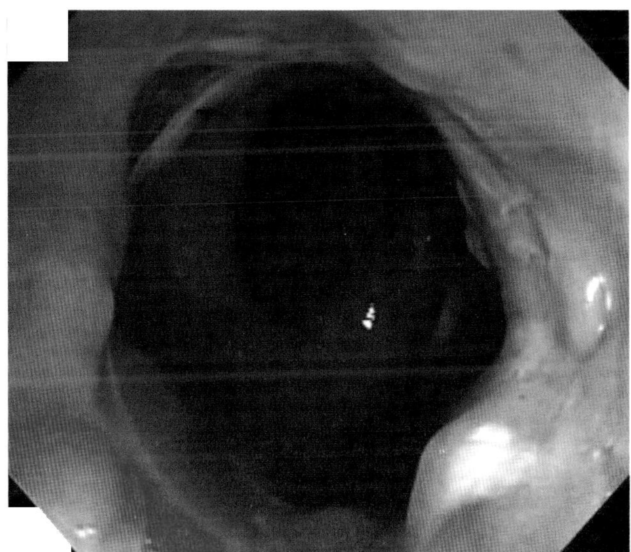

Figure 14 **Appearance of small bowel stricture following balloon dilation.**

RETRIEVAL OF FOREIGN BODIES

Many ingested foreign bodies pass through the gastrointestinal tract uneventfully, but a good number must be removed by endoscopic means—in particular, foreign bodies in the esophagus, sharp objects that are likely to perforate the bowel, and objects that do not progress from the stomach.

If the ingested object is of an unfamiliar type, it is an extremely good idea to practice with a similar object outside the patient before attempting endoscopic retrieval. This preparatory step allows one to select the most appropriate accessory and technique for removing the object.

Technique

Objects with sharp edges should be removed with the sharp end trailing to prevent perforation. In some cases, this means that the object must be pushed into the stomach and turned around before being removed. If multiple foreign bodies are present or if it is highly likely that the foreign body will injure the esophagus if removed in the standard manner, an overtube should be placed over the scope before insertion. The overtube enables one to pass the instrument several times and retrieve any sharp objects without injuring the esophagus; it also helps ensure that the object is not aspirated into the airway. If the patient is a child or there is concern for airway compromise or aspiration, general endotracheal anesthesia may be advisable.

Multiple tools have been used for foreign-body extraction, including snares, nets, biopsy forceps, tripod forceps, suction caps, and baskets. Meat boluses that form in the esophagus or proximal to a gastric band may be extremely difficult to dislodge; the use of a variceal ligator cap to produce a suction chamber can be helpful in such situations. It is imperative to evaluate the site of foreign-body impaction after removal to rule out underlying pathology or resultant trauma, such as ischemic perforation.[11]

Complications

Endoscopic removal of foreign bodies is extremely safe and effective. Care must be taken to ensure that the esophagus is not injured during removal of the object. If the object is deeply embedded or refractory to removal, a surgical approach is preferred.

PERCUTANEOUS ENDOSCOPIC GASTROSTOMY

Since 1980, endoscopically guided placement of a tube gastrostomy has been widely employed to provide access to the gastrointestinal tract for feeding or decompression. Indications for percutaneous endoscopic gastrostomy (PEG) include various disease processes that interfere with swallowing, such as severe neurologic impairment, oropharyngeal tumors, and facial trauma. PEG has also been employed to establish a route for recycling bile in patients with malignant biliary obstruction, to provide supplemental feeding in selected patients with inflammatory bowel disease, and to accomplish gastric decompression in patients with conditions such as carcinomatosis, radiation enteritis, and diabetic gastropathy.

Technique

The patient fasts for 8 hours beforehand, and a single prophylactic dose of an antibiotic is administered just before the procedure is begun. The patient is placed in the supine position, a topical anesthetic is applied to the posterior pharynx, and intravenous sedation is begun. A forward-viewing endoscope is passed into the esophagus and advanced into the stomach. The abdomen is prepared in a sterile fashion and draped. The stomach and the duodenum are then inspected.

The room lights are dimmed, and the light of the endoscope is used to transilluminate the abdominal wall so as to indicate a point where the gastric wall and the abdominal wall are in close proximity. Finger pressure is applied to various areas of the abdomen until a spot is identified at which such pressure produces clear indentation of the gastric wall. An endoscopic snare is deployed through the biopsy channel of the endoscope to cover this spot, and a local anesthetic is infiltrated into the overlying skin [*see Figure 5*]. A 1 cm skin incision is made at the chosen spot, and a needle is passed through the incision and into the gastric lumen. The endoscopic snare is tightened around the needle, and a wire is passed through the needle and into the gastric lumen. The snare is moved so as to surround the wire, which is then pulled out of the patient's mouth. The gastrostomy tube is fastened to the wire and pulled in a retrograde manner down the esophagus and into the stomach. The gastroscope is subsequently reinserted to ensure that the head of the catheter is correctly positioned against the gastric mucosa and there is no evidence of bleeding [*see Figure 6*].

An outer crossbar is put in place to prevent inward migration of the tube and to hold the stomach in approximation to the abdominal wall. The crossbar should remain several millimeters from the skin to prevent excessive tension, which would cause ischemic necrosis of the underlying tissue.

Complications

Local wound infections are the most common complications of PEG. They can be minimized by administering preoperative antibiotics and ensuring that excessive tension is not applied to the crossbar at the end of the procedure. When such infections do occur, they can usually be treated via simple drainage and local wound care; sacrifice of the gastrostomy is rarely necessary. Several other complications, such as early extrusion of the tube, progressive enlargement of the tract, and separation of the gastric and abdominal walls with leakage of feedings into the abdominal cavity, are also most often attributable to excessive crossbar tension and subsequent ischemia. Gastrocolic fistula can occur after PEG. This problem may not be obvious for months afterward, but severe diarrhea after feedings is grounds for suspicion. Once the PEG tract is mature, gastrocolic fistulae usually close quickly after simple removal of the gastrostomy tube.

PEG with Jejunostomy Tube Extension

In patients who fail to tolerate gastric feedings as a result of severe gastroesophageal reflux or gastroparesis, transpyloric feeding can be provided via a jejunostomy tube passed through an existing PEG. PEG-J placement is achieved by passing a jejunal feeding tube through the PEG lumen (a 24 French PEG tube accommodates up to a 12.5 French J tube; a standard 20 French PEG tube accommodates an 8.5 French J tube). Endoscopically, the jejunal tube is guided into the duodenum under direct vision with either a biopsy forceps or an endoscopic clip.

DIRECT PERCUTANEOUS ENDOSCOPIC JEJUNOSTOMY TUBE

Feedings beyond the ligament of Treitz using direct percutaneous endoscopic jejunostomy (PEJ) are associated with a lower incidence of gastroesophageal-induced aspiration compared with simple postpyloric feeding but are associated with increased procedural risks, including bleeding, inadvertent viscus injury, and leakage.[12] Performance of direct PEJ requires both endoscopic and fluoroscopic guidance. Abdominal wall depression with a hemostat is performed at this site to try to identify a loop of small bowel adjacent to the abdominal wall. Safe tract techniques are then used to access the identified bowel, and a "pull" PEJ is performed with either a 16 French or a 20 French tube.

ENDOSCOPIC RETROGRADE CHOLANGIOPANCREATOGRAPHY

Endoscopic retrograde cholangiopancreatography (ERCP) is an advanced procedure that is technically more challenging than standard upper gastrointestinal endoscopy; however, it can be mastered by most endoscopists who are willing to dedicate sufficient time to learning the method. ERCP yields a radiologic image of the pancreatic and biliary trees and, in many cases, provides access for therapy. Indications for ERCP include suspected benign or malignant maladies of the common bile duct (CBD), the ampulla of Vater, or the pancreas. Cholelithiasis per se is not an indication for ERCP unless choledocholithiasis is suspected. Diagnostic ERCP is rarely performed because of the high risks of this procedure. MRCP provides safer radiographic imaging of the pancreaticobiliary trees.[13] The therapeutic potential of ERCP is quite extensive and has supplanted surgical intervention for many diseases of the pancreas and biliary systems.

Technique

As with standard upper gastrointestinal endoscopy, the patient fasts for 6 to 8 hours beforehand. Intravenous sedation is administered, and prophylactic antibiotics are given when biliary obstruction is suspected. The patient is initially placed in the left lateral decubitus position but is later rotated to the prone position after the scope is in place in the second portion of the duodenum. A side-viewing endoscope is employed because it allows the best visualization of the ampulla of Vater. The instrument is passed into the esophagus and maneuvered through the stomach, across the pylorus, and into the duodenum.

Once the endoscope is in the second portion of the duodenum, it is pulled back so that the gastric loop is straightened and the tip of the scope occupies a better position with regard to the papilla. This so-called short scope position is generally best for work in the CBD. The papilla of Vater (also known as the major duodenal papilla) appears as a small, longitudinal nubbin crossing the horizontal semicircular folds of the duodenum, generally in the 12 to 1 o'clock position [*see Figure 15*].

At its tip, a small, soft, reticulated area may be noted; this is the papillary orifice. Often a small mucosal protuberance is seen just proximal and to the right of the papilla of Vater; this is the minor duodenal papilla.

A small plastic cannula is passed through the channel of the endoscope and introduced into the ampullary orifice, and contrast material is injected under fluoroscopic control to provide visualization of the CBD and the pancreatic duct. The two may share a single orifice within the ampulla or may have separate orifices. The CBD exits the papilla in a cephalad direction, tangential to the duodenal wall. The bulge of the ampulla within the duodenum represents the intramural segment of the duct. The orifice of the CBD is typically found at the 11 o'clock position in the ampulla. The pancreatic duct leaves the papilla in a perpendicular fashion. Its orifice is usually in the 1 o'clock area of the papilla.

Therapeutic interventions that may be accomplished at the time of ERCP include sphincterotomy for ductal access, sphincter of Oddi dysfunction, ampullary stenosis, removal of CBD stones, dilation of benign and malignant biliary strictures, and insertion of stents to maintain ductal patency [*see Figure 16*]. Pancreatic duct interventions include removal of stones, bridging of ductal disruptions, and drainage of pseudocysts.

All therapeutic applications of ERCP must begin with selective cannulation of the duct being treated. Frequently, a guide wire is then introduced deep into the duct to provide a means of obtaining access to the duct on an ongoing basis and to ensure correct positioning for intraductal manipulations. After electrosurgical division of the papilla, biliary stones are retrieved with balloons or baskets [*see Figure 17*]. Often large stones can be captured within the duct in mechanical lithotripsy baskets and crushed before removal.

Strictures should be brushed for cytologic evaluation once they have been traversed by a wire, although this carries a very low yield of sensitivity. They may then be dilated with

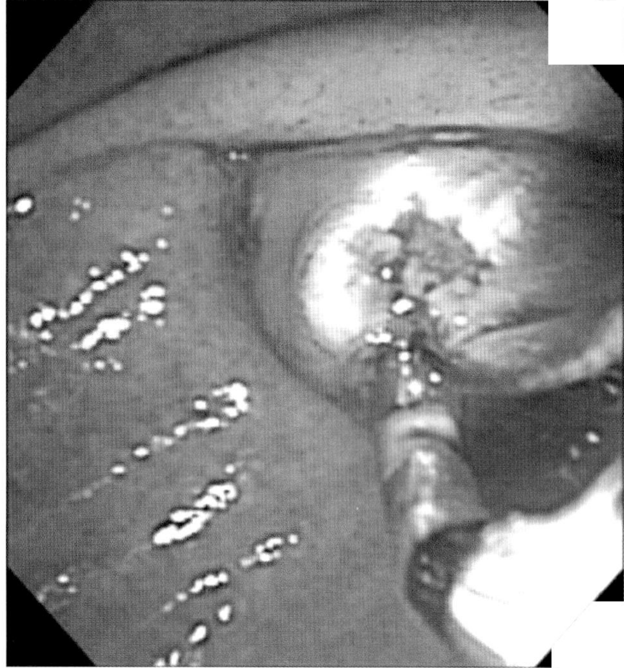

Figure 16 **Electrosurgical division of the ampullary sphincter with a pull-wire sphincterotome.**

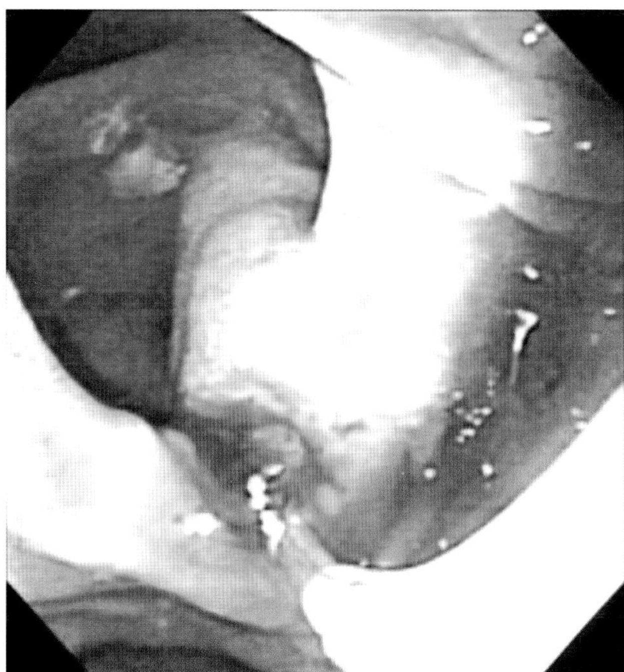

Figure 15 **The appearance of the major papilla with a side-viewing endoscope. A periampullary diverticulum is seen and an endoscopic retrograde cholangiopancreatography catheter is selectively cannulating the common bile duct.**

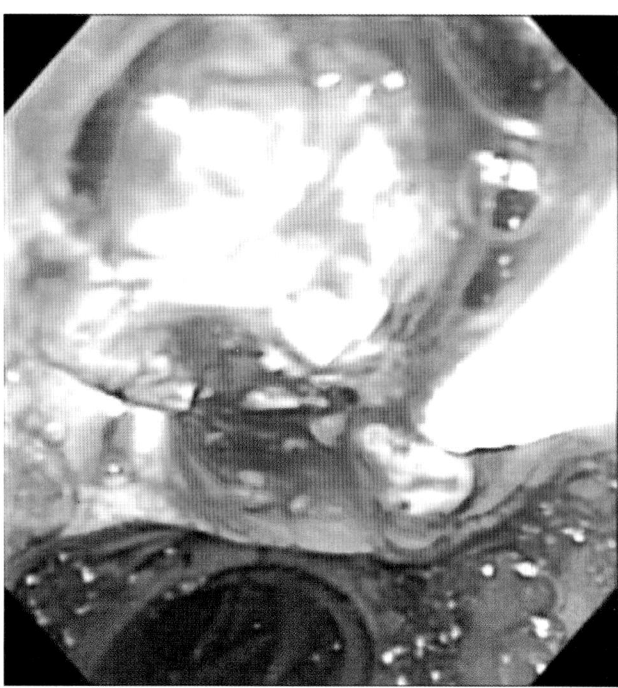

Figure 17 **Following sphincterotomy, stone extraction is performed by withdrawing an extraction balloon.**

hydrostatic balloons under fluoroscopic guidance and stented. Plastic stents are used for most benign and many malignant strictures; however, self-expanding metal stents are now being used more frequently for malignant strictures because they remain patent longer[14] [*see Figure 18, Figure 19, and Figure 20*].

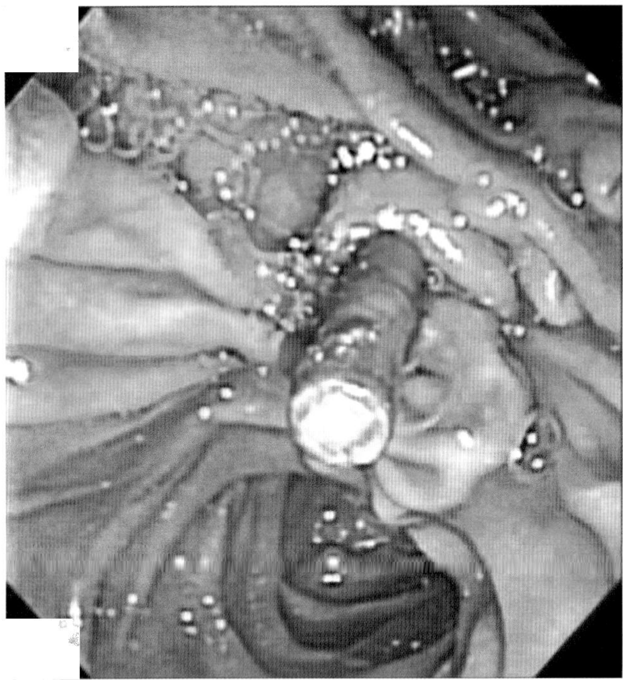

Figure 18 **The appearance of a transpapillary positioned plastic biliary stent.**

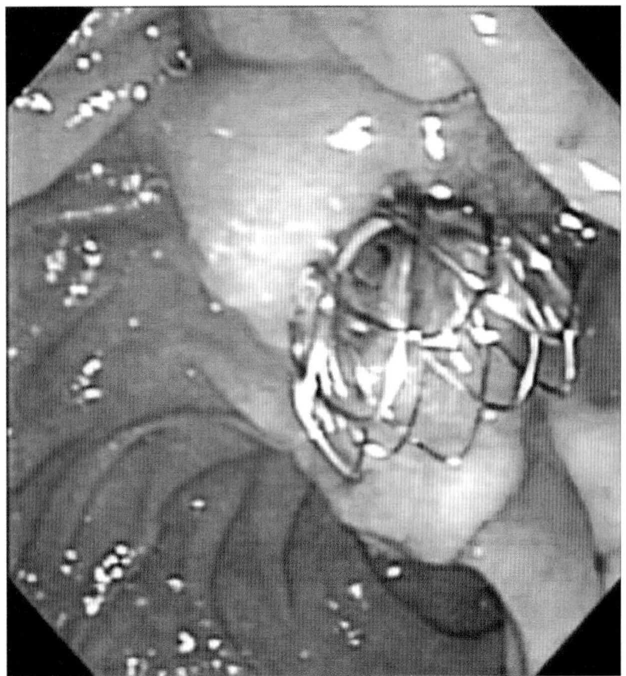

Figure 19 **The appearance of a transpapillary positioned self-expanding metal biliary stent.**

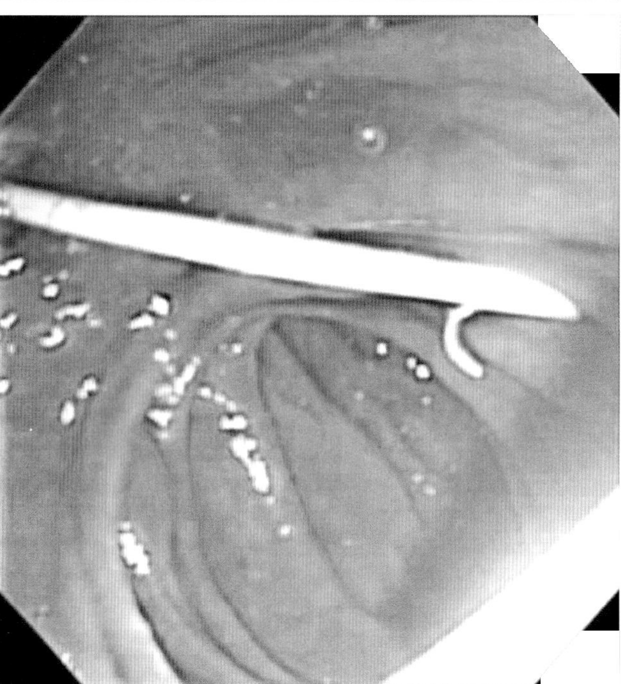

Figure 20 **The appearance of a transpapillary positioned plastic pancreatic stent.**

Complications

Perforation can occur during endoscopic sphincterotomy as a result of extension or tearing of the papilla beyond the junction of the CBD with the duodenal wall. Retroperitoneal or free intraperitoneal air may be seen. In many cases, intravenous antibiotics, hydration, and avoidance of oral intake are sufficient to manage such complications. If the patient's condition deteriorates, surgical exploration is indicated. Bleeding may also occur with endoscopic sphincterotomy at the time of the procedure or in a delayed fashion up to 1 to 2 weeks later. It is usually controllable at the time of the procedure with balloon tamponade, injection sclerotherapy, thermal coagulation, or endoscopic clip placement. If unsuccessful, interventional radiology may be able to provide embolization of the gastroduodenal artery to provide hemostasis.

Pancreatitis is the most common complication and can occur related to contrast injection with overfilling or acinarization of the ducts or rupture of the small ductules, with extravasation of contrast material into the pancreatic parenchyma; pancreatitis is a frequent consequence of acinarization. In addition, sphincterotomy and ampullary dilation are also associated with post-ERCP pancreatitis. Cholangitis may result when contrast is injected proximal to an obstruction of the biliary tree. When obstruction is demonstrated, drainage of the system by means of stone extraction, stenting, or nasobiliary intubation is important to prevent cholangitis.

DEEP SMALL BOWEL ENTEROSCOPY

The small bowel up until recently had been an elusive part of the gastrointestinal tract in terms of diagnostic and therapeutic endoscopic intervention. The advent of capsule endoscopy has permitted the endoscopist to obtain recorded images of the lumen of the small bowel for identification of obscure sites of bleeding, inflammatory changes, and neoplasia, and more recently, specially designed endoscopes have allowed direct access to the entire small bowel via either an antegrade or retrograde fashion. Diagnostic and therapeutic small bowel procedures for processes such as bleeding, obstruction, and occult neoplasia have now been described using double-balloon endsocopy and single-ballon endoscopy. In addition, in select patients following surgical resection and reconstruction (i.e., Roux-en-Y bypass, long afferent limb), balloon enteroscopy can allow access into the desired segment of the small bowel.[15]

Both systems use the principle of scope fixation with a soft balloon that is serially inflated and deflated as the scope is advanced. This permits the endoscopist to pleat the bowel over the endoscope. The use of fluoroscopy is also helpful in guiding the endscopist through the small bowel.

ENDOSCOPIC MUCOSAL RESECTION

The treatment of premalignant as well as superficial cancers can now be managed by endoscopic resective techniques. Endoscopic mucosal resection (EMR) has been employed for adenomas, dysplastic lesions, and early-stage carcinomas, including lateral spreading tumors. Multiple technical variations of EMR for the upper and lower tract have been developed, including submucosal injection, "suck-and-cut," "suck-and-ligate," and strip biopsy.

Saline Lift EMR

The most commonly performed EMR technique employs submucosal injection of a fluid followed by electrosurgical polypectomy. The most commonly used fluid is saline with or without epinephrine, although hyaluronic acid, glycerol, and dextrose have all been described. A bleb is created with the submucosal injection, creating space between the line of resection and the muscularis propria of the organ, and the lesion is resected. One caveat to this technique is that if the submucosal injection does not result in elevation, one must consider that this mass is an invasive lesion and should not be resected endoscopically.

"Suck-and-Cut" EMR

The "suck-and-cut" technique uses a specially designed cap attached to the tip of the endoscope. A submucosal injection may be created initially as with the saline lift EMR, and the lesion is sucked into the cap. A snare affixed inside the cap is used to encircle the lesion and is then resected by application of electrocautery similar to snare polypectomy. Similar to any thermal technique, the risk of perforation exists.

"Suck-and-Ligate" EMR

The "suck-and-ligate" technique transforms a sessile or nodular lesion into an artificial pedunculated polyp, which can then be resected with standard polypectomy techniques. A band ligating device is attached to the tip of the endoscope, the tissue is sucked into the cap, and a band is placed at the base of the lesion. This is done with or without saline lift injections prior to banding. The site is then resected with a snare similar to routine snare polypectomy.

The most frequent complications of EMR are bleeding and perforation. Immediate bleeding can be controlled with endoscopically placed clips or injection of dilute epinephrine. Electrocautery should be used judiciously after EMR because the thin submucosa and serosa are susceptible to full-thickness injury with cautery. Delayed bleeding often requires repeat endoscopy with injection therapy or clip application, although angiography and embolization may be an alternative. Perforations can also be managed endoscopically with endoscopic clips as well as temporary enteral stent placement to cover the site of perforation.

ENDOSCOPIC SUBMUCOSAL DISSECTION

An extension of EMR that has been recently reported for endoscopic resection of more extensive lesions is endoscopic submucosal dissection (ESD). Using a combination of needle cautery and blunt endoscope cap dissection, large segments of tissue can be resected. The potential advantage of ESD is that it represents a more classic oncologic procedure compared with the piecemeal resection that occurs with other EMR techniques in that margins as well as lesion depth can be more accurately pathologically evaluated. Complications may be higher for ESD than for the other EMR techniques, including bleeding, perforation, and stricture formation.

ENDOSCOPIC MUCOSAL ABLATION

Endoluminal therapies for ablation of mucosal based diseases such as Barrett esophagus have recently seen great advances. Endoscopic radiofrequency ablation is a relatively new technology that has recently gained acceptance for treatment of intestinal metaplasia, as seen in Barrett esophagus.[16] A balloon-based system, as well as a directed planar electrode device implementing this technology, has been used in this form of therapy. Several studies have proven feasibility and safety for this novel therapy, with very few documented cases of postprocedural structuring, as had been seen with photodynamic therapy. Further studies documenting the long-term effects of this therapy, as well as the absence of buried submucosal metaplastic glands or cancer, are still necessary.

ENDOSCOPIC ULTRASONOGRAPHY

The 1980s saw the introduction of endoscopic ultrasonography (EUS). Extracavitary ultrasonographic methods have been hampered by the presence of air within the gastrointestinal tract, which precludes high-resolution imaging. Consequently, they had been relegated to gross estimates of disease and detection of displacement of other tissues or fluid accumulation proximal to stenoses, such as ductal dilation in patients with CBD stones.

Three advances have proven invaluable in allowing EUS to carve out a niche in the field of gastrointestinal diagnosis. First is the improvement in endoscopes that allows transducer and receiver channels to traverse a tortuous path. Second is the development of multiple-frequency options in conjunction with circumferential visualization. Higher frequencies provide higher resolutions, allowing useful differentiation of the various layers of the intestinal tract. Third is the evolution of treatment protocols keyed to the accurate staging of tumors—information that is sometimes unobtainable from other imaging techniques.[17]

This technology has now been firmly established as an accurate way to identify carcinoma. More recent developments are allowing EUS to expand from the field of diagnosis into the realm of intervention. Examples of EUS-guided procedures include fine-needle aspiration, lymph node sampling, and drainage of pancreatic pseudocysts.[18]

EUS devices come in both linear and radial transducers.[19] Radial transducers have the advantage of providing circumferential visualization that parallels the standard modes of perceiving the gastrointestinal tract. Linear images allow EUS-directed biopsies and have the potential to provide color and pulsed Doppler imaging. Probes can be mounted on the top of an oblique-viewing fiberoptic scope or come in an over-the-wire format for use in the pancreaticobiliary tree. A series of frequencies are available, with the higher frequencies providing greater resolution but less tissue depth penetration. Lower-frequency probes allow deeper tissue assessment and a broader view, but at the price of reduced resolution. Nevertheless, any form of EUS will provide better resolution than transcutaneous ultrasonography, allowing markedly improved two-point discrimination and hence more accurate tissue diagnosis.

The benefits of accurate staging of gastrointestinal tumors paved the way for EUS development. Tissue sampling techniques are further benefited by this technology. The sensitivity of EUS makes it one of the best modalities for the evaluation and detection of pancreatic tumors. Its sensitivity, which is in excess of 95%, contrasts favorably with those of other modalities, including ultrasonography (75%), computed tomography (CT) (80%), and angiography (89%). The accuracy of T staging by EUS in esophageal cancer (80 to 90%) is greater than that of staging determined by CT scanning (50 to 60%). This finding has led to the development of several staging schemes that are based solely on EUS findings. EUS has established a role in the identification of early pancreatitis; the detection of CBD stones and mediastinal masses; and the assessment of anastomotic strictures, thickened gastric folds, and the integrity of the anal sphincter. It has also proved a useful adjunct in the determination of whether a tumor is amenable to EMR techniques or is better served by adjuvant therapies or surgical interventions.

The sensitivity of EUS is rooted in its ability to delineate the various layers of the alimentary canal. Experienced endoscopists can easily evaluate the submucosa and differentiate intramural from extrinsic masses. Characteristic patterns are readily learned and rapidly recognized, obviating tissue diagnoses in straightforward cases. Criteria have also been established to aid in the differentiation of benign and malignant lesions. With the continued use of this technique, additional algorithms will be established in conjunction with more innovative interventional adjuncts. However, two limitations have caused many practitioners to remain skeptical: cost and training issues. Other imaging modalities, such as CT and magnetic resonance imaging, have also made tremendous strides recently. Although these various modalities are often considered competitors—a view arising from the perceived need for a single imaging modality—the issue of which is superior to the others pales in comparison with the benefits that can be gained from combining imaging techniques in appropriate circumstances.

Future of Endoscopy

The future in endoscopy will be based on advancements of both the tools and the applications available to endoluminal therapy. Intraluminal and transluminal endoscopic techniques are being proposed as potential surgical alternatives, taking on an increasingly more invasive and therapeutic role. Recent interest in NOTES united surgeons and gastroenterologists with the desire to access the abdominal cavity via naturally existing orifices, including the stomach, colon, bladder, and vagina.[20] An appropriate application for this approach is still yet to be elucidated. It is theorized that NOTES may have distinct advantages over laparoscopy in that NOTES may not necessarily require a sterile working environment to perform, and it possibly could also be completed under conscious sedation, similar to other endoscopic procedures.[21]

The obvious limitations to NOTES were based on the lack of adequate and appropriate endoscopic equipment. It was apparent early on that stable platforms would be necessary as well as endoscopic tools for cutting, hemostasis, and tissue manipulation. Transoral and transvaginal multichannel platforms with internal capability for manipulation and fixation are now becoming available. Scissors, suturing devices, bipolar forceps, and grasping devices are a few of the novel instruments soon to be added to the endoscopist's armamentarium.

These tools, however, will have a more likely impact on other endoscopic therapies, including intraluminal endoscopic surgery. Full-thickness resection, intraluminal anastomoses, and closure of perforations are all likely procedures to be seen in the very near future, and it is imperative that surgeons stay attentive to the advancements in these technologies.

Financial Disclosures: None Reported

References

1. Ponsky JL. Endoluminal surgery: past, present and future. Surg Endosc 2006;20 Suppl 2:S500–2.
2. Pearl JP, Marks JM. New technology in endoscopy. In: Soper NJ, editor. Mastery of endoscopic and laparoscopic surgery. 2nd ed. Philadelphia: Lippincott Williams & Wilkins; 2009. p. 17–23.
3. Mannath J, Ragunath K. Narrow band imaging and high resolution endoscopy with magnification could be useful in identifying gastric atrophy. Dis Sci 2009 Oct 3. [Epub ahead of print]
4. Qadeer MA, Rocio Lopez A, Dumot JA, et al. Risk factors for hypoxemia during ambulatory gastrointestinal endoscopy in ASA I-II patients. Dig Dis Sci 2009;54:1035–40.
5. Tang SJ, Lee SY, Hynan LS, et al. Endoscopic hemostasis in nonvariceal upper gastrointestinal bleeding: comparison of physician practice in the east and the west. Dig Dis Sci 2009;54:2418–26.
6. Cappell MS, Friedel D. Acute nonvariceal upper gastrointestinal bleeding: endoscopic diagnosis and therapy. Med Clin North Am 2008;92:511–50.
7. Zepeda-Gómez S, Marcon NE. Endoscopic band ligation for nonvariceal bleeding: a review. Can J Gastroenterol 2008;22:748–52.
8. Yuan Y, Wang C, Hunt RH. Endoscopic clipping for acute nonvariceal upper-GI bleeding: a meta-analysis and critical appraisal of randomized controlled trials. Gastrointest Endosc 2008;68:339–51.
9. Babor R, Talbot M, Tyndal A. Treatment of upper gastrointestinal leaks with a removable, covered, self-expanding metallic stent. Surg Laparosc Endosc Percutan Tech 2009;19(1): e1–4.

10. Huang Q, Dai DK, Qian XJ, et al. Treatment of gastric outlet and duodenal obstructions with uncovered expandable metal stents. World J Gastroenterol 2007;13:5376–9.
11. Prasad GA, Reddy JG, Boyd-Enders FT, et al. Predictors of recurrent esophageal food impaction: a case-control study. J Clin Gastroenterol 2008;42:771–5.
12. DeLegge MH. Small bowel endoscopic enteral access. Gastrointest Endosc Clin N Am 2007;17:663–86.
13. Scaffidi MG, Luigiano C, Consolo P, et al. Magnetic resonance cholangio-pancreatography versus endoscopic retrograde cholangio-pancreatography in the diagnosis of common bile duct stones: a prospective comparative study. Minerva Med 2009;100:341–8.
14. Perdue DG, Freeman ML, DiSario JA, et al. Plastic versus self-expanding metallic stents for malignant hilar biliary obstruction: a prospective multicenter observational cohort study. J Clin Gastroenterol 2008;42:1040–6.
15. Pohl J, May A, Aschmoneit I, et al. Double-balloon endoscopy for retrograde cholangiography in patients with choledochojejunostomy and Roux-en-Y reconstruction. Z Gastroenterol 2009;47:215–9.
16. Fleischer DE, Overholt BF, Sharma VK, et al. Endoscopic ablation of Barrett's esophagus: a multicenter study with 2.5-year follow-up. Gastrointest Endosc 2008;68:867–76.
17. Hunt GC, Faigel DO. Assessment of EUS for diagnosing, staging, and determining respectability of pancreatic cancer: a review. Gastrointest Endosc 2002;55:232–7.
18. Park DH, Lee SS, Moon SH, et al. Endoscopic ultrasound-guided versus conventional transmural drainage for pancreatic pseudocysts: a prospective randomized trial. Endoscopy 2009;41:842–8.
19. Siemsen M, Svendsen LB, Knigge U, et al. A prospective randomized comparison of curved array and radial echoendoscopy in patients with esophageal cancer. Gastrointest Endosc 2003;58:671–6.
20. Pearl JP, Marks JM, Ponsky JL. Hybrid surgery: combined laparoscopy and natural orifice surgery. Gastrointest Endosc Clin N Am 2008;18:325–32.
21. Marks J, Ponsky J, Pearl J, et al. PEG "rescue": a practical NOTES technique. Surg Endosc 2007;21:816–9.

18 LOWER ENDOSCOPY

Brian J. Dunkin, MD, FACS, and Rohan A. Joseph, MD

The lower endoscopy revolution began in 1967 with the development of the first flexible fiberoptic sigmoidoscope by Bergein F. Overholt.[1] Although the idea for fiberoptic examination of the colon was first conceived by Robert Turell in 1963, he failed to pursue it because of skepticism over its potential for success. The breakthroughs in flexible fiberoptic technology by Harold Hopkins and the invention of the first flexible gastroscope by Basil Hirschowitz in 1958 convinced Dr. Overholt of the possibility of endoscopic examination of the colon and enabled him to develop the device for which he is now credited. In 1970, a longer version of the Overholt sigmoidoscope was devised with four-way tip deflection that enabled navigation of the colonic flexures. Between 1970 and 1973, colonoscopy started gathering increased acceptance across the United States as more diagnostic and therapeutic procedures were demonstrated to be safely performed.[1]

Definition

Lower endoscopy includes rigid and flexible sigmoidoscopy, colonoscopy, endoscopic ultrasonography (EUS), and anoscopy. This chapter focuses on the diagnostic and therapeutic maneuvers performed using a colonoscope. A separate section is included at the end to give special attention to the other modalities.

Indications

The indications for performing colonoscopy can be classified into two categories: diagnostic and therapeutic [*see Table 1*]. The most common diagnostic indication is for screening or surveillance of colorectal neoplasms and evaluation of colonic lesions. Investigation of gastrointestinal (GI) blood loss and unexplained abdominal pain are also frequent indications. Therapeutic indications include the removal of polyps, treatment of bleeding, decompression, and stenting. Contraindications to colonoscopy include disease states that increase the risk of perforation, such as recent diverticulitis (within 2 to 4 weeks), suspected perforation, or gangrenous ischemic colitis.

Table 1 Indications for Colonoscopy
Diagnostic
Screening and surveillance of GI neoplasms
GI blood loss
Iron deficiency anemia
Altered bowel habits
Unexplained abdominal pain
Surveillance of inflammatory bowel disease
Intraoperative identification of a lesion
Therapeutic
Removal of GI neoplasms
Treatment of bleeding
Decompression
Dilation of stricture
Placement of stent
Foreign body removal

GI = gastrointestinal.

Diagnostic and Screening Colonoscopy

Colon cancer is the third most common cause of cancer death among men and women in the United States, with approximately 50,000 deaths annually.[2,3] Most cancers arise from adenomatous polyps less than 1 cm in size and take almost 10 years to become invasive cancer. Screening programs have resulted in a decreased incidence of colon cancer as revealed in multiple cohort studies comparing them with patients without any form of screening.[2,3] Interestingly, no current studies have examined whether screening reduces colon cancer related mortality. The ability of colonoscopy to thoroughly visualize the lower GI mucosa, detect lesions, and remove them while obtaining tissue for histologic diagnosis makes it an effective tool for screening and surveillance.

The risk for colon cancer increases with age. Patients who only have age as a risk factor are considered to be at "average risk" [*see Table 2*]. Individuals with personal and familial risk factors are considered to be at "high risk" [*see Table 2*]. The recommendations by the US Multi-Society Task Force for screening and surveillance in colorectal cancer (CRC)[2] are highlighted in Table 2.

A newer technique called virtual colonoscopy (VC) or computed tomographic (CT) colography is finding more acceptance and popularity among providers and patients alike. This technique employs CT, rapid volumetric imaging, and three-dimensional image rendering made possible by contrast differences between intraluminal air, the colonic wall, and the surrounding soft tissues. Patients have to undergo a standard bowel preparation, and images are acquired in the supine and prone positions. Prior to the examination, a soft rubber catheter attached to a bulb syringe is then inserted into the rectum and the bowel is insufflated with either room air or carbon dioxide. The patient's subjective assessment of abdominal discomfort and fullness is a good indicator of bowel distention. Analyses of reports indicate a sensitivity and specificity of 75% and 90%, respectively, for adenomatous polyps larger than 10 mm in diameter, 66% and 63% for adenomas larger than 5 mm, and 45% and 80% for polyps smaller than 5 mm.[4] There are currently no studies that demonstrate a decrease in CRC incidence or mortality using VC, and concerns over radiation exposure have been expressed. VC may be recommended for patients who refuse colonoscopy or have an inadequate bowel preparation but is not currently endorsed by the American Society for

Table 2a Recommendations for Screening and Surveillance in Colorectal Cancer (Average-Risk)

Average-Risk Individual	Preferred Modality	Alternative
Begin screening at 50 yr	Colonoscopy every 10 yr	Annual fecal occult blood test (FOBT) Flexible sigmoidoscopy every 5 yr Annual FOBT and flexible sigmoidoscopy every 5 yr

Table 2b Recommendations for Screening and Surveillance in Colorectal Cancer (High-Risk)

High-Risk Individual with	Screening Strategy
FAP	Annual sigmoidoscopy beginning at 10–12 yr of age followed by colectomy when polyps develop
HNPCC	Colonoscopy beginning at 20–25 yr of age and repeated every 1–2 yr or colonoscopy performed 10 yr earlier than the first known diagnosis of cancer in the family, whichever is earlier Annual colonoscopy is recommended after 40 yr
IBD	Colonoscopy every 1–2 yr after 8–10 yr of the disease
CRC in a first-degree relative younger than 60 yr or two first-degree relatives of any age	Colonoscopy at 40 yr or performed 10 yr earlier than the affected relative, whichever is earlier If screening colonoscopy is normal, follow-up screening examinations are done every 5 yr subsequently
CRC in a first-degree relative older than 60 yr or two second-degree relatives of any age	Colonoscopy at 40 yr If screening colonoscopy is normal, follow-up screening examinations are done every 10 yr subsequently
Personal history of adenomas on previous endoscopy	1–2 tubular adenomas < 1 cm in size: perform surveillance in 5 yr 3 or more adenomas: perform surveillance in 3 yr Advanced adenomas (> 1 cm, high-grade dysplasia or villous elements): perform surveillance in 3 yr
Adenomatous polyp in a first-degree relative younger than 60 yr	Screening colonoscopy at 40 yr or performed 10 yr earlier than the affected relative, whichever is earlier If normal, screening colonoscopy is carried out every 3–5 yr subsequently
Adenomatous polyp in a first-degree relative older than 60 yr	Screening colonoscopy at 40 yr If normal, perform surveillance as for an average-risk individual
After curative surgery for colon cancer	Repeat colonoscopy at 1 and 3 yr and then at 5 yr intervals if normal
After curative surgery for rectal cancer	Repeat colonoscopy at 1 and 4 yr and then at 5 yr intervals if normal

Recommendations by the US Multi-Society Task Force. CRC = colorectal cancer; FAP = familial adenomatous polyposis; HNPCC = hereditary nonpolyposis colon cancer; IBD = inflammatory bowel disease.

Gastrointestinal Endoscopy (ASGE) as a standard screening modality.[2] Patients with lesions detected on VC must undergo a complete colonoscopic examination.

Bowel Preparation for Colonoscopy

A critical element to safe and accurate colonoscopy is the proper cleansing of the colon. To date, no ideal agent has been identified, and the evolution of agents for cleansing reveals a significant transformation with respect to methods used in the past. High-volume gut lavage and rectal pulsed irrigation are only of historic importance today. All patients are advised to take a clear liquid diet on the day prior to the procedure in combination with a bowel cleansing regimen. The use of diet modifications and enemas alone is insufficient to obtain optimal preparation, but they are used as adjuncts to the agents listed below. A joint consensus statement on bowel preparation prior to colonoscopy was published in 2006 by the American Society of Colon and Rectal Surgeons (ASCRS), ASGE, and Society of American Gastrointestinal and Endoscopic Surgeons (SAGES) and is summarized in Table 3.[5]

Patients who present for the procedure without completing their bowel regimen are best managed by rescheduling the procedure for another day. Options for those who have completed the recommended preparation but failed to achieve adequate cleansing include increasing the duration of the dietary modifications, using an alternate compound, and using adjuncts such as bisacodyl and magnesium citrate in combination with the main compound.[5] Pregnant patients may be administered a polyethylene glycol (PEG) solution in the face of data not favoring one agent over another.[5] In pediatric patients, clear data are lacking. A widely used preparation consists of low-volume PEG dosed at 1.25 mg/kg/day for 4 days with the addition of a clear liquid diet on the last day.

Special Considerations for Patients on Anticoagulants and Antiplatelet Agents

Patients on anticoagulant and antiplatelet/antithrombotic therapy for cardiovascular conditions present the usual challenge of balancing the risk of bleeding incurred during the procedure and the risk of thromboembolism from withdrawing these medications. Tailoring of therapeutic strategies to manage these medications must be based on the procedure and patient risk factors to optimize outcomes. The commonly used anticoagulants include warfarin, heparin, and low-molecular-weight heparin. The commonly used antiplatelet

Table 3 **Agents for Bowel Preparation Prior to Colonoscopy**

Agent	Commercial Name	Comments
Polyethylene glycol electrolyte lavage solution (PEG-ELS)	Colyte GoLYTELY	Passes through the colon with no net absorption or secretion Is faster and more effective than diet combined with cathartics, high-volume gut lavage, or mannitol (grade 1A) Is safer than osmotic laxatives/sodium phosphate in patients with fluid and electrolyte disturbances and hence is the preferred agent for patients with cardiac, renal, or liver disease (grade 1A) Is the proven and preferred method for cleansing in infants and children In adults, it is administered as 240 cc every 10 min until rectal output is clear or 4 L is consumed
Sulfate-free ELS	NuLYTELY TriLyte	Safety, effectiveness, and tolerance are comparable to those of PEG-ELS An alternative to PEG-ELS when a PEG-based solution needs to be used (grade 2B)
Low-volume PEG and delayed-release bisacodyl tablets	HalfLytely MiraLAX	Is better tolerated by patients because of the lower volume of fluid consumed and reduces cramping and bloating associated with consumption of 4 L of solution Combining it with bisacodyl improves the efficacy of bowel preparation (grade 1A)
Aqueous sodium phosphate	Fleet	Hyperosmotic bowel preparation that draws plasma water into the colon to induce bowel preparation Can cause fluid shifts and electrolyte derangements such as hyponatremia, hypokalemia, hypocalcemia, and hyperphosphatemia Can also induce phosphate neuropathy and nephrocalcinosis in renal patients In light of the possible fluid and electrolyte derangements, it must be used with caution in pediatric cases, geriatric populations, and patients with cardiac, renal, and hepatic insufficiency Induces mucosal ulcerations and hence must be avoided in patients with ulcerative colitis and Crohn disease Is dosed in 45 cc volumes every 12 h, with the last dose taken the morning of the procedure (grade 2B) Produces cleaning comparable to PEG-ELS (grade 1A)
Enemas	Tap water Soap suds Fleet—bisacodyl Fleet—mineral oil	Does not increase quality of preparation Used today for patients with a poor quality of preparation and those in whom the distal colonic segment is dysfunctional
Bisacodyl and magnesium citrate		Bisacodyl increases colonic motility, whereas magnesium citrate is a hyperosmotic laxative Adjuncts used in combination with PEG to reduce volume of preparation required for cleansing Does not improve quality of the preparation

agents include aspirin, clopidogrel, ticlopidine, dipyridamole, and glycoprotein inhibitors. Screening procedures and the use of "cold" biopsy techniques are considered to be at low risk for bleeding. This risk increases to 1 to 2.5% with snare polypectomies and to approximately 6% with the use of cautery devices and laser ablation. As the population ages, we find more of our patients on anticoagulant and antiplatelet medications. This has prompted the ASGE to publish guidelines for managing anticoagulant and antiplatelet medications based on the patient's risk for developing a thrombotic complication.[6–8] Given that the nature of the procedure to be undertaken is not known a priori, patients may require cessation of their medications for varying lengths of time. These guidelines and treatment strategies are summarized below in Table 4.

Aspirin has been shown to increase mucosal bleeding times, but the significance of this has not been demonstrated clinically. No randomized trials currently exist, and several case control and retrospective analyses have not demonstrated an adverse outcome to continuing aspirin during a procedure. Therefore, the current recommendation is to continue aspirin in the absence of a preexisting bleeding disorder. Those patients taking a combination of clopidogrel and aspirin may be at increased risk for bleeding, and in these circumstances, withholding the clopidogrel while continuing the aspirin may reduce this risk. This increased risk for bleeding, however, is not seen in patients taking the antiplatelet agent dipyridamole either as monotherapy or in combination with aspirin; however, the safety of this combination has not been evaluated in high-risk procedures.[6–8]

An important consideration must be given to those patients who have drug-eluting stents placed for coronary artery disease. The current guidelines advocate continuing dual-antiplatelet therapy (e.g., aspirin and clopidogrel) for a minimum of 1 month after placement of a bare metal stent and 1 year after placement of a drug-eluting stent to allow

Table 4 Guidelines and Strategies for Managing Anticoagulant and Antiplatelet Medication for Lower Endoscopy

Patient	High-Risk Procedure*	
	Warfarin	Antiplatelet Agents
High risk 1. Mechanical valve† in the mitral or aortic position 2. Those with atrial fibrillation and underlying cardiac or valvular disease	Stop warfarin 3–5 days prior. Use heparin (UFH/LMWH) as a bridge to maintain therapeutic anticoagulation. Stop heparin 4–8 hr before the procedure Resume heparin 2–6 hr after the procedure and gradually reinstitute warfarin until INR is in therapeutic range	Consider discontinuation at least 7–10 days before the procedure Reinstitution should be individualized
Low risk 1. Mechanical valves† in other sites 2. Atrial fibrillation without underlying cardiac or valvular disease 3. DVT	Stop warfarin 3–5 days prior and resume within 24 hr postprocedure	Individualize need for therapy based on risk and work with patient's cardiologist
Patient	**Low-Risk Procedure‡**	
	Warfarin	**Antiplatelet Agents**
High risk 1. Mechanical valve† in the mitral or aortic position 2. Those with atrial fibrillation and underlying cardiac or valvular disease	Continue warfarin. Delay procedure while INR is supratherapeutic.	No change in therapy as long as there is no previous issue of bleeding *or* Individualize therapy based on risk and work with patient's cardiologist
Low risk 1. Those with mechanical valves† in other sites 2. Those with atrial fibrillation without underlying cardiac or valvular disease 3. Those with DVT	Continue warfarin. Delay procedure while INR is supratherapeutic.	No change in treatment regimen required *or* Individualize therapy based on risk and work with patient's cardiologist

DVT = deep vein thrombosis; INR = international normalized ratio; LMWH = low-molecular-weight heparin; UFH = unfractionated heparin.
*High-risk procedures: polypectomy, pneumatic or bougie dilation, laser ablation, and coagulation.
†Patients with caged-ball or disk valves have a higher rish than those with bileaflet, tilting, or bioprosthetic valves.
‡Low-risk procedures: screening/surveillance colonoscopy ± biopsy.

reendothelialization and preventing stent thrombosis from premature drug cessation. Elective and semielective procedures should be delayed during this time. At the time of endoscopy, the patient is usually maintained on one agent, usually aspirin because more data are currently available on the safety of aspirin during procedures compared with clopidogrel.

Endocarditis Prophylaxis

It was originally believed that colonoscopy increased the risk of endocarditis as a result of the resulting bacteremia that occurred during the procedure. Contemporary studies cite the risk of bacteremia during colonoscopy to be between 0 and 25%, with a mean frequency of 4.4%.[9] Updated guidelines regarding the indications for antibiotics in patients with prosthetic devices have been published and are based on the American Heart Association (AHA) guidelines. Patients with a history of bacterial endocarditis, vascular grafts placed within 1 year of the procedure, prosthetic cardiac valves including bioprosthetic and homograft valves, and surgically created pulmonary or systemic conduits are considered to be at higher risk for bacterial seeding. These patients may be given antibiotics at the discretion of the endoscopist while undergoing a colonoscopy with or without biopsy or polypectomy. However, antibiotics are recommended should these patients require a dilation of a stricture during colonoscopy.[9] All other subgroups of patients who have prosthetic devices such as joint prostheses, penile prostheses, pacemakers, and implanted defibrillators are considered to be at low risk for infection, and antibiotic prophylaxis is discouraged.[9] Prophylactic antibiotics should be administered as follows: a single dose of 2 g of ampicillin IV and gentamicin (1.5 mg/kg to a maximum of 80 mg) administered 30 minutes prior to the procedure. In the case of a penicillin allergy, vancomycin 1 g IV can be substituted and should be given together with gentamicin.

General Technique

Colonoscopy begins with the proper selection and preparation of the patient. Informed consent should be obtained and a complete history and physical examination done with particular emphasis on the cardiopulmonary system. It is also important to be aware of previous abdominal surgery such as hysterectomy or colon resection as these can alter the anatomy of the colon.

The setup for colonoscopy is depicted in Figure 1a. The procedure is performed with the patient in the left lateral position and with intravenous sedation to increase patient comfort. An adult or pediatric colonoscope may be used. The adult colonoscope has a slightly increased diameter in

a

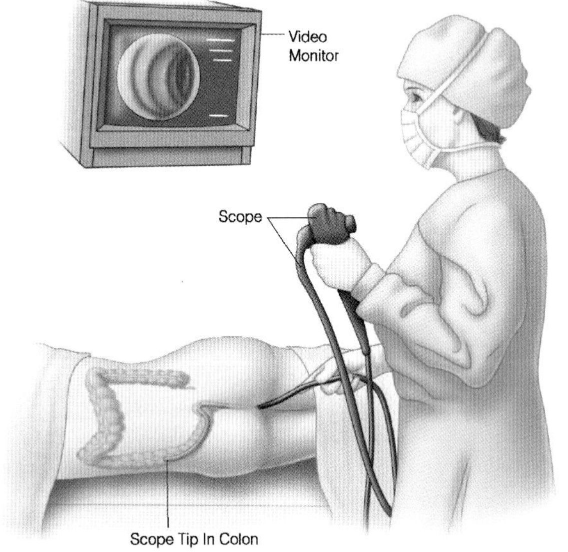

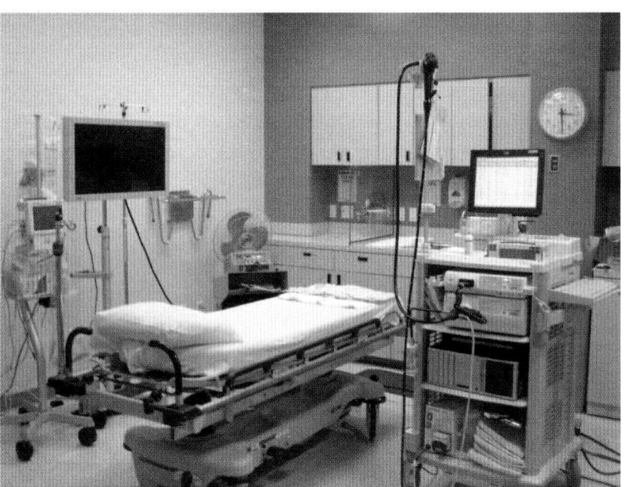

b

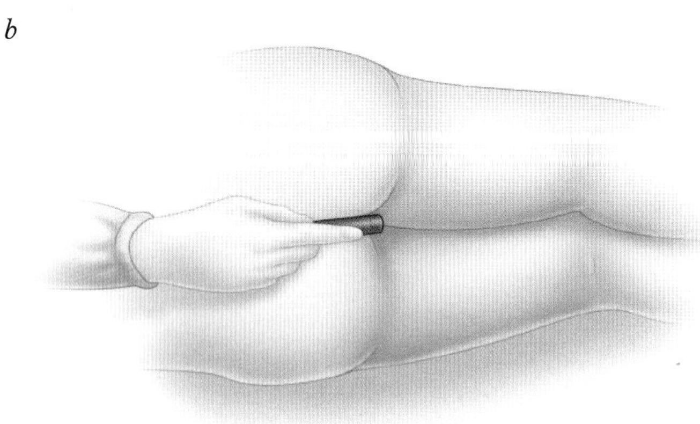

Figure 1 **(*a*) Room setup and patient positioning for colonoscopy. (*b*) Technique for insertion of a colonoscope.**

comparison with the pediatric scope but provides a larger instrument channel and increased shaft stiffness, which may reduce looping. The pediatric scope's smaller diameter may be more comfortable for the patient and allows easier traversal through narrow or angulated areas. It may also improve the endoscopist's ability to traverse the ileocecal valve. The procedure begins with a digital rectal examination to relax the sphincter muscles and screen for anal canal lesions. The well-lubricated colonoscope is then inserted into the anal canal by holding it approximately an inch from the tip and placing it against the patient's perineal body while sliding back and applying pressure toward the anus [*see Figure 1b*]. This maneuver causes the tip of the endoscope to gradually dilate the anus and reduces mechanical trauma to the anal canal during insertion. As the instrument is passed into the rectum, small amounts of air are insufflated and debris is washed from the lens. Traversing the colon expeditiously requires the endoscopist to use the minimum amount of insufflation to maintain visualization while managing the deflection wheels with the left hand and the endoscope shaft with the right. Overinsufflation during entry stretches and elongates the colonic flexures and makes traversal more difficult and uncomfortable. The rectal mucosa is identified by its prominent reticular vascular markings and the semilunar valves of Houston that appear in an alternating fashion [*see Figure 2a*]. As the endoscope is advanced into the sigmoid colon, a combination of tip deflection and shaft torque is used to negotiate this tortuous part of the colon. The long, floppy, and mobile character of the sigmoid colon makes it a common site for loop formation. Further, in patients with previous pelvic surgery, dense peritoneal adhesions to the sigmoid can increase the difficulty of traversal. The endoscope should not be advanced blindly if possible or with excessive force as bowing of the shaft can risk colonic wall perforation. Failure of the tip of the scope to advance while more shaft is introduced transanally is called paradoxical motion and suggests loop formation [*see Figure 2b*]. Such loop formation may be reduced by pulling back on the shaft of the endoscope so as to straighten it. A jiggling motion while pulling back may cause

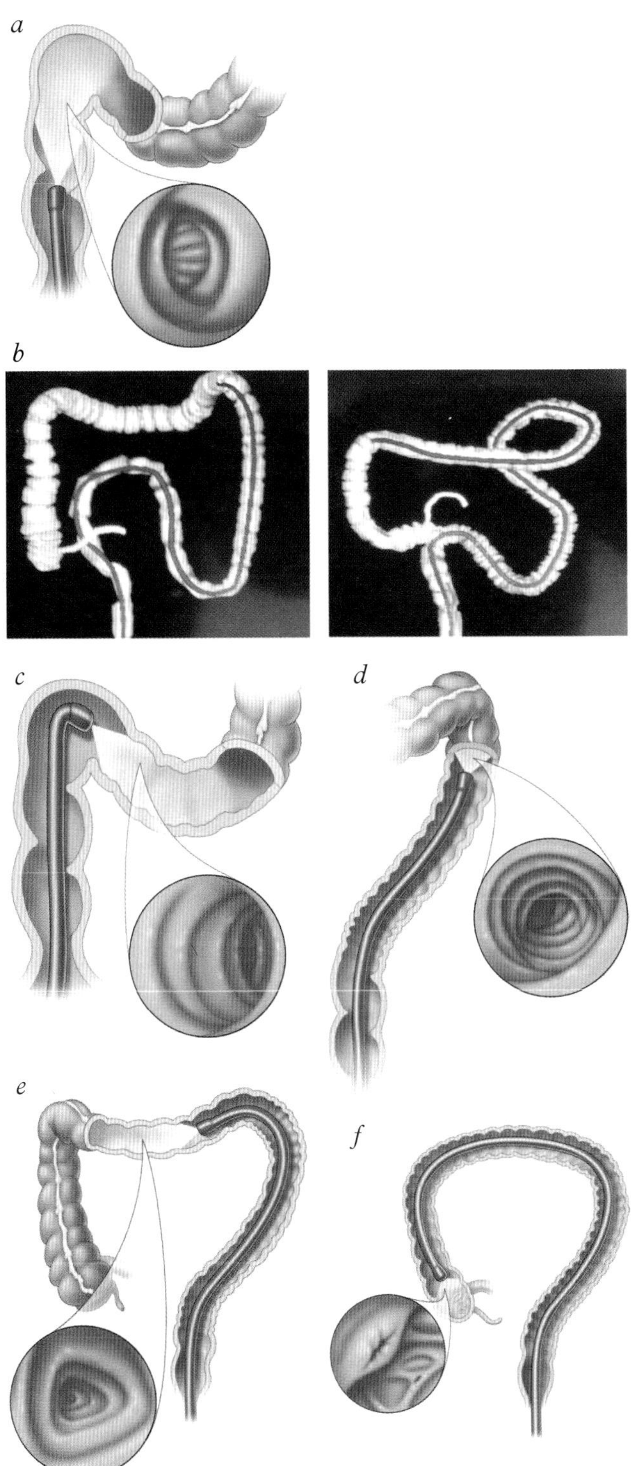

Figure 2 **(*a*) Endoluminal view of rectum with semilunar valves. (*b*) Loop formation during scope advancement. (*c*) Direction of lumen indicated by mucosal concavity. (*d*) Endoluminal view of descending colon. (*e*) Endoluminal view of transverse colon. (*f*) Endoluminal view of cecum.**

the colon to telescope over the instrument and further helps with loop reduction. The scope is then traversed through the sigmoid colon with the direction of the lumen identified by the concavity of the mucosal folds [*see Figure 2c*].

The descending colon is identified by the concentric circular pattern of the mucosa, and traversal to the splenic flexure is usually straightforward [*see Figure 2d*]. The splenic flexure is identified by pooling of fluid and a sharp angulation into the transverse colon. Occasionally, the bluish hue of the spleen can be seen through the colon wall. The transverse colon is identified by the triangular appearance of the lumen formed from omental traction on the tenia [*see Figure 2e*]. The transverse colon is relatively easy to maneuver through, and the appearance of a bluish hue over the mucosa suggests entry into the hepatic flexure. Commonly, entry into the ascending colon must be accompanied with scope withdrawal and left-hand torque to straighten all flexures and allow traversal into the cecum. Moving the patient into a supine position and applying external pressure to the sigmoid colon are adjuncts that can aid cecal intubation. The cecum is identified by the appearance of the convergence of the colonic tenia at the appendiceal orifice, the appearance of which is often called the "Mercedes" sign. Further, the central appendicular orifice and the liplike mucosal folds of the ileocecal valve are seen [*see Figure 2f*]. The valve can be intubated to gain access to the lumen by deflecting toward it while pulling back on the endoscope and insufflating gently. Not all endoscopists intubate the ileum routinely, but it should certainly be done when there are specific indications such as possible inflammatory bowel disease or unexplained iron deficiency anemia.

After successful cecal intubation, the colonic mucosa is carefully inspected during withdrawal of the endoscope. Care is taken to flatten the mucosa and look behind each fold and flexure. Obscuring fluid should be aspirated or the patient position changed to move debris out of the way. Evidence from a study by Barclay and colleagues suggests that scope withdrawals done in less than 8 minutes have an increased propensity to miss subtle adenomas that may harbor neoplasia.[10] The procedure ends with retroflexion in the rectum to inspect the anal canal and area of the dentate line, followed by evacuation of insufflation.

Diagnostic and Therapeutic Techniques during Colonoscopy

During inspection of the colonic mucosa, pathology is often identified that requires sampling, marking, or a therapeutic maneuver such as excision. What follows is a description of techniques available to the endoscopist.

BIOPSY

The most common technique of tissue sampling during colonoscopy is to perform a pinch biopsy. This entails delivering a biopsy forceps to the desired target and taking a sample without applying any electrocautery. Many biopsy forceps have a spike at their base that holds the first "bite" in place and allows obtaining a second "bite" before withdrawing the device [*see Figure 3a*].

POLYPECTOMY

Polypectomy is by far the most common therapeutic procedure performed during colonoscopy. Several techniques have been developed to improve the safety and efficacy of the procedure, and polyps are excised using either a snare or a "hot" biopsy forceps.

a

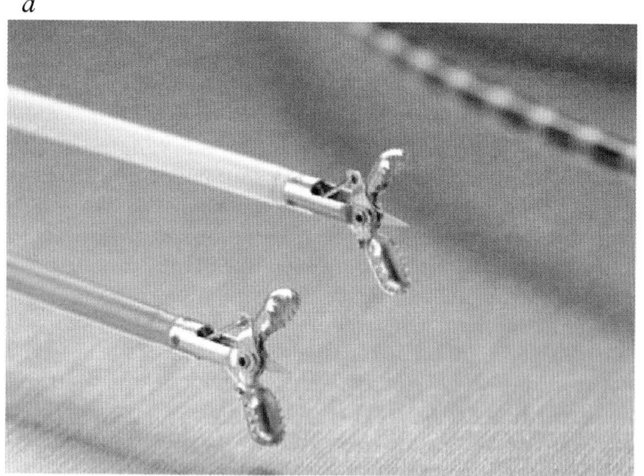

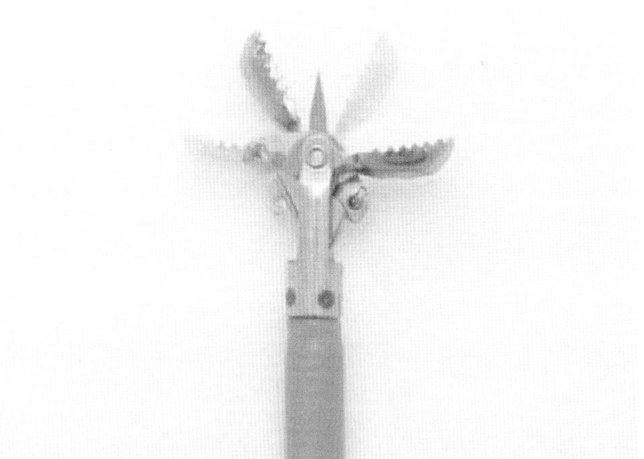

b

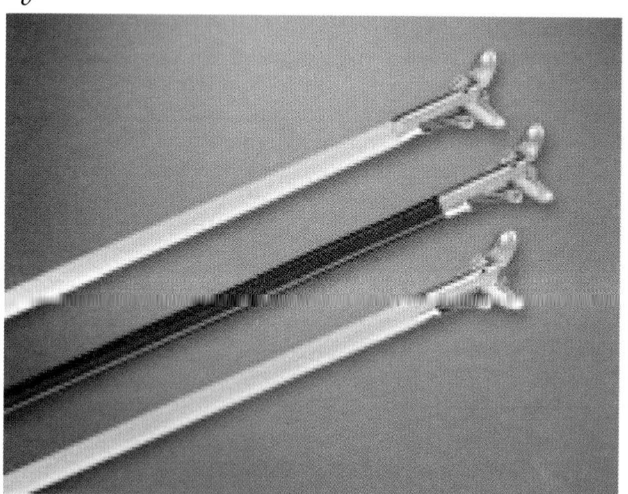

Figure 3 **(*a*) Pinch biopsy forceps. (*b*) Hot biopsy forceps.**

Hot Biopsy

For those polyps less than 3 mm in size, excision with a "hot" biopsy forceps [*see Figure 3b*] can be sufficient. A hot biopsy forceps differs from that used during regular biopsy in that it delivers monopolar electromechanical energy to the jaws to enable tissue destruction. During hot biopsy, the lesion is grasped with the forceps and distracted away from the underlying submucosa. Brief applications of electrocautery are then applied until a white zone of coagulum at the base of the polyp is seen. In theory, this technique allows sampling of the lesion to determine its pathology while destroying any remaining tissue to minimize recurrence or continued growth. Although still practiced, there is controversy about the efficacy of the hot biopsy technique. Gilbert and colleagues reported that hot biopsy techniques failed to reduce the incidence of CRC and were not associated with complete obliteration of the lesion.[11] Further, the procedure risks deep tissue injury, with the consequent complications of bleeding, perforation, and postpolypectomy syndrome [*see* Postpolypectomy Complications, *below*]. In 1992, Tappero and colleagues described a "cold" biopsy technique as an alternative to hot biopsy in 210 consecutive patients in whom 288 polyps less than 5 mm were excised without diathermy.[12] They reported this alternative to be safe and comparable to the conventional hot biopsy technique in adequacy of tissue acquisition for histopathology.

A prospective study by Mönkemüller and colleagues in 2004 asked pathologists blinded to the fashion in which the specimen was acquired (hot versus cold biopsy) to evaluate the specimen quality and found a significant rate of architectural distortion and tissue fragmentation in samples acquired by hot biopsy.[13]

Sessile or pedunculated lesions between 3 mm and 2 cm are snare excised. For pedunculated polyps, it must be borne in mind that the stalk represents an extension of normal mucosa and does not need to be excised completely. The snare is advanced beyond the polyp such that the sheath of the snare rests over the lesion. Gentle drawing back of the snare brings it into position over and around the polyp. Once the snare is tightened, brief bursts of cautery are applied while distracting the lesion away from the submucosa so as to prevent transmural thermal injury [*see Figure 4a*]. The excised polyp must then be retrieved for pathologic examination either by suctioning it through the colonoscope and into a specimen trap (small polyps) or retrieving it directly by attaching it to the tip of the scope (by suction, snare, or basket) and removing it.

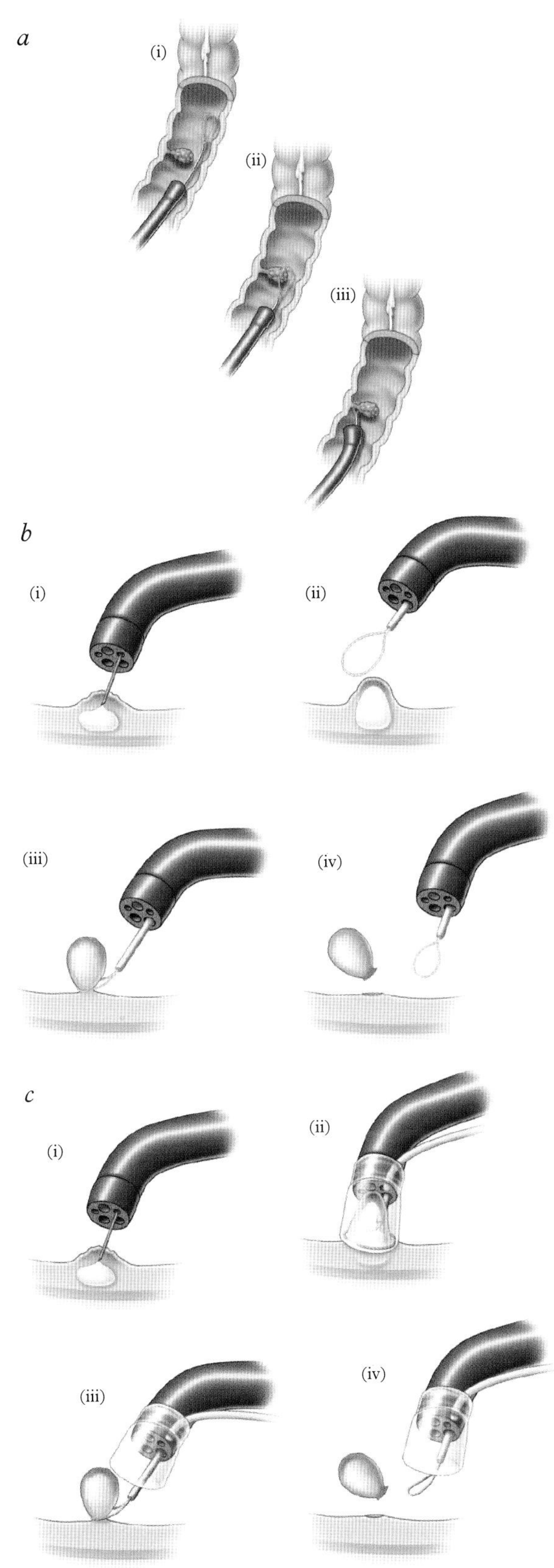

Figure 4 **(*a*) Snare polypectomy of a pedunculated polyp. (*b*) Endoscopic mucosal resection (EMR) of a sessile polyp using the lift and cut technique. (*c*) EMR of a sessile polyp using a suction cap.**

Sessile polyps greater that 2 cm may not be amenable to simple snare excision without risking injury to the colonic wall. This risk can be reduced by resecting the polyp in a piecemeal fashion using endoscopic mucosal resection (EMR). EMR was first described by Tada in 1984 for dealing with giant sessile lesions in the stomach.[14] It has been safely and effectively applied to similar lesions in the colon. EMR begins with a simple saline lift of the submucosa followed by a piecemeal resection of the lesion using a polypectomy snare [*see Figure 4b*].

Alternately, EMR can be performed by mounting a transparent suction cap (EMR-C) to the distal end of the endoscope. After a saline lift is performed, a portion of the lesion is aspirated into this cap, and then an open snare is passed around the base of the lesion. These steps are repeated several times until the entire lesion is excised in a piecemeal fashion [*see Figure 4c*]. EMR affords a greater amount of tissue for resection, thereby optimizing histologic evaluation. Furthermore, lesions located tangentially and those within interhaustral folds are better approached with this technique. EMR-C is a painstaking yet rewarding procedure, with an overall complication rate of 10%, which is comparable to standard snare polypectomy techniques.[15,16]

The treatment strategies for pedunculated polyps excised at polypectomy are best governed by the Haggitt classification.[17] This stratification of treatment depending on the degree of invasiveness of the lesion has demonstrated prognostic importance [*see Figure 5*]. This classification is depicted in Table 5.

Lesions from levels 0 to 2 are treated with polypectomy alone. For a level 3 lesion, polypectomy is adequate as long as a 2 mm negative margin is present, the cancer is not poorly differentiated, and no lymphatic or vascular invasion is present. Level 4 lesions are treated with segmental colectomy because of the higher risk of lymphatic invasion.

It is usually a wise strategy to tattoo lesions that appear suspicious for malignancy. This is often done with a permanent carbon-based dye injected into the submucosa circumferentially in an area proximal to the lesion. These markings are usually visible from the outside of the lumen during surgery. This is an invaluable tool that enables the surgeon to locate the lesion and acquire appropriate operative margins.

Novel approaches to polypectomy using laparoscopic assistance have been described for those polyps that are hard to access endoscopically and for giant sessile polyps. A review of cases done by Franklin and colleagues described the advantages of laparoscopy-assisted endoscopic polypectomy to include the ability to laparoscopically mobilize the colon so as to enable better access to polyps along flexures, the ability to laparoscopically repair a transmural injury should that occur during excision of giant sessile polyps, or the opportunity to perform a colectomy during the same procedure should the frozen section be positive for an invasive carcinoma.[18]

Postpolypectomy Complications

The Munich Polypectomy Study (MUPS), a large, multicenter, prospective trial evaluating risks and complications in 4,000 snare polypectomies, found that the risk of complication increases when polyps are located in the right colon and greater than 1 cm in diameter or located in the left colon and greater than 2 cm in diameter or if multiple polyps are resected.[16] The overall complication rate in this study

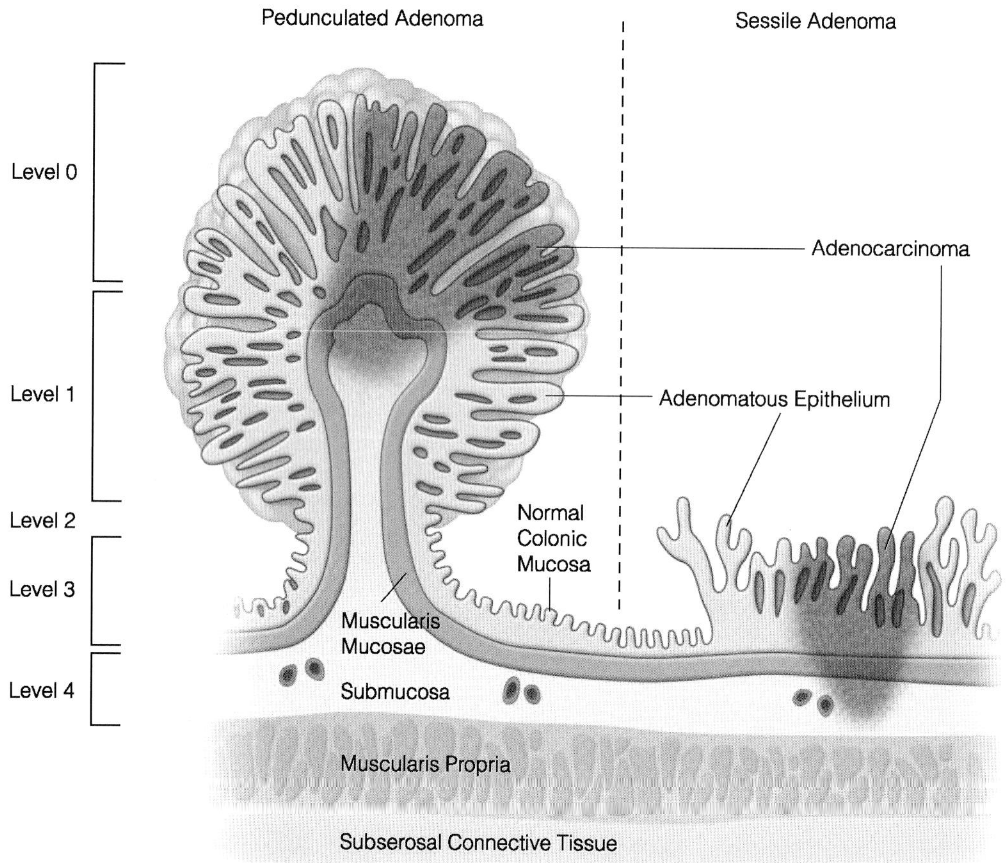

Figure 5 **Haggitt classification of tissue invasion in a pedunculated polyp.**

was 9.7%, with a bleeding risk of 8.6% and a perforation risk of 1.1%.

Postpolypectomy syndrome occurs in 2 to 3% of patients undergoing polypectomy and is the result of a transmural thermal injury with subsequent serosal inflammation. Most patients present with abdominal pain and fever. Workup includes an abdominal and pelvic CT scan to look for evidence of colonic perforation. If there is none, the patient is managed by avoiding oral intake and the administration of parenteral antibiotics along with serial abdominal examinations. Most patients can be managed nonoperatively in this fashion. Those patients who develop signs of peritonitis require surgical exploration and primary repair of the injury. This is usually sufficient because the colon has been recently cleansed and contamination is usually minimal.

Table 5 Haggitt Classification of Tumor Invasiveness in an Adenomatous Polyp

Level	Histology Findings
0	Carcinoma in situ or intramucosal carcinoma. Not invasive.
1	Carcinoma invading through muscularis mucosa into submucosa but limited to the head of the polyp
2	Carcinoma invading the level of the neck of the adenoma
3	Carcinoma invading any part of the stalk
4	Carcinoma invading into the submucosa of the bowel wall below the stalk of the polyp but above the muscularis propria

HEMOSTASIS

Lower endoscopy as a diagnostic and therapeutic tool for management of colonic bleeding is indicated in patients with spontaneous cessation as well as those with ongoing hemorrhage. Although, traditionally, radionucleotide scans and angiography in concert with surgery were the first-line treatments, there is now greater advocacy and acceptance of the use of colonoscopy to manage these cases at the outset. Of course, good clinical judgment should be exerted to identify those patients with massive hemorrhage and hemodynamic instability who would benefit from angiography and/or an early trip to the operating room.

Historically, the role of urgent colonoscopy (defined as a procedure within 12 to 48 hours of admission) for lower GI bleeding has been questioned. This arose due to concerns of inadequate visualization and the fact that most bleeding stops spontaneously. However, several studies have demonstrated that colonoscopy under urgent conditions is safe and feasible after prior rapid cleansing, with a diagnostic yield of between 74 and 90%. This is higher than both radionucleotide scans and angiography, although no studies have compared these procedures head to head in a randomized fashion.[19]

The bowel preparation for the procedure is undertaken simultaneously with the resuscitation efforts and consists of 1 L of PEG administered orally or via a nasogastric tube every 30 to 45 minutes until the stool effluent is relatively clear. The administration of metaclopromide improves gastric emptying and may be a useful adjunct.

The tools for acquiring hemostasis include the following:

- *Vasoconstricting agents.* The most common method of gaining initial hemostasis is by injection of epinephrine, typically in a 1:10,000 concentration. It is injected into the submucosal layer to gain temporary hemostasis and as an adjunct to thermal therapy. Common side effects are transient tachycardia and hypertension. When bleeding obscures the field of view, irrigation with blind injection around an area of clot is considered safe.[19]
- *Thermal devices.* Applying thermal energy to a bleeding lesion either alone or in combination with injection therapy is another common strategy for gaining endoscopic hemostasis. Thorough knowledge of the principles of electrosurgery is critical for this technique. A comprehensive review of this topic is beyond the scope of this chapter, but a basic understanding of the types of electrosurgical energy is reviewed. Cauterizing a lesion with electromechanical energy (electrocautery) is simply the act of applying an alternating electrical current via a device to the desired tissue. Patients are not "shocked" by this energy the way they would be if they came in contact with a common wall outlet because it is delivered at a very high frequency in the radiowave spectrum (radiofrequency). All electrocautery requires a complete circuit to be delivered to the desired tissue. There are essentially two ways to complete this circuit. Monopolar electrocautery completes the circuit by the electrical current passing through the patient. Bipolar electrocautery passes through the affected tissue only. Monopolar electrocautery can penetrate deeply into tissues and is effective for hemostasis but risks deep thermal injury and possible perforation in thin-walled structures. Bipolar energy does not penetrate as deeply but may be less effective in gaining hemostasis. Thorough knowledge of these principles, along with proper energy settings on the generator used for electrocautery, is critical for the safe application of this technology. Argon plasma coagulation (APC) is a special version of monopolar electrocautery that requires additional understanding. Argon gas, when "electrified," is converted to plasma, which conducts monopolar electricity. This principle is very useful in situations where it is desirable to apply electrocautery to large surface areas without risking deep tissue penetration. An additional benefit of the APC probes is that they enable the application of electrocautery without actually touching the tissue, which prevents the buildup of debris on the probe tip and allows for the expeditious "painting" of large surface areas. Understanding the unique energy settings and argon gas flow rates for operating an APC probe is essential. Being mindful to constantly aspirate the argon gas from the GI tract is also important. Another method of applying thermal energy to tissue in the GI tract is through use of a Teflon-tipped probe that is heated to a desired level. This "heater probe" does not apply electrocautery to the tissue but simply cauterizes it by generating heat at its tip. Understanding the energy settings available on this probe and the conformity of its tip is important for its proper use.
- *Endoscopic clips.* Endoscopically placed clips [*see Figure 6*] are an excellent technology used to manage bleeding from discrete sources, such as the mouth of a diverticulum or postpolypectomy bleeding site, and can be applied multiple times. These clips are also excellent for controlling bleeding from a fresh anastomosis when injection and thermal application are undesirable.

DECOMPRESSION

Colonoscopic decompression has been performed in unprepared bowel for sigmoid volvulus and colonic pseudo-obstruction (Ogilvie syndrome). This nonsurgical approach may serve as an invaluable bridge to surgery in those critically ill and elderly patients who may not be able to withstand a surgical operation.

For sigmoid volvulus, the endoscope is advanced beyond the point of torsion gently, without excessive force and while keeping the lumen in sight at all times. Once the bowel is detorsed, contents from the proximal bowel are suction evacuated to decompress it [*see Figure 7, a, b*]. The decompressed state of the colon is maintained by placing a long rubber catheter in the proximal colon using endoscopic guidance [*see Figure 7c*].

STENTING

The first reported use of colonic stenting for treatment of large bowel obstruction was by Spinelli and colleagues in 1992.[20] Several subsequent studies have further validated its efficacy, and indications for their use are as follows:

- *Preoperative decompression.* In patients who present with acute obstruction from a primary colorectal malignancy, use of a stent to relieve the obstruction decreases the likelihood of requiring emergent surgery and the need for a colostomy. A one-stage en bloc resection of the cancer can be performed subsequently once the obstruction is relieved and the patient's condition has optimized. Several prospective and retrospective studies have confirmed this. A large study by Dauphine and colleagues examining the role of stents used for preoperative decompression from 1990 to 2000 revealed that stenting was a successful bridge to surgery in 85% of cases and 95% of patients benefitted from a single-stage procedure.[21] However, data from prospective studies randomizing patients to a stenting versus emergent surgery arm are lacking.
- *Palliation of obstruction.* In those patients with primary or recurrent CRC who are not operative candidates, endoscopic stents can be used as a means of palliation. In the same study by Dauphine and colleagues, stenting averted a colostomy in 90% of the patients.[21]
- *Palliation of malignant fistulas.* Sealing a colovesical or colovaginal fistula for palliation is another indication for stenting, although firm evidence to support this treatment modality is lacking.

Stenting is contraindicated in the presence of a perforation, and this must be definitely excluded prior to the procedure.

a

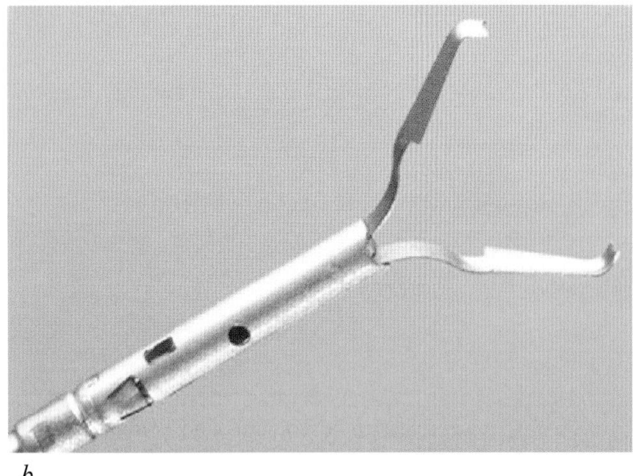

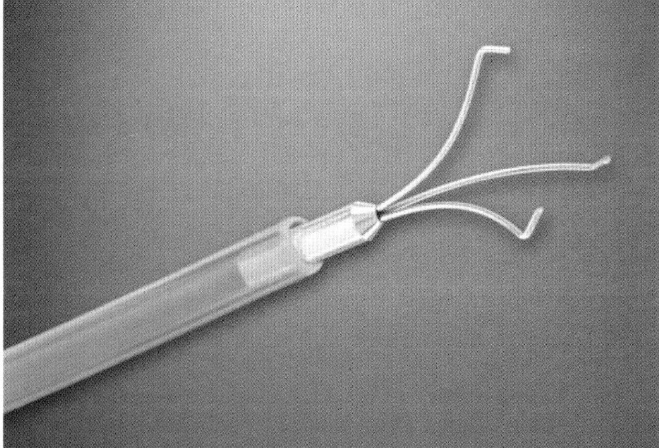

b

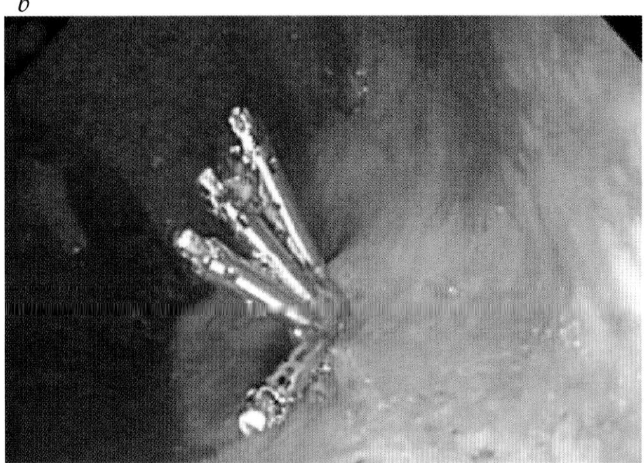

Figure 6 (*a*) **Endoscopic clips.** (*b*) **Endoscopic clip application.**

Similarly, benign strictures are a relative contraindication, although stents have been deployed in these circumstances.

Colonic stents are referred to as self-expanding metal stents and are made of woven, knitted, or laser-cut metal mesh cylinders that exert radially expansive forces when deployed, which helps keep them in position [*see Figure 8a*]. Some stents designed for the esophagus or bile duct are covered with a plastic membrane to prevent tumor ingrowth, but colonic stents are uncovered to allow better fixation and prevent migration. These stents usually foreshorten after deployment, which is an important consideration while choosing the length of stent to be deployed. A variety of stents are available, and their salient features are summarized in Table 6.

These stents are passed over a guide wire and are deployed with or without through-the-scope (TTS) assistance, usually with fluoroscopic guidance. The stents are mounted on delivery systems that differ with regard to the design of their handles and the release of the constricting mechanism. Most delivery systems release the stent at the distal end first.

Prior to stenting a patient with an obstruction, it is important to rule out any other proximal source of obstruction and to characterize the degree and length of the obstruction. An enema may be given prior to the procedure, although most patients with a high-grade obstruction have already evacuated stool below the lesion.

For non-TTS stent placement, a guide wire is passed through the endoscope, across the lesion, and as proximal as possible. The endoscope is withdrawn, and the nondeployed stent is advanced over its delivery system and across the stricture. The endoscope is reinserted to verify optimal positioning of the distal end of the stent and then deployed under direct vision. Positioning of the waist of the stent across the middle of the obstruction indicates optimal placement.

For TTS stent placement, a guide wire is passed across the obstruction and up to 20 cm proximally. The nondeployed stent is placed under direct endoscopic guidance and deployed after confirming optimal positioning [*see Figure 8, b, c, and d*].

Reported complications from stenting include perforation, migration, and bleeding. Perforation is the most devastating complication and negates the reason for the procedure in the first place, which was to avoid a colostomy and facilitate a one-stage resection. The risk of intraprocedural perforation may be reduced by limiting insufflation.[21] Stent migration can be asymptomatic or present with rectal pain, bleeding, tenesmus, or fecal incontinence if the stent migrates distally. Typically, as long as the stent remains 2 cm above the anal canal, it does not produce symptoms and can be easily removed. Obstruction of the stent by tumor ingrowth is usually managed by placement of new stents across the old one. The study by Dauphine and colleagues alluded to earlier in

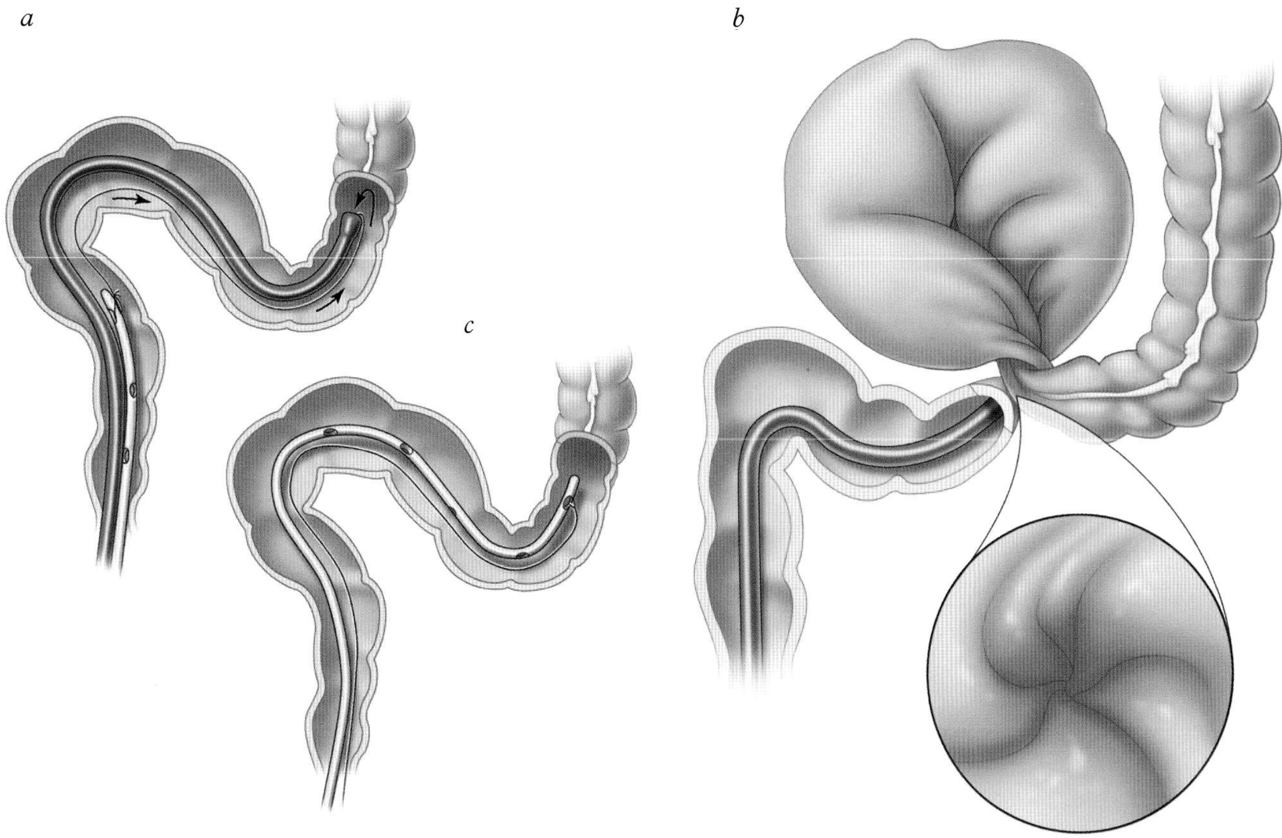

Figure 7 **Colonoscopic decompression.**

this chapter examined all cases of stent placement from 1990 to 2000 and reported a mortality of 1%, a perforation rate of 0 to 7%, a migration rate of 3 to 22%, bleeding in 0 to 5%, and a reobstruction rate of 0 to 15%.[21]

BALLOON DILATION

The endoscopic management of anastomotic and other benign strictures by balloon dilation provides a relatively noninvasive method to a problem that was long managed surgically. Similar to their role in upper endoscopy, endoscopic balloon dilation lends itself well to the management of benign colonic strictures. The procedure is optimally performed under fluoroscopic guidance, and a gentle bowel preparation to cleanse the colon distal to the stricture is recommended. The deflated balloon is passed through the working channel of the endoscope and positioned across the stricture. Under endoscopic and fluoroscopic guidance, the balloon is inflated to its full diameter and left in position for 1 to 2 minutes. It is then deflated and withdrawn, and the area of dilation is endoscopically inspected for evidence of bleeding or perforation. The procedure may be repeated at 2- to 4-week intervals as necessary, and patients should be advised that multiple sessions are frequently required to obtain maximum therapeutic benefit. Although reports indicate a median number of approximately 2.6 dilations to maintain long-term patency, a retrospective review by Araujo and Costa on patients after low anterior resection did not find a relation between the number of dilation sessions and recurrence.[22]

Sigmoidoscopy

The advent of the sigmoidoscope was the first breakthrough in lower endoscopy. Although less in favor and less frequently performed today, it is still a valuable diagnostic and therapeutic tool for conditions of the lower colon and rectum. Indications for its use today include evaluation of a change in bowel habits, bleeding, and lower abdominal pain and as a screening tool for CRC. It is usually performed in the doctor's office after an enema and requires no sedation. Although no prospective studies exist that demonstrate a reduction in CRC mortality from sigmoidoscopy, case control studies have suggested a decrease in the incidence of CRC in the examined areas, with benefits lasting up to 10 years.[23] However, the risk of cancer in the colon beyond the reach of the sigmoidoscope is not reduced, and multiple studies have confirmed that advanced proximal adenomas may exist even in the absence of more distal lesions.[6,23,24] Flexible sigmoidoscopy is currently recommended as an alternative screening tool to colonoscopy every 5 years.

Certain findings on sigmoidoscopy predict a higher risk for proximal advanced neoplasia and warrant a more complete colonoscopic examination. These include villous histology of the distal adenoma, adenomas greater than 1 cm, and multiple adenomas. Adenomas less than 1 cm may be excised using a cold snare technique and can be histologically distinguished as hyperplastic or inflammatory in nature. Electromechanical energy should not be used in the unprepared bowel to avoid explosion.

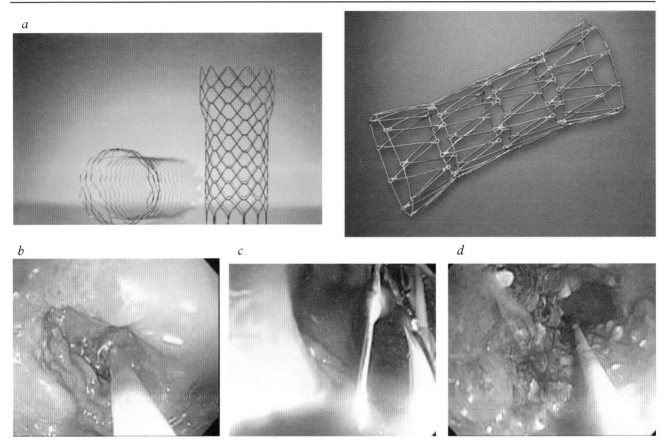

Figure 8 **(*a*) Self-expanding uncovered metal stents. (*b*, *c*, *d*) Self-expanding uncovered metal stent being deployed in a patient with a malignant obstruction. A guide wire is passed through the obstruction. The collapsed stent is passed over the guide wire and across the obstruction. Once optimal position of the stent is confirmed, it is deployed. Luminal caliber is restored once the stent is in position.**

Anoscopy

Anoscopy employs a lubricated speculum [*see Figure 9*] to visually inspect and examine the anal canal. It is performed in the doctor's office or emergency department and may be used to diagnose hemorrhoids, anal fissures, fistulas, abscesses, tumors, and bleeding from the anal canal. Maneuvers such as banding of prolapsed hemorrhoids, biopsies of tumors, fulguration of warts, drainage of small superficial abscesses, and application of silver nitrate to bleeding points may also be safely carried out using anoscopy. Anoscopy requires a minimal preparation such as an enema and produces minimal discomfort. It should be performed carefully after recent anal or rectal surgery.

Table 6 Colonoscopic Stents and Features

Material	Comments
Nitinol	A nickel, titanium alloy that is flexible enough to allow stenting across sharply angulated areas at the cost of reduced radially expansive forces Decreased incidence of migration by creating wider flare at its proximal end Foreshortens by 23% when deployed
Elgiloy	A cobalt, chromium, and nickel alloy that is corrosion resistant and exerts high radial forces when deployed Allows through-the-scope deployment Foreshortens by 39–49% when deployed
Stainless steel	Does not foreshorten when deployed

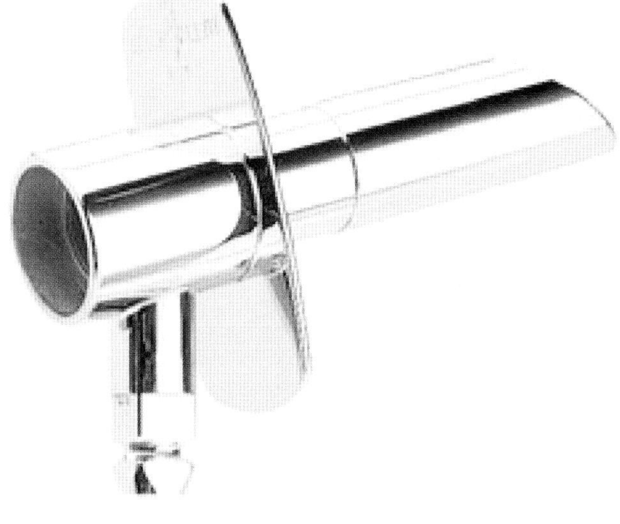

Figure 9 **Anoscope.**

Endoscopic Ultrasonography

The scope of EUS is more limited in lower endoscopy when compared with its application during esophagogastroduodenoscopy (EGD) and endoscopic retrograde cholangiopancreaticography (ERCP). EUS uses rigid endorectal probes [*see Figure 10a*], flexible radial and longitudinal ultrasonographic echoendoscopes, and catheter miniprobes that can be passed through the working channel of the endoscope. A schematic of the endoluminal anatomy as visualized during EUS is depicted in Figure 10b.

Endorectal ultrasonography is an invaluable tool for preoperative staging in rectal cancer [*see Figure 10, c and d*] and helps stratify those patients who would benefit from local excision versus radical resection as well as the need for neoadjuvant chemoradiation. It is also used for surveillance after surgery to detect local recurrence of tumor.

EUS is also used to guide the management of complicated fistulas [*see Figure 10e*] in patients with perianorectal inflammatory bowel disease. Patients with complex perineal fistulas from Crohn disease usually undergo a protracted course of medical and surgical therapy, which is dictated by the clinical discretion of the surgeon. With EUS, superior anatomic delineation of the fistula in relation to the sphincter and identification of occult internal openings and abscesses can guide the surgeon in deciding the optimal course of treatment for these complex problems. A retrospective study by Schwartz and colleagues in 21 patients with complex perineal fistulas treated by a combination of medical and surgical therapy guided by serial EUS revealed that 86% of patients had initial cessation of drainage, whereas 76% had long-term cessation.[25] Furthermore, a small, randomized, prospective study by the same group demonstrated that when EUS was used to guide treatment, 80% of patients responded completely compared with 20% of patients in the control arm, whose management strategy was solely at the clinical discretion of their provider.[26] At this time, the ASCRS recommends the use of EUS as a beneficial adjunct in the management of these patients.[27] The use of EUS requires special training and knowledge of the principles of ultrasonography to avoid misinterpretation.[28]

Lower Endoscopy Training and Innovations on the Horizon

There is currently a deficiency of consistent and curriculum-driven endoscopy training for general surgeons. This has made it difficult for surgeons in training to gain adequate experience in colonoscopy so that they feel confident in performing the procedure. In fact, rural surgeons perform flexible endoscopy more frequently than any other procedure but report a lack of confidence in doing so at the beginning of their practice as a result of either inadequate exposure to the endoscopic platform or lapsed time periods between their rotation as a junior resident and use of the endoscope as a senior resident.[29]

The American Board of Surgery acknowledges the importance of learning colonoscopy during residency and, as part of this acknowledgment, has recently increased the required number of cases for general surgery board certification. Although it is logical to believe that doing more procedures results in better performance, there is considerable debate about what numbers to use and if numbers by themselves are an adequate indicator of competency. Some believe that the real underlying problem in endoscopy training is the lack of a validated assessment tool for measuring procedural competence. Recently, Vassillou and colleagues reported on a score card to measure endoscopic proficiency. This Global Assessment of Gastrointestinal Endoscopic Skills (GAGES) provides the first validated objective measure of specific parameters required for proficiency in flexible GI endoscopy. Preliminary testing using this score card indicates that it is a consistent, reliable, and valid measure of endoscopic skill.[30] Such a score card may eventually replace numbers as a measure of proficiency in endoscopy.

Recognizing the challenges in learning flexible GI endoscopy, the SAGES has worked to develop a validated training and assessment program for GI endoscopy called the Fundamentals of Endoscopic Surgery (FES). This program provides Web-based didactic material on the essentials of flexible GI endoscopy, as well as a validated written examination of knowledge and a hands-on test of skill. FES may become the first "off-the-shelf" validated training and assessment tool for GI endoscopy, and it is hoped that this program will become an integral part of both surgery residency and GI fellowship training.

Over the past decade, the ultimate therapeutic endoscopic procedure has been pioneered, called natural orifice transluminal endoscopic surgery (NOTES). This type of surgery uses a flexible endoscopic platform passed into a natural orifice and across the wall of the GI tract to gain access to the peritoneal cavity. With this approach, all manner of abdominal surgery have been accomplished in animate and cadaver models, and clinical trials are currently under way for NOTES appendectomy and cholecystectomy. The transcolonic route has been described for peritoneoscopy and staging of cancer, drainage of pelvic abscesses, and urologic and gynecologic procedures. Current experiments in NOTES procedures have described using a combination of transgastric, transvaginal, and transcolonic access for full-thickness polyp resection, colostomy, and ileostomy creation, as well as right and left colon resection.[31] These achievements, although exciting, have been limited by inadequacy of instrumentation for retraction, hemostasis and suturing, ergonomic challenges, and the inadequacy of the flexible GI endoscopic platform to perform complex surgical procedures. Lack of definitive closure devices for the colotomy also leaves many surgeons wary of pursuing these new techniques, although novel devices for endoscopic suturing are quickly becoming available, as recently reviewed in an article by Swain.[32] Some of these devices have been used in small clinical trials with success.

Most reports of NOTES procedures are in animal and cadaver models, with few human case reports and even fewer case series. However, some surgeons have used the advent of NOTES to reexamine their practice and try to develop less invasive laparoscopic procedures. One example is the development of a "hybrid" NOTES approach to colon resection, where the dissection and anastomosis are performed laparoscopically, but specimen extraction is done either transanally or transvaginally.[33] Transanal endoscopic microsurgery, a procedure that uses special laparoscopic instrumentation introduced via the anus and into the rectum for transluminal

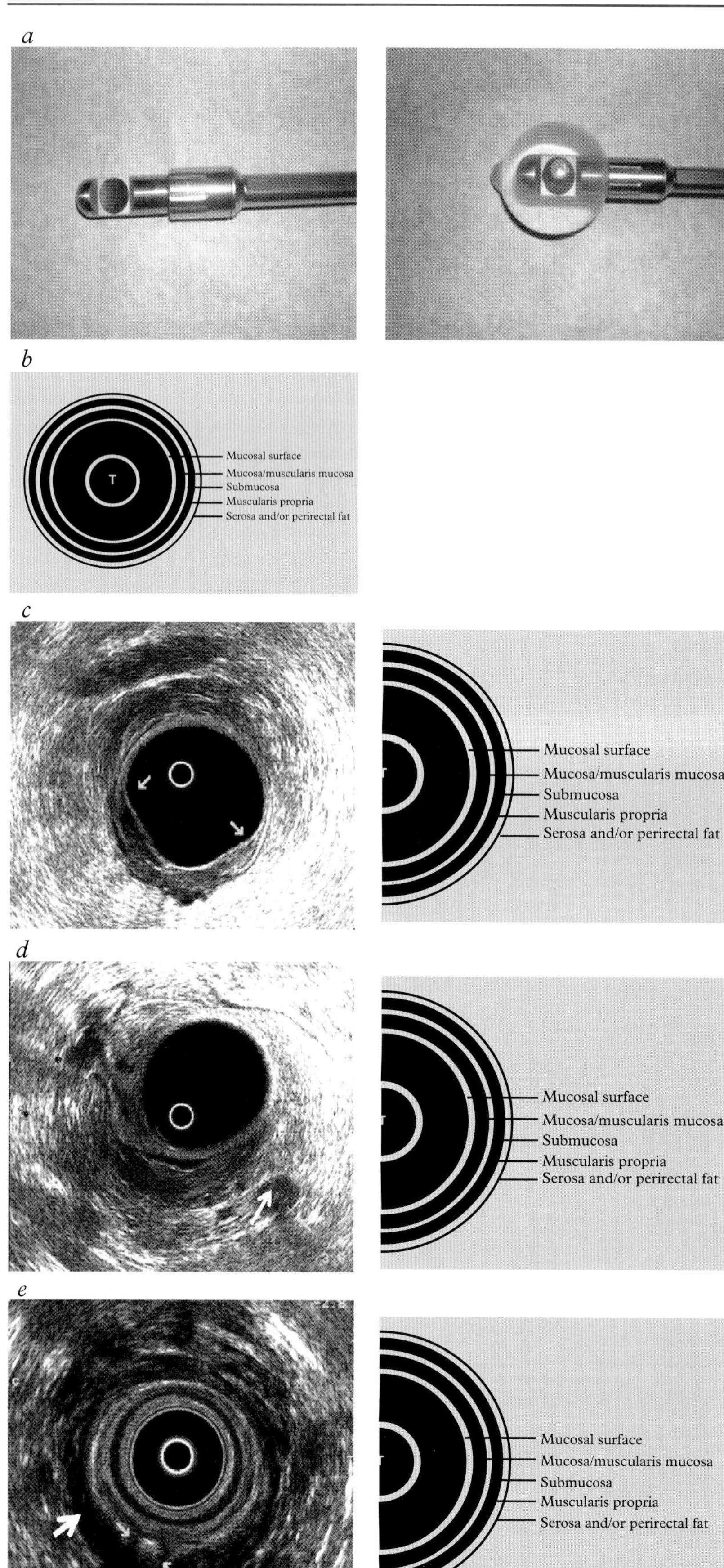

Figure 10 **(*a*) Rigid endorectal probes for endoscopic ultrasonography (EUS). (*b*) Schematic of the endoluminal anatomy visualized on EUS. (*c*) T3 cancer invading the pericolonic fat. *Arrows* indicate lateral limits of tumor extension. (*d*) Presence of lymph node enlargement in a patient with rectal cancer. The *arrow* indicates a 1 cm lymph node. (*e*) Transsphincteric fistula as visualized on EUS. The *larger, thicker arrow* indicates the sphincter complex. The two *smaller arrows* indicate the site of the fistulous opening.**

full-thickness excision of rectal cancer and suture repair of the resultant defect, has been studied as a portal for NOTES surgery on the colon. In a preclinical study on porcine and cadaver specimens, Denk and colleagues demonstrated the feasibility of this platform for colonic excision and extraction using the transrectal route.[34] Technical challenges remain, however. Innovative redesign of instrumentation and the endoscope is currently under way to overcome these ergonomic obstacles and advance its acceptance in the surgical community.

Summary

Whether surgeons perform colonoscopy as part of their practice or work in collaboration with a gastroenterologist to provide the service, it is critical to have a thorough understanding of the technique, the indications and contraindications for its use, and potential complications. Such knowledge will allow surgeons to better use the procedure to the maximum benefit of their patients.

Financial Disclosures: None Reported

References

1. Berci G, Forde KA. History of endoscopy: what lessons have we learned from the past? Surg Endosc 2000;14:5–15.
2. Winawer S, Fletcher R, Rex D, et al. Colorectal cancer screening and surveillance: clinical guidelines and rationale—update based on new evidence. Gastroenterology 2003;124:544–60.
3. Winawer SJ, Zauber AG, Ho MN, et al. Prevention of colorectal cancer by colonoscopic polypectomy. The National Polyp Study Workgroup. N Engl J Med 1993;329:1977–81.
4. Hara AK, Johnson CD, Reed JE, et al. Detection of colorectal polyps with CT colography: initial assessment of sensitivity and specificity. Radiology 1997;205:59–65.
5. Wexner SD, Beck DE, Baron TH, et al. A consensus document on bowel preparation before colonscopy: prepared by a task force from the American Society of Colon and Rectal Surgeons (ASCRS), the American Society for Gastrointestinal Endoscopy (ASGE), and the Society of American Gastrointestinal and Endoscopic Surgeons (SAGES). Surg Endosc 2006;20:1147-60.
6. Eisen GM, Baron TH, Dominitz JA, et al. Guideline on the management of anticoagulation and antiplatelet therapy for endoscopic procedures. Gastrointest Endosc 2002;55:775–9.
7. Kwok A, Faigel DO. Management of anticoagulation before and after gastrointestinal endoscopy. Am J Gastroenterol 2009;104:3055–97.
8. Zuckerman MJ, Hirota WK, Adler DG, et al. ASGE guideline: the management of low-molecular-weight heparin and nonaspirin antiplatelet agents for endoscopic procedures. Gastrointest Endosc 2005;61:189–94.
9. Hirota WK, Petersen K, Baron TH, et al. Guidelines for antibiotic prophylaxis for GI endoscopy. Gastrointest Endosc 2003;58:475–82.
10. Barclay RL, Vicari JJ, Doughty AS, et al. Colonoscopic withdrawal times and adenoma detection during screening colonoscopy. N Engl J Med 2006;355:2533–41.
11. Gilbert DA, DiMarino AJ, Jensen DM, et al. Status evaluation: hot biopsy forceps. American Society for Gastrointestinal Endoscopy. Technology Assessment Committee. Gastrointest Endosc 1992;38:753–6.
12. Tappero G, Gaia E, De Guilli P, et al. Cold snare excision of small colorectal polyps. Gastrointest Endosc 1992;38:310–3.
13. Mönkemüller KE, Fry LC, Jones BH, et al. Histological quality of polyps resected using the cold versus hot biopsy technique. Endoscopy 2004;36:432–6.
14. Tada M, Shimada M, Murakami F, et al. [Development of strip off biopsy.] Gastroenterology Endoscopy 1984;26:533–39. Japanese.
15. Conio M, Repici A, Demarquay JF, et al. EMR of large sessile colorectal polyps. Gastrointest Endosc 2004;60:234–41.
16. Heldwein W, Dollhopf M, Rosch T, et al. The Munich Polypectomy Study (MUPS): prospective analysis of complications and risk factors in 4000 colonic snare polypectomies. Endoscopy 2005;37:1116–22.
17. Haggitt RC, Glotzbach RE, Soffer EE, et al. Prognostic factors in colorectal carcinomas arising in adenomas: implications for lesions removed by endoscopic polypectomy. Gastroenterology 1985;89:328–36.
18. Franklin ME Jr, Díaz JA, Abrego D, et al. Laparoscopic-assisted colonoscopic polypectomy: the Texas Endosurgery Institute experience. Dis Colon Rectum 2000;43:1246–9.
19. Elta GH. Urgent colonoscopy for acute lower-GI bleeding. Gastrointest Endosc 2004;59:402–8.
20. Spinelli P, Dal Fante M, Mancini A, et al. Self-expanding mesh stent for endoscopic palliation of rectal obstructing tumors: a preliminary report. Surg Endosc 1992;6:72–4.
21. Dauphine CE, Tan P, Beart RW Jr, et al. Placement of self-expanding metal stents for acute malignant large-bowel obstruction: a collective review. Ann Surg Oncol 2002;9:574–9.
22. Araujo SE, Costa AF. Efficacy and safety of endoscopic balloon dilation of benign anastomotic strictures after oncologic anterior rectal resection: report on 24 cases. Surg Laparosc Endosc Percutan Tech 2008;18:565–8.
23. Newcomb PA, Storer BE, Morimoto LM, et al. Long-term efficacy of sigmoidoscopy in the reduction of colorectal cancer incidence. J Natl Cancer Inst 2003;95:622–5.
24. Imperiale TF, Wagner DR, Lin CY, et al. Risk of advanced proximal neoplasms in asymptomatic adults according to the distal colorectal findings. N Engl J Med 2000;343:169–74.
25. Schwartz DA, White CM, Wise PE, et al. Use of endoscopic ultrasound to guide combination medical and surgical therapy for patients with Crohn's perianal fistulas. Inflamm Bowel Dis 2005;11:727–32.
26. Spradlin NM, Wise PE, Herline AJ, et al. A randomized prospective trial of endoscopic ultrasound to guide combination medical and surgical treatment for Crohn's perianal fistulas. Am J Gastroenterol 2008;103:2527–35.
27. Whiteford MH, Kilkenny J 3rd, Hyman N, et al. Practice parameters for the treatment of perianal abscess and fistula-in-ano (revised). Dis Colon Rectum 2005;48:1337–42.
28. Bhutani MS. Endoscopic ultrasound in the diagnosis, staging and management of colorectal tumors. Gastroenterol Clin North Am 2008;37:215–27.
29. Asfaha S, Alqahtani S, Hilsden RJ, et al. Assessment of endoscopic training of general surgery residents in a North American health region. Gastrointest Endosc 2008;68:1056–62.
30. Vassillou MC, Stroka G, Dunkin BJ, et al. GAGES: a global assessment tool for evaluation of technical performance during gastrointestinal endoscopy. Gastrointest Endosc 2008;67:AB300.
31. Whiteford MH, Swanstrom LL. Emerging technologies including robotics and natural orifice transluminal endoscopic surgery (NOTES) colorectal surgery. J Surg Oncol 2007;96:678–83.
32. Swain P. Endoscopic suturing: now and incoming. Gastrointest Endosc Clin N Am 2007;17:505–20, vi.
33. Franklin ME Jr, Kelley H, Kelley M, et al. Transvaginal extraction of the specimen after total laparoscopic right hemicolectomy with intracorporeal anastomosis. Surg Laparosc Endosc Percutan Tech 2008;18:294–8.
34. Denk PM, Swanström LL, Whiteford MH, et al. Transanal endoscopic microsurgical platform for natural orifice surgery. Gastrointest Endosc 2008;68:954–9.

19 PROCEDURES FOR BENIGN AND MALIGNANT GASTRIC AND DUODENAL DISEASE

Thomas E. Clancy, MD, FACS, and Stanley W. Ashley, MD, FACS

Procedures for Benign Gastric and Duodenal Disease

Advances in the medical management of peptic ulcer disease, including the use of effective acid-suppressing medications (e.g., histamine receptor antagonists and proton pump inhibitors [PPIs]) and the treatment of *Helicobacter pylori*, have led to a dramatic decrease in the need for elective surgical management of uncomplicated duodenal and gastric ulcers. In the past, surgery was the only effective long-term option for peptic ulcer disease, but over the past two decades, it has become an increasingly rare choice.[1] Currently, operative therapy for peptic ulcer disease is largely reserved for the management of complications such as hemorrhage, perforation, and obstruction. The recognition that medical management successfully prevents ulcer recurrence in most patients has caused surgical management of complicated ulcer disease to evolve into a more minimalist strategy that favors damage control surgery for complications and only infrequently resorts to acid-reducing operations.[2]

In this section of the chapter, we focus primarily on procedures performed to treat peptic ulcer disease, although we also briefly address diverticulectomy for duodenal diverticular disease. Other gastroduodenal procedures for nonmalignant disease are described in more detail elsewhere: gastric restrictive procedures and gastric bypass are discussed in the context of bariatric surgery [*see 6:6 Surgical Treatment of Obesity and Metabolic Syndrome*]; choledochoduodenostomy and transduodenal sphincteroplasty are discussed in the context of biliary tract surgery [*see 6:21 Procedures for Benign and Malignant Biliary Tract Disease*]; cystogastrostomy for intractable pancreatic pseudocysts is discussed in the context of pancreatic surgery [*see 6:23 Procedures for Benign and Malignant Pancreatic Disease*]; and duodenal diverticularization is discussed in the context of pancreatic and duodenal trauma [*see 8:9 Duodenal and Pancreatic Trauma*].

PREOPERATIVE EVALUATION

The appropriate extent of preoperative evaluation for a patient undergoing surgery for a benign gastroduodenal disorder is dictated primarily by the nature of the presenting problem. In the case of gastric outlet obstruction or a rare condition such as intractable peptic ulcer disease that is refractory to medical management, the preoperative workup may be extensive and include detailed endoscopy, contrast studies of the upper abdomen, cross-sectional imaging with computed tomography (CT), and full laboratory panels. In most cases of complicated peptic ulcer disease, however, the emergency nature of the situation necessarily renders an extensive preoperative workup impractical. For instance, patients with perforated duodenal ulcers typically present in distress with an acute abdomen. A chest x-ray that demonstrates free intraperitoneal air is all that is needed before the patient is taken to the operating room; the decision to proceed to operation should not be delayed by waiting for further images (e.g., CT scans).

Patients who are experiencing upper gastrointestinal (GI) hemorrhage secondary to peptic ulcer disease should undergo endoscopy to identify the source of bleeding [*see 6:5 Gastrointestinal Bleeding*]. In many cases, endoscopic management of bleeding ulcers is possible, rendering surgical management unnecessary. Definitive surgical management is indicated, however, if bleeding leads to hemodynamic instability, an extensive transfusion requirement (i.e., more than 6 units), or rebleeding after initial endoscopic management. Objective criteria for surgery must be determined on a patient-by-patient basis. Precise preoperative localization of the bleeding source is essential; a bleeding posterior duodenal ulcer, for example, cannot be managed in the same way as hemorrhage from diffuse severe gastritis. Endoscopy should therefore be performed whenever possible. Alternatively, if brisk bleeding prevents clear intraluminal visualization of a bleeding site, angiographic localization may be attempted.

Occasionally, patients present for surgery with refractory gastric ulcers. If the ulcer has not healed after 12 weeks of optimal medical therapy, resection is indicated to rule out an occult gastric malignancy. In such cases, the preoperative workup should include endoscopic biopsies of the ulcer base and the surrounding gastric mucosa so that a preoperative diagnosis of malignancy can be made if possible. In view of the concern about a possible gastric malignancy, it is reasonable to obtain a preoperative chest x-ray and a CT scan of the abdomen so as to detect possible nodal or distant metastases.

OPERATIVE PLANNING

Patients undergoing gastroduodenal procedures should receive general anesthesia and have a nasogastric tube and Foley catheter in place. The supine position is preferred. The operation is usually done via an upper midline incision or, occasionally, via a bilateral subcostal incision, with fixed retractors used in either case.

The choice of procedure is primarily dictated by the indication for operation. Usually, several options are available. The first priority is to manage complications (e.g., bleeding and perforation); whether an accompanying acid-suppressing procedure is indicated and which one should be done depend on the clinical setting. Most commonly, duodenal perforation is treated with closure and omental patching, with or without an acid-reducing procedure. A bleeding ulcer is treated with oversewing of the bleeding vessel, with or without an acid-reducing vagotomy and pyloroplasty. Gastric outlet obstruction may be managed with several different approaches, including vagotomy with antrectomy and vagotomy with drainage via pyloroplasty or gastroenterostomy. In the rare cases of intractability, highly selective vagotomy (HSV) is the procedure of choice.

An important component of preoperative evaluation is determination of the severity and duration of disease. If symptoms are long-standing or recurrent—particularly when the patient has already received acid-reducing or anti–*H. pylori* therapy—a definitive acid-reducing procedure should be considered. As has been demonstrated,[3] however, ulcer recurrence is significantly reduced even without an acid-reducing procedure when perforated ulcers are managed with anti–*H. pylori* agents in conjunction with a PPI. Therefore, a compliant patient who is presumed to be infected with *H. pylori* may not need to undergo an additional acid-reducing procedure. The evidence for this strategy is less clear with respect to bleeding or obstructing ulcers.

OMENTAL PATCH FOR DUODENAL PERFORATION (GRAHAM PATCH)

Operative Technique

Perforated duodenal ulcers are typically treated by oversewing the perforation and then placing a portion of the greater omentum over the suture line. The duodenal ulcer wall is carefully débrided and closed with three or four interrupted silk sutures; the tails of the sutures may be used to hold the omentum in place. Alternatively, if the ulcer edges are edematous and not expected to close easily, the perforation may be closed with a true Graham patch, which involves plugging the defect with a well-vascularized omental pedicle [*see Figure 1*]. Care should be taken to avoid tying sutures too tightly; this can lead to devascularization of the omental pedicle. Once the operation has been completed, the abdomen is generously irrigated to remove any contamination, and a search is made for occult collections in the subphrenic space and the pelvis.

Troubleshooting

To avoid placing excessive tension on the repair, primary closure should not be attempted if the duodenal wall is overly edematous and thickened. For large perforations that are expected to result in gastric outlet obstruction if closed, consideration should be given to incorporating the closure into a pyloroplasty.

There is some controversy regarding whether an acid-reducing operation should be added to the omental patch procedure. If the patient is stable and has a history of peptic ulcer disease, a definitive ulcer operation is included; HSV may be preferable to truncal vagotomy and pyloroplasty in that it is less likely to give rise to dumping syndrome and postvagotomy diarrhea. If the patient has no history of peptic ulcer disease, has a severe medical illness, is hemodynamically unstable, has a long-standing perforation, or exhibits gross abdominal contamination, a definitive ulcer operation is omitted. In cases

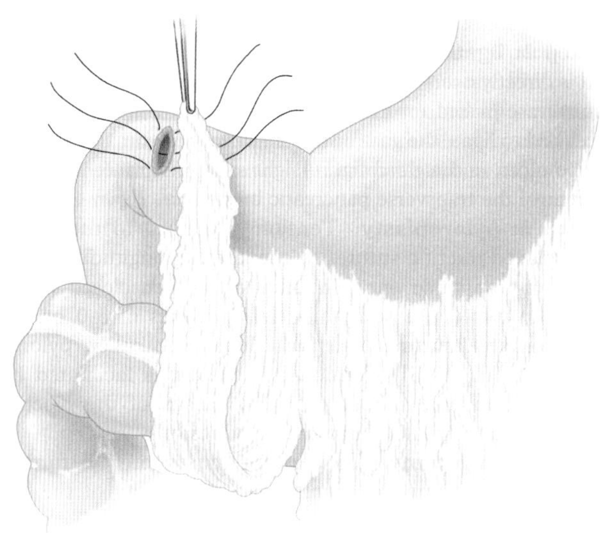

Figure 1 **Omental (Graham) patch. Three or four interrupted sutures are placed along the ulcer edge. If possible, the ulcer is closed primarily and reinforced with omentum. Primary closure may be difficult; in a true Graham patch, primary closure is not attempted, and omentum is used to cover the tissue defect.**

of gross contamination of the abdomen, it is probably inappropriate to divide the peritoneum over the esophagus during vagotomy and thereby expose the mediastinum to infection.

Complications

Persistent leakage should be uncommon after adequate closure. Duodenal scarring at the area of perforation and repair may lead to gastric outlet obstruction. Incomplete exploration and irrigation of the abdomen may result in late infection.

Outcome Evaluation

With adequate acid suppression and anti–*H. pylori* therapy, symptoms of duodenal ulcer are unlikely to recur. The 1-year recurrence rate after omental patching is substantially lower when both therapies are employed than when only a PPI is given (5% versus 38%).[3]

VAGOTOMY AND PYLOROPLASTY FOR BLEEDING DUODENAL ULCER

Truncal vagotomy with pyloric drainage via pyloroplasty is rarely employed as primary therapy for peptic ulcer disease, but it does play a role in emergency management of bleeding duodenal ulcers. This approach to acid suppression fits well with the proximal duodenotomy used to control the hemorrhage. Exposure of the first portion of the duodenum via a longitudinal incision in the pylorus is combined with truncal vagotomy; the pylorus is then closed in a transverse fashion to prevent the development of gastric outlet obstruction.

Operative Technique

Step 1: exposure and pyloric division A Kocher maneuver is performed. The pylorus is identified through palpation and through identification of the pyloric vein as it courses anteriorly. Two traction sutures are placed in the anterior aspect of the pylorus, one superiorly and one inferiorly.

The procedures generally involve either suture closure of the perforation followed by omentopexy or omentopexy alone and should be attempted only by surgeons with advanced laparoscopic skills. The threshold for conversion to an open procedure should be low if the ulcers are particularly large ulcers or prove difficult to localize.

DUODENAL DIVERTICULECTOMY

Incidental duodenal diverticula are common. Such diverticula consist of a sac that includes only mucosa and submucosa, and most occur within 2 cm of the ampulla of Vater. Complications include ulceration and bleeding, compression of the CBD with cholangitis or pancreatitis, and, in cases of perforation, abscess formation with peritonitis. CT scanning is useful for differentiating this condition from cholecystitis or pancreatitis. Surgery is rarely required; it is indicated primarily for complications such as bleeding, perforation, and biliary or duodenal obstruction.

Operative Technique

The main surgical options are simple diverticulectomy with drainage and transduodenal diverticulectomy (as described by Iida[11]). If the duodenum is free of inflammation, the transduodenal approach is preferred because it minimizes the need for dissection of the diverticulum from the surrounding pancreas. However, if the diverticulum does not involve the pancreas, simple excision flush with the duodenal wall, followed by closure in two layers, may be sufficient. The ensuing technical description focuses on transduodenal diverticulectomy.

Step 1: exposure and duodenotomy A generous Kocher maneuver is performed to elevate the head of the duodenum. The duodenum is then opened by making a 4 cm longitudinal incision along the antimesenteric border, and the ampulla is either visualized or palpated. To identify the ampulla, it may be necessary to place a catheter into the CBD via a separate choledochotomy.

Step 2: diverticulectomy The orifice of the diverticulum is identified, and the mucosa is inverted into the lumen of the duodenum. The neck of the diverticulum is transected 2 mm from the junction with the duodenal wall. The diverticular opening is then closed with interrupted seromuscular Lembert sutures of 3-0 silk and interrupted mucosal sutures of 4-0 polyglactin. The duodenum is closed in two layers, also with an inner layer of 4-0 polyglactin and an outer layer of seromuscular Lembert sutures of 3-0 silk. Closed-suction drainage adjacent to the duodenum is indicated.

Special case: perforated duodenal diverticulum In the setting of acute inflammation, duodenotomy is avoided. Instead, the abscess is evacuated, and the diverticulum is excised along with just enough of the adjacent duodenal wall to ensure that only healthy tissue is left. If the resulting duodenal defect is large, either sleeve resection of the duodenum or drainage of the open duodenal defect into a Roux-en-Y jejunal limb may be required.

Troubleshooting

Inadvertent closure of the CBD may be prevented by inserting a catheter into the duct. If the duodenum is markedly inflamed, suture line breakdown is likely, eventually leading to a duodenal fistula. The area can be isolated by means of pyloric exclusion or antrectomy with Billroth II reconstruction. In addition, bile flow can be diverted by performing a choledochojejunostomy to a Roux-en-Y intestinal limb to prevent combined leakage of pancreatic fluid and bile.

Diverticula arising from the third or the fourth portion of the duodenum may be approached via the transverse mesocolon and may be excised either primarily or via a transduodenal approach. Inverting the diverticulum without excising it is not recommended, because it may lead to duodenal obstruction.

Procedures for Gastric Cancer

Surgical resection remains the primary therapeutic modality for gastric cancer [*see 6:7 Tumors of the Stomach, Duodenum, and Small Bowel*]. The diagnosis of gastric cancer is primarily made by means of endoscopy with biopsy. Numerous considerations must be addressed before operation, including the stage of the cancer on diagnostic imaging, the use of staging laparoscopy, the extent of the planned gastrectomy, the extent of the planned lymphadenectomy, the placement of feeding enterostomies, and the patient's overall medical fitness for surgery.

PREOPERATIVE EVALUATION

Endoscopy, with or without endoscopic ultrasonography (EUS), is essential for diagnosis. Preoperative biopsy is helpful for confirming the suspected pathologic process, particularly because the extent of resection will be different if a less common lesion, such as a gastrointestinal stromal tumor (GIST), is identified. Endoscopic localization is critical because the extent of the gastrectomy will depend on the precise location of the tumor. It should be noted, however, that the true location of the tumor, as determined at laparotomy, may differ significantly from the preoperative estimate made on the basis of endoscopy. Abdominal CT and chest radiography are indicated to rule out obvious metastatic disease, which would be an indication for a more conservative surgical approach or even for nonoperative therapy. The preoperative physical examination should also focus on the detection of occult metastatic disease, concentrating on such sites as the supraclavicular lymph nodes and the pouch of Douglas. A bone scan is indicated if metastasis to bone is suspected. Laparoscopic staging (see below) may be performed to identify occult metastatic disease (and, possibly, to prevent an unnecessary laparotomy in an otherwise ill patient).[12] If the tumor is not bleeding or causing an obstruction, palliative resection might be avoided. Generally, curative surgery should be attempted only when the tumor is believed to be limited to the stomach and the perigastric lymph nodes. On occasion, however, curative intent surgery may be considered for tumors that involve nearby resectable structures (e.g., the transverse colon), provided that these structures can be removed en bloc with the primary lesion.

In Japan, where gastric cancer is among the leading causes of cancer-related death, screening endoscopy is widespread and early gastric cancer is identified with some frequency. In Western countries, however, screening endoscopy has not been implemented because of the lower incidence of gastric cancer and hence the lower utility of screening. It is therefore not uncommon for patients to present with more advanced cancers. Accordingly, although procedures such as wedge resection for early gastric cancer have been described, most gastric cancer patients in the United States require formal gastrectomy and lymphadenectomy.

OPERATIVE PLANNING

Extent of Resection

The extent of the resection required for treatment of a gastric malignancy is determined primarily by the preoperative pathologic diagnosis and the site of the tumor. Considerably smaller surgical margins are required for rare mesenchymal tumors (e.g., GISTs) than are necessary for gastric adenocarcinomas, which tend to spread microscopically well beyond the gross extent of the tumor. Most mesenchymal tumors can be adequately treated with a wedge resection or partial gastrectomy that achieves a 1 cm gross margin. Laparoscopic approaches to such tumors have been described that employ either the endoscopic GIA stapler or excision with suture closure [*see* Laparoscopic Resection of Malignant Gastric Tumors, *below*]. Such approaches may be facilitated by endoscopic tattooing of an appropriate margin or by intraoperative endoscopic guidance. For adenocarcinomas, a margin of at least 5 cm is recommended.

A 5 cm margin may be particularly difficult to achieve when the tumor is located along the lesser curvature. In many such cases, although the tumor appears to be distal and possibly amenable to a subtotal gastrectomy, a 5 cm negative margin along the lesser curvature would place the proximal resection margin far above the incisura angularis and near the esophagogastric junction, thus necessitating total or near-total gastrectomy. For lesser-curvature tumors whose location allows adequate margins to be obtained, distal gastrectomy with Billroth II gastrojejunostomy is preferred; for more proximal tumors, total gastrectomy with esophagojejunostomy may be required.

Special consideration must be given to tumors of the esophagogastric junction. In the classification scheme described by Siewert and Stein,[13] such tumors are defined as lying within 5 cm of the anatomic esophagogastric junction in either direction along the craniocaudal axis of the esophagus and the stomach. They are classified into three types as follows:

1. Type I: the center of the tumor lies 1 to 5 cm proximal to the esophagogastric junction
2. Type II: the center of the tumor lies within 1 cm of the esophagogastric junction proximally or within 2 cm distally
3. Type III: the center of the tumor lies 2 to 5 cm distal to the esophagogastric junction

It is generally agreed that total esophagectomy is required for type I esophagogastric junction tumors [*see 5:7 Open Esophageal Procedures*]. The necessary extent of resection for type II and III esophagogastric junction tumors has been more controversial. A microscopically negative (R0) surgical margin is closely associated with survival after resection of esophagogastric junction adenocarcinomas, although R0 resection can be quite difficult to achieve, given the propensity of these tumors for intramural spreading. In our experience, positive margins have not been found in patients with T1 or T2 tumors, even when the margins are smaller than 4 cm. In patients with T3 or T4 tumors, however, proximal margins of at least 6 cm have proved necessary. For T1 and T2 tumors, total gastrectomy without thoracotomy may yield adequate margins. For T3 and T4 tumors, however, extended gastrectomy with thoracotomy or esophagectomy may be required.[14] It is well documented that the margin lengths measured on prefixed esophageal specimens are only about 50% of the corresponding lengths measured in situ before completion of resection.[15] Accordingly, intraoperative decisions about the extent of resection should be based on margin length requirements that may be considerably greater than those derived from resection specimens.

Extent of Lymphadenectomy

The extent of lymphadenectomy with gastrectomy, in terms of not only the gross number of lymph nodes examined but also the particular nodal basins sampled, has been the subject of considerable debate. Regional nodes are classified as N1 (perigastric), N2 (along the splenic and left gastric arteries and at the celiac axis), N3 (along the hepatoduodenal ligament and the root of mesentery), and N4 (para-aortic and middle colic nodes). Alternatively N2 nodes have been variously reported as groups N2–N4 above, including splenic, left gastric, celiac, hepatoduodenal, mesenteric, and para-aortic nodes. Since the 1960s, Japanese surgeons have advocated extended dissection of lymph nodes to improve outcomes in gastric cancer.[16] Whereas a D0 resection represents incomplete dissection of the N1 nodes, D1 resection involves complete resection of the N1 nodes, and D2 involves complete resection of both N1 and N2 nodes. Western and European authors, however, have not demonstrated the benefit of extended lymphadenectomy in gastric cancer.[17] Outside Japan, surgeons have therefore typically limited lymphadenectomy to the perigastric (D1) lymph nodes. Surgeons in Japan, however, have tended to prefer a much more radical lymph node dissection that includes the second-order (D2) nodes [*see Figure 10*]. It has not been clear whether more extensive lymph node dissection actually provides a survival benefit or simply improves surgical staging. To date, four randomized, controlled trials have failed to show any significant benefit from extended lymph node dissection. In the largest such study, performed by the Dutch Gastric Cancer Group, more than 700 patients were randomly assigned to undergo either D1 or D2 lymphadenectomy.[18] The 5-year survival rate was essentially the same in the two groups; perioperative morbidity and mortality were significantly higher after D2 lymphadenectomy.

A subsequent study from the same group found that at 10 years after operation, D2 lymphadenectomy provided a benefit (in terms of lower local recurrence) only in the subgroup with positive second-order nodes; however, these patients could not be identified preoperatively.[19] For the cohort as a whole, extended lymph node dissection generated no long-term survival benefit. Therefore, although some surgeons extend the lymphadenectomy to include lymph nodes along the left gastric, celiac, and common hepatic arteries (a so-called D1+ dissection), the standard of care for surgeons in the United States continues to be a D1 lymphadenectomy that includes all perigastric lymph nodes and the greater omentum.

Furthermore, the minimum number of lymph nodes for gastric cancer staging has been evaluated. It has been suggested

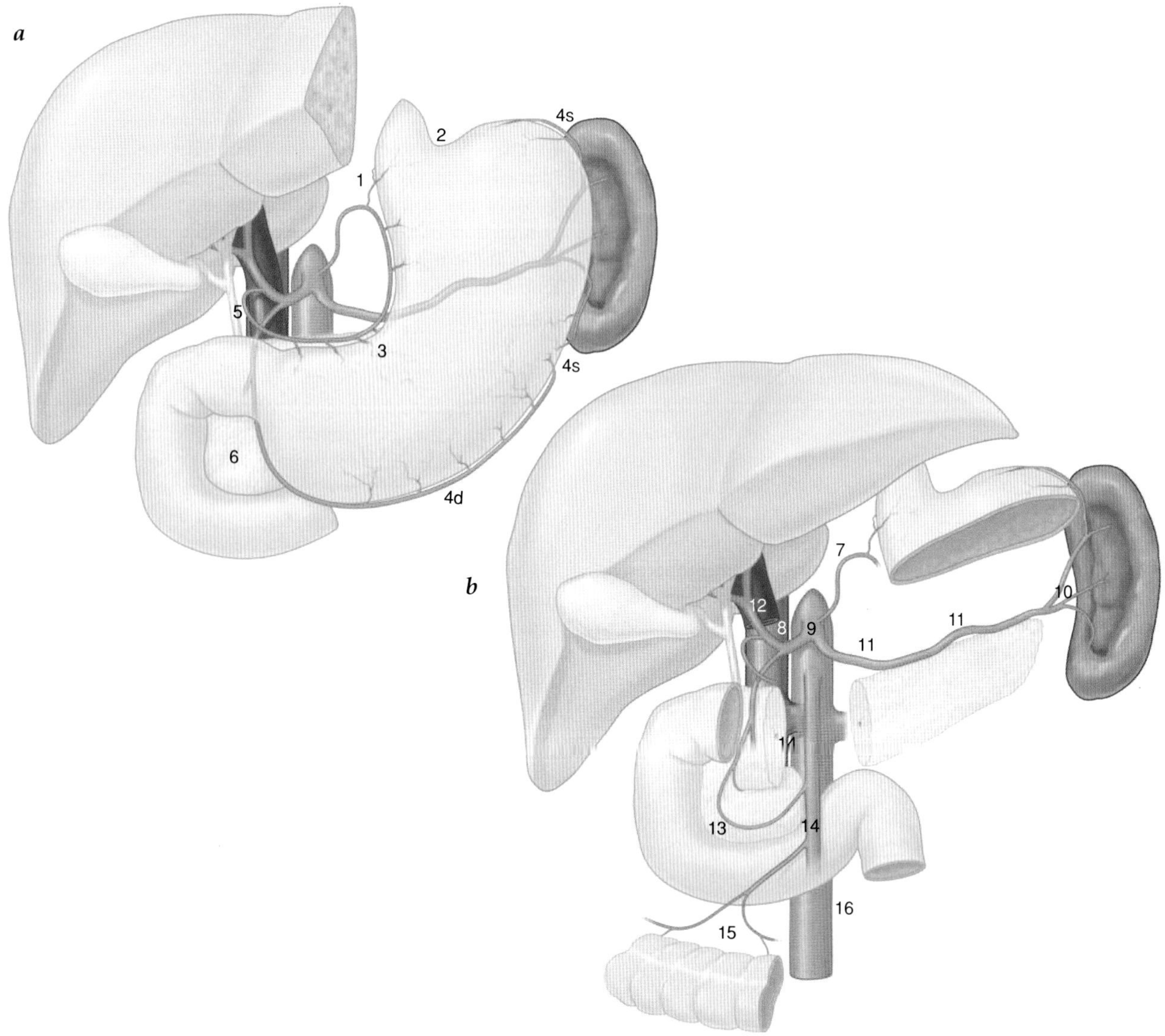

Figure 10 **Illustrated are the differences between a D1 lymphadenectomy and a D2 lymphadenectomy for gastric cancer. (*a*) A D1 lymphadenectomy is accomplished by removing the perigastric lymph nodes with the resection specimen; these nodes include those along the right and left cardia (1, 2), those along the lesser curvature (3), those along the greater curvature (4), the suprapyloric nodes (5), and the infrapyloric nodes (6). (*b*) A D2 lymphadenectomy involves a more radical resection specimen, which includes nodes along the left gastric artery (7), the common hepatic artery (8), the celiac artery (9), the splenic hilum (10), the splenic artery (11), the hepatoduodenal ligament (12), the posterior pancreas (13), the root of the mesentery (14), the transverse mesocolon (15), and the aorta (16).**

that a minimum of 15 lymph nodes must be removed during gastrectomy. In a study published in 2000, 5-year survival rates were significantly lower in patients with fewer than 15 lymph nodes sampled than in those with 15 or more lymph nodes examined.[20] This decreased survival with fewer sampled lymph nodes was attributed primarily to understaging as the result of inadequate lymphadenectomy.

TOTAL GASTRECTOMY

Operative Technique

Step 1: incision and exposure The abdomen is entered via a midline or bilateral subcostal incision. If a subcostal incision is used, it may have to be extended past the xiphoid process in the midline for optimal exposure. Thorough exposure of the peritoneal cavity (including the liver, all peritoneal surfaces, and, in women, the ovaries) is undertaken to search for signs of metastatic disease. If the patient has a proximal lesion near the gastric cardia, a thoracotomy may be needed if the distal thoracic esophagus is to be included in the resection specimen. If an incision into the thoracic cavity is being considered, the left chest should be surgically prepared at the time of initial draping to allow extension of the incision across the lower left costal margin if desired. In this setting, if thoracotomy is possible, preoperative placement of a double-lumen endotracheal tube should be considered. The abdominal portion of a thoracoabdominal incision should be performed first to allow assessment of resectability.

Step 2: dissection of omentum from colon The omentum is separated from the colon with an electrocautery or scissors through the relatively avascular plane. Gentle upward traction is placed on the omentum to facilitate entry into the correct surgical plane [*see Figure 11*]. If the procedure involves a formal D2 lymph node dissection, this is also a convenient time to enter the anterior leaf of the transverse mesocolon, which is resected with the anterior covering of the pancreas. (As noted, most US surgeons perform a D1 resection or some modification thereof and thus do not dissect the anterior peritoneal surface of the mesocolon and pancreas.)

With the dissection starting on the right side, the right gastroepiploic artery is identified and ligated where it originates from the gastroduodenal artery. The short gastric vessels are divided as the dissection proceeds along the greater curvature. The lesser omentum is also divided near the liver and is included with the specimen; care should be taken to identify an aberrant left hepatic artery in the lesser omentum (if present). The dissection is continued onto the peritoneal surface of the distal esophagus.

Step 3: division of duodenum The duodenum is divided just distal to the pyloric ring either with a GIA stapler or with a TA stapler applied twice [*see Figure 12*]. The right gastric artery is identified and ligated near its base. Division of the duodenum allows elevation and rotation of the stomach, thereby facilitating access to the left gastric artery and the surrounding node-bearing tissue.

With the stomach gently retracted upward and anteriorly, dissection identifies the celiac axis and the left gastric artery [*see Figure 13*]. The origin of the left gastric artery is ligated and divided, and a suture ligature is placed on the proximal end.

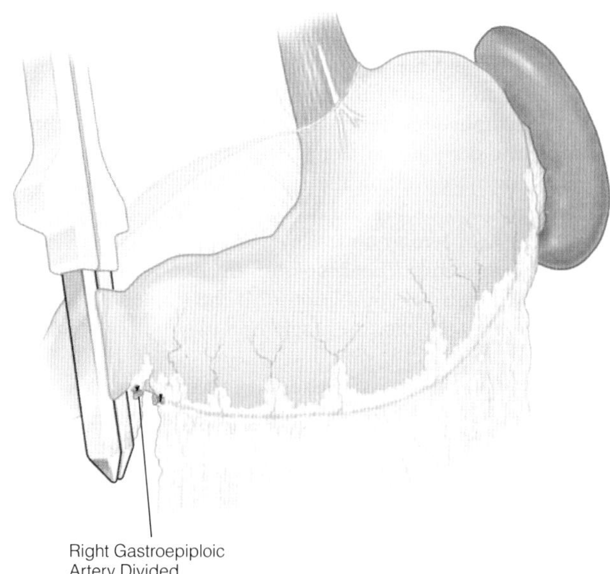

Figure 12 **Total gastrectomy: division of duodenum. The duodenum is divided just beyond the pylorus with a gastrointestinal anastomosis or transverse anastomosis stapler. The duodenal staple line may be reinforced with interrupted Lembert sutures.**

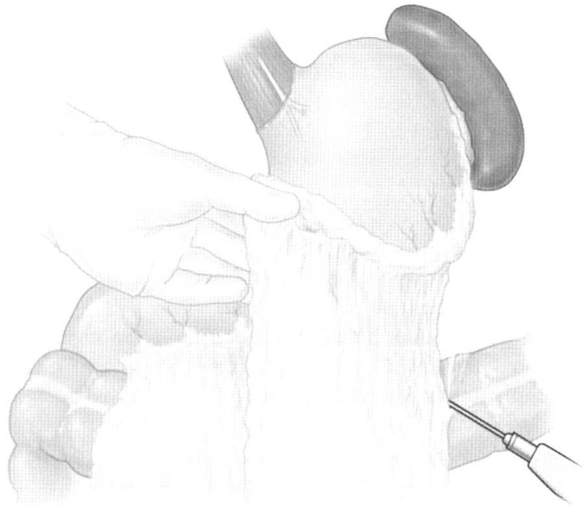

Figure 11 **Total gastrectomy: dissection. The omentum is dissected from the transverse colon with scissors or the electrocautery. In the course of this dissection, the right gastroepiploic artery is encountered near the pylorus and divided near its base at the gastroduodenal artery. The dissection continues along the greater curvature, including ligation of the short gastric vessels. In a formal D2 lymphadenectomy, the anterior leaf of the transverse mesocolon and the anterior capsule of the pancreas are dissected. In a D1 lymphadenectomy, these structures are left intact.**

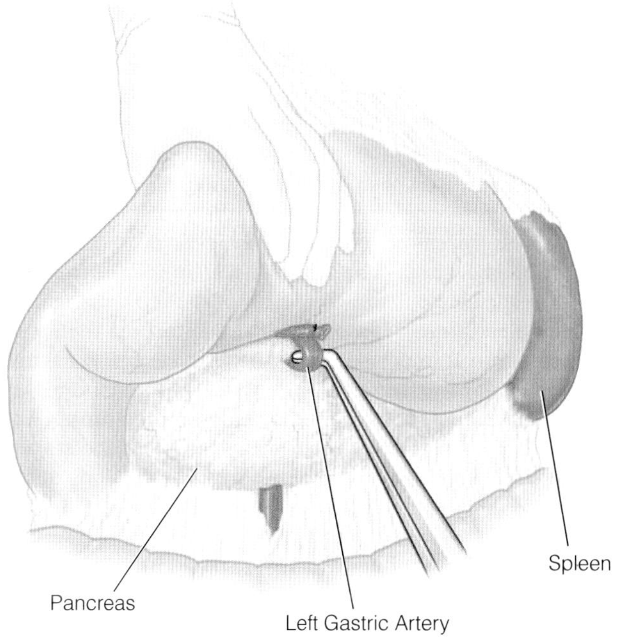

Figure 13 **Total gastrectomy: division of left gastric vessels. The stomach is retracted cephalad to expose the left gastric vessels, which may be divided and suture-ligated on the proximal side. Division of the distal esophagus should be preceded by placement of several stay sutures on the proximal esophagus to prevent it from retracting into the posterior mediastinum.**

A standard D1 lymphadenectomy does not include splenectomy and distal pancreatectomy. The spleen and pancreas are left in situ and are separated from the resection specimen by dividing and ligating the short gastric vessels (see above). The D2 lymphadenectomy as originally described includes stripping the peritoneum along the anterior pancreas, as well as removing nodes along the splenic artery and, if needed, performing splenectomy and distal pancreatectomy to sample the splenic hilar lymph nodes.

Troubleshooting Leakage from the duodenal stump is a potentially disastrous complication. If the stapled duodenum appears to be ischemic, the staple line may be inverted with Lembert sutures of 3-0 silk.

Step 4: inclusion of necessary lymph nodes The degree of dissection to be performed in the porta hepatis depends on the extent of the planned lymphadenectomy. A D1 lymphadenectomy does not require any of the lymph nodes in this area, but a D1+ lymphadenectomy includes lymph nodes along the common hepatic artery. Gentle left lateral traction is placed on the stomach before division of the left gastric artery to apply some tension to the hepatic artery. The dissection proceeds along the celiac and hepatic arteries to the porta hepatis. The tissue surrounding the common hepatic artery and the left gastric artery is swept medially with the specimen. To sample splenic artery nodes, the peritoneum over the anterior border of the pancreas is divided if not previously removed as part of a planned D2 dissection. Nodal tissue along the splenic artery is visualized and sampled.

Step 5: division of esophagus The peritoneum is divided over the anterior esophagus, and the esophagus is completely dissected free of surrounding tissue. The esophagus is then divided either with a TA stapler or with a scalpel after the placement of a noncrushing bowel clamp. To keep the stump from retracting too far proximally, stay sutures of 2-0 silk should be placed in the proximal esophagus before division. Alternatively, the specimen may be left attached and used as a handle to retract the proximal esophagus inferiorly. The esophagus may then be divided after placement of the posterior suture line. Evaluation of the proximal resection margin with frozen-section analysis is advisable.

Troubleshooting The proximal margin may be found to harbor malignancy; if so, reresection of the proximal margin should be performed. Placement of stay sutures in the proximal esophagus is important; if this is not done, the retracting esophagus may migrate into the posterior mediastinum.

Step 6: reconstruction via esophagojejunostomy The options for reconstruction after gastrectomy include stapled end-to-side esophagojejunostomy, hand-sewn end-to-side esophagojejunostomy, side-to-side esophagojejunostomy, and anastomosis to a jejunal pouch. A Roux-en-Y jejunal limb is fashioned; to prevent biliary reflux, it should be at least 40 to 50 cm long. The Roux limb is then brought up behind the colon to the esophagus. Some authors recommend antecolic placement of the Roux limb to prevent obstruction in the setting of recurrent disease; however, retrocolic placement may facilitate a more tension-free anastomosis.

For a stapled end-to-side esophagojejunostomy, a pursestring suture of 3-0 or 2-0 polypropylene is placed in the esophagus and used to secure the anvil of an end-to-end anastomosis stapler. The body of the stapler is placed into the Roux limb, with the tip protruding through the end, and the esophagojejunostomy is created on the antimesenteric border of the jejunum [*see Figure 14a*]. The open end of the Roux limb is then closed with a TA stapler. To reduce tension on the anastomosis, the staple line may be reinforced with interrupted Lembert sutures of 3-0 silk.

A hand-sewn end-to-side esophagojejunostomy is created in a similar fashion at a point near the end of the Roux limb on the antimesenteric border. The posterior row is placed first, with interrupted 3-0 silk sutures as the outer layer and interrupted full-thickness 3-0 absorbable sutures as the inner layer [*see Figure 14b*]. The knots are tied on the inside of the bowel. The anterior row is then placed, with an inner layer of interrupted full-thickness 3-0 absorbable sutures and an outer layer of interrupted 3-0 silk sutures. Some surgeons prefer a single-layer anastomosis, either with a continuous suture or with interrupted full-thickness sutures. The available data do not favor either single- or two-layer anastomosis in this setting.

Side-to-side esophagojejunostomy requires a substantial length of intra-abdominal esophagus and necessitates extensive mobilization of the distal esophagus. The jejunum may be sutured to the underside of the diaphragm to relieve tension on the anastomosis.

Some authors report improved postoperative quality of life with a jejunal pouch reconstruction. Although straight esophagojejunostomy is known to be related to intestinoesophageal reflux, the creation of a gastric reservoir has intrinsic appeal but has not been widely accepted. A recent randomized controlled trial comparing straight Roux-en-Y esophagojejunostomy with a jejunal J-pouch, however, suggested significant benefit to creating a gastric reservoir.[21] Whereas functional results were similar in the first year after surgery, function in years 3 to 5 was significantly improved in patients with a jejunal pouch. For a jejunal pouch, the proximal limb of the Roux-en-Y jejunal limb is folded back on itself for a distance of 10 to 15 cm. The pouch is constructed with an enteric stapling device; esophageal anastomosis may then be constructed via a hand-sewn or stapled technique [*see Figure 14c*].

Drains are not routinely placed after esophagojejunostomy as drain placement may increase the rate of leakage from the esophagojejunostomy.

Troubleshooting Without a sufficient length of intra-abdominal esophagus, primary reconstruction can be difficult. Full mobilization of the intra-abdominal esophagus is essential. Because the esophagus lacks a serosa, transversely oriented Cushing-type sutures may be preferable to Lembert sutures on the anterior and posterior outer layers of a hand-sewn anastomosis.

Step 7 (optional): feeding enterostomy Many patients with gastric adenocarcinoma become significantly malnourished after gastrectomy. The loss of the gastric pouch may adversely affect their ability to fulfill their caloric requirements in the early postoperative period. To prevent further malnutrition, some authors recommend creating a feeding jejunostomy at the time of total gastrectomy with esophagojejunostomy. The jejunostomy should be placed downstream from the jejunojejunostomy (i.e., more than 50 cm distal to

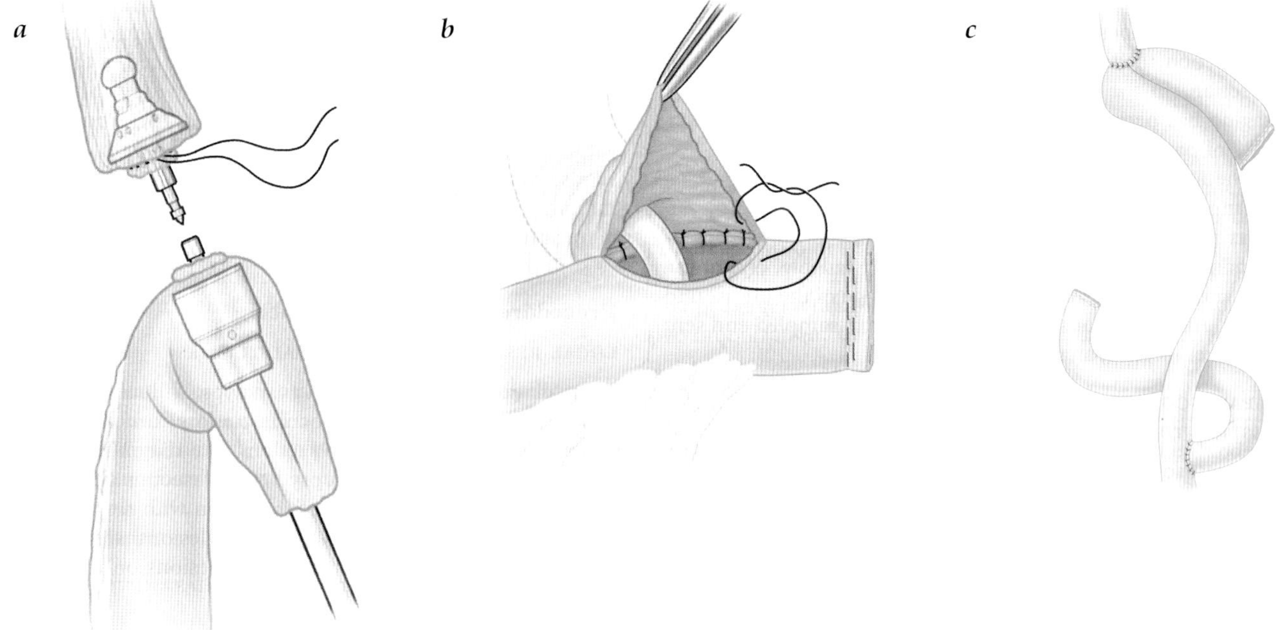

Figure 14 **Total gastrectomy: reconstruction via esophagojejunostomy. Reconstruction via esophagojejunostomy; options include stapled end-to-side esophagojejunostomy, hand-sewn end-to-side esophagojejunostomy, side-to-side esophagojejunostomy, and anastomosis to a jejunal pouch. (*a*) In a stapled esophagojejunostomy, the anvil is secured in the esophagus with a purse-string suture, an end anastomosis stapler is inserted through the distal end of the Roux limb, and the anastomosis is created to the antimesenteric side of the bowel. Once the anastomosis is complete, the end of the Roux limb is amputated with a single firing of a gastrointestinal anastomosis stapler. (*b*) A hand-sewn esophagojejunostomy may be fashioned with interrupted full-thickness sutures (as shown), with a continuous full-thickness suture, or as a two-layer anastomosis. After completion of the posterior row, a sump tube may be placed across the anastomosis into the proximal jejunum. After completion of the anterior row, several reinforcing seromuscular sutures may be placed to reduce tension on the anastomosis. (*c*) Roux-en-Y jejunal pouch. Roux-en-Y reconstruction using a jejunal J pouch is depicted. The antimesenteric sides of two jejunal loops are connected with linear stapling devices for a distance of 10 to 15 cm. The enterotomy is closed with either a hand-sewn or stapled technique. The jejunal pouch may be used for reconstruction via either stapled or hand-sewn esophagojejunostomy.**

the anastomosis). When a feeding enteroenterostomy is indicated, we prefer a Witzel jejunostomy.

Complications

D2 lymphadenectomy has been associated with numerous complications, including increased blood loss, longer operating time, colonic devascularization, pancreatitis, and pancreatic leakage. Although complication rates appear to be acceptably low when the procedure is done by an experienced surgeon, there is still the potential for the benefits of extensive lymphadenectomy to be outweighed by the additional complications. Complications may be reduced by omitting distal pancreatectomy and splenectomy while sampling common hepatic, celiac, and splenic artery nodes (D1+ resection).

Anastomotic leakage at an esophagojejunostomy may lead to postoperative infection. Intra-abdominal leaks may be managed by drainage via percutaneous drains or laparotomy, as well as by proximal nasogastric drainage. High anastomotic leaks may result in contamination of the posterior mediastinum or the pleural space, and thoracotomy or tube thoracostomy may be necessary to achieve external drainage.

Occasionally, bleeding may be substantial enough to necessitate reoperation. In this situation, the gastric remnant may be entered via a transverse incision just proximal to the anastomosis. As a rule, the bleeding can be successfully controlled by placing simple figure-eight sutures.

DISTAL OR SUBTOTAL GASTRECTOMY

Cancers of the distal stomach or antrum may be addressed by means of a distal gastrectomy. Particular attention should be paid to tumors on the lesser curvature, where obtaining an adequate proximal margin may be a problem [*see* Operative Planning, Extent of Resection, *above*]. The dissection proceeds as in a total gastrectomy, but without division of the short gastric vessels. The omentum is separated from the transverse colon with the electrocautery, and the entire omentum is taken with the specimen. A 5 cm proximal margin is ideal. Commonly, the stomach is divided at a point inferior to the short gastric vessels and proximal to the incisura angularis.

Additional operative details and comments on postgastrectomy complications are available elsewhere [*see* Procedures for Benign Gastric and Duodenal Disease, Antrectomy, *above*].

LAPAROSCOPIC STAGING FOR GASTRIC CANCER

The goal of laparoscopic staging before attempted curative resection of gastric carcinoma is to detect occult metastatic disease, the presence of which may affect management. For

the tumor. If pancreatic invasion is identified, pancreaticoduodenectomy should be considered. The distal bowel is brought through the transverse mesocolon, and a side-to-side duodenojejunostomy is created with an outer layer of 3-0 silk and an inner layer of 3-0 polyglactin. Alternatively, the anastomosis may be performed to the second portion of the duodenum.

Troubleshooting

The blood supply to the third portion of the duodenum arises from numerous branches of the inferior pancreaticoduodenal arcade, each of which must be meticulously dissected, divided, and ligated to prevent pancreatic trauma. The distal duodenum receives its blood supply from branches of the superior mesenteric artery.

The duodenum should not be simply closed distally and drained via a gastrojejunostomy; if this is done, the proximal duodenum will not be properly decompressed.

Complications

Delayed gastric emptying is common with duodenojejunostomy; it generally responds to prolonged conservative therapy. A delay in the return of bowel function should generally be treated with nasogastric suction; on occasion, a percutaneous gastrostomy is required for proximal decompression. Postoperative pancreatitis may occur secondary to operative trauma; conservative management is usually sufficient.

AMPULLECTOMY

Local periampullary resection is indicated primarily for rare benign lesions, small neuroendocrine tumors of the pancreas, and small adenomatous or villous polyps. The likelihood of occult malignancy in an adenomatous periampullary tumor is significantly higher when the lesion is larger than 2 cm; caution is therefore indicated in attempting local resection of lesions of this size. The recurrence rate is high after local resection of any periampullary adenocarcinoma. The preoperative workup should include endoscopy with biopsy, EUS or transabdominal ultrasonography, CT scanning, and endoscopic retrograde cholangiopancreatography.

Operative Technique

The ampulla of Vater is resected together with the distal CBD and the distal pancreatic duct [*see Figure 17*]. A Kocher maneuver is performed, and a longitudinal duodenotomy is made to expose the ampulla. Identification of the ampulla may be facilitated by placing a Fogarty catheter in the CBD via the cystic duct after a cholecystectomy. If the ampulla is identified during exploration, it may simply be cannulated. Circumferential stay sutures are placed in the mucosa. The CBD is entered at

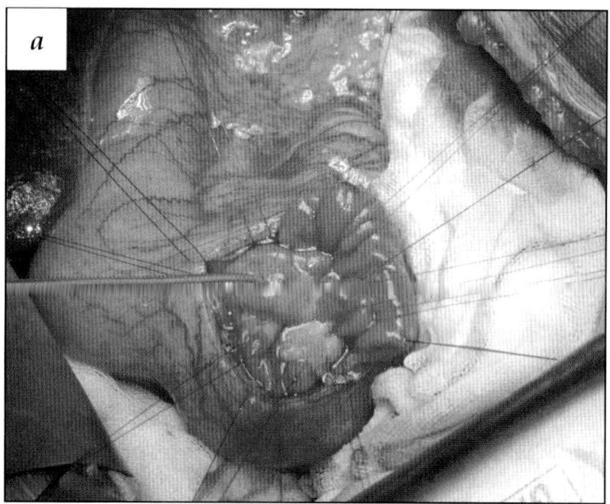

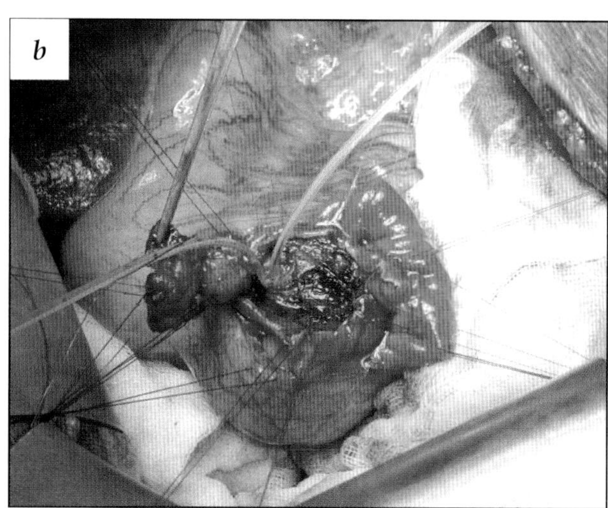

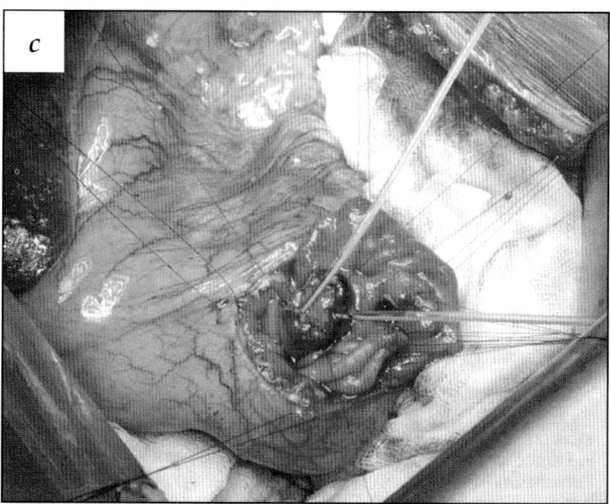

Figure 17 **Ampullectomy. (*a*) After a longitudinal duodenotomy is made, the common bile duct (CBD) is cannulated. Circumferential stay sutures of 4-0 polydioxanone are placed in the duodenal mucosa. A 2 cm periampullary tumor is visualized. (*b*) The ampullary tumor is removed from the underlying duodenum with the electrocautery. The CBD and the pancreatic duct are entered and separately cannulated. The CBD is typically seen at the 11 o'clock position, and the pancreatic duct is typically encountered at the 3 o'clock position. (*c*) The duodenal mucosa is sutured directly to the CBD and the pancreatic duct with 4-0 polydioxanone. In addition, the CBD and pancreatic duct are carefully connected with 4-0 polydioxanone sutures.**

approximately the 11 o'clock position, and duodenal mucosa is reattached to the duct with 4-0 polydioxanone sutures. The pancreatic duct is encountered at approximately the 3 o'clock position; it may be cannulated separately to facilitate identification. The pancreatic duct is approximated to the CBD, and the inferior pancreatic duct is sewn to the duodenal wall. The duodenum is closed transversely in two layers.

Troubleshooting

Frozen-section analysis may identify invasive adenocarcinoma, which is an indication for pancreaticoduodenectomy. This possibility should be carefully considered before the operation.

Financial Disclosures: None Reported

References

1. Schwesinger WH, Page CP, Sirineck KR, et al. Operations for peptic ulcer disease: paradigm lost. J Gastrointest Surg 2001;5:1038.
2. Smith BR, Stablie BE. Emerging trends in peptic ulcer disease and damage control surgery in the *H. pylori* era. Am Surg 2005;71:797.
3. Ng EK, Lam YH, Sung JJ, et al. Eradication of *Helicobacter pylori* prevents recurrence of ulcer after simple closure of duodenal ulcer perforation: randomized controlled trial. Ann Surg 2000;231:153.
4. Tu BN, Sarr MG, Kelly KA. Early clinical results with the uncut Roux reconstruction after gastrectomy; limitations of the stapling technique. Am J Surg 1995;170:262.
5. Eagon JC, Miedema BW, Kelly KA. Postgastrectomy syndromes. Surg Clin North Am 1992;72:445.
6. Amdrup E, Jensen HE. Selective vagotomy of the parietal cell mass preserving innervation of the undrained antrum. Gastroenterology 1970;59:522.
7. Johnston D, Wilkinson AR. Highly selective vagotomy without a drainage procedure in the treatment of duodenal ulcer. Br J Surg 1970;57:289.
8. Adami HO, Enander L-K, Enskog L, et al. Recurrence 1 to 10 years after highly selective vagotomy in prepyloric and duodenal ulcer disease. Ann Surg 1984;199:393.
9. Taylor TV, Bunn AA, MacLeod DAD, et al. Anterior lesser curve seromyotomy and posterior truncal vagotomy in the treatment of chronic duodenal ulcer. Lancet 1982;2:846.
10. Lau H. Laparoscopic repair of perforated peptic ulcer. Surg Endosc 2004;18:1013.
11. Iida F. Transduodenal diverticulectomy for periampullary diverticula. World J Surg 1979;3:103.
12. Burke EC, Karpeh MS, Brennan MF. Laparoscopy in the management of gastric adenocarcinoma. Ann Surg 1997;225:262.
13. Siewert JR, Stein HJ. Classification of adenocarcinoma of the oesophagogastric junction. Br J Surg 1998;85:1457.
14. Ito H, Clancy TE, Osteen RT, et al. Adenocarcinoma of the gastric cardia: what is the optimal surgical approach? J Am Coll Surg 2004;199:880.
15. Siu KF, Cheung HC, Wong J. Shrinkage of the esophagus after resection for carcinoma. Ann Surg 1986;203:173.
16. Jinnai D. Evaluation of extended radical operation for gastric cancer, with regard to lymph node metastasis and follow-up results. Gann Monogr Cancer Res 1968;3:225–31.
17. Roukos DH, Hottenrott C, Lounz M, Koutsogiorgas Couchell S. A critical evaluation of effectivity of extended lymphadenectomy in patients with carcinoma of the stomach. An analysis of early results and long-term survival. J Cancer Res Clin Oncol 1990;116:307–13.
18. Bonekamp JJ, Hermans J, Sasako M, et al; for the Dutch Gastric Cancer Study Group. Extended lymph-node dissection for gastric cancer. N Engl J Med 1999;340:908.
19. Hartgrink HH, van der Velde CJH, Putter H, et al. Extended lymph node dissection for gastric cancer: who may benefit? Final results of the randomized Dutch Gastric Cancer Group trial. J Clin Oncol 2004;22:1.
20. Karpeh MS, Leon L, Klimstra D, et al. Lymph node staging in gastric cancer: is location more important than number? An analysis of 1,038 patients. Ann Surg 2000;232:362.
21. Fein M, Fuchs JH, Thalheimer A, et al. Long-term benefits of Roux-en-Y reconstruction after total gastrectomy. Ann Surg 2008;247:759–65.
22. Kim M-C, Choi H-J, Jung G-J, Kim H-H. Techniques and complications of laparoscopy-assisted distal gastrectomy (LADG) for gastric cancer. Eur J Surg Oncol 2007;33:700–5.

Acknowledgments

Figures 1 through 15 Tom Moore.
Figure 16 Courtesy of Dr. John Windsor and Dr. Yatin Young. Auckland Hospital, Auckland, New Zealand.

20 CHOLECYSTECTOMY AND COMMON BILE DUCT EXPLORATION

Gerald M. Fried, MD, FRCS(C), FACS, Liane S. Feldman, MD, FRCS(C), FACS, and Dennis R. Klassen, MD, FRCS(C), FACS

Cholecystectomy is the treatment of choice for symptomatic gallstones because it removes the organ that contributes to both the formation of gallstones and the complications ensuing from them.[1] The morbidity associated with cholecystectomy is attributable to injury to the abdominal wall in the process of gaining access to the gallbladder (i.e., the incision in the abdominal wall and its closure) or to inadvertent injury to surrounding structures during dissection of the gallbladder. Efforts to diminish the morbidity of open cholecystectomy have led to the development of laparoscopic cholecystectomy, made possible by modern optics and video technology.

Carl Langenbuch performed the first cholecystectomy in Berlin, Germany, in 1882. Erich Mühe performed the first laparoscopic cholecystectomy in Germany in 1985,[2] and by 1992, 90% of cholecystectomies in the United States were being performed laparoscopically. Compared with open cholecystectomy, the laparoscopic approach has dramatically reduced hospital stay, postoperative pain, and convalescent time. However, rapid adoption of laparoscopic cholecystectomy as the so-called gold standard for treatment of symptomatic gallstone disease was associated with complications, including an increased incidence of major bile duct injuries.

Since the early 1990s, considerable advances have been made in instrumentation and equipment, and a great deal of experience with laparoscopic cholecystectomy has been amassed worldwide. Of particular significance is the miniaturization of and improvement in optics and instruments, which have reduced the morbidity of the procedure by making possible ever-smaller incisions. With proper patient selection and preparation, laparoscopic cholecystectomy is being safely performed on an outpatient basis in many centers.[3]

The primary goal of cholecystectomy is removal of the gallbladder with minimal risk of injury to the bile ducts and surrounding structures. Our approach is designed to maximize the safety of both routine and complicated cholecystectomies. In what follows, we describe our approach and discuss current indications and techniques for imaging and exploring the common bile duct (CBD).

Laparoscopic Cholecystectomy

PREOPERATIVE EVALUATION

To plan the surgical procedure, assess the likelihood of conversion to open cholecystectomy, and determine which patients are at high risk for CBD stones, the surgeon must obtain certain data preoperatively. Useful information can be obtained from the patient's history, imaging studies, and laboratory tests.

Preoperative Data

History and physical examination A good medical history provides information about associated medical problems that may affect the patient's tolerance of pneumoperitoneum. Patients with cardiorespiratory disease may have difficulty with the effects of CO_2 pneumoperitoneum on cardiac output, lung inflation pressure, acid-base balance, and the ability of the lungs to eliminate CO_2. Most bleeding disorders can also be identified through the history. A disease-specific history is important in identifying patients in whom previous episodes of acute cholecystitis may make laparoscopic cholecystectomy more difficult, as well as those at increased risk for choledocholithiasis (e.g., those who have had jaundice, pancreatitis, or cholangitis).[4–9]

Physical examination identifies patients whose body habitus is likely to make laparoscopic cholecystectomy difficult and is helpful for determining optimal trocar placement. Abdominal examination also reveals any scars, stomas, or hernias that are likely to necessitate the use of special techniques for trocar insertion.

Imaging studies Ultrasonography is highly operator dependent, but in capable hands, it can provide very useful information. It is the best test for diagnosing cholelithiasis, and it can usually determine the size and number of stones.[4] Large stones indicate that a larger incision in the skin and the fascia will be necessary to retrieve the gallbladder. Multiple small stones suggest that the patient is more likely to require operative cholangiography (if a policy of selective cholangiography is practiced) [*see* Operative Technique, Step 5, *below*]. A shrunken gallbladder, a thickened gallbladder wall, and pericholecystic fluid on ultrasonographic examination are significant predictors of conversion to open cholecystectomy. The presence of a dilated CBD or CBD stones preoperatively is predictive of choledocholithiasis. Other intra-abdominal pathologic conditions, either related to or separate from the hepatic-biliary-pancreatic system, may influence operative planning.

Preoperative imaging studies of the CBD may allow the surgeon to identify patients with CBD stones before surgery. Such imaging may involve endoscopic retrograde cholangiopancreatography (ERCP) [*see 6:17 Upper Gastrointestinal Endoscopy and 6:18 Lower Endoscopy*],[10] magnetic resonance cholangiopancreatography (MRCP) [*see Figure 1*],[11,12] or endoscopic ultrasonography (EUS). These imaging modalities also provide an anatomic map of the extrahepatic biliary tree, identifying unusual anatomy preoperatively and helping the surgeon plan a safe operation. Endoscopic sphincterotomy (ES) is performed during ERCP if stones are identified in the CBD. MRCP has an advantage over ERCP and EUS in that it is noninvasive and does not make use of injected iodinated contrast solutions.[11] Most surgeons would probably recommend that preoperative cholangiography be performed selectively in patients with clinical or biochemical features associated with a high risk of choledocholithiasis. The specific modality used in such a case varies with the technology and expertise available locally.

Laboratory tests Preoperative blood tests should include liver function, renal function, electrolyte, and coagulation studies. Abnormal liver function test results may reflect choledocholithiasis or primary hepatic dysfunction.

a

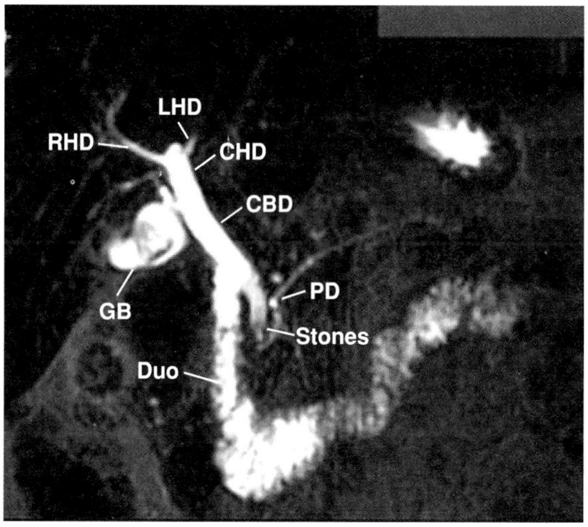

b

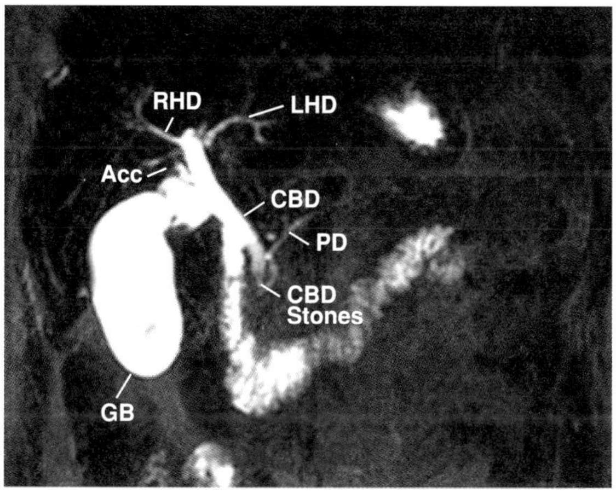

Figure 1 **Laparoscopic cholecystectomy. (*a*) and (*b*) Preoperative magnetic resonance cholangiopancreatography alerts the surgeon to abnormal anatomy and the presence of stones in the distal common bile duct (CBD). Acc = accessory duct entering the common hepatic duct near the neck of the gallbladder; CHD = common hepatic duct; Duo = duodenum; GB = gallbladder, containing stones; LHD = left hepatic duct; PD = pancreatic duct; RHD = right hepatic duct.**

Selection of Patients

Patients eligible for outpatient cholecystectomy Patients in good general health who have a reasonable amount of support from family or friends and who do not live too far away from adequate medical facilities are eligible for outpatient cholecystectomy, especially if they are at low risk for conversion to laparotomy [*see* Special Considerations, Conversion to Laparotomy, *below*].[3] These patients can generally be discharged home from the recovery room 6 to 12 hours after surgery provided that the operation went smoothly, their vital signs are stable, they are able to void, they can manage at least a liquid diet without vomiting, and their pain can be controlled with oral analgesics.

Technically challenging patients Before performing laparoscopic cholecystectomy, the surgeon can often predict which patients are likely to be technically challenging. These include patients who have a particularly unsuitable body habitus, those who are highly likely to have multiple and dense peritoneal adhesions, and those who are likely to have distorted anatomy in the region of the gallbladder.

Morbidly obese patients present specific difficulties [*see* Operative Technique, Step 1, Special Considerations in Obese Patients, *below*].[13] Small, muscular patients have a noncompliant abdominal wall, resulting in a small working space in the abdomen and necessitating high inflation pressures to obtain reasonable exposure.

Patients with a history of multiple abdominal operations, especially in the upper abdomen, and those who have a history of peritonitis are likely to pose difficulties because of peritoneal adhesions.[14] These adhesions make access to the abdomen more risky and exposure of the gallbladder more difficult. Patients who have undergone gastroduodenal surgery, those who have any history of acute cholecystitis, those who have a long history of recurrent gallbladder attacks, and those who have recently had severe pancreatitis are particularly difficult candidates for laparoscopic cholecystectomy. These patients may have dense adhesions in the region of the gallbladder, the anatomy may be distorted, the cystic duct may be foreshortened, and the CBD may be very closely and densely adherent to the gallbladder. Such patients are a challenge to the most experienced laparoscopic surgeon. When such problems are encountered, conversion to open cholecystectomy should be considered early in the operation.[14,15]

Predictors of choledocholithiasis CBD stones may be discovered preoperatively, intraoperatively, or postoperatively. The surgeon's goal is to clear the ducts but to use the smallest number of procedures with the lowest risk of morbidity. Thus, before elective laparoscopic cholecystectomy, it is desirable to classify patients into one of three groups: high risk (those who have clinical jaundice or cholangitis, visible choledocholithiasis, or a dilated CBD on ultrasonography), moderate risk (those who have hyperbilirubinemia, elevated alkaline phosphatase levels, pancreatitis, or multiple small gallstones), and low risk.

In our institution, where MRCP and EUS are available and reliable and where ERCP achieves stone clearance rates higher than 90%, we recommend the following approach: (1) preoperative ERCP and sphincterotomy (if required) for high-risk patients and (2) MRCP, EUS, or intraoperative fluoroscopic cholangiography for moderate-risk patients. Patients at low risk for CBD stones do not routinely undergo cholangiography [*see Figure 2*]. Laparoscopic CBD exploration and postoperative ERCP appear to be equally effective in clearing stones from the CBD.

Ultimately, surgeons and institutions must establish a reasonable approach to choledocholithiasis that takes into account the expertise and equipment locally available.

Contraindications There are few absolute contraindications to laparoscopic cholecystectomy. Certainly, no patient who poses an unacceptable risk for open cholecystectomy should be considered for laparoscopic cholecystectomy, because it is always possible that conversion will become necessary. Of the relative contraindications, surgical inexperience is the most important.

Neither ascites nor hernia is a contraindication to laparoscopic cholecystectomy. Ascites can be drained and the gallbladder visualized. Large hernias may present a problem, however, because with insufflation, the gas preferentially fills the hernia. Patients with large inguinal hernias may require an external support to minimize this problem and the discomfort related to pneumoscrotum. Patients with umbilical hernias can have their hernias repaired while they are undergoing laparoscopic cholecystectomy. For such patients, the initial trocar should be placed by open insertion according to the Hasson technique [*see* Operative Technique, Step 1, *below*], with care taken to avoid injury to the contents of the hernia. The sutures required to close the hernia defect can be placed before insertion of the initial trocar. For patients with small incisional hernias, laparoscopic cholecystectomy can proceed as usual. The hernia may be repaired at the same operation if the cholecystectomy goes smoothly and there is no peritoneal contamination. For large incisional hernias, we would proceed with laparoscopic cholecystectomy, limiting adhesiolysis to that

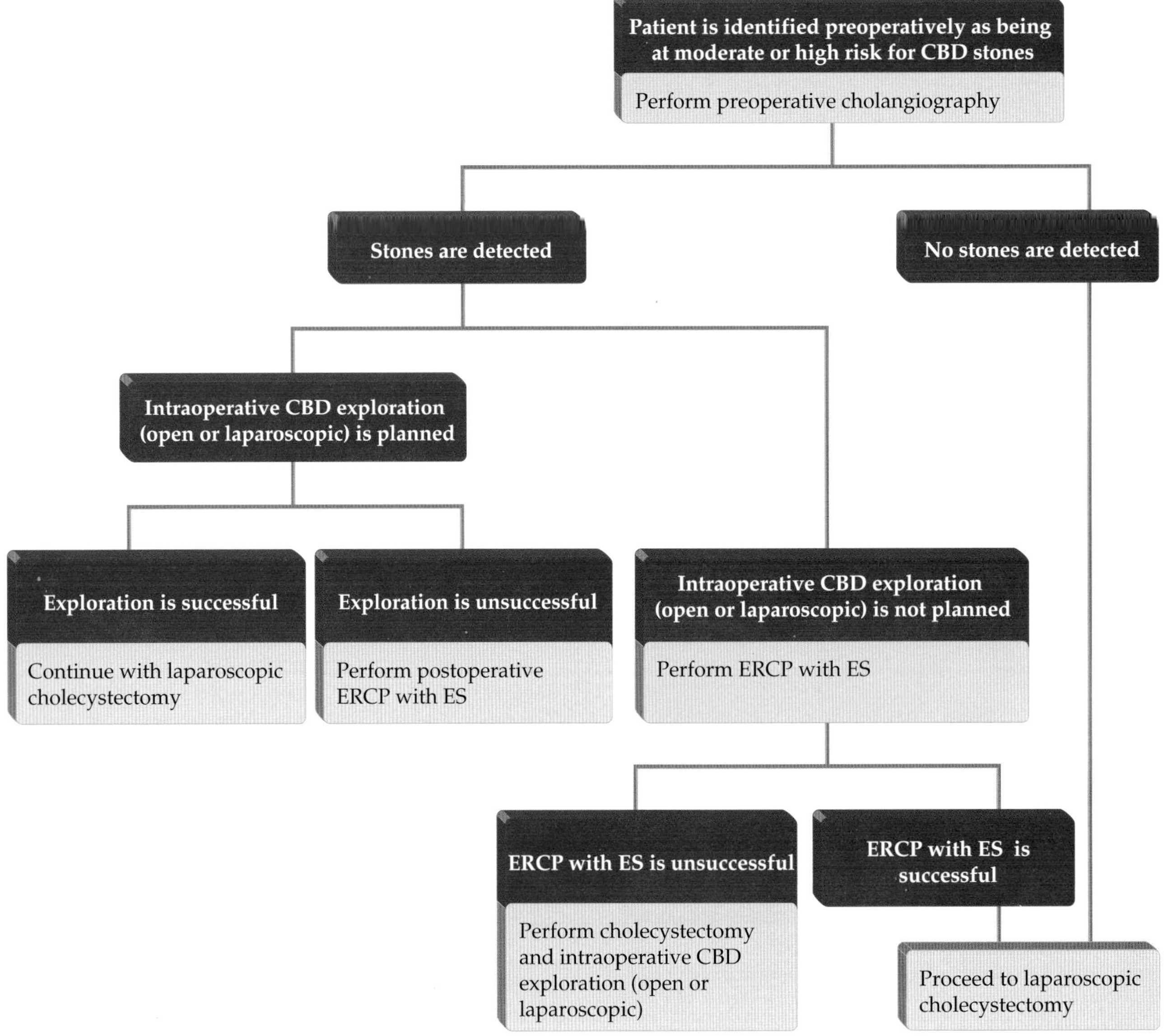

Figure 2 **Laparoscopic cholecystectomy. Shown is an algorithm outlining the use of preoperative cholangiography in patients at moderate or high risk for common bile duct (CBD) stones. ERCP = endoscopic retrograde cholangiopancreatography; ES = endoscopic sphincterotomy.**

required to safely perform the procedure. Patients with stomas may also undergo laparoscopic cholecystectomy provided that the appropriate steps are taken to prevent injury to the bowel during placement of trocars and division of adhesions.

Patients with cirrhosis or portal hypertension are at high risk for morbidity and mortality with open cholecystectomy.[16,17] If absolutely necessary, laparoscopic cholecystectomy may be attempted by an experienced surgeon. The risk of bleeding can be minimized by rigorous preoperative preparation, meticulous dissection with the help of magnification available through the laparoscope, and use of electrocautery and enabling hemostatic devices.

Patients with bleeding diatheses, such as hemophilia, von Willebrand disease, and thrombocytopenia, may undergo laparoscopic cholecystectomy. They require appropriate preoperative and postoperative care and monitoring, and a hematologist should be consulted.

Questions have been raised about whether laparoscopic cholecystectomy should be performed in pregnant patients; it has been argued that the increased intra-abdominal pressure may pose a risk to the fetus. Because of the enlarged uterus, open insertion of the initial trocar is mandatory, and the positioning of other trocars may have to be modified according to the position of the uterus. Inflation pressures should be kept as low as possible, and prophylaxis of deep vein thrombosis (DVT) is recommended. Despite these potential problems, safe performance of laparoscopic cholecystectomy and other laparoscopic procedures in pregnant patients is increasingly being described in the literature. If cholecystectomy is necessary before delivery, the second trimester is the best time for it.[18–21]

Patients in whom preoperative imaging gives rise to a strong suspicion of gallbladder cancer should probably undergo open surgical management.

OPERATIVE PLANNING

Antibiotic Prophylaxis

Some surgeons recommend routine preoperative administration of antibiotics to all patients undergoing cholecystectomy, on the grounds that inadvertent entry into the gallbladder is not uncommon and can lead to spillage of bile or stones into the peritoneal cavity. Other surgeons do not recommend routine prophylaxis. Resolution of this controversy awaits appropriate prospective trials. We recommend selective use of antibiotic prophylaxis for patients at highest risk for bacteria in the bile (including those with acute cholecystitis or CBD stones, those who have previously undergone instrumentation of the biliary tree, and those older than 70 years) and for patients with prosthetic heart valves and joint prostheses.

Prophylaxis of DVT

The reverse Trendelenburg position used during laparoscopic cholecystectomy, coupled with the positive intra-abdominal pressure generated by CO_2 pneumoperitoneum and the vasodilatation induced by general anesthesia, leads to venous pooling in the lower extremities. This consequence may be minimized by using antiembolic stockings or by wrapping the legs with elastic bandages. Subcutaneous heparin and pneumatic compression devices may be employed for patients at increased risk for DVT [*see 7:6 Venous Thromboembolism*]. As yet, however, there is no convincing evidence that the incidence of DVT is higher with laparoscopy than with open surgery.

Patient Positioning

Typically, the patient is positioned supine and the surgeon stands to the patient's left side [*see Figure 3*].

The camera operator usually stands on the patient's left and to the left of the surgeon, while the assistant stands on the patient's right. The video monitor is positioned on the patient's right above the level of the costal margin. If a second monitor is available, it should be positioned on the patient's left to the right of the surgeon, where the assistant can have an unobstructed and comfortable view. Exposure can be improved by tilting the patient in the reverse Trendelenburg position and rotating the table with the patient's right side up. Gravity pulls the duodenum, colon, and omentum away from the gallbladder, thereby increasing the working space available in the upper abdomen.

The operating room (OR) table should allow easy access for a fluoroscopic C arm to facilitate intraoperative cholangiography. The table cover should be radiolucent.

Equipment

The equipment required for laparoscopic cholecystectomy includes an optical system, an electronic insufflator, trocars (cannulas), surgical instruments, and hemostatic devices [*see Table 1*].

Optical system The laparoscope can provide either a straight, end-on (0°) view or an angled (30° or 45°) view. Scopes that provide an end-on view are easier to learn to use,

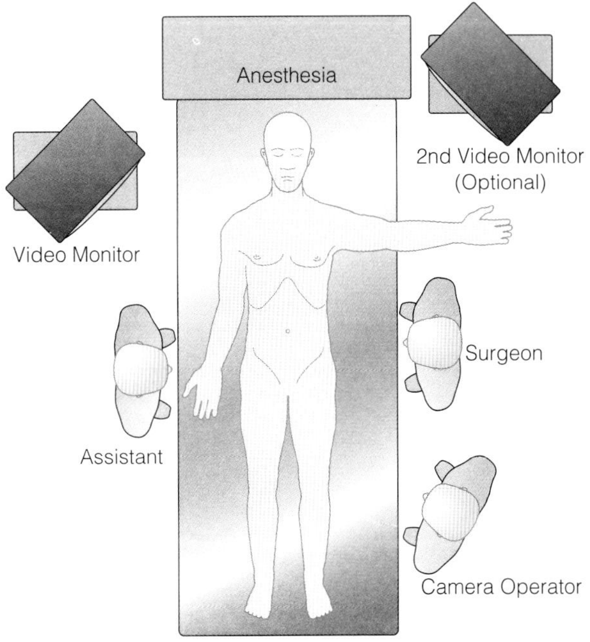

Figure 3 **Laparoscopic cholecystectomy. A patient undergoing laparoscopic cholecystectomy should be positioned so as to allow easy access to the gallbladder and a clear view of the monitors. Shown are the positions of the surgeon, the camera operator, and the assistant in the operating room.**

but angled scopes are more versatile. Scopes with a 30° angle cause less disorientation than those with a 45° angle and are ideal for laparoscopic cholecystectomy. Excellent 30° scopes are currently available in diameters of 10, 5, and 3.5 mm.

Fully digital flat-panel displays are now available that yield better resolution than analog video monitors, take up less space, are less subject to signal interference, and require less power. The introduction of high-definition optics has further improved the quality of the image. The associated 16:9 display increases the width of the field of view.

The resolution and quality of the final image depend on (1) the brightness of the light source; (2) the integrity of the

Table 1 Equipment for Laparoscopic Cholecystectomy

Instrument/Device	Number	Size	Comments
Laparoscopic cart High-intensity halogen light source (150–300 watts) High-flow electronic insufflator (minimum flow rate of 106 L/min) Laparoscopic camera box Videocassette digital video and still image recorder (optional) Digital still image capture system (optional)			
Laparoscope	1	3.5–10 mm	Available in 0° and angled views; we prefer to use a 30° 5 mm diameter laparoscope
Atraumatic grasping forceps	2–4	2–10 mm	Selection of graspers should allow surgeon choice appropriate to thickness and consistency of gallbladder wall; insulation is unnecessary
Large-tooth grasping forceps	1	10 mm	Used to extract gallbladder at end of procedure
Curved dissector	1	2–5 mm	Should have a rotatable shaft; insulation is required
Scissors	[illegible]	[illegible] mm	One curved and one straight scissors with rotating shaft and insulation; additional microscissors may be helpful for incising cystic duct
Clip appliers	1–2	5–10 mm	Either disposable multiple clip applier or 2 manually loaded reusable single clip appliers for small and medium-to-large clips; 5 and 10 mm diameter
Dissecting electrocautery hook or spatula	1	5 mm	Available in various shapes according to surgeon's preference; instrument should have channel for suction and irrigation controlled by trumpet valve(s); insulation required
High-frequency electrical cord	1		Cord should be designed with appropriate connectors for electrosurgical unit and instruments being used
Suction-irrigation probe	1	5–10 mm	Probe should have trumpet valve controls for suction and irrigation; may be used with pump for hydrodissection
10-to-5 mm reducers	2		Allow use of 5 mm instruments in 10 mm trocar without loss of pneumoperitoneum; these are often unncessary with newer disposable trocars and may be built into some reusable trocars
5-to-3 mm reducer	1		Allows use of 2–3 mm instruments and ligating loops in 5 mm trocars
Ligating loops			
Endoscopic needle holders	1–2	5 mm	
Cholangiogram clamp with catheter	1	5 mm	Allow passage of catheter and clamping of catheter in cystic duct
Veress needle	1		Used if initial trocar is inserted by percutaneous technique
Allis or Babcock forceps	1–2	5 mm	Allow atraumatic grasping of bowel or gallbladder
Long spinal needle	1	14 gauge	Useful for aspirating gallbladder percutaneously in cases of acute cholecystitis or hydrops
Retrieval bag	1		Useful for preventing spillage of bile or stones in removal of inflamed or friable gallbladder; facilitates retrieval of spilled stones

fiberoptic cord used to convey the light; (3) clean and secure connections between the light source and the scope; (4) the quality of the laparoscope, the camera, and the monitor; and (5) correct wiring of the components. The distal end of the scope must be kept clean and free of condensation: bile, blood, or fat will reduce brightness and distort the image. Lens fogging can be prevented by immersion in heated water or by antifogging solutions.

Insufflator CO_2 is the preferred insufflating gas for laparoscopic procedures because it is highly soluble in water and does not support combustion when electrocautery is used. The CO_2 should be insufflated with an electronic pump capable of a flow rate of at least 10 L/min; most current systems have a maximum flow rate of 20 L/min or higher. The insufflator is connected to one of the trocars by means of a flexible tube and a stopcock.

Trocars For cholecystectomy, at least one trocar site must be large enough to allow passage of the gallbladder and any stones removed. Most surgeons prefer to use a 10/12 mm trocar at the umbilicus for this purpose. The other trocars can range from 2 to 12 mm, depending on the size of the instruments to be placed through them. The conventional approach is to use a 10/12 mm trocar at the operating port site and 5 mm trocars for the other instruments; however, if a 5 mm laparoscope and a 5 mm clip applier are used, the operating port size can be reduced to 5 mm. Although 2 mm instrumentation is also available, it must be remembered that, as a rule, the smaller the working port, the less versatile the instruments. In our experience, the combination of a 10 mm umbilical trocar, a 5 mm operating port, and 2 mm ports for grasping forceps is a good one: optical quality is maintained, little flexibility is lost with respect to selecting operating instruments, trocar size is minimized, and the cosmetic result is excellent.

Hemostatic devices Hemostasis can be achieved with monopolar or bipolar electrocauterization. A monopolar electrocautery can be connected to most available instruments; however, bipolar electrocauterization may eventually prove safer. With a monopolar electrocautery, depth of burn is less predictable, current can be conducted through noninsulated instruments and trocars, and any area of the instrument that is stripped of insulation may conduct current and result in a burn. Caution is essential when the electrocautery is used near metallic hemostatic clips because delayed sloughing may occur.

Electrocauterization should be avoided near the CBD because delayed bile duct injuries and leaks may occur as a result of sloughing from a burned area and devascularization of the duct. Care must be exercised when cautery is employed near the bowel and when intra-abdominal adhesions are being taken down. The electrocautery can be used with a forceps, scissors, hooks (L or J shaped), a spatula, and other instruments. Some cautery probes incorporate nonstick surfaces to prevent buildup of eschar. The use of hand-activated cautery probes and the presence of a channel that allows suction and irrigation through the cautery probes are especially convenient.

More advanced energy sources and instruments are also available. Bipolar devices designed to weld tissues have proved capable of achieving superb hemostasis. Ultrasonic dissecting shears can also be used to dissect and coagulate tissues effectively and precisely. For laparoscopic cholecystectomy, however, such advanced—and costly—devices are rarely needed.

OPERATIVE TECHNIQUE

Step 1: Placement of Trocars and Accessory Ports

Placement of initial trocar The first step in laparoscopic cholecystectomy is the creation of pneumoperitoneum and the insertion of an initial trocar through which the laparoscope can be passed. This step is critical because complications resulting from improper placement may cause serious morbidity and death. The surgeon may use either a percutaneous technique or an open technique. We prefer the open technique, which eliminates the risks inherent in the blind puncture [*see Figure 4*].[22,23]

Scars Patients who have previously undergone abdominal surgery may have adhesions, both to the undersurface of the abdominal wall and intra-abdominally. Adhesions to the undersurface of the abdominal wall make access to the abdominal cavity potentially hazardous, particularly when the percutaneous method is used for placement of the initial trocar. Scars from previous operations may affect insertion of the initial trocar, depending on its orientation and location. If a patient has a scar in the lower abdomen (e.g., from a Pfannenstiel incision or an incision in the right lower quadrant for an appendectomy), the position of the initial trocar need not be changed. If the scar is in the upper abdomen, the initial trocar may be inserted below the umbilicus in the midline. If there is a long midline scar that is impossible to avoid, careful dissection of the peritoneum through a vertical incision that is somewhat longer than usual affords safe access to the peritoneum in most cases.

An alternative is to insert the initial trocar high in the epigastrium or in the right anterior axillary line, where bowel adhesions are less common. The laparoscope is inserted through this trocar and used to examine the undersurface of the old scar for a clear site near the umbilicus, where a 10 mm trocar can be placed. Previous laparoscopy, which rarely creates significant intra-abdominal adhesions, rarely necessitates modification of trocar insertion.

The surgeon should also consider the reason for the previous surgery. For example, a patient who underwent an appendectomy for perforated appendicitis may have had diffuse peritonitis and may have adhesions well away from the old scar.

Placement of accessory ports In most cases, four ports are necessary. The first port is for the laparoscope; the remaining ports are for grasping forceps, dissectors, and clip appliers. The precise position of the accessory ports depends on the surgeon's preference, the patient's body habitus, and the presence or absence of previous scars or intra-abdominal adhesions [*see Figure 5*]. A rigid approach to port placement is inappropriate: trocar placement determines operative exposure, and improper placement will haunt the surgeon throughout the procedure. In some cases, a fifth trocar is required to elevate a floppy liver or to depress or retract the omentum or a bulky hepatic flexure of the colon [*see Figure 5*].

Most surgeons elect to place one of the grasping forceps on the fundus of the gallbladder through an accessory port placed approximately in the anterior axillary line below the level of the gallbladder. Because the level of the gallbladder varies from patient to patient, the placement of this accessory port should not be decided on until the gallbladder is visualized. If the gallbladder is low lying and the trocar is placed too high, the surgeon will have difficulty achieving the appropriate angle

a

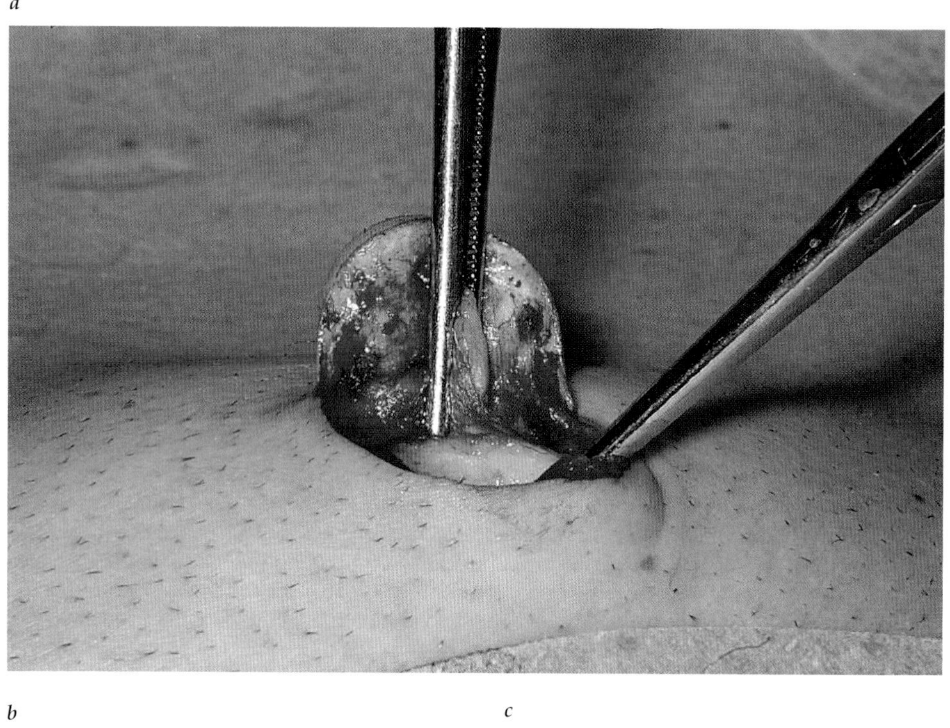

b

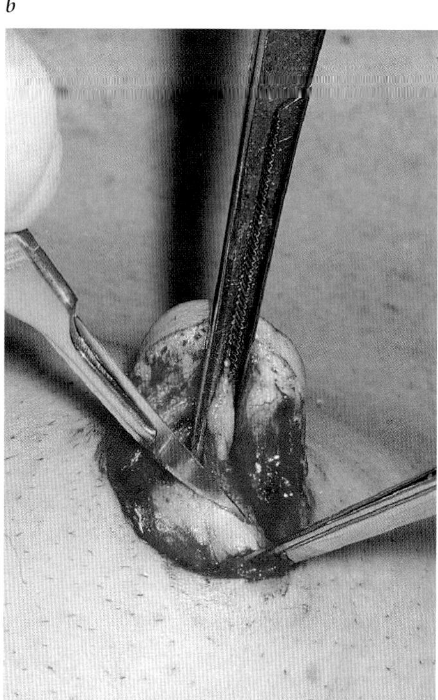

c

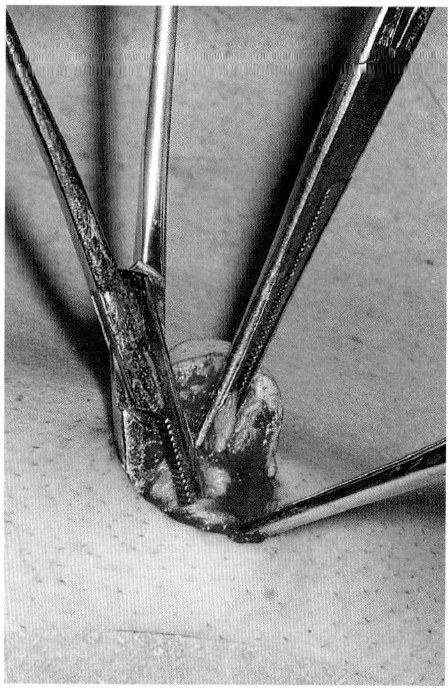

Figure 4 **Laparoscopic cholecystectomy. With the open insertion technique, the initial trocar is placed under direct vision. (*a*) The umbilical skin is elevated with a sharp towel clip. A curvilinear incision is made in the inferior umbilical fold. The skin flap is elevated, and the raphe leading from the dermis to the fascia is thereby exposed. (*b*) The fascia is grasped in the midline between forceps and elevated. The fascia and the underlying peritoneum are incised under direct vision. (*c*) A blunt instrument is placed into the peritoneum to ensure that the undersurface of the peritoneum is free of adhesions. The opening can be enlarged sufficiently to allow placement of a blunt 10/11 mm trocar.**

of retraction. As a general rule, positioning the trocar in the anterior axillary line approximately halfway between the costal margin and the anterosuperior iliac spine provides the appropriate exposure. A 2 to 5 mm port usually suffices at this site because its only likely function is to allow retraction of the gallbladder. In some cases of acute cholecystitis, however, a larger port may be preferable so that a larger grasper can be inserted and used to hold the gallbladder without tearing it.

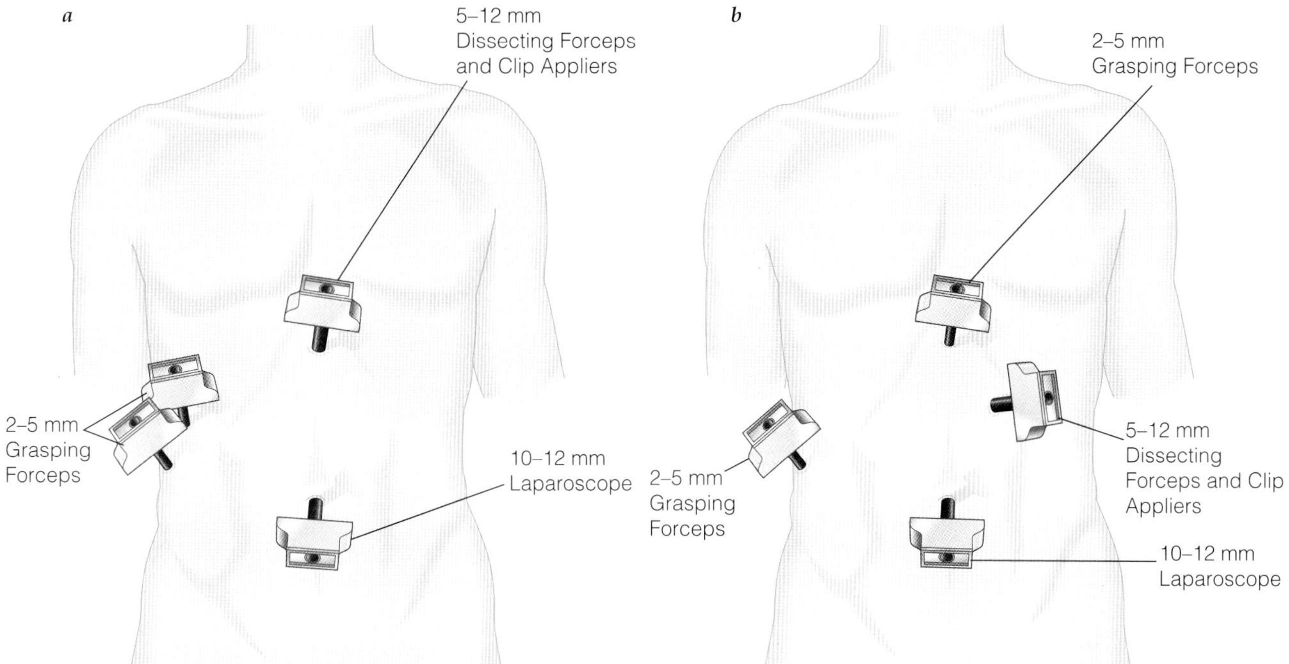

Figure 5 **Laparoscopic cholecystectomy. (*a*) and (*b*) are two popular options for trocar positioning and instrument placement.**

A second accessory port (also 2 to 5 mm) allows the surgeon to grasp the gallbladder in the area of the Hartmann pouch for retraction. This port is usually positioned just beneath the right costal margin. Some surgeons prefer it to be approximately at the midclavicular line; others prefer it to be higher and more medial, just to the right of the falciform ligament.

The main operating port should be 5 or 10 mm in diameter so that clip appliers can be readily placed through it and the laparoscope can be moved to this port at the end of the procedure. The positioning of this port is determined by the surgeon's preference and, in particular, by the patient's body habitus. The optimum placement is at about the same horizontal level as the gallbladder or slightly higher so that during the operation, the laparoscope and the operating instrument form an angle of about 90°. Some surgeons prefer to place the operative port in the midline, to the right of the falciform ligament; others prefer to place it to the left of the falciform ligament, passing the trocar underneath the ligament and elevating it with the trocar.

Surgeons should be encouraged to use both hands when performing laparoscopic cholecystectomy. One hand should control the grasping forceps holding the Hartmann pouch so that the gallbladder can be moved to provide the best possible exposure. The other hand should control the dissecting instruments placed through the operating port.

Special considerations in obese patients Port placement in obese patients may be complicated by the thick abdominal wall, the large amount of intra-abdominal fat, or both. A thick abdominal wall makes it more difficult to rotate the trocar around the normal fulcrum point in the abdominal wall. Consequently, the trocar must be placed at the angle most likely to be used during the procedure. When a trocar is tunneled through the abdominal wall, more of the cannula is within the abdominal wall than if the trocar had been placed perpendicularly; accordingly, the trocar is less mobile. If the trocars are not easily rotated, the instruments placed through them will be difficult to manipulate smoothly. Thus, in the patient with a very thick pannus, a standard-length trocar may be too short. Displacement of trocars can lead to insufflation into the abdominal wall and consequently to subcutaneous emphysema, which further thickens the abdominal wall and hinders exposure.

To prevent such problems, special extra-length trocars designed for morbidly obese patients have been developed. It may also be necessary to place the trocars closer to the area of the gallbladder to ensure that the operating instruments can reach the gallbladder. For example, the initial port may have to be placed above the umbilicus.

In obese patients, the bulky falciform ligament and the large omentum may adversely affect exposure. A 30° laparoscope may help the surgeon see over the omentum and the high-lying hepatic flexure of the colon. In some cases, it is useful to place a fifth port so that the surgeon can retract the hepatic flexure downward. Fat may envelop the cystic duct and artery and the portal structures, obscuring normal anatomic landmarks. When the electrocautery is used, the heat melts the fat and causes it to sizzle and spray onto the lens of the laparoscope, resulting in a blurry image. To prevent this, the camera operator should pull the scope slightly away from the operative field during electrocauterization and then advance the scope during dissection. This should also be done when an ultrasonic dissector is being used.

Given that obese patients are more difficult candidates for open cholecystectomy and have a higher complication rate with laparotomy, the advantages of laparoscopic cholecystectomy in these individuals justify the effort needed to overcome the technical problems.

Step 2: Exposure of the Gallbladder and Calot Triangle

Dissection of adhesions Adhesions must be dissected to provide an unimpeded view of the gallbladder through the laparoscope. Not all intra-abdominal adhesions must be taken down, just enough to allow entry of accessory trocars under direct vision and thus permit access to the gallbladder. This process is facilitated by pneumoperitoneum, which provides traction on adhesions to the abdominal wall, and by the magnification provided by the optical system, which allows identification of the avascular plane of attachment.

The most difficult problem is positioning the dissecting instruments so that they can reach the undersurface of the anterior abdominal wall. A rigid trocar inserted through the anterior abdominal wall cannot be rotated enough to allow scissors passed through this port to cut adhesions to the anterior abdominal wall. In such cases, one or two trocars should be placed laterally, near the anterior axillary or midaxillary line. Instruments passed through these ports can easily be angled parallel to the anterior abdominal wall, and the adhesions can then be dissected without difficulty.

Bowel adhesions should be taken down with endoscopic scissors at their insertion to the abdominal wall, where they are least vascular. Electrocauterization, which is generally unnecessary, should be avoided because of the risk of thermal injury to the bowel. Interloop adhesions, which rarely interfere with exposure of the gallbladder, need not be dissected. Frequently, adhesions to the gallbladder occur as a reaction to inflammatory attacks [*see Figure 6*]. They are usually relatively avascular. Dissection of these adhesions should begin at the fundus of the gallbladder and should then proceed down toward the neck of the gallbladder. The best way to take them down is to grasp the gallbladder with one grasping forceps at the site where the adhesions attach and gradually place traction on the adhesions with the other hand. Usually, the adhesions peel down in an avascular plane. Dissection should continue until all adhesions to the inferolateral aspect of the gallbladder have been taken down. It is not necessary to divide adhesions between the superior surface of the liver and the undersurface of the diaphragm unless they impede superior retraction of the liver.

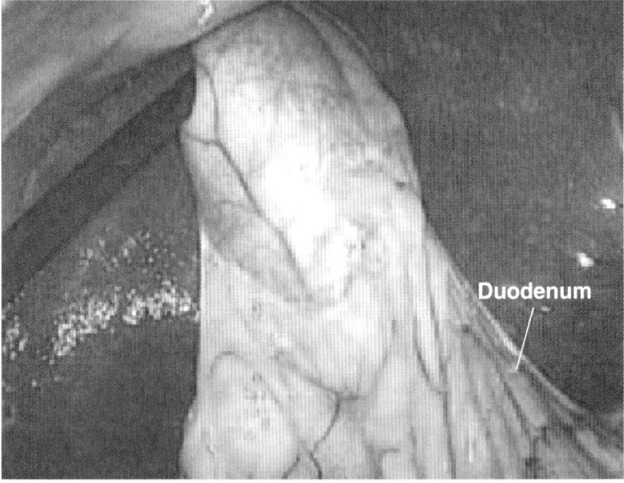

Figure 6 **Laparoscopic cholecystectomy. Adhesions of the duodenum and omentum to the gallbladder wall obscure the view of structures of the Calot triangle.**

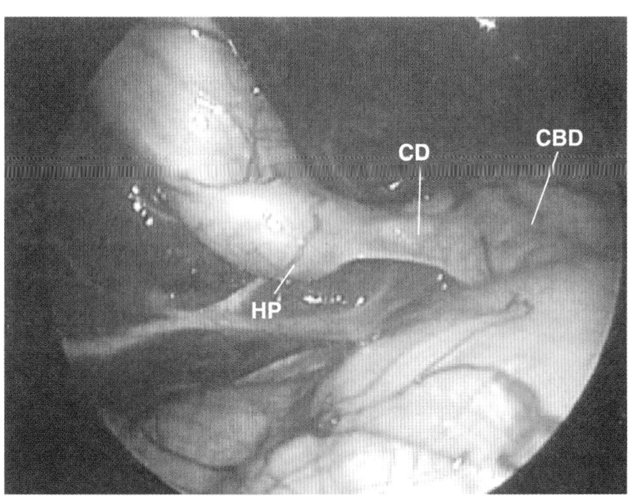

Figure 7 **Laparoscopic cholecystectomy. Initial view of the gallbladder and related structures is facilitated by appropriate tilting of the operating table. The Hartmann pouch (HP), cystic duct (CD), and common bile duct (CBD) can be readily identified before any dissection.**

Exposing the Calot triangle Obtaining adequate exposure of the Calot triangle is a key step. First, the patient is placed in a reverse Trendelenburg position, with the table rotated toward the left side. Next, the fundus of the gallbladder and the right lobe of the liver are elevated toward the patient's right shoulder. One grasping forceps, inserted through the most lateral right-side port and held by an assistant, is placed on the fundus of the gallbladder [*see Figure 7*], and the gallbladder is retracted superiorly and laterally above the right hepatic lobe. This maneuver straightens out folds in the body of the gallbladder and permits initial visualization of the area of the Calot triangle. If the Calot triangle is still obscured, the patient can be placed in a steeper reverse Trendelenburg position, and the stomach can be emptied of air via an orogastric tube inserted by the anesthetist, or, if necessary, a fifth trocar can be inserted on the patient's right side to push down the duodenum.

In some patients, such as those with acute cholecystitis and hydrops of the gallbladder, the gallbladder is tense and distended, making it difficult to grasp and easy to tear. In these patients, retraction of the fundus is difficult, and exposure of the Calot triangle is unsatisfactory. This problem is best managed by aspirating the contents of the gallbladder either percutaneously with a 14- or 16-gauge needle inserted into the fundus of the gallbladder under laparoscopic vision or by using the 5 mm trocar in the right upper abdomen to puncture the fundus and then aspirate with the suction irrigator. After the needle is withdrawn, a large atraumatic grasping forceps can be used to hold the gallbladder and occlude the hole; a 10 mm forceps may be preferred if the wall is markedly thickened. An alternative is to place a stitch or a ligating loop around the fundus of the collapsed gallbladder; the tail of the suture can then be grasped with a forceps to achieve a secure grip and prevent further leakage of gallbladder contents from the needle hole.

Once the fundus of the gallbladder is retracted superiorly by the assistant, the surgeon places a grasping forceps in the area of the Hartmann pouch. Using both hands, the surgeon controls the grasper on the Hartmann pouch and the operating instrument. The surgeon maneuvers the Hartmann pouch to provide various angles for safe dissection of the Calot triangle. Initially, lateral and inferior traction are placed on the Hartmann pouch, opening up the angle between the cystic duct and the common ducts [*see Figure 8*], avoiding their alignment [*see Figure 9*].

A large stone impacted in the gallbladder neck may impede the surgeon's ability to place the forceps on the Hartmann pouch. This problem can usually be managed by dislodging the stone early in the operation, as follows: the gallbladder is grasped as low as possible with one grasping forceps; a widely opening dissecting instrument, such as a right-angle dissector, a Babcock forceps, or a curved dissector, is used to dislodge the stone and milk it up toward the fundus; with the same forceps or another large grasper, the stone is held up and away from the neck of the gallbladder, and appropriate retraction is provided.

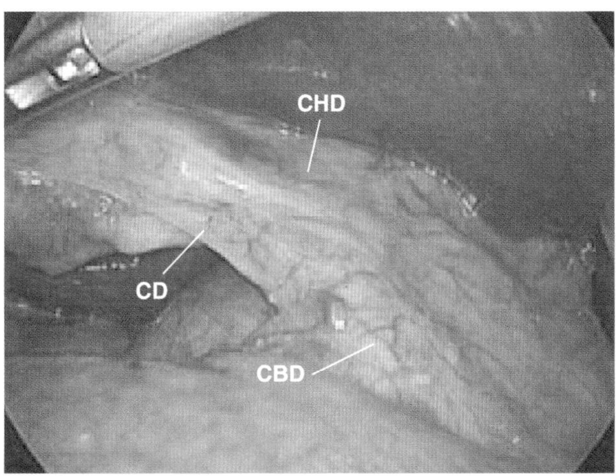

Figure 8 **Laparoscopic cholecystectomy. The area of the Hartmann pouch is retracted laterally. The cystic duct (CD) is seen at an angle to the common hepatic duct (CHD) and the common bile duct (CBD).**

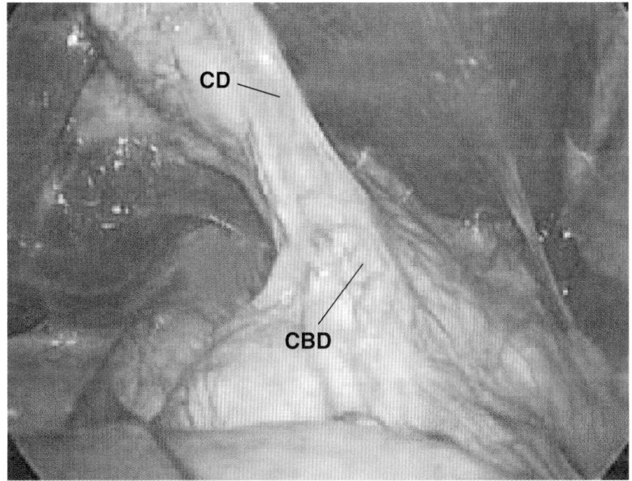

Figure 9 **Laparoscopic cholecystectomy. In this case, the gallbladder is retracted cephalad. The cystic duct (CD) can be seen running in the same direction as the common bile duct (CBD). The CBD may be misinterpreted as being the cystic duct and consequently is at risk for injury.**

If the stone cannot be disimpacted, an instrument can be used to elevate the infundibulum of the gallbladder superiorly, allowing exposure of the Calot triangle. Alternatively, one can attempt to crush the stone, but small pieces of the stone may fall into the cystic duct. A third option is to place a stitch in the Hartmann pouch and grasp the end of the stitch to provide exposure.

Step 3: Stripping of the Peritoneum

The key to avoiding injury to the major ducts during laparoscopic cholecystectomy is accurate identification of the junction between the gallbladder and the cystic duct [*see Figure 10*]. Unless the gallbladder–cystic duct junction is immediately obvious on examination of the Calot triangle anteriorly, our approach is to begin dissection of the Calot triangle posteriorly [*see Figure 11*]. From this approach, the insertion of the gallbladder neck into the cystic duct is usually more clearly identified, especially with the aid of a 30° laparoscope. Exposure is obtained by retracting the Hartmann pouch superomedially and is facilitated by looking from below with a 30° scope.

Dissection should always start high on the gallbladder and hug the gallbladder closely until the anatomy is identified clearly. Using a curved dissector, the surgeon gently teases away peritoneum attaching the neck of the gallbladder to the liver posterolaterally to visualize the funneling of the neck of the gallbladder into the cystic duct [*see Figure 12*]. Only the posterior layer of peritoneum is dissected; care must be taken not to dissect deeply in this area because of the risk of injury to the cystic artery [*see Figure 13*].

In some problem cases, edema, fibrosis, and adhesions make identification of the gallbladder–cystic duct junction very difficult. An anatomic landmark on the liver known as the Rouvier sulcus may be helpful in such circumstances [*see Figure 11*]. This sulcus, or the remnant of it, is present in

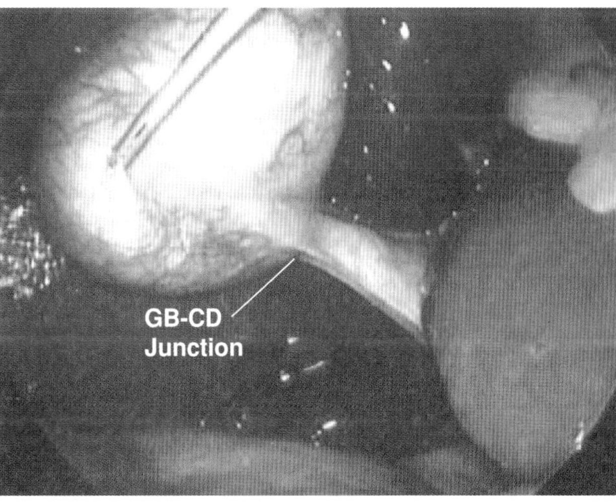

Figure 10 **Laparoscopic cholecystectomy. The gallbladder–cystic duct (GB-CD) junction is clearly seen. This should be dissected circumferentially, allowing a 360° view.**

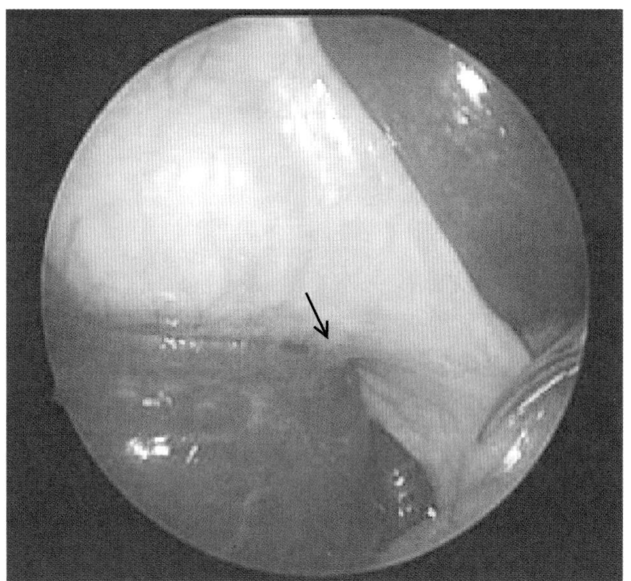

Figure 11 **Laparoscopic cholecystectomy. A view from below with a 30° laparoscope demonstrates the point for beginning dissection (*arrow*), where the gallbladder funnels down to its junction with the cystic duct. Just below this point can be seen a cleft in the liver known as the Rouvier sulcus. This cleft, present in 70 to 80% of livers, reliably indicates the plane of the common bile duct.**

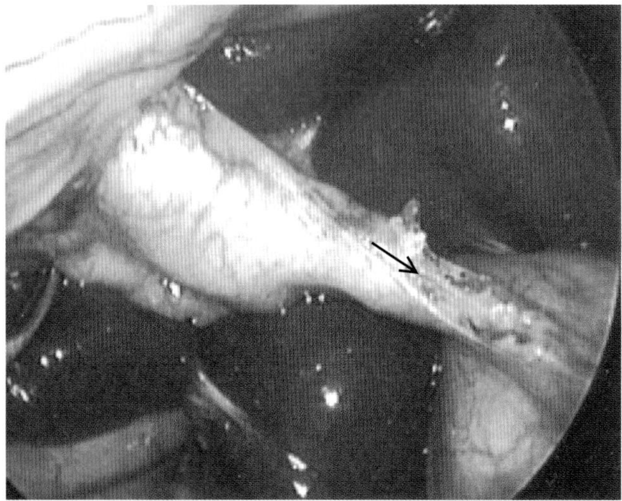

Figure 12 **Laparoscopic cholecystectomy. The peritoneum is dissected from the gallbladder–cystic duct junction (*arrow*), as seen from below through a 30° angled laparoscope.**

70 to 80% of livers and usually contains the right portal triad or its branches. Its location is consistently to the right of the hepatic hilum and anterior to the caudate process (Couinaud segment 1). This landmark reliably indicates the plane of the CBD. Therefore, dissection dorsal to it should be done with caution. Once the funneling of the gallbladder into the cystic duct has been identified, the area of the Hartmann pouch should be again pulled laterally and inferiorly so that the anterior peritoneum can be dissected while the 30° scope is angled to view the area. The two-handed technique facilitates

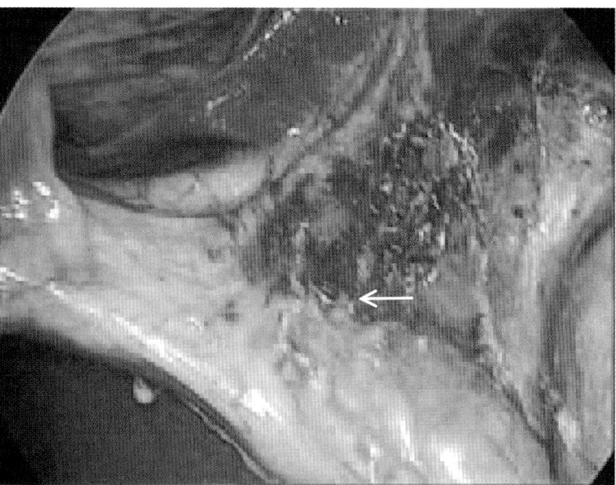

Figure 13 **Laparoscopic cholecystectomy. Arterial bleeding can be seen (*arrow*) from a branch of the cystic artery injured during dissection from the posterior approach.**

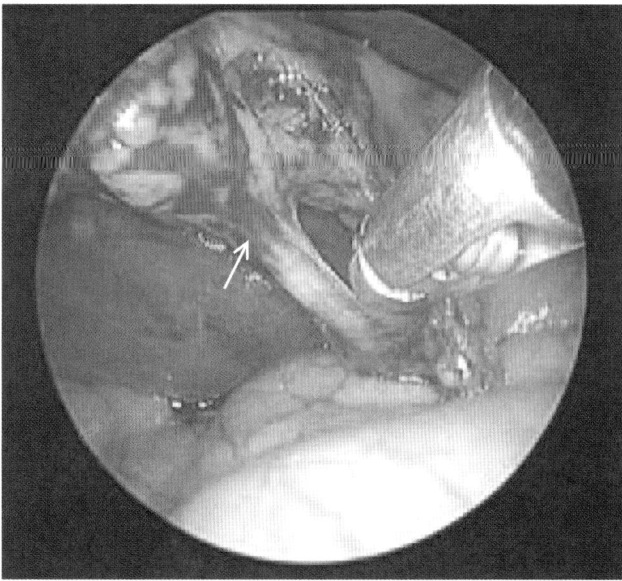

Figure 14 **Laparoscopic cholecystectomy. The superior border of the cystic duct has been dissected. Funneling of the gallbladder into the cystic duct is clearly seen (*arrow*).**

the surgeon's movement between the posterior and anterior aspects of the Calot triangle, providing complete visualization. Dissection should always take place at the gallbladder–cystic duct junction, staying close to the gallbladder to avoid inadvertent injury to the CBD. A curved dissecting forceps is used to strip the fibroareolar tissue just superior to the cystic duct. The superior border of the cystic duct can then be identified and the cystic duct gently and gradually dissected [*see Figure 14*]. The cystic duct lymph node is a useful landmark at this location and may facilitate identification of the gallbladder–cystic duct junction.

When traction is placed as described, the cystic artery tends to run parallel and somewhat cephalad to the cystic duct. This artery can often be identified by noting its close relation to the cystic duct lymph node. Complete dissection of the area between the cystic duct and the artery develops a window through which the liver should be visible. The cystic duct is then encircled with a curved dissecting instrument or an L-shaped hook. Downward traction should be applied to the cystic duct to open this window and ensure that there is no ductal structure running through this space in the Calot triangle to join the cystic duct (i.e., the right hepatic duct).

Dissection of the Calot triangle should be completed before the cystic duct is clipped or divided. This is best accomplished by dissecting the neck of the gallbladder from the liver bed. Unequivocal identification of the gallbladder–cystic duct junction is imperative.[24,25] The cystic duct should be dissected for a length sufficient to permit secure placement of two clips; it is not necessary, and indeed may be hazardous, to attempt to dissect the cystic duct–CBD junction.

The cystic artery is exposed next [*see Figure 15*]. A small vein can usually be identified in the space between the cystic duct and the cystic artery; it can usually be pulled up anteriorly and cauterized. Because dissection is done near the gallbladder, it is not unusual to encounter more than one branch of the cystic artery. Each of these branches should be dissected free of the fibroareolar tissue. Care should also be taken to ensure that the right hepatic artery is not inadvertently injured as a result of being mistaken for the cystic artery.

Step 4: Control and Division of the Cystic Duct and Cystic Artery

At this point, the cystic duct is clipped on the gallbladder side, and a cholangiogram is obtained if desired [*see* Step 5, *below*]. If a cholangiogram is not desired, three or four clips should be placed on the cystic duct and the cystic duct divided between them. Two or three hemostatic clips are placed on the cystic artery, and the vessel is divided. It is prudent to incise the artery partially before transecting it completely to ensure that the clips are secure and that there is no pulsatile bleeding. Once the artery is completely divided, the proximal end will retract medially, making it more difficult to expose and control the artery safely if bleeding occurs. Electrocauterization should be avoided near the cystic duct and all metallic clips. Electric current will be conducted through metallic clips and may result in delayed sloughing of the duct or a clip. Delayed injuries to the CBD may be caused by a direct burn to the duct or by sparking from noninsulated instruments or clips during dissection. An alternative is to use locking polymer clips that fit through 5 mm ports, clip across a greater width of tissue, and do not conduct electricity.

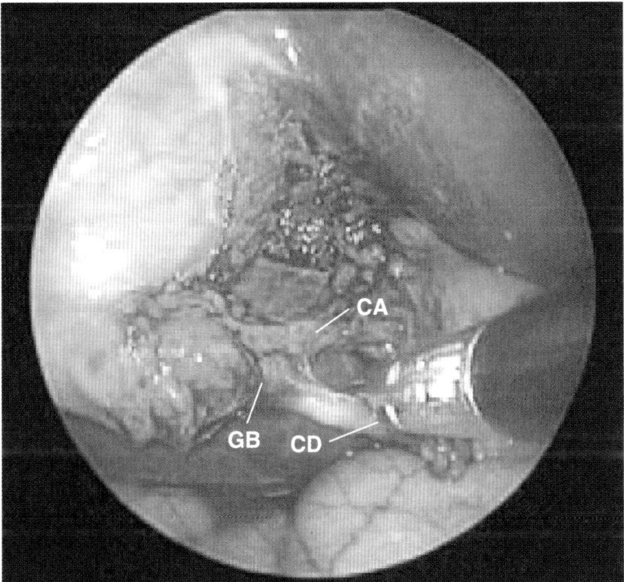

Figure 15 **Laparoscopic cholecystectomy. Dissection of the Calot triangle further exposes the cystic duct (CD) and the cystic artery (CA) near their entry into the gallbladder (GB) in preparation for clipping and division.**

Control of the short or wide cystic duct Edema and acute inflammation may lead to thickening and foreshortening of the cystic duct, with subsequent difficulties in dissection and ligation. If the duct is edematous, clips may cut through it; if the duct is too wide, the clip may not occlude it completely. A modified clipping technique can be employed, with placement of an initial clip to occlude as much of the duct as possible. The occluded portion of the duct is then incised, and a second clip is placed flush with the first so as to occlude the rest of the duct. Alternatively, wider polymer clips may be used.

Because this technique is not always possible, the surgeon should be familiar with techniques for ligating the duct with either intracorporeal or extracorporeal ties. It is extremely helpful to know how to tie extracorporeal ties so that the cystic duct can be ligated in continuity before it is divided. In some cases, the duct can be divided, held with a forceps, and controlled with a ligating loop. If there is concern about secure closure of the cystic duct, a closed suction drain may be placed. If inflammation, as in cholecystitis, has caused the duct to be shorter than usual, dissection must be kept close to the gallbladder to avoid inadvertent injury to the CBD. A short cystic duct is often associated with acute cholecystitis. Patient blunt dissection with the suction-irrigation device may be the safest technique.

Cystic duct stones Stones in the cystic duct may be visualized or felt during laparoscopic cholecystectomy. Every effort should be made to milk them into the gallbladder before applying clips. Placing a clip across a stone may push a fragment of the stone into the CBD and will increase the risk that the clip will become displaced, leading to a bile leak. If the stone cannot be milked into the gallbladder, a small incision can be made in the cystic duct (as is done for cholangiography), and the stone can often be expressed and retrieved. Given that cystic duct stones are predictive of CBD stones, cholangiography or intraoperative ultrasonography is indicated.[26]

Step 5: Intraoperative Cholangiography

Whether intraoperative cholangiography should be performed routinely is still controversial. Advocates believe that this technique enhances understanding of the biliary anatomy, thus reducing the risk of bile duct injury[27,28]; at present, however, there are no objective data to confirm this impression. Cholangiography is not a substitute for meticulous dissection, and injuries to the CBD can occur before cystic duct dissection reaches the point at which cholangiography can be performed. Catheter-induced injuries and perforations of the biliary tree have been reported, and cholangiograms have been misinterpreted. On the other hand, one of the main advantages of cholangiography is that injuries can be

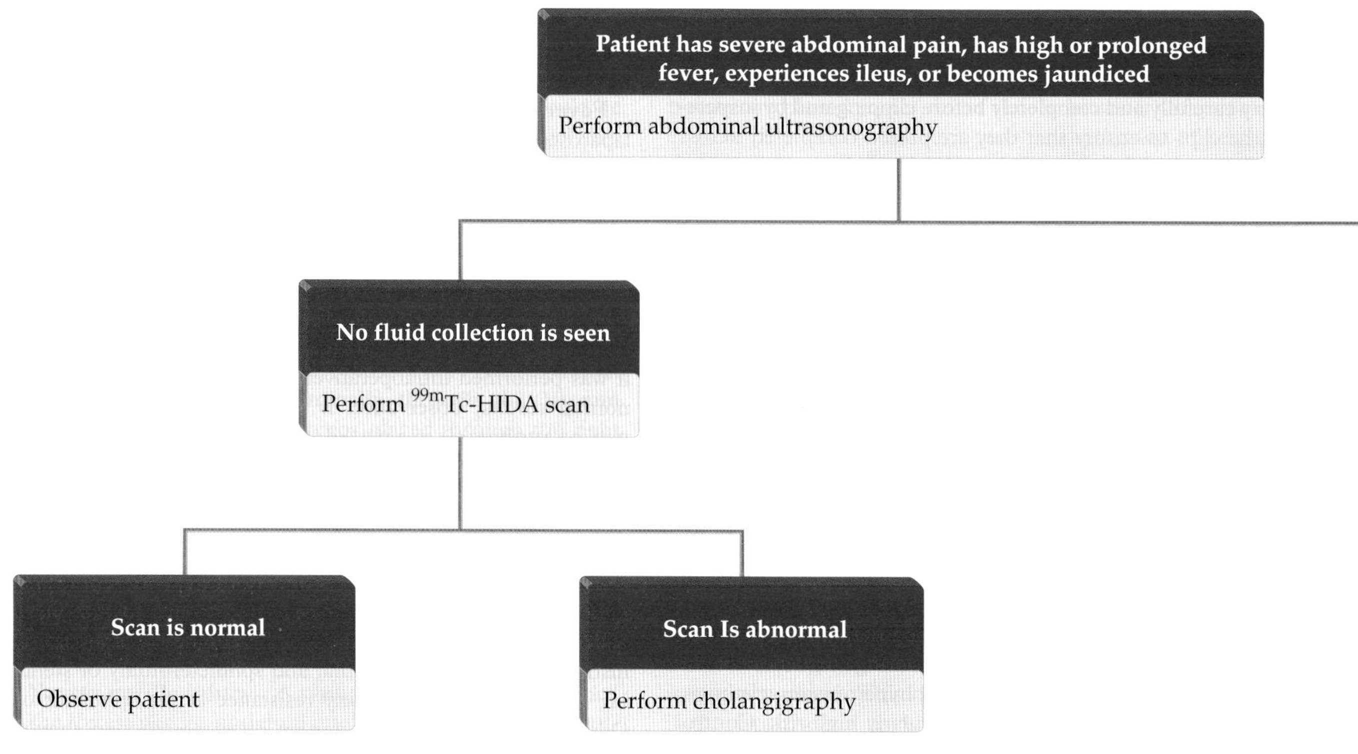

Figure 19 **Laparoscopic cholecystectomy. Shown is an algorithm outlining a screening approach that is often useful when the patient shows signs (e.g., pain, fever, or ileus) that are suggestive of a postoperative intra-abdominal complication, such as fluid collection or bile leakage. ERCP = endoscopic retrograde cholangiopancreatography; MRCP = magnetic resonance cholangiopancreatography.**

ingly, every patient consent obtained for a laparoscopic cholecystectomy must explicitly allow for the possibility of conversion to an open procedure. Attempts have been made to predict the probability of conversion on the basis of preoperative information.[36,37] It is clearly useful to stratify patients according to the likelihood of conversion. This information is helpful in selecting patients for laparoscopic cholecystectomy in an outpatient versus hospital setting, in determining the resources required in the OR, and in assisting patients in planning their work and family needs around the time of surgery.

Factors found to be predictive of an increased probability of conversion include acute cholecystitis, either at the time of surgery or at any point in the past; age greater than 65 years; male sex; and thickening of the gallbladder wall to more than 3 mm as measured by ultrasonography. Other factors more variably associated with an increased likelihood of conversion are obesity, previous upper abdominal operations (especially gastroduodenal), multiple gallbladder attacks over a long period, and severe pancreatitis. Factors not associated with an increased likelihood of conversion are jaundice, previous ES, previous lower abdominal procedures, stomas, mild pancreatitis, and diabetes.

On the basis of our data, a 45-year-old woman with no history of acute cholecystitis and no gallbladder wall thickening has a probability of conversion lower than 1%; such a patient is a good candidate for laparoscopic cholecystectomy in an outpatient setting. Conversely, a 70-year-old man with acute cholecystitis and ultrasonographic evidence of gallbladder wall thickening has a probability of conversion of about 30%; such a patient would be better managed in a traditional hospital environment.

Acute Cholecystitis

Laparoscopic cholecystectomy has been shown to be safe and effective for treating acute cholecystitis.[38,39] There are, however, several technical problems in this setting that must be addressed if the procedure is to be performed with minimal risk. It should also be recognized that the probability of

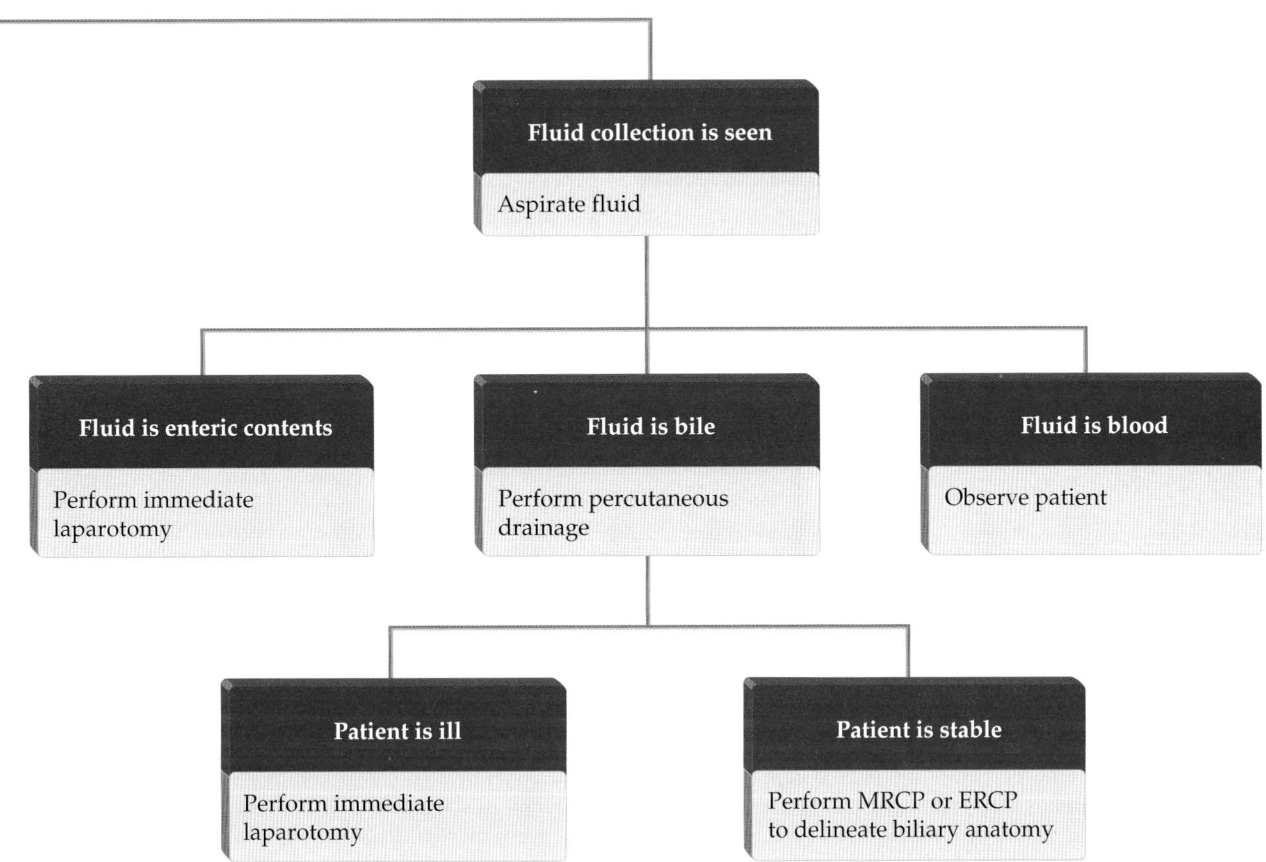

conversion to laparotomy is greatly increased in these circumstances. There appears to be no advantage to delaying surgery in patients with acute cholecystitis, even if rapid improvement is noted with nonoperative management.[40,41] Many patients return within a short time with recurrent attacks, and delaying surgery does not reduce the probability of conversion.

Technical difficulties associated with cholecystectomy for acute cholecystitis include dense adhesions, the increased vascularity of tissues, difficulty in grasping the gallbladder, an impacted stone in the gallbladder neck or the cystic duct, shortening and thickening of the cystic duct, and close approximation of the CBD to the gallbladder wall.

The surgeon should not hesitate to insert additional ports (e.g., for a suction-irrigation apparatus) if necessary. Because the tense, distended gallbladder is difficult to grasp reliably, it should be aspirated through the fundus early in the procedure, as previously described. If the graspers fail to grasp the wall or cause it to tear, exposure of the Calot triangle can be achieved by propping up or levering the neck of the gallbladder and the right liver with a blunt instrument. A sponge can be used for this purpose, thereby reducing the potential trauma of the retraction. This maneuver is also useful when an impacted stone in the neck of the gallbladder prevents the surgeon from grasping the gallbladder in the area of the Hartmann pouch. Dense adhesions that may be present between the gallbladder and the omentum, duodenum, or colon should be dissected bluntly (e.g., with a suction tip). Because the tissues are friable and vascular, oozing may be encountered. Electrocauterization should be only sparingly employed until the vital structures in the Calot triangle are identified. Instead, the surgeon should move to another area of dissection, allowing most of the oozing to coagulate on its own. Liberal use of suction and irrigation will keep the operative field free of blood.

In the identification of anatomic structures, it is important to keep dissection close to the gallbladder wall, working down from the gallbladder toward the Calot triangle. Dissection of the lower part of the gallbladder from the liver bed early in the operation may aid in identification of the gallbladder neck–cystic duct junction (analogous to an open, retrograde dissection). The surgeon should be aware that edema and acute inflammation may cause foreshortening of the cystic duct. If the anatomy cannot be identified, preliminary cholangiography through the emptied gallbladder may indicate the position of the cystic duct and the CBD.

Often the obstructing stone responsible for the acute attack is in the neck of the gallbladder; thus, the cystic duct will be

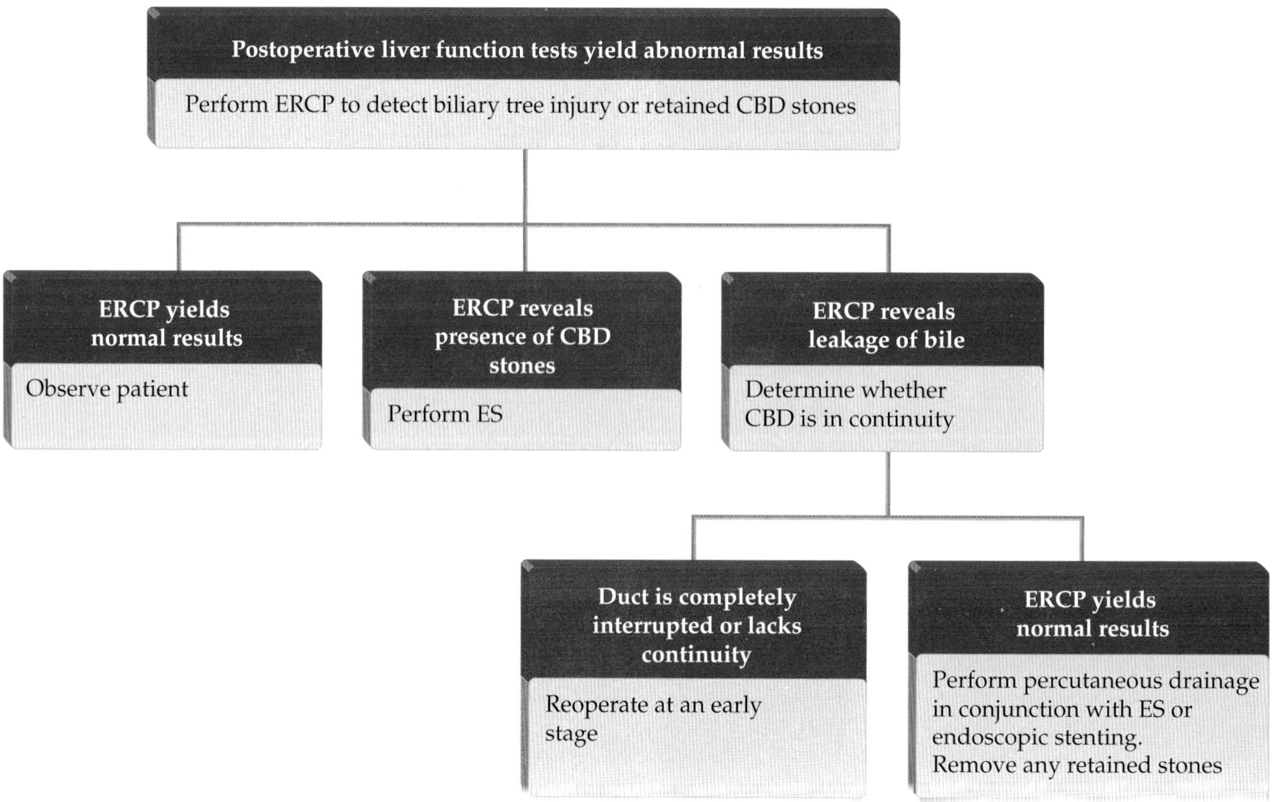

Figure 20 **Laparoscopic cholecystectomy. Shown is an algorithm outlining an approach to abnormal liver function test results after laparoscopic cholecystectomy. CBD = common bile duct; ERCP = endoscopic retrograde cholangiopancreatography; ES = endoscopic sphincterotomy.**

normal and easily secured with clips. If the stone is in the cystic duct, it must be removed before the duct is clipped or ligated. A thickened, edematous cystic duct is better controlled by ligation with an extracorporeal tie or a ligating loop than by clipping. If closure of the cystic duct is tenuous, closed suction drainage is advisable. Obviously, conversion to open cholecystectomy is indicated if the anatomy remains obscure. Conversion should also be considered if no progress is made after a predesignated period (e.g., 15 minutes) because at this point, the surgeon is unlikely to make any headway.

CBD Stones

Identification of patients at risk About 10% of all patients undergoing cholecystectomy for symptomatic gallstones will also have choledocholithiasis. To select from the various diagnostic and therapeutic options for managing choledocholithiasis, it is helpful to know preoperatively whether the patient is at high, moderate, or low risk for stones. Patients with obvious clinical jaundice or cholangitis, a dilated CBD, or stones visualized in the CBD on preoperative ultrasonography are likely to have choledocholithiasis (risk > 50%). Patients who have a history of jaundice or pancreatitis, moderately elevated preoperative levels of alkaline phosphatase or bilirubin, or ultrasonographic evidence of multiple small gallstones are somewhat less likely to have choledocholithiasis (risk 10 to 50%). Patients with large gallstones, no history of jaundice or pancreatitis, and normal liver function are unlikely to have choledocholithiasis (risk < 5%).

Diagnostic and therapeutic options One argument for routine intraoperative cholangiography is that it is a good way of identifying unsuspected CBD stones. However, more selective approaches to diagnosing choledocholithiasis make use of preoperative cholangiography via MRCP, EUS, or, more invasively, ERCP [*see 6:17 Upper Gastrointestinal Endoscopy and 6:18 Lower Endoscopy*]. Preoperative identification of choledocholithiasis allows the surgeon to attempt preoperative clearance of the CBD by means of ES or intraoperative clearance during laparoscopy, depending on his or her expertise. Preoperative cholangiography is suggested when the patient's history and the results of laboratory and diagnostic tests suggest that there is a moderate or high risk of CBD stones. It is our practice to have patients at high risk for CBD stones undergo ERCP and ES if warranted. For patients at moderate risk, MRCP or EUS is done first, followed by therapeutic ERCP if CBD stones are identified. Intraoperative cholangiography can also be used to identify choledocholithiasis. ERCP with ES may result in pancreatitis, perforation, or bleeding and carries a mortality of approximately 0.2%.

When stones are detected during the operation, the options include laparoscopic transcystic duct exploration, laparoscopic choledochotomy and CBD exploration, open CBD exploration, and postoperative ERCP with ES.[10,42] If a single small (≈ 2 mm) stone is visualized, it can probably be flushed into the duodenum by irrigating the CBD via the cholangiogram catheter and administering glucagon, 1 to 2 mg intravenously, to relax the sphincter of Oddi. Even if a stone of this size does not pass intraoperatively, it will usually pass on its own postoperatively.

Laparoscopic transcystic CBD exploration *Access to the biliary tree* The cholangiogram is reviewed; the size of the cystic duct, the site where the cystic duct inserts into the CBD, and the size and location of the CBD stones all contribute to the success or failure of transcystic CBD exploration.[43–45] For example, transcystic exploration is extremely challenging in a patient who has a long, spiraling cystic duct with a medial insertion. The size of the stones to be removed dictates the approach to the CBD: stones smaller than 4 mm can usually be retrieved in fluoroscopically directed baskets and generally do not necessitate cystic duct dilatation; larger stones (4 to 8 mm) are retrieved under direct vision with the choledochoscope.

A hydrophilic guide wire is inserted through the cholangiogram catheter into the CBD under fluoroscopic guidance. The cholangiogram catheter is then removed. If the largest stone is larger than the cystic duct, dilatation of the duct is necessary, not only for passage of the stone but also to allow passage of the choledochoscope, which may be 3 to 5 mm in diameter.

Dilatation is accomplished with either a balloon dilator or sequential plastic dilators. Because plastic dilators may cause the cystic duct to split, balloon dilatation is recommended. A balloon 3 to 5 cm in length is passed over the guide wire and positioned with its distal end just inside the CBD and its proximal end just outside the incision in the cystic duct. The balloon is then inflated to the pressure recommended by the manufacturer and observed closely for evidence of shearing of the cystic duct. The cystic duct should not be dilated to a diameter greater than 8 mm. Larger stones in the CBD may be either fragmented with electrohydraulic or mechanical lithotripsy, if available, or removed via choledochotomy.

Once dilatation is complete, the guide wire may be removed or left in place to guide passage of a choledochoscope or baskets. When the choledochoscope is used, a second incision in the cystic duct, close to the CBD, avoids the Heister valves and allows removal of the guide wire. If baskets are used, a 6 French plastic introducer sheath may be inserted through the trocar used for cholangiography into the cystic duct. This sheath is especially useful if multiple stones must be removed.

Fluoroscopic wire basket transcystic CBD exploration Stones smaller than 2 to 4 mm that do not pass with irrigation through the cholangiocatheter after injection of glucagon can usually be retrieved by using a 4 French or 5 French helical stone basket passed into the CBD over a guide wire under fluoroscopic guidance. The baskets can be passed alongside the cholangiocatheter or inserted via a plastic sheath replacing the cholangiocatheter. The basket is opened in the ampulla of Vater, pulled back into the CBD, and rotated clockwise until the stone is entrapped. The stone and basket are then removed together. A Fogarty catheter should not be used, because the stones are likely to be pulled up into the hepatic ducts, where they are much more difficult to remove.

Endoscopic transcystic CBD exploration When stones are 4 to 8 mm in diameter, the helical stone basket wires are generally too close together to permit retrieval. Hence, choledochoscopic basketing is used. A videocholedochoscope with a working channel is either passed over the guide wire or inserted directly into the cystic duct. Because the usual laparoscopic grasping forceps may damage the choledochoscope, forceps with rubber-covered jaws should be used. The image from the choledochoscope can be displayed on the monitor by means of an audiovisual mixer (i.e., a picture within a picture) or displayed on a separate monitor.

Once the choledochoscope enters the cystic duct, warm saline irrigation is begun under low pressure to distend the CBD and provide a working space. The choledochoscope usually enters the CBD rather than the common hepatic duct. When a stone is seen, a 2.4 French straight four-wire basket is inserted through the operating port. The stones closest to the cystic duct are removed first by advancing the closed basket beyond each stone, opening the basket, and pulling the basket back, thereby trapping the stone. The basket is then closed and pulled up against the choledochoscope so that they can be withdrawn as a unit. Multiple passes may be required until the duct is clear. A completion cholangiogram is done to ensure that the duct is clear and to rule out proximal stones. The dilated, traumatized cystic duct is ligated with a ligating loop rather than a hemostatic clip. If drainage is required, a red rubber catheter can be inserted into the CBD via the cystic duct.

Because of the angle created by the cephalad and superior retraction of the gallbladder, it may be difficult to pass the choledochoscope into the proximal ducts. If a common hepatic duct stone is seen on the cholangiogram, the patient is placed in a steep reverse Trendelenburg position. In this position, any nonimpacted stones may fall into the distal duct for retrieval. It may be possible to pass the choledochoscope into the proximal ducts by applying caudal traction to the cystic duct so as to align it with the common hepatic duct. An additional access port in the right upper quadrant may be needed. If the cystic duct is long or spiraling or inserts medially, this measure may not be feasible, in which case, access must be obtained by means of choledochotomy.

Laparoscopic CBD exploration Large stones (> 1 cm), as well as most stones in the common hepatic ducts, are not retrievable with the techniques described above. Ductal clearance can be achieved via choledochotomy if the duct is dilated and the surgeon is sufficiently experienced.[46,47] The anterior wall of the CBD is bluntly dissected for a distance of 1 to 2 cm. When small vessels are encountered, it is preferable to apply pressure and wait for hemostasis rather than use the electrocautery in this area. Adrenaline-soaked gauzes placed through the 12 mm umbilical port are very effective for this purpose. Two stay sutures are placed in the CBD. An additional 5 mm trocar is placed in the right lower quadrant for insertion of an additional needle driver. A small longitudinal choledochotomy (a few millimeters longer than the circumference of the largest stone) is made with curved microscissors on the anterior aspect of the duct while the stay sutures are elevated. A choledochoscope is then inserted, and warm saline irrigation is initiated. In most cases, baskets should suffice for stone retrieval; however, lithotriptor probes and lasers are available for use through the working channel of the choledochoscope. The choice of approach depends on availability and individual surgical experience.

Subsequently, a 12 or 14 French latex T tube is fashioned with short limbs, placed entirely intraperitoneally to prevent CO_2 from escaping, and positioned in the CBD. The choledochotomy is then closed with fine interrupted absorbable sutures. The first suture is placed right next to the T tube, securing it distally, and the second is placed at the most proximal end of the choledochotomy; lifting these two sutures facilitates placement of additional sutures. Intracorporeal knots are preferred to avoid sawing of the delicate tissues. The end of the T tube is then pulled out through a trocar, and cholangiography is performed after completion of the procedure.

Open Cholecystectomy

Open cholecystectomy is usually reserved for patients in whom the laparoscopic approach is not feasible or is contraindicated. As such, it is typically performed only in the most difficult situations or when additional maneuvers such as CBD exploration are anticipated. Conversion from the laparoscopic to the open approach is not considered a complication and does not represent failure. Rather, conversion to this time-honored and effective procedure represents the prudent judgment of a safe surgeon.

OPERATIVE TECHNIQUE

The choice of incision depends on the surgeon's experience and preference, along with patient factors such as previous surgical procedures and body habitus. Typically, open cholecystectomy is performed through a right subcostal (Kocher) incision, but it can also be approached through an upper midline incision or, less commonly, through a right paramedian or transverse incision. A mechanical retraction system should be used, if available, so that the hands of the participating surgeons are free; there is no good rationale for struggling to perform difficult biliary surgery with handheld retractors.

The abdomen is opened and then explored; the abdominal viscera are inspected and palpated, and a retraction system is put in place. Long curved or angled clamps, such as Kelly or Mixter, are placed on the gallbladder fundus and infundibulum for the application of gentle traction. The fundus is elevated and the infundibulum is pulled laterally and away from the liver [*see Figure 21*]. If the gallbladder is not too inflamed and edematous, the procedure may be performed similarly to the typical laparoscopic approach: the surgeon identifies and ligates the cystic duct and artery and then removes the gallbladder from the liver bed.

With more difficult open cases, the above technique may not be possible. In such cases, a retrograde or so-called fundus down approach is usually employed. Staying as close to the gallbladder wall as is possible, the surgeon uses electrocautery or sharp and digital blunt dissection to remove the gallbladder from the liver bed, continuing downward to the cystic duct and artery [*see Figure 22*]. Anatomic variations of the duct and artery must always be anticipated. These structures can be very difficult to identify and safely dissect in cases of severe inflammation and markedly edematous tissues. In such cases, palpation and gentle digital blunt dissection of the duct and artery between the thumb and index finger is useful [*see Figure 23*]. Opening the gallbladder to remove stones or aspirate bile or pus may be necessary when it is tense and distended or necrotic and gangrenous. As with laparoscopic cholecystectomy, it is critical to identify the cystic duct and artery and their anatomic relations to the gallbladder and CBD before division and to avoid injury to the CBD or common hepatic duct. The cystic duct and artery may be suture ligated or divided between clips. Stones found in the cystic duct should be gently milked back into the gallbladder.

SPECIAL CONSIDERATIONS

Cholangiography

The indications for cholangiography are the same as for laparoscopic cholecystectomy. Several techniques for the performance of cholangiography can be used. Usually, the same technique as for laparoscopic cholecystectomy is employed; the cystic duct is ligated or clipped high near the infundibulum and incised just below this point for insertion of a cholangiography catheter, which is secured against leakage by another

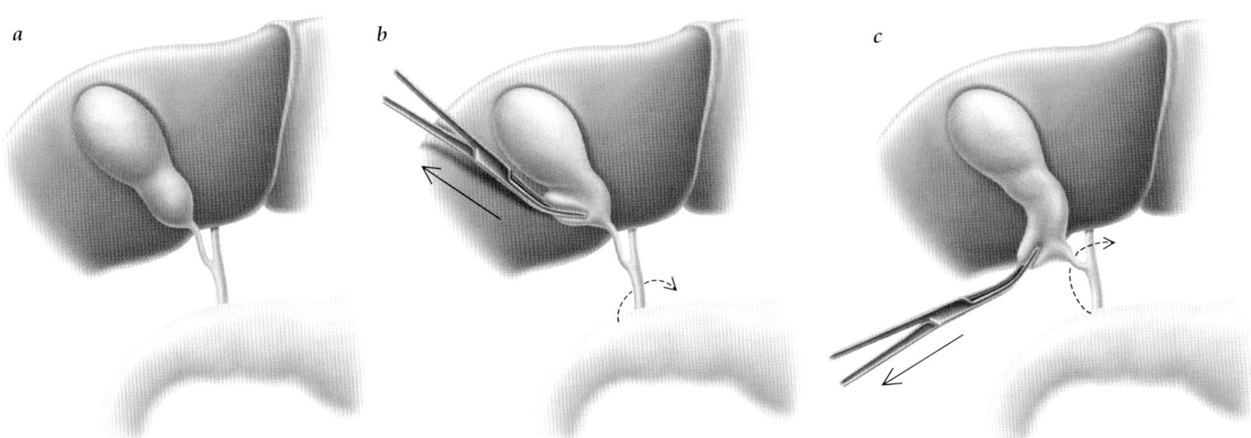

Figure 21 **Open cholecystectomy. (*a*) Shown are the resting positions of the cystic duct and the common bile duct (CBD) (with the Calot triangle closed). (*b*) Improper upward retraction of the Hartmann pouch lines up the CBD and the cystic duct so that one can easily encircle the CBD or clamp the cystic duct and the CBD. (*c*) Correct downward and rightward retraction opens the Calot triangle; dissection proceeds lateral to the CBD.**

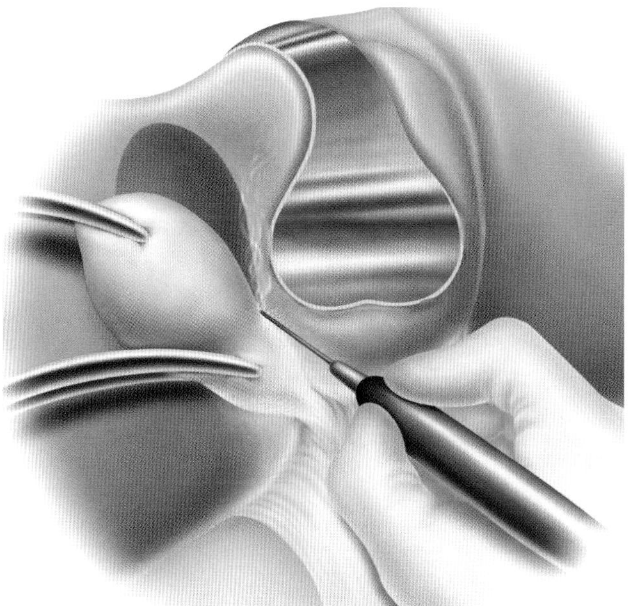

Figure 22 **Open cholecystectomy. In so-called fundus down dissection, the fundus and infundibulum are retracted up and away from the liver while dissection is performed with electrocautery. Sharp dissection with scissors or scalpel and blunt digital dissection all may be used, at the surgeon's discretion.**

clip or ligature. Alternatively, the cystic duct can be divided near the infundibulum and the gallbladder removed; then the cystic duct is cannulated. Needle puncture cholangiography can also be performed via the cystic duct or the common duct. Once cholangiography is complete, the gallbladder is removed and sent for pathologic examination. The operative field is inspected for hemostasis and irrigated. Any bile leak is identified. Drains are not routinely placed but can be used at the surgeon's discretion. If drains are used, a closed suction Jackson-Pratt or similar drain is recommended; the drain should be brought out through a separate stab incision.

Open CBD Exploration

Open CBD exploration has become a rare procedure, but it remains a skill that surgeons require. If ERCP has failed or is not possible, if the surgeon does not have the experience and necessary tools to perform laparoscopic duct exploration, or if laparoscopic efforts have failed, then open exploration becomes necessary. Ductal stones are identified either preoperatively or intraoperatively by ultrasonography, cholangiography, or palpation.

Appropriate retraction and exposure are crucial. The anterior aspect of the duct is exposed over a distance of 1 to 2 cm, avoiding electrocautery during dissection. Two stay sutures of a 3-0 monofilament are placed lateral to the midline of the duct. The common hepatic duct is sharply opened with a No. 11 or No. 15 scalpel and longitudinally incised further with a Potts arteriotomy or similar scissors. When performing these maneuvers, the surgeon must respect the arterial blood supply of the duct, which courses laterally on either side of the duct in the 3 o'clock and 9 o'clock positions [*see Figure 24*]. In some cases, stones are immediately visible and can simply be

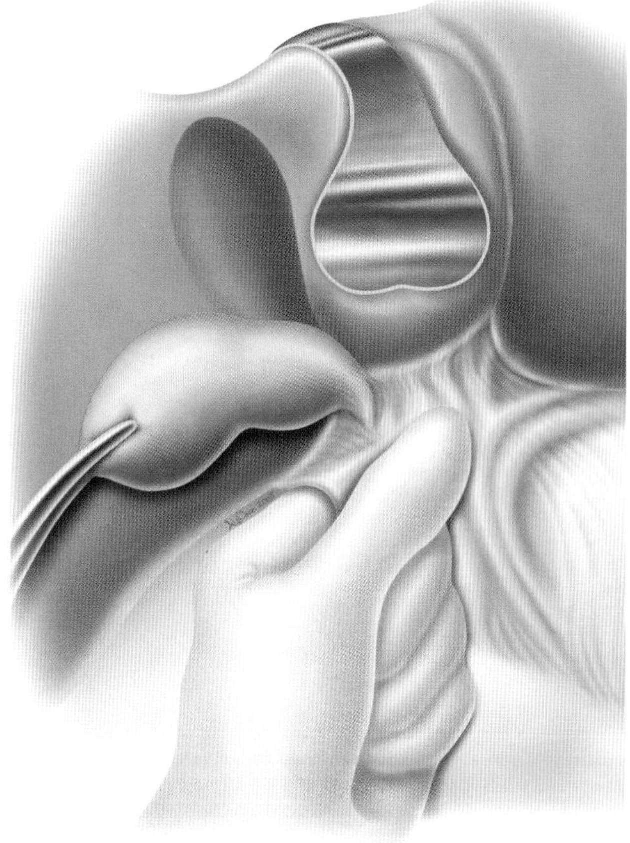

Figure 23 **Open cholecystectomy. In patients with severe inflammation and edema, the surgeon must be cautious when approaching the Calot triangle during fundus down dissection. In such circumstances, digital palpation can be very helpful in safely identifying the cystic duct and artery.**

plucked from the duct once it is opened. Flushing the duct with saline, proximally and then distally, through a 12 or 14 French Foley or red rubber catheter may also clear the duct of stones. The intravenous administration of 1 to 2 mg of glucagon will relax the sphincter of Oddi, which may help in the flushing of stones from the duct. In some cases, stones will be impacted within the duct and will require additional maneuvers. The Kocher maneuver (liberally mobilizing the lateral duodenum and head of the pancreas) will allow the surgeon to hold and palpate the duodenum, the head of the pancreas, and stones within the duct, facilitating instrumentation. Stone retrieval forceps, biliary Fogarty catheters, and wire baskets can all be employed to retrieve stones. A choledochoscope can also be used, either at the outset of exploration or for stone retrieval, if simpler maneuvers are not successful.

Either T tube cholangiography or choledochoscopy may be employed to confirm clearance of ductal stones. If no stones are present, primary closure of the choledochotomy has been successfully employed, although most surgeons will leave in place a 12 or 14 French T tube, which is brought out through a separate stab incision in the right lateral abdominal wall [*see Figure 25*]. If stone clearance is not achieved, a T tube is mandatory for decompression of the biliary tract and to provide a route for future duct instrumentation. The T tube is

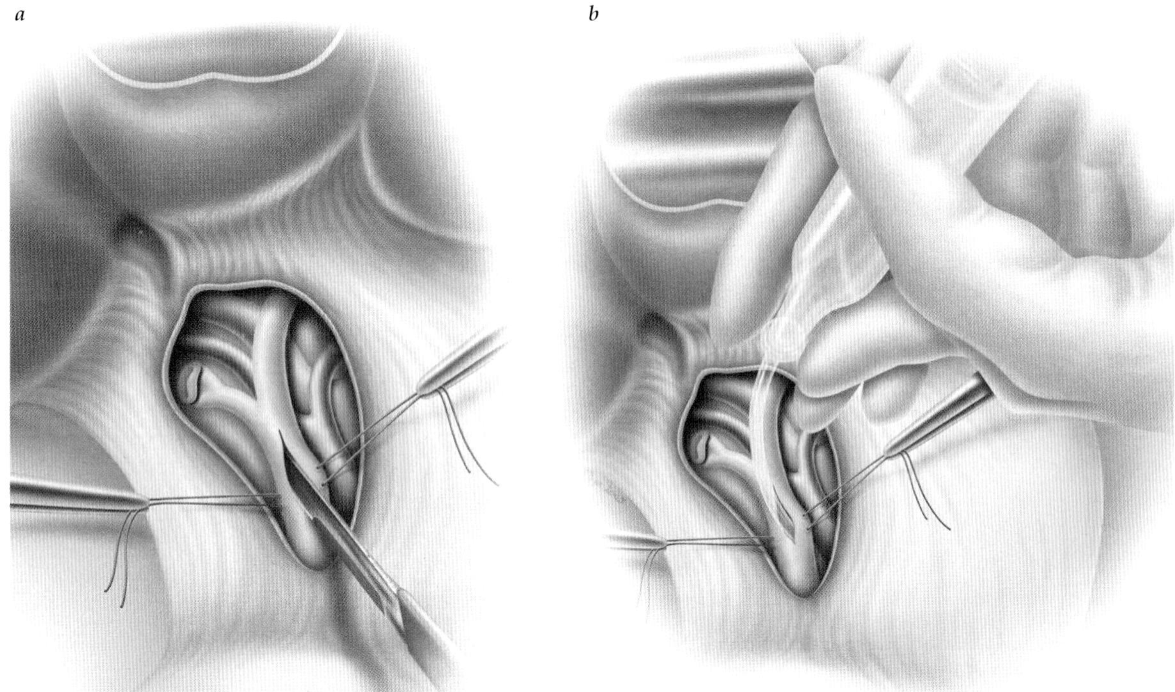

Figure 24 **Open common bile duct exploration. (*a*) The common bile duct is opened vertically between laterally positioned stay sutures. (*b*) A catheter is then used to irrigate and flush stones from the duct. If stones are impacted within the duct, they can be retrieved with Fogarty catheters, wire stone retrieval baskets, or stone retrieval forceps. The choledochoscope can be used if any of these methods fail or as the initial method of exploration.**

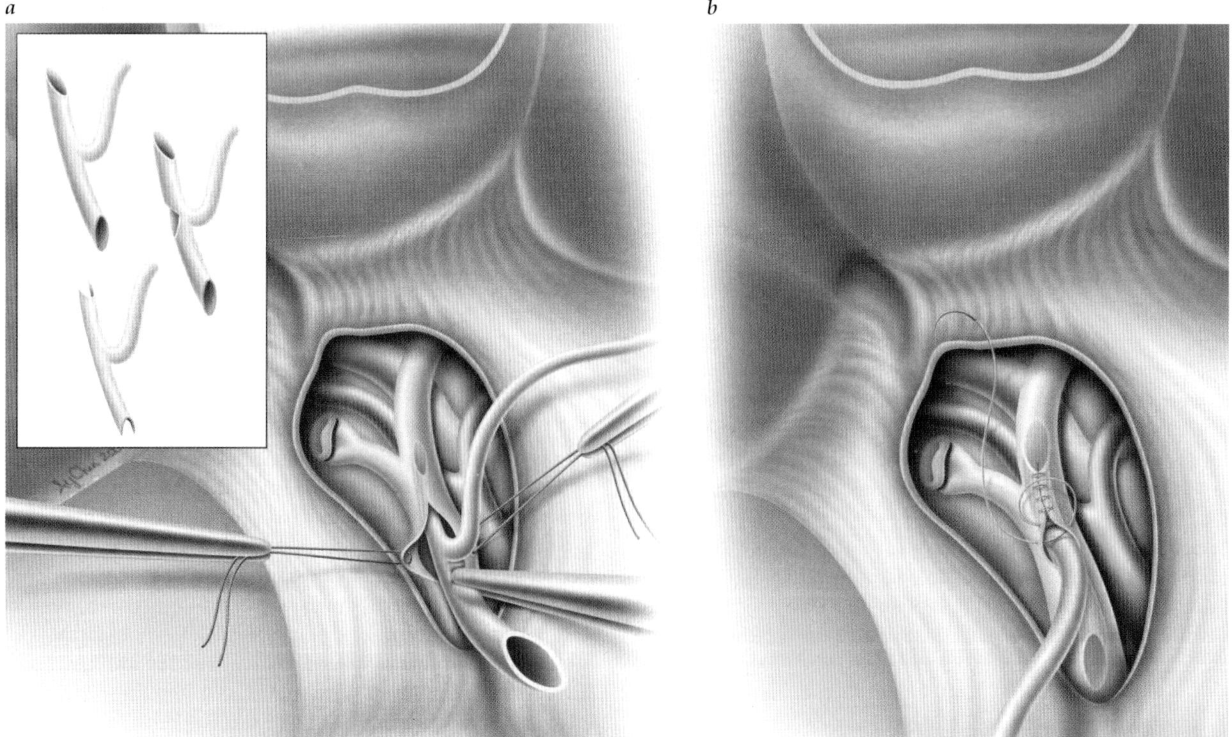

Figure 25 **Open common bile duct exploration. (*a*) After common bile duct exploration, a T tube is fashioned and is placed into the duct. (*b*) Interrupted 4-0 absorbable sutures are used to close the choledochotomy snug around the tube. Completion cholangiography may then be performed. The tube is brought out through the right abdominal wall, through a separate stab incision, and secured to the skin.**

connected to a bag for free drainage. Several days later, cholangiography is repeated. If it shows good flow into the duodenum without obstruction, the tube may be clamped and removed at the 2-week mark. If there are retained stones, a more mature tract must be allowed to develop over 4 to 6 weeks for future instrumentation and stone retrieval. Retained stones may require ERCP, percutaneous transhepatic instrumentation, T tube tract instrumentation, or combinations of these for removal.

Financial Disclosures: None Reported

References

1. McSherry CK. Cholecystectomy: the gold standard. Am J Surg 1989;158:174.
2. Mühe E. Die Erste: Cholecystecktomie durch das Laparoskop. Langenbecks Arch Klin Chir 1986;369:804.
3. Lam D, Miranda R, Hom SJ. Laparoscopic cholecystectomy as an outpatient procedure. J Am Coll Surg 1997;185:152.
4. Abboud PC, Malet PF, Berlin JA, et al. Predictors of common bile duct stones prior to cholecystectomy: a meta-analysis. Gastrointest Endosc 1996;44:450.
5. Barkun AN, Barkun JS, Fried GM, et al. Useful predictors of bile duct stones in patients undergoing laparoscopic cholecystectomy. McGill Gallstone Treatment Group. Ann Surg 1994;220:32.
6. Jones DB, Soper NJ. Common duct stones. In: Cameron JL, editor. Current surgical therapy. 5th ed. St. Louis: Mosby-Year Book; 1995.
7. Paul A, Millat B, Holthhausen U, et al. Diagnosis and treatment of common bile duct stones (CBDS): results of a consensus development conference. Surg Endosc 1998;12:856.
8. Phillips EH. Controversies in the management of common duct calculi. Surg Clin North Am 1994;74:931.
9. Voyles CR, Sanders DL, Hogan R. Common bile duct evaluation in the era of laparoscopic cholecystectomy: 1050 cases later. Ann Surg 1994;219:744.
10. Cohen S, Bacon BR, Berlin JA, et al. National Institutes of Health state-of-the-science conference statement: ERCP for diagnosis and therapy, January 14–16, 2002. Gastrointest Endosc 2002;56:803.
11. Musella M, Barbalace G, Capparelli G, et al. Magnetic resonance imaging in evaluation of the common bile duct. Br J Surg 1998; 85:16.
12. Guibaud L, Bret PM, Reinhold C, et al. Bile duct obstruction and choledocholithiasis: diagnosis with MR cholangiography. Radiology 1995;197:109.
13. Johnson AB, Fink AS. Alternative methods for management of the complicated gallbladder. Semin Laparosc Surg 1998;5:115.
14. Angrisani L, Lorenzo M, De Palma G, et al. Laparoscopic cholecystectomy in obese patients compared with nonobese patients. Surg Laparosc Endosc 1995;5:197.
15. Curet MJ. Special problems in laparoscopic surgery: previous abdominal surgery, obesity, and pregnancy. Surg Clin North Am 2000; 80:1093.
16. Bornman PC, Terblanche J. Subtotal cholecystectomy: for the difficult gallbladder in portal hypertension and cholecystitis. Surgery 1985;98:1
17. Lacy AM, Balaguer C, Andrade E, et al. Laparoscopic cholecystectomy in cirrhotic patients: indication or contraindication? Surg Endosc 1995;9:407.
18. Amos JD, Schorr SJ, Norman PF, et al. Laparoscopic surgery during pregnancy. Am J Surg 1996;171:435.
19. Curet MJ, Allen D, Josloff RK, et al. Laparoscopy during pregnancy. Arch Surg 1996;131:546.
20. SAGES Committee on Standards of Practice. SAGES guidelines for laparoscopic surgery during pregnancy. Santa Monica (CA): Society of American Gastrointestinal Endoscopic Surgeons; 2000. SAGES Publication No.: 0023.
21. Steinbrook RA, Brooks DC, Datta S. Laparoscopic cholecystectomy during pregnancy: review of anesthetic management, surgical considerations. Surg Endosc 1996;10:511.
22. Bhoyrul S, Vierra MA, Nezhat CR, et al. Trocar injuries in laparoscopic surgery. J Am Coll Surg 2001;192:677.
23. Sigman HH, Fried GM, Garzon J, et al. Risks of blind versus open approach to celiotomy for laparoscopic surgery. Surg Laparosc Endosc 1993;3:296.
24. Hunter JG. Avoidance of bile duct injury during laparoscopic cholecystectomy. Am J Surg 1991;162:71.
25. Martin RF, Rossi RL. Bile duct injuries: spectrum, mechanisms of injury, and their prevention. Surg Clin North Am 1994;74:781.
26. Mahmud S, Hamza Y, Nassar AHM. The significance of cystic duct stones encountered during laparoscopic cholecystectomy. Surg Endosc 2001;15:460.
27. Soper NJ, Brunt LM. The case for routine operative cholangiography during laparoscopic cholecystectomy. Surg Clin North Am 1994;74:953.
28. Fletcher DR, Hobbs MST, Tan P, et al. Complications of cholecystectomy: risks of the laparoscopic approach and protective effects of operative cholangiography. Ann Surg 1999;229:449.
29. Wu JS, Dunnegan DL, Soper NJ. The utility of intracorporeal ultrasonography for screening of the bile duct during laparoscopic cholecystectomy. J Gastrointest Surg 1998;2:50.
30. Ohtani T, Kawai C, Shirai Y, et al. Intraoperative ultrasonography versus cholangiography during laparoscopic cholecystectomy: a prospective comparative study. J Am Coll Surg 1997;185:274.
31. Sarli L, Pietra N, Costi R, et al. Gall-bladder perforation during laparoscopic cholecystectomy. World J Surg 1999;23:1186.
32. Schafer M, Suter L, Klaiber C, et al. Spilled gallstones after laparoscopic cholecystectomy. Surg Endosc 1998;12:305.
33. Halevy A, Gold-Deutch R, Negri M, et al. Are elevated liver enzymes and bilirubin levels significant after laparoscopic cholecystectomy in the absence of bile duct injury? Ann Surg 1994;219:362.
34. Ponsky JL. Endoscopic approaches to common bile duct injuries. Surg Clin North Am 1996;76:505.
35. Lillemoe KD, Martin SA, Cameron JL, et al. Major bile duct injuries during laparoscopic cholecystectomy: follow-up after combined surgical and radiologic management. Ann Surg 1997;225:459.
36. Fried GM, Barkun JS, Sigman HH, et al. Factors determining conversion to laparotomy in patients undergoing laparoscopic cholecystectomy. Am J Surg 1994;167:35.
37. Sanabria JR, Gallinger S, Croxford R, et al. Risk factors in elective laparoscopic cholecystectomy for conversion to open cholecystectomy. J Am Coll Surg 1994;179:696.
38. Zucker KA, Flowers JL, Bailey RW, et al. Laparoscopic management of acute cholecystitis. Am J Surg 1993;165:508.
39. Rattner DW, Ferguson C, Warshaw AL. Factors associated with successful laparoscopic cholecystectomy for acute cholecystitis. Ann Surg 1993;217:233.
40. Lo CM, Liu CL, Lai EC, et al. Early versus delayed laparoscopic cholecystectomy for treatment of acute cholecystitis. Ann Surg 1996;223:37.
41. Koo KP, Thirlby RC. Laparoscopic cholecystectomy in acute cholecystitis: what is the optimal timing for operation? Arch Surg 1996;131:540.
42. Park AE, Mastrangelo MJ. Endoscopic retrograde cholangiopancreatography in the management of choledocholithiasis. Surg Endosc 2000;14:219.
43. Petelin JB. Laparoscopic approach to common duct pathology. Am J Surg 1993;165:487.
44. Phillips EH. Laparoscopic transcystic duct common bile duct exploration-outcome and costs. Surg Endosc 1995;9:1240.
45. Rhodes M, Sussman L, Cohen L, et al. Randomized trial of laparoscopic exploration of common bile duct versus postoperative endoscopic retrograde cholangiography for common bile duct stones. Lancet 1998;351:159.
46. Hunter JG, Soper NJ. Laparoscopic management of bile duct stones. Surg Clin North Am 1992;72:1077.
47. Crawford DL, Phillips EH. Laparoscopic common duct exploration. World J Surg 1999;23:343.

Recommended Reading

Asbun HJ, Rossi RL. Techniques of laparoscopic cholecystectomy: the difficult operation. Surg Clin North Am 1994;74:755.

Barkun JS, Barkun AN, Sampalis JS, et al. Randomised controlled trial of laparoscopic versus mini cholecystectomy. The McGill Gallstone Treatment Group. Lancet 1992;340:1116.

Barkun JS, Fried GM, Barkun AN, et al. Cholecystectomy without operative cholangiography: implications for common bile duct injury and retained common bile duct stones. Ann Surg 1993;218:371.

Bass EB, Pitt HA, Lillemoe KD. Cost-effectiveness of laparoscopic cholecystectomy versus open cholecystectomy. Am J Surg 1993;165:466.

Bernard HR, Hartman TW. Complications after laparoscopic cholecystectomy. Am J Surg 1993;165:533.

Branum G, Schmitt C, Baillie J, et al. Management of major biliary complications after laparoscopic cholecystectomy. Ann Surg 1993;217:532.

Clair DG, Brooks DC. Laparoscopic cholangiography: the case for a selective approach. Surg Clin North Am 1994;74:961.

Cotton PB. Endoscopic retrograde cholangiopancreatography and laparoscopic cholecystectomy. Am J Surg 1993;165:474.

Crist DW, Gadacz TR. Laparoscopic anatomy of the biliary tree. Surg Clin North Am 1993;73:785.

Cuschieri A, Lezoche E, Morino M, et al. E.A.E.S. multicenter prospective randomised trial comparing two-stage vs single-stage management of patients with gallstone disease and ductal calculi. Surg Endosc 1999;13:952.

Deziel DJ. Complications of cholecystectomy: incidence, clinical manifestations, and diagnosis. Surg Clin North Am 1994;74:809.

Deziel DJ, Millikan KW, Economou SG, et al. Complications of laparoscopic cholecystectomy: a national survey of 4,292 hospitals and an analysis of 77,604 cases. Am J Surg 1993;165:9.

Freeman ML, Nelson DB, Sherman S, et al. Complications of endoscopic biliary sphincterotomy. N Engl J Med 1996;335:909.

Halpin VJ, Dunnegan D, Soper NJ. Laparoscopic intracorporeal ultrasound vs fluoroscopic intraoperative cholangiography. Surg Endosc 2002;16:336.

Hunter JG, Trus T. Laparoscopic cholecystectomy, intraoperative cholangiography, and common bile duct exploration. In: Nyhus LM, Baker RJ, Fischer JE, editors. Mastery of surgery. 3rd ed. New York: Little, Brown & Co; 1997.

Kane RL, Lurie N, Borbas C, et al. The outcomes of elective laparoscopic and open cholecystectomies. J Am Coll Surg 1995;180:136.

Korman J, Cosgrove J, Furman M, et al. The role of endoscopic retrograde cholangiopancreatography and cholangiography in the laparoscopic era. Ann Surg 1996;223:212.

Liberman MA, Phillips EH, Carroll BJ, et al. Cost-effective management of complicated choledocholithiasis: laparoscopic transcystic duct exploration or endoscopic sphincterotomy. J Am Coll Surg 1996;182:488.

MacFadyen BV, Vecchio R, Ricardo AE, et al. Bile duct injury after laparoscopic cholecystectomy: the United States experience. Surg Endosc 1998;12:315.

McGahan JP, Stein M. Complications of laparoscopic cholecystectomy: imaging and intervention. AJR Am J Roentgenol 1995;165:1089.

Menack MJ, Arregui ME. Laparoscopic sonography of the biliary tree and pancreas. Surg Clin North Am 2000;80:1151.

Millitz K, Moote DJ, Sparrow RK, et al. Pneumoperitoneum after laparoscopic cholecystectomy: frequency and duration as seen on upright chest radiographs. AJR Am J Roentgenol 1994;163:837.

National Institutes of Health Consensus Development Conference Statement on Gallstones and Laparoscopic Cholecystectomy. Am J Surg 1993;165:390.

Olsen D. Bile duct injuries during laparoscopic cholecystectomy. Surg Endosc 1997;11:133.

Phillips EH, Carroll BJ, Pearlstein AR, et al. Laparoscopic choledochoscopy and extraction of common bile duct stones. World J Surg 1993;17:22.

Ress AM, Sarr MG, Nagorney DM, et al. Spectrum and management of major complications of laparoscopic cholecystectomy. Am J Surg 1993;165:655.

Rös A, Gustafsson L, Krook H, et al. Laparoscopic cholecystectomy versus mini-laparotomy cholecystectomy: a prospective, randomized, single-blind study. Ann Surg 2001;234:741.

Schrenk P, Woisetschlager R, Wayand WU. Laparoscopic cholecystectomy: cause of conversions in 1300 patients and analysis of risk factors. Surg Endosc 1995;9:25.

Society of American Gastrointestinal Endoscopic Surgeons. Guidelines for the clinical application of laparoscopic biliary tract surgery. Surg Endosc 1994;8:1457.

Soper NJ, Flye MW, Brunt LM, et al. Diagnosis and management of biliary complications of laparoscopic cholecystectomy. Am J Surg 1993;165:663.

Strasberg SM, Hertl M, Soper NJ. An analysis of the problem of biliary injury during laparoscopic cholecystectomy. J Am Coll Surg 1995;180:101.

Traverso LW, Hargrave K. A prospective cost analysis of laparoscopic cholecystectomy. Am J Surg 1995;169:503.

Wherry DC, Rob CG, Marohn MR, et al. An external audit of laparoscopic cholecystectomy performed in medical treatment facilities of the Department of Defense. Ann Surg 1994;220:626.

Woods MS, Traverso LW, Kozarek RA, et al. Characteristics of biliary tract complications during laparoscopic cholecystectomy: a multi-institutional study. Am J Surg 1994;167:27.

Zucker KA, Josloff RK. Transcystic common bile duct exploration. In: MacFadyen BV, Ponsky JL, editors. Operative laparoscopy and thoracoscopy. Philadelphia: Lippincott-Raven Publishers; 1996.

Acknowledgments

Figures 2, 5 Tom Moore.

Figure 18 Courtesy of Nathaniel J. Soper, MD, Northwestern University Feinberg School of Medicine, Chicago.

Figures 21 through 25 Alice Y. Chen.

21 PROCEDURES FOR BENIGN AND MALIGNANT BILIARY TRACT DISEASE

Susan Logan, MD, MPP, and David Linehan, MD, FACS

Over the past several decades, advances in imaging technology have been made that allow more accurate diagnosis of biliary tract diseases and better planning of surgical procedures and other interventions aimed at managing these conditions. Operative techniques have also improved as a result of a better understanding of biliary and hepatic anatomy and physiology. The role of endoscopists and interventional radiologists in the management of benign conditions, as well as palliation of malignant disease, is also expanding. Accordingly, biliary tract surgery, like many other areas of modern surgery, is constantly changing.

In this chapter, we describe common operations performed to treat diseases of the biliary tract, emphasizing details of operative planning and intraoperative technique and suggesting specific strategies for preventing common problems. Complex biliary tract procedures should be performed only in specialized centers where experienced multidisciplinary teams, including hepatobiliary surgeons, endoscopists, interventional radiologists, and intensivists, collaborate to manage the special problems and requirements of patients undergoing such procedures.

Preoperative Evaluation

ANATOMY

Before embarking on any operation on the biliary tract, the surgeon must accurately define the relevant anatomy and extent of disease. Familiarity with the numerous variations of ductal anatomy is crucial [*see Figure 1a*]. In the prevailing pattern, the segment 6 and 7 ducts coalesce to form the right posterior sectional bile duct, and the segment 5 and 8 ducts join to form the right anterior sectional duct. The right anterior duct is usually oriented vertically, whereas the right posterior duct tends to follow a more horizontal course. The right anterior and posterior sectional ducts unite to form the right hepatic duct. Note that the posterior sectional duct crosses in front of the right anterior portal vein before joining the right anterior bile duct (Hjortsjo crook) [*see Figure 1b*]. Division of the right anterior portal pedicle too close to its origin may result in injury to the right posterior bile duct. The right hepatic duct runs a short extrahepatic course before joining the left hepatic duct at the hepatic confluence, forming the common hepatic duct. Similarly, in the prevailing pattern, the ducts draining segments 2 and 3 join to form the left lateral sectional duct. This duct then crosses behind the ascending portion of the left portal vein and joins the duct from segment 4 (also called the medial sectional bile duct) to form the left hepatic duct. The left hepatic duct runs a longer, usually horizontal, extrahepatic course at the base of segment 4b.

The above description is of the prevailing pattern of biliary anatomy, but the surgeon must be aware of several common variations, particularly those involving the right-sided ducts [*see Figure 1c*]. Not infrequently, one of the right sectional ducts crosses the midplane of the liver to drain directly into the left hepatic duct. If this variation is present and the surgeon performs a standard left hepatectomy, the right-sided duct(s) may be injured. The segment 8 duct may also drain into the posterior sectional duct. Other important variations include a low insertion of the right hepatic duct or an anomalous low insertion of a right sectional, segmental, or subsegmental duct directly into the common hepatic duct, the common bile duct, or even the cystic duct. Variations to the left ductal system most frequently involve variable numbers and sites of insertion of the segment 4 duct(s). Rarely, the segment 4 duct(s) may drain directly into the common hepatic duct or confluence.[1,2]

Finally, familiarity with the plate-sheath system is essential to performing safe dissection at the hepatic hilum [*see Figure 1d*]. This system is composed of four thick, fibrous plates—hilar, umbilical, cystic, and arantian—of which the hilar plate is most important to the liver surgeon. The hilar plate lies mainly in the coronal plane, at the base of segment 4 and posterior to the vasculobiliary structures in the porta. Superiorly, however, the hilar plate curves anteriorly, along the posterior aspect of the quadrate lobe, and here it is superior to all structures in the porta hepatis, including the right and left bile ducts. As the three vasculobiliary structures pass through the hilar plate, they are "sheathed" within the same fibrous tissue and become a single unit above the plate. Identification of these structures as a single unit above the hilar plate is much simpler and safer than individually isolating each structure lower in the porta hepatis. To gain access to these sheathed pedicles above the hilar plate, the surgeon must dissect the upper border of the hilar plate away from the liver, a technique referred to as "lowering the hilar plate."[3]

IMAGING STUDIES

High-quality ultrasonography is useful for confirming the presence of biliary dilatation, and duplex ultrasonography is excellent for assessing vascular involvement. However, ultrasonography is very user dependent and, even in experienced hands, is less helpful for determining resectability or the level or cause of obstruction. Multidetector computed tomography (MDCT) is noninvasive and provides excellent information regarding mass lesions, the presence or absence of ductal dilatation, the extent and level of duct obstruction, and the extent of vessel involvement. Multiphase computed tomography (CT) generates precise and reliable images of the relevant arterial, portal, and venous anatomy. Therefore, conventional

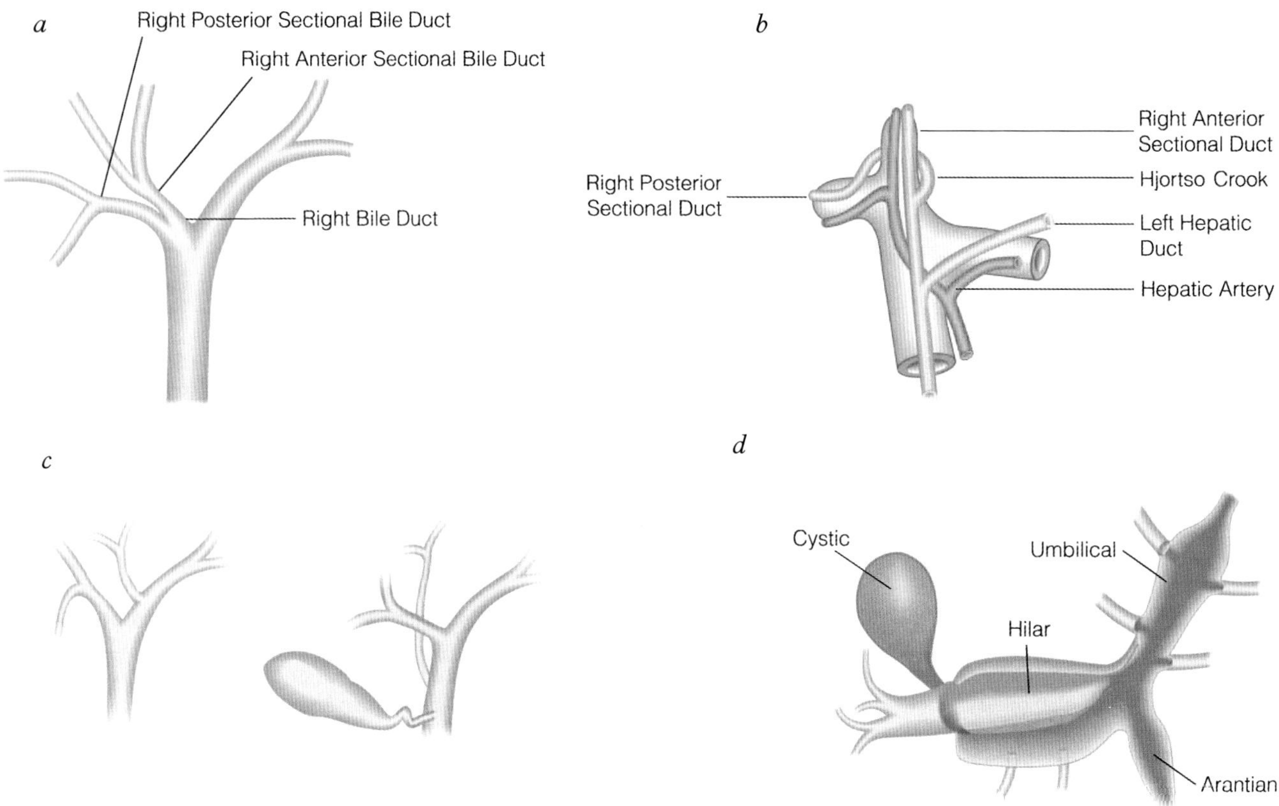

Figure 1 **(*a*) The most common pattern of bile duct anatomy. (*b*) Hjortso crook. (*c*) Common variations of right hepatic duct anatomy: (*left*) right anterior or right posterior duct draining into left hepatic duct; (*right*) low insertion of right sectional duct. (*d*) Plate-sheath system of the liver.**

angiography is no longer used to determine resectability. Magnetic resonance imaging (MRI) and magnetic resonance cholangiopancreatography (MRCP) can provide detailed images of biliary anatomy and have reported accuracy rates of 100% and 95%, respectively, for determining the location and cause of biliary obstruction. Direct cholangiography—percutaneous transhepatic cholangiography (PTC) and endoscopic retrograde cholangiopancreatography (ERCP)—may supply additional information about ductal anatomy, is useful for providing tissue (e.g., brush cytology) for diagnosis, and allows drainage of the biliary tree prior to operation. When major liver resection is anticipated, liver volumetric analysis using three-dimensional reconstruction of axial CT images should also be performed to confirm adequate size of the future remnant liver.[4]

In the case of malignant diseases of the biliary tract, evidence of distant organ metastases remains a contraindication to operation. The resectability of locally advanced hilar cholangiocarcinoma depends on the extent of vasculobiliary involvement, the presence or absence of contralateral lobar atrophy, and the predicted size of the future remnant liver.[5] Repair of biliary injuries should be deferred in the setting of cholangitis, intra-abdominal infection, and sepsis [*see* Repair of Biliary Injuries, *below*].

MANAGEMENT OF BILIARY OBSTRUCTION

Jaundice by itself does not increase operative risk, and we do not routinely perform preoperative biliary drainage in all patients with jaundice.[6] However, long-standing biliary obstruction has secondary effects that may increase perioperative morbidity and mortality. In the presence of these secondary effects, we recommend elective preoperative biliary decompression.

Infection

Patients with cholangitis, whether spontaneous or induced by duct instrumentation (via PTC or ERCP), should be treated with biliary drainage and appropriate antibiotics until they are infection free. We recommend antibiotic treatment and postponement of operation for at least 3 to 4 weeks. Rarely, antibiotics and endoscopic or transhepatic drainage are not immediately effective, and patients with biliary tract infection (e.g., associated with choledocholithiasis) may require urgent surgical decompression. Broad-spectrum antibiotics, including coverage of anaerobic organisms, should be administered preoperatively.

Renal Dysfunction

The pathogenesis of renal failure in the setting of obstructive jaundice is multifactorial. Extracellular water depletion, increased plasma renin and aldosterone activity, a paradoxical increase in atrial natriuretic peptide, and myocardial dysfunction are all thought to contribute to renal insufficiency in jaundiced patients.[7] Because the combination of a high bilirubin level and hypovolemia is a significant risk factor for acute renal failure, patients with biliary obstruction should be well hydrated before receiving intravenous contrast agents or undergoing operative procedures. In patients with acute renal dysfunction secondary to biliary obstruction, decompression of the bile duct until renal function returns to normal is advisable before any major elective procedure for malignant disease.

Impaired Immunologic Function and Malnutrition

In patients with long-standing biliary obstruction, absence of bile salts in the gut lumen may lead to severe malnutrition and contribute to impaired immune function.[8] Decompression of the bile duct until immune function and nutritional status are restored to normal is indicated before any major elective procedure is undertaken. This may take as long as 4 to 6 weeks.

Coagulation Dysfunction

Prolonged bile duct obstruction may lead to significant deficits in vitamin K–dependent clotting factors. These deficits should be corrected with fresh frozen plasma and vitamin K before an operative procedure is begun. Even if there is no measurable coagulation dysfunction, vitamin K should be given to all patients with obstructive jaundice at least 24 hours before operation to replenish their depleted vitamin K stores.

Projected Major Liver Resection

If resection of an obstructing bile duct tumor is likely to necessitate major liver resection (e.g., a right trisectionectomy), we recommend unilateral decompression of the liver segments that are to be retained. Unilateral drainage is usually sufficient to normalize serum bilirubin and allows atrophy of the undrained segments to occur, along with concomitant hypertrophy of the future liver remnant.

Operative Planning

GENERAL TECHNICAL CONSIDERATIONS

Place the patient in the supine position on an operating table that can be rotated, tilted, and elevated. Equipment for fluoroscopy, intraoperative ultrasonography and choledochoscopy should be available during major resections. Access to a pathology department that can perform cytologic or frozen-section examination of tissue is essential in operations for malignant disease.

A right subcostal incision with vertical midline extension provides excellent exposure for most open procedures on the liver and biliary tract. For more extensive resections or reconstructions, the right subcostal incision can be extended laterally below the costal margin and across the midline to the left as a chevron incision. A vertical midline incision may give sufficient exposure in very thin persons. In any case, the incision must be long enough to allow sufficient visualization and as much mobilization of the liver as is necessary for safe performance of the procedure.

Adequate exposure and lighting are essential. The best retractors are those that can be fixed to the table while remaining flexible in terms of placement and angles of retraction. Retractor blades should be positioned to lift the ribcage anteriorly and cephalad and to pull the right abdominal wall laterally.

Locating the hepatoduodenal ligament and dissecting the structures in the porta hepatis are straightforward in patients who have never had an abdominal operation. However, in patients who have undergone previous operations, there may be considerable obliteration of planes. The following are suggestions for gaining access to the subhepatic space in patients who have had previous abdominal procedures:

1. Use the falciform ligament as a landmark. In reoperative surgery, the key to opening up the upper abdomen is the falciform ligament. This structure should be found immediately after the opening of the abdominal wall and retracted superiorly. The omentum, the colon, and the stomach are then dissected inferiorly, and a plane that leads to the hepatoduodenal ligament and the porta hepatis is thereby opened.
2. Take the right posterolateral approach. When the colon and the duodenum are densely adhesed to the undersurface of the right liver, separation may be difficult. In most patients, an open space remains that can be approached by sliding the left hand posteriorly to the right of these adhesions and into the (usually open) subhepatic space in front of the kidney and behind the adhesions. Anterior retraction allows identification of the adherent structures by palpation and permits dissection of the adhesions in a lateral-to-medial direction. The undersurface of the liver is thus cleared, and the hepatoduodenal ligament can be approached.
3. Take the lesser sac approach. Ordinarily, the foramen of Winslow is open, and the left index finger can be passed through it from the right subhepatic space. When the foramen of Winslow is obliterated, however, one should approach it from the left, dividing the lesser omentum and passing an index finger from the lesser sac behind the hepatoduodenal ligament to reopen the foramen of Winslow by blunt dissection.

For a discussion of techniques to aid in the safe exposure of the porta hepatis in patients who have sustained a bile duct injury or have had previous biliary operations, refer to the section below on repair of biliary injuries: exposure of the porta hepatis.

General Guidelines for Biliary Anastomoses

As a rule, biliary anastomoses, whether of duct to bowel or of duct to duct, heal very well provided that the surgeon adheres to the following principles: (1) preservation of adequate blood supply, (2) avoidance of tension, (3) accurate placement of sutures with mucosa-to-mucosa apposition, and (4) construction of anastomoses of adequate caliber. In preparing the bile duct for anastomosis, it is essential to define adequate margins while avoiding excessive dissection that might compromise the blood supply to the duct. In repairs that follow acute injuries, it is important to resect crushed or devascularized tissue; however, in late repairs, it is not necessary to resect all scar tissue as long as an adequate opening can be made in the proximal obstructed duct through normal healthy tissue and as long as mucosa, rather than granulation tissue, is present at the duct margin. The length of the corresponding opening in the jejunal loop should be significantly smaller than the bile duct opening because the bowel opening tends to enlarge during the procedure.

Certain principles of suture placement apply to all biliary anastomoses. Mucosa-to-mucosa apposition is essential for good healing and the prevention of late stricture.[9] Sutures should be of an absorbable, synthetic monofilament material and should be as fine as is practical (e.g., 5-0 for a normal duct and 4-0 for a thickened duct). Because the bile duct wall has only one layer, biliary anastomoses should all be single layer. Sutures should pass through all layers of the bowel, taking sizable bites of the seromuscular layer and much smaller bites of the mucosa, and should take moderate-sized (1 to 3 mm, depending on duct diameter) bites in the bile duct. Interrupted sutures are used when access is difficult or the duct is small; continuous sutures are used when access is easy and the duct is larger. Sutures should be securely placed but should not be so tight as to injure the tissues. Magnification with loupes is useful when anastomosing small ducts. With the exception of repair of high, complex bile duct injuries, we do not routinely place stents for biliary anastomoses. Some studies suggest that placement of drains is not necessary after biliary operations.[10,11] Nevertheless, it is currently our practice to place a drain at the time of the operation and to remove the drain within 2 to 3 days if the output does not show evidence of a bile leak.

When the bile duct opening has a vertical configuration (as in side-to-side choledochoduodenostomy or choledochojejunostomy), we place stay sutures inferiorly and superiorly in the duct and at corresponding points in the intestine. Traction is placed on these sutures to line up the adjacent walls. One side of the anastomosis is done first; the bowel is then rotated 180°, and the other side is completed [*see Figure 2*]. This maneuver may be facilitated by retracting the first interrupted posterior stitch to the opposite side to serve as a pivotal stitch. We recommend sewing about two thirds of the first wall and two thirds of the second, leaving the anterior third of the circumference (the easiest part) to be closed last. For end-to-side choledochojejunostomy, or when the bile duct opening lies transversely, as in bifurcation reconstruction, lateral stay sutures are placed first, and the posterior wall stitches are placed from inside the lumen. If interrupted sutures are used, they are all placed individually before any of them are tied, with the untied tails carefully clamped and arranged in order. When the posterior wall sutures have been tied, the anterior wall can then be sutured with either continuous or interrupted sutures [*see Figure 3*].

When the intended anastomosis will be to a very small-caliber or intrahepatic duct, and access is particularly difficult because of some combination of an unfavorable position, a previous scar, or a stiff liver that is difficult to retract, another technique may be useful. Beginning left to right, place all of the anterior wall stitches (inside to outside) into the duct. Clamp each suture and place them in order on a single retracting forceps with the needles left attached. Retract the sutures superiorly to expose the posterior wall of the duct [*see Figure 3c*]. Again, working left to right, place the posterior stitches inside to outside through the bowel wall and outside to inside into the duct. Remove the needles at the completion of each stitch, clamp each suture, and keep them in order as described for the anterior row. When all of the posterior stitches have been placed, carefully appose the bowel wall to the bile duct, tie all but the two corner stitches in order, and cut the sutures. Leaving the corner stitches (at 3 and 9 o'clock) loose facilitates accurate placement of the lateral and medial stitches of the anterior wall. Finally, place the anterior wall stitches inside to outside on the bowel, sequentially clamp the stitches until the last stitch is placed, and then tie the stitches in order and cut the sutures.[9]

When the duct is very small, three additional techniques may be useful for increasing the size of the lumen:

1. An anterior longitudinal incision can be made in a small common bile duct (CBD) and the sharp corners trimmed to enlarge the opening [*see Figure 4a*].
2. If the cystic duct is present alongside a divided CBD, an incision can be made in the shared wall to create a single larger lumen [*see Figure 4b*].
3. If the bifurcation has been resected, two small ducts can be brought together and sutures placed into their adjoining walls to form a single larger lumen as long as the space between the ducts is small and the ducts can be brought together without tension [*see Figure 4c*]. If the ducts cannot be brought together without tension, more than one anastomosis must be created.

Construction of a Roux Loop

When the jejunum is used for long-term biliary drainage, we prefer a 60 cm Roux loop to prevent reflux of small bowel contents into the biliary system. In the creation of the loop, it is important to select a segment of jejunum with a well-defined vascular arcade that will be long enough to support a tension-free anastomosis. If access to the biliary system will be required in the future (e.g., in an operation for recurrent intrahepatic stones), the loop should be long enough to allow one to place a tube jejunostomy, fixing the loop to the abdominal wall with nonabsorbable sutures. The site of attachment should be marked with metallic clips to facilitate future percutaneous puncture, cannulation, and removal of recurrent or persistent stones. The tube can be removed after postoperative imaging studies confirm that the biliary tree is free of stones.

Choledochoduodenostomy

Choledochoduodenostomy is a relatively straightforward end-to-side (or sometimes side-to-side) biliary-enteric bypass procedure that is useful in certain restricted circumstances. It is most commonly used in patients with multiple bile duct stones when there is concern about leaving residual stones at the time of CBD exploration, as well as in patients with recurrent bile duct stones when endoscopic papillotomy either cannot be done or has been unsuccessful. Choledochoduodenostomy has the advantage of being simpler and safer than transduodenal sphincteroplasty. It is also used in patients with benign distal biliary obstruction (e.g., from chronic pancreatitis or a very low bile duct injury) and occasionally in patients with malignant distal CBD obstruction whose life expectancy is limited. Choledochoduodenostomy works best if the CBD is at least 1 cm in diameter.

CONTRAINDICATIONS

Choledochoduodenostomy should not be used in patients with actual or potential duodenal obstruction.

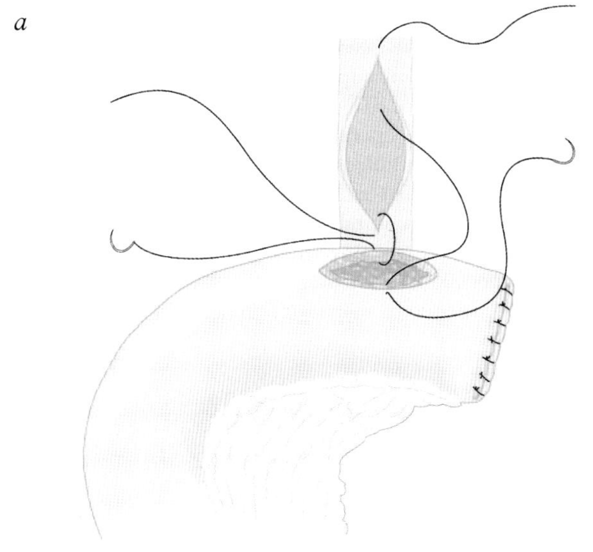

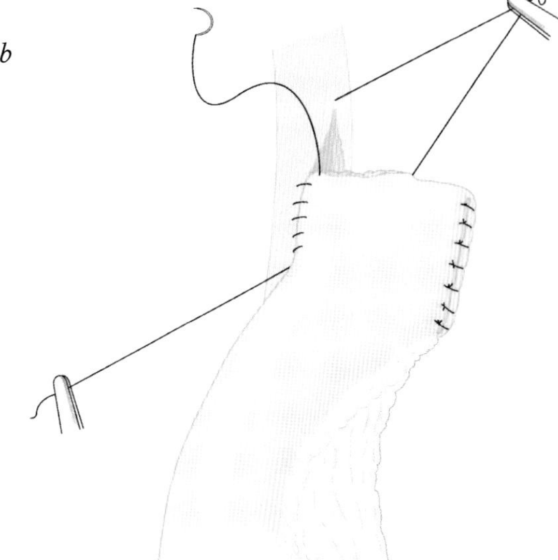

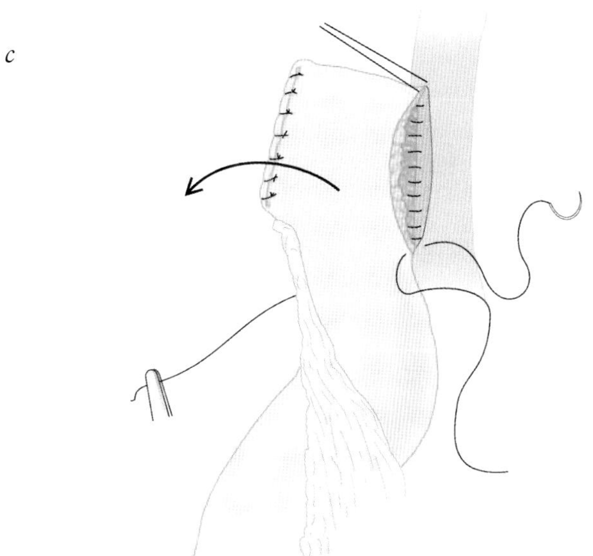

Figure 2 **Technical issues in biliary anastomosis. Shown is a side-to-side choledochojejunostomy using a vertical incision in the bile duct. The same technique can be used for choledochoduodenostomy or end-to-side choledochojejunostomy. (*a*) Inferior and superior corner continuous sutures are placed. (*b*) One side of the anastomosis is sewn first (here, the right side). (*c*) The bowel is rotated 180° so that the other side is exposed. The other side of the anastomosis is then sewn (here, the left side).**

OPERATIVE TECHNIQUE

Mobilize the duodenum to allow approximation to the CBD without tension. Ordinarily, the first part of the duodenum can easily be rolled up against the CBD; however, in patients who have chronic pancreatitis or have previously undergone an abdominal procedure, extensive kocherization may be required. If satisfactory approximation is not achieved with this maneuver, a choledochojejunostomy should be performed instead.

Expose the CBD as described elsewhere. Make longitudinal incisions in both the duodenum and the duct [*see Figure 2*] and create the anastomosis as described previously [*see* Operative Planning, General Technical Considerations, General Guidelines for Biliary Anastomoses, *above*].

COMPLICATIONS

Late closure or stricture of the anastomosis may occur if the CBD is small, has inadequate blood supply, or malignant disease is present. Consider alternative methods of biliary decompression in these situations.

Cholangitis related to the presence of food in the CBD distal to the anastomosis (so-called sump syndrome) is an uncommon occurrence. The larger the anastomosis, the smaller is the likelihood that this complication will occur.

Cholecystojejunostomy

Cholecystojejunostomy may be performed to treat malignant biliary obstruction in selected patients whose lesions are found to be unresectable at operation and whose life expectancy is short.

CONTRAINDICATIONS

Absolute contraindications to this drainage procedure include obstruction above the cystic duct entry point, evidence of cholecystitis, and benign causes of biliary

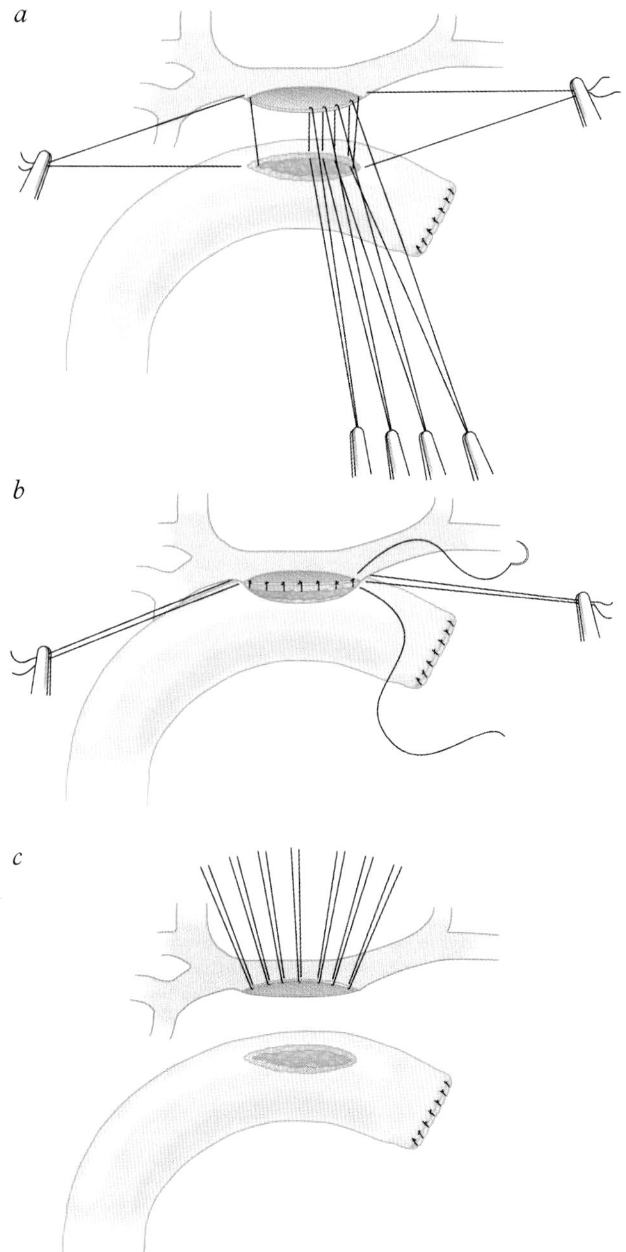

Figure 3 **Technical issues in biliary anastomosis. Shown is an end-to-side choledochojejunostomy using a transverse opening in the bile duct. This technique can be used at any level. (*a*) Corner sutures and posterior wall sutures are all placed before being tied. (*b*) The posterior wall is completed, and the anterior wall is sewn. (*c*) In difficult cases, the anterior wall sutures may be placed first and then retracted superiorly.**

obstruction (i.e., patients with normal life expectancy). This operation is not the preferred procedure for long-term decompression.

OPERATIVE TECHNIQUE

Step 1: Verification of Feasibility of Procedure

The cystic duct must be patent. Its junction with the CBD must be at least 1 cm above the tumor obstruction [*see Figure 5*]. The suitability of the anatomy for cholecystojejunostomy should have been verified by preoperative cholangiography; if not, intraoperative cholangiography via the gallbladder or the CBD is mandatory. If one still cannot be certain that the operation is feasible, the CBD should be opened and a choledochoenterostomy performed. The finding of a bile-filled gallbladder is not sufficient evidence that the patient is a suitable candidate for a cholecystojejunostomy. The gallbladder must be normal: there should be no evidence of cholecystitis or stones. Verify normal status by inspection, palpation, and, if necessary, needle cholecystography.

Step 2: Preparation for Anastomosis

Select a site near the fundus for the anastomosis and anchor an appropriate, tension-free segment of proximal jejunum to the gallbladder with two fine stay sutures. Between the two stay sutures, make a 2 cm transverse opening in the gallbladder and a corresponding longitudinal incision in the antimesenteric border of the bowel.

Step 3: Anastomosis

Create a single-layer anastomosis using a continuous monofilament absorbable suture or a stapler.

COMPLICATIONS

Bile leakage may occur if there is excessive tension on the anastomosis. In addition, jaundice may persist if there is unrecognized cystic duct obstruction resulting from inflammation or an unnoticed stone in the cystic duct or the gallbladder. Recurrent jaundice is usually the result of extension from an obstructing tumor that has involved the cystic duct–CBD junction.

Choledochojejunostomy

Choledochojejunostomy, one of the most commonly performed biliary tract procedures, is done to provide biliary drainage after CBD resection, repair of ductal injury, or relief of obstruction caused by a benign or malignant stricture. To reduce the likelihood of reflux of intestinal contents into the biliary tract, we prefer to use a 60 cm Roux-en-Y jejunal limb for the anastomosis [*see* Operative Planning, General Technical Considerations, Construction of a Roux Loop, *above*].

When the operation is performed after CBD resection, an end-to-side choledochojejunostomy using the proximal transected duct is preferred as long as adequate vascularization of the transected bile duct is confirmed. When the operation is performed for bile duct obstruction resulting from tumor or stricture and no resection has been performed, a side-to-side anastomosis is constructed.

OPERATIVE TECHNIQUE

Step 1: Preparation for Anastomosis

Preparation for an end-to-side anastomosis includes resection of any crushed or devitalized bile duct tissue. The CBD should be trimmed back to healthy, viable, bleeding duct wall.

If a side-to-side anastomosis is being performed for stricture or tumor, the proximal duct is almost always dilated and

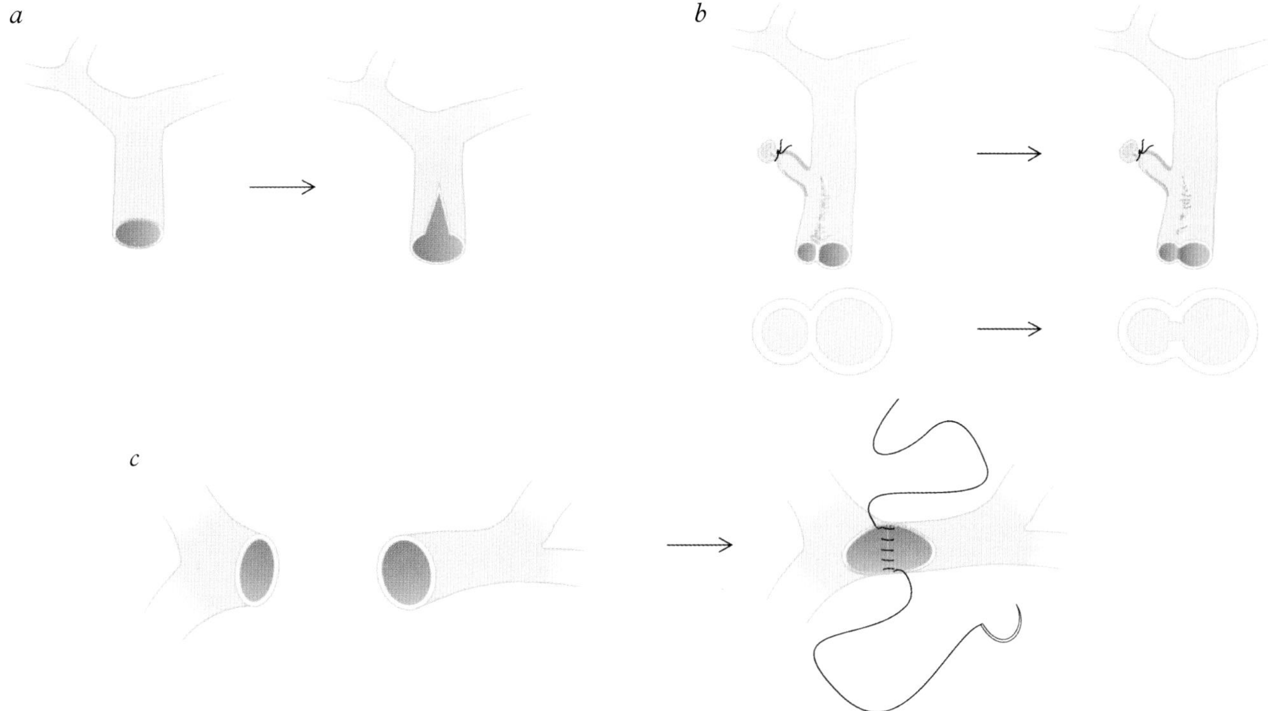

Figure 4 **Technical issues in biliary anastomosis. Shown are three methods of enlarging a small duct. (*a*) An anterior longitudinal incision can be made in the duct wall. (*b*) A wall shared by the common bile duct and the cystic duct can be divided. (*c*) Adjoining walls of two small ducts can be sutured together to make a single opening for anastomosis.**

has thicker walls, facilitating a vertical incision on the anterior surface. When the procedure is being done for malignant disease, the incision should be made as high as possible above the malignancy to delay the eventual obstruction of the anastomosis by tumor growth.

Step 2: Anastomosis

When the duct is large, a secure, tension-free anastomosis is easily constructed by means of the techniques previously illustrated. When the duct is small, extra effort must be made to place sutures carefully to prevent narrowing of the lumen.

TROUBLESHOOTING

Injured ducts must be adequately débrided, even if this means extending the resection of the duct to the bifurcation. However, preservation of the blood supply to the CBD is essential. Avoid extensive mobilization of the duct from the surrounding tissues to prevent injury to the ductal blood supply. Finally, longitudinal incisions should not be made in the medial or lateral (3 and 9 o'clock) portions of the CBD, where the major longitudinal blood supply is located.

Meticulous surgical technique is critical for ensuring good healing and preventing stricture. Use the finest suture material that will do the job and employ magnifying devices to facilitate accurate placement of sutures. Routine postoperative stenting is unnecessary, but stents may be helpful in those very rare cases in which mucosal apposition cannot be accomplished. In these situations, sutures may have to be placed in surrounding liver or scar tissue in much the same way as in a Kasai procedure.[12] In difficult cases of proximal stricture, the surgeon may be forced to incise and lower the liver plate and seek out viable intrahepatic ducts for anastomosis [*see* Repair of Biliary Injuries, *below*].

COMPLICATIONS

The main complications of a choledochojejunostomy are bile leakage, late stricture, and recurrent jaundice as a result of tumor extension [*see* Cholecystojejunostomy *and* Choledochoduodenostomy, *above*].

Choledochal Cyst Resection

Choledochal cysts are generally categorized according to the Todani classification [*see Figure 6*]. More than 80% are type I cysts that involve the CBD in its accessible portion. The following discussion addresses the resection of type I cysts and those type IV cysts that include the proximal right or left hepatic ducts.

Most choledochal cysts are associated with an abnormal junction of the pancreatic duct and the distal CBD. Preoperative cholangiography to clarify the anatomy is important for preventing injury to the pancreatic duct, especially when an intrapancreatic resection is required. Occasionally, intraoperative cholangiography is needed to clarify abnormal anatomy. Patients may be symptomatic as a result of stones within the cyst, infection, or malignancy, any of which is an indication for operation. The increased risk of bile duct malignancy associated with choledochal cysts, and the high mortality associated with cholangiocarcinoma, is justification for prophylactic cyst resection even in asymptomatic patients.

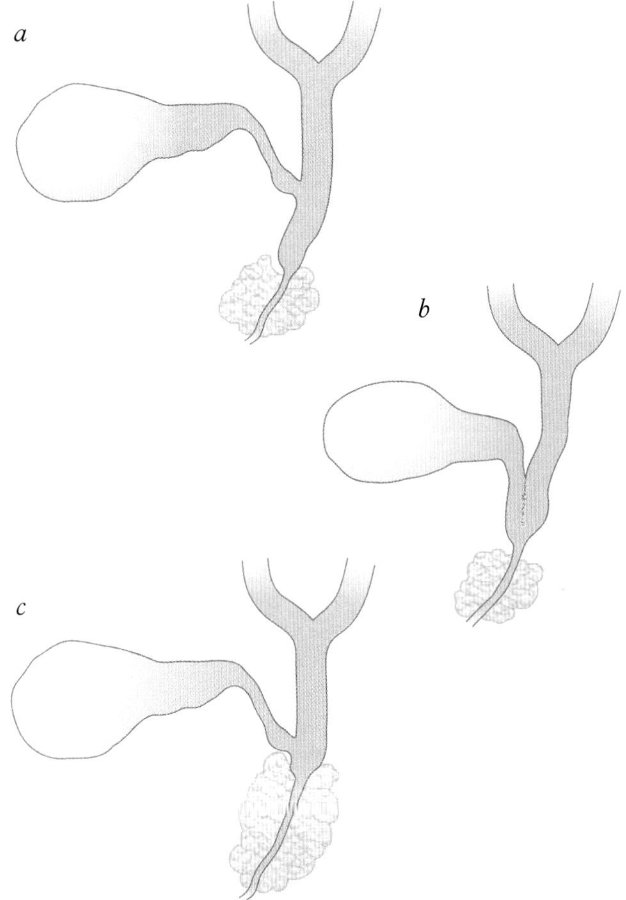

Figure 5 **Cholecystojejunostomy. Cholangiography is essential for determining whether the anatomy is suitable (*a*) or unsuitable (*b*, *c*) for the procedure.**

The objectives of treatment are (1) to remove the cyst completely, along with the gallbladder and any stones that remain in the bile ducts proximal to the cyst, and (2) to restore biliary-enteric drainage. Resection of a choledochal cyst may be made more difficult by several factors, such as previous operations, recurrent bouts of infection and inflammation in the cyst, and portal hypertension, which may develop as a result of long-standing cholangitis or portal vein thrombosis.[13]

OPERATIVE TECHNIQUE

Resection of a choledochal cyst may be difficult, especially if inflammation is present. In addition, dissection of a choledochal cyst in its intrapancreatic portion is hazardous because of the vascularity of this region and the difficulty identifying anatomic structures.

Step 1: Clarification of Anatomy

The proximal and distal extent of the cyst and the presence or absence of stones or tumor may be determined preoperatively, as noted, but in many cases, intraoperative verification of the findings is necessary. Intraoperative cholangiography can be carried out by inserting a catheter through the gallbladder, by directly needling the cyst, or both. If cholangiography does not yield an accurate definition of the anatomy of the cyst, the cyst may then be opened anteriorly and digital exploration and choledochoscopy used to clarify the proximal and distal extent of the cyst.

Step 2: Mobilization of the gallbladder

If the gallbladder is still in place, dissect it free of the liver, leaving it attached to the cyst via the cystic duct, and retract the gallbladder to the right.

Step 3: Distal Dissection

Early distal division of the cyst facilitates the posterior dissection and allows mobilization of the duct to better define the proximal extent of the cyst. Dissect distally along the wall of the cyst until the junction of the cyst with the normal portion of the CBD is reached. If the intrapancreatic portion of the CBD is involved, the cyst must be separated from pancreatic tissue. A number of small vessels must be individually identified and ligated to minimize the risk of early or delayed bleeding. If the cyst is close to the pancreatic duct junction, one must exercise considerable care not to injure the pancreatic duct. Transect the distal bile duct. Place a clamp on the proximal cut end of the duct to assist with retraction and oversew the distal cut end using fine monofilament absorbable suture, being careful not to injure the pancreatic duct.

Step 4: Mobilization of Cyst

Vascularity in the region and the presence of inflammation may render dissection difficult. Rather than cleaning off the hepatic artery and the portal vein and dissecting them off the cyst, find a plane immediately adjacent to the wall of the

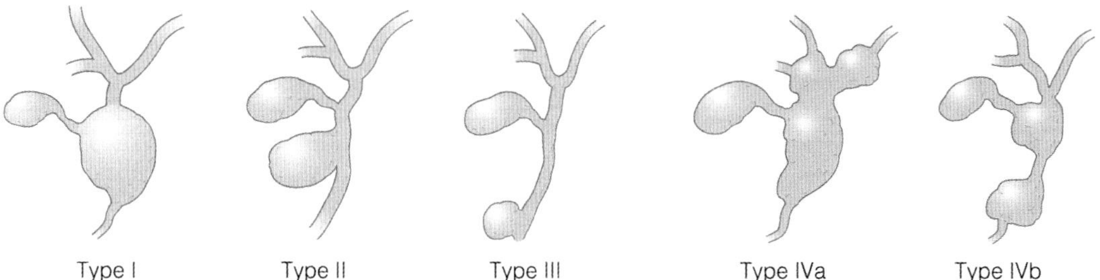

Figure 6 **Choledochal cyst resection. Illustrated is the Todani classification of choledochal cyst.**

cyst and remain close to it [*see Figure 7*]. This approach differs significantly from the corresponding approach in resection of a bile duct malignancy [*see* Resection of Middle-Third and Proximal Bile Duct Tumors, Operative Technique, *below*]. If necessary, open the cyst with a vertical anterior cystotomy and continue the dissection with direct visualization of the inside of the cyst to yield a more accurate definition of its boundaries. Clear the cyst circumferentially, separating the cyst from the hepatic artery, the portal vein, and any remaining soft tissue in the hepatoduodenal ligament.

Step 5: Proximal Dissection

If the proximal common hepatic duct is normal (as in a type I cyst), transect the duct above the cyst. If the cystic dilatation includes the bifurcation (as in a type IVa cyst), a small button of proximal cyst is usually left attached to the intrahepatic ducts [*see Figure 8*].

Step 6: Reconstruction

Reconstruction is accomplished via an end-to-side anastomosis to a Roux jejunal loop to minimize the likelihood of reflux of enteric contents into the biliary tract. Stenting is not required, but we recommend draining the area with closed suction drains, especially if an intrapancreatic resection has been done.

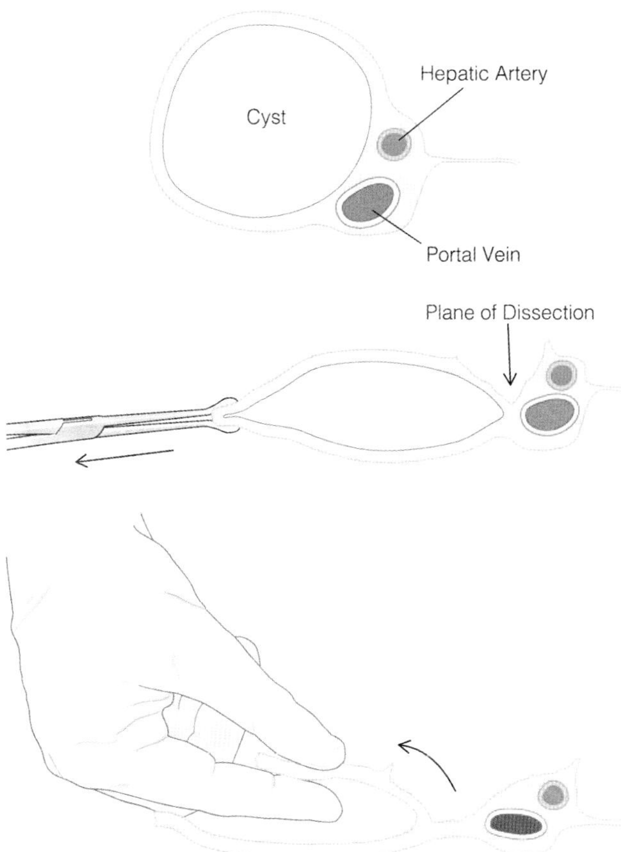

Figure 7 **Choledochal cyst resection. Illustrated is the proper plane of dissection in removal of a choledochal cyst. If necessary, dissection can be done with a finger inside the cyst.**

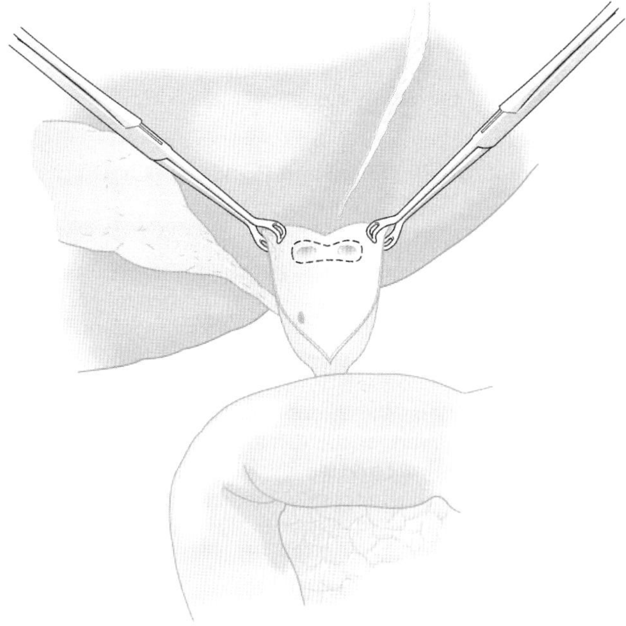

Figure 8 **Choledochal cyst resection. If a cyst extends proximally past the bifurcation (e.g., a type IVa cyst), it may be necessary to open the cyst widely to identify the hepatic duct orifices. A small button of cyst wall is left attached to the hepatic ducts.**

TROUBLESHOOTING

If dissection of the cyst is carried distally into the pancreas, care must be taken to keep from injuring the pancreatic duct. Transect the cyst as distally as possible and carefully oversew the end with absorbable sutures. Intraoperative cholangiography and/or preoperative MRCP are useful to confirm the relationship of the cyst and the CBD to the pancreatic duct.

If the cystic process extends to include the bifurcation (type IVa), the hepatic ducts should be identified from within the cyst and their orifices preserved by leaving a small button of cyst wall in situ; this is preferable to performing an intrahepatic dissection to remove the entire cyst. The presence of this button simplifies and facilitates the anastomosis to the Roux loop. Note that liver resection for choledochal cyst is rarely justified unless there is evidence of a solid mass or papillary excrescence emanating from the cyst mucosa.

COMPLICATIONS

Bleeding and pancreatitis are the main early complications of cystectomy. These can be largely prevented by meticulous dissection and ligation of all fine bleeding vessels as well as tissue adjacent to an intrapancreatic cyst. Late stricture of the anastomosis is an uncommon complication but may occur, especially if a small button of proximal cyst is left in place for the anastomosis; this particular complication is considered an acceptable hazard in a difficult situation.

OUTCOME EVALUATION

The immediate expected outcome is the relief of pain, jaundice, and cholangitis and the return of liver function to normal. The long-term expected outcome is the absence of any recurrence of symptoms of stone disease, cholangitis, or malignancy. Because of the rarity of this condition, no good data on the recurrence rate of problems are available, but in our experience, the need for reintervention is rare.

Resection of Middle-Third and Proximal Bile Duct Tumors

The most common bile duct tumor is adenocarcinoma. Because this tumor responds poorly to irradiation and chemotherapy, surgical resection offers the best opportunity for cure. Unfortunately, many patients present with unresectable local disease and distant metastasis, and only palliative interventions are warranted. The appropriate operative approach depends on the location and extent of the tumor [*see Figure 9*]. Tumors in the distal third of the CBD (the pancreatic portion) are treated by means of a pancreaticoduodenectomy that includes bile duct and periductal tissues right up to the bifurcation. Those in the middle third or the proximal third are treated by means of bile duct resection, often with concurrent liver resection.

Certain basic principles underlying bile duct resection for tumor must be followed. First, the proximal extent of the tumor must be identified so that the correct procedure can be planned. Preoperative PTC is usually not required for staging if high-quality MRI and MRCP are available. With the exception of the clinical circumstances outlined previously [*see* Management of Biliary Obstruction, *above*], we do not routinely place preoperative biliary drainage tubes.

Second, given that bile duct tumors spread by local extension to lymphatics, along perineural spaces, and along the biliary radicles directly into the liver, wide local excision beyond the visible edges of the tumor is required in the performance of curative resections. In proximal tumors, such excision necessitates resection of the adjacent segments of the liver. The principles of en bloc resection beyond tumor margins must be closely adhered to: dissection into or even close to the tumor must be avoided.[14]

Third, intraoperative biopsy of the tumor is unreliable because of the difficulty of making a firm pathologic diagnosis on the basis of frozen-section examination.

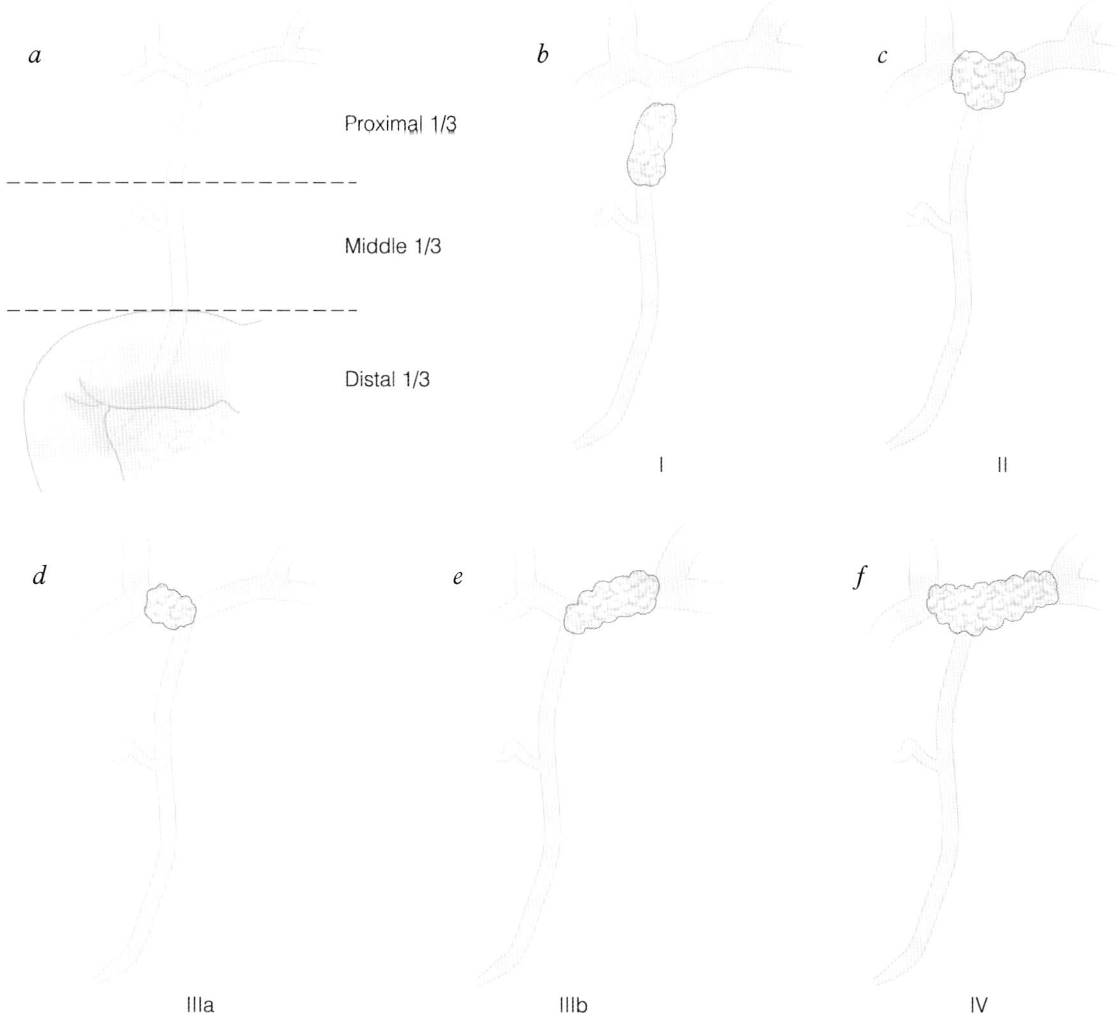

Figure 9 **Resection of middle-third and proximal bile duct tumors. The appropriate operation depends on the location and extent of the tumor. (*a*) Broadly, tumors may be localized to the proximal third, the middle third, or the distal third of the biliary tract. (*b* through *f*) Proximal tumors may be further categorized according to the Bismuth classification.**

Finally, given that liver resection is required in most cases, one must be careful to preserve enough healthy liver tissue to allow regeneration of the remnant.[15] If there has been long-standing obstruction, biliary drainage on the side to be preserved is important for recovery of function in that portion of the liver. Some surgeons advocate preoperative portal vein embolization on the contralateral side to stimulate hepatic regeneration in the segments to be preserved, especially if the future remnant is marginal in size. Often this is unnecessary, however, because of lobar atrophy attributable to ipsilateral portal vein involvement and compensatory contralateral hypertrophy.

On the whole, we are aggressive in treating proximal tumors for two main reasons: (1) the accompanying liver resection can now be done with low morbidity, and (2) this more radical approach has been shown to yield improved long-term results.[5] For middle-third or type I proximal tumors, we favor resection of the bifurcation in conjunction with intrahepatic cholangiojejunostomy. For types II, III, and IV, we recommend additional liver resection: a right trisectionectomy (resection of segments 4, 5, 6, 7, and 8, along with the caudate lobe) for types II, IIIa, and IV and a formal left hepatectomy (resection of segments 1, 2, 3, and 4) for type IIIb. There is some controversy as to whether patients with these complex proximal biliary tumors have a better chance of long-term survival with liver transplantation than with radical resection because of the high incidence of positive microscopic margins. This controversy has yet to be resolved, but we prefer radical resection when feasible. Transplantation for hilar cholangiocarcinoma should be performed only in the context of an approved clinical trial.

OPERATIVE TECHNIQUE

Step 1: Assessment of Resectability

Assessment of resectability begins with an evaluation of the patient's fitness and exclusion of underlying liver disease (i.e., cirrhosis and portal hypertension). The next step is to confirm the radiographic appearance of resectability. Radiographic evidence of metastatic disease is an absolute contraindication to resection. In the absence of metastatic disease, the resectability of hilar cholangiocarcinoma is predicted by the extent of vasculobiliary involvement and the presence or absence of contralateral lobar atrophy. In general, if the tumor involves only the ipsilateral portal vein and/or bile ducts, it may be resectable; if the tumor involves the contralateral portal vein and/or contralateral secondary bile ducts, it is generally not resectable.[5] Finally, if curative resection requires major hepatectomy, the future remnant liver must be of adequate size to prevent postoperative liver failure.

Before any dissection of the tumor or the CBD is done, conduct a careful search for peritoneal metastases. Evaluate spread within the liver by palpation. Palpate for suspicious lymph nodes in the immediate and secondary drainage areas. Biopsy any suspicious areas outside the planned resection margins and send this for frozen-section analysis. If the frozen section confirms that tumor is present outside the planned resection area, palliative stenting or a bypass procedure is indicated.

During dissection, determination of resectability is often difficult, especially with respect to assessment of tumor extension into the liver and the degree of vessel involvement. Therefore, the surgeon should defer any firm commitment to resection (e.g., dividing the blood supply) until resectability is confirmed.

Dissect the gallbladder off the gallbladder fossa, taking care to leave the cystic plate on the liver. The gallbladder can be left attached to the CBD and used as a retractor. Follow the cystic plate down to the hilar plate and lower the hilar plate by dividing its attachment to segment 4B all the way to the umbilical fissure. This allows palpation and inspection of the hilum to determine the extent of tumor involvement into the left and right hepatic ducts.

Dissection is then begun from below. Identify the common hepatic artery and the portal vein just above the neck of the pancreas and circumferentially clear these of all tissue. Continue the dissection proximally, retracting the hepatic artery to the left and the portal vein to the right. Adjacent areolar tissue, nerve trunks, and lymph nodes should be left in place around the CBD and the tumor [*see Figure 10*]. As noted, this approach differs from that used in resection of choledochal cysts [*see* Choledochal Cyst Resection, Operative Technique, *above*].

Step 2: Division of CBD

Once resectability is confirmed, divide the CBD at the level of the pancreas. Place a clamp on the end of the divided duct and use this as a retractor to facilitate the most proximal dissection of the CBD and the tumor away from the hepatic artery and the portal vein [*see Figure 11*].

Step 3: Proximal Dissection

With middle-third tumors or Bismuth type I proximal tumors, it is usually possible to palpate the proximal tumor margin and identify uninvolved right and left hepatic ducts. If this is not the case, the surgeon should consider the possibility of a type II or III tumor and be prepared to completely excise the bifurcation, with or without part of the liver.

Dissect the hepatic artery by retracting the vessel anteriorly and to the left, dividing and ligating the cystic artery where it originates from the right hepatic artery, and clearing all tissue off the right and left branches at least 1 cm proximal to the proximal margin of the tumor. Involvement of the right or left hepatic artery by tumor is a sign of extensive spread on the corresponding side and an indication for resection of that half of the liver.

Dissect the portal vein by retracting the bile duct and the tumor anteriorly and the hepatic artery to the left. All tissue should be cleanly dissected away from the portal vein to expose the bifurcation and the region proximal to it [*see Figure 11*]. At this point, the duct may be tethered down to the caudate lobe. Bile ducts from the caudate lobe may drain into the right or left duct and tumor may extend along these caudate ducts. Therefore, whether or not there is gross tumor in this area, the caudate lobe should be included in the resection.[16]

The level at which the proximal bile ducts are transected depends on the proximal extent of the tumor. For all middle-third or proximal tumors that are at least 1 cm beyond the bifurcation, proximal resection should be above the level of the bifurcation. For type I or type II proximal tumors, proximal resection should always include all of the bifurcation along with the proximal right and left bile ducts out as far as

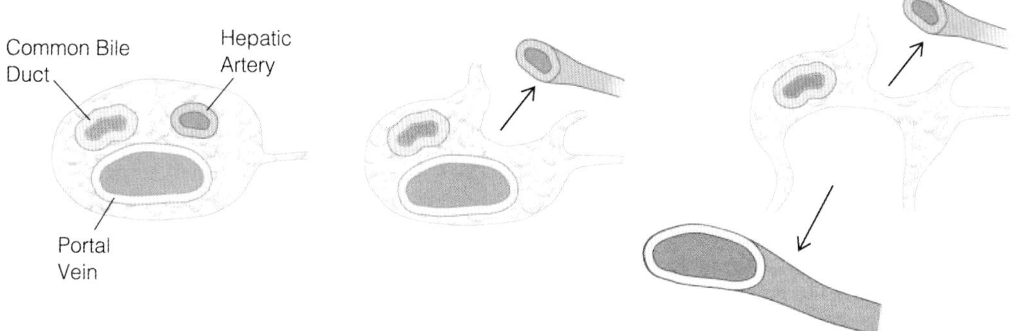

Figure 10 **Resection of middle-third and proximal bile duct tumors. Shown is the proper plane of dissection in the removal of a bile duct cancer. Except for the hepatic artery and the portal vein, all tissue stays with the common bile duct to be resected.**

the first major branch [*see Figure 12*]. With type III or IV proximal tumors, the proximal extent of the tumor cannot be determined in both right and left ducts unless the main pedicles are dissected out of the liver. Because these tumors tend to infiltrate locally, such dissection is not advisable. Instead, concurrent hepatectomy should be performed to optimize the likelihood of curative resection. Intraoperative ultrasonography may help verify the extent of tumor at this point in the operation. Any major liver resection for type III or IV bile duct cancer should include the caudate lobe [*see Figure 13*].

Before committing to a major hepatectomy (i.e., before dividing the blood supply), the tumor must be dissected away from the hepatic artery and portal vein branch supplying the segments of the liver to be preserved. Once this has been accomplished, the hepatic artery and the portal vein branch to the side to be resected can be divided. This allows the tumor to be retracted further and provides better exposure of the duct to the side to be preserved [*see Figure 14 and Figure 15*]. In selected cases, resection of an involved portal vein bifurcation may be carried out at this point [*see Figure 16*]; an end-to-end primary venorrhaphy (without the need for an interposition conduit) can usually be fashioned.

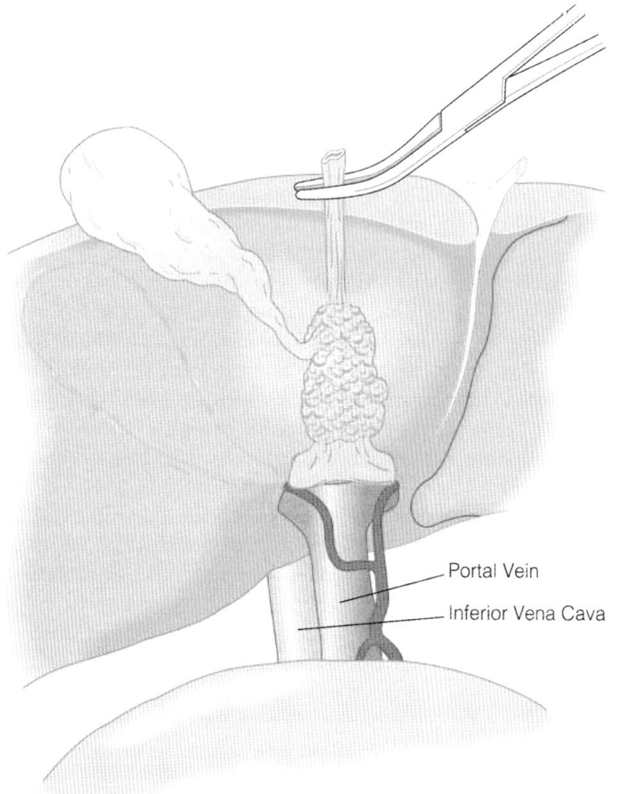

Figure 11 **Resection of middle-third and proximal bile duct tumors. When resectability is confirmed, the common bile duct (CBD) is transected at the duodenum. The proximal portion of the divided duct is retracted anteriorly, and the CBD is cleaned off the portal vein up to a point above the bifurcation.**

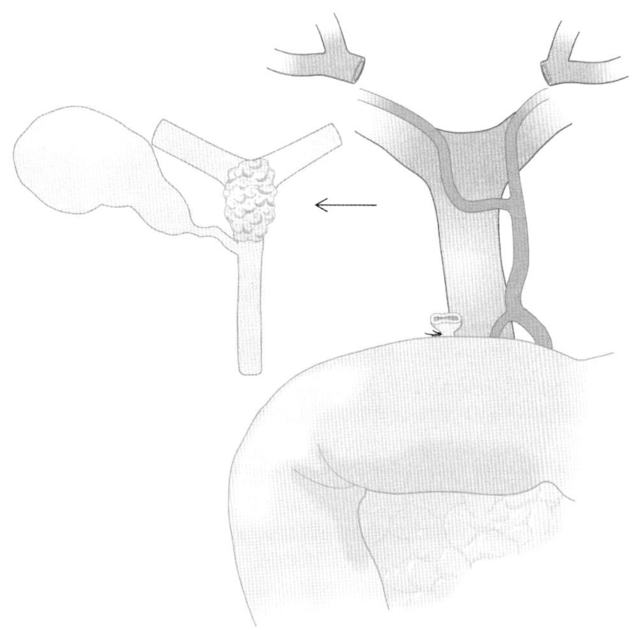

Figure 12 **Resection of middle-third and proximal bile duct tumors. Illustrated is the level of resection for middle-third and type I proximal tumors. The common bile duct is resected from the pancreas to a point above the bifurcation. Reconstruction is accomplished via Roux-en-Y hepaticojejunostomy (involving either one or two separate anastomoses).**

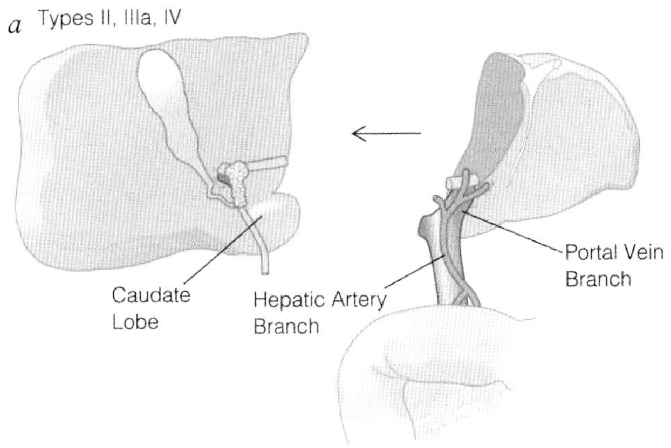

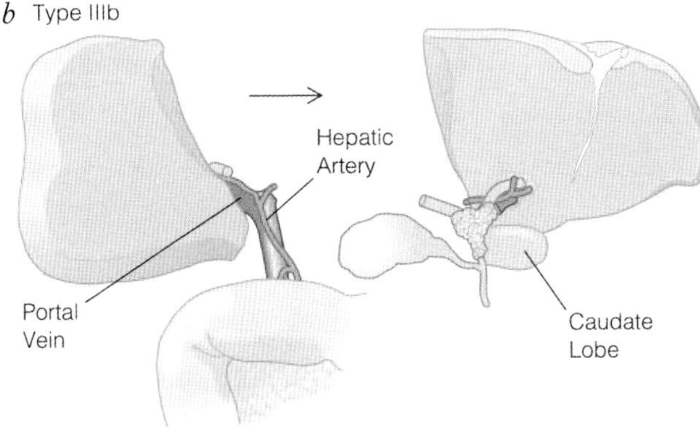

Figure 13 **Resection of middle-third and proximal bile duct tumors. Illustrated are (*a*) a right trisectionectomy (extended right hepatectomy) for type II, IIIa, and IV tumors and (*b*) a left hepatectomy (including the caudate lobe) for type IIIb tumors.**

The point at which the hepatic parenchyma will be divided is marked, and the parenchymal transection is performed. Division of the hepatic duct (or ducts) to the part of the liver being preserved is done as far from the tumor as possible.

Step 4: Reconstruction

After resection of the bifurcation or intrahepatic bile ducts, an intrahepatic cholangiojejunostomy is performed. The duct tissue is usually healthy enough and the duct lumen large enough to allow mucosa-to-mucosa repair without stenting.

Step 5: Closure and Postoperative Care

Close the abdomen in the standard fashion and place closed suction drains. In the early postoperative period, particularly when a major liver resection has been performed, mild abnormalities in coagulation test results are common. In the absence of active bleeding or severe coagulopathy, we do not administer fresh frozen plasma. Drains are removed 2 to 3 days postoperatively if there is no evidence of a bile leak.

COMPLICATIONS

Bile leakage, bleeding, and infection are the most important complications of bile duct resection for tumor. Following major hepatectomy, expect a transient rise in liver function studies. A moderate increase in coagulation studies is also common, and we do not transfuse fresh frozen plasma for an international normalized ratio of 2.0 or less unless clinical bleeding is evident. Nevertheless, these laboratory values should be monitored closely in the early postoperative period as persistent elevation of liver function tests or coagulation studies is an indication of hepatic insufficiency. Parahepatic collections are treated with percutaneous drainage, and significant early postoperative bleeding is usually best managed by reexploration.

Repair of Biliary Injuries

Biliary injuries during laparoscopic cholecystectomy are estimated to occur in only 0.4 to 0.6% of cases, but with approximately 500,000 procedures yearly in the United States, this seemingly low injury rate translates into significantly increased cost, resource use, morbidity, and mortality.[17–21] In as many as 50% of cases, the injury may be discovered at the time of operation, and depending on the type of injury, the surgeon may attempt an immediate repair.[22,23] General surgeons who perform laparoscopic cholecystectomies should be adequately trained to repair Strasberg type A and D injuries [*see Figure 17*]. Strasberg type A injuries include cystic duct stump leaks or leakage from small ducts in the liver bed (e.g., duct of Luschka). If a type A injury is detected during laparoscopic cholecystectomy, oversew the offending duct (laparoscopically or open) and place a drain. A type D injury is a lateral injury to a major duct. One may safely perform a primary repair of the duct at the time of operation under the following conditions: (1) less than 25% of the circumference of the duct is involved, (2) the injury is not thermal (i.e., from a cautery burn), and (3) the duct is of sufficient caliber to allow insertion of a T tube. Place a T tube across the injury (via a separate incision in the duct) and perform a primary repair using fine absorbable monofilament suture. If any one of the above conditions is absent, the surgeon should instead perform a choledochojejunostomy as previously described or refer the patient to a hepatobiliary surgeon if necessary. Type B injuries usually involve ligation of an aberrant right hepatic duct and are rarely detected at the time of surgery. Type C injuries involve transection, but not ligation, of an aberrant (usually right hepatic) duct. If discovered at the time of operation, such injuries are best repaired immediately with cholangiojejunostomy. Strasberg type E injuries parallel the Bismuth classification system of biliary strictures. These injuries occur higher on the biliary tree, may be very complex, and are often accompanied by a vascular component. When such injuries are noted at the time of cholecystectomy, the surgeon must honestly assess his or her expertise in the repair of complex biliary injuries and do nothing that might worsen the injury. In general, this means that once any hemorrhage is carefully controlled, a drain should be placed, the wound should be closed, and the patient should be transferred without delay to the nearest specialty center with provider teams experienced in the management of complex biliary injuries.[24]

Injuries not discovered at the time of initial operation may present days, weeks, or even years later.[25,26] Signs and symptoms of delayed presentation vary depending on the nature of the injury and whether obstruction or bile leakage

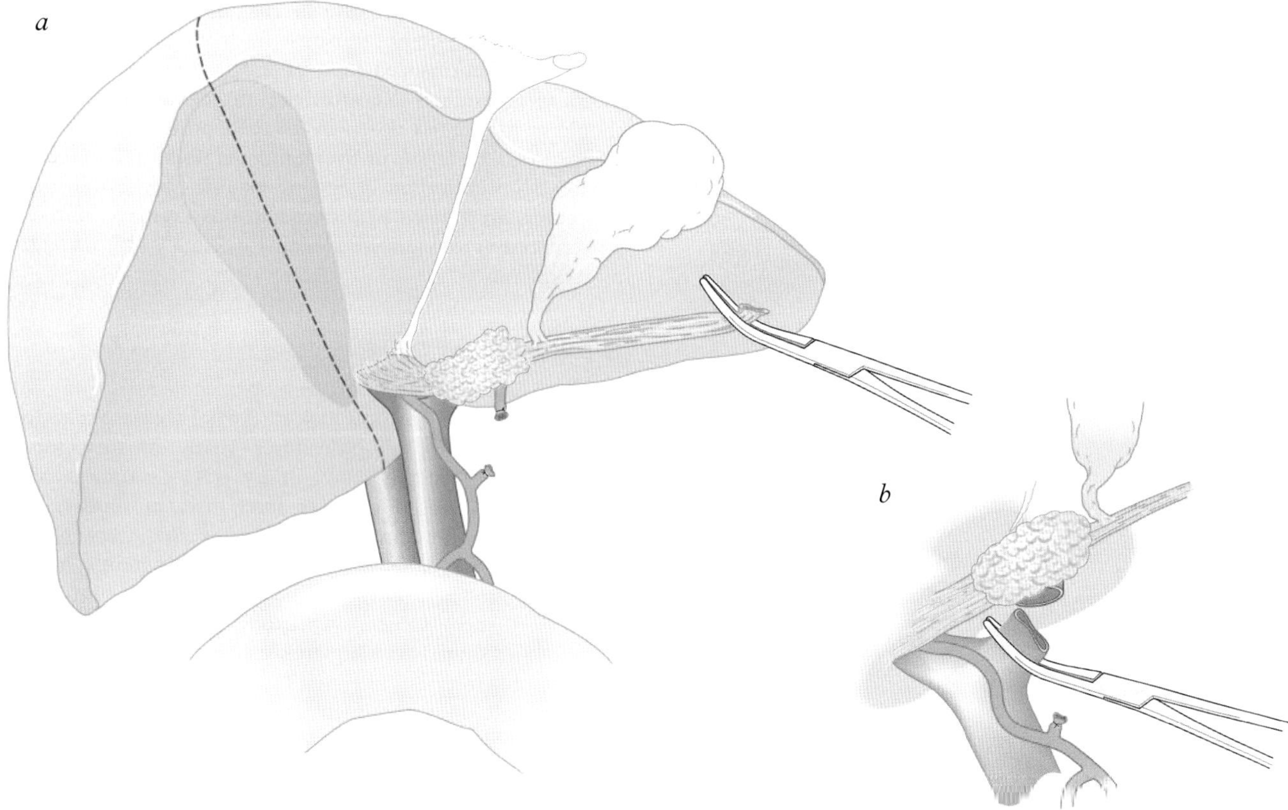

Figure 14 **Resection of middle-third and proximal bile duct tumors. Shown is the resection of type IIIb proximal tumors. (*a*) The common bile duct is retracted upward and to the left; the left hepatic artery is divided; and the right portal vein and the right hepatic artery, which are to be saved, are exposed. (*b*) The left portal vein is divided.**

is the dominant pathology at the time. Persistent but usually mild, unexplained pain and malaise in the postoperative period are the most common initial symptoms, and the nonspecific nature of these symptoms may lead to further delay in diagnosis.[27] Patients may also present with nausea, anorexia, elevated white blood cell count and liver function studies, fever, jaundice, cholangitis, or sepsis. Initial management depends on the clinical state of the patient. Correct any fluid and electrolyte derangements, administer appropriate analgesia to control the pain associated with bile peritonitis, and initiate broad-spectrum antibiotic coverage in any patient with infection. High-quality cross-sectional imaging—multiphase CT, MRI/MRCP, or both—is essential to evaluate the extent of injury and detect abdominal fluid collections or major vascular injury. Patients with signs or symptoms of cholangitis or sepsis should undergo percutaneous drainage of any biloma or abscess seen on imaging, followed by PTC with placement of an external biliary drainage catheter (or bilateral catheters for type E4 injuries). No attempt should be made to internalize the biliary drainage catheter(s) until the patient becomes clinically stable.[28] Stable patients with jaundice and/or biloma may also undergo ERCP, and if a type A injury is clearly demonstrated, then drainage of the biloma and temporary biliary stenting until the leak ceases will usually solve the problem. To adequately define anatomy and plan repair of most other injuries, specifically those involving excluded ducts, requires imaging of both the upper and lower bile ducts with both ERCP and PTC. Failure to adequately define the biliary anatomy and extent of injury by cholangiography predicts eventual failure of any repair.[24] Although there is no level 1 evidence to guide the timing of repair, we generally complete the necessary perioperative imaging studies and repair injuries within 24 hours of transfer under the following conditions: (1) the transfer occurs within 0 to 3 days of the injury, (2) peritoneal contamination is minimal and well drained, (3) the patient has no signs or symptoms of cholangitis or sepsis, and (4) there is no radiographic evidence of major vascular injury. Patients with bile peritonitis, abscesses, and cholangitis are managed as described above, and definitive repair is delayed for at least 3 months. Likewise, repair is delayed 3 months in patients with major vascular injuries to better establish the level of associated ductal ischemia and resulting stricture.

OPERATIVE TECHNIQUE

Step 1: Exposure of the Porta Hepatis

In patients who have sustained a biliary injury, particularly those who have already undergone attempted repair, local inflammation may obliterate the normal tissue planes and lead to significant distortions of the normal portal anatomy. The following are some useful techniques for safely

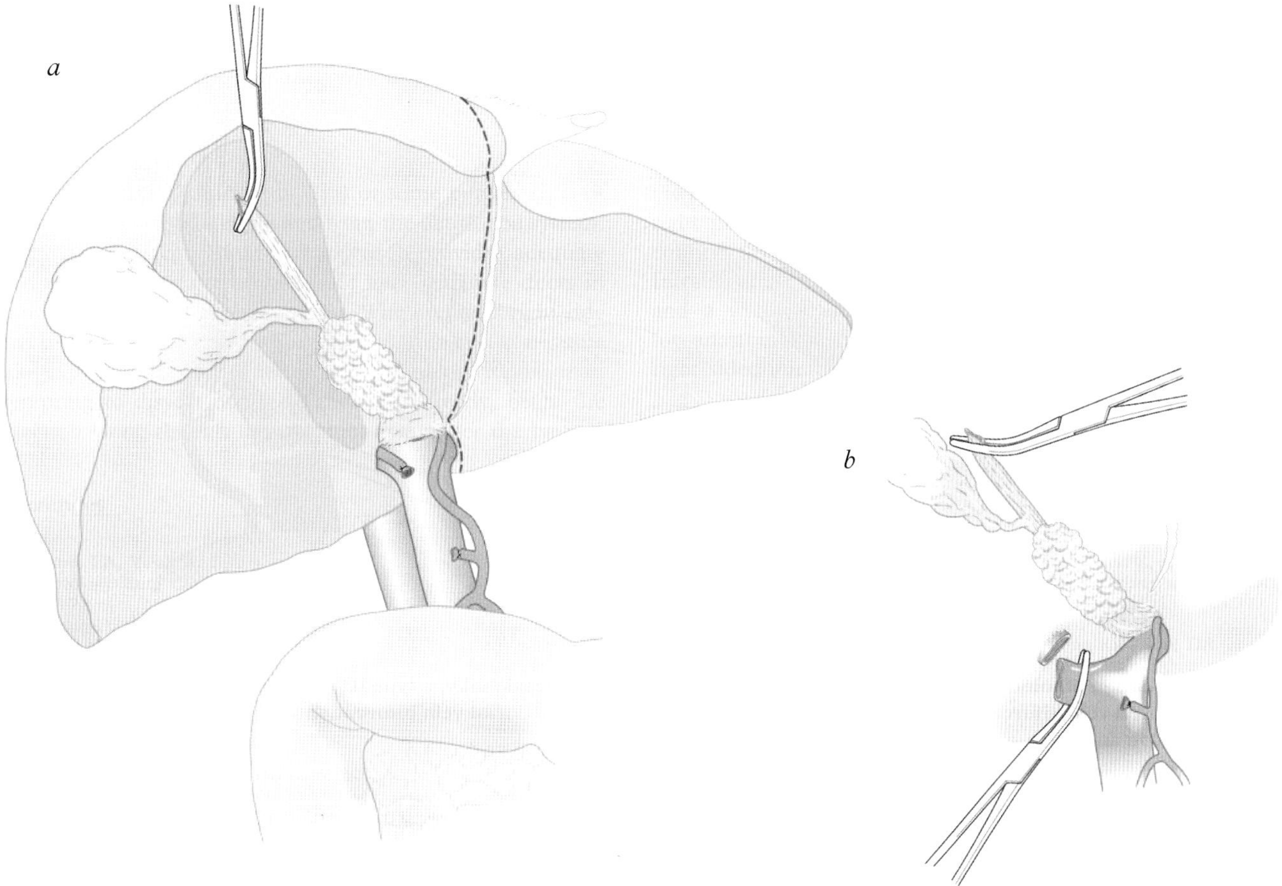

Figure 15 **Resection of middle-third and proximal bile duct tumors. Shown is the resection of type II, IIIa, and IV proximal tumors. (*a*) The CBD is retracted upward and to the right; the right hepatic artery is divided; and the left portal vein and the left hepatic artery, which are to be saved, are exposed. (*b*) The right portal vein is divided.**

defining the anatomy and avoiding potentially devascularizing dissection within the porta hepatis.

1. Use the round ligament to find the true porta hepatis. Patients who have already undergone one or more operations on the bile duct often have adhesions between the hepatoduodenal ligament and segment 4 of the liver. If one dissects this area via the anterior approach, one may think that the actual porta hepatis has been reached but notice that the hepatoduodenal ligament appears unusually short. In most cases, one can safely find the true porta by tracing the round ligament to the point where it joins the left portal pedicle and the umbilical portion (or ascending branch) of the left portal vein. To completely expose the umbilical fissure, the bridge of liver tissue between segment 4b and the left lateral section must first be divided. This tissue is devoid of any major vascular or biliary structures and may be safely divided with electrocautery. One may then follow the pedicle toward the right along the true porta. The adhesions between the hepatoduodenal ligament and segment 4b are more easily divided from the left than from the front.
2. Use aids to dissection. Usually, structures in the hepatoduodenal ligament can be identified by inspection and palpation, especially if a biliary stent is in place. When repairing complex, high biliary injuries (e.g., types E4 and E5), we routinely place percutaneous stents preoperatively for this purpose. Intraoperative Doppler ultrasonography may be useful in identifying the hepatic artery and the portal vein. Intraoperative ultrasonography may also be helpful in identifying the bile duct, and needle aspiration may be used before the duct is incised if there is any doubt about its location. Either blunt or sharp dissection is effective in this area. Our preference is to use a long fine right-angle clamp to obtain exposure in a layer-by-layer fashion. We then carefully cauterize or ligate and divide the exposed tissue.

Step 2: Defining the Duct

Carefully débride crushed, cauterized, or devitalized tissue back to normal healthy tissue. When performing a delayed repair, it is not necessary to resect all scar tissue around the duct. Just be certain that the anastomosis is constructed to healthy duct mucosa proximal to the injury and not to granulation tissue at the opening in the duct.

22 HEPATIC RESECTION

*Clifford S. Cho, MD, and Yuman Fong, MD, FACS**

Although first described centuries ago, the majority of liver resections were performed for management of trauma or infection until the latter half of the 20th century. Today, partial hepatectomy is performed not only for treatment of acute emergencies but also as potentially curative therapy for a variety of benign and malignant hepatic lesions.[1–5]

The first planned anatomic resection of a lobe of a liver is credited to Lortat-Jacob, who performed a right hepatic lobectomy in 1952 as treatment for metastatic colon cancer.[6] However, it was not until the 1980s that major hepatectomies became commonplace. Since that time, the safety of hepatic resection has improved dramatically; moreover, as the safety of the operation has improved, the indications for hepatic resection have broadened. Currently, resection of as much as 85% of functional liver parenchyma is being performed at numerous centers with an operative mortality of less than 2%. The duration of hospitalization is typically well less than 2 weeks, and nearly all patients regain normal hepatic function postoperatively.[7]

In this chapter, we focus on the technical aspects of hepatic resection, emphasizing efficiency and safety and taking into account recent developments, current controversies, and special operative considerations (e.g., the cirrhotic patient and repeat liver resection). Detailed discussions of the indications for hepatic resection are available elsewhere.[8–10]

Hepatic Anatomy

Safe operative conduct during partial hepatectomy demands a close familiarity with the surgical anatomy of the liver.[11] In 1998, in response to the confusion created by various anatomic nomenclatures applied to the liver, the International Hepato-Pancreato-Biliary Association (IHPBA) appointed a committee charged with establishing a universal terminology for hepatic anatomy and hepatic resections. In 2000, the recommendations of this committee were accepted at IHPBA's biannual meeting in Brisbane. Accordingly, this system for naming the anatomic divisions of the liver and their corresponding resections has come to be known as the Brisbane 2000 terminology.[12]

In the Brisbane 2000 system, the anatomy of the liver may be thought of in terms of first-order, second-order, and third-order divisions, all of which are based on the underlying vascular and biliary anatomy and not on surface features [*see Figure 1*]. At the first level, the liver is divided into two hemilivers (right and left). At the second level, it is divided into four sections (right posterior, right anterior, left medial, and left lateral). At the third level, it is divided into nine segments, each of which is a discrete anatomic unit that possesses its own nutrient blood supply and venous and biliary drainage.

The right hemiliver consists of segments V through VIII and is nourished by the right hepatic artery and the right portal vein; the left hemiliver consists of segments II through IV and is nourished by the left hepatic artery and the left portal vein. (The caudate lobe, a portion of the liver that is separate from the two hemilivers, consists of segments I and IX.) The anatomic division between the right hemiliver and the left hemiliver is not at the falciform ligament (the most readily apparent visual landmark on the anterior liver) but follows the principal scissura (or Cantlie line) that runs posterosuperiorly from the medial margin of the gallbladder to the left side of the inferior vena cava.

The venous drainage of the liver consists of multiple small veins draining directly from the back of the right hemiliver and the caudate lobe to the inferior vena cava, along with three major hepatic veins. These major hepatic veins occupy three planes, known as portal scissurae. The three scissurae divide the liver into the four sections, each of which is supplied by a portal pedicle; further branching of the pedicles subdivides the sections into their constituent segments. The right hepatic vein passes between the right anterior section (segments V and VIII) and the right posterior section (segments VI and VII) in the right scissura. This vein empties directly into the vena cava near the atriocaval junction. The middle hepatic vein passes between the right anterior section and the left medial section (segment IV, sometimes subdivided into segments IVa and IVb) in the principal scissura that divides the right and left hemilivers. The left hepatic vein runs in the left scissura between segments II and III (which together comprise the left lateral section). In most persons, the left and middle hepatic veins join to form a common trunk before entering the inferior vena cava. Occasionally, a large inferior right hepatic vein is present that can provide adequate drainage of the right hemiliver after resection of the left even when all three major hepatic veins are ligated.[13]

The portal vein and hepatic artery divide into left and right branches below the hilum of the liver. Unlike the major hepatic veins, which run between segments, the portal venous and hepatic arterial branches, along with the hepatic ducts, typically run centrally within segments [*see Figure 1*]. On the right side, the hepatic artery and the portal vein enter the liver substance almost immediately after branching. The short course of the right-sided extrahepatic vessels and the variable anatomy of the biliary tree make these vessels vulnerable to damage during dissection.[14] In contrast, the left branch of the portal vein and the left hepatic duct take a long extrahepatic course after branching beneath the undersurface of segment IV. When these vessels reach the base of the umbilical fissure, they are joined by the left hepatic artery to form a triad, which

* The authors and editors gratefully acknowledge the contributions of the previous author, James Park, MD, to the development and writing of this chapter.

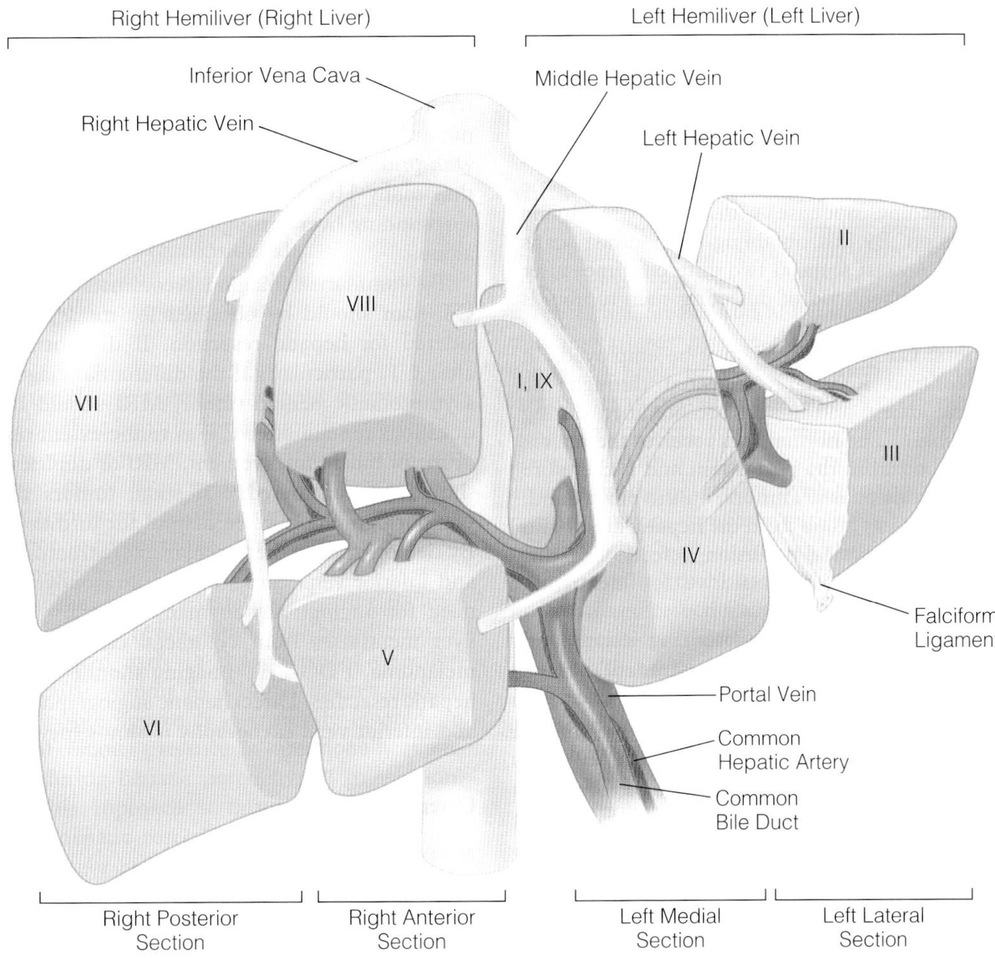

Figure 1 **The liver is separated into nine anatomic segments, each with an independent nutrient blood supply and venous and biliary drainage. Appreciation of this segmental anatomy is the basis of anatomic resection of the liver.**

then enters the substance of the left hemiliver. Importantly, the left-sided structures are not a triad proximal to the base of the umbilical fissure. This long extrahepatic course makes operative exposure of the left-sided structures far easier than on the right. A surgical consequence of this anatomy is that when a choice exists between extended right hepatectomy and extended left hepatectomy [*see* Operative Technique, *below*] for resection of tumors involving the hepatic hilum (e.g., Klatskin tumors), most surgeons choose the former because of the greater ease of dissection and preservation of the left-sided structures. Knowledge of the relative anatomic courses of the portal veins, hepatic arteries, and hepatic ducts is the basis of the classic extrahepatic dissection for control of hepatic inflow [*see* Operative Technique, Right Hepatectomy, Step 6 (Extrahepatic Dissection and Ligation): Control of Inflow Vessels, *below*].

The fibrous capsule surrounding the liver substance was described by Glisson in 1654.[15] It was Couinaud, however, who demonstrated that this fibrous capsule extends to envelop the portal triads as they pass into the liver substance.[16] Thus, within the liver parenchyma, the portal vein, hepatic artery, and hepatic duct running to each segment of the liver lie within a substantive sheath. This dense sheath facilitates rapid control of inflow vessels to specific anatomic units within the liver and permits en masse ligation of these vascular structures in a maneuver known as pedicle ligation [*see* Operative Technique, Right Hepatectomy, Step 6—Alternative (Intrahepatic Pedicle Ligation): Control of Inflow Vessels, *below*].[17]

Preoperative Evaluation

Cross-sectional imaging modalities such as computed tomography (CT), magnetic resonance imaging (MRI), and ultrasonography play important roles in enhancing the safety and efficacy of hepatic resection. These modalities, along with biologic scanning techniques such as positron emission tomography (PET), are also invaluable for staging malignancies so as to improve patient selection and thereby optimize long-term surgical outcomes.[3]

At a minimum, all candidates for hepatic resection should undergo either CT or MRI. These imaging tests not only identify the number and size of mass lesions within the liver but also delineate the relationships of the lesions to the major vasculature—data that are crucial for deciding whether to operate and which operative approach to employ.

Use of contrast enhancement during CT scanning is vital for accurate definition of the vascular anatomy. Data from

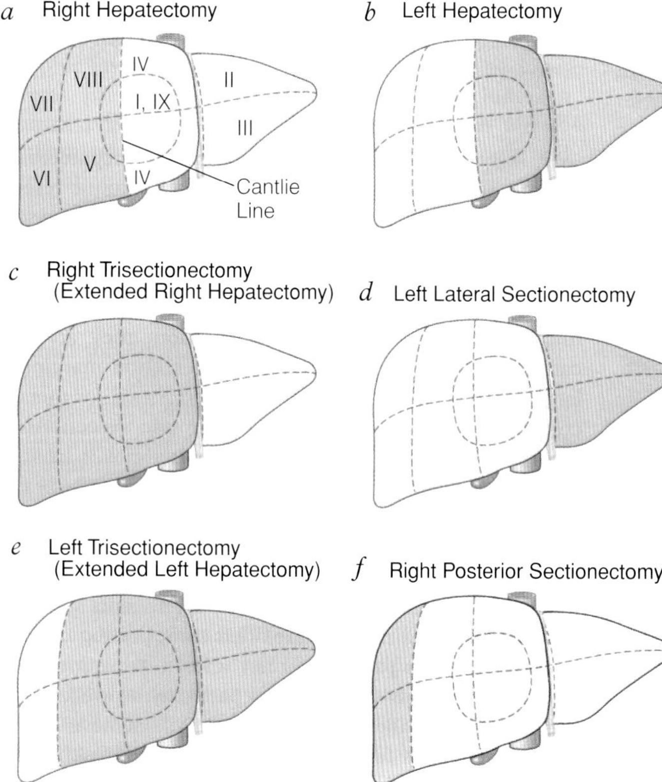

Figure 3 **Shown are schematic illustrations of standard hepatic resections, with the *shaded areas* representing the resected portions: (*a*) right hepatectomy, (*b*) left hepatectomy, (*c*) right trisectionectomy (extended right hepatectomy), (*d*) left lateral sectionectomy, (*e*) left trisegmentectomy (extended left hepatectomy), and (*f*) right posterior sectionectomy.**

RIGHT HEPATECTOMY (RIGHT HEMIHEPATECTOMY)

Step 1: Laparoscopic Inspection

Laparoscopic examination of the peritoneal cavity can detect unresectable metastases that cannot be visualized by cross-sectional imaging, thereby preventing the morbidity associated with a nontherapeutic laparotomy.[37–40] We generally perform laparoscopy immediately before laparotomy during the same period of anesthesia. The laparoscopic port sites are placed in the upper abdomen along the line of the intended incision [*see* Step 2, *below*]. The first two ports are usually 5 or 10 mm ports placed in the right subcostal area along the midclavicular line and along the anterior axillary line. These ports allow inspection of the abdomen and of the entire liver, including the dome and segment VII. A 10 mm port along the right anterior axillary line is particularly suitable for laparoscopic ultrasound devices. If additional ports are necessary, a left subcostal midclavicular port is usually the best choice.

Step 2: Incision

If no evidence of distant or unresectable metastasis is identified at the time of laparoscopy and an open hepatic resection is planned, an incision that will afford optimal exposure of the liver is made. For most hepatic resections, many surgeons use a bilateral subcostal incision extended vertically to the xiphisternum [*see Figure 4*]. Our preference is to use an upper midline incision extending to a point approximately 2 cm above the umbilicus, with a rightward extension to a point in the midaxillary line halfway between the right costal margin and the right anterior superior iliac spine [*see Figure 4*]. This incision provides superb access for both right- and left-sided resections and avoids the wound complications often encountered with trifurcated incisions (e.g., ascites leak, incisional hernia). On rare occasions (e.g., resection of large and rigid posterior tumors of the right hemiliver), a right thoracoabdominal incision may be required. However, in a series of nearly 2,000 resections performed at Memorial Sloan-Kettering Cancer Center, a thoracoabdominal incision was necessary in only 3% of cases, with the most common indication being repeat liver resection after previous right hepatectomy [*see* Repeat Hepatic Resection, *below*].

Step 3: Abdominal Exploration and Intraoperative Ultrasonography

Exploration commences with bimanual palpation of the entire liver. Intraoperative ultrasonography (IOUS) is then performed systemically to identify all lesions and their relation to the major vascular structures. IOUS is capable of identifying small lesions that preoperative imaging studies and palpation of the liver may miss.[41] The lesser omentum is incised to allow examination of the caudate lobe and inspection of the celiac axis nodal metastases. A finger is passed from the lesser sac inferior to the caudate lobe through the foramen of Winslow to permit identification of the portal vein and palpation of the portocaval lymph nodes. The hilar lymph nodes are palpated, and any suspicious nodes may be excised and submitted for frozen-section pathologic analysis. If the operation is being undertaken for malignancy, the entire abdomen is also inspected for evidence of extrahepatic tumors.

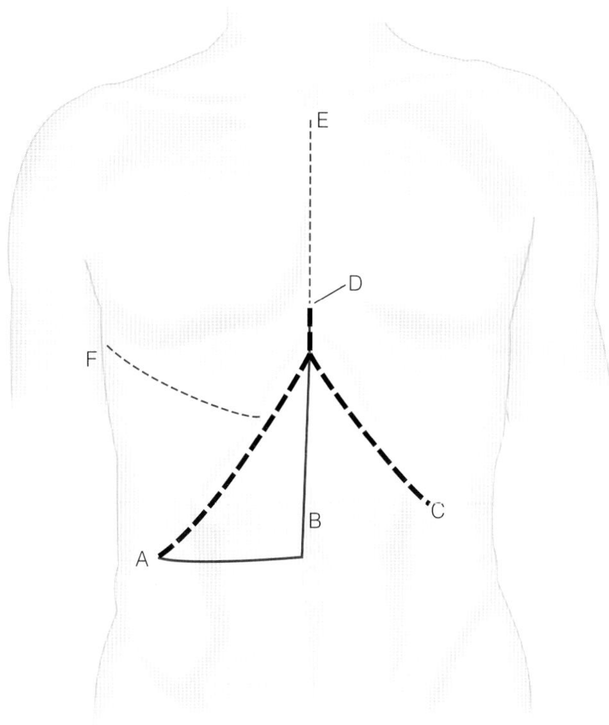

Figure 4 **Right hepatectomy. A right subcostal incision (A) with a midline extension to the xiphoid (D) is the most common choice; an extension to the left subcostal area (C) is sometimes added to provide further operative exposure. We prefer a long midline incision from the xiphoid (D) to a point approximately 2 to 3 cm above the umbilicus (B) along with a rightward extension (A) because this incision provides superb exposure of both the right side and the left without the wound complications of a trifurcated incision. The chest can be entered through either a median sternotomy (E) or an anterolateral right thoracoabdominal incision (F).**

Step 4: Mobilization of Liver

Once the decision is made to proceed with hepatic resection, the liver is fully mobilized by detaching all ligamentous attachments on the side to be resected. (Some surgeons defer completion of mobilization to a later stage in the procedure.) In particular, the falciform ligament is divided and the suprahepatic inferior vena cava and the hepatic veins above the liver are dissected to facilitate the subsequent approach to the hepatic veins [*see* Step 7: Control of Outflow Vessels, *below*]. Early mobilization of the liver will facilitate additional bimanual palpation to detect small lesions that may have been obscured during the initial examination. This additional palpation is particularly important on the right side as the right posterior section cannot be effectively examined prior to mobilization, and IOUS may fail to detect small lesions in this area.[41]

During the course of mobilization, if tumor is found to be attached to the diaphragm, the affected area of diaphragm may be excised and subsequently repaired.

Step 5: Identification of Arterial Anomalies

The presence of possible hepatic arterial anomalies should be verified before resection is initiated. With contemporary imaging techniques, the arterial anatomy can usually be defined with sufficient exactitude prior to laparotomy. However, it is also possible to clarify the arterial anatomy intraoperatively with several simple maneuvers that do not involve major dissection.

The lesser omentum should be examined to determine whether there is a vessel coursing through its middle to the base of the umbilical fissure, and the hepatoduodenal ligament should be palpated with an index finger within the foramen of Winslow to determine whether there is an artery in the gastropancreatic fold along its medial aspect. The usual bifurcation of the hepatic arteries occurs low and medially within the hepatoduodenal ligament, and the left hepatic artery normally travels on the medial aspect of the ligament to reach the base of the umbilical fissure. Therefore, an artery palpable in the medial upper portion of the hepatoduodenal ligament is the main left hepatic artery. If the main left hepatic artery is identified in this manner, any vessel identified in the lesser omentum must be an accessory left artery. If no arterial structure is found in the medial upper portion of the hepatoduodenal ligament, the vessel in the lesser omentum must be a replaced left hepatic artery. The right hepatic artery typically travels transversely behind the common bile duct (CBD) to reach the base of the cystic plate. An artery traversing vertically along the lateral hepatoduodenal ligament must therefore be either a replaced or an accessory right hepatic artery, likely arising from the superior mesenteric artery.

Step 6 (Extrahepatic Dissection and Ligation): Control of Inflow Vessels

The classic approach to controlling the inflow vessels during right hepatectomy involves extrahepatic dissection and ligation [*see Figure 5*]. The cystic duct and the cystic artery are ligated and divided. The gallbladder may be either removed or left attached to the right hemiliver, according to the surgeon's preference. A common practice is to first ligate the right hepatic duct, then the right hepatic artery, and finally the right portal vein, working from anterior to posterior. However, our preference is to work from posterior to anterior.

The sheath of the porta hepatis is opened laterally. Dissection is performed in the plane between the CBD and the portal vein. To facilitate this dissection, the CBD is elevated by applying anterior traction to the ligated cystic duct. The portal vein is followed in a cephalad direction until its bifurcation into the left and right portal veins is visible. Visualization of this bifurcation is critical because the left portal vein arises from the right anterior branch of the portal vein in a small percentage of patients. If the main right portal vein is ligated in a patient with this anatomic variant, portal flow to the entire liver, including the remnant left hemiliver, will be lost. There is usually a small portal branch that passes from the main right portal vein to the caudate process; ligation of this branch will untether an additional 1 to 2 cm of the right portal vein, allowing safer dissection and ligation. The right portal vein can be occluded with vascular clamps, divided, and oversewn with nonabsorbable sutures. Once divided, the right hepatic artery becomes readily visible behind the CBD and can be easily secured and ligated with nonabsorbable sutures. Because of the multitude of biliary anatomic variations, we typically leave the right hepatic duct intact until

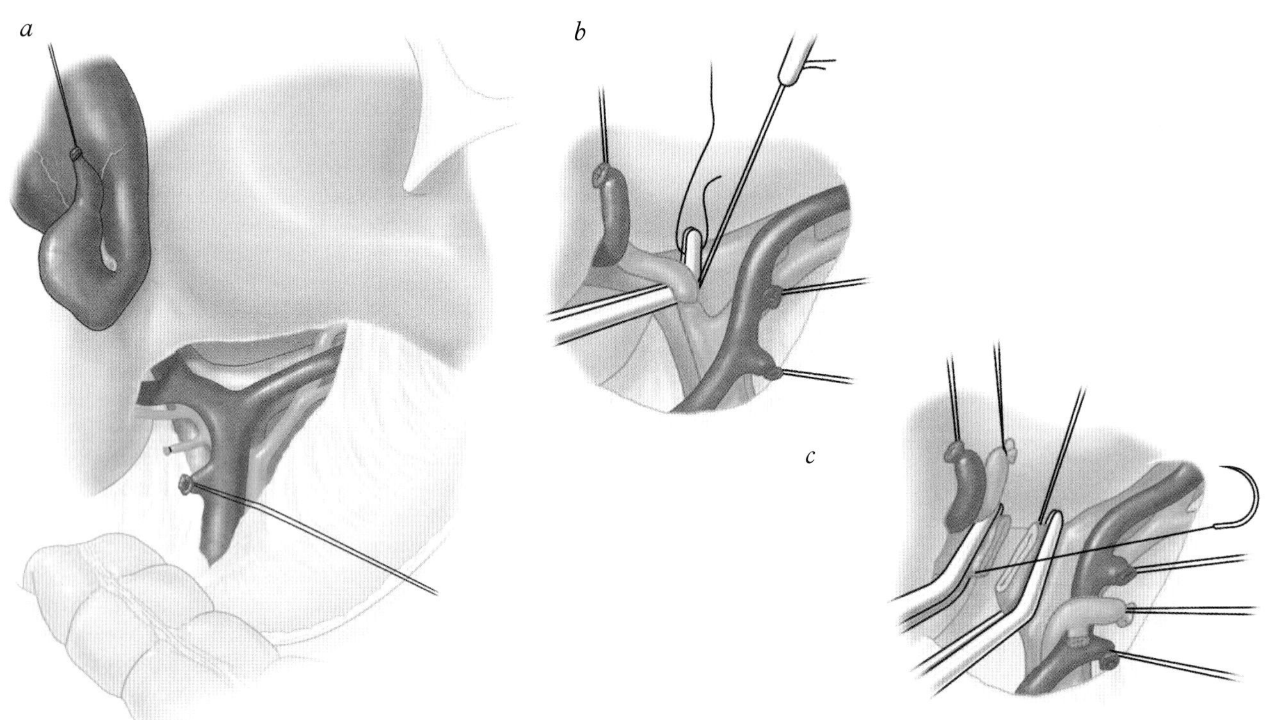

Figure 5 **Right hepatectomy. For control of the inflow vessels of the right hemiliver, the liver is retracted cephalad to allow exposure of the porta hepatis. (*a*) The gallbladder is resected to allow access to the bile duct and hepatic vessels. (*b*) The right hepatic duct is ligated to allow access to the hepatic artery and the portal vein. (*c*) After the right hepatic artery is divided, the right portal vein is controlled and divided. Alternatively, the vessels may be approached from a posterolateral direction and the portal vein and hepatic artery may be divided first, with the hepatic duct left intact until the parenchymal transection.**

parenchymal dissection [*see* Step 8: Parenchymal Dissection, *below*] is begun; this structure can then be divided higher within the hepatic parenchyma to minimize the likelihood of injury to the left ductal system. Once the portal vein and hepatic artery are divided, a clear line of ischemic demarcation of the right hemiliver will be visible along the Cantlie line.

Staple ligation Alternatively, vascular staplers may be used to divide the right or the left portal vein during extrahepatic vascular dissection[42,43]; in most cases, suture ligation of the extrahepatic portal veins is such a straightforward technical exercise that staplers add little except cost.

Step 6—Alternative (Intrahepatic Pedicle Ligation): Control of Inflow Vessels

As stated above, Glisson and Couinaud observed that the nutrient vessels to the liver are contained within a thick connective tissue capsule [*see Figure 6*]; this was the basis for the initial proposal by Launois and Jamieson that intrahepatic vascular pedicle ligation could serve as an alternative to extrahepatic dissection and ligation for controlling vascular inflow to the liver.[17] This alternative technique has the advantages of being rapid and less likely to cause injury to the vasculature or the biliary drainage of the contralateral liver. Using this technique, one can readily access and isolate the major pedicles to the areas of liver to be resected using simple combinations of hepatotomies at specific sites along the inferior surface of the liver [*see Figure 7*].

In this approach, the right hemiliver is completely mobilized from the retroperitoneum. The most inferior small hepatic veins are ligated, and the inferior right hemiliver is mobilized off the vena cava. Incisions are made in the liver capsule at hepatotomy sites A and B [*see Figure 7*]. The first incision is made though the caudate lobe. The full thickness of the caudate lobe is divided with a combination of diathermy, crushing, and ligation. The second incision is made almost vertically in the medial part of the gallbladder bed. Both incisions must be fairly substantive and reasonably deep. Care must be taken to avoid the terminal branches of the middle hepatic vein, particularly along hepatotomy site B, as this is the most common source of bleeding. Using either finger dissection or passage of a large curved clamp (e.g., a renal pedicle clamp), a tape is placed around the right main sheath [*see Figure 8*]. This tape can be pulled medially to provide better exposure of the intrahepatic right pedicle and to retract the left-sided structures away from the area to be clamped and divided. Vascular clamps are applied, the right pedicle is divided, and the stumps are suture-ligated.

In practice, for right hepatectomy, we prefer to isolate the right anterior and posterior pedicles separately [*see Figure 8*] and ligate them individually. By dividing the right inflow structures higher within the liver, this measure ensures that the left-sided structures cannot be injured. Any minor bleeding from a hepatotomy usually ceases spontaneously or with application of Surgicel into the wound.

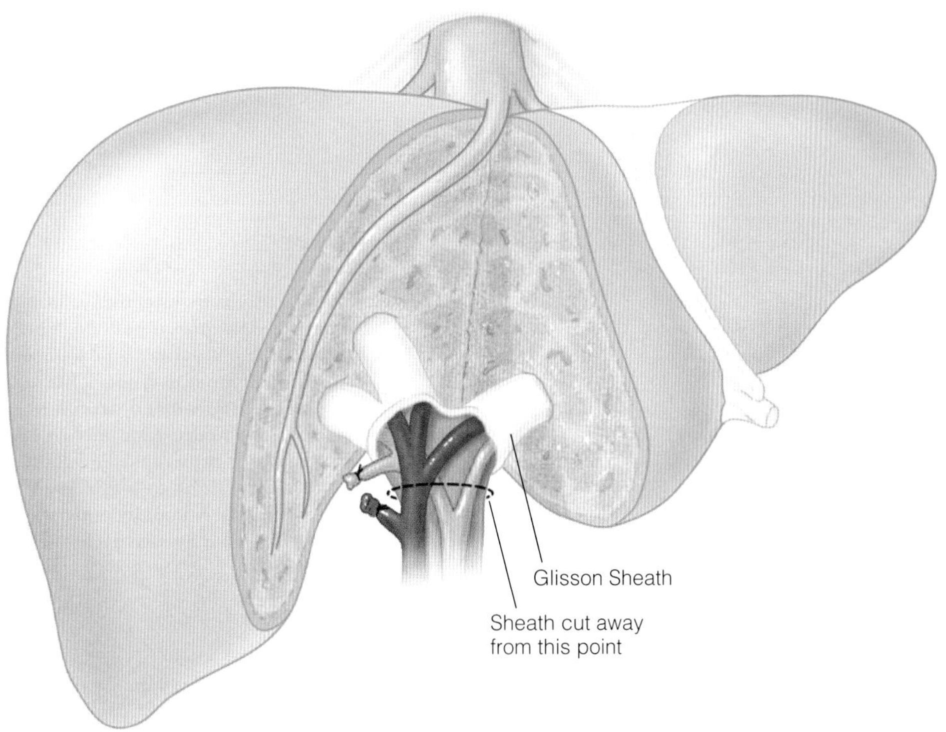

Figure 6 **Right hepatectomy. The Glisson sheath is a vascular and biliary pedicle that contains the portal triad. If this sheath is not violated, the entire pedicle can be suture-ligated or staple-ligated with confidence and safety.**

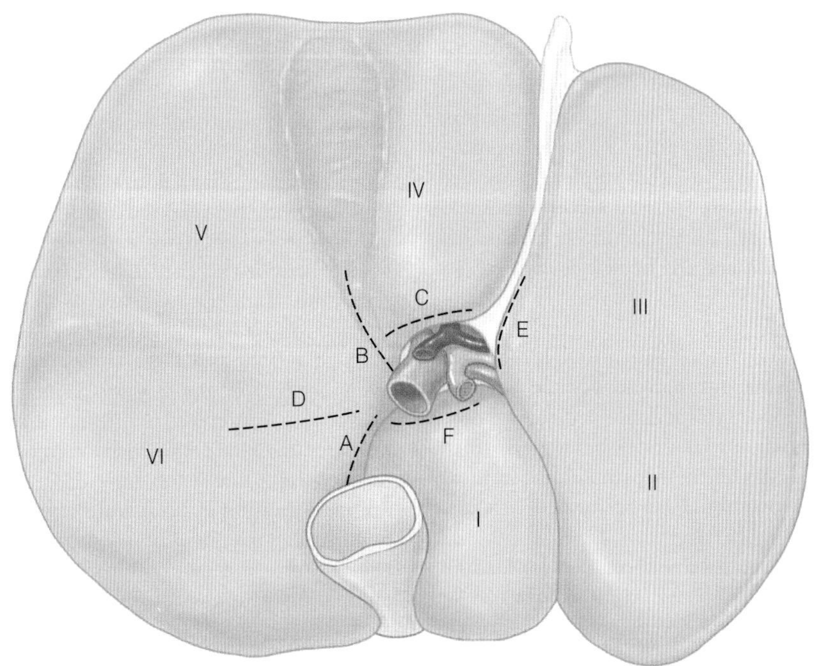

Figure 7 **Right hepatectomy. Depicted are sites where hepatotomies can be made to permit isolation of various vascular pedicles. Incisions at sites A and B allow isolation of the right main portal pedicle. Incisions at sites A and D allow isolation of the right posterior portal pedicle. Incisions at sites B and D allow isolation of the right anterior pedicle. Incisions at sites C and E allow isolation of the left main portal pedicle; if the caudate lobe is to be removed, incisions are made at sites C and F. The Roman numerals refer to the hepatic segments.**

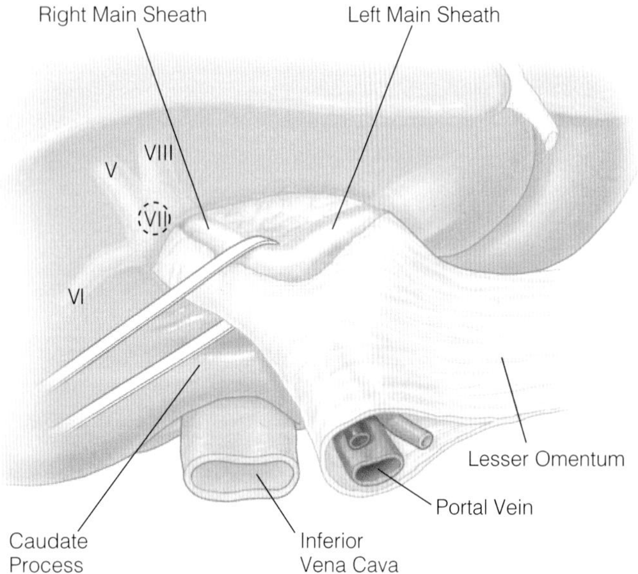

Figure 8 **Right hepatectomy. Depicted is isolation of the main right portal pedicle. The pedicle is controlled with a vascular tape and retracted from within the liver substance. This tape can be used for countertraction when a vascular clamp or stapler is applied. The main right portal pedicle has anterior and posterior branches. The right anterior pedicle consists of pedicles to segments V and VIII. The right posterior pedicle usually consists of only the segment VI pedicle but may also give rise to the segment VII pedicle.**

Staple ligation The use of staplers is now well established for liver resections[42–47]; we have found that staple ligation greatly increases the speed with which intrahepatic portal pedicle ligations can be performed. To control the intrahepatic portal pedicles for a right hepatectomy, incisions are made at hepatotomy sites A and B [*see Figure 7*]. Ultrasonography directed from the inferior aspect of the liver helps determine the depth at which the right pedicle lies, which is usually 1 to 2 cm from the inferior surface. The right main pedicle is secured and encircled with an umbilical tape [*see Figure 9a*]. The hilar plate along the base of segment IV is lowered via an incision at hepatotomy site C [*see Figure 7*] to ensure that the left-sided vascular and biliary structures are mobilized well away from the area of staple ligation. A transverse anastomosis (TA) vascular stapler is applied to the right main pedicle while firm countertraction is applied to the umbilical tape to pull the hilum to the left [*see Figure 9a*]. The stapler is fired, and the pedicle is divided [*see Figure 9b*].

Troubleshooting Several important principles should be followed when considering intrahepatic pedicle ligation. The most important is that intrahepatic pedicle ligation should not be undertaken when resection is being performed for a tumor located within 2 cm of the hepatic hilum. In these cases, extrahepatic dissection should be performed to avoid potential violation of the tumor margin.

From a technical standpoint, removal of the gallbladder greatly facilitates isolation and control of right-sided vascular pedicles in a right hepatectomy. Application of the Pringle maneuver decreases bleeding during hepatotomy and isolation of the pedicle. Also, the lowest hepatic veins behind the liver should be dissected before any attempt is made to isolate the right-sided portal pedicles as incising the caudate lobe without first dividing the small hepatic veins draining this portion of the liver to the inferior vena cava can lead to troublesome hemorrhage.

Step 7: Control of Outflow Vessels

Control of the outflow vessels begins with division of the hepatic veins passing from the posterior aspect of the right hemiliver directly into the inferior vena cava. After the right hemiliver is completely mobilized off the retroperitoneum by dividing the right triangular ligament, it is carefully dissected off the vena cava. Dissection proceeds in a cephalad direction from the inferior border of the liver until the right hepatic vein is exposed. Complete mobilization of the right hemiliver is particularly critical for tumors close to the vena cava. Exposure of the right hepatic vein usually requires division of the inferior vena caval ligament, which connects the right hemiliver to the diaphragm along the right lateral aspect of the right hepatic vein. The right hepatic vein is then isolated, cross-clamped, divided, and oversewn [*see Figure 10*]. Unless the lesion to be resected involves the middle hepatic vein close to its junction with the vena cava, the middle hepatic vein usually is not controlled extrahepatically for right-sided resections and can be easily secured during parenchymal transection.

In cases where a large tumor resides at the dome of the liver, control of the hepatic veins and the vena cava may prove very difficult. In this circumstance, one should not hesitate to extend the incision into the chest with a right thoracoabdominal extension. The morbidity of a thoracoabdominal incision is preferable to the potentially catastrophic hemorrhage that may be encountered when the right hepatic vein is torn during mobilization of a rigid right hemiliver containing a bulky tumor.

Staple ligation Staple ligation has proven very useful for outflow control during partial hepatectomy. When the tumor is in proximity to the hepatic vein–inferior vena cava junction, extrahepatic control of the hepatic veins is essential for excision of the tumor with clear margins, and limits blood loss during parenchymal transection.[48] Ligation of the hepatic veins, particularly when an adjacent large and rigid tumor is

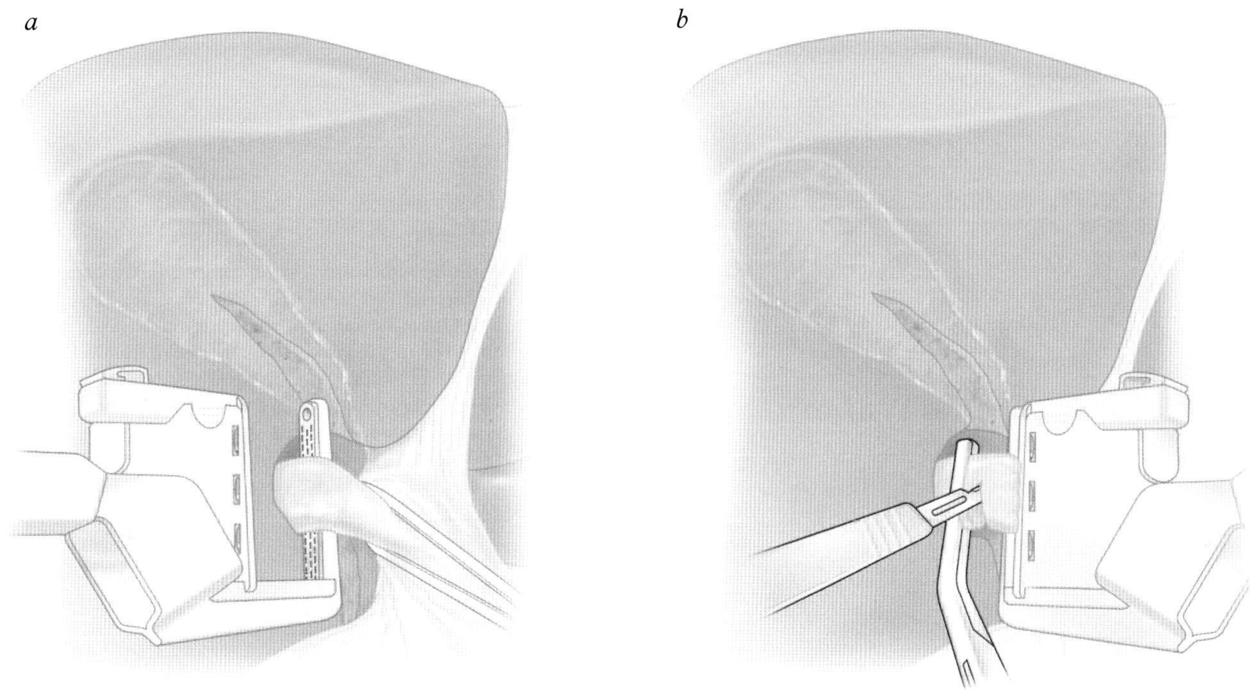

Figure 9 **Right hepatectomy. Shown is staple ligation of the right portal pedicle. (*a*) After the liver is incised across the caudate lobe and along the gallbladder bed, the right main pedicle is isolated and held with an umbilical tape. Countertraction is placed on the umbilical tape while a transverse anastomosis vascular stapler is placed across the pedicle, allowing the left hepatic duct and the left vascular structures to be retracted away from the line of stapling. (*b*) After the stapler is fired, the pedicle is clamped and divided.**

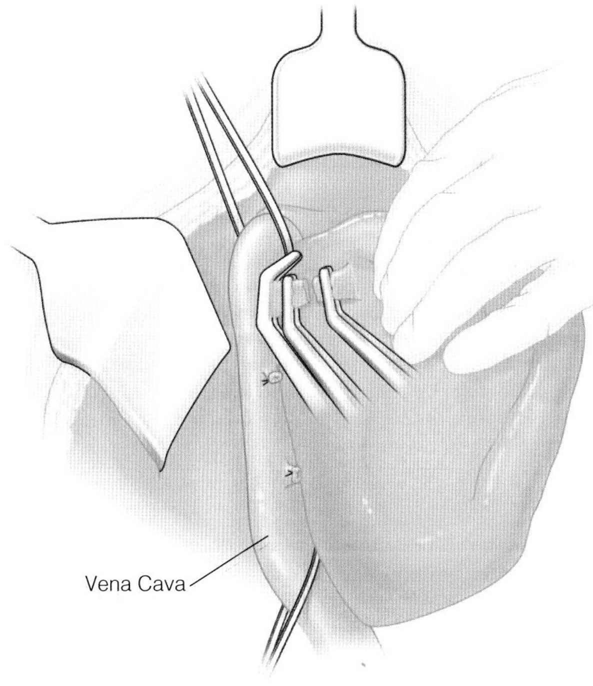

Figure 10 **Right hepatectomy. Once the small perforating vessels to the vena cava have been ligated, further dissection cephalad leads to the right hepatic vein. This vessel is controlled with vascular clamps and divided.**

present, can be a technically demanding and dangerous exercise. Tearing the hepatic vein or the inferior vena cava during this maneuver is the most common cause of major intraoperative hemorrhage.[36] The linear cutting stapler is well suited for ligation of the major hepatic veins because of its low profile and ability to seal the hepatic vein on the inferior vena cava and resection specimen sides simultaneously.

For staple ligation of the right hepatic vein, the right hemiliver is mobilized off the vena cava. Any large accessory right hepatic vein encountered can also be staple-ligated, as can the tongue of liver tissue that often passes from the right hemiliver behind the vena cava to the caudate lobe. The right hepatic vein is then identified and isolated. Although some surgeons introduce the stapler from the top of the liver downward,[43] we find that the location of the liver high in the surgical wound can make this angle of introduction difficult. Rather, we typically introduce the stapler parallel to the vena cava and direct it from below upward [*see Figure 11*]. To ensure that the stapler does not misfire, care should be taken to confirm that no vascular clips are present near the area where the stapler is to be applied.

Step 8: Parenchymal Transection

Inflow to the left hemiliver can be temporarily interrupted by clamping the hepatoduodenal ligament (the Pringle maneuver). The safety of temporary occlusion of the vessels supplying the hepatic remnant is well documented. Even in patients with cirrhosis, the warm ischemia produced by

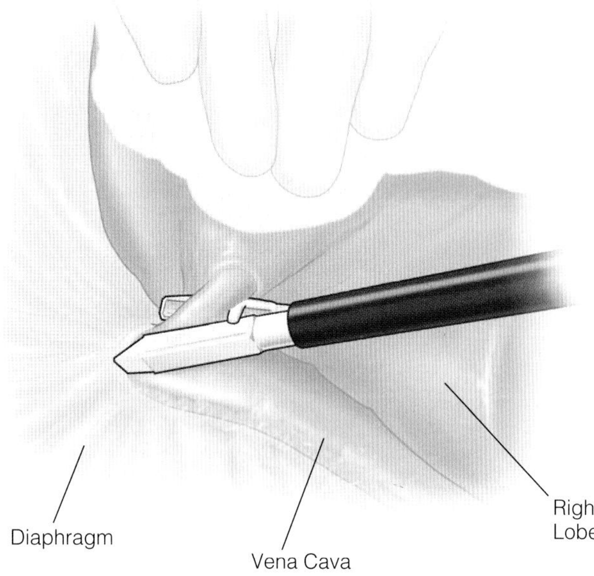

Figure 11 **Right hepatectomy. As an alternative to clamping and division, the right hepatic vein may be staple-ligated. Once the small perforating tributaries from the right hemiliver to the vena cava have been divided, the right hepatic vein is isolated and ligated with an endoscopic gastrointestinal anastomosis (GIA) vascular stapler. The safest method for introducing this stapler is to retract the liver cephalad and to the left while advancing the stapler cephalad in the direction of the vena cava.**

continuous application of the Pringle maneuver is well tolerated for as long as 1 hour.[49] Our practice is to apply the Pringle maneuver intermittently for periods of 10 minutes, with 2 to 5 minutes of perfusion between applications to allow for intestinal venous decompression.

Parenchymal division is then initiated along the line demarcated by devascularization of the right hemiliver. The line of transection along the principal plane is marked with the electrocautery, and the Glisson capsule is cut with scissors. Stay sutures of 0 chromic catgut are placed on either side of the plane of transection and used for traction, separation, and elevation as dissection proceeds.

Many special instruments have been proposed for use in parenchymal transection, including electrocautery, ultrasonic dissectors, and water-jet dissectors. For the majority of hepatic resections, we find that blunt clamp dissection is the most rapid method and is quite safe. In this technique, a large Kelly clamp is used to crush the liver parenchyma [*see Figure 12*]. The relatively soft liver substance dissects away, leaving behind the vascular and biliary structures, which are then ligated with vascular clips. Using this technique, the principal plane of the liver can usually be transected in less than 30 minutes.

In cirrhotic patients, the clamp-crushing technique may not work well because the vessels will often tear before the firm liver parenchyma does. Accordingly, ultrasonic dissectors that coagulate while transecting the parenchyma may be a better choice for cirrhotic patients. Water-jet dissectors may be useful in defining the major intrahepatic vascular pedicles or the junction of the hepatic vein and the vena cava, particularly when the tumor is in close proximity.

After the specimen is removed, the raw surface of the hepatic remnant is carefully examined for hemostasis and bile leakage. Any oozing from the raw surface may be controlled with the argon beam coagulator. Bile leaks should be controlled with clips or suture ligation. The retroperitoneal surfaces should be examined carefully for hemostasis, and the argon beam coagulator can be used where necessary.

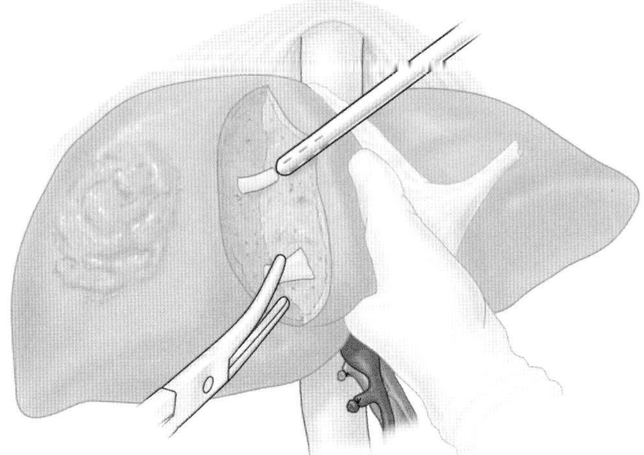

Figure 12 **Right hepatectomy. The parenchyma can be quickly and safely transected by means of the clamp-crushing technique. Large vessels and biliary radicles are visualized and ligated or clipped. This is usually done in tandem with inflow occlusion (i.e., the Pringle maneuver). Alternatively, the parenchyma can be bluntly dissected away by means of the finger-fracture technique.**

Step 9: Closure and Drainage

The abdominal wall is closed in one or two layers with continuous absorbable monofilament sutures. The skin is closed with staples or subcuticular sutures. Drains are unnecessary in most routine cases[50]; in fact, they may introduce harmful effects by promoting ascending infection or fluid management problems if ascites develops postoperatively. We reserve use of drains for four clinical scenarios: (1) evidence of a clear bile leakage, (2) an infected operative field, (3) operations involving a thoracoabdominal incision (in which a drain is used to ensure that any bile leakage does not develop into a peritoneopleural fistula), and (4) operations involving biliary reconstruction.

LEFT HEPATECTOMY (LEFT HEMIHEPATECTOMY)

Steps 1 through 5

Left hepatectomy involves removal of segments II, III, and IV and sometimes I and IX as well. The first five steps of the procedure are much the same as those of a right hepatectomy, except that the left hemiliver is mobilized by dividing the falciform ligament and left triangular ligaments.

Step 6 (Extrahepatic Dissection and Ligation): Control of Inflow Vessels

Extrahepatic control of vascular inflow vessels can be achieved in essentially the same fashion as in a right-sided resection. Our preference is to start the dissection at the base of the umbilical fissure, dividing the left hepatic artery first. The left portal vein is then easily identified at the base of the umbilical fissure. The point at which the left portal vein is to be divided depends on the extent of the planned parenchymal resection [*see Figure 13*]; if the caudate lobe is to be preserved, the left portal vein is divided just distal to its caudate branch (line B); if the caudate lobe is to be removed, the left portal vein is divided proximal to the origins of the portal venous branches to the caudate lobe (line A).

Step 6—Alternative (Intrahepatic Pedicle Ligation): Control of Inflow Vessels

If a left hepatectomy is undertaken to treat benign disease or to remove a malignancy that is remote from the base of the umbilical fissure, we recommend performing stapler-assisted intrahepatic pedicle ligation in preference to extrahepatic dissection and ligation.

The left portal pedicle is identified at the base of the umbilical fissure. The hilar plate is lowered through an incision at hepatotomy site C [*see Figure 7*], and a second incision is made along the back of segment II at hepatotomy site E [*see Figure 7*], permitting isolation of the left portal pedicle with minimal risk of injury to the right-sided inflow vessels at the hilum. If the caudate lobe is to be removed as well, incisions should be made at hepatotomy sites C and F [*see Figure 7*] to allow isolation of the main left portal pedicle proximal to the vessels nourishing the caudate. The portal pedicle is isolated and encircled with an umbilical tape. In the course of dividing the left portal pedicle, the middle hepatic vein, which lies immediately lateral to the left portal pedicle, may be injured. To minimize this risk, firm downward traction is applied to the umbilical tape, and a TA-30 vascular stapler is placed across the left portal pedicle [*see Figure 14*], which is then stapled and divided.

Step 7: Control of Outflow Vessels

The left hemiliver is reflected to the right, and the entire lesser omentum is divided. The ligamentum venosum is identified between the caudate lobe and the back of segment II and is divided near its attachment to the left hepatic vein; this greatly facilitates identification and dissection of the left and middle hepatic veins anterior to the inferior vena cava. The left and middle hepatic veins are isolated in preparation for division.

Control of the left hepatic vein is quickly and safely accomplished with staple ligation. In approximately 60% of patients, the left and middle hepatic veins join to form a single trunk before entering the vena cava. In a left hepatectomy, the middle hepatic vein may be left intact, in which case, it must be protected while ligating the left. After the left hepatic vein is identified, an endoscopic gastrointestinal anastomosis (GIA)-30 vascular stapler is directed from above downward [*see Figure 15*] to divide this vessel. The liver is retracted to the right to permit visualization of the junction of the left and middle hepatic veins. If ligation of the middle hepatic vein is desired as well, as is the case when there is tumor in proximity to the vessel, this can be accomplished with a stapler directed along the same path used for left hepatic vein ligation.

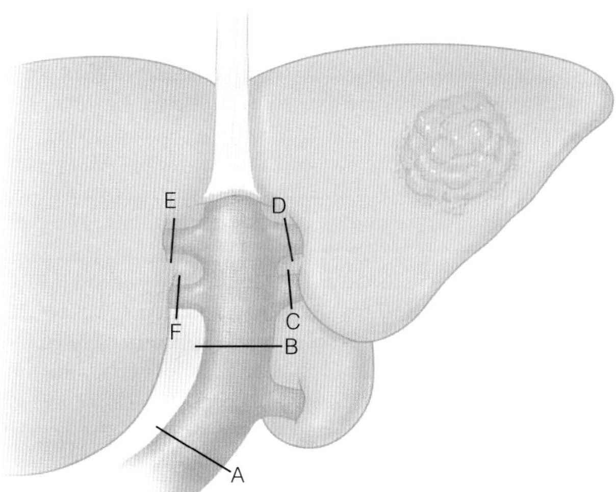

Figure 13 **Left hepatectomy. Ligation of vascular pedicles at specific sites in the left hemiliver interrupts inflow to specific areas. Ligation at A interrupts inflow to the entire left hemiliver, as well as the caudate lobe. Ligation at B interrupts blood flow to the left liver while sparing the caudate lobe. Ligation at C devascularizes segment II, and ligation at D devascularizes segment III. Ligation at E and F devascularizes segment IV.**

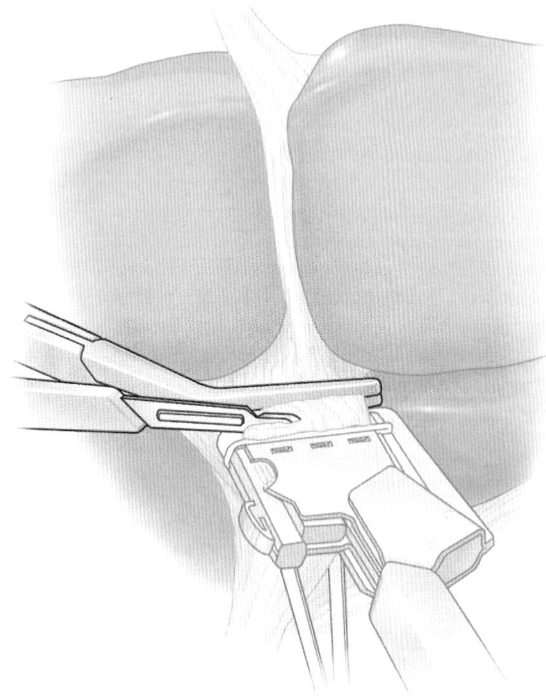

Figure 14 **Left hepatectomy. After hepatotomies in segment IV and in the back of segment II, the left portal pedicle is isolated, stapled, and divided.**

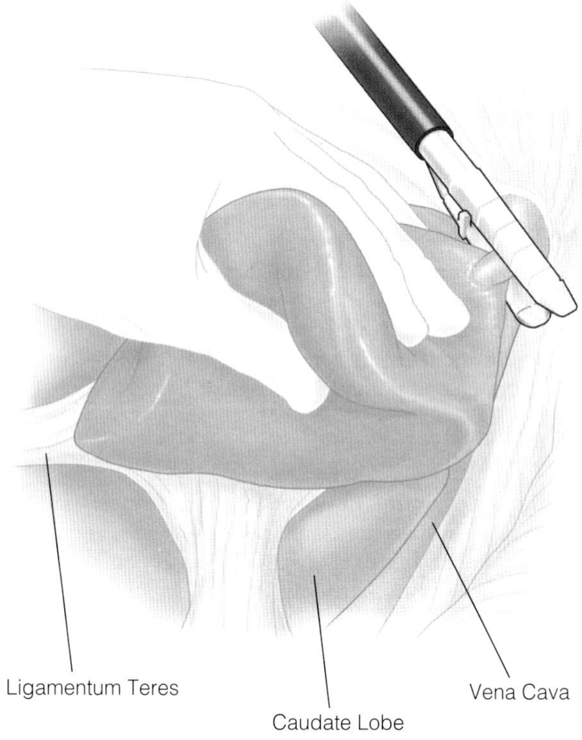

Figure 15 **Left hepatectomy. Staple ligation of the left hepatic vein. After the left hemiliver is completely mobilized through division of the left triangular ligament and the lesser omentum, the left hepatic vein is isolated and ligated with an endoscopic GIA vascular stapler. The best angle for introducing the stapler is from the xiphoid posteriorly and caudad.**

Steps 8 and 9

Parenchymal transection and closure are accomplished in much the same manner in a left hepatectomy as in a right hepatectomy (see above).

OTHER ANATOMIC RESECTIONS

In the following reviews of the other types of major anatomic resections, we focus primarily on the ways in which they differ from right and left hepatectomy. More detailed discussions of these operations are available in specialty texts on liver resection.[35,36]

Right Trisectionectomy (Extended Right Hepatectomy)

Right trisectionectomy (extended right hepatectomy) involves removal of the right hemiliver along with segment IV, thereby resecting all liver tissue to the right of the falciform ligament [*see Figure 3c*]. The initial steps of this operation are the same as those for right hepatectomy, up through division of the right inflow vessels and the right hepatic vein.

The next step is devascularization of segment IV. The umbilical fissure is dissected to permit identification of the vascular pedicles to segments II, III, and IV, which lie within this fissure [*see Figure 13*]. In most patients, the lower part of the umbilical fissure is concealed by a bridge of liver tissue fusing segments II and III to segment IV. After this tissue bridge is divided with diathermy, the ligamentum teres is retracted caudally to reveal the vascular pedicles from the umbilical fissure to segment IV (lines E and F [*see Figure 13*]). We generally suture-ligate these pedicles before dividing them.

The liver tissue is then transected immediately to the right of the falciform ligament, from the anterior surface back toward the divided right hepatic vein. The middle hepatic vein is generally left intact until it is encountered in the upper part of the parenchymal transection, at which point it is either suture- or staple-ligated.

Left Lateral Sectionectomy

A left lateral sectionectomy involves removal of only segments II and III, thereby resecting all liver tissue to the left of the falciform ligament [*see Figure 3d*]. These segments are mobilized by dividing the falciform ligament and left triangular ligaments. As this is done, care is taken to avoid injury to the left hepatic and phrenic veins, which run along the medial portion of the left triangular ligament.

The falciform ligament is retracted caudally, and the bridge of liver tissue between segment IV and segments II and III is divided with diathermy. Dissection is performed along the left of the umbilical fissure. The vascular pedicles to segments II and III are readily dissected and controlled (lines C and D [*see Figure 13*]). Control of these pedicles within the umbilical fissure is particularly important for tumor clearance if tumor is in proximity to the umbilical fissure: if the condition is benign or if tumor is remote from the umbilical fissure, the liver may be split anteroposteriorly just to the left of the ligamentum teres and the falciform ligament, and the vascular pedicles may be identified and ligated as they are encountered during the course of parenchymal transection.

Once the inflow vessels have been ligated, the left hepatic vein is identified and divided either before parenchymal transection or as the vessel is encountered near the completion of parenchymal transection. If there is tumor near the dome, it is particularly important for tumor clearance that the left hepatic vein be controlled and ligated early and outside the liver.

Left Trisectionectomy (Extended Left Hepatectomy)

A left trisectionectomy (extended left hepatectomy) involves resection of segments II, III, IV, V, and VIII and sometimes segments I and IX [*see Figure 3e*]. This is effectively a left hepatectomy combined with a right anterior sectionectomy, with or without resection of the caudate lobe. This complex resection is usually undertaken to excise large tumors occupying the left hemiliver and crossing the principal scissura into the right anterior section.

Throughout this procedure, it is imperative that the right hepatic vein be preserved as it represents the sole venous drainage of the intended hepatic remnant. However, parenchymal transection must often be performed along the course of this vein; therefore, the major risk in the operation is injury to the right hepatic vein, which could result in hemorrhage or hepatic failure from venous congestion of the hepatic remnant. In addition, because the blood supply to segment VII often arises from the right anterior portal pedicle or from the junction of the right anterior and posterior pedicles [*see Figure 8*], there is a risk of devascularization of a large portion of the hepatic remnant. Finally, the enormous variability of biliary anatomy and the extensive intrahepatic dissection required in this procedure increase the risk of biliary complications.[51] For these reasons, left trisectionectomies are rarely performed outside major centers.[52]

When planning a left trisectionectomy, particularly close attention must be paid to preoperative imaging investigations so that the right-sided intrahepatic vessels and biliary structures may be accurately delineated. Thin-slice CT and MRI in the form of arterial, portal venous, and hepatic venous reconstructions [*see Figure 2*] are quite helpful in this regard. For large tumors encroaching on the hepatic hilum or on the junction of the right anterior and posterior pedicles, direct angiography may be helpful on occasion.

The liver is fully mobilized by dividing the peritoneal attachments of the left and right hemilivers. This is essential for identifying the correct plane of parenchymal dissection and for ensuring safe dissection along the right hepatic vein.

The initial dissection is the same as for a left hepatectomy. The liver is turned to the right, the inflow vessels to the left hemiliver are divided, and the left hepatic vein and the subdiaphragmatic inferior vena cava are dissected free. The left and middle hepatic veins are controlled and divided extrahepatically.[52] The left hemiliver is thus freed, facilitating dissection of the right hemiliver.

Next, the plane of transection within the right hemiliver is defined. This plane runs horizontally and lies lateral to the gallbladder fossa and just anterior to the main right hepatic venous trunk in the right scissura, halfway between the right anterior pedicle and the right posterior pedicle. The plane can be approximated by drawing a line from just anterior to the right hepatic vein at its insertion into the vena cava to a point immediately behind the fissure of Gans. This line can also be accurately defined by clamping the portal pedicle to the right anterior section of the liver.[52] If the tumor is remote from the junction of the right anterior and posterior portal pedicles, the anterior pedicle is controlled as outlined earlier [*see* Right Hepatectomy, Step 6—Alternative (Intrahepatic Pedicle Ligation): Control of Inflow Vessels, *above*]. A vascular clamp is placed on the pedicle and the line of demarcation on the liver surface is carefully inspected before the pedicle is divided. If segment VII appears to be ischemic as well, further dissection must be done to identify and protect the origins of the vessels supplying segment VII.

Parenchymal dissection is carried out from below upward, with bleeding controlled by means of low central venous pressure anesthesia and intermittent application of the Pringle maneuver. If the caudate lobe is to be removed as part of the total resection, the veins draining the caudate must be controlled before parenchymal transection.

Segment-Oriented Resection

Each segment of the liver can be resected independently. In addition, right posterior sectionectomy (removal of segments VI and VII) [*see Figure 3f*] and right anterior sectionectomy (removal of segments V and VIII) are not uncommon. Extensive descriptions of so-called segment-oriented hepatic resection are available elsewhere.[53,54]

Postoperative Care

Intravenous fluids administered postoperatively should include phosphorus for support of liver regeneration. For large-volume hepatic resections, electrolyte levels, blood count, and prothrombin time (PT) are checked after the operation and then daily for 3 to 4 days. Packed red blood cells may be administered if the hemoglobin level falls to 8 mg/dL or lower, and fresh frozen plasma may be given if the PT is longer than 17 seconds. Postoperative pain control is best achieved with patient-controlled analgesia or epidural analgesia. Because of the decreased clearance of hepatically metabolized drugs after a major liver resection, selection and dosing of pain medications should be adjusted accordingly. An oral diet can be resumed as early as postoperative day 1 or 2 unless a biliary-enteric anastomosis was performed.

Peripheral edema is common after major hepatic resections and may be treated with spironolactone. Unexplained fevers or isolated hyperbilirubinemia with otherwise normal liver enzymes raises the suspicion for an intra-abdominal biloma, for which CT imaging should be obtained. If a biloma is identified, percutaneous drain placement usually brings about resolution of these collections after a few days, and reoperation is rarely necessary.

Special Considerations

TOTAL VASCULAR ISOLATION FOR CONTROL OF BLEEDING

For control of bleeding during liver parenchymal transection, a technique known as total vascular isolation can be used as an alternative to the Pringle maneuver. In this technique, the liver is isolated by controlling the inferior vena cava (both above and below the liver), portal vein, and hepatic artery. This approach is based on techniques developed for liver transplantation and on the observation that the liver is capable of tolerating total normothermic ischemia for as long as 1 hour.[55] Its primary advantage is that while the liver is isolated, little or no bleeding occurs. It does, however, have disadvantages as well. In some patients, temporary occlusion of the inferior vena cava causes hemodynamic instability resulting from reduced cardiac output coupled with increased systemic vascular resistance.[56] Cardiac failure with marked hypotension, arrhythmia, and even cardiac arrest may ensue. In addition, when hepatic perfusion is restored, the sudden return of stagnant potassium-rich blood to the systemic circulation can aggravate hemodynamic instability. For these reasons, and because bleeding is generally well controlled with low central venous pressure anesthesia, total vascular isolation is useful only in very rare cases. Indeed, one prospective analysis found that total vascular isolation had no major advantages over the approaches described earlier [*see* Operative Technique, Right Hepatectomy, Step 8: Parenchymal Transection, *above*] and was actually associated with greater blood loss.[48]

The one setting in which total vascular isolation may have a significant role is in the resection of very large tumors that compromise the vena cava or the hepatic veins. To extend the duration of vascular isolation in this setting, venovenous bypass that vents the splanchnic blood into the systemic circulation may be used.[57] To further minimize parenchymal injury during vascular isolation, the liver may be perfused with cold organ preservation solutions. For extensive vascular invasion that necessitates major vena cava or hepatic venous reconstruction, some authors have suggested that the liver can be removed during venovenous bypass, with resection and reconstruction performed extracorporeally.[58]

Although there are clinical situations that may call for these measures, they are very rarely necessary. Resection and reconstruction of short lengths of inferior vena cava can be performed quite safely without resorting to them. In fact, involvement of the retrohepatic vena cava at a level below the major hepatic veins can generally be treated with simple excision of the affected segment without replacement,[59] particularly if complete obstruction at this level has already led to established collateral venous circulation.

HANGING MANEUVER IN MAJOR HEPATECTOMY

The classic technique for a right hepatectomy (see above) involves complete mobilization of the right hemiliver before vascular control and parenchymal transection. However, in cases where the tumor has invaded the retroperitoneum or diaphragm, such mobilization may prove exceedingly difficult. Moreover, in cases where the tumor is large, soft, and vascular (e.g., HCC), early mobilization of the right hemiliver may increase the risk of tumor rupture. Finally, division of the vascular inflow and outflow vessels before manipulation of the tumor has the theoretical advantage of preventing vascular dissemination of cancer cells caused by compression of the tumor. For these reasons, some authors have proposed an anterior approach wherein the liver parenchyma is transected from the anterior surface toward the inferior vena cava, with ligation of the inflow and outflow vessels performed before mobilization of the right hemiliver.[60] This approach is now widely followed for resection of HCC.

Subsequently, other authors proposed a modification of this technique, whereby blunt dissection performed along the anterior surface of the vena cava permits passage of a tape that may be used to lift the liver and facilitate parenchymal transection [*see Figure 16*].[61] The first step in this so-called "hanging maneuver" is to dissect the space between the right and middle hepatic veins in a downward direction for approximately 2 cm. Next, dissection is performed between the vena cava and the caudate lobe on the left side of the inferior right hepatic vein. A clamp is then passed along this plane in the notch between the right and middle hepatic veins, and an umbilical tape is passed for suspension of the liver. Transection of the parenchyma is performed in an anterior-to-posterior direction until the vena cava is reached. The right side of the vena cava is then dissected, and the right hepatic vein and the inferior hepatic veins are ligated. The triangular ligament and the retroperitoneal attachments are transected, and the specimen is removed.

THE CIRRHOTIC PATIENT

The reduction in hepatic functional capacity and reserve present in patients with cirrhosis places them at higher risk for posthepatectomy complications. As a result, the cirrhotic patient requires a very careful assessment of liver function, appropriate selection for surgery, possible alteration of operative technique, and closer attention to perioperative care.

Operative Planning

Selection of patients Hepatic failure is the major cause of hospital death and long-term morbidity after hepatic resection in cirrhotic patients.[62–66] Consequently, determination of

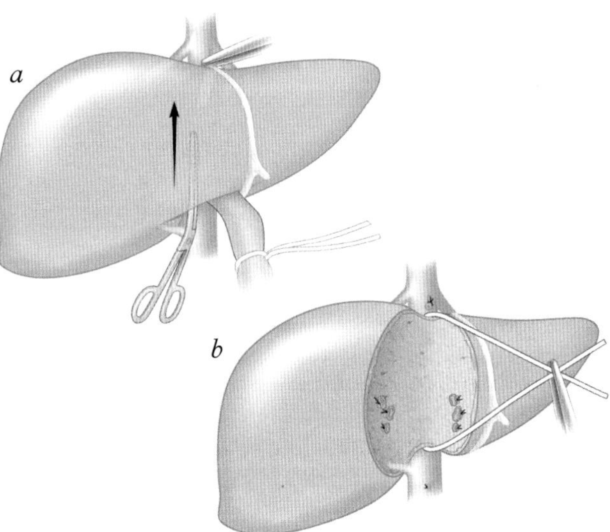

Figure 16 **Illustrated is clamp dissection in preparation for the hanging maneuver. (*a*) A long vascular clamp is passed between the vena cava and the caudate lobe. This clamp is directed at the notch between the right and middle hepatic veins, which has been dissected from above. (*b*) An umbilical tape is then passed to suspend the plane of parenchymal transection.**

a cirrhotic patient's candidacy for hepatectomy is based on a preoperative assessment of baseline liver function.

A variety of tests have been proposed for assessment of hepatic reserve, including measurement of clearance of various dyes and metabolic substrates.[62,65,67–69] Measurement of elevated hepatic portal venous pressure gradients via invasive radiologic techniques and noninvasive Doppler ultrasonography have also been found to predict postoperative hepatic failure.[70,71]

Currently, none of these functional tests are routinely performed at most major liver resection centers. In practice, the Child-Pugh score remains the most commonly employed clinical tool for selection of surgical candidates, with Child-Pugh scores higher than 8 being generally accepted as contraindications to major hepatic resection.[64,66,72–75]

Operative approach The appropriate extent of resection for cirrhotic patients may be quite different from that which may be reasonable for patients without cirrhosis. A guiding principle for hepatectomy in cirrhotic patients is to favor limited resections that spare as much functional parenchyma as possible. In general, even for patients with well-compensated Child class A cirrhosis, we work to limit resections to less than two segments of functional liver. Major hepatic resections involving removal of at least one hemiliver are now reported to carry an operative mortality of less than 10% in cirrhotic patients.[76,77] However, these procedures are usually performed in cirrhotic patients who have large tumors replacing most of one hemiliver, acceptable liver function, and no atrophy of the uninvolved hemiliver. Patients with large and peripheral tumors are more likely to tolerate a major resection because relatively little functional parenchyma is lost after tumor removal. Resection of small and deep-seated tumors can be more challenging; in such patients where resection might require removal of a large amount of functional hepatic parenchyma, an ablative alternative or even transplantation might be more suitable.

The effort to preserve as much functional liver as possible may make the resection more technically challenging. For example, multiple limited resections may be performed to avoid performing a formal hemihepatectomy.[78,79] Some go so far as to reconstruct the right hepatic vein for the purpose of preserving venous outflow in segments V and VI after resection of segments VII and VIII. In cirrhotic patients, hepatectomy is most commonly performed for HCC.[5] For such patients, as long as the resection margin is microscopically clear of cancer, the exact size of the margin does not correlate with the incidence of recurrent disease.[80] The acceptance of limited margins, coupled with the acceptance of nonanatomic resections aimed at preserving as much functional parenchyma as possible, has been responsible for significant improvements in the safety of hepatic resection in cirrhotic patients worldwide.

Operative Technique

A number of specific technical challenges are posed by the cirrhotic liver that substantially increase the complexity of hepatic resection. The parenchyma of the cirrhotic liver is very firm, making retraction and transection of the liver difficult. In addition, anatomic landmarks are distorted and difficult to locate as a consequence of hepatic fibrosis and atrophy-hypertrophy. Finally, portal hypertension and tissue friability contribute to increased blood loss during liver mobilization and parenchymal transection.

Exposure and mobilization Trifurcated incisions and thoracoabdominal incisions should be avoided in cirrhotic patients because of the potential for ascites leak externally or into the chest. The increased firmness of the cirrhotic liver and the consequent difficulty of retraction can lead to significant blood loss from retroperitoneal or phrenic collateral vessels during mobilization. To prevent such bleeding, it may be preferable to use an anterior approach in which the liver parenchyma is split within the principal scissura down to the anterior surface of the vena cava before the right hemiliver is mobilized off the retroperitoneum.[60] The right hemiliver is then mobilized in a medial-to-lateral direction, and the right hepatic vein is secured during mobilization of the right hemiliver off the vena cava.

Inflow control In the past, the safety of the Pringle maneuver in cirrhotic patients has been questioned. More recently, numerous studies have confirmed that hepatic inflow occlusion may be performed for extended periods in cirrhotic patients without increasing operative morbidity or mortality.[81–86] Nevertheless, it is advisable to employ the Pringle maneuver sparingly in this population so as to minimize ischemic stress. Our practice is to clamp the portal triad with a vessel loop tourniquet for 10-minute periods with 5-minute breaks between. We have not found additional protective maneuvers (e.g., topical cooling[87,88]) to be necessary.

Parenchymal transection In patients with normal liver parenchyma, most experienced hepatic surgeons use blunt dissection, with either the clamp-crushing technique or the finger-fracture technique, to transect the liver tissue.[89] In patients with cirrhosis, however, the firmness of the parenchyma makes the clamp-crushing technique less than ideal; because the parenchyma is often harder than the underlying vasculature and biliary radicles, blunt dissection is likely to tear these vessels. As a result, ultrasonic dissectors that coagulate and seal vessels during dissection are more suitable for parenchymal transection in this population.

Closure and drainage Because of the likelihood of postoperative ascites, the abdominal wall is reapproximated with a heavy continuous absorbable monofilament suture to create a watertight closure. To prevent major fluid and protein losses and ascending infections, abdominal drains are generally avoided.[50] Studies specifically examining the role of drainage in cirrhotic patients have documented a much lower incidence of postoperative complications and a shorter hospital stay for patients in whom no drains were placed.[90,91]

Postoperative Care

The focus of postoperative care in cirrhotic patients is on the management of cirrhosis and portal hypertension. In most cirrhotic patients who undergo hepatic resection, transient hepatic insufficiency develops postoperatively, characterized by hyperbilirubinemia, ascites formation, hypoalbuminemia, edema, and worsening of baseline coagulopathy.

In the first 24 hours after the procedure, crystalloid must be administered at a level sufficient to maintain adequate portal perfusion.[92] If patients are stable after the first 24 hours, they are subjected to water and sodium restriction and receive liberal amounts of salt-poor albumin for volume expansion if needed. Spironolactone is started in all patients as soon as an oral diet is resumed, and furosemide is added as needed. On very rare occasions, a peritoneovenous shunt may be employed to control postoperative ascites,[93] but this measure is usually unnecessary if patients are properly selected. The PT or international normalized ratio is checked twice daily during the immediate postoperative period; a PT longer than 17 seconds is corrected by administering fresh frozen plasma.

CHEMOTHERAPY-ASSOCIATED STEATOHEPATITIS

One of the most important advances in the treatment of metastatic colon cancer over the past several years has been the development and approval of a number of newer chemotherapeutic agents such as irinotecan, oxaliplatin, cetuximab, and bevacizumab. These agents target the cancer cell cycle, paracrine growth factors, and angiogenic factors and have led to substantial improvements in survival for patients with hepatic colorectal metastases. They are currently being used not only as effective palliative treatment in cases where resection is not feasible but also to downstage unresectable hepatic tumors to permit effective surgical treatment. Consequently, it is now common for patients to be subjected to intensive chemotherapy prior to partial hepatectomy.[94] Unfortunately, the recognition of hepatotoxic side effects associated with these newer chemotherapeutics has introduced newer challenges in the operative and postoperative management of these patients.[95]

Determination of operative candidacy must therefore include consideration of a condition known as chemotherapy-associated steatohepatitis (CASH).[96] This disease is associated with a characteristic clinical triad consisting of (1) hepatic steatosis, (2) splenomegaly, and (3) thrombocytopenia. Fatty infiltration of the liver is likely if hepatic attenuation is lower than splenic attenuation on CT imaging, but the absence of this finding does not exclude the possibility of clinically significant steatosis.[97] Splenomegaly is a sign of portal hypertension, as is refractory consumptive thrombocytopenia. Because this thrombocytopenia is not related to bone marrow suppression, it is not corrected even after chemotherapy is stopped.

When CASH is documented, patients should be selected for partial hepatectomy according to the same criteria used for patients with early cirrhosis. Consideration should also be given to preoperative portal vein embolization (PVE) (see below) before partial hepatectomy to increase the size of the anticipated hepatic remnant.

PREOPERATIVE PORTAL VEIN EMBOLIZATION

Most liver surgeons would be reluctant to resect more than the equivalent of two segments of functional liver in a patient with documented cirrhosis.[98] Consequently, many cirrhotic patients with technically resectable tumors are relegated to noncurative ablative therapy out of concern for possible postoperative hepatic failure. These limitations may be relieved with the growing use of preoperative PVE, which may extend the opportunities to undertake major hepatic resections in patients with cirrhosis.

In PVE, access to the portal vein on the side of the liver to be resected is gained via a percutaneous transhepatic approach. The vein is embolized approximately 1 month before the planned resection so as to produce ipsilateral atrophy along with compensatory hypertrophy of the contralateral future hepatic remnant.[99] The degree of compensatory hypertrophy can be dramatic [*see Figure 17*] and may modulate postoperative hepatic dysfunction. PVE is also employed in patients with normal parenchyma in whom extensive resection may result in a very small hepatic remnant. In patients undergoing right trisectionectomy, particularly those with a congenitally small left lateral section, the entire area of the extended right hepatectomy, including the main right portal vein and the segmental branches supplying segment IV, can be embolized.[100]

There is substantial evidence that preoperative PVE may be successfully used for patients with cirrhosis or impaired hepatic function; moreover, PVE appears to be generally well tolerated for these patients.[101–103] One immediate benefit of PVE is that it may act as a kind of stress test for the liver, allowing preoperative determination of the likelihood of liver regeneration. If no compensatory hypertrophy is seen 4 weeks after PVE, the decision to perform a major hepatic resection should be reconsidered.

Repeat Hepatic Resection

Since 1984, when one of the earliest descriptions of repeat hepatic resection was published,[104] a number of reports have demonstrated that repeat resection can be performed safely and with good long-term results, even for patients with recurrent malignancy. When appropriately selected, the morbidity and mortality rates associated with repeat partial hepatectomy for metastatic colorectal cancer[105–117] and HCC[118–125] are comparable to those observed after initial hepatectomy. Extended survival has been demonstrated, and in selected cases, survival is at least equivalent to that observed after initial resection.[106,113,120,126] In this section, we concentrate on the key technical aspects of repeat hepatic resection; discussion of indications, patient selection, and outcome are available in other sources.[106,113,120,126]

Repeat hepatic resection poses unique technical difficulties that are not typically encountered during initial resection.[105,127,128] First, adhesions at the previous line of parenchymal transection can make reexposure of the liver difficult. Mobilizing the liver off the vena cava and reexposing the porta hepatis and the hepatic veins can be extremely hazardous if dissection was previously undertaken in these areas. Second, liver regeneration and systemic chemotherapy can induce accumulation of fat within the liver, making it more friable[106]; this increased parenchymal friability further potentiates the difficulties of exposure and predisposes to inadvertent tearing of the Glisson capsule.[127] Third, regeneration alters the normal anatomic configuration of the portal structures [*see Figure 18*].[129] For example, after right hepatectomy, the porta hepatis is rotated posteriorly and to the right. The normal anatomic relations among the portal structures are altered, with the bile duct becoming displaced posteriorly and the portal vein becoming displaced anteriorly.

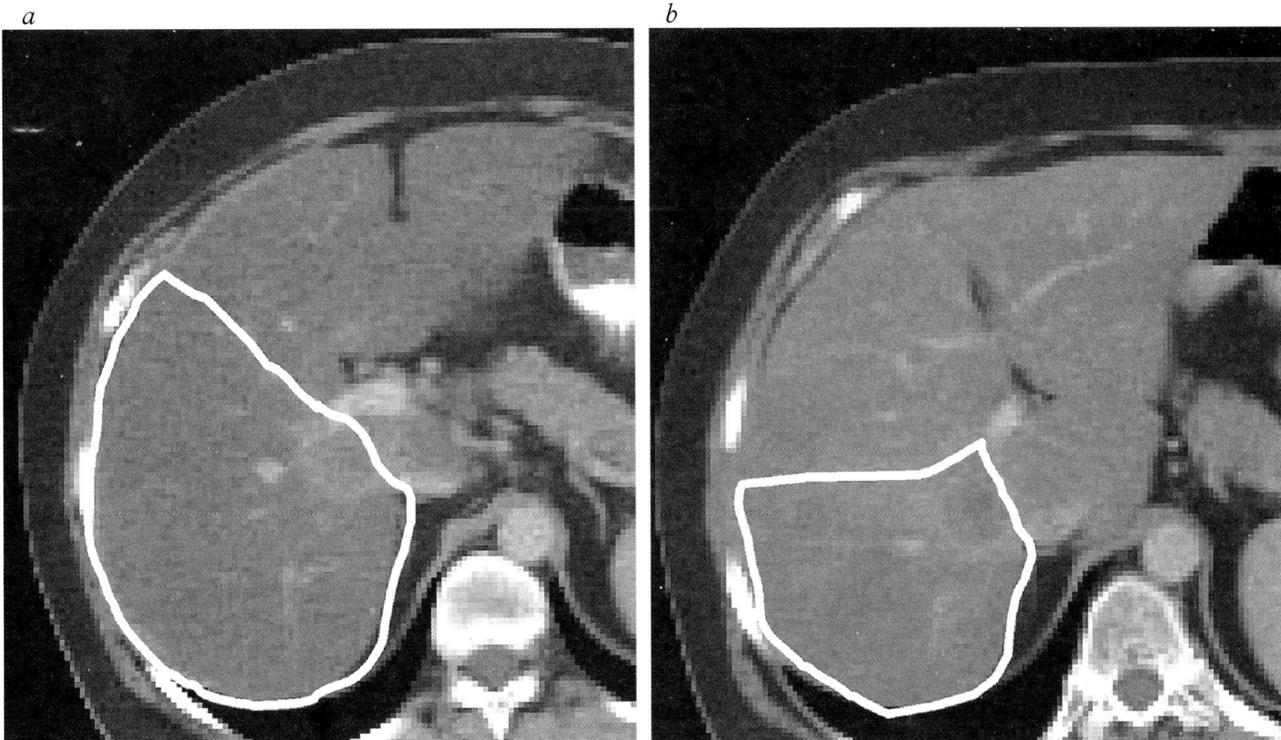

Figure 17 **Liver atrophy and hypertrophy occur after right portal vein embolization. Shown are images of the liver (*a*) at baseline and (*b*) 6 weeks after portal vein embolization. The right hemiliver is outlined in *white*.**

Preoperative imaging is therefore even more important for repeat resections than for primary resections; another reason for this is that postoperative adhesions will limit full access to the liver for intraoperative assessment via palpation or ultrasonography. Before undertaking a repeat resection, it is essential to know the exact number and locations of the lesions to be treated within the regenerated parenchyma. Preoperative imaging also facilitates operative planning by accurately delineating the vasculature within the regenerated liver.

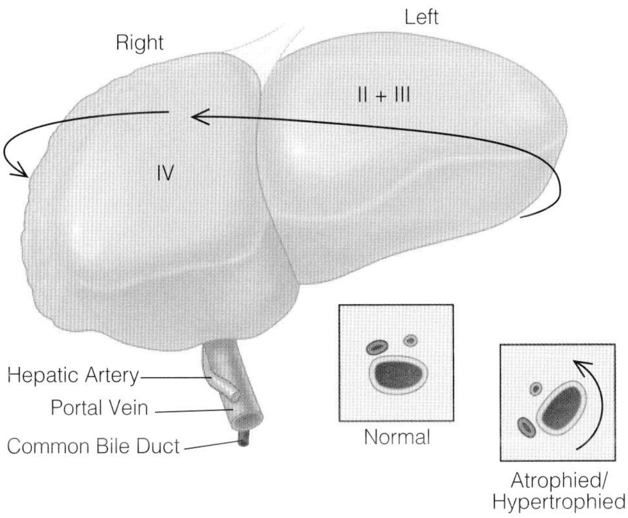

Figure 18 **Repeat hepatic resection. Depicted are the changes in the relations of the portal structures that occur as a result of right-liver atrophy or resection and left-sided hypertrophy. The structures in the porta hepatis rotate to the right, with the common bile duct coming to rest laterally rather than anteriorly. The Roman numerals refer to the hepatic segments.**

During repeat resection after a previous major right hepatectomy, preparations should be in place to convert to a thoracoabdominal incision if necessary. Access through the right chest may be required for mobilization of the liver because of dense adherence of the previous resection margin to the diaphragm; alternatively, it may be required for access to the rotated CBD and portal vasculature at the porta hepatis.

During dissection of the right upper quadrant after a previous right hepatectomy, three landmarks are particularly helpful in defining the anatomic structures within the regenerated left hemiliver. The first landmark is the remnant of the ligamentum teres, which defines the demarcation between the left lateral section (segments II and III) and the left medial section (segment IV); these should be identified early during operative exploration. The ligamentum teres may then be followed to the base of the umbilical fissure to define the location of the left hepatic artery. Regardless of whether this artery arises from the common hepatic artery or from the left gastric artery, it passes into the liver parenchyma at the base of the umbilical fissure. The second landmark is the caudate lobe. The lesser omentum should be opened early on to expose this structure, after which an index finger can then be passed in front of the caudate toward the obliterated foramen of Winslow to define the porta hepatis and the location of the portal vein. The third landmark is the vena cava. Performing a Kocher maneuver to mobilize the duodenum off the vena cava allows this vessel to be dissected, helping to define the portocaval plane. This will define the proper plane for dissection and mobilization of the liver off the vena cava and allows isolation of the hepatoduodenal ligament for application of the Pringle maneuver and for extrahepatic dissection of the inflow vessels.

In a repeat resection after a previous left hepatectomy, the main concern with regard to mobilization of the liver is the anterior displacement of the portal vasculature after right-sided hypertrophy. It is therefore prudent to mobilize the right hemiliver, perform a Kocher maneuver, and follow the vena cava caudally to identify the portal vein from the right. The stomach and the colon are usually adherent against the edge of the previous resection and must be carefully dissected free to allow access to the liver. If the middle hepatic vein was preserved in the earlier left hepatectomy, it will lie immediately deep to the plane of the stomach or the colon and may therefore become a source of hemorrhage during dissection.

Control of the inflow or outflow vasculature may be compromised by scarring resulting from the previous operation. If extensive extrahepatic dissection was performed for control of inflow vasculature in the earlier procedure, control of these vessels in the repeat resection is more safely accomplished via intrahepatic pedicle ligation [*see* Operative Technique, Right Hepatectomy, Step 6—Alternative (Intrahepatic Pedicle Ligation): Control of Inflow Vessels, *above*].

Another major concern with repeat partial hepatectomy is that it is often necessary to perform more limited resections than would be indicated during a primary resection. During primary resections, we typically avoid wedge excisions as these nonanatomic resections are associated with greater blood loss and a higher likelihood of positive margins compared with anatomic resections.[112,130] However, during a repeat partial hepatectomy, the absence of multiple inflow or outflow vessels and other anatomic considerations arising in the regenerated liver may make a wedge resection or ablation the best choice.

With appropriate patient selection and careful operative planning, very favorable perioperative and long-term results can be achieved after repeat hepatic resection. Notably, studies of repeat resection have not documented substantial increases in blood loss, operative duration, or complication rates in comparison with initial resection.[106–110,131]

Laparoscopic Hepatic Resection

In addition to revolutionizing the treatment of gallstone disease,[132] laparoscopic techniques have been used increasingly for fenestration of benign cysts of the liver[133,134] and for staging of hepatobiliary malignancies to prevent unnecessary laparotomies.[38,135–137] Until relatively recently, laparoscopic resection of liver tumors was described only in case reports or small series.[133,138–142] One reason for the strong resistance to laparoscopic hepatic resection has been fear of catastrophic bleeding. If inadvertent damage to a major hepatic vein or the vena cava occurs during an open operation, the bleeding can be temporarily controlled with direct manual compression until the vessel is repaired; however, if such damage occurs during a laparoscopic operation, initial control of the bleeding is considerably more difficult. In addition, damage to a hepatic vein or the vena cava during a laparoscopic procedure may theoretically result in CO_2 embolism. Another concern is that the loss of tactile sensation characteristic of laparoscopic surgery may lead to inadequate tumor clearance. Finally, although there are many liver retractors designed to hold the liver in one position, there is no good retractor for repeatedly moving the liver from side to side, as would be necessary during a laparoscopic hepatectomy. The human hand is still the best tool for this purpose.

Laparoscopic hepatic resection has been greatly facilitated by several recent technologic advances, including the introduction of laparoscopic staplers[143] and ultrasonic dissectors,[144] which can be used for ligation of the hepatic vasculature and transection of liver parenchyma. Another important instrument is the hand access port, a small port through which one hand can be introduced into the abdomen for a hand-assisted laparoscopic resection [*see Figure 19*].[145–147] This approach retains a measure of tactile sensation, permits the employment of the hand for optimal liver retraction, and allows for direct manual compression of any bleeding vessels. Furthermore, the incision made for the hand access port can be used for extraction of the resected specimen.

Appropriate patient selection is essential for safe laparoscopic resection of liver tumors. Resection of any two segments along the lower edge of the liver is easily accomplished laparoscopically. We have laparoscopically resected lesions from all segments.[11] In the following section, we provide a general overview of laparoscopic hepatic resection; more in-depth discussions of the technical aspects of these procedures and the results reported from various centers are available elsewhere.[148]

OPERATIVE TECHNIQUE

The patient is placed on the operating table in a supine position and is securely strapped down to allow for rotation of the table. For a right hepatectomy or resection of segments VII and VIII (bisegmentectomy VII, VIII), the patient may

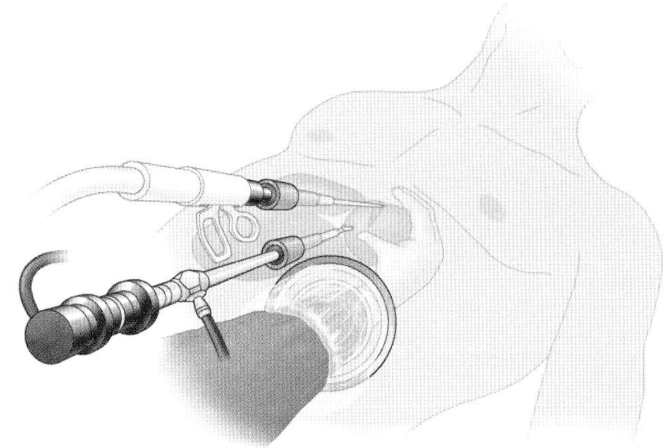

Figure 19 **Laparoscopic hepatic resection: hand assisted. Introduction of the hand within the abdomen restores tactile sensation to the surgeon and facilitates resection of the liver. The hand is the best liver retractor available and can be used to dissect the parenchyma. The specimen can be extracted through the hand access port.**

be positioned in a left lateral decubitus position, although we have not found this to be universally necessary.

As outlined earlier, a hand access port can be of great utility in laparoscopic liver resection. However, care must be taken in placing the hand port in a location that will not impede access of other trocar sites. For left-sided resection, the hand access port can be placed through a transverse incision in the left upper quadrant [*see Figure 19*] or through an upper midline incision. For right-sided resection, the port may be placed in the right lower quadrant [*see Figure 20b*] or through an upper midline incision.

Left-sided resections typically require placement of three to four ports [*see Figure 20a*]. Pneumoperitoneum is established using an initial port placed at the umbilicus; to prevent gas embolism during liver transection, it is maintained at the lowest pressure possible (typically 10 to 12 mm Hg). A 10 to 12 mm port is placed at the intersection of the subcostal and midclavicular lines to permit dissection of the triangular ligament, hepatic vein, and inferior vena cava. An additional 5 mm port may be placed between the previous two ports to facilitate dissection near the porta hepatic and umbilical fissure. A 10 to 12 mm port is placed in the right midclavicular line to permit the introduction of an endovascular stapler for division of the portal structures and liver parenchyma. We generally use the 45 mm rotating articulated stapler loaded with the white 2.5 mm cartridge.

Right-sided resections generally require placement of four ports. Pneumoperitoneum is again established using a port placed at the umbilicus. If the hand access port is placed in the right lower quadrant, a 10 to 12 mm port is placed in a subxiphoid position through which an endovascular stapler may be passed for division of the portal structures, liver parenchyma, and hepatic vein. An additional 5 mm port placed in the midepigastrium will facilitate dissection in the porta hepatis, and a 5 mm port placed in a subcostal location along the anterior axillary line will facilitate mobilization of the right hemiliver off the diaphragm and inferior vena cava.

Laparoscopic partial hepatectomy begins with a staging exploration to confirm that the lesion is resectable and, in cases of malignancy, to exclude the presence of distant extrahepatic metastases. IOUS is especially critical in laparoscopic resections for identification of major inflow and outflow vessels, tumor location, and guidance of parenchymal transection. We place a laparotomy sponge into the abdomen to facilitate retraction, absorb blood, and cleanse the laparoscopic camera as needed. A long bulldog clamp may be inserted into the peritoneal cavity in the event that a Pringle maneuver should prove necessary; a long umbilical tape is tied to the bulldog clamp so that the instrument can be easily located throughout the procedure.

Once the liver is mobilized and the tumor is located, the plane of planned transection is marked with the electrocautery. The liver is manually retracted, and parenchymal transection is initiated using ultrasonic dissection. We typically do not attempt to dissect the inflow and outflow vessels extrahepatically. Rather, when parenchymal dissection approaches the major portal pedicles and hepatic veins, we use an endoscopic GIA vascular stapler for transection. After removal of

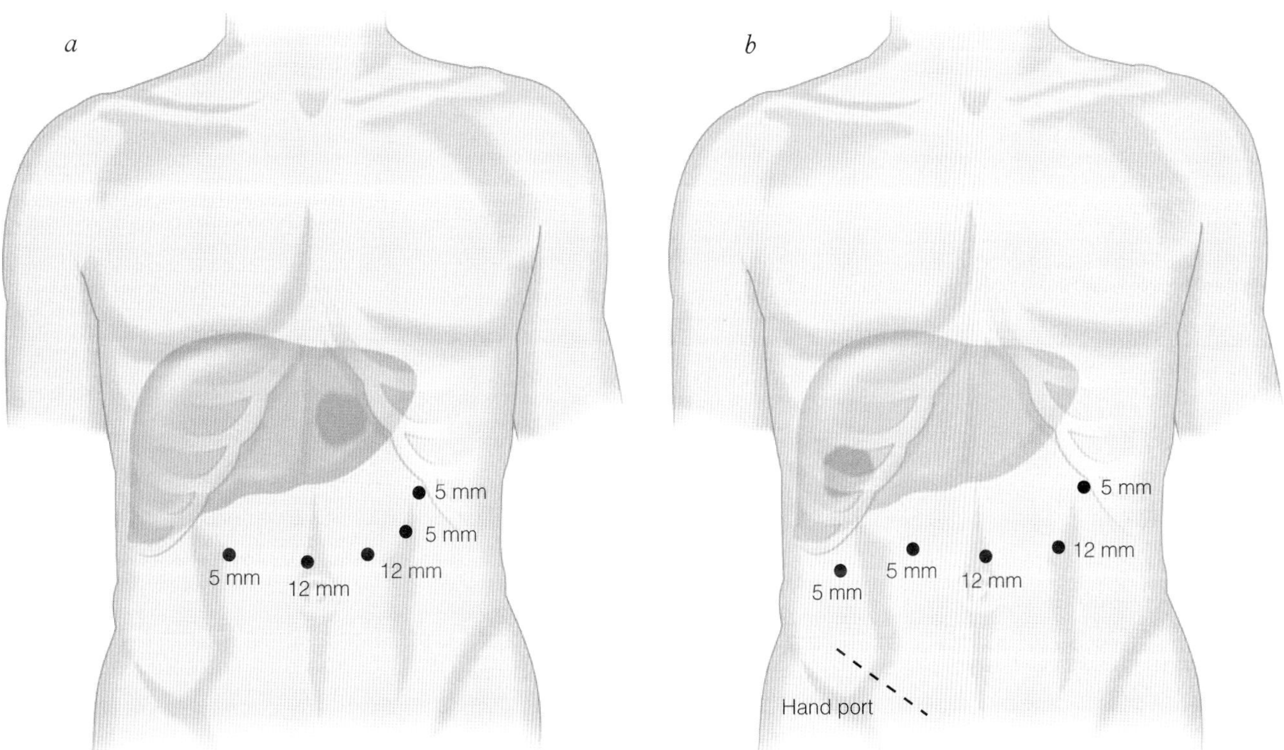

Figure 20 **Shown are the recommended port placements for (*a*) laparoscopic left lateral sectionectomy and (*b*) hand-assisted laparoscopic right hepatectomy.**

the specimen, the laparoscopic argon beam coagulator and topical agents are used to ensure adequate hemostasis.

As experience with laparoscopic partial hepatectomy is increasing, evidence supporting the safety and oncologic efficacy of major laparoscopic hepatic resections is accumulating.[149–151] Ongoing analysis of laparoscopic hepatic resection with respect to long-term measures of quality of life and survival continues.

Financial Disclosures: None Reported

References

1. Weitz J, Klimstra DS, Cymes K, et al. Management of primary liver sarcomas. Cancer 2007;109:1391–6.
2. Weitz J, Blumgart LH, Fong Y, et al. Partial hepatectomy for metastases from noncolorectal, nonneuroendocrine carcinoma. Ann Surg 2005;241:269–76.
3. Charnsangavej C, Clary B, Fong Y, et al. Selection of patients for resection of hepatic colorectal metastases: expert consensus statement. Ann Surg Oncol 2006;13:1261–8.
4. Morris KT, Song TJ, Fong Y. Recent advancements in diagnosis and treatment of metastatic colorectal cancer to the liver. Surg Oncol 2006;15:129–34.
5. Song TJ, Ip EW, Fong Y. Hepatocellular carcinoma: current surgical management. Gastroenterology 2004;127(5 Suppl 1): S248–60.
6. Lortat-Jacob JL, Robert HG. Hepatectomie droite reglee. Presse Med 1952;60:549–51.
7. Fong Y, Gonen M, Rubin D, et al. Long-term survival is superior after resection for cancer in high-volume centers. Ann Surg 2005;242:540–4.
8. Fong Y. Hepatic colorectal metastasis: current surgical therapy, selection criteria for hepatectomy, and role for adjuvant therapy. Adv Surg 2000;34:351–81.
9. Jarnagin WR, Fong Y, Blumgart LH. The current management of hilar cholangiocarcinoma. Adv Surg 1999;33:345–73.
10. Fong Y, Sun RL, Jarnagin W, et al. An analysis of 412 cases of hepatocellular carcinoma at a Western center. Ann Surg 1999;229: 790–9.
11. D'Angelica M, Maddineni S, Fong Y, et al. Optimal abdominal incision for partial hepatectomy: increased late complications with Mercedes-type incisions compared to extended right subcostal incisions. World J Surg 2006;30:410–8.
12. Strasberg SM, Belghiti J, Clavien P-A, et al. The Brisbane 2000 terminology of liver anatomy and resections. HPB 2000;2:333–9.
13. Baer HU, Dennison AR, Maddern GJ, et al. Subtotal hepatectomy: a new procedure based on the inferior right hepatic vein. Br J Surg 1991;78:1221–2.
14. Smadja C, Blumgart LH. The biliary tract and the anatomy of biliary exposure. In: Blumgart LH, editor. Surgery of the liver and biliary tract. 2nd ed. London: Churchill Livingstone; 1994.
15. Glisson F. Anatomia hepatis. London: O Pullein; 1654.
16. Couinaud C. Le foie: etudes anatomiques et chirurgicales. Paris: Masson; 1957.
17. Launois B, Jamieson GG. The importance of Glisson's capsule and its sheaths in the intrahepatic approach to resection of the liver. Surg Gynecol Obstet 1992;174:7–10.
18. Soyer P, Levesque M, Elias D, et al. Preoperative assessment of resectability of hepatic metastases from colonic carcinoma: CT portography vs sonography and dynamic CT. AJR Am J Roentgenol 1992;159:741–4.
19. Hann LE, Schwartz LH, Panicek DM, et al. Tumor involvement in hepatic veins: comparison of MR imaging and US for preoperative assessment. Radiology 1998;206: 651–6.
20. Akhurst T, Kates TJ, Mazumdar M, et al. Recent chemotherapy reduces the sensitivity of [18F]fluorodeoxyglucose positron emission tomography in the detection of colorectal metastases. J Clin Oncol 2005;23: 8713–6.
21. Strasberg SM, Siegal BA. Survival of patients staged by FDG-PET before resection of hepatic metastases from colorectal cancer. Ann Surg 2002;235:308.
22. Hann LE, Fong Y, Shriver CD, et al. Malignant hepatic hilar tumors: can ultrasonography be used as an alternative to angiography with CT arterial portography for determination of resectability? J Ultrasound Med 1996;15:37–45.
23. Gibson RN, Yeung E, Thompson JN, et al. Bile duct obstruction: radiologic evaluation of level, cause and tumor resectability. Radiology 1986;160:43–7.
24. Fortner JG, Lincer RM. Hepatic resection in the elderly. Ann Surg 1990;211:141–5.
25. Karl RC, Smith SK, Fabri PJ. Validity of major cancer operations in elderly patients. Ann Surg Oncol 1995;2:107–13.
26. Mazzoni G, Tocchi A, Miccini M, et al. Surgical treatment of liver metastases from colorectal cancer in elderly patients. Int J Colorectal Dis 2007;22:77–83.
27. Aldrighetti L, Arru M, Catena M, et al. Liver resections in over-75-year-old patients: surgical hazard or current practice? J Surg Oncol 2006;93:186–93.
28. Fong Y, Brennan MF, Cohen AM, et al. Liver resection in the elderly. Br J Surg 1997;84:1386–90.
29. Cunningham JD, Fong Y, Shriver C, et al. One hundred consecutive hepatic resections: blood loss, transfusion and operative technique. Arch Surg 1994;129:1050–6.
30. Melendez J, Ferri E, Zwillman M, et al. Extended hepatic resection: a 6-year retrospective study of risk factors for perioperative mortality. J Am Coll Surg 2001;192: 47–53.
31. Scheele J, Stangl R, Altendorf-Hofmann A, et al. Indicators of prognosis after hepatic resection for colorectal secondaries. Surgery 1991;110:13–29.
32. Weber SM, Jarnagin WR, DeMatteo RP, et al. Survival after resection of multiple hepatic colorectal metastases. Ann Surg Oncol 2000;7:643–50.
33. Cho CS, Labow DM, Tang L, et al. Histologic grade is correlated with outcome after resection of hepatic neuroendocrine neoplasms. Cancer 2008;113:126–34.
34. Allen PJ, Fong Y. Benign and malignant primary liver neoplasms. In: Zinner MJ, Ashley SW, editors. Maingot's abdominal operations. 11th ed. New York: McGraw-Hill; 2010. p. 783–811.
35. Blumgart LH, Jarnagin W, Fong Y. Liver resection for benign disease and for liver and biliary tumors. In: Blumgart LH, Fong Y, editors. Surgery of the liver and biliary tract. 3rd ed. London: WB Saunders; 2000. p. 1639.
36. Blumgart LH, Fong Y. Surgical management of colorectal metastases to the liver. Curr Probl Surg 1995;5:333.
37. Jarnagin WR, Conlon K, Bodniewicz J, et al. A clinical scoring system predicts the yield of diagnostic laparoscopy in patients with potentially resectable hepatic colorectal metastases. Cancer 2001;91:1121–8.
38. Jarnagin WR, Bodniewicz J, Dougherty E, et al. A prospective analysis of staging laparoscopy in patients with primary and secondary hepatobiliary malignancies. J Gastrointest Surg 2000;4:34–43.
39. Lo CM, Lai EC, Liu CL, et al. Laparoscopy and laparoscopic ultrasonography avoid exploratory laparotomy in patients with hepatocellular carcinoma. Ann Surg 1998; 227:527–32.
40. Callery MP, Strasberg SM, Doherty GM, et al. Staging laparoscopy with laparoscopic ultrasonography: optimizing resectability in hepatobiliary and pancreatic malingnancy. J Am Coll Surg 1997;185:33–9.
41. Castaing D, Kunstlinger F, Habib N. Intraoperative ultrasound study of the liver: methodology and anatomical results. Am J Surg 1985;149:676–82.
42. McEntee GP, Nagorney DM. Use of hepatic staplers in major hepatic resections. Br J Surg 1991;78:40–1.
43. Cohen AM. Use of laparoscopic vascular stapler at laparotomy for colorectal cancer. Dis Colon Rectum 1992;35:910–1.
44. Jurim O, Colonna JO II, Colquhoun SD, et al. A stapling technique for hepatic resection. J Am Coll Surg 1994;178:510–1.
45. Yanaga K, Nishizaki T, Yamamoto K, et al. Simplified inflow control using stapling devices for major hepatic resection. Arch Surg 1996;131:104–6.
46. Lefor AT, Flowers JL. Laparoscopic wedge biopsy of the liver. J Am Coll Surg 1994;178: 307–8.
47. Fong Y, Jarnagin W, Conlon KC, et al. Hand-assisted laparoscopic liver resection: lessons from an initial experience. Arch Surg 2000;135:854–9.
48. Belghiti J, Noun R, Zante E, et al. Portal triad clamping or hepatic vascular exclusion for major liver resection. Ann Surg 1996; 224:155–61.
49. Bothe AJ, Steele G Jr. Is there a role for perioperative nutritional support in liver resection? HPB Surg 1997;10:177–9.
50. Fong Y, Brennan MF, Brown K, et al. Drainage is unnecessary after elective liver resection. Am J Surg 1996;171:158–62.
51. Starzl TE, Iwatsuki S, Shaw BW, et al. Left hepatic trisegmentectomy. Surg Gynecol Obstet 1982;155:21–7.
52. Blumgart LH, Baer HU, Czerniak A, et al. Extended left hepatectomy: technical aspects of an evolving procedure. Br J Surg 1993;80: 903–6.
53. Scheele J. Segment oriented resection of the liver: rational and technique. In: Lygidakis NJ, Tytgat GNJ, editors. Hepatobiliary and pancreatic malignancies. Stuttgart: Thieme; 1989.
54. Scheele J, Stangl R. Segment oriented anatomical liver resections. In: Blumgart LH, editor. Surgery of the liver and biliary tract. London: Churchill Livingstone; 1994.
55. Huguet C, Nordlinger B, Gallopin JJ, et al. Normothermic hepatic vascular occlusion

for extensive hepatectomy. Surg Gynecol Obstet 1978;147:689–93.
56. Pappas G, Palmer WM, Martineau GL, et al. Hemodynamic alterations caused during orthotopic liver transplantation in humans. Surgery 1971;70:872–5.
57. Shaw BW, Martin DJ, Marquez JM, et al. Venous bypass in clinical liver transplantation. Ann Surg 1984;200:524–34.
58. Pichlmayr R, Grosse H, Hauss J, et al. Technique and preliminary results of extracorporeal liver surgery (bench procedure) and of surgery on the in situ perfused liver. Br J Surg 1990;77:21–6.
59. Cunci O, Coste T, Vacher B, et al. Resection de la veine cave inferieure retrohepatique au cours d'une hepatectomie pour tumeur. Ann Chir 1983;37:197–201.
60. Lai EC, Fan ST, Lo CM, et al. Anterior approach for difficult major right hepatectomy. World J Surg 1996;20:314–7.
61. Belghiti J, Guevera OA, Noun R, et al. Liver hanging maneuver: a safe approach to right hepatectomy without liver mobilization. J Am Coll Surg 2001;193:109–11.
62. Lau H, Man K, Fan ST, et al. Evaluation of preoperative hepatic function in patients with hepatocellular carcinoma undergoing hepatectomy. Br J Surg 1997;84:1255–9.
63. Takenaka K, Kanematsu T, Fukuzawa K, et al. Can hepatic failure after surgery for hepatocellular carcinoma in cirrhotic patients be prevented? World J Surg 1990;14: 123–7.
64. Nagasue N, Yukaya H, Kohno H, et al. Morbidity and mortality after major hepatic resection in cirrhotic patients with hepatocellular carcinoma. HPB Surg 1988;1: 45–56.
65. Paquet KJ, Koussouris P, Mercado MA, et al. Limited hepatic resection for selected cirrhotic patients with hepatocellular or cholangiocellular carcinoma: a prospective study. Br J Surg 1991;78:459–62.
66. Fan ST, Lai EC, Lo CM, et al. Hospital mortality of major hepatectomy for hepatocellular carcinoma associated with cirrhosis. Arch Surg 1995;130:198–203.
67. Hasegawa H, Yamazaki S, Makuuchi M, et al. [Hepatectomy for hepatocarcinoma on a cirrhotic liver: decision plans and principles of perioperative resuscitation. Experience with 204 cases.] J Chir (Paris) 1987; 124:425–31.
68. Makuuchi M, Kosuge T, Takayama T, et al. Surgery for small liver cancers. Semin Surg Oncol 1993;9:298–304.
69. Ercolani G, Grazi GL, Calliva R, et al. The lidocaine (MEGX) test as an index of hepatic function: its clinical usefulness in liver surgery. Surgery 2000;127:464–71.
70. Bruix J, Castells A, Bosch J, et al. Surgical resection of hepatocellular carcinoma in cirrhotic patients: prognostic value of preoperative portal pressure. Gastroenterology 1996;111:1018–22.
71. Yin XY, Lu MD, Huang JF, et al. Significance of portal hemodynamic investigation in prediction of hepatic functional reserve in patients with hepatocellular carcinoma undergoing operative treatment. Hepatogastroenterology 2001;48:1701–4.
72. Franco D, Capussotti L, Smadja C, et al. Resection of hepatocellular carcinomas: results in 72 European patients with cirrhosis. Gastroenterology 1990;98:733–8.
73. Wu CC, Ho WL, Yeh DC, et al. Hepatic resection of hepatocellular carcinoma in cirrhotic livers: is it unjustified in impaired liver function? Surgery 1996;120:34–9.
74. Noun R, Jagot P, Farges O, et al. High preoperative serum alanine transferase levels: effect on the risk of liver resection in Child grade A cirrhotic patients. World J Surg 1997;21:390–4.
75. Capussotti L, Borgonovo G, Bouzari H, et al. Results of major hepatectomy for large primary liver cancer in patients with cirrhosis. Br J Surg 1994;81:427–31.
76. Vauthey JN, Klimstra D, Franceschi D, et al. Factors affecting long-term outcome after hepatic resection for hepatocellular carcinoma. Am J Surg 1995;169:28–34.
77. Poon RT, Fan ST, Lo CM, et al. Intrahepatic recurrence after curative resection of hepatocellular carcinoma: long-term results of treatment and prognostic factors. Ann Surg 1999;229:216–22.
78. Makuuchi M, Hasegawa H, Yamazaki S, et al. Four new hepatectomy procedures for resection of the right hepatic vein and preservation of the inferior right hepatic vein. Surg Gynecol Obstet 1987;164:68–72.
79. Makuuchi M, Mori T, Gunven P, et al. Safety of hemihepatic vascular occlusion during resection of the liver. Surg Gynecol Obstet 1987;164:155–8.
80. Yoshida Y, Kanematsu T, Matsumata T, et al. Surgical margin and recurrence after resection of hepatocellular carcinoma in patients with cirrhosis: further evaluation of limited hepatic resection. Ann Surg 1989; 209:297–301.
81. Nagasue N, Uchida M, Kubota H, et al. Cirrhotic livers can tolerate 30 minutes ischaemia at normal environmental temperature. Eur J Surg 1995;161:181–6.
82. Wu CC, Hwang CR, Liu TJ, et al. Effects and limitations of prolonged intermittent ischaemia for hepatic resection of the cirrhotic liver. Br J Surg 1996;83:121–4.
83. Kim YI, Kobayashi M, Aramaki M, et al. "Early-stage" cirrhotic liver can withstand 75 minutes of inflow occlusion during resection. Hepatogastroenterology 1994;41: 355–8.
84. Kim YI, Nakashima K, Tada I, et al. Prolonged normothermic ischaemia of human cirrhotic liver during hepatectomy: a preliminary report. Br J Surg 1993;80: 1566–70.
85. Smadja C, Kahwaji F, Berthoux L, et al. [Value of total pedicle clamping in hepatic excision for hepatocellular carcinoma in cirrhotic patients.] Ann Chir 1987;41:639–42.
86. Elias D, Desruennes E, Lasser P. Prolonged intermittent clamping of the portal triad during hepatectomy. Br J Surg 1991;78: 42–4.
87. Yamanaka N, Furukawa K, Tanaka T, et al. Topical cooling-assisted hepatic segmentectomy for cirrhotic liver with hepatocellular carcinoma. J Am Coll Surg 1997;184: 290–6.
88. Kim YI, Kobayashi M, Nakashima K, et al. In situ and surface liver cooling with prolonged inflow occlusion during hepatectomy in patients with chronic liver disease. Arch Surg 1994;129:620–4.
89. Lin TY. A simplified technique for hepatic resection: the crush method. Ann Surg 1974;180:285–90.
90. Smadja C, Berthoux L, Meakins JL, et al. Patterns of improvement in resection of hepatocellular carcinoma in cirrhotic patients: results of a non drainage policy. HPB Surg 1989;1:141–7.
91. Franco D, Smadja C, Meakins JL, et al. Improved early results of elective hepatic resection for liver tumors: one hundred consecutive hepatectomies in cirrhotic and noncirrhotic patients. Arch Surg 1989;124: 1033–7.
92. Tsuge H, Mimura H, Orita K, et al. Evaluation of preoperative and postoperative sodium and water loading in patients undergoing hepatectomy for liver cirrhosis complicated by hepatocellular carcinoma. Hepatogastroenterology 1991;38 Suppl 1:56–62.
93. Maeda T, Shimada M, Shirabe K, et al. Strategies for intractable ascites after hepatic resection: analysis of two cases. Br J Clin Pract 1995;49:149–51.
94. Kornprat P, Jarnagin WR, Gonen M, et al. Outcome after hepatectomy for multiple (four or more) colorectal metastases in the era of effective chemotherapy. Ann Surg Oncol 2007;14:1151–60.
95. Karoui M, Penna C, Amin-Hashem M, et al. Influence of preoperative chemotherapy on the risk of major hepatectomy for colorectal liver metastases. Ann Surg 2006;243: 1–7.
96. Fong Y, Bentrem DJ. CASH (chemotherapy-associated steatohepatitis) costs. Ann Surg 2006;243:8–9.
97. Cho CS, Gonen M, Jarnagin WR, et al. Preoperative radiographic assessment of hepatic steatosis with histologic correlation. J Am Coll Surg 2008;206:480–8.
98. Shirabe K, Shimada M, Gion T, et al. Postoperative liver failure after major hepatic resection for hepatocellular carcinoma in the modern era with special reference to remnant liver volume. J Am Coll Surg 1999; 188:304–9.
99. Makuuchi M, Thai BL, Takayasu K, et al. Properative portal embolization to increase safety of major hepatectomy for hilar bile duct carcinoma: a preliminary report. Surgery 1990;107:521–7.
100. Nagino M, Nimura Y, Kamiya J, et al. Right or left trisegmental portal vein embolization before hepatic trisegmentectomy for hilar bile duct carcinoma. Surgery 1995;117: 677–81.
101. Lee KC, Kinoshita H, Hirohashi K, et al. Extension of surgical indications for hepatocellular carcinoma by portal vein embolization. World J Surg 1993;17:109–15.
102. Azoulay D, Castaing D, Krissat J, et al. Percutaneous portal vein embolization increases the feasibility and safety of major liver resection for hepatocellular carcinoma in injured liver. Ann Surg 2000;232:665–72.
103. Covey AM, Brown KT, Jarnagin WR, et al. Combined portal vein embolization and neoadjuvant chemotherapy as a treatment strategy for resectable hepatic colorectal metastases. Ann Surg 2008;247:451–5.
104. Tomas de la Vega JE, Donahue EJ, Doolas A, et al. A ten year experience with hepatic resection. Surg Gynecol Obstet 1984;159: 223–8.
105. Bismuth H, Adam R, Navarro F. Re-resection for colorectal liver metastasis. Surg Oncol Clin North Am 1996;5:353–64.
106. Adam R, Bismuth H, Castaing D, et al. Repeat hepatectomy for colorectal liver metastases. Ann Surg 1997;225:51–60.
107. Fong Y, Blumgart LH, Cohen A, et al. Repeat hepatic resections for metastatic colorectal cancer. Ann Surg 1994;220: 657–62.
108. Petrowsky H, Gonen M, Jarnagin W, et al. Second liver resections are safe and effective treatment for recurrent hepatic metastases from colorectal cancer: a bi-institutional analysis. Ann Surg 2002;235:863–71.
109. Pinson CW, Wright JK, Chapman WC, et al. Repeat hepatic surgery for colorectal cancer metastases to the liver. Ann Surg 1996;223:765–73.
110. Tuttle TM, Curley SA, Roh MS. Repeat hepatic resection as effective treatment for recurrent colorectal liver metastases. Ann Surg Oncol 1997;4:125–30.
111. Nordlinger B, Vaillant JC, Guiguet M, et al. Survival benefit of repeat liver resections for

procedures in terms of either relative ease of performance or short- or long-term outcome (including survival). The choice between them is usually made on the basis of individual surgeons' preferences (unless there is obvious tumor encroachment on the first portion of the duodenum). In the ensuing technical description, we focus primarily on the pylorus-preserving modification but also refer to certain important components of the classic Whipple resection.

OPERATIVE PLANNING

Operative management of periampullary cancer is carried out in three phases. First, the resectability of the tumor is assessed; then, if the tumor is resectable, a pancreaticoduodenectomy is performed, and, finally, gastrointestinal continuity is restored. Selective use of staging laparoscopy should be considered for patients at high risk for occult metastatic disease, such as patients with large primary tumors; patients with lesions in the neck, body, or tail of the pancreas; patients with equivocal radiographic findings suggestive of occult distant metastatic disease (e.g., low-volume ascites, CT findings indicating possible carcinomatosis, and small hypodense regions in the hepatic parenchyma indicating possible hepatic metastases that are not amenable to percutaneous biopsy); and patients with clinical and laboratory findings suggesting more advanced disease (e.g., marked hypoalbuminemia or weight loss, significant increases in the CA19-9 level, and severe back or abdominal pain).

OPERATIVE TECHNIQUE

The peritoneal cavity is entered through an upper midline or a bilateral subcostal incision. The liver, the omentum, and the peritoneal surfaces are inspected and palpated, and suspicious lesions are biopsied and submitted for frozen-section analysis. Regional lymph nodes are examined for evidence of tumor involvement. The presence of tumor in the periaortic lymph nodes of the celiac axis indicates that the tumor has extended beyond the limits of normal resection; however, the presence of tumor in lymph nodes that normally would be incorporated within the resection specimen does not constitute a contraindication to resection.

Once distant metastases have been excluded, the resectability of the primary tumor is assessed. Various local factors may preclude pancreaticoduodenal resection, including retroperitoneal extension of the tumor to involve the inferior vena cava or the aorta and direct involvement or encasement of the superior mesenteric artery (SMA), the superior mesenteric vein (SMV), or the portal vein. Often the determination of resectability is made on the basis of a careful review of the preoperative imaging (CT plus EUS) in conjunction with operative exploration.

Operative assessment of resectability begins with a Kocher maneuver and mobilization of the duodenum and the head of the pancreas from the underlying inferior vena cava and aorta. When the duodenum and head of the pancreas have been mobilized sufficiently, a hand is placed under the duodenum and the head of the pancreas to palpate the tumor mass and determine its relation to the SMA. Inability to identify a plane of normal tissue between the mass and the arterial pulsation indicates that the tumor directly involves the SMA. In these cases, complete tumor resection is not possible.

The final operative step for determining resectability involves dissection of the SMV and portal vein to rule out tumor invasion. Identification of the portal vein is greatly simplified if the common hepatic duct is divided early in the dissection.[5] Once the hepatic duct has been divided, the anterior surface of the portal vein is easily and quickly identified [*see Figure 1*]. The lymph node tissue lateral to the hepatic duct and the portal vein should be dissected off the structures to be included in the surgical specimen. It must be remembered that important variations in the hepatic arterial anatomy, including a replaced right hepatic artery, may be encountered during this dissection. If the appropriate plane is found along the anterior surface of the portal vein, it should be easy to pass the index finger of the left hand on top of the vessel posterior to the first portion of the duodenum and the neck of the pancreas (because there usually are no veins joining the anterior surface of the portal vein). If this maneuver proves difficult, the gastroduodenal artery should be identified where it comes off the common hepatic artery. Once adequate dissection has been carried out, the artery should first be clamped with a nonoccluding vascular clamp and then, if the hepatic artery pulse is preserved, divided and ligated with 2-0 silk ties. (The initial clamping of the gastroduodenal artery with a vascular clamp confirms that the arterial supply to the liver will not be interrupted should either variations in hepatic arterial anatomy or important collateral circulation be present in the form of celiac artery stenosis.) After the artery has been divided and ligated, an additional ligature of 3-0 polypropylene should be placed on the proximal stump. Division of the gastroduodenal artery unroofs part of the tunnel through which the index finger is slipped, thereby greatly facilitating the separation of the portal vein from the posterior aspect of the first portion of the duodenum and the neck of the pancreas.

Once the anterior surface of the portal vein has been dissected posterior to the neck of the pancreas, the next step is to identify the SMV and dissect its anterior surface. This is most easily accomplished by extending the Kocher maneuver past the second portion of the duodenum to include the third and fourth portions. During this extensive kocherization, the first structure encountered anterior to the third portion of the duodenum is the SMV [*see Figure 2*]. The anterior surface of the vein can then be cleaned and dissected under direct vision by retracting the neck of the pancreas anteriorly. This dissection is continued until it connects to the portal vein dissection from above. If this maneuver can be completed without evidence of SMV or portal vein involvement, the tumor can generally be considered resectable. It is still possible, however, for an uncinate tumor to involve the right lateral surface and the undersurface of the SMV, and this possibility should be carefully evaluated.

If the neck of the pancreas can be successfully dissected off the anterior and lateral surfaces of the portal vein and SMV, most experienced pancreatic surgeons will proceed with pancreaticoduodenectomy without obtaining a tissue diagnosis. In defining the diagnosis of malignancy, an intraoperative biopsy is less conclusive than the combination of the clinical presentation, the results of preoperative CT scanning and cholangiography, and the operative finding of a palpable mass in the head of the pancreas.

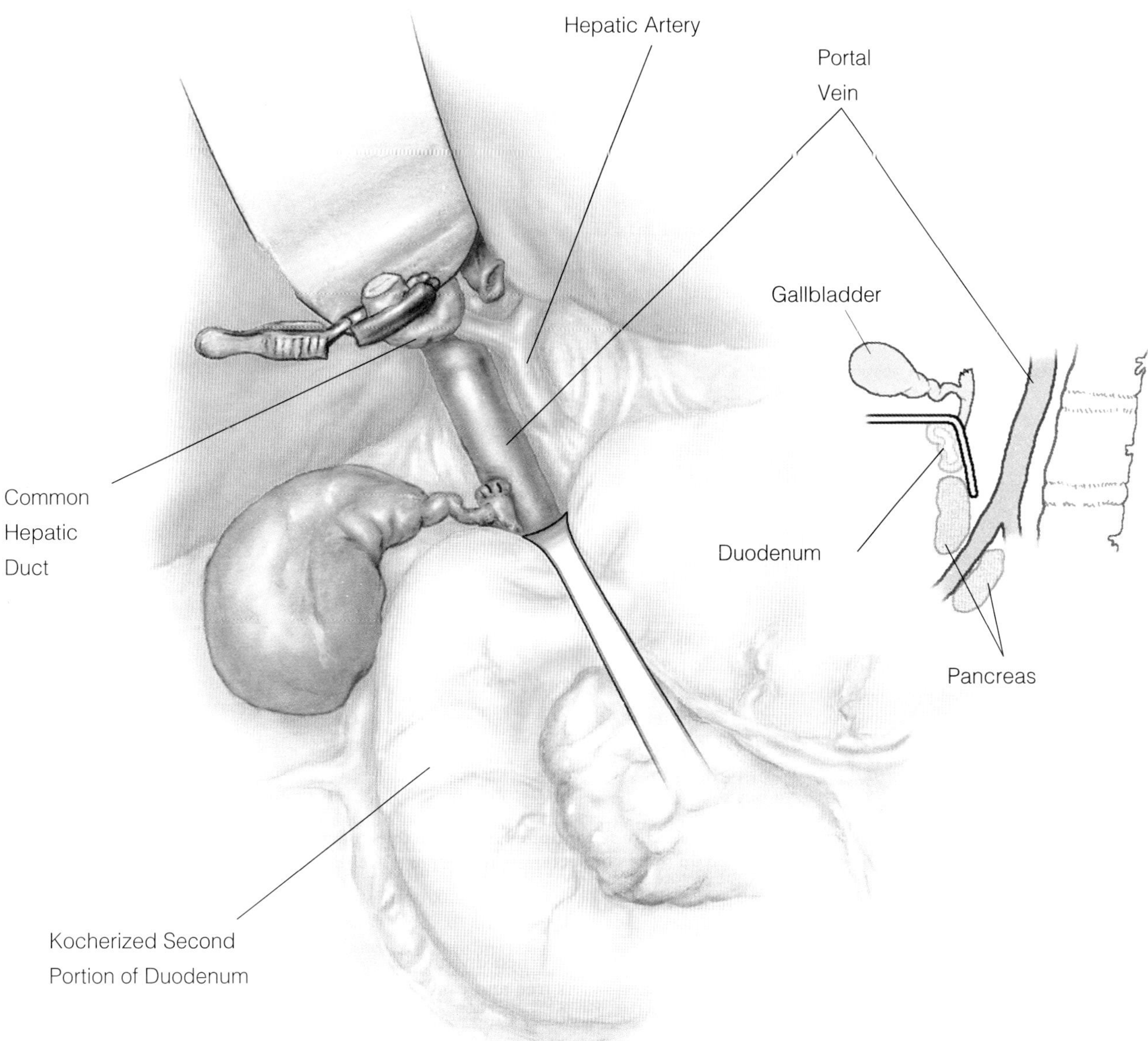

Figure 1 **Whipple procedure. The common hepatic duct is divided at an early stage to facilitate identification of the portal vein. This division also untethers the first portion of the duodenum and allows it to be retracted anteriorly.**

In a PPPD,[6] the duodenum is first mobilized and divided approximately 2 cm distal to the pylorus with a gastrointestinal anastomosis (GIA) stapler. The posterior surface of the proximal first portion of the duodenum is dissected until the lesser sac is entered. At this point, the soft tissue attachments from the inferior border of the duodenum to the inferior border of the pancreas are divided. The right gastroepiploic vessels, which can be sizable, are clamped, divided, and ligated. In a similar fashion, the soft tissue areolar attachments found superiorly are divided with the electrocautery. The right gastric artery, which comes off the common hepatic artery, is also ligated.

In a classic Whipple procedure, an antrectomy is performed. The right gastroepiploic arcade and the right gastric vessels are divided to permit mobilization of the antrum. The stomach is then divided with a GIA stapler, usually at the level of the incisura. At this point, if the gastroduodenal artery was not divided earlier, it is identified, divided, and ligated as described (see above). During this step, particular care must be taken to ensure that the lumen of the common hepatic artery is not encroached on by one of the proximal ties.

The neck of the pancreas is then divided with the electrocautery [*see Figure 3*], with care taken not to injure the underlying SMV and portal vein. These veins are mobilized away from the uncinate process of the pancreas; the dissection should continue until the SMV, clearly palpable with the index finger of the left hand, is visualized. If a replaced right hepatic artery is present, its origin from the SMA will be encountered at this point and must be preserved. The

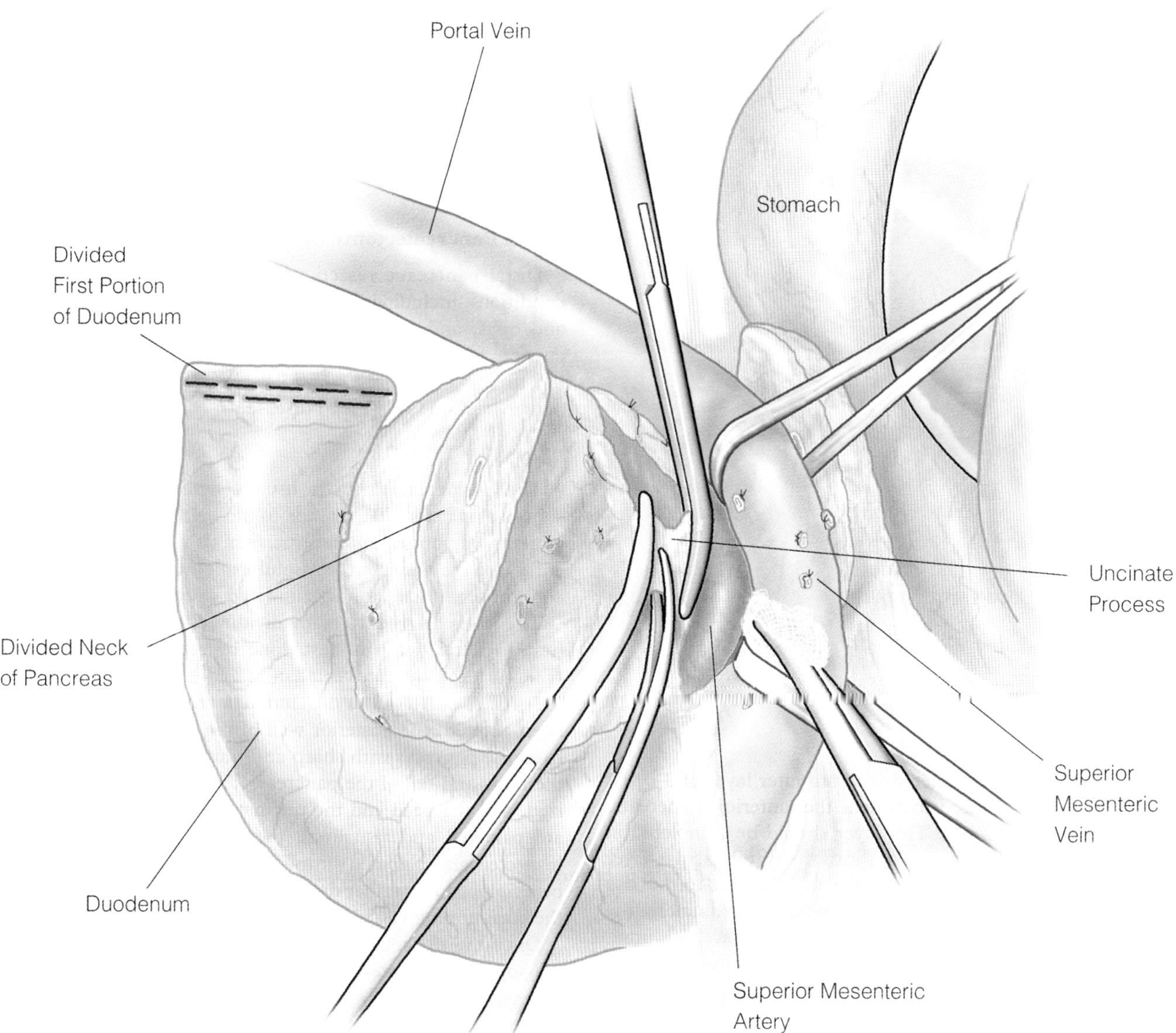

Figure 4 **Whipple procedure. The uncinate process is divided flush with the superior mesenteric artery.**

flexure of the colon is carefully dissected away from the inferior pole of the spleen, and the peritoneal attachments that make up the splenocolic ligament are divided.

The tail and the body of the pancreas are further mobilized out of the retroperitoneum by retracting the spleen and pancreatic tail medially. In the course of this mobilization, care must be taken not to injure the left adrenal gland, which often occupies a fairly superficial position in the retroperitoneum, anterior and medial to the superior pole of the left kidney; care must also be taken not to carry the dissection too deep and thereby risk injuring the kidney or renal vessels. The splenic vein is easily identified in the middle portion of the posterior aspect of the pancreas. The inferior mesenteric vein, which joins the splenic vein at the middle of the body of the pancreas, is identified in the retroperitoneum just lateral to the ligament of Treitz and can be divided at this point.

Further mobilization of the pancreas to the midline exposes the splenic artery where it originates from the celiac axis. As noted (see above), this artery will already have been isolated with a vessel loop. The splenic artery is triply clamped, divided, and triply ligated with 2-0 silk and a 3-0 polypropylene suture near its point of origin.

The SMV can then be identified. A plane is developed by dissecting between the anterior surface of the SMV and the neck of the pancreas; a Penrose drain may be looped around the neck to facilitate exposure. With larger pancreatic cancers, tumor extension into the retroperitoneum may involve the splenic vein. Dividing the pancreatic neck with the electrocautery at this point may facilitate dissection of the splenic vein–portal vein confluence under direct vision. The splenic vein is clamped, divided (without compromising the portal vein–SMV complex), and ligated with 2-0 silk ties

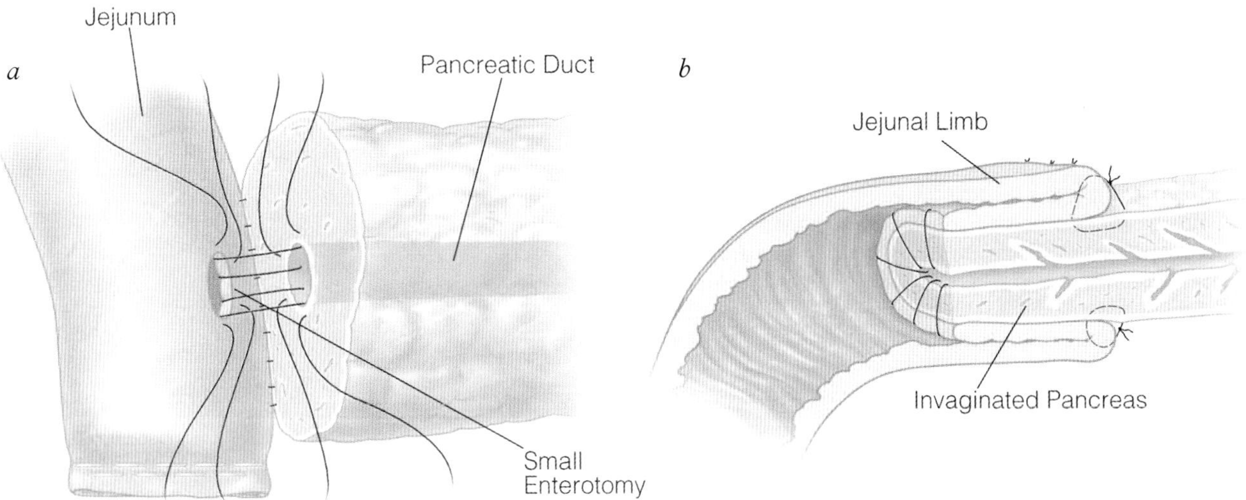

Figure 5 **Whipple procedure. (*a*) An end-to-side mucosa-to-mucosa pancreaticojejunostomy is done in two layers with an outer layer of interrupted 3-0 silk sutures and an inner layer of interrupted 4-0 absorbable synthetic sutures. (*b*) Alternatively, the end of the pancreas can be invaginated into the end of the jejunum for approximately 2 cm. The anastomosis is done with an outer interrupted layer of 3-0 silk and an inner continuous layer of 3-0 absorbable synthetic suture material.**

and a 3-0 polypropylene suture on the proximal stump [*see Figure 8*]. If there is a pancreatic tumor arising from the proximal body of the gland, the splenic vein may be ligated flush with the SMV. At this location, it is best to oversew the vein with a continuous 4-0 polypropylene suture so as not to compromise the portal vein–SMV complex.

The portal vein and the SMV are carefully dissected away from the undersurface of the neck of the pancreas. Stay sutures of 2-0 silk are placed at the superior and inferior edges of the pancreas proximal to the site of transection, and

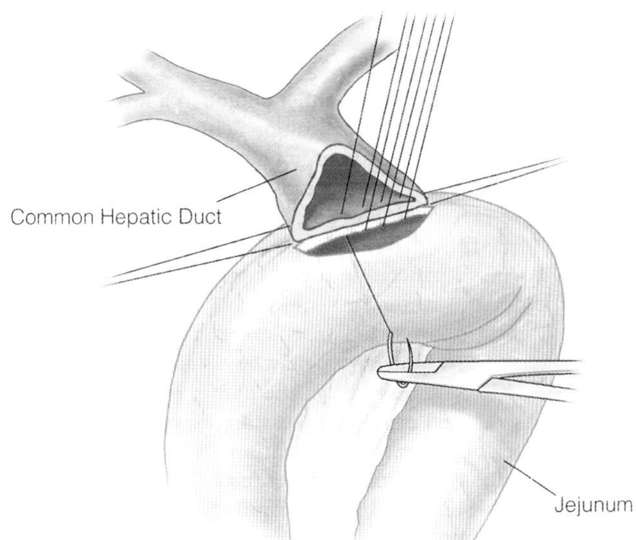

Figure 6 **Whipple procedure. The common hepatic duct is anastomosed to the jejunum in an end-to-side fashion with a single layer of 4-0 interrupted absorbable synthetic sutures.**

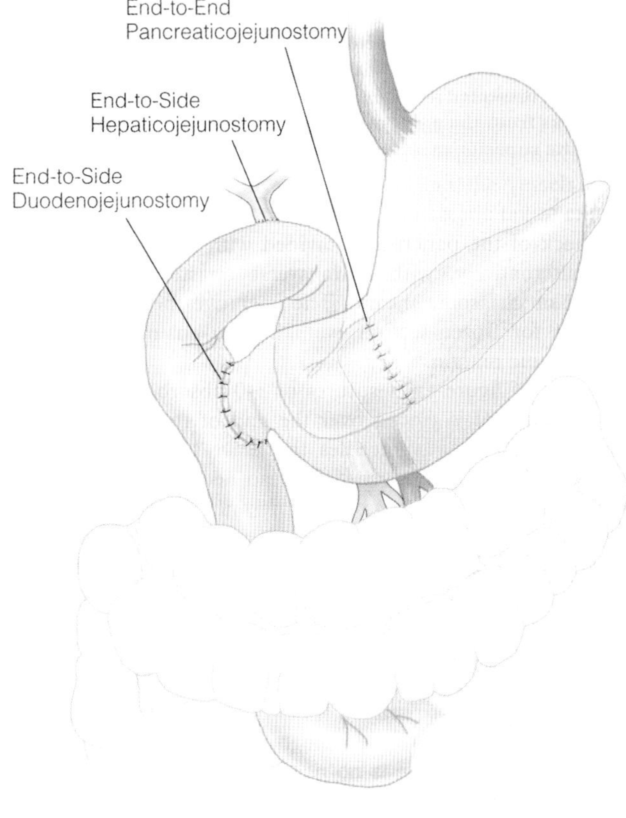

Figure 7 **Whipple procedure. After the end-to-end pancreaticojejunostomy and the end-to-side hepaticojejunostomy, the duodenum is anastomosed to the jejunum in an end-to-side fashion with an inner continuous layer of 3-0 absorbable suture material and an outer interrupted layer of 3-0 silk.**

Roux-en-Y jejunal limb is brought up through a defect in the transverse mesocolon to create a pancreaticojejunostomy. This anastomosis does not have to precisely approximate the pancreatic duct to the jejunal mucosa. It is generally completed in one or two layers using a 3-0 absorbable monofilament suture. The jejunojejunostomy should be constructed in the standard manner to create a 60 cm Roux-en-Y limb. Closed-suction drainage adjacent to the pancreas is optional. The abdomen is closed in a standard fashion.

Duodenum-Preserving Pancreatic Head Resection (Beger Procedure)

The Beger operation begins with the same steps as the Whipple procedure. The peritoneal cavity is entered through either a midline or bilateral subcostal incision, and the abdomen is explored. An extensive Kocher maneuver is completed prior to dividing the gastrocolic ligament to obtain exposure to the anterior surface of the pancreas. The superior mesenteric and portal veins, as well as the common hepatic artery and bile duct, are identified. The portal vein is then dissected off the posterior pancreatic capsule in the same manner as during a Whipple procedure. Caution must be employed during this step, given the frequent inflammatory attachments between the pancreas and the portal vein as a result of chronic pancreatitis. The gastroduodenal artery is doubly ligated once it has been test occluded. The neck of the pancreas is [illegible] identifying the main pancreatic duct during transection. The pancreatic head is then rotated 90° into an anterior-posterior position prior to its complete separation from the portal vein. Mobilizing the portal vein typically entails the ligation of two small branches during this step. The subtotal resection of the pancreatic head is synonymous to that performed during the Frey procedure. Again, a probe inserted into the pancreatic duct toward the ampulla is helpful for identification of the duct trajectory. Reconstruction involves two pancreaticojejunostomies after a Roux-en-Y limb of jejunum is passed to the pancreatic head in a retrocolic manner. The first anastomosis is completed between the remaining left pancreas and the jejunum in a side-to-end manner. This two-layer duct to mucosa anastomosis is the same as during a Whipple procedure. The second anastomosis is a one- or two-layer side-to-end pancreaticojejunostomy approximately 8 cm distal to the left pancreatic anastomosis. The jejunal incision approximates 5 cm in length, and the anastomosis is identical to the one described during the Frey procedure. Finally, a distal jejunojejunostomy is created to complete the 60 cm Roux-en-Y limb. It should also be noted that in patients with multiple stenoses of a dilated main pancreatic duct, the duct can also be opened longitudinally toward the tail of the gland. A side-to-side pancreaticojejunostomy, identical to a Puestow procedure, is then completed.

Drainage of Pancreatic Pseudocyst

OPERATIVE TECHNIQUE

Drainage into Roux-en-Y Jejunal Loop

The peritoneal cavity is entered through a midline incision, and the abdomen is explored. Typically, a substantial mass that is cystic and easily ballotable is palpable posterior to the stomach. The duodenum and the head of the pancreas are kocherized so that the head may be palpated both anteriorly and posteriorly. The physical characteristics of chronic pancreatitis are usually present. The body and the tail of the pancreas are palpated as well; the pancreas is usually fibrotic, firm, and somewhat enlarged. The rest of the abdomen is explored to check for the presence of other pathologic conditions.

At this point, the size and configuration of the cyst are compared with the findings on the preoperative CT scan. If the CT scan shows a unilocular solitary cyst and if, at the time of laparotomy, there appears to be a mass that coincides exactly with what is observed on the CT scan, there is no need to enter the lesser sac. The lesion can be drained into a Roux-en-Y jejunal loop through the transverse mesocolon, and the lesser sac need not be explored. Most pseudocysts are formed by anterior disruptions of the main pancreatic duct. When pancreatic secretions leak out into the lesser sac, the body walls off the leak through an inflammatory response. The transverse mesocolon becomes adherent to the posterior wall of the stomach, which in turn adheres to other adjacent structures in and around the retroperitoneum. As a result, the leak is sealed off. Thus, the transverse mesocolon is usually the inferior and most dependent portion of the pseudocyst, and this site is the ideal location for drainage [*see Figure 16*].

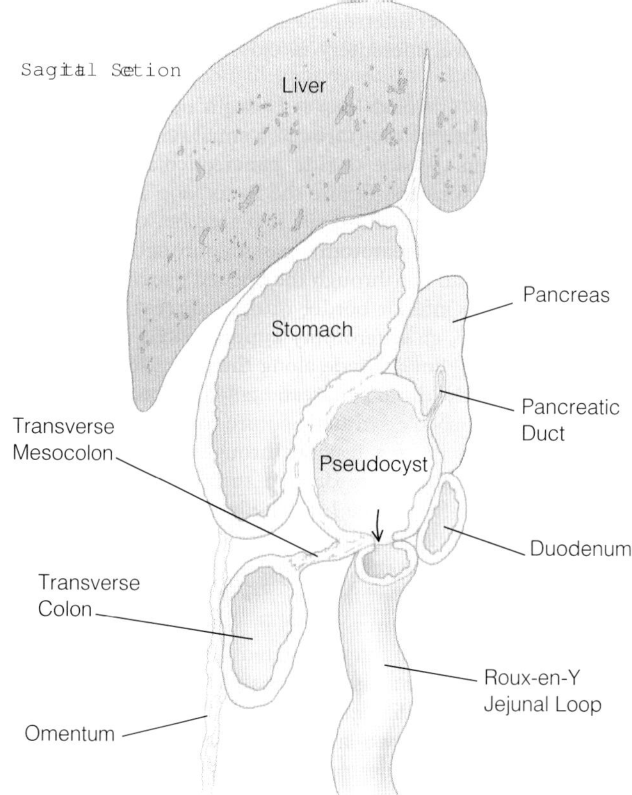

Figure 16 **Drainage of pancreatic pseudocyst into Roux-en-Y jejunal loop. The transverse mesocolon is usually the most inferior and dependent part of a pancreatic pseudocyst; thus, drainage through the transverse mesocolon into a Roux loop is usually the ideal approach.**

The transverse colon is retracted cephalad, and the cyst is easily visualized and palpated through the transverse mesocolon. The location of the cyst is confirmed by aspirating pancreatic juice through the transverse mesocolon with a 10 mL syringe and a 20-gauge needle. The middle colic vessels must be carefully identified and avoided. A 60 cm long Roux-en-Y jejunal loop is constructed. The proximal jejunum is divided with a GIA stapler at the first convenient arcade. The small bowel mesentery is divided down through the arcade. The distal end of the jejunum is inverted with an interrupted layer of 3-0 silk Lembert sutures.

Alimentary tract continuity is reestablished by means of an end-to-side jejunojejunostomy, in which the proximal jejunum is anastomosed to the side of the Roux-en-Y jejunal loop 60 cm from the inverted end. This anastomosis is performed with an inner continuous layer of 3-0 absorbable synthetic suture material and an outer interrupted layer of 3-0 silk. The rent in the small bowel mesentery is closed with a continuous 3-0 silk suture.

A side-to-side cystojejunostomy is performed with an outer interrupted layer of 3-0 silk and an inner continuous layer of 3-0 absorbable synthetic suture material. The posterior outer layer of the anastomosis consists of a series of 3-0 silk sutures passed through and through the jejunal loop and through and through the transverse mesocolon (which is the inferior wall of the pseudocyst) [*see Figure 17*]. The suture line should be approximately 2.5 to 5 cm long. After the posterior layer has been secured, a cystotomy is performed with the electrocautery. An ellipse of cyst wall is removed and sent for frozen-section examination. No matter how clear it seems to be that the lesion is a pseudocyst, a specimen from the cyst wall should always be sent for frozen-section examination. Some of these lesions are cystic neoplasms, which must be resected rather than drained. If no epithelial lining is found on frozen-section examination, it is safe to assume that the lesion is not a cystic neoplasm but a pancreatic pseudocyst and to proceed accordingly.

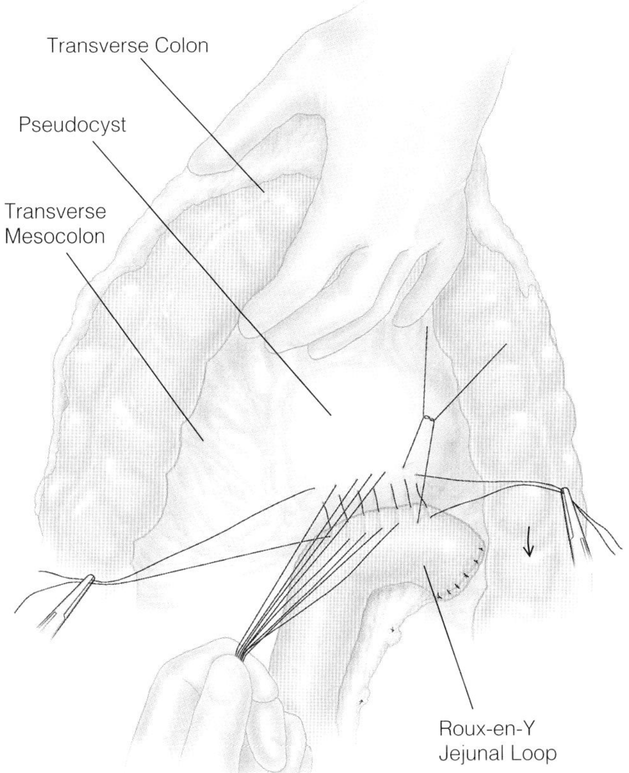

Figure 17 **Drainage of pancreatic pseudocyst into Roux-en-Y jejunal loop. The outer posterior layer of the side-to-side cystojejunostomy comprises a series of 3-0 silk sutures placed through and through the jejunal loop and the transverse mesocolon.**

A parallel enterotomy is made in the jejunum. An inner continuous layer of 3-0 absorbable synthetic suture material is placed inferiorly in a locking fashion and then brought around superiorly in a Connell stitch. An outer interrupted layer of 3-0 silk is placed superiorly. With the cyst decompressed, a sizable lumen should be easily palpable in the anastomosis between the cyst and the jejunal loop.

A closed-suction Silastic drain is left near the anastomosis and brought out through a stab wound in the left upper quadrant. The abdomen is copiously irrigated with an antibiotic solution and closed in a standard fashion.

Drainage into Stomach

The peritoneal cavity is entered through an upper midline incision, and the abdomen is explored. Typically, a pseudocyst that is not amenable to drainage through the transverse mesocolon presents as a mass that is cystic and is palpable through the anterior wall of the stomach and the lesser omentum in the upper abdomen; such a mass is not generally palpable through the root of the transverse mesocolon with the transverse mesocolon reflected cephalad and thus is not easily drained into a Roux-en-Y jejunal loop. The duodenum and the head of the pancreas are kocherized, and the head of the pancreas is palpated. Signs of chronic pancreatitis are invariably present. The rest of the abdomen is explored to check for the presence of other pathologic conditions.

Stay sutures of 3-0 silk are placed in the anterior wall of the body of the stomach. A transverse gastrotomy is made with the electrocautery. The cyst wall is easily palpable through the posterior wall of the stomach. The location of the cyst is confirmed by aspirating pancreatic juice through the back wall of the stomach with a 10 mL syringe and a 20-gauge needle. The mass palpated at the time of operation is compared with the cyst as it appears on the preoperative CT scan. If the CT scan shows a solitary unilocular cyst that corresponds to the palpable mass identified at the time of laparotomy, it is safe to conclude that the cyst is solitary and can be drained effectively into the stomach.

A transverse incision is made with the electrocautery through the posterior wall of the stomach, through the cyst wall, and into the pseudocyst. It is often desirable to leave the 20-gauge needle in place and to perform the posterior wall gastrotomy on either side of the needle. An ellipse of cyst wall is sent for frozen-section examination. Again, this step is mandatory, no matter how obvious it seems that the lesion is an inflammatory cyst. A continuous locking suture of 3-0 absorbable synthetic material is placed through and through the posterior wall of the stomach and the anterior wall of the cyst [*see Figure 18*]. This step may or may not actually be important for achieving long-term patency of the opening

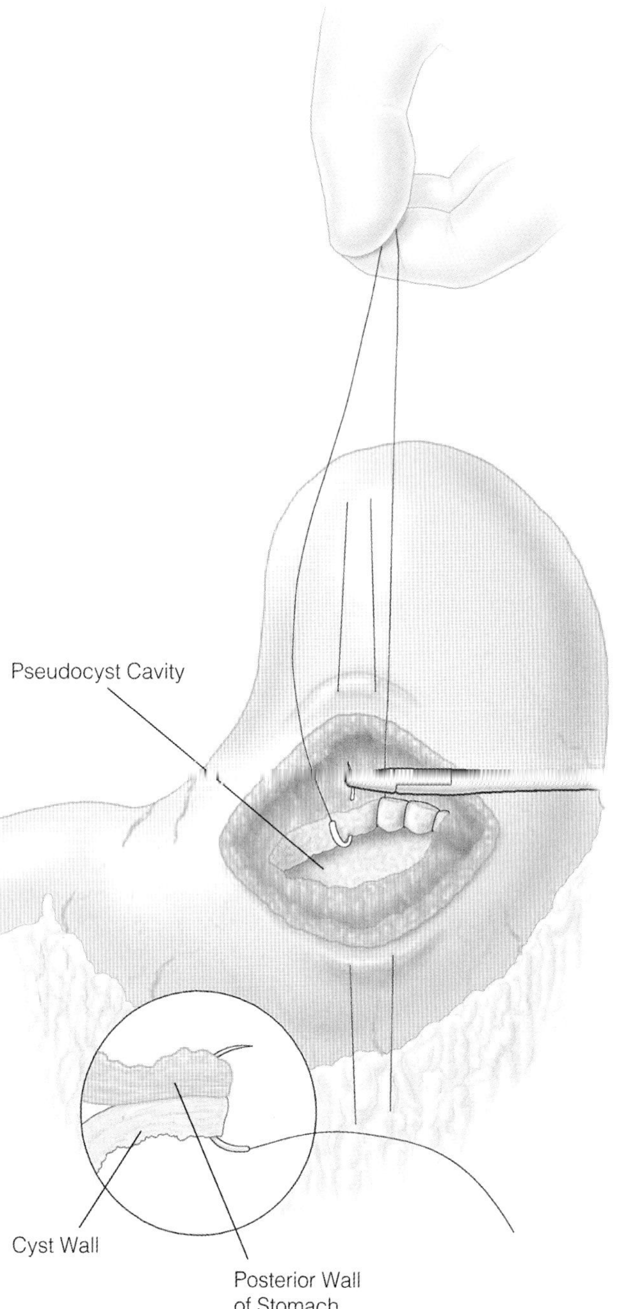

Figure 18 **Drainage of pancreatic pseudocyst into stomach. Once an incision has been made through the posterior wall of the stomach, through the cyst wall, and into the pseudocyst, a continuous locking 3-0 absorbable synthetic suture is placed through and through the posterior wall of the stomach and the cyst wall.**

between the cyst and the posterior wall of the stomach, but it does ensure good hemostasis. The anterior gastrotomy is closed with an inner continuous layer of 3-0 absorbable synthetic suture material in a Connell stitch and an outer interrupted layer of 3-0 silk. The abdomen is closed in a standard fashion. It should also be noted that drainage may be achieved endoscopically in many cases.

Laparoscopic Drainage of Pancreatic Pseudocysts

Five distinct laparoscopic approaches have been described for the treatment of pancreatic pseudocysts: (1) transgastric cystgastrostomy, (2) intragastric cystgastrostomy, (3) minilaparoscopic intragastric cystgastrostomy, (4) cystgastrostomy via the lesser sac approach, and (5) Roux-en-Y cystjejunostomy.

The laparoscopic transgastric cystgastrostomy involves making an anterior gastrotomy, followed by using electrocautery to open the cyst wall through the posterior wall of the stomach. A cystgastrostomy can then be created using an endoscopic stapler or via a handsewn anastomosis with intracorporeal suturing. Intragastric cystgastrostomy involves inserting trocars percutaneously through the abdominal wall and directly into the gastric lumen using simultaneous laparoscopic and gastroscopic guidance. Cautery and sharp dissection are used to create the cystgastrostomy. The minilaparoscopic intraluminal cystgastrostomy is performed in a similar fashion, with the exception that 2 mm intragastric ports are used to minimize invasiveness and trauma to the anterior gastric wall. Laparoscopic cystgastrostomy via the lesser sac approach is becoming the preferred approach when the anatomy is favorable. The advantages of this approach include the avoidance of an anterior gastrotomy, as well as the assurance of a large anastomosis that is not dependent on the adherence of the cyst to the posterior gastric wall. Because the entire anastomosis is either stapled or sutured, the risk of bleeding is minimized. The technique involves creating a window in the gastrocolic omentum through which the lesser sac is entered. The stomach is then elevated, and a cystotomy is made adjacent to a posterior gastric wall gastrotomy. A cystgastrostomy is then created with an endoscopic stapler, followed by a suture closure of the opening.

For large cysts, or those not in direct contact with the posterior wall of the stomach, a laparoscopic Roux-en-Y cyst jejunostomy can be performed. The omentum and transverse colon are retracted cephalad and the pseudocyst can often be visualized through the transverse mesocolon. Laparoscopic ultrasonography can also be used to help identify the location of the cyst. The jejunum is divided approximately 30 cm distal to the ligament of Treitz to create a Roux limb. The pseudocyst is next opened with the Harmonic Scalpel through the transverse mesocolon. A small enterotomy is made in the Roux limb, and a stapled cyst jejunostomy can be performed. The cyst enterostomy is then closed with a running suture. The procedure is completed with the jejunojejunostomy performed at least 30 cm distal to the cyst jejunostomy.

Palliative Bypass for Unresectable Periampullary Cancer

The peritoneal cavity is entered through an upper midline incision, and the abdomen is examined for evidence of liver metastases, serosal spread, carcinomatosis, involvement of regional lymph nodes, and invasion of major vascular structures. Once the tumor has been shown to be unresectable and histologic confirmation of malignancy has been received, a palliative double-bypass procedure is begun, in which the duodenum is bypassed with a retrocolic gastrojejunostomy and the distally obstructed biliary tree is bypassed with a hepaticojejunostomy. A chemical splanchnicectomy is also performed to reduce pain.

Approximately 4 cm of the most dependent portion of the greater curvature of the stomach is cleaned by doubly clamping, dividing, and ligating attachments of the greater omentum. Once this is accomplished, a small rent is made in the transverse mesocolon, and a proximal loop of jejunum is brought up through this rent and anastomosed in an isoperistaltic fashion to the dependent wall of the stomach. The anastomosis is performed with an outer interrupted layer of 3-0 silk and an inner continuous layer of 3-0 absorbable synthetic suture material.

In the past, palliative duodenal bypasses for pancreatic cancer were frequently performed by carrying out an anterior antecolic gastrojejunostomy. Delayed gastric emptying proved to be a common occurrence with this approach. Fortunately, this complication can be virtually eliminated by performing a posterior gastroenterostomy. Once the posterior gastroenterostomy is complete, the anastomosis is tacked to the rent in the transverse mesocolon on the gastric side with interrupted 3-0 silk sutures to prevent the afferent and efferent jejunal limbs from herniating up through the transverse mesocolon [*see Figure 19*].

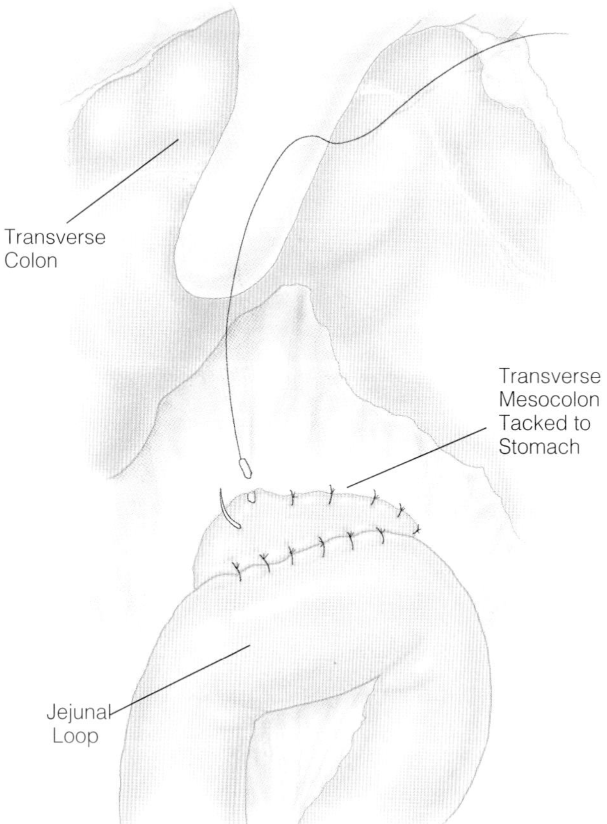

Figure 19 **Palliative double bypass for unresectable pancreatic cancer. Once the retrocolic gastrojejunostomy is complete, the anastomosis is tacked to the rent in the transverse mesocolon on the gastric side with interrupted 3-0 silk sutures.**

The gallbladder is mobilized out of the liver bed in a retrograde fashion and placed on traction to facilitate identification of the common hepatic duct. Once identified, the common hepatic duct is divided just proximal to the cystic duct. The gallbladder is removed, and the distal biliary segment is oversewn with a continuous 3-0 polypropylene suture. The jejunum is divided approximately 30 cm distal to the gastrojejunostomy, and a Roux-en-Y limb is brought up into the right upper quadrant through a second opening in the transverse mesocolon. An end-to-side hepaticojejunostomy is performed with a single layer of interrupted 4-0 absorbable synthetic sutures [*see Figure 20*]. An end-to-side jejunojejunostomy is then performed 60 cm downstream to restore enteric continuity and complete the Roux-en-Y. This anastomosis is performed with an inner continuous layer of 3-0 absorbable synthetic suture material and an outer interrupted layer of 3-0 silk. The Roux-en-Y limb is tacked to the opening in the transverse mesocolon to prevent herniation.

The lesser omentum is divided, and a chemical splanchnicectomy is performed by injecting 20 mL of 50% alcohol into the celiac plexus on each side of the aorta at the level of the celiac axis using a 22-gauge needle. The level of the celiac axis is easily determined by palpating the thrill that is invariably present in the common hepatic artery as it comes off the celiac axis.

A closed-suction Silastic drain may be left posterior to the area of the hepaticojejunostomy and brought out through a stab wound in the right upper quadrant. If tissue confirmation of the presence of adenocarcinoma of the head of

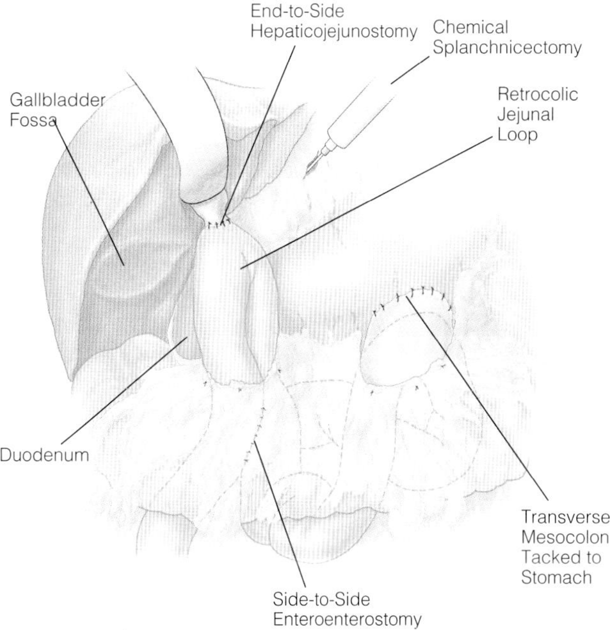

Figure 20 **Palliative double bypass for unresectable pancreatic cancer. An end-to-side hepaticojejunostomy is performed, followed by a side-to-side jejunojejunostomy between the afferent loop leading to the biliary anastomosis and the efferent loop leading from it. An opening is made in the lesser omentum, and a chemical splanchnicectomy is performed by injecting alcohol into the celiac plexus.**

the pancreas was not obtained preoperatively, it should be obtained during the operation. As a rule, this is most easily accomplished by performing a transduodenal needle biopsy (e.g., with a Tru-Cut needle; Cardinal Health, Dublin, Ohio). The abdomen is irrigated with an antibiotic solution and closed in a standard fashion.

Financial Disclosures: None Reported

References

1. Yeo CJ, Cameron JL, Sohn TA, et al. Six hundred fifty consecutive pancreaticoduodenectomies in the 1990s: pathology, complications, and outcomes. Ann Surg 1997;226:248.
2. Trede M, Schwall G, Saeger HD. Survival after pancreatoduodenectomy: 118 consecutive resections without an operative mortality. Ann Surg 1990;211:447.
3. Fernandez-del Castillo C, Rattner DW, Warshaw AL. Standards for pancreatic resection in the 1990s. Arch Surg 1995;130:295.
4. Dye CE, Waxman I. Endoscopic ultrasound. Gastroenterol Clin North Am 2002;31:863.
5. Cameron JL. Rapid exposure of the portal and superior mesenteric veins. Surg Gynecol Obstet 1995;176:395.
6. Traverso LW, Longmire WP Jr. Preservation of the pylorus in pancreaticoduodenectomy. Surg Gynecol Obstet 1978;146:959.

Additional Readings

Cameron JL, Pitt HA, Yeo CJ, et al. One hundred and forty-five consecutive pancreaticoduodenectomies without mortality. Ann Surg 1993;217:430.

Fernandez-Cruz L, Martinez I, Gilabert R, et al. Laparoscopic distal pancreatectomy combined with preservation of the spleen for cystic neoplasms of the pancreas. J Gastrointest Surg 2004;8:493–501.

Fernandez-del Castillo C, Rattner DW, Warshaw AL. Standards for pancreatic resection in the 1990s. Arch Surg 1995;130:295.

Lillemoe KD, Cameron JL, Hardacre JM, et al. Is prophylactic gastrojejunostomy indicated for unresectable periampullary cancer? A prospective randomized trial. Ann Surg 1999;230:322.

Lillemoe KD, Cameron JL, Kaufman HS, et al. Chemical splanchnicectomy in patients with unresectable pancreatic cancer: a prospective randomized trial. Ann Surg 1993;217:447.

Lillemoe KD, Yeo CJ, Cameron JL. Pancreatic cancer: state-of-the-art care. CA Cancer J Clin 2000;50:241.

Sohn TA, Lillemoe KD, Cameron JL, et al. Surgical palliation of unresectable periampullary adenocarcinoma in the 1990s. J Am Coll Surg 1999;188:658.

Trede M, Schwall G, Saeger HD. Survival after pancreatoduodenectomy: 118 consecutive resections without an operative mortality. Ann Surg 1990;211:447.

[illegible] prophylactic octreotide decrease the rates of pancreatic fistula and other complications after pancreaticoduodenectomy? Results of a prospective randomized placebo-controlled trial. Ann Surg 2000;232:419.

Yeo CJ, Cameron JL, Lillemoe KD, et al. Pancreaticoduodenectomy for cancer of the head of the pancreas: 201 patients. Ann Surg 1995;221:721.

Yeo CJ, Cameron JL, Sohn TA, et al. Six hundred fifty consecutive pancreaticoduodenectomies in the 1990s: pathology, complications, and outcomes. Ann Surg 1997;226:248.

Acknowledgments

Figures 1, 2, and 5 Tom Moore
[illegible]
Figures 4, 6, 7, 9, and 14 through 20 Tom Moore. Adapted from originals by Corinne Sandone.

24 SPLENECTOMY

Eric C. Poulin, MD, MSc, FACS, FRCSC, Christopher M. Schlachta, MDCM, FACS, FRSCS, and Joseph Mamazza, MDCM, FRSC

Medicine is not an exact science, and nowhere is this observation more appropriate than in the operating room when a spleen is being removed.[1]

The first reported splenectomy in the Western world was performed by Zacarello in 1549, although the veracity of his operative description has been questioned. Between this initial report and the 1800s, very few cases were recorded. The first reported splenectomy in North America was performed by O'Brien in 1816. The patient was in the act of committing a rape when his victim plunged a large knife into his left side. As in this case, most early splenectomies were done in patients who had undergone penetrating trauma; often the spleen was protruding from the wound, and the surgeon proceeded with en masse ligation. The first elective splenectomy was performed by Quittenbaum in 1826 for sequelae of portal hypertension, and soon afterward, Wells performed one of the first splenectomies using general anesthesia; both patients died. In 1866, Bryant was the first to attempt splenectomy in a patient with leukemia. Over the following 15 years, 14 splenectomies were attempted as therapy for leukemia; none of the patients survived. In a 1908 review of 49 similar cases, Johnston reported a mortality of 87.7%.[2] These dismal results led to the abandonment of splenectomy for leukemia. In 1916, Kaznelson, of Prague, was the first to report good results from splenectomy in patients with thrombocytopenic purpura.

As the 20th century progressed, splenectomy became more common in direct proportion to the increase in the use of the automobile. The eventual recognition of the syndrome known as overwhelming postsplenectomy infection (OPSI) made splenic conservation an important consideration. Partial splenectomy had initially been described by the French surgeon Péan in the 19th century. This procedure received little further study until almost 100 years later, when the Brazilian surgeon Campos Cristo reevaluated Péan's technique in his report of eight trauma patients treated with partial splenectomy.[3] Upadhyaya and Simpson's report on 16 children admitted for splenic trauma to The Hospital for Sick Children in Toronto between 1948 and 1955 was instrumental in establishing the validity of nonoperative treatment of splenic trauma.[4]

In late 1991 and early 1992, four groups working independently—Delaître in Paris, Carroll in Los Angeles, Cushieri in the United Kingdom, and our group in Canada—published the first reports of laparoscopic splenectomy in patients with hematologic disorders.[5–7] Since then, the development of operative techniques for partial laparoscopic splenectomy has tested the limits of minimally invasive surgery and encouraged clinical research into methods of simplifying the execution of the operation.[8–10] The adoption of laparoscopic splenectomy has led to a gradual decrease in the indications for open splenectomy; however, both procedures are still essential components of spleen surgery.

Anatomic Considerations

Most anatomy texts suggest that the splenic artery is constant in its course and branches; however, as the classic essay by Michels made clear, each spleen has its own peculiar pattern of terminal artery branches.[11] SCORE

SPLENIC ARTERY

The celiac axis is the largest but shortest branch of the abdominal aorta: it is only 15 to 20 mm long. The celiac axis arises above the body of the pancreas and, in 82% of specimens, divides into three primary branches: the left gastric artery, which is the first branch, and the hepatic and splenic arteries, which derive from a common stem. In rare instances, the splenic artery originates directly from the aorta; even less often, a second splenic artery arises from the celiac axis. There are numerous other possible variations, in which the splenic artery may originate from the aorta, the superior mesenteric artery, the middle colic artery, the left gastric artery, the left hepatic artery, or the accessory right hepatic artery. As a rule, however, the splenic artery arises from the celiac axis to the right of the midline, which means that the aorta must be crossed to reach the spleen and that selective angiography is likely to be difficult at times. The splenic artery can take a very tortuous course, particularly in patients who are elderly or who have a longer artery.

In his study of 100 cadaver spleens, Michels divided splenic arterial geography into two types, distributed and magistral (or bundled) [*see Figure 1*].[11] In the distributed type, found in 70% of dissections, the splenic trunk is short, and six to 12 long branches enter the spleen over approximately 75% of its medial surface. The branches originate between 3 and 13 cm from the hilum [*see Figure 1a*]. In the bundled type, found in the remaining 30% of dissections, there is a long main splenic artery that divides near the hilum into three or four large, short terminal branches that enter the spleen over only 25 to 35% of its medial surface. These short splenic branches originate, on average, 3.5 cm from the spleen, and they reach the center of the organ as a compact bundle [*see Figure 1b*]. Early identification of the type of splenic blood supply present can help the surgeon estimate how difficult a particular splenectomy is likely to be. Operation on a spleen with a distributed vascular anatomy usually involves dissection of more blood vessels; however, the vessels, being spread over a wider area of the splenic hilum, are relatively easy to deal with. Operation on a spleen with a bundled-type blood supply typically involves dissection of fewer vessels; however, because the

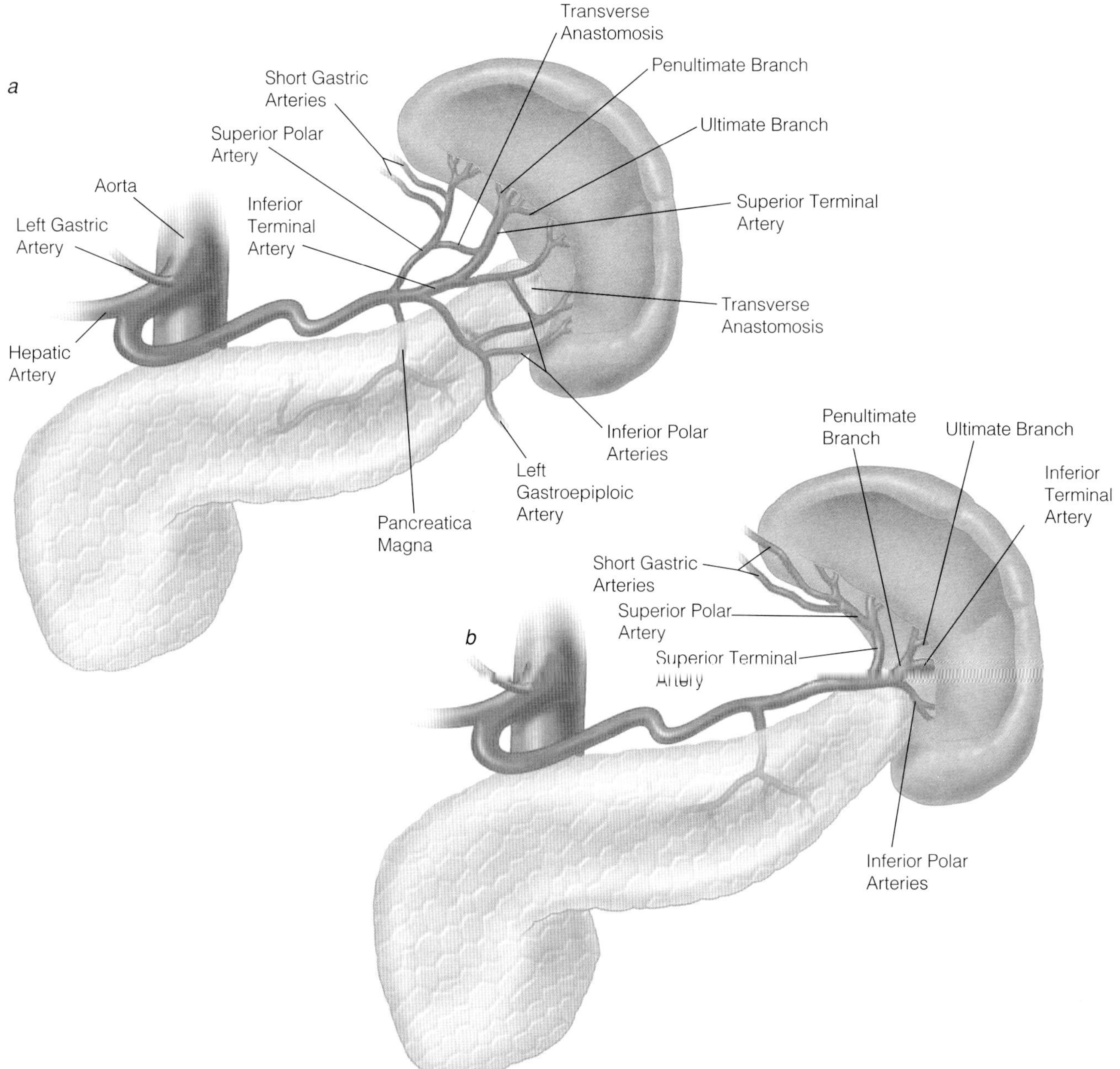

Figure 1 **Splenic vascularization. Shown are (*a*) the distributed type and (*b*) the magistral (bundled) type of splenic vascularization.**

hilum is narrower and more compact, dissection and separation of the vessels are more difficult.

BRANCHES OF SPLENIC ARTERY

The splenic branches vary so markedly in length, size, and origin that no two spleens have the same anatomy. Outside the spleen, the arteries also frequently form transverse anastomoses with each other that, like most collaterals, arise at a 90° angle to the vessels involved [*see Figure 1*].[12] As a consequence, attempts to occlude a branch of the splenic artery by means of clips or embolization, if carried out proximal to such an anastomosis, may fail to devascularize the corresponding splenic segment. Before the splenic trunk divides, it usually gives off a few slender branches to the tail of the pancreas. The most important of these is called the pancreatica magna (a vessel familiar to vascular radiologists); occlusion of this branch with embolic material has been reported to result in pancreatitis. Next, the splenic artery divides into two to six first and second terminal branches, and these branches undergo two further levels of division into two to 12 penultimate and ultimate branches. Segmental and subsegmental division can occur either outside or inside the spleen. The number of arteries entering the spleen ranges from six to 36. The size of the spleen does not determine the number of arteries entering it; however, the presence of notches and tubercles usually correlates well with a higher number of entering arteries.

A reasonable general scheme of splenic artery branches might include as many as seven principal branches at various division levels and in various anatomic arrangements: (1) the superior terminal artery, (2) the inferior terminal artery, (3) the medial terminal artery, (4) the short gastric arteries, (5) the left gastroepiploic artery, (6) the inferior polar artery, and (7) the superior polar artery [*see Figure 2*]. Veins are usually located behind the corresponding arteries, except at the ultimate level of division, where they may be either anterior or posterior.

First Terminal Division Branches

A classic study from 1917 found that 72% of specimens had three terminal branches (superior polar, superior terminal, and inferior terminal) and 28% had two; the medial terminal artery was observed in only 20% of cases.[13] When the superior terminal artery is excessively large, the inferior terminal is rudimentary, with an added blood supply often coming from the left gastroepiploic and polar vessels.

Second Terminal Division Branches

Superior polar artery The superior polar artery is present in 65% of patients. It usually arises from the main splenic trunk (75% of cases) or the superior terminal artery (20% of cases), but, on occasion, it may originate from the inferior terminal artery or separately from the celiac axis (thus providing the spleen with a double splenic artery). In most instances, the superior polar artery gives rise to one or two short gastric branches; rarely, it gives rise to the left inferior phrenic and pancreatic rami. The presence and size of this artery appear to be correlated with tubercle formation in that it is more prominent in spleens with large tubercles. The superior polar artery is frequently very long and slender and thus easily torn during splenectomy; accordingly, it was suggested in 1928 that ligation of splenic branches be started from the inferior pole of the spleen.[14]

Inferior polar artery The inferior polar artery is present in 82% of cases. As many as five collateral branches may arise from the splenic trunk, the inferior terminal artery, or, as noted, the left gastroepiploic artery. Inferior polar branches may have multiple origins, and they tend to be of smaller caliber than the superior polar artery.

Left gastroepiploic artery The left gastroepiploic artery, the most varied of the splenic branches, courses along the left side of the greater curvature in the anterior layer of the greater omentum. In 72% of cases, it arises from the splenic trunk several centimeters from its primary terminal division, and in 22% of cases, it originates from the inferior terminal artery or its branches; however, it may also originate from the middle of the splenic trunk or from the superior terminal artery. Characteristically, the left gastroepiploic artery gives off inferior polar arteries, which vary in number (ranging from one to five), size, and length. Typically, these branches are addressed first during laparoscopic splenectomy. When they are small, they can usually be controlled with the electrocautery.

Collaterals

As many as six short gastric arteries may arise from the fundus of the stomach, but, as a rule, only the one to three

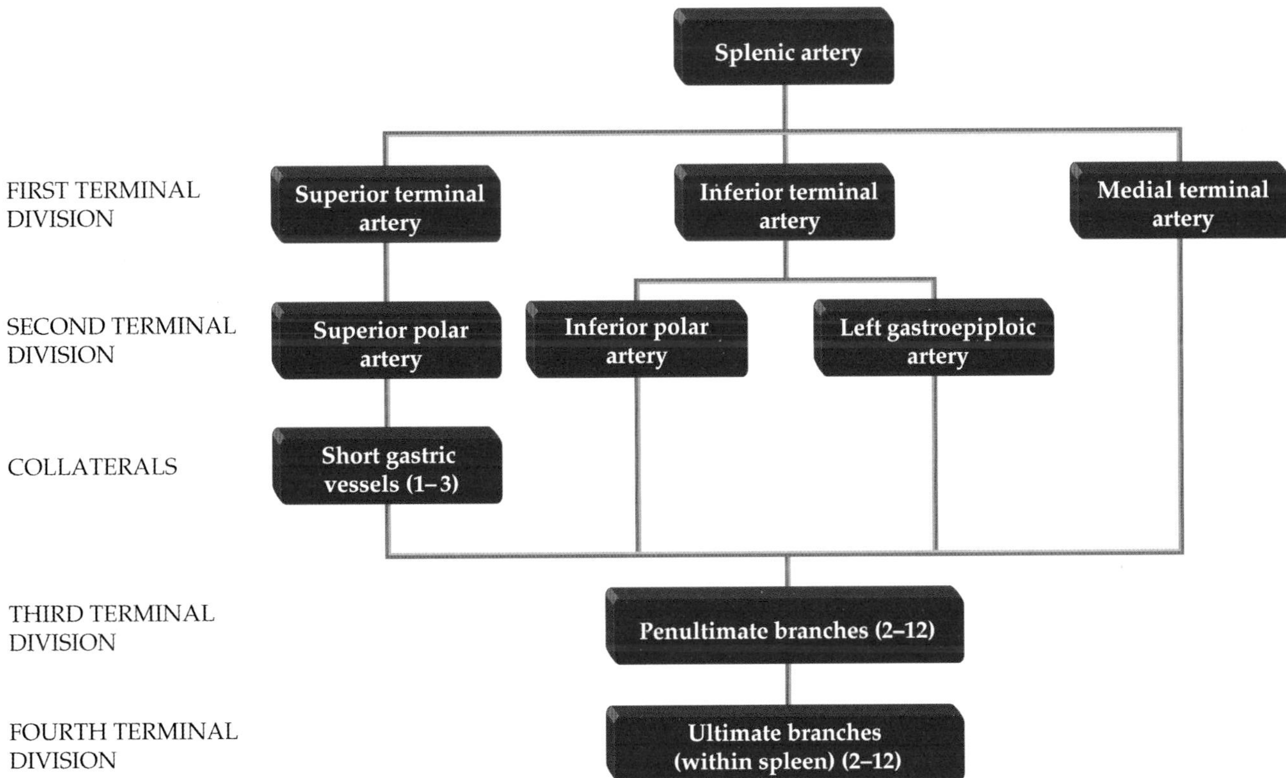

Figure 2 **Division of splenic artery branches. Outlined is a general scheme of the levels of division of the splenic artery branches.**

that open into the superior polar artery must be ligated during laparoscopic splenectomy [*see Figure 1*].

SUSPENSORY LIGAMENTS OF SPLEEN AND TAIL OF PANCREAS

Duplications of the peritoneum form the many suspensory ligaments of the spleen [*see Figure 3*]. Medially and posteriorly, the splenorenal ligament contains the tail of the pancreas and the splenic vessels. Anteriorly, the gastrosplenic ligament contains the short gastric and gastroepiploic arteries. In the lateral approach to laparoscopic splenectomy [*see* Operative Technique, *below*], the splenorenal and gastrosplenic ligaments are easily distinguished, and dissection of the anatomic structures they contain is relatively simple. In the anterior approach, these two ligaments lie on top of each other, and to separate them correctly and safely requires considerable experience with splenic anatomy.

The phrenicocolic ligament courses laterally from the diaphragm to the splenic flexure of the colon; its upper portion is called the phrenicosplenic ligament. The attachment of the lower pole on the internal side is called the splenocolic ligament. Between these two structures, a horizontal shelf of areolar tissue, known as the sustentaculum lienis, is formed on which the inferior pole of the spleen rests. The sustentaculum lienis is often molded into a sac that opens cephalad and acts as a support for the lower pole. This structure, often overlooked during open procedures, is readily visible through a laparoscope. The phrenicocolic ligament, the splenocolic ligament, and the sustentaculum lienis are usually avascular, except in patients who have portal hypertension or myeloid metaplasia.

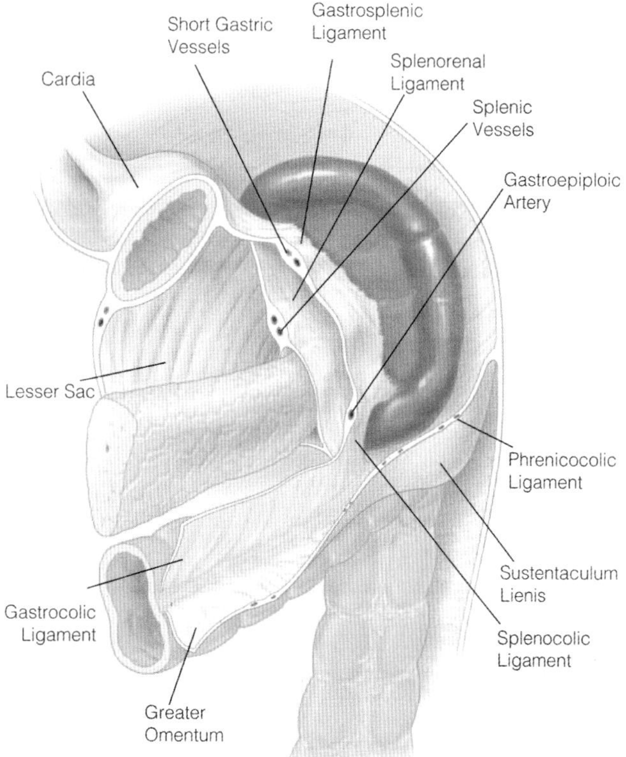

Figure 3 **Suspensory ligaments of the spleen. Depicted are the suspensory ligaments of the spleen.**

A 1937 study found that the tail of the pancreas was in direct contact with the spleen in 30% of cadavers.[15] A subsequent report confirmed this finding and added that in 73% of patients, the distance between the two structures was no more than 1 cm.[16] Although a recent anatomic study based on computed tomography (CT) mapping shows slightly different measures, the message is the same.[17] Care must be exercised to avoid pancreas damage with the electrocautery during dissection as well as damage with the linear stapler in the course of en masse ligation of the splenic hilum (a maneuver more easily performed via the lateral approach to laparoscopic splenectomy).

Laparoscopic Splenectomy

PREOPERATIVE EVALUATION

Currently, we consider all patients evaluated for elective splenectomy to be potential candidates for laparoscopic splenectomy. Contraindications to a laparoscopic approach include severe portal hypertension, uncorrectable coagulopathy, severe ascites, and most traumatic injuries to the spleen. Extreme splenomegaly remains a relative contraindication as well. Because most patients scheduled for laparoscopic splenectomy have hematologic disorders, they undergo the same hematologic preparation that patients scheduled for open surgery do—namely, steroids, γ-globulins, fresh frozen plasma, cryoprecipitate, or platelets when required. Ultrasonography is performed to determine the size of the spleen. Spleen size is expressed in terms of the maximum interpole length (i.e., the length of the line joining the two organ poles) and is generally classified into three categories: (1) normal spleen size (< 11 cm), (2) moderate splenomegaly (11 to 20 cm), and (3) severe splenomegaly (> 20 cm).[18] Because extremely large spleens present special technical problems that test the current limits of laparoscopic surgery, we make use of a fourth category for spleens longer than 30 cm or heavier than 3 kg, which we call megaspleens [*see Table 1*]. The ultrasonographer is also asked to try to identify any accessory spleens that may be present. CT is done when there is doubt about the exactness of the ultrasonographic measurement; such measurement is sometimes inaccurate at the upper pole and with spleens longer than 16 cm.

Patients receive thorough counseling about the consequences of the asplenic state. Polyvalent pneumococcal vaccine is administered at least 2 weeks before operation in all cases with boosters every 5 to 10 years as dictated by the levels of antibody titers;

Table 1 **Classification of Spleens According to Spleen Length***

Spleen Class	Spleen Length (cm)
Normal-size spleen	7–11
Moderate splenomegaly	12–20
Massive splenomegaly	21–30
Megaspleen	> 30

*Spleen length is defined as interpole length, measured along a straight line connecting the two poles.

preoperative vaccination against *Haemophilus influenzae* type B and meningococcus serogroup C is also given. Annual influenza vaccination should also be suggested. Heparin prophylaxis for thrombophlebitis is administered according to standard guidelines provided that there is no hematologic contraindication. Nonsteroidal antiinflammatory drugs (NSAIDs) are often given orally before operation to minimize postoperative pain; however, on empirical grounds, NSAIDs are not used when heparin prophylaxis is employed. Platelets are rarely, if ever, required when laparoscopic splenectomy is performed for idiopathic (immune) thrombocytopenic purpura (ITP).[19]

OPERATIVE PLANNING

Laparoscopic splenectomy presents special problems, such as the necessity of dealing with a fragile and richly vascularized organ that is situated close to the stomach, the colon, and the pancreas and the difficulty of devising an extraction strategy that is compatible with proper histologic confirmation of the pathologic process while maintaining the advantages of minimal access surgery. For successful performance of laparoscopic splenectomy, detailed knowledge of both splenic anatomy and potential complications is essential. The operative strategy is largely determined by the anatomic features, which, as noted [*see* Anatomic Considerations, *above*], may vary considerably from patient to patient.[20]

OPERATIVE TECHNIQUE

Lateral Approach

This approach was first described in connection with laparoscopic adrenalectomy and is currently used for most laparoscopic splenectomies.[21] At present, the only indication for the anterior approach to laparoscopic splenectomy is the presence of massive splenomegaly, a megaspleen, or when a secondary procedure is required, especially in pediatric patients.[22] Typically, this alternative approach is taken when a spleen reaches or exceeds 23 cm in length or 3 kg in weight.

Step 1: placement of trocars The patient is placed in the right lateral decubitus position, much as he or she would be for a left-side posterolateral thoracotomy. The operating table is flexed and the kidney bolster raised to increase the distance between the lower rib and the iliac crest. Usually, four 12 mm trocars are used around the costal margin so that the camera, the clip applier, and the linear stapler can be interchanged with maximum flexibility [*see Figure 4*]. The trocars must be far enough apart to permit good working angles. Some advantage may be gained from tilting the patient slightly backward; this step gives the operating team more freedom in moving the instruments placed along the left costal margins, especially during lifting movements, when it is easy for instrument handles to touch the operating table. For the same reason, it is also advisable to place the anterior or abdominal side of the patient closer to the edge of the operating table.

A local anesthetic is infiltrated into the skin at the midpoint of the anterior costal margin, and a 12 mm incision is made. The first trocar is inserted under direct vision, and a symmetrical 15 mm Hg pneumoperitoneum is created. The locations of the remaining trocars are determined by considering the anatomic configuration in relation to the size of the spleen to be excised. In most cases, the fourth posterior trocar cannot be inserted until the splenic flexure of the colon has been mobilized. Accordingly, the procedure is usually started with three trocars in place. In the end, three trocars are placed anteriorly along the costal margin and one is located in the left flank.

Troubleshooting After years of using the Veress needle, we now prefer the open method of inserting the first trocar. It is true that use of the Veress needle is, for the most part, safe; however, the small number of catastrophic complications that occur with blind methods of first trocar insertion are more and more difficult to justify. Admittedly, these complications are infrequent; thus, it is unlikely that even a large randomized trial would be able to show any significant differences between various methods of first trocar insertion. Nevertheless, even though complications occur with the open method of first trocar insertion as well, they are very uncommon and tend to be limited to trauma to the intestine or the omental blood vessels; they do not have the same serious consequences as the major vessel injury that may arise from blind trocar insertion.

Trocar placements differing from the ones we describe may be considered. More experienced surgeons (or those simply wishing to make the procedure easier) may choose to replace one or two 12 mm trocars with 5 mm trocars [*see Figure 5a*]. The procedure can also be performed with only three trocars. In leaner patients, one of the trocars can be inserted into the umbilicus to gain a cosmetic advantage. The advent of needlescopic techniques has made it possible to replace some of the 5 and 12 mm trocars with 3 mm trocars. The ultimate (i.e., least invasive) technique, usually reserved for lean patients with ITP and normal-size spleens, involves one 12 mm trocar placed in the umbilicus and two 3 mm trocars placed subcostally [*see Figure 5b*]. This approach requires two different camera-laparoscope setups so that a 3 mm laparoscope can be interchanged with a 10 mm laparoscope as necessary to permit application of clips or staplers through the umbilical incision once the dissection is completed. This can also be achieved with a single camera setup using a sterile clip-on camera sleeve with an acrylic window. The specimen is then retrieved through the umbilicus. Because the use of 3 mm laparoscopes is accompanied by a decrease in available intra-abdominal light and focal width, a meticulously bloodless field and sophisticated surgical judgment are critical for successful performance of needlescopic splenectomy.

Step 2: search for and retrieval of accessory spleens The camera is inserted, and the stomach is retracted medially to expose the spleen. Then a fairly standard sequence is followed. A thorough search is then made for accessory spleens. To maximize retrieval, all known locations of accessory spleens should be carefully explored [*see Figure 6*]. Any accessory spleens found should be removed immediately; they are considerably harder to locate once the spleen is removed and the field is stained with blood.

Troubleshooting It is especially important to retrieve accessory spleens from patients with ITP, in whom the presence of overlooked accessory spleens has been associated with recurrence of the disease. Remedial operation for excision of missed accessory spleens has been reported to bring remission of recurrent disease; such an operation can be performed

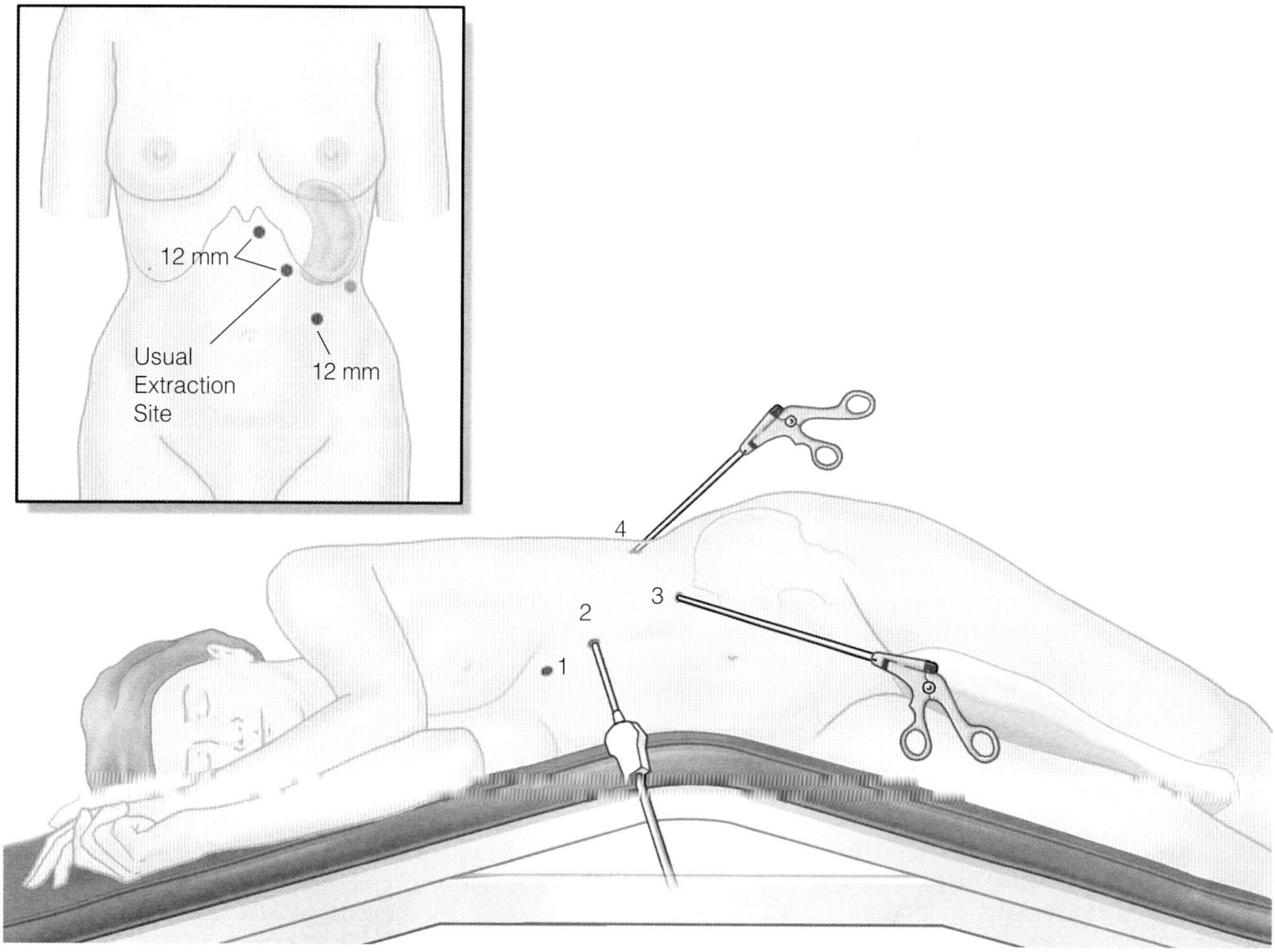

Figure 4 **Laparoscopic splenectomy: lateral approach. Shown is standard trocar placement. Four trocars are used. In most cases, the procedure is begun without the posterior trocar in place.**

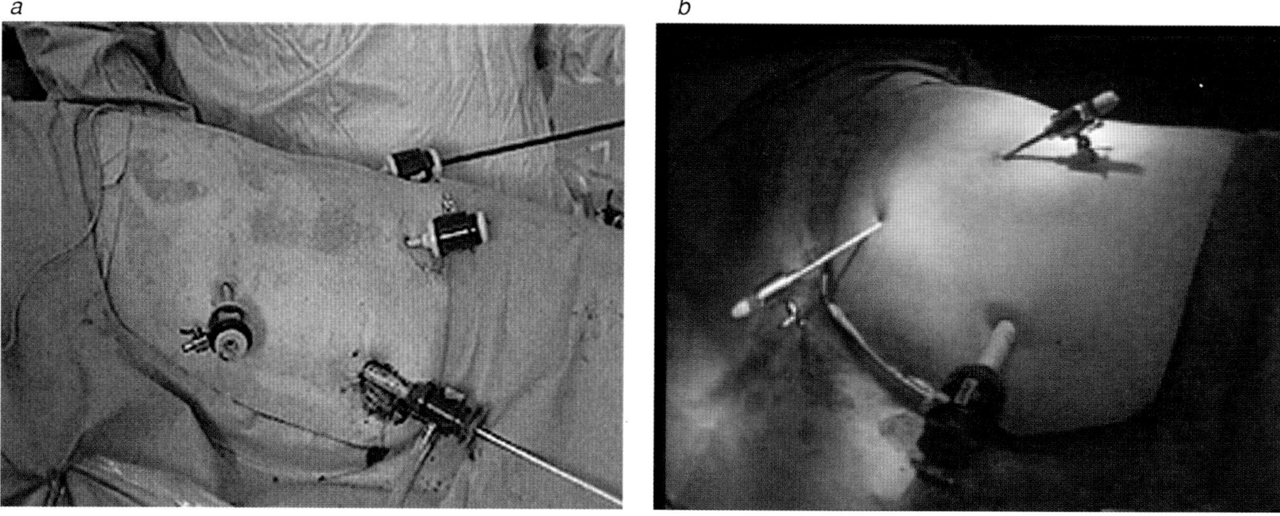

Figure 5 **Laparoscopic splenectomy: lateral approach. Shown are alternative trocar placements. (*a*) In some patients (e.g., thin patients with normal-size spleens), a 12 mm trocar may be placed in the umbilicus to gain a cosmetic advantage, and most of the other trocars may be downsized to 5 mm. (*b*) In the needlescopic approach, only three trocars are placed: a 12 mm trocar in the umbilicus and two 3 mm subcostal trocars. Two camera-laparoscope setups (3 and 10 mm) are required.**

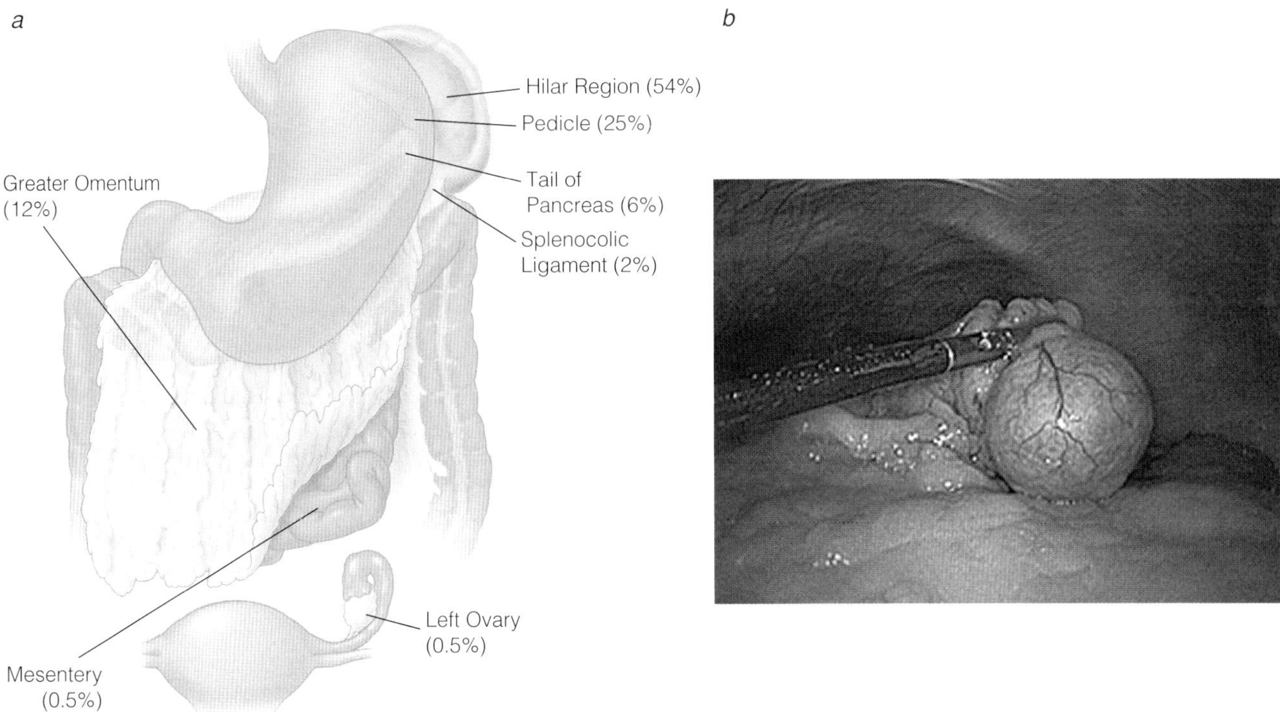

Figure 6 **Laparoscopic splenectomy: lateral approach. (*a*) Accessory spleens are known to occur at specific sites. (*b*) Shown is an accessory spleen.**

laparoscopically, with some authors suggesting the use of a handheld gamma probe and/or CT-guided methylene blue injection for identifying retained accessory spleens.[23] The overall retrieval rate for accessory spleens should fall between 15 and 30%.

Splenic activity has been demonstrated after open and laparoscopic splenectomy for trauma and hematologic disorders[24,25]; accordingly, it is advisable to wash out and recover all splenic fragments resulting from intraoperative trauma at the end of the procedure. This step is particularly important for patients with ITP, in whom intraoperative trauma to the spleen is thought to contribute to postoperative scan-detectable splenic activity.

Step 3: control of vessels at lower pole, demonstration of "splenic tent," and incision of phrenicocolic ligament The splenic flexure is partially mobilized by incising the splenocolic ligament, the lower part of the phrenicocolic ligament, and the sustentaculum lienis. The incision is carried slightly into the left side of the gastrocolic ligament. This step affords access to the gastrosplenic ligament, which can then be readily separated from the splenorenal ligament to create what looks like a tent. This maneuver cannot be accomplished in all cases, but when it can be done, it simplifies the procedure considerably. The walls of this so-called splenic tent are made of the gastrosplenic ligament on the left and the splenorenal ligament on the right, and the floor is made up of the stomach. In fact, this maneuver opens the lesser sac in its lateral portion (a point that is better demonstrated with gentle upward retraction of the splenic tip) [*see Figure 7*].

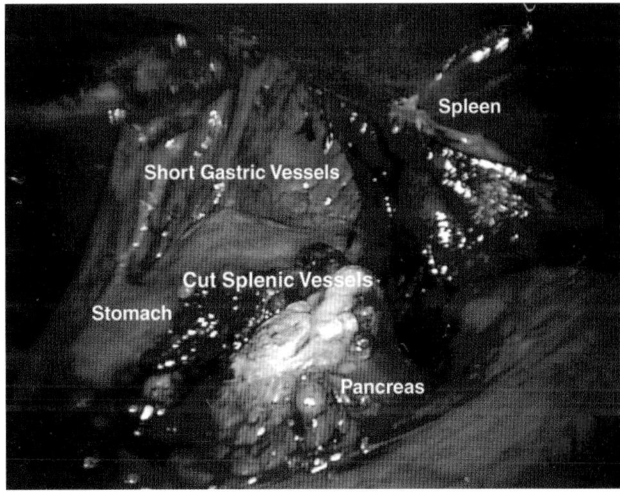

Figure 7 **Laparoscopic splenectomy: lateral approach. The so-called splenic tent is formed by the gastrosplenic and splenorenal ligaments laterally and the stomach below.**

The branches of the left gastroepiploic artery are controlled with the electrocautery or with clips, depending on the size of the branches. The avascular portion of the gastrosplenic ligament, situated between the gastroepiploic artery (and its branches) and the short gastric vessels, is then incised sufficiently to expose the hilar structures in the splenorenal ligament. To accomplish this, the lower pole is gently elevated; in this position, the spleen almost retracts itself as it naturally falls toward the left lobe of the liver. At this point, the surgeon can usually assess the geography of the hilum and determine the degree of difficulty of the operation. The fourth trocar, if needed, is then placed posteriorly under direct vision, with care taken to avoid the left kidney. Caution must also be exercised in placing the trocars situated immediately anterior and posterior to the iliac crest. The iliac crest can impede movement and hinder upward mobilization of structures if the trocars are placed over it rather than in front of or behind it [*see Figure 8*].

Finally, the phrenicocolic ligament is incised all the way to the left crus of the diaphragm, either with a monopolar electrocautery with an L hook or with scissors. A small portion of the ligament is left to keep the spleen suspended and facilitate subsequent bagging. The phrenicocolic ligament is avascular except in patients with portal hypertension or myeloproliferative disorders (e.g., myeloid metaplasia). Leaving 1 to 2 cm of ligament all along the spleen side facilitates retraction and handling of the spleen with instruments.

Troubleshooting Remarkably few instruments are needed for laparoscopic splenectomy: most of the operation is done with three reusable instruments. A dolphin-nose 5 mm atraumatic grasper is used to elevate and hold the spleen. It is also used to separate tissue planes and vessels with blunt dissection because its atraumatic tip is easily insinuated between tissue planes. A gently curved 5 mm fine-tip dissector (Crile or Maryland) and a 10 mm 90° right-angle dissector are the only other tools required for cost-efficient dissection.

When a powered instrument is called for, we use a monopolar electrocautery with an L hook or a gently curved scissors. Alternatively, an ultrasonic dissector or a tissue-welding device may be used, albeit at a much higher cost. We tend to limit the use of these very elegant technologies to cases where some operative difficulty is anticipated.

Step 4: dealing with splenic hilum and tailoring operative strategy to anatomy It is advisable to base one's operative strategy on the specific splenic anatomy. If a

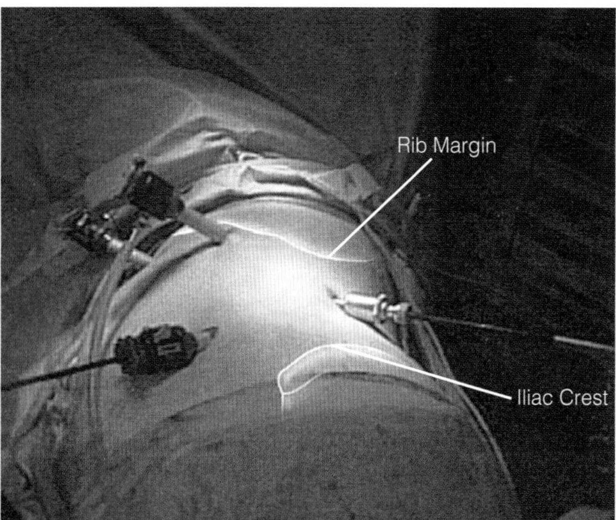

Figure 8 **Laparoscopic splenectomy: lateral approach. Shown is the recommended trocar placement around the iliac crest.**

distributed anatomy is present, the splenic branches are usually dissected and clipped. This is not only the least costly approach but also the simplest, in that the vessels are spread over a wider area of the splenic hilum and are easier to dissect and separate [*see Figure 9*].

A bundled anatomy lends itself more to a single use of the linear stapler provided that the tail of the pancreas is identified and dissected away when required. When possible, a window is created above the hilar pedicle in the splenorenal ligament so that all structures can be included within the markings of the linear stapler under direct vision [*see Figure 10*]. The angles provided by the various trocars make this maneuver much easier via the lateral approach than via the anterior approach. Dissection continues with individual dissection and clipping of the short gastric vessels; occasionally, these vessels can also be taken en masse with the linear stapler. We rarely have had to use intracorporeal sutures in this setting, except occasionally to control a short gastric vessel too short to be clipped safely. This portion of the operation is performed while the spleen is hanging from the upper portion of the phrenicocolic ligament, which has not yet been entirely cut.

Troubleshooting At this point in the procedure, experience in designing the operative strategy pays off in reduced operating time. Because of the many variations in size, shape, vascular patterns, and relations to adjacent organs, spleens are almost as individual as fingerprints. Accordingly, an experienced spleen surgeon learns to keep an open mind with regard to operative strategy and must be able to call on a wide range of skills to facilitate the procedure.

The surgeon should start by looking at the internal surface of the spleen. If the splenic vessels cover more than 75% of the internal surface (as is the case in 70% of patients), a distributed anatomy is present. With a distributed vascular anatomy, the vessels tend to be easier to dissect and isolate and thus can be readily (and cost-effectively) controlled with clips. On the other hand, if the splenic vessels entering the spleen cover only 25 to 35% of the inner surface of the hilum (30% of patients), the pattern is bundled. With a bundled vascular anatomy, the vessels, being fewer and closer together, can usually be controlled with a single application of the vascular stapler across the hilum provided that the tail of the pancreas can be protected.

Experienced surgeons also become very clever in using the position of the operating table to their advantage. The reverse Trendelenburg position (Fowler) allows the spleen to move away from the diaphragm in cases where the dissection of the upper pole is made more difficult by adhesions from previous surgery, large spleens, obesity, or previous infarctions of the spleen. With the patient stabilized by a bean bag, changing the degree of the lateral position is also useful. The surgeon learns to move the spleen back and forth so that it can be observed from an anterior and posterior perspective. The surgeon can then decide whether the approach to the splenic vessels is more appropriate from the front or the back.

Step 5: extraction of spleen A medium-size or large heavy-duty plastic freezer bag, of the sort commercially available in grocery stores, is used to bag the spleen. This bag is sterilized and folded and then introduced into the abdominal cavity through one of the 12 mm trocars [*see Figure 11*]. The

a

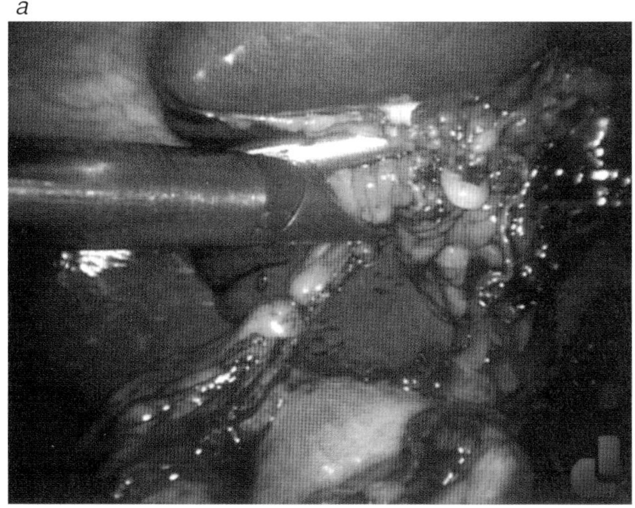

b

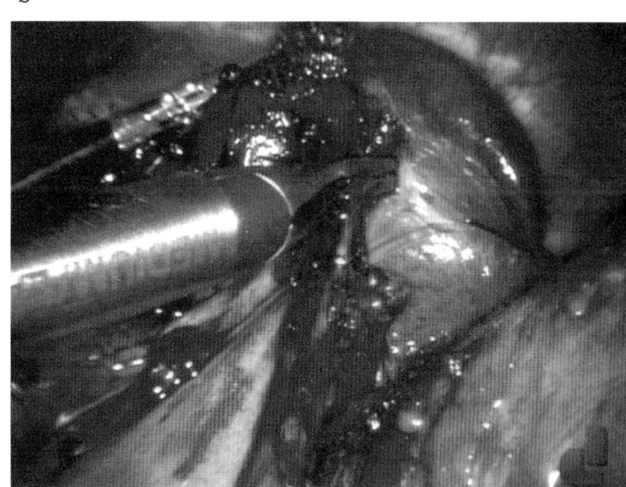

Figure 9 **Laparoscopic splenectomy: lateral approach. (*a, b*) Clipping is well suited to controlling short gastric or gastroepiploic vessels. It is also appropriate for distributed-type splenic vasculatures, in which more splenic vessels are spread over a wider area of the hilum.**

bag is unfolded and the spleen slipped inside to prevent splenosis during the subsequent manipulations. Grasping forceps are used to hold the two rigid edges of the bag and to effect partial closure. Bagging is facilitated by preserving the upper portion of the phrenicocolic ligament. After final section of the phrenicocolic ligament and any diaphragmatic adhesions present, extraction is performed through one of the anterior port sites. Extraction through a posterior site is more difficult because of the thickness of the muscle mass; usually, the incision must be opened, and more muscle must be fulgurated than is desirable.

The subcostal or umbilical incision through which extraction is to take place is extended slightly. Grasping forceps are inserted through the extraction incision to hold the edges of the bag inside the abdomen. Gentle traction on the bag from outside brings the spleen close to the peritoneal surface of the umbilical incision and then out of the wound [*see Figure 12*]. Specimen retrieval bags have been developed that can accommodate a normal-size spleen and thus make bagging much easier, but they are costly.

A biopsy specimen of a size suitable for pathologic identification is obtained by incising the splenic tip. The spleen is then fragmented with finger fracture, and the resulting blood is suctioned. The remaining stromal tissue of the spleen is then extracted through the small incision, hemostasis is again verified, and all trocars are removed. No drains are used. The incisions are closed with absorbable sutures and paper strips.

Troubleshooting The freezer bags can be more easily introduced into the abdomen if they are pulled in rather than pushed in [*see Figure 11*]. This may be accomplished by bringing out a 5 mm toothed grasper through the introduction trocar from another properly angled trocar, grasping the specimen bag, and pulling the bag back down through the trocar. A laparoscopic hernia mesh introducer may also be used.

Slipping the spleen into a freezer bag is also an acquired skill that takes some time to master. It is an important skill that is useful in many other instances where specimen retrieval is needed (e.g., in procedures involving the gallbladder, the appendix, the adrenal glands, or the colon). In addition, it is highly cost-effective in that these commercially available bags cost only a few cents each. Admittedly, laparoscopic retrieval bags are easier to use, but their substantially higher cost can become a factor in a busy minimally invasive surgery unit. A suction machine (–70 mm Hg) and a custom-made sharp beveled 10 mm cannula can be used to suction splenic tissue from the plastic retrieval bag. When extraction is done with the use of any type of forceps or graspers, surgeons have noticed that initially the extracted spleen fragments tend to be small and tedious to extract. As the extraction proceeds, the fragments get bigger and easier to extract. Definitely, imagination and patience are required for this part of the procedure.

Anterior Approach

The anterior approach is seldom used nowadays; however, it remains the preferable approach in some patients with massive splenomegaly (21 to 30 cm long) and all patients with megaspleens (> 30 cm or > 3 kg) with the aid of hand-assisted devices [*see* Special Considerations, Hand-Assisted Laparoscopic Splenectomy, *below*]. Very large spleens are extremely heavy and difficult to manipulate with laparoscopic instruments, and it is complicated to lift them so as to gain access to the phrenicocolic ligament posteriorly. The anterior approach can also be considered if another procedure (e.g., cholecystectomy) is being contemplated; alternatively, in this situation, the lateral approach can be used, and the patient can be repositioned for the secondary procedure.

Step 1: placement of trocars Under general anesthesia, the patient is placed in a modified lithotomy position to allow the surgeon to operate between the patient's legs and to allow the assistants to stand on each side of the patient. The procedure is performed through five trocars in the upper abdomen [*see Figure 13*], with the patient in a steep Fowler position with left-side elevation. A 12 mm trocar is introduced through an

a

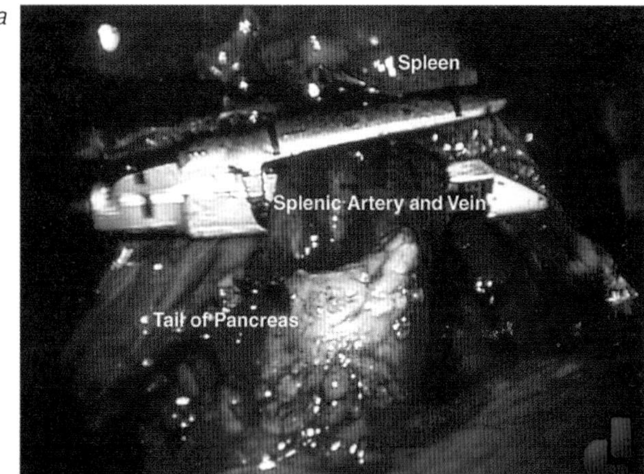

b

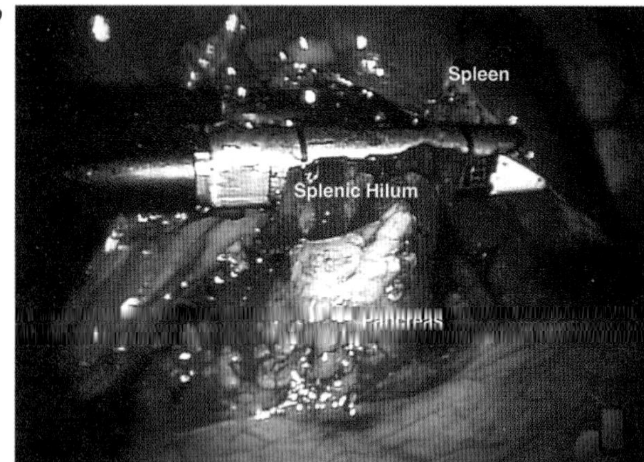

c

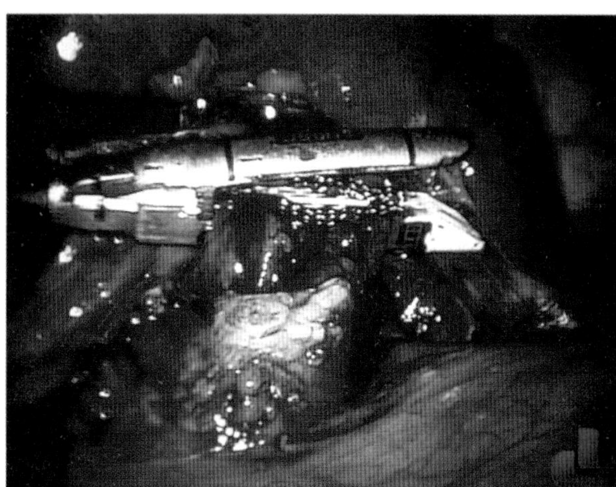

Figure 10 **Laparoscopic splenectomy: lateral approach. (*a* through *c*) Stapling is particularly well suited to the compact hilum found in the magistral-type distribution of splenic vessels. As shown, all of the vascular structures are within the stapler markers, and the tail of the pancreas is well protected.**

umbilical incision, and a 10 mm laparoscope (0° or 30°) is connected to a video system. A 12 mm trocar is placed in each upper quadrant, and two 5 mm trocars are inserted close to the rib margin on the left and right sides of the abdomen.

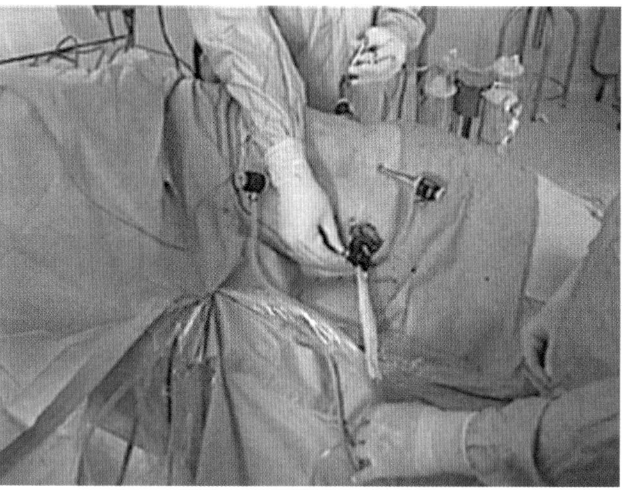

Figure 11 **Laparoscopic splenectomy: lateral approach. Illustrated is the introduction of a sterile freezer bag for specimen extraction via the pull method. A toothed grasper is passed across the abdomen between two trocars and brought out through the 12 mm umbilical trocar site. This grasper is used to pull the extraction bag back into the abdomen.**

Alternatively, trocars can be deployed in a semicircle away from the left upper quadrant. Trocar sites are carefully selected to optimize working angles. The 12 mm ports are used to allow introduction of clip appliers, staplers, or the laparoscope from a variety of angles as needed.

Troubleshooting With increasing experience, we find that we prefer to do as many laparoscopic splenectomies as possible via the lateral approach because it is so much easier, even with spleens that are longer than 20 cm and are readily palpable. The decision is arbitrarily made on the basis of estimated available working space. If the spleen comes too close to the iliac crest or the midline, the anterior approach should be taken instead.

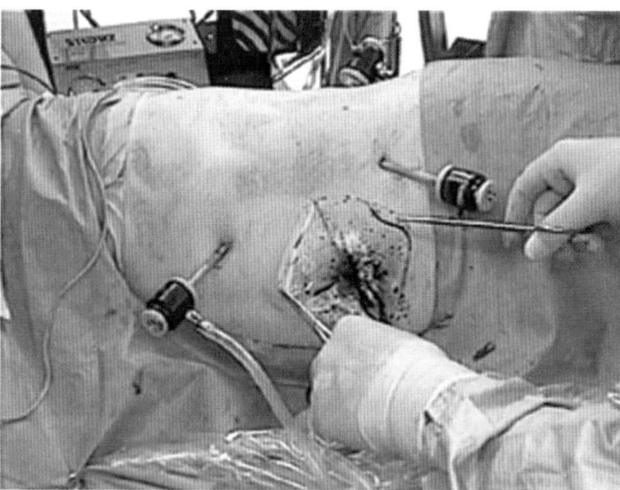

Figure 12 **Laparoscopic splenectomy: lateral approach. Shown is the position of the specimen bag before finger fragmentation or pulp suction.**

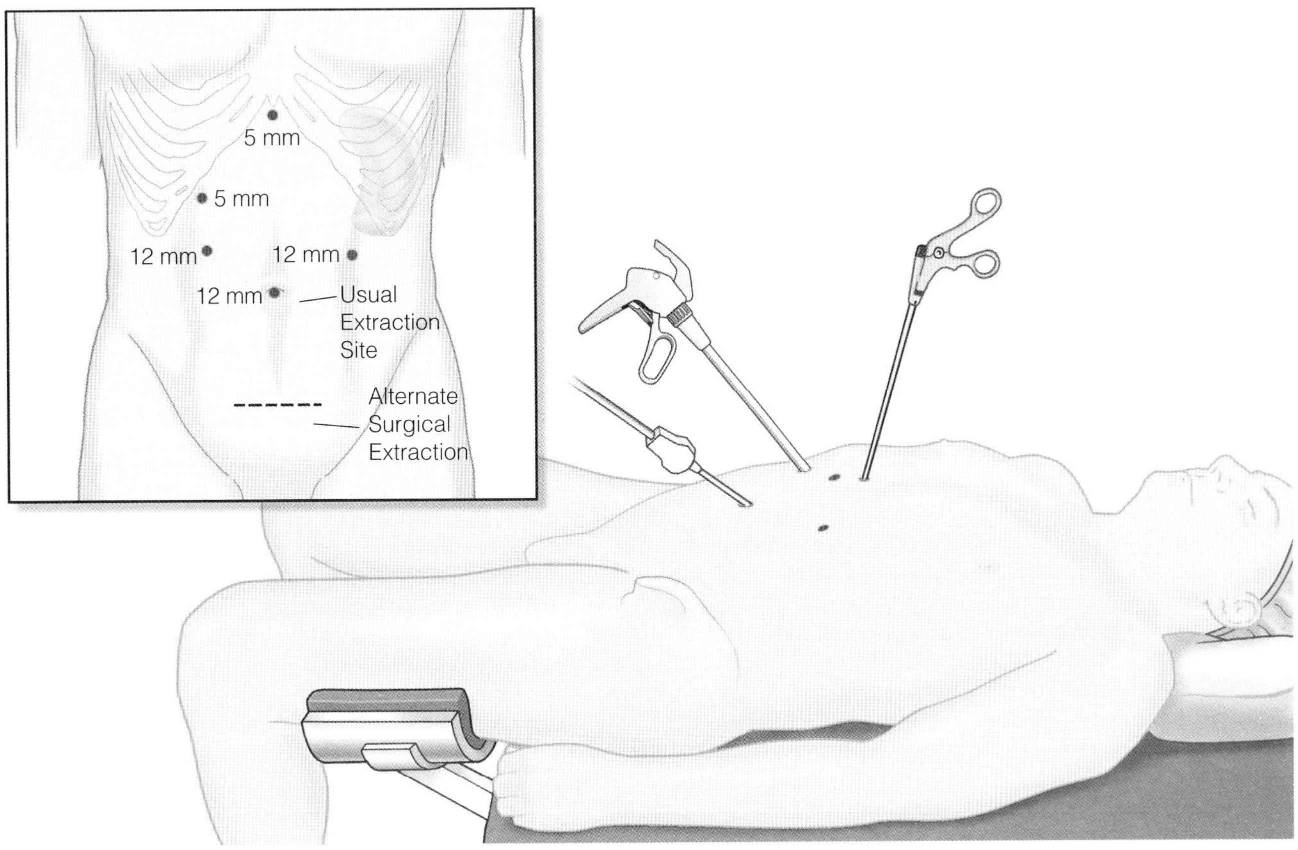

Figure 13 **Laparoscopic splenectomy: anterior approach. Shown is standard trocar placement. The umbilical site is used for the camera. The remaining trocars are placed in the left and right upper quadrants, the epigastrium, and the right subcostal region. Depending on the size of the spleen, the trocars can also be disposed in a semicircle away from the left upper quadrant.**

Step 2: isolation of lower pole and control of blood supply The left hepatic lobe is retracted, and the stomach is retracted medially to expose the spleen. Accessory spleens are searched for, and the phrenicocolic ligament, the splenocolic ligament, and the sustentaculum lienis are incised near the lower pole with an electrocautery and a hook probe or with scissors. Vascular adhesions—frequently found on the medial side of the spleen—are cauterized. They are also called *criminal folds* for their tendency to be avulsed off the spleen during dissection and cause nuisance bleeding from the capsular injury. The gastrocolic ligament is carefully dissected close to the spleen, and the left gastroepiploic vessels are ligated one by one with metallic clips or, if small, simply cauterized. The upper and lower poles of the spleen are gently lifted with one or both palpators (placed through the 5 mm ports) to expose the splenic hilum and the tail of the pancreas within the splenorenal ligament, thereby facilitating individual dissection and clipping of all the branches of the splenic artery and vein close to the spleen. The short gastric vessels are then identified and ligated with clips or, occasionally, with staples. No sutures are used. Alternatively, the splenic artery itself can be isolated and clipped within the lesser sac before extensive dissection of the lower pole and suspensory ligaments.

Because of the segmental and terminal distribution of splenic arteries, it is easy to determine the devascularized portions of the spleen: these segments exhibit a characteristic grayish color, whereas the vascularized segments retain a pinkish hue. When the organ is completely isolated, it is left in its natural cavity, and hemostasis is verified.

Troubleshooting If one elects first to clip the splenic artery within the lesser sac, a few precautions must be taken. First, the clipping must be done distal to the pancreatica magna to prevent pancreatic injury. Second, one must make sure that the splenic artery proper is clipped, not one of its branches (e.g., the superior terminal branch). This is an easy mistake to commit with the distributed type of splenic vasculature [*see Figure 1*] because the splenic artery itself is short and the branches can take off very early. Third, one must always keep in mind the possibility of an anastomotic branch between the major splenic branches, as described by Testut.[12] Should a major terminal branch be clipped rather than the splenic artery proper, there will be no spleen ischemia if such an anastomosis is present [*see Figure 1*].

Yet another challenge posed by the anterior approach is that if bleeding occurs, the blood tends to pool in the area of the hilum and obscure vision even more, whereas in the lateral approach, the blood tends to flow away from the operative field. One quickly learns that there is a steep price to pay for cutting corners during the dissection. The dissection must be meticulous, especially behind branches of the splenic vein.

Step 3: extraction of spleen Given that the anterior approach is now used only in cases of massive splenomegaly or megaspleen, bagging can be problematic. The largest commercially available freezer bag we have seen measures 27 by 28 cm, and the largest spleen we have been able to bag in one of them was 24 cm long. Furthermore, an accessory extraction incision is often required; a Pfannenstiel incision gives better cosmetic results, but a left lower quadrant incision can also be used. Hand-assisted devices are used with increasing frequency in laparoscopic removal of large spleens [*see* Special Considerations, Hand-Assisted Laparoscopic Splenectomy, *below*] and are becoming the preferred method for dealing with massive splenomegaly laparoscopically.

Laparoscopic Partial Splenectomy

Concern regarding the risk of OPSI has encouraged the practice of preserving splenic tissue and function whenever possible. For this reason, partial splenectomy has occasionally been indicated for treatment of benign tumors of the spleen and for excision of cystic lesions.[26] Its use has been described in connection with the management of type I Gaucher disease, cholesteryl ester storage disease, chronic myelogenous leukemia, single metastasis, thalassemia major, staging of Hodgkin disease, and spherocytosis.[27–30] It has also been suggested for some cystic fibrosis patients with hypersplenism. Partial splenectomy is an option in the management of splenic trauma when the patient's condition is stable enough to permit the meticulous dissection required for the operation.[31,32]

Like standard laparoscopic splenectomy, laparoscopic partial splenectomy is performed with the patient in the right lateral decubitus position. Trocar placement is similar as well. The splenocolic ligament and the lower part of the phrenicocolic ligament are incised to permit mobilization of the lower pole of the spleen. If the lower portion of the spleen is to be excised, branches of the gastroepiploic vessels supplying the lower pole are dissected and clipped close to the parenchyma. An appropriate number of penultimate branches of the inferior polar artery are then taken in such a way as to create a clear line of demarcation between normal spleen and devascularized spleen. This process is continued until the desired number of splenic segments are devascularized.

Next, a standard monopolar electrocautery is used to score the splenic capsule circumferentially, with care taken to ensure that a 5 mm rim of devascularized splenic tissue remains in situ; this is the most important technical point for this procedure [*see Figure 14*]. The incision is then carried into the splenic pulp. Atraumatic intestinal graspers are also used to fracture the splenic pulp in a bloodless fashion. The laparoscopic L hook and scissors provide excellent hemostatic control with simple spot coagulation or spray current in the coagulation mode. No drains are used. Alternative methods of hemostatis have also been used, including argon beam coagulators, ultrasonic shears, linear staplers, bipolar tissue welding instruments, and radiofrequency ablation probes.[29]

Once the spleen has been allowed to demarcate, resection is remarkably bloodless, provided that the 5 mm rim of ischemic tissue is left in place. Complete control of the splenic artery is not required before splenic separation, because division occurs in an ischemic segment of spleen.[9] The feasibility of leaving portions of ischemic spleen in situ has been demonstrated in a large prospective, randomized trial involving partial splenic embolization as primary treatment of hematologic disorders.[33]

If the superior pole is to be removed, the phrenicocolic ligament must be incised almost entirely so that the spleen can be easily mobilized and the proper exposure achieved. The short gastric branches are taken first, along with the desired number of superior polar artery branches.

Laparoscopic partial splenectomy can be performed either with or without the aid of selective preoperative arterial embolization (see below). Radiologists are capable of cannulating the desired segmental splenic arterial branch and embolizing the segment that is to be resected. This is well documented in the recent trauma literature.[34]

Preoperative Splenic Artery Embolization

Preoperative splenic artery embolization is used as an adjuvant in a few patients to make laparoscopic splenectomy possible and to reduce blood loss. Although it is now infrequently used, it remains a useful tool in the armamentarium of spleen surgeons.[35]

Generally speaking, the technique involves embolization of the spleen with coils placed proximally in the splenic artery and absorbable gelatin sponges and small coils placed distally in each splenic arterial branch (the double embolization technique), with care taken to spare vessels supplying the tail of the pancreas [*see Figure 15*].

The procedure is ended when it is estimated radiologically that 80% or more of the splenic tissue has been successfully embolized. In most cases, successful embolization is achieved with both proximal and distal emboli; in a minority of cases, it is achieved with proximal emboli alone or with distal emboli alone.[35]

Troubleshooting Preoperative splenic artery embolization is safe provided that two main principles are adhered to. First, embolization must be done distal to the pancreatica magna to avoid damaging the pancreas. Second, neither microspheres nor absorbable gelatin powder should be used, because particles of this small size may migrate to unintended target organ capillaries and cause tissue necrosis; only coils and absorbable gelatin sponge fragments should be used.

POSTOPERATIVE CARE

Postoperative care for patients who have undergone laparoscopic splenectomy is usually simple. The nasogastric tube inserted after induction of general anesthesia is removed either in the recovery room, once stomach emptying has been verified, or the next morning, depending on the duration and the degree of technical difficulty of the procedure. The urinary catheter is usually removed before the patient leaves the recovery room. The patient is allowed to drink clear fluids on the morning after the operation; when clear fluids are well tolerated, the patient is allowed to proceed to a diet of his or her choice.

A proper pain control process is started before the procedure. If the patient has no history of ulcer or dyspepsia, celecoxib, a cyclooxygenase-2 NSAID, is started preoperatively because there is little effect on platelet function. Alternatively, 50 mg of ketorolac can be given 30 minutes before the end of the procedure. All trocar sites are infiltrated with local anesthetic at the start of surgery. This is done to prevent the establishment of peripheral and central sensitization ("wind-up"), conditions that

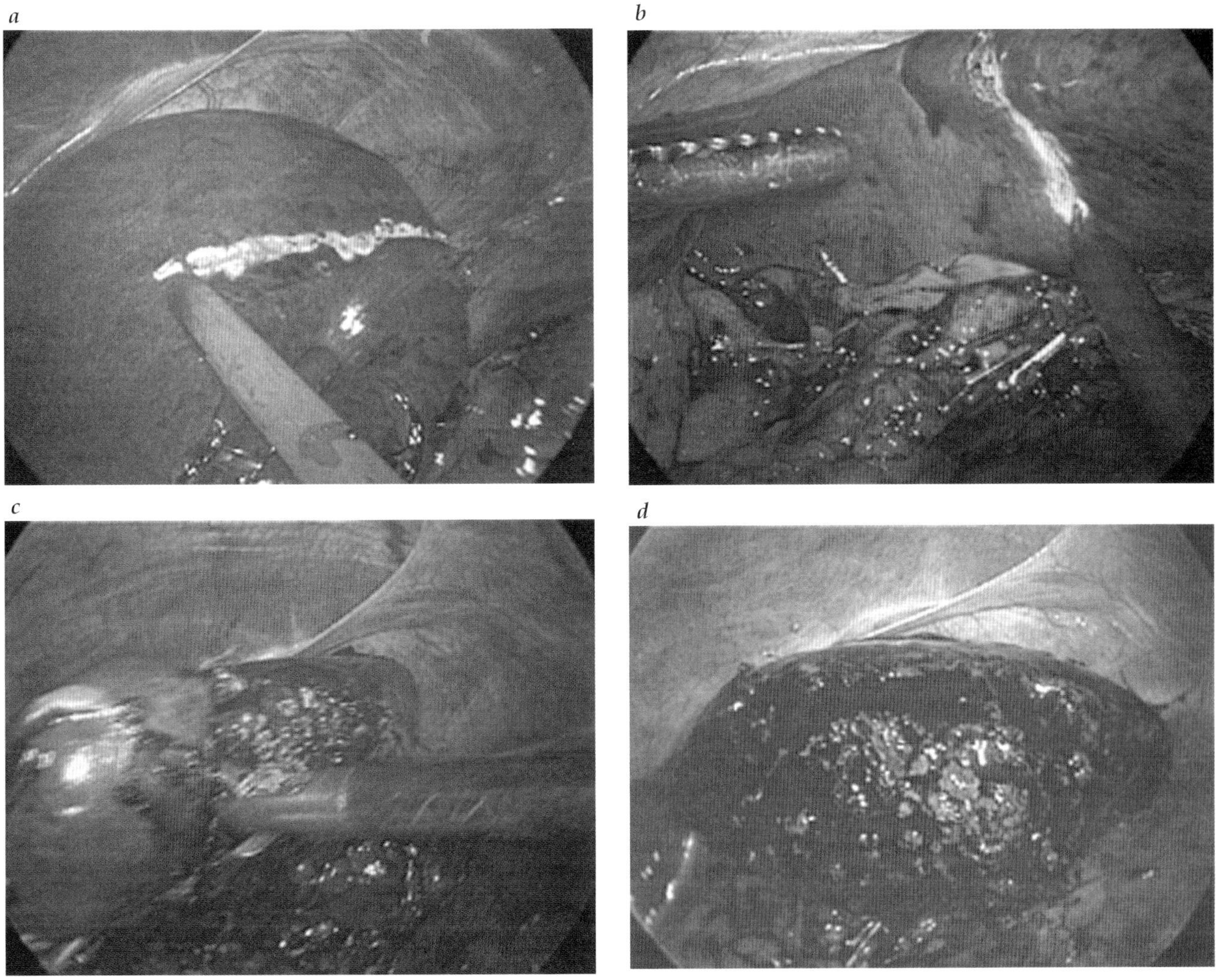

a

b

c

d

Figure 14 **Laparoscopic splenectomy: partial splenectomy. (*a, b*) The splenic capsule is scored with the monopolar cautery, and a 5 mm margin of devitalized tissue is left. (*c*) The splenic pulp is fractured with an atraumatic grasper. The electrocautery with the L hook is also used to control parenchymal bleeding. (*d*) Shown is the cut surface of the spleen after transection. The operative field remains remarkably dry.**

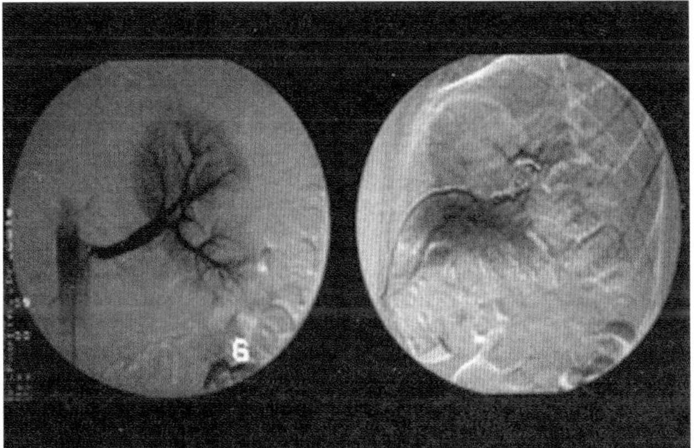

Figure 15 **Laparoscopic splenectomy: splenic artery embolization. Shown are splenic angiograms of a patient with thrombotic thrombocytopenic purpura before (*left*) and after (*right*) splenic artery embolization with 3, 5, and 7 cm coils and absorbable gelatin sponge fragments.**

promote an increased response to pain stimuli. Ketorolac or another NSAID is administered regularly in the postoperative period following the "first in last out" principle of NSAID administration for pain control. NSAIDs have been shown to have a 30 to 50% opioid-sparing effect. Morphine-based patient-controlled analgesia is used the first night after surgery. The following morning, acetaminophen and NSAIDs usually suffice. Oral hydromorphone hydrochloride, 2 to 4 mg, is reserved for breakthrough pain. A prescription for these three oral drugs is given on discharge. Because of its adverse effects of nausea, vomiting, abdominal fullness, and constipation, codeine is avoided. Furthermore, increased reports of codeine intoxication associated with ultrarapid CYP2D6 metabolism make it a poor choice.

Patients receiving intravenous (IV) cortisone are given oral steroids on postoperative day 1 after an overlap IV injection; thereafter, steroids are gradually tapered. Patients are allowed to shower 12 hours after surgery and are advised to keep the paper strips covering the trocar incisions in place for 7 to 10 days. No drains are used. No limitations are imposed on recorded after splenectomy before it would be possible to say that these were not chance events. Some authors feel that so few reports in the literature can only be interpreted as indicating that infection in adults undergoing splenectomy for benign disease is uncommon, and they are reluctant to agree that this number of reports constitutes a proven increased susceptibility to infection after splenectomy in adults. These authors point to the fact that 73% of the pneumococcal infections reported after splenectomy were made up of isolated case reports.[45]

Despite the controversies, the risk of OPSI should be reduced by the measures already described even if accurate data from any of these interventions are scant. Yet in a study at The Hospital for Sick Children in Toronto, children who had splenectomy between 1958 and 1970 (6% infection, 3.9% mortality) were compared with children who had splenectomy between 1971 and 1975. In the latter group, all the children received prophylactic antibiotics and more than two thirds of them were given polyvalent pneumococcal vaccine. In the latter group, the infection rate was reduced by 47% and the mortality by 88%. The use of vaccines against encapsulated organism is thought to have led to a drop in the overall incidence of OPSI to less than 1%.[44,47]

OUTCOME EVALUATION

No randomized, prospective trials comparing open splenectomy with laparoscopic splenectomy have yet been conducted. At present, such trials are unlikely to be held, for a variety of reasons. For one thing, randomization is difficult with procedures that are still in evolution. At one end of the spectrum, laparoscopic splenectomy is done for patients with ITP, who usually are relatively healthy and have normal-size spleens. In many of these patients, needlescopic instruments (< 3 mm) can be used in conjunction with a single 12 mm port site in the umbilicus. This approach permits hospital discharge within 24 hours of operation in a significant number of cases. At the other end of the spectrum, laparoscopic splenectomy is done for patients with myeloid metaplasia and spleens longer than 30 cm. In this setting, a laparoscopic approach poses formidable challenges, and the optimal technique and its justification remain to be determined. The window of opportunity for randomized comparative trials may have been lost.

Large case series and nonrandomized comparative trials, however, have consistently reported better outcomes from laparoscopic splenectomy than from open splenectomy (E.C. Poulin, C.M. Schlachta, J. Mamazza, unpublished data, February 2001).[48–53] For example, in one set of 528 patients [*see Table 2*],[49–51] the rate of postoperative pneumonia was 1.1% (6 of 528), and no subphrenic abscesses occurred as postoperative complications (E.C. Poulin, C.M. Schlachta, J. Mamazza, unpublished data, February 2001). Many surgeons who have completed the learning curve associated with the procedure feel that there is still room for improvement regarding complication rates and length of stay for patients with ITP and other relatively benign conditions necessitating laparoscopic splenectomy. The more serious conditions and the mortality seen in conjunction with the procedure tend to occur in patients with advanced hematologic malignancies or megaspleens. In such cases, most of the adverse results are related to the disease state rather than to the operation, and it remains to be seen whether laparoscopic splenectomy will have a positive effect on outcome.

One of the great attractions of minimally invasive surgery has been the prospect of significant cost reductions. At this point in the development of laparoscopic splenectomy, however, we are reluctant to place too much trust in premature cost analyses that do not take into account the "work in progress" nature of minimally invasive surgery. Most surgeons can now perform most laparoscopic splenectomies with simplified trays of reusable instruments. Our basic laparoscopic tray contains a few instruments and two sizes of reusable clip appliers with inexpensive clips. As noted [*see* Operative Technique, *above*], clips are used for distributed-type spleens, and single-use linear staplers are mostly used for magistral-bundled type spleens. To reduce costs, ultrasonic dissectors are rarely used. In addition, the use of commercially available freezer bags instead of laparoscopic retrieval bags further reduces the cost of specimen extraction. Finally, even if intraoperative costs are higher with laparoscopic splenectomy, our experience is that the increase is offset by reductions in postoperative stay.[19]

We, like most authorities, believe that as a surgeon gains experience with laparoscopic splenectomy, operating time tends to fall until it approaches that of open splenectomy. We also concur with the numerous authors who have suggested that once laparoscopic splenectomy is mastered, use of blood products tends to decrease substantially.

Open Splenectomy

PREOPERATIVE EVALUATION

With the growing acceptance of laparoscopic splenectomy, the indications for open splenectomy have essentially been reduced to (1) elective removal of megaspleens and (2) treatment of splenic trauma when conservative treatment either is not indicated or has failed. In rare cases, open splenectomy may be done for iatrogenic injuries incurred during left upper quadrant surgical procedures.

Preoperative evaluation for elective open splenectomy is similar to that for laparoscopic splenectomy [*see* Laparoscopic Splenectomy, Preoperative Evaluation, *above*]. Preoperative evaluation of trauma patients is covered in more detail elsewhere. Essentially, a coagulogram and blood typing and cross-matching are required. A preoperative CT scan will have established the size of the spleen, the grade of the splenic injury, the presence of other injuries (if any), and, in elective cases, the location and configuration of any masses or cysts.

OPERATIVE PLANNING

Most surgeons would agree that the lessons learned from successful performance of minimally invasive procedures have had a positive impact on the refinement of the corresponding open procedures. The principles of careful appreciation of fine anatomic details (as described for laparoscopic splenectomy) and maximal reduction of tissue trauma from retractors or excessive tissue handling should be incorporated into the planning of open splenectomy.

Total versus Partial Splenectomy

As a consequence of the recognition that splenectomy renders patients susceptible to a lifelong risk of OPSI, it is now

Table 2 Clinical Results of Laparoscopic Splenectomy

Study	N	ITP/ Non-ITP	Conversion Rate (%)	OR Time (min)	Morbidity (%)	Mortality (%)	Length of Stay (days)	Accessory Spleen Present (%)
All diagnoses								
Katkhouda et al (1998)[51]	103	67/36	3.9	161	6	0	2.5	16.5
Targarona et al (2000)[49]	122	54/68	7.4	153	18	0	4.0	12
Park et al (2000)[50]	203	129/74	3.0	145	9	0.5	2.7	12.3
Poulin et al (2001)	100	50/50	8.0	180	15	4	3.0	25
ITP								
Trias et al (2000)[52]	48	—	4.2	142	12	NA	4.0	11
Poulin et al (2001)	51	—	3.9	160	5.9	0	2.0	32
Malignancy								
Schlachta et al (1999)[53]	14	—	21	239	18	9	3.0	—
Trias et al (2000)[52]	28	—	14*	171	28	NA	5.5	—

ITP = idiopathic thrombocytopenic purpura; NA = not available; OR = operating room.
*71% required accessory incision because of spleen size.

routine practice to attempt splenic conservation. Accordingly, saving normally functioning splenic parenchyma has become the most important goal in the management of splenic injuries. In some 50% of adults (and over 80% of children), this goal can be achieved by means of nonoperative treatment. In approximately 20% of adults, splenorrhaphy and partial splenectomy are possible; splenectomy is indicated in the remainder. Partial splenectomy is also favored on occasion when excision of splenic tissue is required for the treatment of other elective conditions.[31]

For the sake of brevity, we describe the surgical technique for total splenectomy and partial splenectomy concurrently, noting differences only where significant.

OPERATIVE TECHNIQUE

Step 1: Incision

The patient is supine, in a reverse Tredelenburg position with a 15° tilt to the right. For maximal exposure, a midline incision is made, starting on the left side of the xiphoid process [*see Figure 17*]. The incision is extended below the umbilicus for a variable distance, depending on circumstances such as the size of the patient, the surgical situation (traumatic versus nontraumatic), the possibility of associated injury, and the size of the spleen. Occasionally, a left subcostal incision may be used for nontraumatic indications in patients with normal-size spleens. This incision may be extended onto the right side to form a chevron incision if necessary; however, this may impede the search for accessory spleens. Some surgeons have performed splenectomy via a thoracoabdominal approach, but most have abandoned this approach. Appropriate retraction of the left lobe of the liver and the abdominal wall is achieved with the help of surgical assistants placed on each side of the table or the use of self-retaining retractors.

Troubleshooting In trauma cases, the anesthetist should always be informed when the peritoneum is opened; release of a tense hemoperitoneum can precipitate hypotension with the loss of tamponade.

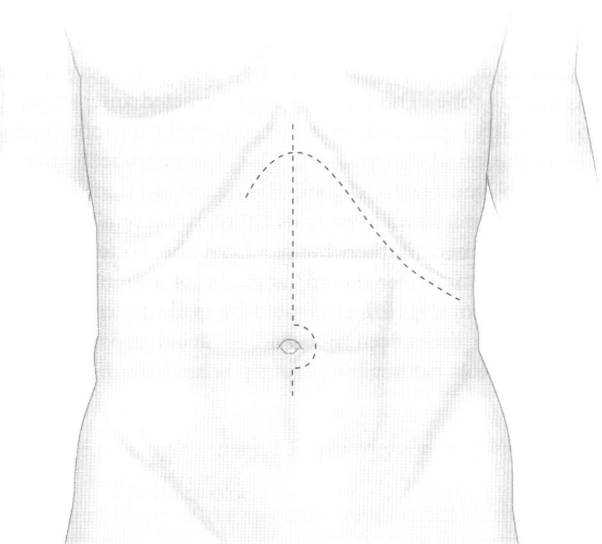

Figure 17 **Open splenectomy. Shown are midline and left subcostal incisions.**

Step 2: Evacuation of Blood and Packing of the Abdomen

In trauma cases, gross blood and clots are evacuated manually with large laparotomy sponges. All quadrants of the abdomen are then packed with laparotomy pads. Standard suction equipment is not very useful for evacuating large quantities of blood from the abdomen.

Step 3: Control of Splenic Artery

Once other major injuries are excluded, the first decision to be made is whether to control the splenic artery first or to proximity. The vessels may be doubly ligated, transfixed, or clipped. If clips are used, care is taken not to dislodge them with inappropriate manipulations. Once the arterial blood supply is controlled, the affected area of the spleen will rapidly become visibly demarcated. If the devitalized area of the spleen corresponds to the intended resection, a similar technique is applied to the venous side. Access to the venous side can also be achieved from the posterior aspect of the spleen. When this approach is followed, it is helpful to identify the tail of the pancreas if possible to avoid inadvertent damage: the tail of the pancreas touches the hilum of the spleen in 30% of cases and lies within 1 cm of the hilum in 70%.

Step 7 (Partial Splenectomy): Incision of Splenic Capsule and Partial Resection of Spleen

The capsule of the spleen is incised circumferentially with a scalpel or a monopolar cautery, and a 5 mm rim of devitalized tissue is left in situ. The splenic fragments may be transected with a scalpel, scissors, a monopolar cautery, or a combination thereof. Various techniques have been used to control residual bleeding, including use of a monopolar cautery on spray current; use of a cutaneous ultrasonic surgical aspirator; use of an argon beam coagulator; suture compression, with or without Teflon pledgets; and omental pedicle packing. One low-tech way of dealing with residual hemostatic requirements is to employ the hollow part of a Poole suction device to aspirate blood while employing a coagulating monopolar current on the suction tip. In some cases, wrapping the splenic remnant in an absorbable polyglycolic mesh is useful. Our experience suggests that when enough residual devitalized tissue (i.e., at least 5 mm) is left behind circumferentially, good hemostasis is easily achieved, typically requiring nothing more than simple measures and topical agents. No drains are used unless the tail of the pancreas has been damaged, in which case a closed-suction drain is placed.

POSTOPERATIVE CARE

The principles of postoperative care are essentially the same for open splenectomy as for laparoscopic splenectomy [*see* Laparoscopic Splenectomy, Postoperative Care, *above*], although most authors agree that the pace of aftercare is slower with the former. It should be kept in mind that acute postoperative gastric distention occurs more frequently in children and may necessitate more prolonged gastric decompression.

COMPLICATIONS

The complications seen after open splenectomy are the same as those seen after its laparoscopic counterpart [*see* Laparoscopic Splenectomy, Complications, *above*]. Hemorrhagic complications may necessitate transfusion, reoperation, or both.

Although the rate of serious postoperative infection after splenic surgery is generally considered to be 8%, it is thought to be lower in patients undergoing splenorrhaphy or partial splenectomy. The lower rate is probably attributable to the presence of less severe underlying injuries rather than to the preservation of splenic tissue. Infectious complications usually manifest themselves between postoperative days 5 and 10 and are typically diagnosed by means of physical examination, chest x-ray, ultrasonography, and CT.

The General Surgery Division at the Ottawa hospital has unrestricted grants from Storz and Covidien. The General Surgery Division at the University of Western Ontario has an unrestricted grant from Johnson and Johnson.

References

1. Cole F. Is splenectomy harmless? Surg Gynecol Obstet 1971;133:98.
2. Johnston GB. Splenectomy. Ann Surg 1908; 48:50.
3. Campos Cristo M. Segmental resections of the spleen: report on the first eight cases operated on. O Hosp (Rio) 1962;62:205.
4. Upadhyaya P, Simpson JS. Splenic trauma in children. Surg Gynecol Obstet 1968;126: 781.
5. Delaitre B, Maignien B. Splénectomie par voie laparoscopique, 1 observation. Presse Med 1991;20:2263.
6. Carroll BJ, Phillips EH, Semel CJ, et al. Laparoscopic splenectomy. Surg Endosc 1992;6:183.
7. Thibault C, Mamazza J, Létourneau R, et al. Laparoscopic splenectomy: operative technique and preliminary report. Surg Laparosc Endosc 1992;2:248.
8. Poulin EC, Thibault C, DesCôteaux JG, et al. Partial laparoscopic splenectomy for trauma: technique and case report. Surg Laparosc Endosc 1995;5:306.
9. Seshadri PA, Poulin EC, Mamazza J, et al. Technique for laparoscopic partial splenectomy. Surg Laparosc Endosc 2000;10:106.
10. Uranues S, Grossman D, Ludwig L, Bergamaschi R. Laparoscopic partial splenectomy. Surg Endosc 2007;21:57–60.
11. Michels NA. The variational anatomy of the spleen and splenic artery. Am J Anat 1942;70:21.
12. Testut L. Traité d'anatomie humaine. 7th ed. Paris: Librairie Octave Doin; 1923. p. 942.
13. Lipshutz B. A composite study of the coeliac axis artery. Ann Surg 1917;65:159.
14. Henschen C. Die chirurgische Anatomie der Milzgefiisse. Schweiz Med Wochenschr 1928; 58:164.
15. Ssoson-Jaroschewitsch A. Zür chirurgischen Anatomie des Milzhilus. Z Anat I Abt 1937; 84:218.
16. Baronofsky ID, Walton W, Noble JF. Occult injury to the pancreas following splenectomy. Surgery 1951;29:852.
17. Saber AA, Hibling B, Khaghang K, et al. Safety zone for splenic hilar control during splenectomy: a computed tomography scan mapping of the tail of the pancreas in relation to the splenic hilum. Am Surg 2007;73: 890–4.
18. Goerg C, Schwerk WB, Goerg K, et al. Sonographic patterns of the affected spleen in malignant lymphoma. J Clin Ultrasound 1990;18:569.
19. Habermalz B, Sauerland S, Decker G, et al. Laparoscopic splenectomy: the clinical practice guidelines of the European Association for Endoscopic Surgery (EAES). Surg Endosc 2008;22:821–48.
20. Poulin EC, Thibault C. The anatomical basis for laparoscopic splenectomy. Can J Surg 1993;36:485.
21. Gagner M, Lacroix A, Bolte E, et al. Laparoscopic adrenalectomy: the importance of a flank approach in the lateral decubitus position. Surg Endosc 1994;8:135.
22. De Lagausie P, Bonnard A, Benkinou M, et al. Pediatric laparoscopic splenectomy: benefits of the anterior approach. Surg Endosc 2004;18:80–2.
23. Altaf AM, Sawatz M, Ellsmere J, et al. Laparoscopic accessory splenectomy: the value of perioperative localization studies. Surg Endosc 2009 Jan 23. [Epub ahead of print]
24. Gigot JF, Jamar F, Ferrant A, et al. Inadequate detection of accessory spleens and splenosis with laparoscopic splenectomy: a shortcoming of the laparoscopic approach in hematologic diseases. Surg Endosc 1998; 12:101.
25. Nielsen JL, Ellegard J, Marqversen J, et al. Detection of splenosis and ectopic spleens with 99mTc-labeled heat damaged autologous erythrocytes in 90 splenectomized patients. Scand J Haematol 1981;27:51.
26. Hansen MB, Moller AC. Splenic cysts. Surg Laparosc Endosc Percutan Tech 2004;14: 316–22.
27. Guzetta PC, Ruley EJ, Merrick HFW, et al. Elective subtotal splenectomy: indications and results in 33 patients. Ann Surg 1990; 211:34.
28. Hoeckstra HJ, Tamminga RY, Timens W. Partial instead of complete splenectomy in children for the pathological staging of Hodgkin's disease. Ned Tijdschr Geneeskd 1993;137:2491.

29. Uranues S, Grossman D, Ludwig L, et al. Laparoscopic partial splenectomy. Surg Endosc 2007;21:57–60.
30. Mertens J, Penninckx F, DeWever I, Topal B. Long-term outcome after surgical treatment of nonparasitic splenic cysts. Surg Endosc 2007;21:206–8. [Epub ahead of print 2006 Nov 23]
31. Sheldon GF, Croom RD, Meyer AA. The spleen. In: Sabiston DC, editor. Textbook of surgery. 14th ed. Philadelphia: WB Saunders; 1991. p. 1108.
32. Jalovec LM, Boe BS, Wyffels PL. The advantages of early operation with splenorrhaphy versus nonoperative management for the blunt splenic trauma patient. Am Surg 1993; 59:698.
33. Mozes MF, Spigos DG, Pollak R, et al. Partial splenic embolization, an alternative to splenectomy: results of a prospective randomized study. Surgery 1984;96:694.
34. Raikhlin A, Baerlocher MO, Asch MR, et al. Imaging and transcatheter arterial embolization for traumatic splenic injuries: review of the literature. Can J Surg 2008;51:464–72.
35. Poulin EC, Mamazza J, Schlachta CM. Splenic artery embolization before laparoscopic splenectomy: an update. Surg Endosc 1998;12:870.
36. Hoeffer RA, Scullin DC, Silver LF, et al. Splenectomy for hematologic disorders: a 20 year experience. J Ky Med Assoc 1991; 89:446.
37. Ly B, Albrechtson D. Therapeutic splenectomy in hematologic disorders. Effects and complications in 221 adult patients. Acta Med Scand 1981;209:21.
38. Macrae HM, Yakimets WW, Reynolds T. Perioperative complications of splenectomy for hematologic disease. Can J Surg 1992; 35:432.
39. Poulin EC, Thibault C. Laparoscopic splenectomy for massive splenomegaly: operative technique and case report. Can J Surg 1995; 38:69.
40. Targarona EM, Balague C, Cerdan G, et al. Hand-assisted laparoscopic splenectomy (HALS) in cases of splenomegaly: a comparison analysis with conventional laparoscopic splenectomy. Surg Endosc 2002;16:426.
41. Ikeda M, Sekimoto M, Takiguchi S, et al. High incidence of thrombosis of the portal veinous system after laparoscopic splenectomy: a prospective study with contrast-enhanced CT scan. Ann Surg 2005;24: 208–16.
42. Targarona E. Portal vein thrombosis after laparoscopic splenectomy: the size of the risk. Surg Innov 2008;15:266–70.
43. Davidson RN, Wall RA. Prevention and management of infections in patients without a spleen. Clin Microbiol Infect 2001;7: 657–60.
44. Park AE, Godivez CT. Spleen. In: Brunicardi FC, Andersen DK, Billiar TR, et al, editors. Schwartz's principles of surgery. 9th ed. New York: McGraw Hill Medical; 2010. p. 1245–65.
45. Holdsworth RJ, Irving AD, Cushieri A. Postsplenectomy sepsis and its mortality rate: actual versus perceived risks. Br J Surg 1991; 78:1031–8.
46. Bisharat N, Omari H, Lavi I, Raz R. Risk of infection and death among post-splenectomy patients. J Infect 2001;43:182–6.
47. Hansen K, Singer DB. Asplenic-hyposplenic overwhelming sepsis: postsplenectomy sepsis revisited. Pediatr Dev Pathol 2001;4: 105–21.
48. Poulin EC, Mamazza J. Laparoscopic splenectomy: lessons from the learning curve. Can J Surg 1998;41:28.
49. Targarona EM, Espert JJ, Bombuy E, et al. Complications of laparoscopic splenectomy. Arch Surg 2000;135:1137.
50. Park AE, Birgisson G, Mastrangelo MJ, et al. Laparoscopic splenectomy: outcomes and lessons learned from over 200 cases. Surgery 2000;128:660.
51. Katkhouda N, Hurwitz MB, Rivera RT, et al. Laparoscopic splenectomy: outcome and efficacy in 103 consecutive patients. Ann Surg 1998;228:568.
52. Trias M, Targarona EM, Espert JJ, et al. Impact of hematological diagnosis on early and late outcome after laparoscopic splenectomy: an analysis of 111 cases. Surg Endosc 2000;14:556.
53. Schlachta CM, Poulin EC, Mamazza J. Laparoscopic splenectomy for hematologic malignancies. Surg Endosc 1999;13:865.

Acknowledgment

Figures 1, 3, 4, 6a, 13, and 17 through 20 Tom Moore

25 REPAIR OF VENTRAL ABDOMINAL WALL HERNIAS

*Karem Harth, MD, MHS, and Michael J. Rosen, MD, FACS**

The repair of noninguinal abdominal wall defects is one of the most common procedures performed by general surgeons. With greater than 200,000 annual operations, there is little agreement or consensus in the literature as to the ideal approach for this difficult problem. In the past, personal recollections and single-center series were the principal data sources that surgeons relied on in choosing the optimum treatment strategy for a patient. In recent years, fortunately, population-based studies have provided better data on the true failure rates associated with the various herniorrhaphies.

In this chapter, we describe different operations for noninguinal abdominal wall hernias. In the repair of abdominal wall defects, the surgeon must consider a multitude of factors to identify the appropriate surgical technique to accomplish the reconstructive goals. Given that a full spectrum of patients develop hernias, it is unlikely that any single technique will be appropriate for all hernias. An individualized approach is needed to find the appropriate procedure. To do this, all surgeons must familiarize themselves with important factors such as patient age, comorbidities, physiologic status, defect size, available local tissue and presence of contamination. Likewise, an understanding of the available reconstructive techniques and an honest assessment of the surgeon's ability to perform each of these techniques should guide the surgeon in establishing the most appropriate repair for the patient. A well-known surgical dictum states that when numerous different operations exist to treat the same disease, the perfect procedure does not exist. This dictum does not hold true for abdominal wall herniorrhaphy, however. Because the disease is so heterogeneous, different techniques are needed to address individual patients' needs.

Epidemiology

In the United States, approximately 1,000,000 abdominal wall herniorrhaphies are performed each year, of which 750,000 are for inguinal hernias, 166,000 for umbilical hernias, 97,000 for incisional hernias, 25,000 for femoral hernias, and 76,000 for miscellaneous hernias.[1] The prevalence of abdominal wall hernias is difficult to determine as the wide range of published figures in the literature illustrates. The major reasons for this difficulty are (1) the lack of standardization in how ventral hernias are defined; (2) the inconsistency of the data sources used (which include self-reporting by patients, audits of routine physical examinations, and insurance company databases, among others); (3) the subjectivity of physical examination, even when performed by trained surgeons; and (4) the lack of long-term follow-up on all patients with prior surgery at risk for developing incisional hernias.

The incidence of the most common type of ventral hernia, incisional hernia, depends on how the condition is defined. The best definition of incisional hernia is any abdominal wall gap, with or without a bulge that is perceptible on clinical examination or diagnostic imaging within 1 year after the index operation. A definition that requires the presence of a visible bulge will lead to underestimation of the true incidence of the condition. The reported incidence of incisional hernia after a midline laparotomy ranges from 3 and 20% and doubles if the index operation was associated with infection. Incisional hernias are most common after midline and transverse incisions but are also well documented after paramedian, subcostal, McBurney (gridiron), and Pfannenstiel incisions.[2] An analysis of 11 publications dealing with ventral hernia incidence after various types of incisions concluded that the risk was 10.5% for midline incisions, 7.5% for transverse incisions, and 2.5% for paramedian incisions.[3] A randomized controlled trial comparing midline versus transverse incisions did not find a difference in analgesia use, pulmonary complications, or hernia recurrence after 1 year but did find increased wound infections in the transverse incision group.[4] Muscle-splitting incisions probably have a lower incidence of incisional hernias, but such incisions restrict access to the abdominal cavity. Given similar recurrence rates between midline and transverse incisions, the operative visualization required should dictate the choice of incision. Most incisional hernias are detected within 1 year of surgery; the most common cause is believed to be separation of aponeurotic edges in the early postoperative period. The male-to-female incidence ratio is 1:1, even though early evisceration is more common in males.

At present, little information is available on the risk of major complications arising from untreated noninguinal abdominal wall hernias. The main reason for this scarcity of data is that surgeons are taught, first, that all hernias, even asymptomatic ones, should be repaired at diagnosis to prevent potential strangulation or bowel obstruction and, second, that herniorrhaphy becomes more difficult the longer the repair is delayed. As a result, it is difficult to find a whole population in which at least some of the members do not routinely have their hernias repaired regardless of symptoms. In these circumstances, accurate estimates of the natural history of the disease are impossible.

* The authors and editors gratefully acknowledge the contributions of the previous authors, Robert J. Fitzgibbons Jr, MD, FACS, Alan T. Richards, MD, FACS, and Thomas H. Quinn, PhD. to the development and writing of this chapter.

Table 1 Zollinger Classification System for Ventral Abdominal Wall Hernias

Type	Examples
Congenital	Omphalocele Gastroschisis Umbilical (infant)

Acquired	Midline
	  Diastasis recti
	  Epigastric
	  Umbilical (adult, acquired, paraumbilical)
	Median
	  Supravesical (anterior, posterior, lateral)
	Paramedian
	  Spigelian
	  Interparietal

Incisional	Midline Paramedian Transverse Special operative sites

Traumatic	Penetrating, autopenetrating*
	Blunt
	  Focal, minimal injury
	  Moderate injury
	  Extensive force or shear
	Destructive

*Penetration from host tissue such as bone.

Classification of Ventral Hernias

A classification system for abdominal wall hernias outside the groin has been proposed by Zollinger [*see Table 1*].[5] Ventral incisional hernias are common enough to warrant their own discrete classification system. The scheme most often used for categorizing incisional hernias [*see Table 2*] was the result of a 1998 consensus conference held in conjunction with the European Hernia Society's annual congress.[6] This system is important in that it affords investigators a reliable means of comparing results between one procedure and another or between one center and another.

Table 2 Classification System for Incisional Hernias

Parameter	Categories

Location	Vertical
	  Midline, above or below umbilicus
	  Midline, including umbilicus
	  Paramedian
	Transverse
	  Above or below umbilicus
	  Crosses midline
	Oblique
	  Above or below umbilicus
	  Combined

Size*	< 5 cm 5–10 cm > 10 cm
Recurrence	Primary Multiply recurrent Stratification for type of previous repair

Reducibility	Yes
	  Obstruction
	  No obstruction
	No
	  Obstruction
	  No obstruction

Symptoms	Asymptomatic Symptomatic

*Difficult to measure consistently.

Abdominal Wall Anatomy

The skin of the lower anterior abdominal wall is innervated by anterior and lateral cutaneous branches of the ventral rami of the seventh through 12th intercostal nerves and by the ventral rami of the first and second lumbar nerves. These nerves course between the lateral flat muscles of the abdominal wall and enter the skin through the subcutaneous tissue.

The first layers encountered beneath the skin are the Camper and Scarpa fasciae in the subcutaneous tissue. The only significance of these layers is that when sufficiently developed, they can be reapproximated to provide another layer between a repaired abdominal wall and the outside. The major blood vessels of this superficial fatty layer are the superficial inferior and superior epigastric vessels, the intercostal vessels, and the superficial circumflex iliac vessels (which are branches of the femoral vessels). These vessels run superficial to the Scarpa fascia.

The external oblique muscle is the most superficial of the great flat muscles of the abdominal wall [*see Figure 1*]. This muscle arises from the posterior aspects of the lower eight ribs and interdigitates with both the serratus anterior and the latissimus dorsi at its origin. The posterior portion of the external oblique muscle is oriented vertically and inserts on the crest of the ilium. The anterior portion of the muscle courses inferiorly and obliquely toward the midline and the pubis. The muscle fibers give way to form its aponeurosis, which occurs well above the inguinal region. The obliquely arranged anterior inferior fibers of the aponeurosis of the external oblique muscle fold back on themselves to form the inguinal ligament, which attaches laterally to the anterior superior iliac spine. In most persons, the medial insertion of the inguinal ligament is dual: one portion of the ligament inserts on the pubic tubercle and the pubic bone, whereas the other portion is fan shaped and spans the distance between the inguinal ligament proper and the pectineal line of the pubis. This fan-shaped portion of the inguinal ligament is called the lacunar ligament. It blends laterally with the Cooper ligament (or, to be anatomically correct, the pectineal ligament). The more medial fibers of the aponeurosis of the external oblique muscle divide into a medial crus and a lateral crus to form the external or superficial inguinal ring, through which the spermatic cord (in females, the round ligament) and branches of the ilioinguinal and genitofemoral nerves pass. The rest of the medial fibers insert into the linea alba after contributing to the anterior portion of the rectus sheath.

Beneath the external oblique muscle is the internal oblique muscle. The fibers of the internal oblique muscle fan out following the shape of the iliac cres so that the superior fibers course obliquely upward toward the distal ends of the lower three or four ribs, whereas the lower fibers orient themselves inferomedially toward the pubis to run parallel to the external oblique aponeurotic fibers. These fibers arch over the round ligament or the spermatic cord, forming the superficial part of the internal (deep) inguinal ring.

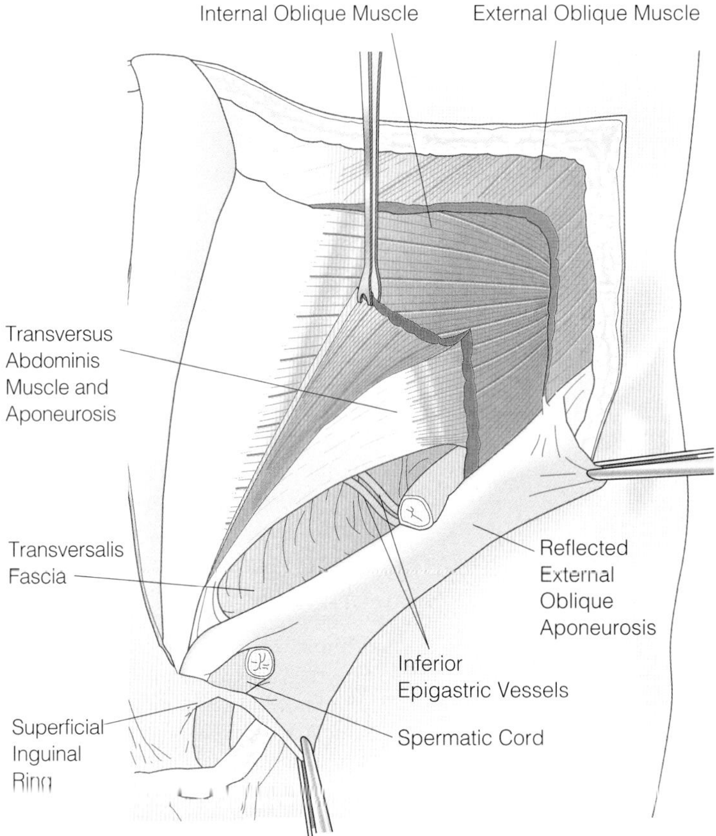

Figure 1 **Shown are the great flat muscles of the abdominal wall, depicting the relationship of the great muscles to the groin.**

Beneath the internal oblique muscle is the transversus abdominis. This muscle arises from the inguinal ligament, the inner side of the iliac crest, the endoabdominal fascia, and the lower six costal cartilages and ribs, where it interdigitates with the lateral diaphragmatic fibers. The medial aponeurotic fibers of the transversus abdominis contribute to the rectus sheath and insert on the pecten ossis pubis and the crest of the pubis, forming the falx inguinalis. Infrequently, these fibers are joined by a portion of the internal oblique aponeurosis; only when this occurs is a true conjoined tendon formed.[7]

Aponeurotic fibers of the transversus abdominis also form the structure known as the aponeurotic arch. It is theorized that contraction of the transversus abdominis causes the arch to move downward toward the inguinal ligament, thereby constituting a form of shutter mechanism that reinforces the weakest area of the groin when intra-abdominal pressure is raised. The area beneath the arch varies. Many authorities believe that a high arch, resulting in a larger area from which the transversus abdominis is, by definition, absent, is a predisposing factor for a direct inguinal hernia. The transverse aponeurotic arch is also important because the term is used by many authors to describe the medial structure that is sewn to the inguinal ligament in many of the older inguinal hernia repairs.

The rectus abdominis forms the central anchoring muscle mass of the anterior abdomen. It arises from the fifth through seventh costal cartilages and inserts on the pubic symphysis and the pubic crest. It is innervated by the seventh through 12th intercostal nerves, which laterally pierce the aponeurotic sheath of the muscle. The semilunar line is the slight depression in the aponeurotic fibers coursing toward the muscle. In a minority of persons, the small pyramidalis muscle accompanies the rectus abdominis at its insertion. This muscle arises from the pubic symphysis. It lies within the rectus sheath and tapers to attach to the linea alba, which represents the conjunction of the two rectus sheaths and is the major site of insertion for three aponeuroses from all three lateral muscle layers. The line of Douglas (i.e., the arcuate line of the rectus sheath) is formed at a variable distance between the umbilicus and the inguinal space because the fasciae of the large flat muscles of the abdominal wall contribute their aponeuroses to the anterior surface of the muscle, leaving only transversalis fascia to cover the posterior surface of the rectus abdominis.

The innervation of the anterior wall muscles is multifaceted. The seventh through 12th intercostal nerves and the first and second lumbar nerves provide most of the innervation of the lateral muscles, as well as of the rectus abdominis and the overlying skin. The nerves pass anteriorly in a plane between the internal oblique muscle and the transversus abdominis, eventually piercing the lateral aspect of the rectus sheath to innervate the muscle therein. The external oblique muscle receives branches of the intercostal nerves, which penetrate the internal oblique muscle to reach it. The anterior ends of the nerves form part of the cutaneous innervation of the abdominal wall. The first lumbar nerve divides into the ilioinguinal nerve and the iliohypogastric nerve [*see Figure 2*]. These important nerves lie in the space between the internal oblique muscle and the external oblique aponeurosis. They may divide within the psoas major or between the internal oblique muscle and the transversus abdominis. The ilioinguinal nerve may communicate with the iliohypogastric nerve before innervating the internal oblique muscle. The ilioinguinal nerve then passes through the external inguinal ring to run parallel to the spermatic cord, whereas the iliohypogastric nerve pierces the external oblique muscle to innervate the skin above the pubis. The cremaster muscle fibers, which are derived from the internal oblique muscle, are innervated by the genitofemoral nerve. There can be considerable variability and overlap.

The blood supply of the lateral muscles of the anterior wall comes primarily from the lower three or four intercostal arteries, the deep circumflex iliac artery, and the lumbar arteries. The rectus abdominis has a complicated blood supply that derives from the superior epigastric artery (a terminal branch of the internal thoracic [internal mammary] artery), the inferior epigastric artery (a branch of the external iliac artery), and the lower intercostal arteries. The lower intercostal arteries enter the sides of the muscle after traveling between the oblique muscles; the superior and the inferior epigastric arteries enter the rectus sheath and anastomose near the umbilicus. During the creation of skin flaps for component separation, preservation of this region has been described as a way to decrease complications such as skin flap necrosis.[8]

The endoabdominal fascia is the deep fascia covering the internal surface of the transversus abdominis, the iliacus, the psoas major and minor, the obturator internus, and portions of the periosteum. It is a continuous sheet that extends throughout the extraperitoneal space and is sometimes referred to as the wallpaper of the abdominal cavity. Commonly, the endoabdominal fascia is subclassified according to the muscle being covered (e.g., iliac fascia or obturator fascia).

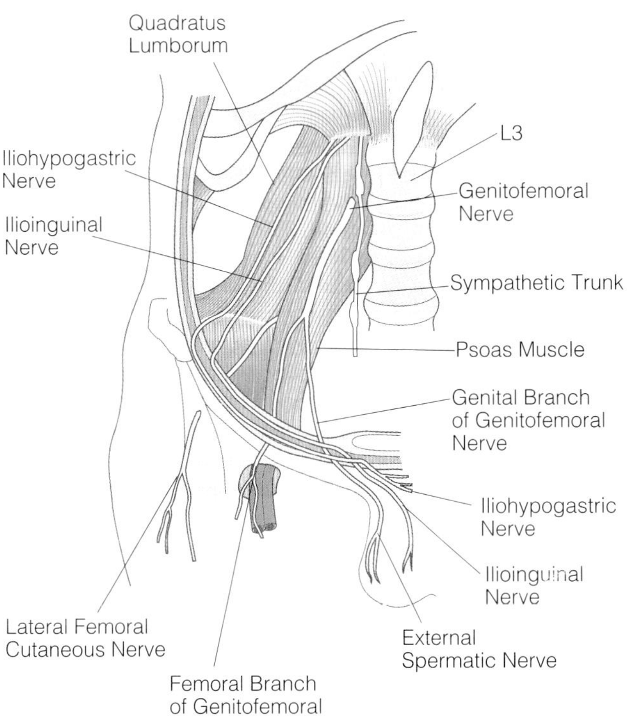

Figure 2 **Shown are the important nerves of the lower abdominal wall.**

Between the transversalis fascia and the peritoneum is the preperitoneal space. In the midline behind the pubis, this space is known as the space of Retzius; laterally, it is referred to as the space of Bogros. The preperitoneal space is of particular importance for surgeons because several hernia repairs (see below) are performed in this area. The inferior epigastric vessels, the deep inferior epigastric vein, the iliopubic vein, the rectusial vein, the retropubic vein, the communicating rectusioepigastric vein, the internal spermatic vessels, and the vas deferens are all encountered in this space.[9]

Choice of Prosthetic Material

For most abdominal wall hernias, the procedure of choice includes the use of a prosthesis. A multitude of prosthetic grafts are currently available, all with their own unique advantages and disadvantages. Most prosthetic grafts can be categorized as derived from polypropylene, polyester, or polytetrafluoroethylene (PTFE). Uscher is credited with developing polypropylene mesh and introduced it in the early 1960s.[10] Since their introduction, there has been an increase in use. An American population-based study of approximately 11,000 patients reflected an increase in mesh use for hernia repair from 35% in 1987 to 65% by 1999.[11] A detailed discussion comparing various prosthetic materials is beyond the scope of this chapter; however, some general statements may be made.

The use of mesh presupposes a situation in which the prosthesis can be isolated from contact with intra-abdominal viscera by one or more layers of human tissue (e.g., peritoneum). In situations where contact with intra-abdominal viscera cannot be avoided, a standard mesh prosthesis should not be used as it causes a significant fibroblastic response and risks subsequent bowel-related complications. Either the prosthesis should be composed of a nonmesh material, such as expanded polytetrafluoroethylene (ePTFE), or a dual-layer prosthesis should be used, with a standard plastic mesh on the side facing the abdominal wall (to encourage an intense fibroplastic response) and an adhesion barrier of some type coating the peritoneal side. Numerous dual-sided prosthetics, incorporating a variety of adhesion barriers, are now available [*see Table 3*]. It has consistently been shown that when these materials are used, adhesions are not only less common but also less tenacious than when mesh alone is used in an intraperitoneal position. Often bowel adhesions can be easily wiped from the peritoneal surface of a dual-layer prosthesis with gentle blunt traction, in sharp contrast to the typically tedious and sometimes impossible dissection of bowel loops from an unprotected mesh prosthesis placed directly on the viscera. Although all of the dual-layer prostheses currently on the market are approved for decreasing adhesions to the adhesion barrier side, no manufacturer has sought approval for complete prevention of adhesions. Consequently, the polydioxanone suture, with stitches placed 1 cm from the fascial edge and 1 cm apart, does as well in terms of hernia recurrence as a continuous monofilament polypropylene suture. The long-term advantages of polydioxanone are its decreased sinus formation and chronic pain.

Other factors should be considered in the closure of midline wounds. To prevent excessive tension, the length of the suture should be four times the length of the wound.[24] Monofilament sutures perform better than braided sutures because bacteria tend to form colonies among the braids of multifilament sutures.[28–31] Nonabsorbable suture material has the advantage of greater longevity than absorbable suture material but is more likely to result in sinus formation and chronic wound pain.[3,24] The incidence of wound infection is not affected by the suture material or the closure method.

Various patient-related risk factors for incisional hernia have been identified [*see Table 6*].[32,33] Although some controversy remains, the current consensus is that there appears to be an association between these comorbid conditions and the incidence of incisional hernia. The type of wound incurred also plays a role. Incisional herniation appears most common after midline laparotomies, especially upper midline incisions, and less common after transverse or oblique incisions.[2] An analysis of 11 publications addressing ventral hernia incidence after various types of incisions found the risk to be 10.5% for midline incisions, 7.5% for transverse incisions, and 2.5% for paramedian incisions.[3] A recent randomized controlled trial evaluating midline versus transverse incisions with a secondary end point of hernia recurrence found no difference between either approach at the 1-year follow-up.[4] However, the authors noted that to truly detect a difference in hernia recurrence between these approaches, nearly 2,500 patients would be required in each group. Thus, the authors recommend that surgeons select the incision that ultimately yields the best exposure.

Over longer periods, the incidence of incisional hernia recurrence increases, with the majority developing in the first 4 years after the sentinel operation.[34] It is anticipated that as the use of minimally invasive surgical techniques increases, the incidence of incisional hernia will drop. Hernias developing within 10 and 12 mm port sites are well documented; hernias in 5 mm port incisions are rare. At present, long-term data on the incidence and natural history of port-site hernias are lacking.[35]

Table 6 Comorbid Factors Associated with Incisional Hernia
Male sex
Old age
Morbid obesity
Abdominal distention
Cigarette smoking
Pulmonary disease
Mechanical ventilation
Type 2 diabetes mellitus
Oral anticoagulants
Malnourishment
Hypoalbuminemia
Anemia/transfusion
Malignancy
Jaundice
Corticosteroid therapy
Chemotherapy
Radiation therapy
Renal failure

Genetic factors are important as well: familial predisposition to incisional hernia has long been recognized as contributory by surgeons caring for patients with this condition. An increased incidence of incisional herniation in patients with certain connective tissue diseases (e.g., osteogenesis imperfecta, Marfan syndrome, and Ehlers-Danlos syndrome) has been documented. Finally, the molecular details of incisional hernia causation are now beginning to be appreciated. Type 1 to type 3 collagen imbalance, abnormal matrix metalloproteinase (MMP) expression, and growth factor relations are among the molecular-level processes that are currently under intense scrutiny by the scientific community with regard to the etiology of incisional hernia.

Not every patient who presents to a surgeon with an incisional hernia is necessarily a candidate for surgical repair. There are three indications for operation: (1) a hernia that is symptomatic, causing pain, discomfort, or changes in bowel habits; (2) a hernia resulting in an unsightly bulge that affects the patient's quality of life; and (3) a hernia that poses a significant risk of bowel obstruction (e.g., a large hernia with a narrow neck). However, the natural history of slow continued growth of incisional hernias attributable to increased intra-abdominal pressure should be taken into consideration. In young patients with moderate-size hernias, a nonoperative approach can result in a more complex reconstruction in the future if the hernia becomes larger and more symptomatic.

The repair of incisional hernias is often more complicated than inguinal repair for several reasons. By definition, all incisional hernias are reoperative cases, demanding careful adhesiolysis and delineation of the anatomy. Additionally, it is important that the patient and the surgeon have a clear understanding of the goals of the procedure. For all ventral hernias, the surgeon must reduce the hernia contents into the abdominal cavity and prevent future migration and recurrent herniation. This can be performed by simply patching a defect with prosthetic material or can similarly be accomplished by reconstructing a functional dynamic abdominal wall via medialization of the rectus muscles with potential prosthetic reinforcement. Each of these approaches has its own unique merits, and careful consideration should be given to each technique to find the ideal reconstruction for the patient.

Open Ventral Hernia Repair: Operative Technique

NONPROSTHETIC REPAIRS

Historically, primary suture repair was the procedure of choice for most incisional hernias; prosthetic material was reserved for particularly difficult cases as a result of the perceived risks of this material. In the latter part of the 20th century, large population-based studies changed this way of thinking, revealing that primary suture repair was associated with a much higher recurrence rate than most surgeons would have assumed (25 to 55%).[6] Studies comparing primary suture with prosthetic repair showed that the recurrence rate was dramatically lower with the latter.[36] In a randomized controlled study from the Netherlands, even small incisional hernias (< 10 cm^2) had a recurrence rate of 67% when primary suture repair was employed.[37] Additionally, a recent Cochrane review of available randomized trials with a minimum of 1-year follow-up showed that suture repair had a recurrence risk of 85% greater compared with mesh repair.[38]

PROSTHETIC REPAIRS

The use of prosthetic material to reduce tension in ventral hernia repair was first described in the 1950s.[10] Since its introduction, inclusion of mesh in ventral hernia repair has unquestionably reduced the recurrence rate. With the addition of synthetic prosthetics to the surgeon's armamentarium, the debate for the ideal surgical approach for placing mesh continues unanswered. Although each approach has its ardent supporters, there are few data carefully evaluating each approach in appropriately designed comparative trials. Given the lack of definitive data, it is difficult to provide a clear, concise recommendation as to the ideal approach. However, certain general guidelines can be stated. Basically, three options exist for mesh placement: as an overlay (onlay), as a bridge secured to the fascial edges (inlay), or as an underlay (sublay) in either a retrorectus, preperitoneal, or intraperitoneal position [*see Figure 3*].

A mesh overlay (onlay) may be placed on top of any of a variety of simple repairs. Although some series have reported that this approach yields acceptable results in selected patients, most surgeons feel that it offers little advantage over the simple repair that the prosthesis overlies and that it is typically associated with a similarly disappointing recurrence rate of up to 25%.[6,39] Additional disadvantages of placing prosthetic material in this position are its close proximity to the skin with higher potential for exposure following a wound infection and the wide skin undermining needed to achieve broad coverage.[40] Wound complications are estimated to be between 4 and 26% using this approach secondary to the creation of skin flaps necessary to secure the mesh.[6] Proponents of this technique claim an advantage of the mesh not being placed in direct contact with the abdominal viscera. However, if the midline fascial closure breaks down, the bowel will interact with an often unprotected macroporous mesh.

Prosthetic inlay (bridging) repair became popular in the 1990s, in keeping with the tension-free ideal for inguinal herniorrhaphy. The principle underlying this technique is that for a prosthetic repair to be truly tension free, the defect should be bridged. Unfortunately, the abdominal wall likely experiences different forces during activity than the groin. In fact, a true tension-free repair might not be ideal in the anterior abdominal wall. Given that contraction of the rectus and lateral abdominal wall muscles that are not joined at the linea alba results in lateral displacement, a constant force of separation is placed on the prosthetic. Coupled with the incidence of some shrinkage of most prosthetics, this has resulted in a predictably high recurrence rate at the mesh–native tissue interface.[41,42] Following a systematic review of 119 studies on ventral hernia repair, the inlay technique was found to have the highest reported rate of recurrence, largely attributed to poor mesh fixation and inadequate lateral overlap.[42] The recurrence rate is especially high in obese patients and greater with increasing hernia size. In a study from the Netherlands,

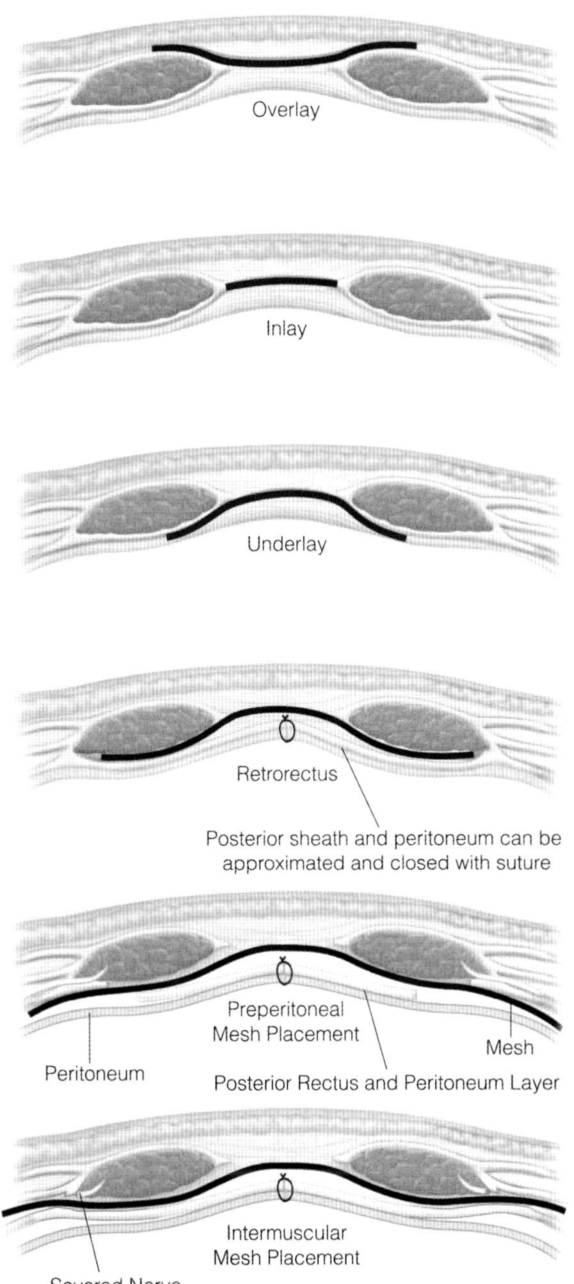

Figure 3 **Incisional hernia repair. Depicted are three potential positions for placement of a prosthesis for repair of ventral abdominal wall defects.**

the recurrence rate even with mesh repairs (mostly onlay and inlay) was 32% for large defects and 17% for small (< 10 cm^2) defects.[37]

Sublay prosthetic repair is sometimes referred to as the retromuscular approach. A sublay prosthetic repair is characterized by the placement of a large prosthesis in the space between the abdominal muscles and the posterior fascia, the transversalis fascia, or the peritoneum, depending on what part of the abdomen is being repaired (there is no posterior fascia inferior to the arcuate line).[43] The technique described

Component Separation Repair

The concept of separating the lateral abdominal wall musculature, allowing medialization of the rectus muscle complex, was first described by Ramirez and colleagues in 1990.[51] Based on cadaveric studies, up to 10 cm of unilateral advancement of the abdominal wall can be achieved with release of the external oblique aponeurosis. A distinct advantage of this approach is the ability to achieve midline closure and recreation of the linea alba. Unlike mesh repair in a bridging fashion, a dynamic abdominal wall can be achieved. A hindrance to broader acceptance of this technique is that the large lipocutaneous flaps created to access the lateral abdominal wall are associated with major wound morbidity.

Historically, component separation has been reserved for complicated hernias when synthetic mesh is contraindicated.[52–54] A recent trial on large midline abdominal wall hernias randomized 39 patients to either component separation or prosthetic repair using antibiotic-impregnated ePTFE.[55] Hernia recurrence was not different between the component separation technique and prosthetic repair (56% versus 58%, respectively; p value > .05) following a 36-month follow-up period.[55] Wound-related complications, including infection and skin necrosis, were also not different between the component separation technique and prosthetic repair (53% versus 72% respectively; p value > .05). However, 54% of infections in the ePTFE group required reoperation for removal of infected mesh. On interim analysis, this latter event caused early cessation of the study. Given the morbidity associated with reoperation in the prosthetic repair group compared with the asymptomatic small hernia recurrences observed in the component separation technique group, the authors concluded that the component separation technique was a favorable repair option for giant midline hernias. Typically, after a component separation, there is still tension on the midline closure. For this reason, most authors advocate reinforcement with a prosthetic. Whether the addition of a prosthetic material (either biologic or synthetic) to reinforce the repair after component separation might reduce recurrence rates further has not been adequately evaluated in the literature.

Patients undergoing abdominal wall reconstruction for massive defects each require individualized preparation and consideration prior to surgery. Physiologic changes occur in both the abdominal and the thoracic cavities following definitive closure of these large defects. In addition to the general preoperative screening, each patient should be assessed for pulmonary status and the potential for return to routine daily activities. Additionally, smoking status is critical as patients who smoke are at significantly higher risk for wound complications. Since its original description in 1990, component separation has undergone several adaptations. We describe the traditional open approach and two newer techniques to achieving a more minimally invasive separation of components.

OPEN COMPONENT SEPARATION

Step 1: Incision

A long midline incision or transverse panniculectomy-type incision is made through the scar to expose the hernia. The hernia sac is dissected up to its neck, deep to the fascial edge.

Step 2: Creation of Flaps

The lipocutaneous flap is dissected away from the anterior sheath of the rectus abdominis and the aponeurosis of the external abdominal oblique muscle. A technique that may help decrease skin flap necrosis is to preserve the periumbilical perforators.[8] There are no exact landmarks to delineate the lateralmost extent of this flap. The surgeon must bimanually assess the rectus muscle belly. Once the lateral edge of the rectus is palpated, the dissection is carried 2 cm lateral to the linea semilunaris.

Step 3: Incising the External Oblique Muscle

The aponeurosis of the external oblique muscle is transected longitudinally about 2 cm lateral to the rectus sheath, with care to avoid cutting into the linea semilunaris [*see Figure 5*]. Transecting the linea semilunaris will result in a

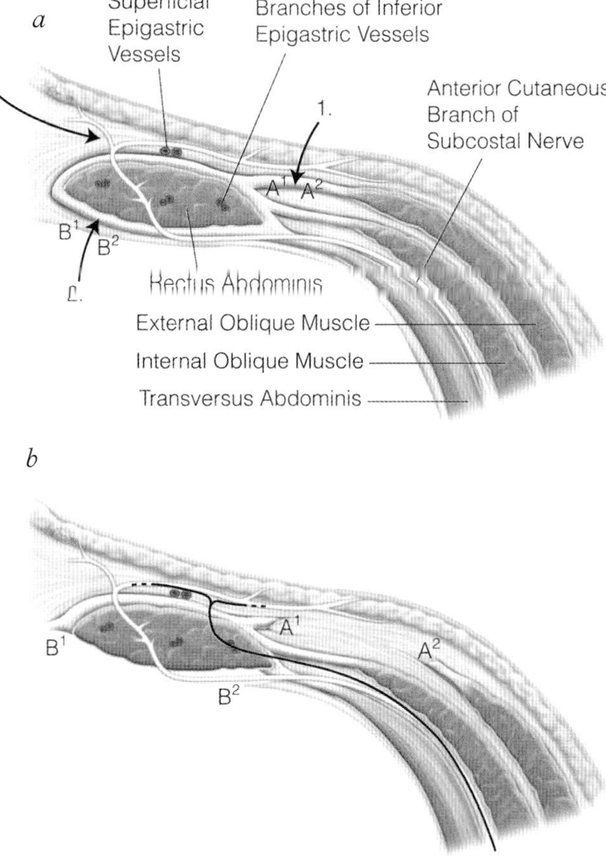

Figure 5 **Component separation repair. Depicted is the technique of component separation, as described by Ramirez and colleagues.[51] (*a*) A longitudinal incision is made in the aponeurosis of the external oblique muscle (1) approximately 2 cm lateral to the rectus sheath, overlapping the hernia defect caudally and extending 5 to 7 cm cranial to the costal margin. Additional length can be gained by incising the posterior rectal sheath (2). (*b*) The external oblique muscle is separated from the internal oblique muscle as far laterally as possible. Care must be taken not to damage the neurovascular structures that run between the internal oblique muscle and the transversus abdominis to enter the rectus sheath on its posterolateral side (*black line*). A^1, A^2 = cut edges of the external oblique aponeurosis; B^1, B^2 = cut edges of the posterior rectus sheath.**

full-thickness defect and a subsequent lateral hernia. If the surgeon inadvertently begins incising the external oblique muscle too medially, he or she runs the risk of potentially transecting the internal oblique fascia too. Transecting the internal oblique muscle will likely result in a lateral abdominal wall bulge. By making the incision lateral on the external oblique muscle, the internal oblique muscle is often muscular and can be clearly delineated from the external oblique. This incision is extended cranially onto the muscular components of the external abdominal oblique to about 5 to 7 cm above the costal margin and caudally to the inguinal ligament. The external oblique muscle is then separated from the internal oblique muscle in the avascular plane to the posterior axillary line.

Step 4: Posterior Rectus Sheath Release

If primary closure is still not possible without undue tension, 2 to 4 cm of additional length can be gained by separating the posterior rectus sheath from the rectus abdominis.

Step 5: Mesh Placement

Depending on the nature of the case (i.e., clean or contaminated), synthetic or biologic mesh, either in the retrorectus or intraperitoneal position, with a minimum 3 to 4 cm of tissue-mesh overlap can be placed. Others have described onlay positioning of the mesh after open component separation.[39,56] Technically, onlay mesh positioning is easier than underlay placement. However, the mesh is then placed in the subcutaneous position, with a fairly high potential for wound breakdown and mesh exposure. Additionally, the mesh is placed below a devascularized subcutaneous fatty tissue, potentially impeding ingrowth.

Step 6: Skin Closure

Excess skin should be liberally resected. Resecting excess skin provides two distinct advantages: the most devascularized tissue is removed and excess dead space is reduced. Finally, the subcutaneous space should be widely drained with the use of Jackson-Pratt drains.

ENDOSCOPIC COMPONENT SEPARATION

In an effort to avoid the significant tissue trauma and the large open surface areas created following the open component separation technique, endoscopic approaches have been described.[57-60] This minimizes the lipocutaneous flaps created in the open approach and can be used in conjunction with a planned laparotomy. Adaptations from its original approach have been made over time. This technique maintains the same principles as the open approach, which is to achieve medialization of the abdominal wall through lateral release of the external abdominal oblique fascia.

Step 1: Incision

In the setting of contaminated single-stage abdominal wall reconstruction, a standard laparotomy incision is commenced and the major infectious issues are addressed, including takedown of fistulas or removing an infected prosthetic. The entire anterior abdominal wall is freed of adhesions, and the defect size is assessed. Those cases that will not close primarily undergo component separation. There is no absolute indication for this as all patients have a different level of compliance to their abdominal wall. A more compliant abdominal wall will come together more easily at the midline than one that is not very compliant. Generally, good surgical judgment, coupled with realistic expectations, should guide the decision-making process.

Step 2: Initial Component Separation Incision

Once a component separation is deemed necessary, a 1 cm incision just inferior to the tip of the 11th rib is made and the external abdominal oblique is identified with blunt dissection and Kocher clamps. The avascular plane between the external abdominal oblique and the internal abdominal oblique is identified by use of retractors. Careful identification of the correct anatomic plane is imperative at this juncture to avoid placing the dissecting balloon in the wrong plane and requiring conversion to an open procedure.

Step 3: Balloon Dissector

A bilateral inguinal hernia balloon dissector is inserted in a caudal direction toward the pubic tubercle. Under direct visualization, the balloon is inflated and the orientation of the muscle fibers is confirmed.[60] A structural balloon port is placed, and insufflation pressures of 10 to 12 mm Hg are maintained. The camera tip bluntly completes the posterior lateral dissection.

Step 4: External Oblique Release

A 5 mm port is placed in the posterior axillary line. This port needs to be quite lateral to obtain the appropriate angle to incise the external oblique fascia. Much like in the open approach, the linea semilunaris should be carefully identified and avoided to prevent a lateral hernia. Anatomically, the linea semilunaris is identified at the junction of the external and internal oblique. Typically, scissors and cautery are used to release the external oblique fascia to the inguinal ligament.

Step 5: Cephalad Dissection

Another 5 mm port is placed medially through this inferior release to be used for the cephalad release of the external abdominal oblique fascia and muscle. The camera is now positioned in the lateral trocar. Given that the external oblique is typically quite muscular at its cephalad extent, some form of ultrasonic dissection is helpful in maintaining hemostasis. The external oblique is then released for at least 5 to 7 cm above the costal margin. Once this is performed bilaterally, it completes the endoscopic component separation and the surgery.

Reinforcement or bridging of a midline defect for both the open and endoscopic approaches can be performed with mesh in the retrorectus or intra-abdominal position with lateral transfascial fixation sutures. The exact technique regarding mesh placement is still under debate. Biologic mesh may be used in the setting of contamination. Synthetic mesh can be used for elective clean cases. If synthetic mesh needs to be placed in the intraperitoneal position, a synthetic mesh of choice with an antiadhesive side should face the bowel.

Three general types of parastomal hernia repairs are currently performed: (1) fascial repair, (2) stoma relocation, and (3) prosthetic repair. Fascial repair involves local exploration around the stoma site, with primary closure of the defect. This approach should be considered of historical interest only because the results are so poor. We reserve this approach for elderly patients or in emergent situations as a bridge to a future definitive repair. Stoma relocation yields much better results and is considered the procedure of choice by many surgeons. This approach is especially appropriate for patients who have other stoma problems, such as skin excoriation or suboptimal stoma construction. The use of a permanent prosthesis with a stoma relocation is not generally recommended because of the inherent danger of contamination. However, biologic mesh reinforcement has shown some promise in reducing recurrence rates. Stoma relocation is a significantly more invasive procedure and subjects patients to a triple threat of hernia recurrence: (1) at the old stoma site, (2) at the new stoma site, and (3) in the laparotomy incision used to move the stoma. Given these risks, we typically place a large sheet of biologic mesh in the retrorectus position. This mesh is keyholed around the new stoma site and is used to reinforce the old stoma site and the midline closure.

Prosthetic repair can provide a reasonable outcome, but it is necessary to accept the complications inherent in the placement of a foreign body. The stoma exit site must be isolated from the surgical field to lower the risk of prosthesis infection. The prosthesis can be placed extraperitoneally by making a hockey-stick incision around the stoma, with care taken to ensure that the incision is outside the periphery of the stoma appliance. Once the subcutaneous tissue is divided, dissection proceeds along the fascia until the sac is identified and removed. The defect is then closed with an overlying prosthesis buttress sutured in place. Alternatively, the fascial defect is bridged with the prosthesis for a tension-free repair.

The extraperitoneal approach seems logical but can be technically demanding in that it is sometimes difficult to define the entire extent of the hernia defect. Moreover, the considerable undermining involved can lead to seroma formation, eventual infection, or peristomal skin necrosis. As an alternative, an intra-abdominal prosthetic approach has been described that is theoretically attractive because it avoids the local complications of the extraperitoneal operation and incorporates the mechanical advantage gained by placing the prosthesis on the peritoneal side of the abdominal wall.[92,93] Intra-abdominal pressure then serves to fuse the prosthetic material to the abdominal wall rather than being a factor in recurrence. Either ePTFE, polypropylene, or polyester mesh with an adhesion barrier can be used for the prosthesis. One technique is to slit the prosthesis and create a keyhole in its center and then suture this directly around the peritoneal side of the stoma so that it widely overlaps the hernia defect. Sugarbaker's practice is to mobilize the bowel thoroughly and then lateralize it with the prosthesis, in effect creating a long tunnel in addition to covering the hernia defect.[93] The detractors of the intra-abdominal approach argue that the risk of complications (e.g., adhesive bowel obstruction and fistula formation) outweighs the advantages. The intra-abdominal approach is particularly well suited for adaptation to laparoscopic methods.[94–96]

SPIGELIAN HERNIA

A spigelian hernia, first described 400 years ago by the Flemish anatomist Adriaan van den Spiegel, is a hernia through a defect in the spigelian fascia.[97] The spigelian fascia is the area between the semilunar line and the lateral border of the rectus abdominis. The majority of spigelian hernias occur just below the arcuate line, where the posterior rectus sheath becomes deficient. This region, known as the spigelian belt, is a band between the iliac crest and a line drawn 6 cm above [*see Figure 6*].[98] These rare hernias are being reported with increasing frequency: there are more than 100 cases in the surgical literature.

A spigelian hernia may present as a bulge lateral to the rectus. However, because many of these hernias are interparietal, they may not be clinically apparent; often they are picked up incidentally during laparoscopy. A significant percentage of patients present with an incarcerated or even strangulated hernia. If such a hernia is interparietal, the diagnosis frequently is not made until a laparotomy is done for treatment of the acute process.

The standard treatment is operative repair.[99] A transverse incision is made over the bulge. The anterior rectus sheath is incised transversely, and the sac is dissected as far as its neck and either excised or inverted. The defect is then repaired with a continuous suture of nonabsorbable material. Alternatively, a mesh may be placed in the defect and sutured to the edges of the defect. Laparoscopic methods are increasingly being employed to repair spigelian hernias.[100]

RICHTER HERNIA

In a Richter hernia, part of the bowel wall herniates through the defect. The herniated bowel wall may become ischemic and gangrenous, but intestinal obstruction does not occur. The overlying skin may be discolored. The herniated bowel wall is exposed by opening the sac, and the neck of the sac is enlarged to allow delivery of the bowel into the wound. The gangrenous patch is excised, and the bowel wall is reconstituted. The hernia is then repaired.

SUPRAVESICAL HERNIA

Supravesical hernias develop anterior to the urinary bladder as a consequence of failure of the integrity of the transversus abdominis and the transversalis fascia, both of which insert into the Cooper ligament. The preperitoneal space is continuous with the retropubic space of Retzius, and the hernia sac protrudes into this area. The sac is directed laterally and emerges at the lateral border of the rectus abdominis in the inguinal region, the femoral region, or the obturator region. It may therefore mimic a hernia from any of these areas and sometimes is associated with a hernia from one of these regions. It is important to recognize this hernia during groin exploration for a suspected groin hernia and then to repair the defect appropriately.

A variant of this hernia, known as an internal supravesical hernia, may also arise. These hernias are classified according to whether they cross in front of, extend beside, or pass behind the bladder. Bowel symptoms predominate in patients with these defects, and urinary tract symptoms may develop in as many as 30%. Treatment is surgical and is accomplished

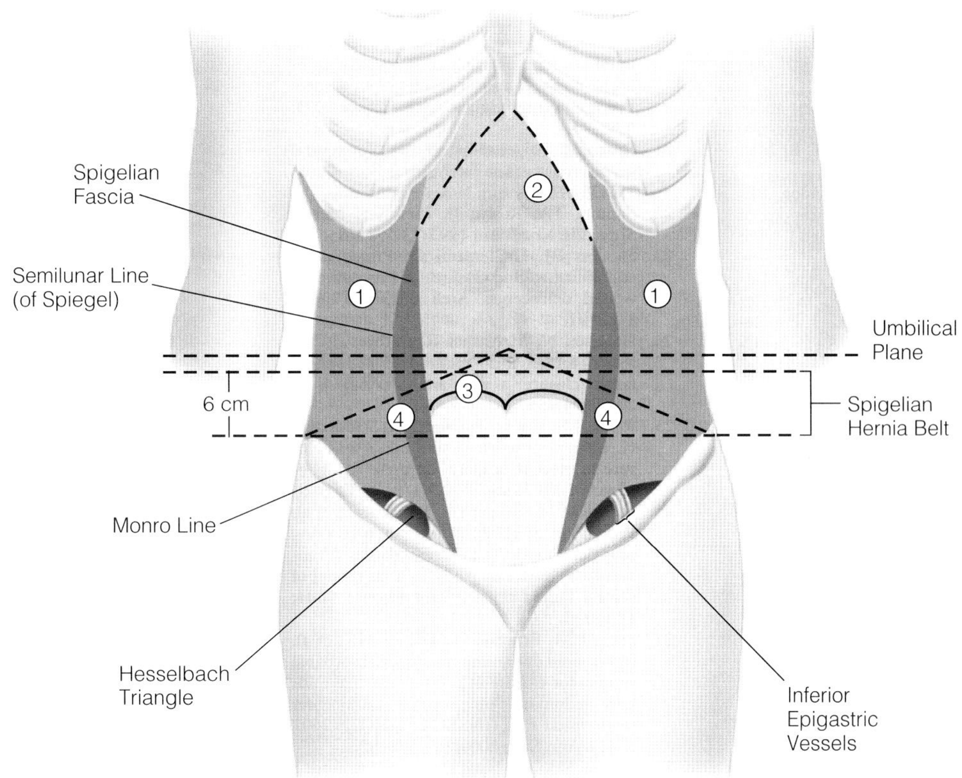

Figure 6 **Depicted is the spigelian hernia belt, with a diagrammatic representation of the relevant components of the anterior abdominal wall, including (1) the transversus abdominis, (2) the dorsal lamella of the rectus sheath (the rectus abdominis itself having been cut away), (3) the semicircular line (of Douglas), and (4) the spigelian aponeurosis.**

transperitoneally via a low midline incision. The sac can usually be reduced without difficulty, and the neck of the sac should be divided and closed.

LUMBAR HERNIA

The lumbar region is the area bounded inferiorly by the iliac crest, superiorly by the 12th rib, posteriorly by the erector spinae group of muscles, and anteriorly by the posterior border of the external oblique muscle as it extends from the 12th rib to the iliac crest. There are three varieties of lumbar hernia:

1. The superior lumbar hernia of Grynfeltt. In this variety, the defect is in a space between the latissimus dorsi, the serratus posterior inferior, and the posterior border of the internal oblique muscle.
2. The inferior lumbar hernia of Petit. Here the defect is in the space bounded by the latissimus dorsi posteriorly, the iliac crest inferiorly, and the posterior border of the external oblique muscle anteriorly.
3. Secondary lumbar hernia that develops as a result of trauma—mostly surgical (e.g., renal surgery)—or infection.[101] In the past, it was encountered relatively frequently as a consequence of spinal tuberculosis with paraspinal abscesses but is less common today. Surgical repair is discouraged because the natural history is more consistent with that of diastasis recti than that of a true hernia. Denervation appears to play a significant role in the pathogenesis. In other words, this "hernia" reflects a weakness in the abdominal wall more than it does a dangerous hernia defect. Therefore, appropriate repair is commonly followed by gradual eventration, which is perceived by the patient as a recurrence.

Lumbar hernias should be repaired if they are large or symptomatic. A prosthesis or a tissue flap of some kind is usually required for a successful repair. A rotation flap of fascia lata can be used for inferior lumbar hernias. Bony landmarks limit anterior open approaches. We typically perform a preperitoneal Stoppa-type repair. If necessary, the mesh can be fixed to the iliac bone with orthopedic bone fixation devices.[102] Laparoscopic repair of lumbar hernias is now being performed with increasing frequency and is proving successful.[103]

Dr. Rosen receives an honorarium as speaker for LifeCell, Gore, and Davol.

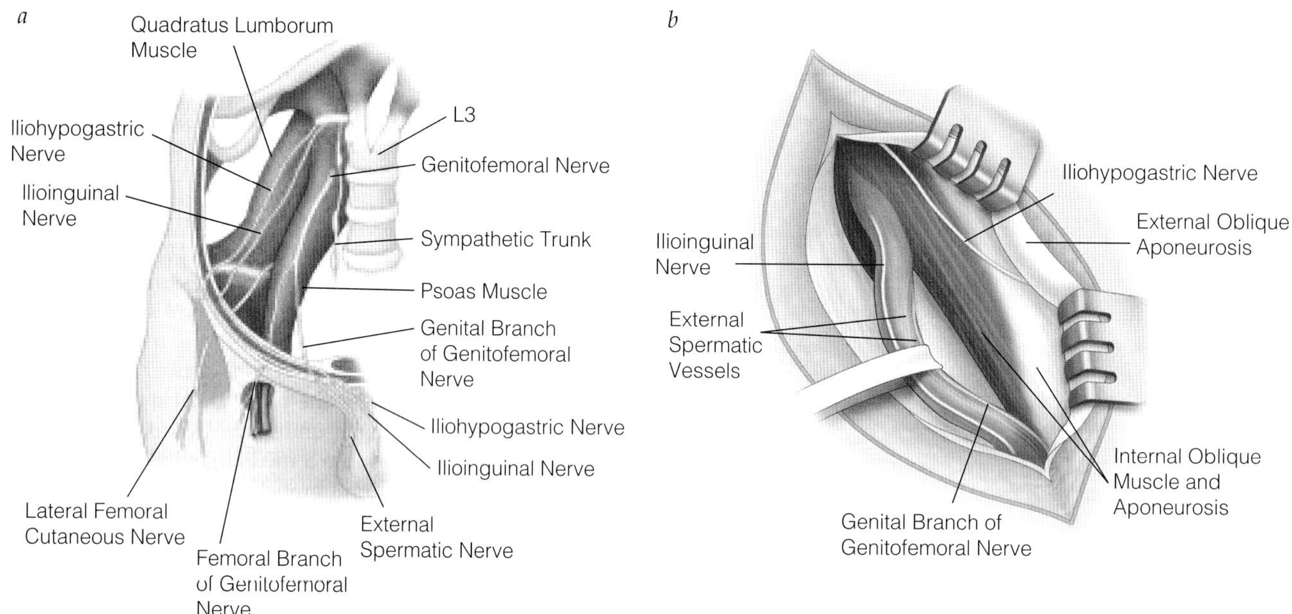

Figure 2 **Shown are the (*a*) important nerves of the lower abdominal wall and (*b*) anatomy of the nerves in the inguinal region as seen during the open anterior approach.**

Medial Umbilical Ligament

The medial umbilical ligament is an unfamiliar but sometimes prominent structure that is seen in the transabdominal preperitoneal (TAPP) approach. It courses along the anterior abdominal wall toward the umbilicus, often with an apparent mesentery. It is most prominent in the region of the medial inguinal space. This ligament is most readily identified when the umbilical laparoscope is directed toward the pelvic midline, where the ligament's bilateral structure is best seen as it is oriented toward the umbilicus. Medial retraction of this structure is usually necessary for full exposure of the medial aspect of the inguinal canal.

Spermatic Cord Structures

The testicular artery and vein descend from the retroperitoneum, travel directly over and slightly lateral to the external iliac artery, and enter the internal spermatic ring posteriorly. These vessels are covered only by the peritoneum and are usually well visualized as flat structures in the abdominal cavity that assume a cordlike appearance when joined by the vas deferens immediately before entering the internal spermatic ring. The vas deferens is best identified where it joins the spermatic vessels. From there, the vas deferens can be traced back medially as it courses over the pelvic brim and falls into the pelvis and behind the bladder.

Inferior Epigastric Vessels

The inferior epigastric artery and vein lie on the medial aspect of the internal inguinal ring and ascend the deep surface of the rectus abdominis. In the TAPP approach, these vessels may be difficult to visualize, particularly in obese patients. They are best identified by locating the internal inguinal ring at the junction of the vas deferens and the testicular artery and vein. At this location, the vessels form the medial margin of the internal ring. However, they can quickly fade from view as they travel superiorly and medially along the anterior abdominal wall. Corona mortis is a vascular communication between the obturator artery and the inferior epigastric artery found in 20% of patients [*see Figure 4*].

Cooper Ligament

The Cooper ligament is a condensation of the transversalis fascia and the periosteum of the superior pubic ramus lateral to the pubic tubercle. It can be seen only in the preperitoneal space. With the peritoneum intact, it is often easier to palpate the ligament than to see it, but once the ligament has been identified and cleaned, its glistening white fibers are apparent. Care must be taken during dissection to avoid the tiny branches of the obturator vein that often run along the ligament's surface. The iliopubic tract inserts into the superior ramus of the pubis just lateral to the Cooper ligament, blending into it.

Internal Inguinal Ring

The medial border of the internal inguinal ring is formed by the transversalis fascia and the inferior epigastric vessels. The inferior border is formed by the iliopubic tract and, anteriorly, is bordered by the transversus abdominis arch, which passes laterally over the internal ring and forms a very well-defined visible edge. The layers of the abdominal wall constituting the lateral border of the internal inguinal ring appear the same as when viewed from the exterior approach. An indirect hernia sac lies anterior and lateral to the spermatic cord at this level as opposed to the familiar medial cord position seen in the classic exterior groin approach to open herniorrhaphy.

a

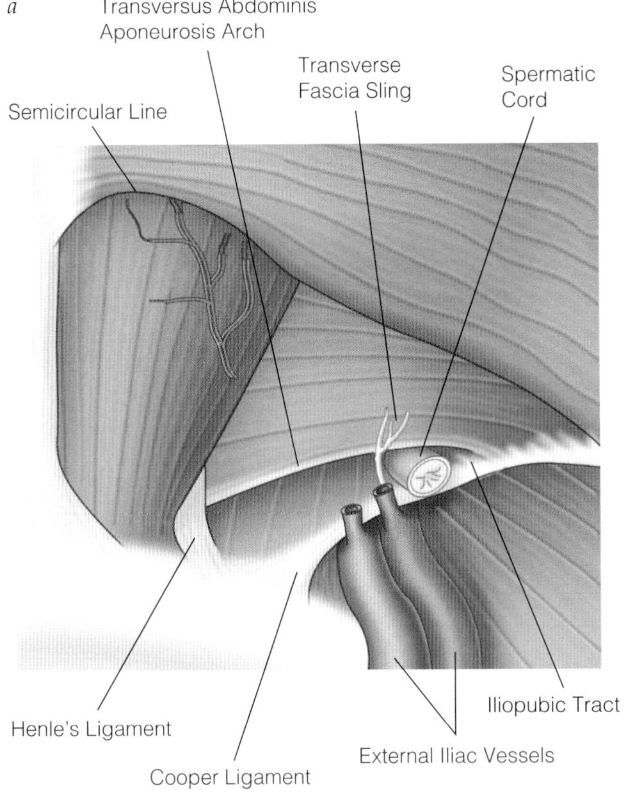

b

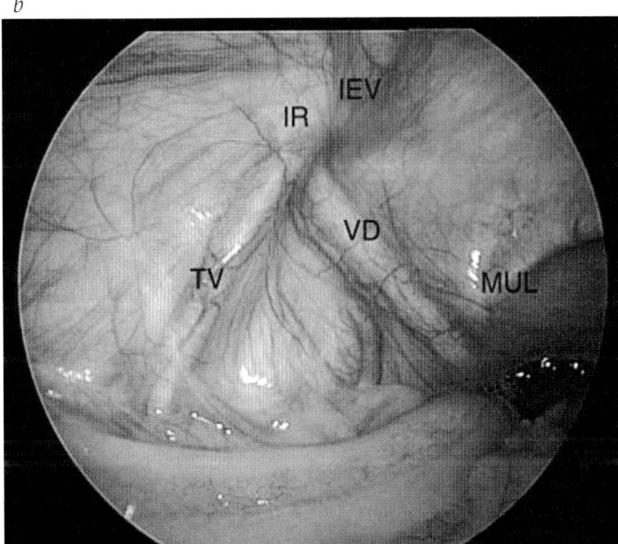

Figure 3 **(*a*) Shown is the anatomy of the right groin from the posterior, or peritoneal, approach. (*b*) Shown is a laparoscopic view of the anatomy of the left groin with the peritoneum intact in a patient without a hernia. IEV = inferior epigastric vessels; IR = internal ring; MUL = medial umbilical ligament; TV = testicular vessels; VD = vas deferens.**

Iliopubic Tract

Frequently confused with the inguinal ligament, which is part of the superficial musculoaponeurotic layer and not seen posteriorly, the iliopubic tract is part of the deep layer. All inguinal hernia defects lie above the iliopubic tract, either anterior or superior to it. Conversely, femoral hernias occur below the tract, either posterior or inferior to it. Fibers of the iliopubic tract extend into the Cooper ligament medially, where they become the medial margin of the femoral canal, also called the lacunar ligament.

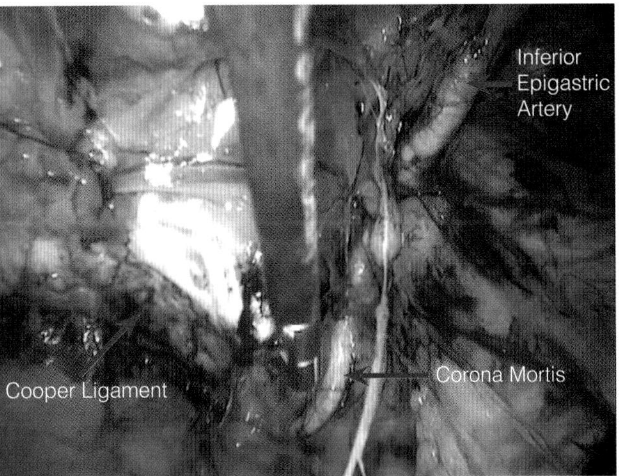

Figure 4 **Laparoscopic view of left groin. The corona mortis is demonstrated here coursing over Cooper ligament.**

Triangle of Doom

The lateral spermatic vessels and the medial vas deferens merge at the internal inguinal ring, where they form the apex of the so-called triangle of doom [*see Figure 5*]. Beneath this triangle lie the external iliac vessels. They are often poorly visualized, and extreme care must be taken not to extend dissection into this area.

Another area worthy of careful attention is the triangle of pain [*see Figure 5*], situated inferior to the iliopubic tract and bordered medially by the spermatic vessels. Using tacks within this triangle risks injury to the genital branch of the genitofemoral, iliohypogastric, and lateral cutaneous nerves of the thigh, a cause of postherniorrhaphy neuralgia.

Operative Planning

CHOICE OF ANESTHETIC

The open approach to inguinal hernia repair lends itself well to many different anesthetic techniques. Depending on the setting and on patient and physician preferences, the procedure can be undertaken under general, regional (spinal or epidural), or local anesthesia. The need for pneumoperitoneum and thus for general anesthesia in laparoscopic herniorrhaphy is sometimes considered a major disadvantage. Nausea, dizziness, and headache are more common in the recovery room after TAPP repair than after Lichtenstein repair.[10] It is not necessarily true, however, that local or regional anesthesia is safer than general anesthesia.[11] For open repair, local anesthesia or general anesthesia with short-acting agents avoids the higher risk of urinary retention associated with spinal anesthesia while maintaining the benefits of rapid recovery.[12] If general or regional anesthesia is chosen, a local anesthetic is injected in the groin incision.

For open anterior repair, local anesthesia combined with intravenous (IV) infusion of a rapid-acting, short-lasting, amnesic, and anxiolytic agent (e.g., propofol) is a popular anesthetic option that may minimize many of the systemic side effects or complications. In addition to a field block injected in the subcutaneous and deeper tissues in the area of the proposed incision, a nerve block is performed by injecting the anesthetic of choice 1 cm medial and 1 cm inferior to the anterosuperior iliac spine, as well as by injecting the areas of the pubic tubercle and the Cooper ligament.

CHOICE OF PROSTHETIC MESH

For most abdominal wall hernias, the procedure of choice includes the use of a prosthetic mesh. A detailed discussion comparing various prosthetic materials is beyond the scope of this chapter; however, some general statements may be made. North American surgeons tend to favor polypropylene, whereas Europeans are more likely to employ polyester mesh, although this distinction has begun to blur. The use of prosthetic mesh presupposes that the prosthesis can be isolated from the intra-abdominal viscera either by human tissue (e.g., peritoneum), by nonmesh material such as expanded polytetrafluoroethylene (ePTFE), or by an added adhesive coating barrier [see *Table 2*]. The standard technique in inguinal hernia repair includes the use of tension-free mesh, which has been shown to minimize recurrences.[13] On the other hand, chronic postoperative pain and dysesthesia remain problematic. Efficacy of mesh repair is based on strengthening of weakened abdominal wall tissue by a strong mesh aponeurosis scar tissue (MAST) complex,[14] through a mesh-induced inflammatory response. The first-generation polypropylene meshes contained too much foreign tissue and led to chronic pain and stiffness in and around the site of foreign mesh placement. This led to the development of lightweight mesh as new studies suggest a correlation between the polypropylene amount, structure of meshes, and postoperative quality of life.[15] Lightweight meshes are associated with less scar tissue, less restriction of abdominal wall movement, and less postoperative pain.[16] The concern with the use of lightweight meshes has been a reported higher recurrence rate. A recent meta-analysis compared the outcome of lightweight mesh and heavyweight mesh in the repair of inguinal hernia and concluded that there was no difference in the incidence of seroma, infection, and testicular atrophy.[17] There was no statistical difference in overall postoperative recurrence between lightweight and heavyweight mesh in inguinal hernia repair according to this meta-analysis, although it was noted that in large indirect and direct hernias, use of lightweight mesh did result in a higher recurrence (six times higher incidence of recurrence with lightweight mesh). This was attributed to the insufficient friction and stiffness of the lightweight mesh, which caused the mesh to slip in larger hernias. The authors of this study pointed out that for larger hernias, reduction of recurrence with the use of lightweight mesh was possible if more fixations were employed. Finally, lightweight mesh was also associated with less chronic postoperative pain and feeling of a foreign body.[18]

Operative Techniques

There are a great deal of described techniques for inguinal hernia repair, both open and laparoscopic, and a degree of controversy remains regarding the ideal approach to and outcome for inguinal hernia repair. The evidence supports the use of mesh as it is associated with a significant reduction in the risk of recurrence between 50 and 75%.[19] With the evolution of the open anterior approach to tension-free

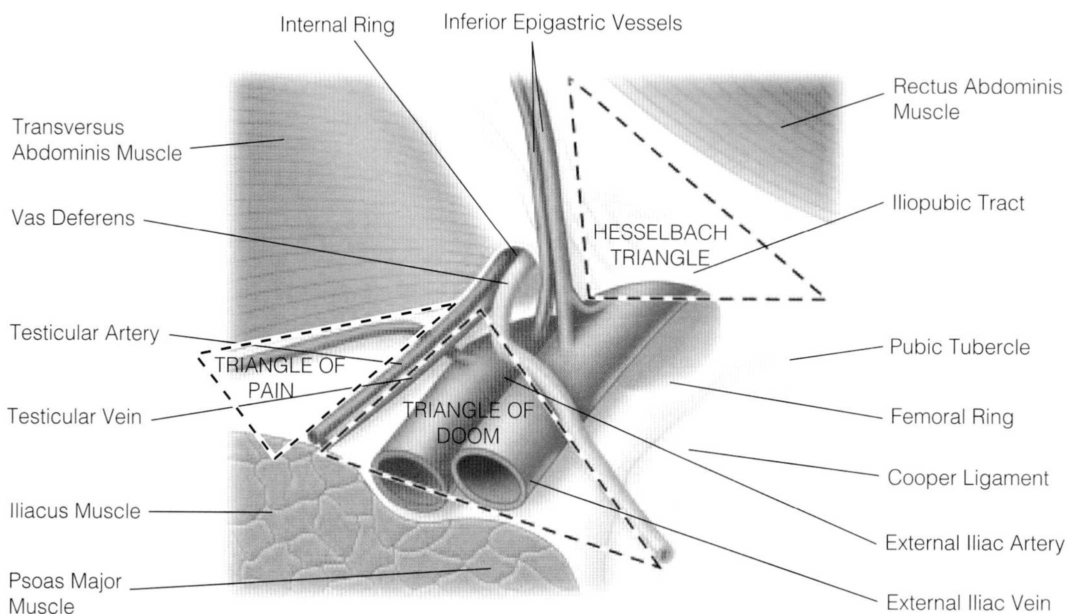

Figure 5 **Shown is the left inguinal region with the peritoneum removed, as seen during laparoscopic inguinal hernia repair. The "triangle of doom" contains the external iliac vessels. The "triangle of pain" is an area that must be paid attention to during repair as multiple sensory nerves run in this area and may cause significant postoperative neuralgia if injured.**

prosthetic mesh repair, determining which patients will benefit significantly from laparoscopic herniorrhaphy has become increasingly important. Patients are well served when a surgeon has several approaches at his or her command that can be applied to and, if necessary, modified for individual circumstances.

Practical considerations do not allow a description of every single named inguinal hernia repair in the literature. The nonprosthetic named repairs alone number more than 70.[20] Rather than address every known variant, we describe the major repairs appropriate for adults on which these variants are based.

GENERAL INDICATIONS FOR SURGICAL REPAIR

The general indications for inguinal hernia repair are the same as for open and laparoscopic approaches, with the alternative to surgical management being watchful waiting. Many surgeons consider the presence of an inguinal hernia to be reason enough to operate; however, recent studies have shown that the presence of a reducible, asymptomatic inguinal hernia in males is not an indication to operate as the incarceration rate is less than 1%.[21] Two trials were conducted to study the effects of watchful waiting for asymptomatic hernias and found that after long-term follow-up, there was no significant difference in hernia-related symptomatology.[22,23] Another long-term follow-up study determined that most patients with an asymptomatic groin hernia eventually develop symptoms and should be offered surgical repair if they are medically fit.[24]

For laparoscopic repair options, the National Institute for Health and Clinical Excellence (NICE) of the United Kingdom's National Health Service has offered a set of guidelines for the use of laparoscopic inguinal hernia repair. Their specific indications for laparoscopy over open repair are recurrent hernias, bilateral hernias, the need for earlier return to full activities, the patient's medical fitness to withstand anesthesia, the personal choice of the patient, and the surgeon's experience.[25] In choosing between open and laparoscopic surgery, the following are considered:

- The suitability of the individual for general anesthesia
- The nature of the presenting hernia
- The suitability of the particular hernia for a laparoscopic or open repair
- The experience and comfort level of the surgeon in the available technique options

Table 2 Commercially Available Synthetic Prostheses for Inguinal Hernia Repair

Polypropylene/polyester
Bard Composix E/X Mesh (PPL + ePTFE)
Sofradim Parietene (PPL + hydrophilic collagen)
Sofradim Parietex (PPL + hydrophilic collagen)
Genzyme Sepramesh (PPL + Seprafilm)
Ethicon Prolene Soft Mesh (PPL)
Ethicon Proceed (PPL + PDS + ORC)
Ethicon Ultrapro (PPL + poliglecaprone 25)
Ethicon Vicryl Knitted Mesh
Gore-Tex Soft Tissue Patch (ePTFE)
Gore-Tex DualMesh (ePTFE)
Gore-Tex DualMesh Plus (ePTFE + silver + chlorhexidine)
Gore-Tex MycroMesh (ePTFE)

ePTFE = expanded polytetrafluoroethylene; ORC = oxidized regenerated cellulose; PPL = polypropylene.

ANTERIOR HERNIORRHAPHY

Step 1: Initial Incision

Traditionally, the skin is opened by making an oblique incision between the anterosuperior iliac spine and the pubic tubercle. For cosmetic reasons, however, many surgeons now prefer a more horizontal skin incision placed in the natural skin lines. In either case, the incision is deepened through Scarpa fasciae and the subcutaneous tissue to expose the external oblique aponeurosis. The external oblique aponeurosis is then opened through the external inguinal ring. If a prosthesis is to be used, a space is created beneath the external oblique aponeurosis from the anterior rectus sheath medially toward the anterosuperior iliac spine laterally. The iliohypogastric, ilioinguinal, and genital nerves should be identified and protected. Efforts to mobilize these structures out of the operative field may increase postoperative groin pain.[20] Although identification of the nerves is important, routine division of the iliohypogastric and ilioinguinal nerves does not seem to be consistently associated with postoperative groin pain either way.[26]

Step 2: Mobilization of the Cord Structures

The cord structures are bluntly dissected away from the inferior flap of the external oblique aponeurosis to expose the inguinal ligament (shelving edge) and the iliopubic tract. This dissection is continued over the pubic tubercle and onto the anterior rectus sheath. The cord structures are then lifted with the fingers of one hand at the pubic tubercle so that the index finger can be passed underneath to meet the ipsilateral thumb or the fingers of the other hand. Mobilization of the cord structures is completed by means of blunt dissection, and a Penrose drain is placed around them so that they can be retracted during the procedure. The cremasteric muscle is then opened longitudinally rather than completely divided; this reduces the chances of damage to the cord and prevents testicular descent.

Step 3: Management of the Hernia Sac

The indirect hernia sac, if present, is located anterior and medial to the cord structures. The sac is dissected free of the cord structures by peeling away or dividing the adhesions between them. The sac can then be ligated and divided but, in adults, is preferably simply reduced into the peritoneal cavity. Proponents of sac inversion believe that this measure results in less pain (because the richly innervated peritoneum is not incised) and may be less likely to cause adhesive complications. Furthermore, sac eversion in lieu of excision protects intra-abdominal viscera in cases of unrecognized incarcerated sac contents or sliding hernia. For large inguinal scrotal hernial sacs, it may be preferential to divide the sac in the middle of the inguinal canal once it is clear that no abdominal contents are present rather than persist at full removal of the sac from the scrotum. The anterior wall of the distal sac is opened as far as possible, and the proximal sac is closed and reduced into the peritoneal cavity.

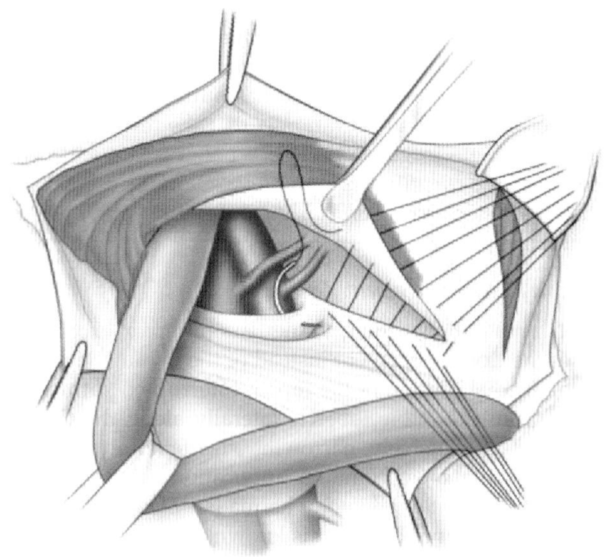

Figure 8 **McVay Cooper ligament repair. The lateral stitch is the transition stitch to the femoral sheath and the inguinal ligament.**

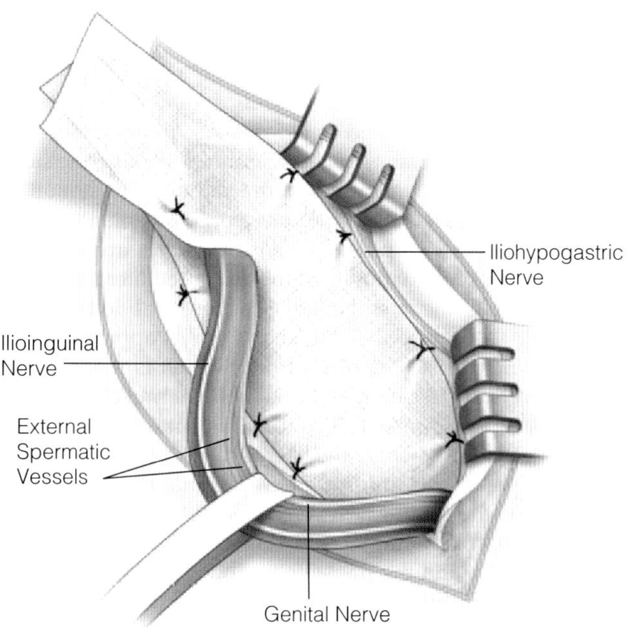

Figure 9 **Lichtenstein repair. A mesh prosthesis is positioned over the inguinal floor to extend approximately 2 cm medial to the pubic tubercle. A slit is made in the mesh to accommodate the cord structures, and the two tails are secured to each other and to the shelving edge of the inguinal ligament with a single interrupted suture. The superior and medial aspects of the prosthesis are secured to the internal oblique muscle and the rectus fascia with a few interrupted sutures.**

in the Bassini repair) should always be used. In the view of many authorities, this tension results in more pain than is noted with other herniorrhaphies and predisposes to recurrence. For this reason, the McVay repair is rarely chosen today, the main exception being for treatment of a patient with a femoral hernia or a patient with specific contraindications to mesh repair.

TENSION-FREE REPAIRS

Lichtenstein Repair

This operation is the current standard for inguinal herniorrhaphy. The initial preparation of the inguinal floor does not differ substantially from that carried out in a nonprosthetic repair. The transversalis fascia is not opened—a practice that has occasionally been criticized on the grounds that it might cause an occult femoral hernia to be missed. To date, however, an excessive incidence of missed femoral hernias has not been reported in men. The situation may be different in women in that femoral recurrence is much more common than one might assume when the entire myopectineal orifice is not addressed (as is the case with the McVay procedure or any of the preperitoneal operations).[27]

The key to the operation is the placement of a large prosthesis (at least 15 × 10 cm for an adult) extending from a point 2 cm medial to the pubic tubercle (to prevent the commonly seen pubic tubercle recurrences) to the anterosuperior iliac spine laterally. The medial end is rounded to correspond to the patient's particular anatomy, and a continuous suture of either nonabsorbable or long-lasting absorbable material is begun between the prosthesis and the anterior rectus sheath 2 cm medial to the pubic tubercle [*see Figure 9*]. The suture is continued laterally, securing the prosthesis to either side of the pubic tubercle (not into it) and then to the shelving edge of the inguinal ligament. The suture is tied at the internal ring.

A slit is made on the lateral side of the prosthesis to create two tails: a wider one (approximately two thirds of the total height) above and a narrower one below. The tails are positioned around the cord structures and placed beneath the external oblique aponeurosis laterally to about the anterosuperior iliac spine, with the upper tail placed on top of the lower. A single interrupted suture is placed to secure the lower edge of the superior tail to the lower edge of the inferior tail and the inguinal ligament—thereby, in effect, creating a shutter valve. This step is considered important for preventing indirect recurrences. The maneuver provides a cradling effect as well, preventing direct contact between the cut edges of the prosthesis and the cord structures, which could result in damage when linear approximation is used. The suture also incorporates the shelving edge of the inguinal ligament so as to create a domelike buckling effect over the direct space, thereby ensuring that there is no tension, especially when the patient assumes an upright position.

Two interrupted sutures are placed to attach the superior aspect of the mesh to the internal oblique aponeurosis and rectus fascia. Care is taken to tie these loosely and to avoid placing them laterally so as to minimize the risk of damaging the intramuscular and therefore invisible portions of the important nerves. The prosthesis should be sutured with enough laxity to allow for the difference between the supine and upright positions and, more importantly, to account for contraction of the mesh.

Plug-and-Patch Repair

The mesh plug technique was first developed by Gilbert and subsequently modified by Millikan and colleagues and Rutkow and Robbins, among others [*see Figure 10*].[28–30] The groin is entered via a standard anterior approach. The hernia sac is dissected away from surrounding structures and reduced into the preperitoneal space. A sheet of polypropylene mesh is formed into a cone, tied, inserted in the defect, and secured with interrupted sutures to either the internal ring (for an indirect hernia) or the neck of the defect (for a direct hernia).

A prefabricated prosthesis that has the configuration of a flower is commercially available and is recommended by Rutkow and Robbins.[30] This prosthesis is tailored to each patient's particular anatomy by removing some of the "petals" to avoid unnecessary bulk. Many surgeons consider this step important for preventing erosion into surrounding structures (e.g., the bladder); indeed, such complications have been reported, albeit rarely.

Millikan and colleagues further modified the procedure by recommending that the inside petals be sewn to the ring of the defect.[29] For an indirect hernia, the inside pedals are sewn to the internal oblique portion of the internal ring; this forces the outside of the prosthesis underneath the inner side of the defect and makes it act like a preperitoneal underlay. For direct hernias, the inside petals are sewn to the Cooper ligament and the shelving edge of the inguinal ligament, as well as to the conjoined tendon; this, again, forces the outside of the prosthesis to act as an underlay.

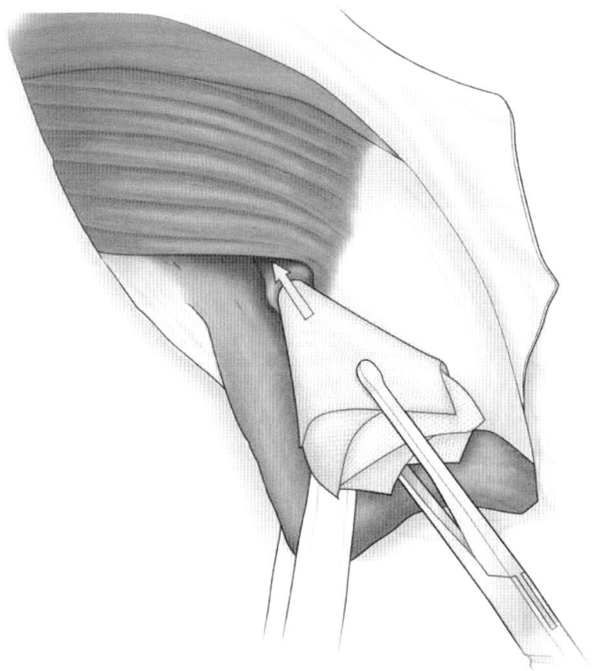

Figure 10 **Gilbert plug-and-patch repair. Depicted is the mesh plug technique for repair of an inguinal hernia. A sheet of polypropylene mesh is formed into a cone (as shown here), inserted into the defect, and secured to either the internal ring (*arrow*) (for an indirect hernia) or the neck of the defect (for a direct hernia) with interrupted sutures. Prefabricated mesh plugs are also available.**

The patch portion of the procedure is optional and involves placing a flat piece of polypropylene in the conventional inguinal space so that it widely overlaps the plug, much as in a Lichtenstein repair. The difference with a plug-and-patch repair is that only one or two sutures—or, sometimes, no sutures—are used to secure the flat prosthesis to the underlying inguinal floor. Some surgeons, however, place so many sutures that they have, in effect, performed a Lichtenstein operation on top of the plug.

The plug-and-patch repair, in all of its varieties, is fast and easy to teach, which has made it popular in both private and academic centers. A randomized, controlled trial has shown it to be equivalent to the Lichtenstein repair in terms of recurrence and morbidity.[31] However, case reports in the literature have described removal of plugs for pain, migration, or erosion, and, as a result, the benefits of the plug-and-patch repair compared with those of the Lichtenstein repair have been scrutinized.

Femoral Hernia Repair

Femoral hernias in females can be approached using a groin incision with dissection beneath the inguinal ligament without opening the external oblique fascia. To facilitate reduction of the contents of the hernia, the femoral canal may need to be opened by dividing the inguinal ligament and/or lacunar ligament. The defect can be closed with sutures or with a mesh plug from below the inguinal ligament [*see Figure 11*]. Larger femoral hernias in females and femoral hernias in males are better repaired using a McVay Cooper ligament repair.

POSTERIOR (PREPERITONEAL) HERNIORRHAPHY

A key technical issue in a preperitoneal hernia repair is how the surgeon chooses to enter the preperitoneal space. In fact, within this general class of repair, the method of entry into this space constitutes the major difference between the various procedures as all the repairs involve placement of a large prosthesis in the preperitoneal space. The theoretical advantage of this measure is that whereas in a conventional repair, abdominal pressure might contribute to recurrence, in a preperitoneal repair, the abdominal pressure would help fix the mesh material against the abdominal wall, thereby adding strength to the repair.

The preperitoneal space may be entered using an open or laparoscopic approach. The two principal laparoscopic techniques are the TAPP and total extraperitoneal (TEP) laparoscopic repairs. Although the laparoscopic repairs are the most prevalent posterior repairs at this time, the major open approaches are also described.

TAPP Repair

Step 1: trocar placement Pneumoperitoneum is established through a small infraumbilical incision. We generally prefer an open technique, in which a blunt-tipped 12 mm trocar is inserted into the peritoneal cavity under direct vision. CO_2 is then insufflated into the abdomen to a pressure of 12 to 15 mm Hg. The angled laparoscope is introduced, and both inguinal areas are inspected. Two 5 mm ports are placed, one at the lateral border of each rectus abdominis at the level of the umbilicus.

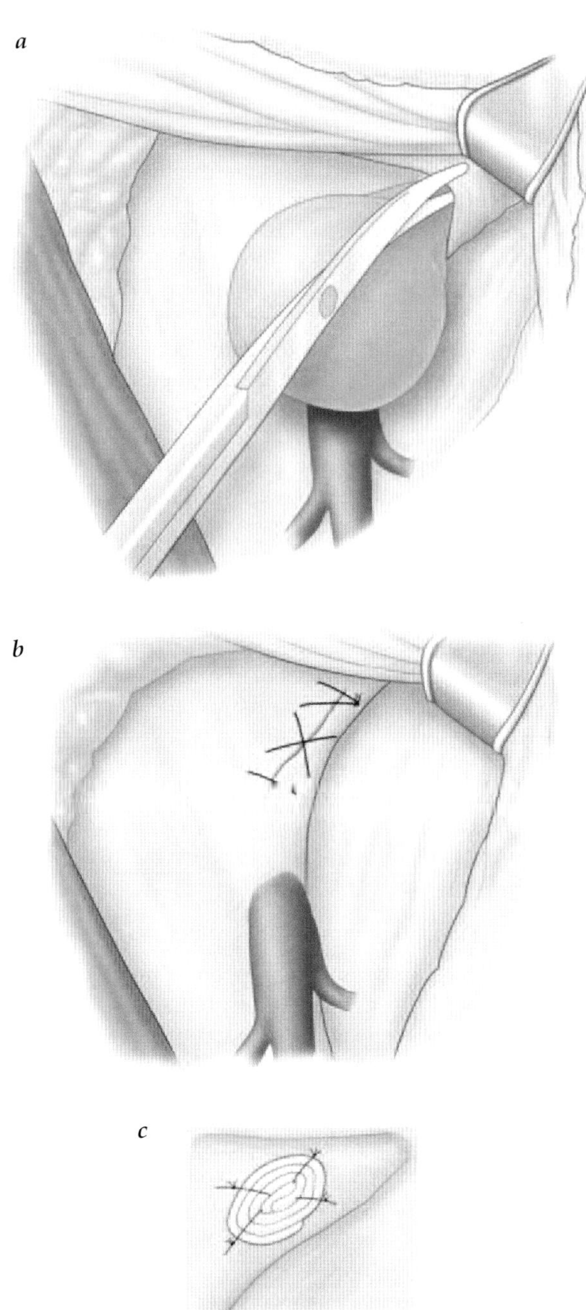

Figure 11 **Femoral hernia repair in females. The femoral canal is opened by dividing the inguinal ligament, the lacunar ligament, or both to allow for reduction of the hernia contents (*a*). The repair is then accomplished with sutures (*b*) or a mesh plug (*c*).**

Step 2: Identification of anatomic landmarks Four important landmarks should be seen initially during laparoscopic inspection of the inguinal region: the spermatic vessels, the obliterated umbilical artery (also referred to as the medial umbilical ligament or the bladder ligament), the inferior epigastric vessels (also referred to as the lateral umbilical ligament), and the external iliac vessels [*see Figure 4*]. In the TAPP approach, an indirect hernia, if present, will be immediately apparent and will have an obvious opening. The internal inguinal ring is then easily identified by the presence of a discrete hole lateral to the junction of the vas deferens, the testicular vessels, and the inferior epigastric vessels. Identification of a direct hernia can be more difficult. Sometimes a direct hernia appears as a complete circle or hole; at other times, it appears as a cleft, medial to the vas deferens–vascular junction; and at still other times, it is completely hidden by preperitoneal fat and the bladder and umbilical ligaments. Visualization can be particularly difficult in obese patients, who may have considerable lipomatous tissue between the peritoneum and the transversalis fascia, or in patients whose hernia consists of a weakness and bulging of the entire inguinal floor rather than a distinct sac.

For adequate definition of this type of hernia and deeper anatomic structures, the peritoneum must be opened, a peritoneal flap developed, and the underlying fatty layer dissected.[32] Traction on the ipsilateral testicle can demonstrate the vas deferens when visualization is obscured by overlying fat or pressure from the pneumoperitoneum.

Step 3: Creation of peritoneal flap The curved scissors or the hook cautery is used to create a peritoneal flap by making a transverse incision along the peritoneum, beginning several centimeters above the upper border of the internal inguinal ring and extending medially above the pubic tubercle and laterally at least 3 cm beyond the internal inguinal ring or to the level of the ipsilateral trocar [*see Figure 12*]. Care must be taken to avoid the inferior epigastric vessels. Bleeding from these vessels can usually be controlled by cauterization, but application of hemostatic clips may be necessary on occasion. Another solution is to pass percutaneously placed sutures above and below the bleeding point while applying pressure to the bleeding vessel so as not to obscure the field of vision. Division of the ipsilateral umbilical ligament may be useful in creating an appropriate medial space; however, the surgeon should be aware that the obliterated umbilical artery may still be patent and that use of the electrocautery or clips is prudent.

The incised peritoneum is grasped along with the attached preperitoneal fat and the peritoneal sac and is dissected cephalad with blunt and sharp instruments to create a lower peritoneal flap. Dissection should stay close to the abdominal wall. A significant amount of preperitoneal fat may be encountered, and this should remain with the peritoneal flap so that the abdominal wall is cleared. When the correct preperitoneal plane is entered, dissection is almost bloodless and is easily carried out.

Step 4: dissection of hernia sac The hernia sac, if present, is removed from the Hesselbach triangle or the spermatic cord and surrounding muscle through inward traction, countertraction, and blunt dissection with progressive inversion of the sac until the musculofascial boundary of the internal inguinal ring and the key deep anatomic structures are identified. In most cases, the hernia sac can be slowly drawn away from the transversalis fascia or the spermatic cord [*see Figure 13*]. The indirect sac may be visualized more easily if it is grasped and retracted medially; this step facilitates its dissection away from the cord structures.

a

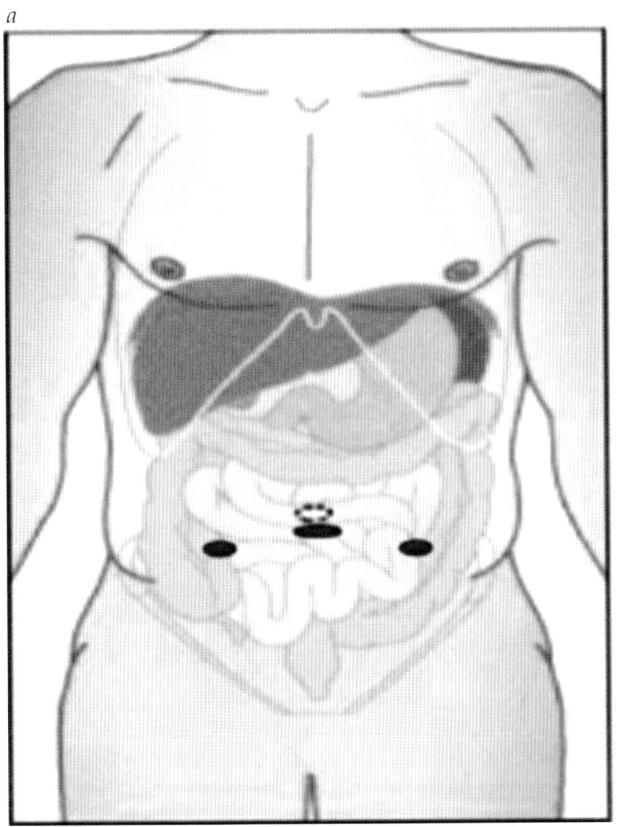

b

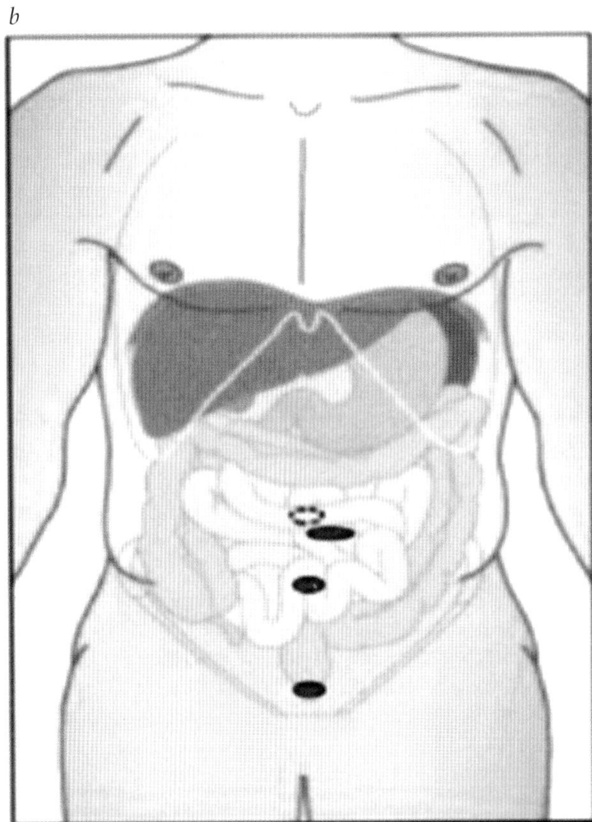

Figure 12 **Shown is the trocar placement for (*a*) laparoscopic transabdominal preperitoneal (TAPP) repair and (*b*) laparoscopic total extraperitoneal (TEP) repair.**

Spermatic cord lipomas usually lie posterolaterally and are extensions of preperitoneal fat. In the presence of an indirect defect, such lipomas should be dissected off the cord along with the peritoneal flap to lie cephalad to the internal inguinal ring and the subsequent repair so that prolapse through the ring can be prevented. A large indirect hernia sac can be divided at the internal ring if it cannot be readily dissected away from the cord structures. This step may prevent cord injury that can result from extensive dissection.

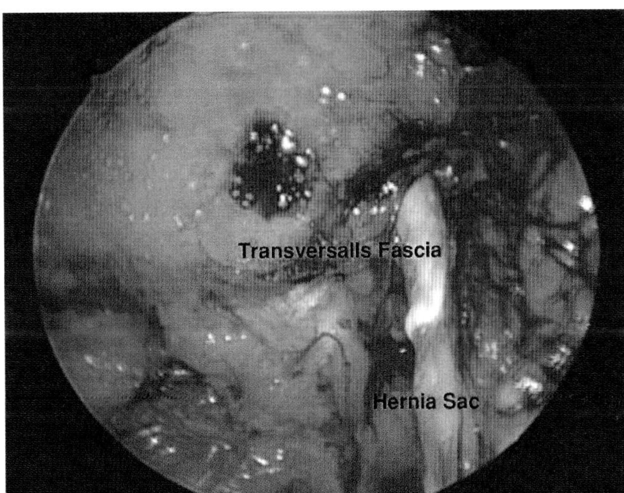

Figure 13 **Laparoscopic inguinal hernia repair: transversalis fascia. The transversalis fascia is seen adherent to the hernia sac. The sac must be separated from the fascia and dissected cephalad.**

The pubic tubercle is often more easily felt than seen. The Cooper ligament is initially felt and subsequently seen along the pectineal prominence of the superior pubic ramus as dissection continues medially and fatty tissue is swept off to expose the glistening white structure. Care must be taken to avoid the numerous small veins that often run on the surface of the ligament, as well as to avoid the occasional aberrant obturator artery. The iliopubic tract is initially identified at the inferior margin of the internal inguinal ring, with the spermatic cord above, and is then followed in both a medial and a lateral direction. Minimal dissection is carried out inferior to the iliopubic tract so as to avoid neurovascular injuries.

Step 5: mesh placement A 15 × 10 cm sheet of polypropylene or polyester mesh is rolled into a tubular shape and introduced into the abdomen through the 10/12 mm umbilical trocar. The mesh is used to cover the direct, indirect, and femoral spaces (i.e., the entire inguinal floor). Some form of mesh fixation should be used, either tacks or fibrin glue. Our preference is to use absorbable tacks. Medially, tacks are placed in the Cooper ligament. A two-handed technique is recommended for lateral tack placement: one hand is on the tacker, and the other is on the abdominal wall, applying external pressure to place the wall against the tacker. Care must be taken not to force the tacker too deeply into the abdominal wall superolateral to the spermatic cord; doing so might lead to inadvertent entrapment of the sensory nerves. The tacker can be moved from the left to the right port, depending on which position more readily allows placement of the staples perpendicular to the mesh and the abdominal wall. Lateral to the cord structures, all tacks are placed superior to the iliopubic tract to prevent subsequent neuralgias involving the lateral cutaneous nerve of the thigh or the branches of the genitofemoral nerve. If the surgeon can palpate the tacker through the abdominal wall with the nondominant hand, the tacker is above the iliopubic tract. The mesh should lie flat.

Step 6: closure The peritoneal flap, including the redundant inverted hernia sac, is placed over the mesh, and the peritoneum is reapproximated with tacks or sutures along its superior edge [*see Figure 14*]. Inferior epigastric vessels must be avoided. Reduction of the intra-abdominal pressure to 8 mm Hg, coupled with external abdominal wall pressure, facilitates a tension-free reapproximation. The peritoneal repair is inspected to ensure that no major gaps might result in exposure of the mesh and subsequent formation of adhesions. The trocars are then removed under direct vision, and the pneumoperitoneum is released. The fascia at the 10/12 mm port sites is sutured closed, and the skin is closed with 4-0 absorbable subcuticular sutures.

TEP Repair

The extra-abdominal preperitoneal approach to laparoscopic hernia repair, developed by McKernan and Laws,[33,34] attempts to duplicate the open preperitoneal repair described by Stoppa and colleagues[35-37] and Wantz.[8,38] In a TEP repair, the trocars are placed preperitoneally in a space created between the fascia and the peritoneum. Ideally, the dissection remains in the extra-abdominal plane at all times, and the peritoneum is never penetrated.

Step 1: creation of preperitoneal space With the patient in the Trendelenburg position, the anterior rectus fascia is opened through a 1 cm infraumbilical transverse incision placed slightly toward the side of the hernia, which helps prevent inadvertent opening of the peritoneum. The rectus is retracted laterally and a narrow retractor is slid over the posterior rectus sheath. In this plane, a preperitoneal tunnel between the rectus muscles and the peritoneum is created in the midline by inserting a dissecting balloon to the level of the symphysis pubis. The preperitoneal working space is developed by gradual inflation of the balloon to a volume of 1 L or until the creases in the balloon are effaced. This is done under direct vision using a 30 or 45 laparoscope as the transparency of the balloon permits constant laparoscopic visualization throughout the distention process. The balloon is then withdrawn and replaced with a 10/12 mm balloon-tipped trocar. Maximal inflation pressure is 10 to 15 mm Hg to prevent disruption of the peritoneum or development of extensive subcutaneous emphysema. Blunt, gentle dissection with the laparoscope can be employed to develop the space sufficiently to allow placement of additional trocars [*see Figure 15*].

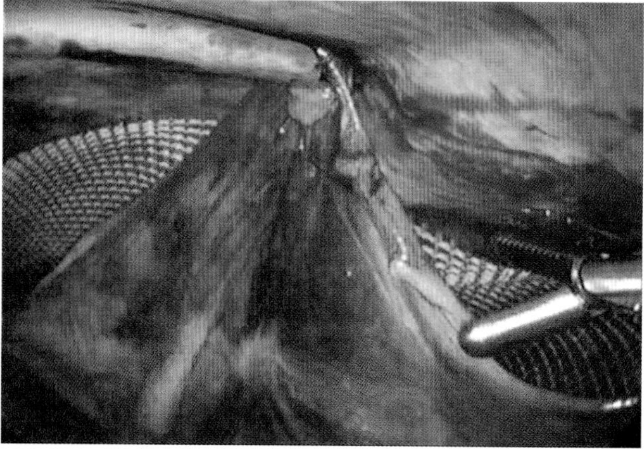

Figure 14 **Laparoscopic inguinal hernia repair: peritoneal flap. The peritoneal flap is placed so as to entirely cover the mesh in the preperitoneal space.**

Step 2: trocar placement [*see Figure 12*] After the peritoneum is dissected away from the rectus abdominis, a midline 5 mm trocar is inserted under direct vision three fingerbreadths below the infraumbilical port. A second 5 mm trocar is then inserted another three fingerbreadths below the first 5 mm trocar. Placement of the working trocars away from the pubis facilitates mesh placement in that the bottom port is not covered by the top of the mesh and thereby rendered nonfunctional. Care must be taken not to penetrate the peritoneum during trocar placement. If the peritoneum is penetrated, the resulting pneumoperitoneum can reduce the already limited working space. If the working space is compromised to the point where the repair cannot continue (which is not always the case), the surgeon can either try to repair the rent with a suture or place a Veress needle or angiocath in the upper abdominal peritoneal cavity. If such maneuvers are unsuccessful, the loss of working space may necessitate conversion to a TAPP or open approach.

Step 3: dissection of hernia sac The inferior epigastric vessels, which help guide lateral dissection and identification of the internal ring, are identified first and are kept up against the abdominal wall during peritoneal dissection. The Cooper ligament is exposed first, during which care must be taken not to injure the obturator branch that crosses it. Wide lateral dissection of the preperitoneal space is then undertaken with blunt graspers in a two-handed technique by bluntly dividing the avascular areolar tissue between the peritoneum and the abdominal wall. Proper lateral dissection is crucial to optimal mesh placement.

If a direct hernia is present medial to the inferior epigastric vessels, it will often be reduced by the balloon dissector. If not, the sac and the preperitoneal contents are carefully dissected away from the fascial defect and swept cephalad as far as possible. Gentle traction is applied to expose and dissect away the attachment of the peritoneum to the transversalis fascia.

The indirect space is then exposed by sweeping off the tissue lateral to the inferior epigastric vessels until the peritoneum is found. If a lipoma of the cord is present, it will be lateral to and covering the peritoneum and should be

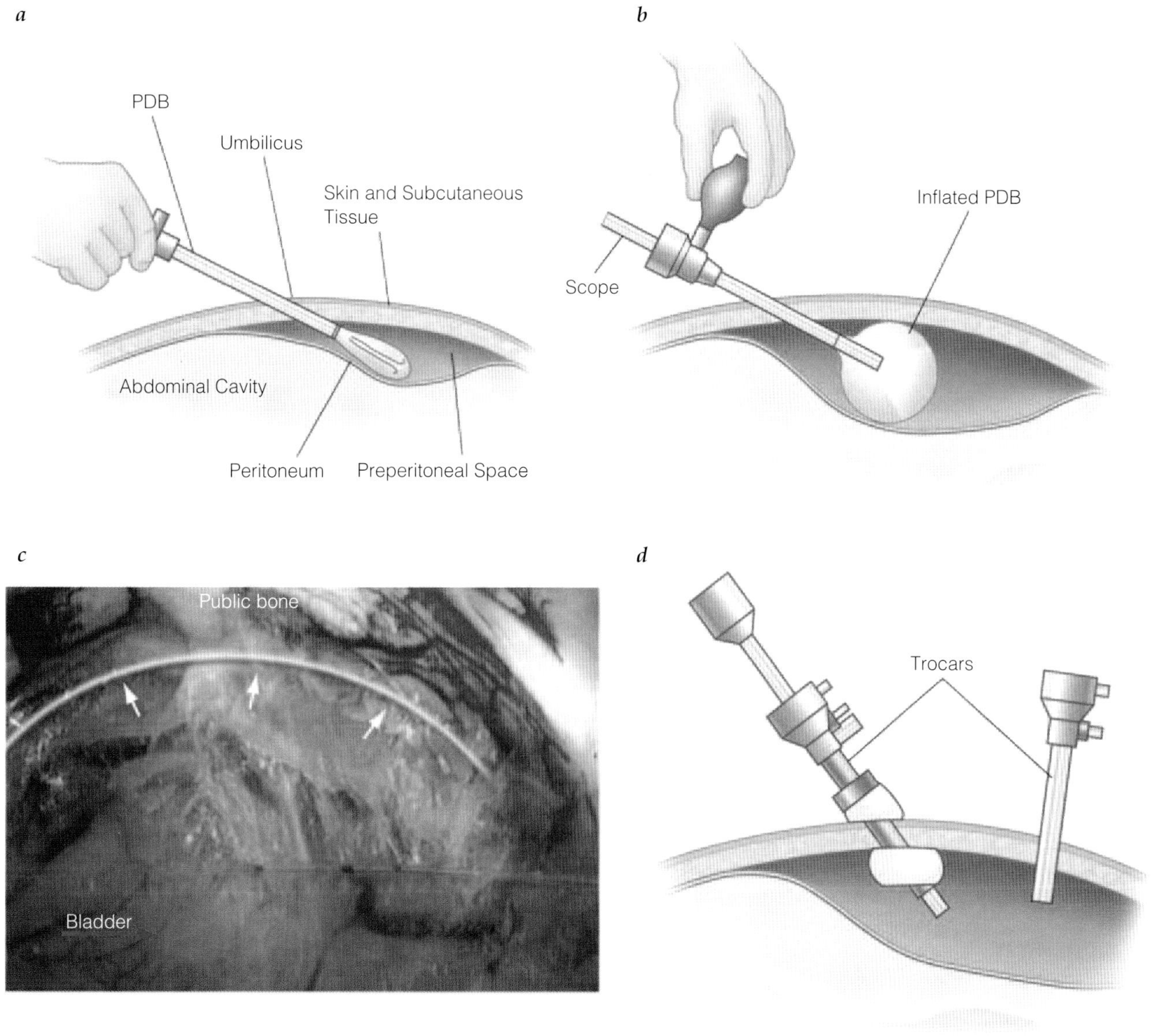

Figure 15 **Laparoscopic inguinal hernia repair: total extraperitoneal (TEP) approach. Shown is the preperitoneal distention balloon (PDB) system. The balloon is introduced into the preperitoneal space (*a*). As it is tunneled inferiorly toward the pubis, the balloon is inflated under laparoscopic vision (*b*). As the balloon is inflated, the pubic bone and peritoneal edge come into view (line and arrows) (*c*). Once the preperitoneal space is created, the balloon is removed and replaced with a blunt-tipped trocar. The preperitoneal space is insufflated under low pressure, additional trocars are placed, and the repair is begun (*d*).**

dissected out of the internal ring in a cephalad direction to prevent it from displacing the mesh.[39] If there is no indirect hernia, the peritoneum will be found cephalad to the internal ring. To ensure secure mesh placement, the peritoneum is bluntly dissected off the cord structures and placed as far cephalad as possible. If an indirect hernia is present, the sac will be lateral and anterior to the cord structures. These must be clearly identified and protected during dissection. A small indirect hernial sac is bluntly dissected off the spermatic cord with a hand-over-hand technique and reduced until an area sufficient for mesh placement is created. To prevent early recurrence, all attachments of the peritoneum should be dissected cephalad to where the inferior edge of the mesh will be. If a large indirect sac is not easily reduced from the scrotum, it may be transected in its superolateral edge, dissected off the cord structures, and closed with clips or a ligating loop. The distal sac is then left in place without ligation.

Unlike a TAPP repair, in which any indirect hernia present is readily apparent at first inspection, a TEP repair always requires that the space lateral to the inferior epigastric vessels be dissected to make sure that there is no indirect component. This dissection should be done even if a direct or femoral hernia is identified.

Step 4: mesh placement A number of different prostheses in a variety of contoured or flat configurations are available, including various forms of polypropylene and several types of polyester. Whichever is chosen, it should be large enough (15 × 10 cm) to provide adequate coverage. A marking suture is placed or a mark is made to identify the inferomedial aspect of the mesh to be placed against the Cooper ligament. The mesh is inserted through the umbilical trocar into the preperitoneal space. Once in the preperitoneal space, the mesh is manipulated to cover the pubic tubercle, the internal ring, the Cooper ligament, the femoral canal, and the rectus abdominis superiorly. The inferior edge of the mesh must be tucked behind the peritoneal reflection to prevent folding of the mesh. Tacks are placed into the Cooper ligament and on the superolateral edge of the mesh on the anterior abdominal wall. To prevent nerve injury, no tacks should be placed inferior to the iliopubic tract lateral to the internal ring.

Mesh fixation options vary and depend on surgeon preference: permanent tacks, absorbable tacks, biologic "glues," or eliminating the use of fixation all together. Early results of a large randomized, controlled trial studying laparoscopic inguinal hernia repair without use of mesh fixation found that it was unnecessary in TEP repair of small hernial defects. Such a strategy was associated with lower operative costs and a lower incidence of chronic groin pain. The omission of mesh fixation did not increase the risk of early hernia recurrence.[40] Another recent meta-analysis compared mesh fixation using a fibrin sealant versus staple fixation in laparoscopic TEP repairs and found less chronic pain and an equivalent recurrence rate in the former.[41]

Step 5: closure The operative site is inspected for hemostasis. The trocars are removed under direct vision. The insufflated CO_2 is slowly released so that the mesh may be visualized as the preperitoneal fat and contents collapse back onto the mesh. The fascia at trocar sites 10 mm or larger is sutured closed, and the skin is closed with subcuticular sutures.

OPEN POSTERIOR PROSTHETIC REPAIRS

For open access, the space can be entered either anteriorly or posteriorly. If an anterior technique is to be used, the initial steps of the operation are similar to those of a conventional anterior herniorrhaphy. If a posterior technique is to be used, any of several incisions (lower midline, paramedian, or Pfannenstiel) will allow an extraperitoneal dissection. The preperitoneal space can also be entered transabdominally. This approach is useful when the patient is undergoing a laparotomy for some other condition and the hernia is to be repaired incidentally.

Read-Rives Repair

The posterior space is accessed directly through the groin; thus, the initial part of a Read-Rives repair, including the opening of the inguinal floor, is much like that of a classic Bassini repair. The inferior epigastric vessels are identified, and the preperitoneal space is completely dissected. The spermatic cord is parietalized by separating the ductus deferens from the spermatic vessels. A 12 × 16 cm piece of mesh is positioned in the preperitoneal space deep to the inferior epigastric vessels and secured with three sutures placed in the pubic tubercle, in the Cooper ligament, and in the psoas muscle laterally. The transversalis fascia is closed over the prosthesis, and the cord structures are replaced.

Stoppa-Rignault-Wantz Repair (Giant Prosthetic Reinforcement of Visceral Sac)

Giant prosthetic reinforcement of the visceral sac (GPRVS) has its roots in the important contribution that Henri Fruchaud, who was Stoppa's mentor, made to herniology. Instead of subdividing hernias into direct, indirect, and femoral and then examining their specific causes, Fruchaud emphasized that the common cause of all inguinal hernias was the failure of the transversalis fascia to retain the peritoneum. This concept led Stoppa to develop GPRVS, which reestablishes the integrity of the peritoneal sac by inserting a large permanent prosthesis that entirely replaces the transversalis fascia over the myopectineal orifice of Fruchaud [*see Figure 16*] with wide overlapping of surrounding tissue. The technique has not gained routine acceptance in North America, however.

Step 1: Skin incision A lower midline, Pfannenstiel, or inguinal incision can be used. The inguinal incision is placed 2 to 3 cm below the level of the anterosuperior iliac spine but above the internal ring; it is begun at the midline and extended laterally for 8 to 9 cm.[42]

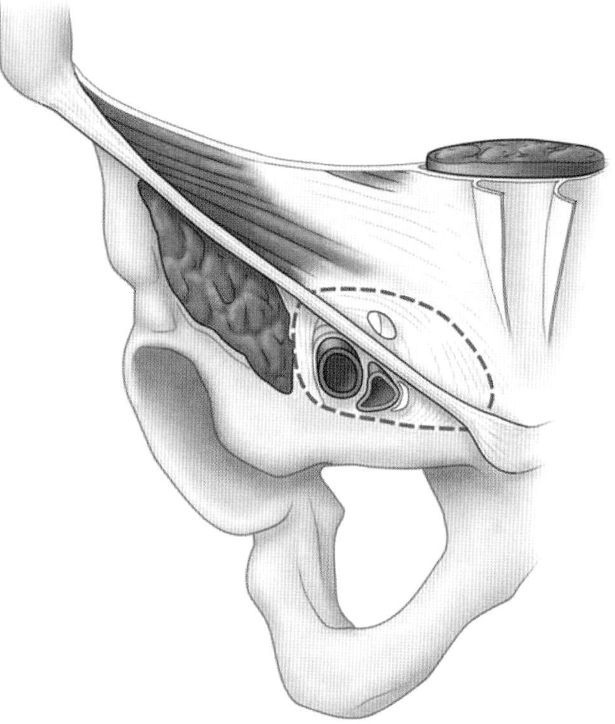

Figure 16 **Depicted is the myopectineal orifice of Fruchaud. The area is bounded superiorly by the internal oblique muscle and the transversus abdominis, medially by the rectus abdominis and the rectus sheath, laterally by the iliopsoas muscle, and inferiorly by the Cooper ligament. Critical anatomic landmarks (e.g., the inguinal ligament, the spermatic cord, and the femoral vessels) are contained within this structure.**

Step 2: preperitoneal dissection The fascia overlying the space of Retzius is opened without violation of the peritoneum. A combination of blunt and sharp dissection is continued laterally posterior to the rectus abdominis and the inferior epigastric vessels. The preperitoneal space is completely dissected to a point lateral to the anterosuperior iliac spine. The symphysis pubis, the Cooper ligament, and the iliopubic tract are identified. Inferiorly, the peritoneum is generously dissected away from the vas deferens and the internal spermatic vessels to create a large pocket, which will eventually accommodate a prosthesis. In the inguinal approach, the anterior rectus sheath and the oblique muscles are incised for the length of the skin incision. The lower flaps of these structures are retracted inferiorly toward the pubis. The transversalis fascia is incised along the lateral edge of the rectus abdominis, and the preperitoneal space is entered; dissection then proceeds as previously indicated.

Step 3: management of hernia sac Direct hernia sacs are reduced during the course of the preperitoneal dissection. Care must be taken to stay in the plane between the peritoneum and the transversalis fascia, allowing the latter structure to retract into the hernia defect toward the skin.

Indirect sacs are more difficult to deal with than direct sacs are in that they often adhere to the cord structures. Trauma to the cord must be minimized to prevent damage to the vas deferens or the testicular blood supply. Small sacs should be mobilized from the cord structures and reduced back into the peritoneal cavity. Large sacs may be difficult to mobilize from the cord without undue trauma if an attempt is made to remove the sac in its entirety. Accordingly, large sacs should be divided, with the distal portion left in situ and the proximal portion dissected away from the cord structures. Division of the sac is most easily accomplished by opening the sac on the side opposite the cord structures. A finger is placed in the sac to facilitate its separation from the cord. Downward traction is then placed on the cord structures to reduce any excessive fatty tissue (so-called lipoma of the cord) back into the preperitoneal space. This step prevents the "pseudorecurrences" that may occur if the abnormality palpated during the preoperative physical examination was not a hernia but a lipoma of the cord.

Step 4: management of abdominal wall defect This step varies most from one author to another. In Nyhus's approach, the defect is formally repaired, and only then is a tailored mesh prosthesis sutured to the Cooper ligament and the transversalis fascia for reinforcement. Rignault prefers to close the defect loosely to prevent an unsightly early postoperative bulge.[43] In Stoppa's and Wantz's techniques,[36,38] the defect is usually left alone, but the transversalis fascia in the defect is occasionally plicated by suturing it to the Cooper ligament to prevent the bulge caused by a seroma in the undisturbed sac.

Step 5: parietalization of spermatic cord The term *parietalization of the spermatic cord*, popularized by Stoppa and Warlaumont,[36] refers to a thorough dissection of the cord aimed at providing sufficient length to permit lateral movement of the structure [*see Figure 17*]. In their view, this step is essential in that it allows a prosthesis to be placed without having to be split laterally to accommodate the cord structures[36]; the keyhole defect created when the prosthesis is split has been linked with recurrences. In Rignault's opinion,[43] creation of a keyhole defect in the mesh to encircle the spermatic cord is preferable, the rationale being that this gives the prosthesis enough security to allow the surgeon to dispense with fixation sutures or tacks. Minimizing fixation in this area is important because of the numerous anatomic elements in the preperitoneal space that can be inadvertently damaged during suture placement.

Step 6: placement of prosthesis Stoppa's technique is most often associated with a single large prosthesis for bilateral hernias.[36] The prosthesis is cut in the shape of a chevron (24 cm in length), and eight clamps are positioned strategically around the prosthesis to facilitate placement into the preperitoneal space.

Unilateral repairs use a prosthesis that is approximately 15 × 12 cm but is cut so that the bottom edge is wider than the top edge and the lateral side is longer than the medial side. In Wantz's technique,[38] three absorbable sutures are used to attach the superior border of the prosthesis to the anterior abdominal wall well above the defect [*see Figure 18*]. The sutures are placed from medial to lateral near the linea alba, the semilunar line, and the anterosuperior iliac spine.

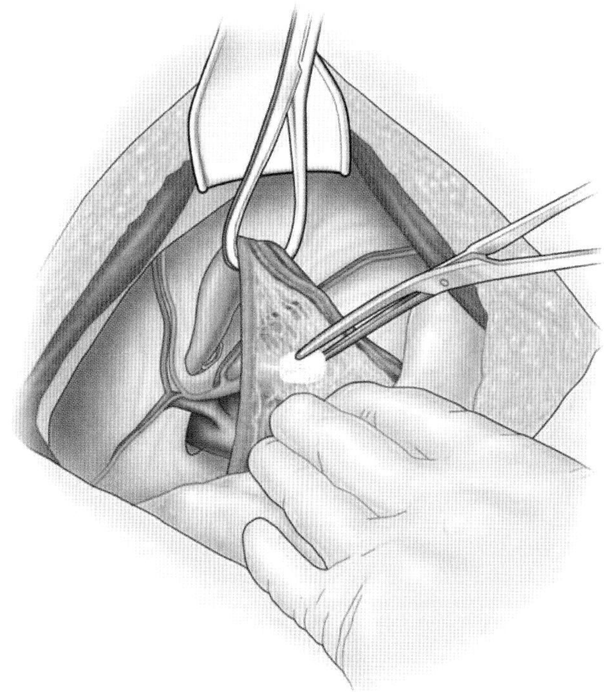

Figure 17 **Preperitoneal inguinal prosthetic herniorrhaphy. Illustrated is parietalization of the spermatic cord. The spermatic vessels and the vas deferens are mobilized so that they move laterally. This step is carried out so that the surgeon can place a large prosthesis that widely overlaps the myopectineal orifice without having to slit the prosthesis to accommodate the cord structures.**

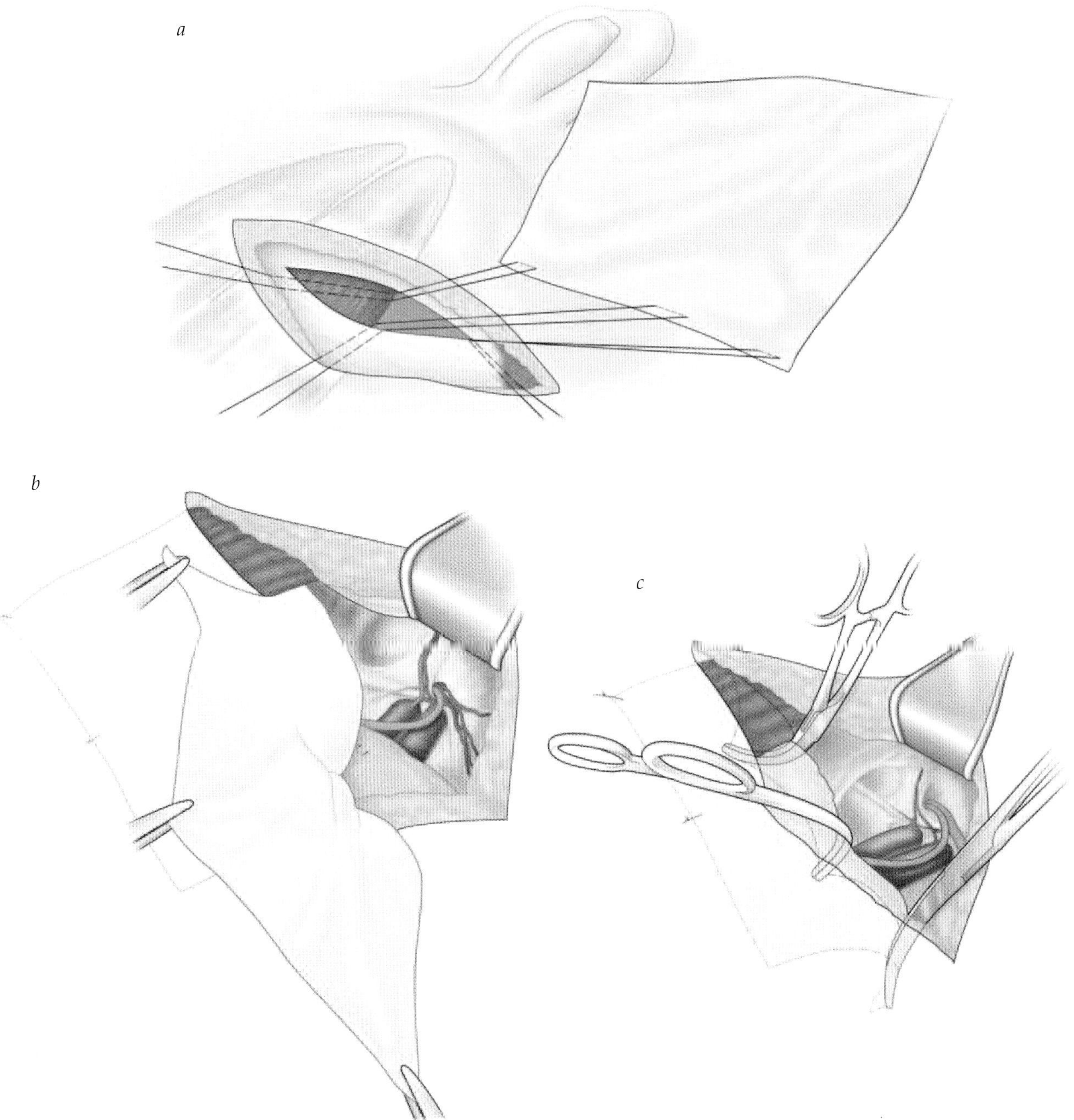

Figure 18 **Unilateral giant prosthetic reinforcement of the visceral sac (Wantz technique). (*a, b*) The prosthesis is cut so that the inferior edge is wider than the superior edge by 2 to 4 cm and the lateral side is longer than the medial side. The width at the superior edge is approximately the distance between the umbilicus and the anterosuperior iliac spine minus 1 cm, and the height is approximately 14 cm. Anteriorly, three sutures are placed—near the linea alba, near the semilunar line, and near the anterosuperior iliac spine—from medial to lateral to fix the superior border. (*c*) Three long clamps on the inferior edge are used to implant the prosthesis deep into the preperitoneal space with the peritoneal sac retracted cranially.**

Three long clamps are then placed on each corner and the middle of the prosthesis of the inferior flap and used to direct the mesh deep into the preperitoneal space with the peritoneal sac pushed cephalad.

Step 7: closure of wound The surgical wound is closed anatomically once the surgeon is assured that there has been no displacement or roll-up of the prosthesis.

Kugel and Ugahary Repairs

The Kugel and Ugahary repairs were developed to compete with laparoscopic repairs. They require only a small (2 to 3 cm) skin incision placed 2 to 3 cm above the internal ring.[44,45] In Kugel's operation, the incision is oriented obliquely, with one third of the incision lateral to a point halfway between the anterosuperior iliac spine and the pubic tubercle and the remaining two thirds medial to this point. The incision is deepened through the external oblique fascia, and the internal oblique muscle is bluntly spread apart. The transversalis fascia is opened vertically for a distance of about 3 cm, but the internal ring is not violated. The preperitoneal space is entered, and a blunt dissection is performed. The inferior epigastric vessels are identified to confirm that the dissection is being done in the correct plane. These vessels should be left adherent to the overlying transversalis fascia and retracted medially and anteriorly. The iliac vessels, the Cooper ligament, the pubic bone, and the hernia defect are identified by palpation. Most hernial sacs are simply reduced; the exceptions are large indirect sacs, which must sometimes be divided, with the distal sac left in situ and the proximal sac closed. To prevent recurrences, the cord structures are thoroughly parietalized to allow adequate posterior dissection.

The key to Kugel's procedure is a specially designed 8 × 12 cm prosthesis. The construction of the prosthesis allows it to be deformed so that it can fit through the small incision; once inserted, it springs open to regain its normal shape, providing a wide overlap of the myopectineal orifice. The prosthesis also has a slit on its anterior surface, through which the surgeon places a finger to facilitate positioning.

Ugahary's operation is similar to Kugel's but does not require a special prosthesis. In what is known as the gridiron technique, the preperitoneal space is prepared through a 3 cm incision, much as in a Kugel repair. The space is held open with a narrow Langenbeck retractor and two ribbon retractors. A 10 × 15 cm piece of polypropylene mesh is rolled onto a long forceps after the edges have been rounded and sutures placed to correspond to various anatomic landmarks. The forceps with the rolled-up mesh on it is introduced into the preperitoneal space, and the mesh is unrolled with the help of clamps and specific movements of the ribbon retractors.

COMBINED ANTERIOR AND POSTERIOR (PREPERITONEAL) HERNIORRHAPHY

Bilayer Prosthetic Repair

The bilayer prosthetic repair involves the use of a dumbbell-shaped prosthesis consisting of two flat pieces of polypropylene mesh connected by a cylinder of the same material. The purpose of this design is to allow the surgeon to take advantage of the presumed benefits of both anterior and posterior approaches by placing prosthetic material in both the preperitoneal space and the extraperitoneal space.

The initial steps are identical to those of a Lichtenstein repair. Once the conventional anterior space has been prepared, the preperitoneal space is entered through the hernia defect. Indirect hernias are reduced, and a gauze sponge is used to develop the preperitoneal space through the internal ring. For direct hernias, the transversalis fascia is opened, and the space between this structure and the peritoneum is developed with a gauze sponge. The deep layer of the prosthesis is deployed in the preperitoneal space, overlapping the direct and indirect spaces and the Cooper ligament. The superficial layer of the device occupies the conventional anterior space, much as in a Lichtenstein repair. It is slit laterally or centrally to accommodate the cord structures and then affixed to the area of the pubic tubercle, the middle of the inguinal ligament, and the internal oblique muscle with three or four interrupted sutures.

Complications

RECURRENCE

An analysis of nearly 18,000 herniorrhaphies in Sweden reported that 15% of operations were performed to treat recurrent hernias.[46] This figure is remarkably consistent with the data from other large population-based series and is influenced by the type of repair, type of hernia (primary versus recurrent), patient characteristics, and surgeon characteristics (hernia specialist or not). The use of mesh is an important factor, with a Cochrane meta-analysis of open mesh inguinal hernia repair versus open nonmesh repair finding that tension-free mesh repair led to a significant reduction in hernia recurrence of between 50 and 75%.[19] Two randomized trials using the Lichtenstein repair as the control operation documented 2-year recurrence rates between 1 and 4%, setting a benchmark for primary inguinal hernia repair.[47,48]

Similar low recurrence rates have been demonstrated regardless of the technique of mesh placement, whether laparoscopic or open.[49,50] On the other hand, a large, randomized, multicenter Veterans Affairs (VA) study found that for primary, unilateral hernias, the laparoscopic approach was associated with a higher overall recurrence rate at 2 years (10%) when compared with open mesh repair (4%).[48] Most reported recurrences after laparoscopic herniorrhaphy come at an early stage in the surgeon's experience with these procedures and arise soon after operation.[48,51] The majority can be attributed to (1) inadequate preperitoneal dissection; (2) use of an inadequately sized patch, which may migrate or fail to support the entire inguinal area, including direct, indirect, and femoral spaces; or (3) staple failure with TAPP repair.

PAIN

Chronic postoperative groin pain is one of the major complications facing patients undergoing inguinal hernia repairs. Although some degree of postoperative groin pain is experienced by as many as 53% of patients,[52] significant long-term pain is probably seen in 5 to 15% of patients,[48,49,53] regardless of whether the nerves were divided or preserved.[54] Persistent pain and burning sensations in the inguinal region, the upper medial thigh, or the spermatic cord and scrotal skin region occur when the genitofemoral nerve or the ilioinguinal nerve is stimulated, entrapped, or unintentionally injured. When the lateral cutaneous nerve is involved, lateral or central upper medial thigh numbness is experienced and often lasts several months or longer. Unlike patients who undergo open anterior herniorrhaphy, in whom discomfort or numbness is usually localized to the operative area, patients who undergo laparoscopic repair occasionally describe unusual but specific symptoms of deep discomfort that are usually positional and are often of a transient, shooting nature suggestive of nerve irritation. Postoperative chronic pain is more likely to be observed in younger patients and in patients who report preoperative pain attributable to their hernia, but other risk factors have also

delayed would experience more complications. The investigators found, however, that postoperative complication rates were the same in patients who underwent immediate surgery as in those who were assigned to WW but had to cross over to surgical treatment.

PRIMARY UNILATERAL HERNIAS

For unilateral primary hernias, the most important consideration in choosing an inguinal hernia procedure may well be the experience of the surgeon, with excellent results demonstrated after both open and laparoscopic mesh repairs in experienced hands. The next consideration should be to tailor the operation to the patient's particular hernia. In infants and young children with indirect hernias, for whom repair of the posterior canal wall is unnecessary, high ligation of the sac via the anterior approach is a sufficient procedure but is not adequate in most adults, where a mesh is recommended to decrease recurrence. Conventional anterior prosthetic repairs are particularly useful in high-risk patients because they can be readily performed with local anesthesia, a safer approach than laparoscopic surgery, for which the pneumoperitoneum could result in adverse events. Similarly, we do not treat acutely incarcerated hernias laparoscopically. Large indirect scrotal hernias are another category of challenging laparoscopic cases. Previous lower abdominal surgery, although not an absolute contraindication, may make laparoscopic dissection difficult. In particular, with respect to TEP repair, previous lower abdominal wall incisions may make it impossible to safely separate the peritoneum from the abdominal parietes for entry into the extraperitoneal plane, and conversion to a TAPP repair or an open repair may be required. Previous surgery in the retropubic space of Retzius, as in prostatic procedures, is a relative contraindication that is associated with an increased risk of bladder injury[60] and other complications.[77] Similarly, previous pelvic irradiation may preclude safe dissection of the peritoneum from the abdominal wall.[42] If local or systemic infection is present, a nonprosthetic repair is usually considered preferable, although the newer biologic prostheses now being evaluated may eventually change this view. A recent meta-analysis of all randomized, controlled trials compared hernia recurrence and surgery-related morbidity between open inguinal hernia repair (OIHR) and laparoscopic inguinal hernia repair (LIHR) for primary unilateral inguinal hernia. The study concluded that TEP repair was associated with an increased risk of recurrence relative to OIHR (relative risk [RR] = 3.72, p = .001) but that TAPP was not (RR = 1.14, p = .001). On the other hand, TAPP repair was associated with increased risk of perioperative complications relative to OIHR. Overall, LIHR was found to cause less chronic groin pain and numbness. The study identified risk factors for recurrence after TEP LIHR: surgeon age under 45 years, presence of postoperative pain, a short operating time, and procedural inexperience.[78]

RECURRENT HERNIAS

In patients with recurrent hernias after previous anterior repair, a laparoscopic or other posterior approach allows the surgeon to avoid the scar tissue and distorted anatomy present in the anterior abdominal wall by performing the repair through unviolated tissue, thereby potentially reducing the risk of damage to the vas deferens or the testicular vessels. This is especially true when mesh has previously been placed anteriorly. Similarly, recurrence following a preperitoneal approach may be more favorably treated with an anterior herniorrhaphy.[79]

BILATERAL HERNIAS

Laparoscopy allows simultaneous exploration of the abdominal cavity (TAPP repair) and diagnosis and treatment of bilateral groin hernias, as well as coexisting femoral hernias (which are often unrecognized preoperatively), potentially without added risk or disability. Bilateral hernias accounted for 9% of the hernias reviewed in the Cochrane database.[49] The operating time was longer in the laparoscopic groups than in the open groups; however, the recovery time, the incidence of persistent numbness, and the risk of wound infection were significantly reduced in the former. These results are consistent with those of a prospective, randomized, controlled trial that compared TAPP repair with open mesh repair for bilateral and recurrent hernias.[80] In this study, TAPP repair not only was less painful and led to an earlier return to work but also was associated with a shorter operating time.

INCARCERATED AND STRANGULATED HERNIAS

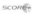

Strangulated groin hernia is a serious surgical emergency associated with high morbidity and mortality (up to 9%). The rate varies between 0.9 and 2.9%, and prompt clinical diagnosis is needed as a delay of 6 to 12 hours increases the likelihood of intestinal necrosis and requires bowel resection in up to 15% of cases.[81] There is no consensus on the preferred surgical approach. The basic surgical principles are as follows: (1) the approach that offers the most optimal exposure and access to the small bowel, should resection be required, should be used; ischemic bowel may be addressed through either the groin incision, a laparotomy, or laparoscopically[82]; (2) the hernia sac should be reduced with minimal trauma to its contents; and (3) synthetic mesh should be avoided in the context of strangulated bowel to avoid mesh infections. Tissue repairs are preferable, and the higher risk of recurrence should not be a deciding factor in the emergency setting.

Financial Disclosures: None Reported

References

1. Rutkow IM. Demographic and socioeconomic aspects of hernia repair in the United States in 2003. Surg Clin North Am 2003;83:1045.
2. Bay-Nielsen M, Kehlet H, Strand L, et al. Quality assessment of 26,304 herniorrhaphies in Denmark: a prospective nationwide study. Lancet 2001;358:1124.
3. Primatesta P, Goldacre MJ. Inguinal hernia repair: incidence of elective and emergency surgery, readmission and mortality. Int J Epidemiol 1996;25:835.
4. Kingsnorth A, LeBlanc K. Hernias: inguinal and incisional. Lancet 2003;362:1561.
5. Zollinger RM Jr. An updated traditional classification of inguinal hernias. Hernia 2004;8:318.

6. Skandalakis JE, Gray SW, Skandalakis LJ, et al. Surgical anatomy of the inguinal area. World J Surg 1989;13:490.
7. Spaw AT, Ennis BW, Spaw LP. Laparoscopic hernia repair: the anatomic basis. J Laparoendosc Surg 1991;1:269.
8. Wantz GE. Atlas of hernia surgery. New York: Raven Press; 1991.
9. Condon RE. The anatomy of the inguinal region and its relation to groin hernia. In: Nyhus LM, Condon RE, editors. Hernia. 3rd ed. Philadelphia: JB Lippincott; 1989. p. 18.
10. Wellwood J, Sculpher MJ, Stoker D, et al. Randomized clinical trial of laparoscopic versus open mesh repair for inguinal hernia: outcome and cost. BMJ 1998;317:103.
11. Amado WJ. Anesthesia for hernia surgery. Surg Clin North Am 1993;73:427.
12. Kehlet H, Aasvang E. Groin hernia repair: anesthesia. World J Surg 2005;29:1058–61.
13. Van Veen RN, Wijsmuller AR, Vrijland WW, et al. Long-term follow-up of a randomized clinical trial of non-mesh versus mesh repair of primary inguinal hernia. Br J Surg 2007;94:506–10.
14. Fitzgibbons RJ Jr. Can we be sure polypropylene mesh causes infertility? Ann Surg 2005;241:559–61.
15. Bringman S, Heikkinen TJ, Wollert S, et al. Early results of a single-blinded, randomized, controlled, Internet-based multicenter trial comparing Prolene and Vypro II mesh in Lichtenstein hernioplasty. Hernia 2004;8:127–34.
16. Nikkolo C, Lepner U, Murruste M, et al. Randomised clinical trial comparing lightweight mesh with heavyweight mesh for inguinal hernioplasty. Hernia 2010;14:253–8.
17. Chowbey PK, Garg N, Sharma A, et al. Prospective randomized clinical trial comparing lightweight mesh and heavyweight polypropylene mesh in endoscopic totally extraperitonel groin hernia repair. Surg Endosc 2010;24: 3073–9.
18. Li J, Ji Z, Cheng T. Lightweight versus heavyweight in inguinal hernia repair: a meta-analysis. Hernia 2012;16:529–39. Epub 2012 Jun 12.
19. Scott NW, McCormack K, Graham P, et al. Open mesh versus non-mesh for groin hernia repair (Cochrane Review). Cochrane Database Syst Rev 2002;(4):CD002197.
20. Amid PK. Groin hernia repair: open techniques. World J Surg 2005;29:1046–51.
21. Chung L, O'Dwyer PJ. Treatment of asymptomatic inguinal hernias. Surgeon 2007;5:95–100.
22. O'Dwyer PJ, Norrie J, Alani A, et al. Observation or operation for patients with an asymptomatic inguinal hernia: a randomized clinical trial. Ann Surg 2006;244:167–73.
23. Fitzgibbons RJ Jr, Giobbie-Hurder A, Gibbs JO, et al. Watchful waiting vs repair of inguinal hernia in minimally symptomatic men: a randomized clinical trial. JAMA 2006; 295:285–92.
24. Chung L, Norrie J, O'Dwyer PJ. Long-term follow-up of patients with a painless inguinal hernia from a randomized clinical trial. Br J Surg 2011;98:596–9.
25. Laproscopic surgery for inguinal hernia repair. Technology Appraisal Guidance 83. National Institute for Clinical Excellence. 2004. Available at: www.nice.org.uk.
26. Wijsmuller AR, van Veen RN, Bosch JL, et al. Nerve management during open hernia repair. Br J Surg 2007;94:17.
27. Koch A, Edwards A, Haapaniemi S, et al. Prospective evaluation of 6895 groin hernia repairs in women. Br J Surg 2005;92:1553.
28. Gilbert AI. Sutureless repair of inguinal hernia. Am J Surg 1992;163:331.
29. Millikan KW, Cummings B, Doolas A. The Millikan modified mesh-plug hernioplasty. Arch Surg 2003;138:525.
30. Rutkow IM, Robbins AW. "Tension-free" inguinal herniorrhaphy: a preliminary report on the "mesh plug" technique. Surgery 1993;114:3.
31. Frey DM, Wildisen A, Hamel CT, et al. Randomized clinical trial of Lichtenstein's operation versus mesh plug for inguinal hernia repair. Br J Surg 2007;94:36.
32. Arregui ME. Transabdominal retroperitoneal inguinal herniorrhaphy. In: MacFayden BV, Ponsky JL, editors. Operative laparoscopy and thoracoscopy. Philadelphia: Lippincott-Raven; 1996. p. 1062–5.
33. McKernan JB, Laws HL. Laparoscopic repair of inguinal hernias using a totally extraperitoneal prosthetic approach. Surg Endosc 1993;7:26.
34. McKernan JB. Extraperitoneal inguinal herniorrhaphy. In: MacFayden BV, Ponsky JL, editors. Operative laparoscopy and thoracoscopy. Philadelphia: Lippincott-Raven; 1996. p. 225–31.
35. Stoppa R, Warlaumont C, Verhaeghe P, et al. Dacron mesh and surgical therapy of inguinal hernia. Chir Patol Sper 1986;34:15.
36. Stoppa R, Warlaumont CR. The preperitoneal approach and prosthetic repair of groin hernias. In: Nyhus LM, Condon RE, editors. Hernia. 3rd ed. Philadelphia: JB Lippincott; 1989. p. 364–78.
37. Stoppa R. The treatment of complicated groin and incisional hernias. World J Surg 1989;13:545.
38. Wantz GE. Giant prosthetic reinforcement of the visceral sac. Surg Gynecol Obstet 1989;169:408.
39. Felix EL. Laparoscopic extraperitoneal hernia repair. In: Eubanks WS, Swanstrom LL, Soper NJ, editors. Mastery of endoscopic and laparoscopic surgery. Philadelphia: Lippincott Williams & Williams; 2000. p. 443–55.
40. Taylor C, Layani L, Liew V, et al. Laparoscopic inguinal hernia repair without mesh fixation, early results of a large randomised clinical trial. Surg Endosc 2008;22:757–62.
41. Kaul A, Hutfless S, Le H, et al. Staple versus fibrin glue fixation in laparoscopic total extraperitoneal repair of inguinal hernia: a systematic review and meta-analysis. Surg Endosc 2012;26:1269–78.
42. Wantz GE, Fischer E. Unilateral giant prosthetic reinforcement of the visceral sac. In: Fitzgibbons RJ Jr, Greenburg AG, editors. Nyhus and Condon's hernia. 5th ed. Philadelphia: Lippincott Williams & Wilkins; 2002. p. 219.
43. Rignault DP. Properitoneal prosthetic inguinal hernioplasty through a Pfannenstiel approach. Surg Gynecol Obstet 1986;163:465.
44. Kugel RD. Minimally invasive, nonlaparoscopic, preperitoneal, and sutureless, inguinal herniorrhaphy. Am J Surg 1999;178:298.
45. Ugahary F. The gridiron hernioplasty. In: Bendavid R, Abrahamson J, Arregui M, et al, editors. Abdominal wall hernias: principles and management. New York: Springer-Verlag; 2001. p. 407.
46. Haapaniemi S, Gunnarsson U, Nordin P, et al. Reoperation after recurrent groin hernia repair. Ann Surg 2001;234:122.
47. Fitzgibbons RJ Jr, Giobbie-Hurder A, Gibbs JO, et al. Watchful waiting vs repair of inguinal hernia in minimally symptomatic men: a randomized clinical trial. JAMA 2006; 295:285.

48. Neumayer L, Giobbie-Hurder A, Jonasson O, et al. Open mesh versus laparoscopic mesh repair of inguinal hernia. N Engl J Med 2004;350:1819.
49. McCormack K, Scott NW, Go PM, et al. Laparoscopic techniques versus open techniques for inguinal hernia repair. Cochrane Database Syst Rev 2003;(1):CD001785.
50. Heikkinein TJ, Bringman S, Ohtonen P, et al. Five-year outcome of laparoscopic and Lichtenstein hernioplasties. Surg Endosc 2004;18:518.
51. Fitzgibbons RJ Jr, Camps J, Cornet DA, et al. Laparoscopic inguinal herniorrhaphy: results of a multicenter trial. Ann Surg 1995;221:3.
52. Poobalan AS, Bruce J, Smith WC, et al. A review of chronic pain after inguinal herniorrhaphy. Clin J Pain 2003;19:48.
53. Bueno J, Serralta A, Planells M, et al. Inguinodynia after two inguinal herniorrhaphy methods. Surg Laparosc Endosc Percutan Tech 2004;14:210.
54. O'Dwyer PJ, Alani A, McConnachie A. Groin hernia repair: postherniorrhaphy pain. World J Surg 2005;29:1062.
55. Johansson B, Hallerbäck B, Glise H, et al. Laparoscopic mesh versus open preperitoneal mesh versus conventional technique for inguinal hernia repair: a randomized multicenter trial (SCUR hernia repair study). Ann Surg 1999;230:225.
56. Heikkinen T, Haukipuro K, Leppälä J, et al. Total costs of laparoscopic and Lichtenstein inguinal hernia repairs: a prospective study. Surg Laparosc Endosc 1997;7:1
57. [illegible] after open versus extra-peritoneal endoscopic tension-free hernioplasty: a randomized clinical trial. Surgery 1996;119:552.
58. Champault GG, Rizk N, Catheline J-M, et al. Inguinal hernia repair: totally preperitoneal laparoscopic approach versus Stoppa operation: randomized trial of 100 cases. Surg Laparosc Endosc 1997;7:445.
59. Khoury N. A randomized prospective controlled trial of laparoscopic extraperitoneal hernia repair and mesh-plug hernioplasty: a study of 315 cases. J Laparoendosc Surg 1998;8:367.
60. Memon MA, Fitzgibbons RJ. Laparoscopic inguinal hernia repair: transabdominal (TAPP) and totally extraperitoneal (TEP). In: Scott-Connor CEH, editor. The SAGES manual. New York: Springer; 1999. p. 365–78.
61. Wantz GE. Ambulatory surgical treatment of groin hernia: prevention and management of complications. Prob Gen Surg 1986;3:311.
62. Heikkinen TJ, Haukipuro K, Halkko A. A cost and outcome comparison between laparoscopic and Lichtenstein hernia operations in a day-case unit: a randomized prospective study. Surg Endosc 1998;12:1199.
63. Laparoscopic versus open repair of groin hernia: a randomized comparison. MRC Laparoscopic Groin Hernia Trial Group. Lancet 1999;354:185.
64. MacFayden BV Jr, Arregui M, Corbitt J, et al. Complications of laparoscopic herniorrhaphy. Surg Endosc 1993;7:155.
65. Sanchez-Manuel FJ, Seco-Gil JL. Antibiotic prophylaxis for hernia repair. Cochrane Database Syst Rev 2004;(4):CD003769.
66. Avtan L, Avci C, Bulut T, et al. Mesh infections after laparoscopic inguinal hernia repair. Surg Laparosc Endosc 1997;7:192.
67. Gray MR, Curtis JM, Elkington JS. Colovesical fistula after laparoscopic inguinal hernia repair. Br J Surg 1994;81:1213.
68. Miller K, Junger W. Ileocutaneous fistula formation following laparoscopic polypropylene mesh hernia repair. Surg Endosc 1997;11:772.
69. Silich RC, McSherry CK. Spermatic granuloma. an uncommon complication of the tension-free hernia repair. Surg Endosc 1996;10:537.
70. Shin D, Lipshultz LI, Goldstein M, et al. Herniorrhaphy with polypropylene mesh causing inguinal vasal obstruction: a preventable cause of obstructive azoospermia. Ann Surg 2005;241:553.
71. Phillips EH, Arregui ME, Carroll BJ, et al. Incidence of complications following laparoscopic hernioplasty. Surg Endosc 1995;9:16.
72. Schneider BE, Castillo JM, Villegas L, et al. Laparoscopic totally extraperitoneal versus Lichtenstein herniorrhaphy: cost comparison at teaching hospitals. Surg Laparosc Endosc Percutan Tech 2003;3:261.
73. Leim MSL, van Steensel CJ, Boelhouwer RU, et al. The learning curve for totally extraperitoneal laparoscopic inguinal hernia repair. Am J Surg 1997;171:281.
74. Pawanindra L, Kajla RK, Chander J, et al. Randomized controlled study of laparoscopic total extraperitoneal vs. open Lichtenstein inguinal hernia repair. Surg Endosc 2003;17:850.
75. Bringman S, Ramel S, Heikkinen T, et al. Tension-free inguinal hernia repair: TEP versus mesh plug versus Lichtenstein: a prospective randomized controlled trial. Ann Surg 2003;237:142.
76. Filipi CJ, Gaston-Johansson F, McBride PJ, et al. An assessment of pain and return to normal activity: laparoscopic herniorrhaphy vs. open tension-free Lichtenstein repair. Surg Endosc 1996;10:983.
77. Ramshaw BJ, Tucker JG, Conner T, et al. A comparison of the approaches to laparoscopic herniorrhaphy. Surg Endosc 1996;10:29.
78. O'Reilly EA, Burke JP, O'Connell PR. A meta-analysis of surgical morbidity and recurrence after laparoscopic and open repair of primary unilateral inguinal hernia. Ann Surg 2012;255:846–53.
79. Neumayer L, Giobie-Hurder A, Jonasson O, et al. Open mesh versus laparoscopic mesh repair of inguinal hernia. N Engl J Med 2004;350:1819–27.
80. Mahon D, Decadt B, Rhodes M. Prospective randomized trial of laparoscopic (transabdominal preperitoneal) vs. open (mesh) repair for bilateral and recurrent inguinal hernia. Surg Endosc 2003;17:1386.
81. Tanaka N, Uchida N, Ogihara H, et al. Clinical study of inguinal and femoral incarcerated hernias. Surg Today 2010;40:1144–7.
82. Romain B, Chemaly R, Meyer N, et al. Prognostic factors of postoperative morbidity and mortality in strangulated groin hernia. Hernia 2012;16:405–10.

Acknowledgments

Figures 2a and 9 Christine Kenney

27 INTESTINAL ANASTOMOSIS

Neil J. Mortensen, MD, and Shazad Ashraf, MD

The creation of a join between two bowel ends is an operative procedure that is of central importance in the practice of a general surgeon. Despite the potentially disastrous consequences that can arise from leakage of an intestinal anastomosis, joining bowel segments is one of the procedures that junior surgeons often perform in the emergency setting. With proper supervision and appreciation of fundamental concerns, however, there is little difference between the outcomes of anastomoses performed by trainees and those performed by established surgeons.[1]

To minimize the risk of potential complications, it is imperative to adhere to several well-established principles [*see Table 1*]. The main ones relate to the creation of a tension-free join with good apposition of the bowel edges in the presence of an excellent blood supply.[2] The importance of surgical technique is underscored by the wide variations of anastomotic leakage rates among surgeons.[3]

The frequency of anastomotic leakage ranges from 1 to 24%.[4–6] The rate of leakage is generally considered to be higher for elective rectal anastomoses (12 to 19%) than for colonic anastomoses (11%).[7–9] The consequences of postoperative dehiscence are dire and include peritonitis, bloodstream infection, further surgery, creation of a defunctioning stoma and death. A threefold rise in mortality was seen (from 7% to 22%) in the St. Mary's Large Bowel Cancer Project, when anastomotic leakage occurred.[7] Also other problems encountered include a significant increase in hospital stay, and there is a proportion of patients who do not go on to have their stomas reversed.[4]

This chapter is divided into three broad sections. The first discusses factors that influence intestinal anastomotic healing. The second analyzes different technical options for creating anastomoses. The third and final section concentrates on the operative techniques that are currently used in constructing intestinal anastomoses.

Intestinal Healing

The process of intestinal anastomotic healing mimics that of wound healing elsewhere in the body in that it can be arbitrarily divided into an acute inflammatory (lag) phase, a proliferative phase, and, finally, a remodeling or maturation phase. Collagen is the single most important molecule for determining intestinal wall strength, which makes its metabolism of particular interest for understanding anastomotic healing. During the proliferative stage, fibroblasts become the predominant cell type, playing an important role in laying down collagen in the extracellular space. At the epithelial level, the crypts undergo division to cover the defect on the luminal surface of the bowel. The density of collagen synthesis is in a constant state of dynamic equilibrium, which is dependent on the balance between the rate of synthesis and that of collagenolysis. After surgery, degradation of mature collagen begins in the first 24 hours and predominates for the first 4 days. This is caused by the upregulation of matrix metalloproteinases (MMPs), which are an important class of enzymes involved in collagen metabolism.[10] This family includes 20 zinc-dependent endopeptidases, among which is collagenase (MMP-1).[10] In vivo use of MMP inhibitors has been found to increase the strength of intestinal anastomoses by up to 48% at postoperative day 3, which suggests that these enzymes may be important in determining the risk of leakage.[11] Sepsis is thought to increase the level of transcription and activity of these enzymes, thereby potentially leading to problems in the early postoperative period. In an animal model where bacterial peritonitis was induced, increased MMP levels were seen on postoperative day 3, coinciding with a fall in the bursting pressure.[10] However, no increase in anastomotic dehiscence was found in comparison with the control group. By postoperative day 7, collagen synthesis becomes the dominant force, particularly proximal to the anastomosis. After 5 to 6 weeks, there is no significant increase in the amount of collagen in a healing wound or anastomosis, though turnover and thus synthesis are extensive. The strength of the scar continues to increase for many months after injury.

The cross-linking between collagen fibers and their orientation are the major factors that determine the tensile strength of tissues. Bursting pressure is used as a quantitative measure to grade the strength of an anastomosis in vivo. This pressure has been found to increase rapidly in the early postoperative period, reaching 60% of the strength of the surrounding bowel by 3 to 4 days and 100% by 1 week.[12,13] The submucosal layer is, in fact, where the tensile strength of the bowel lies, as a consequence of its high content of collagen fibers [*see Figure 1*]. Therefore, in constructing a hand-sewn intestinal anastomosis, it is imperative that this layer is included when extramucosal bites are taken. Collagen synthetic capacity is relatively uniform throughout the large bowel but less so in the small intestine: synthesis is significantly higher in the proximal and distal small intestine than in the midjejunum. Overall collagen synthetic capacity is somewhat less in the small intestine. Although no significant difference has been found between the strength of ileal anastomoses and that of colonic anastomoses at 4 days, colonic collagen formation is much greater in the first 48 hours.[14] It is noteworthy that the synthetic response is not restricted to the anastomotic site but appears to be generalized to a significant extent.[15] The presence of the visceral peritoneum on the bowel wall also has an influence on the ease with which two bowel ends can be joined. This effect is highlighted by the increased technical difficulty of joining extraperitoneal bowel ends, for example the thoracic esophagus and the rectum.

bent or cut staples, the integrity of the anastomosis was not compromised in any way, nor was healing adversely affected.[34,35]

HAND-SEWN VERSUS STAPLED ANASTOMOSES

Titanium staples are ideal for tissue apposition at anastomotic sites because they provoke only a minimal inflammatory response and provide immediate strength to the cut surfaces during the weakest phase of healing. Initially, tissue eversion at the stapled anastomosis was a major concern, given that everted handsewn anastomoses had previously been shown to be inferior to inverted ones; however, the greater support and improved blood supply to the healing tissues associated with stapling tend to counteract the negative effects of eversion. In fact, one study found that bursting strength for canine colonic end-to-end anastomoses was six times greater when the procedure was performed with an EEA stapler than when it was done with interrupted Dacron sutures.[36]

In 1993, a randomized multicenter trial studied 440 patients who had either hand-sewn or stapled anastomoses after ileocolic resection for cancer.[37] The patients were assessed both clinically and by imaging for the presence of a leak (consisting of a contrast enema at about 10 days after the operation). The overall leakage rate in the hand-sewn group was 8.3%, which compared unfavorably with the 2.8% rate in the stapled group. A possible explanation for the higher rate in the hand-sewn group might have been surgical inexperience with the variety of suture techniques used in the study (end-to-end and end-to-side with either continuous or interrupted sutures). In a study from the West of Scotland and Highland Anastomosis Study Group that included data on 732 patients at 5 centers, the rate of radiologically proven leakage was significantly higher in the sutured group (14.4% versus 5.2%); however, no difference was seen with respect to clinical leaks, morbidity, or postoperative mortality.[38] A 1998 meta-analysis comparing the hand-sewn and stapled techniques of intestinal anastomosis addressed 13 trials published from 1980 to 1995.[39] For colorectal anastomoses, no significant differences were seen in mortality, total leakage rate, clinical leakage rate, radiologic leakage rate, tumor recurrence rate, or incidence of wound sepsis. Strictures and technical problems, however, were more common in the stapled group. A subsequent meta-analysis that reviewed data from 955 patients with ileocolic anastomoses reported a significant reduction in the overall leakage rate and the clinical leakage rate when stapling was employed.[40]

Even when the anastomosis had to heal under adverse conditions (e.g., carcinomatosis, malnutrition, previous chemotherapy or radiation therapy, bowel obstruction, anemia, or leukopenia), no significant differences have been demonstrated between stapled and hand-sewn anastomoses. Stapling has, however, been shown to shorten operating time, especially for low pelvic anastomoses. Cancer recurrence rates at the site of the anastomosis have been reported to be higher or lower depending on the technique used. Certainly, suture materials engender a more pronounced cellular proliferative response than titanium staples do, particularly with full-thickness sutures as opposed to seromuscular ones, and malignant cells have been shown to adhere to suture materials.[41,42]

UNUSUAL TECHNIQUES

In 1892, Murphy introduced his button, which consisted of a two-part metal stud that was designed to hold the bowel edges in apposition without suturing until adhesion had occurred.[43] Thereafter, the stud was voided via the rectum. Several modifications of this technique have been described since then, primarily focusing on the composition of the rings or stents. In particular, dissolvable polyglycolic acid systems have been developed. These so-called biofragmentable anastomotic rings leave a gap of 1.5, 2.0, or 2.5 mm between the bowel ends to prevent ischemia of the anastomotic line.

The use of adhesive agents such as methyl-2-cyanoacrylate to approximate the divided ends of intestinal segments has been studied as well.[44] There was only a moderate inflammatory response at the wound, which persisted for 2 to 3 weeks. Leakage rates were high, however, and many technical problems remained (e.g., how to stabilize the bowel edges while they underwent adhesion). Fibrin glues have also been employed in this setting. Although these substances are not strong enough to hold two pieces of bowel in apposition, they have been used to coat a sutured bowel anastomosis in an effort to reduce the risk of anastomotic failure. To date, no controlled clinical trials have confirmed that this approach is worthwhile.

FACTORS CONTRIBUTING TO FAILURE OF ANASTOMOSES

Type and Location of Anastomosis

Since the introduction of stapling, there has been an increase in the number of extremely low anterior resections being performed routinely. The literature seems to suggest that rectal anastomoses are more prone to leakage than more proximal joins are.[7–9] A retrospective review of risk factors in patients undergoing rectal resection for cancer found that low anastomoses, defined as being 5 cm or less from the anal verge, were associated with a 6.5-fold increased risk of leakage when compared to anastomoses that were more than 5 cm from the anal verge.[45] Another study showed that the leakage rate was increased in patients undergoing low colorectal anterior resection in the absence of a proximal stoma (the leakage rate was 17%, which fell to 6% when a stoma was present).[46] The technique of total mesorectal excision (TME), which is now standard for rectal cancer operations, has reduced the local recurrence rate to 5% at 5 years.[47] However, the incidence of anastomotic leakage in patients undergoing TME for low anterior resection is higher in the absence of a defunctioning stoma (25% versus 8%).[48] The Rectal Cancer Trial on Defunctioning Stoma (a randomized multicenter trial) studied the outcomes of 234 patients undergoing low anterior resection with a defunctioning stoma.[4] The overall leakage rate was 19.2%; however, the rate in the group that had a stoma was only 10.3%, compared with 28.0% in the group that did not. Therefore, it is safe practice to cover a low anterior resection with a defunctioning stoma.

Patient Preparation

Patients who present in the emergency setting are usually compromised in terms of hydration status, typically as a consequence of sepsis, obstruction, or a combination of the two. Preoperative fluid optimization is always necessary and may require the aid of intensivists. Before an elective procedure, the patient is assessed with regard to systemic diseases (e.g., cardiovascular, respiratory, or diabetes), and anemia is corrected. Adequate preoperative antibiotic prophylaxis has been shown to reduce the risk of postoperative infection in all types of bowel surgery and must be given at the start of the operation [*see 2:1 Prevention of Postoperative Infection*]. Some patients require additional steroids perioperatively [*see 9:12 Stress Response and Endocrine Deregulation during Critical Illness*].

Mechanical bowel preparation (MBP) has been thought to be an essential component of colorectal surgery for more than 100 years.[49,50] Emptying the bowel before elective operations on the colon was traditional until about 5 years ago, and indeed, this practice was recommended by the Association of Surgeons of Great Britain and Ireland (ASGBI) until relatively recently.[51,52] The evidence for MBP was derived from observational studies showing that mechanical clearance of feces from the bowel was associated with reduced morbidity and mortality in colonic surgery.[53] Proponents of MBP listed several advantages, such as reduction in intraluminal bacterial load, prevention of potential anastomotic disruption by fecal pellets and also easier handling of bowel.[54] In recent years, however, there has been a shift in practice regarding the use of MBP.

A Swiss randomized clinical trial published in 2005 studied the effect of MBP on patients undergoing left-side colorectal resection with primary anastomosis.[54] The anastomotic leakage rate proved to be lower in the group that did not receive MBP than in the group that did. Furthermore, the former group spent less time in hospital and exhibited less extra-abdominal morbidity (e.g., pneumonia and cardiac-related problems). These results seemed to agree with the findings of a Cochrane review.[52] Two large randomized trials published in 2007 compared the outcomes of patients who underwent MBP (with either polyethylene glycol or sodium phosphate) and patients who did not.[55,56] One recruited 1,431 patients undergoing elective colorectal surgery from 13 centers.[55] Leakage was defined by the onset of significant symptoms and corroborated by means of imaging. The rate of leakage was 4.8% in the MBP group, which was not significantly different from the 5.4% rate in the non-MBP group. The other trial examined 1,343 patients from 21 centers and found no significant differences in outcomes (such as cardiovascular problems, general infections and surgical site infections) between the MBP group and the non-MBP group.[56] However, in a a subsequent meta-analysis[57] that examined data from 10 randomized trials conducted over the past 24 years, the rates of both anastomotic leakage and wound infection were significantly higher in the MBP group than in the non-MBP group (5.1 versus 2.6% and 8.2% versus 5.5%, respectively).[57] Possible explanations of these findings include immune changes in the colonic mucosa that might impede wound repair.[57] In view of the currently available evidence, some surgical institutions, including our own, have chosen to adopt a policy of employing fluid restriction and enemas rather than MBP before elective colorectal surgery.[58]

Enemas are given to patients undergoing anterior resections to ensure that fecal matter does not impede the use of stapling devices. It is advisable for patients to stop eating solid food 24 hours before the operation. Many trials have confirmed the benefits of giving IV antibiotics over the perioperative period.[59] However, there is some evidence to suggest that there is an increased risk of *Clostridium difficile*–associated diarrhea with the use of cephalosporin, penicillin, and clindamycin.[60–62] Prophylaxis of thromboembolism [*see 7:6 Venous Thromboembolism*] is mandatory in all patients scheduled to undergo intestinal anastomosis. There is very little evidence in the literature to indicate that thromboembolism has any direct effect on anastomotic leakage rates. However, mesenteric venous thrombosis (MVT) accounts for one-tenth of acute mesenteric ischemic events.[63] The extent of thromboses is variable, with the worst outcome being mesenteric infarction necessitating urgent repeat laparotomy. Inadequate prophylaxis may increase the risk that MVT will occur postoperatively, especially in patients with other risk factors (e.g., a hypercoagulable state, previous thrombosis, or a history of smoking).

Associated Diseases and Systemic Factors

Anemia, diabetes mellitus, previous irradiation or chemotherapy, malnutrition with hypoalbuminemia, and vitamin deficiencies are all associated with poor anastomotic healing. Some of these factors can be corrected preoperatively. Malnourished patients benefit from nutritional support delivered enterally or parenterally before and after operation [*see 11:19 Nutritional Support*]. Well-nourished patients appear not to derive similar benefits from such support.[64]

Resections for Crohn disease appear to carry a significant risk of anastomotic dehiscence (12% in one prospective study) even when macroscopically normal margins are obtained.[65] With the lifetime risk of repeated resections, strictureplasty has therefore become an attractive alternative to resectional management of Crohn disease even in the presence of moderately long strictures, diseased tissue, or sites of previous anastomoses. This approach allows preservation of more of the length of the small intestine.

The glucocorticoid response to injury may attenuate physiologic responses to other mediators whose combined effects could be deleterious to the organism.[66] In animal experiments, wound healing, as measured by the bursting pressure of an ileal anastomosis 1 week after operation, was optimal at a plasma corticosterone level that maintained maximal nitrogen balance and corresponded to the mean corticosterone level of normal animals.[67] Both supranormal and subnormal cortisol levels resulted in significantly impaired wound healing, probably through different mechanisms. It is believed that slow protein turnover is responsible for delayed anastomotic healing in adrenalectomized animals, whereas negative nitrogen metabolic balance is responsible for increased protein breakdown and delayed healing in animals with excess glucocorticoid activity.[67,68]

Lifestyle factors have also been associated with an increased risk of leakage. A Danish prospective study of 333 consecutive patients undergoing colorectal resection collected lifestyle information by means of a questionnaire.[69] The overall leakage rate was 15.9% (53 out of 333). Smoking was found to be associated with an increased risk of anastomotic leakage (relative risk 3.18), as was alcohol consumption exceeding 35 units a week (relative risk 7.18).

CONTROVERSIAL ISSUES IN INTESTINAL ANASTOMOSIS

Inversion versus Eversion

The question of the importance of inversion (as described by Lembert in the early 1800s) versus eversion of the improved functional outcome, especially in the early postoperative period in older patients.[83] A whip-stitch (or purse-string suture) of 2-0 polypropylene is placed around the colotomy, and the anvil from the appropriately sized curved EEA stapler is inserted into the open end and secured in place by tying the suture [*see Figure 7*].The proximal bowel clamp is removed. The assistant—who may also, if desired, gently wash out the rectal stump with a dilute povidone-iodine solution—performs a digital rectal examination.

The stapler, with its trocar attachment in place, is then inserted into the anus under the careful guidance of the surgeon. The pointed shaft is brought out through or adjacent to the linear staple line, and the sharp point is removed. The peg from the anvil in the proximal colon is snapped into the protruding shaft of the stapler, and the two edges are slowly brought together. The colonic mesentery must not be twisted, and the ends must come together without any tension whatsoever. The stapler is fired. In some types of stapling guns, a crunching sound is heard. The anvil is then loosened the appropriate amount, and the entire mechanism is withdrawn through the anus. Finally, the proximal and distal rings of tissue, which remain on the stapler, are carefully inspected to confirm circumferential closure of the staple line.

The pelvis is then filled with body-temperature saline, and a Toomey or bladder syringe is used to insufflate the neorectum with air. The surgeon watches for bubbling in the pelvis as a sign of leakage from the anastomosis. If there is a leak, additional soluble sutures must be placed to close the defect and another air test performed. A rectal tube may then be inserted by the assistant or may be placed at the end of the procedure. When the anastomosis is very low or there is some concern about healing, a drain may be placed in the pelvis behind the staple line; however, as noted [*see* Controversial Issues in Intestinal Anastomosis, *above*], this practice has not been shown to be beneficial and may in fact impair healing.

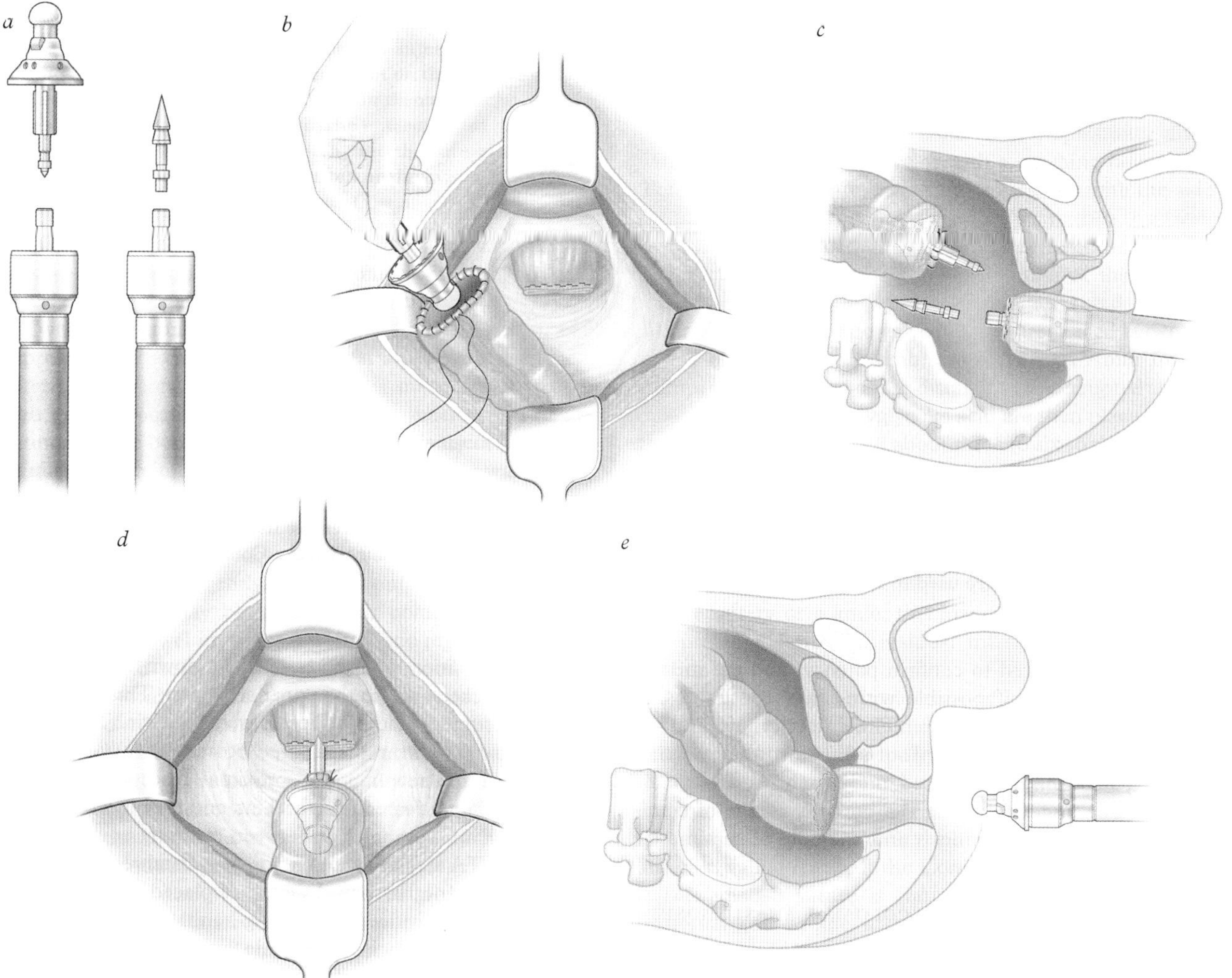

Figure 7 **Double-stapled end-to-end coloanal anastomosis. (*a*) The C-EEA stapler comes with both a standard anvil (left) and a trocar attachment (right). A more recent version of these staplers comes with a trocar in the body rather than in the head of the device. (*b*) The rectal stump is closed with an angled linear noncutting stapler. A purse-string suture is placed around the colotomy, and the anvil of the stapler is placed in the open end and secured. (*c*) The stapler, with the sharp trocar attachment in place, is inserted into the anus, and the trocar is made to pierce the rectal stump at or near the staple line, after which the trocar is removed. (*d*) The anvil in the proximal colon is joined with the stapler in the rectal stump, and the two edges are slowly brought together. (*e*) The stapler is fired and then gently withdrawn.**

As noted (see above), a 1998 meta-analysis by Macrae demonstrated an association between stapled anastomoses and an increased incidence of colorectal anastomotic strictures, in comparison with hand-sewn anastomoses.[39] The cause of this association remains uncertain. Most of these patients were asymptomatic and in those who required treatment, simple dilatation was sufficient to rectify the problem. A 2007 Cochrane review did not find the risk of anastomotic stricture to be increased in patients undergoing ileocolic resection with a linear cutting stapler.[40]

Conclusion

Any anastomosis, no matter how technically sound on creation, may fail. The limiting factor may be the tissue or the resulting inflammatory sequelae that follow closure of the abdominal wall. Therefore, as for ultralow anterior resections, it is important to recognize any potential risk factors and take the measures necessary to prevent any harm that may ensue if leakage results. This may mean giving the patient a temporary stoma. Even if fecal diversion has been carried out, it is important to keep watching closely for any signs of failure and to take prompt action if such signs appear.

Anastomotic failure rates have improved over the past two centuries, and postoperative morbidity and mortality have decreased accordingly. These beneficial developments can be attributed to a combination of factors, such as better appreciation of the principles of healing, improved anesthesia, appropriate antibiotic prophylaxis, and enhanced postoperative monitoring. Currently, with the emergence of laparoscopic colorectal surgery, it is essential that the surgeon continues to practice the same principles of creating a join—good apposition of the edges, without tension and with an optimal blood supply—just as for open colorectal surgery.

Financial Disclosures: None Reported

References

1. Singh K, Aitken RJ. Outcome in patients with colorectal cancer managed by surgical trainees. Br J Surg 1999;86:1332–6.
2. Gillespie IE. Intestinal anastomosis. Br Med J (Clin Res Ed) 1983;286:1002.
3. Smith SRG, Connolly JC, Crane PW. The effect of surgical drainage materials on colonic healing. Br J Surg 1982;69:153.
4. Matthiessen P, Hallbook O, Rutegard J, et al. Defunctioning stoma reduces symptomatic anastomotic leakage after low anterior resection of the rectum for cancer: a randomized multicenter trial. Ann Surg 2007;246: 207–14.
5. Enker WE, Merchant N, Cohen AM, et al. Safety and efficacy of low anterior resection for rectal cancer: 681 consecutive cases from a specialty service. Ann Surg 1999;230: 544–52; discussion 552–4.
6. Matthiessen P, Hallbook O, Andersson M, et al. Risk factors for anastomotic leakage after anterior resection of the rectum. Colorectal Dis 2004;6:462–9.
7. Fielding LP, Stewart-Brown S, Blesovsky L, Kearney G. Anastomotic integrity after operations for large-bowel cancer: a multicentre study. Br Med J 1980;281:411–4.
8. Karanjia ND, Corder AP, Bearn P, Heald RJ. Leakage from stapled low anastomosis after total mesorectal excision for carcinoma of the rectum. Br J Surg 1994;81:1224–6.
9. Pakkastie TE, Luukkonen PE, Jarvinen HJ. Anastomotic leakage after anterior resection of the rectum. Eur J Surg 1994;160:293–7; discussion 299–300.
10. de Hingh IH, de Man BM, Lomme RM, et al. Colonic anastomotic strength and matrix metalloproteinase activity in an experimental model of bacterial peritonitis. Br J Surg 2003; 90:981–8.
11. Syk I, Agren MS, Adawi D, Jeppsson B. Inhibition of matrix metalloproteinases enhances breaking strength of colonic anastomoses in an experimental model. Br J Surg 2001;88: 228–34.
12. Hesp F, Hendriks T, Lubbers E-J. Wound healing in the intestinal wall: a comparison between experimental ileal and colonic anastomoses. Dis Colon Rectum 1984;24: 99.
13. Wise L, McAlister W, Stein T. Studies on the healing of anastomoses of small and large intestines. Surg Gynecol Obstet 1975;141: 190.
14. Martens MF, Hendriks T. Postoperative changes in collagen synthesis in intestinal anastomoses of the rat: differences between small and large bowel. Gut 1991;32:1482–7.
15. Martens MF, de Man BM, Hendriks T, Goris RJ. Collagen synthetic capacity throughout the uninjured and anastomosed intestinal wall. Am J Surg 1992;164:354–60.
16. Khoury GA, Waxman BP. Large bowel anastomosis: I. The healing process and sutured anastomoses: a review. Br J Surg 1983;70:61.
17. Schrock TR, Deveney CW, Dunphy JE. Factors contributing to leakage of colonic anastomoses. Ann Surg 1973;177:513.
18. Daly JM, Vars HM, Dudrick SJ. Effects of protein depletion on strength of colonic anastomoses. Surg Gynecol Obstet 1972;134: 15–21.
19. Hastings JC, Van Winkle W, Barker E. Effects of suture materials on healing of wounds of the stomach and colon. Surg Gynecol Obstet 1975;140:701.
20. Tagart RE. Colorectal anastomosis: factors influencing success. J R Soc Med 1981;74: 111–8.
21. Bissett IP. Ileocolic anastomosis. Br J Surg 2007;94:1447–8.
22. Munday C, McGinn FP. A comparison of polyglycolic acid and catgut sutures in rat colonic anastomoses. Br J Surg 1976;63: 870–2.
23. Koruda MJ, Rolandelli RH. Experimental studies on the healing of colonic anastomoses. J Surg Res 1990;48:504–15.
24. Olsen GB, Letwin E, Williams HT. Clinical experience with the use of a single-layer intestinal anastomosis. Can J Surg 1968;11: 97–100.
25. Irvin TT, Goligher JC. Aetiology of disruption of intestinal anastomoses. Br J Surg 1973;60:461–4.
26. Sarin S, Lightwood RG. Continuous single-layer gastrointestinal anastomosis: a prospective audit. Br J Surg 1989;76:493–5.
27. Shandall A, Lowndes R, Young HL. Colonic anastomotic healing and oxygen tension. Br J Surg 1985;72:606–9.
28. Jiborn H, Ahonen J, Zederfeldt B. Healing of experimental colonic anastomoses: III. Collagen metabolism in the colon after left colon resection. Am J Surg 1980;139: 398–405.
29. Burch JM, Franciose RJ, Moore EE, et al. Single-layer continuous versus two-layer interrupted intestinal anastomosis: a prospective randomized trial. Ann Surg 2000;231: 832–7.
30. Shikata S, Yamagishi H, Taji Y, et al. Single- versus two- layer intestinal anastomosis: a meta-analysis of randomized controlled trials. BMC Surg 2006;6:2.
31. Chassin JL, Rifkind KM, Turner JW. Errors and pitfalls in stapling gastrointestinal tract anastomoses. Surg Clin North Am 1984;64: 441–59.
32. Ravitch MM. Intersecting staple lines in intestinal anastomoses. Surgery 1985;97: 8–15.
33. Chung RS. Blood flow in colonic anastomoses. Effect of stapling and suturing. Ann Surg 1987;206:335–9.
34. Julian TB, Ravitch MM. Evaluation of the safety of end-to-end (EEA) stapling anastomoses across linear stapled closures. Surg Clin North Am 1984;64:567–77.
35. Brennan SS, Pickford IR, Evans M, Pollock AV. Staples or sutures for colonic anastomoses—a controlled clinical trial. Br J Surg 1982; 69:722–4.
36. Greenstein A, Rogers P, Moss G. Doubled fourth-day colorectal anastomotic strength with complete retention of intestinal mature wound collagen and accelerated deposition following immediate full enteral nutrition. Surg Forum 1978;29:78–81.
37. Kracht M, Hay JM, Fagniez PL, Fingerhut A. Ileocolonic anastomosis after right hemicolectomy for carcinoma: stapled or hand-sewn? A prospective, multicenter, randomized trial. Int J Colorectal Dis 1993;8:29–33.
38. Docherty JG, McGregor JR, Akyol AM, et al. Comparison of manually constructed and stapled anastomoses in colorectal surgery. West of Scotland and Highland Anastomosis Study Group. Ann Surg 1995;221:176–84.
39. MacRae HM, McLeod RS. Handsewn vs. stapled anastomoses in colon and rectal surgery: a meta-analysis. Dis Colon Rectum 1998;41:180–9.
40. Choy PYG, Bissett IP, Docherty JG, et al. Stapled versus handsewn methods for ileocolic anastomoses. Cochrane Database Syst Rev 2007;(3):CD004320.
41. Akyol AM, McGregor JR, Galloway DJ, et al. Recurrence of colorectal cancer after sutured and stapled large bowel anastomoses. Br J Surg 1991;78:1297–300.

42. O'Dwyer P, Ravikumar TS, Steele G, Jr. Serum dependent variability in the adherence of tumour cells to surgical sutures. Br J Surg 1985;72:466–9.
43. Murphy JB. A contribution to abdominal surgery, ideal approximation of abdominal viscera without suture. North American Practitioner 1892;4:481.
44. Ballantyne GH. The experimental basis of intestinal suturing. Effect of surgical technique, inflammation, and infection on enteric wound healing. Dis Colon Rectum 1984;27:61–71.
45. Rullier E, Laurent C, Garrelon JL, et al. Risk factors for anastomotic leakage after resection of rectal cancer. Br J Surg 1998;85:355–8.
46. Dehni N, Schlegel RD, Cunningham C, et al. Influence of a defunctioning stoma on leakage rates after low colorectal anastomosis and colonic J pouch–anal anastomosis. Br J Surg 1998;85:1114–7.
47. Heald RJ, Husband EM, Ryall RD. The mesorectum in rectal cancer surgery—the clue to pelvic recurrence? Br J Surg 1982;69:613–6.
48. Carlsen E, Schlichting E, Guldvog I, et al. Effect of the introduction of total mesorectal excison for the treatment of rectal cancer. Br J Surg 1998;85:526–29.
49. Edwards DP. The history of colonic surgery in war. J R Army Med Corps 1999;145:107–8.
50. Halsted WS. Circular suture of the intestine: an experimental study. Am J Med Sci 1887;94:436–61.
51. The Association of Coloproctology of Great Britain and Ireland. Guidelines for the management of colorectal cancer (2001). London: The Association of Coloproctology of Great Britain and Ireland; 2001.
52. Guenaga KF, Matos D, Castro AA, et al. Mechanical bowel preparation for elective colorectal surgery. Cochrane Database Syst Rev 2005;(1):CD001544.
53. Nichols RL, Condon RE. Preoperative preparation of the colon. Surg Gynecol Obstet 1971;132:323–37.
54. Bucher P, Gervaz P, Soravia C, et al. Randomized clinical trial of mechanical bowel preparation versus no preparation before elective left-sided colorectal surgery. Br J Surg 2005;92:409–14.
55. Contant CM, Hop WC, van't Sant HP, et al. Mechanical bowel preparation for elective colorectal surgery: a multicentre randomised trial. Lancet 2007;370:2112–7.
56. Jung B, Pahlman L, Nystrom PO, Nilsson E. Multicentre randomized clinical trial of mechanical bowel preparation in elective colonic resection. Br J Surg 2007;94:689–95.
57. Bucher P, Gervaz P, Morel P. Should preoperative mechanical bowel preparation be abandoned? Ann Surg 2007;245:662.
58. Nichols RL, Gorbach SL, Condon RE. Alteration of intestinal microflora following preoperative mechanical preparation of the colon. Dis Colon Rectum 1971;14:123–7.
59. Jimenez JC, Wilson SE. Prophylaxis of infection for elective colorectal surgery. Surg Infect (Larchmt) 2003;4:273–80.
60. Thomas C, Stevenson M, Riley TV. Antibiotics and hospital-acquired *Clostridium difficile*–associated diarrhoea: a systematic review. J Antimicrob Chemother 2003;51:1339–50.
61. McFarland LV, Surawicz CM, Stamm WE. Risk factors for *Clostridium difficile* carriage and *C. difficile*–associated diarrhea in a cohort of hospitalized patients. J Infect Dis 1990;162:678–84.
62. Chang VT, Nelson K. The role of physical proximity in nosocomial diarrhea. Clin Infect Dis 2000;31:717–22.
63. Millikan KW, Szczerba SM, Dominguez JM, et al. Superior mesenteric and portal vein thrombosis following laparoscopic-assisted right hemicolectomy. Report of a case. Dis Colon Rectum 1996;39:1171–5.
64. Bozzetti F. Perioperative nutrition of patients with gastrointestinal cancer. Br J Surg 2002;89:1201–2.
65. Carty NJ, Keating J, Campbell J, et al. Prospective audit of an extramucosal technique for intestinal anastomosis. Br J Surg 1991;78:1439.
66. Munck A, Guyre PM, Holbrook NJ. Physiological functions of glucocorticoids in stress and their relation to pharmacological actions. Endocr Rev 1984;5:25–44.
67. Matsusue S, Walser M. Healing of intestinal anastomoses in adrenalectomized rats given corticosterone. Am J Physiol 1992;263(1 Pt 2):R164–8.
68. Quan ZY, Walser M. Effect of corticosterone administration at varying levels on leucine oxidation and whole body protein synthesis and breakdown in adrenalectomized rats. Metabolism 1991;40:1263–7.
69. Sorensen LT, Jorgensen T, Kirkeby LT, et al. Smoking and alcohol abuse are major risk factors for anastomotic leakage in colorectal surgery. Br J Surg 1999;86:927–31.
70. Getzen LC. Intestinal suturing: I. The development of intestinal sutures. Curr Probl Surg 1969:3–48.
71. Kratzer GL, Onsanit T. Single layer steel wire anastomosis of the intestine. Surg Gynecol Obstet 1974;139:93–4.
72. Ravitch MM, Steichen FM. Technics of staple suturing in the gastrointestinal tract. Ann Surg 1972;175:815–37.
73. Brunius U, Zederfeldt B. Effects of anti-inflammatory treatment on wound healing. Acta Chir Scand 1965;129:462–7.
74. Goligher J MC, McAdam W. A controlled trial of inverting versus everting intestinal suture in clinical large bowel surgery. Br J Surg 1970;57:817.
75. Burg R, Geigle CF, Faso JM, Theuerkauf FJ Jr. Omission of routine gastric decompression. Dis Colon Rectum 1978;21:98–100.
76. Reasbeck PG, Rice ML, Herbison GP. Nasogastric intubation after intestinal resection. Surg Gynecol Obstet 1984;158:354–8.
77. Argov S, Goldstein I, Barzilai A. Is routine use of the nasogastric tube justified in upper abdominal surgery? Am J Surg 1980;139:849–50.
78. Merad F, Yahchouchi E, Hay JM, Fingerhut A, Laborde Y, Langlois-Zantain O. Prophylactic abdominal drainage after elective colonic resection and suprapromontory anastomosis: a multicenter study controlled by randomization. French Associations for Surgical Research. Arch Surg 1998;133:309–14.
79. Yates JL. An experimental study of the local effects of peritoneal drainage. Surg Gynecol Obstet 1905;1:473.
80. Berliner SD, Burson LC, Lear PE. Use and abuse of intraperitoneal drains in colon surgery. Arch Surg 1964;89:686–9.
81. Merad F, Hay JM, Fingerhut A, et al. Is prophylactic pelvic drainage useful after elective rectal or anal anastomosis? A multicenter controlled randomized trial. French Association for Surgical Research. Surgery 1999;125:529–35.
82. Manz CW, LaTendresse C, Sako Y. The detrimental effects of drains on colonic anastomoses: an experimental study. Dis Colon Rectum 1970;13:17–25.
83. Sailer M, Fuchs KH, Fein M, Thiede A. Randomized clinical trial comparing quality of life after straight and pouch coloanal reconstruction. Br J Surg 2002;89:1108–17.

Acknowledgment

Figures 1 through 7 adapted from Tom Moore.

Portions of this chapter are based on previous iterations written for *ACS Surgery* by Zane Cohen, MD, Barry Sullivan, MD, and Julian Britton. The authors wish to thank Drs. Cohen, Sullivan, and Britton.

28 INTESTINAL STOMAS

J. Graham Williams, MCh, FRCS

Formation of an intestinal stoma is frequently a component of surgical intervention for diseases of the small bowel and the colon. The most common intestinal stomas are the ileostomies (end and loop) and the colostomies (end and loop); the less common stomas, such as cecostomy and appendicostomy, have limited applications and thus are not considered further in this chapter.

For optimal results, it is essential that stoma creation be considered an integral part of the surgical procedure, not merely an irritating and time-consuming addendum at the end of a long operation. Accordingly, the potential requirement for a stoma should be appropriately addressed in the planning of an intestinal procedure. A great effort should be made to counsel the patient before operation as to whether a stoma is likely to be needed, what stoma creation would involve, where the stoma would be situated, and whether the stoma is likely to be permanent or temporary.

Operative Planning

PREOPERATIVE COUNSELING

Ideally, as soon as surgical intervention that may involve a stoma is contemplated, the enterostomal nursing service should become involved, although this may not be possible in an emergency setting. Patients often have misconceptions about the effects a stoma will have on their quality of life and consequently may experience considerable anxiety. Adequate preoperative counseling helps correct these misconceptions and reduce the attendant anxiety. Enough time should be set aside to allow the counselor to explore the patient's knowledge of the disease and understanding of why a stoma may be required. This process involves reviewing the planned operation, describing what the stoma will look like, and explaining how the stoma will function. Visual aids (e.g., videos, CD-ROMs, and booklets) can be very useful in this regard and should be freely available to patients and their families. As simple a measure as showing the patient a stoma appliance and attaching it to the abdominal wall before the procedure can be helpful in preparing the patient for a stoma. Many patients facing the prospect of stoma surgery also derive great benefit from meeting patients of similar age and background who have a stoma.

CHOICE OF PROCEDURE

A number of common indications for stoma formation have been identified [*see Table 1*]. These indications are usually associated with particular types of stoma, but the association is not always a simple or automatic one. In many situations, more than one option exists, and it can be difficult to select the best available option for a particular patient.

Loop Ileostomy versus Loop Colostomy

Defunctioning of a distal anastomosis after rectal excision and anastomosis may be achieved with either a loop ileostomy or a loop transverse colostomy. A number of nonrandomized studies[1–3] and randomized control trials[4–7] have been performed in an effort to determine which of these two approaches is superior. Both types of stoma effectively defunction the distal bowel; however, loop ileostomy appears to be associated with a lower incidence of complications related to stoma formation and closure, although it may also carry a higher risk of postoperative intestinal obstruction.[6] The two types of stoma are comparable with respect to patient quality of life, and the degree of subsequent social restriction is influenced more by the number and type of complications than by the type of stoma formed.[8]

SELECTION OF STOMA SITE

A poorly sited stoma will cause considerable morbidity and adversely affect quality of life. For this reason, great emphasis should be placed on selecting the best site for the stoma on the abdominal wall. In many instances [*see Table 1*], it may not be possible to decide beforehand whether a colostomy or an ileostomy is to be performed. An example would be the case of a patient with a tumor in the lower rectum in which the surgeon's intention is to perform a restorative resection covered by a loop ileostomy. In such a case, the surgeon sometimes finds that restorative resection is not technically possible and elects to perform an abdominoperineal resection or a low Hartmann resection with an end colostomy instead.

A stoma should be brought out through a separate opening in the abdominal wall, not through the main incision: there is a high incidence of wound infection and incisional hernia formation if the main incision is used as a stoma site. In general, ileostomies are sited in the right iliac fossa, sigmoid colostomies (loop or end) in the left iliac fossa, and transverse loop colostomies in either the right or the left upper quadrant. These positions are preferred because they are conveniently close to the particular bowel segments to be used for creating the various stomas. At need, however—as when finding a suitable site proves difficult because of previous scars or deformity—both the ileum and the colon can be mobilized to provide sufficient length to reach most sites on the abdominal wall.

29 APPENDECTOMY

Hung S. Ho, MD, FACS

First depicted in anatomic drawings in 1492 by Leonardo da Vinci, the vermiform appendix was described as an anatomic structure in 1521 by Jacopo Berengari da Carpi, a professor of human anatomy at Bologna. Appendicitis became recognized as a surgical disease when the Harvard University pathologist Reginald Heber Fitz read his analysis of 257 cases of perforating inflammation of the appendix and 209 cases of typhlitis or perityphlitis at the 1886 meeting of the Association of American Physicians. In this landmark report, Fitz correctly pointed out that the frequent abscesses in the right iliac fossa were often attributable to perforation of the vermiform appendix, and he referred to the condition as appendicitis.[1] Among his classic observations of the disease was the emphasis on the "vital importance of early recognition" and its "eventual treatment by laparotomy." It was not until 1894 that Charles McBurney first described the surgical incision that bears his name and the surgical technique that was to become the gold standard for appendectomy.[2]

Although appendectomy has traditionally been done—and largely continues to be done—as an open procedure, there has been increasing interest in laparoscopic appendectomy in the last two decades. At present, however, the only patients for whom laparoscopic appendectomy appears to offer significant advantages are women of childbearing age, obese patients, and patients with an unclear diagnosis [*see Figure 1*]. Accordingly, the gold standard for surgical treatment of acute appendicitis remains open appendectomy as described by McBurney, although the occasional patient with chronic appendicitis can be electively treated with the laparoscopic approach.

Operative Technique

OPEN APPENDECTOMY

With the patient under general anesthesia and in the supine position, the abdomen is prepared and draped in a sterile fashion so as to expose the right lower quadrant. The skin incision is made in an oblique direction, crossing a line drawn between the anterior superior iliac spine and the umbilicus at nearly a right angle at a point about 2 to 3 cm from the iliac spine. This point, the McBurney point, is approximately one third of the way from the iliac spine to the umbilicus [*see Figure 2*]. The subcutaneous fat and fascia are incised to expose the external oblique aponeurosis. A slightly shorter incision is made in this aponeurosis; first, a scalpel is used, and then the incision is extended with scissors in the direction of the fibers of the muscle and its tendon in such a way that the fibers are separated but not cut.

The fibers of the internal oblique muscle and the transversus abdominis are separated with a blunt instrument at nearly a right angle to the incision on the external oblique aponeurosis. The parietal peritoneum is lifted up, with care taken not to include the underlying viscera, and is opened in a transverse fashion with a scalpel. This incision is then enlarged transversely with scissors. When greater exposure is required, the lateral edge of the rectus sheath is incised and the rectus abdominis is retracted medially without being divided [*see Figure 3*].

A foul smell or the presence of pus on entry into the peritoneum is an indication of advanced or perforating appendicitis. The free peritoneal fluid is collected for bacteriologic analysis. The ascending colon or cecum is located, and the appendix is found by following the cecal taeniae distally. The inflamed appendix typically feels firm and turgid. The appendix, together with the cecum, is delivered into the surgical incision and held with a Babcock tissue forceps. If this step proves difficult, the appendix can sometimes be swept into the field with the surgeon's right index finger as gentle traction is maintained on the cecum with a small, moist gauze pad held in the left hand [*see Figure 4*]. Care should be taken at this point not to avulse the friable and possibly necrotic appendix. To deliver a retrocecal appendix, it may be necessary to mobilize the ascending colon partially by sharply dividing the peritoneum on its lateral side, starting from the terminal ileum and proceeding toward the hepatic flexure.

The mesoappendix, containing the appendicular artery, is divided between clamps and ligated with 3-0 absorbable sutures [*see Figure 5*]. The appendix is held up with a Babcock tissue forceps, and its base is gently crushed with a straight mosquito arterial forceps. The mosquito forceps is then opened, moved up the appendix, and closed again. The base of the appendix is doubly ligated with 2-0 absorbable sutures at the point where it was crushed, so that a cuff of about 3 mm is left between the forceps and the tie.

The appendix is divided by running a scalpel along the underside of the forceps. The mucosa of the appendiceal stump is fulgurated with the electrocautery. The stump is not routinely invaginated into the cecum. In those rare cases in which the viability of the appendiceal base is in question, a 2-0 absorbable purse-string suture is placed in the cecum, and the stump is invaginated as the suture is tied. Alternatively, a partial cecectomy is performed using a gastrointestinal anastomosis (GIA) stapler loaded with an intestinal cartridge. If either maneuver is done, palpation for a patent ileocecal valve is indicated. The operative field is then checked for hemostasis, and the ascending colon is returned back to the abdomen. In cases of perforating appendicitis, the right paracolic gutter and pelvis are irrigated and thoroughly aspirated to ensure that any collected pus or particulate material is removed.

The peritoneum is then closed with a continuous 3-0 absorbable suture. The fibers of the transversus abdominis and the internal oblique muscle fall together readily, and their

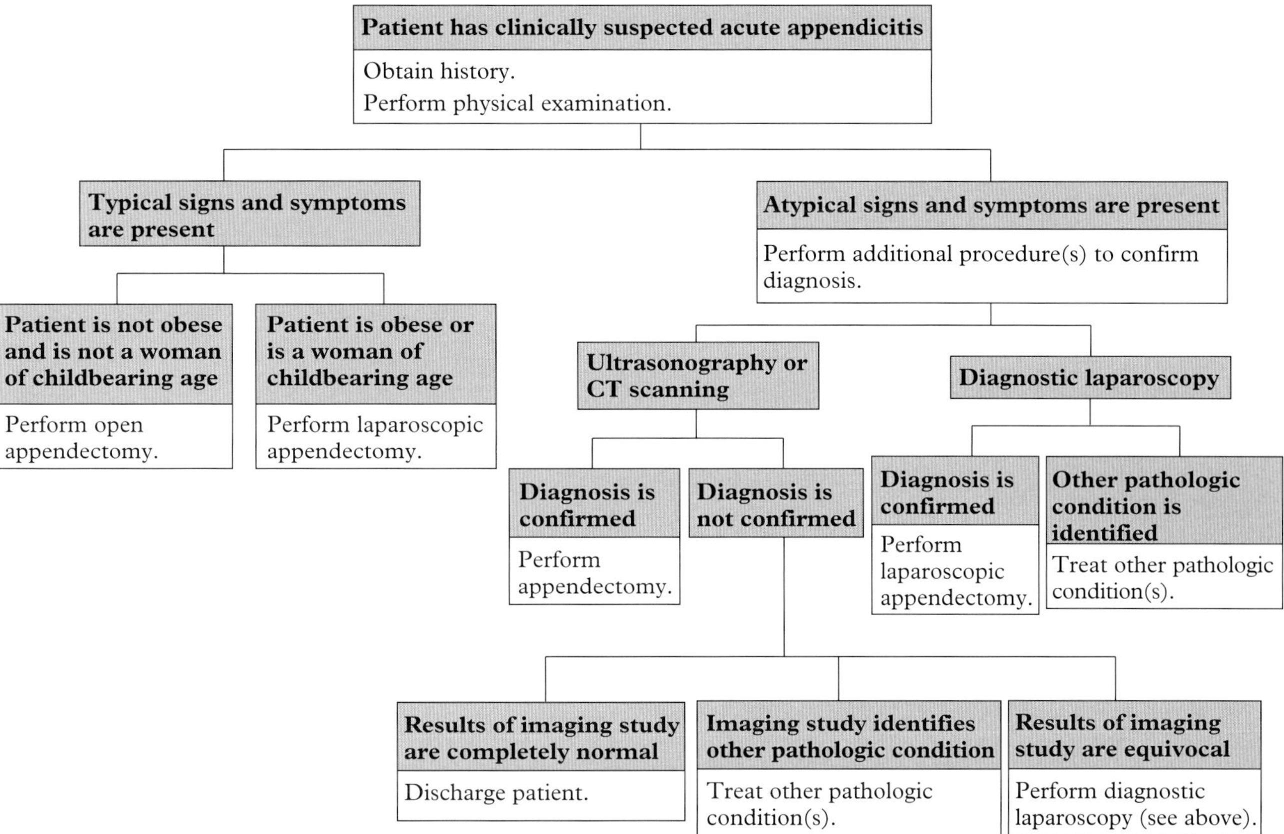

Figure 1 **Shown is an algorithm for choosing between treatment options for patients with suspected acute appendicitis. CT = computed tomographic.**

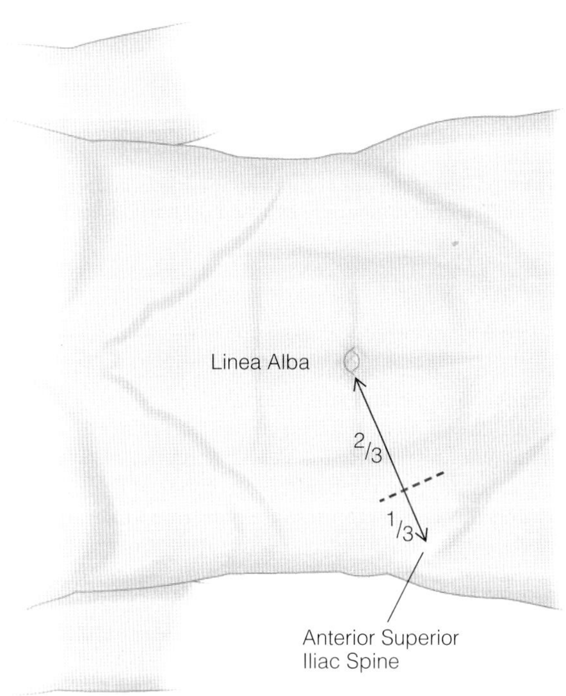

Figure 2 **Open appendectomy. Shown are the McBurney point and the McBurney incision.**

closure can be completed with two interrupted 3-0 absorbable ligatures. The external oblique aponeurosis is closed from end to end with a continuous 2-0 absorbable suture. The Scarpa fascia is approximated with interrupted 3-0 absorbable sutures, and the skin is closed with a continuous subcuticular 4-0 absorbable suture and reinforcing tapes (Steri-Strips, 3M, St. Paul, MN).

If the wound has been grossly contaminated, the fascia and muscles are closed as described, but the skin is loosely approximated with Steri-Strips, which can easily be removed postoperatively if surgical site infection develops. An alternative approach is to leave the skin and the subcutaneous tissue open but dressed with sterile nonadherent material and then to perform delayed primary closure with Steri-Strips on postoperative day 4 or 5. A meta-analysis of 27 studies involving 2,532 patients with gangrenous or perforating appendicitis concluded that the risk of surgical site infection was no higher with primary closure than with delayed primary closure.[3]

LAPAROSCOPIC APPENDECTOMY

The patient is under general anesthesia and in the supine position, with both arms tucked along the sides. Decompression with an orogastric tube should be routine, as should placement of a urinary Foley catheter and use of lower extremity sequential compression devices. The abdomen is prepared and draped in a sterile fashion so as to expose the entire abdomen.

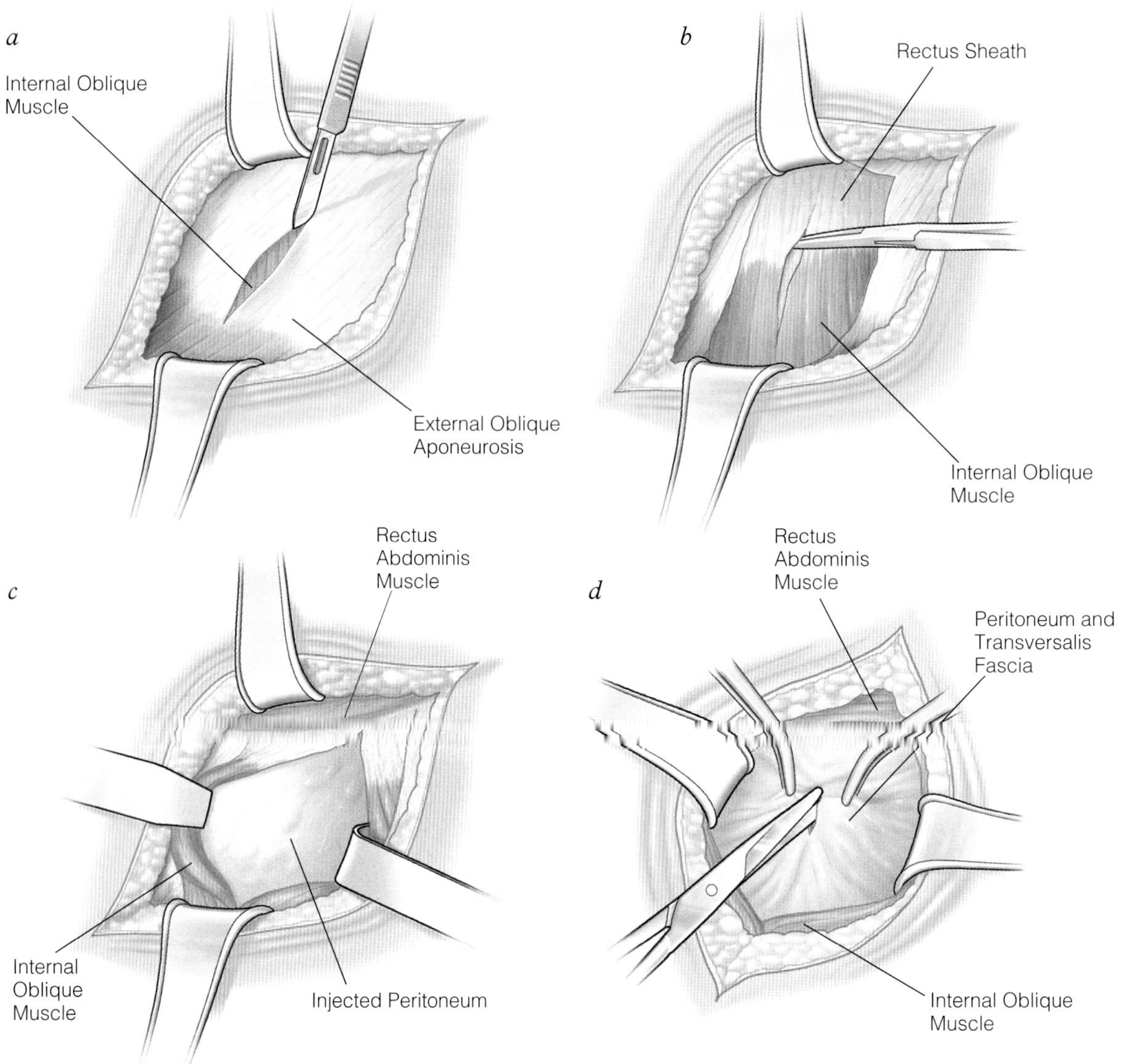

Figure 3 **Open appendectomy. Depicted is exposure of the abdominal cavity. The external oblique aponeurosis is opened (*a*). The fibers of the internal oblique muscle are separated bluntly (*b*). The parietal peritoneum is exposed (*c*) and opened transversely (*d*).**

The surgeon should stand on the patient's left side, with the assistant (who operates the camera) near the patient's left shoulder [*see Figure 6*]. The monitors are placed on the opposite side of the operating table so that both the surgeon and the assistant can view the procedure at all times.

A three-port approach is routinely used [*see Figure 6*]. All skin incisions along the midline are made vertically to allow a more cosmetically acceptable conversion to laparotomy should this become necessary. The midline suprapubic port must be large enough to accommodate the laparoscopic stapler or specimen retrieval bag (usually 12 mm); the other two ports can be smaller (e.g., 5 or 10 mm). The left lower quadrant port is placed as far away from the operative field as possible to permit the application of a two-handed dissection technique. The use of a 30° angled scope facilitates operative viewing and dissection.

With the patient pharmacologically relaxed and in the Trendelenburg position, a Veress needle is inserted into the peritoneal cavity at the base of the umbilical ligament. Aspiration and the saline-drop test are performed to ensure that the tip of the needle is correctly positioned. Pneumoperitoneum is established by insufflating CO_2 to an intra-abdominal pressure of 14 mm Hg. The first port is placed at the infraumbilical skin incision, the laparoscope is inserted, and a complete diagnostic laparoscopy is performed. Once the diagnosis of acute appendicitis is confirmed by inspection, the two remaining ports are placed under direct vision. In many cases, however, the diagnosis cannot be confirmed without

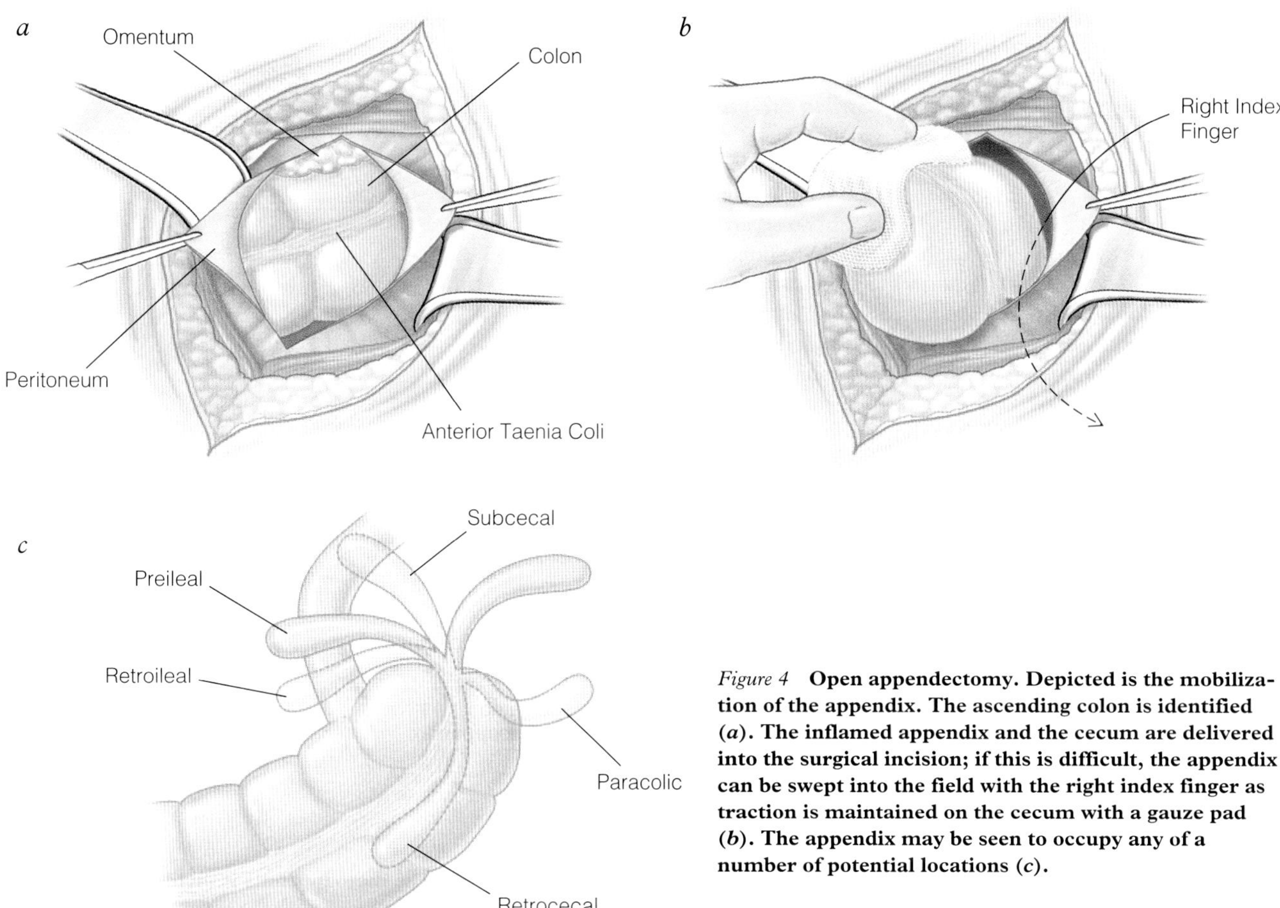

Figure 4 **Open appendectomy. Depicted is the mobilization of the appendix. The ascending colon is identified (*a*). The inflamed appendix and the cecum are delivered into the surgical incision; if this is difficult, the appendix can be swept into the field with the right index finger as traction is maintained on the cecum with a gauze pad (*b*). The appendix may be seen to occupy any of a number of potential locations (*c*).**

first placing the second and third ports and exposing the appendix. If purulent fluid is encountered, it should be carefully aspirated dry without irrigation to ensure that the infected fluid is not disseminated throughout the abdominal cavity.

The patient is tilted toward the left, and the appendix is exposed and traced to its base on the cecum by using an atraumatic retracting forceps. In cases of retrocecal appendix or severe appendiceal inflammation, it is best first to mobilize the cecum medially by taking down the lateral reflection of the peritoneum around the terminal ileum and up the ascending colon with either endoscopic scissors or an ultrasonic scalpel (e.g., the Harmonic Scalpel, Ethicon Endo-Surgery, Inc., Cincinnati, OH). Surrounding structures, such as the iliac and gonadal vessels and the ureter, should be clearly identified to minimize the risk of injury. Dissection of the appendix can then begin.

The tip of the appendix is grasped and retracted anteriorly toward the anterior abdominal wall and slightly toward the pelvis; the mesoappendix is thus exposed in a triangular fashion. A window between the base of the appendix and the blood supply is created with a curved dissecting forceps. The mesoappendix is divided either with hemostatic clips and scissors or with a laparoscopic GIA stapler loaded with a vascular cartridge [*see Figure 7*]. If a window on the mesoappendix cannot be safely created because of intense inflammation, antegrade dissection of the blood supply is necessary. The ultrasonic scalpel is a handy (albeit expensive) instrument for this purpose. Endoscopic hemostatic clips usually suffice to control the small branches of the appendicular artery during the course of this dissection.

The base of the appendix is then cleared circumferentially of any adipose or connective tissue and is divided with a laparoscopic GIA stapler loaded with an intestinal cartridge [*see Figure 8*]. To ensure an adequate closure away from the inflamed appendiceal base, a small portion of the cecum may have to be included within the stapler. To ensure proper placement of the stapler and to prevent injury to the right ureter or the adjacent small bowel, the tips of the stapler must be clearly visualized before the instrument is closed. The use of an angled scope and an articulated rotating laparoscopic GIA stapler (e.g., Roticulator, AutoSuture, Norwalk, CT) will facilitate this maneuver. Once closed, the stapler should be rotated to inspect the back side before firing. A noninflamed or minimally inflamed appendix can be ligated with sutures, as described earlier [*see* Open Appendectomy, *above*].

Table 1 **Results of 31 Prospective, Randomized Trials Comparing Laparoscopic Appendectomy with Open Appendectomy**[31–61]

	Laparoscopic Appendectomy (*n* = 2,194)		Open Appendectomy (*n* = 2,158)	
Variable	***n* (%)**	**Range**	***n* (%)**	**Range**
Negative appendix	314 (14.3)	7.7–36.0%	319 (14.8)	0–35.5%
Conversion to open procedure	223 (10.2)	0–23.9%	NA	NA
Surgical site infection	77 (3.5)	0–18.3%	144 (6.7)	0–17.3%
Intra-abdominal abscess	55 (2.5)	0–7.4%	24 (1.1)	0–4.6%
Days in hospital	2.7	1–4.9	3.2	1.2–5.3

NA = not applicable.

intra-abdominal abscess (2.5% versus 1.1%). The length of stay was slightly shorter after laparoscopic appendectomy (1 to 4.9 days; average 2.7 days) than after open appendectomy (1.2 to 5.3 days; average 3.2 days). There has been no further randomized, controlled trial published since 2005. The inclusion of non-English literature, both in full articles and in abstract reports, by the Cochrane Collaboration[62] has not led to any significant changes in the general statistical picture. In the 2008 update, the authors concluded that laparoscopic appendectomy seems to have various advantages over open appendectomy, but they are small and of limited clinical relevance.

In men and children with suspected acute appendicitis, laparoscopic appendectomy has no major advantage over open appendectomy.[37] In women of childbearing age and in equivocal cases, laparoscopy may be valuable as a diagnostic tool, but the practice of not removing a normal-looking appendix during exploration for right lower quadrant pain remains controversial.[63,64] Laparoscopic appendectomy appears to offer the potential benefit of less postoperative adhesion formation, but the evidence is inconclusive in light of the short follow-up times reported in these trials, and the higher incidence of intra-abdominal abscess formation remains cause for concern. To date, unfortunately, there have been no studies designed specifically to address reduced adhesion formation as a primary end point.

Although laparoscopic appendectomy is being performed with increased frequency, it continues to be used selectively. Laparoscopic appendectomy is at least as safe as the corresponding open procedure, but it is undeniably more time-consuming and more costly. Moreover, it remains questionable whether the benefits of laparoscopic appendectomy—reduced postoperative pain, earlier resumption of oral feeding, shortened hospital stay, quicker return to normal preoperative activities, and lower incidence of surgical site infection—outweigh the higher incidence of postoperative intra-abdominal abscess formation. In clinical settings when the patient is either a woman of childbearing age, is obese, or has an unclear diagnosis and where surgical expertise is available and equipment is affordable, a laparoscopic approach may offer significant advantages over an open procedure. Further randomized clinical studies focusing on the efficacy of laparoscopic appendectomy as a diagnostic tool and on the incidence of postoperative intra-abdominal abscess and adhesion formation are needed, as are additional cost analyses.

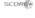

Financial Disclosures: None Reported

References

1. Fitz RH. Perforating inflammation of the vermiform appendix with special reference to its early diagnosis and treatment. Trans Assoc Am Physicians 1886;1:107.
2. McBurney C. The incision made in the abdominal wall in cases of appendicitis, with a description of a new method of operating. Ann Surg 1894;20:38–43.
3. Rucinski J, Fabian T, Panagopoulos G, et al. Gangrenous and perforated appendicitis: a meta-analytic study of 2532 patients indicates that the incision should be closed primarily. Surgery 2000;127:136–41.
4. Flum DR, Morris A, Koepsell T, et al. Has misdiagnosis of appendicitis decreased over time? A population-based analysis. JAMA 2001;286:1748–53.
5. Chang AR. An analysis of the pathology of 3,003 appendices. Aust N Z J Surg 1981;51:169–78.
6. Knight PJ, Vassy LE. Specific diseases mimicking appendicitis in childhood. Arch Surg 1981;116:744–6.
7. Pieper R, Kager L, Nasman P. Acute appendicitis: a clinical study of 1,018 cases of emergency appendectomy. Acta Chir Scand 1982;148:51–62.
8. Arnbjornsson E, Asp NG, Westin SI. Decreasing incidence of acute appendicitis, with special reference to the consumption of dietary fiber. Acta Chir Scand 1982;148:461–4.
9. Blind PJ, Dahlgren ST. The continuing challenge of the negative appendix. Acta Chir Scand 1986;152:623–7.
10. Lau WY. Correlation between gross appearance of the appendix and histological examination. Ann R Coll Surg Engl 1988;70:336–7.
11. Budd JS, Armstrong CP. The correlation between gross appearance at appendix and histological examination. Ann R Coll Surg Engl 1988;70:395–6.
12. Blair PM, Bugis PS, Turner LJ, et al. Review of the pathologic diagnosis of 2,216 appendectomy specimens. Am J Surg 1993;165:618–20.
13. Dahlstom JE, MacArthur EB. Enterobius vermicularis: a possible cause of symptoms resembling appendicitis. Aust N Z J Surg 1994;64:692–4.
14. Pearl RH, Hale DA, Molloy M, et al. Pediatric appendectomy. J Pediatr Surg 1995;30:173–81.
15. Truji M, Puri P, Reen DJ. Characterization of the local inflammatory response in appendicitis. J Pediatr Gastroenterol Nutr 1993;16:43–8.
16. Wang Y, Reen DJ, Puri P. Is a histologically normal appendix following emergency appendicectomy always normal? Lancet 1996;347:1076–9.
17. Grunewald B, Keating J. Should the 'normal' appendix be removed at operation for appendicitis? J R Coll Surg Edinb 1993;38:158–60.
18. Collins DC. 71,000 human appendix specimens: a final report, summarizing 40 years' study. Am J Proctol 1963;14:265–81.
19. Chan W, Fu KH. Value of routine histopathological examination of appendices in Hong Kong. J Clin Pathol 1987;40:429–33.
20. Lenriot JP, Hugier M. Adenocarcinoma of the appendix. Am J Surg 1988;155:470–5.
21. Gupta SC, Gupta AK, Keswani NK, et al. Pathology of tropical appendicitis. J Clin Pathol 1989;42:1169–72.
22. Thomas RM, Sobin LH. Gastrointestinal cancer. Cancer 1995;75:154–70.
23. Modlin IM, Sandor A. An analysis of 8305 cases of carcinoid tumors. Cancer 1997;79:813–29.
24. Moertel CG, Weiland LH, Nagorney DM, et al. Carcinoid tumor of the appendix: treatment and prognosis. N Engl J Med 1987;317:1699–701.

25. Gouzi JL, Laigneau P, Delalande JP, et al. Indications for right hemicolectomy in carcinoid tumors of the appendix. Surg Gynecol Obstet 1993;176:543–7.
26. Nitecki SS, Wolff BG, Schlinkert R, et al. The natural history of surgically treated primary adenocarcinoma of the appendix. Ann Surg 1994;219:51–7.
27. Yang SS, Gibson P, McCaughey RS, et al. Primary Crohn's disease of the appendix. Ann Surg 1979;189:334–9.
28. Jahadi MR, Shaw ML. The pathology of the appendix in ulcerative colitis. Dis Colon Rectum 1976;19:345–9.
29. Ruiz V, Unger SW, Morgan J, et al. Crohn's disease of the appendix. Surgery 1990;107:113–7.
30. Goldblum JR, Appelman HD. Appendiceal involvement in ulcerative colitis. Mod Pathol 1992;5:607–10.
31. Attwood SEA, Hill ADK, Murphy PG, et al. A prospective randomized trial of laparoscopic versus open appendectomy. Surgery 1992;112:497–501.
32. Tate JJT, Dawson JW, Chung SCS, et al. Laparoscopic versus open appendectomy: prospective randomised trial. Lancet 1993;342:633–7.
33. Kum CK, Ngoi SS, Goh PMY, et al. Randomized controlled trial comparing laparoscopic and open appendicectomy. Br J Surg 1993;80:1599–600.
34. Frazee RC, Roberts JW, Symmonds RE, et al. A prospective randomized trial comparing open versus laparoscopic appendectomy. Ann Surg 1994;219:725–8.
35. Ortega AE, Hunter JG, Peters JH, et al. A prospective, randomized comparison of laparoscopic appendectomy with open appendectomy. Am J Surg 1995;169:208–12.
36. Martin LC, Puente I, Sosa JL, et al. Open versus laparoscopic appendectomy: a prospective randomized comparison. Ann Surg 1995;222:256–61.
37. Hansen JB, Smithers BM, Schache D, et al. Laparoscopic versus open appendectomy: prospective randomized trial. World J Surg 1996;20:17–20.
38. Mutter D, Vix M, Bui A, et al. Laparoscopy not recommended for routine appendectomy in men: results of a prospective randomized study. Surgery 1996;120:71–4.
39. Cox MR, McCall JL, Toouli J, et al. Prospective randomized comparison of open versus laparoscopic appendectomy in men. World J Surg 1996;20:263–6.
40. Lejus C, Dellie L, Plattner V, et al. Randomized, single-blinded trial of laparoscopic versus open appendectomy in children. Anesthesiology 1996;84:801–6.
41. Williams MD, Collins JN, Wright TF, et al. Laparoscopic versus open appendectomy. South Med J 1996;89:668–74.
42. Hart R, Rajgopal C, Plewes A, et al. Laparoscopic versus open appendectomy: a prospective randomized trial of 81 patients. Can J Surg 1996;39:457–62.
43. Reiertsen O, Larsen S, Trondsen E, et al. Randomized controlled trial with sequential design of laparoscopic versus conventional appendicectomy. Br J Surg 1997;84:842–7.
44. Laine S, Rantala A, Gullichsen R, et al. Laparoscopic appendectomy—is it worthwhile? A prospective, randomized study in young women. Surg Endosc 1997;11:95–7.
45. Macarulla E, Vallet J, Abad JM, et al. Laparoscopic versus open appendectomy: a prospective randomized trial. Surg Laparosc Endosc 1997;7:335–9.
46. Kazemier G, de Zeeuw GR, Lange JF, et al. Laparoscopic versus open appendectomy: a randomized clinical trial. Surg Endosc 1997;11:336–40.
47. Minne L, Varner D, Burnell A, et al. Laparosopic versus open appendectomy: prospective randomized study of outcomes. Arch Surg 1997;132:708–11.
48. Hay SA. Laparoscopic versus conventional appendectomy in children. Pediatr Surg Int 1998;13:21–3.
49. Klinger A, Henle KP, Beller S, et al. Laparoscopic appendectomy does not change the incidence of postoperative infectious complications. Am J Surg 1998;175:232–5.
50. Hiekkinen TJ, Haukipuro K, Hulkko A. Cost-effective appendectomy: open or laparoscopic? A prospective randomized study. Surg Endosc 1998;12:1204–8.
51. Hellberg A, Rudberg C, Kullman E, et al. Prospective randomized multicentre study of laparoscopic versus open appendicectomy. Br J Surg 1999;86:48–53.
52. Ozmen MM, Zulfikaroglu B, Tanik A, et al. Laparoscopic versus open appendectomy: prospective randomized trial. Surg Laparosc Endosc Percutan Tech 1999;9:187–9.
53. Pedersen AG, Petersen OB, Wara P, et al. Randomized clinical trial of laparoscopic versus open appendicectomy. Br J Surg 2001;88:200–5.
54. Lavonius MI, Liesjarvi S, Ovaska J, et al. Laparoscopic versus open appendectomy in children: a prospective randomised study. Eur J Pediatr Surg 2001;11:235–8.
55. Long KH, Bannon MP, Zietlow SP, et al. A prospective randomized comparison of laparoscopic appendectomy with open appedectomy: clinical and economic analyses. Surgery 2001;129:390–400.
56. Lintula H, Kokki H, Vanamo K. Single-blind randomized clinical trial of laparoscopic versus appendicectomy in children. Br J Surg 2001;88:510–4.
57. Huang MT, Wei PL, Wu CC, et al. Needlescopic, laparoscopic, and open appendectomy: a comparative study. Surg Laparosc Endosc Percutan Tech 2001;11:306–12.
58. Little DC, Custer MD, May BH, et al. Laparoscopic appendectomy: an unnecessary and expensive procedure in children? J Pediatr Surg 2002;37:310–7.
59. Milewczyk M, Michalik M, Ciesielski M. A prospective, randomized, unicenter study comparing laparoscopic and open treatments of acute appendicitis. Surg Endosc 2003;17:1023–8.
60. Ignacio RC, Burke R, Spencer D, et al. Laparoscopic vs open appendectomy: what is the real difference? Results of a prospective randomized double-blinded trial. Surg Endosc 2004;18:334–7.
61. Katkhouda N, Mason RJ, Towfigh S, et al. Laparoscopic versus open appendectomy: a prospective randomized double-blind study. Ann Surg 2005;242:439–48.
62. Sauerland S, Leferung R, Neugebauer EAM. Laparoscopic versus open surgery for suspected appendicitis. Cochrane Database Syst Rev 2004;(4):001546.
63. Van Dalen R, Bagshaw PF, Dobbs BR, et al. The utility of laparoscopy in the diagnosis of acute appendicitis in women of reproductive age: a prospective randomized controlled trial with long-term follow-up. Surg Endosc 2003;17:1311–3.
64. Van den Broek WT, Bijnen AB, De Ruiter P, Gauma DJ. A normal appendix found during diagnostic laparoscopy should not be removed. Br J Surg 2001;88:251–4.

Acknowledgments

Figures 1 and 10 Marcia Kammerer
Figures 2 through 9 Tom Moore

30 PROCEDURES FOR DIVERTICULAR DISEASE

Jeffrey L. Cohen, MD, FACS, FASCRS, John P. Welch, MD, FACS, and Louis Reines, MD, MBA

Preoperative Evaluation

The extent of the preoperative evaluation received by patients undergoing surgical treatment of diverticular disease is dictated predominantly by the urgency of the situation. Whereas patients with recurrent symptoms will undergo repeated assessments with myriad diagnostic tests before the decision is made to proceed with surgical intervention, patients with perforated diverticulitis may have only a chest x-ray documenting free air before they are taken to the operating room. Given the varied complications of diverticular disease and the numerous options for surgical treatment, we believe it is most convenient to divide the relevant operations into emergency procedures and elective procedures. Such a division facilitates discussion of technical issues, preoperative evaluation, and management of complications.

As noted, in the emergency setting, a demonstration of pneumoperitoneum may be the only workup performed. In fact, in most patients with perforated diverticulitis, pneumoperitoneum is the initial presentation.[1,2] In patients who present with massive lower gastrointestinal hemorrhage, angiographic demonstration of the bleeding site is known to reduce operative mortality, even if therapeutic superselective embolization is unsuccessful in controlling the bleeding.[3,4] The other complication of diverticular disease that may necessitate an emergency operation is colonic obstruction. A careful history may reveal progressive obstructive symptoms, but if the patient presents with complete obstruction and cecal dilatation, urgent decompression is required. In this setting, retrograde administration of a water-soluble enema may be very helpful—at least for delineating the level of the obstruction, if not the specific cause.[1,5] Communication with the radiologist should be maintained to prevent both overly forceful instillation of the contrast material and the use of barium, which may cause problems if the agent cannot be evacuated.

When surgical treatment of diverticular disease is to be performed in the elective setting, a detailed preoperative evaluation is imperative. The key point here is that objective evidence of diverticulitis must be obtained at some point in the care of the patient. Too often, symptoms of irritable bowel syndrome are confused with those of diverticulitis, with the result that the patient carries an incorrect diagnosis.[6–9] In the most common scenario, computed tomographic (CT) scanning is performed when a patient is experiencing left-side pain, possibly associated with fever, nausea, anorexia, or abdominal distention. A finding of pericolonic inflammation in an area of diverticulosis is the definitive radiographic presentation.[10,11] Preoperative endoscopic evaluation of the colon, whenever feasible, is extremely valuable not only for confirming the presence of diverticulosis but also for ruling out inflammatory bowel disease or even a neoplastic lesion.

It is possible to expend a great deal of effort on trying to demonstrate a diverticular fistula. In many circumstances, however, this task proves difficult to accomplish. In our view, demonstration of a diverticular fistula should not be considered a mandatory precondition for operative treatment. A strong history of either a colovaginal or a colovesical fistula with suggestive findings on CT scans (e.g., air in the bladder or pericolonic inflammation contiguous with either the bladder or the vagina) constitutes a sufficient indication for surgical resection.[12,13]

Operative Planning

In planning the operative approach to a patient with diverticular disease, the major decision is whether to perform a one-stage or a two-stage procedure. Traditionally, an emergency operation for perforation, obstruction, or massive bleeding includes a temporary stoma procedure to eliminate the risk of anastomotic leakage.[14,15] The operation most commonly performed in this setting is the Hartmann procedure [*see* Emergency Procedures, Hartmann Procedure, *below*], named after Henri Hartmann, who first described the use of this operation to treat colon cancer in 1923.[16] The obvious advantage of the Hartmann procedure is that it removes the inflammatory focus without putting the compromised patient at risk for anastomotic leakage. Unfortunately, to restore intestinal continuity after this procedure, it is necessary to perform a potentially difficult second operation; as many as one third of patients never undergo reversal of their colostomy.[17,18]

Another therapeutic option is to perform a primary anastomosis with a diverting loop ileostomy instead of a colostomy. In this situation, the risk of anastomotic leakage with possible fecal peritonitis is still avoided, but only a relatively minor second procedure is necessary to reverse the ileostomy.[19] Primary anastomosis with a defunctioning stoma may be the optimal strategy for selected patients with diverticular peritonitis (Hinchey III or IV); it may represent a good compromise between postoperative adverse events, long-term quality of life, and risk of a permanent stoma.[20] Occasionally, it may be appropriate to perform on-table colonic lavage with a primary anastomosis. This approach is most useful in the setting of colonic obstruction secondary to a diverticular stricture in a patient who is otherwise hemodynamically stable but has a large fecal load proximal to the intended anastomosis.[21,22]

Laparoscopic intestinal surgery has shown tremendous development of late, benefited both by significant technological improvements and by growing surgical experience with advanced laparoscopic procedures.[23,24] Newer approaches (e.g., hand-assisted techniques) have markedly reduced the learning curve and shortened the operating time.[25,26] Minimum-access techniques have been shown to reduce the risk of postoperative wound infection and hernia formation.[27] Recent literature suggests that fistulizing diverticular disease can be resected safely via a laparoscopic approach with good clinical outcome.[28,29] Moreover, a recent prospective series has described laparoscopic peritoneal lavage with drain placement for complicated perforated sigmoid diverticulitis as a bridge to interval elective laparoscopic resection with primary anastomosis.[30] The newest frontier in elective diverticular resection is single access/port surgery with an operating laparoscope.[31] Consequently, minimal-access surgery is rapidly becoming the approach of choice in the management of nearly all elective diverticular resections.[32–35]

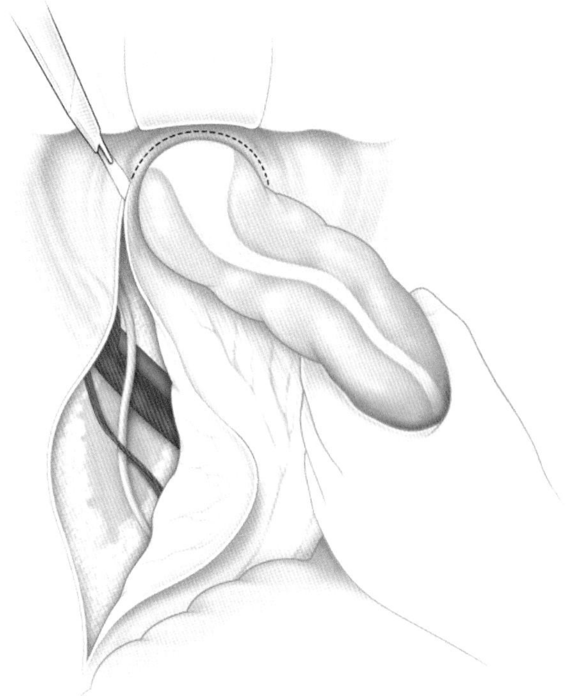

Figure 1 **Hartmann procedure. Illustrated is the relation of the ureter to other structures in the left lower quadrant.**

Emergency Procedures

Patient setup and positioning are similar for all emergency operations. The patient is placed in a modified lithotomy position to facilitate access to the rectum. Urinary drainage with a Foley catheter and temporary gastric decompression with a nasogastric tube is performed. When feasible, the stoma is marked by an enterostomal therapist before operation.

HARTMANN PROCEDURE

Step 1: Incision and Initial Exploration

A lower midline incision is made and extended above the umbilicus as necessary. The abdomen is thoroughly explored to confirm the diagnosis of diverticular disease and to wash out any gross fecal spillage. A self-retaining retractor (e.g., a Bookwalter retractor) is placed, with care taken to pad the abdominal wall.

Step 2: Mobilization and Division of Sigmoid Colon

The patient is placed in the Trendelenburg position, with the small bowel carefully retracted into the upper abdomen. The sigmoid colon is mobilized away from the lateral peritoneal attachments. Mobilization is continued into the pelvis lateral to the upper portion of the rectum.

Troubleshooting If a severe phlegmon is stuck to the pelvic sidewall, it may be helpful at some point in the mobilization to dissect cephalad from below the mass so as to isolate the area from above and below.

Step 3: Identification of Ureter

As the sigmoid colon is retracted medially, the ureter can usually be identified where it crosses over the bifurcation of the iliac vessels. The gonadal vessels are usually identified first; the ureter lies slightly medial and deep to them [*see Figure 1*].

Step 4: Division of Sigmoid Colon

The proximal sigmoid colon is divided through noninflamed tissue with a linear cutting stapler [*see Figure 2a*]. The sigmoid vessels are sequentially divided (with attention paid to their relation to the left ureter) up to the rectosigmoid junction, which is identified by the loss of the taeniae coli. The rectum is then transected through noninflamed tissue with a linear cutting stapler [*see Figure 2b*].

Troubleshooting The top of the rectal stump can be marked with a nonabsorbable suture to facilitate subsequent identification.

Step 5: Construction of Colostomy

The proximal colon is delivered through the previously marked stoma site in the left lower quadrant with a muscle-splitting incision in the rectus abdominis (with care taken not to twist it on its mesentery), and a colostomy is created.

Step 5—Alternative (Primary Anastomosis with Diverting Ileostomy): Creation of Colorectal Anastomosis

As an alternative to a colostomy, the surgeon may elect to perform a primary colorectal anastomosis with a diverting ileostomy. The anvil of a circular stapler is positioned in the proximal colon, and a purse-string suture is placed around it. If there is any gaping of the tissue around the shaft of the anvil, a second suture may be added for reinforcement.

a

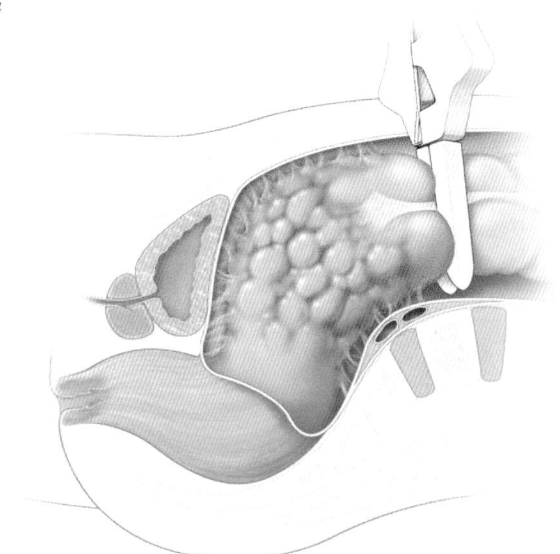

b

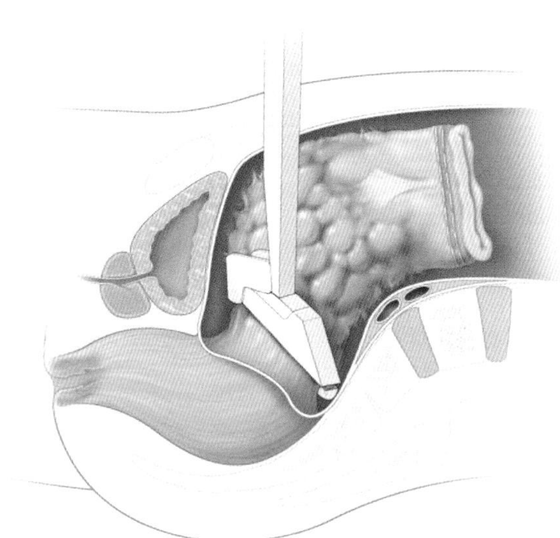

Figure 2 **Hartmann procedure. (*a*) The colon is divided above the level of the inflammatory mass. (*b*) The rectum is divided below the inflammatory mass; division must be through normal tissue.**

The stapler is inserted through the anus, with the shaft being brought out either through the anterior wall of the rectum or through the top of the rectal stump, adjacent to the staple line. The stapler is then engaged, with care taken to ensure that no extraneous tissue is caught between the body of the stapler and the anvil and that the proximal bowel is not twisted on its mesentery. The stapler is fired to create the anastomosis, and the integrity of the anastomosis is tested by occluding the proximal bowel and placing the anastomotic area under water while air is insufflated into the rectum via a rigid proctoscope.

Troubleshooting It is helpful to divide the mesentery where it is draped over the anvil. This measure diminishes the risk of bleeding from the circular staple line while also providing a greater length of colon for the anastomosis. If there is any question regarding possible tension on the anastomosis, the splenic flexure should be fully mobilized.

Step 6—Alternative (Primary Anastomosis with Diverting Ileostomy): Construction of Loop Ileostomy

A loop ileostomy is created in the right lower quadrant using a muscle-splitting incision in the rectus abdominis. Loop ileostomies can usually be designed to be diverting; however, stapling the distal end and leaving it at skin level will ensure complete diversion.

Troubleshooting If there is a column of stool between the ileostomy and the anastomosis, it should be washed out before the ileostomy is completed.

ON-TABLE COLONIC LAVAGE

Steps 1 through 4

Steps 1, 2, 3, and 4 of on-table colonic lavage are the same as the first four steps of the Hartmann procedure.

Step 5: Mobilization of Flexures

After the sigmoid resection, the hepatic flexure and the splenic flexure are carefully mobilized to facilitate the washout process.

Step 6: Placement of Tubing

Corrugated anesthesia tubing is placed in the colon proximal to the resected segment and secured in place with umbilical tape. The distal end of the tubing is passed off the operating table and is connected to a device that collects the effluent [*see Figure 3*].

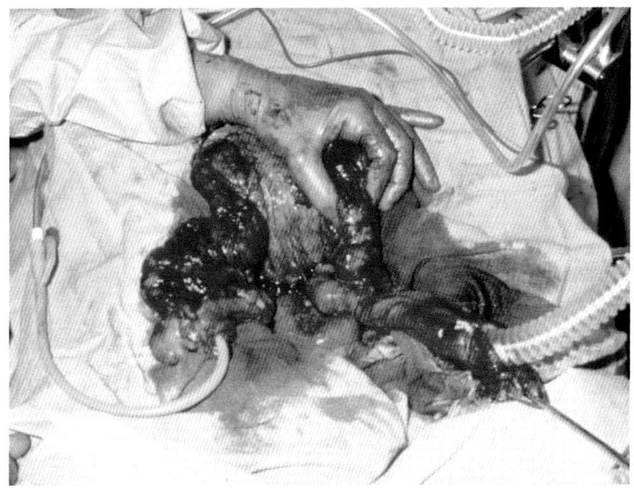

Figure 3 **On-table colonic lavage. Shown is full mobilization of the colon, with corrugated anesthesia tubing secured in the colon and connected to a collection system. A Foley catheter is inserted through an appendicostomy into the base of the cecum.**

Step 7: Construction of Appendicostomy

An appendicostomy is performed, a Foley catheter is placed, and a purse-string suture is tied around the tube with the balloon inflated. If the patient has previously undergone appendectomy, the terminal ileum is used instead.

Step 8: Irrigation of Colon

The colon is washed with an irrigant until the effluent is relatively clear. It may be necessary to manipulate the colon so as to initiate flushing of formed stool.

Step 9: Excision of Appendix and Creation of Colorectal Anastomosis

A formal appendectomy is performed. The corrugated anesthesia tubing is removed from the colon, and a colorectal anastomosis is performed, usually with a circular stapler.

Elective Procedures

OPEN RESECTION

Open resection in the elective setting consists of steps 1 through 4 of the Hartmann procedure, followed by creation of a primary colorectal anastomosis and a diverting loop ileostomy (alternative steps 5 and 6) [*see* Emergency Procedures, Hartmann Procedure, *above*].

LAPAROSCOPIC RESECTION

The patient is placed in a low lithotomy position with minimal hip flexion. The right arm is well padded and tucked at the side because both surgeons will be operating from the right side of the table. Video monitors are placed on both sides of the table. It is beneficial to place the patient on a bean bag because a significant portion of the operation will be performed with the patient in extremes of positioning.

Step 1: Placement of Trocars

The first port is placed at a periumbilical location by means of an open Hasson approach, and a 30° laparoscope is inserted. After pneumoperitoneum is achieved, the other ports are placed under direct vision: 5 and 12 mm ports are placed in the right lower quadrant, and an optional 5 mm port may be placed in the midepigastrium [*see Figure 4*]. The midepigastric port facilitates mobilization of the left colon and is essential for mobilization of the splenic flexure.

Step 2: Mobilization of Sigmoid Colon

After the abdomen has been explored, the patient is placed in a steep Trendelenburg position, with the right side tilted down. This position allows gravity to retract the small bowel into the upper abdomen. The sigmoid colon is mobilized from its lateral peritoneal attachments, and the colon is thereby converted to a midline structure. Mobilization is extended superiorly along the descending colon and inferiorly to the pelvic cul-de-sac. The left ureter is then identified and swept laterally away from the base of the mesentery.

Division of colovaginal or colovesical fistula In most patients, the fistula can be pinched off with no visible defect in either the bladder or vagina or a very small defect. Management

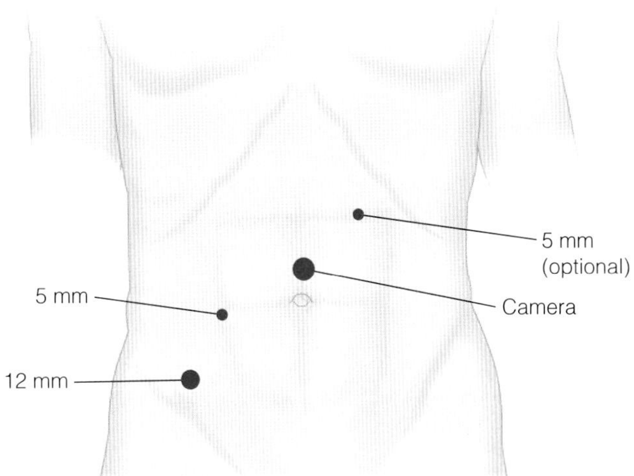

Figure 4 **Laparoscopic sigmoid resection. Shown is recommended port placement. The midepigastric 5 mm port is essential for mobilization of the splenic flexure.**

options include leaving a Foley catheter for 7 to 10 days or placing a few absorbable sutures over the defect and leaving a closed suction drain behind the bladder or vagina.

Alternative approach to colonic mobilization and division In place of the conventional approach (see above), a medial-to-lateral approach can be undertaken. In this approach, the initial dissection proceeds from the right side of the colon, mobilizing the superior rectal vessels from the sacral promontory. The left ureter is then visualized through the window thus created before the sigmoid mesentery is divided. Division of the sigmoid mesentery is performed in a proximal-to-distal direction, with the inferior mesenteric vessels generally divided first. Once the sigmoid mesentery has been completely divided, the bowel is transected with staplers at the rectosigmoid junction.

The advantage of the traditional approach is that surgeons are more familiar with it from corresponding open procedures. In our view, given the difficulty of mastering laparoscopic colon surgery, the medial-to-lateral approach to colonic mobilization only increases the steepness of the learning curve without affording any significant benefit.

Step 3: Division of Rectum and Sigmoid Mesentery

An incision is made in the peritoneum along the right side of the rectosigmoid mesentery and extended inferiorly to the pelvic cul-de-sac. A window is created between the upper rectum and its mesentery and enlarged to allow insertion of an endoscopic gastrointestinal anastomosis (GIA) stapler [*see Figure 5*]. The stapler is then fired once or twice to divide the rectosigmoid bowel. The mesentery of the sigmoid colon is sequentially divided with staplers, clips, an ultrasonic scalpel, or the LigaSure system (Valleylab, Boulder, Colorado).

Step 4: Exteriorization of Sigmoid Colon

Once the colon is mobilized and the blood supply divided, either the Hasson incision is enlarged or a Pfannenstiel incision is made to exteriorize the bowel, which is then divided

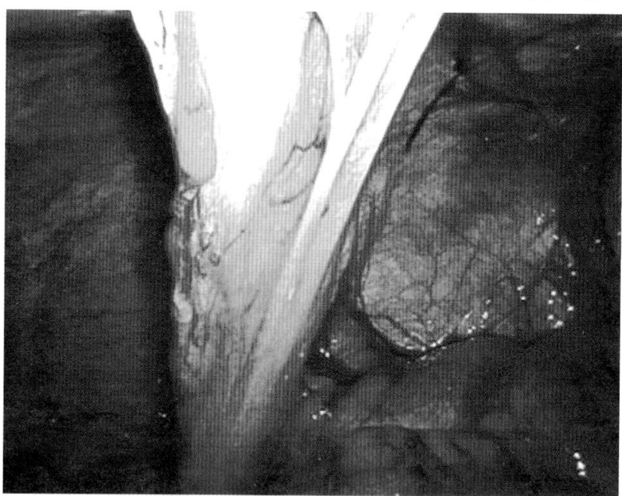

Figure 10 **Laparoscopic Hartmann closure. Shown is a laparoscopic view of the colostomy after intra-abdominal adhesions have been divided.**

engaged and fired while the surgeon's hand keeps any extraneous tissue away from the anastomotic area. The anastomosis is then tested by placing it under water and insufflating air via a proctoscope.

Troubleshooting It is often easier to bring out the shaft of the stapler through the anterior wall of the rectum, especially if there has been a significant inflammatory response around the area of the Hartmann pouch. Occasionally, the end of the Hartmann pouch cannot be reached with the stapler secondary to rectal tortuosity and a lengthy stump. The operator can guide the stapler with his or her hand, attempt further mobilization and resection of the stump, and/or bring the spike through at a more distal location and leave a blind segment of rectum, as long as the distal sigmoid colon is resected.

Complications

Operative management of diverticular disease poses distinct challenges, the level of which is proportional to the degree of inflammation present and to the urgency of the procedure. Whereas many of the complications encountered are not specific to this setting but are common to all abdominal procedures, there are several that warrant particular attention in the context of surgical treatment of diverticular disease.

ANASTOMOTIC LEAKAGE

The most serious and potentially life-threatening complication of procedures for diverticular disease is the development of an anastomotic leak. Many factors contribute to the maintenance of anastomotic integrity, ranging from the surgeon's technical ability to the patient's comorbidities. Of these factors, however, the single most important one is probably the setting in which the operation is carried out. Patients undergoing emergency procedures are at four times higher risk for anastomotic leakage than those undergoing elective procedures.[36,37] Furthermore, mortality is 13% in patients presenting with purulent peritonitis and 43% in those presenting with feculent peritonitis; these figures suggest that performing an anastomosis in these settings is unwise.[14,15,38,39]

As with any anastomosis, the long-established basic technical principles—using healthy, uninflamed tissue; ensuring an adequate blood supply; and avoiding tension on the anastomosis—should be strictly adhered to. If any of these principles cannot be followed, then either the patient should undergo proximal diversion or (preferably) the problem with the anastomosis should be corrected. For instance, in a situation where the sigmoid inflammatory process extends into the rectal mesentery, attempts should be made to resect below the level of the inflammation, even if the process is reaching well into the rectum itself. Another technical point worth mentioning involves preserving the superior rectal vessels, although no randomized, prospective study has yet been performed to determine whether this measure has any significant positive effect.

RECURRENT DISEASE

It is unusual for a recurrent diverticular fistula to develop after takedown with resection of the involved colon. Much more likely than the persistence of a diverticular fistula is the development of a recurrent colovesical or colovaginal fistula secondary to an anastomotic leak with drainage through the point of least resistance (i.e., the anastomosis).

There is some question as to whether a recurrence of diverticulitis after sigmoid resection is actually a complication of the procedure. Although it has been shown that resection of all diverticulum-bearing colon is not required for successful treatment of the disease process, it does appear that the location of any remaining diverticulosis influences the recurrence of the disease. Studies have demonstrated that if a sigmoid resection with a colorectal anastomosis is performed, the recurrence rate is 5%, whereas if the anastomosis is performed to the distal sigmoid colon, the recurrence rate rises to 12%.[40,41] When recurrent diverticulitis develops, it is important to reexamine the histologic findings from the original operation to rule out the possibility that the patient was misdiagnosed. Occasionally, diverticulosis and Crohn disease coexist; recurrence of Crohn disease is much more common than recurrence of diverticulosis and, given a long enough follow-up period, is actually to be expected.

URETERAL INJURY

Ureteral injuries occur in as many as 1% of patients undergoing diverticular resection.[42] Because of the inflammatory process associated with severe diverticular disease, it may be difficult to identify the ureter as it crosses the bifurcation of the iliac vessels; however, it is always possible to identify the ureter more proximally and then follow it down to the inflamed area. If a difficult dissection is anticipated or if technical difficulties are encountered intraoperatively, ureteral stents may be placed. These stents do not prevent injuries from occurring, but they can facilitate early identification of developing problems. Ureteral injuries should always be repaired at the time of operation, in consultation with the urologist.

ANASTOMOTIC STRICTURE

Occasionally, patients may experience feelings of incomplete evacuation, tenesmus, or abdominal bloating. These symptoms may be indicative of an anastomotic stricture. Confirmation may be obtained using a Gastrografin enema or flexible endoscopy. The incidence of symptomatic anastomotic stenosis after elective laparoscopic sigmoidectomy is reported to be as high as 17.6%.[43] Although no single risk factor could be identified, adherence to good surgical principles of a tension-free anastomosis with adequate blood supply is essential. It is our opinion that less than an intraluminal stapler (Ethicon) 29 mm or end-to-end anastomosis 31 mm stapler should never be used to perform the anastomosis The treatment of fibrotic strictures ranges from dilatation or division with electrocautery to resection of the stricture with performance of a new anastomosis.

Financial Disclosures: None Reported

References

1. Hughes LE. Complications of diverticular disease: inflammation, obstruction and bleeding. Clin Gastroenterol 1975;4:147.
2. Dawson JL, Hanon I, Roxburgh RA. Diverticulitis complicated by diffuse peritonitis. Br J Surg 1965;52:354.
3. Browder W, Cerise EJ, Litwin MS. Impact of emergency angiography in massive lower intestinal bleeding. Ann Surg 1986;204:530.
4. Pennoyer WP, Vignati PV, Cohen JL. Mesenteric angiography for lower GI hemorrhage: are there predictors for positive study? Dis Colon Rectum 1997;49:1014.
5. King DW, Lubowski DZ, Armstrong AS. Sigmoid stricture at colonoscopy—an indication for surgery. Int J Colorectal Dis 1990;5:161.
6. Thompson WG. Do colonic diverticula cause symptoms?. Am J Gastroenterol 1986;81:613.
7. Goy JA, Eastwood MA, Mitchell WD, et al. Fecal characteristics contrasted in the irritable bowel syndrome and diverticular disease. Am J Clin Nutr 1976;29:1480.
8. Littlewood ER, Ornstein MH, McLean Baird I, et al. Doubts about diverticular disease. BMJ 1981;283:1524.
9. Francis CY, Whorwell PJ. The irritable bowel syndrome. Postgrad Med J 1997;73:1.
10. Hulnick DH, Megibow AJ, Balthazar EJ, et al. Computed tomography in the evaluation of diverticulitis. Radiology 1984;152:491.
11. Neff CC, van Sonnenberg E. CT of diverticulitis: diagnosis and treatment. Radiol Clin North Am 1989;27:743.
12. Woods RJ, Lavery IC, Fazio VW, et al. Internal fistulas in diverticular disease. Dis Colon Rectum 1988;31:591.
13. Kurtz DI, Mazier P. Diverticular fistulas. Semin Colon Rectal Surg 1994;1:93.
14. Krukowski ZH, Koruth NM, Matheson NA. Evolving practice in acute diverticulitis. Br J Surg 1985;82:684.
15. Hinchey GC, Schall GH, Richards MB. Treatment of perforated diverticulitis of the colon. Adv Surg 1978;12:85.
16. Hartmann H. Nouveau procédé d'ablation des cancers de la partie terminale du côlon pelvien. Cong Franc Chir 1923;30:411.
17. Haas PA, Haas GP. A critical evaluation of the Hartmann's procedure. Am Surg 1988; 54:381.
18. Roe AM, Prabhu S, Ali A, et al. Reversal of Hartmann's procedure: timing and operative technique. Br J Surg 1991;78:1167.
19. Hackford AW, Schoetz DJ, Coller JA, et al. Surgical management of complicated diverticulitis: the Lahey Clinic experience 1967 to 1982. Dis Colon Rectum 1985;28:317.
20. Constantinides VA, Heriot A, Remzi F, et al. Operative strategies for diverticular peritonitis: a decision analysis between primary resection and anastomosis versus Hartmann's procedures. Ann Surg 2007;245:94–103.
21. Murray JJ, Schoetz DJ, Coller JA, et al. Intraoperative colonic lavage and primary anastomosis in nonelective colon resection. Dis Colon Rectum 1991;34:527.
22. Stewart J, Diament RH, Brennan TG. Management of obstructing lesions of the left colon by resection, on-table lavage and primary anastomosis. Surgery 1933;114:502.
23. Ramos JM, Beart RW Jr, Goes R, et al. Role of laparoscopy in colorectal surgery: a prospective evaluation of 200 cases. Dis Colon Rectum 1995;38:494.
24. Ortega AE, Beart RW Jr, Steele GD Jr, et al. Laparoscopic bowel surgery registry: preliminary results. Dis Colon Rectum 1995; 38:681.
25. Mooney MJ, Elliott PL, Galapon DB, et al. Hand-assisted laparoscopic sigmoidectomy for diverticulitis. Dis Colon Rectum 1998; 41:630.
26. Eijsbouts QA, de Haan J, Berends F, et al. Laparoscopic elective treatment of diverticular disease: a comparison between laparoscopic-assisted and resection-facilitated techniques. Surg Endosc 2000;14:726.
27. Leggett PL, Churchmann-Winn R, Miller G. Minimizing ports to improve laparoscopic cholecystectomy. Surg Endosc 2000;14:32–6.
28. Engledow AH, Pakzad F, Ward N, et al. Laparoscopic resection of diverticular fistulae: a 10-year experience. Colorectal Dis 2007; 9:632–4.
29. Bartus CM, Lipof T, Sarwar CMS, et al. Colovesical fistula: not a contraindication to elective laparoscopic colectomy. Dis Colon Rectum 2005;48:233–6.
30. Myers E, Hurley M, O'Sullivan GC, et al. Laparoscopic peritoneal lavage for generalized peritonitis due to perforated diverticulitis. Br J Surg 2008;95:97–101.
31. Leroy J, Cahill RA, Asakuma M, et al. Single-access laparoscopic sigmoidectomy as definitive surgical management of prior diverticulitis in a human patient. Arch Surg 2009;144: 173–9.
32. Berthou JC, Charbonneau P. Elective laparoscopic management of sigmoid diverticulitis. Surg Endosc 1999;13:457.
33. Trebuchet G, Lechaux D, Lecalve JL. Laparoscopic left colon resection for diverticular disease. Surg Endosc 2002;16:18.
34. Kockerling F, Schneider C, Reymond MA, et al. Laparoscopic resection of sigmoid diverticulitis. Surg Endosc 1999;13:567.
35. Senagore AJ, Duepree HJ, Delaney CP, et al. Cost structure of laparoscopic and open sigmoid colectomy for diverticular disease. Dis Colon Rectum 2002;45:485.
36. Irvin TT, Goligher JC. Aetiology and disruption of intestinal anastomosis. Br J Surg 1973;60:461.
37. Krukowski ZH, Matheson NA. Emergency surgery for diverticular disease complicated by generalized fecal peritonitis: a review. Br J Surg 1984;71:921.
38. Shepard A, Keighley MR. Audit of complicated diverticular disease. Ann R Coll Surg Engl 1986;68:8.
39. Sarin S, Poulos PB. Evaluation of current surgical management of acute inflammatory diverticular disease. Ann R Coll Surg Engl 1991;73:278.
40. Benn PL, Wolff BC, Ilstrup DM. Level of anastomosis and recurrent colonic diverticulitis. Am J Surg 1986;151:269.
41. Bell AM, Wolff BG. Progression and recurrence after resection for diverticulitis. Semin Colon Rectal Surg 1990;1:99.
42. Fry DE, Milholen L, Harbrecht PJ. Iatrogenic ureteral injury. Arch Surg 1983; 118:454.
43. Ambrosetti P, Francis K, De Peyer R, Frossard JL. Colorectal anastomotic stenosis after elective laparoscopic sigmoidectomy for diverticular disease: a prospective evaluation of 68 patients. Dis Colon Rectum 2008;51: 1345–9.

Acknowledgments

Figures 1 and 2 Dragonfly Media Group.
Figure 4 Tom Moore.

patient should proceed to surgery. If there is a suspected or known colonic or rectal malignancy, oncologic principles should drive the surgical options. In most patients, except for patients with low rectal cancers or metastatic disease, total colectomy with IPAA is an acceptable surgical treatment modality. In the setting of a rectal cancer, there is a particular concern about performing an IPAA as any required radiation may severely compromise pouch function. In general, CUC patients with malignancies have a stage-for-stage prognosis similar to that of patients without CUC. Those patients who have undergone surgery, particularly with an IPAA, tolerate the chemotherapy as well as cohorts of patients without CUC.[8–10] In general, if oncologic principles are not compromised, then an IPAA can be performed without a deleterious impact on oncologic outcomes or long-term IPAA function.

Surgical Procedures for Ulcerative Colitis

The choice of operation depends on a number of factors that must be individualized to the patient's clinical condition. Currently, there are three major operative approaches used in the treatment of ulcerative colitis: (1) proctocolectomy with an end ileostomy, (2) total colectomy with IPAA, and (3) total abdominal colectomy with ileorectal anastomosis. In general, the operative approach used is dictated by the presentation of the disease either requiring emergency or elective operation.

For those patients who require emergency surgery, are in a poor medical condition because of their underlying disease, or are significantly immunosuppressed, a three-stage procedure is performed. Stage I is total abdominal colectomy with a Hartmann closure and an end ileostomy. This allows the majority of diseased colon to be removed, thus improving the patient's clinical condition while being tapered off of any immunosuppressive medications. Once recovered and clinically ready for another operation, again depending on the patient's condition, stage II entails either a completion proctectomy with end ileostomy or an IPAA with diverting loop ileostomy. In the latter situation, the patient will have to undergo a third stage to reverse the ileostomy. The reason behind not performing a proctectomy in an emergency is that, by leaving the rectum in place, a restorative operation can be performed in the future without having disturbed the dissection planes in the pelvis. In addition, an emergency proctectomy is associated with a higher risk of bleeding and injury to the nerves of the pelvic floor, bladder, and genitalia. Usually, the small amount of diseased tissue left behind does not present a clinical problem. In the nonemergency setting, the procedure of choice in the appropriate patient is the IPAA with a diverting loop ileostomy. However, in some practices, placement of a diverting loop ileostomy is selectively omitted.

ILEAL POUCH-ANAL ANASTOMOSIS

IPAA is considered the standard elective surgical therapy for the treatment of CUC. Parks and Nichols first described the procedure in 1978.[11,12] The decision to proceed with operations other than IPAA is based on individual patient circumstances or preexisting medical or physiologic conditions that are contraindications for this type of restorative procedure. IPAA is the ideal operation for the treatment of CUC because it removes the entire diseased organ while simultaneously preserving the normal anatomic route for defecation. Construction of the ileal pouch is the key to the success of this operation as it provides an adequate fecal reservoir to allow voluntary defecation, albeit at a higher but manageable daily frequency than for patients with an intact rectum.

Since the introduction of IPAA in the early 1980s, the procedure continues to evolve, especially with the application of new technologies such as laparoscopic surgery.[13–15] The operation basically involves four phases: (1) removal of the intra-abdominal colon; (2) dissection and removal of the rectum, sparing the pelvic nerves and the anal sphincter mechanism; (3) construction of an ileal reservoir; and (4) anastomosis of the ileal reservoir to the anal canal.

The general techniques, both open and laparoscopic, used at the Mayo Clinic are described below. Depending on surgeon preference, the patient may receive a bowel preparation the evening before surgery. Oral antibiotics are not used. The patient receives appropriate intravenous antibiotic in the operating room within 1 hour of incision. Once induced into anesthesia, the patient is positioned in the modified lithotomy position, which allows easy access to both the abdomen and the perineum.

For the traditional open technique, the abdomen is entered through a midline vertical incision starting at the pubis and extended as far cephalad as required to remove the colon. The abdomen is thoroughly explored to determine if there are any technical or pathologic contraindications to proceeding with the total colectomy and IPAA. The entire colon is mobilized from its retroperitoneal attachments. The transverse colon is freed from the greater omentum, which is preserved if it is of good quality and quantity. Once the intra-abdominal colon has been mobilized, the terminal ileum is divided from the right colon adjacent to the ileocecal junction using a linear stapling device. The mesentery is divided as close to the right colon as possible to avoid injuring the ileocolic vessels supplying the terminal ileum. Once the right colon has been mobilized, the remainder of the colon is divided from its mesentery in a routine fashion. When the intra-abdominal colon has been fully mobilized and the mesentery has been divided, the patient is placed in a steep Trendelenburg position to facilitate the pelvic dissection of the rectum. The rectum is freed down to the pelvic floor. Great care is taken to avoid the pelvic nerves that lie in the interface between the mesorectum and the presacral fascia. The rectum is divided at the pelvic floor with a stapling device [*see Figure 1*]. The entire colon and rectum is then sent for pathologic evaluation.

After the colon has been removed, the ileal pouch is constructed. The small bowel mesentery is completely mobilized from the retroperitoneum up to the inferior border of the pancreas. It is important to perform this mobilization completely to ensure adequate length for the ileal pouch to reach the pelvic floor. Also, to increase the length, the visceral peritoneum is scored at intervals along the course of the vessels supplying the distal small bowel. Once the mesentery has been mobilized, the pouch is fashioned. It has become our practice to use the J-shaped reservoir constructed from the last 30 to 35 cm of the terminal ileum. The J-shaped reservoir is simpler to construct, uses less intestine length, and is associated with fewer complications related to pouch-emptying

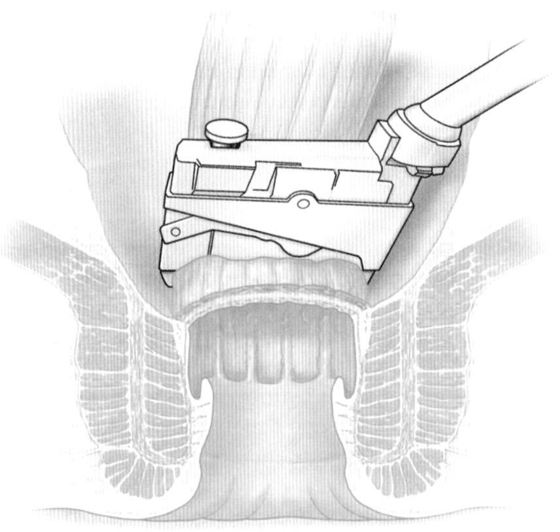

Figure 1 **Once the rectum has been dissected down to the level of the pelvic floor, it is divided with a stapler. The stapler is positioned 1 to 2 cm above the dentate line and fired. This positioning ensures that the final pouch-anal anastomosis is within the anal canal and not in the rectum.**

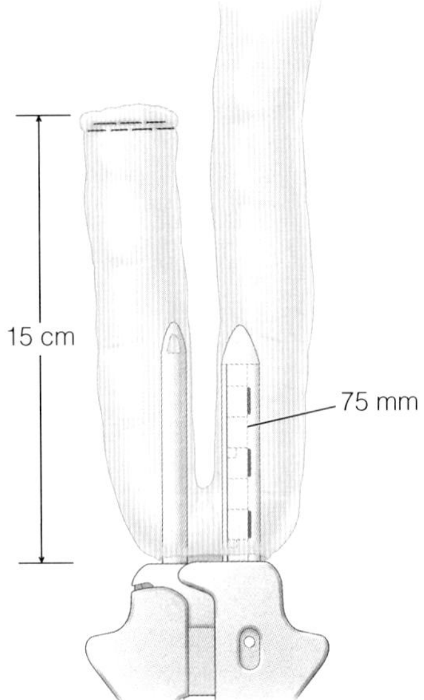

Figure 2 **The ileal pouch is constructed by dividing the common wall of the afferent and efferent limbs of the distal ileum by means of multiple firings of a linear cutting stapler.**

problems than other described W- or S-type reservoirs. To ultimately achieve a pouch with a reservoir capacity of approximately 400 cc, the pouch is constructed by folding the terminal ileum into a J shape. The hook of the "J" should be approximately 15 cm in length. This efferent limb of the J is then loosely secured to the afferent limb of the small bowel.

Prior to forming the reservoir, an adequate length of small bowel has to be determined. To ensure that the pouch will reach the pelvic floor and the region of the anastomosis without tension, the apex of the pouch should be able to be pulled 3 to 5 cm below the upper aspect of the pubic symphysis. If after full mesenteric mobilization and scoring of the visceral peritoneum the pouch does not easily reach the pelvic floor, it may be necessary to divide either the ileocolic vessel or one of the proximal branches of the superior mesenteric vessels. When there is a concern that the J-shaped reservoir will not reach the pelvic floor satisfactorily, one may alternatively construct an S- or W-shaped pouch. If the J pouch will reach the pelvic floor, the reservoir is constructed by two firings of the 75 mm linear cutting stapling device from the apex of the pouch dividing the common wall between the two limbs of the J pouch [*see Figure 2*]. Prior to bringing the pouch down to the anus, it is important to verify that the small intestine from the ligament of Treitz to the ileal pouch is not twisted. At this point in the operation, one of two options is available to perform the anastomosis. The pouch may be secured to the anal canal by performing a double-stapled technique in which the head of the end-to-end anastomosis (EEA) stapling device is secured in the apex of the pouch with a purse-string suture [*see Figure 3*]. The stapling device is then placed into the anus, and the attachment pin is placed through the staple line where the rectum was divided at the level of the pelvic floor. The pouch is then brought down into the pelvis, maintaining the proper orientation, and the stapled anastomosis is performed [*see Figure 4*].

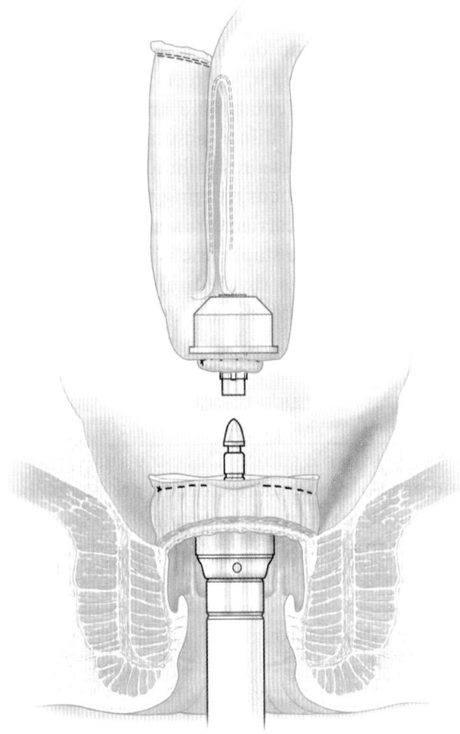

Figure 3 **After the pouch is constructed, the head of an end-to-end anastomosis stapler is secured in the apex of the pouch and connected to the pin of the stapler, which is placed upward through the anus.**

OTHER

Other disease processes appropriate for segmental colectomy include ischemia, volvulus, localized bleeding source, and infectious colitides. Neoplasms in the colon other than colon cancer, such as lipoma, leiomyoma, gastrointestinal stromal tumors, lymphomas, and carcinoid, may also require segmental resection. The diagnosis, evaluation, and treatment algorithms for these relatively infrequent indications for colectomy are beyond the scope of this chapter.

Preoperative Planning

The specific elements of preoperative planning that might be considered appropriate vary widely and are determined by the patient's disease process. Most importantly, pathology and location of disease should be confirmed prior to proceeding with surgery. The informed consent process should involve a discussion of the possibility of anastomotic leak and temporary ostomy (either at the time of surgery or as a result of postoperative complication).

COLONOSCOPY

For a patient with colonic pathology, an endoscopic examination should be considered a natural extension of the physical examination for two main reasons. First, the possibility of previously unsuspected pathology is significant. In one study of patients with obstructing colonic cancers, 58% had adenomas outside the field of resection and 6% had synchronous cancers.[22] Second, it is incumbent upon the operating surgeon to ensure concordance between the suspected and actual location of pathology. Permanent tattooing should be performed routinely except in rare situations where localization is straightforward. Unless clinical circumstances contraindicate such an investigation, any patient for whom a colectomy is planned should undergo a complete colonoscopy. Importantly, mechanical bowel preparation (taken orally) should be considered contraindicated in patients with a significant colonic obstruction.

An adjunct in the management of distal colonic obstruction is endoluminal stenting. Although it is not without significant complications, it can be an excellent bridge to resection in the patient with obstruction secondary to malignancy or benign stricture or as palliation in the patient with advanced disease.[23] In patients for whom resection is planned, decompression of the proximal bowel may facilitate primary anastomosis by minimizing size mismatch and bowel compromise. In addition, this allows for time to correct electrolyte abnormalities and give a bowel preparation if considered necessary. Patients who are candidates for stenting do not need two surgical procedures, with a reported average of 7 days from stenting to operative resection. Approximately 70% of patients with malignant colon obstructions will be successfully managed with a stent and subsequent definitive resection.[24,25] Stenting as a bridge to resection is generally not useful in patients with right-sided colonic obstructions as an ileocolic anastomosis is safe in all but the most advanced cases of obstruction.

COMPUTED TOMOGRAPHY

CT scanning of the abdomen/pelvis is almost universally performed prior to colectomy. In cases of malignancy, CT is an invaluable element of the staging evaluation. Patients with a significant burden of hepatic metastases with replacement of more than 50% of the hepatic parenchyma may be a prohibitive risk for surgery.[26] The direct extension of the tumor into adjacent structures may alter the surgical plan, possibly necessitating the involvement of other surgical disciplines. CT combined with positron emission tomography (PET) is more sensitive for extrahepatic metastases and recurrences and should be strongly considered in preoperative staging.[27] In the setting of diverticular disease, CT is necessary for confirmation of diagnosis and is generally performed prior to surgical evaluation. A close examination of the locations and severity of prior episodes of acute diverticulitis is important to determine the extent of colon resection.

BOWEL PREPARATION

The importance of preoperative mechanical bowel preparation in patients undergoing colectomy is a topic of ongoing debate. Historically, the justification for the exercise has been concern over the risks of surgical site infections and anastomotic leakage. This concern appears to be at least somewhat overstated. The risk of overall complications is similar between patients who had versus those who did not have a mechanical bowel preparation. In the largest randomized trials, however, there is a significantly lower rate of abdominal abscess among patients who underwent preparation, although there is a significantly higher rate of wound infections.[28] These same studies failed to show a significant difference in anastomotic leakage. Notably, fast-track protocols specifically have omitted mechanical bowel preparation as it is thought that this may minimize fluid shifts and the consequences of aggressive fluid resuscitation.[29]

There may be situations in which bowel preparation has particular utility, above and beyond the outcomes mentioned above. When the preoperative localization of a colonic lesion is questionable, an intraoperative endoscopic examination is facilitated by a preoperative mechanical bowel preparation. Laparoscopic manipulation of a colon that is loaded with solid stool can be challenging, and the decompressed colon is easier to exteriorize through a small fascial defect. Colorectal anastomotic techniques using a circular stapler can also be compromised if the distal colorectum is filled with solid stool, thereby impeding the passage of the stapler and the formation of the anastomosis.

The debate regarding bowel preparation goes well beyond what can be covered in this chapter. Given the equivocal evidence regarding the impact of bowel preparation on patient outcomes, the decision should be made on a case-by-case basis by the surgeon based on interpretation of the data and the utility of preparation.

STOMA MARKING

In patients with a high likelihood or certainty of stoma, preoperative marking can assist in planning an appropriate site. Patients who have preoperative education are less likely to have anxiety about caring for a stoma at home. In addition, there are significantly fewer stoma-related complications in patients who have been marked prior to being placed on the operating table.[30]

DEEP VEIN THROMBOSIS PROPHYLAXIS

Patients undergoing colorectal surgery have an increased risk of deep venous thrombosis (DVT) and pulmonary embolism (PE), and without prophylaxis, the rate of DVT is 30%.[31] In addition to routine postoperative therapy, preoperative heparin administration has been shown to decrease venous thromboembolism; heparin three times daily or other chemical DVT prophylaxis should be administered postoperatively, as well as mechanical devices.[32] These regimens have not been associated with any significantly increased risk of bleeding.[33]

PREOPERATIVE ANTIBIOTICS

Preoperative antibiotics with both aerobic and anaerobic coverage should also be given. Current guidelines under the Surgical Care Improvement Project include an appropriate antibiotic (e.g., ertapenem or metronidazole plus a fluoroquinolone, first-generation cephalosporin, or aminoglycoside) started within 1 hour of incision, with hair clipped rather than shaved, urinary catheters removed by postoperative day 2, and normothermia maintained perioperatively. Wound infection rates are decreased by as much as 75% when antibiotics are given preoperatively; the postoperative duration of antibiotic therapy does not impact outcomes, and recommendations are for a single preoperative dose or a total of 24 hours of therapy.[34]

PREOPERATIVE URETERAL STENTING

An in-depth knowledge of colon anatomy and its surrounding relations can prevent inadvertent injuries during the procedure, but the intimate association of both ureters with the colon must be given preoperative consideration. In the setting of bulky tumors or expected severe inflammation in the sigmoid or cecum, ureteral stents may be useful. Ureteral stents offer a means for both visualization and palpation of the ureters to protect them from harm. It is also commonly acknowledged that ureteral stents assist in identifying injury at the time it is caused more so than actually preventing injury[34]; this fact reasserts that there is no substitute for cautious dissection and constant vigilance for the presence of the ureter or other structures, particularly when cautery or transection of tissue occurs.

Technical Considerations

LAPAROSCOPIC VERSUS OPEN SURGERY

Laparoscopic surgical treatment of colon disease is now widely accepted as the standard of care for most colectomies. A growing number of reports have described the short-term benefits of laparoscopy in treating benign conditions of the colon (e.g., diverticulitis, Crohn disease, and ulcerative colitis).[35] Controlled studies performed by experienced surgeons have found laparoscopy to have advantages over open resection in terms of resolution of ileus, duration of hospitalization, level of postoperative pain and narcotic use, recovery of pulmonary function, complication rates, and quality of life in the initial postoperative period.[36–42] Cost analyses also favor laparoscopic colectomy over conventional surgery, finding that the higher costs of the surgical instruments and the potentially longer operating times are outweighed by the shorter duration of hospitalization.[41–44] There also appears to be a lower incidence of surgical site complications after laparoscopy than after open surgery, as well as a lower incidence of postoperative complications.[45,46] Overall complications over time are significantly diminished.[35] There have also been studies suggesting that cosmetic outcome and body image are improved by laparoscopic surgery, although quality of life is generally similar.[47]

Although there was initial concern that pneumoperitoneum and multiple areas of entry might lead to intra-abdominal spread or port site recurrences, wound recurrences are now recognized to be no more common in laparoscopy than in open surgery.[48–50] In addition, the multicenter, randomized, prospective trial carried out by the Clinical Outcomes of Surgical Therapy Study Group showed that survival, recurrence, and complications were not significantly different between laparoscopic and open approaches over long-term follow-up (median 4.4 years).[36,42]

ONCOLOGIC CONSIDERATIONS

When colectomy is performed for an oncologic indication, special deliberation must be given to specific elements of the planned operation. First and foremost, the operation should provide adequate extirpation of the patient's tumor burden and an appropriate mesenteric resection. In general, a proximal and distal margin of at least 5 cm is considered appropriate, although this is further determined by the vascular supply to the colon segment. Usually, the linear margins are easily obtained when an adequate mesenteric resection is executed. When a colon cancer has invaded locally into surrounding structures, an en bloc resection should be planned, with the engagement of other surgical disciplines as required.

In evaluating the appropriateness of a resection for cancer, a significant amount of attention has been paid to the correlation between the number of lymph nodes analyzed and the patient's oncologic outcomes. Greater numbers of lymph nodes analyzed are associated with better survival in stage II and stage III colon cancer, and these findings have led to a belief that an adequate lymph node analysis is a measure of quality of care.[43] The relation between the extent of surgical resection (lymph node harvest), number of nodes analyzed (pathologic examination), and long-term oncologic outcomes is at best speculative at this point.[51,52] Patient quality of care is best served by surgeons and pathologists who are focused on appropriate techniques rather than on achieving a specific lymph node "count."

The extent of resection should encompass one blood vessel proximal and one below the tumor [*see Figure 2*]. Tumors in the cecum or ascending colon require 5 to 10 cm of terminal ileum with ligation of the ileocolic pedicle and right branch of the middle colic vessels, with transection at the level of the proximal to midtransverse colon. A tumor at the hepatic flexure or proximal transverse colon mandates an extended right hemicolectomy, with ligation of the ileocolic, right colic, and middle colic at its origin, with transection at the distal transverse or descending colon. Lesions

A stapled side-to-side anastomosis should be avoided in the left colon as these anastomoses create a reservoir in the middle of a colonic segment, which is prone to stagnation, and anecdotally have a higher leak rate. A handsewn anastomosis is preferred in these circumstances. Colorectal anastomoses can be handsewn or stapled using an end-end-anastomosis (EEA) stapling device.

If the sigmoid colon is resected, an EEA stapler can be used to perform an end-to-end anastomosis into the upper rectum. The largest stapler that will fit is selected; this may be ascertained by placing sizers in the rectum and colon to ensure fit. Prior to suturing the EEA anvil into the colon, the ability of the EEA stapler to reach the top of the rectal stump should be confirmed. When an appropriate size of the EEA is selected, a purse-string or baseball stitch is placed around the cut edge of the colon, and the anvil is tied in place. The stapler is placed through the anus into the rectum and guided such that the spike of the stapler can be protracted adjacent to the staple line rather than through it, which runs the risk of separating the staple line. After docking the anvil to the stapler, the stapler is fired, released, and removed. The donuts are removed from the stapler and examined for completeness; these may be sent for microscopic assessment of margins if warranted. The pelvis is then filled with irrigant, and a rigid proctoscope is inserted. With the colon clamped proximal to the anastomosis, the rectum is insufflated to ascertain if there is any air leak. In cases where an air leak is appreciated, the anastomosis should either be reinforced and reevaluated or completely resected and reconstructed.

LAPAROSCOPIC LEFT COLON RESECTION

After mobilization is completed for a left colectomy, an extraction incision is made and the colon is extracted. The resection and anastomosis are then performed in the same manner employed for the open procedure.

The mobilization and control of vascular pedicles involved in a laproscopic left colectomy vary depending on factors related to tumor location and patient anatomy. As with an open left colectomy, the goal is to fashion a technically sound anastomosis between two portions of colorectum, which are well vascularized and joined without tension, while at the same time respecting oncologic principles (when the operation is performed for cancer). Achieving these goals may require resection of all or part of the rectum, sigmoid colon, descending colon, and transverse colon.

For resections that include the sigmoid colon and/or upper rectum, dissection should proceed distally into the pelvis to mobilize the upper rectum. The mesentery and other fatty tissue are then cleared up to the posterior wall of the rectum/rectosigmoid junction, allowing for division of the bowel in a region that has minimal adherent fat or mesentery. An endoscopic stapling device with a 3.5 mm staple height is placed across this area and fired.

The proximal margin for a laparoscopic resection needs to be planned carefully. Usually, the proximal margin of bowel is divided extracorporeally, but in so doing, the surgeon must ensure that there is enough proximal bowel to fashion a tension-free anastomosis. The marginal arterial circulation from the middle colic vessels is almost always adequate to perfuse the descending colon in cases where the IMA and/or left colic artery are resected.

If a colorectal anastomosis is planned, an EEA anvil is introduced into the proximal colon as previously discussed. Prior to suturing the anvil in place, the surgeon should be confident that the planned EEA stapler will reach the top of the rectal stump. Once this is done, the colon is then returned to the abdomen and the abdominal incision is closed. The EEA stapler is placed transanally and guided to the apex of the rectal stump, where the spike is ejected just above or below the staple line. The anvil is then docked onto the spike, the cut edge of the mesentery is assessed for twisting, and the stapler is closed and fired. After releasing and removing the stapler, the pelvis is filled with irrigant, and the rectum is insufflated to check for air leaks.

Most colocolonic anastomoses cannot be performed with an EEA. In these situations, the sites of proximal and distal transaction should be mobilized sufficiently to allow an extracorporeal handsewn anastomosis. The extraction site should be placed strategically to facilitate construction of the anastomosis.

POSTOPERATIVE CARE

Care after colectomy is primarily a function of three main goals: (1) adequate pain control, (2) awaiting the return of bowel function, and (3) vigilance for complications of surgery. Patient-controlled analgesia is widely accepted as effective management of postoperative pain, although many protocols call for the use of epidural catheters when appropriate. The routine use of nasogastric tubes after colectomy is no longer considered acceptable. Similarly, a course of antibiotics longer than 24 hours postoperatively is also not recommended. Early enteral feeding has been proven to be safe. Once patients are tolerating a low-residue diet, which decreases the local inflammatory response at the anastomosis, and passing flatus or stool, they can be discharged home, with follow-up after 2 weeks.[51]

Fast-track protocols have been developed and studied in multiple institutions in the hope of creating uniformity of care and decreasing postoperative stay. Common characteristics of these protocols are fluid minimization both in the operating room and postoperatively, epidural use, and early enteral feeding.[52] Further components of fast tracking include Foley catheter removal on postoperative day 1, no oral bowel preparation, scheduled nonnarcotic analgesia (e.g., intravenous ketorolac or oral acetaminophen), and early ambulation.[29,56] These strategies have commonly been shown to decrease length of stay by 4 to 6 days without increasing readmissions and potentially decrease complications by nearly 50% in open colorectal surgery.[52,57] The efficacy of fast-track protocols has been demonstrated in laparoscopic surgery as well, with fast-track patients having shorter times to enteral feeding (decreased by 1 day) and first bowel movement (decreased by 1 day), shorter lengths of stay (3 versus 4 to 5 days), and fewer complications (15 to 29% versus 25 to 56%).[29,56]

COMPLICATIONS

As with any major operation, colectomies are associated with a distinct risk of complications. These include those common to any abdominal surgery requiring general anesthesia, such as anesthetic complications, DVT and PE, myocardial infarction, stroke, pneumonia, wound infection, and urinary tract infection. The rates of these complications may be minimized by following national guidelines for prevention and treatment.

Complications specific to colorectal surgery include nerve injury or even compartment syndrome in the extremities secondary to positioning, injury to the spleen mandating splenectomy (approximately 1% of cases), and problems related to the anastomosis. Anastomotic leaks occur on the order of 1 to 5% depending on where in the colon the anastomosis is made; in general, the more distal the anastomosis, the higher the rate of leakage. Significant anastomotic bleeding occurs approximately 1% of the time, and abscesses (1% of cases) and strictures (up to 10% long term) also can occur, which may be related to anastomotic compromise secondary to ischemia, tension, or inflammation.[53,58] Although assessment of blood flow, tension, and bowel appearance makes anastomotic complications less likely, these will still occur. Finally, mortality may occur in 1% or more of cases, although this risk depends heavily on patient preoperative risk factors, emergent indications for surgery, and the complexity of the surgery itself.[58]

One notable theme that has emerged in the recent literature investigating the quality of surgical care is the concept of "rescue." In examining hospitals with widely varying death rates, it has been demonstrated that the underlying rate of serious complications is similar across these hospitals.[54] What is markedly different is the ability of hospitals to respond quickly and adequately to prevent worsened morbidity or mortality from a complication of surgery. This ability to "rescue" patients is an emergent property of various aspects of each hospital, including nursing care, ancillary staff, and culture. It is incumbent on each surgeon who performs colectomies to be part of a system that is focused not only on preventing complications but also on recognizing them and treating them quickly and appropriately.

Financial Disclosures: None Reported

References

1. Etzioni DA, Beart RW Jr, Madoff RD, Ault GT. Impact of the aging population on the demand for colorectal procedures. Dis Colon Rectum 2009;52:583–90; discussion 590–1.
2. Bal DG. Cancer in African Americans. CA Cancer J Clin 1992;42:5–6.
3. Arriaga AF, Lancaster RT, Berry WR, et al. The better colectomy project: association of evidence-based best-practice adherence rates to outcomes in colorectal surgery. Ann Surg 2009;250:507–13.
4. Cohen ME, Bilimoria KY, Ko CY, Hall BL. Development of an American College of Surgeons National Surgery Quality Improvement Program: morbidity and mortality risk calculator for colorectal surgery. J Am Coll Surg 2009;208: 1009–16.
5. Poultsides GA, Servais EL, Saltz LB, et al. Outcome of primary tumor in patients with synchronous stage IV colorectal cancer receiving combination chemotherapy without surgery as initial treatment. J Clin Oncol 2009;27: 3379–84.
6. Kudo S. Endoscopic mucosal resection of flat and depressed types of early colorectal cancer. Endoscopy 1993;25:455–61.
7. Nivatvongs S. Surgical management of malignant colorectal polyps. Surg Clin North Am 2002;82:959–66.
8. Nusko G, Mansmann U, Altendorf-Hofmann A, et al. Risk of invasive carcinoma in colorectal adenomas assessed by size and site. Int J Colorectal Dis 1997;12:267–71.
9. Alder AC, Hamilton EC, Anthony T, Sarosi GA Jr. Cancer risk in endoscopically unresectable colon polyps. Am J Surg 2006;192:644–8.
10. McDonald JM, Moonka R, Bell RH Jr. Pathologic risk factors of occult malignancy in endoscopically unresectable colonic adenomas. Am J Surg 1999;177:384–7.
11. Kronborg O, Fenger C. Clinical evidence for the adenoma-carcinoma sequence. Eur J Cancer Prev 1999;8 Suppl 1:S73–86.
12. Roberts P, Abel M, Rosen L, et al. Practice parameters for sigmoid diverticulitis. The Standards Task Force American Society of Colon and Rectal Surgeons. Dis Colon Rectum 1995;38:125–32.
13. Broderick-Villa G, Burchette RJ, Collins JC, et al. Hospitalization for acute diverticulitis does not mandate routine elective colectomy. Arch Surg 2005;140:576–81; discussion 581–3.
14. Rafferty J, Shellito P, Hyman NH, et al. Practice parameters for sigmoid diverticulitis. Dis Colon Rectum 2006;49: 939–44.
15. Salem L, Veenstra DL, Sullivan SD, Flum DR. The timing of elective colectomy in diverticulitis: a decision analysis. J Am Coll Surg 2004;199:904–12.
16. Gayer C, Chino A, Lucas C, et al. Acute lower gastrointestinal bleeding in 1,112 patients admitted to an urban emergency medical center. Surgery 2009;146:600–6; discussion 606–7.
17. Chintapalli KN, Chopra S, Ghiatas AA, et al. Diverticulitis versus colon cancer: differentiation with helical CT findings. Radiology 1999;210:429–35.
18. Lahat A, Yanai H, Menachem Y, et al. The feasibility and risk of early colonoscopy in acute diverticulitis: a prospective controlled study. Endoscopy 2007;39:521–4.
19. Sakhnini E, Lahat A, Melzer E, et al. Early colonoscopy in patients with acute diverticulitis: results of a prospective pilot study. Endoscopy 2004;36:504–7.
20. Alos R, Hinojosa J. Timing of surgery in Crohn's disease: a key issue in the management. World J Gastroenterol 2008;14:5532–9.
21. Martel P, Betton PO, Gallot D, Malafosse M. Crohn's colitis: experience with segmental resections; results in a series of 84 patients. J Am Coll Surg 2002;194:448–53.
22. Bat L, Neumann G, Shemesh E. The association of synchronous neoplasms with occluding colorectal cancer. Dis Colon Rectum 1985;28:149–51.
23. Small AJ, Coelho-Prabhu N, Baron TH. Endoscopic placement of self-expandable metal stents for malignant colonic obstruction: long-term outcomes and complication factors. Gastrointest Endosc 2010;71:560–72.
24. Sebastian S, Johnston S, Geoghegan T, et al. Pooled analysis of the efficacy and safety of self-expanding metal stenting in malignant colorectal obstruction. Am J Gastroenterol 2004;99:2051–7.

25. Brehant O, Fuks D, Bartoli E, et al. Elective (planned) colectomy in patients with colorectal obstruction after placement of a self-expanding metallic stent as a bridge to surgery: the results of a prospective study. Colorectal Dis 2009;11: 178–83.
26. Liu SK, Church JM, Lavery IC, Fazio VW. Operation in patients with incurable colon cancer—is it worthwhile? Dis Colon Rectum 1997;40:11–4.
27. Selzner M, Hany TF, Wildbrett P, et al. Does the novel PET/CT imaging modality impact on the treatment of patients with metastatic colorectal cancer of the liver? Ann Surg 2004;240:1027–34; discussion 1035–6.
28. Slim K, Vicaut E, Launay-Savary MV, et al. Updated systematic review and meta-analysis of randomized clinical trials on the role of mechanical bowel preparation before colorectal surgery. Ann Surg 2009;249:203–9.
29. Larson DW, Batdorf NJ, Touzios JG, et al. A fast-track recovery protocol improves outcomes in elective laparoscopic colectomy for diverticulitis. J Am Coll Surg 2010; 211:485–9.
30. Millan M, Tegido M, Biondo S, Garcia-Granero E. Preoperative stoma siting and education by stomatherapists of colorectal cancer patients: a descriptive study in twelve Spanish colorectal surgical units. Colorectal Dis 2010;12 (7 Online):e88–92.
31. Alizadeh K, Hyman N. Venous thromboembolism prophylaxis in colorectal surgery. Surg Technol Int 2005;14: 165–70.
32. Geerts WH, Bergqvist D, Pineo GF, et al. Prevention of venous thromboembolism: American College of Chest Physicians Evidence-Based Clinical Practice Guidelines (8th Edition). Chest 2008;133(6 Suppl):381S–453S.
33. Leonardi MJ, McGory ML, Ko CY. A systematic review of deep venous thrombosis prophylaxis in cancer patients: implications for improving quality. Ann Surg Oncol 2007;14:929–36.
34. Nelson RL, Glenny AM, Song F. Antimicrobial prophylaxis for colorectal surgery. Cochrane Database Syst Rev 2009;(1):CD001181.
35. Klarenbeek BR, Bergamaschi R, Veenhof AA, et al. Laparoscopic versus open sigmoid resection for diverticular disease: follow-up assessment of the randomized control Sigma trial. Surg Endosc 2011;25:1121–6.
36. A comparison of laparoscopically assisted and open colectomy for colon cancer. N Engl J Med 2004;350:2050–9.
37. Klarenbeek BR, Veenhof AA, Bergamaschi R, et al. Laparoscopic sigmoid resection for diverticulitis decreases major morbidity rates: a randomized control trial: short-term results of the Sigma Trial. Ann Surg 2009;249:39–44.
38. Faynsod M, Stamos MJ, Arnell T, et al. A case-control study of laparoscopic versus open sigmoid colectomy for diverticulitis. Am Surg 2000;66:841–3.
39. Gonzalez R, Smith CD, Mattar SG, et al. Laparoscopic vs open resection for the treatment of diverticular disease. Surg Endosc 2004;18:276–80.
40. Marcello PW, Milsom JW, Wong SK, et al. Laparoscopic total colectomy for acute colitis: a case-control study. Dis Colon Rectum 2001;44:1441–5.
41. Marcello PW, Milsom JW, Wong SK, et al. Laparoscopic restorative proctocolectomy: case-matched comparative study with open restorative proctocolectomy. Dis Colon Rectum 2000;43:604–8.
42. Fleshman J, Sargent DJ, Green E, et al. Laparoscopic colectomy for cancer is not inferior to open surgery based on 5-year data from the COST Study Group trial. Ann Surg 2007;246:655–62; discussion 662–4.
43. Chang GJ, Rodriguez-Bigas MA, Skibber JM, Moyer VA. Lymph node evaluation and survival after curative resection of colon cancer: systematic review. J Natl Cancer Inst 2007;99:433–41.
44. Grinnell RS. Results of ligation of inferior mesenteric artery at the aorta in resections of carcinoma of the descending and sigmoid colon and rectum. Surg Gynecol Obstet 1965; 120:1031–6.
45. Adachi Y, Inomata M, Miyazaki N, et al. Distribution of lymph node metastasis and level of inferior mesenteric artery ligation in colorectal cancer. J Clin Gastroenterol 1998;26:179–82.
46. Kawamura YJ, Sakuragi M, Togashi K, et al. Distribution of lymph node metastasis in T1 sigmoid colon carcinoma: should we ligate the inferior mesenteric artery? Scand J Gastroenterol 2005;40:858–61.
47. Newcomb WL, Hope WW, Schmelzer TM, et al. Comparison of blood vessel sealing among new electrosurgical and ultrasonic devices. Surg Endosc 2009;23:90–6.
48. Harold KL, Pollinger H, Matthews BD, et al. Comparison of ultrasonic energy, bipolar thermal energy, and vascular clips for the hemostasis of small-, medium-, and large-sized arteries. Surg Endosc 2003;17:1228–30.
49. Campagnacci R, de Sanctis A, Baldarelli M, et al. Electrothermal bipolar vessel sealing device vs. ultrasonic coagulating shears in laparoscopic colectomies: a comparative study. Surg Endosc 2007;21:1526–31.
50. Choy PY, Bissett IP, Docherty JG, et al. Stapled versus handsewn methods for ileocolic anastomoses. Cochrane Database Syst Rev 2007;(3):CD004320.
51. Martinez-Mas E, Vazquez-Prado A, Larrocha-Grau M, et al. The impact of low-residue enteral feeding on the healing of colonic anastomoses. Hepatogastroenterology 1993;40: 481–4.
52. Muller S, Zalunardo MP, Hubner M, et al. A fast-track program reduces complications and length of hospital stay after open colonic surgery. Gastroenterology 2009;136: 842–7.
53. Bernstein J, Holt GB. Paying surgeons less can cost more. J Med Pract Manage 1999;14:282–7.
54. Ghaferi AA, Birkmeyer JD, Dimick JB. Variation in hospital mortality associated with inpatient surgery. N Engl J Med 2009;361:1368–75.
55. Griffiths JD. Surgical anatomy of the blood supply of the distal colon. Ann R Coll Surg Engl 1956;19:241–56.
56. Tsikitis VL, Holubar SD, Dozois EJ, et al. Advantages of fast-track recovery after laparoscopic right hemicolectomy for colon cancer. Surg Endosc 2010;24:1911–6.
57. Basse L, Thorbol JE, Lossl K, Kehlet H. Colonic surgery with accelerated rehabilitation or conventional care. Dis Colon Rectum 2004;47:271–7; discussion 277–8.
58. Killingback M, Barron P, Dent O. Elective resection and anastomosis for colorectal cancer: a prospective audit of mortality and morbidity 1976–1998. Aust N Z J Surg 2002; 72:689–98.

Acknowledgment

Figures 2 through 4 Christine Kenney

33 PROCEDURES FOR RECTAL CANCER

David A. Rothenberger, MD, FACS, Rocco Ricciardi, MD, FACS, and Robert D. Madoff, MD, FACS

Rectal cancer is a common and lethal malignancy diagnosed in over 40,000 Americans each year.[1] Treatment may be undertaken with curative or palliative intent. Cure is almost never achieved without a surgical resection that achieves microscopically clear margins (R0 resection). Other surgical goals are to maintain or restore bowel continuity with normal or near-normal anal continence, preserve sexual and bladder function, and minimize other treatment-associated morbidity and mortality. Low anterior resection (LAR) and abdominoperineal resection (APR) are the most common operations for rectal cancer. Ricciardi and colleagues reported that of 41,631 patients undergoing radical extirpative surgery for rectal cancer in the United States between 1988 and 2003, 60% had sphincter-sacrificing procedures and 40% had sphincter-sparing procedures.[2] Sphincter-sparing operations increased from 27% in 1988 to 48% in 2003. Today, a wide variety of treatment regimens are available to treat rectal cancer spanning the spectrum from simple polypectomy to prolonged and potentially morbid multimodality regimens of neoadjuvant chemoradiation therapy, radical extirpative multivisceral and extended resections, adjuvant chemotherapy, and biologic agents.

Choosing the optimal therapy for rectal cancer is a complex process. Although physicians from different disciplines are increasingly involved, it is the colorectal surgeon who generally directs the initial evaluation of patients with rectal cancer and leads the discussion with a multidisciplinary team and the patient to select a treatment protocol. In this chapter, we examine the surgeon's unique and critical role in the pretreatment evaluation and decisions leading to choice of therapy, review alternative operative approaches, address key technical aspects of the operations performed to treat rectal cancer, and discuss postoperative therapy and follow-up.

Pretreatment Evaluation

The pretreatment evaluation of the patient with a rectal cancer is the basis for rational decision making regarding choice of therapy. Evaluation includes assessment of the patient and the primary cancer as well as a search for metastases and synchronous colonic abnormalities.

PATIENT ASSESSMENT

A complete clinical assessment is done to identify preexisting comorbidities, define operative risk, and explore the patient's psychosocial state and ability to manage the stresses accompanying the diagnosis and treatment of rectal cancer.

Comorbidities

A history and physical examination with standard preoperative blood and urine tests, electrocardiogram, and serum carcinoembryonic antigen (CEA) are obtained. Important general medical issues that the surgeon must review include current medications and allergies; smoking status; use of alcohol or other drugs; major organ dysfunction (cardiopulmonary, renal, and hepatic); hypertension; obesity; anemia; malnutrition; diabetes; deep vein thrombosis; and pulmonary embolism. Knowledge of prior operations (especially those involving the digestive or genitourinary organs), prior infections following surgical procedures, prior pelvic irradiation, baseline bowel and anal sphincter function, a personal history of colorectal polyps or cancers, and a family history suggestive of a hereditary cancer syndrome are vital for the colorectal surgeon. During the physical examination, the surgeon should be especially alert for the presence of liver enlargement, abdominal tenderness or masses, lymphadenopathy, muscle wasting or ascites, and abdominal scars or ventral hernias that may complicate planned surgery. The integrity and function of the anal sphincter are carefully assessed by means of digital rectal examination and, if necessary, by additional physiologic testing and endoanal ultrasonography.

Operative Risk

The risk of postoperative adverse events is important for surgical shared decision making and obtaining informed consent from the patient. In modern series, 30-day postoperative mortality after resection of the rectum ranges from 1.6 to 4.8% and morbidity remains high.[3] Numerous perioperative scoring systems have been developed either to predict the likelihood of postoperative morbidity and mortality or to allow risk-stratified comparison of outcomes between institutions and surgeons.[4] Although none of these scoring systems are specific for the rectal cancer patient, a morbidity and mortality risk calculator for colorectal surgery was recently developed by the American College of Surgeons National Surgery Quality Improvement Program.[5] This tool predicts mortality, overall morbidity, and serious morbidity and provides assessment of hospital effects on adverse outcomes for patients undergoing colorectal surgery.

The influence of age on operative mortality is complex. Although the elderly may tolerate a complex procedure quite well, they often cannot tolerate complications. Thus, prediction of potential morbidity is particularly important in decision making for the elderly patient with rectal cancer. We recently assessed the association between older age (≥ 75 years) and short-term outcomes after major oncologic resections in 8,781 patients, including 485 who underwent proctectomy for rectal cancer with or without total abdominal colectomy.[6] Older patients had increased preoperative comorbidities, higher operative mortality (4.83% if >75 years versus

1.09% if aged 40 to 55 years), higher rates of major complications, and longer hospital stays. Older age is independently associated with worse short-term outcomes after major oncologic resections, but the effect of older age is comparable to other preoperative risks.

Psychosocial Evaluation

The surgeon must understand the patient's desires, knowledge base, expectations, lifestyle, and social support resources. The goal is to obtain information that may impact the treatment plan and identify preexisting conditions that can be addressed and optimized before an elective operation. The needs of a homeless individual or a down-and-out drug addict with no resources, no access to reliable transportation, and no family available for support are quite different from those of a well-educated, upper middle class individual with financial resources and a supportive network of family and friends. Similarly, in some cultures and for some people, a colostomy is worse than death. Each patient deserves optimal care, and the surgeon must recognize and adjust the approach to meet the individual patient's needs. Some patients will require significantly more social resources to help them through the treatment process, whereas others will require more counseling time and direct support from the surgeon or other caregivers.

RECTAL CANCER ASSESSMENT

The gross morphology and histology, precise location, and local extent of the primary rectal cancer are assessed by biopsy, clinical assessment, proctosigmoidoscopy, and imaging studies. The American Joint Committee on Cancer's TNM classification system is clinically useful and accepted worldwide [*see Table 1 and Table 2*].

Gross and Histopathology

The gross morphology is noted. Ulcerated lesions are generally more invasive and aggressive than exophytic lesions. Biopsy (or review of prior biopsies) is an essential first step to confirm the diagnosis of adenocarcinoma and to ascertain the presence of unfavorable histologic features (e.g., mucin production, lymphovascular invasion, or signet cell histology) that may influence choice of therapy.

Location

The precise level and the quadrants and percentage of rectal circumference involved by a rectal cancer are determined by digital rectal examination (DRE) and proctosigmoidoscopy. The surgeon should not rely on the level as determined by another physician as it is often estimated quite inaccurately. Although the level is traditionally measured as centimeters proximal to the anal verge, most experienced rectal cancer surgeons find it more useful to assess the level of a rectal cancer relative to the anal sphincter muscles and anorectal ring and to measure the distance of normal rectum distal to the lower border of the cancer to the dentate line. Such anatomic information is useful to predict whether sphincter-sparing or sphincter-sacrificing resection is likely and whether a temporary diverting ileostomy is likely to be constructed if a low anastomosis is done.

Local Disease

The extent of local spread of rectal cancer includes assessment of four factors: (1) the depth of invasion of the primary lesion (T stage); (2) the presence of local perirectal nodal metastases (N stage); (3) the presence of a threatened or involved mesorectal circumferential resection margin (CRM); and (4) direct intrapelvic spread from the primary.

T staging is generally done by endorectal ultrasonography (ERUS) or magnetic resonance imaging (MRI). Computed tomography (CT) is not able to visualize the layers of the rectal wall and, not surprisingly, is not very useful in determining the T stage of early lesions. In contrast, ERUS is especially useful for assessment of early T-stage tumors.[7] It was found to be 95% accurate in distinguishing cancers confined to the bowel wall (T1 and T2) from those invading through the wall into the perirectal fat (≥ T3).[8] Kim and colleagues reported an overall accuracy in T staging of 81.1% by ERUS, 65.2% by CT, and 81% by endorectal coil MRI.[9]

N staging remains a major challenge despite the many advances in imaging technologies. Overall accuracy for staging lymph node metastases was 63.5% for ERUS, 56.5% for CT, and 63% for MRI.[9] ERUS accuracy for N staging is highly dependent on the operator but has been reported as high as 80 to 85%.[10] MRI accuracy is also variable, but when border contour and signal intensity characteristics of lymph nodes are used to identify lymph node metastases instead of size criteria, the accuracy is significantly improved with a sensitivity of 95% and a specificity of 95%.[11]

CRM clearance by properly performing total mesorectal excision (TME) within the endopelvic fascial plane is critical.[12,13] A positive CRM is highly correlated with high local recurrence rates and worse survival rates. The surgeon has anatomic bony constraints within the pelvis that may make it impossible to get widely around mesorectal nodal or soft tissue spread from a rectal cancer. One of the strategies currently employed to manage the patient with a threatened or involved CRM is to subject such patients to neoadjuvant chemoradiation. Thus, accurate imaging of the mesorectum is essential to select patients who would potentially benefit from this approach. Modern thin-section MRI is extremely accurate in assessing the depth of invasion of a rectal cancer into the mesorectum and can accurately predict an involved margin.[14] The other imaging techniques are not as accurate.

Extrarectal pelvic spread from the primary rectal cancer directly to adjacent structures including the anal sphincters, pelvic sidewall, prostate, seminal vesicles, vagina, bladder, and sacrum may be suspected when tethering or fixation is noted during a DRE. The precise extent of such local invasion is accurately assessed by MRI and pelvic CT. Presacral stranding, obliteration of normal landmarks lateral to the rectum, direct invasion into the bladder or sacrum, and evidence of hydronephrosis are all signs of extensive pelvic disease. Although ERUS may be useful in assessing involvement of the vagina or prostate or seminal vesicles, it is not very effective in assessing other areas of extrarectal spread.[15]

High-spatial resolution surface coil thin-slice MRI has improved in recent years and has essentially replaced the use of endorectal coil MRI for staging rectal cancer. It not only accurately assesses T stage but also has the advantages of being less operator dependent and more useful in stenotic tumors. It is the best method to assess the extent of rectal cancer spread within the mesorectum and can identify tumors with other poor prognostic features, including extramural

Table 1 American Joint Committee on Cancer TNM Clinical Classification of Colorectal Cancer[100]

Stage	Description	
Primary tumor (T)	TX	Primary tumor cannot be assessed
	T0	No evidence of primary tumor
	Tis	Carcinoma in situ; intraepithelial or invasion of lamina propria*
	T1	Tumor invades submucosa
	T2	Tumor invades muscularis propris
	T3	Tumor invades through the muscularis propria into the subserosa or into nonperitonealized pericolic or perirectal tissues
	T4	Tumor directly invades other organs or structures and/or perforates visceral peritoneum†‡
Regional lymph nodes (N)§	NX	Regional lymph nodes cannot be assessed
	N0	No regional lymph node metastasis
	N1	Metastasis in 1 to 3 regional lymph nodes
	N2	Metastasis in 4 or more regional lymph nodes
Distant metastasis (M)	MX	Distant metastasis cannot be assessed
	M0	No distant metastasis
	M1	Distant metastasis

*Tis includes cancer cells confined within the glandular basement membrane (intraepithelial) or lamina propria (intramucosal) with no extension through the muscularis mucosae into the submucosa.
†Direct invasion in T4 includes invasion of other segments of the colorectum by way of the serosa, for example, invasion of the sigmoid colon by a carcinoma of the cecum.
‡Tumor that is adherent to other organs or structures, macroscopically, is classified T4. However, if no tumor is present in the adhesion, microscopically, the classification should be pT3. The V and L substaging should be used to identify the presence or absence of vascular or lymphatic invasion.
§A tumor nodule in the pericolorectal adipose tissue of a primary carcinoma without histologic evidence of residual lymph node in the nodule is classified in the pN category as a regional lymph node metastasis if the nodule has the form and smooth contour of a lymph node. If the nodule has an irregular contour, it should be classified in the T category and coded as V1 (microscopic venous invasion) or as V2 (if it was grossly evident) because there is a strong likelihood that it represents venous invasion.

spread > 5 mm, extramural venous invasion, nodal involvement, and peritoneal infiltration. Importantly, it provides surgeons with anatomic images that define the tumor's location in relation to the anal sphincters, the obturator fossa, and other structures in the pelvis. The MERCURY Research Project demonstrated that high-quality MRI can be performed in routine practice after appropriate training of diagnostic radiologists.[16] Because this information is critical to planning radical resection of the rectum, MRI has increasingly become the diagnostic imaging study of choice for rectal cancer.[17]

Distant Metastases

The presence of distant metastases may completely change the approach to a rectal cancer. The vast majority of distant metastases from a rectal cancer are to the liver and lungs and are generally asymptomatic. Thus, both organ sites should be routinely surveyed by imaging. All patients with rectal cancer are evaluated either with a chest x-ray or CT of the chest to exclude pulmonary metastases. Liver metastases are excluded either by CT or MRI in the United States; abdominal ultrasonography is used in other parts of the world for the same purpose.

If symptoms or findings on physical examination raise suspicion of other sites of spread, appropriate testing is done. The role of positron emission tomography (PET) is not well delineated at this time and remains controversial. It is highly (96%) sensitive in detecting a primary cancer, of limited value in detecting local pelvic lymph node metastases, and possibly of value in detecting distant metastases.[18] Its major current uses are to (1) clarify equivocal findings on other scans and (2) minimize the risk of missing a distant metastasis to an unusual site in a patient being considered for a highly morbid resection of an extensive primary or recurrent rectal cancer. Combined PET-CT has advantages over using either test alone or both tests separately and may be indicated when multivisceral and extended resections are being contemplated to increase the assurance that such a radical procedure can be done with curative intent. Serum CEA may be useful as a baseline study. A CEA that is elevated and drops to normal levels after resection is reassuring. Persistence of an elevated CEA after treatment or a rising CEA should alert the surgeon to the possible presence of a metastasis or incomplete resection of the primary. Prompt additional evaluation is indicated.

Table 2 American Joint Committee on Cancer Staging System for Colorectal Cancer[100]

Stage	T	N	M
0	Tis	N0	M0
I	T1–T2	N0	M0
IIA	T3	N0	M0
IIB	T4	N0	M0
IIIA	T1–T2	N1	M0
IIIB	T3–T4	N1	M0
IIIC	Any T	N2	M0

SYNCHRONOUS COLORECTAL NEOPLASMS AND COLONIC DISEASE

Patients with rectal cancer should undergo colonoscopy not only to assess and biopsy the rectal cancer but also to identify and remove synchronous polyps (13 to 62% of cases) or to localize and biopsy synchronous cancers (2 to 8% of cases).[19,20] The location and nature of a synchronous cancer usually alter the treatment plan for the rectal cancer. Colonoscopy is especially useful to plan the extent of colectomy if the rectal cancer developed in the setting of familial adenomatous polyposis, inflammatory bowel disease, diverticular disease, or other colonic pathologic conditions. If colonoscopy is incomplete, a double-contrast barium enema or virtual colonoscopy with CT colography is a suitable alternative.[20] If preoperative surveillance of the proximal colon is not possible, intraoperative or postoperative colonoscopy should be done.

Choosing a Therapy Protocol

Advances in surgery and anesthesia, medical and radiation oncology, imaging, and staging, as well as improved understanding of the biology of rectal cancer, have all influenced the way we treat the patient with rectal cancer. Ideally, a multidisciplinary team of surgeons, medical oncologists, radiation oncologists, diagnostic radiologists, pathologists, and other caregivers with specific expertise in rectal cancer jointly review the results of the pretreatment evaluation to recommend a specific treatment protocol based on its therapeutic value, that is, the ratio of the relative benefit and the relative harm likely to follow a specific therapy protocol for a specific rectal cancer in a specific patient. Whereas most proximal rectal cancers are treated with LAR regardless of stage, mid- and distal cancers are treated variably, often with multimodality protocols, depending on cancer stage and other factors delineated during the preoperative assessment. Because treatment is so highly individualized, it is difficult to be dogmatic about what constitutes optimal therapy for rectal cancer. Nonetheless, there are certain generally accepted treatment guidelines based on intent of therapy and the perceived role and effectiveness of the components of multimodality therapy including surgical options.[21,22] A frank and honest discussion with the patient is essential for shared decision making and obtaining informed consent.

TREATMENT INTENT

Treatment may be done with curative or palliative intent. On occasion, curative intent therapy may be deliberately compromised either because the patient's comorbidities are so severe that standard resection cannot be safely performed or because the patient refuses to accept a recommended standard curative intent therapy protocol. Curative intent treatment of rectal cancer requires resection and/or ablation of all neoplastic tissue, generally accomplished by an R0 resection usually in the form of a radical resection such as LAR or APR. In the past, stage IV rectal cancer was thought to preclude curative intent therapy, but that dogma was questioned when it was shown that isolated liver or lung metastasis could be safely resected either synchronously with the primary tumor or in sequential operations, with resultant 5-year survival in 25 to 40% of patients.[23] Today, what was once a clear case for palliative care only is now often considered for aggressive, multimodality therapy with the hope of improving the disease state to the point that curative intent surgery can be employed. A multimodality regimen of neoadjuvant chemoradiation plus extended radical resection and intraoperative radiotherapy followed by adjuvant chemotherapy was used for management of 146 patients who presented with unresectable primary colon ($n=40$) or rectal ($n=106$) cancers.[24] This regimen resulted in good local disease control and a 5-year disease-free and overall survival of 43% and 52%, respectively. Similarly, patients who present with advanced or symptomatic distant metastases but have a minimally symptomatic primary rectal cancer are often first treated by aggressive chemotherapy plus biologics. If restaging shows resolution or good local control of the distant metastases, resection of the primary and metastases may then be done. A recent retrospective study reported the outcome of 233 patients who presented with synchronous stage IV colorectal cancer judged not amenable to curative intent therapy but treated instead with modern combination chemotherapy with or without bevacizumab as their initial treatment (unresected primary cancer).[25] In 47 patients (20%), the response was so marked that curative intent resection of the primary cancer and the metastatic disease was possible.

MULTIMODALITY THERAPY OPTIONS

Although surgery remains the dominant form of therapy for rectal cancer, the roles of radiation, chemotherapy, and new biologic agents are expanding.

Surgical Options

The decision to use a standard radical resection, a local or an extended operation, or palliative surgery is primarily based on the pretreatment assessment. Mature judgment is required, and the surgeon's role to select the optimal approach is critical as it is a primary determinant of outcome for patients with rectal cancer. As the multidisciplinary team reviews the workup, the experienced surgeon can identify potential technical challenges and reasonably estimate the likelihood of doing a primary anastomosis with or without temporary proximal diversion versus a permanent colostomy. Most often, a standard radical resection (LAR or APR) is needed, but local approaches are sometimes indicated. Information obtained during the preoperative assessment can alert the surgeon to alter standard approaches to fit the specific features of a rectal cancer. For instance, signet ring histology will increase the standard distal mural margin requirement and synchronous colonic pathology may require an extended colectomy. Multivisceral resections may be indicated based on extent of local spread. Depending on their magnitude, the colorectal surgeon may enlist the expertise of a hepatic, thoracic, plastic, urologic, gynecologic, neurosurgical, or orthopedic surgical colleague. Anticipated impact of contemplated surgery on fecal continence and urinary and sexual function should be considered and discussed honestly with the patient. A patient with preexisting fecal incontinence or sphincter injury may be better served by an APR and colostomy than by a well-intentioned but ill-conceived heroic effort to save the anal sphincter with an extended LAR.

Controversies

Today, the main controversies surrounding the use of multimodality therapy for rectal cancer are (1) the tumor selection criteria (i.e., when will multimodality therapy increase the likelihood of achieving an R0 resection or improve the oncologic, functional, or quality of life outcomes for the patient?); (2) the timing of therapy (i.e., should it be preoperative, postoperative, or both?); (3) the dosing and course of radiation therapy; (4) the choice of chemotherapy and biologic agents; (5) the use of chemoradiation in conjunction with local surgical therapy; (6) whether the surgical distal margin should be based on pretreatment assessment of the level of the cancer or on the post–neoadjuvant chemoradiation assessment; and (7) whether a complete clinical response to neoadjuvant chemoradiation therapy is sufficient to follow the patient without radical surgery being performed. Detailed discussion of these issues is beyond the scope of this chapter, which is focused on surgical approaches, technique, and outcomes. Nonetheless, it is useful to briefly review the evolution and current indications for neoadjuvant therapy and to acknowledge the controversies regarding use of long-course radiation versus short-course therapy.

Neoadjuvant Chemoradiation

In the past, most rectal cancers were treated by radical surgery alone. Patients surviving their operation often died of distant metastases or of locally recurrent cancer in the pelvis. Chemotherapy (primarily 5-fluorouracil) and pelvic radiotherapy (using what is now considered suboptimal doses and less than ideal delivery techniques) were generally ineffective. By the 1980s, local recurrence in the pelvis was reported in up to 40% of patients following "curative intent" rectal cancer excision in some series.[26] In the United States, clinicians and researchers renewed their efforts to improve radiation therapy techniques and to make it a more effective modality by adding "sensitizing" chemotherapy. New and more effective chemotherapy agents for postoperative adjuvant use were developed. This trend to using multimodality therapy gained significant momentum in the United States when a 1990 National Institutes of Health consensus conference endorsed postoperative chemoradiation treatment of all stage II and III rectal cancers generally initiated 4 to 8 weeks following LAR or APR.[27] The consensus statement based on clinical trials suggested that a combination of what is now called "long-course" radiation therapy delivering 50.4 Gy over 6 to 8 weeks to the pelvis coupled with 5-fluorouracil-based chemotherapy would reduce local recurrence rates and prolong survival in patients with stage II and III rectal cancer.

Reports of morbidity from postoperative chemoradiation pushed investigators to propose neoadjuvant (preoperative) chemoradiation as a viable alternative to treat advanced-stage rectal cancers.[28] The same dose was delivered over the same time period, but because preoperative irradiation treats undisturbed, well-oxygenated rectal cancers, it was argued that it would be more effective than postoperative irradiation, resulting in improved local control and better survival. In addition, neoadjuvant therapy should theoretically increase the rate of curative resection and the rate of sphincter preservation by decreasing the size of bulky rectal cancers. It was also thought that a neoadjuvant approach would diminish the incidence of radiation injury seen after postoperative irradiation when small bowel is adherent to the pelvic operative site. Presently, there is considerable evidence that neoadjuvant therapy decreases local recurrence rates for rectal cancer and that it may improve survival and possibly decrease the need for a permanent colostomy. The German Rectal Cancer Study randomly assigned patients with locally advanced rectal cancer to either preoperative or postoperative chemoradiation.[29] Following TME, local recurrence was significantly lower in the preoperative chemoradiotherapy group. In addition, the neoadjuvant therapy group was characterized by significant tumor downstaging. Despite equivalent 5-year disease-free survival and overall survival rates, the decreased local recurrence rate led the National Comprehensive Cancer Network to recommend consideration for preoperative chemoradiation (long course) for all patients with T3 or T4 rectal cancers.[22] New chemotherapy regimens are now being used with high-dose radiation.[30]

Short-Course Radiation

To prevent radiation-related complications and to avoid delaying the timing of surgery for months, many European centers, especially in Scandinavia, developed preoperative "short-course," high-dose, hypofractionation irradiation, which usually delivered 25 Gy over a period of 5 days. This delivers the biologically equivalent dose of that delivered by the long-course chemoradiation protocols (50.4 Gy) typically used in the United States.[31] Radical resection is performed 3 to 4 days after completion of the radiation. Short-course irradiation does not downsize tumors and is not advocated if the CRM is threatened or involved but does appear to be highly effective in many advanced cancers and seems well tolerated.[32] In 2007, Peeters and colleagues published the long-term results of the Dutch study that showed that reduced rates of local recurrence (5.6% after short course versus 10.9% after TME surgery alone, $p = .001$) are maintained after 6 years of follow-up.[33] Unfortunately, no survival benefit was found after short-course radiotherapy. American radiation therapists have been resistant to its use, but that view is now being questioned.[34]

INFORMED CONSENT

After determining whether treatment is offered with curative, compromised, or palliative intent, decisions are made to include or exclude neoadjuvant therapy and to use standard radical resection, local or extended operations, or palliative surgery. Once selected, the treatment protocol must be explained to the patient and consent obtained. The surgeon usually leads this discussion by reviewing the clinical staging information in the context of anticipated operative technical challenges, the likely functional results, operative risk, comorbidities, previous treatments, and specific needs of the patient. Fear of treatment-related morbidity and poor functional outcomes or a misunderstanding of what is to be done and what alternatives are available often underlies the patient's refusal to accept a recommended treatment protocol. This is especially true when the patient is told that a permanent colostomy is needed to achieve optimal control of the rectal cancer. Specific education provided by an ostomy nurse and an honest discussion to ascertain patient preferences and discuss trade-offs between oncologic outcomes, functional outcomes, treatment morbidity, postoperative rehabilitation, and time investment for any particular treatment plan often mitigate the initial refusal. A compromise treatment plan may still be needed even if that choice negatively impacts the oncologic outcome. No matter what treatment protocol is ultimately selected, the experienced surgeon is probably best suited to counsel the patient about therapeutic options, realistic expectations regarding function, and prognosis.

Surgical Approaches and Outcomes

The surgeon's options include local procedures, standard radical resections, extended multivisceral resections, and other less used techniques. The rationale and role for each approach as well as the specific outcomes are detailed below.

LOCAL PROCEDURES

Role of Local Therapy

Today, controversy surrounds the use of local procedures for rectal cancer especially if done with curative intent. Their benefits include minimal morbidity and negligible mortality, rapid postoperative recovery, and preservation of genitourinary and anal sphincter function. In some cases, local therapy is the only alternative to permanent colostomy. Although there is considerable controversy about the role of local therapy for curative intent, almost all surgeons agree that local therapy has a role in compromise situations, that is, for patients who might not tolerate a radical procedure or who refuse a recommended radical resection (usually because of the potential for a permanent colostomy). Local therapy may also be used in select cases for palliation of symptomatic but incurable rectal cancers.

Proponents of curative-intent local therapy argue that in properly selected cases, long-term cancer-free survival is achieved.[35] It is known that the incidence of lymph node metastases correlates most closely with the depth of rectal wall invasion and is especially high if the cancer extends through the wall.[36] Proponents of curative intent local therapy argue that preoperative staging with ERUS or MRI can differentiate intramural (T1 to T2) cancers from transmural (T3) cancers with a high degree of accuracy and can distinguish most of the T1 and T2 cancers in which lymph node metastases are present. In addition, they note that poorly differentiated tumors recur three times more often than well-differentiated to moderately differentiated tumors and that lymph node metastases are more common if preoperative biopsy reveals poor differentiation, lymphovascular invasion, mucin production, or signet cell histology. Proponents of local therapy use these selection criteria to restrict local therapy to the most favorable T1 to T2,N0,M0 rectal cancers.

Critics of local therapy argue that local therapy inevitably compromises oncologic outcomes by not including lymphadenectomy, thus resulting in higher local recurrence rates and decreased survival compared to radical resection.[37,38] They note that occult node-positive disease was found in final pathology specimens in 12% of patients with T1 cancers and 22% of those with T2 cancers who underwent radical resection of lesions that fit the selection criteria for local therapy.[39] Had local therapy been done, such node-positive disease would not have been identified or treated. They conclude that the imaging inaccuracy in detecting lymph nodes prior to instituting treatment inevitably results in worse oncologic outcomes.

Local Therapy Options

Local procedures to treat rectal cancer include surgical excision or ablative techniques of fulguration and endocavitary radiation. Polypectomy is not advised as a planned procedure to treat a known cancer, but as noted below, an unsuspected cancer arising in a polyp can sometimes be cured by polypectomy alone. Excision has the advantage of providing a biopsy specimen that can be examined to determine the depth of tumor invasion and thereby confirm or change the preoperative T stage. If microscopic examination of the specimen shows involvement of the circumferential or deep margins or if the pathologic T stage is more advanced than the preoperative clinical or imaging T stage, radical surgery or chemoradiation may be employed to improve local control. It is not clear whether this approach—excisional biopsy with subsequent additional therapy depending on the final pathologic examination of the specimen—compromises survival in comparison with a more aggressive initial approach. Obviously, this approach is not feasible if local ablative techniques are employed as the primary lesion is destroyed and thus unavailable for pathologic study.

Polypectomy Not infrequently, after snare polypectomy of what was thought to be a benign polyp, the clinician is informed that microscopy reveals the presence of an unsuspected cancer. The first response is to tattoo the polypectomy site if not done initially and the second is to review the pathology. Polypectomy alone is adequate for treating cancer arising in a rectal polyp if the lesion is noninvasive (i.e., confined to the mucosa) or if an invasive cancer is confined to the head, neck, or stalk of a pedunculated polyp and the margins are clear. If tumor is present within 1 to 2 mm of the margin or if the cancer extends into the submucosa of a pedunculated or sessile polyp, additional therapy should be considered. Decision making is based on comparing the risk of local recurrence and of lymph node or distant metastasis with the risk of surgical or other treatment.[40] In general, no further treatment is recommended if the following criteria are fulfilled: (1) the polyp is completely excised and submitted in total for pathologic examination; (2) it is possible to accurately determine the depth of invasion, grade of differentiation, and completeness of excision of the carcinoma; (3) the cancer is not poorly differentiated; (4) there is no vascular or lymphatic involvement; and (5) the margin of excision is not involved. If these criteria are not met, then the patient may be a better candidate for one of the local or radical procedures described below. Professional gastroenterology and surgical societies offer frequently updated guidelines accessible through Web sites to assist decision making in this complex and somewhat controversial area.

Local excision The goal of local excision procedures is to perform a full-thickness resection of the primary lesion with a 1.0 cm margin.[41] Local excision is most often accomplished via a transanal approach under direct vision or by means of transanal endoscopic microsurgery (TEM). The transanal approach is appropriate for tumors up to 7 to 10 cm from the anal verge, whereas TEM can be performed with tumors as high as 20 cm from the anal verge. Visibility with TEM techniques is superior to traditional transanal techniques, but TEM equipment makes it difficult to use for distal tumors close to or overlying the sphincter mechanism. Posterior approaches (transsacral or transsphincteric) have been described for local excision but are rarely used today because of significant associated morbidity (wound infections, bowel fistulas, and impaired continence) and because effective, less morbid transanal techniques are available. Rarely, it is helpful to expose the anorectum via a parasacral incision so as to facilitate local excision of a rectal cancer that is otherwise difficult to access.

Transanal local excision: results Many surgeons predicted that excellent oncologic outcomes could be achieved by restricting curative intent local excision to lesions that are histologically favorable, accessible, small enough to be totally removed, and confined to the bowel wall without sphincter invasion or nodal metastases. Unfortunately, this hope has not been realized. Clinical studies showed that the risk of local recurrence after local excision of selected, presumably favorable lesions is 18% for T1 cancers and 37 to 47% for T2 cancers.[37–39] Although these retrospective studies with relatively short-term follow-up have not demonstrated any impact on cancer-free survival for T1 cancers, some have shown decreased survival in T2 cancers treated by local excision as the only therapy. In addition, a recent study showed that survival is compromised in the setting of rectal cancers with poor histologic markers treated by local excision alone.[42]

Proponents of curative intent local therapy had theorized that close follow-up would detect local recurrence after local therapy at a stage where salvage surgery could be done. However, it appears that although salvage surgery is often possible, the long-term outcome in patients undergoing radical resection after local excision is less than expected, especially considering the early stage of their initial disease. In addition, pelvic recurrence following transanal excision often requires an extended pelvic dissection with en bloc resection of adjacent pelvic organs.

TEM: results A review of TEM in combination with radiotherapy for 137 patients showed this to be a safe technique with 8% minor morbidity, 2% major morbidity, and no mortality. The authors reported a combined 5% recurrence rate for T1 to T3 tumors, but the follow-up was only 6 months.[43] A recently reported Danish multicenter study of 143 consecutive patients with rectal adenocarcinoma treated by TEM showed a cancer-specific survival for T1 tumors to be 94%.[44] In a recent, slightly larger study, 200 patients underwent TEM and the overall and disease-free 5-year survival rates for patients with carcinomas were 76% and 65%, respectively.[45] Further data are needed to draw definitive conclusions regarding the use of TEM for these presumably low-risk tumors.

New approaches to optimize local excision Three approaches have been proposed to overcome the poor outcomes reported after local excision of selected favorable T1 and T2 cancers of the rectum. One approach is to be even more selective by limiting the use of curative intent local therapy to only those T1 lesions that extend into the superficial third or the middle third of the submucosa[46,47] and by using modern MRI to identify lymph node metastases by the criteria of border contour and signal intensity characteristics instead of size criteria.[11,17] Such restricted criteria may prove to be an effective strategy to select the most favorable and least invasive cancers, but further studies are needed.

A second approach is to lower local recurrence rates after local excision by adding adjuvant or neoadjuvant radiation therapy, with or without chemotherapy. Estimated local recurrence rates after local excision followed by adjuvant therapy range from 0 to 9% for T1 tumors and from 0 to 24% for T2 tumors.[35,48] The 5-year survival rate for T2/T3 patients who underwent neoadjuvant therapy prior to local excision was 84%.[49] Local excision may be particularly useful in patients who seem to have evidence of complete pathologic response after neoadjuvant therapy; however, the data supporting this approach are sparse.

A third and recently described approach uses dorsoposterior extraperitoneal pelviscopy to overcome the failure of local excision to remove any of the mesorectal lymph nodes.[50] This hybrid procedure combines local surgery with minimally invasive methods to dissect the mesorectum. The goal is to lower morbidity compared to traditional anterior resection while achieving locoregional control comparable to that of radical surgery. Recently published results reveal that the median number of lymph nodes removed is lower compared to traditional anterior resection. In addition, only two of 25 patients had documented evidence of positive lymph nodes and none of the patients developed locoregional recurrence after a short follow-up period.[51] This technique is still under investigation and requires more supporting data before it can be recommended as a safe option for rectal cancer.

Local ablation techniques

Fulguration (electrocoagulation) In the past, fulguration has been used as curative intent treatment, with reported 5-year survival rates reaching 58%, but it is now used primarily for palliative purposes. The main advantage of fulguration is that it controls bleeding from incurable, bulky rectal cancers with minimal morbidity and is well tolerated by patients who are too ill to undergo radical resection. The disadvantages of this procedure include postoperative fever, the lack of a surgical specimen for staging, the requirement for repeated procedures, and the need to convert to more radical procedures in a large number of patients.

Endocavitary radiation (Papillon technique) This ablative technique has the distinct advantage of being performed in the outpatient setting with local anesthesia and sedation. However, because it requires special equipment and expertise and is dependent on placing the delivery device directly on a small superficial cancer, it is not widely available and used infrequently. Occasionally, it is used in conjunction with local excision. The reported 5-year survival rate is 76%, with a local recurrence rate of 8.3% and a mortality of 7.7%.

RADICAL PROCEDURES

The majority of patients with nonmetastatic rectal cancer require a radical resection, usually an LAR or APR. The primary goal of curative intent radical resection is to perform a resection of the rectal cancer, the rectosigmoid mesentery, and the mesorectum with clear proximal, radial, and distal margins. Radical resections are classified on the basis of the final pathologic assessment as R0 if all margins are clear, R1 if microscopic tumor is present at the margin, and R2 if gross disease is present.

Evolution and Oncologic Outcomes of Radical Surgery

For the first half of the 20th century, APR with permanent end descending colostomy was accepted as the treatment of choice for most rectal cancers including those at the rectosigmoid junction. This highly morbid and not infrequently fatal radical resection was designed to resect the extensive local spread and lymphatic metastases identified at autopsy of patients who had died of advanced-stage rectal cancer. By midcentury, improvements in perioperative care, anesthesia, and surgical technique reduced operative mortality and made laparotomy with colonic anastomosis safer. Studies then revealed that the primary lymphatic spread of most rectal cancers is upward along the inferior mesenteric artery and that distal and lateral spread from all but very distal lesions occurs only after the proximal lymphatics are choked with tumor. This information provided the rationale to pursue LAR and anastomosis whenever technically feasible.

Local recurrence The technical difficulties inherent in hand suturing reliable low colorectal anastomoses and the traditional insistence on achieving a 5.0 cm distal margin were major impediments to routinely doing sphincter-sparing proctectomies for any but the most proximal rectal cancers. The introduction of reliable circular stapling devices in the late 1970s, coupled with knowledge that a distal resection margin of as little as 1.0 to 2.0 cm was oncologically sufficient for most rectal cancers, overcame these impediments.[52,53] Although investigators cautioned that intramural distal margins less than 1.0 cm were associated with increased local recurrence rates and decreased survival, surgeons aggressively pursued lower and lower anastomoses after curative intent proctectomy.[54] By the 1980s, reports appeared noting that local recurrence after "curative intent" proctectomy for rectal cancer was highly variable, ranging from 2 to 40%.[26] It was observed that local recurrence after radical resection correlated not just with the stage of the disease but also with the surgeon performing the operation.

Total mesorectal excision Based on pathology assessment of the mesorectum after proctectomy, Heald and colleagues suggested that local recurrence might be attributable to inadequate resection of nodal or other tumor deposits within the mesorectum.[55,56] After completing studies of the embryology and anatomy of the mesorectum, they popularized a technique now termed TME to decrease local recurrence and optimize outcomes. Sharp dissection in the endopelvic fascial plane, which is virtually bloodless, provided a reliable method to keep the cancer-bearing rectum and its mesorectum intact. Heald and others who adopted TME reported local recurrence rates under 10% following anterior resection without neoadjuvant or adjuvant therapy.[54]

Circumferential resection margin Heald initially believed that optimized proctectomy with TME would obviate the need for chemoradiation as an adjunct to surgery. However, careful analyses showed that local recurrence was still a problem despite optimized technique if the lesion was transmural and in the distal half of the rectum and if the cancer involved or was within 1 to 2 mm of the mesorectal endopelvic fascia. This led to the understanding that the CRM, a pathology variable that had never been properly assessed and reported prior to this time, was critically linked to oncologic outcome. A positive CRM correlates with high local recurrence and shortened survival.[12,13,57] In a recent study, local recurrence occurred in 22% of patients if CRM was positive versus 5% if the CRM was negative for cancer.[58] Such results explain why TME has become the standard method used for radical resection of rectal cancer. Workshops have been held in a variety of European nations for surgeons to acquire the skills needed to perform TME and for pathologists to learn how to properly assess the rectal cancer specimen, including the mesorectum, as described by Quirke and colleagues.[59,60] Marked improvement in oncologic outcomes has resulted.[61,62]

Quality of life and functional outcomes of radical surgery Quality of life is an important factor in the treatment of rectal cancer. Unlike colon cancer treatment, which generally does not have a major impact on bowel function, rectal cancer surgery introduces the real possibility of either a temporary or a permanent stoma. Furthermore, even if a restorative resection is achieved, bowel function can be poor, especially after a very low anastomosis. In addition to bowel dysfunction, pelvic dissection is associated with a risk of sexual or urinary dysfunction because of autonomic nerve injury. Indeed, the combined risk of a stoma, poor functional outcome, and genitourinary function motivates otherwise fit candidates for radical resection to consider local treatment options, despite their higher recurrence risks.

Anastomosis alternatives and bowel function A straight end-to-end colorectal anastomosis is the traditional choice after radical proctectomy for cancers of the proximal half of the rectum. A side-to-end (Baker technique) colorectal anastomosis was an occasionally used alternative. Either anastomosis can be handsewn, but today most surgeons prefer to use a circular stapler. Functional results after such anastomoses are generally good. However, as surgeons developed better means of performing lower colorectal and coloanal anastomoses, two new problems arose: increased anastomotic leaks and anterior resection syndrome.

Anastomotic complications and temporary fecal diversion The incidence of anastomotic complications, including stricture and leakage, is correlated with the level of the anastomosis. In general, the lower the anastomosis, the higher the complication rate is. Other factors, including previous radiation therapy, immunosuppression, underlying vascular insufficiency or diabetes, and technical problems such as tension that cannot be resolved by additional mobilization may also increase the risk of anastomotic complications. The consequences of a leaking anastomosis remain a major source of morbidity and death after surgical resection of rectal cancer. To overcome the problem of leaks, some surgeons advocated for increased use of the side-to-end Baker anastomosis, suggesting that it offered a more reliable blood supply than the traditional end-to-end anastomosis. Many surgeons routinely perform temporary proximal fecal diversion for patients undergoing low anastomoses, especially for those subjected to preoperative irradiation, to mitigate the consequences of a leak.[63] Loop ileostomy is the most commonly performed temporary diversion, although some surgeons prefer proximal loop colostomy. Proximal fecal diversion does not protect against anastomotic leakage or prevent anastomotic complications, but it does diminish the morbidity resulting from leakage and reduce the likelihood of an emergency reoperation.[63] Our practice is to consider diversion for all patients with a low (< 5 cm) colorectal or coloanal anastomosis especially if they have undergone preoperative radiation therapy.

Anterior resection syndrome This syndrome encompasses a variety of bowel functional problems, including frequency, fecal urgency, stool fragmentation (multiple incomplete evacuations), varying degrees of incontinence, or a combination of all of these symptoms. Lange and colleagues reported fecal incontinence in 38.8% of nonirradiated and 61.5% of irradiated patients in the Dutch TME trial.[64] To remedy the problem of anterior resection syndrome, surgeons devised techniques to increase neorectal capacity with a colonic pouch or a coloplasty.[65–67] Initial data indicated that the functional advantages were most discernible early on after operation.[68,69] More recently, however, a randomized, controlled trial comparing functional outcomes of coloplasty, colonic J pouch, or a straight anastomosis revealed significant and lasting benefits for the colonic J pouch compared to the straight anastomosis or coloplasty reconstruction.[70]

A colonic J pouch is considered only for low anastomoses and should be small.[66] If the procedure is performed more proximally than 8 cm from the anal verge, it offers no functional advantages over a straight colorectal anastomosis.[65] In fact, the greatest functional improvements are observed in patients with a colonic J pouch anastomosis 4 cm or less from the anal verge.[70–72] The coloplasty was developed to overcome the difficulty of doing a colonic pouch in a patient with a narrow pelvis and thick mesentery, but a recent trial showed that coloplasty did not improve bowel function over patients with a straight anastomosis,[70] and other data from Singapore reveal an increased incidence of anastomotic leak after coloplasty reconstruction compared to colonic J pouch reconstruction.[69] An end-to-side anastomosis may be optimal as the functional and surgical results are similar to those seen with other colonic pouch anastomoses.[71]

Colostomy Although many assume that avoidance of a stoma is inevitably associated with an improved quality of life, data are conflicting. A Cochrane review of the subject identified studies that both supported and refuted this notion, and its authors concluded that firm conclusions could not be drawn based on currently available data.[73] Patients with the most distal anastomoses tend to have the most functional difficulties postoperatively. Surgeon and patient alike must consider the likely functional outcomes before pursuing a policy of sphincter preservation at any cost. Debilitated patients and individuals with baseline sphincter dysfunction are often best served by creation of a well-constructed stoma rather than an ultralow anastomosis, especially if they have received radiotherapy.

Genitourinary dysfunction In addition to bowel dysfunction, pelvic dissection is associated with a risk of urinary or sexual dysfunction attributable to autonomic nerve injury. Surgical injury to pelvic autonomic nerves is usually the proximate cause of postoperative dysfunction, and this is best avoided by careful anatomic dissection as described below [*see* TME and Preservation of Autonomic Nerves, *below*]. However, other factors play important roles: baseline sexual function, psychological issues (most often related to the presence of a stoma), associated medical disorders (atherosclerotic peripheral vascular disease, diabetes mellitus, hypertension), medications (especially antihypertensives and beta blockers), alcohol use, and pelvic radiation therapy.[64,74]

Widely variable figures for the risk of sexual dysfunction can be cited from the literature. Often these numbers are more a reflection of the stringency of follow-up than the actual incidence of sexual dysfunction, so they must be interpreted with caution. In the 1940s, sexual dysfunction was reported in 95% of male patients after APR.[75] In contrast, Havenga and colleagues reported that 86% of male patients younger than 60 years retain sexual function if TME is done carefully to preserve autonomic nerve function.[76] Conversely, recent data from the Dutch TME trial suggest that approximately 75% of men and 60% of women suffer from sexual dysfunction following TME surgery.[74]

Urinary dysfunction is another common complication of rectal cancer therapy. In the Dutch TME trial, 38.1% of patients complained of urinary incontinence and 30.6% complained of impaired bladder emptying.[77] In contrast to sexual dysfunction, preoperative radiotherapy was not a risk factor for urinary dysfunction.

OTHER OPERATIVE APPROACHES

Extended resection is needed for locally advanced rectal cancer that invades adjacent organs or the sacrum. The prognosis is primarily dependent on achieving an R0 resection. Stoma construction without resection may be needed to control local symptoms caused by obstruction, incontinence, or fistulas to the bladder, the vagina, or other sites. Such an approach may be palliative or part of a staged approach ultimately leading to curative intent therapy.

Local Procedures: Operative Techniques

POLYPECTOMY

Most benign-appearing pedunculated polyps and most small, sessile polyps of the rectum are removed by snare polypectomy or endoscopic excisional biopsy or ablation performed during colonoscopic examination. Polyps larger than 1.0 cm, especially if sessile, villous lesions, and polyps with firm ulcerated edges are those most likely to harbor invasive cancer. If these characteristics are noted, snare polypectomy is not advised. Instead, diagnostic biopsies are done, and if positive, definitive workup and surgery are planned. If biopsies are negative or equivocal, the lesion must be completely removed in one piece to provide the pathologist with an intact specimen that can be properly oriented

44. Baatrup G, Breum B, Qvist N, et al. Transanal endoscopic microsurgery in 143 consecutive patients with rectal adenocarcinoma: results from a Danish multicenter study. Colorectal Dis 2009;11:270–5.
45. Bretagnol F, Merrie A, George B, et al. Local excision of rectal tumours by transanal endoscopic microsurgery. Br J Surg 2007;94:627–33.
46. Kikuchi R, Takano M, Takagi K, et al. Management of early invasive colorectal cancer. Risk of recurrence and clinical guidelines. Dis Colon Rectum 1995;38: 1286–95.
47. Nivatvongs S. Surgical management of malignant colorectal polyps. Surg Clin North Am 2002;82:959–66.
48. Wagman R, Minsky BD, Cohen AM, et al. Conservative management of rectal cancer with local excision and postoperative adjuvant therapy. Int J Radiat Oncol Biol Phys 1999;44:841–6.
49. Kim CJ, Yeatman J, Coppola D, et al. Local excision of T2 and T3 rectal cancers after downstaging chemoradiation. Ann Surg 2001;234:352–8.
50. Tarantino I, Hetzer FH, Warschkow R, et al. Local excision and endoscopic posterior mesorectal resection versus low anterior resection in T1 rectal cancer. Br J Surg 2008;95:375–80.
51. Zerz A, Müller-Stich BP, Beck J, et al. Endoscopic posterior mesorectal resection after transanal local excision of T1 carcinomas of the lower third of the rectum. Dis Colon Rectum 2006;49:919–24.
52. Vernava AM, Moran M. A prospective evaluation of distal margins in carcinoma of the rectum. Surg Gynecol Obstet 1992;175: 333–6.
53. Shirouza K, Isomoto H, Kakegawa T. Distal spread of rectal cancer and optimal margin of resection for sphincter preserving surgery. Cancer 1995;76:388–92.
54. Heald RJ, Moran BJ, Ryall RD, et al. Rectal cancer: the Basingstoke experience of total mesorectal excision, 1978-1997. Arch Surg 1998;133:894–9.
55. Heald RJ. A new approach to rectal cancer. Br J Hosp Med 1979;22:277–81.
56. Heald RJ, Husband EM, Ryall RD. The mesorectum in rectal cancer surgery—the clue to pelvic recurrence? Br J Surg 1982;69: 613–6.
57. Nagtegaal ID, Marijnen CA, Kranenbarg EK, et al. Circumferential margin involvement is still an important predictor of local recurrence in rectal carcinoma: not one millimeter but two millimeters is the limit. Am J Surg Pathol 2002;26:350–7.
58. Wibe A, Rendedal PR, Svensson E, et al. Prognostic significance of the circumferential resection margin following total mesorectal excision for rectal cancer. Br J Surg 2002;89:327–34.
59. Quirke P, Durdey P, Dixon MF, et al. Local recurrence of rectal adenocarcinoma due to inadequate surgical resection. Histopathological study of lateral tumour spread and surgical excision. Lancet 1986;2:996–9.
60. Quirke P, Dixon MF. The prediction of local recurrence of rectal adenocarcinoma by histopathological examination. Int J Colorectal Dis 1998;3:127–31.
61. Martling AL, Holm T, Rutqvist LE, et al. Effect of a surgical training programme on outcome of rectal cancer in the County of Stockholm. Stockholm Colorectal Cancer Study Group, Basingstoke Bowel Cancer Research Project. Lancet 2000;356:93–6.
62. Quirke P. Training and quality assurance for rectal cancer: 20 years of data is enough. Lancet Oncol 2003;4:695–702.
63. Marusch F, Koch A, Schmidt HD, et al. Value of protective stoma in low anterior resections for rectal carcinoma. Dis Colon Rectum 2002;45:1164–71.
64. Lange MM, den Dulk M, Bossema ER, et al. Risk factors for faecal incontinence after rectal cancer treatment. Br J Surg 2007;94:1278–84.
65. Hida J, Yasutomi M, Maruyama T, et al. Indications for colonic J pouch reconstruction after anterior resection for rectal cancer: determining the optimal level of anastomosis. Dis Colon Rectum 1998;41: 558–63.
66. Lazorthes F, Gamagami R, Chiotasso P, et al. Prospective randomized study comparing clinical results between small and large colonic J-pouch following coloanal anastomosis. Dis Colon Rectum 1997;40: 1409–13.
67. Harris GJC, Lavery IJ, Fazio VW. Reasons for failure to construct to colonic J pouch. What can be done to improve the size of the neorectal reservoir should it occur? Dis Colon Rectum 2002;45:1304–8.
68. Sailer M, Fuchs HK, Fein M, et al. Randomized clinical trial comparing quality of life after straight and pouch coloanal reconstruction. Br J Surg 2002;89:1108–17.
69. Ho YH, Brown S, Heah SM, et al. Comparison of J-pouch and coloplasty pouch for low rectal cancers. Ann Surg 2002;236: 49–55.
70. Fazio VW, Zutshi M, Remzi FH, et al. A randomized multicenter trial to compare long-term functional outcome, quality of life, and complications of surgical procedures for low rectal cancers. Ann Surg 2007;246:481–8.
71. Machado M, Nygren J, Goldman S, et al. Similar outcome after colonic pouch and side-to-end anastomosis in low anterior resection for rectal cancer: a prospective randomized trial. Ann Surg 2003;238: 214–20.
72. Brown CJ. Reconstructive techniques after rectal resection for rectal cancer. Cochrane Database Syst Rev 2008;(2):CD006040.
73. Pachler J, Wille-Jørgensen P. Quality of life after rectal resection for cancer, with or without permanent colostomy. Cochrane Database Syst Rev 2005;(18):CD004323.
74. Lange MM, Marijnen CA, Maas CP, et al. Risk factors for sexual dysfunction after rectal cancer treatment. Eur J Cancer 2009; 45:1578–88.
75. Jones TE. Complications of onstage abdominoperineal resection of the rectum. JAMA 1942;120:104–7.
76. Havenga K, Enker WE, McDermott K, et al. Male and female sexual and urinary function after total mesorectal excision with autonomic nerve preservation for carcinoma of the rectum. J Am Coll Surg 1996;182: 495–502.
77. Lange MM, Maas CP, Marijnen CA, et al. Urinary dysfunction after rectal cancer treatment is mainly caused by surgery. Br J Surg 2008;95:1020–8.
78. Cataldo PA Transanal endoscopic microsurgery. Surg Clin North Am 2006;86: 915–25.
79. Wu WX, Sun YM, Hua YB, et al. Laparoscopic versus conventional open resection of rectal carcinoma: a clinical comparative study. World J Gastroenterol 2004;10: 1167–70.
80. Veenhof AA, Engel AF, Craanen ME, et al. Laparoscopic versus open total mesorectal excision: a comparative study on short-term outcomes. A single-institution experience regarding anterior resections and abdominoperineal resections. Dig Surg 2007;24: 367–74.
81. Guillou PJ, Quirke P, Thorpe H, et al. Short-term endpoints of conventional versus laparoscopic-assisted surgery in patients with colorectal cancer (MRC CLASICC trial): multicentre, randomized controlled trial. Lancet 2005;365:1718–26.
82. Jayne DG, Guillou PJ, Thorpe H, et al. Randomized trial of laparoscopic-assisted resection of colorectal carcinoma: 3-year results of the UK MRC CLASICC Trial Group. J Clin Oncol 2007;25:3061–8.
83. Wexner SD, Bergamaschi R, Lacy A, et al. The current status of robotic pelvic surgery: results of a multinational interdisciplinary consensus conference. Surg Endosc 2009; 23:438–43.
84. Rouanet P, Dravet F, Dubois JB, et al. Proctectomy and colo-anal anastomosis after high-dose irradiation of cancers of the lower third of the rectum: functional and oncological results. Ann Chir 1994;48: 512–9.
85. Nagtegaal ID, van de Velde CJ, Marijnen CA, et al. Low rectal cancer: a call for a change of approach in abdominoperineal resection. J Clin Oncol 2005;23:9257–64.
86. Schiessel R, Novi G, Holzer B, et al. Technique and long-term results of intersphincteric resection for low rectal cancer. Dis Colon Rectum 2005;48:1858–67.
87. Wolmark N, Wieand HS, Hyams DM, et al. Randomized trial of postoperative adjuvant chemotherapy with or without radiotherapy for carcinoma of the rectum. National Surgical Adjuvant Breast and Bowel Project, protocol R-02. J Natl Cancer Inst 2000;92: 388–96.
88. Beart RW, Steele GD, Menck HR, et al. Management and survival of patients with adenocarcinoma of the colon and rectum: a national survey of the Commission on Cancer. J Am Coll Surg 1995;181:225–36.
89. Daniels I. MRI predicts surgical resection margin status in patients with rectal cancer: results from the MERCURY Study Group. Clin Oncol 2004;16:S45–6.
90. Eriksen MT, Wibe A, Syse A, et al. Inadvertent perforation during rectal cancer resection in Norway. Br J Surg 2004;91: 210–6.
91. Hojo K, Koyama Y , Moriya Y. Lymphatic spread and its prognostic value in patients with rectal cancer. Am J Surg 1982;144: 350–4.
92. Hermanek P. Current aspects of a new staging classification of colorectal cancer and its clinical consequences. Chirurg 1989; 60:1–7.
93. Salerno G, Chandler I, Wotherspoon A, et al. Sites of surgical waisting in the abdominoperineal specimen. Br J Surg 2008;95: 1147–54.
94. Holm T, Ljung A, Haggmark T, et al. Extended abdominoperineal resection with gluteus maximus flap reconstruction of the pelvic floor for rectal cancer. Br J Surg 2007;94:232–8.
95. Avradopoulos KA, Vezeridis MP, Wanebo HJ. Pelvic exenteration for recurrent rectal cancer. Adv Surg 1996;29:215–33.
96. Sugerbaker PH. Partial sacrectomy for en-bloc excision of rectal cancer with post-

erior fixation. Dis Colon Rectum 1982; 25:708–11.
97. Friel CM, Cromwell JW, Marra C, et al. Salvage radical surgery after failed local excision for early rectal cancer. Dis Colon Rectum 2002;45:875–9.
98. Hahnloser D, Nelson H, Gunderson LL, et al. Curative potential of multimodality therapy for locally recurrent rectal cancer. Ann Surg 2003;237:502–8.
99. Madoff RD. Extended resections for advanced rectal cancer. Br J Surg 2006;93: 1311–2.
100. American Joint Committee on Cancer. Colon and rectum staging schema. In: AJCC Cancer staging manual. 6th ed. New York: Springer Science and Business Media Inc., 2002.

Acknowledgment

Figures 1 through 11. Tom Moore.

Step 2: mobilization of the sigmoid colon The sigmoid colon is mobilized away from the left lateral wall by incising the lateral peritoneal reflection [*see Figure 5a*]. Because the sigmoid colon is redundant in patients with rectal prolapse, minimal mobilization is performed, since acquiring length to perform a tension-free anastomosis is easily accomplished. For the same reasons, the splenic flexure is not mobilized. The gonadal vessels and the ureter are identified and swept posteriorly. The peritoneal incision is continued to the left of the rectum, curving anteriorly in the rectouterine or rectovesical sulcus. The peritoneum at the base of the sigmoid mesentery on the right is also incised, and this incision is continued to the right of the rectum to unite with the previous incision at the anterior rectum.

Step 3: proximal transection of the sigmoid colon and placement of a stapler anvil The proximal point of transection is chosen by finding an area of colon that easily falls into the pelvis and is proximal to the redundant sigmoid colon. This level of the colon, the sigmoid-descending portion, is circumferentially cleaned of surrounding tissue. A straight clamp is placed proximally and an adjacent bowel clamp distally. The bowel is divided with a knife along the straight clamp. The straight clamp is released, and three Babcock forceps are placed to hold open the lumen. A purse-string suture of 2-0 Prolene is placed, and the head of a 33 mm circular stapler is secured in the lumen. Alternatively, a purse-string clamp may be used.

Step 4: division of the sigmoid mesentery The mesentery of the sigmoid colon is clamped, ligated, and divided close to the colon [*see Figure 5b*]. The superior rectal vessels are carefully preserved.

Step 5: mobilization of the rectum and division of the lateral ligaments A Babcock clamp is placed on the rectal stump and lifted upward. The avascular plane of areolar tissue between the mesorectum and the presacral fascia is identified and divided with the electrocautery. A St. Marks' retractor is placed behind the rectum to provide traction and then advanced with dissection distally along the rectum to the level of the coccyx. Again the superior rectal artery is preserved to avoid necrosis of the rectum.

Dissection of the right side of the rectum is performed with the surgeon standing to the patient's left. The left hand places traction on the rectum while the right hand uses the electrocautery to divide the entire lateral stalk in a posterior to anterior direction down to the level of the levators. The St. Marks' retractor is used to retract the tissues of the sidewall away from the rectum.

Dissection of the left side of the rectum is performed with the surgeon on the patient's right. Again, the left hand places traction on the rectum while the right hand performs the dissection in a posterior-to-anterior direction.

Dissection anterior to the rectum is performed by using the retractor to place traction on either the uterus (in women) or the bladder (in men) and then proceeding anterior to the rectum down to the level of the lower third of the vagina (in women) or below the seminal vesicles (in men).

Step 6: placement of sutures for rectopexy With upward traction applied to the rectal stump, horizontal mattress sutures of 2-0 Prolene with a large heavy needle (i.e., CT-1) are placed to perform the rectopexy. Starting on one side, a suture is placed through the peritoneum and the endopelvic fascia adjacent to the rectum, with care taken not to penetrate the rectal wall. The suture is guided through the presacral fascia and the periosteum to the side of the midline and approximately 1 cm below the level of the sacral promontory. A significant amount of force is usually needed to penetrate the bone of the sacrum to ensure stability of the sutures placed. It is then completed by passing it back through the peritoneum and the endopelvic fascia. One or two sutures are placed on each side; they are left untied and are tagged with hemostats.

Step 7: transection of bowel at the upper rectum The rectosigmoid junction is identified on the basis of the splaying of the taeniae coli, the absence of appendices epiploicae, and the proximity to the sacral promontory. This junction marks the site of distal transection. Proctoscopic examination is helpful for determining the appropriate location. Transection may be performed with a stapler, a purse-string suture clamp, or a knife followed by a handsewn purse-string suture.

a

b

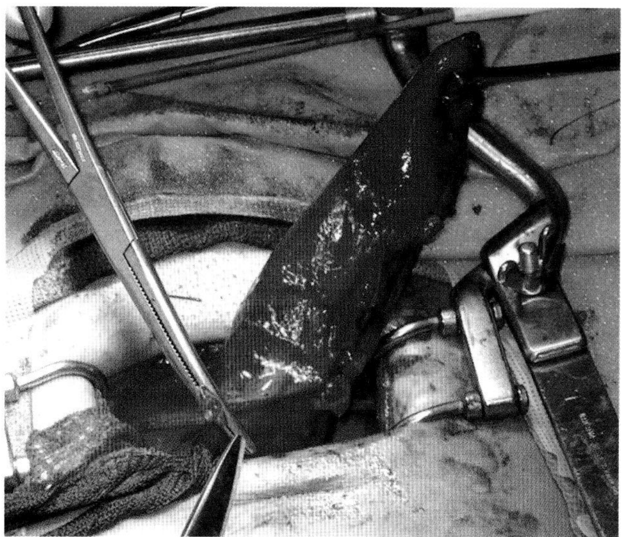

Figure 5 **Open resection rectopexy. (*a*) The redundant sigmoid is mobilized through the abdominal wound. (*b*) The proximal sigmoid is transected, and the sigmoid mesentery is clamped, ligated, and divided.**

Step 8: completion of colorectal anastomosis The circular stapler is advanced through the anus to the rectal stump. Under the manual and visual guidance of the abdominal and perineal operating surgeons, the trocar is advanced and the anvil engaged. The circular stapler is closed and fired. The stapler is then gently removed, and the "doughnuts" are checked for integrity. The anastomosis is tested for leaks by filling the pelvis with irrigant, clamping the colon proximal to the anastomosis, and insufflating air into the rectum. Air bubbles from the anastomosis indicate a leak that requires suture reinforcement or anastomosis reconstruction. The rectopexy sutures are secured snugly to complete the procedure, after which flexible sigmoidoscopy is performed to exclude narrowing of the rectum from the rectopexy sutures. If any narrowing is noted one or more can be removed and replaced as needed so as to prevent narrowing. Ultimately the abdomen is irrigated and closed in the usual fashion.

An alternative approach to this step is to perform endoscopic visualization of the anastomosis while simultaneously insufflating air through either the rigid proctoscope or the flexible sigmoidoscope. This method allows reliable confirmation of mucosal viability and anastomotic integrity. Moreover, if any supplemental anastomotic reinforcement sutures are needed, they can be placed much more easily at this time than after the rectopexy sutures have been secured. Sheets of sodium hyaluronate–based bioresorbable membrane are placed before closure of the fascia to help minimize postoperative adhesion formation; at our institution, these sheets are routinely used during most laparotomies.[18] The abdominal incision is closed in the usual fashion.

Postoperative care After operation, the patient is started on a clear liquid diet and then advanced to a regular diet when bowel function returns. The bladder catheter is removed on postoperative day 1, when ambulation also begins.

Troubleshooting Either suture rectopexy or sigmoid resection can be performed alone by following some of the steps just outlined (see above). Circumferential mobilization of the rectum to the level of the coccyx posteriorly and the upper third of the vagina anteriorly, with division of the lateral ligaments, is advocated to minimize recurrence. Division of the lateral ligaments increases the risk of postoperative constipation; however, inadequate distal mobilization or posterior mobilization performed without lateral ligament division results in laxity of the rectum and the attachments below the level of sacral fixation, which increases the risk of early recurrence. During the sigmoid resection, it is important to remove all redundant bowel; however, it is equally important to ensure that the anastomosis is tension free and well vascularized. During both rectal mobilization and sigmoid resection, careful attention should be paid to preserving the superior rectal artery and the sacral nerves.

Complications Presacral bleeding may result from placement of sutures in the presacral fascia and consequent injury to the presacral veins. It may be controlled by tying down the sutures and applying direct manual pressure. For persistent bleeding, thumbtacks may be required.

Injury to the pelvic nerves and consequent impotence are possibilities with any procedure in which the rectum is mobilized. Performing the dissection close to the bowel wall minimizes the chances that these complications will occur.

Suturing the rectum too close to the sacrum may compress the lumen. This problem may be corrected by removing and replacing the sutures. Any uncertainty about rectal compression can be resolved by means of intraoperative proctoscopy.

The incidence of abdominal sepsis from an anastomotic leak can be minimized by ensuring a well-vascularized and tension-free anastomosis.

LAPAROSCOPIC RECTOPEXY

Laparoscopic Resection Rectopexy

Laparoscopic resection rectopexy is not commonly performed. This procedure necessitates an extraction site in the form of a Pfannenstiel, or lower midline, incision. An entire procedure of open resection rectopexy can also be performed though similarly small incisions making laparoscopic approach unnecessary. In addition, when resection is performed, the rectopexy should be performed with sutures and not mesh to avoid septic complications. Placement of sutures requires significant force to penetrate the sacral bone which cannot usually be accomplished laparoscopically. However, since this procedure is described in the literature, the steps will not be outlined here.

Preoperative management includes full mechanical bowel preparation. In addition, cefotetan, 2 g intravenously, is administered along with heparin, 5,000 units subcutaneously, at the start of the operation.

After the induction of general anesthesia, the patient is placed in the modified lithotomy position with the legs in pneumatic compression stockings and padded stirrups. The arms are tucked at the sides, and extra care is taken to secure the patient to the bed because of the rotation and tilting required during surgery. Two or more monitors are placed on opposite sides of the operating table. The rectum is irrigated with saline through a transanally placed mushroom catheter until the effluent is clear, at which point, additional irrigation is initiated with a povidone-iodine solution. The catheter is left in place for the initial portion of the procedure, and the extra effluent is allowed to drain into a plastic bag secured to the catheter. If requested, bilateral ureteral stents are placed by a urologist, and a urinary catheter and an orogastric tube are inserted. The abdomen is shaved, prepared with povidone-iodine solution, and appropriately draped.

Operative technique *Step 1: placement of ports* A 10 mm trocar is placed infraumbilically or supraumbilically (depending on patient size) by means of the open Hasson technique; this port will be used for the camera. Pneumoperitoneum is established, and two additional 10 mm trocars are placed along the lateral edge of the rectus abdominis in the right midabdomen and the right iliac fossa [*see Figure 6*]. If necessary, one or two additional trocars may be placed laterally on the left of the abdomen to assist with sigmoid retraction.

Step 2: mobilization of the sigmoid colon and rectum The operating table is tilted to the patient's right to facilitate medial retraction of the left colon, which is gently grasped with a Babcock forceps. An ultrasonic scalpel is placed through the right lower port and used to mobilize the sigmoid colon and the descending colon away from the left lateral side wall. Early identification of retroperitoneal structures, includgiven intravenous (IV) narcotics to allow painless injection of local anesthetics, and if any respiratory compromise results because of the prone-flexed position, the patient can quickly be returned to the supine position on the stretcher until respiration resumes without difficulty.

Step 2: Intravenous Sedation and Local Anesthesia

Before administering a local anesthetic, I usually give the following drugs for sedation: midazolam, 2 to 5 mg, given in the holding area for sedation and amnesia; alfentanil, 0.5 to 1 mg, or fentanyl, 50 to 100 mg, for analgesia to help alleviate the discomfort of the local anesthetic injection; and propofol, 20 to 50 mg, or methohexital, 20 to 50 mg, to achieve patient cooperation with the injection. Sedation is followed by the injection into perianal tissue of 40 mL of bupivacaine (0.5%) along with a buffer that is added immediately before injection (0.5 mL of 8.4% sodium bicarbonate [1 mEq/mL] added to 50 mL of local anesthetic). If resection is anticipated, epinephrine (1:200,000) is usually included with the local anesthetic. To achieve adequate local anesthesia, 5 mL of bupivacaine is injected into the subcutaneous tissue in each quadrant of the tissue immediately surrounding the anus [*see Figure 3a*]. Next, 10 mL of local anesthetic is injected deep into the sphincter mechanism on each side of the anal canal [*see Figure 3b*].

Step 3: Anoscopy or Sigmoidoscopy

Anoscopy, sigmoidoscopy, or both should be performed at this point if neither procedure was done before the operation.

Step 4: Sphincterotomy

As noted, sphincterotomy should always be considered, especially if a hypertrophic band of the lower third of the internal sphincter muscle persists after the local anesthetic has been injected and an anoscope has been inserted. It is always best to obtain permission to do this beforehand on the operative consent form.

Step 5: Treatment of Hemorrhoids

Elastic ligation of internal hemorrhoids This is a very safe operation because by the nature of the banding procedure [*see Figure 4*], bridges of normal mucosa are maintained between treated clusters of hemorrhoids. Any clusters of tissue with squamous metaplasia and obviously friable internal hemorrhoids can be treated in this manner. I find that these tissue clusters are not always confined to the three classic positions identified for hemorrhoids and that, in many cases, it is necessary to band three or four clusters. If the bands do not stay on, then the tissue probably need not be treated and no further action need be taken.

a

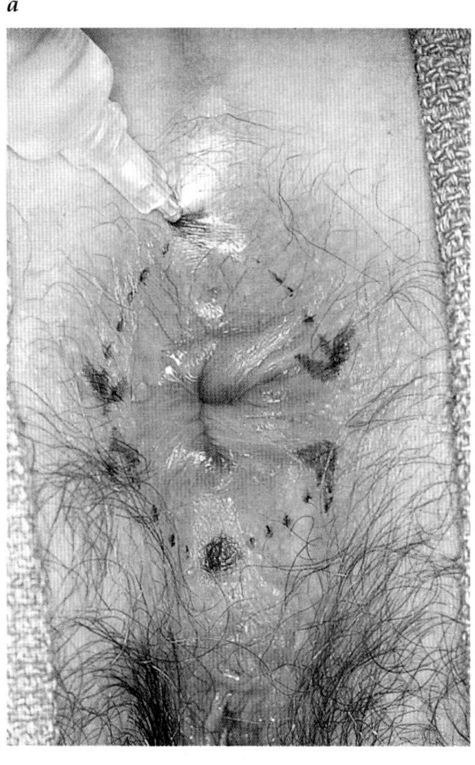

b

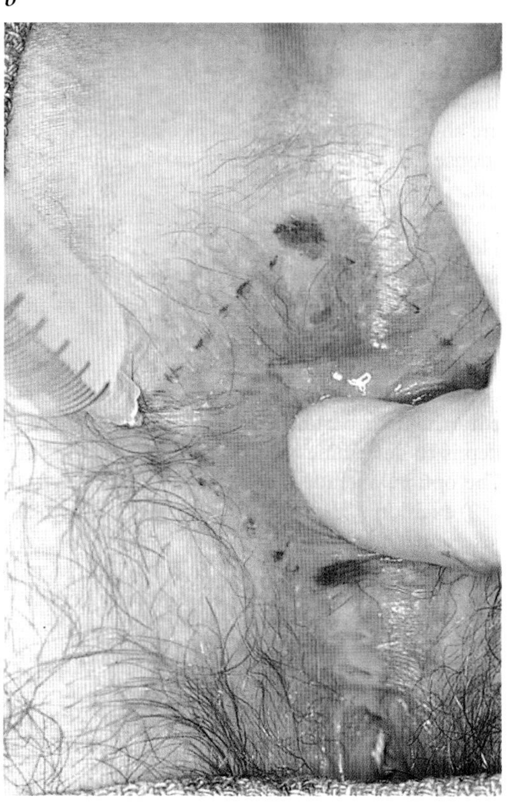

Figure 3 **Operative management of hemorrhoids. (*a*) Five milliliters of bupivacaine is injected into subcutaneous tissue. (*b*) Ten milliliters of local anesthetic is injected deep into the sphincter muscle on each side of the anal canal.**

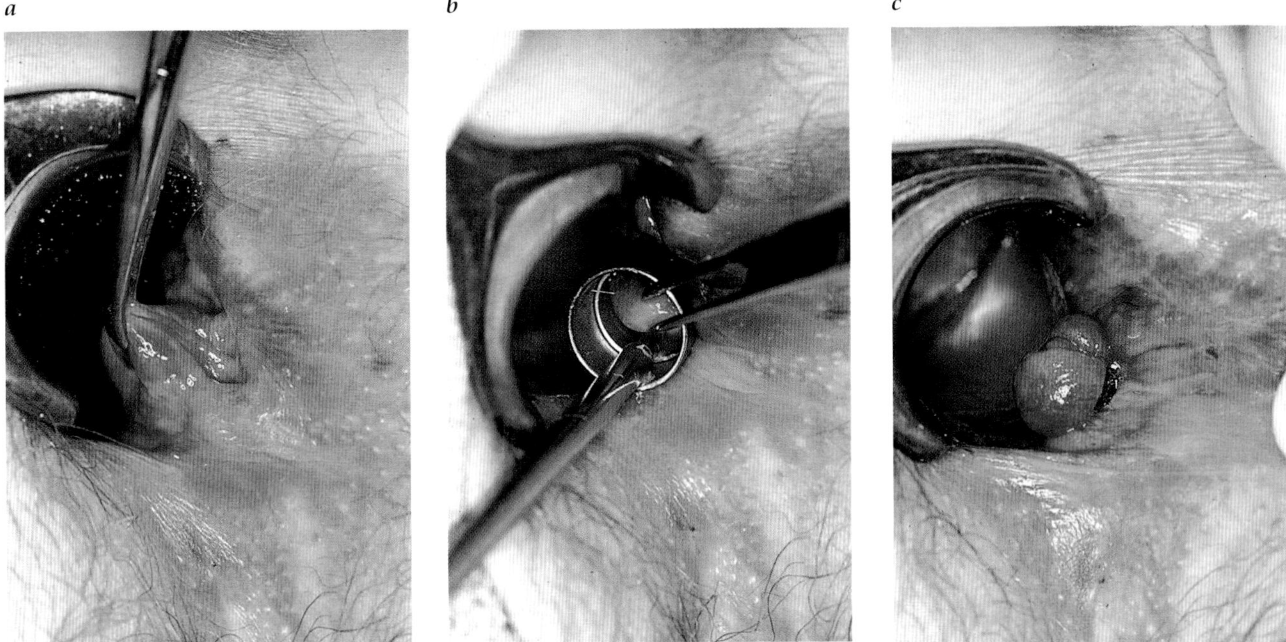

Figure 4 **Operative management of hemorrhoids. Shown is the elastic ligation technique for internal hemorrhoids. (*a*) The hemorrhoidal tissue is identified. (*b*) The hemorrhoid is grasped and pulled through the drum. (*c*) The elastic band is applied to the base of the hemorrhoid.**

I use two rubber bands on each cluster. If one of them breaks, bleeding is unlikely to occur, because the tissue rapidly becomes edematous and necrotic. It is important that the placement of the rubber band be proximal to the mucocutaneous junction; if it is not, the procedure will be too painful, given the extensive innervation of the skin. On the other hand, the band should not be placed so proximally as to incorporate the full thickness of the rectal wall; to do so can be risky for patients in whom difficulties with bowel movements indicate the presence of intussusception or some other pelvic floor abnormality. Occasionally, the friable tissue gives rise to a suspicion of cancer. If this is the case, rubber bands may be placed at the base, and the tip may be excised for biopsy.

Excision of residual external hemorrhoids Residual external hemorrhoids are rarely treated as a primary problem: true symptoms are few, and the main indication for treatment is maintenance of hygiene. In addition, I find that much of the external tissue is pulled in when the internal hemorrhoids are ligated. Accordingly, I do the internal ligation first and then excise any residual symptomatic external tissue. An elliptical incision is made in the perianal skin, with care taken to protect the underlying sphincter muscle and avoid the previously placed elastic band [*see Figure 5a*]. Although the perianal skin is very forgiving, it is essential to protect the anoderm; this is achieved through careful placement of the rubber band. The elliptical defect is then closed with a continuous absorbable suture in a three-point placement to obliterate the underlying dead space [*see Figure 5b and 5c*]. The suture is tied loosely to allow for swelling. There is no need for separate ligation or coagulation of the small bleeding vessels; this problem is obviated by the continuous suture. It is important not to use slowly absorbable suture material because it may give rise to infection in this highly susceptible tissue. I prefer to use 3-0 chromic catgut on an exaggeratedly curved needle.

Complete excisional hemorrhoidectomy This procedure is indicated in patients who have large combined internal and external hemorrhoids, patients who are receiving anticoagulants, and patients who have massive edema and thrombosis, as seen in the postpartum rosette of tissue [*see Figure 6*]. I find that even massive edema generally resolves after the local anesthetic is injected and the muscle is allowed to relax. Resolution of edema then permits identification of the specific clusters of hemorrhoids, which can be isolated with a forceps and excised via an elliptical incision. Care must be taken to preserve the underlying muscle, especially in the anterior region in women. I use 3-0 chromic catgut with a deep stitch at the apex and a continuous three-point suture that is extended on the perianal skin [*see Figure 5b*]. It is important to preserve a bridge of anoderm between the areas of excision. I know of no indications for a radical circumferential procedure (the so-called Whitehead procedure); in fact, I see numerous patients who are seeking a remedy for the stenosis and ectropion that frequently occur after this radical operation [*see Figure 7*].

A newer technique, in which a circumferential band of anorectal mucosa is excised with a special circular stapler, is currently under investigation. This technique is intended for patients who have profound prolapsing internal hemorrhoids without much of an external component. Its proponents claim that it results in minimum postoperative discomfort; however, special training with the instrument is required. European centers have reported excellent success rates, and trials have now been completed in the United States. There appears to be some advantage to this procedure in that patients tend to experience less immediate postoperative pain; however, the

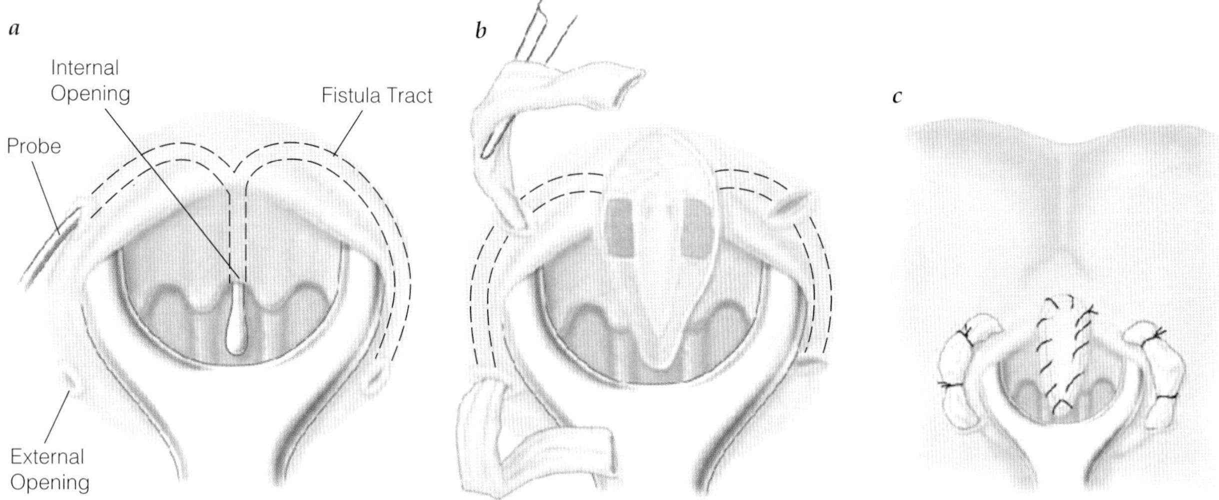

Figure 12 **Operative management of abscess and fistula. Shown is the surgical treatment of a horseshoe fistula. (*a*) The main posterior tract of the fistula is identified by probing. (*b*) The posterior tract is opened, and drains are placed laterally. (*c*) The posterior tract is marsupialized.**

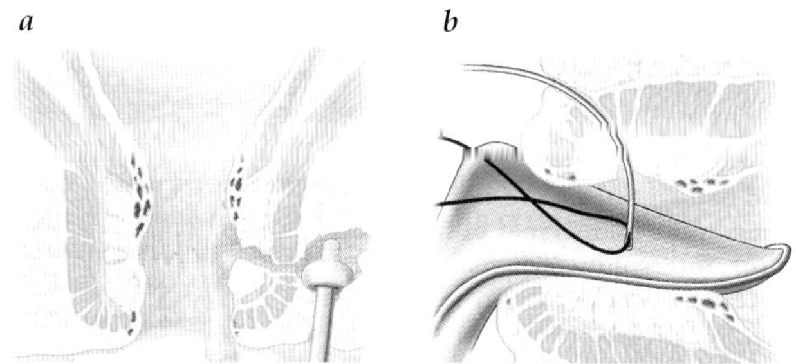

Figure 13 **Operative management of abscess and fistula. Shown are alternatives for treating abscess or fistula associated with Crohn disease. In Crohn disease, multiple perianal and perineal fistulas and abscesses may be seen, often in atypical locations. (*a*) Abscesses may be drained by placing a small mushroom-tipped catheter as close to the anus as possible. A Malecot catheter should not be used. (*b*) In some settings, it is appropriate to place a seton between internal and external openings. This seton may then be left in situ for a time for drainage and for prevention of further disease progression.**

imperative to achieve adequate hemostasis. The disposable suction cautery units currently available can be especially helpful for this purpose. The wounds may be either left open or loosely packed until good granulation tissue forms.

Bathing the perineum, especially after a bowel movement, is helpful. Often showers are better for this purpose than the portable minuscule sitz baths commonly used. For patients who have undergone extensive procedures, twice-daily trips to a whirlpool bath (often located in the physical therapy department) are helpful. Despite the multiple lengthy incisions, there is usually little pain, and most of the postoperative care can be done at home. Adequate follow-up is necessary to treat residual or new areas of disease before the dissection becomes extensive again. Care must be taken, especially in the OR, to search for the infected tracts, which may contain little pus and may be apparent only as indurated cords within the perineal skin.

TROUBLESHOOTING

Most of the important steps for avoiding problems have already been described in the course of addressing preoperative planning and operative technique (see above). The goals in the treatment of all of the processes associated with anorectal abscess and fistula in ano are to preserve sphincter function, to control acute infection, and to eliminate the source of the infection. If it is likely that sphincter function will be compromised at all, a baseline level of sphincter function (including the status of muscles and nerves) must be determined before any surgical procedure is initiated. One should never hesitate to perform an examination with the patient under anesthesia and to inject dilute methylene blue to delineate the extent and location of the infectious process.

Anyone embarking on surgical management of such processes must keep in mind the option of performing an advancement flap procedure to close the internal opening, especially in the anterior region and most particularly in women. If such a procedure is planned, initial drainage should be done external to the rectum with a mushroom catheter rather than through the internal opening with a seton. Simple 3-0 chromic catgut should be used to marsupialize fistula tracts because employing the newer, less quickly absorbable materials may lead to a chronic nidus that gives rise to ongoing infection. Patients should be watched closely in the immediate postoperative period to ensure that all infection is controlled. Not uncommonly, a superficial collection is drained, but a deeper abscess remains that must be sought more aggressively.

One should always take into account the risk of anoperineal infection in immunocompromised patients. Given that the anatomy of the anal tissue planes is complex and can be rendered even more so by multiple surgical procedures, one should not venture beyond one's level of expertise. One should never hesitate to drain an infectious focus with a simple mushroom-tipped catheter and, if appropriate, refer the patient to a colon

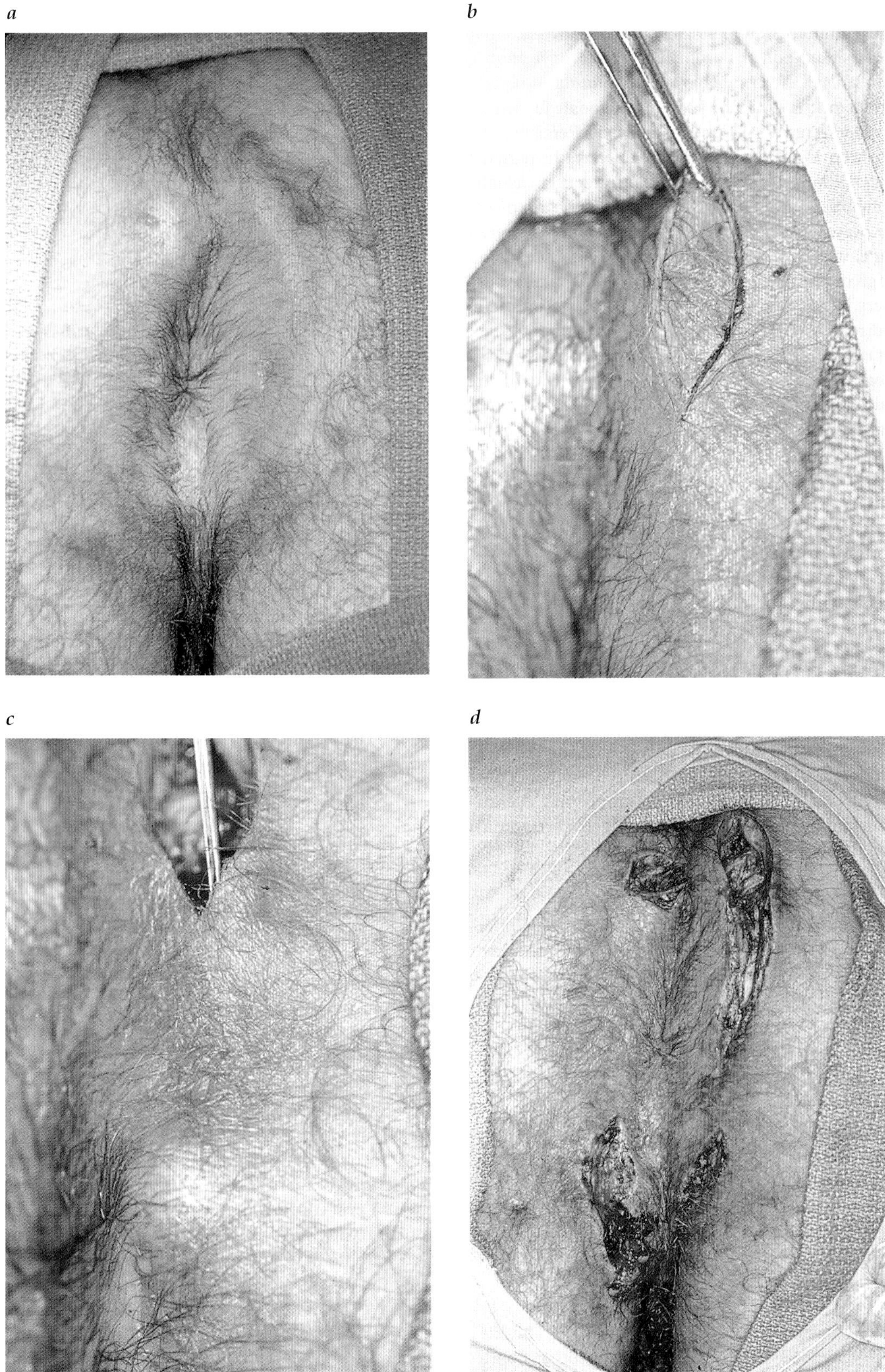

Figure 14 **Operative management of abscess and fistula. In this patient, the causative condition is hidradenitis suppurativa. (*a*) Multiple openings of sinus tracts can be seen and extensive indurated tracts palpated. (*b*) Abscesses are unroofed. (*c*) Indurated tracts are probed. (*d*) All tracts are identified and incised.**

testing is only 70 to 80%. Other tests, such as the CRH stimulation test, are available for differentiating among the possible causes of ACTH-dependent Cushing syndrome, but at present, they are less commonly employed.

Localization Once biochemical evaluation is complete, the next step is radiographic localization of the source of the Cushing syndrome. If adrenal Cushing syndrome is suspected, abdominal cross-sectional imaging with CT is recommended. If a pituitary source is suspected, MRI of the pituitary should be the initial imaging test. Pituitary MRI with gadolinium enhancement will identify an adenoma in more than 60% of patients with pituitary Cushing syndrome. However, as much as 10% of the general population may have an incidental pituitary mass that is not functional, although these lesions are typically small (< 5 mm in diameter). If MRI is not conclusive, measurement of inferior petrosal sinus ACTH levels is recommended as the most direct method of differentiating pituitary from nonpituitary causes of ACTH-dependent Cushing syndrome. In this test, ACTH levels are simultaneously measured peripherally and in the two inferior petrosal sinuses both before and after IV administration of CRH (100 μg). An inferior petrosal sinus–to–periphery ACTH ratio that is higher than 3.0 is diagnostic of pituitary Cushing syndrome; a ratio that is lower than 1.8 is indicative of an ectopic ACTH-secreting tumor.[13] In experienced hands, this procedure has a sensitivity and specificity of 80 to 90%.[illegible] Ectopic ACTH-producing tumors are most often detected by means of CT scanning or radionuclide imaging with indium-111–labeled octreotide analogues, which detect tumors that express somatostatin receptors.

Subclinical Cushing Syndrome

Subclinical Cushing syndrome (SCS) is characterized by abnormalities in cortisol secretion in the absence of overt signs of classic Cushing syndrome. Such findings have been observed in up to 20% of adrenal incidentalomas.[14,15] The array of biochemical abnormalities that define subclinical hypercortisolism include nonsuppressibility of cortisol secretion with dexamethasone, loss of the diurnal variation in cortisol secretion, low or suppressed plasma ACTH levels, and blunted response of ACTH to CRH. Twenty-four-hour urine free cortisol levels are elevated in only about 50% of patients with SCS, and the degree of elevation is usually mild.

The natural history of SCS has not been carefully studied, but these patients do have a higher incidence of hypertension, obesity, and diabetes than controls. In one series, the progression to overt Cushing syndrome at 1 year was 12.5%.[16] Recently, outcomes were compared in 45 patients with SCS randomized to undergo adrenalectomy or conservative management.[17] Assessment was carried out yearly with a mean follow-up of 7.7 years. In the adrenalectomy group, diabetes normalized or improved in 62.5% of patients, hypertension in 67%, hyperlipidemia in 37.5%, and obesity in 50%. In contrast, some worsening of diabetes, hypertension, and hyperlipidemia was observed in the conservatively managed group. No changes in osteoporosis parameters were seen in either group. These results suggest that adrenalectomy results in improved outcomes over conservative management in patients with SCS.

Most patients with SCS are detected during workup of an adrenal incidentaloma, usually by screening with an overnight dexamethasone test. Failure to suppress with dexamethasone should be evaluated further as outlined above for Cushing syndrome. Patients with SCS are at increased risk for AI after adrenalectomy; therefore, they should be given perioperative glucocorticoids intravenously until they can take oral replacement. Replacement therapy may be necessary for up to 6 to 12 months until the pituitary-adrenal axis recovers.

DISORDERS OF EXCESS ADRENAL ANDROGEN PRODUCTION

Excess androgen production may be either acquired (as in Cushing syndrome or ACCA) or congenital (as in congenital adrenal hyperplasia). Congenital adrenal hyperplasia comprises a group of autosomal recessive disorders characterized by defective synthesis of cortisol. This defect in cortisol synthesis results in increased ACTH production, which, in turn, leads to adrenal hyperplasia and increased production of adrenal androgens and androgen precursors. The most common variant of congenital adrenal hyperplasia is 21α-hydroxylase deficiency, which accounts for about 95% of cases. 21α-Hydroxylase deficiency may be divided into three main subtypes: classic salt wasting, classic non–salt wasting, and nonclassic. The two classic subtypes generally are more severe and typically present early in life (i.e., in infancy or early childhood) with virilizing features and AI. The nonclassic subtype tends to be milder: the androgen excess is less pronounced, and there is no cortisol deficiency. As many as 80% of patients with the classic salt-wasting subtype experience severe electrolyte and fluid losses as a result of an associated defect in aldosterone production.

Excess adrenal androgen production from an androgen-secreting tumor can lead to testicular atrophy (in men) or to hirsutism, acne, and irregular or absent menses (in women). Women may also experience other virilizing features, such as male pattern baldness, clitoral enlargement, increased facial hair, and deepening of the voice. Biochemically, the diagnosis is established by measuring plasma levels of androgens, including DHEA, DHEA sulfate, testosterone, and dihydrotestosterone. Other causes of hirsutism and virilism that must be considered in women include the polycystic ovary syndrome and androgen-secreting ovarian tumors.

ADRENOCORTICAL CARCINOMA

ACCA is a rare tumor: the estimated annual incidence ranges from 0.5 to 2 per 1 million adults. The age distribution is bimodal, with peak occurrences noted in childhood and in the fourth and fifth decades of life.[18]

Clinical Evaluation and Investigative Studies

ACCAs are typically large (> 6 to 8 cm) at presentation, and most patients present with advanced (i.e., stage III or IV) disease [*see Table 4*]. In two large series, the mean tumor size at diagnosis was 12 cm and 15 cm.[19,20] The increased use of imaging in clinical practice in recent years has not led to detection of ACCA at an earlier stage or impacted patient survival.[21,22] The clinical presentation may be related to the large size of the tumor (e.g., abdominal or back pain or other mass effects) or to increased secretion of one or more

Table 4 Staging of Adrenocortical Carcinoma[23]	
Stage	*Description*
I	T1 (< 5 cm) N0 M0
II	T2 (> 5 cm) N0 M0
III	T3 (locally invasive) or T1–2 N1 M0
IV	T4 (invasion of adjacent organs) or any T with distant metastases (M1)

steroid hormones. Approximately 60% of ACCAs are hyperfunctioning,[23] about 30% secrete cortisol and give rise to Cushing syndrome, and 20% secrete androgen and have virilizing effects. A mixed hormone secretion pattern is frequently present. Adrenal cancers that secrete estrogen or aldosterone exist but are much less common.

Biochemical evaluation of ACCA patients should consist of testing for hypercortisolism [*see* Cushing Syndrome, *above*] and measurement of adrenal androgens (i.e., DHEA sulfate and testosterone).

Management

ACCA is an aggressive tumor that may spread locally to regional lymph nodes, adjacent organs, and distant sites (including the liver, the lungs, and bones). Complete surgical resection offers the only chance for a cure and is the best predictor of clinical outcome.[18,24] Standardization of surgical resection to include first-order lymph nodes (ipsilateral renal hilar, celiac, and para-aortic and/or paracaval) has been recommended, but nephrectomy is not indicated unless the kidney is directly involved.[25] Overall 5-year actuarial survival rates after complete resection range from 32 to 48%.[18] Patients whose tumors are incompletely resected (i.e., who have residual local or distant gross disease) have a median survival of less than 1 year. The presence of tumor thrombus in the renal vein or IVC is not a contraindication for surgical resection provided that the tumor can be completely excised.[18,23]

Treatment options for patients with unresectable or recurrent ACCA are limited. Locally recurrent tumors may be resected surgically. Radiation therapy is generally ineffective, although a few investigators have reported tumor response rates as high as 42%.[25] Mitotane is toxic for adrenocortical cells and is the most specific chemotherapeutic agent available for the treatment of ACCA. Objective tumor response rates as high as 25% have been reported, but complete responses to mitotane are rare,[23] and treatment is often limited by gastrointestinal and central nervous system side effects. In addition, because of mitotane's toxic effects on normal adrenal cortical function, patients being treated for ACCA with this agent require glucocorticoid replacement. Mitotane has occasionally been used as adjuvant therapy after resection of ACCA, but the data are inconclusive. The results of conventional cytotoxic chemotherapy in ACCA patients have been disappointing. The poor response rates to chemotherapy may be related to high expression of the multiple drug resistance gene *MDR1*; this results in high levels of P-glycoprotein, which acts as a drug efflux pump.[23,26]

ADRENAL INSUFFICIENCY

AI may be either primary or secondary. In industrialized countries, the primary cause of spontaneous AI is autoimmune adrenal disease; in the developing world, it is tuberculosis.[27] Other causes of primary AI include bilateral adrenal hemorrhage, adrenal metastases, adrenal leukodystrophy, and certain viral or fungal infections. The primary cause of secondary AI is suppression of ACTH secretion and normal adrenal cortical function as a result of long-term steroid administration. Several weeks of exogenous administration of glucocorticoids are required before AI develops upon steroid withdrawal.[27]

Clinical Evaluation

Chronic AI (Addison disease) is characterized by weakness, chronic fatigue, anorexia, loss of appetite, abdominal pain, nausea, and diarrhea. Hyperpigmentation of the skin from chronic hypersecretion of melatonin (a product of the ACTH precursor pro-opiomelanocortin) may be apparent as well. Many patients with primary AI also have an associated mineralocorticoid deficiency, the symptoms and signs of which include salt craving, postural hypotension, and electrolyte abnormalities. Because many of the symptoms of AI are nonspecific, patients may go undiagnosed for a long time. The symptoms of primary AI are usually more severe than those of secondary AI.

In patients with inadequate adrenal reserve, an acute adrenal crisis may be precipitated by the stress imposed by surgery, trauma, infection, or dehydration and may result in vascular collapse with hypotension, shock, and, if untreated, death. Consequently, patients with unexplained cardiovascular collapse in whom this diagnosis is suspected should be treated empirically with replacement corticosteroids.

Investigative Studies

Laboratory abnormalities associated with AI include hyponatremia, hyperkalemia (in primary AI), hypoglycemia, and azotemia, with increased blood urea nitrogen and creatinine concentrations. The diagnosis is confirmed by measurement of plasma cortisol and ACTH levels. In primary adrenal insufficiency, 8 am plasma cortisol levels are typically low (< 3 μg/dL)[28] and plasma ACTH levels are high (> 100 pg/mL). Plasma ACTH levels are usually low or inappropriately normal if pituitary failure or hypothalamus pathology is the cause.[27] The ACTH stimulation test may be necessary to establish the diagnosis in patients with partial AI or to assess recovery of the pituitary-adrenal function after treatment of Cushing syndrome. For this test, 250 μg of synthetic ACTH is administered intravenously, and plasma cortisol levels are measured at 0, 30, and 60 minutes. A serum cortisol level higher than 18 μg/dL at either 30 or 60 minutes is considered a normal response.

Management

AI is treated with exogenously administered glucocorticoids [*see Table 5*]. If the patient is in an acute adrenal crisis, hydrocortisone should be given in a dosage of 100 mg IV every 8 hours. If the patient requires oral replacement therapy for chronic AI, hydrocortisone should be given in a dosage of 10 to 12.5 $mg/m^2/day$.[27] Hydrocortisone (20 to 30 mg/day) is often preferred to other steroids because its

Table 5 Equivalent Dosages for Commonly Used Glucocorticoids[21,22]

Glucocorticoid	*Relative Potency*	*Dose Equivalent (mg/day)*	*t½ (hr)*
Hydrocortisone	1	20	8–12
Prednisone	4	5	18–36
Methylprednisolone	5	4	18–36
Dexamethasone	25–50	0.5	36–54

t½ = half-life.

short half-life (8 to 12 hours) more closely mimics the normal circadian rhythm of cortisol secretion; however, it must be administered twice or three times daily, whereas prednisone (equivalent dose, 5 mg/day) may be administered once or twice daily. For patients who are on long-term steroid therapy, outcomes after surgery appear to be essentially the same whether they received their normal replacement doses orally or whether they received stress doses intravenously.[29] Patients who have primary AI or have undergone bilateral adrenalectomy should also receive mineralocorticoid therapy (fludrocortisone 0.05 to 0.2 mg/day).

Disorders of the Adrenal Medulla

PHEOCHROMOCYTOMA

Pheochromocytomas (often referred to as pheos) are catecholamine-producing tumors that arise from chromaffin tissue.[30] The majority (85 to 90%) develop in the adrenal gland, but some occur at extra-adrenal sites. These tumors have their peak incidence during the fourth and fifth decades of life, and they affect males and females with equal frequency. The prevalence of pheochromocytoma in hypertensive patients is approximately 0.1 to 0.5%. Clinically silent pheochromocytomas may be present in as many as 10% of patients who present with an adrenal incidentaloma, and in some series, 30 to 40% of all pheochromocytomas present as incidentalomas.[31,32] Several features of pheochromocytomas have been characterized by a 10% frequency of distribution: 10% are extra-adrenal, 10% are bilateral, 10% occur in children, 10% are familial, and 10% are malignant. Some more recent series, however, have reported lower percentages of malignant pheochromocytomas.[33,34] Because extra-adrenal pheochromocytomas (also referred to as paragangliomas) lack the enzyme phenylethanolamine-*N*-methyltransferase (PNMT), they can secrete norepinephrine but not epinephrine.

Clinical Evaluation

The clinical features of pheochromocytoma are related to the effects of increased secretion of norepinephrine and epinephrine.[30] Hypertension is the most consistent feature and may be either paroxysmal or sustained. Paroxysmal hypertension can be severe and may be associated with "spells" consisting of pounding in the chest, tachycardia, headache, anxiety, and pallor; these spells are related to catecholamine surges. Other symptoms that may be noted include temperature elevation, flushing, and sweating, and some patients experience a feeling of marked anxiety and an impending sense of doom. Most attacks are short and last less than 15 minutes. The paroxysms may occur spontaneously, or they may be precipitated by postural changes, vigorous exercise, sexual intercourse, alcohol, and the use of certain drugs (e.g., histamine, tricyclic antidepressants, and metoclopramide) or anesthetic agents.

Some patients with pheochromocytoma present with an extreme hypertensive crisis that may result in severe headaches, diaphoresis, visual changes, acute myocardial infarction, cardiac dysrhythmias, congestive heart failure, pulmonary edema, or even stroke. Sudden death has been reported in patients with unsuspected pheochromocytomas who have undergone percutaneous biopsy of the tumor[35,36] or surgical procedures for other indications. Hypertensive emergencies are treated with IV esmolol, phentolamine (or sodium nitroprusside), or both.

Pheochromocytoma should be suspected in any patient with severe hypertension, any patient with hypertension that is episodic or associated with spells, any hypertensive pediatric patient, any patient with a family history of pheochromocytoma or multiple endocrine neoplasia type 2A (MEN 2A) or 2B (MEN 2B), and any hypertensive patient with medullary thyroid carcinoma.

Investigative Studies

Laboratory tests The diagnosis of pheochromocytoma is established by demonstrating elevated levels either of catecholamines and metabolites (metanephrines) in urine or of fractionated metanephrines in plasma.[37,38] The urinary vanillylmandelic acid (VMA) concentration is the least specific test because of the frequency of false positive results caused by ingestion of related foods (e.g., coffee, tea, and raw fruits) or drugs (e.g., alpha-methyldopa) and is no longer routinely used. Because the plasma fractionated metanephrine concentration is both sensitive for pheochromocytoma and considerably simpler than a 24-hour urine collection, it is the preferred initial screening test in many institutions; however, some investigators have found that measurement of 24-hour urinary catecholamine and metanephrine levels yields fewer false positive results.[37] In most cases, abnormal plasma metanephrine and norepinephrine levels should be confirmed by measurement of urinary catecholamine and metanephrine concentrations. In the rare case where the biochemical diagnosis is difficult, direct measurement of plasma catecholamine levels during a hypertensive episode may be useful.

Certain agents may interfere with biochemical testing for pheochromocytoma, including iodine-containing contrast media, labetalol, tricyclic antidepressants, and levodopa.[39] Major stress (e.g., from a recent stroke, a major operation, obstructive sleep apnea, or renal failure) may also affect catecholamine and metabolite levels. Because of the sensitivity of current tests and the risk of blood pressure alterations, provocative testing with agents such as glucagon or histamine and suppression testing with clonidine are no longer commonly used for diagnosis of pheochromocytoma.

Imaging Given that only 2 to 3% of pheochromocytomas are found outside the abdomen, localization of suspected tumors should begin with abdominal CT or MRI.[38] The uniquely bright appearance pheochromocytomas typically exhibit on T_2-weighted MRI sequences [see Figure 6] makes MRI the preferred imaging modality in many institutions. Another option is scintigraphy with iodine-labeled metaiodobenzylguanidine (I-MIBG). MIBG labeled with iodine-131 or ^{123}I selectively accumulates in chromaffin tissues but does so more rapidly in pheochromocytomas than in normal adrenal medullary tissue. Multi-institutional experience with ^{131}I-MIBG imaging for pheochromocytomas has found this modality to have an overall sensitivity of 77 to 90% and a specificity of 96 to 100%.[40] ^{123}I-MIBG is now available for use and appears to have greater sensitivity than does ^{131}I-MIBG scintigraphy. Indium-labeled octreotide scintigraphy has also been used to localize pheochromocytomas but has much less sensitivity for benign pheochromocytomas than does MIBG and should be reserved for cases in which all other imaging studies are inconclusive.[41] I-MIBG scintigraphy is most useful for localizing extra-adrenal tumors that are not visualized by conventional imaging modalities and for following patients with malignant pheochromocytomas. Its main disadvantages are its greater complexity and cost (in comparison with other imaging techniques), the need to block thyroid uptake with oral iodine, and the fact that some medications interfere with pharmacologic uptake of the tracer. I-MIBG is not warranted in patients with uncomplicated pheochromocytomas that are localized on CT or MRI as it is expensive and rarely alters treatment in this setting.[42,43]

Pharmacologic Preparation for Operation

Once the diagnosis of pheochromocytoma has been established biochemically and radiographically, the next step is to prepare the patient for adrenalectomy pharmacologically so as to prevent an intraoperative hypertensive crisis. Preoperative alpha blockade with phenoxybenzamine is initiated, usually starting at a dosage of 10 mg twice daily, which is then gradually increased to a total of 60 to 90 mg/day in divided doses until hypertension is controlled and the patient is mildly orthostatic. As alpha blockade progresses, fluids should be administered liberally to fill the expanded intravascular space. If the patient has marked tachycardia or dysrhythmia, beta blockade with atenolol or metoprolol may also be required. Beta blockade should never be initiated until alpha blockade has first been achieved because unopposed alpha-receptor stimulation can induce a hypertensive crisis and acute cardiac failure.

Associated Inherited Syndromes

Pheochromocytomas may occur in the setting of a number of different inherited endocrine tumor syndromes [see Table 6]. Of these, the ones most commonly associated with pheochromocytoma are von Hippel-Lindau (VHL) syndrome and the MEN type 2 syndromes.[44] In addition to pheochromocytoma, VHL syndrome is characterized by bilateral renal tumors and cysts, cerebellar and spinal hemangioblastomas, retinal angiomas, pancreatic cysts and tumors, epididymal cystadenomas, and inner ear canal tumors. MEN 2A and 2B are associated with medullary thyroid carcinoma in 100% of cases. The incidence of pheochromocytomas in MEN 2A and 2B patients ranges from 30 to 50%. MEN type 2 arises from mutations in the *ret* proto-oncogene on chromosome 10. Specific *ret* mutations associated with pheochromocytoma occur predominantly on codons 618 and 634.[44] In addition, familial paragangliomas of the neck are now known to be associated with mutations in the succinate dehydrogenase subunit B (*SDHB*) and succinate dehydrogenase subunit D (*SDHD*) genes,[45,46] which encode mitochondrial enzymes involved in oxidative phosphorylation.[47]

Familial pheochromocytoma may be more common than was previously thought. A 2002 study found mutations in 24% of patients who presented without a known familial pheochromocytoma association: 30 had mutations of the *VHL* gene, 13 of *ret*, 11 of the *SDHD* gene, and 12 of the *SDHB* gene.[48] These findings suggest the need for careful screening for a familial disorder in this setting.

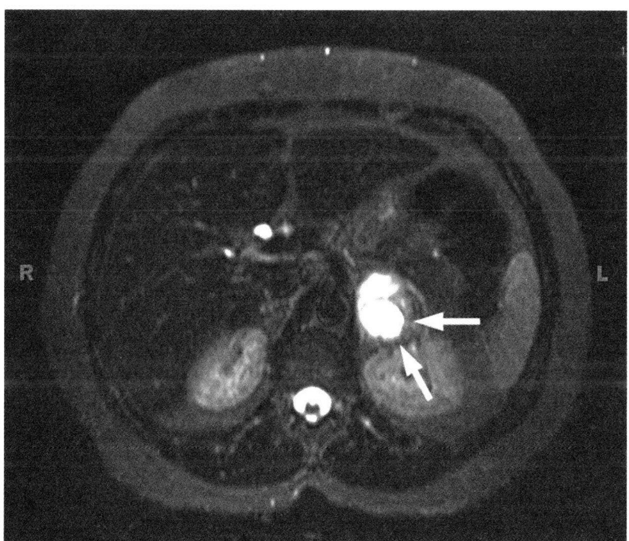

Figure 6 **Magnetic resonance image showing a left adrenal pheochromocytoma (*arrows*). Pheochromocytomas typically appear bright on T_2-weighted images.**

Table 6 Inherited Pheochromocytoma Syndromes

Syndrome	*Mutation*	*Chromosome*	*Frequency (%)**
MEN 2A and 2B	*ret* (proto-oncogene)	10q11	30–50
von Hippel-Lindau syndrome	*VHL* (tumor suppressor gene)	3p25	15–20
Neurofibromatosis	*NF1*	17q11	1–5
Familial paraganglioma and extra-adrenal pheochromocytoma	*SDHD*†	11q23	—
	SDHB†	1p35-36	—
	SDHC†	1q21	—

MEN = multiple endocrine neoplasia.
*Clinical incidence of tumors within persons affected by the mutation.
†*SDHD*, *SDHB*, and *SDHC* designate specific mutations within the succinate dehydrogenase gene (*SDH*). Patients with *SDHD* mutations are more likely to have head and neck paragangliomas, whereas *SDHB* mutations are more likely to be associated with extra-adrenal pheochromocytomas and malignant tumors.

Adrenal metastases occur most commonly in the setting of more widespread metastatic disease. Renal cell cancer, lung cancer, and melanoma are the malignancies that most frequently metastasize to the adrenal gland, but various other tumors (e.g., breast cancers, colon and other gastrointestinal cancers, and lymphomas) may also involve the adrenal. Occasionally, the adrenal gland is the site of an apparent solitary metastasis for which resection is indicated. Imaging characteristics associated with adrenal metastases include larger size (> 3 cm), higher attenuation on CT, and no signal loss on MR chemical shift imaging. PET is often indicated to exclude extra-adrenal metastatic disease that would preclude resection [*see Figure 10*]. Biopsy of a suspected adrenal metastasis should be carried out only if a tissue diagnosis is needed to direct therapy—that is, if the patient is not a surgical candidate either for medical reasons or because of metastases at other sites. Biopsy is not indicated before resection of a solitary resectable lesion, because it could lead to tumor seeding or other complications. Reported 5-year actuarial survival rates after resection of an isolated adrenal metastasis range from 24 to 29%.[57]

Miscellaneous Adrenal Lesions

The adrenal disorders previously described (see above) are the ones most frequently seen and managed by surgeons; however, surgeons may also encounter a number of other adrenal lesions, such as myelolipomas, ganglioneuromas, cysts, and hemorrhage.

Myelolipomas are benign lesions that are composed of fat and bone marrow elements and are usually identified as incidentalomas. In most instances, they can be diagnosed radiographically on the basis of macroscopic fat that is present within the mass [*see Figure 11*]. Myelolipomas may become quite large (> 6 cm), but regardless of their size, they should not be removed unless they are causing symptoms. Ganglioneuromas are benign tumors that may arise either within the adrenal medulla or at an extra-adrenal site. Most adrenal cysts are lymphangiomatous cysts, but pseudocysts from previous hemorrhage may also develop.

Hemorrhage in the adrenal gland is most often the consequence either of trauma or of an underlying adrenal tumor. Accordingly, follow-up imaging should be performed to search for an adrenal mass that may be obscured by the bleeding.

A summary of the above tumors regarding clinical presentation and diagnostic features is given in Table 7.

Indications for Adrenalectomy

Any adrenal lesion that is hyperfunctioning or that is suspected of being malignant or possibly malignant on the basis of imaging criteria discussed above should be removed. Size alone, however, should not be used as the basis for selection for operation because some adrenal lesions (e.g., cortical adenomas, myelolipomas, cysts) may be greater than 4 cm but otherwise have completely benign imaging characteristics and therefore should not be removed.[54] Adrenal metastases should be resected only if they are solitary and appear in the absence of extra-adrenal metastatic disease. Adrenal myelolipomas and cysts should not be removed unless they cause symptoms or if there is uncertainty in the diagnosis.

Most of the adrenal disorders discussed in this chapter are amenable to laparoscopic resection. At present, the only absolute contraindication to laparoscopic adrenalectomy is a tumor with local or regional extension because of the need to perform en bloc resection of the tumor and any adjacent involved structures.

Laparoscopic removal of large (> 6 to 8 cm) or potentially malignant primary adrenal lesions is controversial, as discussed below.[58] Surgeons who attempt laparoscopic adrenalectomy in this setting should be highly experienced with the procedure.

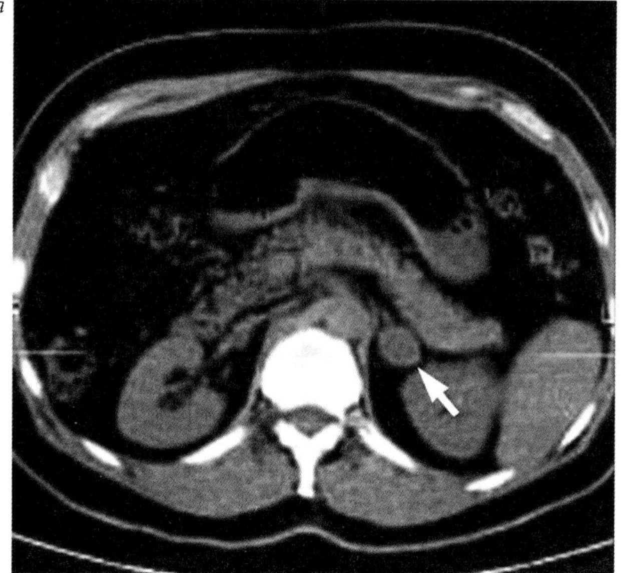

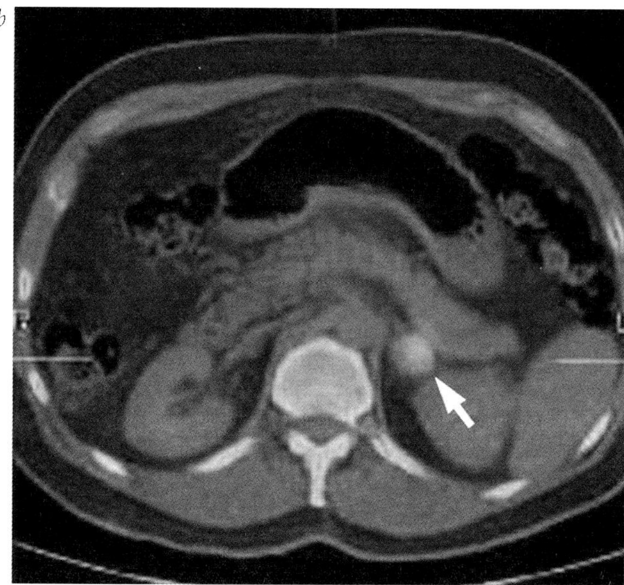

Figure 10 **(*a*) Computed tomographic and (*b*) positron emission tomographic images of a metastasis to the left adrenal gland (*arrows*).**

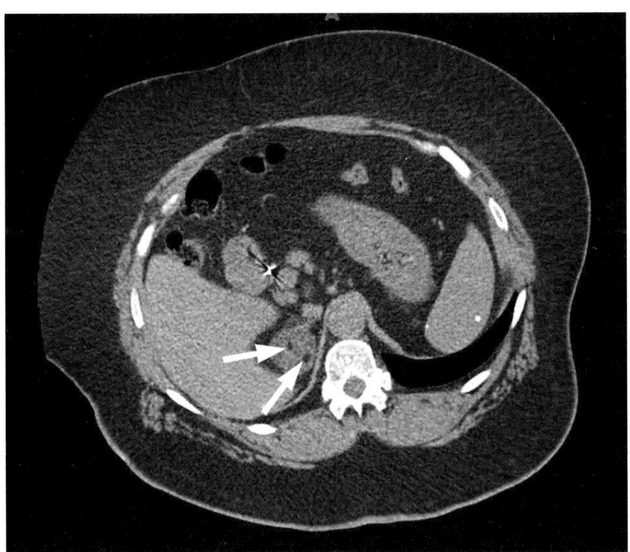

Figure 11 **A myelolipoma of the right adrenal gland. The areas of macroscopic fat (*arrows*) are typical for this lesion.**

Operative Planning

PREPARATION FOR OPERATION

Preoperative preparation of the patient for adrenalectomy entails control of hypertension and correction of any electrolyte imbalances. Patients with a pheochromocytoma should receive 7 to 10 days of alpha-adrenergic blockade with phenoxybenzamine to minimize any exacerbation of hypertension during the operation [*see* Pheochromocytoma, *above*]. Patients with Cushing syndrome or SCS should receive perioperative dosages of stress steroids. Mechanical bowel preparation is not necessary.

CHOICE OF PROCEDURE

The retroperitoneal location of the adrenals renders them accessible via either transabdominal or retroperitoneal approaches.[59,60] The choice of surgical approach in any given patient depends on a number of factors, including the nature of the underlying adrenal pathology, the size of the tumor, the patient's body habitus, and the experience of the operating surgeon. For the vast majority of adrenal lesions, laparoscopic adrenalectomy is preferred. Most centers favor the transabdominal lateral approach to laparoscopic adrenalectomy, which has the advantages of a large working space, familiar anatomic landmarks, and widespread success. Increasingly, however, a number of centers prefer a retroperitoneal endoscopic approach.[61,62] The advantages of this technique are that the peritoneal cavity is not entered, there is no need to retract overlying organs, and the incidence of postoperative ileus may be lower. It may also simplify access in patients who have previously undergone extensive upper abdominal procedures. The disadvantages are that the retroperitoneal approach employs a smaller working space, is more difficult to learn with fewer anatomic landmarks for orientation, and is more difficult in obese patients and those with larger tumors.

Table 7 Clinical and Diagnostic Features of Common Adrenal Tumors

Adrenal Tumor	*Clinical Presentation*	*Biochemical Testing*	*Preferred Method of Imaging/Localization*
Aldosteronoma	Hypertension ± hypokalemia	Elevated PAC with suppressed PRA (PAC:PRA > 20–30)	Thin section (3 mm) adrenal CT
		Urine aldosterone > 12 μg/24 hr	Adrenal vein sampling
		Urine potassium > 30 mEq/24 hr	
Cortisol-producing adenoma (Cushing syndrome)	Centripetal obesity, moon facies, hypertension, purple skin striae, osteopenia, plethora, amenorrhea	Elevated 24 hr urinary free cortisol	Abdominal CT
		Nonsuppressed low-dose dexamethasone test	
		Decreased plasma ACTH	
Pheochromocytoma	Severe episodic hypertension or hypertension with spells of tachycardia, headache, anxiety, and diaphoresis	Elevated plasma fractionated metanephrines or urinary catecholamines and metabolites	MRI (T_2-weighted sequences showing bright-appearing adrenal lesion)
			^{123}I-MIBG scan or Octreoscan reserved for malignant or extra-adrenal tumors not seen on conventional imaging
Adrenal cortical carcinoma	Cushing syndrome, virilizing features, local pain or mass	24 hr urinary free cortisol and metabolites	CT of chest/abdomen/pelvis
		Plasma DHEA sulfate	
Adrenal metastasis	None (often seen on follow-up imaging) or local pain	Plasma fractionated metanephrines and low-dose DM test to exclude functioning lesion	Abdominal CT, PET imaging to evaluate for extra-adrenal metastatic disease as appropriate for the type of tumor
		FNA biopsy only if unresectable	
Myelolipoma	None; occasionally local pain	None if radiographic appearance is unequivocal for myelolipoma	Presence of macroscopic fat on CT or MRI

ACTH = adrenocorticotropic hormone; CT = computed tomography; DHEA = dehydroepiandrosterone; DM = dexamethasone; FNA = fine-needle aspiration; MIBG = metaiodolbenzylguanidine; MRI = magnetic resonance imaging; PAC = plasma aldosterone concentration; PET = positron emission tomography; PRA = plasma renin activity.

The only absolute contraindications to laparoscopic adrenalectomy are local tumor invasion and the presence of regional lymphadenopathy. Cases in which the adrenal tumor is large (> 8 to 10 cm) or is suspected to be a primary adrenal malignancy or in which there is a history of previous nephrectomy, splenectomy, or liver resection on the side of the lesion to be removed should be considered relative contraindications to a laparoscopic approach in all but the most experienced hands. Portal hypertension may also be a contraindication to a laparoscopic approach because of the dilated collateral vessels in the retroperitoneum.

Options for open adrenalectomy include transabdominal, flank, posterior retroperitoneal, and thoracoabdominal approaches. The lateral flank approach and the posterior retroperitoneal approach have been replaced by laparoscopic approaches and are now rarely used. Most large or malignant adrenal tumors that necessitate an open approach can be removed via an anterior abdominal incision, usually a unilateral or bilateral subcostal incision (with subxiphoid extension if necessary); a thoracoabdominal incision is rarely needed.

Operative Technique

LAPAROSCOPIC ADRENALECTOMY

Transabdominal Approach

Patient positioning A gel-padded bean-bag mattress is placed on the operating table before the patient enters the room. The patient is placed in the supine position, general anesthesia is induced, and sequential compression stockings are placed. A urinary catheter may be optional for uncomplicated cases but should be used for all pheochromocytomas and larger tumors. Invasive monitoring is not usually necessary unless the patient has a vasoactive pheochromocytoma, in which case, an arterial line is routinely placed.

Next, the patient is moved into a lateral decubitus position with the affected side up [*see Figure 12*]. A roll is placed underneath the chest wall to protect the axilla. The bean-bag mattress is molded around the patient, and the legs are wrapped in a foam pad to protect all pressure points. The patient is secured to the operating table with tape placed across the padded lower extremities and a safety strap across the pelvis. The operating table is then flexed at the waist. The combination of the lateral position, the flexed operating table, and the reverse Trendelenburg position facilitates placement of the laparoscopic ports and provides optimal access to the superior retroperitoneum.

Initial access and placement of trocars Because of the lateral position, initial access to the peritoneal cavity is usually achieved in a closed fashion with a Veress needle. After insufflation to a pressure of 15 mm Hg, a 5 mm optical view trocar is placed. An open insertion technique may be used instead but requires a larger incision and is hindered somewhat by the bulky overlapping muscle layers in the subcostal region. Open insertion at the umbilicus is an option in nonobese patients.

The initial access site is generally at or somewhat medial to the anterior axillary line about two fingerbreadths below the costal margin [*see Figure 13*]. Subsequent ports should be placed at least 5 cm apart to allow freedom of movement externally. The most dorsal port should be approximately at the posterior axillary line. It is helpful to outline the anterior and posterior axillary lines with a marker before the patient is prepared to ensure that the ports are positioned properly. Whereas four ports are required for a right adrenalectomy, a left adrenalectomy can be done with either three or four ports depending on the surgeon's preference and experience.

Right adrenalectomy *Step 1: exposure of right adrenal gland and vein* The key to exposure of the right adrenal gland is extensive division of the right triangular ligament of the liver. This maneuver should be continued until the liver can be easily elevated and retracted medially and both

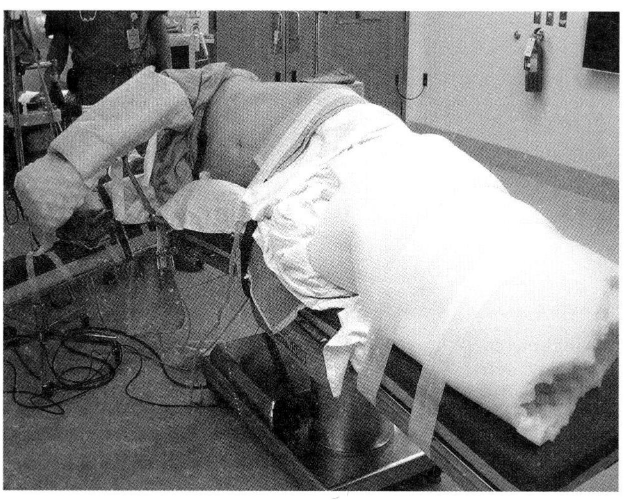

Figure 12 **Laparoscopic adrenalectomy: transabdominal approach. The patient is placed in a lateral decubitus position with the affected side up (here, right lateral decubitus for left adrenalectomy).**

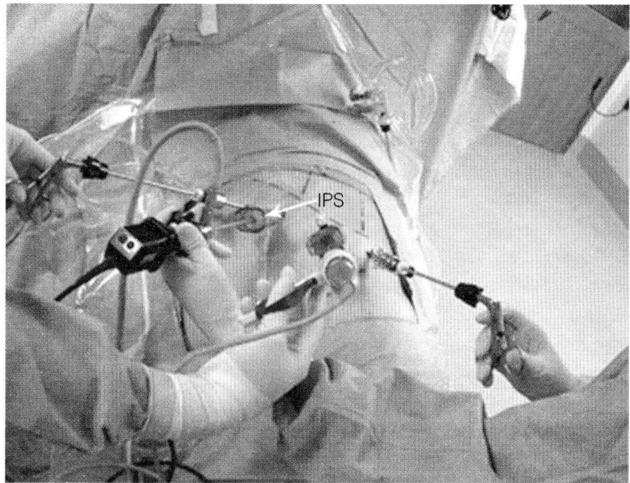

Figure 13 **Laparoscopic adrenalectomy: transabdominal approach. Shown is the recommended port site placement for laparoscopic adrenalectomy (here, left adrenalectomy).** ***Dashed lines*** **indicate the costal margin and the anterior and posterior axillary lines. IPS = initial port site.**

the right adrenal and the IVC are visible. A retractor is then inserted through the most medial port to hold the right lobe of the liver up and away from the operative site.

Next, the plane between the medial border of the adrenal and the lateral aspect of the IVC is developed. An L-hook monopolar instrument is used for gentle elevation and division of the peritoneum and the small arterial branches here [*see Figure 14*]. The adrenal is pushed laterally with an atraumatic grasper to apply traction to the dissection site; however, the gland itself should not be grasped, because it is fragile and the capsule and adrenal parenchyma are easily fractured. At all times, it is imperative to know where the lateral border of the vena cava is, both to ensure that the dissection is extra-adrenal and to avoid injuring it. The right adrenal vein should come into view as the medial border is dissected.

Step 2: isolation, clipping, and division of right adrenal vein The right adrenal vein is first exposed by gentle blunt spreading, and a right-angled dissector is then used to isolate enough of the vein to permit clip placement [*see Figure 15*]. A medium-large clip is usually sufficient for securing the vein, although sometimes it is necessary to use larger clips or even an endovascular stapler. (We use an endovascular stapler primarily in cases in which the tumor is located in the medial area of the adrenal and the vein must be taken along with a portion of the IVC junction.) Usually, two clips are placed on the IVC side and one or two on the adrenal side, depending on the length of vein available.

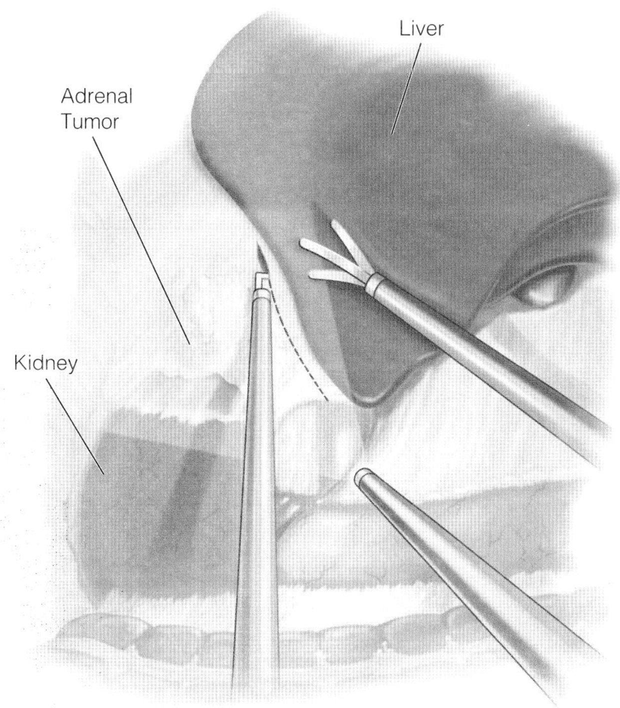

Figure 14 **Laparoscopic right adrenalectomy: transabdominal approach. Depicted is the anatomic exposure for right adrenalectomy. The liver is retracted medially, and the right triangular ligament of the liver is divided with an L-hook electrocautery.**

a

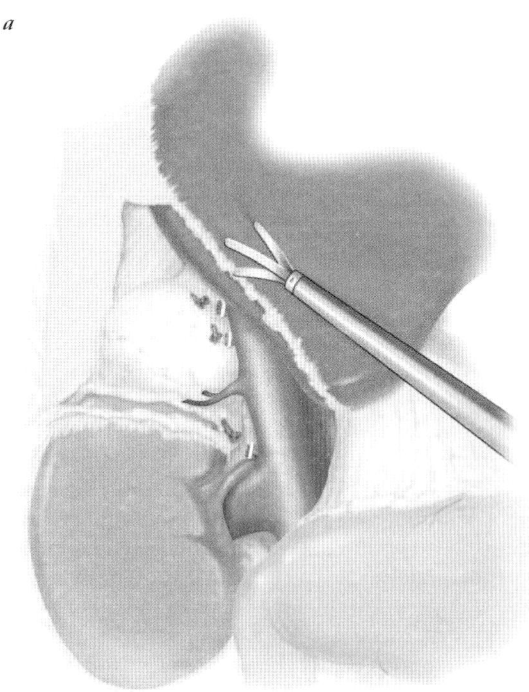

b

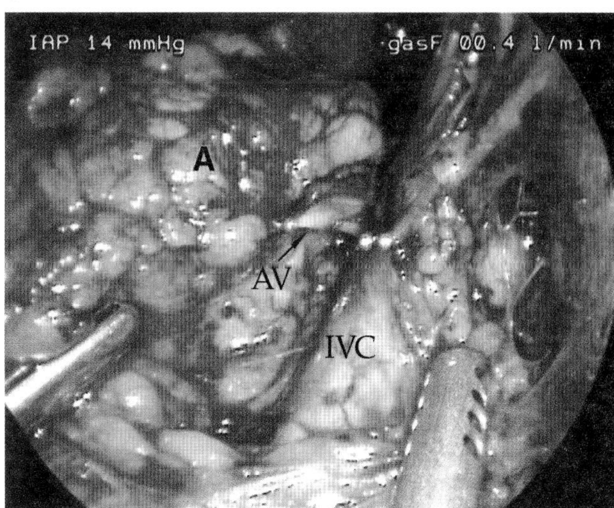

Figure 15 **Laparoscopic right adrenalectomy: transabdominal approach. Once the right adrenal and adrenal vein are exposed, the vein is isolated and clipped. Shown are (*a*) a schematic representation and (*b*) an intraoperative view showing the right adrenal gland/tumor (A), the right adrenal vein (AV), and the inferior vena cava (IVC).**

Meticulous hemostasis throughout the dissection is important: even minimal bleeding will stain the tissue planes and make the dissection more difficult and potentially treacherous.

Step 3: mobilization and detachment of specimen Once the adrenal vein is divided, dissection is continued superiorly and inferiorly with the L-hook. The numerous small arteries that enter the gland at its superior, medial, and inferior margins can be safely bovied, but larger branches should be clipped or taken with an advanced energy device. Superiorly, as the adrenal is mobilized, the musculature of the posterior diaphragm is exposed and serves as a marker of the proper plane for the posterior dissection. Inferiorly, the dissection should stay close to the margin of the adrenal so as not to injure vessels to the superior pole of the kidney. The inferior dissection then proceeds in a medial-to-lateral direction as the gland is elevated off the superior pole of the right kidney. The remaining attachments and retroperitoneal fat are relatively avascular and can be divided as above.

Once the specimen has been detached, it is placed in an impermeable bag. The retroperitoneum is then irrigated and inspected for hemostasis and for secure placement of the clips on the IVC.

Step 4: extraction of specimen The fascial opening at the 10/12 mm port site is enlarged somewhat, and the specimen bag is removed through this site. Large pheochromocytomas may be morcellated within the entrapment bag and removed piecemeal, but, ideally, cortical and other tumors should be extracted intact to permit full pathologic examination.

Left adrenalectomy *Step 1: exposure of left adrenal gland and vein* The splenic flexure of the colon is mobilized, and the colon is then released from the inferior pole of the spleen and away from the left kidney. Next, the splenorenal ligament is incised from the inferior pole of the spleen to the diaphragm to allow full medial rotation of the spleen and provide access to the left retroperitoneum [*see Figure 16*]. It is important not to dissect lateral to the kidney; doing so will cause the kidney to tilt forward and will interfere with exposure. Once the spleen is completely mobilized, it should fall medially, with minimal or no retraction needed to keep it out of the operative field. Division of the ligaments can be accomplished more quickly and with less bleeding if an ultrasonic or advanced bipolar coagulator is used.

At this point in the dissection, the tail of the pancreas should be visible, along with the splenic artery and vein. The plane between the pancreas and the left kidney is then developed, and this key maneuver allows the tail of the pancreas along with the spleen to be retracted medially. The adrenal is located on the superomedial aspect of the kidney just cephalad to the tail of the pancreas and is usually closely applied to the kidney, more so than on the right side. If the adrenal gland is not readily visible (more often a problem in obese patients) laparoscopic ultrasonography should be employed to help locate it and to delineate the surrounding anatomy, upper kidney, and renal hilar vessels. If the dissection starts too low, the renal hilar vessels or the ureter could be injured.

Once the adrenal is visualized, the medial and lateral borders are defined and the dissection is continued inferiorly to locate the adrenal vein as it obliquely exits the inferomedial border of the gland [*see Figure 17*]. The inferior border of the adrenal often sits adjacent to the left renal vein, from which it can be separated by means of gentle blunt dissection.

Step 2: isolation, clipping, and division of left adrenal vein The adrenal vein is isolated, doubly clipped, and divided. Because the adrenal vein is usually joined by the inferior phrenic vein cephalad to its junction with the renal vein, it

a

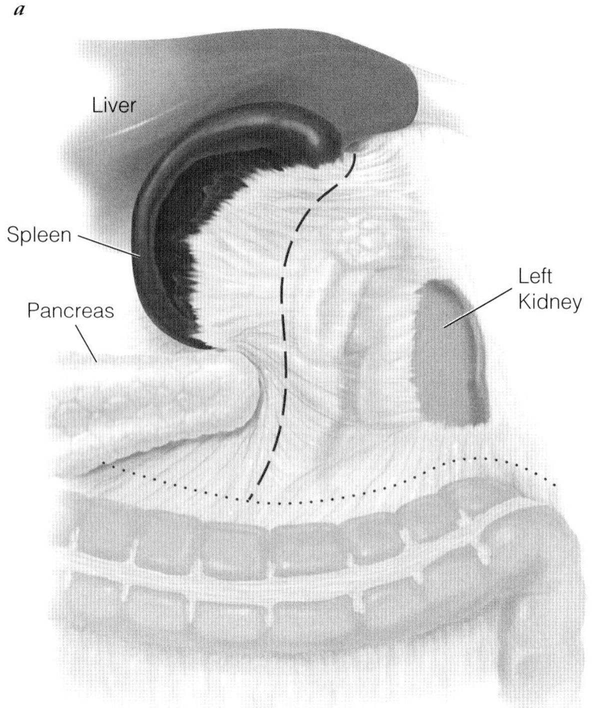

b

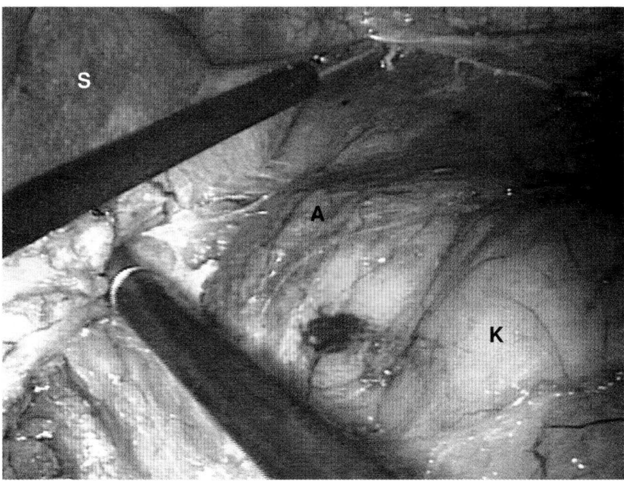

Figure 16 **Laparoscopic left adrenalectomy: transabdominal approach. Depicted is the anatomic exposure for left adrenalectomy. (*a*) The splenic flexure of the colon is divided first (*dotted line*), and the splenorenal ligament is then divided (*dashed line*). (*b*) An intraoperative view. A = adrenal; K = kidney; S = spleen.**

is often necessary to take the inferior phrenic vein again as the dissection proceeds more proximally.

Step 3: mobilization and detachment of specimen The dissection is continued cephalad along both the lateral and the medial borders of the gland. Because of the surrounding retroperitoneal fat, it is advisable to use an advanced energy device for this part of the left-side dissection. One must be careful to stay close to the adrenal until the gland is off the

a

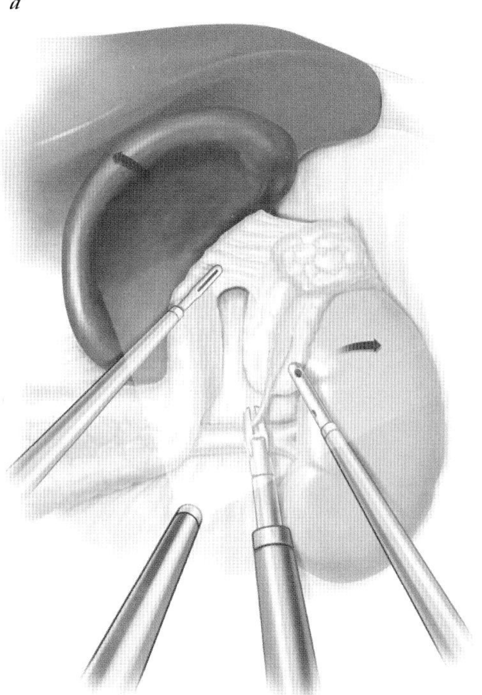

b

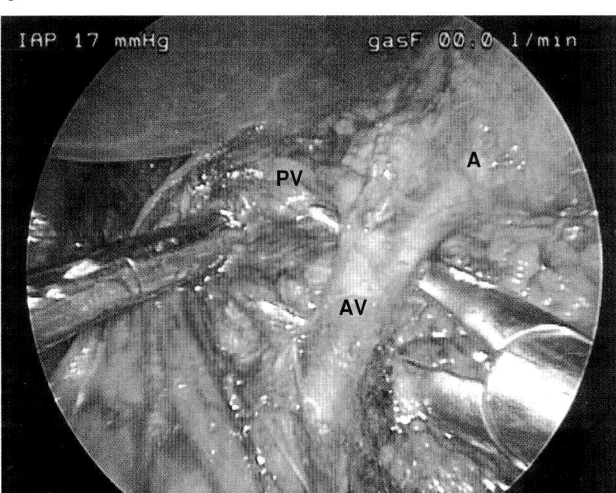

Figure 17 **Laparoscopic left adrenalectomy: transabdominal approach. Once the left adrenal and adrenal vein are exposed, the vein is isolated and clipped. Shown are (*a*) a schematic representation and (*b*) an intraoperative view showing the left adrenal gland/tumor (A), the left adrenal vein (AV), and the phrenic vein (PV). The phrenic vein joins the left adrenal vein above its junction with the renal vein.**

upper kidney to avoid injuring a superior pole renal artery. Finally, the posterior and superior attachments to the diaphragm and the retroperitoneal fat are divided.

Step 4: extraction of specimen The retroperitoneum is inspected and the specimen extracted as in a right adrenalectomy. If there is any possibility that the pancreatic parenchyma may have been violated, a closed-suction drain is left in place.

Retroperitoneal Approach

The technique for performing retroperitoneoscopic adrenalectomy has been well described by Walz and colleagues in over 500 cases.[61] The patient is in a prone position and is lying on a rectangular support that allows the abdominal wall to hang freely so that the retroperitoneum may be more easily expanded by the CO_2 gas [*see Figure 18a*]. The lateral aspect of the working side of the body is at the lateral aspect of the operating table. The 12 mm initial 1.5 to 2 cm access incision is placed just below the tip of the 12th rib and the retroperitoneum is entered under direct visualization. The cavity is developed digitally, and the finger in the retroperitoneal space allows for direct palpation and guidance of the second and third trocars. Both the second and third ports can be 5 mm [*see Figure 18b*]. It is helpful to use an adjustable blunt trocar with an inflatable balloon for the initial access site to maintain a good seal. The retroperitoneal space should be inflated at 20 to 25 mm Hg pressure to aid in both increasing the size of the working space and decreasing the amount of bleeding.

The retroperitoneal approach can be disorienting as most surgeons are not familiar with this viewpoint. When performing a right adrenalectomy, the right lobe of the liver is seen at the right side of the video monitor, with the lateral diaphragm seen at the top side of the screen. The kidney is seen at the bottom of the screen, and the spine is seen on the left side. The upper pole of the kidney should be dissected first, which allows for better visualization of the adrenal gland. The lower pole of the adrenal gland should then be dissected medially to laterally. On the right, the IVC then comes into view medially and deep to the adrenal after the lower pole of the adrenal is dissected. With upward traction of the adrenal, the adrenal vein can be found on the medial-posterior aspect of the gland. With the retroperitoneal approach, the adrenal vein can be secured with an advanced bipolar energy device, and the remaining posterior and lateral attachments can then be divided. As with the transabdominal approach, if the adrenal is difficult to locate, laparoscopic ultrasonography should be used.

During left adrenalectomy, the tail of the pancreas and spleen are deep to the adrenal above the kidney. The steps in exposure of the left adrenal are similar to the right approach, but the adrenal vein is located at the medial/inferior (i.e., right lower) aspect of the gland. The specimen is extracted similar to the transabdominal approach.

Robotic-Assisted Laparoscopic Adrenalectomy

Certain centers have incorporated robotic-assisted laparoscopic adrenalectomies into their practice. The pros and cons of this approach compared with conventional laparoscopy are under investigation.[63] Although the robotic approach has not demonstrated any advantages in operative time, safety, cost, hospital stay, or postoperative complications than laparoscopic surgery, it may provide surgeons with better ergonomics. In experienced hands, the conversion rate from robotics to laparoscopy is about 5 to 7% and to laparotomy is about 1%.[62] Overall, the robotic approach could offer comparable outcomes and feasibility for patients in high-volume centers.

a

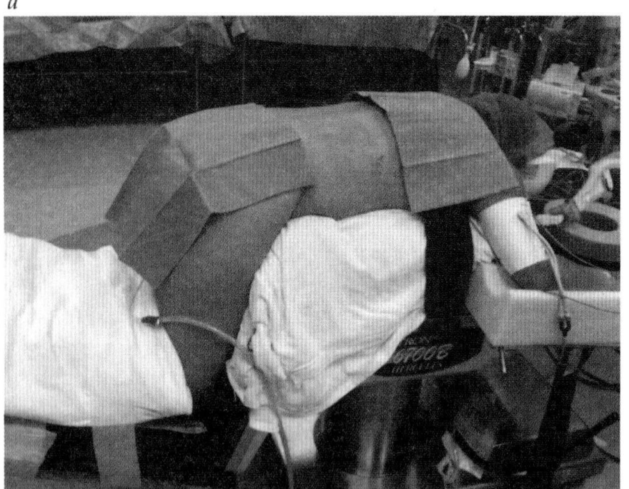

b

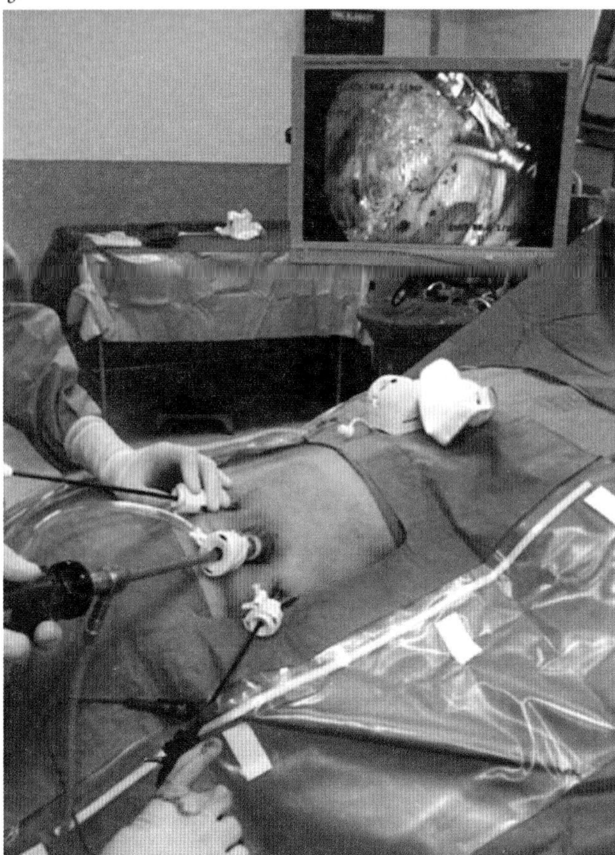

Figure 18 **Laparoscopic left adrenalectomy: retroperitoneal endoscopic approach. Shown are (*a*) patient positioning and (*b*) port site placement.**

OPEN ADRENALECTOMY

Of the four approaches to open adrenalectomy [*see* Operative Planning, Choice of Procedure, *above*], the anterior transabdominal approach is the preferred method for tumors that are too large to be removed laparoscopically and for all invasive adrenal malignancies. The incision most commonly used is an extended unilateral or bilateral subcostal incision, although a midline incision is also an option [*see Figure 19*]. The extended subcostal incision yields exposure of both adrenal glands, as well as the rest of the peritoneal cavity. If necessary, it may be extended superiorly in the midline to the xiphoid to provide better upper abdominal exposure for full mobilization of the liver and access to the hepatic veins and the vena cava. The exposure obtained with this incision is sufficient for all but the most extensive adrenal malignancies. If the tumor involves the vena cava, the incision may be extended into a median sternotomy to provide access to the superior vena cava and the heart. The classic thoracoabdominal incision, which extends from the abdomen up through the seventh or eighth intercostal space and through the diaphragm, provides excellent exposure but is associated with increased incision-related morbidity and is rarely used today.

Much of the exposure and dissection is the same as in a laparoscopic adrenalectomy; however, because open adrenalectomy is often employed for removal of particularly large tumors, some additional maneuvers may be necessary to achieve adequate exposure and vascular control. For example, it may be helpful to elevate the flank with a roll or a bean-bag mattress and then flex the operating table to open up the space between the costal margin and the iliac crest. Once the abdomen is entered, exploration is carried out for the presence of metastatic disease.

Exposure of the adrenal on the right side is similar to the laparoscopic approach. With large tumors, a Kocher maneuver should be performed to afford better exposure

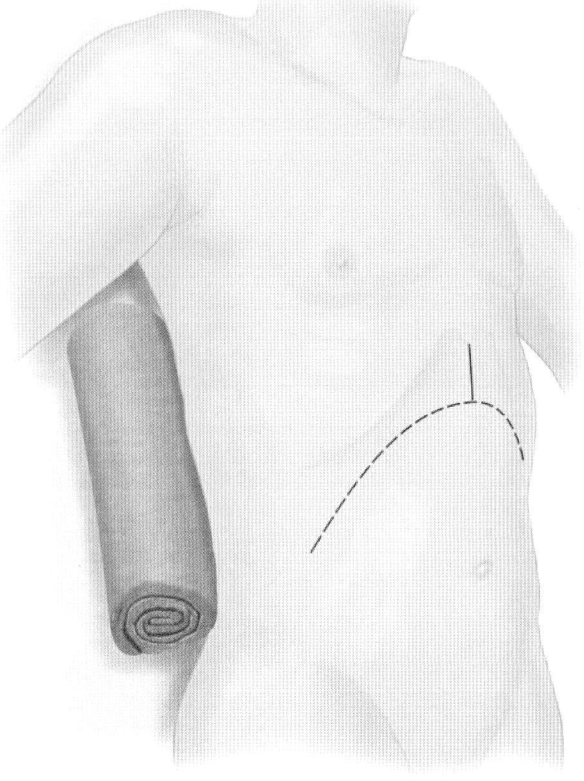

Figure 19 **Open adrenalectomy. The procedure is generally done through a unilateral or bilateral subcostal incision. For better exposure for large adrenal malignancies, the incision may be extended cephalad in the midline.**

of the vena cava and the renal vessels. The remainder of the dissection proceeds in much the same manner as in a laparoscopic right adrenalectomy. For suspected adrenal malignancies, a wide resection should be carried out, with removal of periadrenal fat and lymphatic tissue and any suspicious lymph nodes. For tumors that appear to involve the vena cava, vascular control of both the IVC proximal and distal to the tumor and the renal veins should be achieved before the lesion is removed.

Open left adrenalectomy entails reflection of the spleen, the tail of pancreas, and the stomach medially en bloc to expose the left kidney and the left adrenal. The remainder of the dissection proceeds as in a laparoscopic left adrenalectomy. For left-side primary adrenal malignancies, periaortic lymphatic vessels and lymph nodes should be removed along with the specimen. If a large left-side tumor is invading adjacent structures, removal may require en bloc resection of the spleen, the distal pancreas, and the kidney.

Troubleshooting

INABILITY TO LOCATE ADRENAL

The adrenal is usually not difficult to find on the right side, where it should be visible once the right lobe of the liver has been mobilized. Important landmarks on that side are the IVC, which is medial to the adrenal, and the kidney, which is inferior to the adrenal. Once these structures have been identified, the location of the adrenal should be apparent. In contrast, the adrenal can be difficult to find on the left side, especially if the tumor is small or the patient is obese. To locate the left adrenal, the splenorenal ligament should be fully divided, and then the plane between the kidney and the tail of the pancreas should be developed, with the tail of the pancreas rotated medially. As dissection proceeds superiorly, the adrenal can be visually distinguished from the retroperitoneal fat by its golden-orange appearance. If the adrenal is not yet visualized at this point, laparoscopic ultrasonography should be used to verify the locations of the superior pole of the left kidney and the renal vessels. Ultrasonography should also be able to image the adrenal gland and tumor within the retroperitoneal fat [*see Figure 20*].

CONVERSION TO OPEN ADRENALECTOMY

Conversion to open adrenalectomy may sometimes be necessary because of bleeding, failure to progress with the dissection, or a locally invasive tumor. If the patient is in the lateral decubitus position, conversion may be accomplished by means of a subcostal incision extended into the flank. With the patient on a bean-bag mattress, the operating table can be rotated out of the straight lateral plane so that the patient comes to occupy more of a hemilateral position. If the procedure is a bilateral adrenalectomy, then either a bilateral subcostal incision or a midline incision may be employed after the patient has first been returned to more of a supine position. For this reason, it is important to extend the initial preparation and draping past the midline of the abdomen. Alternatively, if the conversion is not being done on an urgent basis because of bleeding, the port sites may be closed, and the patient may then be moved into the supine position, reprepared, and redraped.

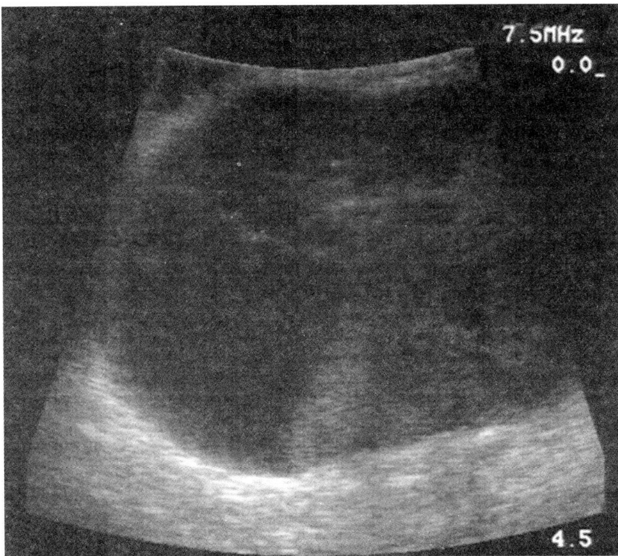

Figure 20 **If the left adrenal proves difficult to find, laparoscopic ultrasonography may be employed to locate the gland and the lesion within the retroperitoneal fat. This laparoscopic ultrasonogram shows an enlarged left adrenal gland secondary to metastatic squamous cell carcinoma of the lung.**

An option that may be considered before conversion to an open procedure is the use of a hand access port. A hand-assisted technique may be particularly useful for larger, noninvasive tumors that are harder to manipulate with laparoscopic instruments. The location of the incision for the hand port may vary according to the patient's body habitus; generally, however, an ipsilateral subcostal or midline location medial to the working ports allows adequate hand access while preserving visualization through the more lateral ports.

LARGE TUMORS

As surgeons become more familiar and proficient with laparoscopic adrenalectomy, the indications for removing large tumors laparoscopically have expanded. Large adrenal tumors (> 6 to 8 cm) are more difficult to remove than smaller ones because they are bulkier and more vascular and because they are harder to manipulate and retract. Accordingly, the dissection should stay extra-adrenal, and care must be exercised during manipulation to avoid entering the tumor. Surgeons should keep in mind that the larger an adrenal tumor is, the more likely it may be malignant. Laparoscopic ultrasonography should also be employed to verify that the tumor is well circumscribed and noninvasive. Surgeons who attempt to remove large adrenal tumors laparoscopically should be highly experienced in laparoscopic adrenalectomy techniques.

For large invasive adrenal malignancies, an open approach, involving a generous bilateral subcostal incision, is indicated, and the chest should be prepared in case a thoracoabdominal or median sternotomy extension proves necessary. The important principles are to obtain wide exposure of the operative field and to control all major vessels that may be involved before removing the tumor.

OBESE PATIENTS

Obese patients present a particular challenge during adrenalectomy, for several reasons: initial access is more difficult; retraction and exposure are more challenging; and the copious amount of retroperitoneal fat makes it difficult to identify the adrenal and to clearly define the margins of the gland within the retroperitoneum. Our practice is to attempt to gain initial access to the peritoneal cavity by using a closed Veress needle technique. Because resting intra-abdominal pressure may be higher in obese patients, especially if they are in the lateral position, it may be necessary to increase the CO_2 pressure to 20 mm Hg temporarily until the first trocar is inserted. If it proves difficult to establish pneumoperitoneum with the Veress needle technique, the initial trocar should be placed at the umbilicus by means of an open insertion technique. On the right side, the presence of a bulky, fatty liver should be anticipated, and the locations of the port sites should be adjusted accordingly by placing them somewhat more caudad. It may be beneficial to place obese patients on a restricted-calorie diet (< 1,400 calories/day) for 2 to 3 weeks before surgery to decrease the extent of fat and thereby overall bulk of the liver. Ample time should be taken to mobilize the liver fully so that the adrenal and the IVC can be safely accessed. On the left, the ports may be placed in the standard locations. Laparoscopic ultrasonography is often needed to locate the gland in the retroperitoneal fat.

Postoperative Care

After laparoscopic adrenalectomy, most patients are admitted to a regular nursing unit, although some patients with pheochromocytomas will need to undergo a short stay in the intensive care unit for invasive monitoring. Patients are started on clear liquids once they are awake and alert, and the diet is advanced as tolerated. A complete blood count is obtained on postoperative day 1 in all patients, and electrolyte levels are monitored in patients with aldosteronomas and hypercortisolism. Patients with Cushing syndrome should be given stress doses of steroids perioperatively and should be discharged on a maintenance prednisone dosage of 10 to 15 mg/day in divided doses. These patients should be advised that it may take 6 to 12 months or longer for the contralateral adrenal to recover to the point where prednisone can be discontinued. Patients undergoing bilateral adrenalectomy will need lifelong replacement therapy with a glucocorticoid (e.g., prednisone) and a mineralocorticoid (e.g., fludrocortisone acetate 0.1 mg/day).

Postoperative management of hypertensive medications depends on the pathology of the underlying adrenal lesion. In patients with aldosteronomas, spironolactone is stopped immediately after adrenalectomy, and the other antihypertensive agents are usually continued while blood pressure is monitored closely on an outpatient basis; further medication reductions are made as clinically warranted. In most patients with Cushing syndrome, antihypertensive medications are continued, whereas in most patients with pheochromocytomas, they are not. In both sets of patients, however, close outpatient monitoring of blood pressure should be carried out in the early postoperative period. Adrenalectomy can have a dramatic impact on hypertensive control and can lead to hypotension if medications are not appropriately adjusted.

In most routine cases, patients can be discharged within 24 hours after laparoscopic adrenalectomy, although some patients require longer in-hospital observation for blood pressure monitoring, for adjustment of steroid replacement therapy, or for resumption of a regular diet. After open adrenalectomy, resumption of an oral diet occurs later, and postoperative hospital stays of 4 to 5 days are more typical.

After discharge, patients are seen in the clinic within 2 to 3 weeks for a wound check, blood pressure evaluation, and a review of antihypertensive medications. In patients who underwent adrenalectomy for an aldosteronoma, electrolyte levels and the creatinine concentration and plasma aldosterone and renin levels should be checked. In patients who underwent adrenalectomy for pheochromocytoma, yearly clinical and biochemical follow-up is indicated, with measurement of plasma fractionated metanephrines (or urine levels of catecholamines and metanephrines). Likewise, patients with ACCA should be followed at regular intervals with periodic cross-sectional imaging and, where appropriate, biochemical testing because of the high recurrence rates. In selected patients on steroid replacement therapy who are proving difficult to wean from prednisone, an ACTH stimulation test may be necessary to assess the responsiveness of the pituitary-adrenal axis.

Complications

It appears that laparoscopic adrenalectomy has a major advantage over open adrenalectomy in terms of the incidence of postoperative complications. In a meta-analysis of 98 adrenalectomy series reported between 1980 and 2000, the overall complication rate was 10.9% with laparoscopic procedures and 25.2% with open procedures.[64] This difference between the complication rates was primarily attributable to the occurrence of fewer wound, pulmonary, and infectious complications in the laparoscopic series. The operative mortality associated with laparoscopic adrenalectomy is about 0.3%.

BLEEDING

The most common complication of laparoscopic adrenalectomy is bleeding, which was reported in 4.7% of patients from the series reviewed in the meta-analysis. Bleeding is also the most common reason for conversion to open adrenalectomy; however, major bleeding that leads to transfusion is relatively uncommon. The most effective strategy for managing bleeding during adrenalectomy is prevention. Important measures for minimizing bleeding risk include obtaining good exposure of the operative field and employing meticulous dissection and gentle handling of the adrenal and surrounding structures. When bleeding does occur, it may be from the adrenal veins, the adrenal gland itself, the IVC, the renal veins, the liver, the pancreas, the spleen, or the kidney. For bleeding during laparoscopic adrenalectomy, the first maneuver should be to tamponade the bleeding site with an atraumatic instrument as the bleeding will often stop with pressure. If this maneuver is successful, dissection should be directed away from the bleeding site for a while, until better exposure of the area can be obtained. Major hemorrhage from the IVC, renal veins, or arterial vessels that is not immediately controlled should be managed by prompt conversion to open adrenalectomy. Lesser bleeding may also be an indication for conversion to open adrenalectomy if it obscures the tissue planes and thereby increases the risk of inadvertent entry into the adrenal gland or tumor.

INJURY TO ADJACENT ORGANS

Other potential complications of adrenalectomy (either laparoscopic or open) include injury to the tail of the pancreas, injury to the diaphragm, and pneumothorax. When performing a left transabdominal adrenalectomy, the tail of the pancreas can be mistaken for the left adrenal, resulting in inadvertent pancreatic resection with pancreatic leak or pancreatitis. This risk may be greater in obese patients due to the abundance of retroperitoneal fat. To avoid this complication, one must be aware of the appearance and texture of the adrenal gland and its anatomic location immediately superior and adherent to the left kidney. It is important to define the plane between the pancreas and left kidney and then to rotate the tail of the pancreas and spleen medially during dissection. One should also see the splenic vein and artery as the pancreas is mobilized to the left. Unusual or large vessels encountered during the dissection should alert the surgeon to the possibility that the dissection plane may not be appropriate. Recently, severe high-grade complications after adrenalectomy have been described, including porta hepatis and hepatic artery injuries that resulted in liver transplantation and injuries to the renal vessels and to the ureter that resulted in a loss of renal function.[65]

RECURRENCE

Several cases of local or regional tumor recurrence have been reported after laparoscopic adrenalectomy. In most of these cases, the tumors removed were either suspected or unsuspected adrenal malignancies, and the extensive nature of the recurrences was probably related to aggressive tumor biology rather than to the minimally invasive surgical technique. In some of these cases, however, the pattern of recurrence, characterized by the development of multiple intraperitoneal or port-site metastases, suggested that laparoscopic dissection and pneumoperitoneum might have contributed to tumor spread.[66–69] One group treated three patients for recurrent pheochromocytomatosis that developed after laparoscopic adrenalectomy.[70] These patients were found to have multiple small tumor nodules in the adrenalectomy bed during open reoperation after removal of apparently benign pheochromocytomas. Fragmentation of the tumor and excessive tumor manipulation during the laparoscopic dissection were considered the probable mechanisms of tumor recurrence.

These reports highlight the need for caution in approaching large, malignant, or potentially malignant adrenal tumors. Surgeons who attempt a laparoscopic approach in this setting should be highly experienced in laparoscopic adrenalectomy techniques, and the tumor should be well circumscribed and not locally invasive. The use of a hand port may be a valuable adjunct to resection in these cases. Regardless of the specific surgical approach followed, wide excision of the lesion along with the surrounding periadrenal fat is crucial for minimizing recurrence rates in this population.

Outcome Evaluation

The safety and efficacy of laparoscopic adrenalectomy for the removal of small, benign adrenal tumors have been clearly established. Rates of conversion to open adrenalectomy in high-volume centers have ranged from 3 to 13%, and operating times have averaged 2 to 3 hours. Most patients are now discharged from the hospital within 24 to 48 hours after operation. Although no prospective, randomized trial comparing laparoscopic with open adrenalectomy has been carried out, several retrospective studies have consistently shown that the laparoscopic approach is associated with decreased pain, a shorter hospital stay, and a faster recovery.[71–74]

The results of a laparoscopic approach in patients with large (> 6 cm) adrenal tumors or malignant primary or metastatic adrenal lesions have been reviewed[58]; generally, the conversion rates for large or malignant tumors have been higher than those reported in other laparoscopic adrenalectomy series. Overall, tumor recurrence rates after laparoscopic adrenalectomy have been low.[75–79] In one series, however, local or regional tumor recurrence developed in three of five patients with adrenocortical carcinomas that were treated laparoscopically.[80] In another series from MD Anderson Cancer Center of patients with local recurrence after adrenalectomy, peritoneal carcinomatosis developed in five of six patients (83%) after laparoscopic resection compared with only 8% of patients with local recurrences after open adrenalectomy.[81] Whether the recurrences in these reported cases were related primarily to the surgical technique employed or to the underlying tumor biology is unclear. It would appear, therefore, that in most cases, primary adrenal malignancies are best approached in an open fashion unless the tumor is small and well circumscribed and the surgeon is highly experienced.

Financial Disclosures: None Reported

References

1. Young WF Jr. Primary aldosteronism: a common and curable form of hypertension. Cardiol Rev 1999;7:207.
2. Mulatero P, Stowasser M, Loh K-C, et al. Increased diagnosis of primary aldosteronism, including surgically correctable forms, in centers from five continents. J Clin Endocrinol Metab 200;89:1045.
3. Funder JW, Carey RM, Fardella C, et al. Case detection, diagnosis, and treatment of patients with primary aldosteronism: an Endocrine Society Clinical Practice Guideline. J Clin Endocrinol Metab 2008;93:3266–81.
4. Young WF, Stanson AW, Thompson GB, et al. Role for adrenal venous sampling in primary aldosteronism. Surgery 2004;136:1227.
5. Mulatero O, Bertello C, Rossato D, et al. Roles of clinical criteria, computed tomography scan, and adrenal vein

poorly defined upper abdominal masses reflect peripancreatic lesser sac fluid collections or pancreatic pseudocysts.

ESTABLISHING THE DIAGNOSIS

Laboratory Tests

Up until this point, the patient's clinical history, signs, and symptoms are suspicious but not diagnostic of AP and, in fact, are consistent with those of many other common surgical illnesses, such as perforated duodenal ulcer, mechanical small bowel obstruction, volvulus, or acute mesenteric ischemia. The diagnosis of AP requires two of the following three features: (1) abdominal pain suspicious for pancreatic origin, (2) serum amylase and/or lipase activity usually at least three times greater than the upper limit of normal, or (3) characteristic findings on contrast-enhanced computed tomography (CECT). Laboratory and\or radiologic investigations are not only essential for diagnosis but also provide important information to allow for risk stratification of disease severity.

Serum pancreatic enzyme measurements are the gold standard for identifying AP. Amylase, lipase, elastase, and trypsin are released into the bloodstream simultaneously at the onset of the disease but are then cleared from the blood at different rates. Amylase is cleared most rapidly (< 48 hours), whereas lipase and elastase remain elevated for over 96 hours. It is because of this differential clearance that the magnitude of elevation for any specific enzyme is dependent on the timing of the blood draw in relation to the onset of disease. In AP, disease onset is defined as the time that the patient's abdominal pain began, not when the patient is first evaluated by medical personnel. Many patients have been home with severe abdominal pain for 24 to 48 hours prior to their presentation in the emergency room, placing them well into the course of their disease process. Amylase traditionally has been the serum test of choice for diagnosis, although its overall sensitivity (83%) is limited by extrapancreatic causes of hyperamylasemia, a short serum half-life, and its unreliability in patients with chronic acinar cell damage (chronic pancreatitis). Currently, serum lipase levels greater than three times normal are the most accurate single test (sensitivity 92%) for diagnosing AP.[3]

A complete blood count (CBC) with differential and platelet count, comprehensive metabolic panel, arterial blood gas, and serum lactate are appropriate laboratory tests to review. The purpose of these is to assess both the degree of systemic inflammatory response and corresponding organ dysfunction in patients with AP. Liver function tests (alanine aminotransferase [ALT], aspartate aminotransferase, alkaline phosphatase, bilirubin) are used primarily to distinguish biliary pancreatitis from other causes of AP and to identify those patients who may have an impacted stone at the ampulla of Vater causing persistent pancreatic and biliary ductal obstruction. A recent meta-analysis showed that a threefold or greater elevation of ALT has a 95% positive predictive value for a gallstone etiology of AP. As a corollary to this statement, only half of all patients with known gallstone pancreatitis have significant elevations of their serum ALT. Therefore, although reasonably specific, an ALT less than three times normal is not particularly sensitive. C-reactive protein levels over 150 mg/L after 72 hours are closely related to necrotizing AP, and these values can be used to follow the clinical disease course over time.

Imaging Studies

CECT is the most accurate single imaging test for establishing the diagnosis, quantifying the inflammatory process, and staging the severity of the disease.[4] Precision in terms is essential in describing the morphology of disease states in AP, and this chapter uses definitions and terminology developed at the Atlanta symposium in 1992 [*see Table 1*].[5] A good-quality chest x-ray is useful to have early in the clinical course to identify a pleural effusion (poor prognostic factor) and to gauge the degree of interstitial pulmonary infiltration. In patients with known or suspected biliary pancreatitis, a right upper quadrant sonogram is useful in both identifying cholelithiasis and providing supportive evidence for choledocholithiasis based on the findings of intra- and/or extrahepatic biliary dilatation.[6,7] Magnetic resonance imaging (MRI) and magnetic resonance cholangiopancreatography (MRCP) have been used extensively in Europe but less so in the United States. The benefits of MRI over computed tomography (CT) are the lack of ionizing radiation, better definition of solid versus liquid components of necrosis, and delineation of ductal structures. The drawbacks are limited image resolution in critically ill patients who cannot follow commands. Endoscopic ultrasonography (EUS) is the most sensitive imaging modality for detecting cholelithiasis and

Table 1 Definitions from the Atlanta Classification of Acute Pancreatitis[5]

Term	Definition
Acute pancreatitis	Acute inflammation of the pancreas
Mild acute pancreatitis	Minimal organ dysfunction response to fluid administration
Severe acute pancreatitis	*One of the following:*
	Local complications (pancreatic necrosis, pancreatic pseudocyst, pancreatic abscess)
	Organ failure ≥ 3 Ranson criteria ≥ 8 APACHE II points
Acute fluid collections	Fluid collection in or near the pancreas, occurring early in clinical course, lacking a defined wall
Pancreatic necrosis	Nonviable pancreatic tissue diagnosed by intravenous contrast-enhanced computed tomographic scan
Acute pseudocyst	Fluid collection containing pancreatic secretions and a defined wall
Pancreatic abscess	Collection of pus, usually near the pancreas

choledocholithiasis and is not limited like transabdominal ultrasonography by intestinal gas or body wall edema.[8]

Risk Stratification

The severity of an episode of AP, as well as the disease-related morbidity and mortality, can be prognosticated based on the etiology [*see Table 2*] and a number of measured clinical and laboratory data points that can be calculated by established scoring systems (APACHE II [Acute Physiology and Chronic Health Evaluation II], Glasgow score, Ranson criteria). Recent observations that obesity is associated with a more severe course of AP have led to the addition of obesity to most scoring systems. Body mass index (BMI) in this application is categorized as normal (score 0), overweight (BMI 26 to 30, score 1), or obese (BMI > 30, score 2). Predicting severity is important for two reasons: (1) it allows patient triage to an appropriate level of hospital care (surgical ward versus intensive care unit [ICU]), and (2) it allows objective quantification of disease severity for both clinical trial recruitment and to compare patient outcomes between different clinical series.

Both the Glasgow and Ranson scoring systems are hampered by requiring 48 hours worth of data collection prior to calculation and are limited to prognosticating at this one point in time. Both scores have a low positive predictive value (below 50%) for disease severity. The APACHE II scoring has sensitivity and specificity similar to those of the Glasgow and Ranson systems but a greater than 90% negative predictive value for disease severity in patients with scores less than or equal to 7. Unfortunately, APACHE II scoring has a low positive predictive value (50%) for disease severity in patients with scores above 7. Although APACHE II can be calculated at any time in the clinical course and sequential scores can reveal trends in the disease state over time, the complexity of its scoring hinders its general clinical applicability.

Table 2 **Etiologic Factors for Acute Pancreatitis**
Common
Gallstone (including microlithiasis)
Alcohol
Hyperlipidemia
Hypercalcemia
Drugs and toxins
Traumatic
Postoperative
Sphincter of Oddi dysfunction
Post–endoscopic retrograde cholangiopancreatography
Uncommon
Pancreatic cancer
Periampullary diverticulum
Pancreas divisum
Vasculitis
Rare
Infection: mumps, coxsackievirus, HIV, parasitic (ascariasis)
Autoimmune: systemic lupus erythromatosus, Sjögren syndrome, autoimmune pancreatitis
α_1-Antitrypsin deficiency

Although of interest, almost all of these scoring systems have fallen out of favor because of the simplicity and directness of measuring the systemic inflammatory response syndrome (SIRS) and/or organ failure. The most accurate and earliest markers of severity in AP are measuring the SIRS or the inflammatory mediators contributing to the systemic effects that are witnessed, such as granulocyte (polymorphonuclear neutrophil) elastase, tumor necrosis factor, interleukin-6, interleukin-8, and C-reactive protein (CRP). The most useful serum test currently available in clinical practice is CRP, with severe pancreatitis defined by a value greater than 150 mg/L within 72 hours after the onset of disease. SIRS is defined by two or more of the following clinical criteria: pulse geater than 90 beats/min; rectal temperature less than 36°C (96.8°F) or greater than 38°C (100.4°F); white blood count less than 4,000 or > 12,000/µL; and respirations greater than 20 breaths/min or carbon dioxide tension less than 32 mm Hg.

Organ failure is most easily and reproducibly defined using the Marshall or Sequential Organ Failure Assessment (SOFA) scoring system [*see Table 3*]. Up to one half of the patients who eventually die of AP do so within the first 7 days of illness from unrelenting multiorgan dysfunction syndrome.[9] The morphologic severity of AP can be defined by the Computed Tomography Severity Index (CTSI) developed by Balthazar and colleagues [*see Table 4*].[4] This system assigns a numeric score to the quantity and location of necrosis to establish disease-related morbidity and mortality [*see Table 4*].

Mild AP Most attacks of AP (80%) are of the mild, edematous variety, consisting of an inflammatory disease state in the pancreatic parenchyma that is self-limited, runs its course over a 5- to 7-day period, and results in complete resolution and full constitutional recovery to the structure and function of the pancreas. The clinician's role in treatment is to provide intravenous fluid hydration, correct electrolyte or blood glucose abnormalities, and provide adequate organ support. Intravascular and interstitial hypovolemia may require 3 to 4 L of a balanced electrolyte solution (9% saline or lactated Ringer solution) over the first 24 hours or correction of deficits. Targeted response to volume resuscitation should include a lowering of the pulse rate, improvement of the blood pressure, and urine output of at least 30 mL/hr. Blood glucose levels tend to rise in AP and may be difficult to control in the initial phases of the disease. Close monitoring and control of blood sugar are essential during the first 24 to 36 hours of a patient's hospitalization, and close control has been found to improve both morbidity and mortality in hospitalized patients. This monitoring can be discontinued in nondiabetic patients as their pancreatitis resolves and they clinically improve. Oxygen saturation should be measured continuously and supplemental oxygen given to maintain an arterial saturation greater than 95%. Any evidence of respiratory insufficiency requires a chest x-ray to assess for pulmonary edema or acute respiratory distress syndrome. Narcotic analgesics are essential in patients with AP, and parenteral administration ensures adequate delivery in patients during their acute illness and period of unreliable gastrointestinal absorption. Patient-controlled analgesia is a safe and effective

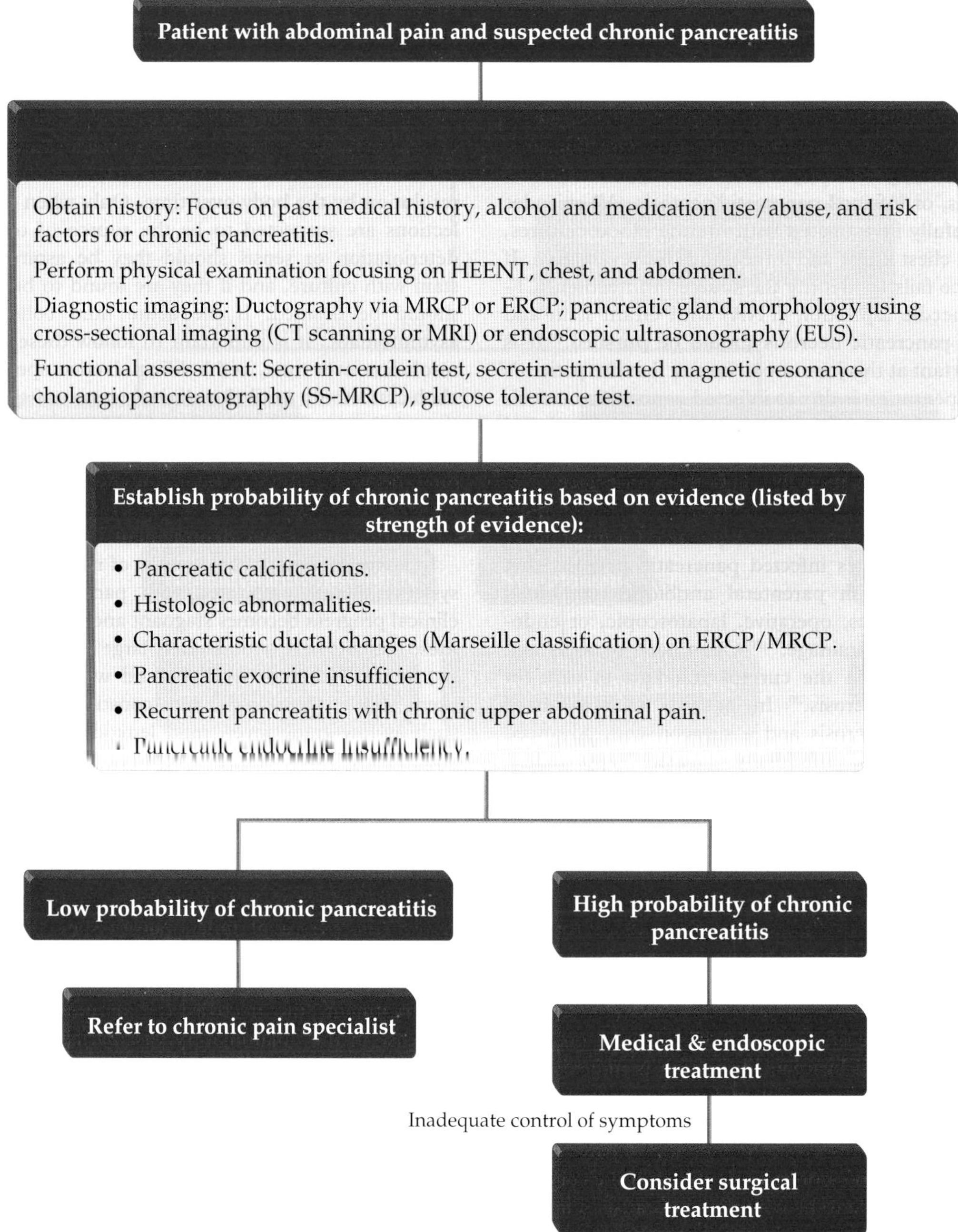

Figure 3 **Diagnosis and treatment of patients with chronic pancreatitis. CT = computed tomography; ERCP = endoscopic retrograde cholangiopancreatography; HEENT = heads, ears, eyes, nose, and throat; MRCP = magnetic resonance cholangiopancreatography; MRI = magnetic resonance imaging.**

Chronic Pancreatitis

Chronic pancreatitis is an inflammatory disorder of the pancreas characterized by glandular fibrosis resulting in permanent structural and functional changes in the organ and leading ultimately to pancreatic endocrine and exocrine failure. Clinical manifestations of this disease are erratic and can range from an asymptomatic state, to circumscribed recurrent bouts of AP (elevated pancreatic enzymes, glandular inflammation), to continuously disabling pain [*see Figure 3*]. Contiguous organ involvement can lead to obstruction of the duodenum (gastric outlet obstruction), distal common bile duct (secondary biliary cirrhosis), or splenic vein (sinistral [left-sided] portal hypertension with isolated gastric varices and hypersplenism). A precise diagnosis can be made only by direct pancreatic biopsy showing fibrosis and a chronic inflammatory cell infiltration. Because of the technical difficulties and potential morbidity associated with this procedure, provisional diagnoses are made using indirect evidence such as pancreatic duct morphology (Cambridge classifications), decreased pancreatic exocrine

Table 5 Summary of the Official International Association of Pancreatology Guidelines for the Surgical Management of Acute Pancreatitis[21]

1. Mild acute pancreatitis is not an indication for pancreatic surgery.
2. The use of prophylactic broad-spectrum antibiotics reduces infection rates in CT-proven necrotizing pancreatitis but may not improve survival.
3. Fine-needle aspiration biopsy (FNAB) should be performed to differentiate between sterile and infected pancreatic necrosis in patients with sepsis syndrome.
4. Infected pancreatic necrosis in patients with clinical signs and symptoms of sepsis is an indication for intervention, including surgery and radiologic drainage.
5. Patients with sterile pancreatic necrosis (FNAB negative) should be managed conservatively, and only selected cases should undergo intervention.
6. Early surgery within 14 days after onset of the disease is not recommended in patients with necrotizing pancreatitis unless there are specific indications.
7. Surgical and other forms of interventional management should favor an organ-preserving approach, which involves débridement or necrosectomy combined with a postoperative management concept that maximizes postoperative evacuation of retroperitoneal debris and exudate.
8. Cholecystectomy should be performed to avoid recurrence of gallstone-associated acute pancreatitis.
9. In mild gallstone-associated acute pancreatitis, cholecystectomy should be performed as soon as the patient has recovered and ideally during the same hospital admission.
10. In severe gallstone-associated acute pancreatitis, cholecystectomy should be delayed until there is sufficient resolution of the inflammatory response and clinical recovery.
11. Endoscopic sphincterotomy is an alternative to cholecystectomy in those who are not fit to undergo surgery to lower the risk of recurrence of gallstone-associated acute pancreatitis. There is, however, a theoretical risk of introducing infection into sterile pancreatic necrosis.

CT = computed tomography.

function (low pancreatic juice HCO_3^- level), or clinical criteria (right upper quadrant abdominal pain with radiation to the back). Recently, advances in imaging (EUS) and molecular genetic techniques have permitted the identification of patients who have subtle, early-stage disease or those patients with a genetic predisposition to eventually develop the disease. Overconsumption of alcohol is the primary etiology for chronic pancreatitis in the developed world with other etiologies, including hereditary pancreatitis, autoimmune pancreatitis, traumatic pancreatitis, post-ERCP pancreatitis, obstructive pancreatitis, or systemic conditions such as hypertriglyceridemia or hypercalcemia contributing to the total population of patients. Chronic pancreatitis is a disease treated primarily by medical therapy, with the surgeon's role limited to the treatment of specific disease complications [*see Table 6*].

INITIAL CLINICAL EVALUATION

History

Abdominal pain is by far the most common complication of chronic pancreatitis for which a patient is referred to a surgeon. Unfortunately, because of the subjective quality of this symptom and our inability to accurately establish causation between a particular patient's pancreas and abdominal complaints, correctly identifying patients in whom an operation will be beneficial is currently more art than science. Classic abdominal pain syndromes (midepigastric radiating to the back) combined with morphologic abnormality of the pancreas (i.e., inflammatory mass in the pancreatic head, pseudocyst, obstructing stone in the pancreatic duct) are more reassuring than patients with atypical pain syndromes and minimal change in the morphology of their pancreas, but these associations still suffer from our inexact understanding of the mechanism of pain in this disease process. Theories as to the pathogenesis of pancreatic pain include high pancreatic tissue or pancreatic duct pressure (compartment syndrome), alteration of sensory nerves with increased transmission as a result of the loss of their myelin sheath, molecular changes within nerve cells surrounding the pancreas, or a relative increase in the size and number of peripancreatic nerves. Despite these theories of pain pathogenesis, current surgical treatment of chronic pancreatitis relies on empirical results from applying a specific type of operation, either resection or drainage procedure, to the dominant anatomic abnormality found in a patient's pancreas.

Table 6 Surgically Remedial Complications of Chronic Pancreatitis
Pain
Relapsing pancreatitis (inflammatory mass in the head, pancreatic duct strictures)
Complicated pancreatic pseudocyst
Biliary obstruction
Duodenal obstruction
Bleeding pseudoaneurysm
Sinistral portal hypertension

All patients with chronic pancreatitis should have a complete medical history and physical examination. The history of present illness should focus on the qualities of their pain: type, location, radiation, chronicity, quality (intermittent or constant), temporal relation to food, and aggregating or alleviating factors. This information is important because when congruent, these clues often lend supporting evidence that the identified anatomic abnormality is related to the patient's pain. For instance, patients with pancreatic head disease should have midepigastric to right upper quadrant pain

Denervation operations Bilateral thoracoscopic splanchnicectomy is a minimally invasive approach to splanchnic denervation used to treat pain in patients with chronic pancreatitis. Candidates are generally patients with no other surgical targets (i.e., minimal change pancreatitis) who have been shown to have a splanchnic-mediated pain pathway based on their response to a differential epidural anesthetic.

Clinical results In measuring the results of surgery in patients with chronic pancreatitis, long-term success is typically defined by a thorough clinical follow-up of at least 5 years' duration. When restricting data to long-term outcome measures, the results for pancreatic head resections are as shown in Table 7. DPPHRs in a recent meta-analysis were shown to be equivalent in outcome to pancreaticoduodenectomy in the outcome variables of pain relief, overall morbidity, and incidence of postoperative endocrine insufficiency.[34] In this same analysis, DPPHRs were judged to be superior to pancreaticoduodenectomy in terms of operative time, postoperative hospital stay, and overall quality of life measures. When one compares the two most common DPPHRs, the Beger operation and the Frey operation, there are no significant differences in a randomized controlled clinical trial when patients were followed for over 8 years [*see Table 7*].[35] Outcomes of patients with chronic pancreatitis treated by longitudinal or lateral pancreaticojejunostomy (drainage operation) are shown in Table 8. After a mean follow-up of 79 months, 72% of patients experienced either complete or partial pain relief following operation, with a mean perioperative mortality in this group of patients of only 1%. A surgical denervation procedure as exemplified by bilateral thoracoscopic splanchnicectomy is a minimally invasive treatment of chronic pancreatitis with low perioperative morbidity and mortality. Based on currently available data, complete or partial pain relief is achieved in only 50% of patients during long-term clinical follow-up [*see Table 9*].

Table 7 Clinical Effectiveness of Pancreatic Head Resection in Patients with Chronic Pancreatitis: Comparison of DPPHR versus PD[34] and Frey Operation versus Beger Operation*[35]

Measured Variable	DPPHR	PD
Pain relief	=	=
Overall morbidity	=	=
Endocrine insufficiency	=	=
Operative time	+++	–
Hospital stay	+	–
Quality of life	++	–
Measured Variable	**Frey Operation (N = 36)**	**Beger Operation (N = 38)**
Quality of life	58.35 (0–100)	66.7 (0–100)
Pain score	11.25 (0–99.75)	11.25 (0–75)
Exocrine insufficiency	78%	88%
Endocrine insufficiency	60%	56%
Late mortality	32% (8/25)	31% (8/26)

DPPHR = duodenum-preserving pancreatic head resection; PD = pancreaticoduodenectomy; = = equal; + = positive; – = negative.
*Median follow-up 102 months.

Table 8 Outcomes of Longitudinal/Lateral Pancreaticojejunostomy in Patients with Chronic Pancreatitis

Study	No. of Patients	Complete or Partial Pain Relief (%)	Mortality (%)	Mean Follow-up (mo)
Greenlee et al[36]	86	80	3	95
Adloff et al[37]	105	93	2	65
Adams et al[38]	85	55	0	76
Sielezneff et al[39]	57	84	0	65
Sakorafas et al[40]	120	81	0	96
Mean results	453	72	1	79

Table 9 Outcome of Bilateral Thoracoscopic Splanchnicectomy in Patients with Chronic Pancreatitis

Study	No. of Patients	Mean Follow-up (mo)	Complete or Partial Pain Relief (%)
Moodley et al[41]	17	12	94
Ihse et al[42]	21	43	50
Buscher et al[43]	44	36	46
Howard[44]	55	32	35
Hammond[45]	20	15	60
Mean results	157	30	50

Pancreatic pseudocysts Complicated pseudocysts frequently occur in patients with chronic pancreatitis in association with an underlying pancreatic duct abnormality, and their surgical treatment should take this into account. Patients with pseudocysts and chronic pancreatitis should not be treated by cyst drainage solely, as is often the case in patients with a pseudocyst following a bout of AP. Patients with chronic pancreatitis frequently require some form of pancreatic duct drainage done and at times a parenchymal resection to treat the underlying anatomic abnormality that contributed to the formation of the pancreatic pseudocyst. Less common complications occur as a consequence of fibrotic stricturing of adjacent organs, including the biliary tract (elevated alkaline phosphatase, transaminases, and a dilated common bile duct) or duodenum (early satiety, weight loss, inability to eat); the majority of these complications can be addressed by the judicious application of one of the aforementioned operative procedures. Pseudoaneurysms occur as a consequence of severe inflammation and are commonly related to a pseudocyst. Angiographic embolization for control is generally the treatment of choice. Following control of hemorrhage, formal resection of the involved pancreas can be carried out.

Financial Disclosures: None Reported

References

1. Yadav D, Lowenfels AB. Trends in the epidemiology of the first attack of acute pancreatitis: a systematic review. Pancreas 2006;33:323–30.
2. Badalov N, Baradarian R, Iswara K, et al. Drug-induced acute pancreatitis: an evidence- based review. Clin Gastroenterol Hepatol 2007;5:648–61.
3. Kwon RS, Banks PA. How should acute pancreatitis be diagnosed in clinical practice? In: Domínguez-Muñoz JE, Malfertheiner P, editors. Clinical pancreatology for practicing gastroenterologists and surgeons. Oxford (UK): Blackwell Publishing; 2005. p. 34–40.
4. Balthazar EJ, Robinson DL, Megibow AJ, Ranson JH. Acute pancreatitis: value of CT in establishing prognosis. Radiology 1990;174: 331–6.
5. Bradley EL III. A clinically based classification system for acute pancreatitis. Summary of the International Symposium on Acute pancreatitis, 11–12 September 1992, Atlanta, GA. Arch Surg 1993;128:586–90.
6. Kelly TR, Wagner DS. Gallstone pancreatitis: a prospective randomized trial of the timing of surgery. Surgery 1988;104:600–5.
7. Behrns KE, Ashley SW, Hunter JG, Carr-Lock D. Early ERCP for gallstone pancreatitis: for whom and when? J Gastrointest Surg 2008;12:629–33.
8. Baron RL, Tublin ME, Peterson MS. Imaging the spectrum of biliary tract disease. Radiol Clin North Am 2002;40:1325–54.
9. Frey C, Zhou H, Harvey DJ, White RH. The incidence and case-fatality rates of acute biliary, alcoholic, and idiopathic pancreatitis in California, 1994–2001. Pancreas 2006;33: 336–44.
10. Rosing DK, de Biergilio C, Yaghoubian A, et al. Early cholecystectomy for mild to moderate gallstone pancreatitis shortens hospital stay. J Am Coll Surg 2007;205:762–6.
11. Uhl W, Warshaw A, Imrie C, et al. IAP guidelines for the surgical management of acute pancreatitis. Pancreatology 2002;2: 565–73.
12. Attasaranya S, Fogel EL, Lehman GA. Choledocholithiasis, ascending cholangitis, and gallstone pancreatitis. Med Clin North Am 2008;92:925–60.
13. Marik PE, Zaloga GP. Meta-analysis of parenteral nutrition versus enteral nutrition in patients with acute pancreatitis. BMJ 2004;12:328:1407.
14. Eatock FC, Haong P, Menezes N, et al. A randomized study of early nasogastric versus nasojejunal feeding in severe acute pancreatitis. Am J Gastroenterol 2005;100: 432–9.
15. Isenmann R, Rünzi M, Kron M, et al. Prophylactic antibiotic treatment in patients with predicted severe acute pancreatitis: a placebo-controlled, double blind trial. Gastroenterology 2004;126:997–1004.
16. Dellinger EP, Tellado JM, Soto NE, et al. Early antibiotic treatment for severe acute necrotizing pancreatitis: a randomized, double-blind, placebo-controlled study. Ann Surg 2007;245:674–83.
17. Casey JE, Porter KA, Langevin RE, Banks PA. Clinical features and natural history of central cavitary necrosis. Pancreas 1993;8: 141–5.
18. Banks PA, Gerzof SG, Langevin RE, et al. CT-guided aspiration of suspected pancreatic infection: bacteriology and clinical outcome. Int J Pancreatol 1995;18:265–70.
19. Kellogg TA, Horvath KD. Minimal-access approaches to complications of acute pancreatitis and benign neoplasms of the pancreas. Surg Endosc 2003;17:1692–704.
20. Büchler MW, Gloor B, Müller CA, et al. Acute necrotizing pancreatitis: treatment strategy according to the status of infection. Ann Surg 2000;232:619–26.
21. Nealon WH, Bawduniak J, Walser EM. Appropriate timing of cholecystectomy in patients who present with moderate to severe gallstone-associated acute pancreatitis with peripancreatic fluid collections. Ann Surg 2004;239:741–9.
22. Mithofer K, Mueller PR, Warshaw AL. Interventional and surgical treatment of pancreatic abscess. World J Surg 1997;21:162–8.
23. Fernandez-del Castillo C, Rattner DW, Makary MA, et al. Debridement and closed packing for the treatment of necrotizing pancreatitis. Ann Surg 1998;228:676–84.
24. Howard TJ, Patel JB, Zyromski N, et al. Declining morbidity and mortality rates in the surgical management of pancreatic necrosis. J Gastrointest Surg 2007;11:43–9.
25. Hartwig W, Maksan S-M, Foitzik T, et al. Reduction in mortality with delayed surgical therapy of severe pancreatitis. J Gastrointest Surg 2002;6:481–7.
26. Broome AH, Eisen GM, Harland RC, et al. Quality of life after treatment for pancreatitis. Ann Surg 1996;223:665–70.
27. Witt H, Apte MV, Keim V, Wilson JS. Chronic pancreatitis: challenges and advances in pathogenesis, genetics, diagnosis, and therapy. Gastroenterology 2007;132:1557–73.
28. Malfertheirner P, Büchler MW, Stanescu A, Ditschuneit H. Pancreatic morphology and function in relationship to pain in chronic pancreatitis. Int J Pancreatol 1987; 1:59–66.
29. Lankisch PG, Andren-Sandberg A. Standards for the diagnosis of chronic pancreatitis and for the evaluation of treatment. Int J Pancreatol 1993;205–12.
30. Etemab B, Whitcomb DC. Chronic pancreatitis: diagnosis, classification, and new genetic developments. Gastroenterology 2001;120: 682–707.
31. Whitcomb DC, Gorry MC, Preston RA, et al. Hereditary pancreatitis is caused by a mutation in the cationic trypsinogen gene. Nat Genet 1996;12:141–5.
32. Erturk SM, Ichikawa T, Motosugi M, et al. Diffusion-weighted MR imaging in the evaluation of pancreatic exocrine function before and after secretin stimulation. Am J Gastroenterol 2006;101(1):133–6.
33. Traverso LW. Pancreaticoduodenectomy for chronic pancreatitis—with or without pyloric preservation. In: Beger HG, Matsunos CJL, Rau BM, et al, editors. Diseases of the pancreas. Berlin: Springer; 2008. p. 414–23.
34. Diener MK, Rahbari NN, Fischer L, et al. Duodenum-preserving pancreatic head resection versus pancreaticoduodenectomy for surgical treatment of chronic pancreatitis: a systematic review and meta-analysis. Ann Surg 2008;247:950–60.
35. Strate T, Taherpour Z, Bloechle C, et al. Long-term follow-up of a randomized trial comparing the Beger and Frey procedures for patients suffering from chronic pancreatitis. Ann Surg 2005;241:591–8.
36. Greenlee HB, Prinz RA, Aranha GV. Long-term results of side-to-side pancreaticojejunostomy. World J Surg 1990;14:70–6.
37. Adloff M, Schloegel M, Arnaud JP, Ollier JC. Role of pancreaticojejunostomy in the treatment of chronic pancreatitis. A study of 105 operated patients. Chirurgie 1991;117: 251–6.
38. Adams DB, Ford MC, Anderson MC. Outcome after lateral pancreaticojejunostomy for chronic pancreatitis. Ann Surg 1994;219: 481–7.
39. Sielezneff I, Malouf A, Salle E, et al. Long term results of lateral pancreaticojejunostomy for chronic alcoholic pancreatitis. Eur J Surg 2000;166:58–64.
40. Sakorafas GH, Farnell MB, Farley DR, et al. Long-term results after surgery for chronic pancreatitis. Int J Pancreatol 2000;27:31–42.
41. Moodley J, Singh B, Shaik AS, et al. Thoracoscopic splanchnicectomy: pilot evaluation of a simple alternative for chronic pancreatic pain control. World J Surg 1999; 23:688–92.
42. Ihse I, Zoucas E, Gylistedt E, et al. Bilateral thoracoscopic splanchnicectomy: effects on pancreatic pain and function. Ann Surg 1999;230:785–91.
43. Buscher HCJL, Jansen JJMB, van Goor H. Bilateral thoracoscopic splanchnicectomy in patients with chronic pancreatitis. Scand J Gastroenterol 1999;34 Suppl 230: 29–34.
44. Howard TJ, Swofford JB, Wagner DL, et al. Quality of life after bilateral thoracoscopic splanchnicectomy: long-term evaluation in patients with chronic pancreatitis. J Gastrointest Surg 2002;6:845–54.
45. Hammond B, Vitale GC, Rangnekar N, et al. Bilateral thoracoscopic splanchnicectomy for pain control in chronic pancreatitis. Am Surg 2004;70:546–9.

Acknowledgment

Figures 5, 6, 7, and 8 Christine Kenney

38 NEUROENDOCRINE TUMORS OF THE PANCREAS

Dina Elaraj, MD, and Cord Sturgeon, MD

The endocrine pancreas is composed of four main cell types, glucagon, insulin, somatostatin, and pancreatic polypeptide (PP) cells, residing within the islets of Langerhans. Neoplasms of these endocrine cell types are a heterogeneous group of benign and malignant tumors that can elaborate hormones of the endocrine pancreas and hormones that are not normally found in the adult pancreas, such as gastrin, growth hormone–releasing factor, adrenocorticotropic hormone (ACTH), and vasoactive intestinal peptide (VIP).

The annual incidence of pancreatic neuroendocrine tumors (PNETs) is approximately 4 to 12 cases per million.[1] Approximately 60% of PNETs secrete a bioactive hormone that leads to a clinical syndrome. For those tumors that produce bioactive hormones, the clinical presentation of disease is usually characteristic of the hormone elaborated by the tumor. The diagnosis is made based on clinical features and through biochemical demonstration of inappropriately elevated hormone levels. Confirmation of disease is usually followed by imaging studies, including cross-sectional imaging, endoscopic ultrasonography (EUS), scintigraphy, and perhaps more invasive testing as detailed below. Treatment is largely surgical, but multimodal therapy is often used, especially to modulate the hormonal effects.

Although rare, the possibility of a syndromic association with multiple endocrine neoplasia type I (MEN I), von Hippel-Lindau (VHL) disease, neurofibromatosis type 1 (NF-1), or tuberous sclerosis should be considered when evaluating patients with PNETs. Patients with MEN I frequently have multiple PNETs, which may or may not be functional.[2] PNETs in patients with VHL disease are usually nonfunctional.[1]

Consensus guidelines for the diagnosis and management of patients with PNETs were published by the National Comprehensive Cancer Network (NCCN) in 2008,[3] the European Neuroendocrine Tumor Society (ENETS) in 2004,[1] and a MEN I international consensus workshop in 2001.[2] The following recommendations are based largely on these consensus guidelines.

General Principles

PRESENTATION

Neuroendocrine tumors can be found incidentally or discovered when searching for the cause of an endocrinopathy or the source of compressive or obstructive symptoms. Likewise, neuroendocrine tumors may be clinically silent or symptomatic as a result of the production of hormones or local mass effect. When an asymptomatic PNET is found incidentally, the main clinical concern is whether it represents benign or malignant disease.

LOCALIZATION PROCEDURES

Imaging studies should be done not only to localize the primary tumor but also to evaluate for metastatic disease. Because malignancy is not accurately predicted from histopathology alone, it is important to evaluate the tumor for clinical, pathologic, or radiographic evidence of invasion into adjacent organs; involvement of regional lymph nodes; or distant metastases. Multiple imaging modalities have been used, including computed tomography (CT), magnetic resonance imaging (MRI), somatostatin receptor scintigraphy (SRS), transabdominal ultrasonography, EUS, visceral angiography, selective arterial injection with hepatic venous sampling, and transhepatic portal venous sampling. Positron emission tomography (PET) with 5-hydroxytryptophan or levodopa has also been used.

Initial imaging of the pancreas is usually done with a high-resolution cross-sectional modality such as helical CT or MRI. EUS is usually the next imaging study employed and can give precise information about the relationship between the tumor and the pancreatic duct. EUS can also be used to guide fine-needle aspiration biopsy of these tumors, if necessary. EUS has a sensitivity of 82 to 93% and a specificity of 95% for the localization of PNETs.[4,5] SRS is highly sensitive for most PNETs other than insulinoma but yields very little anatomic detail. Selective visceral arteriography takes advantage of the hypervascular nature of neuroendocrine tumors but has low sensitivity for small tumors. Selective intra-arterial injection with calcium and measurement of the target hormone from the hepatic veins can be done at the same time as the pancreatic arteriography and has been demonstrated to have higher sensitivity. Portal venous sampling for the target hormone is more invasive and involves transhepatic puncture of the portal vein and selective catheterization of the veins draining the pancreas. These tests can only regionalize the location of the tumor to the head and uncinate region, the neck and body region, and the tail of the pancreas.

PREOPERATIVE MANAGEMENT CONSIDERATIONS

Initial management of a patient with a hormone-producing PNET should focus on pharmacologic control of the effects of hormonal hypersecretion and, in some cases, hydration with correction of electrolyte abnormalities. If an operation is planned that may involve a splenectomy, patients should receive a trivalent vaccine to pneumococcus, *Haemophilus influenzae* b, and meningococcus group C.[3]

Patients should be evaluated for the possibility of an underlying genetic syndrome. MEN I is the most common genetic syndrome associated with PNETs, and additional testing should be done to evaluate for MEN I–associated conditions such as other functional or nonfunctional PNETs, hyperparathyroidism, and pituitary tumors.[3] Genetic counseling should be offered to patients and their first-degree relatives.

SURGICAL RESECTION

Sporadic PNETs with low malignant potential, such as insulinoma, can be treated with enucleation when anatomically feasible based on tumor location and unifocality. Formal pancreatic resection is appropriate for other neuroendocrine tumors because of their higher malignant potential and should also be performed for insulinoma when the anatomic location precludes safe enucleation. Specific surgical techniques for each functional tumor are discussed in greater detail below. It is important to keep in mind that for the malignant islet cell tumors, patients who undergo R0 resection have a better survival than those who undergo R1 or R2 resection.[6]

Surgical management of MEN I–associated PNETs is controversial because these patients usually have multiple synchronous functional and nonfunctional pancreatic or duodenal tumors and are rarely cured by surgery. The ENETS advocates surgery for all PNETs greater than 2 cm to avoid the development of malignancy and recommends distal pancreatectomy combined with intraoperative ultrasonography, bidigital palpation, and enucleation of tumors from the head of the pancreas to remove the bulk of PNETs that are present.[1] Duodenotomy with enucleation of tumors from the duodenal submucosa should be done in patients with concomitant elevated secretin-stimulated gastrin levels.[1,2] Pancreaticoduodenectomy should be considered if the main tumor burden is located in the head of the pancreas.[2] Patients should also undergo dissection of lymph nodes along the celiac trunk and hepatic ligament.[2] The NCCN advocates a similar approach but does not give a specific tumor size criterion.[3] The MEN I international consensus workshop, in contrast, advocates surgery for insulinomas and for most other PNETs except gastrinomas.[2] The management of MEN I–associated gastrinoma is detailed in the gastrinoma section of this chapter.

MANAGEMENT OF METASTATIC DISEASE

PNETs metastasize most commonly to the regional lymph nodes and liver. Regional lymph node metastases should be resected en bloc with the primary tumor. Because neuroendocrine tumors are slow-growing, a reduction in tumor volume can lead to significant palliation of symptoms. Therefore, consideration should be given to a debulking procedure even if the metastases are not completely resectable. Liver metastases can be treated with resection or ablation (radiofrequency ablation or cryotherapy) depending on tumor burden and resectability.[1,3] Cholecystectomy is frequently done prophylactically to eliminate potential gallstone-related complications associated with possible future octreotide therapy. Liver transplantation has been offered as a palliative measure to young patients whose primary tumor is resected but who have developed metastatic disease limited to the liver and debilitating symptoms of hormonal excess.[7] Other treatment options for unresectable liver metastases include hepatic arterial embolization, chemoembolization, and systemic therapy.[1,3]

Systemic treatments for unresectable metastatic disease include octreotide, interferon, chemotherapy, and other investigational agents. Long-acting somatostatin analogues such as octreotide are tumorostatic as a result of an unknown mechanism and take advantage of the expression or overexpression of somatostatin receptors that most neuroendocrine tumors have been shown to have.[8] Octreotide is recommended for patients with positive SRS who have symptomatic or progressing distant metastases or those with large tumor burdens.[3] Interferon therapy has also been shown to stabilize tumor growth, but the mechanism is not well understood.[9]

Other treatment options for patients with distant metastases include systemic chemotherapy[3] or entry onto a clinical trial. The chemotherapeutic agents most commonly used are streptozocin, 5-fluorouracil, and doxorubicin for well- to moderately differentiated tumors and cisplatin or carboplatin and etoposide for poorly differentiated tumors.[1] Although not approved outside of clinical trials, the effects of peptide receptor radionuclide therapy (PRRT) have been reported in several studies.[10–15] PRRT involves administering radiolabeled somatostatin analogues in an attempt to deliver a cytotoxic level of radiation to the neuroendocrine tumor. Although responses have been noted, there have been no reports of improved survival in controlled trials.[9] Inhibitors of vascular endothelial growth factor (VEGF) and multiple tyrosine kinases are currently under investigation. External beam radiotherapy has been effective in the palliation of bony and brain metastases.[16]

STAGING

The World Health Organization (WHO) classifies neuroendocrine tumors as either well-differentiated neuroendocrine tumors, well-differentiated carcinomas, or poorly differentiated carcinomas based on features such as site, size, angioinvasion, proliferative index, and evidence of metastasis.[17] The ENETS has proposed a tumor-node-metastasis (TNM) classification for PNETs.[18] Both of these systems have been found to be reliable and are highly correlated.[19]

LONG-TERM FOLLOW-UP

The malignant potential of an islet cell tumor is not always predictable based on the histopathology. Disease progression can occur late, and surveillance must be lifelong.

For patients with sporadic islet cell tumors, initial surveillance should consist of a history; physical examination; CT of the chest, abdomen, and pelvis; and measurement of tumor markers 3 to 6 months after tumor resection. For patients with gastrinoma, biochemical testing should consist of both a fasting serum gastrin level and a secretin stimulation test.[20] Surveillance by history, physical examination, and measurement of tumor markers should then be done every 6 to 12 months for the first 3 years[3] and annually thereafter. Imaging studies should be ordered as clinically indicated (if the patient is symptomatic or tumor markers are elevated).

Patients with MEN I should have the above tests and serum calcium checked 3 months postresection, followed by clinical and biochemical surveillance every 6 months for the first 3 years and annually thereafter.[3] Imaging studies should be ordered as clinically indicated.

Nonfunctional Pancreatic Neuroendocrine Tumors

EPIDEMIOLOGY

Nonfunctional PNETs represent 30 to 40% of islet cell tumors and have an annual incidence of 1 to 2 per million.[21] Most cases are sporadic, whereas about 20% are associated with MEN I.[21] About 20% of patients with MEN I will develop a nonfunctional PNET by the age of 40.[2] The majority (60 to 90%) of nonfunctional PNETs are malignant.[9]

BIOLOGY OF DISEASE

Nonfunctional PNETs may not secrete anything or may secrete peptides or hormones that fail to result in an overt clinical syndrome. These tumors may elaborate PP, neurotensin, chromogranin A, neuron-specific enolase, or human chorionic gonadotropin subunits.

Most nonfunctional PNETs are malignant, with metastases present in greater than 50% of patients at the time of diagnosis, most commonly to the liver.

CLINICAL FEATURES

Because nonfunctional PNETs do not have a syndrome of hormonal excess, most of these tumors are identified either incidentally or late in the disease course, when they become symptomatic because of a mass effect or metastatic disease. Symptoms and signs can include weight loss, obstructive jaundice, a palpable abdominal mass, hepatomegaly, and bowel obstruction [*see Table 1*].

LOCATION OF PRIMARY TUMOR(S)

Most nonfunctional PNETs are usually larger than 2 cm in size, with the tumors typically measuring between 6.5 and 10 cm in size.[22] Most reside in the head of the pancreas.[22]

LOCALIZATION PROCEDURES

Initial identification is usually by a cross-sectional imaging study such as CT or MRI because of the signs or symptoms with which nonfunctional PNETs present. SRS should be done as clinically warranted, that is, to evaluate for additional tumors in a patient with MEN I or to evaluate for the extent of metastatic disease.[3]

SURGICAL MANAGEMENT OF PRIMARY TUMOR

Patients with locoregional disease should undergo resection. Because of the high malignant potential of nonfunctional PNETs, enucleation should not be done. The NCCN recommends consideration of laparoscopy for staging, followed by resection of the primary tumor with peripancreatic lymph node dissection.[3] Because nonfunctional PNETs are most commonly located in the head of the pancreas, surgical resection usually consists of pancreaticoduodenectomy.

The management of patients with MEN I–associated nonfunctional PNETs is similar to that of patients with sporadic disease but also must take into account the presence of other functional and nonfunctional PNETs that may be present. Consensus guidelines for the treatment of nonfunctional and other PNETs in this context are detailed in the General Principles section of this chapter.[1–3]

PROGNOSIS/OUTCOMES

Despite the predominantly malignant nature of nonfunctional PNETs, they are slow-growing tumors, and long-term survival is possible. Mean survival of patients with nonmetastatic and metastatic nonfunctional PNETs has been reported as 7 years and 5 years, respectively.[23]

Insulinoma

EPIDEMIOLOGY

Insulinomas are rare PNETs with an annual incidence of 1 to 2 per million.[21] They are the most common functional PNETs. Most cases of insulinoma are sporadic, whereas about 5% are associated with MEN I.[21] About 10% of patients with MEN I will develop an insulinoma by the age of 40.[2] Insulinomas are malignant in 5 to 15% of cases.[9,21]

Table 1 Summary of Features of Nonfunctional and Functional Pancreatic Neuroendocrine Tumors

PNET	% Malignant	% Associated with MEN I	Symptoms and Signs	Location	Initial Imaging Studies
Nonfunctional	60–90	20	None or symptoms of local invasion or metastasis	Most in head of pancreas	CT or MRI
Insulinoma	5–15	5	Whipple triad*	Equal distribution throughout pancreas	CT or MRI, EUS
Gastrinoma	60–90	25–40	Triad of abdominal pain, diarrhea, and weight loss in the presence of PUD	Two thirds in gastrinoma triangle	CT or MRI, SRS
Glucagonoma	50–80	10	4 "D's"†	Most in tail of pancreas	CT or MRI, SRS
Somatostatinoma	70–80	45	Cholelithiasis, mild diabetes, malabsorption	Half in duodenum; most pancreatic somatostatinomas in head	CT or MRI, SRS
VIPoma	40–70	5	WDHA syndrome	Three quarters in pancreas, most in body or tail	CT or MRI, SRS

CT = computed tomography; EUS = endoscopic ultrasonography; MEN I = multiple endocrine neoplasia type I; MRI = magnetic resonance imaging; PNET = pancreatic neuroendocrine tumor; PUD = peptic ulcer disease; SRS = somatostatin receptor scintigraphy; WDHA = watery diarrhea, hypokalemia, achlorhydria.
*Whipple triad: fasting hypoglycemia, accompanied by neuroglycopenic symptoms, which are resolved by the administration of glucose.
†4 "D's": dermatitis (necrolytic migratory erythema), diabetes, depression, deep vein thrombosis.

BIOLOGY OF DISEASE

Insulinomas arise from the insulin-secreting beta islet cells located in the pancreas. Beta cells produce proinsulin, which consists of two peptide chains connected by an otherwise inactive C-peptide bridge. Proinsulin is cleaved prior to release from the cell, resulting ultimately in the secretion of equivalent amounts of C-peptide and active insulin. Insulin facilitates the entry of glucose into muscle, adipose, and other tissues and stimulates glycogen and fatty acid synthesis in the liver and glycerol synthesis in adipocytes. Given that insulinomas elaborate excessive amounts of active insulin and C-peptide, both substances are found to be elevated during hypoglycemic episodes. The finding of hyperinsulinism without elevated C-peptide levels indicates an exogenous (factitious) insulin source.

Sporadic insulinomas are usually unifocal and benign. In contrast, insulinomas associated with MEN I are commonly found in the context of other functional and nonfunctional PNETs, making it difficult to diagnose whether one or multiple insulinomas are present.[2]

CLINICAL FEATURES

Insulinoma has been described as causing a classic "Whipple triad" of symptoms (fasting hypoglycemia accompanied by neuroglycopenic symptoms that are then resolved with the administration of glucose) [*see Table 1*].[24] The fasting hypoglycemia is attributed to the release of excessive and unregulated amounts of insulin. The symptoms from profoundly low serum glucose levels may include confusion, combativeness, seizures, visual changes, and loss of consciousness and are collectively described as neuroglycopenic symptoms.

DIAGNOSTIC TESTS AND CONFIRMATION OF DIAGNOSIS

The diagnosis of insulinoma is suspected when the clinical features of hypoglycemia are present. In addition to insulinoma, however, other conditions can cause hypoglycemia, including medications (insulin, oral hypoglycemic, others), alcohol, sepsis or other critical illness, cortisol deficiency, functional beta cell disorders (nesidioblastosis), and insulin autoimmune hypoglycemia (antibodies to insulin or the insulin receptor).[25]

The gold standard diagnostic test for the diagnosis of insulinoma is the 72-hour observed fast,[3,25] although the vast majority of patients will become hypoglycemic within the first 48 hours.[26] Blood is usually drawn for glucose, insulin, C-peptide, proinsulin, and β-hydroxybutyrate every 6 hours or when neuroglycopenic signs and/or symptoms occur. Insulin antibodies should also be measured. A urine sample should be collected and analyzed for oral hypoglycemic agents. Glucose is administered, and the symptomatic response is recorded. Multiple measurements are prudent for confirmation of the biochemical diagnosis. Criteria for the diagnosis of endogenous hyperinsulinism published in a Clinical Practice Guideline from the Endocrine Society in 2009[25] are as follows:

- Signs and/or symptoms of hypoglycemia with a plasma glucose concentration of less than 55 mg/dL (3.0 mmol/L)
- Insulin 3.0 uU/mL (18 pmol/L) or greater
- C-peptide 0.6 ng/mL (0.2 nmol/L) or greater
- Proinsulin 5.0 pmol/L or greater
- β-Hydroxybutyrate 2.7 mmol/L or less
- An increase in plasma glucose of at least 25 mg/dL (1.4 mmol/L) after the intravenous administration of 1.0 mg glucagon

Patients who meet the above criteria who have a negative screening for oral hypoglycemic agents and no circulating insulin antibodies should undergo localization procedures for an insulinoma.

LOCATION OF PRIMARY TUMOR(S)

Approximately 80% of sporadic insulinomas are unifocal. The vast majority of insulinomas are smaller than 2 cm in size. The tumor distribution is equal in frequency between the pancreatic head, body, and tail.

LOCALIZATION PROCEDURES

Initial testing should consist of a cross-sectional imaging study such as triphasic CT or MRI in conjunction with transgastric EUS.[3] Figure 1 shows a 1.2 cm insulinoma in the uncinate process of a 47-year-old man that was seen on EUS but not seen on CT. SRS, although useful for most PNETs, has a lower sensitivity for insulinoma. It does have a role, however, in the workup of a patient with MEN I–associated insulinoma because of the other functional and nonfunctional PNETs that are invariably present.

If the above tests are unable to localize the insulinoma, more invasive testing such as visceral arteriography, selective intra-arterial calcium injection with hepatic venous sampling for insulin, or selective portal venous sampling for insulin can be done. Visceral arteriography has a sensitivity of only 35% as a result of the small nature of insulinomas.[27] Selective intra-arterial calcium injection with hepatic venous sampling for insulin can be used to regionalize the insulinoma to either

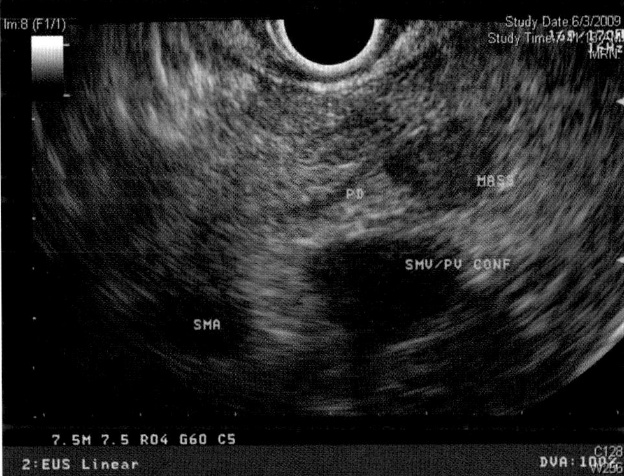

Figure 1 **Endoscopic sonogram demonstrating a 1.2 cm insulinoma in the uncinate process of a 47-year-old man who had negative or equivocal cross-sectional imaging. Because of the location of the tumor, the patient required pancreaticoduodenectomy. PD = pancreatic duct; SMA = superior mesenteric artery; SMV/PV CONF = superior mesenteric vein–portal vein confluence.**

the head, uncinate, or body or tail of the pancreas with a sensitivity of 88%,[27] and portal venous sampling for insulin has a sensitivity of 77 to 81%[28,29] for the regionalization of insulinomas. In addition, intraoperative ultrasonography is very helpful for identifying the tumor location and characterizing the relationship between the tumor and the pancreatic duct and adjacent vessels.

PREOPERATIVE MANAGEMENT CONSIDERATIONS

Initial management of a patient with insulinoma should focus on stabilizing blood glucose levels. This is usually done with diet alone, but in some cases, octreotide and/or diazoxide (an antihypertensive agent that also inhibits insulin release and promotes hyperglycemia by enhancing glycogenolysis) may be necessary.[3,30]

SURGICAL MANAGEMENT

The surgical approach is dictated by the tumor location within the pancreas, clinical suspicion of malignancy, multifocality, and whether it arises sporadically or in association with MEN I.[3] Because sporadic insulinomas are typically solitary and benign, they can usually be treated safely by enucleation, either as an open procedure or laparoscopically. If enucleation results in a disruption of the pancreatic duct, then pancreatic resection may be required. Insulinomas in the tail of the pancreas can be treated with distal pancreatectomy, with splenic preservation, if possible. If the tumor arises in the head or uncinate process and cannot be safely enucleated, pancreaticoduodenectomy may be required. If a malignant insulinoma is suspected, formal resection with peripancreatic lymphadenectomy is required.

The treatment of MEN I–associated insulinomas must take into account the presence of other functional and nonfunctional PNETs that may be present. Consensus guidelines for the treatment of insulinomas and other PNETs in this context are detailed in the General Principles section of this chapter.[1–3]

PROGNOSIS

Benign unifocal insulinoma has an excellent prognosis following surgical resection. Transient mild hyperglycemia is usually observed for several days. There should be no recurrence of neuroglycopenic symptoms in the postoperative setting. If hypoglycemia recurs, there should be suspicion of tumor recurrence at the enucleation site, metastasis from malignant insulinoma, or MEN I. Benign insulinomas that are completely resected should have a 100% long-term recurrence-free survival.[31,32] When elevated preoperatively, neuroendocrine tumor markers such as chromogranin A and neuron-specific enolase may be useful as postoperative markers for tumor recurrence.[9]

Gastrinoma

EPIDEMIOLOGY

Gastrinomas (causing Zollinger-Ellison syndrome) are a rare cause of gastric acid hypersecretion and peptic ulcer disease with an annual incidence of 1 to 2 per million.[21,33] This disease is most commonly diagnosed in the fifth decade of life, with 90% of cases diagnosed between the ages of 20 and 60.[33] Most cases of gastrinomas are sporadic, whereas 25 to 40% are associated with MEN I.[2,21] About 40% of patients with MEN I will develop Zollinger-Ellison syndrome by the age of 40.[2] Gastrinomas have also been reported in association with neurofibromatosis (von Recklinghausen disease).[34] Gastrinomas are malignant in 60 to 90% of cases.[3,35,36]

BIOLOGY OF DISEASE

Gastrinomas predominantly arise from gastrin-secreting G cells located in the duodenal mucosa and pancreas, although most G cells are located in the gastric antrum. Gastrin stimulates acid secretion from parietal cells in the stomach and aids in gastric motility. Hypergastrinemia causes gastric acid hypersecretion, parietal cell hyperplasia, and pancreatic hypersecretion as a result of an increased acid load in the duodenum and the direct trophic effects of gastrin on pancreatic acinar cells.

Gastrinomas are different in sporadic versus MEN I–associated cases; sporadic gastrinomas are monoclonal in etiology, whereas those associated with MEN I have been found to be polyclonal.[33] This may be attributable to a progression from islet cell hyperplasia to microadenosis to neoplasia in MEN I, a hypothesis favored by many authorities.[37] Sporadic and MEN I–associated gastrinomas also differ in the extent of disease at the initial presentation. Sporadic gastrinomas have lymph node metastases in 30 to 50% of cases and have liver metastases at initial presentation in 7 to 22% of cases, whereas MEN I–associated gastrinomas more commonly have lymph node metastases (61 to 80% of cases) but have liver metastases at initial presentation in only 5 to 14% of cases.[35,38,39] Liver metastases correlate with the size of the primary tumor and occur more often with pancreatic versus duodenal primary tumors.[38,40]

CLINICAL FEATURES

Gastrinoma has been described as causing a classic triad of symptoms (abdominal pain, diarrhea, and weight loss) in the presence of peptic ulcer disease [*see Table 1*].[33] There is a mean delay of 5 to 8 years between the onset of symptoms and diagnosis.[39,41] Abdominal pain and diarrhea (as a result of small bowel mucosal injury and increased gastric and pancreatic secretions that may overwhelm the absorptive capacity of the intestine) are the most common symptoms, occurring in 70% of patients, with other symptoms occurring less frequently (heartburn 44%, nausea 33%, vomiting 25%, weight loss 17%).[41] The location or extent of disease does not seem to affect symptom severity.[41] In the current era, complications from peptic ulcer disease such as bleeding or perforation are uncommon. Upper endoscopy usually demonstrates prominent gastric rugal folds, which are attributable to the trophic effects of gastrin on the gastric mucosa.[35]

DIAGNOSTIC TESTS AND CONFIRMATION OF DIAGNOSIS

The diagnosis of gastrinoma is suspected when the clinical features of gastric acid hypersecretion are accompanied by an elevated fasting serum gastrin level. In addition to gastrinoma, however, other conditions can cause hypergastrinemia [*see Table 2*]. The use of proton pump inhibitors or H_2 receptor blockers is associated with elevated gastrin secondary to high gastric pH. To establish a diagnosis of gastrinoma,

Table 2 Differential Diagnosis of Hypergastrinemia
Gastrinoma
Antral G cell hyperplasia
Conditions associated with achlorhydria or reduced gastric acid secretion Pernicious anemia Chronic atrophic gastritis Proton pump inhibitor therapy
Conditions associated with gastric acid hypersecretion *Helicobacter pylori* infection Gastric outlet obstruction
Truncal vagotomy
Retained gastric antrum (in patients who have undergone prior antrectomy)
Short bowel syndrome
Renal failure

however, the hypergastrinemia must accompany low gastric pH or high basal acid output.

A fasting serum gastrin level of more than 1,000 pg/mL (10 times the upper limit of normal) is diagnostic of gastrinoma; however, only one third of patients have gastrin levels this high. The remaining two thirds of patients have fasting serum gastrin levels of 500 to 1,000 pg/mL, values that overlap with the more common conditions associated with hypergastrinemia [*see Table 2*].[42] Gastrinoma can be distinguished from these other conditions by virtue of its paradoxical effect on serum gastrin levels in response to a secretin infusion (secretin stimulation test)[43,44] [*see Table 3*]. Patients who have a strong clinical suspicion of gastrinoma with gastric acid hypersecretion but a negative secretin stimulation test should undergo a calcium infusion test[44] [*see Table 3*]. Criteria for the diagnosis of gastrinoma in patients with a fasting serum gastrin level of less than 1,000 pg/mL include

Table 3 Secretin and Calcium Provocative Testing for Gastrinoma
Withdraw patient from PPIs for at least 3 days, possibly up to 7 days
Withdraw patient from H_2 blocker for at least 30 hours
Overnight fast
Secretin stimulation test Administer 2 U/kg secretin IV bolus Measure serum gastrin levels at 0, 2, 5, 10, 20, 30 min An increase in serum gastrin by more than 200 pg/mL over baseline levels is diagnostic of gastrinoma[44]; new criterion using 120 pg/mL has been found to have increased sensitivity and specificity (sensitivity 94%, specificity 100%)[75]
Calcium infusion test Administer 54 mg/kg/hr of 10% calcium gluconate (5 mg/kg/hr of calcium) by continuous IV infusion for 3 hours Measure serum calcium and serum gastrin levels every 30 min for 3 hours An increase in serum gastrin level by more than 395 pg/mL over baseline levels is diagnostic of gastrinoma[44]

IV = intravenous; PPI = proton pump inhibitor.

a fasting serum gastrin level of more than 200 pg/mL with a basal acid output of greater than 15 mEq/hr (> 5 mEq/hr in a patient who has had an acid-reducing surgical procedure) and a positive secretin or calcium stimulation test.[45]

Although hypercalcemia increases gastrin secretion from gastrinomas, studies differ with respect to gastrin levels in patients with sporadic versus MEN I–associated gastrinomas. Some studies have shown that patients with MEN I–associated gastrinomas do not have higher serum gastrin levels or higher increases in serum gastrin levels with secretin than those with sporadic gastrinomas,[35,42] whereas others have shown higher fasting serum gastrin levels in patients with MEN I.[39]

LOCATION OF PRIMARY TUMOR(S)

Two thirds of gastrinomas are located in the gastrinoma triangle, a triangle bordered by the junction of the cystic and common bile ducts superiorly, the junction of the second and third portions of the duodenum inferiorly, and the junction of the neck and body of the pancreas medially.[46] Large series also report lymph node–only primary gastrinomas in 4 to 13% of patients,[39,47] although these cases may represent lymph node metastases from an occult primary tumor.[48] Other primary sites for gastrinomas have been reported in up to 11% of patients and include the liver, common bile duct, pylorus, jejunum, omentum, heart, and ovary.[39]

Sporadic and MEN I–associated gastrinomas differ with respect to the most common location of the primary tumor; sporadic gastrinomas are located in the duodenum and pancreas with almost equal frequency, whereas MEN I–associated gastrinomas are more commonly located in the duodenum (80%).[35] Furthermore, sporadic gastrinomas tend to be solitary, whereas MEN I–associated gastrinomas are usually multicentric and small (< 0.5 cm).[49,50]

LOCALIZATION STUDIES

Initial testing should consist of a cross-sectional imaging study such as triphasic CT or MRI in conjunction with SRS.[3] The sensitivity of these imaging modalities is related to tumor size. Sensitivity of CT and MRI for the detection of a primary gastrinoma varies from 22 to 90%, with increased sensitivity for the detection of liver metastases (54 to 90%).[21] SRS has a sensitivity of 53 to 72% for the detection of a primary gastrinoma and a sensitivity of 92 to 97% for the detection of liver metastases.[21,36,40]

If these tests are unable to localize the gastrinoma, more invasive testing, such as EUS, selective visceral arteriography, selective intra-arterial secretin or calcium injection with hepatic venous sampling for gastrin, or pancreatic venous sampling for gastrin, can be done. EUS has a sensitivity of 67 to 100%[21,40] for the detection of a primary gastrinoma. Similar to insulinoma, selective visceral arteriography has low sensitivity for the detection of a primary gastrinoma (13 to 28%)[36,51]; therefore, other techniques have been developed. Selective intra-arterial injection of secretin or calcium with hepatic venous sampling for gastrin has a sensitivity of 77 to 93% for the regionalization of a primary gastrinoma,[21,27] whereas pancreatic venous sampling has a similar sensitivity of 94%.[51]

PREOPERATIVE MANAGEMENT CONSIDERATIONS

Initial management of a patient with gastrinoma should focus on pharmacologic control of gastric acid hypersecretion. In the current era, this is most commonly done with proton pump inhibitors.[52] In addition to the known effect of hypercalcemia on serum gastrin levels, hypercalcemia also decreases the effectiveness of the antisecretory drugs by an unknown mechanism.[35] Thus, patients with MEN I–associated gastrinomas should undergo parathyroidectomy both for treatment of their hyperparathyroidism and to allow better pharmacologic control of gastric acid hypersecretion.[53,54]

SURGICAL MANAGEMENT OF PRIMARY TUMOR

Historically, surgery for patients with gastrinoma focused on acid-reducing procedures, including total gastrectomy. With the development of excellent pharmacologic therapy for the control of gastric acid hypersecretion, surgery for gastrinoma has shifted toward tumor localization and resection.

The surgical treatment of the primary tumor can vary depending on if the patient has sporadic versus MEN I–associated gastrinoma. Consensus guidelines recommend surgical resection of sporadic gastrinomas.[1,3] Specific recommendations by the NCCN are as follows.[3] Operative exploration is recommended even if the gastrinoma has not been localized preoperatively; however, observation is an acceptable alternative for these patients with a category 2B recommendation (based on lower level evidence, including clinical experience and nonuniform consensus, but no major disagreement).[3] Intraoperative maneuvers that should be done to localize the tumor include intraoperative ultrasonography, transduodenal palpation, intraoperative upper endoscopy with transduodenal illumination, and duodenotomy with palpation.[55,56] If the tumor is found in the duodenal mucosa, it should undergo enucleation with periduodenal lymph node dissection.[3] Noninvasive tumors 5 cm or smaller that are located in the head of the pancreas should also undergo enucleation and periduodenal lymph node dissection; however, tumors larger than 5 cm or those that are invasive should undergo pancreaticoduodenectomy.[3] Tumors located in the body or tail of the pancreas should undergo enucleation or distal pancreatectomy (spleen preserving, if possible).[3]

There is no consensus as to the best approach to the treatment of MEN I–associated gastrinoma, especially in light of the additional PNETs that are frequently present.[35] Some experts advocate observation with pharmacologic control of gastric hypersecretion, some advocate routine exploration and resection, and others advocate operative exploration based on pancreatic tumor size.[2]

Proponents of observation argue that excellent control of gastric acid hypersecretion can be obtained with medical therapy, identification of the primary gastrinoma(s) may not be possible, and there is a lack of data to support the effectiveness of surgery in altering the natural history of disease in these patients. Most MEN I patients have duodenal gastrinomas, and the pancreatic tumors seen on imaging are usually not the gastrinomas.[49] Furthermore, in MEN I patients who develop liver metastases, it is unclear if these metastases are from the gastrinoma or from the other PNETs, calling into question the utility of resecting primary gastrinomas to prevent metastasis. Finally, studies have shown that very few MEN I patients (< 1 to 16%) are biochemically cured immediately postoperatively,[39,57] and other studies have shown conflicting results with respect to the impact of primary gastrinoma resection on overall survival.

Proponents of surgical resection of MEN I–associated gastrinomas argue that surgery is the only modality that can cure gastrinoma and prevent the later development of malignancy[1,57] and that surgery for curative intent is most effective when tumors are small. Liver metastases, which are the most important predictor of survival, are associated with the increasing size of the primary tumor.[40] Despite these arguments, however, there is no clear consensus as to the timing of surgery for patients with MEN I. The NCCN recommends a similar approach to MEN I–associated gastrinomas as sporadic gastrinomas with the addition of consideration of a distal pancreatectomy (category 2B recommendation) to duodenotomy and enucleation of the primary tumor(s) from the duodenum and/or head of the pancreas to remove the bulk of PNETs that are present.[3] Surgery is likewise advocated by the ENETS and is recommended before tumors become larger than 2 cm.[1] The 2001 MEN I international consensus workshop was unable to come to a consensus with respect to the primacy of surgical versus nonsurgical management in patients with MEN I–associated gastrinomas.[2]

PROGNOSIS/OUTCOMES

The prognosis of patients with gastrinoma depends on the size and location of the primary tumor, the presence of liver metastases, and sporadic versus MEN I–associated disease. The presence of liver metastases is the most important determinant of survival.[40] Other predictors of an aggressive or malignant course include short duration from onset of symptoms to diagnosis, very high gastrin levels, and large primary tumors that are pancreatic in location.[38] Interestingly, lymph node metastases do not appear to be associated with decreased survival,[38] and long-term survival is possible even with lymph node metastases at the initial presentation.

Biochemical cure rates are better for sporadic gastrinoma versus MEN I–associated gastrinoma. Without pancreaticoduodenectomy, 51 to 60% of patients with sporadic gastrinoma are disease-free immediately postoperatively and 30 to 49% are disease-free at 5 years.[39,57] This is in contrast to less than 1 to 16% of patients with MEN I–associated gastrinoma who are disease-free immediately postoperatively and less than 1 to 6% who are disease-free at 5 years.[39,57] Long-term survival is possible, however, even without biochemical cure. Eventually, about one third of patients with both sporadic and MEN I–associated gastrinoma will die of their malignancy.[2]

Glucagonoma

EPIDEMIOLOGY

Glucagonomas are rare PNETs with an annual incidence of 0.1 per million.[21] This disease is most commonly diagnosed in the fourth or fifth decade of life.[58] Most cases of glucagonomas are sporadic, whereas about 10% are associated with MEN I.[21] About 2% of patients with MEN I will develop a glucagonoma by the age of 40.[2] Glucagonomas are malignant in up to 90% of cases.[3,21]

BIOLOGY OF DISEASE

Glucagonomas arise from glucagon-secreting alpha islet cells of the pancreas. In addition to pancreatic alpha cells, glucagon is also produced by some enterochromaffin cells of the gastrointestinal tract and salivary glands. Glucagon is a catabolic hormone that maintains blood glucose levels during periods of hypoglycemia by acting predominantly on hepatocytes and adipocytes to increase gluconeogenesis and glycogenolysis. Glucagon also stimulates insulin release. Normal glucagon release is stimulated by hypoglycemia and vagal nerve stimulation and is inhibited by somatostatin.

Most glucagonomas are malignant. Metastases are present at initial presentation in 78 to 90% of patients,[59,60] most commonly to the liver but also to peripancreatic lymph nodes, bone, adrenal glands, kidney, and lung.[61]

CLINICAL FEATURES

Glucagonomas have been described as causing the 4 "D's": dermatitis, diabetes, depression, and deep vein thrombosis [*see Table 1*]. Patients often also experience hypoproteinemia, malnutrition, and weight loss because the hyperglycemia is a result of the breakdown of protein stores. Anemia is also frequently present and is related to glucagon's effect on suppression of erythropoiesis in the bone marrow.[61] There is a mean delay of 2 years between the onset of symptoms and diagnosis.[58]

Weight loss and a characteristic skin rash (necrolytic migratory erythema) are the most common presenting features, occurring in about 70% of patients, with other symptoms occurring less frequently at initial presentation (diabetes 38%, stomatitis 29%, diarrhea 29%).[61] Necrolytic migratory erythema, which is an intensely pruritic rash that usually presents on the lower abdomen, perineum, perioral area, or lower extremities, may present before any other signs or symptoms and is pathognomonic for glucagonoma. The diabetes is usually mild and eventually develops in 76 to 93% of patients.[58] Neuropsychiatric manifestations occur in about 20% of patients at some point during the course of their illness and can include depression, anxiety, dementia, and psychoses.[58] Thromboembolic events distinguish glucagonomas from other neuroendocrine tumors and occur in up to 30% of patients.[58] The hypercoagulable state is thought to be related to a factor X–like antigen that is secreted by the tumor.[62]

Glucagonomas sometimes secrete secondary hormones and are associated with Zollinger-Ellison syndrome in about 10% of cases.[60,61] Other, less common, secondary hormones secreted by glucagonomas include VIP, pancreatic polypeptide, somatostatin, and ACTH.[58]

DIAGNOSTIC TESTS AND CONFIRMING THE DIAGNOSIS

The diagnosis of glucagonoma is suspected when the fasting serum glucagon level is elevated. In addition to glucagonoma, however, other conditions can cause hyperglucagonemia [*see Table 4*] and are, in fact, more common reasons for an elevated serum glucagon level.

Most glucagonoma patients have glucose intolerance and fasting serum glucagon levels between 1,000 and 5,000 pg/mL (normal < 150 pg/mL).[61,63] Because of the association of glucagonoma with other functional neuroendocrine tumors, fasting levels of other hormones should be measured.[58] Other laboratory abnormalities seen in patients with glucagonomas include hyperglycemia, anemia, and hypoaminoacidemia. Because glucagon stimulates insulin release, patients also often have elevated basal insulin levels.

Table 4 Differential Diagnosis of Hyperglucagonemia[58]

Glucagonoma
Prolonged fasting/starvation
Diabetic ketoacidosis/hyperosmotic nonketotic state
Other endocrine causes Familial hyperglucagonemia Cushing syndrome
Liver disease associated with decreased degradation of glucagon Hepatitis Cirrhosis Hemachromatosis
Conditions associated with a malabsorptive state Pancreatic disease Celiac disease Inflammatory bowel disease
Renal failure
Danazol therapy
Trauma/burns/sepsis

LOCATION OF PRIMARY TUMOR

Most glucagonomas (50 to 75%) are located in the tail of the pancreas, with the remainder distributed throughout the gland.[58] Up to 5% of cases may occur in an extrapancreatic location such as the duodenal wall, accessory pancreatic tissue, or kidney.[64]

LOCALIZATION STUDIES

Initial testing should consist of a cross-sectional imaging study such as triphasic CT or MRI in conjunction with SRS.[3] In the majority of cases, the tumor burden is such that the location of the primary tumor can be identified by noninvasive imaging.

If noninvasive tests are unable to localize the glucagonoma, more invasive testing such as EUS, selective visceral arteriography, or pancreatic venous sampling for glucagon can be done.[63,65]

PREOPERATIVE MANAGEMENT CONSIDERATIONS

Once the biochemical diagnosis is made, the initial management of a patient with glucagonoma should focus on blocking and treating the metabolic effects of glucagon hypersecretion and preventing or treating venous thromboembolism. Octreotide and intravenous fluids should be administered.[3] Octreotide is administered subcutaneously at a dose of 50 μg two to three times daily and titrated to a maximum dose of 500 μg four times daily.[60] Nutrition should be optimized, with total parenteral nutrition, if necessary. Octreotide and total parenteral nutrition have been reported to ameliorate necrolytic migratory erythema. Zinc should be administered orally in the form of zinc sulfate.[3] Hyperglycemia should be controlled. Severe anemia may require transfusion. Because of the hypercoagulable state and predisposition to thromboembolic events, patients should be fully anticoagulated at the time of diagnosis, and an inferior vena cava filter should be considered perioperatively.[3]

SURGICAL MANAGEMENT OF PRIMARY TUMOR

Patients with locoregional disease should undergo resection. Because of the high malignant potential of glucagonoma, enucleation should not be done. The NCCN recommends consideration of laparoscopy for staging, followed by resection of the primary tumor with peripancreatic lymph node dissection.[3] Because glucagonomas are most commonly located in the tail of the pancreas, surgical resection usually consists of distal pancreatectomy with splenectomy. Cholecystectomy should be performed prophylactically to eliminate the potential gallstone-related complications associated with possible future octreotide therapy.[3] The ENETS also recommends radical surgery as the only treatment for cure of glucagonoma.[1]

The management of patients with MEN I–associated glucagonoma is similar to that of patients with sporadic disease but also must take into account the presence of other functional and nonfunctional PNETs that may be present. Consensus guidelines for the treatment of glucagonomas and other PNETs in this context are detailed in the General Principles section of this chapter.[1,3]

PROGNOSIS/OUTCOMES

Glucagonoma is a rare tumor, and there is a paucity of outcomes data. The development of liver metastases is a poor prognostic sign. MEN I patients with glucagonoma, somatostatinoma, and VIPoma were found to have an approximately 54% 10-year survival in a study from the Groupe des Tumeurs Endocrines registry.[66] Glucagonoma is relatively chemoresistant.

Somatostatinoma

EPIDEMIOLOGY

Somatostatinomas are rare neuroendocrine tumors of the pancreas or duodenum with an annual incidence of less than 0.1 per million.[21] Somatostatinomas are most commonly diagnosed in the fifth decade of life, with an equal male to female ratio.[67] Most cases of somatostatinomas are sporadic, whereas about 45% are associated with MEN I.[21] About 2% of patients with MEN I will develop somatostatinomas by the age of 40.[2] Somatostatinomas have also been reported in association with neurofibromatosis (von Recklinghausen disease),[68] and somatostatin expression has also been found in gangliocytic paragangliomas.[69] Somatostatinomas are malignant in 70 to 80% of cases.[3,21]

BIOLOGY OF DISEASE

Somatostatinomas arise from somatostatin-secreting delta islet cells located in the duodenal mucosa and pancreas. Somatostatin has a broad spectrum of inhibitory activity in the gastrointestinal tract, including inhibiting the release of gastric acid, pepsin, pancreatic exocrine secretions, and multiple hormones (insulin, glucagon, gastrin, secretin, VIP, PP, and cholecystokinin). It also inhibits gastrointestinal blood flow and motility.

Most somatostatinomas are malignant. Metastases, most commonly to regional lymph nodes and the liver, are more common in patients with sporadic or neurofibromatosis-associated somatostatinomas and uncommon in MEN I–associated somatostatinoma or gangliocytic paraganglioma.[70]

CLINICAL FEATURES

Pancreatic somatostatinoma has been described as causing a syndrome of cholelithiasis, mild diabetes, malabsorption and steatorrhea [*see Table 1*].[71] Other manifestations of the syndrome include weight loss, anemia, hypochlorhydria.[67] Patients most commonly present with abdominal pain (39%), and cholelithiasis (33%), jaundice (28%), and anemia (28%), with other symptoms occurring less commonly (gastrointestinal bleeding 22%, nausea/vomiting 6%).[70] Duodenal somatostatinomas only rarely lead to a clinically recognized syndrome.

DIAGNOSIS

The diagnosis of somatostatinoma is made on the basis of a pancreatic or duodenal mass and an elevated fasting plasma somatostatin level. There are no provocative tests for somatostatinoma.

LOCATION OF PRIMARY TUMOR

Approximately half of the cases of somatostatinoma arise in the duodenum.[21] Most pancreatic somatostatinomas are located in the head of the gland. Other locations described for primary somatostatinomas include the bile ducts and ovaries.[70] Most somatostatinomas are solitary, whereas those associated with MEN I are usually multiple, very small, and incidental findings in patients undergoing operation for gastrinoma.[70]

LOCALIZATION STUDIES

Initial testing should consist of a cross-sectional imaging study such as triphasic CT or MRI in conjunction with SRS.[1,3]

SURGICAL MANAGEMENT OF PRIMARY TUMOR

Patients with locoregional disease should undergo operation. Similar to glucagonoma, because of the high malignant potential of somatostatinoma, enucleation should not be done. The NCCN recommends consideration of laparoscopy for staging, followed by resection of the primary tumor with peripancreatic lymph node dissection.[3] Because somatostatinomas are most commonly located in the duodenum or head of the pancreas, surgical resection usually consists of pancreaticoduodenectomy. Also similar to glucagonoma, cholecystectomy should be performed prophylactically to eliminate potential gallstone-related complications.[3] The ENETS also recommends radical surgery as the only treatment for cure of somatostatinoma.[1]

The management of patients with MEN I–associated somatostatinoma is similar to that of patients with sporadic disease but also must take into account the presence of other functional and nonfunctional PNETs that may be present. Consensus guidelines for the treatment of somatostatinomas and other PNETs in this context are detailed in the General Principles section of this chapter.[1–3]

PROGNOSIS/OUTCOMES

The 5-year survival for completely resected somatostatinoma without metastasis is 100%. The 5-year survival is approximately 30 to 60% for patients with metastatic disease.[66,72]

VIPoma

EPIDEMIOLOGY

VIPomas (causing Verner-Morrison syndrome, also known as WDHA [watery diarrhea, hypokalemia, and achlorhydria] or pancreatic cholera) are rare neuroendocrine tumors with an annual incidence of 0.1 per million.[21] VIPoma is most commonly diagnosed in the fifth decade of life, with an equal male to female ratio.[73] Patients with VIP-producing neurogenic tumors (ganglioneuromas, ganglioneuroblastomas, neuroblastomas, neurofibromatosis) are usually diagnosed in the first decade of life, although some cases of VIP-producing adrenal neurogenic tumors have been diagnosed in adulthood.[73] Most cases of VIPomas are sporadic, whereas about 5% are associated with MEN I.[21] About 2% of patients with MEN I will develop VIPomas by the age of 40.[2] VIPomas are malignant in 40 to 70% of cases.[3,21]

BIOLOGY OF DISEASE

VIPomas arise from cholinergic nerves that terminate in the pancreatic islets. VIP is a neuropeptide that stimulates the secretion of fluids and electrolytes into the intestinal lumen, causing losses of sodium, chloride, water, and potassium. It also inhibits gastric acid secretion, causing hypo/achlorhydria.

Most VIPomas are malignant, with metastases most commonly to the liver. Metastatic disease occurs more often with pancreatic primary tumors.[73] Pancreatic VIPomas have lymph node metastases in 16% of cases and have liver metastases at the initial presentation in 49% of cases.[73] VIP-producing neurogenic tumors have lymph node metastases as commonly as pancreatic VIPomas but have a lower rate of liver metastases (4%).[73] There is no difference with respect to malignancy rates in sporadic versus MEN I–associated VIPomas.[73]

CLINICAL FEATURES

VIPomas present with a syndrome of profuse watery diarrhea (> 5 L of watery, tea-colored stool/day) with severe hypokalemia and hypo/achlorhydria [*see Table 1*]. The diarrhea is a secretory diarrhea that persists despite fasting and may be intermittent. Diarrhea and hypokalemia (as a result of potassium losses in the stool) are the most common presenting features, occurring in 98% and 89% of patients, respectively, with other signs and symptoms occurring less frequently (hypo/achlorhydria 43%, weight loss 33%, nausea/vomiting 16%, flushing 14%, abdominal pain 10%, anemia 10%).[73] Severe muscle weakness attributable to hypokalemia is also common.

DIAGNOSTIC TESTS

The diagnosis of VIPoma is made on the basis of an elevated fasting serum VIP level when diarrhea is present. VIP secretion may be episodic, and several measurements may be necessary to make the diagnosis. Because the severe diarrhea can cause severe electrolyte derangements, serum electrolytes should be measured.

LOCATION OF PRIMARY TUMOR(S)

Three fourths of VIPomas are located within the pancreas, with the remainder of cases consisting of VIP-producing neurogenic tumors (20%) located in the adrenal gland, retroperitoneum, or mediastinum or nonneurogenic extrapancreatic tumors (5%) located in the small intestine, lung, liver, kidney, or colon.[73] Of the intrapancreatic VIPomas, about 70% are located in the body or tail of the pancreas, with about 30% located in the head.[73] The great majority of VIPomas are solitary, with 4% of cases attributable to multiple tumors.[73]

LOCALIZATION

Initial testing should consist of a cross-sectional imaging study such as triphasic CT or MRI in conjunction with SRS.[3] If noninvasive tests are unable to localize the VIPoma, more invasive testing such as EUS or selective visceral arteriography should be done.[74]

PREOPERATIVE MANAGEMENT CONSIDERATIONS

Initial management of a patient with a VIPoma should focus on blocking and treating the metabolic effects of VIP hypersecretion. Octreotide and intravenous fluids should be administered.[3] Electrolyte imbalances (particularly potassium, magnesium, and bicarbonate) should be corrected.[3]

SURGICAL MANAGEMENT OF PRIMARY TUMOR

Patients with locoregional disease should undergo operation. Similar to glucagonoma and somatostatinoma, enucleation of a VIPoma should not be done. The NCCN recommends consideration of laparoscopy for staging, followed by resection of the primary tumor with peripancreatic lymph node dissection.[3] Depending on the location of the primary tumor, this may consist of distal pancreatectomy with splenectomy or pancreaticoduodenectomy. Also similar to glucagonoma and somatostatinoma, cholecystectomy should be performed prophylactically to eliminate potential gallstone-related complications associated with possible future octreotide therapy.[3] The ENETS also recommends radical surgery as the only treatment for cure of VIPoma.[1]

The management of patients with MEN I–associated VIPoma is similar to that of patients with sporadic disease but also must take into account the presence of other functional and nonfunctional PNETs that may be present. Consensus guidelines for the treatment of somatostatinomas and other PNETs in this context are detailed in the General Principles section of this chapter.[1–3]

PROGNOSIS/OUTCOMES

Five-year survival rates after resection of pancreatic VIPomas are approximately 68%, with better survival for patients without metastatic disease at the initial presentation (94% versus 60%).[73]

Conclusions

PNETs comprise approximately 1 to 2% of all pancreatic tumors. The possibility of a syndromic association with MEN I, VHL disease, NF-1, or tuberous sclerosis should be considered when evaluating patients with PNETs. PNETs are frequently nonfunctional, but a number of bioactive peptides, including insulin, gastrin, glucagon, VIP, somatostatin, parathyroid hormone–related peptide, growth hormone–releasing factor, and others, may be elaborated. For functional tumors, the clinical presentation of disease is usually characteristic of the hormone elaborated by the tumor. The diagnosis is made based on clinical features and biochemical demonstration of inappropriately elevated hormone levels. Confirmation of disease is followed by localizing studies, which may include cross-sectional imaging, EUS, scintigraphy, arteriography, and selective venous sampling. Complete surgical resection offers the only possibility of cure. Treatment, therefore, centers mainly on surgical resection, but multimodal therapy, including biotherapy with somatostatin analogues, is often used in advanced disease, especially for the modulation of debilitating hormonal excess. Adjuvant therapies via PPRT and novel inhibitors of VEGF and tyrosine kinases are being explored.

Financial Disclosures: None Reported

References

1. Plockinger U, Rindi G, Arnold R, et al. Guidelines for the diagnosis and treatment of neuroendocrine gastrointestinal tumours. A consensus statement on behalf of the European Neuroendocrine Tumour Society (ENETS). Neuroendocrinology 2004;80:394–424.
2. Brandi ML, Gagel RF, Angeli A, et al. Guidelines for diagnosis and therapy of MEN type 1 and type 2. J Clin Endocrinol Metab 2001;86:5658–71.
3. Clark OH, Ajani J, Benson AB, et al. Neuroendocrine tumors. NCCN clinical practice guidelines in oncology. Available at: http://www.nccn.org/professionals/physician_gls/PDF/neuroendocrine.pdf (accessed April 10, 2009).
4. Rosch T, Lightdale CJ, Botet JF, et al. Localization of pancreatic endocrine tumors by endoscopic ultrasonography. N Engl J Med 1992;326:1721–6.
5. Anderson MA, Carpenter S, Thompson NW, et al. Endoscopic ultrasound is highly accurate and directs management in patients with neuroendocrine tumors of the pancreas. Am J Gastroenterol 2000;95:2271–7.
6. Casadei R, Ricci C, Pezzilli R, et al. Value of both WHO and TNM classification systems for patients with pancreatic endocrine tumors: results of a single-center series. World J Surg 2009;33:2458–63.
7. Olausson M, Friman S, Herlenius G, et al. Orthotopic liver or multivisceral transplantation as treatment of metastatic neuroendocrine tumors. Liver Transpl 2007;13:327–33.
8. Papotti M, Bongiovanni M, Volante M, et al. Expression of somatostatin receptor types 1-5 in 81 cases of gastrointestinal and pancreatic endocrine tumors. A correlative immunohistochemical and reverse-transcriptase polymerase chain reaction analysis. Virchows Arch 2002;440:461–75.
9. Metz DC, Jensen RT. Gastrointestinal neuroendocrine tumors: pancreatic endocrine tumors. Gastroenterology 2008;135:1469–92.
10. Forrer F, Valkema R, Kwekkeboom DJ, et al. Neuroendocrine tumors. Peptide receptor radionuclide therapy. Best Pract Res Clin Endocrinol Metab 2007;21:111–29.
11. Van Essen M, Krenning EP, De Jong M, et al. Peptide receptor radionuclide therapy with radiolabelled somatostatin analogues in patients with somatostatin receptor positive tumours. Acta Oncol 2007;46:723–34.
12. Kwekkeboom DJ, Teunissen JJ, Kam BL, et al. Treatment of patients who have endocrine gastroenteropancreatic tumors with radiolabeled somatostatin analogues. Hematol Oncol Clin North Am 2007;21:561–73; x.
13. Kwekkeboom DJ, Mueller-Brand J, Paganelli G, et al. Overview of results of peptide receptor radionuclide therapy with 3 radiolabeled somatostatin analogs. J Nucl Med 2005;46 Suppl 1:62S–6S.
14. Kaltsas GA, Papadogias D, Makras P, Grossman AB. Treatment of advanced neuroendocrine tumours with radiolabelled somatostatin analogues. Endocr Relat Cancer 2005;12:683–99.
15. Valkema R, Pauwels S, Kvols LK, et al. Survival and response after peptide receptor radionuclide therapy with [90Y-DOTA0,Tyr3]octreotide in patients with advanced gastroenteropancreatic neuroendocrine tumors. Semin Nucl Med 2006;36:147–56.
16. Strosberg J, Hoffe S, Gardner N, et al. Effective treatment of locally advanced endocrine tumors of the pancreas with chemoradiotherapy. Neuroendocrinology 2007;85:216–20.
17. Solcia E, Kloppel G, Sobin LH. Histological typing of endocrine tumours. In: Sobin LH, editor. World Health Organization international histological classification of tumours. 2nd ed. Berlin: Springer; 2000.
18. Rindi G, Kloppel G, Alhman H, et al. TNM staging of foregut (neuro)endocrine tumors: a consensus proposal including a grading system. Virchows Arch 2006;449:395–401.
19. Casadei R, Ricci C, Pezzilli R, et al. Value of both WHO and TNM classification systems for patients with pancreatic endocrine tumors: results of a single-center series. World J Surg 2009;33:2458–63.
20. Fishbeyn VA, Norton JA, Benya RV, et al. Assessment and prediction of long-term cure in patients with the Zollinger-Ellison syndrome: the best approach. Ann Intern Med 1993;119:199–206.
21. Ramage JK, Davies AH, Ardill J, et al. Guidelines for the management of gastroenteropancreatic neuroendocrine (including carcinoid) tumours. Gut 2005;54 Suppl 4:iv1–16.
22. Azimuddin K, Chamberlain RS. The surgical management of pancreatic neuroendocrine tumors. Surg Clin North Am 2001;81:511–25.
23. Jordan PH Jr. A personal experience with pancreatic and duodenal neuroendocrine tumors. J Am Coll Surg 1999;189:470–82.
24. Whipple A. The surgical therapy of hyperinsulinism. J Int Chir 1938;3:237–76.
25. Cryer PE, Axelrod L, Grossman AB, et al. Evaluation and management of adult hypoglycemic disorders: an Endocrine Society Clinical Practice Guideline. J Clin Endocrinol Metab 2009;94:709–28.
26. Hirshberg B, Livi A, Bartlett DL, et al. Forty-eight-hour fast: the diagnostic test for insulinoma. J Clin Endocrinol Metab 2000;85:3222–6.
27. Doppman JL, Jensen RT. Localization of gastroenteropancreatic tumours by angiography. Ital J Gastroenterol Hepatol 1999;31 Suppl 2:S163–6.
28. Doherty GM, Doppman JL, Shawker TH, et al. Results of a prospective strategy to diagnose, localize, and resect insulinomas. Surgery 1991;110:989–96; discussion 996–7.
29. Vinik AI, Delbridge L, Moattari R, et al. Transhepatic portal vein catheterization for localization of insulinomas: a ten-year experience. Surgery 1991;109:1–11; discussion 111.
30. Goode PN, Farndon JR, Anderson J, et al. Diazoxide in the management of patients with insulinoma. World J Surg 1986;10:586–92.
31. Nikfarjam M, Warshaw AL, Axelrod L, et al. Improved contemporary surgical management of insulinomas: a 25-year experience at the Massachusetts General Hospital. Ann Surg 2008;247:165–72.
32. Grant CS. Insulinoma. Best Pract Res Clin Gastroenterol 2005;19:783–98.
33. Ellison EC, Johnson JA. The Zollinger-Ellison syndrome: a comprehensive review of historical, scientific, and clinical considerations. Curr Probl Surg 2009;46:13–106.
34. Chagnon JP, Barge J, Henin D, Blanc D. [Recklinghausen's disease with digestive localizations associated with gastric acid hypersecretion suggesting Zollinger-Ellison syndrome]. Gastroenterol Clin Biol 1985;9:65–9.
35. Jensen RT. Management of the Zollinger-Ellison syndrome in patients with multiple endocrine neoplasia type 1. J Intern Med 1998;243:477–88.
36. Gibril F, Reynolds JC, Doppman JL, et al. Somatostatin receptor scintigraphy: its sensitivity compared with that of other imaging methods in detecting primary and metastatic gastrinomas. A prospective study. Ann Intern Med 1996;125:26–34.
37. Pritchard DM. Pathogenesis of gastrinomas associated with multiple endocrine neoplasia type 1. Gut 2007;56:606–7.
38. Weber HC, Venzon DJ, Lin JT, et al. Determinants of metastatic rate and survival in patients with Zollinger-Ellison syndrome: a prospective long-term study. Gastroenterology 1995;108:1637–49.
39. Norton JA, Fraker DL, Alexander HR, et al. Surgery to cure the Zollinger-Ellison syndrome. N Engl J Med 1999;341:635–44.
40. Kisker O, Bastian D, Bartsch D, et al. Localization, malignant potential, and surgical management of gastrinomas. World J Surg 1998;22:651–7; discussion 657–8.

41. Roy PK, Venzon DJ, Shojamanesh H, et al. Zollinger-Ellison syndrome. Clinical presentation in 261 patients. Medicine (Baltimore) 2000;79:379–411.
42. Berna MJ, Hoffmann KM, Serrano J, et al. Serum gastrin in Zollinger-Ellison syndrome: I. Prospective study of fasting serum gastrin in 309 patients from the National Institutes of Health and comparison with 2229 cases from the literature. Medicine (Baltimore) 2006;85: 295–330.
43. Isenberg JI, Walsh JH, Passaro E Jr, et al. Unusual effect of secretin on serum gastrin, serum calcium, and gastric acid secretion in a patient with suspected Zollinger-Ellison syndrome. Gastroenterology 1972;62:626–31.
44. Frucht H, Howard JM, Slaff JI, et al. Secretin and calcium provocative tests in the Zollinger-Ellison syndrome. A prospective study. Ann Intern Med 1989;111:713–22.
45. Roy PK, Venzon DJ, Feigenbaum KM, et al. Gastric secretion in Zollinger-Ellison syndrome. Correlation with clinical expression, tumor extent and role in diagnosis—a prospective NIH study of 235 patients and a review of 984 cases in the literature. Medicine (Baltimore) 2001;80:189–222.
46. Stabile BE, Morrow DJ, Passaro E Jr. The gastrinoma triangle: operative implications. Am J Surg 1984;147:25–31.
47. Ellison EC. Forty-year appraisal of gastrinoma. Back to the future. Ann Surg 1995; 222:511–21; discussion 521–4.
48. Anlauf M, Enosawa T, Henopp T, et al. Primary lymph node gastrinoma or occult duodenal microgastrinoma with lymph node metastases in a MEN1 patient: the need for a systematic search for the primary tumor. Am J Surg Pathol 2008;32:1101–5.
49. Donow C, Pipeleers-Marichal M, Schroder S, et al. Surgical pathology of gastrinoma. Site, size, multicentricity, association with multiple endocrine neoplasia type 1, and malignancy. Cancer 1991;68:1329–34.
50. Pipeleers-Marichal M, Somers G, Willems G, et al. Gastrinomas in the duodenums of patients with multiple endocrine neoplasia type 1 and the Zollinger-Ellison syndrome. N Engl J Med 1990;322:723–7.
51. Roche A, Raisonnier A, Gillon-Savouret MC. Pancreatic venous sampling and arteriography in localizing insulinomas and gastrinomas: procedure and results in 55 cases. Radiology 1982;145:621–7.
52. Metz DC, Strader DB, Orbuch M, et al. Use of omeprazole in Zollinger-Ellison syndrome: a prospective nine-year study of efficacy and safety. Aliment Pharmacol Ther 1993;7: 597–610.
53. McCarthy DM, Peikin SR, Lopatin RN, et al. Hyperparathyroidism—a reversible cause of cimetidine-resistant gastric hypersecretion. Br Med J 1979;1:1765–6.
54. Norton JA, Cornelius MJ, Doppman JL, et al. Effect of parathyroidectomy in patients with hyperparathyroidism, Zollinger-Ellison syndrome, and multiple endocrine neoplasia type I: a prospective study. Surgery 1987;102: 958–66.
55. Thompson NW, Vinik AI, Eckhauser FE. Microgastrinomas of the duodenum. A cause of failed operations for the Zollinger-Ellison syndrome. Ann Surg 1989;209:396–404.
56. Norton JA, Alexander HR, Fraker DL, et al. Does the use of routine duodenotomy (DUODX) affect rate of cure, development of liver metastases, or survival in patients with Zollinger-Ellison syndrome? Ann Surg 2004; 239:617–25; discussion 626.
57. Wiedenmann B, Jensen RT, Mignon M, et al. Preoperative diagnosis and surgical management of neuroendocrine gastroenteropancreatic tumors: general recommendations by a consensus workshop. World J Surg 1998;22:309–18.
58. Chastain MA. The glucagonoma syndrome: a review of its features and discussion of new perspectives. Am J Med Sci 2001;321: 306–20.
59. Kindmark H, Sundin A, Granberg D, et al. Endocrine pancreatic tumors with glucagon hypersecretion: a retrospective study of 23 cases during 20 years. Med Oncol 2007;24: 330–7.
60. Frankton S, Bloom SR. Gastrointestinal endocrine tumours. Glucagonomas. Baillieres Clin Gastroenterol 1996;10:697–705.
61. Wermers RA, Fatourechi V, Wynne AG, et al. The glucagonoma syndrome. Clinical and pathologic features in 21 patients. Medicine (Baltimore) 1996;75:53–63.
62. Bordi C, Yu JY, Girolami A, Betterle C. Immunohistochemical localization of factor X-like antigen in pancreatic islets and their tumours. Virchows Arch A Pathol Anat Histopathol 1990;416:397–402.
63. Prinz RA, Dorsch TR, Lawrence AM. Clinical aspects of glucagon-producing islet cell tumors. Am J Gastroenterol 1981;76: 125–31.
64. Weil C. Gastroenteropancreatic endocrine tumors. Klin Wochenschr 1985;63:433–59.
65. Ingemansson S, Holst J, Larsson LI, Lunderquist A. Localization of glucagonomas by catheterization of the pancreatic veins and with glucagon assay. Surg Gynecol Obstet 1977;145:509–16.
66. Levy-Bohbot N, Merle C, Goudet P, et al. Prevalence, characteristics and prognosis of MEN 1-associated glucagonomas, VIPomas, and somatostatinomas: study from the GTE (Groupe des Tumeurs Endocrines) registry. Gastroenterol Clin Biol 2004;28:1075–81.
67. Krejs GJ, Orci L, Conlon JM, et al. Somatostatinoma syndrome. Biochemical, morphologic and clinical features. N Engl J Med 1979;301:285–92.
68. Burke AP, Sobin LH, Shekitka KM, et al. Somatostatin-producing duodenal carcinoids in patients with von Recklinghausen's neurofibromatosis. A predilection for black patients. Cancer 1990;65:1591–5.
69. Hamid QA, Bishop AE, Rode J, et al. Duodenal gangliocytic paragangliomas: a study of 10 cases with immunocytochemical neuroendocrine markers. Hum Pathol 1986;17: 1151–7.
70. Garbrecht N, Anlauf M, Schmitt A, et al. Somatostatin-producing neuroendocrine tumors of the duodenum and pancreas: incidence, types, biological behavior, association with inherited syndromes, and functional activity. Endocr Relat Cancer 2008;15: 229–41.
71. Ganda OP, Weir GC, Soeldner JS, et al. "Somatostatinoma": a somatostatin-containing tumor of the endocrine pancreas. N Engl J Med 1977;296:963–7.
72. Tanaka S, Yamasaki S, Matsushita H, et al. Duodenal somatostatinoma: a case report and review of 31 cases with special reference to the relationship between tumor size and metastasis. Pathol Int 2000;50:146–52.
73. Soga J, Yakuwa Y. Vipoma/diarrheogenic syndrome: a statistical evaluation of 241 reported cases. J Exp Clin Cancer Res 1998;17:389–400.
74. Nikou GC, Toubanakis C, Nikolaou P, et al. VIPomas: an update in diagnosis and management in a series of 11 patients. Hepatogastroenterology 2005;52:1259–65.
75. Berna MJ, Hoffmann KM, Long SH, et al. Serum gastrin in Zollinger-Ellison syndrome: II. Prospective study of gastrin provocative testing in 293 patients from the National Institutes of Health and comparison with 537 cases from the literature. evaluation of diagnostic criteria, proposal of new criteria, and correlations with clinical and tumoral features. Medicine (Baltimore) 2006;85: 331–64.

1 STROKE AND TRANSIENT ISCHEMIC ATTACK

*Billy J. Kim, MD, and Thomas S. Maldonado, MD**

Stroke is defined as any damage to the central nervous system (CNS) caused by an interruption in blood supply. Ischemic strokes result from the failure of oxygen and nutrients to reach the affected brain. Transient ischemic attacks (TIAs) are defined as transient neurologic deficits lasting no longer than 24 hours; longer-lasting deficits are considered to be indicative of a cerebral infarction ("brain attack").

Infarction from ischemia is typically confined to a vascular territory, at whose center can be found the injured or obstructed artery supplying that parenchyma. The full extent of a stroke may not become apparent until days or weeks later, when the tenuous peripheral watershed zone, or penumbra, either survives or succumbs to cell death. Smaller infarcts, adequate collateral circulation, and prompt intervention and resuscitation are associated with improved outcome.

Hemorrhagic stroke damages the brain by cutting off connecting pathways and causing localized or generalized pressure injury. Brain edema and hydrocephalus after hemorrhagic stroke may also be deleterious. In some cases, hemorrhagic stroke can lead to ischemia as a consequence of vasospasm, as seen in the setting of subarachnoid hemorrhage (SAH). Likewise, some ischemic strokes can undergo hemorrhagic transformation.

Incidence and Risk Factors

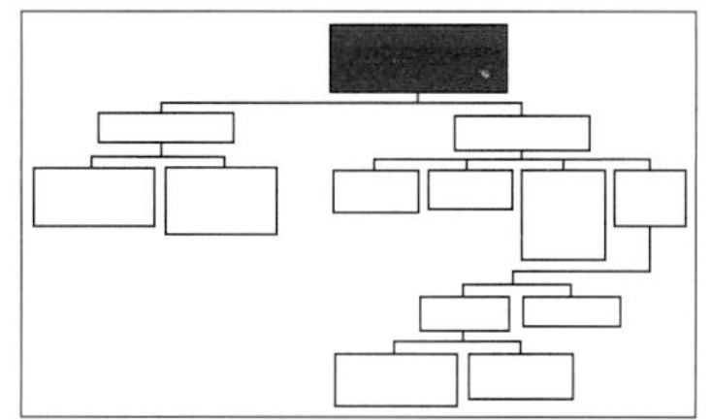

Stroke is the third leading cause of death in the United States with about 137,265 stroke-related deaths each year.[1] Annually, there are greater than 750,000 incident strokes in the United States. In addition, stroke is the leading cause of serious long-term disability in the United States and poses a substantial economic burden. For 2009, US expenditures on stroke-related medical costs and disability amount to roughly $68.9 billion. Although a sharp decline in stroke incidence and mortality was noted throughout most of the 20th century, the decline leveled off in the early 1990s, and stroke incidence and mortality are now rising for the first time since 1915.[2–4]

Numerous population studies and stroke registries have been designed to examine stroke incidence, risk factors, and natural history of stroke.[5–11] Some of the independent risk factors that have been identified—such as age (> 55 years), sex (male), race (African American and American Indian/Alaskan Native), and genetic predisposition—cannot be modified and therefore carry a fixed level of stroke risk. The Rochester (Minnesota) population study demonstrated a marked progressive incidence of cerebral infarction with advancing age, as well as a nearly 1.5 times greater risk of stroke in males.[5] The Lausanne Stroke Registry data confirmed the overall higher incidence of stroke in males, although it also demonstrated a female preponderance in very young (< 30 years) and very old (> 80 years) patients. These latter findings may be attributable to the high frequency of oral contraceptive use in young women in that study, as well as to the lower life expectancy of men, especially those with vascular risk factors.[10] Race and genetic predisposition are also considered independent risk factors, with African Americans having a threefold higher multivariate-adjusted risk ratio of a lacunar stroke than whites.[11,12] The underlying mechanism of stroke appears to vary with race as well: intracranial occlusive disease tends to occur more frequently in African Americans and Asian Americans than in whites or in males as a whole.[13,14] The importance of hereditary risk for stroke has long been recognized. In the Framingham Study, both paternal and maternal histories of stroke were associated with an increased risk of stroke.[11,15]

There are, however, certain risk factors for stroke that are clearly modifiable, including hypertension, smoking, hyperlipidemia, asymptomatic high-grade carotid stenosis, and atrial fibrillation (AF).[16–18] Other purported modifiable risk factors for stroke (e.g., obesity, diabetes, oral contraceptive use, and alcohol intake) are more controversial.[19–22] Hypertension (systolic as well as diastolic) is perhaps the most prominent modifiable risk factor for stroke and is associated with substantial risk of atherothrombotic, lacunar, or subarachnoid hemorrhage. The Systolic Hypertension in the Elderly Program (SHEP) study demonstrated that treating systolic hypertension in patients 60 years of age or older can reduce the incidence of stroke by as much as 36%.[23] Prompt diagnosis and intervention for stroke may be critical, but many authorities feel that primary prevention is the true cornerstone of therapy for this lethal disease.

Clinical Evaluation

When assessing a patient who presents with a neurologic deficit, clinicians must immediately ask themselves the following two questions: (1) what is the mechanism of the

* The authors and editors gratefully acknowledge the contributions of the previous author, Thomas S. Riles, MD, to the development and writing of this chapter.

deficit (i.e., ischemic or hemorrhagic) and (2) where is the lesion (e.g., cerebral lacunae, the territory around a large vessel, or a watershed region)? A thorough history and physical examination, in conjunction with brain imaging studies, usually suffice to guide initial management. Nonvascular conditions that can mimic stroke (e.g., hypoglycemia, migraine, postictal state, encephalopathy, trauma, and brain tumors or abscesses) must be excluded. Although these syndromes can all cause focal findings, they usually lack the abrupt onset of symptoms consistently seen with stroke.

Ischemic and hemorrhagic stroke must be differentiated early on in the course of acute stroke because a number of therapeutic interventions that are beneficial for some subtypes of stroke are potentially catastrophic for others. Approximately 71% of all strokes are ischemic and 26% are hemorrhagic; the remaining 3% are of unknown origin[24] [*see Table 1*]. Hemorrhagic strokes result from subarachnoid or intracerebral bleeding, whereas ischemic strokes result from systemic hypoperfusion, cardioembolism, or atherothrombosis. Although various different laboratory and radiographic tests are available and should be performed, the diagnosis of stroke is primarily a clinical one.

HISTORY

A patient who has suffered a stroke typically presents with a history of sudden onset of a focal brain deficit and a clinical syndrome on neurologic examination. A medical history should elicit any number of risk factors associated with either ischemic or hemorrhagic stroke. For example, hypertension is often associated with deep infarcts and hemorrhages, whereas cigarette smoking and hyperlipidemia are more commonly associated with ischemic infarcts resulting from atherosclerosis.[10] (Hypertension can, however, be associated with infarcts caused by hypertensive arteriolopathy.) The presence of AF, a recent myocardial infarction (MI) (< 6 weeks old), or a prosthetic heart valve suggests a possible cardioembolic mechanism.

The onset and course of neurologic deficit may also be telling. A steady onset is suggestive of hemorrhage, whereas symptoms that progress in stepwise fashion are more likely derived from ischemia. Likewise, accompanying signs are frequently useful in differentiating stroke mechanism subtypes. Headache, vomiting, and loss of consciousness constitute the classic picture of hemorrhagic stroke, whereas a focal deficit preceded by TIAs is more suggestive of ischemic strokes.[25] Although the clinical manifestations are generally helpful in differentiating stroke subtypes, sometimes large infarcts mimic the classic picture of hemorrhage or lobar or small deep hemorrhages resemble infarction resulting from atherosclerosis. Analysis of 1,000 consecutive patients from the Lausanne Stroke Registry who experienced their first stroke confirmed that the classic hemorrhagic picture (headaches, progressive neurologic deficits, and decreased level of consciousness) was indeed more common in patients with hemorrhage but found that only one third of patients with hemorrhagic strokes had this clinical triad.[10]

Table 1 Causes of Stroke as Recorded in the NINCDS Data Bank[24]

Cause	%
Cerebral ischemia	71
Atherosclerosis	10
Larger-artery stenosis	6
Tandem arterial lesions	4
Lacunae	19
Cardioembolism	14
Infarct of undetermined cause	27
Cerebral hemorrhage	26
Parenchymatous	13
Subarachnoid	13
Other	3

NINCDS = National Institute of Neurological and Communicative Disorders and Stroke.

PHYSICAL AND NEUROLOGIC EXAMINATION

A general physical and neurologic examination should detect vascular and cardiac abnormalities and localize the process within the CNS. Heart size and sounds, irregular rhythms or discrepant pulse examinations, and carotid bruits should all be noted. Careful examination of the extremities is essential in that peripheral vascular disease is highly correlated with the presence of atherosclerosis of the carotid and vertebral arteries.[7,26] An ophthalmologic examination should detect subhyaloid hemorrhages, as well as cholesterol emboli (Hollenhorst plaques).

Besides localizing the lesion anatomically, the neurologic examination should be able to identify a probable cause. The absence of major focal neurologic signs is often consistent with SAH; focal deficits localized to the superficial cortex are often attributable to thromboembolism or ischemia. A number of well-described lacunar syndromes also exist; these typically suggest small-vessel disease.

Investigative Studies

IMAGING

Imaging is a mandatory and integral part of evaluation for acute stroke and should be performed expeditiously. Computed tomography (CT) is the initial test of choice; it is readily available in most hospitals and is well tolerated by critically ill patients.[27] CT can promptly identify nonvascular causative conditions (e.g., masses) and can readily diagnose intracerebral hemorrhage (ICH) [*see Figure 1*]. Diagnosis of SAH without intravenous (IV) contrast can be more difficult, especially if bleeding is minor or occurred more than 1 day before; the accuracy of CT in detecting SAH decreases after 24 hours.[28] SAH should appear as an increased density in the cerebrospinal fluid (CSF). If SAH is clinically suspected, lumbar puncture may be necessary for definitive diagnosis.

In cases of acute ischemic stroke, diagnosis of infarction by means of CT can be more difficult. IV contrast CT is of limited value in this setting. Signs of infarction can be absent or subtle in the first few hours after the stroke. A lesion may appear as a slight hypodensity within the infarcted zone or as a loss of definition between gray and white matter.[29] Newer

Algorithm for the Assessment and Management of Stroke and TIA

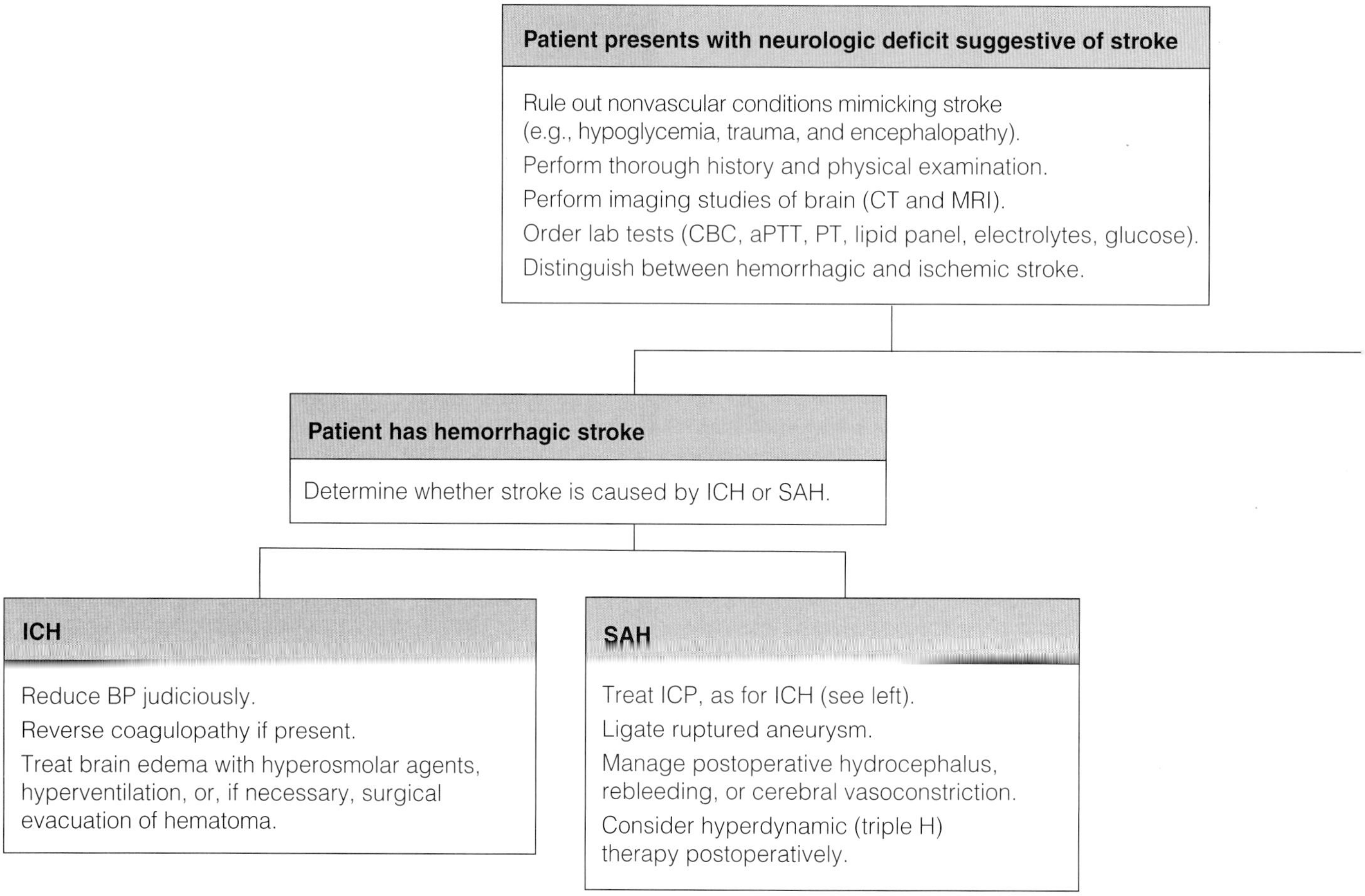

Patient presents with neurologic deficit suggestive of stroke

Rule out nonvascular conditions mimicking stroke (e.g., hypoglycemia, trauma, and encephalopathy).
Perform thorough history and physical examination.
Perform imaging studies of brain (CT and MRI).
Order lab tests (CBC, aPTT, PT, lipid panel, electrolytes, glucose).
Distinguish between hemorrhagic and ischemic stroke.

Patient has hemorrhagic stroke

Determine whether stroke is caused by ICH or SAH.

ICH

Reduce BP judiciously.
Reverse coagulopathy if present.
Treat brain edema with hyperosmolar agents, hyperventilation, or, if necessary, surgical evacuation of hematoma.

SAH

Treat ICP, as for ICH (see left).
Ligate ruptured aneurysm.
Manage postoperative hydrocephalus, rebleeding, or cerebral vasoconstriction.
Consider hyperdynamic (triple H) therapy postoperatively.

ICH = intracerebral hemorrhage; SAH = subarachnoid hemorrhage; BP = blood pressure; ICP = intracranial pressure; TIAs = transient ischemic attacks; CT = computed tomography; MRI = magnetic resonance imaging; CBC = complete blood count; aPTT = activated partial thromboplastin time; PT = prothrombin time; ECG = electrocardiogram; US = ultrasound; MRA = magnetic resonance angiography.

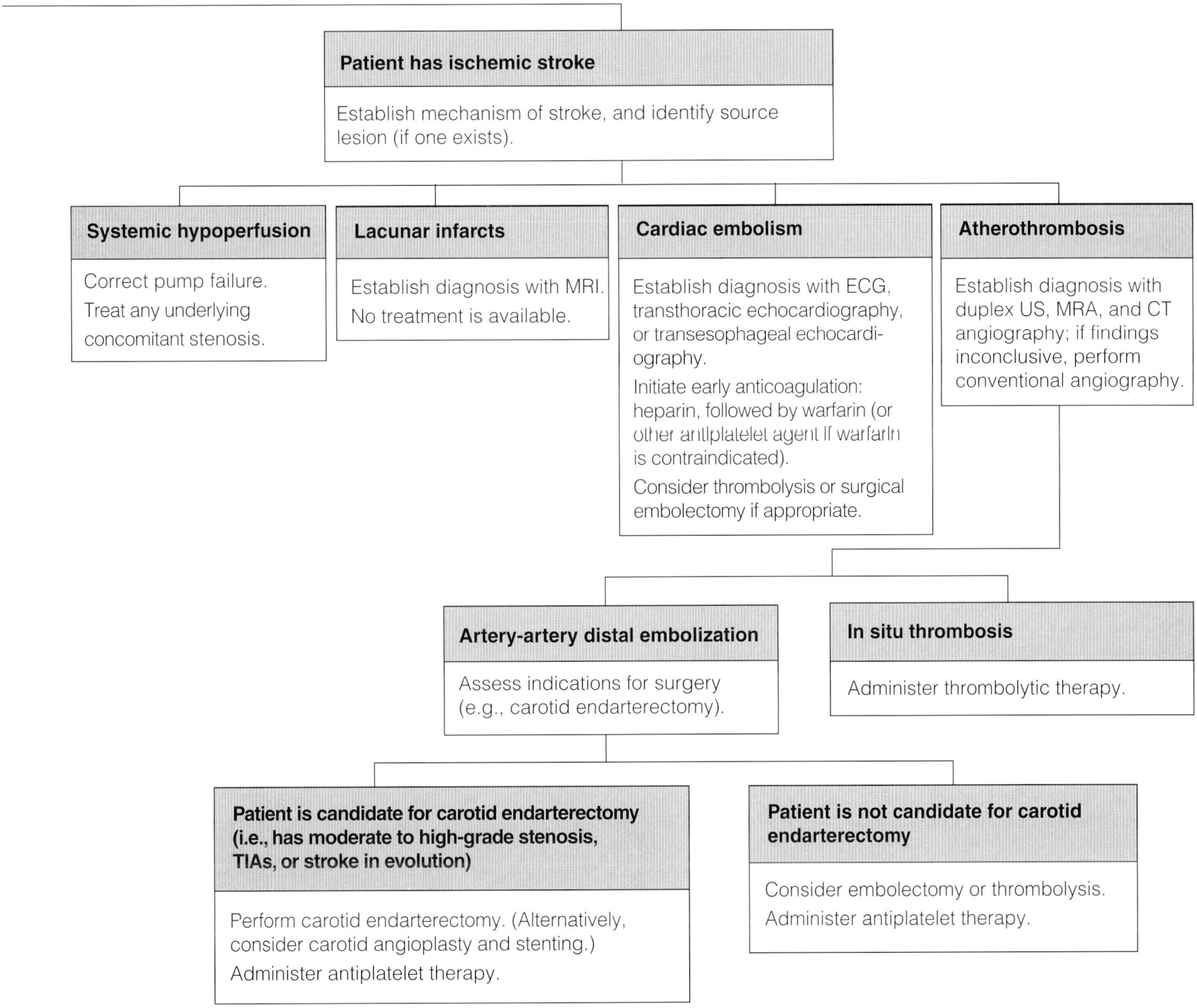

Patient has ischemic stroke

Establish mechanism of stroke, and identify source lesion (if one exists).

Systemic hypoperfusion

Correct pump failure.
Treat any underlying concomitant stenosis.

Lacunar infarcts

Establish diagnosis with MRI.
No treatment is available.

Cardiac embolism

Establish diagnosis with ECG, transthoracic echocardiography, or transesophageal echocardiography.
Initiate early anticoagulation: heparin, followed by warfarin (or other antiplatelet agent if warfarin is contraindicated).
Consider thrombolysis or surgical embolectomy if appropriate.

Atherothrombosis

Establish diagnosis with duplex US, MRA, and CT angiography; if findings inconclusive, perform conventional angiography.

Artery-artery distal embolization

Assess indications for surgery (e.g., carotid endarterectomy).

In situ thrombosis

Administer thrombolytic therapy.

Patient is candidate for carotid endarterectomy (i.e., has moderate to high-grade stenosis, TIAs, or stroke in evolution)

Perform carotid endarterectomy. (Alternatively, consider carotid angioplasty and stenting.)
Administer antiplatelet therapy.

Patient is not candidate for carotid endarterectomy

Consider embolectomy or thrombolysis.
Administer antiplatelet therapy.

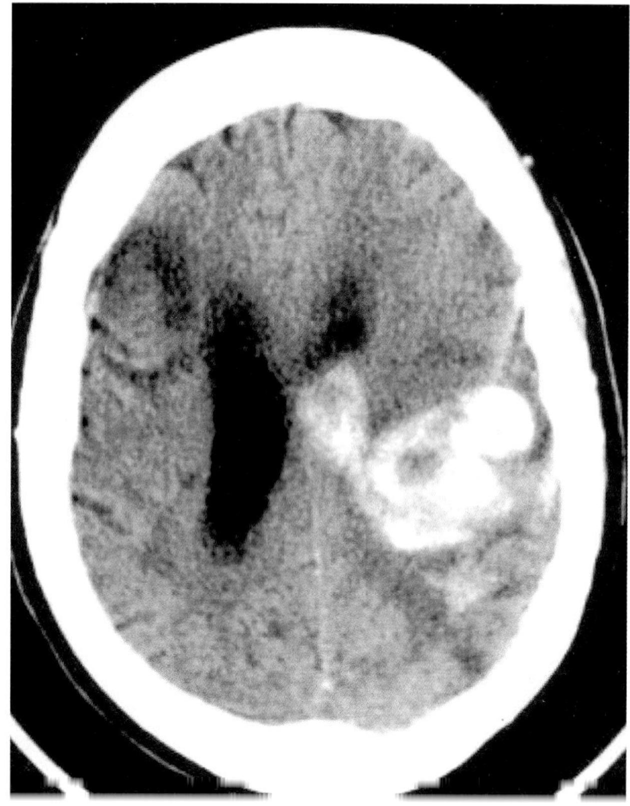

Figure 1 **Shown is a computed tomograpy image of an acute hemorrhagic infarct, with intracerebral bleeding apparent.**

CT scanners may be better at delineating these nuances.[30,31] In the days following an ischemic stroke, an infarct may first appear round or oval and then as a hypodense, dark, or wedge-shaped lesion on CT.

Magnetic resonance imaging (MRI) is more expensive and time-consuming than CT and is less well tolerated by critically ill patients. Nonetheless, MRI is more sensitive than CT in detecting early ischemic changes after a stroke. The speed of MRI acquisition and reconstruction has decreased markedly, the quality of the images has improved, and the diversity of the pulsing sequences has increased significantly. It can be used to distinguish an old stroke from a new one and to assess the size and location of a lesion, especially when the lesion is adjacent to bony structures [*see Figure 2*].[32] The size of the infarct as determined by MRI may be of great importance for prognosis. Although lesion size may not correlate with the severity of the clinical presentation, larger infarcts in the same vascular territory are associated with more severe deficits than smaller infarcts in a similar anatomic location area.

MRI is especially useful for diagnosing lacunar infarcts. In a review of 227 patients with lacunar infarcts, 44% were demonstrated by CT and 78% by MRI.[33] Infarction appears as dark, hypodense areas on T_1-weighted sequences and as bright areas on T_2-weighted sequences. Edema usually develops around the infarct within the first few days and is readily apparent on MRI as a low-density area surrounding the lesion with mass effect. Sometimes the infarct is small but is still associated with substantial edema. Such edema may be insignificant in an older patient with an atrophied brain whose cranium is able to accommodate a mass effect but may be life-threatening in a younger patient with little intracranial room to spare.

The high sensitivity of MRI in detecting infarction has been demonstrated in studies evaluating patients experiencing TIAs. When patients without signs or symptoms of infarction underwent brain imaging after a TIA, 27% were found to have evidence of so-called silent infarcts on CT and 73% on MRI.[34]

Diagnosis of ICH can be a more delicate task with MRI than with CT. Careful scrutiny by an experienced observer using different acquisition techniques is required. The appearance of a cerebral hematoma on T_1- and T_2-weighted sequences varies as the lesion matures and edema resolves. Acute hematomas are black on T_1-weighted images, and chronic hematomas are white on T_1- and T_2-weighted images.

Normal neuroimaging findings are not uncommon in patients presenting with neurologic deficits suggestive of acute stroke. A patient with a neurologic deficit and a negative CT scan should undergo further cerebral imaging with MRI. The absence of ischemic infarction and hemorrhage on both CT and MRI may suggest transient ischemia or persistent ischemia without infarction. In such cases, one may have to rely on signs and symptoms to localize the ischemic lesion responsible for the stroke. Alternatively, electroencephalography (EEG), positron emission tomography (PET), single-photon emission computed tomography (SPECT), or xenon-enhanced computed tomography (XeCT) may be employed to help localize ischemic foci.[35,36]

LABORATORY TESTS

Blood should be sent to the laboratory as part of the initial assessment of a patient with an acute stroke. Measurement of serum electrolyte and glucose levels is essential to rule out nonvascular conditions mimicking stroke (e.g., hypoglycemia and dehydration). A complete blood count (CBC), an activated partial thromboplastin time (aPTT), a prothrombin time (PT), and a lipid panel are likewise essential components of the initial assessment. Severe anemia has the potential to exacerbate or precipitate cerebral ischemia in stroke; although this is an uncommon occurrence, it should be considered and, if present, corrected.[37] Additional laboratory blood tests (e.g., cardiac injury panel to rule out MI or an erythrocyte sedimentation rate to assess the possibility of vasculitis) may be helpful.

Screening should be performed for hematologic disorders that result in hypercoagulable states, including homocystinuria,[38] antiphospholipid antibody syndrome, protein C and S deficiency, antithrombin deficiency, and activated protein C resistance from factor V Leiden mutation.[39,40] Hemoglobinopathies (e.g., sickle cell disease and thalassemia) can also lead to altered blood flow, hypercoagulability, and stroke.[41] Finally, hyperviscosity syndromes (e.g., polycythemia vera, thrombocytosis, myeloproliferative disorders) should be included in the differential diagnosis. If a hyperviscosity syndrome is recognized in the setting of acute stroke, hemodilution therapy may be warranted. Experimental and clinical trials have shown hemodilution to increase blood flow in the ischemic brain; however, other studies have failed to show improvement in neurologic status.[42,43] Hemodilution remains indicated in stroke patients who have a high hematocrit or are

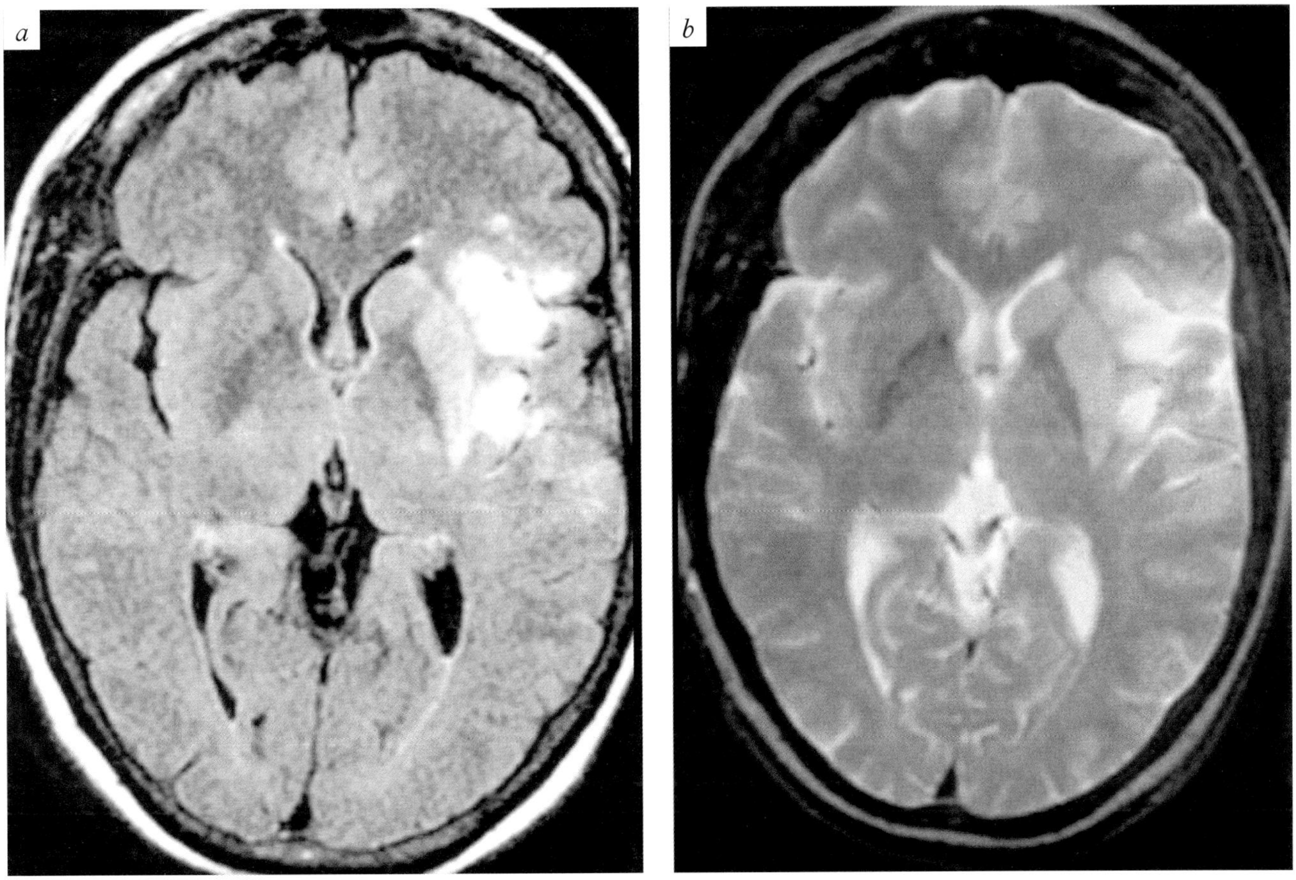

Figure 2 **Shown are (*a*) a fluid-attenuated inversion-recovery (FLAIR) magnetic resonance image (MRI) and (*b*) a T_2-weighted MRI of an acute ischemic infarct in the left middle cerebral artery distribution.**

in a hyperviscosity state; however, close monitoring is required in patients with heart disease or cerebral edema.

Recognition and Management of Specific Stroke Subtypes

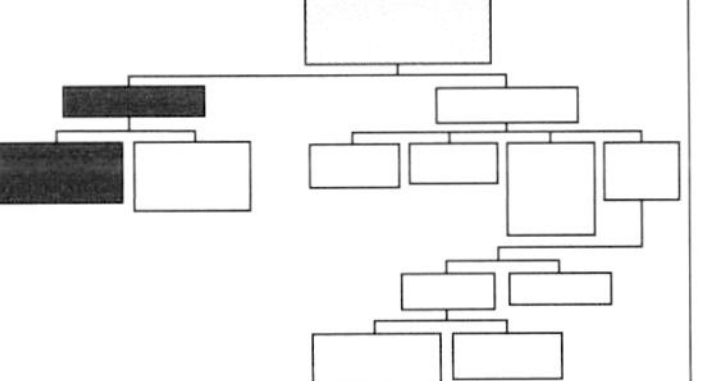

HEMORRHAGIC STROKE

Hemorrhagic stroke can result from ICH or SAH. The consequences of cerebral bleeding can progress rapidly from neurologic deficit to coma to death in a significant number of patients.

Intracerebral Hemorrhage

ICH accounts for approximately 10 to 15% of all strokes in the United States and Europe.[24,44,45] Potential causative mechanisms include hypertension, trauma, arteriovenous malformations, cerebral amyloid angiopathy, brain tumors, blood dyscrasias, and medications (e.g., anticoagulants and thrombolytics). Of these, hypertensive arteriopathy is most commonly responsible for nontraumatic ICH.[24,46,47] Hypertensive brain hemorrhages are usually deep and are typically located in the lateral ganglionic region, subcortex, thalamus, caudate nucleus, pons, or cerebellum. As early as the 1870s, Charcot and Bouchard correctly postulated that such events were the result of microaneurysmal disease of arteries and arterioles penetrating deep in the brain of hypertensive patients.[48,49] These discrete hemorrhages go on to compress neighboring capillary networks, causing them to burst and bringing about a rapid enlargement of the intracerebral hematoma. Indeed, such enlargement is not uncommon: one prospective study found that 38% of patients with ICH had a hematoma that was enlarged at 3 hours in comparison with its size on baseline CT after the initial bleed event.[50] Most hematoma enlargement occurs within 3 hours, although enlargement can occur up to 12 hours after onset.[51] Early large edema volume relative to hematoma volume makes the greatest determination to outcomes.[52] Edema that is initially small can increase in volume in the first 24 hours after hemorrhage.[53]

Patients presenting with sizable ICH often rely on a marked compensatory elevation of blood pressure to maintain a pressure gradient in the setting of acute increases in intracranial pressure (ICP). It is vital to resist the impulse to lower blood pressure aggressively in these patients: a rapid drop in blood pressure may induce brain ischemia. Short-acting antihypertensives should be administered only when the systolic blood pressure is persistently higher than 180 to 200 mm Hg or when there is evidence of active bleeding or enlarging hematoma. Other medical treatment of hemorrhagic stroke from ICH includes reversal of coagulopathies with transfusions of fresh frozen plasma and platelets when appropriate.

Mortality from ICH has plummeted from 90% before the 1970s to less than 50% in the first decade of the 21st century.[2,24,54,55] This precipitous decline probably reflects a decreased prevalence of hypertension, as well as aggressive medical management (e.g., antihypertensive medication) and specialist care in intensive care neurology units.[56,57] Death from ICH most commonly occurs from mass effects resulting from hematomas, edematous tissue surrounding hematomas, and obstructive hydrocephalus with subsequent herniation.[54,58] Monitoring of ICP might identify the risk of neurologic deterioration in patients with impaired consciousness.[59,60] Aggressive care to maintain cerebral perfusion pressure of 50 to 70 mm Hg might improve outcomes.[60] Airway support, blood pressure control, ICP treatment, and anticoagulation reversal are the early steps in management of ICH patients. One of the initial steps in the management of ICH is dealing with brain edema. Corticosteroids, although indicated for reducing cerebral edema in patients with tumors or abscesses, are contraindicated in patients with ICH because they are not beneficial and may, in fact, be injurious, predisposing patients to infection and worsening diabetes.[61] Hyperosmolar agents (e.g., mannitol or glycerol solutions) may be useful for reducing cerebral edema rapidly, yet two randomized trials showed no benefit on regional cerebral blood flow, neurologic improvement, mortality, and functional outcomes from regular use of IV mannitol boluses.[62–64] Only short-term use of mannitol in patients with ICH and special circumstances (e.g., transtentorial herniation or acute neurologic deterioration with high ICP or mass effect) should be considered. Hyperventilation may also reduce ICP through diffuse vasoconstriction in the brain. Likewise, any physiologic perturbation that might increase cerebral blood volume (e.g., hypercarbia, hypoxia, or vasodilation) or reduce cerebral perfusion (e.g., hypotension) should be avoided. The European Stroke Initiative (EUSI) guidelines recommend monitoring ICP for patients who need mechanical ventilation and recommend treatment in patients who have neurologic deterioration or elevated ICPs.[65] Selective use of mannitol, hypertonic saline, and short-term hyperventilation to maintain cerebral perfusion pressure greater than 70 mm Hg is also recommended.[65] Surgical evacuation may prevent expansion, decrease mass effects, block the release of neuropathic products from hematomas, and prevent initiation of pathologic processes. The American Heart Association (AHA)/American Stroke Association Stroke Council and EUSI guidelines do not recommend routine evacuation of supratentorial hemorrhage by standard craniotomy within 96 hours of ictus.[65,66] Both guidelines recommend surgery for patients with good neurologic status deteriorating clinically and presenting with lobar hemorrhage within 1 cm of the surface. However, very early craniotomy might be associated with an increased risk of recurrent bleeding.[67]

Subarachnoid Hemorrhage

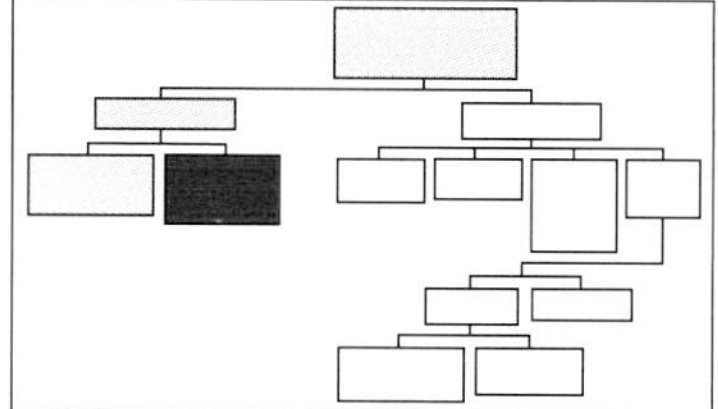

Rupture of saccular or berry aneurysms with subsequent SAH carries significant morbidity and mortality, depending largely on the patient's age, the extent of the hemorrhage, and the presence and severity of rebleeding, cerebral vasospasm, and surgical complications.[68] SAH accounts for approximately 5% of all strokes, yet outcomes for patients are poor, with population-based mortality rates as high as 45% and significant morbidity among survivors.[69] The reported incidence of incidental aneurysms discovered in autopsy studies ranges from 0.8 to 18% and has not changed dramatically over the past four decades.[69–72] The incidence of SAH increases with age and tends to occur in patients aged 40 to 60 years of age and in women more often than men (12.3% versus 7.9%).[73–75] The pathogenesis of saccular aneurysms has not been fully explicated, but the risk factors are well described and include a family history of SAH,[76] hypertension, pregnancy,[77] and black race.[78]

Clinical manifestation of SAH is one of the most distinctive in medicine, by the classic presenting complaint. Awake patients will complain of "the worst headache of my life," described by approximately 80% of patients who can give a history, but warning signs are also described by approximately 20% of patients.[79] Such warning signs include a so-called sentinal headache, oculomotor symptoms, nausea and vomiting, and loss of consciousness.[79] Most intracranial aneurysms remain asymptomatic until they rupture, which can be frequently induced during physical exertion or stress. Nevertheless, SAH can occur at any time.[80] The rupture itself is accompanied by sudden severe headache, nuchal rigidity, back pain, nausea and/or vomiting, photophobia, lethargy, loss of consciousness, and seizure.[77,81] The cornerstone of SAH diagnosis is the noncontrast cranial CT scan.[82] The diagnostic sensitivity of CT scanning is not 100%; therefore, a diagnostic lumbar puncture should be performed if the initial CT scan is negative to evaluate the CSF. A normal CT scan and CSF examination exclude a warning leak in most cases and predict a more favorable prognosis in the setting of a severe and sudden headache.[83,84]

Medical management of SAH is designed to prevent rebleeding. Bedrest with head elevation to 30° alone is not enough to prevent rebleeding after SAH but is an important component of a broader treatment strategy.[85] Blood pressure should be closely monitored and controlled to balance the risk of stroke, hypertension-related rebleeding, and maintenance of cerebral perfusion pressures.[69] Broader treatment management also includes stool softeners, antiemetics, and analgesics, as well as deep vein thrombosis (DVT) prophylaxis using pneumatic compression boots. Management of ICP in SAH patients is similar to that in ICH patients (see above). Furthermore, one must be vigilant for signs of hypothalamic dysfunction manifesting as cardiac dysrhythmias or the syndrome of inappropriate antidiuretic hormone (SIADH).

Surgical or endovascular treatment of ruptured aneurysms in SAH patients includes microsurgical clipping or endovascular coiling, which prevents rebleeding. Aneurysms that are incompletely clipped or coiled have an increased risk of rehemorrhage compared with those that are completely occluded.[69] The International Cooperative Study showed no overall differences in outcome between early surgery (0 to 3 days after SAH) and delayed surgery (11 to 14 days after SAH). Early treatment did reduce the risk of rebleeding after SAH.[69,86] In addition, patients who were alert preoperatively did better with early surgery and demonstrated significantly better rates of good recovery.[86]

Three major neurologic complications affect outcome after surgery for SAH: hydrocephalus, rebleeding, and cerebral vasoconstriction. Hydrocephalus may develop acutely because of obstruction of CSF outflow. Temporary or permanent CSF diversion (e.g., ventriculostomy) can result in immediate decompression of intracerebral pressure and improvement in neurologic symptoms.[87] The risk of rebleeding peaks on postoperative day 1; it is as high as 20% in the first 2 weeks and rises to 50% within 6 months if the aneurysm is not treated.[68] Unlike rebleeding, vasospasm is the delayed narrowing of larger capacitance arteries at the base of the brain after SAH. The typical onset is 3 to 5 days after hemorrhage, maximal narrowing at 5 to 14 days, and a gradual resolution over 2 to 4 weeks.[69] Contemporary series demonstrate 15 to 20% stroke rate or death despite maximal therapy.[86,88] The development of a new focal deficit, unexplained by hydrocephalus or rebleeding, is the first objective sign of symptomatic vasospasm. The diagnosis is initially made with angiography and monitored using transcranial Doppler sonography.[89,90]

Hyperdynamic, or triple H, therapy consists of keeping patients hyperdynamic (to increase cardiac output), hypervolemic-hypertensive (to augment cerebral perfusion pressure), and hemodiluted (to improve cerebral microcirculation by decreasing viscosity). Because of the risk that the aneurysm will rerupture before operation, triple H therapy is reserved for postoperative patients.[91,92] Calcium channel blockers (e.g., nimodipine) may also reduce the incidence of symptoms secondary to vasospasm by cerebral protection, although they most likely have little effect on spasm per se.[93,94]

Ischemic Stroke

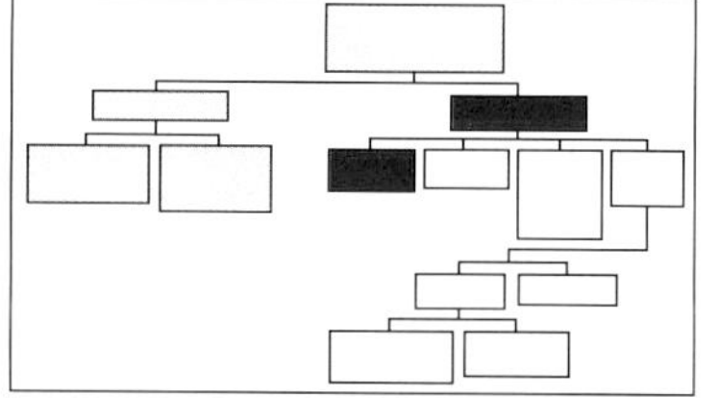

If hemorrhagic stroke is ruled out and ischemic stroke is diagnosed, the next step is to establish the mechanism of the stroke and identify the source lesion responsible (if one exists). Systemic hypoperfusion, cardiac embolism, large-artery atherosclerosis, and small-vessel disease should be systematically examined as potential causes.

SYSTEMIC HYPOPERFUSION

Only a small fraction of all ischemic strokes are attributable to systemic hypoperfusion. A quick assessment of vital signs and symptoms may provide the first clues that a patient is suffering from cerebral ischemia secondary to systemic hypoperfusion. Patients are characteristically either unconscious on arrival in the emergency department or awake but exhibiting neurologic symptoms resembling near-syncope.[95] Generally, they are pale, diaphoretic, and hypotensive. Neurologic signs and symptoms are varied and are explained by ischemia in the border zone (or watershed) between two or three adjacent arterial territories. Difficulty in reading or identifying visual stimuli (or even frank blindness) may be observed; this may be attributed to ischemia between the middle and posterior cerebral arteries. Bilateral arm weakness or cognitive difficulty may suggest ischemia between the middle and anterior cerebral arteries. Global symptoms usually arise from bilateral border-zone infarcts, which can develop in association with prolonged cardiogenic shock, dysrhythmias, or cardiac arrest.[96,97] Alternatively, symptoms may be asymmetrical if they derive from inadequate perfusion distal to a site of severe stenosis or occlusion of major feeding cerebral vessels.

Treatment should focus primarily on correcting the pump failure. Certain patients with concomitant underlying stenosis proximal to border-zone ischemic territories may benefit from treatment of the flow-limiting lesions to eliminate the hemodynamic impairment and thus may do better than patients with systemic hypoperfusion.[98]

Lacunar Infarcts

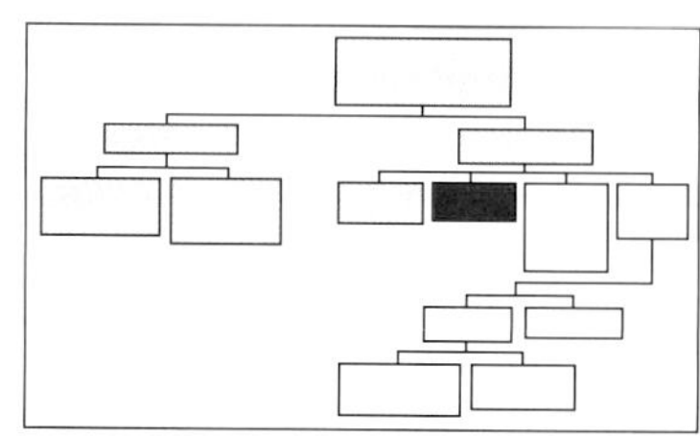

Neurologic examination of a patient believed to have experienced an acute ischemic stroke should be attentive to the possibility of lacunar infarcts, manifested by pure motor hemiparesis, pure sensory syndrome, sensorimotor syndrome, ataxic hemiparesis, and dysarthria–clumsy hand syndrome.[99,100] Lacunae are small (1 to 2 cm) subcortical lesions that result from small-vessel disease deep in the brain. They can either occur alone or in groups and may be present in as many as 23% of persons over the age of 65. Lacunar infarcts, unlike other forms of stroke, do not present with headache and are associated with hypertension and diabetes.[101] Although they are asymptomatic (silent) in as many as 89% of patients, their benignity is currently in some doubt; there is evidence to suggest that they may increase the risk for dementia and cognitive decline.[102,103] Lacunar syndromes are characteristic and highly predictive of the presence of lacunae, but they may be less reliable for excluding other mechanisms of stroke. A review of the Northern Manhattan Stroke Study experience demonstrated that as many as 25% of patients presenting with radiographically confirmed lacunar infarcts were ultimately found to have other mechanisms of ischemic stroke.[104] Thus, MRI should be used to confirm or exclude the presence of lacunar infarct and to screen for nonlacunar mechanisms of stroke.

At present, there is no optimal treatment for lacunar infarcts, but the prognosis is quite good. The survival rate is high, the recurrence rate is low (mean annual stroke rate, 4 to 7%), and the patients generally achieve a relatively good functional recovery, with as many as 74% experiencing mild or no disability at 1 year.[105–108]

Cardiac Embolism

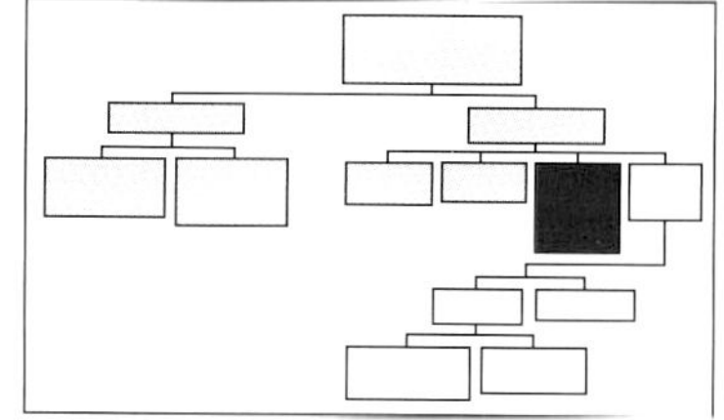

Embolism of cardiac origin accounts for approximately 20% of ischemic strokes [*see Table 1*]. Given that many infarcts of undetermined cause are

Carotid Angioplasty and Stenting

In keeping with the continuing growth of minimally invasive surgery, carotid angioplasty and stenting (CAS) has come to play an emerging role in the management of both symptomatic and asymptomatic carotid stenosis. CAS might avoid the risks associated with CEA, including cranial nerve palsy, MIs, or pulmonary embolism, thus making it especially appealing in patients at high surgical risk. Over the past 10 years, many researchers have tried to add to the wealth of case series, registries, and RCTs to discern the safety and value of CAS compared with CEA. The advent of neuroprotection techniques using distal balloon occlusion and aspiration of debris, filter wires placed distal to the lesion, or reversal-of-flow technology has allowed interventionalists to perform CAS more safely, with complication rates approximating those of CEA.[155,156] Despite the fact that embolic protection device (EPDs) provide additional cerebral protection, there is still a risk of stroke associated with CAS secondary to particle embolization from the aortic arch. In addition, the EPDs have their own inherent risks and complications, such as the inability to cross the target lesion, failure to capture emboli through the filter pores, and vasospasm or injury to the vessel wall.[157] However, EPD use has become standardized and is currently mandated by the Centers for Medicare and Medicaid Services. Even with the routine use of EPDs, the precise role of CAS in the treatment or prevention of stroke has not been completely defined. The two primary questions that remain unresolved are (1) which patients benefit most from CAS as opposed to open surgery and (2) are the immediate and long-term results of CAS as good as those of CEA? Determination of the part CAS will eventually play in the management of cerebrovascular disease awaits the results of ongoing clinical trials comparing CAS with CEA.

Selection of patients Initially, CAS was considered a procedure that would be most beneficial for high-risk patients, for example, patients who were poor surgical candidates because of substantial medical comorbidities and patients with so-called hostile anatomy (such as an extremely high or low bifurcation or a neck that had previously been irradiated or operated on). Indeed, one clear benefit of CAS over CEA is that the risk of nerve injury for patients undergoing the former procedure is 0%. A precise definition of a high-risk patient, however, has proven elusive. One study reviewed CEAs that were performed in 228 patients who, because of their increased level of risk, would not have met the NASCET inclusion criteria.[158] This study was unable to demonstrate that these supposedly high-risk patients actually had inferior outcomes with CEA. A subsequent study that included more than 13,000 CEAs found that cardiopulmonary comorbid conditions did not increase the risk of perioperative stroke, death, or cardiac events.[159] Finally, although many investigators have considered patients over the age of 80 (who were ineligible for NASCET and the Asymptomatic Carotid Atherosclerosis Study [ACAS]) to be at increased risk with open surgery, the interim results from the lead-in phase of the Carotid Revascularization Endarterectomy versus Stent Trial (CREST), which is currently in progress, indicated that the risk of 30-day stroke and death from patients undergoing CAS, surprisingly, was substantially higher (12.1%) in the 99 patients who were over the age of 80 compared with 3.2% among nonoctogenarians.[160] The reason for this increasing risk in older patients is not clear; the CREST results were not affected by adjustment for potential confounding factors such as symptomatic status, the use of EPDs, gender, the degree of carotid stenosis, or the presence of distal arterial tortuosity. Similarly, other studies indicated that CAS in octogenarians was associated with a statistically significant higher rate of adverse events at 30 days and at the 1-year follow-up, which indicates that CAS should be cautiously considered in the elderly population.[161] The etiology of increased adverse event risk for CAS in the elderly remains incompletely understood. Suggestions of adverse vascular anatomy (e.g., aortic arch calcification, common carotid and innominate artery stenosis, and the tortuosity of the common and internal carotid arteries) and lesion characteristics (e.g., severe lesion stenosis greater than 85% and plaque ulceration) that have the potential to increase the technical complexity of CAS may account for this finding.[162–164] However, it is important to note that these anatomic and lesion characteristics (e.g., abnormal arch anatomy, vessel tortuosity, long stenotic lesions greater than 15 mm, involvement of the internal carotid ostium, and plaque echolucency) are thought to be more common in the elderly population; younger patients may also have similar unfavorable risk factors.[165–168] Therefore, the presence of certain anatomic factors that preclude safe passage or proper positioning of EPDs and stents must be considered high risk at any age and thus may not be appropriate candidates for CAS.

The goal of reliably predicting which patients may be at high risk with either stenting or open surgery has impelled some investigators to develop risk stratification scales for CAS. A 2006 prospective study of 606 consecutive patients who underwent CAS identified the following independent risk factors: diabetes mellitus with inadequate glycemic control (hemoglobin A_{1c} level > 7%), advanced age (80 years), ulceration of the carotid artery stenosis, and a significant contralateral stenosis (50%). Patients with two or more of these risk factors had an 11% risk of a periprocedural complication, whereas patients with none or only one had a 2% risk.[169]

Assessment of results The results of various clinical trials comparing CAS with CEA, some already completed and some still under way, will help determine whether there is a clinical equipoise between the two procedures.[160,170–174] The results of early RCTs were mixed. The first RCT comparing endovascular and surgical treatments for carotid artery stenosis, Carotid and Vertebral Artery Transluminal Angioplasty Study (CAVATAS), was designed to compare balloon angioplasty alone without an EPD with CEA in symptomatic patients.[172] The trial randomly assigned 504 patients to the two treatment arms, and the incidence of major stroke or death at 30 days (10.0% for endovascular versus 9.9% CEA) or at 3 years (14.3% endovascular versus 14.2% CEA).[172] This study was, however, criticized for a number of reasons: lack of embolic protection; 26% stent use, which is in contrast to current standard practice; and a substantially higher stroke rate of 9.9% in the CEA arm. The Wallstent trial was the first multicenter RCT designed to compare CAS and CEA equivalence but was stopped early after interim analysis showed worse outcomes in the CAS arm with a combined risk of stroke or death at 30 days of 12.1% versus 4.5% in the CEA group.[175] Once again, EPDs were not used in this trial, which may have contributed in part to the high risk associated with CAS. Single-center RCTs were conducted by Brooks and colleagues, which had encouraging results.[176,177] The trials looked at both symptomatic and asymptomatic patients with extremely low complication rates in both arms, and the results suggested equivalence of CAS to CEA, but these results were criticized because of the small, single-institution studies carried out by a highly select experienced team. The Stenting and Angioplasty with Protection in Patients at High Risk for Endarterectomy (SAPPHIRE) trial was the first randomized trial to use mandatory distal embolic protection and was designed to demonstrate noninferiority of CAS to CEA in 334 patients with coexisting conditions that potentially increased the risk associated with endarterectomy.[171] The 30-day and 1-year outcomes (including death, stroke, and MI) found that CAS was not inferior to CEA.[171] However, the overall risk levels were disturbingly high in both arms of this trial: 12.2% for CAS patients and 20.1% for CEA patients. In addition, the differences in event rates between CAS and CEA were from the greater association of CEA with non–Q wave MI, which is notably a nontraditional surgical end point. Excluding MI, no significant difference was found between CAS (5.5%) and CEA (8.4%) patients. Also, the high event rates in both groups cast serious doubt as to the appropriateness or durability of any intervention in the high-risk, asymptomatic patient population. The Carotid Revascularization using Endarterectomy or Stenting Systems (CaRESS) trial was a multicenter prospective study that compared the two techniques in 397 patients on a nonrandom basis.[173] The results indicated that both the 30-day risk and the 1-year risk of death, stroke, or MI were essentially the same in CAS patients as in CEA patients. Two multicenter, randomized European trials, Stent-Protected Angioplasty Versus Carotid Endarterectomy (SPACE) and Endarterectomy Versus Stenting in Patients with Symptomatic Severe Carotid Stenosis (EVA-3S), sought to establish noninferiority in standard-risk, symptomatic patients.[174,178] The SPACE trial randomly assigned 1,183 patients with symptomatic carotid artery stenosis to either CAS or CEA.[174] At 30 days, the incidence of stroke or death was 6.9% in the CAS group and 6.3% in the CEA group. The difference between the CAS and CEA group was 0.51%, yet the upper 90% confidence limit of this difference between the two groups was 2.9%. This was greater than the predefined equivalence threshold of 2.5%; thus, the one-sided p value for noninferiority is .09 (9% chance of erroneously concluding that CAS is not inferior to CEA). The investigators concluded (1) that the results failed to prove the noninferiority of CAS compared with CEA and (2) that CEA should remain the preferred treatment for patients with symptomatic stenosis. The EVA-3S trial also failed to demonstrate the noninferiority of CAS in symptomatic patients.[178] The study randomized 527 patients and was subsequently ended prematurely for safety reasons after interim results revealed a significantly higher 30-day adverse event rate in the CAS group (9.6%) compared with the CEA group (3.9%). Several criticisms of this trial include the significantly high 30-day stroke rate in the CAS group, lack of initial EPD use, and lack of comparison of physicians with equal experience performing CEA and CAS. The conclusion from the EVA-3S authors essentially supported the notion that CEA remains an excellent option for symptomatic patients with low complication rates that are currently not matched or bested by CAS.

The challenge of interpreting the collective results from the RCTs is attributable to the different conclusions reached by each about the safety and efficacy of CAS versus CEA. Nevertheless, the questions of whether CAS offers an advantage or is equivalent to CEA and which subgroup of patients would most benefit from CAS still remain. While we await the conclusion of the larger RCTs, CAS should be considered for patients with an indication for carotid revascularization and high surgical risk. Currently, the Centers for Medicare and Medicaid Services reimburses the cost of CAS only for patients with symptomatic carotid artery stenosis of a severity of at least 70% who are considered high-risk patients for open surgery. In all other patient categories, the procedure is reimbursed only in the setting of one of the numerous ongoing postmarketing registries or clinical trials.

THROMBOLYTICS

Any patient who presents with an acute ischemic stroke, regardless of subtype, is potentially a candidate for thrombolytic therapy. However, ICH documented on the initial head CT is a clear, absolute contraindication to IV thrombolysis. Other considerations affecting the decision whether to administer thrombolytic agents include a history of gastrointestinal or urologic hemorrhage, recent major surgery, and rapidly improving neurologic signs, any of which may constitute a clinical contraindications to medical treatment. Vigilant monitoring of the aPTT, PT (or the international normalized ratio [INR]), platelet count, and fibrinogen level is essential throughout the course of thrombolytic treatment.

It has been suggested that maximal benefit is derived from IV thrombolytic therapy for acute ischemic stroke when it is delivered within a "golden 3-hour window" starting from the onset of symptoms. The National Institute for Neurological Disorders and Stroke (NINDS) trial (parts 1 and 2) randomly assigned 624 patients to receive either recombinant tissue plasminogen activator (rt-PA), 0.9 mg/kg IV to a maximum of 90 mg/kg, or placebo.[179] Patients with all types of ischemic stroke were eligible provided that they could be treated within 3 hours of the onset of symptoms. Outcome at 3 months was better with rt-PA than with placebo on each of the four outcome measures studied. The odds ratio for a favorable outcome in the rt-PA group was 1.7. The overall rate of symptomatic hemorrhage was 6.4% in the rt-PA group and 0.6% in the placebo group. The beneficial effects of rt-PA were similar for all stroke subtypes and persisted for up to 12 months after the stroke.[180] Patients treated with rt-PA were at least 30% more likely to have minimal or no disability at 12 months than patients treated with placebo were. Mortality at 1 year was comparable in the two groups.

Other randomized, double-blind, placebo-controlled trials of rt-PA for treatment of acute ischemic stroke have examined the effect of thrombolytic therapy given within the first 6 hours after the onset of symptoms. The European Cooperative Acute Stroke Study (ECASS) found no significant differences in functional outcome measures at 90 days between placebo and rt-PA in an intention-to-treat analysis.[181] Similarly, the Alteplase ThromboLysis for Acute Noninterventional Therapy in Ischemic Stroke (ATLANTIS) trial reported no benefit in patients treated with rt-PA within 3 to 5 hours of onset of symptoms.[182,183] However, patients treated within the golden 3-hour window were more likely to have a favorable outcome at 90 days than patients treated with placebo (60.9% versus 26.3%).

Unfortunately, most patients are ineligible for IV rt-PA because of delays in obtaining treatment. Indeed, studies show that only 1 to 2% of ischemic stroke patients receive IV rt-PA.[184,185] The recently published ECASS-3 study results are the first data from a randomized placebo-controlled trial that demonstrated the efficacy of IV rt-PA beyond the established 3-hour time window.[186] This trial randomly assigned 821 stroke patients between placebo and rt-PA in the 3- to 4.5-hour time window. Compared with placebo patients, rt-PA-treated patients experienced a 7.2% absolute increase in the rate of excellent recovery at the 90-day follow-up. A recent meta-analysis was undertaken to determine the efficacy of rt-PA in the 3- to 4.5-hour time window.[187] This meta-analysis evaluated patients in the ECASS-1, ECASS-2, ECASS-3, and ATLANTIS trials, and the rt-PA treatment in the 3- to 4.5-hour window was associated with an increased chance of favorable outcome (odds ratio 1.31) and no significant difference in mortality (odds ratio 1.04) compared to placebo.

Compared to IV thrombolysis, intra-arterial thrombolytic therapy ought, in theory, to be able to deliver a higher local concentration of agent where it is needed while minimizing the systemic concentration. Proponents of intra-arterial thrombolysis hope that it may lengthen the 3-hour treatment window. The PROACT II trial provided the best evidence to date that intra-arterial thrombolysis can improve patient outcomes.[188] This randomized, open-label, multicenter study with blinded follow-up randomly assigned 180 patients with stroke less than 6 hours' duration to receive either heparin with recombinant prourokinase (r-proUK), 9 mg intra-arterially, or heparin alone. Intra-arterial thrombolysis resulted in significantly better recanalization rates than heparin alone did (66% versus 18%). In addition, more of the r-proUK group had no neurologic deficit or only a slight deficit at 90 days (40% versus 25%). However, intra-arterial thrombolysis did result in significantly increased rates of ICH (35% versus 13%). Symptomatic ICH with neurologic deterioration within 24 hours occurred in 10% of r-proUK patients and 2% of control patients. Patients who experienced ICH after r-proUK therapy had a high mortality (83%).[189] It is noteworthy that only 2% (180 of 12,333) of the screened patients in the PROACT II trial were randomized according to inclusion criteria, which suggests that intra-arterial thrombolysis may be of limited applicability. Finally, intra-arterial thrombolysis requires an experienced staff capable of performing cerebral angiography and navigating a microcatheter to the clot. At present, IV thrombolysis is certainly more practical than intra-arterial thrombolysis; more importantly, it can be done earlier in the course of the stroke.

Financial Disclosures: None Reported

References

1. Lloyd-Jones D, Adams R, Carnethon M, et al. Heart disease and stroke statistics—2009 update: a report from the American Heart Association Statistics Committee and Stroke Statistics Subcommittee. Circulation 2009;119:e21–181.
2. Broderick JP, Phillips SJ, Whisnant JP, et al. Incidence rates of stroke in the eighties: the end of the decline in stroke? Stroke 1989;20:577–82.
3. Gillum RF, Sempos CT. The end of the long-term decline in stroke mortality in the United States? Stroke 1997;28:1527–9.
4. Special report from the National Institute of Neurological Disorders and Stroke. Classification of cerebrovascular diseases III. Stroke 1990;21:637–76.
5. Matsumoto N, Whisnant JP, Kurland LT, Okazaki H. Natural history of stroke in Rochester, Minnesota, 1955 through 1969: an extension of a previous study, 1945 through 1954. Stroke 1973;4:20–9.
6. Sacco RL, Wolf PA, Kannel WB, McNamara PM. Survival and recurrence following stroke. The Framingham study. Stroke 1982;13:290–5.
7. Wolf PA, D'Agostino RB, Belanger AJ, Kannel WB. Probability of stroke: a risk profile from the Framingham Study. Stroke 1991;22:312–8.
8. Sobel E, Alter M, Davanipour Z, et al. Stroke in the Lehigh Valley: combined risk factors for recurrent ischemic stroke. Neurology 1989;39:669–72.
9. Mohr JP, Caplan LR, Melski JW, et al. The Harvard Cooperative Stroke Registry: a prospective registry. Neurology 1978;28: 754–62.
10. Bogousslavsky J, Van Melle G, Regli F. The Lausanne Stroke Registry: analysis of 1,000 consecutive patients with first stroke. Stroke 1988;19:1083–92.
11. Sacco RL, Benjamin EJ, Broderick JP, et al. American Heart Association Prevention Conference. IV. Prevention and Rehabilitation of Stroke. Risk factors. Stroke 1997; 28:1507–17.
12. Ohira T, Shahar E, Chambless LE, et al. Risk factors for ischemic stroke subtypes: the Atherosclerosis Risk in Communities study. Stroke 2006;37:2493–8.
13. Wong KS, Huang YN, Gao S, et al. Intracranial stenosis in Chinese patients with acute stroke. Neurology 1998;50: 812–3.
14. Caplan LR, Gorelick PB, Hier DB. Race, sex and occlusive cerebrovascular disease: a review. Stroke 1986;17:648–55.
15. Kiely DK, Wolf PA, Cupples LA, et al. Familial aggregation of stroke. The Framingham Study. Stroke 1993;24:1366–71.
16. Amarenco P. Blood pressure and lipid lowering in the prevention of stroke: a note to neurologists. Cerebrovasc Dis 2003; 16 Suppl 3:33–8.
17. Leys D, Deplanque D, Mounier-Vehier C, et al. Stroke prevention: management of modifiable vascular risk factors. J Neurol 2002;249:507–17.
18. Goldstein LB, Adams R, Becker K, et al. Primary prevention of ischemic stroke: A statement for healthcare professionals from the Stroke Council of the American Heart Association. Stroke 2001;32:280–99.
19. Jorgensen H, Nakayama H, Raaschou HO, Olsen TS. Stroke in patients with diabetes. The Copenhagen Stroke Study. Stroke 1994;25:1977–84.
20. Tegos TJ, Kalodiki E, Daskalopoulou SS, Nicolaides AN. Stroke: epidemiology, clinical picture, and risk factors--Part I of III. Angiology 2000;51:793–808.
21. Stadel BV. Oral contraceptives and cardiovascular disease (first of two parts). N Engl J Med 1981;305:612–618.
22. Gill JS, Zezulka AV, Shipley MJ, et al. Stroke and alcohol consumption. N Engl J Med 1986;315:1041–6.
23. Prevention of stroke by antihypertensive drug treatment in older persons with isolated systolic hypertension. Final results of the Systolic Hypertension in the Elderly Program (SHEP). SHEP Cooperative Research Group. JAMA 1991;265:3255–64.
24. Foulkes MA, Wolf PA, Price TR, et al. The Stroke Data Bank: design, methods, and baseline characteristics. Stroke 1988;19: 547–54.
25. Gorelick PB, Hier DB, Caplan LR, Langenberg P. Headache in acute cerebrovascular disease. Neurology 1986;36:1445–50.
26. Kannel WB, McGee DL. Diabetes and cardiovascular disease. The Framingham study. JAMA 1979;241:2035–8.

27. Welch KM, Levine SR, Ewing JR. Viewing stroke pathophysiology: an analysis of contemporary methods. Stroke 1986;17: 1071–7.
28. Adams HP Jr, Kassell NF, Torner JC, Sahs AL. CT and clinical correlations in recent aneurysmal subarachnoid hemorrhage: a preliminary report of the Cooperative Aneurysm Study. Neurology 1983;33: 981–8.
29. von Kummer R, Nolte PN, Schnittger H, et al. Detectability of cerebral hemisphere ischaemic infarcts by CT within 6 h of stroke. Neuroradiology 1996;38:31–3.
30. Hunter GJ, Hamberg LM, Ponzo JA, et al. Assessment of cerebral perfusion and arterial anatomy in hyperacute stroke with three-dimensional functional CT: early clinical results. AJNR Am J Neuroradiol 1998;19:29–37.
31. von Kummer R, Allen KL, Holle R, et al. Acute stroke: usefulness of early CT findings before thrombolytic therapy. Radiology 1997;205:327–33.
32. Maeda M, Abe H, Yamada H, Ishii Y. Hyperacute infarction: a comparison of CT and MRI, including diffusion-weighted imaging. Neuroradiology 1999;41:175–8.
33. Arboix A, Marti-Vilalta JL, Garcia JH. Clinical study of 227 patients with lacunar infarcts. Stroke 1990;21:842–7.
34. Nicolaides AN, Papadakis K, Grigg M, et al. Amaurosis fugax. Bernstein E, editor. New York: Springer; 1988.
35. Kilpatrick MM, Yonas H, Goldstein S, et al. CT-based assessment of acute stroke: CT, CT angiography, and xenon-enhanced CT cerebral blood flow. Stroke 2001;32: 2543–9.
36. Green JB, Bialy Y, Sora E, Ricamato A. High-resolution EEG in poststroke hemiparesis can identify ipsilateral generators during motor tasks. Stroke 1999;30:2659–65.
37. Kim JS, Kang SY. Bleeding and subsequent anemia: a precipitant for cerebral infarction. Eur Neurol 2000;43:201–8.
38. Eikelboom JW, Hankey GJ, Anand SS, et al. Association between high homocyst(e)ine and ischemic stroke due to large- and small-artery disease but not other etiologic subtypes of ischemic stroke. Stroke 2000; 31:1069–75.
39. Kenet G, Sadetzki S, Murad H, et al. Factor V Leiden and antiphospholipid antibodies are significant risk factors for ischemic stroke in children. Stroke 2000;31:1283–8.
40. Madonna P, de Stefano V, Coppola A, et al. Hyperhomocysteinemia and other inherited prothrombotic conditions in young adults with a history of ischemic stroke. Stroke 2002;33:51–6.
41. Brass LM, Prohovnik I, Pavlakis SG, et al. Middle cerebral artery blood velocity and cerebral blood flow in sickle cell disease. Stroke 1991;22:27–30.
42. Asplund K. Haemodilution for acute ischaemic stroke. Cochrane Database Syst Rev 2002;(4):CD000103.
43. Strand T. Evaluation of long-term outcome and safety after hemodilution therapy in acute ischemic stroke. Stroke 1992;23:657–62.
44. Sivenius J, Heinonen OP, Pyorala K, et al. The incidence of stroke in the Kuopio area of East Finland. Stroke 1985;16:188–92.
45. Sudlow CL, Warlow CP. Comparable studies of the incidence of stroke and its pathological types: results from an international collaboration. International Stroke Incidence Collaboration. Stroke 1997;28: 491–9.
46. Wityk RJ, Caplan LR. Hypertensive intracerebral hemorrhage. Epidemiology and clinical pathology. Neurosurg Clin N Am 1992;3:521–32.
47. Feldmann E, Broderick JP, Kernan WN, et al. Major risk factors for intracerebral hemorrhage in the young are modifiable. Stroke 2005;36:1881–5.
48. Cole FM, Yates P. Intracerebral microaneurysms and small cerebrovascular lesions. Brain 1967;90:759–68.
49. Caplan L. Intracerebral hemorrhage revisited. Neurology 1988;38:624–7.
50. Brott T, Broderick J, Kothari R, et al. Early hemorrhage growth in patients with intracerebral hemorrhage. Stroke 1997;28: 1–5.
51. Qureshi AI, Harris-Lane P, Kirmani JF, et al. Treatment of acute hypertension in patients with intracerebral hemorrhage using American Heart Association guidelines. Crit Care Med 2006;34:1975–80.
52. Gebel JM Jr, Jauch EC, Brott TG, et al. Relative edema volume is a predictor of outcome in patients with hyperacute spontaneous intracerebral hemorrhage. Stroke 2002;33:2636–41.
53. Gebel JM Jr, Jauch EC, Brott TG, et al. Natural history of perihematomal edema in patients with hyperacute spontaneous intracerebral hemorrhage. Stroke 2002;33: 2631–5.
54. Schuetz H, Dommer T, Boedeker RH, et al. Changing pattern of brain hemorrhage during 12 years of computed axial tomography. Stroke 1992;23:653–6.
55. Weimar C, Weber C, Wagner M, et al. Management patterns and health care use after intracerebral hemorrhage. a cost-of-illness study from a societal perspective in Germany. Cerebrovasc Dis 2003;15: 29–36.
56. Ueda K, Hasuo Y, Kiyohara Y, et al. Intracerebral hemorrhage in a Japanese community, Hisayama: incidence, changing pattern during long-term follow-up, and related factors. Stroke 1988;19:48–52.
57. Diringer MN, Edwards DF. Admission to a neurologic/neurosurgical intensive care unit is associated with reduced mortality rate after intracerebral hemorrhage. Crit Care Med 2001;29:635–40.
58. Silver FL, Norris JW, Lewis AJ, Hachinski VC. Early mortality following stroke: a prospective review. Stroke 1984;15:492–6.
59. Broderick JP, Adams HP Jr, Barsan W, et al. Guidelines for the management of spontaneous intracerebral hemorrhage: A statement for healthcare professionals from a special writing group of the Stroke Council, American Heart Association. Stroke 1999;30:905–15.
60. Fernandes HM, Siddique S, Banister K, et al. Continuous monitoring of ICP and CPP following ICH and its relationship to clinical, radiological and surgical parameters. Acta Neurochir Suppl 2000;76:463–6.
61. Poungvarin N, Bhoopat W, Viriyavejakul A, et al. Effects of dexamethasone in primary supratentorial intracerebral hemorrhage. N Engl J Med 1987;316:1229–33.
62. Misra UK, Kalita J, Ranjan P, Mandal SK. Mannitol in intracerebral hemorrhage: a randomized controlled study. J Neurol Sci 2005;234:41–5.
63. Kalita J, Misra UK, Ranjan P, et al. Effect of mannitol on regional cerebral blood flow in patients with intracerebral hemorrhage. J Neurol Sci 2004;224:19–22.
64. Sansing LH, Kaznatcheeva EA, Perkins CJ, et al. Edema after intracerebral hemorrhage: correlations with coagulation parameters and treatment. J Neurosurg 2003;98:985–92.
65. Steiner T, Kaste M, Forsting M, et al. Recommendations for the management of intracranial haemorrhage - part I: spontaneous intracerebral haemorrhage. The European Stroke Initiative Writing Committee and the Writing Committee for the EUSI Executive Committee. Cerebrovasc Dis 2006;22:294–316.
66. Broderick J, Connolly S, Feldmann E, et al. Guidelines for the management of spontaneous intracerebral hemorrhage in adults: 2007 update: a guideline from the American Heart Association/American Stroke Association Stroke Council, High Blood Pressure Research Council, and the Quality of Care and Outcomes in Research Interdisciplinary Working Group. Stroke 2007;38:2001–23.
67. Morgenstern LB, Demchuk AM, Kim DH, et al. Rebleeding leads to poor outcome in ultra-early craniotomy for intracerebral hemorrhage. Neurology 2001;56:1294–9.
68. Kassell NF, Torner JC, Haley EC Jr, et al. The International Cooperative Study on the Timing of Aneurysm Surgery. Part 1: Overall management results. J Neurosurg 1990;73:18–36.
69. Bederson JB, Connolly ES Jr, Batjer HH, et al. Guidelines for the management of aneurysmal subarachnoid hemorrhage: a statement for healthcare professionals from a special writing group of the Stroke Council, American Heart Association. Stroke 2009;40:994–1025.
70. McCormick WF, Acosta-Rua GJ. The size of intracranial saccular aneurysms. An autopsy study. J Neurosurg 1970;33:422–7.
71. Inagawa T, Hirano A. Autopsy study of unruptured incidental intracranial aneurysms. Surg Neurol 1990;34:361–5.
72. Dell S. Asymptomatic cerebral aneurysm: assessment of its risk of rupture. Neurosurgery 1982;10:162–6.
73. van Gijn J, Rinkel GJ. Subarachnoid haemorrhage: diagnosis, causes and management. Brain 2001;124:249–78.
74. Kojima M, Nagasawa S, Lee YE, et al. Asymptomatic familial cerebral aneurysms. Neurosurgery 1998;43:776–81.
75. Rinkel GJ, Djibuti M, Algra A, van Gijn J. Prevalence and risk of rupture of intracranial aneurysms: a systematic review. Stroke 1998;29:251–6.
76. Kissela BM, Sauerbeck L, Woo D, et al. Subarachnoid hemorrhage: a preventable disease with a heritable component. Stroke 2002;33:1321–6.
77. Dias MS, Sekhar LN. Intracranial hemorrhage from aneurysms and arteriovenous malformations during pregnancy and the puerperium. Neurosurgery 1990;27:855–65; discussion 865–56.
78. Broderick JP, Brott T, Tomsick T, et al. The risk of subarachnoid and intracerebral hemorrhages in blacks as compared with whites. N Engl J Med 1992;326:733–6.
79. Bassi P, Bandera R, Loiero M, et al. Warning signs in subarachnoid hemorrhage: a cooperative study. Acta Neurol Scand 1991;84:277–81.
80. Schievink WI. Intracranial aneurysms. N Engl J Med 1997;336:28–40.
81. Hart RG, Byer JA, Slaughter JR, et al. Occurrence and implications of seizures in subarachnoid hemorrhage due to ruptured intracranial aneurysms. Neurosurgery 1981; 8:417–21.
82. Vale FL, Bradley EL, Fisher WS, 3rd. The relationship of subarachnoid hemorrhage and the need for postoperative shunting. J Neurosurg 1997;86:462–6.
83. Wijdicks EF, Kerkhoff H, van Gijn J. Long-term follow-up of 71 patients with thunderclap headache mimicking subarachnoid haemorrhage. Lancet 1988;2:68–70.

84. Markus HS. A prospective follow up of thunderclap headache mimicking subarachnoid haemorrhage. J Neurol Neurosurg Psychiatry 1991;54:1117–8.
85. Torner JC, Kassell NF, Wallace RB, Adams HP Jr. Preoperative prognostic factors for rebleeding and survival in aneurysm patients receiving antifibrinolytic therapy: report of the Cooperative Aneurysm Study. Neurosurgery 1981;9:506–13.
86. Haley EC Jr, Kassell NF, Torner JC. The International Cooperative Study on the Timing of Aneurysm Surgery. The North American experience. Stroke 1992;23:205–14.
87. Pare L, Delfino R, Leblanc R. The relationship of ventricular drainage to aneurysmal rebleeding. J Neurosurg 1992;76:422–7.
88. Longstreth WT Jr, Nelson LM, Koepsell TD, van Belle G. Clinical course of spontaneous subarachnoid hemorrhage: a population-based study in King County, Washington. Neurology 1993;43:712–8.
89. Sloan MA, Burch CM, Wozniak MA, et al. Transcranial Doppler detection of vertebrobasilar vasospasm following subarachnoid hemorrhage. Stroke 1994;25:2187–97.
90. Newell DW, Winn HR. Transcranial Doppler in cerebral vasospasm. Neurosurg Clin N Am 1990;1:319–28.
91. Tommasino C, Picozzi P. Physiopathological criteria of vasospasm treatment. J Neurosurg Sci 1998;42 1 Suppl 1:23–6.
92. Treggiari MM, Walder B, Suter PM, Romand JA. Systematic review of the prevention of delayed ischemic neurological [illegible] and hemodilution therapy following subarachnoid hemorrhage. J Neurosurg 2003; 98:978–84.
93. Feigin VL, Rinkel GJ, Algra A, et al. Calcium antagonists in patients with aneurysmal subarachnoid hemorrhage: a systematic review. Neurology 1998;50:876–83.
94. Allen GS, Ahn HS, Preziosi TJ, et al. Cerebral arterial spasm—a controlled trial of nimodipine in patients with subarachnoid hemorrhage. N Engl J Med 1983;308:619–24.
95. Caplan LR. Diagnosis and treatment of ischemic stroke. JAMA 1991;266:2413–8.
96. Torvik A. The pathogenesis of watershed infarcts in the brain. Stroke 1984;15:221–3.
97. Angeloni U, Bozzao L, Fantozzi L, et al. Internal borderzone infarction following acute middle cerebral artery occlusion. Neurology 1990;40:1196–8.
98. Bogousslavsky J, Regli F. Borderzone infarctions distal to internal carotid artery occlusion: prognostic implications. Ann Neurol 1986;20:346–50.
99. Mori E, Tabuchi M, Yamadori A. Lacunar syndrome due to intracerebral hemorrhage. Stroke 1985;16:454–9.
100. Fisher CM. A lacunar stroke. The dysarthria-clumsy hand syndrome. Neurology 1967;17:614–7.
101. Mast H, Thompson JL, Lee SH, et al. Hypertension and diabetes mellitus as determinants of multiple lacunar infarcts. Stroke 1995;26:30–3.
102. Longstreth WT Jr, Bernick C, Manolio TA, et al. Lacunar infarcts defined by magnetic resonance imaging of 3660 elderly people: the Cardiovascular Health Studsy. Arch Neurol 1998;55:1217–25.
103. Vermeer SE, Prins ND, den Heijer T, et al. Silent brain infarcts and the risk of dementia and cognitive decline. N Engl J Med 2003; 348:1215–22.
104. Gan R, Sacco RL, Kargman DE, et al. Testing the validity of the lacunar hypothesis: the Northern Manhattan Stroke Study experience. Neurology 1997;48:1204–11.
105. Clavier I, Hommel M, Besson G, et al. Long-term prognosis of symptomatic lacunar infarcts. A hospital-based study. Stroke 1994;25:2005–9.
106. Salgado AV, Ferro JM, Gouveia-Oliveira A. Long-term prognosis of first-ever lacunar strokes. A hospital-based study. Stroke 1996;27:661–6.
107. Gandolfo C, Moretti C, Dall'Agata D, et al. Long-term prognosis of patients with lacunar syndromes. Acta Neurol Scand 1986; 74:224–9.
108. Hier DB, Foulkes MA, Swiontoniowski M, et al. Stroke recurrence within 2 years after ischemic infarction. Stroke 1991;22:155–61.
109. Arboix A, Oliveres M, Massons J, et al. Early differentiation of cardioembolic from atherothrombotic cerebral infarction: a multivariate analysis. Eur J Neurol 1999;6: 677–83.
110. Timsit SG, Sacco RL, Mohr JP, et al. Brain infarction severity differs according to cardiac or arterial embolic source. Neurology 1993;43:728–33.
111. Kittner SJ, Sharkness CM, Sloan MA, et al. Infarcts with a cardiac source of embolism in the NINDS Stroke Data Bank: neurologic examination. Neurology 1992;42:299–302.
112. Kelley RE, Minagar A. Cardioembolic stroke: an update. South Med J 2003;96: 343–9.
113. Minematsu K, Yamaguchi T, Omae T. 'Spectacular shrinking deficit': rapid recovery from a major hemispheric syndrome by migration of an embolus. Neurology 1992;42:157–62.
114. Hornig CR, Bauer T, Simon C, et al. Hemorrhagic transformation in cardioembolic cerebral infarction. Stroke 1993;24:465–8.
115. Molina CA, Montaner J, Abilleira S, et al. Timing of spontaneous recanalization and risk of hemorrhagic transformation in acute cardioembolic stroke. Stroke 2001;32:1079–84.
116. Alexandrov AV, Black SE, Ehrlich LE, et al. Predictors of hemorrhagic transformation occurring spontaneously and on anticoagulants in patients with acute ischemic stroke. Stroke 1997;28:1198–202.
117. Laupacis A, Albers G, Dalen J, et al. Antithrombotic therapy in atrial fibrillation. Chest 1995;108 4 Suppl:352S–9S.
118. Kopecky SL, Gersh BJ, McGoon MD, et al. The natural history of lone atrial fibrillation. A population-based study over three decades. N Engl J Med 1987;317:669–74.
119. Wolf PA, Dawber TR, Thomas HE Jr, Kannel WB. Epidemiologic assessment of chronic atrial fibrillation and risk of stroke: the Framingham study. Neurology 1978; 28:973–7.
120. Yamanouchi H, Nagura H, Mizutani T, et al. Embolic brain infarction in nonrheumatic atrial fibrillation: a clinicopathologic study in the elderly. Neurology 1997;48: 1593–7.
121. Peters NS, Schilling RJ, Kanagaratnam P, Markides V. Atrial fibrillation: strategies to control, combat, and cure. Lancet 2002; 359:593–603.
122. Wolf PA, Abbott RD, Kannel WB. Atrial fibrillation as an independent risk factor for stroke: the Framingham Study. Stroke 1991;22:983–8.
123. Saxena R, Lewis S, Berge E, et al. Risk of early death and recurrent stroke and effect of heparin in 3169 patients with acute ischemic stroke and atrial fibrillation in the International Stroke Trial. Stroke 2001;32: 2333–7.
124. Immediate anticoagulation of embolic stroke: a randomized trial. Cerebral Embolism Study Group. Stroke 1983;14:668–76.
125. Cardiogenic brain embolism. Cerebral Embolism Task Force. Arch Neurol 1986; 43:71–84.
126. Cardiogenic brain embolism. The second report of the Cerebral Embolism Task Force. Arch Neurol 1989;46:727–43.
127. Hart RG, Benavente O, McBride R, Pearce LA. Antithrombotic therapy to prevent stroke in patients with atrial fibrillation: a meta-analysis. Ann Intern Med 1999;131: 492–501.
128. Warfarin versus aspirin for prevention of thromboembolism in atrial fibrillation: Stroke Prevention in Atrial Fibrillation II Study. Lancet 1994;343:687–91.
129. Petersen P, Boysen G, Godtfredsen J, et al. Placebo-controlled, randomised trial of warfarin and aspirin for prevention of thromboembolic complications in chronic atrial fibrillation. The Copenhagen AFASAK study. Lancet 1989;1:175–9.
130. Mohr JP, Thompson JL, Lazar RM, et al. A comparison of warfarin and aspirin for the prevention of recurrent ischemic stroke. N Engl J Med 2001;345:1444–51.
131. CAST: randomised placebo-controlled trial of early aspirin use in 20,000 patients with acute ischaemic stroke. CAST (Chinese Acute Stroke Trial) Collaborative Group. Lancet 1997;349:1641–9.
132. The International Stroke Trial (IST): a randomised trial of aspirin, subcutaneous heparin, both, or neither among 19435 patients with acute ischaemic stroke. International Stroke Trial Collaborative Group. Lancet 1997;349:1569–81.
133. Lees RS. The natural history of carotid artery disease. Stroke 1984;15:603–4.
134. Kardoulas DG, Katsamouris AN, Gallis PT, et al. Ultrasonographic and histologic characteristics of symptom-free and symptomatic carotid plaque. Cardiovasc Surg 1996;4:580–90.
135. el-Barghouty N, Nicolaides A, Bahal V, et al. The identification of the high risk carotid plaque. Eur J Vasc Endovasc Surg 1996;11:470–8.
136. Long A, Lepoutre A, Corbillon E, Branchereau A. Critical review of non- or minimally invasive methods (duplex ultrasonography, MR- and CT-angiography) for evaluating stenosis of the proximal internal carotid artery. Eur J Vasc Endovasc Surg 2002;24:43–52.
137. Beneficial effect of carotid endarterectomy in symptomatic patients with high-grade carotid stenosis. North American Symptomatic Carotid Endarterectomy Trial Collaborators. N Engl J Med 1991;325:445–53.
138. MRC European Carotid Surgery Trial: interim results for symptomatic patients with severe (70–99%) or with mild (0–29%) carotid stenosis. European Carotid Surgery Trialists' Collaborative Group. Lancet 1991;337:1235–43.
139. Mayberg MR, Wilson SE, Yatsu F, et al. Carotid endarterectomy and prevention of cerebral ischemia in symptomatic carotid stenosis. Veterans Affairs Cooperative Studies Program 309 Trialist Group. JAMA 1991;266:3289–94.
140. Blaisdell WF, Clauss RH, Galbraith JG, et al. Joint study of extracranial arterial occlusion. IV. A review of surgical considerations. JAMA 1969;209:1889–95.
141. Easton JD, Sherman DG. Stroke and mortality rate in carotid endarterectomy: 228 consecutive operations. Stroke 1977;8:565–8.

142. Sacco RL, Adams R, Albers G, et al. Guidelines for prevention of stroke in patients with ischemic stroke or transient ischemic attack: a statement for healthcare professionals from the American Heart Association/American Stroke Association Council on Stroke: co-sponsored by the Council on Cardiovascular Radiology and Intervention: the American Academy of Neurology affirms the value of this guideline. Circulation 2006; 113:e409–49.
143. Moore WS, Barnett HJ, Beebe HG, et al. Guidelines for carotid endarterectomy. A multidisciplinary consensus statement from the Ad Hoc Committee, American Heart Association. Circulation 1995;91:566–79.
144. Wennberg DE, Lucas FL, Birkmeyer JD, et al. Variation in carotid endarterectomy mortality in the Medicare population: trial hospitals, volume, and patient characteristics. JAMA 1998;279:1278–81.
145. Bruetman M, Fields W, Crawford E, Debakey M. Cerebral hemorrhage in carotid artery surgery. Arch Neurol 1963;9:458–67.
146. Wylie E, Hein M, Adams J. Intracranial hemorrhage following surgical revascularization for treatment of acute strokes. J Neurosurg 1964;21:212–5.
147. Dosick SM, Whalen RC, Gale SS, Brown OW. Carotid endarterectomy in the stroke patient: computerized axial tomography to determine timing. J Vasc Surg 1985;2: 214–9.
148. Whittemore AD, Ruby ST, Couch NP, Mannick JA. Early carotid endarterectomy in patients with small, fixed neurologic deficits. J Vasc Surg 1984;1:795–9.
149. Toni D, Fiorelli M, Bastianello S, et al. Hemorrhagic transformation of brain infarct: predictability in the first 5 hours from stroke onset and influence on clinical outcome. Neurology 1996;46:341–5.
150. Naylor AR. Delay may reduce procedural risk, but at what price to the patient? Eur J Vasc Endovasc Surg 2008;35:383–91.
151. Chobanian AV, Bakris GL, Black HR, et al. The Seventh Report of the Joint National Committee on Prevention, Detection, Evaluation, and Treatment of High Blood Pressure: the JNC 7 report. JAMA 2003; 289:2560–72.
152. Sacco RL, Adams R, Albers G, et al. Guidelines for prevention of stroke in patients with ischemic stroke or transient ischemic attack: a statement for healthcare professionals from the American Heart Association/ American Stroke Association Council on Stroke: co-sponsored by the Council on Cardiovascular Radiology and Intervention: the American Academy of Neurology affirms the value of this guideline. Stroke 2006;37:577–617.
153. Moore WS, Mohr JP, Najafi H, et al. Carotid endarterectomy: practice guidelines. Report of the Ad Hoc Committee to the Joint Council of the Society for Vascular Surgery and the North American Chapter of the International Society for Cardiovascular Surgery. J Vasc Surg 1992;15:469–79.
154. Mentzer RM Jr, Finkelmeier BA, Crosby IK, Wellons HA Jr. Emergency carotid endarterectomy for fluctuating neurologic deficits. Surgery 1981;89:60–66.
155. Ohki T, Veith FJ, Grenell S, et al. Initial experience with cerebral protection devices to prevent embolization during carotid artery stenting. J Vasc Surg 2002;36:1175–85.
156. Parodi JC, Ferreira LM, Sicard G, et al. Cerebral protection during carotid stenting using flow reversal. J Vasc Surg 2005;41: 416–22.
157. Fanelli F, Bezzi M, Boatta E, Passariello R. Techniques in cerebral protection. Eur J Radiol 2006;60:26–36.
158. Gasparis AP, Ricotta L, Cuadra SA, et al. High-risk carotid endarterectomy: fact or fiction. J Vasc Surg 2003;37:40–6.
159. Stoner MC, Abbott WM, Wong DR, et al. Defining the high-risk patient for carotid endarterectomy: an analysis of the prospective National Surgical Quality Improvement Program database. J Vasc Surg 2006; 43:285–95; discussion 295–86.
160. Hobson RW, 2nd, Howard VJ, Roubin GS, et al. Carotid artery stenting is associated with increased complications in octogenarians: 30-day stroke and death rates in the CREST lead-in phase. J Vasc Surg 2004; 40:1106–11.
161. Stanziale SF, Marone LK, Boules TN, et al. Carotid artery stenting in octogenarians is associated with increased adverse outcomes. J Vasc Surg 2006;43:297–304.
162. Lin SC, Trocciola SM, Rhee J, et al. Analysis of anatomic factors and age in patients undergoing carotid angioplasty and stenting. Ann Vasc Surg 2005;19:798–804.
163. Lam RC, Lin SC, DeRubertis B, et al. The impact of increasing age on anatomic factors affecting carotid angioplasty and stenting. J Vasc Surg 2007;45:875–80.
164. Kastrup A, Groschel K, Schnaudigel S, et al. Target lesion ulceration and arch calcification are associated with increased incidence of carotid stenting-associated ischemic lesions in octogenarians. J Vasc Surg 2008;47:88–95.
165. Faggioli GL, Ferri M, Freyrie A, et al. Aortic arch anomalies are associated with increased risk of neurological events in carotid stent procedures. Eur J Vasc Endovasc Surg 2007;33:436–41.
166. Faggioli G, Ferri M, Gargiulo M, et al. Measurement and impact of proximal and distal tortuosity in carotid stenting procedures. J Vasc Surg 2007;46:1119–24.
167. Sayeed S, Stanziale SF, Wholey MH, Makaroun MS. Angiographic lesion characteristics can predict adverse outcomes after carotid artery stenting. J Vasc Surg 2008; 47:81–7.
168. Biasi GM, Froio A, Diethrich EB, et al. Carotid plaque echolucency increases the risk of stroke in carotid stenting: the Imaging in Carotid Angioplasty and Risk of Stroke (ICAROS) study. Circulation 2004;110: 756–62.
169. Hofmann R, Niessner A, Kypta A, et al. Risk score for peri-interventional complications of carotid artery stenting. Stroke 2006;37:2557–61.
170. Gray WA, Hopkins LN, Yadav S, et al. Protected carotid stenting in high-surgical-risk patients: the ARCHeR results. J Vasc Surg 2006;44:258–68.
171. Yadav JS, Wholey MH, Kuntz RE, et al. Protected carotid-artery stenting versus endarterectomy in high-risk patients. N Engl J Med 2004;351:1493–501.
172. Endovascular versus surgical treatment in patients with carotid stenosis in the Carotid and Vertebral Artery Transluminal Angioplasty Study (CAVATAS): a randomised trial. Lancet 2001;357:1729–37.
173. Carotid revascularization using endarterectomy or stenting systems (CARESS): phase I clinical trial. J Endovasc Ther 2003;10: 1021–30.
174. Ringleb PA, Allenberg J, Bruckmann H, et al. 30 day results from the SPACE trial of stent-protected angioplasty versus carotid endarterectomy in symptomatic patients: a randomised non-inferiority trial. Lancet 2006;368:1239–47.
175. Alberts MJ. Results of a Multicenter Prospective Randomized Trial of Carotid Artery Stenting vs. Carotid Endarterectomy. Abstracts of the International Stroke Conference. January 1, 2001. Stroke 2001;32: 325–d.
176. Brooks WH, McClure RR, Jones MR, et al. Carotid angioplasty and stenting versus carotid endarterectomy: randomized trial in a community hospital. J Am Coll Cardiol 2001;38:1589–95.
177. Brooks WH, McClure RR, Jones MR, et al. Carotid angioplasty and stenting versus carotid endarterectomy for treatment of asymptomatic carotid stenosis: a randomized trial in a community hospital. Neurosurgery 2004;54:318–24; discussion 324–15.
178. Mas JL, Chatellier G, Beyssen B, et al. Endarterectomy versus stenting in patients with symptomatic severe carotid stenosis. N Engl J Med 2006;355:1660–71.
179. Tissue plasminogen activator for acute ischemic stroke. The National Institute of Neurological Disorders and Stroke rt-PA Stroke Study Group. N Engl J Med 1995; 333:1581–7.
180. Kwiatkowski TG, Libman RB, Frankel M, et al. Effects of tissue plasminogen activator for acute ischemic stroke at one year. National Institute of Neurological Disorders and Stroke Recombinant Tissue Plasminogen Activator Stroke Study Group. N Engl J Med 1999;340:1781–7.
181. Hacke W, Kaste M, Fieschi C, et al. Intravenous thrombolysis with recombinant tissue plasminogen activator for acute hemispheric stroke. The European Cooperative Acute Stroke Study (ECASS). JAMA 1995; 274:1017–25.
182. Clark WM, Albers GW, Madden KP, Hamilton S. The rtPA (alteplase) 0- to 6-hour acute stroke trial, part A (A0276g): results of a double-blind, placebo-controlled, multicenter study. Thromblytic therapy in acute ischemic stroke study investigators. Stroke 2000;31:811–6.
183. Clark WM, Wissman S, Albers GW, et al. Recombinant tissue-type plasminogen activator (Alteplase) for ischemic stroke 3 to 5 hours after symptom onset. The ATLANTIS Study: a randomized controlled trial. Alteplase Thrombolysis for Acute Noninterventional Therapy in Ischemic Stroke. JAMA 1999;282:2019–26.
184. Hacke W, Brott T, Caplan L, et al. Thrombolysis in acute ischemic stroke: controlled trials and clinical experience. Neurology 1999;53 7 Suppl 4:S3–14.
185. Katzan IL, Furlan AJ, Lloyd LE, et al. Use of tissue-type plasminogen activator for acute ischemic stroke: the Cleveland area experience. JAMA 2000;283:1151–8.
186. Hacke W, Kaste M, Bluhmki E, et al. Thrombolysis with alteplase 3 to 4.5 hours after acute ischemic stroke. N Engl J Med 2008;359:1317–29.
187. Lansberg MG, Bluhmki E, Thijs VN. Efficacy and safety of tissue plasminogen activator 3 to 4.5 hours after acute ischemic stroke: a metaanalysis. Stroke 2009;40: 2438–41.
188. Furlan A, Higashida R, Wechsler L, et al. Intra-arterial prourokinase for acute ischemic stroke. The PROACT II study: a randomized controlled trial. Prolyse in Acute Cerebral Thromboembolism. JAMA 1999; 282:2003–11.
189. Kase CS, Furlan AJ, Wechsler LR, et al. Cerebral hemorrhage after intra-arterial thrombolysis for ischemic stroke: the PROACT II trial. Neurology 2001;57:1603–10.

2 ASYMPTOMATIC CAROTID BRUIT/CAROTID ARTERY STENOSIS

Ali F. Aburahma, MD, and Patrick A. Stone, MD

Stroke is the third leading cause of death in the United States, behind coronary artery disease and cancer. It is also the leading cause of disability. Nearly 80% of strokes are ischemic, and approximately 20% are hemorrhagic.[1] Unfortunately, only 15% of stroke patients have warning transient ischemic attacks (TIAs) prior to stroke, and waiting until symptoms occur is not ideal.[2] Ideally, patients who are at high risk for stroke could be identified and treated prior to permanent neurologic deficit.

The management of patients with asymptomatic carotid stenosis has been controversial over the past few decades because most of the landmark studies comparing best medical therapy with best medical therapy with carotid endarterectomy (CEA) used only aspirin as the antiplatelet agent and occurred prior to the widespread use of statin therapy. In this chapter, we provide a stepwise approach to the evaluation and management of patients with asymptomatic carotid bruit/extracranial carotid artery stenosis.

Clinical Evaluation

It is imperative in evaluating a patient with carotid artery stenosis to determine if the patient is classified as symptomatic or asymptomatic. This requires a careful history and review of the patient's medical records and a detailed neurovascular examination. Most TIAs involve the distribution of the internal carotid arteries, although some may affect the vertebrobasilar system. Typical carotid TIA symptoms include contralateral weakness of the face, arm, and/or leg; contralateral sensory deficit or paresthesia of the face, arm, and/or leg; or transient ipsilateral blindness (amaurosis fugax). If the right cerebral hemisphere is affected, other manifestations may be noted, for example, agnosognosia, asomatognosia, neglect, and sensory or visual extinction. In contrast, if the left hemisphere is affected, patients may show manifestation of alexia, aphasias, agraphesthesia, and anomia. Patients with vertebrobasilar TIAs may have a combination of symptoms, including vertigo, diplopia, ataxia, dysarthria, nausea, vomiting, visual disturbances, decreased consciousness, and weakness, which may include quadriparesis.

Occasionally, patients will present with headache and vague neurologic symptoms and have cerebral imaging, that is, magnetic resonance imaging (MRI) or computed tomographic (CT) scans that show recent cerebral infarcts, which may be the result of carotid pathology. Overall, if these infarcts are old, the patients would be considered asymptomatic. However, Kakkos and colleagues reported a higher stroke rate in patients with more than 60 to 79% asymptomatic stenosis with an annual TIA/stroke rate of 1.3% if there was no silent infarct versus 4.4 if a silent infarct was present.[3]

Physical examination may show signs of stroke: facial/eyelid drooping, sensory or motor deficits, and speech disturbances. Ocular examinations can occasionally identify Hollenhorst plaques, but this generally requires examination by an optometrist or ophthalmologist. Palpation of the carotid artery provides limited data unless there is asymmetry in the pulsation between the two carotids. Neck auscultation may elicit carotid bruit.

CAROTID BRUITS

Carotid bruits may be helpful in detecting asymptomatic carotid artery stenosis. Carotid bruits must be differentiated from venous hums, which are found in one quarter of young adults or in individuals with cardiac murmurs.[4] In contrast to a carotid bruit, the venous hum typically increases in quality with the neck turned away from the auscultated side. Also, the venous hum often disappears with Valsalva maneuver and when the patient lies down. There is no definitive way to differentiate a radiated cardiac murmur or bruit originating from intrathoracic vessels from a carotid bruit, but cardiac murmurs are more frequently bilateral and more audible in the chest and lower neck than in the mid- to upper neck.[5,6] Patients on dialysis can also have bruits that radiate into the neck secondary to arteriovenous fistula placement.[7]

Once a neck bruit is determined to be carotid in origin, the next stage is to determine whether this bruit is asymptomatic or symptomatic. This can be determined by the presence or absence of TIA symptoms or stroke, as indicated earlier. It should be noted that symptoms referable to the contralateral carotid artery, even in the absence of bruit on that side, should prompt evaluation of the patient for stenosis on the contralateral side. Carotid bruit may be absent in patients with severe carotid stenosis in 20 to 35% of patients.[8] In a subset analysis of the North American Symptomatic Carotid Endarterectomy Trial (NASCET), the presence of carotid bruits was compared with angiographic imaging of the carotid system. The presence of focal ipsilateral carotid bruits had a sensitivity of 63% and a specificity of 61% for high-grade carotid stenosis (70 to 99%), and the absence of a bruit did not significantly change the probability of significant stenosis in this group of patients (pretest 52%, posttest 40%).[9]

Several studies have analyzed the significance of carotid bruits. Ratchford and colleagues found in a diverse group of patients that the sensitivity of bruit auscultation to detect a stenosis was low at 56%, but specificity was high at 98%, with positive and negative predictive values of 25% and 99%, respectively.[10] Several conclusions were made from their study, including that the prevalence of carotid bruits is low in the general population. Also, if bruit is heard in an asymptomatic patient, 25% will have a greater than 60% stenosis; however, the ability to predict plaque by ultrasonography was 89%. Asymptomatic carotid bruits have also been associated with an increased risk of ischemic stroke compared with age-matched patients without carotid bruits.[11] Carotid bruits have also been shown in a meta-analysis to be a prognostic indicator of myocardial infarction (MI) and death.[12] MI and death occurred twice as often in patients with versus patients without carotid bruits.[12]

In another prospective clinicopathophysiologic follow-up study of asymptomatic neck bruits, we followed 300 asymptomatic patients with carotid bruits using serial clinical examinations and duplex ultrasonography with Gee/ocular plethysmography (OPG) for a period ranging from 1 to 72 months (mean 32 months). All patients underwent baseline duplex/OPG, which was repeated every 6 months until the end point, TIA or stroke. One hundred seven had arteriograms. Five classes were identified: class I (normal): 96 of 300 (32%) patients, 79 of whom were followed and one had TIA (1 of 79, 1.3%); class II (< 50% stenosis): 118 of 300 (39%) patients, 105 of whom were followed, with three having TIA, and one having stroke (4 of 105, 3.8%); class III (50 to 60% stenosis): 25 of 300 (8%), 21 of whom were followed, with one having TIA (1 of 21, 4.7%); class IV (> 60% stenosis with negative OPG): 39 of 300 (13%), 34 of whom were followed, with three having TIA and one having stroke (4 of 34, 11.7%); and class V (> 60% stenosis with positive OPG): 22 of 300 (7%), 18 of whom were followed, with three having TIA, and one having stroke (4 of 18, 22.2%). From these data, we concluded that in asymptomatic patients with carotid bruits, 32% had no carotid stenosis and 39% had minimal disease with minimal risk of TIA or stroke. Patients with the most severe stenoses (classes IV and V) had a statistically significantly higher likelihood of TIA or stroke occurring during the follow-up period. This last group (class V) would be ideal for prophylactic CEA.[13]

Vascular Risk Evaluation

Vascular risk factors are common in patients with asymptomatic carotid bruits. These patients should be evaluated for the presence of controllable risk factors, including hypertension, diabetes mellitus, hyperlipidemia, and smoking. Hypertension is generally twice as common in these patients than in the general population; similarly, smoking, ischemic heart disease, and peripheral disease are more prevalent.[14–17]

The absolute risk of stroke is generally increased in the presence of carotid bruit. In population-based studies, the annual risk of stroke was 2.1% (95% confidence interval [CI] 0.6 to 8.5) for persons who had a carotid bruit versus 0.86% (95% CI 0.8 to 0.9) for those who did not.[18–20] This represents an absolute risk increase for stroke of 1.24% a year and a relative risk for stroke of 2.4. The presence of a carotid bruit remained an independently significant variable, with a relative risk of 2.0, even after adjustment for various risk factors, including hypertension, age, and sex.[18]

With these facts in mind, and given the low absolute risk of stroke in patients with asymptomatic carotid bruits [see *Table 1*] and the low prevalence of surgically relevant significant carotid stenosis in these patients [see *Table 2*] with a relatively small absolute benefit of CEA, most clinicians pursue further investigations only in patients who carry a high risk of carotid stenosis and stroke and who also carry a low operative risk for CEA.[21,22] Further evaluation in these patients should be done only if the patients prefer to undergo carotid intervention, whether CEA or stenting; otherwise, no further evaluation is indicated.

For any therapy to receive widespread support, the risk attended to this therapy must be significantly less than the actual risk if the disease is not treated. Therefore, carotid intervention must have a significantly lower perioperative complication rate than the natural history of asymptomatic carotid stenosis. This is a particular issue in patients undergoing evaluation for stroke prevention: these patients tend to be elderly, harbor general atherosclerosis, and have concomitant coronary artery disease, hypertension, diabetes mellitus, chronic lung disease, and renal insufficiency. All of these comorbidities may impact the perioperative outcome after CEA or carotid stenting.

A number of caveats must be considered when examining the evidence that carotid artery interventions reduce the risk of stroke and death in patients with carotid disease. First, a significant number of patients were excluded from both the NASCET[23] and the Asymptomatic Carotid Atherosclerosis

Table 1 Annual Risk of Stroke

Patient Population	Annual Risk of Stroke, % (95% CI)
Population without bruits, age > 60 yr[16–18]	0.86 (0.8–0.9)
Population with bruits, age > 60 yr[16,17,59]	2.1 (0.6–8.5)
Male population without bruits, age > 60 yr[14,16]	0.9 (0.1–3.0)
Male population with bruits, age > 60 yr[16]	8.0 (0.2–38.0)
Female population without bruits, age > 60 yr[14]	2.0 (0.8–4.2)
Female population with bruits, age > 60 yr[16]	2.4 (0.7–5.5)

Table 2 Prevalence of Carotid Stenosis in Patients with Bruits and in Healthy Volunteers

Patient Population	Prevalence of Carotid Stenosis, % (95% CI)
Overall population with cervical bruits	
> 35% stenosis[13,59–62]	58 (55–60)
> 60–75% stenosis[13,60,61]	21 (18–24)
Healthy volunteers*	
Age > 70 yr[63]	5.1 (2.6–9.0)
Age ≤ 70 yr[63]	1.5 (0.2–5.3)

*In healthy volunteers, the incidence of asymptomatic carotid stenosis is significantly correlated with age ($p < .01$) and with the presence of hypertension ($p < .005$).

Study (ACAS)[24] because of coexisting medical conditions that could produce significant mortality and/or morbidity. During 6 years of enrolment in the ACAS, 42,000 patients were screened to randomize 1,662 patients. Strict nonneurologic exclusion criteria for ACAS and NASCET included age younger than 40 years or older than 79 years, a less than 5-year life expectancy, or diseases that would seriously complicate surgery, for example, unstable angina, atrial fibrillation, severe diabetes, uncontrolled hypertension, and chronic renal insufficiency. A second caveat is that new lines of medical therapy, such as statins, beta blockers, and modern antiplatelet therapies, were not available at the time of the original ACAS and NASCET. These agents represent current "best medical therapy" and may impact the results comparing interventions with medical therapy alone. Studies such as the Transatlantic Asymptomatic Carotid Intervention Trial (TACIT) may help in determining the outcome of these patients. This ongoing multicenter, prospective, randomized trial involves 100 sites enrolling over 2,000 patients. High- and low-risk individuals with greater than 70% asymptomatic carotid stenosis are randomized into one of three arms: (1) CEA and best medical therapy, (2) carotid artery stenting and best medical therapy, and (3) best medical therapy with antiplatelet, statin, and antihypertensive agents only.[25] Until the trial results are known, our belief is that if these patients have a good likelihood of significant carotid stenosis as evidenced by the presence of other vascular risk factors, have a reasonable life expectancy, and are at low risk for carotid intervention, they should be thoroughly investigated because they will benefit from prophylactic CEA.

Imaging Modalities

Several imaging modalities have been proposed, including carotid duplex ultrasonography, carotid MRI, and CT.

CAROTID DUPLEX ULTRASONOGRAPHY

The initial evaluation of patients with carotid bruit or cerebrovascular symptoms should begin with duplex imaging of the extracranial carotid arteries. Duplex ultrasonography is an accurate and reliable noninvasive tool to determine the degree of carotid stenosis and plaque morphology in most patients. It is important that images be reviewed by the vascular surgeon/vascular interventionalist to understand the quality of the testing. Often duplex ultrasonography performed at nonaccredited facilities provides results that are not acceptable for proceeding with intervention. We continue to use previously validated criteria from our institution to make treatment decisions without secondary imaging prior to carotid intervention [*see Table 3*].[26]

Table 3 Duplex Velocity Criteria for Carotid Stenosis

Stenosis (%)	PSV (cm/s)	EDV (cm/s)
< 30	< 120	< 65
30–50	120–139	< 65
50–60	> 140	< 65
60–70	> 150	> 65
70–99	> 150	> 90

EDV = end diastolic velocity; PSV = peak systolic velocity.

Duplex ultrasonography has been shown to be highly accurate in estimating the degree of carotid stenosis. A meta-analysis conducted in 1995 concluded that for detecting greater than 50% stenosis (determined by arteriography), duplex ultrasonography had a sensitivity of 91% and a specificity of 93%.[27] Given a disease prevalence of about 41% in patients referred for duplex ultrasonography, these findings translated into a positive predictive value of 90% and an overall accuracy of 92%.

In addition to estimating severity of stenosis, duplex ultrasonography can also be used to assess plaque morphology, an important tool that may help predict a patient's future risk of neurologic events. Reilly and colleagues have characterized plaques as homogeneous or heterogeneous.[28] Homogeneous plaques consist of uniform medium- to high-level echoes, whereas heterogeneous plaques consist of a mixture of high-, medium-, and low-level echoes. Homogeneous plaques on duplex ultrasonography have been correlated with fibrous lesions intraplaque hemorrhage on pathologic examination. Pathologic evidence of ulceration and loose stroma-containing lipids and proteinaceous deposits are characteristic of heterogeneous lesions.[28] Heterogeneous plaques [*see Figure 1*] have been shown to increase the risk of neurologic symptoms (TIA/stroke), as previously reported by our group. Heterogeneous plaques were also associated with an incidence of TIA/stroke that was higher than that in homogeneous plaques for all grades of stenosis.[29] Plaque morphology has been shown to be an important predictor of neurologic events using other imaging techniques. Nicolaides used computerized image analysis to assess plaque morphology by quantifying the grayscale median (GSM) of the plaque.[30] The incidence of cerebral infarction in those with GSM of greater than 50 was 9% versus 40% in those with GSM less than 50. Recently, investigators have suggested the importance of normalization of the B-mode value to allow interscan comparison. The Imaging in Carotid Angioplasty and Risk of Stroke (ICAROS) study obtained longitudinal images of the plaque and vessel wall, transferred the images to a workstation, and used commercially available software to normalize the data.[31] They adjusted the GSM of the blood pool to 0 to 5 and the adventitia of the wall to 185 to 195. The region of interest, therefore, was selected and its GSM value was calculated. The investigators of this study demonstrated that GSM values of 25 or less were associated with a stroke risk of 7.1% and GSM values exceeding 25 had a stroke risk of 1.5% during carotid stenting procedures. However, Reiter and colleagues, in a later study, failed to demonstrate the correlation between plaque echogenicity and an increased risk of stroke during carotid stenting.[32]

Recently, intravascular ultrasonography has been used to characterize arterial lesions before intervention, particularly in the evaluation of coronary artery disease. A similar system has also been used for evaluating carotid plaques where tissue characterization algorithms, creating images of "virtual histology" of the arterial wall, are made. These need further validation before having a clinical implication.[33]

Duplex imaging of the carotid artery has a few major limitations. These include quality dependence on the technician's examination and limitations of visualization of the proximal carotid artery and intracranial portions. Although the intracranial cerebral arteries can be assessed with transcranial

a

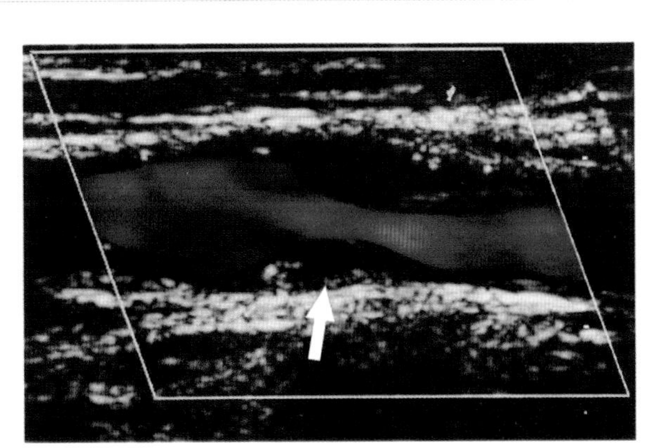

b

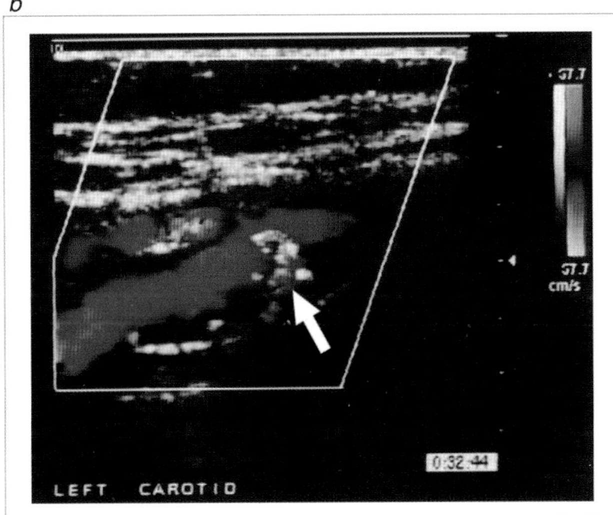

Figure 1 **(*a*) Color duplex ultrasound image of the carotid bifurcation showing a complex heterogeneous plaque at the origin of the internal carotid artery (*arrow*). (*b*) Color duplex ultrasound image of the carotid artery showing a smooth heterogeneous plaque (*arrow*). The dark center of the plaque may represent intraplaque hemorrhage. Reproduced with permission from Duplex scanning of the carotid arteries. In: AbuRahma AF, Bergan JJ, editors. Noninvasive Vascular Diagnosis: a Practical Guide to Therapy. London: Springer; 2007. p. 70.**

Doppler imaging, this technique is not as widely available at most institutions as other imaging modalities. It may also overestimate stenosis contralateral to carotid occlusion due to increased compensatory flow; however, most of the recent studies take this into consideration and adjust velocity thresholds accordingly.[26]

CONTRAST-BASED IMAGING

Magnetic resonance angiography (MRA) and computed tomographic angiography (CTA) are additional tests that can assess the carotid circulation to aid the physician in planning intervention. Compared with catheter-based arteriography, the sensitivity and specificity of MRA in detecting carotid stenosis of 70 to 99% has been 84 to 100% and 75 to 93%, respectively, by using two- and three-dimensional time of flight techniques.[34,35] Proximal lesions (below the clavicle) and intracranial lesions can be assessed when clinically suspected or in cases in which duplex imaging is suggestive. Proximal lesions lead to lower velocities distally with dampened Doppler waveforms. Our group has relied more on CTA when duplex examinations are inconclusive. Rapid acquisition of spiral CT images can allow for excellent timing with contrast administration and provide quality images that can be viewed in multiple plains. Plaque morphology can also be assessed, similar to that of ultrasound-based techniques. The limitations of this technique include cost, contrast exposure, and the added concern of radiation exposure. Additionally, a large calcium burden can limit the ability to distinguish contrast from calcium during postprocessing imaging.

Conventional angiography, once considered the gold standard for carotid imaging, is now reserved for patients with conflicting studies or patients being considered for carotid stenting. Conventional contrast angiography poses a stroke risk of approximately 1% and therefore has a limited role in place of modern MRA and CTA, except in cases of planned carotid stenting. Importantly, in the ACAS study, 1.2% of patients developed a neurologic event following carotid angiography, accounting for 40% of the strokes in the intervention arm.[24] In addition to the neurologic events, access-related complications can occur, increasing the overall morbidity of this invasive diagnostic method.

Natural History of Asymptomatic Carotid Artery Disease

Asymptomatic carotid artery stenosis has been evaluated by multiple investigators over the past several decades. The degree of stenosis, plaque morphology, and development of disease progression have also been correlated to future neurologic event rates. In a group of 121 patients with greater than 75% stenosis determined by duplex ultrasonography, 60% developed a neurologic event during a 5-year follow-up, whereas only 12% of those with less than 75% stenosis developed an event. The plaque morphology was also assessed to determine the effect, if any, on the future risk of stroke. Soft plaques were more frequently associated with events than those with dense calcifications.[36] Roederer and colleagues found a 46% incidence of ischemic symptoms or carotid occlusion 12 months after progression to more than 80% stenosis.[37] This is in comparison with less than 2% of those plaques that did not show progression over a similar period.[37]

The natural history of asymptomatic carotid disease may be altered by the addition of 3-hydroxy-3-methylglutaryl coenzyme A (HMG-CoA) reductase inhibitors. This medication has been shown to reduce neurologic events, even with normal serum cholesterol levels.[38] There has been increasing interest in using statins to slow the progression of carotid disease. In the Asymptomatic Carotid Artery Plaque Study (ACAPS), lovastatin was compared in a double-blinded study to evaluate the effect on intimal medial thickness and cardiovascular events. In men and women with moderately elevated low-density lipoprotein (LDL) levels, the progression of intimal medial thickness in the carotid arteries was reduced compared with placebo, and lovastatin was also associated with reduced cardiovascular events and mortality.[39]

NATURAL HISTORY OF 60% OR GREATER STENOSIS CONTRALATERAL TO CAROTID OCCLUSION

In a study of the natural history of ≥60% asymptomatic carotid stenosis in patients with contralateral carotid occlusion, AbuRahma and colleagues reported that during a 10-year period, patients with 60 to less than 70% asymptomatic carotid stenosis with contralateral carotid occlusion were entered into a protocol of clinical examination and duplex surveillance every 6 months. All patients underwent maximum medical therapy: antiplatelet therapy, primarily an aspirin regimen; risk factor modification, for example, control of high blood pressure, and diabetes mellitus; some had cholesterol-lowering medications. Late CEAs were considered if lesions became symptomatic or progressed to 70% or greater stenosis. Eighty-two patients were enrolled with a mean follow-up of 59.5 months (range 7 to 141 months). Late strokes were noted in 27 of the 82 patients (33%); 19 (23%) were ipsilateral and eight (10%) were contralateral (side of contralateral carotid occlusion). Late TIAs were noted in 22 of 82 (27%, seven ipsilateral and 15 contralateral). The combined neurologic event (TIA/stroke) rate was 60% (49 of 82, 32% ipsilateral and 28% contralateral). Kaplan-Meier life table analysis showed that the rates of freedom from ipsilateral strokes, all strokes, and progression to 70% or greater stenosis at 1, 2, 3, 4, and 5 years were 94%, 90%, 85%, 80%, 73%; 94%, 89%, 84%, 77%, and 67% and 99%, 96%, 92%, 86%, and 82%, respectively. The ipsilateral stroke-free survival rates at 1, 2, 3, 4, and 5 years were 94%, 88%, 78%, 70%, and 63%. Twenty-one late CEAs were performed with no perioperative stroke/deaths (five for ipsilateral TIAs, nine for ipsilateral strokes, and seven for 70% or greater asymptomatic carotid stenosis). Overall, 20 (24%, 11 with symptoms and 9 asymptomatic) progressed to 70% or greater stenosis. We concluded that even with maximal medical therapy, patients with 60 to less than 70% asymptomatic carotid stenosis and contralateral carotid occlusion carry a higher incidence of ipsilateral strokes and all strokes than what was reported by the ACAS; therefore, prophylactic CEA may be justified in these patients.[40]

NATURAL HISTORY OF CAROTID STENOSIS CONTRALATERAL TO CEA

A few nonrandomized studies have reported the natural history of an asymptomatic carotid artery stenosis contralateral to CEA. AbuRahma and colleagues followed the contralateral carotid arteries of 534 patients after CEA.[41] These patients were from two previously reported randomized trials that compared CEA with primary closure versus patching. All patients were followed up clinically and with duplex ultrasound scanning at 1 month and then every 6 months. Progression was defined as progress to a higher category of stenosis. Of 534 patients, 61 had initial contralateral CEA and 53 had contralateral occlusion, leaving 420 patients available for analysis. At baseline, 162 patients had normal carotid arteries, 157 had less than 50% stenosis, and 95 had 50 to 79% stenoses. Six other patients had 80 to 99% or greater stenosis but refused further treatment or follow-up (too sick to undergo intervention). Overall, carotid artery stenosis progressed in 109 of the 420 patients (26%) at a mean follow-up of 41 months. Progression of carotid artery stenosis was noted in five of 162 patients (3%) with baseline normal carotid arteries. Carotid artery stenosis progressed in 56 of 157 patients (36%) with less than 50% stenosis versus 45 of 95 patients (47%) with 50 to 79% stenosis ($p = .003$). The median time to progression was 24 months for less than 50% carotid artery stenosis and 12 months for 50 to 79% carotid artery stenosis ($p = .035$). At 1, 2, 3, 4, and 5 years, freedom from disease progression in patients with baseline carotid artery stenosis less than 50% was 95%, 78%, 69%, 61%, and 48%, respectively, and in patients with 50 to 79% carotid artery stenosis was 75%, 61%, 51%, 43%, and 33%, respectively ($p = .003$). Freedom from progression in patients with baseline normal carotid arteries at 1 through 5 years was 99%, 98%, 96%, 96%, and 94%, respectively. Late neurologic events referable to the contralateral carotid artery were infrequent (28 of 420 [6.7%] in the entire series; 28 of 258 [which included 157 patients with < 50% stenosis, 95 with ≥ 50 to 79% stenosis, and six with ≥ 80 to 99% stenosis; 10.9%] patients with a contralateral carotid artery stenosis at baseline) and included 10 strokes (3.9% of patients with baseline contralateral stenosis, 2.4% of the whole series) and 18 TIAs (7% in patients with baseline contralateral stenosis; 4.3% for the whole series). However, late contralateral CEA was performed in 62 patients (62 of 420 [15%] in the entire series; 24% [62 of 258] patients with initial contralateral carotid artery stenosis). Survival rates were 96%, 92%, 90%, 87%, and 82%, respectively, at 1 through 5 years. Based on these data, the authors concluded that progression of contralateral carotid artery stenosis was noted in a significant number of patients with baseline contralateral carotid artery stenosis after CEA. Serial clinical studies and duplex ultrasound scanning every 6 to 12 months in patients with 50 to 79% carotid artery stenosis and every 12 to 24 months in patients with 50% or less carotid artery stenosis was adequate to detect disease progression in these patients.

Recommendations for Carotid Intervention/Medical Therapy

Patients with carotid plaque and asymptomatic lesions of less than 60% should be managed with medical treatment only. In asymptomatic patients with greater than 60% carotid stenosis, medical treatment and CEA are currently recommended in good surgical risk patients, particularly those who are at high risk for stroke [*see Table 4 and Table 5*], as long as the risk of stroke in the perioperative period is low.[42] Low is defined by the American Heart Association (AHA) as a less than 3% risk of major perioperative morbidity and mortality.[43]

Table 4 lists the primary and secondary risk factors for stroke, and Table 5 ranks the relative increased risk. The following is a brief summary of these risk factors.

Clinical trials confirmed the reduced risk of stroke and coronary artery disease in hypertensive patients who are treated with both diuretics and beta blockers, but not with angiotensin-converting enzymes (ACE) inhibitors or calcium channel blocking agents. A meta-analysis of several trials of blood pressure reduction showed that a 5.8 mm Hg drop in diastolic blood pressure produced a 42% reduction in the incidence of all stroke over a 2- to 3-year period.[44] Paradoxically, it should be noted that aggressive lowering of hypertension in elderly patients may cause an increase in stroke.

Table 4 Risk Factors for Stroke

Primary
- Increasing age
- Male sex
- Family history
- African-American and Asian race
- Smoking*
- Hypertension*
- Cholesterol*
- Diabetes*

Secondary
- Past TIA or stroke
- Carotid artery stenosis
- Previous angina/MI
- Cardiac arrhythmias
- Peripheral vascular disease
- Left ventricular hypertrophy

MI = myocardial infarction; TIA = transient ischemic stroke.
*Can be modified.

Table 5 Ranking of Modifiable Stroke Risk Factors

Factor	Median Risk
Past TIA or stroke	10.0 times
Hypertension	6.0 times
Atrial fibrillation	5.6 times
Carotid bruits	3.0 times
Coronary artery disease	2.2 times
Left ventricular hypertrophy	2.2 times
Hypercholesterolemia	2 times
Smoking	2 times
Diabetes	1.7 times
Congestive heart failure	1.7 times

TIA = transient ischemic attack.

Isolated systolic hypertension, as defined by a systolic blood pressure of greater than 170 mm Hg, should also be treated because an 11 mm Hg decrease in the systolic pressure was associated with a 36% reduction in the stroke risk.[44]

Diabetes mellitus increases the risk of stroke by 2.5 to 3.5 times compared with controls. Insulin resistance is also associated with increased atherosclerosis of the carotid arteries independent of the glucose level, insulin levels, and other major cardiovascular risk factors. However, the ability of oral hypoglycemic medication and insulin to reduce the risk of stroke has yet to be proven in prospective trials.[45]

Cigarette smoking increases the risk of stroke by two times because of accelerated atherosclerosis of the carotid artery, which may be independent of other factors. The risk of stroke decreases rapidly with the cessation of cigarette smoking, regardless of age, compared with a 50% reduction of risk of coronary events in 1 year.[45]

Several studies correlated the relation between cholesterol and stroke risk with variable results. It is generally believed that elevated total cholesterol and LDL are independent risk factors for ischemic events. A pooled meta-analysis of four pravastatin trials documented a 16% reduction in the risk of stroke,[46] and the ACAPS documented fewer strokes in the lovastatin group than in the placebo group (five versus zero).[47]

The AHA guidelines for risk factor modification include the following recommendations concerning tobacco use, hypertension, cholesterol management, and blood glucose goals.[43] Blood pressure should be aggressively lowered to less than 120/80 mm Hg. ACEs and angiotension receptor blockers should be first-line therapy in patients who are diabetic, in addition to lifestyle changes that include diet and exercise. Target levels for the hemoglobin A_{1C} should be less than 7% to reduce the risk of both micro- and macrovascular sequleae of hyperglycemia. Statin agents are recommended to manage hypercholesterolemia with target goals of LDL cholesterol < 100 mg/dL and in patients with multiple risk factors to be lowered to less than 70 mg/dL. In addition to the benefit of stroke reduction, many other benefits of statins have been demonstrated in vascular patients, including reduction of cardiovascular events and overall mortality; this was irrespective of age, gender, or cholesterol level, raising the question of a possible pleiotrophic effect by these agents.[48]

Other studies have continued to accumulate in the literature that have shown a favorable decrease in neurologic event rates of both carotid surgery and stenting with the perioperative administration of statin agents. The Stroke Prevention by Aggressive Reduction in Cholesterol Levels (SPARCL) trial enrolled patients with recent TIA or stroke, and the 5-year risk of stroke was reduced by 16% with statin therapy compared with placebo.[49]

ANTIPLATELET THERAPY IN THE PREVENTION OF STROKE

The current consensus is that patients who have an ischemic cerebral event secondary to atherosclerosis should receive antiplatelet therapy. Several clinical trials have reviewed the efficacy of these medications. The Ticlopidine Aspirin Stroke Study (TASS) was a blinded trial at 56 medical centers that compared the effects of ticlopidine with aspirin.[50] At 3 years, 3,069 patients were evaluated and the rates of fatal and nonfatal stroke were 10% for the ticlopidine and 13% for aspirin, a 21% risk reduction. It should be noted that severe, but reversible, neutropenia developed in less than 1% of patients taking ticlopidine. The Clopidogrel versus Aspirin in Patients at Risk of Ischemic Events (CAPRIE) study randomized 19,185 patients over a 3-year period.[51] Patients treated with clopidogrel experienced a 5.32% annual risk of ischemic stroke, MI, or vascular death versus 5.83% with aspirin, with a relative risk reduction of 8.7% in favor of clopidogrel. Finally, the European Stroke Prevention Study 2 (ESPS-2) was a multicenter, blinded, randomized, placebo-controlled study with four treatment arms consisting of aspirin, dipyridamole, aspirin with dipyridamole, and placebo. This study showed that the combination of extended-release dipyridamole plus aspirin was additive and produced highly sufficient benefits, with a 37% risk reduction for stroke prevention.[52] There is no level 1 evidence to support the use of clopidogrel over aspirin in asymptomatic patients. However, our recommendation is to use one aspirin daily (81 or 325 mg). Clopidogrel (75 mg daily) is used only if aspirin therapy is contraindicated.

LEVEL I EVIDENCE SUPPORTING CEA IN ASYMPTOMATIC PATIENTS

Two large prospective randomized trials [*see Table 6*] have shown the superiority of CEA plus medical treatment versus medical treatment alone.[24,53]

The ACAS was the largest randomized trial to examine the management of asymptomatic carotid stenosis. Patients with 60% or greater asymptomatic carotid artery stenosis (n = 1,662) were randomized to best medical treatment or CEA. After a median follow-up of 2.7 years, the 5-year risk of ipsilateral stroke by Kaplan-Meier projection was 5.1% for CEA and 11% for medically treated patients (p = .004). This showed a relative risk reduction of 53% and an absolute risk reduction of 5.9%. The estimated 5-year event rate was more favorable with surgery for men than women: 4.1% versus 12.1% in men, compared with 7.3% versus 8.7% in women. Part of this was attributed to higher perioperative events in women: 3.6% versus 1.7% in men.

The second largest trial is the UK Medical Research Council Asymptomatic Carotid Surgery Trial (ACST). This was a prospective randomized trial of CEA in asymptomatic patients in which more than 3,000 patients were randomly assigned either to undergo immediate CEA or to be placed on indefinite deferral. For patients who were referred for immediate CEA, half underwent surgery within 1 month of referral: 88% underwent surgery within 1 year. Combining the rate of perioperative events and the nonperioperative strokes, the 5-year results indicate a stroke rate of 6.4% in the group undergoing immediate surgery compared with 11.8% in the deferred group. These findings were similar to the ACAS findings; however, the ACST found a similar benefit for men and women. In addition, no difference was found in the degree of stenosis and the benefit of surgery. Presently, the second ACST-2 is being conducted comparing CEA versus carotid artery stenting for asymptomatic carotid stenosis.

The medical community has questioned the current accuracy of these studies, considering the current improvements in best medical treatment. These two prospective randomized trials were performed prior to widespread use of agents (statins) that have been shown to reduce the risk of stroke. In addition, these studies required surgeons preselected with excellent surgical results and may not be extrapolated to all surgeons performing CEA. As stated earlier, for the patient to derive benefit from prophylactic intervention, the patient's risk of medical therapy alone with the projected natural history for that patient must exceed that of the specific surgeon's intervention. Several patient factors should be considered prior to offering intervention.

Duplex criteria were used for enrolment in the medical treatment arm for the ACAS study and arteriographic confirmation prior to CEA. However, some centers were allowed to do CEA based on duplex ultrasonography if their duplex ultrasonographic findings were validated against angiography. This requirement was associated with a 1.2% combined event rate with angiography, which, if eliminated by imaging today, that is, duplex ultrasonography or noninvasive testing, would have increased the interventional benefit compared with medical therapy at that time.

Table 6 Asymptomatic Randomized Trials Comparing Medical to Medical and Surgical Treatment (Stenosis > 60%)

Trial	n	Perioperative Stroke Rate (%)	5 yr Stroke (Surgery/Medical %)	NNT
ACAS	1,662	2.3	5.1/11	17
ACST	3,120	2.8	6.4/11.8	19

ACAS = Asymptomatic Carotid Atherosclerosis Study; ACST = Asymptomatic Carotid Surgery Trial; NNT = number needed to treat to prevent one stroke.

Decision Making for Medical Therapy Alone versus Intervention

ANATOMIC FACTORS

Asymptomatic lesions that are either higher or lower than can easily be accessed by the surgeon pose specific limitations. High lesions are defined as those at or above the second cervical vertebrae often requiring additional surgical maneuvers to safely remove the lesion. These include but are not limited to dividing external carotid branches, the ansa cervicalis, and the digastric muscle and, rarely, excessive traction and jaw mandibular manipulation. Associated cranial nerve morbidity can be substantial; even if the patient does not have an intraoperative neurologic event, the long-term morbidity may exceed the risk of medical treatment. Similarly for lesions below the clavicle, the natural history has not been well defined, and surgical treatment often requires extra-anatomic bypass or sternotomy. Our group has used retrograde stenting techniques for these proximal lesions as other groups have described, but no prospective studies have shown the best way to treat these combined lesions.

The status of the contralateral carotid artery has also been associated with increased risk of carotid intervention. Contralateral occlusion has been shown to be associated with increased risk of perioperative events with CEA.[23] However, we have not found this to be true in our experience: our perioperative, late stroke, and survival rates of CEA were comparable in patients with and without contralateral occlusion.[54]

An increasing degree of stenosis may also be associated with higher chances of stroke in asymptomatic patients; however, in the ACAS study, there were too few strokes to permit a subgroup analysis of the effect of the degree of stenosis on the ability to benefit from CEA.[24] However, in both the NASCET and the European Carotid Surgery Trialist (ECST) study, a higher degree of stenosis in symptomatic patients was consistently observed to be associated with a higher stroke risk, as well as a greater benefit from surgical therapy. The ECST study, using angiographic data from the asymptomatic carotid arteries from 2,295 patients, reported that the Kaplan-Meier estimate of stroke risk at 3 years was only 2% and remained low, below 2%, in patients with less than 70% stenosis, in contrast to a stroke rate of 9.8% for patients with 70 to 79% stenosis and 14.4% for those with 80 to 99% stenosis.[55]

Recurrent stenosis following CEA has been an exclusion criterion in large prospective randomized trials. The national trend has been to consider carotid stenting (for ≥ 80% asymptomatic recurrent stenosis or ≥ 50% symptomatic recurrent stenosis) in this group secondary to increased risk of perioperative neurologic deficits compared with the initial procedure. Cranial nerve injury also occurs more frequently in the setting of redo surgery and has also been avoided by transcatheter intervention.[56]

The presence of asymptomatic cerebral infarct ipsilateral to the asymptomatic carotid stenosis on a CT scan or MRI may identify patients who would benefit from surgery.[57] In asymptomatic carotid stenosis patients, the incidence of silent strokes demonstrated by CT has been reported to be 10% in patients with 35 to 50% stenosis on duplex ultrasonography, 17% in those with 50 to 75% stenosis, and 50% in those with greater than 75% stenosis. The incidence of silent cerebral infarct demonstrated by MRI in the same type of population has also been reported to be 42%, increasing to 75% for greater than 50% stenosis.[57]

PATIENT FACTORS

As noted, octogenarians were excluded in the ACAS. Increasing age has been associated with overall increased risk of events following surgery. Therefore, prophylactic CEA for asymptomatic stenosis in the elderly should be performed with caution unless the overall medical status is good.

The derived benefit from CEA for women compared with men has also been less in several studies.[24] For uncertain reasons, CEA in women has been associated with increased stroke rates compared with men. Interestingly, women with asymptomatic carotid disease treated medically may do better than their male counterparts. In a subgroup analysis, the ACAS showed that the absolute reduction in the risk of perioperative stroke or death or ipsilateral stroke at 2.7 years was 3.6% (95% CI 1.1 to 9.9) for men and 0.5% (95% CI 0.01 to 2.7) for women. With this combination, a more conservative approach may apply for women, particularly with 60 to 80% asymptomatic stenosis.

The presence of atherosclerosis in other locations appears to carry additional risk. In particular, concomitant severe coronary disease and asymptomatic carotid stenosis has been extensively studied. Perioperative stroke and death have been seen with combined coronary artery bypass grafting (CABG) and CEA, as reported by Naylor and colleagues.[58]

SURGEON FACTORS

Surgeons should use and quote their own perioperative events; not infrequently, surgeons report the risk with major landmark studies and not their personal results. These studies typically have rigorous standards that are required for enrolment. It has been shown in multiple surgical procedures that higher volume surgeons generally have better perioperative results than lower volume surgeons. The American College of Surgeons has stressed personal evaluation of surgical results and has included this in the continued competency guidelines. The AHA currently recommends regular review of independent results and performing combined carotid surgery only when the surgeon's event rate is less than 5%.[13]

Figure 2 summarizes a practical approach for managing patients with asymptomatic carotid bruit/asymptomatic carotid artery stenosis, as follows:

Step 1. This step distinguishes a carotid bruit from a noncarotid bruit, for example, venous hum, cardiac murmur, or intrathoracic vascular structures.

Step 2. This step determines if the carotid bruit is symptomatic or asymptomatic.

Step 3. A carotid duplex sonogram is obtained to determine the severity of the carotid artery stenosis if the patient is felt to have a carotid bruit secondary to carotid stenosis.

Step 4. For patients with less than 60% stenosis, medical therapy, as indicated earlier, with carotid surveillance is recommended.

Step 5. The frequency of surveillance will depend on the severity of the carotid stenosis; that is, patients with less than 50% can be screened every 1 to 2 years, and patients with greater than 50% stenosis can be screened every 6 to 12 months.

Step 6. If the stenosis was 60 to less than 80%, a determination needs to be made whether it was progressive stenosis (stenosis that was < 60% and progressed to < 80%).

Step 7. If not, the patient should be evaluated for stroke risk factors.

Step 8. If the stroke risk is low, medical treatment and surveillance are adequate.

Step 9. If risk factors are present, the patient should be evaluated for his or her life expectancy.

Step 10. If the life expectancy is poor, medical treatment is adequate.

Steps 11 and 12. If the life expectancy is good, the patient should be evaluated for his or her operative risk.

Steps 13 and 14. If the patient is a good surgical candidate, carotid duplex ultrasonography is technically adequate.

Step 15. A CEA may be considered.

Step 16. If carotid duplex ultrasonography is inadequate, other imaging is necessary; however, for patients with poor surgical risk, medical therapy is recommended.

Step 17. Meanwhile, if the stenosis was progressive, and if after evaluation of life expectancy, the patient is felt to be in good condition and a good operative risk, CEA would be recommended; otherwise, medical therapy is adequate.

Step 18. For patients who are poor operative risks, medical therapy is recommended.

Step 19. Patients with 80 to 99% stenosis should be evaluated for their life expectancy, and if it is felt to be good, operative evaluation will follow, and if satisfactory with good quality duplex ultrasonography, they will undergo CEA.

Step 20. In poor surgical risk patients with adequate life expectancy, carotid artery stenting can be an alternative therapy.

Financial Disclosures: None Reported

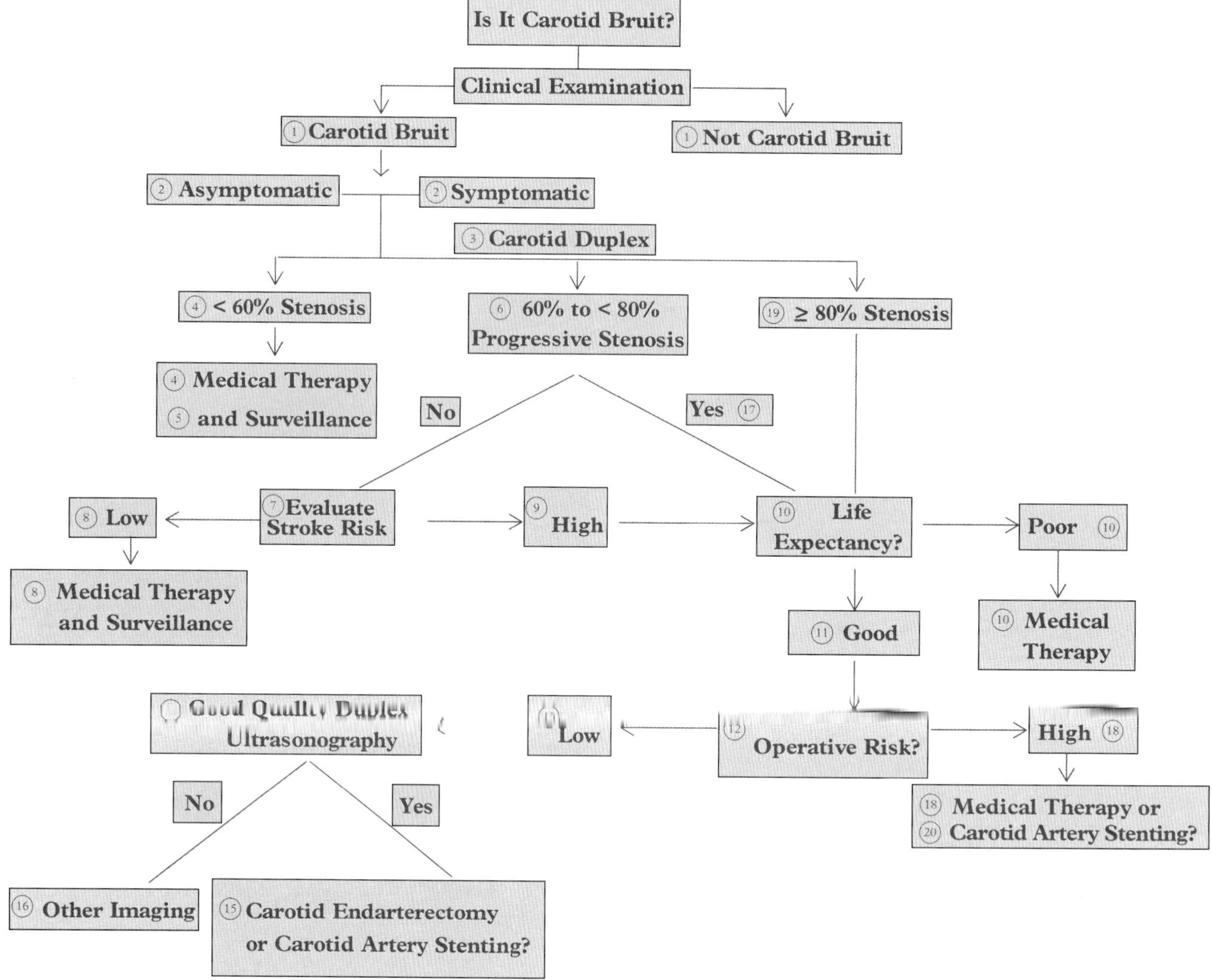

Figure 2 **Protocol of management of asymptomatic carotid bruit/carotid artery stenosis.**

References

1. Warlow CP, Dennis MS, van Gijn J. What caused the tranisent or persisting ischaemic event? In: Warlow CP, Dennis MS, van Gijn J, et al, editors. Stroke: a practical guide to management. Oxford (UK): Blackwell Science; 2001. p. 223–300.
2. Hankey GJ. Impact of treatment of people with transient ischemic attacks on stroke incidence and public health. Cerebrovasc Dis 1996;6 Suppl1:26–33.
3. Kakkos SK, Sabetai M, Tegos T, et al. Asymptomatic Carotid Stenosis and Risk of Stroke (ACSRS) Study Group. Silent embolic infarcts on computed tomography brain scans and risk of ipsilateral hemispheric events in patients with asymptomatic internal carotid artery stenosis. J Vasc Surg 2009;50: 707–8.
4. Jones FL. Frequency, characteristics and importance of the cervical venous hum in adults. N Engl J Med 1962;267:658–60.
5. Sauve JS, Laupacis A, Ostbye T, et al. Does this patient have a clinically important carotid bruit? JAMA 1993;270:2843–5.
6. Caplan LR. Carotid artery disease. N Engl J Med 1986;315:886–8.
7. Messert B, Marra TR, Zerofsky RA. Supraclavicular and carotid bruits in hemodialysis patients. Ann Neurol 1977;2:535–6.
8. Davies KN, Humphrey PRD. Do carotid bruits predict disease of the internal carotid arteries? Postgrad Med J 1994;70:433–5.
9. Sauve JS, Thorpe KE, Sackett DL, et al. Can bruits distinguish high-grade from moderate symptomatic carotid stenosis? The North American Symptomatic Carotid Endarterectomy Trial. Ann Intern Med 1994;120: 633–7.
10. Ratchford EV, Zhezhen J, Di Tullio MR, et al. Carotid bruit for the detection of hemodynamically significant carotid stenosis: the Northern Manhatten Study. Neurol Res 2009;31:748–52.
11. Wiebers DO, Whisnant JP, Sandok BA, O'Fallen WM. Prospective comparison of a cohort with asymptomatic carotid bruit and a population-based cohort without carotid bruit. Stroke 1990;21:984–8.
12. Pickett CI, Jackson JL, Hemann BA, Atwood E. Carotid bruits as a prognostic indicator of cardiovascular death and myocardial infarction: a meta-analysis. Lancet 2008;371: 1587–94.
13. AbuRahma AF, Robinson PA. Prospective clinicopathophysiologic follow-up study of asymptomatic neck bruit. Am Surg 1990;56: 108–13.
14. Anderson KM, Odell PM, Wilson PW, et al. Cardiovascular disease risk profiles. Am Heart J 1991;121:293–8.
15. Anderson KM, Wilson PW, Odell PM, et al. An updated coronary risk profile: a statement for health professionals. Circulation 1991;83: 356–62.
16. Wolf PA, D'Agostino RB, Belanger AJ, et al. Probability of stroke: a risk profile from the Framingham Study. Stroke 1991;22:312–8.
17. Wolf PA, D'Agostino RB, Kannel WB, et al. Cigarette smoking as a risk factor for stroke. The Framingham Study. JAMA 1988;259: 1025–9.
18. Heyman A, Wilkinson WE, Heyden S, et al. Risk of stroke in asymptomatic persons with cervical arterial bruits: a population study in Evans County, Georgia. N Engl J Med 1980;302:838–41.
19. Wiebers DO, Whisnant JP, Sandok BA, et al. Prospective comparison of a cohort with asymptomatic carotid bruit and a

population-based cohort without carotid bruit. Stroke 1990;21:984–8.
20. Shorr RI, Johnson KC, Wan JY, et al. The prognostic significance of asymptomatic carotid bruits in the elderly. J Gen Intern Med 1998;13:86–90.
21. Benavente OR, Moher D, Pham B. Carotid endarterectomy for asymptomatic carotid stenosis: a meta-analysis. BMJ 1998;317: 1477–80.
22. Chambers BR, You RX, Donnan GA. Carotid endarterectomy for asymptomatic carotid stenosis. Cochrane Database Syst Rev 2000;(2):CD001923.
23. North American Symptomatic Carotid Endarterectomy Trial Collaborators (NASCET). Beneficial effect of carotid endarterectomy in symptomatic patients with high-grade carotid stenosis. N Engl J Med 1991;325:445–53.
24. Executive Committee for the Asymptomatic Carotid Atherosclerosis Study. Endarterectomy for asymptomatic patients with high grade stenosis. JAMA 1995;273:1421–8.
25. Veith FJ. Treating carotid plaques in the dark. Vascular Specialist 2007;3.
26. AbuRahma AF, Robinson PA, Stickler DL, et al. Proposed new duplex classification for threshold stenoses used in various symptomatic and asymptomatic carotid endarterectomy trials. Ann Vasc Surg 1998;12: 349–58.
27. Blakeley DD, Oddone EZ, Hasselblad V, et al. Noninvasive carotid artery testing: a meta-analysis review. Ann Intern Med 1997; 122:360–7.
28. Reilly LM, Lusby RJ, Hughes L, et al. Carotid plaque histology using real-time ultrasonography: clinical and therapeutic implications. Am J Surg 1983;146:188–93.
29. AbuRahma AF, Wulu JT, Crotty B. Carotid plaque ultrasonic heterogeneity and severity of stenosis. Stroke 2002;33;1772–5.
30. Nicolaides AN. Asymptomatic carotid stenosis and risk of stroke: identification of a high risk group (ACRS): a natural history study. Int Angiol 1995;14:21–3.
31. Biasi GM, Froio A, Diethrich EB, et al. Carotid plaque echolucency increases the risk of stroke in carotid stenting: the Imaging in Carotid Angioplasty and Risk of Stroke (ICAROS) Study. Circulation 2004;110: 756–62.
32. Reiter M, Bucek RA, Effenberger I, et al. Plaque echolucency is not associated with the risk of stroke in carotid stenting. Stroke 2006;37:2378–80.
33. Rubin BG. Impact of plaque characterization on carotid interventions. Perspect Vasc Surg Endovasc Surg 2006;18:312–5.
34. Young GR, Humphrey PRD, Nixon TE, et al. Variability in measurement of extracranial internal carotid artery stenosis as displayed by both digital subtraction and magnetic resonance angiography: an assessment of three caliper techniques and visual impression of stenosis. Stroke 1996;27: 467–73.
35. Turnipseed WD, Kennell TW, Turski PA, et al. Magnetic resonance angiography and duplex scanning: non-invasive tests for selecting symptomatic carotid endarterectomy candidates. Surgery 1993;114:643–8.
36. O'Halleran LW, Kennely MM, McClurken M, Johnson JM. Natural history of asymptomatic carotid plaque. Am J Surg 1987;154: 659–62.
37. Roederer GK, Langlois YE, Jager KA, et al. The natural history of carotid arterial disease in asymptomatic patients with cervical bruits. Stroke 1984;15:605–13.
38. Crouse JR, Byington RP, Hoen HM, Furberg CD. Reductase inhibitor monotherapy and stroke prevention. Arch Intern Med 1997;157: 1305–10.
39. Furberg CD, Adams HP, Applegate WB, et al. Effect of lovastatin on early carotid atherosclerosis and cardiovascular events. Circulation 1994;90;1679–87.
40. AbuRahma AF, Metz MJ, Robinson PA. Natural history of ≥ 60% asymptomatic carotid stenosis in patients with contralateral carotid occlusion. Ann Surg 2003;238: 551–62.
41. AbuRahma AF, Cook CC, Metz MJ, et al. Natural history of carotid artery stenosis, contralateral to endarterectomy: results from two randomized prospective trials. J Vasc Surg 2003;38:1154–60.
42. Hobson RW, Mackey WC, Ascher E, et al. Management of atherosclerotic carotid artery disease: clinical practice guidelines of the Society for Vascular Surgery. J Vasc Surg 2008;48:480–6.
43. Sacci RL, Adams R, Albers F, et al. Guidelines for the prevention of stroke in patients with ischaemic stroke or transient ischaemic attack: a statement for healthcare professionals from the American Heart Association/ American Stroke Association Council on Stroke, co-sponsored by the Council on Cardiovascular Radiology and Intervention. Stroke 2006;37:577–617.
44. Collins R, Peto R, MacMahon S, et al. Blood pressure, stroke, and coronary heart disease. II. Short-term reductions in blood pressure: overview of randomized drug trials in their epidemiological context. Lancet 1990;335: 827–38.
45. Jichici D. Medical therapy for transient ischemic attacks and ischemic stroke. In: Ernst CB, Stanley JC, editors. Current therapy in vascular surgery. 4th ed. St. Louis, MO: Mosby; 2001. p. 24–30.
46. Byington RP, Jukema JW, Salonen JT, et al. Reduction in cardiovascular events during pravastatin therapy: pooled analysis of clinical events of the Pravastatin Atherosclerosis Intervention Group. Circulation 1995;92: 2419–25.
47. The Scandinavian Simvastatin Survival Study (4S): randomized trial of cholesterol lowering in 4444 patients with coronary heart disease. Lancet 1994;344:1383–9.
48. Heart Protection Study Collaborative Group. MRC/BHF Heart Protection Study of Cholesterol lowering with simvastatin in 20536 high-risk individuals: a randomised placebo controlled trial. Lancet 2002;360: 7–22
49. Goldstein LB, Amarenco P, Zivin J, et al. Statin treatment and stroke outcome in the Stroke Prevention by Aggressive Reduction in Cholesterol Levels (SPARCL) trial. Stroke Prevention by Aggressive Reduction in Cholesterol Levels Investigators. Stroke 2009;40:3526–31.
50. Hass WK, Easton JD, Adams HP Jr, et al. A randomized trial comparing ticlopidine hydrochloride with aspirin for the prevention of stroke in high risk patients. Ticlopidine Aspirin Stroke Study Group. N Engl J Med 1989;321:501–7.
51. CAPRIE Steering Committee: a randomized, blinded trial of clopidogrel versus aspirin in patients at risk of ischaemic events (CAPRIE). Lancet 1996;348:1329–39.
52. Diener HC, Cunha L, Forbes C, et al. Dipyridamole and acetylsalicylic acid in the secondary prevention of stroke: European Stroke Prevention Study 2. J Neurol Sci 1996; 143:1–13.
53. Asymptomatic Carotid Surgery Trial Collaborators. The MRC Asymptomatic Carotid Surgery Trial (ACST): carotid endarterectomy prevents disabling and fatal carotid territory stroke. Lancet 2004;363:1491–502.
54. AbuRahma AF, Holt SM, Herzog TA, Mowery NT. Perioperative and late stroke rates of carotid endarterectomy contralateral to carotid occlusion: results from randomized trial. Stroke 2000;31:1566–71.
55. European Carotid Surgery Trialists' Collaborative Group. Risk of stroke in the distribution of an asymptomatic carotid artery. Lancet 1995;345:209.
56. AbuRahma AF, Abu-Halimah S, Bensenhaver J, et al. Primary carotid artery stenting versus carotid artery stenting for post-carotid endarterectomy stenosis: early and mid-term outcomes. J Vasc Surg 2009;50:1031–9.
57. Hougaku H, Matsumoto M, Handa N, et al. Asymptomatic carotid lesions and silent cerebral infarction. Stroke 1994;25:566–70.
58. Naylor AR, Mehta Z, Rothwell PM, Bell PRF. Carotid artery disease and stroke during coronary artery bypass: a critical review of the literature. Eur J Vasc Endovasc Surg 2002; 23:283–94.
59. Chambers BR, Norris JW. Outcome in patients with asymptomatic neck bruits. N Engl J Med 1986;315:860–5.
60. Zhu CZ, Norris JW. Role of carotid stenosis in ischemic stroke. Stroke 1990;21:1131–4.
61. Lusiani L, Visonà A, Castellani V, et al. Prevalence of atherosclerotic lesions at the carotid bifurcation in patients with asymptomatic bruits: an echo-Doppler (duplex) study. Angiology 1985;36:235–9.
62. Floriani M, Giulini SM, Anzola GP, et al. Predictive value of cervical bruit for the detection of obstructive lesions of the internal carotid artery: data from 2000 patients. Ital J Neurol Sci 1989;10:321–7.
63. Colgan MP, Strode GR, Sommer JD, et al. Prevalence of asymptomatic carotid disease: results of duplex scanning in 348 unselected volunteers. J Vasc Surg 1988;8:674–8.

3 PULSATILE ABDOMINAL MASS

*Guillermo A. Escobar, MD, and Gilbert R. Upchurch Jr, MD**

Assessment of a Pulsatile Abdominal Mass

When a pulsatile abdominal mass is found on physical examination, the location of the mass and the symptoms associated with it become essential clinical clues. The underlying condition may range in severity from benign to life threatening. Pulsatile masses in the abdomen are either attributable to a large blood vessel or from another mass (e.g., lymph node, tumor, abscess) that is simply in close proximity to a blood vessel and the pulsations are transmitted to the skin. Thus, further evaluation is imperative because in certain clinical settings, immediate transport to the operating room will be necessary. Consequentially, inappropriate treatment can be catastrophic, so it is important to base one's approach to assessment and management of a pulsatile abdominal mass as firmly as possible on the available evidence. In what follows, a clinical approach based on relevant evidence is outlined.

Clinical Evaluation

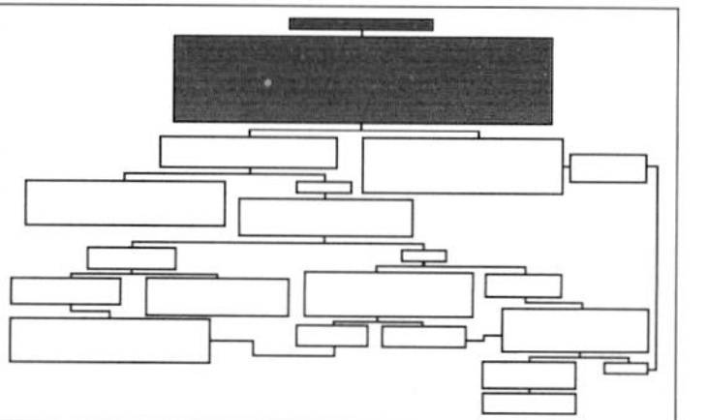

The most feared cause of a pulsatile abdominal mass is an abdominal aortic aneurysm (AAA). In the United States, AAAs are present in 3 to 9% of the population, resulting in approximately 15,000 fatalities each year.[1] The incidence and penetrance of aneurysms are variable according to age and race. As an example, in 2002, AAAs were one of the 10 most common causes of death in Asian or Pacific Islander males 20 to 24 years of age as well as those 65 to 84 years of age![2] Although the number of total aneurysms repaired has remained stable in the last 5 years, the number of deaths from AAA and their rupture has significantly declined over the years.[3,4] On the other hand, with the overall aging of the US population, this disease remains a major threat to public health and should be immediately considered as the diagnosis if the patient is in a high-risk category for AAA.

PRESENTATION

Asymptomatic AAAs are considerably more common than symptomatic AAAs and are often discovered on abdominal or pelvic scans done for other indications (e.g., back pain or renal cysts) rather than on physical examination.[5,6] Plain films of the lumbar region, routinely obtained in patients with back pain, may show a calcified shell of the aorta [*see Figure 1*]. In one review of 31 patients with surgically proven ruptured AAAs, 65% had calcification of the aneurysm that was visible on a plain abdominal radiograph.[7] In addition, ultrasonography (US) and computed tomography (CT) are nearly 100% sensitive in detecting AAAs.[8] In elderly patients, evaluation of the aorta should be routinely included in abdominal US; scanning of the aorta adds, on average, only 43 seconds to the study.[9] If an AAA is unexpectedly found, either the patient is followed or the aneurysm is repaired, depending on the clinical situation and the size of the aneurysm (see below).

Ruptured AAAs, on the other hand, give rise to pronounced symptoms, and the patient's condition may range from hemodynamic stability to class IV shock. When the patient is unstable, further workup is unnecessary and emergency repair is indicated. The situation is less clear when the patient is stable, albeit without normal vital signs. The traditional presentation of a ruptured AAA is a triad comprising hypotension, back or abdominal pain, and a pulsatile abdominal mass. Unfortunately, this traditional presentation occurs less than half of the time. In a study of 116 patients with ruptured AAAs, 45% were hypotensive, 72% had pain, and 83% had a pulsatile abdominal mass.[10] Accordingly, it is essential not to be lulled into a false sense of security when evaluating a hemodynamically stable patient with a pulsatile abdominal mass. Although a ruptured AAA is an uncommon event in a patient with a stable blood pressure and no abdominal pain, the absence of these symptoms does not rule out the possibility. Another misleading scenario occurs when a patient arrives at the hospital several days after the rupture complaining of unrelenting back or abdominal pain and this is disregarded for a musculoskeletal etiology. Bruising may be seen around the pubis, which represents blood in the retroperitoneum that has been there long enough to diffuse to the skin.

Symptomatic or ruptured aneurysms can mimic many other acute medical conditions and therefore are part of multiple differential diagnoses. The following conditions all may be confused with ruptured aneurysms: (1) perforated viscus, (2) mesenteric ischemia, (3) strangulated hernia, (4) ruptured visceral artery aneurysm, (5) acute cholecystitis, (6) acute pancreatitis, (7) acute appendicitis, (8) ruptured necrotic hepatobiliary cancer, (9) lymphoma, and (10) abscess. One must remember that patients with risk factors for AAA are at high risk for other cardiovascular diseases [*see* History, *below*]. A potentially lethal mistake is to rush to operate on a patient who has an AAA that presents with chest pain and hemodynamic instability without considering that the pain and instability may all be attributable to an acute myocardial infarction (MI) or pulmonary embolus rather than a nonruptured AAA. Therefore, care must be taken to thoughtfully and expeditiously evaluate patients with this constellation of signs and symptoms. Fortunately, misdiagnosis of a ruptured AAA is rare, and most patients who make it to the emergency department will allow enough time to undergo proper imaging prior to having to undergo resection.[11,12] One

* The authors and editors gratefully acknowledge the contributions of the previous author, Timothy A. Schaub, MD, to the development and writing of this chapter.

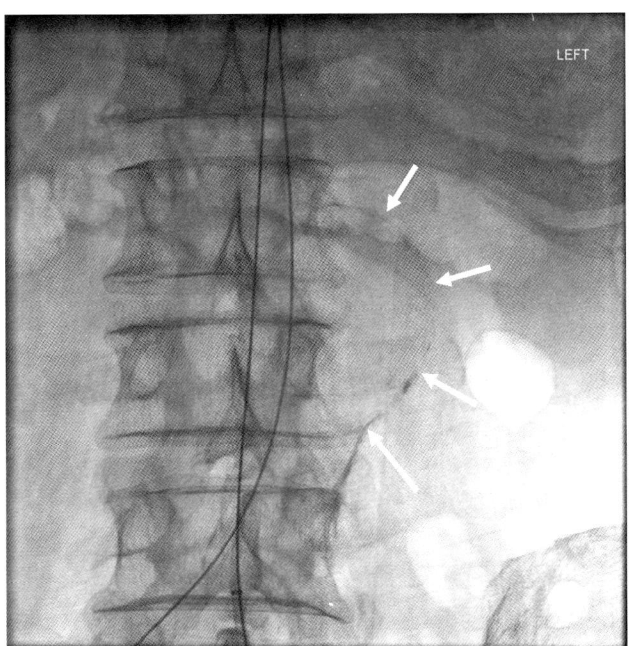

Figure 1 **Plain abdominal x-ray for the diagnosis of aneurysms. Noncontrast x-ray film of the abdomen demonstrating the calcified outline (*arrows*) of an abdominal aortic aneurysm.**

should be exceptionally skeptical of an aneurysm being the cause for instability if the aneurysm is small (< 5 cm). Most patients who do undergo an operation for a misdiagnosis either benefit from or at least are not harmed by the operation as most abdominal catastrophes may benefit from surgical exploration. This alleviates some potential concerns about taking an aggressive approach to a suspected ruptured AAA.[13] Conversely, AAAs can mimic other disease processes. In one study, nearly one in five patients with symptomatic AAAs in an emergency department were originally diagnosed as having nephroureterolithiasis.[14] Patients who have urologic symptoms, but whose urinalysis is normal, may benefit from an AAA workup; radiologic evidence of ureteral involvement is present in as many as 71% of AAAs.[15]

HISTORY

The patient's medical history may be helpful in determining the patient's level of risk for an AAA. Even in the absence of clinical symptoms, knowledge of the risk factors may facilitate earlier diagnosis. The Aneurysm Detection and Management Veterans Affairs Cooperative Study Group trial (commonly referred to as the ADAM trial) found a number of factors to be associated with increased risk for AAA: advanced age, greater height, coronary artery disease (CAD), atherosclerosis, high cholesterol levels, hypertension, and, in particular, smoking.[16] The risk was lower in women, African Americans, and diabetic patients.

AAAs occur almost exclusively in elderly males and are rarely seen in patients younger than 50 years of age. In a 2001 study, the mean age of patients undergoing repair for AAAs in the United States was 72 years.[5] Male patients outnumber female patients by a factor of 4:1 to 6:1 depending on the study cited.[3,17–20] The family members of patients with an AAA are also at significant risk: 12 to 19% of persons undergoing AAA repair have a first-degree relative with an AAA.[21–23] Accordingly, screening is recommended in all men and women older than 50 years who have a family history of AAA.[24] AAAs are over seven times more likely to develop in smokers than in nonsmokers, with the duration of smoking, rather than total number of cigarettes smoked, being the key variable [*see Table 1*].[25]

Of particular importance is identification of risk factors for rupture. The United Kingdom Small Aneurysm (UKSA) trial reported 103 AAA ruptures in 2,257 patients over a period of 7 years, with an annual rupture rate of 2.2%. The factors found to be significantly and independently associated with an increased risk of rupture were female sex, a larger initial AAA diameter, a lower forced expiratory volume in 1 second (FEV_1), a current smoking habit, and a higher mean blood pressure.[25,26] Women are two to four times more likely to experience rupture of an AAA than men are.[27] In a small cohort of 18 patients with aneurysmal aortas greater than 3.5 cm who underwent cardiac and abdominal organ transplantations, seven (41%) of the untreated aortas ruptured and the average growth rate was 1 cm per year. The smallest diameter of a ruptured aorta was 5.1 cm and the mortality of a rupture was 71%. As all eight patients who underwent elective repair survived, aggressive treatment of AAA in patients with or considered for transplantation may be warranted.[28]

The patient's surgical history is also crucial, particularly in that it can shorten the differential diagnosis at presentation by ruling out disease processes (e.g., appendicitis and cholecystitis). In addition, the nature and extent of any previous abdominal procedures may influence the surgeon's operative approach to the AAA repair. When a pulsatile abdominal mass is discovered in a patient who previously underwent open repair of an AAA, it is important to remember that anastomotic pseudoaneurysms[29] or synchronous lesions (e.g., iliac artery aneurysms[30]) can occur at sites remote from the previous repair.

Patients who have undergone endovascular AAA repair may also present with symptoms in the presence or absence of an endoleak. In a 2002 review, most ruptures after endovascular AAA repair occurred with type I endoleaks (lack of a seal with the proximal or distal seal zone of the graft).[31] This clinical scenario is well described and can present as a new pulsatile abdominal mass if the endograft migrates into the aneurysm sac and no longer excludes blood flow from it [*see Figure 2*].[31–33] When this occurs in the proximal seal zone

Table 1 **Risk Factors Associated with AAA Development**
Factors positively associated with development of AAA
Increased age
Increased height
Coronary artery disease
Any atherosclerosis
High cholesterol levels
Hypertension
Smoking
Male sex
Family history (first-degree relative)
Factors negatively associated with development of AAA
Female sex
Black race
Presence of diabetes

AAA = abdominal aortic aneurysm.

Patient Presents with Pulsatile Abdominal Mass

Obtain focused history and physical examination

HPI: Presence or absence of pain, location, associated symptoms

PMH: Associated risk factors for development, risk factors of rupture (see Tables)

PSH: May affect differential diagnosis, potential repair approach

FH: Those patients with relatives with AAA at increased risk for development of AAA

SH: Smoking increases risk of AAA by factor of 7

Physical examination: Examine vital signs for stability, painful aorta(?); palpation of abdomen is safe but alone is a poor method of aneurysm detection and screening

Obtain large-bore peripheral access and crossmatch for blood. Avoid vascular access in groins in case endovascular repair is possible.

Assessment: Stable versus unstable?

Stable

Obtain sonogram for detection of presence of aneurysm

Minimal resuscitation (SBP > 90 mm Hg or enough for normal mental status)

Aneurysm Not Present

Obtain further workup of other complaints

If aortic diameter is normal and patient is older than age 60, no further screening may be needed

If aorta is ectatic, repeat sonogram in 5 to 8 years or if patient is symptomatic

Aneurysm Present

Pain

Assess if patient is having significant pain or discomfort, especially in back, abdomen, legs, or testicles

Palpate aorta and assess for pain

Pain is Absent

Risk of ruptured aneurysm is low

Aneurysm Less than 5.5 cm

Risk of rupture in 1 year less than risk of operative repair

Risk of Rupture Low

Optimize medical management

Follow-up ultrasonography based on initial aortic diameter (3 to 24 months)

If growth accelerated or becomes symptomatic, offer repair

Educate patient on signs and symptoms of symptomatic AAA and AAA rupture

Aneurysm Greater than 5.5 cm

Risk of rupture in 1 year greater than risk of operative repair

Determine if patient willing to undergo evaluation for repair

Go to elective repair algorithm

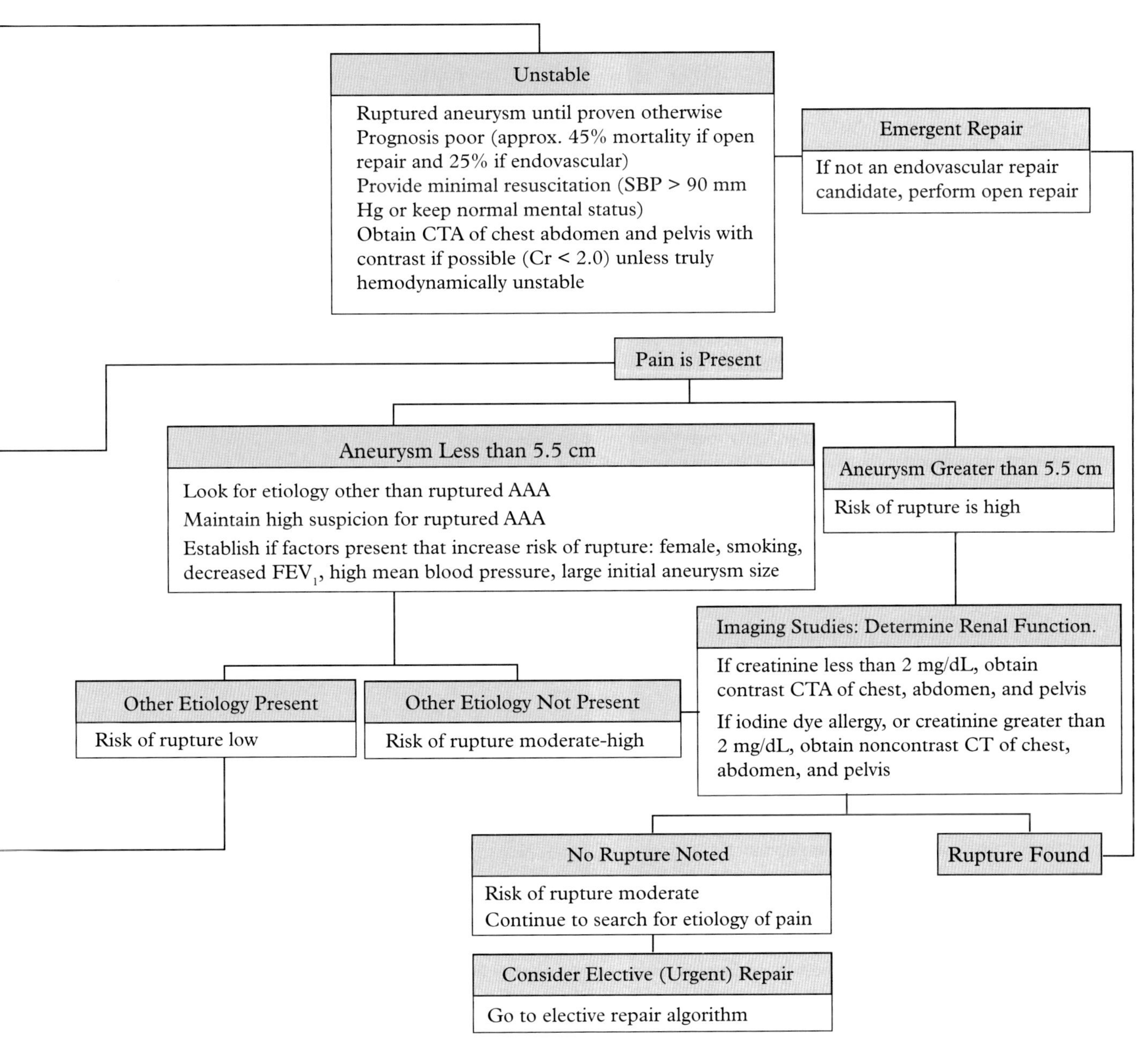
Unstable
Ruptured aneurysm until proven otherwise
Prognosis poor (approx. 45% mortality if open repair and 25% if endovascular)
Provide minimal resuscitation (SBP > 90 mm Hg or keep normal mental status)
Obtain CTA of chest abdomen and pelvis with contrast if possible (Cr < 2.0) unless truly hemodynamically unstable
Emergent Repair
If not an endovascular repair candidate, perform open repair
Pain is Present
Aneurysm Less than 5.5 cm
Look for etiology other than ruptured AAA
Maintain high suspicion for ruptured AAA
Establish if factors present that increase risk of rupture: female, smoking, decreased FEV1, high mean blood pressure, large initial aneurysm size
Aneurysm Greater than 5.5 cm
Risk of rupture is high
Other Etiology Present
Risk of rupture low
Other Etiology Not Present
Risk of rupture moderate-high
Imaging Studies: Determine Renal Function.
If creatinine less than 2 mg/dL, obtain contrast CTA of chest, abdomen, and pelvis
If iodine dye allergy, or creatinine greater than 2 mg/dL, obtain noncontrast CT of chest, abdomen, and pelvis
No Rupture Noted
Risk of rupture moderate
Continue to search for etiology of pain
Rupture Found
Consider Elective (Urgent) Repair
Go to elective repair algorithm

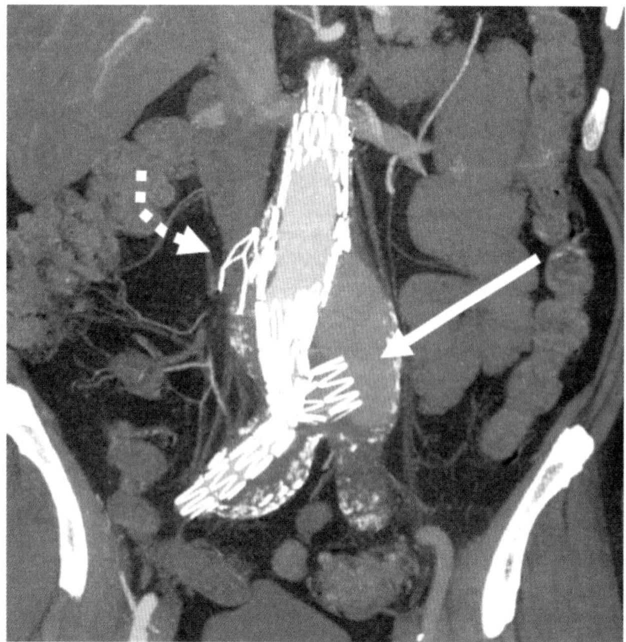

Figure 2 **Type Ib endoleak. A patient who was not followed after placement of an aortic endograft presented with reappearance of a palpable, pulsatile mass. This was secondary to the left limb of the graft migrating into the aneurysm sac (solid arrow) and [illegible] blood pressure into the aneurysm. *Broken arrow* indicates an unassociated inferior vena cava filter.**

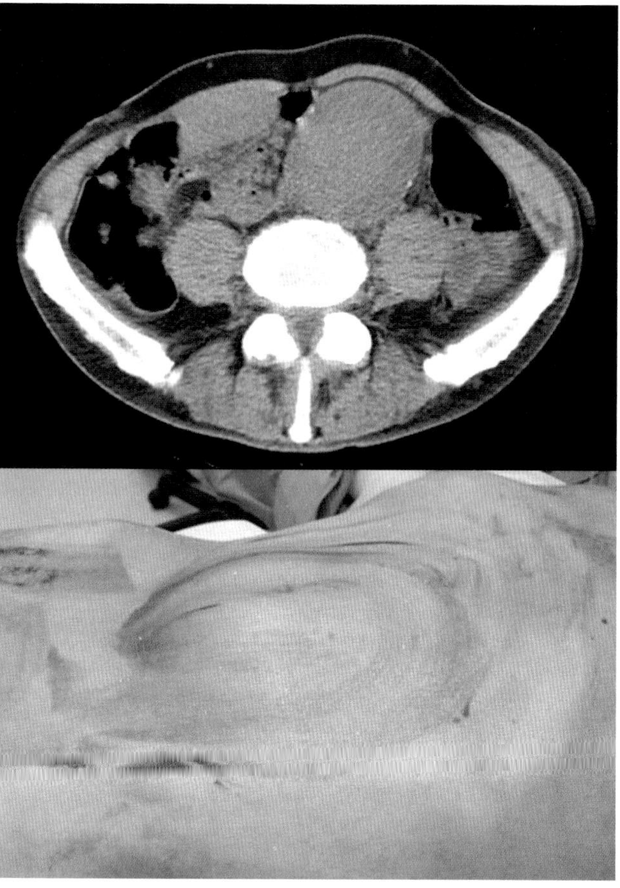

Figure 3 **Visible, palpable abdominal mass. *Top*: Axial computed tomographic scan of the abdomen demonstrating how an abdominal aortic aneurysm can deform the abdominal wall in a thin patient. *Bottom*: Photograph of the same patient demonstrating the visible deformity of the anterior abdominal wall.**

(type Ia endoleak), then blood flows into the sac and has limited outflow, so the risk of rupture may be significant. Type Ib endoleaks occur when the distal fixation site is not sealed and blood flows back into the sac from the graft and may occur from migration of the limb into the aneurysm after deployment. The operative mortality in patients with previous endografts who subsequently rupture is 41% (just like a rupture de novo).[29] Overall, however, the risk of rupture after endovascular repair is small,[31] and over time, survival is no different from that of open repair, although patients will likely undergo several reinterventions during their lifetime.[34]

PHYSICAL EXAMINATION

Before the advent of modern radiologic tests, the abdominal examination was the key to detecting an AAA. The abdominal aorta begins at the level of the diaphragm and the 12th thoracic vertebra and runs in the retroperitoneal space just anterior to and slightly to the left of the spine. At approximately the level of the umbilicus and the fourth lumbar vertebra, it bifurcates into the right and left common iliac arteries. In young, thin individuals, the abdominal aorta runs close to the surface of the abdomen and thus can often be palpated during a normal physical examination. Conversely, in thin patients with AAAs, the aneurysm can also be seen pulsating and deforming the contour of the abdomen [*see Figure 3*]. Palpation of an AAA is safe and has not been reported to precipitate rupture. A 1997 report found, however, that only 31% of the AAAs studied at a major teaching institution were initially detected by physical examination.[35] Nonaneurysmal common iliac arteries also are often difficult to palpate, even in thin individuals. Placing a stethoscope on the abdomen may also detect bruits (manifestations of turbulent blood flow) that may be due to either an aneurysm or from stenosis of visceral arteries—both of which may require some intervention even though it may not be emergent.

There are several methods of conducting a proper physical examination of the abdominal aorta. Our preferred approach resembles that of Lederle and Simel[36]:

1. Have the patient lie supine with the knees raised. Encourage the patient to relax the abdomen. A relaxed abdomen is often obtainable with passive exhalation after a deep inhalation.
2. Beginning a few centimeters cephalad to the umbilicus and just to the left of the midline, palpate deeply for the pulsation of the aorta.
3. To confirm that the aorta is being palpated, place both hands on the abdomen with the palms down in such a way that the pulsation is between the tips of the index fingers. The index fingers should move apart with each heartbeat.
4. Once it is certain that the index fingers are bracketing the aorta, estimate the diameter of the aorta by measuring the distance between the fingertips, taking into account the thickness of the overlying tissue. When evaluating a patient for a possible symptomatic (painful) aneurysm, holding the aorta will be painful and may further strengthen the

diagnosis even before any adjuvant imaging. Although this is not specific for a symptomatic AAA, if compressing the aorta itself is not painful, then the etiology is likely elsewhere.

Unfortunately, physical examination is not very accurate in detecting AAAs: in one study, approximately 62% of known AAAs were missed.[37] Whether an AAA is detectable on physical examination alone depends primarily on the size of the aneurysm. AAAs more than 5 cm in diameter are detectable on physical examination in 76% of the population, whereas those 3 to 3.9 cm in diameter are detectable in only 29%. Palpation of an AAA 3.0 cm in diameter or larger has a positive predictive value of only 43%.[36] In addition, detection of AAAs is significantly limited by truncal obesity.[38,39] Thus, physical examination is clearly insufficient for ruling out or screening for AAAs, but performing a complete abdominal examination will assist in discovering any other sources of pain.[36,39]

In the past, it was considered important to measure the abdominal aorta accurately by means of physical examination. Several studies have been published comparing US, the currently preferred screening method, with physical examination.[38,40] One such study found that abdominal palpation had a poor (14.7%) positive predictive value for detecting AAAs greater than 3.5 cm in diameter.[40] At present, with the wide availability of ultrasound screening, physical examination is playing a smaller role in AAA detection.

Although most AAAs appear supraumbilically, not all pulsatile abdominal masses appear there. In some patients, the abdominal aorta becomes more tortuous and elongated with age. As a result, an AAA may appear infraumbilically or to one side of the abdomen or the other. The abdominal portion that is palpable may also be part of a thoracoabdominal aneurysm for which full imaging of the chest and abdomen is necessary to evaluate the aorta in its entirety. The iliac arteries may become aneurysmal and become palpable in the lower quadrants of the abdomen independently or simultaneously of an aortic aneurysm [*see Figure 4*].[41]

Another indication that an AAA may exist is the presence of a femoral or popliteal artery aneurysm on physical examination. A patient with a femoral artery aneurysm has an 85% chance of having a concomitant AAA, and a patient with a popliteal artery aneurysm has a 62% chance.[42,43] Conversely, in a study evaluating 251 patients with documented AAAs, 14% had either a femoral or a popliteal artery aneurysm.[44] There is a significant male predominance, for unknown reasons.[20,44,45] If a patient has a history of a AAA that was repaired with an endovascular graft and subsequently has a palpable abdominal mass, then you must suspect that the graft may have failed and repressurized the aneurysm and therefore needs emergent repair.

Indications for Emergency Repair versus Further Workup

PATIENT IS UNSTABLE

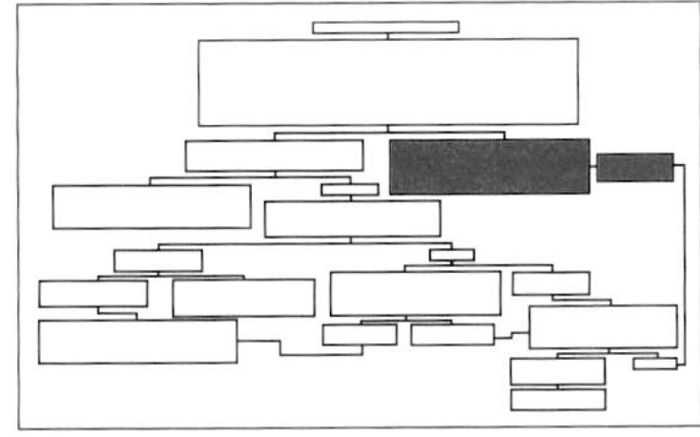

If a patient presents with a painful, pulsatile abdominal mass and is truly unstable, no further study or workup is necessary provided that there is no suspicion of acute MI as the cause: the diagnosis, until proved otherwise, is a ruptured AAA, and the patient should be taken to an operating room with angiographic capabilities. Patients who have stable (but not necessarily normal) vital signs may undergo a computed tomographic angiography (CTA) scan of the abdomen, which will greatly assist not only the diagnosis but also operative planning. The only cure for a ruptured AAA is some sort of emergency repair. Indeed, before the endovascular era, when all patients experiencing a ruptured AAA are taken into account, including both those who arrive at the hospital alive and those who do not, overall mortality is still between 77 and 94%, with over 50% of patients expiring before reaching the hospital.[46,47] Most ruptured AAAs leak into the left retroperitoneum, which may tamponade the bleeding and is referred to as a "contained" rupture.[45] AAAs that rupture freely into the abdominal cavity usually result in death, either at home or en route to the hospital as the volume of blood that can flow into the peritoneum before tamponading is usually lethal. For all patients who have an open repair for a ruptured AAA, the expected mortality exceeds 50% for open repair[48] (although values as low as 15% and as high as 90% have been noted[49]). Mortality after a ruptured AAA has declined since the middle of the 20th century by approximately 3.5% per decade; however, most modern series will report a mortality close to 41% for open repair of ruptured AAA.[50] Although some suggest that patients with predictably high morbidity and mortality from a ruptured AAA may not benefit from open repair,[49] most would still maintain that even in this population, this presentation necessitates operative intervention unless the patient or family feels strongly against it.[51] The high cost of repair and the substantial operative mortality notwithstanding, surgical repair of ruptured AAAs appears to be cost-effective in comparison with no intervention.[52] Thus, cost should not be considered in the management of patients with AAAs, and endovascular repair of ruptured aneurysms may change this paradigm.

Endovascular repair is rapidly becoming the standard of care for ruptured AAAs since the first report by Yusuf and colleagues in 1994.[53] This technique is rapidly becoming standard of care in all patients because the mortality is approaching half of that of open repair, with a dramatically shorter hospital stay. A 2003 study described endovascular repair of 29 ruptured AAAs and reported one of the lowest mortalities (only 11%).[54] As centers have begun to establish protocols for management and experience is much better, the average mortality of endovascular repair likely approaches 25 to 30%.[55-57] The main benefit is that patients can quickly be stabilized and even treated with local anesthesia. This is accomplished by positioning aortic occlusion balloons above the aneurysm percutaneously, thus allowing the patient to be stable much faster than by using conventional, open techniques and, ultimately, be discharged home sooner.[56]

PATIENT IS STABLE

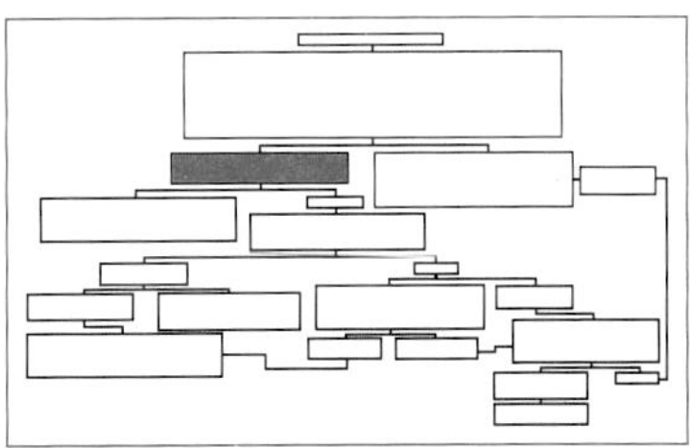

If a patient with a pulsatile abdominal mass is medically stable, further workup is always indicated. As noted, ultrasound imaging is significantly more accurate in detecting an AAA than physical examination alone.[40] Duplex US is used extensively as a primary screening tool for evaluating the size of an abdominal aorta because of certain advantages it possesses over other, more extensive modalities, such as CT,

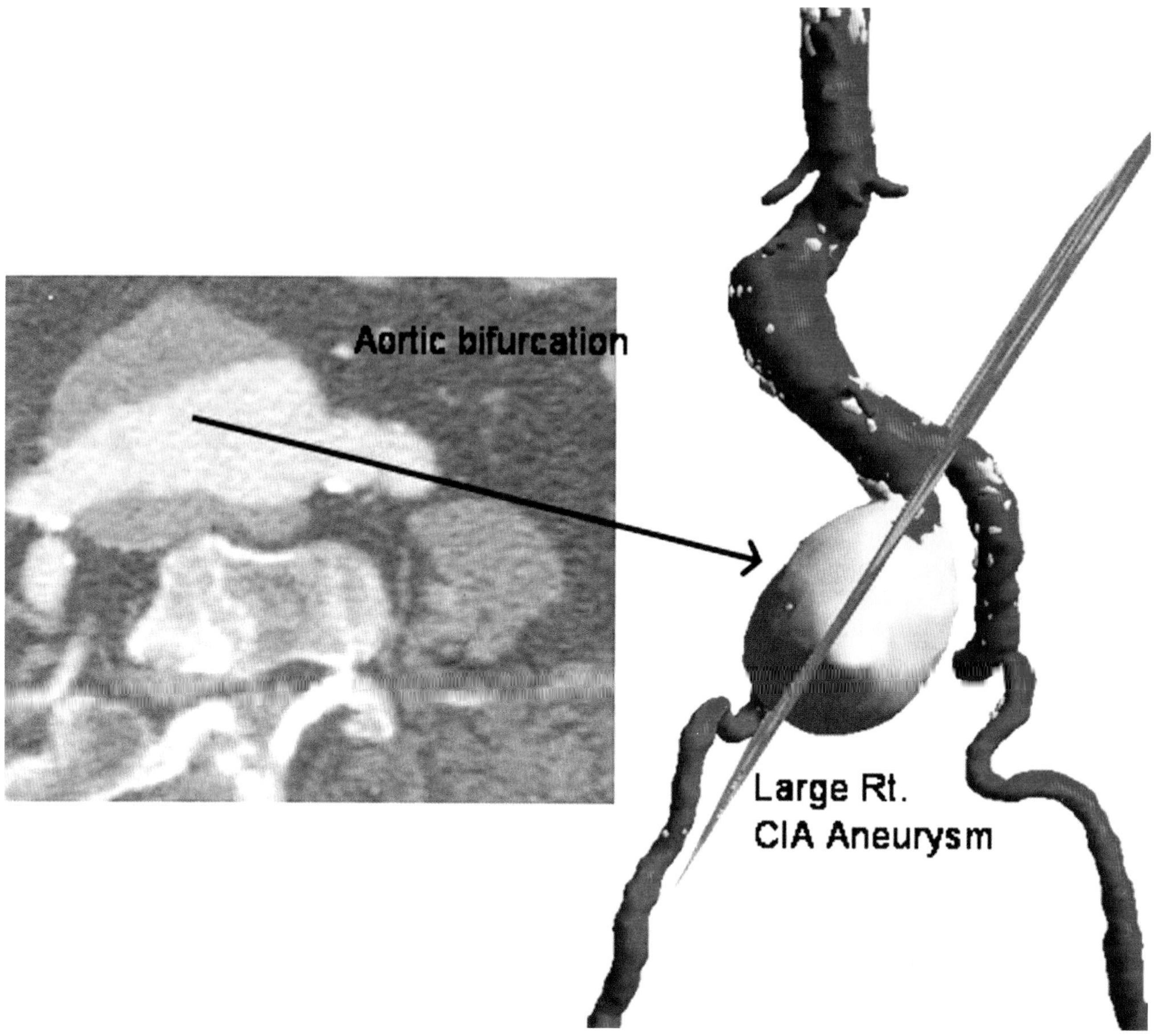

Figure 4 **Right common iliac artery aneurysm. Axial and three-dimensional reconstructions of a computed tomographic angiogram of a right common iliac artery (CIA) aneurysm.**

magnetic resonance angiography (MRA), and conventional angiography. Its main advantages are as follows: (1) it is noninvasive, (2) it is relatively inexpensive, (3) it does not require exposure to radiation, (4) it is portable, and (5) it is as reliable as the other modalities in determining aortic anterior-posterior (AP) diameter. Ultrasound-derived measurements are reproducible to within 3 to 5 mm,[58] and the interobserver variability is less than 5 mm in 84% of AP measurements.[59] On the other hand, in about 75% of cases, US underestimates the size of the aorta. A comparison study found that AAA diameter measurements were consistently and significantly larger with CT than with US (5.69 ± 0.89 cm versus 4.74 ± 0.91 cm).[60] It appears that when radiologists take more care with their measurements (e.g., by using magnifying glasses and calipers), the results correlate better.[61]

Ultrasound measurement of the infrarenal aorta and the common iliac arteries has been evaluated in patients with no known vascular disease. In one study of patients older than 50 years (the age group in which abdominal aortic and iliac artery aneurysms are most common), the aorta measured 1.68 ± 0.29 cm in men and 1.46 ± 0.19 cm in women ($p < .001$).[62] The common iliac arteries measured 1.01 ± 0.20 cm in men and 0.92 ± 0.13 cm in women. An aneurysm is commonly defined as a permanent localized or focal expansion of an artery to 1.5 times its expected diameter.[45] Thus, an infrarenal AAA would generally be considered to be approximately 3 cm in diameter if the average aortic diameter is 2 cm. It must be remembered, however, that infrarenal aortic diameter is affected by height, age, race, body surface area, and sex.[63–65] An aneurysm should be differentiated from arteriomegaly and from arterial or aortic ectasia. Arteriomegaly is a diffuse enlargement of an artery by an amount that is at least 50% of the normal diameter; ectasia is an enlargement of an artery by an amount that is less than 50% of the normal diameter.[66]

The main limitations of US are as follows: (1) the results are highly technician dependent and (2) resolution is dependent on body habitus and intestinal gas.[45] Another limitation is that it is unreliable in detecting rupture [*see Figure 5*]. Because US does not provide an accurate picture of the aorta proximal to the renal arteries and because it is subject to the limitations already mentioned, it cannot be routinely used to differentiate a ruptured AAA from a symptomatic intact AAA. If US is inconclusive in the evaluation of a palpable abdominal mass, then either CT or MRA (see below) is the next step [*see Table 2*].

Once a patient has either undergone screening US or if the patient is deemed to have a pathology that can be differentiated better by a CT scan, then fine-cut CTA will be the best imaging modality. In a patient with a pulsatile abdominal mass and back pain, CTA of the chest, abdomen, and pelvis will greatly assist in differentiating from most abdominal catastrophes that require surgery. Including the chest not only will assist in determining the proximal limit of the aneurysm (which may not be seen if only an abdominal CT scan is obtained and the patient has a thoracoabdominal aneurysm) but will also allow the surgeon to evaluate the aneurysm for possible endovascular repair. Knowing the complete extent of the aneurysm is also critical to appropriately choose the incision (thoracoabdominal, retroperitoneal, or midline laparotomy) if open repair is chosen. If the pelvis is not completely imaged, then potential issues with the iliac and femoral arteries could be missed. The major drawback of CTA is that it requires iodinated contrast, which may precipitate or worsen renal failure. This can be circumvented by even obtaining a noncontrast CTA of the chest, abdomen, and pelvis as this will again help differentiate some diagnoses (e.g., renal stones, free air, bowel obstruction) and also approximate the extent of the aneurysm and degree of calcification.

Management

STABLE PATIENT WITHOUT ANEURYSM

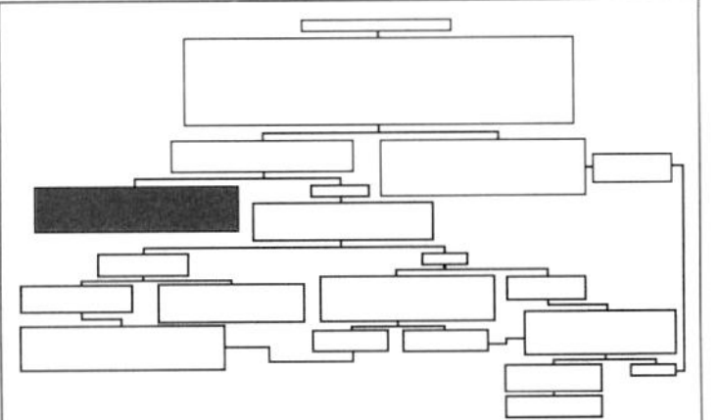

If imaging indicates that a patient with a pulsatile abdominal mass does not have an aneurysm, the risk of aortic or common iliac artery rupture is very low. Consequently, if symptoms (e.g., abdominal pain) persist, another causative condition must be considered.

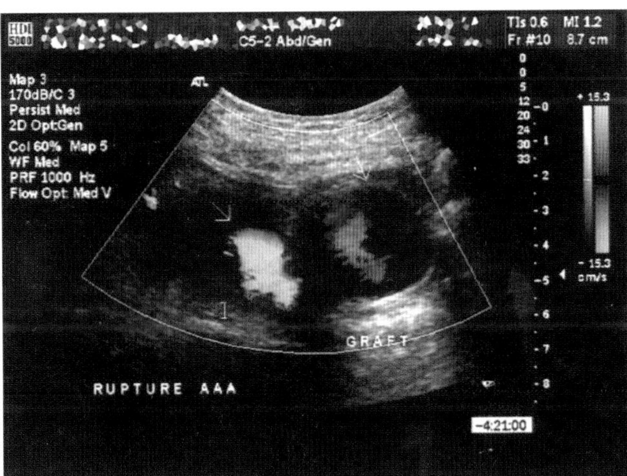

Figure 5 **Ultrasound evaluation of ruptured aneurysms. Color duplex sonogram demonstrating turbulent flow outside an aortic graft wall consistent with extravasation from a ruptured iliac artery aneurysm.**

If arteriomegaly is found to be the cause of the pulsatile abdominal mass and there are no symptoms of occlusion, then no specific treatment is required. Routine ultrasonographic follow-up is indicated because the risk of rupture still applies as the aorta continues to expand. In one study, an aneurysm was present in 1.6% of aortas with arteriomegaly.[67] If aortic ectasia (large aorta less than 1.5 times the normal size—usually 2.5 to 3 cm) is found, follow-up US in 5 to 8 years is recommended.[66,68] It has been suggested that for a 65-year-old man with a normal aortic diameter (defined as less than 2.2 cm), the risk that a significantly dilated aneurysm will develop during the remainder of his life is essentially zero.[69] The distinction between a normal and an ectatic aorta remains something of a gray area, and the preferred follow-up period remains controversial. In general, ectatic infrarenal aortas expand slowly and are not associated with rupture.[66]

In the ADAM trial, independent and significant predictors of a new aneurysm on follow-up US included (1) current smoking (odds ratio 3.09), (2) coexisting CAD (1.81), and, in a separate model with composite variables, (3) any atherosclerosis (1.97).[68] Accordingly, when a patient has any of these risk factors, a lower threshold for follow-up US and a shorter period between examinations may be practical. When patients have a pulsatile mass without a dilated blood vessel, then malignancies or retroperitoneal lymph nodes that envelop surrounding blood vessels may transmit pulsations and explain this physical finding.

STABLE PATIENT WITH ANEURYSM

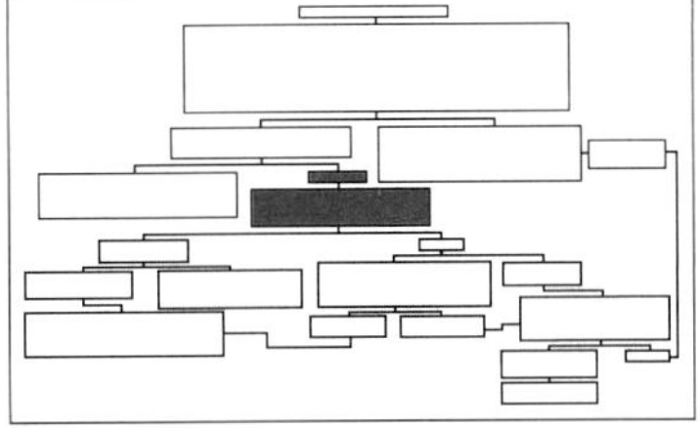

Once the diagnosis of an aneurysm is made in a stable patient, the subsequent course of action is determined by the clinical presentation and the size of the pulsatile abdominal mass. It must be emphasized that if the patient becomes hemodynamically unstable at any point during evaluation, operative intervention is necessary—unless the patient has a terminal condition or has indicated that nothing further should be done to prolong life.

If the patient is experiencing no discomfort and is otherwise stable, the risk of active rupture can be considered extremely low. On the other hand, if the patient is experiencing significant abdominal or back pain and discomfort, AAA rupture should remain a strong diagnostic possibility. Patients with AAA are also at risk for other cardiovascular diseases, so careful evaluation of the patient's signs and symptoms must be done to determine if the patient's presentation is attributable to the AAA or to something else.

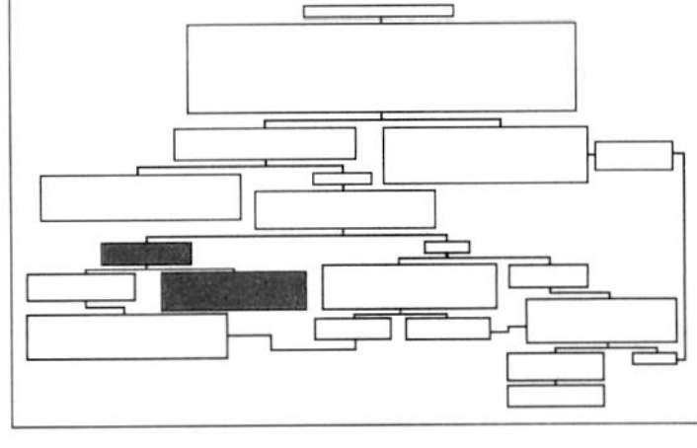

Pain Is Absent

A patient with a pulsatile abdominal mass

Table 2 **Advantages and Disadvantages of Aortic Imaging Techniques**

Imaging Modality	Advantages	Disadvantages
Ultrasonography	1. Noninvasive 2. Relatively inexpensive 3. Does not require radiation exposure 4. Portable 5. Comparable in reliability to other modalities in determining aortic diameter	1. Highly dependent on the skill of the operator 2. Resolution dependent on body habitus and amount of intestinal gas 3. Unreliable in the detection of AAA rupture 4. Poor visualization of the aorta proximal to renal arteries and distal to the iliac arteries 5. Cannot use it to plan operation
Computed tomography (CT)	1. Fast and easy to obtain 2. Highly precise measurements 3. Defines proximal and distal extent of AAAs precisely 4. Delineates the anatomy of the iliac arteries 5. Evaluates AAA wall integrity (notes location and amount of calcification and thrombus) 6. Effective at discovering venous anomalies, retroperitoneal blood, aortic dissection, inflammatory aneurysms, and other intra-abdominal pathology and anomalies 7. Can be done quickly and without contrast to plan for emergent endovascular repair of ruptured AAA	1. Radiation exposure 2. Generally requires iodinated contrast 3. More expensive than ultrasonography
Magnetic resonance angiography	1. Comparable to CT in preoperative evaluation 2. Can be obtained without contrast 3. Highly sensitive and specific in detecting stenoses of the splanchnic, renal, and iliac arteries	1. Not widely available 2. The most expensive 3. Potential claustrophobia in select patients 4. Longer scan time 5. Contraindicated in patients with certain metal foreign bodies (even some endografts)
Angiography	1. Superior in evaluating • Intraluminal characteristics of the aorta • Determining visceral branch involvement • Delineating variations in vascular anatomy 2. Can be done during aortic endograft placement	1. More expensive than CT (3–4 times) 2. Multiple risks, including • Arterial injury • Distal embolization • Local arterial dissection • Risk of renal failure secondary to contrast 3. Only shows luminal characteristics and not mural thrombus or aortic wall diameter

AAA = abdominal aortic aneurysm.

who has a known AAA and who is hemodynamically stable without complaints of pain should be further categorized on the basis of the size of the aneurysm. This categorization is traditionally based on the physics of an expanding aneurysm and on the association between increased risk of rupture and increased aneurysm size. The key considerations in these patients are (1) whether the risk associated with AAA repair exceeds the risk of rupture in a given period and (2) what other factors are present that may affect this decision.

Indications for operative intervention The physics of aneurysm expansion and rupture are probably best understood via the law of Laplace,[9] according to which the tangential stress (t) placed on a cylinder filled with fluid (e.g., a blood vessel) is determined by the equation

$$t = Pr/d$$

where P is the pressure (dynes/cm^2) exerted by the fluid, r is the internal radius (cm) of the cylinder, and d is the thickness (cm) of the cylinder wall. When the aorta expands, its radius increases, whereas its wall thickness decreases; thus, there is a geometric increase in tangential stress. As an aneurysm grows from 2 to 4 cm in diameter, tangential pressure increases not twofold but fourfold. When the increased tangential stress exceeds the elastic capacity of the wall, rupture occurs. Elastic tissue in the abdominal aorta becomes attenuated as a result of age and of certain acquired and genetic factors; thus, a modest degree of expansion over time is not uncommon. An abnormal rate of expansion is usually considered to be greater than 5 mm/yr. Documentation of an accelerated aneurysm growth rate should cause the surgeon to give serious consideration to operative intervention.[45]

The decision on when to operate on patients with AAA began with autopsy studies of individuals with aneurysms who did not have surgery.[70] These autopsy studies also paved the way to try to confirm if it is true that the larger the aneurysm, the higher the risk of rupture and that patients with ruptured aneurysms may live hours to weeks prior to having surgery.[11] This conclusion has been challenged by studies using three-dimensional CT to evaluate wall stress via a mathematical technique called finite element analysis.[71–73] In these studies, maximal wall stress was a better predictor of rupture than maximal AP diameter was. For example, one patient with a ruptured 4.8 cm aneurysm had a wall stress equivalent to that of a patient with an electively repaired 6.3 cm AAA.[72] Future management of AAAs may be based on actual wall stress in addition to maximum AP diameter.

In a 2001 study addressing open operative repair of intact AAAs, increased mortality was associated with increased patient age, female sex, cerebrovascular occlusive disease, preoperative renal insufficiency, and the presence of more than three comorbid conditions before operation.[5] In the UK Small Aneurysm Trial, the 30-day mortality in patients undergoing elective open AAA repair was 5.8%.[74] The point at which the risk of elective repair became acceptable in relation to the risk of rupture with medical management and serial ultrasonographic follow-up was an aneurysm diameter of 5.5 cm. The investigators suggested that in patients with AAAs less than 5.5 cm in diameter, medical management is the best course of action. The operative mortality reported in this study is considered high in that many single-center series have documented mortalities of 1 to 3% after open repair of intact AAAs.[75–77] The ADAM investigators also found that survival was not improved when AAAs smaller than 5.5 cm were repaired electively, even if a low operative mortality was associated with the procedure.[77]

Hospital volume may have a significant effect on patient outcome after elective AAA repair. A 2002 study found that mortality after this procedure was 56% higher at low-volume hospitals than at high-volume hospitals.[78] Moreover, mortality after repair of an intact AAA exhibited a ninefold variation that could be attributed to hospital volume, sex, and age alone. Thus, when a patient is being evaluated for AAA repair, it is important to take into account not only the size of the aneurysm but also age, sex, comorbidities, and hospital volume. In turn, more than half of the effect of hospital volume on operative mortality in elective AAA repair appears to be mediated by surgeon volume.[79] Surgeon specialty also appears to affect operative mortality after elective AAA repair.[80] Outcomes of endovascular repair of ruptured AAAs compared to open repair in the United States using the National Inpatient Sample database documented that the mortality is more than double if the procedure is done at smaller-volume and nonteaching hospitals (55% versus 21%). The outcomes of endovascular repair in teaching hospitals for ruptured aneurysms were even better than those of elective endovascular repair in nonteaching hospitals, all of which strongly support regionalization of AAA repair.[81–83]

Given the various possible complicating factors, it is clear that no single aortic diameter can serve as a definitive indication for operative intervention in every patient. It is well known that ruptures can occur unpredictably at aneurysm diameters smaller than 5.5 cm.[84] Therefore, the timing of AAA repair must be individualized, with the 5.5 cm figure serving as a general guideline in the counseling of patients.

Age has been shown to increase the risk of operative mortality in patients undergoing open repair. The overall operative mortality after elective, open repair of AAA is reported by most series to be less than 5%. However, in the Nationwide Inpatient Sample, if the patients were less than 60 years old, it was 2.2%, whereas it was 9.2% in patients over 80 years old.[82] With regard to endovascular repair, mortality in Medicare patients (all over 65 years old) demonstrated an early mortality benefit in endovascular repair that was consistently better than open repair regardless of the age of the patient, even in those over 85 years of age.[34] Regardless of the technique used, advanced age, terminal conditions, and various end-of-life issues may deter patients from wishing to proceed with operative intervention. In addition, severe coexisting diseases significantly affect the morbidity and mortality associated with AAA repair.[48,85] Accordingly, older patients with multiple comorbidities may be preferentially offered endovascular AAA approach in place of open repair.[32] The surgeon must, however, consider the possibility that any operative intervention will be too risky in this population or that other interventions must be carried out before AAA repair can be attempted. These issues should be addressed via appropriate preoperative evaluation [*see Figure 6*].

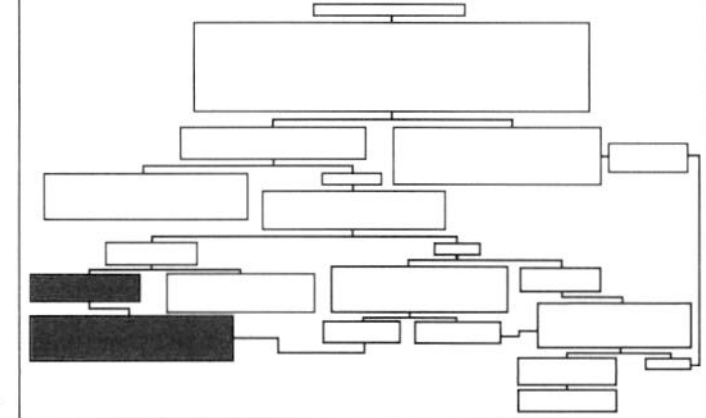

Small AAAs (< 5 cm): medical management and follow-up When a patient with stable vital signs and no abdominal pain is diagnosed as having a small AAA, serial US and optimization of medical management are indicated.[86,87] Small AAAs usually do not rupture.[26,77,86–88] Most small AAAs continue to grow, however, typically by 0.2 to 0.4 cm in diameter per year.[78–80] Small AAAs can also expand rapidly with unpredictable frequency. A rapidly expanding AAA is at high risk for rupture, regardless of how small it may be.[74,77,88,89]

Many risk factors have been identified that may affect the risk of small aneurysm expansion and rupture. For example, one study suggested that diastolic hypertension and chronic

URGENT REPAIR

Known AAA > 5.5 cm or meets other criteria for repair (symptomatic, inflammatory, rapid expansion, etc.)

Preoperative Evaluation

Eagle's criteria: Determine cardiac risk of operative repair, determine need/extent of cardiac workup prior to operative intervention

Comorbid vascular disease (peripheral, carotid, coronary, renal): May affect timing and type of operation chosen

Other medical conditions: Optimize medical management as much as possible (start statin, beta blocker, low dose aspirin, etc.)

Impaired Renal Function?

Yes: Noncontrast CT of chest abdomen and pelvis or MRA with time of flight imaging

No: CTA of chest, abdomen, and pelvis with IV contrast with fine cuts

Indications for Preoperative Arteriography

Inadequate imaging: Perform CO_2 angiography in setting of renal insufficency

Endovascular AAA Repair if Possible and Indicated

Figure 6 **Algorithm for urgent repair of abdominal aortic aneurysm (AAA). CT = computed tomography; CTA = computed tomographic angiography; MRA = magnetic resonance angiography; IV = intravenous.**

obstructive pulmonary disease (COPD) increased the risk that a small AAA would rupture,[84] whereas another found advanced age, severe cardiac disease, previous stroke, and a history of cigarette smoking to be risk factors for rapid expansion.[88] AAAs smaller than 5.5 cm may rupture more frequently in women than in men. A 2002 study found that in almost one quarter of women with ruptured AAAs, the diameter of the aneurysm was less than 5.5 cm at the time of rupture.[47] Currently, the safest and easiest method of following small AAAs is serial US.[14,90] When the diameter of an AAA approaches 5.5 cm, a more detailed study (e.g., CT or MRA) is indicated if repair is being considered.[45]

Over the past several decades, the number of AAAs (especially smaller ones) detected has increased.[91] This increase has been attributed to two causes: (1) increased serendipitous detection in the course of scans done for other indications and (2) the progressive aging of the population.[45,91] There is growing evidence worldwide[92,93] that early screening is cost-effective.[24,94] The U.S. Preventive Services Task Force recommends screening all males 65 to 75 of years who smoked more than 100 cigarettes. This is supported by both Medicare and the Veterans' Administration (among others). Other groups who perhaps will benefit from screening are individuals who have a family history of AAAs.

Basic science studies have helped elucidate the etiology of AAAs in greater detail. In particular, current research is focusing on (1) evaluating the role various proteolytic enzymes, such as matrix metalloproteinases (MMPs), play in processes involving the structural elements in the aortic wall; (2) investigating the importance of the immune system, specifically the macrophage, in the development of AAAs; (3) determining how hemodynamic and biomechanical stress affects aortic wall remodeling; and (4) identifying molecular genetic variables that contribute to AAA development.[95]

Proteolytic enzymes are currently being evaluated as potential predictors of the course of AAA growth.[96] Doxycycline, which decreases MMPs in animal aneurysm models independently of its antibiotic properties, was evaluated in a prospective, randomized phase II trial published in 2002.[97] Although it did not exert a significant effect on aneurysm growth over the short study period (6 months), doxycycline significantly reduced serum levels of MMP9, a gelatinase that plays a central role in degrading elastin and collagen in the abdominal aortic wall. Few side effects were noted, and most of them were easily reversible. These findings, although not conclusive, suggest that the use of doxycycline may one day prove to be a viable medical means of slowing AAA growth.

Control of hypertension would seem to be an obvious approach to medical control of aneurysms as hypertension is a significant risk factor for both development and rupture of AAAs.[20,27,84,87] To this end, various antihypertensive agents, including beta blockers, calcium channel blockers, and angiotensin-converting enzyme (ACE) inhibitors, have been evaluated in patients with AAAs.[25] The results have been somewhat equivocal and continue to be evaluated.

Beta blockers have been shown to reduce the expansion rate of large AAAs (> 5 cm) but not that of smaller AAAs.[98,99] Some of them (e.g., propranolol) may be poorly tolerated at high doses.[98,99] In addition, beta blockers may be contraindicated in patients with severe COPD, although as many as 11% of COPD patients have AAAs.[26] A 1999 study suggested that receiving a calcium channel blocker was an independent risk factor for the presence of an AAA (odds ratio 2.6).[25] The same study also noted, however, that patients receiving calcium channel blockers had stiffer aortic walls. ACE inhibitors, in contrast, were associated with decreased aortic wall stiffness and increased collagen turnover, whereas diuretics and beta blockers had no effect on aortic wall stiffness. None of the medications examined were found to affect the growth rate of AAAs. Aortic stiffness appears to be an important variable: increased aortic wall distensibility is associated with an increased risk of AAA rupture and is almost as powerful a predictor of rupture as actual AAA diameter.[100]

A link between COPD and AAAs is suggested by the presence of a common development pathway: both conditions are associated with elastin breakdown and smoking. A 1999 study argued, however, that the strong association between AAAs and COPD was most likely attributable to coexisting cardiovascular disease and medications.[26] In this study, the average annual aortic diameter expansion rate was 4.7 mm in patients who used oral steroids but only 2.6 mm in those who did not. The use of beta-adrenergic agonists was also a positive predictor of aneurysm expansion. Thus, oral steroids and beta agonists must be used cautiously in COPD patients who have AAAs. If an AAA patient must use one of these medications, close follow-up is indicated to monitor the expansion rate of the aneurysm.

Atherosclerosis is associated with AAAs but is currently believed to be a secondary phenomenon, with inflammation and matrix-degrading enzymes being the primary factors in AAA development.[101] Lipoprotein (a) has been found to be an independent risk factor for atherosclerosis and is elevated in patients with AAAs independently of the patients' cardiovascular risk factors or the extent of atherosclerosis.[102] It seems reasonable that lowering lipid levels would decrease the development of atherosclerosis of the abdominal aorta. This is a potentially important effect because patients with small atherosclerotic AAAs often experience thrombotic complications involving the lower extremities.[103] Levels of apolipoprotein A-I and high-density lipoproteins have also been found to be significantly lower in patients with AAAs.[104] Overall, however, lipids appear to play only a minor role in AAA progression.[105] An animal study suggested that regression of plaque by lowering serum lipid levels after atherosclerotic aneurysm formation may result in increased aneurysm dilation in the abdominal aorta.[106] A subsequent study, however, demonstrated that statins reduce the production of MMPs in the wall of AAAs.[107] The role of lipid-lowering medications in the treatment of AAAs remains to be clarified. Elevated levels of homocysteine in the blood are a recognized independent risk factor for atherosclerosis, and a study of AAA patients has found significantly higher levels of plasma homocysteine, along with lower levels of vitamin B_{12}.[108] Given this finding, and the possible role of vitamin B_{12} in homocysteine regulation, use of supplemental vitamins may theoretically modify AAA progression.[108]

Smoking is an independent risk factor for AAA development,[20,68] expansion,[88,105] and rupture.[27] Current smokers are 7.6 times more likely to have an AAA than nonsmokers are, and ex-smokers are three times more likely to have an AAA.[25] The duration of smoking is the key variable[16,20,25]: the relative risk of AAA development is increased by 4% for each year of smoking.[25] The ADAM trial noted that a longer interval since the cessation of smoking was significantly associated with a decreased risk of AAA formation[16]; however, the decline in risk appears to be slow.[25] The UKSA trial showed that former smokers were at lower risk for death from AAA repair than current smokers were.[74] A 2002 study found that there was an independent association between smoking and high-grade tissue inflammation in AAAs,[109] lending support to the idea that smoking is an initiating event in AAA formation.

At present, intriguing possibilities notwithstanding, few definitive recommendations can be made regarding the use of medical therapy to reduce AAA growth. The indications for perioperative beta blockade are primarily cardioprotective. Administration of antihypertensives may be beneficial from a practical perspective, but current level I data supporting this practice are lacking. If an antihypertensive is given, the choice of agent should be based on associated clinical data (e.g., the presence of coexisting medical conditions, such as angina or renal insufficiency, whose management must be optimized). The administration of lipid-lowering drugs to patients with AAAs also requires further study, although the utility of such agents in the presence of CAD, which is found in almost 50% of AAA patients,[110] is well documented, and long-term statin use after successful AAA surgery has been associated with reduced mortality (both all-cause and cardiovascular).[111] Finally, smoking cessation is clearly mandatory.

Pain Is Present

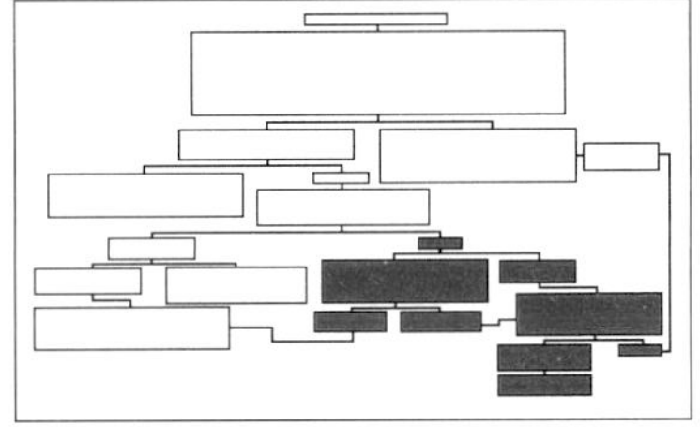

When a patient presenting with a pulsatile abdominal mass is hemodynamically stable but complains of pain in the abdomen, the back, the testicles, or the femoral region, the index of suspicion must be high for a symptomatic or ruptured AAA. Other possible causes should be considered as well. As previously noted above, many abdominal processes may mimic an AAA; however, it is important that recognition of an AAA not be delayed unduly, because the length of the interval between the onset of symptoms and subsequent diagnosis and operation may have a direct bearing on overall survival. The size of the aneurysm is helpful for identifying patients at highest risk for rupture.

In stable patients with AAAs larger than 5.5 cm who are experiencing pain, either CT (faster and more available) or MRA (slower but without contrast nor radiation) may be used to detect AAA rupture; the choice typically depends on the patient's medical history and degree of stability [*see Figure 6*].

After ultrasound evaluation, if an aneurysm smaller than 5.5 cm was found and no associated risk factors for rupture were identified, a search for other possible causes of the pain is reasonable, provided that it is performed expeditiously.

If no other cause for the pain can be found, inflammatory aneurysms or rupture should remain prime considerations, and the next step in evaluation—namely, spiral CTA or MRA—should be implemented. Missing or delaying the diagnosis of a ruptured AAA can be disastrous. If retroperitoneal blood is noted [*see Figure 7*], then the patient should be taken to an operating suite with fluoroscopic capabilities. If the aneurysm is not ruptured, repair should be undertaken with the patient's medical condition optimized to the best extent possible. Precipitous repairs of nonruptured symptomatic AAAs have an operative mortality five times that of elective repairs,[112] for reasons yet unknown. Conversely, if no other source of abdominal pain is found, then treating the aneurysm may resolve the pain, even if done via endovascular repair (and leaving the aneurysm behind) for reasons unknown.

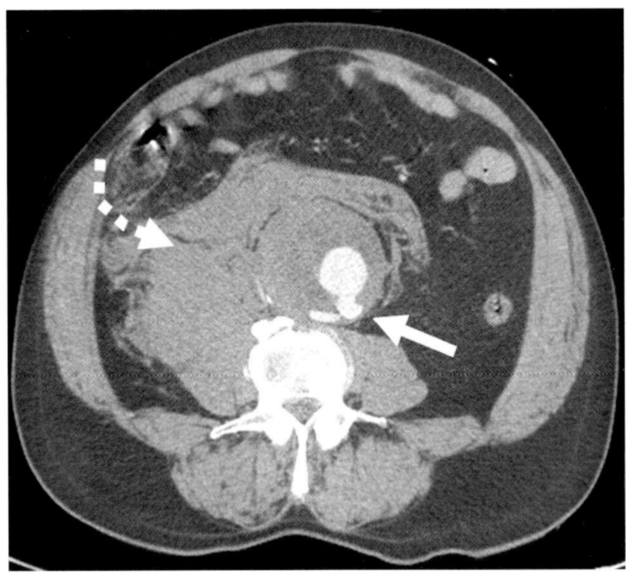

Figure 7 **Ruptured abdominal aortic aneurysm. Computed tomographic angiography of the abdominal aorta demonstrating a large right-sided retroperitoneal hematoma (*broken arrow*) and a 7.9 cm abdominal aortic aneurysm (*solid arrow*).**

Preoperative Evaluation of Nonemergency AAA Repair Candidates

Evaluation of a patient before elective AAA repair begins with assessment of the expected benefit of repair in relation to the estimated risk. If the decision is made to operate, the history and the physical examination should be completed as described earlier [*see* Clinical Evaluation, *above*]. The clinical findings, in conjunction with electrocardiographic (ECG) and routine laboratory test results, provide most of the information that is needed for evaluating a patient's candidacy for AAA repair.

COMORBID CONDITIONS

CAD is common in patients with AAAs and is the leading cause of early and late mortality after AAA repair.[113] Renal insufficiency, COPD, and diabetes mellitus also may influence morbidity and mortality after AAA repair. Accordingly, when any of these disease entities is present, further evaluation before repair may be beneficial. Optimization of perioperative medications is also important for maximizing risk reduction. Finally, adequate preoperative imaging is essential. The decision regarding which type of repair is most appropriate in an AAA patient should be based on the preoperative evaluation.

Coronary Artery Disease

Before elective AAA repair, it is important to identify patients who are at high risk for a perioperative cardiac event and may benefit from preoperative cardiac intervention. It is also important to identify patients who are at low risk so that they are not subjected to unneeded testing. The most recent report from the American College of Cardiology/American Heart Association (ACC/AHA) Task Force on Practice Guidelines is from 2007.[114] It provided useful guidelines for preoperative cardiac evaluation in patients undergoing noncardiac vascular surgery [*see Table 3*], with the express goal of limiting the use of perioperative cardiac procedures in patients at moderate and high risk for complications.[114,115] Use of these guidelines and permutations thereof has proved both safe and effective at reducing resource use and overall costs.[116–118]

According to the ACC/AHA guidelines, patients needing elective AAA repair are stratified first by whether the patient has active cardiac conditions or high-risk factors. If so, and symptoms have not recurred, the patient is cleared for operation. If the patient never underwent coronary revascularization, underwent revascularization more than 5 years before, or is experiencing recurrent symptoms or signs of cardiac ischemia, further evaluation of clinical predictors is necessary.

Clinical predictors of major perioperative cardiovascular risk, defined as MI, congestive heart failure, or death, may be divided into three categories[114]: major, intermediate, and minor. The presence of a major predictor requires that the symptom or disease be managed appropriately before nonemergency surgery. The presence of an intermediate predictor is associated with an increased risk of perioperative cardiac complications and requires that current status be fully investigated. The presence of a minor predictor is indicative of cardiovascular disease but has not been shown to independently increase the risk of perioperative cardiovascular complications.

Once the clinical predictors have been evaluated, additional predictive factors, involving the patient's ability to perform various activities (ranging from minor activities of daily living to strenuous sports), are assessed. The energy required to perform an activity is quantified in terms of metabolic equivalents (METs). The number of METs of which a patient is capable directly correlates with the ability to perform specific tasks [*see Table 4*]. Patients who are unable to attain 4 METs are considered to be at high risk for perioperative cardiac events and long-term complications. Finally, the inherent risk of the procedure to be performed is evaluated. AAA repair is considered high risk.

To date, there have only been two large, controlled, randomized trials including AAA repair to evaluate if preoperative coronary intervention (either coronary artery bypass grafting [CABG] or percutaneous transluminal coronary angioplasty [PTCA]) improved mortality in elective, major vascular surgery. Thirty percent of the 510 patients in the Coronary Artery Revascularization Prophylaxis [CARP] trial were undergoing open AAA repair (70% had peripheral artery disease), and all had at least one significant coronary artery stenosis. They were randomized to either preoperative coronary revascularization or no coronary revascularization procedure. Overall, there was no difference with respect to perioperative (30 days) MI in either group (12% versus 14%. $p = .37$). At 2.7 years after randomization, there was no difference in

Table 3 Risk Stratification Criteria to Determine the Need for Preoperative Cardiac Evaluation for Nonvascular Surgery Patients (Only Indicated for Moderate or High Risk Patients)[114]

1. Major clinical predictor of risk present?	Major clinical predictors include • Unstable coronary syndromes • Decompensated CHF • Significant arrhythmias • Severe valvular disease The presence of these predictors cancels or delays elective intervention until they are ameliorated and/or studied via coronary angiography.
2. Intermediate clinical predictor of risk present?	Intermediate clinical predictors include • Mild angina pectoris • Prior MI • Compensated or prior CHF • Diabetes mellitus • Renal insufficiency, carotid surgery, or aortic endograft Noninvasive testing is unlikely to change management in this risk group; therefore, continue with operation if low risk. If risk is high (several risk factors), then consider stress testing or angiography and go to 4.
3. Minor or no clinical predictors present?	Minor clinical predictors include • Advanced age • Abnormal ECG • Nonsinus rhythm • Low functional capacity • Previous stroke • Uncontrolled systemic hypertension If minor or no clinical predictors are present and the patient can attain 4 METs or more, proceed with surgery. Consider testing when < 4 METs are attained, especially in the presence of multiple minor clinical predictors; then go to 4.
4. Risk after noninvasive testing?	Low risk: Proceed with operation. High risk: Consider coronary angiography.

CHF = congestive heart failure; ECG = electrocardiogram; MET = metabolic equivalent; MI = myocardial infarction.

Table 4 **Estimated Energy Required for Various Activities**[116,156]

Activity Level	METs*	Sample Activities
Mild	1–3	Eating; playing a musical instrument; walking at 2 mph; getting dressed; golfing (with cart)
Moderate	3–5	Calisthenics without weights; climbing a flight of stairs; housework; golfing (without cart); running a short distance
Vigorous	4–12+	Chopping wood; strenuous sports such as football, basketball, singles tennis, karate, or jogging (10 min mile or faster)

*1 MET = 3.5 mL·kg^{-1}·min^{-1} oxygen uptake.

mortality between the groups (23% versus 22%, $p = .92$) and the number of perioperative MIs was also the same (24.2 versus 28.6%; $p = .32$), albeit a predictor of mortality.[119] These data demonstrate that there is no need of preoperative coronary revascularization in patients with stable CAD. Therefore, in stable patients without evidence of heart failure, there may be no role for preoperative intervention as long as aggressive (beta blocker, statin, and aspirin) medical therapy can be initiated (not possible on emergent cases).[119] Of note, this is only one trial, mostly in men, and it should be validated prior to taking these data as absolute recommendations. The DECREASE-V pilot study sought to find if high-risk patients needing vascular surgery would benefit from revascularization or just best medical therapy (beta blockers to a heart rate of 60 to 65 beats/min and aspirin) prior to surgery.[120] The 101 patients who had extensive stress-induced ischemia (≥5 segments or ≥3 walls) were randomized. The results demonstrated no difference in mortality, and one patient in the revascularization-first group died from a ruptured aneurysm. Although ultimately the sample size was small, the results were similar in the two trials; thus, there may not be a benefit to revascularization in the era of modern medical therapy.

Small observational studies have indicated a low cardiac mortality when preoperative PTCA is performed in this setting; complications after PTCA are not infrequent and include the need for emergency CABG. One retrospective review found that patients who underwent prophylactic PTCA before noncardiac surgery were twice as likely to have an adverse cardiac outcome as healthy patients were.[121] This study did not control for CAD severity, medical management, or comorbidities. A later study concluded that both CABG and PTCA offered only modest protection against adverse cardiac events after major arterial surgery (CABG, < 5 years; PTCA, < 2 years).[122] General indications for PTCA use are outlined in the 2001 revision of the 1993 ACC/AHA guidelines for percutaneous coronary intervention.[123] It is recommended that patients wait at least 2 weeks—preferably, 4 to 6 weeks—after PTCA before undergoing AAA repair; this delay allows the plaque to stabilize after stenting and permits full treatment with all antiplatelet agents.

The original ACC/AHA recommendations for supplemental preoperative testing were updated in a 2007 statement.[114] Currently, it is generally agreed that preoperative testing should be limited to patients in whom the results have the potential to alter the current course of management. The following noninvasive tests may be considered in high-risk vascular patients:

Table 5 **ECG Findings as Clinical Predictors of Increased Perioperative Cardiovascular Risk**[155]

Major predictors
High-grade atrioventricular block
Symptomatic ventricular arrhythmias in the presence of underlying heart disease
Supraventricular arrhythmias with uncontrolled ventricular rate
Intermediate predictor
Pathologic Q wave indicating previous myocardial infarction
Minor predictors
Left ventricular hypertrophy
Left bundle branch block
ST-T abnormalities
Rhythm other than sinus (e.g., atrial fibrillation)

ECG = electrocardiogram.

1. *12-lead ECG.* This test is recommended. Certain ECG abnormalities are clinical predictors of perioperative and long-term cardiac risks in patients undergoing high-risk operative procedures [*see Table 5*].
2. *Transthoracic echocardiography to evaluate resting left ventricular function.* This test is indicated in the presence of heart failure. If it was previously done and demonstrated severe left ventricular dysfunction, repeat evaluation is unnecessary. It may be of benefit in patients with prior heart failure and those with dyspnea of unknown etiology. Routine use is not beneficial in the absence of heart failure.
3. *Exercise or pharmacologic stress testing.* Such testing is useful for diagnosing CAD in patients with an intermediate pretest probability of CAD, but its value is less well established in those with a high or low pretest probability. It is a good prognosticator for patients with suspected or proven CAD who are undergoing initial evaluation, for patients whose clinical disposition has changed significantly, and for those who have experienced an acute coronary syndrome.[124] Stress testing is also recommended for demonstrating the presence of myocardial ischemia before coronary revascularization and for evaluating the efficacy of medical therapy. It may be useful in patients whose subjective assessment of exercise tolerance is unreliable and in whom evaluation in terms of METs is therefore impossible. Less clear are the following indications for stress testing: (1) diagnosis of CAD in patients who have resting ST depression of less than 1 mm, are on digitalis, or show evidence of left ventricular hypertrophy on ECG and (2) detection of restenosis in high-risk patients who have recently (i.e., within the past few months) undergone PTCA. Exercise stress testing should not be done (1) to diagnose patients with ECG findings that would prevent adequate assessment, (2) in patients with severe comorbidities that would preclude coronary revascularization,

(3) for routine screening of asymptomatic patients, or (4) to evaluate young patients with isolated ectopic beats on ECG.

If indicated in the very high risk patients, coronary angiography may be performed next. Current indications in patients scheduled to undergo elective AAA repair include (1) a previous history of high-risk status after noninvasive testing, (2) continued angina despite adequate medical therapy, (3) unstable angina, and (4) an equivocal result on noninvasive testing in high-risk patients. Coronary angiography may be beneficial in patients with multiple intermediate clinical risk factors. If noninvasive testing reveals moderate-size to large areas of ischemia in a patient without high-risk criteria and a lower left ventricular ejection fraction, or if testing is nondiagnostic in a patient at intermediate clinical risk, coronary angiography may also be indicated. The indication for coronary angiography is more controversial in patients who have experienced a perioperative MI. Coronary angiography is not indicated in patients who are asymptomatic after coronary revascularization and who are capable of at least 7 METs.

Both CABG and PTCA have been employed to treat CAD before AAA repair. CABG is usually done in this setting only if it has been decided that the patient needs the intervention regardless of the current status of the abdominal aorta. Such patients have a high-risk coronary anatomy and have a long-term prognosis that is generally thought to improve if coronary revascularization is performed. The combination of AAA repair and CABG has been evaluated, and there are some data to support its use in carefully selected patients, but the perioperative mortality may be more than 10%. Although this may be more significant in the era when the AAA repair was exclusively done via a laparotomy and not endovascularly, the mortality is higher when the two procedures are staged (CABG first and then AAA repair), and aneurysms have been reported to rupture in the hospital while recovering from the CABG.[125–127] Surgery should be delayed 2 to 4 weeks after an angioplasty to balance the risk of operating too soon on an unhealed plaque versus too late on a restenosed vessel. Coronary arteries that have bare metal stents should be allowed to heal for 6 to 8 weeks but less than 12 weeks for the same reasons as above. Finally, drug-eluting stents have a very high occlusion rate if the antiplatelet agents are stopped; thus, the current recommendations are to not suspend these for ideally 1 year after placement or at least 1 month without stopping aspirin if absolutely necessary to do the procedure.[114,128]

Pulmonary Disease

Between 7 and 11% of patients with COPD have an AAA.[26] Traditionally, when such patients are to undergo AAA repair, room air arterial blood gas values are determined and pulmonary function tests performed to assess the extent of COPD. If COPD is severe, formal pulmonary consultation may be necessary for prediction of short- and long-term prognoses and optimization of treatment. Several studies have reported that COPD is an independent predictor of operative mortality.[5,76,129] A 2001 study of Veterans Affairs (VA) patients, however, found no significant correlation between the presence of COPD and increased operative mortality (although morbidity was notably higher).[130] A 2003 study evaluating morbidity and mortality after AAA repair in patients with COPD showed that the preoperative factors significantly associated with a poor outcome included (1) suboptimal COPD management, as evidenced by fewer inhalers used, (2) a lower preoperative hematocrit, (3) preoperative renal insufficiency, and (4) the presence of CAD.[131] It is noteworthy that abnormal preoperative pulmonary function tests and arterial blood gas values were not predictive of a poor outcome. Thus, COPD by itself is not a contraindication to AAA repair.

Renal Failure

Preoperative renal insufficiency is known to be a risk factor for a poor outcome after AAA repair[5,76,130,131] and thus should be evaluated and corrected if possible. In certain patients with AAAs, renal artery stenosis may be contributing to impaired renal function; if so, it may be corrected either noninvasively, before AAA repair, or in the course of the repair.[45]

Diabetes Mellitus

Whether diabetes mellitus is truly an independent risk factor for morbidity or mortality after aortic surgery is controversial. Several studies have shown that the risk of death is not increased in diabetic patients, but the risk of perioperative complications may be.[132–134] Most of these studies had small study groups and thus lacked the statistical power needed to demonstrate that diabetes had a significant influence. A 2002 study of patients at VA medical centers who underwent major vascular procedures found that diabetic patients were indeed at higher risk for death and cardiovascular complications. When examined separately, however, patients undergoing AAA repair did not have higher rates of cardiovascular complications or death than patients undergoing other procedures.

PERIOPERATIVE MEDICATIONS

Multiple studies have addressed optimization of medical management in patients with AAAs. Beta blockers, alpha$_2$-adrenergic agonists, nitrates, calcium channel blockers, and insulin infusions have all been evaluated in this setting. Other agents used in the treatment of cardiovascular disease (e.g., aspirin) have not been specifically evaluated in regard to reduction of perioperative cardiac complications in patients undergoing aortic surgery.[114,135]

A review of the literature supporting perioperative beta blockade was published in 2002.[136] Five randomized, controlled trials were evaluated, and the results suggested that this measure had a beneficial effect on perioperative cardiac morbidity. The number needed to treat to prevent one MI was 2.5 to 6.7 patients; the number needed to treat to produce a significant effect on cardiac or all-cause mortality was 3.2 to 8.3 patients. All but one of the studies reported a significant reduction in postoperative MIs after beta blocker use, with the effect being most obvious in high-risk patients. Thus, it appeared that perioperative beta blockade is most likely beneficial for patients at high risk for cardiac events who are to undergo AAA repair, unless it is otherwise contraindicated (e.g., by severe bradycardia or COPD) or if they have only one risk factor (low-risk patients). These data seemed to suggest that a goal should be to attain a resting heart rate of 60 beats/min or lower before operation.[114,135] Since then, a large randomized trial with over 8,000 patients studied the effect of perioperative long-acting metoprolol. The PeriOperative ISchemic Evaluation (POISE) trial found that once again there was a statistical decrease in the rate of perioperative MIs, yet there was an increase in mortality and strokes.[137] This evolving controversy may be substantiated as a recent, large meta-analysis of randomized trials that included perioperative beta blockers in 12,306 patients found again a decrease in MIs but no difference in mortality and a statistically higher risk of strokes.[138] Thus, it is likely that there is a group of high-risk patients with AAA who will benefit, but care must be taken to select the ideal patient to receive perioperative beta blockers, even though their use is listed in the 2007 ACC guidelines.[139]

Alpha$_2$-adrenergic agonists (e.g., clonidine) have not been shown to reduce MI rates or mortality from cardiac causes. In one study, mivazerol did not exert a significant overall effect in patients undergoing major vascular or orthopedic procedures but was associated with a significant reduction in MI rates and mortality from cardiac causes in patients with known CAD.[140] Therefore, when perioperative beta blockade is contraindicated, administration of alpha$_2$-adrenergic agonists may be of benefit in high-risk patients with known CAD undergoing AAA repair.[114]

To date, studies evaluating the perioperative use of nitroglycerin and diltiazem to lower the risk of cardiac events have not found this practice to be beneficial in this regard. It may be best to reserve these agents for patients who need them for angina or ischemic symptoms and for those who have myocardial ischemia after operation.[135]

In the last decade, there has been increasing interest in the role of tight insulin control in critically ill patients and during major surgery. A randomized, controlled trial in 236 patients undergoing vascular surgery (bypass, AAA repair, or amputations) compared continuous insulin infusion versus intermittent dosing in the perioperative period and found that intensive, continuous insulin infusions decreased the all-cause mortality, heart attack, and heart failure rate by a factor of 4.[141]

It is widely accepted that aspirin is beneficial in reducing the risks associated with CAD.[142] Its continued use throughout the perioperative period is controversial in some groups, however, because of the potential complications associated with decreased platelet function.[143] Currently, low doses of aspirin are continued throughout all vascular cases, including aortic surgery. However, clopidogrel should be avoided for at least 10 days prior to aortic surgery attributable to a high risk of bleeding. If an emergent need for surgery arrives, then platelet transfusions should be done prophylactically on the day of surgery.

Statins are an emerging group of medications that seem to dramatically lower all causes of cardiovascular mortality. Their use specifically in aortic surgery should be continued throughout the perioperative period.[114]

FURTHER IMAGING

The methods used to evaluate the aortic anatomy before AAA repair are US, CT, MRA, and aortography. Which method is employed in a given situation depends largely on the clinical presentation, the history, the comorbid conditions present, and the availability of equipment and expertise. Each has its advantages and disadvantages [*see Table 2*].

Ultrasonography

Once the decision has been made to repair a documented AAA, further preoperative ultrasonographic evaluation is no longer needed [*see* Patient Is Stable, *above*].

Computed Tomographic Angiography

The current standard for preoperative imaging of AAAs is contrast-enhanced CTA scanning. This modality is more accurate than aortography at measuring the true AAA diameter and diagnosing ruptures.[58] With CTA, it is possible to obtain a three-dimensional view of the abdominal aorta. CT scanning is highly accurate, with measurements reproducible to less than 1 mm. Historically, measurement variations as great as 5 mm were sometimes seen in older scanners occurring 9 to 17% of the time; however, with the current enhancements in resolution and number of slices, this is no longer the case.[59,60] Such variations may be reduced by standardizing measurements, reducing the number of radiologists reading the images, and using calipers and magnification for greater accuracy.[56,60]

The advantages of CT over US include (1) more precise definition of the proximal and distal extent of AAAs; (2) better delineation of the iliac arterial anatomy; (3) the ability to evaluate AAA wall integrity, noting the location and amount of calcification within vessel walls; and (4) the ability to identify venous anomalies, retroperitoneal blood, aortic dissection, inflammatory aneurysms, and other intra-abdominal pathologic conditions and anomalies (e.g., horseshoe kidney). Therefore, CT is the study of choice for excluding AAA rupture in stable but symptomatic patients.[58,144,145] Thin-cut helical/spiral CTA with multiplanar reconstruction is a recommended study for evaluating patients before endovascular AAA repair; CT arteriography is also preferred for determining whether an endoleak has occurred after endovascular AAA repair.[146] In the near future, US may supplant CT for these applications.

The main drawbacks associated with CT scanning are (1) radiation exposure (which can be substantial as patients undergo multiple in their lifetime)[147] and (2) the requirement for iodinated contrast material, which cannot be used in patients with dye allergies or renal insufficiency. In addition, spiral CTA with three-dimensional reconstruction is relatively expensive. Allergic reactions to the contrast agent can usually be prevented by giving a standard steroid-diphenhydramine preparation. If the patient has renal insufficiency, MRA may be more appropriate, assuming that the patient is stable enough, does not have metal implants that preclude it, and MRA is actually available. Alternatively, CT scanning may be done without contrast to determine whether there is a large retroperitoneal hematoma, which not only is sufficient to diagnose a ruptured AAA but also is useful to determine if the patient can undergo an endovascular repair. For this reason, in patients with renal failure, nonintravenous contrast CT of the chest, abdomen, and pelvis is the preferred test when ruptured aneurysm is high on the list of differential diagnoses.

Magnetic Resonance Angiography

In patients with renal insufficiency who are scheduled for AAA repair, MRA with gadolinium and the breath-hold technique used to be the preoperative study of choice as it was comparable to CT scanning in evaluating elective AAA repair candidates.[96,148] Since then, growing concern for the incidence of nephrogenic fibrosing dermopathy in patients with renal failure exposed to gadolinium has now excluded this patient population from being studied with this contrast agent. In patients who do not have renal failure and are studied with MRA, the main advantages include the following: (1) it does not always require the use of nephrotoxic agents or radiation and (2) it is highly sensitive and specific in detecting stenoses of the splanchnic, renal, and iliac arteries.[95] Its main drawbacks are as follows: (1) it is not widely available, (2) it is expensive, (3) it may cause claustrophobia, and (4) it takes longer to perform than CT. MRA is contraindicated in patients with pacemakers, metallic foreign bodies in the eye, cochlear implants, pulmonary artery catheters, and certain intracranial aneurysm clips, among others.

Aortography

Preoperative digital subtraction angiography of the aorta (aortography) is not routinely used for preoperative diagnosis. In the present era, where CTA and MRA is so often used, rarely is angiography the imaging technique to first discover a AAA. The most common use of aortography in the treatment of AAAs is during the endovascular repair of a known aneurysm. The aortogram is obtained to mark the level of the renal arteries and iliac bifurcation to confirm the appropriate length and positioning of the endograft.

Being an invasive test, aortography carries an added risk over other imaging modalities. Aortography is currently indicated in the preoperative evaluation of an AAA when (1) the extent of the aneurysm may include the juxtarenal or suprarenal aorta; (2) the clinical history is indicative of lower extremity arterial occlusive disease (i.e., claudication or rest pain); (3) renovascular disease may be present, as evidenced by uncontrolled hypertension or azotemia; or (4) the patient has previously undergone arterial reconstruction.[20,90] Aortography is superior at evaluating the intraluminal characteristics of the aorta, determining visceral branch involvement, and delineating variations in the vascular anatomy.[14]

Aortography has a number of important limitations in comparison with CT or MRA starting with the need to gain arterial access with needles and catheters. In particular, it is associated with particular risks not found in CT or MRA, such as infection, arterial thrombosis necessitating emergent thrombectomy and repair, distal embolization, groin hematoma, and local arterial dissection.[149] There is also a 10% risk of renal failure in patients with elevated creatinine levels (≥2.5 mg/dL)[149]; this can often be prevented with adequate hydration before the study or by using carbon dioxide gas as the contrast agent to evaluate the infradiaphragmatic blood vessels. The limitation of carbon dioxide angiography is that the resolution is directly proportional to the quality of the image intensifier and operator, although it is inversely proportional to the surrounding bowel gas and thickness of the patient.[150] Finally, the cost of aortography is three to four times that of spiral CT, which gives health care providers an incentive to replace aortography with spiral CT whenever possible.[151]

Complications of AAAs

Rupture of an AAA is obviously life threatening, but erosion of an aneurysm into adjacent structures may be catastrophic as well. In certain instances, ruptured AAAs may form a continuous luminal connection with a surrounding structure. High-output cardiac failure may result from an arteriovenous shunt between the aorta and the inferior vena cava (aortocaval fistula), which occurs in as many as 2 to 4% of patients with ruptured AAAs.[152,153] AAA patients with intermittent gastrointestinal bleeding may present with so-called herald bleeding from a primary aortoenteric fistula. Most such fistulas occur in the third or fourth part of the duodenum after a repaired aorta, and the graft material can be seen in the duodenum during upper endoscopy.[154] Aorta–inferior vena cava shunts and aortoenteric fistulas are medical emergencies that demand urgent operative attention.

AAAs may also give rise to distal lower extremity atheroemboli. Small AAAs appear to be the most common sources: infrarenal AAAs with mean diameters of [illegible] cm have been linked to lower extremity atheroembolism.[illegible] Thrombosis of an AAA also occurs; if it develops acutely, severe ischemia of the entire lower torso may result, manifested by a bilateral lack of femoral pulses, a drop in skin temperature beginning at the level of the upper thigh, and a change in skin color beginning at the level of the knees.[154] This can also be seen after direct abdominal trauma or after a motor vehicle crash where the seatbelt dislodges aortic thrombus from the AAA to the lower extremities. Recognizing these symptoms as potential complications of AAAs can facilitate diagnosis.

Rare Causes of Pulsatile Abdominal Mass

Finally, when a patient presents with a pulsatile abdominal mass that is suggestive of aneurysmal disease, the most likely diagnosis is an infrarenal AAA as 80 to 90% of aortic aneurysms are found in this location. It is important to keep in mind, however, that various, less common types of aneurysms may also present as a pulsatile abdominal mass, including (but not limited to) iliac artery aneurysms [*see Figure 4*], traumatic pseudoaneurysms, and visceral artery aneurysms.[1]

Financial Disclosures: None Reported

References

1. Upchurch GR. Aortic aneurysms. New Jersey, NJ: Humana Press; 2008.
2. Centers for Disease Control and Prevention. Deaths: leading causes for 2002. Leading causes of death by age group, Asian or Pacific Islander Males—United States, 2002. Available at: http://www.cdc.gov/men/lcod/02asian.pdf (accessed May 12, 2010).
3. Mureebe L, Egorova N, Giacovelli JK, et al. National trends in the repair of ruptured abdominal aortic aneurysms. J Vasc Surg 2008;48:1101–7.
4. Cowan JA Jr, Dimick JB, Henke PK, et al. Epidemiology of aortic aneurysm repair in the United States from 1993 to 2003. Ann N Y Acad Sci 2006;1085:1–10.
5. Huber TS, Wang JG, Derrow AE, et al. Experience in the United States with intact abdominal aortic aneurysm repair. J Vasc Surg 2001;33:304–10; discussion 310–301.
6. Shames ML, Thompson RW. Abdominal aortic aneurysms. Surgical treatment. Cardiol Clin 2002;20:563–78, vi.
7. Loughran CF. A review of the plain abdominal radiograph in acute rupture of abdominal aortic aneurysms. Clin Radiol 1986;37:383–7.
8. LaRoy LL, Cormier PJ, Matalon TA, et al. Imaging of abdominal aortic aneurysms. AJR Am J Roentgenol 1989;152:785–92.

9. Davies AJ, Winter RK, Lewis MH. Prevalence of abdominal aortic aneurysms in urology patients referred for ultrasound. Ann R Coll Surg Engl 1999;81:235–8.
10. Wakefield TW, Whitehouse WM Jr, Wu SC, et al. Abdominal aortic aneurysm rupture: statistical analysis of factors affecting outcome of surgical treatment. Surgery 1982;91:586–96.
11. Darling RC. Ruptured arteriosclerotic abdominal aortic aneurysms. A pathologic and clinical study. Am J Surg 1970;119:397–401.
12. Boyle JR, Gibbs PJ, Kruger A, et al. Existing delays following the presentation of ruptured abdominal aortic aneurysm allow sufficient time to assess patients for endovascular repair. Eur J Vasc Endovasc Surg 2005;29:505–9.
13. Valentine RJ, Barth MJ, Myers SI, Clagett GP. Nonvascular emergencies presenting as ruptured abdominal aortic aneurysms. Surgery 1993;113:286–9.
14. Borrero E, Queral LA. Symptomatic abdominal aortic aneurysm misdiagnosed as nephroureterolithiasis. Ann Vasc Surg 1988; 2:145–9.
15. Hodgson KJ, Webster DJ. Abdominal aortic aneurysm causing duodenal and ureteric obstruction. J Vasc Surg 1986;3:364–8.
16. Lederle FA, Johnson GR, Wilson SE, et al. The Aneurysm Detection and Management Study Screening Program: validation cohort and final results. Aneurysm Detection and Management Veterans Affairs Cooperative Study Investigators. Arch Intern Med 2000; 160:1425–30.
17. Johnston KW. Influence of sex on the results of abdominal aortic aneurysm repair. Canadian Society for Vascular Surgery Aneurysm Study Group. J Vasc Surg 1994;20:914–23; discussion 923–916.
18. Singh K, Bonaa KH, Jacobsen BK, et al. Prevalence of and risk factors for abdominal aortic aneurysms in a population-based study: The Tromso Study. Am J Epidemiol 2001;154:236–44.
19. Steckmeier B. [Epidemiology of aortic disease: aneurysm, dissection, occlusion]. Radiologe 2001;41:624–32.
20. Vardulaki KA, Walker NM, Day NE, et al. Quantifying the risks of hypertension, age, sex and smoking in patients with abdominal aortic aneurysm. Br J Surg 2000;87:195–200.
21. Darling RC 3rd, Brewster DC, Darling RC, et al. Are familial abdominal aortic aneurysms different? J Vasc Surg 1989;10: 39–43.
22. Johansen K, Koepsell T. Familial tendency for abdominal aortic aneurysms. JAMA 1986;256:1934–6.
23. van Vlijmen-van Keulen CJ, Pals G, Rauwerda JA. Familial abdominal aortic aneurysm: a systematic review of a genetic background. Eur J Vasc Endovasc Surg 2002;24:105–16.
24. Kent KC, Zwolak RM, Jaff MR, et al. Screening for abdominal aortic aneurysm: a consensus statement. J Vasc Surg 2004; 39:267–9.
25. Wilmink TB, Quick CR, Day NE. The association between cigarette smoking and abdominal aortic aneurysms. J Vasc Surg 1999;30:1099–105.
26. Brown LC, Powell JT. Risk factors for aneurysm rupture in patients kept under ultrasound surveillance. UK Small Aneurysm Trial Participants. Ann Surg 1999; 230:289–96; discussion 296–287.
27. Brown PM, Zelt DT, Sobolev B. The risk of rupture in untreated aneurysms: the impact of size, gender, and expansion rate. J Vasc Surg 2003;37:280–4.
28. Englesbe MJ, Wu AH, Clowes AW, Zierler RE. The prevalence and natural history of aortic aneurysms in heart and abdominal organ transplant patients. J Vasc Surg 2003;37:27–31.
29. Hallett JW Jr, Marshall DM, Petterson TM, et al. Graft-related complications after abdominal aortic aneurysm repair: reassurance from a 36-year population-based experience. J Vasc Surg 1997;25:277–84; discussion 285–276.
30. Brunkwall J, Hauksson H, Bengtsson H, et al. Solitary aneurysms of the iliac arterial system: an estimate of their frequency of occurrence. J Vasc Surg 1989;10:381–4.
31. Bernhard VM, Mitchell RS, Matsumura JS, et al. Ruptured abdominal aortic aneurysm after endovascular repair. J Vasc Surg 2002; 35:1155–62.
32. Faries PL, Brener BJ, Connelly TL, et al. A multicenter experience with the Talent endovascular graft for the treatment of abdominal aortic aneurysms. J Vasc Surg 2002;35:1123–8.
33. Pearce WH. What's new in vascular surgery. J Am Coll Surg 2003;196:253–66.
34. Schermerhorn ML, O'Malley AJ, Jhaveri A, et al. Endovascular vs. open repair of abdominal aortic aneurysms in the Medicare population. N Engl J Med 2008;358: 464–74.
35. Kiev J, Eckhardt A, Kerstein MD. Reliability and accuracy of physical examination in detection of abdominal aortic aneurysms. Vasc Surg 1997;31:143.
36. Lederle FA, Simel DL. The rational clinical examination. Does this patient have abdominal aortic aneurysm? JAMA 1999;281:77–82.
37. Chervu A, Clagett GP, Valentine RJ, et al. Role of physical examination in detection of abdominal aortic aneurysms. Surgery 1995; 117:454–7.
38. Fink HA, Lederle FA, Roth CS, et al. The accuracy of physical examination to detect abdominal aortic aneurysm. Arch Intern Med 2000;160:833–6.
39. Lederle FA, Walker JM, Reinke DB. Selective screening for abdominal aortic aneurysms with physical examination and ultrasound. Arch Intern Med 1988;148: 1753–6.
40. Beede SD, Ballard DJ, James EM, et al. Positive predictive value of clinical suspicion of abdominal aortic aneurysm. Implications for efficient use of abdominal ultrasonography. Arch Intern Med 1990;150:549–51.
41. Feinberg RL, Trout HH. Isolated iliac artery aneurysm. In: Ernst CB, Stanley JC, editors. Current therapy in vascular surgery, 4th ed. St. Louis: Mosby; 2001. p. 313–6.
42. Graham LM, Zelenock GB, Whitehouse WM Jr, et al. Clinical significance of arteriosclerotic femoral artery aneurysms. Arch Surg 1980;115:502–7.
43. Whitehouse WM Jr, Wakefield TW, Graham LM, et al. Limb-threatening potential of arteriosclerotic popliteal artery aneurysms. Surgery 1983;93:694–9.
44. Diwan A, Sarkar R, Stanley JC, et al. Incidence of femoral and popliteal artery aneurysms in patients with abdominal aortic aneurysms. J Vasc Surg 2000;31:863–9.
45. Ernst CB. Abdominal aortic aneurysm. N Engl J Med 1993;328:1167–72.
46. Chew HF, You CK, Brown MG, et al. Mortality, morbidity, and costs of ruptured and elective abdominal aortic aneurysm repairs in Nova Scotia, Canada. Ann Vasc Surg 2003;17:171–9.
47. Heikkinen M, Salenius JP, Auvinen O. Ruptured abdominal aortic aneurysm in a well-defined geographic area. J Vasc Surg 2002;36:291–6.
48. Cowan JA Jr, Dimick JB, Wainess RM, et al. Ruptured thoracoabdominal aortic aneurysm treatment in the United States: 1988 to 1998. J Vasc Surg 2003;38:319–22.
49. Johansen K, Kohler TR, Nicholls SC, et al. Ruptured abdominal aortic aneurysm: the Harborview experience. J Vasc Surg 1991; 13:240–5; discussion 245–7.
50. Bown MJ, Sutton AJ, Bell PR, Sayers RD. A meta-analysis of 50 years of ruptured abdominal aortic aneurysm repair. Br J Surg 2002;89:714–30.
51. Gloviczki P, Pairolero PC, Mucha P Jr, et al. Ruptured abdominal aortic aneurysms: repair should not be denied. J Vasc Surg 1992;15:851–7; discussion 857–9.
52. Patel ST, Korn P, Haser PB, et al. The cost-effectiveness of repairing ruptured abdominal aortic aneurysms. J Vasc Surg 2000; 32:247–57.
53. Yusuf SW, Baker DM, Chuter TA, et al. Transfemoral endoluminal repair of abdominal aortic aneurysm with bifurcated graft. Lancet 1994;344:650–1.
54. Veith FJ, Ohki T, Lipsitz EC, et al. Treatment of ruptured abdominal aneurysms with stent grafts: a new gold standard? Semin Vasc Surg 2003;16:171–5.
55. Egorova N, Giacovelli J, Greco G, et al. National outcomes for the treatment of ruptured abdominal aortic aneurysm: comparison of open versus endovascular repairs. J Vasc Surg 2008;48:1092–100, 1100 e1091–2.
56. Mayer D, Pfammatter T, Rancic Z, et al. 10 years of emergency endovascular aneurysm repair for ruptured abdominal aortoiliac aneurysms: lessons learned. Ann Surg 2009; 249:510–5.
57. Rayt HS, Sutton AJ, London NJ, et al. A systematic review and meta-analysis of endovascular repair (EVAR) for ruptured abdominal aortic aneurysm. Eur J Vasc Endovasc Surg 2008;36:536–44.
58. Nowygod R. Ultrasonography and computed tomography in the evaluation of abdominal aortic aneurysm. In: Ernst CB, Stanley JC, editors. Current therapy in vascular surgery, 4th ed. St. Louis: Mosby; 2001. p. 221–4.
59. Jaakkola P, Hippelainen M, Farin P, et al. Interobserver variability in measuring the dimensions of the abdominal aorta: comparison of ultrasound and computed tomography. Eur J Vasc Endovasc Surg 1996; 12:230–7.
60. Sprouse LR 2nd, Meier GH 3rd, Lesar CJ, et al. Comparison of abdominal aortic aneurysm diameter measurements obtained with ultrasound and computed tomography: is there a difference? J Vasc Surg 2003;38: 466–71; discussion 471–462.
61. Lederle FA, Wilson SE, Johnson GR, et al. Variability in measurement of abdominal aortic aneurysms. Abdominal Aortic Aneurysm Detection and Management Veterans Administration Cooperative Study Group. J Vasc Surg 1995;21:945–52.
62. Pedersen OM, Aslaksen A, Vik-Mo H. Ultrasound measurement of the luminal diameter of the abdominal aorta and iliac arteries in patients without vascular disease. J Vasc Surg 1993;17:596–601.
63. da Silva ES, Rodrigues AJ Jr, Castro de Tolosa EM, et al. Variation of infrarenal aortic diameter: a necropsy study. J Vasc Surg 1999;29:920–7.
64. Lederle FA, Johnson GR, Wilson SE, et al. Relationship of age, gender, race, and body size to infrarenal aortic diameter. The Aneurysm Detection and Management (ADAM) Veterans Affairs Cooperative Study Investigators. J Vasc Surg 1997; 26:595–601.

65. Pearce WH, Slaughter MS, LeMaire S, et al. Aortic diameter as a function of age, gender, and body surface area. Surgery 1993; 114:691–7.
66. d'Audiffret A, Santilli S, Tretinyak A, Roethle S. Fate of the ectatic infrarenal aorta: expansion rates and outcomes. Ann Vasc Surg 2002;16:534–6.
67. Hollier LH, Stanson AW, Gloviczki P, et al. Arteriomegaly: classification and morbid implications of diffuse aneurysmal disease. Surgery 1983;93:700–8.
68. Lederle FA, Johnson GR, Wilson SE, et al. Yield of repeated screening for abdominal aortic aneurysm after a 4-year interval. Aneurysm Detection and Management Veterans Affairs Cooperative Study Investigators. Arch Intern Med 2000;160:1117–21.
69. Crow P, Shaw E, Earnshaw JJ, et al. A single normal ultrasonographic scan at age 65 years rules out significant aneurysm disease for life in men. Br J Surg 2001;88:941–4.
70. Darling RC, Messina CR, Brewster DC, Ottinger LW. Autopsy study of unoperated abdominal aortic aneurysms. The case for early resection. Circulation 1977;56 (3 Suppl):II161–4.
71. Fillinger MF, Marra SP, Raghavan ML, Kennedy FE. Prediction of rupture risk in abdominal aortic aneurysm during observation: wall stress versus diameter. J Vasc Surg 2003;37:724–32.
72. Fillinger MF, Raghavan ML, Marra SP, et al. In vivo analysis of mechanical wall stress [illegible] abdominal aortic aneurysm rupture risk. J Vasc Surg [illegible]
73. Vorp DA, Raghavan ML, [illegible] MW. Mechanical wall stress in abdominal aortic aneurysm: influence of diameter and asymmetry. J Vasc Surg 1998;27:632–9.
74. Long-term outcomes of immediate repair compared with surveillance of small abdominal aortic aneurysms. N Engl J Med 2002; 346:1445–52.
75. Cruz CP, Drouilhet JC, Southern FN, et al. Abdominal aortic aneurysm repair. Vasc Surg 2001;35:335–44.
76. Hertzer NR, Mascha EJ, Karafa MT, et al. Open infrarenal abdominal aortic aneurysm repair: the Cleveland Clinic experience from 1989 to 1998. J Vasc Surg 2002;35:1145–54.
77. Lederle FA, Wilson SE, Johnson GR, et al. Immediate repair compared with surveillance of small abdominal aortic aneurysms. N Engl J Med 2002;346:1437–44.
78. Dimick JB, Stanley JC, Axelrod DA, et al. Variation in death rate after abdominal aortic aneurysmectomy in the United States: impact of hospital volume, gender, and age. Ann Surg 2002;235:579–85.
79. Birkmeyer JD, Stukel TA, Siewers AE, et al. Surgeon volume and operative mortality in the United States. N Engl J Med 2003; 349:2117–27.
80. Dimick JB, Cowan JA Jr, Stanley JC, et al. Surgeon specialty and provider volumes are related to outcome of intact abdominal aortic aneurysm repair in the United States. J Vasc Surg 2003;38:739–44.
81. McPhee J, Eslami MH, Arous EJ, et al. Endovascular treatment of ruptured abdominal aortic aneurysms in the United States (2001–2006): a significant survival benefit over open repair is independently associated with increased institutional volume. J Vasc Surg 2009;49:817–26.
82. Lesperance K, Andersen C, Singh N, et al. Expanding use of emergency endovascular repair for ruptured abdominal aortic aneurysms: disparities in outcomes from a nationwide perspective. J Vasc Surg 2008;47: 1165–70; discussion 1170–1161.
83. McPhee JT, Hill JS, Eslami MH. The impact of gender on presentation, therapy, and mortality of abdominal aortic aneurysm in the United States, 2001–2004. J Vasc Surg 2007;45:891–9.
84. Cronenwett JL, Murphy TF, Zelenock GB, et al. Actuarial analysis of variables associated with rupture of small abdominal aortic aneurysms. Surgery 1985;98:472–83.
85. Menard MT, Chew DK, Chan RK, et al. Outcome in patients at high risk after open surgical repair of abdominal aortic aneurysm. J Vasc Surg 2003;37:285–92.
86. Biancari F, Mosorin M, Anttila V, et al. Ten-year outcome of patients with very small abdominal aortic aneurysm. Am J Surg 2002;183:53–5.
87. Santilli SM, Littooy FN, Cambria RA, et al. Expansion rates and outcomes for the 3.0-cm to the 3.9-cm infrarenal abdominal aortic aneurysm. J Vasc Surg 2002;35:666–71.
88. Chang JB, Stein TA, Liu JP, Dunn ME. Risk factors associated with rapid growth of small abdominal aortic aneurysms. Surgery 1997;121:117–22.
89. Scott RA, Tisi PV, Ashton HA, Allen DR. Abdominal aortic aneurysm rupture rates: a 7-year follow-up of the entire abdominal aortic aneurysm population detected by screening. J Vasc Surg 1998;28:124–8.
90. Beebe HG, Kritpracha B. Screening and preoperative imaging of candidates for conventional repair of abdominal aortic aneurysm. Semin Vasc Surg 1999;12:300–5.
91. Hallett JW Jr. Management of abdominal aortic aneurysms. Mayo Clin Proc 2000; [illegible]
92. [illegible] Screening for abdominal aortic aneurysm. Cochrane [illegible] Syst Rev. 2007;(2):CD002945.
93. Montreuil B, Brophy J. Screening for abdominal aortic aneurysms in men: a Canadian perspective using Monte Carlo-based estimates. Can J Surg 2008;51:23–34.
94. Multicentre Aneurysm Screening Study (MASS): cost effectiveness analysis of screening for abdominal aortic aneurysms based on four year results from randomised controlled trial. BMJ 2002;325:1135.
95. Wassef M, Baxter BT, Chisholm RL, et al. Pathogenesis of abdominal aortic aneurysms: a multidisciplinary research program supported by the National Heart, Lung, and Blood Institute. J Vasc Surg 2001;34: 730–8.
96. Lindholt JS, Vammen S, Fasting H, et al. The plasma level of matrix metalloproteinase 9 may predict the natural history of small abdominal aortic aneurysms. A preliminary study. Eur J Vasc Endovasc Surg 2000; 20:281–5.
97. Baxter BT, Pearce WH, Waltke EA, et al. Prolonged administration of doxycycline in patients with small asymptomatic abdominal aortic aneurysms: report of a prospective (phase II) multicenter study. J Vasc Surg 2002;36:1–12.
98. Propranolol for small abdominal aortic aneurysms: results of a randomized trial. J Vasc Surg 2002;35:72–9.
99. Gadowski GR, Pilcher DB, Ricci MA. Abdominal aortic aneurysm expansion rate: effect of size and beta-adrenergic blockade. J Vasc Surg 1994;19:727–31.
100. Wilson KA, Lee AJ, Hoskins PR, et al. The relationship between aortic wall distensibility and rupture of infrarenal abdominal aortic aneurysm. J Vasc Surg 2003;37: 112–7.
101. Grange JJ, Davis V, Baxter BT. Pathogenesis of abdominal aortic aneurysm: an update and look toward the future. Cardiovasc Surg 1997;5:256–65.
102. Schillinger M, Domanovits H, Ignatescu M, et al. Lipoprotein (a) in patients with aortic aneurysmal disease. J Vasc Surg 2002;36: 25–30.
103. Keen RR, McCarthy WJ, Shireman PK, et al. Surgical management of atheroembolization. J Vasc Surg 1995;21:773–80; discussion 780–771.
104. Simoni G, Gianotti A, Ardia A, et al. Screening study of abdominal aortic aneurysm in a general population: lipid parameters. Cardiovasc Surg 1996;4:445–8.
105. Lindholt JS, Heegaard NH, Vammen S, et al. Smoking, but not lipids, lipoprotein(a) and antibodies against oxidised LDL, is correlated to the expansion of abdominal aortic aneurysms. Eur J Vasc Endovasc Surg 2001;21:51–6.
106. Zarins CK, Xu CP, Glagov S. Aneurysmal enlargement of the aorta during regression of experimental atherosclerosis. J Vasc Surg 1992;15:90–8; discussion 99–101.
107. Nagashima H, Aoka Y, Sakomura Y, et al. A 3-hydroxy-3-methylglutaryl coenzyme A reductase inhibitor, cerivastatin, suppresses production of matrix metalloproteinase-9 in human abdominal aortic aneurysm wall. J Vasc Surg 2002;36:158–63.
108. Warsi AA, Davies B, Morris-Stiff G, et al. Abdominal aortic aneurysm and its correlation to plasma homocysteine, and vitamins. Eur J Vasc Endovasc Surg 2004;27:75–9.
109. Rasmussen TE, Hallett JW Jr, Tazelaar HD, et al. Human leukocyte antigen class II immune response genes, female gender, and cigarette smoking as risk and modulating factors in abdominal aortic aneurysms. J Vasc Surg 2002;35:988–93.
110. [illegible] EG, Young JR, et al. Coronary [illegible] disease in peripheral vascular patients. A classification of 1000 coronary angiograms and results of surgical management. Ann Surg 1984;199:223–33.
111. Kertai MD, Boersma E, Westerhout CM, et al. Association between long-term statin use and mortality after successful abdominal aortic aneurysm surgery. Am J Med 2004; 116:96–103.
112. Sullivan CA, Rohrer MJ, Cutler BS. Clinical management of the symptomatic but unruptured abdominal aortic aneurysm. J Vasc Surg 1990;11:799–803.
113. Roger VL, Ballard DJ, Hallett JW Jr, et al. Influence of coronary artery disease on morbidity and mortality after abdominal aortic aneurysmectomy: a population-based study, 1971–1987. J Am Coll Cardiol 1989;14: 1245–52.
114. Fleisher LA, Beckman JA, Brown KA, et al. ACC/AHA 2007 guidelines on perioperative cardiovascular evaluation and care for noncardiac surgery: executive summary: a report of the American College of Cardiology/American Heart Association Task Force on Practice Guidelines (Writing Committee to Revise the 2002 Guidelines on Perioperative Cardiovascular Evaluation for Noncardiac Surgery) developed in collaboration with the American Society of Echocardiography, American Society of Nuclear Cardiology, Heart Rhythm Society, Society of Cardiovascular Anesthesiologists, Society for Cardiovascular Angiography and Interventions, Society for Vascular Medicine and Biology, and Society for Vascular Surgery. J Am Coll Cardiol 2007;50:1707–32.
115. Eagle KA, Brundage BH, Chaitman BR, et al. Guidelines for perioperative cardiovascular evaluation for noncardiac surgery. Report of the American College of Cardiology/ American Heart Association Task Force on

Practice Guidelines (Committee on Perioperative Cardiovascular Evaluation for Noncardiac Surgery). J Am Coll Cardiol 1996; 27:910–48.

116. Eagle KA, Berger PB, Calkins H, et al. ACC/AHA guideline update for perioperative cardiovascular evaluation for noncardiac surgery—executive summary: a report of the American College of Cardiology/American Heart Association Task Force on Practice Guidelines (Committee to Update the 1996 Guidelines on Perioperative Cardiovascular Evaluation for Noncardiac Surgery). Circulation 2002;105:1257–67.

117. Froehlich JB, Karavite D, Russman PL, et al. American College of Cardiology/American Heart Association preoperative assessment guidelines reduce resource utilization before aortic surgery. J Vasc Surg 2002;36: 758–63.

118. Samain E, Farah E, Leseche G, Marty J. Guidelines for perioperative cardiac evaluation from the American College of Cardiology/American Heart Association task force are effective for stratifying cardiac risk before aortic surgery. J Vasc Surg 2000;31: 971–9.

119. McFalls EO, Ward HB, Moritz TE, et al. Coronary-artery revascularization before elective major vascular surgery. N Engl J Med 2004;351:2795–804.

120. Poldermans D, Schouten O, Vidakovic R, et al. A clinical randomized trial to evaluate the safety of a noninvasive approach in high-risk patients undergoing major vascular surgery: the DECREASE-V Pilot Study. J Am Coll Cardiol 2007;49:1763–9.

121. Posner KL, Van Norman GA, Chan V. Adverse cardiac outcomes after noncardiac surgery in patients with prior percutaneous transluminal coronary angioplasty. Anesth Analg 1999;89:553–60.

122. Back MR, Stordahl N, Cuthbertson D, et al. Limitations in the cardiac risk reduction provided by coronary revascularization prior to elective vascular surgery. J Vasc Surg 2002;36:526–33.

123. Smith SC Jr, Dove JT, Jacobs AK, et al. ACC/AHA guidelines of percutaneous coronary interventions (revision of the 1993 PTCA guidelines)—executive summary. A report of the American College of Cardiology/American Heart Association Task Force on Practice Guidelines (Committee to Revise the 1993 Guidelines for Percutaneous Transluminal Coronary Angioplasty). J Am Coll Cardiol 2001;37:2215–39.

124. Sicari R, Picano E, Lusa AM, et al. The value of dipyridamole echocardiography in risk stratification before vascular surgery. A multicenter study. The EPIC (Echo Persantine International Study) Group—Subproject: Risk Stratification Before Major Vascular Surgery. Eur Heart J 1995;16: 842–7.

125. Ruddy JM, Yarbrough W, Brothers T, et al. Abdominal aortic aneurysm and significant coronary artery disease: strategies and options. South Med J 2008;101:1113–6.

126. Falk V, Walther T, Mohr FW. Abdominal aortic aneurysm repair during cardiopulmonary bypass: rationale for a combined approach. Cardiovasc Surg 1997;5:271–8.

127. Morimoto K, Taniguchi I, Miyasaka S, et al. Usefulness of one-stage coronary artery bypass grafting on the beating heart and abdominal aortic aneurysm repair. Ann Thorac Cardiovasc Surg 2004;10:29–33.

128. Sun JZ, Maguire D. How to prevent perioperative myocardial injury: the conundrum continues. Am Heart J 2007;154:1021–8.

129. Johnston KW. Multicenter prospective study of nonruptured abdominal aortic aneurysm. Part II. Variables predicting morbidity and mortality. J Vasc Surg 1989; 9:437–47.

130. Axelrod DA, Henke PK, Wakefield TW, et al. Impact of chronic obstructive pulmonary disease on elective and emergency abdominal aortic aneurysm repair. J Vasc Surg 2001;33:72–6.

131. Upchurch GR Jr, Proctor MC, Henke PK, et al. Predictors of severe morbidity and death after elective abdominal aortic aneurysmectomy in patients with chronic obstructive pulmonary disease. J Vasc Surg 2003; 37:594–9.

132. Berry AJ, Smith RB 3rd, Weintraub WS, et al. Age versus comorbidities as risk factors for complications after elective abdominal aortic reconstructive surgery. J Vasc Surg 2001;33:345–52.

133. Dardik A, Lin JW, Gordon TA, et al. Results of elective abdominal aortic aneurysm repair in the 1990s: a population-based analysis of 2335 cases. J Vasc Surg 1999; 30:985–95.

134. Treiman GS, Treiman RL, Foran RF, et al. The influence of diabetes mellitus on the risk of abdominal aortic surgery. Am Surg 1994;60:436–40.

135. Fleisher LA, Eagle KA. Clinical practice. Lowering cardiac risk in noncardiac surgery. N Engl J Med 2001;345:1677–82.

136. Auerbach AD, Goldman L. Beta-blockers and reduction of cardiac events in noncardiac surgery: scientific review. JAMA 2002; 287:1435–44.

137. Devereaux PJ, Yang H, Yusuf S, et al. Effects of extended-release metoprolol succinate in patients undergoing noncardiac surgery (POISE trial): a randomised controlled trial. Lancet 2008;371:1839–47.

138. Bangalore S, Wetterslev J, Pranesh S, et al. Perioperative beta blockers in patients having non-cardiac surgery: a meta-analysis. Lancet 2008;372:1962–76.

139. Chopra V, Plaisance B, Cavusoglu E, et al. Perioperative beta-blockers for major noncardiac surgery: primum non nocere. Am J Med 2009;122:222–9.

140. Oliver MF, Goldman L, Julian DG, Holme I. Effect of mivazerol on perioperative cardiac complications during non-cardiac surgery in patients with coronary heart disease: the European Mivazerol Trial (EMIT). Anesthesiology 1999;91:951–61.

141. Subramaniam B, Panzica PJ, Novack V, et al. Continuous perioperative insulin infusion decreases major cardiovascular events in patients undergoing vascular surgery: a prospective, randomized trial. Anesthesiology 2009;110:970–7.

142. Willard JE, Lange RA, Hillis LD. The use of aspirin in ischemic heart disease. N Engl J Med 1992;327:175–81.

143. Ehlers R, Felbinger TW, Eltzschig HK. Lowering cardiac risk in noncardiac surgery. N Engl J Med 2002;346:1096–7.

144. Cronenwett JL, Krupski WC, Rutherford RB. Abdominal aortic and iliac aneurysms. In: Rutherford RB, editor. Vascular surgery, 5th ed. Philadelphia: W.B. Saunders; 2000. p. 1408–51.

145. Upchurch GR, Wakefield TW, Williams DM. Abdominal aortic aneurysms. In: Eagle KA, Baliga RR, editors. Practical cardiology: evaluation and treatment of common cardiovascular disorders. Philadelphia, PA: Lippincott Williams & Wilkins; 2003. p. 427–40.

146. Geller SC. Imaging guidelines for abdominal aortic aneurysm repair with endovascular stent grafts. J Vasc Interv Radiol 2003; 14(9 Pt 2):S263–4.

147. Sodickson A, Baeyens PF, Andriole KP, et al. Recurrent CT, cumulative radiation exposure, and associated radiation-induced cancer risks from CT of adults. Radiology 2009;251:175–84.

148. Petersen MJ, Cambria RP, Kaufman JA, et al. Magnetic resonance angiography in the preoperative evaluation of abdominal aortic aneurysms. J Vasc Surg 1995;21:891–8; discussion 899.

149. Baker KD, Bandyk DF, Back MR. Arteriography in the evaluation of abdominal aortic aneurysm. In: Ernst CB, Stanley JC, editors. Current therapy in vascular surgery. 4th ed. St. Louis: Mosby; 2001. p. 215–8.

150. Criado E, Kabbani L, Cho K. Catheter-less angiography for endovascular aortic aneurysm repair: a new application of carbon dioxide as a contrast agent. J Vasc Surg 2008;48:527–34.

151. Rubin GD, Armerding MD, Dake MD, Napel S. Cost identification of abdominal aortic aneurysm imaging by using time and motion analyses. Radiology 2000;215: 63–70.

152. Duong C, Atkinson N. Review of aortoiliac aneurysms with spontaneous large vein fistula. Aust N Z J Surg 2001;71:52–5.

153. Rajmohan B. Spontaneous aortocaval fistula. J Postgrad Med 2002;48:203–5.

154. Connolly JE, Kwaan JH, McCart PM, et al. Aortoenteric fistula. Ann Surg 1981;194: 402–12.

155. Messina LM, Sarkar R. Peripheral arterial embolism. In: Mulbolland MW, Lillemore KD, Doherty GM, et al., editors. Surgery: scientific principles and practice. 3rd ed. Philadelphia: Lippincott Williams & Wilkins; 2001. p. 1568–82.

156. Fletcher GF, Balady G, Froelicher VF, et al. Exercise standards. A statement for healthcare professionals from the American Heart Association. Writing Group. Circulation 1995;91:580–615.

4 ACUTE MESENTERIC ISCHEMIA

Melina R. Kibbe, MD, and Heitham T. Hassoun, MD

Diagnosis and Management of Acute Bowel Ischemia

Acute mesenteric ischemia is an uncommon life-threatening clinical entity that ultimately leads to death unless it is diagnosed and treated appropriately. Despite diagnostic and therapeutic advances and an improved understanding of the pathophysiology, the morbidity and mortality associated with acute mesenteric ischemia remain high, having changed relatively little over the past several decades. Accordingly, the index of suspicion for this disease should be high whenever a patient presents with acute-onset severe abdominal pain that is out of proportion to the physical findings. Once the diagnosis is made, prompt intervention is required to minimize morbidity and mortality.

Acute mesenteric ischemia can result from any of four distinct processes: (1) embolic occlusion of the mesenteric circulation (usually the superior mesenteric artery [SMA]), (2) acute thrombosis of the mesenteric circulation; (3) intense splanchnic vasoconstriction—so-called nonocclusive mesenteric ischemia (NOMI)—which is usually associated with a low-flow state or profound hypovolemia; or (4) mesenteric venous thrombosis (MVT).

Clinical Evaluation

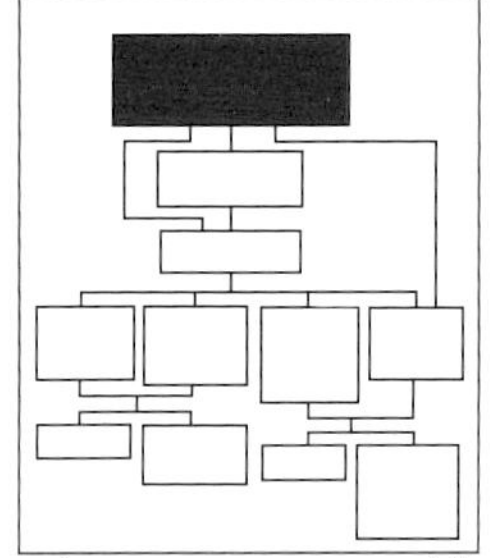

The classic presentation for patients with embolic disease of the mesenteric vessels is sudden-onset midabdominal pain that is described as being out of proportion to the physical findings and is associated with immediate bowel evacuation. In fact, only about one third of patients present with the triad of abdominal pain, fever, and heme-positive stools. A study that considered all causes of acute mesenteric ischemia found that 95% of patients presented with abdominal pain, 44% with nausea, 35% with vomiting, and 35% with diarrhea[1]; only 16% presented with blood per rectum.

Patients with thrombotic mesenteric occlusion also present with sudden-onset severe midabdominal pain that is out of proportion to the physical findings, but unlike patients with acute embolic occlusion, they typically have a history of chronic postprandial abdominal pain and significant weight loss.

Patients with NOMI present somewhat differently. The pain reported is usually not as sudden as that noted with embolic or thrombotic occlusion: it is generally more diffuse and tends to wax and wane, unlike the pain associated with embolic or thrombotic disease, which tends to get progressively worse.

Patients with MVT often present with various nonspecific abdominal complaints; accordingly, this diagnosis may be especially challenging. Common complaints include nausea, vomiting, diarrhea, abdominal cramping, and nonlocalized abdominal pain. As a rule, these symptoms are not acute. A study of MVT patients found that 84% presented with abdominal pain.[2] Of those 84%, only 16% presented with peritoneal signs, whereas 68% presented with vague abdominal pain. Other presenting symptoms included diarrhea (42%), nausea and vomiting (32%), malaise (16%), and upper gastrointestinal bleeding (10%).[2]

In addition to the clinical presentation, risk factors provide essential clues for correct identification of these disease processes. Certain general risk factors for acute mesenteric ischemia have been identified. In one study, 78% of the patients presented with a history of hypertension, 71% with a history of tobacco use, 62% with a history of peripheral vascular disease, and 50% with a history of coronary artery disease (CAD).[1] Acosta-Merida and colleagues found that the presence of cardiac illness, elevated plasma urea levels, and both small and large bowel involvement independently predicted perioperative mortality.[3]

There are also more specific risk factors for individual causes of acute mesenteric ischemia. Patients with embolic occlusion of the mesenteric circulation typically have a history of recent cardiac events (e.g., myocardial infarction, atrial fibrillation, mural thrombus, mitral valve disease, or left ventricular aneurysm) or previous embolic disease. In the study just cited, 50% of the patients who presented with embolic occlusive disease had atrial fibrillation.[1] Patients with acute mesenteric ischemia secondary to thrombotic occlusive disease typically have other manifestations of diffuse atherosclerotic disease (e.g., CAD, peripheral artery disease, and carotid stenosis). The risk factors for NOMI are slightly different. This condition usually occurs during severe low-flow states and represents extreme mesenteric vasoconstriction. It is much more common among severely ill patients in an intensive care unit (ICU) who require vasopressors and among patients undergoing dialysis with excessive fluid removal. The risk factors for MVT include a history of previous venous thrombosis or pulmonary embolism, a known or suspected hypercoagulable state, oral contraception, and estrogen supplementation. In a study of 31 patients who presented with MVT at Northwestern University, 13 (42%) were diagnosed with a hypercoagulable state, six (19%) had a history of previous thrombotic episodes, and four (13%) had a history of cancer.[2]

Diagnosis and Management of Acute Bowel Ischemia

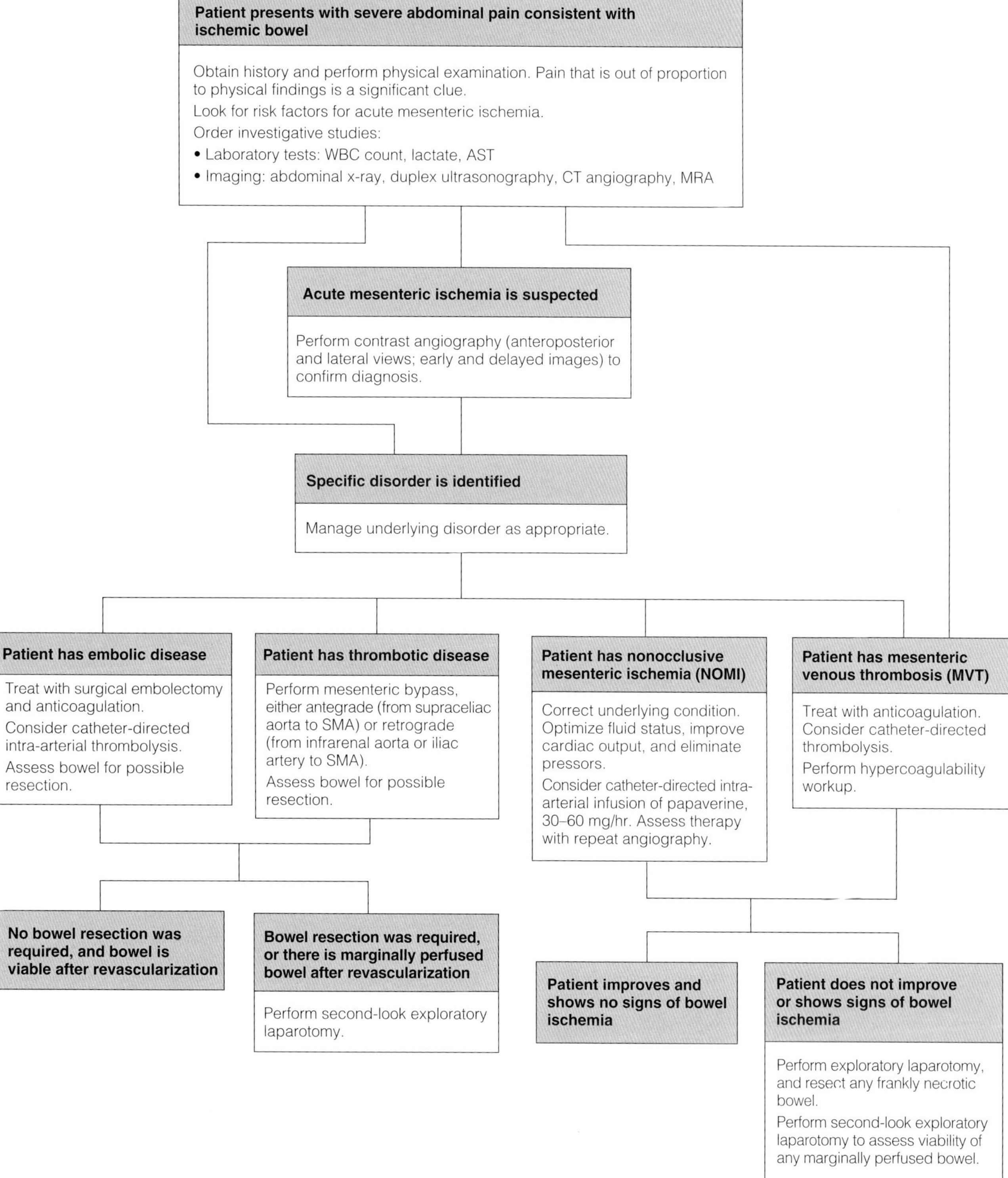

Patient presents with severe abdominal pain consistent with ischemic bowel
Obtain history and perform physical examination. Pain that is out of proportion to physical findings is a significant clue.
Look for risk factors for acute mesenteric ischemia.
Order investigative studies:
• Laboratory tests: WBC count, lactate, AST
• Imaging: abdominal x-ray, duplex ultrasonography, CT angiography, MRA
Acute mesenteric ischemia is suspected
Perform contrast angiography (anteroposterior and lateral views; early and delayed images) to confirm diagnosis.
Specific disorder is identified
Manage underlying disorder as appropriate.
Patient has embolic disease
Treat with surgical embolectomy and anticoagulation.
Consider catheter-directed intra-arterial thrombolysis.
Assess bowel for possible resection.
Patient has thrombotic disease
Perform mesenteric bypass, either antegrade (from supraceliac aorta to SMA) or retrograde (from infrarenal aorta or iliac artery to SMA).
Assess bowel for possible resection.
Patient has nonocclusive mesenteric ischemia (NOMI)
Correct underlying condition. Optimize fluid status, improve cardiac output, and eliminate pressors.
Consider catheter-directed intra-arterial infusion of papaverine, 30–60 mg/hr. Assess therapy with repeat angiography.
Patient has mesenteric venous thrombosis (MVT)
Treat with anticoagulation. Consider catheter-directed thrombolysis.
Perform hypercoagulability workup.
No bowel resection was required, and bowel is viable after revascularization
Bowel resection was required, or there is marginally perfused bowel after revascularization
Perform second-look exploratory laparotomy.
Patient improves and shows no signs of bowel ischemia
Patient does not improve or shows signs of bowel ischemia
Perform exploratory laparotomy, and resect any frankly necrotic bowel.
Perform second-look exploratory laparotomy to assess viability of any marginally perfused bowel.

Lastly, the importance of prompt surgical evaluation and diagnosis cannot be overemphasized. Given the often nonspecific presentation of patients with acute mesenteric ischemia, the diagnosis is delayed in many patients. Eltarawy and colleagues found that a delay in surgical consultation of more than 24 hours after the onset of symptoms resulted in a statistically significant increase in mortality, with an odds ratio of 9.4.[4] Furthermore, a delay in operation of more than 6 hours following surgical consultation was also associated with an increase in mortality, with an odds ratio of 4.9. Interestingly, the authors found that patients who presented with abdominal distention, elevated lactate, acute renal failure, vasopressor administration, and a lack of abdominal pain were more likely to have a delay in surgical consultation. Thus, having a heightened awareness of acute mesenteric ischemia may lead to more prompt surgical consultation, diagnosis, and treatment and may improve patient outcomes.

Investigative Studies

Although there are no basic laboratory or radiographic studies that are diagnostic for acute mesenteric ischemia, such studies can help confirm the diagnosis when it is suspected on the basis of the history and the physical examination.

LABORATORY TESTS

In most cases, the white blood cell count is elevated. In a study from the Mayo Clinic, 98% of patients who presented with acute mesenteric ischemia were found to have an elevation of the leukocyte count, and 50% were found to have counts higher than 20,000/µL.[1] Lactate is another nonspecific indicator of mesenteric bowel ischemia. In the same Mayo Clinic study, approximately 91% of patients had elevated lactate levels, with 61% having levels higher than 3 mmol/L. In addition, 71% of patients presented with an elevated aspartate aminotransferase, whereas 52% presented with an abnormal base deficit.[1] D-dimer is another test that has been suggested to aid in the diagnosis of acute mesenteric ischemia.[5] However, recently Akyildiz and colleagues demonstrated that whereas the sensitivity of D-dimer testing for the diagnosis of acute mesenteric ischemia was 94.7%, the specificity was only 78.6% as many other pathologies may result in a rise in D-dimer levels.[6] Thus, this test should be used with caution.

IMAGING

Abdominal X-rays

Although abdominal radiographic films can neither establish nor exclude the diagnosis of acute mesenteric ischemia, they may reveal signs that are consistent with bowel ischemia. If obtained early, abdominal plain films should show no abnormalities. If obtained late in the presentation, however, they may reveal edematous bowel with thumbprinting. In severe cases, abdominal plain films may reveal gas in the bowel wall and the portal vein. More commonly, however, they reveal a pattern consistent with ileus or are completely unremarkable. In a study of patients operated on for acute mesenteric ischemia, mortality was 29% in patients with normal plain radiographic films, compared to 78% in those with abnormal films.[7] Nevertheless, it must be emphasized that the primary role of abdominal plain radiographic films in this setting is to exclude other identifiable causes of abdominal pain (e.g., obstruction and perforation with free air).

Duplex Ultrasonography

Although duplex ultrasonography does have a definite and well-defined role in the diagnosis of chronic mesenteric ischemia, it plays only a limited role in the management of acute mesenteric ischemia. This is not surprising given the acute nature of the presentation, the accompanying ileus with excessive bowel gas and bowel edema (which hinders visualization of the mesenteric vessels), and the reduced access to the vascular laboratory during off-hours. Furthermore, duplex ultrasonography, although capable of imaging stenotic and occlusive lesions at the origin of a mesenteric vessel, is of little value in detecting emboli beyond the proximal portion of the vessel. Similarly, it has a limited role in the diagnosis of NOMI.

Computed Tomographic Angiography

Computed tomographic (CT) angiography and magnetic resonance angiography (MRA) are more commonly used to confirm the diagnosis of acute mesenteric ischemia than duplex ultrasonography is. Both CT and MRA have undergone significant advances over the past decade. Traditional CT scanning can evaluate arterial patency and anatomy and detect calcifications and aneurysms. In addition, it can evaluate the status of the bowel and help identify other causes of abdominal pain (e.g., pancreatitis, bowel perforation, and bowel obstruction). However, it was not until the advent of helical (spiral) CT scanning—and, subsequently, of multislice, multiarray helical CT scan technology with maximum-intensity projection—that the visceral arterial anatomy could be visualized with three-dimensional spatial resolution [*see Figure 1*]. This technology allows much more rapid acquisition of data and thereby improves the quality of vascular imaging tremendously. A study comparing spiral CT angiography with conventional contrast angiography found that the former had a sensitivity of 75% and a specificity of 100% for the detection of greater than 75% stenosis of the celiac artery.[8] Furthermore, spiral CT angiography had a sensitivity of 100% and a specificity of 91% for the detection of SMA stenosis. More recent studies with multidetector 16-row CT angiography have revealed a sensitivity and specificity of 96.4% and 97.9%, respectively, in diagnosing acute mesenteric ischemia and an overall accuracy of 95.6%.[9,10] Thus, multidetector CT angiography is a useful tool for fast and accurate diagnosis of acute mesenteric ischemia.

Although CT technology has become much more sophisticated and the image clarity and definition have improved greatly, there are still limits that warrant discussion to what can be determined by means of CT in the setting of acute embolic or thrombotic disease. The origins of the celiac artery and the SMA are well visualized with CT, but secondary, tertiary, and smaller branches are less well defined; for visualizing these branches, contrast angiography remains the gold standard [*see* Contrast Angiography, *below*]. Another limitation of current CT scanning technology is the need to administer intravenous (IV) contrast agents, which can be nephrotoxic or, in some patients, trigger contrast allergies.

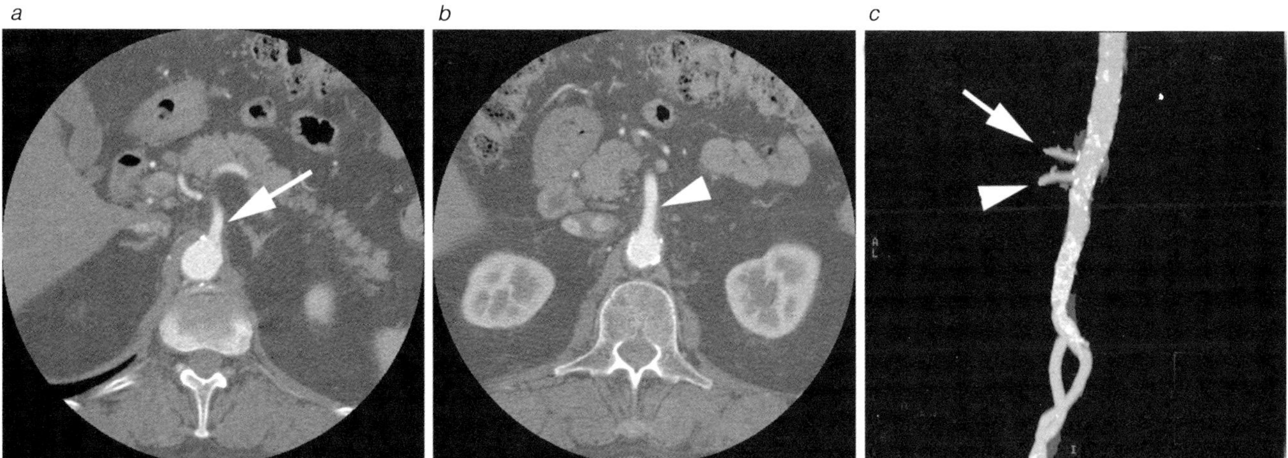

Figure 1 **Shown are computed tomography scans of mesenteric vessels: (*a*) transaxial image of celiac artery (*arrow*); (*b*) transaxial image of the superior mesenteric artery (SMA) (*arrowhead*); and (*c*) three-dimensional reconstruction of aorta and origins of celiac artery (*arrow*) and SMA (*arrowhead*).**

CT angiography also tends to overestimate the degree of critical stenosis when compared with conventional angiography; however, this limitation appears to be less of an issue with the advent of multiarray or multidetector technology, which is more sensitive in detecting arterial stenosis. Finally, significant calcification at the origin of the vessel can make it difficult to determine the true degree of stenosis with CT scanning.

In contrast to its relatively limited role in the diagnosis of acute mesenteric ischemia of embolic or thrombotic origin, CT plays a valuable role in diagnosing MVT and is the preferred diagnostic imaging modality in patients presenting with abdominal pain who have a history of deep vein thrombosis or a known hypercoagulable disorder.[11] CT scanning can readily reveal thrombosis of the superior mesenteric vein (SMV), with or without associated bowel abnormalities [*see Figure 2*]. In fact, CT scans of SMV thrombosis in asymptomatic patients have provided useful information on the pathophysiology of MVT and broadened our understanding of the wide spectrum of this disease entity. In a study from the Mayo Clinic, CT scanning correctly identified 100% of patients who presented with acute MVT and 93% of those who presented with chronic venous thrombosis.[12] In a subsequent study from our institution (Northwestern University), CT scanning identified 100% of MVT patients who presented with vague abdominal pain or diarrhea and 90%

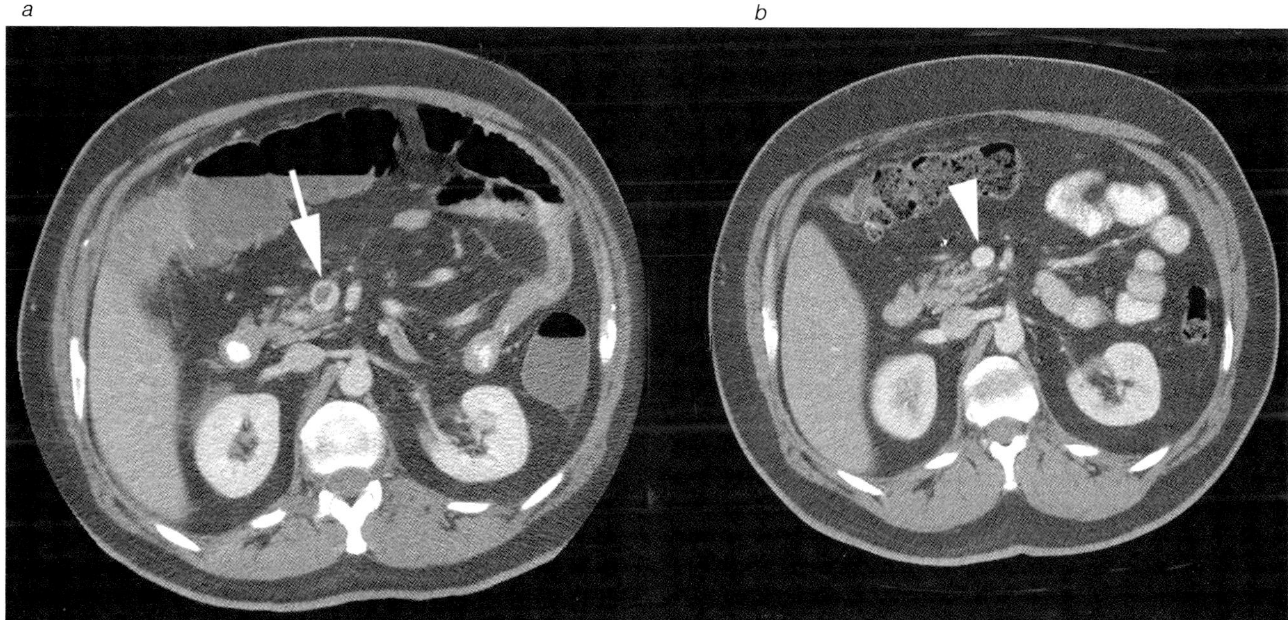

Figure 2 **(*a*) Computed tomography (CT) scan shows partially occluding thrombus in the superior mesenteric vein (SMV) (*arrow*). (*b*) CT scan obtained 4 months later reveals complete resolution of thrombus (*arrowhead*).**

of MVT patients who underwent a CT scan.[2] In contrast, conventional angiography correctly diagnosed MVT in only five of nine patients.[2]

Magnetic Resonance Angiography

Advances in magnetic resonance technology—in particular, the development of contrast-enhanced three-dimensional MRA—have made MRA imaging of visceral vessels much more practical than was once the case. Fast imaging techniques using IV administration of gadolinium over a single breath-hold can provide high-quality three-dimensional images [*see Figure 3*] in axial, sagittal, or oblique planes. An advantage MRA has over CT angiography is that gadolinium is significantly less nephrotoxic than the contrast agents used for CT scans. Like CT angiography, however, MRA does not adequately assess the distal branches of the mesenteric vessels. One study compared contrast-enhanced breath-hold MRA with conventional digital subtraction angiography in 33 patients.[13] There was excellent agreement between the two studies for the celiac artery and the SMA; however, there was poor agreement for the distal branches of the SMA, as well as for the intrahepatic branches of the hepatic artery.

Given the current state of imaging technology, it is possible to confirm the diagnosis of acute mesenteric ischemia with either CT angiography or MRA. If the cause of the ischemia is confirmed—and, in the case of SMA thrombosis, if distal targets are identified for revascularization, it is conceivable that the patient could be explored in the operating room (OR) without undergoing conventional angiography. Many institutions, however, do not have ready access to all of the latest imaging technology. In such situations, contrast angiography remains the best imaging modality for evaluation of the mesenteric vasculature.

Contrast Angiography

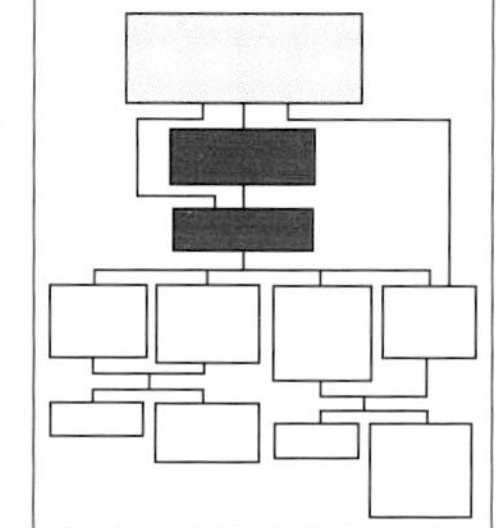

Contrast angiography has long been considered the gold standard for imaging the visceral vessels. This modality can visualize the aorta and the main trunks of the mesenteric vessels and can adequately assess several orders of distal branches. The images obtained with contrast angiography are superior to those obtained with CT angiography or MRA. The procedure is performed in a transfemoral manner by means of the Seldinger technique, with infusion of approximately 60 to 100 mL of contrast material. Arteriography should include both anteroposterior and lateral views of the celiac artery, the SMA, and the inferior mesenteric artery (IMA). The origins of the celiac artery and the SMA are best seen on the lateral view, whereas the middle and distal SMA and the IMA are best seen on the anteroposterior view. Delayed views are useful in evaluating a patient for NOMI.

There are classic angiographic patterns that serve to distinguish mesenteric ischemia of embolic origin from that of thrombotic origin [*see Figure 4*]. Of the three mesenteric vessels, the SMA is most likely to be the site of embolic lodgment because it takes off from the main axis of the aorta at a less sharp angle than the celiac artery and the IMA, which arise from the aorta more perpendicularly. When emboli lodge in the SMA, they usually lodge distal to the middle colic branch and the jejunal branch [*see Figure 5*]. In thrombotic disease, the thrombus usually forms at the atherosclerotic plaque, which, for most patients, is usually at the origin of the mesenteric vessel. Consequently, the angiogram typically demonstrates complete absence of flow in the mesenteric vessel, which often makes it difficult to ascertain the location of the vessel's origin [*see Figure 6*].

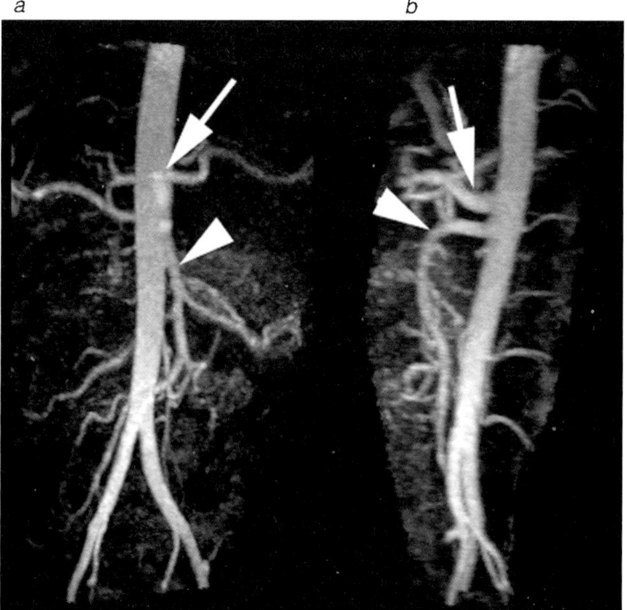

Figure 3 **Shown are contrast-enhanced three-dimensional magnetic resonance angiography images of aorta and mesenteric vessels. (*a*) Anterior projection shows celiac artery (*arrow*) and the superior mesenteric artery (SMA) (*arrowhead*). (*b*) Lateral projection shows celiac artery (*arrow*) and SMA (*arrowhead*).**

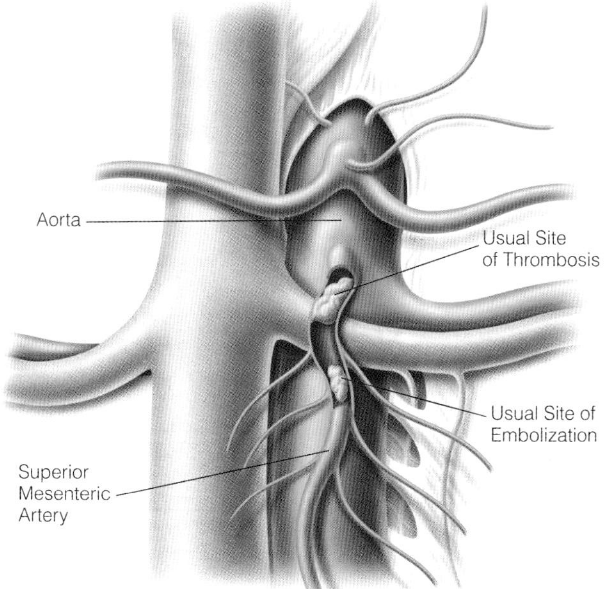

Figure 4 **Schematic drawing demonstrates usual site for superior mesenteric artery (SMA) thrombosis versus that for SMA embolus.**

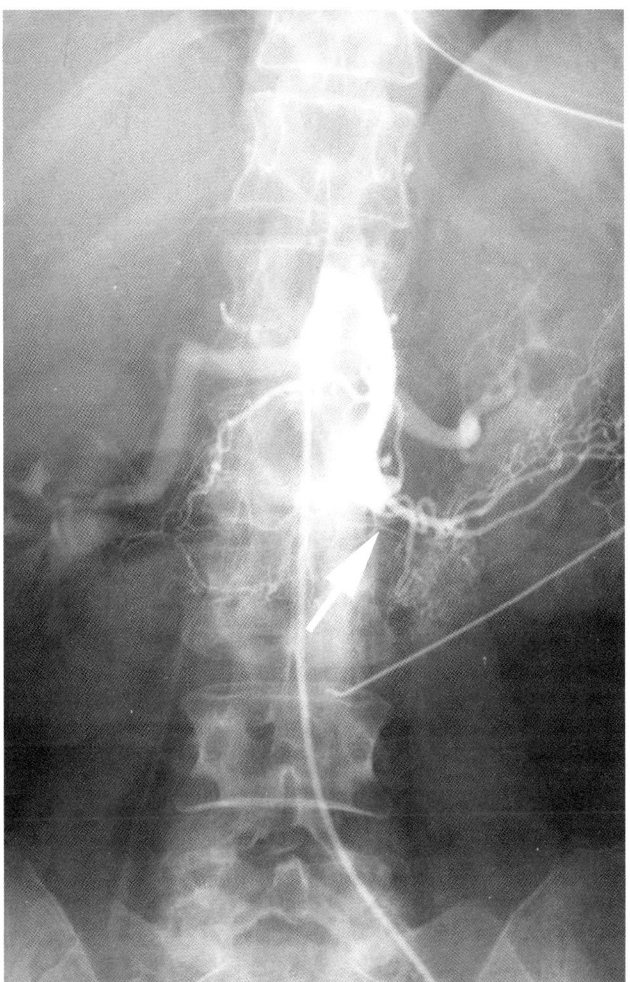

Figure 5 **Selective angiogram of the superior mesenteric artery in anterior projection demonstrates embolus within vessel (*arrow*) at typical location.**

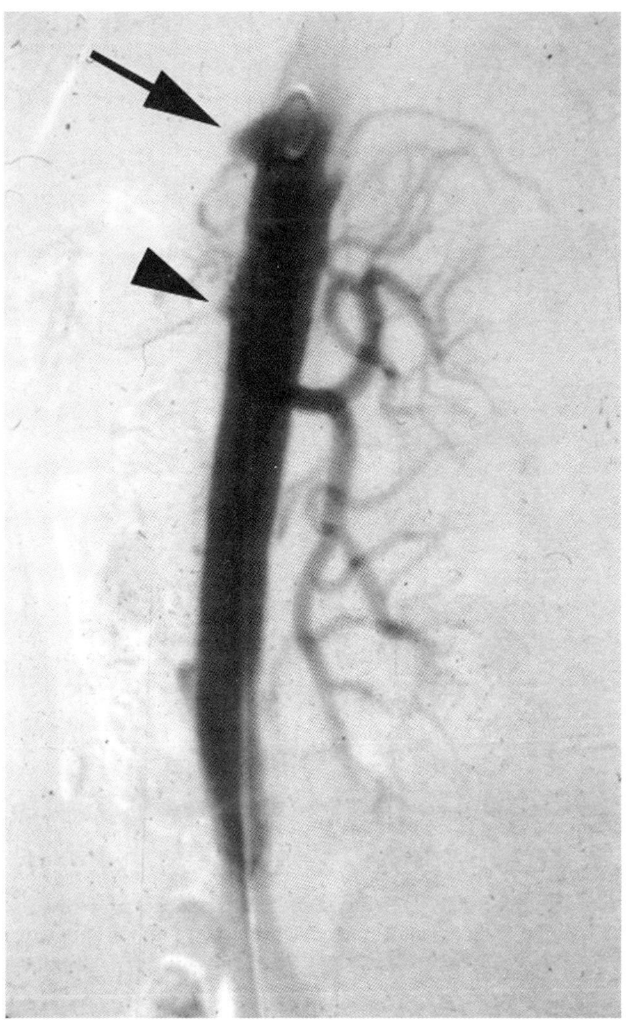

Figure 6 **Lateral contrast angiogram of aorta demonstrates complete occlusion of both celiac artery (*arrow*) and superior mesenteric artery (*arrowhead*) at their origins, consistent with in situ thrombosis. Lack of collaterals suggests an acute process.**

Patients with NOMI typically exhibit angiographic evidence of SMA vasospasm. A small SMA trunk is visualized, with very few branching vessels visible, and the branches that are visualized show a characteristic tapering of the vessel to the point of occlusion [*see Figure 7a*]. These patterns are best seen on the anteroposterior projection.

Angiography is less useful for the diagnosis of MVT. Typically, MVT is diagnosed on the venous phase of the selective arterial contrast injection; however, as noted above [*see* Computed Tomographic Angiography], conventional angiography is less sensitive and specific for MVT than the diagnostic imaging modality of choice—namely, CT.

Besides providing superior image quality, contrast angiography enables the surgeon to perform selective injection of any of the mesenteric vessels and to perform therapeutic intervention. In patients with NOMI, for example, the SMA may be selectively catheterized and papaverine infused directly into the vessel [*see Figure 7b*]. In a stable patient with acute mesenteric ischemia from a partially occluding embolus but no peritoneal signs, selective catheterization of the SMA allows the institution of catheter-directed intra-arterial thrombolytic therapy [*see Figure 8*]. Thus, contrast angiography not only represents the gold standard for diagnostic imaging but also provides important therapeutic options.

Management

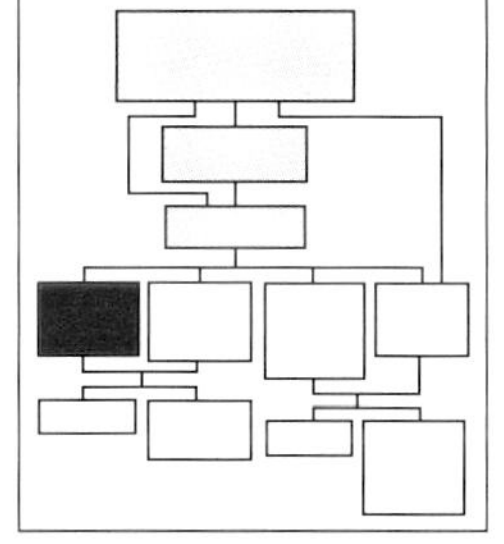

TREATMENT OF SPECIFIC DISORDERS

Embolic Occlusion of Mesenteric Vessels

The goals in the surgical treatment of acute mesenteric ischemia are (1) to restore normal pulsatile flow to the SMA and (2) to resect any nonviable intestine. In general, revascularization precedes resection. The therapeutic approach varies, depending on the specific underlying cause. For embolic disease of the SMA, the standard treatment is surgical embolectomy.

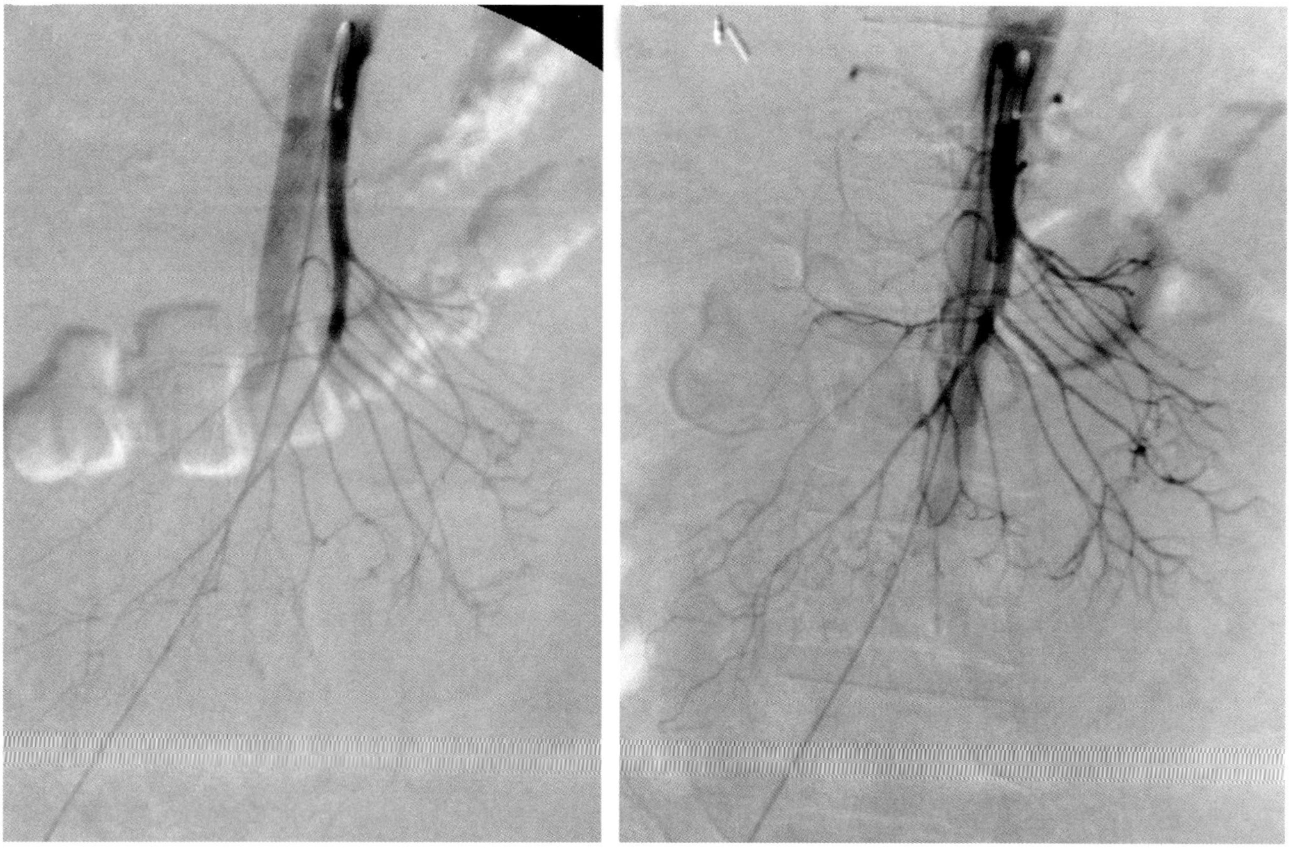

Figure 7 **Shown are contrast angiograms of aorta and mesenteric vessels in a patient with nonocclusive mesenteric ischemia. (*a*) Selective angiogram (anterior projection) of the superior mesenteric artery (SMA) demonstrates distal spasm of SMA. (*b*) Selective angiogram (anterior projection) of SMA after intra-arterial papaverine infusion demonstrates improved filling of distal branches of SMA.**

Percutaneous interventional treatment of acute SMA occlusion has also been described in the literature. At present, however, the applicability of this approach is limited in that most patients present with symptoms that warrant an exploratory laparotomy for evaluation of intestinal viability. In patients who present with abdominal pain, have no peritoneal signs that would necessitate an immediate exploratory laparotomy, and are found to have a partially occluding embolus in the SMA, catheter-directed intra-arterial thrombolytic therapy is worth considering. Demirpolat and colleagues reported performing mechanical thrombus fragmentation in three such patients with good success.[14] We have treated a few patients with partially occlusive emboli and no peritoneal signs on presentation at our institution using endovascular approaches. This route should be used cautiously, however, and if intra-arterial thrombolytic therapy is instituted, the patient should be closely monitored in the ICU with serial abdominal examinations. Even if thrombolytic therapy does restore blood flow to the ischemic intestine, the patient may still experience pain sufficient to necessitate exploration. For these reasons, our use of thrombolytic therapy is highly selective.

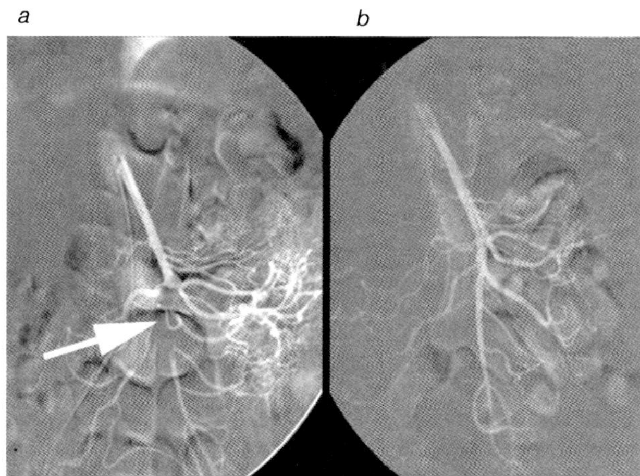

Figure 8 **(*a*) Selective angiogram of the superior mesenteric artery demonstrates partially occluding embolus in distal vessel (*arrow*). (*b*) Selective angiogram after catheter-directed intra-arterial thrombolytic therapy shows resolution of embolus.**

Thrombotic Occlusion of Mesenteric Vessels

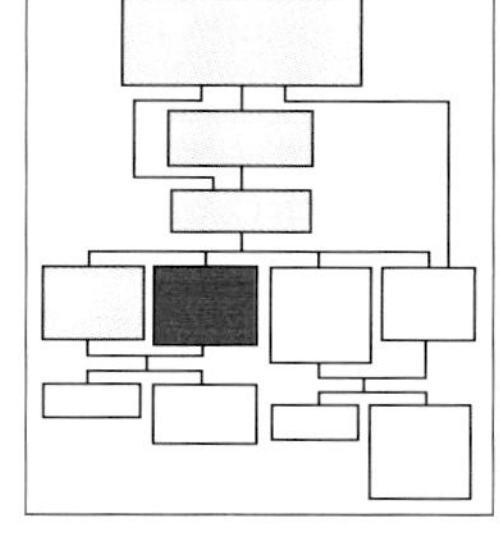

Acute mesenteric ischemia secondary to thrombotic disease occurs in patients with long-standing atherosclerotic disease of the mesenteric vessels. In this situation, the entire midgut is usually involved.

Surgical treatment consists of a bypass procedure, which may be done in either an antegrade or a retrograde manner. The conduit of choice is a reversed autologous great saphenous vein graft. If possible, synthetic graft material should be avoided in the setting of acute bowel ischemia given the high risk of transmural bowel infarction and perforation.

There are several different inflow options for revascularizing the SMA that must be considered carefully. The main choices for inflow are the supraceliac aorta, the infrarenal aorta, and the iliac artery. In cases of acute mesenteric ischemia where time is of the essence and prompt revascularization of the bowel is required, it is often easier to perform a retrograde bypass from the infrarenal aorta or iliac artery in that the exposure is relatively simple and readily familiar to all vascular surgeons. Furthermore, a retrograde bypass yields less hemodynamic compromise because it avoids supraceliac clamping and the associated mesenteric and renal ischemia. Accordingly, retrograde bypass is the preferred approach in our institution. In cases of acute mesenteric ischemia where the suprarenal aorta is easily approachable and not calcified, however, an antegrade vein graft from the suprarenal aorta to the SMA will lie better because it is less susceptible to kinking than a retrograde graft once the bowel is restored to its correct anatomic position.

More recently, a technique that successfully combined an open and endovascular approach for the treatment of thrombotic occlusion of an atherosclerotic SMA lesion has been described.[15,16] In this approach, the infracolic SMA was exposed as usual, and following thrombectomy and patch angioplasty, a sheath was placed in the infracolic SMA through the distal end of the patch for retrograde cannulation and stenting of the culprit lesion. This hybrid technique is an attractive alternative to the traditional surgical approach because it combines open laparotomy and bowel assessment with a rapid approach to revascularization that limits ischemic time.

Nonocclusive Mesenteric Ischemia

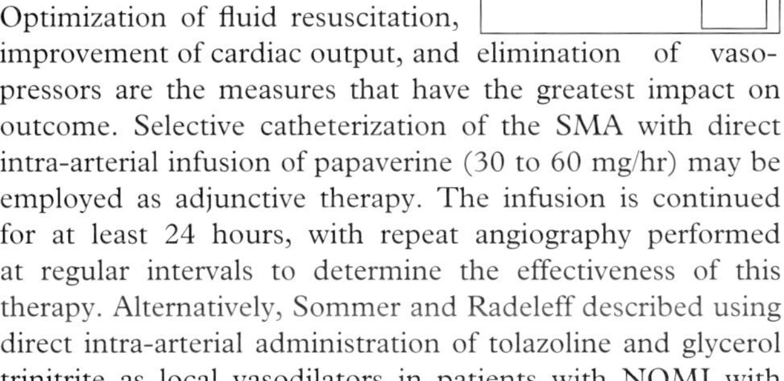

Management of NOMI is largely nonoperative. Once the diagnosis has been established with angiography [*see Figure 7*], treatment of the underlying precipitating cause is the key therapeutic intervention. Optimization of fluid resuscitation, improvement of cardiac output, and elimination of vasopressors are the measures that have the greatest impact on outcome. Selective catheterization of the SMA with direct intra-arterial infusion of papaverine (30 to 60 mg/hr) may be employed as adjunctive therapy. The infusion is continued for at least 24 hours, with repeat angiography performed at regular intervals to determine the effectiveness of this therapy. Alternatively, Sommer and Radeleff described using direct intra-arterial administration of tolazoline and glycerol trinitrite as local vasodilators in patients with NOMI with good clinical success.[17]

If the patient presents with peritoneal signs on physical examination, an exploratory laparotomy will be required for resection of frankly necrotic or gangrenous bowel. If an intra-arterial infusion of papaverine has been initiated, it should be continued throughout the exploratory laparotomy. Given the known propensity of this disease process for waxing and waning, a second-look laparotomy is also imperative [*see* Second-Look Laparotomy, *below*].

Mesenteric Venous Thrombosis

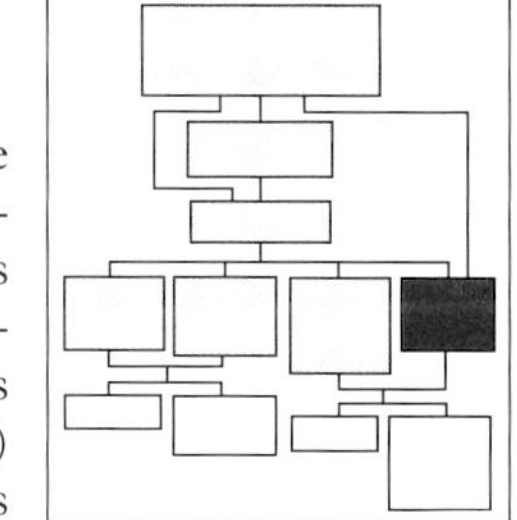

Once MVT is diagnosed, the mainstay of therapy is anticoagulation. If the patient's condition does not improve or worsens after anticoagulation or if signs or symptoms of bowel ischemia (e.g., peritonitis) develop, abdominal exploration is warranted. Typically, the bowel is dusky and edematous. All frankly necrotic bowel should be resected. Within 24 to 48 hours, a second-look laparotomy should be performed to evaluate the viability of any marginally perfused bowel [*see* Second-Look Laparotomy, *below*]. In a study of 31 MVT patients from our institution, the majority were successfully treated with anticoagulation alone and experienced complete resolution of their symptoms; however, 32% did require small bowel resection.[2] Perioperative mortality was 23%. Among those who survived operation, the long-term survival rate was 88%; all of these survivors were symptom free at last follow-up.

Thrombolytic therapy has also been employed to treat MVT. The catheter may be directed into the SMA for lysis of portal vein thrombus.[2] Alternatively, it may be directed into the SMV or the portal vein intraoperatively.[18]

Once the diagnosis of MVT has been established, a hypercoagulability workup should be performed in an effort to identify the underlying cause. If the cause is found to be a hematologic hypercoagulable state, lifelong anticoagulation is recommended. If the cause is reversible, anticoagulation may be discontinued after 3 to 6 months.

SECOND-LOOK LAPAROTOMY

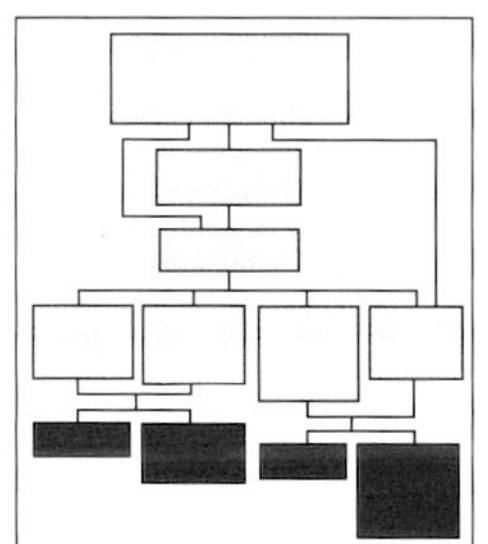

Second-look laparotomy is an essential part of the management of acute mesenteric ischemia. No matter which adjunctive method is used intraoperatively to assess bowel perfusion and viability, second-look laparotomy is the most reliable means of determining the viability of marginally perfused bowel after revascularization. A second-look laparotomy should be preceded by adequate fluid resuscitation and correction of the acid-base imbalance. Furthermore, the decision to perform a second-look laparotomy should be made during the first operation and adhered to no matter what the patient's condition is 24 to 48 hours later. Yanar and colleagues proposed to perform a second-look laparotomy when patients present with a low-flow state, when small bowel is resected and anastomosed during the initial operation, or when a mesenteric thromboembolectomy is performed during the first operation.[19] Occasionally, even though the patient is in better physical condition 24 to 48 hours later—largely because of aggressive fluid resuscitation and correction of the acid-base imbalance—there is still some necrotic bowel that must be resected. Accordingly, we adhere to a strict policy of planned reexploration for acute mesenteric ischemia patients who require bowel resection during the initial operation or who have areas of marginally viable bowel after revascularization.

Intraoperative Consultation

Vascular surgeons are frequently consulted intraoperatively to evaluate a patient for acute mesenteric ischemia. Often the patient has been taken to the OR on an emergency basis for acute abdominal pain with peritoneal signs or hemodynamic instability [see *Figure 9*]. In the OR, acute mesenteric ischemia typically presents as diffuse bowel ischemia. The first decision point in the evaluation is the determination of whether the bowel is salvageable.

Determination of Bowel Viability

If diffuse bowel necrosis exists and the bowel is not salvageable, it is best to close the abdomen without attempting further therapy. Approximately 50 cm of viable bowel is required to sustain life if the ileocecal valve is present, and 100 cm is preferable.[20] Therefore, if it is obvious that no bowel can be preserved, further intervention is pointless. If the bowel is salvageable, blood flow to the bowel is evaluated by assessing the pulses and/or Doppler signals in the SMA. If no pulse can be detected in the SMA, revascularization should be undertaken before bowel resection.

INTRAOPERATIVE EVALUATION OF SMA

SMA pulses are assessed by palpating the root of the mesentery. The transverse colon is reflected superiorly, and the small bowel is reflected to the patient's right. The SMA is then palpated by placing four fingers of the hand behind

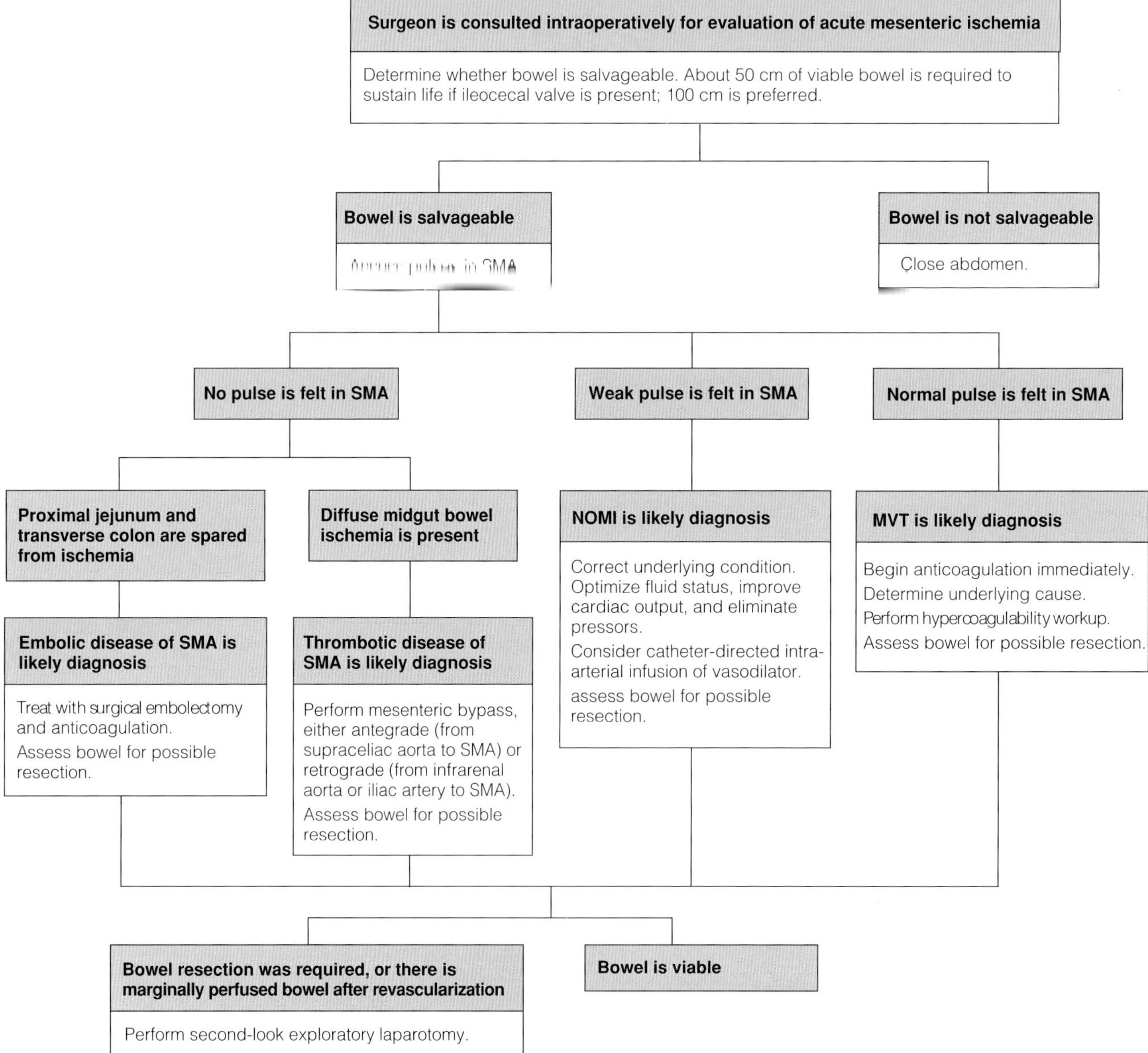
Surgeon is consulted intraoperatively for evaluation of acute mesenteric ischemia
Determine whether bowel is salvageable. About 50 cm of viable bowel is required to sustain life if ileocecal valve is present; 100 cm is preferred.
Bowel is salvageable
Bowel is not salvageable
Close abdomen.
No pulse is felt in SMA
Weak pulse is felt in SMA
Normal pulse is felt in SMA
Proximal jejunum and transverse colon are spared from ischemia
Diffuse midgut bowel ischemia is present
NOMI is likely diagnosis
Correct underlying condition.
Optimize fluid status, improve cardiac output, and eliminate pressors.
Consider catheter-directed intra-arterial infusion of vasodilator.
assess bowel for possible resection.
MVT is likely diagnosis
Begin anticoagulation immediately.
Determine underlying cause.
Perform hypercoagulability workup.
Assess bowel for possible resection.
Embolic disease of SMA is likely diagnosis
Treat with surgical embolectomy and anticoagulation.
Assess bowel for possible resection.
Thrombotic disease of SMA is likely diagnosis
Perform mesenteric bypass, either antegrade (from supraceliac aorta to SMA) or retrograde (from infrarenal aorta or iliac artery to SMA).
Assess bowel for possible resection.
Bowel resection was required, or there is marginally perfused bowel after revascularization
Perform second-look exploratory laparotomy.
Bowel is viable

Figure 9 **Algorithm illustrates intraoperative determination of bowel salvageability, evaluation of the superior mesenteric artery (SMA) pulses, and assessment of bowel viability after revascularization. MVT = mesenteric venous thrombosis; NOMI = nonocclusive mesenteric ischemia.**

the root of the mesentery, with the thumb opposite and anterior to the root. The SMA can also be identified by following the middle colic artery proximally until it enters the SMA. Alternatively, a handheld Doppler device may be employed to listen to the quality and character of the arterial signal at the root of the mesentery. It is important to palpate the SMA pulse distally as well as proximally to ensure that the patient does not have an embolus to the distal SMA. Intraoperative angiography may also be used for evaluation, but it is often difficult to perform in the OR if there has not been adequate preparation and setup ahead of time, and it may not be feasible in some institutions.

If a strong pulse is appreciated throughout the length of the SMA, MVT is the probable cause of the diffuse bowel ischemia. Once MVT is suspected, IV administration of heparin should immediately follow. If the SMA pulse is present but weak, the diagnosis of NOMI should be entertained. However, if there is no SMA pulse at the root of the mesentery, the most likely diagnosis is in situ thrombosis from chronic mesenteric arterial disease [*see Figure 4*]. If the SMA pulse is palpable proximally but not several centimeters distally, the likely diagnosis is an embolus to the SMA [*see Figure 4*]. Distinguishing between these two conditions is important because their surgical treatments differ significantly. To make this distinction correctly, the surgeon should be aware of how the patient presented, whether the patient experienced postprandial abdominal pain for an extended period before the acute presentation, and whether the patient has other risk factors of arterial occlusive disease [*see* Clinical Evaluation, *above*]. In addition, the surgeon should be aware of the specific pattern of bowel ischemia present.

DIFFERENTIATION OF PATTERNS OF BOWEL ISCHEMIA

The different causes of acute mesenteric ischemia are associated with different classic patterns of bowel ischemia, which must be distinguished from one another. The basic distinction between arterial and venous pathologic conditions is relatively simple. In mesenteric ischemia resulting from venous disease, the bowel typically is diffusely edematous, congested, and dilated. In mesenteric ischemia resulting from arterial disease, the small bowel is typically contracted during the early phase of presentation, although it may be dilated and edematous when the patient presents late with frank bowel necrosis.

Within the category of arterial causes of acute mesenteric ischemia, the various underlying conditions are also associated with distinct patterns of bowel ischemia. Typically, in embolic disease, the small bowel and the proximal colon are affected, and the proximal jejunal segment and the transverse colon are spared [*see Figure 10*]; the reason is that the embolus usually lodges just past the middle colic artery and the jejunal branches of the SMA. If the entire small bowel is diffusely affected, as well as the ascending and transverse colon, the origin of the SMA is probably occluded; this disease pattern is consistent with thrombotic occlusion of the vessel by underlying atherosclerotic lesions. In NOMI, the entire small bowel may be affected, but the pattern of ischemia tends to be patchy, with segmental areas of involvement.

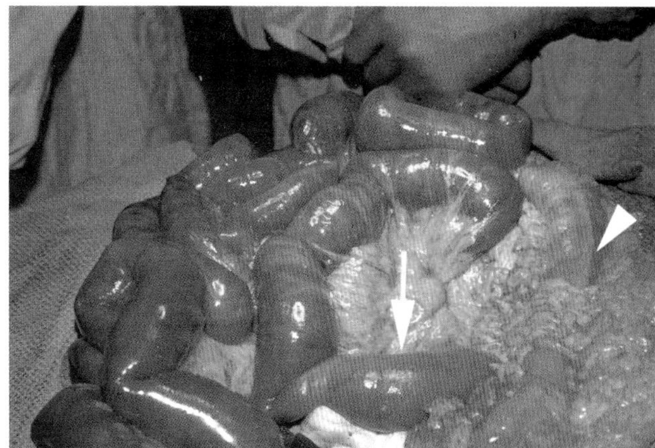

Figure 10 **Intraoperative photograph of patient who presented with acute mesenteric ischemia secondary to embolus of the superior mesenteric artery shows diffuse bowel ischemia with classic sparing of proximal jejunum (*arrow*) and transverse colon (*arrowhead*).**

INTRAOPERATIVE ASSESSMENT OF BOWEL VIABILITY AFTER REVASCULARIZATION

Approximately 10 to 20 minutes after revascularization, the viability of the intestine should be assessed. Waiting until after revascularization to assess the extent of irreversible bowel ischemia or necrosis requiring resection makes it possible to preserve more bowel length. After restoration of flow, the bowel may contain frankly necrotic areas, normal areas, and marginally perfused areas. Obviously, clearly necrotic or nonviable bowel must be resected at the time of the operation. Determination of the viability of marginally perfused bowel is more difficult.

Intraoperatively, the color, motility, and integrity of the bowel should be evaluated. The characteristic appearance of ischemic bowel includes loss of the normal sheen, dull-gray discoloration, and lack of peristalsis. Determination of the character and quality of the pulses in the antimesenteric border and the mesenteric arcades may help determine which areas of the bowel will remain viable once revascularization has been performed. Intraoperative Doppler assessment of bowel perfusion may be performed with a sterilized continuous-wave Doppler ultrasound flow detector. The probe is placed on the antimesenteric border of the intestine to detect pulsatile Doppler signals. Even in the best of hands, however, this technique remains unreliable in predicting subsequent bowel viability.

Other diagnostic options include IV administration of fluorescein, transcutaneous oxygen measurement, and second-look exploratory laparotomy. All of these measures are relatively simple to perform, but each has limitations.

Discussion

Mesenteric Ischemia and Reperfusion

Although acute mesenteric ischemia is initially managed surgically, significant morbidity and mortality remain after treatment, largely resulting from local and systemic inflammation and the subsequent development of multiple organ dysfunction syndrome (MODS). Mesenteric ischemia-reperfusion promotes local synthesis and release of various inflammatory mediators that exacerbate gut injury and prime circulating neutrophils for enhanced superoxide anion production and subsequent remote (i.e., pulmonary and hepatic) injury.[21] At the cellular level, mesenteric ischemia-reperfusion activates a cascade of oxidative stress-sensitive protein kinases that converge on specific transcriptional factors to regulate expression of proinflammatory genes. These gene products include enzymes (e.g., inducible nitric oxide synthase [iNOS], cyclooxygenase, and phospholipase A_2), cytokines (e.g., tumor necrosis factor–α [TNF-α] and interleukin-1 [IL-1]), chemokines (e.g., IL-8), and adhesion molecules (e.g., intercellular adhesion molecule–1 [ICAM-1]).[22–28] Excessive gene activation leads to a maladaptive systemic inflammatory response syndrome that can trigger early MODS. Alternatively, this hyperinflammatory state can cause local gut dysfunction, characterized by histologic evidence of mucosal injury, increased intestinal epithelial and microvascular permeability, and impaired motility; patients become more susceptible to bacteremia and endotoxemia and, eventually, to late MODS.[29]

Experimental work suggests that mesenteric ischemia-reperfusion triggers protein phosphorylation cascades that converge on specific transcription factors to regulate the pattern, timing, and magnitude of expression of not only proinflammatory but also anti-inflammatory gene products.[29] Presumably, this process is mediated by alterations in the cellular redox state induced by the conversion of xanthine dehydrogenase to xanthine oxidase during ischemia, with subsequent production of reactive oxygen metabolites and hydrogen perioxide during reperfusion.[30] Alterations in the cellular redox state activate families of stress-sensitive protein kinases, such as the nonreceptor tyrosine kinases c-Src and Syk, PI3-kinase/Akt, and the mitogen-activated protein kinases. These parallel kinase cascades phosphorylate nascent transcription factors (e.g., nuclear factor–κB [NF-κB] and activator protein-1 [AP-1]), which target genes that encode proteins involved in mediator synthesis.[29,31]

Therapies directed at attenuating these pathways have been successful in laboratory models of mesenteric ischemia-reperfusion and may eventually be able to affect outcome in patients presenting with acute intestinal ischemia.[32–36] However, clinical trials investigating the efficacy of pharmacologic blockade of individual mediators (e.g., TNF-α, IL-1, and iNOS) have found this approach to be largely unsuccessful and sometimes even deleterious in treating patients with sepsis and MODS.[32] The reasons for the failure of these trials are probably multifactorial, but it appears that both the redundancy and breadth of the inflammatory cascade and the poor timing of therapy (i.e., the inability to target early inflammatory events) are major contributing factors. The application of more broad-based therapeutic modalities such as regional controlled hypothermia for organ protection during ischemia may alleviate these aforementioned limitations and prove yet to be efficacious in the clinical setting.[37,38] Nonetheless, it is likely that to achieve any meaningful improvements in our ability to treat patients with acute mesenteric ischemia, we will have to expand our knowledge of the early molecular pathways involved in the activation and proliferation of both local and systemic inflammation.

Outcome after Surgical Treatment

Most studies that include a large number of patients with acute mesenteric ischemia report perioperative mortalities ranging from 32 to 69% and 5-year survival rates ranging from 18 to 50%.[1,39,40] A 2003 study reviewed the institutional experience at Wake Forest University between 1990 and 2000.[37] Seventy-six patients were treated for acute mesenteric ischemia, of whom 42% had embolic disease and 58% had thrombotic disease. Various surgical treatment options were employed, including exploration alone, bowel resection alone, and revascularization with or without bowel resection. Overall perioperative mortality was 62%. When mortality was examined in relation to the cause of ischemia, however, patients with embolic disease tended to fare better: overall perioperative mortality was 62 to 70% for patients with thrombotic disease and 50% for those with embolic disease. None of the patients who underwent exploration alone survived; 33% of those who underwent intestinal resection alone survived. In contrast to perioperative mortality, morbidity was higher in the embolic disease group than in the thrombotic disease group (69% versus 46%). The 5-year survival rates were dismal in both groups (18%). Peritonitis and bowel necrosis at presentation were found to be independent predictors of death or survival dependent on total parenteral nutrition.

In a 10-year institutional review from the Mayo Clinic, 58 patients were treated for acute mesenteric ischemia.[1] Overall 30-day mortality was 32%; however, when the data were further analyzed according to the cause of ischemia, it was found that mortality from embolic disease was 31%, mortality from thrombotic disease was 32%, and mortality from NOMI was 80%. Multiple organ failure was the most frequent cause of death. The 1-year and 3-year cumulative survival rates were 43% and 32%, respectively. Independent predictors of survival included age less than 60 years, bowel resection, and the absence of a recent major cardiovascular procedure.

Schoots and colleagues performed a systematic review of survival after acute mesenteric ischemia according to underlying cause by evaluating available data from the period between 1966 and 2002.[41] The investigators examined 45 observational studies, which included 3,692 patients with acute mesenteric ischemia. They reported that mortality varied substantially according to the cause of the acute mesenteric episode. Overall survival was better for patients with ischemia of venous origin (i.e., MVT) than with ischemia of arterial origin. Within the category of arterial causes, mortality was 54.1% after treatment of arterial embolic disease, 77.4% after treatment of arterial thrombotic disease, and 72.7% after treatment of NOMI. The difference in mortality between embolic and thrombotic disease may be accounted for by the tendency of thrombosis to occur more proximally and thus to be associated with a greater degree of bowel infarction than that of embolic disease, and that patients with thrombotic disease have a greater burden of underlying cardiovascular comorbidity. A recent article highlighted the increasing trend in the United States toward the use of endovascular revascularization for acute mesenteric ischemia and its potential impact on improved outcomes.[42] This study investigated the outcomes of 1,857 patients who underwent SMA percutaneous transluminal angioplasty with or without stenting (PTA/S) versus 3,380 patients who underwent surgical revascularization from the Nationwide Inpatient Sample from 1988 to 2006. In-hospital mortality was significantly less for patients treated with PTA/S (15.6%) versus surgical revascularization (38.6%). Although this large retrospective study certainly has inherent limitations with regard to a comparative effectiveness analysis, novel, less invasive therapies may prove to be effective in reducing the tremendous morbidity and mortality associated with this disease.

Financial Disclosures: None Reported

References

1. Park WM, Gloviczki P, Cherry KJ Jr, et al. Contemporary management of acute mesenteric ischemia: factors associated with survival. J Vasc Surg 2002;35:445.
2. Morasch MD, Ebaugh JL, Chiou AC, et al. Mesenteric venous thrombosis: a changing clinical entity. J Vasc Surg 2001;34:680.
3. Acosta-Merida MA, Marchena-Gomez J, Hemmersbach-Miller M, et al. Identification of risk factors for perioperative mortality in acute mesenteric ischemia. World J Surg 2006;30:1579.
4. Eltarawy IG, Etman YM, Zenati M, et al. Acute mesenteric ischemia: the importance of early surgical consultation. Am Surg 2009; 75:212.
5. Acosta S, Milsson TK, Bjorck M. Preliminary study of D-dimer as a possible marker of acute bowel ischaemia. Br J Surg 2001; 88:385.
6. Akyildiz H, Akcan A, Ozturk A, et al. The correlation of the D-dimer test and biphasic computed tomography with mesenteric computed tomography angiography in the diagnosis of acute mesenteric ischemia. Am J Surg 2009;197:429.
7. Ritz JP, Runkel N, Berger G, et al. [Prognostic factors in mesenteric infarct]. Zentralbl Chir 1997;122:332.
8. Cikrit DF, Harris VJ, Hemmer CG, et al. Comparison of spiral CT scan and arteriography for evaluation of renal and visceral arteries. Ann Vasc Surg 1996;10:109.
9. Aschoff AJ, Stuber G, Becker BW, et al. Evaluation of acute mesenteric ischemia: accuracy of biphasic mesenteric multi-detector CT angiography. Abdom Imaging 2009;34:345.
10. Ofer A, Abadi S, Nitecki S, et al. Multidetector CT angiography in the evaluation of acute mesenteric ischemia. Eur Radiol 2009;19:24.
11. Boley SJ, Kaleya RN, Brandt LJ. Mesenteric venous thrombosis. Surg Clin North Am 1992;72:183.
12. Rhee RY, Gloviczki P, Mendonca CT, et al. Mesenteric venous thrombosis: still a lethal disease in the 1990s. J Vasc Surg 1994; 20:688.
13. Ernst O, Asnar V, Sergent G, et al. Comparing contrast-enhanced breath-hold MR angiography and conventional angiography in the evaluation of mesenteric circulation. AJR Am J Roentgenol 2000;174:433.
14. Demirpolat G, Oran I, Tamsel S, et al. Acute mesenteric ischemia: endovascular therapy. Abdom Imaging 2007;32:299.
15. Wyers MC, Powell RJ, Nolan BW, et al. Retrograde mesenteric stenting during laparotomy for acute occlusive mesenteric ischemia. J Vasc Surg 2007;45:269.
16. Acosta S, Sonesson B, Resch T. Endovascular therapeutic approaches for acute superior mesenteric artery occlusion. Cardiovasc Intervent Radiol 2009;32:896.
17. Sommer CM, Radeleff BA. A novel approach for percutaneous treatment of massive nonocclusive mesenteric ischemia: tolazoline and glycerol trinitrate as effective local vasodilators. Catheter Cardiovasc Intervent 2009;73: 152.
18. Kaplan JL, Weintraub SL, Hunt JP, et al. Treatment of superior mesenteric and portal vein thrombosis with direct thrombolytic infusion via an operatively placed mesenteric catheter. Am Surg 2004;70:600.
19. Yanar H, Taviloglu K, Ertekin C, et al. Planned second-look laparoscopy in the management of acute mesenteric ischemia. World J Gastroenterol 2007;13:3350.
20. Thompson JS, Langnas AN, Pinch LW, et al. Surgical approach to short-bowel syndrome. Experience in a population of 160 patients. Ann Surg 1995;222:600.
21. Moore EE, Moore FA, Franciose RJ, et al. The postischemic gut serves as a priming bed for circulating neutrophils that provoke multiple organ failure. J Trauma 1994;37: 881.
22. Welborn MB III, Douglas WG, Abouhamze Z, et al. Visceral ischemia-reperfusion injury promotes tumor necrosis factor (TNF) and interleukin-1 (IL-1) dependent organ injury in the mouse. Shock 1996;6:171.
23. Tamion F, Richard V, Lyoumi S, et al. Gut ischemia and mesenteric synthesis of inflammatory cytokines after hemorrhagic or endotoxic shock. Am J Physiol 1997;273: G314.
24. Panes J, Granger DN. Leukocyte–endothelial cell interactions: molecular mechanisms and implications in gastrointestinal disease. Gastroenterology 1998;114:1066.
25. Hassoun HT, Weisbrodt NW, Mercer DW, et al. Inducible nitric oxide synthase mediates gut ischemia/reperfusion-induced ileus only after severe insults. J Surg Res 2001;97:150.
26. Sonnino RE, Pigatt L, Schrama A, et al. Phospho-lipase A2 secretion during intestinal graft ischemia. Dig Dis Sci 1997;42:972.
27. Turnage RH, Kadesky KM, Bartula L, et al. Splanchnic PGI2 release and "no reflow" following intestinal reperfusion. J Surg Res 1995;58:558.
28. Salzman AL. Nitric oxide in the gut. New Horiz 1995;3:352.
29. Hassoun HT, Kone BC, Mercer DW, et al. Post-injury multiple organ failure: the role of the gut. Shock 2001;15:1.
30. Granger DN, Hollwarth ME, Parks DA. Ischemia-reperfusion injury: role of oxygen-derived free radicals. Acta Physiol Scand Suppl 1986;548:47.
31. Yeh KY, Yeh M, Glass J, et al. Rapid activation of NF-kappaB and AP-1 and target gene expression in postischemic rat intestine. Gastroenterology 2000;118:525.
32. Huber TS, Gaines GC, Welborn MB III, et al. Anticytokine therapies for acute inflammation and the systemic inflammatory response syndrome: IL-10 and ischemia/reperfusion injury as a new paradigm. Shock 2000;13: 425.
33. Hassoun HT, Zou L, Moore FA, et al. Alpha-melanocyte-stimulating hormone protects against mesenteric ischemia-reperfusion injury. Am J Physiol Gastrointest Liver Physiol 2002;282:G1059.
34. Attuwaybi BO, Kozar RA, Moore-Olufemi SD, et al. Heme oxygenase-1 induction by hemin protects against gut ischemia/reperfusion injury. J Surg Res 2004;118:53.
35. Tadros T, Traber DL, Heggers JP, et al. Effects of interleukin-1alpha administration on intestinal ischemia and reperfusion injury, mucosal permeability, and bacterial translocation in burn and sepsis. Ann Surg 2003; 237:101.
36. Zou L, Attuwaybi B, Kone BC. Effects of NF-kappa B inhibition on mesenteric ischemia-reperfusion injury. Am J Physiol Gastrointest Liver Physiol 2003;284:G713.
37. Hassoun HT, Fischer UM, Attuwaybi BO, et al. Regional hypothermia reduces mucosal NF-kappaB and PMN priming via gut lymph during canine mesenteric ischemia/reperfusion. J Surg Res 2003;115:121.
38. Hassoun HT, Miller CC 3rd, Huynh TT, et al. Cold visceral perfusion improves early survival in patients with acute renal failure after thoracoabdominal aortic aneurysm repair. J Vasc Surg 2004;39:506.
39. Edwards MS, Cherr GS, Craven TE, et al. Acute occlusive mesenteric ischemia: surgical management and outcomes. Ann Vasc Surg 2003;17:72.
40. Klempnauer J, Grothues F, Bektas H, et al. Long-term results after surgery for acute mesenteric ischemia. Surgery 1997;121:239.
41. Schoots IG, Koffeman GI, Legemate DA, et al. Systematic review of survival after acute mesenteric ischaemia according to disease aetiology. Br J Surg 2004;91:17.
42. Schermerhorn ML, Giles KA, Hamdan AD, et al. Mesenteric revascularization: management and outcomes in the United States, 1988-2006. J Vasc Surg 2009;50:341.

Acknowledgment

Figure 4. Alice Y. Chen.

5 ACUTE LIMB ISCHEMIA

*Jovan N. Markovic, MD, and Cynthia K. Shortell, MD, FACS**

Acute limb ischemia (ALI) is one of the most challenging conditions in vascular surgery and carries a high risk of amputation and mortality when treatment is delayed. To emphasize this, the Trans-Atlantic Inter-Society Consensus (TASC II) Working Group defined ALI as "any sudden decrease in limb perfusion causing a potential threat to limb viability."[1] The incidence of ALI in the general population is approximately 1.7 in 10,000 per year.[2] Limb ischemia occurs when there is abrupt interruption of blood supply to an extremity because of either embolic or in situ thrombotic arterial or bypass graft occlusion. The severity of symptoms is directly related to the duration of the hypoperfusion and the abundance of preexisting collateral circulation; the clinical presentation is often complicated by various comorbid conditions typically seen in patients with vascular diseases [*see Table 1*]. The goals of management include limb salvage, minimization of morbidity, and prevention of death. However, given that no objective markers of limb viability are currently available, the initial determination of whether a limb is likely to be viable must be made on clinical grounds by an experienced practitioner with knowledge of the patient's underlying pathophysiology, coexisting comorbidities, and the availability of treatment options.

A study from the 1970s that comprised more than 3,000 patients with ALI from 35 centers documented a mortality of 26% and an amputation rate of 37%.[3] A decade later, a Swedish study showed a mortality rate of 20% in 201 patients with acute arterial embolism or thrombosis treated with thromboembolectomy.[4] Since then, substantial progress in surgical management has been made and major technological advances have occurred, but morbidity and mortality remain high, with death rates approximating 15% and amputation rates ranging from 10 to 30%.[5]

Given the general frailty of ALI patients and the multiplicity of available therapeutic options, it is prudent to take a methodical approach to the management of ALI. Making use of algorithms, decision trees, or clinical pathways can help the clinician visualize and evaluate multiple potential options, which then serve as the basis for selecting the path likely to yield the best outcome.

Table 1 Incidence of Medical Comorbidities in Patients Presenting with Acute Limb Ischemia[155]

	Incidence (%)			
Comorbidity	*Rochester Trial (N = 114)*	*TOPAS-1 Trial (N = 213)*	*TOPAS-2 Trial (N = 544)*	*Total (N = 871)*
Cerebrovascular disease	NR	15.4	11.5	11.6
Congestive heart failure	NR	15.5	12.5	13.3
Coronary artery disease	56.1	47.1	42.5	45.4
Diabetes mellitus	28.1	36.7	29.0	30.8
Hypercholesterolemia	31.6	29.6	23.5	26.0
Hypertension	63.2	60.9	69.6	60.3
Malignancy	NR	11.9	11.5	11.6
Tobacco history	51.8	79.3	77.5	74.6

NR = not reported; TOPAS = Thrombolysis Or Peripheral Arterial Surgery.

* The authors and editors gratefully acknowledge the contributions of the previous author, Sonny Tucker, MD, and Vicken N. Pamoukian, MD, FACS, to the development and writing of this chapter.

CLINICAL EVALUATION

History

An early clinical evaluation is crucial for the diagnosis and identification of the underlying etiology of the ALI. A delay in treatment can result in limb loss, significant morbidity, or death. Because ALI is a clinical diagnosis, a complete history is essential (unless it is unobtainable for some reason). Generally, the dominant symptoms are related to pain (usually the first manifestation) or to loss of motor or sensory function of the affected extremity. The onset and duration of symptoms should be determined, and the location and intensity of any changes should be established. The pain of ALI is often not well localized and is unaffected by gravity. An effort should be made to determine whether the likely cause is embolic or thrombotic: pain of sudden onset suggests an embolic cause, whereas longstanding pain before the acute event suggests a thrombotic cause [*see* Etiology of ALI, *below*].

It is imperative to ask whether the patient experienced pain before the current ischemic episode and whether the current episode is the first. The history should elicit the functional status of the affected extremity prior to the ischemic event. It is also important to ask about previous vascular procedures (including bypass or endovascular interventions), as well as previous or current cardiac disease (e.g., myocardial infarction [MI], atrial fibrillation, or valvular disease), aneurysmal disease, or vasculitis. Finally, inquiries should be made about previous atherosclerotic disease, symptoms of claudication, rest pain, nonhealing ulcers, current risk factors for atherosclerosis (e.g., hypertension, smoking, diabetes, tobacco abuse, hyperlipidemia, and stroke), and previous clotting episodes. The presence of motor or sensory changes in the affected limb is very important in determining the urgency for revascularization.

The characteristic signs of ALI may be summarized as the "six p's": pulselessness, pain, pallor, poikilothermia, paresthesia, and paralysis:

1. Pulses should be palpated and documented. Any previous documentation should be noted and used for comparison. The level at which pulses become absent can predict the site of arterial occlusion. However, fresh clot has a soft, semiliquid consistency that may allow the pulse to be transmitted at the level of obstruction. Only when the thrombus becomes organized and densely compacted is the pulse lost at the site of occlusion. As an example, in a patient with obstruction at the popliteal artery, popliteal pulses remain palpable in the earlier stages of the process, but distal pulses are lost [*see Table 2*]. Intact pulses in the contralateral extremity indicate that an embolic etiology is most likely. Absent pulses in the contralateral extremity suggest underlying peripheral arterial disease and point to in situ thrombosis.
2. Pain is the most common symptom in an ischemic limb, and it progresses along with the ischemia. It must be noted that as ischemia continues to progress, severe pain can be replaced by anesthesia of the limb, which can confound the examiner. Thus, pain should be documented with regard to severity, localization, and progression. In contrast to the rest pain that is limited to the forefoot (pathognomonic for critical limb ischemia), pain associated with ALI is diffuse throughout the entire affected extremity. Pain is usually the first symptom of ALI, with one exception. In acute aortic thrombosis, the first symptom is usually paralysis of the affected extremities rather than pain. Data from a study that evaluated 31 patients who underwent embolectomy for acute embolism of the aortic bifurcation showed that 84% and 14% of patients with acute aortic occlusion presented with paralysis and pain, respectively.[6] The authors of this study emphasized that 55% of patients were referred incorrectly to a neurologist to evaluate paresthesia rather than to a vascular surgeon to treat underlying ALI.
3. Pallor may be seen in the early stages, followed by cyanosis. Pallor develops due to complete empting and/or vasospasm of arteries. As ischemia progresses, the limb will appear mottled, and in early stages, mottling blanches under pressure. Capillary refill on blanching the skin indicates that the affected limb is still retrievable. In patients with thrombosis, initial pallor may be followed by gradual return of skin perfusion and capillary refill over 6 to 12 hours if collaterals are developed.
4. Poikilothermia may propagate the ischemic cascade through its vasoconstrictive effects. The level of coolness and pallor is typically one level below the point of occlusion on the arterial tree and should correlate with the pulses or signals found. As always, baseline documentation should be done so that the progression or resolution of the process can be tracked.
5. Paresthesia is an essential finding. The earliest sign of tissue loss is the loss of light touch, two-point discrimination, vibratory perception, and proprioception, especially in the first dorsal web space of the foot. Proprioception and light touch sensation are lost early in ALI because they are conducted by small myelinated neuron fibers, whereas larger sensory nerves responsible for temperature, pain, and pressure are maintained unless ischemia is prolonged.
6. Paralysis, if present, is an indication of advanced limb-threatening ischemia. The extent of paralysis must be determined. The intrinsic muscles of the foot are affected by ischemia of the vessels around the ankle. Dorsiflexion and plantar flexion of the foot are functions of muscles that rely on blood supplied by the popliteal and superficial femoral arteries. Loss of dorsiflexion and plantar flexion indicates that blood flow is interrupted at a higher level and signals that more tissue may be at risk. Once motor function is lost, limb salvage is more challenging. At this stage, skin mottling is more prominent and nonblanching, representing nonreversible ischemic changes.

Staging of Limb Ischemia

The primary goal of the clinical evaluation is to determine the severity of the disease process so that appropriate management can be rapidly instituted. To this end, the key question that must be answered is whether the limb is viable. Based on a classification system initially proposed by Rutherford and colleagues'[7] in 1997 the Joint Council of the Society for Vascular Surgery and the North American Chapter of the International Society for Cardiovascular Surgery developed reporting standards for ALI and stratified it into three distinct categories on the basis of the severity of the disease process: category I (viable), category II (threatened: marginally and immediately), and category III (irreversible) [*see Table 3*].[8] This staging strategy was also featured in both the TASC I and TASC II documents on peripheral arterial disease.[1,9]

Staging of ALI is based on the clinical assessment of motor and sensory function of the affected limb combined with interrogation of ankle arterial flow velocity signals (as well as venous sounds for category III) using a handheld Doppler ultrasound unit. Terminology in this classification system was used not only to characterize the degree of ischemia but

Table 2 Localization of Arterial Obstruction through Palpation of Peripheral Pulses[164]

Palpable Pulses				
Femoral	*Popliteal*	*Pedal*	*Location of Obstruction*	*Possible Causes*
–	–	–	Aortoiliac segment	Aortoiliac atherosclerosis; embolus to common iliac bifurcation
+	–	–	Femoral segment	Thrombosis, femoral atherosclerosis; common femoral embolus
+	++	–	Distal popliteal ± tibials	Popliteal aneurysm with embolization
+	+	–	Distal popliteal ± tibials	Popliteal embolus; popliteal/tibial atherosclerosis, diabetes

– = no palpable pulse; + = detectable pulse; ++ = bounding pulse.

Table 3 Clinical Categorization of Acute Limb Ischemia[8]

	Findings			*Doppler Signals*	
Category	*Description/Prognosis*	*Sensory Loss*	*Muscle Weakness*	*Arterial*	*Venous*
I. Viable	Not immediately threatened	None	None	Audible	Audible
IIa. Marginally threatened	Salvageable if promptly treated	Minimal (toes) or none	None	(Often) inaudible	Audible
IIb. Immediately threatened	Salvageable with immediate revascularization	More than toes, associated with rest pain	Mild, moderate	(Usually) inaudible	Audible
III. Irreversible*	Major tissue loss or permanent nerve damage inevitable	Profound, anesthetic	Profound, paralysis (rigor)	Inaudible	Inaudible

*When presenting early, category IIb and category III may be difficult to differentiate.

also to predict the need for intervention. In category I (viable), patients present with acute occlusion of an artery that is chronically narrowed. Therefore, abundant collaterals can be found, the limb is viable, and there is no immediate limb threat. In category II ALI, the ischemic limb is threatened but may be salvaged without the need for an amputation if timely revascularization can be achieved. Category II is further subdivided into categories IIa and IIb. Category IIa is named "marginally threatened," which implies a mild to moderate threat to limb viability over time that allows limb salvage if revascularization is performed soon. Thus, category IIa includes patients with mild [illegible] or any lesion for which prompt revascularization of the limb achieves a good result. Category IIb (immediately threatened) includes patients with diminished sensation of the entire foot and weakness of calf muscles whose limb is still salvageable but who require immediate revascularization. In category III (irreversible), ischemia is irreversible, and amputation is required. Clinical features include permanent tissue loss, anesthesia, and paralysis of the limb.

In general, in category I, there is no sensory loss and Doppler signals from ankle arteries are audible. If Doppler signals from ankle arteries are not audible (and sensory functions is preserved), ALI is categorized as IIa. In some patients with IIa stage of the disease, mild sensory loss can be detected that is limited in extent to the toes. Both categories (I and IIa) have preserved motor function. Category IIb is characterized by loss of motor function, prompting immediate revascularization of the affected extremity. Category III represents a nonviable extremity. In these patients, major tissue loss and/or permanent neuromuscular damage are inevitable regardless of revascularization efforts.

INVESTIGATIVE STUDIES

Additional diagnostic tests should be performed to support the clinical evaluation. An electrocardiogram (ECG) should be obtained, and if a cardiac source is suspected, a transesophageal echocardiogram should be obtained as well. A full set of laboratory tests, including a complete blood count and a platelet count, blood chemistries, and coagulation profiles, should be ordered. In addition, chest and abdominal x-rays should be done to look for obvious calcifications. If it appears that a hypercoagulable state may be causing thrombosis, a hypercoagulability profile should be ordered. As recommended in the TASC II report, a thrombophilia screen, which includes anticardiolipin and antiplatelet factor IV antibodies, as well as measurement of homocysteine levels, should be performed, especially in young patients with acute thrombosis or in patients with a significant family history of thrombotic events.[1] If, however, a limb is acutely ischemic and exhibits clear motor or sensory deficits, diagnostic tests other than an ECG and basic hematologic and blood chemistry studies should not be allowed to delay treatment.

Evaluation of Arterial Tree

An objective evaluation of the arterial tree should be performed when feasible. If ischemia is particularly severe and long-lasting, a full angiographic evaluation may not be possible; however, noninvasive duplex studies and, if time permits, angiography should be considered strongly in this setting.

Doppler segmental pressures and ankle-brachial index Evaluation of Doppler segmental pressures should begin at the level of the ankle and should include assessment of arterial signals and venous hums. When arterial signals are found, the ankle-brachial index (ABI) should be measured. The ABI is derived from the ankle systolic pressure and the brachial systolic pressure and is determined as follows. The systolic pressure is measured in each arm, and the higher of the two measurements is taken to be the brachial systolic pressure. A cuff is then placed on each calf, and the examiner listens to signals in the dorsalis pedis and posterior tibial arteries. The cuff is inflated until the signal is no longer heard. At this point, the cuff is slowly released, and the systolic pressure is recorded at the point where the signal is once again audible. Again, the higher of the two systolic measurements is taken to be the ankle systolic pressure. The systolic ankle pressure is then divided by the brachial systolic pressure to yield the ABI. Normally, the ABI is greater than 1.0 because ankle pressures are slightly higher than arm pressures due to gravity.

However, a normal ABI value does not rule out the presence of arterial occlusion. The ABI can be falsely elevated if the distal arteries are not compressible. Falsely elevated ABI can be recorded in diabetic patients, elderly patients, and patients with renal disease due to incompressible calcified lower extremity arteries. When the ABI falls below 0.6, there is a significant difference in blood pressure between the proximal arterial tree and the distal extremity, which usually denotes an occlusive process. An ABI lower than 0.5 is seen in patients with critical ischemia. In these patients, inspection of flow velocity waveform recording the pedal arteries in conjunction with toe pressure measurement can be used to determine the presence and degree of ischemia if the severity of the ischemia is not limb threatening and allows investigative studies. Next, segmental pressures are obtained by placing cuffs at the ankle, below the knee, above the knee, and on the thigh. Systolic blood pressures are measured at each location, and any pressure drop greater than 15 mm Hg is considered significant. When the venous Doppler signal or hum is lost in addition to the arterial Doppler signal, the ischemia is severe. However, the absence of signals does not always signify an irreversibly threatened limb.

Duplex ultrasonography Duplex scanning is a noninvasive imaging modality that can be valuable for localizing the site of occlusion, especially in bypass grafts. In addition, duplex ultrasonography has been useful in assessing the patency of a single arterial segment (i.e., bypass graft or stented superficial femoral artery). Unfortunately, it is not always a practical option in acute circumstances, both because the machine is often unavailable in the emergency setting and because the results of scanning are highly operator dependent. However, in specialized centers where a duplex ultrasound machine is readily available and personnel are experienced in its use, a quick look at the suspected site may yield helpful information.[10] In stenotic regions, the velocities measured across the lesion are greatly increased.[11,12] Duplex ultrasonography can also be used to assess plaque morphology, stenoses, dissections, and thrombi. In some centers, duplex ultrasound technology has obviated the need for lengthy arteriograms and has benefited patients by reducing ischemia time.

Arteriography Arteriography remains the "gold standard" for diagnosis of ALI and may even be a primary tool in its management. An important consideration is whether the delay in performing arteriography can be tolerated in patients with limb-threatening ischemia. In general, in highly specialized centers, patients who require urgent revascularization are evaluated with catheter-based arteriography in operating room angiosuites because it provides detailed and accurate information regarding the etiology, localization, and extent of the lesion as well as adequate visualization of the distal arterial vascular tree without a delay in therapy. In contrast, arteriography in formal angiography suites should be reserved for patients with viable limbs who can tolerate the additional delay before revascularization and should not be performed if doing so would keep a critically ischemic limb from receiving prompt revascularization.

Arteriography should be performed from a site remote from the point of concern. Thus, if lytic therapy is to be administered, entry-site bleeding will be minimized. A complete angiogram that includes the runoff vessels in the foot should be performed to establish the baseline degree of arterial disease and delineate the anatomy of the inflow and outflow vessels. This information facilitates subsequent planning for revascularization should this step prove necessary. Although arteriography is considered to be the "gold standard" in the management of patients with ALI, this imaging modality is invasive and exposes patients to both radiation and potentially nephrotoxic contrast material. Digital subtraction angiography is preferred in that it allows a reduced contrast load and lowers the incidence of contrast-associated renal injury.[13,14] If the patient is allergic to the contrast agent or has renal insufficiency, CO_2 or gadolinium-based angiography may be performed instead. These two modalities have the advantage of minimizing nephrotoxicity but yield poorer suprainguinal arterial visualization compared with standard contrast angiography.[15,16]

Arteriography may help differentiate embolic from thrombotic arterial occlusion and direct proper surgical intervention. Typical arteriographic findings in a patient with arterial embolism include an identifiable source, sharp cutoff, minimal atherosclerosis, a few collateral vessels, and a discrete clot that is clearly visible on contrast studies. If the arteriogram is obtained early following the ALI, acute emboli will appear as a crescent-shaped occlusion at the proximal side of the clot (meniscus sign). Distal to the clot, the artery may appear narrowed secondary to vasospasm. The remaining arteries are typically normal in ALI caused by embolism. In contrast, in a patient with arterial thrombosis, the thrombus has no identifiable source, diffuse atherosclerotic vessel wall disease is present, cutoff is tapered and irregular, and there is ample collateral circulation. Extensive collateralization is pathognomonic because patients with long-standing peripheral arterial disease develop collateral arteries over time to bring blood flow distal to a stenosis of the affected artery. The location of the clot is another feature that can be useful to differentiate embolic versus thrombotic ALI. Emboli frequently lodge at arterial bifurcations, whereas thrombotic clot is usually seen at sites of chronic atherosclerotic disease.

Other modalities Depending on availability within a given institution and the level of quality achievable within the institution, either computed tomographic angiography (CTA) or magnetic resonance angiography (MRA) may be employed as alternative means of evaluating the vasculature of the limb. These two modalities are less invasive than conventional angiography but, depending on the particular information being sought, may yield images of lower resolution than a standard angiogram and may be less diagnostically accurate. Today, MRA is most commonly employed in patients with renal insufficiency to limit the dye load and nephrotoxicity. CTA is characterized by the ability to obtain cross-sectional imaging of the affected artery, speed, and convenience. However, CTA depends on contrast media, preventing its use in patients who require catheter angiography and intervention because this additional load of contrast increases the risk of renal injury. In addition, CTA may fail to demonstrate a target vessel for revascularization distal to an occlusion. Nevertheless, as scanning technology continues to advance, the role of CTA and MRA in the evaluation of limb ischemia will continue to evolve.

was relatively low when cardiopulmonary complications did not occur. The cumulative limb salvage rate was similar in the two groups (82% at 12 months). Total hospital charges were comparable as well, which suggests that at the initial treatment, thrombolytic therapy is as costly as surgery. The median in-hospital cost of treatment in the thrombolytic and open surgery groups was $15,672 and $12,253, respectively. Major bleeding was encountered in 11% of patients.

STILE (Surgery versus Thrombolysis for the Ischemic Lower Extremity) trial This randomized, controlled, multicenter trial was designed to evaluate catheter-directed thrombolysis versus surgery and to determine differences in outcomes between rt-PA and UK in 393 patients.[35] In this study, both patients with chronic limb ischemia and patients with ALI were included. Patients were not stratified based on the duration of ischemia during randomization. The Data and Safety Monitoring Committee stopped the trial early because of an increase in the number of patients with ongoing ischemia in the thrombolysis groups. An ad hoc committee later determined that the reason for this increase was the inclusion of chronically symptomatic patients in the study. In any case, the study clearly demonstrated that patients with less than 14 days of ischemia had a lower amputation rate when treated with thrombolysis (11% versus 30%) but that patients with more than 14 days of ischemia had a lower amputation rate when treated with surgery. A subgroup analysis showed a significantly shorter time of lysis in patients randomized to rt-PA when compared with patients randomized to UK (8 hours versus 16 hours; $p = .01$). Additional analysis did not show any difference in safety and efficacy between rt-PA and UK.

TOPAS (Thrombolysis Or Peripheral Arterial Surgery) trial The preliminary dose-ranging TOPAS trial compared surgery with r-UK thrombolysis in 213 patients with ischemic symptoms of less than 14 days' duration.[36] At the end of 1 year, the amputation rates in the two groups were similar. Bleeding complications were seen only in patients undergoing thrombolysis, four of whom (2.1%) had intracranial hemorrhage. When additional end points were considered, the thrombolysis group was found to require significantly fewer major interventions at the time of discharge and at 12 months. Patients randomized to catheter-directed r-UK received three different dosage regimens (2,000, 4,000, or 6,000 IU/min for 4 hours followed by an infusion of 2,000 IU/min for additional 44 hours, for a maximum of 48 hours). The regimen of 4,000 IU/min seemed to be the most effective when efficacy and safety were considered. Complete lysis (defined as > 95% thrombus extraction) was documented in 71% of patients randomized to a 4,000 IU/min dosage regimen (mean infusion time 23 hours). In contrast, complete lysis was achieved in 67% of patients who received the 2,000 IU/min and 60% of patients who received the 6,000 IU/min dosage regimen. Hemorrhagic complications were documented in 2%, 13%, and 16% of patients who received the 4,000, 2,000, and 6,000 IU/min regimen, respectively. The 1-year mortality rates were not significantly different between the surgical group and the 4,000 IU/min r-UK group (14% versus 16%). Similarly, there was no significant difference in amputation-free survival rates between these two groups (75% versus 65%).

The preliminary dose-ranging TOPAS trial led to a larger trial that compared r-UK with surgical revascularization as initial treatment for acute arterial occlusion of lower extremities. This randomized, multicenter trial conducted at 113 North American and European sites randomized 544 patients into two equal cohorts that underwent either catheter-directed intra-arterial r-UK treatment or surgical revascularization.[37] Both groups of patients had acute arterial obstruction of 14 days or less. In the r-UK group, amputation-free survival rates were 71.8% at 6 months and 65.0% at 1 year compared with respective rates of 74.8% and 69.9% in the group that underwent surgical revascularization. Major hemorrhage was documented in 32 patients (12.5%) in the r-UK group and 14 patients (5.5%) in the surgery group. The authors also documented four episodes (1.4%) of intracranial hemorrhage in the r-UK group (one of which was fatal). There were no episodes of intracranial hemorrhage in the group of patients randomized to the surgical revascularization. Although it was associated with a higher incidence of hemorrhagic complications, r-UK treatment lowered the need for open surgical procedure without a significantly increased risk of amputation and mortality.

Recombinant tissue plasminogen activator versus urokinase A prospective, randomized, multicenter trial evaluated local thrombolysis with either rt-PA or UK in 234 patients with thrombotic femoropopliteal occlusions (223 [95%] native femoral or popliteal arteries, 11 [5%] bypass grafts).[38] Complete reperfusion occurred in 62% of the patients treated with rt-PA and in 50% of the patients treated with UK. However, bleeding was observed in 12.8% of rt-PA-treated patients (including one instance of cerebral hemorrhage) and in 9.1% of UK-treated patients (none of whom experienced cerebral bleeding).

Three additional trials compared UK versus rt-PA for the management of patients with lower extremity arterial occlusion or graft occlusion.[35,39,40] As mentioned above, the STILE trial showed no differences in efficacy or bleeding complications between rt-PA and UK. Data from this study demonstrated a significant difference ($p < .02$) in the speed of lysis favoring rt-PA.[35] In another study that randomized 120 patients with acute or subacute infrainguinal arterial thrombosis (femoral [$n = 21$], femoropopliteal [$n = 33$], popliteal [$n = 13$], and popliteocrural [$n = 53$] artery) to local lysis using UK or rt-PA, Schweizer and colleagues found that patients receiving rt-PA had better lytic success and more rapid lysis with less severe ischemia at 6 months.[40] No major hemorrhages were encountered in either group. Large local hematomas occurred in 8% and 15% of patients treated with UK and rt-PA, respectively. It must be emphasized that the authors of this study compared high doses of rt-PA (5 mg bolus followed by 5 mg/h infusion) with moderate or low doses of UK (60,000 IU/h with no bolus). Both groups of patients were anticoagulated with intravenous heparin (500 IU bolus followed by an infusion of 700 to 750 IU/h) during the treatment.

In another study, from Brigham and Women's Hospital, Myerovitz and colleagues equally randomized 32 patients with peripheral arterial or bypass occlusion to either rt-PA or UK treatment.[39] The cumulative number of patients with successful thrombolysis was eight in the rt-PA group versus six in the UK group at 24 hours. Data from this study showed no apparent differences in 30-day clinical success, save that the end point of 95% clot lysis occurred more rapidly in the rt-PA group (p = .04). The authors also documented major bleeding complications in five rt-PA patients and two UK patients. As in the previous study, the authors of this trial compared high doses of rt-PA (10 mg bolus followed by 5 mg/h for 24 hours) with relatively low doses of UK (60,000 IU bolus followed by 240,000 IU/h for 2 hours, followed by 120,000 IU/h for 2 hours, followed by 60,000 IU/h for 20 hours). Given widely disparate dosing regimens between rt-PA and UK, the data from these trials must be interpreted with caution because the data from several other studies showed that bolus followed with high-dose infusion of rt-PA reduced lysis time and increased the incidence of hemorrhage compared with lower doses.[41,42]

Current recommendations Current data suggest, but do not prove, that thrombolytic therapy is effective as initial therapy for patients with acute arterial and graft occlusions and no sensorimotor deficits. Such an approach, however, is not suitable for patients with common femoral artery emboli, which should be treated surgically, and there are certain patients with sensorimotor deficits (e.g., those without any runoff) for whom the potential benefits of thrombolysis outweigh the risks of delay.

At present, acute thrombotic arterial occlusion in an occluded bypass graft is the area where intra-arterial fibrinolysis may be most useful, permitting better planning of the subsequent operation and resulting in a less extensive procedure. Such therapy, however, does not necessarily yield improvements in major long-term end points. It is important to remember that thrombosis of femoropopliteal or similar bypasses is related to early or late surgical stenosis and atherosclerosis and that restoring flow usually does not suffice to ensure continued patency.

Logistics of thrombolysis In patients with mild or no sensory deficits, angiography is performed first. Depending on the location of the obstruction, the type of clot present, and the level of patient risk, the patient may be offered thrombolysis as initial therapy.

In our practice, the patient is taken from the emergency department to the angiography suite. Informed consent is obtained for diagnostic and therapeutic angiography (including the use of stents, balloon angioplasty, stent grafts, and thrombolysis) and for the performance of an emergency surgical procedure. A discussion is undertaken with the patient to outline the course of treatment and to explain that indwelling catheters may have to be placed and that a stay in the intensive care unit may be required.

Access to the arterial system is gained via a single-wall puncture technique; the risk of posterior wall bleeding associated with a double-wall technique is thereby avoided. Access should be obtained from a site as remote from the intervention site as possible. Generally, this is accomplished by starting from the contralateral groin of the target artery and going up and over the aortic bifurcation and then back to the ipsilateral artery. By removing the puncture site from the side of catheter-directed thrombolysis, the incidence of bleeding and formation of hematomas or pseudoaneurysms is reduced.

After completion of the angiogram and delineation of the pathology, a guide wire is passed into the occluded area. We use a 0.035 in. hydrophilic guide wire, which has a slippery, wet coating that enables it to cross nonhydrophilic lesions. Once in place, the wire is guided through the clot. A multiple -sidehole catheter is placed through the clot, and a hand-injection angiogram is performed to confirm that the catheter tip is in the true lumen. The guide wire is then left within the catheter to occlude the tip so that the lytic agent is preferentially infused through the sideholes. This graded "coaxial" infusion technique allows the agent to reach the greatest possible surface area, maximizes the length of infusion, and enables the surgeon to treat some of the longest bypass grafts. If the guide wire–catheter system cannot be advanced into the clot, it is highly unlikely that thrombolysis will be successful. In a study that included 103 patients with limb-threatening arterial occlusion lasting 14 days or less treated at University of Rochester Medical Center with catheter-directed UK thrombolysis, Ouriel and colleagues demonstrated that the ability to traverse a guide wire through the length of the thrombus within the occluded artery can be used to predict a successful outcome.[43] In 84 (81.6%) patients with successful guide wire traversal, successful lysis was achieved in 89% of cases. In the remaining 19 (18.4%) patients in whom traversal of the thrombus with a guide wire was not possible, clot lysis was achieved in only 16% of cases (p = .003). Another important aspect of thrombolytic procedures that can help predict the success of the intervention determined by the same authors was successful positioning of infusion catheter within the thrombus (p = .001). Successful catheter placement was documented in 89 (86.4%) patients. In this subgroup of patients, successful catheter placement was associated with clot lysis in 88% of cases. In the remaining 14 (13.6%) patients in whom the catheter could not be positioned within the thrombus, lysis was never achieved.

In many cases, mechanical thrombus removal, with or without pulse spray, is employed initially, followed by continuous infusion of a thrombolytic agent. In addition to lytic therapy, administration of heparin is started (200 to 400 IU IV or via sheath) to prevent pericatheter thrombosis. Serial laboratory evaluation is carried out to verify that the patient is not bleeding and that the fibrinogen level is higher than 100 mg/dL. Serial follow-up arteriograms are obtained to monitor progress. It is critically important that successful thrombolysis be followed by treatment, whether endovascular or open, of any lesions uncovered during thrombolysis; if it is not, reocclusion is inevitable. At the conclusion of thrombolysis and before intervention, the patient must be maintained on a heparin drip (or on another anticoagulant) to prevent the formation of a new thrombus. The rate of successful reperfusion is approximately 90 to 95% in most studies.

An important advantage of this selective approach is that it allows simultaneous angiographic definition of the nature of the occlusion (i.e., embolic or thrombotic) and of any vessel wall abnormalities that would lead to rethrombosis if not corrected by means of surgery or balloon angioplasty. A major drawback to this approach is that arterial catheterization is required for prolonged periods (20 hours, on average), leading to major bleeding and thromboembolic this is most easily accomplished in the antecubital fossa. A curvilinear ("lazy S") incision is made that starts on the medial aspect of the upper arm, extends transversely across the antecubital fossa, and ends halfway down the middle of the lower arm. The brachial artery is exposed deep to the bicipital aponeurosis, and a transverse arteriotomy is made proximal to the bifurcation. This incision allows control of the brachial, radial, and ulnar arteries. A 3 French embolectomy catheter is typically used here. If the pulse is not present, the catheter should be passed proximally into the brachial artery first. This is followed by selective embolectomy down the radial and ulnar arteries. Regardless of the clot location, several passes of the balloon catheter are made in each vessel until no more clot can be retrieved and there is brisk back-bleeding from the vessel. A completion angiogram is obtained to visualize the distal vessels and elucidate any anatomic pathology in the native vessels. If distal clot is still present after the completion angiogram, intra-arterial thrombolysis can be employed for a brief period to soften the clot. The multiple sidehole catheter is advanced distally to the location of the clot, the guide wire is passed through the lesion, and the catheter is passed over the wire into the substance of the clot. Infusion of the lytic agent is then started. Repeat angiograms indicate whether the clot has dissolved or is still present. If the clot is still apparent, repeat embolectomy is attempted. If completion arteriography shows successful embolectomy, the arteriotomy is closed using interrupted 6-0 polypropylene suture.

If thrombosis rather than embolism is suspected, an underlying lesion must be sought. Failure to establish inflow via brachial embolectomy should prompt angiographic evaluation of the axillary and subclavian arteries for aneurysm or occlusion. A proximal occlusion of the subclavian artery is most expeditiously treated by stenting via the exposed brachial artery when possible. However, axillary and subclavian aneurysms are often associated with chronic compression by a cervical rib in the thoracic outlet and should be repaired through a separate incision.

Several technical points of balloon embolectomy deserve emphasis. In performing the embolectomy, attention should be paid to the tactile sensations felt as the inflated balloon is withdrawn. Such sensations give the operator a sense of the disease process. When several deflations are needed and the withdrawal path of the balloon feels rough, a long-standing process (e.g., an atherosclerotic calcified vessel with anatomic discrepancies) is likely. If there appears to be no residual clot after embolectomy, then a completion angiogram is sufficient and the artery can be closed primarily. In cases where the source of embolus is not identified or the source cannot be corrected, the patient should be considered for long-term anticoagulation. Heparin is continued into the postoperative period, and the patient is eventually switched to warfarin, which is continued for at least 6 months postoperatively. Data from several studies have demonstrated that postoperative anticoagulation treatment reduces the risk of recurrent thromboembolic events, especially in patients with atrial fibrillation.[67–69] In a study that included 287 patients with acute thromboembolic lower extremity ischemia, Campbell and colleagues demonstrated that recurrent limb ischemia and amputation were less common in patients who received warfarin anticoagulation initially than in patients who were not anticoagulated with warfarin (7% versus 17% and 5% versus 21%, respectively).[70]

The location from which the embolus originated should always be sought and appropriately treated. When an underlying lesion is identified, a decision must be made as to whether it can be treated with angioplasty or stenting or whether a formal bypass is required to correct the problem and salvage the limb. Key to the final management of these patients is assessment of the lower extremities, especially the calves, for compartment syndrome. To minimize the chances that an otherwise successful surgical operation may fail as a consequence of this syndrome, we typically perform prophylactic fasciotomies on the extremity if profound ischemia has been present for several hours.

Cost Considerations

A retrospective study published in 1995 compared thrombolysis with surgical thrombectomy as first-line therapy for ALI.[71] Only the costs of the initial admission were documented. The average charge for the two treatments ranged from $20,000 to $26,000. Economic analysis confirmed that the total economic impact of thrombolysis approximated that of initial operative therapy. The conclusion of the study was that there was no difference between an endovascular approach and an operative approach with respect to cost. A more recent study by Korn and colleagues retrospectively analyzed 100 consecutive cases of acute and subacute lower extremity ischemia in 85 patients treated with UK thrombolysis.[72] The authors documented that the cost of initial hospitalization for thrombolysis approximated $18,500 per patient and concluded that thrombolysis can be as or more costly than traditional surgery. These data show that when acute treatment of ALI is being considered, cost should not be factored into the decision-making process. The choice of treatment strategy should be based on the availability of the equipment, the experience of the surgeon, and the evidence regarding the safety and efficacy of the procedure for each case.

Atheromatous Embolization

Atheroembolism is a condition in which microscopic cholesterol-laden debris travels from proximal arteries to reach the most distal arterial segments, typically in the skin of the lower extremities.[73–76] This debris usually originates from unstable plaque found at inflection points in the arterial tree, especially in the aorta.[77,78] It may also originate from aneurysmal sacs either in the aorta or in the peripheral arteries. The atheromatous embolization can also be a manifestation of a multisystem disorder associated with high mortality and morbidity rates. Although it was first reported more than a century ago (in 1862) by German pathologist Panum,[79] this disorder still remains poorly recognized and underdiagnosed by many practitioners. Much of the confusion can be attributed to the numerous clinical manifestations that are apparent across many different medical specialties, making the differential diagnosis broad and the diagnosis challenging. The confusion has been compounded by the inexact nomenclature that permeates the medical literature. Unfortunately, archaic terms such as "blue toe syndrome," "purple toe syndrome," "cholesterol embolism," "cholesterol crystal embolization," "multiple cholesterol emboli syndrome," or "the pseudovasculitic syndrome" are still frequently used by some specialists.[80–85] Based on data from autopsy studies, the estimated incidence of atheromatous embolization is relatively low and ranges from 0.15 to 3.4%.[86–88] However, data from several clinical studies demonstrated that the incidence is much higher in older patients with atherosclerosis, especially in patients with known atherosclerosis who underwent arteriography or cardiac and/or vascular surgical procedures.[89–93] Thurlbeck and Castleman found that 17 of 22 patients (77.3%) who died after open abdominal aortic aneurysm repair had evidence of atheromatous embolization on a postmortem examination.[93]

CLINICAL EVALUATION

A high index of suspicion for atheromatous embolization should be present in all patients with unexplained MI, stroke, acute renal failure, mesenteric ischemia, cutaneous ischemic manifestations, or limb ischemia, especially following vascular or cardiac surgery, as well as angiographic or endovascular procedures. Patients with atheroembolism of the extremity usually present with focal toe ischemia, the so-called "blue toe syndrome," in conjunction with palpable pulses in the distal extremity [*see Figure 1*]. Acute pain of sudden onset is typically noted in the affected area. The pain can often establish the exact timing of embolization. Cyanosis is present either on the toe or over a more extensive area if the atheroemboli were circulated throughout the extremity.[94] When both lower extremities are involved, the source of the microemboli is commonly found above the aortic bifurcation. Unilateral manifestation implies that atheroemboli most likely originated distal to the bifurcation. The descending thoracic, suprarenal, and infrarenal aortas are common sources of atheromatous embolization to the lower extremities and to the visceral and renal arteries.

A complete vascular examination should be performed and pulses documented. Although a patent arterial tree is the rule, emboli that are sufficiently small may travel through collateral channels. Palpation should be done to detect any aneurysmal disease. A massive proximal atheroembolic event may affect the entire abdominal wall and both extremities, giving the appearance of livedo reticularis.

Livedo reticularis is the most common (present in > 50% of all patients) cutaneous manifestation of atheromatous embolization.[95] It must be noted that livedo reticularis is not pathognomonic for atheromatous embolization as it can be seen in patients with several other disorders, including antiphospholipid antibody syndrome, systemic lupus erythematosus, cryoglobulinemia, and macroglobulinemia. It can also be seen in healthy young women[96] and in patients taking steroids. Livedo reticularis results from delayed venous drainage of the skin secondary to embolic obstruction of capillaries, venules, and small arteries. It frequently involves the lateral aspect of the toes, feet, soles, and calves.[97,98] Less frequently, it is seen on the buttocks or trunk. As the source of the atheroemboli ascends in the arterial tree, more vital organs (e.g., the kidneys and the gastrointestinal tract) may be damaged. Manipulation of an intra-arterial catheter, surgical manipulation of the arterial tree, or clamping in an area of disease can also result in plaque disruption. In these cases, the adverse effects are usually apparent immediately after the procedure.

INVESTIGATIVE STUDIES

A number of noninvasive tests may be used to localize the source of atheroembolization. Doppler segmental pressures may be used to localize the responsible lesion by documenting a significant drop in pressure between measured levels. Duplex ultrasonography can detect aneurysms in the abdominal aorta and femoral or popliteal arteries. It can also be used to define calcified plaques and high-grade stenotic lesions in the lower extremity arteries. B-mode imaging can also provide clues to the morphology of a plaque, such as intraplaque hemorrhage and irregular surfaces. However, as mentioned earlier in the text, the accuracy of duplex ultrasonography is highly operator dependent.

When the aorta is the suspected source of emboli, CTA, magnetic resonance imaging, or MRA should be performed; these modalities provide better visualization of intraluminal disease. In addition to detecting thoracic and abdominal aneurysms, CTA is useful for the detection of iliac artery aneurysms and for identifying concomitant occlusive disease. In patients with atheromatous embolization and non–limb-threatening ischemia, CTA of the thoracic and abdominal aorta should be obtained to evaluate for the underlying source of atheroembolic events. Although more invasive, catheter arteriography also plays a useful role in identifying intraluminal pathology along the entire vascular tree. However, it should be stressed that catheter arteriography can increase the risk of atheroembolic showers; this modality should be used if alternative imaging modalities are not available. Another invasive modality, intravascular ultrasonography, may be performed in the operating room or interventional suite with a guide wire in place to help delineate the extent of the underlying disease.

MANAGEMENT

The two major goals of the management of atheromatous embolization are to treat the end-organ that is affected and to prevent further embolization from occurring. If the atheroembolic events are minor and solitary, conservative medical management is recommended. If, however, the emboli are recurrent or massive, a thorough evaluation should be initiated, followed by urgent treatment.

Medical management of atheroembolism consists primarily of antiplatelet agents and HMG-CoA reductase inhibitors (statins). Given that most patients with atheroemboli are already receiving aspirin, the addition of clopidogrel or ticlopidine is appropriate. In a series of 35 patients, complete recovery of leg ischemia and symptom relief occurred in more than 50% of patients who received antiplatelet therapy.[99] The optimal agents for preventing recurrence of atheroembolism may prove to be lipid-lowering drugs, particularly statins. Cabili and colleagues reported a study that demonstrated improvement in overall lower extremity ischemia caused by atheromatous embolization and no recurrence for 30 months after the initiation of statin therapy.[100] A multivariate analysis from a retrospective study that involved 519 patients with severe thoracic aortic plaque demonstrated that statin therapy was independently protective (p = .0001) against recurrent embolic events.[101] Furthermore, given the goal of preventing recurrence,

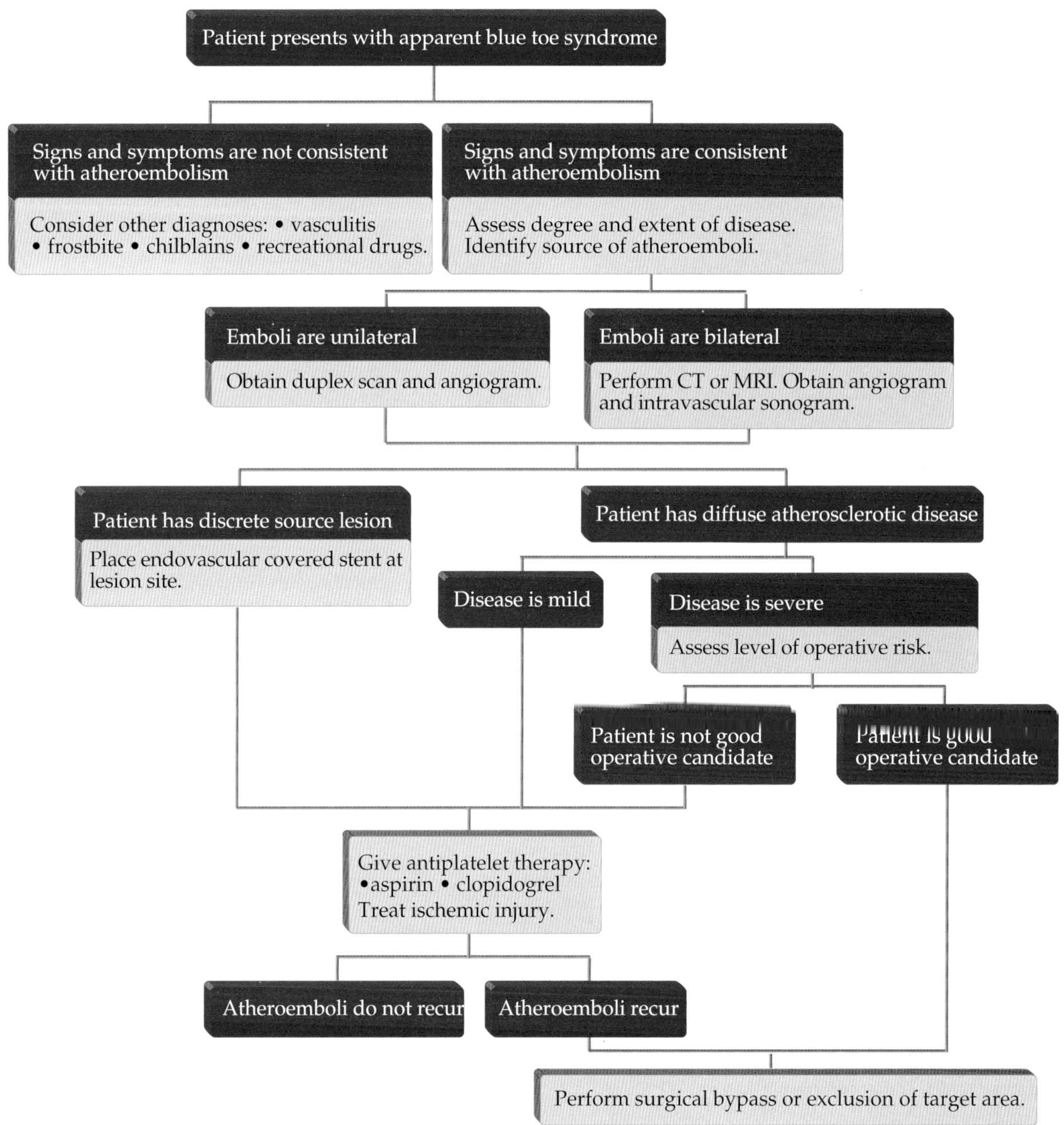

Figure 1 **Algorithm outlining workup of a patient with blue toe syndrome as a result of atheroembolism. CT = computed tomography; MRI = magnetic resonance imaging.**

lifestyle modification should be initiated to minimize preventable risk factors for atheromatous embolization as well as coronary and peripheral arterial disease. All patients should be counseled to stop smoking. Aggressive treatment of diabetes is also warranted. Strict glycemic control should be initiated to achieve recommended hemoglobin A_{1c} levels of less than 6.5 to 7.0%. Tight control of blood pressure is very important as well. The blood pressure goal for nondiabetic and diabetic patients is less than 140/90 mm Hg and less than 130/80 mm Hg, respectively.[102]

The role of warfarin therapy in treating atheroembolic disease has not been established with certainty. Such therapy may even aggravate the disease process by causing intraplaque hemorrhage and increased embolization. The Warfarin Aspirin Recurrent Stroke Study (WARSS), a randomized multicenter study that included 2,206 patients who had recently experienced an ischemic stroke, found no evidence that warfarin is superior to aspirin for preventing recurrent ischemic stroke or death within 2 years.[103] The WARSS also found that there was a significant difference in bleeding risk between warfarin-treated patients and aspirin-treated patients. For patients with diffuse atherosclerotic disease, the mainstay of therapy is an antiplatelet regimen. Traditionally, an atheroembolic source has been treated by surgical excision or by exclusion of the disease process with a bypass graft, either of which provides a good degree of safety from further embolization.[104] With the advent of endovascular surgery, however, the use of covered stents, placed securely and precisely at the site of the offending lesion, appears to be an increasingly effective and popular option [*see Table 5*].[105,106] Dougherty and Calligaro demonstrated successfully treated ulcerated aortic plaques with covered stents in a small series of patients with lower extremity ischemia.[105] In another small series, 19 patients with embolizing abdominal aortic aneurysms were treated with aortic stent grafts. Eight of nine patients (88.9%) with follow-up of 1 year had complete resolution of their ischemic symptoms, with no recurrent manifestations of atheromatous embolization.[107] Despite successful abdominal aortic aneurysm exclusion, one patient in the series had persistent foot ischemia at 1 year of follow-up, but the source of persisting atheromatous embolization was believed to be severe coexisting thoracic aortic disease. Although endovascular treatment for atheromatous embolization is becoming increasingly promising, randomized, controlled trials are needed to accurately assess the safety and efficacy of the different endovascular treatment modalities and compare them with traditional surgery.

Our current approach to treating atheroembolism may be summarized as follows. The source lesion is first identified by means of the modalities already discussed. If embolization is minor, aspirin, clopidogrel, and a statin are started. If embolization is recurrent or massive, an endovascular approach is attempted, involving the placement of a covered stent over the lesion. This approach is indicated for segments of the arterial tree where there are no collaterals so that vital blood flow to organs is not hindered. If aneurysmal disease is present, either conventional or endovascular therapeutic approaches may be applied to exclude any source of emboli. In the case of thoracic aortic disease, covered stents may be placed to push the plaque against the wall and prevent further embolization. If suprarenal plaque cannot be treated with a stented graft, aortic ligation with an axillobifemoral bypass may be performed. Such treatment does not, however, protect the renal and visceral vessels, and these patients require lifelong strict antiplatelet therapy.

Pathophysiology, Etiology, and Complications

PATHOPHYSIOLOGY OF ALI

As mentioned above, ALI begins when arterial embolization, local thrombosis, or arterial trauma results in occlusion of a peripheral artery or bypass graft. The ischemic process may then develop slowly, over an extended period, or quickly, over a few hours. A protracted course leading to thrombosis allows collateral vessels to form, resulting in the gradual onset of symptoms. When occlusion is acute, however, as in trauma, embolization, or acute thrombosis of a vessel or a bypass graft, signs and symptoms of acute ischemia may become rapidly apparent, including excruciating pain, mottling, cyanosis, and, commonly, sensory and motor changes. The magnitude of the ischemic injury is directly proportional to the duration of ischemia and the amount of tissue affected.

The pathophysiology of limb ischemia is related to the progression of tissue infarction and irreversible cell death. Compared with other organs and tissues (e.g., the brain and the heart), the extremities are relatively resistant to ischemia. However, the various tissue types of which an extremity is composed have different metabolic rates. The extent to which each cell type can tolerate ischemia depends on its metabolic rate. Bone and skin are the most resistant to ischemia, nervous tissue is the least resistant, and muscle is somewhere in between. Although nerve tissue is the type that is most sensitive to ischemia, skeletal muscle, the major structural component of an extremity, plays the largest pathophysiologic role in the local and systemic effects of ALI. Initial ischemia leads to a conversion of muscle metabolism from aerobic to anaerobic. This ultimately leads to increased production of lactates and subsequent disruption of acid-base balance characterized by profound metabolic acidosis.[108] In the setting of hypoxia, dysfunction of the calcium-sodium exchanger occurs, resulting in the elevated levels of free calcium within the myocytes. Elevated levels of free calcium interact with muscle fibers, resulting in skeletal muscle fiber necrosis.[109] Cell lysis leads to release of intracellular potassium and free myoglobin, with toxic systemic effects. For muscle tissue, 6 hours is the approximate upper limit of ischemic tolerance; nervous tissue is affected well before this point.[110] Knowledge of the varying degrees of ischemic tolerance helps in determining the viability of the limb.

Hypoperfusion-Reperfusion State

The severity of ALI symptoms is directly related to the duration of ischemia and the effects of reperfusion. Hypoperfusion (ischemia)-reperfusion injury occurs in the settings of reversible diminished or absent blood supply to a tissue followed by the return of oxygenated blood flow. Regardless of the cause of the ischemia, hypoperfusion leads to ischemic infarcts via various mechanisms. In addition to diminished delivery of O_2 to tissues during the hypoperfusion state, three major physiologic events occur. First, movement of blood through the vessels is slowed. As a result, the thrombus is able to grow and propagate, occluding collateral vessels and further decreasing blood flow. Second, ischemic cells swell and accumulate water. The resulting increase in pressure within a fixed space between fascial structures creates an elevation of pressure within the compartment that further decreases flow and exacerbates the injury. Third, the precapillary arteriolar cells swell, narrowing the lumina of distal arterioles, capillaries, and venules and again reducing blood flow. As a result, biotoxic products of anaerobic metabolism accumulate within the ischemic tissues distal to the occlusion with resultant tissue edema, which, if left uncorrected, may progress to compartment syndrome.

Table 5 Surgical Management of Atheroembolism

Source of Emboli	*Treatment*
Upper extremity	Bypass of subclavian or axillary artery First rib or cervical rib resection
Aorta	Focal disease: covered aortic stent Diffuse disease: aortobifemoral bypass
Iliac artery	Covered iliac stent
Popliteal artery	Ligation and bypass of popliteal artery

The reperfusion state that results when flow is restored can be as detrimental to the ischemic extremity as the hypoperfusion state. In addition to local symptoms in the affected extremity, metabolic consequences of reperfusion can have severe systemic effects that are associated with significant morbidity and mortality. In severe cases, systematic involvement may result in systematic inflammatory response syndrome or even in multiple organ dysfunction syndrome, which is often associated with high rates of mortality.[111] During abrupt reperfusion, highly active O_2 metabolites are produced by neutrophils.[112] These free radicals destroy cells by attacking the unsaturated bonds of fatty acids within the phospholipid membrane, thereby disrupting the cell membrane, allowing water to enter the cell, and eventually causing cell lysis. Volume repletion and urinary alkalinization as well as free radical scavengers have been recommended as initial supportive treatment. Free radical scavengers (e.g., mannitol and superoxide dismutase) have a slight protective effect against reperfusion injury when given before large-scale release of these radicals.[113,114] In addition, myoglobin from injured muscle cells is released into the circulation and is cleared via the renal system. Myoglobin may cause renal failure through its direct toxic effect on the renal tubules and through the accumulation of casts in the tubules. Creatine phosphokinase levels may also increase to dramatic levels once perfusion is reestablished. High concentrations of lactic acid, potassium, thromboxane, and cellular enzymes are secreted as a consequence of the rhabdomyolysis; these substances accumulate in the ischemic limb and are released into the systemic circulation on reperfusion.[115] In one study that measured the venous effluent from a series of patients with limb ischemia, the pH was 7.07 and the mean potassium level was 5.7 mEq/L 5 min after surgical embolectomy.[116]

Detrimental physiologic changes are seen when toxic O_2 metabolites are released systemically. Profound acidosis, hyperkalemia, myoglobinuria, renal failure, depression of myocardial function, an increase in cardiac dysrhythmias, and loss of vascular tone may induce shock and even lead to death.[117]

ETIOLOGY OF ALI

The etiology of ALI can be divided into two distinct categories: thrombosis and embolism. A thorough evaluation must be performed to elucidate the precise cause of ischemia in each patient. The two categories are each associated with specific symptoms and signs [*see Table 6*]. Knowledge of these associations helps direct the clinician toward the most appropriate means of accomplishing limb salvage in a given situation.

Thrombosis of a native vessel or bypass graft almost always develops in conjunction with an underlying occlusive lesion in the vessel or graft. The lesion usually has been present for some time, and the thrombosis occurs due to reduced blood flow. In contrast, embolic events occur in smaller-caliber vessels that are not diseased, with emboli commonly resting at or immediately distal to branch points.

Thrombosis

Native artery thrombosis Native artery thrombosis represents the end stage of a long-standing disease process of atheromatous plaque formation at specific sites in the arterial tree. Atherosclerotic plaque begins with the slow deposition of lipids in the intima of the vessel and continues with the deposition of calcium, resulting in an atherosclerotic core.[118] This core has a highly thrombogenic surface that encourages platelet aggregation, which results in disturbances of blood flow.[119] The flow disturbances create a zone of separation, stagnation, turbulence, and distorted velocity vectors. These factors cause low shear rates at inflection points in the arterial tree, and endothelial damage ensues. The endothelial damage activates a repair process that results in intimal hyperplasia, which induces further attraction of platelets and eventual thrombus formation. The process by which occlusion develops from an atheromatous plaque may be more important than the degree of stenosis within the lumen. This would explain why acute occlusion occurs in vessels with minimal (< 50%) stenosis: atheromatous plaque not only reduces blood flow but also represents an irregular surface within the arterial lumen that is prone to thrombus formation. The contact between the atherosclerotic core and the bloodstream leads to platelet aggregation and hence to eventual thrombosis. Occasionally, thrombosis of a native artery occurs without any obvious underlying pathologic condition. In such cases, a thorough investigation should be initiated into other causes of thrombosis (e.g., hypovolemia, malignancy, hypercoagulable states, and blood dyscrasias).

Bypass graft thrombosis Aggressive management of patients with peripheral arterial disease has led to an increase in bypass graft procedures. As a result, graft thrombosis has now become the leading cause of acute lower extremity ischemia. Some patients have graft occlusions without any definable underlying lesion, but most have a definable lesion. In patients with native conduits, intimal hyperplasia leading to the narrowing of the vein graft and valvular hyperplasia are the two leading causes of graft failure.[120] The situation is different in the prosthetic

Table 6 Differentiation of Embolism from Thrombosis

Variable	*Embolism*	*Thrombosis*
Identifiable source	Frequently detected	None
Claudication	Rare	Frequent
Physical findings	Proximal and contralateral pulses normal	Evidence of ipsilateral and contralateral peripheral vascular disease
Angiographic findings	Minimal atherosclerosis; sharp cutoff; few collaterals; multiple occlusions	Diffuse atherosclerotic disease; tapered and irregular cutoff; well-developed collateral circulation

graft population where the graft failure is attributed to one of the following: thrombogenicity of the graft material, kinking of the graft from crossing joints, anastomotic intimal hyperplasia, and progression of atherosclerotic disease proximal or distal to the graft. Among these, anastomotic irregularities probably represent the most common cause of graft thrombosis.[111] Data from the most recent studies suggest that geometric remodeling of the native conduits and decreased vein graft adaptation to the arterial environment are caused by mediators of inflammation.[121] Fortunately, diminished blood flow in the graft can be detected before graft thrombosis occurs. Establishing a policy of routine ultrasound surveillance after bypass procedure and prompt revision of an identified vein graft stenosis is important; if an advanced lesion is not corrected, graft thrombosis leads to acute ischemic events with the possibility of limb loss. Advanced vein graft stenosis should be repaired using open surgical or endovascular techniques prior to occlusion. Most short lesions (< 2 cm in length) can be corrected by percutaneous transluminal angioplasty (PTA). Longer or more complex lesions should be treated with vein patch angioplasty or a short bypass.

Embolism

Peripheral arterial embolization results in the sudden onset of severe ischemia as the absence of collateral vessels compounds the reduction in flow to the extremity. The heart is by far the most common source of spontaneous arterial emboli, accounting for about 90% of cases. The incidence of embolic phenomena has increased as the population has aged, with a corresponding increase in the number of patients with significant cardiac disease. Over the past 25 years, the incidence of embolization has doubled, from 23 to 51 per 100,000 admissions. Atherosclerotic heart disease currently accounts for as many as 60 to 70% of all cases of arterial embolism.[122,123] Atrial fibrillation and rheumatic valvular disease account for the remaining 30 to 40%.[113,124] With respect to peripheral emboli in particular, atrial fibrillation is currently responsible for 65 to 75% of cases. Transthoracic echocardiography is insensitive in visualizing atrial clots, especially in the left atrial appendage, which is the most common cardiac source of emboli.[125,126] Transesophageal echocardiography, however, offers significantly better imaging of all four chambers and thus is considered the superior diagnostic test for suspected cardiac embolic sources.[127–130]

MI is the next most important cause of peripheral emboli. One study from 1986 evaluated 400 patients and found that MI was a causative factor in 20%.[115] A left ventricular wall thrombus is often seen after an acute MI, with or without a left ventricular wall aneurysm; however, only 5% ultimately embolize and result in peripheral ischemia.[131–134] Other studies suggest that day 3 to day 28 is the period during which the risk of embolization is highest for an intracardiac thrombus.[135]

Other cardiac sources of peripheral emboli include the ring portions of prosthetic cardiac valves and biologic xenovalves. Chronic anticoagulation is recommended for prosthetic valves, but the biologic xenovalves do not require anticoagulation.[136,137] Cardiac tumors (e.g., atrial myxomas) are rare sources of peripheral emboli.[126] Cardiac vegetations from bacterial or fungal endocarditis should be considered possible sources of peripheral emboli when intravenous drug abuse is suspected in a patient with no previous history of cardiac disease.[138,139]

Noncardiac sources account for 5 to 10% of peripheral emboli. The majority of these involve upstream atherosclerotic arterial disease (e.g., aneurysms or unstable plaques).[140–143] Unstable plaque is prone to ulceration and rupture, creating a highly thrombogenic surface that promotes platelet aggregation and creates thromboembolic debris that leads to distal arterial embolization. Foreign objects (e.g., missiles) and tumors (e.g., melanoma) can also embolize if they gain access to the arterial tree.[144–147] Paradoxical embolization occurs when a venous thrombus crosses from the right heart circulation to the left, via an atrial or ventricular route such as an atrioseptal defect, a ventricular septal defect, or patent foramen ovale. Once the embolus gains access to the left ventricle, it becomes an arterial embolus.[148–150] About 5 to 10% of emboli remain unidentified despite a thorough diagnostic evaluation[151,152]; some of these are now being attributed to hypercoagulable states and are considered indications for chronic anticoagulation.[153]

Incidence The increase in the number of endovascular interventions has affected the etiology of arterial embolism, with a greater number of embolic episodes now arising from endovascular procedures. A 1996 study found that 45% of all atheroemboli were iatrogenic and that the majority of these (83%) originated during manipulation of the abdominal aorta and the proximal arteries, including the iliac artery and the femoropopliteal artery, with the remainder originating during surgery.[154] Emboli usually lodge at arterial bifurcations and thus cause hypoperfusion of more than one vessel. Axial limb vessels account for 60 to 80% of clinically significant embolic events, with the remainder divided between cerebral vessels (20%) and upper extremity vessels (10 to 20%).[115,126,155] The most common site for embolic lodgment is the common femoral bifurcation [*see Figure 2*]. The aortoiliac region is the next most common site, followed closely by the popliteal artery.[108,114,115,126,156] The presence of normal pulses in the contralateral leg in a patient with an ischemic leg should elicit an aggressive workup to rule out a cardiac embolic source and, as mentioned above, may be a clue that the occlusive event is embolic rather than thrombotic.

Upper extremity emboli Acute ischemia of the upper extremity is usually caused by embolism, usually from a cardiac source. Subclavian aneurysms, arteriovenous fistulas, upper extremity arterial bypasses, and iatrogenic manipulation of the arteries (including axillary bypass procedures and arteriovenous hemodialysis fistulas) are rare causes.[157] As noted above, emboli lodge at bifurcations within the arterial tree. In the upper extremity, the bifurcation of the brachial artery into the radial and ulnar arteries is the most common lodgment site, followed by the takeoff of the deep brachial artery. Adequate exposure of all three arteries can be obtained via an elongated S-shaped incision that runs medially to laterally across the elbow joint. Given that the antecubital region is characterized by an abundant collateral circulation, acute occlusion of the brachial artery is usually well tolerated in regard to limb-threatening distal ischemia

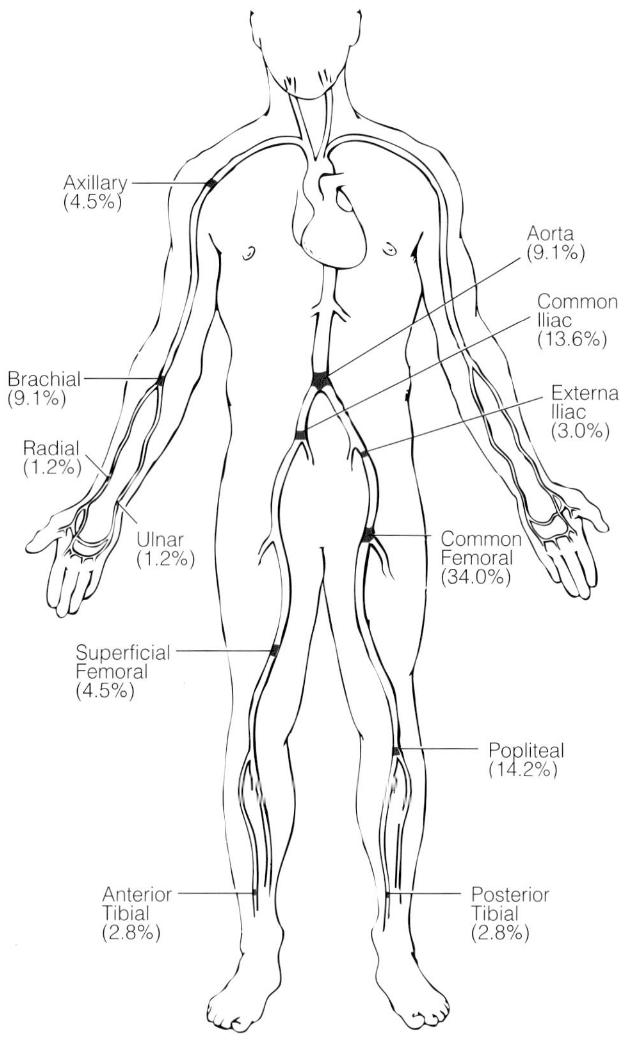

Figure 2 **The most common sites of arterial embolic occlusions.**

and carries a better prognosis than acute occlusion of the popliteal artery. In a study that analyzed 61 patients with acute upper extremity ischemia compared with patients treated for lower extremity ischemia over the same 5-year period, amputation and mortality rates in patients with upper extremity ischemia were reported as 0 and 5% compared with respective rates of 5 and 30% in the patients treated for lower extremity ischemia.[158] Similar to data from the University of Rochester trial,[34] this study demonstrated that the group with the higher mortality rate had the higher incidence of cardiopulmonary complications.

Other causes Sepsis and cardiogenic shock can result in low-flow states that place patients at high risk for thrombosis. Certain vasoconstrictors and recreational drugs are also associated with lower extremity thrombosis.[159,160] Patients with these conditions usually present with bilateral extremity ischemia. Vasculitides (e.g., Takayasu disease) may also cause extremity ischemia.[161] The hypercoagulable states (e.g., AT deficiency, antiphospholipid syndrome, protein C and S deficiencies, activated protein C resistance, and hyperprothrombinemia), usually associated with venous thrombosis, may also be associated with acute arterial thrombosis.[162] The contribution of these states to ALI, with usually devastating consequences, is increasingly being recognized. Another rare but important etiology for ALI is vascular trauma. Although improvements in the management of ALI associated with vascular trauma have reduced the amputation rate to less than 5%, management of these patients is still characterized by long-term disability, which remains a persistent problem for 20 to 50% of patients.[163]

Financial Disclosures: None Reported

References

1. Norgren L, Hiatt WR, Dormandy JA, et al; TASC II Working Group. Inter-Society Consensus for the Management of Peripheral Arterial Disease (TASC II). J Vasc Surg 2007;45 Suppl S:S5–67.
2. Davies B, Braithwaite BD, Birch PA, et al. Acute leg ischaemia in Gloucestershire. Br J Surg 1997;84:504.
3. Blaisdell FW, Steele M, Allen RE. Management of acute lower extremity arterial ischemia due to embolism and thrombosis. Surgery 1978;84:822.
4. Jivegård L, Holm J, Scherstén T. Acute limb ischemia due to arterial embolism or thrombosis: influence of limb ischemia versus pre-existing cardiac disease on postoperative mortality rate. J Cardiovasc Surg 1988;29:32–6.
5. Dormandy J, Heeck L, Vig S. Acute limb ischemia. Semin Vasc Surg 1999;12:148.
6. Batz W, Brückner R. Symptoms and therapy of aortic bifurcation embolism. Chirurg 1985;56:166–9.
7. Rutherford RB, Flanigan DP, Gupta SK, *et al.* Suggested standards for reports dealing with lower extremity ischemia. J Vasc Surg 1986;4:80–94.
8. Rutherford RB, Baker JD, Ernst C, et al. Recommended standards for reports dealing with lower extremity ischemia: revised version. J Vasc Surg 1997;26:517.
9. Dormandy JA, Rutherford RB, TASC Working Group. Management of peripheral arterial disease (PAD). A Trans-Atlantic Inter-Society Consensus (TASC). J Vasc Surg 2000;31 (Suppl):S1–296.
10. Katzenschlager R, Ahmadi A, Atteneder M, et al. Colour duplex sonography-guided local lysis of occlusions in the femoro-popliteal region. Int Angiol 2000;19:250.
11. Mazzariol F, Ascher E, Hingorani A, et al. Lower-extremity revascularization without preoperative contrast arteriography in 185 cases: lessons learned with duplex ultrasound arterial mapping. Eur J Vasc Endovasc Surg 2000;19:509.
12. Hingorani AP, Ascher E, Marks N. Duplex arteriography for lower extremity revascularization. Perspect Vasc Surg Endovasc Ther 2007;19:1.
13. Kim D, Porter DH, Brown R, et al. Renal artery imaging: a prospective comparison of intra-arterial digital subtraction angiography with conventional angiography. Angiology 1991;42:345.
14. Lindholt JS. Radiocontrast induced nephropathy. Eur J Vasc Endovasc Surg 2003;4:296.

15. Kerns SR, Hawkins IFJ, Sabatelli FW. Current status of carbon dioxide angiography. Radiol Clin North Am 1995; 33:15.
16. Waver FA, Pentecoast MJ, Yellin AE, et al. Clinical applications of carbon dioxide/digital subtraction arteriography. J Vasc Surg 1991;13:266.
17. Fogarty T. Historical reflections on the management of acute limb ischemia. Semin Vasc Surg 2009;22(1):3–4.
18. Berridge DC, Hopkinson BR, Makkin GS. Acute lower limb arterial ischemia: a role for continuous oxygen inhalation. Br J Surg 1989;76:1021–3.
19. Bjork I, Lindahl U. Mechanism of the anticoagulant action of heparin. Mol Cell Biochem 1982;48:161.
20. Hirsh J, Dalen J, Deykin D, et al. Heparin, mechanism of action, pharmacokinetics, dosing consideration, monitoring, efficacy and safety. Chest 1992;102:337S.
21. Salzman EW, Deykin D, Shapiro RM, et al. Management of heparin therapy: controlled prospective trial. N Engl J Med 1976;292:1046.
22. Walenga JM, Frenkel EP, Bick RL. Heparin-induced thrombocytopenia, paradoxical thromboembolism, and other adverse effects of heparin-type therapy. Hematol Oncol Clin North Am 2003;7:259.
23. Eisman R, Surrey S, Ramachandran B, et al. Structural and functional comparison of the genes for human platelet factor 4 and PF4alt. Blood 1990;76:336–44.
24. Warkentin TE, Bernstein RA. Delayed-onset heparin-induced thrombocytopenia and cerebral thrombosis after a single administration of unfractionated heparin. N Engl J Med 2003;348:1067.
25. Kelton JG. Heparin-induced thrombocytopenia: an overview. Blood Rev 2002;16:77.
26. Rice L, Attisha WK, Drexler A, et al. Delayed-onset heparin-induced thrombocytopenia. Ann Intern Med 2002; 136:210.
27. Napolitano LM, Warkentin TE, Almahameed A, et al. Heparin-induced thrombocytopenia in the critical care setting: diagnosis and management. Crit Care Med 2006;34: 2898.
28. Dotter C. Selective clot lysis with low-dose streptokinase. Radiology 1974;111:31.
29. Tillett WS, Garner RL. The fibrinolytic activity of hemolytic streptococci. J Exp Med 1933;58:485.
30. Jostring H, Barth U, Naidu R. Changes of antistreptokinase titer following long term streptokinase therapy. In: Martin M, Schoop W, Hirsh J, editors. New concepts of streptokinase dosimetry. Vienna: Hans Huber; 1978. p. 110.
31. Macfarlane RG, Pinot JJ. Fibrinolytic activity of normal urine. Nature 1947;159:779.
32. Sobel GW, Mohler SR, Jones NW, et al. Urokinase: an activator of plasma fibrinolysin extracted from urine. Am J Physiol 1952;171:768–9.
33. Berridge DC, Gregson RHC, Hopkinson BR, et al. Randomized trial of intra-arterial recombinant tissue plasminogen activator, intravenous recombinant tissue plasminogen activator and intra-arterial streptokinase in peripheral arterial thrombolysis. Br J Surg 1991;78:988.
34. Ouriel K, Shortell C, DeWeese JA, et al. A comparison of thrombolytic therapy with operative revascularization in the initial treatment of acute peripheral arterial ischemia. J Vasc Surg 1994;19:1021.
35. Weaver FA, Comerota AJ, Youngblood M, et al. Surgical revascularization vs. thrombolysis for non-embolic lower extremity native artery occlusions: results of a prospective randomized trial. The STILE investigators: Surgery vs. Thrombolysis for Ischemia of the Lower Extremity. J Vasc Surg 1996;24:513.
36. Ouriel K, Veith FJ, Sasahara AA. Thrombolysis or peripheral arterial surgery: phase I results. TOPAS Investigators. J Vasc Surg 1996;23:64.
37. A comparison of recombinant urokinase with vascular surgery as initial treatment for acute arterial occlusion of the legs. Thrombolysis or Peripheral Arterial Surgery (TOPAS) Investigators. N Engl J Med 1998;338:1105.
38. Mahler F, Schneider E, Hess H. Recombinant tissue plasminogen activator versus urokinase for local thrombolysis of femoropopliteal occlusions: a prospective, randomized multicenter trial. J Endovasc Ther 2001;8:638.
39. Myerovitz MF, Goldhaber SZ, Reagan K, et al. Recombinant tissue-type plasminogen activator versus urokinase in peripheral arterial and graft occlusions: a randomized trial. Radiology 1990;175:34.
40. Schweizer J, Altmann E, Stoblein F, et al. Comparison of tissue plasminogen activator and urokinase in the local infiltration thrombolysis of peripheral arterial occlusions. Eur J Radiol 1996;22:129.
41. Braithwaite BD, Buckenham TM, Galland RB, et al. A prospective randomized trial of high dose versus low dose tissue plasminogen activator infusion in the menagement of acute limb ischemia. Br J Surg 1997;84:646.
42. Ward AS, Andaz SK, Bygrave S. Peripheral thrombolysis with tissue plasminogen activator: results of two treatment regimens. Arch Surg 1994;129:861.
43. Ouriel K, Shortell CK, Azodo MW, et al. Acute peripheral arterial occlusion: predictors of success in catheter-directed thrombolytic therapy. Radiology 1994;93:561.
44. Morgan R, Belli AM. Percutaneous thrombectomy: a review. Eur Radiol 2002;12:205.
45. Zehnder T, Birrer M, Do DD, et al. Percutaneous catheter thrombus aspiration for acute or subacute arterial occlusion of the legs: how much thrombolysis is needed? Eur J Vasc Endovasc Surg 2000;20:41.
46. Crain MR. Percutaneous mechanical thrombolysis and thrombectomy. Tech Vasc Interv Radiol 1998;1:235.
47. Demin VV, Zeienin VV, Zheludkov AN, et al. Initial experience of transcutaneous rheolytic thrombectomy for peripheral major arterial lesions. Angiol Vasc Surg 1999; 5:1.
48. Dick A, Neuerburg J, Schmitz-Rode T, et al. Declotting of embolized temporary vena cava filter by ultrasound and the AngioJet: comparative experimental in vitro studies. Invest Radiol 1998;33:91.
49. Douek PC, Gandjbakhche A, Leon MB, et al. Functional properties of a 'prototype rheolytic thrombectomy catheter' for percutaneous thrombectomy—in vitro investigations. Invest Radiol 1994;29:547.
50. Silva JA, Ramee SR, Collins TJ, et al. Rheolytic thrombectomy in the treatment of acute limb-threatening ischemia: immediate results and six-month follow-up of the multicenter AngioJet registry. Possis Peripheral AngioJet Study AngioJet Investigators. Cathet Cardiovasc Diagn 1998;45: 386–93.

51. Kasirajan K, Beavers FP, Clair DG, et al. Rheolytic thrombectomy in the management of acute and subacute limb threatening ischemia. J Vasc Interv Radiol 2001;12:413–20.
52. Tadavarthy SM, Murray PD, Inampudi S, et al. Mechanical thrombectomy with the Amplatz device: human experience. J Vasc Interv Radiol 1994;5:715–24.
53. Müller-Hülsbeck S, Kalinowski M, Heller M, et al. Rheolytic hydrodynamic thrombectomy for percutaneous treatment of acutely occluded infraaortic native arteries and bypass grafts: midterm follow-up results. Invest Radiol 2000;35:131–40.
54. Kasirajan K, Ouriel K. Management of acute lower extremity ischemia; treatment strategies and outcomes. Curr Interv Cardiol Rep 2000;2:119–29.
55. Stahr P, Rupprecht HJ, Voigtländer T, et al. A new thrombectomy catheter device (AngioJet) for the disruption of thrombi: an in vitro study. Catheter Cardiovasc Interv 1999;47:381–9.
56. Wissgott C, Richter A, Kamusella P, et al. Treatment of critical limb ischemia using ultrasound-enhanced thrombolysis (PARES Trial): final results. J Endovasc Ther 2007; 14:438–43.
57. Raabe RD. Ultrasound-accelerated thrombolysis in arterial and venous peripheral occlusions: fibrinogen level effects. J Vasc Interv Radiol 2010;21:1165–72.
58. Motarjeme A. Ultrasound-enhanced thrombolysis. J Endovasc Ther 2007;14:251–6.
59. Parikh S, Motarjeme A, McNamara T, et al. Ultrasound-accelerated thrombolysis for the treatment of deep vein thrombosis: initial clinical experience. J Vasc Interv Radiol 2008;19:521–8.
60. Wormald JR, Lane TR, Herbert PE, et al. Total preservation of patency and valve function after percutaneous pharmacomechanical thrombolysis using the Trellis 8 system for an acute, extensive deep venous thrombosis. Ann R Coll Surg Engl 2012;94:e103–5.
61. Arko FR, Lee E, Zarins CK, Fogarty TJ. Controlled localized thrombolysis with the "turbo" Trellis to treat acute arterial occlusions following major surgery. J Endovasc Ther 2004;11:339–43.
62. Tsetis D, Katsamouris A, Androulakakis Z. Use of the Trellis™ Peripheral Infusion System for enhancement of rt-PA thrombolysis in acute lower limb ischemia. Cardiovasc Intervent Radiol 2003;26:572–5.
63. Kasirajan K, Ramaiah VG, Diethrich EB. The Trellis Thrombectomy System in the treatment of acute limb ischemia. J Endovasc Ther 2003;10:317–21.
64. Daly B, Patel M, Prasad A. The use of the Trellis-6 thrombectomy device in the management of acute limb ischemia due to native vessel occlusion: challenges, tips and limitations. Catheter Cardiovasc Interv. DOI: 10.1002/ccd.24357. [Epub ahead of print]
65. Campbell WB, Ballard PK. Intra-arterial lidocaine in embolectomy. Br J Surg 1996;83:244.
66. Wyffels PL, DeBord JR, Marshall JS, et al. Increased limb salvage with intraoperative and postoperative ankle level urokinase infusion in acute lower extremity ischemia. J Vasc Surg 1992;15:771–9.
67. Hammarsten J, Holm J, Shersten T. Positive and negative effects of anticoagulant treatment during and after arterial embolectomy. J Cardiovasc Surg 1978;19:373–9.
68. Ljungman C, Adami HO, Bergqvist D, et al. Risk factors for early lower limb loss after embolectomy for acute arterial occlusion: a population-based case-control study. Br J Surg 1991;78:1482–5.
69. Connolly SJ. Anticoagulation for patients with atrial fibrillation and risk factors for stroke. BMJ 2000;320:1219–20.
70. Campbell WB, Ridler BM, Szymanska TH. Two year follow-up after acute thromboembolic leg ischaemia: the importance of anticoagulation. Eur J Vasc Endovasc Surg 2000;19:169–73.
71. Ouriel K, Kolassa M, DeWeese JA, et al. Economic implications of thrombolysis or operation as the initial treatment modality in acute peripheral arterial occlusion. Surgery 1995;118:810.
72. Korn P, Khilnani NM, Fellers JC, et al. Thrombolysis for native arterial occlusions of the lower extremities: clinical outcome and cost. J Vasc Surg 2001;33:1148.
73. Carvajal JA, Anderson WR, Weiss L, et al. Atheroembolism: an etiologic factor in renal insufficiency, gastrointestinal hemorrhages, and peripheral vascular diseases. Arch Intern Med 1967;119:593.
74. Karmody AM, Jordan FR, Zaman SM. Left colon gangrene after acute mesenteric artery occlusion. Arch Surg 1976;111: 972.
75. Gore L, Collins DP. Spontaneous atheromatous embolization: review of the literature and a report of 16 additional cases. Am J Clin Pathol 1960;33:416.
76. Ramirez G, O'Neill WM, Lambert R, et al. Cholesterol embolization: a complication of angiography. Arch Intern Med 1966;118:534.
77. Williams GM, Harrington D, Burdick J, et al. Mural thrombus of the aorta: an important, frequently neglected cause of large peripheral emboli. Ann Surg 1981;194:737.
78. Khatibzadeh M, Mitusch R, Stierle U, et al. Aortic atherosclerotic plaques as a source of systemic embolization. J Am Coll Cardiol 1996;27:664.
79. Panum PL. Experimental contributions to the theory of embolism. Virchows Arch Pathol Anat Physiol 1862;25: 308–10.
80. Colt HG, Begg RJ, Saporito JJ, et al. Cholesterol emboli after cardiac catheterization. Eight cases and a review of the literature. Medicine (Baltimore) 1988;67:389–400.
81. Fine MJ, Kapoor W, Falanga V. Cholesterol crystal embolization: a review of 221 cases in the English literature. Angiology 1987;38:769–84.
82. Rosansky SJ. Multiple cholesterol emboli syndrome. South Med J 1982;75:677–80.
83. Feder W, Auerbach R. 'Purple toes': an uncommon sequela of oral coumarin drug therapy. Ann Intern Med 1961;55: 911–7.
84. Baumann DS, McGraw D, Rubin BG, et al. An institutional experience with arterial atheroembolism. Ann Vasc Surg 1994;8:258–65.
85. Cappiello RA, Espinoza LR, Adelman H, et al. Cholesterol embolism: a pseudovasculitic syndrome. Semin Arthritis Rheum 1989;18:240–6.
86. Cross SS. How common is cholesterol embolism? J Clin Pathol 1991;44:859–61.
87. Drost H, Buis B, Haan D, Hillers JA. Cholesterol embolism as a complication of left heart catheterisation. Report of seven cases. Br Heart J 1984;52:339–42.

88. Kealy WF. Atheroembolism. J Clin Pathol 1978;31:984–9.
89. Handler FP. Clinical and pathologic significance of atheromatous embolization, with emphasis on an etiology of renal hypertension. Am J Med 1956;20:366–73.
90. Sieniewicz DJ, Moore S, Moir FD, McDade DF. Atheromatous emboli to the kidneys. Radiology 1969;92:1231–40.
91. Antonucci F, Pizzolitto S, Travaglini M, et al. Atheroembolic renal disease: clinico-pathologic correlations. Adv Exp Med Biol 1989;252:59–64.
92. Blauth CI, Cosgrove DM, Webb BW, et al. Atheroembolism from the ascending aorta. An emerging problem in cardiac surgery. J Thorac Cardiovasc Surg 1992;103:1104–11; discussion 1111–2.
93. Thurlbeck WM, Castleman B. Atheromatous emboli to the kidneys after aortic surgery. N Engl J Med 1957;257:442–7.
94. Karmody AM, Powers SR, Monaco VJ, et al. "Blue toe syndrome": an indication for limb salvage surgery. Arch Surg 1976;111:1263.
95. Falanga V, Fine MJ, Kapoor WN. The cutaneous manifestations of cholesterol crystal embolization. Arch Dermatol 1986;122:1194–8.
96. Sheehan MG, Condemi JJ, Rosenfeld SI. Position dependent livedo reticularis in cholesterol emboli syndrome. J Rheumatol 1993;20:1973–4.
97. Coffman JD. Atheromatous embolism. Vasc Med 1996;1:267–73.
98. Dahlberg PJ, Frecentese DF, Cogbill TH. Cholesterol embolism: experience with 22 histologically proven cases. Surgery 1989;105:737–46.
99. Morris-Jones W, Preston FE, Greaney M, Chatterjee DK. Gangrene of the toes with palpable peripheral pulses. Ann Surg 1981;193:462–6.
100. Cabili S, Hochman I, Goor Y. Reversal of gangrenous lesions in the blue toe syndrome with lovastatin—a case report. Angiology 1993;44:821–5.
101. Tunick PA, Nayar AC, Goodkin GM, et al. Effect of treatment on the incidence of stroke and other emboli in 519 patients with severe thoracic aortic plaque. Am J Cardiol 2002;90:1320–5.
102. The Sixth Report of the Joint National Committee on Prevention, Detection, Evaluation, and Treatment of High Blood Pressure. Arch Intern Med 1997;157:2413–46.
103. Mohr JP, Thompson JL, Lazar RM, et al. A comparison of warfarin and aspirin for the prevention of recurrent ischemic stroke. N Engl J Med 2001;345:1444.
104. Keen RR, McCarthy WJ, Shireman PK, et al. Surgical management of atheroembolism. J Vasc Surg 1995;21:773–80; discussion 780–81.
105. Dougherty MJ, Calligaro KD. Endovascular treatment of embolization of aortic plaque with covered stents. J Vasc Surg 2002;36:727.
106. Kumins NH, Owens EL, Oglevie SB, et al. Early experience using the Wallgraft in the management of distal microembolism from common iliac artery pathology. Ann Vasc Surg 2002;16:181.
107. Carroccio A, Olin JW, Ellozy SH, et al. The role of aortic stent grafting in the treatment of atheromatous embolization syndrome: results after a mean of 15 months follow-up. J Vasc Surg 2004;40:424–9.
108. Knochel JP. Mechanisms of rhabdomyolysis. Curr Opin Rheumatol 1993;5:725–31.
109. Brumback RA, Feeback DL, Leech RW. Rhabdomyolysis in childhood. Pediatr Clin North Am 1992;39:821–58.
110. Blebea J, Kerr JC, Franco CD, et al. Technetium 99m pyrophosphate quantitation of skeletal muscle ischemia and reperfusion injury. J Vasc Surg 1998;8:117.
111. Baue E. MOF, MODS, and SIRS: what is in a name or an acronym? Shock 2006;26:438–49.
112. Quinones-Baldrich WJ, Chervu A, Hernandez JJ, et al. Skeletal muscle function after ischemia: "no reflow" versus reperfusion injury. J Surg Res 1991;51:5.
113. Ricci MA, Graham AM, Corbisiero R, et al. Are free radical scavengers beneficial in the treatment of compartment syndrome after acute arterial ischemia? J Vasc Surg 1989;9:244.
114. Ouriel K, Smedira NG, Ricotta JJ. Protection of the kidney after temporary ischemia: free radical scavengers. J Vasc Surg 1985;2:49.
115. Mathieson MA, Dunham BM, Huval WV, et al. Ischemia of the limb stimulates thromboxane production and myocardial depression. Surg Gynecol Obstet 1983;157:500.
116. Fischer R, Fogarty T, Morrow A. A clinical and biochemical observation of the effect of transient femoral artery occlusion in man. Surgery 1970;68:233.
117. Green RM, DeWeese J, Rob CG. Arterial embolectomy before and after the Fogarty catheter. Surgery 1975;77:24.
118. Stary HC, Chandler AB, Dinsmore RE, et al. A definition of advanced types of atherosclerotic lesions and a histological classification of atherosclerosis: a report from the Committee on Vascular Lesions of the Council on Arteriosclerosis, American Heart Association. Circulation 1995;92:1355.
119. Fernandez-Ortiz A, Badimon JJ, Falk E, et al. Characterization of the relative thrombogenicity of atherosclerotic plaque components: implications for consequences of plaque rupture. J Am Coll Cardiol 1994;23:1562.
120. Ouriel K, Shortell CK, Green RM, et al. Differential mechanisms of failure of autogenous and non-autogenous bypass conduits: an assessment following successful graft thrombolysis. Cardiovasc Surg 1995;3:469.
121. Owens C, Ho K, Conte M. Lower extremity vein graft failure: a translational approach. Vasc Med 2008;13:63–74.
122. Abbott W, Maloney R, McCabe C, et al. Arterial embolism: a 44 year perspective. Am J Surg 1982;143:460.
123. Fogarty T, Daily P, Shumway N, et al. Experience with balloon catheter technique for arterial embolectomy. Am J Surg 1971;122:231.
124. Paneta T, Thomson J, Talkington C, et al. Arterial embolectomy: a 34 year experience with 400 cases. Surg Clin North Am 1986;66:339.
125. Shresta N, Moreno F, Narcisco F, et al. Two dimensional echocardiographic diagnosis of left atrial thrombus in rheumatic heart disease: a clinicopathologic study. Circulation 1983;67:341.
126. Schweizer P, Bardos F, Erbel R. Detection of left atrial thrombi by echocardiography. Br Heart J 1981;45:148.
127. Daniel W, Mugge A. Transesophageal echocardiography. N Engl J Med 1995;332:1268.
128. Husain A, Alter M. Transesophageal echocardiography in diagnosing cardioembolic stroke. Clin Cardiol 1995;18:705.

129. Seward J, Khandheria B, Oh J, et al. Transesophageal echocardiography: technique, anatomic correlations, implementation, and clinical applications. Mayo Clin Proc 1988;63:649.
130. Rubin B, Barzilai B, Allen B, et al. Detection of the source of arterial emboli by transesophageal echocardiography: a case report. J Vasc Surg 1992;15:573.
131. Loop F, Effler D, Navia J, et al. Aneurysms of the left ventricle: survival and results of a ten-year surgical experience. Ann Surg 1973;178:399.
132. Hellerstein H, Martin J. Incidence of thromboembolic lesions accompanying myocardial infarction. Am Heart J 1947;33:443.
133. Keely E, Hillis L. Left ventricular mural thrombus after acute myocardial infarction. Clin Cardiol 1996;19:83.
134. Asinger R, Mikell F, Elsperger J. Incidence of left ventricular thrombosis after acute transmural myocardial infarction. N Engl J Med 1981;305:297.
135. Darling R, Austen W, Linton R. Arterial embolism. Surg Gynecol Obstet 1967;124:106.
136. Perier P, Bessou J, Swanson J, et al. Comparative evaluation of aortic valve replacement with Starr, Bjork, and porcine valve prostheses. Circulation 1985;72:140.
137. Pipkin R, Buch W, Fogart T. Evaluation of aortic valve replacement with porcine xenograft without long-term anticoagulation. J Thorac Cardiovasc Surg 1976;71:179.
138. Kitts D, Bongard F, Klein S. Septic embolism complicating infective endocarditis. J Vasc Surg 1991;14:480.
139. Freischlag J, Asburn H, Sedwitz M, et al. Septic peripheral embolization from bacterial and fungal endocarditis. Ann Vasc Surg 1989;3:318.
140. Lord J Jr, Rossi G, Daliana M, et al. Unsuspected abdominal aortic aneurysm as the cause of peripheral arterial occlusive disease. Ann Surg 1973;177:767.
141. Kempczynski R. Lower extremity emboli from ulcerating atherosclerotic plaque. JAMA 1979;241:807.
142. Kwaan J, Vander Molen R, Stemmer E, et al. Peripheral embolism resulting from unsuspected atheromatous plaques. Surgery 1975;78:583.
143. Machleder H, Takiff H, Lois J, et al. Aortic mural thrombus: an occult source of arterial thromboembolism. J Vasc Surg 1986;4:473.
144. Shannon J, Nghia M, Stanton P Jr, et al. Peripheral arterial missile embolization: a case report and a 22 year review of the literature. J Vasc Surg 1987;5:773.
145. Symbas P, Harlaftis N. Bullet emboli in the pulmonary and systemic arteries. Ann Surg 1977;185:318.
146. Harriss R, Andros G, Dulawa L, et al. Malignant melanoma embolus as a cause of acute aortic occlusion: report of a case. J Vasc Surg 1986;3:550.
147. Morasch MD, Shanik GD. Tumor embolus: a case report and review of the literature. Ann Vasc Surg 2003;17:210.
148. Ward R, Jones D, Haponik E. Paradoxical embolism: an under-recognized problem. Chest 1995;108:549.
149. Katz S, Andros G, Kohl R, et al. Arterial emboli of venous origin. Surg Gynecol Obstet 1992;174:17.
150. Gazzaniga A, Dalen J. Paradoxical embolism: its pathophysiology and clinical recognition. Ann Surg 1970;171: 137.
151. Hight D, Tilney N, Couch N. Changing clinical trends in patients with peripheral emboli. Surgery 1976;79:172.
152. Thompson J, Sigler L, Raut P, et al. Arterial embolectomy: a 20 year experience. Surgery 1970;67:212.
153. Eason J, Mills J, Beckett W. Hypercoagulable states in arterial thromboembolism. Surg Gynecol Obstet 1992;174:211.
154. Sharma P, Babu P, Shah P, et al. Changing patterns of atheroembolism. Cardiovasc Surg 1996;4:573.
155. Elliott J, Hageman J, Szilagyi D. Arterial embolization: problems of source, multiplicity, recurrence, and delayed treatment. Surgery 1980;88:833.
156. Dale W. Differential management of acute peripheral ischemia. J Vasc Surg 1984;1:269.
157. Banis JC Jr, Rich N, Whelan TJ Jr. Ischemia of the upper extremity due to noncardiac emboli. Am J Surg 1977;134: 131.
158. Stonebridge PA, Clason AE, Duncan AJ, et al. Acute ischaemia of the upper limb compared with acute lower limb ischaemia: a 5-year review. Br J Surg 1989;76:515–6.
159. Balbir-Gurman A, Braun-Moscovici Y, Nahir AM. Cocaine-induced Raynaud's phenomenon and ischaemic finger necrosis. Clin Rheumatol 2001;20:376.
160. Disdier P, Granel B, Serratrice J, et al. Cannabis arteritis revisited—ten new case reports. Angiology 2001;52:1.
161. Ishikawa K. Patterns of symptoms and prognosis in occlusive thromboarthropathy (Takayasu's disease). J Am Coll Cardiol 1986;8:1401.
162. Mira Y, Todoli T, Alonso R, et al. Factor V Leiden and prothrombin G20210A in relation to arterial and/or vein rethrombosis: two cases. Clin Appl Thromb Hemost 2001; 7:234.
163. Weaver FA, Papanicolaou G, Yellin AE. Difficult peripheral vascular injuries. Surg Clin North Am 1996;76:843–59.
164. Ouriel K. Acute ischemia and its sequelae. In: Rutherford RB, editor. Vascular surgery. 5th ed. Philadelphia: WB Saunders; 2000. p. 814.
165. Thrombolysis in the management of lower limb peripheral arterial occlusion; a consensus document. Working Party on Thrombosis in the Management of Limb Ischemia. J Vasc Interv Radiol 2003;14(9 Pt 2):5337.

6 VENOUS THROMBOEMBOLISM

Guillermo A. Escobar, MD, Thomas W. Wakefield, MD, FACS, and Peter K. Henke, MD, FACS★

Assessment of a Venous Thromboembolic Event

Deep vein thrombosis (DVT) and pulmonary embolism (PE) comprise venous thromboembolism (VTE). Together, they comprise a serious health problem as there are over 600,000 new cases of VTE in the United States, resulting in a prevalence of one to two per 1,000 individuals, with some studies suggesting that the incidence may even be double that.[1,2] The European Union reports an incidence of VTE of over 760,000 cases a year, with more than 370,000 VTE-related deaths, and one third were sudden deaths.[3] It is estimated that about 10 to 25% of patients with acute PE die from sudden death prior to diagnosis and, thus, do not receive therapy, resulting in approximately 60,000 Americans dying each year from complications associated with VTE[4–6] Postmortem studies have identified that sudden death from PE is misdiagnosed in almost 80% of cases,[7] exemplifying the poor ability we have to identify and prevent it. Of the more than 500,000 patients who survive at least 1 hour to have the opportunity to be diagnosed and treated, only 29% actually receive treatment and 92% of them survive, whereas the untreated 71% have a mortality of 30%.[8] These numbers are staggering when compared with the death rates of other common diseases. Altogether, death from VTE is five times more common than deaths from breast cancer, AIDS, and motor vehicle crashes combined.

The long-term complications of nonfatal DVT are morbid, including one third suffering postthrombotic syndrome (PTS) and another 30% having a recurrent VTE within 10 years of the first.[2,9] Finally, in patients with cancer, VTE-related complications are the second leading cause of death; they increase the mortality associated with increased bleeding complications and the use of health care resources.[10–12]

Patients with PTS may suffer poor quality of life as a result of chronic limb symptoms.[13,14] PTS occurs in up to 30% of patients with DVT at 8-year follow-up, varying in severity from edema to venous claudication and ulcers.[15,16] Risks for PTS include recurrent DVT, a proximal (iliofemoral) DVT, older age, a high body mass index, and female gender.[15] Preventing recurrent DVT is a primary means to decrease PTS. Most of the time, therapy for PTS is palliative, but at times, patients with PTS require (or request) lower extremity amputations because of chronic, unrelenting pain and ulceration. A 12-year review of a Nationwide Inpatient Sample database sampling all hospitalized patients with chronic venous disease found that 1.2% of patients underwent an amputation.[13] This number may be higher at tertiary referral centers, which have a large number of complex venous patients.

Considering that PE and PTS are often preceded by DVT, there is an impetus for prevention, early detection, and aggressive treatment of DVT prior to the presentation of these complications, all while providing appropriate acute management and evaluating the response to treatment. This all begins with a careful history and physical examination.

★ The authors and editors gratefully acknowledge the contributions of the previous author, John T. Owings, MD, FACS, to the development and writing of this chapter.

Clinical Evaluation

The importance of obtaining a good history of present illness and review of systems in patients is critical in the decision tree for the diagnosis and management of patients with acute VTE as subtle clinical findings may dramatically change the treatment plan and are not driven by imaging or laboratory tests alone. For example, a patient with only shortness of breath or tachycardia as a symptom or sign of PE may require a D-dimer prior to receiving any further treatment or imaging, whereas one with tachycardia and leg swelling may benefit from anticoagulation prior to imaging (without needing a D-dimer) because of a higher likelihood of PE.[17]

If a patient presents with a VTE, one must distinguish between those patients who have a temporary risk factor (such as surgery or bed rest) and those who have a lifelong secondary condition, inherited disease, or undefined state that predisposes to thrombosis and may benefit from prolonged anticoagulation after the VTE [*see Table 1*]. This distinction helps determine the long-term treatment and risk of future VTE.

In addition to advancing age, acquired VTE risk factors that are considered lifelong to the patient include a history of previous VTE, active cancer (may be reversible in some cases), extremity paresis or paralysis, medical disorders causing prolonged bed rest, and congenital or autoimmune thrombophilia. Temporary or provoked VTE risk factors include pregnancy, oral contraceptive or hormone therapy, surgery and trauma, central venous catheters, and bed rest or other states of prolonged immobility.

Table 1 **Clinical Scenarios Possibly Benefiting from Prolonged Anticoagulation after VTE[145]**
Antiphospholipid antibody and systemic lupus
Homozygous factor V Leiden mutation
Prothrombin gene mutation (G20210A)
Elevated factor VIII
Protein C or S deficiency
Hyperhomocysteinemia
Cancer (while cancer is active)
Otherwise unexplained, repeated deep vein thrombosis or pulmonary embolus

VTE = venous thromboembolism.

Medical History

THROMBOPHILIC RISK FACTORS

Rudolf Virchow first stated in 1859 that clots in the pulmonary artery originated from the venous circulation and coined the term "embolus." He also described the three components of hypercoagulability that are now referred to as a triad that bears his name: hypercoagulability, stasis, and injury to the vessel wall.[18] These factors are still relevant today.

"Thrombophilia" is defined by the World Health Organization (WHO) as "a tendency towards thrombosis."[19] Thrombophilia, whether acquired or inherited, plays a direct role in about 50% of all VTEs. Most commonly, surgeons evaluate patients for these risks preoperatively. Aggressive screening for VTE risk to provide appropriate prophylaxis or treatment can best be obtained by interviewing the patient. These risks can be determined via group consensus guidelines such as those of the American College of Chest Physicians (ACCP)[20] or via the use of an individualized risk assessment scoring such as the modified Caprini score.[21] The ACCP guidelines account for most risk scenarios by taking into account patient cohorts (e.g., all medical patients, those undergoing hip replacement, patients with cancer, etc.). However, individual patients may overlap into several simultaneous categories. Alternatively, individual risk assessment can be performed by directed intake sheet [*see Figure 1*]. This allows each patient summation and suggests appropriate prophylaxis choices. The questionnaire collects information from the patient's personal (age) and medical history (e.g., family history of VTE, personal history of DVT) and takes into consideration what type of procedure is to be done and the intended mobility status. This system has recently been retrospectively validated.[21]

IRREVERSIBLE RISK FACTORS FOR VTE

Age

Age alone confers an acquired thrombophilic state. Older patients tend to accumulate risk factors such as infections, surgery, and cancer, each of which increases the likelihood of having thrombotic complications. Patients over 50 years of age also have higher concentrations of antiphospholipid antibodies of unknown significance.[22] The older the patient is who suffers a VTE, the lower the likelihood that the VTE was attributable to an inherited etiology and, conversely, the greater the likelihood that it was attributable to an acquired condition.[23] Older patients also have a higher risk of developing limb complications such as PTS[15] as well as PE. Experimental animal data also suggest that age may lead to a higher concentration of P-selectin and impaired fibrinolysis, which may contribute to age-related thrombophilia.[24]

Malignancy

The clinical constellation of asymptomatic cancer and lower extremity deep vein thrombosis (LEDVT) was first described in 1865 by Armand Trousseau,[25] and this syndrome bears his name. The 19th century was also marked by the suggestion by Theodor Billroth that cancer used clot as a mechanism to spread.[26]

Since then, a search for the etiologic factor involved in cancer-related thrombophilia has only been partially fruitful. A "cancer procoagulant" factor was found in 1985 exclusively in amniochorial tissue and associated with multiple malignancies.[27] It is a cysteine protease that specifically activates coagulation factor X. However, even after more than 25 years since this discovery, it has been purified only from several malignant tissue cultures, and no gene has been identified.[28]

Of all types of malignancies, mucin-producing tumors such as adenocarcinomas, small cell lung cancers, gastrointestinal cancer (such as the gastric cancer that led to Trousseau's own DVT),[29] and ovarian cancer are most likely associated with VTE.[30] This notwithstanding, any malignancy increases the risk of VTE. Additional risk factors linked to patients with malignancies are those related to therapy, such as central venous catheters, chemotherapy, and surgical procedures, all of which are independent risk factors for VTE.[31] An additional risk factor found in some cancer patients is an elevated (greater than 75th percentile) soluble P-selectin concentration. It increases the cumulative DVT probability from 3.7 to 11.9% in multiple types of cancer.[32] Whether mucin-producing cancers have increased P-selectin as the mechanism of thrombosis is under investigation.[33]

Inherited Thrombophilia

The WHO defines an inherited thrombophilia as "the presence of an inherited factor that by itself predisposes towards thrombosis but due to the episodic nature of thrombosis, requires interaction with other components . . before onset of the clinical disorder."[19] To evaluate patients with suspected primary thrombophilia, an international consensus was formed to standardize who needs advanced testing. Indications for laboratory investigation of secondary thrombophilia are listed in Table 2, and venous thromboembolic risk according to hypercoagulable state are listed in Table 3.[34,35]

In 1994, the Leiden Institute discovered the point mutation in factor V that explains the most common inheritable thrombophilia. This "factor V Leiden mutation" accounts for up to 25% of secondary thrombophilias.[36] It occurs in 6 to 9% of whites and in up to 50% of families with a history of DVT.[23,37] The G20210A mutation of the prothrombin (coagulation factor II) gene is another common etiology of thrombophilia that is associated with DVT.[36] Impaired fibrinolysis is a hypercoagulable state associated with 4G/5G polymorphisms of the plasminogen activator inhibitor–1 (*PAI-1*) gene. These patients have a threefold increased risk of DVT higher than the general population.[38] As many as one third of non–catheter-related upper extremity deep vein thrombosis (UEDVT) may be due to the above-mentioned inheritable disorders.[39]

Other notable inheritable syndromes include deficiencies of the natural anticoagulants, including antithrombin III and proteins C and S.[40,41] These tend to be more aggressive thrombophilias, with presentation in younger patients. Obtaining a positive screen for these entities directs the long-term anticoagulation strategy for and future risk of VTE.

ANTIBODY-MEDIATED AND RHEUMATOLOGIC RISK FACTORS

The majority of these factors are encountered in rheumatologic disorders. The disease most commonly associated with both arterial and VTE is antiphospholipid syndrome. For decades, clinicians noted that patients with systemic lupus erythematosus (SLE) would present with spontaneous

Deep Vein Thrombosis (DVT)
Prophylaxis Orders
(For use in Elective General Surgery Patients)

Thrombosis Risk Factor Assessment
(Choose all that apply)

BIRTHDATE
NAME
CPI No.
SEX M F VISIT No. ________________

Each Risk Factor Represents 1 Point

- ❑ Age 41-60 years
- ❑ Swollen legs (current)
- ❑ Varicose veins
- ❑ Obesity (BMI >25)
- ❑ Minor surgery planned
- ❑ Sepsis (<1 month)
- ❑ Acute myocardial infarction
- ❑ Congestive heart failure (<1 month)
- ❑ Medical patient currently at bed rest
- ❑ History of inflammatory bowel disease
- ❑ History of prior major surgery (<1 month)
- ❑ Abnormal pulmonary function (COPD)
- ❑ Serious Lung disease including pneumonia (<1 month)
- ❑ Oral contraceptives or hormone replacement therapy
- ❑ Pregnancy or postpartum (<1 month)
- ❑ History of unexplained stillborn infant, recurrent spontaneous abortion ($\geq$ 3), premature birth with toxemia or growth-restricted infant
- ❑ Other risk factors________________

Subtotal:

Each Risk Factor Represents 2 Points

- ❑ Age 61-74 years
- ❑ Arthroscopic surgery
- ❑ Malignancy (present or previous)
- ❑ Laparoscopic surgery (>45 minutes)
- ❑ Patient confined to bed (>72 hours)
- ❑ Immobilizing plaster cast (<1 month)
- ❑ Central venous access
- ❑ Major surgery (>45 minutes)

Subtotal:

Each Risk Factor Represents 3 Points

- ❑ Age 75 years or older
- ❑ History of DVT/PE
- ❑ Positive Factor V Leiden
- ❑ Family History of thrombosis*
- ❑ Positive Prothrombin 20210A
- ❑ Positive Lupus anticoagulant
- ❑ Elevated serum homocysteine
- ❑ Heparin-induced thrombocytopenia (HIT) (Do not use heparin or any low molecular weight heparin)
- ❑ Elevated anticardiolipin antibodies
- ❑ Other congenital or acquired thrombophilia

If yes: Type________________

* most frequently missed risk factor

Subtotal:

Each Risk Factor Represents 5 Points

- ❑ Stroke (<1 month)
- ❑ Multiple trauma (<1 month)
- ❑ Elective major lower extremity arthroplasty
- ❑ Hip, pelvis or leg fracture (<1 month)
- ❑ Acute spinal cord injury (paralysis) (<1 month)

Subtotal:

TOTAL RISK FACTOR SCORE:

FACTORS ASSOCIATED WITH INCREASED BLEEDING

Patient may not be a candidate for anticoagulant therapy & SCDs should be considered.

Active Bleed, Ingestion of Oral Anticoagulants, Administration of glycoprotein IIb/IIIa inhibitors, History of heparin induced thrombocytopenia

CLINICAL CONSIDERATIONS FOR THE USE OF SEQUENTIAL COMPRESSION DEVICES (SCD)

Patient may not be a candidate for SCDs & alternative prophylactic measures should be considered.

Patients with Severe Peripheral Arterial Disease, CHF, Acute Superficial DVT

Total Risk Factor Score	Risk Level	Incidence of DVT	Prophylaxis Regimen
0-1	Low Risk	2%	❑ Early ambulation
2	Moderate Risk	10-20%	Choose the following medication <u>OR</u> compression devices: ❑ Sequential Compression Device (SCD) ❑ Heparin 5000 units SQ BID
3-4	Higher Risk	20-40%	Choose <u>ONE</u> of the following medications + / - compression devices: ❑ Sequential Compression Device (SCD) ❑ Heparin 5000 units SQ TID ❑ Enoxaparin/Lovenox: ❑ 40mg SQ daily (WT < 150kg, CrCl > 30mL/min) ❑ 30mg SQ daily (WT < 150kg, CrCl = 10-29mL/min) ❑ 30mg SQ BID (WT > 150kg, CrCl > 30mL/min) (Please refer to Dosing Guidelines on the back of this form)
5 or more	Highest Risk	40-80%	Choose <u>ONE</u> of the following medications <u>PLUS</u> compression devices: ❑ Sequential Compression Device (SCD) ❑ Heparin 5000 units SQ TID (Preferred with Epidurals) ❑ Enoxaparin/Lovenox (Preferred): ❑ 40mg SQ daily (WT < 150kg, CrCl > 30mL/min) ❑ 30mg SQ daily (WT < 150kg, CrCl = 10-29mL/min) ❑ 30mg SQ BID (WT > 150kg, CrCl > 30mL/min) (Please refer to Dosing Guidelines on the back of this form)

❑ Ambulatory Surgery - No orders for venous thromboembolic prophylaxis required

❑ VTE Prophylaxis Contraindicated, Reason: ________________

Joseph A. Caprini, MD, MS, FACS, RVT
VTE Risk Factor Assessment Tool

Physician Signature | Dr. # | Date | Time

Processed By: | Date/Time:

White-Medical Record
Yellow-MIS Pink-Pharmacy

M University of Michigan Health System

DVT Prophylaxis Regimen

Figure 1 **Modified Caprini score questionnaire used at the University of Michigan to determine individual risk for venous thromboembolism and the indicated prophylaxis regimen.**

Table 2 Indications for Laboratory Investigation of Secondary Thrombophilia[34,35]
Any first, spontaneous VTE without known risk factors
VTE in patients < 50 years, even with a transient predisposing factor
Patients whose only risk factor is estrogen therapy or pregnancy
Recurrent VTE regardless of risk factors (even superficial phlebitis if not associated with cancer or varicosities)
VTE in patients < 50 years in uncommon sites (e.g., intra-abdominal, intracranial, retinal)
Warfarin-induced skin necrosis and purpura fulminans (when not associated with sepsis)
Two consecutive abortions, three nonconsecutive abortions, or one fetal death after 20 wk gestation
Asymptomatic first-degree relatives of a patient with proven thrombophilia
VTE with severe preeclampsia
Children with VTE

VTE = venous thromboembolism.

Table 3 **Venous Thromboembolic Risk Accorded to Hypercoagulable States**

Hypercoagulable Risk Factor	VTE Risk Compared with Unaffected Population
Factor V Leiden mutation	80× in homozygous (5–8× in heterozygous)
Antithrombin III, protein C and S deficiencies	10×
Elevated factor VIII	6×
Prothrombin gene mutation	2.8×
Hyperhomocysteinemia	2.5–4×
Antiphospholipid antibody	Lifetime risk 10% of positive patients

VTE = venous thromboembolism.

clotting yet paradoxically have prolonged activated partial thromboplastin times (aPTTs).[42] This is now known to be attributable to antibodies against the negatively charged phospholipids that interfere with the aPTT assay itself. These antibodies are not specific to lupus as they may be independent (true antiphospholipid antibody syndrome [APS]) or associated with other rheumatologic diseases, such as rheumatoid arthritis, systemic sclerosis, Sjögren syndrome, and systemic vasculitis, among others. The most common antibodies identified are antiphosphatidylserine (lupus anticoagulant), anticardiolipin, anti–β_2-GPI, and sometimes antiprothrombin.[43,44] There is a high IgM anticardiolipin antibody level in females when compared with males[45] and an increased incidence of PE among APS patients. The exact mechanism for thrombophilia in APS is unknown,[46] but it is not simply attributable to antibody- or complement-mediated activation of platelets.[47] This is highlighted by the fact that clinically silent antiphospholipid antibodies may be found in as much as 2% of the population (age related) and that although 30 to 40% of patients with SLE have antiphospholipid antibodies, only 10% will manifest with thrombosis.[48]

Another rheumatologic disorder that confers an increased risk of arterial and venous thrombosis (particularly in the cerebral sinus and lower extremities) is Behçet syndrome. This presents most commonly in patients from the "old silk road" (between China and the Mediterranean Sea) and has yet to have a clear mechanism elucidated.[49,50]

ACQUIRED RISK FACTORS FOR VTE

Immobilization

Stasis is often considered a risk factor for VTE because of sluggish venous flow seen in a spectrum of scenarios ranging from being seated on a transoceanic flight to a paralyzed trauma patient. Although this alone is an inconsistent risk for VTE, even sitting in a chair for 6 to 8 hours may be what unmasks other, more prevalent VTE risk factors by increasing the regional procoagulant factors in the region of stasis.[51] A meta-analysis of medical patients suggests that the risk of VTE in immobilized patients is about twice that of ambulatory patients.[52]

The risk of VTE in those individuals with low or moderate risk after a flight lasting more than 4 hours has been studied and is thought to be 1% or less and 4 to 6% in those who are high risk, presumably from prolonged immobilization.[53,54] Although uncommon, the association of VTE with air travel has been linked to the distance traveled. The lowest risk occurs after flights less than 3,000 miles (0.01 cases per million), and the highest occurs after flights greater than 6,000 miles (4.6 cases per million).[55] Given that these numbers are very small and that there are no control groups, consensus guidelines only recommend frequent ambulation and compression stockings during long flights and reserve pharmacologic prophylaxis for patients with other major risk factors for VTE.[56] Most studies evaluating compression stockings to improve edema after long flights show a benefit, but their role in preventing significant (DVT and PE) VTE depends more on the patient's risk factors than on the length of the flight. It has not been shown that stockings diminish the risk of DVT after prolonged air travel in patients who are low risk, regardless of the length of the flight. Conversely, compression stockings likely reduce the risk of DVT after flights that last more than 8 hours in all patients who are otherwise at high risk for VTE.[54–59] Patients who are at moderate risk for DVT and travel more than 11 hours also may benefit from stockings with compression gradients of 20 to 30 mm Hg, whereas no DVT has been demonstrated in this patient population after flights that last less than this.

Surgery and Trauma

All patients undergoing surgical procedures have an increased risk of thrombosis, with an incidence ranging from 15 to 40% and an odds ratio of more than 10 compared with controls.[60] This may be attributable to accelerated production of procoagulant and inflammatory cytokines that activate platelets, inflammatory cells, and endothelial cells in addition to postoperative inactivity, which increases blood stasis. Although controversial, the incidence may also be attributable to reduced capacity for fibrinolysis during the perioperative period, associated with increased PAI-1 activity.[61,62] Procedures that require prolonged immobility in the postoperative period (such as hip replacements and spine procedures) have the highest risk of DVT (historical prevalence

40 to 60%). Interestingly, decreased concentrations of fibrinolytic enzymes have been documented in patients undergoing orthopedic procedures (compared with general surgical patients) and may partially explain the greater thrombosis risk in these patients.[63]

Although preoperative and operative risk factors are important to predict VTE, the interventions and medical complications associated with the patient's postoperative course also impact the incidence of symptomatic VTE. A cohort study involving over 76,000 patients having surgery in the Veterans Affairs system over a 5-year period found that the strongest predictors of postoperative VTE were myocardial infarction, blood transfusion (> 4 units), pneumonia, and urinary tract infections.[64] This suggests that postoperative systemic inflammatory conditions may substantially contribute to the thrombophilic state. However, the exact mechanism(s) are unknown.

Major trauma patients are also known to be at high risk for VTE (historical prevalence of 40 to 80%),[20] and DVT may occur in up to one third of patients (mostly in the calf of the leg) with a moderate to severe brain injury, especially when associated with extremity injuries.[65,66] For these reasons, prophylaxis with sequential compression devices (SCDs) and eventually heparin or low-molecular-weight heparin (LMWH) when the bleeding risk is deemed safe are strongly encouraged (see below).

Intravenous Catheters

Macroscopically, vessel trauma and foreign bodies placed within veins damage the endothelium and will locally accumulate platelet and coagulation factors. These conditions alone will usually not lead to vessel thrombosis, but when combined with other prothrombotic factors, such as tissue factor, von Willebrand factor, and fibronectin, the likelihood of DVT increases.[67] The conversion from local clot to occlusive thrombus is likely dependent on the time of exposure to the etiologic factor. As such, central venous catheters (including peripherally inserted catheters) have a relatively high rate of thrombosis. Central venous catheters account for two thirds to three quarters of UEDVT and are the strongest independent predictor of UEDVT (7.3-fold increase).[68,69]

Clinical Presentation of VTE

The most common presentation of DVT is limb swelling, calf pain, and discrepant circumference. However, the manifestations of DVT or PE may be subtle and subclinical in many cases. It has been found that over 50% of patients with a DVT may have an unrecognized PE (based on imaging testing)[70] and that over 70% of patients with PE have an undiagnosed LEDVT.[18]

To aid in the appropriate management of PE, Wells and colleagues published clinical criteria that accurately stratify a patient as low, moderate, or high risk and determine who needs further imaging to evaluate for PE.[71] Their 2001 criteria for PE include hemoptysis, malignancy (patients with cancer who are receiving treatment or for whom treatment has been stopped in the previous 6 months or those receiving palliative care), a history of DVT or PE, tachycardia, and no other likely diagnosis. Additional criteria include immobilization for more than 3 consecutive days or surgery less than 30 days from presentation and clinical signs and symptoms of DVT (objectively measured calf swelling and pain with palpation in the deep venous system). Wells and colleagues determined that in cases of low or moderate risk with a normal D-dimer (a serum marker of fibrinolysis), no further imaging was necessary. However, if the D-dimer was positive, then a ventilation-perfusion (V/Q) scan or angiogram was used to confirm the clinical suspicion. In patients with chest symptoms suspicious for PE, the patient should be evaluated for these criteria to determine the need to pursue further imaging or laboratory studies. Patients found to be at intermediate risk or high risk for PE should also be heparinized prior to obtaining imaging.[72]

The first Prospective Investigation of Pulmonary Embolism Diagnosis (PIOPED) study found that of the more than 250 patients with angiographically demonstrated PE, only 11% had physical examinations consistent with DVT.[73] Hemoptysis and pleuritic pain may be present in only about 40% of all patients with PE.[74] Like DVT, patients with clinical manifestations of PE will likely only have nonspecific clinical findings. The most common findings include dyspnea (84%), pleuritic pain (74%), apprehension (63%), and cough (50%). Of these clinically positive patients with PE, dyspnea or tachypnea occurred in 96%, whereas 99% of them demonstrated dyspnea, tachypnea, or DVT.[75] As in other diseases that are shared by the young and old, PIOPED II revealed that dyspnea or tachypnea was less commonly reported in elderly patients.[74]

Rarely, massive iliofemoral DVT may cause phlegmasia alba dolens (swollen white/milk leg), a clinical scenario when arterial inflow becomes obstructed as a result of extreme venous hypertension.[25] Phlegmasia cerulea dolens (swollen blue leg) occurs from severe venous hypertension that occludes the capillaries and may result in venous gangrene. The legs become red or purpuric, and the toes may become cyanotic and often is accompanied by blistering of the skin [*see Figure 2*]. Venous gangrene is always preceded by phlegmasia cerulea dolens, and is often associated with an underlying malignancy.

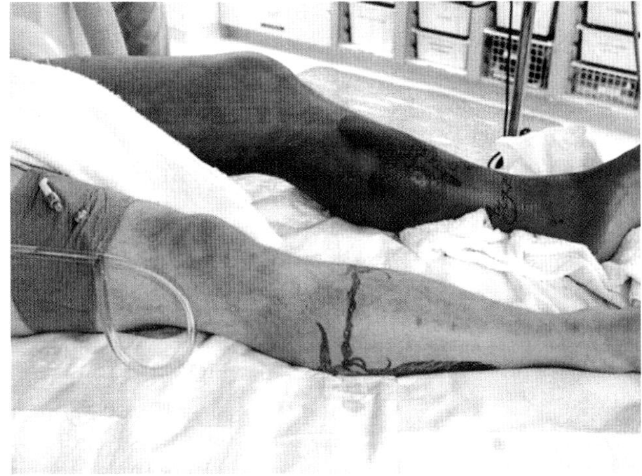

Figure 2 **Phlegmasia cerulea dolens secondary to acute left iliofemoral deep vein thrombosis after thigh trauma. The condition was completely resolved after thrombolysis and stenting of his left common and external iliac veins, followed by anticoagulation and compression stockings.**

Physical Examination

The most common physical findings associated with LEDVT are edema, calf swelling, and tenderness, but these are not specific to DVT. Homan sign (calf pain at dorsiflexion of the foot) and pain on manual compression of the calf muscle against the tibia (Olow sign) are uncommon signs but are suggestive of calf DVT. The extremity may also be warm and ruborous with brisk capillary refill, and care must be taken not to misdiagnose LEDVT for cellulitis. Although the lower leg is the most common site for DVT, thigh pain and arm pain may also be noted in cases of iliofemoral and UEDVT, respectively.

Although physical examination alone is accurate in less than one third of cases,[76] it is critical to determine the next step in the clinical investigation or treatment, particularly in the case of PE,[77] and limb threat, which may mandate urgent therapies (see below). One must remember that unless there is vena cava thrombosis, the clinical findings of DVT are rarely bilateral. This diagnostic rule assists in eliminating other systemic causes of lower extremity edema, such as renal failure or congestive heart failure, which may manifest with edema. Other illnesses that may mimic unilateral leg DVT include popliteal (Baker) cysts, trauma, cellulitis, popliteal aneurysm thrombosis, lymphedema, and muscle strain.

Patients with phlegmasia syndromes will have dramatic swelling associated with tight, plethoric extremities that may be ruborous or pale. A careful evaluation of the motor function of the extremity is necessary to determine which patient has immediate limb threat and requires urgent intervention to resolve the venous hypertension or open the compartment [*see* in Indications for Immediate Intervention (Limb or Life Threat), *below*].

Superficial venous thrombosis may often manifest in the setting of a vessel cannulation. Superficial thrombophlebitis is most often accompanied by pain, an inflamed palpable cord, or both along the axis of the affected vein. Sometimes this may also be accompanied by extremity edema and, if infected, may have purulent discharge at the catheter site.[78]

Laboratory Evaluation

D-dimer is most useful for ruling out a VTE in a low-risk patient. If negative, there is almost no risk for VTE, and no further testing is required. This clinical strategy has been adopted by both the American and European consensus groups as the appropriate workup for a VTE.[56,60] However, D-dimer is not useful for those patients with a high pretest probability of a VTE. We now know that in patients with a high clinical suspicion of VTE, almost 10% may have a false negative D-dimer assay with a VTE, although in those with a low suspicion, it will be accurate nearly 100% of the time. Thus, in a high-risk patient, a D-dimer will not safely rule out a VTE; thus, there is no reason to obtain such a level in a high-risk or even a moderate-risk patient.[79] Furthermore, patients who have undergone surgery or trauma may have an elevated D-dimer from postoperative blood that is being lysed, and this finding may be elevated for over 2 weeks.[80] Thus, D-dimer has less utility in the postoperative period, and reliance on imaging such as computed tomographic angiography (CTA) for PE is important.

Whenever possible, blood screening for patients suspected of thrombophilia should use samples obtained prior to anticoagulation to obtain a baseline partial thromboplastin time, prothrombin time, platelet count, antithrombin, and proteins C and S levels, although with significant thrombosis, these coagulation proteins may be consumed into the thrombus, leading to falsely low levels. Anticoagulation will also change the above-mentioned values. However, accurate results can help predict the etiology of the hypercoagulable state. For example, a prolonged aPTT may be attributable to antiphospholipid antibody syndrome, whereas a low protein C may be attributable to genetic protein C deficiency. The remaining genetic or antibody tests obtained during a thrombophilia evaluation, such as factor V Leiden mutation, factor II G20210A mutation, anticardiolipin, anti–β_2-GPI, and fasting homocysteine, will not be altered by anticoagulation and can be obtained at any time in the patient's course.

Imaging

When used in symptomatic patients, compression duplex ultrasonography (CDU) alone has a sensitivity to detect proximal DVT and calf DVT of 96% and 80%, respectively. In asymptomatic patients, the sensitivity is significantly lower (76% for proximal calf DVT and 11% for isolated calf vein thrombosis).[81] Thus, CDU is the initial screening and diagnostic test of choice in patients with a moderate to high suspicion for DVT or is the second test to be done if a positive D-dimer assay is found when evaluating a low-risk patient for a DVT.

The diagnosis of PE may be further studied with a radionuclide V/Q scan, pulmonary CTA, or pulmonary arteriography. Vena cava or extremity venography is rarely indicated except when combined with a planned catheter-directed fibrinolysis procedure (e.g., May-Thurner or Paget-Schroetter syndrome).

Although V/Q scans do not require radiation or use nephrotoxic contrast agents, they provide a definitive diagnosis in less than half of cases, with a sensitivity of only 41%.[73] Anywhere from 30 to 70% of V/Q scans are interpreted (often erroneously) as "indeterminate," and the management of these patients is unclear, especially as 30 to 40% of these patients may have a PE and are not treated appropriately.[82] This modality has fallen out of favor except where a CTA cannot be obtained and the pulmonary function portion of the test is predicted to be normal. When a patient has other pathologies that alter the ventilatory (such as chronic obstructive pulmonary disease or pneumonia) or perfusion portions (previous infarcts, previous lung resections, or old infarcts) of the test, V/Q imaging is not useful for detecting acute PE.

A prospective multicenter trial evaluating multidetector CTA alone versus CTA combined with venous phase computed tomography (CT) of the pelvic and thigh veins for the diagnosis of acute PE was conducted in the PIOPED II study.[74,83] It revealed that combining pulmonary CTA with CT venography (in the same scan) was more useful in managing suspected PE and DVT than by pulmonary CTA alone. The combination of pulmonary CTA and CT venography for PE yielded a sensitivity and specificity of 90% and 95%, respectively. If the clinical findings correlated with the CT findings, then the positive predictive value is over 92% in all scenarios. Another benefit of the use of CT, even though it requires the infusion of intravenous contrast dye and radiation,[84] is that although it is positive in less than one third of patients who undergo CTA for PE, an alternative diagnosis may be found in more than 70% of those patients.

Of the available imaging modalities, pulmonary arteriography is the most invasive and exposes the patient to potentially nephrotoxic contrast dye. Although historically this was considered the diagnostic test of choice, the use of high-resolution CTA is now the standard for the aforementioned reasons. Angiography is more commonly used when catheter-directed thrombus removal is being contemplated (see below).

Prophylaxis against Perioperative VTE

Without prophylaxis, surgical procedures may have a VTE prevalence of up to 80%.[20] Historically, trials comparing no perioperative VTE prophylaxis with prophylaxis methods ranging from stockings and SCDs or any form of anticoagulation showed that each prophylactic modality could decrease the risk of VTE at least two- to threefold.[85–87] For this reason, every patient undergoing surgery should have some form of prophylaxis unless it is a minor or ambulatory procedure and the patient has no other VTE risk factor other than the procedure (see below).[56] There is no evidence to support the use of inferior vena cava (IVC) filters for perioperative or peritrauma PE prophylaxis without the diagnosis of DVT [*see* Vena Cava Filters, *below*].

As previously stated, one way to determine prophylaxis recommendations is the ACCP consensus guidelines.[20] Whether based on a category or risk score, most at-risk patients who undergo major surgical procedures or suffer significant trauma should receive prophylaxis with an anticoagulant unless they have a high bleeding risk; in these cases, SCDs are recommended until the bleeding risk subsides. In high-risk VTE cases such as in spine injury or hip replacement, stronger pharmacologic agents (LMWH, pentasaccharides, or warfarin) are recommended for prophylaxis, whereas unfractionated heparin (UFH), SCDs, and aspirin alone are not effective prophylaxis [*see Table 4*]. In surgical procedures where the bleeding risk outweighs the benefit of an anticoagulant, such as certain neurologic and vascular procedures, mechanical prophylaxis usually suffices. These include graduated compression stockings and SCDs, which are comparable to low-dose heparin in patients without other risk factors.[88] The caveat is that these devices need to be on the patient's limbs and working, requiring surveillance for compliance.

Indications for Immediate Intervention (Limb or Life Threat)

PULMONARY EMBOLUS

Barring a medical contraindication, full-dose anticoagulation should be started in cases of high clinical suspicion for PE until it is refuted as the cause.[56] If PE is diagnosed, then anticoagulation should be continued with either continuous UFH titrated to an aPTT of 60 to 80 seconds, weight-based, full-dose LMWH, or fondaparinux according to both the American (ACCP) and European (European Society of Cardiology) guidelines.[56,60]

Table 4 Recommended VTE Prophylaxis Stratified by Surgical Procedure and Associated VTE Risk Factors According to the 8th ACCP Consensus Statement[20]

Surgical Procedure	Prophylaxis
Minor general surgery without other risk factors	Early ambulation alone
Major general surgery	LMWH, LDUH, or Fx
High-risk general surgery	LMWH, LDUH, or Fx with SCD or GCS
Major urologic or gynecologic surgery	LMWH, LDUH, Fx, or SCD
Elective hip or knee arthroplasty	LMWH, Fx, or VKA
Hip fracture surgery	Fx, VKA, or LDUH for 10–35 days
Spine surgery without other risk factors	Early ambulation alone
Major trauma and spinal cord injury	LMWH, LDUH, Fx, or SCD
Major vascular surgery without other risk factors	Early ambulation alone
Cancer patient undergoing surgical procedure	Same as above: "high risk"

ACCP = American College of Chest Physicians; Fx = fondaparinux; GCS = graduated compression stocking; LDUH = low-dose unfractionated heparin; LMWH = low-molecular-weight heparin; SCD = sequential compression device; VKA = vitamin K antagonist to international normalized ratio 2.0 to 3.0; VTE = venous thromboembolism.

The management of PE is then determined by the clinical severity, highlighting the importance of a good medical history and physical examination.[77] Massive, unstable PE consists of shock and/or hypotension (systolic blood pressure < 90 mm Hg or drop of 40 mm Hg for > 15 minutes without other cause), usually associated with severe shortness of breath or respiratory insufficiency. Nonmassive PE should be evaluated for echocardiographic signs of right ventricular hypokinesis ("submassive" PE), which may still require thromboreduction of some sort, whereas lack of right heart strain allows for systemic anticoagulation alone. In addition to emergent echocardiography, serum brain naturetic peptide levels and serum troponins may aid in stratifying the severity of PE.

In the case of clinically unstable PE or submassive PE with significant right heart strain, thrombolytics are the treatment of choice (barring contraindication to them). They can be administered systemically if the patient is too unstable for transfer or if the technical requirements are not available for catheter-directed administration. Systemically, tissue plasminogen activator 10 mg bolus followed by a continued infusion of the remaining 90 mg over 2 hours is administered. This may acutely avoid cardiogenic shock and death or, later, the development of chronic thromboembolic pulmonary hypertension.[89]

An evolving treatment option for hemodynamically significant PE is endovascular catheter-directed infusion of lytics into the affected pulmonary vessel or mechanical thrombus reduction. A combination of transjugular, catheter-directed pulmonary embolectomy and thrombofragmentation with fibrinolytics is performed. This technique has been successful in three quarters of cases, with a mortality of 25%.[90] The technology involved in these techniques is still being developed. As a result of the scarcity of both patients with this form of PE and physicians experienced in catheter-directed treatments for PE, the ideal technique is still unclear.[91] In patients with cardiopulmonary instability who either cannot wait for pharmacologic thrombolysis to work or have a contraindication to thrombolytics, open thrombectomy is the only other option. The mortality is high, but in centers with experience, the outcomes are improved over no treatment.

After parenteral anticoagulation has been established, anticoagulation is continued with a vitamin K antagonist (VKA) for 3 to 6 months if the PE was attributable to an isolated or acquired etiology or continued for life if the PE was attributable to a permanent or recurrent etiology.[56]

PHLEGMASIA CERULEA DOLENS AND PHLEGMASIA ALBA DOLENS

As described above, phlegmasia cerulea dolens and phlegmasia alba dolens of the limbs have amputation rates of 20 to 50% (prior to the advent of fibrinolytic therapies) and PE rates of 12 to 40%. Phlegmasia syndromes have a high mortality rate that in addition to the acute, extensive DVT is also likely attributable to the comorbidities that tend to accompany them, such as advanced malignancy and trauma.[92] Phlegmasia syndromes that are associated with acute iliofemoral vein thrombosis have been successfully treated by catheter-directed fibrinolysis. There is no specific endovascular technique shown to be superior to others, but in small series, endovascular techniques show great promise for limb salvage and is the preferred management strategy if the patient still has good motor function and no contraindication to lytics.[93,94] If the patient is not a candidate for fibrinolysis, then open surgical venous thrombectomy and creation of an arteriovenous fistula are necessary to obtain rapid venous decompression and decreased risk of PTS.[95,96]

If the phlegmasia syndrome appears secondary to extensive, microvascular venous thrombosis (and not iliofemoral vein thrombosis), then it is unlikely to benefit from thrombolytic procedures; limb salvage may thus be possible only with fasciotomies. Another scenario potentially requiring fasciotomies for limb salvage occurs if there is evidence of advanced compartment syndrome (motor impairment), although the morbidity of this in the setting of an acutely swollen leg is quite high.

Indications for Urgent Intervention

PRIMARY AXILLARY-SUBCLAVIAN VEIN DVT (EFFORT THROMBOSIS OR PAGET-SCHROETTER SYNDROME)

Primary thrombosis of the axillary-subclavian veins is usually found in young athletes who perform sports with repetitive motion (e.g., baseball, volleyball, swimming) and is known as effort thrombosis or Paget-Schroetter syndrome. It is attributable to hypertrophy and/or a lateral insertion of the subclavius muscle, which compresses the subclavian vein and promotes thrombosis. This syndrome was historically treated with anticoagulation alone with a high rate of pain and swelling, but in the last decade, the treatment has evolved, and patients do better with multimodality treatment.[97]

Current treatment includes early anticoagulation and endovascular thrombolysis and recanalization of the axillary-subclavian vein with balloon venoplasty of the narrowed segment. To return patency to the subclavian vein, thrombolysis may require a several-day infusion of plasminogen activators and/or the use of endovascular devices to fragment clots and aid thrombolysis. If the subclavian vein can be recannulated, then this treatment is followed by removal of the ipsilateral first rib to decompress the thoracic outlet to avoid rethrombosis. The timing for surgical removal of the rib varies by practitioners; some perform it during the same hospitalization, whereas others remove it a few weeks later. Attempts with angioplasty or stenting without prior surgical decompression will invariably fail. Neither can overcome the extrinsic pressure created by the musculoskeletal compression of the vein, and the constant motion of the subclavian vessels at this site will lead to stent fracture.[98,99] If the vein cannot be opened, then the patient can only be anticoagulated and must rely on venous collaterals.

ILIOFEMORAL DVT AND MAY-THURNER SYNDROME

Iliac vein compression syndrome and secondary thrombosis (May-Thurner syndrome) occur when there is an obstruction or thrombosis of the lower left extremity venous outflow as a result of compression by the overlying right iliac artery. They most commonly present spontaneously in the left iliac vein and in young females who may or may not have additional risk factors for DVT, such as factor V Leiden or the use of oral contraceptives.[100,101] They rarely affect the right iliac vein and vena cava but can occur in cases with a high iliac artery bifurcation or left-sided IVC.[102] They can be successfully treated with endovascular venoplasty and stenting [*see Figure 3*] because unlike Paget-Schroetter syndrome, the extrinsic compression to the vein is not attributable to a firm, muscular structure.

Historically, iliofemoral DVT was treated exclusively with anticoagulation or open thrombectomy with subsequent anticoagulation.[96] However, many small series using catheter-directed thrombolysis and mechanical thrombolysis to treat iliofemoral DVT are rapidly demonstrating less PTS than with anticoagulation alone.[103,104] There is a growing consensus that in addition to anticoagulation, primary iliofemoral thrombosis and May-Thurner syndrome should be treated with catheter-directed thrombolysis and placement of a closed-cell stent in the compressed vein (or residual thrombus) to diminish PTS and maintain patency.[56,105] The placement of stents and evaluation of residual stenosis is often guided by the use of intravascular ultrasound probes in addition to venograms to ensure that the confluence of the vena cava is not compromised.[106] The randomized, multicenter Acute Venous Thrombosis: Thrombus Removal With Adjunctive Catheter-Directed Thrombolysis (ATTRACT) trial (ClinicalTrials.gov identifier: NCT00790335)[107] and the European Catheter-directed Venous Thrombolysis in acute iliofemoral vein thrombosis (CaVenT) trial (ClinicalTrials.gov identifier: NCT00251771)[108] are both enrolling patients to evaluate the outcomes of anticoagulation alone versus the use of pharmacomechanical means for thrombus removal in the iliofemoral segment.

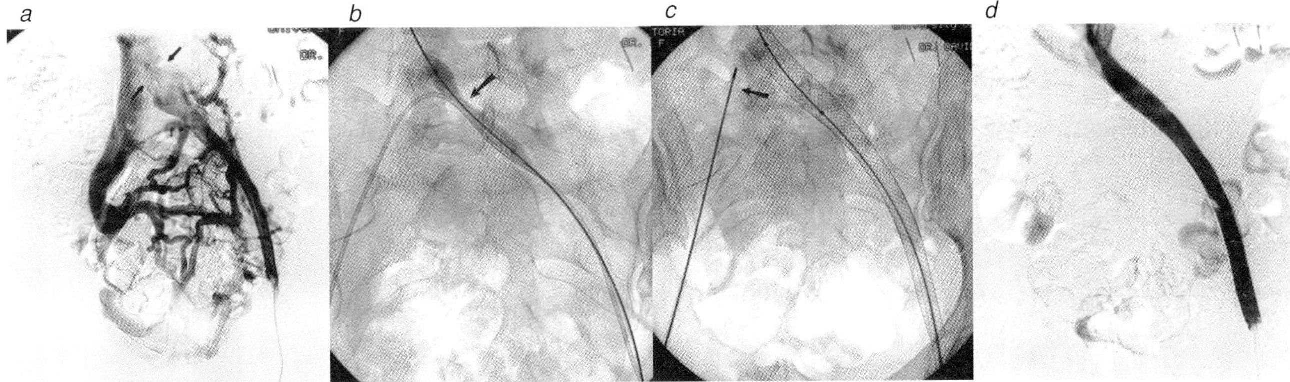

Figure 3 **This panel depicts a lower extremity venogram of a patient with May-Thurner syndrome and its subsequent endovascular treatment. (*a*) Descending venogram demonstrating minimal reflux into the left iliac system and extensive, secondary pelvic collaterals. *Arrows* indicate the area of stenosis of the left common iliac vein. (*b*) Balloon venoplasty of the left common iliac vein. The *arrow* identifies the area of compression on the balloon within the vein. (*c*) Placement of a stent from the common iliac vein to the external iliac vein. The *arrow* demonstrates an intravascular ultrasound probe in the right iliac vein. (*d*) Retrograde venogram after venoplasty and stenting of the left iliac vein demonstrating a patent iliac venous system and resolution of the left-sided pelvic collaterals. Reproduced with permission from Hurst DR et al.[106]**

In addition to the use of plasminogen activator infusions into the thrombus, there are many different types of endovascular devices designed to accelerate the resolution of vessel thrombosis. They range from physically breaking up the clot with a spinning cage to catheters that spray fluid (saline, heparin, or tissue plasminogen activator) from multiple holes at a high pressure to fragment and aspirate the thrombus. None have been compared in a head-to-head randomized study and collectively have variable published effects on the reduction of thrombolysis infusion and final vessel patency. However, small studies seem to show that pharmacomechanical lysis may minimize the amount of thrombolytic administered and the total treatment time required to complete thrombolysis.[109–111]

If the thrombus extends below the inguinal ligament, then open thrombectomy and an arteriovenous fistula may be required to improve the venous inflow and potentially decrease recurrent thrombosis, as well as the sequelae of PTS.[112] All cases are subsequently managed by anticoagulation with a VKA.[56]

Management of Nonemergent VTE

UNCOMPLICATED LOWER AND UPPER EXTREMITY VTE AND FOLLOW-UP

Avoiding the progression and recurrence of DVT is paramount to decrease both the incidence of PE and the occurrence of PTS. The risk of the latter is dramatically increased in the setting of recurrent DVT (hazard ratio 6.4).[16] To avoid this progression, all treatment guidelines recommend that patients with uncomplicated DVT be initially anticoagulated using a parenteral drug (UFH, LMWH, fondaparinux, or hirudin derivative) followed by an oral VKA lasting at least 3 months.[56,60] The VKA is titrated to achieve a target international normalized ratio (INR) between 2.0 and 3.0, and, subsequently, the parenteral drug is ceased.

Almost 90% of patients anticoagulated for only 3 months for VTE will not have a recurrence within 5 years, but because of the morbidity associated with recurrences, much effort has been made to identify patients at risk for recurrences. It has been found that those with an elevated D-dimer or continued scar tissue (from unresolved thrombosis) visualized on CDU seen at the 3-month evaluation should continue their anticoagulation to lower their risk of recurrence.[113,114] For example, if CDU reveals significant residual scar tissue, there is a hazard ratio of 2.4 for recurrent DVT; therefore, these patients may benefit from continued anticoagulation until the risks associated with prolonged anticoagulation are deemed by the clinician to be greater than the risks of recurrent DVT.[113,115]

In patients with DVT and cancer, continued treatment with LMWH is recommended as long as the cancer is active or for at least 3 months of therapy (whichever is longer). This is because the risk of DVT recurrence in these patients is up to 14%, and there is a higher risk of prolonged thrombus resolution (only 23% at 1 year) even with long-term anticoagulation.[16,30,116]

Compression stockings should be worn immediately on starting therapy to decrease the risk of PTS and continued as long as the patient has swelling, usually for at least 2 years.[56] This measure is often forgotten and can significantly reduce the long-term risk of PTS.

Patients with certain inherited or antibody-mediated hypercoagulable states are at high risk for recurrence, and risk assessment needs to be obtained to determine if they require lifelong anticoagulation.[117] There is no indication for anticoagulation with a VKA to an INR over 3, regardless of the risk factor, even in cases of antiphospholipid syndrome that have the highest risk of arterial and venous thrombotic syndromes, as found by both randomized controlled trials and the ACCP guideline statement.[56,118]

General consensus for the management of UEDVT associated with catheter placement is to use anticoagulation, but some controversy exists regarding whether to remove the offending catheter. The 8th ACCP guidelines state that if the catheter is functional, then there is no need to remove it, and anticoagulation therapy is initiated alone as for LEDVT.[56]

A recent study found that when specifically looking at complete thrombus resolution in UEDVT, only removing the catheter had a significant impact on complete thrombus resolution (52% versus 25%, odds ratio 3.25), whereas anticoagulation alone did not have an impact on resolution (36% with anticoagulation versus 56% without any anticoagulation; p = .10).[119] Of note, patients who had a catheter replaced had an increased risk of a new clot, thus highlighting the thrombophilic state of patients with catheter-related DVT.

SUPERFICIAL VEIN THROMBOSIS AND SUPPURATIVE THROMBOPHLEBITIS

Generally, uncomplicated superficial vein thrombosis (particularly when associated with intravenous catheters) can be treated with local warmth and oral or topical antiinflammatory agents to control symptoms.[120] However, there has been growing concern over the rate of underappreciated extension into the deep venous system resulting in PE. The incidence of PE and DVT has been reported as high as 25% with lower extremity superficial vein thrombosis.[121] Thus, duplex ultrasonography is now recommended for cases of superficial vein thrombosis, and if propagation or encroachment into the deep system is seen, then systemic anticoagulation for 3 months is recommended.[56] Surgical excision of superficial vein thrombosis may be indicated if the patient has prolonged or incapacitating pain, if there is no resolution of the acute clot after 3 months of treatment, or as an alternative to anticoagulation if propagation into the deep system is identified.[78,120]

With the advent of great saphenous vein ablations using catheter-delivered energy (laser or radiofrequency thermal energy) for chronic venous insufficiency, an increased number of thrombi have been identified at the saphenofemoral junction. Although there is no consensus for the management of this problem, if clot propagation into the femoral vein is identified during the initial procedure (thrombus "tail"), then we immediately start LMWH and treat for 1 week, although the evidence for the need for this treatment is evolving. Most clots resolve in this short interval of time. However, if a clot continues to be seen near or extending into the deep venous system, then standard DVT treatment guidelines may be followed or surgical thrombus removal and ligation of the saphenous vein can be performed as an alternative (particularly if there is a contraindication to anticoagulation).

Local intravenous catheter-site infections may occur in up to 8% of venous accesses and 18% of arterial catheterizations. Although most do not result in systemic infections, bacteremia can be detected in about one of every 400 intravenous catheterizations and 4% of arterial ones.[122] Localized catheter-site infections may progress to superficial suppurative thrombophlebitis. In these cases, excision or open phlebectomy is indicated to drain all pus, remove the infected hematoma, and control the spread of the thrombosis and infection, removing the entire involved vein. Prevention is best obtained by changing all intravenous sites every 48 to 72 hours.

VENA CAVA FILTERS

IVC filters lower the risk of fatal PE in patients with a DVT who are unable to be anticoagulated or in those who have a recurrence during therapeutic anticoagulation. However, IVC filters are placed in many patients because of the relative ease of the procedure, but often with unfounded indications. A prospective study of over 5,400 patients with DVT in an American registry found that 14% (781) of them had an IVC filter implanted. The indication in one third of these was only "prophylaxis" and not treatment failure.[123] There is evidence that DVT prophylaxis is used in less than half of surgical patients, with a concomitant increase in the placement of IVC filters that may not be indicated.[124]

IVC filters should be placed only in cases where there is a contraindication to anticoagulation or when there is VTE recurrence in the setting of therapeutic anticoagulation. In most instances, IVC filters should not be used in patients without a DVT or PE as a prophylactic measure alone, regardless of the DVT risk factors, including trauma, surgery, and even cancer.[125] Although an example of an indication for a temporary IVC filter may be a trauma patient at high risk for bleeding (contraindication for anticoagulation) with a concomitant DVT or PE, filters are commonly placed as a prophylactic measure (patients without a DVT or PE) in patients undergoing bariatric surgery, after trauma, or with spinal cord injuries even though studies and consensus statements recommend against it.[20,56,60,126]

Patients undergoing bariatric surgery have been undergoing a dramatic increase in the placement of prophylactic IVC filters (from 7 to 55% of patients over the last 10 years).[127] Using only pneumatic compression devices and early ambulation, the risk of DVT in laparoscopic Roux-en-Y gastric bypass is only 0.5%.[128] Studies using IVC filters for primary prophylaxis in bariatric surgery have demonstrated a 2% incidence of PE, in the setting of a 2.5% incidence of IVC filter complications, which include hemopericardium and pneumothorax.[129] The lack of methodologically sound studies and an overall low incidence of VTE (in patients who can usually ambulate and receive all other forms of mechanical and pharmacologic prophylaxis) have led to an overall consensus by the ACCP and others that filters not be used for primary VTE prophylaxis in this or any other surgical procedure.[130]

Deployment of a vena cava filter may be done via the common femoral or the internal jugular veins. Although femoral access is generally used, preplacement imaging of the venous system is imperative to determine if the access route is without thrombus. If clot is identified, then the filter should not be placed through this route to minimize embolization. If there is thrombus in the IVC, then the filter must be placed above it via the internal jugular access. Venography is also done to ensure that the patient has normal venous anatomy (he or she may require two filters if a duplicated vena cava is found), to identify the location of both renal veins to choose the site for deployment, and to measure the diameter of the IVC (it must be less than 30 cm for most filters to minimize their migration). Filters are generally positioned in the IVC with their fixation prongs caudal to the renal veins.

There are two broad types of vena cava filters: permanent and removable. The longest follow-up for a single IVC filter is the permanent, over-the-wire Greenfield filter, which, after more than 20 years, has a very low incidence of IVC thrombosis (< 4%) and migration (only non–clinically significant in 8%)[131] and has not increased the incidence of DVT.[132] The randomized PREPIC trial compared the long-term outcomes of patients with DVT treated with four different permanent filters and anticoagulation with the outcomes of patients treated with anticoagulation alone for 3 months. The authors found that although at 8 years there was a significantly lower incidence of PE (6.2% versus 15.1%, p = .008) in those with IVC filters, no difference in mortality or PTS was found. However, an increased risk of DVT (35.7% versus 27.5%, p = .04) was observed in the group receiving a permanent filter. Of note, almost half of the patients with filters registered to have had a DVT also had filter thrombosis.[133,134] Permanent filters are covered with endothelium and affix into the IVC wall after 2 to 3 weeks, so the risk of attempting to completely remove them in the operating room may be very high.[135] In general, we have found that if IVC filter prongs protruding from the vein wall cause symptoms or bleeding, then the metal that is visible outside the IVC should only be trimmed flush with the vein (in addition to any other repair needed), and the remaining filter should be left in place.

To treat patients with filters only during their acute thrombophilia, optional retrievable filters have become more popular than permanent ones. The theoretical advantage of using retrievable filters for patients with temporary prothrombotic states is often mitigated by poor long-term follow-up, and over 75% are never removed, even in the military experience,[136,137] or may require extreme surgical techniques to remove them when complications arise.[138] These include migration, IVC thrombosis (2 to 14%, especially in biconcave retrievable or bird nest filters),[139] renal vein thrombosis, and erosion into bowel[140] or aorta.[141]

There is no large randomized trial assessing the use of superior vena cava (SVC) filters for UEDVT. Almost two thirds of patients with SVC filters will die of their underlying diseases, and not of PE, within 2 months of placement.[142] SVC perforations from filters with migration may result in a high mortality secondary to tamponade.[143] Once they are in place, it is imperative to adequately warn all practitioners that the SVC filter is there to avoid blind central line placement with standard J wires that may dislodge the filter or entangle themselves in it.[144] Therefore, the benefit of SVC filters is still unclear for patients with UEDVT, and they should be judiciously used for patients whose mortality is high from other causes.

Financial Disclosures: None Reported

References

1. Heit JA, Cohen AT, Anderson, FA Jr. Estimated annual number of incident and recurrent, non-fatal and fatal venous thromboembolism (VTE) events in the US. [abstract] Blood 2005;106:910.
2. Beckman MG, Critchley SE, Hooper WC, et al. CDC Division of Blood Disorders: public health research activities in venous thromboembolism. Arterioscler Thromb Vasc Biol 2008;28:394–5.
3. Cohen AT, Agnelli G, Anderson FA, et al. Venous thromboembolism (VTE) in Europe. The number of VTE events and associated morbidity and mortality. Thromb Haemost 2007;98:756–64.
4. Centers for Disease Control and Prevention. Deep venous thrombosis health care professionals: data & statistics. Available at: http://www.cdc.gov/ncbddd/dvt/hcp_data.htm (accessed Oct 29, 2010).
5. Heit JA. The epidemiology of venous thromboembolism in the community. Arterioscler Thromb Vasc Biol 2008;28:370–2.
6. Nordstrom M, Lindblad B, Bergqvist D, Kjellstrom T. A prospective study of the incidence of deep-vein thrombosis within a defined urban population. J Intern Med 1992;232:155–60.
7. Mandelli V, Schmid C, Zogno C, Morpurgo M. "False negatives" and "false positives" in acute pulmonary embolism: a clinical-postmortem comparison. Cardiologia 1997; 42:205–10.
8. Dalen JE, Alpert JS. Natural history of pulmonary embolism. Prog Cardiovasc Dis 1975;17:259–70.
9. Heit JA, Mohr DN, Silverstein MD, et al. Predictors of recurrence after deep vein thrombosis and pulmonary embolism: a population-based cohort study. Arch Intern Med 2000;160:761–8.
10. Khorana AA, Streiff MB, Farge D, et al. Venous thromboembolism prophylaxis and treatment in cancer: a consensus statement of major guidelines panels and call to action. J Clin Oncol 2009;27:4919–26.
11. Khorana AA, Francis CW, Culakova E, et al. Thromboembolism is a leading cause of death in cancer patients receiving outpatient chemotherapy. J Thromb Haemost 2007;5: 632–4.
12. Chew HK, Wun T, Harvey D, et al. Incidence of venous thromboembolism and its effect on survival among patients with common cancers. Arch Intern Med 2006; 166:458–64.
13. Tsai S, Dubovoy A, Wainess R, et al. Severe chronic venous insufficiency: magnitude of the problem and consequences. Ann Vasc Surg 2005;19:705–11.
14. Prandoni P, Lensing AW, Cogo A, et al. The long-term clinical course of acute deep venous thrombosis. Ann Intern Med 1996; 125:1–7.
15. Kahn SR, Shrier I, Julian JA, et al. Determinants and time course of the post-thrombotic syndrome after acute deep venous thrombosis. Ann Intern Med 2008; 149:698–707.
16. Prandoni P, Lensing AW, Prins MR. Long-term outcomes after deep venous thrombosis of the lower extremities. Vasc Med 1998;3: 57–60.
17. Douma RA, Gibson NS, Gerdes VE, et al. Validity and clinical utility of the simplified Wells rule for assessing clinical probability for the exclusion of pulmonary embolism. Thromb Haemost 2009;101:197–200.
18. Dalen JE. Pulmonary embolism: what have we learned since Virchow? Natural history, pathophysiology, and diagnosis. Chest 2002; 122:1440–56.
19. World Health Organization. Inherited thrombophilia. Presented at the Joint WHO/ International Society of Thrombosis and Haemostasis (ISTH) Meeting; 1995 Nov 6–8; Geneva.
20. Geerts WH, Bergqvist D, Pineo GF, et al. Prevention of venous thromboembolism: American College of Chest Physicians evidence-based clinical practice guidelines (8th Edition). Chest 2008;133(6 Suppl): 381S–453S.
21. Bahl V, Hu HM, Henke PK, et al. A validation study of a retrospective venous thromboembolism risk scoring method. Ann Surg 2010;251:344–50.
22. Favaloro EJ, McDonald D, Lippi G. Laboratory investigation of thrombophilia: the good, the bad, and the ugly. Semin Thromb Hemost 2009;35:695–710.
23. Chan MY, Andreotti F, Becker RC. Hypercoagulable states in cardiovascular disease. Circulation 2008;118:2286–97.
24. McDonald AP, Meier TR, Hawley AE, et al. Aging is associated with impaired thrombus resolution in a mouse model of stasis induced thrombosis. Thromb Res 2010;125(1):72–8. Epub 2009 Jul 18.
25. Trousseau A. Phlegmasia alba dolens. Vol 3. 2nd ed. Paris: Clinique Médicale de l'Hotel Dieu de Paris; 1865.
26. Billroth T. Lectures on surgical pathology and therapeutics: a handbook for students and practitioners. London: New Sydenham Society; 1878.
27. Falanga A, Gordon SG. Isolation and characterization of cancer procoagulant: a cysteine proteinase from malignant tissue. Biochemistry 1985;24:5558–67.
28. Donati MB. Thrombosis and cancer: Trousseau syndrome revisited. Best Pract Res Clin Haematol 2009;22:3–8.
29. Soubiran A. Est-il roi dans quelque ile? Ou le dernier Noël de Trousseau. Presse Med 1967;75:2807–10.
30. Levitan N, Dowlati A, Remick SC, et al. Rates of initial and recurrent thromboembolic disease among patients with malignancy versus those without malignancy. Risk analysis using Medicare claims data. Medicine (Baltimore) 1999;78:285–91.
31. Osborne NH, Wakefield TW, Henke PK. Venous thromboembolism in cancer patients undergoing major surgery. Ann Surg Oncol 2008;15:3567–78.
32. Ay C, Simanek R, Vormittag R, et al. High plasma levels of soluble P-selectin are predictive of venous thromboembolism in cancer patients: results from the Vienna Cancer and Thrombosis Study (CATS). Blood 2008;112: 2703–8.
33. Wahrenbrock M, Borsig L, Le D, et al. Selectin-mucin interactions as a probable molecular explanation for the association of Trousseau syndrome with mucinous adenocarcinomas. J Clin Invest 2003;112: 853–62.
34. Bauer KA, Rosendaal FR, Heit JA. Hypercoagulability: too many tests, too much conflicting data. Hematology Am Soc Hematol Educ Program 2002:353–68.

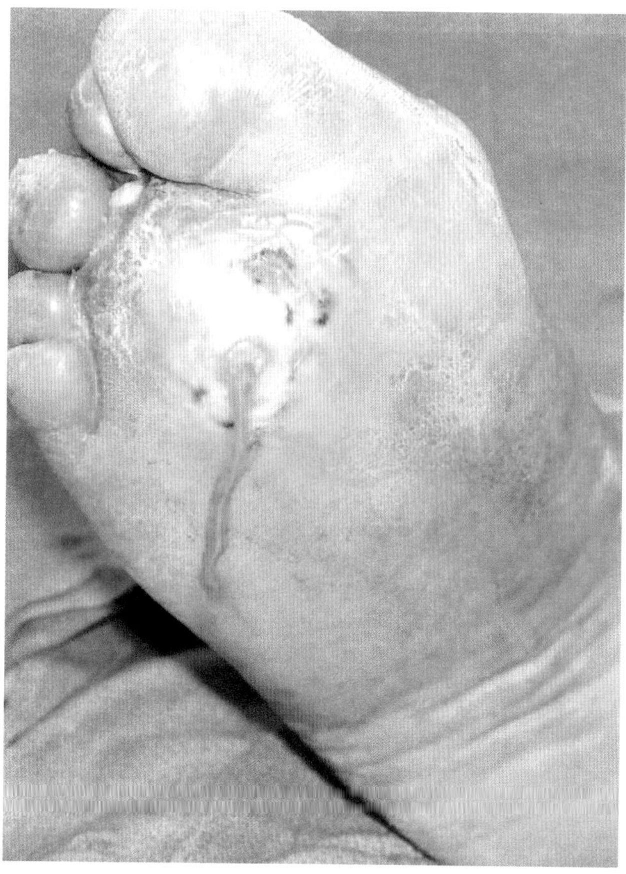

Figure 2 **Purulent drainage is seen from a submetatarsal ulcer on the plantar surface of the foot of a diabetic patient.**

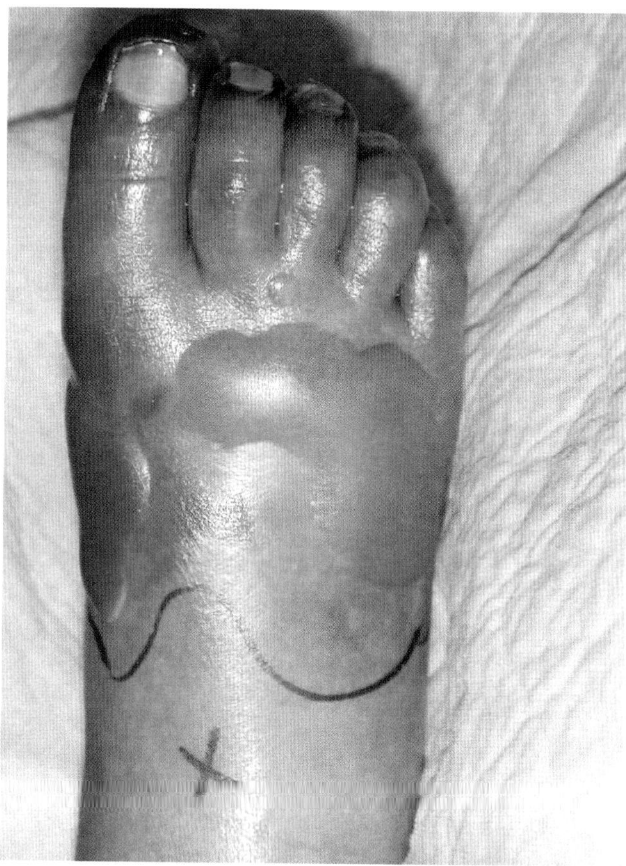

Figure 3 **Wet gangrene with edema and undrained severe infection in the foot of a diabetic patient presenting with hyperglycemia and ketoacidosis.**

slightly aberrant course. A common mistake is to place a single finger at one location on the dorsum of the foot. The posterior tibial artery is typically located in the hollow curve just behind the medial malleolus, approximately halfway between the malleolus and the Achilles tendon. The examiner's hand should be contralateral to the examined foot (i.e., the right hand should be used to palpate the left foot, and vice versa) so that the curvature of the hand naturally follows the contours of the ankle [*see Figure 7*].

Assessment of Clinical Findings

Once the clinical evaluation is complete, the next step is to assess the findings from the history and the physical examination so as to determine the course and urgency of the subsequent workup and treatment. This assessment is made at the bedside, focusing on three main concerns: (1) the presence and severity of infection, (2) the salvageability of the limb, and (3) the presence of ischemia.

PRESENCE OF INFECTION

Evaluation for and treatment of infection are the first priority in the management of any diabetic foot problem.[7,8] Although radiographic tests may confirm initial clinical suspicions, the determination of the severity of infection is almost always made on the basis of clinical findings.

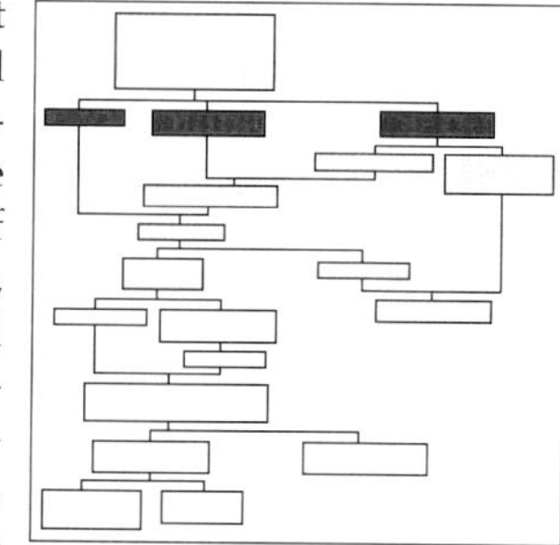

Infection in the diabetic foot may range from a minimal superficial infection to fulminant sepsis with extensive necrosis and destruction of foot tissue. Accordingly, the treatment plan should address the choice of antibiotic (which requires knowledge of the microbiology), the need for drainage, the option of local or even guillotine amputation, and the patient's overall medical condition.

The microbiology of the diabetic foot varies according to the depth and severity of the infection and the nature of the patient's environment (e.g., hospitalized or outpatient). Certain general assumptions can be made about likely causative organisms. Mild localized and superficial ulceration, particularly in outpatients, are usually caused by aerobic gram-positive cocci (e.g., *Staphylococcus aureus* and streptococci). In contrast, deeper ulcers and generalized limb-threatening infections are usually polymicrobial. In addition to gram-positive cocci, potential causative organisms include gram-negative bacilli (e.g., *Escherichia coli*, *Klebsiella*, *Enterobacter aerogenes*, *Proteus mirabilis*, and *Pseudomonas aeruginosa*) and anaerobes (e.g., *Bacteroides fragilis* and

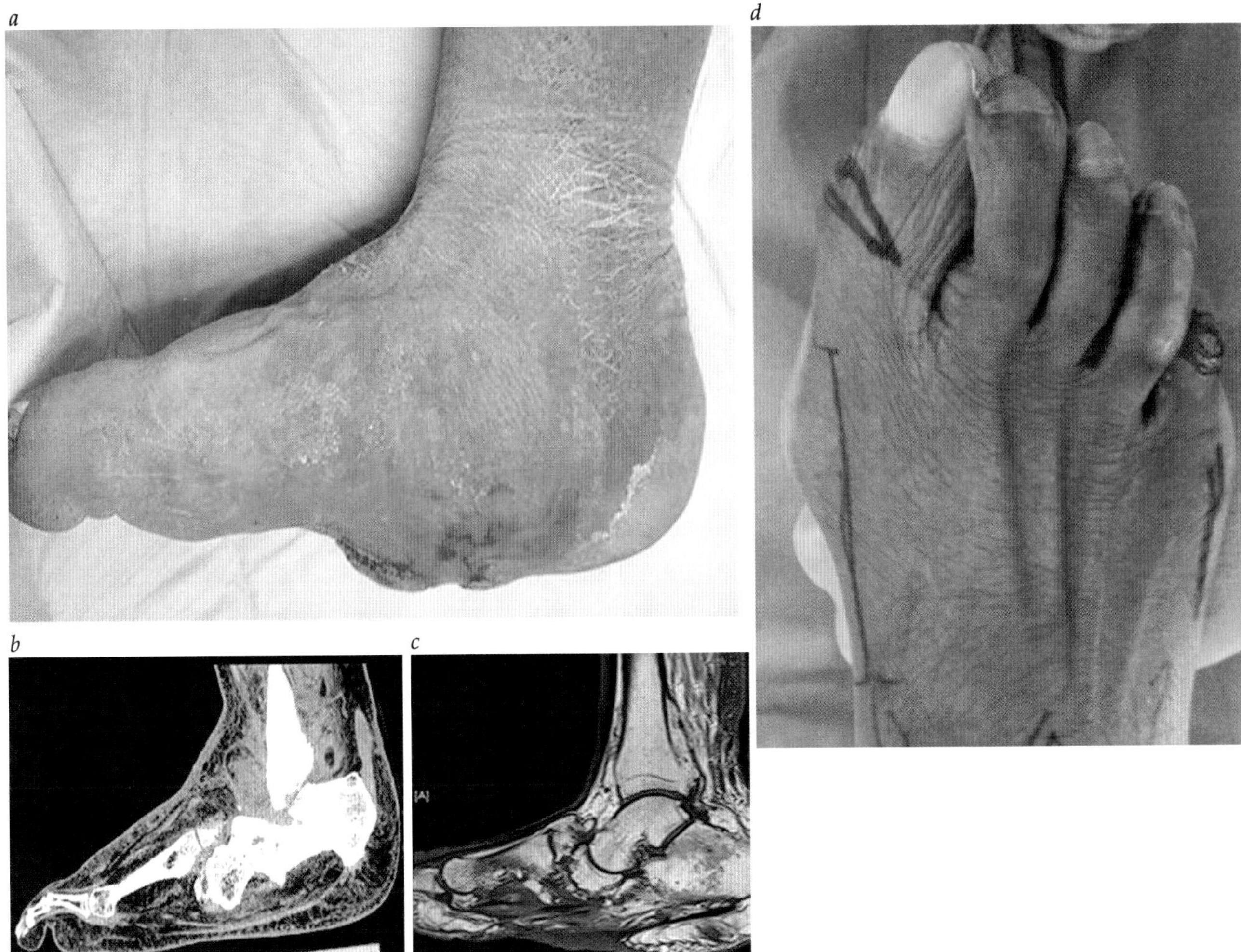

Figure 4 Charcot deformity (*a*) and associated imaging findings on computed tomography (*b*) and magnetic resonance imaging (*c*) illustrating severe bone and joint degeneration and claw foot (*d*) in the feet of diabetic patients. The joint collapse can leave an area of prominent bone more susceptible to ulceration. With advanced sensorimotor dysfunction from diabetes, the imbalance between extrinsic and intrinsic foot muscles results in this permanent claw deformity, where the weakened intrinsic foot muscles can no longer counter the excessive pull of the flexors. This leads to a retrograde buckling and subsequent clawing of the digits with the metatarsophalangeal joints in hyperextension and the interphalangeal joints in excess flexion.

peptostreptococci). Enterococci may also be isolated from the wound, notably in hospitalized patients; in the absence of other cultured virulent organisms, they should probably be considered pathogenic.

Currently, it is clear that resistant organisms, particularly methicillin-resistant *Staphylococcus aureus* (MRSA), are playing a growing role in the development of skin and soft tissue infections. Traditionally arising in patients who had previously been hospitalized and those who had previously received antibiotic therapy, MRSA-associated infections are now frequently encountered in outpatient settings. Indeed, in many US cities, these so-called community-acquired MRSA infections are the most common skin and soft tissue infections seen in patients presenting to the emergency department.[9] Accordingly, in both outpatient and inpatient settings, it is advisable to assume that MRSA is present in a patient with a diabetic foot infection until the culture data suggest otherwise. Awareness of the increasing prevalence of resistant organisms is critical for current management of diabetic foot infections, especially with respect to the initiation of antibiotic coverage.

Initially, the choice of antibiotics is made empirically on the basis of these general assumptions. When the results of the initial cultures become available, antibiotic coverage may be broadened or narrowed as appropriate. In a compliant patient with a small ulcer and no evidence of deep space involvement or systemic infection, treatment may be delivered on an outpatient basis. A dual-antibiotic regimen (pending culture results) is instituted, typically consisting of cephalosporin or a β-lactam antibiotic (for activity against staphylococci and streptococci) and trimethoprim-sulfamethoxazole or a tetracycline (for activity against MRSA). A dual regimen consisting of fluoroquinolone and linezolid is an acceptable alternative that also provides adequate coverage. In addition, the patient is instructed to offload weight from the involved extremity and is taught found to be the superior imaging method to plain radiograph and radionuclide scanning (bone and white blood cell tagging) for diagnosing osteomyelitis in patients with diabetic ulcers.[15] The early diagnosis of osteomyelitis is critical as prompt antibiotic treatment decreases the rate of amputation.[13,16]

In the presence of an abscess or deep space infection, immediate incision and drainage of all infected tissue planes are mandatory. Incisions should be chosen with an eye to the normal anatomy of the foot (including the various compartments) and the need for subsequent secondary (foot salvage) procedures [*see Figure 9*]. Drainage should be complete, with incisions placed to allow for dependent drainage, and all necrotic tissue must be débrided. Repeat cultures (including both aerobes and anaerobes) should be obtained from the deep tissues. Drainage incisions on the dorsum of the foot should be avoided. Abscesses in the medial, central, or lateral compartment should be drained via longitudinal incisions made in the direction of the neurovascular bundle and extending the entire length of the abscess. The medial and central compartments are drained through a medial incision, and the lateral compartment is drained through a lateral incision; both of these incisions are made just above the plantar surface of the forefoot [*see Figure 10*]. Web space infections may be drained similarly through the plantar aspect of the foot. In some instances, open amputation of the foot (e.g., an open toe or transmetatarsal amputation) may be necessary to allow complete drainage and resection of necrotic tissue. Strict adherence to textbook amputations may lead to unnecessary soft tissue removal and possibly to a higher amputation during future closure; therefore, all viable tissue should be conserved.

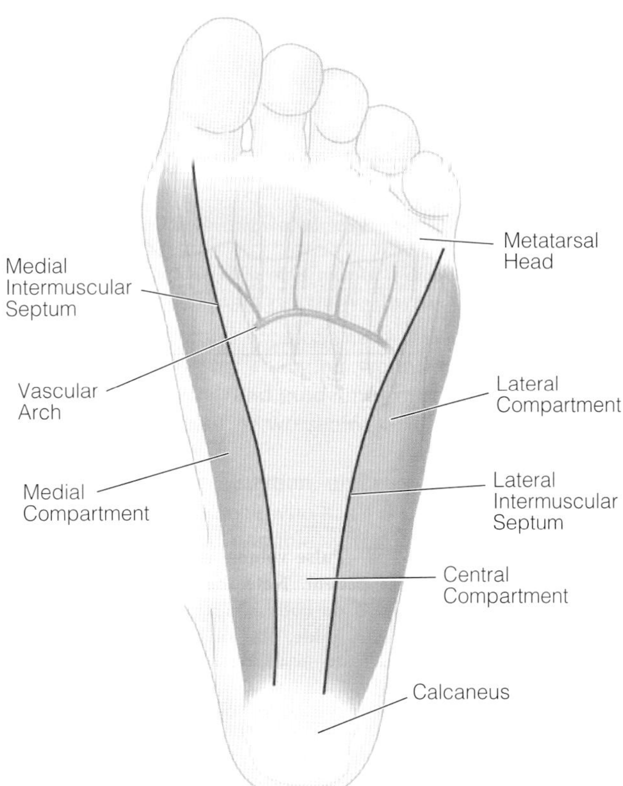

Figure 9 **The foot has three plantar compartments: medial, central, and lateral. The intrinsic muscles of the great toe are in the medial compartment, and those of the fifth toe are in the lateral compartment. The central compartment contains the intrinsic muscles of the second through fourth toes, the extensor flexor tendons of the toes, the plantar nerves, and the plantar vascular structures. The floor of each compartment is the rigid plantar fascia; the roof is composed of the metatarsal bones and interosseous fascia. The medial and central compartments are separated by the medial intermuscular septum, which extends from the medial calcaneal tuberosity to the head of the first metatarsal. The lateral and central compartments are separated by the lateral intermuscular septum, which extends from the calcaneus to the head of the fifth metatarsal.**

A patient with an ongoing undrained infection may present with an unsalvageable foot and fulminant sepsis, manifested by hemodynamic instability, bacteremia, and severe acid-base and electrolyte abnormalities. Such patients should undergo prompt open (guillotine) below-the-knee amputation. This type of amputation is usually performed at the ankle level, with the aim of removing the septic source while allowing for revision and closure at a later date. Administration of IV antibiotics, correction of dehydration and electrolyte abnormalities, and continuous cardiac monitoring are absolutely essential throughout treatment.

Once the infection has been drained and tissue débrided, continued wound inspection and management are essential. Ongoing necrosis should raise the possibility of undrained infection or untreated ischemia, in which case, further débridement and treatment may be necessary. Avoidance of weight bearing should be continued. Neither whirlpool therapy nor soaks are beneficial.

Medical Stabilization

Concomitant with the measures outlined above to control infection, medical stabilization of the diabetic patient must be carried out, and the surgeon must be directly involved in this process. Hyperglycemia is almost always seen when infection is present; it should be gradually corrected. More advanced hyperglycemia leads to ketotic or nonketotic hyperosmolar states, which carry a 10 to 25% mortality. Serum concentrations of electrolytes, magnesium, and creatinine should be obtained and osmolality determined at frequent intervals; any abnormalities should be corrected. Dehydration is common in hyperglycemic patients and should be corrected. A urinary catheter is mandatory to help guide the response to fluid therapy; in unstable patients, a central venous pressure catheter or a pulmonary arterial catheter may be needed. Continuous cardiac monitoring is essential in patients with hyperglycemic hyperosmolar syndrome or ketoacidosis.

SALVAGEABILITY OF LIMB

While the infection is being treated and controlled, the surgeon should determine whether limb salvage is feasible. This determination is based largely on the patient's functional status and the degree of foot destruction. For example, primary limb amputation may be considered in a nonambulatory, bedridden patient or in a patient with severe Charcot destruction and degeneration, for whom no further reconstructive foot surgery is possible. Poor medical condition,

a

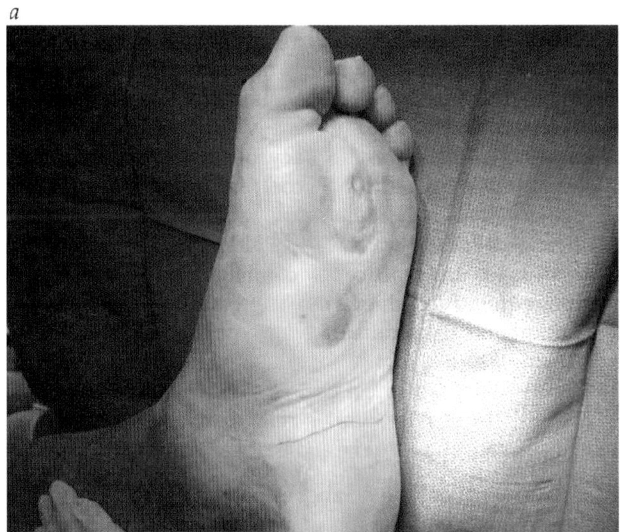

b

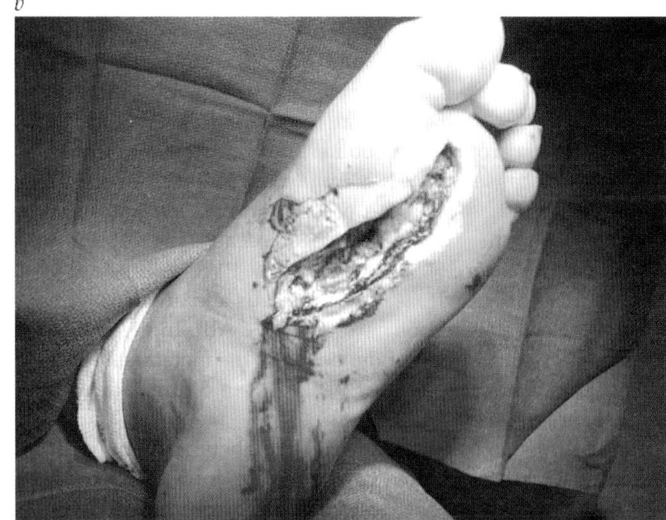

Figure 10 **An infection in the central compartment of the foot from a submetatarsal ulcer that has extended proximally to include the medial compartment (*a*). A plantar incision through the ulcer and both compartments (including the septum) allows complete dependent drainage (*b*).**

by itself, is not necessarily an indication for primary limb amputation given the high perioperative morbidity associated with amputation. Moreover, it is often possible to improve the patient's overall medical status while he or she is being treated for infection and evaluated for ischemia.

Assessment of limb salvageability should be carried out simultaneously with treatment of infection because appropriate drainage and antibiotics can dramatically change the appearance and viability of the foot. If limb salvage is not deemed possible, the patient should undergo formal below-the-knee or above-the-knee amputation. As noted above, a staged procedure beginning with a guillotine amputation is recommended in patients with severe diabetic foot infections.

PRESENCE OF ISCHEMIA

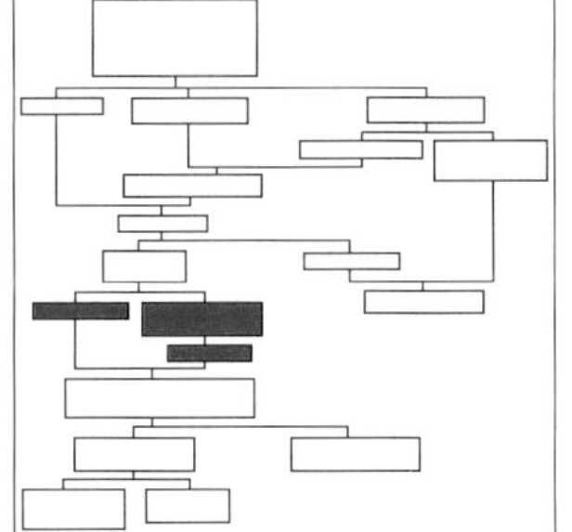

Evaluation of the diabetic foot for ischemia begins with the history and the physical examination. By the conclusion of the clinical evaluation, the surgeon can usually make an accurate assessment of the adequacy of the arterial circulation to the foot. As noted [*see* Clinical Evaluation, Physical Examination, *above*], the absence of a palpable foot pulse strongly suggests ischemia unless proved otherwise. In a patient with a severe foot infection requiring open resection/débridement or in a setting with multiple toe gangrene, just the lack of a foot pulse is enough to proceed to angiography. In more subtle cases, including those with absent foot pulses who have a superficial ulcer with evidence of healing or a previous history of a healed foot ulcer and those without any foot lesions who are scheduled to undergo elective foot surgery, various noninvasive modalities are available to the clinician. The noninvasive arterial study is a first-line test to establish the pattern and severity of arterial ischemia. This examination involves determining segmental pressure measurements, ankle-brachial indices (ABIs), arterial waveforms, and pulse volume recordings (PVRs). Segmental pressures are systolic blood pressure measurements using cuffs at standard locations from thigh to ankle (thigh high and low, below the knee, and at the ankle). In individuals with normal arterial perfusion, the thigh-high value is 30 mm higher, the ankle value is slightly higher, and toe pressures are 80% of brachial. There should not be more than a 20 mm pressure drop between segments. Equally important is a comparison of values between the two legs. An ABI greater than 0.90 indicates normal perfusion, and values less than 0.40 are associated with rest pain and gangrene. In patients with long-standing diabetes mellitus, medial calcinosis occurs and will render the vessels incompressible. Therefore, in diabetic patients, very low ABIs may be presumed to be accurate, whereas normal or high values need validation, such as the presence of a palpable pulse. However, vessels in the diabetic foot are generally spared from the atherosclerotic changes in the more proximal vessels. Vincent and colleagues showed that toe pressure is an "accurate hemodynamic indicator of total peripheral arterial obstructive disease" in diabetics.[17] Toe pressures less than 40 mm Hg predict healing difficulties.

Arterial waveforms are graphic representations of the Doppler shift as erythrocytes flow through the artery being evaluated. High-resistance vessels, such as those found in the lower extremity, should produce a triphasic signal. Forward flow in systole produces a sharp upstroke, followed by reversal of flow in early diastole as reactive vessels recoil from distention. Calcified vessels will lose this small, short notch below the baseline. Then in late diastole, forward flow recurs as vessels contract and pump blood forward, producing a small notch above baseline. These three phases produce the triphasic pattern. Worsening stenoses result in loss of flow reversal and spectral broadening, eventually resulting in a monophasic waveform indicating severe disease.

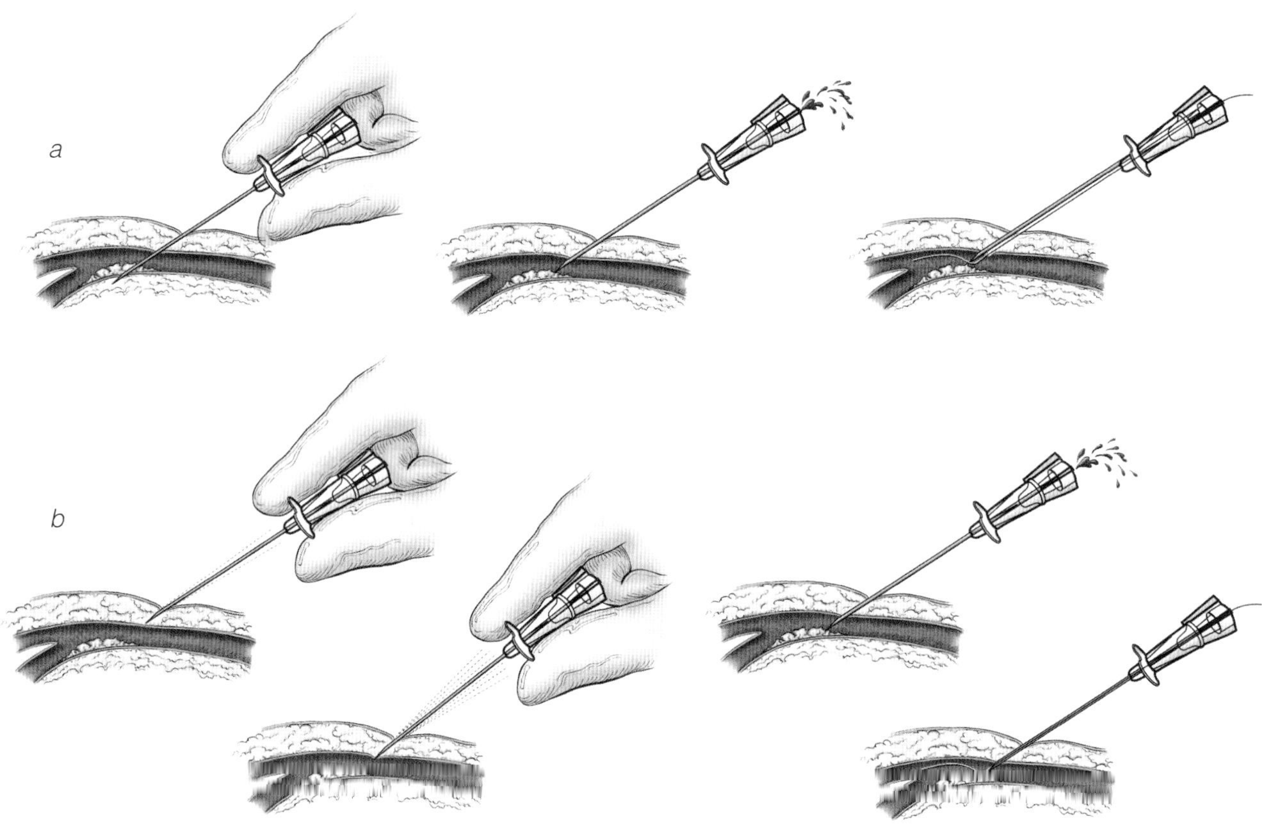

Figure 1 **Shown are the two methods of entry into an artery: (*a*) through-and-through puncture of both walls and (*b*) puncture of the anterior wall only.**

pulsatile back-bleeding. A guide wire is then passed into the needle, and the needle is removed. Immediately after needle removal and prior to catheter or sheath placement, manual compression is held over the puncture site until a catheter or sheath is placed into the access site obtaining hemostasis. This is to prevent periarterial hematomas, which may interfere with vessel closure on completion of the procedure.

Pulsations should be transmitted through the needle shaft in an anterior-to-posterior manner. If the needle is either medial or lateral to the artery, the pulsations may deflect the needle from side to side.[2] Once the needle is in the vessel, the flow pattern should be observed. A barely pulsatile flow may signal occlusive disease, a subintimal location of the needle, or a venous puncture.[2] If the guide wire cannot be passed with minimal resistance after access is obtained, the needle tip may be against the wall or against plaque, or (if the needle tip has already entered the wall) a dissection may have been started. Often the situation can be remedied by making a small change in the needle's insertion angle or by withdrawing the needle slightly.

FEMORAL ARTERY PUNCTURE

As noted, the CFA is the vessel most commonly used for arterial access. It is generally well suited to this purpose, being readily accessible, fairly large, and easily compressible. CFA puncture facilitates study and treatment of a number of key structures, including the lower extremity arteries, the abdominal aorta and its branches, the thoracic aorta, the brachiocephalic vessels, the coronary arteries, and the left ventricle. In addition, CFA puncture is associated with a lower complication rate than puncture of other arteries.[1] The CFA should, however, be avoided when the patient is known to have severe iliofemoral occlusive disease, a local infection, a thrombus-lined femoral artery aneurysm, or marked tortuosity of the iliac arteries that would preclude catheter placement or manipulation.

The CFA runs lateral to the common femoral vein (CFV) and beneath the inguinal ligament. It may be localized by palpation just proximal to its bifurcation into the superficial femoral artery (SFA) and the profunda femoris (PF). The inguinal ligament, which runs from the anterior superior iliac spine to the pubic tubercle, is a convenient landmark for localization of the CFA, but these bony landmarks provide only a rough approximation of the location of the inguinal ligament. The CFA typically lies about two fingerbreadths lateral to the pubic tubercle along the line of the inguinal ligament. The artery should be punctured over the middle of the medial third of the femoral head in the posterior-anterior projection [*see Figure 2*]. The window available for safe CFA puncture is small—only 3 to 5 cm.

Several methods can be used to localize the CFA in patients with difficult anatomy (e.g., those who have previously undergone groin surgery, those who are obese, and those who have a pulseless artery). The bony landmarks are even less

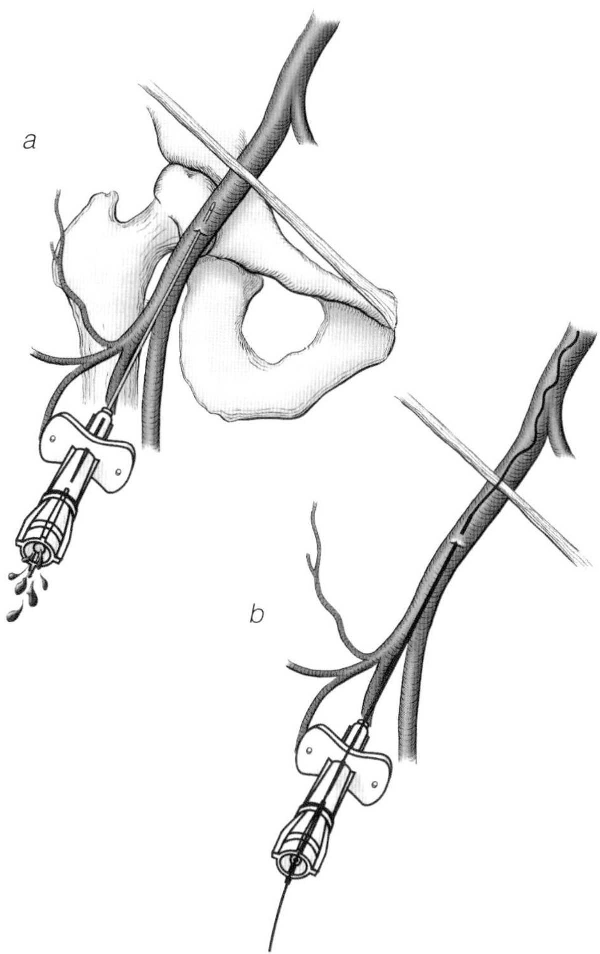

Figure 2 **Shown is a puncture of the common femoral artery. (*a*) The needle enters the common femoral artery. (*b*) The guide wire is passed through the needle.**

reliable guides to the location of the inguinal ligament in these patients. According to a 1993 anatomic study, in the majority of cases, the position of the inguinal ligament is about 1 to 2 cm below where palpation would suggest it to be, and the average position of the ligament is approximately 1.5 cm superior to the midfemoral head.[4]

Fluoroscopy may help localize the CFA over the medial third of the femoral head. The chances of hitting the artery are maximized by aiming for the middle (craniocaudal) portion of the medial third of the femoral head. To minimize parallax errors, the femoral head should be centered in the image intensifier. The anatomic relations of the arteries in this area vary little with body habitus, gender, or age. A 1999 anatomic study showed that the CFA bifurcates into the SFA and the PF approximately 2 cm below the femoral head.[5] Occasionally, calcifications in the arteries may serve as landmarks for locating the CFA.

Another localization approach involves palpation of anatomic landmarks; this approach may be especially useful when the artery is pulseless.[6] With a finger placed immediately lateral to the pubic tubercle and inferior to the inguinal ligament, palpation is carried out to locate the point allowing the greatest degree of posterior depression. Anatomically, this point of maximal depression lies between the iliopsoas muscle laterally and the pectineus muscle medially. The CFV lies in the floor of this depression, and the CFA lies 1.5 cm lateral to the depression.[6]

Ultrasonography has proved useful for finding the CFA. The projection of choice with real-time ultrasonography is the transverse plane. The nonpalpable CFA is identified lateral to the compressible CFV. Occasionally, the artery can be identified on the basis of sonographic shadowing from calcified atheromatous plaques.[7] A second ultrasonographic technique involves the use of a so-called smart needle, which has an ultrasound probe at its tip. The needle emits a signal as it approaches the artery, thereby giving notice of proximity to the vessel. Alternatively, as mentioned above, use of a micropuncture needle with an echogenic tip in conjunction with handheld, B-mode ultrasonography provides added precision.

Another method of localizing and puncturing a pulseless CFA involves performing a contralateral femoral artery puncture, obtaining a diagnostic angiogram, and roadmapping. A similar method that is useful in patients who may be moving or who cannot receive additional contrast material is to pass a guide wire over the aortic bifurcation and then antegrade through the iliac artery into the target femoral artery.[8] Under fluoroscopy, the guide wire becomes a visible target for introduction of the needle into the CFA.

Troubleshooting

The CFA is typically described as lateral to the CFV; however, one study showed that attempts to puncture the CFA frequently result in puncture of the CFV, signaled by the appearance of dark, nonpulsatile venous blood. If this occurs, one should note the position of the original puncture, move the needle 1 to 1.5 cm laterally, and reinsert the needle. It should be noted that when using a micropuncture needle as opposed to a standard entry needle (21-gauge versus 18-gauge, respectively), often, even with arterial puncture, pulsatile back-bleeding is not encountered because of the micropuncture needle's smaller-caliber lumen. At times, especially in emergency procedures, arterial blood may be dark and may resemble venous blood. If it is unclear whether the blood is coming from an artery or a vein, a small amount of a contrast agent should be gently injected into the needle by hand; the source of the blood should then be easily identifiable. When contrast is injected in the femoral sheath outside the artery, the resulting tubular "filling defect" can be used to identify the femoral artery.

If the puncture is done too high (in the external iliac artery), the inguinal ligament and the deeper location of the external iliac artery may make adequate compression of the vessel impossible. Many closure systems will not work in the external iliac artery. High puncture is associated with retroperitoneal bleeding, which should be suspected in any patient with an unexplained drop in the hematocrit, hypotension, or flank pain. Retroperitoneal bleeding is often exacerbated by the use of intra- or periprocedural anticoagulation and antiplatelet agents leading to uncontrollable hemorrhage with devastating outcomes if not recognized early. To minimize this problem, the artery should be entered caudal to the inguinal ligament

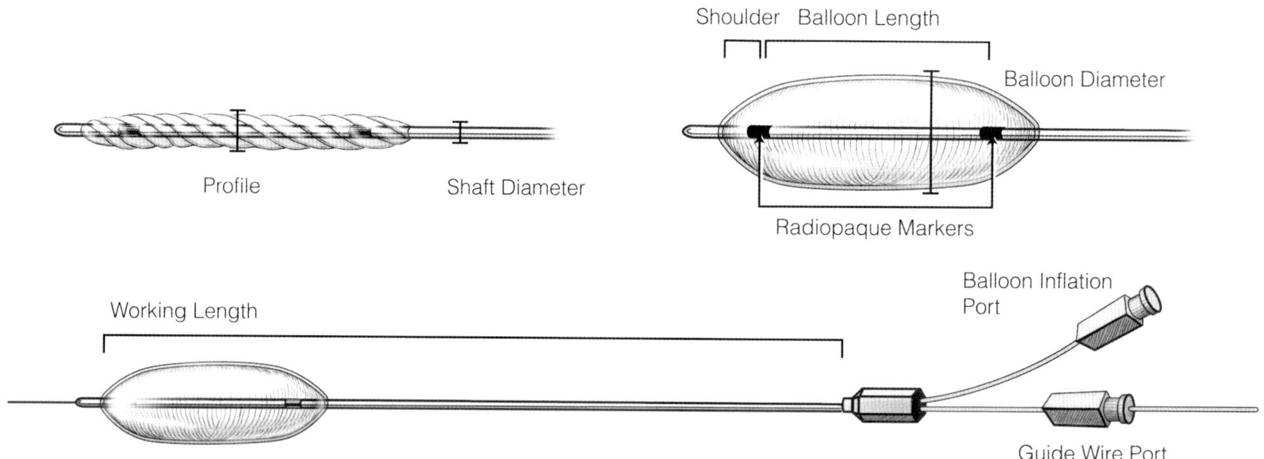

Figure 5 **Shown is a balloon angioplasty catheter.**

with respect to speed and duration of inflation, number of dilatations, and balloon pressure. Typically, the balloon is inflated to a pressure that results in a smooth parallel profile of the balloon walls, held for 20 to 60 seconds (sometimes even prolonged inflation of up to 2 to 3 minutes during tibial artery angioplasty), and then deflated. Short inflations are used for carotid artery stenting to reduce activation of baroreceptors. In most clinical circumstances, the inflation pressure should not exceed rated burst pressures. After dilatation, the balloon catheter is removed, with the guide wire left in place across the lesion (in case stenting proves necessary). Completion angiography is performed for evaluation of the results, including assessment of distal vascular beds.

Dilatation may be considered successful if (1) flow-limiting dissection is absent, (2) residual luminal diameter stenosis is less than 30%, and (3) the systolic pressure gradient is less than 5 to 10 mm Hg. Vasodilators can unmask a significant gradient.

TROUBLESHOOTING

Complications associated with the use of balloon catheters include thrombosis, vessel rupture, embolization, and dissection. The incidence of these complications is influenced by patient selection and by the nature of the lesion being treated. For example, complications may be more likely with treatment of stenoses adjacent to aneurysms, long segments of occlusion, tandem lesions, lesions near major branches, and calcified, eccentric plaques. Even though some degree of dissection is expected after balloon angioplasty, larger flow-limiting dissections may call for further management. This problem can often be solved by placing a stent over the dissection.

Most patients feel discomfort and mild pain during balloon inflation. If a patient experiences severe pain that persists after deflation of the balloon, the possibility of vessel rupture must be considered. If the vessel ruptures, the balloon may be reinflated over the injury to tamponade it. Prolonged balloon inflation often closes the leak, but at the risk of causing thrombosis. If the vessel continues to leak, a covered stent may be placed over the injury, or open vascular repair may be necessary.

If inflation of the balloon fails to dilate the vessel completely, it may be helpful to use a larger-diameter balloon, a less compliant balloon, or a higher inflation pressure. Higher inflation pressures may be cautiously attempted, but the vessel may simply recoil after dilatation.[14] A stent is often useful in this scenario.

If the balloon crosses the lesions only partially, it should not be inflated. The position of the guide wire should be checked: the wire may be in a subintimal location. If the stenosis is very tight, the lesion may be predilated with a smaller-profile balloon catheter.

Placement of Vascular Stents

Intravascular stents are commonly used in endovascular surgery, particularly after failed percutaneous transluminal angioplasty. Placement of an iliac artery stent is indicated when there is significant residual stenosis, flow-limiting dissection, or a persistent pressure gradient. Although angioplasty is often successful, it may fail when there is elastic recoil of the arterial wall or when the lesion is resistant to dilatation because of heavy calcification. Stenting can often remedy these situations by providing physical support to keep the vessel open. Many physicians now regard primary stenting (i.e., routine use of stents) as a preferred approach for many vascular lesions. As mentioned above, the lesion may need to be predilated with a small-profile, small-diameter balloon first to facilitate delivery of the stent across the lesion.

CHOICE OF STENT TYPE

Stents are divided into two categories: balloon-expandable stents and self-expanding stents. They may also be described as being covered (with a graft material), coated (with a therapeutic compound), or absorbable. Stent types differ with respect to hoop strength (for resisting arterial recoil), cell size (open or closed cell), cell structure, shape (e.g., tapered or nontapered), radiopacity, longitudinal flexibility (for crossing tortuous vessels), radial elasticity (for resisting repeated external compression), and profile. Stents come in many different lengths and expanded diameters on a wide variety of deployment catheters.

Balloon-Expandable Stents

Balloon-expandable stents come either premounted on balloon catheters or unmounted; unmounted stents must be manually crimped onto a balloon to be delivered. With unmounted stents, a smaller inventory can be maintained, and a wider range of stent-balloon combinations is available. Premounted stents, however, tend to be more solidly mounted and less likely to be dislodged during delivery. Once the stent is at the desired lesion, the balloon is inflated and the stent expanded.

The main advantage balloon-expandable stents have over self-expanding stents is that they have greater hoop strength, which means that they can better resist the recoil of the vessel after full expansion of the stent. An example of this would be in the treatment of a heavily calcified vessel or in a chronic total iliac occlusion. In addition, many interventionalists feel that balloon-expandable stents can be more precisely placed than self-expanding stents and thus are preferable when accuracy is of high clinical importance. An example of this would be in the treatment of an ostial, visceral vessel lesion where preservation of branches is important. However, older balloon-expandable stents are less flexible than current models, and navigating such older devices in a tortuous vessel can be difficult.

Self-Expanding Stents

Self-expanding stents are placed within a delivery catheter and rely on a self-expansion mechanism for full deployment. A common deployment mechanism involves the use of an outer jacket and a plunger: the jacket is withdrawn while the stent is held in position by the plunger, and the stent then expands to its predetermined diameter. Commonly, a balloon is employed to ensure that the stent is fully expanded and impacted into the plaque.

An advantage self-expanding stents have over balloon-expandable stents is that they offer a greater degree of longitudinal flexibility and thus are more easily tracked into position. Self-expanding stents come in lengths of up to 20 cm, which means that fewer overlap zones and fewer stents are required in the treatment of long lesions. In addition, they may be delivered by catheters with smaller profiles, which may reduce arterial access complications. Self-expanding stents may also be placed in regions of the body where they are subject to crushing forces (e.g., the carotid artery) because they are capable of recovering from the deformation and maintaining the arterial lumen.[15] As noted, however, self-expanding stents have less hoop strength than the balloon-expandable stents.

Covered Stents

Stents may be covered with polyester, polytetrafluoroethylene (with or without a heparin coating), or other materials. Currently, covered stents are being used frequently for treating occlusive lesions, but they are more commonly employed for treating aneurysms, arterial rupture, and arteriovenous fistulas.[15,16]

GENERAL TECHNICAL PRINCIPLES

Conceptually, stent placement is very similar to balloon angioplasty [*see Figure 6*]. Preoperatively, the patient is often given an antiplatelet agent, which may be continued for 4 weeks or longer postoperatively to reduce the risk of thrombosis. In general, the diameter of the fully deployed stent should slightly exceed that of the vessel, although many interventionalists do not fully dilate stents in the aorta and the carotid bifurcation.[11] If occlusion makes the exact diameter of the artery difficult to measure, the vessel's contralateral counterpart can be used as a guide.[16] The stent should also be slightly longer than the lesion to ensure that the entire lesion is covered. In this way, good wall apposition can be achieved and stent migration prevented.

The classic approach is to advance a guide (or a long sheath) across the stenosis over the previously placed guide wire; the vascular stent is then passed through the guide and positioned at the lesion, the guide is withdrawn, and the stent is deployed. With newer stent delivery systems, the leading tip often allows the stent to be delivered without precrossing the lesion with a guide or sheath. Multiple stents are sometimes required to complete the procedure.

TROUBLESHOOTING

It is often helpful to place the leading end of a self-expanding stent slightly beyond the lesion and then draw it back. This measure removes loaded tension from the system; it also allows the stent to be pulled back slightly after the initiation of deployment, at which point various forces sometimes cause the stent to move forward. However, the partially deployed struts of the stent can injure the vessel wall if moved too much or advanced forward. It is also important to keep in mind the potential for foreshortening of the stent during deployment. Failure to cover the entire lesion with the stent results in residual disease after the procedure, which can cause subsequent thrombosis and necessitate the placement of an additional stent. To prevent restenosis, multiple stents should generally be placed so as to overlap one another, but doing so may increase the risk of fatigue fractures. Clearly, the nuances of stent deployment vary according to the system being used; frequent use of a particular system will enhance the surgeon's familiarity with the behavior of the device and improve the subsequent clinical results.

Postprocedural Management of Arterial Access Site

After any endovascular procedure, the arterial access site must be addressed. Manual compression is one of the most common methods of hemostasis and is effective in most instances. The artery often must be compressed for longer than 20 minutes to prevent bleeding complications. If the patient is receiving anticoagulant therapy, it may be necessary to wait until the coagulation parameters have normalized before pulling out the sheath. This can be done when the patient is out of the operating room or the interventional suite and in the recovery room or when the patient has been moved onto the hospital floor. It is important that the person applying manual compression knows to maintain pressure over the actual puncture site in the artery as opposed to the skin incision site. This may be above or below the skin incision site depending on whether an antegrade or retrograde approach is used during the intervention. Failure to do so may lead to bleeding and pseudoaneurysm formation. After hemostasis has been achieved at the access site, the patient should refrain from walking for about 6 hours, after which the

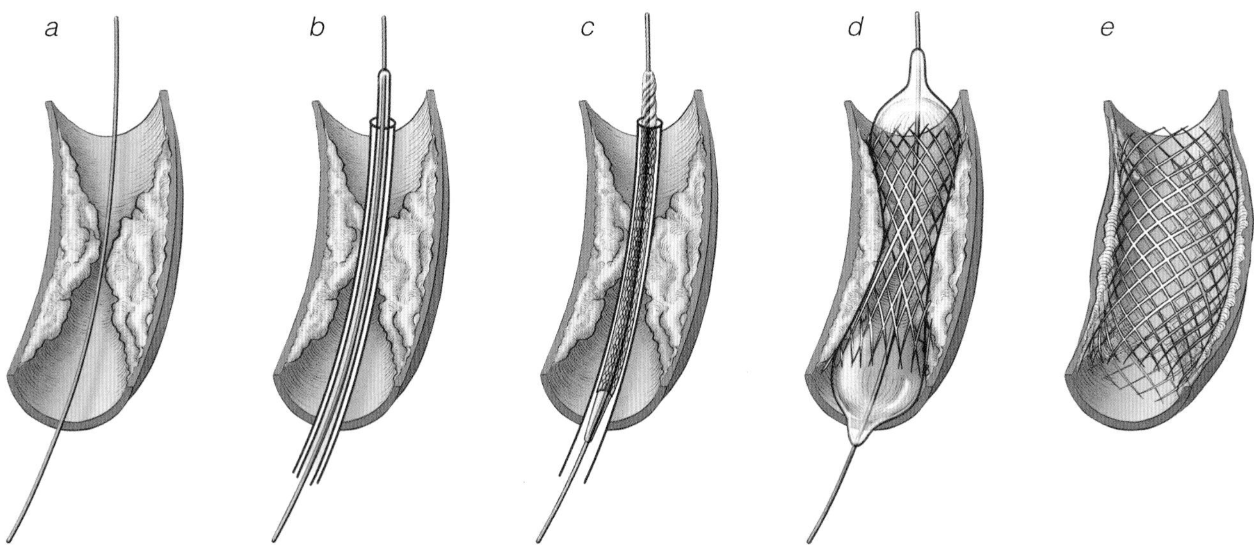

Figure 6 **Shown is the deployment of a balloon-expandable stent. (*a*) The guide wire is passed across the lesion. (*b*) The sheath-dilator combination is passed over the guide wire across the lesion. (*c*) The dilator is removed, and the balloon-expandable stent is advanced. (*d*) The sheath is retracted and the balloon inflated. (*e*) The balloon is deflated and withdrawn, leaving the stent fully deployed.**

puncture site generally is sufficiently stable. After therapeutic procedures involving relatively large devices, use of an arterial closure device may be advantageous. Several such closure devices are now commercially available. These devices are improving in quality and are certain to be used more frequently in the future.

Large Sheath Access during Aortic Interventions

As opposed to most peripheral interventions using 5, 6, or 7 French sheaths, aortic interventions for the treatment of aneurysms or dissections use large sheaths ranging from 12 to 24 French. Often occlusive disease in the iliac arteries makes remote arterial access from a femoral approach much more problematic [*see Figure 7*]. In fact, the EUROSTAR registry reported access-related complications in 13% of patients undergoing endovascular abdominal aortic aneurysm repair.[17] Similarly, large industry-sponsored trials using devices designed to treat thoracic aortic aneurysms have reported that the use of surgically created conduits because of small-caliber or diseased iliac vessels ranges from 9.4 to 21%.[18–20]

Several methods have been developed to overcome unfavorable iliac artery anatomy and to still allow aortic interventions to be performed through remote femoral access. Each of these has its own advantages and disadvantages, and detailed descriptions of their use can be found elsewhere.[21] A creative method has been developed to safely perform aortic interventions requiring large sheaths from a femoral approach using an endoconduit.

The concept behind the endoconduit is to deploy a covered stent across the diseased segment of iliac artery, aggressively balloon within the stent graft, and create a controlled rupture of the iliac artery to allow for passage of the large delivery sheath through the diseased vessel lined by the covered stent [*see Figure 8*]. The rupture occurs in the midportion of the external iliac artery and is controlled because adequate proximal and distal seals are created between the stent graft and a relatively disease-free portion of the common iliac artery and the CFA, respectively. Depending on the size of the delivery sheath needed to accommodate the device or the size of the device itself, the stent graft is ballooned with a 10 or 12 mm noncompliant balloon.

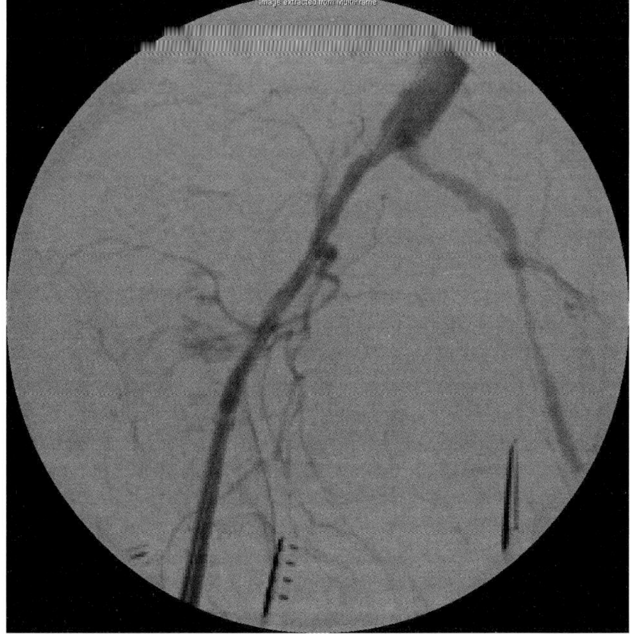

Figure 7 **Aortoiliac angiogram demonstrating a heavily diseased, small-caliber, right external iliac artery. Note that the 18 French sheath in the right external iliac artery is unable to be passed into the aorta.**

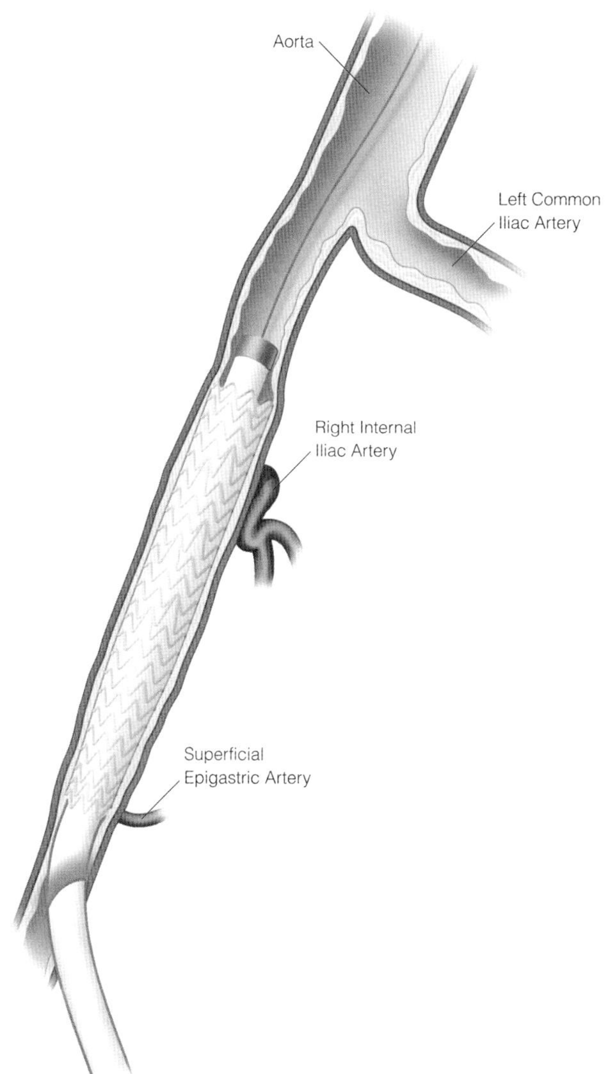

Figure 8 **Shown is a graphic representation of the endoconduit used in the patient whose angiogram is presented in Figure 7: deployment of a covered stent from the right common iliac artery into the common femoral artery and passage of a large delivery sheath through the stent graft after ballooning inside it to create a controlled rupture of a heavily diseased external iliac artery. Note the extension of the endoconduit into the common femoral artery distally.**

TROUBLESHOOTING

This technique has been used safely and effectively without encountering the theoretical complications of hemorrhage from rupture occurring adjacent to a patent internal iliac artery or of paraplegia and buttock ischemia from decrease pelvic perfusion. It is important that the covered stent extend into the CFA to avoid disruption of the vessel between the sheath entry point into the vessel and the end of the stent graft. If vessel rupture does occur in this intervening segment, a short interposition prosthetic graft between the end of the stent graft and the CFA access site is required. This complication shows that emergent surgical repair may still be necessary even with adjunctive access techniques such as the endoconduit. In the future, lower-profile devices may allow less hazardous aortic interventions.

Summary: Basic Steps in Endovascular Procedures

1. Before operation, assess the patient with respect to renal function, medications, allergies, active infections, anticoagulant management, and skin condition (in cases of planned access). Consider prescribing antiplatelet agents.
2. Monitor and sedate the patient as necessary.
3. Prepare and drape the selected arterial access site or sites.
4. Infiltrate a local anesthetic at the selected site.
5. Use a scalpel to nick the skin at the planned needle entry site, a few centimeters remote of the intended arterial puncture site.
6. Cannulate the artery with the entry needle.
7. Pass the guide wire into the needle for at least 20 to 25 cm under direct fluoroscopic guidance. Take care that the wire passes without resistance.
8. Remove the needle while pinning the guide wire in place.
9. Apply manual compression during exchanges to prevent hematoma formation around the artery.
10. Use dilators to create an appropriate tract while pinning the guide wire.
11. Pass a sheath over the pinned guide wire. Often with small sheaths and minimal scarring, the dilator and the sheath are placed simultaneously. Remove the dilator.
12. Administer anticoagulation as indicated.
13. Manipulate the guide wire to the appropriate position past the lesion (in cases of nonselective catheterization).
14. Pass the catheter over the guide wire and through the sheath. Manipulate the catheter to select the branches for guide wire cannulation.
15. Perform angiography through the catheter or the sheath to clarify the anatomy.
16. Remove the catheter while pinning the guide wire.
17. Pass the balloon catheter over the guide wire. Advance the balloon across and center it over the lesion. If indicated, primary stenting may be performed.
18. Inflate the balloon.
19. Deflate the balloon.
20. Remove the balloon catheter while pinning the guide wire.
21. Perform angiography.
22. If necessary, pass the vascular stent over the guide wire and advance it across the lesion.
23. Deploy the stent.
24. Perform completion angiography.
25. If the angiogram is satisfactory, remove the guide wire, the catheter, and the sheath.
26. Apply manual compression to the access site, or use a closure device.

Dr. Matsumura has received grants, research support, or consulting fees from Abbott Laboratories; C. R. Bard, Inc.; Cook Biotech Inc.; Cordis Corp.; ev3 Inc.; Lumen Biomedical, Inc.; W. L. Gore and Associates; and Medtronic, Inc.

Dr. Peterson has received consulting fees from W.L. Gore and Associates.

References

1. Tortorici M. Fundamentals of angiography. St. Louis: CV Mosby; 1982.
2. Johnsrude I, Jackson D, Dunnick N. A practical approach to angiography. 2nd ed. Boston: Little, Brown & Co; 1987.
3. Valji K. Vascular and interventional radiology. Philadelphia: WB Saunders; 1999.
4. Rupp SB, Vogelzang RL, Nemcek AA, et al. Relationship of the inguinal ligament to pelvic radiographic landmarks: anatomic correlation and its role in femoral arteriography. J Vasc Interv Radiol 1993;4:409.
5. Baum PA, Matsumoto AH, Teitelbaum GP, et al. Anatomic relationship between the common femoral artery and vein: CT evaluation and clinical significance. Cardiovasc Radiol 1999;173:775.
6. Millward SF, Burbride BE, Luna G. Puncturing the pulseless femoral artery: a simple technique that uses palpation of anatomic landmarks. J Vasc Interv Radiol 1993;4:415.
7. Jaques PF, Mauro MA, Keefe B. US guidance for vascular access: technical note. J Vasc Interv Radiol 1992;3:427.
8. Khangure MS, Chow KC, Christensen MA. Accurate and safe puncture of a pulseless femoral artery. Radiology 1982;144:927.
9. Spijkerboer AM, Scholten FG, Mali WPTM, et al. Antegrade puncture of the femoral artery: morphologic study. Radiology 1990; 176:57.
10. Grier D, Hartnell G. Percutaneous femoral artery puncture: practice and anatomy. Br J Radiol 1990;63:602.
11. Kandarpa K, Aruny JE. Handbook of interventional radiologic procedures. Philadelphia: Lippincott Williams & Wilkins; 2002.
12. Moore WS, Ahn SS. Endovascular surgery. 3rd ed. Philadelphia: WB Saunders; 2001.
13. Neiman HL, Yao JST. Angiography of vascular disease. New York: Churchill Livingstone; 1985.
14. Hood DB, Hodgson KJ. Percutaneous transluminal angioplasty and stenting for iliac artery occlusive disease. Surg Clin North Am 1999;79:575.
15. Nicholson T. Stents: an overview. Hosp Med 1999;60:571.
16. Henry M, Clonaris C, Amor M, et al. Which stent for which lesion in peripheral interventions? Tex Heart Inst J 2000;27:119.
17. Cuypers PW, Laheij R, Buth J. Which factors increase the risk of conversion to open surgery following endovascular abdominal aortic aneurysm repair? Eur J Vasc Endovasc Surg 2000;20:183–9.
18. Makaroun MS, Dillavou ED, Kee ST, et al. Endovascular treatment of thoracic aortic aneurysms: results of the phase II multicenter trial of the GORE TAG thoracic endoprosthesis. J Vasc Surg 2005;41:1–9.
19. Matsumura JS, Cambria RP, Dake MD, et al, and TX2 Clinical Trial Investigators. International controlled clinical trial of thoracic endovascular aneurysm repair with the Zenith TX2 endovascular graft: 1-year results. J Vasc Surg 2008;47:247–57.
20. Fairman RM, Criado F, Farber M, et al; VALOR Investigators. Pivotal results of the Medtronic Vascular Talent Stent Graft System: the VALOR trial. J Vasc Surg 2008; 48:546–54.
21. Peterson BG, Matsumura JS. Internal endoconduit: an innovative technique to address unfavorable iliac artery anatomy encountered during thoracic endovascular aortic repair. J Vasc Surg 2008;47:441–5.

Acknowledgment

The authors wish to acknowledge Joseph Vijungco, MD for his contributions to the previous rendition of this chapter on which we have based this update.

Figures 1 through 6 Alice Y. Chen.
Figure 8 Tony Stubblefield.

9 SURGICAL TREATMENT OF CAROTID ARTERY DISEASE

Wesley S. Moore, MD, FACS

The rationale for operating on patients with carotid artery disease is to prevent stroke. It has been estimated that in 50 to 80% of patients who experience an ischemic stroke, the underlying cause is a lesion in the distribution of the carotid artery, usually in the vicinity of the carotid bifurcation. It would follow, then, that appropriate identification and intervention could significantly reduce the incidence of ischemic stroke.

Carotid endarterectomy (CEA) for both symptomatic and asymptomatic carotid artery stenosis has been extensively evaluated in prospective, randomized trials. Symptomatic patients have been studied in the North American Symptomatic Carotid Endarterectomy Trial (NASCET),[1] the European Carotid Stenosis Trial (ECST),[2] and the symptomatic carotid stenosis trial from the Veterans Affairs (VA) Cooperative Studies Program.[3] The results of all three trials conclusively demonstrate that symptomatic patients with greater than 50% stenosis on arteriography are at substantially lower risk for stroke after CEA than control subjects receiving medical management alone. Asymptomatic patients with hemodynamically significant stenosis also benefit from surgical treatment: the Asymptomatic Carotid Atherosclerosis Study (ACAS)[4] and the asymptomatic carotid stenosis trial from the VA Cooperative Studies Program[5] showed that the risk of both transient ischemic attacks (TIAs) and stroke is markedly lower in patients treated with CEA and best medical management than in control subjects treated with best medical management alone. The Medical Research Council study of the Asymptomatic Carotid Stenosis Trial (ACST) confirmed the findings of these two studies, citing results virtually identical to those originally reported by the ACAS.[6]

Surgical reconstruction of the carotid artery yields the greatest benefits when done by surgeons who can keep complication rates to an absolute minimum. The majority of complications associated with carotid arterial procedures are either technical or judgmental; accordingly, in what follows, I emphasize the procedural details that I consider particularly important for deriving the best short- and long-term results from surgical intervention.

Preoperative Evaluation

PATIENT SELECTION

Indications for carotid artery surgery can be divided into two major categories: (1) asymptomatic critical stenosis and (2) symptomatic hemodynamically significant stenosis.[7]

Asymptomatic Critical Stenosis

The VA asymptomatic carotid stenosis study, ACAS, and ACST all found that in patients with diameter-reducing stenosis of 60% or greater on angiography, CEA resulted in fewer fatal and nonfatal strokes over a 5-year period than nonoperative treatment with best medical management alone. It is important to keep in mind that there are several different ways of measuring stenosis. The 60% figure cited by the ACAS and the VA study was determined according to the North American method rather than the European method. Moreover, it was determined by means of contrast angiography rather than duplex ultrasonography (DUS) or magnetic resonance imaging (MRI). If the decision for CEA is to be based on DUS, some conversion of values is required. A patient who has an 80 to 99% stenosis on DUS can generally be assumed to have a diameter-reducing stenosis of at least 60% on angiography; a stenosis that is less than 80% on DUS may fall short of a 60% diameter-reducing stenosis on angiography.

Symptomatic Hemodynamically Significant Carotid Stenosis

Both the NASCET and the ECST found that symptomatic patients with hemodynamically significant stenoses experienced fewer fatal and nonfatal strokes after CEA combined with best medical management than after best medical management alone, provided that the perioperative morbidity and mortality from stroke was 6.0% or less. Thus, patients with monocular or hemispheric TIAs are good candidates for CEA. Global ischemic attacks have also been used as an indication for CEA. This practice has not been evalutated in clinical trials; it is usually justified on the basis of the ACAS data alone.

Patients who have previously experienced a hemispheric stroke but who are not disabled and have made a reasonable recovery are also good candidates for CEA if they have a hemodynamically significant stenosis.

IMAGING

Identification of a carotid lesion that can be treated with endarterectomy usually begins with a carotid duplex scan. Indications for carotid duplex scanning fall into three main categories: symptoms, signs, and risk factors. Symptoms include classic TIAs and strokes that give rise to clinical suspicion of carotid bifurcation disease. The primary sign is the presence of a carotid bruit on auscultation. Risk factors include cigarette smoking, hypertension, diabetes mellitus, hypercholesterolemia, peripheral vascular disease, and coronary artery disease. As the number of risk factors present increases, the likelihood of associated carotid bifurcation disease increases exponentially.

Patients who present with focal ischemic symptoms are likely to have associated carotid bifurcation disease; however, other pathologic conditions (e.g., emboli of cardiac origin, aortic arch disease, intracranial vascular disease, coagulopathy, and brain tumors) can also be responsible for focal symptoms. Accordingly, a complete workup of a symptomatic patient should include cardiac evaluation and intracranial imaging.

The accuracy of carotid duplex scanning is highly dependent on the technician performing it and on the laboratory where it is done. A carefully performed carotid duplex scan is often the most accurate indicator of carotid bifurcation disease; however, a hastily or carelessly performed scan can result in overestimation of the extent of the carotid bifurcation disease. For this reason, additional imaging studies (e.g., magnetic resonance angiography, computed tomographic angiography, and, when there is serious doubt, contrast angiography) may be indicated.

Operative Planning

Before operation is scheduled, the general health of the patient must be assessed, with particular attention paid to cardiac and pulmonary status. Given that many patients with carotid artery disease are hypertensive or diabetic, good preoperative control of diabetes mellitus and blood pressure is mandatory. In addition, to reduce the risk of thromboembolic complications, patients should receive antiplatelet drugs (e.g., aspirin) up to and on the day of operation. Finally, it is well documented that the risk of perioperative cardiac complications can be materially reduced by placing patients on a combination regimen that includes a statin and a beta blocker.

ANESTHESIA

Surgery on the cervical portion of the carotid artery may be performed with the patient under either general or cervical block anesthesia. Both techniques have their advocates, their advantages, and their disadvantages.

The advantages of general anesthesia include a quiet operative field, maximal patient comfort, and good airway control. In addition, general anesthesia may lead to improved cerebral blood flow and give better protection against reduced blood flow during carotid clamping. The disadvantages of general anesthesia include blood pressure swings during induction and the inability to monitor the patient's conscious response to carotid clamping. Some reports also suggest that the incidence of cardiac complications is higher during general anesthesia than during cervical block anesthesia, but a meta-analysis of comparative trials failed to show any advantage of cervical block over general anesthesia.

The main advantage of cervical block anesthesia is the ability to monitor cerebral function during carotid clamping: an awake patient can be engaged in conversation and can be asked to carry out motor activities of the extremities. The disadvantages of cervical block anesthesia include possible patient discomfort, restlessness, and intolerance of the longer operations that are sometimes necessary for technical reasons. Another disadvantage is that on occasion, a patient cannot tolerate carotid clamping and demonstrates an immediate neurologic deficit with clamp application. Such an occurrence heightens the anxiety level of the surgical team, thereby increasing the risk that they will commit technical errors in the rush to place an internal shunt.

Besides considering the inherent advantages and disadvantages of these two anesthetic techniques with respect to the patient, it is important to consider their advantages and disadvantages with respect to individual surgical practice. A given surgeon may well work better and achieve better results with one technique or the other.

Whichever anesthetic approach is used, all patients should have a radial arterial line in place to allow continuous blood pressure monitoring and to provide access for determining blood gas levels. As a rule, there is no need to place a central venous line or a right heart catheter, except in patients with marginal cardiac function.

PATIENT POSITIONING

Proper positioning of the patient is necessary to provide optimal exposure of the neck from the clavicle up to the mastoid process on the side of the proposed operation [*see Figure 1*]. The patient is placed in the supine position with a folded sheet under the shoulders to induce a mild degree of neck extension. Excessive neck extension should be avoided, however, because it places tension on the artery and actually hinders rather than facilitates exposure. This potential problem can be addressed by placing one or more towels under the head to adjust the neck to the optimal degree of extension. The patient's head is then turned away from the side of the operation to improve cervical exposure further. Finally, the table top may be rotated slightly away from the side of the operation so as to provide a flat surgical field. The head of the table may be elevated slightly if the patient's blood pressure is adequate; this step helps lower venous pressure and reduce venous bleeding during the operation [*see Figure 1*].

Operative Technique

STEP 1: INITIAL INCISION

Either of two incisions may be used for exposure of the cervical carotid artery. The more common choice is a vertical incision placed along an imaginary line that extends from the sternoclavicular junction to the mastoid process, paralleling the anterior margin of the sternocleidomastoid muscle as well as the course of the carotid artery and the contents of

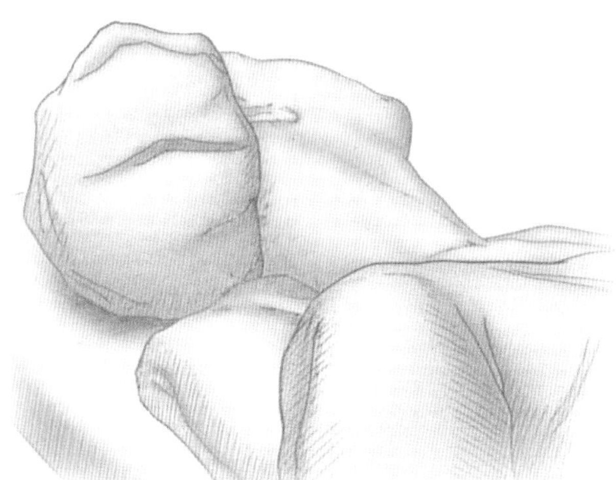

Figure 1 **Carotid arterial procedures. Shown is the recommended patient positioning.**

the carotid sheath [see Figure 2]. The incision is centered over the presumed location of the carotid bifurcation. Placement of the incision can be made more accurate by checking the location of the carotid bifurcation with an ultrasound probe prior to making the incision. The advantage of this incision is that it provides optimal exposure of the cervical carotid artery and can readily be extended either proximally or distally along the aforementioned imaginary line to give additional exposure when needed (e.g., when the carotid bifurcation is unusually high). The disadvantage of this incision is that it runs against the Langer lines; thus, if a keloid occurs, it is likely to be in an unsightly position. In most patients, the incision heals to a fine line and usually is not noticeable once healing is complete.

The alternative to the vertical incision is a transverse incision that is placed in a skin crease on the anterior portion of the neck and then curved toward the mastoid process posteriorly [see Figure 3]. Skin flaps are raised in a subplatysmal layer, and the incision is deepened along the anterior border of the sternocleidomastoid muscle. The advantage of this alternative incision is that it may be more cosmetically acceptable; however, its inferior portion frequently crosses the neck anteriorly, which may make it more visible than an incision confined to the line of the sternocleidomastoid muscle would be. The disadvantage of this incision is that it requires the raising of skin flaps, which takes additional time and may limit the extent of any proximal exposure that may be required.

STEP 2: EXPOSURE OF CAROTID ARTERY

Once the incision through the platysmal layer has been completed, an avascular areolar plane is developed along the anterior border of the sternocleidomastoid muscle for the full length of the incision so as to expose the carotid sheath. The internal jugular vein is usually the most visible vessel, and the carotid sheath is opened along this vessel's anterior border. The common facial vein, which drains into the internal jugular vein, is a relatively constant landmark. Because the common facial vein is the venous analogue of the external carotid artery, it can generally be used as a guide to the position of the carotid bifurcation [see Figure 4]. On occasion, a patient has several accessory facial veins instead of a single common facial vein. The common facial vein or the accessory facial veins are then divided between ligatures so that the jugular vein can be retracted laterally. The common carotid artery and the carotid bifurcation lie immediately beneath the divided facial veins.

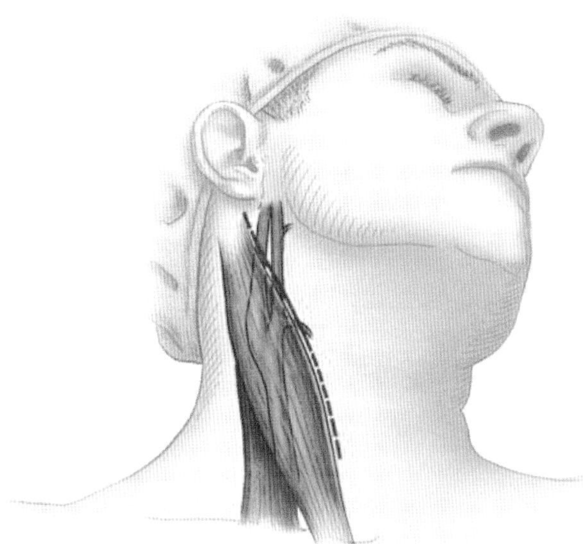

Figure 2 **Carotid arterial procedures. The incision most commonly used to expose the cervical carotid artery is a vertical one placed along the anterior margin of the sternocleidomastoid muscle and centered over the presumed location of the carotid bifurcation. It may be extended proximally or distally, depending on where the carotid bifurcation turns out to be.**

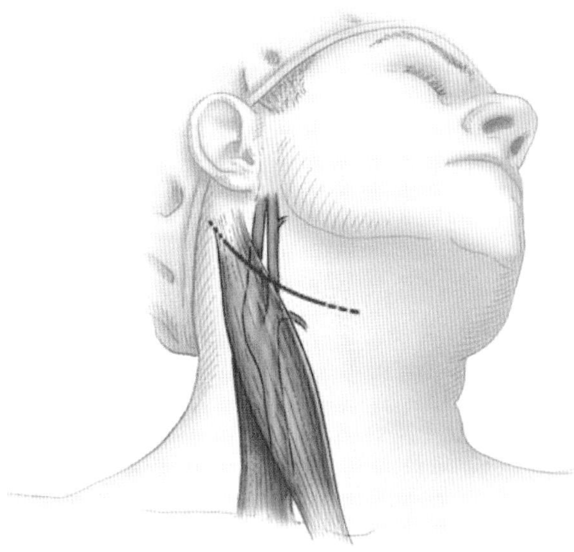

Figure 3 **Carotid arterial procedures. An alternative incision to the vertical incision is a transverse incision along a skin crease in the vicinity of the carotid bifurcation.**

At this point, care must be taken to look for the vagus nerve. This nerve is usually located posterior to the common carotid artery, but it is sometimes rotated into a more superficial position. Another important neurologic structure in this area is the ansa cervicalis, which is formed by the junction of fibers from the hypoglossal (12th cranial) nerve and fibers from the first cervical nerve and which continues inferiorly as a single trunk, providing innervation to the strap muscles. This nerve should be spared if possible, but it can be divided without significant sequelae if it interferes with optimal exposure of the carotid bifurcation. One convenient method of separating the nerve from the artery is to divide the fibers running from the first cervical nerve to the ansa cervicalis; when this is done, the nerve is readily mobilized and retracted anteriorly away from the carotid artery.

The perivascular plane of the common carotid artery is then entered, and the common carotid artery is circumferentially mobilized. The common carotid artery is palpated against a right-angle clamp to determine the proximal extent of the atherosclerotic plaque. If possible, the common carotid artery should be mobilized proximal to the plaque

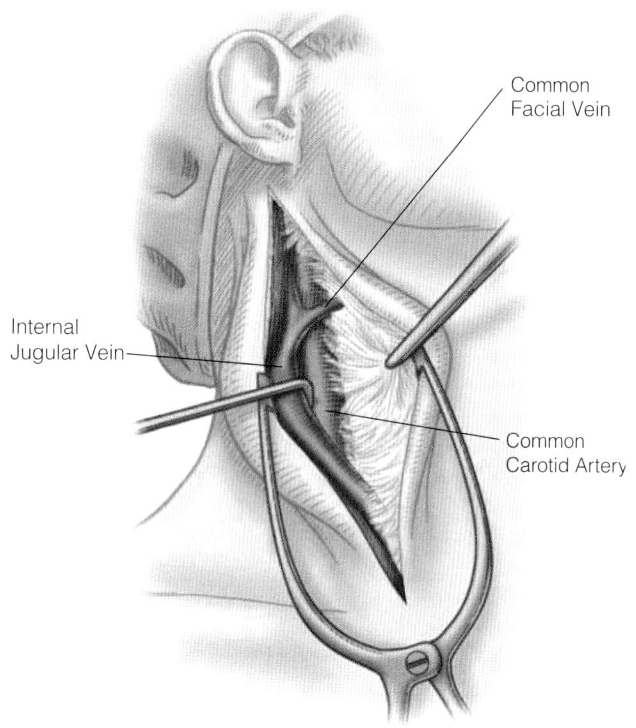

Figure 4 **Carotid arterial procedures. After the [illegible] muscle is mobilized off the carotid sheath, the jugular vein is identified. The perivascular plane along the jugular vein is opened until the common facial vein is exposed.**

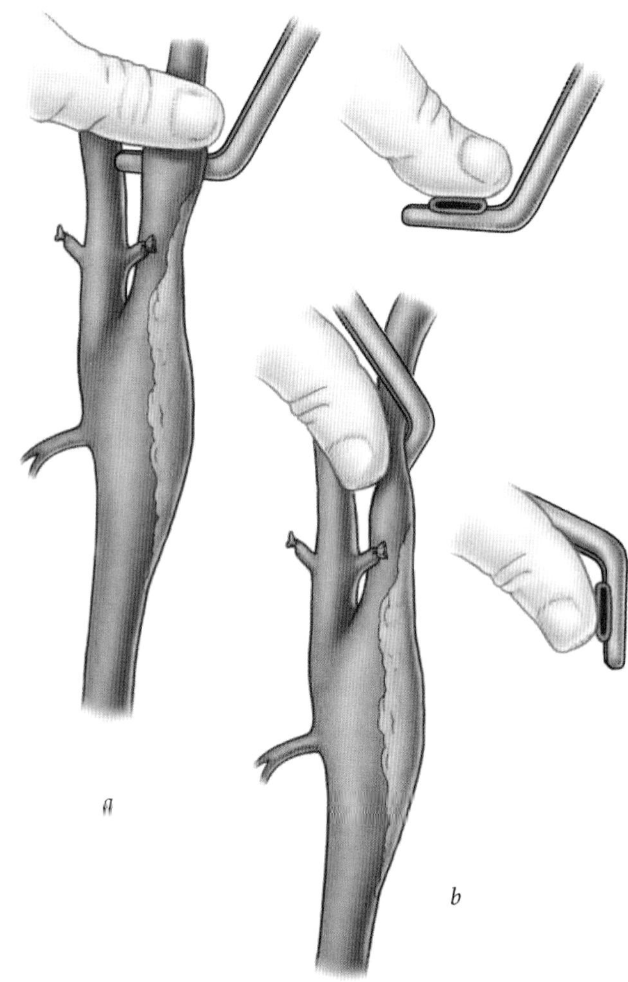

Figure 5 **Carotid arterial procedures. After the common carotid artery and the internal and external carotid arteries have been mobilized, the internal carotid artery is palpated against a right-angle clamp in at least two planes (*a, b*) to confirm that the artery has been freed beyond the end point of the plaque.**

until a circumferentially soft portion of that vessel is reached. During mobilization, the vagus nerve should be identified in its usual location posterior to the vessel and carefully protected; this nerve sometimes spirals anterior to the carotid artery as the vessel is dissected distally.

Dissection is then extended distally toward the carotid bifurcation and continued along both the internal and external carotid arteries. Excessive manipulation of the area around the carotid bifurcation must be avoided. In particular, it is important to be careful around the bulb of the internal carotid artery: this is where the majority of the plaque will be located, and manipulation can easily dislodge plaque or thromboembolic material. With exposure of the carotid bifurcation, the hypoglossal nerve may come into view. Care should be taken not to injure this nerve, although it may have to be mobilized to permit sufficient distal exposure of the internal carotid artery.

Next, dissection is continued distally beyond the bulb of the internal carotid artery to a point where the internal carotid artery is normal. At this point, the relevant portion of the vessel is circumferentially mobilized and palpated against a right-angle clamp in at least two planes to confirm that the atheromatous plaque does not reach up to the level of the proposed clamping [*see Figure 5*]. Once this is accomplished, the external carotid artery is mobilized beyond the end point of plaque extension in a similar manner.

If the patient has a high carotid bifurcation or if the plaque in the internal carotid artery extends further distally than usual, a more extensive exposure of the carotid bifurcation, the internal carotid artery, or both is required. To provide such exposure, the skin incision is extended all the way to the mastoid process. The sternocleidomastoid muscle is fully mobilized up to the mastoid process, with care taken to look for the spinal portion of the accessory (11th cranial) nerve as it enters the sternocleidomastoid muscle on the medial surface. With the sternocleidomastoid muscle fully mobilized and retractors in place, the internal carotid artery can then be further exposed.

The jugular vein is mobilized up toward the base of the skull, with care taken to look for additional accessory facial branches, which must be divided between ligatures so that the jugular vein can be fully mobilized and moved posteriorly. The perivascular plane of the internal carotid artery is carefully defined, and the artery is gently mobilized; the more distal portion of the internal carotid artery can then be mobilized downward. If the vessel is still insufficiently mobile, then the nerve to the carotid body and the ascending pharyngeal artery within the crotch between the internal and external carotid arteries are mobilized and divided between ligatures. These two structures often serve as a de facto suspensory ligament for the carotid bulb; dividing them allows the carotid bifurcation to drop down and permits further downward traction of the internal carotid artery as the vessel is gently mobilized distally [*see Figure 6*].

Once the internal carotid artery is further exposed distally and the hypoglossal nerve is mobilized along its vertical portion and moved anteriorly, the posterior belly of the digastric muscle is encountered. An areolar plane is developed posteriorly and superiorly along the inferior margin of the posterior belly of the digastric muscle, allowing the muscle to be mobilized anteriorly to yield additional exposure of the internal carotid artery. If the resulting exposure is not sufficient, the muscle may be carefully encircled with a right-angle clamp and divided [*see Figure 7*]. In those relatively uncommon cases in which even further distal exposure is required, the styloid process is palpated and the muscular and ligamentous attachments to the styloid process are divided so that the styloid process can be exposed with a periosteal elevator. Once the styloid process has been completely freed of its muscular and ligamentous attachments and the cranial nerves in the vicinity have been identified and carefully protected, the styloid process is cut close to the base of the skull [*see Figure 7*]. This step yields optimal exposure of the internal carotid artery all the way to the base of the skull.

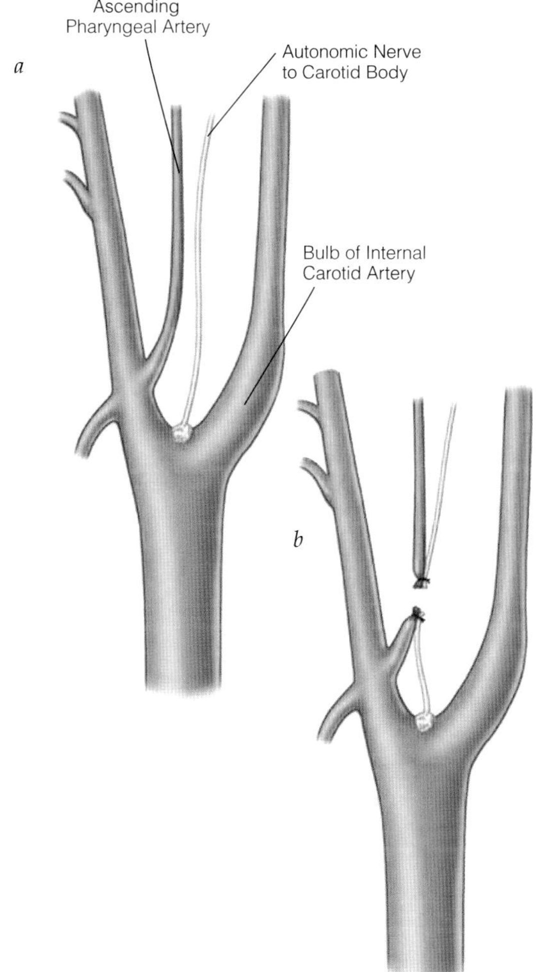

Figure 6 **Carotid arterial procedures. Once the common, internal, and external carotid arteries are fully mobilized, the structures between the internal and external carotid arteries (*a*) are divided (*b*) to allow the carotid bifurcation to drop down.**

Additional adjunctive measures for more extensive exposure of the internal carotid artery have been described. These include subluxation or dislocation of the mandible,[8] wiring of the mandible into a subluxed position, and division of the ramus of the mandible with rotation of the mandible away from the base of the skull. In my view, these measures are unnecessary, provided that the sternocleidomastoid muscle and the jugular vein have been adequately mobilized, the plane around the internal carotid artery has been developed, and the carotid bifurcation has been released.

A significant risk associated with extended exposure of the internal carotid artery is possible injury to the vagus nerve, the accessory nerve, or the hypoglossal nerve. Retraction of the vagus nerve may produce either temporary or permanent vocal cord palsy, and extensive retraction of or injury to the hypoglossal nerve causes denervation of the ipsilateral side of the tongue, manifested by tongue deviation to the ipsilateral side on protrusion or difficulty with mastication or swallowing. In addition, posterior exposure of a high carotid bifurcation may result in injury to branches of the glossopharyngeal (ninth cranial) nerve.

A common error in carotid artery mobilization is failure to recognize that the plaque in the internal carotid artery extends beyond the upper limit of the arterial exposure. It is far better to anticipate this problem before clamping and opening the artery than to discover it afterward and be forced to mobilize the vessel after it has been clamped. Once the common carotid and internal carotid arteries have been mobilized sufficiently, they are encircled with umbilical tapes; Rumel tourniquets are used if an internal shunt is required or desired.

STEP 3: CEREBRAL CIRCULATORY SUPPORT

Clamping of the carotid artery necessarily results in interruption of blood flow through the vessel. Patients who have good collateral circulation via the contralateral carotid artery or the vertebral arteries generally (although not always) tolerate the temporary interruption of flow through the clamped artery well.[9] Patients who have inadequate collateral blood flow require cerebral circulatory support, usually in the form of placement of an internal shunt. There are three basic approaches to shunt use: (1) routine use of an internal shunt, (2) selective use of an internal shunt, and (3) routine avoidance of shunting in an attempt to minimize clamp time.

Shunting Options

Routine shunting In approximately 10% of patients undergoing carotid artery surgery, collateral blood flow is inadequate and temporary use of an indwelling shunt is necessary to prevent brain damage. In the remaining 90%, collateral blood flow is adequate and clamping is generally well tolerated; therefore, shunting is unnecessary. Clearly, routine use of an internal shunt takes care of the 10% of

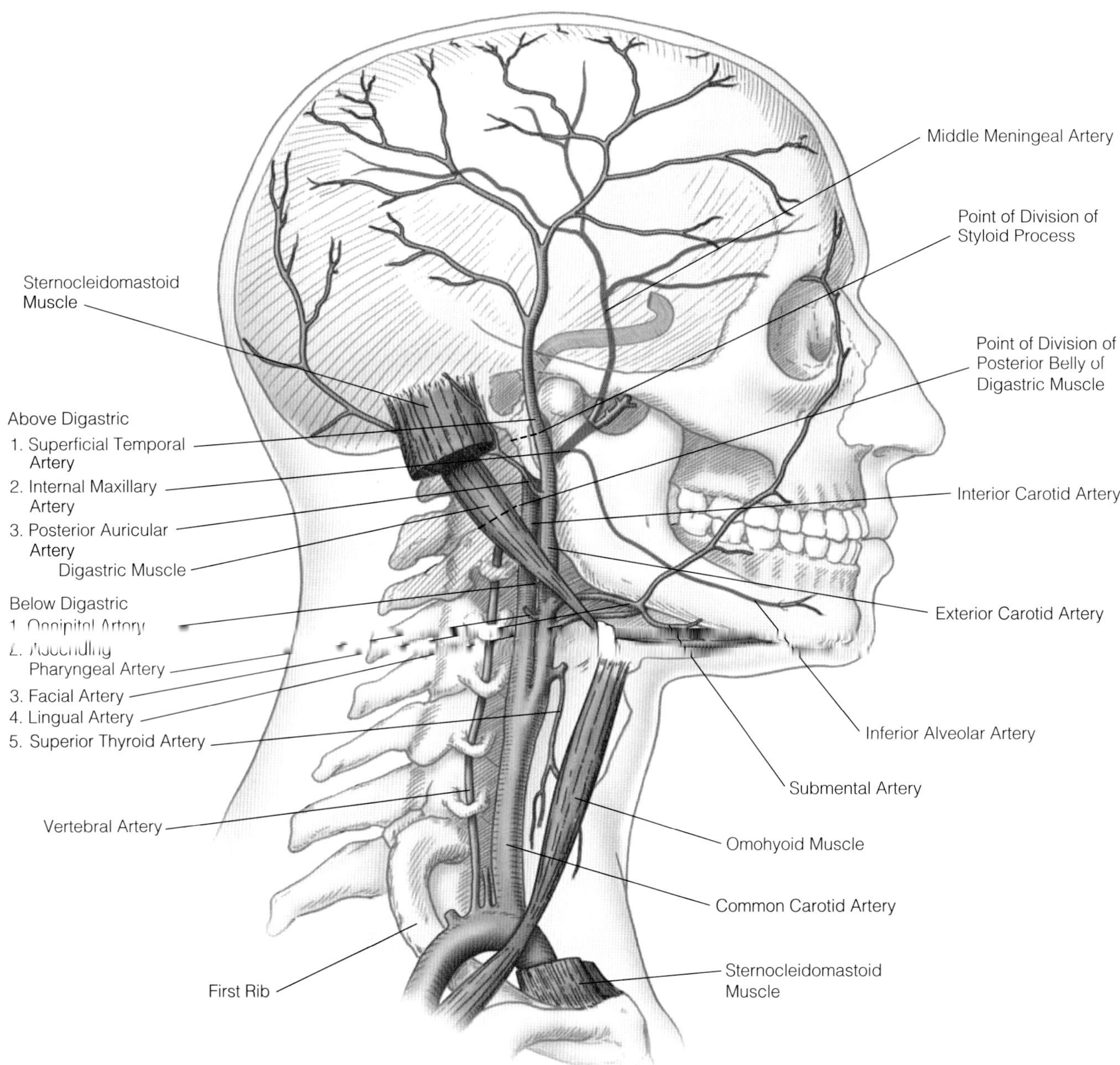

Figure 7 **Carotid arterial procedures. Division of the posterior belly of the digastric muscle yields additional exposure of the internal carotid artery. If the internal carotid artery must be mobilized all the way to the base of the skull, further distal exposure is obtained by separating the attachments of the ligaments to the styloid process and dividing the styloid process.**

patients who require shunts. Its disadvantage is that it is an additional procedure that carries its own complications, to which not only the 10% of patients who require shunting but also the 90% who do not are subjected. The potential complications associated with placement of a shunt include intimal injury (including the raising of an intimal flap), atheroma embolization (if atheromatous material is scooped up during shunt placement), and air embolization (if air bubbles are trapped within the shunt and not recognized).

Selective shunting Selective placement of a shunt has an advantage over routine placement in that the procedure and its potential complications are limited to the 10% of patients who actually require a shunt. Its main disadvantage is that the methods used to identify patients who require shunting may not be entirely reliable.

Selective identification of patients who require shunting can be accomplished in several ways. The most direct—and perhaps safest—method is to employ local or cervical block anesthesia so that the effect of temporary carotid clamping can be assessed in a conscious patient; if clamping leads to a neurologic deficit, then the patient clearly requires an internal shunt. Other methods of identifying patients who require a shunt make use of techniques such as continuous electroencephalographic (EEG) monitoring, measurement of somatosensory evoked potential, and monitoring of middle cerebral blood flow with transcranial Doppler ultrasonography.

A useful method of determining the adequacy of collateral cerebral blood flow is measurement of back-pressure in the internal carotid artery.[10] Back-pressure has been shown to be a good index of the adequacy of collateral blood flow and correlates well with the safety of temporary clamping and thus with the necessity of placing an internal shunt. Back-pressure is measured by placing into the common carotid artery a needle that is connected to pressure tubing and a pressure transducer. The tip of the needle is bent at a 45 angle. Systemic blood pressure is measured, and clamps are placed on the common carotid artery proximal to the needle and on the external carotid artery. The residual pressure in the common carotid artery, which is in continuity with the internal carotid artery, is then allowed to equilibrate; the resulting pressure reading represents internal carotid artery back-pressure [*see Figure 8*]. It has been determined that patients with back-pressures higher than 25 mm Hg can tolerate temporary clamping without incurring brain damage.

The utility of selective shunting in appropriate settings notwithstanding, routine shunting is recommended for patients who have previously had a stroke, regardless of the degree of neurologic recovery. In these patients, a central area of cerebral infarction is surrounded by a zone of relatively ischemic tissue—the so-called ischemic penumbra. The ischemic penumbra is made up of live and potentially functional brain tissue, but its viability is highly dependent on maximization of cerebral perfusion pressure through collateral channels. Accordingly, any interruption of carotid circulation, regardless of the degree of collateral circulation present, may threaten the ischemic penumbra and extend the infarct [*see Figure 9*]. In my opinion, all CEA patients with prior strokes should receive shunts on a routine basis.

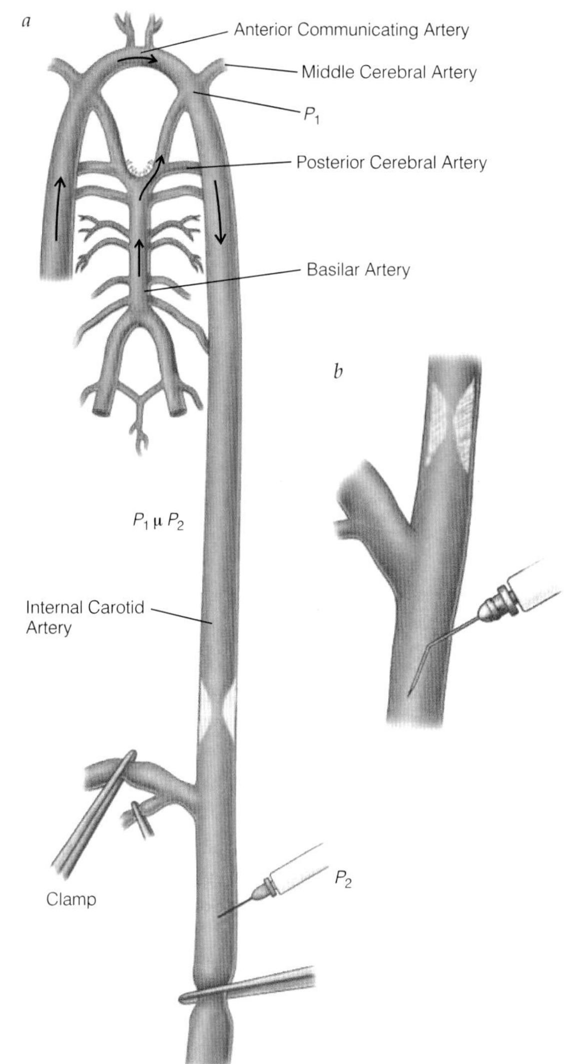

Figure 8 **Carotid arterial procedures. (*a*) A graphic representation of the measurement of internal carotid artery back-pressure. (*b*) The needle is bent at a 45 angle before being inserted into the common carotid artery.**

Routine avoidance of shunting The advantage of routinely avoiding the use of shunts is that the technical issues and potential complications associated with the additional procedure are avoided entirely. The disadvantage is that unshunted patients with poor collateral blood flow may sustain ischemic brain damage, particularly if the clamp time turns out to be longer than was anticipated.

Technique of Shunt Placement

Internal shunts must be placed with great care if shunt-associated complications are to be avoided. Of the various shunts currently available, I prefer the Javid shunt, which is tapered, has smooth leading edges, and possesses external bulbous circumferential extensions that permit it to be held in place with a circumferential Rumel tourniquet, thereby minimizing the chances of inadvertent dislodgment. Optimal placement of an internal shunt may be achieved by means of the following steps [*see Figure 10*].

After the patient has been adequately heparinized and the artery has been clamped and opened, the distal portion of the internal shunt is placed into the internal carotid artery. A clamp is placed on the shunt and briefly opened to allow back-bleeding; good back-bleeding confirms that the shunt is lying free in the lumen of the internal carotid artery. The shunt is then secured by tightening a Rumel tourniquet, and the bulbous portion of the shunt is engaged to prevent dislodgment.

Next, the proximal portion of the shunt is placed into the common carotid artery. As this is done, the clamp is removed from the shunt so that backflow from the shunt will dislodge any loose material and air within the common carotid artery. The shunt is then reclamped, and the clamp is removed from the common carotid artery as the proximal portion of the shunt is passed into that vessel.

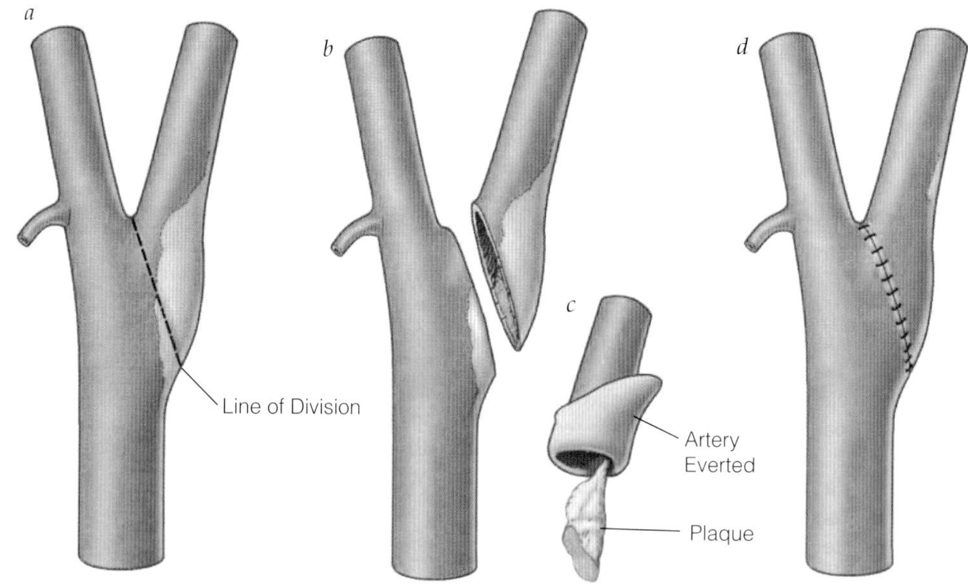

Figure 13 **Carotid arterial procedures: eversion endarterectomy. (*a, b*) The internal carotid artery is divided from the common carotid artery in an oblique line. (*c*) The divided internal carotid artery is everted on itself so that it can be separated from the underlying plaque. Eversion proceeds distally until the plaque end point is encountered, and the plaque is removed from the internal carotid artery. Proximal endarterectomy of the common carotid artery and endarterectomy of the external carotid artery are then carried out. (*d*) Once all of the plaque has been removed, the internal carotid artery is reverted and an end-to-side anastomosis is fashioned between the common carotid artery opening and the internal carotid artery.**

Before completion, the vessels are back-bled and flushed. Once the anastomosis is complete, blood flow is restored, first to the distal subclavian artery and then to the common carotid artery.

Reconstruction for Recurrent Carotid Stenosis

For an initial recurrence of carotid stenosis that primarily results from myointimal hyperplasia, conversion to a patch angioplasty is generally the best treatment. For second or third recurrences or for recurrences that develop in spite of patch angioplasty, resection of the carotid bifurcation with interposition grafting between the common carotid artery and the normal distal internal carotid artery is the best treatment.

Exposure and mobilization Exposure of a carotid bifurcation for treatment of recurrent carotid stenosis can be challenging. The initial skin incision is reopened, and dissection is carried down through the scar tissue to the common carotid artery. The common carotid artery is sharply dissected from the surrounding scar tissue, with the dissection plane kept close to the adventitia to minimize the risk of injury to the vagus nerve and the hypoglossal nerve. Once the common carotid artery has been adequately mobilized, dissection is carried distally to include the carotid bifurcation and the internal carotid artery. In the course of distal dissection, care must be taken to watch for the hypoglossal nerve, which may be incorporated into the scar tissue; this structure must be carefully dissected away from the artery and protected.

Distal dissection continues beyond the end point of the previous closure of the internal carotid artery. Beyond this end point, it is usually possible to enter a previously undissected plane of the internal carotid artery; from here onward, the artery typically is soft around its circumference and is not involved in the recurrent stenosis. The external carotid artery is then mobilized sufficiently to allow the surgeon to control back-bleeding.

Conversion to patch angioplasty If the artery was originally closed primarily, an arteriotomy is made through the old suture line and carried distally through the area of stenosis and onto a relatively normal area of the internal carotid artery. Exploration of the luminal surface usually reveals a smooth, glistening neointima, and observation of the cut section of the artery reveals an area where a whitish, firm thickening of the intimal wall has occurred as a result of myointimal hyperplasia. No attempt should be made to re-endarterectomize the stenotic area, because the intimal lesion is not, in fact, plaque but scar tissue. If the intima is removed, the cascade of events that led to the myointimal hyperplasia will simply be reinitiated. Accordingly, the healed intimal surface should be carefully protected. A patch angioplasty across the stenotic area, extending from the common carotid artery proximally to a relatively normal portion of the internal carotid artery distally, is usually sufficient to treat the lesion.

Resection of carotid bifurcation with interposition grafting If the stenosis is recurring for the second or third time or the artery was originally closed with a patch, the surgeon should proceed with resection and interposition grafting. In most cases, it is necessary to sacrifice the external carotid artery and oversew its origin. The internal carotid artery is divided distal to the intimal hyperplastic lesion, the common carotid artery is divided proximally, and the diseased specimen is removed.

I prefer to use 6.0 mm thin-walled PTFE for the interposition graft. The internal carotid artery distally and the common carotid artery proximally are spatulated by making vertical incisions approximately 6.0 mm in length. The PTFE graft is appropriately beveled both proximally and distally, and beveled or spatulated end-to-end anastomoses are performed, first to the internal carotid artery and then to the common carotid artery.

Before completion, the vessels are back-bled and flushed; once the anastomoses are complete, blood flow is reestablished.

Some surgeons may be tempted to use autogenous saphenous vein for the interposition graft. To use such grafts would appear, on the face of it, to be a good idea; in fact, it is a mistake. For reasons not clearly understood, the use of autogenous saphenous vein in the neck has an extremely poor track record, yielding unacceptably high rates of recurrent stenosis and occlusion in comparison with the use of prosthetic grafts.

Special Considerations

Fibromuscular dysplasia of internal carotid artery Fibromuscular dysplasia of the internal carotid artery is a congenital or acquired lesion that has been subdivided into four pathologic varieties, of which the most common is medial fibroplasia. On contrast angiography, medial fibroplasia has a characteristic appearance, resembling a string of beads in the extracranial portion of the internal carotid artery [*see Figure 14*]. A common initial manifestation is a relatively loud bruit in the neck of a young woman. Fibromuscular dysplasia can cause symptoms of monocular or hemispheric TIAs, or it may go on to cause a stroke, usually as a consequence of a dissection resulting in thrombotic occlusion. If symptoms develop, they can generally be controlled by means of antiplatelet drugs. Currently, the only indication for surgical intervention is the persistence of symptoms despite antiplatelet therapy.

Treatment of fibromuscular dysplasia has evolved over the years. The first attempts at surgical repair involved a total resection of the internal carotid artery coupled with interposition of a graft (usually composed of saphenous vein). This technique has largely been abandoned because of the extensive surgical dissection required and the substantial risk of cranial nerve injury; its only remaining application is in cases where there is associated aneurysmal dilatation in the dysplastic segment that calls for resection and graft interposition. At present, the two most popular modes of therapy both involve intraluminal dilatation with disruption of the small septa within the artery. One mode achieves intraluminal dilatation via an open approach, and the other achieves the same end via a percutaneous approach that includes balloon angioplasty. Dilatation and fracturing of the intraluminal septa often result in the release of particles of septal tissue, which in turn can lead to cerebral embolization and infarction. Consequently, an open approach, which enables the surgeon to flush out the disrupted segments, or balloon angioplasty with cerebral embolic protection is usually favored.

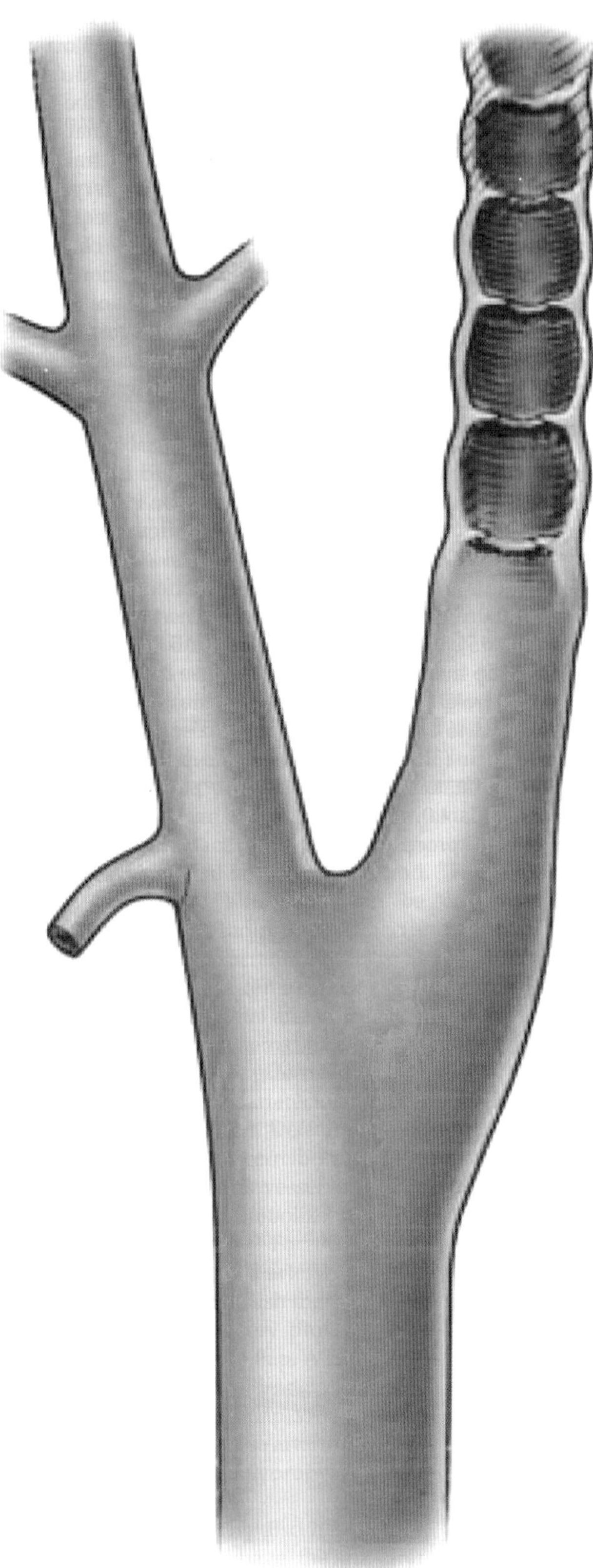

Figure 14 **Carotid arterial procedures: repair of fibromuscular dysplasia. Depicted is the so-called string of beads deformity of the cervical portion of the internal carotid artery, which is characteristic of medial fibroplasia.**

Basic principles of endovascular surgery are discussed more fully elsewhere [*see 7:8 Fundamentals of Endovascular Surgery*]; the following steps focus primarily on the procedural elements specific to CAS.

STEP 1: SECURING OF ARTERIAL ACCESS

Retrograde femoral access is obtained, and a 5 French sheath is inserted. Full heparin anticoagulation (typically 100 mg/kg body mass) is instituted after arterial access is secured and before manipulation of catheters in the aortic arch and the brachiocephalic vessels.

STEP 2: SELECTIVE CAROTID CATHETERIZATION AND ARTERIOGRAPHY

Selective catheterization of the aortic arch vessels is best performed after an arch aortogram in a left anterior oblique projection of 30 to 40 degrees. Although this will usually suffice, when cannulating the right CCA, sometimes it is helpful to image the innominate artery in a right anterior oblique projection. This will allow for a clear delineation of the innominate bifurcation [*see Figure 3*]. After selective catheterization of the midportion of the ipsilateral CCA (typically starting with a simple curved catheter), a selective arteriogram of the carotid bifurcation is obtained, with care taken to choose a view that yields minimal overlapping of the ICA and the ECA and maximal visualization of the target lesion. A cerebral arteriogram with at least anterior posterior and lateral views, if not previously obtained, is obtained at this point to serve as a baseline and to identify any intracranial pathologic conditions (e.g., aneurysms and arteriovenous communications) that may be present.

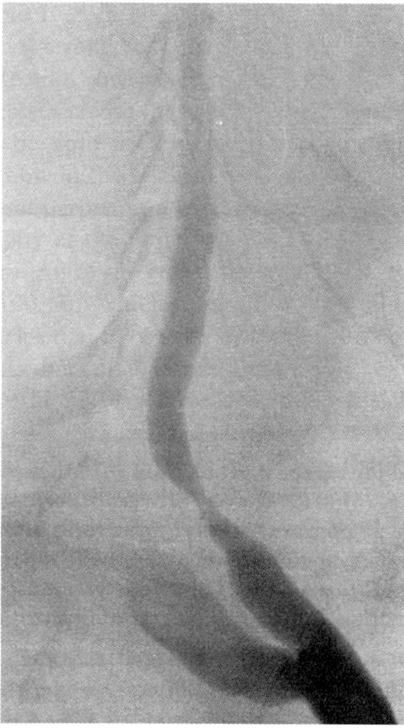

Figure 3 **Right anterior oblique angle angiogram of the right subclavian and common carotid arteries. Note stenosis in the proximal right common carotid artery and the ability to visualize the origins of the two vessels in this projection.**

STEP 3: ADVANCEMENT OF SHEATH AND DILATOR INTO CCA

Two techniques have been employed to advance a sheath into the CCA. The first technique, which is most commonly employed, is to place an exchange-length 0.035-inch guide wire into the terminal branches of the ECA. The diagnostic catheter and the 5 French sheath are removed. Care should be taken to pay close attention to the tip of the stiff wire to ensure that it does not perforate or otherwise traumatize a branch of the ECA. Hematoma formation and airway compromise can be a devastating complication. Sometimes for an angulated CCA, a stiff wire will not successfully pass into the ECA. In these circumstances, the use of a 0.035-inch angled glide wire or stiff angled glide wire will facilitate passage of the diagnostic catheter into the ECA, which will then allow for introduction of stiff wire into the ECA. A long (70 to 90 cm length, depending on patient body habitus) 6 French sheath is then advanced, along with its dilator, into the CCA. Care must be taken to identify the tip of the dilator (which is not radiopaque) because it may extend a significant distance from the end of the sheath, depending on the brand of sheath used. Obviously, inadvertently advancing the dilator into the carotid bulb may have disastrous consequences. In patients with short CCAs or low bifurcations, the sheath can be advanced over the dilator once the sheath edge (a radiopaque marker) is past the origin of the CCA. Generally, the tip of the sheath should be positioned to within 2 cm of the target lesion.

The second technique, often referred to as the "telescoping technique," is to advance the long sheath into the transverse arch over a guide wire. The dilator is removed, and an appropriate selective diagnostic catheter is advanced into the CCA. This catheter must be substantially longer than the sheath, typically more than 100 cm long. A stiff guide wire is then advanced into the ECA. Both the wire and the catheter are pinned at the groin to provide support, and the sheath (without the dilator) is advanced into the CCA. This technique may be advantageous in so-called hostile arches, in that the catheter and the wire provide more support than a wire alone would; however, without the protection of the sheath dilator, there is a risk of "snowplowing" the edge of the sheath at the junction of the aortic arch and the innominate artery or the left CCA, which can cause dissection or distal embolization. The Shuttle Select system by Cook Incorporated has a unified system to accommodate this approach.

The importance of gaining and maintaining sheath access to the distal CCA should not be underestimated: once the 0.035-inch guide wire is removed (and, eventually, exchanged for a 0.014-inch wire), support for angioplasty and stent placement is provided solely by the sheath. If the sheath backs up into the aortic arch during the interventional procedure, it is virtually impossible to advance it into the CCA over a 0.014-inch guide wire or protection device. Appropriate patient selection and accurate recognition of which arches to avoid are essential for success. In particularly difficult arches, deep inspiration or expiration may facilitate sheath advancement by subtly changing the configuration of the brachiocephalic origins once guide-wire access has been obtained. Alternatively, when a sheath cannot be advanced into the CCA, a preshaped guide catheter can be seated in the proximal CCA. Although this maneuver may facilitate an otherwise impossible intervention, it should be kept in mind that guide catheters require a larger arterial puncture and provide a less stable support platform than sheaths do and should be used only if there is no other reasonable alternative [*see Figure 4*].

Troubleshooting

In patients with an occluded ECA, sheath access to the CCA may be difficult to obtain. Two techniques may be employed to overcome this difficulty. The first is to place a stiff 0.035-inch wire with a preshaped J into the distal CCA, taking care to avoid the bulb and the bifurcation. The J configuration keeps the guide wire from crossing the lesion. A stiff wire with a shapeable tip can be used to the same end.

The second technique is to use a variable-diameter wire (0.018 inches at the tip, enlarging to 0.035 inches more proximally) to cross the internal carotid lesion, providing additional guide-wire support to facilitate sheath advancement. This approach is a reasonable option, but it ultimately necessitates crossing the target lesion twice.

STEP 4: REMOVAL OF GUIDE WIRE AND DILATOR AND SELECTIVE ARTERIOGRAPHY OF CAROTID BIFURCATION

Once the sheath is in place, the guide wire and the dilator are removed. The sheath sidearm may be attached to a slow, continuous infusion of heparin-saline solution to keep blood from stagnating in the sheath. Selective angiography of the carotid bifurcation is then performed through the sheath, again demonstrating the area of maximal stenosis, the extent of the lesion, and the normal ICA and CCA above and below the lesion. Roadmapping, if available, is helpful in crossing the lesion with an EPD or guide wire [*see* Step 6, *below*]. The overwhelming majority of procedures are performed with an EPD, typically a distal filter device [*see Figure 5*].

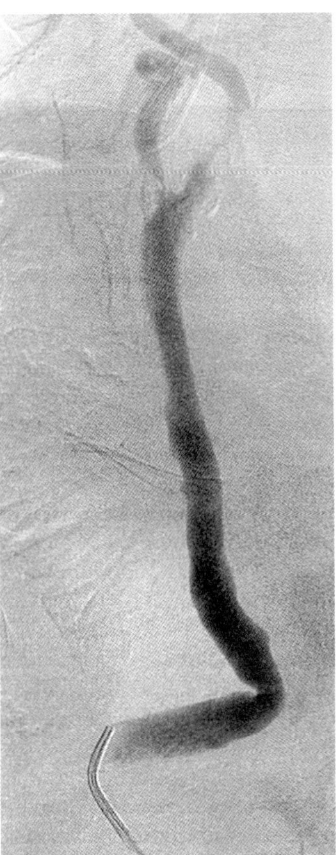

Figure 4 **Selective left common carotid angiogram showing severe angulation (two 90° bends) of the proximal artery and a high-grade stenosis of the external carotid artery.**

STEP 5: MEASUREMENT OF ACTIVATED CLOTTING TIME

It is advisable to measure the activated clotting time (ACT) before crossing the lesion and performing CAS. An ACT of 250 to 300 seconds is generally advised for most instances. The interventional team should discuss, in detail, all of the subsequent steps to be performed. Balloons are flushed and prepared, and special care should be taken to remove all air from the system as a protective measure against the unlikely event of balloon rupture [*see Figure 6*]. The self-expanding stent is opened and placed on the table, and the crossing guide wire or EPD is prepared.

STEP 6: DELIVERY OF EPD ACROSS TARGET LESION

After the target lesion has been clearly identified, the next step is to deliver the constrained filter element across the stenotic target lesion and into the distal normal ICA. If the constrained filter element does not pass because of the severity of stenosis, it may be best to abort the CAS procedure rather than dilate the lesion with a small balloon without distal protection to facilitate passage of the device. If the EPD does not advance beyond the lesion because of angulation of the vessel, the use of a "buddy wire" to straighten the vessel may be employed using a stiffer 0.014-inch wire [*see Figure 7*].

Troubleshooting

Rare complications of filter EPDs have been reported, including filter detachment, filter entanglement with the stent, and iatrogenic ICA dissection, but the more common occurrences are ICA spasm, filter thrombosis, and inability to retrieve the filter. One of the primary problems with distal EPDs when working over long distances—the femoral approach to the carotid artery—is minimizing movement of the filter during the CAS procedure [*see Figure 8*]. Newer filter delivery systems have addressed this to a certain degree by having the filter "free-floating" on a specific wire in the ICA, such as the Emboshield system (Abbott Vascular). Nevertheless, motion of the filter in the distal ICA can induce varying degrees of vasospasm, which may be severe enough to halt flow through the collapsed filter element. Fortunately, this can be easily remedied with an intra-arterial administration of nitroglycerin (100 μg) [*see Figure 9*]. In rare circumstances, vasospasm can be relieved only by removing the filter, but it is important to differentiate spasm from thrombosis of the filter.

Determining the causation for flow arrest at the level of the filter element can be challenging and anxiety provoking. Generally, it is either attributable to intense vasospasm or filter thrombosis. Whereas the former typically improves with nitroglycerin, the latter may require additional maneuvers. A first step is to redose systemic anticoagulation—heparin or angiomax—and recheck the ACT to ensure that it is greater

a

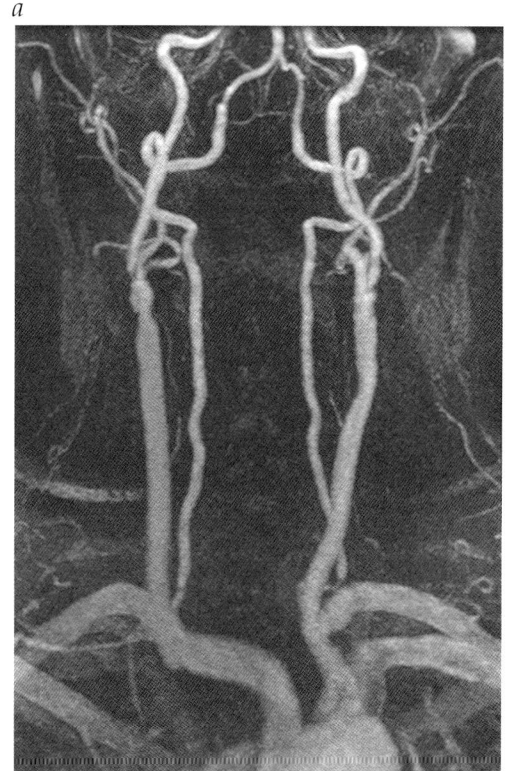

b

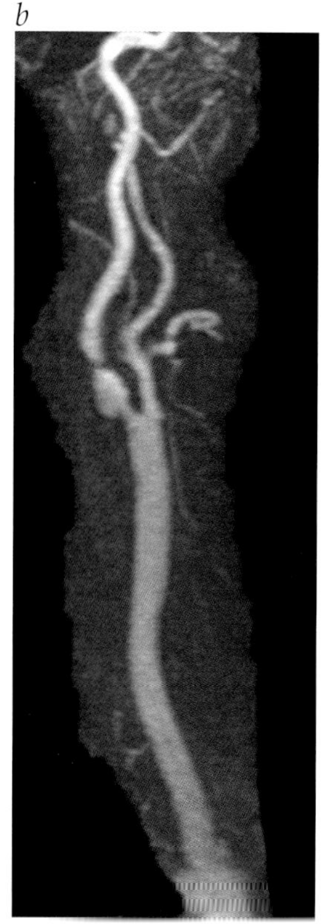

c

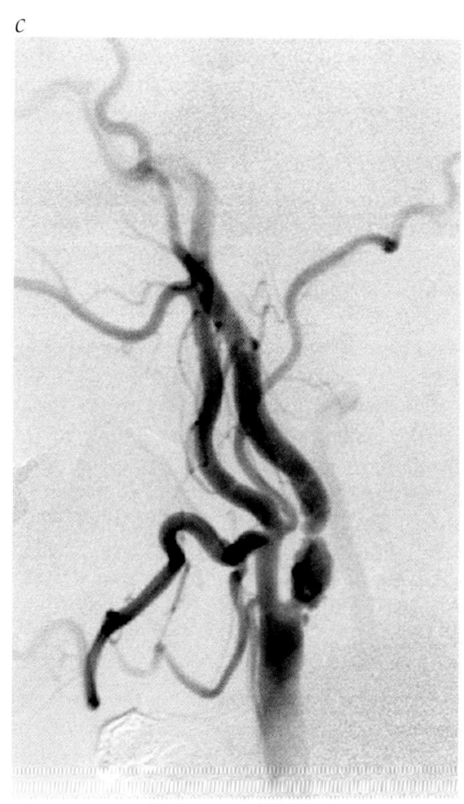

d

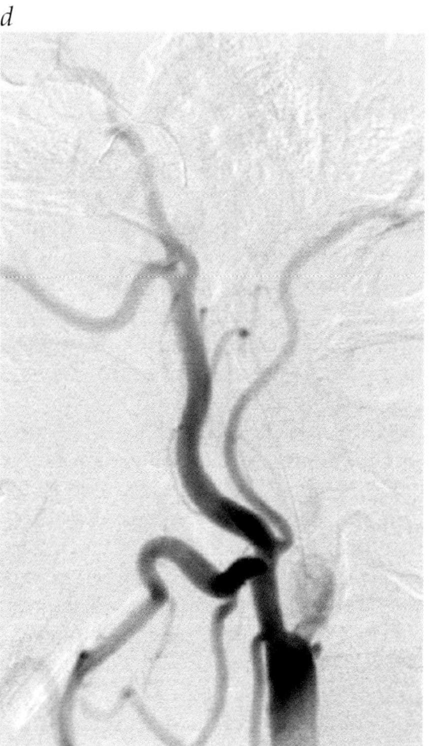

e

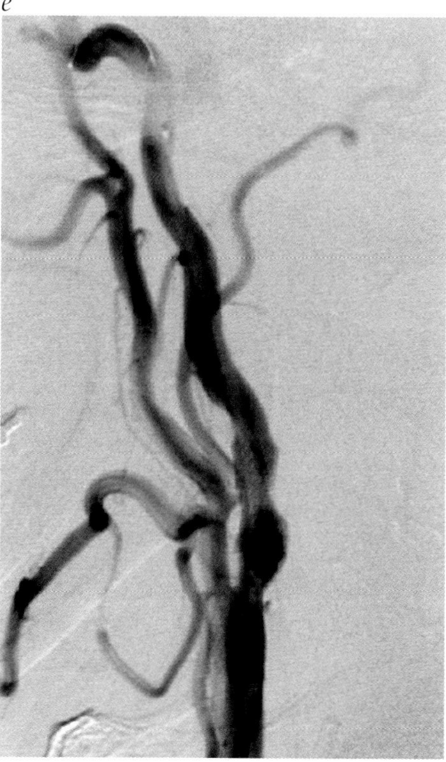

Figure 5 **Carotid angioplasty and stenting. In this example, a balloon occlusion device is used for cerebral protection. (*a*) Magnetic resonance angiography (MRA) shows the aortic arch and cervical carotid and vertebral arteries. (*b*) MRA shows de novo atherosclerotic stenosis of the right internal carotid artery (ICA). (*c*) Diagnostic arteriogram of right carotid bifurcation in a symptomatic patient shows tandem ulcerated stenoses. (*d*) The right ICA is occluded with a PercuSurge GuardWire device. (*e*) Shown is the vessel after angioplasty and placement of a self-expanding nitinol stent.**

than 250 seconds. Next, try intra-arterial nitroglycerin. If these simple steps do not improve the flow, an attempt to aspirate captured debris from inside the filter basket should be made. Available devices to achieve this are the Pronto system (Vascular Solutions) and the Export catheter (Medtronic). After aspirating from the filter down into the CCA with several passes and removal of at least 50 cc of blood, flow should be reassessed. If there is still no improvement, intra-arterial tissue plasminogen activator can be given. Once adequate flow is restored or if all else fails, the filter should then be removed. Luckily, this is an infrequent phenomenon.

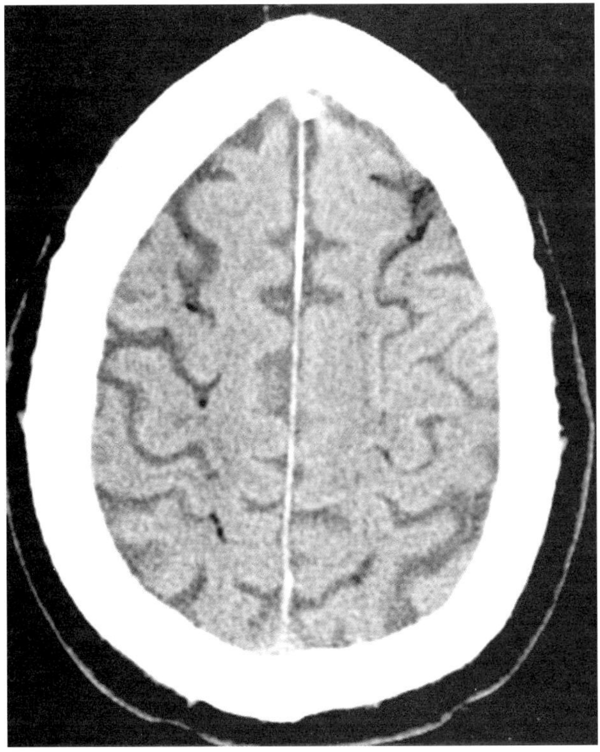

Figure 6 **Noncontrast computed tomographic scan of the brain showing bihemispheric intracerebral air.**

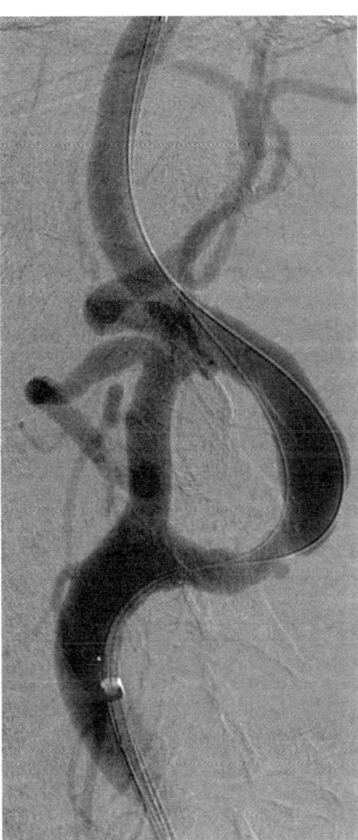

Figure 7 **Use of the "buddy wire" technique to straighten out the carotid bifurcation and allow for delivery of the embolic protection device. Note the two 0.014-inch wires crossing the internal carotid artery lesion.**

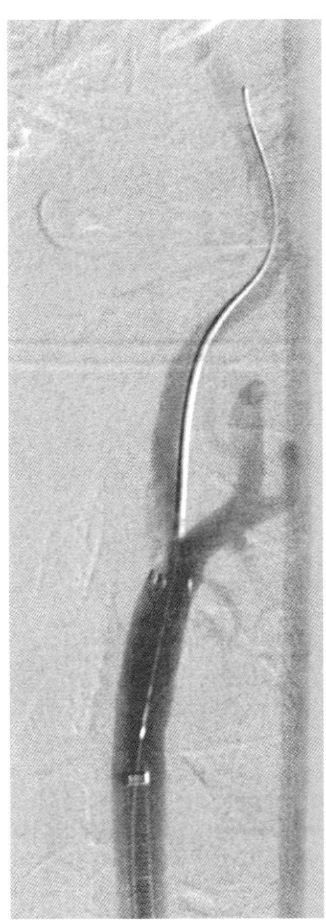

Figure 8 **Deployed distal filter embolic protection device inadvertently pulled down across the target lesion.**

STEP 7: PREDILATION OF LESION

After the EPD has been appropriately deployed in the distal ICA and flow through the filter element is confirmed, the offending lesion is predilated with a 3.5 to 4.0 × 20 mm angioplasty balloon, typically on a monorail or rapid-exchange platform. In most cases, the desired balloon profile can be achieved with relatively low inflation pressures (4 to 6 mm Hg). This balloon angioplasty to the target lesion is performed to allow for easy passage of the stent delivery system across the atherosclerotic plaque. Some data have shown that systemic administration of atropine (0.4 to 1.0 mg) given intravenously prior to balloon angioplasty of the carotid will minimize the effects on the baroreceptors and the clinic manifestation of profound bradycardia or asystole in de novo lesions.[26] After the predilation balloon is removed, another bifurcation angiogram is performed through the sheath to visualize the lesion and confirm continued unimpeded antegrade flow through the filter element.

STEP 8: DEPLOYMENT OF STENT

Once correct positioning has been confirmed, a self-expanding stent is deployed. The diameter of the stent is determined by the diameter of the largest portion of the vessel, which is typically the distal CCA (not the ICA). It is important that there be no unapposed stent in the CCA: any part of the stent that is not apposed to the vessel wall may become a nidus

a *b*

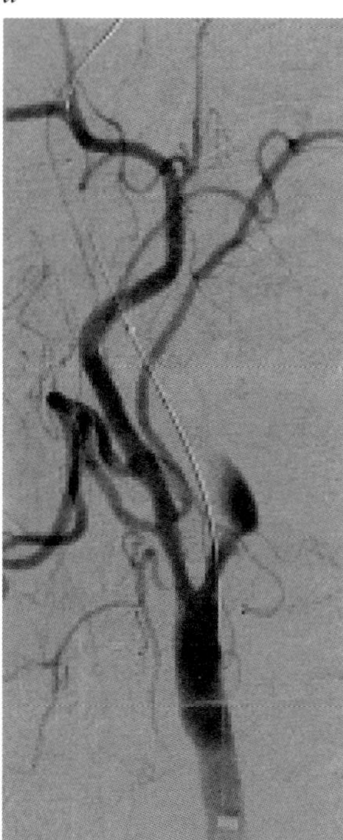

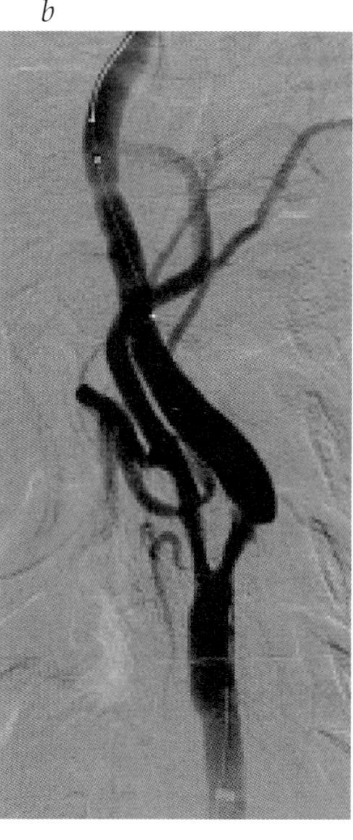

Figure 9 **(*a*) Carotid angiogram after initial angioplasty of the internal carotid artery lesion, showing flow arrest at the level of the embolic protection device (EPD). (*b*) Angiogram after the intra-arterial administration of nitroglycerin to alleviate the severe vasospasm induced by the indwelling EPD. Adequate antegrade flow has been restored through the EPD and the distal internal carotid artery.**

for thrombus formation. The diameter of the unconstrained stent should be at least 10% (approximately 1 to 2 mm) larger than the maximum diameter of the CCA. On occasion, the lesion is limited to the ICA well above the carotid bifurcation; in such cases, a shorter stent confined to the ICA may be used. Current approved self-expanding stents for the carotid artery are either open or closed cell designs. The cell design confers scaffolding and flexibility to the stent such that a closed cell stent is generally more rigid than an open cell stent, but because the stent struts are all interconnected, "fish scaling"—or stent strut protrusion into the lumen—does not occur. Stents also are designed in tapered and nontapered configurations, with the goal of the former being better accommodation to the natural carotid bifurcation. Whether specific stent design systems confer an impact on clinical outcomes remains controversial today, but some speculate that closed cell stents may be associated with a lower periprocedural stroke risk in symptomatic patients treated with CAS.[27]

There are other important points in regard to stent deployment for CAS: (1) a residual stenosis of 10 to 20% is not significant and is best left alone rather than overdilating the vessel; (2) remember that the lesion is longer than what is seen angiographically, so use a longer stent—30 or 40 mm lengths are most commonly used; (3) stenting across the origin of the ECA is very common and will not alter flow into the ECA in the vast majority of cases[28]; and (4) when using a nontapered stent, size the stent according to the CCA so that the stent is not undersized and free-floating in the CCA.

STEP 9: POSTDILATION OF LESION

Generally, the stented lesion is then postdilated with a 5.0 to 5.5 mm × 20 mm balloon; larger balloons are rarely necessary. A residual stenosis of 10 to 20% or so is completely acceptable; the goal of the intervention is protection from embolic stroke, not necessarily a perfect angiographic result.

STEP 10: EPD RETRIEVAL

At the conclusion of the procedure, the filter element needs to be reconstrained and removed. Each manufacturer has a dedicated retrieval device to collapse the filter element and captured debris, which then can be pulled through the stented lesion and removed from the circulation. On occasion, inability to retrieve the filter element can occur because of vessel tortuosity or "fish scaling" of an open cell stent. Some manufacturers provide a catheter with a shapeable tip, whereas others use a tapered tip to allow easy passage through the stented segment. It is important to watch the tip as it passes through the stent to ensure that it does not catch a stent strut and deform the stent or pull down the filter basket. If the catheter does not pass unimpeded, torquing the catheter to alter the tip angle, having the patient turn the head, or advancing the sheath within the stented segment will usually allow the catheter to negotiate through angulated anatomy [*see Figure 10*].

STEP 11: COMPLETION ARTERIOGRAPHY

A completion angiogram of the carotid bulb and bifurcation and the distal extracranial ICA is obtained to verify that no dissection or occlusion has occurred. Severe vasospasm may be encountered (sometimes mimicking dissection); watchful waiting, coupled on occasion with administration of vasodilators through the sheath (e.g., nitroglycerin in 100 μg aliquots), usually resolves this problem. Completion angiography of the carotid bifurcation and intracranial circulation is performed in two views (anterior-posterior and lateral).

STEP 12: ACCESS-SITE HEMOSTASIS

Heparin anticoagulation typically is not reversed. Access-site hemostasis is achieved with a percutaneous closure device or manual compression.

Postoperative Care

After the procedure, the patient is monitored in the recovery area for approximately 30 minutes and then transferred to a monitored floor; admission to an intensive care unit generally is not necessary. In 2 to 3 hours, patients are allowed to ambulate if a closure device was used and are allowed to resume a regular diet. Some patients experience prolonged hypotension from carotid sinus stimulation; this problem can be managed with judicious fluid administration, pharmacologic treatment of bradycardia, and, occasionally, IV infusion of a vasopressor (e.g., dopamine). Rarely, a patient experiences prolonged hypotension that must be treated with an oral agent (e.g., phenylephrine or midodrine).

A duplex ultrasonogram is obtained within the first month of the procedure as a baseline study. Subsequent ultrasound examinations are performed at 6 month and then annually thereafter. Neurologic evaluation is performed according to the same schedule as the duplex

a b

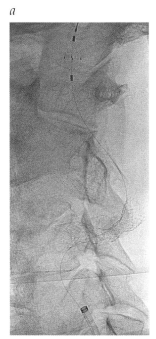

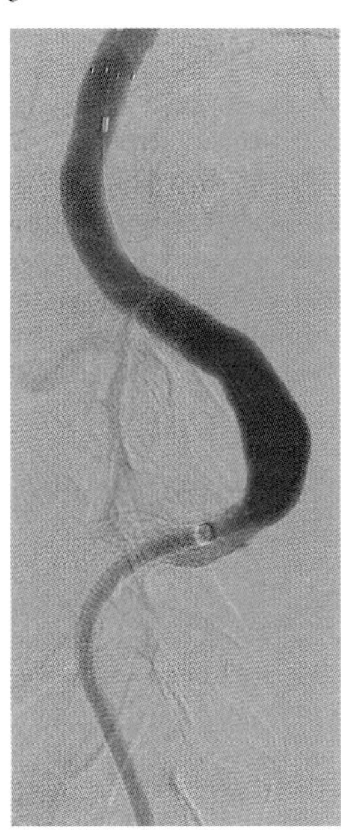

Figure 10 **Severe angulation of the carotid bifurcation. (*a*) X-ray image showing the position of the stent and the distal filter element. (*b*) Advancement of the sheath over the wire and retrieval catheter were necessary to allow for the capture of the embolic protection device.**

studies. Patients are treated with aspirin for life and with clopidogrel for 4 to 6 weeks.

As with CEA, proper patient selection, procedural standardization, and meticulous attention to detail are mandatory for a successful procedure, regardless of the exact technique used for CAS.

Outcome Evaluation

The short-term results of CAS depend largely on the presence or absence of cerebral embolization. It is therefore not surprising that the addition of cerebral protection to CAS appears to have reduced the stroke risk associated with the procedure. Admittedly, however, ongoing technological developments have created something of a moving target, making evaluation of the results of CAS difficult at best.

In a study from the University of Alabama at Birmingham and Lenox Hill Hospital in New York, 604 arteries were treated in 528 consecutive patients over a 5-year period.[29] CAS was performed both with balloon-expandable stents and with self-expanding stents and both with and without cerebral protection devices. The overall 30-day combined stroke-death rate was 8.1% (minor stroke, 5.5%; major stroke, 1.6%; nonneurologic death, 1%). On a year-by-year basis, the risk of stroke and death reached its maximum (12.5%) in the period ending in September 1997 and fell to its minimum (3.2%) the following year. This rather dramatic change in results from one year to the next probably is attributable to technical advances (e.g., in protection devices, stents, and guide wires), as well as to improvements in the investigators' ability to select appropriate patients for intervention.

A subsequent report describes the authors' experience with CAS in a vascular surgery practice.[30] During a 40-month period from 1997 to 2001, 135 procedures were performed in 132 patients, most (60%) of whom were asymptomatic. The rate of complications was acceptable (2%), and only one patient had a significant restenosis at follow-up (mean follow-up interval, 16 months). Perhaps more important, these 132 patients represented 41% of all patients being treated for carotid disease in this practice. This percentage seems extraordinarily high, but it may simply be a bellwether of things to come in the practice of vascular surgery, and it underscores the importance of multispecialty involvement in this new technology.

The results of the SAPPHIRE trial of CAS in high-risk patients were published in 2004.[31] To date, this trial, which included 334 patients randomly assigned to either CAS (n = 167) or CEA (n = 167), is the only industry-sponsored, FDA-approved trial that was actually randomized. A separate registry of nonrandomized patients was compiled that included those who were felt to be at unacceptably high risk for CEA and therefore underwent CAS (n = 406), as well as those who were not suitable candidates for CAS and therefore underwent CEA (n = 7). The goal of the SAPPHIRE trial was to evaluate the combined end point of major adverse events (stroke, death, and MI). Patients were independently evaluated by a certified neurologist before and after the procedure. The majority of the randomized patients were asymptomatic: in the CAS group, only 30% were symptomatic, and in the CEA group, only 28% were symptomatic. A key point to keep in mind is that this trial was designed to test the idea that CAS was not inferior to CEA, not to establish that CAS was superior to CEA or CEA to CAS. At 30 days, the risk of stroke was not significantly different in the two groups (CAS, 3.6%; CEA 3.1%). Two patients in the CAS group (1.2%) and four patients in the CEA group (2.5%) died within 30 days; this difference did not reach statistical significance (p = .39). More patients experienced periprocedural MI in the CEA group (6.1%) than in the CAS group (2.4%), a difference that did not reach statistical significance on the basis of intent to treat. Notably, most of the MIs were non-Q MIs, identified by routine postprocedural laboratory studies. The incidence of the combined end point (stroke-death-MI) was higher in the CEA group (9.8%) than in the CAS group (4.8%), but this difference was statistically insignificant as well. These results have been used to support FDA approval of the stent and filter protection device used in this important study.

Detracting from the growing successful reported outcomes of CAS are two recent prospective randomized European studies evaluating the 30-day death and stroke rates among symptomatic patients treated with either CAS or CEA.[32,33] The first one, Endarterectomy versus Stenting in Patients with Symptomatic Severe Carotid Stenosis (EVA-3S), randomized 527 patients with symptomatic 60% or greater carotid stenosis. The investigators reported a 30-day combined stroke and death rate of 3.9% after CEA compared with 9.6% after CAS. Unfortunately, the conclusions of this study have been heavily criticized because of several flaws: (1) insufficient interventionalist training and experience, (2) lack of mandated periprocedural dual antiplatelet use for CAS, and (3) skewed institutional enrolment. Published in the same year were the results from the Stent-Supported Percutaneous Angioplasty of the Carotid Artery versus Endarterectomy (SPACE) trial, which randomized 1,183 symptomatic patients with 50% or greater carotid stenosis. The reported 30-day ipsilateral stroke and death outcomes were 6.34% following CEA and 6.84% after CAS. Although this study is admirable because of the large number of patients enrolled and the rigorous oversight of both surgeons and interventionalists, two critical design flaws weaken the conclusions: (1) nearly 70% of CAS procedures were performed without the use of an EPD and (2) the category of carotid stenosis (∃ 50%) was rather broad.

As it stands today, CAS with EPD is a useful option for the treatment of symptomatic carotid artery disease in a subset of patients (i.e., recurrent carotid stenosis, prior external beam neck irradiation, class III or IV CHF, or difficult anatomic circumstances). What remains to be determined is the role of CAS in asymptomatic patients, standard-risk patients, and our growing elderly population.

Dr. Eskandari is a consultant for Cordis.

References

1. Beneficial effect of carotid endarterectomy in symptomatic patients with high-grade carotid stenosis. North American Symptomatic Carotid Endarterectomy Trial Collaborators. N Engl J Med 1991;325:445–53.
2. Endarterectomy for asymptomatic carotid artery stenosis. Executive Committee for the Asymptomatic Carotid Atherosclerosis Study. JAMA 1995;273:1421–8.
3. Hobson RW 2nd, Mackey WC, Ascher E, et al. Management of atherosclerotic carotid artery disease: clinical practice guidelines of the Society for Vascular Surgery. J Vasc Surg 2008;48:480–6.
4. Menzoian JO. Presidential address: carotid endarterectomy, under attack again! J Vasc Surg 2003;37:1137–41.
5. [illegible] High-risk carotid endarterectomy: fact or fiction. J Vasc Surg 2003;37:40–6.
6. Jordan WD Jr, Alcocer F, Wirthlin DJ, et al. High-risk carotid endarterectomy: challenges for carotid stent protocols. J Vasc Surg 2002;35:16–21; discussion 22.
7. Mozes G, Sullivan TM, Torres-Russotto DR, et al. Carotid endarterectomy in SAPPHIRE-eligible high-risk patients: implications for selecting patients for carotid angioplasty and stenting. J Vasc Surg 2004;39:958–65; discussion 965–6.
8. Ouriel K, Hertzer NR, Beven EG, et al. Preprocedural risk stratification: identifying an appropriate population for carotid stenting. J Vasc Surg 2001;33:728–32.
9. Eskandari MK, Najjar SF, Matsumura JS, et al. Technical limitations of carotid filter embolic protection devices. Ann Vasc Surg 2007;21:403–7.
10. Gaunt ME, Martin PJ, Smith JL, et al. Clinical relevance of intraoperative embolization detected by transcranial Doppler ultrasonography during carotid endarterectomy: a prospective study of 100 patients. Br J Surg 1994;81:1435–9.
11. Fearn SJ, Pole R, Wesnes K, et al. Cerebral injury during cardiopulmonary bypass: emboli impair memory. J Thorac Cardiovasc Surg 2001;121:1150–60.
12. Rapp JH, Pan XM, Sharp FR, et al. Atheroemboli to the brain: size threshold for causing acute neuronal cell death. J Vasc Surg 2000;32:68–76.
13. Ohki T, Marin ML, Lyon RT, et al. Ex vivo human carotid artery bifurcation stenting: correlation of lesion characteristics with embolic potential. J Vasc Surg 1998;27:463–71.
14. Bicknell CD, Cowling MG, Clark MW, et al. Carotid angioplasty in a pulsatile flow model: factors affecting embolic potential. Eur J Vasc Endovasc Surg 2003;26:22–31.
15. Tubler T, Schluter M, Dirsch O, et al. Balloon-protected carotid artery stenting: relationship of periprocedural neurological complications with the size of particulate debris. Circulation 2001;104:2791–6.
16. Al-Mubarak N, Roubin GS, Vitek JJ, et al. Effect of the distal-balloon protection system on microembolization during carotid stenting. Circulation 2001;104:1999–2002.
17. [illegible] Randomized trial of a distal embolic protection device during percutaneous intervention of saphenous vein aorto-coronary bypass grafts. Circulation 2002;105:1285–90.
18. Coggia M, Goeau-Brissonniere O, Duval JL, et al. Embolic risk of the different stages of carotid bifurcation balloon angioplasty: an experimental study. J Vasc Surg 2000;31:550–7.
19. Eskandari MK. Design and development of mechanical embolic protection devices. Expert Rev Med Devices 2006;3:387–93.
20. Theron J, Raymond J, Casasco A, Courtheoux F. Percutaneous angioplasty of atherosclerotic and postsurgical stenosis of carotid arteries. AJNR Am J Neuroradiol 1987;8:495–500.
21. Theron J, Courtheoux P, Alachkar F, et al. New triple coaxial catheter system for carotid angioplasty with cerebral protection. AJNR Am J Neuroradiol 1990;11:869–74; discussion 875–7.
22. Al-Mubarak N, Vitek JJ, Iyer S, et al. Embolization via collateral circulation during carotid stenting with the distal balloon protection system. J Endovasc Ther 2001;8:354–7.
23. Whitlow PL, Lylyk P, Londero H, et al. Carotid artery stenting protected with an emboli containment system. Stroke 2002;33:1308–14.
24. Reimers B, Corvaja N, Moshiri S, et al. Cerebral protection with filter devices during carotid artery stenting. Circulation 2001;104:12–5.
25. Ohki T, Parodi J, Veith FJ, et al. Efficacy of a proximal occlusion catheter with reversal of flow in the prevention of embolic events during carotid artery stenting: an experimental analysis. J Vasc Surg 2001;33:504–9.
26. Cayne NS, Faries PL, Trocciola SM, et al. Carotid angioplasty and stent-induced bradycardia and hypotension: impact of prophylactic atropine administration and prior carotid endarterectomy. J Vasc Surg 2005;41:956–61.
27. Bosiers M, de Donatoy G, Deloose K, et al. Does free cell area influence the outcome in carotid artery stenting? Eur J Vasc Endovasc Surg 2007;33:135–41; discussion 142–3.
28. Woo EY, Karmacharya J, Velazquez OC, et al. Differential effects of carotid artery stenting versus carotid endarterectomy on [illegible] carotid artery patency. J Endovasc Ther [illegible]
29. Roubin GS, New G, Iyer SS, et al. Immediate and late clinical outcomes of carotid artery stenting in patients with symptomatic and asymptomatic carotid artery stenosis: a 5-year prospective analysis. Circulation 2001;103:532–7.
30. Criado FJ, Lingelbach JM, Ledesma DF, Lucas PR. Carotid artery stenting in a vascular surgery practice. J Vasc Surg 2002;35:430–4.
31. Yadav JS, Wholey MH, Kuntz RE, et al. Protected carotid-artery stenting versus endarterectomy in high-risk patients. N Engl J Med 2004;351:1493–501.
32. Ringleb PA, Allenberg J, Bruckmann H, et al. 30 day results from the SPACE trial of stent-protected angioplasty versus carotid endarterectomy in symptomatic patients: a randomised non-inferiority trial. Lancet 2006;368:1239–47.
33. Mas JL, Chatellier G, Beyssen B, et al. Endarterectomy versus stenting in patients with symptomatic severe carotid stenosis. N Engl J Med 2006;355:1660–71.

Acknowledgment

The author wishes to acknowledge Timothy M. Sullivan, MD, for his contributions to the previous rendition of this chapter on which he has based this update.

11 REPAIR OF INFRARENAL ABDOMINAL AORTIC ANEURYSMS

*James Sampson, MD, and William D. Jordan Jr, MD**

An arterial aneurysm is a permanent localized dilation of an artery having at least a 50% increase in diameter compared with the expected normal diameter of the reference artery.[1] For the infrarenal abdominal aorta, an aneurysm typically equates with a diameter of at least 3 cm. Lesser degrees of enlargement are often referred to as ectasia, whereas arteriomegaly describes diffuse enlargement throughout the arterial tree. Aneurysms may be classified by location, morphology, and etiology. The infrarenal aorta is the most common site of aneurysm development. Most aneurysms are fusiform, involving the entire circumference of the artery, whereas saccular aneurysms are more focal enlargements along one wall of the artery. The etiology may be degenerative, inflammatory, infectious, or congenital. False or pseudoaneurysms are defined by a lack of a complete arterial wall at the location of enlargement and are typically posttraumatic or anastomotic.

Aneurysms are most often sporadic, but familial associations have been noted in 11 to 19% of cases.[2] Aneurysms may also be found in patients with connective tissue disorders such as Marfan syndrome (mutation of the *FBN1* gene on chromosome 15 encoding fibrillin-1), Ehlers-Danlos syndrome type IV (mutation of the *COL3A1* gene on chromosome 2 encoding type III collagen), or Loeys-Dietz syndrome (mutations of genes encoding transforming growth factor–β receptors A and B located on chromosomes 9 and 3). Aneurysms occur with advancing age and are four to five times more common in men than in women. The primary modifiable risk factor for the development of aneurysms is smoking, with the duration of smoking considered to be of the greatest importance. Although aneurysmal disease shares risk factors with atherosclerosis, the pathogenesis is thought to be distinct. Of note, diabetes is associated with a decreased risk of aneurysm development, progression, and/or rupture.[3,4]

Rupture is the feared outcome of abdominal aortic aneurysms (AAAs), resulting in death in the majority of patients who suffer this complication. Aneurysms were accountable for 13,000 deaths in the United States in 2009.[5] The risk of rupture is recognized to be most directly associated with aneurysm size. Laplace's law states that wall tension is exponentially proportional to the radius of the vessel; therefore, as the aneurysm expands, the tension increases as the wall thins and weakens. Additional risk factors for rupture include current smoking, female gender, low forced expiratory volume in 1 second (FEV_1), and increased aneurysm size on initial detection.[6,7] Screening has been shown to reduce aneurysm-related mortality and remain cost-effective over time.[8,9] Although recent epidemiologic evidence suggests that the incidence of aneurysms may be declining,[10] it remains a significant public health issue, such that the U.S. Preventive Services Task Force recommends "one-time screening for abdominal aortic aneurysm by ultrasonography in men aged 65-75 who have ever smoked."[11] This recommendation is further backed by the inclusion of a Medicare benefit to cover one-time screening in men ages 65 to 75 years with a family history of aneurysm or a history of smoking at least 100 cigarettes.

The decision to undertake repair of an AAA is based on a variety of factors. Fundamental to this is an assessment of the relative risks of repair versus the ongoing risk of rupture. In a review of patients who refused or were felt to be unfit for repair, the 1-year rupture risk of aneurysms 5.5 to 5.9 cm in size was found to be 9.2%.[12] Mortality for elective open repair is reported between 3 and 5%, with even better results for endovascular repair. Therefore, there is a general consensus that aneurysms 5.5 cm and larger should be treated in most patients considered fit for surgery. The management of smaller aneurysms, between 4 and 5.5 cm, has been the subject of widespread and intense research over the past two decades. Two studies, the UK Small Aneurysm Trial[13] and the Aneurysm Detection and Management Trial,[14] showed low rupture rates and equivalent long-term survival for both early open repair and surveillance groups. However, in these trials, about half of the patients in the surveillance group developed an indication for intervention such as aneurysm growth to greater than 5.5 cm. Comparisons of endovascular aneurysm repair (EVAR) with surveillance for small aneurysms have also shown equivalent long-term outcomes and frequent progression to repair in those patients in the surveillance groups, especially those with larger aneurysms on initial detection.[15,16] Considering the low morbidity and mortality with endovascular treatment and occasional loss of suitability for endovascular repair in those patients in the surveillance group, these studies prompted consideration of endovascular repair for healthy patients with aneurysms of 5 cm or greater. In light of these findings, the Society for Vascular Surgery recommends surveillance for most patients with aneurysms of 4 to 5.5 cm but considers female, younger, and fit patients most likely to benefit from early intervention and advocates for continued research to identify those groups most likely to benefit from early repair.[17]

The optimal type of repair for each patient also depends on several factors but rests primarily on the anatomic features of the aneurysm and regional vasculature. Randomized trials comparing open and endovascular treatment

* The authors and editors gratefully acknowledge the contributions of the previous authors, Frank R. Arko, MD, Stephen T. Smith, MD, and Christopher K. Zarins, MD, FACS, to the development and writing of this chapter.

have shown early survival advantage to those treated with EVAR,[18,19] and although these studies found convergence of survival through intermediate follow-up, recent publications have reported persistence of this survival advantage beyond 5 years.[20,21] Compared with open aneurysm repair, EVAR is associated with a higher risk of additional procedures to correct aneurysm-related complications such as endoleaks. Fortunately, these complications can usually be treated using endovascular options. On balance, for the majority of patients in whom anatomy is suitable, endovascular repair is the preferred treatment.

Preoperative Evaluation and Optimization

Although aneurysm surveillance is most frequently performed with duplex ultrasonography, computed tomographic (CT) angiography is most useful for detailed anatomic evaluation required for operative planning of both open and endovascular repair. This imaging allows detailed evaluation of the extent of the aneurysm, the presence and extent of thrombus, calcification and burden of disease of the aorta, and characterization of renal, visceral, and iliac arteries. Based on this information, decisions can be made regarding the suitability of endovascular repair and the type and size of device preferred for treatment. If open repair is planned, the approach and extent of exposure, graft size and type, and clamp sites can be planned. Once the decision has been made to pursue treatment, patient optimization should be pursued to limit operative morbidity and mortality. Many patients with an AAA will have concomitant coronary artery disease and chronic obstructive pulmonary disease, and these conditions deserve routine consideration. Chronic kidney disease, diabetes, and anemia/thrombocytopenia have been linked to poor outcomes after AAA repair and, therefore, also require investigation and attention. Current guidelines recommend deferral of aneurysm treatment for active cardiac conditions (unstable angina, recent myocardial infarction, active congestive heart failure, significant arrhythmia, or severe valvular disease). Additional cardiac testing may be considered for those patients with three or more risk factors (previous myocardial infarction, previous congestive heart failure, diabetes mellitus, renal insufficiency, or mild angina pectoris) or those with poor functional capacity in whom the results of testing may alter management.[22] Medical management of cardiac disease in the perioperative period should include continuation of beta blockade in those previously treated and initiation of beta blockade in those patients who have or are at risk for coronary disease.[22–24] Likewise, statins are frequently indicated in patients with aneurysmal disease and have been found to be beneficial in reducing perioperative events in vascular patients.[25–27] Finally, aspirin is generally considered to be safe and beneficial to continue in the perioperative period even considering the potential increased bleeding risk associated with its antiplatelet effects.[23]

Patients with chronic pulmonary disease should be optimized prior to elective aneurysm repair. Room air arterial blood gas and pulmonary function testing may be useful to identify those patients at greatest risk and for whom pulmonary consultation may be helpful. For many, the greatest impact on perioperative pulmonary morbidity would come from cessation of smoking at least 2 weeks prior to repair. Bronchodilator therapy has also been advocated to reduce perioperative pulmonary complications.

Renal dysfunction has been found to be associated with a higher risk of postoperative complications but similar mortality after aneurysm repair.[28] Chronic kidney disease is of additional concern due to the need for intravenous (IV) contrast during preoperative investigation of aneurysms, during endovascular repair, and potentially during surveillance. Although a large review has found no significant increase in the rate of decline of renal function after EVAR versus open surgical repair or observation,[29] measures to limit the impact of aneurysm repair and IV contrast administration should be considered. Specifically, limitation of contrast, preoperative hydration to euvolemia, withholding angiotensin-converting enzyme inhibitors or angiotensin receptor blockers, and avoiding additional nephrotoxic agents in the perioperative period should be routine.

Diabetes mellitus, anemia, and thrombocytopenia have been associated with poor outcomes after aneurysm repair.[30–32] Perioperative management of diabetic patients should follow established guidelines of blood glucose control at or below 180 mg/dL. Anemia and thrombocytopenia should be corrected prior to elective operation.

Operative Planning

Once adequate imaging has been obtained and the patient has been optimized for intervention, decisions can be made regarding the approach to repair. Endovascular suitability depends primarily on the size, length, and quality of the proximal (aortic neck) and distal (iliac arteries) seal zones. The size and quality of the common femoral and iliac arteries must also be suitable for device delivery into the aorta, although most contemporary devices have a small enough delivery profile to deliver through diseased or small iliac access vessels. Multiple endovascular devices exist to allow selection based on aneurysm characteristics or surgeon preference, each with detailed indications for use that describe the anatomic requirements for optimal performance.

Endovascular Repair

TECHNIQUE

After review of appropriate imaging and device selection, an optimized patient may be brought to the operating room for repair. A choice of regional or general anesthesia may be employed, but general anesthesia is typically preferred to ensure patient comfort and optimal imaging. One technique for endovascular repair is described here: femoral access is obtained by percutaneous access or limited exposure of the common femoral arteries, controlling them with umbilical tapes to assist with hemostasis after sheath exchanges. Depending on device characteristics, percutaneous access may be preferred, specifically on the side contralateral to delivery of the main body of the device, where the device profile is likely significantly reduced. Once adequate access has been obtained, the patient is systemically heparinized and sheaths are introduced into the common femoral arteries. A measuring tape is placed on the patient's abdomen, and an aortogram is obtained with a marked pigtail catheter [*see Figure 1*]. In addition to standard angiography, the aorta and iliac arteries may be evaluated with intravascular ultrasonography (IVUS) [*see Figure 2, Figure 3, Figure 4, and Figure 5*]. If employed, this modality allows cross-sectional measurement at the proximal seal zone and again in the distal landing zone [*see Figure 6, Figure 7, Figure 8, Figure 9, and Figure 10*]. Treatment length may also be estimated using the IVUS catheter by marking the catheter position during withdrawal from the aortic neck. Ultimately, a device is chosen and prepared for introduction. The device is introduced over a stiff guide wire under fluoroscopic guidance to ensure smooth advancement through the iliac arteries and into the aorta. The device is advanced to just beyond the anticipated position of deployment, and the fluoroscopy unit is positioned to account for angulation of the aortic neck and orientation of the renal arteries. Magnified aortography is performed to confirm the ideal landing zone and proper device positioning [*see Figure 11*]. The pigtail catheter is withdrawn into the distal aorta, any required positional adjustments are made, and the device is deployed to the level of release of the contralateral gate [*see Figure 12 and Figure 13*]. Next, the pigtail catheter is withdrawn over a guide wire and the contralateral gate is accessed with a wire and catheter. This maneuver can be challenging and typically requires an angled-tip glide wire and a directional catheter. Successful cannulation of the contralateral gate may require adjustments of the fluoroscopy angle and the use of double-curved catheters. Angiography or IVUS should be used to confirm proper positioning within the endograft [*see Figure 14 and Figure 15*]. The contralateral iliac system is then evaluated with either angiography or IVUS to determine limb length and diameter requirements [*see Figure 16*]. Angiography may be performed via retrograde sheath injection [*see Figure 17*]. Contralateral anterior-oblique imaging may be helpful in precisely identifying the origin of the internal iliac artery. Once an appropriate contralateral limb is chosen, it is introduced over a stiff guide wire under fluoroscopic guidance [*see Figure 18*], positioned, and deployed [*see Figure 19*]. Attention then returns to the main body device, and deployment of the ipsilateral limb is completed. The proximal seal zones, device interfaces, and distal seal zones are routinely ballooned to ensure complete expansion and seal [*see Figure 20, Figure 21, Figure 22, and Figure 23*]. Next, the pigtail catheter is positioned just proximal to the graft and completion aortography is performed [*see Figure 24*]. This imaging series is allowed to run for an extended period to detect any late endoleak. If satisfactory, the catheters and wires are removed and a final radiograph is obtained to establish a baseline device position for future comparison during surveillance [*see Figure 25*]. Next, the femoral sheaths are removed; the femoral arteries are flushed and repaired. After the feet are evaluated to ensure good

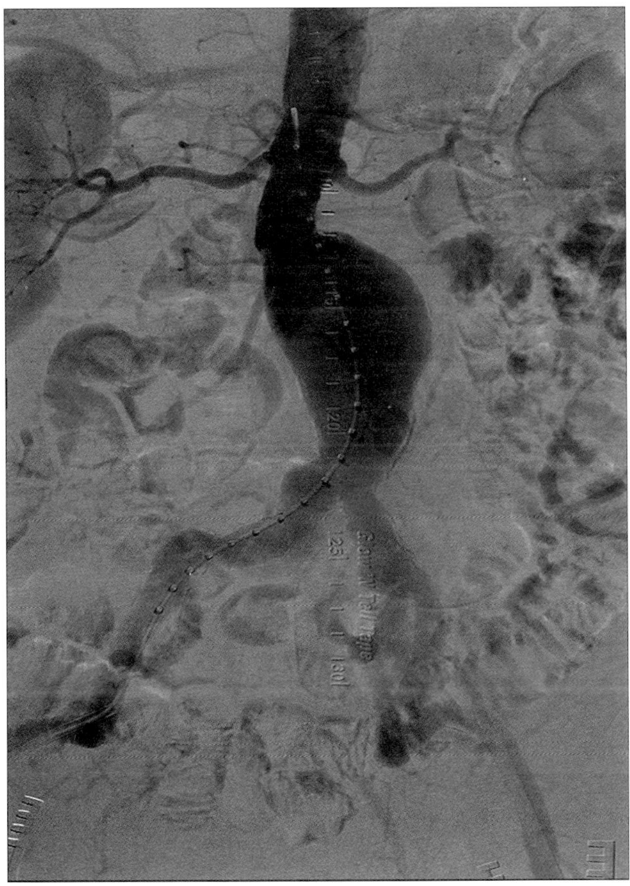

Figure 1 **Aortic angiogram pretreatment.**

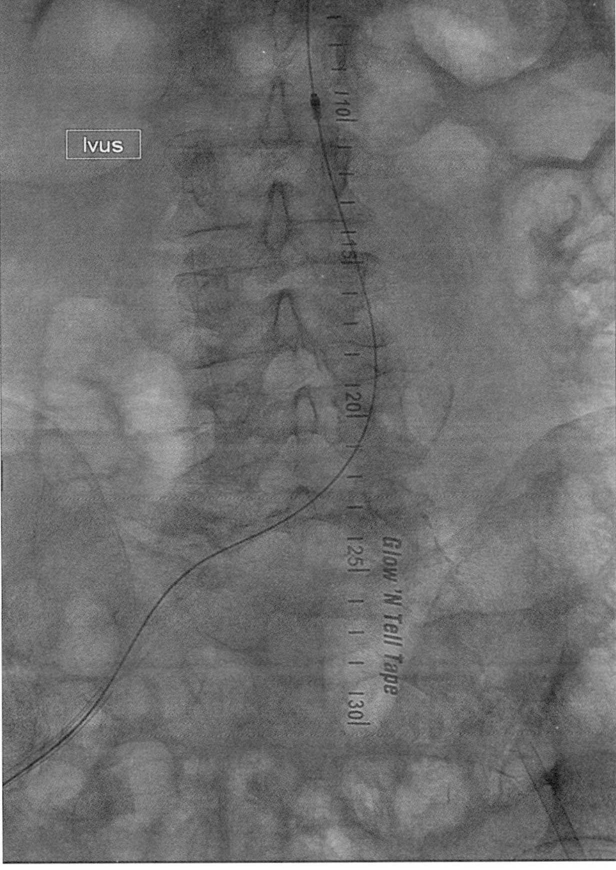

Figure 2 **Angiogram: intravascular ultrasound catheter at the level of the renal arteries.**

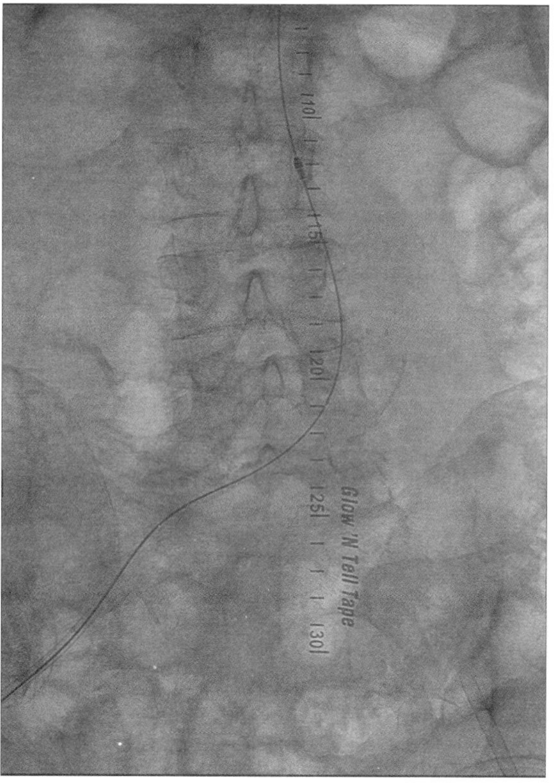

Figure 3 Angiogram: intravascular ultrasound catheter 2 cm distal to the renal arteries.

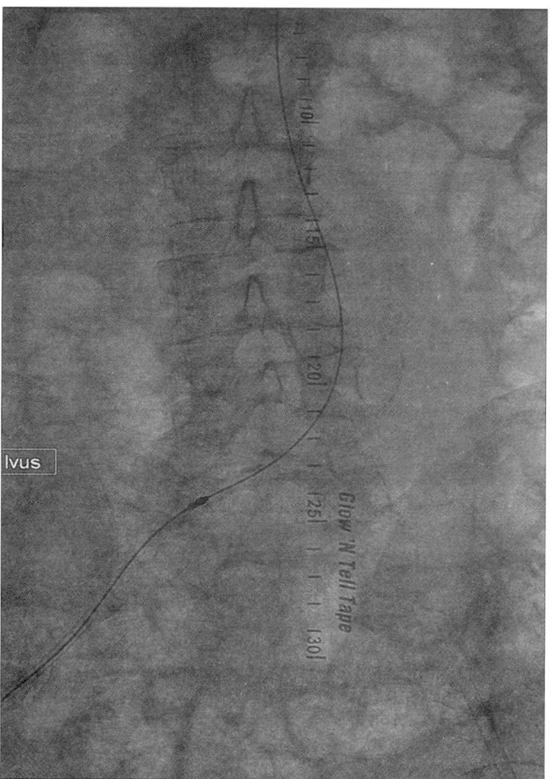

Figure 4 Angiogram: intravascular ultrasound catheter at the right common iliac artery.

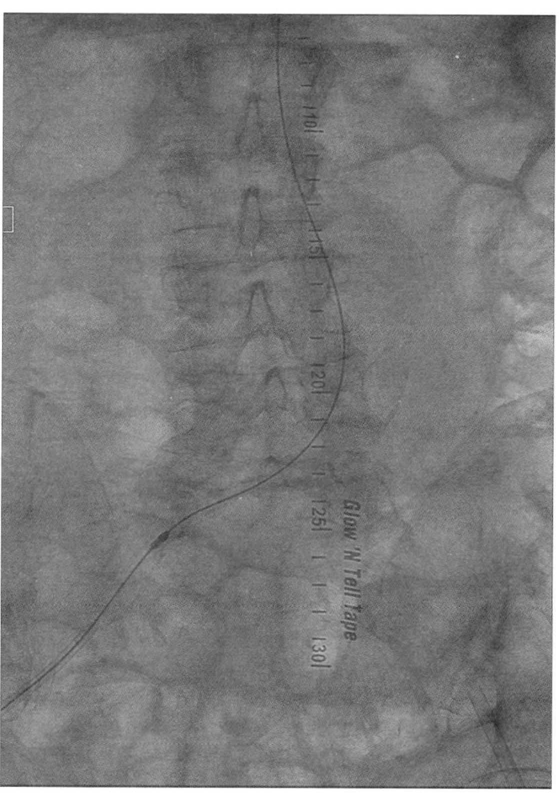

Figure 5 Angiogram: intravascular ultrasound catheter 1 cm distal to the right common iliac artery origin.

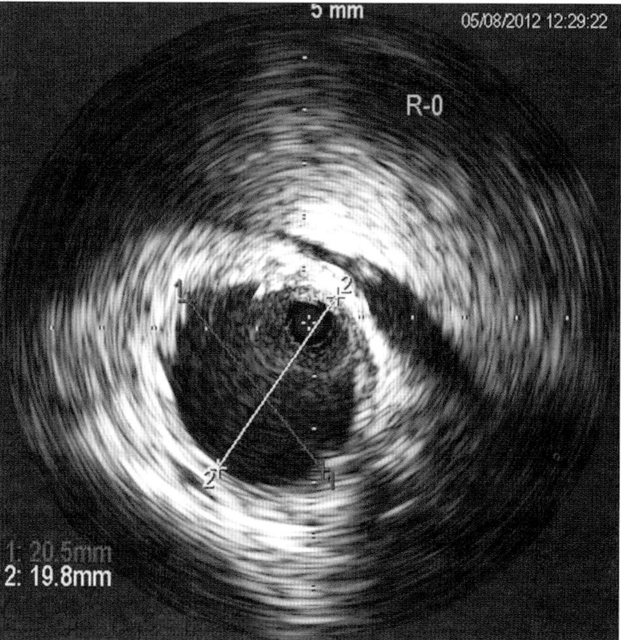

Figure 6 Cross-sectional measurements of the aortic neck at the level of the renal arteries.

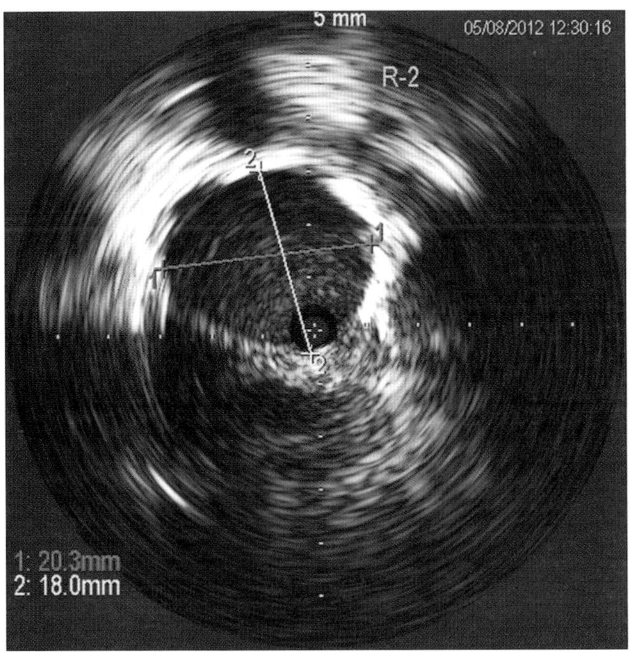

Figure 7 **Cross-sectional measurements of the aortic neck 2 cm distal to the renal arteries.**

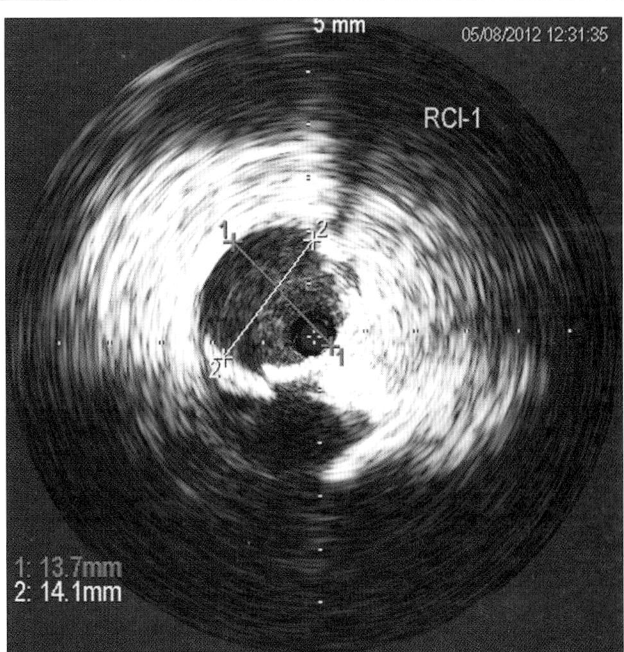

Figure 9 **Intravascular sonogram: cross-sectional measurements of the right common iliac artery.**

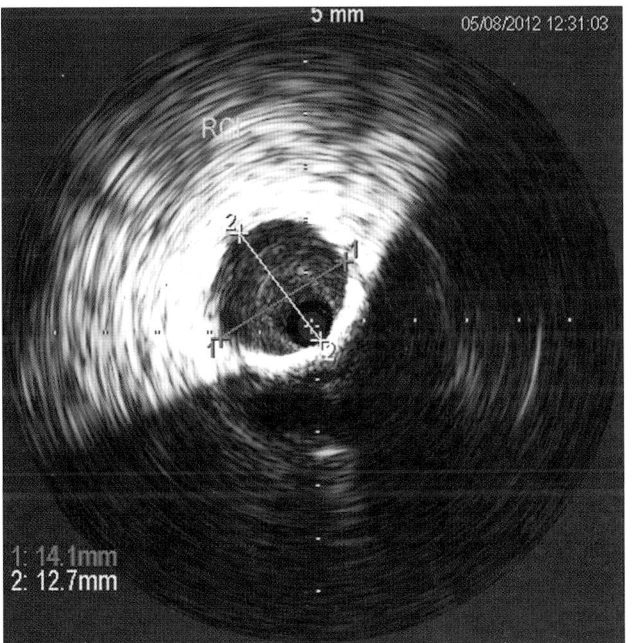

Figure 8 **Intravascular sonogram: cross-sectional measurements of the right common iliac artery.**

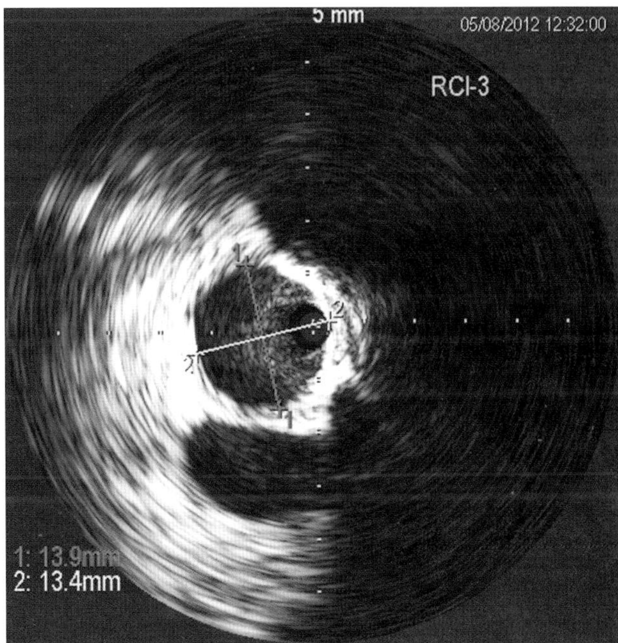

Figure 10 **Intravascular sonogram: cross-sectional measurements of the right common iliac artery.**

distal perfusion and no signs of embolization, heparin may be reversed, the wounds are closed, and the patient is allowed to emerge from anesthesia. Postoperatively, the patient is allowed full mobilization and diet later on the operative day. Discharge criteria are often met on postoperative day 1 or 2.

SPECIAL CONSIDERATIONS

Iliac disease, whether aneurysmal or occlusive, can present special challenges to endovascular repair of aortic aneurysms. Several options exist to meet these challenges. For common and/or internal iliac artery aneurysms, treatment may require embolization of the internal iliac artery

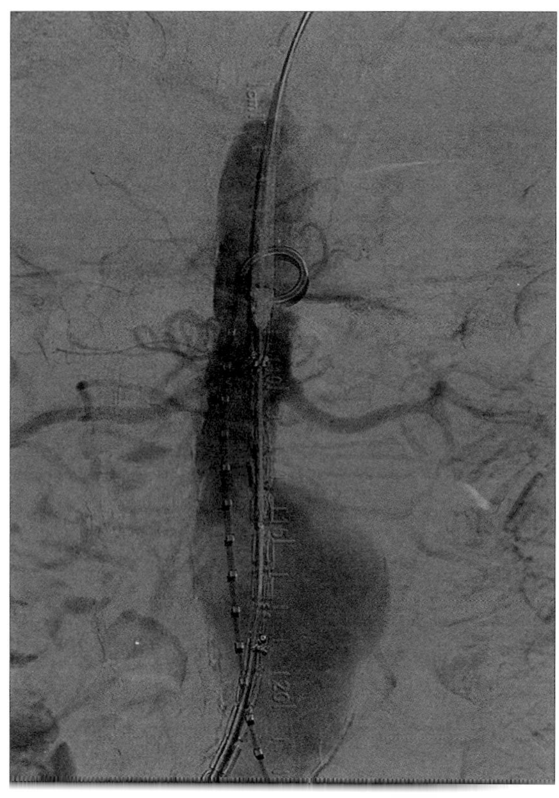

Figure 11 Angiogram: stent graft positioned prior to deployment, magnified view.

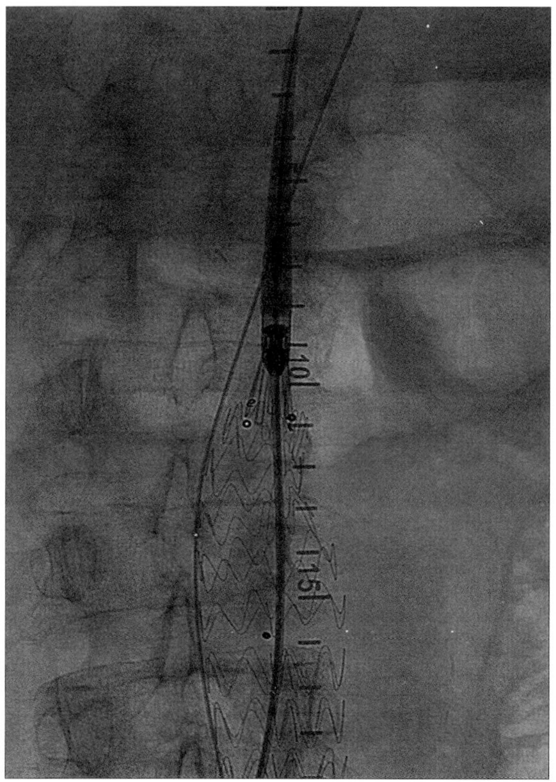

Figure 12 Angiogram: initial stent graft deployment.

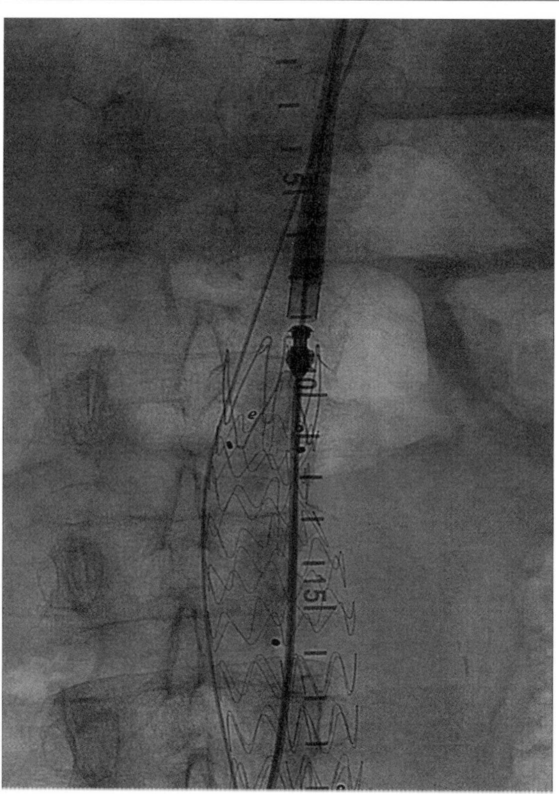

Figure 13 Angiogram: stent graft deployment, release of suprarenal fixation.

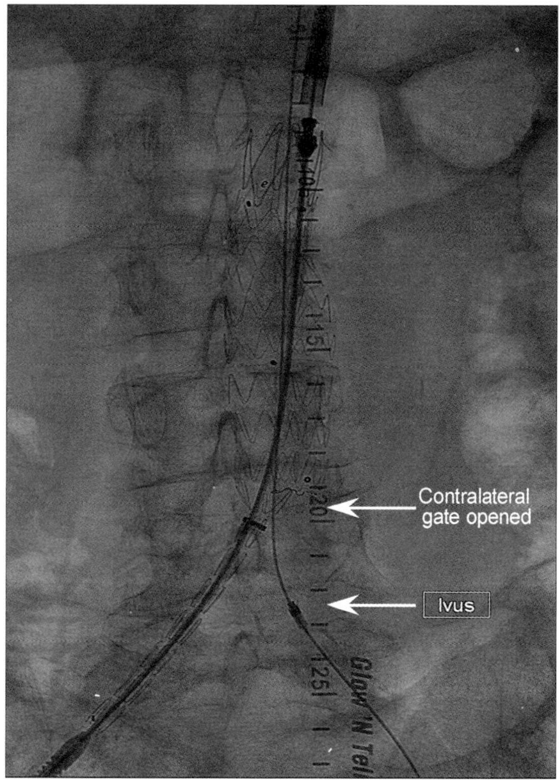

Figure 14 Angiogram: stent graft partially deployed. Contralateral gate access and confirmation with intravascular ultrasonography.

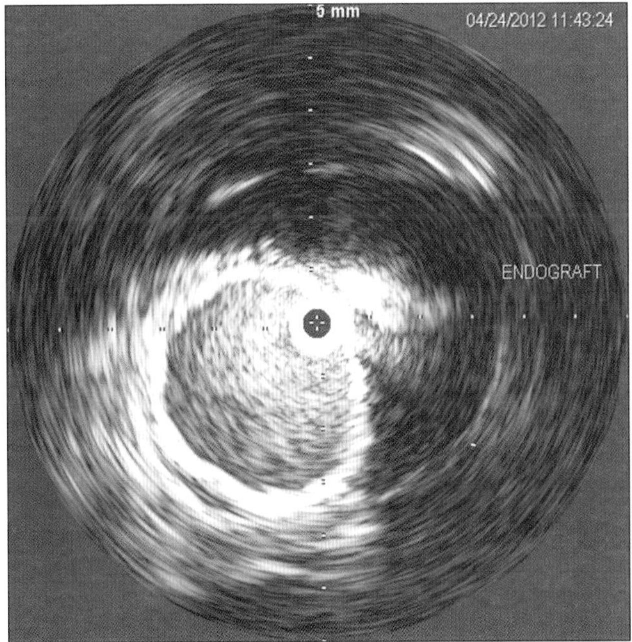

Figure 15 **Intravascular sonogram: confirmation of position within the stent graft.**

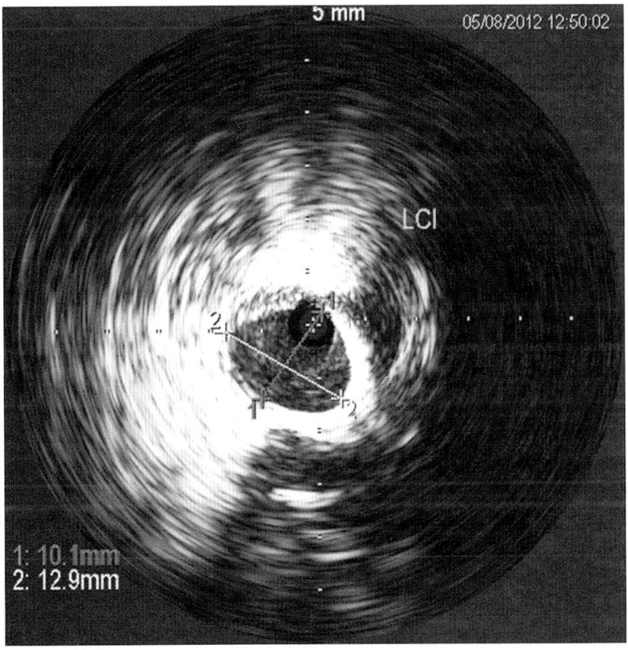

Figure 16 **Intravascular sonogram: cross-sectional measurements of the left common iliac artery.**

and extension of the endograft into the external iliac artery [*see Figure 26, Figure 27, Figure 28, and Figure 29*]. If both sides must be similarly treated, these interventions should be staged over several weeks to limit symptoms and risks from pelvic ischemia. Alternatively, hypogastric flow may be maintained through a "snorkel" technique, where a covered stent is deployed from the external iliac into the internal iliac artery alongside the iliac graft limb, which is deployed

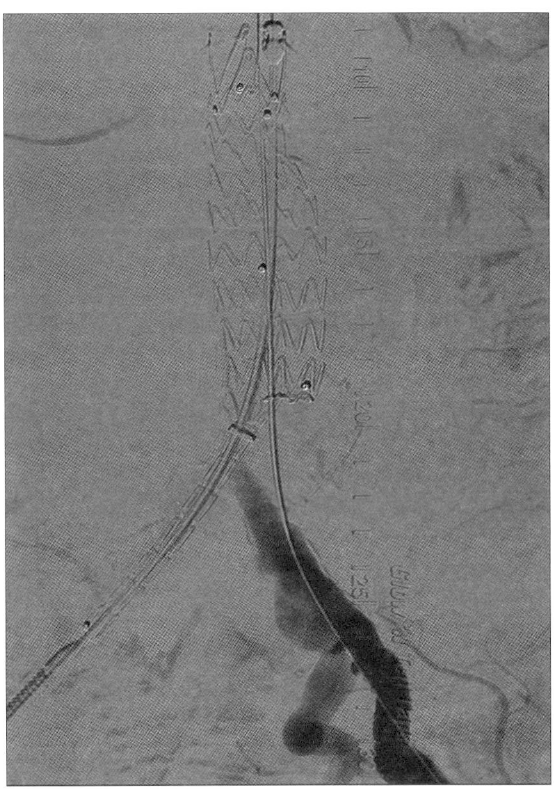

Figure 17 **Angiogram. Retrograde sheath injection into contralateral iliac system after partial deployment of the stent-graft.**

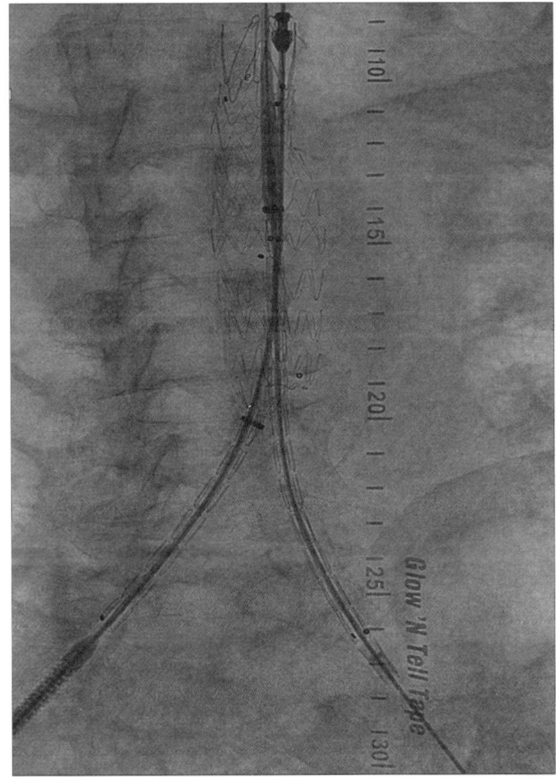

Figure 18 **Angiogram: positioning of the contralateral limb (*left*).**

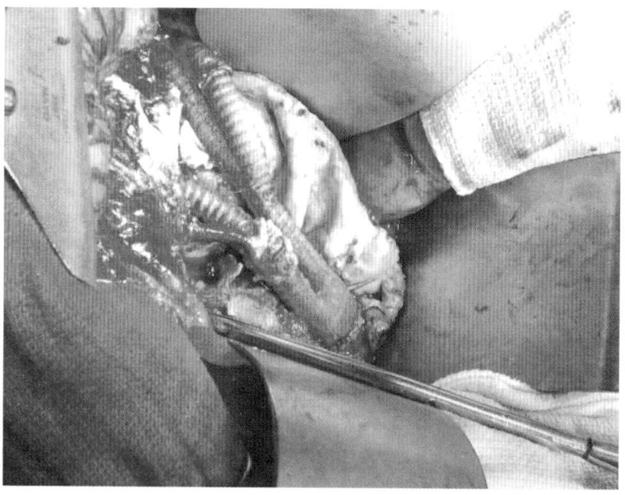

Figure 31 **Open surgical repair of an infrarenal abdominal aortic aneurysm including patch reimplantation of the inferior mesenteric artery. Also note the right external iliac and internal iliac limbs.**

graft, followed by closure of the retroperitoneum to exclude the graft from contact with the bowel [*see Figure 32 and Figure 33*]. If there is insufficient aneurysm sac or retroperitoneal tissue, an omental pedicle may be mobilized and used for graft coverage. The bowel is then returned to its normal anatomic position and inspected to confirm adequate perfusion prior to closure of the abdominal wall. Postoperatively, patients are routinely monitored in the intensive care unit for the initial postoperative period. Epidural analgesia is continued for 48 to 72 hours, and gastric drainage is used selectively beyond the first postoperative day.

SURVEILLANCE

After open repair, patients are typically evaluated in the clinic after several weeks to ensure proper wound healing and progress of recovery. Beyond this, patients may be monitored for the development of incisional hernia and should be considered for imaging with ultrasonography or CT at 5 years to evaluate for the aneurysmal degeneration of other areas of the aortic system such as the visceral aortic segment or iliac degeneration. Continued surveillance for aortic pathology should be considered based on imaging findings and the general clinical status of each patient.

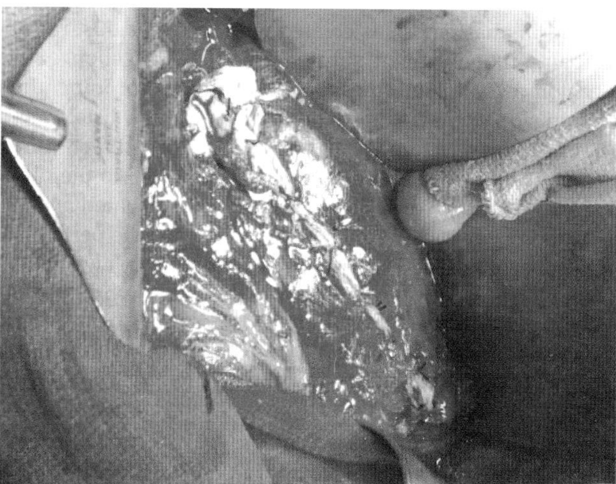

Figure 32 **Closure of the aneurysm sac over the graft.**

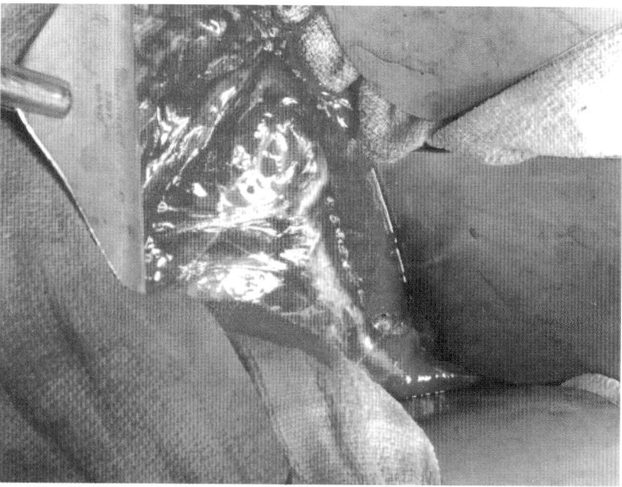

Figure 33 **Retroperitoneal closure.**

Conclusion

Despite steadily increasing knowledge of risk factors and pathogenesis of the disease, AAAs remain a significant public health concern. Screening paradigms continue to evolve to identify affected patients, but, presently, rupture cannot be predicted or prevented; therefore, repair remains the mainstay of treatment. The endovascular approach is now a well-established alternative to open surgical repair of AAAs, with technology and technique advancing rapidly. Alongside our rapidly increasing experience with EVAR, we have been frequently reassured of the excellent outcomes that may be achieved with open surgical repair. Ultimately, the decision to pursue repair depends on a calculated assessment of a patient's rupture risk versus the risks of repair. The method of repair chosen depends on further consideration of the patient's physiologic reserve and arterial anatomy, as well as the expertise of the surgeon and the resources available to him or her. The patient's expectations and desires regarding hospitalization, recovery, and follow-up protocol should also be sought and considered. Open repair should remain an option for all patients; however, it is likely that the endovascular approach will be increasingly sought by patients requiring aortic aneurysm treatment. In either case, the importance of surveillance should only increase as we hope that all of our patients will reap the benefits of comprehensive medical care and test the durability of these repairs for decades to come.

Financial Disclosures: None Reported

References

1. Johnston KW, Rutherford RB, Tilson MD, et al. Ad Hoc Committee on Reporting Standards of the Society for Vascular Surgery. Suggested standards for reporting on arterial aneurysms. J Vasc Surg 1991;13:452–8.

2. Linne A, Lindstrom D, Hultgren R. High prevalence of abdominal aortic aneurysms in brothers and sisters of patients despite a low prevalence in the population. J Vasc Surg 2012 Mar 16. [Epub ahead of print]
3. Shantikumar S, Ajjan R, Porter KE, Scott DJA. Diabetes and the abdominal aortic aneurysm. Eur J Vasc Endovasc Surg 2010;39:200–7.
4. Miyama N, Dua MM, Yeung JJ, et al. Hyperglycemia limits experimental aortic aneurysm progression. J Vasc Surg 2010;52:975–83.
5. Deaths: final data for 2009. Natl Vital Stat Rep 2012;60(3). Available at: http://www.cdc.gov/nchs/deaths.htm (accessed June 2012).
6. UK Small Aneurysm Trial Participants. Risk factors for aneurysm rupture in patients kept under ultrasound surveillance. Ann Surg 1999;230:289–96.
7. Sweetling M, Thompson S, Brown L, Powell J, RESCAN Collaborators. Meta-analysis of individual patient data to examine factors affecting growth and rupture of small abdominal aortic aneurysms. Br J Surg 2012;99:655–65.
8. Ashton H, Buxton M, Day N, et al. Multicentre Aneurysm Screening Study Group. The Multicentre Aneurysm Screening Study (MASS) into the effect of abdominal aortic aneurysm screening on mortality in men: a randomized controlled trial. Lancet 2002;360:1531–9.
9. Thompson S, Ashton H, Gao L, Scott R. Screening men for abdominal aortic aneurysm: 10 year mortality and cost effectiveness results from the randomized Multicentre Aneurysm Screening Study. BMJ 2009;338:b2307.
10. Svensjo S, Bjorck M, Gurtelschmid M, et al. Low prevalence of abdominal aortic aneurysm among 65-year-old Swedish men indicates a change in the epidemiology of the disease. Circulation 2011;124:1118–23.
11. U.S. Preventive Services Task Force. Screening for abdominal aortic aneurysm. February 2005. Available at: http://www.uspreventiveservicestaskforce.org/uspstf/uspsaneu.html (accessed June 2012).
12. Lederle FA, Johnson GR, Wilson SE, et al. Quality of life, impotence and activity level in a randomized trial of immediate repair versus surveillance of small abdominal aortic aneurysm. JAMA 2002;287:2968–72.
13. Powell JT, Brown LC, Forbes JF, et al. Final 12-year follow-up of surgery versus surveillance in the UK Small Aneurysm Trial. Br J Surg 2007;94:702–8.
14. Lederle FA, Wilson SE, Johnson GR, et al. Immediate repair compared with surveillance of small abdominal aortic aneurysms. N Engl J Med 2002;346:1437–44.
15. Ouriel K, Clair DG, Kent KC, Zarins CK; Positive Impact of Endovascular Options for treating Aneurysms Early (PIVOTAL) Investigators. Endovascular repair compared with surveillance for patients with small abdominal aortic aneurysms. J Vasc Surg 2010;51:1081–7.
16. Cao P, De Rango P, Verzini F, et al. CAESAR Trial Group. Comparison of surveillance versus Aortic Endografting for Small Aneurysm Repair (CAESAR): results from a randomized trial. Eur J Vasc Endovasc Surg 2011;41:13–25.
17. Chaikof EL, Brewster DC, Dalman RL, et al. Society for Vascular Surgery. The care of patients with an abdominal aortic aneurysm: the Society for Vascular Surgery practice guidelines. J Vasc Surg 2009;50(4 Suppl):s2–49.
18. Lederle FA, Freischlag JA, Kyriakides TC, et al. Outcomes following endovascular vs open repair of abdominal aortic aneurysm: a randomized trial. JAMA 2009;302:1535–42.
19. United Kingdom EVAR Trial Investigators, Greenhalgh RM, Brown LC, Powell JT, et al. Endovascular versus open repair of abdominal aortic aneurysm. N Engl J Med 2010;362: 1863–71.
20. Jackson RS, Chang DC, Frieschlag JA. Comparison of long-term survival after open vs endovascular repair of intact abdominal aortic aneurysm among Medicare benificiaries. JAMA 2012;307:1621–8.
21. Quinney BE, Parmar GM, Nagre SB, et al. Long-term single institution comparison of endovascular aneurysm repair and open aortic aneurysm repair. J Vasc Surg 2011;54: 1952–7.
22. Fleisher LA, Beckman JA, Vrown KA, et al. ACC/AHA 2007 guidelines on perioperative cardiovascular evaluation and care for noncardiac surgery:executive summary. Circulation 2007;116:1971–96.
23. Feringa HH, Bax JJ, Boersma E, et al. High-dose beta-blocker and tight heart rate control reduce myocardial ischemia and troponin T release in vascular surgery patients. Circulation 2006;114:i344–9.
24. Bauer SM, Cayne NS, Veith FJ. New developments in the preoperative evaluation and perioperative management of coronary disease in patients undergoing vascular surgery. J Vasc Surg 2010;51:242–51.
25. Hindler K, Shaw AD, Samuels J, et al. Improved postoperative outcomes associated with preoperative statin therapy. Anesthesiology 2006;105:1260–72.
26. McNally MM, Agle SC, Parker FM, et al. Preoperative statin therapy is associated with improved outcomes and resource utilization in patients undergoing aortic aneurysm repair. J Vasc Surg 2010;51:1390–6.
27. Paraskevas KI, Veith FJ, Liapis CD, Mikhailidis DP. Perioperative/periprocedural effects of statin treatment for patients undergoing vascular surgery or endovascular procedures: an update. Curr Vasc Pharmacol 2012 Jan 20. [Epub ahead of print]
28. Brown MJ, Norwood MG, Sayers RD. The management of abdominal aortic aneurysms in patients with concurrent renal impairment. Eur J Vasc Endovasc Surg 2005;30:1–11.
29. Brown LC, Brown EA, Greenhalgh RM, et al. UK EVAR Trial Participants. Renal function and abdominal aortic anerusym (AAA): the impact of different management strategies on long-term renal function in the UK EndoVascular Aneurysm Repair (EVAR) Trials. Ann Surg 2010;251: 966–75.
30. Leurs LJ, Laheij JF, Buth J; Eurostar Collaborators. Influence of diabetes mellitus on the endovascular treatment of abdominal aortic aneurysms. J Endovasc Ther 2005;12:228–96.
31. Heller JA, Weinberg A, Arons R, et al. Two decades of abdominal aortic aneurysm repair: have we made any progress? J Vasc Surg 2000;32:1091–101.
32. Matsumura JS, Katzen BT, Sullivan TM, et al. Predictors of survival following open and endovascular repair of abdominal aortic aneurysms. Ann Vasc Surg 2009;23:153–8.

12 AORTOILIAC RECONSTRUCTION

Andrew W. Hoel, MD, and Mark K. Eskandari, MD

The infrarenal aorta and iliac arteries are common sites of atherosclerotic occlusive disease. Although occlusive disease at this level often causes local symptoms and physical findings, it is important to remember that it is part of a systemic disease involving the entire circulatory system. There are multiple techniques for aortoiliac reconstruction that vary in both the physiologic stress to the patient and long-term durability. These treatment options should be individualized based on a patient's anatomy and comorbidities. In this chapter, we focus on open surgical intervention for the treatment of aortoiliac occlusive disease. Endovascular procedures have expanded the treatment options for peripheral arterial occlusive disease and are discussed elsewhere in *ACS Surgery*. Here we detail the preoperative evaluation, clinical decision making, and open surgical treatment options for patients with aortoiliac occlusive disease. The discussion of treatment options includes the potential complications and expected outcomes as well as steps that can be taken to optimize surgical results.

Preoperative Evaluation

HISTORY AND PHYSICAL EXAMINATION

As with all peripheral arterial disease (PAD), a great deal of information can be learned about the anatomic site and severity of aortoiliac disease from the history and physical examination. Although distal lower extremity symptoms (calf claudication) or pain in the forefoot (rest pain) may be elicited on the history, these are nonspecific and may represent multilevel vascular disease involving infrainguinal vessels in addition to the aortoiliac segment. In similar fashion, the physical examination may identify ulceration or gangrene of the distal lower extremity, which is typically a manifestation of multilevel disease. Isolated aortoiliac occlusive disease is more typically associated with claudication symptoms in the buttocks and thigh and with erectile dysfunction because of the proximal location in the arterial tree. The key finding on the physical examination, in addition to findings seen with all forms of PAD, is absent or diminished femoral pulses. The triad of buttock claudication, erectile dysfunction, and absent femoral pulses is often referred to as Leriche syndrome, after the French surgeon who described it in 1948.[1]

NONINVASIVE STUDIES

Following assessment of a patient's symptoms, physical findings, and comorbidities, noninvasive testing is extremely helpful in determining optimal therapy for a patient with suspected aortoiliac occlusive disease. The initial study to objectively quantify the extent of occlusive disease is measuring lower extremity blood flow with arterial waveforms and ankle-brachial indices (ABIs) [*see Figure 1*]. This noninvasive testing provides physiologic information about the severity of the disease and is usually performed at rest. In patients with normal ABIs at rest, ABIs remeasured after a period of exercise (usually walking on a treadmill) may unmask hemodynamically significant occlusive disease warranting treatment.

After determining the physiologic burden of disease, precise understanding of the anatomic location aids surgical planning. Although percutaneous angiography has been widely used for this purpose in the past, technological advances in axial imaging allow noninvasive imaging that is suitable and in some respects superior for surgical planning.

High-quality computed tomographic angiography (CTA) using a multidetector scanner is the current gold standard for preoperative planning. The axial imaging provides detailed information about the location and degree of stenoses as well as specific information about the degree of calcification in the arterial wall—all at submillimeter resolution. In addition, multiplanar reformatting and three-dimensional reconstruction can provide valuable information that can aid preoperative planning.[2,3] However, CTA requires contrast administration and there is some risk of contrast-induced nephropathy, particularly in older patients, those with diabetes, and those with baseline renal insufficiency.[4] In addition, there is some concern about radiation exposure, particularly in young patients and patients undergoing serial imaging studies.[5]

Magnetic resonance angiography (MRA) provides three-dimensional reconstructions of arterial anatomy with high resolution. It has the advantage of avoiding radiation exposure. In addition, time-of-flight, noncontrast imaging can provide reasonable resolution without a risk of contrast nephropathy or nephrogenic systemic sclerosis. However, the diagnostic accuracy of time-of-flight imaging is significantly lower than for contrast-enhanced MRA.[6,7] In addition, it has a number of disadvantages, limiting its usefulness in comparison with CTA. First, it does not show arterial wall architecture; therefore, information about the burden of calcification is limited. Second, stents appear as flow voids in the arterial system, limiting utility in patients who have undergone previous endovascular interventions.[8]

Duplex angiography is a rarely used modality for evaluation of aortoiliac disease. However, in thin patients, it can provide information about the location and severity of stenosis throughout the aortoiliac system to a degree that may be sufficient for surgical planning. It has the advantage of being completely noninvasive and without radiation or contrast exposure, but the overall accuracy is highly dependent on the diligence and skill of the examining technician.[8]

As noted above, diagnostic, catheter-based angiography can provide good-quality information about the anatomy of aortoiliac disease. It is essential during any endovascular aortoiliac intervention [*see Figure 2*]. However, it is an invasive procedure with small but quantifiable risks and,

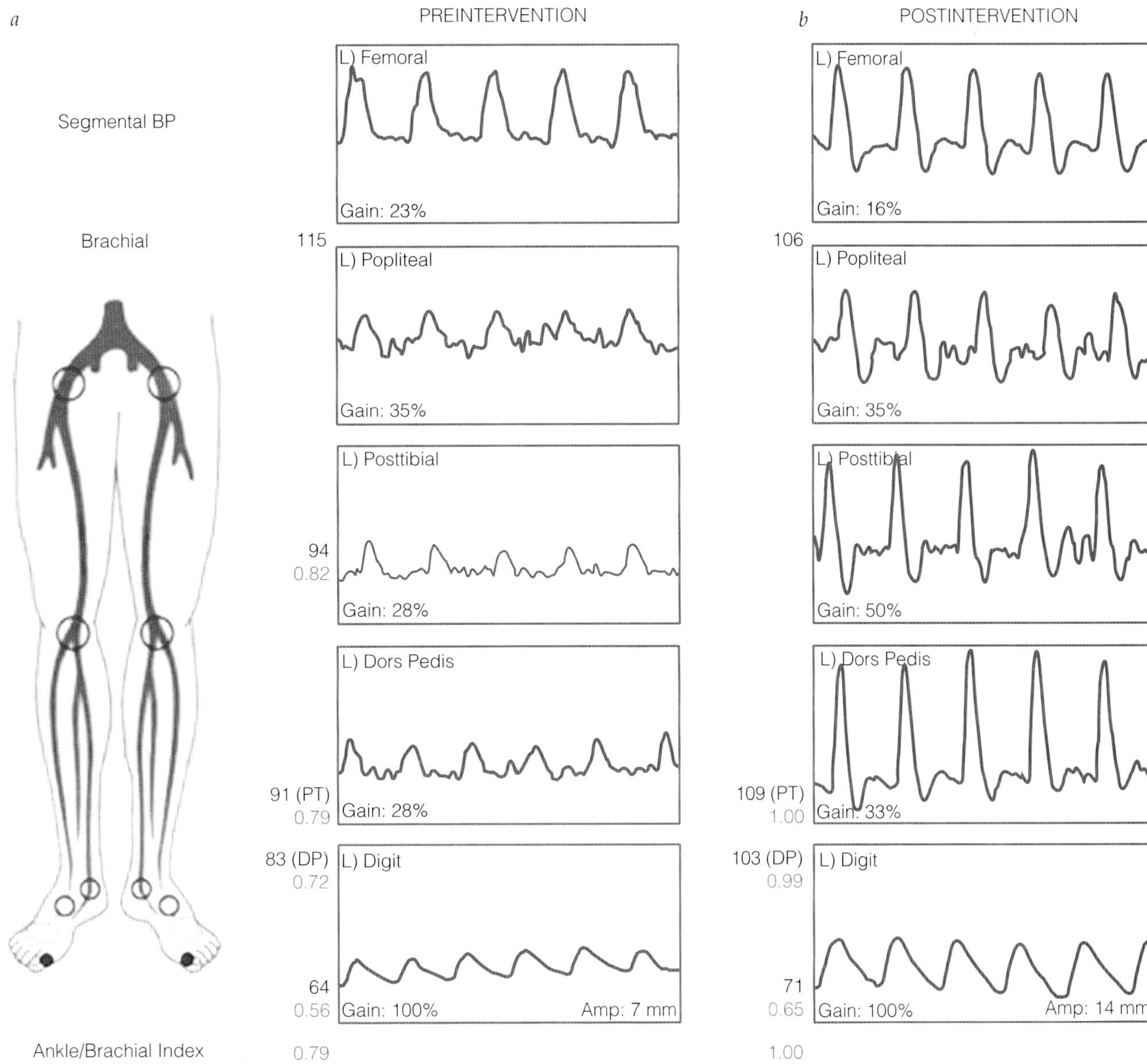

Figure 1 **Noninvasive testing including Doppler waveform at multiple levels and ankle-brachial index (ABI) in a patient with left common iliac artery disease. On the preintervention study (*a*), note the blunted arterial waveform from the left common femoral artery, popliteal artery, and tibial arteries. This patient underwent stenting of a left common femoral artery occlusion. The postintervention study (*b*) demonstrates a (normal) triphasic waveforms throughout the left lower extremity. BP = blood pressure; DP = dorsalis pedis pulse; PT = posterior tibial pulse.**

therefore, has limited utility for aortoiliac occlusive disease as a stand-alone diagnostic procedure given modern axial imaging technology. Furthermore, retrograde diagnostic angiography may have increased risk in the setting of severe femoral and iliac disease. In addition, for patients with aortic occlusion, complete imaging of the aorta and iliac arteries requires access of the descending thoracic aorta from the left brachial or radial artery.

RISK STRATIFICATION

Perioperative risk assessment is critical for any patient with clinically significant aortoiliac occlusive disease. First and foremost, a standard cardiac assessment is necessary because of the systemic nature of atherosclerosis and the likelihood of concomitant coronary disease (CAD), even in patients without cardiac symptoms; CAD may be subclinical in a patient with significant functional impairment due to PAD. Assessment of other potential comorbidities is also important, including but not limited to pulmonary disease, cerebrovascular disease, renal insufficiency, and metabolic abnormalities. These data are used to assess perioperative risk and to tailor therapy based on the significance of a patient's comorbidities, likely functional outcome, and expected long-term survival. For example, a patient with aortoiliac occlusive disease and significant comorbidities may have a better functional outcome with a less invasive procedure such as iliac stenting or axillobifemoral bypass compared with an aortobifemoral bypass. In this respect,

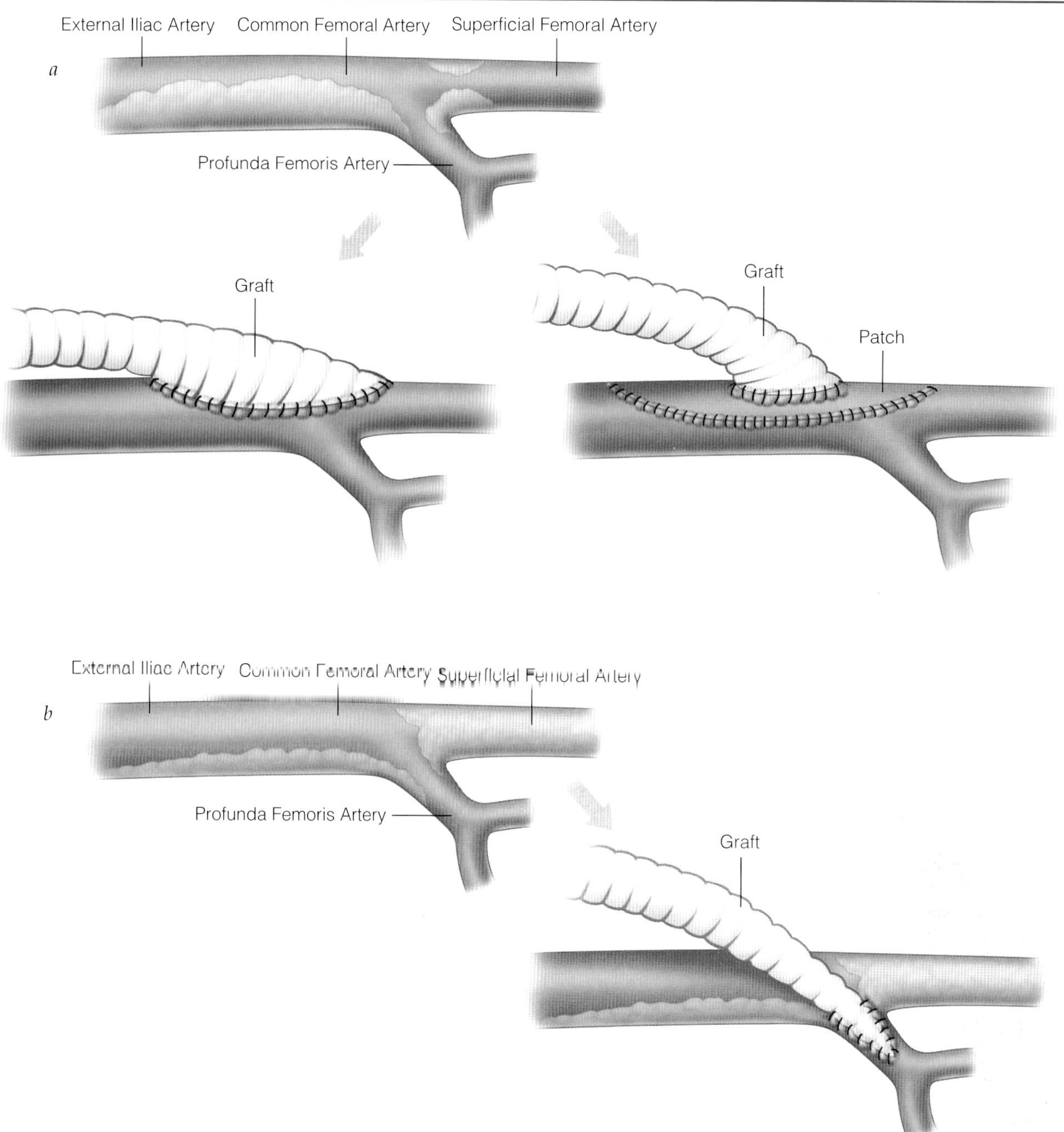

Figure 3 **Techniques for the treatment of femoral artery (outflow) disease. Patients with bulky common femoral artery disease and ostial disease of superficial femoral and profunda femoris arteries should undergo femoral endarterectomy with patch angioplasty. That angioplasty can be created using the hood of the graft or with a separate patch (*a*). If the external iliac artery is open, this configuration also allows retrograde flow to the hypogastric artery. In the setting of severe superficial femoral and external iliac artery disease, a profundaplasty with anastomosis to the profunda femoris artery is indicated. Here the heel of the graft lies in the distal common femoral artery with the toe extending beyond any disease in the profunda femoris artery (*b*).**

femoral artery. This exposure is particularly appropriate when concurrent femoral endarterectomy or profundaplasty is necessary. Alternatively, an oblique incision a fingerbreadth below the inguinal ligament provides good exposure of the common femoral artery and is particularly useful in obese patients and in the absence of significant femoral artery disease. If an oblique incision is used, it is important to open the femoral sheath longitudinally to provide maximum exposure of the femoral artery.

The femoral artery and its branches should be circumferentially dissected and encircled with elastic vessel loops to give the surgeon an unobstructed view for placement of the vascular clamps. The distal external iliac artery is also exposed at this time. This can often be accomplished by retraction and elevation of the inguinal ligament. Occasionally, the inguinal ligament must be divided for adequate exposure and should be reconstructed on completion of the case. Careful ligation of the circumflex iliac vein as it crosses over the external iliac artery prevents inadvertent tearing of the vein when creating the tunnel for the graft conduit or when placing a proximal clamp. Once this portion of the procedure is complete, a moist surgical sponge is placed into each groin, clamps are loosened to minimize tension on the soft tissue, and attention is turned to aortic exposure.

Step 3: Exposure of the Aorta

For a transabdominal approach, the abdominal cavity is entered, the small bowel is reflected to the patient's right, and the fourth portion of the duodenum is dissected free of its retroperitoneal attachments. A self-retaining retractor, such as an Omni (Omni-Tract Surgical, Minneapolis, MN) or a Bookwalter (Cardinal Health, V. Mueller, McGaw Park, IL), is helpful to maintain good exposure. The retroperitoneum overlying the infrarenal aorta is incised in the midline to expose the aorta, ideally in a location that is not heavily diseased or calcified. The aortic dissection should be limited to the segment between the renal arteries and the inferior mesenteric artery. In most cases, the dissection need not be extended downward below the aortic bifurcation into the iliac arteries, where crossing parasympathetic nerves are at risk for injury.

When the aorta is exposed in a retroperitoneal fashion, the incision is extended obliquely from the lateral border of the rectus muscle, at the level of the umbilicus, to the tip of the 11th rib. The dissection is carried through the external oblique, internal oblique, and the transversus abdominis muscles. The retroperitoneum is entered at the costal margin, and the peritoneum is reflected anteriorly. Complete exposure of the infrarenal aorta is obtained by mobilizing the abdominal contents, the left kidney, and the left ureter medially after blunt dissection along the anterior border of the psoas muscle. A large lumbar vein running along the left lateral surface of the aorta and draining into the left renal vein should be carefully ligated and divided as the left kidney is mobilized anteriorly.

Troubleshooting In cases in which aortobifemoral bypass is being performed in a patient with complete infrarenal aortic occlusion, the operative approach is modified to allow placement of a vascular clamp above the renal arteries. In the transabdominal approach, dissection is carried cephalad by retracting the small bowel mesentery and the superior mesenteric artery to the right. The left renal vein is found anterior to the aorta at the level of the renal arteries. Generally, this vein should not be divided to expose the suprarenal aorta. Rather, it should be thoroughly dissected and encircled with a vessel loop so that it can be retracted cephalad and caudad as necessary. Frequently, adrenal, gonadal, or lumbar branches draining into the left renal vein must be ligated and divided to give the renal vein added mobility. With the left renal vein retracted caudad, the suprarenal aorta is dissected.

Step 4: Creating Tunnels Anterior to Iliac Arteries

Once the inflow and outflow vessels are adequately exposed, a tunnel is created through which the bypass graft limbs will be passed from the abdomen to the groins. Its course should pass beneath the ureter and the inguinal ligament. To create the tunnel, one index finger, oriented so that its dorsum faces the vessel wall, is inserted in the midline incision and advanced caudad down to the groin. Simultaneously, the other index finger, oriented so that its volar aspect faces the common femoral artery, is inserted into a groin incision and advanced cephalad until the two fingers meet. With the finger that is dissecting proximally to distally held in place, a long Kelly or aortic clamp is carefully passed from the groin until the tip touches that finger, allowing safe advancement of the clamp proximally. Once these clamps have been passed through the tunnel from each groin, the patient is systemically heparinized in preparation for proximal anastomosis.

Step 5: Proximal Anastomosis to the Aorta

A bifurcated prosthetic graft, typically measuring either 14 × 7 mm or 16 × 8 mm, is selected and prepared for anastomosis. Importantly, the larger diameter end should be trimmed short, leaving the graft bifurcation positioned higher in the retroperitoneum than the native aortic bifurcation. The proximal aortic anastomosis can be done in either an end-to-end or an end-to-side configuration. An end-to-side beveled anastomosis is preferable for (1) patients with a small (< 1.5 cm) infrarenal aorta, (2) patients with severe occlusive disease of both external iliac arteries in whom it is desirable to preserve flow into the pelvic circulation via the internal iliac arteries, and (3) patients with a patent and large-caliber inferior mesenteric artery or accessory renal arteries. An end-to-end anastomosis is preferable for (1) patients with occlusive iliac disease and a concomitant aortic aneurysm—even if the aneurysm is small in diameter—and (2) patients undergoing revascularization for chronic total infrarenal aortic occlusion. The latter configuration is less bulky and easier to cover and isolate from the gastrointestinal (GI) tract at the conclusion of the operation. Ideally, the configuration of the proximal anastomosis should be determined preoperatively based on axial imaging.

After systemic heparin is administered and the graft is appropriately sized and trimmed, the infrarenal aorta is cross-clamped. For an end-to-side anastomosis, most commonly a straight aortic clamp is placed transversely across the aorta in an infrarenal position and a curved DeBakey aortic clamp is placed just proximal to the inferior mesenteric artery with the inner curve facing up to provide adequate exposure of the arteriotomy. The tips of the clamps will typically touch along the posterior wall of the aorta with this technique. This technique should effectively control nuisance back-bleeding from any lumbar arteries at the level of the arteriotomy. A longitudinal aortotomy is then made and the graft is sewn in place in a spatulated fashion. The toe of the graft is oriented cephalad [*see Figure 4*]. The anastomosis should be spatulated steeply so that it is not too bulky in the retroperitoneum and can be covered at the end of the procedure. Before completion of the anastomosis, the graft is flushed and back-bled.

If an end-to-end anastomosis is to be performed, a small portion of the aorta is resected to allow the graft to fit neatly into the retroperitoneum. In some cases, back-bleeding lumbar arteries in the region of the resected aorta must be

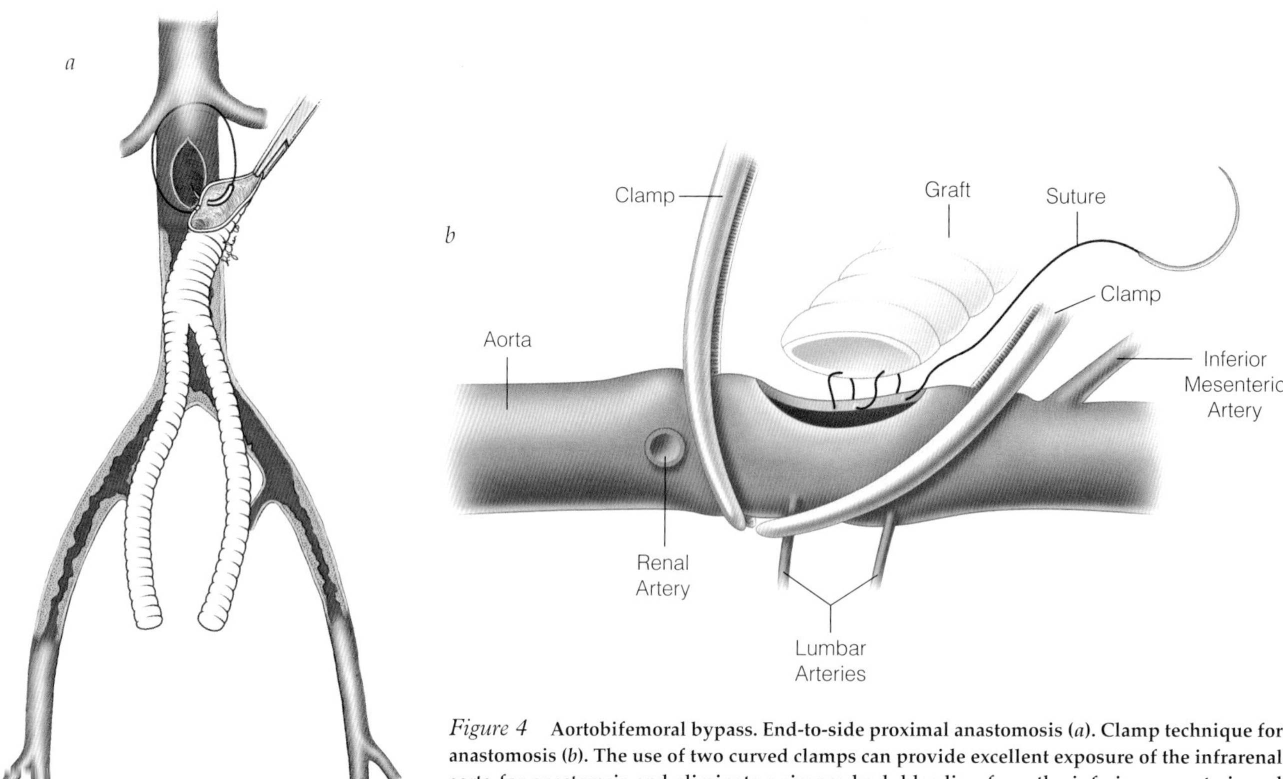

Figure 4 **Aortobifemoral bypass. End-to-side proximal anastomosis (*a*). Clamp technique for anastomosis (*b*). The use of two curved clamps can provide excellent exposure of the infrarenal aorta for anastomsis and eliminate nuisance back-bleeding from the inferior mesenteric and lumbar arteries.**

oversewn. The distal stump is oversewn with 2-0 or 3-0 polypropylene in two rows; the first row is done with a continuous suture in a horizontal mattress stitch and the second with a continuous suture in a baseball stitch [*see Figure 5*].

On completion of the anastomosis, each limb of the bifurcated graft is clamped and the aortic clamps are released. Hemostasis of the proximal anastomosis can be confirmed at this point. It is important to flush the graft at this point by briefly releasing the proximal clamp. This ensures that any debris dislodged by the aortic clamp is removed. At this point, the graft limbs can be passed to the groin by gently pulling the distal ends through the respective tunnels with the clamps left in place from earlier in the procedure. It is important to avoid twisting or kinking the conduit as it is passed.

Vascular control of the aorta is achieved differently when chronic infrarenal aortic occlusion is present. In this setting, placement of a vascular clamp just below the renal arteries may squeeze atherosclerotic debris up into the renal arteries. To prevent this, the vascular clamp should be placed briefly between the superior mesenteric artery and the renal arteries. Once the distal clamp is in place, the aorta is transected 2 cm below the renal arteries and the atherosclerotic plug is removed. A second aortic clamp can then be placed just below the renal arteries, and the suprarenal clamp can be removed. The proximal anastomosis can then be fashioned as described above.

A heavily calcified infrarenal aorta encountered at the time of operation presents a difficult problem. In most cases, the infrarenal aorta can still be used, but the proximal anastomosis should be performed in an end-to-end configuration. Even in the most calcified aortas, the region 1 to 2 cm below the renal arteries is often soft enough to allow an anastomosis to be fashioned. If this is not the case, there are two alternatives: (1) suprarenal aortic control and endarterectomy of the infrarenal aorta just below the renal ostia before the proximal anastomosis and (2) conversion to a thoracobifemoral bypass graft [*see* Thoracobifemoral Bypass, *below*]. Again, this should be determined preoperatively, particularly because conversion of a transabdominal aortobifemoral bypass to a thoracobifemoral bypass is extremely difficult.

Step 6: Distal Anastomosis to the Femoral Artery

Once the graft limbs have been passed to the groins, vascular clamps are placed on the common femoral artery and its branches, and the distal anastomosis is performed. The configuration of the longitudinal arteriotomy depends on the existence of disease in the femoral arteries, as described above [*see* General Principles: Inflow, Outflow, Conduit, *above*].

Before completion of the bypass, the inflow conduit and the proximal and distal native arteries are flushed by briefly releasing their clamps to diminish the risk of distal embolization to the legs.

Step 7: Closure of the Retroperitoneum

Before abdominal closure, the retroperitoneum is closed securely with an absorbable suture to isolate the repair from the GI tract. Careless closure of the retroperitoneum can lead to laceration or entrapment of the ureter, particularly the

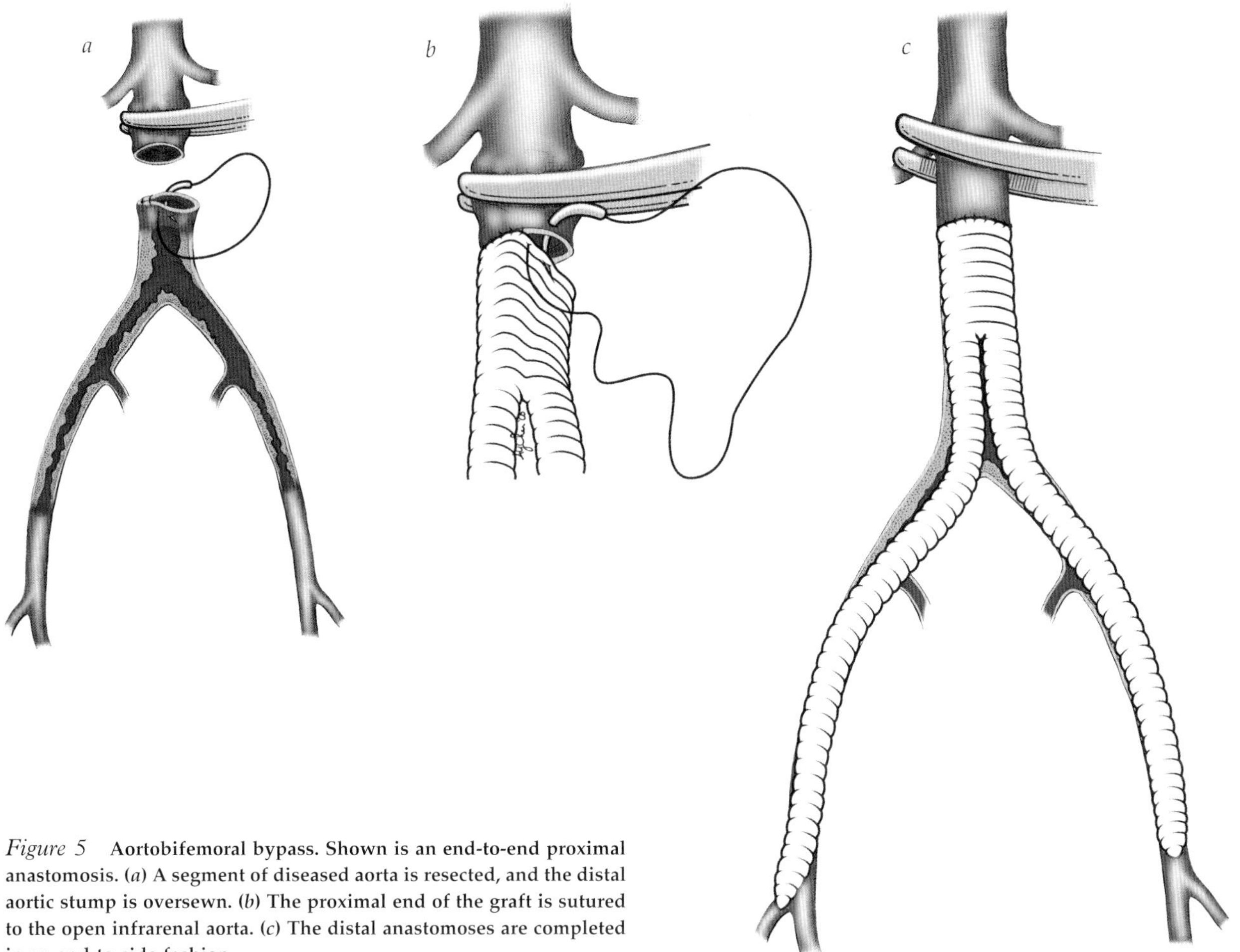

Figure 5 **Aortobifemoral bypass. Shown is an end-to-end proximal anastomosis. (*a*) A segment of diseased aorta is resected, and the distal aortic stump is oversewn. (*b*) The proximal end of the graft is sutured to the open infrarenal aorta. (*c*) The distal anastomoses are completed in an end-to-side fashion.**

right ureter. Every attempt should be made to cover the graft. If the retroperitoneum is too thin or the graft is too bulky, an omental pedicle flap should be used.

Complications

In addition to the complications noted above, a number of complications specific to aortobifemoral bypass are worth mentioning. The retroperitoneal dissection carries a risk of ureteral injury if carried too far laterally or caudally along the iliac arteries. In addition, division of the autonomic nerve fibers overlying the left common iliac artery can lead to sexual dysfunction. These complications can be avoided by limiting dissection only to tissue overlying the aorta and, if possible, between the renal arteries and inferior mesenteric artery.

Aortic cross-clamping adjacent to the renal arteries (either above or below) can cause embolization of debris into the renal arteries, leading to renal failure. This can be anticipated by careful review of the preoperative imaging. In cases in which the infrarenal aorta contains significant mural thrombus or soft atheroma, the renal arteries should be controlled and a suprarenal clamp should be placed until the infrarenal segment can be cleared of this debris after opening the aorta. Once this is done, the infrarenal aorta can be clamped and the suprarenal aortic and renal artery clamps released, preventing migration of debris into the renal arteries.

Finally, a well-described late complication of aortobifemoral bypass is aortoduodenal fistula or erosion between the proximal anastomosis of the aortobifemoral bypass and the third or fourth portion of the duodenum. This complication can be prevented with meticulous closure of the retroperitoneum with absorbable suture, making sure that the duodenum is separated by adequate soft tissue from the prosthetic bypass. If there is inadequate retroperitoneal soft tissue to separate these structures, an omental pedicle flap should be mobilized to cover the graft.

THORACOBIFEMORAL BYPASS

A thoracobifemoral bypass is indicated for a small subgroup of patients, including (1) those with an occluded previous aortobifemoral bypass graft, (2) those with a circumferentially calcified infrarenal aorta that is unusable as an inflow source, and (3) those with a so-called hostile abdomen (i.e., those who have undergone multiple or extensive abdominal procedures; those who have an ileal conduit, ileostomy, or colostomy; or those who have a history of surgery for aortic graft infection). The outcomes from this relatively uncommon procedure are similar in patency to aortobifemoral bypass, with 86% patency at 4 years in one review.[23] Candidates for this procedure must have adequate pulmonary reserve and be able to tolerate a thoracotomy.

The patient is placed in a right semilateral decubitus position so that the hips are nearly flat on the table and the torso is rotated to the patient's right. An axillary roll and an inflatable beanbag will help maintain this position. Because single-lung ventilation will be necessary when the proximal anastomosis is done, either a double-lumen endotracheal tube or a bronchial blocker must be used. Placement of an orogastric tube to decompress the stomach helps keep the diaphragm down during exposure of the descending thoracic aorta.

Step 1: Exposure of the Femoral Artery

Full exposure of the common femoral artery and its bifurcation into the superficial and deep femoral arteries is performed in the same manner as described above for aortobifemoral bypass.

Step 2: Incision and Exposure of the Descending Thoracic Aorta

The descending thoracic aorta is approached through a left posterior lateral thoracotomy at the level of the seventh or eighth interspace. Additional exposure can be gained by resecting part of the rib and by using an Omni retractor. The lung is decompressed and reflected anterior and superior by taking down a portion of the inferior pulmonary ligament. With this exposure, the parietal pleura overlying the descending thoracic aorta is incised. The aorta is cleanly dissected, with care taken not to damage the esophagus, which lies medially. Having a nasogastric tube in place is advantageous in this regard: the esophagus can easily be located by palpating the tube. Any intercostal vessels in the region of the anticipated aortotomy can be preserved and controlled at the time of the anastomosis.

Step 3: Tunneling of the Bypass Graft

Two separate dissection planes are required for this bypass: (1) a tunnel from the thoracic aorta to the left groin and (2) a tunnel from the left side bypass to the right groin. The left retroperitoneal tunnel is started in the chest by making a 2 cm hole in the posterior lateral aspect of the left diaphragm. An index finger is inserted through this hole and advanced caudad into the retroperitoneum as far as it can go. The other index finger is inserted through the left groin incision, oriented directly over the external iliac artery, and advanced cephalad into the retroperitoneum along the iliopsoas muscle [*see Figure 6*]. In most cases, the left retroperitoneal tunnel must then be completed by using a tunneling device such as the Gore Tunneler (W. L. Gore & Associates, Inc., Tempe, AZ). Next, the subcutaneous tunnel from the left groin to the right groin is bluntly fashioned along the lower abdominal wall in the same manner as performed with a femorofemoral bypass, as described below.

Once the tunnels are completed, the graft is fashioned (usually) by suturing a tube graft to a bifurcated graft. It is passed through the tunnel in such a way that the bifurcated limbs are brought caudally down into the left groin wound. The bifurcation of the elongated prosthetic graft should lie just cephalad to the left groin wound. The graft-to-graft anastomosis should remain accessible in the course of this reconstruction to ensure hemostasis at this junction when the graft is perfused. The right limb of the bifurcated graft is then brought through the tunnel from the left groin incision to the right groin incision.

Step 4: Proximal Anastomosis to the Descending Thoracic Aorta

Once the graft has been tunneled, the patient undergoes systemic anticoagulation with IV heparin. The descending thoracic aorta is controlled either with a side-biting clamp or with two completely occluding aortic clamps placed in close proximity to each other. In the latter case, one or two intercostal arteries may have to be temporarily controlled as well. A longitudinal aortotomy is then made along the left lateral aspect of the thoracic aorta, and a beveled end-to-side anastomosis is fashioned. Before completion of the anastomosis, the aorta is flushed and back-bled.

Partial aortic control with a side-biting vascular clamp is successful in most cases, but it is not recommended when the descending thoracic aorta is heavily diseased with calcification or soft atheroma or when mural thrombus is present. This should be determined by preoperative axial imaging. If an intercostal artery cannot be temporarily controlled with clamps, it can be oversewn from the inside of the aorta to prevent nuisance back-bleeding.

Step 5: Distal Anastomosis to the Femoral Artery

Vascular clamps are placed on the common femoral artery and its branches, and an end-to-side anastomosis is fashioned distally. As with infrarenal aortobifemoral bypass, the configuration of the longitudinal arteriotomy and the need for femoral endarterectomy depend on the burden of disease in the femoral arteries, as described above and in Figure 3. Before completion of the bypass, the inflow vessel is flushed and the outflow vessel is back-bled.

Step 6: Closure of the Chest

Once the proximal anastomosis is complete, it should be covered with either parietal pleura or a patch of bovine pericardium. The left lung is then reinflated. At the conclusion of the operation, the chest is closed in a standard fashion over two chest tubes.

Complications

The complications of this procedure are largely the same as those outlined for aortobifemoral bypass. However, this procedure also carries the risk of pulmonary complications related to the thoracotomy, and pulmonary status should be evaluated carefully prior to performing this procedure. Aortopulmonary fistula has also been reported, and careful coverage of the proximal anastomosis with parietal pleura or bovine pericardium minimizes the risk of this complication. Finally, clamping of the thoracic aorta and the oversewing of intercostal arteries at this level are very rarely associated with paraplegia caused by decreasing blood flow to the anterior spinal artery.

ILIOFEMORAL BYPASS

Iliofemoral bypass largely has been supplanted by advances in percutaneous endoluminal techniques. However, there are rare instances in which this procedure is

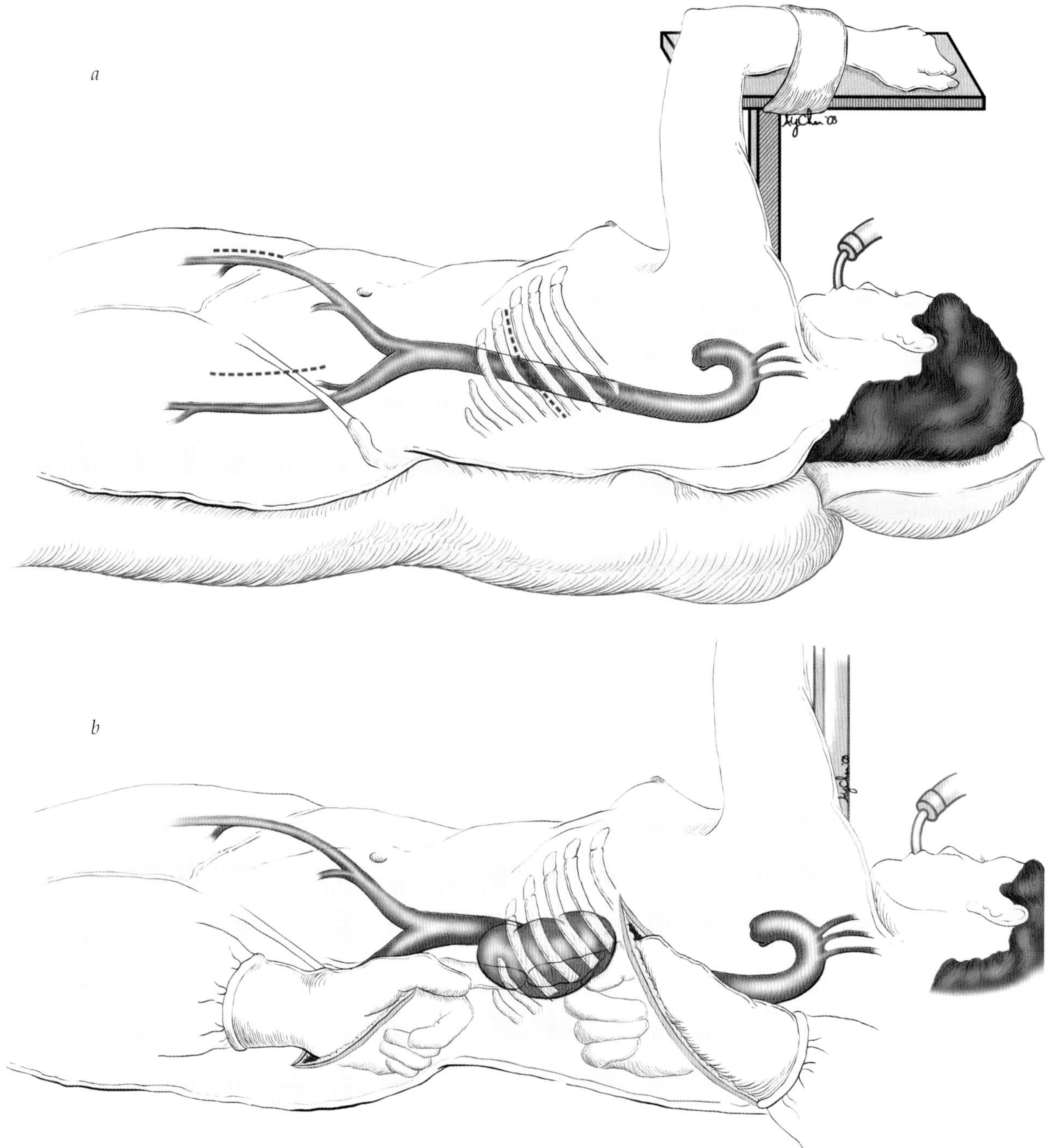

Figure 6 **Thoracobifemoral bypass. The patient is positioned so that the hips are flat, but the torso is slightly rotated to the patient's right (*a*). Three incisions are made: a left posterolateral thoracotomy and two groin incisions. *Dashed lines* denote skin incision. A left retroperitoneal tunnel is fashioned for passage of the prosthetic graft downward to the groin (*b*). (The right arm of the graft is subsequently passed to the right groin via a subcutaneous tunnel anterior to the pubis.)**

indicated. In particular, it is most suitable for patients who have isolated unilateral external iliac artery disease and are good surgical risks. In this situation, the patency of an iliofemoral bypass is superior to that of a femorofemoral bypass, which is the alternative open surgical option in these patients.[24] Iliofemoral bypass also has utility as an adjunct in the endovascular treatment of abdominal aortic aneurysm (EVAR) and thoracic aortic aneurysm (TEVAR) in the setting of concurrent high-grade external iliac artery stenosis. This so-called iliofemoral conduit procedure allows delivery of the large sheaths required for EVAR and TEVAR. The procedure can be done concurrently with the endovascular intervention or can be staged. For this operation to be successful, there must be a relatively disease-free common

tery is controlled with vascular clamps, with care taken not to include any part of the brachial plexus lying nearby. A longitudinal arteriotomy is made along the length of the axillary artery. The proximal anastomosis is then fashioned in an end-to-side configuration. The anastomosis must lie medial to the medial border of the pectoralis minor, and the graft should be positioned so that it lies parallel to the axillary artery for a length of 2 to 3 cm before diving deep and caudad. This is critical for preventing avulsion of the graft from the axillary artery when the patient fully abducts the arm postoperatively. Before the anastomosis is completed, it is flushed and back-bled. The anastomosis is then completed, the graft is clamped just distal to the anastomosis, and the arm is reperfused.

Step 6: Distal Anastomosis to the Femoral Artery

The distal anastomosis to the femoral arteries is performed as described earlier [*see* Aortobifemoral Bypass, *above*]. Some controversy remains over the formation of the short crossover graft from the axillary bypass graft to the contralateral femoral artery. Our practice is to place the proximal anastomosis of the crossover femorofemoral anastomosis just above the distal axillofemoral anastomosis (or just proximal to the "hood" of the bypass) [*see Figure 9*]. Others prefer to use a commercially available bifurcated axillofemoral prosthetic graft or to place the crossover graft more proximally along the length of the axillofemoral graft. Regardless of technique, the second femoral anastomosis is completed in the same manner as the first, the anastomosis is flushed, and the extremities are reperfused. After completion of the bypass, all wounds are closed in standard fashion, as described above.

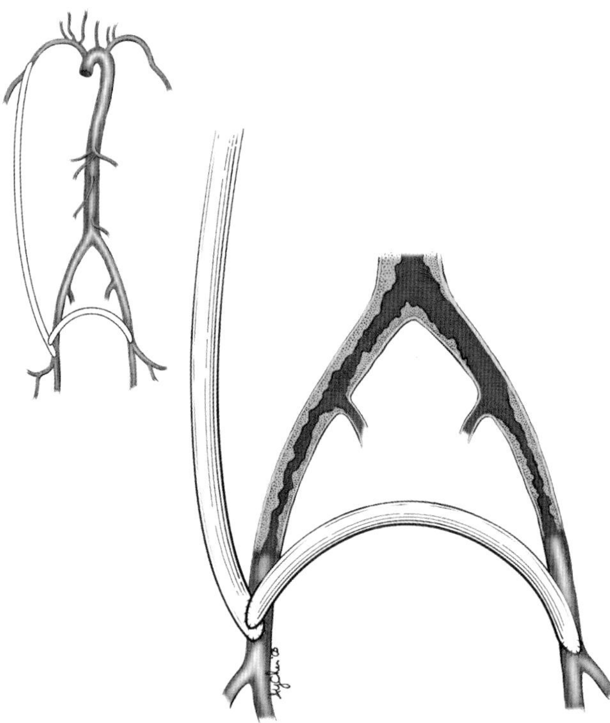

Figure 9 **Axillofemoral bypass. Shown is the recommended configuration for the short femorofemoral crossover graft originating from the long axillofemoral graft. The femorofemoral graft originated from the hood of the axillofemoral graft.**

Complications

The complications associated with this procedure are the same as those associated with the other procedures described here. In addition, albeit rarely, the axillary incision can leave a patient with arm weakness or paresthesias related to injury to the adjacent brachial plexus.

FEMOROFEMORAL BYPASS

A femorofemoral crossover bypass is well suited to patients who have unilateral complete occlusion or a diffusely diseased iliac system but have a relatively normal contralateral iliac system. In this setting, a 5-year patency of 60 to 70% can be expected.[35] In patients with significant inflow disease, stenting of stenosis in the inflow iliac artery [*see* Iliac Stenting and Iliofemoral Endarterectomy, *above*] has demonstrated patency results comparable to those of disease-free inflow patients.[36,37] However, in some patients, the need for inflow stenting is associated with decreased intermediate patency, highlighting the need for good patient selection.[38] If treatment of inflow disease is necessary, it is important to completely treat the inflow, including performing an iliofemoral endarterectomy, if indicated, as described above. Coexistent superficial femoral artery disease in the recipient vessels has a detrimental effect on the long-term patency of these bypasses.[39]

Step 1: Bilateral Femoral Exposure

Bilateral longitudinal groin incisions are made in standard fashion [*see* Aortobifemoral Bypass, *above*]. If there is significant external iliac disease, exposure should include the distal external iliac artery.

Step 2: Prefascial Tunnel

A subcutaneous tunnel is created between the bilateral femoral incisions. Care should be taken to remain in the subcutaneous space just anterior to the abdominal wall. Bladder injury has been reported with this dissection and is avoided by bladder drainage with a Foley catheter and by remaining in the prefascial subcutaneous space. The course of the tunnel should be just superior to the pubic bone in a gentle arc. An 8 mm externally supported PTFE graft is then passed through the tunnel using an aortic clamp. There should be sufficient laxity in the conduit so that it can follow a gentle arc just above the pubis. This is particularly important in obese patients, where an abdominal pannus can stretch an overly tight conduit and put the anastomoses under unnecessary strain, particularly when the patient stands.

Step 3: Anastomosis

After systemic heparinization, the inflow anastomosis is created first by clamping proximally and distally and performing a longitudinal arteriotomy. Care should be taken not to make the arteriotomy too long, particularly in obese patients, to preserve the angle that the conduit comes off the beveled end-to-side anastomosis. An arteriotomy that is too long requires a long graft hood that can fold over on itself when it is angled to the anterior abdominal wall. If a long arteriotomy is necessary to treat significant femoral disease in the inflow artery, a separate patch angioplasty can be performed and subsequently incised for the proximal anastomosis of the femorofemoral bypass. Once the anastomosis is complete, the native artery is forward bled and back-bled into the graft, the graft is clamped just above the anastomosis, and the "donor" extremity is reperfused. The outflow anastomosis is then performed in the same manner.

AORTOILIAC ENDARTERECTOMY

Although localized aortoiliac endarterectomy is rarely performed in modern vascular surgical practice, particularly as endovascular techniques advance, it was once the standard procedure for the treatment of aortoiliac disease. In current practice, it is occasionally useful in patients with few comorbidities who have focal disease at the aortic bifurcation and proximal common iliac arteries, particularly those with a small-caliber aorta and highly calcified atherosclerosis. It is important that patients considered for this procedure have minimally diseased external iliac arteries. The outcomes in this setting are generally excellent, with patency of nearly 90% at 10 years in the lone modern published series.[40] This procedure is also occasionally useful because the aortotomy in some situations can be closed, primarily avoiding leaving prosthetic material in the retroperitoneum.

Step 1: Incision and Approach

A low midline transperitoneal incision allows rapid, direct access. In a nonobese patient, the incision can be performed below the umbilicus and extended to the pubis.

Step 2: Exposure and Control of the Aorta and Iliac Arteries

On entry into the abdominal cavity, exposure of the aortic bifurcation is achieved by retracting the small bowel cephalad and to the patient's right side. A self-retaining retractor is often helpful in maintaining exposure. The retroperitoneum overlying the aortic bifurcation is then incised in the midline, and the aorta is exposed between the bifurcation and the inferior mesenteric artery. Both common iliac arteries are exposed, with care taken not to damage the underlying iliac veins and the overlying ureters, which normally cross at the iliac bifurcation.

Given that this procedure is best suited for treatment of localized disease, exposure beyond the iliac bifurcation is rarely necessary. If it appears that the disease process extends into the external iliac arteries or more proximally in the infrarenal aorta, another form of treatment, such as aortobifemoral bypass, is indicated.

Step 3: Aortoiliac Endarterectomy

Once the aorta and the iliac vessels are exposed, IV heparin is given for systemic anticoagulation. The vessels are then controlled with vascular clamps. As a rule, the iliac vessels should be clamped first to reduce the risk of distal embolization during placement of the aortic cross-clamp. These vessels should be clamped enough only to prevent retrograde bleeding.

Next, the aorta is incised longitudinally from a point just above the bifurcation (where the aorta is soft) and down into the common iliac artery, in which the disease process extends further. Sometimes the middle sacral or lower lumbar arteries must be occluded to control back-bleeding. A dissection plane is developed between the media and the adventitia, and standard endarterectomy of the infrarenal aorta and the more diseased iliac artery is performed. The endarterectomy of the contralateral iliac artery is performed by means of eversion through the aortotomy or through a separate longitudinal incision [*see Figure 10*]. If the distal termination points in the iliac vessels are irregular or have a significant step-off, the plaque should be tacked down with two or three 6-0 polypropylene sutures, with the knots tied on the outside of the vessel wall.

Occasionally, endarterectomy results in a very thin residual wall or the distal termination points are too steep to fix with tacking sutures alone. In such cases, the best recourse is to replace this section of the aorta and the common iliac

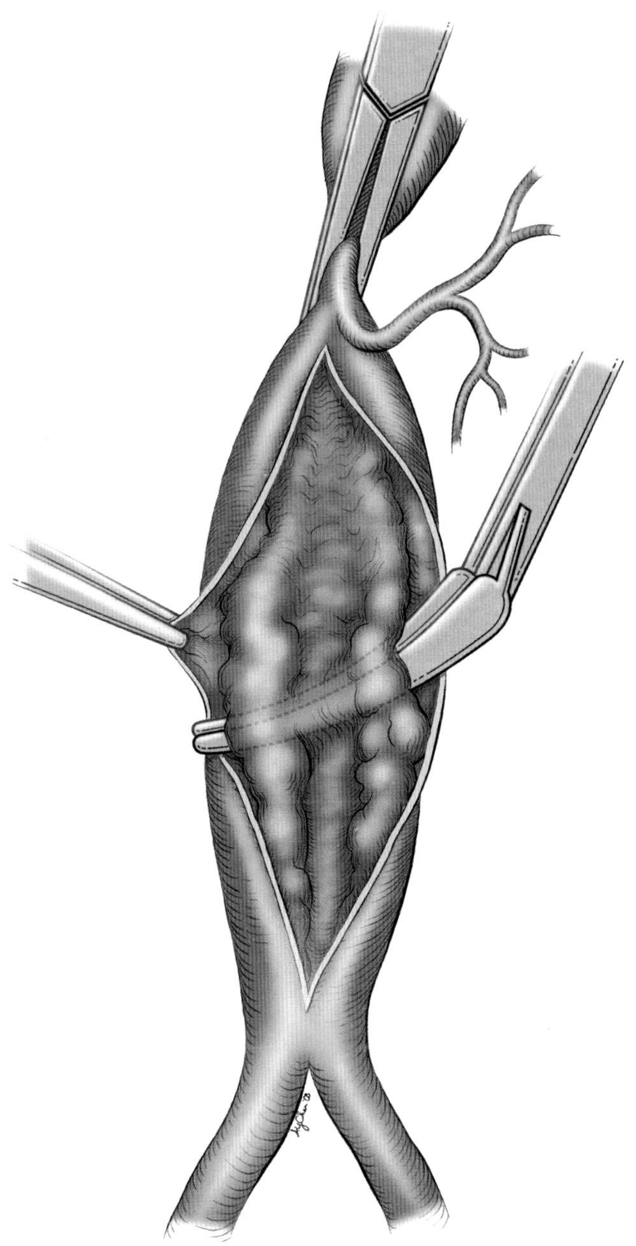

Figure 10 **Aortoiliac endarterectomy. Plaque is removed through a longitudinal arteriotomy.**

vessels with a short standard bifurcated prosthetic interposition graft. Proximally, the graft is sewn to the infrarenal aorta in an end-to-end fashion. Distally, the two limbs are sewn to the two common iliac arteries in the same manner.

Step 4: Repair of Arteriotomy

The arteriotomy can be closed either primarily or with a patch, depending on the size of the aorta and the iliac vessels. Primary closure is preferred, but if it appears that such closure will significantly narrow the aorta or iliac artery, a patch (either prosthetic or autogenous) should be used instead. Before closure is completed, the vessels should be flushed and back-bled to diminish the risk of distal embolization to the legs on reestablishment of inline flow. The adequacy of the repair is confirmed primarily by the palpation of normal femoral pulses in the groins.

Step 5: Closure of the Retroperitoneum

Before abdominal closure, the retroperitoneum is closed with an absorbable suture, as with aortobifemoral bypass above.

Summary

There is a broad spectrum of treatments for aortoiliac occlusive disease. Selection of the most appropriate technique for aortoiliac reconstruction depends significantly on the location and severity of the occlusive disease and on the medical comorbidities of the patient. Although open reconstruction is decreasing in frequency because of expanding technology and advances in endovascular therapy, there will likely always be a group of patients for whom open reconstruction is the best and most durable treatment.

Financial Disclosure: None Reported

References

1. Leriche R, Morel A. The syndrome of thrombotic obliteration of the aortic bifurcation. Ann Surg 1948;127:193–206.
2. Tins B, Oxtoby J, Patel S. Comparison of CT angiography with conventional arterial angiography in aortoiliac occlusive disease. Br J Radiol 2001;74:219–25.
3. Shareghi S, Gopal A, Gul K, et al. Diagnostic accuracy of 64 multidetector computed tomographic angiography in peripheral vascular disease. Catheter Cardiovasc Intervent 2010;75:23–31.
4. Mehran R, Aymong ED, Nikolsky E, et al. A simple risk score for prediction of contrast-induced nephropathy after percutaneous coronary intervention: development and initial validation. J Am Coll Cardiol 2004;44:1393–9.
5. Brenner DJ, Hall EJ. Computed tomography—an increasing source of radiation exposure. N Engl J Med 2007;357:2277–84.
6. Koelemay MJ, Lijmer JG, Stoker J, et al. Magnetic resonance angiography for the evaluation of lower extremity arterial disease: a meta-analysis. JAMA 2001;285:1338–45.
7. Loewe C, Schoder M, Rand T, et al. Peripheral vascular occlusive disease: evaluation with contrast-enhanced moving-bed MR angiography versus digital subtraction angiography in 106 patients. AJR Am J Roentgenol 2002;179:1013–21.
8. Lundin P, Svensson A, Henriksen E, et al. Imaging of aortoiliac arterial disease. Duplex ultrasound and MR angiography versus digital subtraction angiography. Acta Radiol 2000;41:125–32.
9. Willigendael EM, Teijink JA, Bartelink ML, et al. Smoking and the patency of lower extremity bypass grafts: a meta-analysis. J Vasc Surg 2005;42:67–74.
10. Kenfield SA, Stampfer MJ, Rosner BA, Colditz GA. Smoking and smoking cessation in relation to mortality in women. JAMA 2008;299:2037–47.
11. Alonso-Coello P, Bellmunt S, McGorrian C, et al. Antithrombotic therapy in peripheral artery disease: Antithrombotic Therapy and Prevention of Thrombosis, 9th ed: American College of Chest Physicians Evidence-Based Clinical Practice Guidelines. Chest 2012;141:e669S–90S.
12. Collaborative HPS. Randomized trial of the effects of cholesterol-lowering with simvastatin on peripheral vascular and other major vascular outcomes in 20,536 people with peripheral arterial disease and other high-risk conditions. J Vasc Surg 2007;45:645–54; discussion 53–4.
13. Shepherd J, Blauw GJ, Murphy MB, et al. Pravastatin in elderly individuals at risk of vascular disease (PROSPER): a randomised controlled trial. Lancet 2002;360:1623–30.
14. Mohler ER 3rd, Hiatt WR, Creager MA. Cholesterol reduction with atorvastatin improves walking distance in patients with peripheral arterial disease. Circulation 2003;108:1481–6.
15. Feringa HH, Bax JJ, Hoeks S, et al. A prognostic risk index for long-term mortality in patients with peripheral arterial disease. Arch Intern Med 2007;167:2482–9.
16. Fleischmann KE, Beckman JA, Buller CE, et al. 2009 ACCF/AHA focused update on perioperative beta blockade. J Am Coll Cardiol 2009;54:2102–28.
17. de Vries SO, Hunink MG. Results of aortic bifurcation grafts for aortoiliac occlusive disease: a meta-analysis. J Vasc Surg 1997;26:558–69.
18. Feinglass J, McCarthy WJ, Slavensky R, et al. Functional status and walking ability after lower extremity bypass grafting or angioplasty for intermittent claudication: results from a prospective outcomes study. J Vasc Surg 2000;31:93–103.
19. Nguyen LL, Moneta GL, Conte MS, et al. Prospective multicenter study of quality of life before and after lower extremity vein bypass in 1404 patients with critical limb ischemia. J Vasc Surg 2006;44:977–83; discussion 83–4.
20. McDaniel MD, Macdonald PD, Haver RA, Littenberg B. Published results of surgery for aortoiliac occlusive disease. Ann Vasc Surg 1997;11:425–41.
21. Dimick JB, Cowan JA Jr, Henke PK, et al. Hospital volume-related differences in aorto-bifemoral bypass operative mortality in the United States. J Vasc Surg 2003;37:970–5.
22. Danczyk RC, Mitchell EL, Petersen BD, et al. Outcomes of open operation for aortoiliac occlusive disease after failed endovascular therapy. Arch Surg 2012;147:841–5.
23. McCarthy WJ, Mesh CL, McMillan WD, et al. Descending thoracic aorta-to-femoral artery bypass: ten years' experience with a durable procedure. J Vasc Surg 1993;17:336–47; discussion 47–8.
24. Ricco JB. Unilateral iliac artery occlusive disease: a randomized multicenter trial examining direct revascularization versus crossover bypass. Association Universitaire de Recherche en Chirurgie. Ann Vasc Surg 1992;6:209–19.

25. Kashyap VS, Pavkov ML, Bena JF, et al. The management of severe aortoiliac occlusive disease: endovascular therapy rivals open reconstruction. J Vasc Surg 2008;48:1451–7, 7 e1–3.
26. Jongkind V, Akkersdijk GJ, Yeung KK, Wisselink W. A systematic review of endovascular treatment of extensive aortoiliac occlusive disease. J Vasc Surg 2010;52:1376–83.
27. Rzucidlo EM, Powell RJ, Zwolak RM, et al. Early results of stent-grafting to treat diffuse aortoiliac occlusive disease. J Vasc Surg 2003;37:1175–80.
28. Piazza M, Ricotta JJ 2nd, Bower TC, et al. Iliac artery stenting combined with open femoral endarterectomy is as effective as open surgical reconstruction for severe iliac and common femoral occlusive disease. J Vasc Surg 2011;54: 402–11.
29. Chang RW, Goodney PP, Baek JH, et al. Long-term results of combined common femoral endarterectomy and iliac stenting/stent grafting for occlusive disease. J Vasc Surg 2008;48:362–7.
30. Mwipatayi BP, Thomas S, Wong J, et al. A comparison of covered vs bare expandable stents for the treatment of aortoiliac occlusive disease. J Vasc Surg 2011;54:1561–70.
31. Martin D, Katz SG. Axillofemoral bypass for aortoiliac occlusive disease. Am J Surg 2000;180:100–3.
32. Savrin RA, Record GT, McDowell DE. Axillofemoral bypass. Expectations and results. Arch Surg 1986;121:1016–20.
33. Schneider JR, McDaniel MD, Walsh DB, et al. Axillofemoral bypass: outcome and hemodynamic results in high-risk patients. J Vasc Surg 1992;15:952–62; discussion 62–3.
34. Johnson WC, Lee KK. Comparative evaluation of externally supported Dacron and polytetrafluoroethylene prosthetic bypasses for femorofemoral and axillofemoral arterial reconstructions. Veterans Affairs Cooperative Study #141. J Vasc Surg 1999;30:1077–83.
35. Ricco JB, Probst H. Long-term results of a multicenter randomized study on direct versus crossover bypass for unilateral iliac artery occlusive disease. J Vasc Surg 2008;47:45–53; discussion 53–4.
36. Perler BA, Williams GM. Does donor iliac artery percutaneous transluminal angioplasty or stent placement influence the results of femorofemoral bypass? Analysis of 70 consecutive cases with long-term follow-up. J Vasc Surg 1996; 24:363–9; discussion 9–70.
37. Lopez-Galarza LA, Ray LI, Rodriguez-Lopez J, Diethrich EB. Combined percutaneous transluminal angioplasty, iliac stent deployment, and femorofemoral bypass for bilateral aortoiliac occlusive disease. J Am Coll Surg 1997;184: 249–58.
38. Huded CP, Goodney PP, Powell RJ, et al. The impact of adjunctive iliac stenting on femoral-femoral bypass in contemporary practice. J Vasc Surg 2012;55:739–45; discussion 44–5.
39. Criado E, Burnham SJ, Tinsley EA Jr, et al. Femorofemoral bypass graft: analysis of patency and factors influencing long-term outcome. J Vasc Surg 1993;18:495–504; discussion 744–5.
40. Connolly JE, Price T. Aortoiliac endarterectomy: a lost art? Ann Vasc Surg 2006;20:56–62.

Acknowledgments

Figures 3, 4b, and 8 Christine Kenney
Figures 4a, 5, 6, 7, 9, and 10 Alice Y. Chen

13 SURGICAL TREATMENT OF THE INFECTED AORTIC GRAFT

*Sumona V. Smith, MD, and G. Patrick Clagett, MD, FACS**

In dealing with an infected aortic graft, the primary goal of treatment is to save life and limb. This goal is best accomplished by eradicating all infected graft material and maintaining adequate circulation with appropriate vascular reconstruction. Secondary goals are to minimize morbidity, restore normal function and maintain long-term function without the need for repeated intervention or amputation. Despite advances in perioperative critical care and antimicrobial therapy, the morbidity and mortality associated with aortic graft infections remain high.

Before definitive reconstruction, all infected graft material must be débrided, along with any grossly infected vascular tissue and surrounding soft tissue. Once débridement is complete, there are several options for reconstruction, including (1) extra-anatomic bypass, (2) use of an arterial allograft, (3) placement of vascular prostheses treated with or soaked in antibiotic solutions, and (4) in situ replacement with a femoropopliteal vein (FPV) graft. The choice among these options is made on the basis of the specific clinical situation present. The primary focus of the technical description in this chapter, however, is on the fourth option [*see* Operative Technique, *below*].

Choice of Procedure

EXTRA-ANATOMIC BYPASS

Extra-anatomic bypass, usually performed as an axillobifemoral bypass [*see Figure 1*], is a good option for treatment of an infected aortic graft when groin infection is absent and lower extremity runoff is good. The primary advantages of extra-anatomic bypass are that it minimizes lower extremity ischemic time and that it is less of a physiologic insult than an aorta-based bypass procedure (mainly because it is typically done in a staged fashion). The primary disadvantages are that long-term patency is poor and that there is a significant risk of reinfection. In addition, if groin infection is present, the bypass is compromised even further by the need to use vessels such as the profunda femoris artery or the popliteal artery for distal targets. Bilateral axillofemoral bypasses are often required in this situation. Because of these factors, the durability of an extra-anatomic bypass may be limited despite aggressive antithrombotic treatment.

Extra-anatomic bypasses are plagued by sudden thrombotic occlusion, and amputation rates are high. In one large series, one third of patients required a major amputation during long-term follow-up.[1] Reinfection also is a major concern when prosthetic grafts are employed in patients with ongoing infection: it occurs in 10 to 20% of such patients and often proves lethal. A final major concern in patients who undergo excision of an infected aortic graft and extra-anatomic bypass is the possibility of blowout of the aortic stump. This is an infrequent occurrence (incidence < 10%) but one that is almost always fatal.

AORTIC ALLOGRAFT

Several modern reports have confirmed the efficacy of cryopreserved allografts in the treatment of aortic prosthetic graft infection.[2–5] A recent systemic review and meta-analysis suggested that although cryopreserved allografts are not as resistant to infection as an autogenous FPV, the incidence of reinfection after in situ reconstruction with a cryopreserved allograft [illegible] as aneurysmal degeneration and rupture have been reported.[6] Some authors report that the main advantages of cryopreserved vein to replace an infected aortic graft are improved patency rates compared with extra-anatomic bypass and avoidance of the prolonged operating time associated with in situ replacement with FPVs.[7–9] However, because aortic allografts are available in the United States only on a limited basis, this technique is not a useful option in emergency situations.

ANTIBIOTIC-TREATED PROSTHETIC GRAFT

Use of antibiotic-treated prosthetic graft material for reconstruction has the advantage of permitting an expeditious reconstruction that leaves no aortic stump.[7,10–14] However, the reinfection rate is unpredictable, and patients must undergo lifelong antibiotic therapy. Typically, the new prosthetic graft is soaked in rifampin, 60 mg/mL, for 15 minutes before implantation.[12,13]

IN SITU AUTOGENOUS RECONSTRUCTION

Dissatisfaction with the long-term patency of extra-anatomic bypass led to the development of in situ autogenous venous reconstruction.[15–17] Early reconstructive attempts that made use of great saphenous vein grafts proved unsuccessful because the small caliber of the venous conduit resulted in low patency rates. Subsequent attempts that made use of larger-caliber FPV grafts, however, proved highly successful.

FPV grafts have excellent long-term patency and are resistant to reinfection. In addition, they are ideal conduits for patients with extensive multilevel occlusive disease, in whom venous grafts theoretically would have better patency than prosthetic grafts. An analogy would be the superior durability of venous grafts for femoropopliteal bypass in comparison

* The authors and editors gratefully acknowledge the contributions of the previous author, Victor J. D'Addio, MD, FACS, to the development and writing of this chapter.

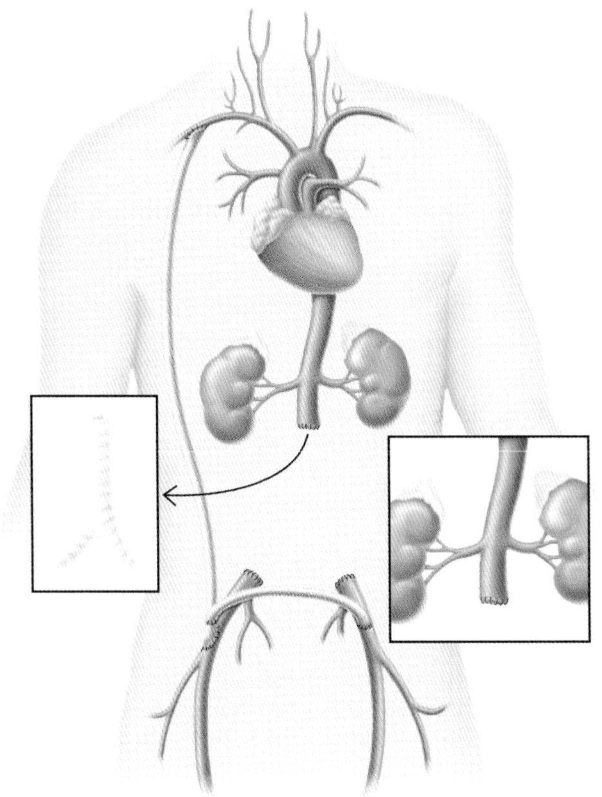

Figure 1 **Standard treatment of aortic graft infection involves axillobifemoral bypass, removal of the infected prosthesis, and oversewing of the aortic stump. This procedure can be performed in either one or two stages. It is most useful in patients who do not have infection extending into the femoral area.**

with prosthetic grafts. The primary disadvantage of reconstruction with FPV grafts is that the procedure is time consuming and technically demanding. In our experience, the mean operating time is about 8 hours. The lower extremity ischemic time is longer than that in patients undergoing extra-anatomic bypass but can be minimized by sequencing the operation so as to shorten the cross-clamp time and by using a two-team approach. Alternatively, FPV harvest can be staged as a separate operation from graft excision and in situ reconstruction.[18] An additional disadvantage of using FPV grafts is the associated short-term venous morbidity. Approximately 12% of patients who undergo FPV harvesting will require fasciotomy, typically performed at the time of vein harvest. The fasciotomy rate is highest in patients who undergo concurrent great saphenous vein harvesting and in those who have severe, preexisting lower extremity ischemia (ankle-brachial index [ABI] < 0.4).[19] Long-term venous morbidity appears to be low, with rare cases of venous ulceration or venous claudication reported in late follow-up.[18] Mild to moderate chronic edema develops in approximately 15% of patients but has been easily controlled with compression stockings. Aneurysmal degeneration of the vein grafts is a theoretical risk but, in practice, is rare. Vein graft stenosis is uncommon but is often amenable to balloon angioplasty to preserve graft patency.[20]

Preoperative Evaluation

The preoperative workup should assess the extent of infection, look for concomitant occlusive disease (indicating a possible need for infrainguinal, visceral, or renal reconstruction), and determine whether there are other associated infectious complications that must be treated surgically (e.g., a psoas abscess, an entrapped ureter with hydronephrosis, or duodenal erosion necessitating duodenal repair). In patients who have previously undergone prosthetic aortofemoral bypass, infection may be limited to one limb of the graft and may be treatable by replacing only that limb. In patients who have previously undergone prosthetic infrainguinal bypass, the prosthetic graft may have to be removed and replaced with an autogenous graft.

Traditionally, the mainstay of the preoperative workup was arteriography complemented by computed tomography (CT), but, currently, the workup is with CT angiography alone. CT angiography is often capable of evaluating the extent of infection, visualizing the sites of previous prosthetic anastomoses, and delineating the arterial anatomy. Magnetic resonance angiography has been a satisfactory alternative, particularly in patients with renal insufficiency. Graft duplex imaging may be useful to diagnose graft infection: the finding of a hypoechoic rim around the graft is indicative of a graft infection. In our experience, tagged white blood cell scanning has rarely been necessary to make the diagnosis of a graft infection and is associated with significant rates of both false positive and false negative results.

When autogenous reconstruction with deep vein grafts is being considered, preoperative assessment of the adequacy of the vein segments must also be performed. This is accomplished by means of venous duplex ultrasonography. Duplex examination of the lower-extremity venous system establishes the diameter and the available length of the deep veins. In addition, the duplex scan can evaluate acute or chronic thrombosis of the deep veins, changes indicative of recanalization, congenital absence or duplication of venous segments, and unusually small deep veins. When the FPV is small (< 6 mm), absent, or incomplete, a dominant profunda femoris vein is usually present. This vein courses posteriorly through the thigh to connect with the popliteal vein and can also be used as a venous autograft. A vein less than 6 mm or a chronically occluded vein is not routinely used. Duplex vein mapping of the great saphenous system is also routinely performed and may provide useful information in the event that concomitant infrainguinal reconstruction is planned or may have to be performed unexpectedly.

Operative Planning

Removal of an infected aortic graft and autogenous reconstruction require prolonged exposure of large portions of the body surface. Significant drops in core body temperature, combined with blood and other fluid losses, may lead to metabolic acidosis, coagulopathy, cardiac dysrhythmia, and immune compromise. Accordingly, core body temperature should be kept above 36°C by applying heated-air warming blankets to the upper body, using warmed fluid for resuscitation, and maintaining a warm ambient temperature in the operating room. Ongoing fluid losses should be anticipated, and aggressive resuscitation should be based on maintaining a normal urine output and/or central venous pressures.

To minimize ischemic time with cross-clamping, the major tasks involved in excision of an infected aortic graft and in situ autogenous reconstruction should be sequenced as follows: (1) dissection of FPVs, which are left in situ until needed; (2) isolation and control of the femoral vessels; (3) entry into the abdomen and control of the aorta; (4) removal of the infected prosthesis; and (5) reconstruction with the deep vein grafts.[21] The entire operation has been termed the creation of a neoaortoiliac system (NAIS).

Operative Technique

STEP 1: THIGH INCISION AND EXPOSURE OF FEMORAL VESSELS

The patient is placed in the supine position with the legs "froglegged" and supported under the thighs. An incision is made on the thigh along the lateral border of the sartorius muscle. This lateral incision not only facilitates vein harvesting but also allows the surgeon to expose the femoral vessels while avoiding the infected femoral incision medially in the groin.

The sartorius is reflected medially so as to preserve the medial segmental blood supply. The subsartorial canal is entered, and the femoral vessels are exposed. The femoral vein is usually located posterior to and slightly lateral to the artery at this level. The entire venous system is then exposed from the distal common femoral vein downward, including the proximal profunda femoris vein through the Hunter canal to the midpopliteal level [*see Figure 2*]. The saphenous nerve is located in this canal and is intimately associated with the femoral vessels. Care must be taken not to injure this nerve either directly or through excessive traction; such an injury will cause irritating postoperative saphenous neuralgia.

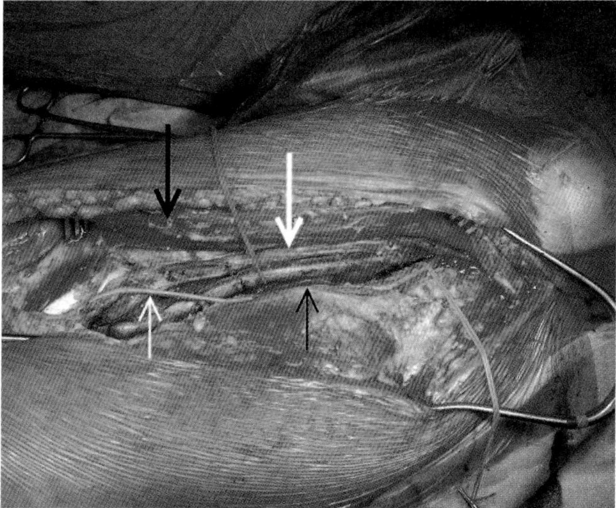

Figure 2 **The femoropopliteal vein (*thin black arrow*), the superficial femoral artery (*thick white arrow*), and the saphenous nerve (*thin white arrow*) lie deep to the sartorius (*thick black arrow*) in the subsartorial canal. The sartorius is reflected medially to expose these structures. The adductor magnus tendon is divided to expose these structures as they traverse the Hunter canal.**

Care must also be taken to preserve major branches of the superficial femoral artery when this vessel is occluded or severely diseased. Interruption of these branches, which may supply collateral circulation to distal beds, may result in unexpected critical ischemia of the lower extremity after completion of the proximal reconstruction, and further infrainguinal arterial reconstruction may be necessary.

STEP 2: DISSECTION OF FPV

The FPV has many large and small side branches. Careful, meticulous, and unhurried ligation of these branches is critical. Most are doubly ligated, with suture ligation reserved for the larger branches. Failure to ligate a branch adequately will result in exsanguinating hemorrhage if a tie loosens and pops off when exposed to aortic pressure. The large diameter of the FPVs, in comparison with the saphenous veins, results in an increase in wall tension that can predispose to a "popped tie." Although, as a rule, the FPV is larger and sturdier than the typical great saphenous vein, it is thin walled in some areas where branches are present. If a branch is avulsed during dissection, suture repair with 6-0 or 7-0 polypropylene is necessary. Branch ligation during FPV harvesting differs from the typical branch ligation during saphenous vein harvesting. The branches of the FPV are ligated close to their base because this is where the vein wall tends to be thin; the larger caliber of the FPV makes this technique possible. In contrast, the branches of the great saphenous vein, which is of smaller caliber, are ligated slightly away from the vessel wall to ensure that the lumen of the vein is not encroached on.

The extent of the harvest depends on the length of venous conduit required for reconstruction. Proximal dissection extends to the level of the junction of the femoral and profunda femoris veins. These veins join to form the common femoral vein, which is also exposed in the dissection. The profunda femoris vein is easily recognizable as a large, posteriorly penetrating vein in the proximal thigh. Distally, dissection is carried through the adductor hiatus by dividing the tendon of the adductor magnus; this measure allows easy access to the proximal portion of the popliteal vein. The popliteal segment of the vein has multiple large branches, which must be carefully ligated. The dissection can easily be taken down to the level of the knee joint. The veins are left in situ until the required length of conduit can be determined.

STEP 3: DISSECTION AND CONTROL OF FEMORAL VESSELS

The femoral vessels can usually be dissected by extending the vein harvest incision cephalad along the lateral border of the sartorius to the level of the anterior superior iliac spine. Through this incision, control of the superficial femoral, profunda femoris, and common femoral vessels is gained. In addition, the distal limbs of the existing aortofemoral graft can be controlled. Occasionally, control is difficult to obtain from a position lateral to the sartorius, in which case, the medial aspect of the muscle may be dissected from the subcutaneous tissue to afford improved exposure. Only rarely is a more medial incision required. As noted [*see* Step 1: Thigh

Incision and Exposure of Femoral Vessels, *above*], the lateral approach allows the surgeon to avoid entering the previous incision, where there may be a draining sinus or cellulitis.

STEP 4: ABDOMINAL INCISION AND DISSECTION OF AORTA

The abdomen is then entered either through a midline abdominal incision or via a retroperitoneal approach; the latter is particularly helpful in avoiding tedious abdominal adhesions. Dissection for control of the aorta above the aortic anastomosis is performed. The anastomosis may be near the level of the renal arteries, in which case, suprarenal or supraceliac aortic control may be required.

STEP 5: REMOVAL AND PREPARATION OF VENOUS GRAFTS

Before cross-clamping, the vein grafts are removed and prepared. The required lengths of each graft are determined by measuring from the aortic anastomosis to the femoral anastomoses on both sides. The femoral vein is divided flush with the profunda femoris vein and oversewn with a 5-0 polypropylene suture. This creates a smooth transition point from the profunda femoris vein to the common femoral vein and leaves no stump in which blood can stagnate and create thrombus. The grafts are then distended in a 4°C solution containing lactated Ringer solution (1 L), heparin (5,000 U), albumin (25 g), and papaverine (60 mg). Any leaks are repaired either with additional silk ties or with figure-eight fine polypropylene sutures. Any adventitial bands that distort the lumen are lysed.

Next, the valves in the grafts must be lysed. This is a critical step because the grafts are placed in a nonreversed fashion to optimize size matching with the aorta for the proximal anastomosis. Valvulotomes have been used for valve lysis in these large-caliber veins, but the results have been unsatisfactory: lysis is often incomplete, and the remnants of the valves may become sites of graft stenosis. Our current practice is to evert the venous grafts completely and to excise all valves under direct vision [*see Figure 3*].

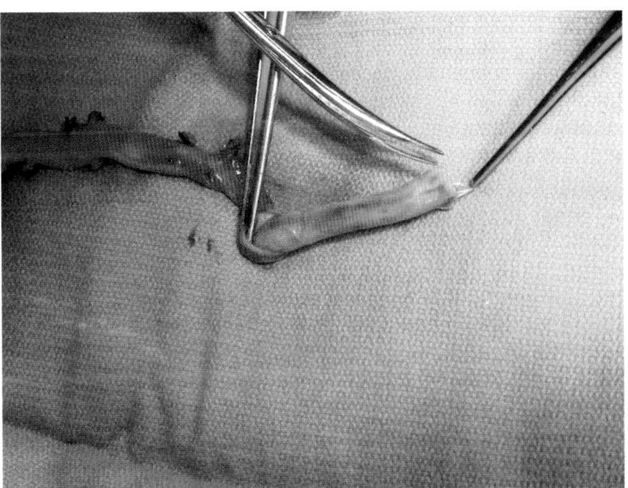

Figure 3 **Use of a valvulotome typically results in incomplete valve lysis. It is preferable to evert the entire venous graft and excise the valves (which usually number three or four) completely with scissors.**

STEP 6: REMOVAL OF BODY OF PREVIOUS GRAFT AND PROXIMAL ANASTOMOSIS OF NEW GRAFT TO AORTA

The patient is systemically heparinized, and the aorta above the anastomosis and both limbs of the graft are cross-clamped. The body of the graft is then excised, with the limbs left in place. All prosthetic material, including sutures, is removed. The previous aortic anastomosis may have been done in either an end-to-end or an end-to-side fashion. If it was an end-to-side anastomosis, the distal end of the aorta will have to be oversewn with a large suture (e.g., 0 or 1-0 polypropylene). Balloon occlusion of the distal lumen is a helpful adjunctive measure before ligation. Regardless of how the previous aortic anastomosis was done, the new anastomosis is typically constructed in an end-to-end fashion. The distal limbs of the existing graft are left in place while the aortic anastomosis is performed so as to decrease the blood loss that typically occurs when the limbs are removed from their tunnels.

Multiple configurations have been successfully employed to reconstruct the distal aortic and iliac-femoral vasculature [*see Figure 4*]. The proximal anastomosis is performed with a continuous 4-0 polypropylene suture. The diameter of the proximal FPV graft is typically about 1.5 cm or a little greater, and the mismatch in diameter between the graft and the aorta is dealt with by taking slightly more advancement (i.e., placing sutures slightly farther apart) on the aortic wall than on the graft wall [*see Figure 5a*]. If the caliber discrepancy between the two structures is too large, other techniques must be employed, such as plication of the aorta, joining of the venous grafts in a pantaloon configuration, or placement of a triangular patch at the proximal aspect of the graft [*see Figure 5, b through d*].

After the proximal anastomosis is complete, the venous graft is distended under aortic pressure, and the side branches are carefully examined to confirm that all ligatures are securely placed. Any questionable areas are repaired. Anastomotic leakage is also repaired with the aorta clamped to ensure that the venous graft is not torn during repair.

STEP 7: REMOVAL OF LIMBS OF PREVIOUS GRAFT AND DISTAL ANASTOMOSES OF NEW GRAFTS TO FEMORAL ARTERIES

The femoral limbs of the prosthetic aortobifemoral grafts are then removed by pulling them through the groin incisions. When the FPV grafts are tunneled to the groins, care must be taken to ensure that ligated side branches are not torn or dislodged. To reduce this risk, we have found it helpful to bring the grafts through the tunnels in the nondistended state. Because it may be difficult to create new tunnels through the scarred retroperitoneum, the vein grafts may be tunneled through the existing tunnels. In many cases, the existing tunnels are smaller in caliber than the new vein grafts, and careful finger dilation of the tunnels is required.

The femoral anastomoses are fashioned in a standard manner. Once again, all prosthetic material and all surrounding infected tissue must be débrided. On occasion, profundaplasty or reimplantation of the profunda femoris may be required. If possible, the femoral anastomoses should be performed in an end-to-side manner to preserve retrograde pelvic perfusion.

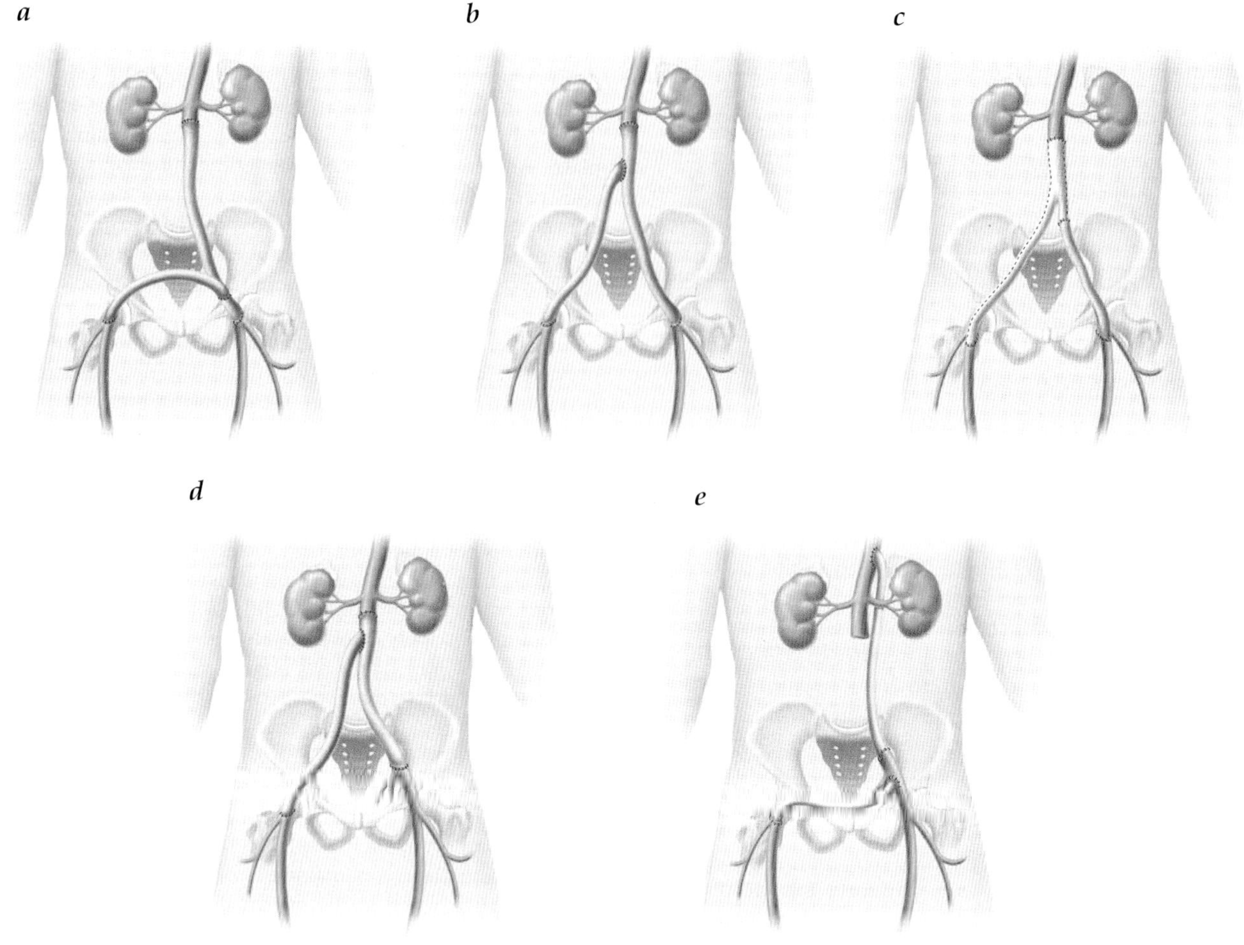

Figure 4 **Multiple anatomic reconstructions have been used to recreate the aorto-iliac-femoral anatomy. (*a*) Shown is an aortounifemoral bypass with a femorofemoral crossover. (*b*) Instead of a femorofemoral bypass, the second limb may be brought off the midportion of the first limb in an end-to-side manner. (*c*) If infection is limited to one limb of an aortofemoral bypass, a femoropopliteal vein graft may be used to replace only the infected portion. (*d*) One segment of vein may be used to replace both segments of an aortoiliac or aortofemoral graft. (*e*) In some instances, it may be easier to approach the paraceliac aorta via a retroperitoneal approach for the proximal anastomosis.**

Perfusion of the extremities must be assessed before the leg wounds are closed. If Doppler arterial signals are absent at the level of the ankle, a femoropopliteal or distal bypass may be necessary. Because the popliteal artery is exposed during FPV harvesting, adjunctive femoropopliteal bypass is easily accomplished in this setting.

STEP 8: CLOSURE

After reversal of heparinization, the thigh wounds are copiously irrigated and closed over closed-suction drains. Placement of drains prevents postoperative seromas and subsequent wound complications. Even though these wounds are contaminated as a consequence of the proximity of the infected graft in the groin wound, infection is rare. Often there are draining sinuses medial to the vein harvest incisions, which are débrided and left open.

Postoperative Care

Parenteral antibiotics are continued for 7 to 10 days, and antibiotic coverage is modified on the basis of intraoperative cultures of the graft material and wound swabs. A longer antibiotic course for up to 6 weeks may be required after incomplete graft removal (because the entire graft was not involved). Patients with associated aortoenteric fistulas (AEFs) are started on antifungal agents in the immediate postoperative period.

Intermittent pneumatic compression and low-dose subcutaneous heparin (5,000 U every 8 to 12 hours) are employed for prevention of deep vein thrombosis. Thrombosis of the residual popliteal vein is common, and aggressive prophylaxis may prevent extension of the thrombus into the calf veins. With the FPV absent, the risk of pulmonary embolism is low. Most of our patients are started on low-dose aspirin as a part of general medical treatment for cardiovascular disease; however, very few require anticoagulation with a vitamin K antagonist.

Outcomes

In our experience, long-term primary patency after NAIS is 81% at 6 years, with secondary patency of 91%.[18] Limb

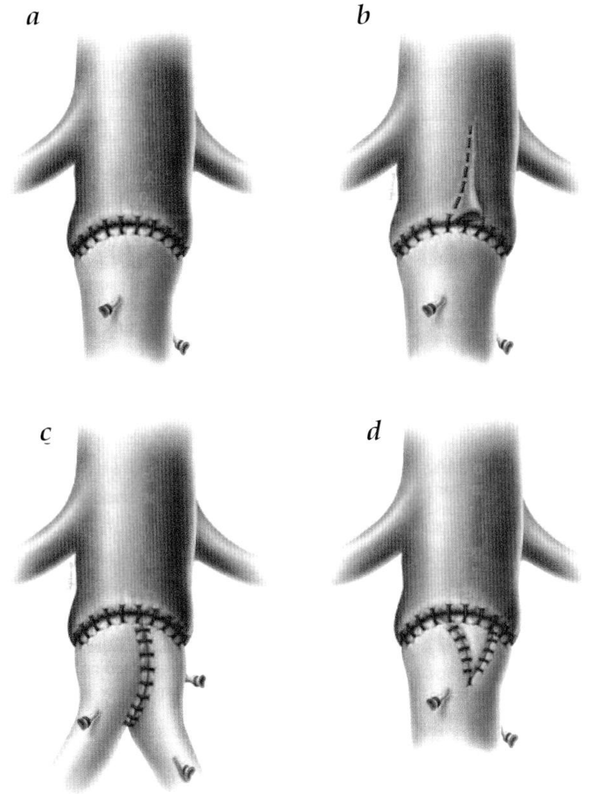

Figure 5 **(*a*) An end-to-end proximal anastomosis is usually possible if the diameter of the femoropopliteal vein (FPV) graft is large enough and the aorta is of normal size. (*b*) If the end of the aorta is significantly larger in diameter than the venous graft, plication of the aorta can be performed. (*c*) A pantaloon technique may also be used to deal with a size mismatch between the aorta and the FPV graft. This technique effectively doubles the circumference of the vein. (*d*) The proximal anastomosis can also be facilitated by incorporating a wedge-shaped portion of vein into the proximal end of the graft.**

salvage and long-term survival have been reported as 89% and 52%, respectively. Most patients die of cardiovascular causes; those who present with aortoduodenal fistula have worse outcomes.[18]

The incidence of graft disruption is about 5%, and most occur within 2 weeks of the initial operation. It is thought that this is secondary to reinfection of the vein graft, usually attributable to virulent organisms or to poor host defenses. This complication has a particularly poor outcome with a high mortality rate.

Complications

The incidence of chronic venous morbidity after FPV harvesting is low, with fewer than 15% of patients demonstrating manifestations of chronic venous insufficiency on long-term follow-up. Very few patients require long-term compression therapy for venous insufficiency. As noted above, the fasciotomy rate is approximately 12% in recent studies. In our practice, the decision to perform a fasciotomy is based primarily on clinical examination of the legs. We specifically assess progressive compartment swelling and firmness on serial examination after reperfusion of the lower extremities. We also consider risk factors in making this decision. Two specific risk factors for fasciotomy are (1) a low preoperative ABI (< 0.4) and (2) concurrent great saphenous vein harvesting.[18,19] Other factors may also help determine the need for fasciotomy, including the indication for operation, the length of vein harvested, the duration of arterial cross-clamping, and the amount of fluid administered intraoperatively.

Special Consideration: Aortoenteric Fistulas

AEF may be classified as primary or secondary, depending on the presence of a previously placed aortic graft. A primary AEF occurs between the native aorta and diseased bowel lumen, whereas a secondary AEF represents a communication between bowel and a previously placed aortic graft. The secondary AEF usually occurs at the third or fourth portion of the duodenum, and the associated graft is considered to be infected. The secondary AEF presents an especially difficult therapeutic challenge because the infected prosthesis must be removed, the distal perfusion preserved, and the gastrointestinal tract repaired. Although AEF may be associated with acute gastrointestinal hemorrhage that requires emergency control, reports suggest that those who present with gastrointestinal bleeding do not have a worse outcome compared with patients who present without bleeding (aortoenteric erosion).[22,23] AEF and aortoenteric erosions have equally high morbidity and mortality rates.[22]

When AEF is suspected, broad-spectrum antibiotics should be initiated immediately. In our experience, a significant percentage of involved grafts have had positive fungal cultures; therefore, we routinely include antifungal agents along with antibiotic therapy. At our institution, the type of repair for secondary AEF is dictated by the presence or absence of active hemorrhage, the hemodynamic stability of the patient, and the degree of retroperitoneal contamination. We prefer in situ replacement with femoropopliteal veins (NAIS) in hemodynamically stable patients without active bleeding. Rifampin-soaked Dacron graft may be an option if there is minimal contamination, particularly in a frail patient. In unstable patients with active bleeding, we perform aortic ligation with extra-anatomic bypass.

The modern era of endovascular therapy has garnered enthusiasm for endovascular aortic repair (EVAR) to treat secondary AEF. Scattered reports suggest early success to control hemorrhage.[24,25] However, reinfection has been reported in several case series, with morbid consequences.[23–25] Use of EVAR to treat AEF violates fundamental principles, especially control of the infectious source and repair of the bowel. In general, EVAR should be considered a temporizing, lifesaving alternative in patients who are hemodynamically unstable from bleeding. EVAR should not be considered a permanent treatment in these circumstances, and more definitive intervention will be necessary as soon as the patient is medically able to tolerate it.

Financial Disclosures: None Reported

prosthetic material or autologous vein, has certain advantages, including a straight graft configuration that minimizes turbulence and graft kinking. Typically, there is also reduced atherosclerotic calcification in the supraceliac aorta.[16] The disadvantages of antegrade bypass are similar to those of visceral endarterectomy and derive from the need to clamp the supraceliac aorta for the proximal anastomosis. As with visceral endarterectomy, partial occlusion clamping is theoretically possible but not always practical. Clamping of the supraceliac aorta may increase the risk of cardiac events, visceral or renal emboli, and ischemia. One prerequisite for use of the supraceliac aorta in an antegrade bypass is that the vessel must be angiographically normal to ensure that it can safely be clamped. It should also be kept in mind that reoperation on the supraceliac aorta is difficult: once this site has been used, reexposure generally is not safe.

Antegrade bypass *Step 1: incision and initial approach* Supraceliac aorta–visceral artery bypass is performed through an upper midline incision. Self-retaining retractors are very helpful.

Step 2: exposure The dissection begins with division of the gastrohepatic ligament and retraction of the left lobe of the liver to the right, followed by incision of the diaphragmatic crus and exposure of the anterior aspect of the aorta.

Step 3: choice of graft In clean cases with no intestinal necrosis or perforation, we use woven Dacron grafts. If a single-vessel bypass is to be performed, a single limb is cut from the bifurcated graft, incorporating a flange of the main body of the bifurcated graft for the proximal anastomosis. Autologous vein grafts are usually reserved for contaminated cases. The femoral vein is an excellent autogenous conduit for mesenteric arterial bypass.

Step 4: anastomosis of graft to supraceliac aorta and visceral artery If the celiac artery alone is to be revascularized, the usual procedure is to perform an end-to-side proximal anastomosis to the aorta, followed by an end-to-side distal anastomosis to the common hepatic artery. If the SMA alone is to be revascularized, it is generally necessary to tunnel the graft beneath the pancreas to the inferior border of the pancreas and then perform an end-to-side anastomosis to the SMA at that level [*see Figure 5a*]. Extreme care must be exercised in developing the retropancreatic tunnel. If this area appears too narrow or is scarred as a result of previous pancreatic inflammation, the graft should be tunneled anterior to the pancreas to ensure that it is not compressed and to avoid causing bleeding from disrupted pancreatic veins.[17] If a prepancreatic tunnel is required, an autogenous conduit should be considered because the graft will be lying adjacent to the posterior wall of the stomach. If both the celiac artery and the SMA are to be revascularized from the supraceliac aorta, a bifurcated prosthetic graft is attached to the supraceliac aorta proximally, with one distal limb anastomosed to the hepatic artery and the other to the SMA [*see Figure 5b*].

Retrograde bypass In a retrograde bypass, the infrarenal aorta or, more commonly, common iliac artery is used as the inflow vessel. One clear advantage of this procedure is that the approach to the infrarenal aorta is more familiar to most surgeons. Another is that dissection and clamping of the infrarenal aorta are less risky than dissection and clamping of the supraceliac aorta. Yet another is that the surgeon can work within a single operative field. Once the self-retaining retractor is placed, the operation on the infrarenal aorta and the SMA can be performed without further adjustment of the retractor. The main disadvantage is the potential for graft kinking.

Step 1: incision and initial approach Here, too, a midline incision and a transperitoneal approach are preferred. The transverse mesocolon is retracted upward, and the ligament of Treitz is divided.

Step 2: exposure After division of the ligament of Treitz, the duodenum and the small bowel are retracted to the right. The SMA may then be identified arising from beneath the inferior border of the pancreas. The retroperitoneum is divided distally along the aorta to a point just beyond the level of the aortic bifurcation. The distal aorta and both common iliac arteries are assessed to allow determination of the optimal location for the proximal anastomosis.

Step 3: choice of graft As a rule, grafts made of Dacron or of ringed, reinforced expanded polytetrafluoroethylene (ePTFE) are preferred. Problems may arise when retrograde bypasses are performed with autologous vein grafts, in that such grafts are prone to kinking when the viscera are replaced. When a retrograde vein bypass is performed, the graft may be brought straight up from the right iliac artery so that it lies between the aorta and the duodenum and then anastomosed to the posteromedial wall of the SMA.

Step 4: anastomosis to infrarenal aorta or common iliac artery and SMA Our preference is to use the area near the junction of the aorta with the right common iliac artery for the proximal anastomosis. (Short grafts originating from the midportion of the infrarenal aorta, although commonly described, are prone to kinking when the viscera are returned to their normal position.) The graft to the SMA is passed cephalad, turned anteriorly and inferiorly 180°, and anastomosed to the anterior wall of the SMA just beyond the inferior border of the pancreas.[17] In this manner, a gentle C loop is formed that, if placed correctly, keeps the graft from kinking when the viscera are restored to their anatomic position after retractor removal [*see Figure 6*]. The ligament of Treitz and the parietal and mesenteric peritoneum are closed over the graft to exclude it from the peritoneal cavity.

Endovascular Techniques

Endovascular techniques, usually a combination of angioplasty and stent placement, are being used with greater frequency for chronic mesenteric ischemia [*see Figure 7*]. By 2002, endovascular procedures (angioplasty/stent) surpassed all surgical procedures performed for chronic mesenteric ischemia, with decreased 30-day mortality compared with open procedures (4 versus 13%).[18] Early reports describing the use of percutaneous transluminal angioplasty (PTA) to treat visceral atherosclerotic lesions indicated that initial technical success rates were as high as 80% but that recurrence rates ranged from 20 to 40%.[17,19] Recent reports of endovascular therapy for chronic mesenteric ischemia showed no difference in in-hospital morbidity or mortality or 2-year survival. Also, there was no difference in symptomatic (23 versus 22%) or radiographic (32 versus 37%) recurrence. However, radiographic primary patency (58 versus 90%) and primary assisted patency (65 versus 96%) were significantly lower

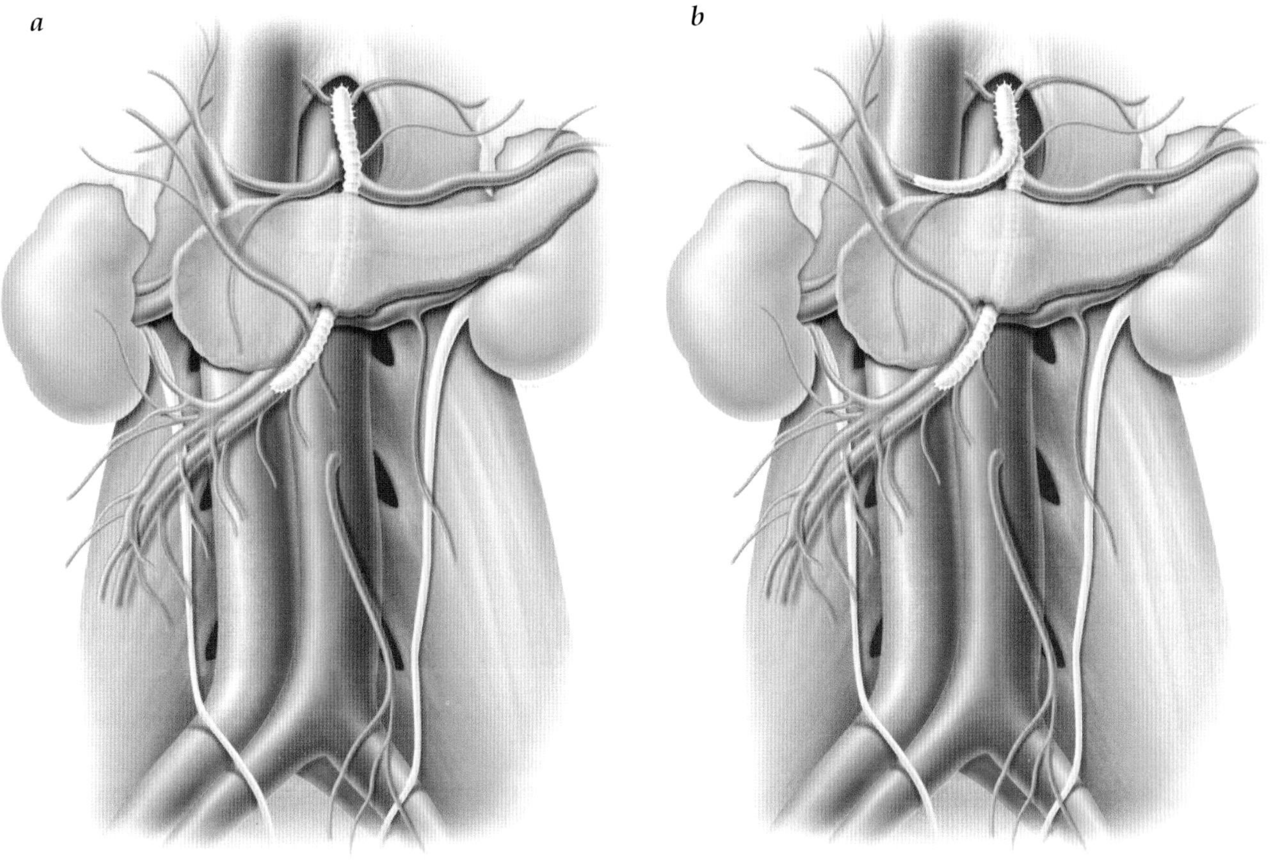

Figure 5 **Arterial bypass: antegrade. Shown is bypass from the supraceliac aorta to the superior mesenteric artery (SMA) alone (*a*) or to the hepatic artery and the SMA (*b*).[39]**

in the patients who received endovascular treatment.[20] Another study with longer follow-up showed 3-year actuarial patency of 63%. About 30% of patients required reintervention for recurrent symptoms. The median time to reintervention for symptom recurrence was 15 months. Because of this high rate of restenosis and symptom recurrence, close follow-up is mandatory in all patients treated with mesenteric artery stents. Most importantly, initial endovascular treatment did not preclude any future surgical bypass options.[21] These early results indicate that an endovascular approach to chronic mesenteric ischemia is a viable option in carefully selected patients.

COMPLICATIONS

Technical

The main technical complication of mesenteric bypass is acute graft thrombosis. This event is rare, but when it occurs, prompt recognition is essential to prevent intestinal infarction. Kinking and compression of the graft are the most common causes of this condition. If the retrograde graft is too long, the redundancy makes it more susceptible to kinking. Similarly, if the graft is not positioned so as to form a gentle C loop, it is at risk for kinking when the viscera are returned to their normal position. An antegrade graft that is too long is equally at risk for kinking and occlusion. When an antegrade bypass is tunneled behind the pancreas, an adequate amount of space must be present to ensure that the graft is not compressed. In general, prosthetic grafts are more resistant to kinking and compression than vein grafts are.

Identification of perioperative graft occlusion is hindered by postoperative incisional pain, fluid shifts, fever, and leukocytosis, all of which are common in the postoperative period and may mask signs of intestinal ischemia. Patients with chronic mesenteric ischemia often have symptoms only when eating and thus may be asymptomatic in the postoperative period until they resume oral feeding. For these reasons, we advocate evaluating the graft early in the postoperative period with either conventional contrast angiography or CT angiography [*see* Outcome Evaluation, *below*].

Additional technical complications may occur as a result of clamp placement. Clamping of the supraceliac aorta can lead to renal atheroemboli or ischemia. These problems can be minimized by using a supraceliac clamp only on an angiographically normal aorta.

Systemic

Myocardial infarction is the most common cause of mortality in patients treated for mesenteric ischemia. Pulmonary compromise is also a common systemic complication of mesenteric revascularization. Renal failure after mesenteric revascularization is more common in patients with preoperative renal insufficiency.[22] Mortality is markedly increased when renal failure occurs postoperatively.[22] Postoperative renal does not appear to correlate with the degree of intestinal infarction.[28] Peritonitis is initially absent, but vomiting and diarrhea may be present, and occult gastric or rectal bleeding may be identified in as many as 25% of patients.[28]

There are no reliable serum markers for acute intestinal ischemia. Leukocytosis, hyperamylasemia, or elevated lactate levels may be present, but these findings are insensitive and inconsistent. Abdominal radiographs may reveal dilated bowel loops and, occasionally, thickened bowel wall, but these findings are similarly inconsistent. In theory, duplex ultrasonography may be helpful, but in practice, its applicability is often limited by the gaseous visceral distention frequently associated with acute intestinal ischemia.

Acute intestinal ischemia is a true surgical emergency. Any evidence of acute abdomen should result in prompt operative intervention. In stable patients suspected of having acute mesenteric ischemia, the paradigm for diagnostic workup has been slowly shifting toward the use of multidetector CT angiography. Multidetector CT angiography uses thinner collimation and overlapping data acquisition, which reduces the amount of volume averaging and creates higher quality volume sets for three-dimensional reconstruction. There are several advantages to CT angiography, including near-universal 24-hour access to a high-resolution scanner. With three-dimensional reconstruction, mesenteric vessels can be evaluated for embolus or thrombotic occlusion with accuracy. Also, bowel can be evaluated concomitantly to support or refute the diagnosis, and other intra-abdominal pathology can be evaluated. A prospective study compared preoperative radiographic findings with operative findings in 62 patients suspected of acute myocardial infarction. Initial radiologist interpretation had a sensitivity of 100% and a specificity of 89%.[29] A subsequent study using CT angiography had similar results in terms of accuracy.[30] Significant limitations include the need for proper timing of the contrast to evaluate the vasculature and that the modality does not offer any therapeutic options.

The use of preoperative arteriography to diagnose acute ischemia is controversial. Delaying treatment to perform arteriography could result in further intestinal infarction. Angiography may be considered in patients who have abdominal pain without any other signs or symptoms of systemic illness [*see Figure 9*]. In patients who have rebound tenderness, rigidity, or evidence of toxicity or shock, emergency exploration is indicated.

OPERATIVE PLANNING

Patients with acute intestinal ischemia who present with evidence of toxicity must be resuscitated expeditiously to ensure that surgical intervention is not delayed. Once it is determined that surgery is indicated, no further delay is justified. The patient is placed supine on the operating table, and the entire abdomen and both legs are prepared. As in operative treatment of chronic intestinal ischemia, the possibility that autologous vein will be needed for bypass grafting must be anticipated.

OPERATIVE TECHNIQUE

Intraoperative Considerations

Mesenteric revascularization and bowel resection The goals of surgical therapy are to restore normal pulsatile

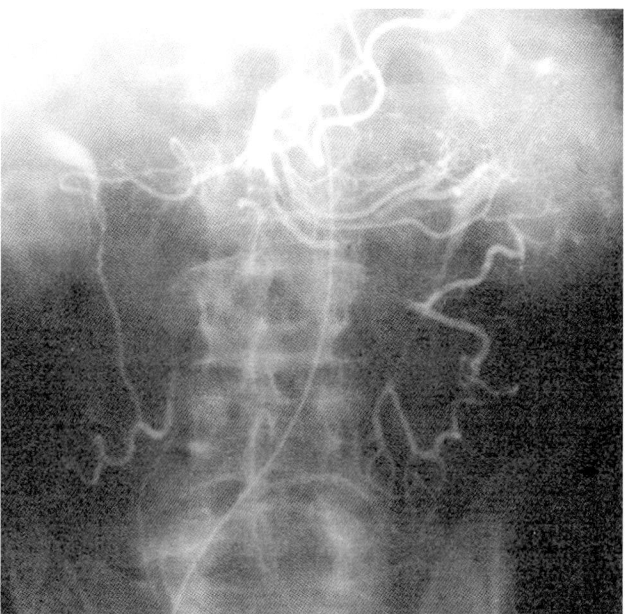

Figure 9 **Preoperative arteriogram shows embolic occlusion of the superior mesenteric artery distal to its origin.**

inflow, to ensure that questionably viable bowel is adequately perfused, and to resect any clearly nonviable bowel. During abdominal exploration, the viability of the intestine and the status of the blood flow to the SMA are assessed with an eye to determining the appropriate treatment. The surgeon should be prepared to perform both intestinal revascularization and intestinal resection. Segments of clearly viable bowel are often interspersed with segments of marginally viable bowel and segments of necrotic bowel. Acutely ischemic bowel that is not yet necrotic may appear deceptively normal. Mildly to moderately ischemic bowel may exhibit loss of normal sheen, absence of peristalsis, and dull-gray discoloration. Other objective signs of ischemia are the absence of a palpable pulse in the SMA or in its distal branches, the absence of visible pulsations in the mesentery, and the absence of flow on continuous-wave Doppler examination of the vessels of the bowel wall. The small bowel may be deeply cyanotic yet still viable. In most cases, bowel resection should not be performed until after revascularization.

The distribution of ischemic changes provides valuable information about the cause of the ischemia. SMA thrombosis often results in ischemia to the entire small bowel, with the stomach, the duodenum, and the distal colon spared; in severe cases, however, the entire foregut may be ischemic. In contrast, ischemia secondary to SMA embolism generally spares the stomach, the duodenum, and the proximal jejunum because the emboli tend to lodge at the level of the middle colic artery rather than at the origin of the SMA. The choice of operation for revascularizing the bowel depends on the underlying causative condition. Embolectomy is indicated for arterial embolism, whereas bypass is indicated for thrombotic occlusion.

Revascularization of the acutely ischemic intestine Patients with very advanced intestinal ischemia may have obvious widespread bowel necrosis. This situation almost invariably proves fatal; thus, revascularization is not likely indicated. In many patients, however, substantial portions of the bowel are ischemic but not frankly necrotic. Whether such bowel segments can be restored to viability cannot be accurately predicted. In most instances, therefore, revascularization should precede resection.

Restoration of normal flow to the SMA can produce remarkable changes in an ischemic bowel. Because these changes do not always occur immediately, it is often necessary to preserve questionably viable portions of the bowel initially and then perform a second-look laparotomy within 12 to 36 hours. If the questionably viable bowel is not in significantly better condition at the time of the second-look operation, it should be resected. Occasionally, however, even a third look is prudent. Revascularized intestine that was profoundly ischemic may swell dramatically. Temporary abdominal closure with mesh or leaving the abdomen open with a temporary closure device may permit tension-free abdominal "closure," prevent abdominal compartment syndrome, and perhaps even improve intestinal perfusion by reducing intra-abdominal pressure.

Superior Mesenteric Artery Embolectomy

Step 1: incision and initial approach A midline incision and transperitoneal approach is used.

Step 2: exposure of SMA at root of mesentery The SMA is exposed after division of the ligament of Treitz at the base of the transverse colon mesentery. The duodenum and the small bowel are retracted to the right [*see Figure 10*]. The visceral peritoneum is incised above the ligament of Treitz, just cephalad to the third portion of the duodenum. The SMA should be readily palpable in this location as it crosses over the third portion of the duodenum. The dissection is continued to obtain sufficient proximal and distal control of the vessel. Heparin is administered, and the vessel is clamped proximally and distally.

Step 3: arteriotomy An arteriotomy is then made in the SMA. The incision may be either transverse or longitudinal. We prefer to perform a longitudinal arteriotomy if there is any possibility that a bypass graft may be needed. The arteriotomy should be made approximately 2 to 3 cm distal to the origin of the SMA, although alternative placements may be appropriate on occasion, depending on the anatomy and the estimated location of the occlusion [*see Figure 11, a and b*].

Step 4: embolectomy Proximal embolectomy should be performed first to ensure adequate inflow. A 3 or 4 French balloon catheter is sufficient in most cases. If very good pulsatile inflow is not achieved after embolectomy, then thrombosis of a stenotic lesion is likely to be the underlying cause of the acute intestinal ischemia, and a bypass graft should be placed. Even when inflow is apparently adequate, a bypass should be strongly considered if the proximal SMA is palpably abnormal.

The narrowness and fragility of the distal SMA and its branches can make distal embolectomy particularly challenging. It is best to use a 2 French embolectomy catheter for this procedure. The catheter must be passed gently, without undue force.

Step 5: closure Once all possible thrombus has been removed, the arteriotomy is closed. A transverse arteriotomy may be closed primarily with interrupted monofilament sutures [*see Figure 11c*]; however, a longitudinal arteriotomy frequently must be closed with an autologous vein patch. If adequate flow is not restored after the clamps are removed, the arteriotomy is used as the distal anastomotic site of a bypass graft.

Superior Mesenteric Artery Bypass

Patients with SMA thrombosis who are seen early enough and who have no intestinal necrosis may undergo SMA bypass grafting with a prosthetic conduit. At exploration, many of these patients have fluid within the peritoneal cavity. This finding is not, in itself, a contraindication to the use of a prosthetic graft. However, if the patient has necrotic bowel that must be resected or if perforation has occurred, a prosthetic graft should not be used. In these situations, an autologous vein graft is preferred. A good-quality vein is mandatory; if the saphenous vein is inadequate, the femoral vein may be used instead.

The techniques of mesenteric bypass for acute intestinal ischemia are identical to those for chronic intestinal ischemia. Because these patients are often acutely ill, it is vital to perform the operation rapidly and efficiently. In the acute setting, bypass to the SMA alone is strongly preferred [*see Figure 12*]. As a rule, a retrograde approach, using the infrarenal aorta or a common iliac artery for inflow, is best; the supraceliac aorta is used for inflow only if the infrarenal vessels are unsuitable for this purpose. Even highly calcified iliac arteries can be used for inflow provided that there is no significant pressure gradient and that the surgeon is familiar with intraluminal balloon occlusion techniques for proximal and distal control.

Hybrid Technique: Retrograde Open Mesenteric Stenting

Recently, a hybrid technique has been described that combines the attributes of both endovascular and open procedures. It allows for both endovascular treatment of mesenteric vessels and thorough assessment of bowel viability. Initial results show a 100% initial success and a lower in-hospital mortality rate of 17% compared with surgical bypass or endovascular treatment.[31,32]

Step 1: Incision and exposure A patient suspected of acute myocardial infarction is brought directly to the operating room with ongoing resuscitation. The left arm is abducted and prepared along with standard preparation for potential brachial access. Once the diagnosis is confirmed, initial midline exploration and control of the infracolic SMA is obtained as described for an SMA embolectomy procedure.

Step 2: Patch angioplasty and cannulation of infracolic SMA Once exposure and control of infracolic SMA are obtained, the patient is fully heparinized to activated clotting time of more than 300 seconds. The artery is incised longitudinally, and a local thromboendarterectomy with patch angioplasty is performed. Either bovine pericardium or saphenous vein can be used for the patch. A purse-string suture is placed in the patch, through which a 6 French sheath is placed into the SMA in retrograde fashion through the distal end of

15 UPPER EXTREMITY REVASCULARIZATION PROCEDURES

John Byrne, MCh, FRCSI (Gen), and R. Clement Darling III, MD

All vascular surgeons are familiar with acute arm ischemia. It is relatively common and amenable, in most cases, to simple embolectomy. Chronic arm ischemia is more infrequent. Even in busier centers, arm revascularization accounts for only 3.2% of elective arterial operations. Its surgical treatment is also more technically demanding. Balloon angioplasty of the subclavian artery was described in 1980.[1,2] Today, endovascular techniques have largely replaced surgical bypass for innominate artery (IA) and subclavian artery (SA) disease. Paradoxically, the exponential growth of endoluminal technology has led to a resurgence in carotid-subclavian bypass due to "prophylactic" debranching of the aortic arch prior to placement of thoracic stents in patients with extensive aneurysms. In addition, the rising incidence of diabetes and longer survival times reported in patients with renal impairment have led to increased use of distal bypass procedures in the arm (analogous to pedal bypass procedures in the leg). Finally, the growing number and increasing complexity of dialysis access procedures has also [illegible]

The consequences of lower limb amputation are serious. Upper extremity amputation is arguably more catastrophic, affecting all aspects of life. In this chapter, we describe a rational approach to emergency and elective arm revascularization, with an emphasis on the technical aspects of these procedures.

Procedures for Acute Arm Ischemia

Acute arm ischemia accounts for one fifth of all episodes of acute limb ischemia. It occurs twice as often in females as males. Brachial embolectomy is the most common treatment. After successful brachial embolectomy, 95% of patients are symptom free[3]; however, the operative mortality may be as high as 12%,[4] although this is slightly higher than in our experience. Most reports that address acute arm ischemia include only those patients who are treated surgically. In fact, between 9 and 30% of patients who present to vascular surgeons with acute arm ischemia are managed conservatively, either because they are unfit for surgery or because they have minimal symptoms. These conservatively managed patients are probably underrepresented in the literature. In the few reported series, assessment of symptoms and disability has been largely inconsistent. However, in a 1964 series that included 95 patients, 32% of those who were managed conservatively were left with abnormal function in their arms after treatment.[5] In a 1977 report, 75% of the conservatively managed patients had poor functional outcomes.[6] In a 1985 study, 50% of conservatively managed patients had persistent forearm claudication.[7] The conclusion to be drawn is that although conservative management is appropriate for some patients presenting with acute arm ischemia, every effort should be made to restore blood flow in patients who have a reasonable life expectancy.

BRACHIAL EMBOLECTOMY

Preoperative Evaluation

Patients presenting with acute arm ischemia tend to be slightly older at presentation than those with leg ischemia (74 versus 70 years).[8] There is often an underlying embolic source, usually left atrial thrombus in patients with atrial fibrillation. Common scenarios include new-onset atrial fibrillation or chronic atrial fibrillation with subtherapeutic anticoagulation. Most arm emboli (75%) are of cardiac origin. Most emboli lodge in the brachial artery (60%), followed by the axillary artery (26%). In situ thrombosis accounts for 5% of episodes of arm ischemia.[9] Patients usually complain of abrupt coldness of the hand but may describe transient pain and paresthesia. Objectively, the hand feels cooler than the healthy limb and may be noticeably paler. Movement is usually preserved, although the affected hand may be a little weaker than normal. Examination confirms absence of the radial, brachial, or axillary pulses depending on the level of occlusion. Usually, within hours of infusing heparin, the hand is appreciably warmer and more erythematous.

Selection of patients All patients with acute-onset arm ischemia are candidates for embolectomy. Most brachial embolectomies are performed under local anesthesia with intravenous sedation. Only a minority of patients require general anesthesia. The duration of surgery is typically short and avoids major cardiovascular compromise. As noted above, conservative management should be considered only for patients who are terminally ill or unfit for surgical intervention.

Alternative therapy Some authors have achieved good results by using thrombolysis to treat occlusion of the axillary or brachial artery.[10] However, in a 2001 series that included 38 patients with 40 occlusions treated with thrombolysis, the success rate of this approach was only 55%, and eight patients required surgical thrombectomy after thrombolysis failed.[11] Excellent outcomes have been reported for the treatment of acute arm ischemia with rotational thrombectomy devices (e.g., Rotarex, Sraub Medical, Wangs, Switzerland). To date, however, no large published studies have evaluated these devices, and clinical experience is limited to case reports.[12]

Operative Planning

In most patients with acute arm ischemia, diagnosis is straightforward and surgical treatment relatively easy. Some instances of acute arm ischemia, however, are caused by an inflow lesion in the SA (e.g., from ulcerated plaques, a thrombosed SA aneurysm, or an arterial thoracic outlet syndrome). In such situations, even a technically perfect embolectomy will fail to restore normal hand perfusion. Even so, angiography is usually unnecessary because more than 90% of patients with acute arm ischemia have an embolus amenable to simple embolectomy. We recommend diagnostic arm angiograms for patients who have undergone axillary or subclavian artery surgery, symptoms suggestive of arterial thoracic outlet syndrome, a history of arm claudication, or clinical evidence of an SA aneurysm. For all others, embolectomy can be performed without imaging.

The majority of brachial embolectomies are performed with local anesthesia, with or without monitored conscious sedation.

Operative Technique

The origins of the ulnar and radial arteries are exposed by means of a so-called lazy S incision [*see Figure 1a*], which prevents the elbow contracture that can occur with a vertical incision. Care is taken to preserve the superficial veins, especially the median antecubital vein, as it may be needed to patch the brachial artery. The bicipital fascia is incised, and the brachial artery is found between the tendon of biceps laterally and the median nerve medially [*see Figure 1b*]. Dissection is continued distally until the ulnar and radial arteries are encountered. The radial artery is considered a continuation of the brachial artery. The ulnar artery, on the other hand, comes off the brachial artery medially and, within 2 to 3 cm, dives beneath the pronator and epitrochlear muscles. It is important to access the origins of both forearm arteries because the embolectomy catheter must be passed down each vessel. If the catheter is blindly passed down the brachial artery, it will probably travel down the radial artery. This will reestablish flow to the hand in the majority of patients. However, it will not restore adequate flow if the ulnar is the dominant artery of the hand or if the catheter passes down the common interosseous artery, which does not provide any flow to the hand.

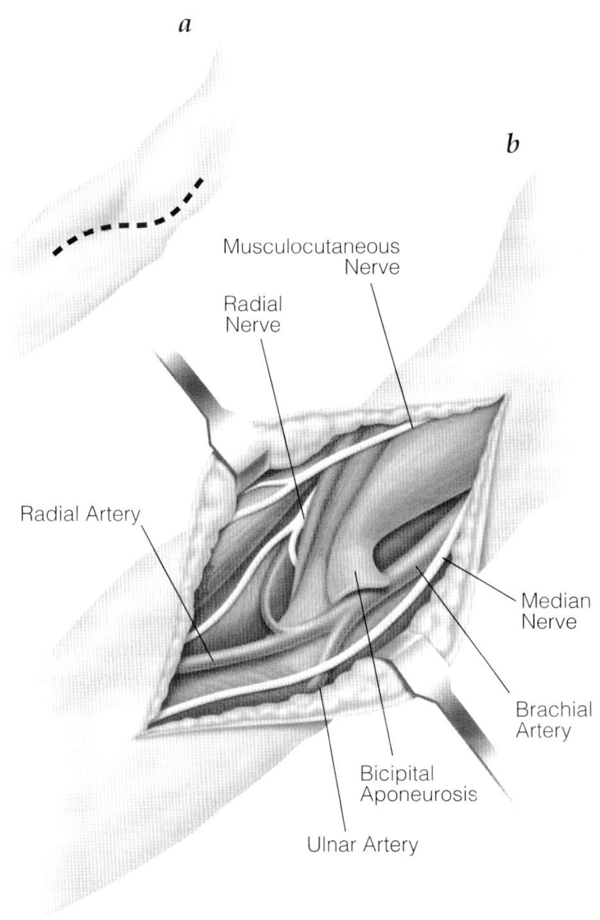

Figure 1 **Brachial embolectomy. Shown are (*a*) a lazy S incision and (*b*) the main nerves and vessels exposed.**

An arteriotomy (usually vertical) is made in the brachial artery. Clot may be encountered at the bifurcation; if so, it is readily removed. In some cases, the brachial artery is pulseless, which indicates that the embolus is lodged more proximally. Once inflow is established, a size 2 or 3 French embolectomy catheter is passed distally down each forearm artery. The arteriotomy is then closed either primarily or with a vein patch. A segment of vein may be harvested from the antecubital fossa. Adequate flow in the radial and ulnar arteries is confirmed by means of an intra-operative Doppler probe.

Occasionally, the hand is still ischemic even after an adequate embolectomy. This persistent ischemia is caused either by an unrecognized inflow lesion or chronic embolization to the digital arteries, which has been occurring over an extended period. In these patients, an arch aortogram with selective views of the affected arm should be performed immediately after the operation or, if the surgery is taking place in a "hybrid" room, prior to closing the surgical incision. Any lesion in the SA or innominate artery can then be treated with angioplasty and stenting.

Postoperative Care

The mainstay of postoperative management is adequate anticoagulation and a search for the source of embolization using noninvasive imaging such as transthoracic echocardiography. Embolization recurs after successful embolectomy in one third of patients if systemic anticoagulation is not instituted. It may recur even in the face of oral anticoagulation: in a 1989 study, 11% of patients given warfarin after embolectomy sustained a further embolic episode, and all had ongoing atrial fibrillation.[8]

After discharge, patients are routinely followed up by means of noninvasive studies of the upper extremity 4 to 6 weeks after operation.

FOREARM FASCIOTOMY

Unlike calf fasciotomies, which are commonly needed for leg ischemia, forearm fasciotomies are rarely required for acute arm ischemia. They are more commonly required for traumatic injuries to the arm (e.g., crush injuries or brachial artery injuries associated with supracondylar fracture of

IA bypass more difficult. In the majority, the IA branches into a right CCA and a right SA, with the left CCA and SA coming directly off the arch. In 16% of patients, however, the IA and the right CCA may have a common ostium. In 8% of patients, the left CCA comes off the IA, leaving the left SA as the only other artery coming off the arch. In 6% of patients, the left vertebral artery comes off the arch between the left CCA and the left SA. In fewer than 1% of patients, the right SA comes off the descending aorta as the last arch branch and then travels behind the esophagus (as the retroesophageal right SA) to reach the right supraclavicular fossa.[15]

Operative technique The IA is approached via a median sternotomy.[16] A sternal retractor is placed and opened. The thymus is divided along its midline with the electrocautery, and the inferior thymic vein is ligated and divided. The brachiocephalic vein is identified as it crosses the IA and then mobilized and placed in a vessel sling. The pericardium is opened from the ventricular surface to a point just below the origin of the IA. It is held away from the operative field with stay sutures. The ascending aorta is then exposed. Fat and visceral pericardium are cleared from the anterior and lateral walls of the aorta to allow placement of a partial occlusion clamp. The brachiocephalic vein is retracted downward, and dissection is continued distally along the IA toward the origins of the right SA and the right CCA. Care must be taken to keep from injuring any major nerves, particularly the right recurrent laryngeal nerve.

Some authors have employed a partial median sternotomy approach to the IA, which is useful when access to the distal half of the IA is required and access to the ascending aorta is not required. The advantage of this approach is that it preserves the lower sternum, thereby enhancing the stability of the chest and reducing postoperative pain. The incision extends only to the fourth intercostal space.

After heparinization, a partial occlusion clamp is placed on the ascending aorta, and an arteriotomy is made. An 8 mm graft is sutured to the aorta in an end-to-side fashion with 3-0 or 4-0 polypropylene. If the IA is occluded, the right CCA and the right SA are clamped, and the IA is divided and oversewn. The graft is then sewn to the common ostium of the SA and the CCA in an end-to-end fashion [*see Figure 4*]. Flow is confirmed with a Doppler probe, as with all the reconstructions we describe in this chapter.

Postoperative care After the operation, patients are observed in the intensive care unit. In general, anticoagulation is not indicated. After recovery, patients are followed by means of noninvasive graft surveillance.

SUBCLAVIAN ARTERY

Most patients with SA stenosis or occlusion require no treatment. In many cases, overt symptoms are absent, and the diagnosis is made serendipitously when a reduced pulse pressure is encountered in one arm. Symptoms affect 5 to 10% of patients with SA lesions causing either arm claudication or vertebrobasilar steal symptoms, manifesting as either "drop attacks" or dizziness on arm exercise (symptomatic subclavian steal syndrome). For patients with symptomatic

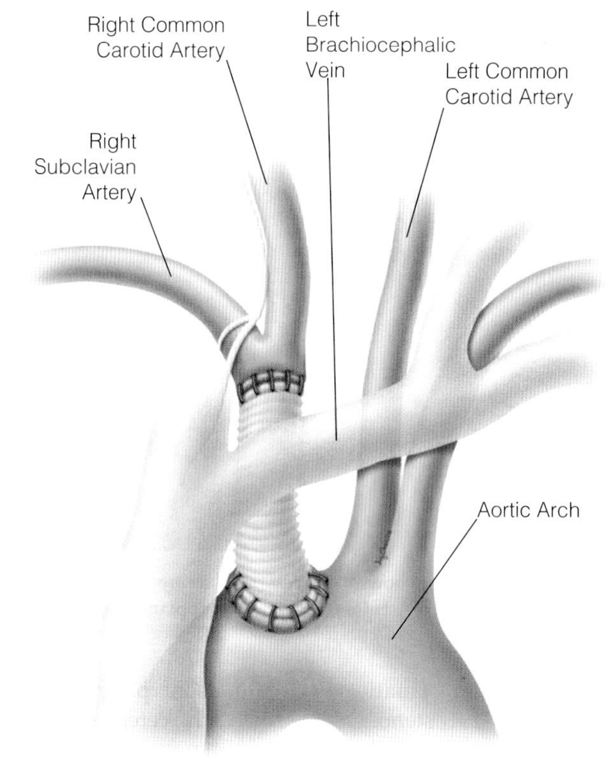

[illegible] to the aorta in an end-to-side fashion, and the other is sewn to the common ostium of the right subclavian artery and the right common carotid artery in an end-to-end fashion.

lesions, balloon angioplasty with stent insertion is currently the treatment of choice.[17,18]

Subclavian Artery Stenting

SA stenting has replaced open surgery for many symptomatic subclavian stenoses. It is usually performed by a femoral approach, although in some circumstances (e.g., an occluded infrarenal aorta), a brachial or retrograde approach may be required. The advantages of a brachial artery approach, however, have to be weighed against the higher likelihood of access-related arterial injuries due to the brachial artery's smaller diameter.

Preoperative evaluation Careful clinical assessment is key. Noninvasive testing will confirm reversal of flow in the vertebral arteries in the case of symptomatic subclavian steal syndrome. PVRs will confirm reduced arterial blood flow in cases of suspected arm claudication. Once the diagnosis is confirmed, all patients undergo arch angiography.

Selection of patients Good candidates for endovascular treatment are those with symptomatic stenoses that do not involve the origins of the vertebral arteries due to the risk of occlusion during balloon angioplasty or stenting.

Alternative therapy Carotid-subclavian bypass and transposition (see below) are excellent alternatives to endovascular approaches in surgically fit candidates. In patients for whom a femoral approach proves difficult, a transbrachial approach may be employed.

Operative planning If possible, we use a femoral approach. The best lesions for endovascular treatment are those several centimeters proximal or distal to the origins of the vertebral artery origins. Those close to or involving the vertebral artery origins are better treated with surgery to avoid stent placement across them. Lesions at the SA origin should be treated with balloon-expandable stents. For those not involving the origin, we choose self-expanding stents followed by balloon angioplasty due to the curvature of the SA. We avoid stenting the junction of the subclavian and axillary arteries at the level of the first rib as these stenoses are usually due to extrinsic compression (arterial thoracic outlet syndrome) rather than primary atherosclerosis. We do not routinely angioplasty SAs prior to stenting, although sometimes we predilate the SA to allow easier passage of the stent device prior to deployment.

Operative technique Using a 5 French sheath for femoral artery access, an arch aortogram is performed using a pigtail catheter. Once the site and extent of the lesion have been confirmed, we exchange the 5 French sheath for a 90 cm long 6 French guiding sheath over an Amplatz wire and administer 50 to 75 units/kg of heparin. A glide wire and glide catheter are then advanced across the lesion. Once across the lesion, the glide wire is exchanged for a Rosen or Amplatz wire. The catheter is removed, and the guiding sheath with its dilator back in place is advanced to the SA origin. The dilator is removed, and the extent and diameter of the lesion are confirmed. Next, either a balloon-expandable (if the lesion is at the origin) or a self-expanding stent is deployed. Self-expanding stents are then dilated with an appropriate balloon (usually 1 mm less than the diameter of the stent). Placement is confirmed, and all catheters and sheaths are removed. We frequently deploy a closure device at this stage in the femoral artery. Typical working lengths for the balloons and stents are 90 to 120 cm, and stent diameters range from 6 to 10 mm.

For a brachial approach, a percutaneous approach is also used. A standard 6 French 12 to 15 cm sheath is used for access. An Amplatz or Rosen wire is advanced beyond the subclavian origin and should be directed into the descending aorta to avoid cerebral embolization.

Postoperative care Patients are pretreated with clopidogrel 75 mg/day for a week prior to the procedure. This is continued for at least 1 month afterward. If patients have not been pretreated, we usually give them a loading dose of 300 mg of clopidogrel immediately after the procedure and continue 75 mg/day for a month.

Carotid-Subclavian Bypass or Transposition

Elective bypass is typically reserved for occlusive lesions that are not amenable to balloon angioplasty. As stenting of thoracic aortic aneurysms has become more common, however, carotid-subclavian transposition or bypass has now become routinely employed to allow aortic stents to be placed across the origin of the left SA to facilitate proximal fixation. Thus, the growth of endovascular surgical treatment of thoracic aortic aneurysms has, paradoxically, created a growing population of patients who require a carotid-subclavian bypass. It is important, therefore, that this procedure remain part of the armamentarium of all vascular surgeons.

Preoperative evaluation A healthy CCA is an excellent inflow source for an SA bypass procedure. Before operation, the CCA should be evaluated with duplex ultrasonography, supplemented by arteriography. Aortic arch anomalies (e.g., the presence of a bovine aortic arch) should be identified.

Selection of patients It is important to confirm that the arm symptoms are caused by subclavian disease. In young patients, the possibility of thoracic outlet syndrome should be considered. In older patients, the differential may include cervical disk problems or osteoarthritis. In patients with descending thoracic aortic aneurysms, our threshold for treatment is a diameter of 5 cm. Given the complexity of the anatomy and the potential for nerve injury, some surgeons are reluctant to perform carotid-subclavian bypass or transposition, instead favoring axilloaxillary crossover grafting. However, axilloaxillary crossover has a lower patency rate than carotid-subclavian bypass or transposition, and its subcutaneous placement and prominence make it less acceptable to most patients. In addition, instances of erosion through the skin have been reported.

Alternative therapy SA balloon stenting is less invasive than surgical bypass and is a durable procedure that is well tolerated by most patients.[19] However, patients who have recurrent stenosis or whose lesions are too close to the vertebral arteries may not be candidates for angioplasty. For such patients, prosthetic bypass or reimplantation of the SA is an ideal option. The temptation to perform a lesser procedure (e.g., axilloaxillary bypass) should be resisted.

Operative planning The two key considerations in the planning of the operation are (1) whether to perform a bypass or a transposition and (2), if a bypass is chosen, whether to use autologous vein or synthetic material as the conduit. For a bypass, prosthetic grafts, being short and of large caliber, are generally considered preferable to autologous vein grafts[20,21]: they are less likely to become kinked or develop intrinsic disease, and the long-term patency of prosthetic reconstructions is excellent.

Transposition of the SA is an excellent alternative to carotid-subclavian bypass, with long-term patency rates approaching 100%.[22] Preoperative consent should include acknowledgment of the potential for injury to the phrenic nerve or the brachial plexus.

Operative technique *Carotid-subclavian bypass* The patient is placed in the supine position, with a towel roll placed between the scapulae. The neck is tilted toward the contralateral shoulder. A transverse incision is made 1 cm superior to the clavicle. The underlying platysma and the lateral portion of the sternocleidomastoid muscle are divided in the line of the incision (an important distinction from the approach for transposition when the incision is between the heads of the sternocleidomastoid). The underlying omohyoid muscle and the external jugular vein are divided, and the scalene fat pad is mobilized and retracted laterally and cephalad. Minor lymphatic vessels are identified and ligated. The internal jugular vein is visible medially in the carotid sheath, and the carotid artery is usually situated posteriorly. Every effort should be made not to injure the vagus nerve and the thoracic duct on the left; the risk of thoracic duct injury may be minimized by not dividing the lymphatic tissue lying between the phrenic nerve and the lateral border of the internal jugular vein. The anterior scalene muscle is divided as far caudal as possible to reveal the SA; care must be taken to avoid injuring the overlying phrenic nerve, which courses diagonally in a lateral-to-medial direction along the anterior surface of the muscle.

A bypass from the CCA to the SA is then performed in an end-to-side fashion with a 6 or 8 mm prosthetic graft [*see Figure 5*]. The graft is usually tunneled under the internal jugular vein. Often the graft-SA anastomosis is constructed first. A clamp is placed on the proximal graft, and the anastomosis to the CCA is constructed. The CCA is mobilized so that once two straight vascular clamps are placed and rotated anteriorly, the graft-CCA anastomosis may be performed more easily. Once the bypass has been completed, flow is restored—first to the arm, then to the proximal SA, and finally to the distal CCA so as to minimize the carriage of embolic debris to the brain. Flow should then be assessed with a pencil Doppler probe.

After completion of the bypass, the scalene fat pad is tacked to its former medial and inferior attachments; failure to do so may leave a visible defect in this area. The wound is drained with a closed-suction apparatus. An upright chest x-ray is obtained to rule out pneumothorax or hemi- [illegible] Postoperative evaluation of bypass patency is accomplished by physical examination with palpation of pulses at the wrist. Further objective documentation of patency is

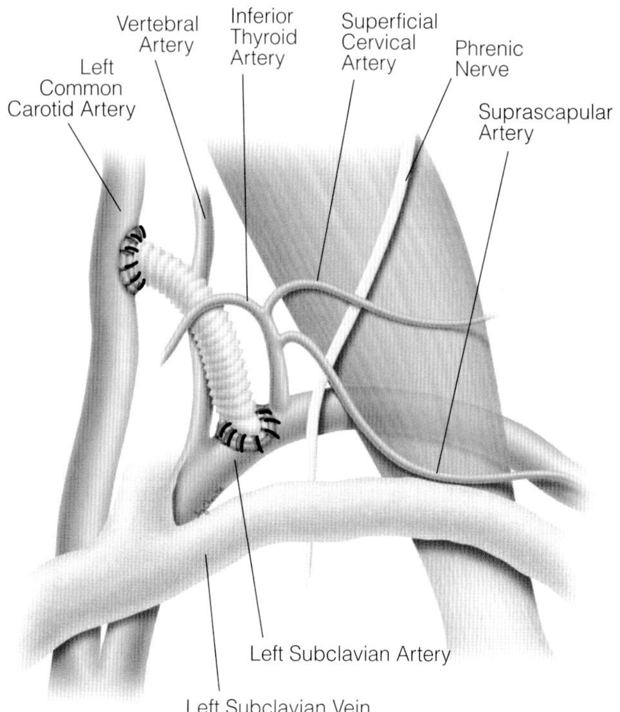

Figure 5 **Carotid-subclavian bypass. One end of the graft is sewn to the left subclavian artery in an end-to-side fashion, and the other is sewn to the left common carotid artery in an end-to-side fashion.**

obtained by means of PVRs, duplex ultrasonography, or both.

Carotid-subclavian transposition A supraclavicular incision is also placed, but, in this case, it is placed between the two heads of the sternocleidomastoid.[23] After division of the platysma muscle, two flaps are created. The omohyoid muscle is divided. Next, the vertebral vein is divided, which allows the SA and its proximal branches to be visualized behind the clavicle. The vertebral artery originates from the posterior aspect of the SA and must be preserved. The internal thoracic artery should also be preserved for possible later use in coronary revascularization. The medial aspect of the anterior scalene muscle may be encountered with more lateral dissection of the SA. Slight lateral reflection of this muscle may be needed to control the SA distal to the thyrocervical trunk. The SA is also dissected as far proximal as possible, well into the mediastinum. It is possible to enter the pleural space anteriorly. This can be avoided by keeping the dissection close to the arterial wall. Care should also be taken to avoid disrupting sympathetic nerve branches as they cross anterior to the SA and ascend in the neck alongside the vertebral vessels. Once heparin has been administered, the SA and its proximal branches are controlled. The vertebral, mammary, and thryocervical trunk are temporarily occluded with Yasargil clips. The distal SA can be controlled with an angled clamp. The proximal SA is then clamped using an angled clamp (e.g., a Martinez clamp) [illegible] important to secure the proximal stump; if control of the transected stump is lost in the chest or mediastinum, the consequences will be disastrous. We oversew the subclavian stump with two rows of running 4-0 polypropylene suture and buttress the anastomosis with two horizontal mattress sutures with Teflon pledgelets. At this point, the carotid artery is slightly rotated to expose the posterior aspect and then clamped proximally and distally. An arteriotomy is made in the CCA, and an end-to-side anastomosis is completed without tension [*see Figure 6*]. Occasionally, some redundant SA must be resected to avoid a kink. Rarely, it may be necessary to endarterectomize the proximal SA. The anastomosis is facilitated by using the parachute technique and by starting the suture line on the posterior wall. Rarely is the SA too short to reach to the side of the carotid. If this problem is encountered, more carotid artery can be mobilized to swing it further lateral to reach the SA. Clamps are removed, and flow is reestablished into the vertebral artery last. Closure is the same as for a carotid-subclavian bypass.

Postoperative care The major postoperative complication is phrenic nerve injury and resulting paralysis of the hemidiaphragm. Another significant complication is lymphatic leakage, which may occur as a result of either minor or major thoracic duct injury. Adequate wound drainage and prompt recognition of the lymphatic leak are the keys to management. Minor leaks usually seal with adequate drainage. If drainage is excessive, the patient will have to be maintained on parenteral nutrition with a formula that includes medium-chain triglycerides. On occasion, thoracic duct ligation via right thoracotomy or thoracoscopy may be necessary. Other complications include pneumothorax, brachial plexus injury, and stroke.

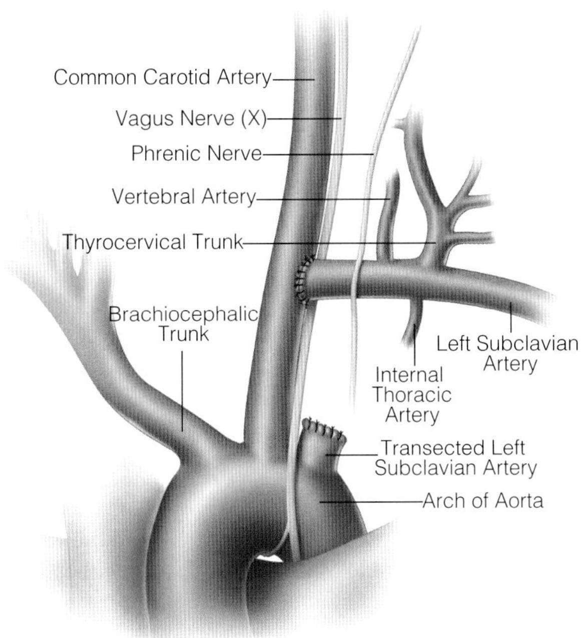

Figure 6 **Carotid-subclavian transposition.**

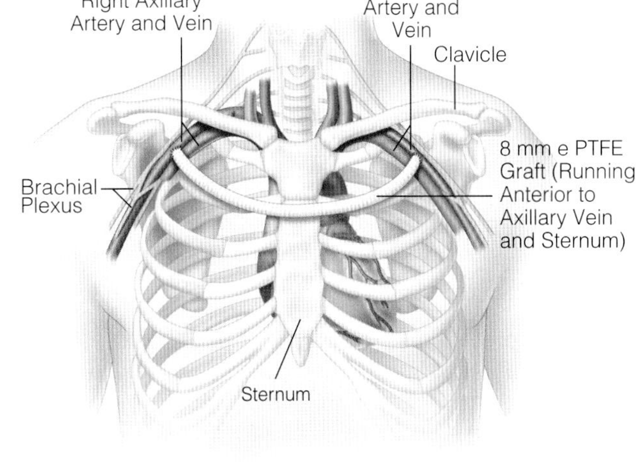

Figure 7 **Axillary-to-axillary artery crossover bypass with a prosthetic graft. ePTFE = expanded polytetrafluoroethylene.**

Patients are followed with serial PVRs of the arm and duplex ultrasonography of the grafts.

Axillary-Axillary Bypass

This operation is rarely performed at our center. We perform it only in extreme situations where there is no other option to preserve life or limb. It is an extra-anatomic bypass that can be performed with low mortality (1.3%) with little or no risk of stroke. However, the patency is as low as 50% at 5 years in some reported series.[24,25] Technically, it is the easiest of the surgical options available for arm revascularization.

Preoperative evaluation All patients should be evaluated with a formal arch angiogram prior to undergoing an elective operation. In the emergency situation, this will obviously not be an option, and clinical evaluation based on a normal pulse examination of the donor limb may have to suffice.

Alternative therapy We recommend all other options, such as subclavian stenting, carotid-subclavian bypass, or transposition or even carotid-carotid crossover, before contemplating this procedure.

Operative planning In all cases, a prosthetic graft, usually an 8 mm expanded polytetrafluoroethylene (ePTFE) graft, is chosen. As the graft will be tunneled subcutaneously across the chest wall [*see Figure 7*], it will obviously pose a problem if coronary artery bypass is being contemplated in the future for these patients. Some patients, especially thin patients, may find the appearances of the graft unsightly.

Operative technique Under general anesthesia, bilateral infraclavicular incisions are made. The pectoralis major muscle is "split" along its line of separation (see below), which exposes the clavipectoral fascia, which is then divided. The axillary artery is identified cephalad to the axillary vein. Next, an 8 mm ePTFE graft is tunneled in a subcutaneous plane. The patient is given a bolus of 3,000 to 5,000 units of heparin, and angled clamps are placed on the axillary artery proximally and distally. A vertical arteriotomy is made, and the graft is sewn with 6-0 polypropylene suture using a parachute technique. At completion of the anastomoses, a Doppler probe confirms flow.

Postoperative care These patients are not routinely anticoagulated, and postoperative care is fairly standard.

THE AXILLARY ARTERY

Axillobrachial Bypass

Axillobrachial bypass may be performed to treat severe occlusive disease in the axillary or proximal brachial arteries. It is infrequently performed for chronic ischemia and more frequently performed for shoulder trauma. In the latter setting, it is often associated with brachial plexus injuries.

Preoperative evaluation Axillobrachial bypass is not commonly performed on an elective basis. The axillary and proximal brachial arteries seem to be remarkably impervious to the effects of systemic atherosclerosis. In those rare cases in which this procedure is indicated, preoperative evaluation of the affected arm with selective angiography is appropriate. Vein mapping should be performed. It is important to confirm that the patient's symptoms derive from arm ischemia and not from other conditions (e.g., neuropathy).

Alternative therapy If arm ischemia is truly symptomatic at this level, sympathectomy may be considered [*see*

Alternative Therapies for Chronic Arm Ischemia, *below*]. Angioplasty may be an option for axillary artery lesions but is infrequently performed in this setting, and data on its effectiveness and durability are relatively sparse.

Operative planning Autogenous vein is the conduit of choice for axillobrachial bypass. Prosthetic bypasses have lower patency rates than venous bypasses in this setting and should therefore be avoided. The great saphenous vein is the preferred source of the venous conduit, although the use of the cephalic vein in situ has also been described.

Operative technique The patient is placed in the supine position, and the arm is draped circumferentially. A previously mapped leg is draped in preparation for vein harvesting. The axillary artery is approached via a transverse incision placed 2 cm below the middle third of the clavicle. The underlying pectoralis major is divided in the line of the decussation between its sternocostal and clavicular portions. Despite the assurances of most operative texts, the decussation is not always readily apparent. Division of the pectoralis major exposes the clavipectoral fascia, which is then divided. The axillary artery is identified cephalad to the axillary vein and is carefully dissected, with care taken not to injure the surrounding branches of the brachial plexus. Dividing the pectoralis minor exposes the second part of the axillary artery.

If necessary, the distal third of the axillary artery may be exposed lateral to the pectoralis minor muscle. An oblique incision is made along the lateral margin of the pectoralis major with the arm abducted 90 relative to the thorax. Once the subcutaneous tissue is divided, the axillary sheath is located near the posteroinferior border of the coracobrachialis muscle. Care should be taken to keep from injuring the medial and lateral cords of the brachial plexus in the medial wound and the median and ulnar nerves in the lateral wound.

By preference, bypasses originating from the axillary artery are tunneled anatomically along the axis of the axillary and brachial arteries. Alternatively, they may be positioned subcutaneously; however, subcutaneous bypasses are more susceptible to distraction injuries caused by forcible abduction of the shoulder. Accordingly, some degree of redundancy should be built into a subcutaneous bypass.

The middle or the distal portion of the brachial artery is exposed as necessary. The proximal or the middle third of the vessel is exposed by making a medial incision over the bicipital groove, with care taken to preserve the basilic vein and the cutaneous nerves located within the subcutaneous tissue. Traction on or transection of the median antebrachial cutaneous nerve may lead to hyperesthesia or anesthesia along the medial dorsal surface of the forearm; these problems occasionally occur after dialysis access procedures (e.g., basilic vein transposition) and can be highly debilitating, sometimes even rendering the fistula unusable. The brachial sheath is then incised longitudinally. The median nerve is the most superficial structure encountered within the sheath. It is gently mobilized and retracted to afford access to the brachial artery. Any venous branches that cross the artery should be divided carefully, and every effort should be made to keep from injuring the posteriorly located ulnar nerve.

In contrast, the distal third of the brachial artery and its bifurcation are exposed in the antecubital fossa. A lazy S or sigmoid incision [*see Figure 1a*] is made to expose the brachial artery while avoiding wound contracture. The bicipital aponeurosis is then incised to expose the brachial artery, which is sandwiched between the biceps tendon laterally and the median nerve medially. Further dissection exposes the origins of the ulnar and radial arteries.

After systemic heparinization, the venous conduit is harvested, and its side branches are ligated with fine polypropylene suture ligatures or silk ties. The vein is distended with a solution containing dextrose 70 (500 mL), heparin (1,000 U), and papaverine (120 mg). The excised vein may be employed in either a reversed or an orthograde (nonreversed) orientation, depending on the taper of the conduit. If the orthograde orientation is used, the proximal anastomosis is performed, the vein is distended, and the valves are lysed with a retrograde Mills valvulotome. In either case, the bypass is tunneled anatomically wherever possible; in this way, it will be less prone to movement, distraction, or distortion. After tunneling, the distal anastomosis is constructed [*see Figure 8*]. Immediately upon completion of the bypass, patency and augmentation of flow are assessed with a pencil Doppler probe.

Major potential complications include injuries to the brachial plexus, the median nerve, or the ulnar nerve. Such injuries are usually caused by traction and may be minimized by careful dissection during operative exposure. The median and ulnar nerves and the brachial plexus are also vulnerable to direct thermal injury; accordingly, dissection with the electrocautery should be avoided.

Postoperative care Postoperatively, the patency of the bypass is documented by surveillance with noninvasive studies. In general, duplex ultrasonography is valuable for determining the patency of the reconstruction and for detecting any early flow abnormalities in the venous conduit. Graft infection should be watched for and appropriately treated if found.

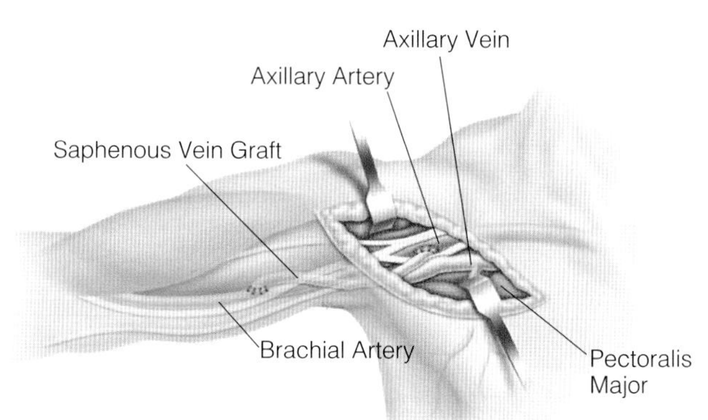

Figure 8 **Axillobrachial bypass. Shown is the completed bypass, with the great saphenous vein tunneled subcutaneously.**

THE BRACHIAL ARTERY

Distal Revascularization–Interval Ligation and Revision Using Distal Inflow

The rising incidence of diabetes in the United States has led to a corresponding rise in the number of patients in whom vascular access is required for hemodialysis.[26,27] As reconstructions become more complex, these patients are increasingly coming under the care of vascular surgeons. An unfortunate consequence of the growing number of upper arm fistulas is that the incidence of dialysis-associated steal syndrome (DASS) is increasing as well. DASS is rare after Cimino or radiocephalic fistula procedures,[28] but it occurs in 6 to 8% of patients who undergo upper arm brachial artery–based fistula or graft procedures.[29,30] DASS may present in either an acute form (characterized by severe rest pain and obvious ischemia developing within 24 to 48 hours after operation) or a chronic form (characterized by symptoms and signs developing several weeks or even months after the original operation), each of which is managed in its own distinct fashion.

In cases of acute ischemia that develops within 24 to 48 hours after an upper arm fistula procedure, the fistula can be ligated to restore flow down the native arteries. In cases of chronic ischemia, however, the aim is to preserve the fistula and avoid ligation. To this end, two main surgical options should be considered. The first option is distal revascularization–interval ligation (DRIL), which involves the creation of a venous bypass from the proximal portion of the brachial artery to the distal portion of the vessel [*see Figure 9*]. The brachial artery distal to the origin of the fistula is ligated, flow to the distal arm is restored, and the fistula is preserved.[31] The second option is revision using distal inflow (RUDI), which involves ligation of the fistula at its origin, followed by reestablishment of the fistula by means of a venous bypass from the radial or the ulnar artery.[32] By using a smaller distal artery as the inflow source, RUDI lengthens the fistula and preserves antegrade flow in the brachial artery.

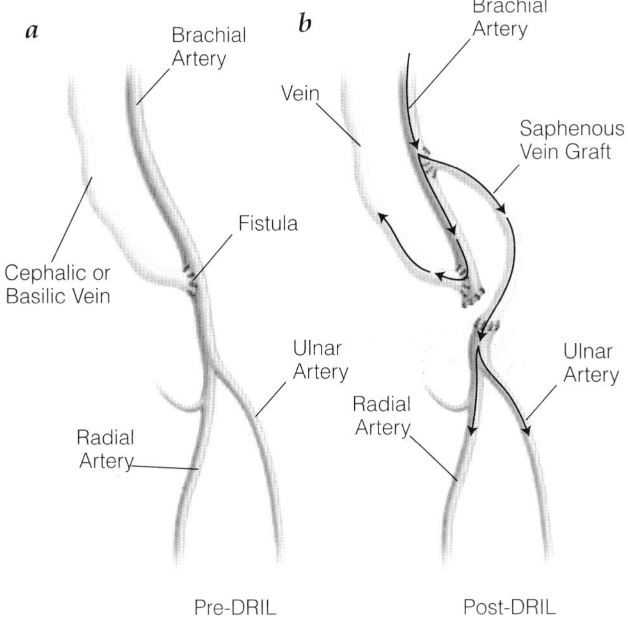

Figure 9 **Distal revascularization–interval ligation (DRIL). In patients with a brachial artery–based fistula (*a*), chronic ischemia may develop weeks or months after the procedure. The best established surgical treatment option is DRIL (*b*), which preserves the fistula by creating a venous bypass between the proximal brachial artery (above the origin of the fistula) and the distal brachial artery.**

Of the two options, DRIL is better established and more widely used at present. It is our preferred option and thus is the primary focus of the ensuing description. Nevertheless, there are aspects of the DRIL procedure that many vascular surgeons find counter intuitive, namely, the ligation of a healthy artery and the bypassing of a normal arterial segment with a venous conduit. There does seem to be a good argument in favor of RUDI. Long-term evaluation of this procedure is awaited.

Preoperative evaluation Preoperative evaluation for DRIL should follow the same pattern as that for any elective procedure performed to treat arm or leg ischemia. Preoperative angiography and vein mapping are performed to rule out a more proximal arterial stenosis and to identify an adequate source of a venous conduit. Cardiac clearance is obtained.

Selection of patients for DRIL is generally reserved for patients with chronic arm ischemia in whom a fistula has been established that must be preserved. If the option of creating a new fistula in the other arm is available, DRIL is probably a less appropriate choice than simply ligating the original fistula.

Alternative therapy Besides simple ligation of the offending fistula, which is an option that should always at least be considered in these patients, there are two techniques that deserve mention as alternatives to DRIL. The first technique is aimed at preventing steal from an upper arm fistula (always a laudable aim). In this technique, the fistula is formed by extending the cephalic vein or the basilic vein down the arm and anastomosing it to the proximal ulnar artery or the radial artery just below the brachial bifurcation so as to preserve part of the blood supply to the hand. The median cubital vein may also be used.[33]

The second technique is RUDI [*see Figure 10*]. This procedure differs from the DRIL in that the fistula, not the native arterial supply, is placed at risk by the surgical revision, so, in the event of graft failure, the fistula is lost, but the arm is not endangered.

Operative planning We do not use prosthetic grafts for this procedure; we prefer to use autogenous vein for the graft, usually a segment of the great saphenous vein from the leg. As a rule, the operation is performed with the patient under general anesthesia. We routinely map the great saphenous vein with ultrasonography prior to surgery.

Operative technique A vertical incision is made in the upper arm at the level of the proximal brachial artery. The skin and the subcutaneous fat are divided, and the proximal brachial artery is sharply dissected free. The portion of the brachial artery distal to the origin of the fistula is also dissected free. An adequately long segment of vein is obtained and prepared. Anticoagulation is initiated, and a proximal

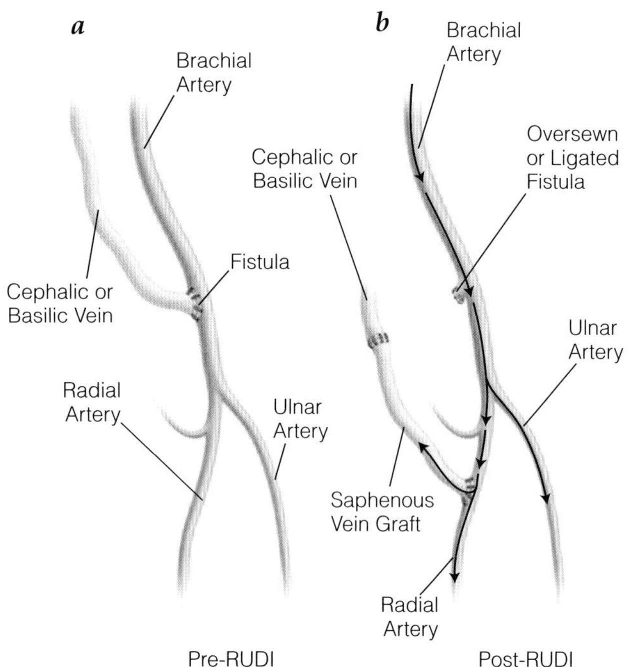

Figure 10 **Revision using distal inflow (RUDI). Another option for patients with a brachial artery–based fistula (*a*) is RUDI (*b*), which involves ligating the fistula at its origin, lengthening the original venous graft with an additional vein segment, and reestablishing the fistula by anastomosing the lengthened graft to the radial artery (as shown) or the ulnar artery.**

end-to-side anastomosis is fashioned with 6-0 polypropylene. The vein graft is tunneled subcutaneously, and a distal end-to-end anastomosis to the distal brachial artery is created. Some surgeons prefer an end-to-side distal anastomosis with ligation of the brachial artery proximal to the anastomosis. Adequate flow is confirmed by means of intraoperative Doppler ultrasonography.

Postoperative care Postoperative anticoagulation is generally not warranted; however, a postoperative graft surveillance protocol is initiated. If the venous graft becomes occluded, the fistula is ligated. This step frequently leads to resolution of the symptoms of arm ischemia. Often, however, the surgeon and patient may wish to preserve the graft and the fistula, and when a graft becomes severely stenotic, revision of the DRIL procedure is performed using excised great saphenous vein.

FOREARM ARTERIES

Hand Revascularization

Patients with rest pain in the hands and digital ulcers often have significant comorbid conditions (e.g., collagen vascular or rheumatologic disorders, end-stage renal disease, or hypercoagulable states). In addition, patients who have received organ transplants and are taking immunosuppressive medications may experience severe occlusion of forearm or palmar arteries. Younger patients with hand ischemia are often manual laborers who have hypothenar hammer syndrome. Patients with established signs and symptoms of hand ischemia have little to lose by undergoing revascularization; there are few viable therapeutic alternatives.

Aggressive treatment of hand ischemia is worthwhile in that it achieves rapid relief of symptoms and offers the opportunity for hand and limb salvage. The techniques resemble those employed for distal bypass in the leg. Early results from several centers indicate that hand bypass procedures can be performed with low morbidity and good long-term patency.[34,35] Postoperative life expectancy, however, is often limited by the comorbid conditions.

Preoperative evaluation Preoperative evaluation for hand bypass should follow the same protocol as that for any elective revascularization: preoperative angiography to delineate anatomy with vein mapping to identify a venous conduit. Many patients with hand ischemia have intractable pain from ulcerative lesions, gangrene, or both. Their main requirement is adequate relief of pain; improved hand function is a secondary consideration. Vascular reconstruction offers a chance to gain both. The alternative to attempted arm salvage is amputation.

Selection of patients At our institution (Albany Medical Center), all patients with rest pain, digital necrosis, or nonhealing ulcers are evaluated for possible palmar artery reconstruction provided that they are surgical candidates. Reconstruction is feasible in approximately half of the patients who have renal disease or diabetes.

Alternative therapy Sympathectomy, in various incarnations, has been employed in the treatment of hand ischemia. Isolated reports of success notwithstanding, the experience of most vascular surgeons with sympathectomy in this setting has not been favorable.

Operative planning Fortunately, exposure of the palmar vessels beyond the wrist is not as difficult as might be imagined [*see* Operative Technique, *below*]. Nevertheless, because hand bypass procedures are relatively new territory for many vascular surgeons, operative planning may benefit from a brief review of the normal anatomy. The hand is supplied with blood by the superficial and deep palmar arches. The superficial palmar arch is supplied by a branch of the radial artery and by the ulnar artery. The deep palmar arch is supplied by the radial artery itself and by a deep branch of the ulnar artery.

Venous grafts are preferred to prosthetic grafts for hand bypasses. All venous grafts are tunneled anatomically. In a radial artery reconstruction, the graft is tunneled over the anatomic snuffbox onto the dorsum of the hand, between the thumb and the index finger, to join the deep palmar arch. In an ulnar artery reconstruction, the venous graft takes a less circuitous course, passing superficial to the flexor retinaculum at the wrist to join the superficial palmar arch.

Operative technique The donor limb that will provide the venous graft is prepared. The brachial artery is exposed as described previously [*see* Procedures for Acute Arm Ischemia, Brachial Embolectomy, Operative Technique, *above*].

The course of the radial artery in the forearm follows an oblique line from the brachial artery pulse medial to the biceps tendon to the styloid process of the radius. In the midforearm, the radial artery is medial to the brachioradialis and lateral to the flexor carpi radialis. A lateral longitudinal incision is made, and the muscles are separated to reveal the radial artery. At the wrist, the radial artery is exposed by making a longitudinal incision between the tendon of the flexor carpi radialis and the tendon of the brachio radialis. This is the site of the radial artery pulse in normal persons. Here the artery is superficial, and exposure is relatively straightforward. Care must be taken, however, not to injure the superficial branch of the radial nerve, which is often located near the lateral aspect of the artery. Injury to this nerve branch can result in troublesome paresthesia along the lateral aspect of the thumb.

The course of the ulnar artery runs from the medial epicondyle of the humerus to the pisiform bone. In the midforearm, the ulnar artery lies beneath the deep fascia between the belly of the flexor digitorum laterally and the belly of the flexor carpi ulnaris medially. The ulnar nerve joins the artery on its lateral aspect for the distal two thirds of the vessel's length; this nerve may be injured if not carefully identified and preserved. At the wrist, the ulnar artery is lateral to the tendon of the flexor carpi ulnaris. It is exposed by locating this tendon (which is the most medial tendon palpable at the wrist) and making a vertical skin incision lateral to it. Although the ulnar artery lies deeper than the radial artery at the wrist, it is just as easily exposed. Superficial to the ulnar artery, palmar cutaneous branches of the ulnar nerve may be identified; these should also be preserved.

Grafts originating from the brachial artery are tunneled in the subcutaneous plane. Subcutaneous tunneling facilitates physical examination to determine the patency of the bypass, as well as surveillance of the bypass with duplex ultrasonography. Alternatively, if good-quality basilic or cephalic veins are present, an in situ bypass may be performed.

Exposure of radial artery and deep palmar arch Exposure of the radial artery is relatively straightforward. Generally, it may be accomplished as previously described (see above). Alternatively, it may be accomplished by making a vertical incision over the anatomic snuffbox (which lies between the extensor pollicis longus tendon posteriorly and the tendons of the extensor pollicis brevis and the abductor pollicis longus anteriorly). This incision is then deepened through the subcutaneous tissues to expose the radial artery in the floor of the snuffbox [*see Figure 11a*]. This area contains no significant nerves and thus is often chosen as a site for hemodialysis access.

The deep palmar arch is much less accessible than the radial artery. Consequently, exposure of this vascular structure is considerably more difficult than exposure of the radial artery. The deep palmar arch extends across the palm, level with the proximal border of the outstretched thumb. To expose it, an incision is made along the medial border of the thenar eminence [*see Figure 11b*]. Extensive dissection of the superficial and deep flexor tendons of the hand and division of the oblique head of the adductor pollicis are then required to provide access to the origin of the deep palmar arch.

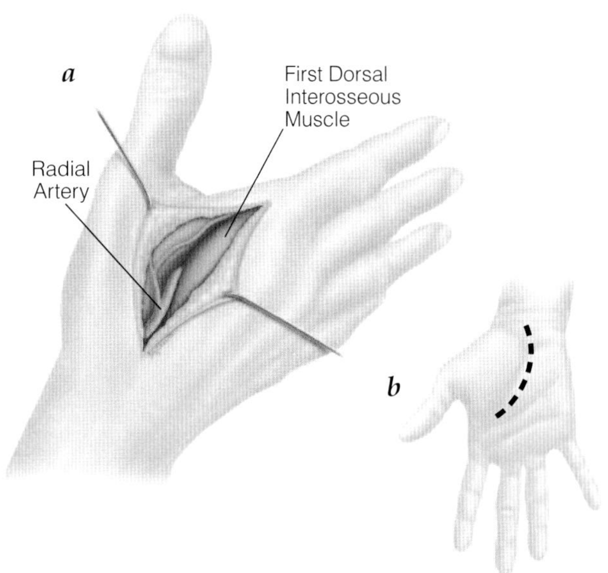

Figure 11 **Hand revascularization. (*a*) Shown is exposure of the distal radial artery. (*b*) The deep palmar arch is exposed via an incision made across the medial border of the thenar eminence.**

Exposure of ulnar artery and superficial palmar arch Like exposure of the radial artery, exposure of the ulnar artery and the superficial palmar arch is fairly straightforward. In reality, these vessels are no smaller than the tibial and pedal vessels in the leg. A curved incision is made along the lateral border of the hypothenar eminence [*see Figure 12a*]. The aponeurotic layer is divided, and the artery is exposed in the upper part of the palm at the origin of the superficial palmar arch. There are no major nerves in the vicinity, and it is usually not difficult to expose a reasonable length of artery for an arterial anastomosis [*see Figure 12b*]. Alternatively, the superficial palmar arch may be exposed in the palm by making an incision along one of the larger vertical or oblique skin creases.

Postoperative care As with all venous grafts, postoperative graft surveillance is essential. Routine postoperative anticoagulation is generally not warranted.

Alternative Therapies for Chronic Arm Ischemia

THORACOSCOPIC SYMPATHECTOMY AND DIGITAL SYMPATHECTOMY

Our experience with sympathectomy in the treatment of patients with critical hand ischemia or digital ulceration has been, frankly, disappointing. When we do perform sympathectomy, we prefer the thoracoscopic approach to the traditional cervical route. Either way, however, the results have been discouraging; any improvements noted prove to be only temporary. Sympathectomy may help alleviate pain in these patients, but even in this regard, the results are, at best, unpredictable. A review of the literature seems to support this conclusion. Admittedly, the available data on thoracoscopic sympathectomy for digital ischemia are

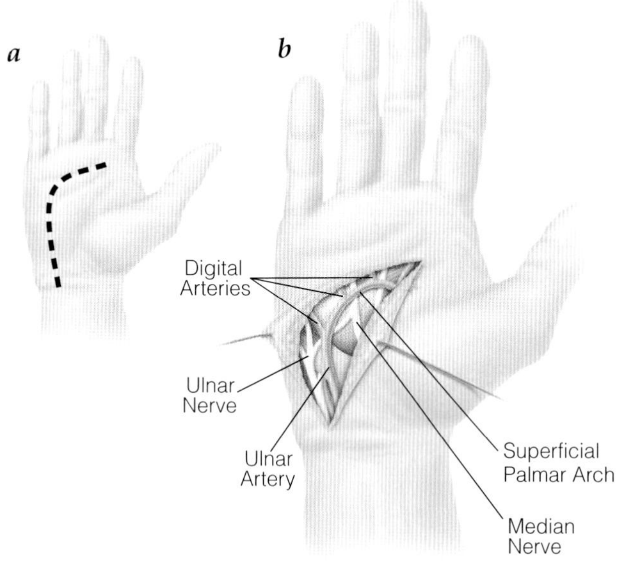

Figure 12 **Hand revascularization. (*a*) The distal ulnar artery and the superficial palmar arch are exposed via a curving incision made along the lateral border of the hypothenar eminence. (*b*) Shown is exposure of the distal ulnar artery and the superficial palmar arch, along with the ulnar and median nerves.**

sparse: to date, only three reports encompassing 21 patients have been published.[36–38] In contrast, there is a wealth of data on thoracoscopic sympathectomy for hyperhidrosis.

An alternative technique has been devised in which a very distal sympathectomy is performed at the level of the origin of the proper digital arteries. The sympathectomy site is exposed via a palmar approach, and a 3 to 4 mm length of the adventitia is removed from the proper digital arteries distal to the junction of the distal perforating artery with the common digital artery. This procedure appears to be well tolerated, and data from small series attest to its value in selected patients with digital ulcers.[39]

Summary

Arm revascularization occupies little space in most vascular surgical textbooks, reflecting its incidence in most vascular surgical practices. Although emergency procedures are relatively frequent, elective procedures are far less common. Whereas prosthetic conduits may be used for reconstruction of inflow disease, autogenous vein is the conduit of choice for more distal procedures.

Nonetheless, there is little doubt that many of these procedures have already been supplanted by endovascular therapies. Elective arm revascularization procedures are more technically challenging due to anatomy and lack of familiarity as they are rarely performed. However, endovascular therapy is not applicable to all, and there are still patients who need open surgical revascularization. Vascular surgeons still need to be aware of these valuable adjuncts, even in the 21st century.

Financial Disclosures: None Reported

References

1. Bachman DM, Kim RM. Transluminal dilatation for subclavian steal syndrome. AJR Am J Roentgenol 1980;135:995–6.
2. Mathias K, Staiger J, Thron A, et al. [Percutaneous transluminal dilatation of the subclavian artery]. Dtsch Med Wochenschr 1980;105:16–8.
3. Hernandez-Richter T, Angele MK, Helmberger T, et al. Acute ischemia of the upper extremity: long-term results following thrombembolectomy with the Fogarty catheter. Langenbecks Arch Surg 2001;386:261–6.
4. Wirsing P, Andriopoulos A, Botticher R. Arterial embolectomies in the upper extremity after acute occlusion. Report on 79 cases. J Cardiovasc Surg (Torino) 1983;24:40–2.
5. Baird RJ, Lajos TZ. Emboli to the arm. Ann Surg 1964;160: 905–9.
6. Savelyev VS, Zatevakhin II, Stepanov NV. Artery embolism of the upper limbs. Surgery 1977;81:367–75.
7. Galbraith K, Collin J, Morris PJ, Wood RF. Recent experience with arterial embolism of the limbs in a vascular unit. Ann R Coll Surg Engl 1985;67:30–3.
8. Stonebridge PA, Clason AE, Duncan AJ, et al. Acute ischaemia of the upper limb compared with acute lower limb ischaemia; a 5-year review. Br J Surg 1989;76:515–6.
9. Eyers P, Earnshaw JJ. Acute non-traumatic arm ischaemia. Br J Surg 1998;85:1340–6.
10. Widlus DM, Venbrux AC, Benenati JF, et al. Fibrinolytic [illegible] 1990;175:393–9.
11. Cejna M, Salomonowitz E, Wohlschlager H, et al. rt-PA thrombolysis in acute thromboembolic upper-extremity arterial occlusion. Cardiovasc Intervent Radiol 2001;24:218–23.
12. Zeller T, Frank U, Burgelin K, et al. Treatment of acute embolic occlusions of the subclavian and axillary arteries using a rotational thrombectomy device. Vasa 2003;32: 111–6.
13. Dente CJ, Feliciano DV, Rozycki GS, et al. A review of upper extremity fasciotomies in a level I trauma center. Am Surg 2004;70:1088–93.
14. Kieffer E, Sabatier J, Koskas F, Bahnini A. Atherosclerotic innominate artery occlusive disease: early and long-term results of surgical reconstruction. J Vasc Surg 1995;21:326–36; discussion 336–7.
15. Daseler EH, Anson BJ. Surgical anatomy of the subclavian artery and its branches. Surg Gynecol Obstet 1959;108: 149–74.
16. Berguer R. Supraaortic trunks. Vascular surgical approaches. In: Branchereau A, Berguer R, editors. New York: Futura Publishing; 1999. p. 93.
17. Woo EY, Fairman RM, Velazquez OC, et al. Endovascular therapy of symptomatic innominate-subclavian arterial occlusive lesions. Vasc Endovascular Surg 2006;40:27–33.
18. Brountzos EN, Petersen B, Binkert C, et al. Primary stenting of subclavian and innominate artery occlusive disease: a single center's experience. Cardiovasc Intervent Radiol 2004;27:616–23.
19. De Vries JP, Jager LC, Van den Berg JC, et al. Durability of percutaneous transluminal angioplasty for obstructive lesions of proximal subclavian artery: long-term results. J Vasc Surg 2005;41:19–23.

20. Law MM, Colburn MD, Moore WS, et al. Carotid-subclavian bypass for brachiocephalic occlusive disease. Choice of conduit and long-term follow-up. Stroke 1995;26:1565–71.
21. AbuRahma AF, Robinson PA, Jennings TG. Carotid-subclavian bypass grafting with polytetrafluoroethylene grafts for symptomatic subclavian artery stenosis or occlusion: a 20-year experience. J Vasc Surg 2000;32:411–8; discussion 418–9.
22. Cina CS, Safar HA, Lagana A, et al. Subclavian carotid transposition and bypass grafting: consecutive cohort study and systematic review. J Vasc Surg 2002;35:422–9.
23. Morasch MD. Technique for subclavian to carotid transposition, tips, and tricks. J Vasc Surg 2009;49:251–4.
24. Brewster DC, Moncure AC, Darling RC, et al. Innominate artery lesions: problems encountered and lessons learned. J Vasc Surg 1985;2:99–112.
25. Schanzer H, Chung-Loy H, Kotok M, et al. Evaluation of axillo-axillary artery bypass for the treatment of subclavian or innominate artery occlusive disease. J Cardiovasc Surg (Torino) 1987;28:258–61.
26. US Department of Health and Human Services, Centers for Disease Control and Prevention, National Center for Chronic Disease and Health Promotion. National Diabetes Surveillance System: state-specific estimates of diagnosed diabetes among adults. Available at: http://www.cdc.gov/diabetes/statistics/prev/state/Methods.htm. (accessed December 20, 2011).
27. U.S. Renal Data System, USRDS 2005 annual data report: atlas of end-stage renal disease in the United States. Bethesda (MD): National Institutes of Health, National Institute of Diabetes and Digestive and Kidney Diseases; 2005.
28. Zibari GB, Rohr MS, Landreneau MD, et al. Complications from permanent hemodialysis vascular access. Surgery 1988;104:681–6.
29. Revanur VK, Jardine AG, Hamilton DH, Jindal RM. Outcome for arterio-venous fistula at the elbow for haemodialysis. Clin Transplant 2000;14(4 Pt 1):318–22.
30. Wolford HY, Hsu J, Rhodes JM, et al. Outcome after autogenous brachial-basilic upper arm transpositions in the post-National Kidney Foundation Dialysis Outcomes Quality Initiative era. J Vasc Surg 2005;42:951–6.
31. Mwipatayi BP, Bowles T, Balakrishnan S, et al. Ischemic steal syndrome: a case series and review of current management. Curr Surg 2006;63:130–5.
32. Minion DJ, Moore E, Endean E. Revision using distal inflow: a novel approach to dialysis-associated steal syndrome. Ann Vasc Surg 2005;19:625–8.
33. Ehsan O, Bhattacharya D, Darwish A, Al-khaffaf H. 'Extension technique': a modified technique for brachio-cephalic fistula to prevent dialysis access-associated steal syndrome. Eur J Vasc Endovasc Surg 2005;29:324–7.
34. Chang BB, Roddy SP, Darling RC 3rd, et al. Upper extremity bypass grafting for limb salvage in end-stage renal failure. J Vasc Surg 2003;38:1313–5.
35. Nehler MR, Dalman RL, Harris EJ, et al. Upper extremity arterial bypass distal to the wrist. J Vasc Surg 1992;16: 633–40.
36. Grigorovici A, Gavrilovici V, Popa R. Thoracoscopic sympathectomy for upper limb ischemic disease. Rev Med Chir Soc Med Nat Iasi 2002;106:817–9.
37. De Giacomo T, Rendina EA, Venuta F, et al. Thoracoscopic sympathectomy for symptomatic arterial obstruction of the upper extremities. Ann Thorac Surg 2002;74:885–8.
38. Ishibashi H, Hayakawa N, Yamamoto H, et al. Thoracoscopic sympathectomy for Buerger's disease: a report on the successful treatment of four patients. Surg Today 1995;25:180–3.
39. el-Gammal TA, Blair WF. Digital periarterial sympathectomy for ischaemic digital pain and ulcers. J Hand Surg [Br] 1991;16:382–5.

Acknowledgments

Figures 1, 2, 4, 5, 8, 9, 10, 12 Alice Y. Chen
Figures 6, 7 Christine Kenney

The graft is brought through the tunnel either by using an aortic clamp or by attaching it to the previously placed red rubber catheter.

Step 6: construction of proximal anastomosis to femoral artery Before the proximal anastomosis is begun, the proper length of the graft should be determined to ensure that there is no redundancy. The proximal end of the graft is split and enlarged in the same fashion as the distal end, and the resulting right-angle corners are similarly trimmed. The graft is then anastomosed to the arteriotomy made in the femoral artery (which, like the popliteal arteriotomy, should be at least twice as long as the vessel is wide). The graft is attached by double-armed needles at its proximal angle and then in a similar fashion at its distal angle. The anastomosis is then completed from each end toward the center, just as the popliteal anastomosis was.

Below-the-Knee Bypass

When occlusion or marked stenosis renders the proximal and middle portions of the popliteal artery unsuitable for graft implantation, the lower portion of the vessel, which is often relatively free of atherosclerosis, may be used for the distal anastomosis instead.

Step 1: exposure of popliteal artery With the knee moderately flexed and supported by a rolled sheet placed under it, a vertical skin incision is made just behind the posteromedial surface of the tibia [*see Figure 5a*], exposing the [illegible] injury to the GSV during the skin incision. When a GSV graft is to be used, the same incision can serve both for harvesting of the vein and for exposure of the artery.

The crural fascia is opened along its fibers [*see Figure 5c*], its distal attachments are separated from the semitendinosus and gracilis tendons, and the two tendons are mobilized proximally and, if necessary, divided. The medial head of the gastrocnemius is retracted posteriorly [*see Figure 5d*] to expose the popliteal artery and vein and the posterior tibial nerve as these structures cross the popliteus posteriorly [*see Figure 5e*].

It should be noted that (1) the distal popliteal artery has few branches below the inferior geniculate arteries, (2) atheromatous plaques are rarely present at this level, and (3) the arterial wall is often more suitable for graft implantation in this portion of the popliteal wall than it is above the knee.

Step 2: exposure of femoral artery This exposure is accomplished in essentially the same way as it would be in an above-the-knee bypass.

Step 3: creation of tunnel Tunneling for a below-the-knee femoropopliteal bypass is carried out through Hunter's canal, through the upper popliteal space, and finally through the region behind the popliteus.

Steps 4 through 6 Steps 4, 5, and 6 of a below-the-knee femoropopliteal bypass—the distal anastomosis of the vein graft to the distal popliteal artery, the placement of the graft in the tunnel, and the proximal anastomosis to the femoral artery—are carried out in much the same way as the corresponding steps in an above-the-knee bypass. A completion angiogram should be obtained to confirm the adequacy of the distal anastomosis and verify the position of the graft in the tunnel [*see Figure 6*].

OUTCOME EVALUATION

Femoropopliteal bypasses performed with segments of the GSV are associated with 4-year primary patency rates ranging from 68% to 80% and limb salvage rates ranging from 75% to 80%.[33] Femoropopliteal bypasses performed with polytetrafluoroethylene (PTFE) grafts yield comparable patency and limb salvage rates above the knee but are significantly less successful below the knee.[34]

Newer vein harvesting techniques may help improve outcome further. The use of endoscopic vein harvesting methods has been shown to reduce the incidence of wound complications associated with femoropopliteal bypass.[35] This approach allows above-the-knee bypasses to be performed through two incisions.

Infrapopliteal Bypass

Bypasses to the small arteries beyond the popliteal artery are performed only when femoropopliteal bypass is contraindicated according to accepted criteria [*see* Femoropopliteal Bypass, *above*]. Infrapopliteal bypasses are performed to the posterior tibial artery, the anterior tibial artery, or the peroneal artery, in that order of preference. As a rule, a tibial artery is used only if its lumen runs without obstruction into the foot, though bypasses to isolated tibial artery segments and other disadvantaged outflow tracts have been performed and have remained patent for more than 4 years.[illegible] Generally, the peroneal artery is used only if it is continuous with one or two of its terminal branches, which communicate with foot arteries [*see Figure 7*]. Neither the absence of a plantar arch nor vascular calcification is considered a contraindication to a reconstruction.[2,7] With both femoropopliteal and infrapopliteal bypasses, stenosis of less than 50% of the diameter of the vessel is acceptable at or distal to the site chosen for the distal anastomosis.

OPERATIVE TECHNIQUE

Bypasses to tibial arteries should be performed with autogenous vein grafts, and either the reversed technique (as previously described [*see* Femoropopliteal Bypass, *above*]) or the in situ technique [*see* In Situ Bypass, *below*] may be used. Placement of a tourniquet above the knee allows the distal anastomosis to be performed without extensive dissection of the tibial vessels or the application of clamps.[36] Exposure of the inflow vessel (i.e., the femoral artery or the popliteal artery) is achieved in the same way as in femoropopliteal bypass. Accordingly, bypasses to tibial and peroneal arteries are best described in terms of the approaches required for exposure of these vessels and the tunnels required for routing the bypass conduits.

Exposure of Posterior Tibial Artery

The very proximal portion of the posterior tibial artery is aproached via a below-the-knee popliteal incision. The deep fascia is incised, and the popliteal space is entered. The gastrocnemius is retracted posteriorly, and the soleus is separated from the posterior surface of the tibia. The distal portion of the posterior tibial artery is approached via a medial

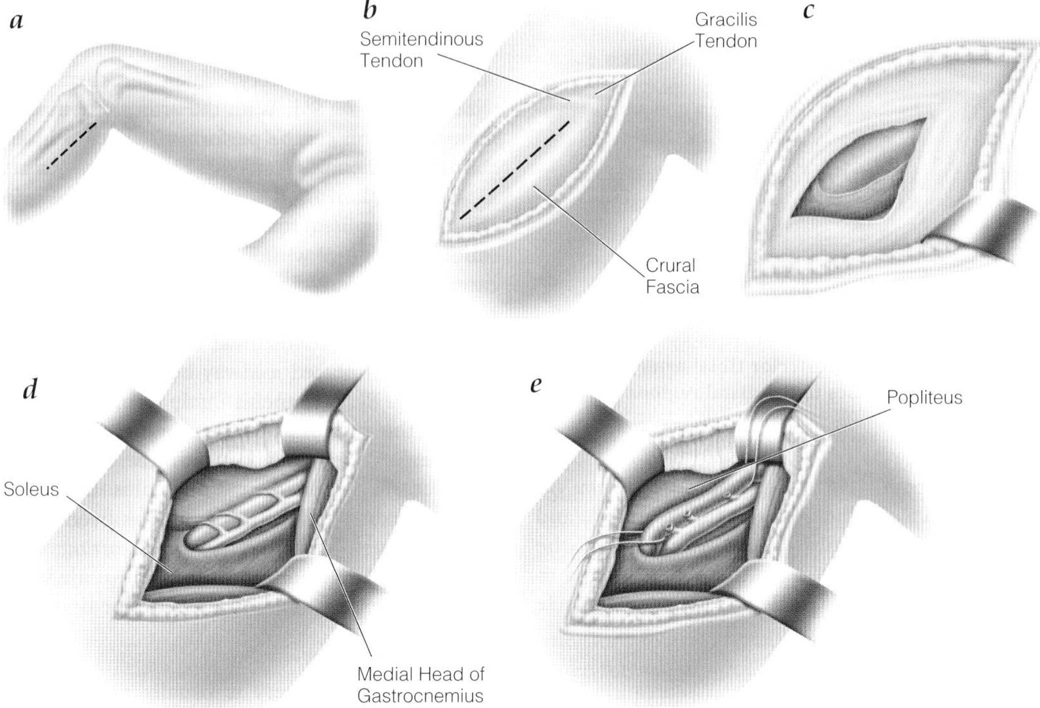

Figure 5 **Femoropopliteal bypass: below knee. Depicted is medial exposure of the distal popliteal artery. (*a*) An incision is made just behind the posteromedial surface of the tibia. (*b*) The crural fascia is exposed. (*c*) The fascia is incised, exposing the vascular bundle. (*d*) The medial head of the gastrocnemius is retracted posteriorly, exposing the distal popliteal vessels and the arcade of the soleus. (*e*) The distal popliteal artery is freed and mobilized between vessel loops.**

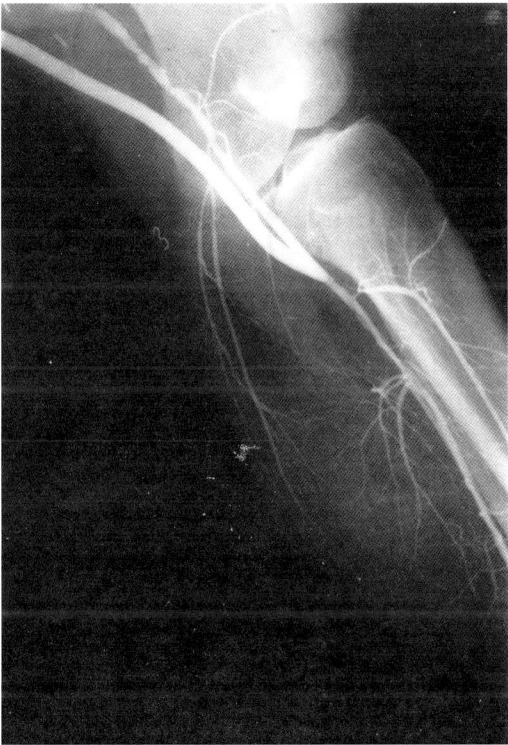

Figure 6 **Femoropopliteal bypass: below knee. A completion arteriogram from a patient who underwent below-the-knee femoropopliteal bypass for a nonhealing toe amputation site shows runoff through all three tibial vessels.**

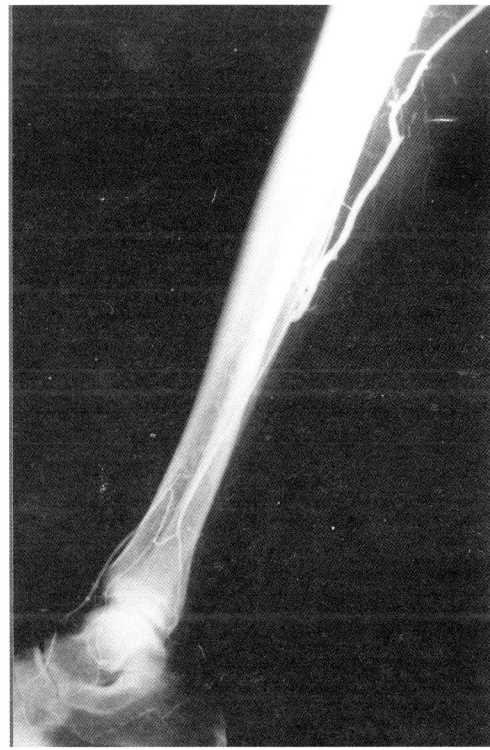

Figure 7 **Infrapopliteal bypass. An arteriogram from a 65-year-old female with rest pain in the right foot who underwent in situ bypass to the middle portion of the peroneal artery shows communication of the peroneal artery with foot arteries and reconstitution of the dorsalis pedis artery.**

18 VARICOSE VEIN SURGERY

John F. Golan, MD, FACS, Donald M. Glenn, PA-C, John J. Bergan, MD, FACS, and Luigi Pascarella, MD

Varicose veins are a common problem, accounting for approximately 85% of the venous conditions treated. Over the past decade, management options for varicose veins and venous insufficiency of the lower extremity have become more diverse. Operative vein stripping is rapidly being replaced with a variety of endovenous techniques, ranging from laser vein obliteration to radiofrequency (RF) closure to foam sclerotherapy. Conventional surgical stripping has a poor image with the public, being associated with large unsightly incisions, severe postoperative pain, and a significant risk of recurrence. Current evidence indicates that patients experience less pain and return to work more quickly after endovenous treatment of varicosities than after surgical vein stripping.[1] In addition, the elimination of the word stripping from the technical description has facilitated the public's growing preference for endovenous therapy over conventional surgical therapy (even though the basic therapeutic principles are essentially similar for the two approaches).

As a consequence of the minimally invasive nature of endovenous therapy, treatment of vein disease is moving from the hospital to the office. This shift has allowed a diverse group of physicians (e.g., dermatologists, gynecologists, and cardiologists) to enter a field that previously had been left to surgeons. Accordingly, to remain up to date with respect to the treatment of vein disease, it is essential for surgeons to acquire the knowledge and skills required to use the new endovenous techniques. In this chapter, we review the procedures, results, and complications associated with endovenous therapy, as well as traditional surgical techniques.

Terminology

All physicians treating lower-extremity venous disease should be familiar with the current names for the veins of the thigh and leg, as specified in the 2001 revision of the official terminologia anatomica by the International Interdisciplinary Consensus Committee on Venous Anatomical Terminology.[2] Failure to employ current standardized terminology can hinder data exchange in translated research studies. In addition, retention of the traditional nomenclature can result in potentially dangerous clinical scenarios. For instance, ultrasonographically diagnosed thrombosis of the superficial femoral vein might, because of the term used for the vein, be erroneously interpreted as superficial thrombophlebitis instead of true deep vein thrombosis (DVT). To prevent these and other errors, a more accurate delineation of the branches of the common femoral vein is required. Thus, the terms femoral vein (instead of superficial femoral vein) and deep femoral vein (instead of profunda femoris) are now employed.

Of particular significance for the purposes of this chapter is that the greater (long) saphenous vein is now referred to as the great saphenous vein (GSV), and the lesser (short) saphenous vein is now referred to as the small saphenous vein (SSV). In addition, the terms saphenofemoral junction and saphenopopliteal junction have been accepted into the official nomenclature—a change that is especially relevant to endovenous treatment of varicose veins. Various other changes in the names of lower-extremity and pelvic veins were also recommended in the Committee's consensus statement; however, these changes have little bearing on the current discussion and thus are not addressed further here.

Indications for Varicose Vein Surgery

The indications for surgical treatment of varicose veins are well established [*see Table 1*]. Although many physicians believe that varicose veins are nothing more than a cosmetic nuisance, this is in fact true only for some men. Women, for the most part, have specific symptoms (e.g., aching, burning pain, and heaviness) that are related to their varicose veins and are exacerbated by the presence of progesterone. Such symptoms develop with prolonged standing or sitting and reach maximal levels on the first day of the menstrual period, when progesterone levels are at their peak. Men, lacking progesterone, have few such symptoms until the varicose veins progress with aging to the point where they press on somatic nerves. In general, the severity of the symptoms bears no relation to the size of the vessels being treated. Telangiectasias can produce symptoms identical to those of varicose veins, and such symptoms can be relieved by simple sclerotherapy [*see 7:25 Sclerotherapy*].

Longitudinal studies have shown that large varicose veins can produce venous ulcerations within 15 years. Given that the incidence of venous ulceration is 20% in patients who are first seen with large varicose veins, large varicosities constitute an indication for surgery. Various skin changes characteristic of chronic venous insufficiency precede the development of venous ulceration.

Varicose thrombophlebitis is followed by recurrent varicose thrombophlebitis in nearly every case, at intervals ranging from a few weeks to many months. Nevertheless, superficial thrombophlebitis, which can be quite disabling, can be prevented by removing varicose vein clusters.

It is true that for many women, the undesirable appearance of varicose veins is a major reason for seeking surgical treatment. When questioned, however, such patients often admit to having symptoms such as pain, heaviness, and fatigue. Typically, they do not relate these symptoms to the varices

Table 1 Indications for Varicose Vein Surgery

Pain: leg aching, leg heaviness
Patchy burning (venous neuropathy)
Swelling: foot, ankle, leg
Dermatitis: focal, extensive
Lipodermatosclerosis
Ulceration: present or healed
Superficial thrombophlebitis
External hemorrhage
Appearance

themselves but instead attribute them to prolonged standing during daily work.

Preoperative Evaluation

DUPLEX MAPPING

Over the years, surgical treatises have devoted a great deal of space to clinical examination of the patient with varicose veins. Numerous clinical tests have been described, many of which carry the names of famous persons interested in venous pathophysiology. This august history notwithstanding, the Trendelenburg test, the Schwartz test, the Perthes test, and the Mahorner and Ochsner modifications of the Trendelenburg test are, for the most part, useless in preoperative evaluation of patients today.[3] There is no doubt that clinical evaluation can be improved by using handheld Doppler devices. In our view, however, preoperative evaluation is best performed by combining duplex scanning with physical examination.[4] Duplex mapping defines individual patient anatomy with considerable precision and provides valuable information that supplements the physician's clinical impression. This information allows the physician to develop a strategy that will treat abnormal refluxing veins while leaving normal portions of the venous system in place, thereby minimizing operative trauma and reducing long-term recurrence.

A protocol for duplex mapping of incompetent superficial veins has been published.[4] In essence, the examination consists of interrogating specific points of reflux with the patient standing [*see Table 2*]. Forward flow is produced with muscular compression, and reverse flow is then assessed in the crucial areas that are important to subsequent procedural planning.

The patient is placed in an upright position so that the leg veins are maximally dilated. No clothing is worn on the lower extremities from the waist down, except for nonconstricting underwear. The patient is instructed to inform the sonographer of any sensation of light-headedness, faintness, dizziness, or nausea. These symptoms seem to be associated with the overall atmosphere of the room and the presence of Doppler velocity signals; they appear to be less likely to occur when the examination itself is performed silently. If a tendency to fainting because of vagovagal reflux is encountered, the examination may have to be modified so that the patient is in a semiupright position instead.

Examination should include both lower extremities, though posttreatment examinations may target a single extremity or a single area of an extremity. The full length of the axial venous system from ankle to groin is examined. The probe is aligned transversely so that specific named veins can be identified and their relations to other limb structures determined. The veins are scanned by moving the probe up and down along their courses. Double segments, sites of tributary confluence, and large perforating veins (along with their deep venous connections) are identified. (Perforating veins are those that course from the subcutaneous tissue through deep fascia to anastomose with one of the named deep venous structures; communicating veins are those that anastomose with one another within a single anatomic plane.) Varicose veins are often arranged in multiple parallel channels. It is unnecessary to follow reflux into all of the varicose clusters, because these are obvious to the treating physician. Augmentation of flow (distal compression) is done sharply, quickly, and aggressively, and pressure is applied to the calf to activate the gastrocnemius-soleus pump. When a color or pulsed-wave Doppler device is used, the probe is angled to provide an insonation angle of 60° or less.

Table 2 Interrogation Points in the Venous Reflux Examination

Common femoral vein
Femoral vein
Upper third
Distal third
Popliteal vein
Sural veins
Saphenofemoral junction*
Saphenous vein, above the knee
Saphenous vein, below the knee
Saphenopopliteal junction†
Mode of termination, lesser saphenous vein

*Record diameter of refluxing long saphenous vein.
†Record distance from floor.

For the anterior examination, the patient faces the sonographer with his or her weight borne on the lower extremity that is not being examined. The non–weight-bearing extremity is then evaluated. The common femoral vein and the saphenofemoral junction are assessed with the Valsalva maneuver and with distal compression and release. If reflux is present, the diameter of the refluxing GSV is noted for subsequent use in selecting the proper endovenous catheter during saphenous ablation.

The GSV is identified on the basis of its relation to the deep and superficial fascia that ensheathe it to form the saphenous compartment. High-resolution B-mode ultrasonographic imaging of the superficial fascia in the transverse plane has shown that this structure reflects ultrasound strongly, yielding a characteristic image of the GSV known as the saphenous eye [*see Figure 1*]. The saphenous eye is a constant marker that is clearly demonstrable in transverse sections of the medial aspect of the thigh and that readily differentiates the GSV from varicose tributaries and other superficial veins. Casual examination of the thigh often reveals an elongated, dilated vein that is incorrectly assumed to be the GSV. This mistaken

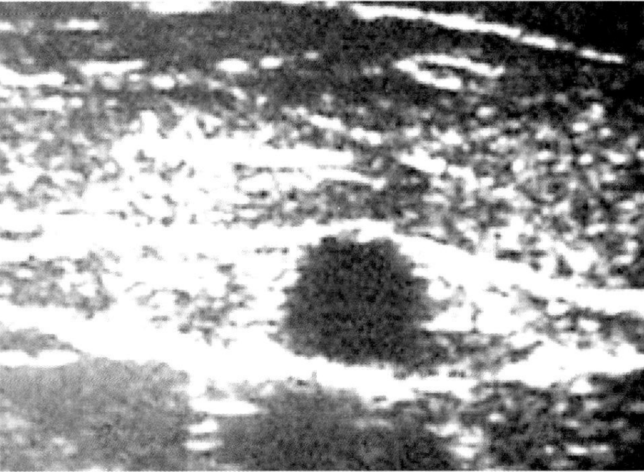

Figure 1 **Shown is an ultrasonographic image of the so-called saphenous eye. Correct identification of this marker is crucial to correct performance of the preoperative ultrasonographic reflux examination.**

assumption can be corrected by means of ultrasound scanning with the saphenous eye as an anatomic marker.

Venous reflux can be elicited manually by calf muscle compression and release, by the Valsalva maneuver, or by pneumatic tourniquet release. In terms of efficacy, there is no difference between pneumatic tourniquet release and manual compression and release. However, pneumatic tourniquet release is cumbersome and requires two vascular sonographers, which makes the manual compression and release method very attractive by comparison. If saphenofemoral reflux lasting longer than 0.5 second is present, the diameter of the GSV is recorded 2.5 cm distal to the saphenofemoral junction.

The examination continues distally along the GSV, with distal augmentation of flow performed at intervals to check for reflux. Reflux frequently ends in the region of the knee. The point at which reflux stops is recorded in terms of distance from the floor in centimeters. The femoral vein (i.e., the vessel formerly termed the superficial femoral vein) is checked at midthigh for reflux and vein wall irregularities.

The posterior examination is also done on the non–weight-bearing lower extremity, with attention paid to reflux in the popliteal vein, the saphenopopliteal junction, and the SSV. The Valsalva maneuver may be used to stimulate reflux, as may distal augmentation and release. Valsalva-induced reflux is halted by competent proximal valves. The SSV is followed from its retromalleolar position on the lateral aspect of the ankle proximally to the saphenopopliteal junction, and augmentation maneuvers are performed every few centimeters.

The termination of the SSV is noted. If the vein terminates proximally in the vein of Giacomini, the femoropopliteal vein, or another vein, a specific check is made for a connection to the popliteal vein. If the SSV shows reflux, the distance from the saphenopopliteal junction to the floor is measured and recorded.

A search for incompetent perforating veins is necessary only in limbs with chronic venous insufficiency (CVI) manifested by hyperpigmentation, atrophie blanche, woody edema, scars from healed ulceration, or actual open ulcers. Incompetent perforating veins in limbs without CVI are associated with varicose veins and can be controlled with varicose phlebectomy. Identification of perforating veins in the lower extremity can be difficult even for the experienced sonographer.

Procedural Planning

For varicose vein treatment to be successful, two goals must be met: (1) reflux must be ablated from the deep veins to the superficial veins, and (2) all branch varicosities must be removed. Reflux must be eliminated from all major problem areas, including the saphenofemoral junction, the saphenopopliteal junction, and the midthigh Hunterian perforator vein. To identify these problem areas, careful preoperative duplex mapping of major superficial venous reflux is essential. All varicose vein clusters are meticulously marked before operation; they may be difficult to identify during the procedure, when the patient is supine.

At present, three techniques are approved for the elimination of axial reflux in the GSV and the SSV: (1) traditional surgical stripping, (2) laser vein ablation (i.e., endovenous laser therapy [EVLT]), and (3) radiofrequency (RF) ablation. Regardless of which technique is employed, the principal goals of treatment (see above) are the same. In addition, the procedure must be done in a manner that optimizes cosmetic results and minimizes complications.

Endovenous Procedures

Current endovenous techniques for treating varicose veins are based on three major developments: (1) the availability of laser and RF probes that deliver heat endovenously, (2) the introduction of tumescent anesthesia, and (3) the evolution of duplex ultrasonography. Tumescent anesthesia allows physicians to use large volumes (500 ml) of dilute (0.1%) lidocaine in a single session while achieving anesthesia levels equivalent to those achieved with 1% lidocaine. In this way, the entire thigh portion of the GSV can be safely anesthetized (and consequently obliterated) at one time. Epinephrine can be added to the solution to improve postoperative hemostasis, increase venous contraction around the heat-generating catheter, and lengthen the duration of postprocedural analgesia. A common formula for the tumescent anesthesia solution is 450 ml of normal saline mixed with 50 ml of 1% lidocaine with epinephrine (1:100,000 dilution) and 10 ml of sodium bicarbonate to buffer the acidity of the lidocaine.

Duplex ultrasonography has revolutionized treatment of varicose veins. It dramatically enhances physicians' ability to evaluate the cause of varicosities and to tailor treatment so that only the diseased vein segments are ablated while the normal segments are preserved. It also serves to guide placement of sheaths and heat-generating catheter tips, allowing these devices to be situated very precisely within the vein.

TECHNIQUE

Laser Vein Ablation

Laser vein ablation [*see Figure 2*] may be performed either in the office or in the hospital. Reimbursement issues make in-office treatment advantageous for most physicians. Neither conscious sedation nor noninvasive monitoring is required. On occasion, a nervous patient may benefit from administration of an oral anxiolytic agent 1 to 2 hours before the procedure.

Standard surgical preparation and draping are indicated, including the use of sterile gowns, masks, drapes and aseptic technique. Depending on the results of the preoperative physical examination and duplex ultrasonography, the GSV, the SSV, the anterior accessory saphenous vein, or the posterior accessory saphenous vein may be treated, either alone or in combination with other vessels as necessary. The GSV is usually treated from the upper third of the calf to the saphenofemoral junction. If the calf portion of the GSV is to be treated, tumescent anesthesia should be liberally employed to reduce the risk of saphenous nerve injury. The SSV is treated from the distal third of the calf to the point where it angles toward the popliteal vein in the popliteal fossa. The relation of the sural nerve to the distal third of the SSV precludes safe treatment of this portion of the vein, and the proximity of the popliteal nerve to the SSV in the popliteal fossa precludes safe treatment of the most proximal portion of the vein. The procedure does not allow flush ligation of the saphenofemoral junction, but current evidence suggests that this measure may not be indicated: flush ligation eliminates normal venous drainage from the saphenofemoral junction and may increase the risk of neovascularization of the saphenofemoral junction and recurrence of varicosities.

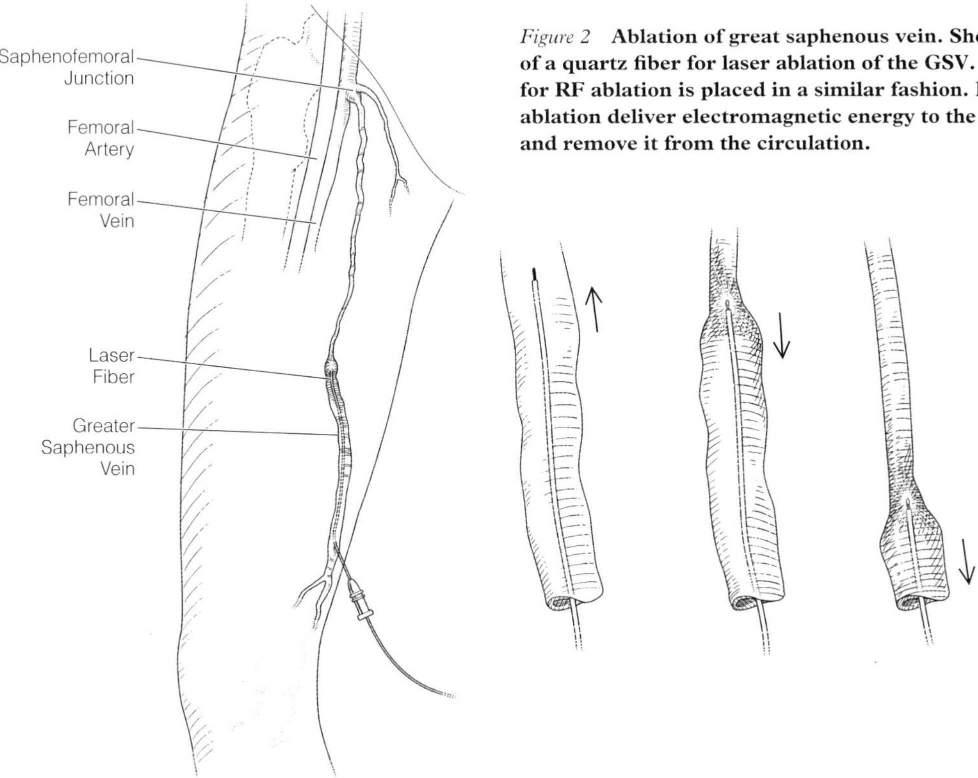

Figure 2 **Ablation of great saphenous vein. Shown is percutaneous placement of a quartz fiber for laser ablation of the GSV. In practice, the catheter used for RF ablation is placed in a similar fashion. Both laser ablation and RF ablation deliver electromagnetic energy to the vein wall to destroy the vessel and remove it from the circulation.**

The saphenous vein being treated is accessed with a micropuncture system after a small amount of lidocaine (sufficient to raise a small skin wheal) is injected into the dermis. The position of the 0.015-in. wire in the saphenous vein is confirmed by means of ultrasonography. A 4 French catheter is then passed over the wire, allowing the placement of a 0.035-in. wire for access to the proximal portion of the saphenous vein. Next, the 0.035-in. wire is positioned at the appropriate saphenous junction, and a 5 French vascular sheath is advanced over the wire to the junction. The sheath is positioned either just below the superior epigastric vein or 1 to 2 cm distal to the junction of the GSV; if the SSV is being treated, the tip is positioned 2 to 3 cm below the junction at the point where the vein makes its transition from an oblique course to a parallel path under the fascia of the leg. The 600 µm laser fiber is then passed to the tip of the sheath, which is pinned and pulled to expose the tip of the laser fiber. The rigidity and sharpness of the laser fiber makes advancing its tip dangerous. Most laser systems allow the fiber to be locked to the sheath, so that the two devices can be advanced and positioned as a single unit.

To this point in the procedure, no anesthesia other than the initial dermal injection has been employed. The next step, accordingly, is to initiate tumescent anesthesia, with or without epinephrine, along the saphenous compartment. The addition of epinephrine to the anesthetic solution results in improved constriction of the vein around the laser sheath, particularly when a saphenous vein larger than 12 mm in diameter is being treated; it also prolongs the analgesic effect of lidocaine, providing pain relief for as long as 6 to 8 hours after the procedure. A particular benefit of tumescent anesthesia is that the large volume of the injectate constitutes a heat sink that absorbs the heat created by the laser, thereby eliminating injury to surrounding soft tissue structures (e.g., nerves, fat, and skin). Further protection against injury is provided by rapid pullback of the laser fiber. As a result, the reported incidence of thermal skin or nerve injuries with laser vein ablation is almost zero.

Administration of the tumescent anesthesia solution starts at the sheath entry site and continues proximally until the entire vein segment to be treated exhibits a circumferential zone of echolucence. The vein is generally treated in the saphenous compartment between the superficial and deep fasciae of the leg. The anesthetic is administered via a 22-gauge needle with a 20 ml syringe or, alternatively, via a 10 ml autofill syringe or a Klein pump (both of which have the advantage of allowing more rapid administration with less risk of needle-stick injury to the staff). The needle is kept in a static position during administration, and the fluid is allowed to dissect up and down the fascial compartment.

Besides providing pain relief, tumescent anesthesia serves to move the saphenous vein being treated away from any structure that might be injured by the heat produced by the laser (e.g., the skin and the femoral vein). A 1 cm distance between the skin and the laser fiber is optimal. More liberal amounts of tumescent anesthesia solution are administered when the vein being treated lies in close proximity to one or more nerves (e.g., the SSV and the calf portion of the GSV). As a rule, we prefer not to treat the subdermal portions of the GSV with laser ablation; the presence of an inflamed and tender vein just beneath the dermis is likely to lead to increased postoperative pain and noticeable skin discoloration. The superficial segments of the GSV are best treated with phlebectomy at the time of laser ablation.

When administration of the tumescent anesthesia solution is complete, the position of the laser fiber's tip is again confirmed. As the vein constricts, it also shortens, and this process may advance the tip of the laser fiber into the saphenofemoral or saphenopopliteal junction. If the tip is found to have moved in this manner, it is withdrawn until it is again 1 to 2 cm below the junction. A quick scan down the vein is done to confirm that the entire vein is surrounded by the anesthetic solution and is at least 1 cm from the skin.

At this point, the laser may be safely activated. The laser is always used in the continuous mode. The power setting may range from 10 to 12 W, depending on the physician's personal preference. We typically employ a 10 W setting for veins smaller than 10 mm and a 12 W setting for veins larger than 10 mm. The essential point is that between 50 and 100 J must be delivered to each centimeter of vein treated; according to one study, 70 J/cm is the ideal amount for reliable long-term vein obliteration.[5] Energy delivery can easily be determined as the laser fiber is withdrawn. Most laser sheaths have markings 1 cm apart, and the laser machines have digital readouts that indicate the total amount of energy (J) delivered in real time. A simple calculation after 10 cm of the catheter has been withdrawn provides instant feedback on the energy delivered per centimeter of vein. On the 12 W power setting, delivery of the recommended amount of energy generally necessitates a pullback rate of 1 cm every 4 to 5 seconds (2.0 to 2.5 mm/sec). One group has advocated delivery of 140 J/cm proximally (pullback rate of 1 mm/sec) and roughly 70 J/cm distally (pullback rate of 3 mm/sec), theorizing that for long-term success, more energy is required proximally.[6] At the completion of the procedure, the laser is deactivated before the fiber is withdrawn from the skin. Ultrasonography is then performed to confirm that the common femoral vein and the superficial epigastric vein are patent and that the GSV is occluded.

An adhesive strip (e.g., Steri-Strip; 3M, St. Paul, Minnesota) covered by a transparent surgical adhesive dressing is applied over the entry site. The patient is then placed in a prescription compression stocking, which is worn for 1 to 2 weeks after the procedure. Whereas most physicians use a class 2 (30 to 40 mm Hg) compression stocking, we have switched to using a class 1 (20 to 30 mm Hg) stocking without observing any changes in complications (e.g., postoperative pain and swelling) or results. This switch has enhanced patient satisfaction, in that a class 1 stocking is easier to don and more comfortable to wear.

A 2003 study that followed 499 limbs over 2 years demonstrated a varicosity recurrence rate of less than 7% after ablation of the GSV with an 810 nm diode laser.[7] This rate is comparable to or lower than those reported after traditional surgical stripping, RF ablation, and ultrasound-guided sclerotherapy. Several smaller studies documented similar outcomes, making it evident that laser vein ablation is both effective and safe when compared to other means of treating varicose veins [*see Table 3*].[1,6,8–11]

At present, the question of how to manage residual varicosities after laser ablation remains controversial. The two main options are (1) to perform phlebectomy simultaneously with laser vein ablation and (2) to perform laser ablation alone, then observe the patient for spontaneous regression of varicosities. When the residual varicosities are left untreated, 10% to 20% of patients show sufficient regression to render further intervention unnecessary; however, 5% to 10% of patients experience superficial thrombophlebitis in the residual varicosities as a consequence of stasis from altered venous drainage. If delayed treatment of residual varicosities proves necessary, it may be accomplished with either phlebectomy or sclerotherapy, depending on the physician's preference. Our treatment of choice is laser vein ablation with concurrent phlebectomy. This approach adds only 10 to 20 minutes to the length of the procedure while offering the patient a more rapid and complete resolution of visible varicose veins and greatly reducing the risk of secondary thrombophlebitis.

Radiofrequency Ablation

In an attempt to minimize postoperative discomfort while maintaining the benefits of saphenous vein ablation, RF alternating current has been employed to effect rapid thermic electrocoagulation of the vein wall and its valves. This approach is exemplified by the Closure procedure (VNUS Medical Technologies, Inc., San Jose, California). Prolonged exposure to the high-frequency energy results in total loss of vessel wall architecture, disintegration, and carbonization.[12] Ultrasonographic follow-up shows that treated saphenous veins disappear after the 2-year point. Clinical observations suggest that patients are much more comfortable after RF ablation than after surgical stripping.[13]

The technique of RF ablation is somewhat similar to that of laser ablation [*see Figure 2*] but differs in several important respects [*see* Laser Vein Ablation, *above*]. After percutaneous access is obtained, either a 6 or an 8 French RF radiofrequency catheter is placed 1 to 2 cm from the saphenofemoral junction, and tumescent anesthesia is instituted. The probe is connected to the RF generator box, the tines of the probe are exposed, and the unit is activated. The catheter is pulled back

Table 3 Complications of Laser Vein Ablation and Radiofrequency (RF) Ablation in Selected Studies[15]

Ablation Method	Study	Limbs Treated (N)	Skin Burn (%)	Paresthesia (%)	Phlebitis (%)	DVT (%)	Recanalization (%)
Laser	Navarro[43]	40	0	0	0	0	0
	Proebstle[44]	109	0	0	10	0	10
	Min[7]	504	0	0	5	0	2
	Perkowski[45]	154	0	0	0	0	3
RF	Weiss[46]	140	0	4	0	0	10
	Merchant[47]	318	4	15	2	1	15
	Hingorani[48]	73	0	0	0.3	16	4
	Merchant[14]	1,078	2	12	3	0.5	11

slowly (1 cm every 30 seconds) while its temperature and impedance are monitored. In the procedure as originally performed, the catheter was heated to 85° C, but current approaches often involve heating the catheter to 90° or 95° C with the aim of shortening the pullback time (to compete with the shorter pullback times characteristic of laser ablation). In general, however, pullback times are still somewhat longer with RF ablation than with laser ablation, allowing more dissemination of heat to surrounding tissue; postprocedural paresthesia continues to be reported in about 12% of cases.[14] The technical results of RF ablation are excellent: with the Closure procedure, the closure rate at 4 years is 89%.[14] However, the continued occurrence of paresthesias and the slower pullback times associated with RF ablation still appear to make laser vein ablation a safer and more rapid procedure.

The issue of recurrent varicosities after obliteration of the GSV without disconnection of the saphenofemoral junction tributaries is unsettled at present. It does appear, however, that endovenous RF ablation of the GSV (e.g., with the Closure procedure) prevents subsequent neovascularization in the groin. Many centers have reported that neovascularization does not occur in the absence of a groin incision.

The specific goal of endoluminal treatment of venous reflux is obliteration of the saphenous vein. Follow-up to 4 years shows that RF ablation with the Closure procedure accomplishes this goal.[14]

OUTCOMES AND COMPLICATIONS

Both EVLT and RF ablation have proved to be effective and safe for the treatment of venous reflux disease. Several studies that followed treated limbs for 2 years or longer have shown that with respect to efficacy, these modalities are equivalent or superior to standard surgical techniques.[7,11,15,16]

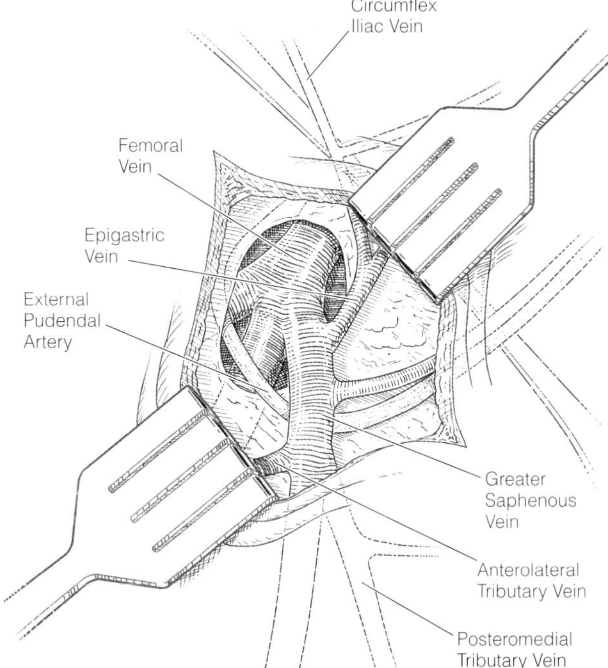

Figure 3 **Shown are a typical saphenofemoral junction and the most important tributary vessels. The classic surgical approach dictates total disconnection of all tributaries at this junction.**

It is noteworthy that neovascularization seems to be almost nonexistent with endovenous procedures; this result appears to be related exclusively to standard ligation surgery.

Multiple studies have reported similar end-point results for EVLT and RF ablation: long-term occlusion of the GSV is consistently achieved at rates approaching or exceeding 90%. In general, EVLT has somewhat better long-term success rates, ranging from 92% to 95%; RF ablation generally yields success rates between 85% and 91%. The incidence of DVT (which is more accurately described as extension of thrombus from the treated vein into the deep venous system) is low with both procedures but is slightly higher with RF ablation. No cases of life-threatening pulmonary embolism have been reported with either EVLT or RF ablation, and both are associated with only negligible rates of superficial thrombophlebitis, cellulitis, (excessive) pain, and transient paresthesias.

A 2006 study stressed the importance of treating the posterior thigh circumflex vein so as to lower the incidence of recanalization.[15] A large posterior thigh circumflex vein can drain cool blood into the segment being ablated, thus inhibiting proper heating of the refluxing segment and making adequate closure more difficult. Accordingly, the authors recommended ablating any posterior thigh circumflex veins larger than 4 mm in tandem with the primary procedure.

Surgical Vein Stripping

Ligation of the GSV at the saphenofemoral junction [*see Figure 3*] has been widely practiced in the belief that it would control gravitational reflux while preserving the vein for subsequent arterial bypass. It is true that the GSV is largely preserved after proximal ligation[17]; however, reflux continues, and hydrostatic forces are not controlled.[18] Recurrent varicose veins are more frequent after saphenous ligation than after stripping.[19] Varicosities also recur more frequently after ligation and sclerotherapy than after stripping and sclerotherapy.[20] A prospective, randomized trial that compared proximal GSV ligation and stab avulsion of varices with stripping of the thigh portion of the GSV and stab avulsion of varices showed the latter approach to be superior.[21,22] Routine GSV stripping reduces the rate of recurrent varicosities and the need for reoperation for recurrent saphenofemoral incompetence.

Although it can be argued that the GSV should be retained for possible use in arterial bypass grafting, the relatively high (> 20%) reoperation rate makes this strategy undesirable. Almost three quarters of limbs that undergo GSV ligation alone have an incompetent GSV on follow-up duplex imaging. Until studies show a clear advantage to retaining the GSV in defined patient populations, surgical stripping should remain a routine part of primary GSV surgery. In several studies, preservation of the patency of the GSV and continuing reflux in this vein were found to be the factors most frequently associated with recurrence of varicosities.[23–25] In one study of patients who underwent reoperation for relief of recurrent variceal symptoms, two thirds of the patients required removal of the GSV as part of the procedure.[23]

Over the past 100 years, ankle-to-groin stripping of the GSV has been the dominant approach to treatment of varicose veins.[26–28] It has been argued, however, that routine stripping of the leg (i.e., ankle-to-knee) portion of the GSV is inadvisable. One argument against this practice is that there is a significant risk of concomitant saphenous nerve injury

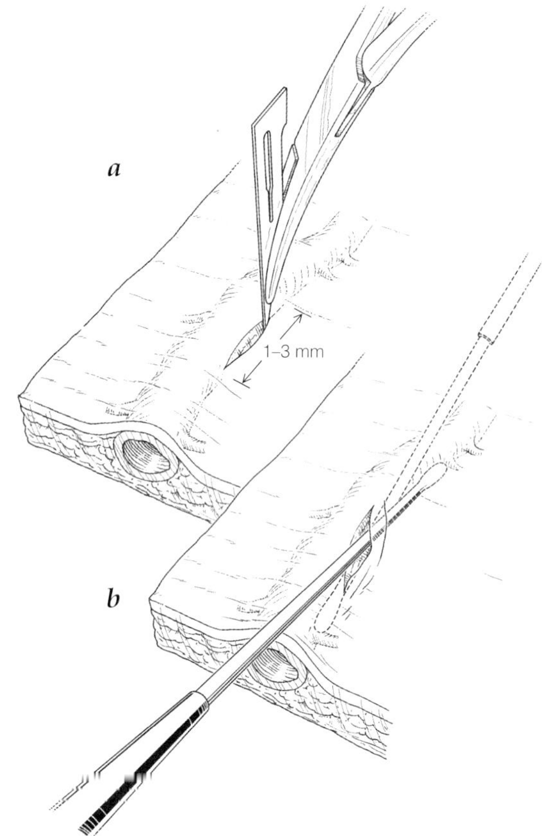

Figure 6 **Surgical stripping of great saphenous vein: phlebectomy for residual varicosities. (*a*) Skin incisions for stab avulsion of varicosities are limited with respect to both length and depth. (*b*) The dissector blade facilitates mobilization of the vein before removal.**

have achieved marked refinements of phlebectomy techniques for varicose clusters.[33]

COMPLICATIONS

Surgical removal of the GSV on an outpatient basis still requires two incisions, one in the groin and the other near the knee. Postoperative compression bandaging is standard, and most patients experience little downtime. Some, however, do experience hematoma, pain, and extensive bruising. These three complications are linked; thus, every effort should be made to prevent oozing. The most feared complication of varicose vein surgery is venous thromboembolism, but the incidence of this complication is quite low (probably about 1%). In countries where postoperative immobilization, hospitalization, and delayed ambulation are employed for patients with varicosities, prophylaxis against venous thromboembolism is common. In the United States, however, this measure is generally considered unnecessary in these patients. The most common complication of varicose vein surgery is recurrence of varicosities, which is experienced by 15% to 30% of patients treated.[24]

To speak of permanent removal of varicosities implies that all potential causes of recurrence have been considered and that surgical management has been planned so as to address them. There are four principal causes of recurrence of varicose veins, three of which can be dealt with at the time of the primary operation.

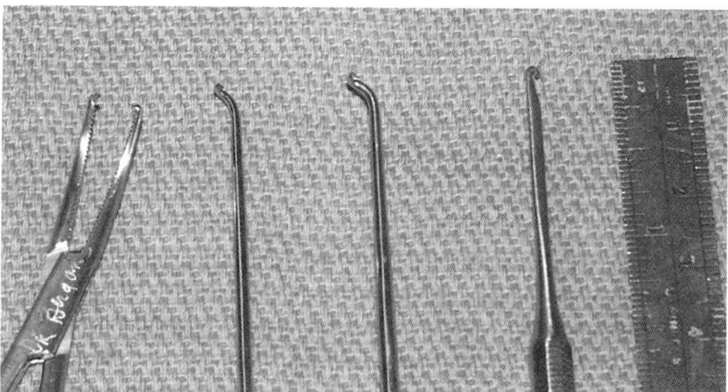

Figure 7 **Surgical stripping of great saphenous vein: phlebectomy for residual varicosities. Shown are tools used for exteriorizing varicosities: a Hartman clamp with its single tooth placed distally, two Muller clamps, and a Varady hook and dissector (left to right).**

One cause of recurrent varicosities is failure to perform the primary operation correctly. Common errors include missing a duplicated saphenous vein and mistaking an anterolateral or accessory saphenous vein for the GSV. Careful and thorough anatomic identification will help minimize such errors. It has long been held that a second cause of recurrent varicose veins is failure to do a proper groin dissection; however, it is now known that such dissection causes neovascularization in the groin, leading to recurrence of varicose veins [*see* Outcome Evaluation, *below*]. A third cause is failure to remove the GSV from the circulation. A reason often cited for this failure is the desire to preserve the GSV for subsequent use as an arterial bypass, but it is clear that the preserved GSV continues to reflux and continues to elongate and dilate its tributaries, thereby producing more varicosities even after primary operative treatment has removed the varicose veins present at the time. A fourth cause of recurrent varicosities is persistence of venous hypertension through nonsaphenous sources—chiefly perforating veins with incompetent valves. Muscular contrac-

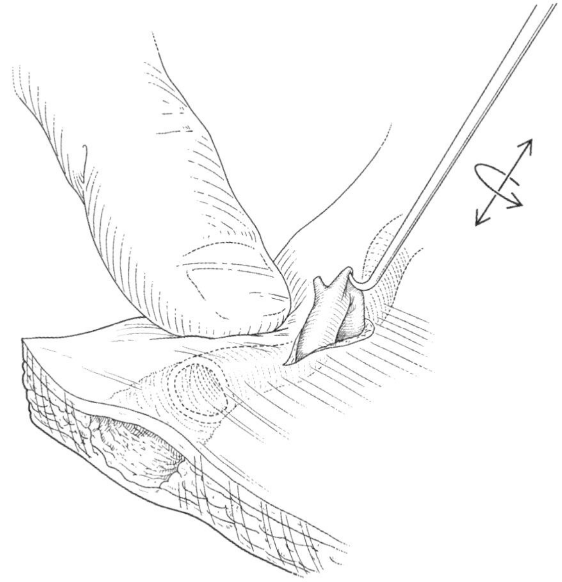

Figure 8 **Surgical stripping of great saphenous vein: phlebectomy for residual varicosities. The varix is exteriorized with a hook, then divided to permit proximal and distal avulsion.**

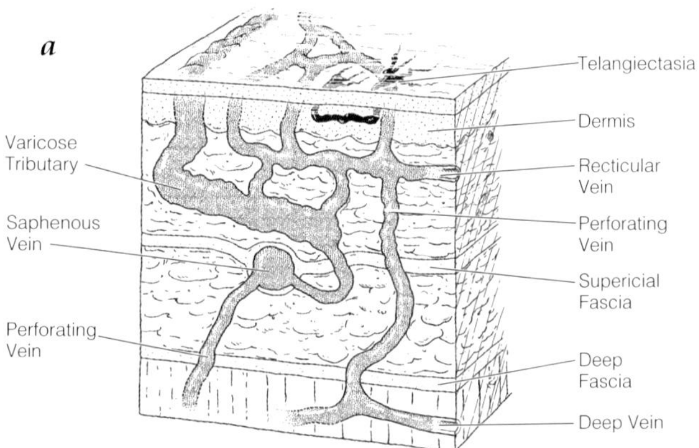

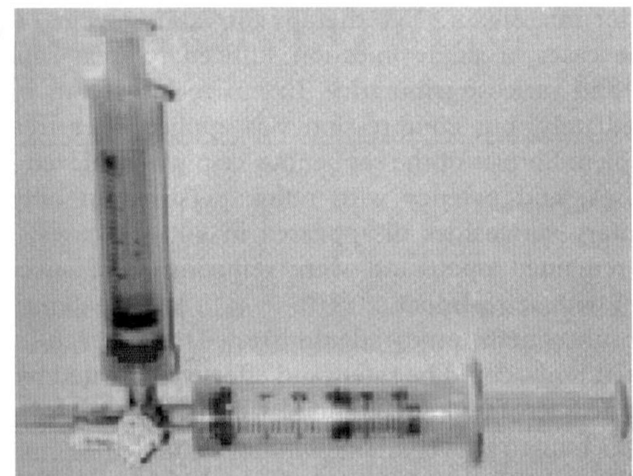

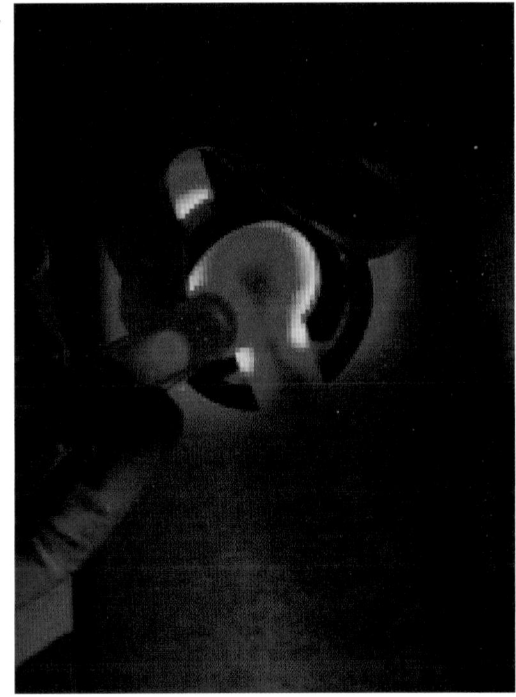

Figure 9 **Microfoam sclerotherapy. (*a*) The relationships among the venous structures in a lower extremity with varicosities explain why microfoam sclerotherapy can succeed. Injections into varices, reticular veins, or perforating veins can place the foam into varicose structures and even into telangiectatic blemishes. (*b*) Sclerosant foam is made by mixing room air with 0.5% sodium tetradecyl sulfate (STS) in a 2:1 ratio via a three-way stopcock. The syringes are emptied 35 times to create a foam that lasts about 5 minutes. (*c*) A halogen light (vein light), as used here during a foam injection, is helpful for treating persistent or ecurrent varices along with the GSV in situations where surgery is undesirable.**

tion generates enormous pressures that are directed against valves in perforating veins. Venous hypertension induces a leukocyte endothelial reaction, which, in turn, incites an inflammatory response that ultimately destroys the venous valves and weakens the venous wall.[34] The perforating veins most commonly associated with recurrent varicosities are the midthigh perforating vein, the distal thigh perforating vein, the proximal anteromedial calf perforating vein, and the lateral thigh perforating vein, which connects the deep femoral vein to surface varicosities.

In addition to the four principal causes of recurrent varicosities, there is a fifth cause, which is beyond the operating surgeon's control—namely, the genetic tendency to form varicosities. This tendency results in the development of localized or generalized venous wall weakness, localized blowouts of venous walls, or stretched, elongated, and floppy venous valves.[35,36]

OUTCOME EVALUATION

As a rule, when undesirable outcomes occur after surgical saphenous vein stripping, they become evident quite early.[21] As noted (*see above*), it has long been accepted practice to dissect tributary vessels at the saphenofemoral junction very carefully, taking each of the vessels back beyond the primary and even the secondary tributaries if possible.[31] In practice, however, such dissection appears to cause neovascularization in the groin[37]; surveillance with duplex ultrasonography supports this finding.[38] It has now been amply confirmed that neovascularization causes recurrent varicose veins. Clearly, this is a significant disadvantage of standard surgical treatment of varicosities. This disadvantage has been a major impetus for the development of less invasive alternatives to surgical saphenous vein stripping [*see* Endovenous Procedures, above, and Foam Sclerotherapy, *below*]. These alternatives are proving to be effective and may be superior to surgical stripping, if only because they are not followed by groin neovascularization.

Foam Sclerotherapy

The prospect of a rapid, minimally invasive, and durable treatment of varicose veins is an attractive one. Current evidence suggests that these objectives may be achieved without operative intervention by using sclerosant microfoam [*see Figure 9*]. In 1944 and 1950, E. J. Orbach introduced the concept of a macrobubble air-block technique to enhance the properties of sclerosants in performing macrosclerotherapy.[39,40] At the time, few clinicians evinced much interest in the subject, and the technique languished.

Half a century later, the work of Juan Cabrera and colleagues in Granada attracted the attention of some phlebologists and reawakened interest in using foam technology for the treatment of venous insufficiency.[41] These investigators showed that foam sclerotherapy was technically simple and worked well in small to moderate-sized varicose veins, and they demonstrated that the limitations of liquid sclerotherapy could be erased by using microfoam. Their 5-year report represents the longest observation period to

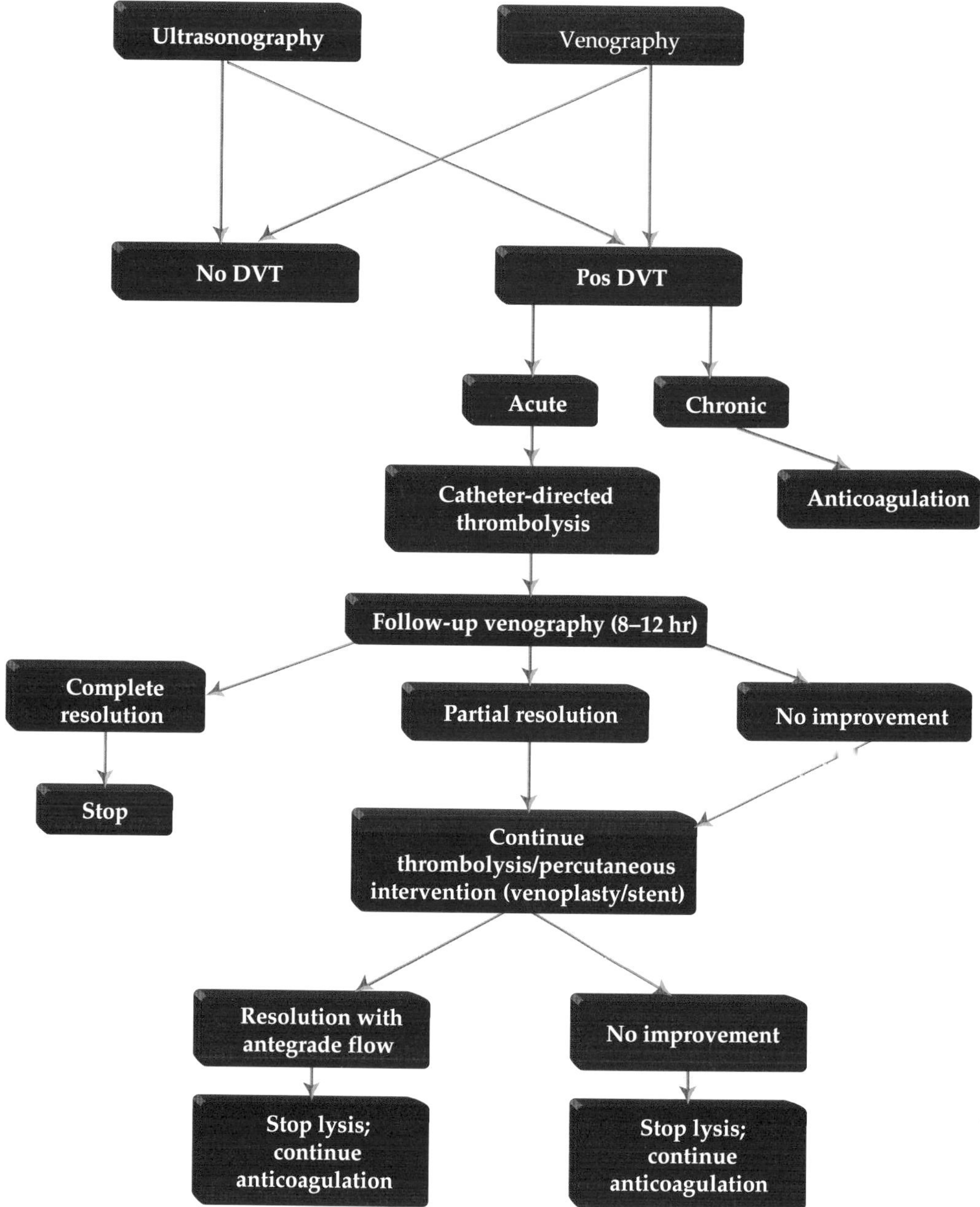

Figure 10 **Algorithm for the treatment of venous thrombolysis.**

The deep venous system must be patent. Patients with ulceration, thrombophlebitis, or bleeding from varicosities are considered symptomatic and suitable for intervention if the GSV is incompetent and meets anatomic criteria.

Preprocedure Planning

GSV ablation procedures may be performed in an office setting or in an operating or procedure room. If an office setting is chosen, patients must be able to tolerate some minimum amount of discomfort with light sedation. The performing physician must be certified to deliver conscious sedation and, in the case of laser therapy, be laser qualified. The procedure room, whether in an office or a medical facility, should be equipped with a procedure table that has the ability to place the patient in the steep Trendelenburg position, a high-resolution duplex ultrasound system, and the appropriate ablation equipment. Nitroglycerin cream can help dilate the vein. Stab avulsions, sometimes needed for more symptomatic side branch varicosities, are generally best done in the operating room if extensive but in the office if localized. Both radiofrequency and laser ablations are effective. If catheter-directed ablation therapy is instituted, then a sheath, a proximal occlusive balloon, and a 3 French microcatheter are used and delivered over wire. If duplex ultrasonography–directed sclerotherapy is performed, then ultrasonography-guided access is obtained, the vein is compressed, and the sclerosant agent is injected into the vein. Available sclerosants are shown in Table 6.

Table 6 Sclerosing Solutions

Vein Diameter	*Sclerosing Solution*
< 0.4 mm	Sodium tetradecyl sulfate 0.1%
	Hypertonic saline 11.7%
0.6–2 mm	Sodium tetradecyl sulfate 0.25%
	Hypertonic saline 23.4%
3–5 mm	Sodium tetradecyl sulfate 0.5–1%
Perforators	Sodium tetradecyl sulfate 2–3%

RFA of the GSV

Development of the Closure device (VNUS Medical Technologies, Inc., San Jose, CA) has allowed the application of RFA to GSV reflux therapy. The GSV is mapped with ultrasonography prior to the procedure. The patients are placed in the Trendelenburg position with a tourniquet around the upper thigh. Access to the GSV is obtained at the knee with an introducer needle and a wire threaded into the vein, and then the needle is replaced with a proprietary sheath. The Closure catheter is threaded through the sheath, and, under ultrasound guidance, the tip is placed just proximal to the takeoff of the superficial epigastric vein at the saphenofemoral junction (SFJ). Tumescent anesthesia (500 cc normal saline, 50 cc of 1% lidocaine with epinephrine, 5 cc of sodium bicarbonate) is injected into the sheath under ultrasound guidance surrounding the saphenous vein to provide anesthesia, improve impedance, and protect the overlying tissues from exposure to the heat. The Closure device is then connected to the RFA delivery system, deployed, and pulled back at a controlled rate (initially 1 cm every 30 seconds) while checking both impedance and temperature. Manual compression, particularly in the high thigh, may aid in obtaining optimal numerical values on the RFA unit and increase ablation efficiency. After the catheter has been withdrawn into the sheath, it is removed, and confirmation of obliteration of the GSV is confirmed by ultrasonography.

Endovenous Laser Treatment of the GSV

Laser therapy has been applied to varicose veins in various forms for the last decade. Access to the GSV is obtained as described above for RFA treatment, and a wire is advanced under ultrasound guidance above the SFJ. A 600 µm laser fiber (AngioDynamics, Latham, NY) is placed over the wire and positioned just distal to the SFJ in the GSV. Tumescent anesthesia is injected (as above). Laser energy is delivered as the laser fiber is pulled back (810 nm diode laser). One advantage of this technique over RFA is that the laser wire can be pulled back relatively quickly, as fast as 18 mm/min.

Catheter-Directed Chemoablation of the GSV

Catheter-directed foam sclerotherapy has been applied to incompetent GSVs and is supported by grade 2B evidence. Access is gained under ultrasound guidance, and a 4 French sheath is placed retrograde. A wire and a microcatheter are delivered, and foam is injected with proximal compression or occlusion with a balloon to prevent embolization.

Duplex Ultrasonography–Directed Chemoablation of the GSV

Duplex ultrasonography–directed foam sclerotherapy for the GSV is widely applied to treat incompetent GSV and accessories. Access is gained under ultrasound guidance, and a series of foam injections are performed to obliterate the GSV. Again, care should be taken to avoid systemic embolization of foam.

Duplex Ultrasonography–Directed Perforator Ablation

Treatment of pathologic perforating veins, defined as outward flow duration 500 ms or greater and vein diameter 3.5 mm or greater, located underneath healed or active ulcers (CEAP class C5 to C6), can be undertaken using endovascular technques. RFA of the perforator vein is performed using a special short RFA catheter and sheath. Local anesthetic is liberally infiltrated. Care should be taken to avoid the deep system and the skin to avoid DVT and burns, respectively.

Complications

The most serious complication associated with any of these endovenous techniques is DVT. There have been several reports of DVT from GSV RFA, with the incidence as high as 16%.[75] Lower extremity DVT has also been reported following endovenous laser therapy. Other problems include saphenous nerve paresthesias along the course of the GSV, bruising, skin burn, and superficial phlebitis. Failure of the GSV to become obliterated can be treated with redo ablation or prompt high ligation at the time of ablation. Clot into the common femoral vein can be treated with standard anticoagulation. Clot abutting the common femoral vein can be treated with clopidogrel 75 mg orally daily for 1 month and serial ultrasonography to ensure no propagation. Care should be taken to quantify the amount of clot in the common femoral vein as there are data to show that there is significant retraction of clot when a patient stands.[75]

Outcomes

Overall, good results are obtained with these endovenous methods of obliterating the GSVs. Two-year data on RFA of the GSV report 85% of patients with complete occlusion of the GSV, with 90% of all patients being free of GSV reflux.[76] Endovenous laser results are similar, with 93% continued vein closure by ultrasound surveillance at 2 years.[77] Above-the-knee GSV ablation improves symptoms regardless of persisting below-the-knee reflux (> 1 s reflux); this reflux can be responsible for residual symptoms and a greater need for sclerotherapy for residual varicosities. It has been shown that following above-the-knee GSV ablation, 40 to 50% of patients have residual varicosities. Extended ablation below the knee is safe, increases spontaneous resolution of varicosities, and has a greater impact on symptom reduction. Similar benefits occurred after concomitant below-the-knee foam sclerotherapy. Application of catheter-directed foamed sclerosant by using a catheter is successful in 90% of cases. A 90% treatment success is predicted for veins less than 6.5 mm.[78,79] A report of percutaneous ablation of perforators showed that 81% of the veins had successful ablation in a 5-year follow-up. A recent review indicated that 90% of remaining outside toes, which can lead to skin ulceration secondary to abnormal pressure points. Finally, loss of several of the metatarsal heads results in abnormal weight bearing on the remaining metatarsal heads, which may give rise to late ulceration.

OPERATIVE TECHNIQUE

Transphalangeal Amputation

Digital block anesthesia is ideal for transphalangeal amputation. A 25-gauge needle is inserted into the skin over the medial aspect of the dorsum of the proximal phalanx and advanced until the bone is encountered. The needle is then withdrawn slightly, and a small amount of fluid is aspirated to confirm that the tip of the needle is not in a blood vessel. Next, 0.5 to 1.0 mL of lidocaine, 0.5 or 1.0% without epinephrine, is slowly injected. The needle is then carefully advanced medial to the bone until the tip can be felt pressing against (but not puncturing) the plantar skin. Again, the needle is withdrawn slightly, fluid is aspirated, and 0.5 to 1.0 mL of lidocaine is injected. The same technique is repeated on the lateral aspect of the proximal phalanx. In this way, all four digital nerve branches are blocked. If multiple toe amputations are required, an ankle block, epidural anesthesia, spinal anesthesia, or general anesthesia can be used.

An incision is made to create dorsal and plantar skin flaps. Typically, these flaps are equal in length; however, depending on the location of the skin lesion, either the dorsal flap or the plantar flap can be left longer [*see Figure 1*]. Care must be taken not to create excessively long flaps, which may lack sufficient perfusion for healing, or to create undermined bevels with the scalpel [*see Figure 2*], which will lead to epidermolysis of the suture line.

The incision is extended down to the phalanx, and the soft tissues are gently separated from the bone with a small periosteal elevator. All tendons and tendon sheaths are débrided because the poor vascularity of these tissues may compromise the healing of the toe. The phalanx is transected at the level of the apices of the skin incisions [*see Figure 1*]. Care must be taken not to leave the remaining bone segment too long: this places undue tension on the skin flaps and is a primary cause of poor healing. The best way of transecting the phalanx is to use a pneumatic oscillating saw. Manual bone cutters can splinter the bone, and manual saws can cause extensive damage to the soft tissues. The bone is always transected across the shaft; because of the poor vascularity of the articular cartilage, disarticulation across a joint typically leads to poor healing.

Hemostasis is achieved with absorbable sutures and limited use of the electrocautery. Excessive tissue manipulation and electrocauterization should be avoided. The skin edges are carefully approximated with simple interrupted nonabsorbable monofilament sutures; perfect apposition is necessary to maximize the potential for primary healing. The sutures must not be placed too close to the skin edges, because the heavily keratinized skin of the foot is easily lacerated. The final step is the application of a soft dressing.

Ray Amputation

For ray amputation [*see Figure 3*], local digital block or spinal, epidural, or general anesthesia can be employed. A so-called tennis-racket incision is made—that is, a straight incision along the dorsal surface of the affected metatarsal bone coupled with a circumferential incision around the base of the toe. The goal is to save all available viable skin on the toe; this skin is used to ensure a tension-free closure,

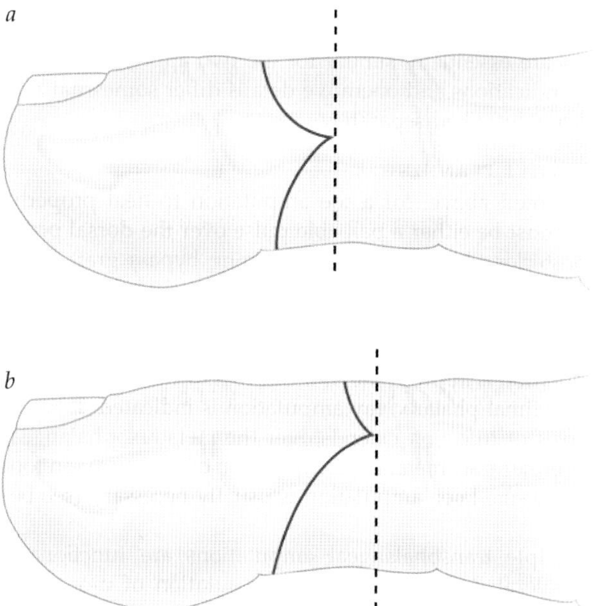

Figure 1 **Toe amputation: transphalangeal amputation. Transphalangeal amputation can be performed with either dorsal and plantar flaps of equal length (*a*) or a plantar flap that is longer than the dorsal flap (*b*). The phalanx is transected at the level of the apex of the skin flaps (*dashed line*). The bone is transected through the shaft of the phalanx, never across the joint.**

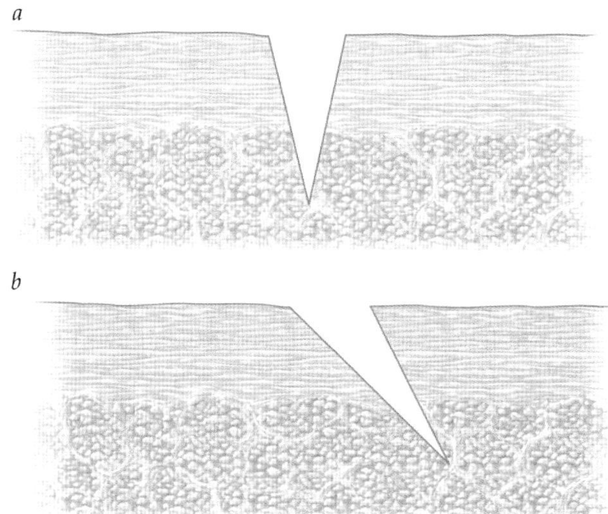

Figure 2 **In a lower extremity amputation, the skin is always incised perpendicular to its surface (*a*). Given the varying contours encountered during extremity amputation, it can be difficult to maintain the perpendicular orientation of the scalpel; however, an incision that undermines the proximal skin flap (*b*) will devascularize the epidermis and lead to necrosis of the suture line.**

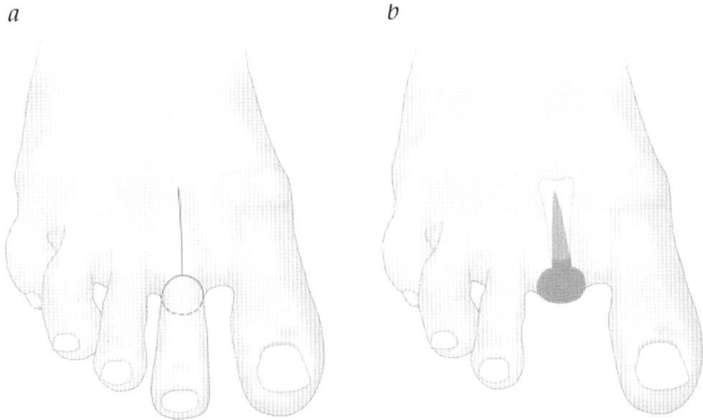

Figure 3 **Toe amputation: ray amputation. (*a*) A longitudinal incision is made along the dorsum of the shaft of the metatarsal bone of the affected toe. A circumferential incision is then made around the phalanx. The circumferential incision should be placed as distal on the toe as there is viable skin so that as much skin as possible is retained for closure of the wound. (*b*) The metatarsal bone is transected across its shaft, proximal to the metatarsal head; the joint is never disarticulated.**

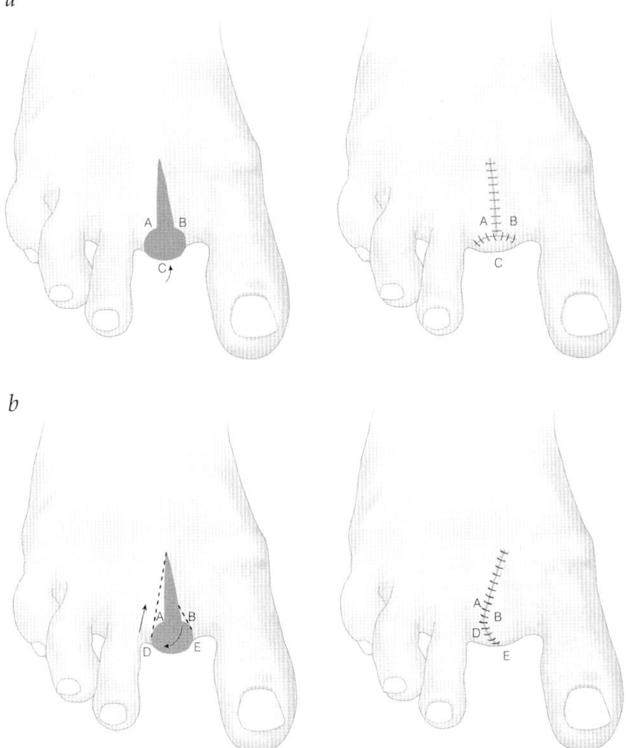

Figure 4 **Toe amputation: ray amputation. (*a*) If adequate skin is available, a plantar flap can be rotated dorsally and the skin closed in a Y configuration. This closure is technically easy to perform; however, there is a risk of skin necrosis at corners A and B. (*b*) Alternatively, the skin can be closed in a linear fashion. Corners A and B are gently trimmed. Corner B is shifted distally toward point D as corner A is shifted proximally. A slight dog-ear will result at point E; however, it will diminish with time.**

and any excess skin can be débrided later, at the time of closure. Again, undermined bevels are avoided. The incision is taken down to the bone, and the soft tissues are separated from the distal metatarsal bone with a periosteal elevator. Dissection must be kept close to the affected metatarsal head to prevent injury to the adjacent metatarsophalangeal joint, which can lead to necrosis of the adjacent toe. The metatarsal bone is transected across the shaft with a pneumatic oscillating saw. Ray amputation of the first toe usually requires fashioning a bevel on the medial and plantar aspects of the transected metatarsal shaft to allow skin closure without tension. The tendons and the tendon sheaths are débrided.

Meticulous hemostasis is achieved with absorbable sutures and limited use of the electrocautery. The skin is approximated with simple interrupted nonabsorbable monofilament sutures [*see Figure 4*]. If sufficient viable skin was preserved, a flap of plantar skin is rotated dorsally, and the incision is closed in the shape of a **Y**. However, necrosis of the corners of the skin is common. Preferably, the medial and lateral edges are shifted (one proximally and the other distally), the corners are trimmed, and the incision is closed in a linear fashion. A soft supportive dressing is applied.

COMPLICATIONS

Complications of toe amputation include bleeding, infection, and failure to heal. Because even a small amount of bleeding under the skin flaps can prevent proper healing, meticulous hemostasis is mandatory. In most cases, infection and failure to heal are attributable to poor patient selection, inadequate arterial perfusion, or poor surgical technique; the usual result is a more proximal amputation.

OUTCOME

For optimal healing, there must be an extended period (2 to 3 weeks) during which no weight is borne by the foot that underwent toe amputation. Once healing is complete, the patient should be able to walk normally, with no need for orthotic or assist devices. Beginning ambulation too early can disrupt healing flaps and necessitate more proximal amputation, which lengthens the hospital stay and increases long-term disability. For these reasons, toe amputation in patients with arterial occlusive disease is not an outpatient procedure. Patients are kept on bed rest and instructed in techniques (e.g., use of a wheelchair, a walker, or crutches) that allow them to function without stepping on the foot with the toe amputation. Hospital discharge is delayed until such techniques are mastered.

Transmetatarsal Amputation

OPERATIVE PLANNING

As noted (see above), transmetatarsal amputation is indicated if there is tissue loss in the forefoot involving more than two metatarsal heads or the dorsal forefoot. It is contraindicated if there is extensive skin loss on the plantar surface of the foot or on the dorsum proximal to the midshaft of the metatarsal bones. The peroneus longus and the peroneus brevis muscles insert on the proximal portions of the fourth and fifth metatarsal bones; if these insertions are sacrificed, inversion of the foot results, eventually leading to chronic skin breakdown from the side of the foot repeatedly striking the ground during ambulation. Transmetatarsal amputation is also contraindicated if there is a preexisting foot drop (peroneal nerve palsy).

OPERATIVE TECHNIQUE

Spinal, epidural, or general anesthesia may be employed for transmetatarsal amputation. Placement of a tourniquet on the calf is a useful adjunctive measure. This step greatly reduces intraoperative blood loss. More important, the bloodless operative field that results allows more accurate assessment of tissue viability and hence more precise selection of the level of amputation; in a field stained with extravasated blood, it is easy to leave behind nonviable tissue that will doom the amputation. Use of a tourniquet is, however, contraindicated in patients who have a functioning infrapopliteal artery bypass graft or recent endovascular reconstruction of the infrapopliteal arteries.

After sterile preparation and draping, the leg is elevated to help drain the venous blood, and a sterile pneumatic tourniquet is placed around the calf, with care taken to pad the skin under the tourniquet and to position the tourniquet over the calf muscles, where it will not apply pressure over the fibular head (and the common peroneal nerve) or other osseous prominences. The tourniquet is then inflated to a pressure higher than the systolic blood pressure. In patients who do not have diabetes mellitus, a tourniquet inflation pressure of 250 mm Hg is typically employed; in patients who have diabetes mellitus and calcified arteries, a pressure of 350 to 400 mm Hg is preferred.

An incision is made across the dorsum of the foot at the level of the middle of the shafts of the metatarsal bones, extending medially and laterally to the level of the center of the first and fifth metatarsal bones, respectively [*see Figure 5*]. The dorsal incision is curved proximally at the medial and lateral edges to ensure that no dog-ears remain at the time of closure. The dorsal incision is continued perpendicularly through the soft tissues on the dorsum down to the metatarsal bones. The plantar incision is extended distally to a point just proximal to the toe crease. Care is taken not to bevel the skin incisions.

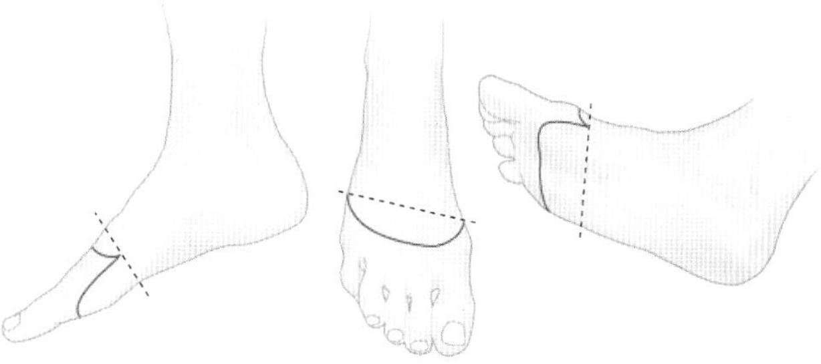

Figure 5 **Transmetatarsal amputation. The skin incisions are shown from various angles. The metatarsal shafts are divided in their midportions (*dashed line*). The metatarsal bone transection is at the level of the apices of the skin incision, and the lateral metatarsal bones are cut slightly more proximally than the medial metatarsal bones, in a pattern reflecting the normal contour of the forefoot.**

A plantar flap is created by making an incision with the scalpel adjacent to the metatarsophalangeal joints; the incision is then carried more deeply to the level of the midshafts of the metatarsal bones on their plantar surfaces. The periosteum of the first metatarsal bone is scored circumferentially with the scalpel, and the soft tissue is dissected away from the first metatarsal bone with a periosteal elevator to a point about 1 cm proximal to the dorsal skin incision. The first metatarsal bone is then transected perpendicular to its shaft at the level 1 cm proximal to the dorsal skin incision with a pneumatic oscillating saw. This process is repeated for each metatarsal bone, with care taken to follow the normal contour of the forefoot by cutting the lateral metatarsal bones at a level slightly proximal to the level at which the more medial bones are transected. All visible digital arteries are clamped and tied with absorbable ligatures. If a tourniquet was used, it is deflated at this time. All tendons and tendon sheaths are débrided from the wound.

Meticulous hemostasis is achieved with absorbable sutures and limited use of the electrocautery. Any sharp edges on the metatarsal bones are smoothed with a rongeur or a rasp. The wound is irrigated to flush out devitalized tissue and thrombus. The plantar flap is trimmed as needed. The dermis is approximated with simple interrupted absorbable sutures, and the knots are buried. Because the edge of the plantar flap is generally longer than the edge of the dorsal flap, the sutures must be placed slightly farther apart on the plantar flap than on the dorsal flap if perfect alignment is to be obtained. It is imperative to achieve the correct skin alignment with the dermal suture layer. Once this is accomplished, the skin edges are gently and perfectly apposed with interrupted vertical mattress sutures of nonabsorbable monofilament material. Finally, a soft supportive dressing with good padding of the heel is applied; casts and splints are avoided because of the risk of ulceration of the heel or over the malleoli.

COMPLICATIONS

If a tourniquet is not used, intraoperative blood loss can be substantial; the blood pools in the sponges and drapes, often out of the anesthesiologist's field of view. Consequently, good communication between the surgeon and the anesthesiologist is crucial for preventing ischemic cardiac complications secondary to hemorrhage.

Postoperative complications include bleeding, infection, and failure to heal, all of which are likely to result in more proximal amputation. They can best be prevented by means of careful patient selection and meticulous surgical technique.

OUTCOME

For proper healing, postoperative edema must be avoided and the plantar flap protected against shear forces. To prevent swelling, the patient is kept on bed rest with the foot elevated for the first 2 to 3 days. This step is particularly important if the transmetatarsal amputation was performed simultaneously with arterial reconstruction, which carries a high risk of reperfusion edema of the foot. After 2 to 3 days, the patient is instructed in techniques for moving in and out of the wheelchair without stepping on the foot. The foot that was operated on should not bear any weight at all for at least 3 weeks; early weight bearing may disrupt the healing of the plantar flap and necessitate more proximal amputation.

Once healed, patients should be able to walk independently with standard shoes with good arch support. There is, however, a risk that they may trip over the unsupported toe of the shoe. In addition, the push-off normally provided by the toes is lost after transmetatarsal amputation, and this change results in a halting, flat-footed gait. These problems can be obviated by using an orthotic shoe with a steel shank (to keep the toe of the shoe from bending and causing tripping) and a rocker bottom (to provide a smooth heel-to-toe motion).

Guillotine Ankle Amputation

OPERATIVE PLANNING

Guillotine amputation across the ankle is indicated when a patient presents with extensive wet gangrene that precludes salvage of a functional foot (e.g., wet gangrene that destroys the heel, the plantar skin of the forefoot, or the dorsal skin of the proximal foot). In such patients, initial guillotine amputation through the ankle is safer than extensive débridement; the operation is shorter, less blood is lost, the risk of bacteremia is reduced, and better control of infection is possible. Guillotine amputation is also indicated in patients with foot infections who have cellulitis extending into the leg. Transection at the ankle, perpendicular to the muscle compartments, tendon sheaths, and lymphatic vessels, allows effective drainage and usually brings about rapid resolution of the cellulitis of the leg, thus permitting salvage of the knee in many cases in which the knee might otherwise be unsalvageable.

OPERATIVE TECHNIQUE

General anesthesia is preferred for guillotine ankle amputation; regional anesthesia is relatively contraindicated for critically ill patients who are in a septic state. Anesthesia is required for no more than 15 to 20 minutes.

A circumferential incision is made at the narrowest part of the ankle (i.e., at the proximal malleoli) regardless of the level of the cellulitis [*see Figure 6*]. This placement takes the line of incision across the tendons, thereby preventing bleeding from transected muscle bellies. The incision is then carried through the skin and soft tissues to the bone. If the arteries are patent, the assistant applies circumferential pressure to the distal calf. The distal tibia and fibula are then divided with a Gigli saw or an oscillating pneumatic saw. Hemostasis is achieved with suture ligation and electrocauterization. A moist dressing is applied.

OUTCOME

After the procedure, the patient is kept on bed rest and given systemic antibiotics. Formal below-the-knee amputation can be performed when the cellulitis resolves, usually within 3 to 5 days. Routine dressing changes are unnecessary—first, because they are painful, and second, because the decision to proceed with formal below-the-knee amputation is based on the extent of the cellulitis in the calf, not on the appearance of the transected ankle.

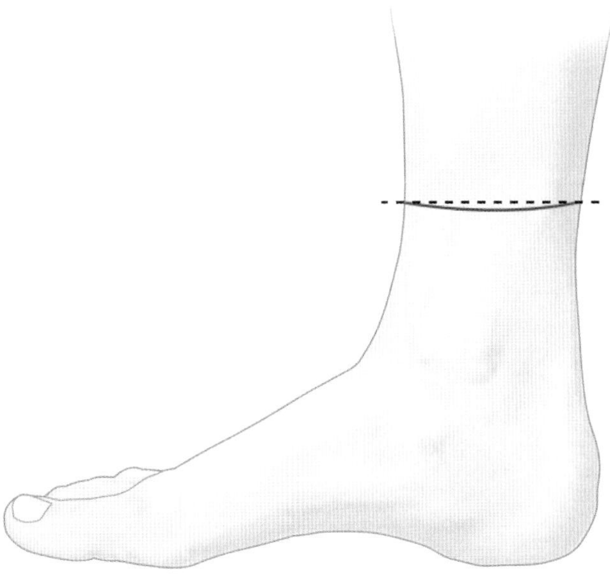

Figure 6 **Guillotine ankle amputation. The skin incision is made circumferentially at the narrowest portion of the ankle. The bones are then transected at the same level (*dashed line*).**

Below-the-Knee Amputation

OPERATIVE PLANNING

Below-the-knee amputation is indicated when the lower extremity is functional but the foot cannot be salvaged by arterial reconstruction or by amputation of one or more of the toes or the forefoot. Healing can be expected if there is a palpable femoral pulse with at least a patent deep femoral artery, provided that the skin is warm and free of lesions at the distal calf. Before formal below-the-knee amputation, infection should be controlled with antibiotic therapy, débridement, and, if indicated, guillotine amputation. It is advisable to obtain consent for possible above-the-knee amputation beforehand in case unexpected muscle necrosis is encountered below the knee.

As with any amputation, the surgeon's preoperative interaction with the patient should be as positive as possible. A constructive perspective to convey is that the amputation, although regrettably necessary, is the first step toward rehabilitation. Although many patients with critical limb ischemia fail to achieve fully independent, community ambulation after below–the-knee amputation, a well-motivated patient whose cardiopulmonary status is not too greatly compromised can generally be expected to achieve some degree of function with a prosthetic limb. In this regard, a preoperative discussion with a physiatrist can be very helpful.

OPERATIVE TECHNIQUE

Epidural, spinal, or general anesthesia is appropriate for below-the-knee amputation. The lines of incision should be marked on the skin. The primary level of amputation is determined by measuring a distance of 10 cm from the tibial tuberosity [*see Figure 7*]. The circumference of the leg at this

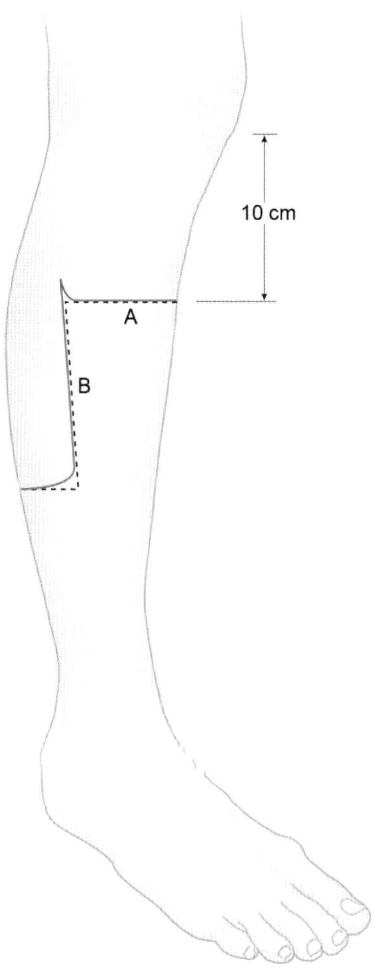

Figure 7 **Below-the-knee amputation. The transverse incision (A) is made 10 cm distal to the tibial tuberosity. Its length is equal to two thirds of the circumference of the leg at that level. The posterior incision (B) is made parallel with the gastrocnemius-soleus muscle complex. The length of the posterior flap is equal to one third of the measured circumference of the leg. The corners of the incisions are curved to avoid dog-ears.**

level is then measured by passing a heavy ligature around the leg and cutting the ligature to a length equal to the circumference. The ligature is folded into thirds and cut once more at one of the folds so that two segments of unequal length remain. The longer segment of the ligature, which is equal in length to two thirds of the leg's circumference 10 cm below the tibial tuberosity, is used to measure the anterior transverse incision; this incision is centered not on the tibial crest but on the gastrocnemius-soleus muscle complex. The shorter segment, which is one third of the leg's circumference at this level, is used to measure the posterior flap; the line of the posterior incision runs parallel to the gastrocnemius-soleus complex. To prevent dog-ears, the medial and lateral ends of the anterior transverse incision are curved cephalad before meeting the posterior incision, and the distal corners of the posterior incision are curved as well.

Blood loss can be reduced by using a sterile pneumatic tourniquet. A gauze roll is passed around the distal thigh. The leg is elevated to drain the venous blood, and the tourniquet is applied over the gauze roll. The tourniquet is inflated to a pressure of 250 mm Hg (350 to 400 mm Hg if the patient has heavily calcified arteries). The assistant elevates the leg, and the incision on the posterior flap is made first, followed by the anterior transverse incision; this sequence helps prevent blood from obscuring the field while the incisions are being made. The incisions are carried fully through the dermis, and the skin edges are allowed to separate and expose the subcutaneous fat. Care is taken to keep the scalpel perpendicular to the skin so as not to bevel the incision, which can lead to necrosis of the epidermal edges [*see Figure 2*].

The anterior muscles are transected with the scalpel in a direction parallel to the transverse skin incision. The tibia is scored circumferentially, and a periosteal elevator is used to dissect the soft tissues away from the tibia for a distance of approximately 3 to 4 cm. The tibia is then transected 1 cm proximal to the transverse skin incision. Dividing the tibia more than 1 cm proximal to the anterior skin incision will cause the thin skin of the anterior leg to be pulled taut over the cut end of the tibia by the weight of the posterior flap, thereby leading to skin ulceration. The tibia is transected perpendicularly, with a cephalad bevel of the anterior 1 cm to keep from creating a sharp point at the tibial crest [*see Figure 8*]. The tibia can be transected with either a Gigli saw or an oscillating saw; because of the unpleasant sound of the

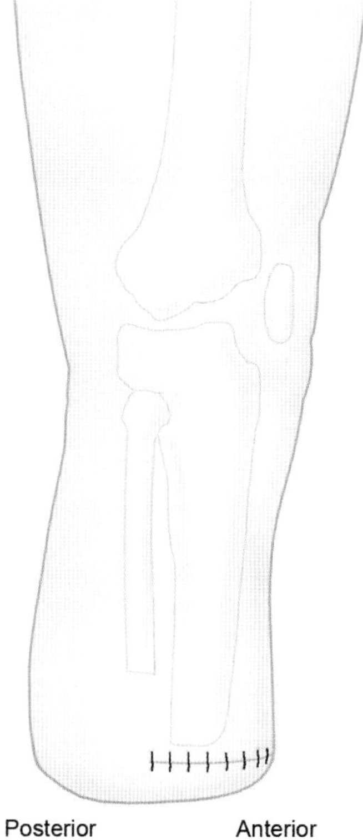

Figure 8 **Below-the-knee amputation. In this lateral view of the right leg, the tibia is beveled anteriorly, and the anterior portion is smoothed with a rasp. The fibula is transected at least 1 cm proximal to the level of transection of the tibia.**

power saw, the Gigli saw is preferred if the patient is under regional anesthesia. Sedation should be augmented in awake patients before division of the tibia. Benzodiazepines provide good sedation and amnesia.

The lateral muscles are divided, and the fibula is scored circumferentially. A periosteal elevator is used to dissect the soft tissues away from the fibula to a point 2 to 3 cm cephalad to the level at which the tibia was transected. The fibula is then transected with a bone cutter at least 1 cm cephalad to the tibial transection level. The distal end of the tibia is lifted with a bone hook, and division of the posterior muscles is completed with an amputation knife. The specimen is then handed off the field.

The anterior tibial, posterior tibial, and peroneal arteries and veins are clamped, and the tourniquet is released. Clamps are placed on all other bleeding vessels. The posterior tibial and sural nerves are placed on gentle traction, clamped proximally, transected, and ligated. The nerves are ligated because their nutrient vessels can bleed significantly. The proximal nerves are allowed to retract into the soft tissues so as to prevent painful pressure points at the end of the stump. All clamped blood vesselss are then ligated with absorbable ligatures. The distal anterior tip of the tibia is smoothed with a rasp to decrease the risk of skin ulceration over this osseous prominence. The stump is gently irrigated to remove all thrombus and devitalized tissue and to reveal any bleeding sites that may have been missed. Electrocauterization is rarely necessary.

The deep muscle fascia—not the Achilles tendon—is approximated with simple interrupted absorbable sutures, with care taken to align the posterior flap with the anterior incision. The skin is approximated with simple interrupted absorbable sutures, with buried knots, at the dermal-epidermal junction (interrupted subcuticular sutures). A carefully padded posterior splint is applied to prevent flexion contracture.

COMPLICATIONS

The most common complications after below-the-knee amputation are bleeding, infection, and failure to heal, all of which are likely to result in a more proximal amputation, frequently accompanied by loss of the knee. Prevention of these complications depends on careful patient selection, preoperative control of infection, and meticulous surgical technique.

To walk with a prosthetic leg, the patient must be able to fully extend and lock the knee; thus, flexion contracture at the knee is a major complication. Such contractures are usually attributable either to poor pain control or to noncompliance with knee extension exercises. Good perioperative analgesia is of vital importance because knee flexion is the position of comfort and the patient will be unwilling to extend the knee if doing so proves too painful. To maintain knee extension, the patient should be placed in a splint in the early postoperative period. Once postoperative pain has abated, the splint can be removed. At this point, the patient must be taught extension exercises, in which the quadriceps muscles are contracted to maintain the length of the hamstring muscles. If a patient spends all of his or her time in a sitting position with the knee flexed, a flexion contracture will quickly develop. Once this happens, the patient may find it very difficult to regain full knee extension, and without full knee extension, prosthetic limb rehabilitation is impossible.

Phantom sensation is common after below-the-knee amputation but is rarely of any consequence. Phantom pain, on the other hand, can be devastating. Sometimes, phantom pain develops as a consequence of unintentional suggestions made to the patient by medical personnel who fail to distinguish between the two entities. For example, a patient remarks to a medical attendant that he or she can still feel the amputated foot and toes, and the attendant suggests in response that the patient has phantom pain; the patient then focuses on the sensation and exaggerates the severity of the foot and toe discomfort, setting up a cycle of ever-worsening pain. Phantom limb pain is more likely if the patient has had prolonged ischemic rest pain before the amputation. Phantom pain can be limited by (1) encouraging early amputation in a patient with a hopelessly ischemic foot, (2) providing good pain control in the early postoperative period, and (3) assuring the patient that phantom sensation after a below-the-knee amputation is common and that any discomfort in the foot immediately after the operation period will improve once he or she begins walking again with a prosthetic leg.

Ulceration of the skin over the transected anterior portion of the tibia is another serious complication that may preclude successful prosthetic limb fitting. This complication is also best managed through prevention, which depends on meticulous surgical technique. As noted (see above), the anterior tibial crest must be carefully beveled and smoothed at the level of transection, and the tibia must not be transected more than 1 cm proximal to the anterior skin incision.

With a standard below-the-knee prosthetic leg, weight is borne on the femoral condyles, the patella, and the tibial tuberosity. Breakdown of the stump can occur if weight is borne on the distal portion of the stump. Several decades ago, Jan Ertl described a tibiofibular synostosis designed to allow distal weight-bearing; however, this technique has not been widely adopted.[11]

OUTCOME

Shortly after the amputation, the patient should be encouraged to start working on strengthening the upper body; upper body strength is critical for making transfers and for using parallel bars, crutches, or a walker. In patients who have preoperative intractable ischemic rest pain, postoperative administration of epidural analgesia can break the cycle of pain. Once postoperative pain is adequately controlled, patients are taught to transfer in and out of a wheelchair. A compression garment is used on the stump once the sutures have been removed and the stump is fully healed.

Prosthetic rehabilitation begins when the stump achieves a conical shape. Unfortunately, a number of patients who have undergone amputation for ischemia are unable to walk with a prosthetic limb because of comorbid medical conditions and general debility. In many cases, however, even if full ambulation is impossible, patients can maintain relative independence if the knee is salvaged by using a combination of a prosthetic leg and a walker for transfers and movement around the house.[6]

Above-the-Knee Amputation

OPERATIVE PLANNING

Above-the-knee amputation is indicated if the lower extremity is unsalvageable and there is no femoral pulse. The presence of pulsatile flow into a well-developed ipsilateral internal iliac artery usually ensures healing, but even when there is more severe arterial occlusive disease in the pelvis, healing can sometimes be achieved. Above-the-knee amputation is also indicated if there is tissue necrosis or uncontrollable infection extending cephalad to the midleg. Above-the-knee amputation is the procedure of choice in the case of gangrene or ulceration of a completely nonfunctional lower extremity.

OPERATIVE TECHNIQUE

Epidural, spinal, or general anesthesia may be used for above-the-knee amputation. For the best functional results, it is desirable to keep the femur as long as possible. A longer stump improves the prognosis for prosthetic limb rehabilitation and provides better balance for sitting and transfers. Healing potential, however, is lower with a longer stump; therefore, if the pelvic circulation is severely compromised, a shorter stump should be fashioned.

Anterior and posterior flaps of equal length are marked on the skin. The flaps should be wide and long [*see Figure 9*], [illegible] should be centered on the line dividing the anterior and posterior muscle compartments. The posterior incision is made first to minimize the presence of blood in the operative field. The anterior incision is made second and carried through the anterior muscles in a plane parallel to the skin incision. The skin incisions are carried through the dermis, and the skin edges are allowed to separate and expose the subcutaneous fat; as in other amputations, they should be perpendicular to the skin surface so as not to undermine the skin.

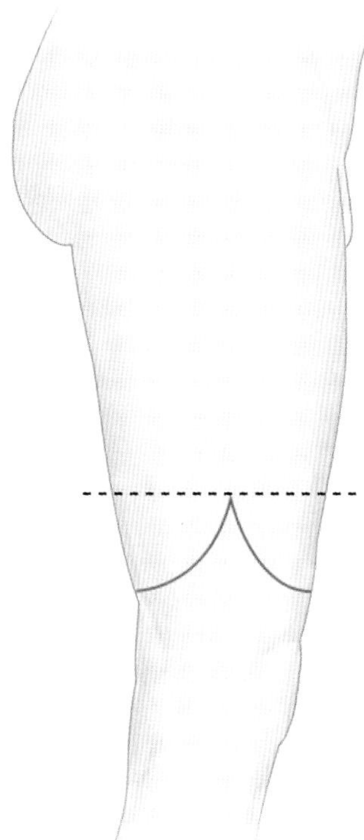

Figure 9 **Above-the-knee amputation. Broadly based anterior and posterior flaps are created. The femur is transected along the *dashed line*, at the apices of the skin flaps. The skin flaps and the level of transection of the femur can be placed more proximally if clinically indicated.**

If the superficial femoral artery is patent, the artery and vein are isolated and clamped after the sartorius muscle is divided but before the remainder of the anterior muscles are divided. The femur is scored circumferentially. The soft tissues are dissected away from the femur to the level of the apices of the flaps, and the femur is divided with an oscillating saw at this level. If the end of the resected femur extends beyond the apices of the flaps, the wound cannot be closed without tension. The posterior flap is completed with an amputation knife, and the specimen is handed off the field.

All bleeding points are clamped and tied with absorbable sutures. The sciatic nerve is placed on gentle traction, clamped, divided, and ligated, and the transected nerve is allowed to retract into the muscles. The deep fascia is approximated with interrupted absorbable sutures, with adjustments made for any discrepancy in length between the two flaps. The skin is approximated with interrupted absorbable sutures, with buried knots, at the dermal-epidermal junction (interrupted subcuticular sutures).

A nonadherent dressing is placed on the [illegible] covered with dry, fluffed gauze bandages. An aerosol tincture of benzoin is sprayed on the thigh, the hip, and the lower abdomen. When the benzoin is dry, a cloth stockinette with a diameter of 4 in. is stretched over the stump [*see Figure 10*]. The cuff of the stockinette is cut medially at the groin, and the stockinette is rolled laterally above the hip, where the cuff is then cut on the midaxillary line. This process yields two strips of cloth, one anterior and one posterior, which are passed around the patient's waist and tied on the anterior midline.

If the patient is a candidate for prosthetic limb rehabilitation, a traction rope is passed through a hole cut in the distal end of the stockinette and tied. The rope is hung over the end of the bed and tied to a 5 lb weight; this step helps prevent flexion contracture at the hip.

The stockinette need not be removed for the wound to be inspected. A window is cut in the distal end of the stockinette, and the gauze is removed. Once the incision has been inspected, fresh gauze is applied, and the window in the stockinette is closed with safety pins.

COMPLICATIONS

Postoperative complications include bleeding, infection, and failure to heal, all of which are likely to result in the need for surgical revision of the amputation stump. Control of preoperative infection and meticulous surgical technique and hemostasis are necessary to prevent these complications.

Flexion contracture of the hip is a major complication of above-the-knee amputation. Such contractures preclude successful prosthetic limb rehabilitation. In dealing with this complication, prevention is far more effective than treatment: once a flexion contracture at the hip becomes fixed,

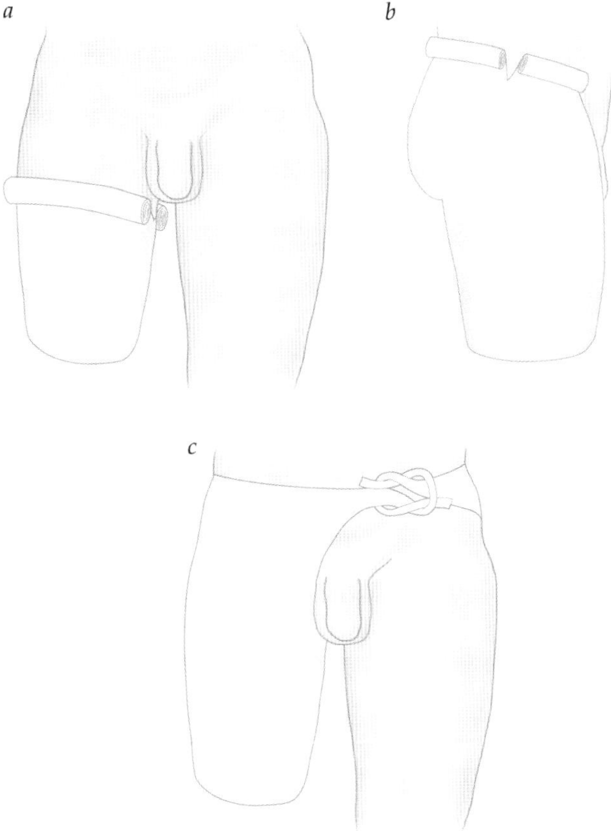

Figure 10 **Above-the-knee amputation. (*a*) After an aerosol tincture of benzoin is applied to the thigh, the hip, and the lower abdomen, a 4 in. wide stockinette is rolled over the amputation stump. The cuff of the stockinette is cut medially at the groin. (*b*) The remainder of the stockinette is then rolled laterally up and over the hip, and the cuff is cut on the lateral midline. (*c*) The two resulting strips of cloth are passed around the waist, one anteriorly and one posteriorly, and these strips are tied on the anterior midline to complete the dressing.**

it is very difficult to reverse. If a patient is a candidate for prosthetic limb rehabilitation, the traction weight mentioned earlier (see above) can be very helpful. As soon as postoperative pain is controlled, the patient should be taught to spend three periods daily in a prone position to help extend the hip. He or she should then be taught exercises for maintaining range of motion in the hip before prosthetic limb rehabilitation is initiated. Flexion contracture of the hip is less of a problem in nonambulatory patients; however, it can still lead to wound breakdown and chronic skin ulceration.

Gottschalk and Stills noted that loss of the adductor magnus leads to abnormal abduction of the femur. Accordingly, they proposed preservation of the adductor magnus and myodesis of the transected muscles to the femur to improve the biomechanics after above-the-knee amputation.[12,13]

OUTCOME

Once postoperative pain has abated, patients are mobilized to wheelchair transfers. The prognosis for successful prosthetic limb ambulation in patients undergoing above-the-knee amputation for ischemia is very poor.

Financial Disclosures: None Reported

References

1. Reichle FA, Rankin KP, Tyson RR, et al. Long-term results of 474 arterial reconstructions for severely ischemic limbs: a fourteen year follow-up. Surgery 1979;85:93.
2. Maini BS, Mannick JA. Effect of arterial reconstruction on limb salvage. Arch Surg 1978;113:1297.
3. Ellitsgaard N, Andersson AP, Fabrin J, et al. Outcome in 282 lower extremity amputations: knee salvage and survival. Acta Orthop Scand 1990;61:140.
4. Stewart CPU, Jain AS, Ogston SA. Lower limb amputee survival. Prosthet Orthot Int 1992;16:11.
5. Inderbitzi R, Buttiker M, Pfluger D, et al. The fate of bilateral lower limb amputees in end-stage vascular disease. Eur Vasc Surg 1992;6:321.
6. Nehler MR, Coll JR, Hiatt WR, et al. Functional outcome in a contemporary series of major lower extremity amputations. J Vasc Surg 2003;38:7.
7. Toursarkissian B, Shireman PK, Harrison A, et al. Major lower extremity amputation: contemporary experience in a single Veterans Affairs institution. Am Surg 2002;68:606.
8. Aulivola B, Hile CN, Hamdan AD, et al. Major lower extremity amputation: outcome of a modern series. Arch Surg 2004;139:395.
9. Ploeg AJ, Lardenoye JW, Vrancken Peeters MP, et al. Contemporary series of morbidity and mortality after lower limb amputation. Eur J Vasc Endovasc Surg 2005;29:633.
10. Hasanadka R, McLafferty RB, Moore CJ, et al. Predictors of wound complications following major amputation for critical limb ischemia. J Vasc Surg 2011;54:1374–82.
11. Pinzur MS, Pinto MA, Smith DG. Controversies in amputation surgery. Instr Course Lect 2003;52:445.
12. Gottschalk F. Transfemoral amputation: biomechanics and surgery. Clin Orthop 1999;361:15.
13. Gottschalk FA, Stills M. The biomechanics of trans-femoral amputation. Prosthet Orthot Int 1994;18:12.

Acknowledgment

Figures 1 through 10 Tom Moore

21 RENOVASCULAR HYPERTENSION AND STENOSIS

J. Gregory Modrall, MD

Renal artery stenosis (RAS) may present clinically as an incidental radiographic finding in an asymptomatic patient or may be the etiology for overt renovascular hypertension or ischemic nephropathy. This chapter outlines the diagnosis and management of renovascular disease and its clinical manifestations. A specific aim is to provide algorithms for evaluating patients with an incidentally identified RAS versus symptomatic RAS. Emphasis is placed on using the data available to refine patient selection for intervention, which is a critical step in optimizing outcomes. The technical details of the endovascular and open surgical management of renovascular disease are discussed in separate chapters.

Pathophysiology of Renovascular Hypertension

Renovascular hypertension involves a complex interplay between the kidney and extrarenal pathways to induce hypertension.[1] The kidney is equipped with sensing organelles in the macula densa and juxtaglomerular apparatus of the afferent arterioles within the kidney that detect changes in luminal sodium concentration and perfusion pressure, respectively. When a RAS narrows the renal artery sufficiently to lower the perfusion pressure or sodium delivery to the kidney, the juxtaglomerular apparatus secretes the enzyme renin to activate the renin-angiotensin system. Activation of the renin-angiotensin-system culminates in release of the octapeptide angiotensin II into the bloodstream and locally within the kidney. Angiotensin II has a number of intrarenal and systemic effects aimed at augmenting blood pressure. Within the kidney, angiotensin II alters intrarenal hemodynamics and promotes sodium reabsorption. Angiotensin II increases vasomotor tone at the afferent and efferent arterioles of glomeruli to decrease glomerular filtration and facilitate fluid retention. Angiotensin II activates multiple tubular sodium transport pathways, including the sodium-hydrogen exchanger NHE3, to promote sodium reabsorption. Outside the kidney, angiotensin II stimulates adrenal cortical secretion of aldosterone, which further promotes sodium retention at the level of the distal tubule. Angiotensin II stimulates antidiuretic hormone secretion from the pituitary gland. Angiotensin II has direct vasoconstrictive activity and increases noradrenergic activity to increase vascular tone. The sum of renal and extrarenal effects is the severe hypertension that characterizes renovascular hypertensions.[1] An additional consequence of sustained exposure to angiotensin II is activation of mitogen-activated protein (MAP) kinase and nuclear factorκB signaling pathways that promote hypertrophy and fibrosis within the kidney, heart, and arteries. The net result of activation of these pathways is nephrosclerosis, cardiac hypertrophy and fibrosis, and progressive arterial wall changes.[2]

Etiology of Renal Artery Stenosis

Renal artery pathologies that may produce RAS include atherosclerosis, fibromuscular dyplasia (FMD), aortic or renal artery dissections, renal artery aneurysm, and Takayasu arteritis. Of these potential etiologies for RAS, atherosclerotic renovascular disease and FMD represent the vast majority of cases. Case series of surgical and endovascular renal artery revascularization indicate that 80 to 91% of RAS are caused by atherosclerosis, whereas FMD accounts for 9 to 14% of RAS.[3,4]

ATHEROSCLEROTIC RENAL ARTERY STENOSIS

Atherosclerotic RAS occurs at the origin of the renal artery [*see Figure 1*] in 49 to 87% of cases and represents "spillover" of aortic atherosclerosis into the orifice of the renal artery.[4,5] Occlusive disease within the main renal artery distal to its origin is less common, whereas renal artery occlusive disease occurs in distal renal artery branches in only 3% of cases.[4,5] The anatomic site of atherosclerotic RAS has direct implications for both open and percutaneous approaches to revascularization of the renal arteries. The

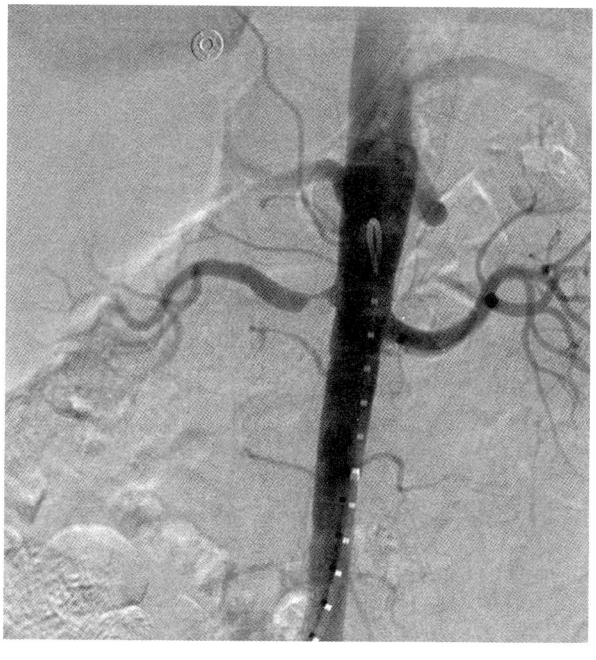

Figure 1 **Aortogram demonstrating a stenosis at the origin of the right renal artery.**

patient population with atherosclerotic RAS is typical of a cohort with significant aortic atherosclerosis. Most patients are older and male with risk factors for atherosclerosis. Many patients with atherosclerotic RAS also have coronary, cerebrovascular, or peripheral arterial disease.

FIBROMUSCULAR DYSPLASIA

FMD most commonly afflicts the mid- and distal renal artery, including the renal artery branches in the hilum of the kidney. The five subtypes of FMD and their incidences are listed in Table 1.[6] The most common subtype of FMD is medial fibroplasia, with its typical arteriographic appearance of a "string of beads" [*see Figure 2*]. This arteriographic appearance is produced by fibrous webs within the renal artery that produce multiple renal artery stenoses in series with intervening post-stenotic dilatations. FMD is usually described as a condition of young females, although the age at eventual diagnosis is 45 to 61 years in most series.[7–9] FMD is bilateral in 35% of cases.[8] FMD may also occur in other arterial beds. The United States Registry for Fibromuscular Dysplasia showed the following distribution of FMD in 447 patients: renal artery (80%), extracranial carotid artery (75%), vertebral artery (37%), mesenteric arteries (26%), lower extremities (60%), intracranial carotid arteries, and upper extremity arteries (16%).[7] In this registry, 35% of patients had FMD in two arterial beds and 22% had FMD in three arterial beds.

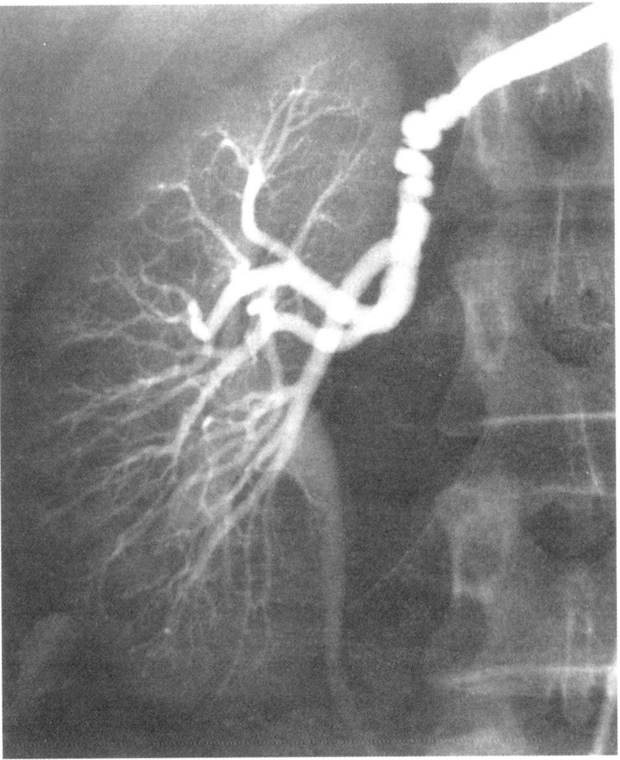

Figure 2 **"String of beads" appearance of the medial fibroplasia subtype of fibromuscular dysplasia on arteriography.**

Prevalence of Renal Artery Stenosis

PREVALENCE IN THE GENERAL POPULATION AND ELDERLY

Data on the prevalence of RAS have been derived primarily from autopsy and imaging studies. Autopsy series found that RAS is not a rare finding in unselected patient populations. In 5,194 consecutive autopsies, Sawicki and colleagues identified RAS in 4.3% of patients.[10] In a series of 870 elderly adults, age 65 years or older, the prevalence of critical RAS by duplex ultrasound screening was 7%.[11] Given that most renal artery lesions are related to atherosclerosis, the prevalence of RAS varies with age. Schwartz and White identified severe RAS (> 50% stenosis) in 7% of autopsy subjects younger than 55 years, which increased to 40% among patients over 75 years of age.[12] Bilateral RAS was present in half of the patients in their series.

Table 1 Pathologic Subtypes of Fibromuscular Dysplasia

Subtype of FMD	*Relative Incidence (%)*
Medial fibroplasia	75–80
Perimedial fibroplasia	10–15
Medial fibroplasia	1–2
Intimal fibroplasia	< 10
Adventitial (periarterial) fibroplasia	< 1

FMD = fibromuscular dysplasia.

PREVALENCE IN HIGH-RISK PATIENT POPULATIONS

The prevalence of RAS increases in patient populations with risk factors for atherosclerosis or manifestations of atherosclerosis in other arterial beds.

Sawicki and colleagues found that the prevalence of RAS in their autopsy series increased from 4.3% in the cohort at large to 8.3% among decedents with diabetes mellitus.[10] Several studies have identified a strong association between symptomatic peripheral arterial disease and RAS.[13–17] In an analysis of pooled data from 12 studies with 2,871 patients who underwent diagnostic arteriography for peripheral arterial disease, de Mast and Beutler found that the prevalence of RAS ranged from 12 to 45% with a pooled prevalence of 25%.[18] The prevalence of RAS among patients with carotid stenosis is similar at 24 to 27%.[19,20]

The association between coronary artery disease and RAS is well documented. In a series of 1,302 patients undergoing diagnostic coronary arteriography at Duke University for suspected or proven coronary artery disease, 30% of patients had some RAS visualized on aortography.[5] Half of these patients (15%) had a stenosis exceeding 50% diameter narrowing and 4% had bilateral RAS. This theme has been recapitulated in numerous other studies. In an analysis of nine studies with 8,011 patients subjected to aortography during coronary arteriography, the pooled prevalence of RAS was 10%.[18] This association is the genesis for the phenomenon of "drive-by" renal arteriography during coronary arteriography. The merit of this practice is discussed later in the chapter [*see* Anatomic Imaging, *below*].

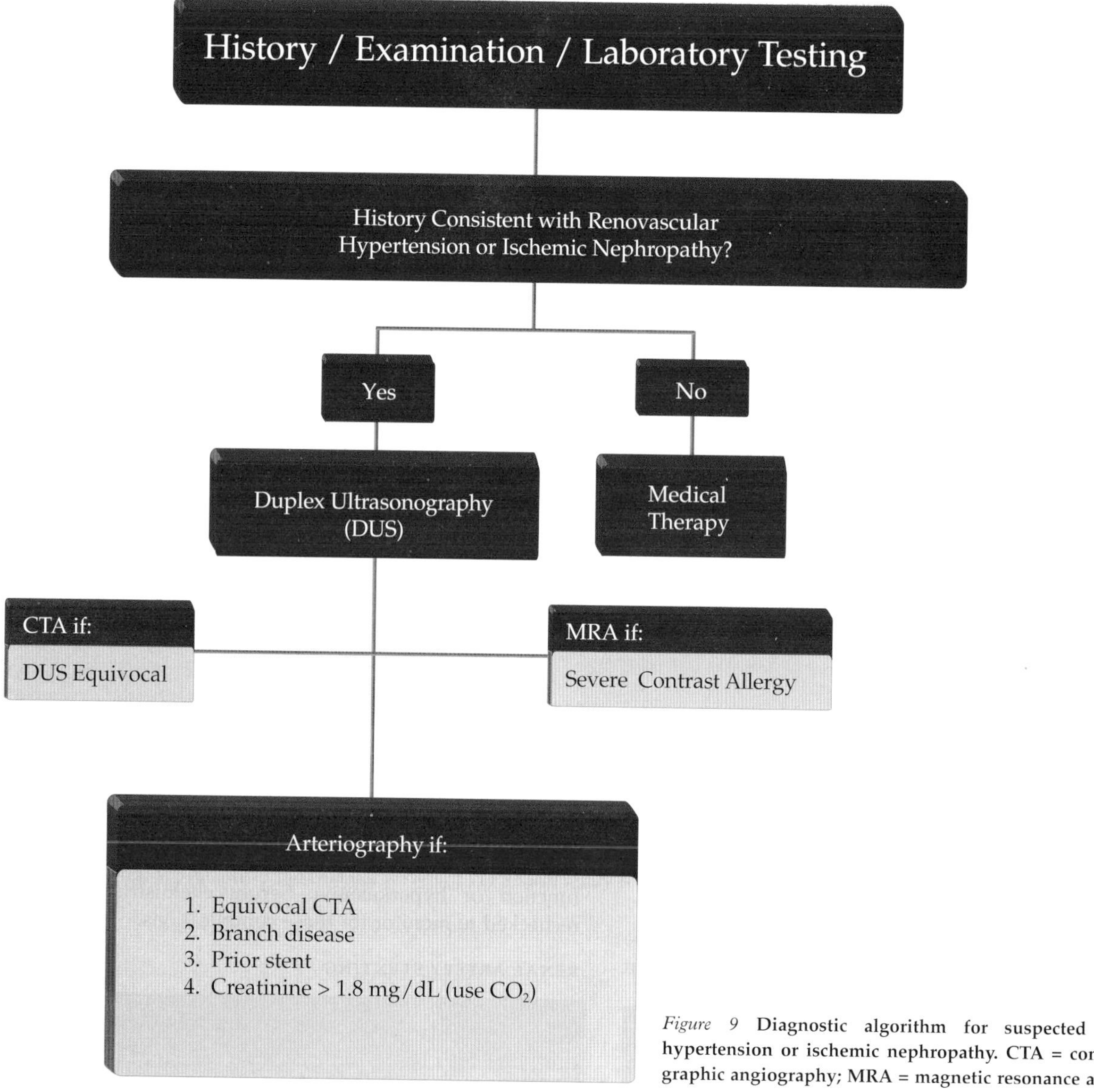

Figure 9 **Diagnostic algorithm for suspected renovascular hypertension or ischemic nephropathy. CTA = computed tomographic angiography; MRA = magnetic resonance angiography.**

stenting is based on a presumptive diagnosis. The American Heart Association practice guidelines suggest that renal artery stenting is "reasonable" in patients with "accelerated hypertension, resistant hypertension, malignant hypertension, hypertension with an unexplained unilateral small kidney, and hypertension with intolerance to medication."[70] These guidelines suggest using three-drug hypertension as the threshold for renal artery stenting, based solely on expert opinion without scientific data. In practice, these guidelines are vague and nonspecific, offering little help in selecting patients for stenting.

In an attempt to improve patient selection for renal artery stenting, we examined our institutional results for 149 renal artery stenting procedures performed for atherosclerotic RAS between 2000 and 2008 by Vascular Surgery and Interventional Radiology at the University of Texas Southwestern Medical Center.[40] The goal of that analysis was to identify preoperative clinical and renal morphologic predictors of a favorable response of blood pressure to renal artery stenting. To analyze patient-specific outcomes, patients were categorized as "responders" or "nonresponders" at late follow-up based on a modification of the American Heart Association reporting guidelines.[71] On multivariate analysis, we identified three preoperative clinical parameters that independently predicted a favorable blood pressure response to renal artery stenting: (1) a requirement for four or more antihypertensive medications; (2) preoperative diastolic blood pressure greater than 90 mm Hg; and (3) preoperative clonidine use. These predictors often occur together in individual patients, and there is a clear "dose-response" effect of having multiple predictors. Patients with one predictor had a 45% probability of a favorable blood pressure response, whereas patients with two or three predictors had a 75% and a 100% response rate, respectively. Pole-to-pole kidney length was not helpful in predicting the response to renal artery stenting, but kidney volume was helpful in discriminating responders with three-drug hypertension. Using CTAs to estimate kidney volume according to a validated formula [kidney length × width × (depth/2)],[72] patients with three-drug hypertension and a kidney volume over 150 cm^3 had a blood pressure response rate of 63%. Patients with three-drug hypertension and smaller kidneys had a response rate of 18%.

Using the data above, we developed an algorithm for patient selection for patients with presumed renovascular hypertension [*see Figure 10*]. We recommend renal artery stenting in patients with three-drug hypertension and preserved renal mass (> 150 cm^3 kidney volume) and all patients with four-drug (or more) hypertension. Patients with one- or two-drug hypertension may be treated if there is persistent diastolic hypertension (> 90 mm Hg). Clonidine is reserved in most institutions for the most resistant hypertension and may also be used to select patients with one- and two-drug hypertension for intervention. These guidelines only apply to patients with atherosclerotic RAS. We advocate angioplasty (without stenting) for any patient with FMD and hypertension because the outcomes for that patient cohort are quite favorable.

A separate study at our institution analyzed 61 patients who underwent renal artery stenting for salvage of renal function.[69] In accordance with the American Heart Association reporting guidelines, patients were categorized as "responders" if the average eGFR at the last follow-up was increased over 20% over the prestenting eGFR.[71] The only independent preoperative predictor of improved renal function after stenting was the rate of decline in renal function prior to stenting. Using a threshold change in the preoperative eGFR over time of −0.46% (the median for the cohort) yielded a sensitivity and a specificity for predicting renal function responders of 88% and 66%, respectively. Those patients with a more rapid decline in eGFR have a higher probability of having improved renal function after stenting. None of the kidney morphologic parameters predicted the response of renal function to stenting. Based on these data, we developed an algorithm for patient selection for patients with presumed ischemic nephropathy [*see Figure 11*].

Outcomes

Immediate complications occur in 1.3 to 7.0% of patients after renal artery stenting.[40,66–68] The most common complications are access-site complications. Renal artery perforations, ruptures, and dissections are less frequent. The late outcomes for renal artery stenting have been sobering. Clinical studies have reported that only 34 to 59% of patients experienced a durable improvement in blood pressure at late follow-up.[40,68] Durable improvements in renal function occurred in 23 to 50% of patients.[37,66,67,69] In our experience,

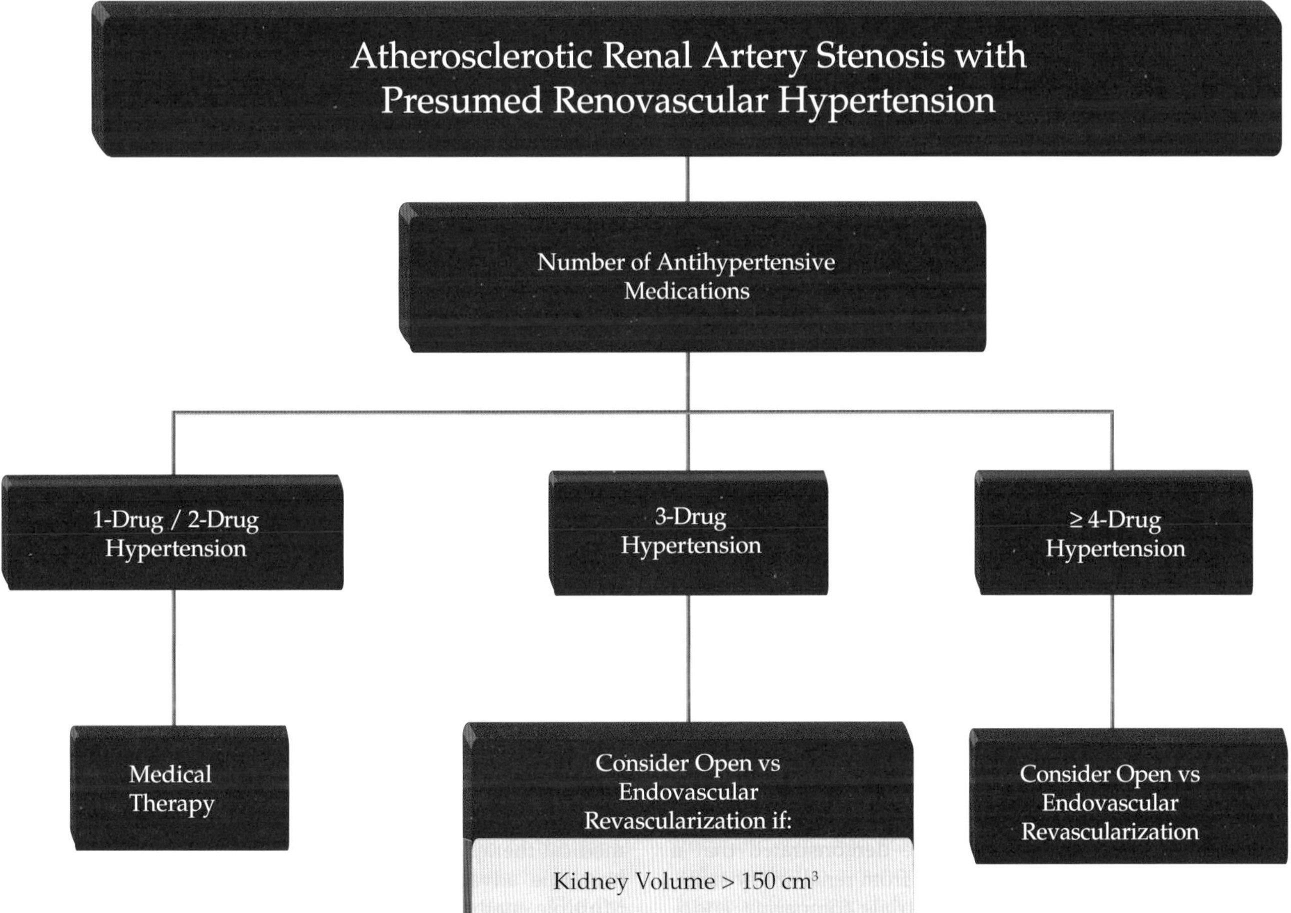

Figure 10 **Algorithm for patient selection for patients with presumed renovascular hypertension.**

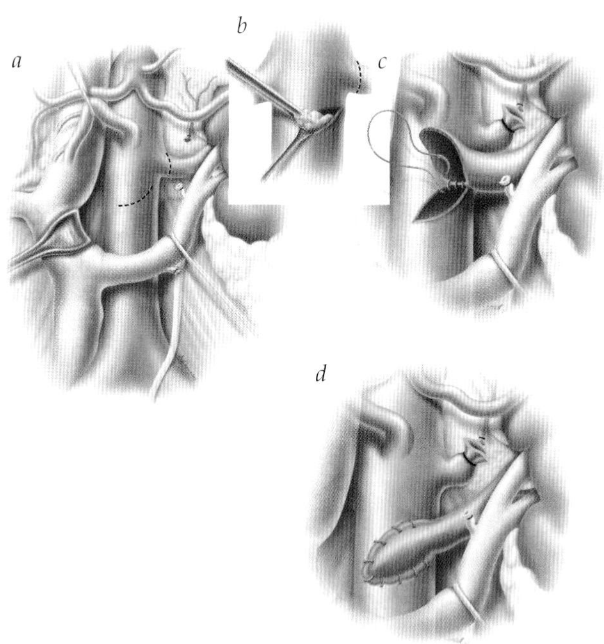

Figure 3 **Renal artery reimplantation.[9] (*a*) When the renal artery is redundant and the disease involves the orifice of the renal artery, it is usually possible to reimplant the vessel at a lower level. The *dotted lines* indicate the location of the aortotomy and the point where the renal artery is divided. (*b*) An elliptical opening is created in the aortic wall, and a local endarterectomy is done as required. (*c*) A monofilament suture is placed in the aortic wall. (*d*) The native renal artery is ligated, proximally spatulated, and reimplanted.**

reimplantation is that it obviates concerns regarding the durability of the renal artery conduit.

EX VIVO RENAL ARTERY RECONSTRUCTION

Due to the widespread use of percutaneous techniques for main renal artery pathologies, a significant proportion of open renal artery reconstructions require branch exposure and branch reconstruction. These procedures may require a complex repair, culminating in prolonged renal ischemia. Available data suggest that when more than 40 minutes of warm renal ischemia is required for renal revascularization, measures to protect renal function should be instituted.

Several pharmacologic therapies have been promoted to provide protection during renal ischemia; however, no therapy to date has surpassed hypothermia for protection when renal ischemia exceeds 1 hour. Surface cooling and hypothermic perfusion have been proposed; however, the advantages of each are not well defined. Renal tolerance to ischemia is, in part, related to the duration of ischemia, to the adequacy of collateral circulation, and to the method of vascular control. Unprotected warm renal ischemia is best tolerated when only the renal artery is controlled. Control of both renal artery and vein is associated with greater dysfunction than isolated arterial control, as is intermittent control with repeated renal perfusion.

Numerous methods for renal cooling and hypothermia during branch renal artery repair have been described; however, our preference has been intermittent hypothermic perfusion with topical ice slush. Otherwise, several steps are common to each branch renal artery reconstruction. To promote renal cortical perfusion, small doses of intravenous mannitol are administered throughout renal artery exposure and reperfusion. Before the division of the renal artery, intravenous heparin (100 units/kg) is administered and monitored as described earlier.

Hypothermia appears to be more important than the composition of perfusate; however, our preference is a perfusate with an intracellular composition of electrolytes. This composition theoretically limits ion exchange and intracellular volume shifts that contribute to organelle dysfunction associated with decreased activity of membrane-bound sodium potassium adenosine triphosphatase. Regardless of whether there is division and reattachment of the renal vein, branch renal artery repairs using cold perfusion preservation are made in an orthotropic fashion, with the kidney returned to the renal fossa rather than autotransplanted into the pelvis.

Several exposures for hypothermic branch renal artery reconstructions are available. When isolated branch renal repair is performed with orthotropic replacement, an extended flank incision is made from the lower rib margin and carried to the posterior axillary line as described earlier. This latter method is our preferred approach for ex vivo reconstruction. The ureter is mobilized to the pelvic brim with a large amount of periureteric soft tissue. An elastic sling is placed around the ureter to control ureteric collaterals and prevent subsequent renal rewarming.[6]

The Gerota fascia is opened with a cruciate incision, the kidney is completely mobilized, and the renal vessels are divided. The kidney is placed in a plastic sling and perfused with a chilled renal preservation solution. Continuous perfusion during the period of total renal ischemia is possible with perfusion pump systems and may be superior for prolonged renal preservation. However, simple intermittent flushing with a chilled preservation solution provides equal protection during the shorter periods (2 to 3 hours) required for ex vivo dissection and branch renal artery reconstructions.[6] For this technique, we refrigerate the preservative overnight, add additional components immediately before use to make up a liter of solution and hang the chilled (5 to 10 C) solution at a height of at least 2 m. Three to 500 milliliters of solution are flushed through the kidney immediately after its removal from the renal fossa until the venous effluent is clear and all segments of the kidney have blanched. As each anastomosis is completed, the kidney is perfused with an additional 100 to 200 mL of chilled solution. In addition to maintaining satisfactory hypothermia, periodic perfusion demonstrates suture line leaks that are repaired prior to reimplantation. With this technique, renal core temperatures are maintained at 10 C or below throughout the period of reconstruction.

Even though it is an accepted method after ex vivo reconstruction, autotransplantation to the iliac fossa is unnecessary for most ex vivo reconstructions. This technique was adopted from renal transplantation. Reduction in the magnitude of the operative exposure, manual palpation of the transplanted kidney, and ease of removal when treatment of rejection fails are all practical reasons for placing the transplanted kidney into the recipient's iliac fossa. However, none of these advantages apply to the patient requiring autogenous ex vivo reconstruction. Because many ex vivo procedures are performed in relatively young patients, the durability of the operation must be measured in terms of decades. For this reason, attachment of the kidney to the iliac arterial system within or below sites that are susceptible to subsequent atherosclerosis subjects the repaired vessels to disease that may threaten their long-term patency. Moreover, subsequent management of peripheral vascular disease may be complicated by the presence of the autotransplanted kidney. Finally, if the kidney is replaced in the renal fossa and the renal artery graft is properly attached to the aorta at a proximal infrarenal site, the result should equal that of the standard aortorenal bypass and thus carry a high probability of technical success and long-term durability.

SPLANCHNORENAL BYPASS

Indirect, or splanchnorenal, bypass [*see Figure 4 and Figure 5*] is an uncommon procedure at our center. In large part, its relative rarity reflects the frequent presence of simultaneous disease of the celiac axis and the frequent need for bilateral renal artery reconstruction in combination with aortic repair. In addition, this approach does not yield long-term patency equivalent to that provided by direct aortorenal reconstruction. Consequently, these indirect bypass techniques are reserved for a selected subgroup of high-risk patients.

Hepatorenal bypass is most frequently performed through a right subcostal incision and splenorenal bypass through a left subcostal incision. In either procedure, the patient is positioned with a roll beneath the ipsilateral flank, with the operating table flexed and the ipsilateral arm padded and tucked to the side. The incision may be extended to the contralateral semilunar line and into the ipsilateral flank as necessary for exposure. In a hepatorenal bypass, a great saphenous vein graft is usually employed, originating from the common hepatic artery and coursing posterior to the portal triad and anterior to the vena cava before the end-to-end renal artery anastomosis [*see Figure 4*]. A splenorenal bypass may be created either in a similar fashion (i.e., with a great saphenous vein graft) or by anastomosing the transected splenic artery directly to the left renal artery [*see Figure 5*]. If the latter approach is taken, the collateral circulation to the spleen is sufficient to maintain splenic viability in most cases.

NEPHRECTOMY

In patients with renovascular renal insufficiency or ischemic nephropathy, an incremental increase in excretory

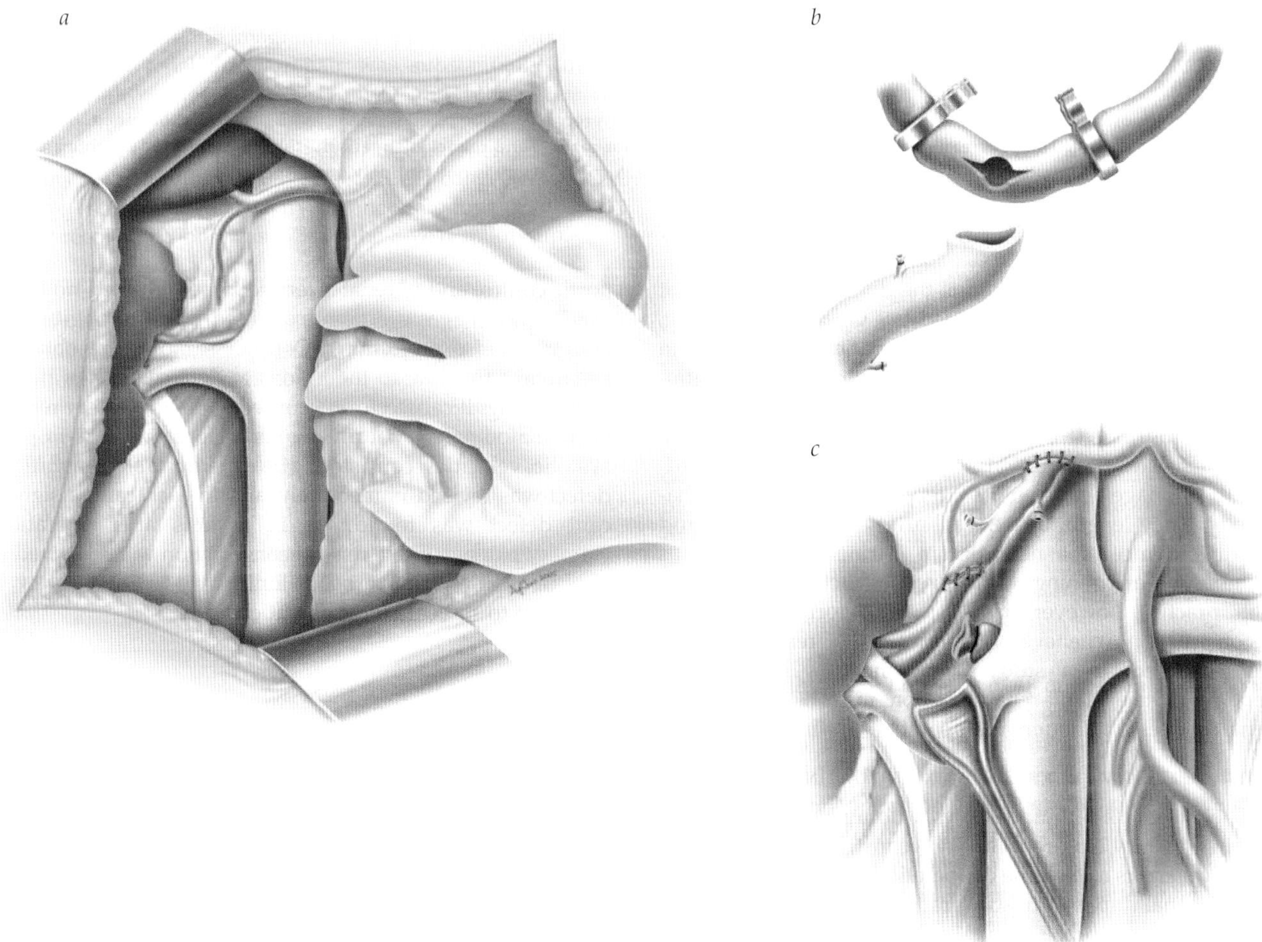

Figure 4 Hepatorenal bypass.[9] (*a*) Exposure of the common hepatic artery and the proximal gastroduodenal artery in the hepatoduodenal ligament in preparation for hepatorenal bypass (typically through a right subcostal skin incision). (*b, c*) The reconstruction is completed by placing a greater saphenous vein interposition graft between the side of the hepatic artery and the distal end of the transected right renal artery.

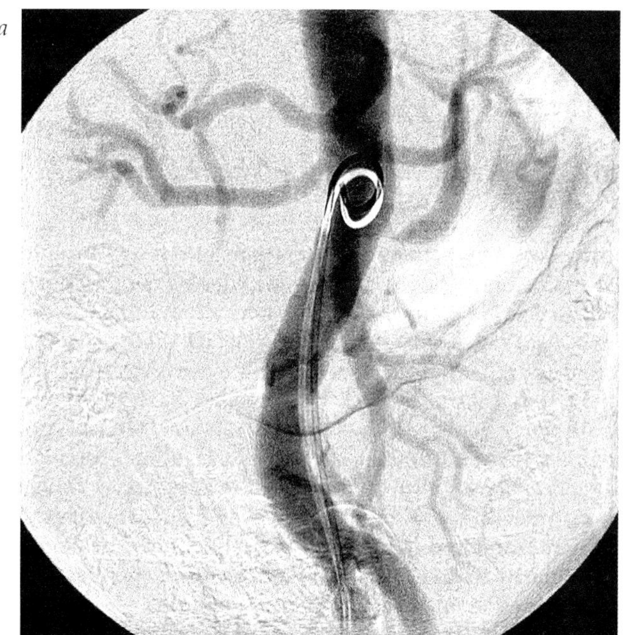

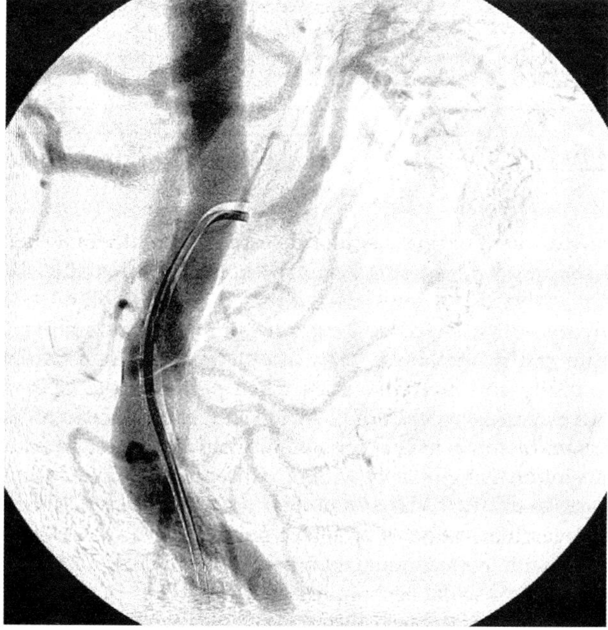

Figure 1 **(*a*) Bilateral high-grade renal artery stenosis visualized by using carbon dioxide angiography to localize the renal ostia. (*b*) Selective right renal artery cannulation with placement of a 6 French left internal mammary artery guide catheter and selective renal arteriography using hand-injected half-strength iso-osmolar contrast material.**

PROJECTIONS

Aortography and selective renal angiography with multiple projections are necessary for full radiographic evaluation of the renal arteries and the juxtarenal aorta. Initial anteroposterior (AP) images of the visceral aorta are obtained by delivering power contrast injections through a flush catheter with multiple side holes positioned at the L1-L2 interspace. These initial AP views provide an overview of the renal artery and the perivisceral aortic anatomy [*see Figure 2*]. Additional nonselective images of the renal arteries should be obtained by moving the catheter to a location below the origin of the superior mesenteric artery to prevent contrast opacification of the visceral vessels, which could obscure the anatomic details of the renal arteries.

The renal arteries usually arise from the anterolateral right or the posterolateral left aspect of the aorta. As a result, lesions within the renal ostia often are not seen or appear insignificant on AP aortograms. Oblique aortography and oblique selective renal arteriography project these portions of the vessel in profile and thus are often better at identifying any renal ostial lesions present. As a rule, the single most useful projection for visualizing the renal ostia is a 15 to 20 left anterior oblique view, although other oblique views may also be necessary.[26,27] Axial images of the renal origins (i.e., computed tomographic scans) may allow estimation of the necessary degree of obliquity and permit the use of smaller amounts of iodinated contrast material and lower doses of ionizing radiation [*see Figure 3*].

For full delineation of lesions within the body of the renal artery, selective arteriographic views may be required. Selective cannulation is usually performed with a configured

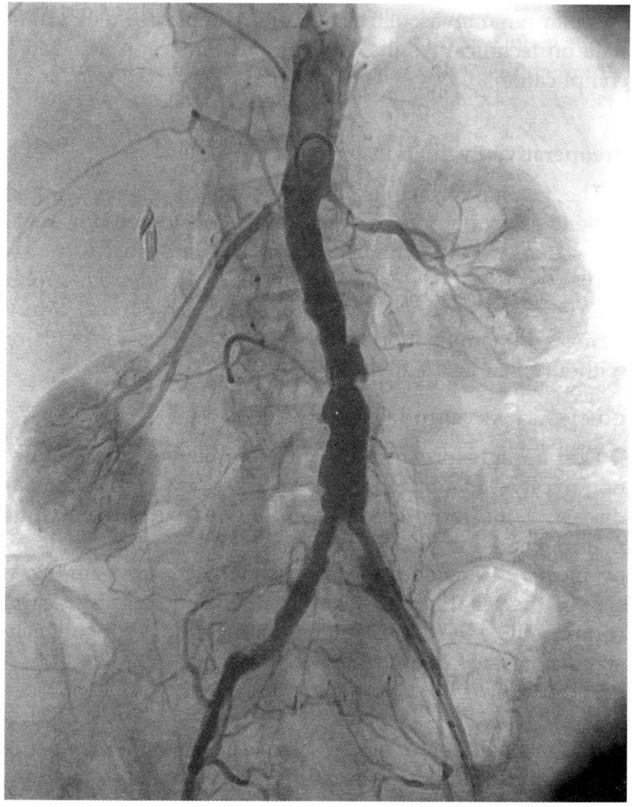

Figure 2 **An anteroposterior aortogram is obtained by delivering a power injection of iso-osmolar iodinated contrast material through a 5 French pigtail catheter positioned at the L1-L2 interspace.**

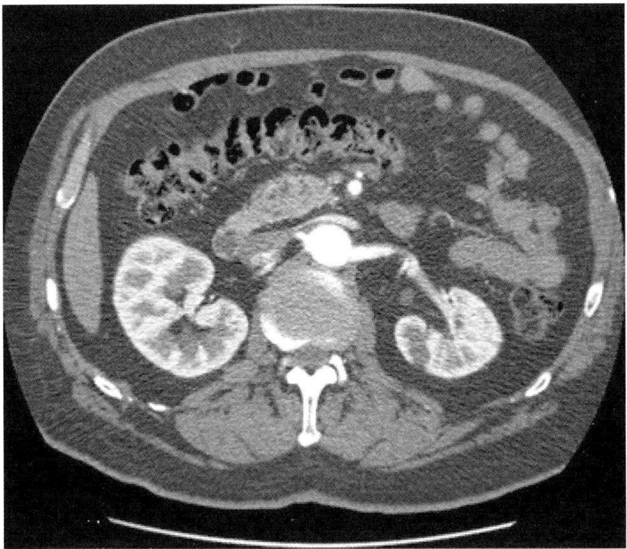

Figure 3 **Axial computed tomographic scan of the renal artery origins allows estimation of the degree of obliquity required for optimal imaging of the renal ostia.**

catheter (e.g., a cobra catheter, a Sos catheter, or a renal double-curve catheter). The varying configurations of available catheters offer specific advantages in particular anatomic situations. Before selective renal artery cannulation, we administer heparin intravenously. Once the guide wire has been gently advanced into the renal artery ostia, contrast material is injected by hand to confirm intraluminal placement. Selective images are then obtained with low-volume power injection or hand injection (our preference) of contrast material [*see Figure 4*]. The proximal third of the left renal artery usually courses anteriorly, the middle third transversely, and the distal third posteriorly; the right renal artery generally pursues a more consistent posterior course. For full delineation of lesions in the various segments, oblique and cranial-caudal projections may be necessary.

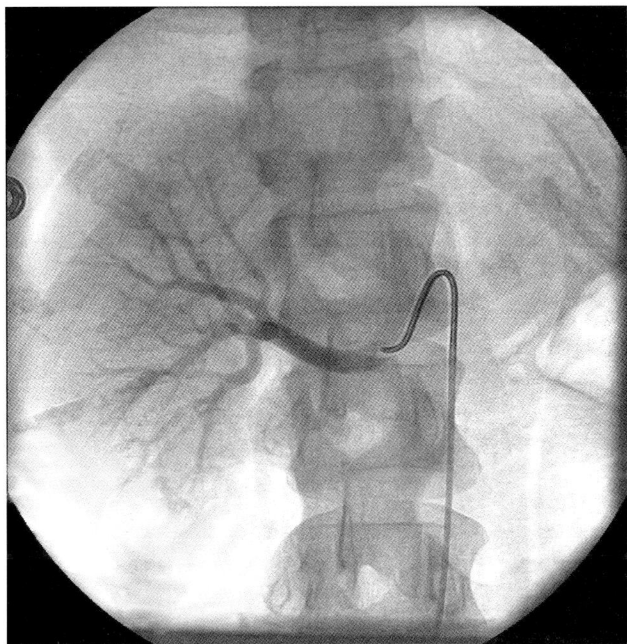

Figure 4 **Selective arteriography of the right renal artery using hand-injected iso-osmolar contrast material through a complexly curved Simmons catheter.**

ADJUNCTIVE MEASURES

Renal artery angiography affords the surgeon the opportunity to employ other measures to characterize a renal artery lesion. For example, the hemodynamic effects of an angiographic stenosis or interaction can be assessed by making direct pressure measurements proximal and distal to the lesion. In general, we consider any pressure gradient greater than 12 mm Hg to be indicative of hemodynamically significant renovascular disease. Additional anatomic information can be obtained by means of intravascular ultrasonography of the renal artery, which can provide detailed information on plaque morphology, vessel size, and potential dissection flaps to complement the data obtained through arteriography.[28,29]

ANGIOGRAPHIC CHARACTERISTICS

Atherosclerotic renovascular disease

Atherosclerosis of the renal artery accounts for approximately 85% of all renovascular lesions. Elderly persons with multiple comorbid medical conditions and manifestations of atherosclerosis are most frequently affected.[30–33] Atherosclerotic renal lesions represent a continuation of a process that begins in the aorta and spills over into the origin of the renal vessels [*see Figure 5*]. These lesions are characterized by an eccentric, irregular narrowing of the ostium and the proximal portion of the renal artery [*see Figure 6*]. In the majority of cases, the lesions are limited to the ostia and the proximal renal artery.[34] The aortic origin of the lesion has important implications for treatment. Placement of an endovascular stent into the proximal renal artery, without covering the aortic origin of the plaque, may result in residual or recurrent disease. Occlusions of the renal artery are also common in patients with clinically significant disease [*see Figure 7*] and frequently occur in the setting of contralateral renal artery stenosis.[2,3]

Fibromuscular dysplasia

Fibromuscular dysplasia (FMD) is a term used to describe a group of histologically distinct pathologic conditions of

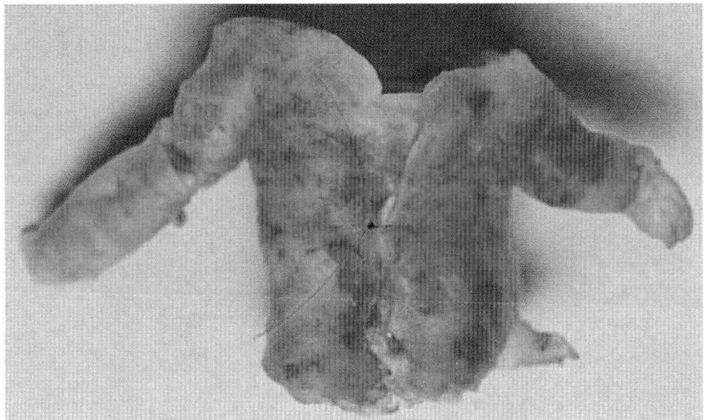

Figure 5 **An aortic endarterectomy specimen demonstrates the pathologic basis of atherosclerotic renovascular disease.**

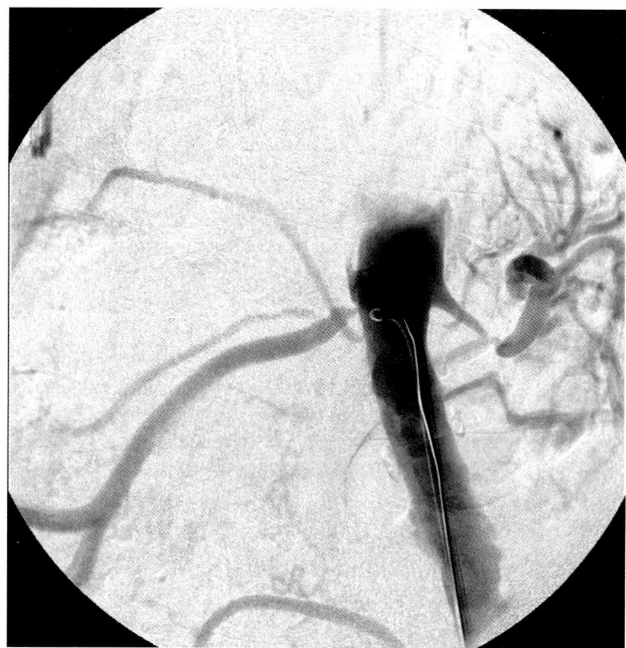

Figure 6 **A magnified preintervention aortogram demonstrates ostial right renal artery atherosclerotic stenosis.**

the arterial wall that most commonly affect the main renal artery and its branches. FMD of the renal artery, with resultant renal artery stenosis, is responsible for approximately 10 to 15% of treated cases of renovascular hypertension.[35] The lesions are categorized according to the layer of the arterial wall involved—hence the terms medial fibroplasia, perimedial dysplasia, and intimal fibroplasia. Medial fibroplasia is the most common variant, representing 85% of recognized cases. It is encountered almost exclusively in women, most commonly in the third or fourth decade of life.[35,36] The arteriographic pattern most frequently associated with medial fibroplasia resembles a string of beads [*see Figure 8*], an appearance created by weblike stenotic areas with intervening areas of poststenotic dilatation. These lesions are frequently bilateral and can be associated with renal artery aneurysm or dissection.[37] Medial fibroplasia of the main renal artery is among the lesions most amenable to endovascular treatment. In our view, however, the presence of branch vessel disease or aneurysms precludes safe treatment.

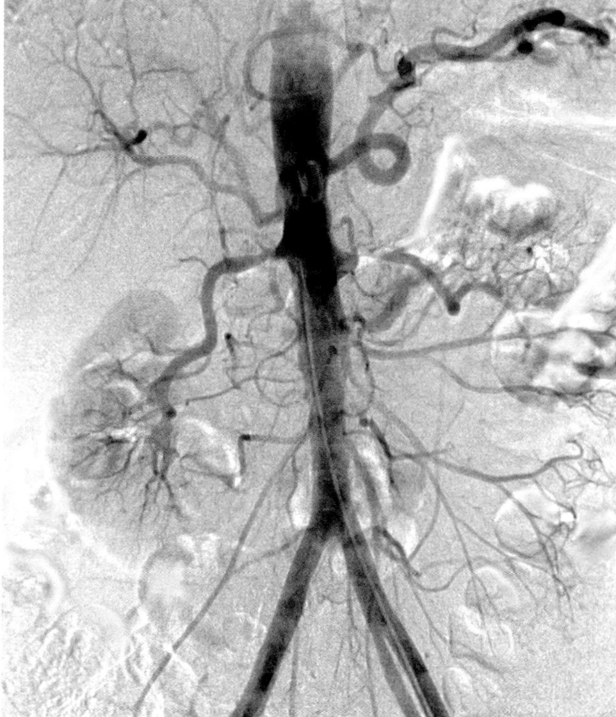

Figure 7 **An aortogram demonstrates right renal artery stenosis and left renal artery occlusion with distal renal artery reconstitution.**

Perimedial dysplasia accounts for approximately 15% of cases of FMD and is most commonly manifested by the appearance of multiple irregular stenoses without microaneurysms.[36] Intimal fibroplasia is the least common variant of FMD, representing fewer than 5% of recognized cases, and the typical lesions are smooth concentric stenoses.[35,36] In general, perimedial dysplasia and intimal fibroplasia tend to respond less well to endovascular treatment than the medial fibroplasia variety.

Procedural Planning

PATIENT PREPARATION

Recently, the use of statins has been associated with a significant and independent decrease in restenosis. Corriere and colleagues reported that patients not receiving statin therapy have a threefold increase in estimated restenosis over time.[38] Consequently, statin therapy is initiated prior to intervention. Patient preparation for renal artery PTAS is similar to that routinely carried out for diagnostic arteriography. Oral intake of food and liquid is stopped at midnight the evening before the procedure. Warfarin is discontinued at least 4 days beforehand; aspirin and clopidogrel are continued. Intravenous fluids and acetylcysteine

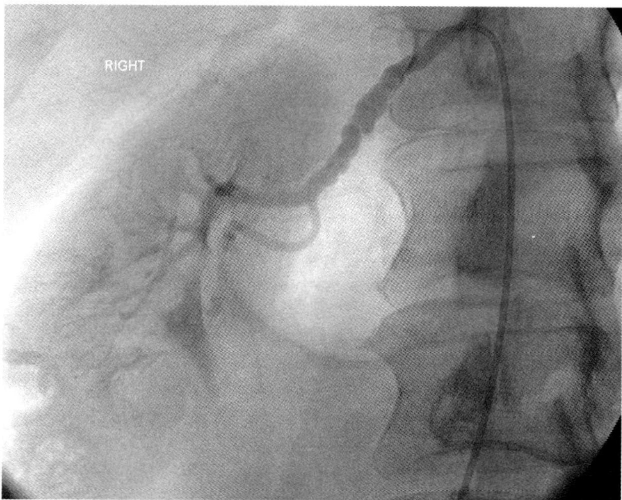

Figure 8 **A selective right renal arteriogram demonstrates findings indicative of medial fibroplasia.**

are administered the evening before the procedure, with care taken to avoid fluid overload in patients with impaired cardiac function. Routine medications, with the exception of angiotensin-converting enzyme inhibitors and angiotensin receptor antagonists, are taken on the morning of the procedure with a sip of water. A first-generation cephalosporin is administered intravenously 30 minutes before the procedure unless the patient is allergic.

After the intervention, the patient is observed in the hospital overnight to check for access-site problems and severe alterations in blood pressure. Acetylcysteine is continued throughout the hospital stay, and oral administration of clopidogrel is initiated the evening after the procedure. The patient continues to take clopidogrel for at least 30 days after revascularization and remains on aspirin therapy indefinitely.

CORRELATION OF DIAGNOSTIC IMAGES WITH CLINICAL FINDINGS

Once the diagnostic portion of the procedure is completed, the images obtained are closely examined and correlated with the patient's clinical presentation. Intra-arterial pressure measurements are occasionally misleading in renal vessels. Because most renal arteries are approximately 5 to 6 mm in diameter, a stenotic lesion that causes a greater than 60% reduction in the luminal diameter leaves only 2.0 to 2.5 mm of patent lumen. A 4 or 5 French diagnostic catheter may completely occlude this narrowed lumen, thus resulting in an inaccurately low pressure measurement distal to the stenosis. Accordingly, it is our practice to assess the anatomic arteriographic information in light of the functional significance of the lesion as determined by either renal vein renin assays or duplex ultrasonography.

MATERIALS AND INSTRUMENTS

The materials commonly used for renal artery PTAS at our center include various guide wires, catheters, sheaths, balloons, and stents [*see Table 1*]. The basic principles underlying the use of these devices are outlined more fully elsewhere [*search* ACS Surgery *for further information on endovascular surgery*].

Procedural Technique

STEP 1: SECURE RENAL ARTERY ACCESS FOR THERAPEUTIC INTERVENTION

Once the decision for endovascular intervention is made, the patient is systemically heparinized, and the 5 French diagnostic catheter and the introducer sheath are exchanged over a 0.035 in. guide wire so that an access platform can be established that will provide secure renal artery access for the therapeutic intervention.

Most angioplasty and stenting devices in current use will pass through a 6 French lumen. Access options include guide sheaths and guide catheters. Common to both of these options is the provision of a long mechanical support segment for guide-wire placement that affords direct access to the renal artery for easy passage of therapeutic devices to the target lesion [*see Figure 9*]. Such systems vary in shape and diameter and come in multiple configurations to facilitate renal artery access in different situations.

After the tip of the guide catheter is positioned at or within the renal artery orifice, guide-wire access across the lesion is obtained. For all subsequent manipulations, the sheath or the guide catheter should not be advanced beyond the orifice, because the nontapered tip may injure the vessel. Depending on the type, severity, and location of the lesion, a 0.35, 0.18, or 0.14 in. guide wire with a floppy radiopaque tip is chosen. The smaller guide-wire systems appear to have inherent advantages, in terms of ability to cross tighter stenoses, limitation of renal artery trauma, and liberation of emboli, but whether these apparent advantages are real remains to be proved. Once the guide wire is in place, the access platform is secured and remains in place until the intervention and any postintervention imaging are complete.

STEP 2: TRANSLUMINAL ANGIOPLASTY

With the guide wire secured distal to the lesion, therapeutic intervention may proceed. Both coaxial systems (in which the entire catheter is exchanged over the wire, so that an assistant is required to control the wire during intervention and catheter exchange) and monorail or rapid-exchange systems (in which only the distal portion of the catheter is over the wire, so that a single operator can control the wire during intervention and catheter exchange) are available for renal artery intervention.

Regardless of the system chosen, the principles of intervention remain the same. Transluminal angioplasty of the renal artery may be performed either as the sole therapy for a renal artery lesion or as a means of predilating a lesion so that an endoluminal stent can be placed. Angioplasty may also be employed to treat recurrent renal artery stenoses after surgical or endovascular therapy. Angioplasty is an effective stand-alone therapy in most cases of main renal artery disease (FMD and nonostial atherosclerosis) but is frequently ineffective for atherosclerotic ostial and proximal renal artery disease.

The angioplasty balloon size is chosen on the basis of quantitative angiographic images. Direct cut-film images with ball-bearing or marker-catheter reference points may be used, as may the quantitative software packages available on most contemporary digital angiographic systems. In general, the angioplasty balloon should be slightly larger than the adjacent normal artery for primary treatment and somewhat smaller for predilation of a stenotic lesion. For predilation before endoluminal stent placement, we usually employ a 3 × 20 mm low-profile angioplasty balloon. This choice tends to make the stent passage less traumatic and helps in estimating the stent diameter and length required.

During inflation of the angioplasty balloon, the aortic origin of most ostial plaques is indicated by the appearance of a visible "waist," and the image can be centered over a bony landmark to facilitate subsequent stent placement. It is not unusual for the patient to experience some discomfort during balloon inflation. This discomfort should resolve quickly when the balloon is deflated; if it does not, renal artery trauma should be suspected. It is our practice to inflate the balloon slowly to its fully inflated profile at the rated nominal pressure and then maintain inflation for 30 to 45 seconds before deflation.

Table 1 Standard Equipment for Renal PTAS

Device Category	*Type*	*Proprietary Name*	*Length*	*Diameter*
Guide wires	Initial	Starter 3 mm J	180 cm	0.035 in.
	Selective	Magic Torque Platinum Plus, V-18 Transend, GuardWire	180 cm 145–180 cm 165–200 cm	0.035 in. 0.018 in. 0.014 in.
Catheters	Flush angiography	Pigtail	70 cm	5 Fr
	Selective: diagnostic	Cobra C1 or C2 Contra 2 VS-1 or Sos Simmons	65 cm 65 cm 65 cm 65 cm	5 Fr 5 Fr 5 Fr 5 Fr
	Selective: guide	Renal Double Curve LIMA JR 4 Hockey Stick	55 cm 55 cm 55 cm 55 cm	6 Fr 6 Fr 6 Fr 6 Fr
	Pressure measuring	Straight Glide, Export	90 cm	4 Fr
Sheaths	Initial access		10 cm	4–5 Fr
	Therapeutic access		10 cm	6 Fr
	Selective: guide	Pinnacle Destination Flexor Check Flow ANL2	45 cm 45 cm	6 Fr 6 Fr
Angioplasty balloons	Predilation	Savoy, Gazelle, Aviator, Symmetry	1.5–2.0 cm balloon 75–90 cm shaft	3 mm balloon 5 Fr sheath
	Therapeutic	Savoy, Gazelle, Aviator, Symmetry	1.5–2.0 cm balloon 75–90 cm shaft	4–7 mm balloon 5 Fr sheath
Stents	Balloon-expandable	Genesis, Express	[illegible] mm stent 75–90 cm shaft	[illegible] mm stent 6 Fr sheath

PTAS = percutaneous transluminal angioplasty with or without endoluminal stent placement.
*None of these stents are approved by the Food and Drug Administration for use in renal arteries.

Once the balloon has been completely deflated, it is removed, and selective angiography is repeated to assess the response of the lesion to angioplasty and check for complications. Guide-wire access must be maintained until the end of the procedure so that complications or unsatisfactory results (e.g., dissection or residual stenosis) can be addressed.

a

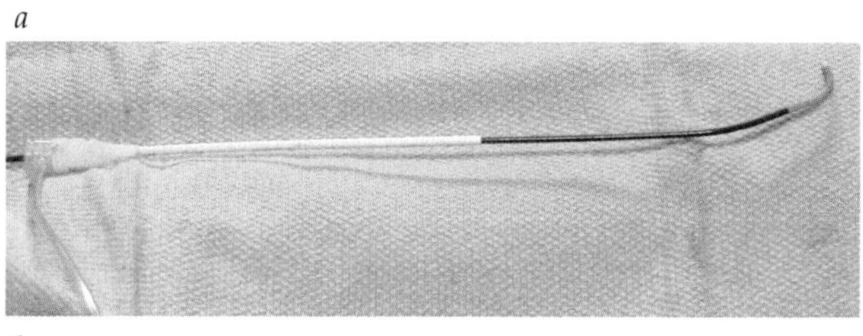

b

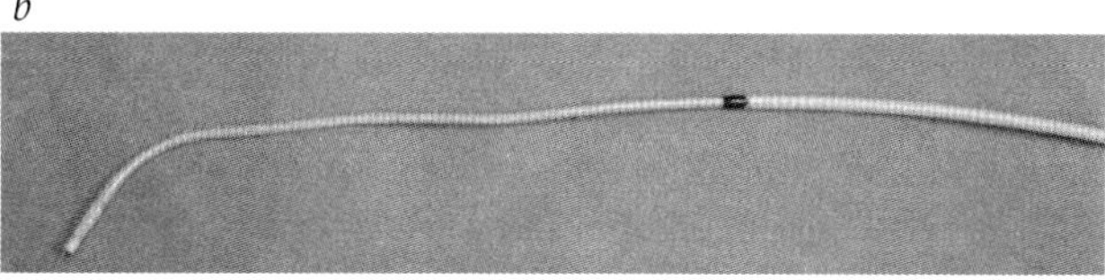

Figure 9 **(*a*) A guide catheter inserted through a short 6 French arterial sheath. (*b*) A diagnostic catheter inserted through a guide sheath.**

STEP 3: ENDOLUMINAL STENTING

Endovascular stent placement may be performed either as a primary procedure or as a secondary procedure in response to suboptimal results from angioplasty. Most FMD lesions and nonostial atherosclerotic lesions respond well to angioplasty alone. Secondary stent placement should, however, be considered for nonostial lesions that do not respond appropriately to angioplasty. Secondary stent placement is typically performed to address elastic recoil, residual stenosis (> 30%), pressure gradients (> 10 mm Hg), and myointimal flaps or dissections. Either balloon-expandable or, less commonly, self-expanding stents may be employed in the renal artery. Typically, balloon-expandable stents have greater radial strength and can be placed more precisely, whereas self-expanding stents are more flexible and conform more readily to the shape of the lumen. We employ balloon-expandable stents primarily in the treatment of ostial atherosclerotic lesions, where their advantages are particularly useful.

In general, the technical aspects of stent placement parallel those of transluminal angioplasty. Frequent hand injections of small amounts of contrast material through the guide sheath or catheter are employed to guide the stent into position across the lesion before deployment [*see Figure 10*]. After the stent has been deployed, completion angiography is performed while guide-wire access to the renal artery is

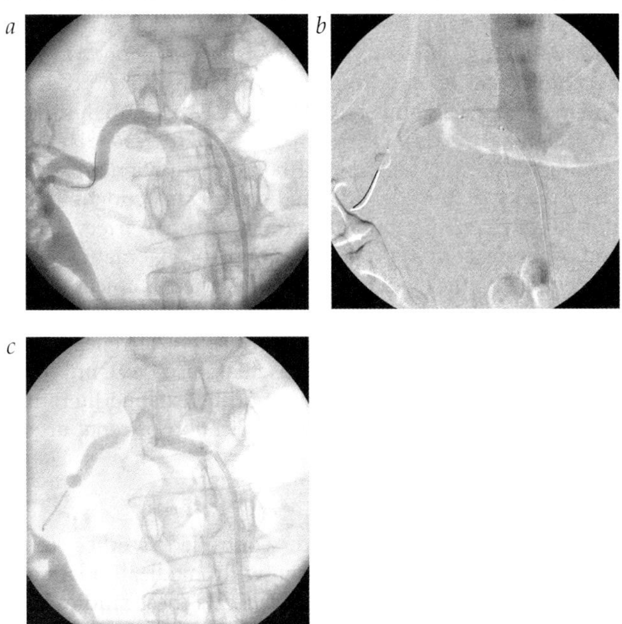

Figure 10 **(*a*) The orifice of a right renal artery with high-grade ostial stenosis is selected with a 5 French cobra catheter, and the lesion is crossed with a 0.014 in. guide wire. (*b*) A balloon-mounted stent is positioned across the renal artery stenosis with the help of intermittent contrast injections and bony landmarks. (*c*) A fully expanded stent is positioned in the renal artery.**

maintained. This is accomplished by hand injection of contrast through the guide sheath or catheter. For the treatment of ostial or proximal renal artery lesions, it is preferable to position the stent with 1 to 2 mm extension into the aorta. Frequent hand injection of contrast material through the guide sheath allows precise placement of the stent and helps prevent misdeployment. If the stent is placed too far into the artery, the true renal orifice is not supported, and there is a greater chance of residual or recurrent disease.[39–43] Such recurrent disease often does not respond to further endovascular attempts; accordingly, it is advisable to use the shortest possible stent that will adequately support the lesion. In addition, a stent that extends well out into the distal renal artery can make later surgical options more difficult[44] and typically carries a higher failure rate.

A balloon-expandable stent is deployed by inflating the angioplasty balloon on which it is mounted. In the past, these stents had to be crimped and hand-mounted on the angioplasty balloon, which made their delivery somewhat insecure. Currently available stents, however, come securely premounted on low-profile delivery systems capable of passing across most lesions with minimal or no predilation. We deploy these stents with 1 to 2 mm extension into the aorta, guided by anatomic information provided by previous positioning over bony landmarks. Self-expanding stents, although not commonly applied to the treatment of renovascular disease, can also be employed in this setting. These devices are deployed by retracting an outer membrane of the delivery device to expose the stent. Care must be taken during deployment to ensure that foreshortening of the stent does not compromise coverage of the lesion.

After a stent is deployed, there may be residual narrow areas within the stent that necessitate balloon dilatation. These areas may be visible on fluoroscopic evaluation of the stent or detected during postdeployment selective renal angiography.

After all therapeutic measures have been completed, the technical result is assessed and undetected defects are sought by means of repeat pressure-gradient measurements, intravascular ultrasonography, or both. When a satisfactory result is obtained, the guide wire and the sheath are removed and hemostasis is secured. Although it is possible to perform bilateral renal interventions in a single procedure, we prefer, when possible, to stage these interventions so as to minimize contrast loads.

Postprocedural Care

Longitudinal follow-up of all patients undergoing renal revascularization is mandatory to check for recurrent disease, contralateral disease, and deterioration of clinical benefit, as well as other preventable cardiovascular and peripheral vascular conditions. Our current approach to follow-up entails clinical visits at 1, 3, 6, 9, 12, 18, and 24 months after renal artery PTAS, with renal duplex ultrasonography, blood pressure measurement, and serum creatinine measurement at each visit. After 24 months, this intensive early follow-up is relaxed to a yearly visit schedule if no conditions necessitating shorter visit intervals have been identified.

Recurrent disease after renal stenting is a significant concern, and disease that recurs within the stent itself can be a particularly challenging problem [*see Figure 11a*]. Because most such recurrences are related to intimal hyperplasia, repeat balloon angioplasty generally does little to improve the situation. Initial dilatation with a Cutting Balloon (Boston Scientific, Natick, MA) is extremely useful for releasing the fibrous scar tissue of the restenotic lesion and allowing subsequent dilatation to a larger diameter with a conventional angioplasty balloon. The Cutting Balloon consists of a noncompliant balloon with three or four atherotomes (microsurgical blades) mounted longitudinally on its outer surface [*see Figure 11b*]. When the device is inflated, the atherotomes score the intimal hyperplasia within the stent; the balloon is then rotated and reinflated to score the lesion in multiple planes. To date, this technique has been used primarily in coronary arteries, but it has also been applied to the treatment of renal artery in-stent restenosis.[45] After the lesion has been scored, a larger balloon is inserted and inflated to redilate the lesion [*see Figure 11c*].

Complications

Potential complications include access-site complications (e.g., hematoma, pseudoaneurysm, retroperitoneal hemorrhage, arteriovenous fistula, and closure-device infection), contrast-mediated allergic reactions or nephrotoxicity, atheroembolism, and direct renovascular trauma. In a meta-analysis published in 2000, the reported complication rate after renal PTAS ranged from 0 to 40% (mean rate 11%).[34]

16. Barrett BJ, Parfrey PS, Mcdonald JR, et al. Nonionic low-osmolality versus ionic high-osmolality contrast material for intravenous use in patients perceived to be at high-risk—randomized trial. Radiology 1992;183:105.
17. Barrett BJ, Parfrey PS, Vavasour HM, et al. A comparison of nonionic, low-osmolality radiocontrast agents with ionic, high-osmolality agents during cardiac-catheterization. N Engl J Med 1992;326:431.
18. Cigarroa RG, Lange RA, Williams RH, et al. Dosing of contrast material to prevent contrast nephropathy in patients with renal disease. Am J Med 1989;86:649.
19. Gomes AS, Baker JD, Martinparedero V, et al. Acute renal dysfunction after major arteriography. AJR Am J Roentgenol 1985;145:1249.
20. Tepel M, van der Giet M, Schwarzfeld C, et al. Prevention of radiographic-contrast-agent-induced reductions in renal function by acetylcysteine. N Engl J Med 2000;343:180.
21. Kay J, Chow WH, Chan TM, et al. Acetylcysteine for prevention of acute deterioration of renal function following elective coronary angiography and intervention—a randomized controlled trial. JAMA 2003;289:553.
22. Merten GJ, Burgess WP, Gray LV, et al. Prevention of contrast-induced nephropathy with sodium bicarbonate—a randomized controlled trial. JAMA 2004;291:2328.
23. Back MR, Caridi JG, Hawkins IF, et al. Angiography with carbon dioxide (CO2). Surg Clin North Am 1998;78:575.
24. Seeger JM, Self S, Harward TRS, et al. Carbon dioxide gas as an arterial contrast agent. Ann Surg 1993;217:688.
25. Grollman JH, Marcus R. Transbrachial arteriography—techniques and complications. Cardiovasc Intervent Radiol 1988;11:32.
26. Verschuyl EJ, Kaatee R, Beek FJA, et al. Renal artery origins: best angiographic projection angles. Radiology 1997;205: 115.
27. Verschuyl EJ, Kaatee R, Beek FJA, et al. Renal artery origins: location and distribution in the transverse plane at CT. Radiology 1997;203:71.
28. Leertouwer TC, Gussenhoven EJ, van Jaarsveld BC, et al. In-vitro validation, with histology, of intravascular ultrasound in renal arteries. J Hypertens 1999;17:271.
29. Sheikh KH, Davidson CJ, Newman GE, et al. Intravascular ultrasound assessment of the renal artery. Ann Intern Med 1991;115:22.
30. Choudhri AH, Cleland JGF, Rowlands PC, et al. Unsuspected renal artery stenosis in peripheral vascular disease. BMJ 1990;301:1197.
31. Hansen KJ, Edwards MS, Craven TE, et al. Prevalence of renovascular disease in the elderly: a population-based study. J Vasc Surg 2002;36:443.
32. Olin JW, Melia M, Young JR, et al. Prevalence of atherosclerotic renal artery stenosis in patients with atherosclerosis elsewhere. Am J Med 1990;88:N46.
33. Valentine RJ, Clagett GP, Miller GL, et al. The coronary risk of unsuspected renal artery stenosis. J Vasc Surg 1993;18: 433.
34. Leertouwer TC, Gussenhoven EJ, Bosch JL, et al. Stent placement for renal arterial stenosis: where do we stand? A meta-analysis. Radiology 2000;216:78.
35. Dean RH, Benjamin ME, Hansen KJ. Surgical management of renovascular hypertension—in brief. Curr Probl Surg 1997;34:214.
36. McCormack LJ, Noto TJ, Meaney TF, et al. Subadventitial fibroplasia of the renal artery, a disease of young women. Am Heart J 1967;73:602.
37. Alimi Y, Mercier C, Pellisier JF, et al. Fibromuscular disease of the renal artery: a new histopathologic classification. Ann Vasc Surg 1992;6:220.
38. Corriere MA, Edwards MS, Pearce JD, et al. Restenosis after renal artery angioplasty and stenting: incidence and risk factors. J Vasc Surg 2009;50:813.
39. Blum U, Krumme B, Flugel P, et al. Treatment of ostial renal-artery stenoses with vascular endoprostheses after unsuccessful balloon angioplasty. N Engl J Med 1997;336: 459.
40. Blum U, Hauer M, Krumme B. Percutaneous revascularization of the kidney: conventional angioplasty versus renal artery stenting. Radiologe 1999;39:135.
41. Rocha-Singh KJ, Ahuja RK, Sung CH, et al. Long-term renal function preservation after renal artery stenting in patients with progressive ischemic nephropathy. Catheter Cardiovasc Interv 2002;57:135.
42. Gill KS, Fowler RC. Atherosclerotic renal arterial stenosis: clinical outcomes of stent placement for hypertension and renal failure. Radiology 2003;226:821.
43. Rundback JH, Jacobs JM. Percutaneous renal artery stent placement for hypertension and azotemia: pilot study. Am J Kidney Dis 1996;28:214.
44. Wong JM, Hansen KJ, Oskin TC, et al. Surgery after failed percutaneous renal artery angioplasty. J Vasc Surg 1999;30: 468.
45. Munneke GJ, Engelke C, Morgan RA, et al. Cutting balloon angioplasty for resistant renal artery in-stent restenosis. J Vasc Intervent Radiol 2002;13:327.
46. Ivanovic V, McKusick MA, Johnson CM, et al. Renal artery stent placement: complications at a single tertiary care center. J Vasc Intervent Radiol 2003;14:217.
47. Plouin P, Chatellier G, Darné B, Raynaud A. Blood pressure outcome of angioplasty in atherosclerotic renal artery stenosis: a randomized trial. Essai Multicentrique Medicaments vs Angioplastie (EMMA) Study Group. Hypertension 1998;31:823.
48. Webster J, Marshall F, Abdalla M, et al. Randomised comparison of percutaneous angioplasty vs continued medical therapy for hypertensive patients with atheromatous renal artery stenosis. J Hum Hypertens 1998;12:329.
49. van Jaarsveld BC, Krijnen P. Prospective studies of diagnosis and intervention: the Dutch experience. Semin Nephrol 2000;20:463.
50. Weibull H, Bergqvist D, Bergentz SE, et al. Percutaneous transluminal renal angioplasty versus surgical reconstruction of atherosclerotic renal artery stenosis—a prospective randomized study. J Vasc Surg 1993;18:841.
51. The ASTRAL Investigators. Revascularization versus medical therapy for renal-artery stenosis. N Engl J Med 2009; 361:1953.
52. Yutan E, Glickerman DJ, Caps MT, et al. Percutaneous transluminal revascularization for renal artery stenosis: Veterans Affairs Puget Sound Health Care System experience. J Vasc Surg 2001;34:685.
53 Corriere MA, Pearce JD, Edwards MS, Stafford JM, Hansen KJ. Endovascular management of atherosclerotic renovascular disease: early results following primary intervention. J Vasc Surg 2008;48:580.

54. Sivamurthy N, Surowiec SM, Culakova E, et al. Divergent outcomes after percutaneous therapy for symptomatic renal artery stenosis. J Vasc Surg 2004;39:565.
55. Tegtmeyer CJ, Selby JB, Hartwell GD, et al. Results and complications of angioplasty in fibromuscular disease. Circulation 1991;83:155.
56. de Fraissinette B, Garcier JM, Dieu V, et al. Percutaneous transluminal angioplasty of dysplastic stenoses of the renal artery: results on 70 adults. Cardiovasc Intervent Radiol 2003;26:46.
57. Dean RH, Kieffer RW, Smith BM, et al. Renovascular hypertension—anatomic and renal function changes during drug therapy. Arch Surg 1981;116:1408.
58. Dean RH, Tribble RW, Hansen KJ, et al. Evolution of renal insufficiency in ischemic nephropathy. Ann Surg 1991;213:446.
59. Krumme B, Schwertfeger E, Donauer J, et al. Intrarenal resistive index (RI) is not useful for the prediction of outcome after stenting in patients with atherosclerotic renal artery stenosis. J Am Soc Nephrol 2002;13:242A.
60. Radermacher J, Weinkove R, Haller H. Techniques for predicting a favourable response to renal angioplasty in patients with renovascular disease. Curr Opin Nephrol Hypertens 2001;10:799.
61. Coh EJ, Benjamin ME, Sandager GP, et al. Can intrarenal duplex waveform analysis predict successful renal artery revascularization? J Vasc Surg 1998;28:471.
62. Henry M, Klonaris C, Henry I, et al. Protected renal stenting with the PercuSurge GuardWire device: a pilot study. J Endovasc Ther 2001;8:227.
63. Henry M, Henry I, Klonaris C, et al. Renal angioplasty and stenting under protection: the way for the future? Catheter Cardiovasc Intervent 2003;60:299.
64. Holden A, Hill A. Renal angioplasty and stenting with distal protection of the main renal artery in ischemic nephropathy: early experience. J Vasc Surg 2003;38:962.
65. Garza L, Aude YW, Saucedo JF. Can we prevent in-stent restenosis? Curr Opin Cardiol 2002;17:518.
66. Burket MW, Cooper CJ, Kennedy DJ, et al. Renal artery angioplasty and stent placement: predictors of a favorable outcome. Am Heart J 2000;139:64.
67. Lederman RJ, Mendelsohn FO, Santos R, et al. Primary renal artery stenting: characteristics and outcomes after 363 procedures. Am Heart J 2001;142:314.
68. Bush RL, Najibi S, MacDonald MJ, Lin PH, Chaikof EL, Martin LG, et al. Endovascular revascularization of renal artery stenosis: technical and clinical results. J Vasc Surg 2001;33:5.
69. Zeller T, Frank U, Muller C, et al. Stent-supported angioplasty of severe atherosclerotic renal artery stenosis preserves renal function and improves blood pressure control: long-term results from a prospective registry of 456 lesions. J Endovasc Ther 2004;11:95.
70. Nolan BW, Schermerhorn ML, Rowell E, et al. Outcomes of renal artery angioplasty and stenting using low-profile systems. J Vasc Surg 2005;41:46.
71. Kashyap VS, Sepulveda RN, Bena JF, et al. The management of renal artery atherosclerosis for renal salvage: does stenting help? J Vasc Surg 2007;45:101.

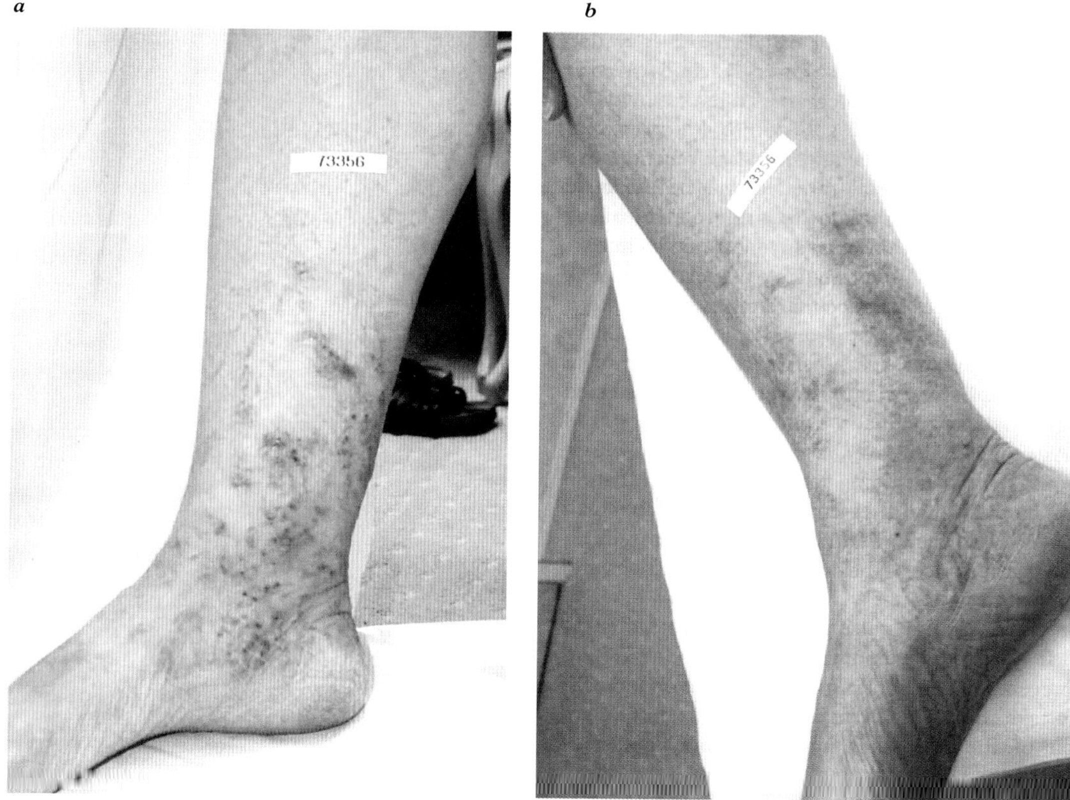

Figure 6 **A 56-year-old woman (*a*) before treatment and (*b*) with residual hyperpigmentation after treatment with 0.2% sodium tetradecyl sulfate.**

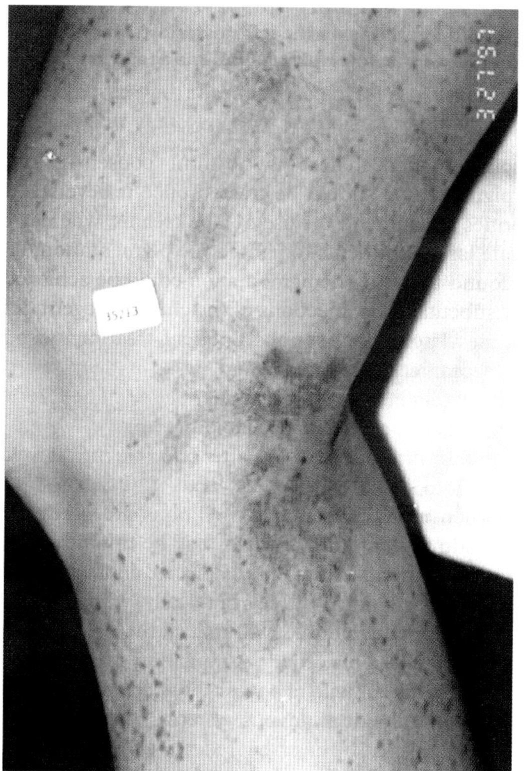

Figure 7 **Telangiectatic matting in a 43-year-old woman after treatment with 0.2% sodium tetradecyl sulfate.**

to treat once it has developed. Occasionally, it resolves spontaneously, but more often, it must be addressed by means of either repeat sclerotherapy with treatment of the feeding reticular vein or laser therapy. Treatment of telangiectatic matting may, in fact, be the one potential efficacious use for laser-type devices in treating diseased leg veins.

Cost Considerations

I strongly believe that all sclerotherapy, with the exception of that performed for spontaneous hemorrhage, is cosmetic. Accordingly, in the practice to which I belong, patients seeking sclerotherapy for reasons other than hemorrhage are informed well in advance that the procedure is cosmetic and not reimbursable, and they receive a good-faith estimate of expected costs in writing. As noted (see above), venous ablation, either open or catheter directed, is the treatment of choice for symptomatic axial reflux and large varicose veins; therefore, sclerotherapy for these conditions is considered medically unnecessary.

Obtaining reimbursement from insurance carriers for sclerotherapy performed to treat small varicose veins or hemorrhage is frustrating at best. Both physicians and patients have contributed to the problem in the past by filing inappropriate claims for reimbursement of cosmetic procedures. This past misuse of insurance coverage has made it difficult to obtain reimbursement even for the one solid medical indication for sclerotherapy, hemorrhage.

Financial Disclosures: None Reported

References

1. Goldman MP, Bergan JJ. Sclerotherapy: treatment of varicose and telangiectatic leg veins. 4th ed. St. Louis: Mosby–Year Book; 2006.
2. Einarsson E, Eklof B, Neglen P. Sclerotherapy or surgery as treatment for varicose veins: a prospective randomized study. Phlebology 1993;8:22.
3. Bishop C, Fronek H, Fronek A, et al. Real-time color duplex scanning after sclerotherapy of the greater saphenous vein. J Vasc Surg 1991;14:505.
4. Goren G. Real-time color duplex scanning after sclerotherapy of the greater saphenous vein [letter]. J Vasc Surg 1992;16:497.
5. Belcaro G, Nicolaides A, Ricci A, et al. Endovascular sclerotherapy, surgery, and surgery plus sclerotherapy in superficial venous incompetence: a randomized, 10-year follow-up trial—final results. Angiology 2000;51:529.
6. Yamaki T, Nozaki M, Sakurai H. Prospective randomized efficacy of ultrasound-guided foam sclerotherapy compared with ultrasound-guided liquid sclerotherapy in the treatment of symptomatic venous malformations. J Vasc Surg 2008;47:578–84.
7. Kanter A, Thibault P. Saphenofemoral incompetence treated by ultrasound-guided sclerotherapy. Dermatol Surg 1996;22:648.
8. Cabrera J, Cabrera J Jr, Garcia-Olmedo MA. Treatment of varicose long saphenous veins with sclerosant in microfoam form: long-term outcomes. Phlebology 2000;15:19.
9. McDonagh B, Huntley DE, Rosenfeld R, et al. Efficacy of the comprehensive objective mapping, precise image-guided injection, anti-reflux positioning, and sequential sclerotherapy technique in the management of greater saphenous varicosities with saphenofemoral incompetence. Phlebology 2002; 17:19.
10. Myers KA, Jolley D, Clough A, et al. Outcome of ultrasound-guided sclerotherapy for varicose veins: medium-term results assessed by ultrasound surveillance. Eur J Vasc Endovasc Surg 2007;33:116–21.
11. Gonzalez-Zeh R, Armisen R, Barahona S. Endovenous laser and echo-guided foam ablation in great saphenous vein reflux: one-year follow-up results. J Vasc Surg 2008; 48:940–6.
12. McCoy S, Evans A, Spurrier N. Sclerotherapy for leg telangiectasia: a blinded comparative trial of polidocanol and hypertonic saline. Dermatol Surg 1999;25:381.
13. Bukhari R, Lohr J, Paget D, et al. Evaluation of lidocaine as an analgesic when added to hypertonic saline for sclerotherapy. J Vasc Surg 1999;29:479.
14. Kern P, Ramelet A, Wutschert R. Single-blind, randomized study comparing chromated glycerin, polidocanol solution, and polidocanol foam for treatment of telangiectatic leg veins. Dermatol Surg 2004;30:367–72.
15. Guex J. Indications for sclerosing agent polidocanol. J Dermatol Surg Oncol 1993; 19:959.
16. Conrad P, Malouf GM, Stacey MC. The Australian polidocanol (aethoxysklerol) study. Dermatol Surg 1995;21:334.
17. Goldman M. Treatment of varicose and telangiectatic leg veins: double-blind prospective comparative trial between aethoxysklerol and sotradecol. Dermatol Surg 2002;28:52.
18. Cavezzi A, Frullini A, Ricci S, et al. Treatment of varicose veins by foam sclerotherapy: two clinical series. Phlebology 2002;17:13.
19. Orbach EJ. Sclerotherapy of varicose veins: utilization of an intravenous air block. Am J Surg 1944;66:362.
20. Frullini A. New technique in producing sclerosing foam in a disposable syringe. Dermatol Surg 2000;26:705.
21. Tessari L, Cavezzi A, Frullini A. Preliminary experience with a new sclerosing foam in the treatment of varicose veins. Dermatol Surg 2001;27:58.
22. Frullini A, Cavezzi A. Sclerosing foam in the treatment of varicose veins and telangiectases: history and analysis of safety and complications. Dermatol Surg 2002;28:1.
23. Raj TB, Goodard M, Makin GS. How long do compression bandages maintain their pressure during ambulatory treatment of varicose veins? Br J Surg 1980;67:122.
24. Smith SL, Belmont JM, Casparian JM. Analysis of pressure achieved by various materials used for pressure dressings. Dermatol Surg 1999;25:931.
25. Goldman MP, Beaudoing D, Marley W, et al. Compression in the treatment of leg telangiectasia. J Dermatol Surg Oncol 1990;16:322.
26. Kern P, Ramelet A, Wutschert R, et al. Compression after sclerotherapy for telangiectasias and reticular leg veins: a randomized controlled study. J Vasc Surg 2007;45: 1212–6.
27. Weiss RA, Sadick NS, Goldman MP, et al. Post-sclerotherapy compression: controlled comparative study of duration of compression and its effects on clinical outcome. Dermatol Surg 1999;25:105.
28. Forlee MV, Grouden M, Moore DJ, et al. Stroke after varicose vein foam injection sclerotherapy. J Vasc Surg 2006;43:162–4.
29. Bihari I, Magyar E. Reasons for ulceration after injection treatment of telangiectasia. Dermatol Surg 2001;27:133.
30. Bergan JJ, Weiss RA, Goldman MP. Extensive tissue necrosis following high-concentration sclerotherapy for varicose veins. Dermatol Surg 2000;26:535.
31. Scultetus A, Villavicencio JL, Kao T. Microthrombectomy reduces postsclerotherapy pigmentation: multicenter randomized trial. J Surg 2003;38:896–903.
32. Lopez L, Dilley R, Henriquez J. Cutaneous hyperpigmentation following venous sclerotherapy treated with deferoxamine mesylate. Dermatol Surg 2001;27:795.

26 MEDICAL MANAGEMENT OF VASCULAR DISEASE

Russell H. Samson, MD, FACS, RVT

Vascular surgery has evolved dramatically with the explosion of noninvasive diagnostic tools and endovascular techniques for the treatment of vascular conditions. Surgeons are now actively involved in all of these technical aspects of care, although many of us still relegate the medical management of the vascular patient to our physician colleagues. Unfortunately, we are also rarely involved in preventive measures. As a result, although we may be able to bypass or open blocked arteries and replace aneurysms with minimally invasive surgery, our patients continue to die from the other cardiovascular consequences of these diseases. The assumption that the family physician, internist, or cardiologist will take care of these issues is not necessarily correct. A number of reports have shown that atherosclerotic risk factors in patients with peripheral arterial disease (PAD) are less intensively treated than in patients with coronary artery disease.[1,2] In a review of 195 PAD patients discharged from a tertiary care hospital in Canada, Anand and colleagues reported that fewer than half were sent home with antiplatelet medication.[2] Only 20% were on beta blockers, and, surprisingly, only 16% were on cholesterol-lowering medications. Clearly, this represents a failure of our responsibility to the patient.

Many factors may explain why surgeons are unwilling to be involved in the nonoperative management of their patients. These include insufficient knowledge, lack of time outside the operating room or endovascular suite, or the surgeon's fear that he or she may alienate a referring medical colleague by becoming involved in that physician's management of the atherosclerotic process. Some of the above-mentioned impediments may be valid in a given surgeon's practice, but surgeons at least should know what appropriate care is for their patients' underlying disease, if only to ensure that it is being appropriately treated. This chapter outlines the medical management of atherosclerosis and its relationship to diabetes and the dysmetabolic syndrome. Medications and lifestyle changes that can improve circulation are also described, as well as therapies to counter the negative effects of platelet activation. Treatment options for hypertension and medications for specific aspects of PAD are also discussed.

Medical Management of Atherosclerosis

Fundamental to all treatment approaches for arterial pathology is an understanding of the role of lipids in atherosclerosis. It is now well known that there is more to cholesterol than good and bad varieties and that medical treatment must be targeted at each abnormality differently. Further, although statins are clearly the dominant medications, not all statins are equal, and other drugs may prove valuable. The beneficial effects of these drugs may go well beyond changes in lipid content. Furthermore, there are patients with asymptomatic PAD who can potentially benefit from these medications even if they have "normal" lipid levels when first screened (especially those with insulin resistance, a family history of atherosclerosis and its complications, truncal obesity, and low high-density lipoprotein [HDL] or high triglycerides). The vascular surgeon, who wishes to be more than a technician and appropriately treat PAD beyond simply intervening for extremity ischemic complications, needs to be aware of such nuances, as well as other key considerations in managing the underlying atherosclerosis process. This includes the value of exercise, good nutrition, and smoking cessation.

There are four major risk factors for the development of atherosclerosis: diabetes, smoking, hypertension, and lipid abnormalities.[3] The management of diabetes and hypertension and techniques for smoking prevention are beyond the scope of this chapter but are briefly outlined.

DIABETES

The development of claudication is five times more frequent in males and three times more frequent in females who suffer from diabetes.[4] Typically, diabetes affects the more distal infrapopliteal arteries, and given that these vessels have the poorest results with revascularization, it is not surprising that diabetics have an increased risk of amputation. Although the degree of glycemic control has never been shown to reliably predict the severity of disease, good control is clearly an important goal of therapy and should be strongly encouraged, although too aggressive control, especially in the elderly, can lead to increased complications.[5]

SMOKING

Cigarette smoking is a major risk factor for the development of PAD. Further, the greater the smoking history, the more likely will be the development and severity of atherosclerotic involvement and subsequent morbidity and mortality. Accordingly, every effort should be made to encourage the patient to quit. Numerous over-the-counter remedies such as nicotine patches have been proposed, as well as some prescription medications, such as the antidepressant bupropion HCl (Wellbutrin, Brentford, Middlesex, England) and the smoking-specific agent varenicline (Chantix, Pfizer, Mission, Kansas).[6]

However, perhaps the single most important treatment that can be offered is simply encouragement by the physician. This should be an integral part of every interaction with the patient. The excess vascular mortality of smoking decreases within 20 years to the level of the never-smoker.[7]

HYPERTENSION

Although hypertension can increase the risk of PAD two- to threefold, it is not as important a risk factor as the others listed above. However, clearly, it will be important to control, if only to prevent the associated cardiac and cerebrovascular morbidity of PAD.[8–10] In clinical trials, antihypertensive therapy has been associated with a 35 to 40% mean reduction in stroke incidence, a 20 to 25% reduction in myocardial infarction, and a more than 50% reduction in heart failure.[11] It is estimated that in patients with stage 1 hypertension and additional risk factors, lowering systolic blood pressure 12 mm Hg for 10 years will prevent one death for every 11 patients treated. If cardiovascular disease or PAD is present or target end-organ damage has occurred, only nine patients would require this treatment to prevent one death.[12]

In our practice treating patients with diagnosed PAD, we have found that only 32% of patients are normotensive during their office visits or vascular laboratory evaluations.[13,14] This may be because patients are anxious and exhibit so-called "white coat" hypertension. To overcome this limitation in pressure measurements, it has been suggested that the blood pressure be taken at the end of the visit, when the patient has had time to relax. The pressure should also be taken in a standard manner with the patient seated comfortably and with the arm resting at heart level. The medical diagnostic workup in patients with hypertension is not germane to this chapter. However, the surgeon should be aware that sudden onset of hypertension or significant exacerbation may be an indication that the patient is suffering from a correctable cause such as renal artery stenosis. If suspected because of the presence of an abdominal bruit, an aneurysm, or aortic atherosclerosis, Doppler ultrasonography will usually be the first-line test. Magnetic resonance angiography or spiral computed tomographic angiography may also obviate the need for arteriography.

Initial blood pressure control will include lifestyle and dietary changes. These should include restriction of sodium, alcohol, and unsaturated fats, as well as increasing daily exercise and intake of fruits and vegetables.[15] There are now a large number of medications to choose from if drug therapy is required, and these fall into the following main groups: diuretics, alpha and beta blockers, direct vasodilators, central agents, calcium channel blockers, angiotensin-converting enzyme (ACE) inhibitors, and angiotensin II receptor blockers. Many are now generic, and different pharmaceutical companies manufacture many very similar drugs. This has led to a great deal of confusion, with multiple studies producing conflicting results. Accordingly, many physicians will follow the guidelines published by the Joint National Committee on the Detection, Evaluation and Treatment of High Blood Pressure.[16] Current recommendations suggest the use of diuretics as the first line of drug therapy. Initial therapy with two drugs should be considered when the blood pressure is 20/10 mm Hg above goal. In patients with diabetes or chronic renal failure, antihypertensive medications should be considered if the blood pressure is greater than 130/80 mm Hg, although a benefit may not be seen in patients excreting more than 1 to 2 g of protein/day. In these patients, three drugs may often be necessary.[16]

In patients with PAD, there has been a historical concern that the use of beta-adrenergic blockers would potentially worsen the symptoms of claudication. However, several studies have shown that this class of drugs is safe in claudicants and is an acceptable choice for lowering blood pressure.[17] However, large reductions of systolic pressure and leg perfusion by any class of antihypertensive agent may result in modest worsening of claudication symptoms.[18] The role of beta blockers in the prevention of perioperative events is discussed later in this chapter.

The ACE inhibitor drugs have also shown benefit beyond blood pressure lowering in high-risk groups. Specifically, in the Heart Outcomes Prevention Evaluation (HOPE) study, results from the study of 4,046 patients with PAD formed a subgroup in which there was a 22% risk reduction in patients randomized to ramipril compared with placebo.[19] This was independent of lowering of blood pressure. Further, it appears from the same HOPE study that these medications may slow or prevent the onset of diabetes.[20] Based on this finding, the Food and Drug Administration (FDA) has now approved ramipril for its cardioprotective benefits in patients at high risk, including those with PAD. Thus, in terms of a drug class, the ACE inhibitors would certainly be recommended in these patients. However, in general, the goals of treating hypertension in patients with PAD should be similar to those of patient populations with other cardiovascular diseases.

HYPERLIPIDEMIA

The term *hyperlipidemia* has the unfortunate connotation that atherosclerosis is a result only of elevated levels of lipid, especially low-density lipoprotein (LDL). However, it is abundantly clear that other abnormalities of plasma lipids, such as triglycerides, can also be deleterious to the arterial wall.[21,22] Further, deficiencies of some of these substances, for example, HDLs, are equally important in the development of atherosclerosis. The simplistic view that LDL is the root cause of atherosclerosis has also undergone reevaluation as research has uncovered moieties of LDL and HDL that may have differing effects on arterial pathology. It is now apparent that there are different fractions of LDL based on particle size, with the smaller particles being more atherogenic. Similarly, some fractions of HDL may be more protective. In PAD, several lipid fractions are critically important in determining the presence and progression of peripheral atherosclerosis. Independent risk factors for PAD include elevations of total cholesterol, LDL cholesterol, triglycerides, and lipoprotein(a).[23] Protective against PAD are increases in HDL cholesterol and apolipoprotein(a-1).[23] For every 10 mg/dL increase in total cholesterol concentration, the risk of PAD increases approximately 10%.[24] Elevations in lipoprotein(a) are also an independent risk factor for PAD, particularly in men.[25,26]

Hyperlipidemia also implies a simplistic etiology to the manifestations of atherosclerosis, that is, that lipids enter the arterial wall and by virtue of the lipid content result in stenosis. However, the actual pathologic process is significantly more complicated, with vascular inflammation playing a critical role. Within several days of a high-cholesterol diet, monocytes adhere to the endothelium, particularly at intercellular junctions.[27] The aberrations of endothelial function represent an oxidative stress to the cells and occur within minutes to hours of exposure to the noxious stimuli. Oxidative stress perturbs the cell membrane and increases endothelial permeability. Monocytes then migrate into the subendothelium, where they begin to accumulate lipid and become foam cells. These activated monocytes (macrophages) release mitogens and chemoattractants that recruit additional macrophages and vascular smooth muscle cells into the lesion. In addition, they generate reactive oxygen species that increase oxidative stress within the vessel wall and that accelerate oxidation of LDL cholesterol trapped in the subintimal space. The oxidation of LDL particles in the subintimal space promotes more foam cell formation.[27,28] This is because the oxidized LDL is taken up via the scavenger receptor. Unlike the receptor for native LDL, intracellular levels of cholesterol do not downregulate the scavenger receptor. Accordingly, oxidized LDL continues to be taken up by the macrophage via the scavenger receptor, with the result that the macrophage becomes swollen with lipid. As foam cells accumulate in the subendothelial space, they distort the overlying endothelium and eventually may even rupture through the endothelial surface.[28] In these areas of endothelial ulceration, platelets adhere to the vessel wall, releasing epidermal growth factor, platelet-derived growth factor, and other mitogens and cytokines that contribute to smooth muscle migration and proliferation. These factors induce smooth muscle cells in the vessel wall to proliferate and migrate into the area of the lesion. These vascular smooth muscle cells undergo a change in phenotype from a "contractile" cell to a "secretory" cell. These secretory vascular smooth muscle cells elaborate extracellular matrix (e.g., elastin), which transforms the lesion into a fibrous plaque. In addition to elaborating extracellular matrix, the smooth muscle cells may also become engorged with lipid to form more foam cells. The lesion grows with the recruitment of more cells, the elaboration of extracellular matrix, and the accumulation of lipid until it is transformed from a fibrous plaque to a complex plaque.

The complex plaque typically is characterized by a fibrous cap that overlies a necrotic core that is composed of cell debris and cholesterol and contains a high concentration of the thrombogenic tissue factor, secreted by macrophages. In later-stage lesions, calcification may occur. Ultimately, the fibrous cap can rupture, leading to distal embolization or the accumulation of platelets on the plaque and subsequent acute arterial occlusion.

As mentioned, inflammation has been associated with the development of atherosclerosis and the risk of cardiovascular events. In particular, C-reactive protein (CRP) is independently associated with PAD,[29] even in patients with normal lipid levels.[30,31] In the Physician's Health Study, an elevated CRP was a risk factor for the development of symptomatic PAD and for peripheral revascularization.[32] In patients with established PAD, an elevated CRP is an independent predictor of future cardiovascular events.[33] The measurement of CRP may also guide lipid therapy in that statin drugs lower CRP levels and the reduction in CRP levels may contribute to the benefits of statin drugs.[34] The JUPITER study (Justification for the Use of Statins in Primary Prevention: An Intervention Trial Evaluating Rosuvastatin) suggested that patients who exhibited elevated levels of CRP despite so-called "normal" cholesterol levels still benefited from statin use.[35] This is important because as many as half of all patients with PAD may present with "normal" lipid levels. However, CRP itself is probably a marker for atherosclerosis rather than a cause. This is evidenced by a study on polymorphisms in the CRP gene, which are associated with marked increases in CRP levels and thus with a theoretically predicted increase in the risk of ischemic vascular disease.[36] However, these polymorphisms were not in themselves associated with an increased risk of ischemic vascular disease.

Treatment of Hyperlipidemia

Based on the knowledge that the effect of lipids on atherosclerosis is more complex than simply a detrimental effect of hypercholesterolemia, treatment programs are now directed at multiple pathways within the development of plaque. However, the dominant treatment remains reducing cholesterol. This is based on a number of large studies conducted on patients with underlying cardiovascular disease or those at risk for developing these conditions. Some of these included patients with so-called "normal" levels of cholesterol. The major studies include the Helsinki Heart Study,[37] the Scandinavian Simvastatin Survival Study (the "4S"),[38] The Cholesterol and Recurring Events (CARE) Trial,[39] the Program on the Surgical Control of Hyperlipidemias (POSCH),[40] the Heart Protection Study (HPS),[41] and, more recently, the JUPITER study.[35]

Diet and exercise There are several methods to alter cholesterol levels, some directed at overall levels, with others more targeted at reducing LDL or triglycerides or elevating HDL. Diet modification has always been a first-line method.[42] Reducing cholesterol and saturated fat intake and weight loss can modestly reduce LDL and can lead to a significant reduction in triglyceride levels. Dietary fiber can assist in these beneficial results. Exercise can also result in a mild reduction in LDL and an increase in HDL.

Lipid-lowering agents Although lifestyle modification by exercise and diet has been shown to be beneficial in altering lipid metabolism, medications are often mandatory additions for the PAD patient. Unfortunately, it is also important to realize that despite the beneficial effects of a lipid-altering diet and medications, many patients are noncompliant, with discontinuance rates as high as 46% being reported.[43]

There are now numerous alternative methods for altering lipid levels. Many of these are nonprescription "remedies," which are, nonetheless, widely used. This chapter deals only with the dominant pharmaceutical agents, the so-called lipid–lowering drugs: statins, fibrates, niacin, ezetimibe, and bile-acid sequestrants.

Statins The statins are the most commonly used medications in the treatment of hypercholesterolemia.[44] They are also the most powerful drugs for lowering LDL cholesterol, with reductions in the range of 20 to 60%.[45,46] Currently available statins include rosuvastatin (Crestor, Astra Zeneca, Wilmington, Delaware), atorvastatin (Lipitor, Pfizer, New York, New York), fluvastatin (Lescol, Novartis Pharmaceuticals Corp., East Hanover, New Jersey), lovastatin (Mevacor, Merck, Whitehouse Station, New Jersey), pravastatin (Pravachol, Bristol-Myers Squibb, New York, New York), and simvastatin (Zocor, Merck, Whitehouse Station, New Jersey). Fluvastatin is somewhat less potent, decreasing LDL levels by 20 to 25% at the maximum recommended dose, whereas rosuvastatin is the most potent, reducing LDL levels by up to 52% and increasing HDL up to 14%. Statins are most effective when taken at night because this is the time when cholesterol production is maximal.

Statins are competitive inhibitors of 3-hydroxy-3-methylglutaryl coenzyme A (HMG-CoA) reductase, the rate-limiting step in cholesterol biosynthesis.[47] A reduction in intrahepatic cholesterol leads to an increase in LDL receptor turnover that results from an enhanced rate of hepatic LDL receptor cycling.[48] An additional benefit is a reduction in the concentration of small, dense LDL, shifting the LDL subfractions to more buoyant, less atherogenic LDL.[49] Interestingly, it is not the baseline LDL level that is the most important factor in predicting the beneficial outcome of statin use. Rather, it is the percentage reduction that seems to be critical. Most of the statins have modest HDL-raising properties (about 5%). Triglyceride concentrations fall by an average of 20% because of a decrease in very low density lipoprotein (VLDL) synthesis and to clearance of VLDL remnant particles by apolipoprotein B/E (LDL) receptors.

Although rosuvastatin would seem to be more efficacious and therefore the statin of choice, subtle differences between the statins and price considerations will impact the decision as to which statin should be used. Claims have been made that water-soluble statins such as rosuvastatin, pravastatin, and fluvastatin are less likely to cause side effects and are, as a result, better tolerated by the patient. They may also have beneficial effects on plaque stability and plasminogen activator inhibitor–1 (PAI-1) that are not seen with the lipid-soluble statins, such as atorvastatin. Also, the metabolism of pravastatin is dual (liver and kidney) and compensatory for the degree of renal insufficiency.[50] This property differs from the other agents in this class; as a result, pravastatin may be safer in patients with renal failure. However, rosuvastatin, atorvastatin, and fluvastatin do not require dose adjustment in renal failure and so may be suitable alternatives.

Side effects Adverse reactions occur less frequently with statins than with the other classes of lipid-lowering agents.

Hepatic dysfunction Although hepatic dysfunction can rarely occur, clinical consequences are exceedingly rare (0.5 to 3% occurrence of persistent elevations in aminotransferases). This primarily occurs during the first 3 months of therapy and is dose dependent. However, two randomized trials have reported no significant difference in the incidence of persistently elevated aminotransferases between statin and placebo therapy.[38,51] The FDA labeling information includes liver function testing before and at 12 weeks following the initiation of statins, at any elevation of dose, and periodically thereafter.[52]

Muscle injury Development of muscle toxicity remains an important concern with the use of the statins.[53] Myopathic syndromes associated with statins span a spectrum of complaints ranging from myalgias (2%), to myositis (0.5%), to overt rhabdomyolysis, which may be associated with acute renal failure (< 0.1%).[54] Enhanced susceptibility to statin-associated myopathy occurs in patients with chronic renal failure, obstructive liver diseases, and untreated hypothyroidism and in patients receiving concurrent therapy with a number of drugs, particularly fibrates and those that inhibit cytochrome CYP3A4. These include cyclosporine, gemfibrozil, nicotinic acid, macrolide antibiotics (e.g., erythromycin), antifungals such as ketoconazole (Nizoral, McNeil-PPC, Fort Washington, Pennsylvania), and HIV protease inhibitors. Unlike other statins, rosuvastatin, pravastatin, and fluvastatin are not extensively metabolized by the CYP3A4 system; as a result, they have few interactions with other drugs. Despite the increased risk of myopathy associated with statin therapy, routine monitoring of serum creatine kinase (CK) levels is not recommended.[52] Patients and clinicians should, however, remain alert for the symptoms of myopathy. In a small number of patients, coenzyme Q_{10} may improve symptoms, but in a systematic review of the literature, there was no level I support for this treatment.[55]

Although several animal studies have suggested that statin therapy is associated with an increased risk of cancer,[56] a meta-analysis of five randomized clinical trials involving 30,817 patients found no association between statin use over a 4- to 6-year period and the risk of fatal or nonfatal cancer.[57] Unusual and as yet unsubstantiated side effects include alopecia and memory disorders.

Although statins are used primarily for the treatment of hypercholesterolemia, there is growing evidence that they increase bone formation, volume, and density and reduce the risk of osteoporotic fractures, particularly in older patients.[58] There is also some evidence that statins may lower blood pressure,[59] prevent Alzheimer disease,[60] and decrease the risk of certain cancers.

Laboratory monitoring of statin therapy Once initiated, a follow-up lipid profile should be performed at 12 weeks and dose adjusted according to the desired reduction. If this cannot be achieved with the original statin, a more powerful dose or drug should be used. In general, although side effects are rare, they do appear to be dose dependent. If necessary, addition of a nonstatin lipid-lowering drug can be considered. At present, the alternative drug of choice would appear to be ezetimibe. Other agents, such as the fibrates and resins, can also be considered.

At the original follow-up, laboratory evaluation of hepatic transaminases can also be evaluated. Subsequent evaluation of hepatic function is unnecessary except if drug interactions are suspected or if transaminases are elevated by more than three times normal. Monitoring should also be considered for patients with preexisting liver disease. There is no benefit to evaluating CK levels unless the patient is symptomatic.[61,62] Further, patients may have symptomatic myalgia but have normal CK levels. If a CK level greater than 10 times normal is encountered, the statin should be discontinued even if the patient is asymptomatic. However, it is also important to realize that CK can be elevated by other conditions, such as hypothyroidism and recent heavy exercise.

Fibrates Fibrates are effective for the treatment of hypertriglyceridemia and combined hyperlipidemia. Four fibrates are currently available in the United States: gemfibrozil, fenofibrate, clofibrate, and fenofibric acid. Clofibrate, however, is now rarely prescribed because it has been associated with cholangiocarcinoma and other gastrointestinal cancers.[63] Other fibrates that are available worldwide include bezafibrate and ciprofibrate.

CLAUDICATION

Although claudication is a manifestation of advanced PAD, it seldom leads to amputation, with the majority of patients staying stable over many years. Accordingly, treatment is usually directed at quality of life. Primarily, treatment should be aimed at lifestyle modification and most importantly at the implementation of a routine walking exercise program to allow improvement in walking distance. Unfortunately, compliance is poor with these methods of management usually because the patient is limited by pain or because of cardiac or respiratory conditions.

Treatment of claudication with medicines may improve both pain-free walking distance (PFWD) and maximal walking distance (MWD), but this should be viewed as supplementary. Currently, FDA approval for the treatment of intermittent claudication is limited to pentoxifylline and cilostazol, with the latter appearing to be more effective in increasing PFWD and MWD. Although many patients will demonstrate an improvement, only half will report subjective improvement in their quality of life following treatment with cilostazol. Further, many patients may simply exhibit a placebo effect.

A number of other medications that are used in Europe, Latin America, and Asia have shown promising results, but further clinical evaluation is necessary. New treatment regimens are under evaluation, and they should be accepted only after they have been proven beneficial and appropriately conducted in scientifically based clinical trials.

Pentoxifylline

Pentoxifylline is a methylxanthine derivative that is now widely available as a generic pharmaceutical. Its primary effect is thought to be an improvement in red blood cell deformability. Other effects include a decrease in blood viscosity, platelet aggregation inhibition, and a reduction in fibrinogen levels.

Although there have been numerous reports of good results concerning pentoxifylline's effects in the treatment of intermittent claudication, two major randomized, double-blind studies have provided conflicting results.[104,105] The first of these two trials compared pentoxifylline with placebo over a 24-week period.[104] The pentoxifylline-treated group had an improvement in PFWD (45% versus a 23% improvement in those given placebo [p = .02]) and MWD (32% improvement versus 20% of those treated with placebo [p = .04]). In common with other claudication studies is the fact that placebo improved PFWD by 23%. Further, despite significant improvements in PFWD and MWD, subjective assessment was not improved in the pentoxifylline group. The second study randomized 150 patients to 1,200 mg a day of pentoxifylline (n = 76) or placebo (n = 74).[105] Differing from the findings of the previous study, these investigators found no improvement in PFWD and only a trend that suggested an improvement in MWD in patients given pentoxifylline (p = .09). However, certain subpopulations of patients showed significant improvement in both PFWD and MWD when compared with placebo. Patients with moderate versus mild disease tended toward significant improvement, and those with chronic duration of the disease (greater than 1 year) also tended toward significance. Unfortunately, the beneficial effects of pentoxifylline may wear off with long-term administration. In a study by Ernst and colleagues, MWD at certain time intervals during the study period did demonstrate significant improvement; however, no significant benefit in PFWD or MWD was observed after 12 weeks of pentoxifylline therapy.[106]

It appears, then, that pentoxifylline may offer a modest improvement in walking distance in some patients, but this may be too small to offer any improvement in quality of life. However, given that this medication is relatively free of side effects and inexpensive, it is frequently used as a first-line medication. The dosage may need to be adjusted if used with other methylxanthine derivatives (e.g., aminophylline or theophylline).

Cilostazol

Cilostazol is a phosphodiesterase type III inhibitor prescribed at a dose of 100 mg twice a day and is now the most widely prescribed medication for improvement in walking distance. It is also available in a generic form and is thought to exert its mechanism of action by inhibiting cyclic adenosine monophosphate (cAMP) phosphodiesterase. By increasing the levels of cAMP in platelets and blood vessels, there is a resultant inhibition of platelet aggregation and a promotion of smooth muscle cell relaxation. Other additional pharmacologic properties include a modest positive lipid effect, mildly increasing HDL cholesterol, and decreasing triglycerides.[107] In vitro studies have shown that there may be a reduction in smooth muscle cell proliferation.[108] As with pentoxifylline, it does not reduce or prevent worsening plaque burden.

Multiple studies have compared cilostazol with placebo with an average improvement in MWD of 140 meters, with 51% of study participants perceiving this improvement versus 30% for those on placebo. Given that this distance may or may not improve quality of life, it is important for the prescribing physician to inform the patient that pain-free walking will be unlikely, and although improved MWD may occur, this may still not be satisfactory.

Given that cilostazol is associated with nausea, diarrhea, palpitations, and headache, it is important that a trial dose of the medicine be prescribed prior to initiating long-term therapy because many patients will not be able to tolerate the medication. In some patients, starting with half the dose and gradually increasing the dose can allow them to take the medication. Cilostazol is contraindicated in patients with congestive heart failure of any severity because other phosphodiesterase inhibitors, but not cilostazol specifically, have been shown to decrease survival rate compared with placebo in patients with class 3 to class 4 (New York Heart Association) congestive heart failure.[109] Further, cilostazol is partially metabolized in the liver by the CYP3A4 or the CYP2C19 enzymes. Because of this, other drugs that rely on these specific hepatic enzymes may increase cilostazol levels. Examples include antifungals, erythromycin, some selective serotonin reuptake inhibitors, and omeprazole. Although the concurrent use of these medications is not discouraged, one may want to consider reducing the daily dose of cilostazol to 50 mg twice a day.

Statins

As mentioned already, all patients with PAD should be considered for a statin irrespective of their underlying cholesterol levels because of the protective effect of statins on cardiovascular morbidity and mortality. However, statins have also been shown to improve walking distance. Mohler and colleagues performed a randomized, double-blind, parallel-design study that included 354 persons with claudication attributable to PAD.[110] Patients were treated with placebo, atorvastatin 10 mg per day, or atorvastatin 80 mg per day for 12 months. The outcome measures included a change in treadmill exercise time and patient-reported measures of physical activity and quality of life based on questionnaires. Maximal walking time after 12 months of treatment with atorvastatin did not change significantly. However, there was improvement in pain-free walking time after 12 months of treatment for the 80 mg ($p = .025$) group compared with the placebo group. A physical activity questionnaire demonstrated improvement in ambulatory ability for the 10 and 80 mg groups ($p = .011$), whereas two quality of life instruments, the Walking Impairment Questionnaire and Short Form 36 Questionnaire, did not show significant change.

Mondillo and colleagues studied 86 patients with PAD, intermittent claudication, and total cholesterol levels greater than 220 mg/dL.[111] Patients were enrolled in a randomized, placebo-controlled, double-blind study. Forty-three patients were assigned to simvastatin (40 mg/day); the remaining 43 patients were assigned to placebo treatment. All patients underwent an exercise test and clinical examination and completed a self-assessment questionnaire at 0, 3, and 6 months. Pain-free and total walking distance, resting and postexercise ankle-brachial indexes, and questionnaire scores were determined at each follow-up. At 6 months, the mean PFWD had increased 90 meters (95% confidence interval [CI] 64 to 116 meters; $p < .005$) more in the simvastatin group than in the placebo group. Similar results were seen for the total walking distance (mean between-group difference in the change, 126 meters; 95% CI 101 to 151 meters; $p < .001$). There was also a greater improvement in claudication symptoms among patients treated with simvastatin. The effects on walking performance and questionnaire scores were also significant at 3 months.

McDermott and colleagues attempted to evaluate whether such improvement was related to achieved cholesterol levels in patients with and without PAD.[112] They found that statin use was associated with superior leg functioning compared with no statin use, independent of cholesterol levels and other potential confounders, such as aspirin, ACE inhibitors, vasodilators, or beta blockers. Their data suggest that the non–cholesterol-lowering properties of statins may favorably influence functioning in persons with and without PAD.

Aspirin

Aspirin has not been demonstrated to improve walking distance or symptoms in patients with intermittent claudication. Further, specific studies in the PAD population using aspirin have not shown a statistically significant reduction in cardiovascular events.[99] Thus, although antiplatelet drugs are clearly indicated in the overall management of PAD, aspirin does not have specific FDA approval for use in this patient population.[113]

Clopidogrel

There is no evidence to suggest that the symptoms of claudication are reduced by long-term treatment with clopidogrel.

STROKE

There is clear evidence that medical management can significantly reduce the occurrence of stroke. Accordingly, it would seem almost mandatory that patients with carotid artery plaque should be treated with a statin and an antiplatelet agent such as aspirin, aspirin and dipyridamole combination, or clopidogrel, although which medication is superior is still a matter of conjecture.[114,115] Current data would suggest that combination therapy of aspirin and dipyridamole may be superior to aspirin alone,[114] but there are no compelling data to suggest that this combination is superior to clopidogrel. Also, warfarin adds no advantage to aspirin in the prevention of recurrent ischemic stroke.[116]

In the HOPE study, the addition of the ACE inhibitor ramipril added stroke protection irrespective of its effects on blood pressure.[19] However, hypertension should be actively and aggressively controlled,[117] except in the very elderly, for whom more moderate control may be safer.

Also, the use of statins perioperatively may reduce the incidence of perioperative stroke.[118] In a nonrandomized retrospective analysis, Kennedy and colleagues found a protective effect of statin therapy in symptomatic patients pretreated at the time of carotid endarterectomy (CEA).[118] This was not seen in asymptomatic patients. The latter finding may be because the plaque of asymptomatic patients is not in a state of inflammation that would be ameliorated by statins. This hypothesis is supported by histologic studies performed by Molloy and colleagues.[119] They performed an observational study on 137 patients undergoing CEA. Patients on statins were less likely to have had symptoms in the 4 weeks before CEA ($p = .0049$) and were less likely to have spontaneous cerebral embolization detected by transcranial Doppler ultrasonography ($p = .0459$).

Beneficial results following CEA were also demonstrated by McGirt and colleagues.[120] Adjusting for all demographics and comorbidities in multivariate analysis, statin use independently reduced the odds of stroke threefold (odds ratio [OR] [95% CI], 0.35 [0.15 to 0.85]; $p < .05$) and death fivefold (OR [95% CI], 0.20 [0.04 to 0.99]; $p < .05$).

There are also data that show that initiating statins after an ischemic stroke can improve recovery.[121–123] Statin use prior to ischemic stroke is also associated with reduced mortality and better recovery.[124] Unfortunately, despite these benefits, statin use remains low (40%) following CEA.[125] The relationship between serum lipid levels and recurrent carotid stenosis has been postulated for many years[126–128] and reconfirmed in recent literature by LaMuraglia and colleagues.[129] These same authors also showed that concurrent administration of a lipid-lowering drug had a profound effect on early recurrent carotid stenosis and that these drugs might have other relevant properties that might promote the anatomic durability of the CEA reconstruction. Such effects may include the decrease in the inflammatory response in the vessel wall, the increase in circulating endothelial progenitor cells, and the promotion of smooth muscle cell apoptosis, all of which have been described with the use of statins and are known to have a role in the restenotic process.[130,131]

Although perioperative clopidogrel may also help reduce postendarterectomy neurologic events, increased bleeding has prompted us to discontinue this medication a week prior to endarterectomy except in patients who are having ongoing symptoms. However, antiplatelet agents such as clopidogrel should be started at least 3 days prior to carotid stenting and continued for at least 3 months thereafter.

Perioperative Medications

Based on evidence that statins may have benefit in reducing early ischemic events following acute coronary syndromes and coronary revascularization,[132] investigators began to evaluate whether similar reductions in cardiac morbidity could be achieved with statins in the vascular patient.[133,134] However, unless LDL levels are driven very low, regression of atherosclerosis occurs only in a minority of patients, if at all, yet clinical benefits of statins are seen often within 6 months of initiating therapy. This suggests that factors other than cholesterol lowering or plaque regression are also important in improving outcome.

The Statins for Risk Reduction in Surgery (StaRRS) study is a retrospective study that recorded patient characteristics, past medical history, and admission medications on all patients undergoing CEA, aortic surgery, or lower extremity revascularization over a 2-year period (January 1999 to December 2000) at a tertiary referral center.[135] Complications occurred in 157 of 1,163 eligible hospitalizations and were significantly fewer in patients receiving statins (9.9%) than in those not receiving statins (16.5%, $p = .001$). The difference was mostly accounted for by reductions in myocardial ischemia and congestive heart failure. After adjusting for other significant predictors of perioperative complications (age, gender, type of surgery, emergent surgery, left ventricular dysfunction, and diabetes mellitus), statins still conferred a highly significant protective effect (OR 0.52, $p = .001$).

Kertai and colleagues studied 570 patients (mean age 69 ± 9 years, 486 males) who underwent abdominal aortic aneurysm (AAA) surgery between 1991 and 2001.[136] The main outcome was a composite of perioperative mortality and myocardial infarction within 30 days of surgery. Perioperative mortality or myocardial infarction occurred in 51 (8.9%) patients. The incidence of the composite end point was significantly lower in statin users compared with nonusers (3.7% versus 11.0%; crude OR 0.31, 95% CI 0.13 to 0.74; $p = .01$). Beta blocker use was also associated with a significant reduction in the composite end point (OR 0.24, 95% CI 0.11 to 0.54). Patients using a combination of statins and beta blockers appeared to be at lower risk for the composite end point across multiple cardiac risk strata; in particular, patients with three or more risk factors experienced significantly lower perioperative events.

Durazzo and colleagues randomly assigned 50 patients to receive atorvastatin and 50 patients to placebo once a day for 45 days, irrespective of their serum cholesterol concentration.[137] Vascular surgery was performed on average 30 days after randomization, and patients were prospectively followed up over 6 months. The incidence of cardiac events was more than three times higher with placebo (26.0%) compared with atorvastatin (8.0%; $p = .031$).

Clearly, the effect of statins on outcome noted in these studies showed that a beneficial effect occurred more rapidly than can be explained by a simple reduction in low-density cholesterol levels. This appears to support the concept that statins have an antiinflammatory effect on coronary vasculature, thus reducing sudden coronary thrombosis.[138,139] It should be noted, however, that not all evaluations prove a beneficial effect of statins on cardiovascular surgery outcomes.[140]

Although commonly used for their cardioprotective effect, perioperative beta blocker use has recently been questioned because of an apparent slight increase in stroke. However, this has not been our experience, and we continue to prescribe these medications prior to and during major intra-abdominal arterial surgery. Antiplatelet agents are routinely avoided for at least a week to 10 days before such procedures, especially if spinal or epidural anesthesia is anticipated.

GRAFT PATENCY

Two articles suggest that statin therapy may also play a role in graft patency,[141,142] and we are currently evaluating the data in the PREVENT III study to see if these data can be confirmed in this large study of infrainguinal vein bypasses.[143]

Henke and colleagues evaluated 293 patients who underwent 338 infrainguinal bypass procedures with autologous veins ($n = 218$), prosthetic grafts ($n = 88$), or composite prosthetic vein grafts ($n = 32$).[141] Statin drugs were taken by 56% of patients, ACE inhibitors by 54% of patients, and antiplatelet agents or warfarin sodium by 93% of patients. Statins were associated with increased graft patency (OR 3.7; 95% CI 2.1 to 6.4) and a lower rate of amputation. Abbruzzese and colleagues performed a retrospective analysis of consecutive 172 patients who underwent [illegible] primary [illegible] infrainguinal reconstructions with a single segment of great saphenous vein.[142] Patients were categorized according to concurrent use of a statin (94 in the statin group, 95 in the control group). Although there was no difference in primary patency, patients on statins had higher primary-revised (94% ± 2% versus 83% ± 5%; $p < .02$) and secondary (97% ± 2% versus 87% ± 4%; $p < .02$) graft patency rates at 2 years. The risk of graft failure was 3.2-fold higher for the control group. Perioperative cholesterol levels (available in 47% of patients) were not statistically different between groups.

AORTIC ANEURYSMS

Given that AAA formation may be a result of inflammation and extracellular matrix remodeling mediated by matrix metalloproteinases (MMPs) and that statins have an antiinflammatory effect, it is not surprising that a possible beneficial effect of statins on decreasing aneurysm development has been investigated. Kalyanasundaram and colleagues studied this in rats and found that AAAs in rats given statins were smaller than in those fed a placebo.[144] MMP-9 and nuclear factor—κB protein levels were also decreased in the aortas of simvastatin-treated animals. Similar findings were also noted by Steinmetz and colleagues, who found that the mechanisms of this effect were independent of lipid lowering and included preservation of medial elastin and smooth muscle cells, as well as altered aortic wall expression of MMPs and their inhibitors.[145] Nagashima and colleagues evaluated the aortic wall in patients, some of whom had been on cerivastatin.[146] Cerivastatin significantly reduced the tissue levels of both total and active MMP-9 in a concentration-dependent manner ($p < .001$) by inhibiting the activation of neutrophils and macrophages. However, cerivastatin has been withdrawn from the US market.

There are also experimental suggestions that doxycycline, a generic tetracycline, may reduce aneurysm growth.[147,148] Given that the side effects of this drug are very rare, except for increased photosensitivity, I routinely use 100 mg daily in the management of small AAAs.

NONATHEROSCLEROTIC VASCULAR DISEASE

The vascular specialist may be confronted with patients suffering from a multitude of nonatherosclerotic conditions affecting the arterial system. These usually will manifest with Raynaud syndrome and, in advanced cases, with digit ischemia and gangrene. In such patients, an attempt should be made to differentiate the underlying etiology and to alleviate the symptoms. In most patients, avoidance of cold and digit injury is all that is required. However, in advanced cases in which ulceration or gangrene is evidenced, medications may be helpful. These will include vasodilators such as calcium channel blockers. Antiplatelet agents as well as pentoxifylline and clopidogrel have been used, but there is no level I evidence supporting their use.

Miscellaneous Medications: Over-the-Counter Medications, Vitamins, and Herbs

Atherosclerosis is a multifactorial process related to interaction between a multitude of genetic processes and environmental pressures. Not surprisingly, many medications, herbs, and vitamins have been suggested to have beneficial effects.[149] For example, homocysteine-lowering vitamin B_{12} compounds and folic acid have been touted as effective. However, although elevated levels of homocysteine are associated with premature development of atherosclerosis and coronary neointimal hyperplasia following stents, lowering homocysteine has not been proven to effect clinical outcome.[85,150] Similarly, antioxidants such as vitamin E have also not been effective.[151] Despite a large amount of literature, very few articles have enough scientific merit to warrant serious consideration, and many offer conflicting results. This accounts for the confusion and suspicion that surround many of these treatments.

Currently, none of the treatment modalities except diet and fish oils[152] can be strongly suggested as beneficial for most patients. However, individual patients may benefit from some of these miscellaneous compounds. Examples would be patients on dialysis or those who are nutritionally deficient, such as the very elderly.

Summary

The ravages of atherosclerosis and other rarer conditions affecting the vascular system continue to account for most deaths in the developed world. Increasingly, vascular surgeons are finding themselves at the forefront of the fight against this scourge. Although advances in the technical method of treatment, such as angioplasty, stents, endografts, atherectomy, and lytic therapy, are all achieving some success in reducing morbidity and mortality, it is anticipated that optimal medical management will have an even more pronounced salutary effect. As such, the modern vascular surgeon must be able not only to operate and dilate but also to medicate.

Financial Disclosures: None Reported

References

1. Bismuth J, Klitford L, Sillesen H. The lack of cardiovascular risk factor management in patients with critical limb ischemia. Eur J Vasc Endovasc Surg 2001;21:143–6.
2. Anand SS, Kundi A, Eikelboom J, et al. Low rates of preventive practices in patients with peripheral vascular disease. Can J Cardiol 1999;15:1259–63.
3. Samson RH. Introduction—risk factors in vascular disease: who is really at risk and what can be done about it? Semin Vasc Surg 2008; 21:117–8.
4. Kannel WB, McGee DL. Diabetes and cardiovascular disease. The Framingham Study. JAMA 1979;241:2035–8.
5. Gerstein HC, Miller ME, Byington RP, et al, for the Action to Control Cardiovascular Risk in Diabetes Study Group. Effects of intensive glucose lowering in type 2 diabetes. N Engl J Med 2008;358:2545–9.
6. Jorenby DE. Smoking cessation strategies for the 21st century. Circulation 2001;104: E51–2.
7. Kenfield SA, Stampfer MJ, Rosner BA, et al. Smoking and smoking cessation in relation to mortality in women. JAMA 2008;299: 2037–47.
8. Franklin SS, Larson MG, Khan SA, et al. Does the relation of blood pressure to coronary heart disease risk change with aging? The Framingham Heart Study. Circulation 2001;103:1245.
9. Benetos A, Thomas F, Bean K, et al. Prognostic value of systolic and diastolic blood pressure in treated hypertensive men. Arch Intern Med 2002;62:577.
10. Strandberg TE, Salomaa VV, Vanhanen HT, et al. Isolated diastolic hypertension, pulse pressure, and mean arterial pressure as predictors of mortality during a follow-up of up to 32 years. Hypertension 2002;20:399.
11. Neal B, MacMahon S, Chapman N. Effects of ACE inhibitors, calcium antagonists, and other blood-pressure-lowering drugs: results of prospectively designed overviews of randomised trials. Blood Pressure Lowering Treatment Trialists' Collaboration. Lancet 2000;356:1955.
12. Ogden LG, He J, Lydick E, et al. Long-term absolute benefit of lowering blood pressure in hypertensive patients according to the JNC VI risk stratification. Hypertension 2000; 35:539.
13. Samson RH, Showalter DP, Liss E. Incidence of hypertension in patients referred for vascular laboratory testing. [In press]
14. Samson RH. Periprocedural hypertension. Current concepts in management for the vascular surgeon. Vasc Endovascular Surg 2004;38:361–6.
15. Lin PH, Appel LJ, Funk K, et al. The PREMIER intervention helps participants follow the Dietary Approaches to Stop Hypertension dietary pattern and the current Dietary Reference Intakes recommendations. J Am Diet Assoc 2007;107: 1541–51.
16. The Seventh Report of the Joint National Committee on Prevention, Detection, Evaluation, and Treatment of High Blood Pressure. The JNC 7 report. JAMA 2003;289: 2560.
17. Hiatt WR, Stoll S, Nies AS. Effect of β-adrenergic blockers on the peripheral circulation in patients with peripheral vascular disease. Circulation 1985;72:1226–31.
18. Solomon SA, Ramsay LE, Yeo WW, et al. β Blockade and intermittent claudication: placebo controlled trial of atenolol and nifedipine and their combination. BMJ 1991; 303:1100–4.
19. Heart Outcomes Prevention Evaluation Study Investigators. Effects of an angiotensin-converting-enzyme inhibitor, ramipril, on cardiovascular events in high-risk patients. N Engl J Med 2000;342:145–53.
20. Yusuf S, Gerstein H, Hoogwerf B, et al; HOPE Study Investigators. Ramipril and the development of diabetes. JAMA 2001;286: 1882–5.

21. Samson RH. Nonoperative management of patients with vascular conditions, pharmaceutical initiatives to combat atherosclerosis—what to do with the good, the bad, and the ugly lipoproteins. Semin Vasc Surg 2002;15:204–15.
22. Brunzell JD. Hypertriglyceridemia. N Engl J Med 2007;357:1009–17.
23. Johansson J, Egberg N, Hohnsson H, et al. Serum lipoproteins and hemostatic function in intermittent claudication. Arterioscler Thromb 1993;13:1441–8.
24. Hiatt WR, Hoag S, Hamman RF. Effect of diagnostic criteria on the prevalence of peripheral arterial disease. The San Luis Valley diabetes study. Circulation 1995;91:1472–9.
25. Lupattelli G, Siepi D, Pasqualini L, et al. Lipoprotein (a) in peripheral arterial occlusive disease. Vasa 1994;23:321–4.
26. Valentine RJ, Kaplan HS, Green R, et al. Lipoprotein (a), homocysteine, and hypercoagulable states in young men with premature peripheral atherosclerosis: a prospective, controlled analysis. J Vasc Surg 1996;23:53–61.
27. Ross R. Cellular and molecular studies of atherosclerosis. Atherosclerosis 1997;131:S3–4.
28. Berliner JA, Navab M, Fogelman AM, et al. Atherosclerosis: basic mechanisms. Oxidation, inflammation, and genetics. Circulation 1995;91:2488–96.
29. Abdellaoui A, Al-Khaffaf H. C-reactive protein (CRP) as a marker in peripheral vascular disease. Eur J Vasc Endovasc Surg 2007;34:18–22.
30. Ridker PM, Hennekens CH, Buring JE, et al. C-reactive protein and other markers of inflammation in the prediction of cardiovascular disease in women. N Engl J Med 2000;342:836–43.
31. Ridker PM, Stampfer MJ, Rifai N. Novel risk factors for systemic atherosclerosis: a comparison of C-reactive protein, fibrinogen, homocysteine, lipoprotein(a), and standard cholesterol screening as predictors of peripheral arterial disease. JAMA 2001;285:2481–5.
32. Ridker PM, Cushman M, Stampfer MJ, et al. Plasma concentration of C-reactive protein and risk of developing peripheral vascular disease. Circulation 1998;97:425–8.
33. Rossi E, Biasucci LM, Citterio F, et al. Risk of myocardial infarction and angina in patients with severe peripheral vascular disease: predictive role of C-reactive protein. Circulation 2002;105:800–3.
34. Ridker PM, Rifai N, Clearfield M, et al. Measurement of C-reactive protein for the targeting of statin therapy in the primary prevention of acute coronary events. N Engl J Med 2001;344:1959–65.
35. Ridker PM, Danielson E, Fonseca FAH, et al. Rosuvastatin to prevent vascular events in men and women with elevated C-reactive protein. N Engl J Med 2008;359:2195–207.
36. Zacho J, Tybjaerg-Hansen A, Jensen JS, et al. Genetically elevated C-reactive protein and ischemic vascular disease. N Engl J Med 2008;359:1897–908.
37. Frick MH, Elo O, Haapa K, et al. Helsinki Heart Study: primary-prevention trial with gemfibrozil in middle-aged men with dyslipidemia. Safety of treatment, changes in risk factors, and incidence of coronary heart disease. N Engl J Med 1987;317:1237–45.
38. Scandinavian Simvastatin Survival Study Group. Randomised trial of cholesterol lowering in 4444 patients with coronary heart disease: the Scandinavian Simvastatin Survival Study (4S). Lancet 1994;344:1383–9.
39. Kramer JR, Proudfit WL, Loop FD, et al. Late follow-up of 781 patients undergoing percutaneous transluminal coronary angioplasty or coronary artery bypass grafting. Am Heart J 1989;118:1144–53.
40. Buchwald H, Bourdages HR, Campos CT, et al. Impact of cholesterol reduction on peripheral arterial disease in the Program on the Surgical Control of the Hyperlipidemias (POSCH). Surgery 1996;120:672–9.
41. MRC/BHF Heart Protection Study of cholesterol lowering with simvastatin in 20,536 high-risk individuals: a randomised placebo-controlled trial. Lancet 2002;360:7–22.
42. Butowski PF, Winder AF. Usual care dietary practice, achievement and implications for medication in the management of hypercholesterolemia: data from the UK Lipid Clinics Programme. Eur Heart J 1998;19:1328–33.
43. Andrade SE, Walerks AM, Gottlieb LK, et al. Discontinuation of antihyperlipidemic drugs: do rates reported in clinical trials reflect rates in primary care settings? N Engl J Med 1995;332:1125–31.
44. Samson RH. The role of statin drugs in the management of the peripheral vascular patient. Vasc Endovasc Surg 2008;42:352–66.
45. Jones P, Kafonek S, Laurora, I, et al, for the CURVES Investigators. Comparative dose efficacy study of atorvastatin versus simvastatin, pravastatin, lovastatin, and fluvastatin in patients with hypercholesterolemia (the CURVES study). Am J Cardiol 1998;81:582–7.
46. Brown AS, Bakker-Arkema RG, Yellen L, et al. Treating patients with documented atherosclerosis to National Cholesterol Education Program recommended low-density-lipoprotein cholesterol goals with atorvastatin, fluvastatin, lovastatin and simvastatin. J Am Coll Cardiol 1998;32:665–72.
47. Istvan ES, Deisenhofer J. Structural mechanism for statin inhibition of HMG-CoA reductase. Science 2001;292:1160–4.
48. Ness GC, Zhao Z, Lopez D. Inhibitors of cholesterol biosynthesis increase hepatic low density lipoprotein receptor protein degradation. Arch Biochem Biophys 1996;325:242–8.
49. Marz W, Scharnagl H, Abletshauser C, et al. Fluvastatin lowers atherogenic dense low-density lipoproteins in postmenopausal women with the atherogenic lipoprotein phenotype. Circulation 2001;103:1942–8.
50. Halstenson CE, Triscari J, DeVault A, et al. Single-dose pharmacokinetics of pravastatin and metabolites in patients with renal impairment. J Clin Pharmacol 1992;32:124–32.
51. Downs JR, Clearfield M, Weis S, et al. Primary prevention of acute coronary events with lovastatin in men and women with average cholesterol levels: results of AFCAPS/TexCAPS. Air Force/Texas Coronary Atherosclerosis Prevention Study. JAMA 1998;279:1615–22.
52. Weismantel D. What laboratory monitoring is appropriate to detect adverse drug reactions in patients on cholesterol-lowering agents? J Fam Pract 2001;50:927–8.
53. Thompson PD, Clarkson P, Karas RH. Statin-associated myopathy. JAMA 2003;289:1681–90.
54. Grundy SM. HMG-CoA reductase inhibitors for treatment of hypercholesterolemia. N Engl J Med 1988;319:24–33.
55. Marcoff L, Thompson PD. The role of coenzyme Q10 in statin-associated myopathy: a systematic review. J Am Coll Cardiol 2007;49:2231–7.
56. Newman TB, Hulley SB. Carcinogenicity of lipid-lowering drugs. JAMA 1996;275:55–60.
57. Bjerre LM, LeLorier J. Do statins cause cancer? A meta-analysis of large randomized clinical trials. Am J Med 2001;110:716–23.
58. Edwards CJ, Russell RG, Spector TD. Statins and bone: myth or reality? Calcif Tissue Int 2001;69:63–6.
59. Sposito AC, Mansur AP, Coelho OR, et al. Additional reduction in blood pressure after cholesterol-lowering treatment by statins (lovastatin or pravastatin) in hypercholesterolemic patients using angiotensin-converting enzyme inhibitors (enalapril or lisinopril). Am J Cardiol 1999;83:1497–9.
60. Scott HD, Laake K. Statins for the prevention of Alzheimer's disease. Cochrane Database Syst Rev 2001;(4):CD003160.
61. Gotto AM Jr. Safety and statin therapy: reconsidering the risks and benefits. Arch Intern Med 2003;163:657–9.
62. Glueck CJ, Rawal B, Khan NA, et al. Should high creatine kinase discourage the initiation or continuance of statins for the treatment of hypercholesterolemia? Metabolism 2009;58:233–8.
63. WHO cooperative trial on primary prevention of ischaemic heart disease with clofibrate to lower serum cholesterol: final mortality follow-up. Report of the Committee of Principal Investigators. Lancet 1984;2:600–4.
64. Staels B, Dallongeville J, Auwerx J, et al. Mechanism of action of fibrates on lipid and lipoprotein metabolism. Circulation 1998;98:2088–93.
65. Vu-Dac N, Schoonjans K, Kosykh V, et al. Fibrates increase human apolipoprotein A-II expression through activation of the peroxisome proliferator-activated receptor. J Clin Invest 1995;96:741–50.
66. Berthou L, Duverger N, Ammanuel F, et al. Opposite regulation of human versus mouse apoprotein A-I by fibrates in human apolipoprotein-A-I transgenic mice. J Clin Invest 1996;97:2408–16.
67. Jin F-Y, Kamanna VS, Chuang M-Y, et al. Gemfibrozil stimulates apolipoprotein A-I synthesis and secretion by stabilization of mRNA transcripts in human hepatoblastoma cell line (Hep G2). Arterioscler Thromb Vasc Biol 1996;16:1052–62.
68. Jones PH, Pownall HJ, Patsch W, et al. Effect of gemfibrozil on levels of lipoprotein(a) in type II hyperlipoproteinemia subjects. J Lipid Res 1996;37:1298–308.
69. Nordt TK, Kornas K, Peter K, et al. Attenuation by gemfibrozil of expression of plasminogen activator inhibitor type 1 induced by insulin and its precursors. Circulation 1997;95:677–83.
70. Westphal S, Dierkes J, Luley C. Effects of fenofibrate and gemfibrozil on plasma homocysteine. Lancet 2001;358:39–40.
71. Dierkes J, Westphal S, Luley C. Serum homocysteine increases after therapy with fenofibrate or bezafibrate. Lancet 1999;354:219–20.
72. Frick MH, Elo O, Haapa K, et al. Helsinki Heart Study: primary prevention trial with gemfibrozil in middle-aged men with dyslipidemia. Safety of treatment, changes in risk factors, and incidence of coronary heart disease. N Engl J Med 1987;317:1237–45.
73. Magarian GJ, Lucas LM, Colley C. Gemfibrozil-induced myopathy. Arch Intern Med 1991;151:1873–4.
74. Pierce LR, Wysowski DK, Gross TP. Myopathy and rhabdomyolysis with lovastatin-gemfibrozil combination therapy. JAMA 1990;264:71–5.
75. Athyros VG, Papageorgiou AA, Hatzikonstandinou HA, et al. Safety and efficacy of long-term statin-fibrate combination in patients with refractory familial combined hyperlipidemia. Am J Cardiol 1997;80:608–13.
76. Miller DB, Spence JD. Clinical pharmacokinetics of fibric acid derivatives (fibrates). Clin Pharmacokinet 1998;34:155–62.

77. Grundy SM, Mok HY, Zech L, et al. Influence of nicotinic acid on metabolism of cholesterol and triglycerides in man. J Lipid Res 1981;22:24–36.
78. Illingworth DR, Stein EA, Mitchel YB, et al. Comparative effects of lovastatin and niacin in primary hypercholesterolemia. A prospective trial. Arch Intern Med 1994;154:1586–95.
79. Philipp CS, Cisar LA, Saidi P, et al. Effect of niacin supplementation on fibrinogen levels in patients with peripheral vascular disease. Am J Cardiol 1998;82:697–9.
80. Probstfield JL, Hunninghake DB. Nicotinic acid as a lipoprotein-altering agent. Therapy directed by the primary physician. Arch Intern Med 1994;154:1557–9.
81. Guyton JR, Goldberg AC, Kreisberg RA, et al. Effectiveness of once-nightly dosing of extended-release niacin alone and in combination for hypercholesterolemia. Am J Cardiol 1998;82:737–43.
82. Etchason JA, Miller TD, Squires RW, et al. Niacin-induced hepatitis: a potential side effect with low-dose time-release niacin. Mayo Clin Proc 1991;66:23–8.
83. Garg A, Grundy SM. Nicotinic acid as therapy for dyslipidemia in non-insulin-dependent diabetes mellitus. JAMA 1990;264:723–6.
84. Pasternak RC, Kolman BS. Unstable myocardial ischemia after the initiation of niacin therapy. Am J Cardiol 1991;67:904–6.
85. Samson RH, Yungst Z, Showalter DP. Homocysteine, a risk factor for carotid atherosclerosis, is not a risk factor for early recurrent carotid stenosis following carotid endarterectomy. Vasc Endovasc Surg 2004;38:345–8.
86. Garg R, Malinow M, Pettinger M, et al. Niacin treatment increases plasma homocyst(e)ine levels. Am Heart J 1999;138:1082–7.
87. Shepherd J, Packard CJ, Morgan HG, et al. The effects of cholestyramine on high density lipoprotein metabolism. Atherosclerosis 1979;33:433–44.
88. Davidson MH, Dillon MA, Gordon B, et al. Colesevelam hydrochloride (cholestagel): a new, potent bile acid sequestrant associated with a low incidence of gastrointestinal side effects. Arch Intern Med 1999;159:1893–900.
89. Insull W Jr, Toth P, Mullican W, et al. Effectiveness of colesevelam hydrochloride in decreasing LDL cholesterol in patients with primary hypercholesterolemia: a 24-week randomized controlled trial. Mayo Clin Proc 2001;76:971–82.
90. Pan HY, DeVault AR, Swites BJ, et al. Pharmacokinetics and pharmacodynamics of pravastatin alone and with cholestyramine in hypercholesterolemia. Clin Pharmacol Ther 1990;48:201–7.
91. Spence JD, Huff MW, Heidenheim P, et al. Combination therapy with colestipol and psyllium mucilloid in patients with hyperlipidemia. Ann Intern Med 1995;123:493–9.
92. Filippatos TD, Mikhailidis DP. Lipid-lowering drugs acting at the level of the gastrointestinal tract. Curr Pharm Des 2009;15:490–516.
93. Gupta EK, Ito MK. Ezetimibe: the first in a novel class of selective cholesterol-absorption inhibitors. Heart Dis 2002;4:399–409.
94. Pandor A, Ara RM, Tumur I, et al. Ezetimibe monotherapy for cholesterol lowering in 2,722 people: systematic review and meta-analysis of randomized controlled trials. J Intern Med 2009;265:568–80.
95. Mitka M. Controversies surround heart drug study questions about Vytorin and trial sponsors' conduct. JAMA 2008;299:885–7.
96. Kastelein JJ, Akdim F, Stroes ES, et al, for the ENHANCE Investigators. Simvastatin with or without ezetimibe in familial hypercholesterolemia. N Engl J Med 2008;358:1431–43.
97. Zusman RM, Chesebro JH, Comerota A, et al. Antiplatelet therapy in the prevention of ischemic vascular events: literature review and evidence-based guidelines for drug selection. Clin Cardiol 1999;22:559–73.
98. Collaborative meta-analysis of randomised trials of antiplatelet therapy for prevention of death, myocardial infarction, and stroke in high risk patients. BMJ 2002;324:71–86.
99. Collaborative overview of randomised trials of antiplatelet therapy—I: prevention of death, myocardial infarction, and stroke by prolonged antiplatelet therapy in various categories of patients. Antiplatelet Trialists' Collaboration. BMJ 1994;308:81–106.
100. Gum PA, Kottke-Marchant K, Welsh PA, et al. A prospective, blinded determination of the natural history of aspirin resistance among stable patients with cardiovascular disease. J Am Coll Cardiol 2003;41:961–5.
101. CAPRIE Steering Committee. A randomized, blinded trial of clopidogrel versus aspirin in patients at risk of ischemic events (CAPRIE). Lancet 1996;348:1329–39.
102. Dunn P, Macaulay TE, Brennan DM, et al. Baseline proton pump inhibitor use is associated with increased cardiovascular events with and without the use of clopidogrel in the CREDO Trial. Circulation 2008;118:S815.
103. Bhatt DL, Fox KA, Hacke W, et al, for the CHARISMA Investigators. Clopidogrel and aspirin versus aspirin alone for the prevention of atherothrombotic events. N Engl J Med 2006;354:1706–17.
104. Porter JM, Culter BS, Lee BY, et al. Pentoxifylline efficacy in the treatment of intermittent claudication: multicenter controlled double blind trial with objective assessment of chronic occlusive arterial disease patients. Am Heart J 1982;104:66–72.
105. Lindgärde F, Jelnes R, Björkman H, et al. Conservative drug treatment in patients with moderately severe chronic occlusive peripheral arterial disease. Circulation 1989;80:1549–56.
106. Ernst E, Kollár L, Resch KL. Does pentoxifylline prolong the walking distance in exercised claudicants? A placebo-controlled double-blind trial. Angiology 1992;42:121–5.
107. Money SR, Herd JA, Isaacsohn JL, et al. Effect of cilostazol on walking distances in patients with intermittent claudication caused by peripheral vascular disease. J Vasc Surg 1998;27:267–75.
108. Takahashi S, Oida K, Fujiwara R, et al. Effect of cilostazol, a cyclic AMP phosphodiesterase inhibitor, on the proliferation of rat aortic smooth muscle cells in culture. J Cardiovasc Pharmacol 1992;20:900–6.
109. Packer M, Carver JR, Rodeheffer RJ, et al. Effect of oral milrinone on mortality in severe chronic heart failure. The PROMISE study research group. N Eng J Med 1991;325:1468–75.
110. Mohler ER 3rd, Hiatt WR, Creager MA. Cholesterol reduction with atorvastatin improves walking distance in patients with peripheral arterial disease. Circulation 2003;108:1481–6.
111. Mondillo S, Ballo P, Barbati R, et al. Effects of simvastatin on walking performance and symptoms of intermittent claudication in hypercholesterolemic patients with peripheral vascular disease. Am J Med 2003;114:359–64.
112. McDermott MM, Guralnik JM, Greenland P, et al. Statin use and leg functioning in patients with and without lower-extremity peripheral arterial disease. Circulation 2003;107:757–61.
113. Food and Drug Administration. Internal analgesic, antipyretic, and antirheumatic drug products for over-the-counter human use; final rule for professional labeling of aspirin, buffered aspirin, and aspirin in combination with antacid drug products. Fed Reg 1998;63:56802–19.
114. ESPRIT Study Group, Halkes PH, van Gijn J, Kappelle LJ, et al. Aspirin plus dipyridamole versus aspirin alone after cerebral ischaemia of arterial origin (ESPRIT): randomised controlled trial. Lancet 2006;367:1665–73.
115. Mohler ER 3rd. Combination antiplatelet therapy in patients with peripheral arterial disease: is the best therapy aspirin, clopidogrel, or both? Catheter Cardiovasc Interv 2009;74 Suppl 1: S1–6.
116. Redman AR, Allen LC. Warfarin versus aspirin in the secondary prevention of stroke: the WARSS study. Curr Atheroscler Rep 2002;4:319–25.
117. Lindholm LH, Ibsen H, Dahlöf B, et al, for the LIFE Study Group. Cardiovascular morbidity and mortality in patients with diabetes in the Losartan Intervention For Endpoint reduction in hypertension study (LIFE): a randomised trial against atenolol. Lancet 2002;359:1004–10.
118. Kennedy J, Quan H, Buchan AM, et al. Statins are associated with better outcomes after carotid endarterectomy in symptomatic patients. Stroke 2005;36:2072–6.
119. Molloy KJ, Thompson MM, Schwalbe EC, et al. Comparison of levels of matrix metalloproteinases, tissue inhibitor of metalloproteinases, interleukins, and tissue necrosis factor in carotid endarterectomy specimens from patients on versus not on statins preoperatively. Am J Cardiol 2004;94:144–6.
120. McGirt MJ, Perler BA, Brooke BS, et al. 3-Hydroxy-3-methylglutaryl coenzyme A reductase inhibitors reduce the risk of perioperative stroke and mortality after carotid endarterectomy. Vasc Surg 2005;42:829–36.
121. Moonis M, Kane K, Schwiderski U, et al. HMG-CoA reductase inhibitors improve acute ischemic stroke outcome. Stroke 2005;36:1298–300.
122. Marti-Fabregas J, Gomis M, Arboix A, et al. Favorable outcome of ischemic stroke in patients pretreated with statins. Stroke 2004;35:1117–21.
123. Elkind MS, Flint AC, Sciacca RR, et al. Lipid-lowering agent use at ischemic stroke onset is associated with decreased mortality. Neurology 2005;65:253–8.
124. Aslanyan S, Weir CJ, McInnes GT, et al. Statin administration prior to ischaemic stroke onset and survival: exploratory evidence from matched treatment-control study. Eur J Neurol 2005;12:493–8.
125. Betancourt M, Van Stavern RB, Share D. Are patients receiving maximal medical therapy following carotid endarterectomy? Perspect Vasc Surg Endovasc Ther 2005;17:272.
126. Rapp JH, Qvarfordt P, Krupski WC, et al. Hypercholesterolemia and early restenosis after carotid endarterectomy. Surgery 1987;101:277–82.
127. Cuming R, Worrell P, Woolcock NE, et al. The influence of smoking and lipids on restenosis after carotid endarterectomy. Eur J Vasc Surg 1993;7:572–6.
128. Colyvas N, Rapp JH, Phillips NR, et al. Relation of plasma lipid and apoprotein levels to progressive intimal hyperplasia after arterial endarterectomy. Circulation 1992;85:1286–92.
129. LaMuraglia GM, Stoner MC, Brewster DC, et al. Determinants of carotid endarterectomy anatomic durability: effects of serum lipids

Table 1 Types and Causes of Lower Extremity Ulcers

Vascular	Venous Arterial Mixed Vascular malformations Lymphatic Primary lymphedema Secondary lymphedema Pyoderma gangrenosum
Vasculitic	Systemic lupus erythematosus Rheumatoid arthritis Wegener granulomatosis Scleroderma Polyarteritis nodosa
Neuropathic	Diabetic neuropathic ulcer Peripheral neuropathy, with or without ischemia
Traumatic	Frostbite Burns Factitious Injury
Radiation-induced	Acute Chronic
Hematologic/dyscrasias	Sickle cell ulcers Polycythemia vera Thalassemia Thrombocythemia
Malignancies	Basal cell carcinoma Squamous cell carcinoma (Marjolin ulcer) Malignant melanoma
Tropical ulcers	Cutaneous tuberculosis Syphilis Parasitic infections Fungal infections
Sarcoidosis	

elevate the leg, the edema will be diminished and local tissue perfusion will be improved. Another step that is often neglected is ensuring adequate hydration, particularly in patients who are hospitalized or have recently undergone surgery. Hydration enhances preload and ensures that arteriovenous shunting does not occur to divert blood away from the cutaneous tissues. Control of pain is also important to minimize sympathetic-induced vasoconstriction. Smoking cessation is beneficial: smoking impairs vascular flow, reduces vasodilatation, and accelerates the formation of atherosclerotic disease in vessels. Counseling should therefore be offered to all patients who use tobacco. The extremity should be kept warm so as to open up capillary beds and enhance tissue perfusion. Supplemental oxygen may be helpful for patients with a regional or systemic malperfusion state.

Chronic Wounds and Problem Wounds

As discussed elsewhere [*see 2:5 Acute Wound Care*], wounds normally progress through several temporally overlapping phases of healing. A chronic wound, however, does not progress through all of these phases but is arrested in one of them, usually the inflammatory phase. For practical purposes, a chronic wound can be defined—and, until comparatively recently, generally has been defined—in strictly temporal terms, as a wound that has not healed after 3 months. This once-standard definition is now being reconsidered, on the grounds that it may subject patients to needlessly prolonged courses of therapy, it may be used to deny advanced treatments to patients, and it fails to take into account the dynamic nature of wound healing, whereby wounds may improve, stall, and then improve again.

A better definition of a chronic wound is one that has fallen off the trajectory of expected healing.[14] This newer definition has implications for clinical practice, in that it emphasizes the importance of measuring the wound periodically. The wound should be measurably smaller during each office visit: typically, an actively healing wound should show a reduction in area or volume of approximately 10% per week.[15] If the wound is healing at a lesser rate or is scarcely healing at all, an immediate effort should be made to investigate the reason for the delay. There is no time for complacency (e.g., "Let's see how it's doing next month"), because the stalled wound is symptomatic of a significant underlying problem. It is imperative for the surgeon to consider possible causes—for example, infection or bacterial colonization. Often, an office debridement is necessary at this stage to reduce the accumulation of tenacious biofilm. If the wound shows no evidence of healing despite vigilant wound care, a biopsy should be considered, particularly if the wound has been present for more than 3 months. Other potential diagnoses besides malignancy should be considered as well, including vasculitis, pyoderma gangrenosum, and fungal or mycobacterial infection.

A number of clinical trials have shown that the rate of healing in the first 30 days after the initiation of good wound care is strongly predictive of an ulcer's ultimate fate, especially in the case of diabetic and venous stasis ulcers: the lesions that eventually heal are the ones that show the highest initial healing rates.[16-20] This observation, though perhaps intuitively obvious, is not always appreciated, nor are its lessons always correctly applied. Part of the problem is that many ulcers are not evaluated frequently enough in the outpatient setting. Weekly measurement is essential for evaluation of healing potential. In fact, it is likely that in the future, the benchmark measured by patients, peers, and insurance companies to evaluate a wound care practitioner's success will be time to ulcer healing. If an ulcer eventually heals after 9 months, this is still a success in some ways, but one may reasonably wonder whether the time away from work, the cost of dressings, and the multiple office visits might have been substantially reduced if the wound care practitioner had more frequently evaluated the rate of healing, had aggressively and preemptively rethought his or her approach, and perhaps had resorted to different therapeutic measures.

Instead of thinking in terms of acute wounds versus chronic wounds, as has been traditional, it may be more useful to think in terms of uncomplicated wounds versus problem wounds.[2] The category of problem wounds encompasses not only chronic wounds but also wounds occurring in persons whose comorbid conditions will almost certainly result in a protracted course of healing. Such persons include most elderly and hospitalized patients, but there are numerous other conditions besides advanced age and hospitalization that can impair healing [*see Table 2*]. For example, a week-old Wagner stage 2 ulcer in a diabetic patient is a problem wound

Table 2 Conditions That Interfere with Healing

Immunosuppressive medications
- Transplant patients
- Arthritic patients
- Autoimmune diseases
- Steroid use, including inhalers

Recent major surgery

Smoking

Malnutrition (particularly acute malnourishment or a recent catabolic state)

Infection

Age

Diminished tissue perfusion

Radiation

and should be treated promptly and comprehensively with offloading, moist wound care, and frequent inspections. A dehiscence at a saphenous vein harvest site in a patient who underwent a cardiac bypass is also a problem wound, both because of the swelling typically present and because of the likelihood of bacterial colonization in the relatively hypovascular subcutaneous tissue of the thigh. The mode of injury also plays a role in determining whether a wound is a problem wound; for example, a heavily devitalized wound in an 18-year-old patient will heal as poorly as a chronic wound if it is not adequately debrided and wound perfusion is not ensured. By preemptively addressing potential impediments to healing, the surgeon can minimize complications, shorten the time to healing, and help the patient return to work in an expeditious fashion.

Incidence and Epidemiology

It is estimated that at any point, the incidence of lower extremity ulcers in the United States may be as high as 1%.[21] The actual number of afflicted patients will rise as a consequence of the extension of the expected average lifespan, the proportional increase in atherosclerotic vascular disease, and the growing epidemic of obesity and associated diabetes mellitus.

The transition of baby boomers from middle age to the ranks of the elderly (over the age of 65) is already occurring, and it is estimated that by 2030, the elderly will constitute 20% of the U.S. population.[22] Persons older than 85 years constitute the most rapidly growing segment of the population. As noted (see above), by far the greatest number of ulcers occur in the elderly, both because of the increased incidence of atherosclerosis and because of the parallel increase in venous stasis disease.

In parallel with the increase in the elderly population, there is also a substantial increase in the diabetic population. The United States is witnessing (and leading) the dual global epidemics of diabetes and obesity. There are nearly 21 million people with diabetes in the United States, 6 million of whom are unaware that they have the disease.[23] Approximately 15% of these 21 million are at significant risk for the development of a foot ulcer. Indeed, 60% of lower extremity amputations unrelated to trauma are performed in diabetic patients.[23] Most of these amputations are preventable. The continuing increases in the incidence of atherosclerotic disease, diabetes, and venous stasis disease make it essential for surgeons to improve their awareness of and competence in the management of wounds in the lower extremity.

Anatomic Considerations

Several unique anatomic and functional factors predispose the lower extremity to ulceration. These factors include the relentless effects of gravity and the repetitive trauma of ambulation. Another factor is the formidable challenges involved in transporting blood from the heart to the foot and back. The vascular tree of the foot is a terminal capillary bed, like that in many other organs, but it is exposed to an enormous pressure gradient that is not present in other parts of the body. In humans, the lower extremities evolved differently from the upper extremities (to enable a bipedal gait), and the limitations and compromises attendant on this evolution are evident in the predisposition of the legs and feet to ulcerate.

The characteristics of the skin of the lower extremity play a role in ulceration. The skin in this area is taut, with minimal intrinsic laxity, and this tautness has implications for flap design.[24] Foot skin is extremely thick, and calluses form readily in response to pressure. Unfortunately, excess callus formation can exacerbate pressure in the sole of a diabetic person's foot. Obesity and lymphedema can alter the barrier function of the skin, as well as diminish cellular perfusion[25]; lymphedema is particularly damaging, in that the accumulation of fluid in the interstitial space causes a relative hypoxia coupled to altered macrophage function in conjunction with the induction of a chronic inflammatory state and tissue fibrosis.[26] Contact sensitivities are common and may influence compliance with the wearing of dressings and compression garments. Lipodermatosclerosis may develop as the result of chronic extravasation of red blood cells into the skin and deposition of hemosiderin within macrophages. Either hypo- or hyperpigmentation may occur, along with the characteristic "woody" firmness of subcutaneous fibrosis.[27–29] Venous eczema is common in patients with venous ulcers; it is probably an inflammatory process and can generally be distinguished from cellulitis on the basis of its chronicity, its poorly demarcated borders, and its pruritic, scaly nature.

The tendons also play a significant role in the etiology of diabetic forefoot ulcers, and their functional relations must be addressed when an amputation is to be performed. Dysregulation of the tendons is a frequent finding in limb ulcer patients. Chronic hyperglycemia leads to glycosylation of collagen, with subsequent loss of elasticity in connective tissues, including muscle, tendons, and skin; an example is glycosylation of the Achilles tendon, which destroys its flexibility and prevents adequate dorsiflexion during normal gait. The forefoot then bears the brunt of the person's weight during walking, and the accumulated stress, particularly in the setting of underlying neuropathy, culminates in a stereotypical diabetic forefoot ulcer (the so-called *mal perforant* ulcer). Correction of underlying biomechanical abnormalities and treatment of underlying medical conditions are as important to the overall treatment plan as debridement and wound care are.

The cutaneous innervation of the leg skin must also be taken into account. The nerves to the lower extremity include the common peroneal nerve, the superficial peroneal nerve, the deep peroneal nerve, the sural nerve, the saphenous nerve, and the tibial nerve. The branches in the foot are the medial plantar nerve, the lateral plantar nerve, and the calcaneal branch. The foot is predisposed to neuropathy for unknown reasons, one of which is almost certainly local-regional ischemia. This predisposition is particularly relevant to the pathogenesis of diabetic neuropathic foot ulcers; chronic

Table 3 Angiosomes (Vascular Territories) of Foot

Artery	Vascular Territory Supplied
Anterior tibial artery	Anterior aspect of lower leg, anterior ankle
Dorsalis pedis artery	Dorsum of foot
Peroneal artery Anterior perforating branch Calcaneal branch	Posterolateral aspect of lower leg Upper portion of lateral ankle Lateral plantar heel
Posterior tibial artery Calcaneal branch	Posteromedial aspect of lower leg Medial heel
Lateral plantar artery	Lateral aspect of plantar foot, plantar forefoot (usually extends to hallux)
Medial plantar artery	Medial instep region between heel and forefoot

tissue hyperglycosylation and fibrosis probably play roles as well. The medial and lateral plantar nerves travel through the tarsal tunnel, a tight anatomic space just under the flexor retinaculum. Division and release of the retinaculum serves a purpose analogous to that served by carpal tunnel release in the hand. In diabetic patients with forefoot ulcers, this procedure can reduce ulceration. Although tarsal tunnel release evolved as a means of treating neuropathic foot pain, it has been shown, in properly selected patients, to prevent foot ulceration by restoring foot sensibility.[30]

A valid grasp of the structural anatomy of the lower extremity vasculature is, of course, essential for surgeons treating patients with leg ulcers. Perhaps even more important, however, is an understanding of precisely how the various blood vessels are related to one another, as well as to the specific structures and areas that they supply. Such an understanding may be facilitated by viewing the blood supply to the foot and lower leg through the concept of angiosomes—that is, the specific vascular beds supplied by major named arteries. Angiosomes have been well described by Taylor,[31] and their application to the foot has been advanced by Attinger and associates.[32,33] The significance of the angiosome concept (which is frequently employed by plastic surgeons but is less familiar to other surgeons) lies in its ability to relate the major nutritive blood vessels to the surface anatomy, to the physical examination, and to the planning of operations. The lower extremity has several angiosomes [*see Table 3*]. Most of them reach watershed status in the ankle and foot, which explains why most ischemic ulcers occur below the midcalf area.

Although the major leg arteries supply distinct angiosomes of the foot and ankle in a consistent manner [*see Figures 1 through 5*], they are not immutably segregated from each other and in fact are linked by anatomically reliable connections. The links are the so-called choke vessels, which represent anastomotic connections between adjacent angiosomes. The significance of these choke vessels is twofold: first, they serve as an alternate route of blood flow from one angiosome to another in situations of low or impaired flow (e.g., stenosis), and second, they can be used by the surgeon in designing flaps and predicting healing status. It is important to be aware of these connections when treating a wound that may be burdened by local ischemia. As an example, the heel is supplied by two distinct angiosomes, the calcaneal branch of the posterior tibial artery and that of the peroneal artery, and native anastomoses exist between these two areas. If there is a necrotic wound in the plantar heel, it follows that both vascular trees must be diseased, because if only one were diseased, the native anastomoses between the two angiosomes would prevent the ulcer from forming.[33] As another example, connections normally exist between the anterior perforating branch of the peroneal artery and the anterior tibial artery at the lateral ankle. The astute surgeon can exploit this knowledge to map blood flow to distinct areas of the foot for the purposes of diagnosis and subsequent reconstructive flap design.[32,33] By alternately compressing flow above and below the arteries, the surgeon can determine whether retrograde blood flow to an adjacent angiosome is occurring (through choke vessels). If it is not, that area should not be used for a distally based flap.

Clinical Evaluation and Investigative Studies

When confronted with a lower extremity ulcer, the surgeon should proceed with the physical examination in a systematic, goal-directed manner. It is important to recognize those

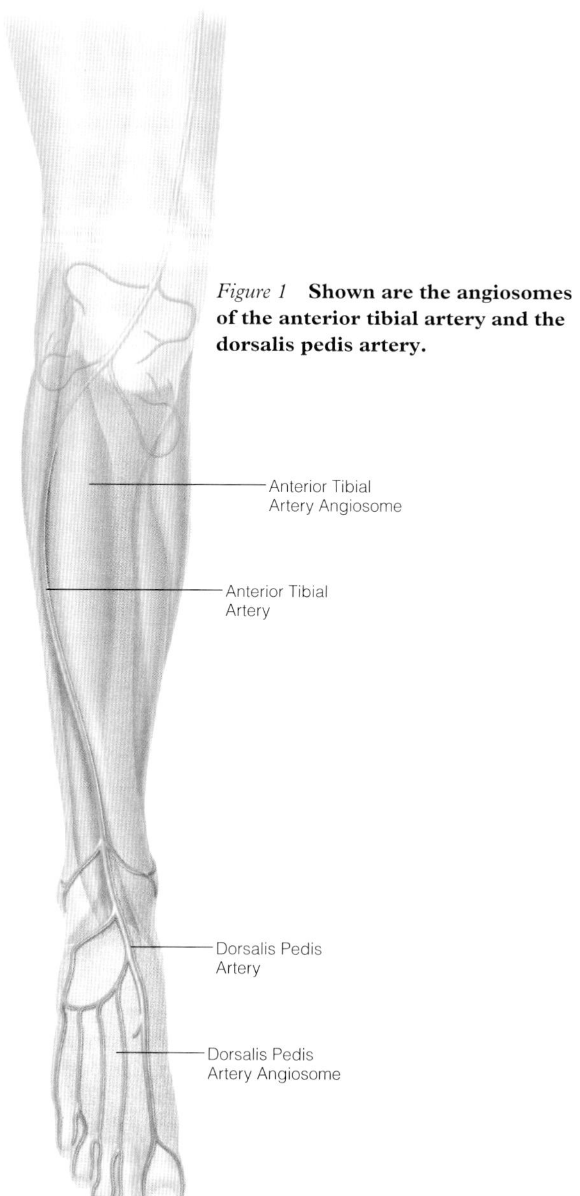

Figure 1 **Shown are the angiosomes of the anterior tibial artery and the dorsalis pedis artery.**

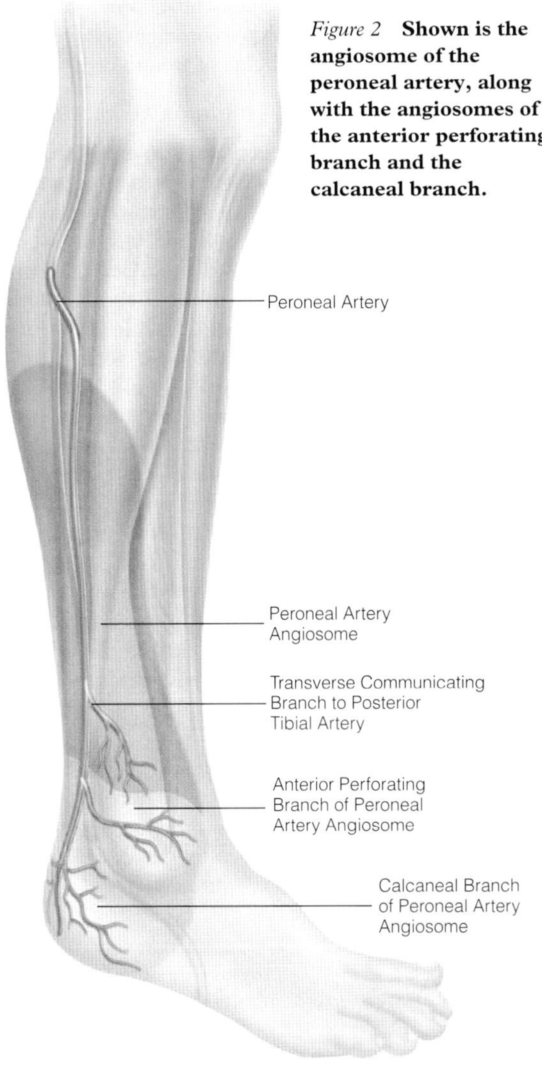

Figure 2 **Shown is the angiosome of the peroneal artery, along with the angiosomes of the anterior perforating branch and the calcaneal branch.**

presentations that call for emergency triage in the operating room. One such surgical emergency is a leg or foot wound that is also acutely ischemic. The priority in this situation is prompt revascularization of the leg. Another emergency is a gangrenous leg or foot wound that has overcome host resistance and is associated with ascending sepsis (often, necrotizing fasciitis). The priority in this situation is urgent debridement of the devitalized and infected tissues; in some cases, emergency guillotine amputation may be required. All other wounds are not emergencies and may be evaluated in a more systematic fashion.

Each patient encounter should commence with a vascular examination. Diligent evaluation of the blood supply to the lower extremity is essential in all patients with problem wounds. Comparison to the contralateral leg (if present) can be very useful. The first step is to assess the appearance of the leg, evaluating such data as color, skin texture, swelling, and temperature. Pulses are then palpated, as is capillary refill. If impaired tissue perfusion seems to be a possibility, these examinations should be supplemented with more objective diagnostic studies. As a practical matter, pulses in the foot are notoriously difficult to evaluate: different examiners not infrequently report different findings. Among other variables, the skin in the area may be edematous or fibrotic, hindering assessment. A pulse may appear diminished to one examiner but normal to another. Finally, blood flow may be impaired distal to the ankle, where pulses are typically evaluated. Various modalities are available for diagnosis in this setting; the following are among the more commonly employed and useful ones.[34,35]

Determination of the ankle-brachial index (ABI) is generally helpful, except in diabetic patients. The reason for the exception is that diabetes is associated with increased calcification of the arterial wall in the calf, which renders the vessel incompressible by the blood pressure cuff. As many as 30% to 40% of diabetic leg ulcer patients have falsely elevated ABIs that may mask an ischemic foot. In nondiabetic patients, an ABI lower than 0.5 mandates further imaging to search for possible stenosis or occlusion. In diabetic patients, measurement of the toe-brachial index (TBI) may be more useful.[36,37] Because toe vessels are less frequently affected by atherosclerotic disease (pedal sparing), toe pressures are a more reliable diagnostic tool in this setting. A value lower than 30 mm Hg is indicative of ischemia.

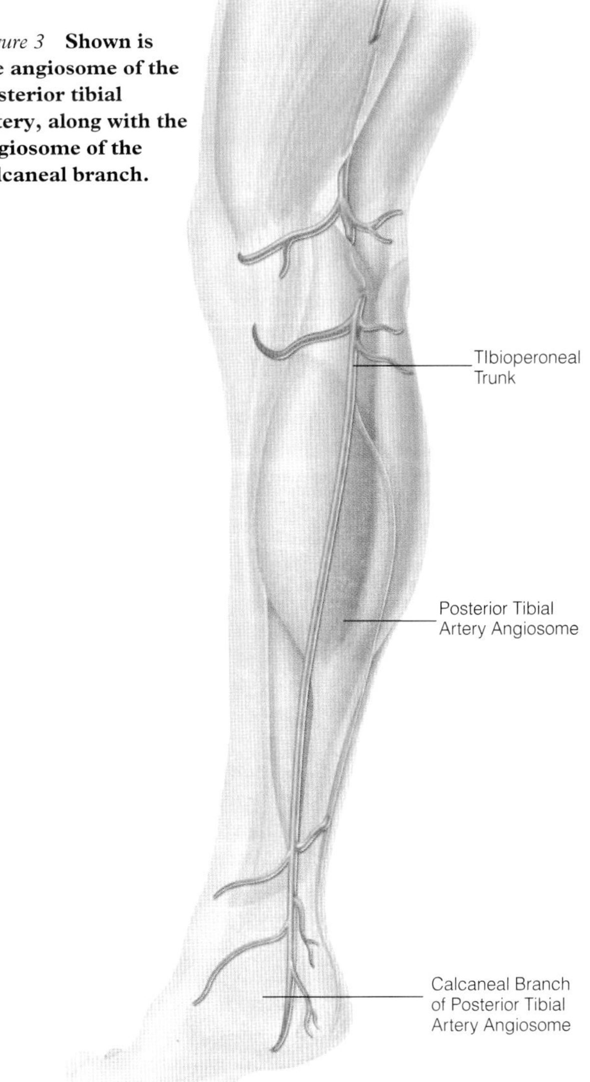

Figure 3 **Shown is the angiosome of the posterior tibial artery, along with the angiosome of the calcaneal branch.**

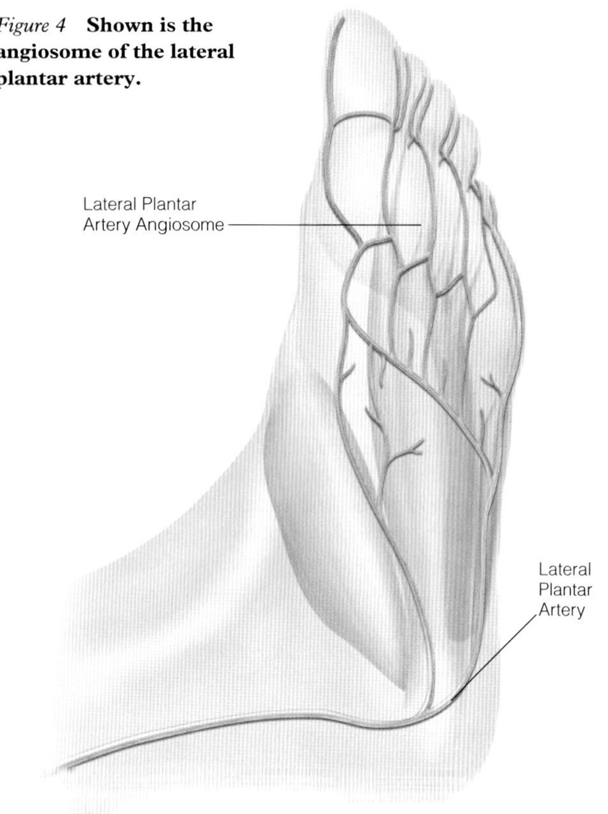

Figure 4 **Shown is the angiosome of the lateral plantar artery.**

In addition, measurement of the transcutaneous oxygen tension ($P_{tc}O_2$) is extremely helpful, particularly for patients with distal foot ulcers that may be prone to impaired oxygenation from local microangiopathy. $P_{tc}O_2$ levels are also useful for evaluating the response to therapy and may help predict healing.[13,38] Ischemia is present if the $P_{tc}O_2$ is lower than 30 mm Hg.

If the quality of the flow is questionable, either a formal noninvasive Doppler evaluation or angiography should be performed. If arterial inflow is found to be inadequate, the patient should be referred to a vascular surgeon—ideally, one who is trained in endovascular techniques and distal revascularizations.

A careful neurologic examination should be done to evaluate sensation and motor function. This is a particularly crucial in the management of a compartment syndrome (whether traumatic or resulting from a vascular accident). In diabetic patients and those with neurologic disorders, the neurologic examination can determine whether neuropathy contributed to the development of the wound. Lack of protective sensation is diagnosed by tonometry: if the patient is unable to feel 10 g of pressure applied by a Semmes-Seinstein 5.07 monofilament, significant sensory loss has occurred. This sensory loss prevents patients from registering skin damage that occurs as a result of excessive local pressure from a prolonged decubitus position; tight shoes, clothes, or dressings; biomechanical abnormalities; or the presence of foreign bodies. In neuropathic patients with biomechanical abnormalities, the repetitive trauma inherent in normal ambulation leads to ulceration as a consequence of the high focal plantar pressures generated during walking.

Management: General Principles

Current surgical education includes little formal training in the proper management of wounds. Accordingly, it is worthwhile to address some of the basic elements of wound care.

PREPARATION OF WOUND FOR HEALING OR RECONSTRUCTION

The first step in wound management is to establish a clean and healthy base. This can be accomplished in a variety of ways. A wound with a heavy eschar and grossly contaminated tissue requires surgical debridement in the OR [*see* Surgical Treatment, Surgical Debridement, *below*]. A wound with a mild amount of slough may be effectively debrided with an enzymatic dressing or even a water jet device (e.g., Waterpik; Water Pik, Inc., Fort Collins, Colorado). All wounds (except arterial and, usually, vasculitic ulcers) should be debrided down to healthy tissue. This measure resets the clock, so to speak, by effectively converting a chronic wound into an acute one. Because debridement is such a basic step, it tends to be underappreciated, even by surgeons.

There are three components of a leg ulcer that must be removed by means of debridement: (1) biofilm and bacteria, (2) callus, and (3) nonviable tissue.[39–41] Whereas the role of bacteria in wound infections has long been recognized, it is only comparatively recently that the contributions of biofilm to wound chronicity have come to be appreciated.[10,42] Biofilm consists of a sessile community of multiple bacteria species encased by a protective carbohydrate-rich polymeric matrix that is resistant to antimicrobial and immune cell penetration.[43] Most wounds are in fact colonized by bacteria that set up residence in a biofilm. Unfortunately, biofilm is exceedingly tenacious and readily reaccumulates after debridement. Thus,

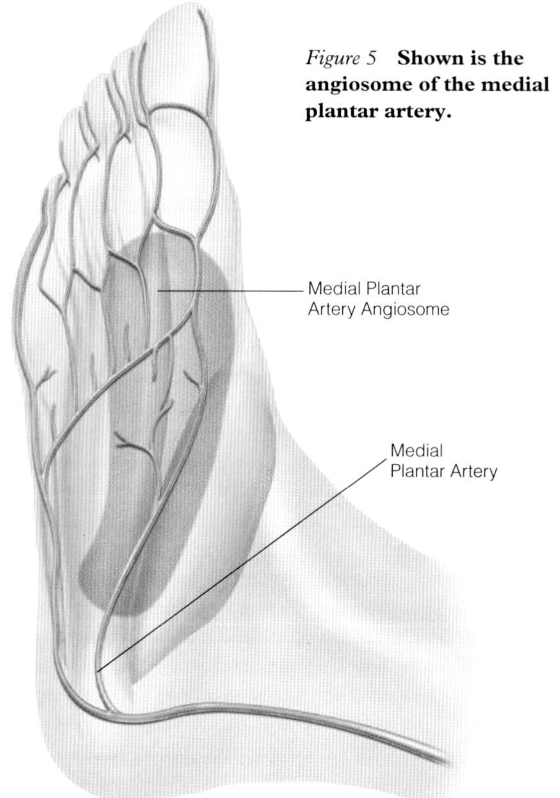

Figure 5 **Shown is the angiosome of the medial plantar artery.**

proper dressing care consists of dressings that both treat the wound and minimize biofilm accumulation.

Bacteria, whether free-floating or (more commonly) incorporated within a biofilm, are extremely detrimental to wound healing, particularly when they reach the level of critical colonization.[44] Wounds may be classified as contaminated, colonized, critically colonized, or infected.[45] These classifications are useful in that they detail the relation between the bacteria and the patient (or host) and define the level of bioburden (i.e., the cost exacted by bacteria from the resources of the wound and the patient). All wounds are contaminated to some degree, either by skin flora or by environmental pathogens. It is likely that this level of bacterial contamination stimulates wound repair mechanisms by upregulating the inflammatory response. When the contaminating bacteria begin to proliferate, the wound is said to be colonized; however, there is still no overt reaction by the host at this point. When the proliferating bacteria begin to overcome host responses, the wound is said to be critically colonized. Finally, when the wound provokes an inflammatory reaction by the host to the proliferating bacteria, the wound is said to be infected. It is important to keep in mind that the host's inflammatory reaction can contribute as much to a wound's failure to heal as the bacteria themselves do [*see Figure 6*].[2,46] Judicious use of antibiotics, adequate debridement, and proper dressing choices can decrease bacterial numbers and reduce the competition for nutrients and resources occurring in wounds contaminated by bacteria.[44] As noted (see above), because most leg wounds are found in ischemic, aged tissue beds, reduction of the bioburden can enable healing by restoring the balance between bacterial numbers and the nutrients available to healing cells.

Callus is formed in response to repetitive high pressure, usually over bony prominences on the foot. Once formed, it can further concentrate and propagate this excessive pressure on the underlying tissues. In addition, the grossly hyperkeratotic skin can act as a functional barrier to dressings and to migrating healthy keratinocytes. Therefore, callus should be removed whenever present. This can be done with a sharp, heavy scissors or a No. 10 blade; anesthesia is not required.

Nonviable tissue plays no necessary role in ulcer healing. The old paradigm of allowing wounds to heal under an eschar is

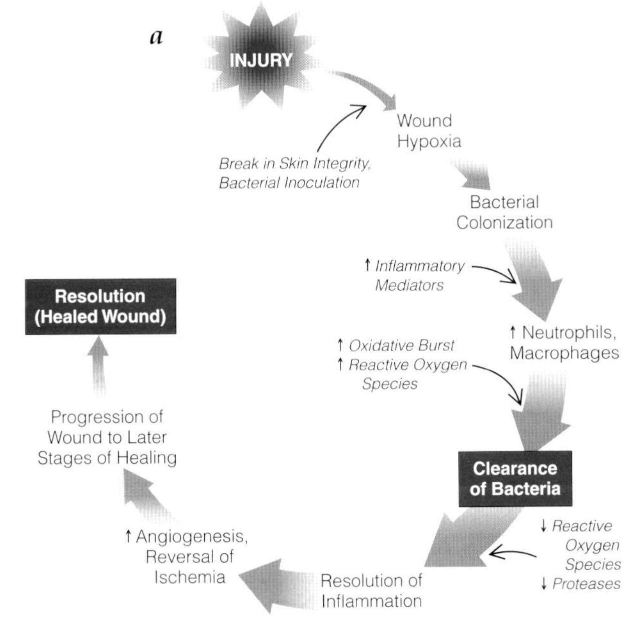

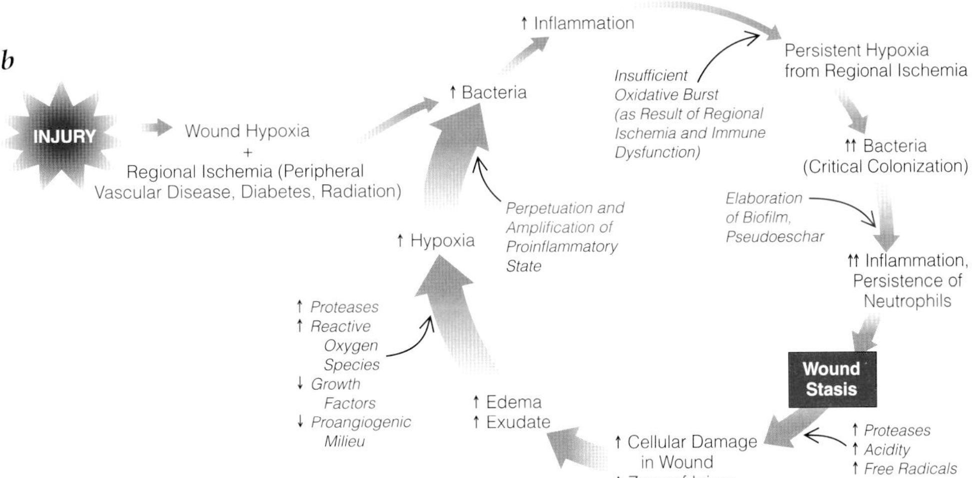

Figure 6 **Schematic representation depicts interplay between bacterial levels, oxidative stress, and parameters of healing in a wound. (*a*) In the typical self-limited inflammatory response in a healthy healing wound, bacteria are cleared rapidly by the body, inflammation is minimized, and the wound progresses to complete healing. (*b*) In states of impaired healing (e.g., from local or regional hypoxia, advanced age, presence of a large eschar, presence of biofilm, or diabetes), bacterial overgrowth occurs, usually in the form of biofilm, and an exaggerated inflammatory response develops that, instead of being self-limited as in (*a*), persists, causing cellular bystander damage and impairing progression of the wound to later stages of healing. A vicious circle often ensues.**

dissected in a distal-to-proximal direction and transposed to cover proximal defects. The donor site is closed primarily and requires a skin graft for coverage.

7. Abductor hallucis brevis flap. With this flap, as with the abductor digiti minimi flap, the dominant arterial pedicle is situated rather proximally, allowing the distal abductor hallucis brevis to be dissected completely free and rotated to cover defects of the medial heel and ankle. Again, a skin graft is required for coverage of the donor site.
8. Extensor digitorum brevis flap. This flap is a multipennate flap consisting of several slips of muscle that inserts via tendons on the second through fifth toes. It is used for coverage of dorsal foot and ankle defects.

Other useful muscle flaps include the flexor digitorum brevis flap (for heel defects) and the flexor digiti minimi musculocutaneous flap.

Free tissue transfers The rich variety of flaps available for coverage of leg and foot wounds has led to a decline in the use of microsurgical free flaps in the lower extremity. The development of NPWT has also contributed to the declining need for free flaps, in that many wounds are currently being downstaged with NPWT to enable eventual closure with a technique farther down the reconstructive ladder. Nevertheless, there remain certain wounds in all areas of the leg and foot for which free flaps may still be useful or even preferable, such as large defects and wounds characterized by significant exposure of bone or hardware. Flow-through free flaps are also commonly used to achieve revascularization and wound coverage simultaneously. Occasionally, free flaps are used for wounds with venous insufficiency or lymphedema in an attempt to improve these conditions by restoring lymphatic channels or competent venous drainage. The free flaps used in the lower extremity may be either fasciocutaneous or muscle flaps. Most studies have not found either type of flap to be superior to the other for treatment of areas of infection. In general, however, fasciocutaneous flaps are preferred for wounds on the sole of the foot, which are exposed to pressure and shearing forces, whereas muscle flaps are preferred for deep wounds.

Amputation

On occasion, amputation proves necessary [*see 7:20 Lower Extremity Amputation for Ischemia*].[76] Factors such as advanced age, uncontrolled diabetes, sepsis and gangrene, unreconstructable blood vessels, and renal failure are all associated with a higher risk of amputation. Nevertheless, a focused, multidisciplinary approach to wound care should be able to reduce amputation levels substantially and achieve limb salvage rates higher than 90%. Overall, the most frequently performed amputations are toetip amputations. Of these procedures, the most common is amputation of the tip of the great toe. This operation is done to treat the claw-type deformity seen in diabetic patients with an intrinsic-minus foot, whereby the toe becomes permanently flexed as a result of the pull of the flexor hallucis longus tendon. The tip amputation may have to be closed with a fishmouth-type incision or a V-Y advancement flap from the plantar surface. In addition, it may be necessary to advance the flexor hallucis longus tendon and perform a volar capsular release to minimize recurrence.

Amputations of the toe rays are frequently performed, most commonly in diabetic patients but also in patients with osteomyelitis of the metatarsal heads. Rebalancing the pull of the extrinsic tendons is crucial for preventing redistribution of the maladaptive forces to adjacent rays and subsequent propagation of serial ulcers in these areas. Therefore, the peroneus brevis and tibialis anterior insertions should be reattached to the cuboid or the cuneiform for proximal fifth and first ray amputations, respectively.[24]

Most amputations of the foot are performed at the transmetatarsal level. Transmetatarsal amputation is a very useful procedure that preserves as much of the foot's length as possible while also maintaining a well-balanced walking surface with thick plantar skin. Fundamentally, it is a reconstructive procedure: the vascular supply to both the plantar and the dorsal flap must be ensured prior to closure, and the balance of the foot tendons must be addressed.[76] The plantar metatarsal arteries, which supply the plantar flap, must be kept intact by avoiding excessive undermining or indiscriminate use of the electrocautery. If the flap appears compromised after closure, the flap sutures should be released, and completion of the flap procedure should be delayed for several days to encourage increased neovascularization. NPWT may be used as a temporizing measure to bridge the wound before formal closure. After a transmetatarsal amputation, the triceps surae may be lengthened to compensate for the loss of ankle dorsiflexion that results from removal of the attachment points to the toe extensor tendons.[24]

Management of Specific Types of Lower Extremity Ulcer

In the early stages of management, it is important to focus on the patient's overall health status, with a particular emphasis on the presence or absence of sepsis. It is also vital to determine whether adequate vascularity is present to enable healing. Most wounds benefit from debridement, whether biologic (i.e., dressings and wound care) or surgical. At the same time, normalization of systemic derangements is undertaken. A decision is made whether to treat the wound surgically. In most instances, this does not have to be done right away. Surgical wound closure, when feasible, is best done after a period of optimization.

In addition to these considerations, which are common to all leg ulcers, there are aspects of care that are specific for different ulcer types. Accordingly, in what follows, I focus on specific care of the most prevalent types of leg ulcer—namely, those resulting from arterial insufficiency, those associated with diabetic neurarthopathy, those resulting from venous stasis, and those of inflammatory origin.

ULCERS RESULTING FROM ARTERIAL INSUFFICIENCY

Most arterial leg ulcers occur in the elderly. A nonhealing ulcer is one of the most common presentations of peripheral vascular disease, the incidence of which is highest in men older than 45 years and women older than 55 years. Modifiable risk factors for peripheral vascular disease include smoking, hyperlipidemia, hypertension, diabetes, and obesity.

In most instances, the diagnosis is suggested by the physical examination. Arterial leg ulcers generally occur in a stereotypical distribution that is well explained by the angiosome concept mentioned earlier [*see* Anatomic Considerations, *above*], most commonly developing over the toes, heels, and bony prominences of the foot. It is worth noting that a heel ulcer typically results if there is disease in the distributions of both the peroneal artery and the posterior tibial artery, as a consequence of the dual blood supply to the posterior heel from these vascular territories.[33] Ulcers in the toes result from the diminished distribution of blood to these terminal vascular beds. An ulcer in the setting of arterial insufficiency is a symptom of the decreased blood flow and may be associated with rest pain or claudication. The metabolic demands of intact skin are less than those of an open wound, but even so, the impaired blood flow renders the skin thin, atrophic, hairless, and dry in the affected extremity. Patients usually experience significant pain, which is relieved by dangling the leg over the bed at night. The ulcer has a sharply demarcated appearance, with a paucity of granulation tissue. The wound bed is pale or pink and typically lacks the red color associated with a hypervascular healing bed. Pulses are usually diminished. Any patient with decreased pulses at the ankle (signaling insufficiency of the dorsalis pedis, the posterior tibial artery, or both) should be referred for vascular studies. In practice, given the wide interindividual variation in the ability to palpate a pulse accurately, it is advisable to set a fairly low threshold for obtaining studies such as an ABI or a TBI. In general, arterial leg ulcer patients with an ABI lower than 0.9 or higher than 1.2 or with a $P_{tc}O_2$ lower than 30 mm Hg should be referred to a vascular surgeon.

Quite often, the etiology of an arterial leg ulcer is not purely ischemic but includes contributions from other conditions, such as diabetes, venous insufficiency, neuropathy, and renal failure. These ulcers of mixed etiology are particularly challenging to treat, and it is all too common to find a supposedly chronic wound whose chronicity actually resulted from an earlier failure to establish the leg's vascular status.

At the cellular level, the cause of an arterial ulcer goes beyond the simple lack of sufficient oxygen supply to a cell. For example, it is known that sublethal ischemia is much more detrimental to aged cells and diabetic cells than to young cells.[77,78] Lack of ATP and inadequate clearance of metabolites result in poor healing and aberrant inflammation. Because healing is an anabolic process, much more energy is needed for healing than for tissue maintenance and homeostasis. The persistence of noxious metabolic byproducts that are not cleared by the circulation may be a cause of the pain commonly associated with these wounds.[79]

At the tissue level, chronic regional ischemia results in atrophic changes to the skin and soft tissues. The terminal nature of the vascular tree in the foot, with the distal foot and toes being less well perfused than the calf and thigh, along with the effects of gravity and the rigors of ambulation, means that these downstream areas bear the brunt of the effects of upstream atherosclerosis. In the setting of a minor injury, the atrophic skin is more liable to progress to a full-thickness injury in the distal foot and toes than in more proximal locations and, indeed, is more likely to tear in the first place. As mentioned (see above), synthesis of new tissues and deposition of matrices and collagen, along with collagen crosslinking, are necessary for ulcer healing. These are all rate-dependent processes, with oxygen being the necessary variable. Unfortunately, the impaired tissue perfusion means that the ulcer bed will not receive an adequate supply of oxygen and nutrients to support tissue growth. In addition, because oxygen is necessary for the neutrophil burst, arterial ulcers are especially predisposed to infection.[11]

These considerations help explain the typical appearance of ulcers resulting from arterial insufficiency: the sharply demarcated boundaries (attributable to the "on/off" borders between the defect and unwounded skin, with a minimal healing interface); the dry wound beds, with minimal transudate and exudate; the pale granulation tissue, indicative of a hypovascular state; the changes in the appearance of the surrounding skin (see above); and the reduced capillary refill time.

In the treatment of a wound with an arterial component [*see Figure 8*], the sine qua non is revascularization: a wound typically will not heal if the leg's blood supply is not improved.[11] Therefore, the urgent decision to be made at this point is whether revascularization is feasible. It should be kept in mind that the decision as to whether an extremity is a candidate for revascularization should be made only by a vascular specialist who is comfortable with or has access to newer modalities and procedures (e.g., distal bypasses and endovascular techniques). Noninvasive means of revascularization are useful in high-risk patients.

After revascularization, there is a lag phase before the ischemia is reversed in the distal leg and foot. Typically, a rise in $P_{tc}O_2$ is seen 1 to 2 weeks after surgical revascularization and is delayed after angioplasty.[15] In patients with foot ulcers, foot pulses must be restored if the ulcers are to heal. The wound must be managed during the weeks after revascularization, and indeed for months to years afterward. It should be noted that techniques associated with lower long-term patency rates can nevertheless be useful if they enable healing of an open wound or amputation site. Once the ulcer is healed, the likelihood that a new wound will develop in the area diminishes (because of the lower energy requirements of healed skin in comparison with those of a healing wound).

Any significant comorbid conditions, such as diabetes or venous stasis disease (see below), should be addressed. Steps must also be taken to prevent or control infection, which can cause rapid deterioration in an arterial ulcer. If signs of local or systemic infection are noted, treatment with systemic antibiotics should be initiated promptly. Unless grossly infected tissue (e.g., wet gangrene) is present, it is best to defer debridement until the vascularity of the area is ensured: debridement while the blood flow to the area is still impaired may promote further ischemia and lead to the formation of a larger ulcer.[11] Dressings applied to ischemic ulcers typically must have moisture added in the form of hydrogels as the hypovascular wound bed desiccates. An enzymatic dressing can also be useful for gentle debridement of nonviable tissue. Systemic factors (e.g., global hypoxia, enhancement of cardiac output, pain control, and warmth) are important as well. In patients who respond to an oxygen challenge, HBO should be considered and offered if available; however, it should not be employed in place of surgical revascularization if the latter is an option.

Final surgical treatment, in the form of flaps or skin grafts, is deferred until blood flow is ensured. Occasionally, it is possible to perform what is termed extended limb salvage, wherein a bypass graft to the leg is performed at the same time that a microvascular free flap is used to cover a large defect.[80–82] With advances in wound care products and the introduction of NPWT, however, most procedures can be staged. Flap procedures are typically undertaken after a period of days to weeks, once the oxygen supply is restored.

These patients are nevertheless at high risk for amputation, typically as a consequence of progressive atherosclerotic disease. Patients with unreconstructable peripheral vascular disease (particularly common in the setting of renal failure) or extensive tissue loss or gangrene usually require a major

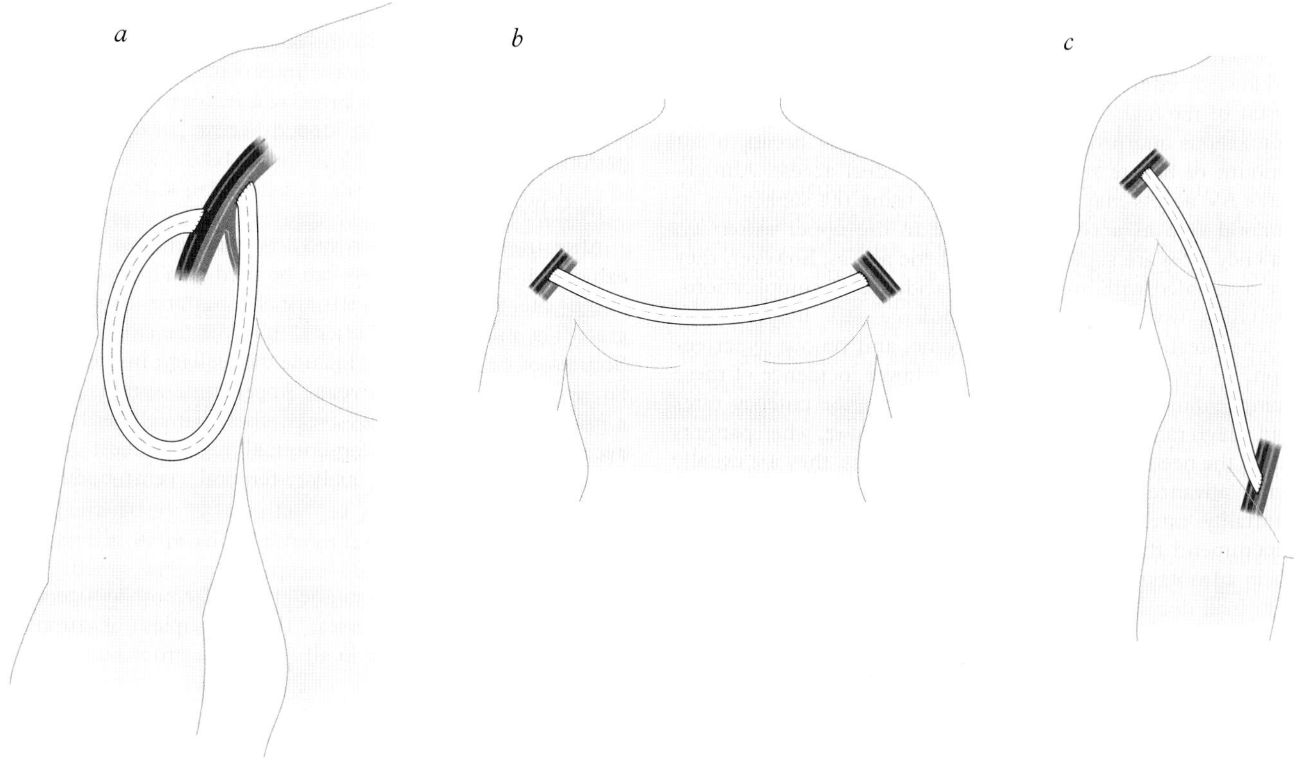

[illegible]
(c) Prosthetic axillary-femoral (vein) body wall straight access.

5. The AV anastomosis is performed between the side of the artery and the end of the vein; this configuration decreases the subsequent risk of venous hypertension.
6. The AV anastomosis is performed using a 6-0 or 7-0 monofilament nonabsorbable continuous suture to avoid subsequent anastomotic dilatation.
7. With nontransposed access, after completion of the anastomosis, large venous branches can be ligated through stab incisions. This encourages flow in the main venous segment, which may promote earlier maturation.
8. The patient is asked to perform hand exercises 24 to 48 hours postoperatively to increase blood flow through the vein and encourage early maturation of the access.

Prosthetic AV Access

A standard 6 mm expanded polytetrafluoroethylene (ePTFE) is our choice for graft material for prosthetic AV accesses. Variations in the standard ePTFE graft include thin-walled, extended stretch, external rings, various tapered configurations, and heparin coating, which are all meant to ease handling, provide external support, and improve patency rates. To date, there is only minimal evidence that any of these variations improve long-term results; therefore, use of any of these variations remains a matter of surgeon preference.[25,26]

The following techniques are common to all prosthetic access:

1. The venous outflow is dissected, examined for appropriate quality and caliber, and controlled with vessel loops.
2. The arterial inflow is dissected and controlled with vessel loops.
3. The subcutaneous tunnel for the prosthetic graft is made with a Kelly-Wick tunneler; the tunnel is made as superficial as possible to allow easy detection by dialysis personnel and as long as possible for a large surface area to prevent repetitive trauma to the same area of the graft and subsequent pseudoaneurysm (PSA) formation.
4. If the venous outflow and arterial inflow are located away from each other, a straight prosthetic AV access configuration is performed. If the venous outflow and arterial inflow are located close to each other, a loop prosthetic AV access configuration is performed; this requires a counterincision at the apex of the loop.
5. The length of the arteriotomy and the venotomy does not need to be limited to 4 to 6 mm. The diameter of the graft will limit the incidence of arterial steal.
6. The artery is flushed proximally and distally with heparinized saline to avoid thrombosis during the anastomosis.
7. The anastomoses are performed using a 6-0 or 7-0 monofilament nonabsorbable suture in a continuous manner.
8. Careful attention to sterile technique is paramount to avoid graft infections.

POSTOPERATIVE FOLLOW-UP

From the time of the access placement, autogenous AV access should be mature and ready for cannulation by 12 weeks postoperatively and prosthetic AV access should be mature and ready for cannulation by as early as 2 weeks postoperatively. Determination of maturity may be done by physical examination alone; the access should have a soft pulse that is easily compressible, a continuous low-pitched bruit, and a thrill near the anastomosis and extending along the outflow vein and should collapse with arm elevation. If the clinical examination remains equivocal after 6 to 8 weeks, the access should be further evaluated with duplex ultrasonography; the outflow vein should have a vein diameter greater than 4 mm and blood flow greater than 500 mL/min. If the access appears to be failing to mature by duplex evaluation, it should be further evaluated with fistulography or venography to identify any underlying problems preventing maturity. Secondary procedures, such as vein patches, interposition vein grafts, vein transposition to proximal arteries, branch ligations, vein superficialization, or endovascular angioplasties, should then be used to salvage the access.[5]

LONG-TERM FOLLOW-UP

After initial maturation, the AV access should be monitored routinely while the patient is on dialysis. The preferred method of monitoring is monthly determinations of access flow by ultrasound dilution, conductance dilution, thermal dilution, or Doppler technique. Access flow less than 600 mL/min or access flow less than 1,000 mL/min that has decreased by 25% over 4 months should be further evaluated with duplex ultrasonography followed by fistulography if further information is needed. Another method of access monitoring that is more useful with prosthetic access is measurement of static venous dialysis pressures; a graft-to-artery ratio of more than 0.75, a graft-to-vein ratio of less than 0.5, or a progressive increase in the venous or arterial segment of more than 0.25 should be further evaluated with duplex ultrasonography followed by fistulography if further information is necessary. Measurements of dynamic venous pressures have been found to be a relatively poor marker of autogenous or prosthetic access function. Other acceptable methods of access surveillance include measurement of prepump arterial dialysis pressure, measurement of access recirculation using urea concentrations or dilution techniques, evaluation of physical findings such as arm edema, altered characteristics of access thrill, and notation of prolonged bleeding after needle removal. Similar to early access failure to mature, after identification, any underlying abnormalities should be treated with secondary procedures to prevent access thrombosis.[3]

COMPLICATIONS OF AV ACCESS

AV Access Failure

Upper extremity autogenous AV access [*see Table 2*] has consistently been shown to have excellent primary and secondary patency rates when compared with prosthetic AV access. One-year primary patency rates of autogenous AV access range from 43 to 85%,[27–34] and 2-year primary patency rates range from 40 to 69%.[28,32,35,36] In comparison, 1-year primary patency rates of prosthetic AV access range from 40 to 54%,[27,28,33,34] and 2-year primary patency rates range from 18 to 30%.[28,35,36] Similarly, secondary patency rates are superior in autogenous access and range from 46 to 90%[27,28,31–33] at 1 year and from 62 to 75%[28,35–37] at 2 years compared with prosthetic access, which ranges from 59 to 65%[27,28,31] at 1 year and from 40 to 60% at 2 years.[28,35,36] Also of note, to maintain these secondary patency rates, prosthetic AV access requires a higher number of interventions than autogenous AV access. These superior patency rates of autogenous access include basilic vein transpositions, which have demonstrated 1-year primary patency rates from 35 to 76%[27,30,32,38,39] and secondary patency rates from 47 to 90%.[27,32,38]

Similar to upper extremity AV access, lower extremity autogenous AV access [*see Table 3*] has consistently been shown to have superior primary and secondary patency rates to prosthetic AV access. One-year primary patency rates of autogenous access average 73% and 2-year primary patency rates average 86%.[21,22] In comparison, 1-year primary patency rates of prosthetic access average 54% and 2-year primary patency rates range from 18 to 47%.[23,24] Similarly, secondary patency rates of autogenous access at 1 year, which average 86%, and at 2 years, which range from 87 to 94%,[21,22] remain superior to secondary patency rates of prosthetic access at 1 year, which average 64%, and at 2 years, which average 18%.[23,24] Also, similar to the upper extremity, to maintain these secondary patency rates, prosthetic AV access requires more revisions.[23,24]

Early AV access thrombosis Early access thrombosis occurs within 30 days of surgery and is attributable to a technical failure. It is most commonly associated with inadequate venous outflow, which may be secondary to inadequate caliber of the outflow vein or central venous stenosis. Other, less common causes include poor arterial inflow and anastomotic stenosis.

Thrombectomies and thrombolysis are rarely successful treatments for autogenous accesses; this situation usually requires complete revision. If early thrombosis is secondary to the small caliber of the outflow vein, the autogenous AV access is redone using a different vein, that is, conversion of an autogenous radial-cephalic direct wrist access to an autogenous radial-basilic forearm transposition or, if no vein is available, a prosthetic AV access. Central venous stenosis is treated with angioplasty and/or stenting or venous bypass, that is, subclavian vein to internal jugular vein bypass [*see* Venous Hypertension, *below*], followed by a new AV access. An arterial inflow stenosis is treated with angioplasty and/or stenting or proximal arterial bypass to restore adequate arterial inflow followed by a new AV access; an alternative approach is to move the AV access either proximally or to another extremity where arterial inflow is adequate. Anastomotic stenosis is a primary technical failure and is redone with close attention to surgical technique.

Table 2 **Autogenous Arteriovenous Access Patency Rates**

Access Location	Primary Patency (%)		Secondary Patency (%)	
	1 yr	2 yr	1 yr	2 yr
Upper extremity	43–85	40–69	46–90	62–75
Basilic vein transposition	35–76	68	47–90	69–75
Lower extremity	73	68	86	87–94

Table 3 **Prosthetic Arteriovenous Access Patency Rates**

Access Location	Primary Patency (%)		Secondary Patency (%)	
	1 yr	2 yr	1 yr	2 yr
Upper extremity	40–54	18–30	59–65	40–60
Lower extremity	54	18–47	64	18

Table 1 Indications for Peritoneal Dialysis
Patient prefers peritoneal dialysis
Patient will not do hemodialysis
Patient cannot tolerate hemodialysis
Patient prefers home dialysis but has no assistance for hemodialysis

avoid catheter stresses and kinks. Preoperative planning should also take into consideration the location of the superior border of the pubic symphysis, the umbilicus, the level of the anterior superior iliac spines, and skin folds.[20] To decrease the risk of contamination, an alternate presternal extension exit site is preferred in individuals with colostomy or urinary stoma, those who are morbidly obese, and those who desire to take tub baths.[23]

With the patient in the upright and supine positions, the incision, intended subcutaneous tract, and exit site of the catheter are marked [*see Figure 1*]. This is especially important in obese patients as a pannus will change position on standing. In a virgin abdomen, the left side is chosen because the right iliac fossa is the preferred site for a first kidney transplant [*see Figure 1*]. Also, as opposed to the right side, the downward intestinal peristalsis of the left colon is thought to maintain proper catheter orientation in the pelvis.

As noted in Table 2, obesity is considered a relative contraindication to PD. This is an important consideration because an estimated 70% of the US population is overweight. In recent years, we have been placing an increasing number of catheters in overweight individuals. PD catheters in obese patients work surprisingly well but require special considerations. As noted above, choosing the exit site in the upper abdomen or on the upper chest using a presternal extension segment is the preferred option in these patients.[23,24]

Table 2 Contraindications for Peritoneal Dialysis
Absolute
Documented loss of peritoneal function or extensive abdominal adhesions that limit dialysate volume or flow
In the absence of a suitable assistant, the patient is physically or mentally unable to perform PD
Uncorrectable mechanical defects that prevent effective PD or increase the risk of infection (e.g., surgically irreparable hernia, omphalocele, gastroschisis, diaphragmatic hernia, and bladder extrophy)
Relative
Fresh intra-abdominal foreign bodies (e.g., VP shunts or vascular prosthesis)
Peritoneal leaks
Body size limitations
Intolerance to volume exchanges needed for adequate PD dose
Inflammatory or ischemic bowel disease
Frequent episodes of diverticulitis
Abdominal wall or skin infection
Morbid obesity
Severe malnutrition

PD = peritoneal dialysis; VP = ventriculoperitoneal.

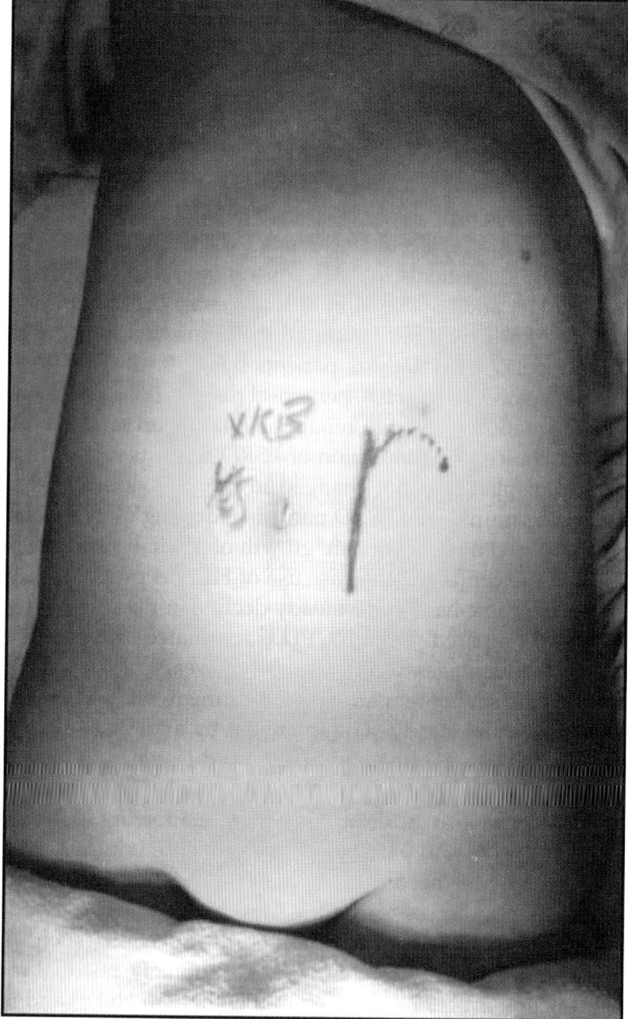

Figure 1 **Skin markings for the placement of a peritoneal dialysis catheter in the open technique. Note the locations of the planned incision, subcutaneous tunnel, and exit site.**

CHOICE OF CATHETER

PD catheters come in a variety of configurations and with one or two Dacron cuffs [*see Figure 2*]. With single-cuff configurations, the Dacron cuff is placed at the posterior rectus fascia; with double-cuff configurations, the second or outer cuff is placed in the subcutaneous space 1.5 to 2.0 cm from the skin exit site. Although this is not borne out in randomized, controlled trials,[25] the double-cuff configuration is thought to provide an additional barrier from bacterial migration along the catheter and may have lower rates of tunnel tract infections and associated peritonitis. Retrospective reviews suggest that double-cuff configurations have a longer catheter survival time, a delayed first episode of peritonitis,[24,26] and a trend toward decreased episodes of peritonitis.[27]

The intraperitoneal and extraperitoneal PD catheter designs vary greatly [*see Figure 2*]. The intraperitoneal segments can be straight, coiled, or weighted (so-called self-locating tips[28]). Catheters with a coiled intraperitoneal

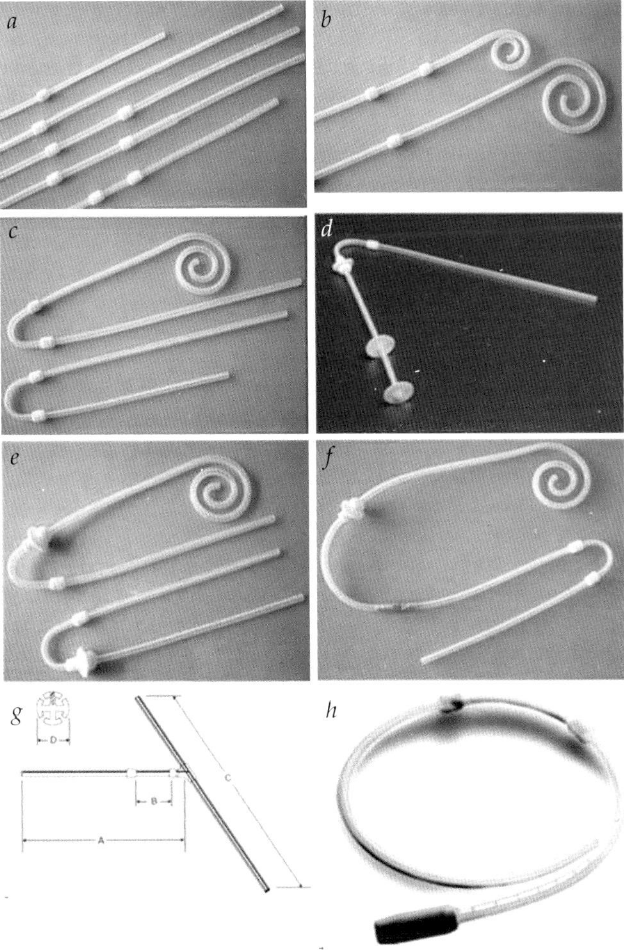

Figure 2 **The different commercially available types of peritoneal dialysis catheters. (*a*) Straight Tenckhoff peritoneal dialysis catheters, in single- and double-cuff configurations. (*b*) Coiled Tenckhoff peritoneal dialysis catheters, in single- and double-cuff configurations. (*c*) Swan neck peritoneal dialysis catheters, with straight and coiled intraperitoneal segments. (*d*) Swan neck Toronto Western Hospital peritoneal dialysis catheter. (*e*) Swan neck Missouri peritoneal dialysis catheter with a straight intraperitoneal segment. (*f*) Swan neck presternal peritoneal dialysis catheter with a coiled intraperitoneal segment. (*g*) T-fluted Ash Advantage peritoneal dialysis catheter. A is the transabdominal tube length, B is the distance between cuffs, C is the overall intraperitoneal length, and D is the flute diameter. (*h*) The "self-locating" Di Paolo peritoneal dialysis catheter. Note the weighted tip at the end of the intraperitoneal segment.**

segment provide greater surface area and more side holes for fluid passage and therefore increased likelihood of success.[26] The coiled segments may be better tolerated than the straight intraperitoneal configurations because the straight tips are thought to produce more pain with instillation of fluid secondary to a "jet" effect.[23]

The extraperitoneal segments can be straight or curved. Because the catheter material has inherent "shape memory," forcing a curve into a straight catheter is thought to increase mechanical complications and infectious complications and cuff extrusion through the skin.[26] We use the double-cuff curled (pigtail) Tenckhoff catheter with straight external configuration.

Surgical Technique/Approach

The choice of surgical approach depends on the experience of the operating surgeon. PD catheters are typically inserted using an open approach or laparoscopic technique. Other methods of placement include the blind Seldinger technique, placement under fluoroscopic guidance, and placement under peritoneoscopic visualization[29]; these methods are strongly discouraged because of the risk of inadvertent bowel injury. The open and laparoscopic techniques of PD catheter placement are discussed here.

Advantages and disadvantages exist for both methods. The open approach is associated with a shorter operating time and can be performed under spinal or local anesthesia, although general anesthesia is preferred. The open approach is also more cost-effective as only basic equipment is required for the procedure.[30] Laparoscopic placement, with the insufflation of carbon dioxide into the peritoneal cavity, requires general anesthesia, which may be precluded in some patients. Laparoscopic placement also requires longer operating times, a finding that has been consistently reported in multiple studies.[30–37] The main advantage of the laparoscopic approach is that it allows for direct visualization and placement of the tip of the catheter, as well as the ability to secure the tip of the dialysis catheter in the pelvis.[35,37] The laparoscopic approach also allows for additional procedures, such as repair of umbilical hernias, lysis of adhesions, or omentopexy.[38,39]

Laparoscopy is the best technique to rescue problem catheters.[38,40] Studies comparing the rates of complications with open versus laparoscopic PD placement have been mixed,[36,37] and one method of placement cannot be recommended over another. The PD catheter surgical approach is greatly influenced by the patient's medical risk, the operating surgeon's training, and institutional resources.

OPERATIVE TECHNIQUE

Open Paramedian Approach

Although open PD catheter placement can be performed under local anesthesia, for patient comfort, general anesthesia is preferred. Preoperative antibiotics, such as first-generation cephalosporin (e.g., cefazolin), are administered prior to skin incision. Patients with penicillin or cephalosporin allergies should receive either clindamycin or vancomycin as alternatives.

The skin incision is placed 2 to 3 cm on either side of the umbilicus, with the left being the preferred side [*see Figure 1*]. The abdominal wall anatomy is shown in Figure 3. The anterior rectus muscle fascia is divided longitudinally. Muscle-sparing technique is used to expose the posterior rectus fascia. Using fine scissors, the posterior rectus fascia and peritoneum are opened for a length of 3 mm. Caution is advised to avoid inadvertent small bowel injury during entry.

A 2-0 polypropylene purse-string suture is placed around the fascial-peritoneal defect [*see Figure 4*]. The suture is placed so that the tie will be located cephalad to the cuff; this suture will also be used to secure the inner Dacron cuff to the posterior rectus fascia. This purse-string suture allows for a watertight seal around the catheter.

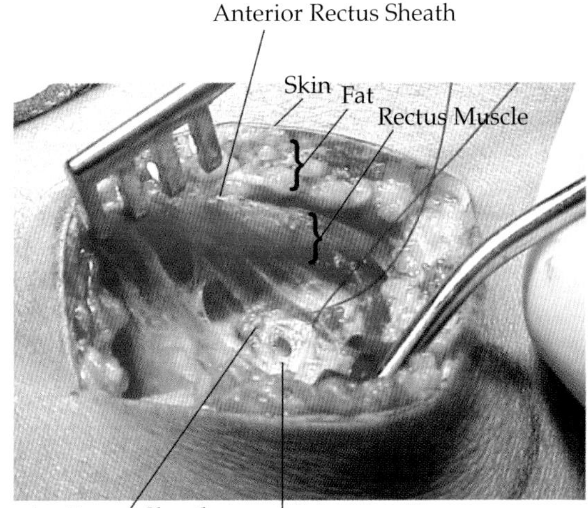

Figure 3 **The abdominal wall anatomy.**

The intra-abdominal catheter placement is facilitated by the use of a stiffening stylet [*see Figure 5*]. The catheter must first be flushed with saline for the stylet to slide freely onto the catheter. The tip of the stylet must not pass outside the tip of the catheter, to minimize the risk of visceral injuries during insertion [*see Figure 6*]. Once inside the abdomen, the stylet is retracted to release the curled end, and the catheter is directed downward along the anterior abdominal wall. Force must not be used. If resistance occurs, redirection of the catheter is attempted until the pelvis is reached. At this point, the stylet is removed with one hand securing the PD catheter at the exit site. Once the catheter is fully inserted, the purse-string suture is tied snugly. The inner Dacron cuff is then secured to the posterior aspect of the posterior rectus fascia with suture [*see Figure 7*]. A second purse-string suture is not required. Next, the catheter is tunneled through the rectus muscle [*see Figure 8*] and pulled through the anterior rectus fascia [*see Figure 9*]. This step secures the craniocaudad direction of the catheter, making malpositioning unlikely.

The sharp, curved subcutaneous Faller tunneler is used to create a smooth, curved subcutaneous tract as the catheter exits through the skin [*see Figure 10 and Figure 11*]. The tunneler is the same diameter as the catheter tubing, making the skin exit site snug [*see Figure 12*]. A snug exit site minimizes irritation from catheter sliding and the risk of infection. The external Dacron cuff is placed 1.5 to 2.0 cm from the exit site.

The tunneler should exit the skin at a 30 to 45 angle to optimize catheter alignment to the skin and comfort for the

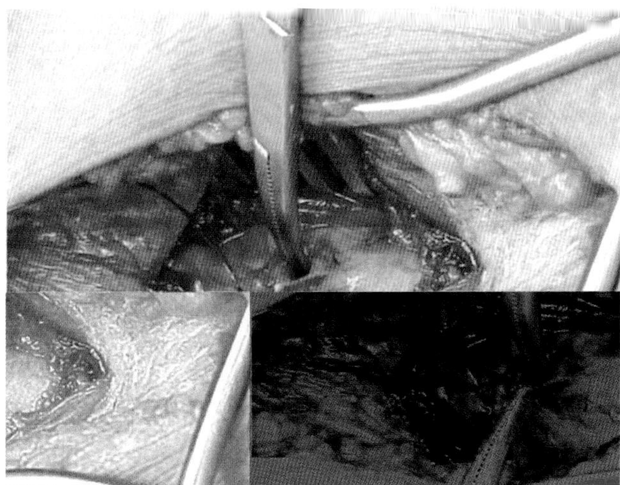

Figure 4 **Several bites (6–8) of suture are placed 5 mm from the edge of the small peritoneal opening circumferentially to form a purse-string closure.**

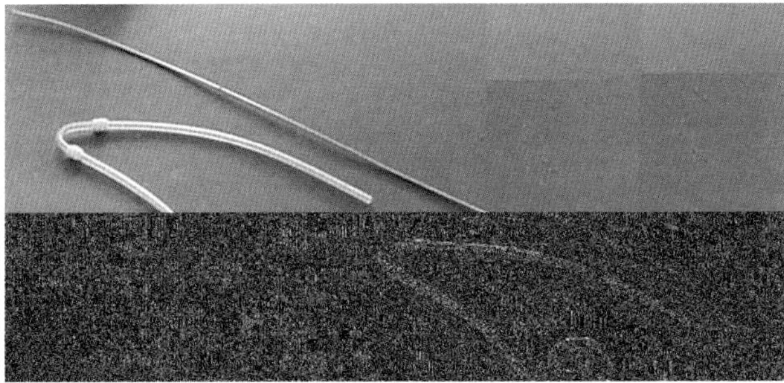

Figure 5 **Catheter and stylet.**

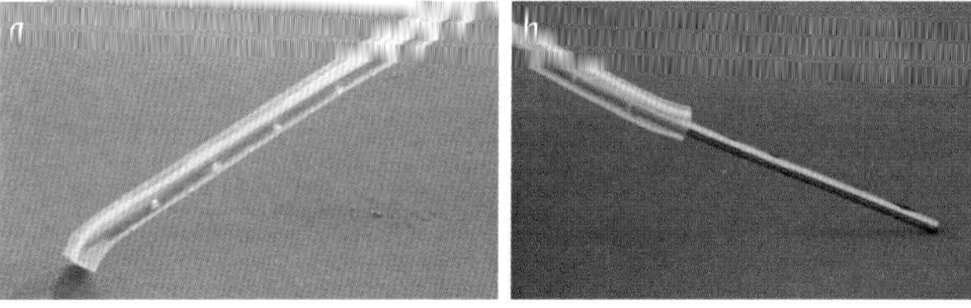

Figure 6 **(*a*) This is the ideal position of the stylet as it is inserted through the small peritoneal incision, minimizing the risk of injuries to visceral structures. (*b*) The catheter with the stylet protruding is dangerous and leads to injuries.**

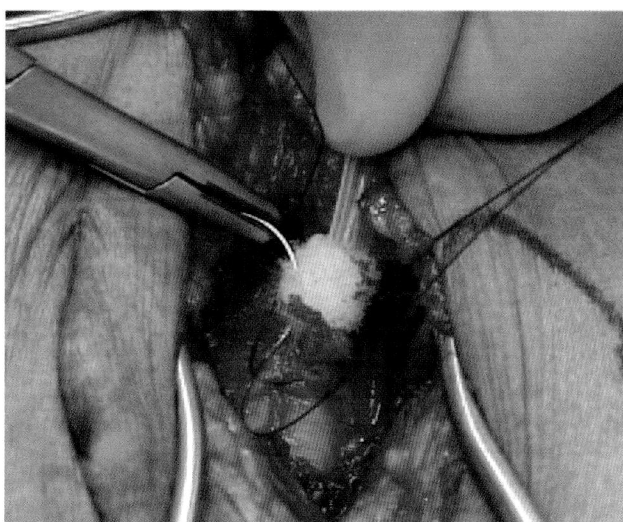

Figure 7 **This image details the placement of suture to secure the inner Dacron cuff. Care should be taken not to inadvertently penetrate the catheter.**

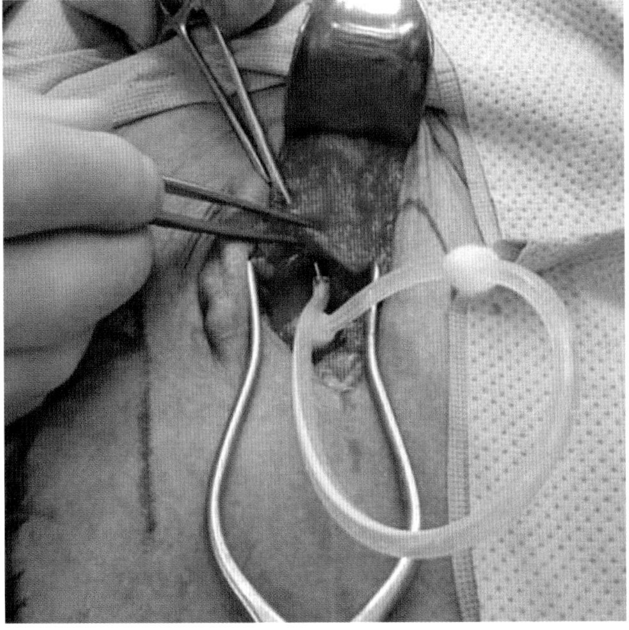

Figure 8 The catheter is tunneled through the rectus muscle and pulled through the anterior rectus fascia.

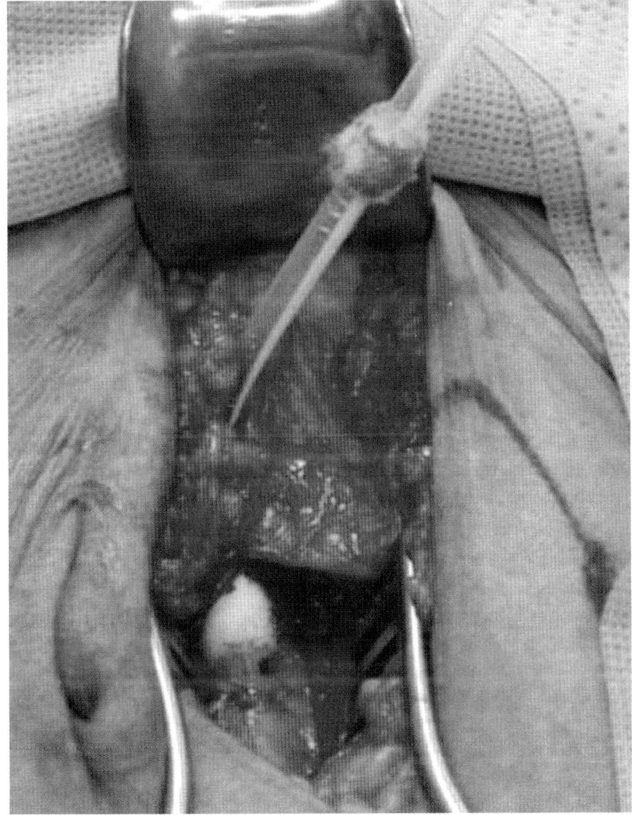

Figure 9 The inner Dacron cuff rests sutured to the posterior rectus muscle fascia. The catheter is aligned in a craniocaudad direction, keeping the coiled portion of the catheter straight down toward the pelvis.

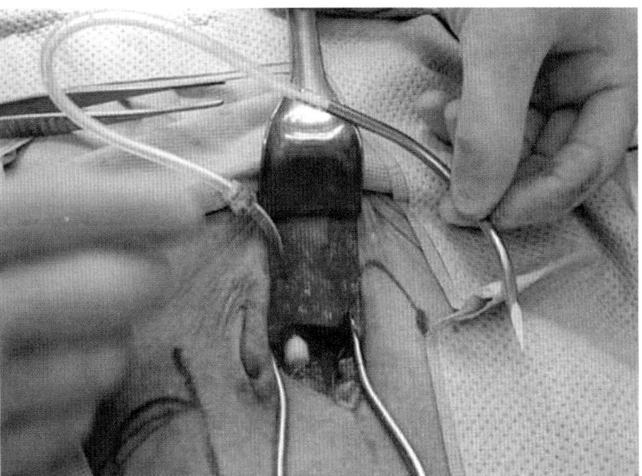

Figure 10 The inner cuff is aligned in a craniocaudad direction. The subcutaneous sharp (Faller) tunneler has now been attached to the catheter.

patient. We strongly advise against the technique of using a skin incision at the exit site and retrograde insertion of a hemostat to catch the PD catheter and pulling through the skin. This technique induces bleeding, is traumatic to the skin, and is prone to complications (mainly infection). The larger skin exit defects (and bleeding) with this technique may require stitching at the skin exit site, which further increases the infection risks and external Dacron cuff migration. Stitches must not be placed at the exit site; sutures here cause trauma and tension and promote infection at the exit site. The anterior fascia is closed in a running fashion with a 2-0 polypropylene suture. The skin is closed with an inverted 4-0 polydioxane or polygalactin subcuticular suture and covered with half-inch SteriStrips and a sterile dressing.

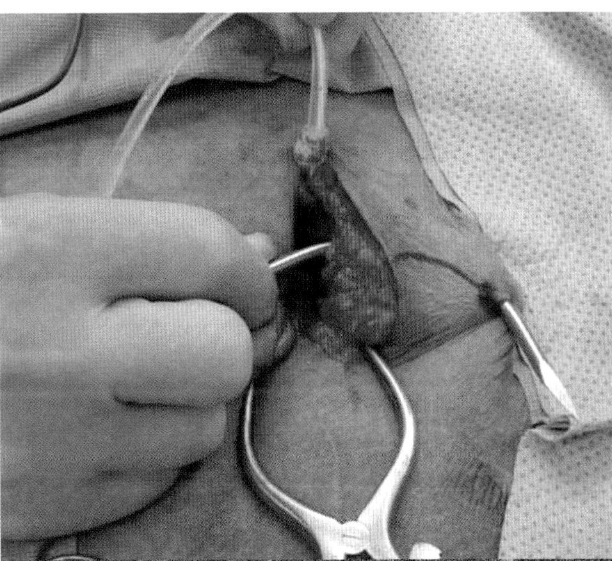

Figure 11 The sharp Faller tunneler has penetrated the skin at the predetermined and marked site. The external cuff ideally will be located 2.0 to 2.5 cm from the skin surface.

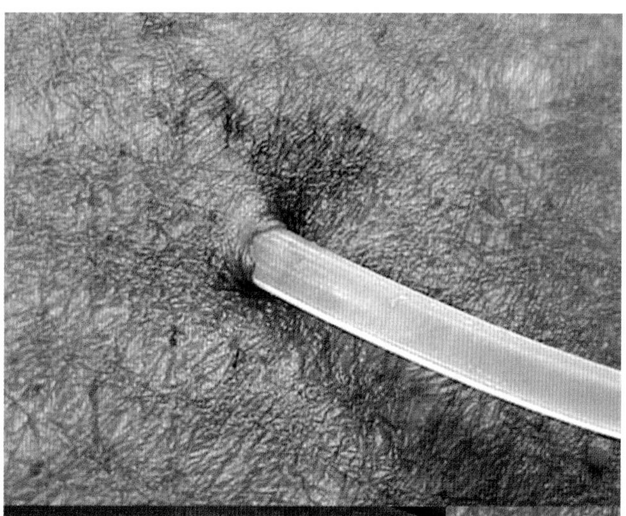

Figure 12 **This close-up image of the catheter skin exit site shows the importance of using the correctly sized and fitted tunneling device.**

Laparoscopic Placement

Although laparoscopic placement of the PD catheter can be performed under local anesthesia and sedation, general anesthesia with endotracheal intubation is safer and preferred for patient comfort. Prophylactic antibiotics are given in the operating room before skin incision, as in the open procedure.

For first-time catheters in a patient with no previous abdominal surgeries, a single camera port and the peel-away catheter sheath are needed. Incidental minor surgical procedures such as small umbilical hernia repairs and omentopexy can also be accomplished with a single port. More complicated and extensive repairs will require additional ports.

The site for Veress needle insufflation should be 1 to 2 inches below the costal margin in the midclavicular line on the ipsilateral side as catheter placement [*see Figure 13*]. Once pneumoperitoneum is established, the Veress needle is exchanged for the camera port. A 5 mm port is placed into the abdomen under direct vision with the camera inside the device. If the patient has had prior abdominal operations or there are concerns for significant adhesions, open Hasson placement in the supraumbilical midline may be used to establish pneumoperitoneum and gain access to the abdominal cavity.

After surveying the abdomen for injury and incidental pathology, the 0 camera is changed to the 30 lens for improved visualization during the PD catheter insertion steps. The desired level of catheter insertion is determined as a location away from the epigastric vessels, or about 3 cm lateral to the midline and 1 to 2 cm above the level of the umbilicus [*see Figure 13*]. A 5 to 7 mm transverse incision is made at the selected catheter insertion site. A slightly larger skin incision is helpful when pulling the catheter with the external cuff to the skin exit site. An 18-gauge needle is inserted through the incision site directed at 45 caudad. As the needle is advanced along and between the peritoneum and the posterior rectus fascia for about 3 to 4 cm, local anesthetic (e.g., bupivacaine 0.25%) is injected along the tract and between the peritoneum and the fascia to create a subperitoneal tunnel and to achieve postoperative pain control. The needle is then used to penetrate the peritoneum about 4 to 5 cm below the level of umbilicus and about 3 cm lateral to the midline in a downward direction.

The syringe is removed and a 0.35-inch internal diameter 50 cm guide wire is inserted. With adequate wire length inside the peritoneal cavity, the needle is also removed, leaving only the guide wire in place. The catheter tract is created using only the stiff dilator inserted over the guide wire with the peel-away sheath off. This facilitates the second pass with the complete peel-away set. While keeping the wire in place, the dilator is removed and inserted into the 22 French peel-away sheath.

The complete set (dilator and peel-away sheath) is now reinserted over the guide wire into the abdomen under direct laparoscopic visualization. When the peel-away sheath is visualized in the abdominal cavity, the inner dilator is removed. The PD catheter is prepared on the back table by inserting the stylet into the PD catheter. The double-cuffed 62 cm long PD catheter with stylet is now inserted into the peel-away sheath, and under direct vision, the PD catheter is advanced until the tip of the guide wire is seen exiting the sheath inside the abdomen.

At this point, the guide is retracted as the catheter is advanced, and the catheter will regain its "pigtail" configuration, which is to be located in the deep pelvis. The catheter is advanced until the inner Dacron cuff is seen. The guide is now completely removed, as is the peel-away sheath. The inner Dacron cuff is pulled back to sit at the posterior rectus muscle fascia or in the rectus muscle. The degree of pull-back is determined based on the length needed to place the external cuff at 1.5 to 2.0 cm from the skin exit site. Next, the curved sharp tunneler is attached to the catheter and penetrated first in an upward and then in a downward curvilinear fashion, out through the skin. This subcutaneous tract step is identical to that in the open procedure. The superficial cuff is placed 1.5 to 2.0 cm from the skin.

Before the camera is removed, the proper position of the curled portion of the catheter in the pelvis is confirmed. Should there be some blood in the abdomen, irrigation through the PD catheter under direct camera vision is performed. After the camera is removed, pneumoperitoneum is released prior to removal of the 5 mm cannula. Port sites are closed with one or two inverted sutures.

Closure and Postoperative Care

With either approach, it is recommended that 40 to 60 mL of saline be left in the abdomen. The newly placed catheter is flushed and aspirated gently with saline or, better, allowed to drain by gravity, ruling out catheter obstruction. Three milliliters of heparin (concentration 1,000 U/mL) is injected into the catheter to avoid catheter obstruction from small blood clots or fibrin. The catheter exit site is covered with 2 × 2–inch gauze wrapped around the catheter to keep the site dry. Dressing changes should be performed in sterile fashion until wound healing is complete. If immediate PD use is required, low-volume exchanges can be initiated within 24 to 48 hours, but it is generally recommended that dialysis be delayed for approximately 2 to 4 weeks, depending on urgency and the postoperative course.

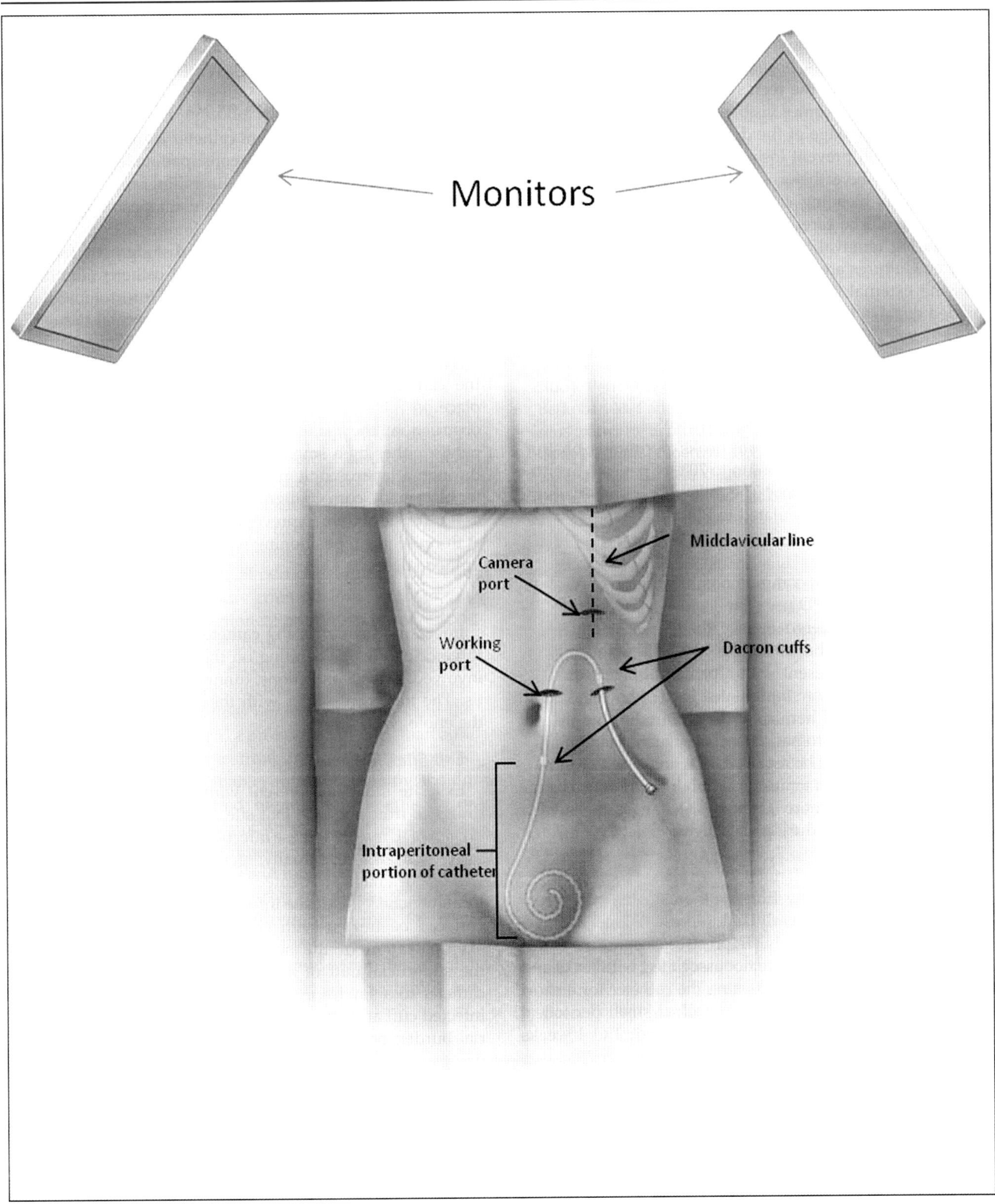

Figure 13 Port locations and final position of the peritoneal dialysis catheter after laparoscopic placement.

Catheter Removal

PD catheters may require removal for various reasons, such as after a successful renal transplantation or after technical malfunctions. During preparation, the catheter should first be clamped next to the skin with a hemostat while the external catheter with the transfer set is removed. The catheter is exposed through the previous incision used

19. Singh N, Davidson I, Minhajuddin A, et al. Risk factors associated with peritoneal dialysis catheter survival: a 9-year single-center study in 315 patients. J Vasc Access 2010;11:316.
20. Crabtree JH, Burchette RJ, Siddiqi NA. Optimal peritoneal dialysis catheter type and exit site location: an anthropometric analysis. ASAIO J 2005;51:743.
21. Crabtree JH, Burchette RJ. Effect of prior abdominal surgery, peritonitis, and adhesions on catheter function and long-term outcomes on peritoneal dialysis. Am Surg 2009;75:140.
22. Saha TC, Singh H. Noninfectious complications of peritoneal dialysis. South Med J 2007;100:54.
23. Davidson IJA. Access for dialysis: surgical and radiologic procedures. 2nd ed. Austin (TX): Landes Bioscience; 2002.
24. Flanigan M, Gokal R. Peritoneal catheters and exit-site practices toward optimum peritoneal access: a review of current developments. Perit Dial Int 2005;25:132.
25. Eklund B, Honkanen E, Kyllonem L, et al. Peritoneal dialysis access: prospective randomized comparison of single-cuff and double-cuff straight Tenckhoff catheters. Nephrol Dial Transplant 1997;12:2664.
26. Gokal R, Alexander S, Ash S, et al. Peritoneal catheters and exit-site practices toward optimum peritoneal access: 1998 update. Perit Dial Int 1998;18:11.
27. Nessim SJ, Bargman JM, Jassal SV. Relationship between double-cuff versus single-cuff peritoneal dialysis catheters and risk of peritonitis. Nephrol Dial Transplant 2010;25:2310.
28. Di Paolo N, Capotondo L, Sansoni E, et al. The self locating catheter: clinical experience and follow-up. Perit Dial Int 2004;24:359.
29. Gadallah MF, Pervez A, El-Shahawy MA, et al. Peritoneoscopic versus surgical placement of peritoneal dialysis catheters: a prospective randomized study of outcome. Am J Kidney Dis 1999;33:118.
30. Jwo SC, Chen KS, Lee CC, et al. Prospective randomized study for comparison of open surgery with laparoscopic-assisted placement of Tenckhoff peritoneal dialysis catheter—a single center experience and literature review. J Surg Res 2010;159:489.
31. Maio R, Figueiredo N, Costa P. Laparoscopic placement of Tenckhoff catheters for peritoneal dialysis: a safe, effective, and reproducible procedure. Perit Dial Int 2008;28:170.
32. Crabtree JH, Fishman A. A laparoscopic method for optimal peritoneal dialysis access. Am Surg 2005;71:135.
33. Crabtree JH, Fishman A. Selective performance of prophylactic omentopexy during laparoscopic implantation of peritoneal dialysis catheters. Surg Laparosc Endosc Percutan Tech 2003;13:180.
34. Dalgic A, Ersoy E, Anderson ME, et al. A novel minimally invasive technique for insertion of peritoneal dialysis catheter. Surg Laparosc Endosc Percutan Tech 2002;12:252.
35. Tsimoyiannis ECT, Siakas P, Glantzounis G, et al. Laparoscopic placement of the Tenckhoff catheter for peritoneal dialysis. Surg Laparosc Endosc Percutan Tech 2000;10:218.
36. Wright MJ, Bel'eed K, Johnson BF, et al. Randomized prospective comparison of laparoscopic and open peritoneal dialysis catheter insertion. Perit Dial Int 1999;19:372.
37. Watson DI, Paterson D, Bannister K. Secure placement of peritoneal dialysis catheters using a laparoscopic technique. Surg Laparosc Endosc 1996;6:35.
38. Santarelli S, Zeiler M, Marinelli R, et al. Videolaparoscopy as rescue therapy and placement of peritoneal dialysis catheters: a thirty-two case single centre experience. Nephrol Dial Transplant 2006;21:1348.
39. Attaluri V, Lebeis C, Brethauer S, et al. Advanced laparoscopic techniques significantly improve function of peritoneal dialysis catheters. J Am Coll Surg 2010;211:699.
40. Zadrozny D, Draczkowski T, Lichodziejewska-Niemierko K. Two millimeter [illegible] mini laparoscopy for rescue of dysfunctional continuous ambulatory peritoneal dialysis catheters. Surg Laparosc Endosc Percutan Tech 1999;9:369–71.
41. Lew SQ, Kaveh K. Dialysis access related infections. ASAIO J 2000;46(6):S6–12.
42. Li PKT, Szeto CC, Piraino B, et al. Peritoneal dialysis-related infections recommendations: 2010 update. Perit Dial Int 2010;30:393.
43. Kern EO, Newman LN, Cacho CP, et al. Abdominal catastrophe revisited: the risk and outcomes of enteric peritoneal contamination. Perit Dial Int 2002;22:323.
44. Figueiredo A, Goh BL, Jenkins S, et al. Clinical practice guidelines for peritoneal access. Perit Dial Int 2010;30:424.

30 DESCENDING THORACIC AND THORACOABDOMINAL AORTIC ANEURYSMS: OPEN AND ENDOVASCULAR REPAIR

*Naveed U. Saqib, MD, and Robert Y. Rhee, MD**

Descending thoracic aortic aneurysms (dTAAs) and thoracoabdominal aortic aneurysms (TAAAs) are localized dilatations in the thoracic and abdominal aorta secondary to weakening and subsequent expansion of the aortic wall. By definition, dTAAs and TAAAs represent dilatation at least 1.5 times the normal diameter of the respective aortic segments.[1] Aortic diseases, including aneurysms, are the 12th leading cause of death in the United States.[2] Although infrarenal abdominal aortic aneurysms (AAAs) and ascending aortic aneurysms are more common, dTAAs and TAAAs are not rare and are estimated to have an incidence of 10 cases per 100,000 persons per year.[3,4] Interestingly, the incidence and prevalence of TAAAs have been increasing over the past several decades.[4] When all of the thoracic aortic aneurysms are considered, the descending thoracic aorta accounts for 35%, whereas aortic arch aneurysms (15%) and TAAAs (10%) account for a smaller proportion.[4,5]

Etiology and Pathogenesis

Most (80%) dTAAs and TAAAs develop secondary to medial degeneration from atherosclerotic disease. Fifteen to 20% of patients develop aneurysms as a consequence of aortic dissection.[6,7] Connective tissue disorders, aortitis (infected or immune related), and trauma constitute the remainder of causes leading to the development of dTAA and TAAA. The aorta in patients with connective tissue disorders such as Marfan syndrome is prone to aortic dissection and subsequent aneurysm formation. Systemic autoimmune disorders such as Takayasu arteritis and chronic nonspecific aortitis are associated with destruction of the aortic media and progressive aneurysm formation.

The pathogenesis of dTAA and TAAA represents a complex interaction of genetic factors, cellular imbalance, and altered hemodynamic stress.[8] The increased incidence of dTAAs and TAAAs in patients with Marfan syndrome and other connective tissue disorders, familial inheritance, marked variability in the age at onset, and decreased penetrance of nonsyndromic aortic aneurysms suggest a varying genetic role along the different segments of the aorta.[9] There is evidence that genetic variation in the extracellular matrix (ECM) actin and myosin may contribute to the development of both dTAA and TAAA.[10] Once the aneurysm formation is initiated through a combination of extracellular and cellular processes, inflammation and pathologic remodeling of the ECM occur in which degradation of the ECM by matrix metalloproteinases (MMPs) exceeds matrix production and repair. Several recently published studies have documented the overexpression and increased activity of a host of ECM proteinases, especially the MMPs, in human dTAAs and TAAAs. An asymmetrical production of MMP-9 in the expanding human TAAA wall is correlated with increased numbers of macrophages; in contrast, MMP-2 is increased in the preserved wall of the TAAA, where smooth muscle cells are predominant and wall is preserved.[11] Investigators studied the role of MMPs in the murine aneurysm model and documented that the *MMP9* gene deletion attenuated the TAAA formation despite increased activity of MMP-2.[12]

Natural History: Risk Factors for Progression and Rupture

The natural history of thoracic aneurysms is not as well defined as the natural history of the isolated infrarenal AAA. Among patients with dTAA and TAAA followed without intervention, nonrandomized studies from earlier decades reported that 40% of the patients died of TAAA rupture and 32% died of cardiovascular diseases. The mean survival in this group of patients was less than 3 years.[13] During observation of patients with dTAA and TAAA, more than 90% of the patients sustained aortic rupture, with 68% of these ruptures occurring more than a month after the diagnosis.[14]

The following have been shown to be risk factors for rupture in patients with dTAA and TAAA: hypertension[15] (in particular, elevated diastolic blood pressure greater than 100 mm Hg), chronic obstructive pulmonary disease (COPD),[16–18] chronic renal failure,[16] coronary artery diseases,[18] absolute aortic diameter (size),[19,20] aneurysm expansion rate more than 1 cm per year,[16,21] uncharacteristic pain,[22] and older age.[22] Among these, aneurysm size is the most important predictor of rupture. The reported risk of rupture in dTAA is varied, but Clouse and colleagues reported the cumulative risk based on size for a 5-year period to be 0% for aneurysms less than 4 cm in diameter, 16% for aneurysms with a diameter between 4 and 5.9 cm, and 31% for an aneurysm larger than 6 cm in diameter.[3] Dapunt and colleagues documented that patients with aneurysms larger than 8 cm in diameter have an 80% risk of rupture within a year.[15] However, as with AAA, the absolute size at which a TAAA will rupture is unpredictable. The average expansion rate of dTAA and TAAA is approximately 0.10 to 0.42 cm per year,[21,23,24] and a faster rate of growth is seen in larger aneurysms. The aneurysm expansion rate of 1 cm annually signals impending rupture.[21] Cambria and colleagues reported an average expansion rate of 0.2 cm annually; although the expansion rate was not influenced by the presence of hypertension, smoking, or renal failure, there was a strong association between increased growth and rupture with COPD.[16]

* The authors and editors gratefully acknowledge the contribution of the previous author, Nathanial Fernandez, MD, to the development and writing of this chapter.

The survival rate in patients diagnosed with dTAA and TAAA is generally poor compared with that for the general population. The 5-year survival rate for dTAA exceeding 6 cm varies between 38 and 64%. The 5-year survival for TAAA exceeding 6 cm in diameter is 54%,[17] with a risk of rupture of 3.7% per year and a risk of death of 12% per year.[17] Aortic rupture is the leading cause of death in this cohort and accounts for 30% of all deaths. Other causes of mortality include cardiac event (25%), pulmonary causes (15%), cancer (10%), and stroke (4%).[3]

Anatomic Classification

Aneurysmal disease can involve all segments of the ascending aorta, aortic arch, and descending thoracic aorta or any combination of these. Morphologically, the aneurysms are either fusiform or saccular. Most dTAAs and TAAAs are fusiform aneurysms, presenting as chronic uniform dilatation involving the whole circumference of the aorta. In contrast, saccular aneurysms represent an eccentric dilatation of the aorta.

dTAAs are classi ed as extent A if they extend from the left subclavian artery (LSA) to the levels of the sixth thoracic vertebrae, extent B if they extend from T6 to the level of the diaphragm, and extent C if they extend from the LSA to the diaphragm [*see Figure 1*].

A different classi cation scheme exists for aneurysms involving the thoracic aorta and visceral segment of the abdominal aorta or TAAA. The full extent of aneurysmal involvement is de ned by proper imaging, most commonly computed tomographic angiography (CTA). TAAAs are normally classi ed according to the extent of aneurysmal involvement of the aorta. Type (extent) I classically involves the descending thoracic aorta distal to the LSA and ends above the renal arteries. Like type (extent) I, type (extent) II involves the thoracic aorta distal to the LSA but extends down to below the renal arteries. Type (extent) III extends from the sixth intercostal space or middescending thoracic aorta to below the renal arteries. Type (extent) IV TAAAs generally involve most if not all of the abdominal aorta, from the 12th intercostal space to the iliac bifurcation. Type (extent) V TAAAs involve the descending aorta below the sixth rib to just above the renal arteries [*see Figure 2*].

Clinical Presentation

The majority of patients with dTAAs are asymptomatic at the time of presentation, and the dTAAs are most commonly an incidental finding during workup and imaging performed for evaluation of another disorder. TAAAs, on the other hand, are more likely to be associated with symptoms at the time of discovery: 49% will present with symptoms other than rupture, 9% will present with a leak or frank rupture, and only 42% will be asymptomatic.[7]

The most common presenting complaint for those symptomatic aneurysms that are not ruptured is ill-de ned chronic back pain that is difficult to differentiate from pain of musculoskeletal origin. Both types of aneurysms may cause symptoms owing to a local mass and pressure effects as well. These may include hoarseness, which can result from vocal cord paralysis secondary to compression of the left recurrent laryngeal or vagus nerves in patients with large aneurysms of the proximal descending thoracic aorta. Patients also may experience dyspnea related to compression of the tracheobronchial tree. Dysphagia can also occur as a result of extrinsic compression of the esophagus by a large aneu-

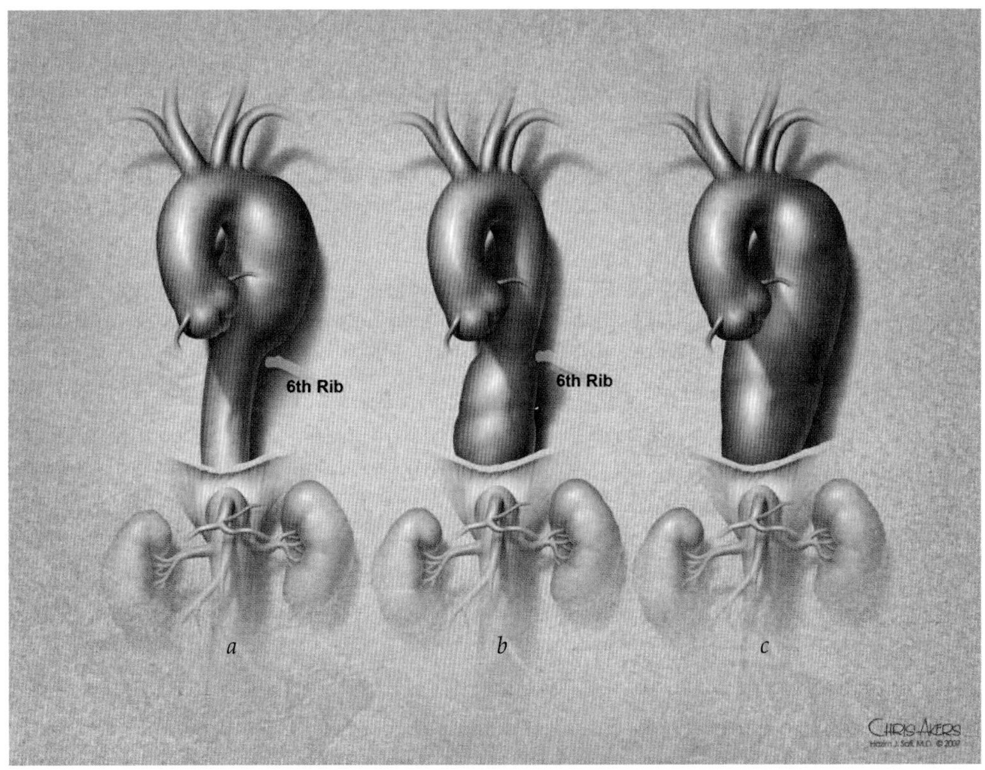

Figure 1 **Classification of descending thoracic aortic aneurysms: (*a*) type A, left subclavian artery to T6; (*b*) type B, T6 to the diaphragm; and (*c*) type C, left subclavian artery to the diaphragm. Adapted from Estrera AL et al.[63]**

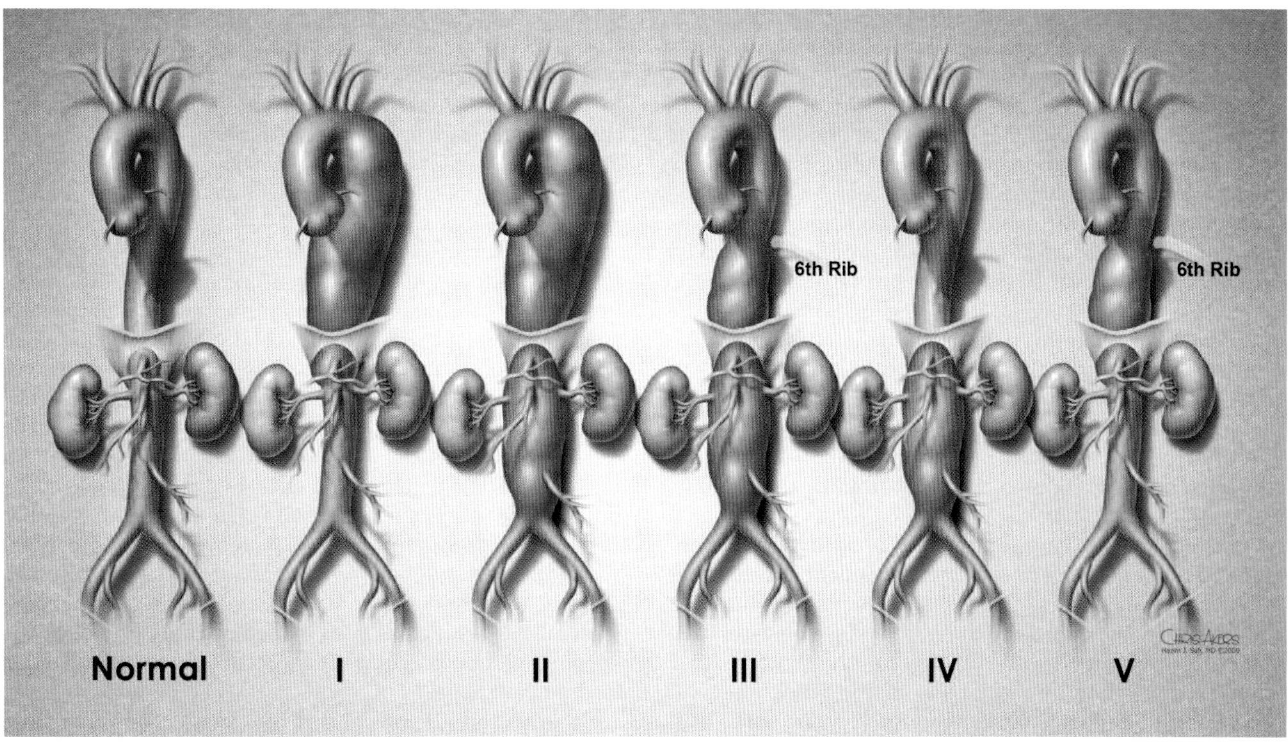

Figure 2 Crawford classification: type I extends from the proximal descending thoracic aorta to the upper abdominal aorta, type II from the proximal descending thoracic aorta to below the renal arteries, type III from the distal half of the descending thoracic aorta to below the renal arteries; type IV involves most of or the entire abdominal aorta; type V extends from the distal descending thoracic aorta to the supra-renal abdominal aorta.

rysm. A large TAAA with an extended paravisceral segment can induce pressure against the duodenum and cause weight loss related to early satiety or obstruction or a vague sensation of "fullness," which may prevent the patient from eating adequately. Rarely, direct erosion of the aneurysm into the adjacent tracheobronchial tree, esophagus, or both can cause exsanguination, presenting as massive hemoptysis or hematemesis or, less frequently, slow, intermittent blood loss [*see Table 1*].

dTAA and TAAA may not be continuous aneurysms. Synchronous discontinuous aneurysms of the abdominal aorta (AAAs), proximal ascending aorta, and aortic arch are present in large numbers of patients recently diagnosed with dTAA and TAAA. Studies examining the natural history of patients with TAAAs indicate that between 20 and 30% will also have an AAA.[13] As many as a third of patients undergoing dTAA or TAAA repair have undergone previous infrarenal AAA repair.[25] Even after repair, at least 10% of patients will require subsequent aneurysm repair in noncontiguous aortic segment.[26]

Regardless of the clinical presentation, patients with dTAA and TAAA frequently have significant coexisting medical conditions, including hypertension, coronary artery disease, COPD, congestive heart failure, cerebrovascular occlusive disease, and peripheral vascular occlusive disease.

Table 1 Symptoms Attributable to Thoracic and Thoracoabdominal Aortic Aneurysms

Symptoms
Back pain
Chronic
Acute change may be sign of impending rupture
Hoarseness
Dyspnea/respiratory dif culty
Dysphagia
Weight loss/early satiety (large TAAA)
Erosion into adjacent structure with bleeding

TAAA = thoracoabdominal aortic aneurysm.

Imaging

For the evaluation of thoracic and thoracoabdominal aortic aneurysms, the most de nitive imaging modality is contrast-enhanced computed tomography (CT) or CTA of the chest, abdomen, and pelvis. CTA is extremely accurate in its ability to de ne the aortic anatomy and the extent of the aneurysm. In addition to providing good spatial resolution, it allows assessment of other intrathoracic, intra-abdominal, or intrapelvic solid organs.[27,28] Evaluation of the aorta for follow-up studies or in patients with renal impairment can be done without contrast if one is interested only in evaluating size progression. CTA is currently the imaging modality of choice for evaluation of the extent of and operative planning for dTAA and TAAA. The 64-slice CT scanner provides fine definition and fast scan times. These scanners also offer three-dimensional volume rendering, as well as maximal intensity projections and sagittal and coronal reconstructions. Third-party software companies such as M2S (Medical Metrx Software, West Lebanon, NH), Vitrea (Vital Images, Minnesota, MN), and Aquarius (TeraRecon,

Inc, San Mateo, CA) offer additional tools, such as orthogonal to the line of flow and virtual grafts, to aid in measurements and preoperative planning.

Magnetic resonance angiography (MRA) is another noninvasive imaging modality that is widely available and can be used to evaluate the aorta and its branches. It has the bene t over CTA of not requiring iodinated contrast and can be used in patients with impaired renal function. Previously, gadolinium-enhanced MRA was used in preference to CTA in patients with renal dysfunction, but recognition of the association between nephrogenic systemic brosis and the use of gadolinium in this patient population has limited the utility of gadolinium and, at least, this theoretical bene t of MRA over CTA.[29] Non–contrast-enhanced MRA can still be performed with good results, but the spatial resolution on a noncontrast MRA is not as precise as with CTA. Additionally, MRA does not show calci cations or mural thrombus as well as CT.

Transesophageal echocardiography is an invasive imaging modality and is more operator dependent than CTA or MRA. It is a useful tool for the evaluation and diagnosis of aortic dissections, especially those involving the ascending aorta. It can provide excellent images of the thoracic aorta but does not allow for evaluation of the whole aorta. It can be useful in the operating room for showing aortic wall disease and assessing cardiac function. Because of the constraints of the chest cavity, standard two dimensional echocardiography or duplex scanning cannot image the descending and ascending aorta adequately to be useful as a routine diagnostic tool.

Decision Making: Timing of Repair and Patient and Treatment Selection

The evaluation and decision-making process for the treatment of DTA are based on prevention of rupture and minimizing the morbidity and mortality associated with repair.

Any symptomatic or ruptured aneurysm mandates urgent repair regardless of the patient's risk factors. Given the fact that the risk of operative intervention in this setting is relatively quite high, the patient and the family must be made fully aware of all of the possible associated morbidities and consequences of an unsuccessful repair attempt.

DESCENDING THORACIC AORTIC ANEURYSM

For asymptomatic patients with nonruptured aneurysms, the decision-making process is slightly complex. Given that the size of the dTAA is the number one predictor of the risk of rupture, ndings on imaging revealing the diameter to be 6 cm or greater are generally considered an indication for repair at our institution provided that the patient is able to physiologically (medically) tolerate such an operation. Additionally, evidence that the aneurysm has grown at a rate of greater than 1 cm per year is a relative indication for repair.

In patients with dTAA of less than 6 cm, observation for a period of 6 months with rigorous follow-up imaging is indicated. Follow-up imaging may be performed with repeat CTA or noncontrasted CT for a patient with renal insuf ciency. If, at any point, the size increases to greater than 6 cm, there is evidence of rapid growth (> 1 cm/year), or the patient has developed any symptoms directly attributable to the aneurysm, we would initiate the process for workup for possible repair [*see Figure 3*]. Patients are instructed that if at any point during the observation period they develop new symptoms attributable to the aneurysm, they should seek medical treatment immediately. If the aneurysm is stable on two consecutive studies, then aneurysm surveillance can be extended to every 12 months.

The main considerations in the preferential choice of thoracic endovascular aneurysm repair (TEVAR) versus open repair are anatomic. If an appropriate landing zone is available both proximally and distally to adequate sealing and exclusion of the aneurysm from the circulation, as well as appropriately sized arterial access to deliver the stent graft to its desired location, patients are preferentially treated with TEVAR at our institution.

The age of the patient and risk assessment also play a significant role in selecting the appropriate treatment modality. We strongly consider open thoracotomy in young patients with low cardiopulmonary risk for surgery even with suitable anatomy for endovascular repair because current endograft fatigue testing has been carried out only to 10 years, in keeping with International Organization for Standardization recommendations.

Other factors to consider in the decision between open and endovascular repair include operative cardiopulmonary risk and incremental risks of branch occlusion or surgical bypass. In the final analysis, [illegible] have suitable anatomy for TEVAR. Hence, TEVAR is usually reserved for poor-risk patients with large aneurysms.

THORACOABDOMINAL AORTIC ANEURYSM

As with dTAA, after the initial evaluation and CTA are completed, the next step in the decision-making process is based on the size of the aneurysm. If the aneurysm is less than 6 cm, then the patient should be observed and seen again in 6 months with a repeat CT scan. If the aneurysm size is stable, without signs of rapid growth (greater than 1 cm per year), and less than 6 cm in diameter, then the plan of observation should be continued. If the TAAA is stable after two consecutive evaluations at 6-month intervals, then this can again be extended to once a year.

If there is continued slow growth of the aneurysm, serial evaluation is undertaken every 6 months until the aneurysm reaches the size of 6 cm, at which point, the patient would undergo assessment of his physiologic status to evaluate tness for possible repair [*see Figure 4*].

All current options for TAAA repair have signi cant morbidity and mortality. The options for management of these patients include open repair with thoracoabdominal incision with adjunct measures, debranching procedure with subsequent endograft repair, branched or fenestrated endograft repair (custom-made or standard off-the-shelf endografts), or continued observation. The selection of type of intervention is individualized to the patient based on the anatomy of the aneurysm and overall functional status, especially related to the patient's pulmonary function and cardiac risk factors. If a patient with a TAAA 6 cm or greater has adequate pulmonary reserve (forced expiratory volume in 1 second [FEV_1] > 70% predicted, FEV_1 > 1.2 L, forced expiratory flow at 25 to 75% of > 40% of predicted) and low

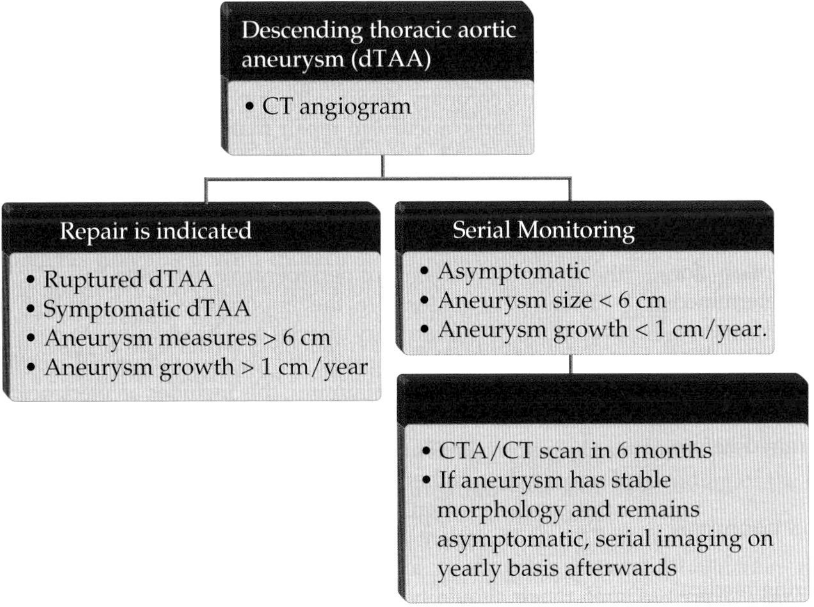

Figure 3 **Evaluation of patient with descending thoracic aortic aneurysm. CT = computed tomography; CTA = computed tomographic angiography.**

cardiac risk, an open thoracoabdominal aneurysm repair is offered as the de nitive primary treatment option. However, if a patient is determined to be at low risk from a pulmonary standpoint but felt to be at high risk from a cardiac perspective, then continued observation is usually recommended. If the patient exhibits continued growth of the aneurysm or has direct aneurysm-related symptoms, appropriate cardiac revascularization may be indicated prior to any type of direct surgical intervention for the TAAA [*see Figure 4*].

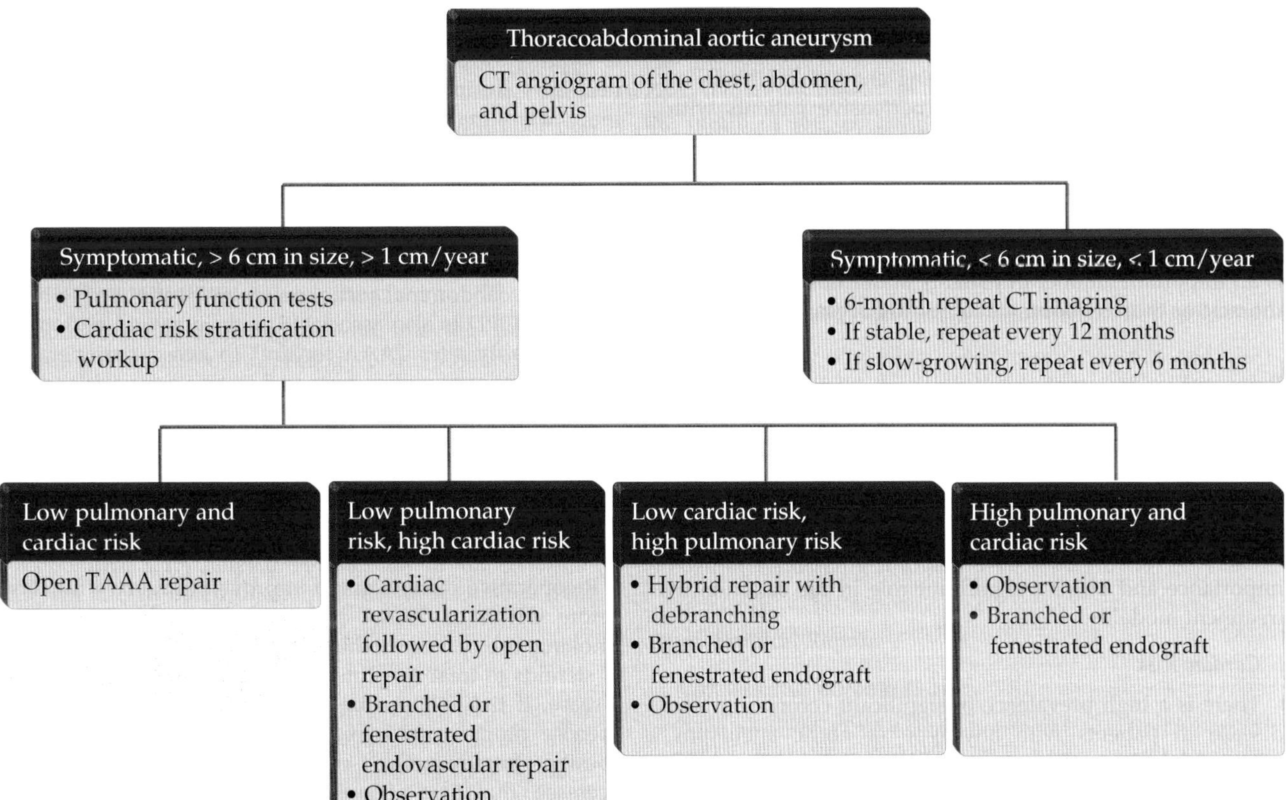

Figure 4 **Evaluation and management algorithm of a patient with a thoracoabdominal aneurysm. CT = computed tomography; TAAA = thoracoabdominal aortic aneurysm.**

the technique for TAAA repair by introducing the principle of inclusion, in which aortic branches are reconstructed from inside the aneurysm, and introduced the concept of reimplantation of intercostal arteries to prevent paraplegia.[53]

Most centers have discarded the simple clamp-and-sew technique advocated by Crawford for its simplicity and its value in hemostasis. Initially, the clamp-and-sew technique was used without adjunctive measures, with subsequent end-organ ischemia being the main postoperative problem. Nowadays, most surgeons have adopted distal aortic perfusion provided by left atriofemoral bypass with a sequential clamping technique.[54] At our institution, we use left atriofemoral bypass for distal aortic perfusion in type I, II, III, and V TAAAs and the majority of dTAAs. The use of adjunctive measures in type IV TAAA remains variable. Approximately, 50% of patients with type IV TAAA can undergo single beveled anastomosis that incorporates the proximal aorta and the visceral vessels without the need for extracorporeal circulation.

Distal aortic perfusion limits end-organ ischemia by maintaining blood flow through the lower extremity, mesenteric, and renal arteries. Distal perfusion also maintains flow to the spinal cord and helps decrease left ventricular afterload, especially in situations needing very proximal aortic cross-clamping.[55] We use partial left heart bypass by venous cannulation of the left inferior pulmonary vein. A centrifugal bypass pump returns blood through a left femoral arterial cannula. The bypass flow rate is set to maintain mean aortic pressure in the distal aorta of approximately 60 mm Hg; however, the mean pressure is raised higher if there is low urine output or a decrease in spinal cord function detected by intraoperative monitoring. Hypothermic circulatory arrest with total cardiopulmonary bypass is required in dTAA and TAAA repairs, where proximal control beyond the left common carotid artery is not feasible.

Monitoring of spinal cord function with evoked potentials, reattachment of large intercostal arteries, distal aortic perfusion, cerebrospinal fluid (CSF) drainage, systemic or local hypothermia, permissive hypertension, and prevention of hypotension are principal adjunct measures in contemporary practice.[55] CSF drainage and intercostal artery reconstruction are measures to preserve cord blood supply. Variations in hypothermia and endorphin receptor blockage are neuroprotective adjunctive measures. Adequate spinal cord perfusion can be assessed by means of monitoring somatosensory evoked potentials (SSEPs) and motor evoked potentials (MEPs).[56,57] SSEPs are known to have longer delay between onset and detection of ischemia compared with MEPs. MEPs are reliable and are used more frequently in current practice; however, MEPs can be influenced by neuromuscular blockade. Changes in spinal cord function as measured by SSEPs and MEPs influence the surgical strategy, including elevation of distal aortic perfusion, increased hypothermia, and reattachment of segmental arteries even outside the standard T8-L1 level.[58] Lowering body temperature significantly decreases the incidence of spinal cord ischemic complications and is thought to be due to decreased tissue metabolism and decreased oxygen requirement.[59] Regional epidural cooling was advocated in the past but has largely been abandoned in favor of systemic hypothermia. CSF drainage during and after open dTAA and TAAA repair decreases CSF pressure and increases the relative spinal cord perfusion pressure. Perioperative CSF drainage has been associated with a significantly lower incidence of spinal cord ischemic events (3% compared with 13%) in a randomized, controlled study of 145 patients with type I and type II TAAA repair.[60] At our institution, a CSF drain is placed in all patients undergoing dTAA and TAAA repair preoperatively and kept in place for 72 hours postoperatively. Delayed paraplegia is treated by increasing blood pressure and replacement of the CSF drain.[61]

During open TAAA repair, we administer local hypothermic perfusion of the renal arteries as an adjunctive measure for renal protection. The perfusate consists of unfractionated heparin, lactated Ringer solution, and mannitol. The hypothermic component is considered the most important one.[62] In dTAA repair, since the distal clamp is above the celiac artery, we use distal aortic perfusion alone.

dTAA Open Repair

After intrathecal CSF drain placement and intubation with a double-lumen endotracheal tube, the patient is put in the right lateral decubitus position with the left hip at 60 to allow access to both groins. A posterolateral thoracotomy at the sixth intercostal space provides excellent exposure to the entire descending thoracic aorta. If more proximal exposure is required, a fifth intercostal space posterolateral thoracotomy is selected. Additional proximal access can be obtained by resection of the sixth rib or dislocation of the rib posteriorly. Adequate preparation of the proximal clamp site is crucial and includes identification of the vagus and recurrent laryngeal nerves followed by transection of the ligamentum arteriosum. If clamping is required proximal to the subclavian artery, the pericardium is opened dorsal to the phrenic nerve and the arch is dissected away from surrounding tissues, including the pulmonary artery. After preparing the proximal clamp site, the esophagus is dissected free and carefully protected to avoid aortoesophageal fistula. Preparation of the distal clamp site at the diaphragm or higher includes opening the parietal pleura. Injury to the accessory hemiazygos vein during distal clamp placement is avoided by direct visualization of the vein and placing the clamp between the vein and the aorta. Distal aortic perfusion is then established, as discussed in the previous section. End-to-end anastomosis of a tube graft using 3-0 or 4-0 monofilament polypropylene suture with or without pledget is performed. Reconstruction of intercostal artery bypass or reimplantation is performed based on the SSEPs and MEPs during the operation. Once hemostasis is achieved, chest tubes are placed, the left atriofemoral bypass is disconnected, and the thoracotomy is closed.

TAAA Repair

The preparation for open TAAA is similar to that for open dTAA repair. In type I, II, and III TAAAs, the posterolateral sixth intercostal space thoracotomy is extended over the costal margin in an oblique line and is continued across the abdomen medially and caudally. The extent of distal incision is dictated by the distal extent of the aneurysm. In type I TAAA, the incision is stopped at the umbilicus. In type IV TAAA repair, the thoracotomy is made in the eighth intercostal space and can be limited to the anterior part of the chest to allow adequate exposure for cross-clamping. The abdominal aorta is exposed via a transperitoneal or retroperitoneal approach. We prefer to divide only the anterior muscular part of the diaphragm to avoid injury to the branches of the phrenic nerve. All para-aortic tissue is transected along the line of the intended aortotomy. We perform left heart bypass in all type I, II, III, and V TAAA operations for distal aortic perfusion. Renal protection by administration of cold perfusate solution is performed by using 12 or 14 French selective perfusion catheters. The sequential clamp-and-sew technique is used for proximal, mesenteric, and renal bypasses. Proximal and distal anastomoses are performed using 3-0 and 4-0 monofilament sutures, and visceral bypasses are performed using 6-0 monofilament sutures. We use prefabricated grafts with 6 or 8 mm prefabricated branches. Due to the high incidence of degeneration and subsequent aneurysm formation in Carrell patches, we have abandoned the Carrell patch for visceral bypass and perform individual visceral and mesenteric bypasses instead. Reimplantation of thoracic segmental arteries and lumbar arteries is performed based on the intraoperative SSEPs and MEPs. After flow has been restored through the graft and hemostasis is ensured, the diaphragm is approximated, chest tubes are placed, the left atriofemoral bypass is disconnected, and the thoracotomy is closed in several layers.

OUTCOMES AND COMPLICATIONS

Open surgical repair of dTAA is a durable option with a low incidence of morbidity and mortality and secondary aortic interventions. Coselli reported an overall paraplegia rate of 2.6% and a 30-day mortality rate of 2.8%, with no reduction in the paraplegia rate even when an adjunctive left heart bypass was performed.[63] Estrera and colleagues demonstrated the beneficial effect of CSF drainage and left heart bypass in open dTAA repair; the authors reported a paraplegia rate of 1.3% with adjunctive measures compared with 6.5% in patients without adjunctive measures ($p < .02$). The 30-day mortality was reported to be 8%.[64] Schermerhorn and colleagues reported an overall mortality of 10% after open dTAA in a Nationwide Inpatient Sample administrative database review.[65] The mortality was 17% in patients above the age of 75 years and 45% in patients with a ruptured dTAA. It has been well known that circumstances other than elective procedures are associated with doubled mortality, even if the patients remain hemodynamically stable. Similarly, in situations involving high proximal clamp placement, such as involvement of the distal aortic arch and proximal descending thoracic aorta, the surgical outcome worsens significantly.

Contemporary series have shown that open repair of TAAAs can be performed with satisfactory results in centers of excellence.[66–68] Mortality and spinal cord injury are the most frequently analyzed outcome measures, but other important end points are renal insufficiency, morbidity, quality of life, and functional status after the operation. Coselli and colleagues reported an operative mortality of 6.6% and spinal cord injury of 4% in a group of 2,286 patients undergoing open TAAA repair.[67] Other reports from large-volume aortic centers have shown mortality in the range of 4.6 to 14.6%.[64] However, real-world data using national and regional data sets have demonstrated more ominous results. In a study by Rigberg and colleagues of 797 Medicare beneficiaries who underwent elective open TAAA repair in California, the mortality was 19% at 30 days and 31% at 1 year.[69] Cowan and colleagues demonstrated significantly higher mortality in low-volume hospitals (27% versus 15%) and when performed by low-volume surgeons (26% versus 11%) in a Nationwide Inpatient Sample administrative database review.[70]

Postoperative cardiac complications, reported in 12 to 25% of patients, include myocardial infarction, arrhythmia, congestive heart failure, and unstable angina. The incidence of pulmonary complications in most recent studies is between 32 and 49%.[68] Respiratory failure is the most common complication after both open dTAA and TAAA repair. The independent predictors of respiratory failure, defined as ventilatory support required beyond 48 hours postoperatively, are COPD, a history of smoking, and cardiac and renal complications.[71] Eight percent of patients ultimately require tracheostomy, and this subgroup has higher mortality (40%). Coselli and colleagues reported overall renal failure requiring dialysis in 5.6% of patients in their series of 2,286 patients.[67] Patients with type II TAAA had an incidence of 8.3%. Using the current classification of acute renal injury, Conrad and colleagues reported renal failure requiring dialysis in 20.9% of patients, compared with 4.6% of patients in whom cold renal perfusion was used intraoperatively.[68] Gastrointestinal complications after open dTAA and TAAA repair are rare. Gastrointestinal complications occur in 7% of patients overall, and these patients have significantly higher mortality (39.5%) compared with patients without gastrointestinal complications (13.5%). Bowel ischemia is the most frequent gastrointestinal complication and is mainly due to embolization secondary to aortic manipulation, cross–clamping, and associated atherosclerotic disease of the visceral vessels. Postoperative pancreatitis is usually secondary to the pancreatic trauma resulting from surgical dissection, hypoperfusion, and embolization. Graft-related complications rarely occur; however, aortoesophageal and aortobronchial fistulas are well-known and feared events.

In open dTAA surgery, the use of adjunctive measures has significantly reduced the incidence of spinal cord ischemia (SCI) and subsequent paraplegia. In centers of excellence, the incidence of immediate paraplegia ranges between 0 and 3% if surgery is performed with the adjunctive measures and the clamp times are kept below 30 minutes.[66]

In open TAAA surgery, the paraplegia rates are higher. In patients who underwent open repair with hypothermic cardiopulmonary arrest and no other adjunct measure, paraplegia was reported in 2.6% with type I TAAA repair, 4.1% with type II, and 5.9% with type III.[72] In patients who underwent open repair with epidural cooling, CSF drainage, and routine reimplantation of intercostal arteries at T9-L1, paraplegia occurred in 9.5% of patients and paresis in 3.7%. The overall incidence of any neurologic deficit was 15.7% in type I, 20.3% in type II, 14% with type III, and 2.9% with type IV TAAA.[68] As previously stated, the incidence of paraplegia in the series published by Coselli and colleagues was 3.8%, with an incidence of 6.3% in patients who underwent

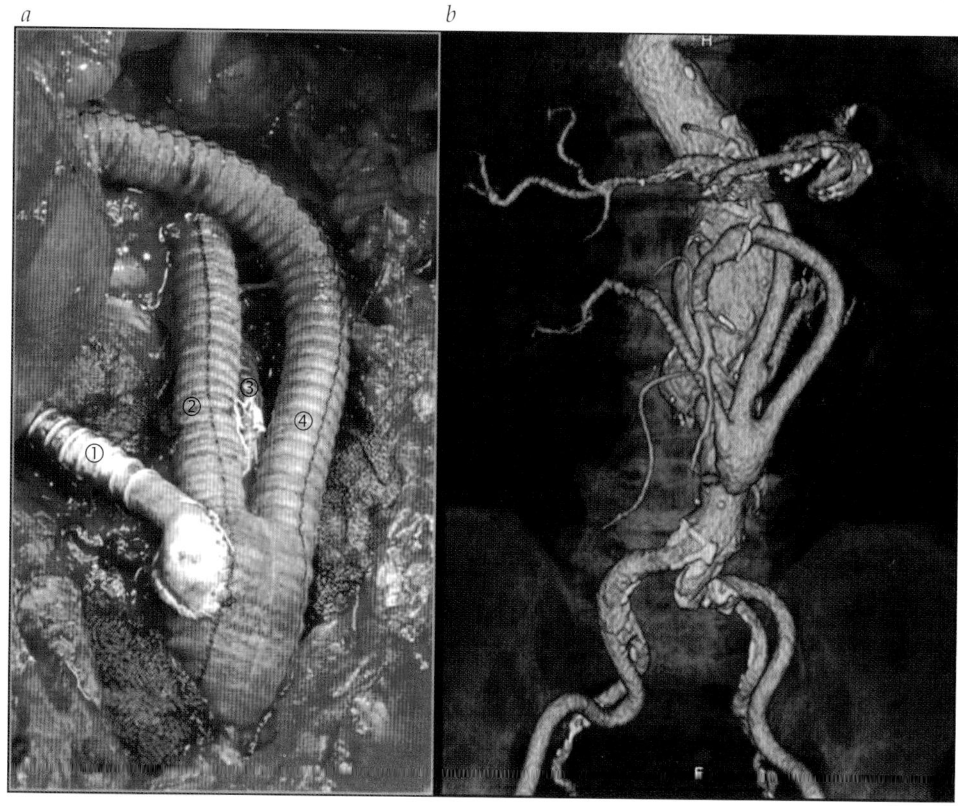

Figure 7 (*a*) **Visceral artery debranching to 1, right renal artery; 2, celiac axis; 3, left renal artery; and 4, superior mesenteric artery. (*b*) Computed tomographic scan showing visceral debranching prior to placement of an endograft.**

At our institution, we use the option for visceral artery debranching followed by exclusion by TEVAR as the rst treatment option for patients with inadequate pulmonary function (FEV_1 < 70% of predicted) but who are at relatively low cardiac risk. The patients are taken to the operating room for the visceral vessel revascularization, given a period of 1 to 2 days to recover physiologically from this operation, and then taken back for the TEVAR procedure. The return for TEVAR can be delayed by 2 to 4 weeks due to postoperative renal insufficiency or delayed recovery from postoperative complications.

Outcomes and Results

Despite perceived advantages over open repair and early reports of successes, enthusiasm for hybrid procedures has been tempered by high morbidity and mortality at several centers.[92–100] The UCLA and University of Michigan groups reported two of the largest experiences, with remarkably low mortality of 0 and 3.4%, respectively.[93,94] Other centers (Cleveland Clinic, Mayo Clinic, Massachusetts General Hospital, and Methodist Hospital, Houston) have shown higher mortality in the range of 10 to 25%.[95,97,101] Spinal cord injury occurs in 2 to 25% of cases and correlates with the extent of aortic coverage, preservation of flow into the subclavian and hypogastric arteries, and periprocedural hypotension.[32,91–95,97–99] Rates of type I and II endoleak have been reported in the range of 3 to 15% and 5 to 25%, respectively.

Bakoyiannis and colleagues reviewed the outcomes of 108 patients from 15 reports between 1999 and 2008.[102] Technical success was achieved in 92% of the reported cases; 30-day mortality was 10%. There was a 17% incidence of primary endoleaks and 3% delayed secondary endoleaks. Spinal cord injury occurred in three patients (3%), and renal insufficiency occurred in 12 patients (11%). After a mean follow-up of 10 months, 97% of the visceral grafts remained patent, and 24% of patients died from unrelated causes.

A more recent meta-analysis by Moulakakis and colleagues included 507 patients from 19 reports published since 1999.[103] There were 319 male (64%) and 188 female patients, with a mean age of 70 years. Aneurysm extent was classified as type I in 14%, type II in 27%, type III in 34%, type IV in 14%, and type V in 11%. A single-stage procedure was used in 55%, and a two-stage procedure was used in 45%, with a mean period of 28 days between the two stages. Thirty-day or in-hospital mortality was 13%, and the most common causes of death were multisystem organ failure, ischemic colitis, respiratory failure, and aneurysm rupture prior to a second-stage procedure. Pooled rates of spinal cord injury were 7.5%, with irreversible paraplegia in 4.5%. After a mean follow-up of 35 months, 111 patients (22%) had endoleaks, and visceral graft patency was 96%.

The preliminary results of the North American Complex Abdominal Aortic Debranching (NACAAD) Registry were presented at the 2011 Vascular Annual Meeting.[104] A total of 208 patients who underwent treatment for complex AAAs at 14 academic centers in North America were included in this study. A total of 659 visceral arteries were reconstructed using single-stage debranching in 92 patients (44%) or a two-stage approach in 116 patients (56%). Arch debranching was needed in 22 patients (11%) to provide an adequate proximal landing zone. The inflow for visceral reconstruction was based on the iliac arteries in 63%, aorta or aortic graft in 29%, or a hepatic or splenic artery in 8%. The extent of visceral reconstruction included one or two vessels in 58 patients (28%) and three or four vessels in 150 patients (72%).

Thirty-day or in-hospital mortality was 14% for all patients, 16% for TAAAs, and 9% for pararenal aneurysms. Mortality ranged from 0 to 21% in centers with more than 10 cases. Any morbidity occurred in 73% of patients, most commonly, pulmonary (22%), renal (19%), and gastrointestinal (14%) complications. Spinal cord injury occurred in 21 patients (10%), and ischemic colitis occurred in 13 patients (6%).

The mean length of hospital stay was 21 days. Patient survival at 1 and 5 years was 77 ± 3% and 61 ± 5%, respectively, and predictors of late mortality included chronic kidney disease (stage > 3), high SVS scores, and more than three-vessel reconstruction. After a median follow-up of 21 months, 70% of patients had repeat aortic imaging. Endoleaks occurred in 23 patients (13%) and were classified as type I in 3%, type II in 8%, and type III in 1%. Primary visceral graft patency and freedom from reinterventions were 90 ± 2% and 85 ± 3% at 1 year, respectively.

Hybrid procedures have several advantages over conventional open repair, including avoiding thoracotomy, single-lung ventilation, aortic cross-clamping, and minimizing end-organ ischemia. The shortcomings are the need for extensive dissection in multiple abdominal areas and prolonged procedure time. Patient selection is a key feature for optimal results. A few centers have adopted hybrid procedures as their primary treatment option in intermediate- and high-risk patients, with good results. However, several centers with large complex aortic volume, systematic reviews, and a national registry have shown that hybrid procedures carry high mortality rates.

Complete Endovascular Repair of TAAA

Endovascular approaches to TAAAs have evolved during the last decade. The initial experiences with fenestrated and branched endografts have shown that total endovascular repair is effective and may reduce morbidity in patients with arch, thoracoabdominal, and pararenal aneurysms.[105] Nonetheless, these devices are not yet widely available and still require a period of customization of 6 to 8 weeks. Although "off-the-shelf" devices are likely to allow treatment of more than 60 to 80% of patients with complex aneurysms, standardized designs have not yet been clinically tested in a large number of patients with longer follow-up.[106,107]

In the absence of widely available endograft designs, a number of centers have reported creative techniques to incorporate the visceral arteries, including chimney, sandwich, octopus, and physician-modified endografts.[101,108] However, these approaches are limited by off-label indication, lack of quality control, violation of basic engineering concepts, and questionable durability.

Parallel Endograft Endovascular Repair

Kolvenbach and colleagues reported their multi-institutional experience of nine thoracoabdominal aneurysms repaired with the "sandwich technique."[109] Three of these TAAAs were type IV. Because endovascular techniques have become routine in the daily practice of vascular surgeons and interventionists, many feel confident using these techniques as a quick bailout procedure in urgent or emergent situations in high-risk patients whose lives may be at risk and are unfit for surgery. Although this treatment option is technically feasible, there are no reported data on mid- or long-term results, making its use in the elective setting questionable. Suprarenal AAA may also be approached in this fashion using "snorkel techniques" for renal and mesenteric preservation.

It must also be emphasized that there is a large difference in the complexity of repair between juxtarenal aneurysms and TAAAs and that a parallel graft repair of a TAAA may require placement of covered stents into all four visceral vessels. The issue of endoleaks associated with these parallel grafts, as well as the durability of the branches, remains unresolved, and their mid- and long-term outcomes are unknown.

Fenestrated and Branched Stent Grafts

Fenestrated and branched stent grafts have been developed as a minimally invasive, total endovascular alternative for the treatment of complex aortic aneurysms in high-risk patients [*see Figure 8*]. The midterm results for treating TAAAs are excellent and demonstrate the benefits of avoiding extensive aortic and visceral vessel surgical exposure and maintaining visceral perfusion during the repair. Successful results with fenestrated and branched endografting have been reported.[79,110–115] Achieving these results requires appropriate patient selection, proper device design, high-resolution imaging, technical expertise with endovascular grafting and visceral vessel cannulation and stenting, and meticulous postoperative follow-up.

Currently, Cook Medical has the only commercially available device outside the United States.[116–118] Their US trial is now complete,[119] and the application for commercial use of the device has been submitted to the FDA. Long-term results and larger series are still needed to further delineate the safety and efficacy of these devices. However, as the technology and technique evolve and become more widely disseminated, fenestrated and branched stent grafts appear destined to play an increasingly important role in the treatment of TAAA, especially type IV TAAA.

Future management and treatment of TAAAs will be driven by evolution in devices and techniques in endovascular repair, in particular with fenestrated and branched stent grafts. However, these advances will not occur just by improving stent grafts and by introducing new devices; rather, the process will be multimodal, including advances in preoperative imaging and peripheral products, as well as adjunctive tools that will facilitate easier and faster visceral access. Most importantly, surgeons will need to become skilled in delivering these complex devices.

The key factor for success is to eliminate issues that may compromise the durability of the repair. Reconstructions need to maintain anatomic fidelity, with branches coming off at smooth angles from the endograft and bridging stents to the aortic branches following the direction of the native artery. Overlap between aortic endograft and branch stents

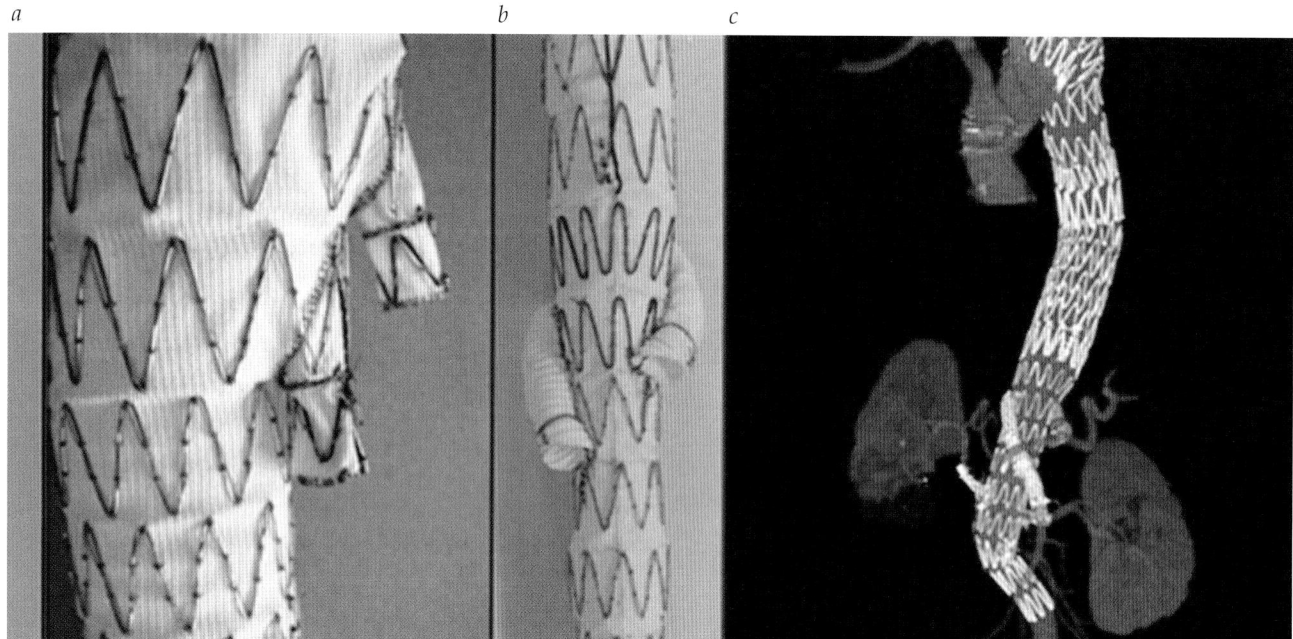

Figure 8 **Branched endograft with cuffs with caudal orientation (*a*) and helical orientation (*b*). Reconstruction of a postoperative computed tomographic scan following branched endovascular repair of a type II thoracoabdominal aortic aneurysm (*c*).**

needs to be maximized to reduce the risk of component separation, type III endoleaks, and protrusion of branch stents into the main stent graft.

Currently, customized devices are available to treat patients in the elective setting, but patients presenting emergently have limited treatment options if they are unfit for open surgery. Although the back-table construction of a surgeon-modified stent graft is currently the most durable and promising endovascular solution to treat such patients,[114,120,121] the introduction of off-the-shelf standardized devices is expected to bring a new push in the field of fenestrated endovascular aneurysm repair (FEVAR). However, standardization should not be allowed to supplant principles such as preservation of all aortic branches with perfectly aligned fenestrations or branches. Finding the balance between standardized and customized stent grafts will be challenging in the coming years.

Key elements in the planning of endovascular TAAA repair are the generation of a centerline path with measurements using centerline of flow analysis, as well as three-dimensional reconstructions. Currently, the TeraRecon Aquarius Workstation is the most widely used in the field. Advances in imaging technology and in available workstations will provide more exact measurements and accurate planning of FEVAR. Improved intraoperative imaging (e.g., the fusion of preoperative CT scans with intraoperative fluoroscopy) will also allow better technical results in shorter operation times, as well as limit radiation exposure and contrast dose.

Devices in the Pipeline

With Cook Medical producing the first fenestrated and branched device for use in pararenal and thoracoabdominal aneurysms, other companies in the field of endovascular surgery have begun to produce their own fenestrated and branched devices [*see Table 3*].[122,123] Most of these devices have approval (or approval is being sought) for pararenal aortic aneurysms; however, iterations of the current devices will be evolved in the near future for use in treating TAAAs.

Stent grafts for FEVAR are currently either fenestrated (typically with reinforcement around the fenestration) or precuffed (with a cuff "branch" coming off the ostium of the fenestrations). The cuffs may be helical or caudally or cranially oriented. The cuffs provide better sealing with the branch stents when compared with the simple fenestrations because the overlap is better and may facilitate easier cannulation of the branch vessels. Typically, the proximity of the fenestration to the ostium of the visceral branch determines whether a fenestration is sufficient or if a cuff should be preferred. Helical cuffs have a more complex multiplanar configuration, with both axial and rotational elements; therefore, side-arm branches are considered to be more efficient in accommodating smooth alignment of the side-arm branch to the target vessel.[124]

Standardized "off-the-shelf" stent grafts Stent grafts that have been manufactured to fit a population with typical visceral vessel anatomy and thus are not patient tailored (custom made) are referred to as standardized grafts. Creating an off-the-shelf, one-size-fits-all device is the "holy grail" for FEVAR and for industry. Currently, patients with complex aortic aneurysms may have to wait up to 8 weeks for their devices to be manufactured and delivered. A standardized stent graft would not only prevent rupture from occurring during this waiting period but would also allow treatment of patients presenting with ruptures and/or symptoms that require urgent or emergent treatment.

Table 3 Overview of Fenestrated and Branched Endograft Devices under Investigation and Current Use

Company	*Device*	*Indication*	*Availability*	*Characteristics*
Cook Medical	Zenith fenestrated	Pararenal AAA TAAA	Available in Europe, Australia, Canada, Brazil, China, New Zealand, Hong Kong	Fenestrations and scallops are premanufactured as ordered according to physician's measurements
	Preloaded fenestrated device	Pararenal AAA	Approved 2012	Fenestrations are preloaded with wires to access visceral arteries
	Standardized off-the-shelf FBSG	Pararenal AAA and TAAA	Under investigation	Standardized locations for fenestrations expected to accommodate > 70% of morphology
Medtronic Inc.	Branch device	Pararenal and suprarenal AAA	In design	Off-the-shelf, precannulated renal branches and SMA scallop
Vascutek Ltd.	Anaconda custom fenestrated	Juxtarenal/ pararenal AAA	Postmarket surveillance registry, custom-made regulations: Europe and Canada	Fenestrations are premanufactured according to individual patient requirements Repositionable stent-free proximal part to provide flexibility
Endologix Inc.	Ventana fenestrated stent graft	Juxtarenal and pararenal AAA	In clinical trial	Off-the-shelf, precannulated, steerable fenestrations
W. L. Gore	Branched Excluder system	Suprarenal AAA, TAAA	In design	Renal, mesenteric branches

AAA = abdominal aortic aneurysm; FBSG = fenestrated/branched stent graft; SMA = superior mesenteric artery; TAAA = thoracoabdominal aortic aneurysm.

Currently, we treat these patients with surgeon-modified grafts.[114,120] Sweet and colleagues demonstrated that 88% of patients treated with stent grafts customized to the patient's anatomy could also have been treated with standardized endografts.[107] The same group continues to report its experience on the transition from customized to standardized stent grafts with excellent outcomes using standardized branched stent grafts.

The off-the-shelf devices currently in the pipeline are aimed at juxtarenal and suprarenal aneurysms (fenestrated design), as well as thoracoabdominal aneurysms (branched design). Although these current designs can theoretically treat up to 80% of these pathologies, the remaining 20% remain outside the current design limits and need custom devices. Due to the way the devices are implanted, they are also generally less suitable for treating ruptured aneurysms, particularly in unstable patients.

Standardized Cook Medical pararenal device Cook Medical's off-the-shelf fenestrated device has a four-piece modular design: a proximal tubular component with fenestrations, a second bifurcated component without a top cap, and two iliac limbs. The device is based on the fenestrated platform for elective patients. The standardized location of the fenestrations is expected to accommodate anatomy for approximately 70% of patients, with less than 10 variations of the proximal piece.

Endovascular Exclusion of TAAA/AAA Utilizing Fenestrated/Branched Stent Grafts is a physician-sponsored clinical trial evaluating a new stent graft design developed in cooperation with Cook Medical. The new device incorporates branches (formed by covered balloon-expandable stents) to both renal arteries and the superior mesenteric artery. The first patient underwent elective endovascular repair, the second patient was treated for a ruptured aneurysm, and the third patient was treated for a type IV TAAA.

Cook Medical preloaded fenestrated device Cook Medical's preloaded device is under consideration as part of the next generation of the Zenith fenestrated endograft in which modifications have been made to the delivery system. A single extra wire was added that runs through the endograft, out one fenestration, through the top of the graft, back through the opposite renal fenestration, and then out through the delivery system. This wire facilitates easier advancement of the sheaths through the fenestrations, which can be one of the most challenging parts of a fenestrated case, thus significantly shortening the duration of the procedure.

Preliminary results of the preloaded fenestrated device demonstrated its feasibility and safety.[123] Studies on this graft are currently ongoing in Europe and the United States.

Endologix Ventana off-the-shelf fenestrated stent graft The Ventana stent graft (Endologix, Inc., Irvine, CA) is an off-the-shelf fenestrated device with steerable fenestrations intended for juxtarenal and pararenal aneurysms. Unlike current fenestrated grafts that are customized for individual patients, the Ventana device has two 3 mm diameter renal fenestrations with renal sheaths preloaded through the fenestrations that can be dilated up to 8 mm in diameter and can be moved up to 15 mm from their nominal locations. The device incorporates a 4 cm deep scallop for celiac and superior mesenteric artery preservation and is used in combination with the Endologix Xpand balloon-expandable renal stent graft. The Ventana fenestrated proximal extension graft is delivered after an AFX bifurcated graft (Endologix, Inc.) has been deployed with anatomic fixation at the aortic bifurcation.

Nevertheless, there are some anatomic eligibility requirements, the most important being an infra-superior mesenteric artery neck length of 15 mm or longer. In January 2012, the device acquired Investigational Device Exemption approval in the United States to begin clinical trials.

Vascutek Anaconda fenestrated stent graft The Anaconda fenestrated stent graft (Vascutek Ltd., Inchinnan, UK) is currently regulated as a custom device within Europe and Canada. The device is not in clinical trials, but there is a postmarket surveillance registry in which data on patients will be captured for up to 5 years. Its primary indication is for juxta- or pararenal aneurysms with an adequate suprarenal neck diameter of 18 to 31 mm. The standard device design has two fenestrations for the renal arteries and two valleys anteriorly and posteriorly. The anteriorly oriented valley is usually used to accommodate the superior mesenteric or celiac artery. Seventy-nine grafts have been implanted to date worldwide, two of which had four fenestrations.

The advantage of this custom-made device is that it can be repositioned by reconstraining the top of the graft, thereby providing more flexibility for alignment of the visceral vessels. The proximal portion of the graft is stent free, which offers flexibility and kink resistance to the graft to better cope with more angulated necks. In addition, the fenestrations are made in unsupported fabric and are therefore not limited in terms of size and position.

Recently, a preliminary report presented four patients undergoing successful repair of pararenal aneurysms with the custom-made Anaconda custom fenestrated device with perfusion of all 12 target vessels and no perioperative adverse events.[122] The Avanta V12 stent graft (Atrium Medical Corporation, Hudson, NJ) was used as a bridging stent to the renal arteries.

Ongoing Clinical Trials

Currently, ongoing registered trials for TAAAs are being conducted in the United States with the fenestrated branched Cook device (trial identifier: NCT00583050) and in France as part of a multicenter clinical trial investigating medical and economical aspects of fenestrated and branched stent grafts (trial identifier: NCT01168037).[125] The French trial is a multicenter, prospective, nonrandomized trial designed to compare the perioperative mortality, severe morbidity, and costs of endovascular versus conventional surgical repair of pararenal, suprarenal, and type IV TAAAs. The primary goal of the study is to demonstrate a significant reduction in 30-day mortality and life-threatening morbidity in the endovascular arm of the study by comparing 220 patients from seven university hospitals with significant experience in fenestrated endografts with 660 similar patients undergoing open repair analyzed from the French national database.

Conclusion

Treatment of dTAA and TAAA has undergone a dramatic change in the past decade. It is now possible to treat many of these complex aortic aneurysms with modified and fully endovascular techniques, promising lower morbidity and mortality. Open repair techniques have also evolved significantly, in parallel with endovascular, minimally invasive techniques. In most large-volume centers, the mortality and paraplegia rates have been reduced to reasonable levels in all fronts. Going forward, it is likely that most aortic aneurysms and other aortic pathologies will be amenable to durable endovascular repair.

Financial Disclosures: None Reported

References

1. Santilli JD, Santilli SM. Diagnosis and treatment of abdominal aortic aneurysms. Am Fam Physician 1997;56:1081–90.
2. National Center for Injury Prevention and Control. WISQARS leading causes of death reports, 1999–2007. Available at: http://webappa.cdc.gov/sasweb/ncipc/leadcaus10.html (accessed July 25, 2012).
3. Clouse WD, Hallet JW, Schaff HV, et al. Improved prognosis of thoracic aortic aneurysms: a population-based study. JAMA 1998;280:1926–9.
4. Bickerstaff LK, Pairolero PC, Hollier LH, et al. Thoracic aortic aneurysms: a population-based study. Surgery 1982; 92:1103–8.
5. Vasan RS, Larson MG, Benjamin EJ, Levy D. Echocardiographic reference values for aortic root size: the Framingham Heart Study. J Am Soc Echocardiogr 1995;8:793–800.
6. Cambria RP, Davison JK, Zanneti S, et al. Thoracoabdominal aortic repair; perspectives over a decade with clamp-and-sew technique. Ann Surg 1997;226:294–305.
7. Panneton JM, Hollier LH. Nondissecting thoracoabdominal aortic aneurysms: part I. Ann Vasc Surg 1995;9:503–14.
8. Barbour JR, Spinale FG, Ikonomidis JS. Proteinase systems and thoracic aortic aneurysm progression. J Surg Res 2007; 139:292–307.
9. Milewicz DM, Chen H, Park ES, et al. Reduced penetrance and variable expressivity of familial thoracic aortic aneurysms/dissections. Am J Cardiol 1998;82:474–9.
10. Guo DC, Pannu H, Tran-Fadulu V, et al. Mutations in smooth muscle alpha-actin (ACTA2) lead to thoracic aortic aneurysms and dissections. Nat Genet 2007;39:1488–93.
11. Sinha I Bethi S, Cronin P, et al. A biologic basis for asymmetric growth in descending thoracic aortic aneurysms: a role for matrix metalloproteinase 9 and 2. J Vasc Surg 2006;43:342–8.
12. Ikonomidis JS, Barbour JR, Amani Z, et al. Effects of deletion of the matrix metalloproteinase 9 gene on development of murine thoracic aortic aneurysms. Circulation 2005;112(9 Suppl):1242–8.
13. McNamara JJ, Pressler VM. Natural history of arteriosclerotic thoracic aortic aneurysms. Ann Thorac Surg 1978;26: 468–73.
14. Pressler V, McNamara JJ. Aneurysm of the thoracic aorta. Review of 260 cases. J Thorac Cardiovasc Surg 1985;89: 50–4.
15. Dapunt OE, Galla JD, Sadeghi AM, et al. The natural history of thoracic aortic aneurysms. J Thorac Cardiovasc Surg 1994;107:1323–32.
16. Cambria RA, Gloviczzki P, Stanson AW, et al. Outcome and expansion rate of 57 thoracoabdominal aortic aneurysms managed nonoperatively. Am J Surg 1995;170: 213–7.

17. Crawford ES, DeNatale RW. Thoracoabdominal aortic aneurysm: observations regarding the natural course of the disease. J Vasc Surg 1986;3:578–82.
18. Griepp RB, Ergin MA, Galla JD, et al. Natural history of descending thoracic and thoracoabdominal aneurysms. Ann Thorac Surg 1999;67:1927–30.
19. Perko MJ, Nørgaard M, Herzog TM, et al. Unoperated aortic aneurysm: a survey of 170 patients. Ann Thorac Surg 1995;59:1204–9.
20. Crawford ES, Hess KR, Cohen ES, et al. Ruptured aneurysm of the descending and thoracocabdominal aorta—analysis according to size and treatment. Ann Surg 1991; 213:417–25.
21. Coady MA, Rizzo JA, Hammond GL, et al. What is the appropriate size criterion for resection of thoracic aortic aneurysms? J Thorac Cardiovasc Surg 1997;113:476–91.
22. Juvonen T, Ergin MA, Galla JD, et al. Risk factors for rupture of chronic type B dissections. J Thorac Cardiovasc Surg 1999;117:776–86.
23. Masuda Y, Takanashi K, Takasu J, et al. Expansion rate of thoracic aortic aneurysms and influencing factors. Chest 1992;102:461–6.
24. Davies RR, Goldstein LJ, Coady MA, et al. Yearly rupture or dissection rates for thoracic aortic aneurysms: simple prediction based on size. Ann Thorac Surg 2002;73:17–27.
25. Coselli JS, Poli de Figueiredo LF, LeMaire SA. Impact of previous thoracic aneurysm repair on thoracoabdominal aortic aneurysm management. Ann Thorac Surg 1997;64: 639–50.
26. Clouse WD, Marone LK, Davison JK, et al. Late aortic and graft-related events after thoracoabdominal aneurysm repair. J Vasc Surg 2003;37:254–61.
27. Loutsidis A, Koukis I, Argiriou M, Bellenis I. Incidental finding of lung cancer in a patient with thoracic aortic aneurysm—simultaneous management. A case report. Eur J Cancer Care 2007;16:387–9.
28. Morimoto Y, Kuratani T, Tanaka Y, Kaneko M. Surgical strategy for advanced gastric cancer with a concomitant thoracoabdominal aortic aneurysm requiring arterial reconstruction of the visceral branches. Surg Today 2007; 37:817–21.
29. Juluru K, Vogel-Claussen J, Macura KJ, et al. MR imaging in patients at risk for developing nephrogenic systemic fibrosis: protocols, practices and imaging techniques to maximize patient safety. Radiographics 2009;29:9–22.
30. Fulton JJ, Farber MA, Marston WA, et al. Endovascular stent-graft repair of pararenal and type IV thoracoabdominal aortic aneurysms with adjunctive visceral reconstruction. J Vasc Surg 2005;41:191–8.
31. Flye MW, Choi ET, Sanchez LA, et al. Retrograde visceral vessel revascularization followed by endovascular aneurysm exclusion as an alternative to open surgical repair of thoracoabdominal aortic aneurysm. J Vasc Surg 2004;39: 454–8.
32. Black SA, Wolfe JH, Clark M, et al. Complex thoracoabdominal aortic aneurysms: endovascular exclusion with visceral revascularization. J Vasc Surg 2006;43:1081–9.
33. Roselli EE, Greenberg RK, Pfaff K, et al. Endovascular treatment of thoracoabdominal aneurysm. J Thorac Cardiovasc Surg 2007;133:1474–82.
34. Chuter TA, Rapp JH, Hiramoto JS, et al. Endovascular treatment of thoracoabdominal aortic aneurysm. J Vasc Surg 2008;47:6–16.
35. Shores J, Berger KR, Murphy EA, Pyeritz RE. Progression of aortic dilatation and the benefit of long-term beta-adrenergic blockade in Marfan's syndrome. N Engl J Med 1994;330:1335–41.
36. Propranolol Aneurygsm Trial Investigators. Propranolol for small abdominal aortic aneurysms: results of a randomized trial. J Vasc Surg 2002;35:72–9.
37. Ejiri J, Inoue N, Tsukube T, et al. Oxidative stress in the pathogenesis of thoracic aortic aneurysm: protective role of statin and angiotensin II type 1 receptor blocker. Cardiovasc Res 2003;59:988–96.
38. Suzuki S, Dravis CA 3rd, Miller CC 3rd, et al. Cardiac function predicts mortality following thoracoabdominal and descending thoracic aortic aneurysm repair. Eur J Cardiothorac Surg 2003;24:119–23.
39. Brooks MJ, Mayet J, Glenville B, et al. Cardiac investigation and intervention prior to thoraco-abdominal aneurysm repair: coronary angiography in 35 patients. Eur J Vasc Endovasc Surg 2001;21:437–44.
40. Hertzer NR, Beven EG, Young JR, et al. Coronary artery disease in peripheral vascular patients. A classification of 1000 coronary angiograms and results of surgical management. Ann Surg 1984;199:223–33.
41. Estrera AL, Rubenstein FG, Miller CC 3rd, et al. Descending thoracic aortic aneurysm: surgical approach and treatment using the adjuncts cerebrospinal fluid drainage and distal aortic perfusion. Ann Thorac Surg 2001;72:481–6.
42. Svensson LG, Hess KR, Coselli JS, et al. A prospective study of respiratory failure after high-risk surgery on the thoracoabdominal aorta. J Vasc Surg 1991;14:271–82.
43. Guo DC, Papke CL, He R, Milewicz DM. Pathogenesis of thoracic and abdominal aortic aneurysms. Ann N Y Acad Sci 2006;1085:339–52.
44. Safi HJ. Vascular surgery. In: Rutherford RB, editor. Rutherford's vascular surgery. Philadelphia (PA): Elsevier Saunders; 2005.
45. Svensson LG, Coselli JS, Safi HJ, et al. Appraisal of adjuncts to prevent acute renal failure after surgery on the thoracic or thoracoabdominal aorta. J Vasc Surg 1989;10:230–9.
46. Cambria RP, Clouse WD, Davison JK, et al. Thoracoabdominal aneurysm repair: results with 337 operations performed over a 15-year interval. Ann Surg 2002;236:471–9.
47. Huynh TT, van Eps RG, Miller CC 3rd, et al. Glomerular filtration rate is superior to serum creatinine for prediction of mortality after thoracoabdominal aortic surgery. J Vasc Surg 2005;42:206–12.
48. Criado FJ, Abdul-Khoudoud OR, Domer GS, et al. Endovascular repair of the thoracic aorta: lessons learned. Ann Thorac Surg 2005;80:857–63.
49. Mitchell RS, Ishimaru S, Ehrlich MP, et al. First International Summit on Thoracic Aortic Endografting: roundtable on thoracic aortic dissection as an indication for endografting. J Endovasc Ther 2002;9 Suppl 2:II:98–105.
50. Lam CR, Aram H. Resection of the descending thoracic aorta for aneurysm; a report of the use of a homograft in a case and an experimental study. Ann Surg 1951;134: 743–52.

117. Haulon S, Amiot S, Magnan PE, et al. An analysis of the French multicentre experience of fenestrated aortic endografts: medium-term outcomes. Ann Surg 2010;251: 357–62.
118. Verhoeven EL, Zeebregts CJ, Kapma MR, et al. Fenestrated and branched endovascular techniques for thoracoabdominal aneurysm repair. J Cardiovasc Surg (Torino). 2005;46: 131–40.
119. Greenberg RK, Haulon S, O'Neill S, et al. Primary endovascular repair of juxtarenal aneurysms with fenestrated endovascular grafting. Eur J Vasc Endovasc Surg 2004;27: 484–91.
120. Lee WA. Endovascular abdominal aortic aneurysm sizing and case planning using the TeraRecon Aquarius workstation. Vasc Endovasc Surg 2007;41:61–7.
121. Oderich GS, Ricotta JJ. Modified fenestrated stent grafts: device design, modifications, implantation, and current applications. Perspect Vasc Surg Endovasc Ther 2009;21: 157–67.
122. Bungay PM, Burfitt N, Sritharan K, et al. Initial experience with a new fenestrated stent graft. J Vasc Surg 2011;54: 1832–8.
123. Manning BJ, Harris PL, Hartley DE, Ivancev K. Preloaded fenestrated stent-grafts for the treatment of juxtarenal aortic aneurysms. J Endovasc Ther 2010;17:449–55.
124. Chuter T, Greenberg RK. Standardized off-the-shelf components for multibranched endovascular repair of thoracoabdominal aortic aneurysms. Perspect Vasc Surg Endovasc Ther 2011;23:195–201.
125. Greenbury RK. Endovascular Exculsion of Thoracoabdorminal Aortic Aneurysms Utilizing Fenestrated/Branched Stent Grafts. Phase I. ClinicalTrials.gov. Available at: http://clinicaltrials.gov/ct2/results?term=fenestrated (accessed November 2012).

Acknowledgments

Figures 1, 2   Chris Akers

31 COMPARTMENT SYNDROME

Neha D. Shah, MD, and Joseph R. Durham, MD, FACS

Disease Definition

Management of compartment syndromes is a vital tool to have in the surgeon's armamentarium. Understanding of the etiologic mechanisms, along with a thorough knowledge of the pertinent pathophysiology and anatomy, will result in timely recognition and treatment. Decreased morbidity and improved patient function are the desired outcomes. Failure to address a compartment syndrome can lead to permanent neurologic damage, loss of function, amputation, and even severe metabolic derangements, leading to permanent renal failure and cardiorespiratory compromise.

Compartment syndrome is defined as an elevation of the interstitial pressure in a closed fascial compartment that results in microvascular compromise. Compartment syndromes can develop anywhere skeletal muscle or abdominal organs are enveloped by a rigid, unyielding fascial layer. Compartments with relatively noncompliant fascial boundaries are most commonly involved, especially the anterior and deep posterior compartments of the leg and the volar compartment of the forearm. Other sites include the buttock, thigh, foot, arm, hand, paraspinous muscles,[1] and abdomen. Increased pressure within these musculoskeletal compartments can result in relative ischemia with neurologic and soft tissue compromise. Once a given increased pressure threshold is reached, arterial perfusion of the soft tissues is diminished, resulting in ischemic damage to the vulnerable nerves and muscles. This can lead to neurologic injury, muscle necrosis, scarring, and contractures. In addition to the local tissue damage, release of abnormal metabolic products can cause significant cardiorespiratory and renal compromise.

Timely diagnosis of a developing or existent compartment syndrome can be a challenging problem. Although such recognition is often straightforward in the awake, alert patient, it can be most difficult in the patient with altered mental or neurologic status, such as a patient already under general or regional anesthesia, a comatose or obtunded patient, a patient with a peripheral nerve injury, a spinal cord injury patient, or a patient under the influence of drugs.

Epidemiology

Compartment syndromes are classified as acute or chronic depending on the etiology of the insult. Acute compartment syndromes typically result from orthopedic or vascular trauma. They may also occur during or following acute ischemic events such as acute arterial thromboembolism, popliteal artery aneurysm thrombosis, or reperfusion following correction of profound limb ischemia. Chronic compartment syndromes are not the result of acute injury or ischemia. They tend to occur in healthy active individuals, resulting from increased compartment pressures during repetitive vigorous exertion. Usually occurring in athletes, this chronic syndrome typically involves the leg or the forearm.[2,3] Chronic exertional compartment syndromes (CECSs) are discussed in more detail below.

There are three basic mechanisms leading to an acute compartment syndrome: increased tissue pressure within the enclosed space, extrinsic compression on the compartment, and decreased volume of the involved compartment. The presence of an existing or a developing acute compartment syndrome is the typical indication for a fasciotomy procedure. Another indication is a clinical situation in which the incipient development of a significant compartment syndrome is very likely, such as prolonged extremity ischemia or combined extremity arterial and venous injuries (especially the popliteal vessels and ligation of the popliteal vein). Other clinical situations that may result in an acute compartment syndrome include severe burns and prolonged limb compression following loss of consciousness from a drug overdose or a stroke. Delayed development of an acute compartment syndrome is common and may be very difficult to document, especially in the patient with altered mental status or the trauma patient with multiple injuries. Development of a compartment syndrome may occur beyond 48 hours after the initial injury.

SCORE The most common cause of the development of an acute compartment syndrome is a bony fracture, especially the tibia; the resultant hemorrhage, soft tissue injury, and edema can lead to increased compartmental pressures. Consequently, these are managed by the orthopedic surgeons in most institutions. Arterial bleeding into rigid, fixed compartments, reperfusion following prolonged extremity ischemia attributable to arterial injury (traumatic or iatrogenic), embolic disease, popliteal aneurysm thrombosis, and failure of an existing bypass often result in compartment syndromes. Not surprisingly, compartment syndrome following penetrating trauma is often attributable to direct vascular injury with resultant ischemia and reperfusion injury; associated soft tissue injury compounds the problem. Blunt trauma typically results in compartment syndrome as a result of musculoskeletal injury or direct tissue damage. Development of a clinically relevant compartment syndrome following elective extremity revascularization for chronic extremity ischemia may occur but is distinctly uncommon.

Another common cause of an acute compartment syndrome is reperfusion of an ischemic limb following an acute thromboembolic event or repair of a vascular injury, especially if the ischemia is profound and exceeds 6 hours. The combination of arterial and venous injuries significantly increases the risk of developing this disorder. Iatrogenic extravasation of intravenous fluids into a compartment can result in increased compartmental pressures, especially if the infused agent is caustic to the local tissues. Increased edema and compartment pressures can also result from electrical or thermal injuries, especially if associated with rigid, circumferential eschars. Venous outflow obstruction from advanced deep vein thrombosis can result in phlegmasia cerulea dolens, increased compartmental pressures, and venous gangrene; this is usually associated with a malignant process or other hypercoagulable state.

Extrinsic compression of muscle compartments can also result in significant compartment syndromes. First recognized during the bombing of Britain during World War II, crush injuries from being trapped in the rubble led to muscle compromise from the unyielding weight of collapsed building materials; those lucky enough to survive the initial insult often died from renal failure resulting from myoglobinemia as a consequence of the muscle ischemia. Although still occurring in combat and earthquake casualties, this extrinsic compression mechanism is more often seen in the comatose drug overdose victim who collapsed on a hard floor surface for many hours before discovery and rescue. Unfortunately, this mechanism can also affect the elderly person with prolonged immobility on the floor after a fall or stroke. A preventable iatrogenic cause of compartment syndrome from extrinsic pressure is inadequate padding of vulnerable pressure points during a prolonged surgical procedure under general or regional anesthesia. Finally, compartment syndromes can result from extrinsic compression from burn eschars, tight casts, or constricting bandaging.

Pathophysiology

The pathophysiology of compartment syndrome involves an insult to normal local tissue homeostasis that results in increased tissue pressure, decreased capillary blood flow, and local tissue necrosis because of a lack of adequate oxygen delivery.[3] Local tissue blood flow (LBF) is equal to the arteriovenous pressure gradient (Pa-Pv) divided by the local vascular resistance (R): LBF = (Pa-Pv)/R. In the usual setting, tissue ischemia results in vasodilation with decreased vascular resistance, leading to recruitment of increased blood flow. Elevated compartmental pressures can effectively shut down capillary flow, even in the patient with no intrinsic peripheral vascular disease. This can result in significant muscle necrosis if the intracompartmental pressure exceeds 30 mm Hg for more than 8 hours.[3] Certainly, significant neuromuscular injury can be expected to occur in a shorter time frame in the settings of even higher compartment pressures, preexisting chronic ischemia from peripheral vascular disease, hypovolemic shock from trauma, cardiogenic shock, or severe soft tissue damage from a crush injury.

Compartment syndrome results from inadequate perfusion of the soft tissues; this process begins when the pressure within the compartment meets or exceeds the perfusion pressure within the capillary beds of the nerves and muscles. Normal compartment tissue pressures range from 0 to 10 mm Hg. Arteriolar and capillary blood flows are very sensitive to changes in compartment pressures. Critical closing pressures have been shown to be 21 mm Hg in the leg and 33 mm Hg in the arm.[4] When the compartment pressure exceeds these values, arterial perfusion is reduced, resulting in ischemic changes. In the patient with systemic hypotension, compartmental pressures as low as 20 to 40 mm Hg can result in diminished tissue perfusion and tissue injury. At this point, microcapillary flow ceases and the onset of anaerobic metabolism begins, resulting in lactic acidosis. Inflammatory mediators are activated, and free radicals are released. Cellular damage ensues. Neutrophils are recruited and adhere to vascular endothelium, stimulating the release of more free radicals and proteases. The inflammatory mediators cause cell wall lipid peroxidation, which, in turn, increases basement membrane permeability. Leakage from capillaries further increases tissue edema and, therefore, tissue pressure. This sets in play a vicious cycle of progressive muscle edema, actual closure of the capillary beds, increased capillary permeability, and further soft tissue swelling. Eventually, the pressure becomes great enough to reduce arterial inflow and mechanically compress veins and nerves, resulting in nerve injury and myonecrosis; rarely does the compartment pressure increase sufficiently to compress major arteries. Hence, the patient's pulses will usually remain intact during the development of compartment syndrome.

Diagnosis

The diagnosis of a compartment syndrome is based on clinical suspicion, the mechanism and location of injury, physical examination findings, and objective compartment pressure measurements [*see Figure 1*]. It cannot be overemphasized that a high level of suspicion must be held for compartment syndrome, especially in trauma victims and patients with vascular disease undergoing revascularization. The clinical presentation may be subtle in the early stage of compartment syndrome, but early diagnosis is critical so that therapy can be initiated prior to the onset of irreversible tissue ischemia.

The most important initial symptom is pain out of proportion to that expected from the injury. Severe tenderness and pain on passive stretching of the musculature are also suggestive of an existing compartment syndrome. Possible neurologic findings are hypesthesia, paresthesia, or decreased motor function (e.g., peroneal nerve involvement and decreased foot dorsiflexion). Diminished sensation in the distribution of relevant nerves within the compartment in question may be an early finding attributable to ischemia of the nerves [*see Table 1 and Table 2*]; sensory loss usually precedes any compromise of motor function. The neurologic sensory examination should include testing with pinprick, light touch, and two-point discrimination. These diminished sensory findings are often the first abnormality noted with a developing compartment syndrome. Muscle weakness with eventual paralysis follows if the compartment is not promptly released.

These findings are often straightforward and readily evident in the awake and alert patient. The diagnosis of compartment syndrome is straightforward and is based on physical findings and the mechanism of injury. Diagnosis is much more challenging in the patient with an altered mental state or neurologic deficit, as may be seen with alcohol or drug influence, general or regional anesthesia, spinal cord injury, peripheral nerve injury, or unconsciousness. In these instances, compartment pressure measurements are invaluable in the decision-making process. Diagnosis may

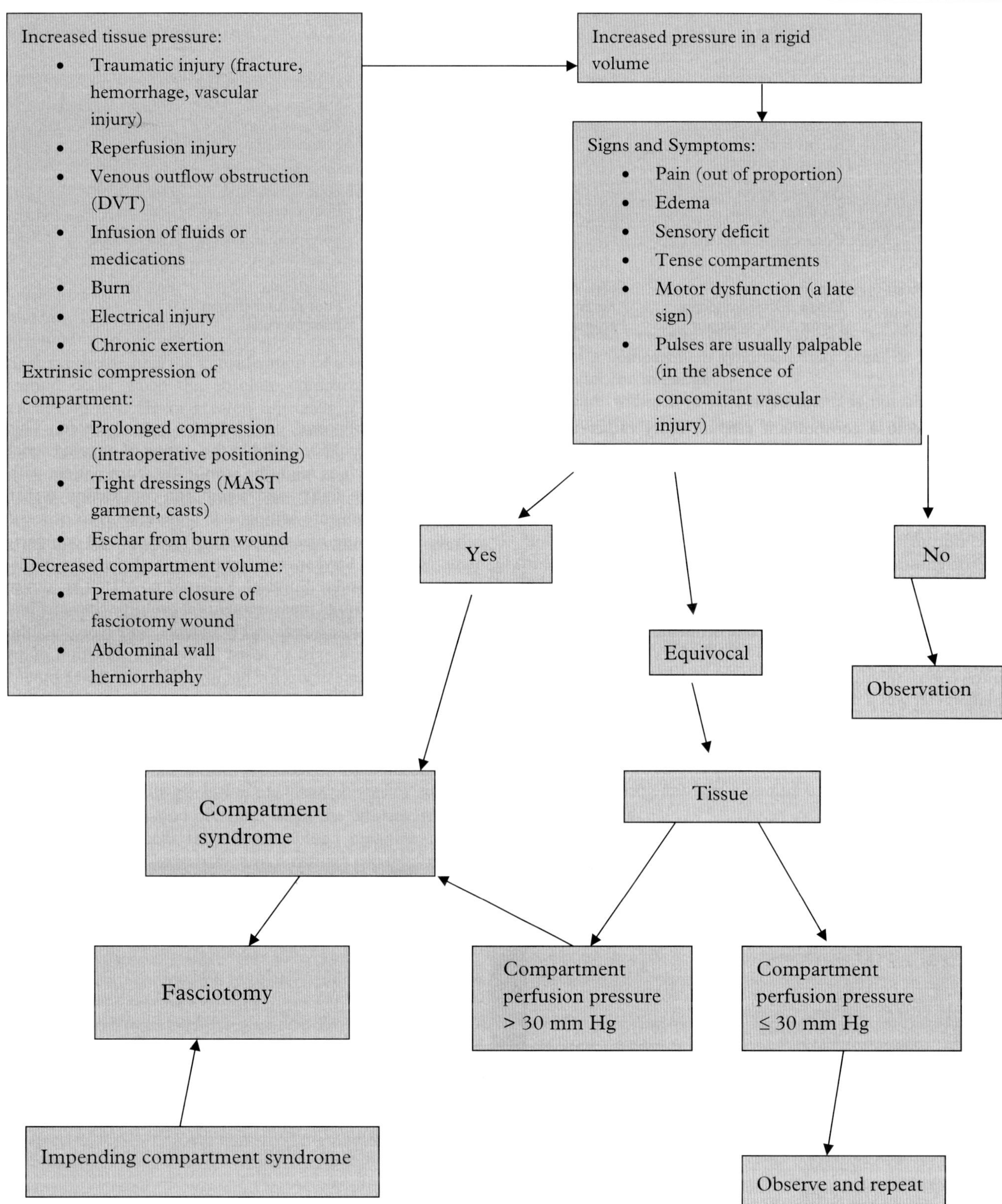

Figure 1 **The algorithmic approach to management of compartment syndrome. MAST = military anti-shock trousers; DVT = deep vein thrombosis.**

also be quite difficult in the young child as a result of agitation, fear, communication challenges, and lack of cooperation. Appropriate pressure analysis can prevent unnecessary procedures and, at the same time, allow appropriate timely action when a compartment syndrome is documented.

Physical examination findings suggestive of an advanced acute compartment syndrome typically include rigidity and tenderness of muscles in the involved compartment, pallor or mottling of the skin, or neurologic motor deficits. Loss of arterial pulses may be a late sign but is more likely

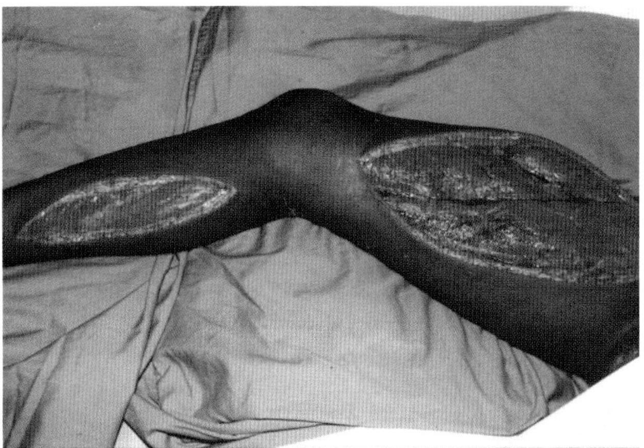

Figure 6 **Photograph of the large skin defects of the medial leg and thigh fasciotomy wounds following a gunshot wound with superficial femoral arterial and venous injury, second postoperative day.**

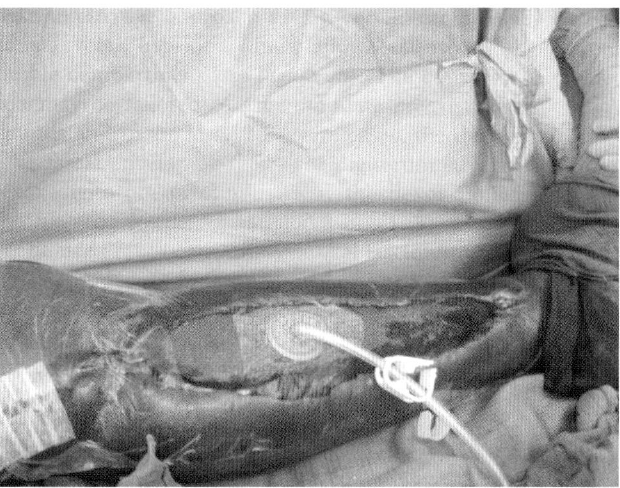

Figure 8 **Photograph of vacuum dressing for a fasciotomy wound.**

of closure must be individualized based on patient compliance, equipment availability, cost, and wound factors such as tension and amount of myonecrosis. It is important that the surgeon be familiar with the various closure techniques so that the particular method used optimizes the functional outcome of the fasciotomy procedure for that individual patient.

Chronic Exertional Compartment Syndrome

CECS is a well-recognized entity that tends to occur in relatively young athletes. CECSs arise from repetitive exertion and exercise. Vigorous exercise can increase muscle volume by 20%, causing an increase in pressure within the fixed compartment. Chronically recurring increased pressure within the closed space can cause debilitating symptoms in the athlete; this is most often seen in long-distance runners and military recruits and usually involves the anterior or deep posterior compartment of the leg.[2] Weight lifters may also develop this chronic disorder, especially in the forearm.[3]

Potential causes of CECS include hypertrophy from aggressive training, altered fascial compliance, and myofascial scarring associated with repetitive impact stress and inflammation.[2] Involvement of the leg is more common, typically affecting runners and soccer players. CECS of the forearm is less common and is seen in competitive motorcyclists,[30] weight lifters, and manual laborers. Previous orthopedic trauma is common for both locations. In both sites, diagnosis is based on symptoms and measurement of compartment pressures.

THE FOREARM

Typical symptoms suggestive of CECS of the forearm include forearm pain with exertion that disappears with rest.

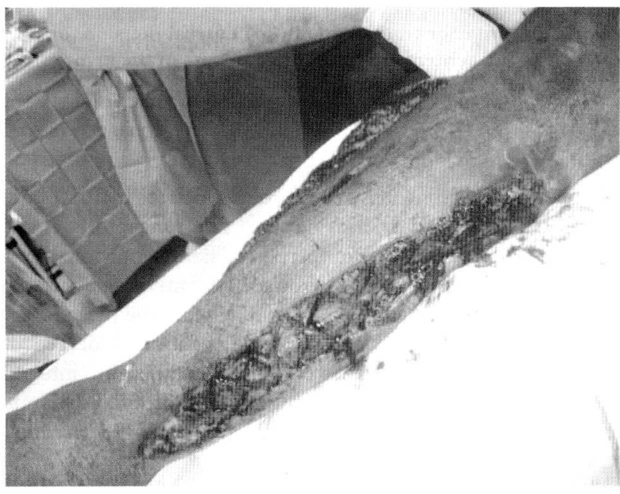

Figure 7 **Photograph of leg fasciotomy wound approximation using the shoelace technique.**

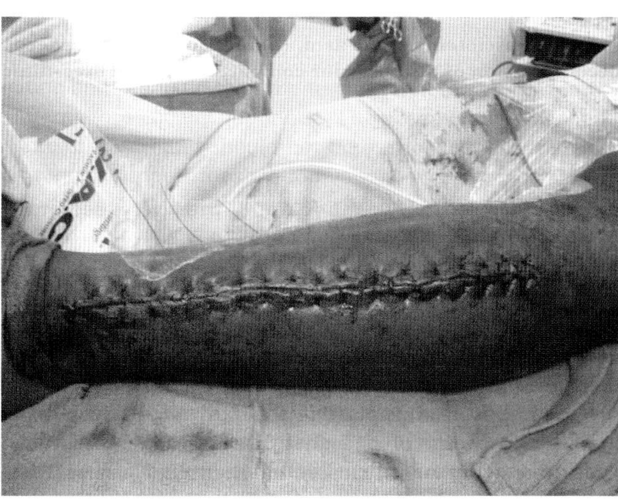

Figure 9 **Photograph of delayed primary closure of fasciotomy wounds after vacuum dressing therapy.**

Paresthesias are often felt in the fingers. Transient hand dysfunction or cramping has also been described. Examination at the time of symptoms usually reveals a firm, stiff compartment. Diagnosis is confirmed by direct dynamic measurement of compartment pressures using the Stryker STIC device. Measurements are obtained with the patient at rest, during exertion, and following the exercise stress. A finding of a compartment pressure greater than 30 mm Hg in any compartment is abnormal. No further studies are required.[30] Treatment requires complete release of involved compartments. Release of the forearm compartments may be performed as an outpatient procedure using a tourniquet under general anesthesia. Release of the compartments is performed using either two volar incisions or two dorsal incisions depending on the compartments involved. Details of the surgical technique are outlined in Croutzet and colleagues' study.[30] Sutures are removed at 2 weeks, with initiation of normal daily activities and an exercise program. Full exertional activity is typically reached at 6 weeks following operation.[30]

THE LEG

CECS involving the leg typically results in atypical claudication symptoms characterized by isolated muscle cramping or swelling with occasional paresthesias localized to the dorsal or plantar surface of the foot. The onset of symptoms is fixed and reproducible but usually occurs at a very long exercise distance, often measured in miles rather than city blocks. Although symptoms may abate with rest, they quickly return with resumption of exertion. These symptoms rarely respond to nonsteroidal antiinflammatory drugs (NSAIDs) or physical therapy. A consistent pattern of failed medical management is characteristic.

Initially noted to be more common in men, the gender profile has shifted dramatically over the past 20 years. Women now comprise more than 70% of patients in Turnipseed's comprehensive analysis of 28 years of experience.[2] Initially more common in runners, the most common sport associated with CECS of the leg is now soccer. The average age of patients is 32 years. Symptoms are unilateral in 44% of patients.

The most commonly affected lower extremity muscle groups are in the anterolateral (72%), deep posterior (16%), and superficial posterior (12%) compartments. Plantar foot paresthesia is most commonly associated with the deep posterior compartment; dorsal foot paresthesia results from involvement of the anterolateral compartments. Diagnosis is confirmed by measurement of compartment pressures at rest and following exercise. Normal resting pressure within the leg compartments is less than 15 mm Hg. Resting pressures ranging from 16 to 24 mm Hg are suggestive of CECS, whereas pressures greater than 25 mm Hg are considered diagnostic. Those patients with borderline resting compartment pressures (16 to 24 mm Hg) are retested following exercise stress. Postexercise compartment pressure usually returns to baseline within 3 minutes. If the compartment pressure remains elevated (> 25 mm Hg) for more than 10 minutes after exercise, this is considered a positive provocative stress test result.[2]

Initial treatment of CECS of the leg may include rest, along with modification of the intensity and duration of workouts; however, most high-level athletes are not willing or are unable to adjust their training schedules as a permanent means of controlling symptoms. Failure to respond to nonsurgical treatment or the inability to pursue a noninvasive treatment regimen leads to the need for surgical intervention.

The surgical approach to CECS involves either a fasciotomy or fasciectomy procedure. Whereas fasciotomy is probably a more common procedure, fasciectomy with open technique seems to yield more durable positive results with fewer complications. As described by Turnipseed, the open procedure is performed through a 2.5 to 3.0 cm incision, an ellipse of the fascia encasing the involved compartments is excised, and then, under direct vision, the fascia can be released from the level of the tibial plateau down to about 2 cm above the ankle level.[2] The small incisions (< 3 cm) required for this approach yield acceptable cosmetic outcomes with fewer postoperative complications than semiclosed methods with limited incisions and exposure. Either method can be performed in the ambulatory setting using local anesthesia with intravenous sedation. Structured rehabilitation programs allow a graduated return to full activity over 3 months.

Abdominal Compartment Syndrome

The physiology of abdominal compartment syndrome is consistent with that of extremity compartment syndrome in that increased pressure in a rigid volume causes tissue ischemia. Abdominal compartment syndrome can occur postoperatively after abdominal operations (e.g., tight closure after abdominal wall herniorrhaphy, aortic cross-clamping), and secondary abdominal compartment syndrome can result from massive fluid resuscitation. The signs and symptoms of abdominal compartment syndrome differ from those of extremity compartment syndrome because of the contents of the abdominal compartment. Compression of the inferior vena cava results in diminished preload and decreased cardiac output, which may cause hypotension. Decreased venous return of intra-abdominal organs contributes further to organ ischemia, resulting in bowel necrosis and hepatic ischemia. The compliance of the thoracic cavity is decreased, resulting in hypoventilation as a result of the inability to expand the thoracic cavity and elevation in airway pressure. Intra-abdominal hypertension also results in compression of kidneys, resulting in oliguria attributable to mechanisms not yet defined.

In contrast to extremity compartment syndrome, abdominal compartment syndrome is very difficult to diagnose by physical examination. Manometry for the diagnosis of abdominal compartment syndrome should be performed and can be accomplished by the measurement of bladder pressure. Twenty-five milliliters of normal saline solution is instilled in the bladder via a Foley catheter. The catheter is connected to a transducer device, which should be positioned at the level of the midaxillary line. The pressure is measured at end-expiration. For accuracy, multiple measurements are taken. Normal intra-abdominal pressure (IAP) is 5 to 7 mm Hg. Intra-abdominal hypertension is defined as IAP greater than 11 mm Hg.[31] Abdominal perfusion pressure can also be measured by subtracting the IAP from the systemic mean arterial pressure. However, the diagnostic value of this has not been confirmed by prospective studies. Therefore, the current standard of diagnosis is the IAP. The grading system instated by the World Congress on Abdominal Compartment Syndrome is as follows: grade I, IAP 12 to 15 mm Hg; grade II, IAP 16 to 20 mm Hg; grade III, IAP 21 to 25 mm Hg; and grade IV, IAP > 25 mm Hg. Those patients in grades I and II can be managed medically with gastric decompression, sedation, diuresis or ultrafiltration. Patients falling within grade III should be clinically evaluated for signs of end-organ failure. If those signs are present, decompressive laparotomy is indicated. For grade III patients without evidence of organ failure, close monitoring is essential. Neuromuscular blockade for relaxation of the abdominal wall musculature may decrease IAP. For those patients in grade IV, decompressive laparotomy is usually necessary. Failure of medical therapy and signs of end-organ ischemia mandate decompression. For those patients with intra-abdominal fluid, blood, or abscess causing compartment syndrome, catheter drainage is acceptable.[32]

After laparotomy for decompression, temporary abdominal closure can be achieved with either a Bogota bag sutured to the skin or a vacuum-assisted device for closure. Primary closure is usually possible within 5 to 7 days of decompression. After closure, the patient must be monitored for recurrent abdominal compartment syndrome.

Financial Disclosures: None Reported

References

1. Mubarak SJ, Hargens AR. Compartment syndromes and Volkmann's contracture. Philadelphia: W.B. Saunders; 1981.
2. Turnipseed WD. Clinical review of patients treated for atypical claudication: a 28-year experience. J Vasc Surg 2004;40:79–85.
3. Azar FM. Traumatic disorders. In: Canale ST, Beatty JH, editors. Campbell's operative orthopaedics. 11th ed. St. Louis: Mosby; 2008. p. 2737–88.
4. Padberg F Jr, Duran WN. Metabolic and systemic consequences of acute limb ischemia. In: Hallett JW, Mills JL, Earnshaw JJ, et al, [illegible] vascular surgery. 2nd ed. St. Louis: Mosby; 2009. p. 278–90.
5. Whitesides T, Haney T, Morimoto K. Tissue pressure measurement as a determinant for the need for fasciotomy. Clin Orthop 1975; 113:43–51.
6. Modrall JG. Compartment syndrome. In: Cronenwett JL, Johnston KW, editors. Rutherford's vascular surgery. 7th ed. Philadelphia: Saunders Elsevier; 2010. p. 2412–21.
7. Boland MR, Heck C. Acute exercise-induced bilateral thigh compartment syndrome. Orthopedics 2009;32:218.
8. Spinner M, Aiache A, Silver L, Barsky A. Impending ischemic contracture of the hand. Plast Reconstr Surg 1972;50:341.
9. Ascer E, Strauch B, Calligaro KD, et al. Ankle and foot fasciotomy: an adjunctive technique to optimize limb salvage after revascularization for acute ischemia. J Vasc Surg 1989;9:594–7.
10. Manoli A II. Compartment releases of the foot. In: Johnson KA, editor. Master techniques in orthopaedic surgery: the foot and ankle. New York: Raven Press; 1994. p. 257–67.
11. Maurel B, Brilhault J, Martinez R, Lermusiaux P. Compartment syndrome with foot ischemia after inversion injury of the ankle. J Vasc Surg 2007;46:369–71.
12. Nypaver TJ. Fasciotomy in vascular trauma and compartment syndrome. In: Ernst CB, Stanley JC, editors. Current therapy in vascular surgery. 4th ed. St Louis: Mosby; 2001. p. 624–8.
13. Bermudez K, Knudson MM, Morabito D, et al. Fasciotomy, chronic venous insufficiency, and the calf muscle pump. Arch Surg 1998;133:1356–61.
14. Ritenour AE, Dorlac WC, Fang R, et al. Complications after fasciotomy revision and delayed compartment release in combat patients. J Trauma 2008;64(2 Suppl):S153–62.
15. [illegible] Starnes BW, [illegible] Lessons learned from modern military surgery. Surg Clin North Am 2007;87:157–84.
16. Watson JC, Johansen KH. Compartment syndrome: pathophysiology, recognition, and management. In: Rutherford RB, editor. Vascular surgery. 6th ed. Philadelphia: Elsevier Saunders; 2005. p. 1058–65.
17. Gonzalez RP, Scott W, Wright A, et al. Anatomic location of penetrating lower-extremity trauma predicts compartment syndrome development. Am J Surg 2009;197: 371–5.
18. Grossman MD, Reilly P, McMahan D, et al. Gunshot wounds below the popliteal fossa: a contemporary review. Am Surg 1999;65: 360–5.
19. Asensio JA, Kuncir EJ, Garcia-Nunez LM, Petrone P. Femoral vessel injuries: analysis of factors predictive of outcomes. J Am Coll Surg 2006;203:512–20.
20. Huynh TTT, Pham M, Griffin LW, et al. Management of distal femoral and popliteal arterial injuries: an update. Am J Surg 2006; 192:773–8.
21. Woodman G, Croce MA, Fabian TC. Iliac artery ischemia: analysis of risks for ischemic complications. Am Surg 1998;64:833–7.
22. Tarlow, SD, Achterman CA, Hayhurst J, Ovadia DN. Acute compartment syndrome in the thigh complicating fracture of the femur: a report of three cases. J Bone Joint Surg Am 1986;68A:1439–43.
23. Hill SL, Bianchi J. The gluteal compartment syndrome. Am Surg 1997;9:823–6.
24. Schwartz JT Jr, Brumback RJ, Lakatos R, et al. Acute compartment syndrome of the thigh, a spectrum of injury. J Bone Joint Surg Am 1989;71A:392–400.
25. Friedrich JB, Shin AY. Management of forearm compartment syndrome. Hand Clin 2007;23:245–54.
26. Doyle J. Anatomy of the upper extremity muscle compartments. Hand Clin 1998;14: 343–64.
27. Morin RJ, Swan KG, Tan V. Acute forearm [illegible] syndrome secondary to local arterial injury after penetrating trauma. J Trauma 2009;66:989–93.
28. Dente CJ, Feliciano DV, Rozycki GS, et al. A review of upper extremity fasciotomies in a level I trauma center. Am Surg 2004;70: 1088–93.
29. Zannis J, Angobaldo J, Marks M, et al. Comparison of fasciotomy wound closures using traditional dressing changes and the vacuum-assisted closure device. Ann Plast Surg 2009;62:407–9.
30. Croutzet P, Chassat R, Masmejean EH. Mini-invasive surgery for chronic exertional compartment syndrome of the forearm. Tech Hand Surg 2009;13:137–40.
31. Malbrain MLNG, Cheatham ML, Kirkpatrick A, et al. Results from the conference of experts on intra-abdominal hypertension and abdominal compartment syndrome. Part I: definitions. Intensive Care Med 2006;32: 1722–32.
32. Cheatham ML, Malbrain MLNG, Kirkpatrick A, et al. Results from the conference of experts on intra-abdominal hypertension and abdominal compartment syndrome. Part II: recommendations. Intensive Care Med 2007; 33:951–62.

Acknowledgments

Figures 2 through 5 Christine Kenney

32 CURRENT MODALITIES FOR IMAGING THE VASCULAR SYSTEM

Aoife N. Keeling, FFRRCSI, and Peter A. Naughton, MD

Over the last two decades, there has been a paradigm shift for both the diagnosis and the treatment of many vascular pathologies. Noninvasive imaging using duplex ultrasonography (US), computed tomography (CT), and magnetic resonance angiography (MRA) is now often preferred to digital subtraction angiography (DSA) for diagnosis, and endovascular intervention has emerged as an attractive alternative to open surgery for the treatment of many vascular conditions. This chapter focuses on the noninvasive imaging modalities currently used in the investigation and diagnosis of both arterial and venous disorders, covering both technical factors and clinical applications with a number of case-based examples.

Plain Film

Previously, prior to the widespread use of computed tomographic angiography (CTA) and MRA, plain film could be used to assist in the diagnosis of certain vascular pathologies, including aneurysmal disease, atherosclerosis, trauma, and postoperative follow-up. Now with the many other imaging modalities available, the emphasis has moved away from plain film radiography. However, vascular specialists should be aware of their current role in vascular diagnosis, often incidentally, and in postprocedural follow-up.

Aneurysms, particularly abdominal aortic aneurysms (AAAs), can be diagnosed incidentally on an abdominal radiograph manifested by the presence of retroperitoneal linear calcification representing the calcified atherosclerotic aortic wall. Similarly, mesenteric arterial aneurysms can also be identified as concentric or curvilinear calcification within the right or left upper quadrant. This finding should prompt further investigation with US or CTA. Thoracic aortic aneurysms and pseudoaneurysms may also be incidentally diagnosed on chest radiographs, usually manifesting as a widened mediastinum. Ascending thoracic aortic aneurysms/pseudoaneurysms can produce a right sided mediastinal mass on CXR, with descending thoracic aortic aneurysms/pseudoaneurysms causing a left sided mediastinal mass. Linear calcification along the aneurysmal aortic wall or within the rim of a pseudoaneurysm can be identified on CXR. CXR may also reveal mass effect from the aneurysms/pseudoaneurysms, manifested by downward displacement of the left mainstem bronchus. Similarly, unrecognized thoracic aortic coarctations can present incidentally on a chest x-ray in teenagers or young adults with the classical rib notching and small mediastinum [*see Figure 1*].

Prior to the widespread use and availability of CTA in the emergency setting, a small study demonstrated that the diagnosis of an AAA contained rupture could be made in a large proportion (90%) of patients on the basis of plain abdominal radiograph findings.[1] Plain film findings including the presence of aortic rim calcification (65%), soft tissue mass (67%), loss of psoas muscle (75%) or renal (78%) outlines, renal displacement (25%), and properitoneal flank stripe changes (19%) were all associated with an AAA rupture in the correct clinical context.[1] Acute thoracic aortic injury including transection has a number of classical findings on plain chest radiograph, including signs of mediastinal hematoma—widened mediastinum, deviation of the trachea to the right of the T4 spinous process, deviation of a nasogastric tube to the right of the T4 spinous process, obscuration of the margin of the aortic arch, left apical cap, depression of the left mainstem bronchus, and loss of the aortopulmonary window—and associated signs, including fractured first and/or second rib, left pleural effusion from hemothorax, and left pneumothorax or hemopneumothorax. However, these plain film findings are not specific; thus, CTA is required for definitive diagnosis and preprocedural planning.[2]

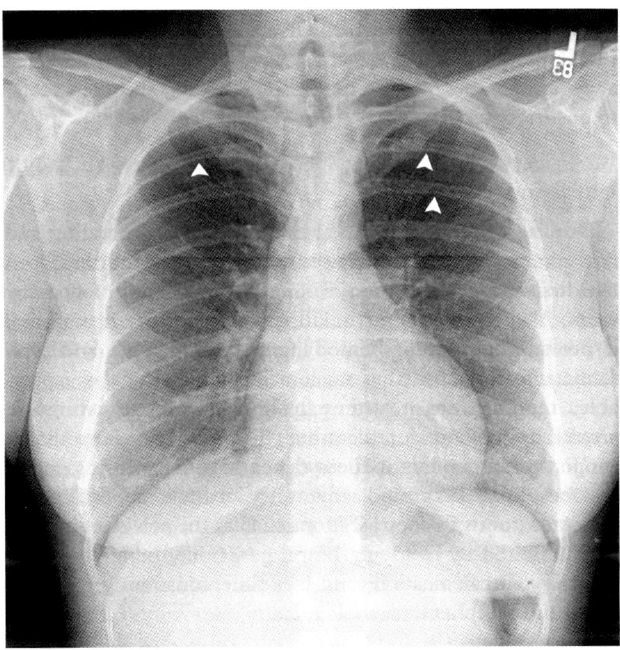

Figure 1 **A 21-year-old female with a cough and fever underwent a chest radiograph to evaluate for pneumonia. Incidental note was made of bilateral rib notching (*arrows*). This was confirmed at time-resolved magnetic resonance angiography to be an aortic coarctation with multiple arterial collaterals resulting in the bilateral rib notching.**

can eloquently diagnose many other aortic pathologies, including dissection; atherosclerosis causing stenosis, occlusion, or ulceration; and pseudoaneuryms and mycotic aneurysms.

Patients treated with EVAR undergo frequent imaging by CTA to monitor for endoleak, stent migration or fracture, and stability of aneurysm size.[42] An increase in the diameter of an aneurysmal sac is associated with endoleak. Evaluation of an endoleak requires an unenhanced CT scan, as well as imaging during arterial and venous phases of contrast enhancement. Unenhanced images are used to detect artifact from calcification or embolization material that may mimic endoleak on the enhanced images and to evaluate stent graft material for any infolding or migration. Arterial phase imaging enables assessment of stent graft patency and endoleak identification. Delayed venous phase images have been shown to enhance the detection rate of endoleaks as some may not be appreciated in the arterial phase.

The CT scanning volume for imaging the abdominal aorta usually starts at the diaphragm and extends caudally to the symphysis pubis. Bolus tracking triggering can reliably obtain the optimal arterial phase by placing a region of interest (ROI) on the aorta at the level of the celiac artery. An injection volume of 100 mL of high-concentration contrast agent (350 mg iodine/mL) at a flow rate of 5 mL/s is typically used. Images are acquired in the cranial to caudal direction with a slice thickness of 2.0 mm, a slice interval of 2.0 mm, and 0.6 mm of collimation.

PERIPHERAL ARTERIAL CTA

The most common indication for peripheral CTA in many centers is for further evaluation of PAD. The diagnosis has already been established clinically and with ABIs, but the extent and severity of arterial involvement are of interest to the vascular surgeon or interventional radiologist. The TransAtlantic Inter-Society Consensus (TASC) guidelines recommend appropriate endovascular or surgical treatment of PAD based on lesion location, number, severity, length, and morphology.[11] Peripheral CTA is well positioned to evaluate all of these criteria to enable appropriate treatment planning. MRA is also a useful modality for diagnosing the extent and severity of PAD; however, cost, scanner availability, patient contraindications, local expertise, and the risk of nephrogenic systemic fibrosis can limit this tool.[43] CTA can also be employed to perform bypass or vein graft surveillance[44] or follow-up of lesions treated with percutaneous transluminal angioplasty.[45] Availability and rapid access place CTA at the forefront for fast and complete arterial assessment in lower limb injury, in both trauma settings and iatrogenic events.[46,47] Lower limb aneurysmal and pseudoaneurysmal disease can be eloquently evaluated with CTA as sac size, relation to parent vessel, thrombus load, and distal runoff can all be demonstrated prior to covered stent placement or surgical repair.[45] Rarer indications encountered include vasculitis,[47] arteriovenous malformations (AVMs),[44] and popliteal entrapment syndrome.[48]

Most institutions will initially perform a scout view from the diaphragm to the feet, an optional noncontrast acquisition from the celiac axis to the feet, and an arterial phase timed acquisition from the celiac axis to the feet, with the option of a second limited acquisition from the lower thighs to the feet in the event that the contrast has a slower transit time on the symptomatic side.

Bolus tracking triggering can reliably obtain the optimal arterial phase by placing a ROI on the aorta at the level of the celiac artery. An injection volume of 150 mL of high-concentration contrast agents (350 mg iodine/mL) at a flow rate of 5 mL/s is typically used. Images are acquired in the cranial to caudal direction with a slice thickness of 1.0 mm, a slice interval of 1.0 mm, and 0.6 mm of collimation.

CAROTID CTA

In the United States, stroke is the leading cause of adult disability and the third leading cause of death. About 80% of strokes are ischemic strokes. Conventional DSA remains the reference standard for the evaluation of carotid artery disease; however, DSA has significant risks. Thus, noninvasive methods are now widely used, usually in combination at present, with initial duplex US performed followed by cross-sectional imaging with CTA or MRA prior to intervention. There is an emerging role for CTA in the evaluation of carotid disease likely attributable to continued advances in CT technology, its noninvasive nature, and its lower cost than DSA. A recent meta-analysis assessed the accuracy of CTA versus DSA for assessment of symptomatic carotid artery disease.[49] Sensitivity and specificity for detection of a 70 to 99% carotid artery stenosis were 85% and 93%, respectively, rising to 97% and 99%, respectively, for 100% stenosis detection.[49] However, another meta-analysis comparing US, CTA, and MRA to DSA determined that contrast-enhanced MRA was the most accurate for assessing a 70 to 99% symptomatic carotid stenosis with sensitivity and specificity of 86% and 91%, respectively.[50] In this study, CTA performed poorly and was the least accurate noninvasive modality, with sensitivity and specificity for detection of 70 to 99% carotid artery stenosis of 68% and 77%, respectively, compared with 82% and 77%, respectively, for Doppler US.[50] These conflicting results from two meta-analyses should prompt further evaluation into the role of CTA in assessing carotid artery disease and should caution surgeons on the decision to proceed with intervention based solely on one noninvasive imaging modality of the carotid artery. Plaque composition can be evaluated by CTA, which is an important indicator of plaque stability and helps with the assessment of risk factors for thromboembolic events and in monitoring the effects of best medical therapy.

Other carotid pathologies can be eloquently diagnosed with CTA, including aneurysm disease [*see Figure 11*], dissection, vasculitis, and postoperative complications such as para-anastomotic aneurysms and infections. The scanning volume of carotid CTA is determined based on the initial anteroposterior and lateral topograms. The volume should include all the vascular structures from the aortic arch to the entire intracranial circulation to the level of the skull vault. This scan volume also serves to diagnose any preexisting cerebral infarcts. Automated bolus tracking or test bolus triggering techniques can reliably obtain the optimal arterial phase by placing an ROI on the aortic arch. An injection volume of 75 mL of high-concentration contrast agent (350 mg iodine/mL) at a flow rate of 5 mL/s is typically used. Images are acquired in the caudal to cranial direction with

a

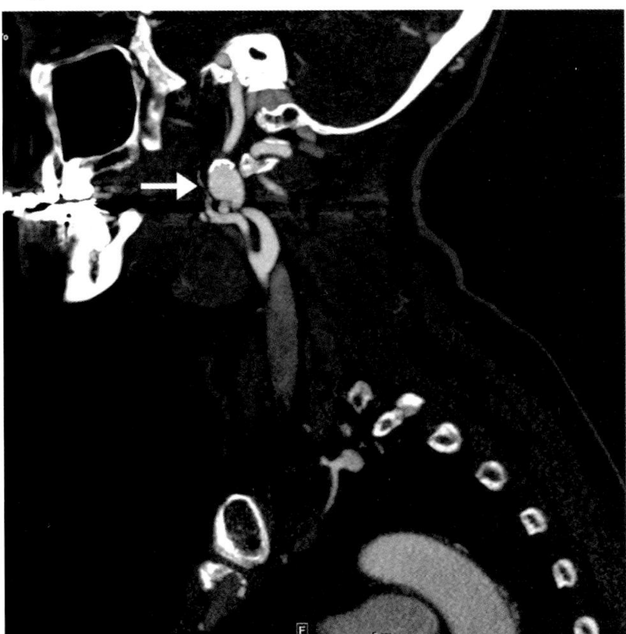

b

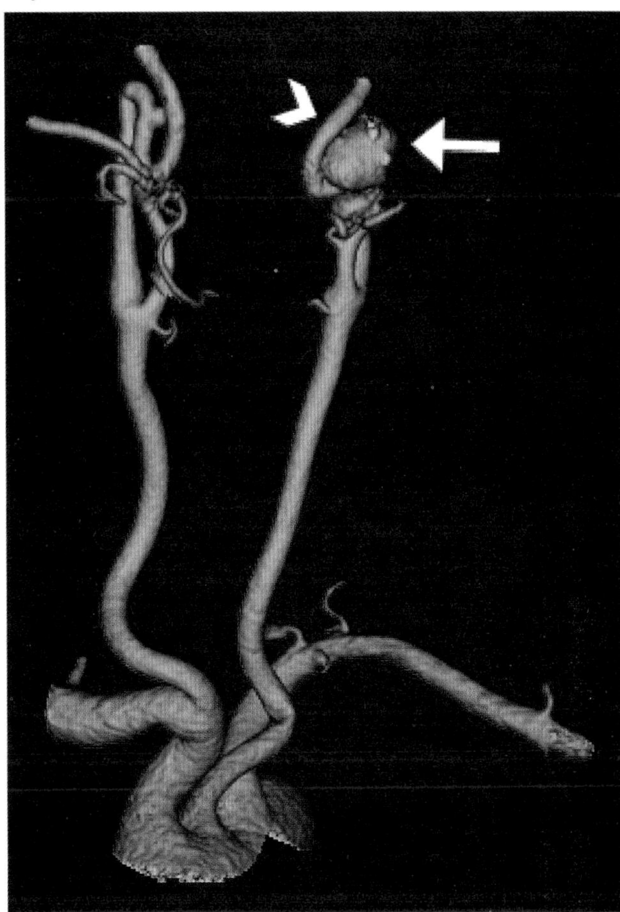

Figure 11 **A 48-year-old female presented with a pulsatile lump within her left neck that she discovered herself. (*a*) Sagittal reconstruction from a multidetector computed tomographic angiogram of the carotid arteries demonstrates a fusiform focal aneurysm of the left internal carotid artery (*arrow*). The internal carotid was very tortuous. (*b*) A volume-rendered view of both carotid arteries demonstrates the left internal carotid (*arrowhead*) fusiform aneurysm (*arrow*). Because of the tortuosity of the internal carotid artery, the aneurysm was surgically resected.**

a slice thickness of 1 mm, a slice interval of 0.5 mm, and 0.6 mm of collimation.

THORACIC CTA

The disease processes affecting the aortic root and thoracic aorta include aneurysmal dilatation and rupture, aortic dissection, intramural hematoma and penetrating ulcer, traumatic injury presenting early as transection or late as a pseudoaneurysm formation, inflammatory processes that can extend into the arch vessels, and congenital malformations. The diagnosis, surveillance, and monitoring with MDCTA play an important role in determining the timing and role for endovascular and surgical intervention.

Conventional DSA is regarded as the reference standard for evaluation of the thoracic arterial system. CTA of the thoracic aorta is currently the preferred method, however, for follow-up of patients with thoracic aortic aneurysms.[51] In addition to evaluating luminal disease, CTA can also assess the vessel wall for plaque composition, hematoma, and dissections. The wall of the aneurysm is easily identified by intramural calcifications allowing for accurate size measurement. CT also allows for evaluation of the extent of mural thrombus and aneurysm wall for a contained leak, as well as any associated dissection, distal embolization, or pleural

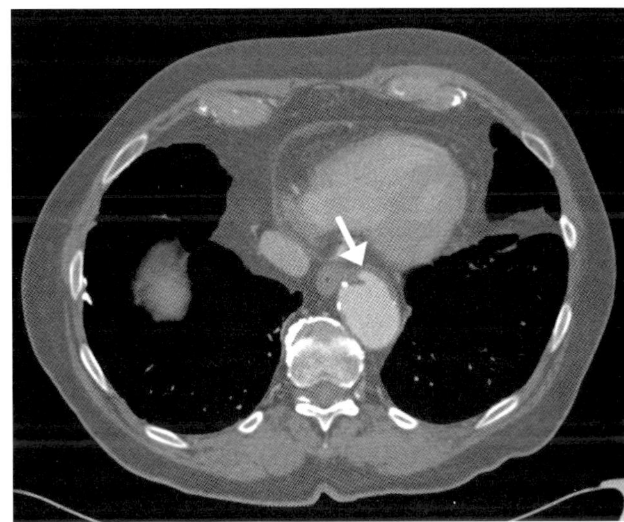

Figure 12 **A 74-year-old male undergoing computed tomography for abdominal pain. Axial multidetector computed tomographic angiography through the lower descending thoracic aorta demonstrates a small outpouching from the thoracic aorta into the aortic wall consistent with an anterior small penetrating ulcer (*arrow*).**

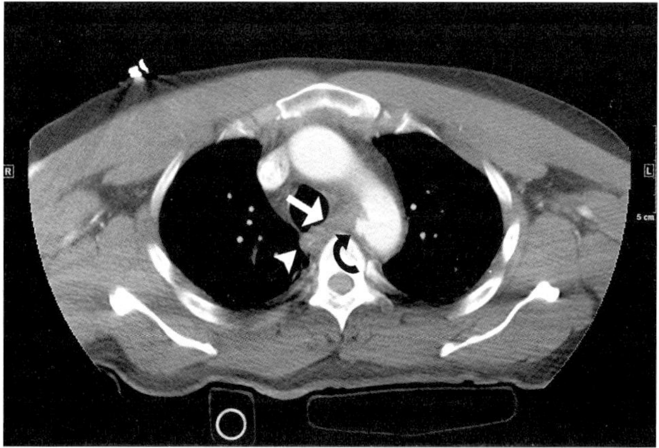

Figure 13 **A 40-year-old male who presented to the emergency department following a high-velocity motor vehicle accident with crushing central chest pain. An axial multidetector computed tomographic angiogram at the level of the aortic arch demonstrates increased attenuation material (*white arrow*) within the mediastinum displacing the esophagus (*arrowhead*) to the right. On the medial aspect of the undersurface of the aortic arch, at the level of the relatively fixed aortic isthmus, there is a disruption in the smooth contour of the aortic wall (*curved black arrow*), with a small area of outpouching of contrast. The finding of mediastinal hematoma (*white arrow*), along with aortic disruption in the setting of a motor vehicle accident, is consistent with acute aortic injury known as aortic transection. This requires emergent repair, with many centers now favoring endovascular and/or hybrid methods. This patient underwent a left subclavian arterial transposition. The transposition was performed before covering the transection with a stent graft to preserve the dominant left vertebral artery.**

effusion. Three-dimensional images demonstrate the normal anatomic relationship of the branch vessels, the mediastinal structures, and the extent of the disease process.

MDCTA has become the imaging modality of choice for the evaluation of thoracic aortic dissection at most medical centers. Magnetic resonance imaging (MRI) and transesophageal echocardiography (TEE) are widely used with sensitivities and specificities similar to those of MDCTA; however, ease of availability, lower cost, ability to evaluate arch vessels and the abdominal aorta, increased spatial resolution, nonoperator dependence, and no limited acoustic windows mean that MDCTA is preferred by many. The pathognomonic imaging finding for thoracic aortic dissection on CT is two adjacent contrast-filled lumens, which represent a patent true lumen and the false lumen. The two lumens are separated by a thin band known as the intimal flap. The intimal flap can have unusual characteristics, which are detected by CT, including partial thrombosis, a circular or spiral orientation down the aorta, or multiple fenestrations. CT is also effective for visualizing more subtle signs of dissection such as internal displacement of intimal calcium, mural thickening, ischemia of end-organs supplied by aortic branches, or a left pleural effusion. CT also demonstrates the start point, course, and extent of the intimal flap in relation to the ascending aorta, aortic arch, abdominal aorta, and branch vessel ostia, which is vital for planning surgical or endovascular repair. The major limitations of CT for thoracic aortic dissection are technical factors that can cause a false positive reading. These include improper timing of contrast bolus injection, aortic wall or cardiac motion, streak artifacts, and periaortic structures. Motion or pulsation artifact in the region of the aortic root can be misinterpreted as the flap of an aortic dissection. Aortic motion from pulsation artifact has now been virtually

a

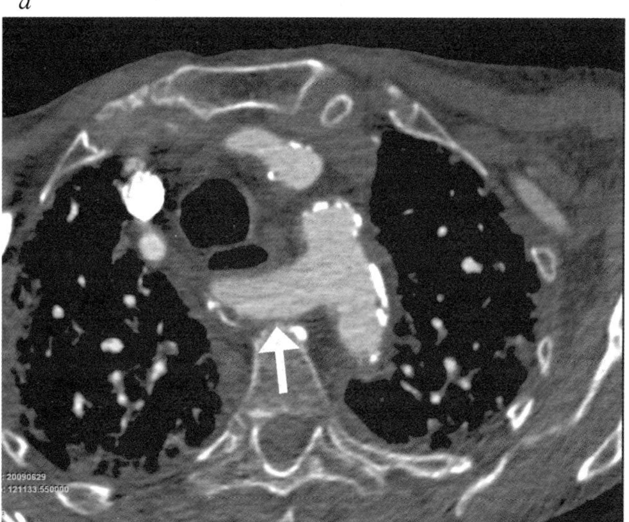

b

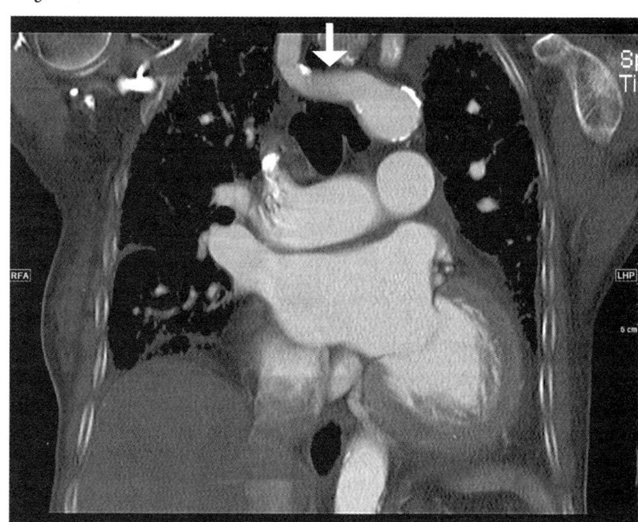

Figure 14 **A 63-year-old female presented with dysphagia for solids with no significant weight loss. (*a*) An axial multidetector computed tomographic angiogram demonstrates an artery arising from the medial aspect of the aortic arch and coursing posterior to the esophagus consistent with an aberrant right subclavian artery (*arrow*). (*b*) Coronal maximum-intensity projection demonstrates the aberrant right subclavian artery (*arrow*) passing posterior to the esophagus, causing posterior indentation on the esophagus. The dysphagia associated with this anatomic variant is classically known as dysphagia lusoria. This is the most common embryologic abnormality of the aortic arch, occurring in up to 1.8% of the population.**

a

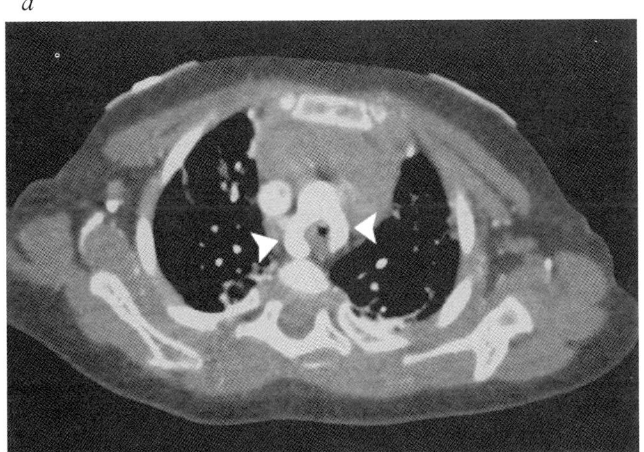

b

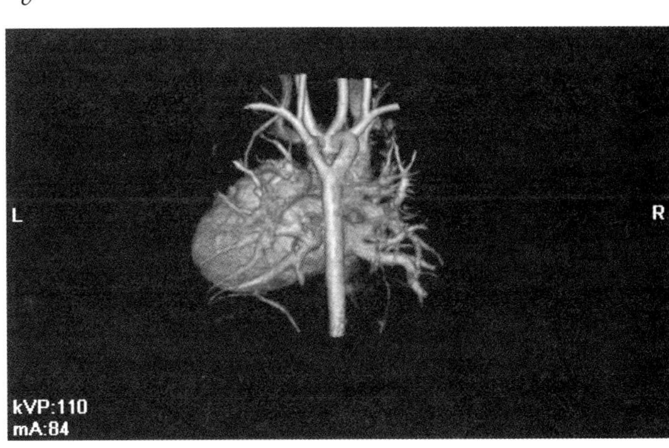

Figure 15 **A 4-year-old male child with episodes of dyspnea and intermittent cyanosis and a widened mediastinum on a chest radiograph was referred for computed tomographic angiography. (*a*) Axial view from a multidetector computed tomographic angiogram shows a crescentic vascular ring (*arrowheads*) surrounding the trachea and esophagus. (*b*) A posterior coronal volume-rendered view demonstrates a complete vascular ring consistent with a double aortic arch with the right arch of larger caliber. The carotid arteries arise anteriorly from the common arch, and a subclavian artery arises from each of the right and left arches. This patient went on to have surgical correction because of the respiratory symptoms.**

eliminated with the advent of electrocardiographic (ECG) gating and faster acquisition times, allowing for near-complete suppression of cardiac and thoracic aortic motion. ECG gating consists of image acquisition only in the diastolic phase of the cardiac cycle when the heart, and consequently the ascending thoracic aorta, is in its most quiescent phase.

Intramural hematoma, which can also cause an acute aortic syndrome similar to dissection, may be overlooked if an initial

a

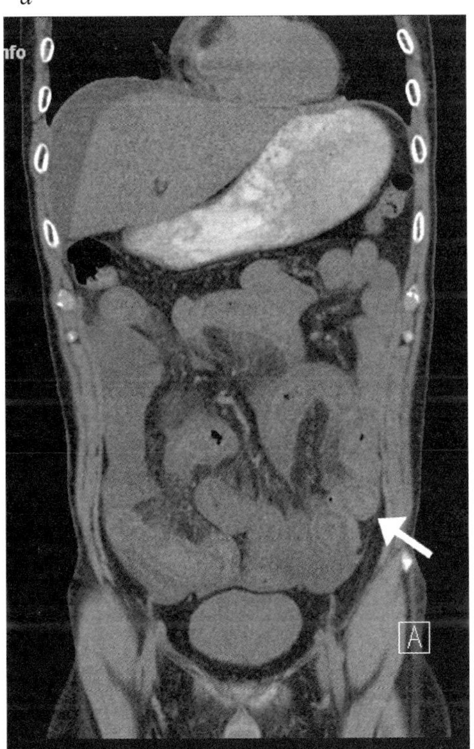

b

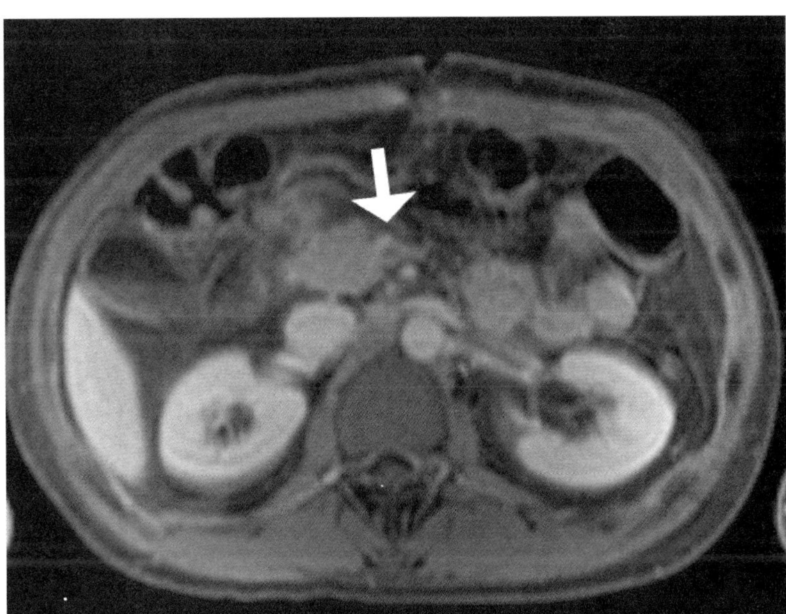

Figure 16 **A 78-year-old male presented with acute-onset abdominal pain and one episode of diarrhea. (*a*) Coronal reconstruction of a noncontrast abdominal computed tomographic (CT) scan demonstrates thickened loops of small bowel (*arrow*). (*b*) An axial postcontrast T_1 fat saturation magnetic resonance image demonstrates a filling defect within the superior mesenteric vein (SMV) with expansion of the SMV (*arrow*) consistent with SMV thrombus, which correlates with the noncontrast CT findings.**

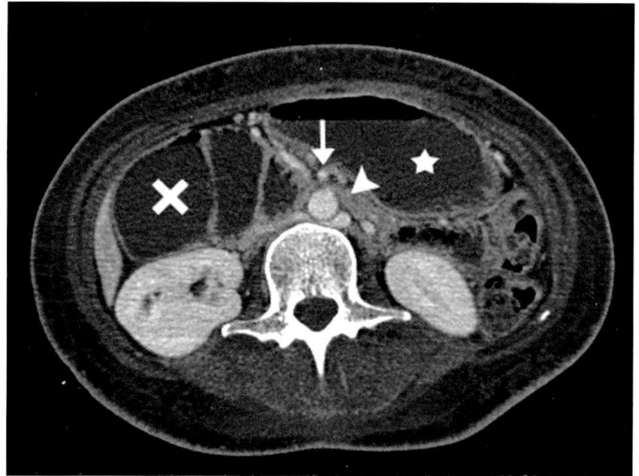

Figure 17 **A 36-year-old female presented with intermittent midline abdominal pain, weight loss, postprandial vomiting, and food avoidance. Despite her young age, symptoms were suggestive of mesenteric ischemia; thus, multidetector computed tomographic angiography (MDCTA) was performed. An axial image from the MDCTA demonstrates dilatation of the stomach (*star*) and the first and second parts of the duodenum (*x*), with a compressed third part of the duodenum (*arrowhead*) crossing the midline between the aorta and the superior mesenteric artery (SMA) (*arrow*). Note the presence of little intraperitoneal fat. The entity where the duodenum is compressed between the SMA and the aorta is known as SMA syndrome.**

noncontrast scan of the thoracic aorta is not performed. This hematoma is usually attributable to bleeding of the vasa vasorum within the aortic media and results in chest pain radiating to the back, with a clinical history almost identical to dissection. The imaging features of intramural hematoma are a crescentic area of high attenuation within the aortic wall extending longitudinally and nonspirally on the noncontrast scan, which simply looks like a thickened aortic wall with a preserved lumen on the CTA. The imaging features, however, may be identical in the setting of a dissection with a small thrombosed false lumen. Also, the noncontrast images for intramural hematoma may be identical to those of a penetrating ulcer; however, the CTA will differentiate these two conditions as a penetrating ulcer appears as a contrast-filled outpouching, diverticulum-like structure penetrating into the aortic wall [*see Figure 12*]. Many authors regard intramural hematoma, penetrating ulcer, and aortic dissection as a spectrum of the same disease process.

CTA is now regarded as the first-line modality for evaluating traumatic disruption or transection of the thoracic aorta, replacing DSA. CTA is the cornerstone diagnostic tool because of its accessibility, noninvasiveness, rapid acquisition, and ability to evaluate the entire thorax and other body regions in a single examination.[52] MDCTA has been shown to be nearly 100% sensitive, with, accordingly, high negative predictive value for the detection of acute thoracic injury.[53] CTAs can be used to plan appropriate intervention for acute thoracic transaction, with many centers now advocating endovascular repair as first line treatment[*see Figure 13*].

Some congenital variant anatomy can be eloquently demonstrated with thoracic MDCTA, often incidentally diagnosed [*see Figure 14 and Figure 15*].

The scanning volume of CTA is determined by the indication. It is typical to start at the lung apices, which provides adequate coverage of the supra-aortic vessels. The end position is typically at the level of the midkidney; however, if a dissection is suspected, the coverage can be extended to the groin. Full assessment of aortic dissection by CT requires unenhanced CT followed by arterial phase contrast-enhanced CT. The unenhanced CT is useful for detection of dense intramural hematoma that may be mistaken for chronic thrombus on the enhanced images. ECG gating is usually reserved for the evaluation of aortic dissections, along with aortic root and ascending thoracic aortic aneurysmal disease,

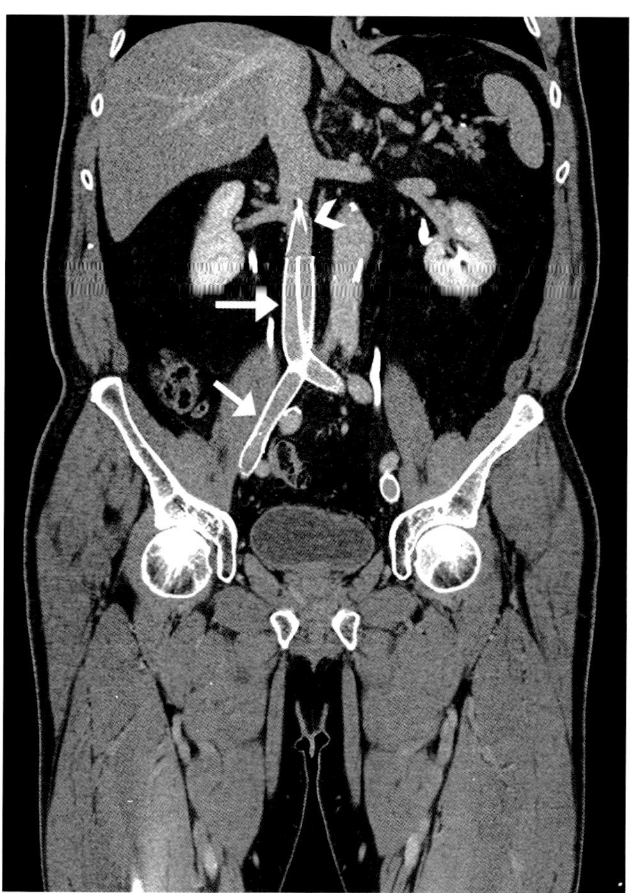

Figure 18 **A 45-year-old male presented with bilateral lower limb swelling and tenderness. Duplex ultrasonography diagnosed bilateral deep vein thrombosis extending above the inguinal ligaments. Because of the severity of limb symptoms, catheter-directed lysis was initiated, with a safety retrievable caval filter also inserted. On check venography, cavoileal stenosis was unmasked. A coronal computed tomographic scan acquired during the portovenous phase following iodinated contrast administration demonstrates the postprocedure result. There are bilateral kissing cavoileal stents in situ (*arrows*), along with the caval filter (*arrowhead*). Note that the thrombus has completely cleared following lysis.**

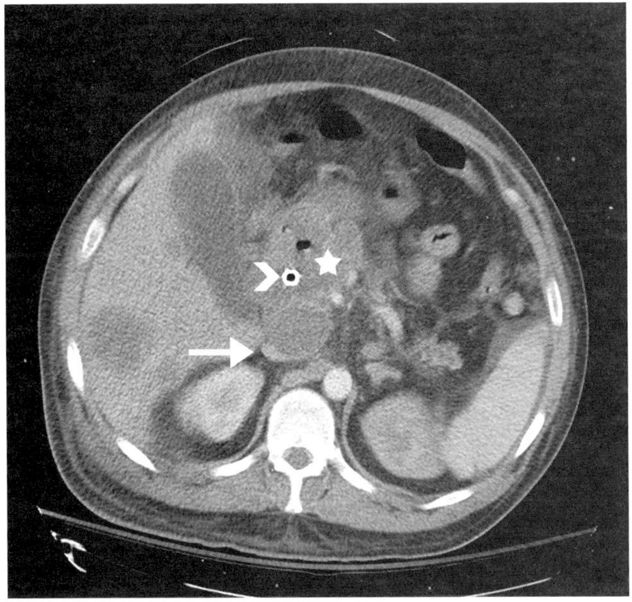

Figure 19 **A 36-year-old male with metastatic pancreatic cancer undergoing palliative care presented with gross bilateral lower limb painful edema. Duplex ultrasonography showed no evidence of deep vein thrombosis. An axial multidetector computed tomographic scan acquired in the portovenous phase demonstrates a metal biliary stent (*arrowhead*) in situ passing through the large pancreatic malignancy (*star*). There is marked anterior extrinsic compression of the inferior vena cava by the pancreatic tumor, with only a small residual caval lumen remaining (*arrow*).**

as gating reduces cardiac and aortic motion and therefore reduces pulsation artifact.

Automated bolus tracking or test bolus triggering techniques can reliably obtain the optimal arterial phase by placing an ROI on the ascending thoracic aorta. An injection volume of 100 mL of high-concentration contrast agent (350 mg iodine/mL) at a flow rate of 5 mL/s is typically used. Images are acquired in the cranial to caudal direction with a slice thickness of 1.5 mm, a slice interval of 1.0 mm, and 0.6 mm of collimation.

CTA OF THE MESENTERIC ARTERIES

CTA allows excellent visualization of the mesenteric vasculature.[54] Aneurysms, thrombosis, stenosis or occlusion, dissection, and inflammatory processes affecting the mesenteric vasculature have been evaluated by MDCTA.

Mesenteric ischemia comprises three categories: acute arterial occlusion, nonocclusive ischemia (mesenteric angina), and venous thrombosis. Acute mesenteric ischemia is a life-threatening event that may be caused by a variety of etiologies. These include embolic phenomenon, severe hypoperfusion, thrombosis of an underlying arterial stenosis, dissection, hypercoagulable states (in situ thrombosis formation), and vasculitis. MDCTA with optimally timed contrast bolus can often readily delineate the site of arterial occlusion manifested by an abrupt cutoff of arterial contrast enhancement with complete occlusion or thrombus identified as a filling defect with contrast surrounding it in a nonocclusive thrombus. A combination of imaging planes, including the axial source images and the sagittal and coronal reformatted images, together with some curved multiplanar reformatted images, can increase the diagnostic yield. Although DSA remains the gold standard, it is usually reserved for cases

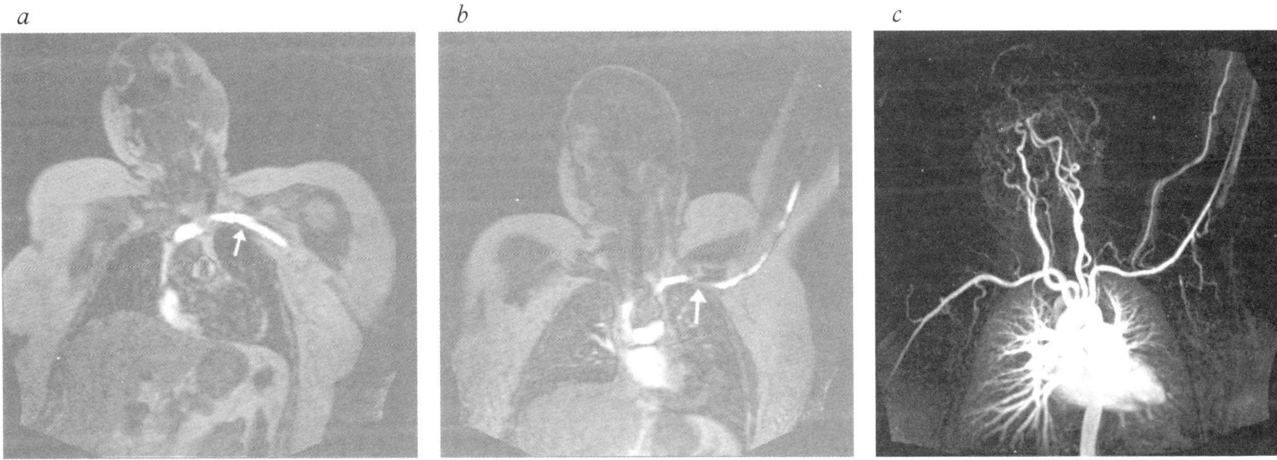

Figure 20 **A 29-year-old female swimmer presented with left arm pain and intermittent swelling. (*a*) Coronal image from a direct magnetic resonance venogram (MRV) with injection of dilute gadolinium contrast via a left peripheral intravenous canula with the left arm adducted. There is no evidence of subclavian venous compromise at the level of the thoracic outlet (*arrow*). (*b*) Coronal image from a direct MRV with the left arm abducted demonstrates subclavian venous compromise with luminal narrowing at the level of the thoracic outlet (*arrow*). (*c*) Coronal maximum-intensity projection from a high-resolution magnetic resonance angiogram demonstrates no arterial compromise with the left arm abducted. Incidental note is made of a four-vessel aortic arch, with the right subclavian and the right common carotid arteries arising separately from the aortic arch.**

requiring concurrent endovascular intervention, which is less likely in the acute setting as open surgery with embolectomy and bowel inspection is more desirable to restore mesenteric perfusion as rapidly as possible. CT accurately visualizes the portal, splenic, and superior mesenteric veins and can be used to diagnose mesenteric venous thrombosis.[55] Diagnosis of mesenteric venous thrombosis requires delayed images in the venous phase to avoid unopacified mesenteric veins, which can mimic thrombosis. Unenhanced images are also beneficial because they may show a hyperdense thrombus.[56] A pathognomonic finding of mesenteric venous thrombosis on CT includes an enlarged mesenteric vein with a low-density center surrounded by an enhancing wall along with marked edema of the mesentery with bowel wall thickening [*see Figure 16*]. When evaluating for mesenteric vascular pathology, close attention to the morphology of the bowel is important as thickened bowel loops with thumbprinting, the presence of a sentinel loop or an ileus, secondary bowel wall hemorrhage or edema, pneumatosis (air within the bowel wall—a late sign that usually indicates dead infarcted bowel), and altered enhancement (either hyper- or hypoenhancement of the affected bowel) are signs of ischemia or infarction. Portal venous air is a late and often premorbid sign that can occur with a long segment of infarcted bowel.

a

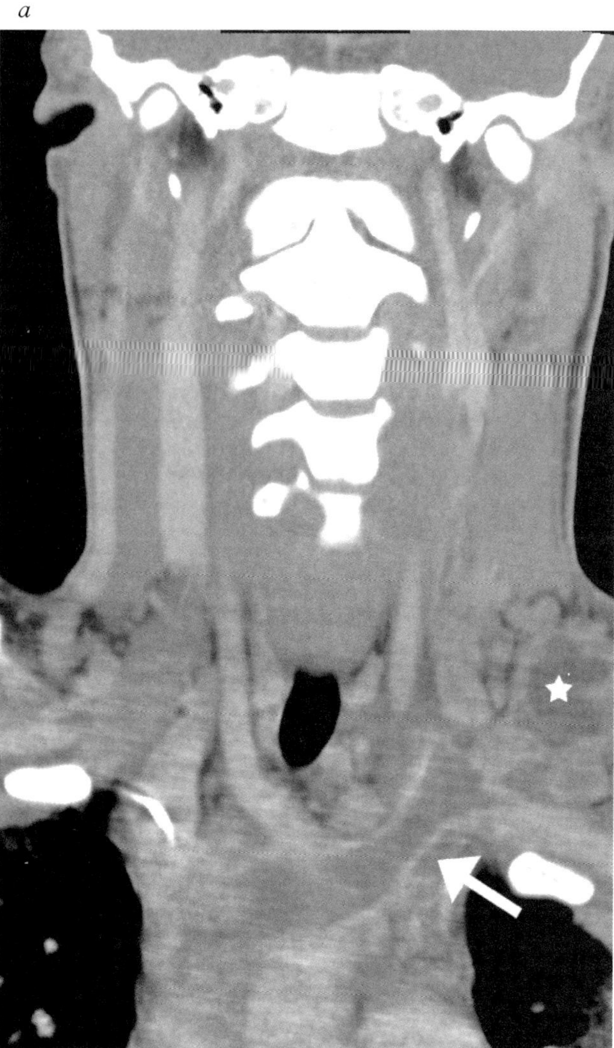

b

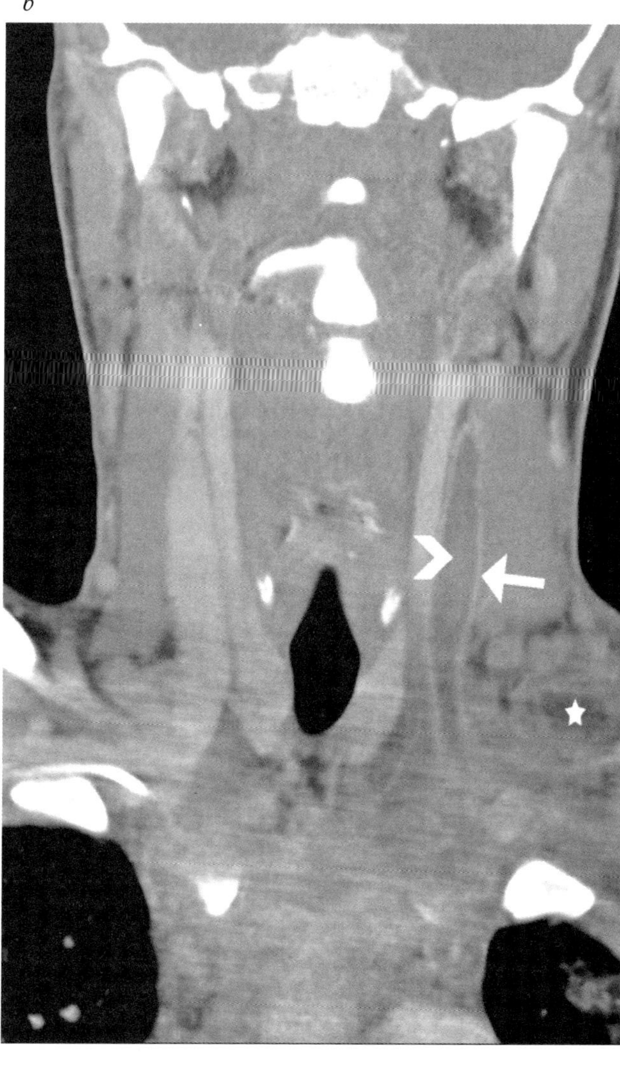

Figure 21 **An 18-year-old male presented with a painful mass in the left side of his neck and low-grade fevers. (*a*) Coronal reconstruction of a multidetector computed tomographic venogram was obtained and demonstrates a focal mass in the left supraclavicular region with a low-attenuation center (*star*) and an enhancing rim. There is extensive low-attenuation material within an expanded left brachiocephalic vein (*arrow*). (*b*) More posterior coronal reconstruction demonstrates further low-attenuation material within an expanded left internal jugular vein (LIJV) (*arrow*). Note that the material is also enhancing within the vein lumen (*arrowhead*). The focal mass in the left supraclavicular region with a low-attenuation center (*star*) and an enhancing rim is also seen. These findings are consistent with a septic thrombus within the LIJV extending into the left brachiocephalic vein as a result of the left supraclavicular abscess. This constellation of findings is known as Lemierre syndrome. The neck abscess was drained percutaneously under ultrasound guidance, and the patient was treated with intravenous antibiotics, with resolution of fevers.**

Chronic mesenteric ischemia classically manifests clinically with the triad of postprandial abdominal pain, weight loss, and food avoidance. Atherosclerosis, causing severe stenosis or occlusion in at least two mesenteric arteries, is the usual etiology. CTA can accurately demonstrate the stenoses or occlusions, degree of calcification, and number of mesenteric vessels involved and serves as a pretreatment roadmap prior to stenting or bypass. The advantage of CTA over MRA is in the follow-up of stented patients as a result of the superior spatial resolution and lack of stent-related artifacts with CTA to determine stent patency and detect any in-stent restenosis. Other etiologies of chronic mesenteric angina can also be diagnosed with CTA, including fibromuscular dysplasia, vasculitis, radiation arteritis, and, albeit rarely, SMA syndrome [*see Figure 17*].

Celiac axis compression by the median arcuate ligament is known as median arcuate ligament syndrome and can lead to mesenteric angina; however, it is often asymptomatic. Additionally, this entity has been reported to predispose patients who have undergone orthotopic liver transplantation to hepatic artery thrombosis. If median arcuate ligament syndrome is suspected, imaging should be obtained during full inspiration to avoid artifactual stenosis.[57] Celiac and mesenteric stenoses are best visualized by sagittal thin-slab MIP or volume-rendered images. However, a thin-slab coronal MIP image also provides an excellent overview of the mesenteric vascular structures and the bowel loops. Treatment is surgical, consisting of release of the ligament, with no real role for an endovascular option as a result of stent compression or even fracture. Although surgical treatment can lead to clinical improvement in symptomatic patients, the importance of celiac artery compression in asymptomatic patients is not established.

Most institutions will initially perform an arterial phase scan from the lower third of the chest above the diaphragm to the pubic symphysis; an optional initial noncontrast acquisition may be useful to see a high-attenuation thrombus, and venous phase timed acquisition covering the same scan range should also be obtained. Bolus tracking triggering can reliably obtain the optimal arterial phase by placing an ROI on the descending thoracic aorta above the diaphragm. An injection volume of 150 mL of high-concentration contrast agent (350 mg iodine/mL) at a flow rate of 5 mL/s is typically used. Images are acquired in the cranial to caudal direction with a slice thickness of 1.0 mm, a slice interval of 1.0 mm, and 0.6 mm of collimation.

COMPUTED TOMOGRAPHIC VENOGRAPHY

Duplex US is regarded as the first-line tool for diagnosis of lower and upper limb deep vein thrombosis (DVT); however, in certain clinical scenarios, particularly when interrogating the pelvic veins, computed tomographic venography (CTV) may be necessary to aid diagnosis for suprainguinal DVT. Venous phase contrast-enhanced CT can also be valuable in cases of May-Thurner syndrome with extensive thrombus prior to intervention with pharmacologic or mechanical

a

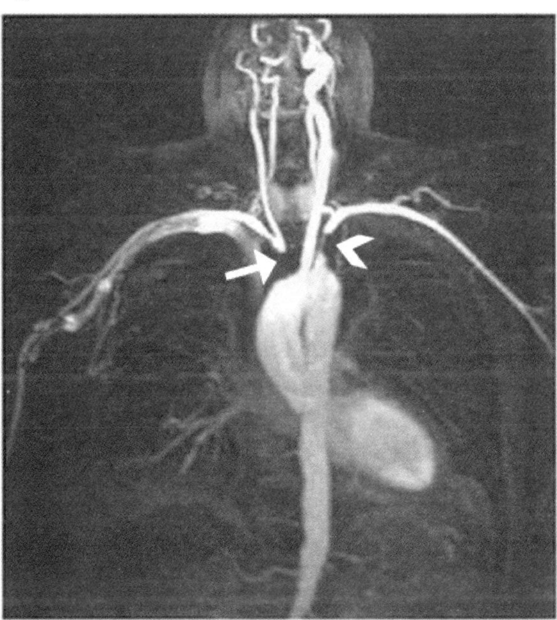

b

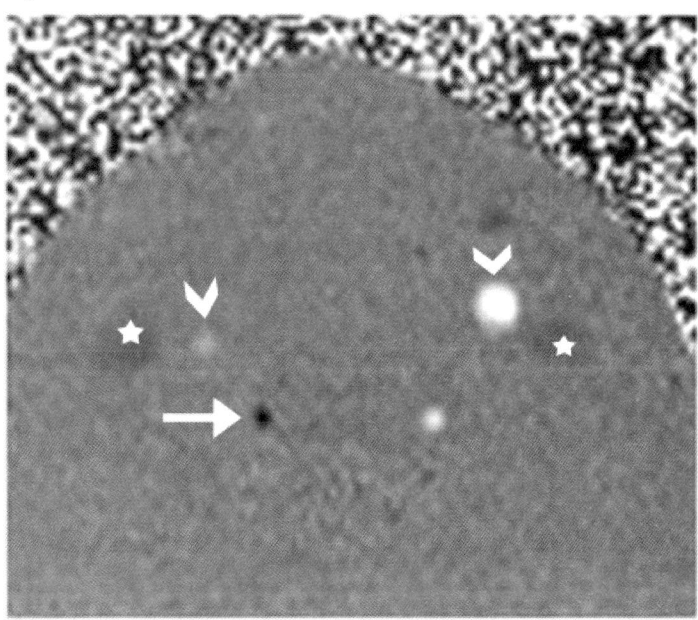

Figure 22 **A 63-year-old female presents with lightheadedness and dizziness, particularly when grocery shopping. (*a*) Coronal maximum-intensity projection from a high-resolution contrast-enhanced thoracic aortic magnetic resonance angiogram demonstrates an occlusion of the right innominate artery (*arrow*) and a focal tight stenosis of the left subclavian artery (*arrowhead*). (*b*) Axial phase contrast magnetic resonance image obtained for flow directional information. Note that the antegrade flow is white in color and retrograde flow is black in color. There is forward flow (*white*) within both carotid arteries (*arrowheads*); note the smaller caliber of the right carotid artery compared with the left. There is reverse or retrograde flow (*black*) within the right vertebral artery (*arrow*) consistent with a right subclavian artery steal phenomenon. Note the normal retrograde flow within both internal jugular veins (*stars*).**

MR fluoroscopy. Contrast volume is determined on an individual patient basis per weight, with a single dose being 0.1 mmol/kg; for CE-MRA, at least double the dose is usually administered. Based on the Fourier nature of MRI data acquisition, image contrast depends mainly on central k-space data; thus, collection of the central lines of k-space during the plateau phase of arterial enhancement is essential for optimal CE-MRA. Image fine detail depends on peripheral k-space data, which may be collected before and/or after the gadolinium peak to enhance MRA image resolution.

Repetition times (TRs) used for CE-MRA are approximately 5 milliseconds or less, with echo times (TEs) of 1 to 2 milliseconds and total scan times ranging from 10 to 30 seconds, thus fast enough to acquire all of the data in one breath-hold. Many other tricks can be employed to perform time-resolved MRA, which is a dynamic MRA technique almost analogous to the concept of rapid imaging frames obtained during DSA. A combination of ultra-short TR, parallel imaging, partial Fourier transform, sharing of peripheral k-space data, and sliding window reconstruction with radial or spiral trajectories makes time-resolved (TR) CE-MRA possible at subsecond temporal resolution. TR-MRA is particularly useful in evaluating the peripheral runoff arteries, where traditional high-resolution CE-MRA can be limited by discordant flow bilaterally, contrast bolus timing issues, and consequent venous overlay [*see Figure 23*].

Postprocessing of the CE-MRA source data is somewhat easier and less time consuming than that of CTA data as the contrast-filled vessel is the brightest structure for the MRA MIP image because the calcium is of low signal on MR, unlike the high attenuation of calcified plaque and bone on CT. As with CTA, image interpretation is performed on a computer workstation, where the source images are analyzed and postprocessing techniques, including multiplanar reformation, MIP reformation, and volume rendering, are used.

THORACIC AORTIC MRA

Thoracic aortic aneurysmal disease is particularly suited to diagnosis and follow-up with CE-MRA as MRA is highly accurate, is reproducible, and incurs no radiation dose for

a

b

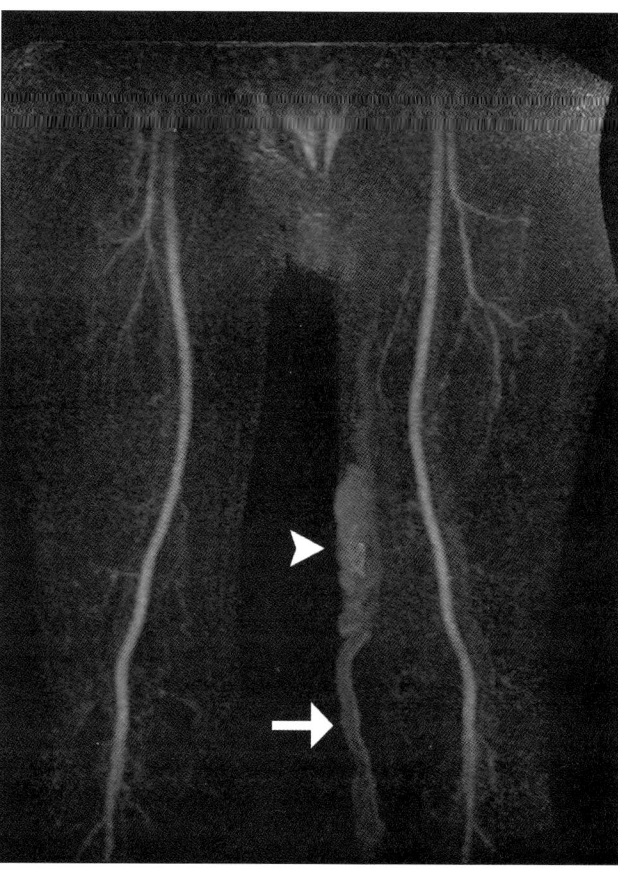

Figure 32 **A 29-year-old male presented with a painful left lower limb with some skin discoloration. (*a*) Coronal maximum-intensity projection (MIP) from a time-resolved peripheral magnetic resonance angiogram (MRA) demonstrating both lower limb runoff vessels. Although this is within the arterial phase of contrast injection, early draining veins are identified on the medial aspect of the left lower limb with a small nidus (*arrowhead*). (*b*) Coronal arterial phase time-resolved MIP more proximal within the thighs demonstrates a large left great saphenous vein (*arrow*) with varicosity (*arrowhead*). As directionality of the flow can be determined with dynamic time-resolved MRA, it was noted that the direction of flow was from the nidus in the cephalad direction, confirming arteriovenous malformation with varicosity, as opposed to reflux from the saphenofemoral junction or perforators, which would result in flow in a caudal direction and manifest as venous insufficiency with varicose veins.**

the patient. Also, MRI can be used to evaluate the adjacent aortic valve for anatomy (bicuspid or trileaflet), stenosis, or regurgitation, all of which are vital to know prior to an ascending aortic aneurysm repair to determine if the surgery is valve sparing or necessitates a concomitant aortic valve replacement. Acquiring the CE-MRA images in the oblique sagittal plane allows for almost the entire aorta to be visualized, which is useful for thoracoabdominal aneurysms and type B dissections.

Aortic dissection, along with its complications of coronary artery involvement, aortic valve rupture, pericardial hemorrhage with tamponade, branch vessel involvement, visceral ischemia, and peripheral ischemia, can be reliably diagnosed with MR using both noncontrast bright blood imaging techniques—mainly the new steady-state free procession (SSFP) techniques such as FISP, FIESTA, and FFE—and CE-MRA. Techniques such as FISP can rapidly diagnose and determine the extent of aortic dissection in a few minutes, without the need for breath-hold, contrast, or radiation. Cine FISP through the aortic valve can rapidly assess function, and a stack of short axis slices through the heart can determine any ventricular wall motion abnormalities that may be seen with coronary artery involvement resulting in myocardial infarction, along with tamponade physiology; however, there are obviously other methods to diagnose these complications, such as transthoracic or transesophageal echocardiography. Previously, SE black blood sequences were also used to demonstrate the intimal flap, usual signal void in the true lumen, and high signal attributable to slow flow or thrombus within the false lumen. CE-MRA can eloquently confirm the diagnosis, differentiate thrombus from slow flow within the false lumen, and diagnose complicated type B dissection with visceral or peripheral ischemia that may need endovascular or surgical intervention.

The limitations of MRI are availability, MR-compatible vital sign monitoring equipment, and fear of placing an unstable patient in the magnet. However, in high-volume centers with 24-hour access to magnets and staff experienced in monitoring unstable patients within the MRI scanner, this modality offers a viable alternative to CTA and TEE, especially in the setting of an iodinated contrast allergy or renal impairment.

Intramural hematoma, regarded by many as a spectrum in the same disease process as dissection, can be differentiated from dissection with thrombosis of the false lumen with the use of different sequences, namely cine GRE. SE can be used to age the thrombus with intermediate signal attributable to oxyhemoglobin in the acute setting and high signal attributable to methemoglobin in the more subacute setting.

Large vessel vasculitides such as Takayasu arteritis and giant cell arteritis are well suited to evaluation with MRI and CE-MRA. Aortic and branch vessel wall thickening can be diagnosed even before the occurrence of luminal compromise and/or dilatation. Aortic wall thickness can be demonstrated readily on fat-suppressed T_1-weighted (T_1W) MRI, and edema is seen as a hyperintense intramural signal on T_2-weighted (T_2W) imaging. Mural hyperenhancement of the aortic or arch vessel wall on fat saturation T_1W images after injection of contrast material is considered to indicate active inflammation; thus, a delayed postcontrast T_1W image is obtained after the CE-MRA portion when considering large vessel vasculitis. The CE-MRA portion of the study identifies the involved segments of the aorta and its branch arteries. Takayasu arteritis classically causes proliferation of the intima, with medial and advential fibrosis, which subsequently leads to segments of arterial stenosis, occlusion, and/or poststenotic dilatation, usually affecting the aorta and its arch branches in a patchy distribution [*see Figure 24*].

Coarctation usually presents in childhood but occasionally can present in adulthood or recur in adulthood. MRA is an eloquent way to demonstrate the coarctation or the previous repair [*see Figure 25a, Figure 26, and Figure 27*]. However, once a coarctation is stented, MRA becomes limited in its ability to follow up the patient because of the susceptibility artifact encountered [*see Figure 25b*].

ABDOMINAL AORTIC MRA

CE-MRA has been shown by a number of authors to have a high sensitivity and specificity, both 100%, for the diagnosis of AAA.[63] The important information for preprocedural planning can be gleaned from MRA, including location, size, extent, adjacent arterial branch anatomy, thrombus load, and 3D spatial relations. Importantly, when measuring the size of an AAA on MRA, the source images and not the MIP images should be used to see the wall of the aorta and thus not underestimate the size of the aneurysm on the MIPs. However, to date, most centers continue to perform pre-EVAR planning with CTA. Post-EVAR follow-up can be performed with CE-MRA to detect endoleaks and monitor sac size; however, the stainless steel stent grafts cause marked susceptibility artifact and are contraindicated for MRI per the manufacturer's guidelines. Open aneurysm repair is not without its flaws, and CE-MRA can be used to detect potential complications such as para-anastomotic aneurysms, infections, graft occlusions, and venous or enteric fistulae. Graft infections, when confirmed, usually require complex surgical intervention with removal of the graft material and extra-anatomic bypass grafting; however, infection can often be difficult to diagnose. MRI can aid in the diagnosis by using fat-suppressed T_1W and T_2W imaging, along with delayed contrast enhanced fat-suppressed T_1W images. The presence of fluid surrounding the graft (bright on T_2W, dark on T_1W), surrounding muscle edema (bright on T_2W), and delayed peripheral contrast enhancement on fat-suppressed T_1W images are all signs of graft infection.[63]

MRI is rarely used in the acute setting of suspected AAA rupture, again for the reasons outlined in the section on thoracic aortic MRA above.

CAROTID MRA

A recent meta-analysis examining noninvasive imaging modalities for diagnosis of carotid artery stenosis determined that contrast-enhanced MRA seems to be the most accurate noninvasive imaging test,[50] compared with US and MDCTA, and this finding is concordant with that of an earlier systematic review.[64] Sensitivity and specificity for CE-MRA for the diagnosis of 70 to 99% NASCET stenosis were in the order of 85% (95% CI 0.69 to 0.93) and 85% (95% CI 0.76 to 0.92), respectively,[50] and 94% (95% CI 0.88 to 0.97) and 93% (95% CI 0.89 to 0.96), respectively.[64] The results were not as accurate, in either meta-analysis, in the diagnosis of

43. Met R, Bipat S, Legemate DA, et al. Diagnostic performance of computed tomography angiography in peripheral arterial disease: a systematic review and meta-analysis. JAMA 2009;301:415–24.
44. Willmann JK, Mayer D, Banyai M, et al. Evaluation of peripheral arterial bypass grafts with multi-detector row CT angiography: comparison with duplex US and digital subtraction angiography. Radiology 2003;229:465–74.
45. Fleischmann D, Hallett RL, Rubin GD. CT angiography of peripheral arterial disease. J Vasc Interv Radiol 2006;17:3–26.
46. Soto JA, Munera F, Morales C, et al. Focal arterial injuries of the proximal extremities: helical CT arteriography as the initial method of diagnosis. Radiology 2001;218:188–94.
47. Karcaaltincaba M, Akata D, Aydingoz U, et al. Three-dimensional MDCT angiography of the extremities: clinical applications with emphasis on musculoskeletal uses. AJR Am J Roentgenol 2004;183:113–7.
48. Takase K, Imakita S, Kuribayashi S, et al. Popliteal artery entrapment syndrome: aberrant origin of gastrocnemius muscle shown by 3D CT. J Comput Assist Tomogr 1997;21:523–8.
49. Koelemay MJ, Nederkoorn PJ, Reitsma JB, Majoie CB. Systematic review of computed tomographic angiography for assessment of carotid artery disease. Stroke 2004;35:2306–12.
50. Chappell FM, Wardlaw JM, Young GR, et al. Carotid artery stenosis: accuracy of noninvasive tests—individual patient data meta-analysis. Radiology 2009;251:493–502.
51. Chiles C, Carr JJ. Vascular diseases of the thorax: evaluation with multidetector CT. Radiol Clin North Am 2005;43:543–69, viii.
52. Alkadhi H, Wildermuth S, Desbiolles L, et al. Vascular emergencies of the thorax after blunt and iatrogenic trauma: multi-detector row CT and three-dimensional imaging. Radiographics 2004;24:1239–55.
53. Mirvis SE, Shanmuganathan K, Miller BH, et al. Traumatic aortic injury: diagnosis with contrast-enhanced thoracic CT—five-year experience at a major trauma center. Radiology 1996;200:413–22.
54. Laghi A, Iannaccone R, Catalano C, Passariello R. Multislice spiral computed tomography angiography of mesenteric arteries. Lancet 2001;358:638–9.
55. Morasch MD, Ebaugh JL, Chiou AC, et al. Mesenteric venous thrombosis: a changing clinical entity. J Vasc Surg 2001;34:680–4.
56. Bradbury MS, Kavanagh PV, Bechtold RE, et al. Mesenteric venous thrombosis: diagnosis and noninvasive imaging. Radiographics 2002;22:527–41.
57. Horton KM, Talamini MA, Fishman EK. Median arcuate ligament syndrome: evaluation with CT angiography. Radiographics 2005;25:1177–82.
58. Oguzkurt L, Tercan F, Pourbagher MA, et al. Computed tomography findings in 10 cases of iliac vein compression (May-Thurner) syndrome. Eur J Radiol 2005;55:421–5.
59. Matsumura JS, Rilling WS, Pearce WH, et al. Helical computed tomography of the normal thoracic outlet. J Vasc Surg 1997;26:727–35.
60. Charles K, Flinn WR, Neschis DG. Lemierre's syndrome: a potentially fatal complication that may require vascular surgical intervention. J Vasc Surg 2005;42:1023–5.
61. Lauenstein TC, Salman K, Morreira R, et al. Nephrogenic systemic fibrosis: center case review. J Magn Reson Imaging 2007;26:1198–203.
62. Spuentrup E, Ruebben A, Mahnken A, et al. Artifact-free coronary magnetic resonance angiography and coronary vessel wall imaging in the presence of a new, metallic, coronary magnetic resonance imaging stent. Circulation 2005;111:1019–26.
63. Grist TM. MRA of the abdominal aorta and lower extremities. J Magn Reson Imaging 2000;11:32–43.
64. Wardlaw JM, Chappell FM, Best JJ, et al. Non-invasive imaging compared with intra-arterial angiography in the diagnosis of symptomatic carotid stenosis: a meta-analysis. Lancet 2006;367:1503–12.
65. Fayad LM, Hazirolan T, Bluemke D, Mitchell S. Vascular malformations in the extremities: emphasis on MR imaging features that guide treatment options. Skeletal Radiol 2006;35:127–37.
66. Meaney JF, Prince MR, Nostrant TT, Stanley JC. Gadolinium-enhanced MR angiography of visceral arteries in patients with suspected chronic mesenteric ischemia. J Magn Reson Imaging 1997;7:171–6.
67. Vasbinder GB, Nelemans PJ, Kessels AG, et al. Diagnostic tests for renal artery stenosis in patients suspected of having renovascular hypertension: a meta-analysis. Ann Intern Med 2001;135:401–11.
68. Vasbinder GB, Nelemans PJ, Kessels AG, et al. Accuracy of computed tomographic angiography and magnetic resonance angiography for diagnosing renal artery stenosis. Ann Intern Med 2004;141:674–82; discussion 82.
69. Wheatley K, Ives N, Gray R, et al. Revascularization versus medical therapy for renal-artery stenosis. N Engl J Med 2009;361:1953–62.
70. Kreft B, Strunk H, Flacke S, et al. Detection of thrombosis in the portal venous system: comparison of contrast-enhanced MR angiography with intraarterial digital subtraction angiography. Radiology 2000;216:86–92.

33 ANTERIOR RETROPERITONEAL SPINE EXPOSURE

Theodore H. Teruya, MD, and Ahmed M. Abou-Zamzam Jr, MD

Anterior surgical exposure of the lumbar spine is a technique that has been increasingly performed by a host of general and vascular surgeons over the past decade to aid spinal surgeons. Whereas anterior spinal approaches were once reserved for rare spinal disorders such as tumors or infections, the development of spinal instrumentation has led to many commonly encountered spinal disorders, such as lumbar disk disease and spondylolisthesis, being treated through an anterior approach. Owing to the predominance of spinal pathology at the lower lumbar levels and the spinal surgeons' need for assistance with anterior approaches, the "exposure surgeon" has emerged.

The knowledge and expertise in dealing with the structures encountered in the anterior exposures lie within the field of general surgery. Manipulation of diverse structures, including the small bowel, colon, ureter, aorta, and iliac vessels, must be done with precision and is an excellent opportunity for the surgeon to provide added expertise to aid the spinal surgeon in obtaining a successful outcome.

This chapter covers the aspects of anterior surgical exposure of the spine relevant to the exposure surgeon. A brief review of the background, pathophysiology, and clinical presentation of lumbar spine disease is presented, followed by a review of the treatment options and preoperative evaluation. The technical aspects, including the relevant anatomy, exposure techniques, and conduct of the operation, are presented. The routine postoperative management of these patients and frequently encountered complications are reviewed. Important but rare situations, such as redo anterior approaches, are discussed. These areas are all important for the exposure surgeon to understand and master to safely provide optimal anterior spinal exposures and offer an important avenue for the surgical trainee to gain experience with open surgical techniques.

Background

Anterior lumbar interbody fusion was first described for Pott disease of the spine.[1] This approach has gained popularity in treating a variety of diseases of the spine. Over the past decade, a broad range of lumbar pathology has been treated with instrumentation requiring an anterior approach. General, vascular, and trauma surgeons are often enlisted to provide exposure of the spine. Anterior fusion and disk replacement procedures have become common, especially with the development of anterior lumbar interbody fusion and total disk arthroplasty. The spinal pathology addressed during the anterior exposures may be divided into diseases that affect the intervertebral disk and diseases that involve the vertebral bodies along with the disk. The most common sites of involvement are the fourth and fifth lumbar vertebrae and the intervertebral disks between L4 and L5 and L5 and the sacrum (S1).

Knowledge of retroperitoneal anatomy is essential to the successful performance of these procedures. The iliac vessels will often need to be mobilized to gain access to the anterior aspect of the lumbar spine. During this mobilization, injury to the vessels may occur. Injuries to the iliac vessels are uncommon; however, when these injuries occur, life-threatening hemorrhage may result. Having a surgeon who can repair these injuries and perform the exposure can potentially reduce the chances of complications and optimize patient outcomes.

Pathophysiology

Isolated intervertebral disk disease is believed to be a major cause of chronic low back pain. The intervertebral disk is generally an avascular, fluid-rich structure that consists of the outer collagenous annulus fibrosus and the inner gelatinous nucleus pulposus. The intervertebral disk serves to absorb and dissipate loads on the spinal column and allows motion. With aging, desiccation and loss of disk height are universal. Back pain may result from internal disk disruption (IDD), disk herniation, or degenerative disk disease (DDD).

Discogenic pain is primarily attributable to IDD and DDD. IDD is marked by the presence of normal disk anatomy. This generally affects younger patients who present with back pain without radiculopathy. As the intervertebral disk is avascular and poorly innervated, pain is postulated to result from the leak of noxious chemicals.[2] In this manner, the disk serves as a "pain generator," and removal of the disk can lead to relief of pain. In contrast, DDD is marked by changes in the intervertebral disk architecture. In this setting, neurovascular ingrowth into the degenerated disk may lead to pain. The adjacent end plates and vertebral bodies may also serve as pain generators. Mechanical changes occur with DDD, which can lead to pain as a result of loading and alignment changes.

Bony abnormalities of the lumbar spine frequently treated by the exposure surgeon include lumbar spondylolisthesis. Spondylolisthesis exists when there is actual forward translation of one vertebral body over another with an intact neural arch. This misalignment and change in mechanical stress can lead to back pain secondary to muscular strain as well as potential nerve impingement with radicular pain. Often with these processes, the changes in alignment can lead to a change in disk structure and worsening pain. The pain is mechanical and aggravated by back extension or on arising from a bent posture. Radicular leg pain or neurogenic claudication may exist. For spondylolisthesis to exist, there must be both disk disruption and ligamentous disruption. Therefore, therapies to treat this address both the disk and the vertebral alignment.

Clinical Presentation

Most of the types of lumbar spine pathology discussed above typically present with back pain. Radicular pain indicates nerve root impingement. These processes are more common in women and present in the fourth decade.[2] Back pain without radiculopathy, sitting intolerance, and increased pain with flexion, rotation, and bending are common complaints. Symptoms include low back pain, which is often made worse with long periods of standing or sitting. The postural relation and alleviating factors are important in differentiating lumbar disease from other pathologies. DDD may be accompanied by radiation to the sacroiliac joints, buttocks, and thighs. Spinal stenosis attributable to disk herniation may lead to lower extremity complaints but can be differentiated from vascular claudication by (1) the long time needed for recovery and (2) alleviation of pain by leaning forward and removing pressure on the spine. The presence of any atherosclerotic risk factor is a very important historical consideration. Physical examination in a patient with spinal stenosis may reveal pain with straight leg elevation, limited mobility, [illegible]

Imaging modalities play a large role in the diagnosis of lumbar pathology. Plain x-rays may demonstrate a loss of disk height, bony abnormalities, and spondylolisthesis. Flexion and extension views are important. Magnetic resonance imaging (MRI) may demonstrate the "black disk" phenomenon. The significance of this finding is debated as this may often be seen in asymptomatic patients.[2] Discography is frequently performed to elicit the pain and to correlate the findings with other imaging studies. A computed tomographic (CT) scan can be combined with the discogram for additional information on disk architecture, and spinal stenosis. Imaging abnormalities may have a high false positive rate as 30% of asymptomatic patients will have abnormal imaging. Therefore, the diagnosis of lumbar spine disease must be based on sound clinical judgment, taking into account the history and physical examination and all imaging studies.

Treatment Options

Although the treatment of lumbar disk disease and spondylolisthesis has undergone significant evolution, the stepwise approach is needed. Nonoperative therapy is an essential first step. Patient education and activity modification are important initial treatments. Physical therapy and antiinflammatory medications are important cornerstones in patient management. The importance of appropriate pain control is clear; escalation of therapy is dependent on the response of the patient. Surgical therapy is reserved for failures of all less invasive therapies. Several less invasive surgical procedures may be offered to the patient, such as intradiscal electrothermal therapy, nucleus replacement, kyphoplasty, and other evolving treatments within the armamentarium of the spinal surgeon. However, the most invasive treatments, such as anterior lumbar interbody fusion and disk arthroplasty, are the procedures of interest to the exposure surgeon.

Intervertebral disk disease is approached with two options: motion preservation or fusion. Lumbar fusion has been traditionally performed with a posterior approach. However, with new developments in instrumentation, the fusion can also be performed with an anterior approach.[2,3] The anterior approach offers several advantages over posterior instrumentation and fusion. Anterior lumbar interbody fusion (ALIF) avoids the disruption of the muscular stability of the back and potential nerve root injury. Anterior fusion also produces a larger fusion surface, more complete disk decompression, and improved outcomes. ALIF was initially reserved for failures of posterior fusion, but with the improved results, ALIF may now be offered as the primary surgical treatment. The goal of all fusion procedures is to eliminate motion at the intervertebral space, restore alignment, and alleviate pain.

Although fusion has been successful in treating isolated intervertebral disk disease, recent investigations have established the options for motion-preserving therapy in affected patients.[4] The development of total disk replacement (TDR) has the potential to preserve motion at the treated disk space while eliminating the disk as a source of pain. Preservation of motion at the disk space can avoid the late sequelae of adjacent-level degeneration seen above a previous spinal fusion. Prospective, randomized trials have demonstrated the superiority of TDR to ALIF in selected patients.[5–8] This has [illegible] fusions may be performed from a posterior approach, all currently available TDR systems in the United States require an anterior approach to the lumbar spine.

The treatments available for spondylolisthesis include decompression alone and decompression with fusion. Simple decompression may be chosen in high-risk patients and those with limited slip. However, prospective, randomized trials have demonstrated that the addition of fusion to decompression leads to improved outcomes.[9] This has led to increased use of fusion for the treatment of spondylolisthesis, with anterior fusion demonstrating greater success than posterior fusion. Along with the fusion, anterior instrumentation with plates and screws is necessary when anterior columnar support is inadequate.[3]

Preoperative Evaluation

A thorough understanding of the background and treatment options for lumbar spine disease enables the exposure surgeon to fully participate in the treatment of these patients and not function as a mere technician. The importance of teaming with an experienced spinal surgeon with sound judgment cannot be overemphasized. Exposure surgeons must develop their own preoperative approach to the patient that maximizes the opportunity for success.

Once a patient has been selected as a candidate for anterior spinal surgery, a thorough evaluation by the exposure surgeon should be performed in a preoperative office visit. Given the magnitude of the operation and the central role the exposure surgeon plays, establishing a relationship with the patient is very important. Given the different perspectives of the spine and exposure surgeons, important additional information may be gleaned from the exposure surgeon's assessment.

A thorough medical history is an essential first step. Most patients who require this type of surgery tend to be young and otherwise healthy. Some patients will be overweight because of inactivity from their spine disease. Significant comorbidities that may place the patient at high risk for surgery must be considered at this point. General health issues, with an emphasis on atherosclerotic risk factors such as diabetes, hypertension, and tobacco use, should be queried. Previous surgical interventions, including previous abdominal operations, must be reviewed. Previous spinal surgery, even procedures from a posterior approach, can have implications related to scarring, instrumentation, and infection that can complicate an anterior approach.

A physical examination with special attention to body habitus, planned incision site, and previous surgical incisions should be performed. In all patients, a thorough pulse examination must be documented. The presence of significant vascular disease should be a relative contraindication to any anterior approach given the potential for vascular calcification and injury. If aortoiliac occlusive disease is suspected, noninvasive vascular studies may aid in the evaluation of patients with the potential presence of vascular disease by history or physical examination.

A review of all available imaging studies should be performed by the exposure surgeon. This will ensure that the approach surgeon understands and reviews the relevant anatomy. Available x-rays will demonstrate any vascular calcification, which may then suggest the need for further vascular imaging. The relevant vascular anatomy demonstrating the relation of the lumbar level of interest and the aortic bifurcation, confluence of iliac veins, and course of the iliac arteries and veins can often be determined from MRIs or CT scans. These scans can also demonstrate the presence of arterial calcification, surgical clips from previous operations, and other findings that may alter the considered approach. This will allow the exposure surgeon to have the clearest understanding possible to formulate an effective surgical plan.

A key part of any surgical procedure involving more than one specialist is communication. After the preoperative visit, the exposure surgeon should contact the spine specialist and review the case. This will minimize any potential for confusion at the time of surgery. At all stages, the exposure surgeon must be open and forthcoming, with both the patient and the spine surgeon, regarding expectations of the proposed surgery. It is important to remember that not all patients are good candidates for anterior spinal surgery. Previous colon surgery, retroperitoneal dissection, pelvic irradiation, or the presence of aortoiliac occlusive disease should be considered relative contraindications. Overall physiologic status is important and should be carefully considered prior to committing the patient to any major operation. The spine disorders treated via the anterior retroperitoneal approach are almost never life threatening; therefore, if the surgeon performing the exposure feels that the surgery will carry excessive risk, the procedure should be reconsidered.

Vascular Anatomy and Variations

The arterial anatomy is relatively simple, and variations rarely pose any difficulty in exposure of the disk levels. The arterial structures of importance include the aorta and the bilateral common iliac arteries. Most mobilization involves the left common iliac artery, but exposure usually does not require division of any significant branches. If exposure of the disk levels cephalad to the L4-L5 level is necessary, then division of segmental lumbar arteries may be required.

Although the arterial anatomy is simple, the venous anatomy will require intraoperative assessment to determine the best method for exposure. At certain levels, typically L4-L5, mobilization of the iliac veins is essential to gain proper exposure to the lumbosacral spine. The venous anatomy in this area can be variable, and if there is improper mobilization of the veins, injury can occur, and this can lead to large blood loss.

The inferior vena cava originates at the confluence of the left and right common iliac veins. This usually occurs at the L4-L5 disk level; however, this can be variable. The left common iliac vein has tributaries that are known as the ascending lumbar vein (ALV) and the iliolumbar vein (ILV) [*see Figure 1*]. The ALV commonly arises from the lateral aspect of the common iliac vein. This vein will need to be divided to properly mobilize the left common iliac vein. The ILV can arise near the ALV or may arise more distally. Unruh and colleagues demonstrated that the venous anatomy can be variable and categorized the tributaries of the left common iliac vein into three types.[10] More than half of the patients will have a common origin of a venous branch from the left common iliac vein, which then divides into the ALV and ILV. The other common variants both include two distinct origins for the ALV and ILV. The authors have proposed referring to these veins as the lateral lumbosacral veins because of the variation often encountered.[10] The importance of this anatomy lies in the fact that these veins can be easily torn with medial retraction of the left common iliac vein and result in severe hemorrhage that is difficult to control. Mobilization and division of these key branches are necessary for full retraction of the left common iliac vein. It is important to note that although there can be significant variation of the venous anatomy in this area, careful dissection can avoid serious venous injuries in nearly all cases, and usually no more than two veins in this area need to be divided.

Operative Approach

GENERAL CONSIDERATIONS

The lumbar spine is most frequently diseased at the levels of the fourth lumbar vertebra through the sacrum (L4-S1). The anterior approach to the spine at these levels will therefore have to address the peritoneal and retroperitoneal structures overlying the spine at these levels. Employing an extraperitoneal approach can minimize the need to directly address the intraperitoneal structures. The external landmark for the aortic bifurcation is generally the umbilicus, although this can vary with age and body habitus. The L4-L5 disk space is generally located near the aortic bifurcation [*see Figure 1*]. The L4-L5 disk lies in a plane that is generally axial but may be angulated in a slightly caudal direction. In a thin person, the step-off between L5 and S1 can be palpated and identifies the L5-S1 disk space. In the supine patient, the L5-S1 disk lies roughly halfway between the umbilicus and the pubis. However, the L5-S1 disk space is often angulated

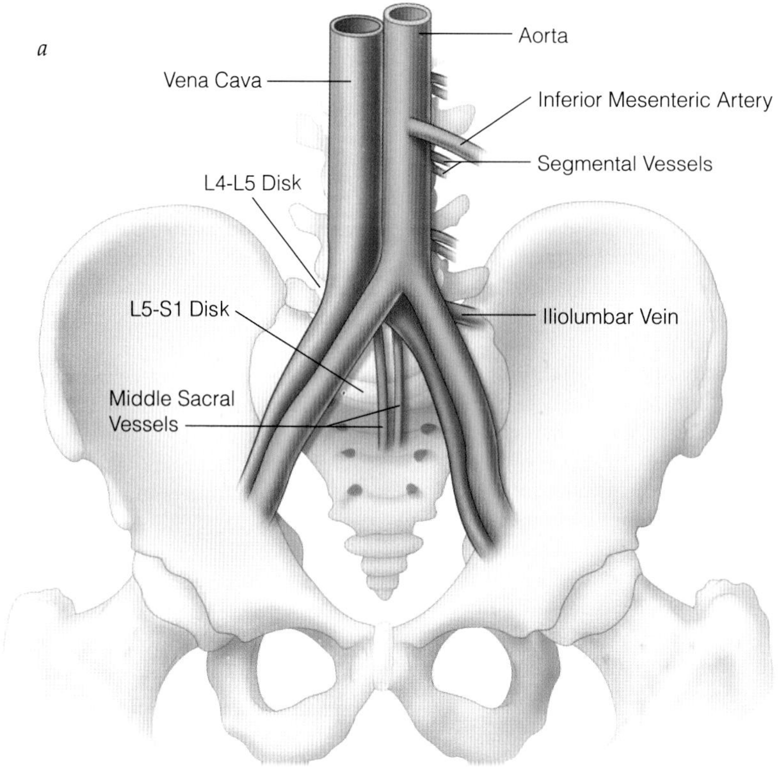

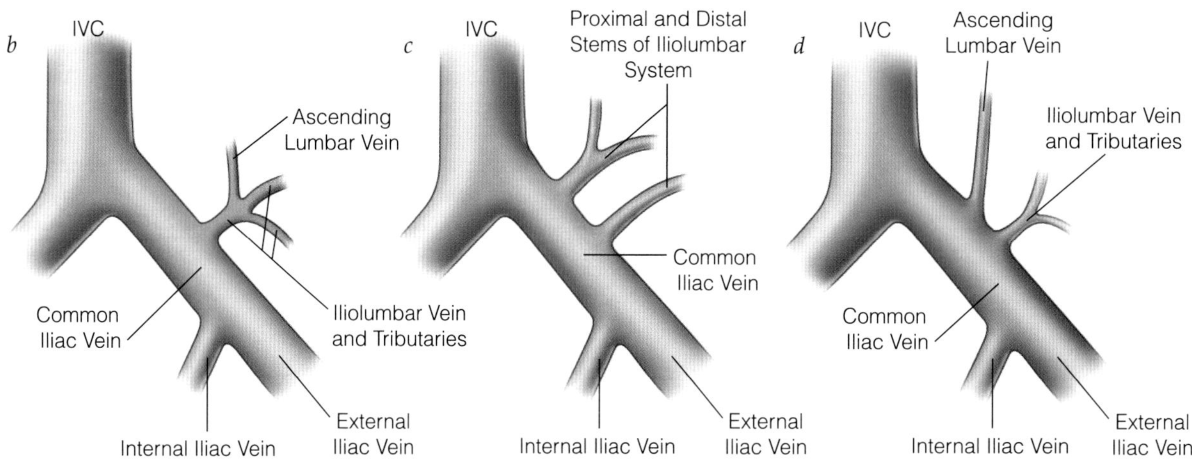

Figure 1 **(*a*) The important anatomic relations of the disk spaces to the aorta, vena cava, and iliac arteries and veins are depicted. (*b to d*) The three differing patterns of venous tributaries into the left common iliac vein are demonstrated. IVC = inferior vena cava.**

in a more caudally directed plane than L4-L5. These are all important aspects to keep in mind when planning the surgical approach.

The vascular manipulations necessary during exposures of the lumbar spine are the most critical aspects of the exposure. Exposure at L4-L5 generally involves mobilization of the left common iliac artery and vein. The disk space may be exposed above the vessels, between the vessels, or below the vessels [*see Figure 2*]. Chiriano and colleagues reviewed 243 cases of L4-L5 exposure.[11] The exposure was achieved superolateral to the left common iliac artery in 44% of cases. Mobilization of the left common iliac artery laterally and left common iliac vein medially was necessary in 45% of cases. The ALV and/or ILV will have to be divided to mobilize the vein medially. In 11% of cases, the exposure was achieved between left and right common iliac veins as described for L5-S1.[11] The

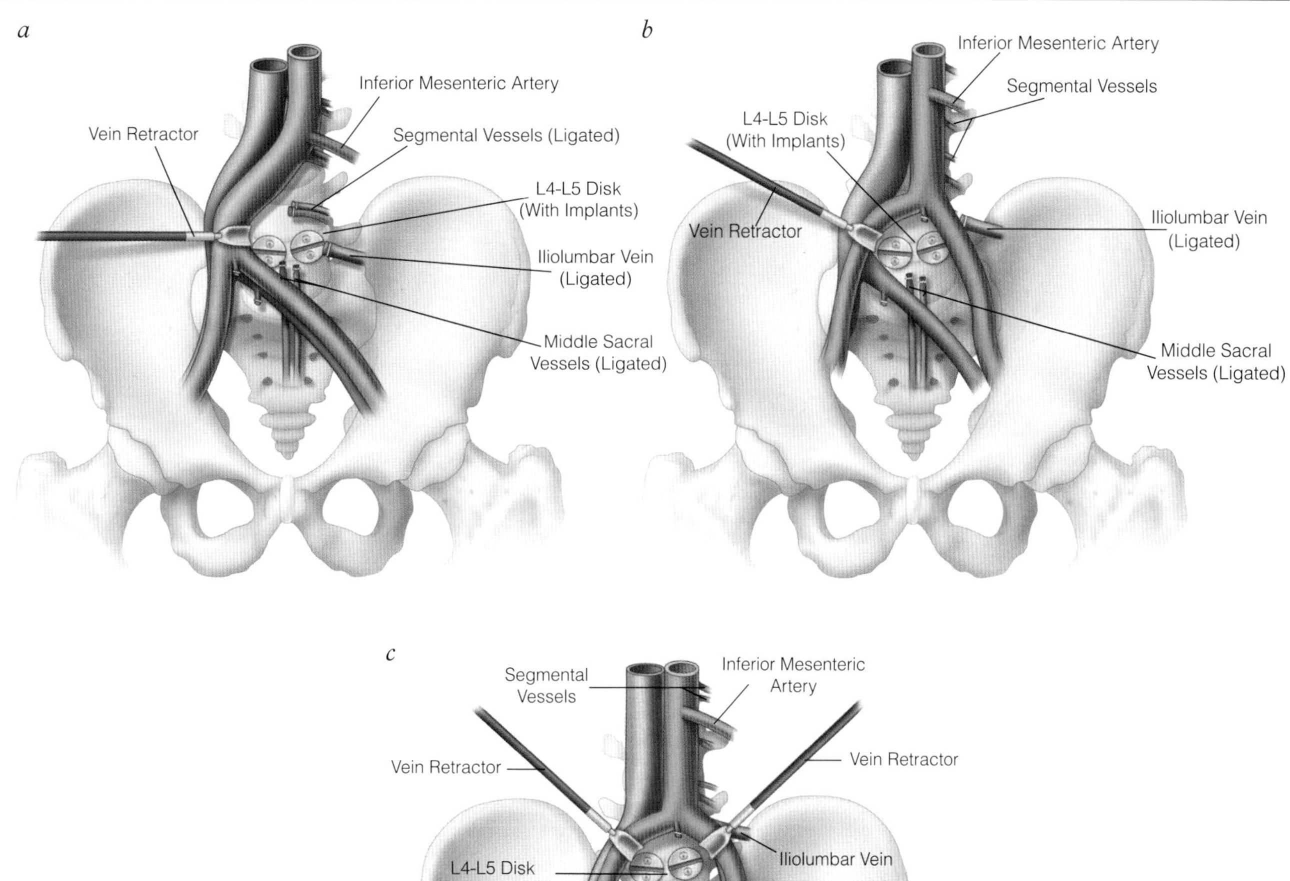

Figure 2 **The manipulations necessary ation of the disk space to the iliac vessels. (*a*) Exposure obtained above the left common iliac artery and vein. (*b*) Exposure obtained between the left common iliac artery and vein. (*c*) Exposure obtained below the left common iliac vein.**

exposure of the L5-S1 disk space is typically obtained between the right and left iliac veins without the need for significant vascular mobilization [*see Figure 1*]. The median sacral vessels serve as a consistent landmark on the anterior disk surface for the centerpoint of the disk.

Overlying nervous structures within the area of the aortic bifurcation include the sympathetic plexus, which often lies over the origin of the left common iliac artery. Care in this area is important to prevent damage and preserve sexual function, primarily ejaculatory function, in the patient. Also in this area, the ureter must be identified and protected from injury.

CONDUCT OF OPERATION

Anterior approaches are all performed with the patient placed supine on a radiolucent table. Care must be taken to ensure that the patient is not rotated as this will affect the ability to accurately place the instrumentation. The patient's arms are placed on armboards extending out at a 90° angle as arms tucked at the sides will interfere with lateral fluoroscopic imaging. Appropriate monitoring lines are placed by the anesthesia and neurology services. Prior to preparing the operative field, fluoroscopy is performed to identify the levels of interest and mark the level on the skin [*see Figure 3*]. This simple step avoids malpositioning of the incision and limits

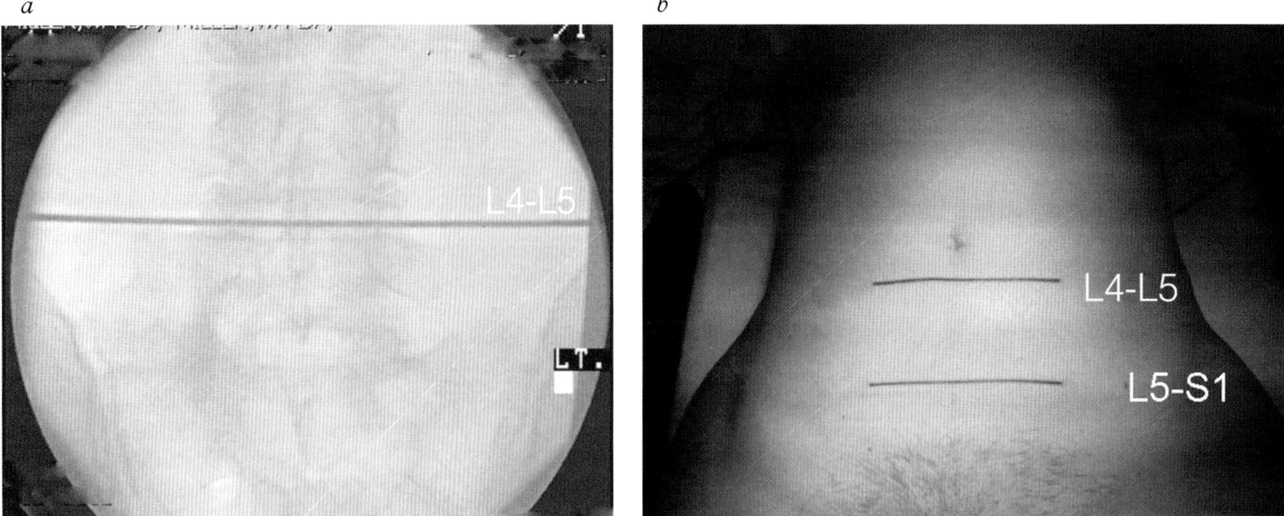

Figure 3 **Intraoperative incision planning: (*a*) fluoroscopy is used to identify the disk space, and (*b*) the level is marked on the skin.**

the size of the incision. The choice of a lower transverse abdominal or vertical paramedian incision typically depends on two factors: the upper level of exposure necessary and the number of levels to be exposed. For exposures involving L4-L5 and/or L5-S1, we prefer a lower abdominal transverse incision. For exposures involving L3-L4 or higher or for all three-level approaches, we prefer a left vertical paramedian incision [*see Figure 4*]. Both incisions allow for excellent extraperitoneal exposure.

When a transverse incision is made, the incision is generally approximately 3 cm below the umbilicus when the L4-L5 disk is to be exposed. Because of the more caudal angulation of the L5-S1 disk space, isolated L5-S1 exposure can be obtained with a transverse incision a few fingerbreadths above the pubis. When both L4-L5 and L5-S1 are to be exposed, the incision generally is made slightly favoring the upper level because of the importance of adequate exposure to address vascular manipulations, which are frequently required at L4-L5. The soft tissues are divided with cautery down to the anterior rectus sheath. The sheath is divided transversely, with the lateral aspect extending no further than the lateral aspect of the rectus muscles. The anterior rectus sheath is then mobilized away from the rectus muscles in a cephalad and caudal direction. This will allow lateral retraction of the muscles and superior-inferior retraction of the fascia. The muscle bellies are separated in the midline, and the muscles are mobilized laterally. The midline plane may be somewhat scarred if the patient has had a previous cesarean section

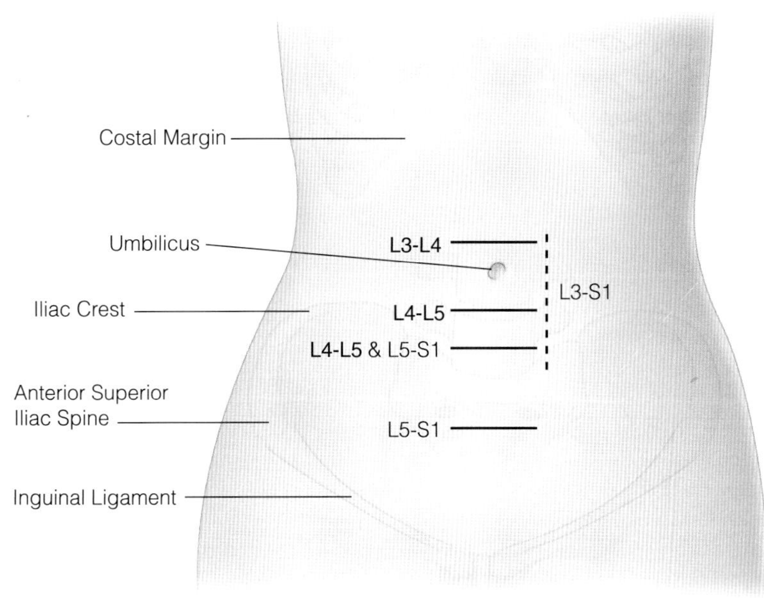

Figure 4 **General guideline for planning skin incision.**

or hysterectomy, but these muscles can almost always be separated and retracted. The extraperitoneal plane is then developed, with dissection being carried out behind the rectus muscles. The inferior portion of the posterior rectus sheath may be encountered and is divided in a vertical direction to then allow entry into the extraperitoneal plane. In the midline, the peritoneum may be adherent to the linea alba, and careful sharp dissection is necessary. When there has been a previous lower midline or Pfannenstiel incision, the extraperitoneal plane can generally be developed slightly laterally toward the left, away from any scarring. Dissection can then be carried back toward and across the midline. At any point, if a hole is made in the peritoneum, dissection can be carried out in another location and the extraperitoneal plane developed while keeping the peritoneum mostly intact. The dissection proceeds downward and toward the patient's left with mobilization of the peritoneum and its contents toward the right.

When a left paramedian incision is chosen, the dissection begins as above. Once the anterior rectus sheath is identified, the sheath is incised vertically 2 to 3 cm lateral to the midline. The fascia is mobilized away from the left rectus abdominus muscle. The left rectus is then dissected to the midline and mobilized laterally. The posterior rectus sheath is then identified and incised vertically. The extraperitoneal plane is then entered. Given the vertical orientation, this incision allows for more optimal access when three-level exposures are necessary and is favored for any lumbar exposure above L4-L5.

Once the extraperitoneal plane is developed via either the transverse or paramedian approach, dissection is generally unencumbered downward and to the patient's left [*see Figure 5*]. Care should be taken to avoid injury to the inferior epigastric vessels, which should be left anteriorly attached to the posterior aspect of the rectus. The round ligament may be identified and divided during this portion of the procedure. In males, the spermatic cord is mobilized and retracted inferomedially. The psoas muscle can be identified at this point.

Blunt dissection is used to mobilize the peritoneal contents medially while keeping the peritoneum intact. Cephalad dissection in a retronephric plane will allow creation of a larger dissection space. The ureter is identified and rotated medially along with the peritoneal structures. The external iliac artery will be seen and can be traced to the left common iliac artery and the aorta. This dissection anterior to the arteries can be done bluntly, but there may be some small veins coursing anteriorly that can be cauterized. The distal dissection typically then occurs medial to the iliac vessels. Occasionally, the obliterated umbilical artery (a branch of the internal iliac artery) will be encountered and should be ligated and divided. The bladder is typically caudal to the area of dissection and is not directly identified. At this point, a self-retaining retractor system is essential. We prefer the Omni-Tract surgical retractor system (St. Paul, MN) with radiolucent blades. This allows the maintenance of exposure throughout the instrumentation process with minimal interference.

Often multilevel exposures are required, and exposure of the disk spaces usually proceeds in a cephalad to caudal direction. When multiple disk levels need to be treated, it is safer to expose one level at a time. Adequate exposure often requires retraction of the vessels, and optimal exposure of one level may compromise the exposure of the other disk levels. The dissection at each level should be carried out sequentially. After one level has been adequately exposed, the retractors can then be adjusted to expose the subsequent (typically more caudal) level. For proper instrumentation to take place, wide exposure of the anterior aspect of the intervertebral disk must be achieved. The placement of an artificial disk requires clear identification of the midline of the disk and extensive side-to-side exposure of the anterior aspect of the disk. The performance of fusion with anterior instrumentation typically involves less side-to-side exposure of the disk but does require exposure of several millimeters of the vertebral bodies adjacent to the disk. Thus, it is important for the exposure surgeon to be aware of the surgical plan.

The most common intervertebral disk levels that require exposure are the L4-L5 and the L5-S1 disks. The L4-L5 disk level will often be more difficult to expose. The key intraoperative decision is what relation the disk space holds to the iliac vessels [*see Figure 2*]. This can often be anticipated in light of preoperative imaging (when available). Palpation of the disk will often clearly identify the important relations determining whether the window should be created above the left common iliac artery, between the left common iliac artery and vein, or below the left common iliac vein. During all manipulations of the left common iliac vein, careful dissection and control of the iliolumbar and ascending lumbar veins are key.

For exposure of the L5-S1 disk, the sacral promontory can be easily palpated in the retroperitoneal space. Dissection is carried out medially to the left common iliac vessels. The left common iliac vein can generally be carefully retracted laterally, and the soft tissues over the L5-S1 disk can be divided. The middle sacral artery will be identified and serves as an excellent mark for the midline of the disk. The middle sacral artery and vein can be divided with ligature, the harmonic scalpel, electrocautery, or clips. Blunt dissection can then be used to retract the tissues toward the right, medial to the right common iliac vein, and complete the exposure of the anterior aspect of the disk.

Once all levels have been exposed, radiopaque markers are placed in the disk spaces. This allows confirmation of the appropriate level by the exposure surgeon and confirmation by the spine surgeon [*see Figure 6*]. By obtaining anteroposterior and lateral views, this also allows the identification of the centerline, which is very important during instrumentation.

Instrumentation is then performed by the spinal surgeon. Clearly orienting the spinal surgeon about the relevant anatomy, retractor positioning, and centerline will help avoid any potential for injury. As a result of the observation that nearly all serious vascular injuries occur during the instrumentation portion of the procedure, we have adopted the policy of remaining scrubbed and assisting with the instrumentation. Often at L4-L5, compression of vascular structures is necessary to obtain adequate exposure [*see Figure 7*]. Periodic relief of compressing retractors will help avoid any thrombotic complications. Compression of vascular structures is rarely necessary at L5-S1 [*see Figure 8*]. Following completion of instrumentation at each level, the retractors should be readjusted to optimize exposure.

preliminary results. Spine (Phila Pa 1976) 1995;20:2029–34.

26. Shen FH, Samartzis D, Khanna AJ, et al. Minimally invasive techniques for lumbar interbody fusions. Orthop Clin North Am 2007;38:373–86.
27. Kaiser MG, Haid RW Jr, Subach BR, et al. Comparison of the mini-open versus laparoscopic approach for anterior lumbar interbody fusion: a retrospective review. Neurosurgery 2002;51:97–103.
28. Kleeman TJ, Michael Ahn U, Clutterbuck WB, et al. Laparoscopic anterior lumbar interbody fusion at L4-L5: an anatomic evaluation and approach classification. Spine (Phila Pa 1976) 2002;27:1390–5.
29. Zdeblick TA, David SM. A prospective comparison of surgical approach for anterior L4-L5 fusion: laparoscopic versus mini anterior lumbar interbody fusion. Spine (Phila Pa 1976) 2000;25:2682–7.
30. Lieberman IH, Willsher PC, Litwin DE, et al. Transperitoneal laparoscopic exposure for lumbar interbody fusion. Spine (Phila Pa 1976) 2000;25:509–14.
31. Regan JJ, Yuan H, McAfee PC. Laparoscopic fusion of the lumbar spine: minimally invasive spine surgery. A prospective multicenter study evaluating open and laparoscopic lumbar fusion. Spine (Phila Pa 1976) 1999; 24:402–11.
32. Mahvi DM, Zdeblick T. A prospective study of laparoscopic spinal fusion: technique and operative complications. Ann Surg 1996;224: 85–90.
33. Mathews HH, Evans MT, Molligan HJ, et al. Laparoscopic discectomy with anterior lumbar interbody fusion: a preliminary review. Spine (Phila Pa 1976) 1995;20:1797–802.
34. Gumbs AA, Bloom ND, Bitan FD, et al. Open anterior approaches for lumbar spine procedures. Am J Surg 2007;194:98–102.

34 AORTIC DISSECTION

Mark F. Conrad, MD, MMSc, and Richard P. Cambria, MD

Acute aortic dissection is the most common catastrophic event affecting the aorta. However, its overall prevalence is rare, occurring in three of every 1,000 patients who present to the emergency department with chest and/or back pain.[1] Acute aortic dissection is a lethal disease: early studies showed that in the absence of treatment, the majority of patients died within 3 months of presentation. Reported mortality rates of untreated patients approached 75% within the first 2 weeks after the onset of symptoms.[2] Few survived the chronic phase more than 5 years as a result of progressive aneurysmal degeneration and rupture of the outer wall of the false lumen.[3,4] Despite improvements in both medical and surgical therapies, overall mortality associated with acute dissection in contemporary practice remains significant: mortality was 27% in a recent report from the International Registry of Acute Aortic Dissections (IRAD).[5] Early death attributable to an acute dissection of the ascending aorta is usually secondary to the central cardioaortic complications of aortic rupture into the pericardium, acute aortic regurgitation, and coronary ostia compromise,[6,7] whereas descending aortic dissections are more commonly associated with death from end-organ compromise attributable to visceral or extremity malperfusion.[8,9]

General Features

CLASSIFICATION

Aortic dissections are classified according to the anatomic location of the entry tear and the time between onset of symptoms and patient presentation. A dissection is considered acute when the diagnosis is made within 2 weeks of the initial onset of symptoms and thereafter becomes chronic. Although such a designation appears arbitrary, it is based on autopsy studies that showed that 74% of patients who die from aortic dissections do so in the first 14 days.[10]

Anatomically, aortic dissection is classified based on the location of the intimal tear and the extent of the dissection along the aorta. Two classification schemes are used to describe aortic dissections. The DeBakey classification delineates both the origin of the entry tear and the extent of the descending aortic dissection as follows [*see Figure 1*]:[11]

- Type I: dissection originates in the ascending aorta and extends through the aortic arch and into the descending aorta and/or abdominal aorta for a varying distance
- Type II: dissection originates in and is confined to the ascending aorta
- Type IIIa: dissection originates in the descending aorta and is limited to the same
- Type IIIb: dissection involves descending and variable extents of the abdominal aorta

The Stanford classification simplified the anatomic classification according to the origin of the entry tear alone. A Stanford type A dissection originates in the ascending aorta and therefore encompasses DeBakey type I and II dissections, whereas a Stanford type B dissection originates in the descending aorta distal to the origin of the left subclavian artery and includes DeBakey types IIIa and IIIb [*see Figure 1*].

INCIDENCE AND EPIDEMIOLOGY

Recent population-based studies have estimated the incidence of acute aortic dissection to range from 2.9 to 3.5 per 100,000 person-years.[12,13] Men are more frequently affected, with a male-to-female ratio of 4:1 reported in a recent IRAD series.[14] In our cumulative experience, type A dissections account for 60% of cases, and this is consistent with the IRAD data, wherein 62.5% of 1,417 patients presented with a type A dissection.[15] The incidence of type A dissection peaks between 50 and 60 years of age, whereas type B dissections occur more frequently in older patients, between 60 and 70 years of age.[5]

Hypertension is common and was present in 70% of patients in the IRAD database [*see Table 1*].[14] Aortic wall structural abnormalities and the presence of a bicuspid aortic valve with or without its accompanying aortic root dilatation are well-established risk factors for ascending aortic dissections. Indeed, the presence of a bicuspid aortic valve has been documented in 7 to 14% of all aortic dissections.[5,16] Other aortic diseases, such as coarctation of the aorta, annuloaortic ectasia, chromosomal abnormalities (Turner syndrome, and Noonan syndrome), aortic arch hypoplasia, and hereditary conditions (Marfan syndrome and Ehlers-Danlos syndrome), are also risk factors for the development of acute aortic dissection.[17] Marfan syndrome accounts for 50% of cases of acute aortic dissection in patients under 40 years of age.[14]

It has been previously reported that in women under 40 years of age, 13 to 50% of aortic dissections occur during pregnancy.[14,18] Preeclampsia with resultant hypertension is the most common etiology of peripartum aortic dissection, but pregnant women with Marfan syndrome are also at high risk. The presence of a dilated aortic root (> 4 cm) is the best predictor of dissection in the pregnant patient with Marfan syndrome.[19] Cocaine ingestion is a rare cause of acute aortic dissection in otherwise healthy individuals, with an incidence as high as 37% in an urban setting but less than 1% in the IRAD population.[14,20,21] These patients are typically young (average age 47 years), male (75%), and smokers (100%) with a history of hypertension (70%) and no particular trend toward dissection type.[21]

Pathologic Anatomy

INTIMAL TEAR

The process of aortic dissection is dynamic and can occur anywhere along the course of the aorta, resulting in a wide considered to be an important etiologic feature of acute aortic dissection and was present in only 31% of patients in the IRAD.[27] However, Jex and colleagues noted either gross or microscopic atheroma in 83% of patients in their series.[28] The presence of an atherosclerotic aneurysm presenting with concurrent aortic dissection is uncommon, occurring in only 14 to 15% of patients in recent series.[27,29] The unusual coexistence of an aortic dissection that originates in and/or involves a preexistent atherosclerotic aneurysm appears to change the natural history; rupture is the likely scenario. To wit, in a review of 325 patients with aortic dissection, rupture in the abdomen occurred only in the setting of antecedent degenerative, atherosclerotic aneurysm.[30] These findings support the posture of treating such type B dissections as "complicated," and initial surgical priority should be given to the aorta where both entities are present (usually the infrarenal abdominal aorta).

Malperfusion Syndromes

Malperfusion syndrome occurs when there is end-organ ischemia secondary to aortic branch compromise from the dissecting process. This can involve one or more vascular beds simultaneously. Early symptoms are often subtle and of varying severity over the hours and days after the initial onset of symptoms. Consistent over several series, aortic branch compromise is present in up to 31% of patients with acute aortic dissection,[9,27,31,32] with progression to the malperfusion syndrome correlating with early mortality.[8,9,27] Virtually any aortic branch can be affected, and as intuitively suspected, the morbid clinical events will vary as a function of the vascular territory involved.

Identifying the mechanisms of branch compromise is a critical step in formulating effective treatment plans. The anatomic and physiologic variables underpinning any compromised vascular bed include (1) the percentage of aortic circumference dissected, (2) the presence of a distal reentrant focus in the false lumen or true lumen outflow, and (3) the topography of branch ostia to the true versus the false lumen.[6] In the minutes after an aortic dissection is initiated, the true lumen (representing the remnant of the original aortic lumen) collapses to a variable degree and the false lumen expands.[33] The adventitially bound outer wall of the false lumen must expand to a larger diameter to accommodate the same wall tension at a given blood pressure, as governed by the law of LaPlace. In contrast, the true lumen, which contains the majority of the elastic components of the aortic wall, undergoes radial elastic collapse.[33] Therefore, the degree to which the true lumen recoils and the false lumen expands (i.e., their respective cross-sectional area) is dependent on the percentage of the total aortic circumference involved with the dissection. In the presence of a deep proximal tear and the absence of distal fenestrations, the mean false lumen pressure increases, leading to compression of the true lumen[34] [*see Figure 2*]. A compressed true lumen will lead to impaired perfusion of distal structures and should increase the index of suspicion for visceral and renal ischemia. Two mechanisms for aortic branch vessel compromise have been identified, each of which has specific treatment implications in the management of malperfusion syndromes.[33]

DYNAMIC OBSTRUCTION

In dynamic obstruction, the dissection flap prolapses into the vessel ostium and impedes blood flow with each cardiac cycle [*see Figure 3*]. This is the more common mechanism of branch compromise and is responsible at least in part for some 80% of malperfusion syndromes.[35] The severity of the true lumen collapse and the degree of aortic-level ostial vessel occlusion are determined by the circumference of the dissected aorta, cardiac output, blood pressure, heart rate, and peripheral resistance of the outflow vessel.[36] Pulse deficits based on dynamic obstruction may wax and wane over time bcause of variability in the aforementioned

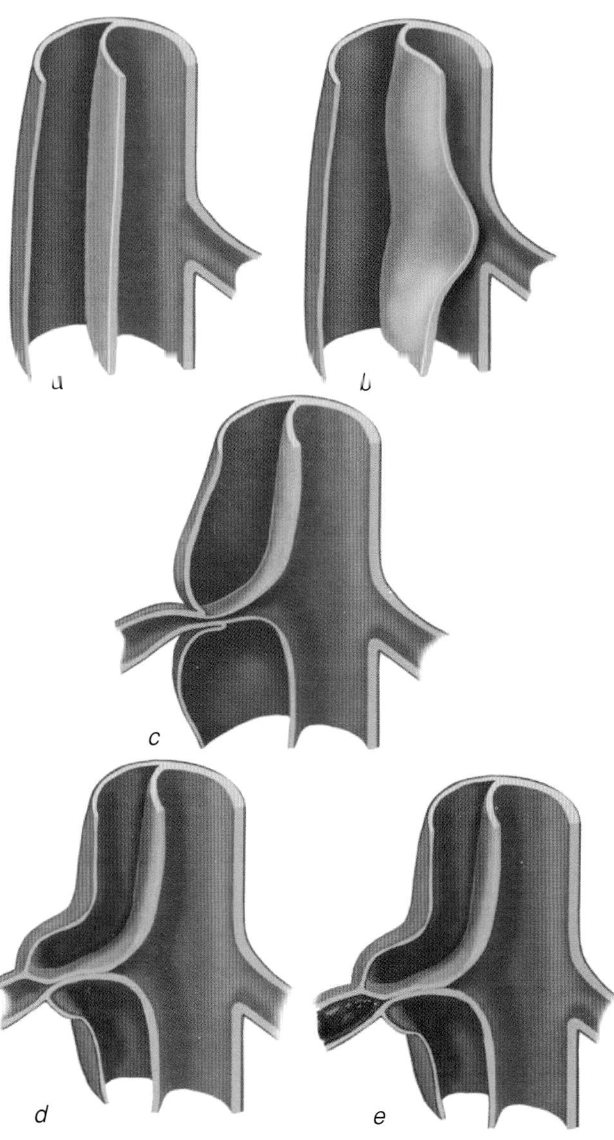

Figure 3 **Mechanisms of aortic branch obstruction in acute dissection. (*a* and *b*) In dynamic obstruction, the septum may prolapse into the vessel ostium during the cardiac cycle, and the compressed true lumen flow is inadequate to perfuse branch vessel ostia, which remain anatomically intact. (*c*, *d*, and *e*) Near-complete circumferential dissection with static obstruction; the cleavage plane of the dissection extends into the ostium and compromises inflow. Thrombosis beyond the compromised ostia may further worsen perfusion.**

factors.[6,37] Chung and colleagues modeled the anatomy and physiologic conditions of a Stanford type B aortic dissection in vitro and concluded that the movement of the dissection flap to produce dynamic obstruction of any branch vessel is related to the size of the entry tear, the limitation of false lumen outflow, and increased true lumen outflow produced by falling peripheral resistance.[36]

STATIC OBSTRUCTION

In acute dissection, the false lumen is highly thrombogenic as a result of the exposed adventitial and medial layers. Thrombus formation may occur in the blind end of the dissection column; more often, "reentrant" foci maintain false lumen flow.[38] If the blind end or the propagating end of the dissection column enters and constricts the ostia of a branch vessel, organ injury can occur by thrombosis or hypoperfusion of the involved vessel. This mechanism for malperfusion syndrome involves the dissecting process extending into the branch vessel proper, narrowing it to a variable degree, and has been termed *static obstruction*.[35] This obstruction is unlikely to resolve with restoration of aortic true lumen flow alone, and some manipulation of the vessel itself (e.g., stent, bypass graft) will typically be required [*see Figure 3*].

Clinical Presentation

PAIN

The most common presenting symptom of acute aortic dissection is pain (located in the back, abdomen, or chest), reported in over 93% of patients, with 85% specifying an abrupt onset.[5,39] Whereas the pain is typically described as anterior in location in type A dissections, for type B dissections, pain is more often experienced in the back (78% versus 64%, respectively).[5,16] The classic presentation of an "acute aortic syndrome" is severe chest or back pain that causes the patient to seek medical attention within minutes to hours of onset and has been described as "the worst ever" by nearly 90% of patients.[5]

HYPERTENSION

On initial physical examination, arterial hypertension is present in 70% of type B dissections but only in 25 to 35% of type A dissections. The presence of hypotension complicating a type B dissection is rare (< 5% of patients) but may be present in 25% of dissections that involve the ascending aorta, potentially as a result of aortic valve disruption or cardiac tamponade.[5] The malperfusion of brachiocephalic arteries by the dissection may falsely depress brachial cuff pressures.[40] Hypertension that is refractory to medical management is common in type B dissections, occurring in 64% of patients.[41] However, as this refractory hypertension is usually not associated with renal artery compromise or aortic dilatation, continued medical management is warranted.

PERIPHERAL VASCULAR COMPLICATIONS

Peripheral vascular complications are common and occur in 30 to 50% of patients in whom the aortic arch and/or the thoracoabdominal aorta is involved.[9,31,32] In patients with peripheral vascular complications not involving the ascending aorta, the brachiocephalic trunk is involved in 15% patients, the common carotid arteries in 20%, the left subclavian artery in 15%, and the ileofemoral arteries in 35%.[9,42] In this population, mortality is clearly linked to the number of pulse deficits at the time of presentation. Indeed, within the first 24 hours, the mortality increases from 9.4% in patients with no deficits to 35.3% in patients with three or more deficits.[42] Although it is uncommon for isolated lower extremity pulse deficits to cause mortality as a result of lower extremity ischemia or its sequelae, leg ischemia remains a marker of extensive dissection.[9]

OTHER COMPLICATIONS

Syncope may complicate the presentation of acute aortic dissection in 5 to 10% of patients, and its presence often indicates the development of cardiac tamponade or involvement of the brachiocephalic vessels.[43] Overall, patients in the IRAD who presented with syncope were more likely to have a type A dissection than a type B (19% versus 3%, $p < .001$), more likely to have cardiac tamponade (28% versus 8%, $p < .001$), and more likely to die in the hospital (34% versus 23%, $p = .01$).[44] Spinal cord ischemia from the interruption of intercostal vessels is clearly more common with type B aortic dissections, occurring in 2 to 10% of all patients.[45] In addition, direct compression of any peripheral nerve can occur, albeit rarely, resulting in paresthesia (lumbar plexopathy), hoarseness of voice (compression of recurrent laryngeal nerve), or Horner syndrome (compression of sympathetic ganglion).[46–48]

Diagnosis

In the United States, acute chest pain is the chief complaint in 8.2% of all emergency department visits. This translates to almost 4.6 million patients annually.[49] The majority of these patients do not have an aortic dissection, and it would be inefficient, unrealistic, and costly to obtain axial imaging on all patients with acute chest pain. Indeed, the indiscriminate application of thoracic imaging to patients with a low pretest probability of having an aortic dissection has been predicted to yield an 85% false positive rate.[50] However, aortic dissection often affects younger patients (in their 50s) and thus is often not readily apparent. Indeed, physicians correctly suspect the entity in only 15 to 43% of presentations as aortic dissection is often identified as an incidental finding during evaluation of another pathologic process.[13,51] A recent review of the IRAD population showed that the average time between presentation and confirmation of the diagnosis was 24 to 34 hours depending on the patient's age.[14] This underscores the importance of clinical suspicion for early identification, and aortic dissection should be considered in patients who present with persistent chest pain, a normal chest x-ray, and a negative cardiac workup.

IMAGING

The goal of imaging is to first confirm the diagnosis of acute aortic dissection and then determine the extent of dissection, the potential involvement of branch vessels, and the presence of immediate life-threatening complications,

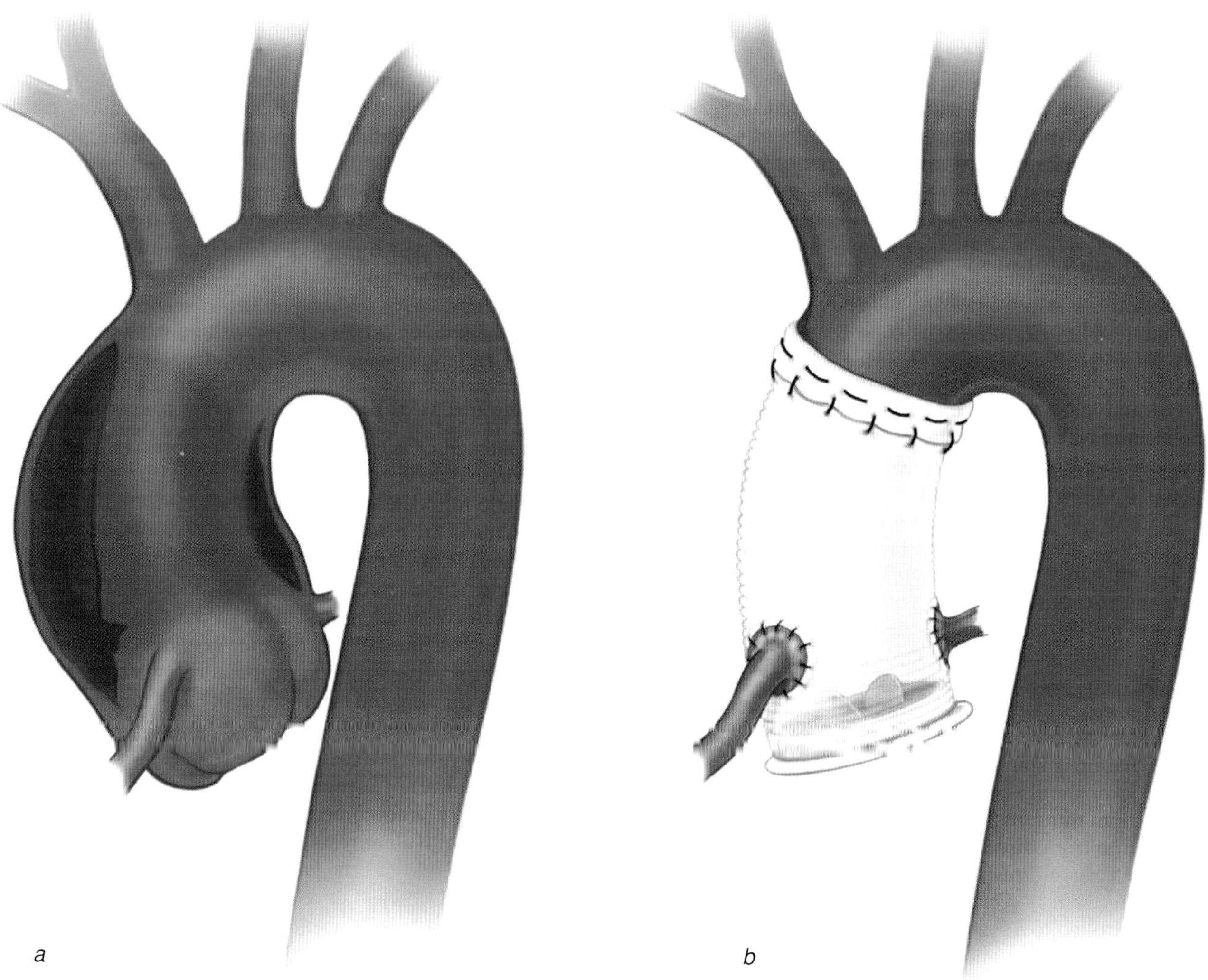

Figure 4 (*a*) **Cartoon depicition of type A dissection limited to the ascending aorta. (*b*) Repair of type A dissection with replacement of the ascending aorta. Anatomic goals of replacement include (1) resection of aortic tear, (2) resuspension/repair or replacement of the aortic valve as necessary, (3) routine use of circulatory arrest to perform at least the distal anastomosis, and (4) reconstruction of the aortic layers so as to redirect flow into the true lumen and eliminate false lumen flow (this is successful only 50% of time).**

ENDOVASCULAR TREATMENT OF AORTIC DISSECTION

Although medical therapy remains the current standard of care for uncomplicated type B aortic dissections, stent graft coverage of the aortic entry tear may ultimately prove to be the best solution to correct malperfusion syndromes in the acute phase and reduce late aortic-related complications by minimizing aneurysmal degeneration of the false lumen. When indicated, the goals of TEVAR for acute type B dissection include coverage of the proximal entry tear, expansion of the true lumen with restoration of flow to the visceral vessels, and obliteration of false lumen flow with subsequent complete thrombosis [*see Figure 5*]. When these components of therapy are successfully achieved, aortic remodeling should occur with subsequent prevention of future aneurysmal degeneration of the outer wall of the false lumen.

There are particular technical points of stent graft repair of aortic dissection that deserve emphasis. First, the placement of uncovered stents over the entry tear within the proximal true aortic lumen is ill advised as this may lead to a retrograde dissection into the arch or ascending aorta.[86–88] If a patient is to be considered a candidate for stent graft treatment, the location of the entry tear and proper recognition of the proximal zone of fixation are fundamental to procedural success, and the operator should have definitive knowledge of the three-dimensional aortic topography displayed on the preintervention CT scan prior to embarking on endovascular therapy. Endovascular repair of acute aortic dissection should be performed in an operating room with adequate fluoroscopic imaging. True lumen access should be obtained from either a brachial or femoral approach; typically, since the tear in type B dissection is distal to the left subclavian artery, rapid true lumen access is easily obtained through a right brachial approach. The proper true lumen position should then be confirmed

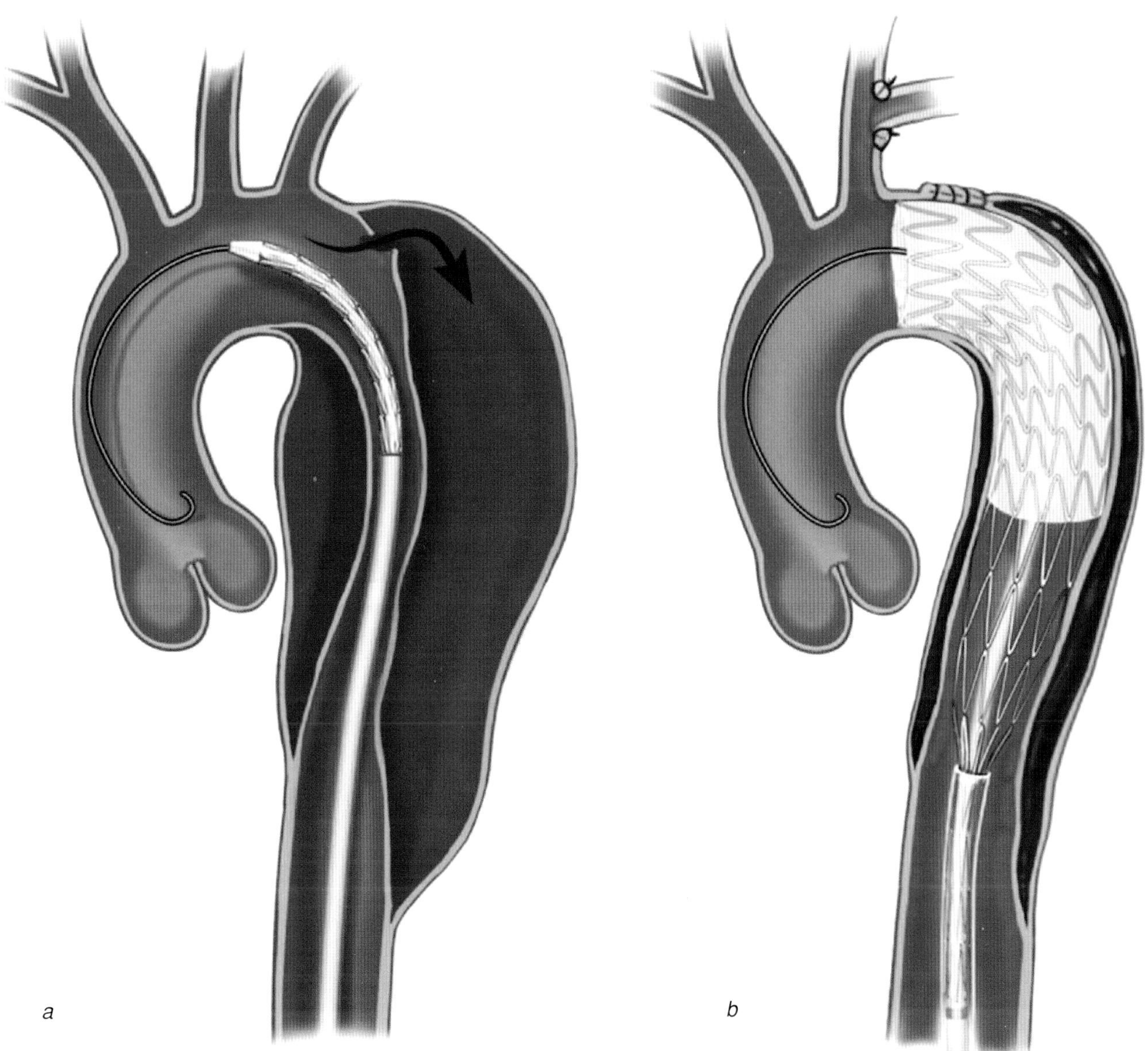

Figure 5 **(*a*) Cartoon depiction of type B dissection with undeployed stent graft advanced to the level of the left carotid artery to ensure appropriate coverage of the entry tear. (*b*) Stent graft deployment to cover the proximal entry tear in the hope of inducing false lumen thrombosis and true lumen reexpansion. The latter should also alleviate "downstream" branch compromise caused by dynamic obstruction mechanisms. False lumen thrombosis in the thoracic aorta should, in theory, minimize subsequent aneurysmal expansion of the outer wall of the false lumen.**

using intravascular ultrasonography to avoid inadvertent deployment of the stent in the false lumen [see *Figure 6*].

The Eurostar/United Kingdom registry report is the largest compendium of patients treated with thoracic aortic stent grafts to date.[89] In the combined registry, 131 patients with aortic dissection (5% proximal, 81% distal, 14% not classified) were treated with stent grafts; 57% had symptoms of rupture, aortic expansion, or side branch occlusion. Although no meaningful long-term data are available, primary technical success was achieved in 89% and 30-day mortality was 8.4%. Paraplegia occurred in 0.8% of those treated, and survival at 1 year after treatment was reported in 90% of 67 patients who had such follow-up.

A recent meta-analysis of stent graft repair for aortic dissection prior to 2005 identified 609 patients with a procedural success of 98.2%.[90] The 30-day mortality was 5.3% and was threefold higher in patients with acute dissection. The neurologic complication rate was 2.9%. A more recent review of the Nationwide Inpatient Sample (from 2005 to 2007) identified 5,000 patients who underwent repair of type B aortic dissections (3,619 open versus 1,381 TEVAR) and found that the TEVAR group had a significantly lower 30-day mortality (10.6% versus 19% for open repair).[91]

The Investigation of Stent-grafts in Aortic Dissection (INSTEAD) trial was a prospective, randomized, multicenter trial of stent grafting versus medical therapy for the treatment

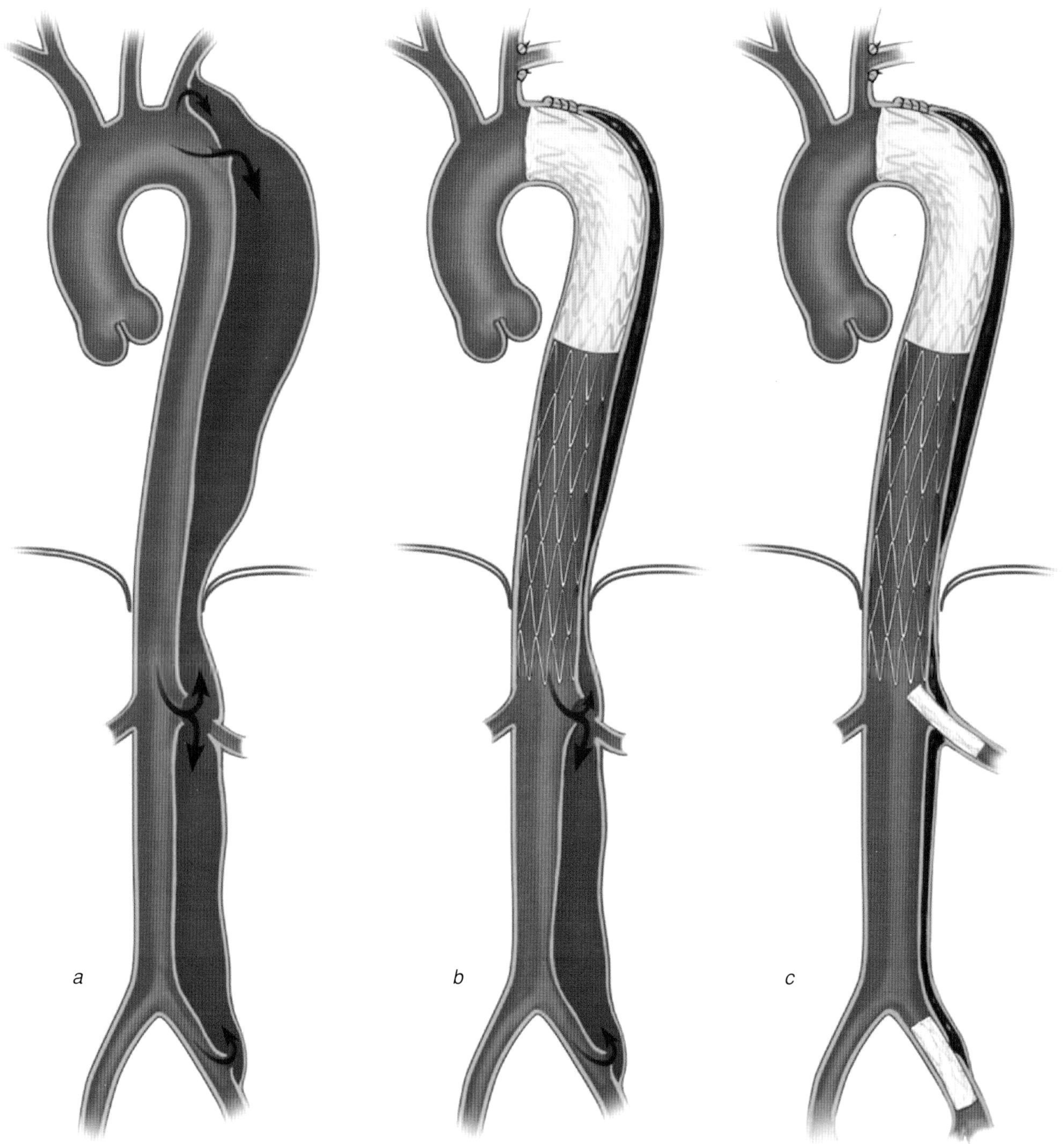

Figure 7 **Cartoon depiction of the use of a combination of covered and bare metal stents to completely obliterate the false lumen in acute type B dissection. (*a*) Stanford type B dissection with entry tear distal to the left subclavian artery and fenestrations at branch artery ostea. (*b*) Covered stent graft used to seal the proximal entry tear (with coverage of the left subclavian artery to obtain adequate seal). Bare metal stents then obliterate the thoracic false lumen to the level of the renal arteries. False lumen flow remains in the abdominal portion of the dissection as a result of multiple entry points. (*c*) Interval placement of covered stents over false lumen entry points with complete obliteration of the false lumen.**

permitting direct inspection or repair of the ostia of the mesenteric and renal vessels.[102] Experience has demonstrated that the duration of supraceliac clamping can be limited to the 20-minute range, with repositioning of the clamp to an infrarenal location following closure of the visceral segment aortotomy. Interposition of a short segment polyester graft in the infrarenal aorta facilitates reconstruction of the aortic layers at the distal anastomosis with the double-layer polytetrafluoroethylene felt technique. Our posture relative to extending the fenestration or septectomy into the visceral aortic segment is dictated by the anatomic complexity displayed on the CT scan. Small aortic diameter, total absence of visceral artery flow, the dissected septum extending directly to or beyond a vital branch orifice, and radiographic

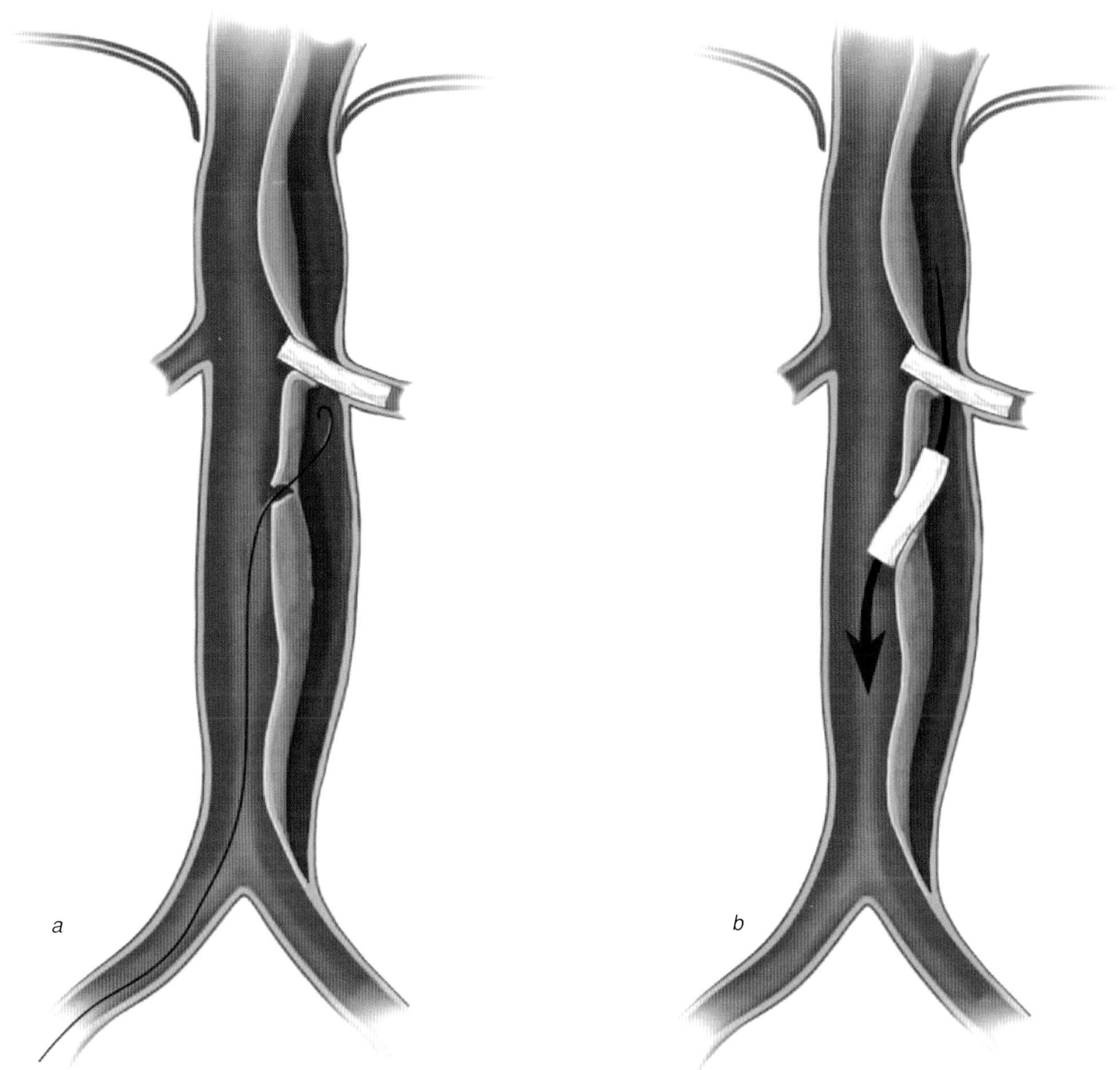

Figure 8 **Cartoon depiction of endovascular fenestration. (*a*) The left renal artery (coming off the false lumen) made to originate from the true lumen. This requires stenting using either a covered or bare metal stent. (*b*) A balloon is then used to enlarge natural fenestrations in the dissection flap, and a stent can be used to keep this fenestration open.**

evidence of intussuscepted septum into a renal/mesenteric vessel are all considerations that prompt extension of the aortotomy into the visceral segment. Such an approach also permits direct repair of a static obstruction, that is, where the branch vessel itself is dissected. This can be accomplished by circumferential suture of the vessel intima to the aortic wall at the ostia. Since continuous exposure of the visceral segment is desirable in surgical treatment of malperfusion syndrome, we prefer left flank approaches for this procedure. Depending on body habitus, a ninth or 10th interspace thoracoabdominal approach is used to allow for complete infradiaphragmatic aortic exposure and transperitoneal inspection of the viscera and palpation of the superior mesenteric artery pulse caudal to the mesocolon. At a median follow-up of 19 months, no significant aortic dilatation occurred with such aortic tailoring as a surgical technique.[102]

Advocates of surgical fenestration for malperfusion syndromes have asserted that the "surgical" morbidity and mortality rates quoted to support endovascular therapies are outdated and strongly influenced by delays in diagnosis and treatment.[103] Elefteriades and colleagues reported a survival of 65% at 1 year, 57% at 3 years, 50% at 5 years, and 28% at 10 years for patients treated with a "complication-specific" approach.[104] Overall, of the 14 patients in the total experience treated by open fenestration, their actuarial survival was 77%, 77%, and 53% at 1, 3, and 5 years, respectively. None of the surgically fenestrated patients were noted to have expansion of their aortic diameters on follow-up.

102. Webb TH, Williams GM. Abdominal aortic tailoring for renal, visceral, and lower extremity malperfusion resulting from acute aortic dissection. J Vasc Surg 1997;26:474–80; discussion 480–471.
103. Oderich GS, Panneton JM. Acute aortic dissection with side branch vessel occlusion: open surgical options. Semin Vasc Surg 2002;15:89–96.
104. Elefteriades JA, Hartleroad J, Gusberg RJ, et al. Long-term experience with descending aortic dissection: the complication-specific approach. Ann Thorac Surg 1992;53:11–20; discussion 20–11.
105. Panneton JM, Teh SH, Cherry KJ Jr, et al. Aortic fenestration for acute or chronic aortic dissection: an uncommon but effective procedure. J Vasc Surg 2000;32:711–21.
106. Panneton JM, Hollier LH. Dissecting descending thoracic and thoracoabdominal aortic aneurysms: part II. Ann Vasc Surg 1995;9:596–605.
107. Hollier LH, Symmonds JB, Pairolero PC, et al. Thoracoabdominal aortic aneurysm repair. Analysis of postoperative morbidity. Arch Surg 1988;123:871–5.
108. Cambria RP, Davison JK, Zannetti S, et al. Thoracoabdominal aneurysm repair: perspectives over a decade with the clamp-and-sew technique. Ann Surg 1997;226:294–303; discussion 303–295.
109. White RA, Donayre CE, Walot I, Kopchok GE. Intraprocedural imaging: thoracic aortography techniques, intravascular ultrasound, and special equipment. J Vasc Surg 2006; 43 Suppl A:53A–61A.
110. Bernard Y, Zimmermann H, Chocron S, et al. False lumen patency as a predictor of late outcome in aortic dissection. Am J Cardiol 2001;87:1378–82.
111. Tsai TT, Fattori R, Trimarchi S, et al, International Registry of Acute Aortic Dissections. Long-term survival in patients presenting with type B acute aortic dissection: insights from the International Registry of Acute Aortic Dissection. Circulation 2006;114:2226–31.
112. Shores J, Berger KR, Murphy EA, Pyeritz RE. Progression of aortic dilatation and the benefit of long-term beta-adrenergic blockade in Marfan's syndrome. N Engl J Med 1994;330:1335–41.
113. Chuter T, Hartley D, Rapp J, et al. Totally endovascular thoracoabdominal aneurysm repair. In: Society for Vascular Surgery Annual Meeting; 2007. p. 106–7.
114. Nienaber CA, von Kodolitsch Y, Petersen B, et al. Intramural hemorrhage of the thoracic aorta. Diagnostic and therapeutic implications. Circulation 1995;92:1465–72.
115. von Kodolitsch Y, Csosz SK, Koschyk DH, et al. Intramural hematoma of the aorta: predictors of progression to dissection and rupture. Circulation 2003;107:1158–63.
116. Muluk SC, Kaufman JA, Torchiana DF, et al. Diagnosis and treatment of thoracic aortic intramural hematoma. J Vasc Surg 1996;24:1022–9.
117. Cho KR, Stanson AW, Potter DD, et al. Penetrating atherosclerotic ulcer of the descending thoracic aorta and arch. J Thorac Cardiovasc Surg 2004;127:1393–9; discussion 1399–401.
118. Sundt TM. Intramural hematoma and penetrating atherosclerotic ulcer of the aorta. Ann Thorac Surg 2007;83(2):S835–41; discussion S846–50.
119. Ohmi M, Tabayashi K, Moizumi Y, et al. Extremely rapid regression of aortic intramural hematoma. J Thorac Cardiovasc Surg 1999;118:968–9.
120. Evangelista A, Mukherjee D, Mehta RH, et al. Acute intramural hematoma of the aorta: a mystery in evolution. Circulation 2005;111:1063–70.
121. Sueyoshi E, Imada T, Sakamoto I, et al. Analysis of predictive factors for progression of type B aortic intramural hematoma with computed tomography. J Vasc Surg 2002; 35:1179–83.
122. Tittle SL, Lynch RJ, Cole PE, et al. Midterm follow-up of penetrating ulcer and intramural hematoma of the aorta. J Thorac Cardiovasc Surg 2002;123:1051–9.

INDEX

Note: Page numbers followed by t indicate tables; numbers followed by f indicate figures.

A

E

H

M

Q

R

S

T

W

XYZ